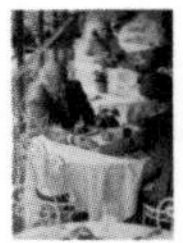

SECTION 8

PROBLEMS OF INGESTION, DIGESTION, ABSORPTION, AND ELIMINATION

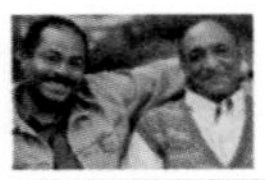

SECTION 9

PROBLEMS OF URINARY FUNCTION

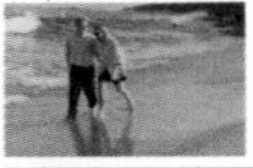

SECTION 10

PROBLEMS RELATED TO REGULATORY MECHANISMS

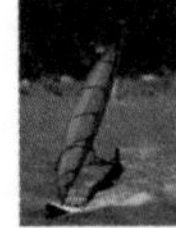

SECTION 11

PROBLEMS RELATED TO MOVEMENT AND COORDINATION

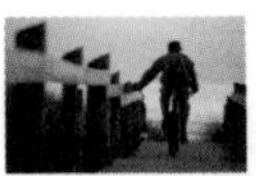

SECTION 12

NURSING CARE IN SPECIALIZED SETTINGS

APPENDIXES

CONGRATULATIONS

You now have access to Mosby's "Get Smart" Bonus Package!

Here's what's included to help you "Get Smart"

sign on at:

http://www.mosby.com/MERLIN/medsurg_lewis/

A Web site just for you as you learn medical-surgical nursing with the new 5th edition of **Medical-Surgical Nursing: Assessment and Management of Clinical Problems**

what you will receive:

Whether you're a student, an instructor, or a clinician, you'll find information just for you. Things like:

- Content Updates
- Links to Related Products
- Author Information . . . and more

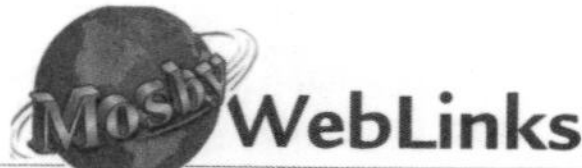

An exciting new program that allows you to directly access hundreds of active Web sites keyed specifically to the content of this book. The WebLinks are continually updated, with new ones added as they develop.

Free CD-ROM

with every copy of **Medical-Surgical Nursing**, 5th Edition

This valuable CD-ROM Features:

Overviews of Common Diseases
Key Terms
Case Studies
Review Questions

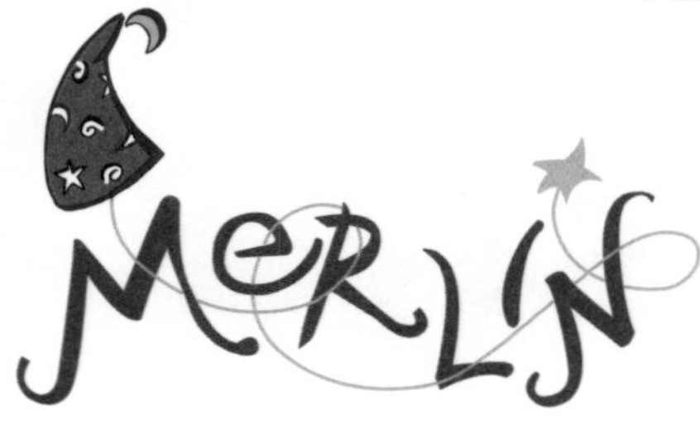

Mosby's Electronic Resource Links & Information Network

Mosby

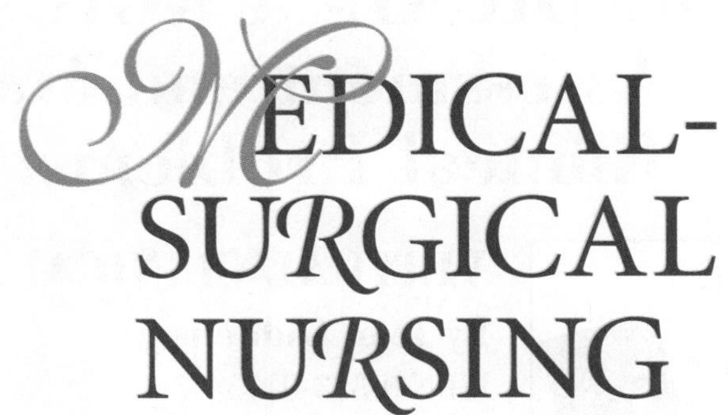

ASSESSMENT and **MANAGEMENT** of
CLINICAL PROBLEMS

Superb resources to accompany

MEDICAL-SURGICAL NURSING: Assessment and Management of Clinical Problems, 5th Edition!

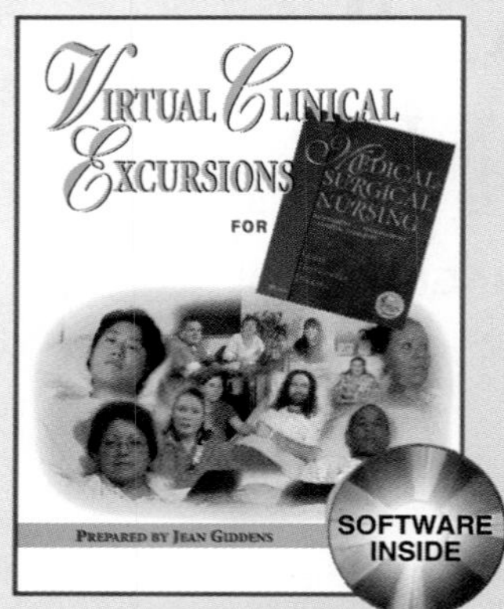

VIRTUAL CLINICAL EXCURSIONS

By **Jean Giddens**

ISBN 0-323-01734-7

- A multi-media CD-ROM features a virtual hospital with five true-to-life patients.
- Workbook exercises send you into this interactive clinical simulation to observe the application of important concepts and make appropriate clinical choices.
- The virtual clinical environment offers you an ideal, safe setting in which to "practice" what you've learned in the text.

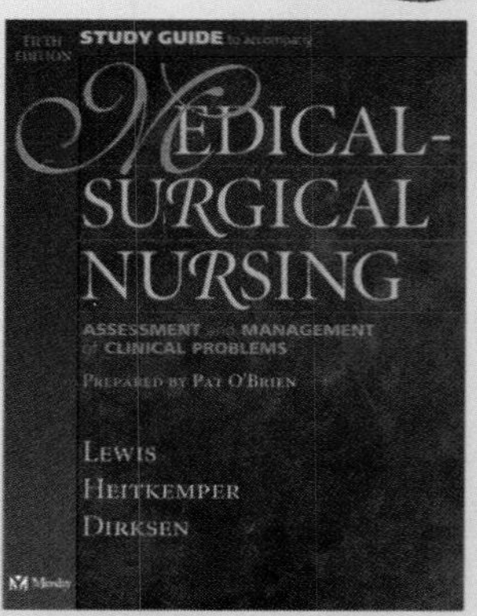

STUDY GUIDE

By **Patricia O'Brien**

ISBN 0-323-00258-7

- Over 400 pages of valuable review and testing material.
- Wide variety of exercises and activities includes multiple-choice questions in NCLEX format, case studies, crossword puzzles, matching exercises, fill-in-the-blank questions, and much more.
- Answers to all exercises included in the back to facilitate self-study.

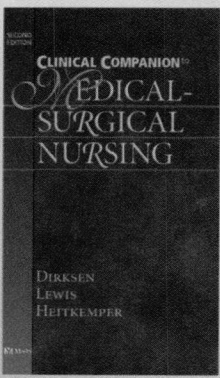

CLINICAL COMPANION

By **Shannon Ruff Dirksen**

ISBN 0-323-00404-0

- More than 200 disorders organized alphabetically for quick reference.
- Need-to-know information formatted for practical use in clinical settings.
- Patient education points are highlighted with a special icon.
- New attractive and functional two-color design.

Please check with your local bookstore to order copies of these helpful study tools.

www.mosby.com
A Division of Elsevier Science

FIFTH EDITION

MEDICAL-SURGICAL NURSING

ASSESSMENT and MANAGEMENT of CLINICAL PROBLEMS

SHARON MANTIK LEWIS, RN, PHD, FAAN
Professor, College of Nursing
Research Associate Professor, Department of Pathology
University of New Mexico
Albuquerque, New Mexico

MARGARET MCLEAN HEITKEMPER, RN, PHD, FAAN
Professor, Biobehavioral Nursing and Health Systems
School of Nursing
University of Washington
Seattle, Washington

SHANNON RUFF DIRKSEN, RN, PHD
Associate Professor, College of Nursing
Arizona State University
Tempe, Arizona

with 845 *illustrations*

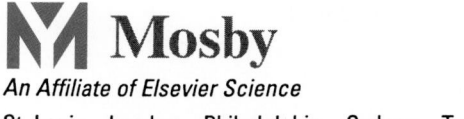

St. Louis London Philadelphia Sydney Toronto

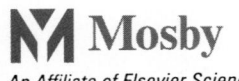

An Affiliate of Elsevier Science

Editor-in-Chief Sally Schrefer
Developmental Editor Kristin Geen
Project Manager Dana Peick
Project Specialist Catherine Albright Jackson
Designer Amy Buxton

FIFTH EDITION

NOTICE

Pharmacology is an ever-changing field. Standard safety precautions must be followed, but as new research and clinical experience broaden our knowledge, changes in treatment and drug therapy may become necessary or appropriate. Readers are advised to check the most current product information provided by the manufacturer of each drug to be administered to verify the recommended dose, the method and duration of administration, and contraindications. It is the responsibility of the treating physician, relying on experience and knowledge of the patient, to determine dosages and the best treatment for each individual patient. Neither the Publisher nor the editor assume any liability for any injury and/or damage to persons or property arising from this publication.

Mosby, Inc.
An Affiliate of Elsevier Science
11830 Westline Industrial Drive
St. Louis, Missouri 63146

Printed in the United States of America.

Library of Congress Cataloging-in-Publication Data

Medical-surgical nursing : assessment and management of clinical problems / [edited by] Sharon Mantik Lewis, Margaret McLean Heitkemper, Shannon Ruff Dirksen. -- 5th ed.
p. cm.
Includes bibliographical references and index.
ISBN 1-55664-430-2 (alk. paper)
1. Nursing. 2. Surgical nursing. I. Lewis, Sharon Mantik. II. Heitkemper, Margaret M. (Margaret McLean) III. Dirksen, Shannon Ruff.
[DNLM: 1. Nursing Care. 2. Nursing Assessment. 3. Perioperative Nursing. WY 100 M489 2000]
RT41.M488 2000
610.73--dc21
DNLM/DLC

99-23884

02 03 / 9 8 7 6 5

ABOUT THE AUTHORS

Sharon Mantik Lewis, RN, PhD, FAAN

Sharon Lewis received her Bachelor of Science in nursing from the University of Wisconsin-Madison, Master of Science in nursing with a minor in biological sciences from the University of Colorado, and PhD in immunology from the Department of Pathology at the University of New Mexico School of Medicine. She had a 2-year postdoctoral fellowship from the National Kidney Foundation. Her more than 25 years of teaching experience include inservice education and teaching in associate, baccalaureate, and master's degree programs in Maryland, Illinois, Wisconsin, and New Mexico. Favorite teaching areas are pathophysiology, immunology, and renal failure. She has been actively involved in clinical research for the last 18 years, investigating altered immune responses in patients with chronic renal failure and other chronic illnesses. Currently she is using biofeedback and immune parameters to study the effects of relaxation therapy for caregivers of Alzheimer's patients.

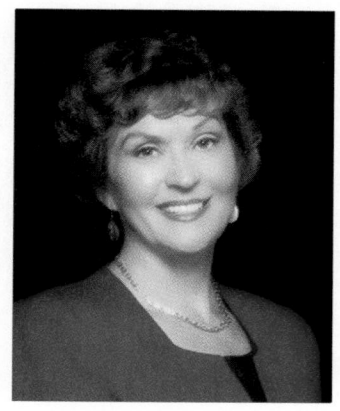

Margaret McLean Heitkemper, RN, PhD, FAAN

Margaret Heitkemper received her Bachelor of Science in nursing from Seattle University, Master of Science in gerontologic nursing from the University of Washington, and PhD in physiology and biophysics from the University of Illinois. She was a research associate on an NIH research grant project related to problems with enteral nutrition where she developed an interest in gastrointestinal problems. She has experience as a staff nurse and has worked in an acute geriatric care facility associated with Rush-St. Luke's Presbyterian Medical Center. Since 1981, she has been on the faculty at the University of Washington where she is department chairperson and teaches at all levels—undergraduate and graduate. She currently teaches medical-surgical nursing theory and pharmacology for nurses.

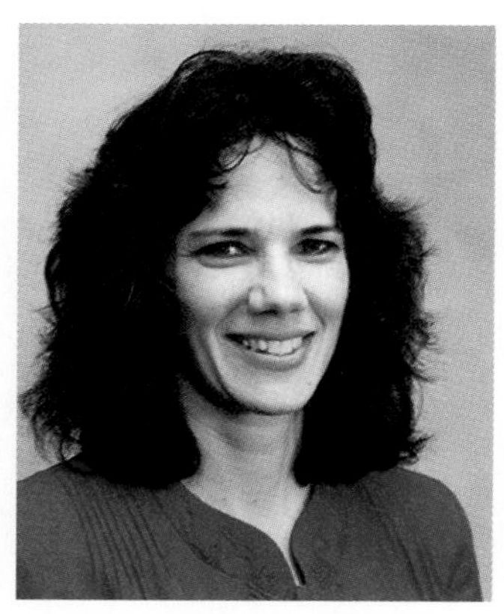

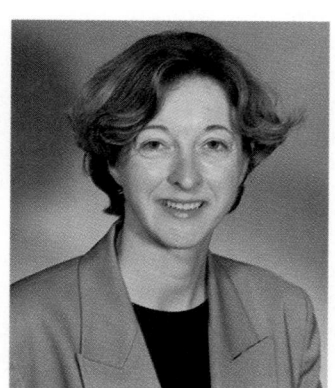

Shannon Ruff Dirksen, RN, PhD

Shannon Dirksen received her Bachelor of Science in nursing from Arizona State University and Master of Science and PhD in nursing from the University of Arizona. In her 12 years of teaching at the graduate and undergraduate levels, she has taught at Edith Cowan University (Western Australia), Intercollegiate Center for Nursing Education (Spokane, Washington), University of New Mexico, and Arizona State University. She currently teaches nursing research and management and leadership. For the past 14 years, she has been actively involved in oncology research, focusing on adjustment in Caucasian and Hispanic patients with melanoma and breast cancer and cancer prevention in the community. She is the primary author of the *Clinical Companion to Medical-Surgical Nursing,* which accompanies this book.

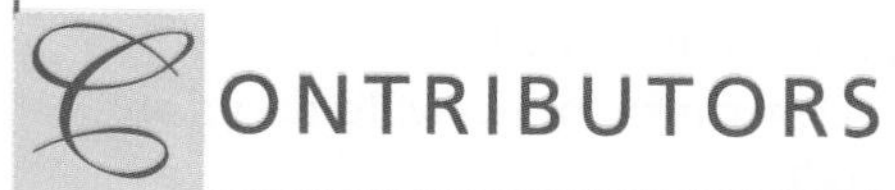

CONTRIBUTORS

Charlotte R. Abbink, RN, PhD
Professor Emeritus
University of New Mexico College of Nursing
Albuquerque, New Mexico

Elizabeth A. Ayello, RN, PhD, CS, CETN
Clinical Assistant Professor
Division of Nursing
New York University
New York, New York

Marilyn Rossman Bartucci, MSN, RN, CS, CCTC
Head Nurse Manager, Transplant Center
University Hospitals of Cleveland
Cleveland, Ohio

Patricia Bates, RN, BSN, CURN
Staff Nurse, Urology
Kaiser Permanente
Portland, Oregon

Catherine M. Bender, RN, PhD
Assistant Professor
University of Pittsburgh School of Nursing/
University of Pittsburgh Cancer Institute
Pittsburgh, Pennsylvania

Chuck Biddle, RN, CRNA, PhD
Associate Professor
Department of Anesthesiology
Dartmouth Hitchcock Medical Center
Lebanon, New Hampshire

Donna Zimmaro Bliss, PhD, RN, CCRN
Assistant Professor, School of Nursing
University of Minnesota
Minneapolis, Minnesota

Eleanor F. Bond, PhD, RN
Associate Professor, School of Nursing
University of Washington
Seattle, Washington

Lucy A. Bradley-Springer, RN, PhD
Co-Director, New Mexico AIDS Education and Training Center
Assistant Professor
University of New Mexico School of Medicine
Albuquerque, New Mexico

Barbara Brillhart, RN, PhD, CRRN, FNP-C
Associate Professor, College of Nursing
Arizona State University
Tempe, Arizona

Gillian Brunier, RN, MScN, CNeph(C)
Clinical Nurse Specialist/Nurse Practitioner, Nephrology
Sunnybrook and Women's College Health Science Centre
Toronto, Ontario
Canada

Melissa Bush, RN, MSN
Nurse Practitioner
Dr. Gary J. Silverman
Scottsdale, Arizona

Kathryn Ann Caudell, RN, PhD, OCN
Assistant Professor
University of New Mexico College of Nursing
Albuquerque, New Mexico

Cecilia C. Dail, BS, MT (ASCP)
Instructor, Medical Laboratory Sciences
Department of Pathology, School of Medicine
University of New Mexico
Albuquerque, New Mexico

Lee Danielson, BS, MT (ASCP)
Instructor, Medical Laboratory Sciences
Department of Pathology, School of Medicine
University of New Mexico
Albuquerque, New Mexico

Jennie Daugherty, MSN, RN, CS
Clinical Nurse Specialist
Edwards Eve Clinic
Nashville, Tennessee

Patricia J. Davies, RN, MSN
Pulmonary Clinical Nurse Specialist
Primary Teacher/Instructor
University of Pittsburgh School of Nursing
Pittsburgh, Pennsylvania

Julie M. Dax, MSN, RN
Critical Care Nurse Educator
University Hospital
Albuquerque, New Mexico

Anne M. Devney, EdD, RN
Director, Health Services
College of Lake County
Grayslake, Illinois

Shannon Ruff Dirksen, RN, PhD
Associate Professor
College of Nursing
Arizona State University
Tempe, Arizona

Ellen Stoetzner Duke, RN, MSN
Nursing Instructor
Angelina College Nursing Program
Lufkin, Texas

Laura Dulski, RN, MSN
Staff Nurse
Rush-Presbyterian St. Luke's Medical Center
Chicago, Illinois

Patsy Orth Duphorne, RN, MN
Assistant Professor
College of Nursing
University of New Mexico
Albuquerque, New Mexico

Tana Durnbaugh, RNCS, EdD
Professor of Nursing
College of Lake County
Grayslake, Illinois

Rachel Elrod, RN, MS
Professor of Nursing
Front Range Community College
Westminster, Colorado
University of Phoenix-Colorado Campus
Aurora, Colorado

Susan Flagler, DNS, RNC (WHCNP)
Associate Professor
School of Nursing
University of Washington
Seattle, Washington

Linda B. Haas, PhC, RN, CDE
Endocrinology Clinical Nurse Specialist
VA Puget Sound HCS, Seattle Division
Seattle, Washington

Margaret McLean Heitkemper, RN, PhD, FAAN
Professor, Biobehavioral Nursing and Health Systems
School of Nursing
University of Washington
Seattle, Washington

Patricia Robertson Hercules, RN, MS
Director, Nursing Support and Patient Education Department
The Methodist Hospital
Houston, Texas

Cynthia L. Hermey, RN, MN, CCRN
Manager of Cardiac and Intensive Care Services
Oconee Memorial Hosptial
Seneca, South Carolina

Margaret M. Hickey, RN, MSN, MS, OCN, CORLN
Clinical Director
Tulane University Comprehensive Cancer Center
New Orleans, Louisiana

Leslie A. Hoffman, RN, PhD, FAAN
Professor and Chair, Department of Acute/Tertiary Care
University of Pittsburgh
Pittsburgh, Pennsylvania

Mima M. Horne, RN, MSN, CDE
Diabetes Clinical Nurse Specialist
New Hanover Regional Medical Center
Wilmington, North Carolina

Mary Ann House-Fancher, RN, ARNP, MSN
Nurse Practitioner, Cardiothoracic Surgery
University of Florida
Gainesville, Florida

Bettyann Hutchisson, RN, BSN, CNOR
Nurse Clinician, Perioperative Education
The Methodist Hospital
Houston, Texas

Linda Witek Janusek, RN, PhD
Professor, School of Nursing
Loyola University of Chicago
Chicago, Illinois

Carolyn I. Johns, RN, CANP, MS
Adult Nurse Practitioner, Cardiology
Lovelace Health Systems
Albuquerque, New Mexico

Anne M. Jones, MN, RNC
Medical Surgical Clinical Nurse Specialist
Providence Saint Joseph Medical Center
Burbank, California

The Reverend Barbara Gail Jorelman, BA, MDiv
President, New Mexico Health Decisions
Albuquerque, New Mexico

Mary Kerr, RN, PhD, FAAN
Associate Professor, School of Nursing
Director for Center for Nursing Research
University of Pittsburgh
Pittsburgh, Pennsylvania

Cindy J. Knipe, RN
Care Delivery Director
Wishard Regional Burn Center
Wishard Memorial Hospital
Indianapolis, Indiana

Nancy Stoetzner Kupper, RN, MSN
Associate Professor
Tarrant County Junior College
Fort Worth, Texas

Barbara S. Levine, PhD, RN, CRNP, CS
Clinical Director
Gerontological Nursing
Assistant Professor
School of Nursing
University of Pennsylvania Health System
Philadelphia, Pennsylvania

Sharon Mantik Lewis, RN, PhD, FAAN
Professor, College of Nursing
Research Associate Professor, Department of Pathology
University of New Mexico
Albuquerque, New Mexico

Kathleen Oare Lindell, RN, MSN
Pulmonary Clinical Nurse Specialist
University of Pennsylvania Health System
Philadelphia, Pennsylvania

Phyllis Lisanti, RN, PhD
Undergraduate Program Director
Clinical Associate Professor
New York University-Division of Nursing
New York, New York

Kim Litwack, PhD, RN, FAAN, CFNP
Associate Professor
University of New Mexico College of Nursing
Albuquerque, New Mexico

Carol O. Long, RN, PhD
Assistant Professor
College of Nursing
Arizona State University
Tempe, Arizona

Janis Luft, RN, MSN
UCSF/Stanford Women's Health
San Francisco, California

Nancy J. MacMullen, RNC, PhD
Associate Professor
Rush University College of Nursing
Chicago, Illinois

Linda C. Griego Martinez, MSN, RN, CS, CCRN
Cardiology Care Manager
Presbyterian Heart Group
Albuquerque, New Mexico

Katheryn E. McCash, RNC, MSN
Instructor
University of New Mexico College of Nursing
Albuquerque, NM

Cindy Meredith, RN, MSN
Adjunct Lecturer in Nursing
Jackson Community College
Jackson, Michigan

Diane H. Michalec, RN, MSN, CCRN, CNRN
Clinical Systems Analyst IV
University of Pittsburgh Medical Center
Pittsburgh, Pennsylvania

Lorene Newberry, RN, MS, CEN
Clinical Nurse Specialist—Emergency Services
WellStar Health System
Marietta, Georgia

Noreen Heer Nicol, RN, MS, FNP
Director of Nursing
Dermatology Clinical Specialist/Nurse Practitioner
National Jewish Medical and Research Center;
Clinical Senior Instructor
University of Colorado, School of Nursing
Denver, Colorado

Ann M. O'Mara, RN, PhD, AOCN
Fellow, Division of Cancer Prevention and Control
National Cancer Institute, National Institutes of Health
Bethesda, Maryland;
Assistant Professor, University of Maryland School of Nursing
Baltimore, Maryland

Judy Ozuna, RN, MN, ARNP, CNRN
Clinical Nurse Specialist in Neurology
Veterans Affairs Medical Center
Clinical Assistant Professor
Biobehavioral Nursing and Health Systems
University of Washington School of Nursing
Seattle, Washington

Anita M. Ralstin, RN, MS, CS, CNP
Family Nurse Practitioner
New Mexico Heart Institute, Surgery Division
Albuquerque, New Mexico

Lynn F. Reinke, RN-CS, MSN
Adult Nurse Practitioner, Pulmonary
VA Medical Center
Milwaukee, Wisconsin

Susan C. Ruda, RN, MS, ONC
Clinical Nurse Specialist
Parkview Musculoskeletal Institute
Palos Heights, Illinois

Anne Marie Ruszkowski, RN, BSN
Director of Nursing
Deparment of Dermatology
Columbia University
New York, New York

Linda Sawchuk, RN, ARNP, CETN
Enterostomal Therapy Nurse
Virginia Mason Medical Center
Seattle, Washington

Sarah C. Smith, RN, MA, CRNO
Educational Associate/Advanced Practice Nurse
Department of Ophthalmology
The University of Iowa Hospitals and Clinics
Iowa City, Iowa

Laurie A. Soine, RN, MN, ARNP
Clinical Nurse Specialist/Nurse Practitioner
University of Washington Medical Center
Seattle, Washington

Kathleen C. Solotkin, RN, MSN
Trauma Nurse Coordinator
Wishard Memorial Hospital
Indianapolis, Indiana

Sally Sperry Steen, BS, MT (ASCP)
Instructor, Medical Laboratory Sciences
Department of Pathology, School of Medicine
University of New Mexico
Albuquerque, New Mexico

Roberta A. Strohl, RN, MN, AOCN
Clinical Associate Professor
Department of Radiation Oncology
University of Maryland at Baltimore
Baltimore, Maryland

Virginia Valentine, RN, MSN, CDE
CEO and Clinical Specialist
Diabetes Network, Inc.
Albuquerque, New Mexico

Trisch Van Sciver, RN, MS, PCNS, CFNP, DOM
Nurse Practitioner
Lovelace Health Systems
Albuquerque, New Mexico

Joan Stehle Werner, RN, DNS
Professor, Department of Adult Health and Illness
Oregon Health Sciences University
School of Nursing
Portland, Oregon

Una E. Westfall, PhD, RN
Professor, School of Nursing
Oregon Health Sciences University
Portland, Oregon

Marie Bakitas Whedon, RN, MS, AOCN, FAAN
Research Assistant Professor
Norris Cotton Cancer Center
Dartmouth-Hitchcock Medical Center
Lebanon, New Hampshire

Mary E. Wilbur, RN, MSN
Continuum of Care Manager
Medical University of South Carolina
Charleston, South Carolina

Diana J. Wilkie, PhD, RN, AOCN, FAAN
Associate Professor
School of Nursing
University of Washington
Seattle, Washington

Joyce M. Yasko, RN, PhD, FAAN
Associate Director for Clinical Network Administration
University of Pittsburgh Cancer Institute
Professor of Oncology Nursing
University of Pittsburgh School of Nursing
Pittsburgh, Pennsylvania

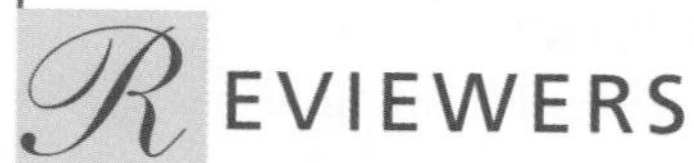

REVIEWERS

Aris Andrews, RN, MS
Hastings, Nebraska

Kathleen C. Ashton, RN, PhD, CS
Camden, New Jersey

Mary Baird, RN, MN, ARNP
Seattle, Washington

Debra A. Bancroft, RN, MSN, FNP-C
Milwaukee, Wisconsin

Linda Bernard, RN, MS
Chicago, Illinois

Donna Berry, RN, PhD, AOCN
Seattle, Washington

Carol Blainey, RN, MN
Seattle, Washington

Patricia A. Blissitt, RN, MSN, CCRN, CNRN, CCM
Seattle, Washington

Diane Britt, RN, MN, CS, CDE
Seattle, Washington

Gillian Brunier, MScN, RN, CNeph (C)
Toronto, Ontario, Canada

Kathryn Ann Caudell, RN, PhD, OCN
Albuquerque, New Mexico

Ann Tyler Chadwick, MN, RN, CCRN
Seattle, Washington

Elizabeth Chapman, RN, MS, CCRN
Long Beach, Mississippi

Kerry H. Cheever, RN, PhD, CEN
Milwaukee, Wisconsin

Sharon G. Childs, RN, MS, CRNP, CS, CEN, ONC
Baltimore, Maryland

Christine Chmielewski, RN, MS, CRNP
Philadelphia, Pennsylvania

Evelyn M. Clingerman, RN, MS
Rochester, Michigan

Rebecca Crane, RN, PhD, AOCN
Santa Monica, California

Janet T. Crimlisk, RN, MS, NP, CS
Boston, Massachusetts

Marjorie Cypress, C-ANP, CDE, RN
Albuquerque, New Mexico

Deborah K. Drummonds, RN, MN, CCRN, CEN
Milledgeville, Georgia

Sheila A. Dunn, RN, MSN, C-ANP
St. Louis, Missouri

Sheena Ferguson, RN, MSN, CCRN
Albuquerque, New Mexico

Diane M. Fesler, RN, MSN, PhD Candidate
DeKalb, Illinois

Linda Monfore Fluke, RN, MN, ARNP
Seattle, Washington

Rebecca Fruge, RN, MN
San Juan, Puerto Rico

Michele Geiger-Bronsky, RN, MSN, CS, FAACVPR
Manitowoc, Wisconsin

Margaret Grady, RN, MS
Albuquerque, New Mexico

Mikel Gray, RN, PhD, CUNP, CCCN, FAAN
Charlottesville, Virginia

Pauline McKinney Green, RN, PhD
Washington, DC

Shirley M. Gullo, RN, MSN, OCN
Cleveland, Ohio

James P. Halloran, RN, MSN, OCN, ANP
Houston, Texas

Susan Harrington, RN, MN, ARNP
Seattle, Washington

Stephine Heitkemper, RN, ARNP
Olympia, Washington

Kathryn Hennessy, RN, MS, CNSN
Deerfield, Illinois

Mary Jo Holechek, RN, MS, CRNP, CS, CNN
Baltimore, Maryland

Alicia M. Horkan, RN, MSN, CEN
Moultrie, Georgia

Katherine A. Howe, RN, MSN, MEd
Toledo, Ohio

Marguerite Jackson, RN, PhD, CIC, FAAN
San Diego, California

Monica Jarrett, RN, PhD
Seattle, Washington

Janet Katz, RNC, MSN
Spokane, Washington

Judy Kaye, RN, CNRN, CCRN, ANP, GNP, CS, PhDc
Augusta, Georgia

Judy Knighton, RN, MScN
Toronto, Ontario, Canada

Joy Knopp, RN, MN, ARNP
Seattle, Washington

Barbara S. Levine, RN, PhD, CRNP, CS
Philadelphia, Pennsylvania

Kim Litwack, PhD, RN, FAAN, CFNP
Albuquerque, New Mexico

Carol O. Long, RN, PhD
Tempe, Arizona

Marci Lovett, RN, MN, FNP, CS
Los Angeles, California

Margaret Lunney, PhD, RN, CS
Staten Island, New York

Holly Evans Madison, RN, MS
Manchester, Vermont

Elyse B. Mandell, MSN, RNCS
Boston, Massachusetts

Karen March, RN, MN, CNRN, CCRN
Seattle, Washington

Deborah L. Martin, RN, MN
Austin, Texas

Katherine E. Matas, RN, PhD
Kalamazoo, Michigan

Martha A. Melcher, RN, GNP
Port Angeles, Washington

Mary S. Merchant, RN, MSN, FNP
Charleston, South Carolina

Carmella Moran, RN, MSN
Naperville, Illinois

Mary Lou Muwaswes, RN, MS
San Francisco, California

Betsy Nielsen-Omeis, RN, BSN
San Antonio, Texas

Jane Parks, RN, MSN
Hastings, Nebraska

Jill H. Pendarvis, RNC, MA, CNOR
Fort Walton Beach, Florida

Janice Post-White, RN, PhD
Minneapolis, Minnesota

Virginia Printz-Feddersen, RNC, MSN, CNS, CNOR, CNRN
Albuquerque, New Mexico

Kimberly L. Quinn, RN, MS, CCRN
Baltimore, Maryland

Dennis Ross, RN, PhD
Castleton, Vermont

Deborah L. Roush, RN, MSN
Valdosta, Georgia

Paul Ruston, RN, BS
Warrenville, Illinois

Linda Schakenbach, RN, MSN, CS, CCRN, CETN
Annandale, Virginia

Darlene F. Schelper, RN, MSN, CEN, RNC
Hershey, Pennsylvania

Suzanne Shaffer, MN, RN, AOCN
Kansas City, Kansas

Lisa Anderson Shaw, RNC, MSN, MA
Chicago, Illinois

Geoff Shuster, RN, PhD
Albuquerque, New Mexico

Sandra Somma, RN, BSN
New Haven, Connecticut

Susan B. Stillwell, RN, MSN
Tempe, Arizona

Priscilla Ann Taylor, RN, MN, CGRN
Tacoma, Washington

Trisch Van Sciver, RN, MS, PCNS, CFNP, DOM
Albuquerque, New Mexico

Kathleen Dorman Wagner, RN, MSN, CS
Lexington, Kentucky

Eileen Walsh, RN, MSN, CVN
Toledo, Ohio

Joyce S. Willens, PhD, RN
Villanova, Pennsylvania

To the profession of nursing

and

to the important people in our lives

PREFACE TO THE INSTRUCTOR

The fifth edition of *Medical-Surgical Nursing: Assessment and Management of Clinical Problems* has been extensively revised to incorporate the most recent medical-surgical nursing information in an attractive, easy-to-use format. More than just a textbook, this is a comprehensive resource containing essential information that students need to prepare for lectures, classroom activities, examinations, clinical assignments, and comprehensive care of patients. In addition to the readable writing style and full-color illustrations, the text includes many special features to help students learn the most important medical-surgical nursing content. This edition highlights this content for today's nursing students, including patient teaching, gerontology, collaborative care, cultural and ethnic considerations, nutrition, community and home care, nursing research, and much more.

The comprehensive and accurate content, special features, attractive layout, and student-friendly writing style have combined to make this the number one medical-surgical nursing textbook used in more nursing schools around the country than any other medical-surgical textbook.

The strengths of the first four editions have been retained, including the use of the nursing process as an organizational theme for nursing management and a commitment to support the role of nurses on the home health care team. Numerous new features have been added to address some of the rapid changes in practice. Contributors have again been selected for their acknowledged excellence in specific content areas; one or more specialists in the subject area have thoroughly reviewed each chapter to increase accuracy. The editors have undertaken final rewriting and editing to achieve internal consistency. All efforts were directed toward building on the strengths of the previous edition while preparing an even more effective new edition.

ORGANIZATION

Content is organized into two major divisions. The first division, Section One (Chapters 1 through 10), discusses general concepts related to adult patients. The second division, Sections Two through Twelve (Chapters 11 through 64), presents nursing assessment and nursing management of medical-surgical problems.

The various body systems are grouped to reflect their interrelated functions. Each section is organized around two central themes: assessment and management. Chapters dealing with assessment of a body system include a discussion of the following:

1. A brief review of anatomy and physiology, focusing on information that will promote understanding of nursing care
2. Health history and noninvasive physical assessment skills to expand the knowledge base on which decisions are made
3. Common diagnostic studies, expected results, and related nursing responsibilities to provide easily accessible information

Chapters dealing with management of the various diseases and disorders focus on the etiology and pathophysiologic bases, clinical manifestations, diagnostic study results, collaborative care, and nursing management of diseases and disorders. The nursing management sections are organized into nursing assessment, nursing diagnoses, planning, nursing implementation, and evaluation. To emphasize the importance of patient care in various clinical settings, nursing implementation of all major health problems is organized by the following levels of care:

1. Health Promotion
2. Acute Intervention
3. Ambulatory and Home Care

SPECIAL FEATURES

- **Home health care/community-based care** is an ongoing theme throughout the text. Coverage has been significantly increased in the fifth edition, including a new chapter (Chapter 2: Community-Based Nursing and Home Health Care) and Patient and Family Home Care Guides appearing throughout the text. Ambulatory and Home Care headings appear in Nursing Implementation sections. In addition, there are examples of clinical pathways—home care of diabetes mellitus and ostomy—that focus specifically on home health care.
- **Patient teaching** has also been emphasized in this edition. Coverage includes a new chapter (Chapter 6: Patient Teaching) and more than 50 Patient Teaching Guides and Patient and Family Teaching Guides throughout the text.
- **Collaborative care** is highlighted in this revision, including new Collaborative Care sections in all management chapters and more than 80 Collaborative Care tables throughout the text.
- **Gerontology** coverage includes Chapter 3: Adult Development and Chapter 4: Gerontologic Considerations and appears throughout the text under Gerontologic Considerations headings and in Gerontologic Differences in Assessment and Effects of Aging tables.
- **Nutrition** is highlighted throughout the book. Nutritional Therapy tables summarize nutritional interventions

and promote healthy lifestyles in patients with various conditions.

- **Nursing management** is presented in a consistent and comprehensive format, which now includes Evaluation headings where appropriate. In addition, 78 Nursing Care Plans appear in management chapters. These are thoroughly updated to incorporate (1) current NANDA nursing diagnoses, including the problem, etiologic statement, and defining characteristics; (2) specific nursing interventions with rationales; (3) expected patient outcomes; and (4) collaborative problems.
- A new chapter on **alternative and complementary therapies** addresses timely issues in today's health care settings related to nontraditional therapies.
- **Nursing research** encourages application of research into clinical practice. Research Implications for Nursing Practice boxes appear throughout the text, and Nursing Research Issues at the end of management chapters present possible research questions to be used for research studies.
- **Cultural and ethnic considerations** information is integrated into the text and appears in special boxes highlighting important issues related to the nursing care of various ethnic populations.
- **Ethical Dilemmas** boxes appear in management chapters to promote critical thinking for timely and sensitive issues that nursing students may deal with in practice. Each box contains a discussion of ethical and legal principles.
- **Clinical Pathways** for selected medical-surgical disorders show how hospitals and home health agencies are implementing collaborative care.
- **Emergency Management** tables outline the emergency treatment of health problems most likely to require emergency intervention.
- **Common Assessment Abnormalities** tables in assessment chapters alert the nurse to frequently encountered abnormalities and their possible etiologies.
- **Nursing Assessment** tables summarize the key subjective and objective data related to common diseases. Subjective data are organized by functional health patterns.
- **Health History** tables in assessment chapters present key questions to ask patients related to a specific disease or disorder.

LEARNING AIDS

- ✔ Learning Objectives beginning each chapter help students focus on the key information for that body system or disorder.
- ✔ Review Questions at the end of each chapter help students learn the important points in the chapter. Answers are provided in an appendix so that the review questions serve as a self-study tool.
- ✔ Critical Thinking Exercises appearing at the end of nursing management chapters include Case Studies with Critical Thinking Questions for clinical application, as well as Nursing Research Issues.
- ✔ Resources at the end of each chapter contain information about nursing and health care organizations that provide patient teaching and disease and disorder information. Resources include Internet sites to help students find current information online.

Media learning tools provided free with the text include the following:

- ✔ The CD-ROM packaged with this text contains overviews of common diseases and disorders, key terms, case studies, and review questions to help students apply this challenging content. This special icon appears in the margin of the text to designate content areas where students are encouraged to use their free CD-ROM for further self-study.
- ✔ MERLIN The MERLIN website customized for this book features WebLinks for each chapter of the book and Content Updates by the authors to keep students and instructors informed on the most current medical-surgical nursing information. Be sure to visit the site at www.mosby.com/MERLIN/medsurg_lewis

ANCILLARIES

The fifth edition ancillary package has been extensively revised to include even more creative and comprehensive materials to aid instructors and students.

- **Clinical Companion to Medical-Surgical Nursing,** 2nd edition, presents more than 300 common medical-surgical conditions and procedures in a concise, alphabetical format for quick clinical reference. Designed for portability, this valuable reference includes the essential, need-to-know information for medical-surgical nursing practice. This edition features an attractive and functional two-color internal design, as well as an increased emphasis on patient teaching.
- **Instructor's Resource Kit** remains the most comprehensive set of instructor's materials available, containing suggested lecture strategies, case studies with critical thinking questions, answers to worksheets included in the *Study Guide*, a test bank with more than 1000 questions with coded answers, and worksheets to accompany *Mosby's Medical-Surgical Nursing Video Series.*
- **Test Bank** includes more than 1200 questions with NCLEX-coded answers.
- **Electronic Image Collection** is a CD-ROM containing hundreds of full-color images from the text for use in lectures and to import into PowerPoint.
- **Study Guide** contains extensive review and testing material that has been thoroughly updated to reflect the revision of the textbook. It features a wide variety of clinically

relevant exercises and activities, including fill-in-the-blank worksheets, anatomy identification review, true-false questions, critical thinking activities, crossword puzzles, case studies, matching exercises, word scrambles, and multiple-choice questions in NCLEX format. Answers to all questions are included in the back of the *Study Guide* to provide students with immediate feedback as they study.

- **Virtual Clinical Excursions** is an exciting and innovative new teaching and learning tool. The dynamic CD-ROM presents true-to-life simulations of clinical practice in a "virtual hospital" setting. The accompanying workbook contains case-based activities prepared specifically for this text. This is an excellent way for students to apply what they learn from the text and to foster critical thinking skills.

ACKNOWLEDGMENTS

The editors are especially grateful to many people at Mosby who assisted with this major revision effort. In particular, we wish to thank the team of Sally Schrefer, Jeanne Allison, Kristin Geen, Dana Peick, Catherine Albright, and Amy Buxton. In addition, we want to thank the marketing team of Janet Blanner and Tom Wilhelm.

We would like to thank Idolia Cox Collier for her ideas, creativity, and hard work as co-editor on the first four editions of this book.

Our persevering typists have earned our special thanks and include Christa Cooper and Elizabeth Miller. Kay McCash provided invaluable assistance as a consultant on nursing diagnoses and revision of the nursing care plans. Pat O'Brien worked diligently on the *Study Guide* and provided excellent new material for the *Test Bank, Instructor's Resource Kit,* and CD-ROM to accompany the text.

We are particularly indebted to the nurses and student nurses who have put their faith in our book to assist them on their path to excellence. The increasing use of this book throughout the United States and Canada has been gratifying. We appreciate the many users who have shared their comments and suggestions on the previous editions.

We also wish to thank our contributors and reviewers for their conscientious attention to detail throughout the revision process. We sincerely hope that this book will assist both students and clinicians in practicing truly professional nursing.

Sharon Lewis

Margaret McLean Heitkemper

Shannon Ruff Dirksen

PREFACE TO THE STUDENT

Medical-Surgical Nursing: Assessment and Management of Clinical Problems was developed to provide you, today's busy nursing student, with the most important medical-surgical nursing information in an attractive, easy-to-use format. The authors know how important it is that you have a resource containing the essential information you need to prepare for lectures, classroom activities, examinations, clinical assignments, and overall care of your patients. This bestselling text is carefully designed to meet these needs.

Not only will this book help you to succeed in your studies, it will also prepare you for advanced study and practice in clinical settings. In addition to the readable writing style and full-color illustrations, it includes many special features to help you study and learn the most important medical-surgical nursing concepts. Some of these features include:

- ✔ **Learning Objectives** beginning each chapter to help you focus on the key information.
- ✔ **Review Questions** at the end of each chapter to help you learn the important points in the chapter. Answers are provided in an appendix so that the review questions serve as a self-study tool.
- ✔ **Critical Thinking Exercises** at the end of nursing management chapters include Case Studies with Critical Thinking Questions useful for clinical application and Nursing Research Issues useful for research projects.
- ✔ **Special tables and boxes** summarizing information that is key to understanding disease management and providing effective patient care. These features include:
  - **Patient Teaching Guides**
  - **Patient & Family Home Care Guides**
  - **Ethical Dilemmas**
  - **Research Implications for Nursing Practice**
  - **Cultural & Ethnic Considerations**
  - **Nursing Care Plans** and many others.
- ✔ **Resources at the end of each chapter** containing information about nursing and health care organizations that provide patient teaching and disease and disorder information. Resources include Internet sites to help you find current information online.

In addition to the text, here are some additional learning tools provided free:

- ✔ **CD-ROM** packaged with this text containing overviews of common diseases, key terms, case studies, and review questions to help you apply this challenging content. This special icon appears in the margins of the text to indicate areas where you may want to access your CD-ROM for further content review.
- ✔ MERLIN **MERLIN website** customized for this book featuring WebLinks for each chapter of the book and Content Updates by the authors to keep you informed on the most current medical-surgical nursing information. Be sure to visit the site at www.mosby.com/MERLIN/medsurg_lewis

And do not forget the **Study Guide** to accompany this book. This valuable study tool contains extensive review and testing material that has been thoroughly updated to reflect the revision of the book. It features a wide variety of clinically relevant exercises and activities, including:

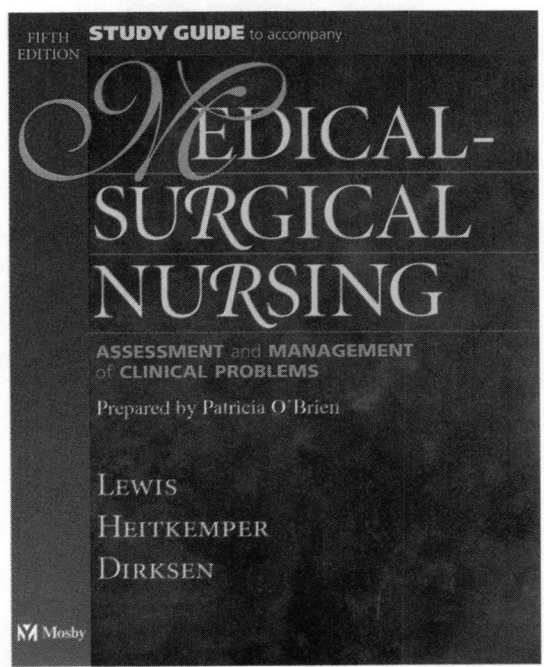

- ✔ Fill-in-the-blank worksheets
- ✔ Anatomy identification review
- ✔ True-false questions
- ✔ Critical thinking activities
- ✔ Crossword puzzles
- ✔ Case studies
- ✔ Matching exercises
- ✔ Word scrambles
- ✔ Multiple-choice questions in NCLEX format

Answers to all questions are included in the back of the *Study Guide* to provide immediate feedback as you study.

Also accompanying this text is the ***Clinical Companion to Medical-Surgical Nursing,*** 2nd edition. This handy reference presents more than 300 common medical-surgical conditions and procedures in a concise, alphabetical format for quick clinical reference. Designed for portability, it includes the essential, need-to-know information for medical-surgical nursing practice.

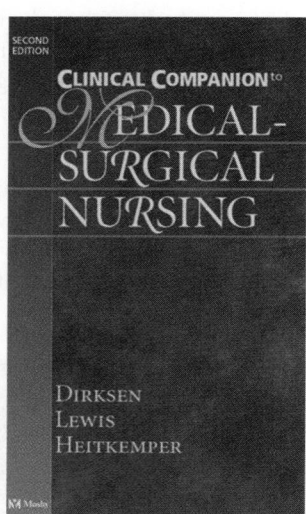

Be sure to check out **Virtual Clinical Excursions,** an exciting and innovative new study tool. The CD-ROM presents true-to-life simulations of clinical practice in a "virtual hospital" setting. The accompanying workbook contains case-based activities prepared specifically for this text. This is an excellent way to practice what you are learning in the text, and to apply your knowledge to clinical settings.

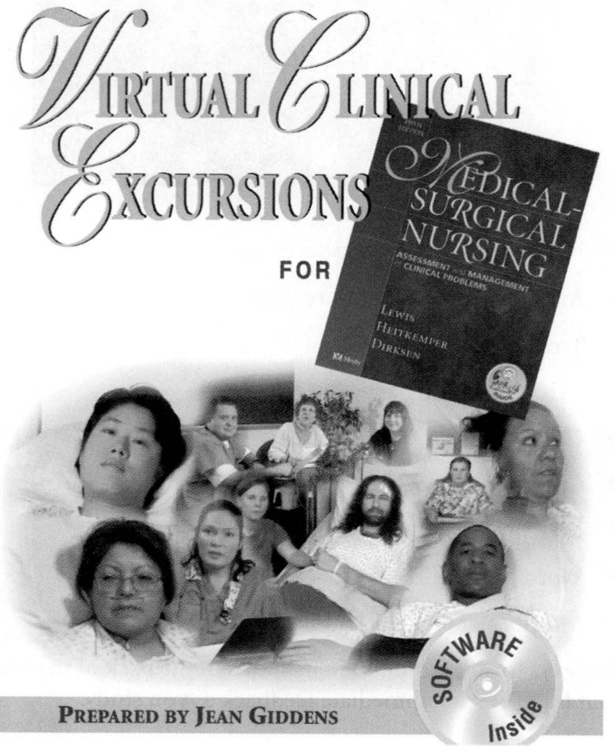

■■■

The authors and Mosby hope that you find this book helpful as you continue your nursing education! Please feel free to contact us anytime with feedback about the book.

DETAILED CONTENTS

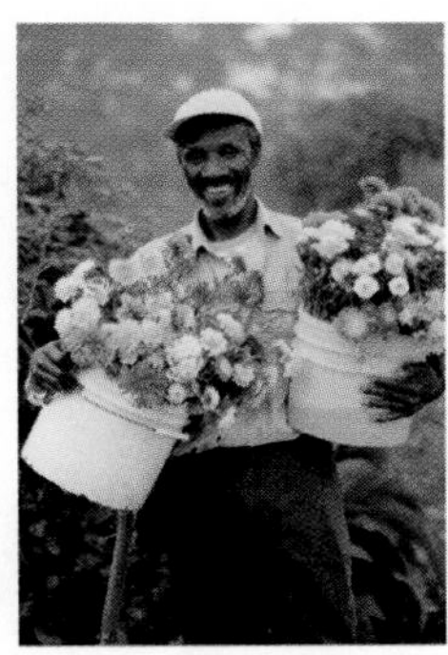

SECTION 1

GENERAL CONCEPTS OF NURSING PRACTICE

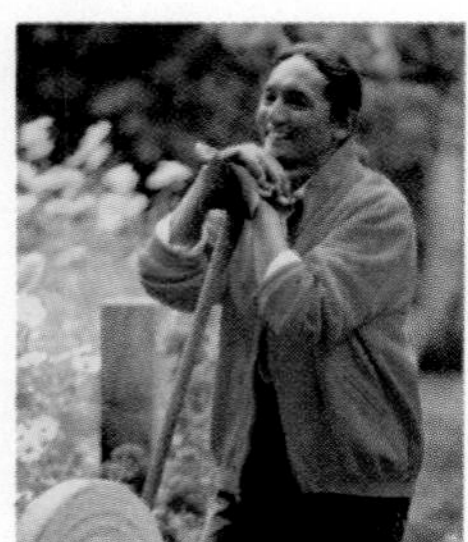

SECTION 2

PATHOPHYSIOLOGIC MECHANISMS OF DISEASE

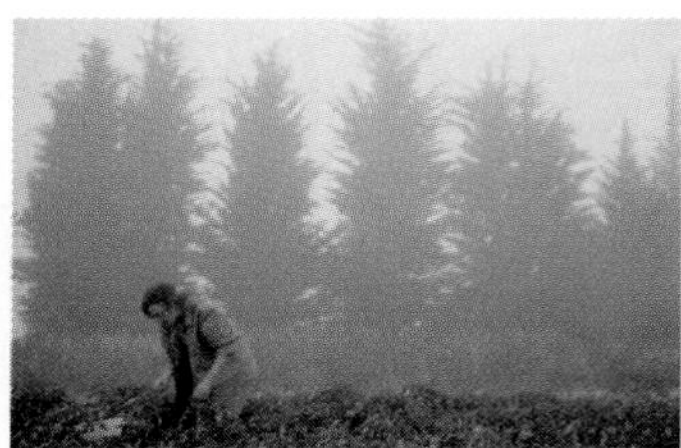

SECTION 3

THE SURGICAL EXPERIENCE

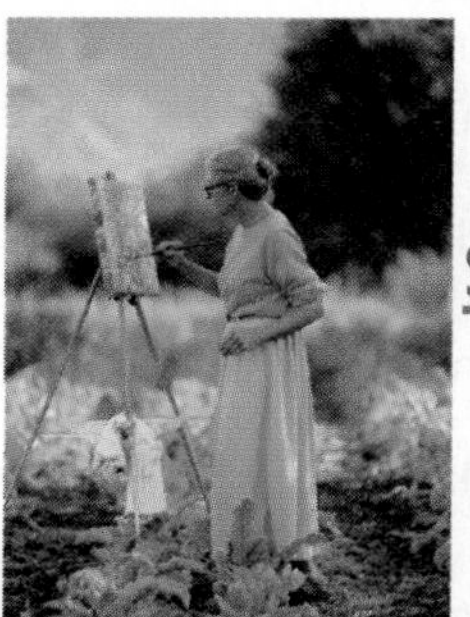

SECTION 4

PROBLEMS RELATED TO ALTERED SENSORY INPUT

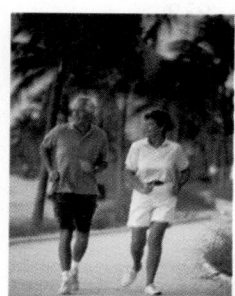

SECTION 5

PROBLEMS OF OXYGENATION: VENTILATION

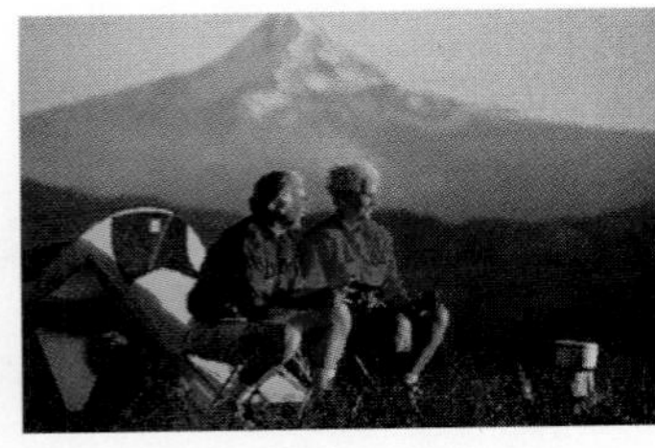

SECTION 6

PROBLEMS OF OXYGENATION: TRANSPORT

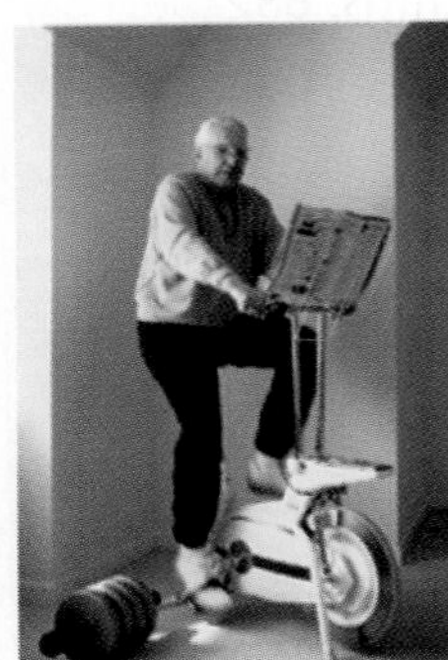

SECTION 7

PROBLEMS OF OXYGENATION: PERFUSION

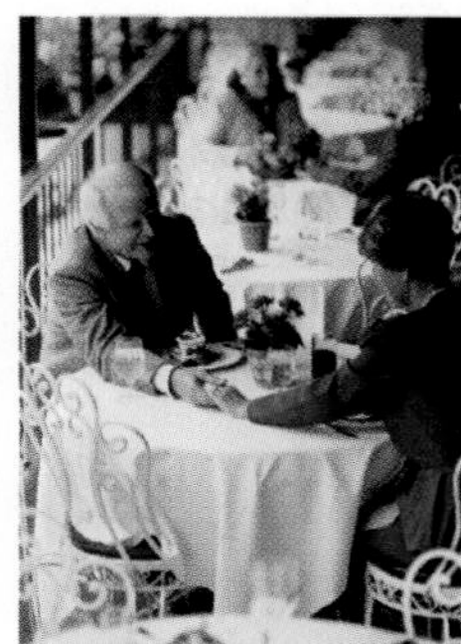

SECTION 8

PROBLEMS OF INGESTION, DIGESTION, ABSORPTION, AND ELIMINATION

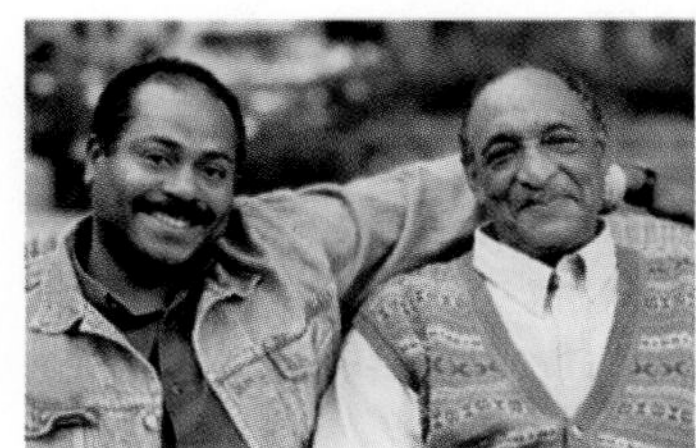

SECTION 9

PROBLEMS OF URINARY FUNCTION

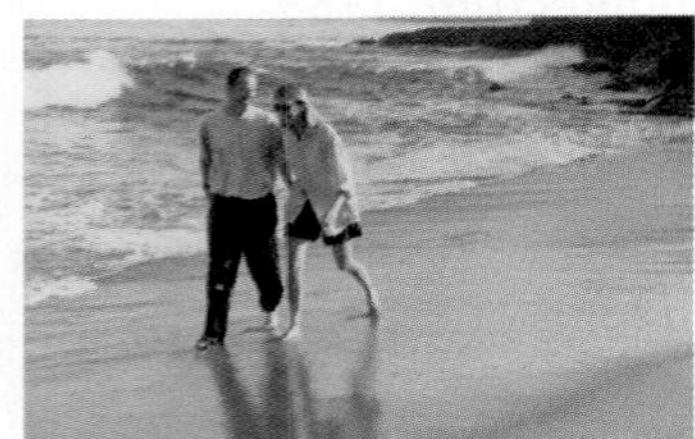

SECTION 10

PROBLEMS RELATED TO REGULATORY MECHANISMS

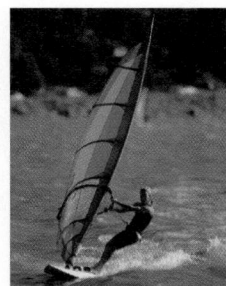

SECTION 11

PROBLEMS RELATED TO MOVEMENT AND COORDINATION

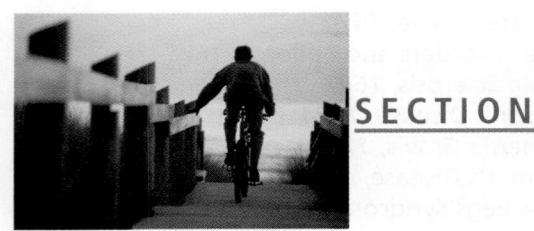

SECTION 12

NURSING CARE IN SPECIALIZED SETTINGS

Nursing Care Plans

SECTION

1

GENERAL CONCEPTS OF NURSING PRACTICE

SECTION OUTLINE

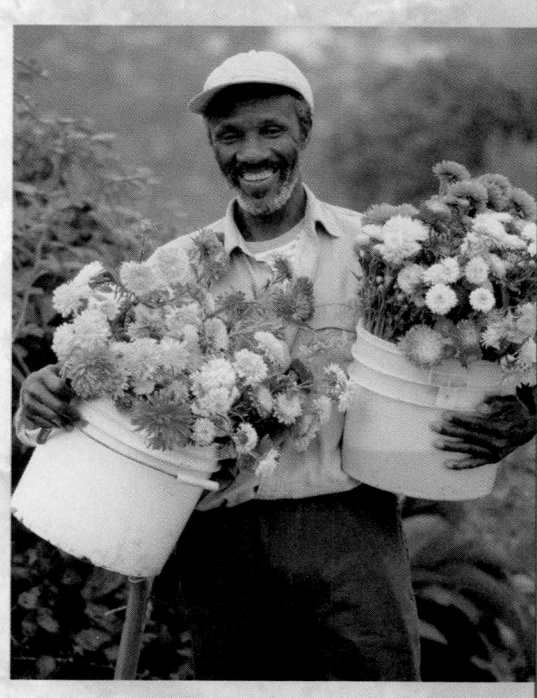

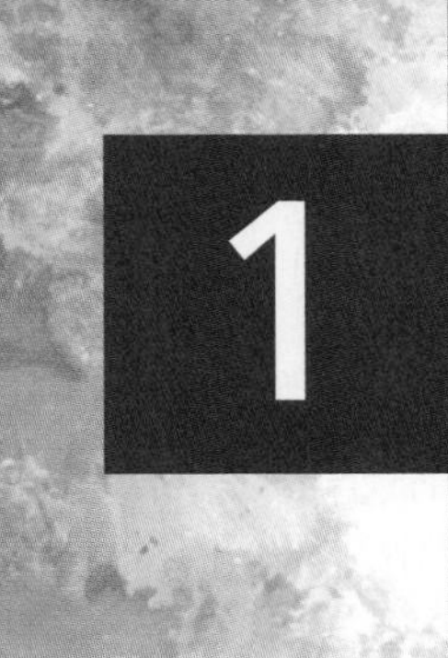

REMEMBER to check out your companion CD-ROM

1 Applying Critical Thinking to the Nursing Process

Katheryn Ellen McCash

www.mosby.com/MERLIN/medsurg_lewis

LEARNING OBJECTIVES

1. Describe the basic focus of the domain of nursing.
2. Distinguish among the independent, dependent, and collaborative functions of nursing practice.
3. Describe the five phases of the nursing process.
4. Differentiate between the process of making a nursing diagnosis and a nursing diagnosis as a form of diagnostic nomenclature.
5. Describe the criteria for writing expected patient outcomes.
6. Identify the types of interventions a nurse can use to implement the plan.
7. Identify the places in the nursing process where evaluation is appropriate.
8. Describe the importance of documentation to the nursing process.

The nursing process is a framework used by the nurse to organize thinking about the health care needs of individuals, families, and communities and to organize and deliver nursing care. The nursing process is an inherent part of nursing care and is actualized in the unique style of each nurse.

NURSING YESTERDAY AND TODAY

In primitive times, there was no distinction between nursing and medicine. The sick and injured were merely cared for by those with nurturant instincts.[1] Today there is a clearer delineation between nursing and medical practice.

Nurses deal with "the diagnosis and treatment of human responses to actual or potential health problems,"[2] whereas medicine is primarily concerned with the diagnosis and treatment of illness or injury. The unique nursing focus is on the response of an individual or group to an actual or potential health problem rather than on the disease process itself. For example, in caring for a person with a fractured hip, the nurse focuses on the self-care restrictions and the effects of immobility and pain. The surgeon is primarily concerned with the type of surgery and prosthesis to use in doing the surgical repair.

Many modern theorists, such as Neuman, Orem, and Rodgers, have attempted to precisely define nursing's domain.[3] Although much work is needed in testing nursing theories, many of the current issues in nursing today were concerns of Florence Nightingale. In 1893 she addressed holistic health when she emphasized that one must nurse the whole person rather than the disease.[4] Current emphases in nursing practice, such as health promotion, patient and family teaching, family and community nursing, establishment of trust, use of good communication skills, and stress reduction techniques, were all an integral part of nursing as defined by Florence Nightingale.

Historically, nursing care has been delivered using a variety of models. Team nursing was the model of care used in the 1960s and 1970s. Primary nursing was the model of the 1970s and 1980s. In this model there was a primary nurse who ensured that all the basic needs of the patient were met. Managed care is a new health care delivery concept that evolved from the health care reform movement of the 1990s (see Chapter 2). Interdisciplinary or collaborative care, as well as renewed appreciation of the joint contributions of various disciplines, is the current trend. In the current health care system, case management is an approach that coordinates and links health care services to patients and their families. As a member of the interdisciplinary health care team, the nurse case manager coordinates the clinical care of the patient across care settings, from admission through discharge from the hospital, and back home in an effort to achieve optimal outcomes. (Case management is discussed in Chapter 2.)

Advanced Practice Nursing

Advanced practice nursing roles emphasize health assessment, diagnosis, and treatment of conditions previously considered only within the physician's domain. Examples of the advanced practice nursing roles are clinical nurse specialist, nurse practitioner, nurse midwife, and nurse anesthetist. They

Reviewed by Pauline McKinney Green, RN, PhD, Associate Professor, Howard University College of Pharmacy, Nursing, and Allied Health Sciences, Washington, DC.

are considered advanced practice nurses because of their advanced education. These nurses may work in hospitals, but they also may work in a variety of settings, such as outpatient clinics, physician's offices, independent practice, nursing homes, schools, and industry.

Nurses have always assessed their patients' health status. Today, however, as a result of scientific and technologic advances, there are new methods available requiring new equipment and skills. Today, nurses are asserting their right to learn and apply skills that enhance their abilities to determine the health status of their patients. By increasing their assessment skills, nurses increase their database on which they make sound judgments. The stethoscope was at one time used only by the physician. Today, no one questions whether the nurse should use this instrument in patient care activities.

By expanding their scientific understanding of pathophysiology, psychopathology, and pharmacology, nurses are better able to understand the scientific basis of assessment findings that indicate various levels of health or disease. Incorporating the sciences and humanities into nursing education has broadened and deepened the knowledge base of nursing practice. Nurses continuously face the challenge of keeping current with developments in science and technology.

Scientific and technologic advances have made an impact on health care and care of the sick. In response to these advances, nursing is in a state of evolution. Increasing emphasis on accountability, assertiveness, persistence, risk taking, and decision making are essential if nursing is to "get somewhere else." In its attempt to keep pace, nursing would do well to remember what the Queen in *Through the Looking Glass* said to Alice: "Now here, you see, it takes all the running you can do to keep in the same place. If you want to get somewhere else, you must run at least twice as fast as that."[5]

Definitions of Nursing

A basic question revolves around how the profession of nursing views itself. Several well-known definitions of nursing indicate that a basic theme of health, illness, and caring has existed since Florence Nightingale. Following are two such examples:

> The unique function of the nurse is to assist the individual, sick or well, in the performance of those activities contributing to health or its recovery (or to peaceful death) that he would perform unaided if he had the necessary strength, will, or knowledge. And to do this in such a way as to help him gain independence as rapidly as possible.[6]
>
> Nursing is putting the patient in the best condition for nature to act.[4]

In this textbook the American Nurses' Association's definition of nursing is used:

> Nursing is the diagnosis and treatment of human responses to actual and potential health problems.[2]

Nursing's View of Humanity

Nursing's view of humanity must be considered when describing nursing. Although different terms have been used, there is widespread agreement among nursing theorists that an individual has physiologic (or biophysical), psychologic (or emotional), sociocultural (or interpersonal), spiritual, and environmental components or dimensions. In this text the human individual is considered "a biopsychosocial being in constant interaction with a changing environment."[7] The individual is composed of dimensions that are interrelated and not separate entities. Thus a problem in one dimension generally affects one or more of the other dimensions. Psychologic anxiety, for instance, affects the autonomic nervous system, a part of the biophysical dimension.

Growth and development are influenced by interactions with others. No two individuals are exactly alike. No one individual remains the same from moment to moment. Therefore each individual has value as an irreplaceable member of humanity. Inherent in this individuality is the right to develop one's unique potential according to a personal value system to the extent that the exercise of this right does not deny it to others.

The behavior of the individual is meaningful and oriented toward fulfilling needs and coping with environmental stresses. At times, however, an individual needs assistance to meet these needs and to cope successfully.

NURSING PROCESS

Nursing accomplishes its goal of assisting others to resolve actual or potential problems by the use of the nursing process. The nursing process is an assertive, problem-solving approach to the identification and treatment of patient problems. It provides an organizing framework for the knowledge, thoughts, and actions that nurses bring to patient care.[8] Using the nursing process, the nurse can focus on the unique responses of patients to actual or potential health problems. The nursing process is operationalized by means of cognitive (thinking, reasoning), psychomotor (doing), and affective (feelings, values) skills and abilities of the nurse to plan and implement patient care.

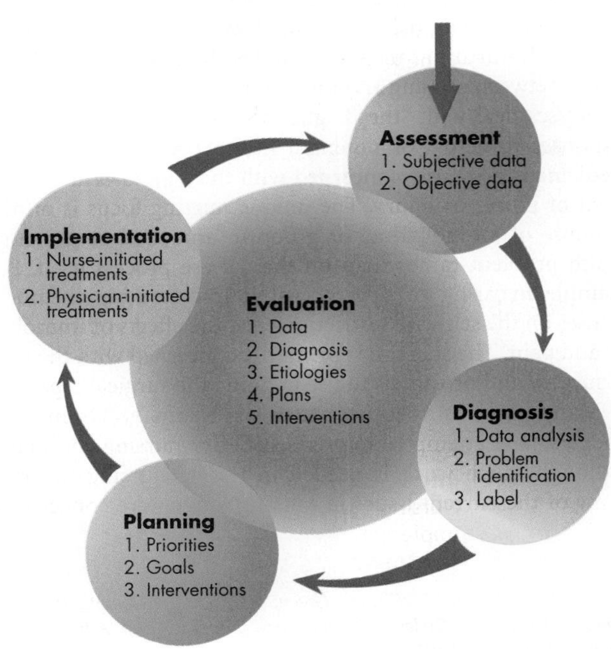

Fig. 1-1 The nursing process.

Phases of the Nursing Process

The nursing process consists of five phases: assessment, diagnosis, planning, implementation, and evaluation (Fig. 1-1). However, numerous other terms or phrases are used in nursing to describe the steps of the nursing process (Table 1-1). Assessment involves collecting subjective and objective information about the patient. The diagnosis phase involves analyzing the information, drawing conclusions from the information, and labeling the human response. Planning consists of setting goals with the patient and family, when feasible, and determining strategies for accomplishing the goals. Implementation involves the use of interventions to activate the plan. Evaluation is the analysis of the effectiveness of the assessment, diagnosis, planning, and implementation phases.

Table 1-1 Commonly Used Terms for Components of the Nursing Process

Assessment Phase		
		Data collection
		Data gathering
		Assessment
		Collection of information
		History and physical examination
Diagnosis Phase		
	Step I:	Data analysis
		Assessment
		Judgment
		Decision making
		Clustering information
		Determination of strengths and weaknesses
		Determination of unmet needs
		Determination of assets and limitations
	Step II:	Nursing diagnosis
		Problem identification
		Etiology determination
		Labeling the problem
		Naming the problem
Planning Phase		
	Step I:	Priority setting
	Step II:	Expected outcome
		Goal setting
		Objective setting, subgoals
		Desired behaviors
		Outcome criteria
	Step III:	Planning interventions
		Planning nursing actions
		Nursing orders
		Planning strategies of care
Implementation		
		Application
		Intervention
		Nursing care
		Implementation
		Treatment
Evaluation		
		Reassessment
		Audit

Interrelatedness of Phases

The five phases of the nursing process do not occur in isolation from one another. For example, nurses may gather data about the wound condition (assessment) as they change the soiled dressing (implementation). There is, however, a basic order to the nursing process, beginning with assessment. This provides the data on which to base the plan. A judgment about the nature of the assessment data usually follows immediately. Implementation follows a careful plan based on the nursing diagnosis. Evaluation continues throughout the cycle. This continuous evaluation provides feedback on the effectiveness of the plan or the need for revision. Revision may be needed in the data collection method, the diagnosis, the goals, the plan, or the intervention method. Once begun, the nursing process is not only continuous but also cyclic in nature. There is no limit to the number of times the cycle can be reinitiated. Application of the nursing process requires sound knowledge of the physical and behavioral sciences and a repertoire of intellectual, interpersonal, and technical skills.

The nursing profession and the medical profession use a problem-solving process in caring for a patient. The uniqueness of nursing's problem-solving approach stems from the goals of nursing and the means of accomplishing these goals. A comparison of the goals of medicine and nursing is made in Table 1-2.

Independent and Collaborative Functions

Nursing practice has independent, dependent, and collaborative functions. As the profession becomes more autonomous, nurse-initiated (independent) interventions, such as health teaching, counseling, and other measures that assist the patient in meeting basic needs, are carried out to manage the nursing diagnosis.[9]

The nurse functions dependently when a nurse carries out medical orders. Physician-initiated functions may include administering medications, performing or assisting with certain medical treatments, and assisting with diagnostic tests and procedures. The exact roles are often determined by state and agency policies. The nurse's role in most cases is one of "interdependence and coparticipation" with the patient and other health team members.

In the collaborative role, the nurse is primarily responsible for monitoring for possible or actual complications and for treating the patient to prevent or manage the complication. In

Table 1-2 Comparison of Primary Goals: Nursing and Medicine

Nursing	Medicine
Determines responses to health problems, level of wellness, and need for assistance	Determines etiology of illness or injury
Provides physical care, emotional care, teaching, guidance, and counseling	Provides medical treatments and surgery
Interventions aimed at prevention and assisting the patient to meet his or her own needs	Interventions aimed at preventing and curing injury or illness

this role the nurse may use either physician-prescribed or nurse-prescribed interventions. The collaborative role is frequently demonstrated in the intensive care unit as the nurse monitors patients for complications of acute illness, administers intravenous fluids and medications per physician orders, and implements nursing interventions such as providing emotional support or teaching about specific procedures.

The nurse is expected to have a variety of skills and abilities that are required during various phases of the nursing process. These include the following:

Administrative	History taking
Analytic	Leadership and management
Communication	Physical examination
Counseling and referral	Improvisation
Creativity	Psychosocial assessment
Decision making	Recording and reporting
Diagnostic	Research
Group leadership	Teaching
Health assessment	Technical
Health teaching	Therapeutic

ASSESSMENT PHASE

Data Collection

A sound database is the foundation for the entire nursing process. Collection of data is a prerequisite to diagnosis, planning, and intervention. A human being as a biopsychosocial being has needs and problems in all dimensions: biophysical, psychologic, sociocultural, spiritual, and environmental. A nursing diagnosis made without supporting data in all dimensions can lead to incorrect conclusions and depersonalized care. For example, a hospitalized patient who does not sleep all night may be mistakenly diagnosed as having a sleep pattern disturbance. In fact the patient may have worked nights his entire adult life, and it is normal for him to be awake at night. Information concerning his sleeping habits is necessary to individualize his care so that he does not routinely receive a sleep medication at 10 PM. The importance of assessment in the process of clinical decision making cannot be overemphasized. The use of a nursing database is recommended to facilitate the collection of data. Chapter 5 provides a detailed discussion of the nursing database.

Because nursing interventions are only as sound as the database on which they are formulated, it is critical that the database be accurate and complete. When possible, information gained from sources such as the patient's record, other health care workers, the patient's family, and the nurse's observations should be validated with the patient. Likewise, when possible, questionable statements by the patient should be validated by a knowledgeable person.

DIAGNOSIS PHASE

Data Analysis and Problem Identification

The diagnostic phase begins with the clustering of information and ends with an evaluative judgment about a patient's health status. This evaluative judgment is reached after analysis of the assessment data. Analysis involves sorting through and organizing or clustering the information and determining unmet needs, as well as patient strengths. The findings are then compared with documented norms to determine whether anything is interfering or could interfere with the patient's needs or ability to maintain his or her usual health pattern.

After a thorough analysis of all available information, one of two possible conclusions results. Either there are no problems that require nursing intervention or the patient needs nursing assistance to solve a potential or actual problem. The statements of final conclusions about the problems are the nursing diagnoses.

Nursing Diagnosis

The term *nursing diagnosis* has many different meanings. To some it merely connotes the identification of a health problem. More commonly, a nursing diagnosis is viewed as the conclusion about an identified cluster of signs and symptoms. The diagnosis is generally expressed as concisely as possible according to specific guidelines.

Diagnosis is the act of identifying and labeling human responses to actual or potential health problems or stressors. Throughout this book, the term *nursing diagnosis* will mean (1) the process of identifying actual and potential health problems and (2) the label or concise statement that describes "a clinical judgment about an individual, family, or community response to actual or potential health problems and life processes. Nursing diagnoses provide the basis for the selection of nursing interventions to achieve outcomes for which the nurse is accountable."[10] The human responses identified, however, frequently result from the disease process. For example, a patient may have the medical diagnosis of chronic obstructive pulmonary disease (COPD). However, the nursing diagnosis will focus on how the COPD affects daily functioning (e.g., activity intolerance *related to* imbalance between oxygen supply and demand).

A number of other terms or situations are not nursing diagnoses but are often mislabeled as such.[11] These include the following:

Medical pathologic conditions (coronary artery disease)
Diagnostic tests or studies (upper gastrointestinal series)
Equipment (nasogastric tube)
Signs (restlessness)
Surgical procedures (hysterectomy)
Treatments (pressure ulcer care)
Therapeutic goals (perform own oral care)
Nursing problems (difficult to turn)
Therapeutic needs (needs more rest)
Staff problems (Mr. Jones is too demanding)

Collaborative Problems. Collaborative problems are potential or actual complications of disease or treatment that nurses treat with other health care providers, most frequently physicians.[11] A look at the primary goals of nursing helps in differentiating between nursing and medical diagnoses (see Table 1-2). Collaborative problem statements are usually written as potential complication: _____ without a "related to" statement. When potential complications are used in this textbook, "related to" statements have been added to increase understanding and relate the potential complication to possible causes. The focus of nursing interventions for collaborative problems is to reduce the severity of complications or to prevent them from occurring.[11]

North American Nursing Diagnosis Association. Nursing is moving toward a common language for classifying patients' responses or problems. The identification and development of a classification system of nursing diagnoses formally began in 1973 when Kristine Gebbie and Mary Ann Lavin of St. Louis University called the First National Conference on Classification of Nursing Diagnosis. National conferences have been held regularly since 1973. Since the Fifth National Conference, the National Group for the Classification of Nursing Diagnosis has evolved into a formal organization and has been renamed the North American Nursing Diagnosis Association (NANDA). The two main purposes of NANDA are to develop a diagnostic classification system (taxonomy) and to identify and approve nursing diagnoses. A list of diagnoses accepted by NANDA for clinical testing is found in Appendix A.

The nursing diagnoses used in this textbook are NANDA approved. However, it is acceptable to use non–NANDA approved nursing diagnoses whenever a new label is identified because the NANDA list is continually expanding. The accepted NANDA nursing diagnoses are evolving as research results are interpreted and as nurses identify new human responses. Therefore the nurse may encounter diagnoses in clinical practice that are not cited on the list. Nurses are encouraged to submit refinements of accepted diagnoses and new submissions to NANDA (NANDA, c/o NURSECOM, 1211 Locust St., Philadelphia, PA 19107).

In addition to the NANDA classification, several other individuals and groups are working to identify, standardize, and disseminate nursing's language, including Home Health Care Classification (Virginia Saba), Omaha System (Karen Martin), Oxbolt System (Judy Oxbolt), Nursing Intervention and Lexicon Terminology (Susan Grobe), Nursing Intervention Classification (Joanne McCloskey and Gloria Bulechek), Nursing Outcome Classification (Marian Johnson and Meridean Maas), and International Classification of Nursing Practice (International Council of Nursing). The outcome of all these efforts will be a universal nursing language system.

Diagnostic Process

Nursing diagnostic statements are acceptable when written as two-part or three-part statements. A two-part statement is acceptable if the signs and symptoms data are easily accessible to other nurses caring for the patient through such means as the nursing history or progress note. Use of a three-part statement is recommended during the learning process. When written as a three-part statement, the problem–etiology–signs and symptoms (PES) format is used.[12]

- Problem (P): a brief statement of the patient's potential or actual health problem (e.g., pain)
- Etiology (E): a brief description of the probable cause of the problem; contributing or related factors (e.g., related to surgical incision, localized pressure, edema)
- Signs and symptoms (S): a list of the cluster of the objective and subjective data that lead the nurse to pinpoint a problem; critical, major, or minor defining characteristics (e.g., as manifested by verbalization of pain, isolation, withdrawal)

It is important to remember that gathering the "S" comes first in the diagnostic process, even though the format has been described as PES.

Identifying the Problem. The NANDA list of accepted nursing diagnoses has been grouped using Marjory Gordon's 11 functional health patterns (see Appendix A). This framework is extremely useful when analyzing the data for actual, at risk, and possible nursing diagnoses. Clinically relevant cues are clustered into the functional health patterns. (The 11 functional health patterns are discussed in Chapter 5.) The process of making a nursing diagnosis from clustered cues begins with the recognition of general patient problems.[8] From the general problem area, the nurse identifies nursing diagnoses and collaborative problems that are tested for accuracy before final selection as the patient's nursing diagnosis or collaborative problem. The most accurate nursing diagnosis is based on the individual patient's data.

Etiology. The etiology of a nursing diagnosis should be included in the diagnostic statement and separated from the defining characteristics. Taking time to refine the problem with its proper etiology directs the nurse to the correct interventions. Interventions are planned to manage the problem by directing nursing efforts toward the etiology. The etiology can be a pathophysiologic, maturational, situational, or treatment-related factor.[11] The etiology is written after the diagnostic label. These two components are separated by the statement "related to." For example, a correctly written nursing diagnosis might be, "Feeding self-care deficit *related to* upper limb weakness." The etiology directs the nurse to select the appropriate interventions to modify the factor of upper limb weakness. When the etiology is not included in the diagnosis, the nurse is not able to plan the correct intervention to treat the specific cause of the problem. When possible, the etiology should be validated with the patient. When the etiology is unknown, the statement reads, "*related to* unknown etiology."

Multiple etiologies become more common as expertise in the use of nursing diagnoses increases. There is often no single cause of a problem. Most nursing diagnoses presented in the general nursing care plans of this book contain multiple etiologies. They can be used as a checklist of possible related factors to be considered when determining the nursing diagnosis specific to an individual patient.

Signs and Symptoms. Signs and symptoms, also called *defining characteristics,* are the clinical cues that, in a cluster, point to the nursing diagnosis.[10] Critical defining characteristics must be present in the database to make an accurate nursing diagnosis. Major defining characteristics are those signs or symptoms that are usually present when the diagnosis exists. At least one critical defining characteristic or one major defining characteristic must be present to have an actual nursing diagnosis. Minor defining characteristics have also been identified and are evidence of a possible nursing diagnosis. The signs and symptoms are included in the diagnostic statement using the phrase "as manifested by." A correctly written nursing diagnostic statement would be, "Feeding self-care deficit *related to* upper limb weakness *as manifested by* inability to bring food to mouth."

PLANNING PHASE

Priority Setting

After the nursing diagnoses and collaborative problems are identified, the nurse must decide on the urgency of intervention needed. Diagnoses of the highest priority require immediate intervention. Those of lower priority can be addressed at a later time. When setting priorities, the nurse should first intervene for life-threatening problems involving airway, breathing, or circulation.

Maslow's hierarchy of needs also acts as a useful guide in determining priorities. These needs include physical, safety, love and belonging, esteem, and self-actualization.[13] Lower level needs must be reached before a higher level can be attained.

Another guideline in setting priorities is to determine the patient's perception of what is important. When the patient's priorities are not congruent with the actual situation, the nurse may need to give explanations or do some teaching to help the patient understand the need to do one thing before another. Often it is more efficient to meet the patient's priority need before moving on to other priorities.

Another suggestion is to identify nursing diagnoses that may be managed simultaneously. For example, the nurse may assess the condition of a pressure ulcer (impaired skin integrity) while giving morning care (bathing self-care deficit).

Identified priorities change as a patient's level of wellness fluctuates. For example, the patient's highest priority in the morning may be a need for information about diabetes because she is going home and must care for herself. During the teaching session, the patient shows signs of a hypoglycemic reaction. The nurse would interrupt the teaching session to provide a glass of orange juice to avoid a progression of the hypoglycemia to a dangerous level. In this instance risk problems may have a higher priority than existing (actual) problems.

Identifying Outcomes

After priorities are established, goals or outcomes are written. The terms *goals* and *outcomes* are often used interchangeably. Goals are either long term or short term (Fig. 1-2). Once goals are set, the nurse can identify the more specific expected patient outcomes, which will assist in the evaluation of nursing interventions. Although the ultimate goal for the patient is to maintain or attain a state of dynamic equilibrium at the highest possible level of wellness, the setting of more specific goals, both short term and long term, is necessary for systematic evaluation of the patient's progress. Short-term goals may be met relatively quickly (i.e., in less than 24 to 48 hours). Long-term goals may take weeks or months to achieve. In today's acute care setting where the length of stay is often short, there is a predominance of short-term goals. Long-term goals may be addressed by a community-based nurse. Short-term goals may also be small steps toward achieving a long-term goal. For example, a short-term goal may be, "Mr. S. will ambulate with crutches 1 day postoperatively," whereas a long-term goal may be, "Mr. S. will ambulate unassisted by discharge."

In this textbook goals will be worded as expected patient outcomes. They should be specific enough so that everyone caring for the patient will be able to agree on whether the outcomes have been achieved. Writing the expected patient outcomes in terms of desired, measurable behaviors and specifying a date when the expected outcome should be accomplished facilitates this process. To be worthwhile, expected patient outcomes should fit the following criteria:

1. Realistic and achievable
2. Behavioral, measurable, observable
3. Patient centered (patient's expected outcome)
4. Time designated (by end of shift)
5. Mutually set

Short-term expected outcomes can serve as motivators for the patient and nurse, especially when long-term expected outcomes take significant time and effort to reach or when the patient is poorly motivated. For example, for the nursing diagnosis "altered health maintenance *related to* lack of knowledge regarding oral hygiene," the outcome for the patient is to attain healthy gums and teeth. Short-term expected outcomes may be that after teaching sessions the patient does the following:

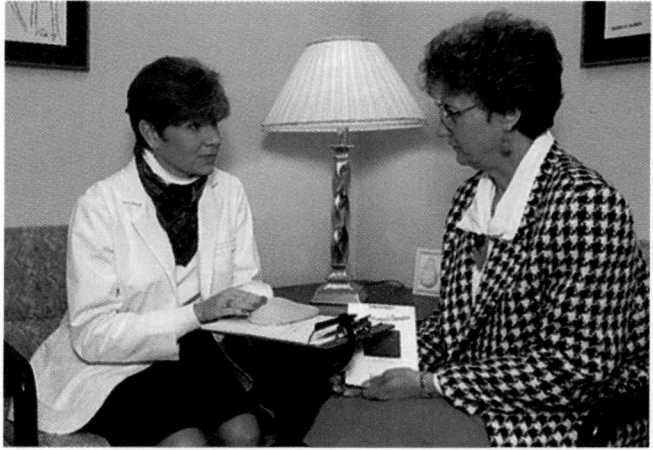

Fig. 1-2 Cooperation between the patient and the nurse is necessary in setting goals.

1. Demonstrates proper brushing technique after each meal
2. Demonstrates proper flossing of teeth before going to bed at night
3. Permanently refrains from chewing gum containing sugar
4. Visits the dentist by November 9

Planning Interventions

After expected patient outcomes are determined, nursing actions to accomplish these desired behaviors should be planned. The nurse should use available resources when determining possible nursing interventions. The patient often has a wealth of information about measures that were successful or unsuccessful in the past. Significant time and effort are saved by asking the patient what has been tried and discarded as ineffective. In addition, the patient's family can be consulted regarding the feasibility of the plan.

Other nurses and health care providers can be valuable sources for intervention ideas. Because members of the health team share common goals or expected outcomes for the patient, sharing ideas to reach these goals or expected outcomes should be encouraged. A patient-centered interdisciplinary conference is an effective way to foster such sharing.

Literature and research provide valuable suggestions and information that can facilitate the process of determining a means to accomplish the expected outcomes. The nurse should foster the use of a research-based approach to interventions.

Sound knowledge, good judgment, and decision-making ability are required to effectively choose the interventions that the nurse will use. Interventions should be based on sound rationales from the behavioral and biologic sciences. In addition, the nurse must use ingenuity, intuition, creativity, and past experience when tailoring a plan to meet a patient's needs. The benefits of the intervention must outweigh the disadvantages. Factors such as availability of help, equipment, time, money, and other resources must also be considered. As in the case of the determination of expected outcomes, the final selection of strategies remains the choice of the patient when the patient is able.

When recording the plan on the patient's written record, computer-based record, or Kardex, the nurse needs to be specific. Specificity in documenting outcomes enables everyone concerned with the patient to understand precisely what is to be accomplished. The plan should be tailored to meet each patient's needs and should note particulars, such as how, when, how long, how often, where, by whom, and with what. For example, "Wound care qid" is not an adequate plan. The following plan communicates much more: "The nurse (who) is to irrigate the right leg wound (where) with 200 ml normal saline (with what); @ 9-1-5-9 (how often)." These specific, individualized interventions may be called nursing orders.

Nursing Outcomes Classification

One of the newest classifications is the Nursing Outcomes Classification (NOC). The Nursing Outcomes Classification NOC is a published list of 190 outcomes that are responsive to nursing intervention.[14] This classification is in the early stages of development. As the NOC continues to evolve, the nurse will use it to develop the plan and to assess the effects of nursing interventions used to treat nursing diagnoses.

IMPLEMENTATION PHASE

Carrying out a specific, individualized plan constitutes the implementation phase. The planned activities that the nurse performs to accomplish the implementation phase are called nursing interventions. The Nursing Interventions Classification (NIC) is a comprehensive standardized language being developed at the University of Iowa School of Nursing to describe the treatments that nurses perform.[9] Table 1-3 presents the NIC Taxonomy. The NIC is one tool to assist the nurse in using a standardized language to document the treatments performed by the nurse. The NANDA and NOC are tools used to document the nursing diagnoses of patients and the resulting patient outcome. The nurse may carry out the interventions or designate others who are qualified to intervene. Listed in the sample Nursing Care Plan on p. 11 are five nursing diagnosis statements followed by examples of some appropriate NIC and NOC statements.

A nursing intervention is any direct action that a nurse performs (or designates others to perform) on behalf of a patient. These actions include nurse-initiated treatments resulting from nursing diagnoses; physician-initiated treatments resulting from medical diagnoses; and daily, essential activities that the patient cannot perform independently (Table 1-4). When choosing an intervention, the nurse considers the following:

1. Appropriateness of the nursing diagnosis
2. Research base associated with the intervention
3. Feasibility of successfully implementing the intervention
4. Acceptability of the intervention to the patient
5. Capability of the nurse[9]

There are a variety of nursing interventions from which to choose. Examples include the following:

1. Directly performing an activity for a patient
2. Assisting the patient
3. Supervising the patient and family
4. Teaching
5. Counseling
6. Monitoring[9]

Throughout the implementation phase the nurse must evaluate the effectiveness of the method chosen to implement the plan. For example, the nurse may determine that the nursing assistant caring for a patient with a mastectomy should not continue to be the person who implements the patient's exercise plan. Perhaps the patient is more depressed than anticipated and would benefit from contact with a nurse who is knowledgeable about changes in body image and sensitive to patient cues that may indicate body image disturbance. The exercise plan might essentially remain the same, but the implementor of the plan would be different and would use different skills to carry out the plan. Referrals to other professionals may also be made when the nurse anticipates that expertise in specialized areas is required to help the patient.

EVALUATION PHASE

The diagram of the nursing process (see Fig. 1-1) indicates that all phases must be evaluated. Evaluation not only occurs after implementation of the plan but is ongoing throughout the process.

The nurse evaluates whether sufficient assessment data have been obtained to allow a nursing diagnosis to be made. The diagnosis is, in turn, evaluated for accuracy. For example, was the pain actually related to the wound itself or related to pressure from a constricting dressing?

Next the nurse evaluates whether the expected patient outcomes and interventions are realistic and achievable. If not, a new plan should be formulated. This may involve revision of expected patient outcomes and interventions. Consideration must be given to whether the plan should be maintained, modified, totally revised, or discontinued in light of the patient's status.

The effectiveness of each intervention and its contribution to progress toward the expected patient outcome are also evaluated. In addition, the nurse considers whether a different method of implementation of the same plan will provide better results.

Documentation

It is critical that the patient's progress be documented in a systematic way. Many documentation methods are used, depending on personal preference and agency policy. Methods of documentation include SOAP charting, clinical pathways, FOCUS charting, and computer-based charting.

SOAP Charting. One method of evaluating and recording patient progress is the problem-oriented progress note, referred to as the subjective-objective-assessment plan (SOAP) method. This type of progress note is problem specific and incorporates the components described in Table 1-5. In some institutions, SOAP notes constitute the "Nurses' Notes" portion of the nurses' charting.

The process of SOAP documentation is as follows:

1. Additional subjective and objective data are gathered concerning the area of concern.
2. Based on old and new data, an assessment of the patient's progress toward the expected patient outcome and the effectiveness of each intervention is made.
3. Based on the reassessment of the situation, the initial plan is maintained, revised, or discontinued.

Table 1-3 Nursing Intervention Classification Taxonomy

	Domain 1	Domain 2	Domain 3	Domain 4	Domain 5	Domain 6
Level 1 Domains	**1. Physiologic: Basic** Care that supports physical functioning	**2. Physiologic: Complex** Care that supports homeostatic regulation	**3. Behavioral** Care that supports psychosocial functioning and facilitates lifestyle changes	**4. Safety** Care that supports protection against harm	**5. Family** Care that supports the family unit	**6. Health System** Care that supports effective use of the health care delivery system
Level 2 Classes	A. *Activity and Exercise Management:* Interventions to organize or assist with physical activity and energy conservation and expenditure B. *Elimination Management:* Interventions to establish and maintain regular bowel and urinary elimination patterns and manage complications due to altered patterns C. *Immobility Management:* Interventions to manage restricted body movement and the sequelae D. *Nutrition Support:* Interventions to modify or maintain nutritional status E. *Physical Comfort Promotion:* Interventions to promote comfort using physical techniques F. *Self-Care Facilitation:* Interventions to provide or assist with routine activities of daily living	G. *Electrolyte and Acid-Base Management:* Interventions to regulate electrolyte/acid-base balance and prevent complications H. *Drug Management:* Interventions to facilitate desired effects of pharmacologic agents I. *Neurologic Management:* Interventions to optimize neurologic functions J. *Perioperative Care:* Interventions to provide care before, during, and immediately after surgery K. *Respiratory Management:* Interventions to promote airway patency and gas exchange L. *Skin/Wound Management:* Interventions to maintain or restore tissue integrity M. *Thermoregulation:* Interventions to maintain body temperature within a normal range N. *Tissue Perfusion Management:* Interventions to optimize circulation of blood and fluids to the tissue	O. *Behavior Therapy:* Interventions to reinforce or promote desirable behaviors or alter undesirable behaviors P. *Cognitive Therapy:* Interventions to reinforce or promote desirable cognitive functioning or alter undesirable cognitive functioning Q. *Communication Enhancement:* Interventions to facilitate delivering and receiving verbal and nonverbal messages R. *Coping Assistance:* Interventions to assist another to build on own strengths, to adapt to a change in function, or to achieve a higher level of function S. *Patient Education:* Interventions to facilitate learning T. *Psychologic Comfort Promotion:* Interventions to promote comfort using psychologic techniques	U. *Crisis Management:* Interventions to provide immediate short-term help in both psychologic and physiologic crises V. *Risk Management:* Interventions to initiate risk-reduction activities and continue monitoring risks over time	W. *Childbearing Care:* Interventions to assist in understanding and coping with the psychologic and physiologic changes during the child-bearing period X. *Life Span Care:* Interventions to facilitate family unit functioning and promote the health and welfare of family members throughout the life span	Y. *Health System Mediation:* Interventions to facilitate the interface between patient/family and the health care system a. *Health System Management:* Interventions to provide and enhance support services for the delivery of care b. *Information Management:* Interventions to facilitate communication among health care providers

NURSING CARE PLAN CONGESTIVE HEART FAILURE

Expected Patient Outcomes	Nursing Interventions‡
NURSING DIAGNOSIS **Activity intolerance** *related to* fatigue secondary to cardiac insufficiency, pulmonary congestion, and inadequate nutrition *as manifested by* dyspnea, shortness of breath, increase/decrease in pulse on exertion.	
▪ Cardiac pump effectiveness (0400*). ▪ Endurance (0001*). ▪ Energy conservation (0002*).	▪ Energy management (0180†). ▪ Teaching: prescribed activity/exercise (551†).
NURSING DIAGNOSIS **Sleep pattern disturbance** *related to* nocturnal dyspnea, inability to assume favored sleep position, and nocturia *as manifested by* inability to sleep through night.	
▪ Sleep (0004*).	▪ Sleep enhancement (513†). ▪ Teaching: procedure/treatment (555†).
NURSING DIAGNOSIS **Risk for impaired skin integrity** *related to* edema or immobility.	
▪ Tissue integrity: skin and mucous membranes (1101*).	▪ Pressure management (3500†). ▪ Pressure ulcer prevention (3540†). ▪ Skin surveillance (3590†).
NURSING DIAGNOSIS **Impaired gas exchange** *related to* increased preload, mechanical failure, or immobility *as manifested by* increased respiratory rate, shortness of breath, dyspnea on exertion.	
▪ Respiratory status: gas exchange (0402*).	▪ Respiratory monitoring (3350†). ▪ Airway management (3140†).
NURSING DIAGNOSIS **Ineffective management of therapeutic regimen** *related to* lack of knowledge regarding signs and symptoms of CHF, proper diet, and medications *as manifested by* lack of adherence to low-sodium diet and questioning about disease, diet, and medications.	
▪ Knowledge: disease process (1803*). ▪ Knowledge: diet (1802*). ▪ Knowledge: medication (1808*). ▪ Knowledge: treatment regimen (1813*).	▪ Teaching: disease process (5602†). ▪ Teaching: prescribed diet (5614†). ▪ Teaching: prescribed medication (5616†). ▪ Teaching: procedure/treatment (5618†).

*Represents the classification code in the NOC for this expected outcome.
†Represents the classification code in the NIC for this intervention.
‡Select specific activities from each intervention believed to be most effective for the patient.

Table 1-4 Examples of Nursing Activities to Treat Patients' Health Care Problems

Intervention	Nursing Activities
Nurse-initiated treatments	Encourage patient to cough and deep breathe
Physician-initiated treatments	Administer medications
Essential activity patient cannot perform independently	Provide range-of-motion exercise

The following is an example of SOAP charting for the nursing diagnosis "risk for infection *related to* traumatized tissue secondary to surgery:"

S: Wound is more painful today
O: Temperature of 103° F, facial grimacing in response to movement, dressing saturated with purulent drainage
A: Risk for wound infection
P: Notify surgeon, take temperature q2hr, reinforce dressing, obtain wound culture

Table 1-5 Components of a Problem-Oriented Progress Note

SOAP	Explanation
Subjective (S)	Information supplied by patient or knowledgeable other
Objective (O)	Information obtained by nurse directly by observation or measurement, from patient records, or through diagnostic studies
Assessment (A)	Nursing diagnosis or problem based on subjective and objective data
Plan (P)	Specific interventions related to a diagnosis or problem considering diagnostic, therapeutic, and patient education needs

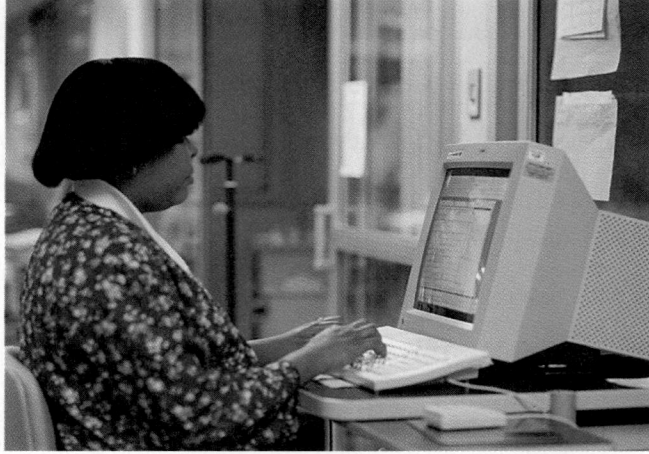

Fig. 1-3 Computerized documentation systems allow nurses to be more productive and ensure comprehensive recording of patient information.

Clinical Pathways. The clinical (critical) pathway, or care map, is a guide specifically designed to direct the health care team in the daily care goals for select health care problems. It includes a care plan, interventions specific for each day of hospitalization, and a documentation tool.[15] Samples of clinical pathways are included throughout this textbook for selected health problems (see inside back cover).

The clinical pathway is part of a case management system that organizes and sequences the caregiving process at the patient level to better achieve quality and cost outcomes. It is a cyclic process organized for specific case types by all related health care departments. The case types selected for clinical pathways are usually those that occur in high volume and are highly predictable, such as myocardial infarction, cerebrovascular accident, and angina.

The clinical pathway describes the patient care required at specific times in the treatment. A multidisciplinary approach moves the patient toward desired outcomes within an estimated length of stay. The exact contents and format of these clinical pathways vary among institutions.

FOCUS Charting. FOCUS charting is a method of documentation that structures the nurse's note according to the focus of the note, such as a sign or symptom, a condition, or a nursing diagnosis. Charting by exception is a shorthand method for documenting normal findings and routine care based on clearly defined standards of practice and predetermined criteria for nursing assessments and interventions.[16]

Computer-Based Charting. As technologies are rapidly developing, the computer-based patient record (CPR) is becoming more common (Fig. 1-3). The CPR maintains the traditional components of the paper-based patient record such as the physician's orders and the history but also offers many benefits for the nurse's direct patient care such as rapid data entry and retrieval and enhanced clinical decision-making capabilities. Documenting on the CPR is easier and faster. Software programs allow nurses to quickly enter specific assessment data one time, and the information is automatically transferred to different reports. Instead of writing lengthy nursing notes, nurses can select choices on a screen that are used to build a comprehensive patient record. Computerized patient records help reduce errors, standardize nursing care plans, and increase nursing satisfaction and productivity.

WRITTEN CARE PLANS

An individualized nursing care plan is recorded to facilitate continuity of care and to help avoid duplication of services. When kept as a permanent part of the patient's record, the care plan can aid in the evaluation of nursing care. It also documents the patient's nursing care requirements and directs nursing care. Generally only the more unusual or unexpected problems are addressed in the care plan. Predictable routine problems experienced by many patients with the same diagnosis should be planned for but not necessarily recorded on the care plan. These routine problems are covered by unit policies or protocols.

Sometimes the care plan is written in pencil so that the outdated interventions can be erased; the current plan remains, avoiding confusion. However, this method should not be used without some kind of permanent record of the plan because the nurse also needs a source of information on which interventions were unsuccessful to avoid repeating them. The permanent care plan is considered a part of the legal medical record. Some nurses use a highlighting marker over completed or changed items, leaving current plans readable in ink while preserving a record of outdated care plans. Care planning on the CPR should be much easier to maintain.

There are various methods of recording the nursing care plan, and there are many formats available. An example of a format for a nursing care plan for the patient with postoperative pain is shown in NCP 1-1. This example shows the incorporation of NANDA, NIC, and NOC into a nursing care plan.

Some institutions write the care plan in ink and retain the entire plan as a part of the patient's record. This kind of care plan often has a column for evaluation, where comments are recorded on the progress toward the expected patient outcomes and the effectiveness of the interventions.

1-1 NURSING CARE PLAN SAMPLE

Expected Patient Outcomes	Nursing Interventions and *Rationales*
NURSING DIAGNOSIS	**Pain** *related to* surgical incision and localized pressure and edema *as manifested by* verbalization of pain, isolation, withdrawal.
▪ Verbalization of satisfaction with pain relief.	▪ Assess degree of pain *to plan appropriate intervention.* ▪ Administer analgesics as needed *to relieve pain.* ▪ Encourage patient to avoid sudden movements *to prevent an increase in pain.* ▪ Do not position patient on operative side *to avoid accumulation of fluid and subsequent increase in pain.*
USING *NIC* AND *NOC*	
NURSING DIAGNOSIS	**Pain** *related to* surgical incision and localized pressure and edema *as manifested by* verbalization of pain, isolation, withdrawal.
▪ Pain control behavior (1605*).	▪ Pain Management (1400†) Activities: Nurse selects specific activities believed to be most effective for the patient.

*Represents the classification code in the NOC for this expected outcome.
†Represents the classification code in the NIC for this intervention.

Standardized care plans are often used as guides for routine nursing care and for developing individualized care plans. The care plans throughout this textbook are general or standardized. This type of plan lists nursing actions, or broad interventions, that are applicable to any number of patients having the particular problem. When planning individualized care, a standardized care plan should be personalized and made specific based on the unique needs of the patient.

SUMMARY

Nursing roles continually evolve as our society changes and we learn to apply new technology. Although nursing is defined in different ways, the various definitions of nursing have commonalities of health, illness, and caring.

Nursing care is provided through the application of the nursing process: assessment, diagnosis, planning, implementation, and evaluation. Assessment involves collecting data by patient record review, taking a nursing history, and performing a physical examination. The nurse's skill at collecting subjective and objective data affects the quality of the database.

There are two major steps to the diagnosis phase: data analysis and nursing diagnosis (or problem identification). The planning phase has three major steps: priority setting, identification of expected patient outcomes, and planning interventions. The plan of action must be founded on a sound database. Implementation, the actual carrying out of the plan, may be performed by the nurse or by someone the nurse designates. It continues throughout the nursing process. Evaluation of each step of the nursing process fosters timely revisions of the nursing care plan.

Several methods of record keeping are used to promote continuity of patient care and facilitate the nursing process. These documentation methods include SOAP charting, clinical pathways, FOCUS charting, and computer-based charting.

The nursing process requires the use of reasoning, analytic thinking skills, and synthesis of information. It differs from medicine's problem-solving approach and means of accomplishing its goals. Knowledge of the biologic and behavioral sciences and specific skills such as critical thinking, teaching, counseling, and technical skills are required to apply the nursing process. Through the systematic use of the nursing process, nursing can best accomplish its goal of assisting others to maintain or attain optimal health.

REVIEW QUESTIONS

The number of the question corresponds to the same-numbered objective at the beginning of the chapter.

1. An example of a nursing activity that reflects the American Nurses' Association's definition of nursing is
   a. establishing the cause of hepatitis in a patient who is jaundiced.
   b. determining the cause of hemorrhage in a postoperative patient based on vital signs.
   c. identifying and treating arrhythmias that occur in a patient in the coronary care unit.
   d. diagnosing that a patient with pneumonia cannot effectively cough up pulmonary secretions.
2. An example of an independent nursing intervention is
   a. administering blood.
   b. starting an intravenous fluid.
   c. teaching a patient to self-administer insulin.
   d. administering medication per physician's order.
3. When the nurse interviews a patient to determine if the patient's pain is relieved following repositioning, the phase of the nursing process that is being used is
   a. assessment.
   b. diagnosis.
   c. implementation.
   d. evaluation.

4. The process of making a nursing diagnosis differs from a diagnostic statement in that the diagnostic process involves
   a. stating what needs the patient has.
   b. identifying pathologic effects of a disease process.
   c. analyzing assessment data to identify health problems.
   d. identifying the diagnosis, related factors, and signs and symptoms.
5. Which of the following expected patient outcomes is most complete?
   a. The patient ambulates independently.
   b. The patient maintains oral intake of at least 1500 ml/day.
   c. The patient will be turned and repositioned every 2 hours.
   d. The patient will experience less anxiety about having surgery.
6. An example of an appropriate nursing intervention based on a nursing diagnosis is
   a. administering blood to a patient who is hemorrhaging.
   b. ordering laboratory tests for a patient who is dehydrated.
   c. listening to a patient express her grief following a mastectomy.
   d. inserting a nasogastric tube to suction for a patient with vomiting.
7. The main purpose of the evaluation phase of the nursing process is to
   a. assess the patient's strengths.
   b. identify progress toward goals.
   c. describe new nursing diagnoses.
   d. implement new nursing strategies.
8. The primary purpose of the nurse documenting all steps of the nursing process is to
   a. validate performance of nursing services for reimbursement.
   b. record the nursing plan, its implementation, and the patient's response.
   c. communicate the status of the patient's progress to the health care team.
   d. provide evidence that high standards of care are met in providing patient care.

References

1. Goodnow M: *Outlines of nursing history,* ed 6, Philadelphia, 1938, Saunders.
2. American Nurses' Association: *Nursing: a social policy statement,* Kansas City, Mo, 1995, The Association.
3. Fawcett J: *Analysis and evaluation of nursing theories,* Philadelphia, 1993, FA Davis.
4. Nightingale F: *Notes on nursing: what it is and what it is not, facsimile edition,* Philadelphia, 1946, Lippincott.
5. Carroll L: *Alice's adventures in wonderland and through the looking glass,* New York, 1973, Collier Books.
6. Henderson V: *The nature of nursing,* New York, 1966, Macmillan.
7. Roy S: *The Roy adaptation model: the definitive statement,* Norwalk, Conn, 1991, Appleton & Lange.
8. Collier I, McCash K, Bartram J: *Writing nursing diagnoses: a critical thinking approach,* St Louis, 1996, Mosby.
9. Bulechek G, McCloskey J: *Nursing interventions classification,* ed 2, St Louis, 1996, Mosby.
10. North American Nursing Diagnosis Association: *Nursing diagnoses: definitions and classifications,* Philadelphia, 1999.
11. Carpenito L: *Nursing diagnosis: application to clinical practice,* ed 7, Philadelphia, 1997, Lippincott.
12. Gordon M: *Nursing diagnosis: process and application, 1997-1998,* ed 8, St Louis, 1997, Mosby.
13. Maslow A: *Motivation and personality,* New York, 1954, Harper & Row.
14. Johnson M, Maas M: *Nursing outcomes classification (NOC),* St Louis, 1997, Mosby.
15. Cohen E, Cesta T: *Nursing case management: from concept to evaluation,* ed 2, St Louis, 1997, Mosby.
16. Eggland ET, Heinemann DS: *Nursing documentation: charting, recording, and reporting,* Philadelphia, 1997, Lippincott.

Resources

American Medical Association (AMA)
515 North State Street
Chicago, IL 60610
312-464-5000
http://www.ama-assn.org

American Nurses' Association
600 Maryland Avenue SW
Suite 100 West
Washington, DC 20024
202-651-7012
800-274-4ANA
Fax: 202-651-7006
http://www.ana.org/

Canadian Nurses' Association
50 The Driveway
Ottawa, Ontario
K2P 1E2 CANADA
613-237-2133
800-361-8404
Fax: 613-237-3520
http://www.cna-nurses.ca/

Lippincott's Nursing Center-Nursing Links
http://www.ajn.org/people/pp_norgs.cfm

National Association of Hispanic Nurses
1501 16th Street NW
Washington, DC 20036
202-387-2477
Fax: 202-483-7183
http://www.incacorp.com/nahn

National Black Nurses' Association, Inc.
1511 K Street NW, Suite 415
Washington, DC 20005
202-393-6870
Fax: 202-347-3808

National Institute of Health
Bethesda, MD 20892
http://www.nih.gov/

National Institute of Nursing Research
31 Center Drive, Room 5B09, MSC 2178
Bethesda, MD 20892-2178
310-496-0207
http://www.nih.gov/ninr/

National League for Nursing
350 Hudson Street
New York, NY 10014
212-989-9393
800-669-9656
http://www.nln.org

National Student Nurses' Association
555 West 57th Street, Suite 1327
New York, NY 10019
212-581-2211
Fax: 212-581-2368
http://www.nsna.org

North American Nursing Diagnosis Association (NANDA)
1211 Locust Street
Philadelphia, PA 19107
800-647-9002
215-545-8105
Fax: 215-545-8107
http://www.virtualer.com/

Sigma Theta Tau
550 West North Street
Indianapolis, IN 46202
317-634-8171
1-888-634-7575
Fax: 317-634-8188
http://stti-web.iupui.edu/

World Health Organization
525 23rd Street, NW
Washington, DC 20037
202-974-3000
Fax: 202-974-3663
http://www.who.ch

For additional Internet resources, see the website for this book at www.mosby.com/MERLIN/medsurg_lewis

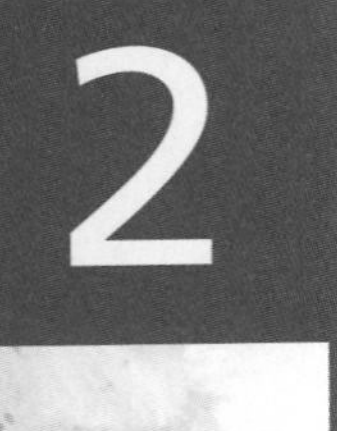

REMEMBER to check out your **companion CD-ROM**

2 Community-Based Nursing and Home Health Care

Carol O. Long & Anne M. Jones

www.mosby.com/MERLIN/medsurg_lewis

LEARNING OBJECTIVES

1. Describe how changes in the health care system have affected the delivery of patient care.
2. Compare patient care settings and levels of intensity of nursing care.
3. Describe the purposes and services provided by home health care and hospice.
4. Describe the roles and challenges of nurses working in community-based and home health care settings.

CHANGING HEALTH CARE SYSTEM

The health care delivery system has significantly changed in recent years, with a shift in patient care from hospitals to community-based settings. In response to this changing health care environment, the practice of professional nursing also is evolving because of the changing and complex health care system. Today, nurses have career opportunities that extend beyond the hospital setting to community-based settings and the home. Nurses can choose to work in a variety of health care settings, allowing for increased diversity in both patient contact and nursing practice. Nurses working in community-based care settings require a different set of skills, depending on the intensity of patient care and the practice setting.

The changes in health care have been largely initiated by the continued efforts of the government, employers, insurance companies, and regulating agencies to provide health care in the most cost-effective manner. Historically, the most notable event related to changing reimbursement patterns was the institution of prospective payment systems and the use of diagnosis-related groups (DRGs) in the Medicare program. With DRGs, hospitals were no longer reimbursed for all costs; rather, payment for hospital services to Medicare patients was based on flat fees per admission based on DRGs. DRGs have shifted patient care from acute care settings to other settings, such as home health. The prospective payment system has been and continues to be one of the most significant factors affecting health care. These policies, combined with recent advances in technology, allow nurses to care for increasingly complex patients in community and home settings.

Reviewed by Katherine E. Matas, RN, PhD, Associate Professor, Western Michigan University, Kalamazoo, MI, and Geoff Shuster, RN, PhD, Associate Professor, College of Nursing, University of New Mexico, Albuquerque, NM.

In recent years, the increase in the managed care market through health maintenance organizations (HMOs) and preferred provider organizations (PPOs) has shifted care from expensive acute care settings to ones that are less costly but equally qualified to care for patients. Charges are negotiated in advance of the delivery of care using predetermined reimbursement rates or capitation fees for medical care, hospitalization, and other health care services. Not only are cost savings anticipated, but there has also been a shift to less expensive community-based health care for patients.

Changes in nursing practice and patient care also have occurred because of increasing patient consumerism, changing demographics, and the introduction of sophisticated technology. Health care is becoming a consumer-focused business. Because patients are more interested in their health care, they are becoming active participants rather than passive bystanders. Patients eagerly seek out information about their health. They expect that information will be provided so that they may collaborate with care providers in making the right decisions about their health care. In addition, the public has come to view health care as an entitlement or a human right. Health care legislation emphasizes equal access to health care services, regardless of the ability to pay. As increasing demands are made on scarce and costly health care resources, nurses are becoming more active partners with patients in promoting self-care through education and advocacy.

The average age of people in North America is increasing. The cohort of Americans over age 75 years is increasing even more rapidly than the general population. As a result of these demographic trends, health care needs and demands have changed. Our aging population is demanding more health care and straining the financial resources that fund it, such as the Medicare program. Aging Americans have disabilities that may compromise their ability to remain functional in their own homes and at times without supportive community or professional help. The elderly also have complex medical and health care needs, often having multiple chronic conditions that may compromise their independence. Physical and functional problems, dementia, fixed incomes, and limited family or community support all put the elderly at an increased need for social and health care assistance.

Surgical innovations, such as advances in cardiac surgery, and medical interventions, such as new medications for cystic fibrosis, have allowed individuals to live longer, shifting both acute and long-term chronic care to community-based settings and the home. Advances in technology have also significantly affected the work of nurses in terms of performance, productivity, and patient care interventions. New technology has improved diagnostic procedures and management of patient care. Computers, lasers, and lifesaving drugs have simplified diagnosis and treatment and shortened hospital stays.

Patient care has also moved to outpatient settings such as surgical centers, providing services that have been traditionally delivered only in hospitals. Patient care treatments, such as IV antibiotic therapy, are also increasingly being delivered in the home care setting. Evolving technology, the interest in less costly care, and the patient preference to be at home have simultaneously stimulated the movement to provide health care in the community and home health care settings.

Patients today can be treated in a multitude of settings, opting for the one most appropriate for their health care needs but within the constraints of health care insurance plans and the cost of care. Today health care is increasingly constrained by third-party payer cost containment efforts. At the same time third-party payers are demanding outcome-based quality care. Although the hospital remains the mainstay for acute care interventions, settings such as extended care facilities, assisted living centers, and home health care offer patients the opportunity to live or recover in settings that maximize their independence and preserve human dignity. The professional nurse has an increasingly important role in facilitating the patient's independence and movement through the continuum of care. Today's health care system requires experienced, flexible, broad-based nurses to oversee patient care in a variety of practice settings.

Case Management

Case management is a central focus of community-based and home health care. The focus of case management is on the coordination of patient care during the entire episode of illness across every setting where the patient receives care.[1] The goals of case management are the provision of quality care along a continuum, decreased fragmentation of care across many settings, enhancement of the patient's quality of life, and cost containment.[2]

As the health care environment continues to change, case management coordinates and links health care services to patients and their families. Case managers are an extremely important part of managed care.[3] The case manager is accountable for short- and long-term outcomes, as well as overall financial outcomes.

Case management involves managing the patient's care across the continuum of care. The case manager establishes a plan of care with the patient and family, coordinates consultations, updates the patient and family on progress of care, and facilitates discharge to an appropriate community-based care setting or the home. For example, a patient with severe coronary artery disease may be assigned a nurse as a case manager in the medicine outpatient clinic. When the patient is hospitalized for coronary bypass surgery, the same case manager coordinates care so that all health care providers understand the patient's unique needs. When the patient is discharged, the case manager determines whether home health care or other services are necessary for the patient. The case manager may visit the patient in the home to ensure that appropriate health care measures are being implemented.

CONTINUUM OF PATIENT CARE

Depending on an individual's health status and often the cost of care required, patients can move among different health care settings. There is a continuum of care whereby different settings accommodate the varying needs of the patient. For example, a person may be hospitalized in a trauma unit following a motor vehicle accident. After the person is stabilized, he or she may be transferred to a general medical-surgical unit and then to an acute rehabilitation facility. After months of rehabilitation, the person may be discharged to his or her home to be followed up by home health care nurses.

This section provides an overview of selected patient care settings within the patient care continuum (Table 2-1). The emerging roles for nurses are described in relation to patient needs and the variety of acute care and community-based care settings. Home health care and hospice are also discussed, along with the challenges faced by nurses who are employed in these care settings.

Acute Care

Acute care refers to medical and nursing care delivered to patients in controlled settings, such as hospitals, where continuous monitoring and interventions are required. By definition, acutely ill patients are unable to care for themselves. Their condition dictates that they receive specialized medical treatments or procedures in a hospital setting. Acute care is the most expensive kind of care, and it accounts for the greatest portion of health care expense in the United States.[4] Different levels of care exist within acute care settings based on the severity of the patient's condition, such as critical or intensive care units, definitive observation or telemetry observation units, and general or specialty nursing units.

Critical Care. *Critical care* encompasses medical and surgical intensive care units (ICUs), trauma and emergency care services, neonatal and pediatric ICUs, and coronary care units (CCUs). Patients most often seen in critical care units have multiple complex physiologic needs.

Nurses working in CCUs must be familiar with advanced cardiac life support, ventilators, and hemodynamic monitoring. The nurse continually observes the patient and frequently documents the patient's status. Since the patient's condition is highly unstable, critical care nurses follow medically approved protocols that allow them to proceed quickly with lifesaving interventions as needed. Critical care nursing is fast paced, dynamic, and independent. Care is highly focused, with one professional nurse performing most of the nursing care for one or two critically ill patients.

Definitive Observation Units. *Definitive observation units,* or telemetry observation units, are considered step-down units from the critical care or intensive care areas. At this level of care, patients require frequent monitoring with or

Table 2-1 Comparison of Patient Care Settings

	Acute Care	Transitional Care	Long-Term Care	Home Health Care	Hospice	Ambulatory
Examples	Hospital	Subacute Rehabilitation Skilled nursing facilities	Nursing facilities	Formal and informal Primarily in the home	Home Inpatient	Physician or nurse practitioner office Surgicenter Clinic
Emphasis	Cure Lifesaving Surgical care	Stabilization Rehabilitation	Restoration Support	Teaching Rehabilitation Independence	Care of the dying Bereavement	Diagnosis Outpatient surgery Prevention Maintenance Treatment
Financing	All payers	Medicare	Medicaid Out-of-pocket	Medicare Medicaid Commercial insurance	Medicare Medicaid Commercial insurance Charity	All payers
Patient Care	Acute, short length of stay	Short- to long-term care	Long length of stay	Short to long length of stay Part-time intermittent	Until death	Episodic
Nursing Practice	Acute and critical care skills Specialty practice	Rehabilitation	Maintenance Health promotion	Skilled care	Palliation Symptom control	Education Procedures Advanced practice care

without advanced life support until they are stable. One nurse may care for three to four very ill patients. Patients in these units may typically have cardiac arrhythmias, recent trauma, drug toxicities, and otherwise serious and complex conditions that require additional stabilization and monitoring before being transferred to a general medical-surgical unit.

Nurses working in definitive observation units need to combine critical assessment skills with quick intervention strategies for potentially unstable patients. Nurses must be able to recognize subtle changes in neurologic, cardiovascular, and respiratory status for patients in these units. Similarly, nurses can prepare patients for the next stage of their recovery as they progress to the general nursing unit or a community-based setting.

General Nursing Units. *General nursing units* may be referred to as medical-surgical nursing care areas. Patients on the medical-surgical unit do not require advanced hemodynamic or cardiac monitoring. The typical patient in this area may require intravenous therapy, may require treatments for wounds or postoperative care, or may have a medical condition, such as an acute episode of a chronic condition (e.g., diabetes, congestive heart failure). Surgical patients require close monitoring following invasive procedures and anesthesia. Medical patients may require frequent monitoring and laboratory tests with diagnoses such as diabetes mellitus, pneumonia, congestive heart failure, chronic obstructive pulmonary disease, vascular disease, cancer, and immune disorders.

The nurse working in medical-surgical units may typically oversee the care of six or more patients with the help of a nursing assistant or trained technician. Personal care activities may be delegated to ancillary support personnel, with supervision by the registered nurse. Nursing assessment, planning, and interventions; medication administration; patient and family education; and discharge planning are the general responsibilities of the medical-surgical nurse.

Transitional Care

Transitional care refers to intermediary care between the acute care setting and the home. Patients who have recently been admitted to the acute care hospital but who cannot take care of themselves, or who are too sick to go to a nursing home, may be placed for a short time in a transitional care setting.[5] Transitional care may take place in a distinct part of a hospital or nursing home or in a separate, freestanding facility. Different levels of transitional care that exist within the health care settings are described.

Subacute Care. *Subacute care* is post-acute care designed for patients who need a greater intensity of care than that generally provided in a skilled nursing facility but no longer require acute care. Typical patients requiring subacute care are chronically ill, ventilator dependent, or those needing specialized monitoring, equipment, and nursing care. Many of the patients who require subacute care are outliers (those who have exhausted their inpatient DRG days). Subacute care settings may exist in a distinct section of a hospital or in long-term care settings, such as nursing or skilled nursing facilities. Nurses working in subacute care need to be familiar with tracheostomy care, ventilators, complex wound management, and care of the terminally ill. Although subacute patients are usually medically stable, they require multiple and complex treatments. The nurse in subacute care generally gives primary care for five to seven patients with the assistance of other nursing personnel.

Acute Rehabilitation. *Acute rehabilitation* is a postacute level of care specializing in therapies for patients with neurologic or physical injuries, such as those with head trauma, spinal cord injury, or cerebrovascular accident (CVA). Acute rehabilitation settings may be in separate units of a hospital or in freestanding facilities in the community. The patient in acute rehabilitation may receive several hours of exercise and other rehabilitative training or therapy daily. Patients learn to use assistive devices and need time and encouragement to perform activities of daily living and other aspects of self-care. Patients may need weeks to months of rehabilitative care before they can return home.

When rehabilitation is the focus of care, nurses work closely with other disciplines such as dietary, social work, physical therapy, occupational therapy, and speech therapy to develop a plan of care that advances the patient toward independence. The team approach involves frequent, collaborative patient care conferences that include the patient and the family or significant others in the plan of care.

Long-Term Care

Long-term care refers to the care of patients for a time period greater than 30 days. Long-term care takes place in nursing homes, convalescent centers, rehabilitation hospitals, and housing facilities designed for persons with functional self-care deficits. Long-term care may be required for individuals who are severely developmentally disabled, are mentally impaired, or have physical deficits requiring continuous medical or nursing management, such as those who are ventilator dependent or those with Alzheimer's disease. The person being cared for in these settings is referred to as a resident. Long-term care settings may be classified as nursing facilities or skilled nursing facilities.[6] Long-term care facilities, specifically nursing homes (currently known as nursing facilities), provide different levels of nursing care, including skilled nursing, extended or intermediate care, or personal care.

The emphasis of care for nursing facilities is on attaining the highest level of functioning for the individual with services provided based on an interdisciplinary assessment of the resident's needs. The needs of the individual determine which setting would be most appropriate. Skilled nursing facilities provide the same services with increased emphasis on rehabilitative therapies for convalescing patients.

Nurses working in long-term care facilities generally provide care for large numbers of residents with different levels of acuity often dependent on the kind of setting in which the nurse is employed. Professional nurses are responsible for the supervision of many nursing personnel. Licensed practical nurses administer routine medications and treatments, and most of the physical care needs are provided by certified nursing assistants. Recreational activities are offered several times per week. Family members and guests are encouraged to visit regularly, sometimes participating in social events and meals offered by the facility. Since physicians rarely visit, nurses often

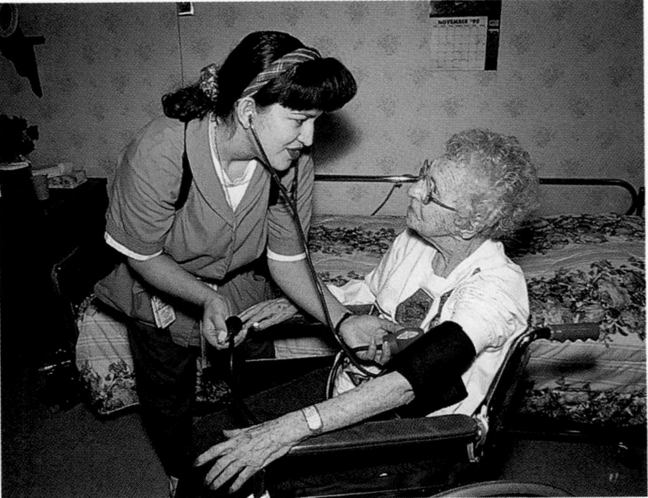

Fig. 2-1 Nurse taking blood pressure for patient in an extended care facility.

need to obtain verbal orders and report patient concerns via the telephone. Nurse practitioners frequently are responsible for patient care in long-term care facilities. Nurses involved in long-term care require special organizational and leadership skills to manage resident care and activities and other health care workers employed in these settings. These skills are needed in long-term care facilities whether they are skilled nursing facilities, extended care/intermediate care facilities, nursing homes, or residential care facilities.

Skilled Nursing Facilities. *Skilled nursing facilities,* or nursing centers, provide care for patients who require 24-hour nursing supervision, many of whom are confined to bed for some portion of the day or are incontinent. These facilities offer treatment under the supervision of licensed nurses and at least one registered nurse who must be on duty during the day. Like other long-term care settings, skilled nursing facilities are licensed by state licensing authorities.

Skilled nursing facilities offer a transitional level of postacute care in which the patient requires specified nursing skills and therapeutic support. These patients may be too weak or ill to tolerate rapid rehabilitation. Patients in skilled care may need IV medications, aggressive anticoagulant therapy, renal dialysis, or programmed pain management. Some patients are terminally ill or disabled to the degree that continuous nursing support is required.

As in acute rehabilitation or subacute settings, the skilled care nurse collaborates with rehabilitation professionals to create a patient-centered, comprehensive, interdisciplinary plan of care. Nurses who work in these settings require skills in complex wound management, intravenous therapy, care of ostomies and feeding tubes, orthopedic care for patients with joint replacement or arthritis, and care for patients with chronic pulmonary and cardiovascular disorders.

Extended Care/Intermediate Care. An *extended care facility* or *intermediate care facility* provides convalescent care and regular medical, nursing, social, and rehabilitative services in addition to room and board for people not capable of independent living (Fig. 2-1). Residents in these facilities require less

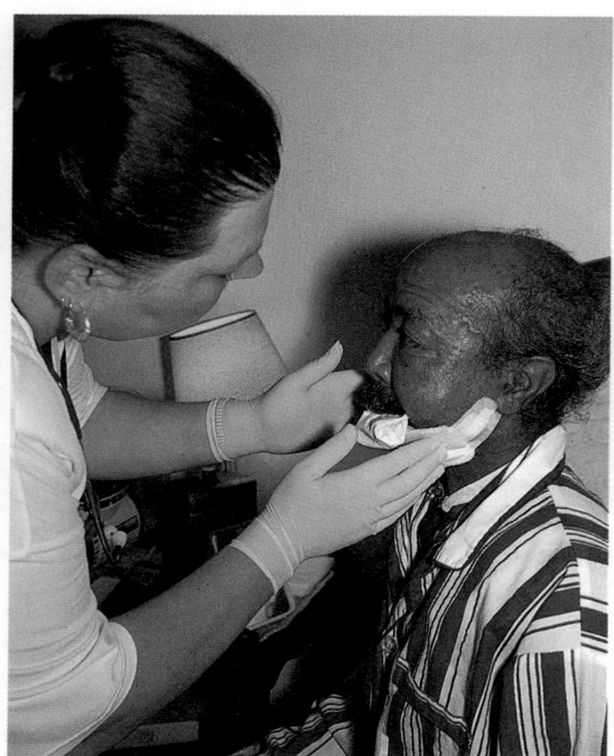

Fig. 2-2 Care provided in a nursing home.

intensive nursing care than that provided by skilled nursing facilities. Extended care can be temporary care for individuals recovering from an acute illness or injury, and often for those who have been discharged from the hospital. Specialized intermediate care facilities for those who are mentally impaired or for those with developmental disabilities are also available.[6] Residents may receive care in extended or intermediate care facilities for several weeks to years or from youth to old age, making these facilities a permanent home and staff a second family. Common goals of these facilities are to assess what individuals are capable of doing and to help them achieve their potential by teaching and training them to achieve maximum independence.

Nurses working in extended care settings take care of a large group of residents, providing routine medications and treatments on a scheduled basis. Most of the physical care needs for residents are provided by certified nursing assistants working under the supervision of a licensed nurse. Special nursing skills required for those working in extended and intermediate care facilities include long-term planning to meet developmental, physical, spiritual, and psychosocial needs of the residents.

Nursing Homes and Residential Care. Personal care assistance is generally provided in two formal health care settings: *nursing homes,* or the previously described nursing facilities, and *residential care facilities.* Residential care facilities may be referred to as supervisory care homes or assisted living arrangements.[7] Both settings are generally licensed by the state to ensure that quality living, safety, and health care standards are met. Often the nursing homes may provide one or more of the other specified levels of care, such as skilled nursing or intermediate care (Fig. 2-2). The dominant trend, however, is to provide more acute services in nursing facilities while basic custodial and residential services are provided in assisted living situations. Residents often live in nursing homes or supervisory care homes in order to obtain additional assistance for their activities of daily living, such as grooming and meal preparation, or supervision with their medications. Residents generally must be able to care for themselves and move about without the help of another person.

Residents may also reside in a *continuing care retirement community,* which is a blend of several options, including housing complex, activity center, and health care system. Continuing care retirement communities differ from other retirement options by providing a continuum of housing, services, and health care. There is a written agreement or contract between the resident and the continuing care retirement community and is generally intended to last the resident's lifetime or for a specific period of time.[8]

Nurses may work intermittently in these facilities as supervisors for specific care needs for residents, such as monitoring medical treatment, taking blood pressures, or administering insulin. If more extensive care is required, patients may transfer to other care settings that provide the nursing or personal care that is required. If specific treatments, such as wound care, skilled monitoring, or teaching, are required, home health care nurses may visit patients intermittently in supervisory care homes to provide nursing care. Many of these facilities also have a skilled nursing facility. This enables residents who temporarily need skilled nursing care to receive it until they can return to their own residence.

Home Health Care

Home health care refers to care delivered in the home setting, most often in the patient's own residence. The National Association for Home Care (NAHC) defines home care as the broad spectrum of health care and social services provided in the home environment to recovering, disabled, or chronically ill patients.[9] Home health care may include health maintenance, education, illness prevention, diagnosis and treatment of disease, palliation, and rehabilitation. Care may be delivered in assisted living situations when no other skilled nursing professional is available for patient care needs. Patients receiving home health care may require intermittent services or full-time, 24-hours-a-day assistance to remain in their home.[10]

Home health care has its roots in community health nursing.[11] In fact, until hospitals became the predominant source of health care, nurses often made visits to the patient's home to teach and provide skilled care. At one time, home health care was one aspect of public health nursing, along with other community health services such as immunizations, well child care, and communicable disease control. It was not until the mid-1960s that home health care became established on its own. With the inception of Medicare (Title XVIII of the Social Security Act) and Medicaid (Title XIX), provisions were made for the federal government to reimburse home health care services through fiscal intermediaries. Over the years other forms of insurance have become available for the payment of home health care (Table 2-2).

Over the past decade there has been an explosive growth in home health care services, coupled with a steady decline in hospital bed occupancy and length of hospital stay. The growth in

Table 2-2 Funding Mechanisms for Home Health Care

1. Title programs under the Social Security Act of 1965
   - Medicare or Title XVIII
   - Medicaid or Title XIX
2. Title program under the Social Services Amendment of the Social Security Act of 1975
   - Title XX for homemaking and chore service for low-income persons
3. Older Americans Act of 1965
   - Title III, governed by the Area Agencies on Aging, for homemaker services, home health aide, nutrition, home-delivered meals, legal services
   - Title IV, research and demonstration projects for frail elderly who are at risk for institutionalization
4. Title V—maternal, child health, and crippled children services
5. Private or commercial insurance
6. Managed care arrangements, such as through preferred provider organizations (PPOs) or health maintenance organizations (HMOs)
7. Veterans benefits through the Veterans Administration
8. Private pay or out-of-pocket
9. No-fault insurance
10. Charity organizations and foundations, such as the United Way

home health care has been stimulated by DRGs, the increase in managed care, and often the patient's preference to be cared for at home. Home health care is one of the most rapidly growing segments in health care today, with the primary motivation being to shift health care to less costly services.[8]

Formal home health care can be provided to patients by many different types of licensed or accredited agencies. These different types of agencies can be grouped together in a number of different ways. Three types of distinctions used to group agencies are (1) certified or noncertified agencies, (2) for-profit or not-for-profit agencies, and (3) organizational structure. The first distinction is whether an agency is certified for Medicare payments. In 1994 over half of the home health agencies were certified for Medicare reimbursement. A second distinction is based on tax status. Some home health care agencies are proprietary or for-profit agencies; others are voluntary or private non-profit agencies. A third distinction is based on organizational structure of the home health agency. Some home health agencies are hospital-based, some are official agencies operated by state or local governments such as health departments, and others are freestanding home health agencies. Freestanding home health agencies are not affiliated with one particular hospital or governmental agency. Although all of these agencies have different organizational structures and different purposes, they must all meet specific similar standards for certification, licensure, or accreditation.

In 1966 there were only 1200 home health care agencies. Recent reports indicate there are over 18,000 home care organizations, which include home health care agencies, home care aide organizations, and hospices.[8] Hospital-based and proprietary agencies have grown faster than any other segment of the home care industry.

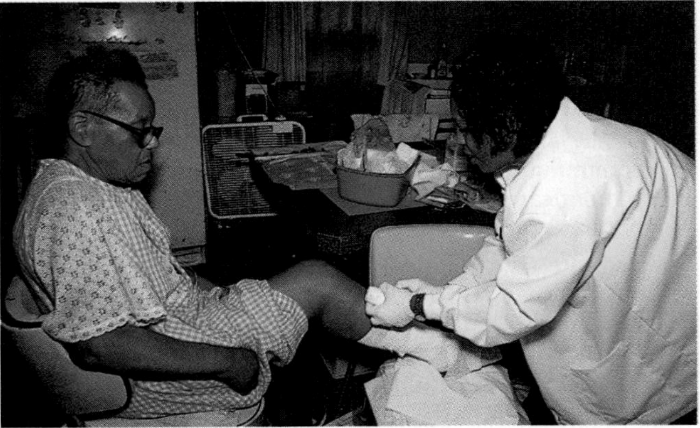

Fig. 2-3 Educating patient in home setting.

Home health care that is paid for privately provides a substantial amount of care in the home. Individuals may pay for their own care if it is not covered by their insurance plan. Private care may also supplement home health care that may be paid for by a patient's insurance plan. Grants may be secured by home health agencies to provide homemaking or home health aide services for select patient groups, such as through the Area Agency on Aging. Often a combination of services, provided by formal home health agencies, registry services or private-duty care, and the community are used to facilitate the patient's ability to remain at home.

Home health agencies may be licensed by state licensing bureaus and certified to receive reimbursement for care to Medicare beneficiaries. They may also be accredited by the Joint Commission on Accreditation of Healthcare Organizations, the Community Health Accreditation Program sponsored by the National League for Nursing, or the Accreditation Commission for Home Care, Inc.[12] Certification requires that home health agencies adhere to the Conditions of Participation as set forth by Medicare. The Conditions of Participation provide the rules that agencies must adhere to in order to receive reimbursement from Medicare through fiscal intermediaries. These rules are the minimum criteria or standards for agency operation, maintenance of patient records, supervision of patient care, and qualifications of personnel, such as nursing. Nursing care is the central component of the regulations, and nurses provide most home health care services.[8] The Conditions of Participation stipulate that registered nurses are the coordinators of patient care, being both accountable for the supervision of personal care services by home health aides and for case management services, including all aspects of care in the home.

Patient Care in the Home. Patients admitted to home care may have a length of stay anywhere from one visit to many visits lasting over years. The most common admission diagnoses are congestive heart failure, wound care, diabetes, chronic obstructive pulmonary disease, and cancer.[13] Skilled nursing care may include observation and assessment, management and evaluation, teaching and training (Fig. 2-3), the administration

Table 2-3 Examples of Home Health Care Nursing Activities

Activity	Description
Assessment	Performance of in-depth holistic assessment of patient, family, and home environment. Assessment of community services as a source of referral for patient/caregiver needs. Ongoing evaluation of patient's progress.
Wound Care	Dressing changes. Observation, assessment, and culture of wounds. Debridement and irrigation of wounds. Instructing patients and families in wound care.
Respiratory Care	Management of oxygen therapy, mechanical ventilation, chest physiotherapy. Suctioning and care of tracheostomies.
Vital Signs	Monitoring blood pressure and cardiopulmonary status. Instructing patients and families in taking of blood pressure and pulse.
Elimination	Assistance with colostomy irrigation and skin care procedures. Insertion of urinary catheters, irrigation, and observation for infection. Instruction of family in intermittent catheterization. Insertion, replacement, and sterile irrigation of urethral and suprapubic catheters. Bowel and bladder training.
Nutrition	Assessment of nutrition and hydration status. Instruction on prescribed diet. Administration of nasogastric and percutaneous tube feedings, including gastrostomy and jejunostomy tubes and instructing families in tube feedings. Placement and replacement of tubes and ongoing management and evaluation.
Rehabilitation	Instructing patients and families in the use of devices, range-of-motion exercises, ambulation, and transfer techniques.
Medications	Instructing patients and families on medication actions, administration, and side effects. Monitoring compliance and effectiveness of prescribed medications. Administration and teaching of insulin injections.
Intravenous Therapy	Assessment and management of dehydration. Giving antibiotic medications, parenteral nutrition, blood products, and analgesic and chemotherapeutic agents. Use of peripheral and central lines.
Pain Management	Assessment of pain, including location, characteristics, precipitating factors, and impact on life. Instructing patient and family on nonpharmacologic techniques (e.g., relaxation, imagery) for pain management. Providing optimal pain relief with prescribed analgesics.
Selected Laboratory Studies	Drawing blood for studies related to disease processes or therapy.

of medications, wound care, tube feedings, catheter care, and behavioral health interventions (Table 2-3). Commonly performed treatments in the home include administration of infusion therapy, such as antibiotic administration, patient-controlled analgesia for pain control, enteral feedings, parenteral nutrition, chemotherapy, and hydration therapy.[14] The nurse and a rehabilitation team member may also provide home medical equipment in the home to facilitate medical treatment and safety. These may include electrical beds, wheelchairs, commodes, walkers, and other assistive devices.

Patients have benefited from the influx and sophistication of technology in the home health care setting. The miniaturization of infusion pumps makes it possible for patients to go to work while receiving antibiotics or total parenteral nutrition. The use of central venous catheter devices and peripherally inserted central catheters has eliminated many problems associated with short-term and less reliable IV therapy. Tabletop ventilators allow patients who are dependent on mechanical ventilation to be cared for in the home setting, allowing for even greater mobility when the equipment is strapped onto the back of a wheelchair.

Concerns of patients requiring home health care are presented in Table 2-4. Examples of nursing diagnoses for patients requiring home health care are presented in Table 2-5.

Although the patient is the center of care and visit reimbursement is based on what is done for the identified patient, nursing care must be family-centered. Families usually help in decision making and provide care for the patient. Often teaching is directed at both the patient and the family. For example, diet modification is a cornerstone of diabetes management, and although an elderly male diabetic may be the identified patient, it may be the patient's wife who does the grocery shopping and cooking. Any dietary teaching that does not include the wife will not be successful.

Family-centered care also means that the home health nurse helps family members understand and cope with changing roles, responsibilities, and stresses, because an illness experienced by one family member will affect the entire family and drastically alter family interactions.

Home Health Care Team. Home health agencies provide part-time, intermittent, skilled nursing care and often provide at least one therapy service in the patient's home. Coverage for home health care varies depending on whether the patient is covered by Medicare, an HMO, or an insurance company. In general, to qualify for coverage, patients have to be confined to the home, known as "homebound status," and in need of professional skilled care such as nursing. Depending on the needs of the patient, home health visits

Table 2-4 Concerns of Patients Requiring Home Health Care Organized by Functional Health Patterns

Health Perception–Health Management Pattern ▪ Self-care capability ▪ Maintenance of safety ▪ Adherence to prescribed therapy	**Self-Perception/Self-Concept Pattern** ▪ Body image disturbances ▪ Feelings of self-worth ▪ Feelings of powerlessness
Nutritional-Metabolic Pattern ▪ Suitability of diet ▪ Integrity of skin ▪ Energy for daily activities	**Role-Relationship Pattern** ▪ Altered family/living arrangements ▪ Capability for vocation/employment ▪ Social contact and involvement ▪ Altered family roles
Elimination Pattern ▪ Bowel control ▪ Bladder control ▪ Use of medications	**Sexuality-Reproductive Pattern** ▪ Methods of contraception ▪ Facilitation of conception ▪ Alternative means of sexual activity
Activity-Exercise Pattern ▪ Endurance for or in activities ▪ Impairments in mobility ▪ Home maintenance management	**Coping–Stress Tolerance Pattern** ▪ Perception of intense stressors ▪ Dealing with change and loss ▪ Exhaustion of adaptive abilities ▪ Management of stress ▪ Sources of formal and informal support
Sleep-Rest Pattern ▪ Decreased daytime altertness ▪ Interference with or interrupted sleep ▪ Sleep/activity asynchrony	**Value-Belief Pattern** ▪ Maintenance of the human spirit ▪ Holistic well-being ▪ Worth of life and health ▪ Desire to maintain independence
Cognitive-Perceptual Pattern ▪ Capacity to learn ▪ Acute pain and chronic pain ▪ Sensory impairments ▪ Complaints or discomforts	

Source: Potter PA, Perry AG: *Fundamentals of nursing: concepts, process, and practice*, St Louis, 1997, Mosby, p 89.

may be as frequent as twice daily or as infrequent as only once a month. Visits may be extensive and require significant time, such as the initial admissions visit, or they may be shorter in length, such as visits to check a healing wound. These visits may be characterized by a predetermined routine or treatment regimen, such as insulin administration and blood glucose monitoring or noncomplicated wound care dressings.

Patients may also benefit from the management and evaluation aspect of home health care programs. Under this program, skilled nursing visits are allowed for nurses to function as case managers in the home for a longer duration of care. Reimbursement is allowed for prevention, health promotion, and the ongoing management of the chronic care needs of patients.[15]

Nursing is one of the primary services in the home health care setting. Skilled nursing in home health care refers to the care by a registered nurse that requires the knowledge, assessment, execution of clinical skills, and judgment to evaluate the process and outcome of care on the basis of nursing intervention. The home health care team may be composed of many members, including the patient, family, nurse, physician, social worker, physical therapist, occupational therapist, speech therapist, social worker, home health aide, pharmacist, respiratory therapist, and dietitian. Physical conditions or diagnoses that may trigger a referral to a physical therapist include orthopedic conditions, such as hip or knee surgeries or neuromuscular deterioration commonly seen with multiple sclerosis, amyotrophic lateral sclerosis, and cerebrovascular accidents (CVAs). The physical therapist will work with patients on strengthening and endurance, gait training, transfer training, and developing a patient education program. Occupational therapists may assist the patient with fine motor coordination, performance of the activities of daily living, cognitive-perceptual skills, sensory testing, and the construction or use of assistive or adaptive equipment. Speech therapists focus on various speech pathologies for those who have suffered speech or swallowing disorders seen in patients with a CVA, laryngectomy, or progressive neuromuscular diseases.

The social worker assists patients with coping skills, caregiver concerns, securing adequate financial resources or housing assistance, or making referrals to social service or volunteer agencies. Home health aides assist patients with their personal care needs, such as bathing, dressing, hair washing, or some homemaking activities, such as meal preparation or light housekeeping. Other members of the home health care team may include pharmacists, who are involved in the preparation of infusion products; respiratory therapists, who may assist in oxygen therapy in the home; and dietitians for dietary consultation. The members of the home health care team work collaboratively with the home health care nurse to plan and evaluate the patient's progress on a regular basis with a significant emphasis placed on home education programs.

Table 2-5 Examples of Nursing Diagnoses for Patients Requiring Home Health Care

Altered nurition *related to* inability to ingest or digest food, inability to absorb nutrients

Caregiver role strain *related to* assuming total care of patient

Constipation *related to* decreased fluid intake, lack of mobility, narcotic analgesics

Fatigue *related to* disease process and therapy

Fluid volume deficit *related to* poor nutrition and hydration, dysphagia, and confusion

Impaired home maintenance management *related to* decreased mobility, decreased endurance

Impaired skin integrity *related to* physical immobility, radiation, pressure

Pain *related to* disease process, therapy, decreased joint mobility

Risk for aspiration *related to* enteral tube feedings, impaired gag reflex, inability to expectorate sputum

Risk for infection *related to* inadequate primary or secondary defenses, impaired immune status, malnutrition

Risk for injury *related to* altered mobility, confusion, fatigue

Self-care deficit *related to* pain, musculoskeletal impairment, decreased endurance

Social isolation *related to* physical immobility, alteration in physical appearance

Third-party covered home health care is given only with a physician's order, and a plan of treatment is written for each patient. Physicians authorize the plan of care, requiring a review of the treatment plan at a minimum of every 60 days. Qualified nurses and therapists provide and supervise all of the care. Patients seen by home health care nurses are most often discharged from hospital settings but may also be referred directly from a physician's office or nursing facilities, or they may be requested by the patient. At times, costly hospitalizations can be prevented by skilled nursing personnel who can monitor, teach, administer treatments, and perform procedures that may be otherwise performed in an acute care setting.

Role and Skills of Home Health Nurse. Home care nurses must have expert organizational skills, be able to make independent decisions, and know how to set priorities and respond to problems promptly.[16] They must adapt to a variety of circumstances that challenge their assessment, planning, and intervention abilities. For example, the nurse may need to modify the technique for dressing changes for a patient with limited manual dexterity and no running water in his or her home. Nurses who work in home care require additional skills in time and case management, communication, assessment and diagnosis, community resource identification, teaching, and discharge planning. Attributes of home health care nurses include flexibility, empathy, patient advocacy, and the ability to function independently in the home setting. Nurses need to balance administrative and agency demands and productivity standards with patient care needs.

A holistic, nonjudgmental, and family-centered philosophy is essential for the nurse in the home. In addition to drawing on distinct knowledge, home care nursing also calls for a different process of decision making. Home care nurses focus on empowering the patient and family to meet their own needs so they can feel in control of their lives. Goals aim for long-term rather than short-term results. Decision making and priority setting become shared activities among the patient, family, and nurse.[17]

Projected planning to meet patient needs that may span from several visits to many weeks or months requires creative problem-solving skills and care planning that is definitive, yet adaptable to changing situations and conditions. Clinical or critical pathways (care maps) and standard care plans often guide patient care and assist the nurse in setting up a plan of care that covers a span of time. Clinical paths are designed to streamline patient care, emphasize the achievement of predetermined expected outcomes, and control costs while maintaining acceptable quality. Long-term planning and progressive monitoring toward patient independence are often included in the plan of care.

Documentation is the key to continuing services in the patient's home. Reimbursement for nursing visits is retroactive based on documentation. Nurses must use concise and accurate documentation to ensure both legal and professional accountability. Documentation is the only way to substantiate recommendations about the patient's needs, the care provided, and the patient's response. These are all necessary to meet reimbursement criteria for the services rendered.[18]

Home health care nurses must be knowledgeable in the adaptive equipment or assistive devises used in the patient's home to promote independent functioning. Understanding rehabilitation terminology is helpful in collaborating with therapists and evaluating the patient's plan of care. Medical supplies provided through most home health care agencies include urinary catheters, wound care products, and IV therapy supplies. Nurses need to be knowledgeable and organized to secure needed supplies in the home on a timely basis.

Continuous quality improvement is a mandate for home health care agencies and nurses.[11] Patient care monitoring of infection control rates, readmissions to hospitals, and other facets of clinical care are evaluated with respect to quality care and patient outcomes. With the influx of managed care in home health care, nurses are expected to provide the maximum amount of quality care in a shorter period of time. The recent emphasis on outcome management requires home health care nurses to monitor patient progress toward realistic goals in a timely fashion. Federal regulations are being proposed to require patient outcome monitoring by home health care agencies.[19]

Informal Home Health Care. Many patients rely on the provision of supportive health care through a system of informal home care. Patients may need some assistance in their own home to maintain functional independence that may otherwise require placement in a long-term care facility. The assistance required may include assisted meal preparation, meals brought in by family and friends, or the organized delivery of meals to the home, often known as meals-on-wheels. Other arrangements necessary to maximize independence in the home setting may include housekeeping, food deliveries, friendly visiting, homemaker services, or personal care assistance by home health aides. Many church, charity, or community organizations offer assistance to those in need in the form of food, service, or transportation.

This type of care and support in the home does not require the direct services of the professional nurse. Rather, nurses may oversee the case management of individuals who may require these services in the home as a part of federal, state, or locally funded programs targeted to assist the elderly and disabled at home. Nurses may also supervise trained nursing assistants as part of a formal home health care agency if care is paid for out-of-pocket by the patient. Nurses may also direct the care for homebound or at-risk elderly through parish nursing partnerships, community-sponsored programs, or area aging agencies. Nurses in these settings require skills in case management, assessment of activities of daily living, and community resource identification and referral.

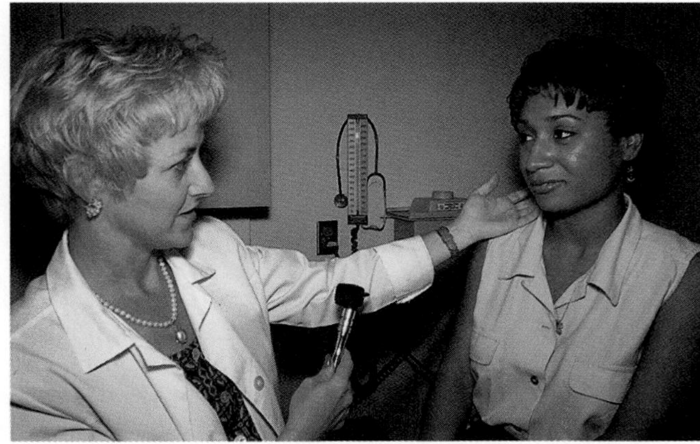

Fig. 2-4 Advance practice nurses play an important role in primary care delivery.

Ambulatory Care

The predominant source of health care today occurs in ambulatory care settings. Patients may be seen in physician and nurse practitioner offices, clinics, freestanding surgical centers, schools, churches, and adult or child day care centers. A wide range of medical and nursing services are available, with most care being delivered in a one-time encounter.

Nurses in ambulatory care settings may assist in a physician practice or with additional training assume nurse practitioner or advanced practice roles. Nurses in ambulatory care settings assess patients' problems, evaluate the need for resources and information, and provide the appropriate interventions that allow patients to care for themselves. Patient teaching and telephone follow-up are routine practices in ambulatory care settings. Nurses may perform phlebotomy service, administer medications, counsel and teach patients and families, immunize children, or lead support groups. Nurses in freestanding surgical centers may assist with the preoperative and postoperative care for patients who will be discharged home the same day. Advanced practice nurses may work in gerontologic, adult health, pediatrics, women's health, and family practice settings assessing and treating patients requiring their services (Fig. 2-4).

Hospice

Many people choose to die at home in the comfort of their own home and surrounded by family and friends. Terminally ill patients may die in dignity at home without the heroic measures commonly seen in acute care settings. Hospice exists to provide support and care for persons in the last phases of incurable diseases so that they might live as fully and as comfortably as possible. The term *hospice* is derived from a medieval word that means a place of shelter for people on a difficult journey. Hospice is not a place but a concept of care that provides compassion, concern, and support for the dying. Hospice care represents a return to previous times when dying individuals were helped to remain at home and to die at home, if possible, surrounded by familiar sights, sounds, and smells and by the love of those who care.

Overview of Hospice Care. The hospice concept of care has existed in England for many years. During the 1970s the concept of hospice was integrated into health care in the United States, and by the end of the decade, every state had existing hospice programs. Currently, there are over 2600 hospice programs in all 50 states, the District of Columbia, and Puerto Rico.[20] Like home health care, hospice programs are organized under a variety of models. Some are hospital based, others are part of existing home health care agencies, and others are freestanding or community-based, volunteer-intensive programs.[21] However, regardless of their organization, all hospices emphasize palliative rather than curative care.

Admission to a hospice program is voluntary and based on patient and family need. Patients with terminal conditions such as cancer, acquired immunodeficiency syndrome, chronic obstructive pulmonary disease, and end-stage cardiovascular or renal disease may qualify for hospice care.[19] Hospice care is generally provided in the home, with inpatient care generally reserved for acute pain management or respite care for families or caregivers in need of a break. Home care is provided on a part-time, intermittent, on-call, regularly scheduled, or continuous basis. Hospice services are available 24 hours a day and 7 days a week to provide help to patients and families in their homes. The inpatient settings have been deinstitutionalized to make the atmosphere as relaxed and homelike as possible. Staff and volunteers are available to the patient and family. A multidisciplinary team approach often provides holistic health care.

Reimbursement for hospice care is as varied as for home health care. Section 122 of the Tax Equity and Fiscal Responsibility Act of 1982 created the hospice Medicare benefit. Hospice services may be provided to terminally ill Medicare beneficiaries with a life expectancy of 6 months or less with four benefit periods (Table 2-6). In addition to the usual services covered by Medicare, the hospice benefit also covers medications, home medical equipment, counseling, bereavement, and homemaker services. Commercial insurance, Medicaid, and other charitable sources may also reimburse for hospice services.

Patient Care in Hospice. There is often a point in terminal disease when curative treatment is no longer possible. At this time the hospice philosophy of promoting the patient's quality of life and providing palliative care is appropriate. Hospices provide a means by which individuals can receive supportive physical, emotional, and spiritual care in their dying days. Hospice care ensures that patient and family needs are the focus of any intervention.

Table 2-6 Medicare Hospice Benefit Periods

Initial 90-day period
Subsequent 90-day period
Subsequent 30-day period
Subsequent fourth and final extension period of indefinite duration

Hospice care is not technology oriented. Rather, it is intensive personal care that provides skilled bedside nursing and focuses attention on the emotional, social, spiritual, and familial aspects of the patient. Hospice offers the opportunity to work with patients and families to achieve mutually agreed on goals.

Pain is a common concern among terminally ill patients. In hospice, pain is considered a total experience rather than a physiologic event. Adequate medication and adjunctive therapy are used to provide relief. The "prn" (as needed) order for pain is not found in hospice. Analgesia is routinely given in an attempt to eliminate pain and, more important, to prevent its recurrence and to erase the memory of pain. Attention is also given to other factors that may contribute to a patient's pain, including fear, loneliness, anxiety, insomnia, spiritual doubts or concerns, financial worries, and depression.

Hospice Team. Services are provided by a medically supervised interdisciplinary team of professionals and volunteers. The hospice nurse is an integral part of the hospice team. Hospice nurses work collaboratively with hospice physicians, social workers, certified nursing assistants, clergy, and volunteers to provide care and support to the patient and family members. Hospice nurses are specially trained in pain control and symptom management. As with home health care, hospice care requires excellent teaching skills, compassion, flexibility, and adaptability to patient needs.

Bereavement counseling is another aspect of the hospice program. Because the patient and family are the focus of hospice care, grief support to family members and significant others during the illness, as well as after the death of the patient, is incorporated into the organizational structure and treatment plan. The objective of a bereavement program is to provide support and to assist survivors in the transition to a life without the deceased person.

Support groups are available to help hospice staff and volunteers. Crises and grief result in varying forms of stress for caregivers. To give to patients and families, the staff and volunteers must also have a means to be nourished and refreshed. Various means of stress relief may be used for staff members and volunteers, including professional-assisted groups, informal discussion sessions, flexible time schedules, and additional time off. The needs of the caregiver must be considered important or the care receiver will receive less of what is needed.

SUMMARY

Many changes are occurring within the health care delivery system. Patient care settings are becoming highly diversified. The evolving structure of health care is in flux, but it is becoming more focused on providing patient care in the community. Acute care needs of patients are provided in hospitals and settings that are equipped to handle unstable and critically ill patients. Transitional care settings are permitting the movement of patients to settings where specific care needs can be met. The increasing number of home health care and hospice settings allow patients to receive technical nursing care, education, and support in the home environment. Multiple professional, accrediting, and trade associations are available to nursing and other interested individuals to support home health care and hospice (Table 2-7).

Table 2-7 National Home Health Care or Hospice Organizations or Affiliations and Accrediting Agencies

Accreditation Commission for Home Care, Inc. 3325 Executive Drive, Suite 150 Raleigh, NC 27609 (919) 872-8608 (Home care agency accreditation in AL, FL, GA, KY, NC, SC, MS, TN, VA)
American Hospital Association 840 North Lake Shore Drive Chicago, IL 60611 (302) 280-6000
Community Health Accreditation Program, Inc. 350 Hudson Street New York, NY 10014 (800)-669-1656
Home Health Nurses' Association 437 Twin Bay Drive Pensacola, FL 32534-1350 (904) 474-1066
Hospice Association of America 519 C. St., N.E. Washington, DC 20002-5809
Hospice Foundation of America 2001 S. Street, N.W. Suite 300 Washington, DC 20009 (202) 638-5419
Hospice Nurses' Association Medical Center East, Suite 375 211 N. Whitfield Street Pittsburgh, PA 15206 (412) 361-2470
Joint Commission of Accreditation of Health Care Organizations 875 North Michigan Avenue Chicago, IL 60611 (312) 642-6061
National Association for Home Care 228 Seventh Street, S.E. Washington, DC 20003-4306 (202) 547-7424
National Hospice Organization 1901 N. Moore Street, Suite 901 Arlington, VA 22209 (703) 243-5900

CRITICAL THINKING EXERCISES

CASE STUDY

Home Health Care for Cardiac Patient

Patient Profile

José, 72 years old, was discharged from the hospital 4 days after a myocardial infarction. He and his wife live in an apartment five miles from the hospital. His case manager at the hospital referred him to the home health care agency for follow-up care. Neither he nor his wife are able to drive.

Subjective Data

- Has history of hypertension
- Had heart attack 3 years ago
- Cannot walk one block without getting short of breath
- Has swollen feet and cannot wear shoes
- Had fractured hip that was surgically repaired 6 months ago

Collaborative Care

- O_2 at 3 L/min
- Furosemide (Lasix) 40 mg bid
- Captopril (Capoten) 50 mg bid
- 2 g sodium diet
- Assessment of home environment
- Patient education program

Critical Thinking Questions

1. What are the initial priorities for the home health nurse?
2. What other members of the home health team should be involved in the care of José? What are their roles and responsibilities?
3. What type of patient education program should be implemented? What are the priority teaching goals?
4. What types of medical equipment will José need? What teaching should accompany the use of this equipment?
5. José's wife inquires about an outpatient cardiac rehabilitation program. What would be an appropriate response from the home health nurse?
6. What are the long-term expected outcomes for José?

Nursing is also diversifying, adapting, and moving into a variety of patient care settings. As nursing's role continues to expand, patients are expecting advanced clinical skills within a complex health care environment. Cost-containment strategies and quality assurance will remain a priority in the health care system. More nurses are working in collaborative or independent roles administering direct care to patients or directing care by team members. Nurses are called on to maintain clinical proficiency and critical thinking skills and to become proficient in problem solving, teaching, management, and promoting wellness for patients in all settings along the continuum of patient care.

REVIEW QUESTIONS

The number of the question corresponds to the same-numbered objective at the beginning of the chapter.

1. Recent changes in the health care delivery system are largely attributed to
   a. changing demographics and an aging society.
   b. more insurance payment for health care services.
   c. desires of patients to be in more restrictive settings.
   d. diagnosis-related groups and the influx of managed care.
2. Patients may move among different care settings to
   a. maintain psychologic integrity.
   b. adhere to physician orders for treatment.
   c. maximize dependence on health care providers.
   d. ensure that physical, emotional, and psychosocial care needs are met.
3. Home health care has emerged as a significant segment in the health care delivery system primarily because of
   a. improved funding for care.
   b. efforts to contain and control health care costs.
   c. deregulation of home health and hospice care services.
   d. recent advances in computer and medical technology.
4. Nurses working in community-based and home health care settings
   a. utilize case management skills along the continuum of care.
   b. focus only on patient needs specific to the setting.
   c. function autonomously in meeting patient needs.
   d. use the same skills as in acute care or critical care settings.

References

1. Zander K: Responsive restructuring. IV. Care management and case management, *New Definition* 9:1, 1994.
2. *Standards of home health nursing practice,* Kansas City, Mo, 1986, American Nurses' Association.
3. Molloy SP: Defining case management, *Home Health Nurse* 12:51, 1994.
4. Stanhope M, Lancaster J: *Community health nursing: process and practice for promoting health,* ed 4, St Louis, 1996, Mosby.
5. Jones AM, Foster N: Transitional care: bridging the gap, *Medsurg Nurs* 6:32, 1997.
6. American Health Care Association: Consumer information. In the American Health Care Association, 1997. Available Internet http://www.ahca.org
7. American Association of Homes and Services for the Aging: Consumer information. In the American Association of Homes and Services for the Aging, 1997. Available Internet http://www.aahsa.org
8. National Association for Home Care: Basic statistics about home care 1996. In the National Association for Home Care Consumer Information, 1997. Available Internet http://www.nahc.org
9. National Association for Home Health Care: *A providers guide to a Medicare home health certification process,* ed 3, Washington, DC, 1994, National Association for Home Health Care.
10. Marosy JP: Assisted living: opportunities for partnerships in caring, *Caring* 16:72, 1997.
11. Mosby: *Mosby's home health nursing pocket consultant,* St Louis, 1995, Mosby.
12. Zang SM, Bailey NC: *Home care manual: making the transition,* Philadelphia, 1997, Lippincott.

13. United States Department of Health and Human Services: Health United States 1995, Hyattsville, Md, 1996, Public Health Service.
14. Humphrey CJ, Milone-Nuzzo P: *Home care nursing. An orientation to practice,* Norwalk, Conn, 1991, Appleton & Lange.
15. Allen S: Medicare case management, *Home Healthc Nurse* 12:21, 1994.
16. Benefield LE: Making the transitions to home care nursing, *AJN* 96:47, 1996.
17. O'Neill ES, Pennington EA: Preparing acute care nurses for community-based care, *NSHC: Perspectives on Community* 17:62, 1996.
18. Rice R: *Home health nursing practice: concepts and application,* ed 2, St Louis, 1996, Mosby.
19. United States Department of Health and Human Services, Health Care Financing Administration: Medicare and Medicaid programs; review of the conditions of participation for home health agencies and the use of the outcomes and assessment information set (OASIS) as part of the revised conditions of participation for home health agencies, *Federal Register* (62)46:11004, 1997.
20. National Hospice Organization: Hospice facts sheet. In the National Hospice Organization, 1997. Available Internet http://www.nho.org
21. National Association for Home Care. Hospice facts and statistics 1996. In the National Association for Home Care Consumer Information, 1997. Available Internet http://www.nahc.org

Resources

American Association for Continuity of Care
638 Prospect Avenue
Hartford, CT 06105-4250
860-586-7525
Fax: 860-586-7550

American Association of Ambulatory Care Nursing
E. Holly Avenue, Box 56
Pitman, NJ 08071-0056
609-256-2350
800-262-6877
Fax: 609-589-7463
http://www.inurse.com/~AAACN

American Association of Occupational Health Nurses, Inc.
50 Lenox Pointe
Atlanta, GA 30324
404-262-1162
800-241-8014
Fax: 404-262-1165
http://www.aaohn.org

American Society for Long-Term Care Nurses
660 Lonely Cottage Drive
Upper Black Eddy, PA 18972-9313
610-847-5396
Fax: 610-847-5063

Foundation for Hospice & Home Care
513 C Street NE
Washington, DC 20002
202-547-6586
202-546-8968
http://www.aoa.dhhs.gov/aoa/dir/100.html

Home Health Care Nurse's Association
http://junior.apk.net/~nurse/

Home Healthcare Nurses' Association
7794 Grow Drive
Pensacola, FL 32514
904-474-1066
800-558-4462

Hospice Association of America
519 C Street NE
Washington, DC 20002
202-546-4759
Fax: 202-546-9312
http://www.nahc.org/HAA/consumer.html

Hospice Education Institute
190 Westbrook Road
Essex, CT 06426
800-331-1620

Hospice Foundation of America
2001 S Street NW, Suite 300
Washington, DC 20009
202-638-5419
Fax: 202-638-5312
http://www.hospicefoundation.org/page3.htm

Hospice Nurses' Association
Medical Center East, Suite 375
211 North Whitfield Street
Pittsburgh, PA 15206-3031
412-361-2470
Fax: 412-361-2425
http://www.roxane.com/hpna.org

National Association for Home Care
228 7th Street SE
Washington, DC 20003
202-547-7424
http://www.nahc.org

National Association for Senior Living Industries
184 Duke of Gloucester Street
Annapolis, MD 21401-2523
410-263-0991
Fax: 410-263-1262
http://www.desert.net/nasli/index.html

National Gerontological Nursing Association
7250 Parkway Drive, Suite 510
Hanover, MD 21076
800-723-0560
http://www.nursingcenter.com/people/nrsorgs/ngna/apply.html

National Hospice Organization (NHO)
1901 North Moore Street, Suite 901
Arlington, VA 22209
800-658-8898
http://www.nho.org/

For additional Internet resources, see the website for this book at www.mosby.com/MERLIN/medsurg_lewis

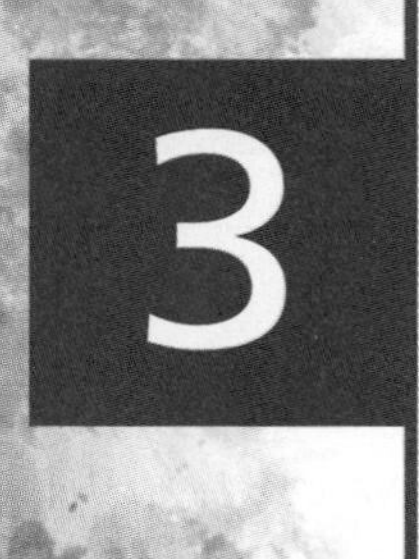

REMEMBER to check out your companion CD-ROM

3 Adult Development

Anne M. Devney & Charlotte R. Abbink

www.mosby.com/MERLIN/medsurg_lewis

LEARNING OBJECTIVES

1. Explain the major concepts of biologic and psychologic theories of aging.
2. Explain the major concepts in adult developmental theories proposed by Erikson, Peck, Havighurst, and Levinson.
3. Describe the major psychodynamic concerns of young, middle, and older adults in terms of self-concept, concept of death, intellectual processes, and sexuality.
4. List the major family developmental tasks for young, middle, and older adults.
5. Describe important health promotion concerns for young, middle, and older adults related to changes resulting from the process of aging.
6. Describe the impact of illness on young, middle, and older adults related to their developmental status.

The entire human life span is a dynamic sequence of chronologic, functional, biologic, psychologic, and social changes that occur in predictable patterns. Knowledge of an adult's growth and development status is as crucial in planning appropriate nursing care as it is for a child. Separation of a patient's illness experience from the patient's other life experiences can result in nursing care that is superficial and incomplete. Incorporating principles of adult growth and development into the assessment process gives the nurse insight into what may be happening in a patient's life at given points in the life cycle. Like childhood, adulthood can be divided into developmental stages, although adult stages have not been as comprehensively described or studied as childhood stages.

AGING

Adult development can be viewed within the larger framework of aging. As a continuation of the childhood process, adult development is commonly thought of as aging in the chronologic sense. Chronologic age is simply the number of years that the person has lived. It is used as a benchmark to denote processes that occur over time, such as becoming of legal age at age 21. Functional age refers to the person's ability to function effectively within the environment or society. This concept can apply, for example, in the determination of whether people can live on their own and be self-sufficient and not require the assistance of others for mobility or personal activities of daily living.

As the mean age of the population increases, more research regarding characteristics of successful aging is needed. Currently, research has focused on biologic and psychologic factors that contribute to the physical and mental changes associated with aging. However, it is important to point out that it is difficult, if not impossible, to separate or isolate physical, sociocultural, and psychologic factors when studying adult development. Adulthood therefore reflects the interrelationships of all factors. Although the emphasis of this chapter is on adult development, it is important to consider factors that may account for biologic and psychologic aging because of their impact on development.

Biologic Aging Theories

Biologic aging occurs in all organisms. Despite this universality, the exact etiology of biologic aging remains to be determined. Several theories regarding this phenomenon are currently proposed. One way to categorize theories related to biologic aging is to designate those that propose that aging is due to chance (stochastic) and those that propose that aging is not related to chance (nonstochastic).[1] A nonstochastic theory hypothesizes that events that occur at the molecular and cellular levels are programmed by genes.[1] Proposed theories of aging are shown in Table 3-1.

Stochastic Theories. The somatic mutation and intrinsic mutagenesis theories postulate that aging is a result of lifelong genetic damage.[2] This damage may include the progressive accumulation of faulty copying in dividing cells or the accumulation of errors in information-containing molecules. According to somatic mutation theory, body cells develop spontaneous mutations in the same way germ cells do. These mutations are presumably a result of lifelong background radiation of various types. Subsequent cell divisions perpetuate the mutations until organs become inefficient and ultimately fail. The intrinsic mutagenesis theory suggests that the increase in mutational cells occurs because of a breakdown of genetic regulatory mechanisms. The basic premise is that the regulatory capacity of the human genetic constitution diminishes throughout life, and thus more mutations occur

Reviewed by Holly Evans Madison, RN, MS, Southern Vermont College, Manchester, Vt.

Table 3-1 Summary of Biologic Theories of Aging

Theory	Dynamics
Stochastic Theories	
Error	Faulty synthesis of DNA, RNA, or both.
Somatic	Alteration in RNA/DNA; protein or enzyme synthesis causes defective structure or function.
Transcription	Failure of transcription or translation between cells; malfunctions of RNA or related enzymes.
Free Radical	Oxidation of fats, proteins, and carbohydrates creates free electrons that attach to other molecules, altering cellular function.
Cross-link	Lipids, proteins, carbohydrates, and nucleic acid react with chemicals or radiation to form bonds that cause an increase in cell rigidity and instability.
Nonstochastic Theories	
Programmed	Biologic clock triggers specific cell behavior at specific time. Organism capable of specific number of cell divisions and specific life span.
Neuroendocrine	Control mechanisms (pituitary and hypothalamus) regulate interplay between various organs and tissues; efficiency of signals between mechanisms is altered or lost.
Immunologic/Autoimmune	Alteration of B and T cells leads to loss of capacity for self-regulation; normal or age-related cells recognized as foreign matter; system reacts by forming antibodies to destroy these cells.
Telomere-telomerase Hypothesis	With aging there is a loss of telomeres (repeated sequences at the ends of DNA). This loss limits the number of times cells can divide.

with aging that will ultimately result in functional failure. Although both theories are attractive, little evidence exists to support or deny them.

The free radical theory was initially proposed in 1956 by Harman but in recent years has become the focus of new research.[3,4] A free radical is a highly reactive atom or molecule that carries an unpaired electron and thus seeks to combine with another molecule, causing an oxidative process. This process can ultimately disrupt cell membranes and alter DNA and protein synthesis. Cellular integrity, function, and regeneration mechanisms are injured. Free radicals are natural by-products of many normal cellular processes and are also created by such environmental factors as smog, tobacco smoke, and radiation.[4] Recent research has focused on the roles of various antioxidants, including vitamins C, E, and niacin, as well as β-carotene and selenium, to slow down the oxidative process and ultimately the aging process.[5] However, optimal doses of these substances have not been established. These substances are being investigated for their usefulness in preventing diseases related to aging, such as oral, esophageal, and reproductive cancers; coronary artery disease; and cataracts.

Another stochastic theory is the cross-link theory, which postulates that over time and as a result of exposure to chemicals and radiation in the environment, cross links form between lipids, proteins, and carbohydrates, as well as nucleic acids. These cross links result in decreased flexibility and elasticity, and this increases rigidity in tissues. Such changes in cell structure may explain the observable cosmetic changes associated with aging, such as wrinkles of the skin. However, it is unlikely that such changes account for all of the detrimental physical events associated with aging.

Nonstochastic Theories. For many years it was believed that cells had the capability to reproduce for an infinite amount of time. However, in the 1950s Hayflick in a series of classic experiments demonstrated that culture skin fibroblasts would reproduce or divide a finite number of times. From these observations rose the programmed theory of cell death.[6] In this theory it is proposed that there is an impairment in the ability of the cell to continue dividing. Others have suggested that a "biologic clock" may reside not within each individual cell but centrally, such as in the central nervous system or immune system, where multiple organs can be affected.[7]

The neuroendocrine theory proposes that aging occurs because of functional decrements in neurons and associated hormones.[2] It suggests that neural and endocrine changes may be pacemakers for many cellular and physiologic aspects of aging. This approach relates aging to the organism's loss of responsiveness of neuroendocrine tissue to various signals. In some cases this is a result of a loss of receptors, but in others, it is caused by changes in neurotransmission beyond the receptors. An important focus of this theory is the functional changes of the hypothalamic-pituitary system, which are accompanied by a decline in functional capacity in other endocrine organs, such as the adrenal and thyroid glands, ovaries, and testes.

The immunologic theory proposes declining functional capacity of the immune system as the basis for the aging process.[1] It suggests that aging is not a passive wearing out of systems but an active self-destruction mediated by the immune system. This theory is based on observing an age-associated decline in T cell functioning, accompanied by a decrease in resistance and an increase in autoimmune diseases with aging. Whether the immunologic changes are genetically determined, regulated by environment, or influenced by endocrine factors remains to be defined. However, some studies of cell division suggest that the cells of the immune system become more diversified with age and demonstrate a progressive loss of self-regulatory patterns. The result is an autoimmune phenomenon

Table 3-2 Adult Developmental Stage Theories

Theorist	Young Adulthood	Middle Adulthood	Older Adulthood
▪ Erikson	Intimacy versus isolation	Generativity versus self-absorption	Ego integrity versus despair
▪ Peck		Valuing wisdom versus physical power Socializing versus sexualizing relationships Emotional flexibility versus emotional impoverishment Mental flexibility versus mental rigidity	Ego differentiation versus work role preoccupation Body transcendence versus body preoccupation Ego transcendence versus ego preoccupation
▪ Havighurst	Mate selection and marriage adjustments Establishing family and child rearing Home management Occupation launching Beginning civic responsibility	Launching teenage children Maturing relationship with spouse Adjusting to aging parents Career and occupational maturity Adult social and civic responsibility Developing leisure activities Adjusting to physiologic changes	Adjusting to health decline Adjusting to retirement Adjusting to social role changes Establishing satisfactory living arrangements Adjusting to death of spouse
▪ Levinson	Early adult transition Entering the adult world Thirties transition Settling down	Midlife transition Payoff years	

in which cells normal to the body are mistaken as foreign and are attacked by the person's own immune system.

A more recent theory of aging is the telomere-telomerase hypothesis. Telomeres are specialized repeated sequences that are present at the ends of DNA strands. Telomerase is the enzyme that synthesizes these repeat sequences. With aging there is loss of these strands and a decrease in telomerase activity, both of which affect the number of times a cell can divide.[8]

Psychologic Theories of Aging

Several theories have been proposed to define and describe adult development from a psychologic perspective. These theories emphasize the sequential patterns within age and stage, life events and transition, and individual timing and variability.[9,10] Models within these perspectives have been generated in terms of personal development, including the theories of ego development,[10,11] general personality development,[12-14] moral development,[15] and faith development.[16]

Although predictable developmental patterns exist, caution must be used in imposing these patterns on a patient before first validating the unique developmental processes that the patient is experiencing. The nurse also must be sensitive to the impact that culture has on developmental expectations and norms. Although there are common assumptions that are applicable to most Western societies, the nurse should not assume that developmental theories fit universally across all cultures. Societal disruptions that occur with war, famine, or poverty can dramatically alter adult life patterns and development.

CONCEPTUAL APPROACHES TO ADULT DEVELOPMENT

Adult growth and development have been approached in several ways, and despite rigorous attempts no single theory has been universally accepted to explain the process. In fact, there is no way to isolate physical, sociocultural, and psychologic factors to study adult development. Adulthood therefore reflects the interrelationship of all factors. Therefore the best approach toward holistic care incorporates the psychologic, biologic, and spiritual aspects of the unique person.

Theorists have explained adult development based on the following premises:

1. Adult development continues to occur in definable, predictable, and sequential patterns.
2. Critical periods occur throughout the life span when physical and psychosocial growth undergo reorganization.
3. In each stage of development, there are certain normative activities or tasks to be accomplished.
4. Mastering the tasks of preceding stages is fundamental to transition and mastery of tasks in future stages.[17]

The adult development models of Erikson, Peck, Levinson, and Havighurst are summarized in Table 3-2.

Erikson's Theory: Psychosocial Developmental Conflicts

Erikson[10] views personality development as resulting from the confrontations between ego and social milieu. He identifies points in the life cycle when specific developmental conflicts become paramount because a person's capacities or experiences dictate that a major self-adjustment and adjustment to the environment must be made. In the process of making this adjustment, the individual moves toward one of two opposing positions, such as toward intimacy or toward isolation. When a person successfully masters a core conflict (such as intimacy), the negative sense (isolation) remains as a dynamic counterpart

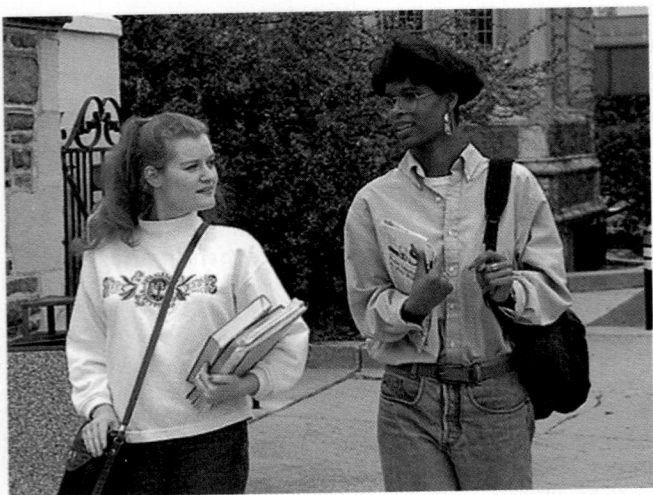

Fig. 3-1 The building of friendships is an important task for young adults.

and may be demonstrated in new situations in which this conflict must be mastered again at a higher level. Although critical times for mastery of each core conflict exist, all conflicts are present throughout the life span. For example, autonomy is especially important to a toddler; however, adolescents striving for identity need some independent space, and older adults frequently suffer loss of autonomy when limitations are placed on their decision making.

Intimacy versus Isolation. In Erikson's model, the young adult task is intimacy (Fig. 3-1). This involves fusing self-identity with the identities of others in friendships, for causes or creative efforts, or in close personal relationships, including sexual union. Intimacy requires a degree of commitment that necessitates sacrifice, compromise, and self-abandonment for the benefit of others. The young adult who avoids making this commitment to others, fearing the loss of self-identity, will experience a sense of isolation and consequently self-absorption.

Generativity versus Stagnation. During middle adulthood, the primary task is generativity. Generative adults are concerned with establishing the next generation by nurturing and guiding either their children or other young people. A sense of productivity in work and creativity in living are also important components of this task. This core conflict probably arises out of an altruistic need to leave some mark that will make the world a better place in which to live. If generativity does not occur, adults experience a sense of stagnation and turn inward, becoming self-preoccupied and overly concerned with physical and psychologic health needs. The focus of self-absorbed people on physical changes of middle age may result in either invalidism or inappropriate youthfulness in an attempt to stay young. Regression to an obsessive need for pseudointimacy may occur, which may be expressed through affairs with younger members of the opposite sex.

Ego Integrity versus Despair. Older adulthood is a time for reviewing the past and rearranging the "photo album of life." This bringing together of all the previous life stages should result in a sense of wholeness, purpose, and a life well lived, or a sense of ego integrity, according to Erikson. When a person accepts and approves of a unique life, death also can be accepted as a meaningful part of life. However, if the life review is laden with opportunities missed or wrong directions taken, a sense of despair arises. At this point the person knows life is too short to correct the failures. Death is faced with anxiety because it steals away the chance to make changes. In this last stage of ego integrity versus despair, each person must face adjustments and come to a final conflict resolution that is the product of all previous developmental conflict resolutions.

Peck's Theory: Developmental Tasks

Based on Erikson's work, Peck further defined psychosocial tasks of middle and older adulthood.[10,17] With a general decline in physical and sexual functioning, the middle-aged adult's self-esteem can suffer if it is heavily based on such changes. However, judgmental abilities tend to increase with experience, so valuing the use of one's "head" becomes a positive alternative for maintaining self-esteem. People need flexibility to shift attachments and reinvest emotions in other people and pursuits. People also need the mental flexibility to allow for new solutions to life problems, rather than being dogmatic and governed by past experiences.

Havighurst's Theory: Developmental Tasks

Havighurst also proposed specific developmental tasks for each life stage.[18] Like Erikson, he contends that there are optimal points in life to master these tasks, and the mastery level depends on the success of previous life stages. Notably, he includes family-oriented tasks that are significant to individual development. In addition, Havighurst proposed that "successful achievement of [a task] leads to happiness and to success with later tasks, while failure leads to unhappiness in the individual, disapproval by the society, and difficulty with later tasks."[18]

Levinson's Theory: Evolution of Life Structures

Levinson's theory describes the evolution of life structures. Although men and women go through similar stages of development, women may have more difficulty planning a life course if the themes of family and career are viewed as mutually exclusive choices. Levinson's basic concept, individual life structure, is the pattern of a given life at any point in time. Any change in the person's self-system (e.g., judgments, motives, values) and his or her interactions with other systems (such as the social and cultural context of life within the family, ethnicity, religion, occupation, and social events), and the particular set of roles he or she assumes, will disrupt the components. Such disruptions call for reorganizing of the life structure (Fig. 3-2).[14]

Life structure is dynamic, with predictable changes occurring as individuals move through life. The four major periods in adult life are early adulthood (ages 21 through 40), middle adulthood (ages 41 through 60), late adulthood (ages 61 through 80), and late-late adulthood (beyond 80). Within each of the four stages in adult life, individuals face transitions and stability (Fig. 3-3). Transitions are a time to make changes and redirect growth toward personal goals and objective. Stable times present opportunities to build and maintain the intact life structures necessary to pursue those goals and objectives.

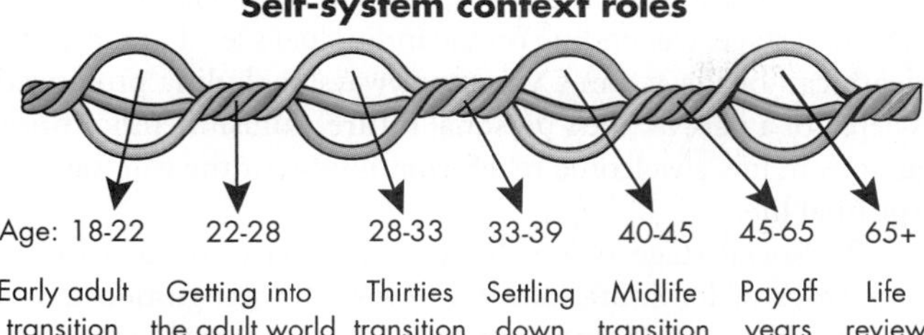

Fig. 3-2 An individual's life structure. According to Levinson's theory, life structure may be seen as a "life rope" in which the interacting strands are taken apart and individually reviewed during transition periods and are then rewoven into stable periods.

Other Theories of Development

Other theorists have used life event and transition perspectives to describe adult development. To these theorists major life events are more important than chronologic age in assessing and understanding adult behaviors.[19] Activities within one's life such as being newly married, starting a job, middle-age parenting, divorce, retirement, illness, job-related pressures, adolescent children, and parenting one's parents provide stresses of varying degrees, not always associated with a specific age.[19]

Another component of development is the individual's perception and reaction to the expected or unexpected timing of life events and the aging process. In this model one's life experiences are viewed within the appropriate time context: historical time (calendar time), life time (chronologic age), and socially defined time (as related to age norms and expectations).[20]

Courtenay[21] reviewed adult development models and found four characteristics that are common to all models. All models focus on self-identity and growth through developmental tasks. An individual's psychologic identity is closely related to personal growth and the achievement of tasks that extend his or her capabilities.[21] Another characteristic common among the models is that individuals move through hierarchic stages that range from the simple to the complex, from rigidity to flexibility, and from narrow to comprehensive perspectives.[13]

The belief that human development occurs throughout the life span is a third characteristic. The vast variety and complexity of proficiencies faced by adults require constant evolution and lifelong pursuit. Today's increasing life span offers adults multiple opportunities for continued development. The fourth characteristic of these models is that the ultimate goal of adult development is to achieve autonomy, separateness, and independence.[21]

Attention has been directed toward increasing research to answer questions of gender differences and the effects of sociocultural and environmental factors on adulthood. Early research was conducted primarily with males, and thus there is less information related to women. Gilligan[22] noted that women tend to value relationships, attachments, and interdependence to a greater degree than men.

PSYCHODYNAMIC ISSUES OF ADULTHOOD

Psychodynamic issues arise from confrontation between inner development and the demands of the social world. Individuals

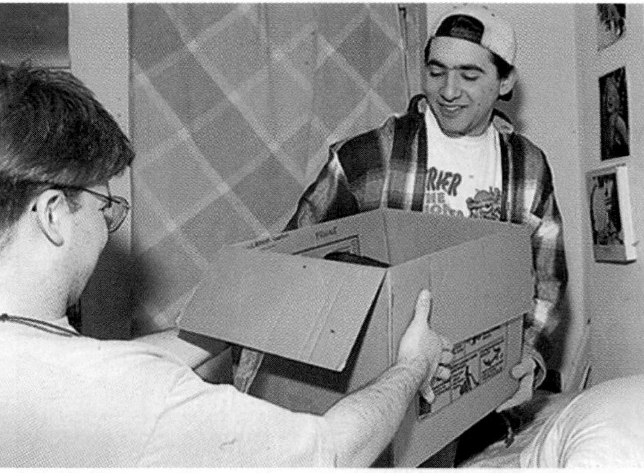

Fig. 3-3 The move from home to college is an external sign of early adult transition.

continually try to find a comfortable fit between themselves and their world, attempting to integrate their sense of who they are and who they are becoming.

Self-Concept and Self-Esteem

Self-concept and self-esteem are interdependent constructs. Self-concept may be defined as the totality of ideas people hold about themselves, and self-esteem is self-evaluation, that is, satisfaction or dissatisfaction with these ideas.

Young Adulthood. During the young adult years, a strong theme in self-concept is "I can handle it." A sense of mastery and self-control over life events and the environment prevails. The actions of young adults convey the attitude that self-will and boldness are the components of success. This confidence is a reflection of the high energy levels and increasing power and control young adults experience over life when moving out of adolescence.

Middle Adulthood. During the middle adult years, self-concept may vary greatly, depending on the perceived balance between positive and negative aspects of middle age. This stage is partially determined by culture, social class, personality, and health status. In some cultures, people are programmed to consider themselves "old" at the age of 40; in other groups, people have just "made it" at this age. For example, a blue-collar worker may consider himself old at 40, whereas a white-collar professional may perceive age 70 as old. Some middle-aged people have the "time of their life," with an increased sense of self-approval because of peak family and career investments in terms of power, prestige, and income and continued good health. In contrast, if people experience a decline in career or health, self-esteem may also decline.

The sense of self-control continues into middle age; however, during middle adulthood, people recognize the finiteness of life and shift to a more realistic appraisal of the limits of self-will. Recognizing that willpower alone does not overcome life circumstances, people become aware that help and advice from others can be valuable. With this new insight, middle-aged adults may also reevaluate a personal spiritual position (Fig. 3-4). This may become evident through participation in church activities.

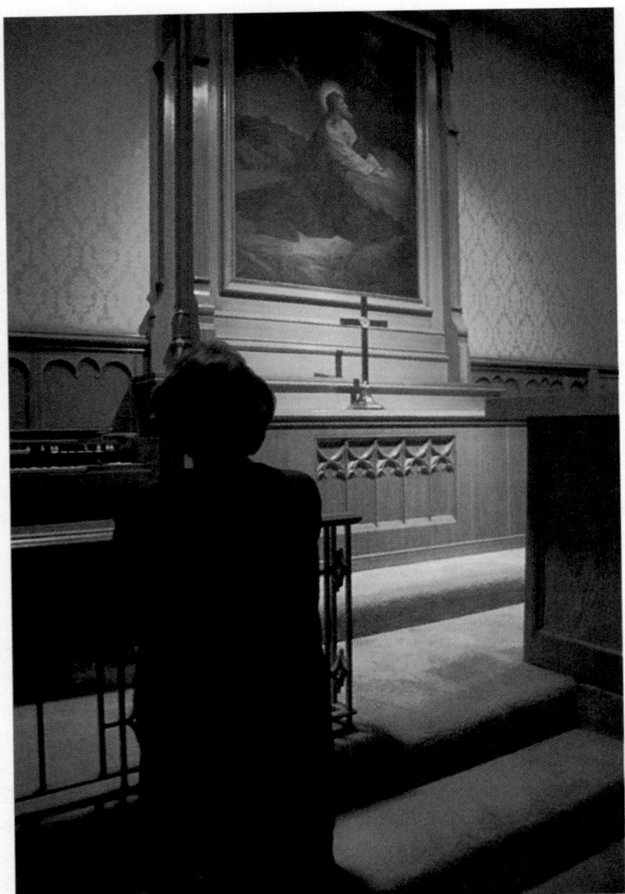

Fig. 3-4 An increasing awareness of spiritual needs often occurs in the middle years.

Older Adulthood. Although self-concept is usually stable from middle age to old age, it is not static. Life events experienced with aging (poor health, loss of income, loss of roles, isolation, relocation, and institutionalization) all serve to decrease the older adult's sense of control and may threaten self-esteem. However, it has been found that older people have compensatory mechanisms to offset some threats brought on by aging changes. A paradox exists in that age perception decreases with age. Older adults may think of age peers as old, according to social stereotypes attributed to older people. However, they may not perceive themselves as old and will refuse to respond to the suggestions of others that they are aging or need help or care. Another compensatory mechanism is that many older adults retain their middle-age self-concepts by thinking of themselves in their former roles. A retired farmer still may think of himself as a farmer, or a schoolteacher as a teacher. Maintaining a consistent sense of self, making decisions, and managing life are clearly important to well-being at this stage of life. Autonomy and dignity are essential elements to an older adult's positive self-esteem.

Concepts of Death and Dying

Death is more than a biologic event; it is also a social phenomenon. Rooted in religious, cultural, and societal context, people have viewed death with a variety of attitudes. It has been conceptualized as a life course or "career" with a social stage and a terminal stage. Depending on the individual's level of maturity, death can be viewed in a variety of ways, including prolonged sleep, not a part of one's personal future, punishment for one's actions in life, a welcome relief from illness, or the gateway to a spiritual life.

The social stage of death can begin early in life with an awareness of its limitations. However, this recognition is not real to most people until later in life. (Most theorists suggest that it occurs at midlife or later.) A heightened awareness of one's mortality is associated with the societal experiences of death, such as death of age peers, attainment of parent's age at death, close personal experiences or encounters, and personal deterioration in social activity, mobility, and physical and mental functioning. Awareness of one's mortality comes not only from within but from society by subtle, and some not so subtle, messages that the older person has less to contribute as compared with younger adults.

Anticipated losses associated with death include not only the cessation of relationships but also loss of the future and ability to complete projects and plans. Studies have shown that when asked to report anticipated important future events in life, older persons project a more limited time frame than younger persons project. They also are less likely to indicate that their activities would change if they knew they would die in 6 months.[23] Because of a heightened awareness of finiteness, older persons often engage in social remembrances with others. This talking about the past brings the past and present together as an integrated whole life. Success in legitimating life and death is associated with satisfaction and finding meaning in death.

The terminal stage of dying occurs with the news that one "is dying." People facing death confront the task of making sense of death itself. Factors such as culture, religion, race, and socioeconomic status are important in determining the meaning of death. Kubler-Ross[24] described five stages of coping with the dying process: denial, anger, bargaining, depression, and acceptance. These stages have not been empirically demonstrated to occur in this order or that all individuals react in this fashion. Because her sample represented mostly young and middle-aged adults, the results may not be generalizable to older persons. The assumption that people instinctively fear death and respond with anger and bargaining may be a more common reaction for younger rather than older adults.[25] Comparative data indicate a growing evidence that the fear of death diminishes with advancing age. Shneidman[26] found that some people regress back through the stages as described by Kubler-Ross. Older adult communal settings and hospice settings, where people are frequently reminded of death, facilitate the development of social conventions to deal routinely with death.

Mental Functioning

Intelligence. Traditionally it has been held that intelligence declines after age 30. However, longitudinal research indicates that intellectual abilities can be improved or at least sustained until late adulthood.[27] Much of the observed intellectual loss in persons as old as the eighties and nineties occurs primarily in unfamiliar, complex, or stressful situations. In the months before death an older adult's intellectual

Table 3-3 **Effects of Aging on Adult Mental Functioning**

Function	Effect of Aging
Fluid intelligence	Declines during middle age
Crystallized intelligence	Improves
Vocabulary and verbal reasoning	Improves
Spatial perception	Constant or improves
Synthesis of new information	Declines during middle age
Mental performance speed	Declines during middle age
Short-term recall memory	Declines during old age
Long-term recall memory	Constant

abilities may decrease sharply. This change is part of a complex phenomenon called terminal decline.

The patterns of change in adult intelligence vary with the specific mental abilities measured (Table 3-3). Cattell[28] conceptualized intelligence in two ways, each with a different origin: fluid intelligence and crystallized intelligence. Fluid intelligence consists of those abilities that are related to neurologic development and includes associative power, memory, figural relationships, and visual-motor flexibility. Because of degenerative neurologic changes, fluid intelligence may decline during middle age. Crystallized intelligence consists of those abilities that arise out of experience and the accumulation of learning and includes verbal comprehension, formal reasoning, and general information. Crystallized intelligence improves with age.[28]

Several environmental and individual variables such as education, social class, illness, personality, and motivation affect adult intelligence. Generally, individuals who have above-average intelligence as young adults, who have obtained more years of formal education, and who have continued to use intellectual processes demonstrate greater increases in intelligence throughout adulthood.[28] In addition, those who keep mentally active with a variety of thinking challenges and exercises (such as crossword puzzles and word games) have greater success in keeping degenerative changes from happening. Nurses must recognize that speed in mental functioning may be a major problem for older adults. Because of central nervous system decline and sensory deficits such as poor eyesight, some older persons have trouble with quick thinking and quick performance. Older people perform equally as well as younger people when time is not a factor. Because of this, any teaching or skills practice should be planned carefully to allow the older patient adequate time for comprehension and performance without the pressure of hurrying.

Memory. Although many middle adults fear becoming forgetful, no real decline in memory has been demonstrated until old age. Short-term memory deteriorates first. This refers to immediate recall that requires information retention for a few seconds to a few minutes. An example is remembering how to dial an unfamiliar phone number after having read it in the phone book. The decline in short-term memory may be related to neurotransmission interference or temporary storage integration problems. Because neurotransmission is slower, older adults become vulnerable to interference from other stimuli, which impede acquisition and storage of information. Thus information cannot be retrieved later because it was inadequately registered. This short-term memory problem can have significant effects on the learning process, since learning new material often requires speed in acquisition, comprehension, and registration.

Long-term memory seems highly resistant to aging. It is often noted that older adults can describe in minute detail past life events yet forget recent ones. This recall ability for past events may be attributed to the fact that once information is registered, people retain a sound memory for it. It is also likely that the memory for past events is firmly consolidated because the details have been previously recalled and rehearsed by the person.

Another memory difficulty in older adults is the inability to recall specifics after recognizing a person or a place. For example, a grandmother may recognize her grandchild but call him by another family member's name. In this case, she has placed the child in the family, recognizing the person, but cannot recall the name. This problem seems to be in the retrieval process rather than in registration of information.

In addition to aging changes, the memory of an older adult is affected by health status, drugs, education, amount of stimulation, motivation, and the meaningfulness of the material.

Sexuality

Sexuality is a broad concept that incorporates physiologic characteristics, attitudes, values, and behaviors related to gender perceptions. The task of developing a compatibility between gender identity and self-expression of sex-related roles is vital to self-concept integration during adulthood. This is an ongoing task that pervades practically all aspects of adult life, including mate selection, career choices, friendships, and all forms of self-expression.

Young Adulthood. For the young adult, gender identity and sexual relationships are primary concerns in achieving a sexual self-concept and sense of intimacy. Although intimacy transcends a sexual relationship to include affiliative sharing, for the sexually active young adult intimacy is usually established by commitment to a relationship that includes an expression of affection and physical sexuality. Sexual performance in a marriage relationship represents more than physical pleasure. It becomes an expression of caring and closeness, which helps the couple find satisfaction in sharing their work, play, childbearing, and child-rearing activities. It has been found that young couples who are satisfied with their sexual relationship are most often satisfied with their overall marriage, and vice versa. For some, a homosexual relationship provides a feeling of intimacy and comfort. Just as in heterosexual individuals, homosexual men and women vary greatly in their emotional and social adjustments.

Young adults are in the prime of physical and reproductive performance. Many of their biosocial concerns center around sexual activity, including cyclic changes in sexual arousal and orgasm, use and selection of contraceptives, sexual changes with pregnancy and postpartum, abortion, infertility, and sexually transmitted diseases. It has been found that the peak sexual drive and responsiveness in men occurs during the late teens and early twenties, whereas this peak occurs between the ages of 30 and 45 in women. However, most healthy adults maintain a strong sex drive beyond the age of 70.

Middle Adulthood. During the middle years, both men and women experience hormonal declines that produce physiologic changes that may affect sexual desire and responsiveness. However, more important than the physiologic changes are the psychologic expectations related to these changes. It has been found that menopausal and postmenopausal women have fewer fears and negative feelings about the effects of menopause on their sexuality than young adult women. Rather than experiencing a decline in sexual capacity, postmenopausal women frequently experience an increased libido and greater enjoyment. With the male climacteric, the decline in testosterone may result in a decreased libido and a slower sexual arousal and climax, but these changes do not necessarily lessen the pleasure of sexual intercourse.

Factors probably more important than hormonal changes that negatively affect sexual activity in the middle years include monotony in a repetitious sexual pattern, boredom with a relationship, career and economic preoccupation, mental and physical fatigue, excessive eating or drinking, and fear of sexual failure. Becoming a victim to the myth that a youthful body is equated with sexual desirability and potency also negatively affects sexual activity. Middle-aged adults are at risk for the potential onset of chronic illnesses that may affect libido and performance, and they may be taking a variety of prescribed drugs that can reduce sexual interest and responsiveness.

Sexual activity continues to be a very important part of middle adult life. Satisfaction with sexual life in the middle years is not as related to frequency of intercourse as to vitality in the relationship and enjoyment derived from all sexual experiences in younger years.

Older Adulthood. Although our society attributes sexlessness to the older adult, people are sexual beings throughout their lives. Most studies attest to continued sexual activity well into the last decades of life for men and women who have been sexually active as young and middle adults. Physical changes in the sexual organs should not be considered as biologic limitations of sexual activity, nor should they reduce the satisfaction experienced by sexual partners. The most important criteria for remaining sexually active in old age are a receptive partner, reasonable physical health, and a positive attitude about sexual activity.

Because society has been slow to recognize the sexual needs of older adults and most older adults have been socialized not to talk about sex, identifying and intervening in sex-related problems is difficult for caregivers. It has been suggested that sex education programs be developed for older adults to inform them of normal changes and to help them cope with unmet sexual needs and with social and familial attitudes about continued sexual activity.

Intimacy. In a broad context, intimacy incorporates the concept of attachment or seeking a relationship in which an individual can maintain contact or proximity to the object of attachment. Throughout life, touch plays an important role in receiving and expressing intimacy. However, as hearing and sight decline with age, reaching out to touch becomes an even more important way to make intimate physical contact (Fig. 3-5). Elderly people often attempt to touch and be touched by others to experience a sense of physical closeness. The response to their touch communicates a message of acceptance or nonacceptance that may never have been expressed verbally.

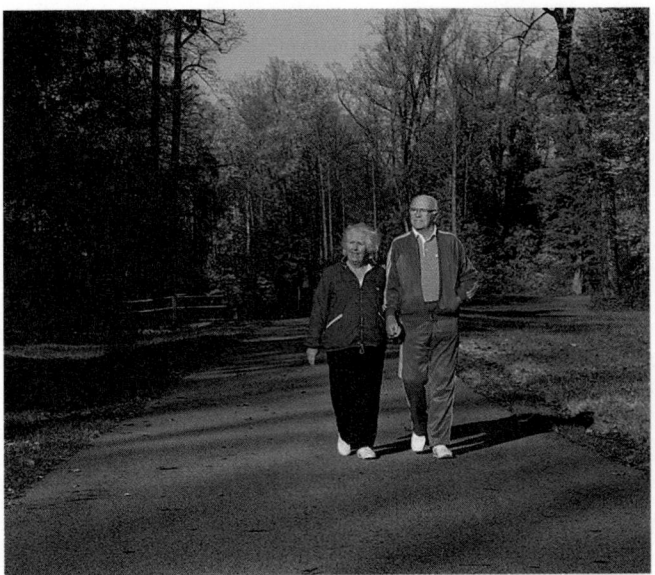

Fig. 3-5 Intimacy and physical touch are important to the older adult.

The need for expressing physical intimacy in behaviors having sexual connotations is often disregarded for older adults. Although these expressions are accepted as normal in younger adults, they may be viewed with disdain and disapproval or as an amusing and childish behavior when expressed by older people. This disregard is seen in some institutional structures and policies. Many nursing homes provide little opportunity for expression of sexual needs. Private rooms and locked doors often are neither provided nor respected. Older adult couples may be segregated and placed on separate men's and women's units or, if in the same room, may have single beds. This may explain why an older person, who has for years shared a bed with a spouse, becomes disoriented at night and wanders around or gets into bed with someone else.

SOCIAL PROCESSES IN ADULTHOOD

Adulthood is lived out in a social context with major developmental tasks being determined by the interaction of individuals with their social systems. Adult social concerns primarily involve the family, work and leisure, and community responsibilities.

Family and Adult Development

Throughout life the family is the major socializing institution for its members. A global survey of people representing 70 nations found that family life is overwhelmingly the greatest source of satisfaction and happiness for most people.[29] The family is a focal source for adults in meeting their needs for emotional security, belonging, love, companionship, esteem, and approval from others. The process of family development reflects the developmental changes occurring in the adult members. (See Table 3-4 for a summary of family tasks during adulthood.)

Young Adulthood. Emancipation from the family of origin is the first family task of young adulthood. This

Table 3-4 **Family Tasks in Adult Development**

Young Adulthood	Middle Adulthood	Older Adulthood
Emancipating from family of origin Establishing interdependent adult relationship with parents Selecting mate and adjusting to intimate relationship Adapting family system to demands of childbearing Finding balance to family, work, and social demands	Assisting teenage children to become responsible adults Restructuring relationship with spouse as children leave home Restructuring relationship with aging parents Adjusting to death of parents Defining roles and responsibilities of grandparent	Establishing satisfactory living arrangements with limited income Restructuring family roles and responsibilities after retirement Adapting living arrangements to meet problems caused by physical decline Adjusting to death of spouse

usually occurs as a gradual process that includes physical, economic, and emotional independence from parents. However, emancipation is not the end of a relationship with the family but rather the first step in establishing an interdependent adult relationship between young adults and their parents. Often concurrent with emancipation from the family of origin, the young adult establishes a new family system in which roles, relationships, and expectations are being determined. This usually includes adjusting to an intimate relationship and adapting to the predictable crises of childbearing. Stress is frequently high in the emerging young adult family because of changing relationships and support structures. Also, the work trajectories for both partners are often launched, and new outside demands are placed on adult family members. The stress of such demands is reflected in the fact that the highest divorce rate occurs during the first 3 to 5 years of marriage for young adults under the age of 30.

Middle Adulthood. Middle adults find themselves caught in the "family sandwich" between the needs of their children and those of their aging parents. Family life can be stressful because it is a complex chore to concurrently work through a midlife identity transition, the identity confusion of teenagers, and the redefinition of family roles and relationships in both the families of origin and marriage and parenthood.

Disenchantment with the marital relationship is frequently experienced by middle-aged adults. Married couples are least satisfied with each other when they are between the ages of 40 and 50. There are multiple contributing factors to this dissatisfaction, including the preoccupation or confusion about occupational goals and the financial and emotional strain of having adolescent children. Although the divorce rate is not as high during middle adulthood as during early adulthood, it does increase again during the years shortly after children leave home.

Middle-aged couples who recommit themselves to their spouses and a continuing marriage find that marital satisfaction frequently hits a new high. Although much discussion has been heard about the crisis of the "empty nest," many middle-aged men and women experience a new sense of self and unity as a couple after the children leave home. They again define their relationship as lovers and companions, rather than as parents.

During middle age, adults often come to appreciate their parents and understand the problems of old people in a new way. When the aging parent is in good health and basically self-reliant, the parent-child relationship is usually characterized by

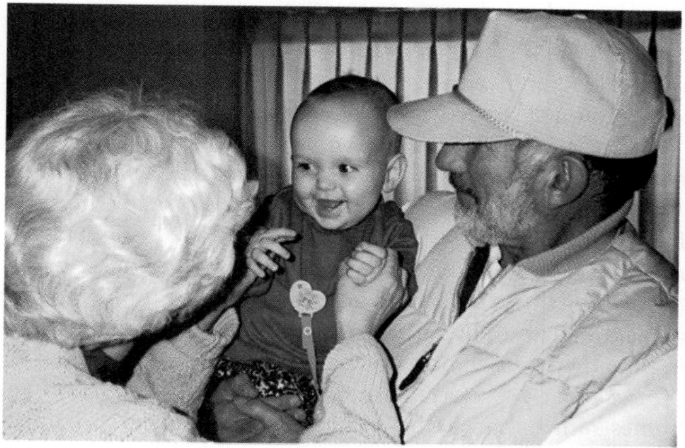

Fig. 3-6 The active grandparent plays a positive role in the lives of the child and the grandchild.

a friendship that is satisfactory to both. If aging parents are confronted with problems such as inadequate finances, ill health, or death of a spouse that make it impossible for them to remain independent, the parent-child relationship and roles may be restructured. A difficult but sometimes necessary role reversal occurs when a middle-aged adult must become the "parent" to his or her parent. This requires giving up feelings of dependency on the parent and often assuming an uncomfortable authority role, which the older adult parent may find difficult to relinquish. The manner in which the middle-aged adult responds to the parent's dependency needs will be determined by the previous relationship, available resources, and the other responsibilities of the middle-aged adult. Eventually, many middle-aged adults must deal with their feelings about the death of parents. Although little has been done to study the family changes at this time, becoming a member of the family's oldest generation because of the death of parents is an important phase in family life.

Grandparenting. Many adults become grandparents during middle adulthood (Fig. 3-6). This new social role may have a positive or negative impact on the grandparent's self-esteem. To some it is met with excitement and anticipation; for others it represents "growing old," which conflicts with how the grandparent wants to feel. Birth of children to teenagers also may spark unwelcome early transitions to grandparenthood. Because teenage parents are often unwilling or unable to

Table 3-5 **Living Arrangements for Persons More Than 65 Years of Age (1995)**

	Percentage of Men	Percentage of Women
Living in household	99.7	99.8
Living alone	16.3	41.8
Spouse present	73.8	39.8
Living with someone else	9.6	18.0
Not in household (e.g., institutions)	0.3	0.2

From US Bureau of Census, Current Population Reports: *Statistical abstract of the United States,* 1995, Washington, DC.

assume the responsibilities of parenthood, many grandparents are becoming the primary caregivers to their young grandchildren. This family arrangement can cause significant physical and emotional stress to grandparents in middle adulthood.

Older Adulthood. The onset of this final period in family life is generally considered to be marked by retirement and poses new and unique developmental tasks for the aging family. The first task is to establish satisfactory living arrangements within a limited income, considering the role changes brought on by retirement and the physical limitations of aging. In terms of living arrangements, most older adults live in their own households[30] (Table 3-5). In a recent survey, 87% of the elderly preferred independent living in their own homes rather than living with children.[30] However, contact with children is frequent; 73% of older adults have at least one child living less than 30 minutes away, and 77% have contact with a child each week.[30] For older adults who are in relatively good health and have an adequate income, living in their own homes rather than with family members allows them to maintain a sense of privacy, competency, and independence.

Being able to adjust family responsibilities and routines becomes an important part of the adaptation a couple must make following retirement. Schedules and activities are readjusted, and a retiree will frequently turn to family members to meet self-esteem needs that were previously met by the referent work group.

Loss of spouse. The loss of a spouse is a major crisis at any stage in life. Currently women are more likely than men to experience the loss of a spouse through death. The reaction to a spouse's death may vary, depending on the compatibility of the relationship; circumstances of the death; the available support systems, including family and religious beliefs; the physiologic independence of the survivor; and the adequacy of financial resources. Although the degree of marital happiness varies for older adults, couples who have had a long marriage have generally established an interdependent symbiotic relationship that gives them a great deal of pleasure during their later years.

Developing a new social identity and adjusting living arrangements are major tasks of adjusting to loss of a spouse. For many, this is a time when they are socially isolated unless they actively seek out activities they can participate in without a spouse. Some older adults choose to move in with family members; others move to smaller apartments, condominiums, or a community for older adults. In any case, relocation may be an additional trauma.

Remarriage becomes an alternative to living alone or to living with children or friends. Most older adults remarry for companionship, and although there is the danger of idealizing the deceased mate and making unrealistic comparisons with the new spouse, most of these remarriages are happy.

PHYSIOLOGIC PROCESSES IN ADULTHOOD

Physiologic Changes During Adulthood

The young adult body is generally at its peak of health and performance. Physical changes associated with aging are just beginning at this time. Extrinsic factors such as accidents and physical stressors such as lack of sleep and substance abuse are the most common sources of disabling biophysical problems in young adults.

Structural and functional body changes that were unnoticed in young adulthood may begin to be apparent during middle age. The rate and expression of physiologic aging changes are highly individual. Frequently, changes in physical appearance such as dry skin, wrinkles, thinning and graying hair, and added inches on the waist and hips are the first noticeable signs of aging. Sometime during the middle years, most adults notice that muscle strength and agility are declining, but on a day-to-day basis, most people make small compensations that minimize the effects of these changes. Because age-related changes are due to aging rather than a pathologic process, they begin insidiously in young adulthood and become more apparent in middle adulthood.

Although many older people remain vigorous beyond the age of 80, the general decline in all systems and reduction of normally functioning cells caused by aging decrease the older person's overall ability to withstand and adapt to physical or emotional stress. When one system is placed under stress, there is a domino effect; without the ability to compensate, all systems may collapse. Thus maintaining physical and emotional integrity in the older person can be precarious. However, continued physical exercise, balanced nutrition, and active mental pursuits result in many positive outcomes (Fig. 3-7). For a more complete discussion of physiologic changes related to the aging process, see Table 4-1.

Considerations for Health Promotion

Young Adulthood. Although the young adult years are a time of generally good physical and emotional health, the young adult lifestyle may have potential health hazards. Accidents, human immunodeficiency virus (HIV) infection, acquired immunodeficiency syndrome (AIDS), sexually transmitted disease (STD), substance abuse, sleep deprivation, inactivity, obesity, exposure to environmental and occupational hazards, and stress-related illnesses such as ulcers, depression, and suicide are important health problems during this time of life. Chronic illnesses such as hypertension, coronary artery disease, and diabetes may have their onset in young adulthood without being known to the young adult but may become serious health problems later in life.

Middle Adulthood. For the individual during the middle adult years, lifestyle factors are assessed for ones that are detrimental to health. With a decline in strength and stamina, daily exercise is essential; however, sporadic weekend exercise or competitive physical overexertion can lead to injury. Reducing caloric intake is often necessary to prevent weight gain. This may be particularly difficult for middle-

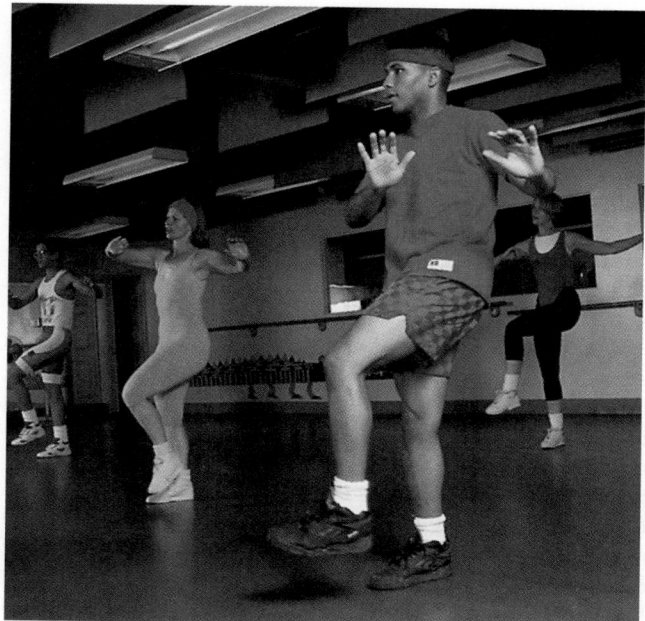

Fig. 3-7 Both young and middle-aged adults are subject to injuries associated with sporadic activity.

aged adults whose social and business lifestyles encourage overindulgence at dinners and parties. Life pressures frequently mount during middle age, and a variety of substances may be used and overconsumed to cope, including cigarettes, alcohol, food, and tranquilizers (Fig. 3-8). Rather than relying on these substances, the individual may need assistance to deal with the sources of stress.

Middle-aged adults should be encouraged to seek routine medical and dental examinations directed toward disease prevention and early treatment of problems. *Healthy People 2000* recommends annual dental and biannual physical examinations for healthy middle-aged adults.[31] The American Cancer Society recommends that all women who are or have been sexually active or have reached the age of 18 should have an annual Pap smear and pelvic examination. After three consecutive satisfactory normal examinations, the Pap smear may be performed less frequently at the discretion of the physician. For early detection of breast cancer the American Cancer Society recommends monthly breast self-examination, a baseline mammogram between 40 and 49 years of age, and then every 1 to 2 years until age 49. After the age of 50, mammography is recommended along with a breast examination by a health care provider. Nurses have a fundamental role in health promotion by educating and promoting self-care responsibility among middle-aged adults.

Although many middle-aged adults feel that they are in the prime of life, a rising incidence of chronic illnesses is associated with middle age. Some major health concerns are cardiovascular disease, cancer, liver cirrhosis, diabetes, and sexual dysfunctions.

Older Adulthood. An estimated 86% of the population over age 65 have one or more chronic conditions with varying degrees of disability.[32] The health problems of older people reflect past health and lifestyle influences. The major problems include chronic or recurrent conditions from earlier adult stages, chronic brain syndrome, degenerative bone and joint diseases, malnutrition, acute and chronic respiratory diseases, renal diseases, drug-induced problems, and mental disorders.

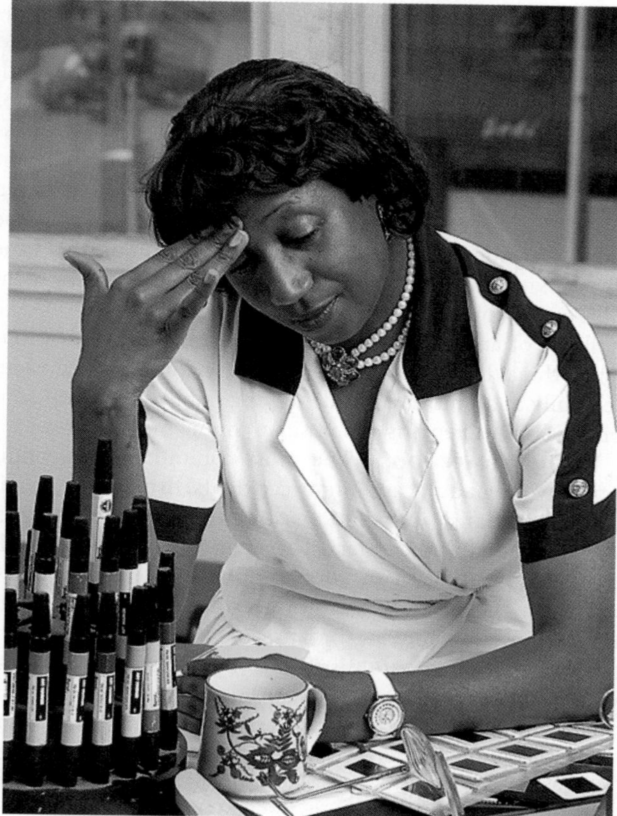

Fig. 3-8 The middle-aged woman may experience the same work-related pressures as a man because of economic concerns and increased life choices.

The health of older adults is influenced not only by disease processes but also by the process of aging. Although the aging process cannot be stopped, the effects can be reduced by good health habits, including proper nutrition, activity and rest, safety, and correct drug usage.

Stress of Illness During Adulthood

Illness is a situational crisis that can disrupt adult life at any time. The extent of the disruption may vary from a minor annoyance to a complete lifestyle change. The significance that "being ill" holds for an individual is determined by multiple variables: the type of illness and its perceived threat, the personality type, socioeconomic resources, family or significant other support, and possible restrictions on current lifestyle or structure.

Based on Levinson's model, the impact of illness will differ depending on whether the individual is in a transitional or stable period of development. During stable periods when life is generally going smoothly, people have more energy to cope with illness. In contrast, with the changes being made in overall life structure during transitional periods, there is less energy to cope with illness, and illness and its potential effects add new variables to consider in the restructuring process. Because transitional stages represent a time of uncertainty, role changes, and anxiety, the individual is also more vulnerable to becoming ill. Conversely, the stable periods, which are typically times of commitment, confidence, and success, foster health. The presence of illness, either personal illness or illness in a significant other, can also trigger movement from a stable period into a transitional stage. This may be characteristically seen in the midlife transition during which an illness can initiate the "time left" thinking that is fundamental to the profound reassessment of life at this time.

Illness of an individual member may also pose a developmental threat to the family's integrity. The nurse must consider the family as a unit of care, identifying family needs and supporting family strengths and positive coping mechanisms.

Young Adulthood. The most common acute conditions in young adults are minor accidents, drug abuse, respiratory infections, influenza, gastroenteritis, urinary tract infections, and minor surgery. These conditions may be developmentally significant to young adults for several reasons. First, with the hectic schedules of young adults, an acute minor illness is annoying because of the disruption in life activities. With an acute disability, young adults may know that the effects are short term; however, they may be impatient with the healing process and concerned that long-term problems will result. Family rearrangements can be stressful, especially when hospitalization is required. Hospitalization is also frustrating because of forced dependency and limitations posed by treatment regimens. Maintaining control is important for young adults, so they need to be informed and involved with decisions about care. Young adults are generally strongly motivated toward recuperation to resume life activities.

Although chronic conditions are not common in young adulthood, they can occur. Disabilities caused by accidents, multiple sclerosis, rheumatoid arthritis, AIDS, and cancer are the common long-term conditions faced by young adults. Chronic illness and disability in young adulthood strike at the very core of developmental tasks and can result in delayed development. With the onset of chronic illness or disability, the threat to the young adult's independence may precipitate multiple crises when personal, family, and career goals need to change. The nurse must identify and direct nursing intervention toward potential developmental problems in the areas of identity reorganization; establishment of independence; and reorganization of intimate relationships, family structure, and launching of a chosen career.

Middle Adulthood. The characteristics of acute illness are much the same in middle adulthood as in young adulthood. However, recuperative power in middle adulthood slows. Injuries and acute conditions that were rapidly resolved in young adulthood may have a longer recovery period and are more likely to become chronic problems.

Chronic conditions during middle age interfere with the individual's sense of generativity. This task requires outward-directed concerns and activities. Long-term recurrent illness often forces an inferiority that can lead to physical and psychologic self-absorption. When middle-aged adults develop a chronic illness or disability, they may feel unable to influence their destiny, let alone influence and provide for others. The impact on generativity includes changes in family, job, and community involvement.

With the onset of chronic illness in middle age, established family roles are often forced to change. The psychologic trauma of these role changes is caused by the strong emotional component to roles, which is based on the value placed on a role as a part of self-identity and the vested power the role holds. The nurse should be perceptive to the potential for family dysfunction and should serve as a resource to the entire family, helping them seek counseling and therapy as necessary.

Career or occupational orientation may need to change as a result of chronic illness. This is particularly stressful during the middle years because it confounds the career timing and readjustment of goals that occur with the midlife occupational crisis. When the illness is severely disruptive, the person may need to change occupations or jobs or may need to face an early forced retirement. Both these options may be a source of great stress and a threat to generativity because of occupational regression or being denied the gratification that comes from closing a career with the feeling of a job well done.

Older Adulthood. The distinction between acute and chronic illness in older adults is less precise, since acute conditions may become chronic or may be an exacerbation of chronic problems. However, acute problems such as gastroenteritis, pneumonia, tumors, and noncomplicated accidental injuries can have a short course with complete recovery. The difficulties such illnesses pose for older adults are that they add stress to a body system with a decreased physiologic and psychologic ability to compensate for stress. The ability to perform self-care is an important problem for older adults when an acute illness occurs (Fig. 3-9). If the person lives alone or with a frail spouse or housemate and does not have adequate support systems, an acute illness can precipitate a life disorganization that results in a move from the home and toward dependency.

When an older adult is hospitalized, many situations occur that threaten ego integrity and cause the hospitalization to be a very disrupting experience. New situations and environments often normally produce anxiety, and when combined with the stress of being sick, the unfamiliar becomes confusing. When giving care, the nurse should carefully orient and reorient the older adult to the hospital environment. Allowing the older adult patient to keep personal belongings within reach and visible will also help maintain a sense of orientation, as well as reduce the depersonalized feeling that accompanies hospitalization. Nursing care should be paced to allow older adult patients an opportunity to participate without hurrying so that they can maintain control and have time to understand and cooperate with what is being done.

Family situations are an important concern in caring for the hospitalized older adult. The nurse must recognize when role reversals are occurring between an older parent and the adult children. Children who have problems with this reversal may respond by withdrawing or by becoming overprotective and smothering. In either case, the parent's self-worth is threatened. The nurse should also be perceptive to other family concerns of the hospitalized older adult, such as worry over a spouse being

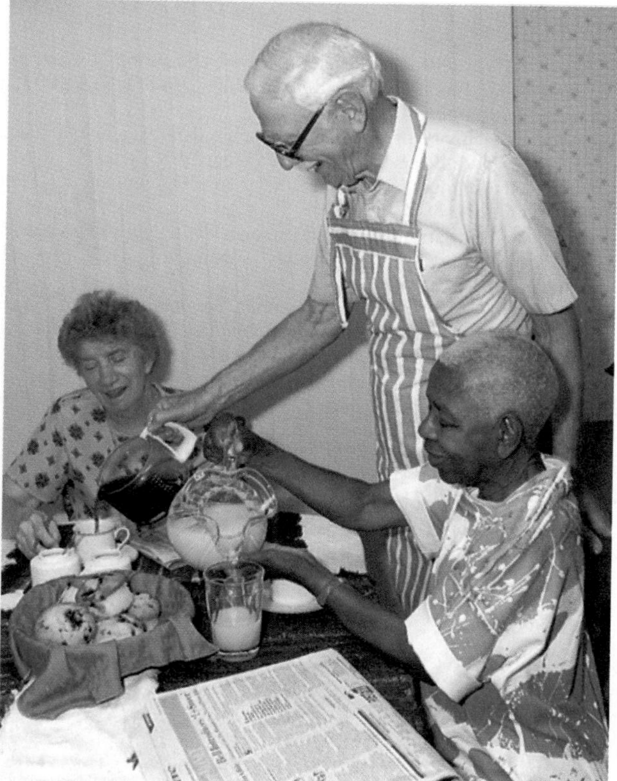

Fig. 3-9 Good friends and pleasant activities help fill the lives of active older adults.

home alone or concern for pets and plants or household maintenance if the patient lives alone.

Chronic conditions are common health problems that older adults can learn to manage. Part of this process includes incorporating support devices such as canes, wheelchairs, dentures, and hearing aids into a healthy self-esteem. Chronic conditions also have social implications if the illness imposes an involuntary disengagement process. When this occurs, transcending the physical problems is increasingly difficult. The social isolation that is experienced may reduce self-esteem and the physical and emotional strength needed to cope with the stresses of disease and aging.

REVIEW QUESTIONS

The number of the question corresponds to the same-numbered objective at the beginning of the chapter.

1. Which description of his lifestyle by an older adult patient is most characteristic of the identity continuity theory of psychosocial aging?
   a. "I think it is important to frequently visit with my friends and family."
   b. "After years of struggle I am happy to sit in my rocking chair and watch the world go by."
   c. "I go to the senior center every day and do what volunteer work I can manage physically."
   d. "Although I am retired, I get up every day and follow the same routine I have all my life."
2. A 45-year-old patient newly diagnosed with diabetes responds by telling the nurse that she must reevaluate what things in life are most important to her and focus her activities around these priorities. This response is most consistent with
   a. Peck's middle-age task of valuing wisdom versus physical power.
   b. the adjustment to declining health reflective of Havighurst's developmental tasks.
   c. a sense of wholeness and purpose to life described by Erikson's sense of ego integrity.
   d. Levinson's midlife transition, which involves the changing of life structures toward identified values.
3. In teaching an older adult patient how to modify her diet to reduce fat and sodium intake, the nurse recognizes that the intellectual ability necessary for this type of learning
   a. declines during middle age.
   b. continues to improve with aging.
   c. is impaired by long-term memory loss.
   d. is at its highest peak during young adulthood.
4. The most likely cause of stress in a typical young adult family is
   a. role reversal in caring for aging parents.
   b. identity confusion of the adult family members.
   c. health problems that threaten the career timetable.
   d. multiplicity of changing relationships and social demands.
5. Health maintenance during middle adulthood should be directed toward
   a. preventing illnesses that are due to lifestyle.
   b. halting the physiologic aging changes.
   c. preparing for the inevitable physical decline.
   d. maintaining stamina and strength at a young adult level.
6. For the elderly adult, hospitalization can be a disrupting experience resulting in confusion because
   a. hospitalization forces dependency and self-absorption.
   b. poor ego integrity is characteristic of this age-group.
   c. unfamiliar, stressful surroundings can cause loss of control.
   d. adult children assume parenting roles that threaten self-esteem of the patient.

References

1. Ebersole P, Hess P: *Toward healthy aging,* ed 5, St Louis, 1998, Mosby.
2. Hampton J, Craven R, Heitkemper M: *The biology of human aging,* ed 2, Chicago, 1997, Wm C Brown.
3. Birren JE, Bengston V: *Emergent theories of aging,* New York, 1988, Springer.
4. Harman D: Aging: a theory based on free radical and radiation chemistry, *J Gerontol* 11:298, 1956.
5. Byers T, Perry G: Dietary carotenes, vitamin C, and vitamin E as protective antioxidants in human cancers, *Annu Rev Nutr* 12:139, 1992.
6. Hayflick L: *How and why we age,* New York, 1994, Ballantine Books.
7. Cristofalo VJ: An overview of the theories of biological aging. In Birren JE, Bengston VL, editors: *Emergent theories of aging,* New York, 1988, Springer.
8. Shay JW: Telomerase in human development and cancer, *J Cell Phys* 173:266, 1997.
9. Schlossberg NK: *Counseling adults in transition,* New York, 1984, Springer.
10. Erikson EH: *Childhood and society,* ed 2, New York, 1963, Norton.
11. Loevinger J: *Ego development: conceptions and theories,* San Francisco, 1976, Jossey-Bass.
12. Vaillant GE: *Adaptation to life,* Boston, 1984, Little, Brown.
13. Gould R: *Transformations: growth and change in adult life,* New York, 1978, Simon & Schuster.
14. Levinson DH and others: *The season's of a man's life,* New York, 1978, Knopf.
15. Kohlberg L: Continuities in childhood and adult moral development. In Baltes P, Schaie K, editors: *Life-span developmental psychology: personality and socialization,* New York, 1973, Academic Press.

16. Fowler J: *Stages of faith: the psychology of human development and the quest for meaning,* New York, 1981, Harper & Row.
17. Peck TA: Women's self-definition in adulthood: from a different model, *Psychology of Women Quarterly* 10:274, 1986.
18. Havighurst RJ: *Developmental tasks and education,* ed 3, New York, 1972, McKay.
19. Lowenthal MF, Thurnher M, Chiriboga D: *Four stages of life: a comparative study of men and women facing transitions,* San Francisco, 1975, Jossey-Bass.
20. Neugarten B: Adaptation and the life cycle, *Counseling Psychologist* 6:16, 1976.
21. Courtenay B: Are psychological models of adult development still important? *Adult Education Quarterly* 44:145, 1994.
22. Gilligan C: *In a different voice: psychological theory and women's development,* Cambridge, Mass, 1982, Harvard University Press.
23. Kart CS, Metress ES: Death and dying. In Kart CS, editor: *The realities of aging: an introduction to gerontology,* ed 3, Boston, 1990, Allyn & Bacon.
24. Kubler-Ross E: *On death and dying,* New York, 1969, Macmillan.
25. Marshall V, Levy J: Aging and dying. In Binstock RH, George LK, editors: *Handbook of aging and the social sciences,* ed 3, San Diego, 1990, Academic Press.
26. Shneidman E: *Death: current perspectives,* ed 3, Mountain View, Calif, 1976, Mayfield.
27. Schaie KW: Intellectual development in adulthood. In Birren J, Schaie KW, editors: *Handbook of the psychology of aging,* ed 3, San Diego, 1990, Academic Press.
28. Cattell RB: Theory of fluid and crystallized intelligence: a critical approach, *Journal of Educational Psychology* 54:1, 1986.
29. Gallup GH: Human needs and satisfaction: a global survey, *Public Opinion Quarterly* 40:459, 1976.
30. American Association of Retired Persons: *Home equity conversion for the elderly: an analysis for lenders,* Washington, DC, 1989, The Association.
31. US Department of Health and Human Services, Office of Disease Prevention and Health Promotion: *Healthy People 2000: national health promotion and disease promotion objectives,* pub no 017-001-00473, Washington, DC, 1990, US Government Printing Office.
32. Rybash JM, Roodin PA, Hoyer WJ: *Adult development and aging,* ed 3, Chicago, 1995, Brown & Benchmark.

Resources

Resources for this chapter are listed after Chapter 4 on p. 64.

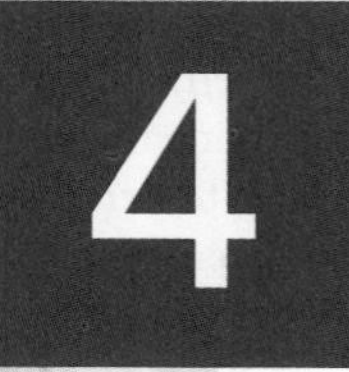

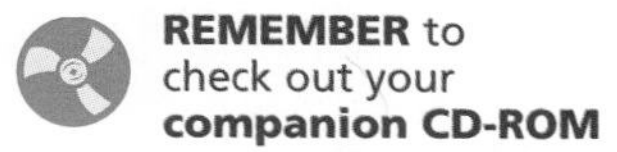

4 Gerontologic Considerations

Tana Durnbaugh

www.mosby.com/MERLIN/medsurg_lewis

LEARNING OBJECTIVES

1. Describe the impact of older adults on the health care system.
2. Describe the effects of ageism on care of older adults.
3. Describe clinical manifestations related to specific age-related physiologic changes.
4. Describe the nursing interventions and needs of special populations of older adults.
5. Identify the effects of culture on aging.
6. Identify differences in health status and disease manifestation between older and younger adults.
7. Identify the role of the nurse in health screening and promotion and disease prevention for older adults.
8. Describe the tasks of chronically ill older adults and the nursing interventions needed to assist them in the accomplishment of these tasks.
9. Describe common problems of older adults related to hospitalization and acute illness and the role of the nurse in assisting them with selected care problems.
10. Describe social support alternatives for older adults.
11. Identify care alternatives to meet patient-specific needs of older adults.
12. Identify the legal and ethical issues related to older adults.

Care of older adults is based on the specialty body of knowledge of gerontologic nursing. The nurse approaches the patient with a whole-person (physical, psychologic, socioeconomic) perspective. This chapter presents specific information about older adults that will assist the nurse in providing care to groups of individuals. Additional information about developmental issues related to the older adult is discussed in Chapter 3. Gerontologic considerations present challenges to nurses that require skilled assessment and creative adaptations of nursing interventions.

In the last two decades the older adult population (those 65 years of age and older) has grown twice as fast as the rest of the population. This growth is expected to continue into the next century (Fig. 4-1). Several factors have led to this increase. The large post–World War II immigrant population has now grown older. Common diseases of the early 1900s, such as influenza and diarrhea, that killed many older adults are now less common, and people are living longer.

People born today have a life expectancy 26 years longer than those born in 1900. The U.S. Census Bureau predicts life expectancy to continue to increase for both men and women. The life expectancy of women in the United States is 79.6 years, and for men it is 72.7 years. For Canadian women it is 78 years, and for Canadian men it is 71 years. In both the United States and Canada, 12% of the Caucasian population is 65 years of age and older. In the United States, only 8% of African-Americans and 3.5% of all Hispanic-Americans are older than 65.[1,2]

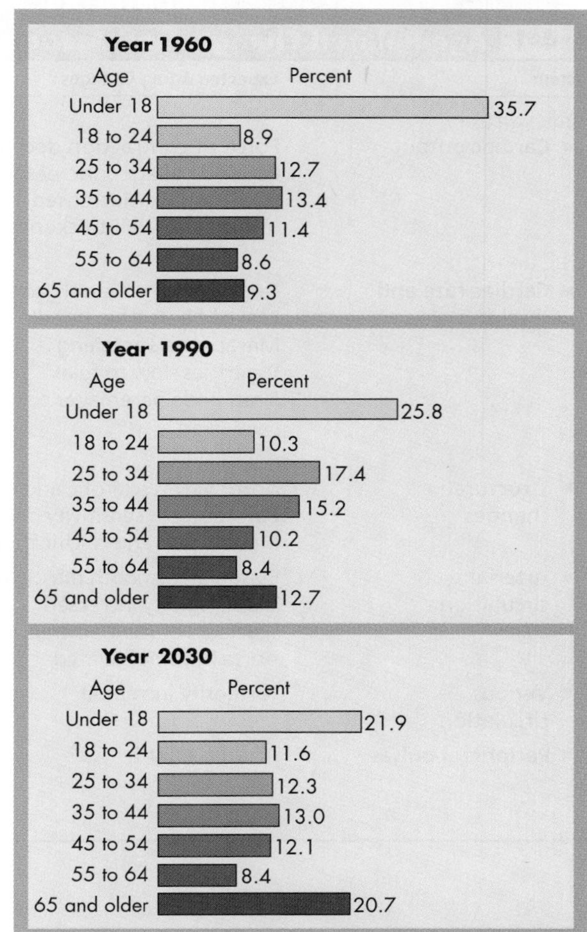

Fig. 4-1 Age distribution of total U.S. population.

Reviewed by Martha A. Melcher, RN, GNP, Advanced Registered Nurse Practitioner, Virginia Mason Medical Center, Port Angeles, Wash.

The most rapidly increasing population age group is composed of those persons 85 years of age and older. The terms *young-old* (55 to 75 years of age) and *old-old* (75 years of age and older) were introduced in 1978.[3] These two groups represent chronologic ranges that often present different characteristics and needs. The term *frail elderly* has been suggested to represent those 75 years of age and older with a variety of ongoing and accumulating health concerns.[4]

ATTITUDES TOWARD AGING

Who is old? The answer to this question often depends on the age and attitude of the respondent. It is important that the nurse maintains the position that aging is normal and is not related to disease. Age is a date in time and is influenced by many factors, including emotional and physical health, developmental stage, socioeconomic status, culture, and ethnicity.

As people age, they are exposed to more and different life experiences. The accumulation of these differences makes older adults more diverse than any other age-group.[5] As the nurse assesses the older adult, it is important to consider this diversity. The nurse should assess the patient for perceptions of age. Older adults with poor health report a higher perceived age and lower sense of psychologic well-being.[6] Age is important, but it may not be the most relevant data for determining appropriate care of an individual patient.

Myths and stereotypes about aging, found throughout society, are supported by media reports of needy, problematic older adults. Myths and stereotypes regarding aging provide the basis of commonly held misconceptions that may lead to errors in assessments and unnecessary limitations to interventions. For example, if the nurse thinks all old people are rigid, new ideas will not be presented to the patient.

Ageism is a negative attitude based on age. It leads to discrimination in the care given to the older adult. The nurse who demonstrates negative attitudes may fear his or her own aging process or be misinformed about aging and the health care needs of the older adult. The nurse may benefit from gaining knowledge about normal aging; increasing contact with the healthy, independent older adult; and participating in simulation life experiences of the older adult.

AGE-RELATED PHYSIOLOGIC CHANGES

Age-related changes affect every body system. These changes are normal and occur as people age. However, the age at which specific changes become evident differs from person to person and within the same person. For instance, a person may have gray hair at age 45 but relatively unwrinkled skin at age 80. The nurse should assess for these age-related changes. Table 4-1 presents gerontologic differences in assessment based on age-related changes and associated clinical manifestations.

GERONTOLOGIC DIFFERENCES IN ASSESSMENT

Table 4-1 Age-Related Changes and Associated Clinical Manfestations

System	Expected Aging Changes	Clinical Manifestations
Cardiovascular		
▪ Cardiac output	Force of contraction decreased Fat and collagen increased Heart muscle decreased Ventricular wall thickened	Myocardial oxygen demand increased Stroke volume and CO decreased Fatigue, shortness of breath, tachycardia occur Blood flow to vital organs and periphery decreased
▪ Cardiac rate and rhythm	Dependence on atrial contraction increased Loss of fibers from bundle of His Mitral valve stretching Ventricles slow to relax Sinus node pacemaker cells decreased	HR slow to increase with stress Decrease in maximum HR (e.g., 80-year-old person, 120 bpm; 20-year-old person, 200 bpm) Possible AV block Resting HR constant Recovery time from tachycardia prolonged Premature beats increased
▪ Structural changes	Aortic valves sclerotic and calcified Baroreceptor sensitivity decreased Mild fibrosis and calcification of valves	Diastolic murmur present in 50% of older patients Heart position landmarks change
▪ Arterial circulation	Elastin and smooth muscle reduced Vessel rigidity increased Vascular resistance increased Aorta becomes dilated	Modest increase in systolic BP (e.g., 160/90) Rigid arteries contribute to coronary artery and peripheral vascular disease
▪ Venous circulation	Tortuosity increased	Inflamed, painful, or cordlike varicosities
▪ Peripheral pulses	Arteries rigid	Pulses weaker but equal Circulation slowed to periphery Cold feet and hands

Continued

GERONTOLOGIC DIFFERENCES IN ASSESSMENT

Table 4-1 Age-Related Changes and Associated Clinical Manfestations—cont'd

System	Expected Aging Changes	Clinical Manifestations
Respiratory		
▪ Structures	Cartilage degeneration Vertebrae rigid Strength of muscles decreased Respiratory muscles atrophy Thoracic wall increased ridigity Ciliary action decreased	Kyphosis Anterior-posterior diameter increased Use of accessory muscles decreased Chest rigid and barrel-shaped Respiratory excursion decreased Cough and deep breathing diminished
▪ Change in ventilation and perfusion	Pulmonary vascular bed decreased Alveoli decreased Thickened alveolar walls Elastic recoil decreased	Lung compliance decreased Total lung volume not changed Vital capacity decreased Residual lung volume increased Mucus thickens PaO_2 and oxygen saturation decreased Hyperresonance
▪ Ventilation control	Response to hypoxia and hypercarbia decreased	Ability to maintain acid-base balance decreased Respiratory rate 12-24/min
Integumentary		
▪ Skin	Collagen and subcutaneous fat decreased Sweat glands decreased Epidermal cell turnover slowed Skin tissue fluid decreased Capillary fragility increased Pigment cells decreased Sebaceous gland activity decreased Sensory receptors decreased Thresholds for touch, vibration, heat, pain increased	Skin less elastic Wrinkles and folds increased Extremity fat lost; fat on trunk increased Skin heals slowly Skin dry Skin tears and bruises easily Skin color uneven Multiple senile lentigines Normal skin lesions increased Ability to respond to heat and cold decreased Ability to feel light touch decreased Cutaneous pain sensitivity declines
▪ Hair	Melanin decreased Germ center and hair follicle decreased	Gray or white hair Hair quantity decreased and thinner Scalp, pubic, axillary hair decreased Facial hair on men decreased Facial hair on women increased
▪ Nails	Blood supply to nail bed decreased Longitudinal striations increased	Growth slowed Nails thickened and brittle Split easily Potential for fungal infection increased
Urinary		
▪ Kidney	Renal mass decreased Number of functioning nephrons decreased Glomerular filtration rate decreased Renal plasma flow decreased	Protein in urine increased Potential for dehydration increased Creatinine clearance decreased Serum creatinine and BUN increased Excretion of toxins and drugs decreased Nocturia increased
▪ Bladder	Bladder smooth muscle and elastic tissue decreased	Capacity decreased Less control; stress incontinence
▪ Micturition	Sphincter control decreased	Frequency, urgency, and nocturia increased
Reproductive		
▪ Male structures	Prostatic enlargement Testicular volume decreased Sperm count decreased Seminal vesicles atrophy Serum testosterone constant Estrogen level increased	Sexual response less intense Longer to achieve erection Erection maintained without ejaculation Force of ejaculation decreased

Continued

GERONTOLOGIC DIFFERENCES IN ASSESSMENT

Table 4-1 Age-Related Changes and Associated Clinical Manfestations—cont'd

System	Expected Aging Changes	Clinical Manifestations
Reproductive—cont'd		
■ Female structures	Estradiol, prolactin, progesterone diminished Size of ovaries, uterus, cervix, fallopian tubes, labia decreased Associated glands and epithelium atrophied Elasticity in the pelvic area decreased Breast tissue decreased Vaginal pH becomes alkaline	Responses to changing hormone levels altered Cervical, vaginal secretions decreased Intensity of sexual response gradually decreased Potential for vaginal infections increased Potential for vaginal and uterine prolapse increased
Gastrointestinal		
■ Oral cavity	Dentine decreased Gingival retraction Bone density lost Papillae of tongue decreased Taste threshold for salt and sugar increased Salivary secretions decreased	Taste changes Potential loss of teeth Gingivitis Bleeding gums and dry mouth Oral mucosa dry
■ Esophagus	Lower esophageal sphincter pressure decreased Motility decreased	Epigastric distress Dysphagia Potential for hiatal hernia and aspiration
■ Stomach	Gastric mucosa atrophy Blood flow decreased	Food intolerance
■ Small intestine	Intestinal villae decreased Enzyme secretions decreased Motility decreased	Absorption of nutrients diminished Absorption of fat-soluble vitamins delayed
■ Large intestine	Blood flow decreased Motility decreased Sensation to defecation decreased	Potential for constipation and fecal impaction
■ Pancreas	Pancreatic ducts distend Lipase production decreased Pancreatic reserve impaired	Impaired fat absorption Decreased glucose tolerance
■ Liver	Number and size of cells decreased Hepatic protein synthesis impaired Ability to regenerate decreased	Lower border extends past costal margin Decreased drug metabolism
Musculoskeletal		
■ Skeleton	Intervertebral disks narrowed Cartilage of nose and ears increased	Height diminished 1-4 in (2.5-10 cm) Nose and ears lengthen Kyphosis Pelvis wider
■ Bone	Cortical and trabecular bone decreased	Bone resorption exceeds bone formation Potential for osteoporotic fractures
■ Muscles	Number of muscle fibers decreased Muscle fibers atrophy Muscle regeneration slowed Contraction time and latency period prolonged Flexion of joints increased Ligaments stiffening Sclerosis of tendons Tendon flexor reflexes decreased	Strength decreased Agility decreased Rigidity in neck, shoulders, hips, and knees increased Potential restless leg syndrome
■ Joints	Cartilage erosion Calcium deposits increased Water in cartilage decreased	Mobility decreased ROM limited Osteoarthritis

Continued

GERONTOLOGIC DIFFERENCES IN ASSESSMENT

Table 4-1 Age-Related Changes and Associated Clinical Manfestations —cont'd

System	Expected Aging Changes	Clinical Manifestations
Nervous		
▪ Structure	Loss of neurons in brain and spinal cord Brain size decreased Dendrites atrophy Major neurotransmitters decreased Size of ventricles increased	Conduction of nerve impulses slowed Peripheral nerve function lost Reaction time decreased Response time precise and slowed Potential for altered balance, vertigo, syncope Postural hypotension increased Proprioception diminished Sensory input decreased EEG alpha waves decreased
▪ Sleep	Deep sleep decreased	Difficulty remembering dreams Difficulty falling asleep Periods of wakefulness increased Sleeptime averages 6 hr
Visual		
▪ Eye structure	Orbital fat lost Eyebrows and eyelashes gray Elasticity of eyelid muscles decreased Tear production decreased	Eyes sunken Eyes dry Potential ectropion and entropion Potential conjunctivitis
▪ Cornea	Corneal sensitivity decreased Corneal reflex decreased Arcus senilis	Potential corneal abrasion
▪ Ciliary	Aqueous humor secretion decreased Ciliary muscle atrophy	Ability of lens to accommodate declines Potential presbyopia Peripheral vision decreased
▪ Lens	Less elastic, more dense Blue-green color discrimination decreased	Lens yellow and opaque Less ability to adapt to light and dark Tolerance to glare decreased Incidence of cataracts increased Night vision impaired
▪ Iris and pupil	Pigment lost Smaller pupil Vitreous gel debris increased	Visual acuity decreased Pupils appear constricted Floaters
Auditory		
▪ Structure	Hairs in external auditory canals of men increased Ceruminal glands decreased	Potential conductive hearing loss Cerumen more dry
▪ Middle ear	Middle ear bone joints degenerate Ear drum thickens	Sound conduction decreased
▪ Inner ear	Vestibular structures decline Hair cells lost Cochlea atrophies Organ of Corti atrophies	Sensitivity to high tones: "s," "t," "f," "g" decreased Understanding of speech decreased Discrimination of background voice decreased Equilibrium-balance deficits Potential for tinnitus
Immune System	Secretory immunoglobulin (IgA) declines Thymus gland involuted Thymopoietin decreased Lymphoid tissue decreased Antibody production impaired T lymphocytes decreased Autoantibodies increased	Potential increase for infection on mucosal surfaces Impaired cell-mediated immune response Malignancy incidence increased Response to acute infection reduced Potential recurrence of latent herpes zoster and tuberculosis Autoimmune disease increased

AV, atrioventricular; *BP,* blood pressure; *bpm,* beats per minute; *BUN,* blood urea nitrogen; *CO,* cardiac output; *EEG,* electroencephalogram; *HR,* heart rate; *REM,* rapid eye movement; *ROM,* range of motion.

SPECIAL POPULATIONS

Older Adult Women

For the aging woman, the impact of an aging body and being a woman is considered a double jeopardy. Women are often discriminated against for being older and female. Table 4-2 lists numerous factors that have had a significant negative impact on the health of the older woman. Gender-based inequities in health care can be seen in the emphasis on (1) Medicare coverage of acute care conditions that occur more frequently in men, such as coronary artery disease; (2) high out-of-pocket costs for depression, arthritis, and hypertension, which occur more often in women; (3) lack of research on diseases for which women are at risk, such as breast cancer; and (4) less aggressive diagnostic workup for anxiety, depression, and cardiac disease in women.[7]

The nurse is in an excellent position to be an advocate for health equity for the older woman in the health care system. Advocacy organizations, such as the Older Women's League (OWL), can be helpful in this process.

Cognitively Impaired Older Adults

For the majority of healthy older adults, there is no noticeable decline in mental abilities. The older adult may experience a memory lapse or benign forgetfulness that is significantly different from cognitive impairment (Table 4-3).

The older adult who is forgetful should be encouraged to use memory aids to attempt recall in a calm and quiet environment, and actively engage in memory improvement techniques. Memory aids include clocks, calendars, notes, marked pillboxes, safety alarms on stoves, and identity necklaces or bracelets. Memory techniques include word association, mental imaging, and mnemonics.

Declining physical health is an important factor that influences cognitive impairment. The older adult who experiences sensory loss, cardiovascular disease, or hypertension shows a decline in cognitive functioning. Although intelligence quotient (IQ) is important, the nurse needs to assess functional use of information. An appropriate cognitive assessment includes functional ability, memory recall, orientation, use of judgment, and appropriate emotional state. Standard mental status examinations and behavioral descriptions provide data for determining cognitive status. The three most common cognitive problems of the elderly are compared in Table 4-4. (See Chapter 56 for a discussion of Alzheimer's disease.)

Table 4-2 Factors Negatively Affecting Health of Older Women

1. A disproportionately higher number of women than men live in poverty.
2. Minority women have the highest poverty rates.
3. Lack of formal work experience of older women leads to low incomes.
4. More older women rely on social security as a major source of income than men.
5. Older women more frequently live alone than men.
6. Traditional caregiving and homemaking roles increase women's economic insecurity.
7. Older women have less access to health insurance.
8. Older women have a higher incidence of chronic health problems, such as arthritis, hypertension, strokes, and diabetes.
9. Older women who are married are likely to be caregivers for ill husbands.

Compiled from Hooyman NR, Kiyak HA: *Social gerontology: a multidisciplinary perspective,* ed 4, Boston, 1996, Allyn and Bacon.

Rural Older Adults

Approximately one half of all persons 65 years of age and older live in nonmetropolitan areas (Fig. 4-2). The older adult tends to move to these areas because living costs are reduced, communities are less complex, and crime is less common. Statistically, the rural older adult is most frequently Caucasian, male, married, and has a higher poverty rate.[8]

Because of geographic isolation and a higher poverty level, the rural older adult is highly stressed by changing financial resources and declining self-care abilities.[9] Although the rural older adult fears dependence on others, symptoms of ill health are greater than those found in urban peers. These concerns may be related to two factors: the rural older adult is less likely to engage in health-promoting activities, and the rural community is underserved by health care workers.[10]

The nurse working with the rural older adult must clearly define the lifestyle values and practices of rural life. Health care providers should consider transportation as a possible barrier to service. Alternative service approaches such as videotapes, radio, and church social events should be used to promote healthful practices or to conduct health screening. Innovative models of nursing practice must be developed to assist the rural older adult.

Frail Older Adults

The old-old population (75 years of age and older) is steadily increasing in number. Since the 1960s this group has increased 250%. The old-old adult is usually a widowed woman dependent on family or kinship support. Many have outlived children, spouses, and siblings. The old-old adult is often char-

Table 4-3 Forgetfulness versus Cognitive Impairment

Benign—Forgetfulness	Pathology—Cognitive Impairment
Forgets, then remembers	Forgets important people
When item is lost, mental retracing occurs	Unable to mentally retrace
Forgets unimportant events	Forgets entire recent events
Forgets long-ago events	Forgets events minutes ago
Uses reminders and notes	Cannot use reminders consistently
Oriented to self as a person	May be disoriented to self
May repeat stories over time	Repeats same question in a short time

acterized as a hardy, elite survivor. Because the old-old adult has lived so long, she may have become the family icon, the symbol of family tradition and legacy. Approximately one fourth are in nursing homes or other institutions. In this old-old population, ethnic group members often live with extended family and often continue to speak their native language.

The old-old adult has difficulty coping with declining functional abilities and decreasing daily energy. When stressful life events (e.g., the death of a pet) and daily strain (such as caring for an ill spouse) occur, the old-old individual often cannot alleviate the effects of stress and, as a result, may become ill. Common health problems of the frail older adult include mobility limitations, sensory impairment, cognitive decline, falls, and increasing frailty.

The frail older adult is at particular risk for malnutrition. Malnutrition is related to sociopsychologic factors such as living alone, depression, and low income. Physical factors such as declining cognitive status, inadequate dental care, sensory limitation, physical fatigue, and limited mobility also add to the risk of malnutrition. Because many frail older adults have therapeutic diets and multiple drug regimens, their nutritional state may be altered. It is important for the nurse to monitor the frail older adult for adequate calorie, protein, iron, calcium, and vitamin D intake.

The acronym SCALES can remind the nurse to assess important nutritional indicators:

Sadness, or mood change
Cholesterol, high
Albumin, low
Loss or gain of weight
Eating problems
Shopping and food preparation problems

Once the older adult's nutritional needs are identified, common interventions include home-delivered meals, dietary supplements, food stamps, dental referrals, and vitamin supplements.

The nurse should remember that the frail older adult tires easily, has little physical reserve, and is at risk for disability, elder abuse, and institutionalization. This older adult is dependent on a delicate network of family, individual, and social support that should be respected and supported.

Sick Older Adults

The older adult population has a higher rate of hospitalization, home care, day surgery, and physician visits than any other age-group. Eighty percent of all older adults have at least one chronic disease. The older adult is more likely than the adult in a younger age-group to have days of restricted activity as a result of acute illness. Although health status refers to acute and chronic illness, it also includes an individual's level of daily

Table 4-4 A Comparison of the Clinical Features of Acute Confusion, Dementia, and Depression

Feature	Acute Confusion (Delirium)	Dementia	Depression
Onset	Rapid, often at night	Usually insidious	Coincides with life changes; often abrupt
Course	Fluctuates, worse at night; lucid intervals	Long; symptoms progressive yet relatively stable over time	Diurnal effects, typically worse in the morning; situational fluctuations
Progression	Abrupt	Slow but even	Variable, rapid-slow but uneven
Duration	Hours to less than 1 month	Months to years	At least 2 weeks, but can be several months to years
Awareness	Reduced	Clear	Clear
Alertness	Fluctuates, lethargic or hypervigilant	Generally normal	Normal
Orientation	Fluctuates in severity, generally impaired	May be impaired	Selective disorientation
Memory	Recent and immediate impaired	Recent and remote impaired	Selective or patchy impairment, "islands" of intact memory
Thinking	Disorganized, distorted, fragmented; slow or accelerated incoherent speech	Difficulty with abstraction, thoughts impoverished, judgment impaired, words difficult to find	Intact but with themes of hopelessness, helplessness, or self-deprecation
Perception	Distorted; illusions, delusions, and hallucinations	Misperceptions often present; delusions and hallucinations absent except in severe cases	
Psychomotor behavior	Variable; hypokinetic, hyperkinetic, or mixed	Normal, may have apraxia	Variable; psychomotor retardation or agitation
Sleep-wake cycle	Disturbed, cycle reversed	Fragmented	Disturbed, often early morning awakening
Mental status testing	Distracted from task; poor performance; improves when patient recovers	Frequent "near miss" answers, struggles with test, great effort to find an appropriate reply; consistently poor performances	Frequent "don't know" answers, little effort, frequently gives up, indifferent

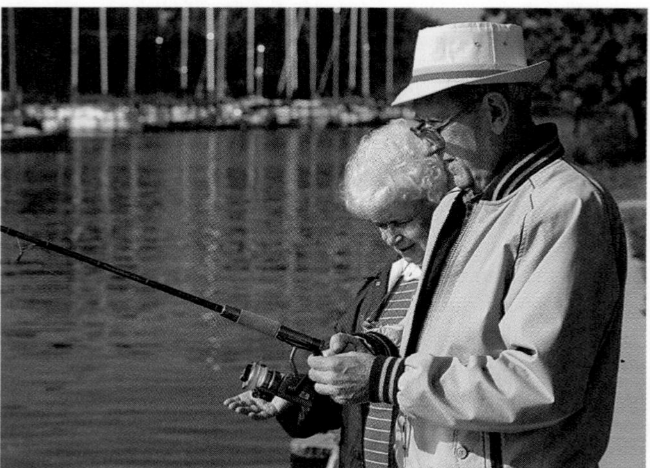

Fig. 4-2 Many older adults live in rural areas.

functioning. *Functional health* includes activities of daily living (ADLs), such as bathing, dressing, eating, toileting, and transfer. Instrumental ADLs, such as using a telephone, shopping, preparing food, housekeeping, doing laundry, arranging transportation, taking medication, and handling finances, are also included in functional health assessment.

As age increases, a pattern of declining functional health and increasing disability is seen. The nurse caring for the older adult can advocate accurate, comprehensive assessment in which health and disease states are diagnosed accurately and can actively teach health promotion strategies.

Disease in the older adult is often difficult to accurately diagnose. The older adult tends to underreport symptoms and to treat these symptoms by altering functional status. The older adult eats less, sleeps more, or "waits it out." The older adult often attributes a new symptom to "old age" and will ignore it.

Disease in the older adult may vary greatly. As one disease is treated, another may be affected. For example, the use of an anticholinergic medication may cause urinary retention. In the older adult, disease symptoms are atypical, and complaints of "aching in the joint" may actually be a broken hip. Silent asymptomatic pathology frequently occurs. Cardiac disease may be diagnosed when the patient is being treated for a urinary tract infection. Pathologies with similar symptoms are often confused. Depression may be mistreated as dementia. A cascade disease pattern may occur. An example of cascade would occur when the patient who experiences insomnia treats the condition with a hypnotic medication, becomes lethargic and confused, falls, and breaks a hip.

ETHNICITY AND AGING

The older adult who identifies with a certain ethnic group presents a particular challenge to the nurse (Fig. 4-3). Ethnic identity can be determined by asking the following questions:

1. Does this person identify with an ethnic or racial group?
2. Do others identify this person with an ethnic or racial group?
3. Does this person show behavioral patterns that are unique to the ethnic group?

Ethnic identity is often found in certain religious groups, nations, and minorities. As American society changes, ethnic

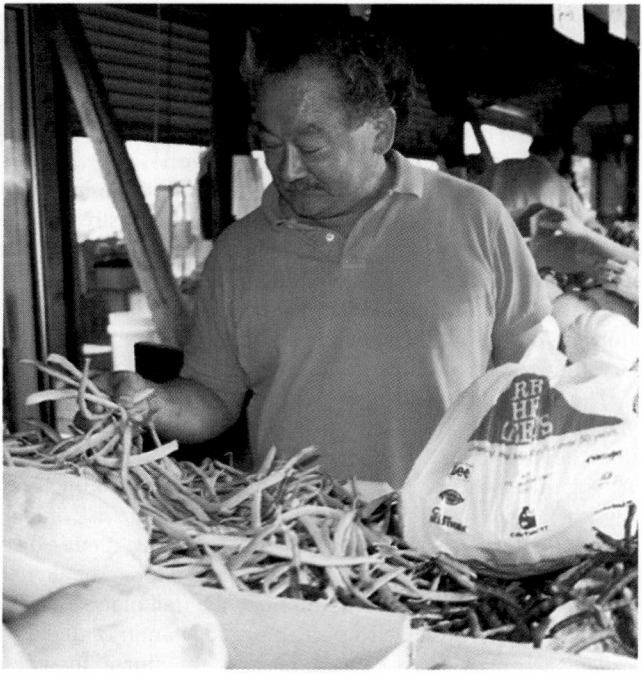

Fig. 4-3 Ethnic elders need special consideration.

institutions and neighborhoods may be altered. For the older adult with strong ethnic roots, the loss of friends who speak the "mother tongue," the loss of the church that supports social ethnic activities, and the loss of stores that carry desired ethnic foods may present situational crises that emphasize and diminish a sense of self-worth and personhood. This loss of self is increased when children and others deny or ignore ethnic practices and behaviors. Support for the ethnic older adult is most frequently found in family, religious practices, and isolated geographic or community ethnic clusters.

The ethnic older adult is faced with specific problems. Because the ethnic older adult often lives in older neighborhoods, physical security and personal safety related to high crime rates become a concern. Because the individual with an ethnic identity often has a disproportionately low income, Medicare deductibles or medications needed to treat chronic illnesses may not be affordable.

For the nurse to be effective with the ethnic older adult, a sense of respect and clear communication is critical. The nurse must identify self-behaviors that could be interpreted as noncaring or disrespectful, such as a refusal to allow a patient to display an item considered important for healing. Nursing interventions to assist in meeting the needs of the ethnic older adult are described in Table 4-5. Questions to ask the ethnic older adult about health-related practices include the following:

1. What makes people ill?
2. When do you know someone is sick?
3. What helps people get better?
4. Who can assist people to get well?
5. Do you believe this will help you get well?

American culture is changing. For some older adults, ethnic identity is also changing. The nurse should not assume that ethnic identity is or is not of value to the patient and the patient's family. The nurse must assess each older adult's ethnic orientation.[11,12]

Table 4-5 Nursing Interventions to Assist in Meeting the Needs of Ethnic Older Adults

1. Identify health practices, rituals, and food patterns that are central to an ethnic identity.
2. Identify stereotypic attitudes in the ethnic older adult that interfere with multiethnic group participation.
3. Inform ethnic older adult about services available.
4. Support the ethnic older adult who is fearful about traveling outside the accepted neighborhood for services.
5. Advocate for ethnic older adult to receive services that provide special attention to language limitations and cultural health practices.
6. Use strategies specific to an ethnic group. For example, African-Americans may respond to themes such as "do it for your loved ones." Asians may respond to fear of dependency themes.
7. Learn about services and programs that focus on specific ethnic groups. Examples include home-meal services that serve ethnic foods or nursing homes that include specific ethnic or religious preferences.

NURSING PROCESS AND THE OLDER ADULT

Establishing a Therapeutic Environment

The older adult may face a developing health problem with fear and anxiety. Health workers may be perceived as helpful, but institutions may be perceived as negative, potentially harmful places. The nurse can communicate a sense of concern and care by careful use of direct and simple statements, appropriate eye contact, direct touch, and gentle humor. These actions assist the older adult to relax in this stressful situation.

Before beginning the interview the nurse should attend to primary needs first, ensuring that the patient is pain-free and does not need to urinate. All assistive devices such as glasses and hearing aids should be in place. The interview should be short so the patient is not fatigued. The interviewer should allow adequate time for response to questions. The older adult and caregiver should be interviewed separately, unless the patient is cognitively impaired or specifically requests the caregiver's presence. Medical history may be lengthy. The nurse must determine what is relevant information. Old medical records should be obtained and available for review.

Assessment

As with all age-groups, assessment of the older adult provides the database for the rest of the nursing process. The focus of a geriatric assessment is to determine appropriate interventions to maintain and enhance the functional abilities of the older adult. Cure is often not possible because of the complexity and chronicity of the health problems that commonly affect the older adult. Consequently, the nurse directs the planning and implementation of those actions that assist the older adult in remaining as functionally independent as possible.

Elements in a comprehensive assessment include a history using a functional health pattern format (see Chapter 5), physical assessment, assessment of ADLs and instrumental activities of daily living (IADLs), mental status evaluation, and a social-environmental assessment. Evaluation of mental status is particularly important for the older adult because results often determine the patient's potential for independent living. Evaluation of the results of a comprehensive assessment helps determine the service and placement needs of the older adult patient. A good match between needs and services should be the goal of a geriatric assessment.

Clinical assessment should be based on instruments specific to the older adult population (Table 4-6). Interpretation of laboratory results can be problematic because many values change with age, and parameters are not well defined for the older adult, particularly the old-old patient.[13] The healthy adult may have age-related changes that may be considered abnormal in a younger population but are normal for an older adult. An appropriate reference book should be consulted for the correct ranges of laboratory values for the older adult. The nurse is in an important position to recognize and correct inaccurate interpretation of laboratory tests.[14]

The comprehensive geriatric assessment is often conducted at a geriatric evaluation unit (GEU) by an interdisciplinary geriatric assessment team. The interdisciplinary team may include many disciplines, but the minimum components include the nurse, the physician, and the social worker. After the assessment is complete, the interdisciplinary team meets with the patient and family to present the team's findings and recommendations. These assessment centers are often affiliated with large medical complexes.

Nursing Diagnoses

With few exceptions the same nursing diagnoses apply to the older adult as to a younger person. Often, however, the etiology and defining characteristics are related to age and unique to the older adult. Table 4-7 lists nursing diagnoses that are commonly associated with specific age-related changes. The identification and management of nursing diagnoses result in improved patient function and quality patient care for the older adult.

Planning

When setting goals with the older adult, it is helpful to identify the strengths and abilities that the patient demonstrates. Personal characteristics such as hardiness, persistence, and the ability to laugh and learn are positive factors in goal setting. Caregivers should be included in goal development. The older adult who perceives increasing dependence and learned helplessness as an appropriate response may be resistant to self-care. Priority goals for the older adult may be gaining a sense of control, feeling safe, and reducing stress.

Implementation

When carrying out a plan of action, the nurse may need to modify the approach and techniques used on the basis of the physical and mental status of the elderly patient. Small body size, common in the frail older adult, may necessitate the use of smaller pediatric equipment. Bone and joint changes often require transfer assistance, altered positioning, and use of gait belts and lift devices. The older adult with declining energy reserves requires extra rest periods alternated with short periods of exertion. A slower approach, restricted scheduling, and the use of a bedside commode or other adaptive equipment may be necessary.

GERONTOLOGIC DIFFERENCES IN ASSESSMENT

Table 4-6 Geriatric Assessment Instruments

Area of Concern	Example of Assessment Instrument	What Is Tested
Mental status	Folstein Mini-Mental State[1]	Tests orientation, memory, attention, language, recall Low score = cognitive impairment—general
Mood state	Geriatric Depression Scale[2]	30 affective items test for depression
Functional ability	Katz Index of Activities of Daily Living[3]	Tests bathing, dressing, toileting, transfer, continence, feeding Coded as: Independent—Assistance—Dependent
Functional ability	Lawton Instrumental Activities of Daily Living[4]	Tests telephone usage, traveling, shopping, meal preparation, housework, medication, money Coded as: Independent—Assistance—Dependent
Dementia indicators	Set Test[5]	Tests ability to name up to 10 items in 4 sets: *Fruits, Animals, Colors, Towns (FACT)* Score maximum = 40
Social support	Zarit Burden Interview[6]	Tests for feelings of burden in caregiving
Alcohol usage	CAGE[7]	Tests for alcohol abuse 4 items; response of yes in 2 or more = problem
	Michigan Alcohol[8] Screening Test—Geriatric Version	Tests for alcohol use
Falls assessment	Get Up and Go Test[9]	Tests balance and sway as risk for fall

1. Folstein MF, Folstein SE, McHugh PR: Mini-mental state: a practical method for grading the cognitive state of patients for the clinician, *J Psychiatr Res* 12:189, 1975.
2. Yesavage JA, Brink TL: Development and validation of a geriatric depression screening scale: a preliminary paper, *J Psychiatr Res* 17:41, 1983.
3. Katz S and others: Studies of illness in the aged. The index of ADL: a standardized measure of biological and psychological function, *JAMA* 185:914, 1963.
4. Lawton H, Brody E: Assessment of older people: self-maintaining and instrumental activities of daily living, *Gerontologist* 9:179, 1969.
5. Isaacs B, Kennie AT: The Set Test as an aid to the detection of dementia in old people, *Br J Psychiatry* 123:467,1973.
6. Zarit SH: Relatives of impaired elderly: correlates of feelings of burden, *Gerontologist* 20:699, 1980.
7. Mayfield D, Mcleod G, Hall P: The CAGE questionnaire: validation of a new alcoholism screening instrument, *Am J Psychiatry* 131:10, 1974.
8. Gurnedi AM: *Older adults' measure of alcohol, medicines, and other drugs,* New York, 1997, Springer.
9. Mathias S, Nayok U, Isaacs B: Balance in elderly patients: the "get up and go" test, *Arch Phys Med Rehabil* 67:387, 1986.

Cognitive impairment, if present, requires the nurse to offer careful explanations and a calm approach to avoid producing anxiety and resistance in the patient. Depression can result in apathy and poor cooperation with the treatment plan.

Evaluation

The evaluation phase of the nursing process is similar for all patients. Evaluation is ongoing throughout the nursing process. The results of evaluation direct the nurse to continue the plan of care or revise as indicated. Often the change in health status is not as dramatic in the older adult as it is in the younger patient. Because of this, the nurse needs to be cautious in changing plans prematurely.

When evaluating nursing care with the older adult, the nurse should focus on functional improvement, rather than cure. Useful questions to consider when evaluating the plan of care for an older adult are included in Table 4-8.

TEACHING OLDER ADULTS

The nurse is involved in teaching the older adult self-care practices to enhance health and modify disease processes (Fig. 4-4). The older adult presents the following challenges to learning: (1) time needed to learn is increased, (2) new learning must relate to the patient's actual experience, (3) anxiety and distractions decrease learning, (4) lack of risk taking and cautiousness decrease motivation to learn, and (5) sensory-perceptual deficits and cognitive decline require modified teaching techniques.

Specific approaches that increase the level of learning in the older adult include (1) the use of peer educators, (2) the use of simplicity and repetition, and (3) the support of the belief that change in behavior is both helpful and worth the effort of increased learning.[15] (Patient teaching is discussed in Chapter 6.)

HEALTH PROMOTION AND SCREENING

Health promotion and prevention of health problems in the older adult are focused in three areas: reduction in diseases and problems, increased participation in health promotion activities (Fig. 4-5), and increased targeted services that reduce health hazards. These goals are central to three major health initiatives currently guiding services for the older adult: (1) *The Healthy People 2000* national health objectives, (2) the recommendations of the U.S. Preventive Services Task Force Guide to Clinical Preventive Services, and (3) the Nutrition Screening Initiative.[16,17]

The nurse places a high value on health promotion and positive health behaviors. Programs have been successfully developed for screening for chronic health conditions, smoking cessation, geriatric foot care, vision and hearing screening,

Table 4-7 Nursing Diagnoses Associated with Age-Related Physiologic Changes

Cardiovascular System
- Decreased cardiac output
- Activity intolerance
- Fatigue

Respiratory System
- Ineffective breathing pattern
- Impaired gas exchange
- Ineffective airway clearance
- Risk for infection
- Risk for aspiration

Integumentary System
- Impaired skin integrity

Urinary System
- Fluid volume deficit
- Altered urinary elimination

Reproductive System
- Altered sexuality patterns
- Body image disturbance
- Sexual dysfunction

Gastrointestinal System
- Altered nutrition
- Constipation
- Altered oral mucous membrane

Musculoskeletal System
- Risk for injury
- Self-care deficit
- Pain
- Impaired physical mobility

Nervous System
- Altered thought processes
- Sensory-perceptual alteration
- Sleep pattern disturbance
- Hypothermia
- Hyperthermia

Senses
- Body image disturbance
- Impaired verbal communication
- Social isolation

Immune System
- Risk for infection

stress reduction, exercise programs, medication usage, crime prevention, and home hazards assessment. The nurse can carry out and teach the older adult about the need for specific preventive services.

Health promotion and prevention can be included in nursing interventions at any location or level where the nurse and the older adult interact. The nurse can use health promotion activities to strengthen self-care, increase personal responsibility for health, and increase independent functioning that will enhance the well-being of the older adult.[18]

Table 4-8 Evaluating Nursing Care for Older Adults

Evaluation questions may include the following:
1. Is there an identifiable change in ADLs, IADLs, mental status, or disease signs and symptoms?
2. Does the patient identify a better health state?
3. Does the patient think the treatment is helpful?
4. Do the patient and caregiver think the care is worth the time and cost?
5. Can the nurse document positive changes that support interventions?
6. Does change adequately meet the required mandates for reimbursement?

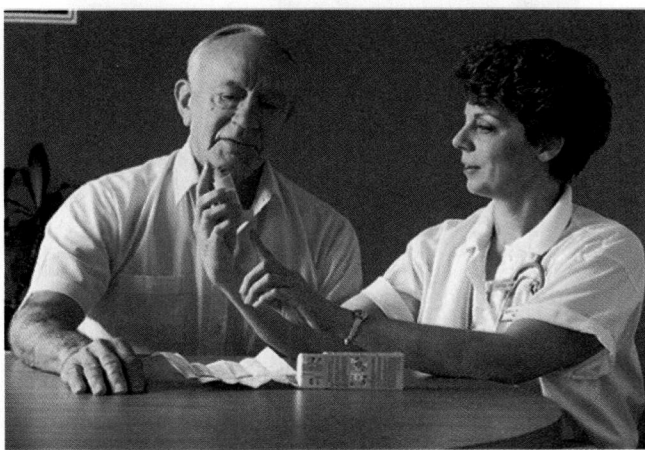

Fig. 4-4 Careful patient teaching increases the possibility of successful discharge of the older adult patient.

The nurse interested in older adult health promotion can contact the following organizations:

National Center for Health Promotion
National Council on the Aging
600 Maryland Avenue SW
West Wing 100
Washington, DC 20024

Health Promotion Interest Group
Gerontological Society of America
1275 K Street NW
Suite 350
Washington, DC 20005-4006

CHRONIC ILLNESS

Although the U.S. health care system is dominated by an acute illness focus, daily living with chronic illness is a reality for many older adults. Although persons of all ages have chronic health problems, chronic illness is most common in the older adult. Eighty-five percent of persons 65 years of age and older have at least one chronic condition. The twelve most common chronic conditions present in the older adult are visual impairment, diabetes, heart disease, deafness and hearing

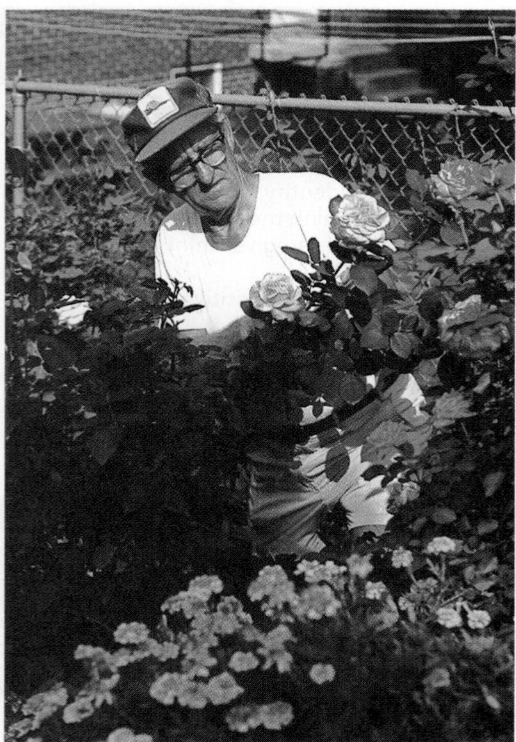

Fig. 4-5 Gardening is an example of a health promotion activity.

impairment, arthritis, Alzheimer's, osteoporosis, hip fractures, urinary incontinence, stroke, Parkinson's disease, and depression.[19]

Often, chronic illness is composed of multiple health problems that have a protracted, unpredictable course. Diagnosis and an acute phase of a chronic illness are often managed in a hospital. All other phases of a chronic illness are usually managed at home. The management of a chronic illness can profoundly affect the lives and identities of the patient, caregiver, and family.

Tasks required for daily living with chronic illness include (1) preventing and managing crisis, (2) carrying out prescribed regimens, (3) controlling symptoms, (4) reordering time, (5) adjusting to changes in the course of the disease, (6) preventing social isolation, and (7) attempting to normalize interactions with others.[20] Both the patient and the nurse must practice behaviors different from that required of patients with an acute illness if the older adult is to accomplish the tasks associated with a chronic disease.

GERIATRIC REHABILITATION

Older adults make up the majority of the disabled population yet receive less than the majority of all services. Rehabilitation interventions are focused toward adapting to or recovering from disability. With proper training, assistive equipment, and attendant personal care, the patient with disabilities can often live an independent life. For the younger disabled adult, the approach of personal attendant care with a focus on independent living stimulated the 1990 Americans with Disabilities Act. Advocates suggest that the elimination of environmental barriers allows the disabled to function normally in society. The older adult, primarily through Medicare reimbursement, receives rehabilitative assistance through post-incident, inpatient rehabilitation (limited days) and home care programs. These health care services are extensions of medical services. Reliance on unpaid family caregivers and a focus on patient limitations restrict the rehabilitation potential for the older adult.[21]

The nurse must understand physical disability in the older adult. The older person with cerebrovascular disease, arthritis, and coronary artery disease has a risk of becoming functionally limited within 4 years. Hip fracture, amputation, and stroke occur at higher rates in the older adult population. These disabilities lead to increased mortality rates, decreased life span, and increased rates of institutionalization. Reducing residual disability through geriatric rehabilitation is important to the quality of life of the older adult.

Rehabilitation of the older adult is influenced by several factors. First, the older patient shows greater initial variability in functional capacity than an adult at any other age. Preexisting problems associated with reaction time, visual acuity, fine motor ability, physical strength, cognitive function, and motivation affect the rehabilitation potential of the older adult.

Also, the older adult often loses functioning because of inactivity and immobility. This deconditioning can occur as a result of unstable acute medical conditions, environmental barriers that limit mobility, and a lack of motivation to stay in condition. The effect of inactivity clearly leads to "use it or lose it" consequences. The older adult can improve flexibility, strength, and aerobic capacity even into very old age. The nurse must use passive and active range-of-motion exercises with all older adults to prevent deconditioning and subsequent functional decline.

Last, the goal of geriatric rehabilitation is to strive for maximal function and physical capabilities considering the individual's current health status. When a patient demonstrates suboptimal health, the nurse screens and evaluates for risk behaviors. For example, a woman with a history of osteoporosis should be given a fall-risk appraisal, and the older adult diabetic patient should receive a geriatric foot assessment.

Rehabilitation is directed at preventing permanent disability. Therefore rehabilitation interventions emphasize four areas: (1) functional activity to increase capacity and mobility, (2) balance improvement, (3) good nutrition, and (4) social and emotional support.

Often the older adult has specific fears and anxieties related to falling and fatigue. The older adult is limited in the rehabilitation process by sensory-perceptual deficits, other disease states, slowed cognition, poor nutrition, and funding problems. Disability can be diminished by using appropriate assistive devices and adapting the environment to support function. Supportive and concerned caregivers are critical to the success of these modifications. Nurse and caregiver encouragement, support, and acceptance assist the older adult in remaining motivated for the hard work of rehabilitation.[22]

HOSPITALIZATION AND ACUTE ILLNESS

Frequently the hospital is the first point of contact for the older adult and the formal health care system. Approximately 20% of all Medicare recipients are hospitalized annually. The hospitalized older adult is often experiencing multisystem failure. Illnesses that most commonly result in hospitalization include arrhythmia, heart failure, cerebrovascular accidents, fluid and electrolyte imbalances, dehydration, hyponatremia, pneumonia, and hip fractures.[23] The complexity of the acute situation often results in a loss of the whole-person perspective and focuses care on the diseased part. Because the nurse provides an integrated approach, care that is individualized and helpful to the older adult can be reestablished.

The outcome of hospitalization for the older adult varies. Of particular concern are the problems of high surgical risk, acute confusional state, nosocomial infection, and premature discharge with an unstable condition.

High Surgical Risk

Age-related body changes, chronic illness, and declining physical reserve place the older adult at an increased surgical risk. Other key factors that increase surgical risk include age older than 75 years, emergency operations, use of spinal anesthesia, and thrombolytic complications. The risk of surgery should be balanced against the benefit and appropriateness of surgery for the older adult patient. (See Chapters 14, 15, and 16 for additional surgical considerations for the older adult.)

Acute Confusional State

The sudden onset of an acute confusional state (delirium) occurs in 18% to 38% of hospitalized older adults.[24] Although delirium is usually a transient condition that lasts from 1 to 7 days, research indicates that some delirium symptoms may persist up to discharge. Delirium is one of the most frequent consequences of unscheduled surgery because the older adult has not been stabilized physically or prepared emotionally. The patient who experiences delirium will exhibit a decline in ability to perform ADLs.[25]

Nosocomial Infections

Nosocomial (hospital-acquired) infections occur at higher rates in older adults. For the old-old patient, the rate is two to five times the rate of a younger person. Age-related changes of decreased immunocompetence, the presence of pathologic conditions, and an increase in disability all contribute to higher infection rates. Infections common to the older adult include pneumonia, urinary tract infections, and skin infections.[26] Tuberculosis is disproportionately high in the older adult population.[27] These infections often have atypical presentations showing cognitive and behavioral changes before alterations occur in laboratory values or temperature.

Hospital Discharge

At the time of hospital discharge, 17% to 38% of older adults are considered to be in an unstable condition. The frail older adult and the old-old patient are particularly vulnerable. Most of these patients are discharged under Medicare regulations that require a registered nurse or qualified person to develop a plan for discharge. The discharge plan should be periodically reassessed, and caregivers and patients must be counseled to prepare the patient for posthospital care.

The nurse can use screening inventories to identify at-risk patients.[28] The postdischarge assistance needed by at-risk patients includes bathing, taking medications, housekeeping, shopping, preparing meals, and making satisfactory transportation arrangements.[29] Risk of unstable discharge increases in the patient who experiences greater length of stay and who is dependent for meals.[30] Early hospital discharge is most successful when patients have had little change in functional status or are returning to a place with a high level of assistance, such as a nursing home.[30]

Nursing Role in Hospital Care

When caring for the hospitalized older adult, both patient and caregivers are assisted when the nurse performs the following:

1. Identifies the frail and old-old patients at risk for the iatrogenic effects of hospitalization
2. Considers discharge needs early in the hospital stay, especially assistance with ADLs, IADLs, and medications
3. Encourages the development and use of interdisciplinary teams, special care units, and individuals who focus on the special needs of gerontologic patients[31]
4. Develops standard protocols to screen for at-risk conditions commonly present in the hospitalized older adult patient, such as urinary tract infection and delirium
5. Advocates for referral of the patient to appropriate community-based formal care services (see Chapter 2)

GENERAL GERONTOLOGIC CARE CONSIDERATIONS

Environmental Considerations

As people age, the environment in which they live can be adapted to increase safety and comfort. Uncluttered floor space, railings, increased lighting and night-lights, and clearly marked stair edges are some of the easiest and most practical adaptations.

The older adult in an inpatient or long-term care setting needs a thorough orientation to the environment. The nurse should repeatedly reassure the patient that he or she is safe and attempt to answer all questions. The unit should foster patient orientation by displaying large-print clocks, avoiding complex or visually confusing wall designs, clearly designating doors, and using simple bed and nurse-call controls. Lighting should be adequate while avoiding glare. Beds should be close to the floor with four side rails that can be modified to individual needs. Environments that provide consistent caregivers and an established daily routine assist the older adult patient.

Assistive Devices

The use of assistive devices should be considered as an intervention for the older adult. Many older adults use or could benefit from the use of assistive devices such as dentures, glasses, hearing aids, walkers, wheelchairs, adult briefs or protectors, adaptive utensils, elevated toilet seats, and skin protective devices. These tools and devices should be included in the patient's care plan when appropriate. The nurse is in a position to ensure the correct and consistent use of these devices.

Pain Management

The older adult may not ask for pain relief. When pain is a known complication of a particular condition, the nurse should offer pain medication at regular intervals. Pain assessment in the elderly may be complicated by cognitive decline, sensory-perceptual deficits, and age-related changes. The use of verbal and visual pain scales can assist in correct assessment of

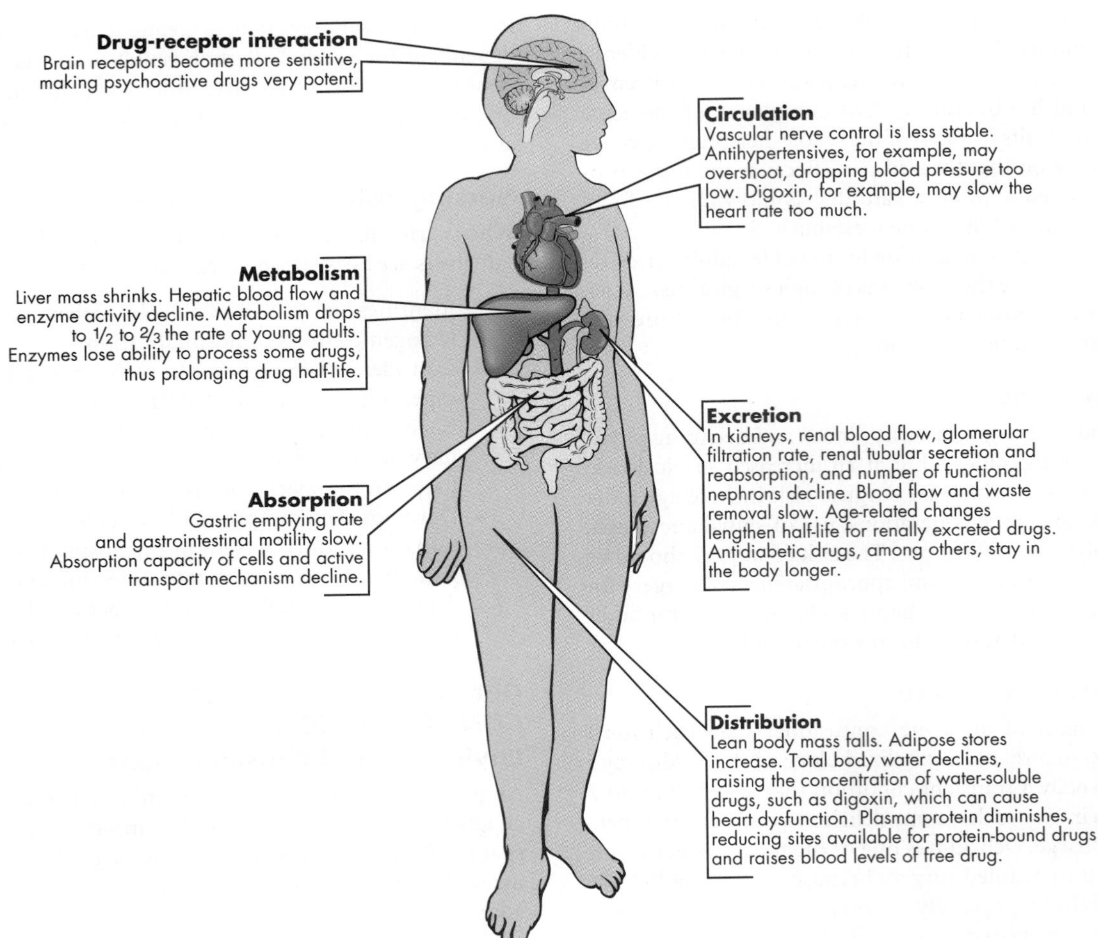

Drug-receptor interaction
Brain receptors become more sensitive, making psychoactive drugs very potent.
Circulation
Vascular nerve control is less stable. Antihypertensives, for example, may overshoot, dropping blood pressure too low. Digoxin, for example, may slow the heart rate too much.
Metabolism
Liver mass shrinks. Hepatic blood flow and enzyme activity decline. Metabolism drops to 1/2 to 2/3 the rate of young adults. Enzymes lose ability to process some drugs, thus prolonging drug half-life.
Excretion
In kidneys, renal blood flow, glomerular filtration rate, renal tubular secretion and reabsorption, and number of functional nephrons decline. Blood flow and waste removal slow. Age-related changes lengthen half-life for renally excreted drugs. Antidiabetic drugs, among others, stay in the body longer.
Absorption
Gastric emptying rate and gastrointestinal motility slow. Absorption capacity of cells and active transport mechanism decline.
Distribution
Lean body mass falls. Adipose stores increase. Total body water declines, raising the concentration of water-soluble drugs, such as digoxin, which can cause heart dysfunction. Plasma protein diminishes, reducing sites available for protein-bound drugs and raises blood levels of free drug.

Fig. 4-6 The effects of aging on drug metabolism.

pain. For the patient with ongoing pain, a pain diary may be helpful in identifying activities that relieve or increase pain.[32] Because the older adult may believe that pain is something that must be endured, creative methods may be developed to deal with it. The nurse should ask the patient to describe techniques used to reduce pain. Change in body position, heat, exercise, distraction, and rest may help alleviate pain. Mental imaging, positive thinking, and prayer and other spiritual interventions are also used. Poor pain management may lead to reduced socialization, limited mobility, impaired posture, sleep disturbances, depression, anxiety, and constipation.[33] (See Chapter 9 for additional discussion of pain.)

Medication Use

Medication usage in the older adult requires thorough and regular assessment and care planning. The use and abuse of medication by the older adult is supported by the following facts:

1. The older adult woman may take as many as five prescription drugs and three or more over-the-counter medications at the same time.
2. The old-old patient takes an average of 12 prescribed medications.
3. The frequency of adverse drug reactions increases as the number of prescribed drugs increases.
4. Twelve percent of older adult hospital admissions occur because of drug reactions.
5. After discharge from a hospital, even one unnecessary medication may put the older adult at risk for adverse drug reaction.[34]

Age-related changes alter the pharmacodynamics and pharmacokinetics of drugs. Drug-drug, drug-food, and drug-disease interactions all influence the absorption, distribution, metabolism, and excretion of drugs. Figure 4-6 illustrates the effects of aging on drug metabolism.

In addition to changes in the metabolism of drugs, the older adult may have difficulty as a result of cognitive decline, altered sensory perceptions, limited hand mobility, and the high cost of many prescriptions. Common medication errors made by the older adult include (1) forgetting to take drugs, (2) failing to understand instructions or the importance of drug treatment, (3) taking over-the-counter drugs, (4) taking out-of-date drugs, (5) taking drugs prescribed for someone else, and (6) refusing to take medication because of undesirable side effects such as nausea and impotence. Polypharmacy, overdose, and addiction to prescription drugs are recognized as major causes of illness in the older adult.

To accurately assess drug use and knowledge, many nurses ask their older adult patients to bring to the health care appointment all medications (both over-the-counter and prescription) that they take regularly or occasionally. The nurse can then accurately assess *all* medications the older adult is taking, including drugs that the patient may have omitted or thought unimportant. Additional nursing interventions to assist the older adult in following a safe medication routine are listed in Table 4-9.

Depression

Depression, seen in 7% to 11% of community-based elderly, is the most common emotional problem of the older adult.[36] Rates of depressive symptoms in institutionalized older adults are high. Although depressive symptoms occur frequently, marked mood alteration is not common. Depression in the older adult tends to arise from a loss of self-esteem and may be related to life situations such as loss of a spouse or retirement. Problems such as hypochondriac complaints, insomnia, lethargy, agitation, decreased memory, and inability to concentrate are common. Feelings of guilt are seldom present with depression in the older adult.

Late-life depression is often accompanied by physical illness. It is important that assessment include physical examination and laboratory testing for physical disorders that may have symptoms similar to depression. Diseases of concern are thyroid disorders and vitamin deficiencies. The older adult who exhibits depressive symptoms should be encouraged to seek treatment.

Because a patient often feels unworthy and may withdraw and become isolated, the nurse may need to seek the support of the family to assist in helping the older adult seek treatment. The depressed older adult who is involved in caregiving should seek respite and reevaluate the caregiving role.

Of all suicides, older adults commit 20.6% in the United States and 12.4% in Canada.[36] The nurse should take seriously comments such as "ending this life." Suicide precautions should be followed. The low-income older man who is divorced or widowed with a history of substance abuse is at greatest risk for suicide.

Nutritional Therapy

Maintaining adequate nutrition can be a problem for the older adult for physical and social reasons. Physiologically, food may be less appealing with the decline in taste and smell, and chewing is more difficult with dentures or loss of teeth. Swallowing and digestive problems may also result because of a decrease in saliva, gastric motility, and enzyme production. Socially, if a person eats alone, snacking on fast foods is easier than preparing meals. The lack of transportation or access to a grocery store, inability to see the merchandise, and poverty may be additional factors in poor nutrition. However, obesity may be a problem for some older adults. Normally this problem has arisen earlier in adulthood and continues because of difficulty in changing lifelong eating patterns.

The nurse can have the patient keep a 3-day dietary history. Analysis of this record is helpful in determining dietary adequacy. When appropriate the nurse can arrange for transportation to a senior meal site or delivery of home meals. Attention to and correction of the many reasons for poor nutrition in the elderly person is an important nursing responsibility.

Table 4-9 Nursing Interventions Related to the Uses of Medications by Older Adults

1. Emphasize medications that are essential.
2. Attempt to reduce medication usage that is not essential for minor symptoms.
3. Screen medication usage using a standard assessment tool—including over-the-counter drugs, eyedrops and eardrops, antihistamines, and cough syrups.
4. Assess alcohol usage.
5. Encourage the use of written or medication-reminder systems.
6. Monitor medication dosage strength; normally the strength should be 30-50% less than that of the younger person.
7. Encourage the use of one pharmacy.
8. Work with physicians and pharmacists to establish routine drug profiles on all older adult patients.
9. Advocate (with drug companies) for low-income prescription support services and dosage routines that are simple once-a-day time-release forms.

Sleep

Adequacy of sleep is often a concern of the older adult because of changed sleep patterns. Older people experience a marked decrease in stage IV deep sleep and are easily aroused. As a result they have difficulty maintaining prolonged sleep. Although the demand for sleep decreases with age, older adults may be disturbed by insomnia and complain that they spend more time in bed but still feel tired. Frequently, the older person prefers to spread sleep throughout 24 hours with short naps that provide adequate rest. Often, assurance from the nurse that this type of sleep pattern is adequate and normal for the patient's age will relieve anxiety concerning sleep. Many times a later bedtime will promote a better night's sleep and a feeling of being refreshed on awakening.

Safety

Environmental safety is crucial in the health maintenance of the older person. With normal sensory changes, slowed reaction time, decreased thermal and pain sensitivity, changes in gait and balance, and medication effects, the older adult is prone to accidents. Most accidents occur in or around the home. Falls, motor vehicle accidents, and fires are the common causes of accidental death in older adults.[37] Another environmental problem arises from an impaired thermoregulating system that cannot adapt to extremes in environmental temperatures. The body of an older adult can neither conserve nor dissipate heat efficiently. Therefore both hypothermia and heat prostration occur more readily. This age-group accounts for the majority of mortality statistics during severe cold spells and heat waves.

The nurse can provide valuable counsel regarding environmental changes, which may improve safety for the older adult. Measures such as stronger lighting, colored step strips, tub and toilet grab bars, and stairway handrails can be effective in "safety-proofing" the living quarters of the older adult. The nurse can also advocate for home fire and security alarms.

Behavioral Management

When patient behaviors such as agitation, anxiety, resisting care, and wandering become problematic, the nurse must plan nursing interventions carefully. Initially the patient's physical status must be assessed. The patient should be checked for changes in vital signs, urinary patterns, or constipation, which could be responsible for behavioral problems. Disruptive behaviors can be interrupted and redirected by encouraging the patient to participate in activities such as stacking papers, singing, playing music, exercising, or walking with the nurse.

When the patient is agitated by the environment, either the patient or the stimulus should be moved. The patient can be assisted to call family members if this is reassuring. When a patient resists or pulls tubes or dressings, these items can be covered with stretch tube gauze or removed from the visual field.[38] The older adult with behavioral problems should be reassured that the nurse is present to keep him or her safe. Reality orientation can be used to orient to time, place, and person. The confused or agitated patient should not be asked challenging "why" questions. If the patient cannot verbalize distress, his or her mood should be validated. The patient's emotional state should be closely observed. The patient's statement can be rephrased to validate its meaning.

When dealing with the difficult patient, the nurse's frustration should be acknowledged. The nurse should not threaten to restrain the patient or threaten to call the physician. A calming family member can be requested to stay with the patient until the person becomes more calm. The patient should be monitored frequently, and all interventions should be documented. The use of positive nurse actions can reduce the use of physical and chemical (drug therapy) restraints.[39]

Use of Restraints

Chemical and physical restraints should be a last resort in the care of the older patient. The nurse should clearly document restraint use and the behaviors that require this intervention. Research indicates that nurses are unclear about the use of restraint measures.[40] It is not appropriate to use restraints on a patient whom the nurse assumes will fall or on the patient who demonstrates irritating behaviors such as calling out. The use of restraints makes care more time consuming and complex. Restraints do not reduce falls but do increase potential patient confusion and the severity of injury when falls occur. Restraint alternatives require vigilant, creative nursing care. Restraint alternatives include wedge cushions, low beds, body props, and bed alarm signaling devices.[41] The nurse can avoid chemical restraint by using early interventions as discussed in the section on behavioral management. The use of restraints must follow rigid and explicit criteria. Long-term care regulations and the Joint Commission on Accreditation of Healthcare Organizations set standards for restraint usage. The movement to "restraint-free" environments is supporting restraint use decline.[42]

Elder Abuse

Elder abuse occurs in approximately 2% of the general older adult population.[43] The abuse is seldom reported to authorities even though it shows a repetitive pattern. The typical victim is an older woman with at least one limitation in ADLs. Most of these women are widowed, Caucasian, low income, and dependent on the abuser for some aspect of care. Elder abuse is often associated with substance abuse, caregiver strain, and depression. The lack of reporting abuse may be related to the older adult's feeling of vulnerability, lack of self-worth, impaired cognitive functioning, and sense of isolation.

Table 4-10 Types of Elderly Abuse

Type	Example
Violation of individual rights	Lack of privacy; unwanted visitors
Exploitation	Taking a social security check or property
Physical abuse	Shaking or hitting
Psychologic neglect	Isolating or locking the person in a room
Psychologic abuse	Swearing at person; displaying threatening behavior
Physical neglect	Not providing correct medications or proper physical care

Elder abuse can occur in a variety of forms (Table 4-10). Self-neglect is also a form of elder abuse when the older adult is no longer competent to perform self-care or when the older adult has severe psychologic impairments.

In assessing elder abuse the nurse must understand the legal limits of practice within state mandates. With a competent, older adult victim, the nurse may be limited in intervention because of patient resistance. In some situations health care workers are seen as interferences and opportunists. There are several elder abuse assessment instruments that include basic information, signs of maltreatment, severity of signs, and response of abuser.[44] If the nurse suspects abuse, an appropriate assessment protocol should be carried out, and consultation should be obtained based on agency policy. Follow-up actions for the nurse may include consultation with adult protective services and potential court testimony. In most situations, nurses are mandated to report abuse.

SOCIAL SUPPORT AND THE OLDER ADULT

Social support for the older adult occurs at three levels. Family and kinship relations are the first and preferred providers of social support. Second, a semiformal level of support is found in clubs, churches, neighborhoods, and senior citizen centers. Last, the older adult may be linked to a formal system of social welfare agencies, health facilities, and government support. Generally the nurse is part of the formal support system.

Caregivers

More than 80% of care is provided by a family caregiver who lives with the patient. A caregiver is usually a married woman who is often old herself, has chronic diseases and disabilities, and is often poor. Ethnic background influences the type of caregiving network. Italian-American, Polish-American, Irish-American, and African-American people most commonly use extended family networks for caregiving.[45] A caregiver provides supervision, provides direct care, and coordinates services. The tasks of caregiving include (1) assisting with ADLs and IADLs,

(2) providing emotional and social support, and (3) managing health care.

Caregiver Problems. Caregiver concerns change as the intensity of the caregiving role changes. For example, a caregiver may need to adjust work schedules to accommodate patient health care appointments, or the caregiver may need to be available to monitor the cognitively impaired patient's safety 24 hours a day.

Common problems facing the caregiver include the following: (1) a lack of understanding of the time and energy needed for caregiving; (2) a lack of information about specific tasks of caregiving, such as bathing or medication administration; (3) a lack of respite or relief from caregiving; (4) an inability to meet personal self-care needs, such as socialization and rest; (5) conflict in the family unit related to decisions about caregiving; and (6) financial depletion of resources as a result of a caregiver's inability to work and the increased cost of health care.[46]

The intensity and complexity of caregiving places the caregiver at risk for high levels of stress; the caregiver may develop a sense of being overwhelmed with feelings of inadequacy, powerlessness, and depression.[47] Although most older adults deny loneliness even when they spend much time alone, the caregiver often lacks sufficient social exchange. The primary caregiver is often at risk for social isolation; the burden of caregiving separates the individual from others who provide social, emotional, and interactional involvement. Time commitments, fatigue, and, at times, socially inappropriate behaviors of the dependent older adult contribute to social isolation. The socially isolated caregiver needs to be identified, and plans should be designed to meet the needs for social support and exchange.

The burden of caregiving may result in the nursing diagnosis of caregiver role strain. The escalating incidence of caregiving sets the stage for increased incidences of elder abuse. Physical, financial, psychologic, or sexual abuse and neglect may occur in families ill equipped to handle caregiving. The nurse should assess the caregiver and the patient for the possibility of caregiver role strain and elder abuse.

Emotional Problems of Caregivers. The stress of caregiving may result in emotional problems such as depression, anger, and resentment and feelings of hopelessness and powerlessness. The nurse should consider the caregiver as a patient and plan behaviors to reduce caregiver role strain. The nurse should communicate a sense of empathy to the caregiver while allowing discussion about the burdens and joys of caregiving. The caregiver can be taught about age-related changes and diseases and specific caregiving techniques. Attendance at a support group should be encouraged by the nurse. The nurse can also assist the caregiver in seeking help from the formal social support system regarding matters such as respite care, housing, health coverage, and finances. Finally, the nurse should monitor the caregiver for indications of declining health, emotional distress, and caregiver role strain.[48,49]

Older Adult Network

A network of services supports the older adult both in the community and in health care facilities. Most older adults are involved in at least one social or governmental service. This is true in both Canada and the United States. To understand the older adult situation, the nurse should know the government structures that fund and regulate the older adult programs.

In the United States the Department of Health and Human Services is the responsible federal agency for many older adult programs. In 1958 interest in the older citizen inspired the formation of the President's Council on Aging. From this beginning the Administration on Aging (AOA) has evolved. The general goal of AOA is to include older people wherever programs exist by cooperating and consulting with other agencies or organizations. There are several major grant programs under AOA. Title III of the Older Americans Act funds comprehensive, community-based service systems. Title IV funds the training of persons who are employed or preparing for employment in the field of aging. Funding from the AOA is funneled to state and local area agencies on aging.

Concurrent with the founding of AOA was the establishment of the White House Conferences on Aging, a forum for issue debate and policy recommendation. These conferences, held approximately every 10 years, have fostered decision making at a grass roots level for the good of older adults. Older adult delegates from all over the United States represent their home communities.

The legislative action that has evolved from this process is dramatic. At the 1951 exploratory conference the AOA had its roots. As a result of the 1961 conference, legislative action included the Older Americans Act, Medicare, Medicaid, and the Age Discrimination Act. From the 1972 conference the National Nutrition Program and Multipurpose Senior Centers were developed. In later conferences the federal, state, and local networks on aging were established, and the National Institute on Aging was designed. More than a dozen federal agencies are involved in programs for the elderly.

In Canada the Department of National Health and Welfare is the responsible federal agency for many older adult programs. The policies of the federal and provincial governments cannot be easily separated. Policy often results in an intermingling of activities through shared jurisdiction and cost sharing. This shared role has been changing during the last 30 years. Before 1950 the provincial government's responsibility ended with assistance to the aged poor. Since that time a wide range of federal and provincial programs has evolved. The role of the government has changed from that of regulator to provider.[50]

Medicare

Almost all U.S. citizens older than 65 years of age have Medicare coverage. Medicare also covers persons who receive social security disability benefits and persons with end-stage renal disease. Medicare is designed for acute illness care. Reimbursement is based on daily documentation that indicates a patient is improving in function. This nursing documentation process is complex and critical for adequate reimbursement.

Medicare is composed of two parts, A and B. Part A covers inpatient hospital care. Medicare A pays reasonable charges on the basis of the diagnosis, not on the length of stay. Skilled nursing facility care in a hospital or long-term care facility is paid if the stay results in an improved or rehabilitated condition. These skilled nursing benefit days are limited. The percentage of coverage changes each year. Medicare A pays for home care if it requires skilled nursing or rehabilitation intervention and is needed on a part-time basis. The patient must be homebound.

Durable medical equipment used daily is covered, but home safety equipment is not. Hospice care is covered under Medicare A. When hospice care is elected, the patient no longer qualifies for the condition to be treated in the standard Medicare program.

Part B covers outpatient treatment and physician's services. Medicare B is voluntary and has a monthly premium and an annual deductible before payment begins.

Medicare does not cover long-term nursing home care, custodial ADLs or IADLs care, dental care or dentures, preventive health care, prescription drugs, routine foot care, hearing aids, or eyeglasses. These costs plus the Medicare deductible costs account for the fact that most older adults pay for 50% of all acquired health care costs yearly. Analysis of chronic health care needs in the United States continues to indicate widespread unmet needs.[51]

General Support Services

Services for the older adult in the United States and Canada include hospital and medical benefits, community-based services, long-term institutional care, house and shelter assistance, transportation, employment programs, and income maintenance and support. These services are diverse and complex. Eligibility is limited and requires a subtle understanding of the rules. The older adult is often too frail, undereducated, or uninformed about these services to evaluate eligibility.

The nurse can assist the elderly patient and the caregiver by acknowledging the complexity of the health care system and empathizing with anger and frustration about regulations that seem unfair or inadequate. The nurse can assist the older adult to access the appropriate service or refer the patient to a case manager or other health care expert when appropriate.

CARE ALTERNATIVES FOR OLDER ADULTS

Housing

Most older adults are aging in place. Most do not move or return to the geographic location of childhood when health becomes frail. The community becomes important to the older adult as an environment that is safe from crime and accidents. The older adult needs privacy and companionship, as well as a sense of belonging. The community needs to be accessible. The older adult may need housing assistance through property tax relief, assistance with home repair, and fuel payment. A variety of subsidized, low-income housing arrangements are available for older adults.

For the older adult who chooses to remain in the home as functional abilities decline, home adaptations and modifications can be made. Homes can be made wheelchair accessible. Lighting can be increased and adjusted. Safety devices can be installed in bathrooms and kitchens. Alarms and assistive listening devices can be used.

Retirement communities may be an option for some older adults (Fig. 4-7). These communities are age-segregated, self-contained developments and provide social activities, security, and recreational facilities. When retirement communities offer expanded health care and social support services, including nursing home care, they become continuing care retirement communities (CCRCs). The CCRCs require an entrance fee and monthly fees for continuing care.

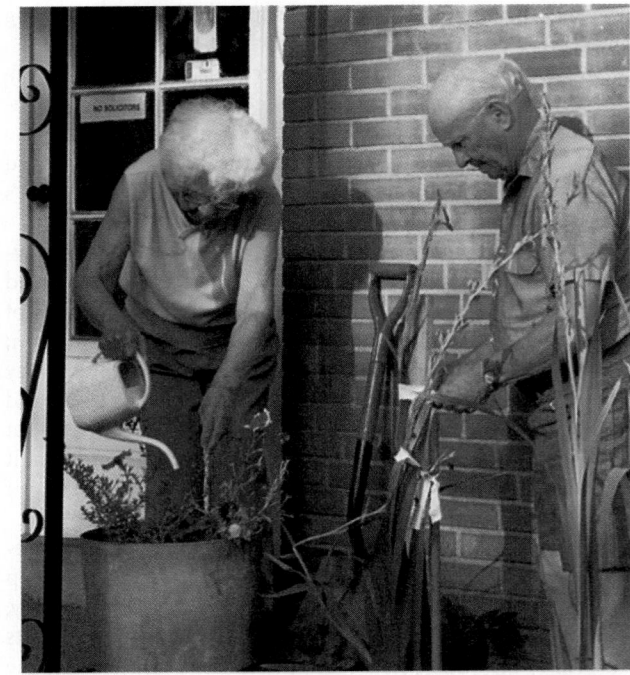

Fig. 4-7 This older couple works together to stay in their home.

Congregate housing provides services to the older adult at two levels: independent and assisted living. Independent living facilities provide housing and congregate meals but no supervision. Other home maintenance and care services can be purchased from these facilities. Board and care homes provide housing and meals in small congregate home environments.

Assisted-living facilities are designed to provide housing and personalized health care. Because over half of community-based older adults require assistance with ADLs or IADLs, this is the most rapidly developing area of long-term care. Services vary from state to state. Nurses provide care to or manage assisted-living facilities and services. Nurses working in this area are challenged by questions related to regulations, use of unlicensed assistive workers, assessment to ensure safe "fit of resident to facility," and shared resident decision making.[52]

Creative housing options are being developed by home sharing, the use of "granny flats," and apartment rentals in established older homes. The nurse can play a role in meeting the housing needs of older adults by identifying housing preferences and by advocating community housing changes that create a safe, liveable community.

Community-Based Older Adults with Special Needs

Older adults with special care needs include homeless persons, persons who need constant assistance with ADLs, persons who are home bound, and persons who can no longer live at home. The older adult may be served by adult day care, home health care, and nursing home care.

Homeless Older Adults. In areas where homelessness is increasing, the older adult is at additional risk because many aging network services are not designed to reach out to homeless persons. It is estimated that between 14% and 50% of

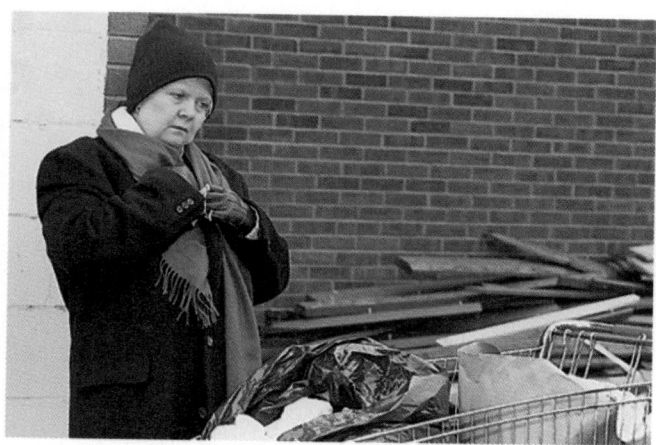

Fig. 4-8 Elderly homeless person.

homeless persons are older adults (Fig. 4-8). Street surveys suggest that most older homeless people are transient men. The older homeless person is less likely to use shelters or meal sites. The low-income older adult often becomes homeless because of a lack of affordable housing. Key factors that are associated with homelessness include (1) having a low income, (2) reduced cognitive capacity, and (3) living alone.[53] Nursing home placement is often an alternative to homelessness. Fear of institutionalization may explain the reason the older homeless adult does not use shelter and meal site services.

The older homeless person needs affordable housing. When cognitively impaired and alone, the older person needs financial management assistance. Solutions to the problem of homelessness among the elderly require more research and intervention studies.

Adult Day Care Programs. Adult day care (ADC) programs provide daily supervision, social activities, and ADLs assistance for two major groups of older adults—persons who are cognitively impaired and persons who have ADLs management problems. The services offered in the ADC programs are based on patient needs. Restorative programs for persons with problems of ADLs management offer health monitoring, therapeutic activities, one-to-one ADLs training, individualized care planning, and personal care services. Programs designed for the cognitively impaired offer therapeutic recreation, support for family, family counseling, and social involvement. Patient characteristics in the cognitively impaired group include a high number of persons with Alzheimer's disease. In this group, incontinence is a common problem. Patient characteristics in the restorative care group include a large number of wheelchair users, problems with incontinence, and some depression.

Day care centers provide relief to the caregiver, allow continued employment for the caregiver, and delay institutionalization for the patient. Centers are regulated and standards are set by the state. Costs are $25 to $50 per day and are not covered by Medicare. Adult day care is tax deductible as dependent care. Appropriate placement in a day care program that matches the patient's needs is important. The nurse can assist by knowing the available day care services and assessing the needs of the patient. The nurse is then in a position to aid the patient and family in making a good placement decision. The caregiver and the patient are often uninformed about day care and its services as an alternative care option.

Home Health Care. Home health care can be a cost-effective care alternative for the older adult patient who is homebound, has health needs that are intermittent or acute, and has supportive caregiver involvement. Home health care is not an alternative for the patient in need of 24-hour ADLs assistance or continuous safety supervision. Home health care services require physician recommendation and skilled nursing care for Medicare reimbursement. Unless these requirements are met, assistance by a home health aide for ADLs management or assistance by a homemaker for IADLs management will not be paid by Medicare. (Home health care is discussed in Chapter 2.)

Nursing Home Care

Nursing home care is a placement alternative for the older adult who can no longer live alone, who needs continuous supervision, who has three or more ADLs disabilities, or who is frail. The cost of nursing home care is high. These costs are paid privately for 50% of all patients and by state-funded public assistance programs (Medicaid) for 40% of all patients. This public assistance support for nursing home care accounts for more than 50% of all Medicaid care costs. When nursing home patients receive Medicaid, they contribute all their personal income to pay their expenses, except for a small amount per month kept as a personal needs allowance. Managed care affects both nursing homes and Medicaid enrollees. This trend will alter nursing home care.[54] (Nursing home care is discussed in Chapter 2.)

Placement Issues. Three factors appear to precipitate nursing home placement: (1) rapid patient deterioration, (2) caregiver inability to continue care as a result of "burnout"—too much and too long, and (3) an alteration in or loss of family support system. Physical changes of confusion, incontinence, or a major health event (e.g., stroke) can accelerate placement.[55]

The conflicts and fears faced by the family and patient make nursing home placement a transition time. Common caregiver concerns include the following: (1) the process of admission will be resisted by the patient; (2) the level of care given by staff will be insufficient; (3) the patient will be lonely; and (4) the financing of nursing care will not be adequate.[56]

This time of disruption is increased by the physical relocation of the patient. Research indicates that the process of physical relocation results in adverse health effects for the older adult.[57] The crisis of relocation syndrome should be anticipated by the nurse, and appropriate interventions to reduce the effects of relocation should be used. Whenever possible the older adult should be involved in the decision to move and should be fully informed about the location. The caregiver can share information, pictures, or a videotape of the new location. New health personnel can send a welcome message. On arrival the new patient can be greeted by a staff member to orient the older adult. To bridge the relocation the new patient can be "buddied" with a seasoned patient.

The satisfied nursing home patient tends to show a variety of behaviors indicating adjustment (Fig. 4-9). The patient is assertive and self-reliant; keeps active, follows a routine, keeps

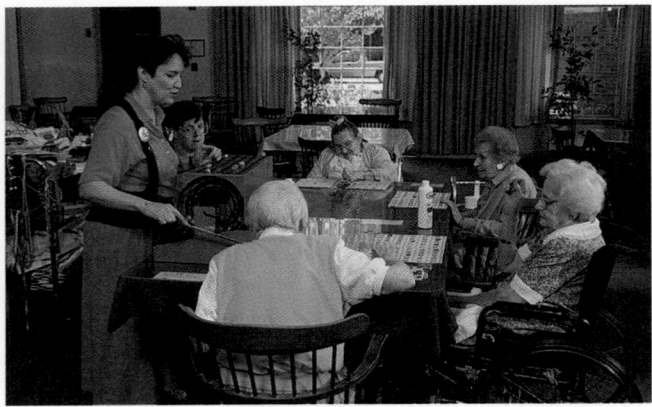

Fig. 4-9 Social interaction and acceptance is an important aspect of nursing home care for the elderly.

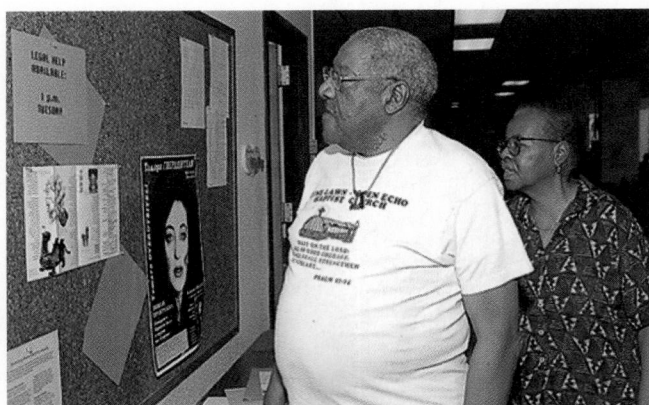

Fig. 4-10 Bulletin board at a senior center showing time legal help is available.

mentally involved, and is sociable; maintains family interaction; and shows a level of acceptance. The satisfied patient also expresses a determined, positive perspective. The satisfied patient uses coping strategies that increase control and management of her or his life.[58] The nurse can encourage and enable the use of these strategies for the nursing home patient.

Case Management

Matching older adult social support services to the needs of the older adult is complex. For family members who live out of town and cannot provide direct caregiving, the use of a case manager may be helpful. This is a new and developing role that the nurse is well suited to assume. The case manager supervises and manages care to ensure continuity of care for the older adult. The process of locating and organizing older adult services is time consuming. The use of the Elder Care Locator program (800-677-1116), a national telephone resource for older adult services, is available toll free. A written directory of nationwide services (A National Eldercare Directory of Information and Referral) is available from the National Association of Area Agencies on Aging (202-296-8130) for approximately $30.

LEGAL AND ETHICAL ISSUES

Patient Concerns

Legal assistance is a concern for many older adults. Legal concerns center on advance directives, estate planning, taxation issues, and appeals for denied services. Legal aid is available to the low-income older adult by contacting a local multipurpose senior center (Fig. 4-10). This service is supported by funds authorized through Title III of the Older Americans Act.

Advance directives are mandated on admission to a health care facility by the Patient Self-Determination Act of 1991. There are primarily two types: a living will and a durable power of attorney for health. A living will is a directive that permits an individual to direct his or her health care in the event of a terminal or irreversible condition. Most living wills direct that in the event of a terminal illness, extraordinary medical care should not be initiated or should be withdrawn so that the process of dying will not be artificially prolonged. A living will is directive but not legally binding. A durable power of attorney for health is another form of advance directive that designates another person to voice health care decisions when the patient is unable to do so personally. A durable power of attorney for health is directive and legally binding. In most states it includes the naming of an individual to carry out directives when the patient cannot make choices.[59] Discussion of estate planning, taxation issues, and appeals for denied services is beyond the scope of this text.

Nursing Concerns

The nurse who works with the older adult identifies areas of ethical concern that influence practice. This nurse identifies that these issues center around the following: (1) to restrain or not restrain and (2) to evaluate the patient's ability to make decisions. Other ethical concerns related to (1) resuscitation, (2) treatment of infections, (3) issues of nutrition and hydration, and (4) transfer to more intensive treatment units are all a part of long-term care.[60]

These situations are often complex and emotionally charged. The nurse can assist the patient, family, and other health care workers by acknowledging when an ethical dilemma is present, by keeping current on the ethical implications of new biotechnology, and by advocating for an institutional ethics committee to help in the decision-making process.

REVIEW QUESTIONS

The number of the question corresponds to the same-numbered objective at the beginning of the chapter.

1. The impact that older adults have on the health care system is illustrated by the fact that
   a. the aging population is growing faster than any other age-group.
   b. all persons over the age of 65 have at least two chronic diseases requiring medical care.
   c. older adults have a lower rate of hospitalization, home care, and physician visits than any other group.
   d. older adults tend to over-report symptoms and cannot distinguish normal changes of aging from symptoms of disease.

2. Ageism is characterized by
   a. negative attitudes toward the elderly based on age.
   b. negative attitudes toward the elderly based on physical disability.
   c. denial of negative stereotypes regarding aging
   d. positive attitudes toward the elderly based on age.
3. A 78-year-old patient has a blood pressure of 158/88. The nurse recognizes that
   a. the patient has hypertension and should follow up with the physician.
   b. blood pressure should decrease with age because of decreased heart rate and cardiac output.
   c. the systolic blood pressure tends to rise with aging because of loss of elasticity of the arteries.
   d. dilation of the aorta and rigid arterial pulses make the blood pressure more difficult to accurately measure.
4. To differentiate depression from dementia in an older adult the nurse recognizes that
   a. the progression of dementia is variable and uneven.
   b. judgment and thoughts are more impaired in dementia.
   c. awareness and alertness are impaired in both problems.
   d. a patient with depression is motivated to perform well on mental status testing.
5. An ethnic older adult may experience a loss of self-worth when the nurse
   a. informs the patient about ethnic support services.
   b. has to use an interpreter to provide explanations and teaching.
   c. allows a patient to rely on ethnic health beliefs and practices.
   d. emphasizes that a therapeutic diet does not allow ethnic foods.
6. When older adults become ill they are more likely than younger adults to
   a. complain about the symptoms of their problems.
   b. alter their daily living activities to accomodate new symptoms.
   c. seek medical attention because of limitations on their lifestyle.
   d. refuse to carry out lifestyle changes to promote recovery.
7. Nursing interventions directed at health promotion in the older adult are primarily focused on
   a. disease management.
   b. controlling symptoms of illness.
   c. teaching positive health behaviors.
   d. providing a sense of control over health problems.
8. An important nursing action helpful to a chronically ill older adult is to
   a. avoid discussing future lifestyle changes.
   b. assure the patient that the condition is stable.
   c. treat the patient as a competent manager of the disease.
   d. encourage the patient to "fight" the disease as long as possible.
9. Delirium can be defined as
   a. an acute confusional state with a sudden onset.
   b. a prolonged state of confusion related to dementia.
   c. a confusional state that lasts only minutes to hours.
   d. a condition that is directly related to medication use.
10. An important fact for the nurse to know about caregivers is that they
    a. can often share the burden of caregiving with other family members.
    b. frequently require nursing to assist them in reducing caregiver strain.
    c. are usually trained health care workers who do not live with the patient.
    d. are generally strong and healthy but need teaching to carry out care activities.
11. An appropriate care choice for an older adult living with an employed daughter, but who requires constant assistance with activities of daily living, is
    a. adult day care.
    b. nursing home care.
    c. a retirement center.
    d. an assisted-living home.
12. A living will is an advance directive that
    a. is legally binding.
    b. encourages the use of artificial means to prolong life.
    c. allows a person to direct his or her health care in the event of terminal illness.
    d. designates who can act for the patient when the patient is unable to do so personally.

References

1. Edmondson B: The facts of death, *American Demographics* 19:46, 1997.
2. *Statistics Canada. A portrait of seniors in Canada, target group project,* Ottawa, 1990, Ministry of Supply and Services, Canada.
3. Neugarten B: The future and the young-old. In Jarvik LF, editor: *Aging into the 21st century: middle ages today,* New York, 1978, Gardner Press.
4. Burke M, Walsh M: *Gerontologic nursing: wholistic care of the older adult,* ed 2, St Louis, 1997, Mosby.
5. Neugarten BL, editor: *The meaning of age: selected papers of Bernice L. Neugarten,* Chicago, 1996, University of Chicago Press.
6. Smith MA and others: Age and health perception among elderly blacks, *J Gerontol Nurs* 17:13, 1991.
7. Ebersole B: Aging and gender issues, *Geriatr Nurs* 17:149, 1996.
8. Coward RT and others: An overview of health and aging in rural America. In Coward RT and others, editors: *Health services for rural elders,* New York, 1994, Springer.
9. Vrabec N: Implications of U.S. health care reform for the rural elderly, *Nursing Outlook* 43:260, 1995.
10. Armer J: An exploration of factors influencing adjustment among relocating rural elders, *Image J Nurs Sch* 28:35, 1996.
11. Gelfand A: *Aging and ethnicity,* New York, 1994, Springer.
12. White EC: *The black women's health book,* Seattle, 1994, Seal.
13. Lueckenotte A: Laboratory and diagnostic tests. In Lueckenotte A, editor: *Textbook of gerontologic nursing,* St Louis, 1996, Mosby.
14. Martin J and others: Interpreting laboratory values in elderly surgical patients, *AORN* 65:621, 1997.
15. Dellasya C and others: Nursing process: teaching elderly clients, *J Gerontol Nurs* 20:31, 1994.
16. US Department of Health and Human Services, Office of Disease Prevention and Health Promotion: *Healthy People 2000: national health promotion and disease prevention objectives,* pub no 017-001-00473, Washington, DC, 1990, US Government Printing Office.
17. *Report of nutrition screening I: toward a common view,* Washington, DC, 1991, Nutrition Screening Initiative.
18. Daly D, Mitchell R: Case management in the community setting, *Nurs Clin North Am* 31:527, 1996.
19. *Putting aging on hold: delaying the diseases of old age,* Washington, DC, 1995, American Federation for Aging Research and the Alliance for Aging Research.
20. Robinson LA and others: Operationalizing the Corbin and Strauss trajectory model for elderly clients with chronic illness, *Sch Inq Nurs Pract* 7:253, 1993.
21. Lohr KN: Improving health care outcomes through geriatric rehabilitation. Conference summary, *Med Care* 35:JS/21, 1997.
22. Bottomley JM: Principles and practice in geriatric rehabilitation. In Satin DG, editor: *The clinical care of the aged person,* New York, 1994, Oxford University Press.
23. Kelly M: Surgery, anesthesia, and the geriatric patient, *Geriatr Nurs* 16:213, 1995.

24. Shedd P and others: Confused patients in the acute care setting: prevalence, interventions and outcomes, *J Gerontol Nurs* 21:5, 1995.
25. Simon L and others: Management of acute delirium in hospitalized elderly: a process improvement project, *Geriatr Nurs* 18:150, 1997.
26. Hofland SL, Mort J: Infections in long-term care facilities: issues for practice, *Geriatr Nurs* 15:260, 1994.
27. Tuberculosis morbidity—United States, 1996, *MMWR Morb Mortal Wkly Rep* 46:695, 1997.
28. Holloway C, Pokorny M: Early hospital discharge and independence: what happens to the elderly, *Geriatr Nurs* 15:24, 1994.
29. Hester L: Coordinating a successful discharge plan, *AJN* 6:35, 1996.
30. Hammer B: Improved coordination of care for elderly patients, *Geriatr Nurs* 17:286, 1996.
31. Rock BD and others: Research changes a health care delivery system: a biopsychosocial approach to predicting resource reutilization in hospital care of the frail elderly, *Soc Work Health Care* 22:21, 1996.
32. Dubin S: Geriatric assessment, *AJN* 5:49, 1996.
33. Fulmer T and others: Pain management protocol, *Geriatr Nurs* 17:222, 1996.
34. DeMaajd G: High-risk drugs in the elderly population, *Geriatr Nurs* 16:198, 1995.
35. Roberts RE and others: Prevalence and correlates of depression in an aging cohort: the Alameda County study, *J Geront B Psychol Sci Soc Sci* 52:S252, 1997.
36. Adamek ME, Kaplan M: Managing elder suicides: a profile of American and Canadian preventive centers, *Suicide Life Threat Behav* 26:122, 1996.
37. Lange M: The challenge of fall prevention in home care: a review of the literature, *Home Healthc Nurse* 14:198, 1996.
38. Special issue: disruptive behavior, *J Gerontol Nurs* 22:5, 1996.
39. Garrad J: The impact of the 1987 federal regulation on the use of psychotropic drugs in Minnesota nursing homes, *Am J Public Health* 85:771, 1995.
40. Bryant H, Fernald L: Nursing knowledge and use of restraint alternatives: acute and chronic care, *Geriatr Nurs* 18:57, 1997.
41. Burke M, Walsh M: *Gerontologic nursing: wholistic care of the older adult,* ed 2, St Louis, 1997, Mosby.
42. Stolley J: Freeing your patients from restraints, *AJN* 2:27, 1995.
43. Lachs MS and others: Risk factors for reported elder abuse and neglect: a nine-year observational cohort study, *Gerontologist* 37:460, 1997.
44. Special issue: elder abuse, *Aging* 367:4, 1996.
45. Nielsen J and others: Characteristics of caregivers and factors contributing to institutionalization, *Geriatr Nurs* 17:24, 1996.
46. Kelechi T, Lukas K: Meeting the needs of home care givers: a family caregiver checklist, *J Gerontol Nurs* 2:50, 1995.
47. Wykle M: The physical and mental health of women caregivers of older adults, *J Gerontol Nurs* 3:48, 1994.
48. Kroch P, Brooks J: Identifying the responsibilities and needs of working adults who are primary caregivers, *J Gerontol Nurs* 10:41, 1995.
49. Calkins M and others: *Key elements of dementia care,* Chicago, 1997, Alzheimer's Disease and Related Disorders Association.
50. Welch WP and others: A detailed comparison of physician services for the elderly in the United States and Canada, *JAMA* 275:1410, 1996.
51. *Chronic care in America: a 21st century challenge,* Princeton, NJ, 1996, The Robert Wood Johnson Foundation.
52. Just G and others: Assisted living: challenges for nursing practice, *Geriatr Nurs* 16:165, 1995.
53. Payne D, Coombes R: Old, down and out, *Nurs Times* 93:16, 1997.
54. Scruggs D: *Operating in a managed care environment,* Washington, DC, 1995, American Association of Homes and Services for the Aging.
55. Montgomery R, Kosloski, K: A longitudinal analysis of nursing home placement for dependent elders cared for by spouses vs adult children, *J Gerontol* 49:562, 1994.
56. Kaisik B, Ceslowitz S: Easing the fear of nursing home placement: the value of stress inoculation, *Geriatr Nurs* 17:182, 1996.
57. Johnson RA, Hlava C: Translocation of elders: maintaining the spirit. Nurses can build interventions into translocation plans to minimize the negative effects, *Geriatr Nurs* 15:209, 1994.
58. Allen L, Coeling H: Quality of life: its meaning to the long-term care resident, *J Gerontol Nurs* 2:20, 1995.
59. Mezey M and others: Advance directives protocol: nurses helping to protect patient's rights, *Geriatr Nurs* 17:204, 1996.
60. Special Issue: End-of-life decisions, *J Gerontol Nurs* 23:7, 1997.

Resources

Administration on Aging
330 Independence Avenue SW, Suite 4760
Washington, DC 20201
202-619-0556
http://www.aoa.dhhs.gov/

American Association of Homes and Services for the Aging
901 E Street NW, Suite 500
Washington, DC 20004
202-738-2242
Fax: 202-783-2255
http://www.aahsa.org

American Association for International Aging
1900 L Street NW, Suite 510
Washington, DC 20036-5002
202-833-8893
Fax: 202-833-8762
http://www.unm.edu/~aging/AAIAInf.html

American Association of Retired Persons (AARP)
601 E Street NW
Washington, DC 20049
202-434-2277
Fax: 202-434-2320
http://www.aarp.org/index.html

American Geriatrics Society
770 Lexington Avenue, Suite 300
New York, NY 10021
212-308-1414
800-247-4779
Fax: 212-832-8646
http://www.americangeriatrics.org

American Society on Aging
833 Market Street, Suite 516
San Francisco, CA 94130
415-974-9600
Fax: 415-974-0300
http://www.asaging.org/

Association for Adult Development & Aging
c/o American Counseling Association
5999 Stevenson Avenue
Alexandria, VA 22304-3300
703-823-9800
800-347-6647
Fax: 703-823-0252
http://www.aoa.dhhs.gov/aoa/dir/63.html

Canadian Association on Gerontology
1306 Wellington Street, Suite 500
Ottawa, ON, Canada K1Y 3B2
613-728-9347
Fax: 613-728-8913
http://www.mbnet.mb.ca/crm/ca/advoc/cag1eng.html

Canadian Coalition on Medication Use & the Elderly
1565 Carling Ave, Suite 400
Ottawa, ON K1Z 8R1 CANADA
613-725-3769

Eldercare Web
http://www.ice.net/~kstevens/living.htm

Gerontological Society of America
1275 K Street NW, Suite 350
Washington, DC 20005-4006
202-842-1275
Fax: 202-842-1150
http://www.geron.org

Geroweb
Institute of Gerontology
Wayne State University
87 East Ferry Street
Detroit, MI 48202
313-577-2297
Fax: 313-875-0127
http://www.iog.wayne.edu/IOGlinks.html

GoldenAge Net
http://elo.mediasrv.swt.edu/goldenage/Script.htm

Health After 50
http://www.enews.com/magazines/jhml

International Federation on Aging
Secretariat—Canada
380 St. Antoine St. W, Suite 3200
Montreal, Quebec, Canada H2Y 3X7
514-287-9679
Fax: 514-987-1567

International Senior Citizens Association, Inc.
255 S Hill Street, Suite 409
Los Angeles, CA 90012
213-625-5008
Fax: 213-625-7115

Meals on Wheels America
280 Broadway, Suite 214
New York, NY 10007
212-964-5700
Fax: 212-442-3162

Medicare/Medicaid
7500 Security Boulevard
Baltimore, MD 21244
410-786-3000
http://www.hcfa.gov/

National Alliance of Senior Citizens
101 Park Washington Court, Suite 125
Falls Church, VA 22046
202-986-0117
Fax: 202-986-2974

National Association of Area Agencies on Aging
1112 16th Street NW, Suite 100
Washington, DC 20036
202-296-8130
Fax: 202-296-8134
http://www.aoa.dhhs.gov/aoa/dir/132.html

National Association for Hispanic Elderly
Asociacion Nacional Por Personas Mayores
3325 Wilshire Blvd., Suite 800
Los Angeles, CA 90010
213-487-1922
Fax: 213-385-3014
http://www.aoa.dhhs.gov/aoa/dir/127.html

National Caucus & Center on Black Aged
1424 K Street NW, Suite 500
Washington, DC 20005
202-637-8400
Fax: 202-347-0895
http://www.aoa.dhhs.gov/aoa/dir/140.html

National Council on the Aging, Inc.
409 Third Street SW, Suite 200
Washington, DC 20024
202-479-1200
http://www.ncoa.org

National Council of Senior Citizens
8403 Colesville Road, Suite 1200
Silver Spring, MD 20910
301-578-8800
Fax: 301-578-8911
http://www.aoa.dhhs.gov/aoa/dir/149.html

National Gerontological Association
7250 Parkway Drive, Suite 510
Hanover, MD 21076
800-723-0560

National Gerontological Nursing Association
7250 Parkway Drive, Suite 510
Hanover, MD 21076
800-723-0560
http://www.nursingcenter.com/people/nrsorgs/ngna/page1.html

National Hispanic Council on Aging
2713 Ontario Road NW
Washington, DC 20009
202-265-1288
Fax: 202-745-2522
http://www.aoa.dhhs.gov/aoa/dir/122.html

National Indian Council on Aging
City Center, Suite 510-W
6400 Uptown Blvd NE
Albuquerque, NM 87110
505-888-3302
Fax: 505-888-3276
http://www.aoa.dhhs.gov/aoa/dir/214.html

National Institute on Aging Information Center
PO Box 8057
Gaithersburg, MD 20870-8057

Older Women's League (OWL)
666 11th Street NW, Suite 700
Washington, DC 20001
202-783-6686
Fax: 202-638-2356

U.S. Administration on Aging: Directory of Web & Gopher Aging Sites
http://www.aoa/dhhs/gov/aoa/webres/craig.htm

Action Without Borders
http://www.idealist.org

***For additional Internet resources, see the website for this book at* www.mosby.com/MERLIN/medsurg_lewis**

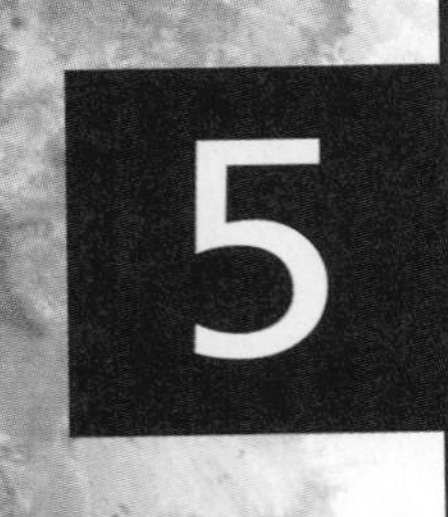

REMEMBER to check out your companion CD-ROM

5 Health History and Physical Examination

Katheryn Ellen McCash

www.mosby.com/MERLIN/medsurg_lewis

LEARNING OBJECTIVES

1. Explain the purpose, components, and techniques related to the patient history and physical examination.
2. Obtain a nursing history using a functional health pattern format.
3. Describe the appropriate use and techniques of inspection, palpation, percussion, and auscultation.
4. Identify the equipment needed to perform a physical examination.
5. Describe the indications, purposes, and components of the branching or regional examination.
6. Record a nursing history and physical examination using a standard format.

The patient history and physical examination are part of the assessment phase of the nursing process. This information provides a database about a patient's health, including potential and actual health problems, on which the other phases of the nursing process are based.[1] Numerous formats exist for taking histories in the various health care settings. These histories are described as *medical history* and *nursing history.*

Both subjective and objective information is collected. A nursing history provides subjective data about the state of the patient's health. Subjective data are supplied by the patient either as spontaneously offered information or as a response to direct questioning by the nurse. Knowledgeable others, such as family members and caregivers, can also contribute subjective data about the patient. The *general survey* statement provides a comprehensive descriptive statement about the patient. The *physical examination* provides objective data related to the health status of the patient. Objective data are gathered by the nurse through inspection, palpation, percussion, and auscultation. Additional sources of objective data include the findings of other health care providers and the results of diagnostic studies.

INTERVIEWING CONSIDERATIONS

Effective communication is a key factor in the interview process. Creating a climate of trust and respect is critical to establishing a therapeutic relationship.[2] Nurses should remember that individuals communicate not only through language but in their manner of dress, gestures, and body language. Sitting with arms crossed and a downward gaze is an example of body language that suggests an unwillingness to communicate.

Collection of data assists the examiner and the patient in identifying health problems, as well as patient strengths and resources. The nurse can use the data to identify areas where the patient may be unable to meet personal needs and therefore requires nursing assistance. The patient perceives this encounter as an indication of how the health care system will provide assistance. A direct interview technique, which is more structured, is used to collect factual, easily categorized information. Closed questions (e.g., "Have you had surgery before?") that require brief, specific responses are used.

The amount of time needed to complete a nursing history may vary with the format used and the experience of the nurse. It may be completed in one or several sessions, depending on the setting and the patient. In the case of an older adult patient with a low energy level, several short sessions may need to be scheduled. Allowing time for the patient to volunteer information about particular areas of concern enables the nurse to work with the patient to identify existing and potential health problems. When a patient is unable to provide the necessary data (e.g., is unconscious or aphasic), the nurse should ask the person who has assumed responsibility for the patient's welfare to provide as much information as possible.

Before beginning the nursing history, the nurse should explain to the patient that the purpose of a detailed history is to collect information that will provide a health profile for comprehensive health care, including health promotion. This detailed information is collected during entry into the health care system, and, subsequently, only updates are needed. The nurse should explain that personal and social data are needed

Reviewed by Sheila Dunn, RN, MSN, C-ANP, Nurse Practitioner, John Cochran Veterans Administration Medical Center, St. Louis, Mo.

to individualize the plan of care. This explanation is necessary because the patient may not be accustomed to sharing personal information and may need to know the purpose of such questioning. The nurse should assure the patient that all information will be kept confidential.

A nursing history form indicates *what to ask*, not *how to ask it*. In addition to understanding the principles of effective communication, each nurse must develop a personal style of relating to patients. Although no single style fits all people, wording specific questions in certain ways will increase the probability of eliciting the needed information. Ease at asking questions, particularly those related to sensitive areas such as sexual functioning and income, comes with experience. Videotaping and reviewing the health history interview is an effective method to use in evaluating communication techniques and identifying areas needing improvement.

To obtain accurate social and personal information, the nurse must communicate acceptance of the patient as an individual. When asking sensitive questions, the nurse can communicate the acceptance or normalcy of behaviors by prefacing questions with phrases such as "most people" or "frequently." For example, stating, "Most people have sexual concerns; do you have any you would like to discuss?" shows the patient that a particular situation may not be unique to that patient. Another method of putting the patient at ease is to word the question so that an affirmative answer appears expected. An example of this technique is to ask "What do you like to drink at a party?" instead of "Do you drink?" "How often do you drink alcohol?" is another way of obtaining information related to alcohol intake. These questions are open ended, encouraging the patient to discuss the issue in the patient's own words and at his or her own pace.[3]

The nurse must judge the reliability of the patient as a historian. An older adult may give a false impression about his or her mental status because of a prolonged response time or visual and hearing impairment. The complexity and long duration of health problems may also make it difficult for an older adult to be an accurate, orderly historian.

It is important that the nurse determine the patient's priority concerns and expectations from the present encounter. Often there is a lack of congruency between the priorities of the patient and the nurse. For example, the priority for the nurse might be to get a consent form signed, whereas the patient is interested only in getting relief from pain. Until the patient's priority need is met, the nurse will probably be unsuccessful in meeting the priority goal.

The amount of information that should be collected on initial contact with the patient is a nursing judgment based on the patient, the problem, and the setting. Interviews with older adult patients, patients with long-term chronic disease, and emergency department admissions are examples of situations in which the nurse must use this judgment. The nurse may choose to ask only those questions that are pertinent to a specific problem and to defer the complete history interview until a more appropriate time.

Medical History

The nurse and physician use different formats and analyze the data differently because of each discipline's different focus. A medical history is a standard format designed to collect data to be used primarily by the physician to diagnose a health problem (Table 5-1). However, this history is also used by nurses and other health care providers. In an inpatient setting, members of the medical team (physician, resident, and medical student) usually collect the medical history. In other settings, such as clinics and physicians' offices, the nurse may be primarily responsible for collecting the medical history.

Table 5-1 Medical History Format

Demographic data	Past health history
Chief complaint	Family health history
History of present illness	Review of systems

Nursing History—Subjective Data

A nursing history has a different focus than a medical history. Nursing is concerned with "the diagnosis and treatment of human responses to actual or potential health problems."[4] During a nursing history interview the nurse should ask questions that elicit information related to individual responses to actual or potential problems. Information obtained from this questioning will provide the necessary data to support the identification of nursing diagnoses.

The format used in this text for gathering a nursing history is based on a patient's functional health patterns (Table 5-2). Gordon[1] has described an assessment format, which specifies functional areas that are collected regardless of the conceptual framework being used. Analysis of each functional health pattern facilitates the nursing diagnosis process. The format is designed to gather information systematically to determine the presence of actual, risk, or possible nursing diagnoses. Subjective data are collected related to each functional health pattern. Objective data are collected using a systems approach.

At any time during the history or physical examination the patient may relate a symptom such as pain, fatigue, or weakness. Because symptoms are directly experienced by the patient and not observable to the nurse, the symptom must be investigated. Table 5-3 lists eight areas that should be investigated if a symptom is present. The information that is obtained may help determine the cause of the symptom. For example, if a patient states that he has "pain in his leg at times," the provider may obtain and record the following information:

> Has right midcalf pain *(location)*, described as "like being stabbed with a knife" *(quality)*. Pain is so severe that it is not possible for the patient to continue walking *(quantity)*. Onset is abrupt, lasting for 1 to 2 minutes; it occurs once or twice daily, and it last occurred on 5/5/99 *(chronology)*. Generally occurs at work when climbing stairs after lunch, but last occurred when cutting lawn *(setting)*. Pain is alleviated by rest for 2 to 3 minutes. The patient has been salting his food "more heavily" than he used to, but "it doesn't help" *(alleviating factor)*. Leg pain is at times accompanied by chest pain that causes some nausea *(associated manifestations)*. The patient has not altered his lifestyle because of the intermittent pain. He thinks it is caused by "muscle cramps from lack of salt" *(personal meaning)*.

Important Health Information. Important health information provides an overview of past and present medical conditions and treatments. Past health history, medications, and surgery or other treatments are included in this part of the history.

Table 5-2 Nursing History: Functional Health Pattern Format

Demographic Data
Name, address, age, occupation

Important Health Information
Past health history
Medications
Surgery or other treatments

Functional Health Patterns

Health Perception–Health Management Pattern
1. Reason for visit?
2. General state of health?
3. Any colds in past year?
4. Most important things done to keep healthy? Breast self-exam? Testicular self-exam? Other routine screening?
5. Health compliance problems?
6. Cause of illness? Action taken? Results?
7. Things important to you while here?
8. Family health history?
9. Illness and injury risk factors: use of cigarettes, alcohol, drugs?
10. Allergies? Immunizations?

Nutritional-Metabolic Pattern
1. Typical daily food intake (describe)? Supplements?
2. Typical daily fluid intake (describe)?
3. Weight loss or gain (amount, time span)?
4. Desired weight?
5. Appetite?
6. Food or eating: Discomfort? Diet restrictions?
7. Appetite?
8. Heal well or poorly?
9. Skin problems: Lesions? Dryness?
10. Dental problems?
11. Change in appetite with anxiety?
12. Food preferences?
13. Food allergies?

Elimination Pattern
1. Bowel elimination pattern (describe): Frequency? Character? Discomfort? Laxatives? Enemas?
2. Urinary elimination pattern (describe): Frequency? Problem in control? Diuretics?
3. Any external devices?
4. Excess perspiration? Odor problems? Itching?

Activity-Exercise Pattern
1. Sufficient energy for desired or required activities?
2. Exercise pattern? Type? Regularity?
3. Spare time (leisure) activities?
4. Dyspnea? Chest pain? Palpitations? Stiffness? Aching? Weakness?
5. Perceived ability for (code for level):
   Feeding ______ Cooking ______
   Grooming ______ Bed mobility ______
   Bathing ______ Home maintenance ______
   General mobility ______ Dressing ______
   Toileting ______ Shopping ______

Sleep-Rest Pattern
1. Generally rested and ready for daily activities after sleep?
2. Sleep onset problems? Aids? Dreams (nightmares)? Early awakening?
3. Usual sleep rituals?
4. Usual sleep pattern?

Cognitive-Perceptual Pattern
1. Hearing difficulty? Aid?
2. Vision? Wear glasses? Last checked?
3. Any change in taste? Any change in smell?
4. Any recent change in memory?
5. Easiest way to learn things?
6. Any discomfort? Pain? How managed?
7. Ability to communicate?
8. Understanding of illness?
9. Understanding of treatments?

Self-Perception–Self-Concept Pattern
1. Self-description? Self-perception?
2. Effect of illness on self-image?
3. Relieving factors?

Role-Relationship Pattern
1. Live alone? Family? Family structure diagram?
2. Difficult family problems?
3. Family problem solving?
4. Family dependence on you for things? How managing?
5. Family's and others' feelings about illness/hospitalization?*
6. Problems with children? Difficulty handling?*
7. Belong to social groups? Have close friends? Feel lonely (frequency)?
8. Work satisfaction (school)? Income sufficient for needs?*
9. Feel part of or isolated to neighborhood where living?

Sexuality-Reproductive Pattern
1. Any changes or problems in sexual relations?*
2. Effect of illness?
3. Use of contraceptives? Problems?
4. When menstruation started? Last menstrual period? Menstrual problems? Gravida?† Para?
5. Effect of present condition or treatment on sexuality?
6. Sexually transmitted diseases?

Coping–Stress Tolerance Pattern
1. Tense a lot of the time? What helps? Use any medicines, drugs, alcohol?
2. Have someone to confide in? Available to you now?
3. Recent life changes?
4. Problem-solving techniques? Effective?

Value-Belief Pattern
1. Satisfied with life?
2. Religion important in your life?
3. Conflict between treatment and beliefs?

Other
1. Other important issues?
2. Questions?

Functional levels code
Level 0: Full self-care
Level I: Requires use of equipment or device
Level II: Requires assistance or supervision from another person
Level III: Is dependent and does not participate

Modified from Fuller J, Schaller-Ayers J: *Health assessment, a nursing approach,* ed 3, Philadelphia, 1998, JB Lippincott.
*If appropriate.
†For women.

Table 5-3 Investigation of a Symptom

Location	
Ask:	"Where do you feel it? Where is it located?"
Record:	Region of the body Local or radiating, superficial or deep
Quality	
Ask:	"What does it (feel, look) like?"
Record:	The patient's analogy (e.g., "Like being burned")
Quantity	
Ask:	"How often do you have this feeling? How bad is it? How much is it? How big is it?"
Record:	Frequency (mild, moderate, severe), volume, size, extent, number
Chronology	
Ask:	"When was the first time it occurred? Any particular time of day, week, month, or year?"
Record:	Time of onset, duration, periodicity and frequency, course of symptoms
Setting	
Ask:	"Where are you when this occurs? What are you doing?"
Record:	Where patient is when symptom occurs, what patient is doing, if symptom is related to anything
Aggravating or Alleviating Factors	
Ask:	"What makes it better? Worse? Is there any activity that seems to cause it? What have you done for it? Did it help? Was there some reason you didn't do anything about it?"
Record:	Influence of physical and emotional activities, patient's attempts to alleviate (or treat) the symptom
Associated Manifestations	
Ask:	"What other things do you see or feel when it occurs? Has it affected your appetite? Elimination? Sleeping?"
Record:	Other symptoms
Meaning of the Symptom to the Patient	
Ask:	"How has it affected your life? Why have you sought care now? What do you think may be the cause?"
Record:	Patient's statements about the effect of the symptom and the cause of the symptom

Past health history. The past health history provides information about the patient's prior state of health. The patient is specifically asked about major childhood and adult illnesses, injuries, hospitalizations, operations, therapeutic regimens, travel, habits, and the use of supportive devices. Specific questioning is more effective than simply asking if the patient has had any illness or health problems in the past.

Medications. Specific details related to past or present medications are obtained. This includes the use of prescription medications, over-the-counter medications, and any vitamins or herbal substances. Examples of specific medications to ask about include steroids, birth control pills, antibiotics, diuretics, aspirin, antacids, and laxatives. Older adult patients, in particular, should be questioned about medication routines. Changes in absorption, metabolism, reaction to drugs, and elimination of drugs, as well as surgery and concurrent disease, make drug-related concerns a serious potential problem for older adults.[5]

Surgery or other treatments. All injuries, hospitalizations, and surgeries are recorded along with the date of the event, the treatment, and the outcome (whether the problem was completely resolved). Blood transfusions received by the patient also are noted.

Functional Health Patterns. The nurse assesses the patient's functional patterns (strengths), dysfunctional health patterns (nursing diagnoses), and potential dysfunctional patterns (risk conditions). Use of the functional health pattern framework for assessment assists the nurse in differentiating between areas for independent nursing intervention and areas requiring collaboration or referral. Table 5-4 presents an overview of the content usually included in each functional health pattern.

Health perception–health management pattern. Assessment of the health perception–health management functional health pattern focuses on the patient's perceived level of health and well-being and on personal practices for maintaining health. This includes preventive screening activities, such as breast and testicular examinations; colorectal cancer, hypertension, and cardiac risk factor screening; and Papanicolaou's (Pap) test.

The questions for this pattern also seek to identify risk factors by obtaining a family history, history of health habits (e.g., smoking, alcohol, and drug use), and exposure to environmental hazards.

There are several ways to identify the patient's perceived level of health and well-being. First, when questioning the patient, the nurse determines the patient's feelings of effectiveness at staying healthy by asking what helps and what hinders.

Next, the patient is asked to describe personal health and any concerns about it. This information should be recorded in

Table 5-4 Overview of Functional Health Patterns

Health Perception–Health Management Pattern
- Description of health (usual); description of present illness (onset, course, treatment)
- Relevance of health to activities
- Preventive measures, general health care behavior
- Previous hospitalizations, expectations of this hospitalization
- Potential self-care problems

Nutritional-Metabolic Pattern
- Usual food and fluid intake; appetite
- Daily eating times
- Recent weight change and reason
- Food restrictions or preferences, food supplements
- Swallowing, chewing, eating problems, food allergies
- Skin lesions and general ability to heal
- Condition of skin, hair, nails, mucous membranes, and teeth
- Temperature, pulse, respiration, height, weight

Elimination Pattern

Bowel
- Usual time, frequency, color, consistency
- Assistive devices (laxatives, suppositories, enemas)
- Constipation, diarrhea

Bladder
- Usual frequency
- Problems with dysuria or polyuria
- Assistive devices

Skin condition
- Color, temperature
- Turgor, lesions, edema, pruritus

Activity-Exercise Pattern
- Exercise, activity, leisure, and recreation patterns
- Limitations in activities of daily living

Sleep-Rest Pattern
- Usual sleep routine, sleep pattern
- Perception of quality and quantity of sleep

Cognitive-Perceptual Pattern
- Sensory adequacy—hearing, sight, smell, touch, taste
- Prosthetic devices (glasses, hearing aids)
- Pain
- Problems with vertigo
- Heat or cold sensitivity
- Language, understanding, memory abilities

Self-Perception–Self-Concept Pattern
- Self-description
- Effects of illness on self
- Perception, body image, identity, self-esteem
- Posture, eye contact, voice and speech patterns

Role-Relationship Pattern
- Life roles and responsibilities
- Satisfaction or dissatisfaction in family, work, and social relationships

Sexuality-Reproductive Pattern
- Sexuality patterns and satisfaction or dissatisfaction with
- Adequacy of sexual knowledge
- Reproductive state (female—premenopausal or postmenopausal)

Coping–Stress Tolerance Pattern
- General coping strategies
- Stress tolerance, stress reduction behaviors
- Support systems
- Ability to manage situations

Value-Belief Pattern
- Values, goals, beliefs that are basis for decisions
- Value or belief conflict
- Spiritual practices

the patient's own words. It often is useful to determine whether the patient considers his or her health to be excellent, good, fair, or poor.

In addition, the patient is asked about a family history of major problems, such as cardiovascular disease, hypertension, cancer, diabetes mellitus, psychiatric illness, and genetic disorders. Information about sexual abuse, violence, and drug and alcohol abuse should also be obtained. The patient should be asked about immunization history and allergies. One of the objectives in this pattern is to identify any preventive measures used by the patient to promote personal health.

If the patient is hospitalized, expectations of this hospitalization should be determined. A description of the patient's understanding of the current health problem, including a description of its onset, course, and treatment, should be obtained. Determining what the patient does when not well is important. These questions elicit information about a patient's knowledge of the health problem, awareness of what should be done, and ability to use appropriate resources to manage the problem.

The nurse also assesses the patient's developmental stage in this pattern. This ensures that care appropriate for the developmental capabilities of the patient is planned.

Nutritional-metabolic pattern. The processes of ingestion, digestion, absorption, transport, and metabolism are assessed in this pattern. A 24-hour dietary recall should be obtained from the patient. From this information the nurse can evaluate the quantity and quality of foods and fluids consumed. If a problem is identified, the nurse may request that the patient keep a 3-day food diary for a more careful analysis of dietary intake. Food frequency questionnaires are also available to obtain information from the person. Questions regarding weight gain, weight loss, and energy level should be asked to evaluate metabolism.

The impact of psychologic factors such as depression, anxiety, and self-concept on nutrition is assessed. For example, "How is your appetite affected by anxiety?" is an appropriate question. Sociocultural factors such as food budget, who prepares the meals, and food preferences are also assessed.

Determining how the patient's present condition has interfered with eating and appetite is important. If the patient's present condition has produced symptoms such as nausea, gas, or pain, the effect of these symptoms on appetite should be determined. Food allergies and the need for a special or restricted diet should be noted. Additional information about the person's nutritional status can be determined by asking specific questions such as the following:

"How many fruits and vegetables do you eat a day?"
"Give me an example of your usual intake of meat."
"How well do you heal from a wound?"

Elimination pattern. The nurse assesses bowel, bladder, and skin function in this pattern. The nurse asks about the frequency of bowel and bladder activity. A description of consistency, amount, color, and unusual odor should be elicited. The patient should be asked if loss of control or pain are associated with defecating or urinating. If laxatives or enemas are used, the frequency, type, and results should be noted. If any collecting devices are used, such as catheter or colostomy equipment, the nurse asks about their care.

The skin is also assessed in this pattern in terms of its excretory function. The patient should be asked about the condition of his or her skin, the presence of any lesions, and whether edema or pruritus are problematic.

Activity-exercise pattern. The patient's usual pattern of exercise, activity, leisure, and recreation is assessed by the nurse. The patient should be questioned about his or her ability to perform activities of daily living. Table 5-2 includes the grading scale for self-care abilities under the activity-exercise pattern. If the patient is unable to perform activities of daily living, such as toileting, eating, and moving independently, the specific problems that limit an activity should be noted. Chest pain, dyspnea, dizziness, claudication, musculoskeletal pain, fatigue, and weakness are problems that commonly result in some degree of self-care deficit.

Sleep-rest pattern. This pattern describes the patient's pattern of sleep, rest, and relaxation in a 24-hour period. The individual's perception of the effectiveness of sleep and relaxation is pertinent. This information can be elicited by asking, "Do you feel rested when you wake up?" Most people take sleep for granted unless they have a problem with sleeping.

The patient's usual activities related to bedtime and the usual sleep pattern should be determined. Particular routines, position, and environmental factors used to foster sleep should also be elicited.

Cognitive-perceptual pattern. Assessment of this pattern involves a description of all senses (vision, hearing, taste, touch, and smell) and the cognitive functions such as communication, memory, and decision making. The patient should be asked about any sensory deficits that affect the ability to perform activities of daily living. Routine eye care, including the date of the last examination, should be elicited. Ways in which the patient compensates for any sensory-perceptual problems should be discussed and noted. Patients should be asked how they communicate best and about their understanding of their illness and treatments. This information is used by the nurse in planning for patient education.

In addition, pain is assessed in this pattern. See Chapter 9 for details on pain assessment.

Self-perception–self-concept pattern. This pattern describes the patient's self-concept, which is critical in determining the way the person interacts with others. Included are attitudes about self, perception of personal abilities, body image, and general sense of worth.[6]

The nurse should ask the patient for a self-description and how the health condition affects self-attitude. Nurses should avoid making value judgments about how people perceive themselves. What concerns the patient about a personal situation may differ from what concerns the nurse. For example, the patient may feel cheated by the system when denied disability benefits. The nurse may feel the patient was not eligible for the benefit.

Role-relationship pattern. This pattern describes the roles and relationships of the patient, including major responsibilities. It also examines the patient's self-evaluation of his or her performance of the expected behaviors related to these roles.

The patient should be asked to describe family, social, and work relationships. The nurse should determine if patterns in these relationships are satisfactory or if strain is evident. The nurse should note the patient's feelings about his or her role in these relationships and the effect the present condition has on his or her role and relationship.

Sexuality-reproductive pattern. This pattern describes satisfaction or dissatisfaction with personal sexuality and describes the reproductive pattern. Assessing this pattern is important because many illnesses, surgical procedures, and medications affect sexual function. A patient's sexual and reproductive concerns may be expressed, teaching needs and treatable problems may be identified, and normal growth and development may be monitored through information obtained in this pattern.

The interview should be appropriate to the sex, age, and developmental stage of the patient. For example, a 60-year-old widowed female patient might be asked if she has any problems related to her genital area, such as vaginal discharge. However, a 25-year-old single male patient might be asked about his knowledge and use of condoms.

Obtaining information related to sexuality often is difficult for the inexperienced nurse. However, a beginning nurse, with no advanced education or experience related to sexual issues, should take a health history and screen for sexual function and dysfunction. Based on the complexity of the problem, this nurse may be able to provide limited information or refer the patient to a more experienced professional.

Specifically, the nurse should determine if there is a lack of knowledge in relation to sexuality and reproduction. Whether the patient perceives a problem in the area of sexuality should also be determined. The effect of the patient's present condition or treatment on personal sexuality should be noted.

Coping–stress tolerance pattern. This pattern describes the general coping pattern and the effectiveness of the coping mechanisms. Assessment of this pattern involves analyzing the specific stressors or problems that confront the patient, the patient's perception of the stressor, and the patient's response to the stressor.

The major losses or changes experienced by the patient in the previous year are important to document. Current major stressors confronting the patient are also important. The strategies used by the patient to deal with stressors and relieve tension should be noted. The person on whom the patient can rely when problems arise should be recorded.

Value-belief pattern. This pattern describes the values, goals, and beliefs (including spiritual) that guide health-related choices.[1] The patient's ethnic background and the effects of culture and beliefs on health practices should be noted. The patient's beliefs about health and illness should be documented. The patient's wishes about continuation of religious practices and the use of religious articles should be noted and honored. The possibility of a conflict in values or beliefs can be determined by asking a question such as, "Does your plan of care cause any conflict in your value or belief system?"

Objective Data

General Survey. Following the nursing history, a general survey statement is made. The general survey is a statement of the provider's general impression of a patient, including behavioral observations. This initial survey is considered a scanning procedure and begins with the provider's first encounter with the patient and continues during the health history interview.

Although the provider may include other data that seem pertinent, the major areas usually included in the general survey statement are (1) body features, (2) state of consciousness and arousal, (3) speech, (4) body movements, (5) obvious physical signs, (6) nutritional status, and (7) behavior. Vital signs, height, and weight are often included in the general survey statement. Observations of these areas provide the data for the general survey statement. The following is a sample of a general survey statement:

> Mrs. H. is a 34-year-old Hispanic woman, BP 130/84/80, P 88, R 18. No distinguishing body features. Alert but anxious. Speech rapid with trailing thoughts. Wringing hands and shuffling feet during interview. Skin flushed, hands clammy. Overweight relative to height. Sits with eyes downcast and shoulders slumped and avoids eye contact.

Physical Examination. The physical examination is the systematic assessment of the physical and mental status of a patient and is considered objective data. During the physical examination, additional subjective data may be obtained from the patient. This may occur as a result of direct questioning by the nurse in response to a finding or as a result of the patient remembering a forgotten piece of information.

Throughout the history and physical examination, any positive findings are explored using the same criteria as the investigation of a symptom (see Table 5-3). A positive finding indicates that the patient has or had the particular problem or symptom under discussion. For example, if the patient answers "yes" to a question about chest pain, it is a positive finding. Relevant information about this problem should then be gathered.

Negative findings may also be significant. A negative finding is the absence of a symptom usually associated with a problem. For example, peripheral edema is common with congestive heart failure. If edema is not present in a patient with congestive heart failure, this should be specifically noted as "no peripheral edema." Another type of negative finding is the absence of usual health promotion practices. Lack of tetanus immunization is an example of a negative finding that should be recorded.

Types. There are two types of physical examinations: the screening physical examination and the branching or regional examination. The screening physical examination is performed for screening situations, health surveillance, and health maintenance purposes. It is an organized, purposeful check of major body systems to detect any possible problems. If a problem is detected in the course of the screening physical examination, a more detailed branching examination of the involved system should be done.

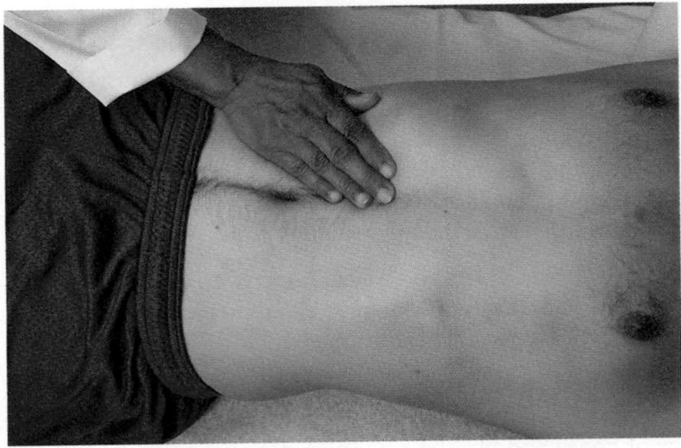

Fig. 5-1 Palpation is the examination of the body through the use of touch.

A branching or regional examination is a more detailed assessment of a particular body system. The patient's clinical manifestations should alert the nurse to the appropriate branching examination. For example, abdominal pain indicates the need to do a branching examination of the abdomen. Some problems necessitate more than one branching examination. A complaint of headache indicates the need to do musculoskeletal, neurologic, head and neck, and psychiatric examinations.

Techniques. Four major techniques are used in performing the physical examination: inspection, palpation, percussion, and auscultation.

Inspection. Inspection is the visual examination of a part or region of the body to assess normal conditions or deviations from normal. Inspection is more than just looking. This technique is deliberate, systematic, and focused. The nurse needs to compare what is seen with the known, generally visible characteristics of the body part being inspected. For example, most 30-year-old men have hair on their legs. Absence of hair may indicate a vascular problem and signals the need for further investigation. This same absence of hair in a 70-year-old man may represent a normal skin change of aging.

Palpation. Palpation is the examination of the body through the use of touch. The use of light and deep palpation can yield information related to masses, pulsations, organ enlargement, tenderness or pain, swelling, muscular spasm or rigidity, elasticity, vibration of voice sounds, crepitus, moisture, and differences in texture.[7] The nurse will learn that different parts of the hand are more sensitive for specific assessments. For example, the tips of the fingers are used to palpate lymph nodes, the dorsa of hands and fingers are used to assess temperatures, and the palmar surface is best suited for feeling vibrations (Fig. 5-1).

Percussion. Percussion is an assessment technique involving the production of sound to obtain information about the underlying area. The percussion sound may be produced directly or indirectly. Direct percussion is performed by directly tapping the body with one or two fingers to elicit a sound.

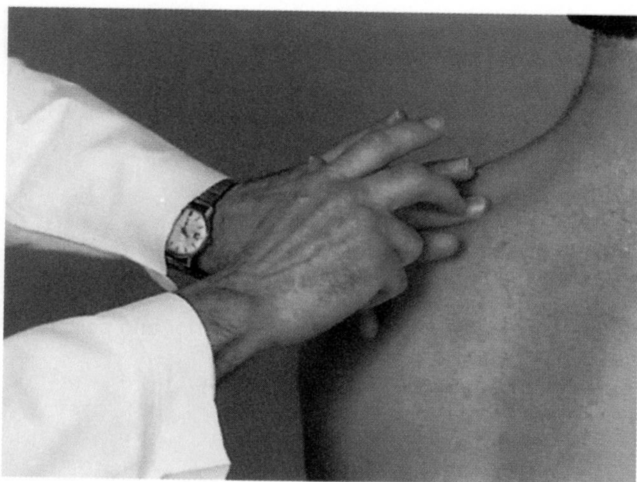

Fig. 5-2 Percussion technique: tapping the interphalangeal joint. Only the middle finger of the nondominant hand should be in contact with the skin surface.

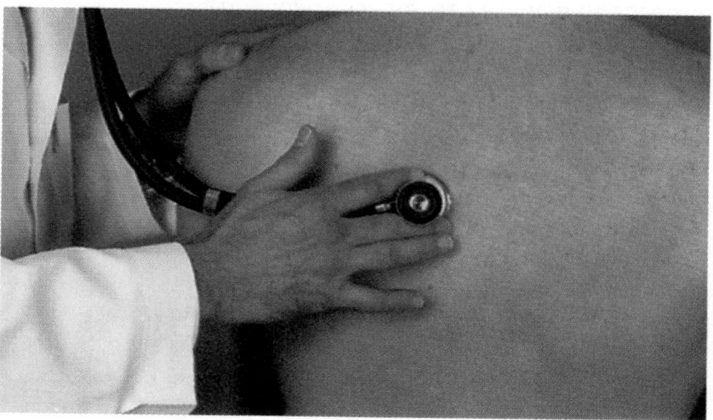

Fig. 5-3 Auscultation is listening to sounds produced by the body to assess normal conditions and deviations from normal.

Indirect or mediated percussion is the more common percussion technique. The middle finger (pleximeter) of the nondominant hand is placed firmly against the body surface. The tip of the middle finger of the dominant hand (plexor) strikes the distal phalanx of the pleximeter finger (Fig. 5-2). A relaxed wrist and rapid strike produce the best sounds. The sounds and the vibrations produced are evaluated relative to the underlying structures. Deviation from an expected sound may indicate a problem. For example, the usual percussion sound in the right lower quadrant of the abdomen is tympany. Dullness in this area may indicate a problem that should be investigated. (Specific percussion sounds of various body parts and regions are discussed in the appropriate assessment chapters.)

Auscultation. Auscultation is listening to sounds produced by the body to assess normal conditions and deviations from normal. Auscultation is usually indirect, using a stethoscope to amplify sounds (Fig. 5-3). The bell of the stethoscope is more sensitive to low-pitched sounds. The diaphragm of the stethoscope is more sensitive to high-pitched sounds. Auscultation is particularly useful in evaluating sounds from the heart, lungs, abdomen, and vascular system. (Specific auscultatory sounds are discussed in the appropriate assessment chapters.)

Table 5-5 Equipment for Screening Physical Examination
Stethoscope (with bell and diaphragm, tubing 15-18 in [38-46 cm])
Wristwatch (with second hand or digitalized)
Blood pressure cuff
Ophthalmoscope/otoscope set
Eye chart (wall chart or Snellen pocket eye card)
Pocket flashlight
Tongue blades
Cotton balls
Percussion hammer
Tuning fork
Alcohol swabs
Patient gown
Paper cup with water
Examining table or bed

Not all assessment techniques are appropriate for all body parts and systems. The nurse will learn which technique to use to elicit the most information. The physical assessment techniques are usually performed in the sequence of inspection, palpation, percussion, and auscultation. The only exception to this sequence is for the abdominal examination. In this situation the sequence is inspection, auscultation, percussion, and palpation. Palpation and percussion of the abdomen before auscultation can alter bowel sounds and produce false findings.

Equipment. The equipment needed for the physical examination should be easily accessible during the examination (Table 5-5). Organizing equipment before the examination saves the time and energy of the patient and the nurse. Lack of organization can discourage the patient from the trust and confidence the nurse needs to collect the database. (The use of specific pieces of equipment is discussed in the appropriate assessment chapters.)

Developing a system. The physical examination should be performed systematically and efficiently. Explanations should be given to the patient as the examination proceeds. The factors to be considered are the nurse's efficiency and the patient's comfort, safety, and privacy. The examiner is less likely to forget a procedure, a step in the sequence, or a portion of the body if the same sequence is followed every time. Table 5-6 presents an outline for the screening physical examination that is organized, logical, and complete. Adaptations of the physical examination often are useful for the older adult patient who may have age-related problems such as decreased mobility, limited energy, and perceptual changes.[8] An outline listing some of the useful adaptations is found in Table 5-7.

Recording the screening physical examination. Only abnormal findings should be recorded during the actual examination. This prevents needless interruptions in the examination to write lengthy normal findings. At the conclusion of the examination, the nurse should combine the normal and abnormal findings in a carefully recorded physical examination. Table 5-8 is an example of how to record a screening physical on a healthy adult. Table 4-1, Age-Related Changes in Assessment, and the age-related assessment findings in each assessment chapter are helpful references in recording age-related assessment differences.

Table 5-6 Outline for Screening Physical Examination

1. General Survey

Observe general state of health (patient is seated)

- Body features
- State of consciousness and arousal
- Speech
- Body movements
- Physical signs
- Nutritional status
- Stature

2. Vital Signs

Record vital signs:

- Blood pressure
- Radial pulse
- Respiration

Record height and weight

3. Integument

Inspect and palpate skin for the following:

- Color
- Lesions
- Scars
- Bruises
- Edema
- Moisture
- Texture
- Temperature
- Turgor
- Vascularity

Inspect and palpate nails for the following:

- Color
- Lesions
- Size
- Flexibility
- Shape
- Angle

4. Head and Neck

Inspect and palpate head for the following:

- Shape and symmetry of skull
- Masses
- Tenderness
- Hair
- Scalp
- Skin
- Temporal arteries
- Temporomandibular joint
- Sensory (CN V, light touch, pain)
- Motor (CN VII, shows teeth, purses lips, raises eyebrows)
- Looks up, wrinkles forehead (CN VII)
- Raises shoulders against resistance (CN XI)

Inspect and palpate (occasionally auscultate) neck for the following:

- Skin (vascularity and visible pulsations)
- Symmetry
- Postural alignment
- Range of motion
- Pulses and bruits (carotid)
- Midline structure (trachea, thyroid gland, cartilage)
- Lymph nodes (preauricular, postauricular, occipital, mandibular, tonsillar, submental, anterior and posterior cervical, infraclavicular, supraclavicular)

Inspect and palpate eyes for the following:

- Visual acuity
- Eyebrows
- Position and movement of eyelids
- Visual fields
- Extraocular movements (CN III, IV, VI)
- Cornea, sclera, conjunctiva
- Pupillary response
- Red reflex
- Eyeball tension

Inspect and palpate ears for the following:

- Placement
- Pinna
- Auditory acuity (Weber's or Rinne, whispered voice, ticking watch)
- Mastoid process
- Auditory canal
- Tympanic membrane

Inspect and palpate nose and sinuses for the following:

- External nose
  - Shape
  - Blockage
- Internal nose
  - Patency of nasal passages
  - Shape
  - Turbinates or polyps
  - Discharge
- Frontal and maxillary sinuses

Inspect and palpate mouth for the following:

- Lips (symmetry, lesions, color)
- Buccal mucosa (Stensen's and Wharton's ducts)
- Teeth (absence, state of repair, color)
- Gums
- Tongue for strength (asymmetry, ability to stick out tongue, side to side, fasciculations)
- Palates
- Tonsils and pillars
- Uvular elevation (CN IX)
- Posterior pharynx
- Gag reflex (CN X)
- Jaw strength (CN XI)
- Moisture
- Color
- Floor of mouth

Continued

Table 5-6 Outline for Screening Physical Examination—cont'd

5. Extremities
Observe size and shape, symmetry and deformity, involuntary movements
Inspect and palpate arms, fingers, wrists, elbows, shoulders for the following:
- Strength
- Range of motion
- Crepitus
- Joint pain
- Swelling
- Fluid

Test reflexes:
- Biceps
- Triceps
- Brachioradialis
- Patellar
- Achilles
- Plantar

Inspect and palpate legs for the following:
- Strength of hips
- Edema
- Hair distribution
- Pulses (dorsalis pedis, posterior tibialis)

6. Posterior Thorax
Inspect for muscular development, respiratory movement, approximation of AP diameter
- Palpate for symmetry of respiratory movement, tenderness of CVA, spinous processes, tumors or swelling, tactile fremitus
- Percuss for pulmonary resonance
- Auscultate for breath sounds

7. Anterior Thorax
- Assess breasts for configuration, symmetry, dimpling of skin
- Assess nipples for rash, direction, inversion, retraction
- Initiate teaching or review of breast self-exam
- Inspect for PMI, other precordial pulsations
- Palpate for thrills, lifts, heaves, tenderness over precordium
- Inspect neck for venous distention, pulsations, waves
- Palpate axillae
- Palpate breasts
- Auscultate for rate and rhythm, character of S_1 and S_2 in the aortic, pulmonic, Erb's point, tricuspid, mitral areas; bruits at carotid, epigastrium; breath sounds at RML

8. Abdomen
- Inspect for scars, shape, symmetry, bulging, muscular position and condition of umbilicus, movements (respiratory, pulsations, presence of peristaltic waves)
- Auscultate for peristalsis, bruits
- Percuss border of liver, four abdominal quadrants
- Palpate to confirm positive findings; check liver (size, surface contour, tenderness); spleen; kidney (size, contour, consistency, tenderness, mobility); urinary bladder (distention); femoral pulses; inguinofemoral nodes

9. Completion of Examinations of Extremities
Observe the following:
- Range of motion of hips, knees, ankles, feet
- Crepitus
- Joint pain
- Swelling
- Fluid
- Muscle development
- Coordination (heel to shin)
- Homan's sign
- Proprioception (position sense of great toe)

10. Neurologic
- Motor status observations
  - Gait
  - Toe walk
  - Heel walk
  - Drift
- Coordination
  - Finger to nose
  - Romberg's sign
- Spine (scoliosis)

11. Genitalia*
Male external genitalia
- Inspect penis, noting hair distribution, prepuce, glans, urethral meatus, scars, ulcers, eruptions, structural alterations
- Inspect epidermis of perineum, rectum
- Inspect skin of scrotum; palpate for descended testes, masses, pain

Female external genitalia
- Inspect hair distribution; mons pubis, labia (minora and majora); urethral meatus; Bartholin's, urethral, Skene's glands (may also be palpated, if indicated); introitus
- Assess for presence of cystocele, rectocele, prolapse
- Inspect perineum, rectum

*If the nurse has the appropriate training, the speculum and bimanual examination of women and the prostate gland examination of men should be performed after this inspection.
AP, anteroposterior; *CVA,* costovertebral angle; *PMI,* point of maximal impulse; *RML,* right middle lobe.

GERONTOLOGIC DIFFERENCES IN ASSESSMENT

Table 5-7 Adaptations in Physical Assessment Techniques

General Approach
Keep patient warm and comfortable, because loss of subcutaneous fat decreases ability to stay warm. Adapt positioning to physical limitations. Avoid unnecessary changes in position. Perform as many activities as possible in the position of comfort for the patient.

Skin
Handle with care because of fragility and loss of subcutaneous fat.

Head and Neck
Provide a quiet environment free from distraction because of patient's sensory deficits (e.g., decreased vision, touch, hearing).

Extremities
Use nonvigorous movements and reinforcement techniques. Avoid having patient hop on one foot or perform deep knee bends because of patient's limited range of motion of the extremities, decreased reflexes, and diminished sense of balance.

Thorax
Adapt examination for changes due to decrease in force of expiration, weakened cough reflex, and shortness of breath.

Abdomen
Be cautious in palpating patient's liver because it is easily palpated with increased size. The older adult patient may have diminished pain perception in abdominal wall.

Genitalia
Use a well-lubricated, smaller speculum for vaginal examination because dryness and atrophy of the female genitalia may cause discomfort.

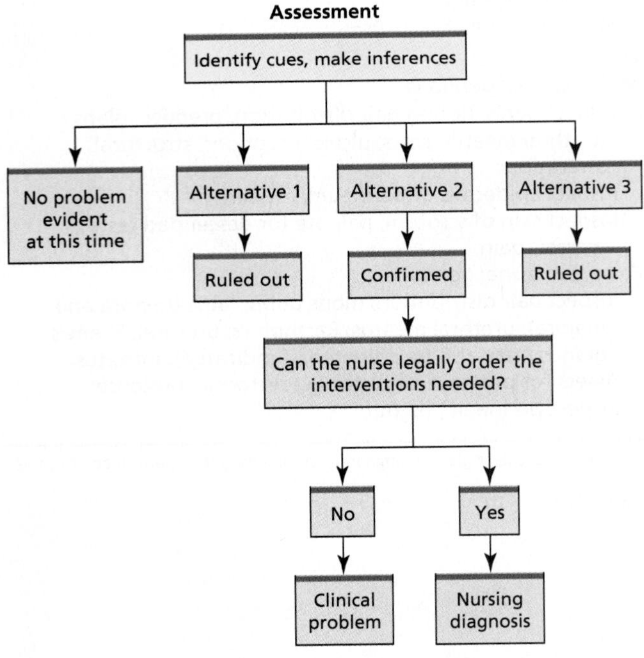

Fig. 5-4 Problem identification phase of the nursing process.

PROBLEM IDENTIFICATION AND NURSING DIAGNOSES

After completing the history and physical examination, the nurse is ready to develop a list of nursing diagnoses and collaborative problems. Figure 5-4 illustrates the problem identification phase of the nursing process.

Nursing diagnoses are health-related problems that are managed primarily by nursing care. (Chapter 1 explains the process of establishing nursing diagnoses.)

REVIEW QUESTIONS

The number of the question corresponds to the same-numbered objective at the beginning of the chapter.

1. The nursing history provides information to assist the nurse primarily in
   a. diagnosing a medical problem.
   b. investigating patient's symptoms.
   c. classifying subjective and objective data.
   d. supporting identification of nursing diagnoses.
2. The nurse would place information that the patient revealed about his concern that his illness is threatening his job security in which of the following functional health patterns?
   a. health perception–health management
   b. cognitive-perceptual
   c. role-relationship
   d. coping–stress tolerance

Table 5-8 Recording a Screening Physical Examination

Patient's Name ______________________

Age _______

General Status

Well-nourished, well-hydrated, well-developed Caucasian (woman) or (man) in NAD, appears stated age, looks pleasant, smiles readily, speech clear and evenly paced; is alert and oriented × 3; cooperative, calm

Skin

Clear s̄ lesions, warm and dry, trunk warmer than extremities, turgor returns quickly, no ↑ vascularity, no varicose veins

Nails

Well-groomed, round 160-degree angle s̄ lesions, nail beds pink, nails flexible

Hair

Thick, brown, shiny, normal (male, female) distribution

Head

Normocephalic, sinuses nontender

Eyes

Visual fields intact on gross confrontation

VA: OD 20/20
OS 20/20
OU 20/20
s̄ glasses

EOM: Intact on all gazes s̄ ptosis, nystagmus

Fundi: Red reflex present bilat no opacities, fundi WNL

Pupils: PERRLA, negative cover and uncover tests, negative Hirschberg test

Ears

Pinna intact, in proper alignment; external canal patent; small amount cerumen present; TMs intact; pearly gray LM, LR visible, not bulging; Rinne: AC>BC; Weber's: does not lateralize, whisper heard at 3 ft

Nose

Patent bilaterally; turbinates pink, no swelling

Mouth

Moist and pink, soft and hard palates intact, uvula rises midline on "ahh," 24 teeth present and in good repair

Throat

Tonsils surgically removed, no redness

Tongue

Moist, pink, size appropriate for mouth

Neck

Supple, s̄ masses, s̄ bruits, lymph nodes nonpalpable and nontender

Thyroid: Palpable, smooth, not enlarged

ROM: Full, intact, strong

Trachea: Midline, nontender

Breasts

Soft, nonpendulous, s̄ venous pattern, s̄ dimpling, puckering

Nipples: s̄ inversion, point in same direction, areola dark and symmetric, no discharge, no masses, nontender

Axilla

Hair present, shaved, no lesions, nontender

Lungs

No increase in AP diameter, resp rate 18, reg rhythm, no ↑ in tactile fremitus, no tenderness, lungs resonant throughout, diaphragmatic excursion 4 cm bilaterally, lung fields clear throughout

Heart

Rate 82, reg rate and rhythm; no lifts, heaves

PMI: 5th ICS at MCL; nonpalpable thrills; S_1, S_2 louder, softer in appropriate locations; no S_3, S_4; no murmurs, rubs, clicks

Carotid, femoral, pedal, and radial pulses present; equal, strong bilaterally

Continued

3. To examine the skin of a patient who has a full-thickness burn, the nurse primarily uses the technique of
   a. inspection
   b. palpation
   c. percussion
   d. auscultation
4. A penlight or pocket flashlight is used during physical examination to determine the
   a. presence of a gag reflex.
   b. character of the oral mucosa.
   c. presence of extraocular movements.
   d. character of the tympanic membranes.
5. A branching examination is performed when
   a. the patient denies a health problem.
   b. a baseline health maintenance examination is required.
   c. a specific problem is identified during physical examination.
   d. the medical diagnosis directs attention to a specific problem area.
6. After performing a screening history and physical, the first information the nurse records is the
   a. general survey.
   b. health history.
   c. patient symptoms.
   d. abnormal findings.

Table 5-8 Recording a Screening Physical Examination—cont'd

Abdomen
No pulsations visible, rounded, active bowel sounds, no bruits or CVA tenderness, no palpable masses

Liver
Lower border percussed at costal margin, smooth, nontender; approx 9 cm span

Spleen
Nonpalpable, nontender

Neurologic System
Cranial nerves I-XII intact
Motor (drift, toe stand) intact
Coord (FN, Romberg) intact
Reflexes: See diagram
Sensation (touch, vibration, prop) intact
Grading Scale
0 No response
1+ Diminished
2+ Normal
3+ Increased
4+ Hyperactive

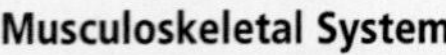

Musculoskeletal System
Well developed, no muscle wasting; s̄ crepitus, nodules, swelling
ROM: Full, intact, and equal bilaterally; no scoliosis
Strength: Equal, strong bilaterally
Gait: Walks erect 2-foot steps, arms swinging at side s̄ staggering

Female Genitalia
External genitalia: No swelling, redness, tenderness in BUS; normal hair distribution, no cysts, rectocele
Vagina: No lesions, discharge; pink
Cervix: Os closed; pink, no lesions, erosions, nontender
Uterus: Small, firm, nontender
Adnexa: No enlargement; nontender
Rectovaginal: Sphincter intact; confirms above findings

Male Genitalia
Normal male hair distribution, negative inguinal hernia
Penis: Urethral opening patent; no redness, swelling, discharge; no lesions, structural alterations
Scrotum: Testes descended; no redness, masses, tenderness
Rectal: No lesions, redness; sphincter intact; prostate small, nontender

Psychologic Status
Affect appropriate; eye contact
Orientation: Oriented × 3
Mood: Pleasant, appropriate
Thought content: Intelligent, coherent
Memory: Remote and recent intact
Serial sevens: Not done or intact

Signature ______________________

AC>BC, air conduction greater than bone conduction; *BUS,* Bartholin's gland, urethral meatus, Skene's duct; *coord,* coordination; *EOM,* extraocular movements; *FN,* finger to nose; *LM,* landmarks; *LR,* light reflex; *MCL,* midclavicular line; *NAD,* no acute distress; *PERRLA,* pupils equal, round, reactive to light and accommodation; *prop,* proprioception; *ROM,* range of motion; s̄, without; *TM,* tympanic membrane; *VA,* visual acuity; *WNL,* within normal limits.

References

1. Gordon M: *Manual of nursing diagnosis, 1997-1998,* ed 8, St Louis, 1997, Mosby.
2. Barkauskas V and others: *Health and physical assessment,* St Louis, 1998, Mosby.
3. Thompson J, Wilson S: *Health assessment for nursing practice,* St Louis, 1996, Mosby.
4. American Nurses' Association, Congress for Nursing Practice: *Nursing: a social policy statement,* Kansas City, Mo, 1995, The Association.
5. Eliopoulos C: *Gerontological nursing,* ed 4, Philadelphia, 1997, Lippincott.
6. Fuller J, Schaller-Ayers J: *Health assessment: a nursing approach,* ed 2, Philadelphia, 1994, Lippincott.
7. Weber J, Kelley J: *Health assessment in nursing,* Philadelphia, 1998, Lippincott.
8. Burke M, Walsh M: *Gerontologic nursing: wholistic care of the older adult,* ed 2, St Louis, 1997, Mosby.

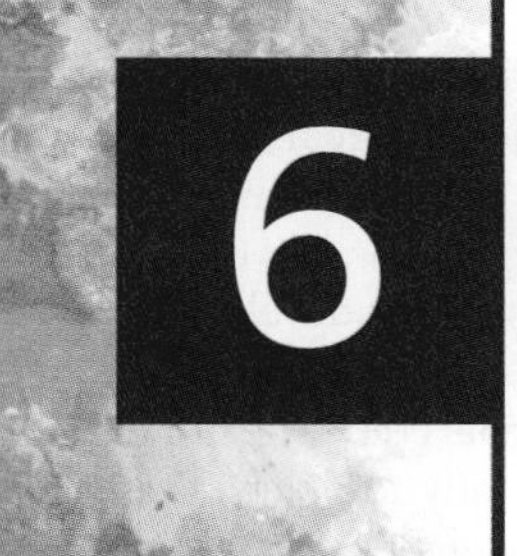

REMEMBER to check out your companion CD-ROM

6 Patient Teaching

Laurie A. Soine

www.mosby.com/MERLIN/medsurg_lewis

LEARNING OBJECTIVES

1. Identify four specific goals of patient teaching.
2. Discuss stressors facing the nurse-teacher.
3. Identify four common characteristics of the adult learner.
4. Identify factors that contribute to successful learning for the adult patient, including implications for nursing interventions.
5. Explain the basic steps in the teaching-learning process.
6. Explain the components of a correctly written learning objective.
7. Describe the seven basic teaching strategies.
8. Describe common methods of short- and long-term evaluation.

ROLE OF PATIENT TEACHING

Overview

Patient education is a planned learning experience using methods such as teaching, counseling, advising, demonstrations, and discussion to positively affect patient outcomes. Patient education is a critical part of nursing care and has proven benefits to patients and their caregivers. The Joint Commission on Accreditation of Healthcare Organizations (JCAHO), the body that accredits and oversees delivery of health care in the United States, mandates that nurses offer patient and family education that includes an assessment of need, ability, and readiness to learn.[1] In addition to assessment, nurses develop an educational plan, deliver the educational intervention, and evaluate the effectiveness of the teaching.

This chapter describes the steps involved in patient education. This chapter also emphasizes factors that contribute to successful patient teaching and demonstrates how to develop a patient and family teaching plan.

Goals of Patient Education

The goal of patient education is to help patients and their families cope with acute and chronic health problems. More specific goals include maintenance of health, prevention of disease, living with illness, and appropriate selection and use of treatment options. Through education nurses have the ability to dramatically affect the lives of their patients and families. The nurse has many teaching opportunities in the community, schools, industry, ambulatory care centers, clinics, hospitals, and homes. Every interaction the nurse has with a patient or the family member can be viewed as an opportunity to supply information that alters patients' outcomes.

Reviewed by Janet Katz, RN, MSN, Spokane Cardio-Pulmonary Rehabilitation, Spokane, Wash.

EDUCATION PROCESS

In nursing, patient education is guided by an underlying philosophy or an approach to modifying patient behavior. Two common philosophies are used to guide patient education. The traditional *compliance* approach to educating the patient asserts that the nurse independently develops, implements, and evaluates a teaching plan. The patient is a passive recipient of the teaching experience. In contrast, the *empowerment* approach encourages patients and their families to identify and articulate personal and health-related goals. This approach is particularly effective when caring for a patient with a chronic condition, such as diabetes mellitus, heart failure, or arthritis. The nurse assists the patient in developing a plan to attain his or her individual goals. The empowerment approach seeks to optimize patient knowledge and autonomy within the context of the patient's illness. In this approach patients are the writers of their own stories. The nurse is an editor, providing guidance, information, and insight while assisting the patient in living out his or her life story.[2] Success with both approaches is measured by adherence to a standard regimen, measured by objective data (e.g., pill counts, blood glucose levels, smoking cessation).

The education process involves the educator, in this case the nurse, the patient, and the patient's family and social support system. The complex nature of each of these variables must be taken into account when planning and implementing the education process.

Nurse

To be effective educators, nurses must develop skills that enable them to help patients in an efficient manner. These skills are discussed in the next section.

Knowledge of the Subject Matter. Because nurses practice in a variety of health care settings, ranging from intensive care units in large, tertiary care hospitals to rural home care settings, the scope of practice is large and diverse.

Although it is impossible to be an expert in all areas, nurses have the educational background to understand many aspects of health and illness. Lack of confidence in their own knowledge base may be a reason why nurses shy away from the role of educator. A first step for the nurse to increase understanding is to read the materials that will be distributed to patients.[3] Most institutions have pamphlets related to the common diseases, diagnostic tests, or treatments. These materials should be read by the nurse before their distribution to the patient or family member. However, it is equally important for the nurse who is not sure of an answer to not hesitate to tell the patient and to follow through with seeking additional information to answer the questions.

Communication Skills. Patient education is an interactive process. It is dependent on communication between the nurse and patient or family member. It is a process of mutual influence. Communication includes both verbal and nonverbal forms.

Verbal communication. The words used to communicate information should be chosen carefully. Simple factual information is most effective. Most written health care information is aimed at the tenth-grade reading level. Verbal communication should match this level.

Medical jargon is inherently intimidating and frightening to most patients and their families. Patients can feel alienated when large, complex medical terms are used in their presence without an understanding of what the terms mean. This can be particularly distressing to the patient who is ill, scared, and aware that his or her illness is being discussed. The nurse should begin by defining the medical words or terms that are necessary to understanding the content to be taught. For example, if a patient is told that he has idiopathic dilated cardiomyopathy, he most likely will need the nurse to interpret this diagnosis in words that mean something to him. The nurse can explain that the term *idiopathic* is a scientific way of saying "for an unknown reason," dilated means enlarged, and cardiomyopathy describes a heart muscle not pumping with full force. Therefore the patient has an enlarged heart that is not working properly for an unknown reason. With this one sentence interpretation the nurse has enhanced the education process.

The speed at which words are delivered, the tone of the voice, and voice modulation are also important to consider. It is important to allow time at the end of an interaction for questions. The nurse should always ask patients if they understood the words that the nurse used.

Nonverbal communication. The importance of nonverbal communication in the teaching process should also be considered. It has been suggested that up to 65% of perceived meaning of a message is carried by nonverbal cues.[4] Some nonverbal cues are obvious, such as tone of voice, rate of speaking, amount and type of gesturing, touch, and proximity. Examples of other nonverbal cues include the speed at which the nurse enters a patient's room, where the nurse chooses to sit or stand, and whether the nurse crosses his or her legs or arms. These nonverbal cues can affect the interpretation of the message.

To provide positive nonverbal messages it is important for the nurse to sit facing the patient. If possible, raise the bed or sit in a chair so that the nurse's and patient's eyes are level. Open body gestures communicate an interest and a willingness to share. If time is limited, the nurse should tell the patient at the beginning of the interaction how much time the nurse can devote to the session. This will allow both the patient and nurse to both set priorities on what needs to be taught during the allotted time.

Active listening. It is important for the nurse to develop the art of active listening. This means paying attention to what is said, as well as observing the patient's nonverbal cues. The nurse must be prepared both physically and mentally to listen. This includes sitting directly in front of the patient, getting rid of distractions, and trying to dismiss personal worries. The nurse concentrates on the patient as a communicator of vital information and allows the patient full hearing by not interrupting. Giving the impression of impatience can often lead to misunderstanding. To allow time for listening without appearing in a hurry requires thoughtful organization and planning on the part of the nurse. Attentive listening provides important information needed for the assessment phase of the teaching process.

Empathy. *Empathy* can be defined as having the courage to enter into the world of another in a manner that does not judge, sympathize, or correct, but in a manner where the goal is creative understanding. Empathy means putting aside one's own self for a moment and stepping into the shoes of the patient. With regard to patient teaching, empathy means assessing the patient's needs before planning the teaching plan. For example, the nurse who is working in a rural outpatient clinic is asked to teach a newly diagnosed diabetic patient the symptoms of hypoglycemia. The nurse enters the room with the packet of written information and finds the patient sitting very still, with gaze fixed, mouth slightly ajar, and appearing anxious. The empathetic approach to this situation may include entering the room, sitting down in a chair next to the patient, pausing for a moment, and respecting the myriad of feelings that the patient may be experiencing before starting the discussion of educational materials.

Stressors. Lack of time and insecurity about knowledge and competence are two stressors that can detract from the effectiveness of the teaching effort. A third potential stressor is disagreement between nurse and patient regarding the expectations of teaching.

Perhaps the most difficult problem faced by the nurse is accepting that some patients or families may not be willing to talk about the illness or its implications. The patient or family may hold preset ideas that override the nurse's efforts. Sometimes the nurse may face hostility, resentment, or even verbal abuse.

Another important stressor for the nurse who is attempting to provide patient education is the current health care system. Shortened lengths of inpatient hospitalizations have resulted in patients being discharged into the community with only the basic elements of the educational plan established. Medicine is offering more and complex treatment options, and the educational needs of the patient and family are also increasing. Nurses must be aware that the health care system can also affect the patient's and family's ability to utilize resources. Strategies that can be used to manage or overcome these stressors are presented in Table 6-1.

Patient

The overall teaching plan and goals are dependent on the individual characteristics of the patient and her or his health care

Table 6-1 Suggested Approaches to Overcoming Nurse-Teacher Stressors

Lack of time	Preplan. Set realistic goals. Use time with patient efficiently. Break teaching and practice into small time periods.
Lack of knowledge	Broaden knowledge base. Read, study, ask questions. Screen teaching materials, participate in other teaching sessions, observe more experienced nurse-teachers, attend classes.
Disagreement with patient	Establish agreed-on, written goals. Develop a plan and discuss with patient before teaching begins. Introduce a role model to help illustrate therapeutic expectations. Enlist the aid of significant others. Revise expectations; learn to be satisfied with small achievements.
Powerlessness, frustration	Recognize how you react to stress. Develop a support system. Rely on friends and family for positive encouragement. Join a nurse-oriented support group. Express your feelings to others, but avoid griping and other negative interactions. Improve communications with other professionals.

problems. Important variables include age, culture, educational level, occupation, self-efficacy, and psychologic state.

Age. The age of a patient affects the teaching plan. For example, a man in his twenties who has never thought about his own mortality may be unable to deal with the long-term implications of a current unhealthy practice (e.g., smoking) and may be able to process only the immediate effects (e.g., asthma). An elderly person with impaired cognitive ability may need simple explanations followed by specific written instructions. A patient's age is useful information in planning educational activities, yet the nurse is cautioned against using age alone to guide the approach taken. Although hearing and vision problems increase with aging, it cannot be assumed that all older adults have these problems. Thus it is important to look at each patient's specific cognitive and physical abilities and needs.

Culture. *Culture* is defined as a "learned, shared, and symbolically transmitted design for living."[5] It is a design for living in that it provides meaning and values to patients' lives. Many cultural groups hold specific beliefs related to health that will affect the teaching plan. Culture is learned, so it cannot be assumed that all members of an ethnic group will share the same culture. It is important not to stereotype patients or their families.

The nurse has several points to consider in providing culture-sensitive care. The first is knowledge, which includes both knowledge of the patient's culture and knowledge of self. If the nurse is unsure of a patient's cultural background, it is important to ask if there is a cultural group with which the patient identifies.[5] Patients may also be asked to share beliefs that their culture ascribes regarding health and illness. Second, nurses should be aware of their own biases when delivering care to a patient from a different culture. Ethnocentrism, the belief that one's own culture holds the best and right way, is at times difficult to avoid. Nurses need to avoid reactions such as anger, laughter, or shock when faced with differing values and beliefs. Third, mutual respect, which is based on reciprocal knowledge and underlies negotiation, is important. This is achieved through recognizing the common humanity of all people. The nurse may encounter patients who practice health behaviors that the nurse does not agree with or understand. Fourth, negotiation is achieved through development of a mutually accepted plan that promotes the values and beliefs of the patient. This involves the merging of two perspectives: that of the nurse, whose understanding of health and illness are physiologically based, and that of the patient, whose understanding of the world may be quite different.[6]

Educational Level. The nurse should not "speak down" to the patient, yet the nurse must speak at a level that promotes understanding. A person's level of formal education may help the nurse determine appropriate literature selections and the vocabulary to use when speaking with the patient. However, this assumes that patients will read or comprehend at the level of their formal education. Asking patients about their education background is useful, but it does not always reflect what the patient knows or understands. Thus each patient should be assessed for his or her ability to comprehend the materials provided.

Reading ability. Printed educational materials are extensively used for the purpose of informing patients and families. If this is the primary route of teaching, the patient's reading level should be evaluated. In a recent study of 202 patients treated at the emergency room or walk-in clinic of a large public hospital in the southeastern United States, it was found that up to 42% of the patients interviewed had marginal functional literacy. In this study, low literacy level was associated with a sense of shame.[7] This sense of shame could decrease the likelihood that the individual would admit to having a reading problem or seek educational help. Other factors that may decrease reading ability include poor or failing eyesight and failure to wear eyeglasses or contacts. If the patient has a low literacy level or is unable to read, a family member or support person may help. For example, a patient may say, "I don't read much, but my sister does." This opens the door for the nurse to involve other family members in the teaching process.

Cognitive ability. Decreases in cognitive function can impair the person's ability to read and to comprehend oral instructions. Some patients may simply be too ill or in too much discomfort to concentrate. The nurse assesses this by asking questions such as, "Do you like to read?" The response might be, "Yes, but my head hurts so bad today that I just can't focus on the page," or, "No, I really don't."

Occupation. Knowing a patient's present or past occupation may assist the nurse in determining the vocabulary to use during teaching. For example, an auto mechanic might understand the volume overload associated with heart failure as a flooding of an engine that at baseline is not functioning at full force. This technique of teaching requires creativity but can facilitate a patient's understanding of advanced pathophysiologic processes.

Self-Efficacy. Illness poses many challenges for patients. Adopting new health behaviors and eliminating unhealthy behaviors are difficult tasks for most patients. One important determinant of successful adoption of new behaviors is a patient's sense of self-efficacy. *Self-efficacy* is a person's belief in his or her ability to understand and follow a regimen, advice, or recommendation. A strong sense of self-efficacy has been shown to predict adherence to diet[8] and an involvement in an exercise program[9] in patients with coronary artery disease. Self-efficacy can be increased in some patients through techniques such as rehearsing new behaviors (role playing) and learning from peers.

Psychologic State. Anxiety and depression are common reactions to illness. Anxiety can be due to a sense of loss of control or a perception that life may be significantly altered by the illness. It is well known that anxiety and depression produce functional disability and decreased quality of life in patients with medical problems. Both short- and long-term depression can also affect functional ability. In fact, depression has been found to be an independent risk factor for poor outcomes following hospitalization in the elderly population.[10] Both anxiety and depression can negatively affect the patient's motivation and readiness to learn. For example, the newly diagnosed diabetic patient who is depressed about his or her diagnosis may not be able to learn about blood glucose testing. Discussions with the patient about his or her concerns or connecting the patient with an appropriate support group may enhance the patient's ability to learn self-care strategies.

Hope is another psychologic factor that can affect the teaching process. Hope can positively affect patient readiness to learn and compliance with instructions. Nurses promote hope through verbal and nonverbal communication, promotion of self-efficacy, and empathetic listening.

Denial is a simple and common defense mechanism used to cope with stress. In denial there is distortion of what the individual sees, thinks, feels, or perceives when encountering a stressful situation. For example, the patient who denies having cancer will not be receptive to information related to treatment options.

Rationalization is another psychologic response to stress that can affect the teaching process. In this response the patient imagines a number of reasons for avoiding change or for rejecting advice. For example, a patient who wants to continue eating a diet high in saturated fat will relate stories of persons she or he has known who have eaten eggs and bacon every morning for years and lived to be 100 years of age.

Humor is used by some patients to filter or avoid reality. Making light of a situation keeps reality from setting in. Laughter is sometimes used to cover up anxiety or to escape from the experience of facing threatening situations. Humor in the teaching process is important and useful, but be aware of humor being used to mask a patient's or family's anxieties regarding a health crisis.

Family and Social Support

What defines a family? Traditionally, families have consisted of a mother, father, and children living together in a home. Variations of this structure are many and include single-parent homes, couples with no children, children living with grandparents, and same-sex couples. The common thread through all of these is that a family infers a strong sense of kinship that arises from either a biologic or psychologic basis.[11] Maintaining a sense of family is important to a patient's sense of physical, psychologic, and spiritual well-being.[12] As a result, teaching plans often involve working with identified family members.

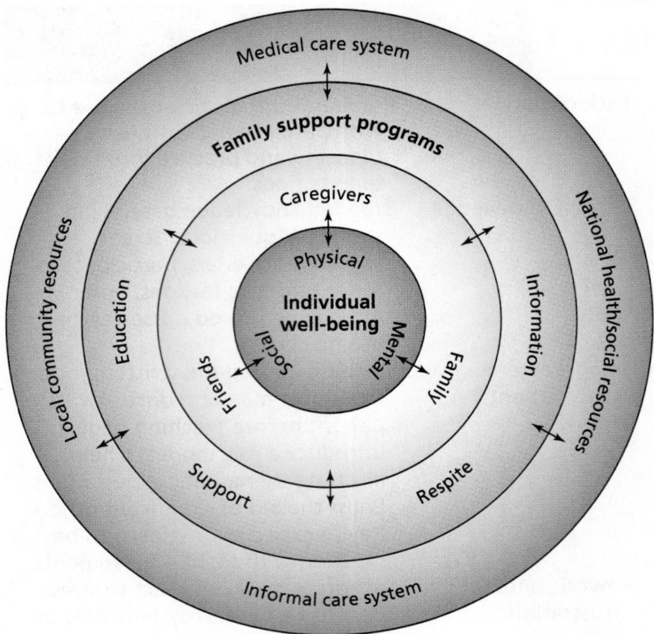

Fig. 6-1 Family support model.

In the family support model (Fig. 6-1), the patient's ultimate well-being is composed of his or her ability to perform self-care activities in and through both formal and informal support systems.[13] In this model no part of the system is an independent agent because the well-being of the individual depends on support from family, community resources, and the medical care system.[13] The support, provided by the family unit, greatly affects a patient's health outcome. Studies have demonstrated that having little emotional support[14] or living alone[15] increases mortality rates in the 6 months after a myocardial infarction. Identifying patients with minimal support and working collaboratively with other health care professionals to develop networks for these patients may improve the patients' long-term outcomes.

Patients and families may have different educational needs; therefore the nurse must take this into account when gathering assessment data. For example, the first priority of an elderly diabetic patient with a large ulcer on the back of his leg may be to learn how to rise from a chair in the least painful manner. On the other hand, family members may be most concerned about learning clean technique for dressing changes. Both the patient's and the family's learning needs are important. The patient and family may have differing or conflicting views of the illness and of treatment options. Frequently the health problem has effects on family roles and functions. Developing a successful teaching plan requires the nurse to view the patient's needs within the context of the family's needs. For example, the nurse may spend time discussing low-potassium meal preparation with a female patient in renal failure, only to have the patient come to the emergency room 3 days after discharge with a severely elevated serum potassium level. When the nurse inquires whether she is following her low-potassium meal plan, it is learned that her husband does most of the cooking, and he did not receive the information.

FACTORS CONTRIBUTING TO SUCCESSFUL ADULT LEARNING

Respect

Respect is the foundation on which adult learning is based. Adults want to be decision makers in their own lives and wish to decide, insofar as they can, what occurs during the learning experience. The learning process is enhanced when the nurse has established a trusting, nonthreatening relationship with the patient. When this occurs, the patient is likely to feel valued and is better prepared to learn. Respect for the patient can be reflected in questions such as "What do you feel you need to learn about this topic?"[16] In doing this the nurse conveys respect for the patient's input as an active participant.

The nurse, patient, and family must discuss and agree on desired outcomes. For example, working with a patient postoperatively following bowel resection and colostomy placement, the nurse might begin the interaction by asking what the patient thinks he needs to know before being discharged from the hospital. Soliciting input shows respect for the patient's needs, and together the patient and nurse can develop a plan to accomplish the task. The nurse might also ask what time of day the patient would like the teaching to occur and which members of his family he would like involved in the experience. Offering control and self-direction will increase the patient's sense of responsibility, and thus involvement, in the education process.

It will also enhance the learning process if the teaching builds on the patient's life experiences. Patients will be more motivated to learn if they feel that they already know something about the subject from past experience. It is important for the nurse to remember that new experiences can be threatening. By finding familiar ground the nurse helps build confidence in the patient.

Relevance

The second factor contributing to successful teaching is appreciating that an adult's readiness to learn depends on the perceived need to learn. Adults learn and remember what they perceive is useful and relevant to their life's experience. Therefore the nurse should select subject material that relates directly to the patient or family needs.

There will be times when the patient does not appreciate the relevance of a topic to his or her overall health. This then becomes an important part of the nurse's discussion with the patient. For example, teaching a preoperative patient how to use an incentive spirometer to decrease the possibility of postoperative pneumonia may not seem relevant to the patient. Many patients do not understand that bed rest and surgical procedures put all individuals at risk for developing atelectasis and pneumonia. However, if the person correctly uses the incentive spirometer every 2 hours postoperatively, this complication can be prevented.

Suggestions for pointing out the relevance of a topic include (1) building on previous knowledge; (2) organizing the material and presenting it in logical order from simple to complex; (3) presenting a warm, caring, nonthreatening image to the patient; (4) using positive, supportive verbal and nonverbal communication; and (5) providing frequent measures of success. Patients who know that they are learning and succeeding are strongly motivated to learn more. Immediate, genuine experiences of success in the learning process help overcome the fear of failure, which is a learning block for many adults.

The nurse should use written or audiovisual materials that target the specific problem or circumstance. The discussion and demonstrations should be limited to necessary content. Nurses are experts in the management of health and illness, but they must be aware that they may overwhelm a patient with too much information about a subject. If overwhelmed the patient may not be able to determine which information is critical for his or her particular situation.

Immediacy

The third factor contributing to successfully teaching the adult learner is the need to apply learning immediately. Long-term goals may have little appeal. The nurse should provide short-term, realistic goals. For example, patients with heart failure must follow their volume status by weighing themselves daily and compliantly taking diuretics. These behaviors result in less shortness of breath and decrease the chance of multiple hospitalization for heart failure. The nurse should present this information to the patient in a format so that the patient can appreciate its relevance to her or his life. An adult is more likely to learn when presented with a persuasive explanation than when told what to do.

Learning Environment

Another factor contributing to successful learning is the learning environment. From the moment the patient enters the hospital until he or she is discharged, even before the initial assessment is complete, the nurse works to develop a feeling of trust, respect, and support. The patient will learn best in an atmosphere of warmth, comfort, and caring. When the nurse and patient establish rapport, the teaching-learning transaction will be more successful.

The learning environment is also a physical climate. Since distractions can reduce the efficiency of teaching and learning, the nurse should eliminate, rearrange, or control noise, lighting, ventilation, and odors. The window should be closed if too much traffic noise is coming from the street. The office door should be shut to eliminate visual distractions from passersby. The television set or radio should be turned off and the privacy curtain pulled.

Process of Change

Patients and their families may progress through a series of steps before they are able or willing to accept a change in health behaviors. Five stages of change have been identified and are described in Table 6-2.[17] It is important to note that individuals progress through these stages at their own pace. Some patients may get stalled in the early stages and need assistance

Table 6-2 Stages of Change

Stages	Patient Behavior	Nurse Behavior
1. Precontemplation	Refuses to see need for change	Provides support to patient Does not argue
2. Contemplation	Considers change in behavior	Describes positive outcomes Provides encouragement, information, support
3. Preparation	Exhibits active interest, gathers information Participates in self-inquiry	Assists patient or family Devises strategies to achieve change
4. Action	Implements new behavior Experiences possible relapses	Encourages and provides information Develops plan to deal with potential relapses
5. Maintenance	Incorporates new behavior	Provides support

From Prochaska J and others: *Changing for good,* New York, 1994, William Morrow. Copyright 1994 by the authors. By permission of William Morrow & Co., Inc.

to move further in the process. Recidivism or relapse is another problem associated with changing health behaviors. Understanding these stages will allow the nurse to better guide patients through the process of change.

TEACHING PROCESS

The teaching process can be likened to assembling a huge puzzle. It begins with identification of individual pieces, followed by a calculated plan, thoughtful implementation, and evaluation of outcomes.

Assessment

Assessment is a process of gathering relevant information about the patient for the purpose of developing a teaching plan. It encompasses a patient's readiness to learn, and biophysical, psychologic, socioeconomic, and sociocultural characteristics. Assessment can also include the family or caregiver to determine their abilities to care for the patient at home. A thoughtful approach to assessment is important to the ultimate success of the education plan. The more complete the assessment, the more effective the teaching plan is likely to be. Table 6-3 lists questions that can be asked to determine information relevant to planning teaching activities. Consistent with the idea that change involves several steps or phases as outlined in Table 6-2, the nurse first determines which phase the patient is at in the process.[18] Such information assists the nurse in targeting the teaching plan.

Biophysical Characteristics. The nurse first assesses the patient's physical and mental state of health. The answers to these questions affect the development of a teaching plan and the timing for its implementation. For example, if a patient with poor vision is given only written medication instructions, the likelihood that she will learn and comply with the new medication regimen is decreased.

Sensory impairments, such as hearing or vision loss, alter sensory input and can impair the patient's ability to learn. Learning requires an adequately functioning central nervous system (CNS). Therefore patients with pathophysiologic states that decrease CNS function, such as cerebrovascular accident, poor perfusion, or nervous system trauma, may require small amounts of information repeated frequently. It is important to recognize the patient's physical abilities and limitations.

Pain and fatigue also influence a patient's ability to learn. No one can learn effectively when in severe pain. When the patient is experiencing pain, the nurse might choose only brief explanations and follow up with more detailed instruction when the pain has been managed.

A patient's energy level is also an important variable. A fatigued and weak patient cannot learn effectively because of the inability to concentrate. Sleep disruption is a common problem in hospitalized or acutely ill patients, and this also affects the ability to concentrate. Historically, hospital stays were lengthy, which allowed for patients to more fully recover and regain strength before discharge. This is no longer the case. With an increase in the number of short stays, patients may still be tired and fatigued at the time of hospital discharge. Thus the nurse's teaching plan must take this into account, setting goals that are need based and realistic in expectations.

Medications may also influence a patient's ability to retain information. For example, barbiturates, tranquilizers, and narcotic analgesics cause drowsiness and a general decrease in mental alertness. Many chemotherapeutic agents cause nausea, vomiting, and headaches, which can affect the patient's ability to assimilate new information.

The assessment of the patient's physiologic state involves looking at the patient's medical chart for information about past medical history, current medical diagnosis, treatment plan, medication record, and expected outcomes. The chart may also contain information related to the patient's functional status. Other care providers and family members are also sources of information.

Assessment of the patient's knowledge related to the topic to be taught is also important. This is done by asking questions related to understanding of the problem and the therapies and medications, sources of previous information, and understanding of resources from which to obtain information.

Psychologic Characteristics. A second area of assessment is the psychologic dimension. This information may not be in the patient's chart and is best collected in person. The nurse evaluates the patient's mood. Although mild anxiety increases the learner's perceptual and learning abilities, severe anxiety decreases learning.

Other psychologic variables that influence learning have been discussed previously and include self-efficacy, hope, denial, and rationalization. Individual personality characteristics can also influence the learning process. Some patients acclimate easily to illness and treatment in a complex, structured, multidisciplinary health care system while others do not.

Table 6-3 Assessment of Characteristics That Affect Patient Teaching

Characteristic	Key Questions
Readiness to learn	What has your physician or nurse practitioner told you about your health problem? What behaviors could make your problem better or worse?
Biophysical	What is the primary diagnosis? Are there additional diagnoses? Is the patient acutely ill? How old is the patient? What is the patient's current mental status? What is the patient's hearing ability? Visual ability? Motor ability? Is the patient fatigued? In pain? What medications is the patient on? How might these affect learning?
Psychologic	Does the patient appear anxious? Afraid? Depressed? Defensive? Is the patient in a state of denial?
Sociocultural	Does the patient have family or close friends? What is the patient's belief regarding his or her illness or treatment? Is the proposed change consistent with the patient's cultural values?
Socioeconomic	Does the patient work? What is the patient's occupation? What is the patient's living arrangement?
Learning style	Does the patient "learn best" through visual (reading), auditory (tape or lecture), or physical stimuli (demonstration)? In what kind of environment does the patient learn best? Formal classroom? Informal setting, such as home or office? Alone or among peers? What prior learning experiences were helpful?

Sociocultural and Socioeconomic Characteristics. The patient's social and cultural network also should be assessed. This network influences a patient's perception of health, illness, health care system, life, and death and thus affects the learning process. Socioeconomic elements include occupation, educational level, income, housing arrangement, and living location (rural, urban, etc.). Sociocultural elements include dietary and sleep patterns, exercise, sexuality, language, values, and beliefs. All of these variables influence how a patient responds to the teaching-learning process. For example, a patient who values a trim figure can be taught to diet and exercise to retain that figure while at the same time bringing his blood pressure under better control. However, in other cultures, being heavy is a sign of financial success and sexuality. A patient from such a culture may have a more difficult time accepting the concept of diet and exercise for weight control.

Learning is closely related to the wider culture and the subculture to which a patient belongs. Health practices, beliefs, and behaviors vary by religious, ethnic, and family group. The nurse must appreciate the impact that a patient's cultural background has on the development of a teaching plan. This information is not always readily available. Many of the subculture and social implications of health and illness are subtle. Observing a patient's verbal and nonverbal interactions within his or her family and social circle may give clues to practices and beliefs. For example, a middle-age, upper-income woman may belong to a subculture in which taking pills is widely accepted. She may therefore be willing to take prescribed medications but unwilling to learn to self-administer an injection. The nurse, in assessing the patient's attitude toward this skill, must take a holistic approach and see the patient as a total person within her subculture. The teaching plan should include information attempting to adjust the patient's attitude, as well as showing the patient how this new skill will fit into her existing lifestyle.

Learning Style. The nurse should assess the patient's learning style. Each person has a distinct style of learning, as individual as his or her personality. The three learning styles are (1) visual (reading), (2) auditory (listening), and (3) physical (doing things). People often use more than one learning style.

Based on the assessment information, the nurse may make the nursing diagnosis of *knowledge deficit.* This refers to the state in which the individual experiences a deficiency in cognitive knowledge or psychomotor skills that alters or may alter health maintenance. If a knowledge deficit is identified, it is important to specify the exact nature of the deficit so that objectives, strategies, implementation, and evaluation relate to the identified problem. For example, the nursing diagnosis of knowledge deficit related to inability to recognize symptoms of drug overdose provides the nurse with a clear direction for the teaching-learning process.

Planning

Following a detailed assessment the second step in the education process is setting goals, determining objectives for the learner, and planning the learning experience. Information obtained from the assessment related to what the patient knows, believes, and is able to do is compared with what the patient needs to know, understand, and be able to do. Identifying the gap between the known and unknown helps focus the teaching process.

Individuals tend to feel more committed to a decision or activity when they participate in making or planning it. Therefore the patient and nurse should mutually agree on learning objectives. If the biophysical or psychologic condition of the patient is such that she or he cannot actively participate, the patient's family or significant other can assist the nurse in the planning phase.

Writing clear, specific, and measurable learning objectives is important. Learning objectives describe the intended result of the learning process, guide the selection of teaching strategies and materials, and help evaluate patient and teacher progress. Objectives should be written down and made readily available to all members of the health care team.

Writing Specific Learning Objectives. Learning objectives are written statements that define exactly what patients are able to do to show that they have mastered the content. The objectives contain the following four elements:

1. Who will perform the activity or acquire the desired behavior?
   Examples: I (the patient) will . . .
   I (the spouse) will . . .
   We (the patient's family) will . . .
2. The actual behavior that the learner will exhibit to demonstrate mastery of the objective.
   Examples: List the symptoms
   Self-administer an insulin injection
   Identify from a hospital menu
3. The conditions under which the behavior is to be demonstrated.
   Examples: In front of the nurse
   In own house
   Select from a random list
   Choose from a restaurant menu
4. The specific criteria that will be used to measure the patient's success, such as time and degree of accuracy.
   Examples: With 100% accuracy
   Using correct technique
   Within 3 minutes

Note that well-written learning objectives have precise descriptions using terms with few interpretations. When writing objectives the nurse uses verbs such as "identify," "list," "describe," "demonstrate," "name," "recognize," and "compare and contrast," and avoids terms with vague, ambiguous meanings, such as "appreciate," "learn," "understand," "enjoy," "feel," or "value."

An example of a poorly written learning objective is, "The patient will appreciate the importance of foot care." In this objective it is not clear how the patient will demonstrate that he "appreciates" the importance of foot care, when and to whom he will demonstrate this behavior, or what criteria will be used to determine whether the objective has been met.

The following are examples of well-written learning objectives:

- The patient will be able to demonstrate to the nurse the correct technique for changing his colostomy bag.
- The patient will administer in front of the nurse a subcutaneous injection of insulin to herself using correct technique.
- The patient will select a 2000 mg sodium diet from the hospital menu for breakfast, lunch, and dinner for 3 consecutive days with 90% accuracy.
- Given a list of symptoms of heart failure, the patient will identify the early symptoms of heart failure with 80% accuracy before discharge from the hospital.

When learning objectives are clear and specific and when they are written down and available in the patient record, all members of the health care team can work together to accomplish the same objectives. This type of communication will ensure optimal results. Once the objectives are clearly stated, the nurse and patient can develop the teaching plan. The following section outlines several teaching strategies. The nurse, patient, and patient's family should choose the strategy or strategies that are most appropriate and beneficial to meet the objectives of the learning process.

Teaching Strategies

Once the objectives are clearly stated, the nurse and patient can develop the teaching plan. The following section outlines several teaching strategies. The nurse, patient, and patient's family should choose the strategy or strategies that are most appropriate and beneficial to meet the objectives of the learning process.

Selecting a particular strategy is determined by at least three factors: (1) patient characteristics (e.g., age, educational background, degree of illness, culture); (2) the subject matter; and (3) available resources. Listed next are teaching strategies that can be employed to achieve learning objectives. Each has advantages and disadvantages that make it more or less suitable to a particular patient and learning situation (Fig. 6-2).

Lecture. The lecture format is an efficient, versatile, and economical teaching strategy that can be used when the amount of time is limited. The nurse presents a series of related ideas or facts to one person or to a group. Usually, the lecture is short, from 15 to 20 minutes, and some visual reinforcement, such as a diagram on a blackboard, emphasizes key points. It is important to remember that the average adult learner can remember five to seven points at a time. Disadvantages of the lecture format are that it often has negative "school learning" connotations, and individual learning is difficult to evaluate. The nurse is active, but the patients are passive unless they are allowed to participate or ask questions.

Lecture-Discussion. A second teaching strategy is the lecture-discussion, which can overcome some of the disadvantages of the lecture only. With this strategy, the nurse presents specific information by using the lecture technique, followed by a period during which patients and their families ask questions and exchange points of view with the nurse. This strategy assists the patient in becoming an active participant in the learning process and creates a more informal give-and-take learning environment.

Discussion. A third strategy is discussion, and its purpose may be to exchange points of view concerning a topic or questions or to arrive at a decision or conclusion. The nurse can discuss content with an individual or with a group, keeping the specific learning objectives in mind and clarifying information as needed. This strategy is a good choice when the patient or patients have previous experience with a subject and have information to share, such as smoking cessation, post–coronary artery bypass grafting, or preoperative teaching classes. The discussion allows the patient or family members

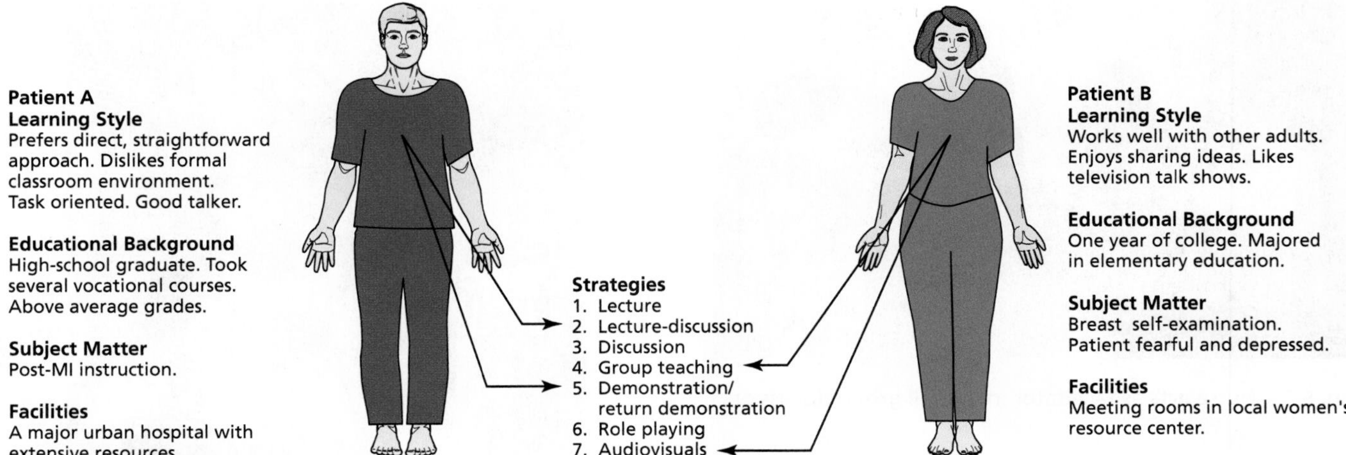
Patient A
Learning Style
Prefers direct, straightforward approach. Dislikes formal classroom environment. Task oriented. Good talker.
Educational Background
High-school graduate. Took several vocational courses. Above average grades.
Subject Matter
Post-MI instruction.
Facilities
A major urban hospital with extensive resources.
Strategies
1. Lecture
2. Lecture-discussion
3. Discussion
4. Group teaching
5. Demonstration/ return demonstration
6. Role playing
7. Audiovisuals
Patient B
Learning Style
Works well with other adults. Enjoys sharing ideas. Likes television talk shows.
Educational Background
One year of college. Majored in elementary education.
Subject Matter
Breast self-examination. Patient fearful and depressed.
Facilities
Meeting rooms in local women's resource center.

Fig. 6-2 Selecting learning strategies.

to actively participate and to apply their own experiences and observation to the learning process. However, one disadvantage must be remembered: The discussion will take longer to cover a given amount of material than some other methods. The informal sharing and nonthreatening environment of discussions are positive factors, but the time and difficulty of reaching desired objectives is a negative feature.

Group Teaching. There are two kinds of group teaching. In the first, the nurse acts as a facilitator, or helper, for group sharing about a common problem. Figure 6-3 shows the nurse acting as a facilitator in small group discussion. The nurse does not teach or participate but keeps information moving among all group members. The nurse may introduce the patient to an existing group or may form a group of patients with similar problems, such as women whose elderly parents live at home with them.

A second kind of group teaching involves peer teaching as found in support groups. A support group is a self-help organization that can provide continuing information, shared experiences, acceptance, understanding, and useful suggestions about a problem or concern. Patients with problems such as impotence, suicide, cancer, alcoholism, Parkinson's disease, compulsive overeating, diabetes, or heart surgery can benefit from the support group approach. In many cases, support groups have proved to be an effective form of teaching. Therefore the nurse should actively look for opportunities to refer a patient or family to a support group. This action should be taken in addition to, not instead of, the nurse's planned teaching sessions.

Demonstration/Return Demonstration. The demonstration/return demonstration is probably the most common strategy a nurse uses. The purpose is to show how something works and the procedure to follow when doing it. Another purpose is to illustrate to the patient or family how a skill is performed or to demonstrate ideas, problem solving, or motor skills. The focus is on correct procedure and application. To handle this strategy correctly, the nurse tells the patient the purpose of the demonstration and makes sure that the patient can see and hear clearly. Then the nurse presents the demonstration in an informal manner, defines unfamiliar terms, and watches for signs of confusion from the patient. The nurse clarifies and repeats as needed, and then the patient returns the demonstration with the nurse as observer. The entire process should last no more than 15 to 20 minutes and should be briefly repeated during the nurse's next teaching session with the patient. Reviewing material over time enhances compliance. Another factor that enhances retention and compliance is to help the patient identify "rewards" that can be used when a behavior or skill is consistently performed.

Role Playing. Role playing is another strategy that the nurse might employ depending on teaching objectives. This format is most often used when patients need to examine their attitudes and behaviors, when they need to understand the viewpoints and attitudes of others, or when they need to practice carrying out thoughts, ideas, or decisions. This strategy is challenging for the nurse because he or she is responsible for defining the problems, determining the goals, setting the climate, and determining the situation and roles to be played. The nurse gives information and clear instructions to role players and observers and provides time for feedback and evaluation. Role playing requires maturity, confidence, and flexibility on the part of the participants. It is important to remember that some patients may feel uncomfortable and inhibited with this method. Role playing takes time, and this must be factored into the teaching plan. An example of the use of role playing is a wife who needs to rehearse how to talk with her husband about his need to quit smoking. In this case, "play acting" the discussion ahead of time may be a helpful strategy.

Audiovisual Material. A final strategy for the nurse to consider is the use of audiovisual materials, including movies, videotapes, slides, posters, computer-based programs, charts, audiotapes, or simple transparencies. This strategy can be used to effectively present most types of information in a more interesting manner than a straight lecture format. The reason is that more than one sense is being used. To use this strategy, the nurse must know what materials are available within the care facility, from support agencies, and from professional groups. These materials are previewed and evaluated for accuracy, completeness, and appropriateness to the learning objectives before being shown to the patient and family.

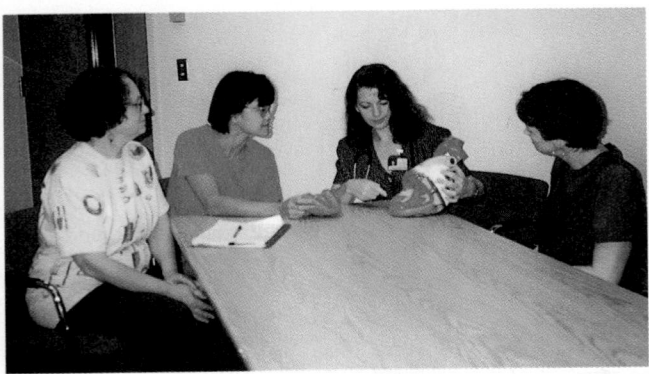

Fig. 6-3 Nurse acts as facilitator in a small group discussion.

Audiotapes are relatively easy to use and can be inexpensive. The use of audiovisual materials can be extremely beneficial, particularly when teaching content that is largely visual, such as the steps, processes, or results of a surgical procedure. However, audiovisual equipment such as televisions, projectors, computers, or viewers must be kept in good repair and available for the nurse to use. Figure 6-4 shows a nurse working with a patient to select learning activities and materials.

Use of Printed Material. A wealth of printed health-related material is available. These are considered for use in combination with each of the previously presented teaching strategies. For instance, following a lecture on the physiologic effects of smoking, the nurse could distribute a pamphlet from the American Cancer Society that reviews and reinforces the topic. Or the nurse might select a book or magazine article written by a woman who has had a mastectomy and suggest that the patient read this material before viewing a video on the same topic.

It is important to remember the learning style of the patient. Many people prefer to read material in private at their own pace, before or after a learning experience. Major resources for acquiring relevant printed material include the hospital or care facility library, the pharmacy, members of the health care team, the public library, federal and state agencies, universities, and research centers. Three factors that influence a patient's or family's interpretation of written material are (1) their literacy level, (2) cultural influences, and (3) prior life or health care experiences. These variables act as filters through which the new information flows.[19]

Written materials, including computer-based programs, should be reviewed by the nurse before their use. The following criteria for review have been suggested: (1) accuracy, (2) completeness, (3) whether the material meets specific learning goals, (4) vocabulary and sentence length suitable to the patient's reading ability, (5) use of pictures and diagrams to stimulate interest, (6) use of one main idea or concept per pamphlet or program, (7) use of terminology that the patient would understand, (8) whether the material contains information the patient would like to know, and (9) whether the material is culturally and gender sensitive and appropriate.[20] The nurse must remember that adult patients may have reduced visual ability and should provide clear visual cues (adequate illumination, larger print, reduced glare) and adequate auditory cues (speak clearly, face the patient, slightly increase the volume of speech).

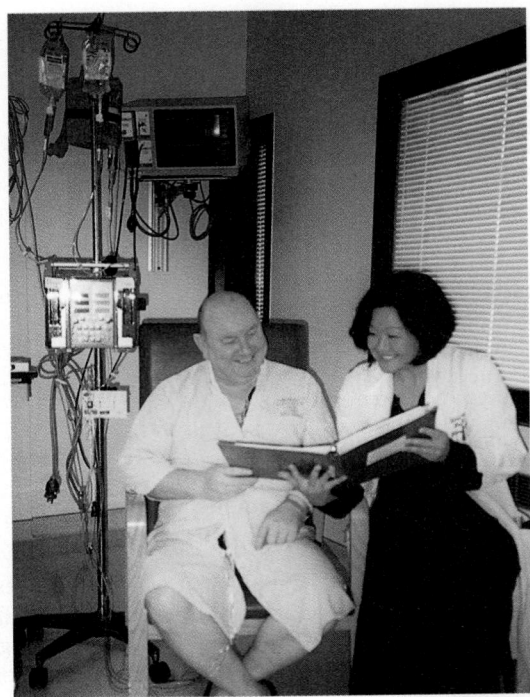

Fig. 6-4 Medication teaching with intensive care unit patient.

Implementation

During the implementation phase presentation of learning materials occurs. The nurse uses verbal and nonverbal communication skills to present the materials. Active listening, empathy, and respect are incorporated into the process. Based on the assessment of the patient's physical and psychologic condition, the nurse can determine how much active participation the patient can assume.

In implementing the teaching plan the nurse should remember the important elements of successful adult learning: respect, relevance, and immediacy. Strategies to enhance the teaching process are shown in Table 6-4.

Evaluation

Evaluation is the final step in the learning process and is a measure of the degree to which the patient has mastered the learning objectives. The nurse monitors the performance level of the patient so that changes can be made as needed. The nurse may find that the patient has achieved the goals; however, if certain goals were not reached, the nurse may need to develop a new teaching plan. If the patient has developed new needs, the nurse then plans new goals, content, and strategies.

For example, an elderly man with diabetes mellitus enters the hospital with a blood glucose level of 550 mg/dl (30.53 mmol/L). When the student nurse began to prepare his insulin injection, the nurse asked, "Are you going to have him give his own insulin and observe his technique?" "Oh, no," replied the student nurse, "He has been a diabetic for 20 years!" The assumption was that a patient with diabetes would know how

Table 6-4 Strategies to Enhance Patient Learning

- Keep the physical environment relaxed and nonthreatening.
- Identify what the patient wants to learn first to provide direction for learning activities.
- Maintain a respectful, warm, and enthusiastic attitude.
- Involve the patient and family in the process; emphasize active participation.
- Build on the patient's previous experience.
- Emphasize the relevancy of the learned material to the patient's lifestyle, and suggest an immediate solution to a problem.
- Time learning according to the patient's needs.
- Individualize the teaching plan, even if standardized plans are used.
- Emphasize helping the patient to learn, not just transmitting subject matter. Don't tell, explain.
- Allow the patient and family to pace their own learning when possible.

to perform this task correctly. The two nurses returned to the patient's room and asked him to prepare an insulin injection. The patient filled the syringe with 20 units of insulin and 20 units of air, instead of 40 units of insulin. After correcting the dosage and questioning the patient more fully, the nurses concluded that the patient could not accurately see the markings on the syringe and that the patient may have been administering insufficient insulin to himself for a long period of time. The patient's vision was not as good as it had been 20 years ago, and special equipment was now necessary for him to safely and accurately administer the insulin.

Evaluation techniques may be short- or long-term. Short-term evaluation techniques are used to quickly evaluate the patient's mastery of a concept, skill, or behavior change and can be accomplished in the following ways:

1. Observe the patient directly. "Show me how you will change your dressing." "Let me see how you administer your injection." By observation, the nurse determines if a task has been mastered, if further instruction is needed, or if the patient is ready for new or additional content. If a task is mastered, it is vital that the nurse affirms the patient's newly acquired skill. Affirmation is a strong motivating factor for continued learning.
2. Observe verbal and nonverbal cues. If the patient asks the nurse to repeat instruction, asks questions, shakes his or her head, loses eye contact, slumps or droops in the chair or bed, becomes restless and fidgety, or otherwise expresses doubt about understanding, the patient may be indicating that further instruction is needed or an alternative approach should be taken. The nurse must be alert to the patient's nonverbal as well as verbal cues.
3. Ask direct questions. "What are the major food groups?" "How often must you change your dressing?" "What should you do if you develop chest pain after returning home?" Open-ended questions will provide more information about the patient's understanding than questions that require a "yes" or "no" answer.
4. Use a written measurement tool, graded for accuracy. Paper and pencil tests may increase anxiety in patients. Adults may "freeze" when given a test, or "go blank" when asked to write something that will be graded. Assess the patient's comfort or learning style before using this method of evaluation.
5. Talk with a member of the patient's family or support system. "Is he eating regularly?" "How is he handling the walker?" "When is she taking her medications?" Since the nurse cannot be with the patient 24 hours a day, utilize other people who have contact with the patient.
6. Seek the patient's self-evaluation of progress. What evidence does the patient have that the objectives are being met? How does the patient feel—confident or unsure? Apprehensive or ready to go forward with new material? Remember that self-direction is important in adult learning. By seeking out a patient's opinion the nurse is allowing the patient input into the evaluation process.

These short-term evaluation techniques can be used frequently and interchangeably to keep informed of the patient's progress and assess changing needs.

Long-term evaluation requires follow-up by the nurse, outpatient clinic, or outside agency. The nurse's role is to explain to the patient the positive outcomes associated with regular reevaluation by someone familiar with the patient's needs. The nurse should set up a schedule of visits for the patient before the patient leaves the hospital or clinic or refer the patient to the proper agencies. The nurse keeps written documentation of follow-up telephone calls or mailed, written reminders to urge the patient to maintain the follow-up schedule. The patient's family or support person should be familiar with the follow-up plan, so that everyone is involved in the patient's long-term progress.

The nurse takes the initiative in contacting persons or agencies involved in the patient's long-term follow-up. The nurse should telephone, visit, or write these health professionals and supply them with the education plan, including learning objectives, teaching plan, and short-term evaluation measures. These data are charted in the patient's medical records for further use.

Documentation is an essential component of the entire learning transaction. The nurse records everything from the assessment through short- and long-term plans for evaluation. As mentioned, the documentation should be forwarded to the agency or health professional providing long-term follow-up. Since many different members of the health care team will use these records on different shifts, in different places, and for different reasons, the teaching objectives, content, strategies, and evaluation results should be written clearly and completely. Team members are encouraged to add comments and observations to these records.

The standardized teaching plans, often included in care maps and clinical pathways, used for common health problems or treatment plans have become an accepted method of developing a teaching plan. Standardized teaching plans contain widely accepted knowledge, understanding, and skills that a patient and family need to know concerning a specific diagnosis or procedure. The nurse should individualize these plans to meet the patient's specific needs.

CRITICAL THINKING EXERCISES

CASE STUDY

Example of the Teaching Process

Jane is admitted to the hospital for preliminary testing and preparation for a hysterectomy. The nurse is aware that a patient undergoing a hysterectomy is often deeply concerned about her self-concept as a woman. The nurse also knows that such patients need to express their feelings in an atmosphere of support and understanding. Therefore the nurse has sought to listen attentively and ask questions carefully in order to assess the patient's feelings about and knowledge of her surgical procedure. The nurse has asked open-ended questions, such as "How do you feel about having the surgery?" and "What concerns do you have about undergoing a hysterectomy?" By establishing a climate of trust and a counseling relationship, the nurse has completed the following assessment:

Biophysical Dimension

Age 44, white female, high school English teacher and coaches girls' varsity basketball team; good general health. Height and weight proportional and average for age. Patient reports that she jogs five evenings a week. No sensory impairment; vision, hearing, and reaction time seem normal.

Psychologic Dimension

Patient appears mildly anxious about surgery and worried about her husband's acceptance of her sexuality. She is also worried about missing work and leaving her classes to a substitute teacher. She states that she does not "let physical problems get me down," and that she dislikes "pills and hospitals." She states that she is used to "teaching" and not being "taught," and she tries to dominate any conversation or input from the nurse.

Sociocultural Dimension

Married with one child (son) age 23. Mother had a mastectomy at age 51; father healthy. Two younger sisters; both experienced difficult pregnancies but are otherwise healthy. Patient describes family communication as very good. She describes her lifestyle as work oriented and that her friends are primarily teaching associates. Her Norwegian and Lutheran heritage places a high priority on work and family. One of her close friends has previously undergone this procedure.

Learning Style

Responds well to formal lectures. Enjoys reading and group discussions.

Determine Objectives

After a brief period of rest and adjustment to the unfamiliar hospital environment, Jane states that she would like to learn more about the details of the upcoming planned surgical procedure. Together Jane and the nurse identify the following objectives.
Following the teaching session, I (Jane) will be able to:

1. Describe to the nurse the surgical procedure (hysterectomy).
2. Express to the nurse and my husband my feelings about maintaining an active and fulfilling sex life.
3. Complete arrangements with my family and school principal for convalescence and return to normal activities.
4. List the general recovery experiences that are expected and under what circumstances to seek medical advice.
5. Discuss "old wives' tales" regarding hysterectomy and verbalize concerns regarding undergoing the hysterectomy.
6. Identify ways to avoid constipation, weight gain, and potential periods of depression during the recovery period.
7. Identify ways to comfortably return to baseline sexual activities.

REVIEW QUESTIONS

The number of the question corresponds to the same-numbered objective at the beginning of the chapter.

1. Which is not a realistic goal of patient teaching?
   a. Prepare patient for postoperative experiences
   b. Teach and practice skills needed for home care
   c. Alter patient's cultural belief regarding diet
   d. Explain medical terminology
2. Which of these statements concerning nurse-teacher stressors is most accurate?
   a. Most nurses believe teaching should be done by the physician.
   b. Establishing agreed on, written goals can reduce disagreement with the patient.
   c. For teaching, the nurse should rely only on her or his basic understanding or knowledge.
   d. Family members should not be used in the teaching process.
3. A characteristic of an adult learner is that
   a. adults do not need to practice a skill until they are in their home environment.
   b. most adults prefer lecture presentations.
   c. adults can often learn best from other adults with similar experiences.
   d. adults enjoy learning regardless of the relevance to their personal lives.
4. Considering the factors contributing to successful teaching, the nurse should
   a. plan teaching sessions when the work schedule permits.
   b. not involve family members in planning teaching activities.
   c. avoid reviewing content because this can be discouraging to patients.
   d. individualize the teaching plan.
5. Which of the following is *not* a basic step in the teaching process?
   a. Assessment
   b. Planning

c. Implementation
d. Evaluation
e. All of the above are basic steps in the teaching process

6. Which of the following learning objectives is correctly written?
   a. The patient should understand the implications of the condition.
   b. The patient will read two pamphlets on the subject of breast self-examination.
   c. The patient's spouse will demonstrate to the nurse how to correctly change a gastrostomy bag before drainage.
   d. The patient will lose 25 pounds in 6 weeks.
7. Which of the following is *not* true concerning teaching strategies?
   a. The most effective strategy is role playing.
   b. Audiovisual materials provide multisensory learning experiences, increasing the patient's confusion.
   c. For group discussions to be effective, they must be led by a nurse.
   d. Lecture-discussion can be more effective than lecture alone because it allows for the patient to participate.
8. Short-term evaluation of teaching effectiveness includes
   a. observing the patient and asking direct questions.
   b. following the patient through the medical chart for 3 to 6 months after the teaching.
   c. asking the patient what he or she found helpful about the teaching experience.
   d. monitoring for the behavior change for up to 6 weeks following discharge.

References

1. *Comprehensive accreditation manual for hospitals,* Oakbrook Terrace, Ill, 1997, Joint Commission on Accreditation of Healthcare Organizations.
2. Feste C, Anderson RM: Empowerment: from philosophy to practice, *Patient Educ Couns* 26:139, 1995.
3. Winthrop E: *Patient teaching tips,* St Louis, 1995, Mosby.
4. Stewart J: *Bridges not walls,* Mass, 1982, Addison-Wesley.
5. Chrisman N: The multicultural challenge, *J Multicult Nurs Health* 1:6, 1995.
6. Chachkes E, Christ G: Cross cultural issues in patient education, *Patient Educ Couns* 27:13, 1996.
7. Parikh NS and others: Shame and health literacy: the unspoken connection, *Patient Educ Couns* 27:33, 1996.
8. Platnikoff RC, Higgenbotham N: Predicting low-fat intentions and behaviors for the prevention of coronary artery disease, *Psychol Health* 10:397, 1995.
9. Ewart CK and others: Self-efficacy mediates strength gains during circuit training in men with coronary artery disease, *Med Sci Sports Exer* 18:531, 1986.
10. Covinsky KE and others: Relation between symptoms of depression and health status outcomes in acutely ill hospitalized older persons, *Ann Intern Med,* 126:417, 1997.
11. Grieco AJ: The importance of the family in patient education and care, *Patient Educ Couns* 27:1, 1996.
12. Bailey KG, Wood HE, Nava GR: What do clients want? Role of psychological kinship in professional helping, *Patient Educ Couns* 2:125, 1992.
13. Boise L, Heagerty B, Eskenazi: Facing chronic illness: The family support model and its benefits, *Patient Educ Couns* 27:75, 1996.
14. Berkman LF, Leo-Summers L, Hoewitz RI: Emotional support and survival after myocardial infarction, *Ann Intern Med,* 117:1003, 1992.
15. Case RB, Modd AJ, Case N, McDemott M, Eberly S: Living alone after myocardial infarction, *JAMA* 267:515, 1992.
16. Vella J: *Learning to listen, learning to teach,* San Francisco, 1994, Jossey-Bass.
17. Prochaska J, Norcross J, Declemente C: *Changing for good,* New York, 1994, William Morrow.
18. Katz JR: Providing effective patient teaching, *AJN* 97:33, 1997.
19. Hussey LC: Strategies for effective patient education material design, *J Cardiovasc Nurs* 11:37, 1997
20. Redman BK: *The practice of patient education,* St Louis, 1997, Mosby.

Resources

Achoo (Medical information directory)
http://www.achoo.com/

American Running & Fitness Association
4405 East West Highway, Suite 405
Bethesda, MD 20814
301-913-9517
Fax: 301-913-9520
http://www.arfa.org/

Asthma & Allergy Foundation of America
1125 15th Street NW, Suite 502
Washington, DC 20005
202-466-7643
Fax: 202-466-8940
http://www.aafa.org/

Choice In Dying
1035 30th Street, NW
Washington, DC 20007
202-338-9790
Fax: 202-338-0242
http://www.choices.org/

Disabled Sports/USA
451 Hungerford Drive, Suite 100
Rockville, MD 20850
301-217-0960
Fax: 301-217-0968
http://www.dsusa.org/~dsusa/

HealthAnswers (Orbis Broadcast Group)
http://www.healthanswers.com/

Healthfinder
http://www.healthfinder.gov/

The Health Manual (Columbia/HCA Healthcare Corp.)
http://www.columbia.net/consumer/consumer.html

Healthtouch (Medical Strategies, Inc.)
http://www.healthtouch.com/

InteliHealth (Johns Hopkins)
http://www.intelihealth.com

MedicineNet (Information Network, Inc.)
http://www.medicinenet.com

Meducation
http://www.meducation.com/patient.html

National Hospice Organization (NHO)
1901 North Moore Street, Suite 901
Arlington, VA 22209
800-658-8898
http://www.nho.org/

National Wellness Institute
1045 Clark Street, Suite 210
PO Box 827
Stevens Point, WI 54481
715-342-2969
http://www.wellnessnwi.org/

Office of Disease Prevention & Health Promotion (ODPHP)
National Health Information Center
PO Box 1133
Washington, DC 20013-1133
http://odphp.osophs.dhhs.gov/

On Health (IVI Publishing, Inc.)
http://www.onhealth.com

For additional Internet resources, see the website for this book at www.mosby.com/MERLIN/medsurg_lewis

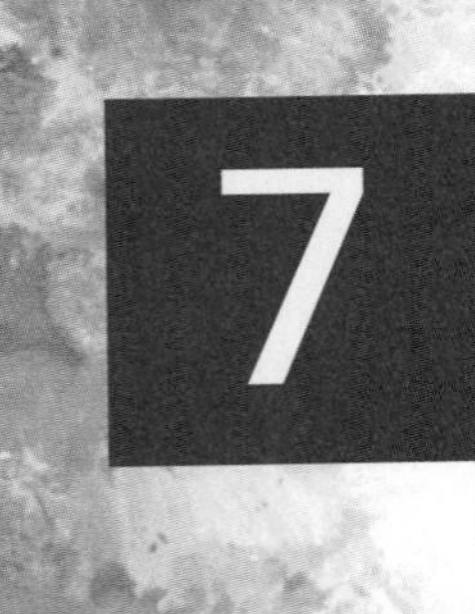

REMEMBER to check out your companion CD-ROM

7 NURSING MANAGEMENT Stress

Linda Witek-Janusek & Joan Stehle Werner

www.mosby.com/MERLIN/medsurg_lewis

LEARNING OBJECTIVES

1. Define the terms *stressor, stress, demands, primary appraisal, secondary appraisal, coping,* and *adaptation.*
2. Describe the three stages of Selye's general adaptation syndrome.
3. Describe the role of cognitive appraisal in the stress process.
4. Describe the role of the nervous and endocrine systems in the stress process.
5. Describe the effects of stress on the immune system.
6. Describe the coping behaviors used by a patient experiencing stress.
7. List the variables that may influence the response to stress.
8. Describe the nursing assessment and management of a patient experiencing stress.

THEORIES OF STRESS

Interest in the study of stress has intensified as investigators have begun to identify its role in relation to physical and emotional health. Most contemporary approaches to the study of stress have been influenced by three different but complementary stress theories. The first theory conceptualizes stress as a response to an environmental stressor. This theory was first proposed by Selye, who identified stress as a nonspecific response of the body to any demand made on it.[1] Selye referred to these stress-inducing demands as stressors. Stressors can be physical or emotional and pleasant or unpleasant, as long as they require the individual to adapt (Table 7-1). In response to either physical (e.g., burns) or psychologic (e.g., death of a loved one) stressors, a series of physiologic changes occur. Selye called this pattern of responses the general adaptation syndrome (GAS).

A second stress theory views stress as a stimulus that causes a response. This theory originated with Holmes, Rahe, and Masuda, who developed a tool (Table 7-2) to assess the effects of life changes on health.[2,3] Life changes are defined as conditions ranging from minor violations of the law to death of a loved one. The major assumption of this theory is that frequent life changes make people more vulnerable to illness (Table 7-3).

A third stress theory focuses on person-environment transactions and is referred to as the transaction or interaction theory.[4] A proponent of this theory is Lazarus, who emphasized the role of cognitive appraisal in assessing stressful situations and selecting coping options. Lazarus and Folkman[5] defined *psychologic stress* as a particular relationship between the person and the environment that is appraised by the person as taxing or exceeding his or her resources and endangering his or her well-being. These three stress theories are discussed in more detail in this chapter.

Reviewed by Monica Jarrett, RN, PhD, Research Associate Professor, University of Washington, Seattle, Wash.

STRESS AS A RESPONSE

Historically, Selye's early research using animals supported his theory that stressors from different sources produce a similar physical response pattern. He termed these physical responses to stress the *general adaptation syndrome.* The GAS is composed of three stages: alarm reaction, stage of resistance, and stage of exhaustion. Once the stressor or stimulus is integrated into the central nervous system (CNS), multiple responses occur because of activation of the hypothalamic-pituitary-adrenal axis and autonomic nervous system. The nature of these responses, in which the stimulus successively causes changes in the nervous, endocrine, and immune systems, is fundamental to understanding the physiologic and behavioral changes that occur in an individual experiencing stress.

Stage of Alarm Reaction

The first stage of the stress response is the alarm reaction of the GAS, in which the individual perceives a stressor physically or mentally, and the fight-or-flight response is initiated. When the stressor is of sufficient intensity to threaten the steady state of the individual, it requires a reallocation of energy so that adaptation can occur. This temporarily decreases the individual's resistance and may even result in disease or death if the stress is prolonged and severe.

Physical signs and symptoms of the alarm reaction are generally those of sympathetic nervous system stimulation. These signs include increased blood pressure, increased heart and respiratory rate, decreased gastrointestinal (GI) motility, pupil dilation, and increased perspiration. The patient may complain of such symptoms as increased anxiety, nausea, and anorexia.

Table 7-1 Examples of Stressors

Physical	Emotional
Noise	Diagnosis of cancer
Amphetamines	Promotion at work
Burns	Watching a loved one die
Running a marathon	Failing an examination
Infectious diseases	Financial loss
Pain	Winning a beauty contest

Stage of Resistance

Ideally the individual quickly moves from the alarm reaction to the stage of resistance in which physiologic reserves are mobilized to increase the resistance to stress. At this time adaptation may occur. The amount of resistance to the stressor varies among individuals, depending on the level of physical functioning, coping abilities, and total number and intensity of stressors experienced. For example, a person who has been exercising regularly and is physically fit will have greater ability to adapt to the stress of emergency surgery

Table 7-2 Social Readjustment Rating Scale

No.	Life Event	Mean Value
1	Death of spouse	100
2	Divorce	73
3	Marital separation from mate	65
4	Detention in jail or other institution	63
5	Death of a close family member	63
6	Major personal injury or illness	53
7	Marriage	50
8	Being fired at work	47
9	Marital reconciliation with mate	45
10	Retirement from work	45
11	Major change in health of a family member	44
12	Pregnancy	40
13	Sexual difficulties	39
14	Gaining a new family member (e.g., through birth, adoption, moving in)	39
15	Major business readjustment (e.g., merger, reorganization, bankruptcy)	39
16	Major change in financial state (e.g., a lot worse off or a lot better than usual)	38
17	Death of a close friend	37
18	Changing to different line of work	36
19	Major change in number of arguments with spouse (e.g., either a lot more or a lot less than usual regarding child rearing, personal habits)	35
20	Taking out a mortgage or loan for a major purchase (e.g., for a home, business)	31
21	Foreclosure on a mortgage or loan	30
22	Major change in responsibilities at work (e.g., promotion, demotion, lateral transfer)	29
23	Son or daughter leaving home (e.g., marriage, attending college)	29
24	Trouble with in-laws	29
25	Outstanding personal achievement	28
26	Spouse beginning or ceasing work outside the home	26
27	Beginning or ceasing normal schooling	26
28	Major change in living conditions (e.g., building a new home, remodeling, deterioration of home or neighborhood)	25
29	Revision of personal habits (e.g., dress, manners, associations)	24
30	Trouble with boss	23
31	Major change in working hours or conditions	20
32	Change in residence	20
33	Changing to a new school	20
34	Major change in usual type or amount of recreation	19
35	Major change in church activities (e.g., a lot more or a lot less than usual)	19
36	Major change in social activities (e.g., clubs, dancing, movies, visiting)	18
37	Taking out a mortgage or loan for a lesser purchase (e.g., for a car, TV, freezer)	17
38	Major change in sleeping habits (a lot more or a lot less sleep, or change in part of day when asleep)	16
39	Major change in number of family get-togethers (e.g., a lot more or a lot less than usual)	15
40	Major change in eating habits (a lot more or a lot less food intake, or very different meal hours or surroundings)	15
41	Vacation	13
42	Christmas	12
43	Minor violation of law (e.g., traffic tickets, jaywalking, disturbing the peace)	11

Source: Holmes TH, Rahe RH: Social readjustment rating scale, *J Psychosom Res* 11:216, 1967.

Table 7-3 Life Change Units and Incidence of Major Illness*

Number	Amount of Change	Incidence of Major Illness
0-149	Insignificant	Minimal
150-199	Mild	33%
200-299	Moderate	50%
300+	Major	80%

Source: Holmes T, Rahe E: The social readjustment rating scale, *J Psychosom Res* 11:213, 1967.
*This table describes the amount of stress as measured by LCUs (life change units), followed by the statistical incidence of disease according to the number of LCUs. The chance of illness is based on the number of LCUs during 1 to 2 years.

Table 7-4 Examples of Disorders and Diseases of Adaptation

Angina	Impotence
Carpal tunnel syndrome	Insomnia
Depression	Irritable bowel syndrome
Dyspepsia	Low back pain
Eating disorders	Myocardial infarction
Fatigue	Peptic ulcer disease
Headaches	Sexual dysfunction
Hypertension	

than a person who is deconditioned and leads a sedentary lifestyle.

Although few overt physical signs and symptoms occur in this stage as compared with the alarm stage, the person is expending energy in an attempt to adapt. This adaptive energy is limited by the resources available to the individual. These resources include not only the individual's internal physical and psychologic reserves, but also external resources such as social support from family, friends, and health care workers. When resources are adequate, the individual may successfully recover from a stressor such as surgery and return to his or her baseline (presurgery) state. If adaptation does not occur, the person may move to the next phase of the GAS, which is the stage of exhaustion.

Stage of Exhaustion

The stage of exhaustion is the final stage of the GAS. It occurs when all the energy for adaptation has been expended. Physical symptoms of the alarm reaction may briefly reappear in a final effort by the body to survive. This is exemplified by a terminally ill person who becomes alert and has stronger vital signs shortly before death. The individual in the stage of exhaustion usually becomes ill and may die if assistance from outside sources is not available. This stage can often be reversed by external sources of adaptive energy, such as medication, blood transfusions, or psychotherapy.

Refinements in Selye's Stress Theory

Selye's work addressed the importance of conditioning factors that may affect the stress response. These internal conditioning factors include age, genetic makeup, and previous experience with the stressors, and external conditioning factors such as diet and climate.[6] Selye coined the term *eustress* to refer to stress associated with positive events such as winning a tennis match. However, he never fully explained the health consequences of eustress versus stress. This relationship is currently under investigation by others, as exemplified by studies in which not only "daily hassles" but also positive events or "uplifts" experienced by an individual are measured.

Selye's description of stress focuses on the physiologic changes of the nervous, immune, gastrointestinal, and endocrine systems that occur as an organism responds to a specific stressor. In his original work, Selye described a triad of responses that occur during stress: (1) adrenocortical activation, (2) thymic involution, and (3) GI ulceration. His work indicates that there is a predictable uniform pattern in the physiologic response to various stressors. This emphasis is due in part to the fact that Selye used animal models that were not capable of complex psychologic processing of a stressor. As stress researchers began to study humans, the individual variations and psychologic modification of the stress response became apparent.

Human research supports different patterns of physiologic responses that occur during stress. Illustrating this view is an early classic study conducted by Lacey and Lacey[7] in 1958. These investigators subjected 42 participants to four mild stressors. Stressors included (1) the cold pressor test, in which one arm is placed in ice water; (2) anticipating the cold pressor test; (3) a mental math problem; and (4) a test of word fluency. A number of physiologic stress responses were assessed. The investigators found substantial variability in blood pressure, heart rate, pulse pressure, and other measures among subjects in response to the same stressor. More recently, individual differences in the cellular immune response to acute psychologic stress have been described.[8] Thus stressors are likely to produce complex and varying profiles of hormonal and immunologic changes in different individuals. This may help explain why a variety of the diseases or disorders of adaptation exist (Table 7-4) and also why there are differences in susceptibility to stress-related disease.

Selye's studies employed acute and intense physical stressors, such as cold, electric shock, and injection of toxic agents.[6] Today researchers are finding differences in the behavioral and physiologic adaptive response to a stressor based on duration of a stressor (i.e., if it is acute or chronic) as well as the intensity (i.e., mild, moderate, severe). For example, an individual dealing with the chronic stress of caring for a loved one may also be exposed to a multitude of acute episodic stressors. Researchers are finding that the processes underlying acute versus chronic stress are not always the same.[9] Therefore the duration or chronicity of exposure to a stressor is an important variable that can influence an individual's adaptive response.

STRESS AS A STIMULUS

Life Events

Another approach to the study of stress is to view stress as a stimulus or event that disturbs an individual's homeostatic balance. Stress defined in this way is similar to Selye's definition of a stressor. Historically this approach stems from attempts to develop questionnaires to measure stress in terms of life changes or life events.[2,3] Two such questionnaires are the Social Readjustment Rating Scale (SRRS) (see Table 7-2) and the Schedule of Recent Experiences (SRE). Life events questionnaires such as the SRRS and the SRE were developed in an attempt to numerically weight the impact (stress) of various life changes (e.g., death of a spouse, financial changes). A life event is regarded as stressful if it is associated with some adaptive or coping behavior on the part of the involved individual.[3] Each event, whether desirable or not, is indicative of the amount of change it produces in the ongoing life pattern of the individual.

It was originally theorized that the more stressful life events occurring throughout a specific period of time, the greater the vulnerability to illness. Of particular interest was the research that reported an association between the number and intensity of life events and the resulting probability of physical and emotional illness following the events (see Table 7-3).[10] Although several studies have shown statistically significant relationships between stressful life events and illness onset, these relationships are often weak. Life-events scaling has raised methodologic issues regarding additional factors (e.g., age, perception, previous experiences, health) that must be taken into account when considering life events. Further, stressful life events may prove to have a greater impact on illness progression as opposed to illness onset.

Refinements in the Stress as a Stimulus Theory

Factors that affect an individual's response to life events include cultural influences, personality, clustering of events, biologic variables, socioeconomic status, timing, and interpersonal support systems. These factors indicate the importance of using a holistic approach when assessing the patient.

Hardiness and Sense of Coherence. An interesting aspect of research focused on life events is the identification of some individuals who experience significant life events but do not succumb to illness. *Hardiness* is a mediating factor in the stress-illness relationship.[11] The hardy person has (1) a clear sense of personal values and goals, (2) a strong tendency toward interaction with the environment, (3) a sense of meaningfulness, and (4) an internal rather than external locus of control.

Sense of coherence (SOC), a concept closely related to hardiness, has been defined and developed by Antonovsky.[12] It has been shown that SOC is a more powerful mediator of stress and illness than hardiness.[13] In general, SOC refers to how an individual sees the world and one's life in it. It is a personality characteristic or coping style rather than a response to a specific situation. The three components of SOC are comprehensibility (stimuli derived from one's internal and external environments are structured, predictable, and explicable), manageability (resources are available to meet the demands posed by these stimuli), and meaningfulness (demands are challenges worthy of investment and engagement). An individual with a strong SOC has an enduring tendency to see one's life as ordered, predictable, and manageable. Resilience is another personality characteristic that is believed to moderate the negative effects of stress. Resilience is defined as being resourceful, flexible, and having an available source of problem-solving strategies. Individuals who possess a high degree of resilience are not as likely to perceive an event as stressful or taxing.[14]

Hassles and Uplifts. Daily-hassle scores have been found to be an important supplement to the life-events approach in predicting health and illness outcomes related to the impact of a stressor. *Daily hassles* are experiences and conditions of daily living that have been appraised as harmful or threatening to an individual's well-being.[15] The frequency and intensity of daily hassles have a stronger relationship with somatic illness than the life-events scale.[5] Items addressed on the daily hassles scale reflect the content areas of work, family, social activities, environment, practical considerations, finances, and health (Table 7-5).[15] Recent research in this area has shown that an increase in daily hassles is implicated in the onset of migraine headaches.[16]

Table 7-5 Examples of Daily Hassles

Misplacing or losing things	Chronic pain
Inconsiderate smokers	Inadequate financial resources
Planning meals	Job dissatisfaction
Concerns about job security	Caring for disabled child
Difficulties with friends	Marital problems
Waiting	

As an adjunct to hassles, *uplifts* are defined as positive experiences that are likely to occur in everyday life.[5] This concept seems comparable with the term *eustress* described earlier by Selye. Further investigation is needed to determine the effects of positive experiences on health outcomes.

STRESS AS A TRANSACTION

Appraisal

In contrast to theories of stress as a response or stimulus, Lazarus's theory focuses on the person-environment transaction and the cognitive appraisal of demands and coping options.[5] A multitude of internal and external data are received at the neurocognitive level. Lazarus proposed that these data are interpreted during the process of cognitive appraisal. *Appraisal* is a judgment process that includes recognizing the degree of demands, or stressors, placed on the individual (Fig. 7-1). The appraisal process also involves the recognition of available resources or options that help when dealing with potential or actual demands.

During primary appraisal, demands are assessed according to the possible impact on the individual's well-being (i.e., what is at stake). Demands can be judged as irrelevant, benign-positive, or stressful. If demands are appraised as stressful, they can be classified as representing harm or loss, threat, or challenge. Harm or loss demands involve actual damage, and threat demands involve anticipated harm or loss. Challenge demands differ from threat and harm or loss demands because they are viewed as a potential for personal gain or growth. For example, hiking in the wilderness may place demands on the individual that will provide an opportunity to test and exhibit strength and endurance. Therefore stress is a situation in which demands exceed the individual's adaptive resources. If an adaptive response to these demands does not occur, negative consequences will result.[17]

Secondary appraisal refers to the process of recognizing the coping resources and options that are available. Primary and secondary appraisal often occur simultaneously and interact with each other in determining stress. Cognitive reappraisal is the process of continuously relabeling cognitive appraisals. Certain factors influence the labeling of appraisals.[5] Situational factors include the intensity of the external demands, the immediacy of the expected impact, and ambiguity. Person-related

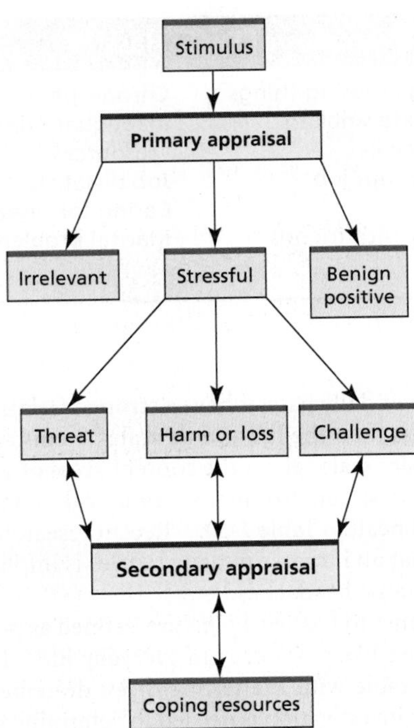

Fig. 7-1 Cognitive appraisal process.

factors include motivational characteristics, belief systems, and intellectual resources and skills.

Theoretic Summary

The role of perception is the key to understanding the difference between the three major stress theories presented. In Selye's stress response theory, all demands are stressors with the capacity to elicit the GAS. Conditioning factors in individuals influence the stress response. In the life-change theory, perceived stressfulness of the event is not considered because each individual receives the same score for a certain stressor. In the Lazarus transaction theory, the cognitive appraisal process determines whether the demands will be assessed as stressful. Through cognitive appraisal, individuals experience different outcomes in dealing with demands, not only because of conditioning factors, but also as a result of how the demand is perceived and labeled during the person-stressor interaction. An event that is stressful to one individual may not be stressful to another.

PHYSIOLOGIC RESPONSE TO STRESS

To simplify the description of the physiologic response to stress, the following discussion is divided into the roles of the nervous system, the endocrine system, and the immune system. However, these systems are interrelated, and thus the ultimate response of the person to stress reflects the integration of the three systems (Fig. 7-2). Further, stress-activation of these systems affects other physiologic systems, such as the cardiovascular, respiratory, gastrointestinal, renal, and reproductive systems. As a result, an individual's response to stress has the potential to lead to diseases of adaptation in any physiologic system. Understanding the physiologic changes associated with stress will help provide the foundation for the assessment of the patient experiencing stress and the implications for health outcomes.

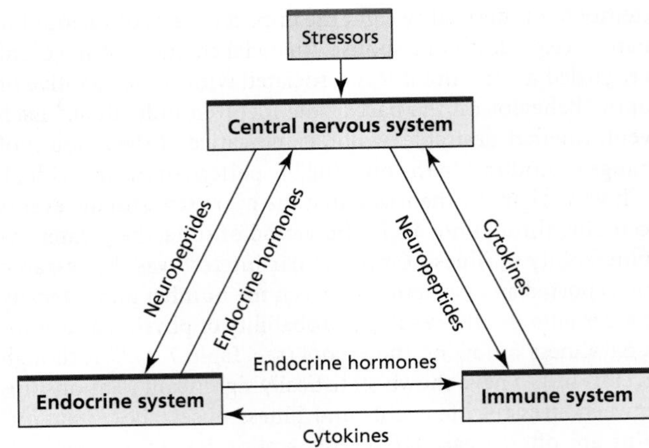

Fig. 7-2 Neurochemical links among the nervous, endocrine, and immune systems. The communication among these three systems is bidirectional.

Nervous System

Stressors, or demands, may be physical, psychologic, or social. The body will respond physiologically to both actual and potential stressors. The complex process by which an event is perceived as a stressor and by which the body responds is not fully understood. The hypothalamus participates in both the emotional and physiologic responses to stressors. This control is significant because most stressors precipitate an emotional reaction. In addition to the hypothalamus, other parts of the CNS, including the cerebral cortex, limbic system, and reticular formation, are involved in the neural control of emotions and the physiologic response to stress (Figs. 7-3 and 7-4). The functions of these structures are closely interrelated.

Cerebral Cortex. After an external event has occurred, afferent input is sent to the cerebral cortex via sensory impulses from the peripheral nervous system, including the eyes and the ears. For example, the pressure of a restraint on an arm or leg that is applied too tightly will act as a stressor. Afferent impulses that travel to the cortex from the periphery via the spinal cord (spinothalamic pathways) also activate the reticular formation in the area of the brainstem. The reticular formation then relays input to the thalamus and from the thalamus to the cerebral cortex. This network of neurons, which is involved with arousal and consciousness, is called the reticular activating system (RAS). The RAS functions to maintain wakefulness and alertness.

The somatic, auditory, and visual associative areas of the cerebral cortex receive input from the peripheral sensory fibers and then interpret it. The prefrontal area serves to reduce the speed of the associative functions so that the person has time to evaluate the information in light of past experiences and future consequences (primary and secondary appraisal) and to plan a course of action. All these functions are involved in the perception of a stressor.

The temporal lobes of the cerebral cortex contain the auditory association areas, which, when stimulated, produce the sensation of fear. Stimulation of the temporal lobes can result in sounds that seem louder or softer, visual displays that seem nearer or farther, and experiences that seem familiar or strange. These effects modify the perception of stress.

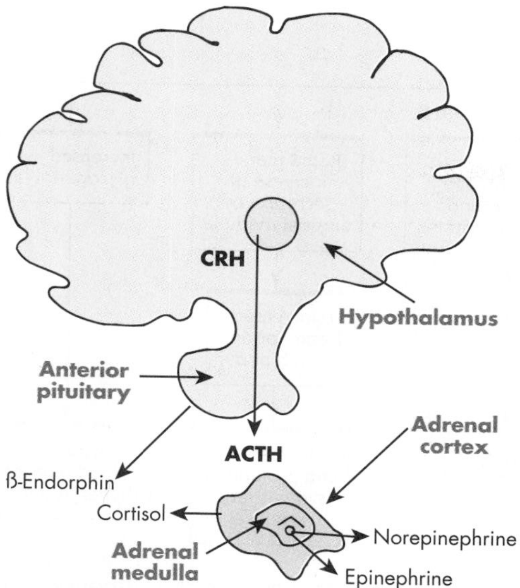

Fig. 7-3 Hypothalamic-pituitary-adrenal axis. *ACTH,* adrenocorticotropic hormone; *CRH,* corticotropin-releasing hormone.

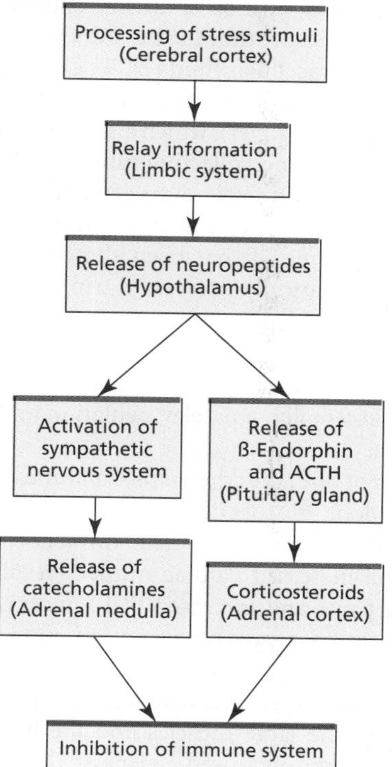

Fig. 7-4 The cerebral cortex processes stressful stimuli and relays the information via the limbic system to the hypothalamus. Corticotropin-releasing hormone (CRH) stimulates the release of adrenocorticotropic hormone (ACTH) from the pituitary gland. ACTH stimulates the adrenal cortex to release corticosteroids. The sympathetic nervous system is also stimulated, resulting in the release of epinephrine and norepinephrine.

Table 7-6 Hypothalamic Functions

Coordinates Impulses
Autonomic nervous system
Body temperature regulation
Food intake
Water balance
Urine formation
Cardiovascular function
Secretes Releasing Factors
Regulation of anterior and posterior pituitary hormones
Affects Behavior
Emotion
Alertness

Limbic System. The limbic system, which lies in the inner midportion of the brain near the base, includes the septum, cingulate gyrus, amygdala, hippocampus, and anterior nuclei of the thalamus. (The hypothalamus is located in the center of these structures but is not considered a part of the limbic system.) The function of the limbic system is thought to be involved primarily with emotions and behavior. When these structures are stimulated, emotions, feelings, and behaviors can occur that ensure survival and self-preservation, such as feeding, sociability, and sexuality. The cerebral cortex and limbic system interact to serve the experiential and executive functions of emotion. Endorphins are found in structures of the limbic system and in the thalamus, brain, and spinal cord. They are known to reduce the perception of painful stimuli. Endogenous opioids have also been shown to increase in response to stress in the absence of pain.

Reticular Formation. The reticular formation is located between the lower end of the brainstem and the thalamus. It contains the RAS, which sends impulses contributing to alertness to the limbic system and to the cerebral cortex and thalamus. In addition to receiving input from the periphery, the RAS also receives impulses from the hypothalamus. When the RAS is stimulated, it increases its output of impulses leading to wakefulness. Both physiologic and perceived stress usually increase the degree of wakefulness and can lead to sleep disturbances.

Hypothalamus. The hypothalamus, which lies just above the pituitary gland, has many functions (Table 7-6). The hypothalamus receives information regarding traumatic stimuli via the spinothalamic pathway, pressure-sensitive input from the baroreceptors via the brainstem, and emotional stimuli via the limbic system. Because the hypothalamus secretes peptide hormones and factors that regulate the release of hormones by the anterior pituitary, it is central to the connection between the nervous and endocrine systems in responding to stress (see Fig. 7-3).

In addition, the hypothalamus regulates the function of both the sympathetic and parasympathetic branches of the autonomic nervous system. Thus when an individual perceives the existence of a stressor, the hypothalamus mediates both the neural and endocrine responses. It does this primarily by activating the sympathetic nervous system and by releasing corticotropin-releasing hormone (CRH), which stimulates the pituitary to release adrenocorticotropic hormone (ACTH) (see Chapters 45 and 47). In response to certain stress

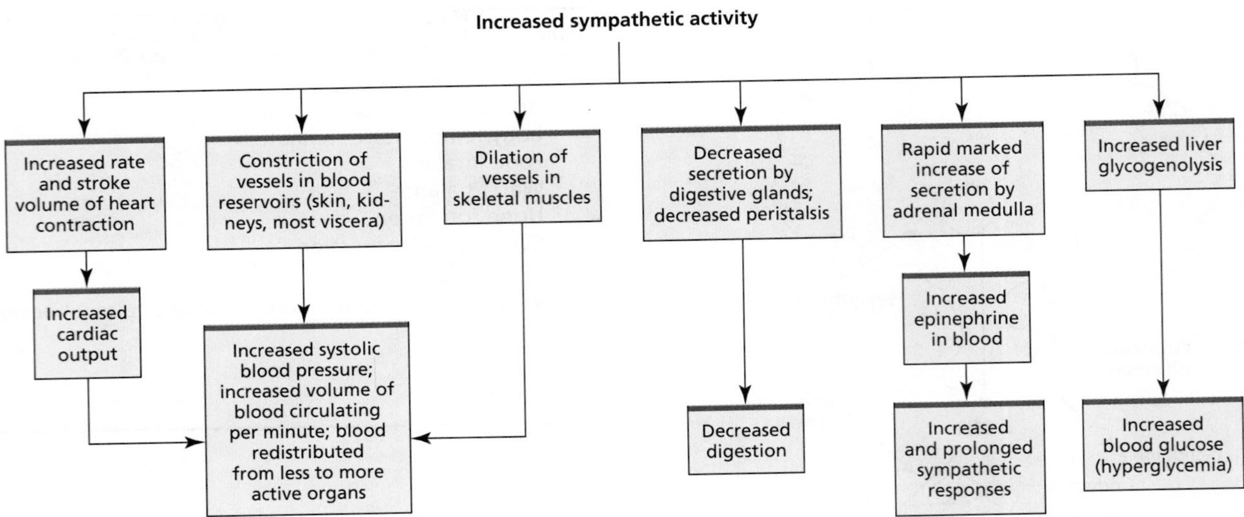

Fig. 7-5 Alarm reaction responses resulting from increased sympathetic activity. Note that these are the responses commonly referred to as the fight-or-flight reaction.

conditions, the parasympathetic nervous system is stimulated. This may be manifested as increased GI motility, flushing, or bronchial constriction.

Endocrine System

Once the hypothalamus is activated in response to stress, the endocrine system becomes involved. The sympathetic nervous system stimulates the adrenal medulla to release the hormones epinephrine and norepinephrine (catecholamines). The effect of catecholamines and the sympathetic nervous system, including the adrenal medulla, is referred to as the sympathoadrenal response. These hormones prepare the body for the fight-or-flight response (Fig. 7-5). This response is activated by physical stressors such as hypovolemia and hypoxia and emotional states, particularly anger, excitement, and fear. Catecholamines can be measured in the blood or urine; as a result, numerous research studies have used them to determine the impact of various stressors.

Both acute situational stress and chronic stress activate the hypothalamic-pituitary-adrenal (HPA) axis. It is noteworthy, however, that the HPA axis is especially sensitive to situations marked by novelty, uncertainty, frustration, conflict, and lack of control. In response to perceived stress, the hypothalamus releases CRH, which stimulates the anterior pituitary to release pro-opiomelanocortin (POMC). Both ACTH and β-endorphin are derived from POMC. Endorphins have analgesic-like effects and blunt pain perception during stress situations involving pain stimuli. ACTH, in turn, stimulates the adrenal cortex to synthesize and secrete glucocorticoids (e.g., cortisol) and, to a lesser degree, aldosterone. Glucocorticoids are essential for the stress response. Cortisol produces a number of physiologic effects that include increasing blood glucose levels, potentiating the action of catecholamines on blood vessels, and inhibiting the inflammatory response. Glucocorticoids play an important role in "turning off" or blunting aspects of the stress response, which can become self-destructive. This is best exemplified by the ability of glucocorticoids to suppress the release of proinflammatory mediators, such as tumor necrosis factor (TNF) and interleukin-1 (IL-1). The persistent release of such mediators is believed to initiate organ dysfunction in conditions such as sepsis. Hence glucocorticoids act not only to support the adaptive response of the body to a stressor, but also act to suppress an overzealous and potentially self-destructive response. Cortisol is commonly measured in studies of stress and can be measured in plasma, urine, or saliva. Aldosterone acts to increase sodium reabsorption in the kidney tubules and, as a result, increases extracellular fluid (ECF). During stress, neural stimulation of the posterior pituitary results in the secretion of antidiuretic hormone (ADH), which also promotes water reabsorption by the distal and collecting tubules of the kidney.

The secretion of adrenal androgens (dehydroepiandrosterone [DHEA]), as well as testicular androgens, is typically decreased during stress. It has been shown that testosterone levels in men dramatically decrease during physical stressors, such as surgery, and also in response to psychologic stressors, such as anticipation of parachute jumping.[18] Stress effects on female reproductive hormones is harder to measure; however, intense stress in females can delay ovulation and at times lead to amenorrhea.[19]

Stimulation of both the adrenal medulla and cortex results in an increased blood glucose level. This elevation provides the additional fuel for the increased metabolism needed for fighting or fleeing. The increased cardiac output (resulting from the increased heart rate and increased ECF), increased blood glucose levels, increased oxygen consumption, and increased metabolic rate make the physical responses possible. In addition, dilation of skeletal muscle blood vessels and resulting increased blood supply to the large muscles and the brain provide for quick movement and increased alertness. The increased blood volume (from increased ECF and the shunting of blood from the GI system) and increased clotting time function to help maintain adequate circulation to vital organs in case of traumatic blood loss. These responses to stress illustrate the complexity and interrelated nature of the processes involved (Fig. 7-6).

The physiologic responses to stressors seem better suited to persons living in a primitive society than in the industrialized societies of today. Because of social conventions, many of the physiologic responses to stress are internalized and produce

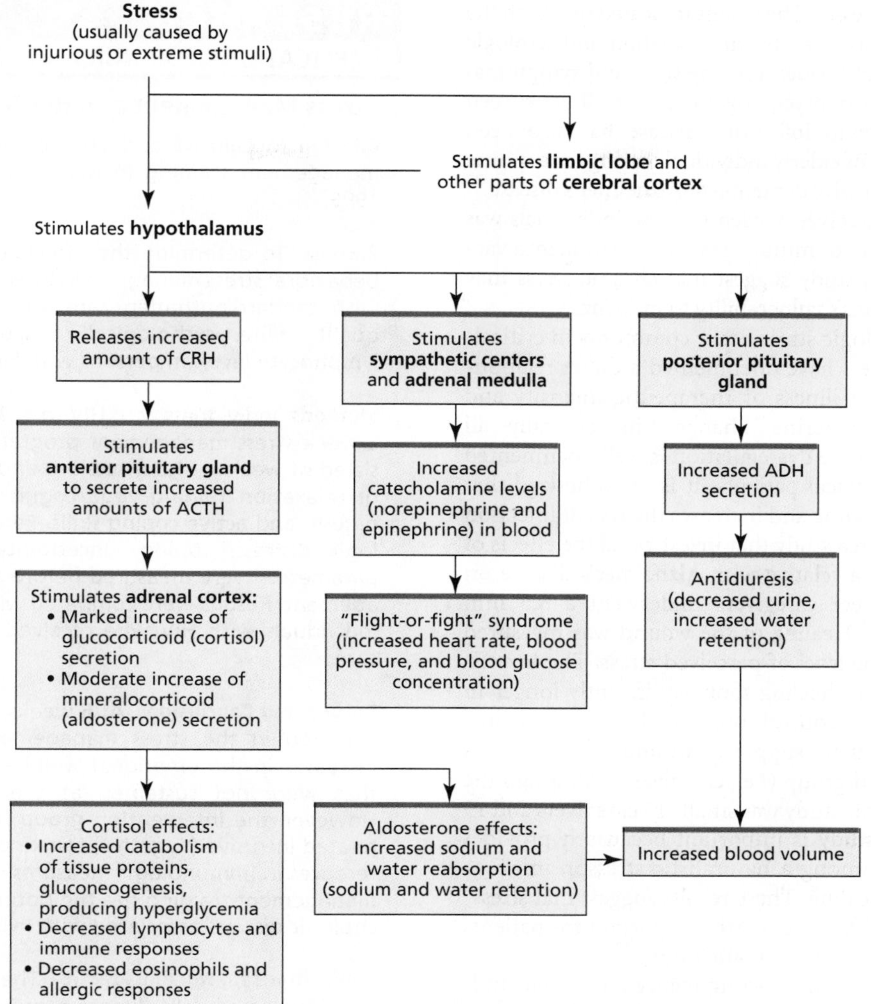

Fig. 7-6 Current concepts of the stress syndrome. *ACTH,* adrenocorticotropic hormone; *ADH,* antidiuretic hormone; *CRH,* corticotropin-releasing hormone.

wear and tear on the body. As a result, many diseases (the diseases of adaptation) experienced by modern people are considered maladaptations to stress.

Immune System

Recently there has been a major focus on understanding the potential impact of stress on immune function.[20] Negative stressors lead to alterations in immune function in humans through processes involving the hypothalamic-pituitary-adrenal axis and the autonomic nervous system that affect immune function (see Fig. 7-4). In return, the immune system also affects endocrine and CNS responses (see Fig. 7-2). Both corticosteroids and catecholamines are known to suppress immune function. Interleukin-1 (which is released by activated macrophages), one type of cytokine, may directly stimulate the release of ACTH and thus initiate the stress response. It is now known that there are multiple complex interactions between the endocrine and the immune system. This includes not only adrenocortical hormones but also endorphins, thyroid hormones, reproductive hormones, growth hormone, and prolactin. Although most stress hormones suppress the immune system, some, such as prolactin, stimulate certain aspects of immunity.[20]

There is now a large body of literature that suggests a relationship between stress and immune-based illness.[20-22] This has led to the development of the discipline of psychoneuroimmunology (PNI), which is an interdisciplinary science that seeks to understand the relationship among the brain, behavior, and immunity. Multiple studies have shown that both acute and chronic stress can affect immune function, including decreased number and function of natural killer cells, altered lymphocyte proliferation, decreased production of cytokines by lymphocytes, and decreased phagocytosis by neutrophils and monocytes.[20,23] Most of these studies have shown that stress induces immunosuppression. Although these are definite in vitro findings, it is not known how much stress is needed to cause these changes or how much of an alteration in the immune system is necessary before disease susceptibility occurs. The current task of researchers in the field of PNI is to link stress-induced immune changes to illness.[22]

A recent study demonstrated a relationship between psychologic stress and the common cold.[24] In this study healthy volunteers were inoculated intranasally with low doses of upper respiratory viruses. The subjects underwent psychologic testing to determine the occurrence of stressful events in their lives and their reactions to such stresses. The results indicated that both the rates of viral infection (assessed by viral isolation and serologic response) and clinical colds (identified by signs and symptoms) increased with the degree of psychologic stress. The link between stress and susceptibility to infectious disease has also been demonstrated in a study of elderly individuals caring for a spouse suffering from the progressive dementia of Alzheimer's disease.[25] The chronic stress of caregiver burden in these individuals was associated with an impaired immune response to influenza vaccine. The results of this study suggest that chronic stress may increase an elderly persons's vulnerability to influenza.

Physical and psychologic stress occur commonly in critically ill patients. Researchers have documented a direct relationship between severity of illness or therapeutic intensity and stress-induced neuroendocrine changes in critically ill patients.[26] Because immune dysregulation is well documented in both injured and surgical patients, it is hypothesized that stress impairs wound healing and increases the risk of infection in the critically ill.[26,27] In a study that investigated the effects of the stress of caring for a relative with Alzheimer's disease on wound healing, volunteer caregivers underwent a 3.5 mm punch biopsy wound.[27] Healing of the wound was measured over time along with the level of perceived stress. The investigators found that wound healing took significantly longer in stressed caregivers than in control subjects. Also, IL-1 beta production, a cytokine that supports wound healing, was depressed in the stressed group (i.e., caregivers). Although the number of subjects in this study was small (13 caregivers and 13 control subjects), the study is important because it provides evidence of a linkage among a naturalistic stressor, immune response, and wound healing. These results suggest that stress-related delays in wound healing may be important for patients recovering from surgery and traumatic injury.[27]

Strategies to enhance immunocompetence have been studied, and results are promising. These strategies include relaxation and imagery techniques, biofeedback-assisted relaxation strategies, humor, exercise, and social support.[28] An important study in this area showed that patients with metastatic breast cancer who were involved in a weekly support group lived longer (an average of 18 months) than patients in the control group.[29] Recently, these investigators made a final evaluation of the subjects from this study and showed that the difference in survival could not be explained by a difference in medical treatment between the two groups, thus further strengthening the importance of their findings.[30] Although few studies document the importance of psychologic interventions on survival, research in this area has intensified and now not only includes studies of individuals with cancer but also individuals with human immunodeficiency virus (HIV).[28]

RESEARCH
IMPLICATIONS FOR NURSING PRACTICE

Stress Management and HIV Disease

Citation McCain NL and others: The influence of stress management training in HIV disease, *Nurs Res* 45:246, 1996.

Purpose To determine the effectiveness of a cognitive-behavioral stress management intervention, as compared with standard outpatient care, on stress, coping patterns, quality of life, psychologic distress, uncertainty, and CD4$^+$ lymphocyte levels in persons with HIV disease.

Methods Individuals with HIV (n = 30) were enrolled in a 6-week stress management program. The program consisted of weekly 1-hour sessions and included instruction on relaxation training, yoga, cognitive restructuring techniques, and active coping skills. Perceived stress, psychologic distress, coping, uncertainty, and immunologic parameters were measured before and after stress management. Results were compared with a control group of individuals with HIV who received standard outpatient care.

Results and Conclusions At 6 weeks, individuals who participated in the stress management intervention had increases in the emotional well-being of quality of life that were not sustained at the 6-month follow-up. However, the intervention group had a decline in HIV-related intrusive (negative) thinking at 6 months. No differences in immunologic measures were observed. Stress management training has the potential to decrease psychologic distress associated with living with HIV.

Implications for Nursing Practice The psychologic needs of individuals with HIV disease require careful assessment. Stress management intervention can be used by nurses to improve the psychologic well-being of persons with HIV; however, these individuals should be encouraged to independently practice these techniques. Future studies are needed to determine the potential of more intensive stress management interventions on immune status in individuals with HIV.

IDENTIFYING STRESSORS OR DEMANDS

Work-Related Stressors

The nurse should become familiar with the types of stressors experienced by various populations and individuals in particular circumstances. For example, work-related stressors are common.[31] Some demands are intrinsic to the job, such as poor working conditions, work overload, and time pressures. Other demands stem from the individual's role in the organization (role conflict), career development (overpromotion or underpromotion), relationships at work (difficulties in delegating responsibilities), and the organizational climate (restrictions on behavior). The extensive research on these factors and their effects validates inclusion of occupation and work experience as essential factors in assessment.[32]

Nurses and student nurses have been extensively studied as groups experiencing high levels of stress and burnout. Stressors such as heavy workload, lack of adequate rewards, and lack of participation in decision making have been identified in various practice settings. Knowledge of these stressors is important if nurses do not want to become victims of stress and burnout in the work environment.

Illness-Related Stressors

Another major source of stress relates to illness experienced by a patient, which often causes stress for family members as well as the patient. The nurse should assess what aspects of the illness are the most stressful for the patient. These may include

Table 7-7 Examples of Coping Resources

Coping Resources in the Person	
Health, Energy, Morale	**Problem-solving Skills**
Robust health	Collection of information
High energy level	Identification of problem
High morale	Generation of alternatives
Positive Beliefs	**Social Skills**
Self-efficacy	Communication skills
Spiritual faith	Compatibility
Coping Resources in the Environment	
Social Networks	**Utilitarian Resources**
Family members	Finances
Co-workers	Instructional manuals
Social contacts	Social agencies

Table 7-8 Examples of Demands and Coping

Demands	Coping
Being diagnosed with diabetes	Attending diabetic education classes (P-S) Taking a short vacation (E-R)
Failing an examination	Obtaining a tutor (P-S) Having dinner with friends (E-R)
Being told that more work will be required as part of the job	Learning to use a word processor (P-S) Venting negative feelings about paperwork to spouse (E-R)
Being notified of an appointment for an IRS audit	Reviewing tax records with accountant (P-S) Practicing deep breathing exercises (E-R)
Giving a public speech for the first time	Practicing in front of family members (P-S) Jogging the morning of the speech (E-R)

E-R, emotion-regulating efforts; *P-S,* problem-solving skills.

such factors as physical health, job responsibilities, finances, and children. This information is valuable because it gives the nurse the patient's perspective on stressors.

Although the nurse and patient generally agree on what stressors are experienced by the patient, the nurse generally rates all items as significantly more stressful than the patient does.[33] These findings emphasize the need for understanding the patient's perception of the situation.

A hospital stress rating scale has been developed based on stressors identified by medical-surgical patients.[34] The five most stressful events in descending order of stressfulness are (1) the possibility of losing sight, (2) the anticipated diagnosis of cancer, (3) the possibility of losing a kidney or other organ, (4) knowing the illness is serious, and (5) the possibility of losing one's sense of hearing.

A powerful case-study report of the perceptions of a critically ill patient experiencing therapeutic paralysis in an intensive care unit (ICU) was based on interviewing the patient after recovery.[35] The perceptions are especially poignant because the patient was a former ICU nurse. She recounted the intense stress she felt caused by feelings of powerlessness that accompanied her paralysis, her desperation due to the severity of her illness, and her lack of control and uncertainty about her prognosis. Providing information, control, and reassurance are important nursing interventions that can have a significant impact on decreasing a patient's perception of stress. Another study identified hospital stressors of patients with acquired immunodeficiency syndrome (AIDS). Major stressors for this group of patients were loss of independence, separation from significant others, and medication problems.[36] Knowledge of stressors and the feelings these stressors invoke can further assist the nurse in identifying potential and actual sources of stress and assessing the impact these stressors have on the hospitalized patient.

COPING

The term *coping* has been defined as constantly changing cognitive and behavioral efforts to manage specific external or internal demands that are appraised as taxing or exceeding the resources of the person.[5] Defense processes, such as denial, may also be included as coping processes, since both defensive and coping processes intertwine and are intrinsic to the psychologic integrity of the individual. *Coping resources,* defined as characteristics or actions drawn on to manage stress (Table 7-7), include factors in the person or environment that encompass categories such as (1) health, energy, and morale; (2) positive beliefs; (3) problem-solving skills; (4) social skills; (5) social networks; and (6) material resources.

Coping efforts function broadly in two ways: as problem-solving (problem-focused) and emotion-regulating (emotion-focused) efforts (Table 7-8). As an individual attempts to deal with demands (internal or environmental) or obstacles that create the demands, the person is said to be using the problem-focused coping efforts. When the individual's effort is concentrated on methods of regulating the emotional response to the problem, the person is using emotion-focused coping efforts. For example, a patient with diabetes mellitus who learns to give injections is engaged in problem-focused coping. This patient is using emotion-focused coping when the distress of being diagnosed with diabetes is lessened by the thought that it would be worse if the diagnosis had been cancer. Combinations of emotion-focused and problem-focused coping can be used in dealing with the same stressor. An individual who has flexibility in coping or the ability to change coping strategies over time and across different stressful conditions is better equipped to handle stressful circumstances.

As an individual begins to deal with a stressor, modes of coping may include the following:

1. Information seeking (gathering data about the problem and possible solutions to the problem)
2. Direct actions (performing concrete acts to alter self or environment)
3. Inhibition of action (refraining from any action)
4. Intrapsychic processes (reappraising the situation; initiating cognitive activity aimed at improving feelings)
5. Turning to others (obtaining social support)
6. Escaping or avoiding

The choice of coping strategies depends on various factors. Variables that affect an individual's choice of coping strategies include degrees of uncertainty, threat, or helplessness and the presence of conflict.[37] If uncertainty is high, direct action is less likely to be selected as a coping strategy. If the degree of appraised threat is severe, more primitive coping modes such as panic are more likely to occur. In the presence of conflict, an individual may not be able to take direct actions. Helplessness promotes immobilization. The strategy chosen may also be influenced by the outcome of the cognitive appraisal that categorizes the stressor as harm or loss, threat, or challenge.

Specific strategies termed *coping activities* or *processes* have been identified by studying groups of individuals assumed to be dealing with specific stressors. In a study of women with cancer, four problem-focused coping modes were identified: (1) bargaining, (2) focusing on the positive, (3) social support, and (4) concentrated efforts. Three emotion-focused coping processes were also determined: (1) wishful thinking, (2) detachment, and (3) acceptance. The emotion-focused strategies of detachment and wishful thinking and the problem-focused strategy of focusing on the positive were shown to significantly affect various types of emotional distress. Detachment and focusing on the positive helped mitigate distress, whereas wishful thinking increased emotional distress.[38] Optimistic coping strategies were also perceived to be most effective in individuals with rheumatoid arthritis, who are dealing with the stressors of pain and limitation of mobility.[39]

Spirituality has been found to be beneficial for individuals dealing with acute and chronic illness. In a study of elderly people coping with cancer, spiritual well-being was associated with hope and positive mood states.[40] Spirituality can relieve anxiety, provide a sense of purpose, and help cope with illness and approaching death. Nurses can assess the importance of spirituality and if appropriate support this method of coping. Additionally, hope has been found to offset feelings of despair and can empower an individual to cope with stress, chronic illness, and pain. Indeed, feelings of hopelessness and helplessness often characterize individuals overwhelmed by stress and lack of control. Various strategies that nurses can use to support hope in individuals with congestive heart failure have recently been described.[41]

Most of the research to date has focused on types of coping strategies. Findings about which coping strategies are the most beneficial or adaptive are inconclusive.

NURSING MANAGEMENT: STRESS

■ Nursing Assessment

The patient faces an array of potential stressors, or demands, that can have health consequences. The nurse must be aware of situations that are likely to result in stress and must also assess the patient's appraisal of the situation. In addition to the stress itself, specific coping mechanisms have health consequences and therefore must be included in the assessment.

Although the manifestations of stress may vary from person to person, the nurse should assess the patient for the signs and symptoms of the stress response that occur as a result of changes in the nervous, endocrine, and immune systems (see Chapters 53, 45, and 12, respectively).

Three major areas are important in assessment of stress: demands, human responses to stress, and coping. These areas provide the nurse with a useful guide in the assessment process.

Demands. Stressors, or demands, on the patient may include major life changes, events, or situations, such as changes in family constellation or daily hassles the patient is experiencing. Demands may be categorized as external (environmental) or internal (e.g., perceived tasks, goals, and commitments). Internal demands may also include physical demands resulting from disease or injury. In addition, the number of simultaneous demands, the duration of these demands, and previous experience with similar demands should be assessed. Specific assessment guides for particular types of patients are also available.

Primary appraisal or perception of the demands should be assessed. Demands may be categorized as representing harm or loss, threat, or challenge. Family responses to demands on the patient should also be assessed.[42]

Human Responses to Stress. Physiologic effects of demands that are appraised as stressful are mediated primarily via the sympathetic nervous system and the hypothalamic-pituitary-adrenal system. Responses such as increased heart rate, increased blood pressure, loss of appetite, sweating, and dilated pupils are included. In addition, the patient may exhibit some of the diseases of adaptation (see Table 7-4).

Behavioral human responses include observable actions and cognitions of the patient. Behavioral effects may include responses such as inability to concentrate, accident proneness, impaired speech, anxiety, crying, and shouting. Behavior in other aspects of life such as occupation may include absenteeism or tardiness at work, lowered productivity, and job dissatisfaction. Observable cognitive responses include self-reports of excessive demand, inability to make decisions, and forgetfulness. Some of these responses may also be apparent in significant others.

Coping. Secondary appraisal by the patient, or the patient's evaluation of coping resources and options, should be assessed. Resources such as supportive family members, adequate finances, and the ability to solve problems are examples of positive resources (see Table 7-7).

Coping strategies include cognitive and behavioral efforts to meet demands. The use and effectiveness of problem-focused and emotion-focused coping efforts should be addressed (see Table 7-8). These efforts may be categorized as direct action, avoidance of action, seeking information, defense mechanisms, and seeking assistance of others. The probability that a certain coping strategy will bring about the desired result is another important aspect to be assessed.[37]

■ Nursing Diagnoses

The importance of stress and coping to the nurse is shown by the amount of attention these concepts have received related to nursing diagnoses. A coping–stress tolerance pattern has been identified as 1 of 11 functional health patterns.[43] This pattern includes the diagnoses presented in Table 7-9. Assessment of the health pattern results in a description of the coping–stress tolerance patterns of a patient. Stressors can be identified at the individual or family level.

Table 7-9 Nursing Diagnoses in Coping–Stress Tolerance Pattern

Nursing Diagnoses
Impaired adjustment
Caregiver role strain
Ineffective individual coping
Defensive coping
Ineffective denial
Ineffective family coping: compromised
Ineffective family coping: disabling
Ineffective community coping
Family coping: potential for growth
Post-trauma syndrome
Rape trauma syndrome
Relocation stress syndrome
Risk for self-mutilation
Risk for violence

Two specific nursing diagnoses have been identified related to stress: ineffective individual coping and ineffective family coping. *Ineffective individual coping* is defined as the inability to form a valid appraisal of the stressors, inadequate choices of practiced responses, and/or inability to use available resources.[43] Potential etiologies include inadequate level of confidence in ability to cope, uncertainty, inadequate social support, inadequate resources, and high degree of threat. *Ineffective family coping: compromised* refers to the usually supportive primary person (family member or close friend) providing insufficient, ineffective, or compromised support, comfort, assistance, or encouragement, which may be needed by the patient to manage or master adaptive tasks related to health challenge.[43]

Nursing Implementation

The first step in managing stress is to become aware of its presence. This includes identifying and expressing stressful feelings. The role of the nurse is to facilitate and enhance the processes of coping and adaptation. Nursing interventions depend on the severity of the stress experience or demand. In the multiple trauma patient, the person expends energy in an attempt to physically survive. The nurse's efforts are directed to life-supporting interventions and to the inclusion of approaches aimed at the reduction of additional stressors to the patient. For example, the multiple trauma patient is much less likely to adapt or recover if faced with additional stressors such as sleep deprivation or an infection.

The importance of cognitive appraisal in the stress experience should prompt the nurse to assess if changes in the way the patient perceives and labels particular events or situations (cognitive reappraisal) are possible. Some experts also propose that the nurse consider the positive effects that result from successfully meeting stressful demands. Greater emphasis should also be placed on the part of cultural values and beliefs enhancing or constraining various coping options.

Because dealing with physical, social, and psychologic demands is an integral part of daily experiences, the coping behaviors that are used should be adaptive and should not be a source of additional stress to the individual. Generalizing about which coping strategies are the most adaptive is not yet possible. However, in evaluating coping behaviors, the nurse should look at the short-term outcomes (i.e., the impact of the strategy on the reduction or mastery of the demands and the regulation of the emotional response) and the long-term outcomes that relate to health, morale, and social and psychologic functioning.

Table 7-10 Conditioning Factors Altering the Stress Response

Age	Personality
Nutrition	Circadian rhythms
Heredity	Previous experiences
Social support	Socioeconomic status
Health	Financial resources

Conditioning factors affect the response to various stressors (Table 7-10). Resistance to stress can be increased with a healthy lifestyle. Some behaviors seem to promote and maintain health. These include the following:

1. Sleeping regularly 7 to 8 hours per night
2. Eating breakfast
3. Eating regular meals with minimal or no snacking
4. Eating moderately to maintain an ideal weight
5. Exercising moderately
6. Drinking alcohol moderately if drinking
7. Not smoking (best if have never smoked)

These behaviors help people maintain good health regardless of sex, age, and economic status. These behaviors are also cumulative; that is, the greater the number of these factors habitually practiced by the individual, the better the health.

Good mental health practices are important for good health as well. These practices primarily result in a realistic, positive self-conception, and the ability to solve problems. Teaching problem-solving skills can equip individuals to better handle present and future encounters with stressful circumstances.

Stress-reducing activities can be incorporated into nursing practice. The activities suggested can also be viewed as conditioning factors, because the patient is developing a sense of control with an increase in self-esteem as the practices are incorporated into daily activities. A sense of control is an important mediator in the stress process.[44]

The nurse can assume a primary role in planning stress-reducing interventions. Specific stress-reducing activities within the scope of nursing practice (some of which may require additional training) include relaxation training, cognitive reappraisal, music therapy, exercise, decisional control, assertiveness training, massage, and humor (Table 7-11). Specific relaxation strategies are presented in Table 8-2.

In summary, a knowledge of stress and coping theories provides the nurse with useful concepts that are applicable to all phases of the nursing process. Keeping abreast of the current research on this topic is a challenge. The models and concepts proposed are useful to the nurse who chooses to establish a research- and theory-based practice that recognizes the relationships among stress, coping, and health. The nurse should recognize when the patient or family needs to be referred to a professional with advanced training in counseling.

Table 7-11 Examples of Stress Management Techniques

Techniques	Descriptions
Progressive relaxation	Self-taught or instructor-directed exercise that involves learning to contract and relax muscles in a systematic way, beginning with the face and ending with the feet. The exercise may be combined with breathing exercises that focus on inner self.
Guided imagery	Purposeful use of one's imagination to achieve relaxation and control. An individual concentrates on images and mentally pictures oneself in the scene.
Thought stopping	Self-directed behavioral approach used to gain control of self-defeating thoughts. When these thoughts occur, the individual stops the thought process and focuses on conscious relaxation.
Exercise	Regular exercise, especially aerobic movement, results in improved circulation, increased release of endorphins, and an enhanced sense of well-being.
Humor	Humor in the form of laughter, cartoons, funny movies, riddles, audiocassettes, comic books, and joke books can be used for both the nurse and patient.
Assertive behavior	Open, honest sharing of feelings, desires, and opinions in a controlled way. The individual who has control over one's life is less subject to stress.
Social support	This may take the form of organized support and self-help groups, relationships with family and friends, and professional help.

CRITICAL THINKING EXERCISES

CASE STUDY

Stress During Hospitalization

Patient Profile

Ms. R. White, a 20-year-old college student and starting soccer forward, was admitted for an emergency appendectomy the night before her soccer team entered the final playoffs.

Subjective Data

- Has exertional asthma that has been controlled with medication
- Has primarily been eating pizza and doughnuts and drinking coffee and sodas
- Does not want her family or friends to visit

Critical Thinking Questions

1. Explain the physiologic changes that would be expected in Ms. White during the first 24 hours postoperatively as a result of the demand of surgery.
2. Explain how Ms. White's previous diet may affect her current adaptability.
3. What physiologic and psychologic stressors can be identified or predicted in Ms. White's situation? Describe the possible effects of these stressors on her asthma.
4. What factors will Ms. White's secondary appraisal process focus on?
5. What specific nursing interventions can be included in Ms. White's management that will enhance her adaptability?
6. Based on the assessment data provided, write one or more nursing diagnoses. Are there any collaborative problems?

NURSING RESEARCH ISSUES

1. Does preoperative stress level correlate with postoperative complications (e.g., pneumonia, delayed wound healing)?
2. Will interventions to reduce stress (e.g., stress management, exercise) improve patient outcomes following surgery?

REVIEW QUESTIONS

The number of the question corresponds to the same-numbered objective at the beginning of the chapter.

1. According to Selye, stress is defined as
   a. any stimulus that causes a response in an individual.
   b. a response of an individual to environmental demands.
   c. a physical or psychologic adaptation to internal or external demands.
   d. the result of a relationship between an individual and the environment that exceeds the individual's resources.
2. A patient who has undergone extensive surgery for multiple injuries has a period of increasing blood pressure, heart rate, and alertness. The nurse recognizes that these changes are most typical of
   a. the alarm reaction of the GAS.
   b. the resistance state of GAS.
   c. the stage of exhaustion of GAS.
   d. an individual response stereotype.
3. The nurse recognizes that cognitive appraisal is most evident when a patient facing surgery says,
   a. "I don't think I'm strong enough to undergo surgery tomorrow."
   b. "I have too many changes in my life to deal with surgery right now."
   c. "I am so anxious about this my heart is about to leap out of my chest."

d. "I'm just going to trust the surgeon and put my life in his hands."

4. The nurse would expect which of the following findings in a patient as a result of the physiologic effect of stress on the limbic system?
   a. an episode of diarrhea while awaiting painful dressing changes
   b. refusing to communicate with nurses while awaiting a cardiac catheterization
   c. inability to sleep the night before beginning to self-administer insulin injections
   d. increased blood pressure, decreased urine output, and hyperglycemia following a car accident
5. The nurse utilizes knowledge of the effects of stress on the immune system by encouraging patients to
   a. avoid stress when they are ill.
   b. receive regular immunizations when they are stressed.
   c. use humor and social support systems to maintain wellness.
   d. avoid exposure to upper respiratory infections when physically stressed.
6. The nurse recognizes that a patient with newly diagnosed cancer of the breast is using an emotion-focused coping process when she
   a. joins a support group for women with breast cancer.
   b. considers the pros and cons of the various treatment options.
   c. tells the nurse that she has a good prognosis because the tumor is small.
   d. delays treatment until her family can take a weekend trip together.
7. During assessment, the nurse recognizes that a patient is more likely to have a greater response when stressed when the patient
   a. feels that the situation is directing his life.
   b. sees the situation as a challenge to be addressed.
   c. has a clear understanding of his values and goals.
   d. uses more emotion-regulating than problem-solving coping mechanisms.
8. An appropriate nursing intervention for a patient who has a nursing diagnosis of ineffective individual coping related to inadequate psychologic resources is
   a. controlling the environment to prevent sensory overload and promote sleep.
   b. encouraging the patient's family to offer emotional support by frequent visiting.
   c. arranging for the patient to phone family and friends to maintain emotional bonds.
   d. asking the patient to describe previous stressful situations and how she managed to resolve them.

References

1. Selye H: The stress concept: past, present, and future. In Cooper CL, editor: *Stress research: issues for the eighties,* New York, 1983, Wiley.
2. Holmes T, Masuda M: Magnitude estimations of social readjustments, *J Psychosom Res* 11:219, 1966.
3. Holmes T, Rahe R: The social readjustment rating scale, *J Psychosom Res* 12:213, 1967.
4. Derogatis LR, Coons H: Self-report measures of stress. In Goldberger L, Breznitz S, editors: *Handbook of stress: theoretical and clinical aspects,* ed 2, New York, 1993, Free Press.
5. Lazarus R, Folkman S: *Stress, appraisal, and coping,* New York, 1984, Springer.
6. Selye H: *The stress of life,* New York, 1956, McGraw-Hill.
7. Lacey JI, Lacey BC: Verification and extension of the principle of autonomic response stereotype, *Am J Psychol* 71:50, 1958.
8. Marsland AL, Manuck SB, Fazzari TV, Stewart CJ, Rabin BS: Stability of individual differences in cellular immune responses to acute psychological stress, *Psychosomatic Med* 57:295, 1995.
9. O'Keefe MK, Baum A: Conceptual and methodological issues in the study of chronic stress, *Stress Med* 6:105, 1990.
10. Holmes TH, Masuda M: Life change and illness susceptibility. In Dohrenwend BA, Dohrenwend BP, editors: *Stressful life events: their nature and effects,* New York, 1974, Wiley.
11. Ouellette SC: Inquiries into hardiness. In Goldberger L, Breznitz S, editors: *Handbook of stress: theoretical and clinical aspects,* ed 2, New York, 1993, Free Press.
12. Antonovsky AA: *Unraveling the mystery of health: how people manage stress and stay well,* San Francisco, 1987, Jossey-Bass.
13. Williams SJ: The relationship among stress, hardiness, sense of coherence, and illness in critical care nurses, *Medical Psychotherapy* 3:171, 1990.
14. Wagnild GM, Young HM: Development and psychometric evaluation of the resilience scale, *J Nurs Meas* 1:165, 1993.
15. Kanner AD and others: Comparison of two modes of stress measurement: daily hassles and uplifts versus major life events, *J Behav Med* 4:1, 1981.
16. Sorbi MJ, Maassen GH, Spierings EL: A time series analysis of daily hassles and mood changes in the 3 days before the migraine attack, *Behav Med* 22:103, 1996.
17. Lazarus RS, Launier R: Stress-related transactions between person and environment. In Pervin LA, Lewis M, editors: *Perspectives in international psychology,* New York, 1978, Plenum.
18. Chatterton RT, Vogelsong KM, Lu YC, Hudgens GA: Hormonal responses to psychological stress in men preparing for skydiving, *J Clin Endocrinol Metab* 82:2503, 1997.
19. Magiakou MA, Mastorakos G, Webster E, Chrousos GP: The hypothalamic-pituitary-adrenal axis and the female reproductive system, *Ann N Y Acad Sci* 816:42, 1997.
20. Savino W, Dardenne M: Immune-neuroendocrine interactions, *Immunol Today* 16:318, 1995.
21. Andersen BL, Kiecolt-Glaser JK, Glaser R: A biobehavioral model of cancer stress and disease course, *Am Psychol* 49:389, 1994.
22. Kiecolt-Glaser JK, Glaser R: Psychoneuroimmunology and health consequences: data and shared mechanisms, *Psychosom Med* 57:269, 1995.
23. Cohen S, Herbert TB: Health psychology: psychological factors and physical disease from the perspective of human psychoneuroimmunology, *Ann Rev Psychol* 47:113, 1996.
24. Cohen S and others: Psychological stress and susceptibility to the common cold, *N Engl J Med* 325:606, 1991.
25. Kiecolt-Glaser JK, Glaser R, Gravenstein S, Malarkey WB, Sheridan J: Chronic stress alters the immune response to influenza virus vaccine in older adults, *Proc Natl Acad Sci U S A* 93:3043, 1996.
26. Witek-Janusek L, Cusack C, Mathews HL: Trauma-induced immune dysfunction: a challenge for critical care, *DCCN* 17:187, 1998.
27. Kiecolt-Glaser JK, Marucha PT, Malarky WB, Mercado AM, Glaser R: Slowing of wound healing by psychological stress, *Lancet* 346:1194, 1995.
28. Ironson G, Antoni M, Lutgendorf S: Can psychological interventions affect immunity and survival? Present findings and suggested targets with a focus on cancer and human immunodeficiency virus, *Mind/Body Med* 1:85, 1995.
29. Spiegel D and others: Effect of psychosocial treatment on survival of patients with metastatic breast cancer, *Lancet* 2:881, 1989.
30. Kogon MM, Biswas A, Pearl D, Carlson RW, Spiegel D: Effects of medical and psychotherapeutic treatment on the survival of women with metastatic breast carcinoma, *Cancer* 80:225, 1997.
31. Holt RR: Occupational stress. In Goldberger L, Breznitz S, editors: *Handbook of stress: theoretical and clinical aspects,* ed 2, New York, 1993, Free Press.
32. Repetti RL: The effects of work load and the social environment at work on health. In Goldberger L, Breznitz S, editors: *Handbook of stress: theoretical and clinical aspects,* ed 2, New York, 1993, Free Press.

33. Werner JS: Stressors and health outcomes: synthesis of nursing research, 1980-1990. In Barnfather JS, Lyon BL, editors: *Stress and coping: state of the science and implications for nursing theory, research, and practice,* Indianapolis, 1993, Sigma Theta Tau Center Press.
34. Volicer BJ, Bohannon MW: A hospital stress rating scale, *Nurs Res* 24:352, 1975.
35. Parker MM, Schubert W, Shelhamer JH, Parrillo JE: Perceptions of a critically ill patient experiencing therapeutic paralysis in an ICU, *Crit Care Med* 12:69, 1984.
36. Van Servellen G, Lewis CE, Leake B: The stresses of hospitalization among AIDS patients on integrated and special care units, *Int J Nurs Stud* 27:235, 1990.
37. Moos RH, Schaefer J: Coping resources and processes: current concepts and measures. In Goldberger L, Breznitz S, editors: *Handbook of stress: theoretical and clinical aspects,* ed 2, New York, 1993, Free Press.
38. Mishel MH, Sorenson D: Revision of the ways of coping checklist for a clinical population, *West J Nurs Res* 15:59, 1993.
39. Mahat G: Perceived stressors and coping strategies among individuals with rheumatoid arthritis, *J Adv Nurs Sci* 25:1144, 1997.
40. Fehring RJ, Miller JF, Snow C: Spiritual well-being, religiosity, hope, depression, and other mood states in elderly people coping with cancer, *Oncol Nurs Forum* 24:663, 1997.
41. Johnson LH, Dahlen R, Roberts SL: Supporting hope in congestive heart failure patients, *DCCN* 16:65, 1997.
42. Halm MA and others: Behavioral responses of family members during critical illness, *Clin Nurs Res* 2:414, 1993.
43. The Association: Nursing diagnoses: definitions and classifications 1999-2000, Philadelphia, 1999. North American Nursing Diagnoses Association.

Resources

Stress Information Site
McKinley Health Center
University of Illinois at Urbana-Champaign
http://www.uiuc.edu/departments/mckinley/health-info/stress/stress.html

Stress Links—Michigan Electronic Library
http://mel.lib.mi.us/health/health-stress.html

For additional Internet resources, see the website for this book at **www.mosby.com/MERLIN/medsurg_lewis**

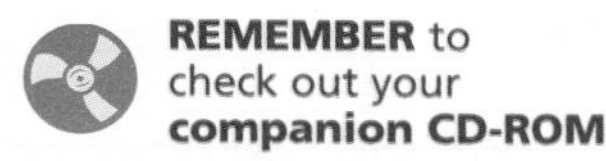

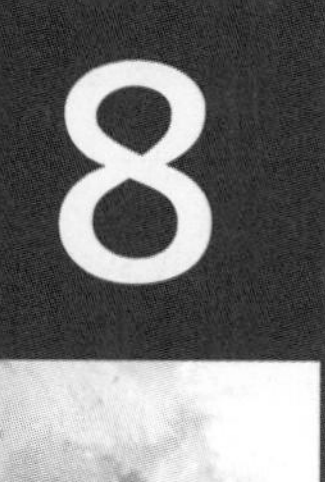

8 Complementary and Alternative Therapies

Kathryn Ann Caudell

www.mosby.com/MERLIN/medsurg_lewis

LEARNING OBJECTIVES

1. Differentiate between complementary and alternative therapies.
2. Describe the clinical applications of relaxation therapies.
3. Discuss the relaxation response and its effect on somatic ailments.
4. Describe the purpose and principles of biofeedback.
5. Identify the principles and effectiveness of imagery, meditation, and hypnotherapy.
6. Describe the methods of and the psychophysiologic responses to therapeutic touch.
7. Explain the scope of practice of chiropractic therapy.
8. Discuss the principles and applications of acupuncture.
9. Describe the types and advantages and disadvantages of herbal therapy.

The general health of North American people has steadily improved over the course of the last century as evidenced by lower mortality rates and increased life expectancies. Changes in science and medicine have provided the knowledge and technology that have successfully altered the course of many illnesses. Despite the success of allopathic (traditional Western) medicine, many conditions, such as arthritis, chronic back pain, gastrointestinal problems, allergies, headache, and insomnia, have been difficult to treat, and more patients are exploring alternative methods to relieve their symptom distress.[1] It is estimated that up to 75% of patients seek care from their primary care practitioners for stress, pain, and health conditions for which there are no known causes or cures.[2] Although allopathic medicine is effective in treating numerous physical ailments (e.g., bacterial infections, structural abnormalities, acute emergencies), it is less effective in preventing disease, decreasing stress-induced illnesses, managing chronic disease, and caring for the emotional and spiritual needs of individuals.

The number of patients seeking unconventional treatments has risen considerably. In part this increase is due to (1) the perception that the treatments offered by the medical profession do not provide relief for a variety of common illnesses, (2) the increasing interest by patients to become more educated about their health and the need to take a more active role in their treatment, and (3) the increased number of magazine articles and television programs.[3]

Unconventional therapies are frequently referred to as either complementary or alternative medicine (CAM) therapies. Complementary therapies are those therapies used in addition to conventional treatment prescribed by the person's health care provider. As the name implies, complementary therapies complement the conventional treatment. Complementary therapies include relaxation, exercise, massage, prayer, biofeedback, hypnosis, acupuncture, meditation, chiropractic therapy, herbal therapy, and homeopathy. Alternative therapies, on the other hand, may include the same interventions as complementary therapies but frequently become the primary treatment modality that replaces allopathic medical care. Types of complementary and alternative therapies are presented in Table 8-1.

Between one third and one half of the population in the United States uses one or more forms of CAM.[2] Between 1986 and 1991 there was a 70% increase in people in the United Kingdom using complementary medicine, and similar increases have been observed in Holland and France.[3] Because of this increased interest in and use of CAM, many institutions, including some mainstream medical schools, are establishing training programs that incorporate CAM philosophy and content into the curriculum. Integrative medical programs are being developed that allow health care consumers the opportunity to be treated by a team of providers consisting of both allopathic and complementary practitioners. Furthermore, an increasing number of insurance companies are now covering costs for certain types of CAM therapies such as herbal therapy, biofeedback, chiropractic medicine, megavitamin therapy, and acupuncture.[2]

The interest in CAM is also evident in the increased number of publications in respected medical journals and the development of several journals that specifically focus on complementary and alternative medicine. The Office of Alternative Medicine was established in 1992 as a part of the

Reviewed by Trisch Van Sciver, RN, MS, PCNS, CFNP, DOM, Nurse Practitioner, Lovelace Health Systems, Albuquerque, NM, and Janice Post-White, RN, PhD, Assistant Professor, Cancer Society; Professor of Oncology Nursing, University of Minnesota, Minneapolis, Minn.

Table 8-1 Complementary and Alternative Therapies

Type	Description
Traditional and Ethnomedicine Therapies	
Acupuncture	A traditional Chinese method of producing analgesia or altering the function of a body system by inserting thin needles along a series of lines or channels, called meridians. Direct needle manipulation of energetic meridians influences deeper internal organs.
Ayurveda	Traditional Hindu system of medicine practiced in India since the first century AD. Combination of herbs, purgatives, rubbing oils, etc. used in treating disease.
Homeopathic medicine	System of medical treatment based on the theory that certain diseases can be cured by giving small doses of drugs that in a healthy person would produce symptoms like those of the disease. Remedies or medicines are made from naturally occurring plant, animal, or mineral substances.
Latin-American practices	Curanderismo medical system that includes a humoral model for classifying food, activity, drugs, and illnesses and a series of folk illnesses.
Native-American practices	Therapies include sweating and purging, herbal remedies, and shamanic healing (healer makes contact with spirits to ask their direction in bringing healing to people).
Naturopathic medicine	System of therapeutics based on natural foods, light, warmth, massage, fresh air, regular exercise, and avoidance of medications. Recognition of inherent healing ability of the body. Treatments integrate traditional natural therapies with modern diagnostic science; includes botanical medicine.
Traditional Chinese (Oriental) medicine	Set of systematic techniques and methods including acupuncture, herbal medicines, massage, acupressure, moxibustion, Qigong, and oriental massage. Fundamental concepts embedded in Taoism, Confucianism, and Buddhism.
Bioelectromagnetic Applications	
Electroacupuncture	Electrical stimulation via acupuncture needles to enhance or replace manual needles. Technique has been used to treat chemotherapy-induced symptom distress, renal colic, and postoperative pain and induce uterine contractions in post-term pregnancy.
Electromagnetic fields	Use of relatively large levels of electrical and magnetic energy. Therapy used to promote healing of bone fractures, nerve stimulation, wound healing, treatment of osteoarthritis, tissue regeneration, immune system stimulation, and neuroendocrine modulation.
Diet Therapies	
Gerson therapy	Integrated set of treatments that includes primarily raw vegetables and fruit; salt, fat, and protein restriction, potassium and thyroid supplementation; and coffee enemas.
Kelly regimen	Dietary program that includes carrot juice, vegetarian diet, coffee enemas, and pancreatic enzymes. Diet used in treatment of cancer patients.
Macrobiotic diet	Predominantly a vegan diet (no animal products except fish) initially used in the management of a variety of cancers. Emphasis placed on whole cereal grains, vegetables, and unprocessed foods.
Orthomolecular medicine (Megavitamin)	Increased intake of nutrients such as vitamin C and beta carotene. Diet used in treatment of cancer, schizophrenia, and certain chronic diseases such as hypercholesterolemia and coronary artery disease.
Herbal Therapies	
European phytomedicines	Products developed under strict quality control in sophisticated pharmaceutical factories, packaged professionally, tablets or capsules. Examples of well-studied herbal medicines include Ginkgo biloba, milk thistle, and bilberry. Herbs have a wide variety of uses (see Table 8-10).
Traditional Chinese herbal remedies	Over 50,000 medicinal plant species, many of which have been studied extensively. Herbs considered the backbone of medicine. Examples include *Panax ginseng* (ginseng root) for treatment of asthma and stomach disorders, lowering stress, reducing hypoxia, improving cardiac performance, and inhibiting platelet aggregation; fresh ginger rhizome for treatment of acute dysentery and acute orchitis; Chinese foxglove root for treatment of hepatitis and rheumatoid arthritis.
Ayurvedic herbs	Herbs used for over 2000 years. Examples include *Eclipta alba* for the treatment of liver cirrhosis and infectious hepatitis; *Commophora mukul* for reducing serum cholesterol; *Picrorhiza kurroa* for fever and dyspepsia; and *Curcuma longa* (turmeric) for healing chronic ulcers and scabies.
Manual Healing Therapies	
Acupressure	Therapeutic technique of applying digital pressure in a specified way on designated points on the body to relieve pain, produce analgesia, or regulate a body function.

Continued

Table 8-1 Complementary and Alternative Therapies—cont'd

Type	Description
Manual Healing Therapies—cont'd	
Chiropractic therapy	System of therapy based on the theory that state of person's health is determined by condition of nervous system. Application of the knowledge of the relationship between structure and function to diagnose and treat structural dysfunctions that affect the nervous system. Treatment frequently involves manipulation of spinal column and may also include physiotherapy and diet therapy.
Feldenkrais method	Alternative therapy based on establishment of good self-image through awareness and correction of body movements. Technique integrates the understanding of the physics of the body's movement patterns with an awareness of the way people learn to move, behave, and interact.
Qigong	Technique that incorporates breath, movement, and meditation to cleanse, strengthen, and circulate vital life energy and blood. Therapy used to stimulate immune system and maintain external and internal balance.
Massage therapy (See Fig. 8-1)	Manipulation of soft tissue through stroking, rubbing, or kneading to increase circulation, improve muscle tone, and relax patient.
Osteopathy	Therapeutic approach that uses all forms of medical diagnosis and therapy but places greater emphasis on the influence of the relationship between the organs and musculoskeletal system than conventional medicine.
Reiki therapy	Therapy derived from ancient Buddhist practices in which practitioner places hands on or above a body area and transfers "universal life energy" to the patient. This energy provides strength, harmony, and balance to treat health disturbances.
Rolfing (structural integration)	Technique of deep massage intended to realign the body by altering the length and tone of myofascial tissue. Basis of practice is the belief that misalignment of myofascial tissue may have detrimental effect on person's energy level, self-image, muscular efficiency, and general health.
Therapeutic touch	Practitioner directs own interpersonal energy to flow through hands to help or heal another. Practitioner restores correct vibrational component to the patient's universal unitary field.
Biobehavioral Therapies	
Art therapy	Use of art to reconcile emotional conflicts, foster self-awareness, and express unspoken and frequently unconscious concerns.
Biofeedback	A process providing a person with visual or auditory information about autonomic physiologic functions of the body, such as muscle tension, skin temperature, and brain wave activity, through the use of instruments. Used for treatment of anxiety disorders, Raynaud's syndrome, hypertension, and temporomandibular joint dysfunction (see Table 8-4).
Dance therapy (See Fig. 8-2)	Intimate and powerful medium for therapy because it is a direct expression of the mind and body. Therapy used to treat persons with social, emotional, cognitive, or physical problems.
Imagery	Formation of mental concepts, figures, and ideas applied therapeutically to decrease anxiety. Mental process and a variety of procedures to encourage changes in attitudes, behavior, or physiologic reactions.
Guided imagery	Therapeutic technique used for relieving pain or discomfort in which the person is encouraged to concentrate on an image that helps relieve pain or discomfort.
Hypnotherapy	The induction of trance states and therapeutic suggestion for treatment of paralysis, headaches, joint pains, addictions, pain control, and phobias.
Meditation	Self-directed practice for relaxing the body and calming the mind. State of consciousness in which individual eliminates environmental stimuli from awareness, producing a state of relaxation and stress relief.
Music therapy	Use of music to address physical, psychologic, cognitive, and social needs of individuals with disabilities and illnesses. Therapy used to improve physical movement for people with impaired movement, improve communication in people with communication disorders, develop emotional expression for people with mental health problems, evoke memories for persons with memory impairment, and distract people who are in pain or having painful treatments or chemotherapy.
Prayer therapies	Variety of techniques used in multiple cultures that incorporate caring, compassion, love, or empathy with the target of prayer.
Psychotherapy	Treatment of emotional and mental disorders by psychologic techniques.
Relaxation therapy	Variety of techniques that may be used to elicit the relaxation response, a protective mechanism against stress that decreases heart rate, lowers metabolism, decreases respiratory rate, and decreases muscle tension.

Continued

Table 8-1 Complementary and Alternative Therapies—cont'd

Type	Description
Biobehavioral Therapies—Cont'd	
Yoga	Discipline that focuses on the body's musculature, posture, breathing mechanisms, and consciousness. Goal of yoga is attainment of physical and mental well-being through mastery of body achieved through exercise, holding of postures, proper breathing, and meditation.
Pharmacologic and Biologic Treatments	
Antioxidizing agents	Use of vitamins A, C, E, selenium, and beta carotene to treat and prevent a variety of disorders.
Cartilage products	Cartilage preparations from a variety of animals and fish used to treat several skin disorders, accelerate wound healing, and provide antiinflammatory effects.
Chelation therapy	Use of ethylenediaminetetraacetic acid (EDTA) to remove toxic metals and substances from the body. Suggested benefits for heart disease, circulatory problems, and rheumatoid arthritis.

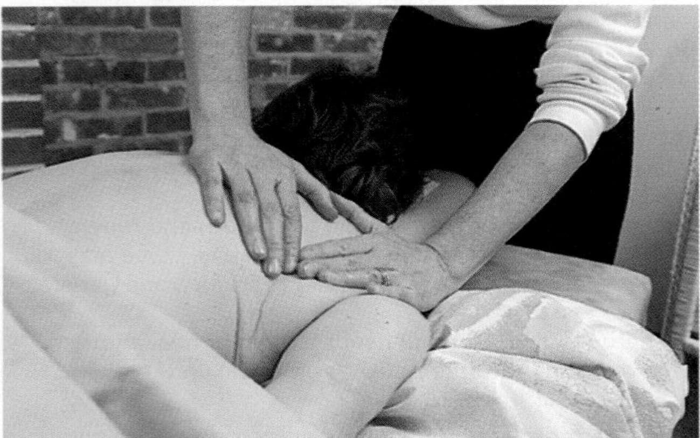

Fig. 8-1 Massage therapy can be effectively used to relieve tension.

National Institutes of Health. The goals of this office are to facilitate the evaluation of alternative medical treatment modalities, specifically acting as a clearinghouse to disseminate information to the public, media, and professionals and supporting, coordinating, and conducting research and research training in the area of alternative medicine.[4]

This chapter discusses several types of complementary and alternative medicine therapies. A description, clinical applications, and limitations of each therapy are presented.

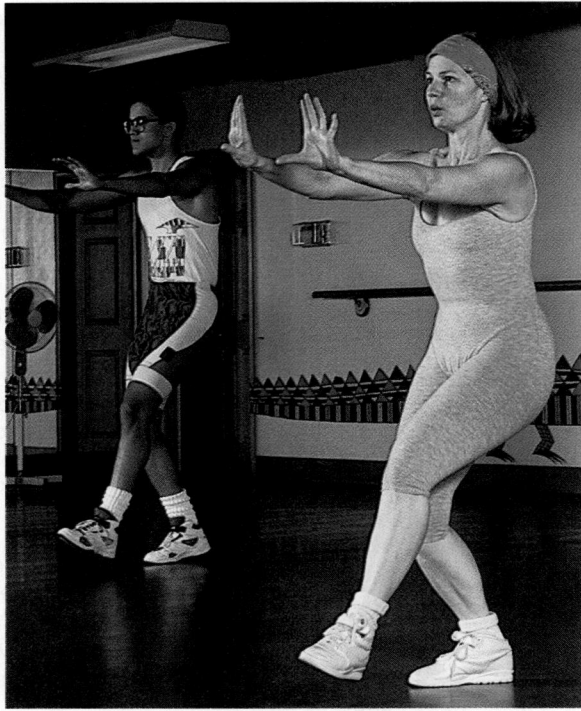

Fig. 8-2 Dance therapy.

BIOBEHAVIORAL THERAPIES

Biobehavioral therapy is designed to teach individuals ways in which to change their behavior in order to alter physical responses to stress and improve symptoms such as muscle tension, gastrointestinal discomfort, pain, or sleep disturbances. One of the principles of biobehavioral therapy is that the individual becomes actively involved in the treatment. Individuals achieve better responses if they practice the techniques or exercises daily. Types of biobehavioral therapies include relaxation, imagery, biofeedback, hypnosis, and meditation (see Table 8-1).

Relaxation Therapy

People are exposed to stressful situations in everyday life that evoke the stress response. During the stress response, the musculature reacts immediately by tightening. If the individual does not learn how to reduce the muscle tension, a condition of chronic overtension and continued hyperactivity of the autonomic nervous system may occur, leading to pathophysiologic changes in the endocrine, cardiovascular, and immune systems.[5,6] (The stress response is discussed in Chapter 7.)

Relaxation is the state of generalized low cognitive, physiologic, or behavioral arousal. Relaxation is also defined as arousal reduction. The process of relaxation elongates the muscle fibers, reduces the neural impulses sent to the brain, and thus decreases the activity of brain and other body systems. The relaxation response is characterized by decreased heart and respiratory rates, blood pressure, and oxygen consumption and increased alpha brain activity and peripheral skin temperature. The relaxation response can be obtained through a variety of techniques that incorporate a repetitive mental focus and the adoption of a calm, peaceful attitude.[7] Relaxation strategies are listed in Table 8-2.

Table 8-2 Relaxation Strategies

Rhythmic Breathing*

1. Provide a quiet environment.
2. Help the patient get comfortable by elevating the legs with the knees bent (relaxing the leg, back, and abdominal muscles) or supporting the neck with a pillow. Check to see that arms and legs are not crossed.
3. Instruct patient to close eyes and to breathe in and out slowly, saying, "Breathe in, 2, 3, 4; breathe out, 2, 3, 4."
4. Once rhythmic breathing is established, instruct patient to listen to your voice, and with a low and steady voice, instruct patient to do the following:
   Breathe in and out slowly and deeply.
   Try to breathe from the abdomen.
   Feel more relaxed with each exhalation.
   Try to identify your own special feeling of relaxation (e.g., light and weightless or very heavy).
   While you are breathing, let your imagination take you to a place you remember as peaceful and pleasant; look around, listen to the sounds, feel the air, notice the smells.
   When you are ready to end this relaxation exercise, count silently from 1 to 3; on 1, move your lower body; on 2, move your upper body; on 3, breathe in deeply, open your eyes, and while breathing out slowly, say silently: "I am relaxed and alert." Stretch as if just waking up.

Progressive Relaxation*

1. Follow steps 1, 2, and 3 of rhythmic breathing.
2. Once the patient is breathing slowly and comfortably, instruct patient to tighten and relax an ordered succession of muscle groups, tensing and then relaxing them, while *feeling* the part relax.
3. Instruct patient to tense and then relax the calves, knees, and so on.

Relaxation by Sensory Pacing

1. Follow steps 1 and 2 of rhythmic breathing.
2. Instruct patient to slowly repeat and finish either in a low voice or to self each of the following sentences:
   Now I am aware of seeing . . .
   Now I am aware of feeling . . .
   Now I am aware of hearing . . .
   Instruct patient to repeat and complete each sentence 4 times, then 3 times, then twice, and finally once.
3. Instruct patient to allow the eyes to close when they feel heavy.

Relaxation by Color Exchange

1. Follow steps 1, 2, and 3 of rhythmic breathing.
2. Instruct patient to notice any tension, tightness, aches, or pains in the body and to give that sensation the first color that comes to mind.
3. Instruct patient to breathe in pure white light from the universe and send the light to the tense or painful place in the body, letting the white light surround the color of the discomfort.
4. Instruct patient to exhale the color of the discomfort and let the white light take its place.
5. Instruct patient to continue breathing in the white light and exhaling the color of the discomfort, allowing the white light to fill the entire body and bring about a sense of peace, well-being, and energy.

Modified Autogenic Relaxation

1. Follow steps 1, 2, and 3 of rhythmic breathing.
2. Instruct patient to repeat each of the following phrases to self 4 times, saying the first part of the phrase while breathing in for 2 to 3 sec, holding the breath for 2 to 3 sec, then saying the last part of the phrase while breathing out for 2 to 3 sec:

Breathing in	*Breathing out*
I am	relaxed
My arm and legs	are heavy and warm
My heartbeat	is calm and regular
My breathing	is free and easy
My abdomen	is loose and warm
My forehead	is cool
My mind	is quiet and still

Relaxing with Music

1. Provide patient with a tape recorder and headset.
2. Ask patient to select a favorite cassette of slow, quiet music.
3. Instruct patient to get into a comfortable position (either sitting or lying down but with arms and legs uncrossed) and to close eyes and listen to the music through the headset.
4. Instruct patient to imagine floating or drifting with the music while listening.

Rhythmic Massage

1. Massage near the area of tension in a circular, firm manner.
2. Avoid tender, red, or swollen areas.

*In conditioning of a relaxation response, a "signal breath" involving deep inhalation through the nose and forceful exhalation through the mouth is the key. The signal breath precedes and follows each run through the exercise.

Relaxation involves the cognitive skills that people develop during relaxation training to help them reduce the negative ways in which they respond to situations within their environment. The cognitive skills include focusing (the ability to identify, differentiate, maintain attention on, and return attention to simple stimuli for an extended period), passivity (the ability to stop unnecessary goal-directed and analytic activity), and receptivity (the ability to tolerate and accept experiences that may be uncertain, unfamiliar, or paradoxic).[8] In addition, the individual experiences cognitive restructuring during which negative thoughts are replaced with positive ones.[9] The long-term goal of relaxation therapy is for the person to continually self-monitor for indicators of tension and to consciously let go and release the tension contained in various body parts.

Progressive relaxation training helps teach the individual how to effectively rest and reduce tension in the body. One initially learns to detect subtle localized sensations of muscle tension in one muscle group (e.g., the forearm muscle). Using the method of diminishing tensions, the individual learns to differentiate between high-intensity tension (strong fist clenching) and very subtle tension.[10] This activity is then practiced using multiple muscle groups. One active progressive relaxation technique involves the use of slow, deep abdominal breathing while tightening and relaxing an ordered succession of muscle groups. The practitioner may elect to begin with the muscles in the face, followed by those in the arms, hands, abdomen, legs, and feet.

Another important component of progressive relaxation is reducing cognitive or mental activity by having the person focus on muscle contraction and relaxation. If cognitive activities correspond with muscle activity (and energy expenditure), by reducing the muscle tension through relaxation techniques, unwanted cognitive activities and emotions can be reduced.[10]

Passive relaxation involves teaching the individual to relax individual muscle groups passively (i.e., without actively contracting the muscles). One passive relaxation technique incorporates slow, abdominal breathing exercises in addition to the person imagining warmth and relaxation flowing through specific muscle groups during inspiration while letting go of muscle tension during expiration. Passive relaxation is useful for persons for whom the effort and energy expenditure of active muscle contracting leads to discomfort or exhaustion.

Clinical Applications of Relaxation Therapy. Relaxation techniques are effective in lowering heart rate and blood pressure, decreasing muscle tension, improving well-being, and reducing symptom distress in persons experiencing a variety of situations (e.g., complications from medical treatment or disease, bereaving the loss of a significant other). The type of relaxation intervention should be matched to the individual's functional status, the energy expenditure of the relaxation technique, and the motivation of the individual for frequent practice.

Relaxation, alone or in combination with deep breathing, imagery, yoga (Fig. 8-3), and music, has been shown to reduce pain,[9] improve emotional well-being[11] and immune function,[12,13] reduce heart rate and blood pressure, and reduce cancer treatment–related nausea and vomiting in a number of patient populations.[14-17] More well-controlled studies are needed to validate the effects of relaxation therapy.

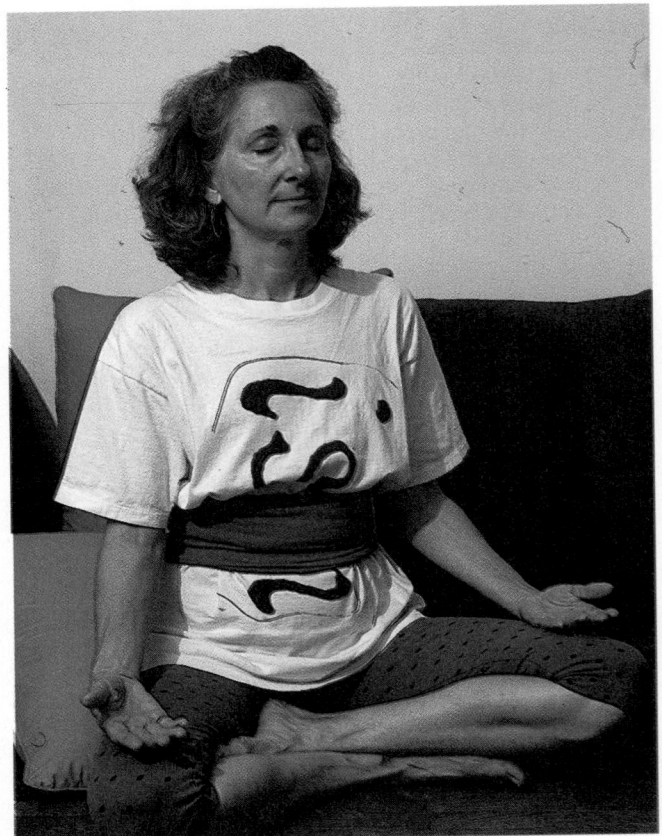

Fig. 8-3 Yoga is a discipline that focuses on muscles, posture, breathing, and consciousness.

Relaxation is a valuable technique because it empowers individuals and allows them to exert some control over their lives. The person may experience a diminished feeling of helplessness and a more positive psychologic state overall, which helps the person have a less negative view of his or her situation.

Limitations of Relaxation Therapy. Individuals undergoing relaxation training have reported fearing loss of control, feeling like they are floating, and experiencing relaxation-induced anxiety related to these feelings. During relaxation training, individuals are taught to differentiate between low and high levels of muscle tension. During the first 1 or 2 months of training sessions when the person is learning how to focus on body sensations and tensions, there have been reports of increased sensitivity in detecting muscle tension. Usually these feelings are minor and resolve as the person continues with the relaxation training.[18] However, practitioners must be aware that on occasion some relaxation techniques may result in continued intensification of symptoms or the development of altogether new symptoms.[19]

Another physiologic event that occasionally occurs early in relaxation training is the "predormescent start" in which the trunk and limbs of the individual jerk during the process of falling asleep. This muscle spasm is seen in people who have been very tense during the day or who are experiencing major traumatic events. It will usually disappear as the relaxation training progresses.[18]

An important consideration when choosing the type of relaxation technique is the physiologic and psychologic status of the individual. Patients with advanced disease such as cancer may seek relaxation training in order to reduce their stress response. However, techniques such as active progressive relaxation training require a moderate expenditure of energy, which can amplify a person's existing fatigue and limit his or her ability to complete individual relaxation sessions and practice. Therefore active progressive relaxation would not be appropriate for patients with advanced disease or those who have decreased energy reserves. Passive relaxation or imagery is more appropriate for these individuals.[20]

Imagery

Imagery, or visualization, techniques use the conscious mind to create mental images to evoke physical changes in the body, improve perceived well-being, and enhance self-awareness. Frequently imagery is combined with some form of relaxation training to facilitate the effect of the relaxation technique. Imagery can be self-directed, in which the individual creates his or her own mental images, or guided, during which a practitioner leads the individual through a particular scenario.[21] For example, the patient may be directed to begin slow, abdominal breathing while focusing on the rhythm of breathing, then instructed to visualize ocean waves coming to shore with each inspiration, then receding with each expiration. The patient is then instructed to take notice of the smells, sounds, and temperatures that he or she is experiencing. As the imagery session progresses, the patient may be instructed to visualize warmth entering the body during inspiration and tension leaving the body during expiration. Imagery scenarios should be individualized for each patient or left up to the patient to develop.

Imagery can evoke powerful psychophysiologic responses. Many imagery techniques involve visual imagery, but they can also include the auditory, proprioceptive, gustatory, and olfactory senses. An example of this involves visualizing a lemon being sliced in half and squeezing the lemon juice under the tongue. This visualization has been observed to produce increased salivation as effectively as the actual event. People typically respond to their environment according to the way they perceive it as well as by their own visualizations and expectancies. Therefore individuals can learn to regulate themselves by selecting appropriate visualizations and expectations.[22]

Creative visualization is a form of self-directed imagery that is based on the principle of mind-body connectivity (i.e., every mental image leads to physical or emotional changes).[23] The steps of creative visualization are listed in Table 8-3.

Clinical Applications of Imagery. Imagery has applications in a number of patient populations. Imagery has been used to visualize cancer cells being destroyed by cells of the immune system, control or relieve pain, and achieve calmness and serenity. It has also been used in the treatment of chronic conditions such as asthma, hypertension, functional urinary disorders, menstrual and premenstrual syndromes, gastrointestinal disorders such as irritable bowel syndrome and ulcerative colitis, and rheumatoid arthritis.[21]

Limitations of Imagery. Imagery, for the most part, is a behavioral intervention that has few side effects. However, it is probably one of the least clearly defined interventions and can range from being highly structured and practitioner led to consisting of spontaneous daydreams by the individual.[8]

Table 8-3 Four Basic Steps of Creative Visualization

1. Set goals that can be accomplished, because confidence and increased self-esteem are achieved through success.
2. Create the image clearly. Although it may be difficult to develop a visual image, if the goals of the imagery are viewed with clear thoughts and in the present tense, the individual may be more successful in creating an effective image.
3. Frequently visualize the image. This visualization should be done during relaxing states as well as throughout the day, but particularly before bedtime or on wakening when the person's mind is usually more relaxed.
4. While focusing on the image, repeat encouraging statements, such as positive affirmations. Alleviate any doubts about one's ability to achieve the goals.

Biofeedback

Biofeedback techniques are frequently used in addition to relaxation interventions to assist individuals in learning how to control specific autonomic nervous system responses. Biofeedback is a group of therapeutic procedures that uses electronic or electromechanical instruments to measure, process, and provide information to persons about their neuromuscular and autonomic nervous system activity (Fig. 8-4). The information or feedback is given in the form of analog or binary and auditory or visual feedback signals. Practitioners, usually credentialed in biofeedback, help persons develop greater awareness and resulting voluntary control over their physiologic responses of which they are otherwise unaware.[24]

Biofeedback is considered an adjuvant to more traditional relaxation programs because it can immediately demonstrate to the patient his or her ability to control physiologic responses. It can also focus on and monitor specific body parts. By providing immediate feedback in terms of what stress relaxation behaviors work most effectively, it helps the patient control physiologic functions that are most difficult for the patient to control. Eventually, the patient will be able to notice positive physiologic changes without the need for instrument feedback. Finally, biofeedback demonstrates to the patient the relationship among thoughts, feelings, and physiologic responses.[25]

Clinical Applications of Biofeedback. Biofeedback has application in a number of situations (Table 8-4). Stroke patients who experience injury to the brain often find that the recovery of their muscle groups occurs at different rates. During the period of inactivity in some muscles, the patient may learn to not use muscles that are temporarily paralyzed. When the muscle paralysis decreases over time, the patient may not know how to use the muscle in the correct manner. Biofeedback assists in this muscle rehabilitation because it provides the patient with information about how much muscle tension is generated when the patient attempts to contract a specific muscle group. With continued practice using these muscle groups and the feedback, the patient is able to see progress and avoid discouragement. Furthermore, even if

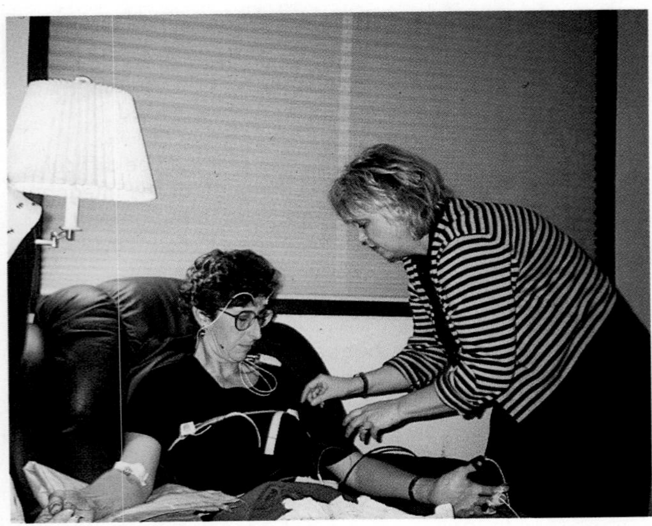

Fig. 8-4 Biofeedback monitoring. Electrodes are placed on the frontalis and trapezius muscles as well as the fingers on the left hand. Pneumograph measurements are also made.

the muscle has atropied, patients can learn exercises to strengthen the muscle, thus achieving a return of function.[5]

Biofeedback therapy is also used to treat Raynaud's syndrome, which appears to be mediated by stress as evidenced by the relationship between decreased peripheral skin temperature and increased affective states such as fear.[37] Biofeedback can also be used in autogenic training, during which patients are taught to relax and warm their hands or feet, usually the nondominant side initially. The patient is directed to repeat the phrase "My left hand is feeling warm and heavy." Biofeedback is used to provide immediate information to the patient regarding the effectiveness of the relaxation/autogenic training. This technique has been effectively used to increase skin temperature. Furthermore, temperature differences can be observed from one side of the body to the other, indicating that the individual is learning to control the body's response.[31]

One of the most critical components of any behavioral program is adherence to the treatment regimen.[38] Patients who are compliant with appointments, practice times, and goal setting and take responsibility for their treatment tend to be the most successful.

When investigating the effectiveness of an intervention on a population of patients, it is important to be aware of differences in responses between genders. For example, on the average males have higher baseline skin temperature levels than females, and can, during autogenic sessions, increase their skin temperature higher than females. It is also important to note that physiologic responses may not correspond with reported anxiety and that women frequently report higher levels of psychologic distress than do men.[39] Furthermore, if the goal of the intervention is to elevate skin temperature, for example, a small or insignificant response would be expected if the beginning temperature was elevated. On the other hand, if the skin temperature is low, one would expect to see a marked increase if the individual achieved a state of relaxation.

Limitations of Biofeedback. Although biofeedback has demonstrated effectiveness in a number of patient populations, several precautions should be discussed. During relaxation therapy or biofeedback sessions repressed emotions or feelings may be uncovered that patients cannot cope with by themselves. For this reason, it is recommended that practitioners who offer biofeedback should either be trained in more traditional psychologic methods or have qualified professionals available for referral. Although biofeedback is indicated in the treatment of psychosomatic disorders such as phobias, insomnia, and cardiac neurosis, it is not recommended for individuals who have bipolar disease or psychosis such as schizophrenia.[40]

Hypnotherapy

Hypnotherapy did not gain medical approval until the middle of the twentieth century when both the British Medical Association and the American Medical Association approved its use for certain medical problems. Hypnosis is defined as a trance-like state of heightened susceptibility. The purpose of hypnosis is to induce a hypnotic state during which posthypnotic suggestions are implanted.[21] These suggestions usually relate to a change in behavior desired by the patient. Three levels of trance have been identified (Table 8-5).

Hypnosis is a process whereby the individual relaxes followed by a shift in focus of the conscious mind from the external environment to ideas suggested by either the practitioner or the individual (self-hypnosis). The success of hypnotherapy depends on the extent to which individuals can retain a suggestion in a wakeful state. Hypnosis sessions usually last from 60 to 90 minutes, and between 6 and 12 sessions are needed for results to occur.[41]

Many physiologic and psychologic responses have been observed during hypnotic trances, depending on the emotion introduced to the person. Tachycardia frequently occurs during the initial stage of the trance. Decreases in cortisol, respiratory rate, sensitivity to pain, temperature, pressure, or touch have been observed in deeper hypnotic states. Changes in senses can occur depending on the suggestion. In addition to these physiologic changes, hypnosis can change thought processes, produce feelings of relaxation and calmness, or enhance certain emotional states. For example, a pessimistic person may be given the suggestion of focusing on feelings of optimism.[42]

Clinical Applications of Hypnosis. Hypnosis has been used to treat asthmatic patients, particularly children with asthma, because they have a greater ability to be hypnotized, resulting in a better response to treatment.[42] Hypnosis also has been used to reduce examination stress,[43] facilitate smoking cessation, induce deep relaxation, manage chronic pain for a variety of illnesses, treat irritable bowel syndrome, and relieve symptoms of fibromyalgia.[21]

Limitations of Hypnosis. The success of hypnotherapy depends on the ability of the individual to become hypnotized. The World Health Organization (WHO) proposes that 90% of the general population can be hypnotized to some extent. The degree of response relates to the suggestibility of the individual to enter the hypnotic state. The WHO also recommends that hypnosis not be used as a treatment for psychosis, organic psychiatric conditions, and antisocial personality disorders. Another potential limitation to hypnosis is that patients may have negative expectations or fears regarding hypnosis such as undesirable outcomes. Irregularities in

Table 8-4 Types of Biofeedback for Specific Health Problems

Health Problem	Type of Biofeedback	Outcome	Reference
Anxiety	EMG	↓ Anxiety, heart rate, blood pressure ↑ Skin temperature	Taylor[26]
Fecal incontinence	Double-balloon devices to measure pressure	↓ Incontinence	Ko and others[27]
Gastrointestional motility disorders (reflux)	Motility recordings using open-tipped catheters	Learned contraction of lower esophageal sphincter, ↓ reflux	Soykan and others[28]
Migraine headaches	EEG	EEG: small to moderate ↓ in headache	Lewis and Solomon[29]
Parkinsonian symptoms	EMG	Facial muscles relaxed ↓ Hand tremor spike amplitudes	Cleeland[30]
Raynaud's disease	Autogenic training, peripheral skin temperature, EMG, breathing	↑ Skin temperature ↑ Feeling of warmth ↓ Vasospasm	Miller and Morgan[31]
Speech-language pathology	EMG	↓ Stuttering Improvement of voice quality	Blood[32] McGillivray and others[33]
Supraventricular arrhythmias	ECG amplifier	Heart rates controlled and lowered	Schaldach[34]
Tension headaches	EMG	↓ Headaches	Arena and others[35]
Temporomandibular joint dysfunction	EMG	↓ Jaw tension, ↓ pain	Turk and others[36]

ECG, electrocardiogram; *EEG,* electroencephalogram; *EMG,* electromyogram.

Table 8-5 Three Levels of Hypnotic Trance

1. *Light trance,* in which the person's eyes are closed; deeply relaxed and accepts suggestions
2. *Medium trance,* in which physiologic processes are decreased; partial sensitivity to pain with total cessation of allergic reactions
3. *Deep trance,* in which total anesthesia can occur; eyes are open and most posthypnotic suggestions are successful

heart rhythm and increased respiratory rate have been observed when thoughts of fear or anger are introduced. Patients also have reported numbness, tingling, itching, coldness or warmth, and burning sensations.[21]

Meditation

Meditation is any activity that limits stimulus input by directing attention to a single unchanging or repetitive stimulus.[44] Many different forms of meditation have been used by a number of societies to alter consciousness and evoke beneficial responses. Transcendental meditation (TM), mindfulness meditation, Chinese Tao, gnyana yoga, Japanese Zen, Buddhist meditation, Christian prayer, and Moslem Sufism are all methods of meditation. Clinically standardized meditation is a technique that was developed with specific clinical objectives in mind. The individual chooses a sound or creates one, then repeats the sound mentally. The Respiratory One method is another clinical meditation that also requires the individual to repeat a sound, but while doing so links the repetition of the sound with breathing.[44] Regardless of the type of meditation used, they all evoke a restful state, a lower oxygen consumption, a reduction in respiratory and heart rates, and subjective reports of reduced anxiety (Fig. 8-5).

Clinical Applications of Meditation. There are many indications for meditation (Table 8-6). There is some evidence that meditation improves stress-related illnesses and breathing patterns in asthmatics, lowers blood pressure in hypertensive patients and blood glucose levels in diabetics, reduces anxiety in some individuals, decreases episodes of angina pectoris, lowers cholesterol in hypercholesterolemic patients, improves sleep-onset insomnia and stuttering, decreases the central nervous system reactivity, and indirectly reduces the incidence of dental caries by lowering salivary bacteria. Meditation has also increased productivity, improved mood, increased sense of identity, and lowered irritability.[44]

Although practitioners and researchers have attempted to determine which type of person is more appropriate for meditative therapy, the data are inconclusive at this point. Other considerations for the appropriateness of meditation include the degree of self-discipline. Meditation can be easily learned and does not require memorization or particular procedures. It actually requires less self-discipline than most other behavioral therapies. Another consideration involves the self-reinforcing properties that meditation offers. Meditation can induce a peaceful, drifting mental state that is unusually pleasurable and provides an incentive for individuals to continue.

Limitations of Meditation. Although meditation has demonstrated improvement in a variety of physiologic and psychologic ailments, it may be contraindicated in some people. For example, if a person has a strong fear of losing control, he may perceive meditation as a form of mind control and thus may be resistant to learning the technique. Some individuals may also be hypersensitive to meditation and require a much shorter

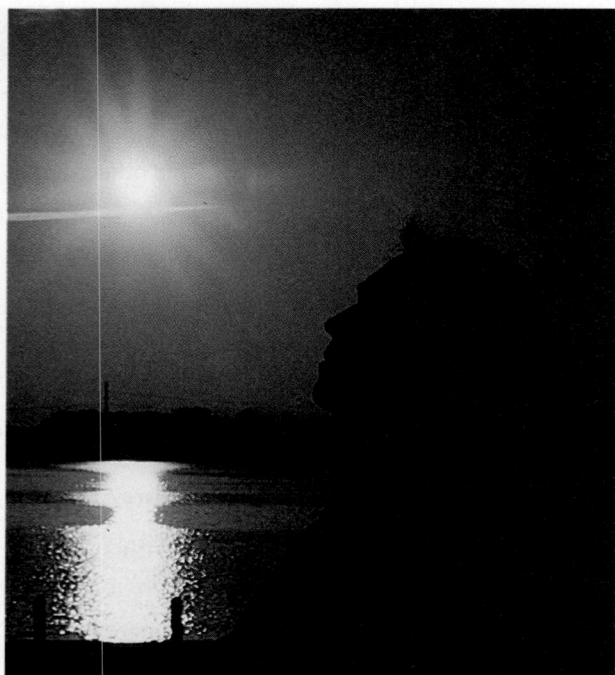

Fig. 8-5 Meditation can be used to relax the body and calm the mind.

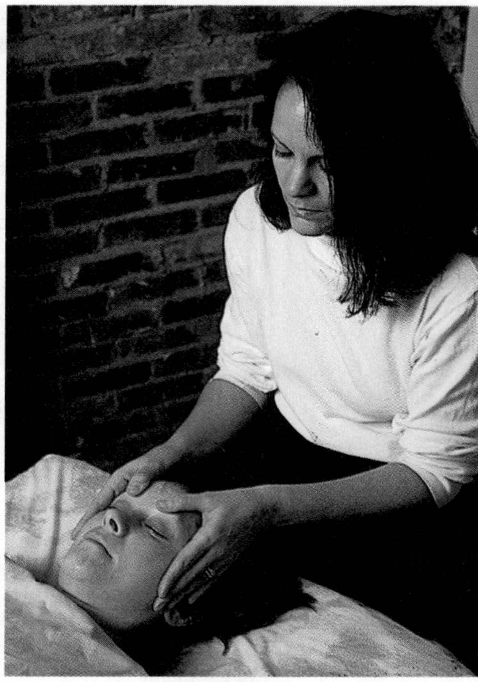

Fig. 8-6 In therapeutic touch the practitioner directs her own interpersonal energy to help or heal another.

Table 8-6 Indications for Meditation

Indications for Meditation
Anxiety or tension states
Chronic bereavement
Chronic fatigue syndrome
Chronic pain
Drug abuse (alcohol or tobacco)
Hypertension
Irritability
Low self-esteem or self-blame
Mild depression
Psychophysiologic disorders
Sleep disorders

session than the average 15- to 20-minute session. Overmeditation should also be avoided. The individual who overmeditates may experience the release of emotional material that may be difficult for the person to cope with. Also, overmeditation in an individual with a history of psychoses may precipitate psychotic episodes. Meditation may also augment the effects of certain drugs. For example, individuals taking antihypertensive medications or thyroid-regulating, antidepressive, or antianxiety drugs should be monitored. Prolonged practice of meditation techniques may, in some instances, lead to the reduced need for certain medications such as antihypertensive drugs. Whatever the case, individuals learning meditation should be monitored closely for physiologic changes with respect to their medications, and adjustment of the medication may be needed.[44]

MANUAL HEALING THERAPIES

Manual healing therapies (see Table 8-1) are based on the theory that energy systems in the body need to be balanced in an effort to enhance healing. A number of manual healing therapies originated from ancient Chinese healing disciplines such as Qigong. In Qigong, trained practitioners learn to emit vital energy of the body, or Qi, for the purpose of healing another person.[45,46]

Therapeutic Touch

A more contemporary manual healing therapy is therapeutic touch.[47] Although the philosophic and religious assumptions between Qigong and other Eastern healing modalities are different from that of therapeutic touch, it is similar to Qigong in that it involves trained practitioners who attempt to direct their excess energies in an intentional and motivated manner toward that of the patient.

Therapeutic touch is a natural human potential that consists of placing the practitioner's hands either on or close to the body of a person (Fig. 8-6). The process of therapeutic touch involves the practitioner scanning the body of the patient and diagnosing areas of accumulated tensions. The practitioner then attempts to redirect these energies to bring the person back into energy balance.[47,48] Therapeutic touch consists of five phases: centering, assessment, unruffling, treatment, and evaluation. Centering is the process whereby the practitioner becomes aware and fully present during the entire treatment. The next phase involves the assessment of the patient, in which the practitioner moves his or her hands (roughly 2 to 6 inches from the body) in a rhythmic and symmetric movement from the head to the toes. During this phase the practitioner notices the quality of energy flow and detects accumulations of energy. The

Table 8-7 Effects of Therapeutic Touch on Outcome Variables

Outcome Variable	Population	Findings	Author
Hemoglobin (Hb)	Ill people	↓ Hb	Krieger[47,48]
Anxiety	Cardiovascular patients	↓ Anxiety	Heidt[50] Quinn[51]
Tension headache pain	Outpatient adults	↓ Headache	Keller and Bzdek[52]
Anxiety and mood	TT practitioners Bereaved adults	↑ Positive mood ↓ Negative mood ↓ Anxiety	Quinn and Strelkauskas[53]

TT, therapeutic touch

physiologic indicators of energy imbalance are perceived as feelings of congestion, pressure, warmth, coolness, blockage, pulling or drawing, or static or tingling.[49] During the third phase, the practitioner unruffles the energy flow or facilitates the symmetric and rhythmic flow of energy through the body. This technique is accomplished by long downward strokes over the energy field located over the entire body. During the actual treatment the practitioner directs and modulates the energy, attempting to rebalance the energy flow. This remodulation of energy is achieved either by the practitioner touching the body or maintaining the hands in a position a few inches away from the body. The final phase consists of an evaluation of the patient and a reassessment of the energy field. If a rebalance has occurred, the practitioner detects a more symmetric, freely flowing energy field.[49]

Clinical Applications of Therapeutic Touch. Some of the earliest studies found that therapeutic touch was able to increase hemoglobin levels in several patients.[47,48] Other studies have found that therapeutic touch was effective in reducing anxiety levels in hospitalized patients with cardiovascular disease, reducing headache pain, and improving mood in bereaved adults[50-53] (Table 8-7). Anecdotal clinical reports have also suggested that therapeutic touch is useful in facilitating healing of traumatic injuries such as sprains, fractures, burns, and wounds; managing suicidal tendencies; reducing chemotherapy-related nausea and vomiting; and facilitating recovery from incest and abuse.[49]

Limitations of Therapeutic Touch. Although some studies have demonstrated that therapeutic touch produced positive outcomes, others have not. Suggestions for this lack of response include an absence of eye and facial contact during the therapeutic session and too brief of a session. Therapeutic touch may be contraindicated in certain patient populations. For example, persons who are sensitive to human interaction and touch (e.g., those who have been physically abused or have psychiatric disorders) may misinterpret the intent of the treatment and may feel threatened by the treatment. Other patients who are sensitive to energy repatterning may also need to avoid therapeutic touch. These include premature infants, newborns, children, pregnant women, older or debilitated people, and those in critical or unstable conditions.[49]

Chiropractic Therapy

Chiropractic therapy, a manual healing art, was developed in 1895 in Iowa. Of the independently practicing health professions, it is the third largest in the Western world.[54] The central tenet of the chiropractic profession is intervertebral manipulation characterized by short-lever, specific, high-velocity, controlled forceful thrusts directed at certain joints by the practitioner either using the hand or an instrument. Manipulation is defined as the forceful passive movement of a joint beyond its active limit of motion.[50] Chiropractic practice does not typically include drug therapy or surgery.

Spinal manipulation received an endorsement from the U.S. Department of Health and Human Services Agency for Health Care Policy and Research in 1994. The agency concluded that spinal manual therapy provides symptomatic relief and functional improvement. The basic principles of chiropractic therapy incorporate the idea that human beings have an innate healing potential, and the goal of healing professions is to access this potential. Drug therapy may compromise the body's natural healing ability, and because of this, natural, nonpharmaceutical therapies should be the first line of treatment. Finally, both a natural diet and regular exercise are critical components for the body to function properly.[55]

Clinical Applications of Chiropractic Therapy. The basic goals of chiropractic therapy focus on restoring the structural and functional imbalances that may result in pain. It is believed that structure and function coexist with one another, and that alterations or distortions in structure can ultimately lead to abnormalities in function. One of the major structural distortions that chiropractors treat is vertebral subluxation in which the motion of the joints is decreased because of slight changes in the position of the articulating bones and subjective symptoms such as pain.[55] A more severe form of subluxation, called fixation, exists when joint motion is restricted.

Chiropractic interventions are used to treat not only musculoskeletal abnormalities, but headaches, dysmenorrhea, blood pressure, vertigo, tinnitus, and visual disorders. In one study chiropractic therapy has also been shown to increase the activity of polymorphonuclear cells and monocytes.[56]

Limitations of Chiropractic Therapy. Several diseases or joint conditions should not be treated with manipulation. If a malignancy is suspected or determined through diagnostic testing, the patient should be referred to a medical physician for further evaluation and treatment. Bone and joint infections also require pharmaceutical or surgical intervention, and the structural integrity of the bone may be compromised if excessive force is used. Contraindications for chiropractic therapy include acute myelopathy, fractures, dislocations, and rheumatoid arthropathies.

Table 8-8 Three Causes of Disease According to Traditional Chinese Medicine

Cause of Disease	Influences
External causes, or "the six evils"	Wind, cold, fire, damp, summer heat, dryness
Internal causes, or internal damage by seven affects	Joy, anger, anxiety, thought, sorrow, fear, fright
Nonexternal, noninternal causes	Dietary irregularities, excessive sexual activity, taxation fatigue, trauma, parasites

From Ergil KV: China's traditional medicine. In Micozzi MS, editor: *Fundamentals of complementary and alternative therapy,* New York, 1996, Churchill Livingstone.

Table 8-9 Types of Qi

Type	Function
Ying qi (construction qi)	Supports and nourishes the body
Wei qi (defense qi)	Protects and warms the body
Jing qi (channel qi)	Flows in the channels (felt during acupuncture)
Zang qi (organ qi)	Flows in the organs (physiologic function of the organs)
Zong qi (ancestral qi)	Responsible for respiration and circulation

From Ergil KV: China's traditional medicine. In Micozzi MS, editor: *Fundamentals of complementary and alternative therapy,* New York, 1996, Churchill Livingstone.

TRADITIONAL AND ETHNOMEDICINE THERAPIES

Traditional Chinese Medicine

Traditional Chinese medicine (TCM) comprises a variety of healing modalities, including herbs, acupuncture, moxibustion, diet, exercise, and meditation. TCM is several thousand years old and has its roots in Taoism. There are several major concepts that constitute Chinese medicine. The most important of these are the concepts of yin and yang, which represent opposing yet complementary phenomena that exist in a state of dynamic equilibrium. Examples are night/day, hot/cold, and shady/sunny. Yin represents shade, cold, and inhibition; yang represents fire, light, and excitement. Yin also represents the inner part of the body, specifically the viscera, liver, heart, spleen, lung, and kidney; yang represents the outer part, specifically the bowels, stomach, and bladder. When there is an imbalance in these two paired opposites, it is thought that disease occurs.[57]

Qi is defined as the vital energy of the human body. Disease is classified into three major categories: external causes, internal causes, and neither internal nor external causes (Table 8-8). Regardless of the cause, it is thought that yin and yang go out of balance, thus altering the movement of Qi. The body consists of several forms of this energy that directly influence physiologic functions of the body and help maintain homeostasis (Table 8-9).

Channels of energy run in regular patterns through the body and over its surface. These channels, called meridians, are like rivers flowing through the body. An obstruction in the movement of these energy rivers is like a dam that backs up the flow in one part of the body and restricts it in others. Any obstruction and blockages or deficiencies of energy would eventually lead to disease. Research has been done to identify and systematize the meridians or channels through which Qi flows. Twelve primary and eight secondary or extra channels have been identified. Located along the channels are acupoints, or holes through which Qi can be influenced by the insertion of needles, a process known as acupuncture.

Another important component of Chinese medicine involves five elements. The five elements consist of earth, metal, water, wood, and fire. Various health phenomena are organized according to these phases and interact with each other.[57]

In Chinese medicine, outward manifestations are reflective of the internal environment. Two primary areas are assessed in Chinese medicine: the tongue and several pulses. The color, shape, and coating of the tongue reflect the general condition of the internal organs. The pulses provide information about the condition and balance of Qi, blood, yin and yang, and the internal organs.[21]

Acupuncture

Acupuncture is a method of stimulating certain points (acupoints) on the body by the insertion of special needles to modify the perception of pain, normalize physiologic functions, or treat or prevent disease (Fig. 8-7).[21] Acupuncture is used to regulate the flow of Qi. The acupuncture needles unblock the obstruction of energy and reestablish the flow of Qi through the meridians, thereby stimulating and activating the body's self-healing mechanism.

There are several types of acupuncture. Auricular acupuncture is based on the perspective that regions of the body are parallel to sites on the ear. Auricular acupuncture is frequently indicated for conditions that are painful and acute, such as renal colic. The therapeutic effect from this method is usually quick, but the duration is not as long as body acupuncture. For this reason, occasionally semipermanent needles may be left in the tissue until the treatment is terminated. Electroacupuncture is another type of acupuncture in which electrical currents are applied to the needles. Different frequencies of electrical stimulation result in the release of different neuropeptides within the central nervous system.[58]

Clinical Applications of Acupuncture. Acupuncture is the primary treatment modality used by physicians of Chinese medicine. Many allopathic physicians and health care professionals are also being trained and certified in acupuncture. Many states now have regulations and licensure requirements to practice as an acupuncturist.

The most common problems for which acupuncture is used include low-back pain, myofascial pain, simple and migraine headaches, sciatica, shoulder pain, tennis elbow, osteoarthritis, whiplash, and musculoskeletal sprains. Other problems that have been successfully treated include sinusitis, gastrointestinal disorders, perimenstrual symptoms, neurologic disorders, chronic pulmonary diseases (including asthma), hypertension, smoking and other addictions, and clinical depression.[58,59]

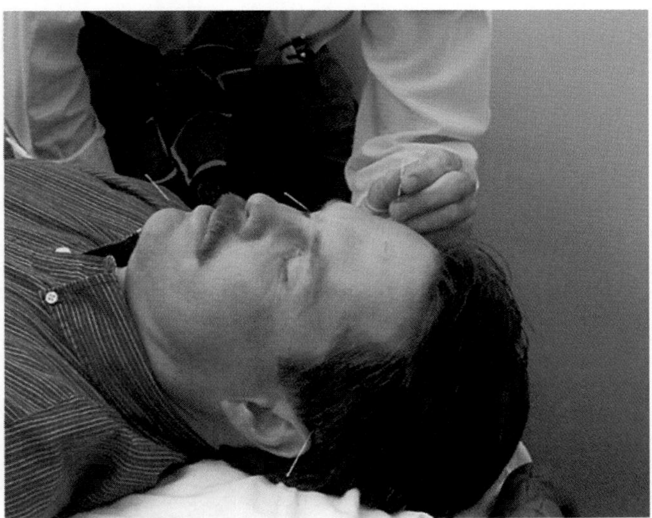

Fig. 8-7 Acupuncture.

Limitations of Acupuncture. Acupuncture is considered a safe therapy when the practitioner has been appropriately trained and uses sterilized needles. Although complications have been noted, they are rare if appropriate steps are taken to ensure the safety of equipment and the patient. These complications include (1) infections resulting from inadequately sterilized needles or those that are left in place for an extended length of time, (2) broken needles, (3) puncture of an internal organ, (4) bleeding, (5) fainting, (6) seizures, (7) miscarriage, and (8) post-treatment drowsiness.[21] To prevent fainting, it is recommended that patients be treated lying down. For patients who become drowsy after treatment, care should be taken to ensure their safe return to home.

Acupuncture should be used with caution and performed by trained practitioners in pregnant patients, those who have a history of seizures, are carriers of hepatitis, or have human immunodeficiency viral infection, bleeding disorders, thrombocytopenia, or skin infections. The semipermanent needles should not be used with persons who have valvular heart disease because of the increased risk of infection. Electroacupuncture should be avoided in persons with a pacemaker, those who have cardiac arrhythmias or epilepsy, and those who are pregnant.[21]

HERBAL THERAPIES

It is estimated that approximately 25,000 plant species are used medicinally throughout the world. It is the oldest known form of medicine, and archaeologic evidence suggests that herbal remedies were used 60,000 years ago by Neanderthals. Use of herbal therapy gained widespread popularity in many countries as early as 3000 BC but began to decline with the development of modern scientific medicine in the early eighteenth century. However, approximately 80% of the world's population lives in developing countries, and herbal medicine constitutes a prominent part of health care in these countries. Furthermore, a resurgence in interest has developed in countries whose health care is dominated by allopathic medicine. The increase in herbal medicine has occurred because of a growing concern by the general public about the complications and limitations of modern scientific medicine and consumer interest in "natural" foods.[21]

The federal Food, Drug, and Cosmetic Act mandates that all drugs must be proven safe and effective before being sold to the public. Because herbal medicines have not undergone the same rigorous research as have pharmaceuticals, the majority have not received approval for use as drugs. For this reason many herbal medicines are sold as foods or food supplements in health food stores and through private companies. The Dietary Supplement Health and Education Act passed in 1994 now allows herbs to be sold as dietary supplements as long as there are no health claims written on their labels.[60]

Herbal substances used in Chinese medicine are taken from plants, animals, or minerals; those used in Western herbal medicine are primarily prepared from plant materials. The active ingredients are "packaged" in tinctures or extracts, elixirs, syrups, capsules, pills, tablets, lozenges, powders, ointments or creams, drops, and suppositories. Many people tend to think that because herbs are natural plants they will not cause harm or side effects. Many herbs are also sold with claims that they can "cure" certain ailments, despite the fact that their efficacy has not been determined through clinical trials. Herbs are generally classified as beneficial, harmful, or neutral, in which case they have no effects on the specific ailment.

The philosophy of herbal therapy is also different from that of conventional drug therapy. The goal of herbal therapy is to restore balance within the individual by facilitating the person's self-healing ability. Drug therapy, on the other hand, is aimed at the treatment of specific diseases or symptoms. Herbal therapy is also prescribed on an individual basis with unique herbal concoctions tailored for each person.

Clinical Applications of Herbal Therapy

A number of herbs have been determined to be safe and effective for a variety of conditions (Table 8-10). Milk thistle, for example, has been observed to be effective in treating a number of liver and gallbladder conditions. It is thought to protect the liver through its antioxidant properties and by facilitating regeneration of liver cells. St. John's Wort has effectiveness as a mild antidepressant and mild sedative. Hypericin and pseudohypericin, major constituents of the drug, have also been shown to have potent action against viruses. Clinical trials investigating the effectiveness of St. John's Wort against acquired immunodeficiency syndrome have begun.[21]

Limitations of Herbal Therapy

Although herbal medicine has been shown to provide beneficial effects for a variety of conditions, a number of problems may exist. When herbal medicines are developed, concentrations of the active ingredients have been found to vary considerably. Contamination with other herbs or chemicals, including pesticides and heavy metals, may also occur. Not all companies follow strict quality control and manufacturing guidelines, which set standards for acceptable levels of pesticides, residual solvents, bacterial levels, and heavy metals.[21] For this reason, herbal medicine should be purchased only from reputable manufacturers. In addition, labels on herbal products should

Table 8-10 Safe or Effective Herbs Determined by Non-U.S. Regulatory Authorities

Common Name	Effects	Examples of Uses
Aloe	Antiinflammatory Acceleration of wound healing Alkalinization of digestive juices	■ Minor burns ■ Wound healing ■ Gastrointestinal disorders
Astralagus	Stimulant of immune system	■ Cancer
Bilberry	Improvement of microcirculation in eyes Mild antiinflammatory	■ Myopia ■ Retinal problems ■ GI disorders
Cat's claw	Stimulant of immune system Antioxidant Antiinflammatory Lowering of blood pressure	■ Cancer ■ GI disorders ■ Hypertension ■ Infections
Chamomile	Antiinflammatory Antispasmodic Antiinfective	■ Inflammatory diseases of GI and upper respiratory tracts ■ Inflammation of skin and mucous membranes ■ GI spasms
Dong quai	Antispasmodic Vasodilatation Balancing effects of estrogen Mild sedative effect	■ Menstrual cramps ■ Premenstrual syndrome ■ Menstrual irregularities ■ Hot flashes ■ Vaginal dryness
Echinacea	Stimulant of immune system Antiinflammatory Antibacterial	■ Upper respiratory tract infections ■ Allergic rhinitis ■ Wound healing
Feverfew	Antiinflammatory Inhibition of serotonin and prostaglandins Vasodilator	■ Migraine headaches ■ Arthritis
Garlic	Lowering of lipids Inhibition of platelet aggregation Antibacterial	■ Elevated cholesterol levels ■ Hypertension ■ Diabetes ■ Infections
Ginger	Antiemetic	■ Nausea and vomiting ■ Motion sickness
Gingko biloba	Memory improvement Increasing blood flow Antioxidant Increased metabolism efficiency	■ Alzheimer's disease ■ Dementia ■ Eye disease ■ Heart disease ■ Poor circulation ■ Varicose veins ■ Anxiety ■ Age-related diseases
Ginseng	Increased physical endurance "Balancing" of body Resistance to stress	■ Fatigue ■ Headaches ■ Decreased libido ■ Hot flashes
Goldenseal	Antiinflammatory Antibacterial Laxative	■ Respiratory and GI infections ■ Gallbladder inflammation ■ Cirrhosis of liver
Hawthorn	Increased O_2 utilization by heart Lowering of cholesterol Peripheral vasodilator	■ Angina ■ Coronary artery disease
Milk thistle	Stimulation of production of new liver cells Protection of liver from damage	■ Liver disease

Continued

Table 8-10 Safe or Effective Herbs Determined by Non-U.S. Regulatory Authorities—cont'd

Common Name	Effects	Examples of Uses
St. John's Wort (hypericum)	Inhibition of monoamine oxidase (MAO) and serotonin reuptake	▪ Mild to moderate depression
	Antiviral	▪ Viral infections
	Antibacterial	▪ Wound healing
	Warning: Avoid foods containing tyramine, such as aged cheese, red wine, etc.	
Saw palmetto	Prevention of conversion of testosterone to dihydrotesterone (needed for prostate cell multiplication)	▪ Benign prostatic hyperplasia ▪ Urinary problems
	Balancing of sex hormones	
Valerian	Minor tranquilizer CNS depression	▪ Sleep disorders ▪ Restlessness

CNS, central nervous system; *GI*, gastrointestinal.

Table 8-11 Unsafe Herbs

Common Name	Use/Effect	Comments
Borage	Diuretic Antidiarrheal	Contains toxic pyrrolizidine alkaloids
Calamus	Fever Digestive aid	Contains varying amounts of carcinogenic *cis*-isoasarone; Indian type most toxic; North American type nontoxic
Chaparral	Anticancer	No proven efficacy; may induce severe liver toxicity
Coltsfoot	Antitussive Demulcent	Contains carcinogenic pyrrolizidine alkaloids
Comfrey	Wound healing	Contains large number of toxic pyrrolizidine alkaloids; may induce veno-occlusive disease
Ephedra (Ma Huang)	CNS stimulant Anorectic Bronchodilator Cardiac stimulation	Unsafe for people with hypertension, diabetes, or thyroid disease; avoid consumption with caffeine
Germander	Anorectic	Causes hepatotoxicity because of diterpenoid derivatives
Life root	Menstrual flow stimulant	Hepatotoxic; contains toxic pyrrolizidine alkaloids
Pokeroot	Antirheumatic Anticancer	May be fatal in children
Sassafras	Stimulant Antispasmodic Antirheumatic	Volatile oil contains carcinogenic safrole

contain the scientific name of the botanical, the name and address of the actual manufacturer, a batch or lot number, the date of manufacture, and the expiration date.[60]

Some herbs have also been found to contain toxic products and can cause cancer. Comfrey, for example, has been used for its wound-healing properties. However, various species of comfrey contain certain pyrrolizidine alkaloids that are highly carcinogenic. Comfrey has been shown to produce liver cancer in small animals and fatal veno-occlusive disease in humans. For this reason comfrey should not be used internally and, as a poultice, should be used only on intact skin.[60] Other unsafe herbs are listed in Table 8-11.

Despite the increased use of herbal products, there has not been a parallel increase in reports of toxicity. Nonetheless, herbal products should be used with caution in pregnant women, nursing mothers, infants and young children, and the elderly with liver or cardiovascular disease.[60]

NURSING ROLE IN COMPLEMENTARY AND ALTERNATIVE THERAPIES

The interest in CAM therapies has increased significantly in the last 15 years. The majority of people using and seeking information about complementary and alternative therapies are well educated and have a strong desire to actively participate in the decision making about their health care. This increased interest comes not only from health care consumers, but also from allopathic physicians who have increasing concerns that current Western medicine is not meeting the needs of their patients. Many allopathic physicians do not refer their patients for CAM therapies because they are not familiar with the therapies and have had little, if any, education and training in complementary and alternative medicine. Many physicians have reservations about CAM therapies because they have not been appropriately tested in clinical trials in which other factors that may influence the outcomes are strictly controlled.

In North America and in the United Kingdom many professional groups are exploring the use of CAM and facilitating and monitoring research being conducted in this area. Proposals put forth by several of these groups include assessing the need by the public for CAM therapies, incorporating CAM educational components in the curriculum for all health care programs, providing appropriate information to the public, and encouraging and facilitating communication between CAM practitioners and allopathic physicians so each can be open to the other's approaches and values.[61] For example, if CAM therapies are to be accepted and incorporated into Western medicine as a more integrative medical approach, practitioners of CAM should realize the advantages of their therapies being researched more rigorously. On the other hand, allopathic physicians and more conventional practitioners should also begin to understand the benefits of therapies that encourage active participation by their patients in illness prevention or managing chronic illness rather than relying solely on surgery or drugs.

Integrative medicine, a health care strategy that is gaining popularity, involves a multiple-practitioner treatment group in which a patient seeks care simultaneously from more than one type of practitioner. The patients are given the option to choose the kind of practitioner they feel would benefit their particular health problem. Patients who may benefit from these groups are those who have health problems that have historically been difficult to treat using traditional allopathic medicine, such as fibromyalgia or chronic fatigue syndrome. This represents a pluralistic and truly complementary health care system in which both alternative and allopathic practitioners work side-by-side to improve the well-being of their patients.

The integrative medicine approach is consistent with the holistic approach nurses are taught to practice. Nurses have the potential for becoming essential participants in this type of health care philosophy. Many nurses already practice forms of CAM by offering relaxation, imagery, massage, and therapeutic touch to their patients (Fig. 8-8). Nurses should be knowledgeable of CAM therapies in order to make appropriate recommendations to allopathic primary care providers about which therapies may be useful for patients. Nurses should also be able to provide advice to patients regarding when to seek conventional therapy rather than CAM therapy. For example, if a patient complains of right lower abdominal pain, nausea, and vomiting, the nurse should be suspicious of appendicitis and recommend that the patient be assessed by an allopathic physician. However, if the patient has a chronic gastrointestinal disorder and has been diagnosed with irritable bowel syndrome, the patient may benefit from relaxation and herbal therapy.

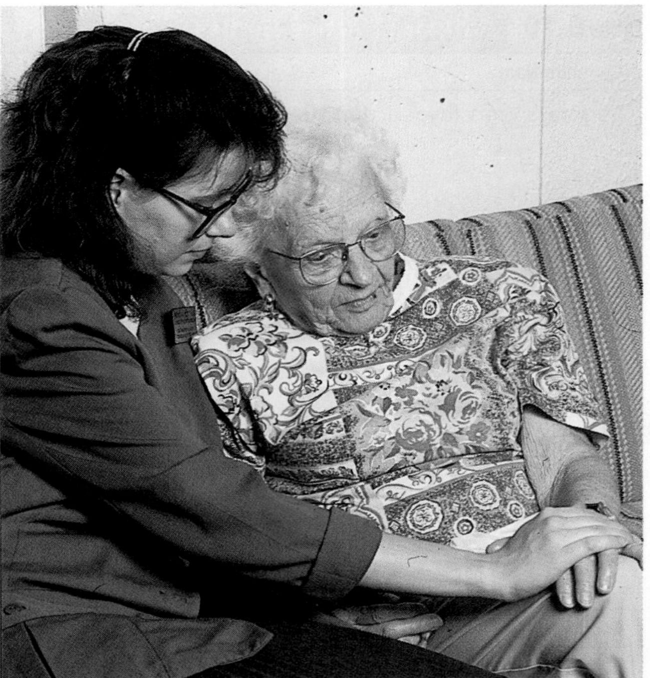

Fig. 8-8 The nurse encourages the patient to use imagery to relax and relieve pain.

Nurses work very closely with their patients and are in the unique position of becoming familiar with the patient's religious and cultural viewpoints and existential issues. Nurses may be able to determine which CAM therapies would be more appropriately aligned with these beliefs and offer recommendations accordingly.

Patient interest and participation in CAM therapies is increasing. Therefore it is important for nurses to be knowledgeable of the multiple CAM therapies available and the use of these therapies by their patients. It is also important for nurses to keep abreast of the current research being done in this area in order to provide accurate information, not only to the patients, but to other health care professionals. Many studies related to CAM therapies have involved small numbers of subjects and were not well controlled. More studies are needed to validate the effectiveness of CAM therapies.

CRITICAL THINKING EXERCISES

CASE STUDY

College Student with Abdominal Distress

Patient Profile

Jane, a 21-year-old college student, was seen in the student health center for increasing episodes of abdominal fullness and discomfort with alternating diarrhea and constipation.

Subjective Data

- Reports being diagnosed with irritable bowel syndrome several years ago
- Was told to eat more fiber, but nothing has seemed to be effective in reducing her abdominal distress
- Is taking a heavy course load this semester
- Has to work 20 hours each week for her work-study contract
- Eats mainly fast foods and drinks several colas daily

Critical Thinking Questions

1. Explain the psychologic stressors that may be contributing to Jane's abdominal discomfort.
2. Describe how her current diet may be affecting her both physiologically and psychologically.
3. What complementary and alternative therapy (or therapies) would be appropriate for Jane?
4. How would you recommend complementary therapies to her physician? What arguments could you use to support their use?

REVIEW QUESTIONS

The number of the question corresponds to the same-numbered objective at the beginning of the chapter.

1. One of the primary differences between alternative and complementary therapy is
   a. alternative therapies offer distinctly different therapies than complementary therapies.
   b. complementary therapies are used in addition to the primary medical treatment while alternative therapies become the primary treatment.
   c. complementary therapies have proven effectiveness in treating acute emergencies and bacterial infections while alternative therapies do not.
   d. complementary therapies usually are ordered by the physician while alternative therapies are not.
2. The type of relaxation intervention (progressive, active, or passive) should be chosen based on
   a. age and gender of the person.
   b. susceptibility of the person to relax.
   c. functional status and energy expenditure required.
   d. physician or health care provider.
3. Relaxation is a state of generalized low cognitive, physiologic, or behavioral arousal during which
   a. muscle fibers lengthen and neural impulses to the brain decrease.
   b. alpha brain activity decreases.
   c. peripheral skin temperature decreases.
   d. heart and respiratory rates increase.
4. Biofeedback is frequently used in addition to relaxation therapy because
   a. it provides immediate feedback regarding the ability to control physiologic responses.
   b. it is viewed among allopathic practitioners as more scientific than relaxation alone.
   c. it is more difficult for patients to obtain a relaxed state without it.
   d. insurance companies are more likely to reimburse for biofeedback.
5. Any activity that limits stimulus input by directing attention to a single unchanging or repetitive stimulus is
   a. imagery.
   b. hypnosis.
   c. meditation.
   d. relaxation.
6. The basis for therapeutic touch involves the
   a. acquisition of the relaxation response.
   b. stimulation of peripheral nerves to reduce pain.
   c. remodulation of energy by a trained practitioner in an attempt to rebalance the patient's energy field.
   d. the emission of vital energy by a trained practitioner for the purpose of healing another person.
7. The primary goals of chiropractic therapy focus on
   a. reducing muscle tension that produces spinal instability.
   b. increasing spinal flexibility and muscle tone.
   c. restoring the structural and functional vertebral imbalances that cause pain.
   d. combining vertebral manipulation and drug therapy for the treatment of chronic back pain.
8. Critical components in the treatment of acupuncture include all of the following except
   a. Qi.
   b. yin and yang.
   c. channels or meridians
   d. muscular manipulation.
9. Herbal therapy is different from drug therapy in that
   a. only organic plant materials are used in herbal therapy.
   b. the goal of herbal therapy is to restore balance by facilitating the person's self-healing ability.
   c. herbal therapy is available only in teas and tinctures while drug therapy is available in multiple forms.
   d. it is safe to use because herbal therapy is more organic and natural.

References

1. Eisenberg DM and others: Unconventional medicine in the United States—prevalence, costs, and patterns of use, *N Engl J Med* 328:246, 1993.
2. Taylor E, Lee CT, Young JDE: Bringing mind-body medicine into the mainstream, *Hosp Pract* 32:183, 1997.

3. Alternative Medicine. Expanding Medical Horizons. Workshop on alternative medicine, Chantilly, Va, Sept 14-16. US Government Printing Office, 1992.
4. Mandle CL, Jacobs SC, Arcaro PM, Domar AD: The efficacy of relaxation response interventions with adult patients: a review of the literature, *J Cardiovasc Nurs* 10:4, 1996.
5. Miller NE: Biomedical foundations for biofeedback as a part of behavioral medicine. In Basmajian JV, editor: *Biofeedback: principles and practice for clinicians,* Baltimore, 1989, Williams & Wilkins.
6. Rabin BS and others: Mechanistic aspects of stressor-induced immune alteration. In Glaser R , Kiecolt-Glaser J, editors: *Human stress and immunity,* San Diego, 1994, Academic Press.
7. Benson H, Beary J, Carol M: The relaxation response, *Psychiatry* 37:37, 1974.
8. Smith JC and others: Relaxation: mapping an uncharted world, *Biofeedback Self Regul* 21:63, 1996.
9. Syrjala KL and others: Relaxation and imagery and cognitive-behavioral training reduce pain during cancer treatment: a controlled clinical trial, *Pain* 63:189, 1995.
10. Good M: Effects of relaxation and music on postoperative pain: a review, *J Adv Nur* 24:905, 1996.
11. McCain NL and others: The influence of stress management training in HIV disease, *Nurs Res* 45:246, 1996.
12. Houldin AD, McCorkle R, Lowery BJ: Relaxation training and psychoimmunological status of bereaved spouses, *Cancer Nurs* 16:47, 1993.
13. Van Rood YR and others: The effects of stress and relaxation on the in vitro immune response in man: a meta-analytic study, *J Behav Med* 16:163, 1993.
14. Holland JD and others: A randomized clinical trial of alprazolam versus progressive muscle relaxation in cancer patients with anxiety and depressive symptoms, *J Clin Oncol* 9:1004, 1991.
15. Burish TG and others: Conditioned side effects induced by cancer chemotherapy: prevention through behavioral treatment, *J Consult Clin Psychol* 55:42, 1987.
16. Carey MP, Burish TG: Providing relaxation training to cancer chemotherapy patients: a comparison of three delivery techniques, *J Consult Clin Psychol* 55:732, 1987.
17. Burish, TG, Snyder SL, Jenkins RA: Preparing patients for cancer chemotherapy: effect of coping preparation and relaxation interventions, *J Consult Clin Psychol* 59:518, 1991.
18. McGuigan FJ: Progressive relaxation: origins, principles, and clinical applications. In Lehrer PM, Woolfolk RL, editors: *Principles and practice of stress management,* ed 2, New York, 1993, Guilford Press.
19. Carlson CR, Nitz AJ: Negative side effects of self-regulation training: relaxation and the role of the professional in service delivery, *Biofeedback Self Regul* 16:191, 1991.
20. Kaempfer SH: Relaxation training reconsidered, *Oncol Nurs Forum* 9:15, 1982.
21. Lewith G, Kenyon J, Lewis P, editors: *Complementary medicine: an integrated approach,* Oxford, 1996, Oxford University Press.
22. Norris PA, Fahrion SL: Autogenic biofeedback in psychophysiological therapy and stress management. In Lehrer PM, Woolfolk RL, editors: *Principles and practice of stress management,* ed 2, New York, 1993, Guilford Press.
23. Patel C: Yoga-based therapy. In Lehrer PM, Woolfolk RL, editors: *Principles and practice of stress management,* ed 2, New York, 1993, Guilford Press.
24. Olson RP: Definitions of biofeedback. In Schwartz MS and others, editors: *Biofeedback: a practitioner's guide,* New York, 1987, Guilford Press.
25. Adler CS, Adler SM: Biofeedback and psychosomatic disorders. In Basmajian JV, editor: *Biofeedback: principles and practice for clinicians,* Baltimore, 1989, Williams & Wilkins.
26. Taylor DN: Effects of a behavioral stress-management program on anxiety, mood, self-esteem, and T-cell count in HIV positive men, *Psychol Rep* 76:451, 1995.
27. Ko CY and others: Biofeedback is effective therapy for fecal incontinence and constipation, *Arch Surg* 132:829, 1997.
28. Soykan I, Chen J, Kendall BJ, McCallum RW: The rumination syndrome: clinical and manometric profile, therapy, and long-term outcome, *Dig Dis Sci* 41:1866, 1995.
29. Lewis TA, Solomon GD: Advances in migraine management, *Cleve Clin J Med* 62:148, 1995.
30. Cleeland CS: Biofeedback and other behavioral techniques in the treatment of disorders of voluntary movement. In Basmajian JV, editor: *Biofeedback: principles and practice for clinicians,* ed 3, Baltimore, 1989, Williams & Wilkins.
31. Miller LM, Morgan RF: Vasospastic disorders: etiology, recognition, and treatment, *Hand Clin* 9:171, 1993.
32. Blood GW: A behavioral-cognitive therapy program for adults who stutter: computers and counseling, *J Commun Dis* 28:165, 1995.
33. McGillivray R, Proctor-Williams K, McLister B: Simple biofeedback device to reduce excessive vocal intensity, *Med Biol Eng* 32:348, 1994.
34. Schaldach M: New aspects in electrostimulation of the heart, *Med Prog Technol* 21:1, 1995.
35. Arena JG and others: A comparison of frontal electromyographic biofeedback training, trapezius electromyographic biofeedback training, and progressive muscle relaxation therapy in the treatment of tension headache, *Headache* 35:411, 1995.
36. Turk DC and others: Dysfunctional patients with temporomandibular disorders: evaluating the efficacy of a tailored treatment protocol, *J Consult Clin Psychol* 64:139, 1996.
37. Sedlacek K: Biofeedback treatment of primary Raynaud's disease. In Basmajian JV, editor: *Biofeedback: principles and practice for clinicians,* Baltimore, 1989, Williams & Wilkins.
38. McGrady A: Good news—bad press: applied psychophysiology in cardiovascular disorders, *Biofeedback Self Regul* 21:335, 1996.
39. Roberts G, McGrady A : Racial and gender effects on the relaxation response: implications for the development of hypertension, *Biofeedback Self Regul* 21:51, 1996.
40. Adler CS, Adler SM: Strategies in general psychiatry. In Basmajian JV, editor: *Biofeedback: principles and practice for clinicians,* Baltimore, 1989, Williams & Wilkins.
41. DeBetz B, Sunnen G: *A primer of clinical hypnosis,* Littleton, Mass, 1985, PSG.
42. Lewith GT, Watkins AD: Unconventional therapies in asthma: an overview, *Allergy* 51:761, 1996.
43. Whitehouse WG and others: Psychological and immune effects of self-hypnosis training for stress management throughout the first semester of medical school, *Psychosom Med* 58:249, 1996.
44. Carrington P: Modern forms of meditation. In Lehrer PM, Woolfolk RL, editors: *Principles and practice of stress management,* ed 2, New York, 1993, Guilford Press.
45. Sheng-han X: Psychophysiological reactions associated with Qigong therapy, *Chinese Med J* 107:230, 1994.
46. Sancier KM: Medical applications of Qigong, *Altern Ther* 2:40, 1996.
47. Krieger D: Searching for evidence of physiological change, *AJN* 79:660, 1979.
48. Krieger D: Therapeutic touch: the imprimatur of nursing, *AJN* 75:784, 1975.
49. Mulloney SS, Wells-Federman C: Therapeutic touch: a healing modality, *J Cardiovasc Nurs* 10:27, 1996.
50. Heidt P: Effect of therapeutic touch on anxiety level of hospitalized patients, *Nurs Res* 30:32, 1980.
51. Quinn JF: Therapeutic touch an energy exchange: testing the theory, *Adv Nurs Sci* 6:42, 1984.
52. Keller E, Bzdek VM: Effects of therapeutic touch on tension headache pain, *Nurs Res* 35:101, 1986.
53. Quinn JF, Strelkauskas AJ: Psychoimmunologic effects of therapeutic touch on practitioners and recently bereaved recipients: a pilot study, *Adv Nurs Sci* 15:13, 1993.
54. Manipulation terminology in the chiropractic, osteopathic, and medical literature. In Leach RA, editor: *The chiropractic theories,* Baltimore, 1986, Williams & Wilkins.
55. Redwood D: Chiropractic. In Micozzi MS, editor: *Fundamentals of complementary and alternative therapy,* New York, 1996, Churchill Livingstone.
56. Brennan PC and others: Enhanced phagocytic cell respiratory burst induced by spinal manipulation: potential role of substance P, *J Manipulation Physiol Ther* 14:399, 1992.
57. Ergil KV: China's traditional medicine. In Micozzi MS, editor: *Fundamentals of complementary and alternative therapy,* New York, 1996, Churchill Livingstone.

58. Ulett GA: Conditioned healing with electroacupuncture, *Altern Ther* 2:56, 1996.
59. Diehl DL and others: Use of acupuncture by American physicians, *J Altern Comple Med* 3:119, 1997.
60. Tyler VE: What pharmacists should know about herbal remedies, *J Am Pharm Assoc* NS36:29, 1996.
61. Foundation of integrated medicine, 1997, Steering Committee for Prince of Wales' Initiative on Integrated Medicine.

Resources

Acupuncture.com
http://www.acupuncture.com

American Holistic Nurses' Association
PO Box 2130
Flagstaff, AZ 86003-2130
800-278-AHNA
Fax: 520-526-2752
http://www.ahna.org

Association for Applied Psychophysiology and Biofeedback
10200 W. 44th Avenue, Suite 304
Wheat Ridge, CO 80033-2840
800-477-8892
303-422-8436
Fax: 303-422-8894
http://www.aapb.org

Colorado Center for Healing Touch, Inc.
198 Union Boulevard, Suite 204
Lakewood, CO 80228
303-989-0581
Fax: 303-985-9702
http://www.healingtouch.net

Council of Colleges of Acupuncture and Oriental Medicine
1424 16th Street NW, Suite 501
Washington, DC 20036-2211
202-265-3370

Henriette's Herbal Homepage
http://sunsite.unc.edu/herbmed

Holistic Alliance of Professional Practitioners, Entrepreneurs, Networkers, Inc. (HAPPEN)
PO Box 90177
Gainesville, FL 32607
888-8HAPPEN
Fax: 352-379-3055
http://www.toolcity.net/~kauffeld/happen

Holistic Healing Homepage
http://www.holisticmed.com

Homeopathy Home Page
http://www.homeopathyhome.com/

National Commission for the Certification of Acupuncturists
1424 16th Street NW, Suite 501
Washington, DC 20036
202-232-1404
Fax: 202-462-6157

Office of Alternative Medicine
OAM Clearinghouse
PO Box 8218
Silver Spring, MD 20907-8218
888-644-6226
301-495-4957
http://altmed.od.nih.gov

Sivananda Yoga Vedanta Centers
http://www.sivananda.org/

For additional Internet resources, see the website for this book at **www.mosby.com/MERLIN/medsurg_lewis**

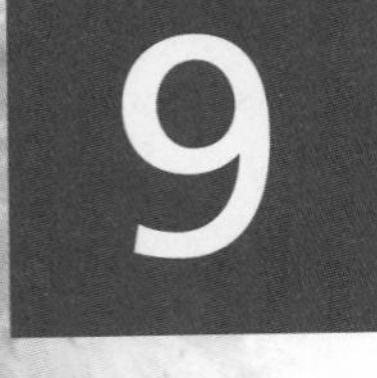

REMEMBER to check out your companion CD-ROM

9 NURSING MANAGEMENT Pain

Diana J. Wilkie

www.mosby.com/MERLIN/medsurg_lewis

LEARNING OBJECTIVES

1. Describe the neural mechanisms of pain and pain modulation.
2. Differentiate between nociceptive and neuropathic types of pain.
3. Recognize the physical and psychologic effects of unrelieved pain.
4. Interpret the subjective and objective data that are obtained when a pain assessment is conducted.
5. Describe collaborative care pain management techniques.
6. Describe pharmacologic and nonpharmacologic methods of pain relief.
7. Explain the nurse's role and responsibility in pain management.
8. Discuss ethical and legal issues in the management of pain.
9. Evaluate the influence of one's own knowledge, beliefs, and attitudes about pain assessment and management.

Pain is a complex, multidimensional phenomenon. The understanding of this phenomenon is evolving as research is conducted by scientists from many disciplines, including nursing. Increased knowledge provides health care professionals with many strategies for pain management. In choosing the most effective strategy, it is important to approach the patient experiencing pain from a holistic perspective. This chapter presents current knowledge about pain and pain management to enable the nurse to collaborate with other health care professionals in the assessment and management of pain.

DEFINITIONS OF PAIN

Pain is defined as whatever the person experiencing the pain says it is, existing whenever the person says it does.[1] This clinical definition recognizes pain as a personal, private experience. Scientists at the International Association for the Study of Pain (IASP) have proposed another definition. This definition states that pain is an unpleasant sensory and emotional experience associated with actual or potential tissue damage, or it is described in terms of such damage.[2] It is important to note that both definitions indicate that pain is a subjective experience.

The first definition, however, does not allow the nurse to adequately distinguish between the statement "I have pain in my heart" made by a person who has just experienced the loss of a loved one or by a person who is experiencing angina related to cardiac disease. In both situations the nurse using the clinical definition would diagnose chest pain but would not be correct in providing pain medications to the first person without further assessment. Based on further assessment appropriate interventions for these two people would be quite different.

Reviewed by Joyce S. Willens, PhD, RN, Associate Professor, College of Nursing, Villanova University, Villanova, Penn.

If the IASP definition of pain is used to guide practice, the nurse is less likely to provide inappropriate interventions to these two people. The nurse would investigate the patient's statement and would consider the potential for the stimulus to cause tissue damage. This consideration would prompt further assessment to determine the cause of the problem, and, from that information, appropriate therapy would be initiated.

In considering the IASP definition, it is also important to note that not all potentially tissue-damaging (noxious) stimuli result in pain. For this reason, it is critical for the nurse to differentiate pain from nociception. *Nociception* is the activation of the primary afferent nerves with peripheral terminals (free nerve endings) that respond differently to noxious (tissue-damaging) stimuli. Nociceptors function primarily to sense and transmit pain signals. Nociception may or may not be perceived as pain, depending on a complex interaction within the nociceptive pathways. If nociceptive stimuli are blocked, pain is not perceived.

Finally, it is important to distinguish pain or nociception from suffering. *Suffering* has been defined as the state of severe distress associated with events that threaten the intactness of the person.[3] Suffering is an emotion that evolves from the meaning attached to an event.[4] Pain and suffering are not the same experiences. The person who complains of pain in the heart because of the death of a loved one is suffering rather than sensing pain as it is defined by the IASP. It is clear that suffering can occur in the presence of pain; suffering can occur when pain is not present; and pain can occur when suffering is not present. For example, the woman awaiting breast biopsy may suffer because of anticipated loss of her breast. After the biopsy, she may have pain without suffering if the biopsy is negative or pain with suffering if the biopsy is positive for malignancy. Interventions aimed at relieving pain and suffering may have some commonalities, but clearly some interventions for suffer-

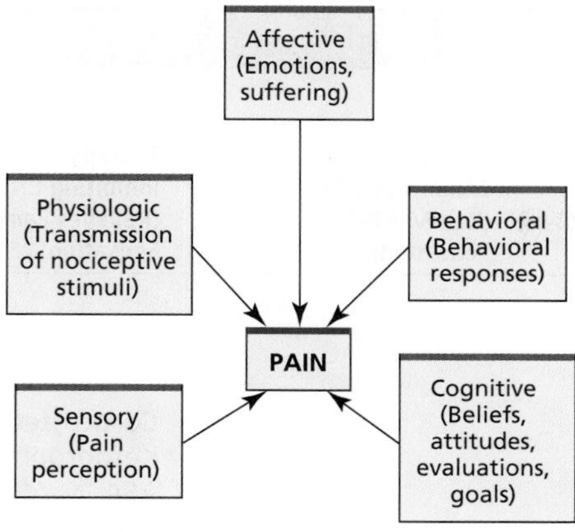

Fig. 9-1 The five components of pain.

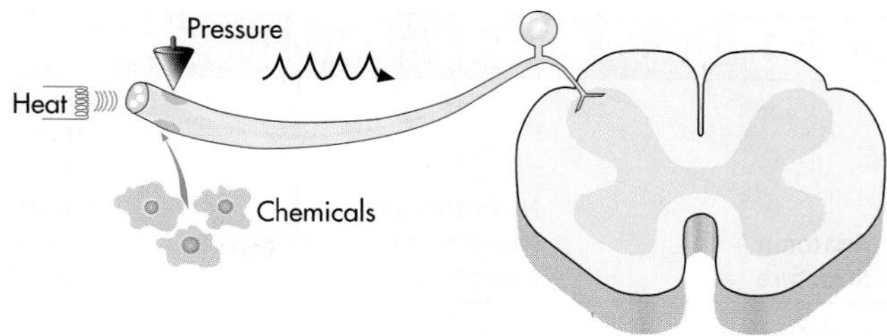

Fig. 9-2 Peripheral terminals are sensitive to direct heat, mechanical pressure, and chemicals released in response to tissue damage.

ing will be inadequate for pain, just as some interventions for pain are inadequate for suffering. Therefore it is crucial to correctly diagnose alterations in comfort that are caused by pain and alterations in comfort that result from suffering. Pain, not suffering, is the focus of this chapter.

MAGNITUDE OF THE PAIN PROBLEM

Pain is one of the most common reasons patients seek health care. Annually 15% to 20% of the nearly 270 million Americans have acute pain and about 25% to 30% have chronic pain.[5] More than 23 million people have operations each year and experience pain.[6] Of the nearly 1.4 million Americans diagnosed annually with cancer, 70% have moderate to severe pain.[7] Canadians experience these various types of pain in similar proportions.

A significant number of people with pain are disabled by their pain, resulting in a serious economic problem in society, as well as a major health problem. For example, most workers (80% to 90%) return to work within 3 weeks of an injury, but the pain may persist or result in prolonged work absences. Adding to the problems of patients with acute pain, especially cancer pain, is a tendency for health care providers to prescribe small, insufficient doses of analgesics to control the pain. Also, nurses tend to routinely administer the smallest prescribed analgesic dose when a range of doses is prescribed.[8] Such practices do little to provide relief from unremitting pain and are not consistent with current pain management guidelines.[6,7,9,10]

DIMENSIONS OF PAIN

As a multidimensional phenomenon, pain consists of five components: affective, behavioral, cognitive, sensory, and physiologic (Fig. 9-1). These are also termed the *ABCs of pain.* The emotions related to the pain (affective component), the behavioral responses to the pain (behavioral component), and the beliefs, attitudes, evaluations, and goals about the pain and pain control (cognitive component) alter how the pain is perceived (sensory component) by modifying the transmission of nociceptive stimuli to the brain (physiologic component). Therefore each dimension is important in the assessment and management of pain. Pain results from complex interactions among these dimensions and can be understood by considering first the physiologic and then the sensory, affective, behavioral, and cognitive dimensions.

Physiologic Dimension of Pain*

Understanding the physiologic dimension of pain requires knowledge of neural anatomy and physiology. The neural mechanism by which pain is perceived is composed of four major steps: transduction, transmission, perception, and modulation. Transduction and transmission involve processing nociceptive stimuli. However, depending on the type and degree of modulation, a nociceptive stimuli may or may not be perceived as pain.[11] If there is no perception of nociception, there is no pain. Perception and modulation are crucial to the sensation of pain.

Transduction. Transduction, the first step of the pain process, occurs at the level of the peripheral nerves. Transduction is the conversion of a mechanic, thermal, or chemical stimulus into a neuronal action potential[12] (Fig. 9-2). Noxious (tissue-damaging) pressure, heat, or chemical forces trigger an action potential, causing the peripheral nerve fiber to become activated. After an action potential is initiated, the information is then transmitted to the central nervous system (CNS).

Chemical activation. In understanding transduction of chemical nociceptive stimuli, it is helpful to consider the microenvironment around each primary afferent nociceptor (PAN). When tissue trauma occurs and cells are damaged, a number of chemicals are released into the area around the PAN. Some of these chemicals activate (e.g., bradykinin, serotonin, histamine, potassium, norepinephrine) or sensitize (e.g., leukotrienes, prostaglandins, substance P) the PAN to send a signal to the spinal cord. In other words, the chemicals cause the PAN to be excited and fire an action potential toward the spinal cord. Several details are helpful in fully understanding this process, and they are summarized in Table 9-1.

If the PAN is activated and fires an action potential, the PAN itself releases chemicals into the peripheral tissues. Substance P is an example of a chemical stored in the distal terminals of the PAN. When substance P is released from the PAN, it sensitizes the PAN, dilates nearby blood vessels with subsequent production of edema, and causes release of histamine from mast cells.[13]

Finally, activation of the autonomic nervous system (ANS) contributes to PAN transduction through release of norepinephrine and synthesis of prostaglandins. Norepinephrine, the

*Parts of this section are copyrighted material by DJ Wilkie, 1994.

Table 9-1 Neural Mechanisms of Pain: Facilitating and Inhibiting Factors

Anatomic Structure	Neurotransmittors, Neurochemicals, or Receptors	Modulatory Effect on Transduction or Transmission—Facilitates (F), Inhibits (I)	Therapy-Enhancing Effect (Relieves Pain Sensation)	Therapy-Inhibiting Effect (Relieves Pain Sensation)
Peripheral Nervous System				
PAN Terminal		**Transduction**		
	Leukotrienes	F, sensitizes		Corticosteroids Ketoprophen
	Prostaglandins	F, sensitizes		ASA, NSAIDs
	Potassium	F, activates		n/a
	Histamine, bradykinin	F, activates		Antihistamines
	Serotonin	F, activates		n/a
	Substance P	F, activates		n/a
		F, sensitizes		Capsaicin
	Endorphins	I	Opioids	
Fiber		**Transmission**		
	Na^+, K^+ exchange across the cellular membrane	F, of action potential to CNS		Mexiletine, Mexitil Tocainide, EMLA
Autonomic Nervous System		**Transduction**		
	Norepinephrine	F, sensitizes Nociceptive state F, activates Neuropathic state		Anxiolytics, relaxation
Spinal Cord		**Transmission**		
	Substance P, glutamate, others	F, to projection cell (second-order neuron)		Opioids
	NMDA	F, with windup		Ketamine
	Serotonin ($5HT_{1B}$ and $5HT_3$)	I	TCAs TCAs	
	Norepinephrine	I	TCAs, clonidine	
	Mu	I	Opioid agonists (e.g., morphine)	
	Delta	I	Opioid agonists	
	Kappa	I	Opioid antagonist-agonists	
	$GABA_A$	I	Baclophen	
	$GABA_B$	I	Benzodiazepines	
Brain	Substance P, glutamate, others	F, **transmission** to third- or fourth-order neuron		Opioids

ASA, aspirin; *CNS,* central nervous system; *EMLA,* eutectic mixture of local anesthetics; *K^+,* potassium; *n/a,* not available or not applicable; *Na^+,* sodium; *NSAIDs,* nonsteroidal antiinflammatory drugs; *PAN,* primary afferent nociceptor; *TCAs,* tricyclic antidepressant drugs or other reuptake inhibitor drugs.

primary neurotransmitter of the sympathetic nervous system, activates a PAN on contact, if the PAN has been injured.[13] Therefore emotional responses mediated by the ANS can increase pain through physiologic mechanisms.

Types of peripheral nerve fibers. Peripheral sensory nerves conduct either nonpainful or noxious (tissue-damaging, painful) signals to the spinal cord. The A-delta fibers and C fibers conduct noxious signals and are known as PANs.[12] These neurons, which project from the periphery to the spinal cord, are also known as first-order neurons. Many nociceptors do not respond to noxious stimuli until there is an inflammatory response in the surrounding tissue. These "silent" or "sleeping" nociceptors respond to both noxious and non-noxious signals when the tissue is inflamed.[13]

Different fibers have different characteristics (Table 9-2). A-alpha and A-beta fibers are large and enclosed by myelin

Table **9-2** Characteristics of Peripheral Nerve Fibers

Type of Fiber	Size	Myelinization	Conduction Velocity*
A-alpha	Large	Myelinated	Rapid
A-beta	Large	Myelinated	Rapid
A-delta	Small	Myelinated	Medium
C	Smallest	Not myelinated	Slow

*The conduction rates are important because information carried to the spinal cord by the more rapid nerve fibers will communicate with dorsal horn cells sooner than information carried by the slower fibers.

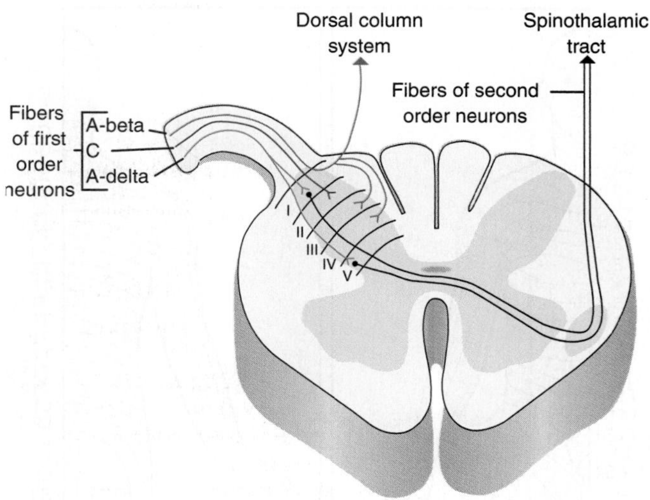

Fig. 9-3 Primary afferent neurons project to the dorsal horn (laminae I to V) of the spinal cord. These afferent fibers synapse on projection cells and interneurons.

sheaths, which allows them to conduct at a rapid rate. A-delta fibers are smaller fibers also with myelin sheaths. Because of their smaller size, A-delta fibers conduct at a slower rate than the larger A-alpha and A-beta fibers. C fibers, in comparison, are the smallest fibers and are unmyelinated. C fibers conduct at the slowest rate. The conduction rates are important because information carried to the spinal cord by the A-alpha and A-beta fibers will communicate with dorsal horn cells sooner than will information carried by A-delta or C fibers. This conduction rate has important implications for the modulation of noxious information from A-delta and C fibers, as will be discussed later.

Stimulation of different fibers results in different sensations. A-delta fiber pain is described as pricking, sharp, well localized, and short in duration. C fiber pain is described as dull, aching, burning sensations and is characterized by its diffuse nature, slow onset, and relatively long duration. The A-alpha (sensory muscle) and A-beta (sensory skin) fibers typically transmit nonpainful sensations such as light pressure to deep muscles, soft touch to skin, and vibration. All of these fibers extend through the dorsal root ganglia into the dorsal horn of the spinal cord where various connections are made (Fig. 9-3).

The A-beta fibers make connections (synapses) in the spinal dorsal horn close to synapses of the A-delta and C fibers (see Fig. 9-3). This dorsal horn connection means that input from touch fibers can enter the spinal cord and synapse or communicate with cells carrying nociceptive input, a fact important to nonpharmacologic management of pain, as will be discussed later.

Transmission. Once the PAN has been transduced, the neuronal action potential must be transmitted to and through the CNS before pain is perceived. Three steps are involved in nociceptive signal transmission: (1) projection to the CNS, (2) processing within the dorsal horn of the spinal cord, and (3) transmission to the brain (i.e., through the brainstem and the thalamus to the cortex). Each step in the transmission process is important in pain perception.

Projection to the central nervous system. When the PAN terminal is transduced, the PAN membrane becomes depolarized, sodium enters the cell, and potassium exits the cell to generate an action potential. The action potential rapidly spreads along the neuron, more rapidly for myelinated than unmyelinated axons. The transmission of the action potential along the entire length of the neuron is necessary for the cell to deliver the nociceptive signal to cells in the spinal cord.

The action potential can be inhibited, however, if the ion channels are inactivated. Drugs known as membrane stabilizers inactivate the sodium channels and disrupt the transmission of the action potential along the PAN axon.[14] Some adjuvant drugs, such as local anesthetics (e.g., lidocaine, bupivacaine, tocainide, mexiletine) and antiseizure drugs (e.g., phenytoin [Dilantin], carbamazepine [Tegretol], clonazepam [Klonopin]), prevent transmission via this type of mechanism. In diluted concentrations, local anesthetics are effective in blocking small fiber transmission without affecting nonpainful sensation or motor function. Larger concentrations of local anesthetics are required to block larger fibers.

It is important to understand that one nerve cell extends the entire distance from the periphery to the dorsal horn of the spinal cord with no synapses. For example, an afferent fiber from the great toe travels from the toe through the fifth lumbar nerve root into the spinal cord; it is one cell. Once generated, an action potential travels all the way to the spinal cord unless it is blocked by a sodium channel inhibitor or disrupted by a lesion at the central terminal of the fiber (e.g., by a dorsal root entry zone [DREZ] lesion). For this reason, therapies directed at altering the PAN environment and sensitivity of the PAN and thus preventing the initiation of the action potential are frequently used.

The A-alpha, A-beta, A-delta, and C fibers extend from the peripheral tissues through the dorsal root ganglia to the dorsal horn of the spinal cord (see Fig. 9-3). The manner in which nerve fibers enter the spinal cord is central to the notion of spinal dermatomes (Fig. 9-4). Each nerve root innervates a specific segment of the body, sometimes far removed from the area in which the nerve enters the spinal cord. Although fibers enter the spinal segment associated with the nerve root in which they travel to the spinal cord, the A-delta and C fibers send dendrites up toward the brain or downward for two to four spinal segments. Therefore one fiber can communicate with as many as nine spinal segments.

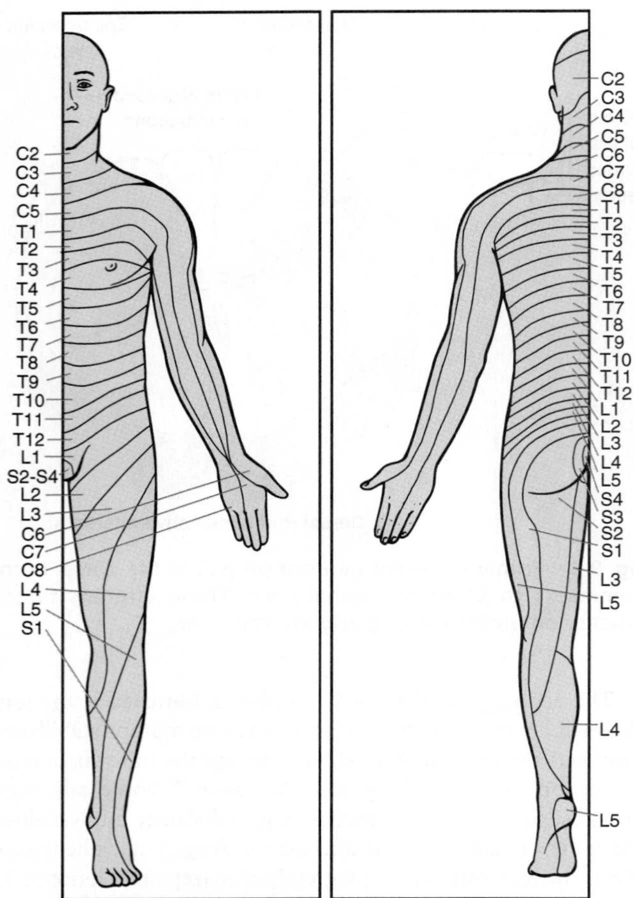

Fig. 9-4 Spinal dermatomes representing organized sensory input carried via specific spinal nerve roots. *C*, cervical; *L*, lumbar; *S*, sacral; *T*, thoracic.

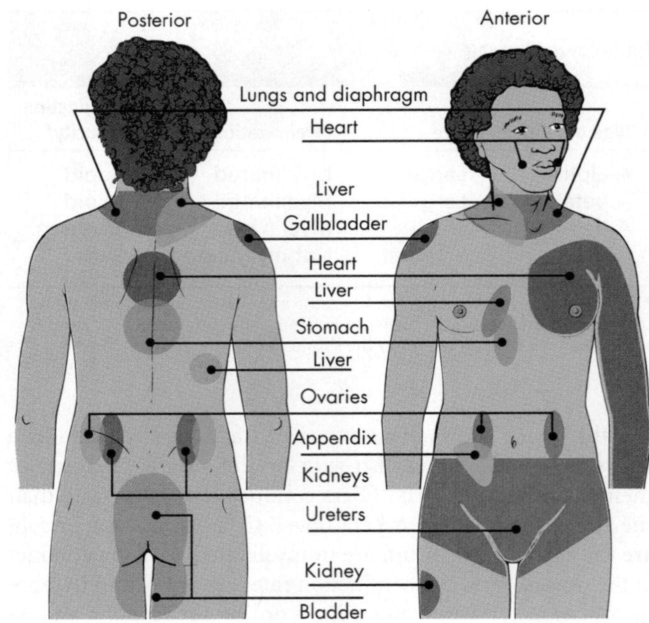

Fig. 9-5 Typical areas of referred pain.

Dorsal horn processing. Once the nociceptive signal arrives in the CNS, it is processed within the dorsal horn of the spinal cord. This processing includes releasing neurotransmitters from the PAN into the synaptic cleft. These neurotransmitters bind to receptors on nearby cell bodies and dendrites of cells that may be located elsewhere in the dorsal horn. Some of these PAN neurotransmitters produce activation whereas others inhibit activation of nearby cells. Cells excited by PAN input release other neurotransmitters. The effects of the complex neurotransmitter release can facilitate or inhibit transmission of nociceptive stimuli.[11]

Most projection cells send axons to the brain on the opposite side of the body. They receive excitatory and inhibitory messages, the net sum of which determines whether the PAN message will be transmitted to the brain. These projection neurons are also referred to as second-order neurons.

Interneurons can be either excitatory or inhibitory. The concept of excitatory and inhibitory interneurons is important because it helps explain why some nonpharmacologic therapies are effective. Although the exact mechanisms have not been determined, it is known that stimulation of large sensory fibers (A-beta) can have an inhibitory effect on cells that project nociceptive signals to the brain.

Wide dynamic range (WDR) neurons receive input from noxious stimuli primarily carried by A-delta and C fiber afferents (especially from viscera), non-noxious stimuli from A-beta fibers, and indirect input from dendritic projections.[13]

Discovery that WDR neurons receive input from noxious as well as innocuous stimuli from distant areas provides a neural explanation for referred pain. Inputs from nociceptive fibers and A-beta fibers converge on the WDR neuron, and, when the message is transmitted to the brain, the originating area of the body is poorly localized. Pain is therefore perceived in the body part presumably innervated by the A-beta fiber rather than from the visceral A-delta or C fibers. The concept of referred pain must be considered when interpreting the location of pain reported by the person with injury to or disease involving visceral organs. The location of a tumor may be distant from the pain location reported by the patient (Fig. 9-5). For example, pain from liver disease is located in the right upper abdominal quadrant, but it frequently is referred to the anterior and posterior neck region and to a posterior flank area. If referred pain is not considered when evaluating a pain location report, therapy could be misdirected.

N-methyl-d-aspartate (NMDA) and non-NMDA receptors have been implicated in dorsal horn processing.[12,15] The NMDA receptors produce alterations in neural processing of afferent stimuli that can persist for long periods of time. For this reason, an important goal of therapy is to prevent pain and avoid adverse neural plasticity. Although research is being conducted to develop NMDA antagonist drugs for clinical use, the only NMDA antagonist currently available is ketamine, a drug occasionally used in anesthesia.[12]

Pain Pathways

Transmission to the brain. With adequate summation (net excitatory effects) on projection cells, nociceptive stimuli are communicated to the third-order neuron, primarily in the thalamus and several other areas of the brain. Fibers of dorsal horn projection cells enter the brain through several pathways, including the spinothalamic tract (STT), spinoreticular tract

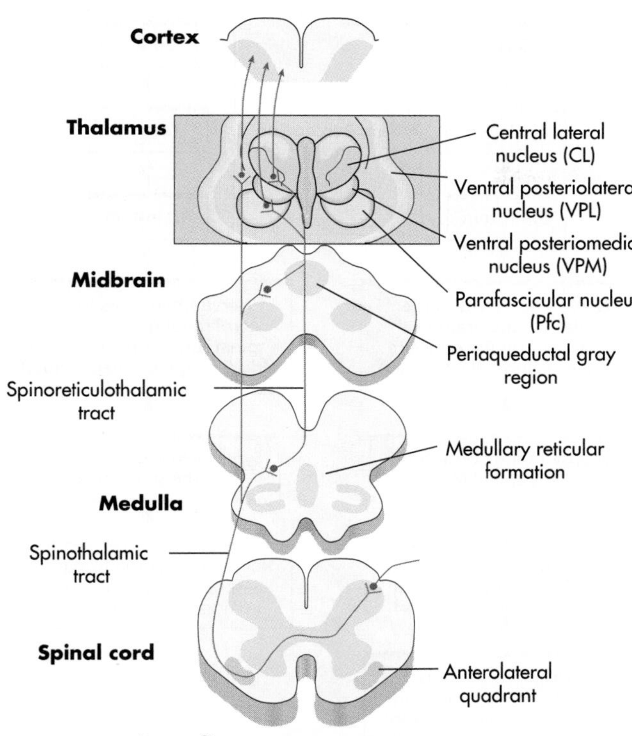

Fig. 9-6 Nociceptive pathways and synaptic connections of selected pain pathways.

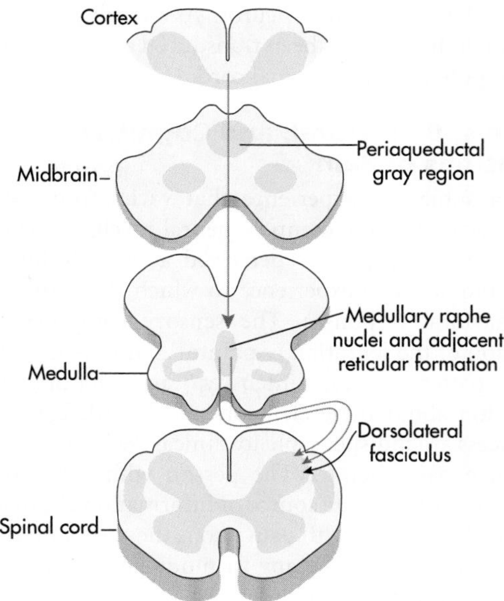

Fig. 9-7 Example of the descending pain-modulation system at receptors in the dorsal horn of the spinal cord.

(SRT), spinomesencephalic tract (SMT), spinocervical tract, second-order dorsal column tract (SDCT), and spinohypothalamic tract.[13] The nociceptive pathways and synaptic connections of each of these pathways are summarized in Fig. 9-6.

Distinct thalamic nuclei receive nociceptive input from the spinal cord and have projections to the cerebral cortex, the anterior cingulate cortex, or the insula (see Fig. 9-6). The primary somatosensory cortex responds selectively to nociceptive input. Recent studies with positron emission tomography (PET) imaging show that the somatosensory cortex is important for interpretation of pain location, pattern, and possibly intensity.[16] PET studies show the frontal cortex and especially the anterior cingulate cortex to be involved in affective components of pain. The insula has been shown to be involved in the suffering components of pain.[17]

Pain Perception. In the brain, nociceptive input is perceived as pain. There is no single, precise location where pain perception occurs. Instead, pain perception involves several brain structures.[16] It is known that the brain is necessary for pain perception; hence no brain, no pain. Until it is understood clearly where pain is perceived, prudent nursing practice involves treatment of any noxious stimulus as potentially painful, even in the comatose patient who does not appear to respond to noxious stimuli. Lack of a behavioral response to a noxious stimulus does *not* indicate that the person lacks pain perception. Therefore it is important for the nurse to provide pain therapies to the person receiving any nociceptive input, even though the person cannot report pain perception or show behaviors indicative of pain.

Modulation. Transmission of nociceptive stimuli and pain perception can be changed by descending (efferent) mechanisms (Fig. 9-7). Modulation may include both inhibition and facilitation of nociceptive signals.[18] Modulation of pain signals can occur at the peripheral, spinal cord, and brain levels.

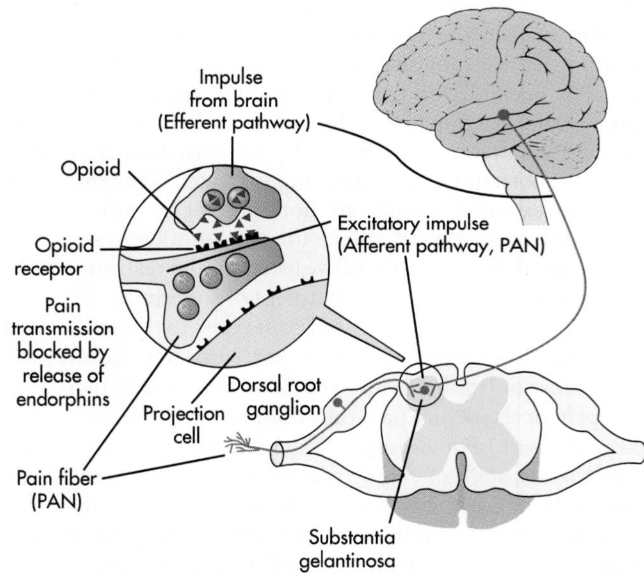

Fig. 9-8 Descending pathway and endorphin response. The biologic receptors of the enkephalins and endorphins are located close to pain receptors in the peripheral primary afferent nociceptor (PAN) and ascending and descending pain pathways.

Figure 9-8 provides a summary of the descending inhibitory mechanisms. Once nociceptive information is perceived as pain, inhibition can occur at any of the synapses in the ascending pathways. For example, neurotransmitters released by descending fibers in the spinal dorsal horn can keep the PAN from communicating its information about the nociceptive stimuli to the second-order neuron. As a result pain is blocked even though the PAN has been transduced and has transmitted an action potential to the spinal cord.

Affective, Behavioral, and Cognitive Dimensions of Pain

Pain is a subjective experience that varies from person to person. Because of the complex neural mechanisms of nociceptive processing, pain is perceived as a multidimensional sensory and affective experience to which there are cognitive and behavioral responses. The sensory component is the recognition of the sensation as painful. Sensory-pain elements include pattern, area, intensity, and nature (PAIN). Information about these elements and knowledge about the pain process are indispensable to clinical decisions that lead to appropriate pain therapy. The person with the pain is the expert and most accurate source of information about the pain sensation. The person with pain also is the expert on the effectiveness of prescribed therapy to modulate the pain process and block pain perception.

The affective component of pain refers to the feelings and emotions that affect the experience of pain. A patient with unrelieved pain often has concurrent emotional responses, such as anger, fear, depression, and anxiety, that can increase sympathetic nervous system release of norepinephrine and thereby intensify the pain sensation. In addition, simultaneous emotions such as joy may decrease the amount of pain perceived by persons with pain. Evaluation of emotions that activate or control sympathetic discharge can help determine the amount of suffering experienced by patients. This determination is important because suffering is treated differently than pain. For example, opioids are not effective for suffering but can be the treatment of choice for pain. Antidepressant and antianxiety drugs, as well as active listening and relaxation techniques, may be useful in the treatment of suffering.

The behavioral component of pain refers to the actions and posturing of a patient to express the pain or to control the pain. Pain control behaviors are those that reduce pain, prevent pain onset, reduce pain duration, and help the patient tolerate the pain. For example, watching television or talking with friends, staff, or family members helps distract patients from pain and can be effective in helping control pain.[19,20] How the patient complies with or adjusts analgesic therapy plans is also an important aspect of the patient's pain behavior. Pain may interfere with usual behaviors that bring the patient joy and satisfaction. Inability to perform activities because of pain has been associated with increased negative emotions, such as anxiety.[19]

The cognitive component of pain refers to the meanings, beliefs, attitudes, past experiences, and expectations about the illness (e.g., elective surgery) or disease (e.g., cancer) and about the pain that influence the patient's response to pain therapy. A patient's goal for and expectations about pain relief and treatment outcomes are crucial to understanding cognitive aspects of pain. Goals of treatment, however, must be realistic and attainable given the patient, health care providers, and environment. Determining the optimal goal (usually 0 pain) as well as the goal with which the patient will be satisfied (usually 1 to 4 on a scale of 0 to 10) helps evaluate progress toward pain relief. Level of consciousness (sedation level), dementia, memory of past pain, source of motivation (internal versus external locus of control), and cognitive resources to cope with the pain can dramatically influence the pain the person experiences.

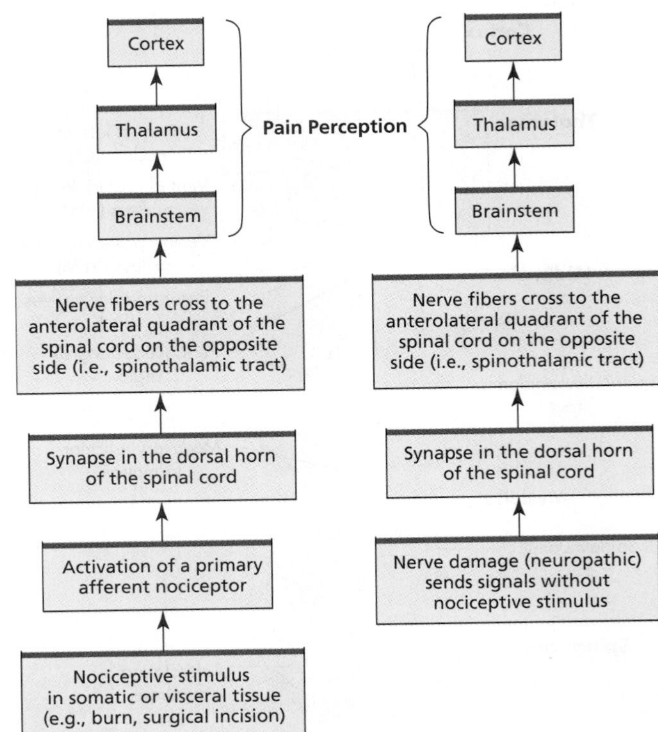

Fig. 9-9 Mechanisms of nociceptive and neuropathic pain.

Summary of Pain Process. The pain process includes neural mechanisms related to transduction, transmission, perception, and modulation (Fig. 9-9). These mechanisms represent complex, not fully understood systems, but they begin to explain the tremendous variability in pain reported by persons experiencing similar degrees of tissue damage. The idea for these mechanisms was previously described in 1965 by the gate control theory of pain, which emphasizes that the outcome of activation of nociceptive receptors is not totally predictable. The amount of pain perceived by a patient may vary tremendously depending on the context of the situation. The context of the situation may include other physiologic, sensory, affective, cognitive, or behavioral variables, the effects of which cannot be physiologically measured today.

ETIOLOGY AND TYPE OF PAIN

When a patient is experiencing pain, the cause of the pain should be sought so that it can be removed if possible. The nurse should observe for physical signs of the source of pain, including trauma, inflammation, ischemia, distention or perforation of a visceral organ, and muscle spasm. In many cases there may be a secondary pain source. For example, the postoperative patient may have, in addition to the surgical incision (involving somatic tissue), a distended bladder. Searching for the cause of pain is especially important with the onset of a new or recurrent episode of acute pain. It must be remembered that persons with chronic nonmalignant or cancer pain also may have related or unrelated acute pain. If

Table 9-3 Dangers of Unrelieved Acute Pain

Body System	Pathophysiologic Responses to Unrelieved Acute Pain	Complications
Respiratory	Reflex muscle spasms and muscle splinting leads to decreased tidal volume, vital capacity, functional residual capacity, and alveolar ventilation	Atelectasis and impaired oxygen and carbon dioxide exchange lead to hypoxemia and pneumonia
Cardiovascular	Sympathetic overactivity leads to increased heart rate, peripheral resistence, blood pressure, and cardiac output; decreased diastolic filling time; and coronary vasoconstriction	Increased cardiac work and myocardial oxygen use and decreased oxygen delivery to myocardium lead to increased risk of hypoxemia, myocardial ischemia, and myocardial infarction
Gastrointestinal	Increased sympathetic activity leads to increased intestinal secretions and smooth muscle sphincter tone and to decreased intestinal motility	Gastric stasis, paralytic ileus
Immune	Decreased natural killer cell number and function	Host resistance decreased, especially to cancer metastasis
Neurologic	Primary and secondary hyperalgesia with changes in primary afferent nociceptor responses at peripheral terminal and changes in the communication patterns of central nervous system cells	Neuropathic pain can occur and may persist for long periods of time after healing has occurred
Musculoskeletal	Muscle spasms increase pain leading to increased sympathetic activity, which increases sensitivity of nociceptors	Impaired muscle metabolism and muscle atrophy

Sources: Cousins M: Acute and postoperative pain. In Wall PD, Melzack, R, editors: *Textbook of pain,* ed 3, New York, 1994, Churchill Livingstone; Page GG, Ben Eliyahu S: The immune-suppressive nature of pain, *Semin Oncol Nurs* 13:10, 1997; and Willis WD, Westlund KN: Neuroanatomy of the pain system and of the pathways that modulate pain, *J Clin Neurophysiol* 14:2, 1997.

the etiology of the pain cannot be determined from physical signs or diagnostic tests, it is important that the patient's pain report not be dismissed. Pain should be assessed completely and treated.

Type of Pain

The etiology of the pain may dramatically influence the affective, behavioral, and cognitive responses, and therefore the pain experience. Patients can experience pain caused by acute, chronic nonmalignant, or malignant conditions. Causes can be grouped as two different types of pain: nociceptive and neuropathic. Nocicepetive pain is caused by damage to somatic or visceral tissue. Neuropathic pain is caused by damage to nerve cells or changes in spinal cord processing. Some causes of pain can be cured because the damage can be determined and repaired or healed. Other causes of pain cannot be cured, but the pain can be palliated, helping the patient to feel more comfortable.

Acute Pain. Acute nociceptive pain occurs abruptly after an injury or disease, persists until healing occurs, and often is intensified by anxiety or fear. Sprains, bone fractures, burns, sickle cell crisis, tension headaches, unstable angina, and incisions are examples of conditions causing acute nociceptive pain. Without pretreatment, acute pain increases during wound care, turning, ambulation, coughing, and deep breathing. If acute pain is not effectively managed, it may progress to acute neuropathic pain or a chronic nocioceptive pain.

Chronic Nonmalignant Pain. Chronic nonmalignant pain lasts for a prolonged period of time, and its cause is not amenable to specific treatment.[2] Chronic nociceptive pain is associated with prolonged tissue pathology or pain that persists beyond the normal healing period for an acute injury or disease. Stable angina, gout, bursitis, diverticulitis, gastritis, and pancreatitis are examples of conditions causing chronic nociceptive pain. Chronic neuropathic pain is associated with abnormalities in the peripheral nervous system or CNS that result in pain long after the original injury has healed. Low back pain, diabetic neuropathy, fibromyalgia, and phantom limb pain are examples of chronic neuropathic pain. Many times the abnormalities are not detectable with current diagnostic techniques. Depression, frustration, anger, and fear related to chronic pain are common.

Malignant Pain. Malignant pain often is a complex, progressive process. It can be acute, chronic, or both acute and chronic in nature. The causes of malignant pain are often resistant to cure. Arthritis and cancer are examples of diseases that produce malignant types of pain. Tumor involvement of a nerve root or plexus (e.g., brachial, sacral) is a common cause of malignant neuropathic pain. Malignant nociceptive pain is more responsive to palliative treatments than malignant neuropathic pain. All types of malignant pain may be described as intractable, but each can be relieved. The patient with unrelieved malignant pain often describes it as all-consuming and interfering with mood, family relationships, and quality of life.

Unrelieved pain from either a nociceptive or neuropathic process is potentially dangerous to a person's well-being. Unrelieved pain can result in many physical, psychologic, social, and economic consequences.[21] Some of the effects of unrelieved pain are listed in Table 9-3. An important nursing role is to recognize the life-threatening dangers of unrelieved pain; it is more than an annoying, unpleasant sensation. The nurse helps prevent the consequences of unrelieved pain by assessing the pain and using the information from the assessment to implement pain relief therapies.

ASSESSMENT OF PAIN

The goals of pain assessment are (1) to identify the etiology of the pain; (2) to understand the patient's sensory, affective, behavioral, and cognitive pain experience for the purpose of implementing pain management techniques; and (3) to identify the patient's goal for therapy and resources for self-management of the pain. Often it is the nurse who is responsible for gathering and documenting assessment data and for making collaborative decisions with the patient and other health care providers about pain management.

Pain Expert

The person with the pain, not health professionals, is the expert about the pattern, area, intensity, and nature of the pain, as well as the degree of pain relief obtained from therapy. A patient often does not recognize that health professionals cannot tell how much pain is experienced. The nurse must assist the patient to recognize his or her expertise about the pain and that, when the expertise is shared in partnership with health professionals, better pain management can be obtained. Empowering the patient to be an active partner in reporting information about the pain is an important nursing therapy. Persons from different racial or cultural backgrounds are consistent about the level of stimulus that is perceived as painful; pain threshold does not vary in persons.[22] The amount of pain that is tolerated (pain tolerance) by a person, however, varies widely among individuals, probably because of variability in pain modulation.[18]

Assessment Process

The nature of pain is efficiently assessed by a three-step process. The steps provide a method by which to triage the information collected based on the patient's condition and ability to tell the nurse about his or her pain.

Step One: Assessment of Sensory Component. The first step is to assess the sensory components of pain. The number of components essential to assessment varies by the nursing care setting. In critical situations such as in the emergency department or critical care unit, each patient should be questioned about pain location and intensity. Vital signs and gross body activities often are used to assess pain. However, changes in these indicators are difficult to attribute specifically to the pain or pain therapy because these indicators may be affected by other therapies used in critical situations. Vital signs used in isolation are unreliable indicators of the amount of pain experienced by a patient.[23] Abnormally high values may be an indicator of increased pain, but normal or low values may also be present when a patient has excruciating pain. *Pain reporting is the single best measure of pain* for the person able to communicate. Even critically ill patients can report the location and intensity of their pain.[24]

Sensory components of *every* pain assessment in noncritical situations should include pattern, area, intensity, and nature (PAIN) of the pain (Table 9-4). Each component is briefly discussed considering the type of pain and how the nurse uses the information to make clinical decisions about pain management.

Pattern of pain. Pain onset (when it starts) and duration (how long it lasts) are components of the pain pattern. Acute pain consistently increases during wound care, ambulation, coughing, and deep breathing. Acute pain associated with surgery or injury tends to diminish over time with recovery as tissues heal. Like chronic and cancer pain, acute pain often increases at night. A patient may have pain all the time (constant, around-the-clock pain), incident or procedural pain (pain with movement or specific procedures [e.g., lumbar punctures]), or breakthrough pain (pain that returns before the regularly scheduled analgesic dose). Pain pattern can be used to determine the appropriate dosing schedule and medication preparation (immediate release versus long acting). Return of pain before the end of analgesic duration of a drug suggests the need for an increased amount of drug or more frequent dosing intervals (dosing frequency). The nurse makes many decisions that can be guided by knowing the pattern of a patient's pain.

Table 9-4 Important Pain Qualifiers

Qualifier	Description
Pattern	How pain changes with time; its onset (when it starts) and its duration (how long it lasts)
Area	Place on the body where pain is felt
Intensity	Amount of pain felt
Nature	How the pain feels to the patient

Area of pain. For the person with acute pain, the area of pain draws attention to a new injury or process and may indicate damage to deep structures. A patient with chronic pain may be able to pinpoint a specific location. However, it is common for a patient with chronic pain to locate the pain in several areas. A patient with cancer pain also may have pain in multiple sites of the body, usually two to four sites, but up to 14 sites have been reported.[20] Pain area helps identify the site and spinal dermatome of an injury or a tumor. For example, back pain frequently is felt by the patient with cancer months before sensory or bladder dysfunction would indicate that tumor growth has caused compression of the spinal cord.

Intensity of pain. A new pathologic condition must be ruled out when there is a sudden increase in pain intensity. Pain treatment, however, should not be withheld pending comprehensive evaluation of the patient. The nurse should ask the question, "Will the differential diagnosis or medical treatment be altered if pain is obscured by pain therapy?" If not, there is no ethical reason not to provide pain treatment. It is also important to evaluate how intense the pain is when it is least (lowest intensity) and when it is worst (highest intensity). Wide variation in pain intensity and analgesic requirements may exist between patients despite similar tissue damage and type of injury, procedure, or disease process.

The intensity of chronic pain can range from 0 to 10, just like acute or cancer pain. Patients with pain may not use the term *pain* to refer to mild or small amounts of pain; they may save the word *pain* to refer to the strong or really intense sensation.[21] Level of pain intensity can be used to select appropriate analgesic medications and to increase dosages until pain is relieved. The nurse measures and documents pain intensity before and after each analgesic therapy. The nurse also uses this pain intensity level to guide the next nursing decision that he or she will make to help the patient obtain pain relief.

RESEARCH
IMPLICATIONS FOR NURSING PRACTICE

Differences in Patients' and Family Caregivers' Perceptions of Pain Experience

Citation Miaskowski C and others: Differences in patients' and family caregivers' perceptions of the pain experience influence patient and caregiver outcomes, *Pain* 72:217, 1997.

Purpose The first aim was to determine the congruence of pain intensity and duration scores between oncology outpatients and their family caregivers. The second aim was to determine whether the congruence or noncongruence of pain ratings between patient and caregiver were associated with differences in mood states, quality of life, and caregiver strain.

Methods Descriptive study using oncology patient-caregiver dyads (n = 78). Patients completed a Cancer Pain Questionnaire, the Profile of Mood States (POMS), and the Multidimensional Quality of Life Scale—Cancer 2. Caregivers completed the POMS, the Caregiver Strain Index, and the Medical Outcome Study Short-Form Health Survey. Both patients and family rated the patient's pain intensity with the Visual Analog Scale.

Results and Conclusions Patients in the noncongruent dyad had significantly greater mood disturbance and a poorer quality of life relative to patients in whom the ratings were congruent with that of their caregiver. Family caregivers in the noncongruent dyads reported greater caregiver strain compared with those in the congruent dyads. The results suggest that differences in perception of pain intensity between patients and their caregivers are associated with deleterious outcomes for the patient and caregiver.

Implications for Nursing Practice Family caregiver evaluation of the patient's pain may not be the most reliable source for determining pain intensity and duration. When the caregiver's perception of the patient's pain differs from the patient, lack of congruence affects both the patient and the caregiver.

Nature of pain. The nature of the pain is how the pain feels to the patient. Patients given lists of pain descriptors frequently use words such as aching, burning, gnawing, heavy, sharp, shooting, stabbing, tender, throbbing, exhausting, sickening, terrifying, tiring, intense, unbearable, nagging, tight, or torturing to describe how their pain feels. The nature of acute and chronic pain provides information regarding the type of the pain. For example, a burning, hypersensitive area or a sharp, shooting pain may indicate neuropathic pain from nerve damage. The nature and location both can be used to select adjuvant analgesic agents to help control pain. Some types of pain respond to treatment with certain drugs (i.e., burning pain often responds to tricyclic antidepressants; shooting pain often responds to phenytoin [Dilantin] or carbamazepine [Tegretol]).[7] The nurse helps the patient find the words describing the nature of the pain, documents the words for colleagues, and makes decisions about administration of therapies likely to be effective, based on the nature of the pain.

After the sensory components of pain have been assessed, it is important to provide therapy for the pain. If pain relief is not at the level expected following therapy, the second step of the assessment process should be undertaken.

Step Two: Comprehensive Assessment. The second step of the pain assessment is begun if the expected level of pain relief is not obtained by the patient (i.e., initial pain treatments do not provide the anticipated pain relief). The second step includes comprehensive assessment of pain difficult to manage in noncritical situations. In addition to the sensory components, a comprehensive pain assessment includes evaluation of the affective, behavioral, and cognitive aspects of pain.

Step Three: Follow-up Assessment. The third step of the pain assessment process is doing follow-up assessments. The nurse assesses the sensory components of pain (pattern, area, intensity, and nature) when initial care is provided to the patient. Pain intensity is reassessed at the analgesic action onset, peak, and duration time points until pain relief has been stabilized. Pain intensity values at onset indicate initiation of analgesic effect; at peak they determine maximum relief obtained; and at duration they reveal length of analgesic effect. The nurse can use these three pieces of information to show the physician the actual effect of the prescribed drug, dose, and interval. If the patient's pain is not relieved, the nurse uses these numbers to communicate with the physician regarding the need to alter the dose, interval, or drug.

The nurse also evaluates the patient's goals for pain relief, the pain at rest, with activity, and when painful procedures are performed (e.g., when wound care is provided). Also, assessment of the highest pain intensity, lowest pain intensity, and present pain intensity provides a perspective on how the pain fluctuates with time. Each new pain, particularly unexpected, intense pain, must be evaluated and reported promptly. Follow-up assessment of chronic nonmalignant pain and cancer should be conducted regularly to ensure that pain relief is continuous.

Measurement of Pain

A common belief is that pain can be assessed but not measured. Assessment has been defined as the act of determining the importance, size, or value of something. In contrast, measurement is the act or process of applying a metric to gauge something. Because pain is a subjective phenomenon, many health professionals believe that pain cannot be measured; it can only be assessed. Other subjective phenomena, however, are considered to be measurable. For example, vision is a subjective phenomenon, yet a metric can be applied to determine visual acuity (e.g., Snellen's chart) and ability to see color. The concept of measuring pain can be applied in a similar fashion by using valid and reliable metrics (tools) for components of the pain experience.

Many tools are available to measure the sensory components of pain (pattern, area, intensity, and nature). Fewer tools are available to measure the affective, behavioral, and cognitive pain components in clinical practice. Therefore nurses can *measure* pain pattern, area, intensity, and nature and *assess* affective, behavioral, and cognitive pain components.

There is no one best tool to measure sensory pain components, although some are easier to use than others. The nurse

Table 9-5 **Pain Pattern Descriptors from the McGill Pain Questionnaire**

How does your pain change with time? Circle the words you would use to describe the pattern of your pain.

1	2	3
Continuous	Rhythmic	Brief
Steady	Periodic	Momentary
Constant	Intermittent	Transient

From Melzack R: The McGill Pain Questionnaire: major properties and scoring methods, *Pain* 1:277, 1975.

should choose a tool and use it consistently. The patient and family need to understand the pain measurement tool that is used to ensure a valid measurement. If different pain tools are used by staff working throughout an organization (e.g., in home care or on an inpatient unit), the patient and family may have difficulty reporting pain to different professionals. Also colleagues may misinterpret pain information unless there is documentation about which tool has been used. If the agency does not have a specific pain assessment tool, the following are suggested because they have been tested for validity, reliability, and feasibility and include instructions for use.

Pain Pattern. Pain pattern is measured by the use of words listed in Table 9-5 to describe how the pain changes with time, activity, or other factors. The patient is asked to describe the pain as variations of a constant, intermittent, or transient pattern. The patient is also asked the date or time that the pain started and how long the pain lasts to measure the onset and duration of a painful episode.

Figure 9-10 shows another method for the patient to document the pattern of the pain. This method allows the patient to report how the intensity of the pain changes with time. A similar method could be used to document the changes in the area or nature of the pain.

Pain Area. The nurse can determine pain location by asking the patient to show all painful areas on a drawing of the body (Fig. 9-11). Another method is to ask the patient to point to the places where pain is felt, and the nurse can document those places on either a body outline or descriptively in the medical record and on the care plan. New pain sites should be reported, because they may signal complications.

Pain Intensity. Pain intensity can be measured using the numbers 0 through 10 as a scale to report the pain magnitude.[6,7] A patient may not intuitively know how to use numbers to measure pain. The script shown in Table 9-6 has been useful even with children as young as 8 years[25] and with elderly patients.[19] The use of a pain scale is also very effective in monitoring the effects of pain treatment.

The visual analog scale is a variation of the verbal scale. It usually consists of a straight line that represents a continuum of pain intensity. Verbal anchors—no pain to the worst pain possible—are placed at either end of the scale (Fig. 9-12). The length of the line may vary, but it is most commonly set at 4 inches (10 cm).

Verbal descriptors of pain intensity, such as the present pain intensity (PPI) scale from the McGill Pain Questionnaire, are commonly used by patients to describe the strength of their pain. These words mean different levels of pain to individual

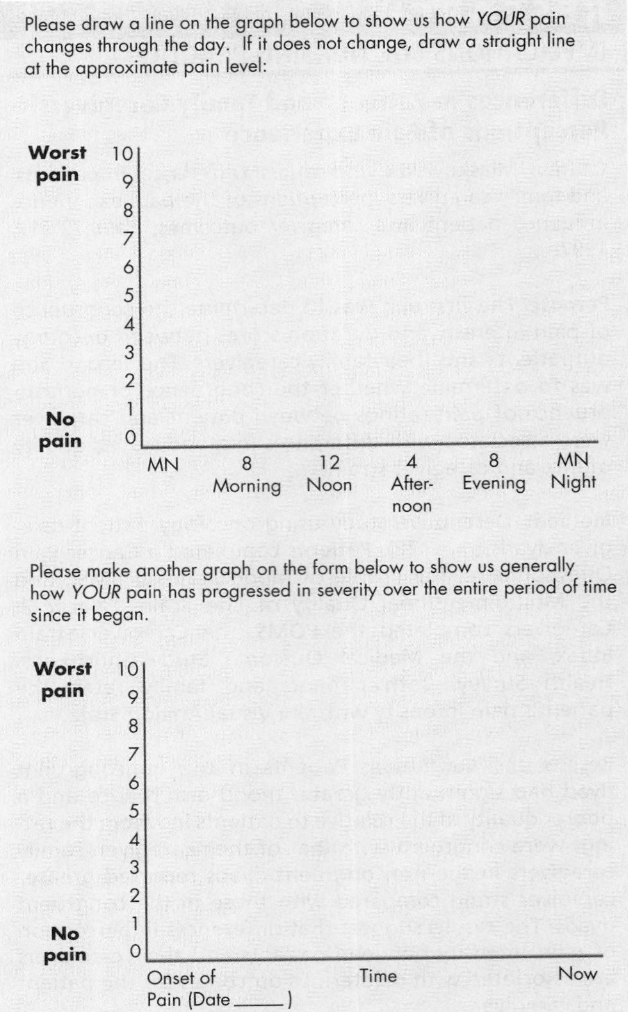

Fig. 9-10 A method for tracking pain over time.

patients.[26] The nurse may use these values to clarify the ambiguous language of pain intensity and better understand the level the patient is likely to be feeling when a particular word is used to describe the pain.

Pain intensity scales can also be used to help a patient identify a goal for pain therapy. The patient can be asked what amount of pain is desired (usually 0, a small number, or no pain) and what is acceptable (often a higher number than what is desired). This information is useful to both the patient and the nurse in planning and evaluating pain interventions.

Pain Nature. Pain quality is measured using a verbal descriptor list, such as the words listed in Table 9-7.[27] These words represent those most commonly used to describe the nature of pain and are derived from a more comprehensive list included in the McGill Pain Questionnaire.[28] The patient is asked to select the word or words that best describe the pain. If the patient has pain in more than one site, often several words per group will be selected, and the patient will indicate that some words describe one pain site and the other words describe another pain site. The number of the words selected are counted with a possible score of 0 to 19. Research indicates

Fig. 9-11 Body outline—a method of documenting pain location. The patient is instructed to place a mark on the figures to indicate all the currently painful places. The patient is also instructed to indicate where the pain is generally located.

Table 9-6 Standardized Instructions for Using the Pain Intensity Number Scale

"I need to know how much pain you have. Because I can't feel your pain, I want you to use a scale to let me know how much pain you have right now. The numbers between 0 and 10 represent *all* the pain a person could have. Zero means no pain and 10 means pain as bad as it could be. You can use *any* number between 0 and 10 to let me know how much pain you have right now. ***Call your pain** a number between 0 and 10 so I will know the intensity of the pain you feel now."

**Note:* Use the phrase "call your pain" rather than "rate your pain" because patients have difficulty knowing what is expected of them when asked to rate their pain. They easily "call" their pain a number.

that complex pain quality, as reflected by a higher score, is associated with increased patient attempts to engage in pain control behaviors.[19]

Documentation of Pain

Pain assessment information should be documented in a part of the medical record that is easy to access by all health care providers, such as on the bedside vital signs form.[29] Even the best pain measurement or assessment conducted by one nurse is of limited value, unless the information is shared with other nurses and health professionals responsible for the care of the patient with pain. Until standardized documentation forms are available in all health care institutions, the progress notes and flow sheets can be used to document pain measurement information. Usually blank sections on flow sheets can be modified to document the type of pain pattern words selected by the patient, the area and number of pain sites, intensity numbers, and number of pain nature words selected. Computerized tools for pain measurement are being developed with hopes of simplifying the process for the patient and health professionals.

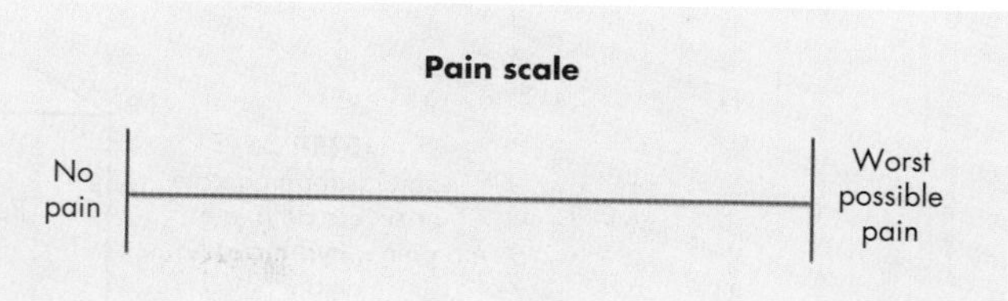

Fig. 9-12 Visual analog scale for measuring pain intensity.

Table 9-7 Pain Quality Descriptors Most Commonly Used to Describe the Nature of Pain

Some of the words below describe your *present* pain. Circle *only* those words that best describe it.

1	2
Throbbing	Tiring
Shooting	Exhausting
Stabbing	Sickening
Sharp	Terrifying
Gnawing	Torturing
Burning	3
Aching	Nagging
Tender	Annoying
Heavy	Intense
Tight	Unbearable

From Wilkie DJ and others: Use of the McGill Pain Questionnaire to measure pain: a meta-analysis, *Nurs Res* 39:36, 1990.

DRUG THERAPY FOR PAIN

Although a physician or an advanced nurse practitioner prescribes the drugs, it is usually the nurse's responsibility to evaluate the effectiveness and side effects of prescribed medications. It is also a nursing responsibility to communicate the effectiveness of the medication regimen to the prescriber and suggest changes when appropriate. As the nurse implements these roles, he or she applies knowledge and skill related to several pharmacologic concepts: calculating equianalgesic doses, scheduling analgesic doses, titrating opioids, and selecting from the prescribed analgesic drugs.

Equianalgesic Dose

The term *equianalgesic dose* refers to a dose of one analgesic that is equivalent in pain-relieving effects to another analgesic. This equivalence permits substitution of medications to relieve the pain and avoid possible adverse effects of one of the drugs. The tables describing step 1, 2, and 3 drugs have columns indicating the approximate equivalent analgesic dose of common drugs of each class (see Tables 9-8, 9-9, 9-10, and 9-11 later in this chapter). The nurse uses standard drug calculation formulas to determine the equianalgesic dose needed by a patient when the drug or route is changed.

Scheduling Analgesic Doses

A preventive approach to pain is crucial. A patient should be medicated before painful procedures and activities that can be expected to produce pain. If these procedures or activities are planned so that they occur when the patient's analgesic has reached its peak effectiveness, the pain will be decreased and

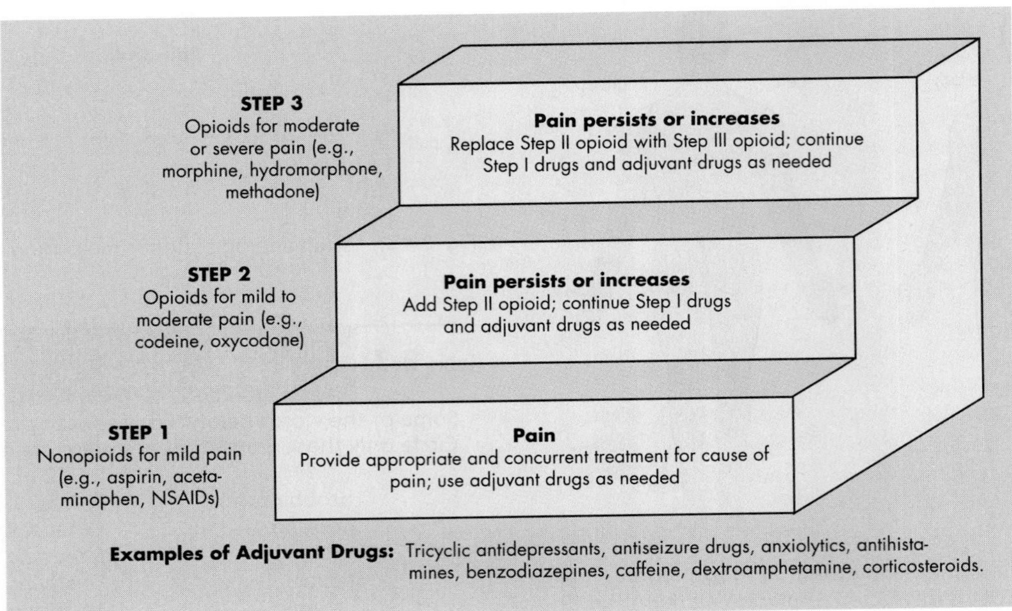
STEP 3
Opioids for moderate or severe pain (e.g., morphine, hydromorphone, methadone)
Pain persists or increases
Replace Step II opioid with Step III opioid; continue Step I drugs and adjuvant drugs as needed
STEP 2
Opioids for mild to moderate pain (e.g., codeine, oxycodone)
Pain persists or increases
Add Step II opioid; continue Step I drugs and adjuvant drugs as needed
STEP 1
Nonopioids for mild pain (e.g., aspirin, acetaminophen, NSAIDs)
Pain
Provide appropriate and concurrent treatment for cause of pain; use adjuvant drugs as needed
Examples of Adjuvant Drugs: Tricyclic antidepressants, antiseizure drugs, anxiolytics, antihistamines, benzodiazepines, caffeine, dextroamphetamine, corticosteroids.

Fig. 9-13 The analgesic ladder proposed by the World Health Organization. *NSAIDs,* nonsteroidal antiinflammatory drugs (e.g., ibuprofen, naproxen, ketorolac).

the patient's ability to participate will be increased. Moreover, if the patient is medicated before the pain begins to increase rather than once it has become severe, far less medication is required. The patient and the family should be taught when to ask for pain medication. Administration may also be time-controlled, with the medication given on a set schedule regardless of the presence or absence of pain. Analgesic doses scheduled around the clock are particularly helpful if the patient has constant pain.

Titration of Opioids

One of the most important aspects of pain management is to titrate the analgesic dose to effect. *Analgesic titration* is dose adjustment based on decision making about the adequacy of analgesic effect versus the side effects produced. For example, a patient at home titrates to effect when following a prescription, such as Percodan 1 to 2 tablets every 3 to 4 hours as needed. The patient evaluates how much pain relief was obtained 3 hours after 1 tablet was taken. If the patient continues to have good pain relief, he or she would not take another Percodan. If very little pain relief was obtained, the patient would decide to take 2 tablets and after an additional 3 hours evaluate if more tablets should be taken at that time or at 4 hours. A patient with constant pain relieved by 2 tablets for 4 hours could effectively manage the pain by scheduling the Percodan to be taken every 4 hours around the clock.

The nurse often assists the patient to make decisions about titrating analgesics. Titration requires pain assessment to evaluate the desired effect of the analgesic and the side effects produced by the analgesic. There is no set amount of an opioid that will produce pain relief for every patient; the right dose is the dose that works and helps the patient achieve the pain intensity goal. Morphine 0.05 to 0.1 mg/kg IV every 2 hours can be used as a formula to determine the size of the dose to begin titration.[6,7] Skillful titration results in the optimal dose of an analgesic being given and helps the nurse identify conditions when additional or alternative drugs might be helpful. Consultation with the physician provides the patient with the appropriate prescription to effectively continue dose titration.

The dose required to relieve a person's pain can vary tremendously. Differences in pain levels, drug metabolism, drug interactions, and other responses to specific drugs can affect the dose needed to relieve pain. Larger doses may be required if the pain is out of control. The person with a smoking history may require larger doses of morphine, meperidine, pentazocine, and propoxyphene to obtain pain control.[30] Genetic factors can also affect analgesic responses. The nurse plays an important role in recognizing the variable responses to pain medications by titrating the analgesic drug to the dose that relieves the patient's pain.

Selecting Analgesics

Several national and international groups have published practice guidelines recommending a systematic plan for using analgesic medications.[6,7,9,10] The analgesic ladder proposed by the World Health Organization (WHO) is shown in Fig. 9-13. The systematic plan calls for concurrent treatment of the cause of the pain when possible and use of a three-step ladder approach. If pain persists or increases, drugs from the next higher step are used to control the pain. For chronic nonmalignant pain and cancer pain, drug use is recommended from the bottom of the ladder to the top (i.e., up the ladder from step 1 to step 2 to step 3). For acute pain, the steps can be reversed in order from the top step to the bottom step (i.e., down the ladder from step 3 to step 2 to step 1) as recovery occurs and pain decreases. The WHO, the American Pain Society, and the United States Agency for Health Care Research all have supported this plan.[7,9,10]

Analgesic Ladder

Step 1 Drugs. When pain is mild (1 to 3 on a scale of 0 to 10), step 1 nonopioid drugs, aspirin and other salicylates,

DRUG THERAPY

Table 9-8 Step 1 Analgesics: Pharmacokinetics

Generic Drug (Trade Drug)	Typical Dose (Maximum Dose)	Approximate Equivalent	Onset Effect (min)	Peak Effect (min)	Duration Effect (hr)
▪ Acetaminophen (Tylenol, Tempra, others)	600 mg PO 600 mg PR (4000-6000 mg/day)	Aspirin 600 mg	30	60	3-4
▪ Acetylsalicylic acid (aspirin)	600 mg PO 600 mg PR (5200 mg/day)	Morphine 2 mg IM	30	60	3-4
▪ Ibuprophen (Motrin, Advil, others)	200 mg PO (3200 mg/day)	Aspirin 650 mg	30	60-120	4
▪ Choline magnesium trisalicylate (Trilisate)	2000-3000 mg PO (3000 mg/day)		5-30	60-180	3-6
▪ Diflunisal (Dolobid)	500 mg PO (1500 mg/day)	Aspirin 650 mg	60	120-180	8-12
▪ Ketoprofen (Orudis)	25 mg PO (300 mg/day)	Aspirin 650 mg	30	30-120	6
▪ Naproxen (Naprosyn)	250 mg PO (1250 mg/day)	Aspirin 650 mg	60	120-240	6-8
▪ Ketorolac (Toradol)	30-60 mg IM initially (120 mg IM/day × 5 day, max 30 mg IM × 20 doses over 5 days)	Morphine 6-12 mg IM	10	60	3-6
▪ Piroxicam (Feldene)	20 mg/day		60	180-300	>12
▪ Sulindac (Clinoril)	200 mg/day		1-2 days	60-120	Unknown
▪ Indomethacin (Indocin)	25 mg PO (100 mg/day)	Aspirin 650 mg	60	60-120	4
▪ Nabumetone (Relafen)	1000 mg PO (2000 mg/day)	Aspirin 3600 mg/day	1-2 days	Days-2 wk	Unknown
▪ Etodolac (Lodine)	200-400 mg PO (1200 mg/day)	Aspirin 650 mg	30	60-120	4-12

IM, intramuscular; *IV,* intravenous; *PO,* oral; *PR,* rectal.

other nonsteroidal antiinflammatory drugs (NSAIDs), and acetaminophen are used with or without adjuvant drugs to control the pain. Step 1 drugs can be very effective for pain; they provide adequate analgesia until death for nearly one third of patients with mild to moderate cancer pain. Aspirin-like drugs and NSAIDs provide analgesia by blocking prostaglandin synthesis. Acetaminophen (Tylenol) does not block this synthesis but instead produces pain relief through central mechanisms that are not clearly understood. Pharmacokinetic properties of common step 1 drugs are listed in Table 9-8.

A number of nonopioid analgesics (e.g., acetylsalicylic acid, NSAIDs) inhibit the chemicals that activate the PAN as shown in Fig. 9-14. Thus when these agents are used the PAN is transduced less often or a larger stimulus is needed to produce transduction.

Many of these drugs are available over the counter (OTC) without prescription. The patient can use these drugs without any type of medical supervision. Although effective for alleviation of mild pain, OTCs can cause serious problems related to drug interactions, side effects, and overdose.[31]

Adjuvant drugs have been shown to provide analgesia but traditionally have not been used as analgesics. Adjuvant drugs act in many different ways. Some actions are central and some are peripheral, but adjuvant drugs work differently than acetaminophen, aspirin, NSAIDs, or opioids. Therefore it is a rational approach to combine selected adjuvants (e.g., tricyclic

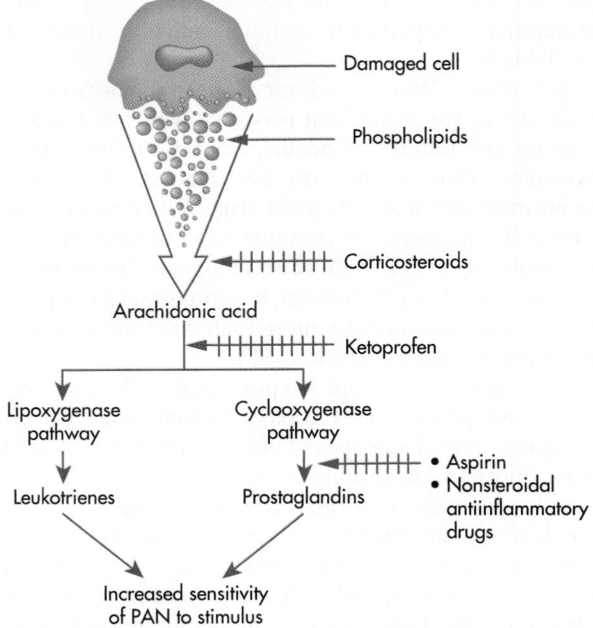

Fig. 9-14 Schematic representation of two pathways that lead to the production of chemicals that cause the peripheral afferent nociceptors (PAN) to be more easily excited. Drugs that block the synthesis of these chemicals are also shown.

DRUG THERAPY

Table 9-9 Step 1 Adjuvant Drugs: Pharmacokinetics

Generic Drug (Trade Drug)	Approximate Daily Dose	Onset Effect	Peak Effect	Duration Effect (hr)
▪ Carbamazepine (Tegretol, Epitol)	200-1600 mg PO	8-72 hr	2-12	Unknown
▪ Phenytoin (Dilantin)	300-500 mg PO	2-24 hr	1.5-3	6-12
▪ Gabapentin (Neurontin)	900-1800 mg PO	60-120 min	2-4 hr	Up to 24 hr
▪ Sumatriptan (Imitrex)	6-12 mg SC	30 min	Up to 2 hr	Up to 24 hr
▪ Amitriptyline (Elavil and others)	10-150 mg PO	3-4 days	1-2 wk	Days-weeks
▪ Doxepin (Sinequan, Adapin)	25-150 mg PO	3-4 days	1-2 wk	Days-weeks
▪ Imipramine (Tofranil and others)	20-100 mg PO	60 min	2-6 wk	Weeks
▪ Trazodone (Desyrel and others)	75-225 mg PO	2 wk	2-4 wk	Weeks
▪ Paroxetine (Paxil)	20-50 mg PO	3-4 days	1-2 wk	Days-weeks
▪ Hydroxyzine (Vistaril, Atarax, and others)	300-450 mg IM	15-30 min	2-4 hr	4-6 hr
▪ Lidocaine	5 mg/kg IV	2 min	2 min	10-20 min
▪ Mexiletine (Mexitil)	200-400 mg PO	30-120 min	2-3 hr	8-12 hr
▪ Dexamethasone (Decadron and others)	16-96 mg PO/IV	2-4 days	1-2 hr	2.75 days
▪ Dextroamphetamine (Dexedrine and others)	10-15 mg PO	1-2 hr	Unknown	2-10 hr
▪ Methylphenidate (Methidate, Ritalin)	10-15 mg PO	Unknown	1-3 hr	4-6 hr
▪ Nefazodone (Serzone)	200-600 mg PO	3-4 days	1-2 wk	Days-weeks

antidepressants and anxiolytics) with step 1 drugs and continue the adjuvants when moving to step 2 or step 3 drugs. Generally, adjuvants are more effective as analgesics for neuropathic rather than nociceptive types of pain. Pharmacokinetic properties of common adjuvant drugs are listed in Table 9-9.

Step 2 Drugs. When pain is moderate in intensity (4 to 6 on a scale of 0 to 10) or mild but persistent with step 1 drugs, step 2 drugs are indicated. Codeine, oxycodone (Percodan), propoxyphene (Darvon), pentazocine (Talwin), and hydrocodone are examples of step 2 opioid drugs. When progressing up to step 2, it is important to continue step 1 drugs, including the adjuvants. If drugs with acetaminophen (Percocet or Vicodin) are used at step 2, however, it is important to stop the step 1 acetaminophen because more than 4000 mg of acetaminophen per day can be toxic to the liver.

Step 2 drugs bind to opioid receptors in the CNS and perhaps on the peripheral nerves to block transmission of nociceptive signals. Several subtypes of opioid receptors are found in differing proportions throughout the nervous system. Mu, delta, and kappa receptors are associated with analgesia.[32]

Opioids mimic the descending inhibitory system by binding to endogenous endorphin receptors (mu, delta, kappa) in the brain, brainstem, spinal cord, and peripheral tissues. Opioids act by hyperpolarizing the cell membrane and thereby inhibiting generation of an action potential. Opioids effectively inhibit A-delta and C fibers, but are less effective in states of NMDA receptor activation. Administered intrathecally in small volumes, opioids exert powerful analgesic action at spinal cord synapses with limited rostral spread. In contrast, opioids delivered by the epidural route exert action not only at spinal cord sites, but also brain sites, because a substantial portion of the dose is absorbed by epidural blood vessels. Opioids administered systemically (oral, transdermal, rectal, vaginal, subcutaneous, intramuscular, or intravenous) cross the blood-brain barrier, enter the cerebrospinal fluid, and bind to opioid receptors throughout the brain and the spinal cord. Systemic opioids can also bind to opioid receptors on peripheral nerves. Opioids have shown powerful analgesic effects when bound to peripheral receptors in inflamed tissues but not in uninjured tissue.[33]

Some opioids bind to receptors and produce an effect at some but not all of the receptors. Agonist opioids, such as oxycodone and hydrocodone, are believed to bind to mu, delta, and kappa receptors and produce effects at each receptor. Agonists fit into a receptor site, "turn on" the site, and the drug effect occurs. Agonist-antagonist opioids, such as pentazocine, bind to mu and kappa receptors and produce an effect at the kappa receptor (agonist) but block the drug's effect at the mu receptors (antagonist). Partial agonist drugs bind to opioid receptors but produce a submaximal bodily response.

A drug acting as an antagonist binds to a receptor site without activating it. This binding blocks other drugs or neurotransmitters from activating the site. An antagonist can also dislodge an agonist from its receptor site, counteracting the agonist's effects. Naloxone is an example of an opioid antagonist (Fig. 9-15).

Drugs classified as agonist-antagonists or partial agonists have an analgesic ceiling (larger doses do not produce greater

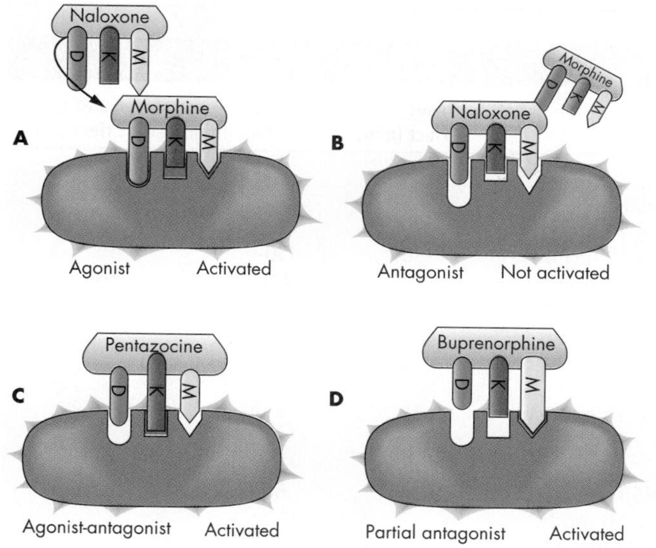

Fig. 9-15 Opioid receptor subtypes. **A,** Agonist action. **B,** Antagonist action. **C,** Agonist-antagonist action. **D,** Partial agonist action. *M,* mu receptor; *K,* kappa receptor; *D,* delta receptor.

analgesic effects) and can produce a withdrawal syndrome if used in a patient physically dependent on agonist drugs. In contrast, agonist drugs do not have an analgesic ceiling. Doses of agonist drugs can be titrated as high as needed to relieve pain. Table 9-10 lists the classifications of commonly prescribed step 2 opioid drugs.

Step 3 Drugs. Step 3 drugs are recommended for moderate to severe pain (7 to 10 on a scale of 0 to 10) or when step 2 drugs do not produce effective pain relief. Step 3 drugs include opioid drugs, such as morphine, hydromorphone, and methadone. Meperidine (Demerol) could be considered a step 3 opioid, but the high incidence of neurotoxicity (e.g., seizures) associated with its metabolite, normeperidine, limits its use. Use of meperidine is contraindicated for more than 2 days or in large doses (more than 600 mg per 24 hours).[10] Step 3 drugs produce a desired effect—analgesia—by binding to opioid receptors in the CNS and in the peripheral nervous system if tissues are inflamed. Pharmacokinetic properties of step 3 opioids are listed in Table 9-11.

Recommended Drug and Route

Morphine has been recommended as the drug of choice for the patient with pain and oral administration as the route of choice for the person with a functioning GI system.[6,7,9,10] Intramuscular (IM) opioid administration produces pain on injection and unreliable pain relief because of variable drug absorption. Other administration routes for opioid drugs, such as epidural, intrathecal, transdermal, and transmucosal, have been developed, but achieving pain relief by these routes is generally more expensive than by the oral route. In cancer pain management, federal guidelines recommend that these routes be used only when oral administration is not possible.[7]

Morphine is a very effective drug; however, recent evidence raises questions about its use as the drug of choice when high doses are needed and for use in the patient with compromised renal function.[34] Levorphanol, oxycodone, methadone, and fentanyl are examples of alternative opioids that may be used by the person with compromised renal function.[35]

Adjuvant Therapy. Tricyclic antidepressants, which appear to enhance the descending inhibitory system by preventing the cellular reuptake of serotonin and norepinephrine, are classified as adjuvant analgesics according to the WHO analgesic ladder (see Fig. 9-13). These neurotransmitters typically are released from the cell and are rapidly taken back up by the cell and stored for rerelease. Rapid reuptake limits the time serotonin and norepinephrine are available for receptor binding and inhibits transmission of nociceptive signals in the CNS.

Alpha$_2$-adrenergic agonists (e.g., clonidine [Catapres]), calcitonin, somatostatin, and baclofen are other agents known to provide analgesia. The exact location where these agents act is known for some drugs but not others. Although not specifically mentioned by the WHO, these agents could be classified as adjuvant drugs. Figure 9-16 shows the sites of actions of pharmacologic and nonpharmacologic therapies for pain.

Administration Routes

Oral. Many opioids are available in oral preparations, such as liquid and tablet formulations. Equianalgesic doses for oral opioids are larger than for doses administered IM or IV (see Table 9-11). The reason larger doses are required is related to the first-pass effect of hepatic metabolism. This means that oral opioids are absorbed from the GI tract into the portal circulation and shunted to the liver. Partial metabolism in the liver occurs before the drug enters systemic circulation and becomes available to peripheral receptors or to cross the blood-brain barrier and access CNS opioid receptors, which is necessary to produce analgesia. Oral opioids are as effective as parenteral opioids if the dose administered is sufficiently large to compensate for the first-pass metabolism.

Transmucosal: sublingual. Opioids administered under the tongue and absorbed into systemic circulation are exempt from the first-pass effect. Although morphine is commonly administered to persons with cancer pain via the sublingual route, little of the drug is absorbed from the sublingual tissue.[36] Most probably, morphine administered sublingually is dissolved in saliva and swallowed, making its metabolism similar to oral morphine. In contrast, fentanyl and buprenorphine are readily absorbed from the sublingual tissue. A fentanyl preparation is available as a premedication before surgery and for use in monitored anesthesia care and in management of breakthrough cancer pain.[37] Sublingual delivery systems for buprenorphine are under investigation.

Transmucosal: transnasal. When the patient is not able to tolerate oral opioids, the transnasal route may be an alternative delivery method that allows rapid absorption by the nasal mucosal blood vessels. Currently, butorphanol (Stadol) is the only transnasal opioid commercially available in the United States; it is not available in Canada. Several transnasal opioid agents are being investigated. Butorphanol is classified as an agonist-antagonist, which limits its use in patients dependent on agonist opioids. This drug is indicated for acute headache and other intense, recurrent types of pain.

Transmucosal: rectal. The rectal route is often overlooked but is particularly useful when the patient cannot take an analgesic by mouth. Rectal suppositories that are effective for pain

DRUG THERAPY

Table 9-10 Step 2 Analgesics: Pharmacokinetics

Generic Drug (Trade Drug)	Typical Dose (Maximum Dose)	Approximate Equivalent	Onset Effect (min)	Peak Effect (min)	Duration Effect (hr)
Step 2 Opioid-Agonist Drugs					
▪ Codeine	30-60 mg PO (200 mg PO)	Aspirin 650 mg Morphine 10 mg IM	30-45	20-120	4
Immediate release	15-60 mg IM	Morphine 10 mg IM	10-30	30-60	4
▪ Oxycodone (Roxicodone, w/aspirin—Percodan, w/acetaminophen—Percocet)	5 mg PO (30 mg PO)	Codeine 60 mg PO Morphine 10 mg IM	10-15	60	3-4
▪ Hydrocodone (Vicodin, Lortab, Lorcet, and others)	5 mg PO (30 mg PO)	Morphine 10 mg IM	10-30	3-60	4-6
▪ Meperidine (Demerol, Pethidine)	50 mg PO (300 mg PO)	Aspirin 650 mg Morphine 10 mg IM Demerol 75 mg IM	15	60-90	2-4
	75 mg IM	Morphine 10 mg IM	10-15	30-60	2-4
	50 mg IV	Morphine 10 mg IM	1	5-7	2-3
▪ Propoxyphene HCl (Darvon, Dolene);	65 mg PO	Aspirin 600 mg	15-60	120	4-6
▪ Propoxyphene napsylate (w/aspirin—Darvon-N, w/acetaminophen—Darvocet-N)	100 mg PO	Aspirin 600 mg			
▪ Tramadol (Ultram)	50-100 mg	Codeine 60 mg PO	60	2 hr	4-6
Step 2 Agonist-Antagonist Drugs					
▪ Pentazocine HCl (Talwin)	60 mg IM	Morphine 10 mg IM	15-20	30-60	2-3
	30 mg PO (180 mg PO)	Aspirin 600 mg Morphine 10 mg IM or Talwin 60 mg IM	15-30	60-90	3

relief include hydromorphone (Dilaudid), oxymorphone (Numorphan), and morphine.

Transdermal. Fentanyl also is available as a transdermal patch system for application to nonhairy skin. This delivery system is useful for the patient who cannot tolerate oral analgesic medications. Absorption from the patch is slow. Therefore transdermal fentanyl is not suitable for rapid dose titration but can be effective if the patient's pain is stable and the dose required to control it is known. Patches may need to be changed every 48 hours rather than the recommended 72 hours based on individual patient responses.[38]

Currently, creams and lotions containing 10% trolamine salicylate (Aspercreme, Myoflex cream) are available. These agents have been recommended by the manufacturers for joint and muscle pain. The aspirin-like substance is absorbed locally. This route of administration avoids gastric irritation, but the other side effects of high-dose salicylate are not necessarily prevented.

Ointments, lotions, gels, liniments, and balms (most of which are OTC products), are sometimes applied to the skin to achieve pain relief. Although these agents contain various substances, two common ingredients are menthol and methyl salicylate (wintergreen oil). The salicylate component is absorbed from the skin. On application, these agents usually produce a strong hot or cold sensation and should not be used after massage or a heat treatment when blood vessels are already dilated. Skin testing is advisable when the patient has not used the particular agent before, because the strengths of the agents vary and different intensities of sensation are produced. Relief of pain is reported for muscle pain, joint pain, headache, and visceral pain associated with gas, distention, and endometriosis.

Other topical analgesic agents, such as capsaicin (Zostrix), and local anesthetic agents, such as lidocaine and prilocaine (EMLA), also provide analgesia. Capsaicin has been useful in controlling pain associated with postherpetic neuralgia, diabetic neuropathy, and arthritis. EMLA is useful for control of pain associated with venipunctures, ulcer debridement, and postherpetic neuralgia. The area to which EMLA is applied should be covered with a plastic wrap for 30 to 60 minutes before beginning a painful procedure.

Infusions

Subcutaneous, intravenous, epidural, and intrathecal routes. These routes are used for administration of continuous infusions of analgesic medications. A continuous infusion technique provides a relatively stable plasma or cerebrospinal fluid (CSF) concentration. The portion of the total analgesic requirement administered as a continuous infusion depends on the patient's situation. It is important to provide a loading dose (a dose that provides comfort) before starting a continuous infusion. This loading is accomplished by giving a bolus equivalent to the hourly dose of the medication to be used in the con-

DRUG THERAPY

Table 9-11 **Step 3 Analgesics: Pharmacokinetics**

Generic Drug (Trade Drug)	Typical Dose	Approximate Equivalent	Onset Effect (min)	Peak Effect (min)	Duration Effect (hr)
Step 3 Agonist Drugs					
■ Morphine sulfate	30 mg PO	Morphine 10 mg IM	20-60	120	4-5
Immediate release tablets and liquids	30 mg PR	Morphine 10 mg IM			
Sustained release (MS Contin, Oramorph SR)	30 mg PO	Morphine 10 mg IM	-	210	8-12
Injectable (Astramorph PF, Duramorph, Infumorph)	10 mg IM	Morphine 10 mg IM	10-30	60	4-5
	5 mg IV	Morphine 10 mg IM	5	20	2-4
■ Oxycodone					
Immediate release (Roxicodone)	5 mg PO	Codeine 60 mg PO	0-15	60	3-4
	30 mg PO	Morphine 10 mg IM			
		Morphine 30 mg PO			
Controlled release (OxyContin)	30 mg PO	Morphine 30-60 mg PO	30-60	60, 420	12
■ Methadone (Dolphine)	20 mg PO	Morphine 10 mg IM	30-60	90-120	4-6
		Methadone 10 mg IM			
	10 mg IM	Morphine 10 mg IM	10-20	60-120	4-5
	5 mg IV	Morphine 10 mg IM	5	15-30	3-4
■ Hydromorphone	7.5 mg PO	Morphine 10 mg IM	30	90-120	4
(Dilaudid)	3 mg PR	Hydromorphone 1.5 mg IM	15-30	30-90	4-5
	1.5 mg IM	Morphine 10 mg IM	15	30-60	4-5
	1 mg IV	Morphine 10 mg IM	10-15	15-30	2-3
■ Oxymorphone	1 mg IM	Morphine 10 mg IM	10-15	30-90	3-6
(Numorphan)	0.5 mg IV	Morphine 10 mg IM	5-10	15-30	3-4
	10 mg PR	Oxymorphone 1 mg IM	15-30	60	3-6
■ Levorphanol	4 mg PO	Morphine 10 mg IM	10-60	90-120	4-5
(Levo-Dromoran)		Levorphanol 2 mg IM		60	4-5
	2 mg IM	Morphine 10 mg IM	10-15	15	3-4
	1 mg IV	Morphine 10 mg IM			
■ Fentanyl	0.1 mg IM	Morphine 10 mg IM	7-15	20-30	1-2
(Sublimaze, Duragesic)	25-50 μg/hr transdermal	Morphine 30 mg sustained-release q8hr	6 hr	12-24 hr	72
Step 3 Agonist-Antagonist Drugs					
■ Butorphanol (Stadol); see pentazocine	2 mg IM	Morphine 10 mg IM	10-30	30-60	3-4
	2 mg IV	Morphine 10 mg IM	2-3	30	2-4
■ Nalbuphine (Nubain); see pentazocine	10 mg IM	Morphine 10 mg IM	15	60	3-6
	10 mg IV	Pentazocine 60 mg IM	2-3	30	3-4
■ Dezocine (Dalgan)	10 mg IM	Morphine 10 mg IM	30	60-120	3-6
Step 3 Partial Agonist Drugs					
■ Buprenorphine (Buprenex)	0.4 mg IM	Morphine 10 mg IM	15	60	6

tinuous infusion. Pain unrelieved by the continuous infusion must be reevaluated and appropriate treatment instituted. If the patient requires frequent additional doses of medication for pain relief, and the pain is not expected to diminish abruptly, the continuous infusion may need to be adjusted upward.

Patient-controlled analgesia. Another type of delivery system is patient-controlled analgesia (PCA), or demand analgesia. With PCA a dose of opioid is delivered when the patient decides a dose is needed. PCA may be accomplished using oral medications or an infusion system in which the patient pushes a button to receive a bolus infusion of an analgesic into the subcutaneous tissue, a vein, or the epidural or intrathecal spaces. Ability to deliver a dose when needed places the patient in control and eliminates waiting for medication to be brought and

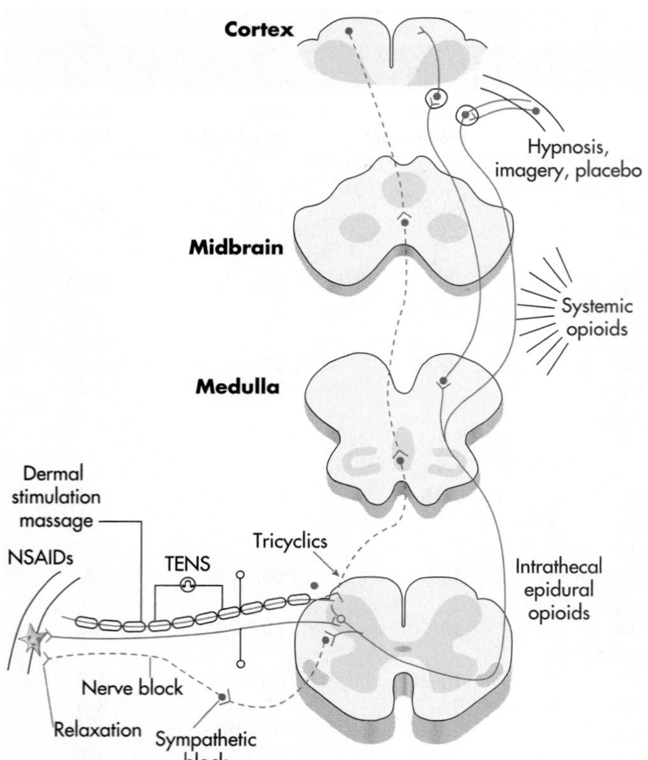

Fig. 9-16 The sites of commonly used pharmacologic and nonpharmacologic analgesic therapies. *NSAIDs,* nonsteroidal antiinflammatory drugs; *TENS,* transcutaneous electrical nerve stimulation.

given. Infusion pumps, however, deliver the drug only as frequently as the preset interval allows. PCA has rapidly gained acceptance for use in the management of acute pain, including postoperative pain, and cancer pain. The addition of a continuous infusion to a PCA regimen will improve nighttime pain relief and promote sleep, because PCA administration naturally decreases at night because the patient is sleeping and cannot self-administer doses.

Use of PCA begins with patient education. The patient needs to understand the mechanics of getting a medication dose and how to titrate the medication to achieve good pain relief. The patient should be guided to take another dose before pain intensity is greater than the patient's desired pain intensity goal (a cognitive aspect of pain). The effectiveness of the initial PCA programming must be assessed. If the patient reports pain that is intolerable, the nurse can request an order to give the patient bolus doses (titrate) until comfort is achieved. The nurse can then make adjustments in the PCA settings. A routine order for the loading process is as follows: give 1.5 to 2 times the PCA dose, evaluate pain relief at the time peak analgesic effect is expected (specific for each drug and route), and repeat the loading dose if the pain is unrelieved. This process should be continued until the patient reports either comfort or unacceptable side effects. If there are no orders for management of breakthrough pain (pain unrelieved by the prescribed pain management regimen), the patient's report of breakthrough pain must be communicated to the physician for a change in the orders. In a patient whose pain is steady and predictable, the majority of the patient's requirements can be met with a background infusion plus an occasional bolus (e.g., once an hour).

If the patient experiences side effects or toxic effects of PCA therapy, the specific symptom (e.g., nausea) should be treated. Ineffective symptom relief may require either a dose adjustment or an alternate drug.

To make a smooth transition from infusion PCA to oral medications, it may be helpful to start the oral regimen before discontinuing the PCA or at least to give the first oral dose at the time PCA is discontinued. Another method is to replace the continuous infusion and a portion of the PCA dose requirement with an around-the-clock, equally potent oral medication while continuing the PCA for another 24 hours.[9] When there is a transition in the pain management plan, a consistent approach to the assessment of pain is vital to pain relief.

Other injections and infusions. Intraspinal (epidural, intrathecal, or regional) opioid therapy is extremely effective. In particular, epidural analgesia is effective in the management of acute, chronic nonmalignant, and cancer pain. Epidural catheters may be surgically implanted or placed percutaneously (through a needle). Although the lumbar region is the most common site of placement, epidural catheters may be placed at any point along the neuroaxis (cervical, thoracic, lumbar, or caudal). When choosing the epidural opioid dose, the site of pain in relation to the position of the epidural catheter and the age of the patient are considered.

Epidural drugs may be given as an intermittent bolus injection or as a continuous infusion. There is great variability in response to given doses. An elderly patient may be more sensitive to epidural opioids because of slowed or altered metabolism and excretion. Timing, frequency, and type of the assessment (e.g., sensory and motor effects) depend on the drug being delivered. Opioids with diluted concentrations (0.125% or less) of local anesthetics, such as bupivacaine (Sensorcaine), are examples of drugs used epidurally. Fentanyl is the ideal drug for treatment of breakthrough pain because of its rapid onset (4 to 10 minutes) and short duration of action (2.6 to 4 hours).

The American Nurses Association (ANA) has established practice guidelines for the role of the registered nurse in management of the patient receiving analgesia by catheter techniques.[39] Prompt recognition and treatment of side effects and complications are necessary, and meticulous catheter care is required. The patient's skin must be assessed regularly and frequent position changes made to prevent skin breakdown if a local anesthetic is used because it can cause altered sensation with numbing. Intrathecal (into the CSF) administration and monitoring guidelines are similar to epidural administration. Doses administered, however, are much lower because the entire dose reaches the spinal cord (i.e., is not influenced by the dura and high vascularity of the epidural space).

Other regional sites for infusions of local anesthetics or analgesics include the brachial plexus, celiac plexus, and lumbar sympathetic chain and along a nerve. This type of infusion has been used for both acute and chronic pain. The drug concentration varies with each patient. The anesthetic or analgesic agent is usually delivered in 300 ml of normal saline solution with an infusion rate adjusted to the degree of pain and to the physiologic responses to the medication, such as hypotension, bradycardia, or respiratory depression, during the first 24 hours. After that time, the dosage is gradually titrated downward.

Side Effects of Step 2 and Step 3 Drugs. In addition to producing analgesia, step 2 and step 3 drugs produce side effects, such as constipation, sedation, nausea, vomiting, itching, and respiratory depression. Constipation is common when repeated opioid doses are administered. It is necessary to prevent this type of constipation by giving laxatives (e.g., senna) and stool softeners (e.g., docusate sodium [Colace]) early in the course of opioid therapy. For example, stool softeners and laxatives should be started immediately if long-term treatment is expected in chronic and cancer pain or if frequent doses are required to control acute pain. Stool softeners alone are insufficient to overcome the constipating effects of opioids.

Sedation can be effectively treated with stimulants (caffeine, dextroamphetamine, methylphenidate [Ritalin]). Metoclopramide (Reglan), transdermal scopolamine, hydroxyzine (Vistaril), or a phenothiazine (Compazine) antiemetic can be used to treat opioid-related nausea and vomiting. Metoclopramide is particularly effective when a patient complains of gastric fullness, because opioids delay gastric emptying and this effect is reversed by metoclopramide.

Respiratory depression is rare when opioids are titrated to analgesic effect. A patient who is awake does not succumb to respiratory depression.[9] A patient is most at risk for respiratory depression when asleep. For this reason, it is important to observe rate and depth of respirations of the sleeping patient for 3 to 4 hours past the expected time for peak blood concentrations based on the route of administration. If severe respiratory depression occurs and stimulation of the patient (calling and shaking patient) does not reverse the somnolence or increase the respiratory rate and depth, naloxone (Narcan, 0.4 mg in 10 ml saline) in 0.5 ml increments every 2 minutes can be administered.[9] The naloxone dose should be titrated to avoid precipitation of profound withdrawal, seizures, and severe pain. Naloxone can be administered SQ, IV, or PO, but *never* by the spinal route.

Itching is another common side effect of opioids. An antihistamine or a low-dose oral or IV opioid antagonist (e.g., naloxone) can be used to treat itching.

NONPHARMACOLOGIC THERAPY FOR PAIN

In addition to the pharmacologic analgesics described, a number of nonpharmacologic strategies provide analgesia and can be used alone or in combination with pain medications. Use of nonpharmacologic pain management strategies can reduce the dose of an analgesic required to control pain and thereby minimize side effects of drug therapy. Some strategies are believed to alter ascending nociceptive input or stimulate descending pain modulation mechanisms. The exact mechanisms by which some nonpharmacologic therapies exert analgesia are not known. It has been demonstrated, however, that placebo response probably is mediated by endogenous opioid systems. The placebo somehow causes the individual to mobilize endogenous opioids. Placebo response can be reversed by naloxone (Narcan), indicating that its mechanism involves endogenous opioid systems.[32] It is possible that other nonpharmacologic therapies, such as counterirritation, hypnosis, imagery, and distraction, also act via endogenous opioid or possibly nonopioid inhibitory systems.

Categorizing the nonpharmacologic pain relief methods as physical or cognitive-behavioral strategies is a helpful way of considering the potential mechanisms by which they provide pain relief.

Physical Pain Relief Strategies

Physical methods of producing analgesia include noninvasive and invasive techniques. The nurse can prescribe and administer many of the noninvasive therapies and can monitor and provide patient education when invasive techniques are prescribed by the physician.

Noninvasive Pain Relief Strategies

Positioning. Institution of preventive measures to minimize joint and muscle stiffness is important to the pain-management regimen, especially when the patient immobilizes or guards painful body parts in an attempt to control the pain. Establishment of a passive range-of-motion program and, if not contraindicated by the patient's condition, an active exercise regimen for the patient can reduce joint and muscle stiffness. These strategies are particularly beneficial when timed to coincide with the peak analgesic effect of the drug therapy. The exercise program reduces the stiffness and helps release any muscle spasms that may be present. Both patient and family should be taught the exercise regimen. The patient should be encouraged to move about as much as possible within the medically prescribed activity order.

The nurse must also prevent painful complications that result from immobility, including pressure ulcers, contractures, and thrombophlebitis. Because pain can be intensified by distention of an internal organ, constipation should be prevented by ensuring that the patient is mobilized as soon as possible and given laxatives as necessary. Because urinary retention can cause or increase pain, intake and output should be monitored and the bladder percussed to assess the degree of distention. An indwelling catheter, if present, should be checked frequently to ensure patency and free flow of urine. The patient should be helped to identify the precipitating physical factors that cause pain. Measures to prevent the pain should then be instituted and taught to the patient and family.

Pain management must include methods to promote rest and sleep. The person deprived of sleep becomes irritable and fatigued and has an increased sensitivity to pain. The patient must be allowed to sleep undisturbed for at least 2 hours at a time. Comfort measures, analgesics and hypnotics, and relaxation techniques should be used as appropriate to promote sleep.

Dermal stimulation. Dermal (cutaneous) stimulation to produce analgesia is defined as noninjurious stimulation of the patient's skin for the purpose of pain relief.[1] Dermal stimulation may be provided by the patient or someone else. Dermal stimulation methods differ in relation to convenience, cost, need for a physician's prescription, precautions, contraindications, and the availability of trained health care professionals who may provide the intervention.

Pressure. Application of pressure is an instinctual response to pain. An injured part is reflexively clutched and pressure is applied. Dermal stimulation that uses a pressure method takes advantage of this automatic response in a deliberate fashion. Pressure may be applied with the fingertips, the ball of the thumb, knuckles, heel of the hand, entire hand, or both hands. Occasionally a hard but smooth object, such as a sandbag, may be used to apply pressure. Pressure applied to a trigger point is effective in some instances. A *trigger point* is a small hyperirritable area with a taut band in the muscle or connective tissue, often just below the skin, that causes pain when it is stimulated sufficiently. Trigger points may be present in the painful area or at a point distant from the actual pain. There is a strong association between trigger points and acupuncture points for pain. Although pressure on a trigger point may produce a dull, aching discomfort, continued pressure may relieve the pain. Certified massage therapists are trained in these techniques.

Acupressure. *Acupressure* is a specific pressure technique that involves application of pressure, massage, or both to specified points on the skin. These points are the same as the traditional acupuncture points. Pressure is applied with the thumb, the tip of the index finger, or the palm of the hand.

Massage. Massage of an injured body part with rubbing is also an instinctual response. This response can be deliberately tapped to manage pain. Many massage techniques exist. Examples include moving the hands or fingers over the skin slowly or briskly with long strokes or in circles (superficial massage) or applying firm pressure to the skin to maintain contact while massaging the underlying tissues (deep massage). Specific massage techniques are involved in some forms of acupressure and in trigger point massage. Cold massage to trigger points is also used.

Cutaneous vibration. The application of cutaneous vibration and high-frequency energy, such as by ultrasound, short-wave and long-wave diathermy, and microwave, is used to provide pain relief.[40] The pain relief may be immediate, or it may require several minutes to occur. The duration of the pain relief is highly variable. Many different vibration devices exist, varying in size and shape to meet individual needs. A physician's prescription is not necessary for the purchase of a vibratory device. Cutaneous vibration is often done in an outpatient physical therapy department.

Transcutaneous electrical nerve stimulation (TENS). TENS involves the delivery of an electric current through electrodes applied to the skin surface over the painful region, at trigger points, or over a peripheral nerve. A TENS system consists of two or more electrodes connected by lead wires to a small, battery-operated stimulator (Fig. 9-17). Most stimulators may be worn and used 24 hours a day. The system can also be disassembled for intermittent use by detaching the stimulator and wires while leaving the electrodes in place. Pain relief with TENS has been reported in low-back pain, cervical (neck) syndrome, arthritis, sciatica, tic douloureux, postherpetic neuralgia, peripheral nerve injuries, brachial plexus injuries, and stump and phantom limb pain and during childbirth labor.[18] During the actual application of TENS, acute postoperative pain is reduced. Postoperative pulmonary and GI tract complications can also be minimized with the use of TENS. Pain relief after discontinuance of TENS varies. A physician's order is required to initiate this therapy.

Physical therapists often apply the TENS, but application and patient education can be done by a nurse. Experimentation with different stimulators, different electrode placements, and different frequency settings is often necessary to achieve therapeutic results with TENS. If one stimulator is not effective in providing pain relief, another should be tried. Multiple sites of stimulation, based on spinal dermatomes, may also be tried during successive trials to determine the most effective site for pain modulation.

Conventional (high-frequency) TENS units that use alternating currents set at a rate of 40 to 400 Hz (cycles per second)

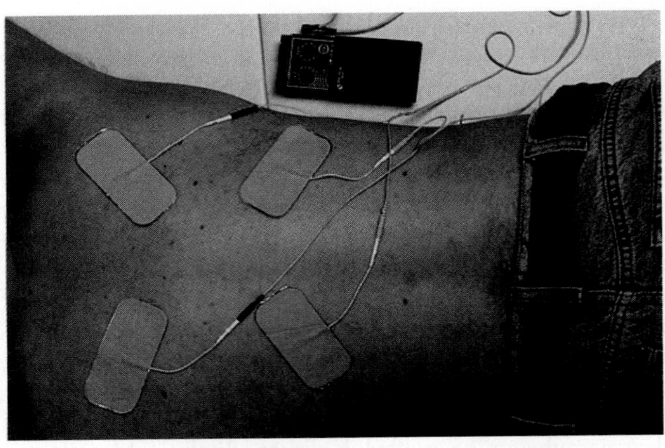

Fig. 9-17 Initial TENS treatment being given by physical therapy department to assess value in pain relief.

typically produce rapid analgesia (within 20 minutes). The person receiving high-frequency TENS experiences paresthesias (subjective sensation of numbness or tingling) during the treatments. The voltage and the rate of stimulation are altered according to the patient's response to the paresthesias.

Contraindications for the use of TENS are not firmly established. TENS is not currently recommended for patients with cardiac pacemakers or with a history of myocardial ischemia or arrhythmias. TENS is not applied over a pregnant uterus, broken skin, or anesthetic areas; in areas of the carotid sinuses or laryngeal and pharyngeal muscles; or on the eyes.

Heat therapy. Heat therapy is the application of either moist or dry heat to the skin. Heat therapy can be either superficial or deep. Superficial dry heat can be applied by means of an electrical device, such as a heating pad, a heat cradle, or a gooseneck or infrared lamp, or by nonelectric means, such as hot-water bottles and exposure to the sun. Superficial moist heat can be obtained nonelectrically from hydrocollator (moist heat) packs, soaks, showers, baths, whirlpools, and Hubbard tanks and by wrapping the body part in plastic to trap body heat. Electric heating pads designed to provide moist heat are also available. Physical therapy departments provide deep-heat therapy through such techniques as short-wave diathermy, microwave diathermy, and ultrasound therapy. Heat therapy generally involves intermittent applications of heat for short periods of time (5 minutes for acute pain and 20 to 30 minutes for chronic pain), but some therapy methods, such as trapping of body heat, may be continued for prolonged periods or may be continuous.[40]

Cold therapy. Cold therapy involves the application of either moist or dry cold to the skin. Dry cold can be applied by means of an ice bag, moist cold by means of towels soaked in ice water, cold hydrocollator packs, or immersion in a bath or under running cold water. Icing, with ice cubes or blocks of ice made to resemble Popsicles, is another technique used for pain relief. Ice massage is a technique combining cold therapy and massage; the ice is applied evenly over the area of pain with slow up-and-down strokes for 10 to 30 minutes. Physical therapists sometimes use ethyl chloride or "vasocoolant" sprays as part of a cold-therapy regimen.

Cold therapy is used for a variety of painful conditions, including posttraumatic pain and postoperative pain (especially following orthopedic procedures) and with bursitis, osteomyelitis, and muscle spasms. In addition, contrast baths (alternating hot and cold applications) and hydrotherapy used in conjunction with relaxation, passive movement exercises, and breathing exercises may be used to treat pain.

Guidelines for dermal stimulation. Any type of dermal stimulation should initially be of moderate intensity and then increased or decreased to achieve optimal pain relief. The most effective intensity for dermal stimulation is slightly less than the intensity that produces discomfort in persons with normal skin—frequently a stimulation of slightly above moderate intensity.[40] Dermal stimulation may be continuous or intermittent. The duration of most cutaneous stimulation is 10 to 30 minutes; however, ice massage rarely lasts longer than 10 minutes. Cold therapy is contraindicated in the person with hypersensitivity to cold. When firm pressure is applied to trigger points or acupuncture points, steady pressure is usually not maintained for more than a few seconds. The frequency of dermal stimulation should be determined by how long the pain relief lasts following stimulation. When the pain recurs, the dermal stimulation is reapplied. An arbitrary schedule (such as tid or qid) may be established in an institutional setting. On an outpatient basis, dermal stimulation that requires professional supervision is scheduled by appointment, usually with a physical therapy department. Continuous application of most dermal stimulation methods is impractical. If the patient needs continuous stimulation to achieve pain relief, TENS or a menthol product may be the most practical solution.

Generally, dermal stimulation is applied directly over the painful area, around the painful site, or just proximal and distal to the painful area. Another possible area of stimulation is over peripheral nerves that innervate the painful area. This type of stimulation is most readily accomplished by TENS. Contralateral stimulation may be necessary when a painful area is too sensitive to be directly stimulated or when the painful area is not accessible because of a covering. The reason for the effectiveness of contralateral stimulation is not known. Contralateral stimulation is also used with phantom limb pain. Use of cutaneous stimulation techniques must be individualized to the patient and the particular type of pain. The patient may have strong preferences regarding the type of dermal stimulation used and the area to be stimulated. Individual concerns include cost, convenience, and intensity and duration of the stimulation.

Many different persons may be able to administer the dermal stimulation techniques. The nurse, physical therapists, certified massage therapists, the patient, and family members may be able to perform the prescribed technique. Often, the patient and family members can be taught the effective technique after the therapy has been initiated by a trained person. Some of the techniques require purchasing or renting equipment (e.g., TENS) or using a physical therapy department (e.g., ultrasound). Some treatments are covered by insurance; others are not. The practical aspects of dermal stimulation must be considered if this method of treatment is to provide long-term relief.

Invasive Pain Relief Strategies

Acupuncture. *Acupuncture* is used to provide pain relief (see Chapter 8). It is unknown at this time if acupuncture analgesia is superior to placebo analgesia or other types of hyperstimulation procedures. It is important to point out that extensive education is necessary to become certified to perform acupuncture.

Percutaneous electrical nerve stimulation. Deeper peripheral tissues can be stimulated through percutaneous electrical nerve stimulation. Percutaneous electrical nerve stimulation is a preliminary step designed to evaluate the potential usefulness of a permanently implanted device. It is accomplished by inserting a needle, to which a stimulator is attached, near a large peripheral or spinal nerve. The amount of electric current is regulated to provide maximum pain relief. If the percutaneous stimulation successfully reduces the patient's pain, a permanent peripheral nerve stimulator is surgically implanted. A special electrode is placed around the nerve, and an internal receiver is implanted subcutaneously at waist level on the anterior chest wall. The patient activates the receiver by means of a special transmitter and antenna as needed for optimal pain relief.

Dorsal cord or deep brain stimulation. CNS stimulation can be achieved through dorsal cord stimulation or deep brain stimulation.[41,42] Dorsal cord stimulation is an alternative pain-management technique to percutaneous electrical nerve stimulation when the pain involves large areas, such as the lower extremities or the back. During a laminectomy, electrodes are implanted intradurally in the dorsal aspect of the spinal cord. The level of implantation is determined by the pain location. A receiver is implanted subcutaneously on the anterior chest wall at waist level. The antenna and the transmitter system are similar to those used in permanent peripheral nerve stimulation.

Electrical stimulation of certain regions of the brain, including areas of the frontal lobes, thalamus, midbrain, lower brainstem, caudate nucleus of the basal ganglion, and internal capsule, produces long-lasting analgesia. Motor function, affect, and other behavior responses are unaffected.

Nerve blocks. Nerve blocks are used to reduce pain by temporarily or permanently interrupting transmission of nociceptive input by application of local anesthetics or neurolytic agents (e.g., alcohol, phenol). Initially, temporary nerve blocks with local anesthetics are used to isolate the involved pain pathway and to determine the possible effectiveness of a permanent blocking procedure for the particular individual. Typically, the local anesthetic effects last for only a few hours. The effects of neurolytic agents last for weeks to months; therefore these agents are used for a more long-lasting effect.

Nerve blocks have been a successful pain-management technique for more localized chronic pain states, such as peripheral vascular disease, trigeminal neuralgia, causalgia, and some cancer pain. A nerve block was formerly considered advantageous in managing localized pain caused by malignancy and in debilitated patients who could not withstand a surgical procedure for pain relief. This use is currently being reevaluated in view of the increasing life expectancy of persons being treated for malignancies and the availability of other therapeutic modalities.

Neurosurgical interventions. Neurosurgical interventions are accomplished by surgical resection or thermocoagulation, including radio-frequency coagulation. Interventions that destroy the sensory division of a peripheral or spinal nerve are classified as neurectomies, rhizotomies, and sympathectomies. Neurosurgical procedures that ablate the lateral spinothalamic tract are classified as cordotomies if the tract is interrupted in the spinal cord, or tractotomies if the interruption is in the

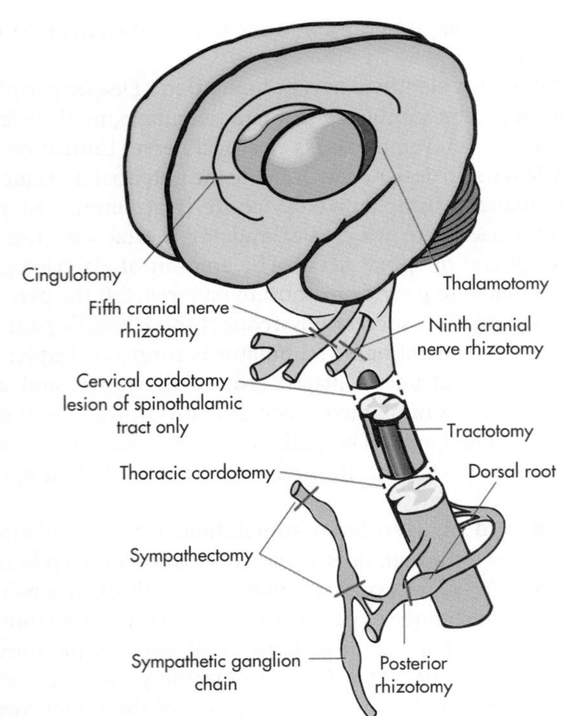

Fig. 9-18 Sites of neurosurgical procedures for pain relief.

medulla or the midbrain of the brainstem. Figure 9-18 identifies the sites of neurosurgical procedures for pain relief. Surgical resection of the lateral spinothalamic tract is rare today because a percutaneous approach is available. Both cordotomy and tractotomy can be performed with the aid of local anesthesia by a percutaneous technique in which the pain fibers are isolated by fluoroscopy and a radio-frequency lesion is created.

Neurosurgical interventions involving the thalamus or frontal lobe region of the brain are carried out through a stereotactic procedure. Long electrodes or other probes are inserted deep into the brain tissue and positioned by the use of external points or landmarks of the skull. The tissue is destroyed by thermocoagulation or other means.

Ablative procedures of the CNS or peripheral nervous system are used less frequently today because of the availability of good analgesic methods to control pain and new concerns about the lesion creating a long-lasting neuropathic pain syndrome.

Cognitive-Behavioral Therapies

Techniques to alter the affective, cognitive, and behavioral components of pain include a variety of cognitive strategies and behavioral approaches. Many cognitive-behavioral techniques elicit emotions, behaviors, and thoughts that are incompatible with pain. For example, relaxation is incompatible with muscle tension. Thinking or talking about a scenic view is incompatible with thinking about pain. Rhythmic breathing is incompatible with the holding one's breath and gasping that are associated with pain. Eliciting behaviors that are incompatible with pain is part of the nursing management of the patient experiencing pain. Providing periods of rest and sleep may also be necessary to conserve the energy needed for those activities the patient considers important.

Anticipatory Guidance. The patient should be prepared as much as possible regarding pain experiences. This is termed *anticipatory guidance.* Preparing the patient for what to expect allows the nurse to help reduce anxiety and clarify misinformation and misinterpretation. Knowing what to expect helps the patient cope. In the anticipatory phase of the pain experience some anxiety mobilizes the development of coping strategies. This is an important point when the nurse is dealing with a patient who is to have a painful experience. Such a patient cannot be reassured that there will be little or no pain, but instead must be helped to identify ways to cope with the expected pain.

Distraction. Distraction involves redirection of attention on something away from the pain. The distraction stimuli may be external events, internal activities, or bodily sensations. Distraction techniques help the patient cope with the pain being experienced. When assisting the patient to use cognitive strategies, the nurse must remember that the patient's ability to use distraction effectively to decrease the pain experience does not mean that the pain is not severe. Distraction techniques remove pain from the center of attention, thereby increasing pain tolerance and decreasing the response to the pain experience. The pain, however, is real.

Part of the nurse's role is to encourage the patient to use the distraction techniques that have been found helpful in the past. The nurse should also assist the patient to use these distraction techniques. Family members also need to be taught how to assist the patient to use these techniques effectively. Both patient and family need support in adopting them.

Imagery and Hypnosis. For pain relief the individual's own imagination is used to develop sensory images that focus away from the pain sensation and emphasize other sensory experiences and pleasant memories. Guided imagery provides a mental substitute for the pain. Although it requires training, hypnosis can be used successfully for a person whose pain syndrome involves a strong affective component.[43] These strategies are discussed in Chapter 8 (see Table 8-2).

Conditioning. Certain pain-relief measures result in relief frequently enough for classic conditioning to take place. The nurse can help the patient benefit from this phenomenon by deliberately pairing relief methods. For example, the nurse should teach a relaxation technique to be used each time a pain medication is given. One result of this is the additive effect gained from two measures used simultaneously.

Behavior modification (operant conditioning) is based on the principle that the frequency of a behavior may be increased or decreased by the use of reinforcement. Positive reinforcement results in an increase in the frequency of the behavior. The nurse can use behavior modification by giving praise and attention to the patient who is willing to try new pain relief methods or who engages in behaviors incompatible with pain. The patient's attempts to progress toward recovery should be praised and noticed. Silence or ignoring nonbeneficial behavior is also important. The family should be taught to provide positive reinforcement, ignore nonbeneficial behavior, and use silence.

Stress inoculation training involves a three-stage approach to behavioral change. First, the meaning of the clinical manifestations is taught. Second, the patient is taught coping strategies that are incompatible with the pain experience and pain behavior. Third, the patient is taught how to use this new knowledge and awareness in the pain situation. The nurse participates in all phases of stress inoculation training, assisting the patient to progress through the stages.

Relaxation. The positive effects of relaxation include reducing the effects of stress, decreasing acute anxiety, distracting from the pain, alleviating skeletal muscle tension or contraction, combating fatigue, facilitating sleep, and enhancing the effectiveness of other pain-relief measures.[6,7] Elicitation of the relaxation response requires a quiet environment, a comfortable position, and a mental device as a focus of concentration (e.g., a word, a sound, the heartbeat, or the person's breathing). Relaxation strategies include deep-breathing regimens, heartbeat breathing, music, slow and rhythmic breathing, and progressive relaxation exercises with a trainer. These strategies are also described in Chapter 8.

NURSING AND COLLABORATIVE MANAGEMENT: PAIN

Therapeutic techniques to manage pain syndromes are generally directed at altering either the physiologic-sensory or the affective, behavioral, and cognitive components of pain. Comprehensive, holistic pain-management programs use a multidisciplinary approach including a combination of techniques directed at all components of pain. Most comprehensive pain-management programs began in the early 1970s. This approach involves comprehensive assessment and problem identification by an interdisciplinary team. The treatment plan includes elimination of unnecessary drug dependence, therapeutic measures to reduce the pain, physical rehabilitation, psychologic rehabilitation for the patient and family, and the return of control over the pain-management program to the patient. A comprehensive multidisciplinary pain assessment and pain profile, along with a complete physical and laboratory evaluation, are the first steps.

Generally, treatment is aimed at achieving maximum mobilization and relief of pain with the use of physical and psychologic treatment techniques. Physical reconditioning is initiated slowly. A sound and reasonably vigorous exercise program is gradually established. Physical treatment modalities may include massage, pressure, heat therapy, cold therapy, vibration, TENS, and acupuncture. An equally important component of chronic pain management is psychotherapy and cognitive-behavioral approaches. The patient is taught skills to help cope with the pain while cognitive restructuring is addressed. Biofeedback training is often used (see Chapter 8). Psychologic counseling for both the patient and the family is a critical component. A person who has been in pain for a prolonged time may have greatly altered interpersonal relationships and communication patterns with family, friends, and health care personnel. The chronic stress of the pain may have left the person's life in shambles. Most authorities recommend an intensive program of psychologic therapy over a short time, dealing with issues in the present, rather than the more traditional prolonged therapy.

In a holistic pain-management program, the patient learns to draw on inner resources and to assume responsibility for practicing skills that will help the patient cope with the pain. The person is taught how to use pain medication, as well as the support from family and significant others, effectively.

The nurse is an important member of the multidisciplinary pain-management team. The nurse acts as planner, educator, patient advocate, interpreter, and supporter of the patient in pain and the patient's family. Because pain can be present in any patient in a wide variety of care settings—home, hospital, clinic—the nurse must be knowledgeable about current therapies and flexible in trying new approaches to pain management. The extent of the nurse's involvement depends on the unique factors associated with the patient, the setting, and the cause of the pain.

A critical element in the nursing management of a patient with pain is the establishment of a trusting relationship and a good rapport with the patient and the family. The patient and the family need to know that the nurse considers the pain significant and understands that pain may totally disrupt a person's life. The nurse's goal is to help the patient obtain pain relief. The nurse's secondary goal is to help the patient cope with any unrelieved pain. These goals are achieved through use of pharmacologic and nonpharmacologic interventions.

Nursing actions that promote the establishment of an effective relationship with the person who is experiencing pain and with the family should include the following:

1. *Believe the patient.* The patient needs to be able to trust the nurse to believe that the pain exists. This message can be conveyed verbally to the patient by saying "I know you are in pain." The nurse may need to help the family believe the patient.
2. *Clarify responsibilities in pain relief.* Discuss what the nurse is going to do and what the patient and the family are expected to do.
3. *Respect the patient's response to pain.* The nurse should accept the right of the patient to respond to the pain in the necessary manner. The family also needs help in this area. The patient may need help to accept the response to the pain; the behavior may be less than is expected by the patient and the family.
4. *Collaborate with the patient.* The patient and the family should be helped to participate actively in setting goals for pain relief. The patient should be encouraged to use coping techniques that have been effective in the past. The patient and the family should be assisted to use personal resources more effectively. The patient's expectations of a nurse must be met or clarified, if those expectations are not consistent with professional practice.
5. *Explore the pain with the patient.* The nurse needs to find out the meaning of the pain to the person enduring the pain and to the family.
6. *Be with the patient often.* The nurse's physical presence may reassure or distract the patient, or it may offer variety, thus relieving the pain.

Because pain has such a pervasive impact on the lives of the patient and family, many possible nursing diagnoses must be considered. Table 9-12 lists possible nursing diagnoses that may be appropriate for the patient in pain.

Barriers to Effective Pain Management

Although pain is a complex, subjective experience, pain management can be either facilitated or constrained by the environment, including social and political factors. These factors include emotions, behaviors, beliefs, and attitudes of family members, health professionals, health agencies, and society about pain and use of pain therapies. Planning pain management with the patient as a partner requires careful consideration of the influence of these factors.

Table 9-12 Possible Nursing Diagnoses for the Patient with Pain

Activity intolerance
Altered family processes
Altered thought processes
Anxiety
Chronic pain
Constipation
Fear
Hopelessness
Ineffective individual coping
Pain
Powerlessness
Risk for self-mutilation
Sleep pattern disturbance

Table 9-13 Manifestations of Withdrawal Syndrome from Short-acting Opioids

	Early Responses (6-12 hr)	Late Responses (48-72 hr)
Psychosocial	Anxiety	Excitation
Secretions	Lacrimation	Diarrhea
	Rhinorrhea	
	Diaphoresis	
Other	Yawning	Restlessness
	Piloerection	Fever
	Shaking chills	Nausea and vomiting
	Dilated pupils	Abdominal cramps
	Anorexia	Hypertension
	Tremor	Tachycardia
		Insomnia

Concerns regarding tolerance, dependence, addiction, assisted suicide, and euthanasia often serve as barriers to effective pain management. These concerns are shared by the patient, family members, and health care providers. It is important that the nurse understand and be able to explain the differences among these various concepts.

Tolerance. Tolerance occurs with chronic exposure to a variety of drugs. In the case of opioids, tolerance is characterized by the need for an increased opioid dose to maintain the same degree of analgesia. Every patient does not experience tolerance, but patients with a past or current substance abuse history are likely to do so. The need for an increase in the analgesic dose may reflect other factors, such as disease progression (e.g., cancer progression), or a new pathologic condition (e.g., pulmonary embolus), rather than tolerance. The patient's reports of increased pain should not be ignored; the increased pain should be treated while the cause is pursued. One of the ways tolerance is managed is by drug titration to balance desired effects and side effects while maintaining patient comfort. Other approaches include changing to another drug in the same class or adding a nonopioid drug such as ibuprofen. It is important to note that there is no ceiling effect (increased dosing provides additional pain relief) for opioid-agonist drugs. As tolerance increases, doses can be increased.

Patients often worry about tolerance, especially if they expect their pain to increase or persist. The nurse can ease this worry by explaining that numerous pain medicines are available and that many have no maximum dose.

Dependence. Dependence is an expected physiologic response to ongoing exposure to pharmacologic agents that can produce a withdrawal syndrome when exposure is abruptly stopped. Withdrawal from opioids is characterized by symptoms such as chills alternating with hot flashes, salivation, sweating, runny nose, anxiety, irritability, insomnia, abdominal cramps, vomiting, and diarrhea when the drug dosage is markedly decreased or abruptly discontinued[9] (Table 9-13). Dependence appears to be highly individualized. Some patients will gradually decrease their use of pain medication as the pain decreases. Other patients require a tapering schedule. For example, to withdraw a patient from morphine, the total 24-hour dose used by the patient is calculated and decreased by 50%. Of this decreased amount, 25% is given every 6 hours.[9] After 2 days, the daily dose is reduced by an additional 25% every 2 days until the 24-hour oral dose is 30 mg per day. The morphine is then discontinued.

Addiction. *Addiction* is a psychologic condition characterized by a drive to obtain and take substances for other than the prescribed therapeutic value (see Chapter 10). Less than 0.1% of those who receive analgesics as a part of their medical treatment regimen become addicted.[44] In populations of patients with a substance abuse history, this percentage may be higher. A previous or present substance abuse problem can be identified during the initial pain assessment. Two examples of behavior suggestive of addiction are patients receiving pain medications from multiple physicians and reporting that pain prescriptions have been lost or stolen. Other types of behavior may be incorrectly interpreted as signs of addiction, such as clock watching by the person undertreated for the pain. Addiction cannot be verified in the person with pain until the etiology of the pain has been eliminated, physical dependence has been eliminated through detoxification, and the patient seeks and takes the substance again. The patient who is physically dependent on the drug will seek and take the drug but may not be addicted. Often the term *addiction* is inappropriately applied to a patient, and the label can be a barrier to pain relief for that person. It is important for the nurse to recognize that opioid tolerance and physical dependence are expected with long-term opioid treatment and should not be confused with addiction.[6,7]

Assisted Suicide and Euthanasia. It is not uncommon for the health professional, patient, and family members to be concerned that the effect of providing sufficient medication to relieve pain will precipitate the death of a terminally ill person. When large doses of opioids are required to control pain, often both the physician and nurse will hesitate in their respective roles to prescribe and administer the dose, because they are concerned that the actions will be considered performing euthanasia or assisting the patient to commit suicide. Relieving pain, even if it hastens the death of a terminally ill person, is considered the ethical and moral obligation of the professional nurse; it is not euthanasia or assisted suicide.[39,45,46] When consistent with the patient's wishes, the position of the ANA is as follows: "Nurses should not hesitate to use full and effective doses of pain medication for the proper management of pain in the dying patient. The increasing titration of medication to achieve adequate symptom control, even at the expense of life, thus hastening death, is ethically justified."[45] Relief of pain, not death, is the objective of the intervention.

Unfortunately, inadequate pain relief and intolerable suffering have been cited by many patients as reasons for seeking assisted suicide. The nurse is responsible for assisting the patient to obtain pain relief satisfactory to him or her. Aggressive management of pain is essential and may limit the number of people who seek assisted suicide. The ANA and other nursing organizations have taken the position that nurses should not participate in assisted suicide or euthanasia. Assisting a patient to commit suicide is in violation of the Code for Nurses.[46] Professional nurses, however, have a responsibility to provide analgesia to patients with pain.[46]

Evaluation of the Pain-Management Plan

In acute and chronic pain situations, the nurse should evaluate the effectiveness of the pain-relief measures taken by the patient, nurses, and other health care personnel. The judgments about effectiveness are made by comparing the patient's self-report of pain pattern, area, intensity, and nature and the affective, behavioral, and cognitive responses before the intervention with additional reports and responses after the intervention. Both subjective and objective data enter into the evaluation, but it must be remembered that the patient is the final judge.

If the patient says that the relief measures are not adequate, the nurse should reassess the pain and also consider the following questions:[1]

1. Are a variety of pain-relief measures being used? (If not, additional measures should be added.)
2. Are the pain-relief measures being used before the pain becomes severe? (If not, an anticipatory analgesia regimen should be implemented.)
3. Is what the patient believes will be effective included in the pain-management protocol? (If not, the reasons should be determined.) Can classic conditioning be used if the patient cannot keep receiving what is perceived as most effective?
4. Is the patient willing and able to be a more active participant in the pain management? (If not, the reasons should be determined.) How can the patient be helped to become more active?
5. Can the patient be encouraged to try the pain-relief measure one or two more times, especially if some additional measures are implemented? A revised pain-management plan should then be formulated and implemented.

NEEDS OF PATIENT CAREGIVERS

Working with the patient who is experiencing pain generates stress in the nurse and in other health care personnel. Pain, like death, is one of the most universally frightening experiences, not only for those experiencing it but also for those witnessing it. The patient's fear of the pain and feelings of powerlessness to control the pain elicit an awareness of the nurse's own vulnerability and limitations. Fear and a sense of powerlessness may be evoked. These affective experiences and the stress they engender may elicit defense mechanisms and inappropriate coping behaviors, such as alienation from or avoidance of the patient and the family and denial of the severity of the pain experience or of the fact that the patient has any pain at all.

The nurse working with the patient experiencing pain needs self-insight and value clarification. The nurse needs peer group involvement, not only to assist with value clarification but to offer support, guidance, and perhaps counseling on an ongoing informal and formal basis. In addition, consultation from experts in the area of pain management may be necessary. The nurse also needs to keep abreast of the rapidly expanding knowledge in pain and pain management.

Family teaching and the family-nurse relationship are extremely important. Assessment of the family and friends and their interaction with the patient is essential in the presence of a pain syndrome. Relationships are often inappropriate and stressful. Nursing interventions to teach the family and friends and to provide information on more effective coping techniques for themselves, as well as strategies to help the patient, are essential.

GERONTOLOGIC CONSIDERATIONS

Pain

The effects of aging on the pain process may be confounded in an older adult who has a chronic illness that affects the nervous system. An older person who is well instructed in use of pain measurement tools and without diseases (e.g., diabetes) affecting the nervous system tends to report pain intensity similar to a younger person.[47] Peripheral nerve disease (e.g., diabetic neuropathy), however, can interfere with an elderly person's ability to sense pain related to tissue injury.

Older age is associated with chronic health problems, increased risk for musculoskeletal pain, depression, and limitations in activities of daily living. For many elderly people, pain is a constant companion. Increased pain intensity has been noted in older individuals, particularly when adequate treatment is not provided for chronic and recurrent pain. Treatment of pain in the older adult is as likely to be successful as that for a younger person.[47]

Older individuals may have fear that use of pain medications will result in drug addiction and oversedation.[48] Nurses play a key role in teaching patients and their family members regarding the importance of pain management and factual information to address their concerns.

A condition that would produce acute pain in some younger people may remain virtually undetected in some older people until complications occur. For example, an older person experiencing a myocardial infarction may complain of excess gas, an upset stomach, or extreme fatigue rather than the crushing chest pain identified by a younger adult. In this situation, the complication of congestive heart failure may be the first indicator of the older individual's primary problem. It is important to recognize, however, that pain is the most frequent presenting symptom of acute myocardial infarction in both older and younger patients. The frequency of silent myocardial infarctions in older adults has been overestimated.[47]

CRITICAL THINKING EXERCISES

CASE STUDY

Pain

Patient Profile

Mrs. C. is a 280-pound (112 kg) 48-year-old African-American woman admitted for an incision and drainage of a right renal abscess.

Subjective Data

- RN for 20 years
- Lives alone
- Desires 0 pain during therapy but will accept 1-2 on a 0-10 scale
- Reports incision area pain as a 2-3 between dressing changes and as a 10 during dressing changes
- States sharp, pulling pain persists 1-2 hr after dressing change
- Reports pain between dressing changes controlled by two tablets of Percocet
- Reports morphine 2 mg IV barely touches pain during dressing changes

Objective Data

- Requires qid dry-to-dry dressing changes for 1 week
- Morphine 4-15 mg IV every 1-2 hr

Critical Thinking Questions

1. Initially, what dose of IV morphine should be given?
2. Describe the assessment data that support the dose selected in question 1.
3. How long should the nurse wait after the IV morphine dose to begin the dressing change?
4. If an initial dose of 6 mg IV morphine reduces the pain to a 6 mid-dressing change, what nursing action is indicated?
5. What dose should be administered for subsequent dressing changes?
6. What additional pain therapies might the nurse plan to help Mrs. C. through the dressing change?
7. When Mrs. C. is discharged needing dressing changes for 3 days at home, how would the home care nurse organize her care? The nurse knows that Mrs. C. has obtained adequate pain relief with 8 mg IV morphine.
8. Based on the data presented, write one or more appropriate nursing diagnoses. Are there any collaborative problems?

NURSING RESEARCH ISSUES

1. Does a person with acute, chronic nonmalignant, or cancer pain spontaneously tell others about the pain?
2. What information (location, intensity, quality, pattern) does the patient with pain tell others?
3. What is the most effective and efficient way to overcome misconceptions the patient has about addiction, dependence, and tolerance to opioid drugs?
4. Based on the patient's usual methods of coping with pain, what nonpharmacologic pain-management strategies are most effective in promoting pain relief?
5. What is the onset of action, peak action, and duration of action for specific nonpharmacologic pain-management strategies?

REVIEW QUESTIONS

The number of the question corresponds to the same-numbered objective at the beginning of the chapter.

1. The single most important component of the pain process that determines the amount and character of experienced pain is
   a. the A-delta and C fibers.
   b. transmission of nociceptive signals.
   c. facilitation and inhibition of nociceptive signals.
   d. transduction of mechanical, thermal, or chemical stimuli.
2. The typical dose of opioids drugs is most likely to be effective for treatment of
   a. acute neuropathic pain.
   b. chronic neuropathic pain.
   c. neuropathic pain in opioid-naive patients.
   d. acute or chronic nociceptive pain with tissue inflammation.
3. Unrelieved pain is
   a. to be expected after major surgery.
   b. to be expected in a person with cancer.
   c. dangerous and can lead to many physical and psychologic complications.
   d. an annoying sensation, but it is not as important as other physical care needs.
4. An activity appropriate for the nurse during the initial pain assessment process is to
   a. assess critical sensory components.
   b. teach the patient about pain therapies.
   c. conduct a comprehensive pain assessment.
   d. provide appropriate treatment and evaluate its effect.
5. Drugs that are considered as adjuvant analgesics according to the WHO analgesic ladder include
   a. nonopioid analgesics.
   b. tricyclic antidepressants.
   c. agonist-antagonist drugs.
   d. opioid-agonist drugs.
6. In the person with an intact GI system, the recommended route of administration for morphine is
   a. IM.
   b. oral.
   c. IV.
   d. sublingual.
7. An important nursing responsibility related to pain is to
   a. leave the patient alone to rest.
   b. help the patient appear to not be in pain.
   c. believe what the patient says about the pain.
   d. assume responsibility for eliminating the patient's pain.
8. A nurse administering a prescribed, very large dose of an IV opioid that was titrated for a person with severe pain related to a terminal illness would be considered to be participating in

a. the patient's addiction.
b. palliative pain management.
c. euthanasia, an unethical activity for nurses.
d. assisted suicide, an unethical activity for nurses.

9. A nurse believes that patients with the same type of tissue injury should have the same amount of pain. This statement reflects
   a. a belief that will contribute to appropriate pain management.
   b. the nurse's belief will have no effect on the type of care provided to people in pain.
   c. an accurate statement about pain mechanisms and an expected goal of pain therapy.
   d. the nurse's lack of knowledge about pain mechanisms and is likely to contribute to poor pain management.

References

1. McCaffery M, Beebe A: *Pain: a clinical manual for nursing practice,* ed 2, St Louis, 1998, Mosby.
2. Merskey H, Bogduk N: *Classification of chronic pain: descriptions of chronic pain syndromes and definitions of pain terms,* Seattle, 1994, IASP Press.
3. Cassell EJ: The nature of suffering and the goals of medicine, *N Engl J Med* 306:639, 1982.
*4. Kahn DL, Steeves RH: An understanding of suffering grounded in clinical practice and research. In Ferrell BR, editor: *Suffering,* Boston, 1996, Jones & Bartlett.
5. Bonica JJ, editor: *The management of pain,* ed 2, Philadelphia, 1990, Lea & Febiger.
6. Agency for Health Care Policy and Research: *Clinical practice guideline. Acute pain management: operative or medical procedures and trauma,* Rockville, Md, 1992, US Department of Health and Human Services.
7. Agency for Health Care Policy and Research: *Clinical practice guideline. Management of cancer pain,* Rockville, Md, 1994, US Department of Health and Human Services.
*8. Maxam-Moore VV, Wilkie DJ, Woods SL: Analgesics for cardiac surgery patients in critical care: describing current practice, *Am J Crit Care* 3:31, 1994.
9. American Pain Society: *Principles of analgesic use in the treatment of acute pain and chronic cancer pain: a concise guide to medical practice,* ed 4, Skokie, Ill, 1997.
10. World Health Organization: *Cancer pain relief,* ed 2, Geneva, 1996, World Health Organization.
11. Dickenson AH: Central acute pain mechanisms, *Ann Med* 27:223, 1995.
12. Sidedall PJ, Cousins MJ: Spine update: spinal pain mechanisms, *Spine* 22:98, 1997.
13. Willis WD, Westlund KN: Neuroanatomy of the pain system and of the pathways that modulate pain, *J Clin Neurophysiol* 14(1):2, 1997.
14. Woolf CJ, Wiesenfield-Hallin Z: The systemic administration of local anaesthetics produce a selective depression of C-afferent fiber evoked activity in the spinal cord, *Pain* 23:361, 1985.
15. Coderre TJ and others: Contribution of central neuroplasticity to pathological pain: review of clinical and experimental evidence, *Pain* 54:363, 1993.
16. Casey KL and others: Comparison of human cerebral activation pattern during cutaneous warmth, heat pain, and deep cold pain, *J Neurophysiol* 76:571, 1996.
17. Jones AKP: Pain, its perception, and pain imaging, *IASP Newsletter* May/June:3, 1997.
18. Fields HL, Basbaum AL: Central nervous system mechanisms of pain modulation. In Wall PD, Melzack R, editors: *Textbook of pain,* ed 3, New York, 1994, Churchill Livingstone.
*19. Wilkie DJ and others: Behavior of patients with lung cancer: description and associations with oncologic and pain variables, *Pain* 51:231, 1992.
*20. Wilkie DJ and others: Cancer pain control behaviors: description and correlation with pain intensity, *Oncol Nurs Forum* 15:723, 1988.
*21. Page GG, Ben Eliyahu S: The immune-suppressive nature of pain, *Semin Oncol Nurs* 13:10, 1997.
*22. Gaston-Johansson F, Albert M, Fagan E: Similarities in pain descriptions of four different ethnic-culture groups, *J Pain Symptom Manage* 5:94, 1990.
23. McCaffery M, Ferrell BR: Influence of professional vs. personal role on pain assessment and use of opioids, *J Contin Educ Nurs* 28:69, 1997.
*24. Puntillo KA: Pain: its mediators and associated morbidity in critically ill cardiovascular surgical patients, *Nurs Res* 43:31, 1994.
*25. Tesler MD and others: Postoperative analgesics for children and adolescents: prescription and administration, *J Pain Symptom Manage* 9:85, 1994.
*26. Myklebust EK and others: Measurement of pain: quantifying pain intensity word descriptors. Manuscript submitted for publication.
*27. Wilkie DJ and others: Use of the McGill pain questionnaire to measure pain: a meta-analysis, *Nurs Res* 39:36, 1990.
28. Melzack R: The McGill pain questionnaire: major properties and scoring methods, *Pain* 1:277, 1975.
29. American Pain Society Quality of Care Committee: Quality improvement guidelines for the treatment of acute pain and cancer pain, *JAMA* 274:1874, 1995.
30. Porter J, Jick H: Addiction rare in patients treated with narcotics, *N Engl J Med* 302:123, 1980.
31. Garnett WR: GI effects of OTC analgesics: implications for product selection, *J Am Pharm Assoc Wash* NS36:565:1996.
32. Levine JD, Gordon NC, Fields HL: The mechanism of placebo analgesia, *Lancet* 2:654, 1978.
33. Herz A: Peripheral opioid analgesia—facts and mechanisms, *Prog Brain Res* 110:95, 1996.
34. Portenoy RK and others: Plasma morphine and morphine-6-glucuronide during chronic morphine therapy for cancer pain: plasma profiles, steady-state concentrations, and the consequences of renal failure, *Pain* 47:13, 1991.
35. Mercadante S and others: Subcutaneous fentanyl infusion in a patient with bowel obstruction and renal failure, *J Pain Symptom Manage* 13:241, 1997.
*36. Robison JM and others: Sublingual and oral morphine administration: review and new findings, *Nurs Clin North Am* 30:725, 1995.
37. Fine PG: Fentanyl in the treatment of cancer pain, *Semin Oncol* 24:S16, 1997.
38. Cherny NJ and others: Opioid pharmacotherapy in the management of cancer pain: a survey of strategies used by pain physicians for the selection of analgesic drugs and routes of administration, *Cancer* 76:1283, 1995.
39. American Nurses' Association: *Position statement on the role of the registered nurse (RN) in the management of analgesia by catheter techniques (epidural, intrathecal, intrapleural, or peripheral nerve catheters),* Washington, DC, 1990, The Association.
40. Lehmann JF, de Lateur B: Ultrasound, shortwave, microwave, laser, superficial heat and cold in the treatment of pain. In Wall PD, Melzack R, editors, *Textbook of pain,* ed 3, New York, 1994, Churchill Livingstone.
41. Krainick FU, Thoden U: Spinal cord stimulation. In Wall PD, Melzack R, editors: *Textbook of pain,* ed 3, New York, 1994, Churchill Livingstone.
42. Young RF, Rinaldi PC: Brain stimulation for relief of chronic pain. In Wall PD, Melzack R, editors: *Textbook of pain,* ed 3, New York, 1994, Churchill Livingstone.
43. Chaves JF, Dworkin SF: Hypnotic control of pain: historical perspectives and future prospects, *Int J Clin Exp Hypn* 45:356, 1997.
44. Miller LG: Cigarettes and drug therapy: pharmacokinetic and pharmacodynamic considerations, *Clin Pharm* 9:125, 1990.
45. American Nurses' Association: *Compendium of position statements on the nurse's role in end-of-life decisions,* Washington, DC, 1992, The Association.
46. American Nurses' Association: ANA's position on assisted suicide, *Am Nurse* 28(4):9, 1996.
47. Harkins SW and others: Geriatric pain. In Wall PD, Melzack R, editors: *Textbook of pain,* ed 3, New York, Churchill Livingstone, 1994.
48. Pasero CL, McCaffery M. Pain in the elderly. *AJN* 96:39-45, 1996.

*Nursing research-based articles or chapters.

Resources

American Academy of Pain Management (ACPM)
13947 Mono Way No. A
Sonora, CA 95370
209-533-9744
http://www.aapainmanage.org/index.html

American Academy of Pain Medicine (AAPM)
4700 W. Lake Avenue
Glenview, IL 60025
847-375-4731
Fax: 847-375-4777
http://www.painmed.org/

American Chronic Pain Association
PO Box 850
Rocklin, CA 95677
916-632-0922

American Society of Pain Management Nurses
2755 Bristol Street, Suite 110
Costa Mesa, CA 92626
714-545-1305
Fax: 714-545-3643
http://www.nursingcenter.com/people/nrsorgs/aspmn/

Association for Applied Psychophysiology and Biofeedback
10200 W. 44th Avenue, Suite 304
Wheat Ridge, CO 80033-2840
USA 800-477-8892
303-422-8436
Fax: 303-422-8894
http://www.aapb.org/

International Association for the Study of Pain (IASP)
909 NE 43rd Street, Suite 306
Seattle, WA 98105
206-547-6409
Fax: 206-547-1703
http://www.halcyon.com/iasp/

National Committee on Treatment of Intractable Pain
PO Box 9553
Friendship Station
Washington, DC 20016
202-965-6717
Fax: 202-293-4827

North American Chronic Pain Association of Canada
150 Central Park Drive, Unit 105
Brampton, Ontario L6T 2T9
CANADA
905-793-5230
800-616-PAIN
Fax: 905-793-8781
http://www3.sympatico.ca/nacpac/nacpac14.htm

Roxane Pain Institute
c/o Roxane Laboratories, Inc.
PO Box 16532
Columbus, OH 43216
http://pain.roxane.com/main.html

***For additional Internet resources, see the website for this book at* www.mosby.com/MERLIN/medsurg_lewis**

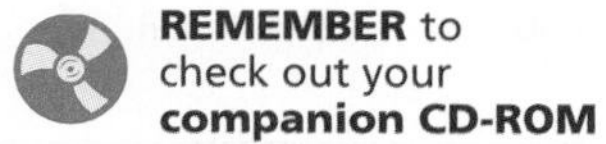

NURSING MANAGEMENT Substance Abuse and Dependence

Patsy L. Orth Duphorne & Phyllis Lisanti

www.mosby.com/MERLIN/medsurg_lewis

LEARNING OBJECTIVES

1. Define addiction, abuse, craving, loss of control, dependence, tolerance, withdrawal, abstinence, sobriety, detoxification, and relapse.
2. Identify risk factors associated with substance abuse.
3. Describe the process of addiction.
4. List common characteristics of substance abusers.
5. Recognize the effects of use of stimulants, depressants, and hallucinogenic drugs.
6. Describe acute care nursing interventions for patients who experience withdrawal, overdose, or intoxication from stimulants, depressants, or hallucinogens.
7. Describe nursing management of the surgical patient who abuses drugs.
8. Describe the nursing role in primary, secondary, and tertiary prevention activities.
9. Identify health promotion strategies to support drug-free lifestyles that the nurse can use in a variety of settings.
10. Discuss the long-term nursing management of the patient with substance abuse problems.
11. Discuss substance abuse problems of the older adult.
12. Describe signs and symptoms of chemical dependence among nurses.

Individuals who abuse substances typically use the health care system more than non–substance-abusing individuals for both acute and chronic problems. It is estimated that one third of all patients hospitalized have alcohol-related illnesses.[1] One out of every five patients cared for in ambulatory settings is anticipated to have a problem with alcohol.[2] The elderly, women, minorities, and dual-diagnosis patients (having concurrent psychiatric disorder and substance dependence) are predicted to be at a higher risk for substance abuse and related health problems.[3]

Nurses provide care across a continuum of services and are therefore in key positions to identify patients who are abusing or addicted to substances. This chapter addresses the nursing role in identifying and managing the substance-abusing patient in a variety of care settings. Promotion of health and long-term care of the chronic substance abuser are also presented. Special consideration is given to two high-risk groups: the elderly and nurses.

OVERVIEW OF SUBSTANCE ABUSE

Terminology of Substance Abuse

Commonly used terms in the diagnosis and treatment of substance abuse are presented in Table 10-1. These terms are applicable to all abused substances, including those substances intended to be helpful, such as prescribed and over-the-counter medications.

Patterns of Substance Use and Abuse

There are various patterns of substance use and abuse, including a tendency among substance abusers to take a variety of drugs simultaneously or in a sequence to obtain specific effects. Patterns of use generally fall along a continuum ranging from experimental to compulsive use. Although an individual may move back and forth among patterns, compulsive use is indicative of addiction, and only abstinence or a drug-free status can break this pattern (Fig. 10-1).

Risk Factors Associated with Substance Abuse

Although numerous studies have focused on the problem of substance abuse, the cause (or causes) remains unknown or unclear. Substance abuse is a multidimensional phenomenon with a multifactorial etiology. However, a variety of factors can increase an individual's vulnerability or risk for developing problems of substance abuse. Several risk factors are presented in Table 10-2.

Addictive Process

The length of time that passes from casual use to dependence is a function of many factors related to the host (individual), agent (drug), and environment as explained by the public health model (Fig. 10-2). The type of drug, frequency of use, amount of drug used, route of administration, health of the user, and support for drug use (enabling) from friends or family members affect the development of an addiction. The typical progression of drug use begins with cigarettes and alcohol and moves to marijuana, cocaine, hallucinogens, and opiates. Repeated IV use of heroin or cocaine can produce addiction in a few days or weeks, although it generally takes years and heavy periods of drinking to develop an addiction to

Table 10-1 Terminology of Substance Abuse

Term	Definition
▪ Substance	Drug, chemical, or biologic entity that is self-administered.
▪ Habituation	Pattern of repeated drug use in the absence of an actual physical need for the drug. There is no desire for increased use. There may be withdrawal manifestations.
▪ Misuse	Drug used for purposes other than those for which it is intended. Common among people, especially the elderly, who self-medicate for a variety of reasons.
▪ Abuse	Drug use patterns that lie outside the limits acceptable by society and that have a negative impact on psychologic, physiologic, and social functioning of an individual. Drug abuse may be combined with misuse.
▪ Dependence	Reliance on a substance that has reached the level that absence of it will cause an impairment in function.
Psychologic	Compulsive need to experience pleasurable response from the substance.
Physical	Altered physiologic state from prolonged substance use; regular use is necessary to prevent withdrawal.
▪ Tolerance	Decreased effect of a substance that results from repeated exposure. It is possible to develop cross-tolerance to other substances in same category.
▪ Withdrawal	Constellation of physiologic and psychologic responses that occur when there is abrupt cessation or reduced intake of a substance on which an individual is dependent or when the effect is counteracted by a specific antagonist.
▪ Addiction	Compulsive substance use that exists for both physical and psychologic reasons.
Dual	Simultaneous dependence on substances that have similar effects, such as barbiturates and alcohol.
Mixed	Dependence on more than one substance not necessarily similar in effect, such as alcohol and cocaine.
▪ Craving	Subjective need for a substance, usually experienced after decreased use or abstinence.
▪ Loss of control	Inability to quit after just one drink or substance use ("one drink, one drunk"). Substance takes control of person's life.
▪ Abstinence	Refrain from substance use.
▪ Sobriety	Complete abstinence practiced within a balanced, healthy lifestyle.
▪ Detoxification	Process of removing the substance and its effects from the individual's body.
▪ Relapse	Process of readdiction during sobriety.
▪ Binge	Consumptions of large quantities of a substance on occasion to the point of excess.

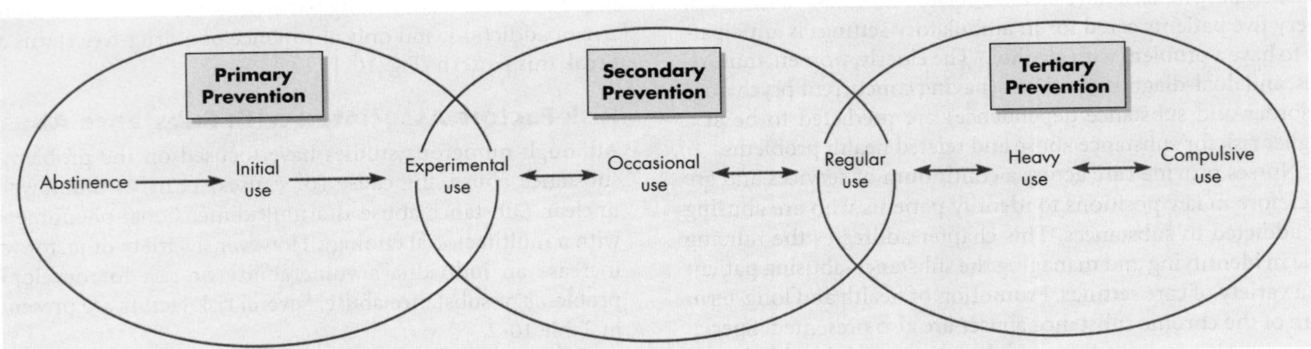

Fig. 10-1 Drug use patterns and prevention framework.

alcohol. The development of alcoholism in women occurs more rapidly than in men (telescoping effect).

The process of addiction may be thought of as a cycle that is self-reinforcing (Fig. 10-3). Interruptions in the cycle occur because of inaccessibility of the substance, decrease in the amount used, attempts to control drug use, or entry into treatment. These factors may precipitate withdrawal symptoms in the physically dependent individual. Substance use may be reinitiated to ward off withdrawal symptoms and leads to rapid reinstatement of the cycle, or relapse.

Characteristics of Substance Abusers

Substance abusers have certain common characteristics that may influence the initiation or maintenance of patterns of abuse and dependence. The nurse should recognize the importance of these features that contribute to the complex problems of addiction. These characteristics include excessive or compulsive use, impulsive behaviors, and low frustration tolerance. Feelings of depression and helplessness are common, along with low self-esteem. Rationalization, denial, projection, and

Table 10-2 Risk Factors Associated with Substance Abuse

Risk Factors	Comments
Availability and encouragement	▪ Advertising campaigns make the use of chemical substances appealing and socially acceptable. ▪ Sedatives and antianxiety agents are prescribed excessively for a variety of reasons.
Adverse social conditions	▪ Poverty, unemployment, discrimination, homelessness, and lack of social and educational opportunities contribute to high rates of substance abuse.
Environmental or biologic factors	▪ Abuse patterns occur in families (e.g., heavy smoking and drinking).
Psychologic influence	▪ Certain personality traits (e.g., low frustration tolerance, risk-taking behavior, impulsivity) may make the development of substance abuse more likely. ▪ Psychodynamic factors, such as anxiety or panic disorders, mood disorders, and personality disorders, are linked with substance abuse.
Disabilities	▪ Physically disabled individuals have higher rates of alcoholism and problems with other substances. ▪ Many individuals with disabilities have low self-esteem, chronic medical problems, and high incidence of depression.
Developmental influence	▪ Individuals who sustain parental loss (through death, divorce, abandonment) may be predisposed to substance abuse problems. ▪ Children of substance-abusing parents are at greater risk for becoming substance abusers.
Cultural influence	▪ Cultural beliefs influence religious rituals and practices that support or inhibit substance use and abuse. ▪ Alcoholism is a major problem among Native-Americans and Alaskan Natives. Hispanics may also have high rates of alcohol abuse. ▪ Type of abuse varies with age, gender, and specific minority subgroup.

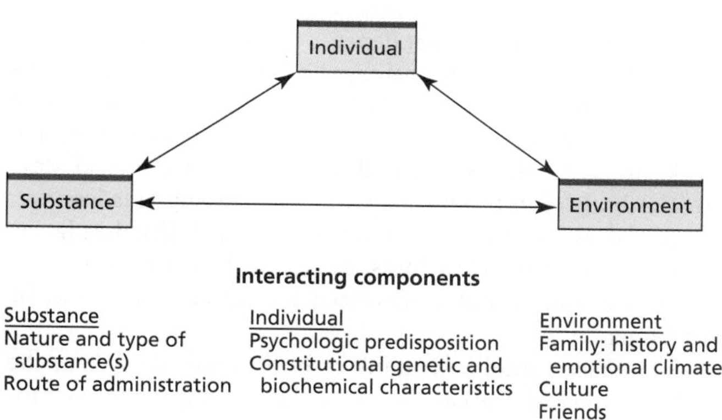

Fig. 10-2 Public health model.

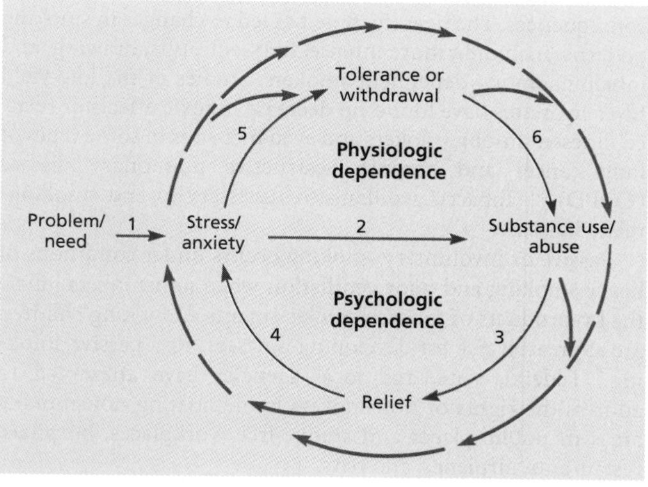

Fig. 10-3 The addictive cycle. *Step 1,* The problem or need arouses stress or anxiety and is dealt with through substance use. *Steps 2 through 4,* The cycle of substance use, relief, and recurring stress or anxiety is repeated until psychologic dependence is established. Interrupting the cycle brings about anxiety but not physical symptoms. *Steps 5 and 6,* Physiologic dependence usually follows psychologic dependence. Withdrawal symptoms follow abstinence. Interruptions in the cycle are indicated by a *broken line.*

manipulation are frequently found. Family dysfunction and lack of social support are also common.

STIMULANTS

While the two most frequently used stimulants are nicotine and caffeine, amphetamines and cocaine are the stimulants that lead to the most serious types of abuse. The most potent stimulant of natural origin is cocaine.

Nicotine (Tobacco Abuse)

Characteristics

Nicotine, an alkaloid found in tobacco, is the component of tobacco that causes dependence. Nicotine dependence is the most common form of chemical dependence in the United States. It is particularly prevalent among alcoholics and other drug users.[4]

Cigarette smoking is the predominant form of tobacco abuse in the United States, involving over 25% of the adult population.[5] Smokeless tobacco, popular with young people, includes chewing a plug of tobacco or snuffing tobacco powder intranasally. Because a greater number of harmful substances

MYTHS ABOUT SUBSTANCE ABUSE

Myths	Truths
Narcotic users are sociopaths who frequently commit murder, rape, and other crimes of violence while under the influence of drugs.	Narcotic users, alone or in groups, prefer a quiet, secluded place where they can enjoy the drugs' effects in peace and quiet.
Narcotic parties are characterized by highly stimulating sexual activities.	Narcotics reduce sexual drives.
Drug addicts are easily distinguished from other people by their appearance and behavior.	It is often difficult for police and medical experts to identify a user without specific medical tests or interviews.
Professional pushers hang around schools and street corners waiting to introduce innocent victims to narcotics.	Individuals are generally introduced to the use of narcotics through their friends.
Marijuana use inevitably leads to physical dependence.	Marijuana does not usually produce physical dependence; it can lead to emotional dependence, which can be equally habit forming.
Users can control casual use of narcotics without becoming dependent.	No one can predict at which point an individual can or will lose control. The occasional user is highly vulnerable to becoming addicted.
Beer drinkers do not become alcoholics. Only people who drink "hard" liquor become alcoholics.	Any form of alcohol, if frequently consumed in large quantities over a period of years, may lead to alcoholism.

are released during the smoking process, more attention has been focused on cigarette smoking.

The only "safe" cigarette is no cigarette. The low-yield filter cigarette is an attempt to produce a "safe" cigarette that reduces tar and nicotine levels to decrease its toxic effects and health consequences. The new cigarette has led to changes in smoking patterns, including more intense, frequent puffs, drawing, and inhaling, among dependent smokers. Studies of the low-yield filter cigarettes have found no decrease in toxic effects or related illnesses among smokers and even increases in some types of lung cancer and chronic obstructive pulmonary disease (COPD).[6,7] Tobacco avoidance is necessary to end smoking-related disease.

Passive or involuntary smoking occurs under conditions of heavy smoking and poor ventilation when nonsmokers inhale the by-products of tobacco smoke. Infants and young children are at greatest risk for developing illnesses from passive smoking.[8] Federal, state, and local agencies have attempted to address the rights of nonsmokers by mandating nonsmoking areas in public places and smoke-free workplaces, hospitals, restaurants, airplanes, and bars.

Effects of Use

Smoking is a powerful self-reinforcing behavior that decreases stress and tension. Tobacco contains more than 100 known chemical compounds, including at least 15 known carcinogens and a number of hydrocarbons or solvents that may cause death. Three of the most damaging substances are nicotine, carbon monoxide, and tar.

Nicotine is a mild stimulant that has no therapeutic value. It has a unique biphasic effect on the peripheral and central nervous systems. It initially acts as a stimulant, followed by a depressant effect, which may be associated with fatigue. The amount or dose of nicotine varies with the form and method of ingestion. In general, cigarettes contain about 1 mg of nicotine.[8] The effects of nicotine appear to be dose related. Nicotine is absorbed through the lungs in smoking, through the buccal mucosa in chewing, and through the nasal mucosa in snuffing. When taken by these routes, nicotine initially bypasses the liver and goes directly to the brain and other parts of the body. The effects of smoking are listed in Table 10-3.

The strong psychologic dependency associated with nicotine use is supported by the fact that it acts on the brain within seconds. Physiologic dependence occurs with regular heavy use and is evidenced by increased tolerance and withdrawal symptoms following attempts to stop smoking. Withdrawal symptoms may occur within the first few hours after stopping, peak in 24 to 48 hours, and may last from several days to a month. Symptoms may include craving, restlessness, decreased ability to concentrate, hyperirritability, headache, insomnia, anxiety, drowsiness, decreased blood pressure and heart rate, and an initial increased appetite that may not be permanent.

All tobacco smoke contains carbon monoxide. When the smoke is inhaled, the carbon monoxide combines with hemoglobin and prevents the hemoglobin from carrying oxygen, which may explain the smoker's shortness of breath during exertion.

Tar contains several hundred chemicals, some of which are carcinogenic. The small particles of tar are trapped inside the lung where they damage the tissue. Tar is considered a major contributor to cardiovascular diseases, COPD, and lung cancer.[7]

Complications

A major concern related to smoking involves accidental death resulting from fires caused by carelessness, especially smoking in bed. Smoking predisposes a person to respiratory disease (especially COPD), cardiovascular disease, and increased incidence of cancer of the lungs, urinary bladder, prostate, and pancreas. Upper respiratory tract cancers (mouth, larynx, esophagus) are associated with an increased incidence of mortality for pipe and cigar smokers along with cigarette smokers.[8] The risk of myocardial infarction is higher among women who smoke than among men who smoke.[9] Nicotine abuse contributes to delayed wound healing, reproductive disorders, peptic ulcer disease, and gastroesophageal reflux.[10,11,12]

Table 10-3 Effects of Smoking (Nicotine Related)*

Raised arousal level
Decreased attention to extraneous stimuli
Decreased muscle tone
Stress reduction
Performance enhancement
Fine tremor (nicotine tremor)
Shortness of breath
Decreased appetite
Antidiuretic effect
Decreased aggressiveness
Increased gastrointestinal motility

*Found in varying degrees in nicotine users.

Table 10-4 Effects of Caffeine*

Increased alertness and thinking
Increased respirations
Relaxation of smooth visceral muscles
Decreased peristalsis
Possible interference with REM and deep sleep
Increased speed of motor tasks
Increased force of myocardial contraction
Increased heart rate
Diuresis
Jitteriness
Nervousness
Gastrointestinal upset

REM, rapid eye movement.
*Found in varying degrees in caffeine users.

Collaborative Care

Pharmacologic aids to control symptoms of nicotine withdrawal include nicotine gum (Nicorette), a nicotine transdermal system or patches (Habitrol, Nicoderm, Prostep), nasal spray, nicotine inhalers, and clonidine (Catapres) to suppress craving. Bupropion (Zyban), an antidepressant, has been approved as a smoking cessation aid. It is the first non-nicotine product and is particularly appealing to individuals who object to using nicotine-based products to quit smoking.

A combination of medications, behavioral approaches, and support is believed to be most effective in long-term smoking cessation.[5] Formal or community-based behavioral smoking cessation programs that promote alternative tension-relieving and leisure activities are valuable aids to the nicotine-dependent person. (Patient teaching guide for smoking cessation is presented in Table 26-19).

Caffeine Abuse

Characteristics

Caffeine use is integral to the American culture and is the most widely consumed psychoactive agent in the world.[13] As a result of mass marketing, coffee is promoted for use to wake up in the morning and to enhance work performance during the day. Although its acceptance as a social drug implies that it has few negative effects on health, caffeine has many significant physiologic effects.

One cup of coffee contains approximately 100 to 150 mg of caffeine, which is considered a therapeutic dose. The content of caffeine in tea varies according to how it is brewed. A cup of tea averages 60 to 75 mg caffeine, and a glass of cola averages 40 to 60 mg caffeine. Brewed coffee contains the highest level of caffeine. Decaffeinated coffee, tea, and cola drinks have become more popular, which indicates that caffeine may not be necessary to maintain consumption of these drinks.[8]

Caffeine is a xanthine derivative that occurs naturally in a number of plants such as coffee beans, tea leaves, cocoa, and cola nuts. It is also found in medications such as No Doz, Vivarin, Excedrin, Vanquish, Anacin, Bromo-Seltzer, cold preparations, appetite suppressants, and some prescription medications.

Effects of Use

Caffeine is one of the most widely used stimulant drugs. It is a relatively weak CNS stimulant. It is a diuretic and a myocardial stimulant, relaxes smooth muscles, promotes vasodilation, constricts cerebral arteries, and enhances contraction of skeletal muscles. Caffeine is absorbed by the gastrointestinal (GI) tract and is rapidly distributed throughout the body. Peak blood plasma levels occur within 30 minutes after ingestion. Stimulant effects may last from 3 to 5 hours.

The effects of caffeine are listed in Table 10-4. Some of the physiologic actions help explain caffeine's effectiveness in increasing work output and prolonging the time one can perform physically exhausting work. The effects of caffeine are dose related. Oral doses of 200 mg (two cups of coffee) can elevate mood, produce insomnia, increase irritability, cause anxiety, and offset fatigue. Heavy doses of 500 mg or more are known to cause tachycardia and respiratory stimulation. Ingestion of a lethal dose is extremely rare but could occur with caffeine-containing drugs or the oral ingestion of 10 g (70 to 100 cups of coffee).

Caffeine interferes with sleep by increasing sleep onset time, decreasing dreaming (rapid eye movement [REM]) sleep, and decreasing deep sleep time. Coffee taken in the evening is more likely to have adverse effects on light users than on regular or heavy users (five to six cups or more per day). Coffee taken in the morning by regular or heavy users is required to avoid morning tiredness and irritability.

Tolerance to caffeine's stimulant effects develops slowly but may be overcome by increasing the amount consumed. Physical and psychologic dependence have been found with chronic heavy use (more than five cups per day). The most common and best-substantiated withdrawal symptoms are headache, irritability, and nervousness. They occur within 12 to 24 hours, peak at 20 to 48 hours, and last for about 1 week. Other effects of withdrawal include sleepiness and feelings of decreased contentment that may be mistaken for depression.

Complications

Caffeine is contraindicated in the patient with glaucoma. It can significantly raise the intraocular pressure when the glaucoma is uncontrolled, resulting in a caffeine-induced headache. It is thought that caffeine withdrawal could account for many of the cases of headaches that occur following general anesthesia.[13]

Toxic effects of caffeine include ringing in the ears, flashes of light, insomnia, increased sensitivity, tachycardia, and arrhythmias. In heavy coffee drinkers, blood lipid levels may be increased, which may lead to an increased incidence of angina and myocardial infarction. Habitual users are reported to have slightly higher blood pressure, increased basal metabolic rates, and increased blood glucose levels. In high doses, caffeine influences behavior patterns and may precipitate anxiety states. In susceptible individuals, lower doses of caffeine may result in tachycardia, tremors, and rebound hypoglycemia.

Amphetamines

Characteristics

Amphetamines, developed in the 1930s as a substitute for ephedrine, were found to be potent bronchodilators and useful in asthma. Amphetamines have been found to be effective in the treatment of narcolepsy. The amphetamine group includes amphetamine (Benzedrine), dextroamphetamine (Dexedrine), and methamphetamine (Desoxyn), also known as "speed" or "ice" (pure form). Phenmetrazine (Preludin) and methylphenidate (Ritalin) are also stimulants that may be abused. Other drugs in this category are benzphetamine (Didrex), diethylpropion (Tenuate), fenfluramine (Pondimin), mazindol (Sanorex), phendimetrazine (Anorex, Adphen), and phentermine (Fastin, Ionamin), which are used as anorectic drugs. Currently, methylphenidate is primarily used in the treatment of attention-deficit disorders in children, and phenmetrazine is used as an appetite suppressant. Fenfluramine and dexfenfluramine (Redux) have been withdrawn from the U.S. market because of increased risk of valvular heart disease. (These drugs are discussed in Chapter 38.)

As amphetamine use has become more tightly controlled through prescriptions, "look-alike" pills that are identical in appearance and illicit methamphetamine (e.g., "crank," "crystal") have been illegally produced.

Effects of Use

Amphetamines act primarily by stimulating the central and peripheral nervous systems and the cardiovascular system. Manifestations initially begin with feelings of euphoria and excitement and continue with effects on the cardiovascular and respiratory systems. These drugs result in excess catecholamine release that leads to a "fight or flight" reaction.

The primary effects of stimulants are listed in Table 10-5. Initial use results in increased alertness or concentration, improved performance, relief of fatigue, or weight control. The user comes to rely on the euphoric effects and the feeling of power. With continued use these drugs may also lead to unpleasant feelings of irritability, fear, and anxiety. Chronic consumption may lead to stereotyped behavior, paranoia, and possible aggression and sudden violent outbursts. Compulsive use often leads to decreased sleep and eating and exhaustion when the individual "crashes" (suddenly falling asleep after heavy use) or experiences withdrawal symptoms.[8]

Amphetamines are primarily taken orally; peak effects occur within 2 to 3 hours with complete elimination occurring within 2 days. Effects are generally intensified by inhaling (smoking) or IV injection of the drug, which produces a "rush" or "flash," an almost immediate, intense burst of energy. A "run" is similar to a binge when large doses of a drug are smoked or injected over a prolonged period.[8]

Complications

Toxic reactions to stimulants are usually dose related and include increased levels of stimulation, sometimes described as "overamping," which may culminate in paranoia, severe brain damage, massive overdose, and death (Table 10-6, p. 163). Without medical intervention, death may occur as a result of seizures, cardiovascular collapse, hyperthermia, and cerebral hemorrhage.

Collaborative Care

Patients generally seek treatment for complications such as panic reactions or temporary psychosis related to intoxication, overdose, or withdrawal. Intoxication is a reversible substance-specific syndrome resulting from the ingestion of or exposure to a substance. Overdose has also been termed *acute poisoning* or *toxicity*. Emergency management of drug overdose is presented in Table 10-7 on p. 164.

Drugs that may be helpful during withdrawal of amphetamines include dopaminergic agents, including amantadine (Symadine), bromocriptine (Parlodel), and levodopa (L-Dopa) to decrease craving; neuroleptics or some benzodiazepines to relieve "crash" symptoms; and antidepressants, such as desipramine (Norpramin), imipramine (Tofranil), and trazodone (Desyrel), to prevent relapse.

Cocaine

Characteristics

Cocaine is an extract of the leaves of the coca plant. It is now the most abused major stimulant in the United States and Canada. "Crack," a cocaine alkaloid that gets its name from the popping sound the crystals make when heated, is also popular because it is inexpensive, readily available, easy to use, and has an increased purity over cocaine.

Effects of Use

Cocaine is a potent stimulant of the central and peripheral nervous, cardiovascular, and respiratory systems and has potentially fatal effects[14] (Table 10-8, p. 164). The most common route of administration is intranasal, although it may be used parenterally, orally, vaginally, sublingually, and rectally; it may also be smoked. The most rapid routes of administration are IV and inhalation. When taken IV or inhaled, cocaine's effects are felt within 1 minute and last about 20 minutes.

Addiction can develop from any route of administration. Collapse and scarring of the veins at the injection site may occur as a result of "shooting up" (See Fig. 10-4, p. 165). With intranasal use, the nasal septum and mucosa may be damaged, leading to nasal sores, decreased smell, chronic sinusitis, perforation, and collapse of the nose or septal necrosis. Cocaine "runny nose" or chronic rhinitis is common with long-term intranasal use. Frequent sniffing and increased susceptibility to upper respiratory infections are common symptoms of cocaine abuse.[15]

Users who experience personality changes are described as being "coked out." Anxiety, restlessness, and extreme irritability may signal the onset of a toxic psychosis. Cocaine psychosis is characterized by tactile hallucinations of bugs crawling under the skin and scratches on the arms, legs, or chest, which may indicate attempts to dig out the bugs, or visual hallucinations of bright lights or "snow lights." This psychosis is shorter in duration than the psychosis observed with amphetamine abuse.

Crack in the form of chips, chunks, or rocks is the most potent form of the drug and produces the most dramatic "high" and the most rapid addiction. Because crack is inhaled, it is absorbed more rapidly (2 to 3 seconds) as a result of the larger

Table 10-5 **Effects of Frequently Abused Substances**

Substance	Street Names	Effects	Length of Effects
Stimulants			
Amphetamine (Benzedrine)	Bennie, uppers	Euphoria, mood swings, hyperactivity, hyperalertness, anorexia, insomnia, hypertension, tachycardia, tremor, restlessness, arrhythmias, seizures, sexual arousal, dilated pupils, diaphoresis	Onset: route related; 10-30 min (nicotine: immediate) Duration: drug related (caffeine: 3-7 hr; nicotine: 5-15 min)
Chlorphentermine (Pre-sate)			
Dextroamphetamine (Dexedrine)	Dexies, speed, crystal, meth		
Methamphetamine (Desoxyn)			
Methylphenidate (Ritalin)			
Phenmetrazine (Preludin)			
Cocaine	Coke, snow, flake, rock, superblow, topot		
Caffeine			
Nicotine			
Depressants			
Alcohol		Initial euphoria, decreased inhibitions, drowsiness, lack of coordination, impaired judgment, slurred speech, hypotension, bradycardia, bradypnea, emotional lability, decreased urinary output, constricted pupils	Onset: route related; 30-40 min (alcohol: 20 min-1 hr) Duration: 4-5 hr
Barbiturates	Barbs, goofballs		
Secobarbital (Seconal)	Red devil, seggy		
Phenobarbital (Luminal)	Phennie		
Pentobarbital (Nembutal)	Yellow jacket, nembies		
Amobarbital (Amytal)	Blue devil, blue bird		
Methaqualone (Quaalude)	Ludes, wallbangers		
Chloral hydrate (Noctec)	Peter, Mickey Finn		
Meprobamate (Miltown, Equanil)			
Diazepam (Valium)			
Chlordiazepoxide (Librium)	Roaches, Tranqs		
Narcotics			
Heroin	Horse, junk, H. brown, scat M, microdots, poppy, tar, black smack	Analgesia, drowsiness ("nod out"), relaxation, constricted pupils, constipation, nausea, slurred speech, impaired judgment, decreased sexual and aggressive drives, hypertension, euphoria/detachment	Onset: 20-30 min Duration: 4-8 hr
Morphine			
Opium			
Codeine			
Meperidine (Demerol)			
Hydromorphone (Dilaudid)	Pinks and grays		
Propoxyphene (Darvon)			
Pentazocine (Talwin)			
Oxycodone (Percodan)			
Methadone (Dolophine)	Dollies		
Hallucinogens			
Lysergic acid diethylamide (LSD)	Acid, cube D, window pane sugar, sunshine, blue dots	Perceptual distortions, hallucinations, delusions (PCP), depersonalization, heightened sensory perception, euphoria, mood swings, suspiciousness, panic, impaired judgment, increased body temperature, hypertension, flushed face, tremor, dilated pupils, constricted pupils (PCP), nystagmus (PCP), violence (PCP)	Onset: 40-60 min (PCP 2-3 min) Duration: 6-12 hr
Psilocybin (mushrooms)	Shroom, magic (exotic) mushroom		
Dimethyltryptamine (DMT)			
Diethyltryptamine (DET)			
3,4-Methylendioxyamphetamine (MDA)	Love drug, ecstasy		
Mescaline (peyote)	Cactus, mescal, button		
Pencyclidine (PCP)	Angel dust, hog, peace pill, rocket fluid		

Continued

Table 10-5 Effects of Frequently Abused Substances—cont'd

Substance	Street Names	Effects	Length of Effects
Cannabis			
Marijuana	Pot, reefer, grass, weed	Relaxation, euphoria, amotivation, slowed time sensation, sexual arousal, abrupt mood changes, impaired memory and attention, impaired judgment, reddened eyes, dry mouth, lack of coordination, tachycardia, increased appetite	Onset: 20-30 min Duration: 3-7 hr
Hashish	Hash, rope		
Inhalants			
Aerosol propellants Fluorinated hydrocarbons Nitrous oxide (in deodorants, hair spray, pesticide, whipped cream spray, spray paint, cookware coating products) Solvents Gasoline, kerosene, nail polish remover, typewriter correction fluid, cleaning solutions, lighter fluid, paint, paint thinner, glue Anesthetic agents Nitrous oxide, chloroform		Euphoria, decreased inhibitions, giddiness, slurred speech, illusions, drowsiness, clouded sensorium, tinnitis, nystagmus, arrhythmias, cough, nausea, vomiting, diarrhea, irritation to eyes, nose, mouth	Onset: immediate Duration: 20-45 min

surface area in the lungs compared with that of the nasal mucosa. Consequently, crack produces a more intense effect and withdrawal. Pulmonary damage from smoking crack may be evident with black or dark brown sputum.[15]

Frequently users consume both alcohol and cocaine. Cocaethylene is a metabolite of concurrent cocaine and alcohol use. Alcohol boosts and prolongs the euphoria produced by cocaine while decreasing the paranoia and agitation. It is considered one of the most dangerous combinations because it increases the risk of liver injury and sudden death.[16]

Complications

Complications are directly related to the route of administration, type of cocaine, dose, and individual vulnerabilities. They may include cellulitis, wound abscess, hepatitis, HIV infection, seizures, myocardial ischemia and infarction, cardiac arrhythmias, sudden cardiac death, acute renal failure, acute respiratory distress, pulmonary edema, asthma, and bilateral loss of eyebrow and eyelash hair (from inhalation of hot vapors). "Crack lung," which manifests as pneumonia without supporting x-ray findings, has recently been reported.[17]

Acute cocaine toxicity may be manifested by forceful cardiac palpitations with feelings of impending doom, tachycardia, hypertension, myocardial ischemia or infarction, rhabdomyolysis (muscle wasting), seizures, agitated delirium, hallucinations, confusion, paranoia, aggressive behavior, electrolyte imbalances, and fever (see Table 10-6). An overdose is an exaggerated version of the classic physical and psychologic response to cocaine use. In severe cocaine intoxication, termed *Casey Jones reaction,* the patient progresses rapidly through stages of stimulation and depression, which may result in death.[15] There is no margin of safety with the use of cocaine, and there is no antidote for toxicity.

Overdose occurs more frequently with IV use, smoking "freebase," or "body packing." Freebasing is the process of extracting the alkaloid form from cocaine hydrochloride, producing crack and rock. Freebase can be smoked in a cigarette with tobacco or heated and inhaled through a water pipe. Body packing is a form of smuggling packets of cocaine in the intestines. If the packets burst, a toxic reaction and death occur unless immediate medical intervention is available.

Collaborative Care

Cocaine abuse and dependence have become growing concerns in emergency departments and drug treatment programs. The picture of the addict may be complicated by the cocaine abuser's frequent use of alcohol, marijuana, or heroin. Cocaine combined with heroin is termed *speedball,* and cocaine combined with phencyclidine hydrochloride (PCP) is termed *space base.*

Emergency management of cocaine intoxication is presented in Table 10-9. Emergency management of overdose is presented in Table 10-7.

An individual who is addicted to cocaine usually does not initially seek treatment for drug abuse but rather for problems with sleep, appetite, depression, sinusitis, respiratory infections, chest pain, or migraine-like headaches. Specific clues that should alert the nurse to cocaine abuse or dependence are included in Table 10-8.

Engaging an individual who is addicted to cocaine in treatment is difficult because of the intense craving for the drug and a strong denial that cocaine is addicting or that the individual

Table 10-6 **Signs and Symptoms of Overdose and Withdrawal of Abused Substances**

Substance Category	Overdose	Withdrawal
Stimulants		
Cocaine, amphetamines, methylpenidate, phenmetrazine, chlorphentermine,dextroamphetamine, caffeine, nicotine	Agitation Increased temperature, pulse, respiratory rate, blood pressure Cardiac arrhythmias Myocardial infarction Hallucinations Seizures Possible death	Severely depressed mood Prolonged sleep Apathy Irritability Disorientation Anxiety
Depressants		
Alcohol, barbiturates, benzodiazepines, methaqualone, chloral hydrate, meprobamate	Shallow respirations Cold, clammy skin Weak, rapid pulse Constricted pupils Hyporeflexia Coma Possible death	Anxiety Agitation Insomnia Diaphoresis Tremors Delirium Seizures Possible death
Narcotics		
Opium, morphine, codeine, heroin, methadone, oxycodone, meperidine, hydromorphone, propoxyphene, pentazocine	Slow, shallow respirations Hypotension Clammy skin Constricted pupils Coma Possible death	Watery eyes Dilated pupils Runny nose Yawning Loss of appetite Tremors Panic Chills, fever, diaphoresis Cramps Nausea, vomiting, diarrhea Achiness Piloerection
Hallucinogens		
LSD, psilocybin, mescaline, amphetamine variants, phencyclidine	More prolonged episodes possibly resembling psychotic states Panic Agitation Anxiety Self-destructive behavior Flashbacks	None
Cannabis		
Marijuana, hashish, tetrahydrocannabinol	Fatigue Paranoia Anxiety Confusion Hallucinations	None except for rare syndrome Insomnia Hyperactivity
Inhalants		
Glues, aerosols, cleaning solutions, nail polish removers, lighter fluids, paint, paint thinners, gasoline, halothane, nitrous oxide, amyl nitrite, butyl nitrite	Anxiety Blurred vision Excessive tearing Nasal secretions Nausea, vomiting, diarrhea Loss of appetite Chest pain Seizures Depressed repiration Cardiac arrhythmias Sudden death	None

cannot control it. Often various forms of leverage such as family threats, loss of job or professional license, legal action, or major health consequences provide sufficient motivation for an individual to enter a treatment program.

DEPRESSANTS

Drugs categorized as depressants have common psychologic effects and the ability to produce sedation and other major depressant effects. Drugs in this category include sedative-hypnotics, alcohol, and opioid narcotics.

With the exception of alcohol and some federally regulated drugs, most CNS depressants are medically useful. They can be used for relief of anxiety, insomnia, pain, symptoms of withdrawal from alcohol, or as antiseizure or anesthetic agents. These drugs are also widely recognized for their abuse potential, which leads to rapid tolerance, dependence, and medical emergencies involving overdoses and withdrawal.

Alcohol is a major depressant and the most widely used substance in this category. It is frequently used in combination with barbiturates or benzodiazepines, as well as with stimulants

+EMERGENCY MANAGEMENT

Table 10-7 Drug Overdose

Etiology	Assessment Findings	Interventions
Ingestion, inhalation, or injection of drugs—accidental or intentional	▪ Aggressive behavior ▪ Agitation ▪ Confusion ▪ Lethargy ▪ Stupor ▪ Hallucinations ▪ Depression ▪ Slurred speech ▪ Pinpoint pupils ▪ Nystagmus ▪ Seizures ▪ Needle tracks ▪ Cold, clammy skin ▪ Rapid, weak pulse ▪ Slow or rapid shallow respirations ▪ Decreased O_2 saturation ▪ Hypotension ▪ Arrhythmia ▪ ECG changes ▪ Cardiac or respiratory arrest	**Initial** ▪ Ensure patent airway. ▪ Anticipate intubation if respiratory distress evident. ▪ Establish IV access. ▪ Obtain temperature. ▪ Obtain 12-lead ECG. ▪ Obtain information about substance (e.g., name, route, when taken, amount). ▪ Obtain specific drug levels or comprehensive toxicology screen. ▪ Obtain a health history including drug use and allergies. ▪ Administer antidotes as appropriate. ▪ Perform gastric lavage if necessary. ▪ Administer activated charcoal and cathartics as appropriate. **Ongoing** ▪ Monitor vital signs, temperature, level of consciousness, O_2 saturation, cardiac rhythm.

Table 10-8 Effects of Cocaine Use

	Early Effects	Long-term Effects
Central nervous system	Excitation, euphoria, restlessness, talkativeness	Depression, hallucinations, tremors, visual disturbances, dysarthria, seizure activity, headaches, insomnia, stroke
Cardiovascular system	Tachycardia, hypertension, angina, arrhythmias, palpitations	Ventricular arrhythmias, hypotension, congestive heart failure, myocardial infarction, cardiomyopathy
Respiratory system	Increased respiratory rate, dyspnea, chest pain, epistaxis	Chronic cough, inflamed throat, congestion of lungs, brown or black sputum production, pneumonia, respiratory distress or arrest, pulmonary edema, rhinorrhea, rhinitis, erosion and perforation of the nasal septum
Reproductive system	Heightened sexual desire, delayed orgasm and ejaculation; women may have difficulty achieving orgasm	Difficulty in maintaining erection and ejaculation, loss of interest in sexual activity; women may develop abnormal sexual behavior
Gastrointestinal system	Decreased appetite	Dehydration, weight loss, nausea, intestinal ischemia may cause gangrene
Psychologic	Behavior changes or mood swings	Depression or suicidal thoughts

and hallucinogens. Depressants have been used frequently with stimulants to produce an "upper-downer" effect or to "mellow out" the effect of stimulants.

Sedative-Hypnotics

Characteristics

Chloral hydrate and paraldehyde were two of the earliest drugs in this category used for their sedating effects. They were generally replaced when barbiturates were introduced. The barbiturates are frequently responsible for accidental overdoses and are often used to commit suicide, especially in combination with alcohol. Benzodiazepines are considered more selective as antianxiety agents with less drowsiness and a larger margin of safety than the barbiturates. Chlordiazepoxide (Librium), diazepam (Valium), and alprazolam (Xanax) have been the most commonly used benzodiazepines.

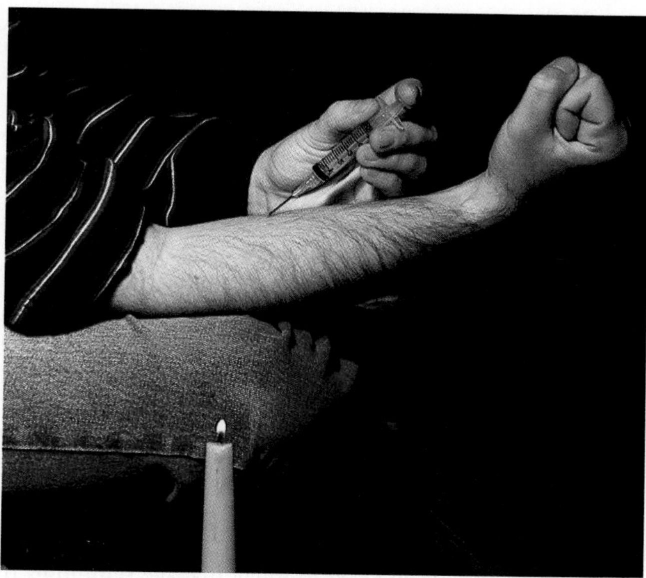

Fig. 10-4 Shooting up. Sharing needles and syringes and other contaminated "works" has increased the spread of human immunodeficiency virus and hepatitis B and C.

Two patterns of abuse and dependence have been recognized with sedative-hypnotic drugs. The first pattern begins with prescription use of the drug for the treatment of anxiety or insomnia. Subsequently, the patient may become tolerant to the effects and increase the dose and frequency of use without medical advice or indication. The second and more common pattern involves illegal sources, which often begins with intermittent use by teenagers or young adults at parties and leads to daily use to achieve sedation.

Effects of Use

Sedative-hypnotic drugs act primarily on the central nervous system (CNS) by depressing cardiac and respiratory function (see Table 10-5). They are largely metabolized in the liver and excreted in the urine. The effects of this group of drugs are dose related. With low doses, sedation and calming effects occur; with high doses, they act as hypnotics, and sleep is induced. They decrease the time needed to fall asleep and increase total sleep time but decrease the amount of REM sleep or dream sleep. Excessive amounts produce an initial euphoria and a state of intoxication similar to alcohol intoxication, including impaired judgment, slurred speech, and loss of motor coordination.

Tolerance develops rapidly with a narrow margin of safety between intoxicating effects and lethal dose. Tolerance develops

+EMERGENCY MANAGEMENT

Table 10-9 Cocaine Toxicity

Etiology	Assessment Findings	Interventions
Intranasal, inhalation, parenteral, oral, vaginal, rectal, or sublingual administration of cocaine	**Cardiovascular** ▪ Palpitations ▪ Tachycardia ▪ Hypertension ▪ Arrhythmias ▪ Myocardial ischemia or infarction **Central Nervous System** ▪ Feeling of impending doom ▪ Euphoria ▪ Agitation ▪ Combativeness ▪ Seizures ▪ Hallucinations ▪ Confusion ▪ Paranoia ▪ Fever **Other** ▪ Track marks ▪ Consumption of bags of cocaine	**Initial** ▪ Ensure patent airway ▪ Anticipate need for intubation if respiratory distress evident ▪ Establish IV access and initiate fluid replacement as appropriate ▪ Obtain 12-lead ECG ▪ Treat ventricular arrhythmias as appropriate with lidocaine, bretylium, or procainamide (Pronestyl) ▪ Administer haloperidol IV for psychosis ▪ Administer diazepam (Valium) or lorazepam (Ativan) IV for seizures ▪ Naloxone IV should be given if CNS depression is present and concurrent opiate use is suspected ▪ Anticipate the need for propranolol (Inderal) or labetalol for hypertension and tachycardia **Ongoing** ▪ Monitor vital signs, level of consciousness, cardiac rhythm ▪ Use restraints only if needed to protect the patient and staff

RESEARCH

IMPLICATIONS FOR NURSING PRACTICE

Informal vs. Formal Reporting of Nurses Suspected of Substance Abuse

Citation Hood JC, Duphorne PL: To report or not to report: nurses' attitudes toward reporting co-workers suspected of substance abuse, *J Drug Issues* 25:313, 1995.

Purpose To examine the effects of moralistic attitudes, knowledge of a diversion program, gender, type of license (RN/LPN), years in nursing, and managerial status on the choice of formal or informal reporting strategies when confronted with substance-abusing co-workers.

Methods Survey data using a stratified, random sample of male and female RNs and LPNs ($n = 498$) were collected 2 years after a diversion program for substance-abusing nurses was established. Data from the questionnaires were analyzed to test three explanatory models and interrelationships among different factors and reporting measures. A combination of analysis of variance, multiple regression, and logistic regression was done to analyze the data and interpret the findings.

Results and Conclusions The best predictors of reporting measures are years in nursing, working alone, and beliefs about what will happen to the co-worker. The longer nurses have been on the job, the more willing they are to use formal reporting measures. Nurses who have not been in positions long, are male, or work alone are more vulnerable and tend to avoid formal reporting, which follows the vulnerability model. The nurse administrator's desire to maintain control over the workplace and handle problems internally and informally was supported by the occupational hegemony model. Nurses who believed that the reported worker would be punished were generally more reluctant to use formal measures of reporting, which supports the diffusion model.

Implications for Nursing Practice Nurses' beliefs and moralistic attitudes, lack of knowledge about programs and resources for substance-abusing co-workers, and experiences with other substance abusers may be barriers in helping other nurses with substance abuse problems. Nurses must be aware of these factors, gain knowledge about diversion programs and resources, and recognize their own workplace position and vulnerability. Nurses need to know how the occupational culture handles problems informally in their workplace setting and when formal reporting measures must be used.

to the sedative effects, requiring higher doses to achieve euphoria. The tolerance may not develop to the brainstem-depressant effects, so an increased dose may trigger hypotension and respiratory depression, resulting in death.

The benzodiazepines affect the limbic system and decrease anxiety without producing sedation at low doses. Although they are believed to have a wide margin of safety, they are not without adverse reactions, including rebound anxiety and insomnia with short-acting drugs and confusion and memory loss with long-acting drugs.

Complications

The symptoms of mild to moderate overdose are listed in Table 10-6. Manifestations of withdrawal from benzodiazepines include nausea and vomiting, muscle cramps, diaphoresis, increased sensitivity to light and sound, anxiety, dysphoria, tachycardia, hypertension, seizures, and coarse tremors of the hands, tongue, and eyelids. The withdrawal syndrome may be a medical emergency, because it may progress from minor symptoms within the first 24 hours and lead to convulsions, delirium, psychoses, and respiratory and cardiac arrest. Symptoms of major withdrawal peak on the second or third day for short-acting barbiturates, benzodiazepines, and meprobamate (Equanil) and on the seventh or eighth day for long-acting drugs.

Collaborative Care

There are no known antagonists to counteract the effects of these drugs. Emergency life support measures must be taken in cases of overdose. In addition to the symptoms associated with overdose and withdrawal, there can be complications associated with the route of administration. These may include cellulitis, vascular complications, hepatitis B and C, endocarditis, pneumonia, bacterial infections, and human immunodeficiency virus (HIV) infection. Treatment of a drug-dependent individual must include a gradual withdrawal of the drug. Most individuals who have been abusing large amounts of these drugs need to be hospitalized to safely manage symptoms of withdrawal.

Alcohol

Characteristics

Millions of people worldwide are dependent on alcohol (Fig. 10-5). The degree of dependence varies, but all either feel that they have to drink or have a physical need to do so. It is estimated that 65% to 70% of Americans use alcohol, and that more than 10 million are alcohol dependent.[2] Additionally, 10 million more Americans are subject to the negative consequences of alcohol abuse, including automobile accidents, arrests, violence, occupational injuries, and negative effects on job performances.[2] Almost one half of all fatal motor vehicle accidents are alcohol related, and as many as 37% of all emergency department trauma admissions involve alcohol use. These dramatic statistics indicate that the nurse must become knowledgeable about the acute and chronic effects of alcohol use and be able to recognize the subtle cues of alcohol abuse.

Alcoholism is currently viewed as a chronic, progressive, potentially fatal disease if left untreated. Numerous factors appear to be interrelated in the development of alcohol abuse. Currently, there are no clearcut explanations for its development. Alcohol dependence may be related to a combination of risk factors, including genetic and biologic factors, psychosocial factors, and cultural-environmental background (see Table 10-2).

There are several patterns of alcohol abuse and dependence: (1) large amounts daily, (2) large amounts on weekends, and (3) binge drinking for weeks or months with periods

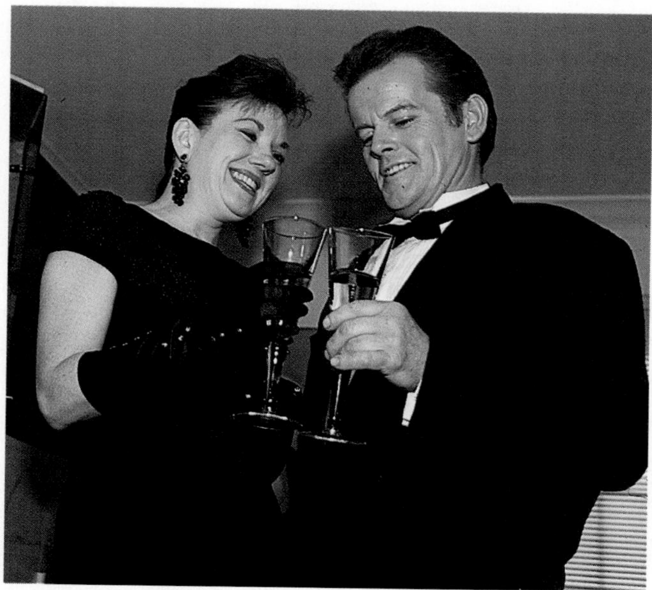

Fig. 10-5 Alcohol abuse is not easy to identify in our society.

of sobriety. Alcohol dependence generally occurs over a period of years and may be preceded by heavy social drinking and progress to abuse. Alcohol is frequently used by individuals with bipolar disorders or schizophrenia to self-medicate. This may result in the patient having a dual diagnosis, which indicates a concurrent diagnosis of substance dependence and a psychiatric disorder.

Effects of Use

Alcohol affects almost all cells of the body and depresses all areas and functions of the CNS. Alcohol requires no digestion because it is absorbed directly from the stomach and the small intestine. The absorption rate can be decreased by food in the stomach, especially protein and fats or plain water mixed with alcohol. The rate is increased by mixing alcohol with soda water or by strong emotions. Alcohol is almost completely metabolized in the body and has a slow oxidation rate. The liver is the site of oxidation. The alcohol dehydrogenase system breaks down alcohol. If the enzymes are blocked by drugs such as disulfiram (Antabuse) or unable to work, acetaldehyde builds up in the system, and a disulfiram ethanol reaction, or Antabuse reaction, occurs. (Antabuse reaction is explained in the next section.) The rate of oxidation is approximately one drink per hour (7 g equals 7 ml of 100% alcohol). Alcohol (5% to 15%) is also excreted directly through the lungs, perspiration, and urine.

Alcohol's effects are directly proportional to the blood alcohol concentration (BAC). Because alcohol is evenly distributed in the body through the bloodstream, the BAC can be correlated with psychophysiologic effects on the body. Alcohol has a biphasic effect; at low doses it acts as a behavioral stimulant, and at high doses it acts as a depressant. Alcohol may be measured within 15 to 20 minutes of ingestion, peaks in 60 to 90 minutes, and is excreted in 12 to 24 hours. BAC is affected by the amount consumed, drinking rate, body size and composition (percentage of fat content), drink concentration, and hormones. For the nonalcoholic drinker, the BAC is fairly predictable. At higher levels of BAC, there is a narrow margin of safety between anesthesia and death (Table 10-10). The relationship between BAC and behavior is thought to be different in a person who has developed tolerance to alcohol and its effects. This individual is commonly able to drink large amounts without obvious impairment and perform complex tasks without problems at BAC levels several times higher than levels that would produce obvious impairment in the nontolerant drinker.

Drug Interactions with Alcohol. Antagonistic effects are seen within 5 to 10 minutes of drinking alcohol in the individual taking disulfiram (Antabuse). Flushing, headache, bounding pulse, diaphoresis, nausea, vomiting, and vasomotor collapse with orthostatic hypotension may occur.

Drugs that interact with alcohol in an additive manner include antihypertensives, antihistamines, marijuana, antianginals (nitrates), and analgesics (salicylates). Alcohol taken with aspirin may exacerbate GI bleeding. Alcohol taken with acetaminophen may result in more liver damage. Alcohol and nitrates may lead to postural hypotension, faintness, and loss of consciousness.

Substances that interact in a synergistic manner with alcohol include barbiturates, benzodiazepines, meprobamate, chloral hydrate, paraldehyde, narcotics, and anesthetics. Most of these substances potentiate depressant effects and often lead to respiratory failure and death. Alcohol may produce either a synergistic or an antagonistic effect when used with antidepressants.

Complications

Alcohol has a direct or an indirect effect on every organ and system within the body (Table 10-11). Intoxication is evidenced with increasing BAC. Intoxication may be mild, moderate, or severe, and it may result in coma. Intoxication is also evident in behavioral and physical changes. Behavioral changes include aggressiveness, impaired judgment, impaired attention, irritability, euphoria, depression, and emotional lability. Physical signs include slurred speech, incoordination, unsteady gait, nystagmus, and flushed face. In long-term alcoholics the signs are less evident because of developed tolerance.

A blackout (period for which an individual has no memory but was conscious) is an early sign of abuse and a probable sign of alcoholism. Reported signs of alcoholism include depression, frequent references to drinking, drinking to relieve negative feelings or physical or social discomforts, and the use of defense mechanisms, such as denial, projection, rationalization, "all-or-nothing" thinking, and avoidance to minimize the consequences and to maintain the drinking behavior. Behavioral signs associated with alcoholism reflect impaired functioning in the areas of family relationships, employment, and legal or social situations. As the disease progresses, the individual becomes more focused on drinking activities to the exclusion of everything else, with resulting isolation and frequent consumption of large amounts of alcohol.

Alcohol withdrawal is a state of hyperactivity and irritability in response to a marked decrease in consumption or cessation of alcohol use after periods of frequent or prolonged heavy drinking. Withdrawal should be anticipated if the individual reports consumption of over 10 ounces every day for a period

Table 10-10 Blood Alcohol Concentration and Related Effects

BAC (mg%)*	Psychophysiologic Effect
20	Light and moderate drinkers begin to feel some effects. Approximate BAC is reached after one drink.[†]
40	Most people begin to feel relaxed.
60	Judgment is mildly impaired. People are less able to make rational decisions about their capabilities (e.g., driving skills).
80	Definite impairment of muscle coordination and driving skills occurs. Person is legally drunk in some states.
100	Clear deterioration of reaction time and control is observed. Person is legally drunk in most states.
120	Vomiting occurs unless this level is reached slowly.
150	Balance and movement are impaired. Equivalent of one-half pint of whiskey is circulating in the bloodstream.
300	Many people lose consciousness.
400	Most people lose consciousness, and some die.
450	Breathing stops; person eventually dies.

*Blood alcohol concentration (BAC) is generally recorded in milligrams of alcohol per deciliter (mg/dl) of blood, or milligrams percent (mg%). BAC is determined by how much alcohol is consumed, how fast it is consumed, and the person's weight.
[†]One drink is 12 oz of beer, 5 oz of wine, or 1 oz of distilled spirits, which provide the same amount of alcohol.

Table 10-11 Effects of Chronic Alcohol Abuse

Body Systems	Effects
▪ Central nervous system	Alcoholic dementia; Wernicke's encephalopathy (confusion, nystagmus, paralysis of ocular muscles, ataxia); Korsakoff's psychosis (confabulation, amnesic disorder); impairment of cognitive function, psychomotor skills, abstract thinking, and memory; depression, attention deficit, labile moods, seizures, sleep disturbances
▪ Peripheral nervous system	Peripheral neuropathy including pain, paresthesias, weakness
▪ Immune system	Increased risk for tuberculosis and viral infections; increased risk for cancer of oral cavity, pharynx, esophagus, liver, colon, rectum, and possibly breast
▪ Hematologic system	Bone marrow depression, anemia, leukopenia, thrombocytopenia, blood clotting abnormalities
▪ Musculoskeletal system	Painful, tender swelling of large muscle groups; painless progressive muscle weakness and wasting; osteoporosis
▪ Cardiovascular system	Elevated pulse and BP, decreased exercise tolerance, cardiomyopathy (irreversible), increased risk for hemorrhagic stroke, coronary artery disease, hypertension, sudden cardiac death
▪ Hepatic system	Steatosis (reversible)—nausea, vomiting, hepatomegaly; alcoholic hepatitis (reversible)—anorexia, nausea, vomiting, fever, chills, abdominal pain; cirrhosis; cancer
▪ Gastrointestinal system	Gastritis, peptic ulcer, esophagitis, esophageal varices, enteritis, colitis, Mallory-Weiss syndrome, pancreatitis
▪ Nutrition	Decreased appetite, indigestion, malabsorption, vitamin deficiencies
▪ Urinary system	Diuretic effect from inhibition of antidiuretic hormone
▪ Endocrine and reproductive systems	Altered gonadal function, testicular atrophy, decreased beard growth, decreased libido, diminished sperm count, gynecomastia, glucose intolerance
▪ Integumentary system	Palmar erythema, spider angiomas, rosacea, rhinophyma

of 2 weeks. Hangovers, which appear early in alcohol use, are replaced by symptoms of withdrawal. Four characteristic signs of withdrawal are gross tremors, seizures, hallucinations, and delirium tremens (DTs) (Table 10-12).

Most alcoholics experience a mild or minor withdrawal syndrome in the first 10 to 12 hours after the last drink, which peaks at 24 to 48 hours and may last up to 5 days. The symptoms are manifestations of CNS hyperactivity resulting from a rebound from the depressant effects of alcohol. Characteristic symptoms include tremulousness, anxiety, increased heart rate, increased blood pressure, sweating, nausea, hyperreflexia, and insomnia. These manifestations vary in intensity and will depend on the severity of the alcoholic problem and general physical condition of the patient.

An alcohol withdrawal seizure is most likely to occur 7 to 48 hours after the last drink. Alcohol withdrawal delirium, or DTs, is considered a major withdrawal symptom occurring from 30 to 120 hours after the last drink. This is a serious complication and can be life threatening if untreated.[18] Delirium components include disorientation, visual or auditory hallucinations, and increased hyperactivity without seizures. Death may be caused by hyperthermia, peripheral vascular collapse, or cardiac failure.

Collaborative Care

Initial treatment of alcoholism is aimed at detoxification as necessary and stabilization of the patient's condition. The most common emergency problems related to alcohol are accidents and toxic reactions. Toxic reactions occur as the result of com-

Table 10-12 Clinical Manifestations of Alcohol Withdrawal with Suggested Drug Treatment

Clinical Manifestations	Medications
Gross tremors Seizures Hallucinations Delirium tremens (DTs) Minor withdrawal syndrome: Tremulousness, anxiety Increased heart rate Increased blood pressure Sweating Nausea Hyperreflexia Insomnia Major withdrawal (DTs): Disorientation Visual/auditory hallucinations Increased hyperactivity without seizures	Benzodiazepines (e.g., chlordiazepoxide [Librium]) Thiamine (prevention of Wernicke's encephalopathy) Multivitamins (folic acid, B vitamins) Phenytoin (Dilantin)—for seizures or past history of seizures Magnesium sulfate (if serum magnesium is low) Temazepan (Restoril) Haloperidol (Haldol) for hallucinations For DTs: may need IV fluids (do not overhydrate), cooling blanket, well-lighted quiet room, consistent staff, frequent vital signs, check for hypoglycemia, assessment of any other health problems

bining alcohol with another drug and may lead to respiratory and circulatory arrest without adequate intervention. Naloxone (Narcan), an opiate antagonist, may be given if opiates have been used with alcohol. Toxicology screening identifies types of drugs (including alcohol) and levels present. Methanol (wood alcohol), ethylene glycol (antifreeze), and isopropyl alcohol (rubbing alcohol) may be found in accidental overdoses or suicide attempts.

Medications may be useful in treating withdrawal by decreasing symptoms, increasing levels of comfort, and decreasing the risk of convulsions and DTs (see Table 10-12). Benzodiazepines are the most effective agents in preventing and treating alcohol withdrawal seizures and DTs. Other agents may include beta-adrenergic blockers (e.g., atenolol [Tenormin]), clonidine (Catapres), and calcium channel blockers. The patient who is intoxicated with rising BACs should not be given other depressants because of their additive effects. Inadequate treatment of alcohol withdrawal may precipitate more severe stages.

Some useful screening tools for alcohol abuse include the Alcohol Use Disorders Identification Test (AUDIT) (a 10-item questionnaire to identify early-stage problem drinkers), the CAGEAID questionnaire (a four-item mnemonic tool) (Table 10-13), and the Short Michigan Alcoholism Screening Test (MAST) (a 13-item tool) (Table 10-14).

Laboratory tests that may provide evidence of alcoholism are liver function tests and a complete blood count. Liver function tests include gamma-glutamyltransferase (GGT), aspartate aminotransferase (AST), alanine aminotransferase (ALT), and alkaline phosphatase.

Although cessation of drinking is the short-term goal that is accomplished through detoxification, rehabilitation and sustained abstinence are the primary long-term goals. The aim of intervention is to assist the patient to see the adverse consequences of drinking and to make appropriate lifestyle changes. The earlier an individual engages in treatment, the greater the chances of a more complete recovery.

Inpatient or intensive outpatient treatment programs, aftercare services, and community support groups such as Alcoholics Anonymous (AA) are essential for long-term sobriety. AA is based on the 12 steps (Table 10-15) and is designed to help the individual cope with problems. The group support is a key element in the success of AA. Alateen is available for teenagers and Al-Anon for families and friends of alcoholics. Other programs such as Women in Sobriety and Smart Recovery can be helpful to people who do not attend programs in the AA model. A number of drugs have been used as adjuncts in aftercare programs, including agents that repress the desire to drink, such as naltrexone (Trexan), and agents that prevent drinking by causing aversive consequences when alcohol is consumed, such as disulfiram (Antabuse).

Table 10-13 The CAGE Questionnaire

CAGE Questions Adapted to Include Drugs (CAGEAID)

Have you felt you ought to cut down on your drinking *(or drug use)*?

_____ Yes _____ No

Have people annoyed you by criticizing your drinking *(or drug use)*?

_____ Yes _____ No

Have you felt bad or guilty about your drinking *(or drug use)*?

_____ Yes _____ No

Have you ever had a drink *(or used drugs)* first thing in the morning to steady your nerves or get rid of a hangover *(or to get the day started)*?

_____ Yes _____ No

From Fleming MF, Barry KL: *Addictive disorders,* St Louis, 1992, Mosby; and Ewing JA: Detecting alcoholism: the CAGE questionnaire, *JAMA* 252:1905, 1984.
NOTE: Boldface text shows the original CAGE questions; boldface italic text shows modifications of the CAGE questions used to screen for drug disorders. In a general population, two or more positive answers indicate a need for more in-depth assessment.

Opiates

Characteristics

Opium is a natural poppy extract. Nonsynthetic narcotics that are alkaloids of opium include morphine and codeine. Thebaine is a major alkaloid of another variety of poppy and is converted

Table 10-14 Short Michigan Alcoholism Screen Test

1. Do you feel you are a normal drinker? (By normal, do you drink less than or as much as most other people.) (No)*	No ______	Yes ______
2. Does your wife, husband, a parent, or other near relative ever worry or complain about your drinking? (Yes)	No ______	Yes ______
3. Do you ever feel guilty about your drinking? (Yes)	No ______	Yes ______
4. Do friends or relatives think you are a normal drinker? (No)	No ______	Yes ______
5. Are you able to stop drinking when you want to? (No)	No ______	Yes ______
6. Have you ever attended a meeting of Alcoholics Anonymous? (Yes)	No ______	Yes ______
7. Has drinking ever created problems between you and your wife, husband, a parent, or other near relative? (Yes)	No ______	Yes ______
8. Have you ever gotten into trouble at work because of drinking? (Yes)	No ______	Yes ______
9. Have you ever neglected your obligations, your family, or your work for 2 or more days in a row because you were drinking? (Yes)	No ______	Yes ______
10. Have you ever gone to anyone for help about your drinking? (Yes)	No ______	Yes ______
11. Have you ever been in a hospital because of your drinking? (Yes)	No ______	Yes ______
12. Have you ever been arrested for drunken driving, driving while intoxicated, or driving under the influence of alcohol? (Yes)	No ______	Yes ______
13. Have you ever been arrested, even for a few hours, because of other drunken behavior? (Yes)	No ______	Yes ______

*Alcoholism-indicating responses appear in parentheses.

Scoring: 0-1, nonalcoholic; 2, possibly alcoholic; 3 or more, alcoholic.

Table 10-15 Twelve Steps of Alcoholics Anonymous

1. We admitted we were powerless over alcohol—that our lives had become unmanageable.
2. We came to believe that a Power greater than ourselves could restore us to sanity.
3. We made a decision to turn our wills and our lives over to the care of God as we understood Him.
4. We made a searching and fearless moral inventory of ourselves.
5. We admitted to God, to ourselves, and to another human being the exact nature of our wrongs.
6. We were entirely ready to have God remove all these defects of character.
7. We humbly asked Him to remove our shortcomings.
8. We made a list of all persons we had harmed, and became willing to make amends to them all.
9. We made direct amends to such people whenever possible, except when to do so would injure them or others.
10. We continued to take personal inventory and, when we were wrong, promptly admitted it.
11. We sought through prayer and meditation to improve our conscious contact with God as we understood Him, praying only for knowledge of His will for us and the power to carry that out.
12. Having had a spiritual awakening as the result of these steps, we tried to carry this message to alcoholics, and to practice these principles in all our affairs.

From Alcoholics Anonymous: *The twelve steps of alcoholics anonymous,* New York, 1939, Works Publishers.

to codeine, hydrocodone, oxycodone, oxymorphone, nalbuphine, naloxone, and the Bentley compounds. Semisynthetic narcotics include heroin, hydromorphone (Dilaudid), and oxycodone. Synthetic narcotics include meperidine (Demerol), methadone, and propoxyphene (Darvon). Narcotic antagonists include naloxone (Narcan) and nalorphine (Nalline).

Individuals who abuse drugs are most frequently identified in medical settings. People who combine alcohol with other drugs are often middle class, females, and individuals with chronic pain who are frequently taking more than one prescription drug.[18] Health care professionals have the highest rate of abuse of narcotics of any middle-class population.[2,18] Job stresses, interference of work with family life, long hours, and availability of drugs are considered contributing factors.

Effects of Use

Opiates are CNS depressants and are detoxified in the liver and excreted in urine and stool. Most of the metabolites, with the exception of methadone, are excreted in 24 to 48 hours.

Narcotics are the most effective medicines for relief of intense pain, cough suppression (antitussives), and treatment of intestinal disorders such as colic and diarrhea. As drugs of abuse, they are sniffed, smoked, or self-administered by subcutaneous ("skin-popping") or IV ("mainlining") injection (see Fig. 10-4).

Heroin is rapidly converted to morphine in the body. Hydromorphone is shorter acting and more sedating than morphine and 2 to 10 times as potent. Percodan is aspirin plus oxycodone. Percocet is acetominophen plus oxycodone.

The primary effects of narcotics are analgesia, drowsiness, changes in mood, and, at high doses, clouding of mental functioning (see Table 10-5). IV use usually causes a "kick" or "rush" of feelings in the lower abdomen, along with warm skin flushing, an intoxicated feeling, euphoria, and decreased respiratory rate, peristalsis, and pupil size. Narcotics lead to a rapid tolerance and physical dependence after short-term use. Cross tolerance is common among the opiates.

The signs of opiate intoxication may be seen within 2 to 5 minutes of IV use, beginning with euphoria and progressing to lethargy, somnolence, apathy, and dysphoria. Unintentional overdose frequently occurs with recreational use of narcotics because of the unpredictability in potency and purity. Some narcotic overdoses may be suicide attempts. Signs of overdose are presented in Table 10-6.

Withdrawal from opiates occurs with decreased amounts or cessation of the drug after prolonged moderate to heavy use. The administration of an antagonist (e.g., naloxone) will trigger withdrawal symptoms in dependent individuals. Manifestations of withdrawal include craving, nausea or vomiting, muscle aches, tearing or rhinorrhea, pupillary dilation, piloerection ("gooseflesh"), perspiration, diarrhea, yawning, fever, nightmares, or insomnia. Generally within 12 hours of the last dose there is physical discomfort followed by a restless sleep, flu-like symptoms, and craving. The onset of withdrawal begins at the time of the next usual dose and ranges from 4 to 6 hours for heroin to 1 day or longer for methadone. The kicking movements sometimes observed in a patient during withdrawal are responsible for the phrase "kicking the habit." The individual may be suicidal during withdrawal. The severity of withdrawal is related to the degree of dependence, but it usually runs its course in 96 hours. Symptoms may recur for 6 to 10 months.

Complications

Medical complications are linked with the routes of administration. Street heroin, which is often cut with quinine, has vasodilator effects when given IV and may lead to tissue abscesses if administered subcutaneously. Heroin users have been found to have a higher incidence of infections, especially those associated with needle use. Drug use tends to reduce safe sex practices, which also increases the risk of contracting HIV.

Other complications that are associated with opiate addiction include hepatitis B and C, peptic ulcer disease, arrhythmias, endocarditis, anemias, electrolyte abnormalities, bone and joint infections, kidney failure, muscle destruction, pneumonia, lung abscesses, tuberculosis, bronchospasm and wheezing, stroke, abnormal sexual function, and depression.

Collaborative Care

The short-term prognosis for narcotic addicts is poor because of high relapse rates. The long-term prognosis is better because addicts in their thirties and forties tend to stop drug use.

Overdose of opiates can precipitate a medical emergency (see Table 10-7). Laboratory analysis must be performed to identify the drug ingested. A narcotic antagonist such as naloxone, nalorphine, or levallorphan should be given before any irreversible brain anoxia develops. Prophylactic tetanus immunizations are often given. If a suicide attempt is suspected, the individual should be evaluated by a psychiatric/mental health professional before discharge.

Treatment of withdrawal is symptom based and may not require the use of medication. One of the goals of treatment for an opiate addict is to maintain a relative comfort level and use motivational counseling so the patient is more likely to consider entering a rehabilitation program.

Methadone is a federally regulated synthetic narcotic that may be used in detoxification and maintenance programs for heroin addicts. Methadone maintenance is supportive therapy that is most effective when provided in addition to education, counseling, and vocational training programs. Methadone has been beneficial for some individuals and is the most effective method of decreasing the risk of heroin use and the most promising available treatment for IV narcotic users seeking treatment.

HALLUCINOGENS

A number of psychoactive substances, either natural or synthetic, act to produce a change in level of consciousness, alter mood, and induce hallucinations. These drugs are classified as hallucinogens (see Table 10-5).

Cannabis

Characteristics

The cannabis group includes substances with psychoactive ingredients derived from the cannabis or hemp plant, or chemically similar synthetic substances. The three drugs of this group that are most commonly found in the United States and Canada are marijuana, hashish, and hashish oil. Tetrahydrocannabinol (THC) is believed to be responsible for most of the psychoactive effects. Marijuana, which is derived from the dried leaves and flowering tops of the cannabis plant, is a less potent source of THC than hashish, which is a rich resinous secretion of the plant. Hashish oil, a dark viscous extraction of the plant, has a much higher percentage of THC. A drop or two of hashish oil on a cigarette has the same effect as a marijuana "joint." Although a number of potential benefits of THC have been reported, the only demonstrated benefits are for resistant glaucoma and for the control of nausea from cancer chemotherapy.

Patterns of use vary from occasional to long-term, habitual use. Generally it is the first illegal drug that is used by young people and follows use of alcohol. Peer influence is considered the strongest predictor of use. Occasional users are more common, and they tend to smoke in groups. Daily use may lead to compulsive or everyday use.

Effects of Use

The mechanism of pharmacologic action of cannabis is uncertain. It is fat soluble, is stored in body fats, is metabolized in the liver, and has a half-life of 7 to 10 days. It is excreted as metabolites in feces and urine. Metabolites may be detectable days to weeks after brief exposure to marijuana. Marijuana is usually smoked, and peak plasma level occurs within 10 minutes. The most prominent effects occur in 20 to 30 minutes, and intoxication lasts from 2 to 3 hours. Tolerance of many effects occurs. Physiologic dependence does not usually develop even with long-term heavy use. A mild cross-tolerance to alcohol develops. Marijuana has low toxicity, and there is no known level of lethal dose.

The most commonly affected organs are the brain, cardiovascular system, and lungs. Most changes are reversible. Signs of intoxication include euphoria, anxiety, suspiciousness or paranoid ideation, sensation of slowed time, impaired judgment, social withdrawal, redness of conjunctiva, increased appetite for sweets, dry mouth, and tachycardia. Problems of habitual users include impaired short-term memory, visual hallucinations (from high doses), decreased motor coordination, tremors, increased heart and respiratory rates, increased sexual arousal, and sleepiness. Marijuana use may precipitate seizures in persons with epilepsy, psychotic episodes in persons with schizophrenia, and ketoacidosis in persons with diabetes mellitus.

Medical problems associated with marijuana use are generally mild and transient. More serious potential problems have been reported with heavy use. These include bronchitis, increased rates of precancerous lesions in the lungs, sinusitis, pharyngitis, acute memory impairment, increased risk of cardiac problems for individuals with heart disease, depression of the immune system, and alterations in the reproductive and endocrine systems.

Collaborative Care

Acute reactions, including intoxication and withdrawal, are usually mild and time limited. An individual may be treated for toxic reactions to a combination of drugs that includes marijuana or may seek treatment for panic reactions. Most therapeutic approaches depend on the characteristics and severity of symptoms. Treatment is directed toward relief of symptoms, and the administration of drugs is avoided if possible.

Inhalants

Inhalants first received attention in the United States in the 1950s with "glue sniffing." Since then a wide variety of volatile substances have been inhaled to produce a "high." They are also known as "unheated vapors" to differentiate them from cocaine and other narcotic inhaling. Forms of use include sniffing, bagging (emptying contents into a plastic bag and inhaling), huffing (soaking a rag with solution, putting in mouth, inhaling) or directly spraying the substance in the oral cavities and inhaling. Because of the strong odors and stains left by these substances, the user is easily identified.

Because inhalants are readily accessible, widely available, inexpensive, legally purchased, and produce a rapid high, they are particularly appealing for use among younger age-groups with higher incidence for young boys between the ages of 10 and 15 years.[8] There are four main classes of inhalants: volatile solvents, aerosols, anesthetic agents, and nitrites (amyl, butyl, isobutyl). They act as CNS depressants exhibiting stimulant effects at low doses and leading to depression and death at high doses (see Table 10-5). Death, which may be sudden, is due to direct toxic effects, inhalation of gastric contents, trauma, and suffocation.[8,19,20]

NURSING MANAGEMENT: SUBSTANCE ABUSE

■ Nursing Assessment

The nurse must be alert to the subtle and overt cues of substance use and the implications for nursing management. Possible behaviors suggesting substance dependence are listed in Table 10-16. Early recognition and identification of a patient with substance-related problems is crucial to successful treatment outcomes. The nurse must recognize patient behaviors that influence the history taking such as efforts at manipulation, denial, impulsiveness, avoidance, underreporting or minimizing substance use, giving inaccurate information, and inaccurate self-reporting. These behaviors are common in substance-abusing patients. Reframing questions to make them more open and not "yes or no" responses (e.g., "how much or how often do you drink?") and providing information about the effects of substance use may facilitate more honest responses and build a therapeutic relationship.

If the nurse is to obtain an accurate and thorough patient assessment, there are certain essential nursing behaviors that can facilitate the patient's accurate self-disclosure. The nurse must be aware of personal feelings and attitudes about substance abuse that may affect one's ability to be open and nonjudgmental. Addicted patients often evoke hostility from a health care worker when help is needed. Some health professionals may view the substance-abusing patient as emotionally weak and irresponsible. Such an individual is frequently seen as not contributing to society or as one who inflicts harm on society and drains social and economic resources. It is important for the nurse to be aware that negative feelings may be inadvertently communicated to the patient. The nurse may also fail to recognize signs and symptoms of abuse in a patient or coworker who does not fit the stereotype of an "addict." The nurse may also fail to recognize the substance abuser because of enabling behaviors that minimize symptoms or clues or

Table 10-16 Symptoms and Behaviors That May Suggest Dependence on Substances

- Trauma secondary to falls, auto accidents, fights, and burns
- Fatigue
- Insomnia
- Headaches
- Vague physical complaints
- Sexual dysfunction, decreased libido, erectile dysfunction
- Anorexia, weight loss
- Seizure disorder
- Appearance older than stated age
- Problems in areas of life function
  - Frequent job changes
  - Marital conflict, separation, or divorce
  - Work-related accidents, tardiness, absenteeism
  - Legal problems, including arrest
  - Social isolation, estrangement from friends or family
- Driving while intoxicated (more than one citation suggests dependence)
- Leisure activities that involve alcohol or other drugs
- Financial problems, including those related to spending for substances
- Failure of standard doses of sedatives to have a therapeutic effect
- Changes in mood, especially before and after visiting hours
- Overabundant use of mouthwash or toiletries
- Frequent references to alcohol or alcohol use indicating a preoccupation with the importance of alcohol in the patient's life

Table 10-17 Diagnoses Related to Substance Use

Nursing Diagnosis	Examples of Complete Diagnosis
Sensory/perceptual alteration	Sensory/perceptual alteration *related to* hallucinogen ingestion *as manifested by* visual hallucination of snakes in the bed
Altered thought processes	Altered thought processes *related to* alcohol withdrawal *as manifested by* disorientation to time, person, and place
Ineffective individual coping	Ineffective individual coping *related to* cocaine abuse of 6 months' duration *as manifested by* loss of job and lack of personal goals
Altered family processes: alcoholism	Altered family processes *related to* alcoholism *as manifested by* marital conflict and avoidance of the family and home by the children
DSM-IV Diagnosis	**Essential Features***
Substance dependence	Maladaptive pattern of substance use characterized by any three of the following within 12 months: tolerance; withdrawal; using more of the substance or using for longer than planned; persistent desire or unsuccessful efforts to cut down or control use; much time spent in efforts to obtain, use, or recover from use; interference with social, occupational, or recreational activities; continued use despite knowledge of use-related recurrent physical or psychologic problems
Substance abuse	Maladaptive pattern of substance use characterized by one or more of the following within 12 months: recurrent use resulting in failure to meet role obligations, recurrent use in physically hazardous situations, recurrent use-related legal problems, continued use despite persistent or recurrent use-related social or interpersonal problems, has never met the criteria for dependence for this class of substance

conspire with the patient by agreeing with excuses or promises to change.

During assessment the nurse must (1) facilitate privacy and avoid or minimize interruptions, (2) stress the importance of an accurate and thorough substance use history to provide appropriate care and prevent complications, and (3) be aware of the concerns of the substance-abusing patient. Such a patient is fearful and distressed over loss of control of self-medicating and is concerned that withdrawal may not be treated or will be treated inadequately. There may also be concerns that the health professional will report the patient to legal authorities.

The nurse must operate from a high level of suspicion to accurately and promptly identify the substance-abusing patient. A brief assessment of substance-related emergency conditions is essential for any patient newly admitted, regardless of age or condition and especially for a trauma or accident patient. It is necessary to obtain current and past substance use information and patterns. Inquiries should be made about recreational drugs, over-the-counter drugs, alcohol, nicotine, caffeine, and prescription drugs. This information is necessary to avoid withdrawal syndromes, acute intoxication, overdose, or drug interactions that may be life threatening. A thorough psychosocial assessment can be done when indicated to document other health-related, social, financial, and legal consequences of substance use.

Nursing Diagnoses

Nursing diagnoses assist nurses in the management of patient problems. Specific nursing diagnoses are useful in caring for an individual who has problems related to substance abuse. Several relevant nursing diagnoses have been identified along with the American Psychiatric Association (APA) Diagnostic and Statistical Manual's (DSM IV) medical diagnostic criteria for substance abuse and dependence (Table 10-17). Nursing diagnoses related to the individual with a substance abuse problem are also presented in NCP 10-1.

Planning

The overall goals are that the patient with a substance abuse problem will (1) abstain from the use of addicting substances, (2) cooperate with the proposed treatment plan, (3) make appropriate lifestyle adjustments to support abstinence, and (4) practice healthy lifestyle behaviors to foster sobriety.

Nursing Implementation

Health Promotion. A prevention framework (see Fig. 10-1) considers that as patterns of dependence become firmly established, individuals have fewer options for reversing these without treatment and rehabilitation for addiction. Preventing drug use and implementing early interventions when patterns of use are too frequent or dysfunctional may avoid later problems. The nurse must understand each level of prevention, its focus, and the nursing management and role of the nurse in primary, secondary, and tertiary prevention (Table 10-18). Health promotion strategies begin with the nurse's own recognition of attitudes, values, and substance use patterns and continue with activities that influence patients, families, and co-workers and can result in social change (Table 10-19).

Acute Intervention. Acute care situations precipitated by substance abuse involve withdrawal, overdose, or acute intoxication (see Table 10-6).

10-1 NURSING CARE PLAN PATIENT WITH SUBSTANCE ABUSE PROBLEM

Expected Patient Outcomes	Nursing Interventions and *Rationales*
NURSING DIAGNOSIS	**Ineffective denial** *related to* refusal to acknowledge substance abuse or dependency *as manifested by* delay in seeking or refusal of health care to detriment of health, lack of perception of personal relevance of symptoms, self-treatment, minimization of symptoms, denial of impact of disease on life, blaming of others for problems, use of rationalization or intellectualization.
▪ Able to explain psychologic and physiologic effects of alcohol and drug use. ▪ Admission of alcohol or drug abuse problem. ▪ Use of alternative positive coping skills to relieve stress. ▪ Recognition of need for continued treatment.	▪ Educate patient about alcohol's or other drug's psychologic and physiologic impact on health, as well as other ways in which it affects one's life *to lay the groundwork for change.* ▪ Link health-related and other drug use consequences with substance abuse problem *to facilitate acceptance of responsibility for behaviors.* ▪ Assist patient in identifying and altering patterns of substance abuse *to assist patient to develop new healthy coping skills.* ▪ Do *not* argue about whether patient is an "alcoholic" or "abuser" or allow patient to use blame of others, rationalization, or intellectualization *to confront maladaptive defense mechanisms.* ▪ Assist patient to improve self-esteem *because low self-esteem is a common characteristic of the substance abuser.* ▪ Assist patient in resocialization and building support system, including self-help groups (e.g., Alcoholics Anonymous, Narcotics Anonymous) *to provide patient with a new and healthier support system.* ▪ Initiate referral to addiction specialist or substance abuse treatment program as indicated *because the emotional problems and recovery issues often associated with substance abuse may be beyond the scope of a nurse without special training.*
NURSING DIAGNOSIS	**Altered health maintenance** *related to* lack of knowledge of progression of substance abuse and its effects and relapse prevention *as manifested by* inappropriate use of alcohol and other drugs; inaccurate or lack of knowledge of signs and symptoms of abused substance, nature of disease, effect on body; repeated relapses.
▪ Recognition of signs and symptoms of disease. ▪ Knowledge of warning signs of relapse. ▪ Plan for seeking help at first sign of relapse. ▪ Abstinence from alcohol/drugs. ▪ Regular participation in support groups.	▪ Provide educational information to patient and family about substance abuse (e.g., development, effects, and consequences) *to enable them to be informed and to encourage active participation in treatment.* ▪ Teach early warning signs of relapse *so immediate intervention is possible.* ▪ Assist patient in developing a specific plan regarding person to contact and rehearsing responses to stressful situations or triggers to substance abuse *to facilitate effective coping and prevent relapse.* ▪ Support abstinence and participation in support groups (e.g., Alcoholics Anonymous) *because these groups are known to be helpful in maintaining sobriety.* ▪ Refer to substance abuse treatment program or counseling (if indicated) *to foster ongoing treatment.*
NURSING DIAGNOSIS	**Ineffective individual coping** *related to* lack of knowledge of problem-solving and assertiveness skills *as manifested by* inappropriate use of alcohol and other drugs, inability to problem solve, depression, suicidal thoughts.
▪ Decrease in depression. ▪ Increase in expression of thoughts and feelings, problem-solving ability, and assertiveness.	▪ Assist patient to express negative thoughts and feelings (sadness, hopelessness, anger, guilt) *to clarify thoughts and begin problem-solving process.* ▪ Assess degree of depression and suicidal or homicidal thoughts or poor impulse control *to determine degree of danger to self or others.* ▪ Assist patient in defining problems, planning problem-solving approaches, implementing solutions, and evaluating the process *to develop problem-solving ability.* ▪ Assist patient in practicing assertive responses to stressful situations *to develop confidence in ability to use alternative ways of responding to stress.*

Continued

10-1 NURSING CARE PLAN PATIENT WITH SUBSTANCE ABUSE PROBLEM —continued

Expected Patient Outcomes	Nursing Interventions and *Rationales*
NURSING DIAGNOSIS **Altered nutrition: less than body requirements** *related to* history of poor nutrition *as manifested by* body weight 20% below normal for height and age and hair loss.	
▪ Steady gain in weight until proper weight achieved. ▪ No signs or symptoms of malnutrition.	▪ Monitor patient's weight, albumin, and prealbumin *to determine extent of problem and plan appropriate interventions.* ▪ Encourage patient to abstain from alcohol and other drugs *because they interfere with absorption and utilization of nutrients.* ▪ Provide frequent, small, nourishing meals *to improve caloric intake and enhance tolerance of food.* ▪ Teach patient to take vitamins, including thiamine, *to correct deficiencies and reduce neurologic complications.* ▪ Explain need to take nothing by mouth (NPO) if gastritis or bleeding is present *to reduce gastric stimulation.*
NURSING DIAGNOSIS **Ineffective family coping: disabling** *related to* substance abuse problem *as manifested by* abusive treatment and neglect and general intolerance of affected family member, denial about the problem's existence.	
▪ Identification of need to establish effective communication and living skills with family.	▪ Assess coping skills of patient and individual family members *to determine extent of problem.* ▪ Foster discussion of family coping skills and explore relationship problems *to increase awareness of need for long-term family counseling.* ▪ Explore abusive treatment *to identify need for immediate intervention.* ▪ Refer patient and family to qualified family or addiction counselor *because a specialist is required to treat this complex problem.*

Withdrawal. In general, withdrawal signs and symptoms are somewhat opposite in nature from the direct effects of the drug. Withdrawal from all classes of drugs is similar in producing symptoms of acute anxiety and protracted depression. Withdrawal from CNS depressants, including alcohol, is the most dangerous withdrawal syndrome. Abrupt withdrawal may be life threatening. Management of withdrawal from CNS depressants is symptomatic and includes a gradual reduction in drug dosage. Although withdrawal from narcotics is the least life threatening, symptoms are dramatic, temporarily disabling, and painful. Nursing management includes ensuring safety, preventing injury, and halting the progression of symptoms. Specific nursing approaches include careful monitoring of vital signs and level of consciousness and providing reassurance and orientation as needed. Methadone is often recommended for treating withdrawal from narcotics, but any opiate may be administered. Symptoms of withdrawal may be reduced by administering the drug of choice in decreasing amounts over 2 weeks. Nonopiates may also be administered for detoxification and include clonidine (Catapres) and benzodiazepines.

Alcohol withdrawal. Management goals for alcohol withdrawal are to prevent the progression of symptoms, provide for the patient's safety and comfort, and motivate the patient to engage in long-term treatment (see Table 10-12). The patient must be carefully assessed because alcohol withdrawal may be life threatening. Most of the life-threatening conditions occur during the first few days of withdrawal. Generally, acute alcohol withdrawal lasts for 3 to 5 days.

An individual who is experiencing alcohol withdrawal may also be suffering from other illnesses, health conditions, or trauma. The most common severe manifestations are hallucinations and seizures. The progression of symptoms to DTs can be prevented by prompt early treatment. A quiet, calm environment is important to prevent exacerbation of symptoms. The use of restraints and IVs should be avoided whenever possible. Supportive care is needed to ensure adequate rest and nutrition. It is important not to overhydrate the patient, particularly if the patient has renal or cardiac disease, because overhydration can lead to sudden arrhythmias. The majority of patients improve without medical treatment. The nursing care for the patient in withdrawal is presented in NCP 10-2.

Management of amphetamine and cocaine withdrawal involves assessment and monitoring of symptoms with particular attention to suicidal thoughts and complications from multiple drug use (see Table 10-6). The primary goals are to control symptoms, decrease craving, and establish a basis for recovery. Specific approaches to managing withdrawal include providing active support, encouraging adequate nutrition (including vitamin supplements), maintaining adequate fluid balance, recommending aerobic exercise if there are no medical contraindications, and teaching relaxation techniques and measures to promote sleep.

Table 10-18 Nursing Role in Substance Abuse Prevention

Level of Prevention	Nursing Role
Primary prevention	Teaching and counseling nonusers and occasional users Education on immediate effects of substances on body, long-term negative outcomes, effects of experimentation and continued use Adolescents and young adults are target groups
Secondary prevention	Education, case finding, early intervention Detection through health screening clinics Intervention through peer or employee assistance programs Support and teach substance-free alternatives and stress management techniques
Tertiary prevention	Engaging and motivating in treatment Education regarding relapse, identification of precipitating factors, high-risk situations, triggers of use Referral to treatment, support groups, relapse prevention programs

Overdose. Management of a drug overdose is based on the type of the substance involved. Drug overdose can be accidental or intentional. Accidental overdose usually involves only one substance, whereas intentional overdose is more likely to involve multiple substances and results in a complex and potentially confusing clinical picture.[21] The first priority of care in overdose is always the patient's ABCs (see Table 10-7 and NCP 10-3). As soon as the patient is stable, a thorough history and physical examination must be completed.[22] When the patient is unwilling or unable to give a history, a collateral history should be obtained from the patient's significant others. A patient who intentionally overdoses should not be allowed to return home until seen by a psychiatric professional.

The patient who has overdosed on depressants must be treated aggressively and may require dialysis to decrease the drug level and to prevent irreversible CNS depressant effects and death. It is important to avoid the use of any CNS stimulants in the treatment of overdose. Nursing management of individuals who have overdosed involves closely monitoring the neurologic status, level of consciousness, and respiratory status in addition to continuous physical assessment.

Intoxication. Acute alcohol intoxication may manifest as an emergency. It is important to obtain as accurate a history as possible, utilizing collateral information as necessary, and assess for injuries, trauma, diseases, and hypoglycemia. The basic principles of airway, breathing, and circulation (ABC) must be implemented. Vital signs and level of consciousness should be monitored. Generally, the pulse rate is normal in

Table 10-19 Health Promotion Strategies Related to Substance Abuse

- Recognition of nurse's attitudes, beliefs, and values related to addiction
- Assessment of nurse's patterns of substance use
- Teaching patient and family about substance abuse
- Education of public, nurses, and co-workers about substance use
- Identification of individuals at risk
- Identification of early signs and symptoms of substance abuse
- Initiation of activities to effect social change, legislation, and public policy

uncomplicated intoxication but elevated in withdrawal. The patient who is hypoglycemic should be given thiamine before receiving dextrose to prevent Wernicke's encephalopathy. Seizures may occur and are managed with an antiseizure drug. It is critical to continue assessments until the BAC has decreased to at least 100 mg% and until any associated disorders or injuries have been ruled out. A satisfactory BAC is usually reached within 6 to 10 hours.

In acute reactions to marijuana, it is important for the nurse to perform a physical examination, a toxicology screen, and a thorough history. The approach is basically the same for treating panic, flashbacks, and toxic reactions. The main interventions are to provide support and reassurance to the patient by explaining what is happening. The patient should understand that the level of intoxication may fluctuate over several days as metabolites are released.

An individual with cannabis intoxication or other acute problems related to cannabis use is seldom hospitalized and may be assisted in recovery by providing a quiet environment and adequate support and reassurance. Long-term users usually seek treatment for annoying symptoms rather than drug use. A long-term user may need assistance in achieving abstinence and may experience changes in mental functioning, alertness, memory, and motivation. As with other drug use, maintaining abstinence usually involves changes in values, lifestyles, and friends.

Substance abusers requiring surgery. Because of substance abuse, this individual is more likely to have accidents and injuries that require surgery. A large number of trauma victims may be under the influence of drugs and must be carefully assessed for signs and symptoms of overdose, withdrawal, and medical complications that could lead to adverse interactions with drugs used in the management of pain or administration of anesthesia. Special nursing considerations for the substance-abusing patient undergoing surgery are presented in Table 10-18. During the surgical recovery period, the nurse should be alert for the patient who may exhibit signs and symptoms of drug interactions with pain medications or anesthesia or who may exhibit signs of withdrawal.

Because the substance-abusing patient is at high risk for postoperative complications and death, a thorough health history and assessment of substance use is critical. This includes questions related to nicotine and caffeine use. Smoking makes the airway more irritable to the introduction of suction

10-2 NURSING CARE PLAN PATIENT IN ALCOHOL WITHDRAWAL

Expected Patient Outcomes	Nursing Interventions and *Rationales*
NURSING DIAGNOSIS **Risk for injury** *related to* sensorimotor deficits, seizure activity, and confusion.	
▪ No falls or injuries. ▪ Decrease in tremors and psychomotor activity. ▪ No seizures. ▪ Able to verbalize risk for injury associated with alcohol use before discharge.	▪ Assess for risk factors such as impaired mobility (e.g., unsteady gait), sensory deficits, tremors, impaired judgment, confusion, seizure activity *to plan appropriate preventive measures.* ▪ Assess for signs of injury such as lacerations, bruises, or burns *to treat appropriately.* ▪ Monitor vital signs frequently, especially increased pulse rate, *because prompt recognition of extreme autonomic nervous system response is necessary for early intervention to prevent progression of signs and symptoms.* ▪ Administer benzodiazepines as ordered *to control hyperactivity;* B vitamins (especially thiamine) *to reduce neurologic complications (e.g., Wernicke's encephalopathy)*; and antiseizure agents as ordered *to prevent seizures.* ▪ Use protective devices or restraints *to prevent injury of patient or others.* ▪ Use seizure precautions *to prevent injury.* ▪ Encourage verbalization of consequences of alcohol use related to physical injuries.
NURSING DIAGNOSIS **Sensory/perceptual alterations** *related to* sensory overload *as manifested by* inaccurate interpretation of environmental stimuli, disorientation, auditory or visual hallucinations.	
▪ No hallucinations. ▪ Oriented to person, place, time.	▪ Assess patient's orientation to reality *to determine appropriate interventions.* ▪ Provide quiet, nonstimulating, well-lit environment *to reduce external stimuli and calm overactive CNS.* ▪ Orient to nurse and environment with each contact; use calm, matter-of-fact approach; provide consistent staff; explain procedures and what is expected *to assist in reality orientation and decrease anxiety.* ▪ Do not reinforce fears or hallucinations by agreeing or disagreeing *because this does not facilitate reality orientation.* ▪ Administer benzodiazepines if ordered *to reduce CNS stimulation.* ▪ Administer antipsychotic medication (e.g., haloperidol [Haldol]) if ordered *to reduce severity of hallucinations.*
NURSING DIAGNOSIS **Sleep pattern disturbance** *related to* increased CNS stimulation *as manifested by* agitation, mood alterations, fatigue, dozing, difficulty falling or remaining asleep.	
▪ Able to describe factors including alcohol withdrawal that prevent or inhibit sleep. ▪ Use of techniques to induce or maintain sleep. ▪ Normal sleep patterns and rested feeling after sleep.	▪ Monitor sleep pattern *to individualize interventions to patient's unique problems.* ▪ Educate on alcohol withdrawal effects on sleep pattern. ▪ Identify contributing factors *so they may be corrected when possible.* ▪ Reduce or eliminate environmental stimuli (extremes of temperature, noise) and interruptions *to promote restful environment.* ▪ Provide comfort measures including bedtime routine, bathing, snacks, massage, music, reading *to promote sleep and show a caring attitude.* ▪ Assist with relaxation activities (e.g., walking, rhythmic deep breathing) *to encourage sleep by decreasing agitation and anxiety through light physical exertion.* ▪ Substitute decaffeinated products for coffee, tea, soda. Discourage use of chocolate and cocoa *to decrease stimulant effects.* ▪ Assist to decrease nicotine use (smoking) especially 30 min before bedtime *to decrease stimulant effects.*

Continued

10-2 NURSING CARE PLAN PATIENT IN ALCOHOL WITHDRAWAL—continued

Expected Patient Outcomes	Nursing Interventions and *Rationales*
NURSING DIAGNOSIS **Risk for violence** *related to* withdrawal from alcohol and/or accompanying depression.	
▪ No self-destructive or violent behavior. ▪ Control over behavior.	▪ Assess level of risk as evidenced by feelings of fear, suicidal or homicidal thoughts, hallucinations, environmental misperceptions, poor impulse control, panic *to ensure early recognition of violence potential and plan appropriate interventions.* ▪ Provide safe environment on the basis of risk level, including informing staff of risk, *to prevent injury to self or others.* ▪ Use medications or restraints if necessary *to prevent escalation of activity to violence.* ▪ Communicate expectation of need to maintain control of behavior (no harm to self or others) in clear, simple language and contract for "no harm" *so patient can compare present behavior with expected behavior and accept responsibility to maintain control.*
NURSING DIAGNOSIS **Ineffective breathing pattern** *related to* alcohol toxicity, airway obstruction, complicating respiratory diseases *as manifested by* shortness of breath, dyspnea, use of accessory muscles to breathe.	
▪ Maintenance of effective breathing. ▪ No indications of hypoxia.	▪ Monitor respiratory rate, depth, and pattern *so appropriate interventions may be taken.* ▪ Position patient on side and in semi-Fowler's position *to reduce possibility of aspiration and to enhance lung expansion by lowering diaphragm.* ▪ Monitor effects of medications given for withdrawal *to detect respiratory depression.* ▪ Encourage coughing and deep breathing *to prevent complications of hypoventilation.* ▪ Administer supplemental oxygen *to treat hypoxia.*

catheters and endotracheal tubes and increases risks for respiratory problems because of chronic bronchitis, pulmonary emphysema, and thick secretions. Heavy caffeine consumption may lead to postoperative headaches.[19]

Special precautions must be taken for the patient who is intoxicated or alcohol dependent and requires surgery (Table 10-20). Alcoholic shock as a cause of decreased pulse and high BAC may be overlooked in an accident victim. Many persons are undiagnosed as alcoholics at the time of admission for surgery. Optimally, health problems such as malnutrition, dehydration, and infection may need to be treated before surgery can be performed. The patient who is alcohol dependent but currently has no BAC usually requires an increased level of anesthesia because of cross-tolerance. The intoxicated individual needs a decreased level of anesthesia because of the synergistic effect of the alcohol present in the system.

Whenever possible, surgery is postponed until the BAC is less than 200 mg%. In individuals with a BAC over 150 mg% a synergistic effect occurs with anesthesia. A patient with a BAC over 250 mg% presents a significantly increased surgical risk and mortality rate. Acute withdrawal and DTs may be triggered by surgery and the cessation of alcohol consumption. Surgery should be delayed for at least 48 to 72 hours, if possible, or IV alcohol may be given to avoid this reaction if immediate surgery is required. Alcohol interferes with pulmonary function and may be associated with an increased incidence of hepatic dysfunction, esophageal varices, coagulation problems, poor wound healing, and metabolic abnormalities that can affect the outcome of surgery. Vital signs, including body temperature, must be closely monitored to identify signs of withdrawal, possible infections, and respiratory or cardiac problems. Postoperative patients may need benzodiazepines (e.g., chlordiazepoxide [Librium]) to control restlessness.

Pain management. Pain management for the substance-abusing patient is challenging. The nurse must consider the issue of cross-tolerance. It is important to know that the therapeutic doses of pain medication for a nonaddicted patient may not be adequate for a substance-abusing patient. Undermedication may also be caused by fear of addiction. In fact, inadequate pain management may lead to pseudoaddiction, which is characterized by increasing demands for pain medication, efforts to convince others of the severity of pain, and mistrust between the patient and nurse. Another issue is whether the patient is actually experiencing pain or just wants the medication to relieve a craving or prevent withdrawal symptoms.

It is important for the nurse to differentiate between drug-seeking behaviors and pain avoidance behaviors.[19] Although the nurse can ask the patient to rate the pain, the existence and severity of pain is based on the patient's perception. The nurse should evaluate the pain as objectively as possible and accept and respect the patient's report of pain as an indication of the patient's experience.[23] The nurse needs accurate knowledge of equianalgesic doses and opioid dosing and the likelihood of dependence resulting from narcotic use for pain control.[24] The acute medical-surgical problem must be managed first and the patient safely detoxified. Rehabilitation and treatment for problems with substance abuse remain long-term goals when an acute condition exists.

Ambulatory and Home Care. Before rehabilitation and treatment are considered, all acute medical-surgical

10-3 NURSING CARE PLAN PATIENT WITH COCAINE TOXICITY

Expected Patient Outcomes	Nursing Interventions and *Rationales*
NURSING DIAGNOSIS **Anxiety** *related to* increased CNS stimulation *as manifested by* increased pulse rate, palpitations, hyperventilation, talkativeness, fearfulness, tremor, confusion, feelings of losing control.	
▪ Decreased physiologic and psychologic manifestations of anxiety. ▪ Able to verbalize feelings of anxiety, dread, helplessness.	▪ Continuously monitor vital signs *to detect indicators of effects of cocaine use and subsequent anxiety.* ▪ Explain procedures using short, simple, clear statements in a calm manner *to reduce patient's agitation and increase cooperation and understanding of situation.* ▪ Provide safe, secure environment *to prevent anxiety related to unfamiliar or threatening events.* ▪ Decrease stimuli (if possible) *to decrease delusions and agitation.* Reinforce reality orientation *because disorientation and confusion increase anxiety.* ▪ Encourage verbal expression of feelings. Link response to effects of cocaine use *to provide recognition and acceptance of feelings and understanding of the consequences of use.* ▪ Encourage participation in relaxation exercises if possible, including deep breathing and progressive muscle relaxation *to provide effective, nonchemical ways to reduce anxiety and to exert some conscious control over behavior.*
NURSING DIAGNOSIS **Self-care deficit: bathing/hygiene, dressing/grooming, feeding** *related to* extreme CNS stimulation progressing to CNS depression *as manifested by* inability to perform any self-care activities.	
▪ Care needs met by self or others to patient's satisfaction. ▪ Increasing ability to meet personal care needs.	▪ Assess self-care deficits *to initiate appropriate treatment plan.* ▪ Provide assistance as needed and explain procedures *to meet patient's care requirements.* ▪ Monitor vital signs *to identify patient's response to care activities.* ▪ As patient recovers, reassess ability to participate in self-care *to make appropriate changes in care plan and allow as much self-care as possible.*
NURSING DIAGNOSIS **Fluid volume deficit** *related to* diaphoresis and hypermetabolic state *as manifested by* thirst, decreased urinary output, dry skin and mucous membranes, decreased skin turgor, decreased blood pressure.	
▪ No manifestations of dehydration. ▪ Intake of at least 1500 ml/day (oral fluids) and output of at least 1000-1500 ml/day. ▪ Vital signs and lab work within normal limits.	▪ Monitor fluid intake and output *to plan for adequate fluid replacement.* ▪ Assess for dehydration *to ensure early identification and treatment.* ▪ Start IV lines with large-bore needles for one or more fluid resuscitations with normal saline and lactated Ringer's solution *for rapid infusion of large volume of fluid.* ▪ Monitor vital signs *because decreasing blood pressure (BP) and increasing pulse and respiratory rate can indicate hypovolemia.* ▪ Monitor serum electrolytes, creatinine, blood urea nitrogen (BUN), urine and serum osmolalities, hematocrit, and hemoglobin levels *to detect hypovolemia and dehydration.* ▪ Consider additional fluid losses associated with vomiting, diarrhea, fever *to increase the accuracy of monitoring output.* ▪ Give sips of 5% glucose solution *to meet some of patient's requirements for both calories and fluid.* ▪ Administer IV ammonium chloride *to acidify urine and to increase rate of cocaine excretion.*
NURSING DIAGNOSIS **Situational low self-esteem** *related to* addictive behavior *as manifested by* self-destructive behavior associated with cocaine abuse, negative self-talk, helplessness, sadness, depression, self-neglect, apathy.	
▪ Verbalization of feelings of self-worth and identification of both positive and negative aspects of self. ▪ Able to analyze own behavior associated with cocaine abuse and its consequences.	▪ Assess emotional status *to determine patient's perception of situation and to plan appropriate interventions.* ▪ Assist patient in identifying and expressing feelings, including strengths and weaknesses *to enable patient to begin to accept responsibility for self.* ▪ Support use of effective coping mechanisms to deal with crisis *to reinforce new behaviors.* ▪ Assist patient in identifying own responsibility and control in situation *because these insights are necessary before dealing with an addiction.* ▪ Refer to treatment program, counseling, support group, or other resources *because these are often required to provide patient new skills and hope.*

Continued

10-3 NURSING CARE PLAN PATIENT WITH COCAINE TOXICITY —continued

Expected Patient Outcomes	Nursing Interventions and *Rationales*
NURSING DIAGNOSIS **Risk for self-directed violence** *related to* cocaine abuse.	
▪ Abstinence from further drug use. ▪ Treatment for cocaine abuse. ▪ No apparent risk of self-harm or harm to others.	▪ Assess risk for self-destruction as evidenced by compulsive focus of attention on cocaine, low self-esteem, hopelessness, acute agitation, depression, suicidal thoughts, poor impulse control, helplessness, lack of support systems, hallucinations, proneness to violence *to initiate appropriate plan of care.* ▪ Assist patient in building self-esteem with caring, empathic approach *because improved self-esteem will decrease impulse for self-destruction.* ▪ Assess support systems *as possible resources in preventing self-destructive behavior.* ▪ Ask patient to report suicidal or homicidal thoughts immediately *to prevent destructive behavior to self/other.* ▪ Assist patient in contacting members of support systems *because patient may not be motivated to do independently.* ▪ Initiate health teaching and referral for treatment or counseling when crisis is resolved *to ensure knowledge of positive health practices and adequate assistance with follow-up planning.*
NURSING DIAGNOSIS **Altered health maintenance** *related to* practices of behaviors/activities associated with cocaine use *as manifested by* reported or observed inability to take responsibility for basic needs.	
▪ Long-term abstinence from cocaine. ▪ Participation in recovery program that encourages a drug-free lifestyle.	▪ Assess patient's lifestyle *to determine thoughts, feelings, activities, or situations that are likely to trigger relapse.* ▪ Assist patient to make specific plans *to avoid such activities or situations and to constructively deal with thoughts and feelings.* ▪ Encourage appropriate inpatient or outpatient treatment *to meet patient's specific treatment needs.* ▪ Teach patient early warning signs *to prevent relapse.* ▪ Assist patient in learning positive ways to deal with stress and to live a balanced lifestyle *to reduce need to use drugs.*

COLLABORATIVE PROBLEMS

POTENTIAL COMPLICATIONS **Neurologic, cardiovascular, and respiratory problems** *related to* the toxic effects of cocaine.

Nursing Goals	Nursing Interventions and *Rationales*
▪ Monitor neurologic, cardiovascular, and respiratory functions. ▪ Report abnormal findings. ▪ Initiate appropriate medical and nursing interventions.	▪ Assess for neurologic, cardiovascular, and respiratory problems such as compromised vital signs, seizures, altered level of consciousness and motor activity, arrhythmias, vascular collapse, cerebrovascular accident, congestive heart failure, hypoxia, acute respiratory distress syndrome, cardiopulmonary arrest *to initiate immediate medical and nursing interventions if indicated.* ▪ Take seizure precautions *because cocaine poisoning can precipitate seizures.* ▪ Provide airway management and ventilation support *to treat respiratory failure.* ▪ Keep open IV lines *to provide immediate access to vascular system for IV fluids or medications.* ▪ Administer medications aggressively as indicated *to treat specific problems.* ▪ Employ cardiac life support measures (if indicated) *to treat cardiac or respiratory arrest.*

Table 10-20 Considerations for Substance-Abusing Patients Undergoing Surgery

- Standard amounts of anesthetic and analgesic medication may not be sufficient if patient is cross-tolerant.
- Increased doses of pain medication may be required if patient is cross-tolerant.
- Anesthetic agents may have a prolonged sedative effect if the patient has liver dysfunction. This situation requires an extended observation period.
- Patients have an increased susceptibility to cardiac and respiratory depression.
- Patients have an increased risk for bleeding, postoperative complications, and infection.
- Withdrawal from substances may be delayed for up to 5 days because of cross-tolerance with anesthetics and pain medications.
- Dosage of pain medications must be reduced gradually.

Table 10-21 Warning Signs of Relapse

Apprehension about well-being
Defensiveness and denial
Loneliness and isolation
Periods of confusion and restlessness
Readiness to anger
Irregular eating and sleeping habits
Feelings of powerlessness, helplessness, depression
Development of "don't care" attitude
Wishful thinking and fantasizing
Loss of daily structure

problems must be resolved. The patient must recognize and show initial understanding of the substance problem and be willing to accept long-term treatment. Outcomes are more positive when the nurse can work closely with the family and significant others as well as the substance-abusing patient in planning long-term care. Rehabilitation may be available for the patient in private or public psychiatric hospitals or in facilities specifically designed to meet the health care needs of the substance-abusing patient. It is important that a multidisciplinary team of nurses, physicians, social workers, and recreational therapists collaborate with the patient in planning care and in providing a therapeutic environment.

Although many drug abusers can be effectively treated in outpatient programs, inpatient programs should be recommended when resources and accessibility increase the likelihood of use and when social, family, or work environments do not promote abstinence. A structured inpatient program may be desirable during early recovery to provide a support system until the individual is able to develop coping skills and resources to resist drug use and begin working toward a drug-free lifestyle. The patient may progress from hospitalization to halfway houses, therapeutic communities, or other community-based programs.

Treatment modalities for the substance-abusing patient include counseling and psychotherapy, pharmacotherapy, and professional peer groups. Self-help groups are not considered treatment but are helpful adjuncts to treatment. They are usually based on 12-step programs and include AA, Cocaine Anonymous, and Narcotics Anonymous. Counseling and psychotherapy are helpful approaches for both the substance-abusing individual and his or her family. These approaches are thought to be most effective when combined with self-help groups.

Pharmacologic approaches include the use of disulfiram (Antabuse) for the alcoholic patient and the use of methadone in the treatment of opiate dependence. Antabuse, an alcohol antagonist or antialcohol, may be given orally over an extended period of time up to 1 year. Antabuse cannot be given to a patient with serious medical problems such as diabetes, cirrhosis, hypertension, and heart disease. If alcohol is in the system, the use of Antabuse may result in facial flushing, palpitations, rapid heart rate, difficulty in breathing, a possible serious drop in blood pressure, and nausea and vomiting. The patient must be taught about the effects of Antabuse, its purpose, and the highly unpleasant reactions that will occur if alcohol in any form is ingested. Alcohol ingestion can induce the uncomfortable symptoms for up to 1 week after use is discontinued.

Methadone is used both for detoxification and maintenance to help the patient develop a lifestyle free of street drugs and to improve family and job functioning, improve health, and decrease legal problems. The drug is administered in an oral liquid once a day at a licensed clinic or designated center; weekend doses are taken by the patient at home.

Complete abstinence from drugs is important because the use of another drug can impair judgment and trigger a craving for the abused substance, resulting in relapse. A conscious commitment is required not to use drugs and to initiate lifestyle changes that protect against persons, places, and circumstances that induce or contribute to drug use.

Addiction is a health problem that is chronic in nature and characterized by relapses. The nurse must be alert for signs of relapse (Table 10-21). Relapse prevention is a behavioral approach that identifies environmental cues that trigger relapses. It is an essential component of any recovery program and includes behavioral, cognitive, educational, and self-control techniques. The individual needs to identify specific increased risk situations or triggers that are likely to lead to substance use and to practice ways to avoid or deal with these situations. Programs that include relapse prevention strategies assist the recovering individual in the development of coping strategies and increased personal confidence (self-efficacy) for managing high-risk situations. Cravings can be diminished and eventually eliminated by ongoing counseling and substituting other activities for drug use. Negative consequences of the substances should be recalled to counteract distorted memories of the drug euphoria. Temporary relapses should be viewed as learning opportunities to minimize feelings of failure and to assist the patient to continue recovery. The nurse can guide the patient in learning stress management techniques for promoting a healthy lifestyle.

SPECIAL POPULATIONS WITH SUBSTANCE ABUSE PROBLEMS

GERONTOLOGIC CONSIDERATIONS

Patterns of substance use in older persons are considerably different from younger groups. The elderly, more than any other age group, have the highest use of over-the-counter (OTC) and prescription drugs. The simultaneous use of OTC drugs, prescription drugs, and alcohol occurs in many older adults. In the acute care setting, the prevalence of alcoholism is estimated to be as high as 20% in individuals over age 65, with higher rates occurring in nursing homes and psychiatric settings.[25] Illegal drug use is minimal in the elderly except for long-term addicts. However, it is expected that this pattern may change given the drug-using patterns now seen in the middle-aged population.

The most commonly used OTC drugs are analgesics; laxatives and antidiarrheals; vitamins, minerals, and iron; antacids; sedatives; cold and cough medications; antiemetics; hemorrhoidal preparations; and ophthalmic preparations. Among the most frequently prescribed drugs are anxiolytics, sedatives, hypnotics, and analgesics, as well as those prescribed for multiple chronic conditions (e.g., hypertension, COPD). An individual with a long history of heavy alcohol consumption and abuse often demonstrates complications as changes associated with aging occur. Daily drinking is more common among the elderly than binge drinking.

Two patterns of alcohol abuse have been identified: early-onset abuse and late-onset abuse. Early-onset abuse originating in the thirties or forties is a more chronic and debilitating course. Late-onset abuse is a reaction to a stressful late-life event or loss and generally causes fewer physical problems.[26,27]

Losses associated with aging pose stressful adjustments. Deaths of friends and spouse, retirement, relocation to new communities or supervised care facilities, lifestyle changes resulting from economic constraints, and declining health including hearing and vision losses create cumulative emotional strain. Late-onset alcoholism may emerge as attempts to cope with perceived life stresses or as possible passive suicide attempts in individuals for whom life has lost meaning.

The adverse effects of interaction of alcohol and other drugs are increased with aging. Ethanol may accelerate or inhibit the metabolism of other drugs at any age. When taken with alcohol, sedative-hypnotic drugs, minor tranquilizers, and CNS depressants have additive and synergistic effects, to which the older person is particularly sensitive. Other changes include impaired drug absorption, reduced blood circulation, and declining metabolic and excretion rates.

The interaction of physiologic and psychologic effects and drug actions results in behavioral patterns particular to the older patient. These include both acute and chronic responses to drug intake. Drug-induced memory deficits may precipitate drug misuse. Social problems, particularly isolation secondary to intoxication, may occur. Confusion, disorientation, delirium, memory loss, and neuromuscular problems are effects of the interaction of alcohol, drug misuse, and normal aging. Substance abuse problems in the elderly do not present a clear picture. Nonspecific indicators of alcohol abuse may include malnutrition, falls, frequent accidents, incontinence, decreased attention to self-care, mood swings, depression, confusion, and uncharacteristic reactions to prescribed medication.

Interventions targeted at substance abuse by the older adult include recognizing alcoholism as a separate chronic illness, treating the person in familiar places, using therapies known to be helpful with older people (e.g., socialization), and peer groups. A simple tool for recognizing alcohol problems in older adults is HEAT (how, excess, anyone else, trouble): *How* do you use alcohol? Have you ever thought you used alcohol to *excess*? Has *anyone else* ever thought you used too much? Have you ever had any *trouble* resulting from your use? Positive responses to any question should be followed up. Another instrument for screening alcoholism among the elderly is the MAST-G (Michigan Alcohol Screening Test—Geriatric Version).[26] Therapy must be aimed at identifying and reducing environmental stressors that may trigger alcohol and drug use. The basic needs of food and shelter must be adequately met. Home visits provide a good source of direct assessment data.

Patient education for the older adult includes teaching about the desired effects, possible side effects, and appropriate storage of prescribed and OTC medications. The patient's knowledge of medications that are currently being taken (both prescription and OTC) should be assessed. The patient should be advised to use only one pharmacy because many pharmacies maintain a medication profile, which may prevent problems with drug interactions. The patient should be advised not to drink alcohol when using prescribed medications and OTC drugs. Family members and significant others must be informed about the medication regimen, drug interactions, and the effects of alcohol on drugs.

CHEMICAL DEPENDENCE IN NURSES

The prevalence of chemical dependence among nurses is unknown but is estimated at 6% to 8%. Alcohol is the most common substance abused among nurses, at least initially.[28] A number of contributing factors have been identified. Specific stressors that are commonly thought to contribute to this problem include fatigue, responsibility for patient care, having responsibility without authority within a physician-dominated environment, access to drugs, exposure to death and illness, downsizing and cost containment, being sole providers with career and child care responsibilities, and the final common pathway—physical and emotional pain.[28] Nurses with addictive problems frequently operate with a number of false perceptions and beliefs, such as taking drugs solves problems or knowledge of drugs provides immunity to drug problems.

Nurses frequently lack the knowledge and understanding of addiction and the ability to recognize early behavioral clues. Nursing education may not provide adequate knowledge about substance abuse problems. The working knowledge of many nurses is based on public stereotypes and clinical experiences with difficult alcohol and drug abusers.

Signs of chemical dependence related to work performance may be apparent by changes in personality and behavior, job performance, and attendance (Table 10-22). Nurses often *enable* chemical dependence to continue among co-workers by covering their mistakes or tardiness, excusing another nurse's behavior, repeatedly helping someone complete an assignment, or simply ignoring obvious signs and symptoms (see the Ethical Dilemmas box on p. 183). Helping chemically dependent nurses requires sharing observations and concerns with the nurse and supervisor to provide the means for rehabilitation. Caring about the nurse who is in trouble because of drug

Table 10-22 Signs of Chemical Dependence Among Nurses

Job Performance Changes

Controlled Drug Handling/Records (Potential Drug Diversion)
- Drug counts incorrect
- Excessive errors
- Excessive wastage, often not countersigned
- Medicine signed out to patient who has not been in pain
- Two strengths of drug signed out to same patient, same time
- Packaging appears to be tampered with
- Patient complaints of ineffective pain control
- Volunteers to give controlled drugs
- Comes in early or stays late
- Disappears into the bathroom after handling controlled drugs
- Unexplained absences from the unit

General Performance
- Medication errors
- Poor judgment
- Euphoric recall for involvement in unpleasant situations, or confrontations on the job
- Illogical or sloppy charting
- Absenteeism, especially in conjunction with days off
- Requesting leave time just before the assigned shift
- Lateness with elaborate excuses
- Job shrinkage (does the minimum work required to get by)
- Missed deadlines

Behavior/Personality Changes
- Sudden changes in mood
- Periods of irritability
- Forgetfulness
- Wears long sleeves even in hot weather
- Socially isolates from co-workers
- Inappropriate behavior
- Has chronic pain condition
- History of pain treatment with controlled substances

Signs of Use
- Alcohol on the breath
- Constant use of perfumes, mouthwash, and breath mints
- Flushed face, reddened eyes, unsteady gait, slurred speech
- Hyperactivity, accelerated speech
- Increasing family problems that interfere with work

Signs of Withdrawal
- Tremors, restlessness, diaphoresis, pupil changes
- Watery eyes, runny nose, stomach aches, joint pains, gooseflesh

From Stuart GW, Laraia MT: *Principles and practices of psychiatric nursing,* ed 6, St Louis, 1998, Mosby, p 518.

ETHICAL DILEMMAS

Impaired Providers

SITUATION

The nurses in the geriatric unit know that one of their colleagues has undergone treatment for prescription drug addiction. She seemed to be doing well until recently, when she has been totally focused on her separation and subsequent divorce. Her colleagues suspect that she is using drugs again and worry that it will affect her patient care. How should they handle this situation?

DISCUSSION

These nurses have responsibilities to their patients, colleague, and profession. Knowing their colleague's past history of drug problems, they have been especially concerned about her. Reporting her to the administration may cost her her job and license. However, her patients may be endangered by her carelessness and inability to function in a crisis. If the nurses agree not to report her, they would be in collusion with her and might be held legally liable for any harm she causes to patients. These nurses will also be damaging the profession by putting a colleague's interests before their duty to their patients. These nurses have the responsibility of documenting observed behaviors and confronting their colleague personally in some cases, as well as reporting her to a supervisor and the state board of nursing. They can help best by getting her the help she needs, not by covering up for her or hoping that she will not harm patients.

ETHICAL AND LEGAL PRINCIPLES

- In cases of impaired nurses, whistle-blowing is protected under most nurse practice acts, which require mandatory reporting in some states. Anonymous contacts with the board may be possible, especially if the reporting nurse is concerned about retaliation. Confidentiality is maintained during the reporting process.
- Nurses have a duty to be loyal to their colleagues. However, they also have a professional obligation to protect the safety of patients who might be adversely affected by the incompetence of any health care professional.
- Nonmaleficence—not doing harm and protecting from harm—is a primary ethical principle. According to the American Nurses' Association Code, one's primary loyalty is to patients.

and alcohol abuse may be a painful process for the co-worker. It involves self-awareness, confrontation, patience, support, and belief in the nurse's recovery.

Because of widespread denial and the "conspiracy of silence," chemical dependence in nurses has not been addressed as a professional issue until the 1980s. The American Nurses' Association responded to nurses' need for help by passing a resolution in 1982 that advocates rehabilitation for nurses who are chemically dependent and the establishment of assistance programs by state nurses' associations.

The National Nurses' Society on Addictions (NNSA) produced a position paper on impaired nurses, established a national network of resources, and created a model diversion program to assist states in developing programs. The goals of these programs are to protect the safety of the public, to maintain the integrity of the profession, and to ensure that the nurse is offered the possibility of treatment and rehabilitation before the license to practice is revoked or the job is terminated. Essential components of these programs include education, intervention, referral to appropriate treatment, monitoring of

CRITICAL THINKING EXERCISES

CASE STUDY

Cocaine Toxicity

Patient Profile

Mr. C. is a 34-year-old man who was admitted to the emergency department with chest pain, tachycardia, dizziness, nausea, and severe migraine-like headache.

Subjective Data

- Is extremely nervous and irritable
- Thinks he is having a heart attack
- Admits that he was at a party earlier in the evening drinking alcohol, smoking pot, and snorting cocaine
- Noted a change in personality, including irritability and restlessness
- Experienced an increased need for cocaine in the past few months

Objective Data

Physical Examination

- Appears pale and diaphoretic
- Has tremors
- BP 210/110, pulse 100 beats/min, respiratory rate 30/min

Critical Thinking Questions

1. What other information is needed to assess Mr. C.'s condition?
2. How should questions regarding these areas be addressed?
3. What other clues should the nurse be alert for in assessing his drug use?
4. What emergency conditions must be carefully monitored?
5. What nursing interventions are appropriate?
6. What is the best way to approach Mr. C. to engage him in a treatment program?
7. Based on the assessment data presented, write one or more nursing diagnoses. Are there any collaborative problems?

recovery, and support for reentry into practice. Types of programs include diversion programs associated with the state board of nursing, which allow nurses to maintain their licenses and practice while being monitored through recovery, state nurses' association peer assistance programs, and employee assistance programs.

REVIEW QUESTIONS

The number of the question corresponds to the same-numbered objective at the beginning of the chapter.

1. A pattern of abnormal or pathologic use resulting in physical, emotional, or social impairment is known as
   a. abuse.
   b. addiction.
   c. habituation.
   d. dependence.
2. One of the most compelling reasons leading to continued drug use is
   a. poor social skills.
   b. poor body image.
   c. family dysfunction.
   d. powerful immediate gratification.
3. A nurse caring for a patient who has had an interruption in the addictive cycle after the development of tolerance would expect to see
   a. loss of control.
   b. decreased dependence.
   c. withdrawal symptoms.
   d. no change in condition.
4. A common characteristic of substance abusers is
   a. high frustration tolerance.
   b. impulsive behaviors.
   c. precocious sexual behavior.
   d. enabling behavior.
5. Which of the following combinations is used to prolong euphoria and decrease paranoia and agitation but greatly increases the risk of liver injury and sudden death?
   a. heroin and cocaine
   b. cocaine and alcohol
   c. PCP and cocaine
   d. marijuana and alcohol
6. A withdrawal syndrome that is characterized by stomach cramps, diaphoresis, gooseflesh, rhinorrhea, anxiety, and restlessness is associated with dependence on
   a. alcohol.
   b. narcotics.
   c. cannabis.
   d. stimulants.
7. Pain management of patients with drug-related problems in the postoperative period requires that the nurse
   a. avoid narcotics.
   b. induce withdrawal.
   c. provide patient-controlled analgesia.
   d. accept and respect the patient's report of pain.
8. Secondary prevention activities for substance abuse are aimed at
   a. control and monitoring of addicted persons.
   b. prevention of relapse for recovering persons.
   c. early identification and intervention in a health problem.
   d. collective action to influence social policy and develop social responsibility.
9. The nurse's assessment of personal patterns of drug use is a health promotion strategy that primarily supports the nurse's role as
   a. educator.
   b. resource.
   c. case finder.
   d. change agent.

10. The nursing management of a patient in long-term rehabilitation for substance abuse includes
    a. observing for withdrawal symptoms.
    b. administering drugs prescribed during detoxification.
    c. providing a safe, drug-free environment.
    d. assisting the patient to recognize early triggers of relapse.
11. Substance abuse problems in older adults most commonly are related to
    a. use of drugs and alcohol as a social activity.
    b. misuse of prescribed and over-the-counter drugs.
    c. binge drinking for weeks or months with periods of sobriety.
    d. continuing the use of illegal drugs initiated during middle age.
12. One factor contributing to chemical dependence among nurses is
    a. denial of substance abuse among their peers by nurses.
    b. unimpaired access to a wide variety of mood-altering drugs.
    c. an increased knowledge of the effects of addiction and how to control addictive behavior.
    d. the development of diversion programs that support treatment and rehabilitation of nurses with dependency.

References

1. Tweed SH: Identifying the alcoholic patient, *Nurs Clin North Am* 24:13, 1989.
2. Kinney J: *Clinical manual of substance abuse,* ed 2, St Louis, 1996, Mosby.
3. Westermeyer J: Substance use disorders: predictions for the 1990s, *Am J Drug Alcohol Abuse* 18:1, 1992.
4. American Society of Addiction Medicine: Public policy statement on nicotine dependence and tobacco, *J Addict Dis* 16:99, 1997.
5. Schmitz JM, Schneider NG, Jarvik ME: Nicotine. In Lowinson JH and others, editors: *Substance abuse: a comprehensive textbook,* ed 3, Baltimore, 1997, Williams & Wilkins.
6. Thun MJ, Heath CW: Changes in mortality from smoking in two American Cancer Society prospective studies since 1959, *Prev Med* 26:422, 1997.
7. Hoffmann D, Djordjevic MV, Hoffmann I: The changing cigarette, *Prev Med* 26:427, 1997.
8. Winger G, Hofmann FG, Wood JH: *A handbook on drug and alcohol abuse: the biomedical aspects,* ed 3, New York, 1992, Oxford University Press.
9. Vriz O and others: Smoking is associated with higher cardiovascular risk in young women than in men: the Tecumseh blood pressure study, *J Hypertens* 15:127, 1997.
10. Benowitz NL: The role of nicotine in smoking-related cardiovascular disease, *Prev Med* 26:412, 1997.
11. Wise RA: Changing smoking patterns and mortality from chronic obstructive pulmonary disease, *Prev Med* 26:418, 1997.
12. Svanes C and others: Smoking and ulcer perforation, *Gut* 41:177, 1997.
13. Greden JF, Walters A: Caffeine. In Lowinson JH and others, editors: *Substance abuse: a comprehensive textbook,* ed 3, Baltimore, 1997, Williams & Wilkins.
14. Verderber A, Fitzsimmons L, Shively M: Cocaine abuse, *J Cardiovasc Nurs* 6:43, 1992.
15. Zafar H, Vaz A, Carlson RW: Acute complications of cocaine intoxication, *Hosp Pract* 32:167, 1997.
16. Andrews P: Cocaethylene toxicity, *J Addict Dis* 16:75, 1997.
17. Gold MS: Cocaine. In Lowinson JH and others, editors: *Substance abuse: a comprehensive textbook,* ed 3, Baltimore, 1997, Williams & Wilkins.
18. Schuckit MA: *Drug and alcohol abuse: a clinical guide to diagnosis and treatment,* ed 4, New York, 1995, Plenum.
19. Sullivan EJ: *Nursing care of clients with substance abuse,* St Louis, 1995, Mosby.
20. Sharp CW, Rosenberg NL: Inhalants. In Lowinson JH and others, editors: *Substance abuse: a comprehensive textbook,* ed 3, Baltimore, 1997, Williams & Wilkins.
21. Weinman SA: Emergency management of drug overdose, *Crit Care Nurse* 13:45, 1993.
22. Soloway RA: Street-smart advice on treating drug overdoses, *Am J Nurs* 93:9, 1993.
23. Salerno E, Wilkens J: *Pain management handbook: an interdisciplinary approach,* St Louis, 1996, Mosby.
24. Ferrell BR, McCaffery M: Nurses' knowledge about equianalgesia and opioid dosing, *Cancer Nurs* 20:201, 1997.
25. Adams W and others: Alcohol-related hospitalizations of elderly people, *JAMA* 270:1222, 1993.
26. Gurnack AM, editor: *Older adults' misuse of alcohol, medicines, and other drugs,* New York, 1997, Springer.
27. Bailes BK: Chronic alcohol abuse in elderly surgical patients, *AORN J* 65:963, 1997.
28. Nace EP: *Achievement and addiction: a guide to the treatment of professionals,* New York, 1995, Brunner/Mazel.

Resources

Action on Smoking & Health
2013 H Street NW
Washington, DC 20006
202-659-4310

Al-Anon Family Group Headquarters, Inc.
1600 Corporate Landing Parkway
Virginia Beach, VA 23454-5617
757-563-1600
Fax: 757-563-1655
800-344-2666
http://www.al-anon-alateen.org/

Alcoholics Anonymous
P.O. Box 459
New York, NY 10163
212-870-3400
Fax: 212-870-3003
http://www.alcoholics-anonymous.org/

American Psychiatric Nurses' Association
200 19th Street NW, Suite 300
Washington, DC 20036-2422
202-857-1133
Fax: 202-223-4579
http://www.apna.org/

American Society of Addiction Medicine
4601 North Park Ave
Arcade Suite 101
Chevy Chase, MD 20815
301-656-3920
http://www.asam.org/asam50.htm

Another Empty Bottle
http://www.alcoholismhelp.com/help/

Cocaine Anonymous World Services
P.O. Box 2000
Los Angeles, CA 90049-8000
310-559-5833
Fax: 310-559-2554
http://www.ca.org/

Cocaine/Crack Action Helpline
1-800-888-9383

Drug & Alcohol Nursing Association, Inc.
660 Lonely Cottage Drive
Upper Black Eddy, PA 18972-9313
610-847-5396
Fax: 610-847-5063

Drugs Anonymous
P.O. Box 473
Ansonia Station
New York, NY 10023

Institute of Addiction Awareness
31878 Del Obispo No. 118, Suite 433
San Juan Capistrano, CA 92675
714-830-4866 (phone/fax)

National Association of Alcoholism & Drug Abuse Counselors
1911 N. Fort Myer Drive, Suite 900
Arlington, VA 22209
703-741-7686
Fax: 703-741-7698
http://www.naadac.org/

National Clearinghouse for Alcohol & Drug Information
11426 Rockville Pike, Suite 200
Rockville, MD 20852
800-729-6686
http://www.health.org/aboutn.htm

National Consortium of Chemical Dependency Nurses
1720 Willow Creek Circle, Suite 519
Eugene, OR 97402
800-876-2236
Fax: 503-485-7372

National Council on Alcoholism & Drug Dependence, Inc.
12 W 21st Street
New York, NY 10010
212-206-6770
Fax: 212-645-1690
800-NCA-CALL
http://www.ncadd.org

National Institute on Drug Abuse
5600 Fishers Lane, Room 10A-39
Rockville, MD 20857
301-443-6245
http://www.nida.nih.gov/

National Nurses' Society on Addictions
4101 Lake Boone Trail, Suite 201
Raleigh, NC 27607
919-783-5871
Fax: 919-787-4916
http://www.nnsa.org/

Substance Abuse & Mental Health Services Administration
Department of Health and Human Services
The U.S. Department of Health and Human Services
200 Independence Avenue SW
Washington, DC 20201
202-619-0257
http://www.samhsa.gov/

For additional internet resources, see the website for this book at www.mosby.com/MERLIN/medsurg_lewis

SECTION

2

PATHOPHYSIOLOGIC MECHANISMS OF DISEASE

SECTION OUTLINE

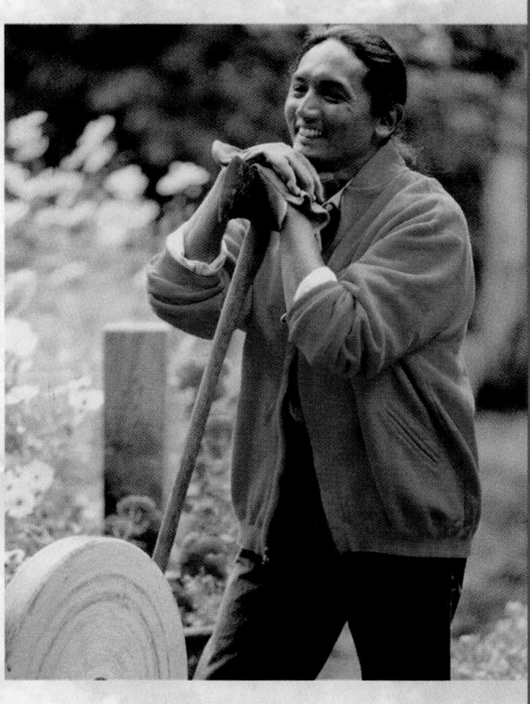

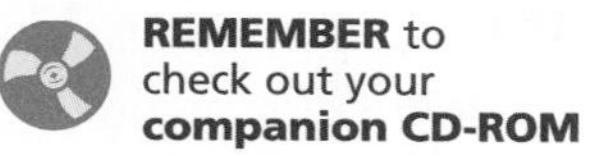

11 NURSING MANAGEMENT Inflammation and Infection

Sharon Mantik Lewis

www.mosby.com/MERLIN/medsurg_lewis

LEARNING OBJECTIVES

1. Explain the cellular adaptive mechanisms to sublethal injury.
2. Describe the causes and mechanisms of lethal cell injury.
3. Differentiate among types of cell necrosis.
4. Describe the components and functions of the mononuclear phagocyte system.
5. Describe the inflammatory response, including vascular and cellular responses and exudate formation.
6. Explain local and systemic manifestations of inflammation and their physiologic bases.
7. Differentiate among healing by primary, secondary, and tertiary intention.
8. Describe the factors that delay wound healing and common complications of wound healing.
9. Describe the pharmacologic, dietary, and nursing management of inflammation.

CELL INJURY

Cell injury can be sublethal or lethal. Sublethal injury alters function without causing cell death. The changes caused by this type of injury are potentially reversible if the injurious stimulus is removed. Lethal injury is an irreversible process that causes cell death.

Cell Adaptation to Sublethal Injury

Cell adaptations to sublethal injuries are common and are part of many physiologic and disease processes. For example, prolonged exposure to sunlight stimulates melanin production and thus provides protection of deeper skin layers by tanning the skin. Lack of muscular activity can lead to atrophy and decreased muscle tone. Adaptive processes of the cell include hypertrophy, hyperplasia, atrophy, and metaplasia (Fig. 11-1). Other responses that are considered maladaptive are dysplasia and anaplasia.

Hypertrophy. *Hypertrophy* is an increase in the size of cells without cell division. For example, the uterus during pregnancy enlarges from hormonal stimulation. The heart of a person with severe hypertension enlarges to compensate for the increased resistance to its pumping action. Removal of one kidney results in an increase in the size of the remaining kidney due to the increased work demand. Muscle hypertrophy results from an increase in the size of muscle fibers due to an increase in cellular protein, as would occur in an individual who does weight training.

Reviewed by Ann Caudell, RN, PhD, OCN, Assistant Professor, College of Nursing, University of New Mexico, Albuquerque, NM, and Marguerite Jackson, RN, PhD, CIC, FAAN, Administrative Director, Epidemiology Unit and Nursing and Research Education; Associate Clinical Professor of Family and Preventive Medicine, Division of Epidemiology, University of California-San Diego, San Diego, Calif.

Hyperplasia. *Hyperplasia* is an increase in the number of cells due to increased cellular division. This process is reversible when the stimulus is removed. *Compensatory hyperplasia* is an adaptive process whereby cells of certain organs regenerate. For example, if portions of the liver are removed, the remaining cells will undergo increased mitosis in order to compensate for the cells removed. Hormonal hyperplasia occurs primarily in organs responsive to estrogen, such as the breast and uterus. For example, the female breast experiences hyperplasia during lactation.

Atrophy. *Atrophy* is a decrease in the size of a tissue or organ caused by a decreased number of cells or reduction in the size of the individual cells. It frequently occurs as a result of disease (e.g., musculoskeletal disease), lack of blood supply (e.g., thrombus formation), natural aging process (e.g., decreased breast size after menopause), inactivity (e.g., decreased muscle size), and nutritional deficiency.

Metaplasia. *Metaplasia* is the reversible transformation of one cell type into another. An example of physiologic metaplasia is when circulating monocytes change to macrophages as they migrate into inflamed tissues. An example of pathophysiologic metaplasia is when the normal pseudostratified columnar epithelium of the bronchi changes to squamous epithelium in response to chronic cigarette smoking. If the irritating stimulus (the cigarette smoke) is removed, the bronchial metaplasia may be reversible.

Dysplasia. *Dysplasia* is an abnormal differentiation of dividing cells resulting in changes in the size, shape, and appearance of the cells. Minor dysplasia is found in some areas of inflammation. Dysplasia is potentially reversible if the stimulus is removed. Frequently, dysplasia can be a precursor of malignancy as in cervical dysplasia.

Anaplasia. *Anaplasia* is cell differentiation to a more immature or embryonic form. Malignant tumors are often characterized by anaplastic cell growth.

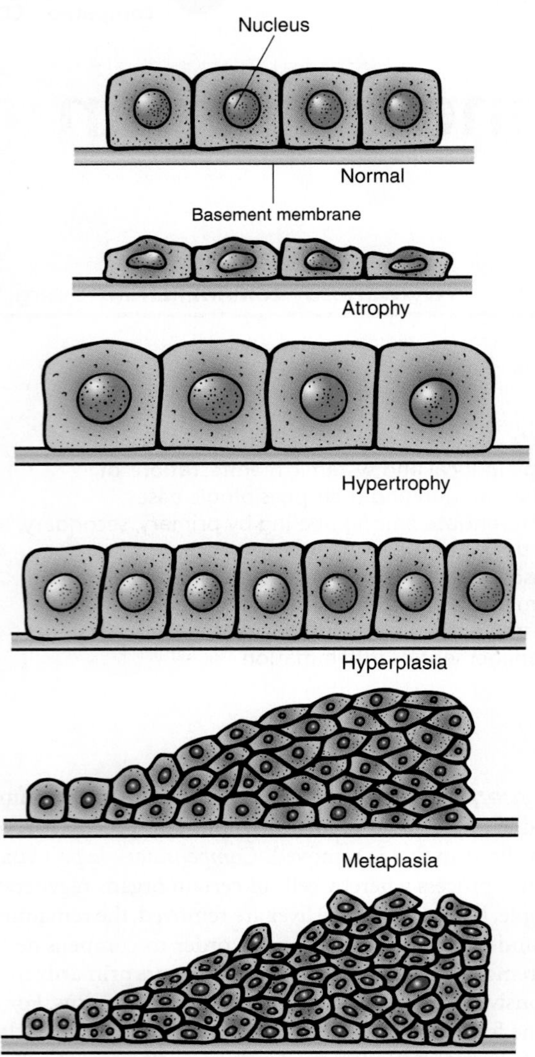

Fig. 11-1 Adaptive alterations in simple cuboidal epithelial cells.

Causes of Lethal Cell Injury

Many different agents and factors can cause lethal cell injury (Table 11-1). The mechanism of actual cell death varies. Examples include deterioration of the nucleus, such as *pyknosis* (nuclear condensation and shrinking) and *karyolysis* (dissolution of nucleus and contents), disruption of cell metabolism, and rupture of the cell membrane.

Microbial invasion frequently, but not always, results in cell injury and death. Infection occurs when *pathogens* (microorganisms capable of producing disease) invade and multiply in body tissues. (Common viruses and bacteria that cause diseases in humans are listed in Tables 11-2 and 11-3.) *Opportunistic* organisms are microorganisms that are not usually considered pathogens. However, they may cause infection if the resistance of the host is decreased from events such as immunosuppression, trauma, or illness.

Cell Necrosis

Necrosis is the death of cells within a living organism. Different types of necrosis tend to occur in different organs or tissues (Table 11-4, p. 193).

DEFENSE AGAINST INJURY

To protect against injury and infection, the body has various defense mechanisms. These defense mechanisms are (1) the skin and mucous membranes, which are the first lines of defense (see Chapter 21); (2) the mononuclear phagocyte system; (3) the inflammatory response; and (4) the immune system (see Chapter 12).

Mononuclear Phagocyte System

The mononuclear phagocyte system (MPS) consists of monocytes and macrophages and their precursor cells. In the past, the MPS system was called the reticuloendothelial system (RES). However, it is not a body system with distinctly defined tissues and organs. Rather, it consists of phagocytic cells located in various tissues and organs (Table 11-5, p. 193). The phagocytic cells are either fixed or free (mobile). The macrophages of the liver, spleen, bone marrow, lungs, lymph nodes, and nervous system (microglial cells) are fixed phagocytes. The monocytes (in blood) and the macrophages found in connective tissue, termed *histiocytes,* are mobile or wandering phagocytes.

Monocytes and macrophages originate in the bone marrow. Monocytes spend a few days in the blood and then enter tissues and change into macrophages. Tissue macrophages are larger and more phagocytic than monocytes.

The functions of the macrophage system include recognition and phagocytosis of foreign material such as microorganisms, removal of old or damaged cells from circulation, and participation in the immune response (see Chapter 12).

Inflammatory Response

The inflammatory response is a sequential reaction to cell injury. It neutralizes and dilutes the inflammatory agent, removes necrotic materials, and establishes an environment suitable for healing and repair. The term *inflammation* is often but incorrectly used as a synonym for the term *infection.* Inflammation is always present with infection, but infection is not always present with inflammation. However, a person who is neutropenic may not be able to mount an inflammatory response. An infection involves invasion of tissues or cells by microorganisms such as bacteria, fungi, and viruses. In contrast, inflammation can also be caused by nonliving agents such as heat, radiation, trauma, and allergens (see Table 11-1). If infection is also present, it is from a superimposed invasion of microorganisms.

The mechanism of inflammation is basically the same regardless of the injuring agent. The intensity of the response depends on the extent and severity of injury and on the reactive capacity of the victim. The inflammatory response can be divided into a vascular response, a cellular response, formation of exudate, and healing.

Vascular Response. After cell injury, arterioles in the area briefly undergo transient vasoconstriction. After release of histamine and other chemicals by the injured cells, the vessels dilate. This vasodilation results in *hyperemia* (increased blood flow in the area), which raises filtration pressure. Vasodilation and chemical mediators cause endothelial cell retraction, which increases capillary permeability. Movement of fluid from capillaries into tissue spaces is thus facilitated. Initially composed of serous fluid, this inflammatory exudate

Table 11-1 Causes of Lethal Cell Injury

Cause	Effect on Cell
Physical Agents	
▪ Heat	Denaturation of protein, acceleration of metabolic reactions
▪ Cold	Decreased blood flow from vasoconstriction, slowed metabolic reactions, thrombosis of blood vessels, freezing of cell content that forms crystals and can burst cell
▪ Radiation	Alteration of cell structure and activity, alteration of enzyme systems, mutations
▪ Electrothermal injury	Interruption of neural conduction, fibrillation of cardiac muscle, coagulative necrosis of skin and skeletal muscle
▪ Mechanical trauma	Transfer of excess kinetic energy to cells causing rupture of cells, blood vessels, tissue; examples include: *Abrasion:* scraping of skin or mucous membrane *Laceration:* severing of vessels and tissue *Contusion (bruise):* crushing of tissue cells causing hemorrhage into skin *Puncture:* piercing of body structure or organ *Incision:* surgical cutting
Chemical Injury	Alteration of cell metabolism, interference with normal enzymatic action within cells
Microbial Injury	
▪ Viruses	Taking over of cell metabolism and synthesis of new particles that may cause cell rupture, cumulative effect possibly producing clinical disease
▪ Bacteria*	Destruction of cell membrane or cell nucleus, production of lethal toxins
Ischemic Injury	Compromised cell metabolism, acute or gradual cell death
Immunologic†	
▪ Antigen-antibody response	Release of substances (histamine, complement) that can injure and damage cells
▪ Autoimmune	Activation of complement, which destroys normal cells and produces inflammation
Neoplastic Growth	Cell destruction from abnormal and uncontrolled cell growth
Normal Substances (e.g., digestive enzymes, uric acid)	Release into abdomen causing peritonitis, crystallization of excess accumulation in joints and renal tissue

*Bacteria are commonly classified as gram-negative or gram-positive bacteria.
†See Chapter 12 for a more detailed discussion.

later contains plasma proteins, primarily albumin. The proteins exert oncotic pressure that further draws fluid from blood vessels. The tissue becomes edematous. This response is illustrated in Fig. 11-3.

As the plasma protein fibrinogen leaves the blood, it is activated to fibrin by the products of the injured cells. Fibrin strengthens a blood clot formed by platelets. In tissue the clot functions to trap bacteria, to prevent their spread, and to serve as a framework for the healing process.

Cellular Response. The cellular response to injury is illustrated in Fig. 11-4 on p. 194. The blood flow through capillaries in the area slows as fluid is lost and viscosity increases. Neutrophils and monocytes move to the inner surface of the capillaries (margination) and then, in ameboid fashion, through the capillary wall (diapedesis) to the site of injury (Fig. 11-5, p. 194).

Chemotaxis is the directional migration of white blood cells (WBCs) along a concentration gradient of chemotactic factors, which are substances that attract leukocytes to the site of inflammation. Chemotaxis is the mechanism for ensuring accumulation of neutrophils and monocytes at the focus of injury. Chemotactic factors include bacterial-derived chemotactic factors, complement-derived chemotactic factor (C5a), lipid-derived chemotactic factors (leukotriene B_4, 5-HETE, platelet-activating factor), platelet-derived chemotactic factors, and coagulation-related chemotactic factors.

Neutrophils. Neutrophils are the first leukocytes to arrive (usually within 6 to 12 hours). They phagocytize (engulf) bacteria, other foreign material, and damaged cells. With their short life span (24 to 48 hours), dead neutrophils soon accumulate. In time the mixture of dead neutrophils, digested bacteria, and other cell debris accumulates as a creamy substance termed *pus.*

To keep up with the demand for neutrophils, the bone marrow releases more neutrophils into circulation. This results in an elevated WBC count (especially the neutrophil count).[1] Sometimes the demand for neutrophils increases to the extent that the bone marrow releases immature forms of neutrophils (bands) into circulation. (Mature neutrophils are called segmented neutrophils.) The finding of increased numbers of band neutrophils in circulation is called a shift to the left, which is commonly found in patients with acute bacterial infections.

Monocytes. Monocytes are the second type of phagocytic cells that migrate from circulating blood. They are attracted to the site by chemotactic factors and usually arrive at the site within 3 to 7 days after the onset of inflammation. On entering the tissue spaces, monocytes transform into macrophages. Together with the tissue macrophages, these macrophages assist in phagocytosis of the inflammatory debris. The macrophage role is important in cleaning the area before healing can occur. Macrophages have a long life span; they can multiply and may

Table 11-2 Common Viruses Causing Disease

Type	Disease Caused
■ Adenoviruses	Upper respiratory tract infection, pneumonia
■ Arbovirus	Syndrome of fever, malaise, headache, myalgia; aseptic meningitis; encephalitis
■ Coronavirus	Upper respiratory tract infection
■ Coxsackie viruses A and B	Upper respiratory tract infection, gastroenteritis, acute myocarditis, aseptic meningitis
■ Echoviruses	Upper respiratory tract infection, gastroenteritis, aseptic meningitis
■ Hepatitis	
A	Viral hepatitis
B	Viral hepatitis
C	Viral hepatitis
■ Herpesviruses	
Varicella-zoster	Chickenpox; shingles
Herpes simplex	
Type 1	Herpes labialis ("fever blisters"), genital herpes infection
Type 2	Genital herpes infection
Epstein-Barr	Mononucleosis, Burkitt's lymphoma (possibly)
Cytomegalovirus (CMV)	Pneumonia in immunosuppressed individuals, infectious mononucleosis–like syndrome
■ Human immuno-deficiency virus (HIV)	HIV infection, acquired immunodeficiency syndrome (AIDS)
■ Influenza A, B, C	Upper respiratory tract infection
■ Mumps	Parotitis, orchitis in postpubertal males
■ Papovavirus	Warts
■ Parainfluenza 1-4	Upper respiratory tract infection
■ Parvovirus	Gastroenteritis
■ Poliovirus	Poliomyelitis
■ Pox viruses	Smallpox
■ Reoviruses 1, 2, 3	Upper respiratory tract infection
■ Respiratory syncytia virus	Gastroenteritis, respiratory tract infection
■ Rhabdovirus	Rabies
■ Rhinovirus	Upper respiratory tract infection, pneumonia
■ Rotaviruses	Gastroenteritis
■ Rubella	German measles
■ Rubeola	Measles

Table 11-3 Common Bacteria Causing Disease

Type	Diseases Caused
■ Clostridia	Tetanus (lockjaw)
C. tetani	Food poisoning with progressive muscle paralysis
C. botulinum	Diphtheria
■ *Corynebacterium diphtheriae*	Urinary tract infections, peritonitis
■ *Escherichia coli*	Urinary tract infections
■ *Haemophilus* organisms	
H. influenzae	Nasopharyngitis, meningitis, pneumonia
H. pertussis	Whooping cough
■ *Helicobacter pylori*	Peptic ulcers
■ *Klebsiella-Enterobacter* organisms	Urinary tract infections, peritonitis, pneumonia
■ *Legionella pneumophila*	Pneumonia (Legionnaires' disease)
■ Mycobacteria	
M. tuberculosis	Tuberculosis
M. leprae	Leprosy (Hansen's disease)
■ Neisseriae	
N. meningitidis	Meningococcemia, meningitis
N. gonorrhoeae	Gonorrhea, pelvic inflammatory disease
■ *Proteus* species	Urinary tract infections, peritonitis
■ *Pseudomonas aeruginosa*	Urinary tract infections, meningitis
■ *Salmonella* species	
S. typhi	Typhoid fever
Other *Salmonella* organisms	Food poisoning, gastroenteritis
■ *Shigella species*	Shigellosis, diarrhea with abdominal pain and fever (dysentery)
■ *Staphylococcus aureus*	Skin infections, pneumonia, urinary tract infections, acute osteomyelitis, toxic shock syndrome
■ Streptococci	
S. pyogenes (group A β-hemolytic streptococci)	Pharyngitis, scarlet fever, rheumatic fever, acute glomerulonephritis, erysipelas, pneumonia
S. pyogenes (group B β-hemolytic streptococci)	Urinary tract infections
S. pneumoniae	Pneumococcal pneumonia
S. viridans	Bacterial endocarditis
S. faecalis	Genitourinary infection, infection of surgical wounds
■ *Treponema pallidum*	Syphilis

stay in the damaged tissues for weeks. These long-lived cells are important in orchestrating the healing process.

In some cases, macrophages perform tasks other than phagocytosis. They may accumulate and fuse to form a multinucleated giant cell. The giant cell attempts to phagocytize particles too large for macrophages. The giant cell is then encapsulated by collagen leading to the formation of a granuloma. A classic example of this process occurs with the tubercle bacillus in the lung. While the bacillus is walled off, a chronic state of inflammation exists. The granuloma formed is a cavity of necrotic tissue.

Lymphocytes. Lymphocytes arrive later at the site of injury. Their primary role is related to humoral and cell-mediated immunity (see Chapter 12).

Table **11-4** Types of Necrosis

Type	Description
Coagulative necrosis	Necrotic cells maintain their outline. Lytic enzymes are somewhat inhibited. Proteins are denatured. Enzymes lose their function. Commonly caused by a lack of blood supply.
Liquefactive necrosis	Necrotic cells rapidly disappear as lytic enzymes digest tissues. This type commonly occurs in the brain where the supply of lytic enzymes is abundant.
Caseous necrosis	Necrotic cells disintegrate, but cell fragments remain for long periods of time. This type is called caseous (cheeselike) necrosis because of its crumbly appearance. It is frequently found in tuberculosis of the lung.
Gangrenous necrosis	Necrotic cells result from severe hypoxia and subsequent ischemic injury, which is common after impaired circulation in the lower legs. Dry gangrene refers to the dry, shriveled, darkened area (Fig. 11-2), and wet gangrene refers to the liquefied underlying necrotic tissue.

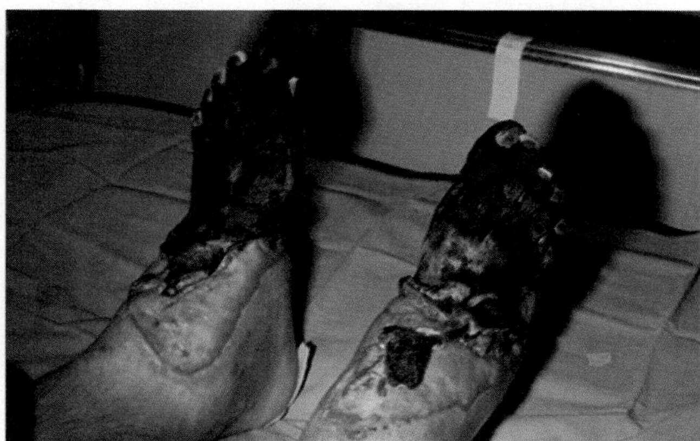

Fig. 11-2 Gangrene of the toes.

Table **11-5** Location and Name of Macrophages*

Location	Name
Connective tissue	Histiocytes
Liver	Kupffer cells
Lung	Alveolar macrophages
Spleen	Free and fixed macrophages
Bone marrow	Fixed macrophages
Lymph nodes	Free and fixed macrophages
Bone tissue	Osteoclasts
Central nervous system	Microglial cells
Peritoneal cavity	Peritoneal macrophages
Pleural cavity	Pleural macrophages
Skin	Histiocyte, Langerhans' cells
Synovium	Type A cells

*In addition, monocytes become macrophages once they leave the blood and enter the tissues.

Eosinophils and basophils. Eosinophils and basophils have a more selective role in inflammation. Eosinophils are released in large quantities during an allergic reaction. They release chemicals that act to control the effects of histamine and serotonin. They are also involved in phagocytosis of the allergen-antibody complex. The histamine and heparin that basophils carry in their granules are released during inflammation. Eosinophils also contain very caustic chemicals that are capable of destroying a parasite's cell surfaces.

Chemical Mediators. Mediators of the inflammatory response are presented in Table 11-6.

Complement system. The complement system is a major mediator of the inflammatory response. Major functions of the complement system are enhanced phagocytosis, increased vascular permeability, chemotaxis, and cellular lysis. All of these activities are important in the inflammatory response.

When activated, the components occur in the sequential order of C1, C4, C2, C3, C5, C6, C7, C8, and C9 (Fig. 11-6). The numbering reflects the order of their discovery. Some components have subparts designated by lowercase letters, such as C3a, C3b, and C5a. The primary pathway for activation of the complement system is through fixation of component C1 to an antigen-antibody complex. The immunoglobulins IgG and IgM are responsible for fixing complement. Each activated complex can act on the next component, creating a cascade effect.

An alternative pathway exists in which C3 is activated without prior antigen-antibody fixation. Bacterial products, lipopolysaccharides, plasmin, and neutrophil proteases can stimulate the complement sequence at the C3 level with activation of C5 through C9.

Complement activation increases phagocytosis through opsonization and chemotaxis. Opsonization occurs when the antigen, in combination with complement factor C3b and immunoglobulin, sticks to the surface of phagocytic cells. This leads to more rapid phagocytosis. In addition, complement component C5a promotes chemotaxis.

The components C3a, C5a, and C4a are termed *anaphylatoxins* and bind to receptors on mast cells and basophils, thus triggering histamine release. Histamine causes smooth muscle contraction, vascular dilation, and an increase in vascular permeability.

The entire complement sequence of C1 to C9 must be activated for cell lysis to occur. The final components (C8, C9) act on the cell surface, causing rupture of the cell membrane and lysis. Bacteria, red blood cells (RBCs), and nucleated cells are susceptible to the lysis.

Prostaglandins and leukotrienes. Prostaglandins (PGs) are substances that can be synthesized from the phospholipids of cell membranes of most body tissues, including blood cells. On stimulation by chemotactic factors or phagocytosis or after cell injury, phospholipids can be converted to arachidonic acid (a 20-carbon polyunsaturated fatty acid), which is then oxidized by two different pathways (Fig. 11-7).

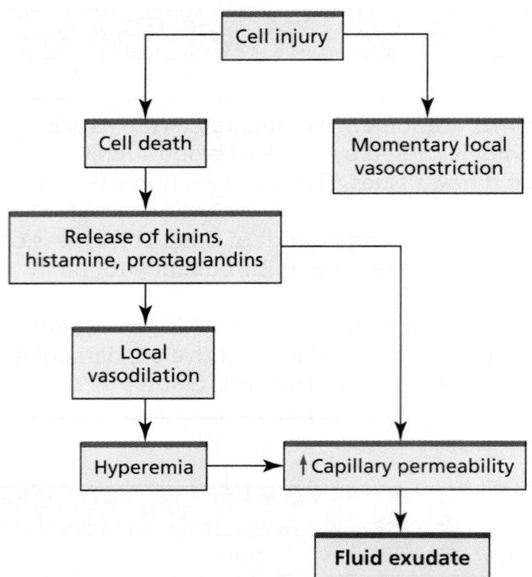

Fig. 11-3 Vascular response in inflammation.

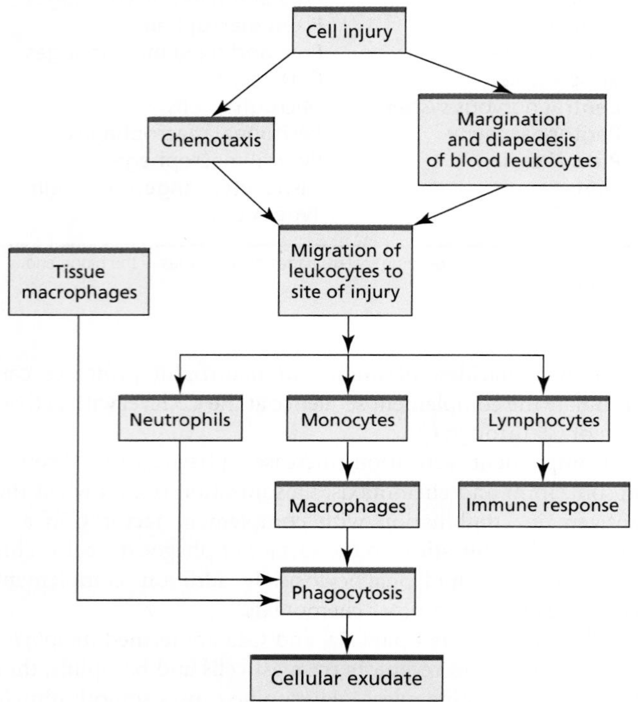

Fig. 11-4 Cellular response in inflammation.

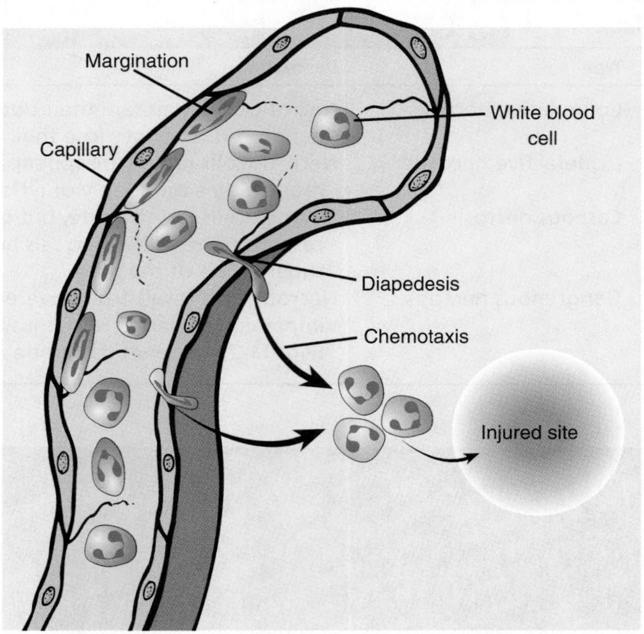

Fig. 11-5 Margination, diapedesis, and chemotaxis of white blood cells.

The cyclooxygenase metabolic pathway leads to the production of PGs of the D, E, F, and I series and thromboxanes (formed on activation of platelets). PGs of the E and I series are potent vasodilators and inhibit platelet and neutrophil aggregation. PGE_2 can also sensitize pain receptors to arousal by stimuli that would normally be painless. PGE_2 is also a potent pyrogen, acting on the temperature-regulating area of the hypothalamus. Thromboxane A_2 is a potent vasoconstrictor and platelet-aggregating agent. PGs are generally considered proinflammatory, contributing to increased blood flow, edema, and pain. Metabolism of arachidonic acid by the lipoxygenase pathway leads to the production of leukotrienes (LTs). LTB_4 is a potent chemotactic factor. LTC_4, LTD_4, and LTE_4 form the slow-reacting substance of anaphylaxis (SRS-A), which constricts smooth muscles of bronchi and increases capillary permeability.

Drugs that inhibit PG synthesis are useful clinically. Nonsteroidal antiinflammatory drugs (NSAIDs), one type of these drugs, are a prototype drug treatment for many acute and chronic inflammatory conditions. Acetylsalicylic acid (ASA) blocks platelet aggregation; it also has antiinflammatory action. Prostacyclin (PGI_2) has been used to prevent platelet deposition in extracorporeal systems, such as hemodialysis and heart-lung bypass oxygenators.

Another group of drugs that inhibit PGs are corticosteroids. They are valuable in the treatment of asthma because they inhibit leukotriene production and thus prevent bronchoconstriction. (Other mediators of the inflammatory response are described in Table 11-6.)

Exudate Formation. Exudate consists of fluid and leukocytes that move from the circulation to the site of injury. The nature and quantity of exudate depend on the type and severity of the injury and the tissues involved (Table 11-7).

Clinical Manifestations. The local response to inflammation includes the manifestations of redness, heat, pain, swelling, and loss of function (Table 11-8).

Systemic manifestations of inflammation include leukocytosis with a shift to the left, malaise, nausea and anorexia, increased pulse and respiratory rate, and fever.

Leukocytosis results from the increased release of leukocytes from the bone marrow. An increase in the circulating number of one or more types of leukocytes may be found. Inflammatory reactions are accompanied by the vaguely defined constitutional symptoms of malaise, nausea, anorexia, and fatigue. The causes of these systemic changes are poorly understood but are

Table **11-6** **Mediators of Inflammation**

Mediator	Source	Mechanisms of Action
Histamine	Stored in granules of basophils, mast cells, platelets	Causes vasodilation and increased vascular permeability by stimulating contraction of endothelial cells and creating widened gaps between cells
Serotonin	Stored in platelets, mast cells, enterochromaffin cells of GI tract	Causes vasodilation and increased vascular permeability by stimulating contraction of endothelial cells and creating widened gaps between cells; stimulates smooth muscle contraction
Kinins (e.g., bradykinin)	Produced from precursor factor kininogen as a result of activation of Hageman factor (XII) of clotting system	Cause contraction of smooth muscle and dilation of blood vessels; result in stimulation of pain
Complement components (C3a, C4a, C5a)	Anaphylatoxic agents generated from complement pathway activation	Stimulate histamine release; stimulate chemotaxis
Fibrinopeptides	Produced from activation of the clotting system	Increase vascular permeability; stimulate chemotaxis for neutrophils
Prostaglandins and leukotrienes	Produced from arachidonic acid (Fig. 11-7)	PGE_1 and PGE_2 cause vasodilation; LTB_4 stimulates chemotaxis
Lymphokines	For information on lymphokines, see Table 12-4.	

LT, leukotrienes; *PG,* prostaglandin.

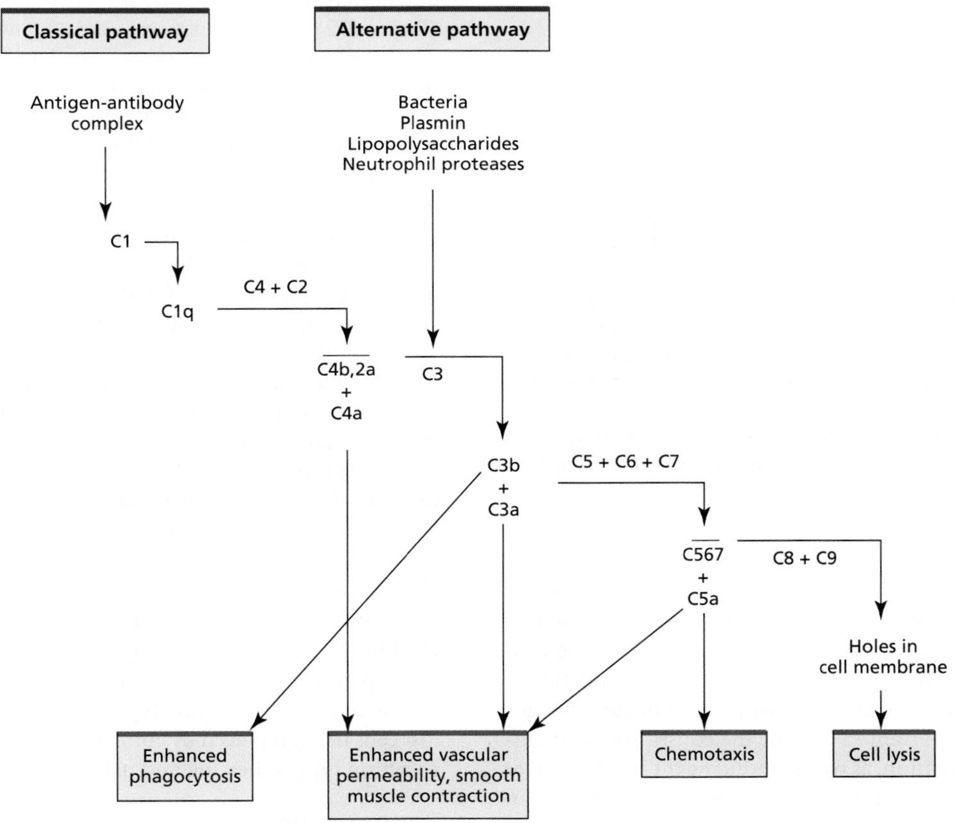

Fig. 11-6 Sequential activation and biologic effects of the complement system.

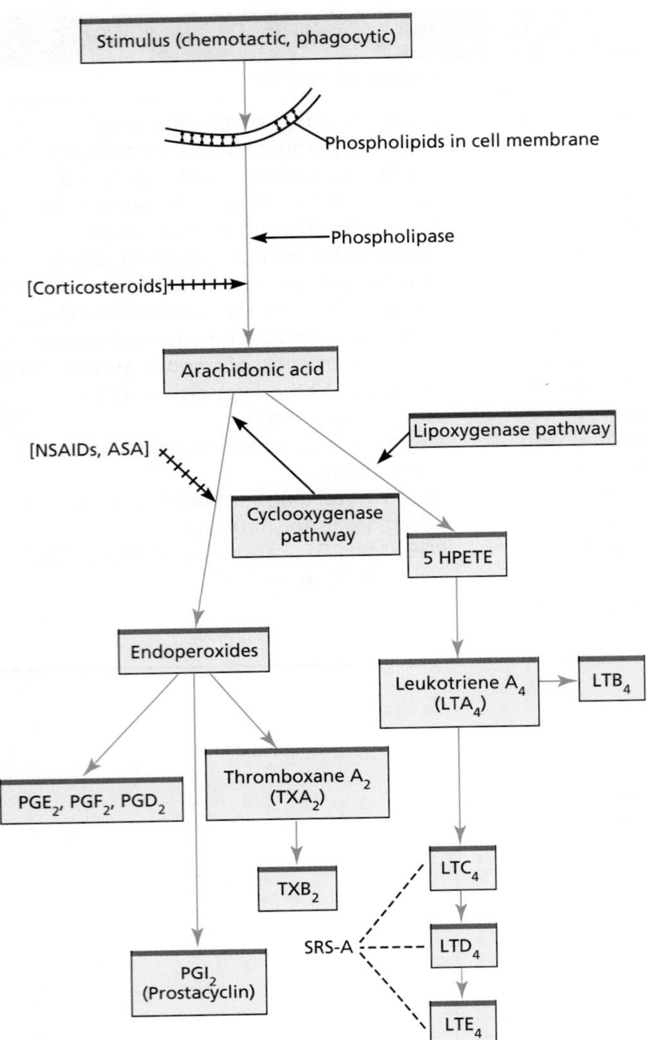

Fig. 11-7 Pathway of arachidonic acid oxygenation and generation of prostaglandins and leukotrienes. Corticosteroids, nonsteroidal antiinflammatory drugs, and acetylsalicylic acid act to inhibit various steps in this pathway. LTC_4, LTD_4, and LTE_4 form the slow-reacting substance of anaphylaxis (SRS-A), an important mediator of allergic responses, by causing bronchoconstriction and increased vascular permeability. *5-HPETE,* 5-hydroperoxyeicosatetraenoic acid.

probably due to complement activation and the production of factors released from stimulated WBCs. Collectively, these factors are termed *cytokines* and function as intercellular messengers. Two of these cytokines, interleukin-1 (IL-1) and tumor necrosis factor (TNF), are released from mononuclear phagocyte cells and are important in causing the constitutional manifestations of inflammation, as well as inducing the production of fever. An increase in pulse and respiration follows the rise in metabolism as a result of an increase in body temperature.

Fever. Fever is caused by endogenous pyrogenic cytokines.[2] The most potent of these cytokines are IL-1 and TNF. Interferon-α (IFN-α), interferon-β (IFN-β), and interferon-γ (IFN-γ) are also pyrogenic cytokines. These pyrogenic cytokines cause fever by their ability to initiate metabolic changes in the temperature-regulating center[3] (Fig. 11-8). Of the metabolic changes the synthesis of prostaglandin E_2 (PGE_2) is the most critical. PGE_2 acts directly to increase the thermostatic set point. The hypothalamus then activates the sympathetic branch of the autonomic nervous system to stimulate increased muscle tone and shivering and decreased perspiration and blood flow to the periphery. Epinephrine released from the adrenal medulla increases the metabolic rate. The net result is fever.

With the physiologic thermostat fixed at a higher-than-normal temperature, the rate of heat production is increased until the body temperature reaches the new set point. As the set point is raised, the hypothalamus signals an increase in heat production and conservation to raise the body temperature to the new level. At this point the individual feels chilled and shivers. The shivering response is the body's method of raising the body's temperature until the new set point is attained. This seeming paradox is quite dramatic: the body is hot yet an individual piles on blankets and may go to bed to get warm. When the circulating body temperature reaches the set point of the core body temperature, the chills and warmth-seeking behavior ceases. The febrile response is classified into four stages (Table 11-9).

Endogenous pyrogenic cytokines and the fever they trigger activate the body's defense mechanisms. Beneficial aspects of fever include increased killing of microorganisms, increased phagocytosis by neutrophils, and increased proliferation of T cells.[4] Higher body temperatures may also enhance the activity of interferon, the body's natural virus-fighting substance (see Chapter 12).

Types of Inflammation. The basic types of inflammation are acute, subacute, and chronic. In acute inflammation the healing occurs in 2 to 3 weeks and usually leaves no residual damage. Neutrophils are the predominant cell type. A subacute inflammation has the features of the acute process but lasts longer. For example, infective endocarditis is a smoldering infection with acute inflammation, but it persists throughout weeks or months (see Chapter 35).

Chronic inflammation lasts for weeks, months, or even years. The injurious agent persists or repeatedly injures tissue. The predominant cell types are lymphocytes, plasma cells, and macrophages. Examples of chronic inflammation include rheumatoid arthritis and tuberculosis. Tuberculosis is a type of chronic granulomatous inflammation. A chronic inflammatory process is debilitating and can be devastating. The prolongation and chronicity of any inflammation may be the result of an alteration in the immune response.

HEALING PROCESS

The final phase of the inflammatory response is healing. Healing includes the two major components of regeneration and repair. *Regeneration* is the replacement of lost cells and tissues with cells of the same type. *Repair* is healing as a result of lost cells being replaced by connective tissue. Repair is the more common type of healing and usually results in scar formation.

Regeneration

The ability of cells to regenerate depends on the cell type (Table 11-10). Labile cells, such as cells of the skin, lymphoid organs, bone marrow, and mucous membranes of the GI, urinary, and reproductive tracts, divide constantly. Injury to these organs is followed by rapid regeneration.

Table 11-7 Types of Inflammatory Exudate

Type	Description	Examples
Serous	Serous exudate results from outpouring of fluid that has low cell and protein content; it is seen in early stages of inflammation or when injury is mild.	Skin blisters, pleural effusion
Catarrhal	Catarrhal exudate is found in tissues where cells produce mucus. Mucus production is accelerated by inflammatory response.	Runny nose associated with upper respiratory tract infection
Fibrinous	Fibrinous exudate occurs with increasing vascular permeability and fibrinogen leakage into interstitial spaces. Excessive amounts of fibrin coating tissue surfaces may cause them to adhere.	Adhesions
Purulent (pus)	Purulent exudate consists of WBCs, microorganisms (dead and alive), liquefied dead cells, and other debris.	Furuncle (boil), abscess, cellulitis (diffuse inflammation in connective tissue)
Hemorrhagic	Hemorrhagic exudate results from rupture or necrosis of blood vessel walls; it consists of RBCs that escape into tissue.	Hematoma

RBC, red blood cell; *WBC,* white blood cell.

Table 11-8 Local Manifestations of Inflammation

Manifestations	Cause
Redness (rubor)	Hyperemia from vasodilation
Heat (color)	Increased metabolism at inflammatory site
Pain (dolor)	Change in pH; change in local ionic concentration; nerve stimulation by chemicals (e.g., histamine, prostaglandins); pressure from fluid exudate
Swelling (tumor)	Fluid shift to interstitial spaces; fluid exudate accumulation
Loss of function (functio laesa)	Swelling and pain

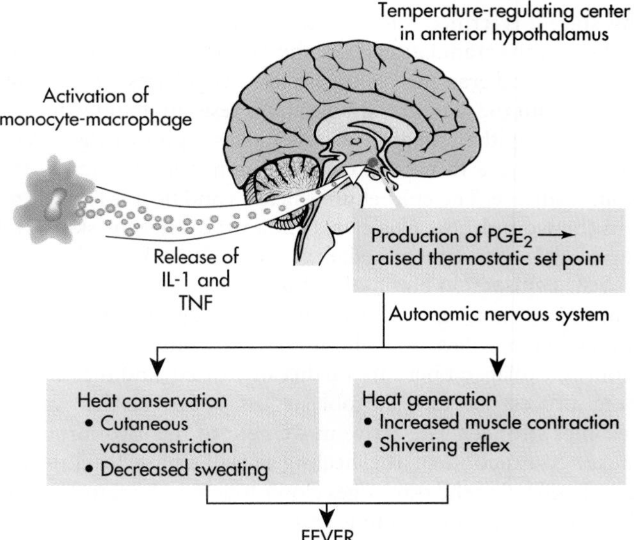

Fig. 11-8 Production of fever. When monocytes/macrophages are activated, they secrete endogenous pyrogenic cytokines such as interleukin-1 (IL-1) and tumor necrosis factor (TNF), which reach the hypothalamic temperature-regulating center. These cytokines promote the synthesis and secretion of prostaglandin E_2 (PGE_2) in the anterior hypothalamus. PGE_2 increases the thermostatic set point, and the autonomic nervous system is stimulated, resulting in shivering, muscle contraction, and peripheral vasoconstriction.

Stable cells retain their ability to regenerate but do so only if the organ is injured. Examples of stable cells are liver, pancreas, kidney, and bone cells.

Permanent cells do not regenerate. Examples of these cells are neurons of the central nervous system (CNS) and cardiac muscle cells. Damage to heart muscle or CNS neurons leads to permanent loss. Healing will occur by repair with scar tissue.

Repair

Repair is a more complex process than regeneration. Most injuries heal by connective tissue repair. Repair healing occurs by primary, secondary, or tertiary intention (Fig. 11-9).

Primary Intention. Primary intention healing takes place when wound margins are neatly approximated, such as in a surgical incision or a paper cut. A continuum of processes is associated with primary healing (Table 11-11). These processes include three phases.

Initial phase. The initial phase lasts for 3 to 5 days. The edges of the incision are first aligned and sutured in place. The incision area fills with blood from the cut blood vessels, and blood clots form. An acute inflammatory reaction occurs. The area of injury is composed of fibrin clots, erythrocytes, neutrophils (both dead and dying), and other debris. Macrophages ingest and digest cellular debris, fibrin fragments, and RBCs. Extracellular enzymes derived from macrophages and neutrophils help digest fibrin. As the wound debris is removed, the fibrin clot serves as a meshwork for future capillary growth and migration of epithelial cells.

Granulation phase. The granulation (fibroplasia) phase is the second step and lasts from 5 days to 4 weeks. The components of granulation tissue include proliferating fibroblasts; proliferating capillary sprouts (angioblasts); various types of WBCs; exudate; and loose, semifluid, ground substance.

Table 11-9 Stages of the Febrile Response

Stage	Characteristics
Prodromal	Nonspecific complaints such as mild headache, fatigue, general malaise, muscle aches
Chill	Cutaneous vasoconstriction, "goose pimples," pale skin; feeling of being cold; generalized, shaking chill; shivering causing body to reach new temperature set by control center in hypothalamus
Flush	Sensation of warmth throughout body; cutaneous vasodilation; warming and flushing of skin
Defervescence	Sweating; decrease in body temperature

Fibroblasts are immature connective tissue cells that migrate into the healing site and secrete collagen. In time the collagen is organized and restructured to strengthen the healing site. At this stage it is termed *fibrous* or *scar tissue.*

During the granulation phase the wound is pink and vascular. Numerous red granules (young budding capillaries) are present. At this point the wound is friable and is resistant to infection.

Surface epithelium at the wound edges begins to regenerate. In a few days a thin layer of epithelium migrates across the wound surface. The epithelium thickens and begins to mature, and the wound now closely resembles the adjacent skin. In a superficial wound, reepithelialization may take 3 to 5 days.

Scar contraction and maturation phase. The scar contraction and maturation phase overlaps with the granulation phase. It may begin 7 days after the injury and continue for several months. Collagen fibers are further organized, and the remodeling process occurs. Fibroblasts disappear as the wound becomes stronger. The active movement of the myofibroblasts causes contraction of the healing area, helping to close the defect and bring the skin edges closer together. A mature scar is then formed. In contrast to granulation tissue, a mature scar is virtually avascular and pale, and it may be more painful at this phase than in the granulation phase.

Secondary Intention. Wounds that occur from trauma, ulceration, and infection and have large amounts of exudate and wide, irregular wound margins may not have edges that can be approximated. The inflammatory reaction may be greater than in primary healing. This results in more debris, cells, and exudate. The debris may have to be cleaned away (debrided) before healing can take place.

In some instances a primary incision may become infected, creating additional inflammation. The wound may reopen, and healing by secondary intention takes place.

The process of healing by secondary intention is essentially the same as by primary healing. The major differences are the greater defect and the gaping wound edges. Healing and granulation take place from the edges inward and from the bottom of the wound upward until the defect is filled. There is more granulation tissue, and the result is a much larger scar.

Wound classification. The red-yellow-black concept is sometimes used to describe open wounds. This concept is based on the color of the open wound (red, yellow, black) rather than on the depth of tissue destruction (Table 11-12 and Fig. 11-10).

Table 11-10 Regenerative Ability of Different Types of Tissues

Tissue Type	Regenerative Ability
Epithelial	
Skin, linings of blood vessels, mucous membranes	Cells readily divide and regenerate
Connective Tissue	
Bone	Active tissue heals rapidly
Cartilage	Regeneration possible but slow
Tendons and ligaments	Regeneration possible but slow
Blood	Cells actively regenerate
Muscle	
Smooth	Regeneration usually possible (particularly in GI tract)
Cardiac	Damaged muscle replaced by connective tissue
Skeletal	Connective tissue replaces severely damaged muscle; some regeneration in moderately damaged muscle occurs
Nerve	
Neuron	Cells do not divide; cells regenerate only if cell body not injured
Glial	Cells regenerate; scar tissue often formed when neurons are damaged.

GI, gastrointestinal.

It can be applied to any wound allowed to heal by secondary intention, including surgically induced wounds left to heal without skin closure because of a risk for infection. A wound may have two or three colors at the same time. In this situation the wound is classified according to the least-desirable color present.

Tertiary Intention. Tertiary intention (delayed primary intention) occurs with delayed suturing of a wound in which two layers of granulation tissue are sutured together. This occurs when a contaminated wound is left open and sutured closed after the infection is controlled. It also occurs when a primary wound becomes infected, is opened, is allowed to granulate, and is then sutured. Tertiary intention results in a larger and deeper scar than primary or secondary intention.

Delay of Healing

In a healthy person, wounds heal at a normal, predictable rate. Little can be done to accelerate this process. However, some factors delay wound healing. These are summarized in Table 11-13 on p. 201.

Complications of Healing

The shape and location of the wound determine how well the wound will heal. Complications result from interference with wound healing. These factors may include malnutrition, obesity, decreased blood supply, tissue trauma, denervation, and infection.[5] Complications that may result include hypertrophic scars and keloids, contracture, dehiscence, excess granulation tissue, adhesions, and major organ dysfunction.

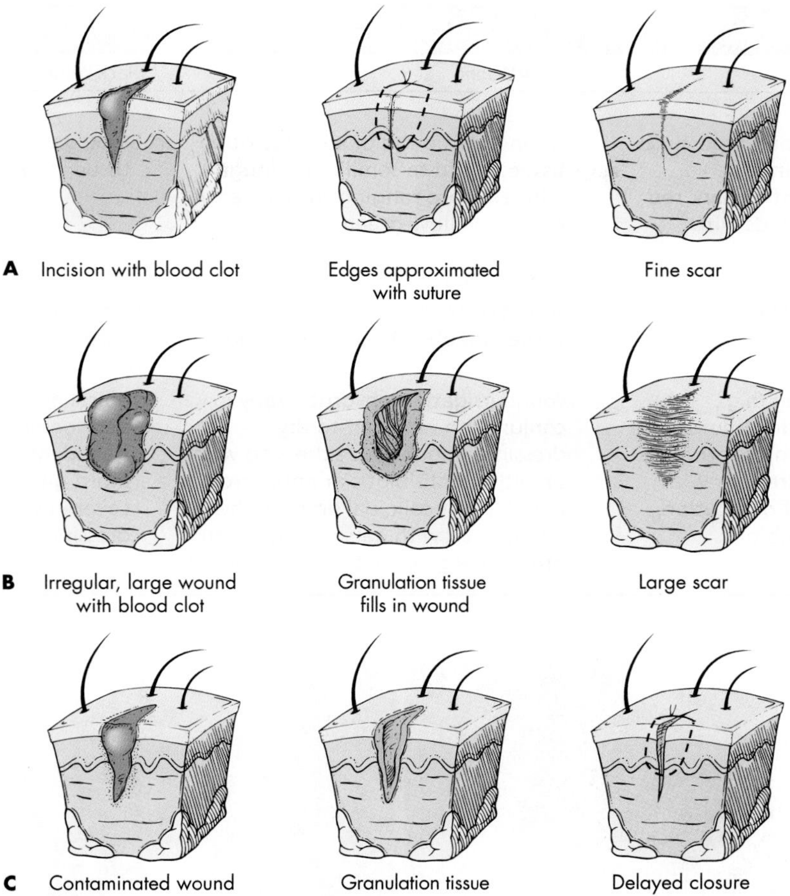

Fig. 11-9 Types of wound healing. **A,** Primary intention. **B,** Secondary intention. **C,** Tertiary intention.

Table 11-11 Phases in Primary Intention Healing

Phase	Activity
Initial (3 to 5 days)	Approximation of incision edges; migration of epithelial cells; clot serving as meshwork for starting capillary growth
Granulation (5 days to 4 weeks)	Migration of fibroblasts; secretion of collagen; abundance of capillary buds; fragility of wound
Scar contracture (7 days to several months)	Remodeling of collagen; strengthening of scar

Hypertrophic Scars and Keloid Formation. Hypertrophic scars and keloid formation occur when the body produces an excess of collagen tissue. A hypertrophic scar is inappropriately large, red, raised, and hard. However, it remains confined to the wound edges and regresses in time. In contrast, a keloid is an even greater protrusion of scar tissue that extends beyond the wound edges and may assume tumorlike masses (Fig. 11-11). In addition, keloids are permanent, without any tendency to subside. The patient with keloids often complains of tenderness, pain, and hyperesthesia, particularly in the early stages of development. A predisposition to keloid formation is thought to be hereditary and occurs more often in dark-skinned people, particularly African-Americans. Neither complication is life threatening, but both can have serious cosmetic implications.

Contracture. Wound contraction is necessary for healing. This process may become abnormal when there is excessive contraction resulting in deformity or contracture. A shortening of muscle or scar tissue results from excessive fibrous formation, especially if the wound is near a joint (see Fig. 23-13). Contracture frequently occurs in burns in which a great loss of skin and subcutaneous tissue occurs (see Chapter 23).

Dehiscence. Dehiscence is the separation and disruption of previously joined wound edges. It usually occurs when a primary healing site bursts. There are three possible contributing causes of dehiscence. First, an infection may cause an inflammatory process. Second, the granulation tissue may not be strong enough to withstand the forces imposed on the wound. Third, obese individuals are at a higher risk for dehiscence because adipose tissue interferes with healing. Evisceration occurs when wound edges separate to the extent that intestinal contents protrude through the wound.

Table 11-12 Red-Yellow-Black Concept of Wound Care

Red Wound	Yellow Wound	Black Wound
Characteristics		
Traumatic or surgical wound, possible presence of serosanguineous drainage, pink to bright or dark red healing or chronic wounds with granulating tissue	Presence of slough or soft necrotic tissue, liquid to semiliquid slough with exudate ranging from creamy ivory to yellow-green	Black, gray, or brown adherent necrotic tissue; possible presence of pus
Purpose of Treatment		
Protection and gentle atraumatic cleansing	Wound cleansing to remove nonviable tissue and absorb excess drainage	Debridement of eschar and nonviable tissue
Dressings and Therapy		
Transparent film dressing (e.g., Tegaderm, Opsite), hydrocolloid dressing (e.g., Duoderm), hydrogels (e.g., Vigilon), gauze dressing with antimicrobial ointment or solution, Telfa dressing with antibiotic ointment	Wound irrigations, hydrotherapy in conjunction with wet-to-dry dressings, moist gauze dressing with or without antibiotic or antimicrobial agent, hydrocolloidal dressing, hydrogel covered with gauze, absorption dressing (e.g., Debrisan beads, paste)	Topical enzyme debridement, surgical debridement, hydrotherapy, chemical debridement (e.g., Dakin's solution), moist gauze dressing, hydrogel covered with gauze, absorption dressing covered with gauze

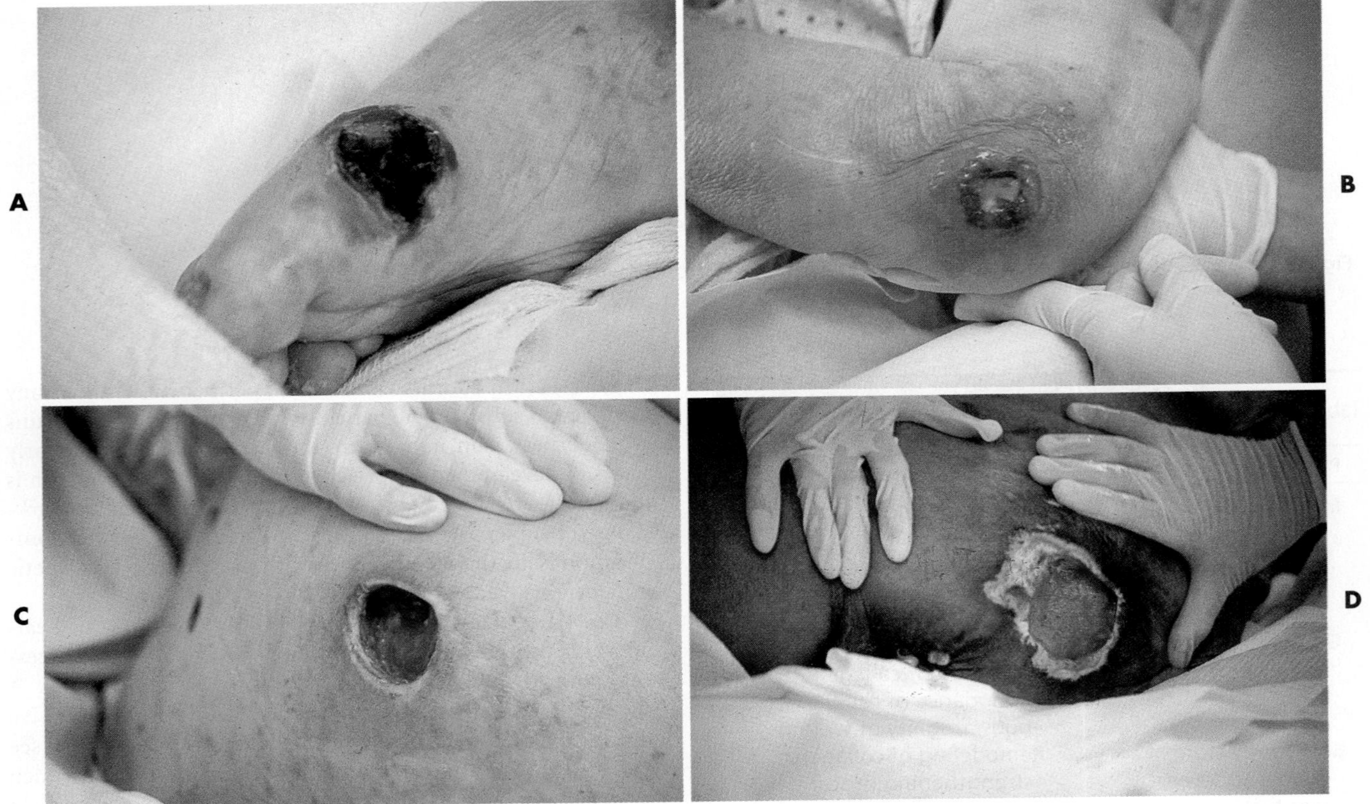

Fig. 11-10 Wounds classified by color assessment. **A,** A black wound. **B,** A yellow wound. **C,** A red wound. **D,** A mixed-color wound.

Excess Granulation Tissue. Excess granulation tissue ("proud flesh") may protrude above the surface of the healing wound. If the granulation tissue is cauterized or cut off, healing continues in a normal manner.

Adhesions. Adhesions are bands of scar tissue between or around organs. Adhesions may occur in the abdominal cavity or between the lungs and pleura. Adhesions in the abdomen may cause an intestinal obstruction. Adhesions between the lungs and pleura require *decortication,* or stripping of pleura, to permit normal ventilation.

Collaborative Care

Collaborative care related to inflammation and infection is highly variable. It depends on the causative agent, the degree of

Table 11-13 Factors Delaying Wound Healing

Factor	Effect on Wound Healing
Nutritional deficiencies	
Vitamin C	Delays formation of collagen fibers and capillary development
Protein	Decreases supply of amino acids for tissue repair
Zinc	Impairs epithelialization
Inadequate blood supply	Decreases supply of nutrients to injured area, decreases removal of exudative debris, inhibits inflammatory response
Corticosteroid drugs	Impair phagocytosis by WBCs, inhibit fibroblast proliferation and function, depress formation of granulation tissue, inhibit wound contraction
Infection	Increases inflammatory response and tissue destruction
Mechanical friction on wound	Destroys granulation tissue, prevents apposition of wound edges
Advanced age	Slows collagen synthesis by fibroblasts, impairs circulation, requires longer time for epithelialization of skin, alters phagocytic and immune responses
Obesity	Decreases blood supply in fatty tissue
Diabetes mellitus	Decreases collagen synthesis, retards early capillary growth, impairs phagocytosis (result of hyperglycemia)
Poor general health	Causes generalized absence of factors necessary to promote wound healing
Anemia	Supplies less oxygen at tissue level

WBCs, white blood cells.

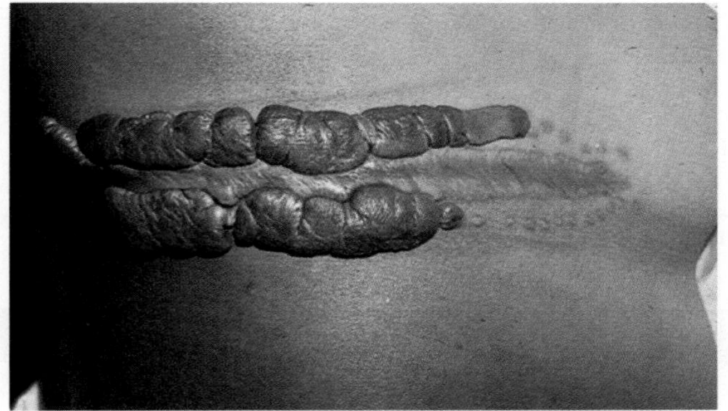

Fig. 11-11 Keloid formation resulting from suture marks.

injury, and the patient's condition. Superficial skin injuries may only need cleansing. Deeper skin wounds can be closed by suturing the edges together. Adhesive strips may be used instead of sutures. If the wound is contaminated, it must be converted into a clean wound before healing can occur normally. Surgical debridement of a wound that has multiple fragments or devitalized tissue may be necessary. If the source of inflammation is an internal organ (e.g., appendix, ruptured spleen), surgical removal of the organ is the treatment of choice.

Drug Therapy. Pharmacologic agents are used in all types of inflammation. Drugs are used to decrease the inflammatory response (antiinflammatory agents) and destroy the infectious agent (antibiotics) (Table 11-14). Antihistamine drugs may also be used to inhibit the action of histamine. (Antihistamines are discussed in Chapter 12).

Antibiotic-resistant organisms. Organisms that have become resistant to antibiotics are becoming an ever-increasing problem in the treatment of infections. Approximately 2 million nosocomial (hospital-acquired) infections occur in the United States each year with one half caused by antibiotic-resistant organisms.[6] Organisms that consistently had been susceptible to all antimicrobial agents for years now have developed resistance not only to the classic agents but to newer agents as well. Methicillin-resistant *Staphylococcus aureus* (MRSA), vancomycin-resistant enterococci (VRE), and penicillin-resistant *Streptococcus pneumoniae* (PRSP) are three of the most troublesome bacterial strains of present concern (Table 11-15).

These bacteria are highly adaptable organisms that have acquired resistance through clever mechanisms to evade pharmacologic innovations.[7] Bacteria have evolved genetic and biochemical ways of resisting antimicrobial actions. Genetic mechanisms include mutation and acquisition of new DNA.[8] Biochemically the bacteria resist antibiotics by producing enzymes that destroy or inactivate the drugs, altering drug target sites so the antibiotic cannot bind to the bacteria, and changing their cell walls to keep drugs out.[6]

Inappropriate antibiotic use has been one of the major factors contributing to the development of drug-resistant organisms. Health care providers often administer antibiotics for viral infections, are pressured by the patient to provide unnecessary antibiotic therapy, inadequately treat established infections, and use broad-spectrum or combination agents for infections that should be treated with first-line antibiotics.

For therapy of resistant organisms, various strategies can be used, including larger doses of antibiotics, other routes of administration, combinations of antibiotics, and alternative antibiotics. Recommended alternative antibiotics for treatment of serious infections caused by resistant organisms are vancomycin for MRSA; ceftriaxone (Rocephin), cefotaxime (Claforan), cefepime (Maxipime), or vancomycin for PRSP; and combined β-lactam and aminoglycoside therapy for VRE.

As the magnitude of the problem continues to increase, nurses must become familiar with ways in which the emergence of resistance in bacteria can be prevented or minimized. Patients and their families should be taught the proper use of antibiotics (Table 11-16). Appropriate use of antibiotics is crucial to treatment success and reduction in the emergence of resistant pathogens.

Nutritional Therapy. There are special nutritional measures to consider to facilitate wound healing.[9] A high fluid

DRUG THERAPY

Table 11-14 Pharmacologic Agents Used to Treat Inflammation

Drug	Mechanisms of Action
Antipyretic Drugs	
Salicylates (aspirin)	Lower temperature by action on heat-regulating center in hypothalamus, resulting in peripheral dilation and heat loss; interfere with formation and release of PGs; selectively depress CNS
Acetaminophen (Tylenol)	Lowers temperature by action in heat-regulating center in hypothalamus
NSAIDs (e.g., ibuprofen [Motrin, Advil])	Inhibit synthesis of PGs
Antiinflammatory Drugs	
Salicylates	Inhibit synthesis of PGs, reduce capillary permeability
Corticosteroids	Interfere with tissue granulation, induce immunosuppressive effects (decreased synthesis of lymphocytes), prevent liberation of lysosomes
NSAIDs (e.g., ibuprofen [Motrin], piroxicam [Feldene])	Inhibit synthesis of PGs
Antibiotic and Antimicrobial Drugs	
Penicillin	Interferes with formation of bacteria cell wall, is bacteriostatic and bactericidal
Cephalosporins	Interfere with formation of bacteria cell wall, are bactericidal
Erythromycin	Inhibits synthesis of bacterial protein, is bacteriostatic
Tetracycline	Inhibits synthesis of bacterial protein, is bacteriostatic
Aminoglycosides	Inhibit synthesis of bacterial protein, are bactericidal
Sulfonamides	Interfere with incorporation of PABA into folic acid, are bacteriostatic
Vitamins	
Vitamin A	Accelerates epithelialization
Vitamin B complex	Acts as coenzymes
Vitamin C	Assists in synthesis of collagen and angiogenesis
Vitamin D	Facilitates calcium absorption

CNS, central nervous system; *NSAIDs,* nonsteroidal antiinflammatory drugs; *PABA,* paraaminobenzoic acid.

Table 11-15 Antibiotic-Resistant Organisms

	Methicillin-resistant *Staphylococcus aureus* (MRSA)	Vancomycin-resistant enterococci (VRE)	Penicillin-resistant *Streptococcus pneumoniae* (PRSP)
Location	Nasal secretions, skin	GI tract, female genital tract	Respiratory tract
Mode of transmission	Contact; person to person, contact with contaminated surfaces	Contact; person to person, contact with contaminated equipment	Droplets from respiratory tract
Nursing considerations	Wash hands with antiseptic soap Wear gloves for patient contact Isolate patient in private room Wear gown if soiling is likely	Wash hands with antiseptic soap Wear gloves for patient contact Isolate patient in private room Wear gown if soiling is likely Wear gown for patient contact	Wash hands with antiseptic soap Wear mask if coming in close contact with patient Isolate patient in private room

intake is needed to replace fluid loss from perspiration and exudate formation. An increased metabolic rate intensifies water loss. There is a 7% increase in metabolism for every 1° F increase in temperature above 100° F (37.8° C) or a 13% increase for every 1° C increase.

A diet high in protein, carbohydrate, and vitamins with moderate fat intake is necessary to promote healing. Protein is needed to correct the negative nitrogen balance resulting from the increased metabolic rate. Protein is also necessary for synthesis of immune factors, leukocytes, fibroblasts, and collagen. Carbohydrate is needed for the increased metabolic energy required in inflammation and healing. If there is a carbohydrate deficit, the body will break down protein for the needed energy. Fats are also a necessary component in the diet to help in the synthesis of fatty acids and triglycerides, which are part of the cellular membrane. Vitamin C is needed for capillary synthesis, capillary formation, and resistance to infection. The B-complex vitamins are necessary as coen-

PATIENT & FAMILY HOME CARE GUIDE

Table 11-16 Steps to Reduce Risk for Antibiotic-Resistant Infection

1. **Do not take antibiotics to prevent illness.** Doing this increases your risk for developing resistant infection. Exceptions include taking antibiotics before certain surgeries and taking antibiotics before dental work if you have a heart valve disorder.
2. **Wash your hands frequently.** Hand washing is the single most important thing you can do to prevent an infection.
3. **Follow directions.** Not taking your antibiotic as prescribed or skipping doses can encourage the development of antibiotic-resistant bacteria.
4. **Finish your medication.** Do not stop taking your medication as soon as you feel better. By stopping your medication early, the hardiest bacteria survive and multiply. Eventually you could develop an infection resistant to many antibiotics.
5. **Do not request an antibiotic for flu or colds.** If your health care provider says that you do not need an antibiotic, chances are you do not. Antibiotics are effective against bacterial infections but not viruses, which cause colds and flus.
6. **Do not take leftover antibiotics.** People often save unfinished antibiotics for later use or borrow leftover drugs from family or friends. This is dangerous because (1) the leftover antibiotic may not be appropriate for you, (2) your illness may not be a bacterial infection, and (3) old antibiotics can lose their effectiveness and in some cases can even be fatal.

Adapted from September 1997 *Mayo Clinic Health Letter* with permission of Mayo Foundation for Medical Education and Research, Rochester, MN 55905.

zymes for many metabolic reactions. If a vitamin B deficiency develops, a disruption of protein, fat, and carbohydrate metabolism will occur. Vitamin A is also needed in healing because it aids in the process of epithelialization. It increases collagen synthesis and tensile strength of the healing wound.

If the patient is unable to eat, enteral feedings should be the first choice if the GI tract is functional. Parenteral nutrition is indicated when enteral feedings are contraindicated or not tolerated. (Enteral and parenteral nutrition are discussed in Chapter 38.)

NURSING MANAGEMENT: INFLAMMATION AND INFECTION

Health Promotion. The best management of inflammation is the prevention of infection, trauma, surgery, and contact with potentially harmful agents. This is not always possible. A simple mosquito bite causes an inflammatory response. Because occasional injury is inevitable, concerted efforts to minimize inflammation and infection are needed.

Adequate nutrition is essential so that the body has the necessary factors to promote healing when injury occurs. Individuals at risk for wound-healing problems are those with malabsorption problems (e.g., Crohn's disease, GI surgery, liver disease), deficient intake or high energy demands (e.g., malignancy, major trauma or surgery, sepsis, fever), and diabetes. An individual should always be considered at risk for wound-healing problems if the following have occurred: (1) loss of 20% or more of total body weight in the preceding 6 months or (2) 10% loss of total body weight in the preceding 2 months.[10]

Early recognition of the manifestations of inflammation and infection is necessary so that appropriate treatment can begin. This may be rest, pharmacologic treatment, or specific treatment of the injured site. Immediate treatment may prevent the extension and complications of inflammation.

Acute Intervention

Observation and vital signs. The ability to recognize the clinical manifestations of inflammation is important. In the individual who is immunosuppressed (e.g., taking corticosteroids or receiving chemotherapy), the classical manifestations of inflammation may be masked. In this individual, early symptoms of inflammation may be malaise or "just not feeling well."

Observation and recording of wound healing are essential. The consistency, color, and odor of any drainage should be recorded and reported if abnormal for the situation. *Staphylococcus* and *Pseudomonas* species are common organisms that cause purulent, draining wounds.

Vital signs are important to note with any inflammation and especially when an infectious process is present. When infection is present, temperature may rise, and pulse and respiration rates may increase. If a wound infection develops in a postoperative patient, vital signs will show a change in 3 to 5 days after surgery.

Fever. The most important aspect of fever management should be determining its cause.[11] Although fever is usually regarded as harmful, an increase in body temperature is an important host defense mechanism. In the seventeenth century, Thomas Sydenham noted that "fever is a mighty engine which nature brings into the world for the conquest of her enemies."[12] Steps are frequently taken to lower body temperature to relieve the anxiety of the patient and medical personnel. Because mild to moderate fever usually does little harm, imposes no great discomfort, and may benefit host defense mechanisms, antipyretic drugs are rarely essential to patient welfare.[3] Moderate fevers (up to 103° F [39.5° C]) usually produce few problems in most patients. However, if the patient is very young or very old, is extremely uncomfortable, or has a significant medical problem (e.g., severe cardiopulmonary disease, brain injury), the use of antipyretics should be considered. Fevers in immunosuppressed patients should be treated rapidly and antibiotic therapy begun because infections can rapidly progress to septicemia.

Fever (especially if greater than 104° F [40° C]) can be damaging to body cells, and delirium and seizures can occur. At temperatures greater than 105.8° F (41° C), regulation by the hypothalamic temperature control center becomes impaired, and damage can occur to the internal structures of many cells, including those in the brain.

Several drugs are commonly used to lower the body temperature set point in the hypothalamus. Aspirin specifically blocks PG synthesis in the hypothalamus and elsewhere in the body. Acetaminophen acts on the heat-regulating center in the hypothalamus. Some NSAIDs (e.g., ibuprofen [Motrin, Advil]) have antipyretic effects (see Fig. 11-7). Corticosteroids

11-1 NURSING CARE PLAN PATIENT WITH A FEVER

Expected Patient Outcomes	Nursing Interventions and *Rationales*
NURSING DIAGNOSIS	**Hyperthermia** *related to* infection *as manifested by* increased body temperature and increased heart and respiratory rate.
▪ Body temperature below 100° F (37.8° C).	▪ Assess patient's temperature every 2-4 hr *to monitor temperature.* ▪ Administer antipyretic drugs q3-4hr if ordered. ▪ Keep environmental temperature at 70° F (21.1° C). ▪ Avoid heavy layers of clothing or bed covers *to aid in lowering body temperature.* ▪ Change linen frequently if patient is diaphoretic *to prevent shivering and subsequent rise in body temperature from muscular activity.*
NURSING DIAGNOSIS	**Risk for fluid volume deficit** *related to* increased metabolic rate, diaphoresis, and decreased oral intake.
▪ No signs of dehydration.	▪ Assess for rapid respirations and pulse; damp skin, clothing, and bed clothes; unwillingness or inability to ingest fluids; signs of dehydration such as dry lips and tongue, poor skin turgor, sunken eyes *to determine risk for or presence of fluid volume deficit.* ▪ Encourage fluid intake of 3-4 L/day if tolerated *to replace fluid lost as a result of fever and diaphoresis.* ▪ Monitor vital signs q2-4hr *because increasing pulse and respirations and decreasing blood pressure can indicate hypovolemia.* ▪ Administer IV fluids if necessary *to replace fluid loss if oral intake is inadequate.* ▪ Monitor intake and output accurately and carefully estimate insensible losses *to evaluate need for replacement.*

are antipyretic through the dual mechanisms of inhibiting IL-1 production and preventing PG synthesis. The action of these drugs results in dilation of superficial blood vessels, increased skin temperatures, and sweating.

Antipyretics should be given around the clock to prevent acute swings in temperature. Chills may be evoked or perpetuated by the intermittent administration of antipyretics. These agents cause a sharp decrease in temperature. When the antipyretic wears off, the body may initiate a compensatory involuntary muscular contraction (i.e., chill) to raise the body temperature back up to its previous level. This unpleasant side effect of antipyretic drugs can be prevented by administering these agents regularly and frequently at 2- to 4-hour intervals. Although sponge baths increase evaporative heat loss, there is no evidence that they decrease the body temperature unless antipyretic medications have been given to lower the set point; otherwise, the body will initiate compensatory mechanisms (e.g., shivering) to restore body heat. The same principle applies to the use of cooling blankets; they are most effective in lowering body temperature when the set point has also been lowered. The nursing care of the patient with a fever is presented in NCP 11-1.

Rest and immobilization. Rest and immobilization of the inflamed area promote healing by decreasing the inflammatory process, assisting in the repair process, and decreasing metabolic needs. Immobilization with a cast, splint, or bandage lessens wound debris and the possibility of hemorrhage. The repair process is facilitated by allowing fibrin and collagen to form across the wound edges with little disruption. Rest helps the body better use its nutrients and oxygen for the healing process.

Elevation. Elevating the injured extremity will reduce the edema at the inflammatory site and increase venous return. Elevation helps reduce pain and improve the circulation of blood, which provides the oxygen and nutrients needed for healing.

Oxygenation. Adequate oxygenation of the inflamed area is essential because oxygen promotes the differentiation of fibroblasts and collagen synthesis. Oxygen is also essential for cell growth and division. A person with arterial disease, hypovolemia, or hypotension is at great risk for infection and may benefit from oxygen administration.

Heat and cold. Applications of heat and cold are somewhat controversial interventions. Cold application is usually appropriate at the time of the initial trauma to cause vasoconstriction and decrease swelling, pain, and congestion from increased metabolism in the area of inflammation. Heat may be used later (e.g., after 24 to 48 hours) and when swelling has subsided, to promote healing by increasing the circulation to the inflamed site and subsequent removal of debris. Heat is also used to localize the inflammatory agents. Warm, moist heat may help debride the wound site if necrotic material is present.

Wound management. The type of wound management and dressings required depend on the type, extent, and characteristics of the wound.[14,15] The purposes of wound management include cleaning a dirty, infected wound to prepare it for healing and protecting a clean wound until it can heal normally. Emergency care of the patient with a skin wound is

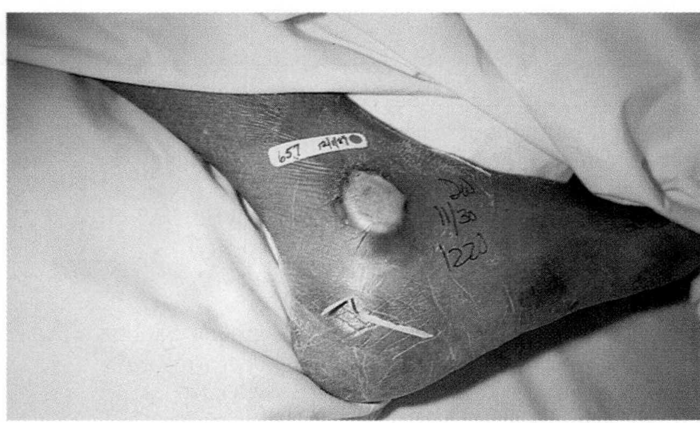

Fig. 11-12 Transparent film dressing.

presented in Table 22-7. Pressure ulcers are discussed in Chapter 22.

Sutures and fibrin sealant are used to facilitate wound closure and create an optimal setting for wound healing. Most commonly sutures are used to close wounds because suture material provides the mechanical support necessary to sustain closure. A wide variety of suturing material is available. Fibrin sealant, in contrast, is a biologic tissue adhesive that can function as a useful adjunct to sutures. Fibrin sealant can be used in conjunction with sutures or tape to promote optimal wound integrity, or it can be used independently to seal wound sites where sutures cannot control bleeding or would aggravate bleeding. This adhesive can effectively seal tissue and eliminate potential spaces. Clinically, fibrin sealant has resulted in a low rate of infection and has promoted healing. Further study is needed to determine the best fibrin sealant mixtures both to achieve hemostasis and to encourage healing.[13]

For wounds that heal by primary intention, it is common to cover the incision with a dry, sterile dressing that is removed as soon as the drainage stops or in 2 to 3 days. Medicated sprays that form a transparent film on the skin may be used for dressings on a clean incision or injury. Transparent film dressings are also commonly used (Fig. 11-12). Sometimes a surgeon will leave a surgical wound uncovered.

Wound healing management by secondary intention can be described as the red-yellow-black concept of wound care (see Table 11-12 and Fig. 11-10). Types of wound dressings are presented in Table 11-17.

Red wound. A red wound can be a superficial wound if it is clean and pink in appearance. Examples include skin tears, pressure necrosis sores (stage 2), partial-thickness or second-degree burns, and wounds created surgically that are allowed to heal by secondary intention. The purpose of treatment is protection of the wound and gentle cleansing (if indicated). Clean wounds that are granulating and reepithelializing should be kept slightly moist and protected from further trauma until they heal naturally. A dressing material that keeps the wound surface clean and slightly moist is optimal to promote epithelialization. Transparent film or adhesive semipermeable dressings (e.g., Opsite, Tegaderm) are occlusive dressings that are permeable to oxygen.[14] Antimicrobials such as bacitracin, neomycin, and povidone-iodine ointment can be used for application on clean wounds, which are then usually covered with a sterile dressing. Unnecessary manipulation during dressing changes may destroy new granulation tissue and break down fibrin formation.

Yellow wound. This type of wound results from surgical or traumatic injuries or after eschar (thick necrotic tissue) is removed. The moist environment resulting from wound drainage creates an ideal situation for bacterial growth. The purpose of treatment is continual cleansing to remove nonviable tissue and to absorb excessive drainage. A type of dressing used in yellow wounds is an absorption dressing (e.g., Debrisan), which absorbs exudate and cleanses the wound surface. Absorption dressings work by drawing excess drainage from the wound surface. After these preparations are saturated with exudate, they should be removed by washing with sterile saline or water. The amount of wound secretions determines the number of dressing changes (usually two to three daily).

Hydrocolloid dressings such as Duoderm are also used to treat yellow wounds. The inner part of these dressings interacts with the exudate, forming a hydrated gel over the wound. When the dressing is removed, the gel separates and stays over the wound, thus preventing damage to newly formed tissue. These types of dressings are designed to be left in place for up to 7 days or until leakage occurs around the dressing.

Black wound. A black wound is covered with thick necrotic tissue (eschar). Examples of black wounds include full-thickness or third-degree burns, pressure necrosis sores (stages 3 or 4), and gangrenous ulcers. The risk of wound infection increases in proportion to the amount of necrotic tissue present. The immediate treatment is debridement of the eschar and nonviable tissue. The debridement method used depends on the amount of debris and the condition of the wound tissue.[16] There are three approaches to debridement:

1. *Surgical debridement.* This method is indicated when large amounts of nonviable tissue are present.
2. *Mechanical debridement.* This method is used when minimal debris is present. A common form of mechanical debridement is wet-to-dry dressings in which open-mesh gauze is moistened with normal saline or an antimicrobial solution, packed on or into the wound surface, and allowed to dry. Wound debris adheres to the dressing. When the dressing is removed, the coarse debris is entrapped in the gauze. One disadvantage to this method is that it is nonselective and will also debride healthy tissue. Topical antimicrobials and antibactericidals used on wet-to-dry dressings include povidone-iodine (Betadine), Dakin's solution (sodium hypochlorite), hydrogen peroxide (H_2O_2), and chlorhexidine (Hibiclens). Topical antimicrobials should be used with caution in wound care, because they can damage healing tissue (e.g., H_2O_2 damages new epithelium). Semiocclusive or occlusive dressings (see Table 11-17) may be used to promote eschar softening by autolysis. These types of dressings are used in open wounds with minimal necrotic debris and no contamination. Another method of mechanical debridement is wound irrigation. This method may be appropriate when wounds are contaminated. However, irrigation should be used with caution because high pressure can interfere with fibroblast formation and macrophage function.

Table 11-17 Types of Wound Dressings

	Description	Examples
Gauze	Provides absorption of exudate. Supports debridement if applied and kept moist. Can be used to maintain moist wound surface. Can be used as filler dressings in sinus tracts.	Numerous products available
Nonadherent dressings	Woven or nonwoven dressings may be impregnated with saline, petrolatum, or antimicrobials. Are minimally absorbent.	Adaptic Exu-Dry Sofsorb Telfa Vaseline gauze Xeroform
Transparent film	Semipermeable membrane that permits gaseous exchange between wound bed and environment. Minimally absorbent so fluid environment is created in presence of exudate. Bacteria do not penetrate membrane. Used for dry noninfected wounds or wounds with minimal drainage.	AcuDerm Biocclusive Blisterfilm OpSite Polyskin Tegaderm Transeal
Hydrocolloid	Occlusive dressing does not allow O_2 to diffuse from atmosphere to wound bed. Occlusion does not interfere with wound healing. Not used in infected wounds. Supports debridement and prevents secondary infections. Used for superficial and partial-thickness wounds with light to moderate drainage.	Comfeel DuoDerm Intact IntraSite Restore Tegasorb Ultec
Polyurethane foams	Moderate to heavy amounts of exudate can be absorbed. Can be used on infected wounds. Used for partial- or full-thickness wounds with minimal to heavy drainage.	Allevyn Epilock Hydrasorb Lyofoam Mitraflex Synthaderm
Absorption dressing	Large volumes of exudate can be absorbed. Supports debridement. Maintains moist wound surface. Placed into wounds and can obliterate dead space. For partial- or full-thickness wounds or infected wounds.	AlgiDERM Bard Absorption Debrisan Duoderm Paste Hydragan Kaltostat Sorbsan
Hydrogel	Debridement because of moisturizing effects. Maintains moist wound surface. Provides limited absorption of exudate. Available as sheet or gel. Most require a secondary dressing. Used for partial- or full-thickness wounds, deep wounds with minimal drainage, and necrotic wounds.	Aquasorb ClearSite Elastogel Geliperm IntraSite Gel Normlgel Transorb Vigilon

3. *Enzymatic debridement.* This method uses agents such as sutilains (Travase) and fibrinolysin/desoxyribonuclease (Elase) in conjunction with normal, saline-moistened dressings.

Infection prevention and control. The nurse and the patient must scrupulously follow aseptic procedures for keeping the wound free from infection. The patient should not be allowed to touch a recently injured area. The patient's environment should be as free as possible from contamination from items introduced by roommates and visitors. Antibiotics may be administered prophylactically to some patients. If an infection develops, a culture and sensitivity test should be done to determine the organism and most effective antibiotic for that specific organism. The culture should be taken before the first dose of antibiotic is given.[17]

OSHA guidelines. The Occupational Safety and Health Administration (OSHA) standard for preventing occupational transmission of blood-borne pathogens was implemented in 1992. The ruling mandated that employers provide at-risk employees with appropriate personal protective equipment (PPE). The nurse needs to minimize or eliminate exposure to infectious material. When that is not possible, appropriate PPE must be selected. These include gloves, clothing, and facial pro-

Table 11-18 Occupational Safety and Health Administration (OSHA) Requirements for Personal Protective Apparel to Minimize Exposure to Blood-borne Pathogens*

Equipment	Indications for Use	Must Be
Gloves	When contact with infectious material is likely During all vascular procedures Before contact with mucous membranes and nonintact skin	Suitable for task: general patient care, sterile surgical procedures Individualized: various sizes, hypoallergenic, powderless
Clothing (gowns, aprons, shoe covers, hats, hoods)	When splattering of clothing with body substances is likely	Suitable for task: prevent blood, infectious materials from penetrating and reaching employee's skin or clothes
Facial protection (masks, face shields, eyewear including glasses with side shields, goggles)	When splattering, splashing, or spraying of eyes, nose, or mouth with blood or other potentially infectious body substances is likely	Effective: in preventing infectious material from penetrating around or under barriers

From Occupational Safety and Health Administration: *Federal Register* 56:64003, 1991.
*All personal protective equipment must be conveniently located, accessible, and provided free to employee. Employer is responsible for purchasing, repairing, and laundering as appropriate.

tection (Table 11-18). Appropriate PPE will vary depending on the situation.

Infection precautions. If the patient develops an infection that is considered a risk to others, infection precautions may be needed. The purpose of these precautions is to prevent the transmission of organisms from patients to health care providers, from health care providers to patients, and from one patient to another. Four precaution systems were commonly used until recently: (1) category-specific precautions, (2) disease-specific precautions, (3) universal precautions, and (4) body substance isolation.

Category-specific precautions are recommended to prevent transmission of the most infectious diseases in each category (e.g., respiratory isolation, enteric isolation). This system frequently means more isolation precautions than necessary are required to prevent transmission of a certain organism.

Disease-specific precautions handle each infectious disease or condition separately. With this system, it is possible to list only those precautions necessary to interrupt transmission of the specific organism.

Universal precautions recommend that blood and body fluid precautions be consistently used for all patients, regardless of blood-borne infection status. Universal precautions are intended to prevent parenteral, mucous membrane, and nonintact skin exposure of health care workers to blood-borne pathogens. In addition, immunization with hepatitis B vaccine is recommended as an important adjunct to universal precautions for health care workers who are exposed to blood and blood products.

The body substance isolation (BSI) system was first described in 1984 and revised in 1990. It is intended to reduce nosocomial transmission of infectious agents among patients and to reduce the risk of transmission of infectious agents to health care personnel.

Some facilities continue to use one of these systems even though the Centers for Disease Control and Prevention (CDC) revised their guidelines for isolation precautions to incorporate features of all of these systems into a single easy-to-understand system.[19,20] The 1996 guidelines contain two levels of precautions (Table 11-19): *Standard Precautions,* which are designed for the care of all patients in hospitals and health care facilities regardless of their diagnosis or presumed infection status; and *Transmission-based Precautions,* which are used for patients known to be or suspected of being infected with epidemiologically important pathogens that can be transmitted by airborne or droplet transmission or by contact with dry skin or contaminated surfaces.

The 1996 Standard Precautions system synthesizes the major features of universal precautions and BSI and applies to (1) blood; (2) all body fluids, secretions, and excretions regardless of whether they contain visible blood; (3) nonintact skin; and (4) mucous membranes. Standard Precautions are designed to reduce the risk of transmission of microorganisms from both recognized and unrecognized sources of infection in hospitals. Standard Precautions should be applied to all patients regardless of diagnosis or infection status.

Transmission-based Precautions are designed for patients documented or suspected to be infected with highly transmissable or epidemiologically important pathogens for which additional precautions beyond Standard Precautions are needed to interrupt transmission in hospitals. The three types of Transmission-based Precautions are *airborne precautions, droplet precautions,* and *contact precautions.* They may be combined together for diseases that have multiple routes of transmission. When used either by themselves or in combination these precautions are used in addition to Standard Precautions.

All hospitals are encouraged to review and consider adoption of Standard Precautions and Transmission-based Precautions and discontinue use of the older forms of isolation precautions. The CDC offers hospitals the option of modifying the recommendations according to their needs and circumstances and as directed by federal, state, or local regulations. For example, OSHA's requirements are still operable, and all facilities are required to comply with these provisions. The CDC's 1996 Standard Precautions incorporate all requirements of OSHA's Bloodborne Pathogens Standard.

Protective isolation. A low WBC count and depressed immune responses (e.g., in patient undergoing cancer chemotherapy, patient with neutropenia, or patient with

Table 11-19 CDC Recommendations for Isolation Precautions in Health Care Facilities*

	Standard Precautions	Transmission-based Precautions: Airborne	Transmission-based Precautions: Droplet	Transmission-based Precautions: Contact
When to use	All patients	Use in addition to Standard Precautions for patients known to be or suspected of being infected with microorganisms transmitted by airborne droplet (e.g., measles, varicella, tuberculosis).	Use in addition to Standard Precautions for patient known to be or suspected of being infected with microorganisms transmitted by droplets (e.g., *Haemophilus influenzae, Neisseria meningitidis, Streptococcus pneumoniae,* Mycoplasma pneumoniae).	Use in addition to Standard Precautions for specified patients known to be or suspected of being infected with epidemiologically important microorganisms that can be transmitted by direct contact with patient (e.g., enteric pathogens, multidrug-resistant bacteria, *Staphylococcus aureus, Clostridium difficile,* herpes simplex) or in direct contact with environmental surface or patient care items in the patient's environment.
Hand washing	Wash hands after touching blood, body fluids, secretions, excretions, and contaminated items, regardless of whether gloves are worn; wash hands immediately after gloves are removed, between patient contacts, and to prevent transfer of microorganisms to other patients or environments.	Same as Standard Precautions.	Same as Standard Precautions.	Same as Standard Precautions.
Gloves	Wear nonsterile gloves when touching blood, body fluids, secretions, excretions, and contaminated items; put on clean gloves just before touching mucous membranes and nonintact skin; remove gloves promptly after use, before touching noncontaminated items, environmental surfaces, or going to another patient.	Same as Standard Precautions.	Same as Standard Precautions.	In addition to glove use as described in Standard Precautions, wear gloves when entering the room whenever providing direct patient care or having hand contact with potentially contaminated surfaces or items in patient's environment.
Mask, eye protection, face shield	Wear mask and eye protection or face shield to protect mucous membranes of eyes, nose, and mouth during procedures and patient care activities likely to generate splashes or sprays of blood, body fluids, secretions, and excretions.	In addition to Standard Precautions, wear respiratory protection when entering room of patient known to have or suspected of having tuberculosis.	In addition to Standard Precautions, wear a mask when working within 3 ft of patient.	Same as Standard Precautions.

Continued

Table 11-19 CDC Recommendations for Isolation Precautions in Health Care Facilities*—cont'd

	Standard Precautions	Transmission-based Precautions: Airborne	Transmission-based Precautions: Droplet	Transmission-based Precautions: Contact
Gown	Wear clean, nonsterile gown to protect skin and prevent soiling of clothing during procedures and patient care activities likely to generate splashes or sprays of blood, body fluids, secretions, or excretions or likely to cause soiling of clothing; remove gown promptly when tasks are completed; wash hands.	Same as Standard Precautions.	Same as Standard Precautions.	Wear clean, nonsterile gown if substantial contact is anticipated with patient, surfaces, or items in environment; wear gown if patient is incontinent or has diarrhea, an ileostomy, a colostomy, or uncontained wound drainage; remove gown carefully when tasks are completed; wash hands.
Linen	Handle, transport, and process used linen in manner that prevents skin and mucous membrane exposure, contamination of clothing, and environmental soiling.	Same as Standard Precautions.	Same as Standard Precautions.	Same as Standard Precautions.
Patient transport		Limit movement and transport of patient from room to essential purposes only; if transport or movement is necessary, minimize patient dispersal of droplet nuclei by placing surgical mask on patient, if possible.	Limit movement and transport of patient from room to essential purposes only; if transport or movement is necessary, minimize patient dispersal of droplet nuclei by masking patient, if possible.	Limit movement and transport of patient from room to essential purposes only; if transport is necessary, ensure that precautions are maintained to minimize contamination of environmental surfaces or equipment.

*A complete listing of recommendations is published in Garner J: Guidelines for isolation precautions in hospitals, *Infect Control Hosp Epidemiol* 17:53, 1996.
CDC, Centers for Disease Control and Prevention.

leukemia or lymphoma) may in some facilities be placed on another type of isolation termed *protective (reverse) isolation.* The purpose of protective isolation is to protect the vulnerable patient from environmental sources of infection. However, some studies have not definitively proven that protective isolation is of value, and the use of this form of isolation is controversial. Institutional policies related to protective isolation vary considerably, and if they exist, they should be followed when the patient's condition warrants this intervention. (Protective isolation is discussed in Chapter 29.)

Psychologic implications. The patient may be distressed at the thought or sight of an incision or wound because of fear of scarring or disfigurement. Drainage from a wound often causes increased alarm. The patient needs to understand the healing process and the normal changes that occur as the wound heals. When a nurse is changing a dressing, inappropriate facial expressions can alert the patient to problems with the wound or the nurse's ability to care for it. Wrinkling of the nose by the nurse may convey disgust to the patient. A nurse should also be careful not to focus on the wound to the extent that the patient is not treated as a total person.

Ambulatory and Home Care. Because patients are being discharged earlier after surgery and many have sugery as outpatients, it is important that the patient, the family, or both know how to care for the wound and perform dressing changes. Wound healing may not be complete for 4 to 6 weeks or longer. Adequate rest and good nutrition should be continued throughout this time. Physical and emotional stress should be minimal. Observing the wound for complications such as contractures, adhesions, and secondary infection is important. The patient should understand the signs and symptoms of infection. The patient should note changes in wound color and the amount of drainage. The health care provider should be notified of any signs of abnormal wound healing.

Medications will often be taken for a period of time after recovery from the acute infection. Drug-specific side effects and adverse effects should be reviewed with the patient; the patient should be instructed to contact the health care

CRITICAL THINKING EXERCISES

CASE STUDY

Inflammation and Infection

Patient Profile

Roger, a 20-year-old man, was admitted to the hospital emergency department with partial-thickness burns that involved his face, neck, and upper trunk. He also had a lacerated right leg. His injuries occurred about 24 hours earlier.

Subjective Data

- Complains of slightly hoarse voice and irritated throat
- States that he tried to treat himself because he does not have health insurance
- Has been coughing up sooty sputum
- Has been a model for athletic clothing

Objective Data

Physical Examination

- Leg wound is gaping and looks infected, temperature 101.1° F (38.4° C)

X-ray

- Reveals a fractured tibia

Laboratory Studies

- WBC count 26,400/µl (26.4 × 10^9/L) with 80% neutrophils (10% bands)

Critical Thinking Questions

1. What clinical manifestations of inflammation did Roger exhibit, and what are their pathophysiologic mechanisms?
2. What type of exudate formation did he develop?
3. What is the basis for the development of the temperature?
4. What is the significance of his WBC count and differential?
5. Because his wound was deep, primary tissue healing was not possible. How would you expect healing to take place?
6. What problems might Roger have with self-concept or body image? What concerns or problems might a nurse have in caring for Roger?
7. Based on the assessment data provided, write one or more appropriate nursing diagnoses. Are there any collaborative problems?

provider if any of these effects occur. Awareness of the necessity to continue the drugs for the specified time is an important point to teach the patient. For example, a patient who is instructed to take an antibiotic for 10 days may stop taking the medication after 5 days because of decreased or absent symptoms. However, the organism may not be entirely eliminated, and it may also become resistant to the antibiotic if the medication is not continued (see Table 11-16).

REVIEW QUESTIONS

The number of the question corresponds to the same-numbered objective at the beginning of the chapter.

1. Physiologic hyperplasia is commonly found in
   a. a distended urinary bladder.
   b. the female breast during lactation.
   c. the bronchi of a chronic cigarette smoker.
   d. an enlarged myocardium in congestive heart failure.
2. When radiation therapy is used in the treatment of cancer the desired effect is death of cancer cells by
   a. altering cellular metabolism and activity.
   b. producing mutations that interfere with only cancer cell function.
   c. accelerating metabolic reactions to reduce the normal life span of cells.
   d. stimulating synthesis of new particles that cause cell rupture and death.
3. A common cause of coagulation necrosis is
   a. autophagocytosis.
   b. pulmonary embolus.
   c. malignant brain tumor.
   d. peripheral vascular disease.
4. A patient with an impaired mononuclear phagocyte system will have
   a. increased circulation of histamine.
   b. decreased susceptibility to infection.
   c. decreased vascular response to cell injury.
   d. decreased surveillance for damaged or mutated cells.
5. The role of the complement system in opsonization affects which response of the inflammatory process?
   a. vascular
   b. cellular
   c. formation of exudate
   d. healing
6. Fever that accompanies inflammation is most likely caused by
   a. activation of the complement system.
   b. release of IL-1 and TNF from white blood cells.
   c. increased production and activity of neutrophils.
   d. massive vasodilation during the vascular response.
7. A patient has an open, infected surgical wound that is treated with irrigations and moist gauze dressings. The nurse expects that this wound will
   a. be classified as a black wound.
   b. have to heal by tertiary intention.
   c. heal by regeneration of epithelial cells.
   d. heal by the same processes as an uninfected deep wound.
8. Contractures frequently occur after burn healing because of
   a. secondary infection.
   b. lack of adequate blood supply.
   c. excess fibrous tissue formation.
   d. weakness of connective tissue.
9. Rest and immobilization are important measures of acute care for wound healing because they
   a. prevent swelling and congestion.
   b. increase the circulation to the area.
   c. increase the body's production of corticosteroids.
   d. are known mechanisms to increase the rate of healing.

References

1. Borton D: WBC count and differential, *Nursing* 26:26, 1996.
2. Dinarello CA: Thermoregulation and the pathogenesis of fever, *Infect Dis Clin North Am* 10:433, 1996.
3. Kluger MJ: Cytokines and the pathogenesis of fever, *Physiologist* 37:A28, 1994.
4. Letizia M, Janusek L: The self-defense mechanism of fever, *Medsurg Nurs* 3:373, 1994.
5. Beck VP: On the lookout for impaired wound healing, *Nursing* 28:1, 1998.
6. Tenover FC, McGowan JE: Antimicrobial resistance, *Infect Dis Clin North Am* 10:433, 1996.
7. Capriotti T: Emerging antibiotic resistance among community-acquired and nosocomial bacterial pathogens, *Medsurg Nurs* 6:296, 1997.
8. McManus MC: Mechanisms of bacterial resistance to antimicrobial agents, *Am J Health-System Pharm* 54:1420, 1997.
9. Pontieri-Lewis V: The role of nutrition in wound healing, *Medsurg Nurs* 6:187, 1997.
10. Meser MS: Wound care, *Crit Care Nurs Q* 11:17, 1989.
11. Klein NC, Cunha BA: Treatment of fever, *Infect Dis Clin North Am* 10:211, 1997.
12. Atkins E: Fever: its history, cause, and function, *Yale J Biol Med* 55:283, 1982.
13. Spotnitz WD, Falstrom JK, Rodeheaver GT: The role of sutures and fibrin sealant in wound healing, *Surg Clin North Am* 77:651, 1997.
14. Rolstad BS: Wound dressings: making the right match, *Nursing* 27:32hn1, 1997.
15. Erwin-Toth P, Hocevar BJ: Wound care: selecting the right dressing, *AJN* 95:46, 1995.
16. Walker D: Choosing the correct wound dressing, *AJN* 96:35, 1996.
17. DeGroot-Kosolcharoen J: Culture and sensitivity testing, *AJN* 96:33, 1996.
18. Eggleston B: Infection control update, *Nursing* 24:70, 1994.
19. Garner J: Guideline for isolation precautions in hospitals, *Infect Control Hosp Epidemiol* 17:53, 1996.
20. Borton D: Isolation precautions: clearing up the confusion, *Nursing* 27:49, 1997.

Resources

Association for Professionals in Infection Control and Epidemiology (APIC)
1275 K St, NW, Suite 1000
Washington, DC 20005-4006
202-789-1890
Fax: 202-789-1899
http://www.apic.org/

For additional Internet resources, see the website for this book at **www.mosby.com/MERLIN/medsurg_lewis**

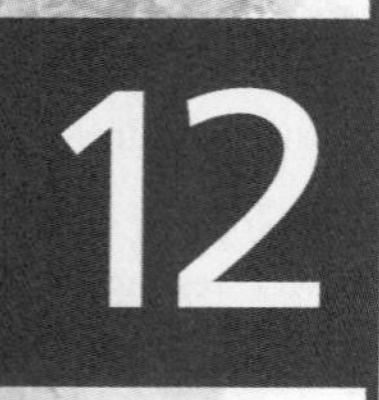

12 NURSING MANAGEMENT Altered Immune Responses

Sharon Mantik Lewis

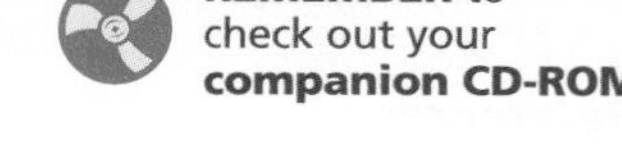

REMEMBER to check out your **companion CD-ROM**

www.mosby.com/MERLIN/medsurg_lewis

LEARNING OBJECTIVES

1. Describe the functions and components of the immune system.
2. Differentiate between natural and acquired immunity.
3. Compare and contrast humoral and cell-mediated immunity regarding lymphocytes involved, types of reactions, and effects on antigens.
4. Identify the five types of immunoglobulins and their characteristics.
5. Differentiate among the four types of hypersensitivity reactions in terms of immunologic mechanisms and resulting alterations.
6. Identify the clinical manifestations and emergency management of a systemic anaphylactic reaction.
7. Describe the assessment and collaborative care of a patient with chronic allergies.
8. Describe the drug therapy used for patients with allergies.
9. Describe the etiologic factors, clinical manifestations, and treatment modalities of autoimmune diseases.
10. Explain the relationship between the human leukocyte antigen system and certain diseases.
11. Describe the etiologic factors, categories, and treatment of immunodeficiency disorders.
12. Describe new technologies in immunology, including hybridoma technology, recombinant DNA technology, and gene therapy.

The human body has always had to protect itself from invasion by foreign substances such as microorganisms. A complex defense system has evolved to withstand these constant attacks. The defense system in humans consists of nonspecific protective mechanisms and responses (including the skin, tears, sneezing, and phagocytosis by some types of white blood cells) and a specific immune response (humoral immunity and cell-mediated immunity). (The inflammatory response is discussed in Chapter 11.)

Immunocompetence exists when the body's immune system can identify and inactivate or destroy foreign substances. When the immune system is incompetent or underresponsive, severe infections, immunodeficiency diseases, and malignancies may occur. When the immune system overreacts, hypersensitivity disorders such as allergies and autoimmune diseases may occur.

NORMAL IMMUNE RESPONSE

Immunity

Immunity is a state of responsiveness to foreign substances such as microorganisms and tumor proteins. Immune responses serve three functions (Table 12-1):

1. *Defense.* The body protects against invasions by microorganisms and prevents the development of infection by attacking foreign antigens and pathogens.
2. *Homeostasis.* Damaged cellular substances are digested and removed. Through this mechanism the body's different cell types remain uniform and unchanged.
3. *Surveillance.* Mutations continually arise in the body but are normally recognized as foreign cells and destroyed.

Properties of the Immune Response

The immune system has five important properties that make its protection diverse and long lasting while not being harmful to the person:

1. *Specificity.* When a foreign antigen (substance capable of stimulating an immune response) enters the body, a series of cellular changes occurs. These changes result in the formation of a specific antibody or sensitized lymphocyte that attaches to the specific antigen.
2. *Memory.* The immune system has the unique ability to remember the antigen. Therefore a secondary immune response is faster and stronger.
3. *Self-recognition.* Because there frequently is little difference between the body's own proteins and foreign proteins, the body must distinguish between the two. When the body fails to recognize self-proteins, autoantibodies develop, leading to tissue destruction.
4. *Self-limitation.* After the antigen is eliminated, the stimuli for the immune response is decreased, thereby decreasing and eventually eliminating the immune response. The self-limiting aspect of the immune response prevents damage to cells that would result from a prolonged response.
5. *Specialization.* The immune system reacts in different ways to various antigens and microorganisms.

Reviewed by Kathryn Ann Caudell, RN, PhD, OCN, Assistant Professor, College of Nursing, University of New Mexico, Albuquerque, NM.

Table 12-1 Functions of the Immune System

Function	Adaptive Response	Maladaptive Response: Hyper	Maladaptive Response: Hypo
Defense	Destruction of viruses, bacteria, fungi	Allergic disorders	Immunodeficiency disorders
Homeostasis	Removal of damaged cells	Autoimmune diseases	—
Surveillance	Removal of mutated cells	—	Malignant diseases

Table 12-2 Types of Acquired Specific Immunity

Acquisition of Immunity	Protection
Active	
Natural Natural contact with antigen through clinical or subclinical infection; for example, recovery from childhood diseases (e.g., chickenpox, measles, mumps)	**Development** Develops slowly; protective levels reached in a few weeks **Duration** Long-term, often lifetime **Spectrum** Specific to antigen contacted
Artificial Immunization with antigen (e.g., immunization with live or killed vaccines, toxoid immunization)	**Development** Develops slowly; protective levels reached in few weeks **Duration** Several years; extended protection with "booster" doses **Spectrum** Specific to antigen targeted by immunization
Passive	
Natural Transplacental and colostrum transfer from mother (source) to child (e.g., maternal immunoglobulins in neonate)	**Development** Immediate **Duration** Temporary; several months **Spectrum** All antigens to which source has immunity
Artificial Injection of serum from immune human or animal (source) (e.g., injection of pooled human γ-globulin)	**Development** Immediate **Duration** Temporary; several weeks **Spectrum** All antigens to which source has immunity

Types of Immunity. Immunity is classified as natural or acquired. *Natural (innate) immunity* is not produced by an immune response. Natural immunity exists in a person without prior contact with an antigen. One type of natural immunity present at birth is species specificity of infectious agents. Humans are naturally immune to some of the infectious agents that cause illnesses in other species. *Acquired immunity* is the development of immunity, either actively or passively (Table 12-2).

Active acquired immunity. Active acquired immunity results from the invasion of the body by foreign substances such as microorganisms and subsequent development of antibodies and sensitized lymphocytes. With each reinvasion of the microorganisms, the body responds more rapidly and vigorously to fight off the invader. Active acquired immunity may result naturally from a disease or artificially through inoculation of a less virulent antigen (e.g., immunizations). Because antibodies are synthesized, immunity takes time to develop but is long lasting.

Passive acquired immunity. Passive acquired immunity implies that the host receives antibodies to an antigen rather than synthesizing them. This may take place naturally through the transfer of immunoglobulins across the placental membrane from mother to fetus. Artificial passive acquired immunity occurs through injection with gamma-globulin (serum antibodies). The benefit of this immunity is its immediate effect. Unfortunately, passive immunity is short lived, because the host did not synthesize the antibodies and consequently does not retain memory cells for the antigen.

Antigens

An *antigen* is a substance that elicits an immune response. Most antigens are composed of protein. However, other substances

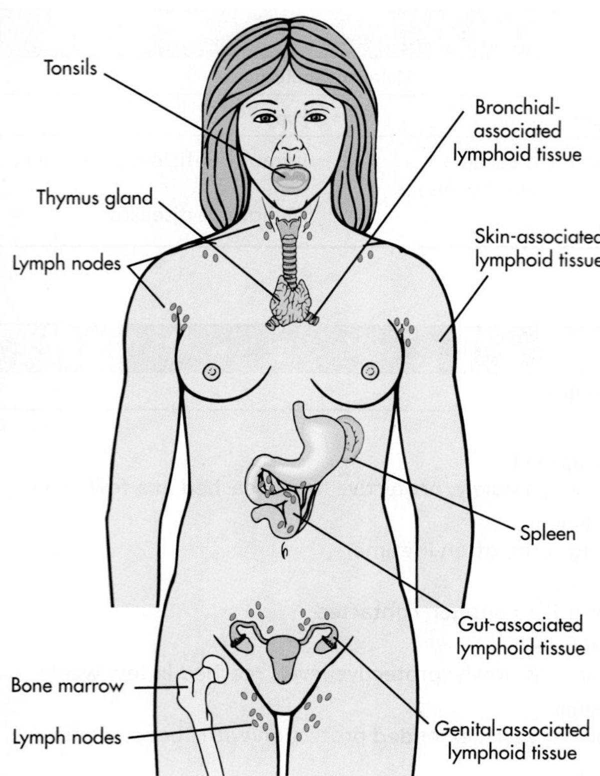

Fig. 12-1 Organs of the immune system.

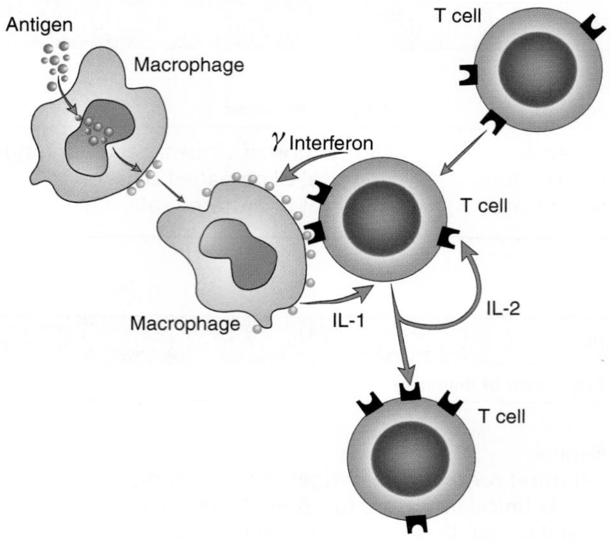

Fig. 12-2 Schematic representation of the cellular events involved in T cell activation. In the early phase of the immune response, foreign antigen is taken up by macrophages, processed, and reexpressed on the macrophage cell membrane where it is recognized by specific T cells. In the presence of monocyte-derived mediators, such as interleukin-1, this series of events leads to proliferation and activation of T cells. The activated T cells secrete various lymphokines (e.g., interleukin-2, γ-interferon) that mediate responses involving lymphocytes and mononuclear phagocytes.

such as large-size polysaccharides, lipoproteins, and nucleic acids can act as antigens. All of the body's cells have antigens on their surface that are unique to that person and enable the body to recognize self. The immune system becomes "tolerant" to the body's own molecules and therefore is nonresponsive to self.[1]

Most foreign antigens are not chemically pure substances but rather have multiple antigenic determinants with which antibodies can combine. Small variations in cell surface antigens will elicit an immune response. This is the basis of transplant rejection if the donor organ is not a perfect match with the recipient.

Haptens are low-molecular-weight substances that by themselves are harmless. However, they can form complexes with larger molecules called carriers that are antigenic. Once antibodies are produced, future exposure to the hapten alone can elicit an immune response. Common haptens include dust, animal danders, drugs, and industrial chemicals. Immune responses to haptens are the basis for many common allergies.

Physical or chemical damage to cell membranes may expose other cell structures to the immune system. The "new" antigens can stimulate the immune system to react against the body's own tissues. This process results in autoimmunity, which is discussed later in this chapter.

Components of the Immune System

Lymphoid organs function in production of lymphocytes, one of the essential cells of the immune response. The mononuclear phagocyte system (discussed in Chapter 11) is also involved in the production of a normal immune response.

Lymphoid Organs. The lymphoid system is composed of central (or primary) and peripheral lymphoid organs. The *central lymphoid organs* are the thymus gland and bone marrow. The *peripheral lymphoid organs* are the tonsils; gut-, genital-, bronchial-, and skin-associated lymphoid tissues; lymph nodes; and spleen (Fig. 12-1).

Lymphocytes are produced in the bone marrow and eventually migrate to the peripheral organs. The thymus is important in the differentiation and maturation of T lymphocytes and is therefore essential for a cell-mediated immune response. During childhood the gland is large. The gland shrinks with age and is a collection of reticular fibers, lymphocytes, and connective tissue in older persons.

Lymphoid tissue is found in the submucosa of the respiratory (bronchial-associated), genitourinary (genital-associated), and gastrointestinal (gut-associated) tracts. This tissue protects the body surface from external microorganisms. The tonsils are a typical example of lymphoid tissue.

The skin-associated lymph tissue primarily consists of lymphocytes and Langerhans' cells (a type of resident macrophage) found in the epidermis of skin. When Langerhans' cells are depleted, the skin can neither initiate an immune response nor support a skin-localized delayed hypersensitivity response.

When antigens are introduced into the body, they may be carried by the bloodstream or lymph channels to regional lymph nodes. The antigens interact with B and T lymphocytes and macrophages in the lymph node. The two important functions of lymph nodes are (1) filtration of foreign material brought to the site and (2) circulation of lymphocytes.

The spleen is important as the primary site for filtering foreign substances from the blood. It consists of two kinds of tissue: white pulp containing B and T lymphocytes and red pulp containing erythrocytes. Macrophages line the pulp and

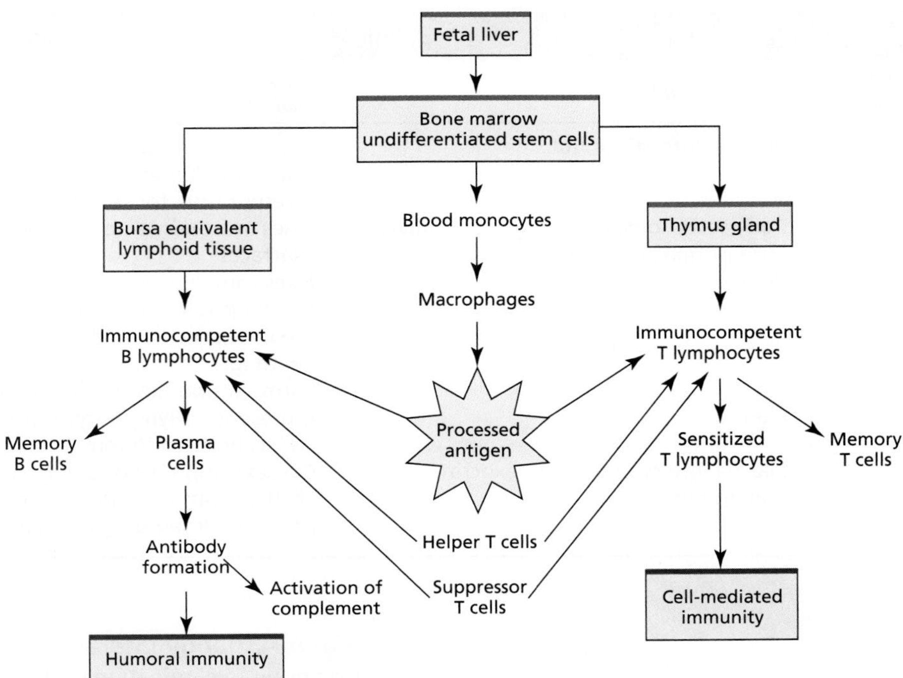

Fig. 12-3 Relationships and functions of macrophages, B lymphocytes, and T lymphocytes in an immune response.

sinuses of the spleen. The spleen is the major site of immune responses to blood-borne antigens. If the spleen is removed in children, it can predispose them to life-threatening septicemia.

Mononuclear Phagocyte System. The mononuclear phagocyte system includes monocytes in the blood and macrophages found throughout the body. (See Chapter 11 for a more complete description.) Mononuclear phagocytes have a critical role in the immune system. They are responsible for capturing, processing, and presenting the antigen to the lymphocytes. This stimulates a humoral or cell-mediated immune response. Capturing is accomplished through phagocytosis. The macrophage-bound antigen, which is highly immunogenic, is presented to circulating T or B lymphocytes and thus triggers an immune response (Fig. 12-2).

Lymphocyte Production

Lymphocytes arise from undifferentiated stem cells in the fetal liver and later from the bone marrow (Fig. 12-3). Lymphocytes differentiate into B and T lymphocytes.

In birds, B lymphocytes (bursa-equivalent or thymus-independent cells) mature under the influence of the bursa of Fabricius. However, this lymphoid organ does not exist in humans. The bursa-equivalent tissue in humans is the bone marrow.

Cells that migrate from the bone marrow to the thymus differentiate into T lymphocytes (thymus-dependent cells). The thymus secretes hormones, including thymosin, that stimulate the maturation and differentiation of T lymphocytes. T cells compose 70% to 80% of the circulating lymphocytes and are primarily responsible for immunity to intracellular viruses, tumor cells, and fungi. These T cells live from a few months to the life span of an individual and account for long-term immunity.

Humoral Immunity

Humoral immunity consists of antibody-mediated immunity. The term *humoral* comes from the Greek word *humor,* which means body fluid. Antibodies are proteins produced by B cells and found in plasma; therefore the term *humoral immunity* is used. Production of antibodies (immunoglobulins) is an essential component in a humoral immune response. Immunoglobulins are composed of amino acids arranged on two light and two heavy polypeptide chains. Differences in the heavy chain configuration differentiate the five classes of immunoglobulins, which are IgG, IgA, IgM, IgD, and IgE. Each class of immunoglobulins has specific characteristics (Table 12-3).

Humoral Immune Response. When a pathogen (especially bacteria) enters the body, it may encounter a B lymphocyte specific for antigens located on that bacterial cell wall. In addition, a monocyte or macrophage may phagocytize the bacteria and present its antigens to a B lymphocyte. The B lymphocyte recognizes the antigen because it has receptors on its cell surface specific for that antigen. When the antigen comes in contact with the cell surface receptor, the B cell becomes activated, and most B cells will differentiate into plasma cells (see Fig. 12-3). The mature plasma cell secretes immunoglobulins. Some stimulated B lymphocytes remain as memory cells.

The *primary immune response* is evident 4 to 8 days after initial exposure to the antigen (Fig. 12-4). IgM is the first type of antibody formed. Because of the large size of the IgM molecule, this immunoglobulin is confined to the intravascular space. As the immune response progresses, IgG is produced and can move from intravascular to extravascular spaces.

When the individual is exposed to the antigen the second time, a *secondary antibody response* occurs. This response occurs faster (1 to 3 days), is stronger, and lasts for a longer time

Table **12-3** Characteristics of Immunoglobulins

Class	Relative Serum Concentration (%)	Location	Characteristics
IgG	76	Plasma, interstitial fluid	Is only immunoglobulin that crosses placenta Fixes complement Is responsible for secondary immune response
IgA	15	Body secretions, including tears, saliva, breast milk, colostrum	Lines mucous membranes and protects body surfaces
IgM	8	Plasma	Fixes complement Is responsible for primary immune response Provides specific antitoxin action when combined with IgG Forms antibodies to ABO blood antigens
IgD	1	Plasma	Is present on lymphocyte surface Assists in the differentiation of B lymphocytes
IgE	0.002	Plasma, interstitial fluids, exocrine secretions	Causes symptoms of allergic reactions Fixes to mast cells and basophils Assists in defense against parasitic infections

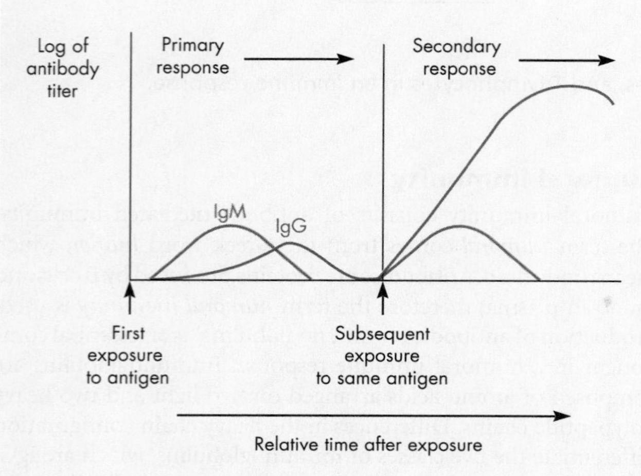

Fig. 12-4 Primary and secondary immune responses. The introduction of antigen induces a response dominated by two classes of immunoglobulins, IgM and IgG. IgM predominates in the primary response, with some IgG appearing later. After the host's immune system is primed, another challenge with the same antigen induces the secondary response, in which some IgM and large amounts of IgG are produced.

than a primary response. Memory cells account for the memory of the first exposure to the antigen and the more rapid production of antibodies. IgG is the primary antibody found in a secondary immune response.

During gestation, the fetus has some immunity to protect against in utero infections. However, the lymph nodes and spleen are underdeveloped in the neonate. Fortunately, IgG crosses the placental membrane and provides the newborn with passive acquired immunity for at least 3 months. Infants may also get some passive immunity from IgA in breast milk and colostrum. By 9 months of age, a baby's IgM level is at a normal concentration and the lymph nodes and spleen are well developed.

Antigen-Antibody Interactions. Antigen-antibody interactions result in elimination or destruction of the antigen. The five kinds of interactions are the following:

1. *Precipitation.* Soluble antigens combine with antibodies to form a lattice formation of insoluble complexes that precipitate and are eventually eliminated.
2. *Agglutination.* Particulate antigens (e.g., red blood cells [RBCs]) may combine with antibodies to form clumps.
3. *Opsonization.* Bacteria are coated with molecules that allow them to be more easily recognized and ingested by neutrophils and monocytes. The opsonization mechanism involves IgG and complement-derived C3b. Opsonized particles attach to receptors on the surface of neutrophils and monocytes.
4. *Lysis.* Lysis occurs after complement acts on the cell membrane of the antigen to cause rupture and leakage of cell contents. (The complement system is discussed in Chapter 11.)
5. *Neutralization.* Antibodies neutralize some toxins released from bacteria. The mononuclear phagocyte system phagocytizes the antigen-antibody complex and removes it from the body.

Cell-Mediated Immunity

Immune responses that are initiated through specific antigen recognition by T cells are termed *cell-mediated immunity.* Although these reactions were initially considered to be solely mediated by T cells, several cell types and factors are involved in cell-mediated immunity. The cell types involved include T lymphocytes, macrophages, and natural killer cells. Cell-mediated immunity is of primary importance in (1) immunity against pathogens that survive inside of cells, including viruses and some bacteria (e.g., *Mycobacterium*); (2) fungal infections; (3) rejection of transplanted tissues; (4) contact hypersensitivity reactions; and (5) tumor immunity.

T Lymphocytes. T lymphocytes can be categorized into T-cytotoxic, T-helper, and T-suppressor cells. Antigenic characteristics of white blood cells (WBCs) have now been classified using monoclonal antibodies. These antigens are classified as clusters of differentiation or CD antigens. Many types of WBCs, especially lymphocytes, are referred to by their CD designations. All mature T cells have the CD3 antigen.

T-cytotoxic cells. T-cytotoxic cells are involved in attacking antigens on the cell membrane of foreign pathogens and releasing cytolytic substances that destroy the pathogen. These cells have antigen specificity and are sensitized by exposure to the antigen. Similar to B lymphocytes, some sensitized T cells do not attack the antigen but remain as memory T cells. As in the humoral immune response, a second exposure to the antigen will result in a more intense and rapid cell-mediated immune response.

T-helper and T-suppressor cells. T-helper (CD4) cells and T-suppressor (CD8) cells are involved in the regulation of the humoral antibody response and cell-mediated immunity, providing a positive and a negative signal, respectively. These two cell types are often referred to as *immunoregulatory* cells. With many autoimmune diseases the number of T-suppressor cells decreases in proportion to the number of T-helper cells, thus resulting in an overaggressive immune response. The human immunodeficiency virus (HIV) invades T-helper cells, thus decreasing their number and function. Therefore individuals with HIV infection do not mount an aggressive immune response and are at an increased risk for opportunistic infections and malignancies.

Natural Killer Cells. Natural killer (NK) cells are also involved in cell-mediated immunity. These cells are not T or B cells, but are large lymphocytes with numerous granules in the cytoplasm. Thus they are often referred to as *large granular lymphocytes.* NK cells do not require prior sensitization for their generation. These cells are involved in recognition and killing of virus-infected cells, tumor cells, and transplanted grafts. The mechanism of recognition is not fully understood.[2] NK cells have a significant role in immune surveillance for malignant cell changes.

Cytokines. The immune response involves complex interactions of T cells, B cells, monocytes, and neutrophils. These interactions depend on *cytokines* (soluble factors secreted by these cells) acting as messengers between the cell types. These cytokines can be classified as *lymphokines* (secreted by lymphocytes) and *monokines* (secreted by monocytes or macrophages). Cytokines instruct cells to alter their proliferation, differentiation, secretion, or activity. There are currently at least 60 different cytokines, and they can be classified into distinct categories. Some of these cytokines are listed in Table 12-4.

In general, the interleukins and colony-stimulating factors act as immunomodulatory and growth-regulating factors for hematopoietic cells. The interferons are antiviral and immunomodulatory.

Cytokines have a beneficial role in hematopoiesis and immune function. They can also have detrimental effects in inflammation, autoimmunity, and infection. Cytokines such as erythropoietin (see Chapter 44), colony-stimulating factors (see Chapters 14 and 29), interferons (see Chapters 14 and 41), and interleukin-2 (see Chapter 14) are used clinically either to stimulate hematopoiesis or to modulate tumor immunity. In addition, inhibitors of cytokines such as tumor necrosis factor and interleukin-1 are being used in clinical trials as antiinflammatory agents.

Interferon. Interferon, one type of lymphokine, was identified in 1957 as a substance that helps the body's natural defenses attack tumors and viruses. Three types of interferon have now been identified (see Table 12-4). In addition to their direct antiviral properties, interferons have immunoregulatory functions (e.g., enhancement of NK cell production and activation, as well as inhibition of tumor cell growth).

Interferon is not directly antiviral but produces an antiviral effect in cells by reacting with them and inducing the formation of a second protein termed *antiviral protein* (Fig. 12-5). This protein mediates the antiviral action of interferon by altering the cell's protein synthesis and preventing new viruses from becoming assembled.

Macrophages. Cytokines attract and activate macrophages in the area of the immune reaction. These macrophages secrete cytokines that further modulate the immune response. In addition, they can release lysosomal enzymes that damage surrounding tissues. (Macrophages are discussed in Chapter 11.)

Summary of Immune Responses

Humans need both humoral and cell-mediated immunity to remain healthy. Each type of immunity has unique properties and different methods of action; each reacts against particular antigens. Table 12-5 compares humoral and cell-mediated immunity.

GERONTOLOGIC CONSIDERATIONS

Effects of Aging on the Immune System

With advancing age there is a decline in the immune system (Table 12-6, p. 219). The primary clinical evidence for this immunosenescence is the high incidence of tumors in older adults. A greater susceptibility also occurs to infections (such as influenza and pneumonia) from pathogens that an older person has been relatively immunocompetent against earlier in life.[3]

Aging does not affect all aspects of the immune system. The bone marrow is relatively unaffected by increasing age. However, aging has a pronounced effect on the thymus, which decreases in size and activity with aging. These changes in the thymus are probably a primary cause of immunosenescence. Both T and B cells show deficiencies in activation, transit time through the cell cycle, and subsequent differentiation. However, the most significant alterations seem to involve T cells.[4] As thymic output of T cells diminishes, the differentiation of T cells in peripheral lymphoid structures increases. Consequently, there is an accumulation of memory cells rather than new precursor cells responsive to previously unencountered antigens.

Delayed hypersensitivity response, as determined by skin testing with injected antigens, is frequently decreased or absent in older adults. This altered response reflects *anergy* (immunodeficient condition characterized by lack of or diminished reaction to an antigen or group of antigens). The clinical consequences of a decline in cell-mediated immunity are evident. Anergic responses to delayed hypersensitivity skin tests in older

Table 12-4 Types and Functions of Cytokines

Type	Primary Functions
Interleukins (IL)	
IL-1	▪ Augments the immune response; inflammatory mediator; activates T cells; activates phagocytes; induces a fever
IL-2	▪ Activates T lymphocytes and NK cells; promotes proliferation and growth of T cells
IL-3 (multi-CSF)	▪ Hematopoietic growth factor for hematopoietic precursor cells
IL-4	▪ Growth factor for T cells, B cells, mast cells, and eosinophils
IL-5	▪ Promotes growth and function of B cells and eosinophils
IL-6	▪ B cell stimulation and differentiation factor; enhances the inflammatory response, induces fever, synergistic effects with IL-1 and TNF
IL-7	▪ Promotes growth of T and B cells
IL-8	▪ Chemoattractant for neutrophils and T cells
IL-9	▪ Some hematopoietic and thymopoietic effects
IL-10	▪ Inhibits cytokine production by T cells and NK cells; promotion of B cell proliferation and antibody responses
IL-11	▪ Is a multifunctional regulator of hematopoiesis and lymphopoiesis
IL-12	▪ Stimulates proliferation of activated T and NK cells; promotes gamma interferon production; promotion of cell-mediated immune responses
IL-13	▪ Inhibits activation and release of inflammatory cytokines; important regulator of inflammatory response
IL-14	▪ Proliferation of activated B cells
IL-15	▪ Mimics IL-2 effects; stimulates proliferation of T cells
IL-16	▪ Chemoattractant for T cells, eosinophils, and monocytes
IL-17	▪ Promotes release of IL-6, IL-8, and G-CSF
IL-18	▪ Induces production of gamma-interferon; enhances NK activity
Interferons	
Alpha-interferon	▪ Inhibits viral replication; activates NK cells
Beta-interferon	▪ Inhibits viral replication
Gamma-interferon	▪ Activates macrophages; stimulates NK cell activity; promotes B cell differentiation; inhibits viral replication
Tumor Necrosis Factor (TNF)	Activates macrophages and granulocytes; promotes the immune and inflammatory responses; kills tumor cells; is responsible for extensive weight loss associated with chronic inflammation and cancer
Colony-Stimulating Factors (CSF)	
Granulocyte colony–stimulating factor (G-CSF)	Stimulates proliferation and differentiation of neutrophils and affects functional activity of mature neutrophils
Granulocyte-macrophage colony–stimulating factor (GM-CSF)	Stimulates proliferation and differentiation of granulocytes and monocytes
Macrophage colony–stimulating factor (M-CSF)	Promotes the proliferation, differentiation, and activation of monocytes and macrophages
Erythropoietin (EPO)	Stimulates erythroid progenitor cells to produce red blood cells

HLA, human leukocyte antigen; *NK*, natural killer.

adults are related to an increased risk of cancer mortality, as well as mortality in general.[5]

ALTERED IMMUNE RESPONSE

The immune system normally reacts protectively against the presence of foreign antigens. However, sometimes the response is overreactive against foreign antigens or fails to maintain self-tolerance, and this results in tissue damage. This is termed a *hypersensitivity reaction.* A type of hypersensitivity response occurs when the body fails to recognize self-proteins and reacts against its own protein. The diseases that occur as a result of immune responses against self-antigens are termed *autoimmune diseases.* Finally, tissue damage may occur if the immune system is deficient. The immunodeficiency state may be primary or secondary to other diseases.

Hypersensitivity Reactions

Classification of hypersensitivity reactions may be done according to the source of the antigen, time sequence (immediate or delayed), or the basic immunologic mechanisms causing the injury. Basically, four types of hypersensitivity reactions exist. Types I, II, and III are immediate and are examples of humoral immunity. Type IV is a delayed hypersensitivity reaction and is related to cell-mediated immunity. Table 12-7 on p. 220 presents a summary of the four types of hypersensitivity reactions.

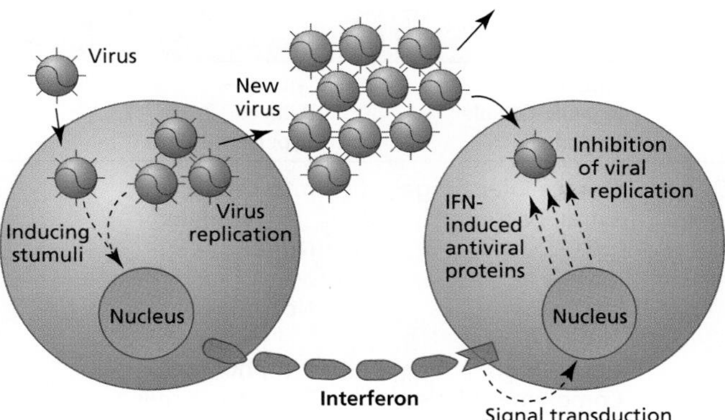

Fig. 12-5 Mechanism of action of interferon. Virus attacks a cell. The cell begins to synthesize new viruses and interferon. Interferon serves as an intercellular messenger. Interferon induces the production of antiviral proteins. Virus is not able to replicate in the cell.

Type I: Anaphylactoid Reactions. Anaphylactoid reactions are type I reactions that occur *only* in susceptible persons who are highly sensitized to specific allergens. IgE antibodies, produced in response to the allergen, have a characteristic property of attaching to mast cells and basophils (see Fig. 27-1). Within these cells are granules containing potent chemical mediators (histamine, serotonin, slow-reacting substance of anaphylaxis [SRS-A], eosinophil chemotactic factor of anaphylaxis [ECF-A], kinins, and bradykinin). (Leukotriene components [LTC_4, LTD_4, and LTE_4] of slow-reacting substance of SRS-A are discussed in Chapter 11 and Fig. 11-7.) On the first exposure to the allergen, IgE antibodies are produced and bind to mast cells and basophils. On any subsequent exposures, the allergen links with the IgE bound to mast cells or basophils and triggers degranulation of the cells and the release of chemical mediators from the granules. In this process, the mediators that are released attack target organs, causing clinical allergy symptoms (Fig. 12-6). These effects include smooth muscle contraction, increased vascular permeability, vasodilation, hypotension, increased secretion of mucus, and itching. Fortunately, the mediators are short acting and their effects are reversible. (The mediators and their effects are summarized in Table 12-8 on p. 221.)

A genetic predisposition for the development of allergic diseases exists. The capacity to become sensitized to an allergen appears to be the inherited trait rather than the specific allergic disorder. For example, a father with asthma may have a son who has allergic rhinitis.[6]

The clinical manifestations of an anaphylactoid reaction depend on whether the mediators remain local or become systemic or whether they affect particular organs. When the mediators remain localized, a cutaneous response termed the *wheal-and-flare reaction* occurs. This reaction is characterized by a pale wheal containing edematous fluid surrounded by a red flare from the hyperemia. The reaction occurs in minutes or hours and is usually not dangerous. A classic example of a wheal-and-flare reaction is the mosquito bite. The wheal-and-flare reaction serves a diagnostic purpose as a means of demonstrating allergic reactions to specific allergens during skin tests.

Table 12-5 Comparison of Humoral Immunity and Cell-Mediated Immunity

Characteristics	Humoral Immunity	Cell-Mediated Immunity
Cells involved	B lymphocytes	T-lymphocytes, macrophages
Products	Antibodies	Sensitized T cells, lymphokines
Memory cells	Present	Present
Reaction	Immediate	Delayed
Protection	Bacteria	Fungus
	Viruses (extracellular)	Viruses (intracellular)
	Respiratory and gastrointestinal pathogens	Tumor cells
Examples	Anaphylactic shock	Tuberculosis
	Atopic diseases	Fungal infections
	Transfusion reaction	Contact dermatitis
	Neutralization of exotoxins	Graft rejection
	Bacterial infections	Destruction of cancer cells

Table 12-6 Effects of Aging on the Immune System

Thymic involution
↓ Percentage of T cells
↓ Percentage of T-helper cells
↓ Percentage of T-suppressor cells
↓ Delayed hypersensitivity response
↓ Interleukin-1 synthesis
↓ Interleukin-2 synthesis
↓ Expression of interleukin-2 receptors
↓ Activation potential of T and B cells
↓ Proliferative response of T and B cells
↓ Primary and secondary antibody responses
↑ Autoantibodies

Common allergic reactions include anaphylactic shock (anaphylaxis) and atopic reactions.

Anaphylactic shock. Anaphylactic shock (anaphylaxis) occurs when mediators are released systemically (e.g., after injection of a drug or after an insect sting). The reaction occurs within minutes and is life threatening because of bronchial constriction and subsequent airway obstruction and vascular collapse. The target organs affected are seen in Fig. 12-7 on p. 222. Initial symptoms include edema and itching at the site of the exposure to the allergen. Shock can occur rapidly and is manifested by rapid, weak pulse; hypotension; dilated pupils; dyspnea; and possibly cyanosis. This is compounded by bronchial edema and angioedema. Death will occur if emergency treatment is not initiated. Some of the important allergens leading to anaphylactic shock in hypersensitive persons are listed in Table 12-9 on p. 222.

Table 12-7 Types of Hypersensitivity Reactions

	Type I—Anaphylactic	Type II—Cytotoxic	Type III—Immune-Complex Mediated	Type IV—Delayed Hypersensitivity
Antigen	Exogenous pollen, food, drugs, dust	Cell surface of RBC Basement membrane	Extracellular fungal, viral, bacterial	Intracellular or extracellular
Antibody involved	IgE	IgG IgM	IgG IgM	None
Complement involved	No	Yes	Yes	No
Mediators of injury	Histamine SRS-A	Complement lysis Neutrophils	Neutrophils Complement lysis	Lymphokines T-cytotoxic cells Monocytes/macrophages Lysosomal enzymes
Examples	Allergic rhinitis Asthma	Transfusion reaction Goodpasture's syndrome	Serum sickness Systemic lupus erythematosus Rheumatoid arthritis	Contact dermatitis Tumor rejection Transplant rejection
Skin test	Wheal and flare	None	Erythema and edema in 3 to 8 hours	Erythema and edema in 24 to 48 hours (e.g., TB test)

RBC, red blood cell; *SRS-A,* slow-reacting substance of anaphylaxis; *TB,* tuberculosis.

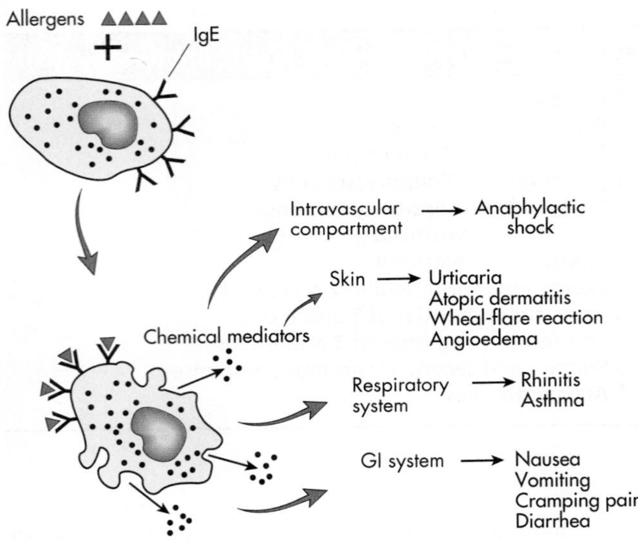

Fig. 12-6 Steps in an allergic type I reaction.

Atopic reactions. An estimated 20% of the population is *atopic,* an inherited tendency to become sensitive to environmental allergens.[7,8] The atopic diseases that can result are allergic rhinitis, asthma, atopic dermatitis, urticaria, and angioedema.

Allergic rhinitis, or hay fever, is the most common type I hypersensitivity reaction.[9] It may occur year-round (perennial allergic rhinitis), or it may be seasonal (seasonal allergic rhinitis). Airborne substances such as pollens, dust, or molds are the primary cause of allergic rhinitis. Perennial allergic rhinitis may be caused by dust, molds, and animal dander. Seasonal allergic rhinitis is commonly caused by trees, weeds, or grasses. The target areas affected are the conjunctiva of the eyes and the mucosa of the upper respiratory tract. Symptoms include nasal discharge, sneezing, lacrimation, mucosal swelling with airway obstruction, and pruritus around the eyes, nose, throat, and mouth. (Treatment of allergic rhinitis is discussed in Chapter 25.)

Many patients with asthma have an allergic component to their disease. These patients frequently have a history of atopic disorders (e.g., infantile eczema, allergic rhinitis, or food intolerances). In asthma, SRS-A and histamine are primarily responsible for action on the bronchioles (see Fig. 27-1). These mediators produce bronchial smooth muscle constriction, excessive secretion of viscoid mucus, edema of the mucous membranes of the bronchi, and decreased lung compliance. Because of these physiologic alterations, patients manifest dyspnea, wheezing, coughing, tightness in the chest, and thick sputum. (Pathophysiology and management of asthma are discussed in Chapter 27.)

Atopic dermatitis is a chronic, inherited skin disorder characterized by exacerbations and remissions. It is caused by several environmental allergens that are difficult to identify. Children with infantile eczema frequently have allergic respiratory disorders, although the relationship between the two is not fully understood. Although patients with atopic dermatitis have elevated IgE levels and positive skin tests, the histopathologic features do not represent the typical, localized wheal-and-flare type I reactions. The skin lesions are more generalized and involve vasodilation of blood vessels, resulting in interstitial edema with vesicle formation (Fig. 12-8, p. 222). (Dermatitis is discussed in Chapter 22.)

Urticaria (hives) is a cutaneous reaction against systemic allergens occurring in atopic persons. It is characterized by transient wheals (pink, raised, edematous, pruritic areas) that vary in size and shape and may occur throughout the body.

Table 12-8 Mediators of Allergic Response

Source and Storage	Biologic Activity	Pathologic Outcomes
Histamine		
Mast cell and basophil granules	Increases vascular permeability; constricts smooth muscle; stimulates irritant receptors	Edema of airways and larynx; bronchial constriction; urticaria, angioedema, pruritus; nausea, vomiting, diarrhea; shock
Leukotrienes		
Metabolites of arachidonic acid by lipoxygenase pathway*	Constrict bronchial smooth muscle; increase vascular permeability	Bronchial constriction; enhanced effect of histamine on smooth muscle
Prostaglandins		
Metabolites of arachidonic acid by cyclooxygenase pathway*	Stimulate vasodilation; constrict smooth muscle	Wheal-and-flare reaction on skin; hypotension; bronchospasm
Platelet-Activating Factor		
Mast cell	Aggregates platelets; stimulates vasodilation	Increase in pulmonary artery pressure; systemic hypotension
Kinins		
Kininogen	Stimulate slow, sustained smooth muscle contraction; increase vascular permeability; stimulate secretion of mucus; stimulate pain receptors	Angioedema with painful swelling; bronchial constriction
Serotonin		
Platelets	Increases vascular permeability; stimulates smooth muscle contraction	Mucosal edema; bronchial constriction
Eosinophil Chemotactic Factor		
Mast cells	Promotes chemotaxis of eosinophils	Influx of eosinophils
Anaphylatoxins		
C3a, C4a, C5a from complement activation	Stimulate histamine release	Same as for histamine

*See Fig. 11-7.

Urticaria develops rapidly after exposure to an allergen and may last minutes or hours. Histamine causes localized vasodilation (erythema), transudation of fluid (wheal), and flaring. Flaring is due to blood vessels on the edge of the wheal dilating in response to a reaction augmented by the sympathetic nervous system. Internal urticaria is characterized by edema in internal organs. Histamine is also responsible for the numbness and pruritus associated with the lesions. (Urticaria is discussed in Chapter 22.)

Angioedema is a localized cutaneous lesion similar to urticaria but involving deeper layers of the skin and the submucosa. The principal areas of involvement include the eyelids, lips, tongue, larynx, hands, feet, gastrointestinal (GI) tract, and genitalia. Swelling usually begins in the face and then progresses to the airways and other parts of the body. Dilation and engorgement of the capillaries secondary to release of histamine cause the diffuse swelling. Welts are not apparent as in urticaria; the outer skin appears normal or has a reddish hue. The lesions may burn, sting, or itch and can cause acute abdominal pain if in the GI tract. The swelling may occur suddenly or over several hours and usually lasts for 24 hours.

Type II: Cytotoxic and Cytolytic Reactions. Cytotoxic and cytolytic reactions are type II hypersensitivity reactions involving the direct binding of IgG or IgM antibodies to an antigen on the cell surface. Antigen-antibody complexes activate the complement system, which mediates the reaction. Cellular tissue is destroyed in one of two ways: (1) activation of the complement cascade resulting in cytolysis, and (2) enhanced phagocytosis.

Target cells frequently destroyed in type II reactions are erythrocytes, platelets, and leukocytes. Some of the antigens involved are the ABO blood group, Rh factor, and drug haptens such as chloramphenicol. Pathophysiologic disorders characteristic of type II reactions include ABO incompatibility transfusion reaction, Rh incompatibility transfusion reaction, autoimmune and drug-related hemolytic anemias, leukopenias, thrombocytopenias, erythroblastosis fetalis (hemolytic disease of the newborn), and Goodpasture's syndrome. The tissue damage usually occurs rapidly.

Hemolytic transfusion reactions. A classic type II reaction occurs when a recipient receives ABO-incompatible blood from a donor. Naturally acquired antibodies to antigens of the ABO blood group are within the recipient's serum but are not present on the erythrocyte membranes (see Table 28-8). For example, a person with type A blood has anti-B antibodies, a person with type B blood has anti-A antibodies, a person with type AB blood has no antibodies, and a person with type O blood has both anti-A and anti-B antibodies.

If the recipient is transfused with incompatible blood, antibodies immediately coat the foreign erythrocytes, causing agglutination (clumping). The clumping of cells blocks small blood vessels in the body, uses existing clotting factors, and

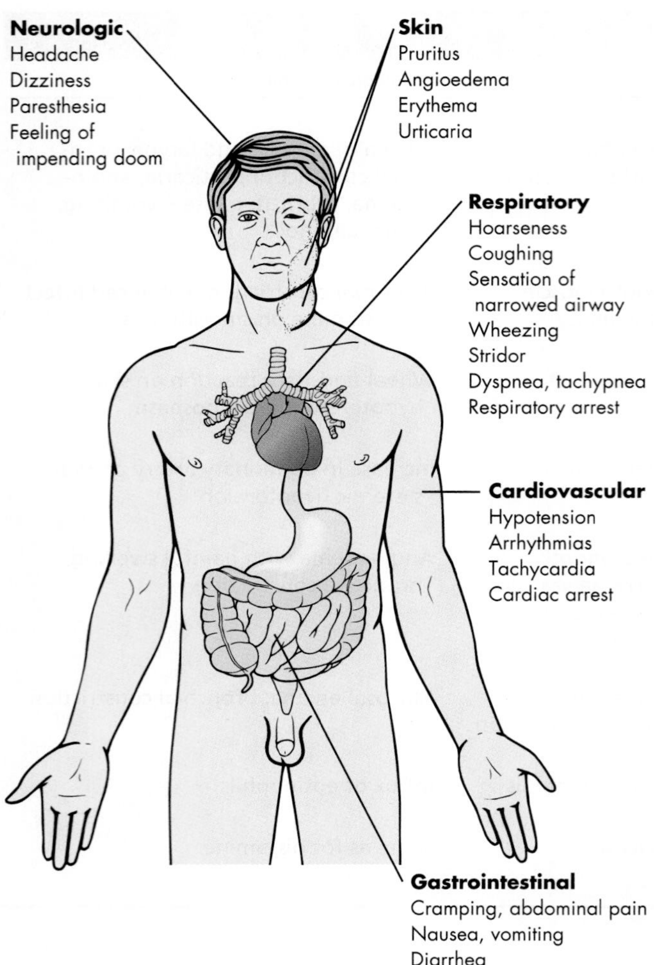

Fig. 12-7 Clinical manifestations of a systemic anaphylactic reaction.

Table 12-9 Allergens Causing Anaphylactic Shock

Drugs	
Penicillins	Sulfonamides
Insulins	Aspirin
Tetracycline	Local anesthetics
Chemotherapeutic agents	Cephalosporins
Nonsteroidal antiinflammatory agents	
Insect Venoms	
Hymenoptera*	
Foods	
Eggs	Milk
Nuts	Peanuts
Shellfish	Fish
Chocolate	Strawberries
Animal Serums	
Tetanus antitoxin	Rabies antitoxin
Diphtheria antitoxin	Snake venom antitoxin
Treatment Measures	
Blood products (whole blood and components)	Iodine-contrast media dye for IVP or angiogram test
Allergenic extracts in hyposensitization therapy	

*Wasps, hornets, yellow jackets, bumblebees, and ants.
IVP, intravenous pyelography.

depletes them, leading to bleeding. Within hours, neutrophils and macrophages phagocytize the agglutinated cells. As complement is fixed to the antigen, cytolysis occurs. Cellular lysis causes the release of hemoglobin into the urine and plasma. In addition, a cytotoxic reaction causes vascular spasms in the kidney that further block the renal tubules. Acute renal failure can result from the hemoglobinuria. (Blood transfusions are discussed in Chapter 29.)

Goodpasture's syndrome. Goodpasture's syndrome is a rare disorder involving the lungs and kidneys. An antibody-mediated autoimmune reaction occurs with the glomerular and alveolar basement membranes. The circulating antibodies combine with tissue antigen to activate complement, which causes deposits of IgG to form along the basement membranes of the lungs or kidney. This reaction may result in pulmonary hemorrhage and glomerulonephritis. The disease is usually rapidly progressive. Corticosteroids, immunosuppressive drugs (e.g., cyclophosphamide [Cytoxan]), and plasmapheresis have been used effectively to slow the progression of the disease. (Goodpasture's syndrome is discussed in more detail in Chapter 43.)

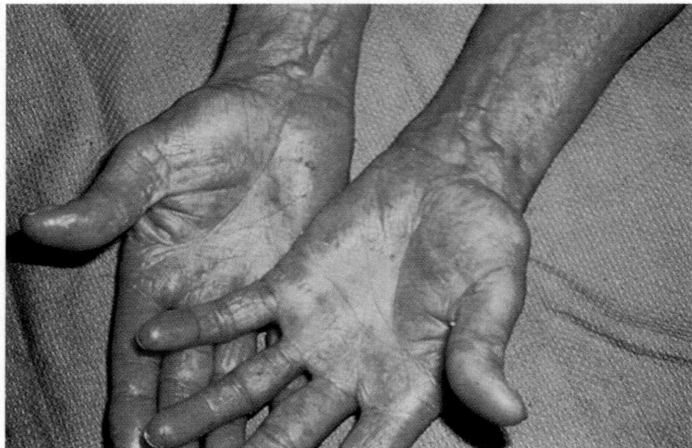

Fig. 12-8 Chronic lesions of atopic dermatitis on the hands of a woman; erythema, papules, bullae, and weeping vesicles.

Type III: Immune-Complex Reactions. Tissue damage in immune-complex reactions, which are type III reactions, occurs secondary to antigen-antibody complexes. Soluble antigens combine with immunoglobulins of the IgG and IgM classes to form complexes that are too small to be effectively removed by the mononuclear phagocyte system. Therefore the complexes deposit in tissue or small blood vessels. They cause the fixation of complement and the release of chemotactic factors that lead to inflammation and destruction of the involved tissue.

Type III reactions may be local or systemic and immediate or delayed. The clinical manifestations depend on the number of complexes and the location in the body. Common sites for deposit are the kidneys, skin, joints, blood vessels, and lungs. Severe type III reactions are associated with autoimmune disorders such as systemic lupus erythematosus, acute glomerulonephritis, and rheumatoid arthritis. Two classic disorders that illustrate type III reactions are the Arthus reaction and serum sickness.

Arthus reaction. The Arthus reaction is a localized inflammatory response resulting from antigen-antibody complexes deposited in the small vessels of the skin and is caused by repeated exposure to an exogenous antigen. It may occur from inhalation of dust or spores, resulting in pneumonitis or farmer's lung. The underlying defect that triggers an Arthus reaction appears to be the production of excess IgG to specific antigens. On subsequent exposure to soluble antigens, antigen-antibody complexes form, leading to a type III reaction. Because of the chemotactic substances released by complement activation, neutrophils infiltrate to the site of the complex. These neutrophils are the primary factor responsible for tissue damage.

Arthus reactions are manifested by edematous, hemorrhagic, and necrotic lesions that begin within 1 hour and peak 6 to 12 hours later. Most classic Arthus reactions are not clinically significant because strong antigenic substances are not ordinarily given repeatedly to a hypersensitive individual. However, allergic vasculitis resulting from drugs (e.g., penicillin, sulfonamides) resembles the Arthus reaction.

Serum sickness. Serum sickness is another type III reaction that involves deposits of antigen-antibody complexes in blood vessel walls of the skin, joints, and especially the renal glomeruli. In contrast to an Arthus reaction, this disorder is systemic. It develops slowly, 10 to 14 days after exposure to an antigen, and is self-limiting.

The critical factor in serum sickness is the presence of excess soluble antigen. Common antigens triggering the reaction are horse antitoxin serums and certain drugs (e.g., penicillins, sulfonamides). Unlike patients with a type I reaction, the person does not need to be previously sensitized to react to the antigen. Rather, a single dose of the antigen that remains at high levels in the body for several days reacts with antibodies formed about 2 weeks after initial exposure to the antigen. The antigen-antibody complex then triggers complement to deposit in vessels, resulting in an intravascular inflammation. The predominant signs and symptoms of serum sickness are urticaria, angioedema, fever, muscle soreness, malaise, lymphadenopathy, joint pain, polyarthritis, and nephritis.

Fortunately, serum sickness reactions from the use of horse antitoxin serum can be avoided by using human serums. However, watching for drug sensitivities is still critical. The actual treatment of serum sickness depends on the severity of the reaction. For mild reactions, aspirin is prescribed for the fever and arthritis, and antihistamines are given for urticaria and angioedema. Corticosteroids are prescribed for more severe reactions, especially when renal or neurologic changes are present.

Type IV: Delayed Hypersensitivity Reactions.

A delayed hypersensitivity reaction—a type IV reaction—is also termed a *cell-mediated immune response.* Although cell-mediated responses are usually protective mechanisms, tissue damage occurs in delayed hypersensitivity reactions.

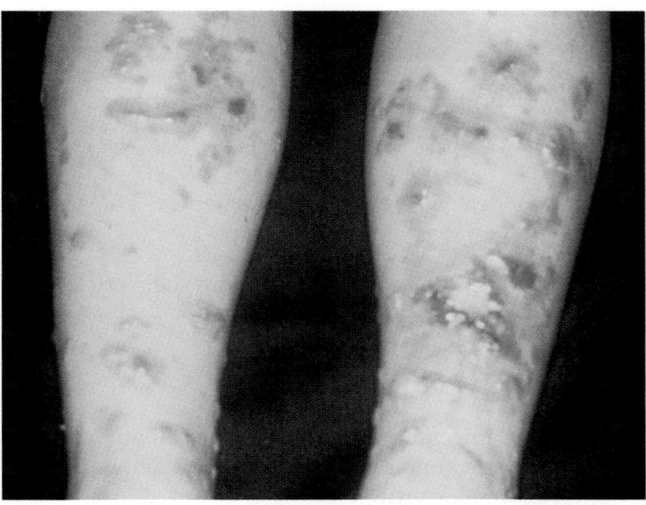

Fig. 12-9 Acute contact dermatitis on lower extremities. Note the edema, erythema, papules, bullae, and weeping vesicles.

The tissue damage in a type IV reaction does not occur in the presence of antibodies or complement. Rather, sensitized T lymphocytes attack antigens or release cytokines. Some of these cytokines attract macrophages into the area. The macrophages and enzymes released by them are responsible for most of the tissue destruction. The delayed hypersensitivity response takes 24 to 48 hours for a reaction to occur.

Clinical examples of a delayed hypersensitivity reaction include contact dermatitis; hypersensitivity reactions to bacterial, fungal, and viral infections; and transplant rejections. Some drug sensitivity reactions also fit this category.

Contact dermatitis. Allergic contact dermatitis is an example of a delayed hypersensitivity reaction involving the skin. The reaction occurs when the skin is exposed to haptens. The haptens easily penetrate the skin to combine with epidermal proteins. The hapten-carrier substance then becomes antigenic. Over a period of 7 to 14 days, memory cells form to the antigen. On subsequent exposure to the hapten, a sensitized person develops eczematous skin lesions within 48 hours. The most common haptens encountered are metal compounds (e.g., nickel, mercury); rubber compounds; catechols present in poison ivy, poison oak, and sumac; cosmetics; and some dyes.

In acute contact dermatitis the skin lesions appear erythematous and edematous and are covered with papules, vesicles, and bullae (Fig. 12-9). The involved area is very pruritic but may also burn or sting. When contact dermatitis becomes chronic, the lesions resemble atopic dermatitis because they are thickened, scaly, and lichenified. The main difference between contact dermatitis and atopic dermatitis is that contact dermatitis is localized and restricted to the area exposed to the allergens, whereas atopic dermatitis is usually widespread.

Microbial hypersensitivity reactions. Although cell-mediated immunity plays an important defensive role in destroying viruses, bacteria, and fungi, delayed hypersensitivity reactions do occur as the surrounding tissue is damaged.

Table **12-10** Categories of Allergens

Inhalants	Contactants	Ingestants	Injectables
Pollens Molds Spores Animal dander House dust Mites	Plants Drugs Metals Cosmetics Dyes Fibers Various chemicals	Food Food additives Drugs	Drugs Vaccines Insect stings

Examples of infectious delayed hypersensitivity reactions include skin rashes of measles and smallpox, lesions of leprosy and herpes simplex virus, and the generalized toxemia and caseous necrosis with tuberculosis.

The classic example of a bacterial cell-mediated immune reaction is the body's defense against the tubercle bacillus. Tuberculosis results from invasion of lung tissue by the highly resistant tubercle bacillus. The organism itself does not directly damage the lung tissue and may live in the host for some time before signs and symptoms appear. However, antigenic material released from the tubercle bacilli reacts with T lymphocytes over time, initiating a cell-mediated response. The resulting lymphocytotoxicity causes extensive caseous necrosis of the lung.

After the initial cell-mediated reaction, memory cells persist, so subsequent contact with the tubercle bacillus or an extract of purified protein from the organism causes a delayed hypersensitivity reaction. This is the basis for the purified protein derivative (PPD) tuberculosis skin test read 48 to 72 hours after the injection. (Tuberculosis is discussed in Chapter 26.)

Transplant rejection. Rejection of organs occurs by cell-mediated immunity if the donor organ does not perfectly match the recipient's human leukocyte antigens [HLAs], also termed *histocompatibility antigens.* The rejection can be prevented by closely matching ABO, Rh, and HLA antigens between donor and recipient. Unfortunately, many different HLA antigens exist, and a perfect match is nearly impossible unless the tissue is from oneself or an identical twin.

Graft rejection is a complicated process that involves sensitized T lymphocytes (see Fig. 44-17). If the tissue is mismatched, sensitized T lymphocytes arrive at regional lymph nodes within 6 to 10 days. The clinical signs of rejection appear in about 14 days when sensitized T lymphocytes attack the graft. At this time the vascularization stops and the tissue becomes necrosed. Common manifestations of transplant rejection include fever, malaise, localized graft tenderness, hypertension, leukocytosis, and elevated sedimentation rate. Transplant rejection is discussed in Chapter 44.

Drugs that interfere with cell-mediated immune responses are given to recipients of transplanted organs. (Some of the agents used are summarized in Table 44-12.) Unfortunately, the use of immunosuppressant drugs can result in major complications, including increased susceptibility to infection, increased risk of developing cancer, and graft-versus-host disease.

ALLERGIC DISORDERS

Although an alteration of the immune system may be manifested in many ways, allergies or type I hypersensitivity reactions are seen most frequently.

Assessment

For a thorough assessment of a patient with allergies, a complete database must be obtained. This consists of a comprehensive patient history, physical examination, diagnostic workup, and skin testing for allergens.

Health History. A comprehensive history that covers family allergies, past and present allergies, and social and environmental factors is essential. The information may be obtained from the patient or the patient's caregiver.

Family history, including information about atopic reactions in relatives, is especially important in identifying at-risk patients. The specific disorder, clinical manifestations, and treatments prescribed should be assessed.

Past and present allergies must be noted. Identifying the allergens that may have triggered a reaction is essential to control allergic reactions. Table 12-10 lists four major categories of allergens that should be evaluated. Determination of the time of year that an allergic reaction occurs can be a clue to a seasonal allergen. Information should also be obtained about any over-the-counter or prescription medications used to treat the allergies.

In addition to identification of the allergen, information about the clinical manifestations and course of allergic reaction should be obtained. If the patient is a woman, assessment of symptoms during pregnancy, menstruation, or menopause may be important.

Social and environmental factors, especially the physical environment, are important. Questions about pets, trees, and plants on property; pollutants in the air; and floor coverings, house plants, and cooling and heating systems in the home and workplace can provide valuable information about allergens. In addition, a daily or weekly food diary with a description of any untoward reactions is important. Of particular interest is a screening for any reaction to medication. Finally, questions about the patient's lifestyle and stress level should be reviewed in connection with the appearance of allergic symptoms.

Physical Examination. A comprehensive head-to-toe physical examination should be given to a patient with allergies, with particular attention focused on the site of the allergic manifestations. A comprehensive assessment that includes

NURSING ASSESSMENT

Table 12-11 Allergies

Subjective Data

Important Health Information

Past health history: Recurrent respiratory problems, seasonal exacerbations; unusual reactions to insect bites or stings; past and present allergies

Medications: Unusual reactions to any drugs or medications; use of over-the-counter medication, use of medications for allergies

Functional Health Patterns

Health perception–health management: Family history of allergies; malaise

Nutritional-metabolic: Food intolerances; vomiting

Elimination: Abdominal cramps, diarrhea

Activity-exercise: Fatigue; hoarseness, cough, dyspnea

Cognitive-perceptual: Itching, burning, stinging of eyes, nose, throat, or skin; chest tightness

Role-relationship: Altered home and work environment, presence of pets

Objective Data

Integumentary

Rashes, including urticaria, wheal and flare, papules, vesicles, bullae; dryness, scaliness, scratches, irritation

Eyes, Ears, Nose, and Throat

Eyes: Conjunctivitis; lacrimation; rubbing or excessive blinking; dark circles under the eyes ("allergic shiner")

Ears: Diminished hearing; immobile or scarred tympanic membranes; recurrent ear infections

Nose: Nasal polyps; nasal voice; nose twitching; itchy nose; rhinitis; pale, boggy mucous membranes; sniffling; repeated sneezing; swollen nasal passages; recurrent, unexplained nosebleeds; crease across the bridge of nose ("allergic salute")

Throat: Continual throat clearing; swollen lips or tongue; red throat; palpable neck lymph nodes

Respiratory

Wheezing, stridor; thick sputum

Possible Findings

Eosinophilia of serum, sputum, or nasal and bronchial secretions; elevated serum IgE levels; positive skin tests; abnormal chest and sinus x-rays

subjective and objective data should be obtained from the patient (Table 12-11).

Diagnostic Studies

Many specialized immunologic techniques can be performed to detect abnormalities of lymphocytes, eosinophils, and immunoglobulins. A complete blood count (CBC) and serology tests are commonly done.

A CBC with WBC differential is required with an absolute lymphocyte count and eosinophil count. Cellular immunodeficiency is diagnosed if the lymphocyte count is below 1200/μl (1.2×10^9/L). T cell and B cell quantification is used to diagnose immunodeficiency syndromes. The eosinophil count is elevated with type I hypersensitivity reactions involving IgE immunoglobulins. Serum IgE level is also generally elevated in type I hypersensitivity reactions and serves as a diagnostic indicator of atopic diseases.

Radioallergosorbent test (RAST) is an in vitro diagnostic test for IgE antibodies to specific allergens. Although expensive, it is safe but less sensitive and takes longer than skin tests for detecting allergens. RAST is helpful in confirming reactivity to various foods or drugs in individuals who give a history of severe anaphylactic reactions.

Sputum, nasal, and bronchial secretions also may be tested for the presence of eosinophils. If asthma is suspected, pulmonary function tests for vital capacity, forced expiratory volume, and maximum midexpiratory flow rates are helpful.

Skin Tests. Skin testing is generally used to confirm specific sensitivity in patients with atopic disease after the history has suggested possible allergens for testing.

Procedure. Skin testing may be done by one of two methods: (1) a cutaneous scratch or prick or (2) an intracutaneous injection. The areas of the body usually used in testing are the arms and back. Allergen extracts are applied to the skin in rows with a corresponding control site opposite the test site. Saline or another diluent is applied to the control site. In the scratch test the epidermal skin layer is scratched with a lancet and the allergen extract is applied at the site. The prick test involves placing a drop of allergen extract on the skin and then piercing the underlying epidermis with a needle. In the intracutaneous method the allergen extract is injected intradermally in rows, usually on the arm. Since the allergic reaction is more severe with this method, the test is used only for persons who did not react to cutaneous methods.

Results. If the person is hypersensitive to the allergen, a positive reaction will occur within minutes after insertion in the skin and may last for 8 to 12 hours. A positive reaction is manifested by a local wheal-and-flare response. The size of the positive reaction does not always correlate with the severity of allergy symptoms. False-positive and false-negative results may occur. Negative results from skin testing do not necessarily mean the person does not have an allergic disorder, and positive results do not necessarily mean that the allergen was causing the clinical manifestations. Positive results imply that the person is sensitized to that allergen. Therefore correlating skin test results with the patient's history is important.

Precautions. A highly sensitive person is always at risk for developing an anaphylactic reaction to skin tests. Therefore a patient should never be left alone during the testing period. Sometimes skin testing is completely contraindicated and the RAST test is used. If a severe reaction does occur with a cutaneous test, the extract is immediately removed and antiinflammatory topical cream is applied to the site. For intracutaneous testing, the arm is used so that a tourniquet can be applied during a severe reaction. A subcutaneous injection of epinephrine may also be necessary.

Collaborative Care

After an allergic disorder is diagnosed, the therapeutic treatment is aimed at reducing exposure to the offending allergen,

✚ EMERGENCY MANAGEMENT

Table **12-12** Anaphylactic Shock

Etiology	Assessment Findings	Interventions
Injection, inhalation, ingestion, or topical exposure to substance that produces profound allergic response Refer to Table 12-9 for more complete listing	■ See Fig. 12-7.	**Initial** ■ Ensure patent airway. ■ Remove stinger if an insect sting. ■ Epinephrine 1:1000, 0.2-0.5 ml SC for mild symptoms. ■ Repeat at 20 min intervals if necessary. ■ Epinephrine 1:10,000, 0.5 ml IV at 5-10 min intervals for severe reaction. ■ Administer high-flow oxygen via non-rebreather mask. ■ Place recumbent and elevate legs. ■ Keep warm. ■ Administer diphenhydramine (Benadryl) IM or IV. ■ Administer histamine H_2 blockers such as cimetidine (Tagamet). ■ Maintain blood pressure with fluids, volume expanders, vasopressors (e.g., dopamine [Intropin], levarterenol [Levophed]). **Ongoing Monitoring** ■ Monitor vital signs, respiratory effort, oxygen saturation, level of consciousness, and cardiac rhythm. ■ Anticipate intubation with severe respiratory distress. ■ Anticipate cricothyrotomy or tracheostomy with severe laryngeal edema.

SC, subcutaneous.

treating the symptoms, and if necessary desensitizing the person through immunotherapy. All health care workers must be prepared for the rare but life-threatening anaphylactic reaction, which requires immediate medical and nursing interventions. It is extremely important that all of a patient's allergies be listed on the chart, the nursing care plan, and the medication record.

Anaphylaxis. Anaphylactic reactions occur suddenly in hypersensitive patients after exposure to the offending allergen. They may occur following parenteral injection of drugs (especially antibiotics), blood products, and insect stings. The cardinal principle in therapeutic management is *speed* in (1) recognition of signs and symptoms of an anaphylactic reaction, (2) maintenance of a patent airway, (3) prevention of spread of the allergen by using a tourniquet, (4) administration of drugs, and (5) treatment for shock. Table 12-12 summarizes the emergency treatment of anaphylactic shock.

Mild symptoms such as pruritis and urticaria can be controlled by administration of 0.2 to 0.5 ml of epinephrine, diluted 1:1000, given subcutaneously every 20 minutes according to the physician's orders or a hospital emergency drug protocol. An intravenous infusion should be initiated to provide a route for administration of 0.5 ml of epinephrine, diluted 1:10,000, at 5- to 10-minute intervals; volume expanders; and vasopressor agents such as dopamine if intractable hypotension occurs.

Oxygen via a non-rebreather mask should be administered. Endotracheal intubation or a tracheostomy is mandatory for O_2 delivery if progressive hypoxia exists. Other agents are used, including an antihistamine such as diphenhydramine (Benadryl) intravenously or intramuscularly for urticaria and angioedema.

In more severe cases of anaphylaxis, hypovolemic shock may occur because of the loss of intravascular fluid into interstitial spaces that occurs secondary to increased capillary permeability. Peripheral vasoconstriction and stimulation of the sympathetic nervous system occur to compensate for the fluid shift. However, unless shock is treated early, the body will no longer be able to compensate, and irreversible tissue damage will occur, leading to death. (Hypovolemic shock is discussed in Chapter 61.)

Chronic Allergies. Most allergic reactions are chronic and are characterized by remissions and exacerbations of symptoms. Treatment focuses on identification and control of allergens, relief of symptoms through pharmacologic interventions, and hyposensitization of a patient to an offending allergen.

Allergen recognition and control. The nurse plays an important role in helping the patient make lifestyle adjustments so that there is minimal exposure to offending allergens. The nurse must reinforce that, even with drug therapy and immunotherapy, the patient will never be desensitized or completely symptom free. The nurse can initiate various preventive measures that will help control the allergic symptoms.

Of primary importance is the need to identify the offending allergen. Sometimes this is done through skin testing. In the case of food allergies, an elimination diet is sometimes valuable. If an allergic reaction occurs, all food eaten should be eliminated and gradually reintroduced one at a time until the offending food is detected.

Many allergic reactions, especially asthma and urticaria, may be aggravated by fatigue and emotional stress. The nurse

DRUG THERAPY

Table 12-13 Allergic Rhinitis

Generic Name	Trade Name
Antihistamines	
Diphenhydramine	Benadryl
Azatadine maleate	Optimine
Carbinoxamine maleate	Clistin, Histadyl
Triprolidine	Actidil
Brompheniramine maleate	Dimetane
Chlorpheniramine maleate	Coricidine, Chlor-Trimeton, Teldrin
Clemastine	Tavist
Cetirizine*	Zyrtec
Astemizole*	Hismanal
Loratadine*	Claritin
Fexofenadine*	Allegra
Decongestants	
Pseudoephedrine	Sudafed
Phenylephrine	Neo-Synephrine, Alconefrin, Sinex
Oxymetazoline	Afrin, Dristan
Antihistamine/Decongestant	
Clemastine/phenylpropanolamine	Tavist D
Triprolidine/pseudoephedrine	Actifed
Brompheniramine/phenylpropanolamine	Dimetapp
Chlorpheniramine/pseudoephedrine	Novafed A
Fexofenadine/pseudoephedrine	Allegra-D
Intranasal Corticosteroids	
Beclomethasone	Beconase, Vancenase
Flunisolide	Nasalide
Mometasone	Nasonex
Triamcinolone	Nasacort
Fluticasone	Flonase
Budesonide	Rhinocort
Mast-Cell Stablizer	
Cromolyn	Intal, Nasalcrom, Rynacrom
Nedocromil	Tilade
Antipruritics	
Diphenhydramine	Benadryl
$ZnCO_3$	Calamine lotion
Methdilazine	Tacaryl

*Second-generation antihistamines, generally less sedating.

can be instrumental in initiating a stress management program with the patient. Relaxation techniques can be practiced when the patient comes for frequent immunotherapy treatments.

Sometimes control of allergic symptoms requires environmental control, including changing an occupation, moving to a different climate, or giving up a favorite pet. In the case of airborne allergens, sleeping in an air-conditioned room, damp dusting daily, covering mattresses and pillows with hypoallergenic covers, and wearing a mask outdoors may be helpful.

If the allergen is a drug, the patient should be instructed to avoid the drug. The patient also has the responsibility to make the drug intolerance well known to all health care providers. The patient should wear a Medic Alert bracelet listing the particular drug allergy and have the offending drug listed on all medical and dental records.

For a patient allergic to insect stings, commercial bee-sting kits containing preinjectable epinephrine and a tourniquet are available. The nurse has the responsibility to instruct the patient about the technique of applying the tourniquet and self-injecting the subcutaneous epinephrine. This patient also should wear a Medic Alert bracelet and carry a bee-sting kit whenever going outdoors.

Drug Therapy. The major categories of drugs used for symptomatic relief of chronic allergic disorders include antihistamines, sympathomimetic/decongestant drugs, corticosteroids, antipruritic drugs, and mast cell stabilizing drugs. Many of these drugs may be obtained over the counter and are often misused by patients.

Antihistamines. Antihistamines are the best drugs for treatment of allergic rhinitis and urticaria (Table 12-13). They are less effective for severe allergic reactions. The drugs may be given intravenously or orally, applied topically, inhaled, or used as a nasal spray. They act by competing with histamine for H_1-receptor sites and thus blocking the effect of histamine.

Best results are achieved if they are taken immediately after allergy signs and symptoms appear. Antihistamines can be used effectively to treat edema and pruritus but are relatively ineffective in preventing bronchoconstriction. With seasonal rhinitis, antihistamines should be taken during peak pollen seasons.

Side effects of many antihistamines are drowsiness, sedation, and disturbed coordination. Therefore patients should be cautioned about driving and operating machinery. Other side effects include dryness of mouth, GI upset, blurred vision, and dizziness.

Because of the difficulties with side effects, a new generation of antihistamines has been developed. Astemizole (Hismanal), loratadine (Claritin), cetirizine (Zyrtec), and fexofenadine (Allegra) do not readily cross the blood-brain barrier. Therefore the central nervous system depression and anticholinergic side effects seen with other types of antihistamines are not frequently observed with these newer antihistamines. In addition, these drugs require administration only once or twice per day.

Sympathomimetic/decongestant drugs. The major sympathomimetic drug is epinephrine (Adrenalin), which is the drug of choice to treat an anaphylactic reaction. Epinephrine is a hormone produced by the adrenal medulla that stimulates alpha- and beta-adrenergic receptors. Stimulation of the α-adrenergic receptors causes vasoconstriction of peripheral blood vessels. β-Receptor stimulation relaxes bronchial smooth muscle spasms. Epinephrine also acts directly on mast cells to stabilize them against further degranulation. The action of epinephrine lasts only a few minutes. For the treatment of anaphylaxis the drug must be given parenterally (usually subcutaneously).

Several specific, minor sympathomimetic drugs differ from epinephrine because they can be taken orally or nasally and last for several hours. Included in this category are phenylephrine (Neo-Synephrine) and pseudoephedrine (Sudafed). The minor sympathomimetic drugs are used primarily to treat allergic rhinitis. The action of these drugs includes nasal decongestion, reduction in nasal edema, elevation of blood pressure, and cardiac stimulation.

Of the drugs used in the management of chronic allergies, phenylephrine and pseudoephedrine are abused most frequently. Because these drugs may be bought over the counter, patients tend to overmedicate themselves. *Rhinitis medicamentosa,* a rebound effect in which nasal mucosa becomes more edematous and congested after medicating, may develop from the local overuse of nasal sprays containing ephedrine.

Corticosteroids. Nasal corticosteroid sprays are very effective in relieving the symptoms of allergic rhinitis (see Chapter 25 and Table 25-2). Occasionally patients have such severe manifestations of allergies that they are truly incapacitated. In these situations, a brief course of oral corticosteroids can be used.

Antipruritic drugs. Topically applied antipruritic drugs are most effective when the skin is not broken. These drugs protect the skin and provide relief from itching. Common over-the-counter drugs include calamine lotion, coal tar solutions, and camphor. Menthol and phenol may be added to other lotions to produce an antipruritic effect. Some more potent drugs that require a prescription include methdilazine (Tacaryl) and trimeprazine (Temaril). These drugs should be used with great caution because of the associated risk of agranulocytosis.

Mast cell–stabilizing drugs. Cromolyn (Intal, Nasalcrom, Rynacrom) and nedocromil (Tilade) are mast cell–stabilizing agents that inhibit the release of histamines, leukotrienes, and other agents from the mast cell after antigen-IgE interaction. They are available as an inhalant nebulizer solution, a nasal spray, or an oral pill. They are used in the management of asthma (see Chapter 27) and in the treatment of allergic rhinitis (see Chapter 25). An important feature of these drugs is a very low incidence of side effects.

Immunotherapy. Immunotherapy is the recommended treatment for control of allergic symptoms when the allergen cannot be avoided and drug therapy is not effective.[10] Relatively few patients with allergies have symptoms so intolerable that they require allergy immunotherapy. Immunotherapy is absolutely indicated only in individuals with anaphylactic reactions to insect venom. It involves administration of small titers of an allergen extract in increasing strengths until hyposensitivity to the specific allergen is achieved. For best results the patient should continue to avoid the offending allergen whenever possible because complete desensitization is impossible.

Mechanism of action. IgE immunoglobulin level is elevated in atopic individuals. When IgE combines with an allergen in a hypersensitive person, a reaction occurs, releasing histamine in various body tissues. Allergens more readily combine with IgG immunoglobulin than with other immunoglobulins. Therefore immunotherapy involves injecting allergen extracts that will stimulate increased IgG levels. The binding of IgG to allergen-reactive sites interferes with allergen binding to mast cell–bound IgE, preventing mast cell degranulation, and thus reduces the number of reactions that cause tissue damage. The goal of long-term immunotherapy is to keep "blocking" IgG levels high. In addition, allergen-specific T-suppressor cells develop in individuals receiving immunotherapy.[11]

Method of administration. The allergens included in immunotherapy are chosen on the basis of the results of skin testing with a panel of allergens found in the local geographic area. Immunotherapy involves the subcutaneous injection of titrated amounts of allergen extracts biweekly or weekly. The dose is small at first and is increased slowly until a maintenance dosage is reached. Generally it takes 1 to 2 years of immunotherapy to reach the maximal therapeutic effect. Therapy may be continued for about 5 years. After that, consideration is given to discontinuing therapy. In many patients a decrease in symptoms is sustained after the treatment is discontinued.[9] For patients with severe allergies or sensitivity to insect stings, maintenance therapy is continued indefinitely. Best results are achieved when immunotherapy is administered throughout the year.

NURSING MANAGEMENT: IMMUNOTHERAPY

The nurse is often primarily responsible for giving immunotherapy. Adverse reactions should always be anticipated, especially when using a new-strength dose, after a previous reaction, or after a missed dose. Early signs and symptoms indicative of a systemic reaction include pruritus, urticaria, sneezing, laryngeal edema, and hypotension. Emergency measures for anaphylactic shock should be initiated immediately. A local reaction should be described according to the degree of redness and swelling at the injection site. If the area is greater than the size of a 50-cent piece in an adult, the reaction should be reported to the physician so that the allergen dosage may be decreased.

Immunotherapy always carries the risk of a severe anaphylactic reaction. Therefore a physician, emergency equipment, and essential drugs should be available whenever injections are given.

Record keeping must be accurate and can be invaluable in preventing an adverse reaction to the allergen extract. Before giving an injection, the nurse should check the patient's name with the name on the vial. Next, the vial strength, amount of last dose, date of last dose, and any reaction information should be screened.

The nurse should always administer the allergen extract in an extremity away from a joint so that a tourniquet can be applied for a severe reaction. The site should be rotated for each injection. The nurse must aspirate for blood before giving an injection to ensure that the allergen extract is not injected into a blood vessel. An injection directly into the bloodstream can potentiate an anaphylactic reaction. After the injection is given, the patient should be carefully observed for 20 minutes because systemic reactions are most likely to occur immediately. However, the patient should be warned that a delayed reaction can occur as long as 24 hours later.

Latex Allergies

Allergies to latex products have become a problem of increasing proportion, affecting both patients and health care professionals.[12] The increase in allergic reactions has coincided with the sharp increase in glove use related to the introduction of universal precautions against infectious diseases in 1987.[13] It is estimated that 8% to 17% of health care workers regularly exposed to latex are sensitized.[14] The more frequent and prolonged the exposure to latex, the greater the likelihood of developing a latex allergy.[12,13] In addition to gloves, many latex-containing products are used in health care, such as blood pressure cuffs, stethoscopes, tourniquets, IV tubing, syringes, electrode pads, O_2 masks, tracheal tubes, colostomy and ileostomy pouches, urinary catheters, anesthetic masks, and adhesive tape. Latex proteins can become aerosolized through powder on gloves and can result in serious reactions when inhaled by sensitized individuals.

Types of Latex Allergies. Two types of latex allergies that can occur are type IV allergic contact dermatitis and type I allergic reactions. Type IV contact dermatitis is caused by the chemicals used in the manufacturing process of latex gloves. It is a delayed reaction that occurs within 6 to 48 hours. Typically the person first has dryness, pruritis, fissuring, and cracking of the skin, followed by redness, swelling, and crusting at 24 to 48 hours. Chronic exposure can lead to lichenification, scaling, and hyperpigmentation. The dermatitis may extend beyond the area of physical contact with the allergen.

A type I allergic reaction is a response to the natural rubber latex proteins and occurs within minutes of contact with the proteins. These types of allergic reactions can manifest as various reactions ranging from skin redness, urticaria, rhinitis, conjunctivitis, or asthma to full-blown anaphylactic shock. Systemic reactions to latex may result from exposure to latex protein via various routes, including the skin, mucous membranes, inhalation, or blood.

NURSING AND COLLABORATIVE MANAGEMENT: LATEX ALLERGIES

The identification of patients and health care workers sensitive to latex is crucial in the prevention of adverse reactions. A thorough health history and history of any allergies should be collected, especially on patients with any complaints of latex contact symptoms. Not all latex-sensitive individuals can be identified, even with a careful and thorough history. Risk factors include long-term multiple exposures to latex products (e.g., health care personnel, individuals who have had multiple surgeries, rubber industry workers). Additional risk factors include a patient history of hay fever, asthma, and allergies to certain foods (e.g., avocados, guava, kiwi, bananas, water chestnuts, hazelnuts, tomatoes, potatoes, peaches, grapes, apricots). Latex-sensitive individuals should wear a Medic Alert bracelet and carry an epinephrine kit.

The National Institute for Occupational Safety and Health (NIOSH) has published recommendations for preventing allergic reactions to latex in the workplace. This free publication (No. 97-135) can be obtained from NIOSH (phone 800-356-4674; e-mail: pubstaft@niosdt1.em.cdc.gov). In summary they include the following:

1. Use nonlatex gloves for activities that are not likely to involve contact with infectious materials (e.g., food preparation, housekeeping).
2. Use powder-free gloves with reduced protein content.
3. Do not use oil-based hand creams or lotions when wearing gloves.
4. Frequently clean work areas that are contaminated with latex dust.
5. Know the symptoms of latex allergy, including skin rash; hives; flushing; itching; nasal, eye, or sinus symptoms; asthma; and shock.
6. If symptoms of latex allergy develop, avoid direct contact with latex gloves and products.

Latex precaution protocols should be used for those patients identified as having a positive latex allergy test or a history of signs and symptoms related to latex exposure. Many health care facilities have created latex-free product carts that can follow patients with latex allergies. (Latex allergies are also discussed in Chapters 16 and 18.)

AUTOIMMUNE PHENOMENA

Autoimmunity is an inappropriate reaction to self-proteins; the immune system no longer differentiates self from nonself with respect to these substances. For some unknown reason, immune cells that are normally unresponsive (tolerant to self-antigens) are activated. Both T cells and B cells have the ability for tolerance to self-antigens. Therefore an alteration in T cells alone or in both B cells and T cells can produce autoantibodies and autosensitized T cells to cause pathophysiologic tissue damage. The particular autoimmune disease manifested depends on which self-antigen is involved.[15]

Autoimmune diseases tend to cluster so that a given person may have more than one autoimmune disease (e.g., rheumatoid arthritis and Addison's disease), or the same or related autoimmune diseases may be found in other members of the same family. This observation has led to the concept of genetic predisposition to autoimmune disease.

Theories of Causation

The cause of autoimmune diseases is still unknown. Age plays some role, since the number of circulating autoantibodies increases in persons over age 50. It appears that no one theory is conclusive. A combination of etiologic factors may be involved.

Forbidden Clone Theory. Maturing lymphocytes in the central lymphoid organs encounter self-antigens during embryogenesis, and as lymphocytes reactive against self-antigens develop their clones are prevented or forbidden from maturing. Autoimmunity may result from the survival of a forbidden clone and its proliferation later in life. These clones may become reactive against the body's own tissue, resulting in an autoimmune process.

Sequestered Antigen Theory. During embryonic development (when immune tolerance develops), certain tissues are normally separated or sequestered from the circulatory and lymph systems. These tissues include the lens of the eye, thyroid, testes, and central nervous system. If later trauma, infection, or chemical exposure results in the cells' release into circulation, these cells will not be recognized as self and an autoimmune response will occur. Examples of this reaction include Hashimoto's thyroiditis and autoantibody formation against sperm after vasectomy and cardiac muscle after myocardial infarction.

Tissue Injury/Infections Theory. After severe trauma, necrosis, radiation, drugs, and infections, the body tissue is sometimes altered so that the body no longer recognizes it as self. An example of this is hemolytic anemia secondary to methyldopa (Aldomet) administration.

Viral infections can cause an alteration of tissues that are not normally antigenic. There is some evidence that viruses may be involved in the development of multiple sclerosis and type 1 diabetes mellitus.

Cross-reacting Antigen Theory. Autoimmunity sometimes develops because of the close structural resemblance between the body's own antigens and foreign antigens. The antibodies synthesized in response to the foreign invasion cross-react with healthy tissue. This appears to be the cause of rheumatic heart disease. Antibodies developed against group A beta-hemolytic streptococcus cross-react with heart muscle, heart valves, and synovial membranes, causing tissue damage.

Genetic Instruction Theory. For an unknown reason the genetic instruction for antibody production is altered. There appears to be a genetic predisposition to develop autoimmune diseases within some families. Most of the research work in this area correlates certain HLA types with an autoimmune condition (discussed later in this chapter).

Diminished T-Suppressor Cell Function Theory. Decreased levels of T-suppressor cells have been noted in individuals with autoimmune disease. Suppressor cells are short lived and may become less numerous with aging. The incidence of autoantibodies increases with age, presumably because atrophy of the thymus results in a decreased ability to produce new T-suppressor cells. If T-suppressor cells are decreased, immunoregulation is altered and antibody levels or T cell responses are increased.

Autoimmune Diseases

Generally, autoimmune diseases are grouped according to organ-specific and systemic diseases. (See Table 12-14 for a summary of autoimmune diseases.)

Autoimmune Hemolytic Anemia. Autoimmune hemolytic anemia is an organ-specific disease involving the erythrocytes. The autoimmune disease may be primary or secondary to other diseases such as systemic lupus erythematosus and lymphocytic leukemia. Regardless of the cause, the immune response is similar. The cause is unknown, but drugs and viruses may alter the antigenic structure of the erythrocyte membrane, making it more susceptible to hemolysis. In addition, some people appear to have a genetically determined susceptibility to form autoantibodies. Patients with hemolytic anemia have signs and symptoms of pallor, fatigue, fever, jaundice, splenomegaly, and hepatomegaly. (Hemolytic anemia is discussed in Chapter 29.)

Systemic Lupus Erythematosus. Systemic lupus erythematosus (SLE) is a classic example of a systemic autoimmune disease characterized by damage to multiple organs. It occurs most frequently in women ages 20 to 40 years. The etiology is unknown, but there appears to be a loss of self-tolerance for the body's own DNA antigens. Viruses, drugs, and genetic factors are believed to affect the self-tolerance.[16]

Systemic lupus erythematosus meets the criteria of an autoimmune disease. Laboratory analysis reveals (1) elevated serum immunoglobulins because of hyperactive humoral immunity, (2) defective T cell function, (3) deposition of antigen-antibody complexes in small blood vessels of various target organs, and (4) low serum-complement levels.

In systemic lupus erythematosus, tissue injury appears to be the result of the formation of antinuclear antibodies. For some reason (possibly a viral infection), the cell membrane is damaged and DNA is released into the systemic circulation where it is viewed as nonself. This DNA is normally sequestered inside the nucleus of cells. On release into circulation the DNA antigen reacts with an antibody. Some antibodies are involved in immune complex formation, and others may cause damage directly. Once the complexes are deposited, complement is activated and further damages the tissue, especially the renal glomerulus. (Systemic lupus erythematosus is discussed in more detail in Chapter 60.)

Apheresis

Apheresis has been effectively used to treat autoimmune diseases and other diseases and disorders. Apheresis is the use of a procedure to separate components of the blood followed by the removal of one or more of these components. Compound words are often used to describe any particular apheresis procedure, depending on the blood components being collected. *Cytapheresis* is a general term for cell separation and removal. *Plateletpheresis* is the removal of platelets, usually for collection from normal individuals to infuse into patients with low platelet counts (e.g., chemotherapy patients). *Leukocytapheresis*

Table 12-14 Examples of Autoimmune Diseases

Disease	Autoantigen	Comments
Systemic Diseases		
Systemic lupus erythematosus	DNA, DNA proteins	Circulating antinuclear antibodies attack DNA. See Chapter 60
Rheumatoid arthritis	IgG	See Chapter 60
Progressive systemic sclerosis or scleroderma	DNA proteins	See Chapter 60
Mixed connective tissue disease	DNA proteins	See Chapter 60
Organ-Specific Diseases		
Blood		
Autoimmune hemolytic anemia	RBC surface	Drugs and trauma may alter the RBC surface antigens. See Chapter 29
Immune thrombocytopenic purpura	Platelet surface	See Chapter 29
Central Nervous System		
Multiple sclerosis	Myelin sheath around nervous tissue	See Chapter 56
Guillain-Barré syndrome	Myelin sheath	See Chapter 56
Muscle		
Myasthenia gravis	Muscle cells and thymus cells	See Chapter 56
Heart		
Rheumatic fever	Cross-reactive streptoccocal antigens	Occurs secondary to strep throat infection. See Chapter 35
Endocrine System		
Addison's disease	Adrenal cell	See Chapter 47
Thyroiditis	Thyroid cell surface	See Chapter 47
Hypothyroidism	Thyroid globulin	See Chapter 47
Type 1 diabetes mellitus	Islet cell antigens	See Chapter 46
Gastrointestinal Tract		
Pernicious anemia	Intrinsic factor of parietal cells	See Chapter 29
Ulcerative colitis	Colon mucosal cells	See Chapter 40
Kidney		
Goodpasture's syndrome	Glomerular basement membrane	See Chapter 43
Glomerulonephritis	Cross-reactive streptococcal antigens	See Chapter 43
Liver		
Primary biliary cirrhosis	Mitochondria	See Chapter 41
Autoimmune hepatitis	Virally infected liver cells	See Chapter 41
Eye		
Uveitis	Uvea	See Chapter 20

is a general term indicating the removal of WBCs and is used in chronic myelogenous leukemia to remove high numbers of leukemic cells. *Lymphocytapheresis* is used to decrease high lymphocyte counts such as in individuals with chronic lymphocytic leukemia. *Lipid apheresis* is being used to treat patients with hypercholesterolemia.

Plasmapheresis. *Plasmapheresis* is the removal of plasma containing components causing or thought to cause disease. When plasma is removed, it is replaced by substitution fluids such as saline or albumin. Therefore the term *plasma exchange* more accurately describes this procedure.[17]

Plasmapheresis has been used to treat autoimmune diseases such as systemic lupus erythematosus, glomerulonephritis, Goodpasture's syndrome, myasthenia gravis, thrombocytopenic purpura, rheumatoid arthritis, and Guillain-Barré syndrome. Apheresis procedures are also done on healthy donors to obtain plasma and selected blood components to administer as replacement therapy for patients.

The rationale for performing therapeutic plasmapheresis in autoimmune disorders is to remove pathologic substances present in plasma. Many disorders for which plasmapheresis is being used are characterized by circulating autoantibodies (usually of the IgG class) and antigen-antibody complexes. Immunosuppressive therapy has been used to prevent recovery of IgG production, and plasmapheresis has been used to prevent antibody rebound.

In addition to removing antibodies and antigen-antibody complexes, plasmapheresis may also remove inflammatory mediators (e.g., complement) that are responsible for tissue damage.[18] In the treatment of systemic lupus erythematosus,

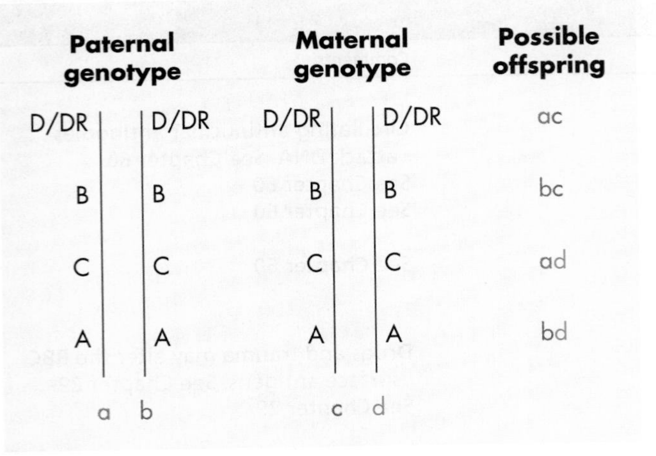

Paternal genotype		Maternal genotype		Possible offspring
D/DR	D/DR	D/DR	D/DR	ac
B	B	B	B	bc
C	C	C	C	ad
A	A	A	A	bd
a	b	c	d	

Fig. 12-10 Patterns of HLA inheritance. The two haplotypes of the father are labeled *a* and *b,* and the haplotypes of the mother are labeled *c* and *d.* Each child inherits two haplotypes, one from each parent. Therefore only four combinations—*ac, bc, ad,* and *bd*—are possible, and 25% of the offspring will have identical HLA haplotypes.

plasmapheresis is usually reserved for the patient in an acute attack who is unresponsive to conventional therapy.

Plasmapheresis involves the removal of whole blood through a needle inserted in one arm and circulation of the blood through a cell separator. Inside the separator the blood is divided into plasma and its cellular components by centrifugation or membrane filtration. A needle is inserted into the opposite arm for return of the blood to the patient. Plasma, platelets, WBCs, or RBCs can be separated selectively. The undesirable component is removed, and the remainder is returned to the patient. The plasma is generally replaced with normal saline, lactated Ringer's solution, fresh frozen plasma, plasma protein fractions, or albumin. When blood is manually removed, only 500 ml may be taken at one time. However, with the use of apheresis procedures, over 4 L of plasma can be pheresed in 2 to 3 hours.

As with administration of other blood products, nurses must be aware of side effects associated with plasmapheresis. The most common complications are hypotension and citrate toxicity. Hypotension is usually the result of vasovagal reaction or transient volume changes. Citrate is used as an anticoagulant and may cause hypocalcemia, which may manifest as headache, paresthesias, and dizziness.

Human Leukocyte Antigen System

The HLA system consists of a series of linked genes that occur together on the sixth chromosome in humans.[19] The products of these genes include the cell membrane antigens of the HLA series. Because of its importance in the study of tissue matching in transplant rejection, the chromosomal region incorporating the HLA genes is termed the *major histocompatibility complex.* The genes determining the products recognized as the HLA-A, HLA-B, HLA-C, HLA-D, and HLA-DR antigens are clustered together (Fig. 12-10). HLA antigens are present on all nucleated cells and platelets.

Table 12-15 Characteristics of Diseases Showing HLA Associations

1. Hereditary or familial tendencies
2. Immune or autoimmune features
3. Poorly understood etiology and pathophysiology
4. Subacute or chronic course
5. Little or no effect on reproductive capacity
6. Association with HLA-B or HLA-DR loci

HLA, human leukocyte antigen.

An important characteristic of HLA genes is that they are highly polymorphic. Each HLA locus can have many different possible alleles (antigens). The specific allele is identified by a number. For example, a person could be A6, B7, C8, D1, DR7. With many alleles possible at each HLA locus, many combinations exist. Each person has two antigens for each locus. Both antigens of a locus are expressed independently (i.e., they are codominant). The entire set of A, B, C, D, and DR antigens located on one chromosome is termed a *haplotype.* A complete set of antigens located on a chromosome is usually inherited as a unit (haplotype). Figure 12-10 illustrates the inheritance of HLA haplotypes in a family.

Because of the polymorphic nature of the HLA system, it is an ideal marker for genetic studies. This characteristic also makes it a useful tool in settling paternity disputes. The frequencies of HLA antigens vary considerably among different races. For example, HLA-B8 is relatively high in American Caucasians, but it is very low in Native-American and Japanese persons.

Human Leukocyte Antigen and Disease Associations. The early interest in HLA was stimulated by its potential role in matching donors and recipients of organ transplants. (Its role in transplantation is discussed in Chapter 44.) During the last few years, interest in the association between HLA and disease has grown (Table 12-15). Strong associations between HLA type and susceptibility to certain diseases have been demonstrated (Table 12-16). HLA disease associations mean that the frequency of a defined HLA allele is significantly increased in patients with a certain disease when compared with ethnically matched controls. Most of the HLA-associated diseases are classified as autoimmune disorders. The discovery of HLA associations with certain diseases is a major breakthrough in understanding the genetic bases of these diseases. It is now known that at least part of the genetic bases of HLA-associated diseases lies in the HLA region, but the actual mechanism or mechanisms involved in these associations are still unknown. However, most individuals who inherit an HLA type associated with a disease will never develop the disease.

The association between HLA and certain diseases is presently of little practical clinical importance. Nevertheless, there is promise for the development of clinical applications in the future. For example, with certain autoimmune diseases it may be possible to identify members of a family at greatest risk for developing the same or a related autoimmune disease. These persons would need close medical supervision, preventive measures implemented (if possible), and early diagnosis and treatment instituted to prevent chronic complications.

Table 12-16 Examples of HLA Types and Disease Associations

Disease	HLA Type
Addison's disease	DR3
Ankylosing spondylitis	B27
Celiac disease	DR3
Chronic active hepatitis	DR3
Diabetes mellitus, type 1	DR3 DR4
Goodpasture's syndrome	DR2
Graves' disease	B35 DR3
Hashimoto's thyroiditis	DR3
Multiple sclerosis	DR2
Myasthenia gravis	B8 DR3
Narcolepsy	DR2
Reiter's syndrome	B27
Rheumatoid arthritis	DR3 DR4
Sjögren's syndrome	DR3
Systemic lupus erythematosus	DR2 DR3

IMMUNODEFICIENCY DISORDERS

When the immune system does not adequately protect the body, an immunodeficient state exists. The immunodeficiency disorders involve an impairment of one or more immune mechanisms, which include (1) phagocytosis, (2) humoral response, (3) cell-mediated response, (4) complement, and (5) a combined humoral and cell-mediated deficiency. Immunodeficiency disorders are primary if the immune cells are improperly developed or absent and secondary if the deficiency is caused by illnesses or treatment. Primary immunodeficiency disorders are rare and often serious, whereas secondary disorders are more common and less severe.

Primary Immunodeficiency Disorders

The basic categories of primary immunodeficiency disorders include (1) phagocytic defects, (2) B cell deficiency, (3) T cell deficiency, and (4) a combined B cell and T cell deficiency (Table 12-17).

Hypogammaglobulinemia. The defect in B cells can range from the complete absence of all immunoglobulin classes (agammaglobulinemia) to a defect in only one immunoglobulin class. Hypogammaglobulinemia refers to a decreased level of the circulating immunoglobulins. The disorder may be congenital or acquired. Congenital hypogammaglobulinemia (Bruton's disease) is a rare sex-linked recessive disorder that occurs only in males. It is characterized by a deficiency of B cells and immunoglobulins and an intact thymus gland and normal T cell immune response. The disorder usually first manifests in the infant at approximately 3 months of age when the IgG antibody from the mother is depleted and the infant develops recurrent respiratory tract and pyrogenic bacterial infections.

Acquired hypogammaglobulinemia (common variable hypogammaglobulinemia) is a more common disorder that is characterized by the presence of T and B cells but no plasma cells. There appears to be a defect in differentiation of B cells to plasma cells, which results in an absence of plasma cells. A possible cause of acquired hypogammaglobulinemia is an abundance of T-suppressor cells that suppress B cell maturation into plasma cells. The disorder resembles Bruton's disease except that the recurrent bacterial infections (primarily of the respiratory tract) do not occur until patients are 15 to 35 years of age. The treatment includes gamma-globulin injections or transfusions of plasma.

DiGeorge's Syndrome. DiGeorge's syndrome (also known as congenital thymic hypoplasia) is a condition in which neither the thymus nor the parathyroid gland develops. B cell function is normal, but T cell function is absent. The disorder manifests as recurrent viral, fungal, and protozoan infections and inability to react in a delayed hypersensitivity skin test. Symptoms of oral candidiasis and chronic diarrhea develop in the first year of life. Microscopically, no thymus-dependent areas in the spleen or lymph nodes are seen. Because T-helper cells are missing, the circulation levels of some antibodies may also be reduced. Hypocalcemic tetany is also present because of the absence of parathyroid hormone from the parathyroid gland. Treatment consists of administration of calcium in combination with vitamin D. Fetal thymus transplant (from a fetus less than 14 weeks of gestational age) and HLA-matched bone marrow transplant have been successfully used in the treatment of DiGeorge's syndrome.

Severe Combined Immunodeficiency Disease. This condition includes a group of inherited disorders in which B cell and T cell functions are abnormal. The most common form of severe combined immunodeficiency disease is sex-linked. The etiology of the disorder is unknown but seems to represent a bone marrow stem defect or a failure in normal development of thymus and bursa-equivalent tissue. Microscopically, the thymus gland is hypoplastic and lymph nodes contain no B and T cells. The disorder manifests as severe viral, bacterial, fungal, or protozoan infections that occur within the first 2 years of life. Treatment consists of controlling the infection with antibiotics and placing the patient in protective isolation. HLA-matched bone marrow transplant is the definitive treatment. Intravenous immunoglobulin injections are also used.

Secondary Immunodeficiency Disorders

Some of the important factors that may cause secondary immunodeficiency disorders are listed in Table 12-18. Drug-induced immunosuppression is the most common. Immunosuppressive therapy is prescribed for patients to treat autoimmune disorders and to prevent transplant rejection. In addition, immunosuppression is a serious side effect of cytotoxic drugs used in cancer chemotherapy. Generalized leukopenia often results, leading to a decreased humoral and cell-mediated response. Therefore secondary infections are common in immunosuppressed patients. (Refer to Table 44-12 for a summary of the specific actions of the various drugs on the immune system.)

Stress may alter the immune response. This response involves interrelationships among the nervous, endocrine, and immune systems (see Chapter 7).

A hypofunctional state of the immune system exists in young children and older adults. Laboratory studies have

Table 12-17 Primary Immunodeficiency Disorders

Disorder	Affected Cells	Genetic Basis
Chronic granulomatous disease	PMN, monocytes	Sex-linked
Job's syndrome	PMN, monocytes	
Bruton's X-linked hypogammaglobulinemia	B	Sex-linked
Common variable hypogammaglobulinemia	B	
Selective IgA, IgM, or IgG deficiency	B	Some sex-linked
DiGeorge's syndrome (thymic hypoplasia)	T	
Severe combined immunodeficiency disease	Stem, B, T	Sex-linked or autosomal recessive
Ataxia telangiectasia	B, T	Autosomal recessive
Wiskott-Aldrich syndrome	B, T	Sex-linked
Graft-versus-host disease	B, T	

Table 12-18 Causes of Secondary Immunodeficiency

Drug-induced	Surgery and trauma
Antineoplastic agents	Infections
Corticosteroids	Burns
Stress	Chronic renal failure
Age	Diabetes mellitus
Infants	Alcoholic cirrhosis
Older adults	Systemic lupus erythematosus
Malnutrition	Anesthesia
Dietary deficiency	Malignancies
Cirrhosis	Acquired immunodeficiency syndrome
Cancer cachexia	
Radiation	

demonstrated that immunoglobulin levels decrease with age and therefore lead to a suppressed humoral immune response in older adults. Thymic involution occurs with aging along with decreased numbers of T cells. The incidence of malignancies and autoimmune diseases increases with aging and may be related to immunologic deterioration.

Malnutrition alters cell-mediated immune responses. When protein is deficient over a prolonged period, atrophy of the thymus gland occurs and lymphoid tissue decreases. In addition, an increased susceptibility to infections always exists.

Radiation destroys lymphocytes either directly or through depletion of stem cells. As the radiation dose is increased, more bone marrow atrophies, leading to severe pancytopenia and severe suppression of immune function.

Surgical removal of lymph nodes, thymus, or spleen can suppress the immune response. Splenectomy in children is especially dangerous and may lead to septicemia from simple respiratory infections.

Hodgkin's disease greatly impairs the cell-mediated immune response, and patients may die from severe viral or fungal infections. (Hodgkin's disease is discussed in Chapter 29.) Viruses, especially rubella, may cause immunodeficiency by direct cytotoxic damage to lymphoid cells. Systemic infections can place such a demand on the immune system that resistance to a secondary or subsequent infection is impaired.

Graft-versus-Host Disease

Graft-versus-host (GVH) disease occurs when an immunoincompetent (immunodeficient) patient is transfused or transplanted with immunocompetent cells. A GVH response may result from the infusion of any blood product containing viable lymphocytes, such as in therapeutic blood transfusions, and from the transplantation of fetal thymus, fetal liver, or bone marrow. In most transplantation situations, the biggest concern is the host's rejection of the graft. However, in GVH disease the graft rejects the host or recipient tissue.

The GVH response may have its onset 7 to 30 days after transplant. Once the reaction is started, little can be done to modify its course. The exact mechanism involved in this reaction is not completely understood. However, it involves donor T cells attacking and destroying vulnerable host cells.

The target organs for the GVH phenomenon are the skin, GI tract, and liver. The skin disease may be a maculopapular rash, which may be pruritic or painful. It initially involves the palms and soles of the feet but can progress to a generalized erythema with bullous formation and desquamation. The liver disease may manifest as mild jaundice with elevated liver enzymes ranging to hepatic coma. The intestinal disease may be manifested by mild to severe diarrhea, severe abdominal pain, GI bleeding, and malabsorption. The biggest problem with GVH disease is infection, with different types of infections seen in different periods. Bacterial and fungal infections predominate immediately after transplantation when granulocytopenia exists. The development of interstitial pneumonitis is the predominant later problem.

There is no adequate treatment of GVH disease once it is established. Although corticosteroids are often used, they enhance the susceptibility to infection. The use of immunosuppressive agents (e.g., methotrexate, cyclosporine) have been most effective as preventive rather than treatment measures. Radiation of blood products before they are administered is another measure to prevent T cell replication.

IMMUNE-RELATED DISEASES

Mononucleosis

Mononucleosis, often referred to as "mono" or the "kissing disease," is a benign, self-limiting disease characterized by lymph node enlargement, lymphocytosis, and elevated temperature. The peak incidence of mononucleosis occurs between 14 and 18 years of age. It may occur in isolated cases or in epidemics.

Although benign, the disease may incapacitate patients because of the extreme fatigue associated with it.

Etiology and Pathophysiology. Mononucleosis is caused by the Epstein-Barr virus (EBV), a type of herpesvirus, which is primarily transmitted in saliva. The virus grows productively in B lymphocytes and oropharyngeal epithelial cells. Once exposed, susceptible patients manifest symptoms of disease after a 4- to 8-week incubation period. Symptoms evolve gradually, intensifying as the disease becomes apparent. After causing mononucleosis, the EBV may lie dormant in lymphocytes and other lymphatic tissue. The virus can be shed for up to 18 months following primary infection.

In the United States and Canada 50% of the population have experienced a primary EBV infection by adolescence. These early infections are usually mild, nonspecific, and clinically inapparent. By adulthood, most individuals have antibodies to EBV.

Clinical Manifestations. Prodromal symptoms of headache, fatigue, malaise, chills, puffy eyelids, anorexia, arthralgia, and a distaste for smoking cigarettes may occur. As the disease becomes more acute, most patients have a triad of symptoms, including fever, painful lymph node enlargement (especially cervical, axillary, and groin nodes), and sore throat. The sore throat may be severe enough to cause dysphagia. If the spleen is enlarged by massive lymphocyte infiltration, pain will occur in the left upper quadrant.

Infectious mononucleosis is a self-limiting disease in the majority of cases, rarely lasting more than 2 to 3 weeks. The most persistent symptom is malaise. It is rare for significant complications to develop from mononucleosis. The problems that may occur include pneumonia, neurologic changes (e.g., encephalitis), splenic rupture, hepatitis, thrombocytopenia, hemolytic anemia, airway obstruction, myocarditis, pericarditis, Guillain-Barré syndrome, and Bell's palsy.

Diagnostic Studies. Initially the WBC and differential cell counts are normal, but within 1 week a leukocytosis (WBC $> 20{,}000/\mu l$ [$20 \times 10^9/L$]) will occur. There is a rise in lymphocytes and monocytes, with 10% to 20% atypical lymphocytes, which are predominantly activated T lymphocytes. Heterophilic antibodies are found in the majority of individuals. The "monospot" test, which uses a commercial kit to assay these antibodies, is available and easily performed. However, specificity for mononucleosis is limited with this test because cytomegalovirus, adenovirus, and toxoplasmosis may also produce heterophilic antibodies. Antibodies to EBV can also be measured. The presence of IgM antibodies to EBV is diagnostic of a primary EBV infection. Liver function studies may be used to ascertain whether any liver involvement exists. Since beta-hemolytic streptococci can be isolated from the throat in up to 30% of patients with mononucleosis, isolation of this organism does not rule out the diagnosis of mononucleosis.

NURSING AND COLLABORATIVE MANAGEMENT: MONONUCLEOSIS

There is no specific therapeutic protocol for patients with mononucleosis. Patients must rest for 2 to 3 weeks and get adequate nutrition and fluids. Fever and sore throat can be treated with acetaminophen. Isolation procedures are not required because mononucleosis is minimally contagious in adults. Antibiotics have not proved useful unless the throat culture is positive for beta-hemolytic streptococci. Corticosteroids may be used to treat airway obstruction, hemolytic anemia, and thrombocytopenia. Recovery is gradual, and malaise may occur intermittently for some time.

Nursing interventions are most appropriate when the disease is actually present. Helping the patient comply with the prescribed rest may prove challenging if fatigue is negligible. Saline solution mouthwashes may ease sore throat pain. The nurse should be observant for the development of complications. For the patient with splenomegaly, the nurse must emphasize the need to avoid any possible activities that can lead to splenic rupture. For example, the patient should avoid Valsalva's maneuver with bowel movements, and abdominal trauma from lifting or from sports must be avoided until the splenic enlargement resolves.

The need for ongoing care after mononucleosis is uncommon. After 2 to 3 weeks, the patient can usually return to a normal lifestyle. If mononucleosis occurs in older adults, complications may be more common and complete disease resolution may take longer.

Chronic Fatigue Syndrome

Chronic fatigue syndrome (CFS) is a disorder characterized by debilitating fatigue and a variety of associated complaints (Table 12-19). CFS is three times more common in women than in men, and onset typically occurs between the ages of 25 and 45. Its prevalence is difficult to determine but is less than 1% in the United States.[20] CFS is a poorly understood condition. Although some health care providers doubt the existence of this disorder, it does exist and can have a devastating impact on the lives of patients.

Etiology and Pathophysiology. Despite numerous attempts to determine the etiology and pathology of CFS, the precise mechanisms remain unknown. However, there are many theories about the etiology of chronic fatigue syndrome. It is often postinfectious, frequently follows a viral infection, and is associated with immune alterations. A dysfunction may exist in the hypothalamus-pituitary-adrenal axis. Several viruses have been investigated as etiologic agents, including herpesviruses (e.g., EBV, cytomegalovirus), retroviruses, and enteroviruses. Antibody titers to many infectious agents are elevated in patients with CFS. It is known that viruses can precipitate the syndrome, but whether they can cause the long-term features is unknown.[21]

Abnormal immune system activation appears to be a central event in CFS. Immune alterations that have been shown to occur with CFS include decreased immunoglobulin production in vitro, reduced NK cell activity, decreased lymphocyte proliferation, increased CD4/CD8 ratio, and increased percentage of activated T cells.[20] If the mechanism of CFS involves a continuing immune response to an initial viral infection, the symptoms may be due in part to the production of cytokines. These immune mediators can cause muscle and central nervous system manifestations, including fatigue. However, immune alterations do not occur in all patients and have not been shown to correlate with the severity of the disease.

Table 12-19 Diagnostic Criteria for Chronic Fatigue Syndrome*

Major Criteria
1. Unexplained, persistent, or relapsing chronic fatigue that is of new and definite onset (not lifelong)
2. Fatigue is not due to ongoing exertion
3. Fatigue is not substantially alleviated by rest
4. Fatigue results in substantial reduction in occupational, educational, social, or personal activities

Minor Criteria
1. Substantial impairment in short-term memory or concentration
2. Sore throat
3. Tender cervical or axillary lymph nodes
4. Muscle pain
5. Multijoint pain without joint swelling or tenderness
6. Headaches of a new type, pattern, or severity
7. Unrefreshing sleep
8. Postexertional malaise lasting more than 24 hours

Adapted from Fukuda K and others (International Chronic Fatigue Syndrome Study Group): The chronic fatigue syndrome: a comprehensive approach to its definition and study, *Ann Intern Med* 121:953, 1994.
*For a diagnosis to be made, the patient must fulfill all the major criteria, plus four or more of the minor criteria. Each minor criterion must have persisted or recurred during 6 or more consecutive months of illness and must not have predated the fatigue. These criteria were prepared by the Centers for Disease Control and Prevention, National Institutes of Health, and International Chronic Fatigue Syndrome Study Group.

Neuroendocrine regulation may be altered in CFS. There may be reduced production of corticotropin-releasing hormone in the hypothalamus. Serum cortisol levels are low, and adrenocorticotropic hormone levels are correspondingly high. These changes could cause decreased energy and altered mood states in patients with CFS.

Because mild to moderate depression occurs in about 70% of these patients, it has been proposed that CFS is a psychiatric disorder. However, it is difficult to determine if depression is a cause or an effect of debilitating chronic fatigue.

Clinical Manifestations. Incapacitating fatigue is the most common symptom of CFS and is the problem that causes the patient to seek health care. Associated symptoms (see Table 12-19) may fluctuate in intensity over time. In about one half of the cases, CFS develops insidiously, or the patient may have intermittent episodes that gradually become chronic. In other situations CFS arises suddenly in a previously active, healthy individual. An unremarkable flulike illness or other acute stress is often identified as a triggering event. Cases of CFS typically occur in isolation, but there are reports of clusters, in which a number of patients have developed chronic fatigue after the same viral infection.[19]

The patient may become angry and frustrated with the inability of physicians to diagnose a problem. The disorder may have a major impact on work and family responsibilities. Some individuals may even need help with activities of daily living.

Diagnostic Studies. Physical examination and diagnostic studies can be used to rule out other possible causes of the patient's symptoms. No laboratory test can diagnose CFS or measure its severity. In general, it remains a diagnosis of exclusion.

NURSING AND COLLABORATIVE MANAGEMENT: CHRONIC FATIGUE SYNDROME

Because there is no definitive treatment for CFS, supportive management is essential.[20] The patient should be informed about what is known about the disease, and all complaints should be taken seriously. Nonsteroidal antiinflammatory drugs can be used to treat headaches, muscle and joint aches, and fever. Antihistamines and decongestants can be used to treat allergic symptoms. Antidepressants (e.g., fluoxetine [Prozac], paroxetine [Paxil]) can improve mood and sleep problems. Clonazepam (Klonopin) can also be used to treat sleep disorders.

Total rest is not advised because it can potentiate the self-image of being an invalid. On the other hand, strenuous exertion can exacerbate the exhaustion. Therefore it is important to plan a carefully graduated exercise program. Behavioral therapy may be used to promote a positive outlook, as well as improve overall disability, fatigue, and other symptoms.

One of the major problems facing many CFS patients is financial. When the illness strikes, they cannot work or must decrease the amount of time working. Loss of a job often leads to loss of medical insurance. Obtaining disability benefits can be frustrating because of the difficulty of establishing a diagnosis of CFS.

Chronic fatigue syndrome does not appear to progress. Although most patients recover or at least improve over time, some never show improvement. Recovery is more common in individuals with a sudden onset of CFS. Patients with CFS suffer from substantial occupational and psychosocial impairments and loss, including the social pressure and isolation from being characterized as lazy or "crazy."

NEW TECHNOLOGIES IN IMMUNOLOGY

Hybridoma Technology: Monoclonal Antibodies

Monoclonal antibodies are homogeneous populations of identical antibody molecules produced by specialized tissue cell culture lines. The procedure uses cell fusion techniques and standard in vitro tissue culture systems (Fig. 12-11). The two essential biologic components are immunized mice or rats and myeloma tumor cell lines, which are of lymphoid origin. Single antibody-forming cells (lymphocytes) from rodents previously immunized with antigen are fused with myeloma cells to create hybrid cells with properties of both parent cell types. The hybrids have an unlimited capacity to grow similar to that of the myeloma parent cell. The hybrids produce the single type of antibody molecule that they inherited from the normal, antibody-forming parent cell. Hybrid cells derived in this way can produce unlimited quantities of specific antibodies. With appropriate selection techniques, producing monoclonal antibodies to virtually any antigen is possible. Because the monoclonal antibodies are a completely homogeneous population, their use incurs fewer problems than conventional polyclonal antisera.

Monoclonal antibodies are finding wide application in many areas of medicine and biologic science.[2] Thousands of monoclonal antibodies have been made against many different types of antigens. Monoclonal antibodies have begun to replace conventional antibodies in blood banking and are used in the identification of organisms in the bacteriology laboratory.

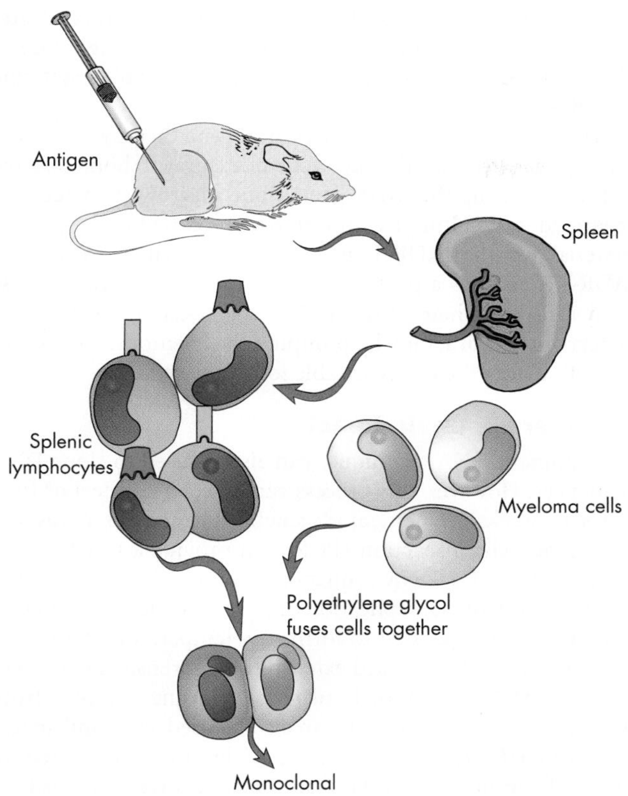

Fig. 12-11 Monoclonal antibodies are identical antibodies made by clones of a single antibody-producing cell. The target antigen is injected into a mouse. The spleen cells, which contain plasma cells, are harvested and fused with myeloma cells using polyethylene glycol. The fused cells, or hybridomas, are then cloned. A clone can secrete monoclonal antibodies over a long period of time.

Monoclonal antibodies have also been extensively used in radioimmunoassays to measure serum levels of various substances (e.g., parathyroid hormone). They have been useful in quantitating types of WBCs and subgroups of lymphocytes. They are also used in the diagnosis of leukemia. More recently, monoclonal antibodies have been used in the treatment of malignancies (see Chapter 14). They have been used to treat transplant rejection episodes (see Chapter 44), purge bone marrow of tumor cells in bone marrow transplants, and remove mature T cells that cause graft-versus-host (GVH) disease in bone marrow transplants.

A major limitation of these monoclonal antibodies is that they are mouse antibodies and therefore can elicit an antibody response by the host against the foreign agent. Recently, human hybridomas have been produced using human myelomas. These hybrids synthesize human monoclonals and are therefore advantageous for in vivo use in diagnosis and therapy.

Recombinant DNA Technology

Recombinant DNA technology, a form of genetic engineering, involves taking segments of DNA from one type of organism and combining them with genes from a second organism (Fig. 12-12). When the cell divides, the DNA is transcribed and a specific protein coded by the DNA is made. In this way relatively simple organisms such as *Escherichia coli*, yeast, or mammalian tissue culture cells can be used to make large quantities of human proteins. This process is used to make human insulin and cytokines (e.g., alpha-interferon, interleukin-2), as well as many other substances.

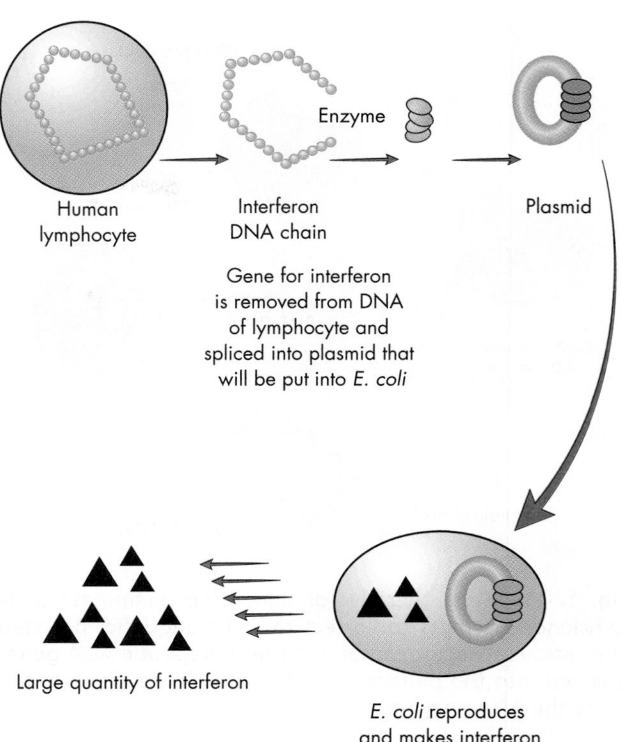

Fig. 12-12 Mass production of interferon by recombinant gene technology.

Gene Therapy

A facet of recombinant DNA technology involves gene therapy, which can be used to replace or repair defective or missing genes with normal genes. Using recombinant DNA methods, a normal gene can be inserted into a human chromosome to counteract the effects of a missing or abnormal gene.

The first approved gene therapy trials involved children with severe combined immunodeficiency disease caused by adenosine deaminase deficiency.[22] T lymphocytes from these children were obtained, and the missing gene was inserted into these T cells (Fig. 12-13). The new T cells were then reinjected into the children's bloodstreams. The gene signaled the cells to produce the missing enzyme, and these children developed a functioning immune system.

The success of these efforts has led scientists to try gene therapy for a variety of other genetic disorders, including cystic fibrosis, Gaucher's disease, familial hypercholesterolemia, alpha-1-antitrypsin deficiency, and Fanconi's anemia. Gene therapy is also being investigated in different types of cancer, including melanoma, renal cell, and hematologic malignancies. In cancer patients gene therapy ideally involves the inhibition of oncogene function or restoration of tumor suppressor function.[23] Gene therapy is also being used in viral infections, including acquired immunodeficiency syndrome and hepatitis B and C.

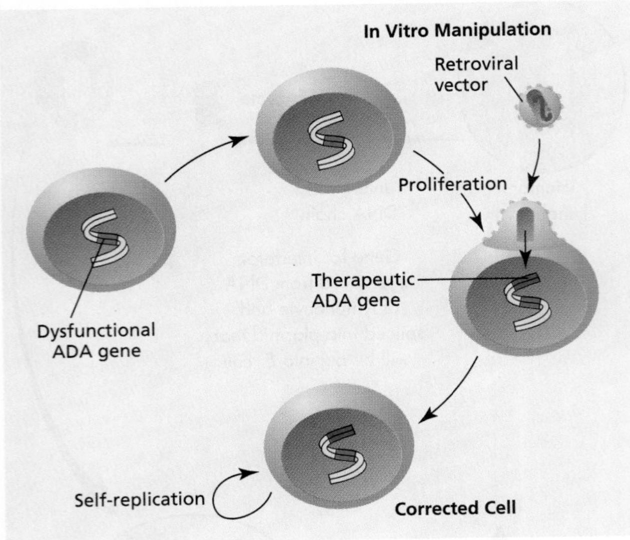

Fig. 12-13 Gene therapy for adenosine deaminase (ADA) deficiency attempts to correct this immunodeficiency state. The retroviral vector containing the therapeutic ADA gene is inserted into the patient's lymphocytes. These cells can then make the ADA enzyme.

Gene therapy has great promise for treating a wide array of problems, both inherited and acquired, that do not respond to conventional methods of intervention. Although gene therapy is still experimental, the impact of adding another treatment option has created excitement and hope for future health care.

Methods of Gene Delivery. Currently the only gene therapy approved for clinical trials involves gene transfer in which corrected genetic materials are placed in the body's cells (e.g., bone marrow cells) for correction of nonreproductive cells. By preventing delivery of the therapeutic gene to the patient's reproductive tissues, it avoids modifying the heritable gene pool.

Gene therapy can be done using in vitro methods or an in vivo method. The in vitro method, which is used most commonly, involves removal of target cells from the body to be altered genetically and then reinfused. This method has been used with lymphocytes, hepatocytes, skin keratinocytes, fibroblasts, and bone marrow cells. The disadvantage of this method is that nondividing cells (e.g., kidney, brain cells) are not easily grown in vitro. In this approach a vector, usually an altered (cannot cause disease) retrovirus, carries the desired therapeutic gene into the human cell. The transduced cells are then reinfused back into the patient.[24] Nonviral methods can also be used and usually involve physical transfection of the genetic material. One method involves direct microinjection of DNA into cells by particle acceleration.

In the in vivo method the altered gene and its vector is directly instilled into the patient. This approach allows more promise for its potential to directly affect disease sites, minimize risks to the individual, and potentially decrease expense.[23]

Examples of Gene Therapy for Cancer. One of the first gene therapy protocols used in treating cancer patients involved the addition of a gene for tumor necrosis factor (TNF). TNF is a powerful anticancer agent. The vector with the gene for TNF was inserted into lymphocytes aimed at sites of malignant melanoma. This approach allows a high dose of TNF to be delivered to the tumor only and avoids systemic side effects.

The purpose of the MDR-1 clinical gene therapy trials is to modify the effects of high-dose chemotherapy in bone marrow cells by inserting the MDR gene. Bone marrow stem cells are separated and cultured with a retrovirus carrying the genetic material for the MDR-1 gene. The retrovirus transfers the MDR-1 gene into a portion of the patient's stem cells. These stem cells and their offspring become resistant to the toxic effects of chemotherapy by pumping the chemotherapy out of the cells before the drugs are able to kill the cells.[23]

Polymerase Chain Reaction

Recombinant DNA techniques can also be used to clone DNA sequences. However, this process can take a great deal of time (days to weeks). When rapid genetic diagnosis is necessary, polymerase chain reaction (PCR) can provide a way to make many copies of a DNA sequence in only a few hours. PCR involves the artificial replication of a DNA sequence. The DNA strands can be separated to form new templates that are used for replication. PCR is used extensively in forensic medicine to identify DNA of criminal suspects by using samples from blood, hair, and semen. PCR can also be used as a confirmatory test in HIV testing. This is especially important when an infant of a mother who is HIV-antibody positive also tests HIV positive. In this situation it is not known whether the antibodies from the infant's blood are from the baby or the mother. PCR techniques can be used on the baby's lymphocytes to determine whether the baby is infected with HIV.

REVIEW QUESTIONS

The number of the question corresponds to the same-numbered objective at the beginning of the chapter.

1. The function of monocytes in immunity is related to their ability to
   a. produce antibodies on exposure to foreign substances.
   b. capture antigens by phagocytosis and present them to lymphocytes.
   c. stimulate the production of T and B lymphocytes by the bone marrow.
   d. bind antigens and stimulate natural killer cell activation.
2. Administration of the MMR (mumps, measles, rubella) vaccine will promote
   a. active natural immunity.
   b. active artificial immunity.
   c. passive natural immunity.
   d. passive artificial immunity.
3. One function of cell-mediated immunity is
   a. formation of antibodies.
   b. activation of the complement system.
   c. surveillance for malignant cell changes.
   d. opsonization of antigens to allow phagocytosis by neutrophils.
4. The reason newborns are protected for the first 6 months of life from bacterial infections is because of the maternal transmission of
   a. IgG.
   b. IgA.
   c. IgM.
   d. IgE.

5. In a type I hypersensitivity reaction the primary immunologic disorder appears to be
   a. binding of IgG to an antigen on a cell surface.
   b. deposit of antigen-antibody complexes in small vessels.
   c. release of lymphokines to interact with specific antigens.
   d. release of chemical mediators from IgE-bound mast cells and basophils.
6. The nurse is alerted to possible anaphylactic shock immediately after a patient has received intramuscular penicillin by the development of
   a. edema and itching at the injection site.
   b. sneezing and itching of the nose and eyes.
   c. a wheal-and-flare reaction at the injection site.
   d. chest tightness and production of thick sputum.
7. The nurse advises a friend who asks him to administer his allergy shots that
   a. it is illegal for nurses to administer injections outside of a medical setting.
   b. he is qualified to do it if the friend has epinephrine in an injectible syringe provided with his extract.
   c. avoiding the allergens is a more effective way of controlling allergies and allergy shots are not usually effective.
   d. immunotherapy should only be administered in a setting where emergency equipment and drugs are available.
8. In teaching a patient about using the new generation of antihistamines the nurse emphasizes that
   a. these drugs are indicated for all type I hypersensitivity reactions.
   b. the drugs should be taken routinely during times of high exposure to allergens.
   c. the drugs cause vasoconstriction relieving nasal congestion and edema.
   d. the patient should limit critical activities such as driving because of sedative side effects.
9. A patient is undergoing plasmapheresis for treatment of systemic lupus erythematosus. The nurse explains that plasmaphersis is used in her treatment to
   a. remove T lymphocytes in her blood that are producing antinuclear antibodies.
   b. remove normal particles in her blood that are being damaged by autoantibodies.
   c. exchange her plasma that contains antinuclear antibodies with a substitute fluid.
   d. replace viral-damaged cellular components of her blood with replacement whole blood.
10. Association between HLA antigens and diseases is most commonly found in what disease conditions?
    a. malignancies
    b. infectious diseases
    c. neurologic diseases
    d. autoimmune disorders
11. Gamma-globulin injections are indicated in the treatment of
    a. Bruton's disease.
    b. DiGeorge's syndrome.
    c. chronic granulomatous disease.
    d. acquired immunodeficiency syndrome.
12. Which of the following techniques can be used to modify an individual's genetic structure?
    a. gene therapy
    b. polymerase chain reaction
    c. monoclonal antibody production
    d. recombinant RNA technology

References

1. Roitt I, Brostoff J, Male D: *Immunology,* ed 5, St Louis, 1998, Mosby.
2. Kuby J: *Immunology,* ed 3, New York, 1997, WH Freeman.
3. Proceedings of the 1st International Conference on Immunology and Aging, Bethesda, Md, June 16-19, 1996, *Mech Ageing Dev* 94:1, 1997.
4. Weksler ME: Immunology and the elderly: an historical perspective for future international action, *Mech Ageing Dev* 93:1, 1997.
5. Miller RA: Aging and immune function: cellular and biochemical analyses, *Exp Gerontol* 29:21, 1994.
6. Hanson L, Telemo E: The growing allergy problem, *Acta Paediatr* 86:916, 1997.
7. Donohoe MR: Allergic diseases, *Lippincott's Primary Care Practice* 1:117, 1997.
8. Ruffilli A, Bonini S: Susceptibility genes for allergy and asthma, *Allergy* 52:256, 1997.
9. Hollingsworth HM: Allergic rhinoconjunctivitis: current therapy, *Hosp Pract* 31:61, 1996.
10. Norman PS: Current status of immunotherapy for allergies and anaphylactic reactions, *Adv Intern Med* 41:681, 1996.
11. Wheeler AW, Drachenberg KJ: New routes and formulations for allergen-specific immunotherapy, *Allergy* 52:602, 1997.
12. Kam PCA, Lee MSM, Thompson JF: Latex allergy: an emerging clinical and occupational health problem, *Anaesthesia* 52:570, 1997.
13. Shoup AJ: Guidelines for the management of latex allergies and safe use of latex in perioperative practice settings, *AORN J* 66:726, 1997.
14. National Institute for Occupational Safety and Health, Department of Health and Human Services, NIOSH Alert: *Preventing allergic reactions to natural rubber latex in the workplace,* pub no 97-135, 1997.
15. Rose NR: Autoimmune diseases: tracing the shared threads, *Hosp Pract* 32:147, 1997.
16. Roberts WN: Keys to managing systemic lupus erythematosus, *Hosp Pract* 32:113, 1997.
17. Rock G, Buskard NA: Therapeutic plasmapheresis, *Curr Opin Hematol* 3:504, 1996.
18. Bartges JW: Therapeutic plasmapheresis, *Semin Vet Med Surg* 12:170, 1997.
19. Stites DP, Terr AI, Parslow TG: *Medical immunology,* ed 9, Stamford, Conn, 1997, Appleton & Lange.
20. Plioplys AV, Plioplys S: Meeting the frustrations of chronic fatigue syndrome, *Hosp Pract* 32:147, 1997.
21. *Chronic fatigue syndrome,* Bethesda, Md, National Institute of Allergy and Infectious Diseases, National Institutes of Health, 1997.
22. Blaese RM: Steps toward gene therapy: 1. The initial trials, *Hosp Pract* 30:33, 1995.
23. Lea DH: Gene therapy: current and future implications for oncology nursing practice, *Semin Oncol Nurs* 13:115, 1997.
24. Richter J: Gene transfer to hematopoietic cells—the clinical experience, *Eur J Haematol* 59:67, 1997.

Resources

American Academy of Allergy, Asthma, and Immunology (AAAAI)
800-822-2762
http://www.aaaai.org/

American Association for Chronic Fatigue Syndrome
c/o Harborview Medical Center
325 Ninth Avenue
Box 359780
Seattle, WA 98104
206-521-1932
800-232-8710
Fax: 206-521-1930
http://weber.u.washington.edu/~dedra/aacfs1.html

American Association of Immunologists
9650 Rockville Pike
Bethesda, MD 20814-3994
301-530-7178
Fax: 301-571-1816
http://www.scienceXchange.com/aai

American Public Health Association
1015 15th Street NW
Washington, DC 20005-2605
202-789-5600
Fax: 202-789-5661
http://www.apha.org/

American Society for Microbiology
1325 Massachusetts Avenue
Washington, DC 20005
202-737-3600
http://www.asmusa.org/

Asthma and Allergy Foundation of America
1125 15th Street NW, Suite 502
Washington, DC 20005
202-466-7643
Fax: 202-466-8940
http://www.aafa.org

National Allergy Bureau
611 East Wells Street
Milwaukee, WI 53202
http://www.aaaai.org/

National Center for Infectious Diseases (NCID)
Centers for Disease Control and Prevention
1600 Clifton Road NE
Atlanta, GA 30333
404-639-3311
http://www.cdc.gov/ncidod/ncid.htm

National Foundation for Infectious Diseases
4733 Bethesda Avenue, Suite 750
Bethesda, MD 20814
301-656-0003
Fax: 301-907-0878
http://www.nfid.org/

National Institute for Allergy and Infectious Diseases
Building 31, Room 7A-50
31 Center Drive MSC 2520
Bethesda, MD 20892-2520
301-496-2263
http://www.niaid.nih.gov

***For additional Internet resources, see the website for this book at* www.mosby.com/MERLIN/medsurg_lewis**

REMEMBER to check out your companion CD-ROM

13 NURSING MANAGEMENT Human Immunodeficiency Virus Infection

Lucy Bradley-Springer

www.mosby.com/MERLIN/medsurg_lewis

LEARNING OBJECTIVES

1. List the modes of transmission for the human immunodeficiency virus (HIV) and variables involved in the transmission of HIV.
2. Describe the pathophysiology HIV infection.
3. Outline HIV disease progression in the spectrum of HIV infection.
4. List the diagnostic criteria for acquired immunodeficiency syndrome (AIDS).
5. Explain the methods of testing for HIV infection.
6. Discuss the collaborative management of HIV infection.
7. Specify the characteristics of opportunistic diseases associated with AIDS.
8. Compare and contrast the methods of HIV prevention that eliminate risk and those that decrease risk.
9. Describe nursing management principles for HIV-infected patients and HIV-at-risk patients.

HUMAN IMMUNODEFICIENCY VIRUS INFECTION

The history of the human immunodeficiency virus (HIV) epidemic in the United States and Canada is relatively short. Although it obviously had been present for a number of years before 1981, it was not until that year that physicians and public health officials documented the presence of a new disease that would become known as the *acquired immunodeficiency syndrome (AIDS)*.[1] By 1985 the causative agent, HIV, had been identified, and AIDS was determined to be the end stage of a chronic infection with HIV. In addition, an antibody test was developed and routes of transmission determined. Drug therapy to treat the infection became available in 1987 with the release of zidovudine (ZDV, AZT, Retrovir) and has since expanded.[2] Since 1994 several important advances have been made, including the development of laboratory tests to assess viral levels in the blood, the production of new groups of antiretroviral agents, multidrug therapy, and treatment to decrease the risk of perinatal transmission.[3] These important advances have made it possible to improve the quality and quantity of life for many people living with HIV disease. Unfortunately, these advances are not effective or available for all those who need them. Although great progress has been made, the HIV epidemic is not over, and nursing care continues to be a critical need.

Significance of Problem

By the end of June 1998, over 665,000 cases of AIDS had been diagnosed and over 401,000 AIDS-related deaths had been reported in the United States and its territories.[4] An estimated 650,000 to 900,000 people in the United States are infected with HIV. The fastest growing groups of people with HIV are women and adolescents.[3] In addition, 10% of people with AIDS in the United States are 50 years of age or older.[5] AIDS in the United States is not only changing related to gender and age, it is also becoming an increasing problem for people of color, people who live in poverty, people who live in rural areas,[3] and people who deal with violence in their lives.[6] HIV infection patterns in Canada and western Europe resemble those in the United States.[3]

Globally, HIV is even more devastating, with an estimate of over 29 million infected people. Worldwide, more than 8500 people become infected with HIV every day.[7] By 1997, approximately 29.4 million people in the world had been infected with HIV,[7] and in the year 2006, when HIV-related deaths are expected to peak, 1.7 million people will die from the disease.[8] By 2020, HIV will be the tenth leading cause of disease in the world, increasing from its twenty-eighth ranking in 1990.[8]

Transmission of HIV

HIV is a fragile virus that can only be transmitted under specific conditions that allow contact with infected body fluids, including blood, semen, vaginal secretions, and breast milk. Transmission of HIV has occurred through sexual intercourse with an infected partner, internalized exposure to HIV-infected blood or blood products, and perinatal transmission during pregnancy, at the time of delivery, or through breastfeeding.[9,10]

HIV-infected individuals can transmit HIV to others within a few days after initial infection. After that, the ability to transmit HIV is lifelong. Transmission of HIV is subject to the same requirements as other microorganisms: a sufficient amount of

Reviewed by James P. Halloran, RN, MSN, OCN, ANP, Clinical Director, Clinical Partners, Inc., Houston, Tex.

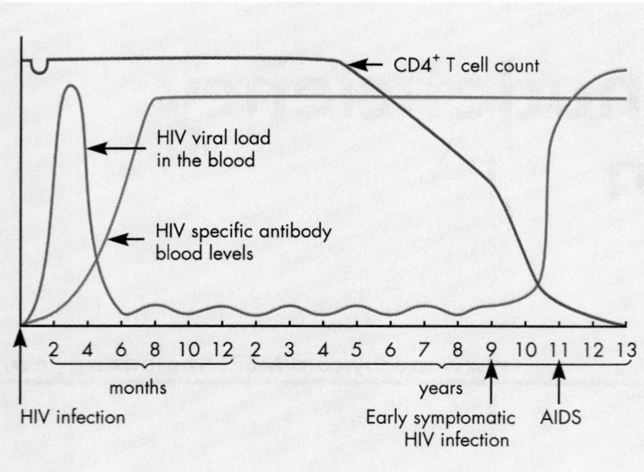

Fig. 13-1 Viral load in the blood and CD4$^+$ T cell counts over the spectrum of human immunodeficiency virus (HIV) infection.

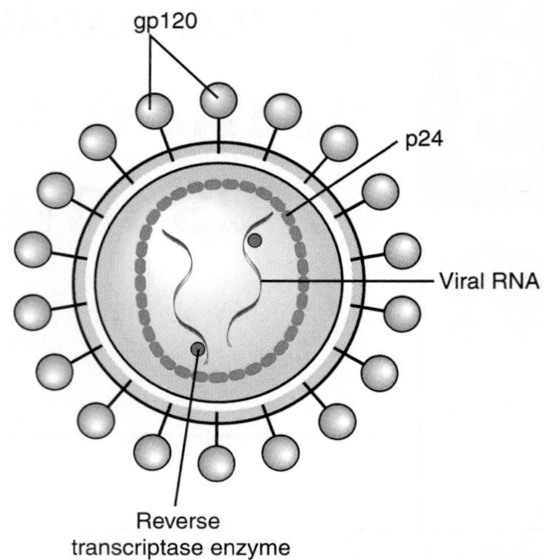

Fig. 13-2 HIV is surrounded by an envelope made up of proteins (including gp120) and contains a core of viral RNA and proteins (including p24).

the infectious agent must be introduced through an appropriate portal of entry into a susceptible host. Duration and frequency of contact, volume of fluid in exposure, virulence and concentration of the organism, and host immune defense capability all affect whether infection actually occurs after an exposure. The number of viral particles in the blood, semen, vaginal secretions, or breast milk of the "donor" is an important variable. In HIV infection large amounts of virus are detected in the blood during the first 2 to 6 months after initial infection and again during the late stages of the disease (Fig. 13-1). Unprotected sexual or blood exposure to an infected individual is more risky during these periods, although HIV can be transmitted during all phases of the disease.[11]

HIV is not spread casually. The virus cannot be transmitted through hugging, dry kissing, shaking hands, sharing eating utensils, attending school, or working with an HIV-infected person. It is not transmitted through tears, saliva, urine, emesis, sputum, feces, or sweat. In addition, there is no evidence that the virus can be transmitted by insects or fomites. Repeated studies have failed to demonstrate transmission of the virus by respiratory droplets, enteric routes, or casual encounters in any setting.[10] Health care workers have a real, but very low, occupational risk of acquiring the virus, even with needle-stick injury.[3]

Sexual Transmission. Sexual contact with an HIV-infected partner is the most common method of transmission. Sexual activity provides an opportunity for contact with semen, vaginal secretions, and/or blood, all of which contain the lymphocytes that harbor HIV and allow HIV replication. The most important variable is whether HIV is present in one of the sexual partners, not whether the partners are of the same or opposite sexes. Although men who have sex with men (MSM) initially accounted for most cases of HIV in the United States and Canada, heterosexual transmission is becoming more prevalent and is now the most common method of infection for women.[4] The most risky form of sexual intercourse is unprotected anal intercourse.[12]

During any form of sexual intercourse (anal, vaginal, or oral), the risk of infection is considerably greater for the partner who receives the semen, although infection also can be transmitted to an inserting partner. This increased risk occurs because the receiver has prolonged contact with the semen. This helps to explain why women are more easily infected than men during heterosexual intercourse.[11] Sexual activities that involve blood, such as during menstruation or as a result of trauma to tissues, also increase the risk of transmission. In addition, the presence of genital lesions caused by other STDs (e.g., herpes, syphilis) increases the likelihood of infection after exposure to HIV.[13]

Contact with Blood and Blood Products. HIV is transmitted by exposure to contaminated blood through the accidental or intended sharing of injection equipment. Sharing equipment to inject illegal drugs is a major means of transmission in many large metropolitan areas and is becoming more common in smaller cities and rural areas. It is important to remember that equipment used to inject any drug, whether prescribed or not, is contaminated after use. It does not matter what substance has been injected. Used equipment is potentially contaminated with HIV and/or other blood-borne organisms, and sharing can result in disease transmission.[10]

In the United States, transfusion of infected blood and blood products has caused 2% of adult AIDS cases and 8% of pediatric AIDS cases.[4] In 1985 routine screening of blood donors to identify at-risk individuals and testing donated blood for the presence of HIV antibodies were implemented, thereby improving the safety of the blood supply. HIV infection as a result of blood transfusions is now unlikely, but still possible because blood donated during the first few months of infection (Fig. 13-1) will not be positive for HIV antibodies on testing.[13] No new cases of HIV related to the use of clotting factor by people with hemophilia are expected because these products are now treated with heat or chemicals that kill HIV as well as other blood-borne viruses.[14]

By the end of June 1998, 54 health care workers in the United States had been shown to have been infected with HIV through occupational exposure and the Centers for Disease Control and Prevention (CDC) was following 133 more who may have been infected at work. Of these 30% are nurses.[4] HIV can be occupationally transmitted during exposure to HIV-infected fluids

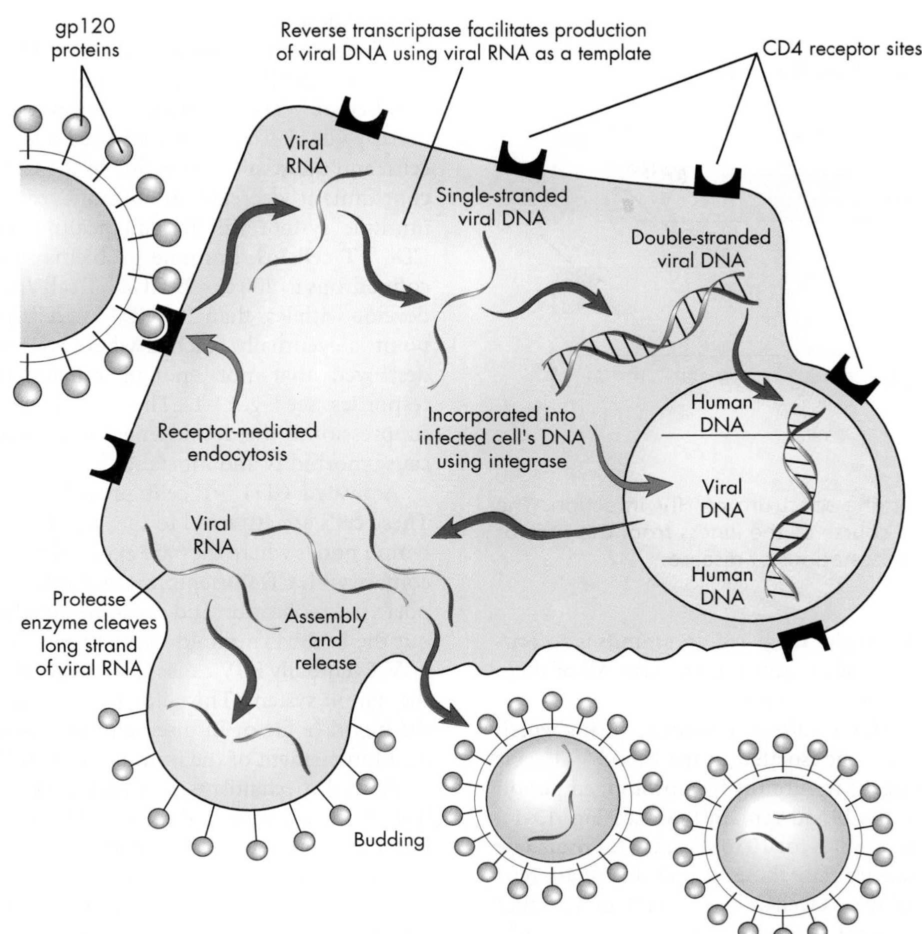

Fig. 13-3 HIV has gp120 proteins that attach to the CD4 receptors on the surface of $CD4^+$ T cells. The viral RNA then enters the cell, produces viral DNA in the presence of reverse transcriptase, and incorporates itself into the cellular genome in the presence of integrase, causing permanent cellular infection and the production of new virions. New viral RNA develops initially in long strands that are cut in the presence of protease and leave the cell through a budding process that ultimately contributes to cellular destruction.

through percutaneous injury or nonintact skin and mucous membranes. The greatest risk for occupational transmission of HIV occurs through puncture wounds. The risk of infection after a needle-stick exposure to HIV-infected blood is 0.3% to 0.4%. The risk is higher if the exposure is caused by blood from a patient with a high viral load, if the puncture wound is deep, if the needle is hollow bore with visible blood, if the device provided venous or arterial access, or if the patient dies within 60 days. Splash exposures of blood on skin with an open lesion also present some risk, although the risk is much lower than from a puncture wound.[3,15,16]

Perinatal Transmission. Transmission from an HIV-infected mother to her infant can occur during pregnancy, at the time of delivery, or after birth through breastfeeding.[17] Studies in various countries have found that 14% to 45% of infants born to HIV-infected women will be born with HIV.[15] This means that 55% to 86% of these infants will not be infected. Among children with AIDS in the United States who are less than 13 years of age, 91% were infected at birth.[4] AIDS is now among the top 10 leading causes of death among children aged 1 to 4.[10]

Pathophysiology

HIV is an RNA virus that was discovered in 1983. RNA viruses are called retroviruses because they replicate in a "backward" manner (going from RNA to DNA). Like all viruses, HIV is an obligate parasite: it cannot replicate unless it is inside a living cell. HIV can enter a cell when the gp120 "knobs" (Fig. 13-2) on the viral envelope bind to specific CD4 receptor sites on the cell's surface (Fig. 13-3). Once bound, the genetic material of the virus enters the cell. In the cell, viral RNA is transcribed into a single strand of viral DNA with the assistance of *reverse transcriptase,* an enzyme made by HIV. This strand replicates itself, becoming double stranded viral DNA. At this point, viral DNA can enter the cell's nucleus and, using an enzyme called *integrase,* splice itself into the genome, becoming a permanent part of the cell's genetic structure. There are two consequences of this action: (1) because all genetic material is replicated during cellular division, all daughter cells from the infected cell will also be infected; and (2) because the genome now contains viral DNA, the cell's genetic codes can direct the cell to make HIV. Production of HIV within the cell is a complicated process that results in long strands of HIV RNA that must be cut into

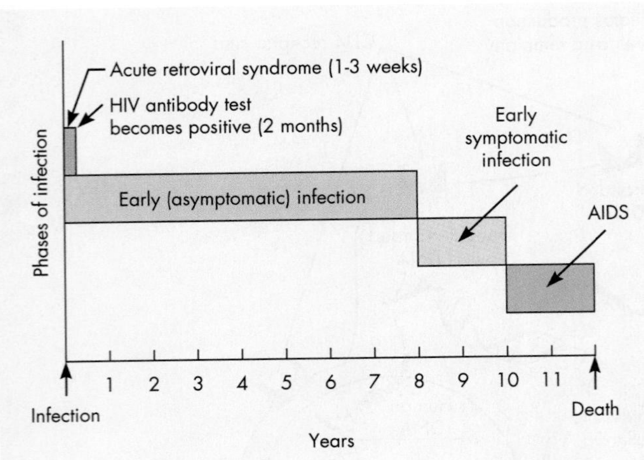

Fig. 13-4 Timeline for the spectrum of HIV infection. The timeline represents the course of the illness from the time of infection to clinical manifestations of disease.

appropriate lengths. Cleaving of these genetic strands is accomplished with the assistance of the enzyme *protease.* All of these steps are required to produce new virions.[9]

Initial infection with HIV results in a viremia, during which large amounts of virus can be isolated in the blood.[18] This is followed within a few weeks to months by a prolonged period in which HIV levels in the blood remain low (see Fig. 13-1). During this time, which may last for 10 to 12 years, there are few clinical symptoms. It was initially thought that this phase represented a period of biologic as well as clinical latency, and that viral replication was minimal. It is now known that HIV replication occurs at rapid and constant rates in the blood and lymph tissues from early in the infection. A steady-state viral load is achieved and maintained in the body of infected individuals for many years. In order to do this, 10^8 to 10^9 new viruses are produced each day.[11] A major consequence of rapid replication is that replication errors are made, causing mutations that can lead to difficulties in treatment and vaccine development.[3]

In a normal immune response, foreign antigens interact with B cells, which initiate the process of antibody development, and with T cells, which initiate a cellular immune response. In the initial stages of HIV infection these cells respond and function normally. B cells make HIV-specific antibodies that are effective in reducing viral loads in the blood, and activated T cells respond to the site when viruses are trapped in the lymph nodes.[9]

HIV can infect human cells that have CD4 receptors on their surfaces. These include lymphocytes, monocytes/macrophages, astrocytes, and oligodendrocytes. Immune dysfunction in HIV disease is caused predominantly by the dysregulation and destruction of *$CD4^+$ T cells* (also known as T helper cells or $CD4^+$ lymphocytes). These cells are targeted because they have more CD4 receptors on their surfaces than other CD4 receptor-bearing cells. The $CD4^+$ T cell plays a pivotal role in the ability of the immune system to recognize and defend against pathogens. Adults normally have 800 to 1200 $CD4^+$ T cells per microliter (μl) of blood. The normal life span of a $CD4^+$ T cell is about 100 days, but HIV-infected cells will die after an average life span of only 2 days.[11]

Viral activity destroys about 1 billion $CD4^+$ T cells every day. Fortunately the bone marrow and thymus are able to produce enough $CD4^+$ T cells to replace the destroyed cells for a number of years. Eventually, however, the ability of HIV to destroy $CD4^+$ T cells exceeds the body's ability to replace the cells, and the result is a decline in the $CD4^+$ T cell count and a concomitant decrease in immune capability. Generally the immune system will remain healthy with greater than 500 $CD4^+$ T cells/μl. Immune problems start to occur when the count drops to 200 to 499 $CD4^+$ T cells/μl, and severe problems develop with less than 200 $CD4^+$ T cells/μl. In HIV infection, a point is eventually reached where so many $CD4^+$ T cells are destroyed that not enough remain to regulate immune responses (see Fig. 13-1). The major concern related to immune suppression is the development of infections and cancers that cause morbidity and mortality.[9]

Activated $CD4^+$ T cells provide an ideal target for HIV. These cells are attracted to the site of concentrated HIV in the lymph nodes where they are exposed to infection through viral contact with CD4 receptors. Once infected, activated cells support viral replication and assist in spreading infection throughout the body. Lymphoid tissue becomes an early reservoir for HIV. Eventually HIV causes significant degenerative changes in the lymph system. This allows viral particles to spill over into the blood (a factor in disease progression) and causes significant impairment of the immune system.[18]

Several mechanisms by which HIV destroys $CD4^+$ T cells have been identified. Viral replication includes a process of budding, which results in increased permeability of the cell's membrane and an eventual loss of cellular integrity (see Fig. 13-3). Another destructive mechanism occurs when infected cells fuse with other cells. This fusion process continues until many cells, some of which are not infected, combine into a multinucleated nonviable mass called a *syncytium* that destroys all affected cells. A third process of destruction is initiated by the infected person's immune system and the antibodies that are produced against HIV. These antibodies bind to the surface of infected cells and activate the complement system, which ultimately promotes lysis of the infected cells. Other theories about $CD4^+$ T cell destruction during HIV infection include initiation of apoptosis (programmed cell death), the development of "superantigens," autoimmune mechanisms, and increased production of cytokines.[11]

HIV also can infect monocytes by attaching to CD4 receptors or by phagocytic ingestion. Infected monocytes move into body tissues where they differentiate into macrophages. Although HIV replicates in infected macrophages, no external budding occurs. This allows the cell to remain intact while becoming an "HIV factory." A local inflammatory process may cause the infected macrophage to rupture, distributing newly formed HIV into surrounding tissues. Skin, lymph node, lung, central nervous system, and possibly bone marrow tissues have been directly infected in this manner.[19]

Clinical Manifestations and Complications

The typical course of untreated HIV infection follows the pattern shown in Fig. 13-4. However, it is important to remember that HIV is highly individualized. The information depicted in Fig. 13-4 represents data from large groups of people and should not be used to predict an individual's life span after HIV infection.

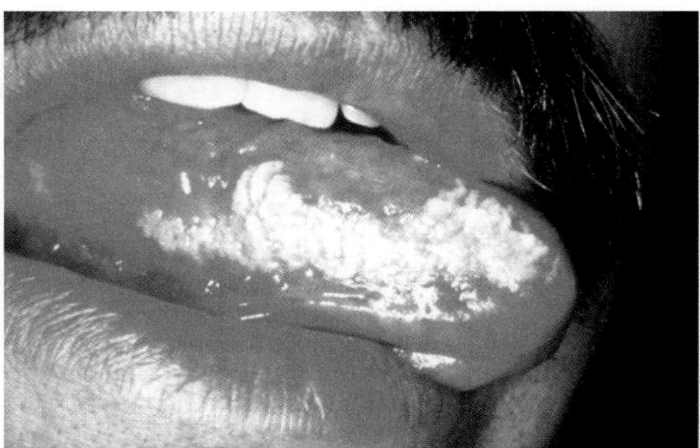

Fig. 13-5 Oral hairy leukoplakia on the tongue.

Acute Retroviral Syndrome. The development of HIV-specific antibodies (or *seroconversion*) is frequently accompanied by a flu- or mononucleosis-like syndrome of fever, lymphadenopathy, pharyngitis, headache, malaise, nausea, muscle and joint pain, diarrhea, photophobia, and/or a diffuse rash.[9,19] These symptoms, called *acute retroviral syndrome,* generally occur 1 to 3 weeks after initial infection and last for 1 to 2 weeks, although some of the symptoms may persist for several months. $CD4^+$ T cell counts will fall temporarily during this time but quickly return to baseline.[11] This temporary decrease is a typical healthy immune response to acute illness.[9] In most people, acute retroviral symptoms are mild and may be mistaken for a cold or flu. In a few people neurologic complications, such as aseptic meningitis, peripheral neuropathy, facial palsy, or Guillain-Barré syndrome, have developed.[20]

Early Infection. The median interval between HIV infection and a diagnosis of AIDS is about 10 years. During this time T cell counts remain normal or slightly decreased. This phase is referred to as *asymptomatic disease* but vague symptoms, including fatigue, headache, low grade fever, and night sweats, may occur.[10]

Because most of the symptoms during early infection are vague and nonspecific for HIV, people can remain unaware that they are infected for a decade or more.[11] During this time, infected people continue activities that may include high risk sexual and drug-using behaviors, creating a public health problem because infected people can transmit HIV to others even if they have no symptoms. Personal health also is affected because people who do not know they are infected have no motivation to seek treatment or to make changes in health habits that could beneficially alter the quality and quantity of their lives.[14]

Early Symptomatic Disease. Toward the end of the asymptomatic phase and before a diagnosis of AIDS, the $CD4^+$ T cell count drops below 500 to 600 cells/μl and early symptomatic disease develops. Early symptoms can include constitutional problems such as persistent fever, recurrent drenching night sweats, chronic diarrhea, headaches, and fatigue. These may be severe enough to interrupt normal routines. Other problems that may occur at this time include localized infections, lymphadenopathy, and neurologic manifestations.[11,19]

The most common infection associated with early symptomatic HIV disease is oropharyngeal candidiasis or thrush.

Table 13-1 Diagnostic Criteria for AIDS

AIDS is diagnosed when an individual with HIV develops at least one of these additional conditions:

1. $CD4^+$ T cell count drops below 200/μl.
2. Development of one of the following opportunistic infections (OIs):
   Fungal: candidiasis of bronchi, trachea, lungs, or esophagus; *Pneumocystis carinii* pneumonia (PCP); disseminated or extrapulmonary histoplasmosis
   Viral: cytomegalovirus (CMV) disease other than liver, spleen, or nodes; CMV retinitis (with loss of vision); herpes simplex with chronic ulcer(s) or bronchitis, pneumonitis, or esophagitis; progressive multifocal leukoencephalopathy (PML); extrapulmonary cryptococcosis
   Protozoal: disseminated or extrapulmonary coccidioidomycosis, toxoplasmosis of the brain, chronic intestinal isosporiasis; chronic intestinal cryptosporidiosis
   Bacterial: Mycobacterium tuberculosis (any site); any disseminated or extrapulmonary *Mycobacterium,* including *M. avium* complex or *M. kansasii;* recurrent pneumonia; recurrent *Salmonella* septicemia
3. Development of one of the following opportunistic cancers:
   Invasive cervical cancer, Kaposi's sarcoma (KS), Burkitt's lymphoma, immunoblastic lymphoma, or primary lymphoma of the brain
4. Wasting syndrome occurs. Wasting syndrome is defined as a loss of 10% or more of ideal body mass.
5. Dementia develops.

Modified from Centers for Disease Control and Prevention (CDC): Recommendations and Reports: 1993 revised classification system for HIV infection and expanded surveillance case definition for AIDS among adolescents and adults, *MMWR* 41 (RR-17):1, 1992.

Candida rarely causes problems in healthy adults, but occurs in more than 90% of HIV-infected people at some time during their lives.[9] Other infections that can occur at this time include shingles (caused by the varicella zoster virus), persistent vaginal candida infections, and outbreaks of oral or genital herpes. Oral hairy leukoplakia, an Epstein-Barr virus infection that causes painless, white, raised lesions on the lateral aspect of the tongue, can also occur (Fig. 13-5). Oral lesions such as those seen in candidiasis and hairy leukoplakia may provide the earliest indications of HIV infection. Oral hairy leukoplakia is also a prognostic indicator of disease progression.[9]

Neurologic manifestations can occur at any time during the spectrum of HIV infection but may become more problematic during this phase. Common neurologic symptoms include headache, aseptic meningitis, cranial nerve palsy, myopathy, and painful peripheral neuropathies that may be related to HIV, other infections, neoplasms, or medication side effects.[9] Abnormal neurologic findings can also develop during this phase, including alterations in the cerebrospinal fluid (CSF), central nervous system production of HIV-specific antibodies, and CSF that is HIV-culture positive.[21]

AIDS. A diagnosis of AIDS cannot be made until the HIV-infected patient meets case definition criteria established by the CDC.[22] These criteria (listed in Table 13-1) are more likely to occur when the immune system becomes severely compromised. As the disease progresses, the $CD4^+$ T cell count decreases and

DRUG THERAPY

Table 13-2 **Common Opportunistic Diseases Associated with AIDS***

Organism/Disease	Clinical Manifestations	Diagnostic Tests	Treatment
Respiratory System			
Pneumocystis carinii pneumonia (PCP)	Nonproductive cough, hypoxemia, progressive shortness of breath, fever, night sweats, fatigue	Chest x-ray, induced sputum for culture, bronchoalveolar lavage	Trimethoprim-sulfamethoxazole (Bactrim), pentamidine, dapsone+ trimethoprim, clindamycin (Cleocin) + primaquine, atovaquone (Mepron), trimetrexate (Neutrexin) + folinic acid+/− dapsone, corticosteroids
Histoplasma capsulatum	Pneumonia, fever, cough, weight loss; disseminated disease	Sputum culture, serum or urine antigen assay	Amphotericin B, itroconazole (Sporanox), fluconazole (Diflucan)
Mycobacterium tuberculosis	Productive cough, fever, night sweats, weight loss	Chest x-ray, sputum for AFB stain and culture	Isoniazid (INH), ethambutol (Myambutol), rifampin (Rifadin), pyrazinamide, streptomycin
Coccidioides immitis	Fever, weight loss, cough	Sputum culture, serology	Amphotericin B, fluconazole (Diflucan), itroconazole (Sporanox)
Kaposi's sarcoma (KS)	Dyspnea, respiratory failure	Chest x-ray, biopsy	Cancer chemotherapy, alpha-interferon, radiation
Integumentary System			
Herpes simplex, type 1 (HSV1) and type 2 (HSV2)	Orolabial mucocutaneous ulcerative lesions (type 1), genital and perianal mucocutaneous ulcerative lesions (type 2)	Viral culture	Acyclovir (Zovirax), famciclovir (Famvir), valacyclovir (Valtrex), foscarnet (Foscavir)
Varicella zoster virus (VZV)	Shingles, erythematous maculopapular rash along dermatomal planes, pain, pruritis	Viral culture	Acyclovir, famciclovir, valacyclovir, foscarnet
Kaposi's sarcoma (KS)	Firm, flat, raised or nodular, hyperpigmented, multicentric lesions	Biopsy of lesions	Cancer chemotherapy, alpha-interferon, radiation of lesions
Bacillary angiomatosis	Erythematous vascular papules, subcutaneous nodules	Biopsy of lesions	Erythromycin, doxycycline
Eye			
Cytomegalovirus (CMV) retinitis	Lesions on the retina, blurred vision, loss of vision	Ophthalmoscopic exam	Ganciclovir (Cytovene), foscarnet, cidofovir (Vistide)
Herpes virus, type 1 (HSV1)	Blurred vision, corneal lesions, acute retinal necrosis	Ophthalmoscopic exam	Acyclovir, famciclovir, valacyclovir, foscarnet
Varicella zoster virus (VZV)	Ocular lesions, acute retinal necrosis	Ophthalmoscopic exam	Acyclovir, famciclovir, valacyclovir, foscarnet
Gastrointestinal System			
Cryptosporidium muris	Watery diarrhea, abdominal pain, weight loss, nausea	Stool exam, small bowel or colon biopsy	Antidiarrheals, paromomycin (Humatin), azithromycin (Zithromax), atovaquone (Mepron), octreotide (Sandostatin)
Cytomegalovirus (CMV)	Stomatitis, esophagitis, gastritis, colitis, bloody diarrhea, pain, weight loss	Endoscopic visualization, culture, biopsy, rule out other causes	Ganciclovir (Cytovene), foscarnet, cidofovir
Herpes simplex, type 1 (HSV1)	Vesicular eruptions on tongue, buccal, pharyngeal, or perioral esophageal mucosa	Viral culture	Acyclovir, famciclovir, valacyclovir, foscarnet
Candida albicans	Whitish-yellow patches in mouth, esophagus, GI tract	Microscopic exam of scraping from lesion, culture	Fluconazole, nystatin, clotrimazole (Lotrimin), itroconazole, Amphotericin B

Continued

DRUG THERAPY

Table 13-2 Common Opportunistic Diseases Associated with AIDS*—cont'd

Organism/Disease	Clinical Manifestations	Diagnostic Tests	Treatment
Gastrointestinal System—cont'd			
Mycobacterium avium complex (MAC)	Watery diarrhea, weight loss	Small bowel biopsy with AFB stain and culture	Clarithromycin (Biaxin), rifampin (Rifadin), ciprofloxacin (Cipro), Rifabutin (Mycobutin), amikacin, azithromycin
Isospora belli	Diarrhea, weight loss, nausea, abdominal pain	Stool exam, small-bowel or colon biopsy	Trimethoprim-sulfamethoxazole, pyrimethamine + folinic acid
Salmonella	Gastroenteritis, fever, diarrhea	Blood and stool culture	Ciprofloxacin, ampicillin, amoxicillin, trimethoprim-sulfamethoxazole
Kaposi's sarcoma (KS)	Diarrhea, hyperpigmented lesions of mouth and GI tract	GI series, biopsy	Cancer chemotherapy, alpha-interferon, radiation
Non-Hodgkin's lymphoma	Abdominal pain, fever, night sweats, weight loss	Lymph node biopsy	Chemotherapy
Neurologic System			
Toxoplasma gondii	Cognitive dysfunction, motor impairment, fever, altered mental status, headache, seizures, sensory abnormalities	MRI, CT scan, toxoplasma serology, brain biopsy (usually deferred)	Pyrimethamine + folinic acid + sulfadiazine, clindamycin , azithromycin,clarithromycin
JC papovavirus	Progressive multifocal leukoencephalopathy (PML) mental and motor declines	MRI, CT scan, brain biopsy	Effective antiretroviral therapy may help
Cryptococcal meningitis	Cognitive impairment, motor dysfunction, fever, seizures, headache	CT scan, serum antigen test, CSF analysis	Amphotericin B, flucytosine (Ancobon), fluconazole, itroconazole
CNS lymphomas	Cognitive dysfunction, motor impairment, aphasia, seizures, personality changes, headache	MRI, CT scan	Radiation, chemotherapy
AIDS-dementia complex (ADC)	Insidious onset of progressive dementia	CT scan	Effective antiretroviral therapy may help

Sources: Bartlett JG: *Medical management of HIV infection,* Baltimore, Md, 1998, Johns Hopkins University; and Sande MA, Volberding PA: *The medical management of AIDS,* ed 5, Philadelphia, 1997, Saunders.
*Opportunistic diseases are reported in this table by systems frequently affected. However, it is important to note that in HIV infection dissemination is common.
AFB, acid-fast bacilli; *CNS,* central nervous system; *CSF,* cerebrospinal fluid; *CT* scan, computed tomography; *GI,* gastrointestinal; *MRI,* magnetic resonance imaging.

the ratio of $CD4^+$ to $CD8^+$ cells (T helper to T suppressor cells), which is usually about 2:1, gradually reverses. The amount of HIV that can be detected in the blood is increased. Decreases in the absolute number of lymphocytes as well as the percent of lymphocytes, may occur. Delayed hypersensitivity skin reactions are decreased or absent.[23]

The median time for survival after a diagnosis of AIDS is 2 years, but this varies greatly. Some people with AIDS live for 6 or more years, while others survive for only a few months. There is also a wide variation in morbidity. Some people with AIDS are severely (and often terminally) ill, yet others are able to continue usual routines with lifestyle adjustments to obtain health care and cope with symptoms such as fatigue. Advances in the treatment and diagnosis of HIV infection, opportunistic diseases, and constitutional symptoms have increased survival times, but AIDS fatality rates remain high.[11]

Opportunistic disease. Opportunistic diseases, commonly a reactivation of a prior infection, generally do not occur in the presence of a functioning immune system. Numerous infections, a variety of malignancies, wasting, and dementia can result from HIV-related immune impairment. Organisms that are nonvirulent or cause limited or localized diseases in immunocompetent individuals can cause severe, debilitating, disseminated, and life-threatening opportunistic infections in AIDS patients (Table 13-2). Unfortunately multiple opportunistic diseases tend to occur at the same time, further compounding the difficulties of diagnosis and treatment.[9,19]

Diagnostic Studies

Diagnosis of HIV Infection. The most useful screening tests for HIV are those that detect HIV-specific antibodies. The major problem with these tests is a median delay of 2 months after infection before detectable antibodies are produced (see Fig. 13-1). This creates a *window period* during which an infected individual will not test HIV-antibody positive. HIV-antibody screening is generally done in the sequence shown in Table 13-3. This process has been found to

Table 13-3 HIV Antibody Test Screening Process

The following steps are used in the process of testing blood for antibodies to HIV:

1. A highly sensitive enzyme immunoassay (EIA, ELISA) is done to detect serum antibodies that bind to HIV antigens on test plates. Blood samples that are negative on this test are reported as negative.
2. If the blood is EIA reactive, the test is repeated.
3. If the blood is repeatedly EIA reactive, a more specific confirming test, such as the Western blot (WB) or immunofluorescence assay (IFA), is done.
   - WB testing uses purified HIV antigens electrophoresed on gels. These are incubated with serum samples. If antibody in the serum is present, it can be detected.
   - IFA is used to identify HIV in infected cells. Blood is treated with a fluorescent antibody against p17 or p24 antigen and then examined using a fluorescent microscope.
4. Blood that is reactive in all of the first three steps is reported as HIV-antibody positive.
5. If the results are indeterminant, testing should be repeated within 6 months. Consistently indeterminant test results require the use of polymerase chain reaction (PCR), viral culture, and other diagnostic measures.
   - PCR analyzes DNA extracted from lymphocytes and/or HIV from serum using an *in vitro* amplification procedure.
   - A cell culture system can be used to grow viruses from infected lymphocytes.

Because these tests are expensive and difficult to do, they are usually not used for screening purposes, but may be done in situations where the index of suspicion is high and antibody tests are negative.

produce highly accurate results. HIV antibody testing can now be done on saliva and with home testing kits.[24]

Diagnosis of HIV in newborns can be problematic. All infants born to HIV-infected mothers will be positive on the HIV antibody test because maternal antibodies cross the placental barrier and these antibodies remain present in the infant for up to 18 months. For that reason, early detection of HIV infection in infants depends on testing for HIV antigen through the use of polymerase chain reaction (PCR) or viral culture (see Table 13-3). These tests can definitively diagnose HIV in infected infants by age 4 weeks.[10]

Laboratory Studies in HIV Infection. The progression of HIV infection has been monitored by $CD4^+$ T cell counts for many years. As the disease progresses, there is usually a decrease in the number of $CD4^+$ T cells, a marker for decreased immune function (see Fig. 13-1). However, $CD4^+$ T cell counts, while extremely important, reveal only part of the clinical picture.[24] Recently improved technologies that quantitate viral activity have resulted in the ability to better assess clinical status and disease progression. *Viral load* (also referred to as viral burden and HIV RNA level) quantifies viral particles in a biologic sample (usually serum). Viral loads can be determined with quantitative competitive PCR (RT-PCR) and branched-chain DNA (bDNA) techniques.[24] These tests provide information that help to determine when to initiate therapy, the efficacy of therapy, and whether clinical goals are being met.[25,26]

Hematologic abnormalities are common in HIV infection and may be caused by HIV, opportunistic diseases, or complications of drug or radiation therapy. A decreased white blood cell (WBC) count is often seen, usually with concomitant absolute lymphopenia. Thrombocytopenia may be caused by antiplatelet antibodies or drug therapy. Anemia is associated

Table 13-4 Baseline and Follow-Up Assessment Parameters in HIV Infection

Parameters	Initial Visit	CD4 >500	CD4 <500	CD4 <200	CD4 <100
Office visit	Follow-up in 2 weeks	q 3-6 mos	q 2-3 mos	q 1-2 mos	prn
CBC with differential and platelet count		q 3-6 mos	q 2-3 mos	q 1-2 mos	prn
Chemistry panel (SMA 12, 14, or 20)		q 3-6 mos	q 2-3 mos	q 1-2 mos	prn
Amylase		Monthly if patient is on didanosine			
RPR or VDRL	✓	Annually as long as patient is sexually active			
$CD4^+$ T cell count	✓	q 3-6 mos	q 2-3 mos	q 2-3 mos	prn
Viral load assessment (bDNA or PCR)*	✓	q 3-4 mos	q 3-4 mos	q 3-4 mos	q 3-4 mos
Hepatitis B serology	✓				
Toxoplasma and CMV serologies (IgG)	✓			✓	
AFB, blood culture				✓	✓
Chest x-ray	✓			✓	prn
PPD skin test by Mantoux method	✓	If negative at baseline, repeat annually; consider q 6 mo testing in high prevalence areas			
Family planning/contraception	✓	With each visit as needed			
Pelvic with Pap/colposcopy	✓	annual	q 6 mos	q 6 mos/prn	q 6 mos/prn
Mammogram	✓	annually for rest of life			
Eye exam by ophthalmologic consult	✓	annual	annual	q 6 mos	q 4-6 mos
Dental exam/prophylaxis	Oral exam at each visit; dental care q 3-6 mo for cleaning and as needed				

Adapted from Bradley-Springer LA, Fendrick R: *HIV instant instructor cards,* El Paso, Tex, 1994, Skidmore-Roth.

*Viral loads should be assessed immediately before and 4 weeks after initiation or change in antiretroviral therapy. A greater than tenfold decrease (1 $\log_{10}$) in viral load will indicate successful therapy. With optimal therapy, viral load should be undetectable at 6

CBC, complete blood count; *PCR,* polymerase chain reaction; *PPD,* purified protein derivative; *RPR,* rapid plasma reagin; *VDRL,* Venereal Disease Research Laboratories.

with the chronic disease process as well as with common adverse effects of some antiretroviral agents.[24]

Alterations in liver function tests are not uncommon. These may be caused by disease processes or drug therapy and may be more common with newer drug therapy. Early identification of co-infection with hepatitis B virus and/or hepatitis C virus is important because these infections may have a more serious course in the patient with HIV infection and may ultimately limit options for drug therapy.[24]

Collaborative Care

Collaborative management of the HIV-infected patient focuses on monitoring HIV disease progression and immune function, initiating and monitoring antiretroviral therapy, preventing the development of opportunistic diseases, detecting and treating opportunistic diseases, managing symptoms, and preventing complications of treatment. Ongoing assessment and clinician-patient interactions are required to accomplish these objectives.[13,24] See Table 13-4 for a summary of assessment parameters that need to be accomplished during the course of HIV disease.

The initial visit provides an opportunity to gather baseline data and to establish rapport. A complete history and physical examination, including an immunization history and psychosocial and dietary evaluations, should be conducted. Findings from the history, assessment, and laboratory tests help to determine the patient's needs. This is a good time to initiate patient education related to the spectrum of HIV disease, treatments, preventing transmission to others, improving health, and family planning. Patient input should be used to develop a plan of care, and necessary referrals can be made. It is important to remember that a newly diagnosed patient may be in a state of shock or denial[13] and unable to retain or synthesize information.[27] The nurse should be prepared to repeat and clarify information over the course of several months. If case reports are required by the State Health Department, they should be completed at this time.

Drug Therapy for HIV Infection. The goals of drug therapy in HIV infection are to (1) decrease HIV RNA levels to <5000 copies/μl (undetectable HIV RNA levels are possible and preferred), (2) maintain or raise $CD4^+$ T cell counts to >500 cells/μl (a range of 800 to 1200 cells/μl is preferred), and (3) delay the development of HIV-related symptoms, including a wide range of opportunistic diseases. A variety of drug therapies is now available to help patients meet these goals. Because of the rapidity with which new therapies are evolving, there has been considerable confusion about how and when to use antiretroviral therapy. The National Institutes of Health (NIH) has published a report on the principles of therapy (Table 13-5).[28] Guidelines on the use of antiretroviral agents have also been published.[20] Recommendations for the initiation of therapy in the chronically infected patient are summarized in Table 13-6. A major goal of these recommendations is to prevent the development of viral resistance to the available drugs. This can happen rapidly when patients miss or delay dosages. For this reason, strict adherence to treatment protocols is extremely important.

Table 13-5 Summary of Principles of Therapy of HIV Infection

1. Ongoing HIV replication leads to immune system damage and progression to AIDS. HIV infection is always harmful, and true long-term survival free of clinically significant immune dysfunction is unusual.
2. Plasma HIV RNA levels indicate the magnitude of HIV replication and its associated rate of $CD4^+$ T cell destruction, while $CD4^+$ T cell counts indicate the extent of HIV-induced immune damage already suffered. Regular, periodic measurement of plasma HIV RNA levels and $CD4^+$ T cell counts is necessary to determine the risk of disease progression in an HIV-infected individual and to determine when to initiate or modify antiretroviral treatment regimens.
3. As rates of disease progression differ among individuals, treatment decisions should be individualized by level of risk indicated by plasma HIV RNA levels and $CD4^+$ T cell counts.
4. The use of potent combination antiretroviral therapy to suppress HIV replication to below the levels of detection of sensitive plasma HIV RNA assays limits the potential for selection of antiretroviral-resistant HIV variants, the major factor limiting the ability of antiretroviral drugs to inhibit virus replication and delay disease progression. Therefore maximum achievable suppression of HIV replication should be the goal of therapy.
5. The most effective means to accomplish durable suppression of HIV replication is the simultaneous initiation of combinations of effective anti-HIV drugs with which the patient has not been previously treated and that are not cross-resistant with antiretroviral agents with which the patient has been previously treated.
6. Each of the antiretroviral drugs used in combination therapy regimens should always be used according to optimum schedules and dosages.
7. The available effective antiretroviral drugs are limited in number and mechanism of action and cross-resistance between specific drugs has been documented. Therefore any change in antiretroviral therapy increases future therapeutic constraints.
8. Women should receive optimal antiretroviral therapy regardless of pregnancy status.
9. The same principles of antiretroviral therapy apply to both HIV-infected children and adults, although the treatment of HIV-infected children involves unique pharmacologic, virologic, and immunologic considerations.
10. Persons with acute primary HIV infections should be treated with combination antiretroviral therapy to suppress virus replication to levels below the limit of detection of sensitive plasma HIV RNA assays.
11. HIV-infected persons, even those with viral loads below detectable limits, should be considered infectious and should be counseled to avoid sexual and drug-use behaviors that are associated with transmission or acquisition of HIV and other infectious pathogens.

Revised from *Report of the NIH Panel to Define Principles of Therapy of HIV Infection,* National Institutes of Health, 1997.

DRUG THERAPY

Table 13-6 Indications for the Initiation of Antiretroviral Therapy in the Chronically HIV-Infected Patient

Clinical Category	$CD4^+$ T Cell Count and HIV RNA Level	Recommendation
Symptomatic (AIDS diagnosis, thrush, or unexplained fever)	Any value	Treat
Asymptomatic	$CD4^+$ T cells <500/μl or HIV RNA > 10,000 (dDNA) or > 20,000 (RT-PCR)	Treatment should be offered. Strength of recommendation is based on prognosis for disease-free survival as demonstrated in research and willingness of the patient to accept and adhere to therapy.*
Asymptomatic	$CD4^+$ T Cells >500/μl and HIV RNA <10,000 (bDNA) or <20,000 (RT-PCR)	Some experts would delay therapy and observe; however, some experts would treat.

Revised from *Guidelines for the Use of Antiretroviral Agents in HIV-Infected Adults and Adolescents,* Department of Health and Human Services (DHHS), 1997.
*Some experts would observe patients with $CD4^+$ T cell counts between 350-500/μl and HIV RNA levels <10,000 (bDNA) or <20,000 (RT-PCR).

Drugs in three different pharmacologic groups have now been approved to treat HIV infection. Research is progressing rapidly to develop new groups of drugs as well as new drugs in the established categories. No drug or combination of drugs can cure HIV, but new therapies can decrease viral replication and delay progression of disease in many patients. The major advantage of having antiretroviral drugs from different drug groups is that combination therapy, which decreases the likelihood of drug resistance, is now available.[29] An additional advantage is that alternatives now exist for those patients who fail to respond to a specific drug regimen.[3,20]

The three currently approved groups of drugs include two types that inhibit the ability of HIV to make a DNA copy early in replication and one type that inhibits the ability of the virus to produce viable virions in the late stages of replication (Table 13-7). Nucleoside reverse transcriptase inhibitors (NRTIs) and non-nucleoside reverse transcriptase inhibitors (NNRTIs) both work by inhibiting the activity of the enzyme reverse transcriptase, while protease inhibitors (PIs) work by interfering with the activity of the protease enzyme.[30] A major problem with PIs is that resistance develops rapidly when they are used alone. For that reason PIs must always be used in combination with other drugs and must be taken on a strictly adhered to schedule.[2,31] PIs and NNRTIs also have a number of dangerous and potentially lethal interactions with commonly used drugs.[9,20]

Because treatment with new drug combinations has resulted in dramatic improvements in many HIV-infected patients, current therapeutic recommendations are for combination antiretroviral therapy with at least three drugs, preferably two NRTIs and one PI.[22] Monotherapy is not recommended unless extenuating circumstances are documented. While the research on these treatment protocols is generally very good, with viral loads being reduced by 90% to 99% in many cases,[20] there are some problems. Up to 50% of patients with HIV will not experience a dramatic response to the drugs, causing feelings of guilt, despair, and futility. In addition, many patients will not be able to use combination therapies because of the expense, side effects and drug reactions, or inability to adhere to stringent schedules and dietary prescriptions required with these therapies. Expense is an important concern for many, although economic analysis suggests that combination antiretroviral therapy is more cost effective than the cost of advancing disease.[32] Although the outlook is improving, there is, as yet, "no magic bullet."[33]

Drug Therapy for Opportunistic Diseases. The management of HIV is complicated by the many opportunistic diseases that can develop as the immune system deteriorates. Although it is usually not possible to eradicate these diseases, treatments that can control them are available. Suppressive therapy must continue for life or the diseases will return.[34] Advances in the diagnosis and treatment of opportunistic diseases have contributed significantly to increased life expectancy. Table 13-2 lists treatments for common opportunistic diseases in HIV-infected individuals.

A preferred approach to opportunistic diseases is to prevent their occurrences in the first place. A number of opportunistic diseases associated with HIV can be delayed or prevented through the use of adequate antiretroviral management and disease-specific prophylactic interventions. Prophylaxis contributes significantly to the decreased morbidity and mortality associated with HIV infection and is recommended according to established criteria (Table 13-8).[24,34]

Vaccination. Early in the HIV epidemic there was optimism that a vaccine would be quickly developed.[35] Despite considerable research and development, a vaccine still eludes scientists, but there is hope for an effective preventive vaccine within the next decade.[7] The problems that impede HIV vaccine development are numerous. Because HIV is an intracellular pathogen, it can hide from circulating immune factors. HIV also mutates rapidly, so that infected individuals develop HIV variants that may not all respond to a simple vaccine. In addition, two strains of HIV (HIV-1 and HIV-2) cause AIDS

DRUG THERAPY

Table 13-7 Antiretroviral Agents Used in HIV Infection*,†

Drug/Administration	Adverse Effects
Nucleoside Reverse Transcriptase Inhibitors (NRTI)	
Zidovudine (AZT, ZDV, Retrovir)	Fatigue, malaise, headache, GI intolerance, nausea, insomnia, asthenia, hepatitis, myalgias; bone marrow suppression: anemia, neutropenia, granulocytopenia
Didanosine (ddl, Videx) Dose must be provided in 2 tablets to ensure adequate buffer for absorption. Tablets must be chewed or dissolved to release buffer.	Pancreatitis, painful peripheral neuropathy (dose related and reversible), GI intolerance, rash, bone marrow suppression, hyperuricemia, hepatitis
Zalcitabine (ddC, HIVID)	Painful peripheral neuropathy (dose related and reversible), stomatitis, oral/esophageal ulcers, pancreatitis, nausea, diarrhea, hepatitis
Stavudine (d4T, Zerit)	Painful peripheral neuropathy, ALT elevations, anemia, headache
Lamivudine (3TC, Epivir)	Minimal toxicity; headache, malaise, diarrhea, insomnia, nausea, abdominal pain
Abacavir (Ziagen)	Hypersensitivity, fever, nausea, vomiting, malaise, rash; may produce life-threatening event if hypersensitivity is re-challenged
Adefovir dipivoxil (Preveon)	Fanconi syndrome and renal failure; requires careful monitoring of renal function; nausea, vomiting, anorexia
Combivir (lamivudine and zidovudine combination)	Combines side effects of lamivudine and zidovudine
Non-nucleoside Reverse Transcriptase Inhibitors (NNRTI)	
Nevirapine (Viramune)	Rash, Stevens-Johnson syndrome, fever, nausea, headache, increased liver enzymes
Delavirdine (Rescriptor) Mix tablets in 3 or more oz of water to produce a slurry. May be given with or without food.	Rash, pruritis, headache, fatigue, nausea, vomiting, diarrhea, conjunctivitis
Efavirenz (Sustiva) Take at bedtime to help with side effects; pregnant women should not take this drug.	Dizziness, disconnected feeling, insomnia, nightmares, usually resolve within 2 wk; rash, nausea, diarrhea, headache
Protease Inhibitors (PI)	
Saquinovir (Fortovase) Take with meals or within 2 hr of a full meal.	Diarrhea, abdominal pain, nausea, headache, elevated transaminase enzymes
Indinavir (Crixivan) Ensure adequate hydration during therapy; patient should drink 2-4 L of fluid a day. Administer 1 hr before or after eating. Do not take in conjunction with grapefruit juice.	Kidney stones (flank pain with or without hematuria), asymptomatic hyperbilirubinemia, headache, blurred vision, dizziness, nausea, vomiting, diarrhea, rash, fatigue, insomnia, thrombocytopenia, metallic taste
Ritonivir (Norvir) Preferable to give with food, but not required. Keep capsules refrigerated. (Single dose may be kept at room temperature for up to 12 hr.) Taking with chocolate milk decreases bitter aftertaste.	Nausea, diarrhea, vomiting, anorexia, abdominal pain, taste perversion, circumoral and peripheral paresthesias, asthenia; elevations in triglycerides, transaminase levels, CK, and uric acid
Nelfinavir (Viracept) Take with meal or light snack.	Diarrhea, nausea, back pain, fever, headache, malaise, anorexia, anemia
Amprenavir (Agenerase)	Diarrhea, wekaness, headache, nausea, abdominal pain

Sources: Bartlett J: *Medical management of HIV infection,* Baltimore, Md, 1998, Johns Hopkins University; and *Guidelines for the use of antiretroviral agents in HIV-infected adults and adolescents,* 1997.

*Current recommendations for therapy encourage combinations of these drugs. The following should never be used as monotherapy: lamivadine or any of the NNRTIs or PIs.

†Many of these drugs, especially the NNRTIs and PIs, cause serious and potentially fatal interactions when used in combination with other commonly used drugs, some of which are available over the counter.

ALT, alanine aminotransferase; *CK,* creatine kinase; *GI,* gastrointestinal.

DRUG THERAPY

Table 13-8 Prophylactic Interventions for Patients with HIV Infection

Problem	Prophylactic Interventions	Comments
Hepatitis B virus (HBV)	Hepatitis B vaccine series; screen and vaccinate those who show no evidence of previous HBV infection	Provide as soon as possible during course of infection. Encourage vaccine in injecting drug users, sexually active gay men, and sex partners or household contacts of HBV-infected individuals.
Influenza virus	Whole or split virus influenza vaccine	Provide annually, before influenza virus season.
Mycobacterium avium complex (MAC)	Clarithromycin (Biaxin) or azithromycin (Zithromax) (preferred); rifabutin (Mycobutin)	Initiate when $CD4^+$ T cells go below 50/μl. Rule out disseminated disease or tuberculosis. Rifabutin has caused dose-related uveitis (above 600 mg/day) that is reversible with drug withdrawal or dose reduction.
Mycobacterium tuberculosis (TB)	Treat if PPD is >5 mm reactive, after high risk exposure, or if prior positive PPD without treatment. Isoniazid (INH) + pyridoxine for 12 mo. Consider directly observed therapy.	Rule out active disease, extrapulmonary disease, or drug resistant strain, all of which require multidrug therapy. Remember that a negative PPD in the presence of HIV does not exclude a diagnosis of TB. Provide ongoing assessment and intervention.
Pneumococcal pneumonia	Pneumococcal vaccine	Provide as soon as possible during course of infection. Antibody response is optimal when $CD4^+$ T cells are > 350/μl.
Pneumocystis carinii pneumonia (PCP)	Trimethoprim-sulfamethoxazole (TMP-SMX) (preferred) or dapsone, dapsone with pyrimethamine + folinic acid, aerosolized pentamidine	Initiate when $CD4^+$ T cells go below 200/μl. Offer to any patient with a history of PCP, fever of undetermined origin for 2 or more wk, or oropharyngeal candidiasis regardless of $CD4^+$ T cell count. Oral drugs that provide systemic effect are preferred. Side effects of TMP-SMX and dapsone, especially rash and fever, are common and may limit use.
Toxoplasmosis	Trimethoprim-sulfamethoxazole (TMP-SMX) or dapsone with pyrimethamine + folinic acid	Initiate with positive toxoplasmosis IgG titer when $CD4^+$ T cells go below 100/μl.
Varicella zoster virus (VZV)	Varicella zoster immune globulin (VZIG) administered within 96 hr after an exposure	Only after significant exposure to chicken pox or shingles for patients with no history of disease or negative on a VZV antibody test.

Sources: Bartlett J: *Medical management of HIV infection*, Baltimore, Md, 1998, Johns Hopkins University; Masci JR: *Outpatient management of HIV infection*, ed 2, St Louis, 1996, Mosby; CDC: *1997 USPHS/IDSA guidelines for the prevention of opportunistic infections in persons infected with human immunodeficiency virus*, 46(RR-12):1, 1997.

and at least ten clades (or families) of HIV-1 exist around the world.[1,3] Development of an effective vaccine for Clade B (the predominant group in the Americas and Western Europe) may not prove effective in developing countries where the need is even greater.[7] A major problem for vaccine development is that the correlates of protective immunity for HIV are unknown. Antibody development after vaccination usually indicates immunity, but HIV-infected patients produce an antibody that does not prevent active disease or confer immunity. In addition, HIV is frequently transmitted through mucosal contact, so a successful vaccine would need to induce mucosal as well as systemic protection.[36,37]

There are also social, ethical, and economic issues related to vaccination. Because no known animal model for HIV exists, vaccine efficacy can be established only through human testing. How will volunteers be recruited? How will true protection be determined? Will volunteers be exposed to HIV after immunization to test immunity? Because HIV is a global problem, with developing countries bearing the brunt of the epidemic, is it possible to develop a vaccine that can be widely distributed in a short amount of time at an acceptable cost?[37]

Despite the overwhelming nature of these issues, considerable research is in progress. Vaccines in various stages of development have been tested in animals, and a few have progressed to human trials.[3,7,36,37] However, authorities warn that the development of a successful vaccine will not replace current prevention methods based on education to decrease risk behaviors, because no vaccine is likely to be 100% effective.[7]

NURSING ASSESSMENT

Table 13-9 HIV-Infected Patient

Subjective Data

Important Health Information

Past health history: Route of infection; hepatitis; other STDs; tuberculosis; foreign travel; frequent viral, fungal, and/or bacterial infections

Medications: Use of immunosuppressive drugs

Functional Health Patterns

Health perception–health management: Perception of illness; alcohol and drug use; malaise

Nutritional-metabolic: Weight loss, anorexia, nausea, vomiting; lesions, bleeding, or ulcerations of lips, mouth, gums, tongue, or throat; sensitivity to acidic, salty, or spicy foods; difficulty swallowing; abdominal cramping; skin rashes, lesions, or color changes; nonhealing wounds

Elimination: Persistent diarrhea, change in character of stools; painful urination

Activity-exercise: Chronic fatigue, muscle weakness, difficulty walking; cough, shortness of breath

Sleep-rest: Insomnia; night sweats

Cognitive-perceptual: Headaches, stiff neck, chest pain, rectal pain, retrosternal pain; blurred vision, photophobia, diplopia, loss of vision; hearing impairment; confusion, forgetfulness, attention deficit, changes in mental status, memory loss, personality changes; paresthesias, hypersensitivity in feet, pruritis

Role-relationship: Support system, financial resources

Sexuality-reproductive: Lesions on genitalia (internal or external), pruritis or burning in vagina, painful sexual intercourse, changes in menstruation, vaginal or penile discharge

Coping-stress tolerance: Stress levels, previous losses, coping patterns, self-concept

Objective Data

General

Lethargy, persistent fever, lymphadenopathy, wasting; social withdrawal

Integumentary

Decreased skin turgor, dry skin, or diaphoresis; pallor, cyanosis; lesions, eruptions, discolorations, or bruises of skin and mucous membranes; vaginal or perianal excoriation; alopecia, delayed wound healing

Eyes

Presence of exudate; retinal lesions or hemorrhage; papilledema

Respiratory

Tachypnea, dyspnea, intercostal retractions; crackles, wheezing, productive or nonproductive cough

Cardiovascular

Pericardial friction rub, murmur, bradycardia, tachycardia

Gastrointestinal

Mouth lesions including blisters (HSV), white-gray patches (candida), painless white lesions on lateral aspect of the tongue (hairy leukoplakia), discolorations (KS); gingivitis, tooth decay or loosening; redness or white patchy lesions of throat; vomiting, diarrhea, incontinence; rectal lesions; hyperactive bowel sounds, abdominal masses, hepatosplenomegaly, guarding

Musculoskeletal

Muscle wasting

Neurologic

Ataxia, tremors, lack of coordination; sensory loss; slurred speech, aphasia; memory loss, apathy, agitation, depression, inappropriate behavior; decreasing levels of consciousness, seizures, paralysis, coma

Reproductive

Genital lesions or discharge, abdominal tenderness secondary to pelvic inflammatory disease (PID)

Possible Findings

Positive HIV antibody assay (EIA or ELISA, confirmed by WB or IFA); positive HIV culture or PCR; detectable viral load levels by bDNA or PCR, decreased CD4 lymphocytes, reversal of CD4 : CD8 ratio; decreased WBC, lymphopenia, anemia, thrombocytopenia; electrolyte imbalances; abnormal liver function tests

EIA, enzyme immunoassay; *ELISA,* enzyme-linked immunosorbent assay; *HSV,* herpes simplex virus; *IFA,* immunofluorescence assay; *KS,* Kaposi's sarcoma; *PCR,* polymerase chain reaction; *STDs,* sexually transmitted diseases; *WB,* Western blot; *WBC,* white blood cells.

NURSING MANAGEMENT: HIV INFECTION

■ Nursing Assessment

Nursing assessment for individuals not known to be infected with HIV should include a focus on behaviors that put the person at risk for HIV infection and other sexually transmitted and blood-borne diseases. Nurses can help individuals assess risks by asking basic questions such as (1) Have you ever had a blood transfusion or used clotting factor? Was it before 1985? (2) Have you ever shared needles, syringes, or other injecting equipment with another person? (3) Have you ever had a sexual experience in which your penis, vagina, rectum, or mouth came into contact with another person's penis, vagina, rectum, or mouth? and (4) Have you ever had an STD? These questions provide the minimum data needed to initiate a risk assessment. They should be modified to meet the needs of the person and the situation. A positive response to any of these questions requires an in-depth exploration of the issues specific to the identified risk.[38]

Further assessment is needed when an individual has been diagnosed with HIV infection. Subjective and objective data that should be obtained are presented in Table 13-9. Ongoing nursing assessments are essential because early recognition

Table 13-10 Nursing Diagnoses Commonly Used in HIV Infection

Altered family processes
Altered nutrition: less than body requirements
Altered oral mucous membrane
Altered sexuality patterns
Altered thought processes
Anticipatory grieving
Anxiety
Body image disturbance
Caregiver role strain
Chronic low self-esteem
Decisional conflict
Diarrhea
Fatigue
Fear
Hyperthermia
Ineffective denial
Ineffective individual coping
Ineffective management of therapeutic regimen
Noncompliance
Pain
Powerlessness
Relocation stress syndrome
Risk for disuse syndrome
Self-care deficit
Situational low self-esteem
Sleep pattern disturbance
Social isolation
Spiritual distress

and treatment of problems can decrease morbidity and mortality related to HIV infection. A complete history and thorough systems review can help the nurse identify problems in a timely manner.[9]

Nursing Diagnoses

Nursing diagnoses related to HIV infection are dictated by several variables: the stage (e.g., is prevention of HIV infection the issue? Are there concerns related to ongoing infection? Is the patient in terminal phases of the disease?); presence of specific etiologic problems (e.g., respiratory distress, depression, wasting); and social factors (e.g., issues related to self-esteem, sexuality, family interactions, finances).[38] Because HIV infection is a complex and individually experienced disease, a broad spectrum of nursing diagnoses may be required, including, but not limited to, those presented in Table 13-10.

Planning

Infection with HIV results in a devastating disease that affects the entire range of a person's life from physical health to social, emotional, economic, and spiritual well-being.[39,40] Prevention of the infection also presents a number of difficulties for the patient. Nurses can be instrumental in this process. Nursing interventions to help in the prevention of disease transmission depend on assessment of the patient's individual risk behaviors and knowledge and skill deficits. Nursing orders provide education to help the patient learn safer, healthier, and less risky behaviors.[43]

Once HIV infection is established, the overriding goals are to keep the viral load as low as possible and to maintain a functioning immune system.[20] Nursing orders to assist in meeting these goals focus on (1) adherence to medication regimens, (2) health promotion activities, and (3) prevention of opportunistic disease. Additional nursing activities encourage the HIV-infected patient to (1) protect others from HIV, (2) maintain or develop healthy, supportive relationships, (3) maintain activities and productivity for as long as possible, and (4) come to terms with issues related to disease, death, and spirituality. Goals are individualized and change as new treatment protocols develop and/or as HIV disease progresses.[38,41]

Nursing Implementation

The complexity of HIV disease is related to its chronic nature. As with most chronic and infectious disease processes, primary prevention and health promotion are the most effective health care strategies.[38,41] When prevention fails, however, disease results. Chronic diseases have no cure, continue for life, cause increasing physical disability and dysfunction, and ultimately contribute to morbidity and mortality. This is compounded by a health care system that deals better with acute problems than with chronic disorders and the many losses that accompany these diseases.[42]

Nursing interventions at every stage of HIV disease can be instrumental in improving the quality and quantity of the patient's life. Nurses who emphasize a holistic and individualized approach to care are well suited to and capable of providing optimal care to these patients. Table 13-11 presents a synopsis of nursing goals, assessments, and interventions at each stage of HIV infection.

Health Promotion. A major goal of health promotion is to prevent disease. Even with recent successes in the treatment of HIV, prevention is crucial for control of the epidemic. A secondary goal of health promotion is to detect disease early so that, if primary prevention has failed, early intervention can be implemented to decrease morbidity and mortality.[14]

Prevention of HIV infection. HIV infection is preventable. Until a vaccine is available, education and behavior change are the only effective prevention tools. Educational messages should be specific to the patient's need, culturally sensitive, language appropriate, and age-specific.[3] Nurses are excellent resources for this type of education, but nurses must be comfortable with and knowledgeable about sensitive topics such as sexuality and drug use.

Specific protective behaviors have been known and recommended since the mid-1980s. It is important to remember that a range of activities can reduce the risk of HIV infection and that individuals will choose different techniques. The goal is for the person to develop safer, healthier, and less risky behav-

Table 13-11 Nursing Interventions in HIV Disease

Levels of Care/Goals	Assess	Interventions
Health Promotion		
1. Prevent HIV infection 2. Detect HIV infection early	Risk factors: What behaviors or social, physical, emotional, pathologic, and immune factors place the patient at risk? Does the patient need to be tested?	Education, including knowledge, attitudes and behaviors with an emphasis on risk reduction to: General population: cover general information Pregnant women: general information and information specific to HIV infection and pregnancy Individual patient: specific to assessed need Empower patients to take control of prevention measures. Provide HIV antibody testing with pre- and post-test counseling.
Acute Intervention		
1. Promote health and limit disability 2. Manage problems caused by HIV infection	Physical health: Is patient experiencing problems? Mental health status: How is the patient coping? Resources: Does the patient have family/social support? Is the patient accessing community services? Is money/insurance a problem? Does the patient have access to spiritual support?	Provide case management. Educate regarding HIV, the spectrum of infection, options for care, signs and symptoms to watch for, treatment options, immune enhancement, harm reduction, and ways to adhere to treatment regimens. Refer to needed resources. Establish long-term, trusting relationship with patient, family, and significant others. Provide emotional and spiritual support. Provide care during acute exacerbations: recognition of life-threatening developments, life support, rapid intervention with treatments and medications, patient and family emotional support during crisis, comfort, and hygiene needs. Develop resources for legal needs: discrimination prevention, wills and powers of attorney, child care wishes. Empower patient to identify needs, direct care, seek services.
Ambulatory and Home Care		
1. Maximize quality of life 2. Resolve life and death issues	Physical health: Are new symptoms developing? Is the patient experiencing drug side effects or interactions? Mental health status: How is the patient coping? What adjustments have been made? Finances: Can the patient maintain health care and basic standards of living? Family/social/community supports: Are these available? Is the patient using supports in an effective manner? Spirituality issues: Does the patient desire support from an established religious organization? Are spirituality issues private and personal? What assistance does the patient need?	Continue case management. Educate about changing treatment options and continued adherence. Empower patient to continue to direct care and to make desires known to family members and significant others. Continue physical care for chronic disease process: treatments, medications, comfort, and hygiene needs. Support patient and family/significant others in a trusting relationship. Refer to resources that will assist in meeting identified needs. Promote health maintenance measures. Assist with end of life issues: resuscitation orders, funeral plans, estate planning, child care continuation, etc.

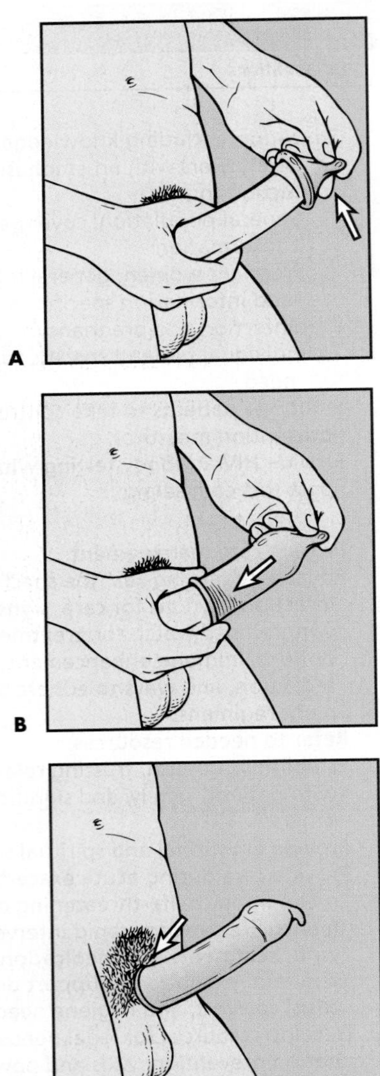

Fig. 13-6 Proper placement of the male condom. **A,** The condom is placed over the glans of the erect penis, being careful to squeeze air out of the reservoir. **B** and **C,** The condom is then rolled down the shaft of the penis to the hair line.

PATIENT TEACHING GUIDE

Table 13-12 Proper Use of the Male Condom

- Use only condoms (rubbers) that are made out of latex or polyurethane.
  - ✓ "Natural skin" condoms have pores that are large enough for HIV to penetrate.
- Store condoms in a cool, dry place and protect them from trauma. The friction caused by carrying them in a back pocket, for instance, can wear down the latex.
- Do not use a condom if the expiration date has passed or if the package looks worn or punctured.
- Lubricants used in conjunction with condoms must be water soluble.
  - ✓ Oil-based lubricants can weaken latex and increase the risk of tearing or breaking.
  - ✓ Non-lubricated, flavored condoms can provide protection during oral intercourse.
- The condom must be placed on the erect penis before any contact is made with the partner's mouth, vagina, or rectum to prevent exposure to pre-ejaculatory secretions that may contain HIV.
- See Fig. 13-6 for proper steps in male condom placement.
- Remove the penis and condom from the partner's body immediately after ejaculation and before the erection is lost.
  - ✓ Hold the condom at the base of the penis and remove both at the same time.
  - ✓ This keeps semen from leaking around the condom as the penis becomes flaccid.
- Remove the condom after use, wrap in tissue, and discard. Do not flush down the toilet, as this can cause plumbing problems.
- Condoms are not reuseable! A new condom must be used for every act of intercourse.

iors than are currently being used.[43] These techniques can be divided into safe activities (those that eliminate risk) and risk-reducing activities (those that decrease risk, but do not eliminate it). The more consistently and correctly prevention methods are used, the more effective they are in preventing HIV infection.[38]

Decreasing risks related to sexual intercourse. Safe activities eliminate the risk of exposure to HIV in semen and vaginal secretions. Abstaining from all sexual activity is the most effective way to accomplish this goal, but there are safe options for those who cannot or do not wish to abstain. *Outercourse,* or limiting sexual behavior to activities in which the mouth, penis, vagina, or rectum does not come into contact with a partner's mouth, penis, vagina, or rectum, is safe because there is no contact with blood, semen, or vaginal secretions. These activities include massage, masturbation, mutual masturbation ("hand job"), telephone sex, and other activities that meet the "no contact" requirements. Insertive sex is considered to be safe only in a mutually monogamous relationship between partners who are not infected with HIV or not at risk of becoming infected with HIV.

Risk-reducing sexual activities decrease the risk of contact with HIV through the use of barriers. Barriers should be used when engaging in insertive sexual activity (oral, vaginal, or anal) with a partner who is known to be HIV infected or with a partner whose HIV status is not known. The most commonly used barrier is the male condom (Fig. 13-6). Male condoms have been shown to be up to 100% effective in preventing the transmission of HIV when used correctly and consistently.[44,45] Major points for correct use of male condoms are discussed in Table 13-12. Female condoms are also available (Fig. 13-7). Use can be complicated, so careful instructions and practice are required (Table 13-13). In addition, squares of

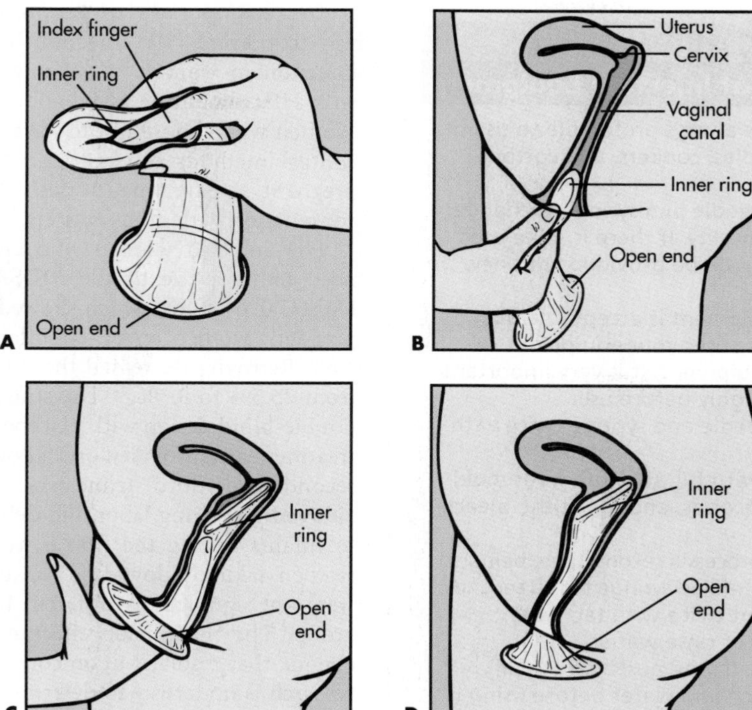

Fig. 13-7 Proper placement of the female condom. **A,** Inner ring is squeezed for insertion. **B,** Sheath is inserted similarly to a diaphragm. **C,** Inner ring is pushed up as far as it can go with the index finger. **D,** Proper placement of female condom.

PATIENT TEACHING GUIDE

Table 13-13 Proper Use of the Female Condom

- Female condoms consist of a polyurethane sheath with two spring form rings.
  - The smaller ring is inserted into the vagina and holds the condom in place internally. This ring can be removed if the condom is to be used for anal intercourse. It **should not be removed** if the condom is to be used for vaginal intercourse.
  - The larger ring surrounds the opening to the condom. It functions to keep the condom in place externally while protecting the external genitalia.
- Use only water-soluble lubricants with female condoms.
  - Female condoms come pre-lubricated and with a tube of additional lubricant.
  - Lubrication is needed to protect the condom from tearing during sexual intercourse and can also decrease the noise that results from friction of the penis against the condom.
- Some men have reported that the female condom feels better than the male condom. Other men like male condoms better. The only way to find out which type of condom works best is to try them both.
- Practice inserting the female condom. The steps for proper insertion are shown in Fig. 13-7. Lubrication makes the condom slippery, but do not get discouraged, just keep trying.
- During sexual intercourse, ensure that the penis is inserted into the female condom through the outer ring. It is possible for the penis to miss the opening, thus making contact with the vagina and defeating the purpose of the condom.
- Do not use a male condom at the same time as a female condom.
- After intercourse, remove the condom before standing up.
  - Twist the outer ring to keep the semen inside, gently pull the condom out of the vagina, and discard.
  - Do not flush down the toilet, as this can cause plumbing problems.
- Do not reuse a female condom.

latex (known as dental dams) or plastic wrapping paper can be used to cover the external female genitalia during oral sexual activity.[38]

Decreasing risks related to drug use. Illicit drug use is harmful. It can cause immune suppression and malnutrition as well as a host of psychosocial problems. However, drug use in and of itself does not cause HIV infection. The major risk for HIV infection is related to sharing injecting equipment and/or having unsafe sexual experiences while under the influence of drugs. The basic rules are (1) do not use drugs,

PATIENT TEACHING GUIDE

Table 13-14 Proper Use of Injection Equipment

- When injecting drugs, it is always preferable to use new, sterile syringes, needles, cookers, and cotton (works).
  - ✔ Find out if there is a needle and syringe exchange program in your community. If there is, take used equipment in and you will be provided with new works.
  - ✔ Reusing your own equipment is acceptable. Just ensure that no one else uses your equipment.
- If you must share your equipment, it is very important to clean the works thoroughly before use.
  - ✔ First, rinse the used needle and syringe twice with tap water.
  - ✔ Then, fill the syringe with full strength household bleach, shake for 30 seconds, and squirt the bleach out.
  - ✔ Repeat the bleaching process a second time, being sure to shake the bleach-filled syringe for 30 seconds.
  - ✔ Finally, rinse equipment twice with tap water.
- Do not share your bleach or rinse water.
- Do not share your cooker. If you must share your cooker, clean it with bleach and water before using it again.

(2) if you use drugs, do not share equipment, and (3) do not have sexual intercourse when under the influence of any drug (including alcohol) that impairs decision-making ability.[38]

The safest mechanism is to abstain from drugs. Although this is the best option for those who do not currently use drugs, it may not be a viable alternative for users who choose not to quit or for those who have no access to drug treatment services. The risk of HIV for these individuals can be eliminated if they use alternatives to injecting, such as smoking, snorting, or ingesting the drug. Risk for HIV can also be eliminated if users do not share injecting equipment. Injecting equipment (works) include needles, syringes, cookers (spoons or bottle caps used to mix the drug), cotton, and rinse water. None of this equipment should be shared.[38] Another safe tactic is for the user to have ready access to sterile equipment. This can be accomplished through community needle and syringe exchange programs that provide sterile equipment to users in exchange for used equipment. Opposition to these programs is supported by the fear that ready access to injecting supplies will increase drug use. However, studies have shown that in communities where exchange programs have been established, drug use does not increase,[46] rates of HIV infection are controlled,[47] and an overall cost benefit results.[48,49]

Cleaning equipment before use is a risk-reducing activity. It decreases the risk for those who share equipment (Table 13-14). This process takes time and may be difficult for a person in drug withdrawal.[49]

Decreasing risks of perinatal transmission. The best way to prevent HIV infection in infants is to prevent HIV infection in women.[50,51] Women who are already infected with HIV should be asked about their reproductive desires. Women who choose not to have children need to have birth control methods discussed in detail. Should they become pregnant, abortion may be desired and should be discussed in conjunction with other options.[38]

HIV-infected women who choose to become pregnant need to be aware of the AIDS Clinical Trials Group 076 (ACTG 076) study, which showed that treating HIV-infected pregnant women and their infants with zidovudine (ZDV, AZT, Retrovir) decreased the rate of perinatal transmission from 25.5% to 8.3%.[52] The study was a randomly assigned, double-blind design with placebo and treatment groups. The treatment arm provided oral zidovudine to women during the second and third trimesters of pregnancy, intravenous zidovudine during labor and delivery, and zidovudine syrup to infants during the first 6 weeks of life. Side effects for women taking zidovudine (headache, nausea, and fatigue) were not significantly different from women in the placebo group. The major side effect for infants was a transitory anemia that resolved upon completion of therapy.[52] Further research is underway to determine long-term effects in these children, efficacy of focused therapy (i.e., during one specific phase of reproduction), and benefits and risks (if any) of combination antiretroviral therapy in pregnancy. The major conclusion that comes from ACTG 076 is that women who are pregnant or contemplating pregnancy should be counseled about HIV infection, informed of their choices, routinely offered access to voluntary HIV antibody testing, and provided with optimal antiretroviral therapy if desired.[52]

Decreasing risks at work. The risk of infection from occupational exposure to HIV is small but real. The CDC and the Occupational Safety and Health Administration (OSHA) have instituted policies to ensure that employees are protected from exposure to blood and other potentially infectious fluids.[53] Precautions and safety devices decrease the risk of direct contact with blood and body fluids,[54] thereby decreasing the risk of infection with all blood-borne pathogens. Precautions for the prevention of occupational exposure to blood-borne disease are discussed in Chapter 11. Should exposure to HIV-infected fluids occur, research now confirms that postexposure prophylaxis with zidovudine (ZDV, AZT, Retrovir) reduces the rate of infection from 0.3% to 0.1%,[16] and the CDC now recommends antiretroviral postexposure prophylaxis based on the nature of the exposure and the broader range of antiretroviral drugs (Table 13-15). The possibility of treatment makes the reporting of all blood exposures even more critical.[15,16]

HIV testing and counseling. Individuals who are at risk of HIV infection should be encouraged to be tested because testing is the only definitive way to determine if infection has occurred. Testing for HIV is an important part of the public health response to HIV. When negative, testing can relieve anxieties about past behaviors and provide opportunities for prevention education; when positive, testing provides the needed

DRUG THERAPY

Table 13-15 Provisional Public Health Service Recommendations for Chemoprophylaxis after Occupational Exposure to HIV, by Type of Exposure and Source Material, 1996

Type of Exposure	Source Material[1]	Antiretroviral Prophylaxis[2]	Antiretroviral Regimen[3]
Percutaneous	Blood[4]		
	Highest risk	Recommend	ZDV plus 3TC plus IDV
	Increased risk	Recommend	ZDV plus 3TC +/− IDV[6]
	No increased risk	Offer	ZDV plus 3TC
	Fluid containing visible blood, other potentially infectious fluid,[5] or tissue.	Offer	ZDV plus 3TC
	Other body fluid (e.g., urine)	Not offer	none
Mucous membrane	Blood	Offer	ZDV plus 3TC +/− IDV[6]
	Fluid containing visible blood, other potentially infectious fluid,[5] or tissue.	Offer	ZDV plus 3TC
	Other body fluid (e.g., urine)	Not offer	none
Skin, increased risk[7]	Blood	Offer	ZDV plus 3TC +/− IDV[6]
	Fluid containing visible blood, other potentially infectious fluid,[5] or tissue.	Offer	ZDV plus 3TC
	Other body fluid (e.g., urine)	Not offer	none

Source: Update: Provisional Public Health Service recommendations for chemoprophylaxis after occupational exposure to HIV, *MMWR* 45:468, 1996.
Current updates on postexposure prophylaxis can be found at the website for this book at www.mosby.com/MERLIN/medsurg_lewis.
[1]Any exposure to concentrated HIV (e.g., in a research laboratory or production facility) is treated as percutaneous exposure to blood with highest risk.
[2]*Recommend:* Postexposure prophylaxis (PEP) should be recommended to the exposed worker with counseling (see *MMWR*). *Offer:* PEP should be offered to the exposed worker with counseling. *Not offer:* PEP should not be offered because these are not occupational exposures to HIV.
[3]Regimens: zidovudine (ZVD), 200 mg. PO tid; lamivudine (3TC), 150 mg. PO bid; indinavir (IDV), 800 mg. PO tid (if IDV is not available, saquinovir may be used, 600 mg. PO tid). Prophylaxis is given for 4 weeks. For full prescribing information, see package inserts.
[4]*Highest risk:* Both larger volume of blood (e.g., deep injury with a large diameter hollow needle previously in source patient's vein or artery, especially involving an injection of source-patient's blood) and blood containing a high titer of HIV (e.g., source with acute retroviral illness or end-stage AIDS; viral load measurement may be considered, but its use in relation to PEP has not been evaluated). *Increased risk:* either exposure to larger volume of blood or blood with a higher titer of HIV. *No increased risk:* Neither exposure to larger volume of blood nor blood with a high titer of HIV (e.g., solid suture needle injury from source patient with asymptomatic HIV infection).
[5]Includes semen; vaginal secretions; cerebrospinal, synovial, pleural, pericardial, and amniotic fluids.
[6]Possible toxicity of additional drug may not be warranted (see *MMWR*)
[7]For skin, risk is increased for exposures involving a high titer of HIV, prolonged contact, an extensive area, or an area in which skin integrity is visibly compromised. For skin exposures without increased risk, the risk of drug toxicity outweighs the benefit of PEP.

impetus to seek treatment and to protect sex and drug using partners. All testing for HIV should be accompanied by pre- and post-test counseling.[14] Table 13-16 summarizes the basic components of counseling related to HIV testing.

Acute Intervention

Early intervention. Early intervention after detection of HIV infection can promote health and limit or delay disability. Because the course of HIV is variable, assessment attains primary importance.[41] Nursing interventions are based on and tailored to patient needs noted during assessment. The nursing assessment in HIV disease should focus on early detection of symptoms, opportunistic diseases, and psychosocial problems.[38] See Table 13-9 for information on nursing assessment.

Reactions to a positive HIV-antibody test are similar to the reactions of people who are diagnosed with any life-threatening, debilitating illness. They include anxiety, panic, fear, depression, denial, hopelessness, suicidal ideation, anger, and guilt.[27] Many of these reactions also extend to the patient's family members, friends, and caregivers.[55,56] As time passes, patients and their loved ones must confront common issues associated with life-threatening illness, including (1) making difficult treatment decisions; (2) feelings of loss, anger, powerlessness, depression, and grief; (3) social isolation, imposed by self or others; (4) altered concept of the physical, social, emotional, and creative self; (5) thoughts of suicide; and (6) the possibility of death. The nurse needs to help the patient gain control. Facilitating empowerment is particularly important because the individual with HIV infection often experiences multiple losses, including an overwhelming feeling of loss of control. Empowerment is facilitated by education and honest discussions about the patient's health status and treatment options.[38,57]

Newly developed multidrug therapy protocols (sometimes called cocktails) have been shown to significantly reduce viral loads in HIV-infected patients.[25,26] Many cases of undetectable viral loads and reversals in clinical progression of HIV have been documented.[30] Nurses must be aware, however, that the protocols are complex, the drugs have side effects and interactions, and they do not work for everyone. All of these factors can contribute to problems with adherence to treatment protocols, a dangerous situation for these patients.

Table 13-16 Pre- and Post-test Counseling Associated with HIV-Antibody Testing

General Guidelines

People who are being tested for HIV are frequently fearful about the test results.
- Establish rapport with the patient.
- Assess patient's ability to understand counseling.
- Determine the patient's ability to access support systems.

Explain the benefits of testing.
- Testing provides an opportunity for education that can decrease the risk of new infections.
- Infected individuals can be referred for early intervention and support programs.

Discuss negative aspects of testing.
- Confidentiality issues: breeches of confidentiality have led to discrimination.
- A positive test affects all aspects of the patient's life (personal, social, economic, etc.) and can raise difficult emotions (anger, anxiety, guilt, and thoughts of suicide).

Pre-test Counseling

Determine the patient's risk factors and when the last risk occurred. Counseling should be individualized according to these parameters.

Provide education to decrease future risk of exposure.

Provide education that will help the patient protect sex and drug-sharing partners.

Discuss problems related to the delay between infection and an accurate test. Testing will need to be repeated at intervals for 6 months after each possible exposure. Discuss the need to abstain from further risky behaviors during that interval. Discuss the need to protect partners during that interval.

Discuss the possibility of false negative tests, which are most likely to occur during the window period.

Explain that a positive test shows *HIV infection* and not *AIDS*.

Explain that the test *does not establish immunity*, regardless of the results.

Assess support systems. Provide telephone numbers and resources as needed.

Discuss patient's personally anticipated responses to test results (positive and negative).

Outline assistance that will be offered if the test is positive.

Post-test Counseling

If the test is negative, reinforce pre-test counseling and prevention education. Remind patient that test needs to be repeated at intervals for 6 months after the most recent exposure risk.

If the test is positive, understand that the patient may be in shock and not hear much of what you say.
- Provide resources for medical and emotional support and help the patient get immediate assistance.
- Evaluate suicide risk and follow up as needed.
- Determine need to test others who have had risky contact with the patient.
- Discuss retesting to verify results. This tactic supports hope for the patient, but more importantly, it keeps the patient in the system. While waiting for the second test result, the patient has time to think about and adjust to the possibility of being HIV infected.
- Encourage optimism.
  —Remind patient that effective treatments are available.
  —Review health habits that can improve the immune system.
  —Arrange for patient to speak to HIV-infected people who are willing to share and assist newly diagnosed patients during the transition period.
  —Reinforce that an HIV positive test means that the patient is infected, but does not necessarily mean that the patient has AIDS.
- Educate to prevent new infections. HIV-infected people should be instructed to avoid donating blood, organs, or semen; sharing razors, toothbrushes, or other household items that may contain blood or other body fluids; and infecting sex-sharing and needle-sharing partners.

Adapted from Bradley-Springer L: *HIV/AIDS care plans,* ed 2, El Paso, Tex, 1999, Skidmore-Roth.

Frequently, nurses are the health care providers who work most closely with patients who are trying to cope with these issues. Interventions include education about (1) the advantages and disadvantages of new treatments, (2) the dangers of nonadherence to therapeutic regimens, (3) how and when to take each medication, (4) drug interactions to avoid, and (5) side effects that need to be reported to the primary care provider.[3] Table 13-17 provides guidance for patient education in these areas.

HIV disease progression also can be delayed by promoting a healthy immune system. Useful interventions for HIV-infected patients include (1) nutritional support to maintain lean body mass and ensure appropriate levels of vitamins and micronutrients, (2) smoking and drug-use cessation interventions, (3) moderation or elimination of alcohol intake, (4) regular exercise, (5) adequate rest, (6) stress reduction, (7) avoidance of exposure to new infectious agents, (8) mental health counseling, and (9) involvement in support groups and community activities.[14,58]

Patients should be taught to recognize clinical manifestations that may indicate progression of the disease so that prompt medical care can be initiated. Table 13-18 provides an overview of symptoms that patients should report. In general, patients should have as much information as needed to make informed decisions about health care. These decisions then dictate the appropriate interventions.[41]

PATIENT & FAMILY TEACHING GUIDE

Table 13-17 Use of Antiretroviral Drugs

- Resistance to antiretroviral drugs is a major problem in treating HIV infection. To decrease the risk of developing resistance:
  - Take three different antiretroviral drugs at a time; discuss other options with your physician or nurse practitioner.
  - Know what you are taking and how to take them (some have to be taken with food, some must be taken on an empty stomach, some cannot be taken together). If you do not understand, ask. Get your nurse to write the instructions clearly for you.
  - Take the full dose prescribed and take it on schedule. If you cannot take the drug because of side effects or other problems, report to your physician or nurse practitioner.
  - Take all of the drugs prescribed. Do not quit taking one drug while continuing the others. If you cannot tolerate one of your drugs, your physician or nurse practitioner will recommend a completely new set of drugs.
  - Many of the antiretroviral drugs interact with other drugs, including a number of common drugs you can buy without a prescription. Be sure your physician, pharmacist, or nurse practitioner knows *all* of the drugs you are taking and do not take any new drugs without checking for possible interactions.
- The goal of antiretroviral therapy is to decrease the number of viruses in your blood. This is called your viral load.
  - Viral load can be determined by tests such as the PCR or bDNA. The results are reported in absolute numbers. The goal is to get your viral load to an undetectable level. Most physicians and nurse practitioners will check this number on a regular basis whether you are taking antiretroviral agents or not.
  - Two to four weeks after you start on drug therapy (or change your therapy), your physician or nurse practitioner will test your viral load to find out if the drugs are working. These results are reported in logs (a mathematical concept). All you have to know is that you want to see the viral load drop by at least 1 log, which means that 90% of your viral load has been eliminated. If your viral load drops by 2 logs, your viral load will have decreased by 95%. If your viral load drops by 3 logs, your viral load will have decreased by 99%.

PCR, polymerase chain reaction.

Acute exacerbations. Chronic diseases are characterized by acute exacerbations of cyclical problems.[42] This is especially true in HIV disease where infections, cancers, debility, and psychosocial/economic issues interact to tax the patient's ability to cope. Nursing care becomes more complicated if the patient's immune system deteriorates and new problems arise to compound existing difficulties. When opportunistic diseases develop, symptomatic nursing care, education, and emotional support are necessary.[59]

***Pneumocystis carinii* pneumonia.** *Pneumocystis carinii pneumonia (PCP)* is caused by a fungus that is so common that most of us develop antibodies to it by the age of three.[9] A healthy immune system keeps *P. carinii* from causing disease, but an HIV-infected patient is at risk for PCP when the $CD4^+$ cell count is less than 200/μl (Fig 13-8).[60] The most common symptoms of PCP include shortness of breath, fever, night sweats, fatigue, and weight loss. It is frequently accompanied by oropharyngeal candida and a nonproductive cough that may progress to a productive cough.[60] An acute case of PCP requires intensive nursing intervention. Nursing care includes monitoring respiratory status, assessing fever and fever symptoms, administering medications and oxygen, positioning to facilitate breathing, guiding relaxation exercises to decrease anxiety, promoting nutritional support and fluid replacement, and conserving energy to decrease oxygen demand.[9] Because a high mortality rate is associated with the disease, emotional support for the patient and caregiver is particularly important.

Cryptococcal meningitis. *Cryptococcus neoformans* is a yeast that causes disease in 6% to 10% of all HIV-infected patients. When it causes meningitis, the symptoms tend to be vague, including a prolonged waxing and waning period of fever, headache, and malaise, followed by nausea and vomiting, altered mental status, stiff neck, visual disturbances, papilledema, ataxia, seizures, aphasia, and photophobia.[9,21] Nursing care includes providing medications for acute episodes and ensuring that patients understand the need to continue lifelong maintenance therapy after acute disease. Without this, 50% to 75% of patients with a history of cryptococcal meningitis will relapse within a year.[9] Additional nursing care requirements include frequent assessments of neurologic and mental status to detect subtle changes that can affect adherence to treatment regimens. In addition, nurses need to help patients prepare for and tolerate the lumbar punctures required for diagnosis and evaluation of the disease.[60]

Cytomegalovirus retinitis. *Cytomegalovirus (CMV)* is a common organism that can cause esophagitis, colitis, pneumonia, and several neurologic problems, including retinitis. Ocular disease generally will not appear until there is severe immune suppression (Fig. 13-9). Common symptoms of retinal disease include decreased visual acuity, complaints of "floaters," and unilateral visual field loss.[61] Left untreated, CMV retinitis leads to blindness. Because symptoms occur relatively late, periodic ophthalmologic examinations are recommended for early identification and treatment. Nursing care focuses on teaching the patient and caregiver about the drug therapy that needs to continue for life (see Table 13-2). The goal is to prevent vision loss, but there may be progression despite treatment. Nursing assistance can help patients cope with vision loss by altering activities of daily living, arranging referrals to agencies that provide services for vision-impaired patients, teaching about assistive devices, and providing support for loss-related grief.[38,60]

PATIENT & FAMILY TEACHING GUIDE

Table 13-18 Signs and Symptoms to Report

- Report the following signs and symptoms immediately:
  - Any change in level of consciousness: lethargy, hard to arouse, unable to arouse, unresponsive, unconscious
  - Headache accompanied by nausea and vomiting, changes in vision, changes in ability to perform coordinated activities, or after any head trauma
  - Vision changes: blurry or black areas in vision field, new floaters
  - Persistent shortness of breath related to activity and not relieved by a short rest period
  - Nausea and vomiting accompanied by abdominal pain
  - Dehydration: unable to eat or drink because of nausea, diarrhea, or mouth lesions; severe diarrhea or vomiting; dizziness when standing
  - Yellow discoloration of the skin
  - Any bleeding from the rectum that is not related to hemorrhoids
  - Pain in the flank with fever and unable to urinate for more than 6 hours
  - New onset of weakness in any part of the body, new onset of numbness that is not obviously related to pressure, new onset of difficulty speaking
  - Chest pain not obviously related to cough
  - Seizures
  - New rash accompanied by fever
  - New oral lesions accompanied by fever
  - Severe depression, anxiety, hallucinations, delusions, or possible danger to self or others
- Report the following signs and symptoms within 24 hours:
  - New or different headache; constant headache not relieved by aspirin or acetaminophen
  - Headache accompanied by fever, nasal congestion, or cough
  - Burning, itching, or discharge from the eyes
  - New or productive cough
  - Vomiting 2-3 times a day
  - Vomiting accompanied by fever
  - New, significant, or watery diarrhea (more than 6 times a day)
  - Painful urination, bloody urine, urethral discharge
  - New, significant rash (widespread, painful, itchy, or following a path down the leg or arm, around the chest, or on the face)
  - Difficulty eating because of mouth lesions
  - Vaginal discharge, pain, or itching

Mycobacterium avium complex. *Mycobacterium avium complex (MAC)* is a mycobacteria that frequently causes gastrointestinal tract problems for HIV-infected patients.[62] It is also capable of causing widely disseminated infection, invading the blood, spleen, lymph nodes, bone marrow, and liver. The signs and symptoms of MAC infection include chronic diarrhea and abdominal pain, fever, malaise, weight loss, anemia and neutropenia, malabsorption syndrome, and obstructive jaundice.[63] A major task of nursing care for patients with MAC is to teach them about the complicated drug therapy (see Table 13-2). Nurses also help patients deal with problems caused by diarrhea (see section on diarrhea later in this chapter).[60]

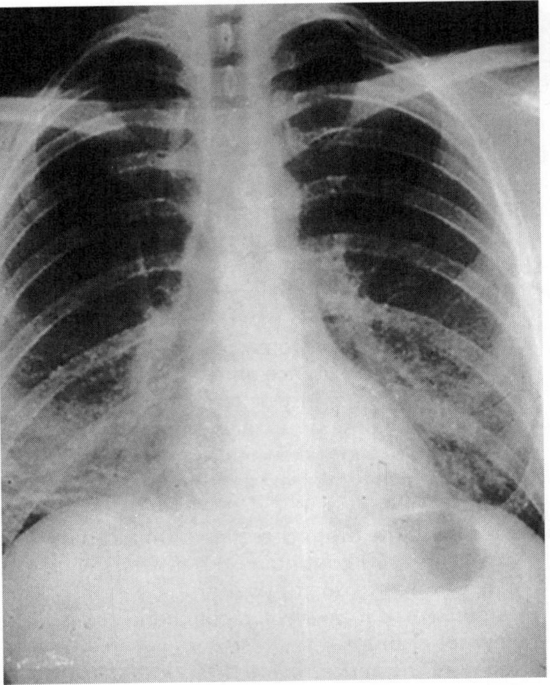

Fig. 13-8 Chest x-ray showing interstitial infiltrates as the result of *Pneumocystis carinii* pneumonia.

Ambulatory and Home Care

Ongoing care. HIV-infected patients share problems experienced by all individuals with chronic diseases, but these problems are exacerbated by social constructs surrounding HIV. Chronic diseases are characterized by negative social attitudes that label the patient as weak-willed or immoral for being sick.[42] In HIV this stigma is compounded by several factors. HIV-infected people may be seen as lacking control over urges to have sex or use drugs. It is then easy to jump to the conclusion that they brought the disease on themselves and, therefore, somehow deserve to be sick. The behaviors associated with HIV infection may be viewed as immoral (e.g., homosexuality, having many sexual partners) and are sometimes illegal (e.g., injecting heroin, sex work). The fact that infected individuals can transmit the virus to others further entrenches the negative, stigmatizing social concept of HIV. Social stigmatization supports discrimination in all facets of life.[14] HIV-infected people, for instance, have lost jobs, families, homes, and insurance because of such discrimination, even though some forms of discrimination are now illegal in the United States because of the Americans with Disabilities Act (ADA).[64]

The chronic nature of HIV infection results in the consequences seen in all such diseases: family stress, social isolation,

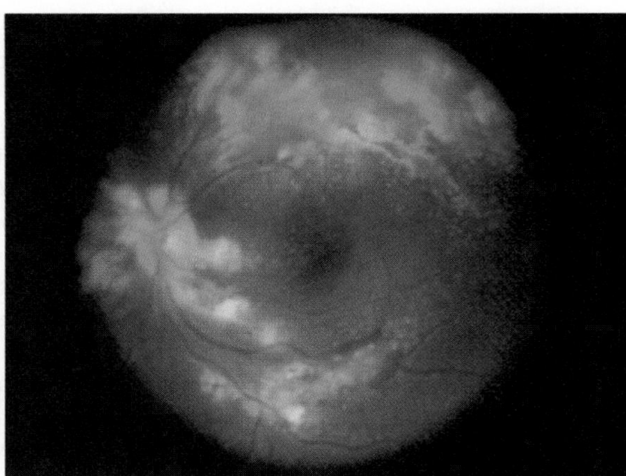

Fig. 13-9 The retina with "cottage cheese and ketchup" findings caused by cytomegalovirus (CMV) retinitis.

dependence, frustration, lowered self-image, loss of control, and economic pressures.[42,43,55,56] An interesting observation is that all of these variables may have contributed to the patient's infection in the first place. Low self-esteem, searching for social contact, frustration, and economic difficulties are all contributors to drug use and risky sexual behaviors.

Physical problems that may persist even during relatively healthy periods include diarrhea and fatigue. Diarrhea is often a continuing problem that affects as many as 60% of patients with HIV. Causes include pathogens such as CMV, herpes simplex virus, *Isospora belli, Microsporidium,* MAC, *Salmonella, Shigella,* and HIV itself. Other causes of diarrhea include some cancers, side effects of drugs, and malabsorption. The consequences of prolonged diarrhea include weight loss, dehydration, malnutrition, electrolyte imbalances, and skin breakdown, as well as social and emotional problems.[38,65]

Nursing management includes recommending dietary interventions, encouraging fluid and electrolyte replacement, instructing the patient about skin care, and managing excoriation around the perianal area. The nurse can recommend the use of incontinent products to prevent soiling of the clothes and can help patients manage antidiarrheal medications. In addition, nurses should assess for factors that may trigger the diarrhea, such as anxiety, medications, caffeine, or lactose intolerance. Relaxation techniques and alterations in the diet may provide some relief and help patients maintain control.[38,65]

Fatigue is a common symptom that can affect HIV-infected patients at any time in the spectrum of disease. It is caused by a variety of factors including chronic HIV infection, opportunistic diseases, anemia, malnutrition, diarrhea, decreased activity, and psychosocial variables. Helpful nursing interventions include education and encouraging treatment for underlying causes. Patients should be taught to assess fatigue patterns, determine contributing factors, set activity priorities, conserve energy, and schedule rest periods during the day. Exercise can improve sleep patterns, while certain substances such as caffeine, nicotine, alcohol, and other drugs may disturb sleep, adding to the fatigue.[38,41]

ETHICAL DILEMMAS

Duty to Treat

SITUATION

A nurse on a medical unit has just discovered that a patient with respiratory problems is HIV-positive. The nurse is concerned about contact with this patient and his bodily fluids, and requests she not be assigned to his care. The nurse believes that she has her own family to support and protect.

DISCUSSION

A nurse's professional obligation to treat patients in need transcends concerns about the diseases or conditions of those patients. As infectious disease health care providers often note, it is not the known HIV-positive patient who is of concern, but the one whose HIV or infectious status is *not* known that presents the greatest risk to health care providers. If a nurse's primary concern is her personal safety, she needs to reexamine her commitment to her profession. This patient can provide valuable lessons in issues related to infectious disease control, stereotyping patients, and understanding the dedication of health care providers.

ETHICAL AND LEGAL PRINCIPLES

- The Rehabilitation Act and the Americans with Disabilities Act prohibit discrimination against the handicapped and disabled. People who are HIV-infected or who have AIDS are included under these acts.
- Refusal to treat or care for people who are HIV-infected or have AIDS, when that refusal is not based on medical judgment, is as unethical as discrimination against a person based on race, gender, or any other characteristic.
- Health care professionals may not pick and choose their patients if they are true to their professional codes to provide care to all those in need.

Terminal care. Despite exciting new developments in the treatment of HIV infection, many patients will experience disease progression, disability, and death. Sometimes these occur simply because the patient fails to respond to the available therapy or becomes resistant to it. This can be devastating because of the media hype related to "miracle" recoveries among those for whom the drug protocols work. In other cases, patients may make a calculated decision to forego further treatment, allowing the disease to progress toward death. This may be especially difficult for family members and loved ones to accept. Nursing care during the terminal phase of any disease needs to focus on keeping the patient comfortable, facilitating emotional and spiritual acceptance of the finite nature of life, and helping the patient's significant others deal with grief and loss. Nurses become pivotal care providers during the terminal phase of illness, especially in HIV disease where patients and families often choose terminal care at home.

Wasting and dementia are two especially bothersome problems that frequently accompany the final stages of HIV disease. Nursing interventions can help alleviate patient discomfort and family concerns related to these problems.

Wasting, defined as a loss of 10% or more of ideal body weight, occurs in many people as death approaches. The major HIV-related nutritional problems are related to decreased nutrient intake, malabsorption, and metabolic disturbances. These problems can be caused by HIV infection itself, opportunistic diseases, therapeutic interventions, and psychosocial or economic problems. Wasting contributes to delayed recovery from infection, impaired wound healing, increased risk of secondary infection, impaired cardiopulmonary function, and early death.[66] HIV infection contributes to wasting, while wasting hastens the negative immune consequences of HIV infection, causing an insidious downward clinical spiral.[67]

Patients with wasting syndrome begin to take on the characteristics of frail, older adults. As emaciation occurs, the hair turns gray and becomes thinner, the posture slumps, and the gait becomes unsteady. Caring for the person with wasting is a tremendous nursing challenge. Interventions need to be initiated at the first sign of the problem, and include diet modifications, enteral supplements (either oral or through gastric tubes), and/or intravenous nutrition.[60] Useful interventions for wasting-related disturbances in self-concept and self-image include creating an atmosphere of acceptance and reassurance, encouraging a focus on past accomplishments and personal strengths, and facilitating the use of positive affirmations.

AIDS-dementia complex (ADC), also called HIV encephalopathy, is caused by HIV infection in the brain, but similar symptoms may result from other HIV-related central nervous system problems caused by lymphoma, toxoplasmosis, CMV, herpes virus, *Cryptococcus,* progressive multifocal leukoencephalopathy (PML), dehydration, or medication side effects. Dementia symptoms are sometimes reversible if a treatable cause is diagnosed. Treatable causes include dehydration, depression, some opportunistic diseases, and medication side effects. In addition, adequate antiretroviral drug therapy has been instrumental in decreasing the rates of HIV dementia.[21,60]

The clinical manifestations of ADC include cognitive, behavioral, and motor abnormalities. Symptoms of ADC include decreased ability to concentrate, apathy, depression, inattention, forgetfulness, social withdrawal, personality change, reduced sleep, confusion, hallucinations, slowed response rates, clumsiness, and ataxia. ADC can progress from minor symptoms to global dementia, paraplegia, incontinence, and coma.[9] Nursing interventions focus on safety, including issues related to assistance devices, home environment, and smoking. Nurses need to encourage patients to continue self-care and help caregivers support those activities, even as the patient loses the ability for total self-care. Preventing confusion

CRITICAL THINKING EXERCISES

CASE STUDY

At Risk for HIV Disease

Patient Profile

Emilio, a 20-year-old male college student, presents at the student health center with pain on urination.

Subjective Data

- Describes pain as "Just like it felt when I had the clap last year"
- Provides a history of sexual activity since age 15, reports life-time sexual partners as 6 women and 2 men
- Denies injected drug use, tobacco use, or steroid therapy
- Uses alcohol (mainly beer) at weekend parties and has smoked marijuana, but not recently
- Recent sexual activity has been on weekends during or after beer parties

Objective Data

Physical Examination

5′11″ tall, 168 lbs, temp 100.4° F (38° C), purulent urethral discharge noted

Laboratory Studies

Urethral swab positive for *Neisseria gonorrhoeae*

Collaborative Care

- IM injection with 250 mg ceftriaxone (Rocephin)
- Doxycycline 100 mg PO bid for 7 days

Critical Thinking Questions

1. Why should Emilio be encouraged to be tested for HIV?
2. How will you counsel Emilio about the testing process? How can you help him prepare for the test and the test results?
3. What further questions will you need to ask Emilio before you can determine his education needs?
4. Ask a classmate to be "Emilio" and role play HIV risk assessment, risk reduction counseling, and pre- and post-test counseling.
5. What are the main considerations to cover when teaching about barrier methods of protection?
6. How will you discuss the issue of partner notification with Emilio?
7. If Emilio's HIV test is positive, what nursing diagnoses most likely apply? If his HIV test is negative, what nursing diagnoses most likely apply?

and disorientation requires maintaining a meaningful environment, frequent reorientation, and stress reduction measures. A major emphasis also should be placed on providing support to family members and significant others who may have difficulty dealing with the patient's deteriorating mental and physical status.

Evaluation

The expected outcomes are that the patient at risk for HIV infection will

- analyze personal risk factors
- develop a personal plan to decrease risks

The expected outcomes are that the patient with HIV infection will

- describe basic aspects of the affect of HIV on the human immune system
- relate various treatment options for HIV disease
- work with a team of health care providers to achieve optimal health

CRITICAL THINKING EXERCISES—continued

CASE STUDY

Symptomatic HIV Disease

Patient Profile

Teresa, a 35-year-old single mother, was admitted to the hospital with AIDS and CMV retinitis that were diagnosed 2 days ago.

Subjective Data

- Was initially seen by a doctor 6 years ago for retrosternal pain and dysphagia, which was diagnosed as esophageal candidiasis
- Had a positive HIV antibody test at that time
- Has consistently refused antiretroviral drug therapy because "It's poison, I've seen how sick it makes other people, and besides, we can't afford it"
- Married to Jim, a former IV drug user, for 10 years until his recent death from AIDS-related complications
- Has two children, ages 6 and 8, who are both HIV-antibody negative
- Experiences fatigue and frequent oral and vaginal candidiasis outbreaks
- Expresses concern about welfare of children who are at home with her sister and says, "Maybe I should take better care of myself for them"

Objective Data

Physical Examination

5′6″ tall, 100 lbs, temp 99.8° F (37.7° C)

Laboratory Studies

$CD4^+$ T cell count — 185/μl
Viral load = 25,328 (by bDNA)
Hematocrit 30%

Collaborative Care

- Insertion of central venous catheter to be used for CMV treatment
- Trimethoprim-sulfamethoxazole
- Triple antiretroviral therapy: zidovudine (AZT, ZDV, Retrovir), lamivudine (3TC, Zerit), and indinavir (Crixivan)

Critical Thinking Questions

1. Why was Teresa's initial medical problem (esophageal candidiasis) unusual for a young, healthy woman?
2. Why is Teresa taking trimethoprim-sulfamethoxazole, and what are its common side effects?
3. What drugs are used to treat CMV retinitis? What side effects do they have, and what problems are associated with their administration?
4. Is there a potential advantage to Teresa's refusal to take antiretroviral medications in the past?
5. What teaching needs to be done before Teresa is allowed to return home after this hospitalization? What referrals need to be made?
6. What psychosocial and legal issues need to be assessed? What interventions might be appropriate?
7. What nursing interventions are immediately appropriate? What plans need to be made for continued nursing care after discharge?
8. Based on the assessment data presented, choose at least three appropriate nursing diagnoses. Are there any collaborative problems?

NURSING RESEARCH ISSUES

1. What types of interventions most influence people to change risky behaviors?
2. How can nurses help patients consistently adhere to complicated treatment regimens? What factors place patients at risk for poor adherence to drug therapy?
3. What measures can the nurse institute that will positively affect the self-esteem of patients with HIV infection?
4. What effect do relaxation exercises have on pain relief in patients with HIV infection?
5. What are the psychosocial variables that influence the ability of the family or significant other to adapt to HIV infection in a loved one?
6. What procedures, techniques, or equipment can decrease the nurse's risk of exposure to blood in a health-care setting?
7. Which oral hygiene protocols provide the best relief for HIV-infected patients with oral lesions?
8. What dietary interventions may reduce wasting?

REVIEW QUESTIONS

The number of the question corresponds to the same-numbered objective at the beginning of the chapter.

1. Transmission of HIV from an infected individual to another occurs
   a. most commonly as a result of sexual contact.
   b. in all infants born to women with HIV infection.
   c. only when there is a large viral load in the blood.
   d. frequently in health care workers with needle-stick exposures.
2. Following infection with HIV
   a. the virus replicates mainly in B lymphocytes before spreading to $CD4^+$ T cells in lymph nodes.
   b. the immune system is impaired predominantly by infection and destruction of $CD4^+$ T cells.
   c. infection of monocytes may occur, but these cells are destroyed by antibodies produced by oligodendrocytes.
   d. within weeks a long period develops during which the virus is not found in the blood and there is little viral replication.
3. In which of the following ways does HIV disease progress?
   a. seroconversion illness, latent disease, AIDS, viral depletion
   b. AIDS, acute viral loading, stage of chronicity, terminal phase
   c. asymptomatic disease, AIDS, acute retroviral reaction, latent chronic disease
   d. acute retroviral syndrome, asymptomatic infection, early symptomatic infection, AIDS
4. A diagnosis of AIDS is made when an HIV-infected patient has
   a. a $CD4^+$ T cell count $<200/\mu l$.
   b. an increasing amount of HIV in the blood.
   c. a reversal of the CD4:CD8 ratio to less than 2:1.
   d. oral hairy leukoplakia, an infection caused by Epstein-Barr virus.
5. Testing for HIV infection generally involves
   a. laboratory analysis of blood to detect HIV antigen.
   b. electrophorectic analysis of HIV antigen in plasma.
   c. laboratory analysis of blood to detect HIV antibodies.
   d. analysis of lymph tissues for the presence of HIV RNA.
6. Antiretroviral drugs are used to
   a. cure acute HIV infection.
   b. treat opportunistic diseases.
   c. supplement radiation and surgery.
   d. decrease viral RNA levels in the blood.
7. Opportunistic diseases in HIV infection
   a. usually occur one at a time.
   b. are generally slow to develop and progress.
   c. occur in the presence of immunosuppression.
   d. are curable with appropriate pharmacologic intervention.
8. Which of the following eliminates the risk of transmission of HIV?
   a. using sterile equipment to inject drugs
   b. cleaning equipment used to inject drugs
   c. taking zidovudine (AZT, ZDV, Retrovir) during pregnancy
   d. using latex barriers to cover genitals during sexual contact
9. An appropriate nursing intervention for the patient with HIV infection at risk for infection transmission would be to
   a. implement isolation procedures on all HIV-infected inpatients.
   b. monitor for signs of infection, such as fever and fatigue, to allow early detection.
   c. teach the patient about risk behaviors and risk reduction measures for transmission.
   d. evaluate the need for measures to decrease fatigue, such as frequent rest periods during eating and bathing.

References

1. Garrett L: *The coming plague: newly emerging diseases in a world out of balance*, New York, 1994, Penguin Books.
2. Wilson BA: Understanding strategies for treating HIV, *MEDSURG Nursing* 6:109, 1997.
3. Ungvarski PJ: Update on HIV infection, *AJN* 97:44, 1997.
4. U.S. Department of Health and Human Services, Centers for Disease Control and Prevention (CDC): *HIV/AIDS surveillance report* 10:12, 1998.
5. Whipple B, Scura KW: The overlooked epidemic: HIV in older adults, *AJN* 96:23, 1996.
6. Seals BF: Viewpoint: The overlapping epidemics of violence and HIV, *J Assoc Nurses AIDS Care* 7:91, 1996.
7. Johnston MI: HIV vaccines: problems and prospects, *Hosp Pract* 32:125, 1997.
8. Murray JL, Lopez AD, editors: *The global burden of disease*, Cambridge, Mass, 1996, Harvard University Press.
9. Lisanti P, Zwolski K: Understanding the devastation of AIDS, *AJN Nurs* 97:26, 1997.
10. Casey KM and others, editors: *ANAC's core curriculum for HIV/AIDS nursing*, Philadelphia, 1996, Nursecom.
11. Staprans SI, Feinberg MB: Natural history and immunopathogenesis of HIV-1 disease. In Sande MA, Volberding PA, editors: *The medical management of AIDS*, ed 5, Philadelphia, 1997, Saunders.
12. Sullivan AK, Atkins MC, Boag F: Factors facilitating the sexual transmission of HIV-1, *AIDS Patient Care and STDs* 11:167, 1997.
13. Masci JR: *Outpatient management of HIV infection*, ed 2, St Louis, 1996, Mosby.
14. Flaskerud JH: Health promotion and disease prevention. In Flaskerud JH, Ungvarski PJ, editors: *HIV/AIDS: a guide to nursing care*, ed 3, Philadelphia, 1995, Saunders.
15. Porche DJ: Postexposure prophylaxis after an occupational exposure to HIV, *J Assoc Nurses AIDS Care* 8:83, 1997.
16. Centers for Disease Control and Prevention (CDC): Update: Provisional Public Health Service recommendations for chemoprophylaxis after occupational exposure to HIV, *MMWR* 45:468, 1996.
17. Mandelbrot L: Timing of *in utero* HIV infection: implications for prenatal diagnosis and management of pregnancy, *AIDS Patient Care and STDs* 11:139, 1997.
18. Fauci AS and others: Immunopathogenic mechanisms of HIV infection, *Ann Intern Med* 124:654, 1996.
19. Casey KM: Pathophysiology of HIV-1, clinical course, and treatment. In Flaskerud JH, Ungvarski PJ, editors: *HIV/AIDS: a guide to nursing care*, ed 3, Philadelphia, 1995, Saunders.
20. Panel on Clinical Practices for the Treatment of HIV Infection: Guidelines for the use of antiretroviral agents in HIV-infected adults and adolescents, 1997, available: http://www.hivatis.org/upguidaa.html
21. Price RW: Management of the neurologic complications of HIV-1 infection and AIDS. In Sande MA, Volberding PA, editors: *The medical management of AIDS*, ed 5, Philadelphia, 1997, Saunders.
22. Centers for Disease Control and Prevention (CDC): Recommendations and Reports: 1993 revised classification system for HIV infection and expanded surveillance case definition for AIDS among adolescents and adults, *MMWR* 41:1, 1992.

23. Saag MS: Quantitation of HIV viral load: a tool for clinical practice. In Sande MA, Volberding PA, editors: *The medical management of AIDS,* ed 5, Philadelphia, 1997, Saunders.
24. Bartlett JG: *Medical management of HIV infection,* Baltimore, Md, 1998, Johns Hopkins University.
25. Saag MS: Use of HIV viral load in clinical practice: back to the future, *Ann Intern Med* 126:983, 1997.
26. O'Brien WA and others: Changes in plasma HIV RNA levels and $CD4^+$ lymphocyte counts predict both response to antiretroviral therapy and therapeutic failure, *Ann Intern Med* 126:939, 1997.
27. Flaskerud JH: Psychosocial and psychiatric aspects. In Flaskerud JH, Ungvarski PJ, editors: *HIV/AIDS: a guide to nursing care,* ed 3, Philadelphia, 1995, Saunders.
28. National Institutes of Health: Report of the NIH panel to define principles of therapy of HIV infection, 1997, available: http://www.hivatis.org/upguidaa.html
29. Richman DD: New strategies to combat HIV drug resistance, *Hosp Pract* 31:47, 1996.
30. Phillips KD: Protease inhibitors: a new weapon and a new strategy against HIV, *J Assoc Nurses AIDS Care* 7:57, 1996.
31. Mellors JW: Clinical implications of resistance and cross-resistance to HIV protease inhibitors, *Infections in Medicine* suppl:32, 1996.
32. Moore RD, Bartlett JG: Combination antiretroviral therapy in HIV infection: an economic perspective, *PharmacoEconomics* 10:109, 1996.
33. Bradley-Springer L: Prevention vs. treatment: an ongoing dilemma, *J Assoc Nurses AIDS Care* 8:87, 1997.
34. Centers for Disease Control and Prevention (CDC): Recommendations and Reports: 1997 USPHS/IDSA guidelines for the prevention of opportunistic infections in persons infected with human immunodeficiency virus, *MMWR* 46 (RR-12):1, 1997.
35. Caldwell M: The long shot, *Discover* 14:60, August 1993.
36. Grady C, Kelly G: HIV vaccine development, *Nurs Clin North Am,* 31:25, 1996.
37. Mascola JR, McNeil JG, Burke DS: AIDS vaccines: are we ready for human efficacy trials? *JAMA* 272:488, 1994.
38. Bradley-Springer L: *HIV/AIDS care plans,* ed 2, El Paso, Tex, 1999, Skidmore-Roth.
*39. Gray J: Spiritual perspective and social support in women with HIV infection: pilot study, *Image* 29:97, 1997.
*40. Sharts-Hopko NC and others: Problem-focused coping in HIV-infected mothers in relation to self-efficacy, uncertainty, social support, and psychological distress, *Image* 28:107, 1996.
41. Ungvarski PJ, Schmidt J: Nursing management of the adult client. In Flaskerud JH, Ungvarski PJ, editors: *HIV/AIDS: a guide to nursing care,* ed 3, Philadelphia, 1995, Saunders.
*42. Michael SR: Integrating chronic illness into one's life: a phenomenological inquiry, *J Holistic Nursing* 14:251, 1996.
43. Bradley-Springer L: Patient education for behavior change: help from the transtheoretical and harm reduction models, *J Assoc Nurses AIDS Care 7:* 23, 1996.
44. DeVincenzi I and others: A longitudinal study of human immunodeficiency virus transmission by heterosexual partners, *N Engl J Med* 331:341, 1994.
45. Messiah A and others: Condom breakage and slippage in heterosexual intercourse: a French national survey, *Am J Public Health,* 87:421, 1997.
46. Normand J, Vlahov D, Moses LE, editors: *Preventing HIV transmission: the role of sterile needle and bleach,* Washington, DC, 1995, National Academy Press.
47. Watters JK and others: Syringe and needle exchange as HIV/AIDS prevention for injection drug users, *JAMA* 27:115, 1994.
48. Lurie P, Drucker E: An opportunity lost: HIV infections associated with lack of a national needle-exchange program in the USA, *Lancet* 349:604, 1997.
*49. Bradley-Springer L: Needle and syringe exchange: pride and prejudice, *J Assoc Nurses AIDS Care* 8:3, 1997.
*50. Lauver D and others: HIV risk status and preventive behaviors among 17,619 women, *JOGNN* 24:33, 1995.
51. Kinsey KK: "But I know my man!" HIV/AIDS risk appraisal and heuristical reasoning patterns among childbearing women, *Holistic Nurs Pract* 8:79, 1994.
52. Centers for Disease Control and Prevention (CDC): Recommendations for the use of zidovudine to reduce perinatal transmission of human immunodeficiency virus, *MMWR* 43(RR-11):1, 1994.
53. Occupational exposure to bloodborne pathogens: Final Rule, *Federal Register* 235:64175, Dec 6,1991.
54. Centers for Disease Control and Prevention (CDC): Evaluation of safety devices for preventing percutaneous injuries among health-care workers during phlebotomy procedures, *MMWR* 46:1, 1996.
*55. Powell-Cope GM: HIV disease symptom management in the context of committed relationships, *J Assoc Nurses AIDS Care* 7:19, 1996.
*56. Phillips KD, Thomas SP: Extrapunitive and intropunitive anger of HIV caregivers: nursing implications, *J Assoc Nurses AIDS Care* 7:17, 1996.
*57. Stevens PE: Struggles with symptoms: women's narratives of managing HIV illness, *J Holistic Nursing* 14:142, 1996.
*58. McCain NL, Cella DF: Correlates of stress in HIV disease, *West J Nursing Research* 17:141, 1995.
59. Kenny P: Managing HIV infection: how to bolster your patient's fragile health, *Nursing96* 26:26, 1996.
60. Ungvarski PJ, Staats JA: Clinical manifestations of AIDS in adults. In Flaskerud JH, Ungvarski PJ, editors: *HIV/AIDS: a guide to nursing care,* ed 3, Philadelphia, 1995, Saunders.
61. Drew WL, Stempien MJ, Erlich KS: Management of herpesvirus infections (CMV, HSV, VZV). In Sande MA, Volberding PA, editors: *The medical management of AIDS,* ed 5, Philadelphia, 1997, Saunders.
62. Cello JP: Gastrointestinal tract manifestations of AIDS. In Sande MA, Volberding PA, editors: *The medical management of AIDS,* ed 5, Philadelphia, 1997, Saunders.
63. Jacobson MA: Disseminated *Mycobacterium avium* complex and other bacterial infections. In Sande MA, Volberding PA, editors: *The medical management of AIDS,* ed 5, Philadelphia, 1997, Saunders.
64. The Americans with Disabilities Act, 42 U.S.C. s. 1201 et seq. (1992 and 1994).
65. Anastasi JK, Sun V: Controlling diarrhea in the HIV patient. *Am J Nurs* 96:35, 1996.
66. Beal JA, Martin BM: The clinical management of wasting and malnutrition in HIV/AIDS, *AIDS Patient Care* 9:66, 1995.
67. Kotler DP and others: Magnitude of body-cell-mass depletion and the timing of death from wasting in AIDS, *Am J Clin Nutr* 50:444, 1989.

* Nursing research-based articles.

Resources

AIDS Action Council
1875 Connecticut Avenue, Suite 700
Washington, DC 20009
202-986-1300
http://www.aidsaction.org/

AIDS Clinical Trials Information Service
PO Box 6003
Rockville, MD 20849-6003
800-874-2572 (800-TRIALS-A)
Fax: 301-738-6616
http://www.atis.org

AIDS Education & Training Centers
5600 Fishers Lane
Room 4C-03
Rockville, MD 20857
301-443-6364
Fax: 301-443-8890

AIDS Hotline for the Hearing Impaired
800-243-7889

AIDS Infonet
http://www.aidsinfonet.org

American Foundation for AIDS Research
120 Wall Street, 13th Floor
New York, NY 10005
800-39-AMFAR
Fax: 212-682-9812
http://www.amfar.org

Association of Nurses in AIDS Care
11250 Roger Bacon Drive, Suite 8
Reston, VA 20190-5202
800-260-6780
703-925-0081
Fax: 703-435-4390
http://www.anacnet.org/aids/

CDC National AIDS Clearinghouse
PO Box 6003
Rockville, MD 20849-6003
800-458-5231
800-243-7012-TTY/TDD
Fax: 888-282-7681
http://www.cdcnac.org/

Center for AIDS Prevention Studies
74 New Montgomery, Suite 600
San Francisco, CA 94105
415-597-9100
Fax: 415-597-9213
http://www.caps.ucsf.edu/

HIV Information Web
http://www.infoweb.org/

Joint United Nations Programme on HIV/AIDS
http://www.unaids.org

National Association of People with AIDS
1413 K Street NW, 7th Floor
Washington, DC 20005
202-898-0414
Fax: 202-898-0435
703-998-3144 (BBS)
http://www.napwa.org/

National Institute for Allergy & Infectious Diseases
Building 31, Room 7A-50
31 Center Drive MSC 2520
Bethesda, MD 20892-2520
301-496-2263
http://www.niaid.nih.gov

National Minority AIDS Council
1931 13th Street NW, Suite 400
Washington, DC 20009-4432
202-483-6622
Fax: 202-544-0378
http://www.nmac.org

Safer Sex Pages
http://www.safersex.org/

San Francisco AIDS Foundation
PO Box 426182
San Francisco, CA 94142-6182
415-863-AIDS
http://www.sfaf.org/

Spanish AIDS Hotline
800-344-7432

For additional Internet resources, see the website for this book at www.mosby.com/MERLIN/medsurg_lewis

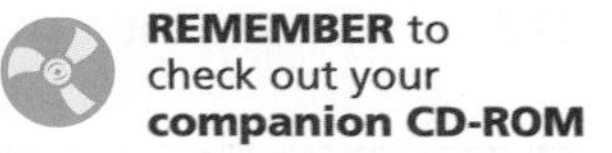

REMEMBER to check out your companion CD-ROM

14 NURSING MANAGEMENT Cancer

Catherine M. Bender, Joyce M. Yasko, & Roberta A. Strohl*

www.mosby.com/MERLIN/medsurg_lewis

LEARNING OBJECTIVES

1. Describe the prevalence and incidence of cancer in the United States.
2. Describe the processes involved in the biology of cancer.
3. Differentiate the three phases of the development of cancer.
4. Describe the role of the immune system related to cancer.
5. Describe the use of the classification systems for cancer.
6. Explain the role of the nurse in the prevention and detection of cancer.
7. Explain the use of surgery, radiation therapy, chemotherapy, and biologic therapy in the treatment of cancer.
8. Differentiate between external beam radiation and brachytherapy.
9. Identify the classifications of chemotherapeutic agents and methods of administration.
10. Describe the effects of radiation therapy and chemotherapy on normal tissues.
11. Identify the types and effects of biologic therapy agents.
12. Describe the nursing management of the patient receiving radiation therapy, chemotherapy, and biologic therapy.
13. Describe the nutritional therapy for patients with cancer.
14. Explain the role of the nurse related to unproven methods of cancer treatment.
15. Describe the complications that can occur in advanced cancer.
16. Describe the appropriate psychologic support of the patient with cancer and the patient's family.

SIGNIFICANCE

It is believed that all multicellular organisms have the potential to develop cancer at some point in their lifetime. Hippocrates coined the word *carcinoma,* meaning a tumor that spreads and destroys the host. However, the ancient Egyptians and later Galen described cancer as being crablike in nature.

Cancer is a group of more than 200 diseases characterized by unregulated growth of cells. It can occur in persons of all ages and all races and is a major health problem in the United States. An estimated 30% of Americans now living will experience cancer at some point in their lives. The overall incidence of cancer has been steadily increasing since 1970. An estimated 1,228,600 persons were diagnosed with cancer in 1998 (excluding nonmelanoma skin cancer and carcinoma in situ).[1] Some cancers, such as cancer of the stomach and uterus, have decreased in incidence in recent times whereas others, such as cancer of the lung, have increased in incidence.[2] A most notable increase in the incidence of melanoma is occurring at a rate of 3.4% per year.[1] Differences are noted in the incidence of certain cancers in men and women (Table 14-1).

Considerable progress has been made in controlling cancer for long periods of time. More than 8 million Americans alive today have a history of cancer; in 5 million of these the cancer was initially diagnosed 5 or more years ago. Many of these 5 million persons now show no evidence of disease (NED). NED usually means that the person has remained free of disease and has the same life expectancy as a person who has never had cancer.[1] This term is frequently substituted for the term *cured,* which is used cautiously because of the slow-developing nature of some forms of cancer.

Cancer is the second most common cause of death in the United States (heart disease is the most common). One of every five deaths is caused by cancer, with one half of these deaths occurring before the age of 65. The death rate as a result of cancer is leveling off or decreasing except for an increasing rate of deaths from lung cancer in women (Table 14-2). In 1998 an estimated 564,800 Americans died from cancer—more than 1500 people per day. About 175,000 of these cancer deaths were caused by tobacco use and an additional 19,000 cancer deaths were related to excessive alcohol use, frequently in combination with tobacco use.

Reviewed by Evelyn M. Clingerman, RN, MS, Visiting Professor, Oakland University, Rochester, Mich; and Shirley M. Gullo, RN, MSN, OCN, Oncology Clinical Nurse Specialist, Cleveland Clinic Cancer Center, Cleveland, Ohio.

*Contributed section on radiation therapy.

Table 14-1 Cancer Incidence by Site and Sex in 1998*

Male		Female	
Type	Percentage	Type	Percentage
Prostate	29	Breast	30
Lung	15	Lung	13
Colon/rectum	10	Colon/rectum	11
Urinary tract	9	Uterus	8
Leukemia/ lymphoma	8	Leukemia/ lymphoma	7

From *Cancer statistics 1998,* Atlanta, Ga, 1998, American Cancer Society.
*Excluding basal and squamous cell skin cancers and carcinoma in situ.

Table 14-2 Estimates of Cancer Deaths by Site and Sex in 1998

Male		Female	
Type	Percentage	Type	Percentage
Lung	32	Lung	25
Prostate	13	Breast	16
Colon/rectum	9	Colon/rectum	11
Leukemia/ lymphoma	9	Leukemia/ lymphoma	8

From *Cancer statistics 1998,* Atlanta, Ga, 1998, American Cancer Society.

The cancer incidence and death rate are higher in African-Americans than in Caucasians. This rate is especially higher among African-American males. Most of the differences in cancer rates between African-Americans and Caucasians are attributed to environmental and social rather than biologic factors.[1]

Statistics cannot reveal the physiologic, psychologic, and sociologic impact of cancer. Cancer is known to be the most feared of all diseases, feared far more than heart disease. The word *cancer* is viewed as being synonymous with death, pain, disfigurement, and dependency. However, attitudes toward cancer do not fit today's status of the treatment and control of cancer. Education of health professionals and the public is essential if current attitudes surrounding cancer and cancer care are to become more positive and realistic.

BIOLOGY OF CANCER

Cancer is a group of many diseases of multiple causes that can arise in any cell of the body capable of evading regulatory controls over proliferation and differentiation. Two major dysfunctions present in the process of cancer are defective cellular proliferation (growth) and defective cellular differentiation.

Defect in Cellular Proliferation

Normally, most tissues of the human adult contain a population of predetermined, undifferentiated cells known as stem cells. Predetermined means that the stem cells of a particular tissue will ultimately differentiate and become mature, functioning cells of that tissue and only that tissue.

Cell proliferation originates in the stem cell and begins when the stem cell enters the cell cycle (Fig. 14-1). The time from when a cell enters the cell cycle to the time the cell divides into two identical cells is called the generation time of the cell. A mature cell continues to function until it degenerates and dies.

All cells of a tissue are controlled by an intracellular mechanism that determines when cellular proliferation is necessary. Under normal conditions, a state of dynamic equilibrium is constantly maintained (i.e., cellular proliferation equals cellular degeneration or death). The process of cellular division and proliferation is activated only in the presence of cellular degeneration or death. Cellular proliferation will also occur if the body has a physiologic need for more cells. For example, a normal increase in white blood cell (WBC) count occurs in the presence of infection.

Another explanation for the phenomenon of proliferation control of normal cells is contact inhibition. Normal cells respect the boundaries and territory of the cells surrounding them. They will not invade a territory that is not their own. The neighboring cells are thought to inhibit cellular growth through the physical contact of the surrounding cell membranes.

The rate of normal cellular proliferation (from the time of cellular birth to the time of cellular death) differs in each body tissue. In some tissues, such as bone marrow, hair follicles, and epithelial lining of the gastrointestinal (GI) tract, the rate of cellular proliferation is rapid. In other tissues, such as myocardium, neurons, and cartilage, cellular proliferation does not occur.

Cancer cells usually proliferate in the manner and at the same rate of the normal cells of the tissue from which they arise. However, cancer cells respond differently than normal cells to the intracellular signals that regulate the state of dynamic equilibrium. Cancer cells divide indiscriminately and haphazardly. Sometimes they produce more than two cells at the time of mitosis. The loss of intracellular control of proliferation may be a result of a mutation of the stem cells.[3] The stem cells are viewed as the target or the origin of cancer development. The deoxyribonucleic acid (DNA) of the stem cell is substituted or permanently rearranged. When this happens the stem cell is mutated and has the potential to become malignant. It will usually proliferate at the rate of the tissue of origin, and some subpopulations can promote tumor progression to gen-

CULTURAL & ETHNIC CONSIDERATIONS

Cancer

- African-Americans have a higher incidence of cancer than Caucasians.
- Death rates related to cancer are higher for African-Americans than Caucasians.
- Native Americans have a lower incidence of cancer than any other group in the United States but have the poorest survival rate when they do get cancer.

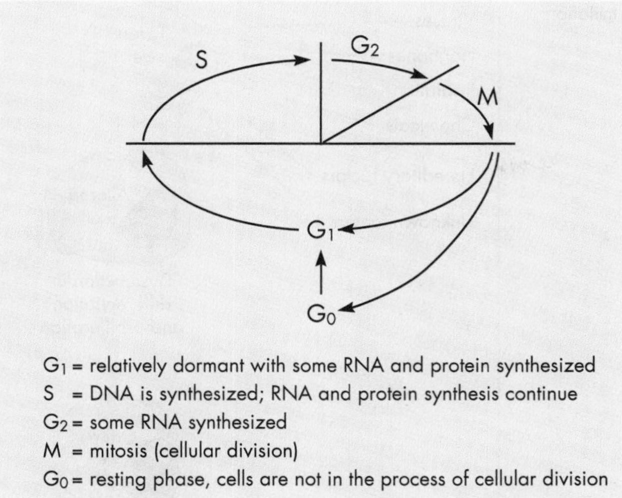

Fig. 14-1 Cell life cycle and metabolic activity. Generation time is the period from *M* phase to *M* phase. Cells not in the cycle but capable of division are in the resting phase (G_0).

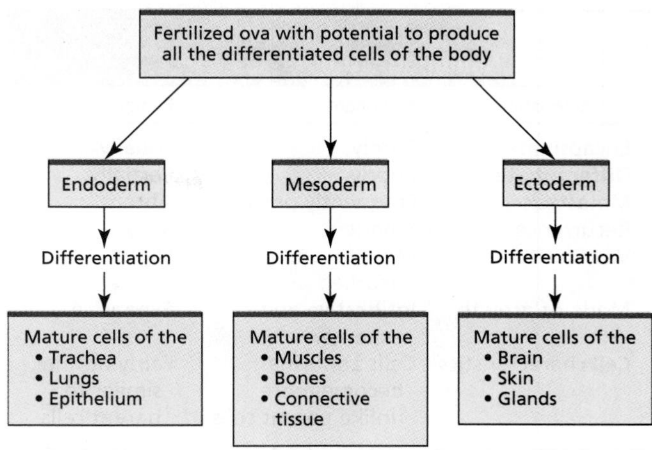

Fig. 14-2 Normal cellular differentiation.

erate malignant cells (i.e., cells with invasive and metastatic potential). The stem cell theory of cancer development is not complete, because it has been noted that malignant stem cells can differentiate to form normal tissue cells.[3]

A common misconception regarding the characteristics of cancer cells is that the rate of proliferation is more rapid than that of any normal body cell. In most situations, cancer cells proliferate at the same rate as the normal cells of the tissue from which they originate. The difference is that proliferation of the cancer cells is indiscriminate and continuous. In this way, with each cell division creating two or more offspring cells, there is continuous growth of a tumor mass: 1→2→4→8→16; and so on. This is termed the *pyramid effect.* The time required for a tumor mass to double in size is known as its doubling time.

Cancer cells grown in tissue culture are also characterized by loss of contact inhibition. These cells have no regard for cellular boundaries and will grow on top of one another and also on top of or between normal cells.

Defect in Cellular Differentiation

Cellular differentiation is normally an orderly process that progresses from a state of immaturity to a state of maturity. Because all body cells are derived from the fertilized ova, all cells have the potential to perform all body functions. As cells differentiate, this potential is repressed and the mature cell is capable of performing only specific functions (Fig. 14-2).

With cellular differentiation there is a stable and orderly phasing out of cellular potential. Under normal conditions the differentiated cell is stable and will not dedifferentiate (that is, revert to a previous undifferentiated state).

The exact mechanism that controls cellular differentiation and proliferation is not completely understood. Genes that are important regulators of normal cellular processes are proto-oncogenes. Mutations that alter the expression of these genes or their products can activate proto-oncogenes to function as *oncogenes* (tumor-inducing genes) by inducing mitosis but inhibiting differentiation of the cell.

The proto-oncogene has been described as the genetic lock that keeps the cell in its mature functioning state. When this lock is "unlocked," as may occur through exposure to carcinogens (agents that cause cancer) or oncogenic viruses, genetic alterations and mutations occur. The abilities and properties that the cell had in fetal development are again expressed. Oncogenes interfere with normal cell expression under some conditions, causing the cell to become malignant. This cell regains a fetal appearance and function. For example, some cancer cells produce new proteins, such as those characteristic of the embryonic and fetal periods of life. These proteins located on the cell membrane include carcinoembryonic antigen (CEA) and alpha-fetoprotein (AFP). They can be detected in human blood by laboratory studies (see under Role of the Immune System, later in this chapter). Other cancer cells, such as small (oat) cell carcinoma of the lung, produce hormones (see under Complications Resulting from Cancer, later in this chapter) that are ordinarily produced by cells arising from the same germ cell layer as the tumor cells.

Tumors can be classified as benign or malignant. In general, benign neoplasms are well differentiated, and malignant neoplasms range from well differentiated to undifferentiated. The ability of malignant tumor cells to invade and metastasize is the major difference between benign and malignant cells. Other differences between benign and malignant cells are presented in Table 14-3.

Development of Cancer

The following is a theoretic model of the development of cancer. The cause and development of each type of cancer are likely to be multifactorial. It is not known how many tumors have a chemical, environmental, genetic, immunologic, or viral origin. Cancers may arise spontaneously from causes that are thus far unexplained.

It is a common belief that the development of cancer is a rapid, haphazard event. However, the natural history of cancer is an orderly process comprising several stages and occurring

Table 14-3 Comparison of Benign and Malignant Tumors

Characteristic	Malignant	Benign
Encapsulated	Rarely	Usually
Differentiated	Poorly	Partially
Metastasis	Frequently present	Absent
Recurrence	Frequent	Rare
Vascularity	Moderate to marked	Slight
Mode of growth	Infiltrative and expansive	Expansive
Cell characteristics	Cells abnormal, become more unlike parent cells	Fairly normal; similar to parent cells

over a period of time. These stages include initiation, promotion, and progression (Fig. 14-3).

Initiation. The first stage, *initiation,* is an irreversible alteration in the cell's genetic structure resulting from the action of a chemical, physical, or biologic agent. This altered cell has the potential for developing into a clone of neoplastic cells.[4] Many carcinogens (agents capable of producing these cellular alterations) are detoxified by protective enzymes and are harmlessly excreted. If this protective mechanism fails, carcinogens can enter the cell's nucleus and may irreversibly bind to DNA. DNA repair is possible. However, if repair does not occur before cell division, the cell will replicate into daughter cells, each with the same genetic alteration.[4]

Carcinogens may be chemical, physical, or genetic in nature. Common characteristics of carcinogens are that their effects in the stage of initiation are irreversible and additive.

Chemical carcinogens. Chemicals were identified as cancer-causing agents in the latter part of the eighteenth century when Percival Pott noted that chimney sweeps had a higher incidence of cancer of the scrotum associated with exposure to soot residues in chimneys. As the years passed, more chemical agents were identified as actual and potential carcinogens as evidence indicated that persons exposed to certain chemicals over a period of time had a greater incidence of certain cancers than others. The long latency period from the time of exposure to the development of cancer makes it difficult to identify cancer-causing chemicals. Also, those chemicals that cause cancer in animals may or may not cause the same specific cancer in humans. Some chemicals are cancer causative in their environmental form, but others must first undergo certain metabolic changes. Chemical carcinogens thought to cause cancer in humans are listed in Table 14-4.

Certain drugs have also been identified as carcinogens (Table 14-5). Drugs that are capable of interacting with DNA (e.g., alkylating agents), as well as immunosuppressive agents, have the potential to cause neoplasms in humans. The use of alkylating agents (e.g., cyclophosphamide [Cytoxan] and nitrogen mustard), either alone or in combination with radiation therapy, has been associated with an increased incidence of acute myelogenous leukemia in persons treated for Hodgkin's disease, non-Hodgkin's lymphomas, and multiple myeloma.

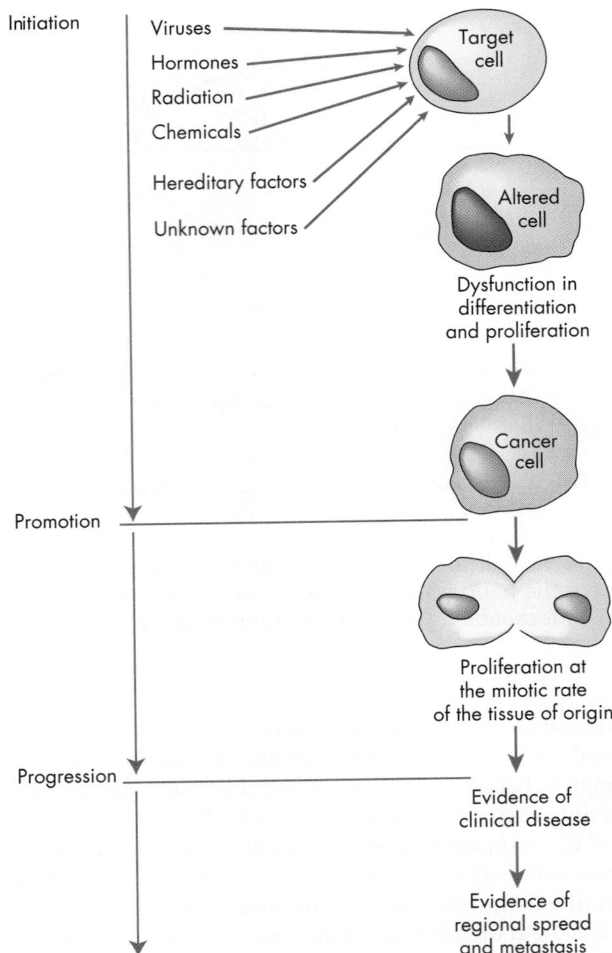

Fig. 14-3 Process of cancer development.

These secondary leukemias are relatively refractory to induction of remission with combination chemotherapy. Secondary leukemia has also been observed in persons who have undergone transplant surgery and who have taken immunosuppressive drugs.

The administration of estrogens to women has also been linked to the development of cancer. Although the use of estrogen as an oral contraceptive has not been shown to increase a woman's risk of developing cancer, the use of estrogen replacement therapy has been associated with the development of endometrial and breast cancer. Additionally, the past administration of diethylstilbestrol (DES) as an attempt to prevent miscarriages has led to an increased risk for the development of vaginal cancers in female offspring exposed to DES in utero.[4]

Chemical carcinogens associated with lifestyle have also been identified. For example, dietary factors have been demonstrated to play a role in the development of cancer. Persons who are overweight have a higher incidence of certain malignant conditions, such as colon cancer. Although evidence does not support dietary factors as capable of genetic alteration, their role is believed to be one of tumor promotion.[2]

Table 14-4 Chemical Carcinogens

Carcinogen	Associated Neoplasm
Cigarette smoke	Lung, upper respiratory tract, bladder, cervix, and other cancers
Asbestos	Mesothelioma, lung
Acrylonitrile	Lung, colon, prostate
Arsenic	Skin, lung, liver
Benzene	Leukemia
Cadmium	Prostate, kidney
Chromium compounds	Lung
Nickel	Lung, nasal sinuses
Uranium	Lung
Aflatoxin	Liver
Nitrites	Stomach
Chloromethyl ethers	Lung
Isopropyl oil	Nasal sinuses
Benzidine	Bladder
Vinyl chloride	Angiosarcoma of liver
Radiation	Numerous locations
Polycyclic hydrocarbons	Lung, skin
Mustard gas	Lung

Table 14-5 Cancers Related to Drug Exposures in Humans

Drug	Associated Neoplasm
Radioisotopes	
Phosphorus (^{32}P)	Acute leukemia
Radium, mesothorium	Osteosarcoma and sinus carcinoma
Thorotrast	Hemangioendothelioma of liver
Immunosuppressive Agents	
Antilymphocyte serum Antimetabolites Alkylating agents Corticosteroids	Reticulum-cell sarcoma, epithelial cancer of skin and viscera, acute myelogenous leukemia
Azathioprine	Lymphoma, reticulum cell carcinoma, skin cancer Kaposi's sarcoma
Cytotoxic Drugs	
Phenylalanine mustard	Bladder cancer
Cyclophosphamide	Acute myelogenous leukemia
Hormones	
Synthetic estrogens	
Prenatal	Vaginal and cervical adenocarcinoma (clear-cell type)
Postnatal	Endometrial carcinoma (adenosquamous type)
Androgenic-anabolic steroids	Hepatocellular carcinoma
Diethylstilbestrol (DES)	Vaginal cancer
Others	
Arsenic	Skin, liver cancer
Phenacetin-containing drugs	Renal pelvis carcinoma
Coal for ointments	Skin cancer
Diphenylhydantoin(?)	Lymphoma
Chloramphenicol(?)	Leukemia
Amphetamines(?)	Hodgkin's disease

Physical carcinogens. Three classifications of physical carcinogens exist: (1) ionizing radiation, (2) ultraviolet (UV) radiation, and (3) foreign bodies. Since the turn of the century, it has been known that ionizing radiation can cause cancer in almost any human body tissue. Presently, the dose of radiation that causes cancer is not known, and there is considerable debate surrounding the effect of exposure to low-dose radiation over a period of time.[2] When cells are exposed to a source of radiation, damage occurs to one or both strands of DNA. Certain malignancies have been correlated with radiation as a carcinogenic agent:

1. Leukemia, lymphoma, thyroid cancer, and other cancers increased in incidence in the general population of Hiroshima and Nagasaki after the atomic bomb explosions.
2. A higher incidence of bone cancer occurs in persons exposed to radiation in certain occupations, such as radiologists, radiation chemists, and uranium miners.
3. Thyroid cancer has a higher incidence in those persons who have received radiation to the head and neck area for treatment of a variety of disorders, such as acne, tonsillitis, sore throat, or enlarged thyroid gland.
4. A higher incidence of childhood cancer occurs in children exposed to radiation during fetal life.

UV radiation has long been associated with squamous or basal cell carcinoma of the skin. Skin cancer is the most common type of cancer among Caucasians in the United States. Of concern is the relatively recent increase in the incidence of melanoma, a skin cancer that is much less responsive to treatment. It is the second most rapidly increasing cancer in the United States.[1] Although the cause of melanoma is probably multifactorial, mounting evidence suggests that UV radiation secondary to sunlight exposure is linked to the development of melanoma.[5]

Foreign bodies that are not biodegradable, such as asbestos fibers and Bakelite disk and cellophane implants, can induce the development of cancer by stimulating reactions to constant tissue damage such as scar formation, thus increasing the probability of neoplastic formations. The exact mechanism of this neoplastic transformation is as yet unknown. However, in general, the greater the surface area exposure of the foreign body, the greater the probability of neoplastic transformation.

Certain DNA and ribonucleic acid (RNA) viruses, termed *oncogenic,* can transform the cells they infect and induce malignant transformation. Viruses have been identified as causative agents of cancer in animals and humans. One cancer found in human beings, Burkitt's lymphoma, has consistently shown evidence of the presence of the Epstein-Barr virus (EBV) in vitro.[4] This virus is also present in infectious mononucleosis, but the explanation of why an infectious disease develops in some

Table 14-6 Factors Promoting Cancer Development

Factor	Effect
Age	↑ Incidence of cancer in the young and in persons >55 yr of age
Hormones	↑ Progression of endometrial cancer in the presence of estrogen ↓ Progression of certain cancers with removal of the thyroid, adrenals, ovaries, and pituitary gland
Coping potential	↑ Progression of cancer in person with inadequate coping who exhibits feelings of hopelessness, helplessness, and being out of control (not scientifically proven at the present time)
Dietary fat, high-caloric intake	↑ Incidence and progession of cancer in persons ≥25% their recommended weight ↑ Incidence and progression of breast and gallbladder cancers in the presence of a high-fat diet ↑ Incidence and progression of colon cancer in the presence of a low-fiber diet ↑ Progression of cancer in persons with protein deficiency
Cigarette smoke	↑ Incidence of bronchogenic, esophageal, and bladder cancers
Alcoholic beverages	↑ Incidence of oral, liver, and esophageal cancers
Combination of alcohol consumption and cigarette smoke	↑ Incidence of head, neck, esophageal, and bladder cancers

persons and a lymphoma in others is not known. Persons with acquired immunodeficiency syndrome (AIDS), which is caused by a virus, have a high incidence of Kaposi's sarcoma (see Chapter 13). Other viruses that have been linked to the development of cancer include hepatitis B virus, associated with hepatocellular carcinoma, and human papillomavirus, which is believed to be capable of inducing lesions that progress to squamous cell carcinomas, such as cervical cancers.[4]

Genetic susceptibility. Few types of cancer are considered hereditary in the mendelian sense. However, what is inherited in a few cases is a strong predisposition to cancer. An example of such an inherited predisposing condition is familial polyposis coli. The incidence of carcinoma of the colon in persons with such a syndrome is 1000 times the average incidence. Several preneoplastic syndromes can be inherited and can increase the probability of certain cancers. Xeroderma pigmentosum is a preneoplastic syndrome that can be a precursor of certain skin cancers, especially with exposure to sunlight.

"Cancer families" have also been identified in which several family members develop one or several specific cancers at an early age. The specific cancers usually involve the colon and uterus. Multiple-site cancers or cancers that occur at an early age are thought to have a genetic link. The occurrence of cancer in these instances is probably a result of inherited chromosomal abnormalities.

For many years scientists have searched for genetic patterns in the most common cancer sites. The following patterns have emerged:

1. The incidence of postmenopausal breast cancer is three times higher and the incidence of premenopausal breast cancer is five times higher in women with a family history of this disease. Breast cancer is rare in Asian women and common in Caucasian women.
2. The incidence of lung cancer is greater in smokers with a family history of this disease than in smokers without a family history of the disease.
3. The incidence of leukemia is greater in an identical twin of a person with the disease.
4. Neuroblastoma occurs with increased frequency among siblings.
5. Colon cancer is more likely to occur in women who have a history of breast cancer.

Promotion. A single alteration of the genetic structure of the cell is not sufficient to result in cancer. At least one more mutation must occur in cells in which a mutation has already occurred. The chances of this occurring, given the billions of cells in the human body, seem highly unlikely. However, the odds of cancer development are increased with the presence of promoting agents.[2] *Promotion,* the second stage in the development of cancer, is characterized by the reversible proliferation of the altered, initiated cells; consequently, with an increase in the initiated cell population, the likelihood of a second cell mutation is increased.

An important distinction between initiation and promotion is that the activity of promoters is reversible. This is a key concept in cancer prevention. Promoting factors include such agents as dietary fat, obesity, cigarette smoking, and alcohol consumption (Table 14-6). Prolonged, severe stress may also be a promoter. (For a complete discussion of stress, see Chapter 7.) The withdrawal of these factors can reduce the risk of neoplastic formation.

Several promoting agents exert activity against specific types of body tissues or organs. Therefore these agents tend to promote specific kinds of cancer. For example, cigarette smoke is a promoting agent in bronchogenic carcinoma and, in conjunction with alcohol intake, promotes esophageal and bladder cancers. Some carcinogens (complete carcinogens) are capable of both initiating and promoting the development of cancer. Cigarette smoke is an example of a complete carcinogen capable of initiating and promoting cancer.

A period of time, ranging from 1 to 40 years, elapses between the initial genetic alteration and the actual clinical evidence of cancer. This period, called the *latent period,* is now theorized to comprise both the initiation and the promotion stages in the natural history of cancer.[2] The variation in the length of time that elapses before the cancer becomes clinically evident is as-

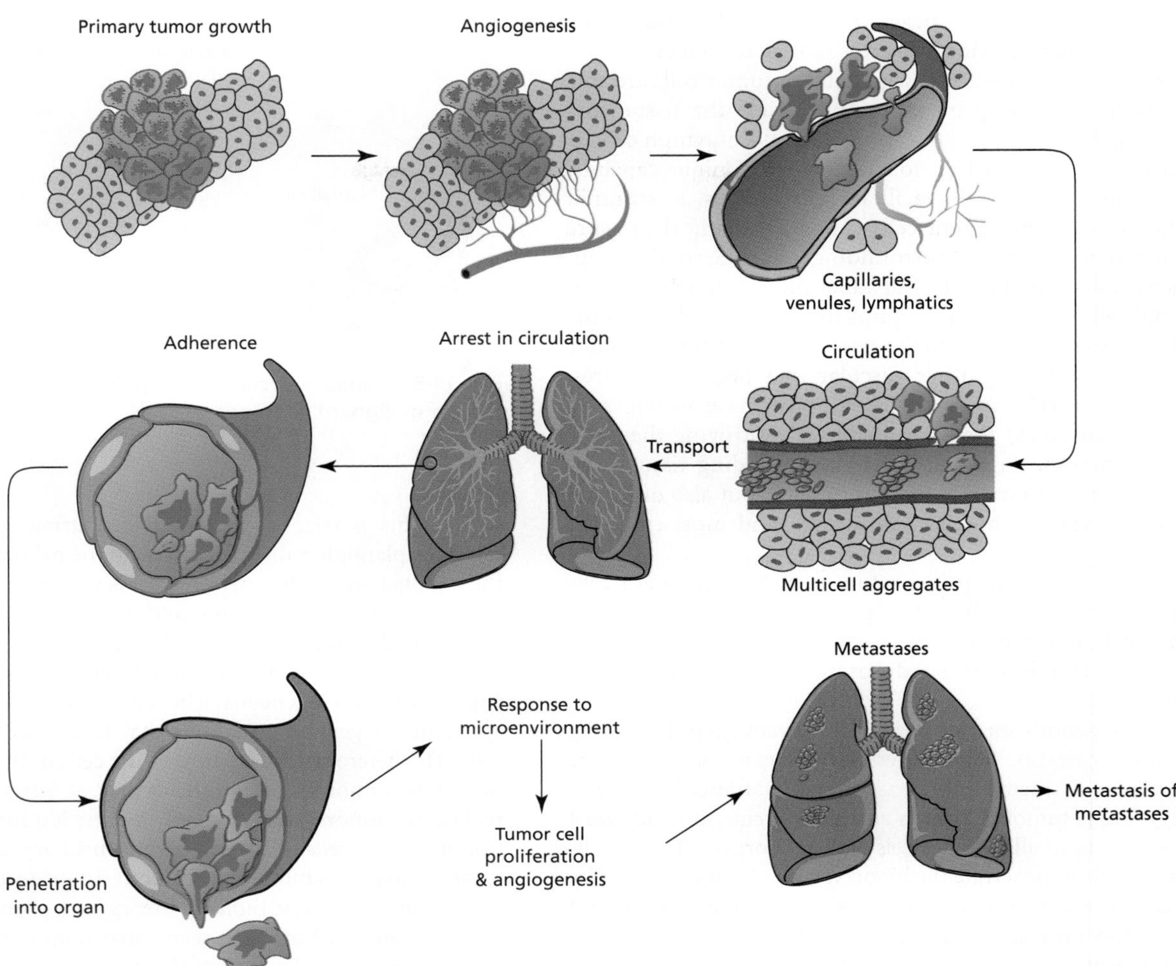

Fig. 14-4 The pathogenesis of cancer metastasis. To produce metastases, tumor cells must detach from the primary tumor and enter the circulation, survive in the circulation to arrest in the capillary bed, adhere to basement membrane, gain entrance into the organ parenchyma, respond to growth factors, proliferate and induce angiogenesis, and evade host defenses.

sociated with the mitotic rate of the tissue of origin and environmental factors.

For the disease process to become clinically evident, the cells must reach a critical mass. A 1 cm tumor (the size usually detectable by palpation) contains 1 billion cancer cells. A 0.5 cm tumor is the smallest that can be detected by current diagnostic measures, such as magnetic resonance imaging (MRI).

Progression. *Progression* is the final stage in the natural history of a cancer. This stage is characterized by increased growth rate of the tumor, as well as by increased invasiveness and metastasis. Certain biochemical and morphologic alterations also take place during this stage, enabling the tumor to survive and thrive in this primary environment and throughout the process of metastasis.

Some cancers metastasize early in the process of development (e.g., premenopausal breast cancer), whereas others spread regionally and rarely metastasize (e.g., glioblastoma multiforme and basal cell carcinoma of the skin). Certain cancers seem to have an affinity for a particular tissue or organ as a site of metastasis; other cancers are unpredictable in their pattern of metastasis (melanoma). Certain cancers ("seed") require a particular site for proliferation ("soil"). The most frequent sites of metastasis are the lungs, brain, bone, and liver. Most metastatic lesions are multiple and widely disseminated, but a few cancers such as adenocarcinoma of the kidney usually produce a single metastatic lesion.

Metastasis is a multistep process beginning with the rapid growth of the primary tumor (Fig. 14-4). This rapid growth is facilitated by the production of growth factor by tumor cells and development of a vascular system in the primary tumor. The growth of the primary tumor may cause damage within the organ, thus causing the release of growth factors. Additional nutrients are supplied by the microenvironment of the organ surrounding the tumor. As the tumor increases in size, development of its own blood supply is critical to its survival and growth. The process of the formation of blood vessels within the tumor itself is termed *tumor angiogenesis* and is facilitated by tumor angiogenesis factor produced by the cancer cells. As the tumor grows, it can begin to mechanically invade surrounding tissues, growing into areas of least resistance.[6]

Certain subpopulations (segments) of tumor cells are able to detach from the primary tumor, invade the tissue surrounding the tumor, and penetrate the walls of lymph or vascular vessels for metastasis to a distant site. Unique capabilities of some tumor cells facilitate this process. First, rapid proliferation of malignant cells causes mechanical pressure leading to penetration of surrounding tissues. Second, certain cells have decreased cell-to-cell adhesion in comparison with normal cells. This property equips these cancer cells with the mobility needed to move to the exterior of the primary tumor and to move within other vascular and organ structures. Some cancer cells produce metalloproteinase enzymes (a family of enzymes) that are capable of destroying the basement membrane (a tough barrier surrounding tissues and blood vessels) of not only the tumor itself, but also of lymph and blood vessels, muscles, and nerves, and most epithelial boundaries.[6]

Once free from the primary tumor, metastatic tumor cells frequently travel to distant organ sites via lymphatic and hematogenous routes. These two routes of metastasis are interconnected. Thus it is theorized that tumor cells metastasize via both routes.

Hematogenous metastasis involves several steps beginning with the penetration of blood vessels by primary tumor cells via the release of metalloproteinase enzymes (described previously). These tumor cells then enter the circulation and arrest and adhere to small blood vessels of distant organs. Tumor cells are then able to penetrate the blood vessels of distant organs by releasing the same types of enzymes. Most tumor cells do not survive this process and are destroyed by mechanical mechanisms (turbulence of blood flow) and cells of the immune system. However, the formation of a combination of tumor cells, platelets, and fibrin deposits may protect some tumor cells from destruction in blood vessels.

In the lymphatic system, tumor cells may be "trapped" in the first lymph node confronted or they may bypass initial lymph nodes (regional lymph nodes) and travel to more distant lymph nodes, a phenomenon termed *skip metastasis.* This phenomenon is exhibited in malignancies such as esophageal cancers and is the basis for questions about the effectiveness of dissection of regional lymph nodes for the prevention of some distant metastasis.[7]

Tumor cells that do survive the process of metastasis must create an environment in the distant organ site that is conducive to their growth and development. This growth and development is facilitated by the ability of tumor cells to evade cells of the immune system and to produce a vascular supply within the metastatic site similar to that developed in the primary tumor site. Vascularization is critical to the supply of nutrients to the metastatic tumor and to the removal of waste products. Vascularization of the metastatic site is also facilitated by tumor angiogenesis factor produced by the cancer cells.[8,9] Ultimately, metastases can occur from the initial site of metastasis to secondary sites. The processes involved in the development of secondary metastases are similar to those of the initial metastatic process.

Some cancer cells become embedded along the serosal surfaces of body organs, such as the peritoneal cavity or the pleural cavity. This is termed *implantation.* During surgical procedures, implantation may also occur in the primary organ or in the regional area if the environment is suitable.

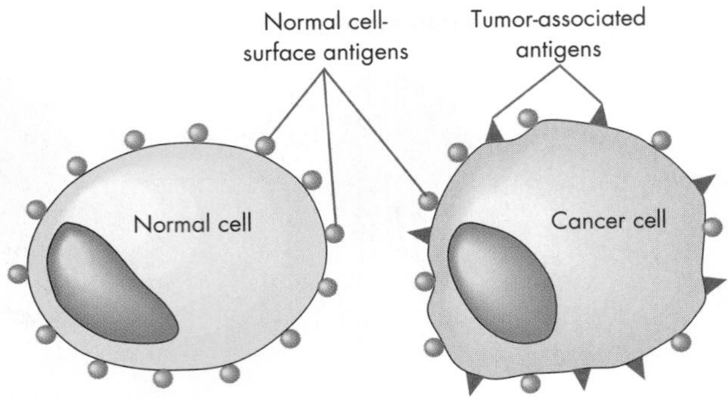

Fig. 14-5 Tumor-associated antigens appear on the cell surface of malignant cells.

Cells of the primary tumor and metastatic site may develop from a single cell or a group of identical cells (clone). However, as the primary and metastatic sites develop, the cells quickly become more heterogeneous. This change occurs as a result of spontaneous genetic mutations that take place in the tumor cells. The heterogeneous nature of the cells in the primary and metastatic tumor makes it difficult to treat. Surgical removal of metastatic tumors is of value only if there is a small number of tumors. Some cells of heterogeneous, primary, and metastatic tumors have the ability to become resistant to chemotherapy and radiation therapy. Biologic therapy is a promising form of cancer treatment because it seems that tumor cells do not develop resistance to this type of therapy.

Role of the Immune System

This section is limited to a discussion of the role of the immune system in the recognition and destruction of tumor cells. (For a detailed discussion of immune system function, see Chapter 12.)

Both the normal and abnormal cell have a complex array of antigenic determinants (markers) on the surface of the cell membrane and within the cell itself. These antigenic determinants differ from one cell type to another. When foreign cells are transplanted from one individual to another individual, these antigenic determinants elicit an immunologic response. This is the basis for rejection of a transplanted organ.

Some cancer cells have changes on their cell surface antigens as a result of malignant transformation. These antigens are termed *tumor-associated antigens* (TAAs) (Fig. 14-5). TAAs are antigens found on tumor cells and undetected on the cells of a normal adult, but they may be found on normal cells under special circumstances (e.g., fetal antigens that are normally expressed during embryonic development). In addition to the retrogenetic expression of oncofetal antigens, TAAs may result from mutations in the cell's DNA (e.g., by chemical carcinogens) or the expression of new genetic material introduced by a virus (e.g., oncogenic DNA or RNA viruses).[10]

It is believed that one of the functions of the immune system is to respond to TAAs. The response of the immune system to antigens of the malignant cells is termed *immunologic surveil-*

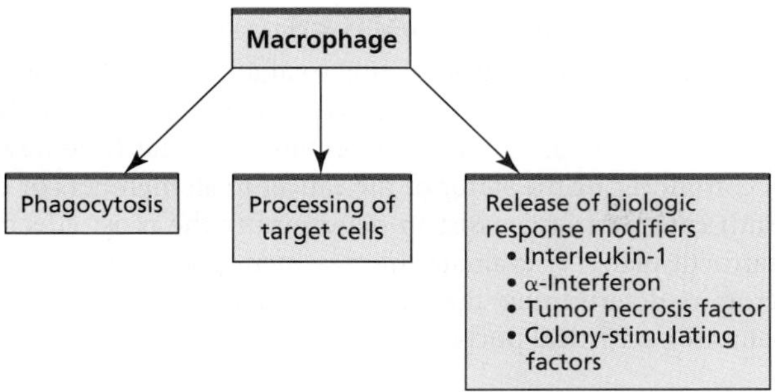

Fig. 14-6 Macrophage functioning in response to malignant target cells.

lance. Lymphocytes continually check cell surface antigens and detect and destroy cells with abnormal or altered antigenic determinants. It has been proposed that malignant transformation occurs continuously and that the malignant cells are destroyed by the immune response. Under most circumstances, immune surveillance will prevent these transformed cells from developing into clinically detectable tumors.[11]

Virtually every cell type involved in normal immune responses and every effector function used to inactivate or remove antigens has been demonstrated in immune responses to tumors. These immune responses involve cytotoxic T cells, natural killer cells, macrophages, and B lymphocytes.

Cytotoxic T cells are thought to play a dominant role in resisting tumor growth. These cells are capable of killing tumor cells. T cells are also important in the production of cytokines (e.g., interleukin-2 [IL-2] and γ-interferon), which stimulate T cells, natural killer cells, B cells, and macrophages.

Natural killer (NK) cells are able to directly lyse tumor cells spontaneously without any prior sensitization. These cells are stimulated by γ-interferon and IL-2 (released from T cells), resulting in increased cytotoxic activity.

Monocytes and macrophages have several important roles in tumor immunity (Fig. 14-6). Macrophages can be activated by γ-interferon (produced by T cells) to become nonspecifically lytic for tumor cells. Macrophages also secrete cytokines including (1) IL-1, (2) α-interferon, (3) tumor necrosis factor (TNF), and (4) colony-stimulating factors. The release of IL-1, coupled with the presentation of the processed antigen, stimulates T lymphocyte activation and production. α-Interferon augments the killing ability of NK cells. TNF causes hemorrhagic necrosis of tumors and exerts cytocidal or cytostatic actions against tumor cells. Colony-stimulating factors regulate the production of various blood cells in the bone marrow and stimulate the function of various WBCs.

B lymphocytes can produce specific antibodies that bind to tumor cells and can kill these cells by complement fixation and lysis (see Chapter 11). These antibodies are often detectable in the serum and saliva of the patient. In some persons, antibodies that are apparently specific for both the person's own tumor and a similar tumor in other persons have been found.[11]

Certain groups of people have a higher incidence of cancer than the general population. Cancer occurs in approximately 10% of children with congenital immunodeficiencies. These cancers are derived primarily from cells of the lymphoid system. The person who receives high doses of immunosuppressive drugs has an 80- to 100-fold increased risk of developing cancer. The types of cancer found in immunosuppressed persons are primarily epithelial or lymphoid. These findings are mostly reported in patients treated with immunosuppressive agents for organ transplantation, in patients with autoimmune diseases such as rheumatoid arthritis and systemic lupus erythematosus, and in patients with human immunodeficiency virus (HIV) infection.[10]

Other groups at an increased risk of cancer include very young persons and older adults. In the very young person the immune system is immature. The incidence of cancer increases dramatically in persons 40 to 60 years of age; the reasons for this are not known. It is possible that the immunologic surveillance system of the older adult works less effectively. It is also known that the thymus undergoes involution and atrophy with aging. In addition, the functional efficiency of T cells decreases with aging.

Escape Mechanisms from Immunologic Surveillance. Tumor development has been termed *immunologic escape.* In many persons with cancer there is evidence of an active immunologic response, yet the tumor survives. Theoretic explanations for immunologic escape that have been proposed follow.

Sneaking through. The process of sneaking through is thought to occur when the cell-surface antigens are weak. Cancer cells in the early phase of growth may not excite an immunologic response because the transformed cell-surface markers are of low antigenicity. By the time the immune system is alerted, the cancer is well established and too large for the immune system to destroy.

Antigenic modulation. The malignant cell has the ability to change or lose antigenic determinants during or after a response by the immune system. The cell may then express a new set of antigens. This process is termed *antigenic modulation.* The new set of antigens on the malignant cell fails to adequately stimulate the immune system.

Overwhelming antigen exposure. Cancers may escape attack by flooding the body with tumor antigen. The antigens bind to specific antibodies or to receptors on lymphocytes and prevent them from recognizing and destroying the cancer cells. The excess of antigens paralyzes the host immune system, enhancing tumor growth.

Blocking factors. Blocking factors can prevent the attack of the TAAs by T lymphocytes. For example, blocking antibodies may bind with TAAs and prevent their recognition by T cells (Fig. 14-7). Another possibility is that free antigen produced and released by the malignant cell may bind with the T cell and prevent it from recognizing the malignant cell. These blocking factors related to the immune system can actually enhance tumor growth. This is termed *immunologic enhancement.*

Oncofetal Antigens. Oncofetal antigens, also called carcinofetal antigens, are a type of tumor antigen. They are found on both the surfaces and the inside of cancer cells, as well as fetal cells. These antigens are an expression of the shift of cancerous cells to a more immature metabolic pathway, an expression usually associated with embryonic or fetal periods of life. The reappearance of fetal antigens in malignant disease

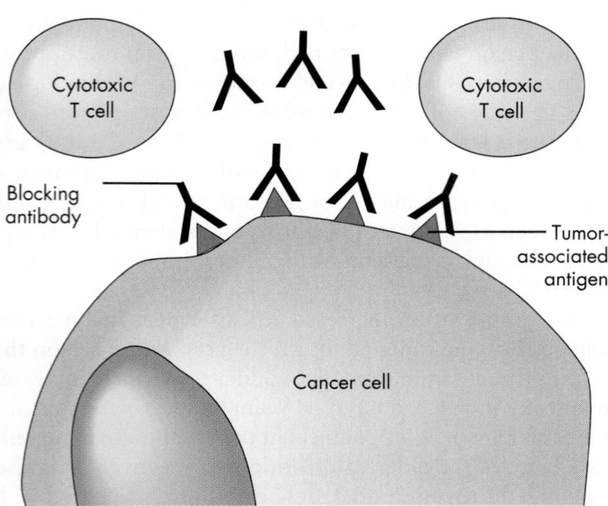

Fig. 14-7 Blocking antibodies prevent T cells from interacting with tumor-associated antigens and from destroying the malignant cell.

is not well understood, but it is believed to occur as a result of the cell regaining the cellular potential that it once had.

Examples of oncofetal antigens are CEA and AFP. CEA is found on the surfaces of cancer cells derived from the GI tract and from normal cells from the fetal gut, liver, and pancreas. Normally, it disappears during the last 3 months of fetal life. CEA was originally isolated from colon cancer cells. However, elevated CEA levels have also been found in nonmalignant conditions (e.g., cirrhosis of the liver, ulcerative colitis, and heavy smoking). Presently, the major value of CEA is its use as an indicator of the success of cancer treatment. For example, the persistence of elevated preoperative CEA titers after surgery indicates that the tumor is not completely removed. A rise in CEA levels after chemotherapy or radiation therapy may indicate recurrence or spread of the cancer.

AFP is produced by malignant liver cells, as well as fetal liver cells. AFP levels have also been found to be elevated in some cases of testicular carcinoma, viral hepatitis, and nonmalignant liver disorders. AFP has diagnostic value in primary cancer of the liver (hepatoma), but it is also produced when metastatic liver growth occurs. The detection of AFP is of value in tumor detection and determination of tumor progression.

Other examples of oncofetal antigens currently being studied are CA-125, found in ovarian carcinoma; CA-19-9, found in pancreatic, colon, and breast cancer; and prostate-specific antigen (PSA), found in prostate cancer.

Virus-induced Antigens. TAA may be induced by certain viruses. In experimental animals, DNA and RNA viruses induce unique nuclear and cell-surface antigens in cells. Establishing these findings in humans is difficult. The DNA viruses include adenovirus and various herpesviruses. Three major human DNA virus-induced tumors are Burkitt's lymphoma, nasopharyngeal carcinoma, and cancer of the cervix. RNA viruses have been correlated with leukemia in mice and other animals, as well as with mouse mammary tumors. Presently, conclusive evidence that human leukemia is a virus-induced disease does not exist.[2]

CLASSIFICATION OF CANCER

Tumors can be classified according to anatomic site, histologic analysis (grading), and extent of disease (staging). Tumor classification systems are intended to provide a standardized way to (1) communicate the status of the cancer to all members of the health care team, (2) assist in determining the most effective treatment plan, (3) evaluate the treatment plan, (4) serve as a factor in determining the prognosis, and (5) compare like groups for statistical purposes.

Anatomic Site Classification

In the anatomic classification of tumors, the tumor is identified by the tissue of origin, the anatomic site, and the behavior of the tumor (i.e., benign or malignant) (Table 14-7). Carcinomas originate from embryonal ectoderm (skin and glands) and endoderm (mucous membrane linings of the respiratory tract, GI tract, and genitourinary [GU] tract). Sarcomas originate from embryonal mesoderm (connective tissue, muscle, bone, and fat). Lymphomas and leukemias originate from the hematopoietic system.

Histologic Analysis Classification

In histologic grading of tumors, the appearance of cells and the degree of differentiation are evaluated. For many tumor cells, four grades are used:

Grade I. Cells differ slightly from normal cells (mild dysplasia) and are well differentiated.
Grade II. Cells are more abnormal (moderate dysplasia) and moderately differentiated.
Grade III. Cells are very abnormal (severe dysplasia) and poorly differentiated.
Grade IV. Cells are immature and primitive (anaplasia) and undifferentiated; cell of origin is difficult to determine.

Extent of Disease Classification

The extent of disease classification is termed *staging.* This classification system is based on a description of the extent of the disease rather than on cell appearance. Although there are similarities in the staging of cancers, there are many differences based on a thorough knowledge of the natural history of each specific type of cancer.

Clinical Staging. The clinical staging classification system determines the extent of the disease process of cancer by stages:

Stage 0: cancer in situ
Stage I: tumor limited to the tissue of origin; localized tumor growth
Stage II: limited local spread
Stage III: extensive local and regional spread
Stage IV: metastasis

This classification system has been used as a basis for staging in cancer of the cervix (see Table 51-13 and Hodgkin's disease (see Fig. 29-14).

TNM Classification System. The TNM classification system represents the standardization of the clinical staging of cancer by the International Union Against Cancer (IUCC).

Table 14-7 Anatomic Classification of Tumors

Site	Benign	Malignant
Epithelial Tissue Tumors*	-oma	-carcinoma
Surface epithelium	Papilloma	Carcinoma
Glandular epithelium	Adenoma	Adenocarcinoma
Connective Tissue Tumors†	-oma	-sarcoma
Fibrous tissue	Fibroma	Fibrosarcoma
Cartilage	Chondroma	Chondrosarcoma
Striated muscle	Rhabdomyoma	Rhabdomyosarcoma
Bone	Osteoma	Osteosarcoma
Nervous Tissue Tumors	-oma	-oma
Meninges	Meningioma	Meningeal sarcoma
Nerve cells	Ganglioneuroma	Neuroblastoma
Hematopoietic Tissue Tumors		
Lymphoid tissue	—	Hodgkin's disease, non-Hodgkin's lymphoma
Plasma cells		Multiple myeloma
Bone marrow		Lymphocytic and myelogenous leukemia

*Body surfaces, lining of body cavities, and glandular stuctures.
†Supporting tissue, fibrotic tissue, and blood vessels.

Table 14-8 TNM Classification System

Primary Tumor (T)	
T_0	No evidence of primary tumor
T_{is}	Carcinoma in situ
$T_{1\text{-}4}$	Ascending degrees of increase in tumor size and involvement
Regional Lymph Nodes (N)	
N_0	No evidence of disease in lymph nodes
$N_{1\text{-}4}$	Ascending degrees of nodal involvement
N_x	Regional lymph nodes unable to be assessed clinically
Distant Metastases (M)	
M_0	No evidence of distant metastases
$M_{1\text{-}4}$	Ascending degrees of metastatic involvement of the host, including distant nodes

This classification system (Table 14-8) is used to determine the extent of the disease process of cancer according to three parameters: tumor size (T), degree of regional spread to the lymph nodes (N), and metastasis (M). (This system has been applied to cancer of the breast in Chapter 49.)

Staging of the disease can be done initially and at several intervals. Clinical diagnostic staging is done at the time of diagnosis to determine the most effective treatment plan. Examples of diagnostic studies that may be performed to assess for spread of disease include bone and liver scans, ultrasonography, computerized tomography (CT), and MRI.

Surgical evaluative staging is used to describe the extent of the disease process after biopsy or surgical exploration. For example, a laparotomy and a splenectomy may be performed in staging of Hodgkin's disease. During a staging laparotomy, areas of lymph node biopsy and margins of any masses may be marked with metal clips. These clips are used as markers when radiotherapy is used as a treatment modality.

Postsurgical treatment pathologic staging is used after pathologic examination of the surgical specimen. The presence of residual tumor should be recorded at this time. The stages are R_0 (no residual tumor), R_1 (microscopic residual tumor), and R_2 (macroscopic residual tumor).

After the extent of the disease is determined, the stage classification is not changed. The original description of the extent of the tumor remains part of the original record. If additional treatment is needed, or if treatment fails, retreatment staging is done to determine the extent of the disease process at the time of retreatment.

Carcinoma in situ is a commonly used term in classification of cancer. It is defined as a lesion with all the histologic features of cancer except invasion. If left untreated, carcinoma in situ will eventually become invasive.

In addition to tumor classification systems, there are also classification systems used to describe the status of the patient with cancer. The status of the patient is recorded at the time of diagnosis, treatment, and retreatment and at each follow-up examination. The Karnofsky functional performance scale is an example of a method used to evaluate the performance status of the patient (Table 14-9).

PREVENTION AND DETECTION OF CANCER

The nurse plays a prominent role in the prevention and detection of cancer. Early detection and prompt treatment are directly responsible for increased survival rates in patients with cancer. One important aspect is to educate the public to do the following:

1. Reduce or avoid exposure to known or suspected carcinogens and cancer-promoting agents, including cigarette smoke and sun exposure.
2. Eat a balanced diet that includes vegetables (green, yellow, and orange), fresh fruits, whole grains, and adequate amounts of fiber, and reduce the amount of fat and preservatives, including smoked and salt-cured meats.

Table 14-9 Karnofsky Performance Scale

100	Normal; no complaints; no evidence of disease
90	Ability to carry on normal activity; minor signs or symptoms of disease
80	Normal activity with effort; some signs or symptoms of disease
70	Ability to care for self; inability to carry on normal activity or do active work
60	Occasional assistance necessary but ability to care for most needs
50	Considerable assistance and frequent medical care necessary
40	Disabled; special care and assistance necessary
30	Severely disabled; indication for hospitalization although death not imminent
20	Very sick; hospitalization necessary; active supportive treatment necessary
10	Moribund; fatal processes progressing rapidly
0	Dead

3. Participate in a regular exercise regimen.
4. Obtain adequate, consistent periods of rest (at least 6 to 8 hours per night).
5. Have a health examination on a regular basis that includes a health history, a physical examination, and specific diagnostic tests for common cancers in accordance with the guidelines published by the American Cancer Society[12] (Table 14-10).
6. Eliminate, reduce, or change the perceptions of stressors and enhance the ability to effectively cope with stressors (see Chapter 7).
7. Enjoy consistent periods of relaxation and leisure.
8. Know the seven warning signs of cancer as identified by the American Cancer Society (Table 14-11).
9. Learn and practice self-examination (e.g., breast self-examination and testicular self-examination).
10. Seek immediate medical care if cancer is suspected. Early detection of cancer has a positive impact on prognosis.

When the public is educated regarding the disease process of cancer, care should be taken to minimize the fear that surrounds the diagnosis of cancer. Tactics that increase fear should never be used. The facts should be taught in an accurate, low-key manner at the level of the learner. The goal of public education is to motivate the learner to change the pattern of behavior as necessary to achieve and maintain an optimal state of health. The nurse can play a significant role in meeting this goal. Although the general public must be taught, those who are at an increased risk of cancer are the target population for effective cancer control (see Table 14-10). The nurse can have a definite impact in convincing people that a change in lifestyle patterns will have a positive influence on health. If the nurse is to have a significant impact, the challenge must be recognized and strategies must be developed to teach cancer control effectively.

RESEARCH

IMPLICATIONS FOR NURSING PRACTICE

Cancer Detection

Citation Nichols BS, Misra R, Alexy B: Cancer detection: how effective is public education? *Cancer Nurs* 19:98, 1996.

Purpose To examine the attitudes, knowledge, and belief of laypersons regarding cancer prevention and detection methods.

Methods A convenience sample of 172 laypersons ages 18 to 80 years old completed a four-part questionnaire. The first section contained questions about the individual, health practices, and risk status. The second section obtained information on the subject's ability to identify the seven warning signs of cancer. Attitudes toward cancer detection methods were evaluated in the third section. The fourth section asked the subjects to respond to 24 statements indicating their beliefs about the importance of cancer detection.

Results and Conclusions Although the sample was predominantly white and middle class, 19% of the sample could not identify any of the cancer warning signs. The median number of warning signs correctly identified was 3. Gender was not related to scores on attitudes or beliefs about cancer detection. Race was significantly related to scores on the attitudes toward cancer detection. Level of education was positively related to scores on attitudes.

Implications for Nursing Practice The key to early detection of cancer is an informed public who recognize warning signs of cancer. Survival of cancer is linked to early detection. Nurses must know the seven warning signs so they can teach others. Community awareness programs should be organized and implemented to educate the public about the warning signs of cancer. Educational packages for children using the acronym of CAUTION could result in more effective learning and a better educated public.

Diagnosis of Cancer

When a patient has a possible diagnosis of cancer, it is a stressful time for the patient and the family. The patient typically undergoes several days to weeks of diagnostic studies. During this time the fear of the unknown may be more stressful than ultimately being told of a positive diagnosis of cancer.

During the time the patient is waiting for the results of the diagnostic studies, the nurse should be available to actively listen to the patient's concerns. False reassurance that everything will be all right is inappropriate and may shut off further communication with the patient. During this time of high anxiety the patient may need repeated explanations regarding the

Table **14-10** Screening for Specific Cancer Sites

High-Risk Profile	Screening	Medium- and Low-Risk Profile	Screening
Lung Cancer			
History of 20 pack-years of smoking (1 pack a day for 20 years); exposure to airborne carcinogens, especially asbestos, uranium, hydrocarbons; age range 40 to 80 years; chronic lung disease	Early detection method not available; annual chest x-rays (advised by some physicians); observation by patient for change in respiratory status; increased frequency of infections and change in cough, sputum, breathing, voice	History of less than 20 pack-years of smoking, nonsmokers exposed to passive cigarette smoke from smokers, nonsmokers, former smokers after 10 years	Early detection method not available
Colon and Rectal Cancer			
History of familial polypopsis, ulcerative colitis, Crohn's disease; personal or family history of colon or rectal cancer; diet high in fat and low in fiber; age range 40 to 75 years	Guaiac test on stools and digital rectal examination annually after age 40; sigmoidoscopic examination every 3 to 5 years with beginning age based on advice of physician; observation by patient for changes in bowel pattern: diarrhea, constipation, pain, flatus, black tarry stools, bleeding	Persons with no known risk factors	Guaiac test on stools and digital rectal examination annually after age 40; sigmoidoscopy, preferably flexible, as a baseline at age 50; after two normal examinations, repeated proctosigmoidoscopic examination every 3 to 5 years
Prostatic Cancer			
Presence of prostatic hyperplasia, presence of prostatic infection, African-American, increased risk with age	Digital rectal examination and prostate-specific antigen blood test annually age 50 and over; observation by patient for dysuria, blood in urine, difficulty in producing stream of urine	Presence of one risk factor, excluding age	Digital rectal examination and prostate-specific antigen blood test annually age 50 and over
Cervical Cancer			
Early intercourse (before age 18) with multiple partners or with partners who have had multiple partners, poor personal hygiene, infected with human immunodeficiency virus (HIV), genital warts, chlamydia, gonorrhea, cervical dysplasia, smoking	Pap test and pelvic examination every year for women who are or have been sexually active or who have reached age 18; colposcopy if suspicious area is noted; observation by patient for abnormal vaginal bleeding or discharge, pain or bleeding with sexual intercourse	No known risk factors	Pap test and pelvic examination every year after age 18; after 3 or more normal examinations in a row, at least every 3 years. Pap test may be performed less frequently at the discretion of the physician.
Endometrial Cancer			
Infertility, never having children, early menarche, late menopause, ovarian dysfunction, obesity, uterine bleeding, estrogen replacement therapy and tamoxifen over long period of time, diabetes, hypertension, gallbladder disease, exposure to pelvic radiation, over age 50	Pap test every year; pelvic examination every year; endometrial biopsy for women at menopause and at high risk; observation by patient for abnormal uterine bleeding, pain, change in menstrual pattern	Presence of one risk factor, excluding estrogen therapy, over long period of time	Pap test and pelvic examination, observation by patient for abnormal uterine bleeding, pain, change in menstrual pattern

Source: Based on the American Cancer Society 1996 Recommendations.

Continued

Table 14-10 Screening for Specific Cancer Sites—cont'd

High-Risk Profile	Screening	Medium- and Low-Risk Profile	Screening
Skin Cancer			
Prolonged exposure to sun; three or more blistering sunburns during adolescence; previous radiation exposure; fair, thin skin; positive family history of dysplastic nevus syndrome (DNS)	Self-examination monthly; physical examination every year; observation by patient for sore that does not heal, change in size, shape, or color of wart or mole	Presence of one risk factor, excluding prolonged exposure to sun	Self-examination, physical examination each year; observation by patient for sore that does not heal, change in size, shape, or color of wart or mole
Breast Cancer			
Caucasian, early menarche, late menopause, fibrocystic breast disease, infertility, over age 30 for first pregnancy, personal history of breast cancer, mother or sister with history of breast cancer, obesity, age range 35 to 65	Monthly breast self-examination; breast examination by health professional every 3 years for women age 20 to 40 and every year after age 40; baseline mammogram at age 40, every 1 to 2 years between ages 40 and 49, and every year after age 49; observation by patient for lump or thickening discharge from nipple, pain in breast	Excluding family history of breast cancer, fewer than two risk factors	Monthly breast self-examination; breast examination by health professional every 3 years for women age 20 to 40 and every year after age 40; baseline mammogram at age 40, every 1 to 2 years between ages 40 and 49, and every year after age 49; observation by patient for lump or thickening discharge from nipple, pain in breast

Table 14-11 Seven Warning Signs of Cancer

C	hange in bowel or bladder habits
A	sore that does not heal
U	nusual bleeding or discharge from any body orifice
T	hickening or a lump in the breast or elsewhere
I	ndigestion or difficulty in swallowing
O	bvious change in a wart or mole
N	agging cough or hoarseness

diagnostic workup. Explanations should include as much information as needed by the patient and the family; the information should be given in clear, understandable terms and should be reinforced as necessary. Written information is helpful for reinforcement of verbal information.

A diagnostic plan for the person in whom cancer is suspected includes health history, identification of risk factors, physical examination, and specific diagnostic studies. (The specifics of the health history and the screening physical examination are presented in Chapter 5.)

The health history includes particular emphasis on risk factors, such as family history of cancer, exposure to or use of known carcinogens (e.g., cigarette smoking and exposure to occupational pollutants or chemicals), diseases characterized by chronic inflammation (e.g., ulcerative colitis), and drug ingestion (e.g., hormone therapy). Other important information relates to dietary habits, ingestion of alcohol, lifestyle, and patterns and degree of coping with perceived stressors.

The physical examination should be thorough, and particular attention should be given to the respiratory system, the GI system (including colon, rectum, and liver), the lymphatic system (including the spleen), the breasts, the skin, the reproductive system of the male (testicles, prostate gland) and of the female (cervix, uterus, ovary), and the musculoskeletal and neurologic systems.

Diagnostic studies to be performed will depend on the suspected primary or metastatic site(s) of the cancer. (Specific procedures as they relate to each body system are discussed in the respective assessment chapters.) Examples of studies that may be included in the process of diagnosing cancer include the following:

1. Cytology studies (e.g., Pap smear)
2. Chest x-ray
3. Complete blood count
4. Proctoscopic examination (including guaiac for occult blood)
5. Liver function studies
6. Radiographic studies (e.g., mammogram)
7. Radioisotope scans (liver, brain, bone, lung)
8. CT
9. MRI
10. Presence of oncofetal antigens such as CEA and AFP
11. Bone marrow examination (if a hematolymphoid malignancy is suspected)
12. Biopsy

Biopsy. The biopsy procedure is the definitive means of diagnosing cancer. It involves the histologic examination by a pathologist of a piece of tissue from the suspicious area. A biopsy is essential in planning a treatment regimen for the patient. A biopsy will determine whether the tissue is benign or

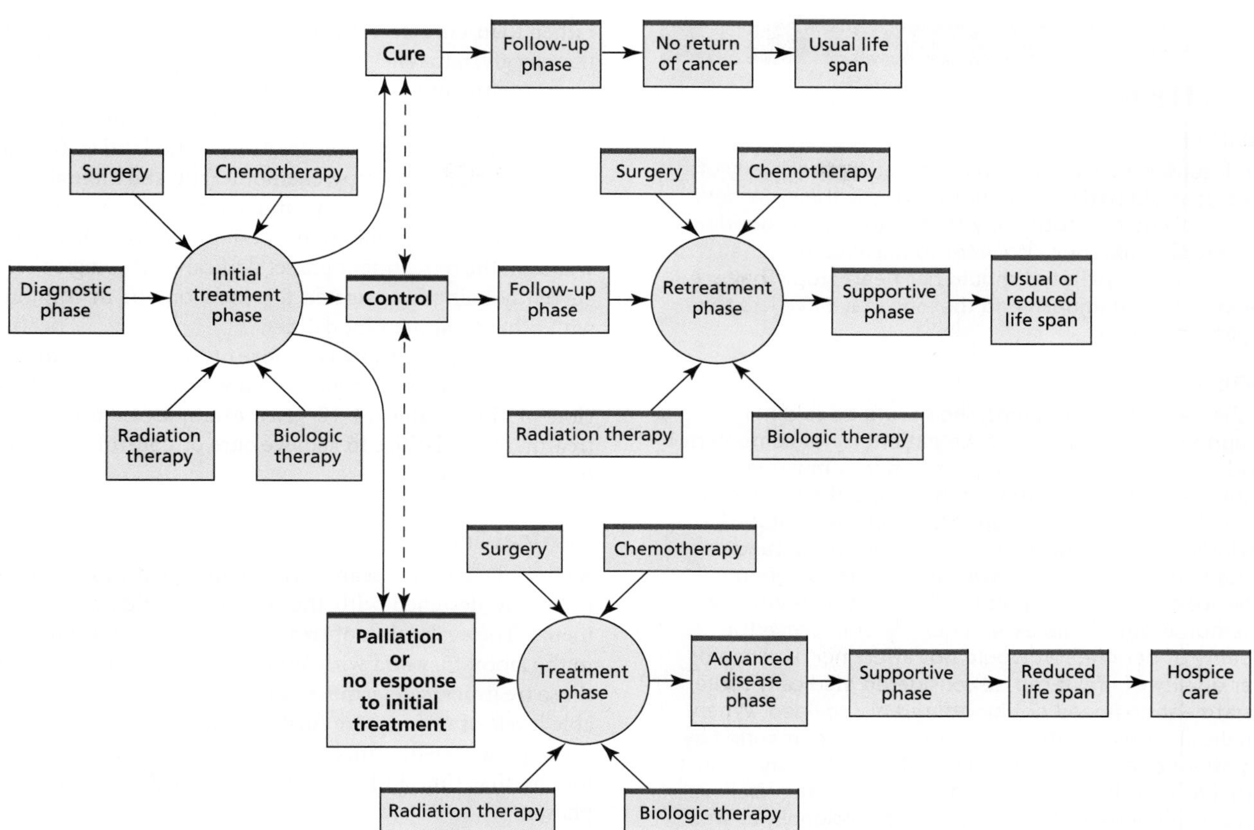

Fig. 14-8 Goals of cancer treatment.

malignant, the anatomic tissue from which the tumor arises, and the degree of cellular differentiation of the cancer cells present in the tumor.

The procedure may be a needle biopsy, an incisional biopsy, or an excisional biopsy. A needle biopsy specimen can be obtained by aspiration (e.g., bone marrow aspiration) or by the use of a large-bore needle. These needles are used in obtaining samples of prostate gland, breast, liver, and kidney tissues.

Incisional biopsy performed with a scalpel or dermal punch is a common technique used for obtaining a tissue sample for making a diagnosis of cancer. The premise that incisional biopsy may contribute to the spread of cancer has not been proven.

Excisional biopsy involves removal of the entire tumor. It is usually used for small tumors (smaller than 2 cm), skin lesions, intestinal polyps, and breast tumors. This procedure can be considered therapeutic, as well as diagnostic. Often when a tumor is not easily accessible, a major surgical procedure (laparotomy, thoracotomy, craniotomy) is necessary to obtain a piece of the tumor tissue. Biopsy specimens of the GI, respiratory, and GU systems can usually be obtained by endoscopic procedures.

COLLABORATIVE CARE

Goals and Modalities

The goal of cancer treatment is cure, control, or palliation (Fig. 14-8). Factors that determine the treatment modality are the cell type of the cancer, the location and size of the tumor, and the extent of the disease. The physiologic and psychologic status and the expressed needs of the patient also have an important part in determining the treatment plan. These factors influence the modalities chosen for treatment and the length of time the treatment is administered.

When caring for the patient with cancer, the nurse should know the goals of the treatment plan to appropriately communicate with and support the patient. When cure is the goal, it is expected that after treatment the patient will be free of disease and will have a normal life span. Many kinds of cancer have the potential to go into permanent remission with an initial course of treatment or with treatment that extends for several weeks, months, or years. Basal cell carcinoma of the skin is usually cured by surgical removal of the lesion or by several weeks of radiation therapy. Acute lymphocytic leukemia (ALL) in children has the potential for cure. The treatment plan for ALL includes the administration of several chemotherapy drugs on a scheduled basis over a time span of 6 months to several years. Some forms of testicular cancer are also treated for cure.

Until a few years ago, a 5-year disease-free period was thought to be indicative of a cancer cure. This is not true for all cancers. The patient with a tumor that has a rapid mitotic rate (e.g., testicular cancer) is considered in remission if cancer is not detected in a 2-year time span. The patient with a tumor that has a slower mitotic rate (e.g., postmenopausal breast cancer) needs 20 or more disease-free years before she can be considered cured of cancer.

Control is the goal of the treatment plan for many cancers considered to be chronic. The patient undergoes the initial

ETHICAL DILEMMAS

Medical Futility

SITUATION

An intensive care nurse is approached by the family of a 65-year-old patient who question why their mother is not receiving chemotherapy for the tumor surrounding her esophagus. They also want to make certain that she will be resuscitated should her heart stop. They are aware of the diagnosis and that she may have less than 1 year to live.

DISCUSSION

If the patient is competent, she should be told her diagnosis and prognosis. If the patient is not competent and has no advance directives, the family must be consulted about both the diagnosis and the prognosis. If the patient wants life support measures instituted, including resuscitation, she must be given the range of treatment alternatives as well as information about hospice care. A crucial piece of information is whether chemotherapy would extend her life or improve the quality of her life. If it would not affect her life span or her quality of life, it can be considered medically futile treatment and need not be offered or provided. When medically futile treatment is requested or demanded by a patient or a patient's family, health professionals must provide very clear explanations about why they believe it to be inappropriate. The health professionals, as well as the patient and family, are always free to seek additional medical consultation or to transfer care to another physician or hospital.

ETHICAL AND LEGAL PRINCIPLES

- Definitions of *medically futile* range from medically inappropriate to a small likelihood of success to failure to achieve intended results in the last 95 of 100 similar cases. Health care providers usually do not provide patients and their families with treatment options that they consider to be medically futile.
- *Scientific futility,* based on medical records and scientific experience, may not be the same as *ethical futility,* which is care that would be incompatible with dignity.
- Patient autonomy allows the refusal of treatment. It does not, however, have an ethical and legal counterpart that would allow the patient to demand treatment.

course of therapy and is continued on maintenance therapy for a period of time or is followed closely so that early signs and symptoms of recurrence can be detected. These cancers are usually not cured, but they are controlled by therapy for long periods of time. They are controlled in a manner similar to other chronic illnesses, such as diabetes mellitus, chronic lung disease, and congestive heart failure. An example of this type of cancer is chronic lymphocytic leukemia (see Chapter 29).

Palliation can also be a goal of the treatment plan. With this treatment goal, relief or control of symptoms and the maintenance of a satisfactory quality of life are the primary goals rather than cure or control of the disease process. Radiation therapy given to relieve the pain of bone metastasis is an example of treatment with a goal of palliation.

The goals of cure, control, and palliation are achieved through the use of four treatment modalities for cancer: surgery, radiation therapy, chemotherapy, and biologic therapy. Surgery, radiation therapy, and chemotherapy can be used alone or in any combination in the initial treatment phase, as well as in the retreatment phase(s) of cancer. Biologic therapy is currently being investigated for use alone or in combination with other treatment modalities.

For many cancers, two or more of the treatment modalities are used to achieve the goal of cure or control for a long period of time. Table 14-12 gives examples of the use of the treatment modalities to achieve cure or control of the disease process of cancer.

Clinical Trials

A clinical trial is a research study conducted with patients and is usually designed with the intent of evaluating new treatments. The evaluation of treatments in cancer research begins in the laboratory and with animal studies. From these studies, those treatments determined to be most effective, with reasonable levels of toxicity, are further evaluated in a series of studies on patients with cancer. New drugs or treatments, evaluated for the first time in human beings, usually go through three phases:

Phase I clinical trials. Determine dosage and route of administration of an agent and assess potential toxicities.

Phase II clinical trials. Evaluate the effect of a particular treatment on various types of cancer.

Phase III clinical trials. Compare the new treatment with standard therapy to determine which is more effective and which is associated with less morbidity.

The rights of the patient who participates in clinical trials are closely guarded by institutional review boards (IRBs) in each agency conducting research. IRBs not only review clinical trials at their inception but continue to review and monitor the study until its completion. Informed consent is a process in which information is fully disclosed to the patient by a physician and a nurse regarding the nature of the treatment being evaluated and the potential risks and benefits of entering the clinical trial. The patient must understand that she or he may elect to leave a clinical trial at any time.

Surgical Interventions

Surgery is the oldest form of cancer treatment, and for many years it was the only effective method of cancer diagnosis and treatment. The treatment of choice for many years was to remove the cancer and as much of the surrounding normal tissue as possible. Therefore most of the surgical procedures used were considered to be radical in nature. In the mid-1950s it was observed that even though the radical procedures were technically sophisticated, the mortality rates associated with certain cancer sites were not improving (e.g., breast cancer). Many cancers that were thought to be local disease processes were found to be systemic diseases with metastatic lesions located in anatomic sites other than the site of the primary disease. On

Table 14-12 Treatment Modalities Used in Cancer

Original Cancer	Surgery	Radiotherapy	Chemotherapy	Biologic Therapy
Breast (stage I)	P	Adj, I	Adj, I	I
Ovary (stage I)	P	Adj, I	Adj, I	I
Uterine cervix (stage II)	P	P	I	ND
Lung				
Small (oat) cell	NU	Adj, I	P	I
Non–small cell	P	P, Adj	P, Adj	I
Gastrointestinal				
Colon	P	Adj, I	Adj, I	I
Stomach	P	Adj, I	Adj	I
Melanoma	P	I	I	Adj, I
Head and neck	P	P	I	I
Testes seminoma (stage I)	P	P	Adj	ND
Prostate	P	Alt	I	I
Kidney	P	Adj, I	I	Adj, I
Brain	P	Alt, I	I	I
Lymphomas				
Hodgkin's disease				
Stage I	NU	P	Adj	ND
Stage II	NU	Adj	P	ND

Adj, adjuvant therapy used after localized tumor is treated by a primary method; routine use is not considered essential. *Alt,* an alternate, although less commonly used, method of primary treatment for which data are already available indicating results equivalent to more common approaches. *I,* investigational. The role in treatment is under examination in controlled clinical trials. Either a new approach to treatment or an older approach, which in the absence of sufficient data to support its frequent use, is being evaluated in controlled clinical trials. *ND,* no data are available to evaluate this form of treatment. *NU,* no use in the primary treatment program. Control rate of the tumor in question may be sufficiently high with other forms of treatment to preclude the testing of this modality. *P,* considered an integral part of standard primary treatment programs.

analysis of these findings, it became obvious that surgery alone, regardless of the extent of the procedure, was not an effective treatment for every type of cancer. Currently, surgery plays several roles in the diagnosis and treatment of cancer (Fig. 14-9).

Cure and Control. Several principles are applicable when surgery is used to cure or control the disease process of cancer:

1. Cancer that arises from a tissue with a slow rate of cellular proliferation or replication is the most amenable to surgical treatment.
2. A margin of normal tissue must surround the tumor at the time of resection.
3. Only as much tissue as necessary is removed, and adjuvant therapy is used. The current trend among health care professionals is toward less radical surgery.
4. Preventive measures are used to reduce the surgical seeding of cancer cells.
5. The usual sites of regional spread may be surgically removed.

Examples of surgical procedures used for cure or control of cancer include radical neck dissection, lumpectomy, mastectomy, pneumonectomy, orchiectomy, thyroidectomy, and bowel resection.

A debulking procedure may be used if the tumor cannot be completely removed (e.g., attached to a vital organ). When this occurs, as much tumor as possible is removed, and the patient may be given chemotherapy or radiation therapy. This type of surgical procedure makes the adjuvant therapy more effective.

Supportive Care. Surgical procedures can also be used to provide supportive care throughout the disease process of cancer. Examples of supportive surgical procedures include the following:

1. Insertion of feeding tubes in the stomach
2. Creation of a colostomy to allow a rectal abscess to heal
3. Suprapubic cystostomy for the patient with advanced prostatic cancer

Palliation of Symptoms. When cure or control of cancer is no longer possible, the quality of life must be maintained at the highest possible level for the longest possible period of time. Examples of surgical procedures performed for palliative care include the following:

1. Cordotomy or rhizotomy for relief of pain (see Chapter 9)
2. Colostomy for the relief of a bowel obstruction (see Chapter 40)
3. Laminectomy for the relief of a spinal cord compression (see Chapter 57)

Rehabilitative Management. Cancer surgery often mutilates and produces a change in the body image. It is often difficult for the patient to cope with this while attempting to maintain usual lifestyle patterns. As the treatment for certain cancers becomes more effective, the length of time the patient must live with an alteration created by surgery will be increased. If quality of life is to be maintained, the body image must be one that the patient is able to accept and cope with on a daily basis. A greater emphasis has been placed on the rehabilitative role of surgery in cancer care to increase the quality of life. Mammoplasty after a mastectomy is an example of a rehabilitative surgical procedure. The new appliances and the care of ostomies are other major focuses of rehabilitative management.

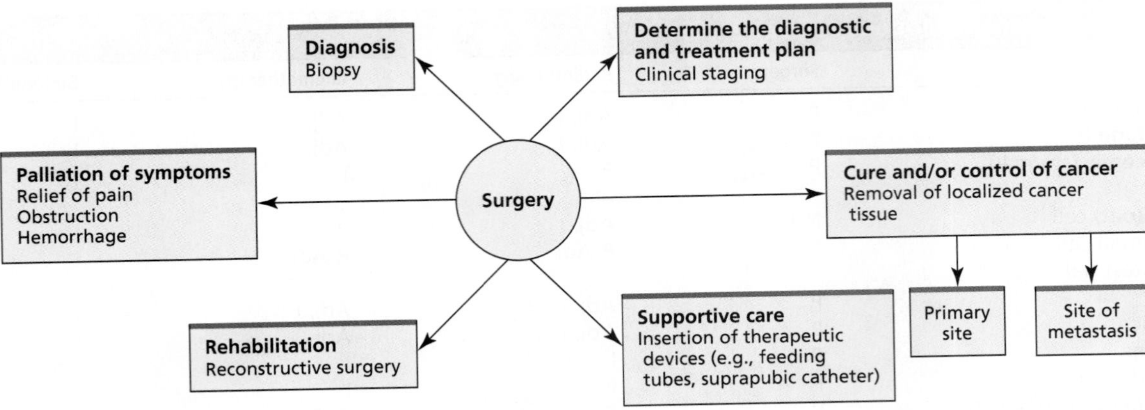

Fig. 14-9 Role of surgery in the treatment of cancer.

Table 14-13 Tumor Radiosensitivity

High Radiosensitivity	Moderate Radiosensitivity	Mild Radiosensitivity	Poor Radiosensitivity
Ovarian dysgerminoma Testicular seminoma Hodgkin's disease Non-Hodgkin's lymphoma Wilms' tumor Neuroblastoma	Skin carcinoma Oropharyngeal carcinoma Esophageal carcinoma Breast adenocarcinoma Uterine and cervical carcinoma Prostate carcinoma Bladder carcinoma	Soft tissue sarcomas (e.g., chondrosarcoma) Gastric adenocarcinoma Renal adenocarcinoma Colon adenocarcinoma	Osteosarcoma Malignant melanoma Malignant gliomas Testicular nonseminoma

A nursing challenge is to assist the patient to think of cancer as a chronic rather than a terminal illness. Many people with chronic illnesses, such as arthritis and diabetes mellitus, learn to cope with their disease and have a high quality of life. This is also the goal for the person with cancer.

Radiation Therapy

Radiation therapy is a local treatment modality for cancer. It is one of the oldest methods of cancer treatment. From the time that Wilhelm Roentgen discovered x-rays in 1895, the Curies discovered radium in 1898, and Henri Becquerel discovered radioactivity in 1896, the role of radiation in the management of cancers has been explored. Early radiation workers, unaware of the properties of these materials, often handled radioactive sources unprotected. These workers experienced skin desquamation and developed carcinomas of the fingers. Marie and Pierre Curie both developed leukemia related to radiation exposure.[13,14]

These experiences led scientists to explore the use of radiation to treat tumors. The correlation made was that if radiation resulted in the destruction of the highly mitotic skin cells of workers it could be used in a controlled way to prevent the continued growth of highly mitotic cancer cells. Early therapeutic use of radiation was hampered by inadequate equipment and lack of knowledge of the effects of radiation on cancer and normal tissues. It was not until the 1960s that highly sophisticated equipment and treatment planning facilitated the delivery of adequate radiation doses to tumors and tolerable doses to normal tissues.[15] It is estimated in current practice that up to 60% of all persons with cancer will receive radiation therapy at some point in the treatment of their disease.

Effects of Radiation. Radiation is the emission and distribution of energy through space or a material medium. The energy produced by radiation, when absorbed into tissue, produces ionization and excitation. This local energy is sufficient to break chemical bonds in DNA, which leads to a biologic effect. The major target of the radiation effect is DNA. The ionization that occurs eventually causes damage to DNA, which renders cells incapable of surviving mitosis. Loss of proliferative capacity results in cellular death at the time of division. Cellular death is dependent on the cell going through its mitotic cycle. Thus death occurs at different rates for different cell types. This is true for both normal cells and cancer cells. However, cancer cells are more likely to be dividing because of the loss of control of cellular division. Furthermore, these cells are unable to repair the radiation damage to DNA. Therefore cancer cells are more likely to be permanently damaged by cumulative doses of radiation. Normal tissues are usually able to recover from radiation damage if therapeutic doses are kept within certain ranges.[16]

Cellular death and tissue reactions. Cellular death related to radiation is defined as an irreversible loss of proliferative capacity. Cells may undergo several mitoses and then die. A cell that retains its proliferative capacity is a clonogenic cell because it is able to produce new clones or colonies of similar cells. Local control of a cancer occurs after radiation if the cells that remain are nonclonogenic.

Cellular sensitivity to radiation varies throughout the cell cycle with cells being most sensitive in the M and G_2 phases and least sensitive during the S or synthesis phase (see Fig. 14-1). Cells treated during the M and G_2 phase of the cell cycle are more likely to suffer lethal damage. The damage to DNA in cells that are not in the M phase will be expressed when division occurs.

The amount of time that is required for the manifestation of radiation damage is determined by the mitotic rate of the tissue. Sufficient cells within the tissue must be killed to establish a noticeable effect. This is true in both normal and cancer cells. The time for this process to occur is measured in hours for intestinal epithelium and bone marrow and in months for slowly proliferating tissues such as the kidney and lung. In nonproliferating tissues such as nerves, the damage may take years to be expressed.[17]

Normal cells within the radiation field will also be affected by treatment. For each normal cell type there is a maximally tolerated radiation dose. Administration of radiation above the maximally tolerated doses results in limited ability of normal cells to recover from damage and potentially irreversible side effects. Treatment planning and computerized dosimetry ensure that normal tissue tolerance is not exceeded.[18,19]

The manifestation of side effects of radiation therapy may be divided into phases. Acute effects occur during treatment and for up to 6 months following the completion of radiation therapy. Subacute effects occur in the next 6 months following the completion of radiation therapy, and late effects occur 1 year and beyond. The severity of acute effects does not predict the occurrence of late effects.[20]

Actively proliferating tissue, such as GI mucosa, esophageal and oropharyngeal mucosa, and bone marrow, exhibit early, acute responses to radiation therapy. Cartilage, bone, kidney, and central and peripheral nervous tissue manifest subacute or late responses. Tumors derived from proliferating cell types, such as lymphomas and leukemias, exhibit a rapid response to therapy at relatively low doses. These are mitotically active cells yielding a rapid expression of radiation damage. Tumors derived from more slowly growing cell types, such as rhabdomyosarcoma and leiomyosarcoma, take a higher dose of radiation and a longer period of time to respond because the mitotic rate of the tumor is slower, and many tumor cells must attempt mitosis for the damage to be expressed. Table 14-13 describes the relative radiosensitivity of a variety of tumors. In responsive tumors, even a large tumor burden will be affected by therapy. (Figure 14-10, parts *A, B,* and *C,* shows a patient with Hodgkin's disease before therapy and 6 years after therapy.) In less responsive tumors a large tumor burden may result in a slower and perhaps incomplete response. Late effects of radiation therapy are partially related to vascular changes that decrease circulation to tissues and lead to depletion of target cells, such as Schwann cells in peripheral nerves, tubule epithelium in the kidney, and oligodendrocytes in the central nervous system (CNS).[20]

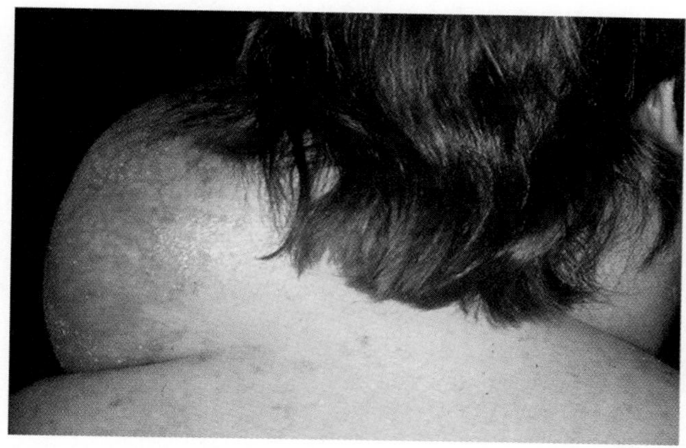

A

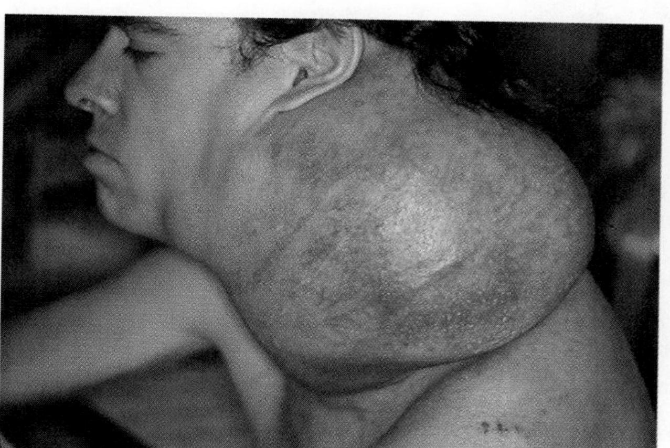

B

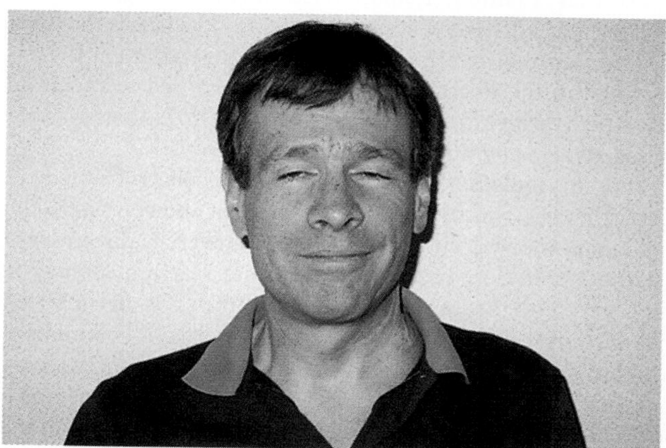

C

Fig. 14-10 **A, B,** Patient with Hodgkin's disease before radiation therapy. **C,** Patient 6 years after radiation therapy.

Simulation and Treatment. Simulation is a part of radiation treatment planning used to determine the optimal treatment method. The patient lies on a table in the treatment position. Under fluoroscopy the critical normal structures that will be included in the treatment field or portal are identified. A film is taken to verify the field, and marks are placed on the skin so that the field can be reproduced on a daily basis. Figures 14-11 and 14-12 illustrate the simulator and a simulation film. Computerized dosimetry using CT scanning is used to produce a treatment plan that delivers the maximum amount of radiation to the tumor within the acceptable dose to normal tissue.[21]

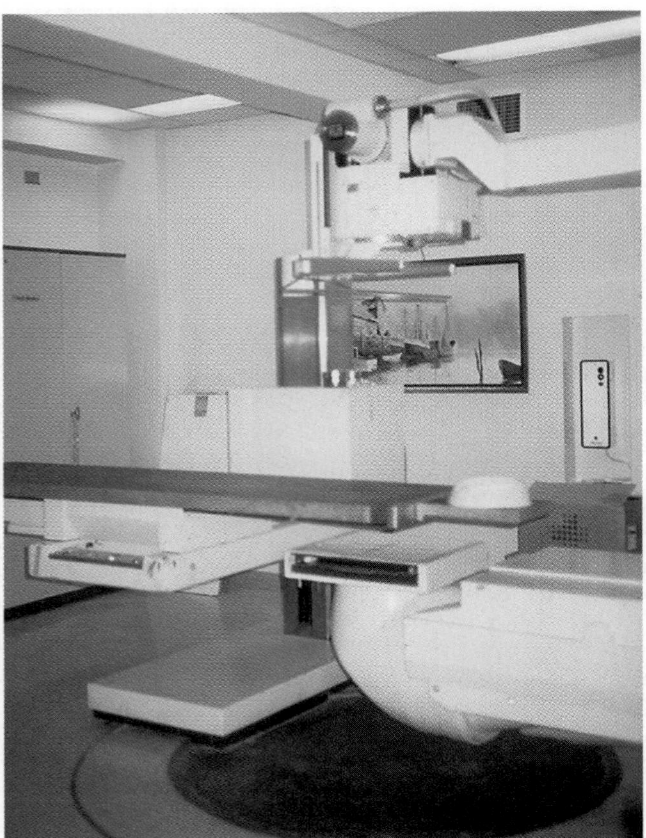

Fig. 14-11 Radiation simulator.

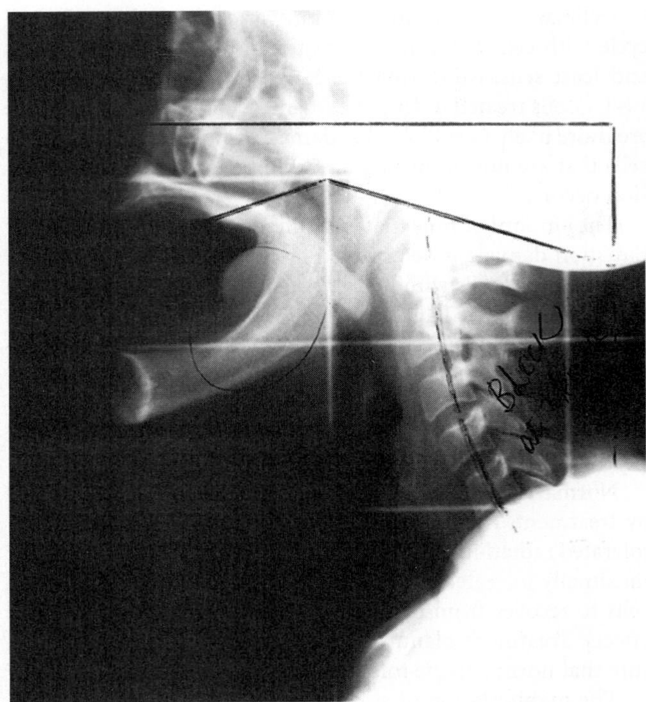

Fig. 14-12 Radiation simulation film.

External radiation. Radiation treatment can be given by external beam radiation therapy (teletherapy), which is the most common form of treatment delivery. In this treatment the patient lies on the treatment couch and is exposed to radiation from the treatment machine (Fig. 14-13). The patient is never radioactive during this treatment.

Internal radiation. Another radiation delivery system is brachytherapy. This means "close" treatment and consists of the implantation or insertion of radioactive materials directly into the tumor or in close proximity to the tumor. An implant may be temporary with the source placed into a catheter or tube inserted into the tumor area and left in place for several days. This method is commonly used for tumors of the head and neck and gynecologic malignancies. Implants, such as prostate implants, may also be permanent with insertion of radioactive seeds into tumors. Figures 14-14 and 14-15 illustrate the applicator and a simulation film of a gynecologic implant. Brachytherapy is used in the clinical situation where the tumor dose must be high to eradicate the tumor. However, this dose is too high for the tolerance of nearby normal tissues. The sources used in brachytherapy are not as energetic or penetrating as those used in the external beam machines and thus deliver most of the dose locally. Often external beam radiation and brachytherapy will be used in combination.

Caring for the person with an implant requires that the nurse be aware that the patient is radioactive. If a patient has a temporary implant, the patient is radioactive during the time the source is in place. If the patient has a permanent implant, the radioactive exposure to the outside and others is low, and the patient may be discharged with precautions. For example, the person with a permanent radioactive ^{125}I seed implant for prostate cancer may be told to double flush the toilet and not to allow children to sit on his lap for a specified period of time after the implant.

The principles of *time, distance,* and *shielding* are used when caring for the person with an implant. Nursing care should be organized so that a limited amount of time is spent with the patient. The patient should be prepared for the implant before the procedure and be aware of time limitations. The radiation safety officer will indicate how much time at a specific distance can be spent with the patient. This is determined by the dose delivered by the implant. Because the source is nonpenetrating, small differences in distance are critical. Only care that must be delivered near the source, such as checking placement of the implant, is performed in close proximity. Shielding, if available, should be used, and no care should be delivered without wearing a film badge. This badge will indicate any radiation exposure. The film badge should not be shared, should not be worn other than at work, and should be returned according to the agency's protocol.

Measurement of Radiation. Several different units are used to measure radiation (Table 14-14). Grays and centigrays are the units currently used in clinical practice.

Goals of Radiation Treatment. The goals of radiation therapy are cure, control, or palliation. To accomplish these treatment goals, radiation therapy can be used alone or as an adjuvant treatment modality in combination with surgery, chemotherapy, and biologic therapy.

Cure is the goal when radiation therapy is used alone as a curative modality for treating patients with basal cell carcinoma of the skin, tumors confined to the vocal cords, and stage I or IIA Hodgkin's disease. Radiation therapy can be combined with

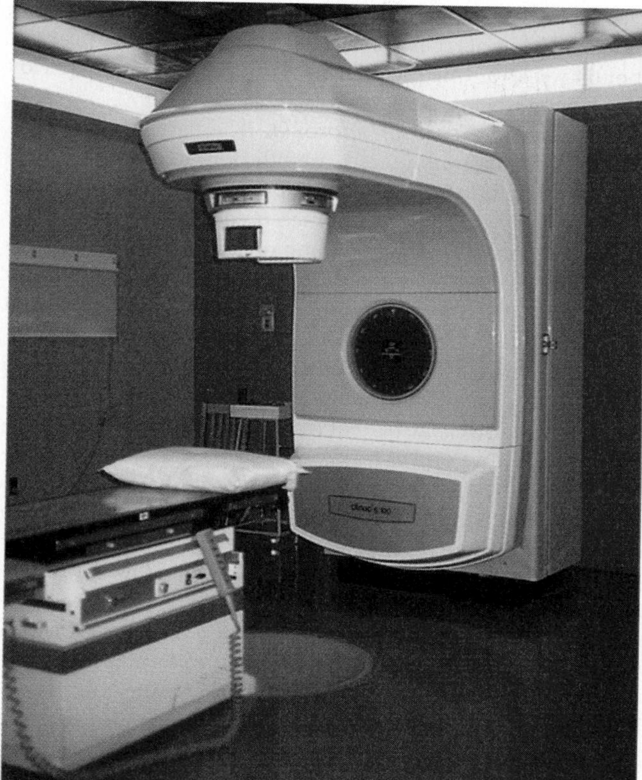

Fig. 14-13 Radiation treatment machine.

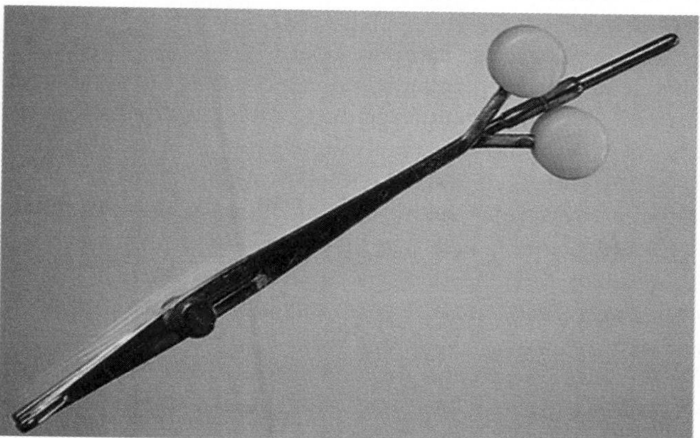

Fig. 14-14 Applicator for gynecologic implant.

surgery and chemotherapy to cure certain cancers such as (1) stage IIB, IIIA, and IIIB Hodgkin's disease in combination with chemotherapy; (2) Wilms' tumor in combination with surgery and chemotherapy; (3) Ewing's sarcoma in combination with chemotherapy; (4) head and neck cancer in combination with surgery and chemotherapy; and (5) stage I and II breast cancer.

Control of the disease process of cancer for a period of time is considered to be a reasonable goal in some situations. Initial treatment is offered at the time of diagnosis, and additional treatment is instituted each time symptoms of disease recur. Most patients enjoy a satisfactory quality of life during the

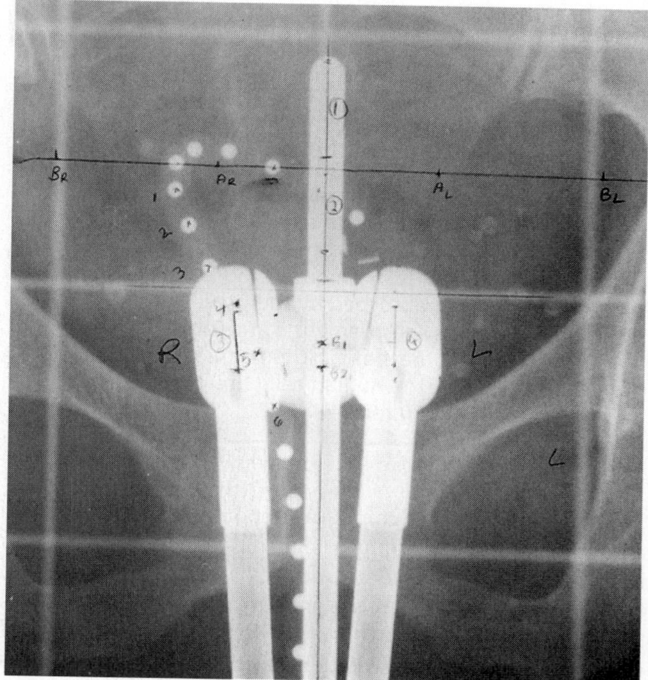

Fig. 14-15 Simulation film of a gynecologic implant.

symptom-free period. Radiation therapy can be combined with surgery to further enhance the local control of cancer. It can be given preoperatively to reduce the size of the tumor so that it can be more easily resected, or it can be given postoperatively to destroy any remaining tumor cells. Intraoperative radiation therapy is now being given at some research centers. In this procedure, radiation is administered directly to the site of the tumor during surgery.

Inoperable tumors can be treated with radiation therapy. These tumors are large and have extended regionally. An example of an inoperable cancer treated for control with radiation therapy is small (oat) cell cancer of the lung.

Palliation is often the goal of radiation therapy. The patient can be treated to control the distressing symptoms that are occurring as a result of the disease process. Tumors can be reduced in size to relieve symptoms such as pain and obstruction. Examples of the use of radiation therapy for palliation include relief of the following:

1. Pain associated with bone metastasis
2. Pain and neurologic symptoms associated with brain metastasis
3. Spinal cord compression
4. Intestinal obstruction
5. Superior vena cava obstruction
6. Bronchial or tracheal obstruction
7. Bleeding (e.g., bladder and intrabronchial)

Side Effects of Radiation Therapy. Common side effects of radiation therapy are presented in Table 14-15. Fatigue, anorexia, bone marrow suppression, skin reactions, and mucosal reactions, as well as pulmonary, GI, and reproduction effects, are discussed in this section.

Table 14-14 Measurement of Radiation

Unit	Definition
Curie (Ci)	A measure of the number of atoms of a particular radioisotope that disintegrate in 1 sec
Roentgen (R)	A measure of the radiation required to produce a standard number of ions in air; a unit of exposure to radiation
Rad	Measurement of radiation dosage absorbed by the tissues
Rem	Measurement of the biologic effectiveness of various forms of radiation on the human cell (1 rem = 1 rad)
Gray (Gy)	100 rads = 1 Gy

Fatigue. Fatigue is a commonly reported side effect of radiation therapy. The pathophysiologic mechanisms that result in radiation-induced fatigue are unclear, because it is not believed to be a result of loss of the cell's proliferative ability. Delay in the cell cycle may partially explain the fatigue. Accumulation of metabolites from the destruction of cells during treatment is another probable cause. The metabolites include lactate, hydrogen ions, and other end products of cellular destruction and result in decreased muscle strength. Alterations in energy production in the patient with cancer may also result from cachexia, anorexia, fever, and infection. Fatigue generally begins during the third to fourth week of treatment, persists after treatment ends, and then gradually subsides. Factors such as weight loss, anemia, depression, nausea, and other symptoms exacerbate the sensation of fatigue.

Collaborative care of fatigue. The patient must recognize that fatigue is an expected side effect of radiation therapy. Otherwise the patient may interpret fatigue as a sign that the treatment is not effective and that the cancer must be spreading. A patient may report more energy on some days than on others. Encouraging the individual to identify days or times during the day when feeling better may allow the patient to remain more active. Resting before activity and having others assist with work or home management may be necessary. Ignoring the fatigue or overstressing the body when fatigue is tolerable leads to an increase in symptoms. Maintaining nutritional status and managing other symptoms also help the problem. Walking programs are a way of keeping the patient active. Most patients are able to participate in walking programs.[22] Fatigue is one symptom that shows improvement during walking programs. Walking programs have also been found to lessen anxiety, fatigue, and difficulty sleeping in women receiving radiation for breast cancer.[23] The ability to remain active has been shown to improve mood and avoid the debilitating cycle of fatigue-depression-fatigue that can occur.

Anorexia. Anorexia may develop as a general reaction to treatment. The mechanisms for anorexia are unclear, but several theories exist. Macrophages release TNF and IL-1 in an attempt to fight the cancer. Both TNF and IL-1 have an appetite-suppressing (anorectic) effect. As tumors are destroyed by therapy, it is proposed that increased levels of these factors may be released into the system and cross the blood-brain barrier, exerting an influence on the satiety center. Large tumors produce more of these factors, thus resulting in the cachexia seen in advanced cancer. In addition, treatment to the head and neck and GI areas exacerbate eating difficulties. Anorexia peaks at about 4 weeks of treatment and seems to resolve more quickly than fatigue when treatment ends.

Collaborative care of anorexia. The patient with anorexia will need to be monitored carefully during treatment to ensure that weight loss does not become excessive. At least twice weekly, body weight should be measured. The individual may assume responsibility for weighing once a return demonstration indicates the patient is able to do so accurately. Laboratory values such as serum prealbumin and albumin are monitored to assess nutritional status. Small, frequent meals of high-protein, high-calorie foods are better tolerated than large meals. Family members should be supported if they are in the position of assisting the patient to eat. Anger and frustration related to the entire cancer trajectory often seem to find expression in arguments related to eating. Nutritional supplements are indicated if anorexia is severe or other factors contribute to difficulty in eating.

Bone Marrow Suppression. Bone marrow within the treatment field will be affected by radiation at a rate commensurate with the turnover rate of cells. WBCs are affected within 1 week, platelets in 2 to 3 weeks, and red blood cells (RBCs) in 2 to 3 months. The degree of the acute effect is determined by the amount of proliferating bone marrow tissue in the treatment field. In the adult about 40% of active marrow is in the pelvis, and 25% is in the thoracic and lumbar vertebrae. When the marrow is irradiated, eradication of blood cells occurs within the treatment field. As a consequence, the nonirradiated marrow becomes more active in an attempt to compensate.

The experience of immunosuppression is not clinically as significant a problem in radiation as it is in the patient receiving certain chemotherapeutic agents. Combination radiation and chemotherapy may cause precipitous drops in WBC, RBC, and platelet counts as does radiation following chemotherapy when bone marrow reserves are limited. Blood counts, including WBC, RBC, and platelets, in these individuals must be closely monitored. Bleeding and infection as consequences of immunosuppression are rare when radiation therapy is delivered alone.

If anemia occurs and the hemoglobin level drops below 10 g/dl (100 g/L), the patient may require blood transfusions. Radiation therapy is more effective against well-oxygenated cells. Therefore there is a concern that a hemoglobin level below 10 g/dl (100 g/L) does not provide for adequate oxygenation of cells in the treatment field.

Skin Reactions. Skin reactions develop within the radiation field. The skin-sparing property of modern radiation equipment limits the severity of these reactions. Both acute and chronic changes occur in the skin. Although the skin reaction begins as early as the first treatment, it is usually transitory at first. Erythema may develop 1 to 24 hours after a single treatment. The true radiation reaction usually begins later at a dose of approximately 800 cGy. The skin cells are mitotically active and exhibit early response to treatment. Erythema is an acute response followed by desquamation. Cells become dark before they slough off because radiation stimulates the melanocytes. The basal cells of the epidermis begin to peel. A dry desquamation results when cells are shed. This dry reaction occurs when cells are shed at a rate that allows new cells

Table 14-15 Problems Caused by Radiation Therapy and Chemotherapy

Problem	Etiology and Comments
Gastrointestinal System	
Dryness of the mucous membranes of the mouth	When salivary glands are located in the radiation treatment field, they are frequently damaged. This may be a permanent side effect of radiation therapy, and it can be quite disturbing because it is difficult to eat, swallow, and talk when the mucous membranes are dry. Artificial saliva is available.
Stomatitis and mucositis	This problem occurs when epithelial cells of the oral mucosa and intraoral soft tissue structures are destroyed by chemotherapy or radiation therapy. These cells are extremely sensitive because of their normal high cell turnover rate. Mucositis can precipitate complications of infection and hemorrhage.
Esophagitis	Inflammation and ulceration of mucous membranes of esophagus as a result of rapid cell destruction occur as a side effect of chemotherapy and radiation therapy to the area of the neck, chest, and back.
Nausea and vomiting	The vomiting center in the brain is stimulated by products of cellular breakdown that occur in response to chemotherapy and radiation therapy. The drugs used in chemotherapy also stimulate the vomiting center. Destruction of the epithelial lining of the gastrointestinal tract occurs in response to chemotherapy and radiation therapy to chest, abdomen, and back. A strong psychologic impact is associated with nausea and vomiting and the high stress level associated with cancer and cancer treatment.
Anorexia	Site-specific side effects of radiation therapy—dry mouth, mucositis, esophagitis, nausea, vomiting, and diarrhea occur. Side effects of chemotherapy include nausea, vomiting, stomatitis, esophagitis, and diarrhea. Fatigue, pain, and infection are present. Alteration in the sensation of taste occurs when tumors release waste products into the bloodstream. Psychologic and social impact of cancer and cancer therapy result in an increased level of stress and changes in the usual lifestyle pattern.
Altered taste sensation	Destruction of the taste buds in the treatment field occurs with radiation therapy. The amount of taste alteration or loss depends on the radiation dosage and the extent of the treatment field. Complete loss of taste often occurs. Taste changes may be a permanent outcome of therapy. Waste products occur in response to cellular destruction from radiation therapy and chemotherapy. These waste products are thought to be responsible for alterations in taste sensation. Reduction in the amount of saliva occurs because of the location of the salivary glands in the treatment field. Food must be in solution to be tasted.
Diarrhea	Denuding of the epithelial lining of the small intestines occurs as a side effect of chemotherapy and radiation therapy to the abdomen or the lower back.
Constipation	Dysfunction of the autonomic nervous system from neurotoxic effects of plant alkaloids (vincristine, vinblastine) occurs.
Hepatotoxicity	Toxic effects of certain chemotherapy drugs such as methotrexate, mitomycin, 6-MP, and cytosine arabinoside are present.
Hematopoietic System	
Anemia	Depressant effect on bone marrow function occurs because of chemotherapy and radiation therapy. Malignant infiltration of bone marrow by cancer occurs. Ulceration, necrosis, and bleeding of neoplastic growth occur.
Leukopenia	Depressant effect on bone marrow activity is present as a result of chemotherapy and radiation therapy. The effect is especially significant because of the short life span of white blood cells. Infection is the most frequent cause of morbidity and death in the patient with cancer. Usual sites of infection are the respiratory and genitourinary systems.
Thrombocytopenia	Depressant effect on bone marrow function is present as a result of chemotherapy and radiation therapy. Malignant infiltration of the bone marrow occurs. Abnormal destruction of circulating platelets is present. When the platelet count is less than 20,000/μl, spontaneous bleeding can occur.
Integumentary System	
Alopecia	Alopecia occurs as a side effect of some chemotherapy agents and radiation therapy to the skull. Hair loss that occurs in response to chemotherapy is usually temporary, and hair loss that occurs in response to radiation therapy is usually permanent. The hair begins to fall out during the first week of therapy, and this may progress to complete hair loss.
Skin reactions	Extravasation of vesicant chemotherapeutic drugs (e.g., doxorubicin) given intravenously causes severe necrosis of tissues exposed to the drug. This can also occur with implantable access devices if needle is not in septum (see later in chapter).

Continued

Table 14-15 Problems Caused by Radiation Therapy and Chemotherapy—cont'd

Problem	Etiology and Comments
Genitourinary Tract	
Cystitis	This problem occurs when the epithelial cells of the lining of the bladder are destroyed as a side effect of chemotherapy (e.g., cyclophosphamide) and as a side effect of radiation therapy when the bladder is located in the treatment field. Clinical manifestations of urgency, frequency, and hematuria are present.
Reproductive dysfunction	This problem occurs as a result of the effect of chemotherapy on the cells of the testes or ova or as a result of the effects of radiation therapy when the cells of the testes or ova are located in the treatment field. Symptoms of cancer and cancer therapy include fatigue, diarrhea, nausea, vomiting, anxiety, fear, and pain.
Nephrotoxicity	Necrosis of proximal renal tubules is present as a result of an accumulation of drugs (e.g., cisplatin) in the kidney and tumor lysis.
Nervous System	
Increased intracranial pressure	This problem may result from radiation edema in the central nervous system. This phenomenon is not well understood but is easily controlled with steroids and pain medication.
Peripheral neuropathy	Paresthesias, areflexia, skeletal muscle weakness, and smooth muscle dysfunction (e.g., paralytic ileus, constipation) can occur as a side effect of the plant alkaloids (e.g., vinblastine, vincristine) and cisplatin.
Respiratory System	
Pneumonitis	When the lungs are located in the treatment field, radiation pneumonitis may develop 2-3 mo after the start of treatment. It is characterized by a dry, hacking cough, fever, and exertional dyspnea. After 6-12 mo, fibrosis will occur and will be persistently evident on x-ray. The patient with fibrosis is more susceptible to respiratory infection. This problem can also occur as a result of chemotherapy (e.g., bleomycin, busulfan).
Cardiovascular System	
Pericarditis and myocarditis	This problem is an infrequent complication when the chest wall is radiated. It may occur up to 1 yr after treatment.
Cardiotoxicity	Chemotherapeutic agents such as doxorubicin and daunorubicin can cause nonspecific electrical changes (i.e., low voltage) and rapidly progressive heart failure. The drug therapy must be modified if these effects occur.
Biochemical	
Hyperuricemia	An increase in uric acid levels occurs because of cell destruction by chemotherapy. This problem can cause a secondary form of gout.
Hypomagnesemia	This problem occurs with cisplatin therapy.
Psychoemotional	
Fatigue	Increase in the metabolic rate occurs when cancer is present with resultant increase in the amount of energy used. Destruction of cancer cells and normal cells by chemotherapy and radiation therapy occurs with the release of waste products into the bloodstream. Increase in anabolic processes of cellular proliferation and differentiation is necessary to repair the normal cells and tissue destroyed by chemotherapy and radiation therapy.
Pain	Compression or infiltration of the blood vessels, the lymphatic vessels, and the nerves occurs. Obstruction of the gastrointestinal or genitourinary system occurs. Inflammation, ulceration, or necrosis of the tissues or organs is present. Fear, anxiety, and depression are often experienced in response to the diagnosis and treatment of cancer.

to be available to replace the lost cells (Fig. 14-16). If the rate of cellular sloughing is faster than the ability of the new epidermal cells to replace dead cells, a wet desquamation occurs with exposure of the dermis and oozing of serum (Fig. 14-17). Surviving cells will form islands of new cells that eventually grow together to repair the damage. The effect of megavoltage radiation on the dermis may be greater than in the epidermis. Skin reactions are particularly evident in areas subjected to pressure such as behind the ear and in gluteal folds, perineum, breast, collar line, and bony prominences.

Late effects in the skin are related to the total radiation dose. The epidermis in the field is thinner and smoother than nonradiated skin and may be unable to form pigment. The skin in the treated area may contain no hair and few or no sweat or sebaceous glands. This thin epidermis will be more vulnerable to damage from trauma, and wound healing is delayed. Late reactions in the dermis may lead to fibrosis and fibrous hyperplasia in vessels with resultant telangiectasia. These are the dilated spidery vessels that may be seen in the treated area.[24]

Collaborative care of skin reactions. Although there is a lack of consistency in protocols for the management of radiated skin in terms of products used, there are basic principles of skin care.[19] Dry reactions are uncomfortable and result in pruritus. Wet reactions result in discomfort and drainage. Dry skin

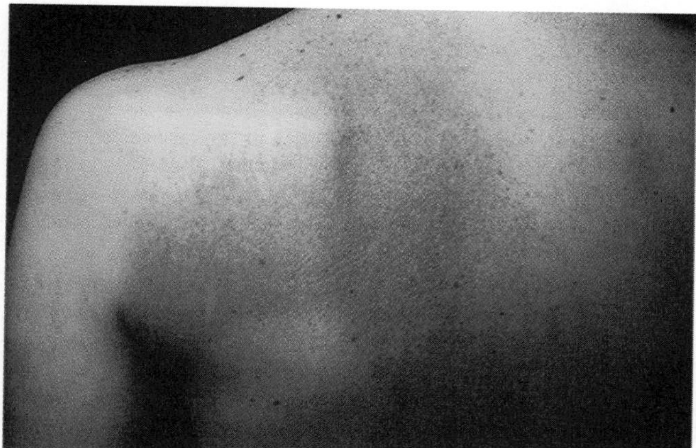

Fig. 14-16 Dry desquamation.

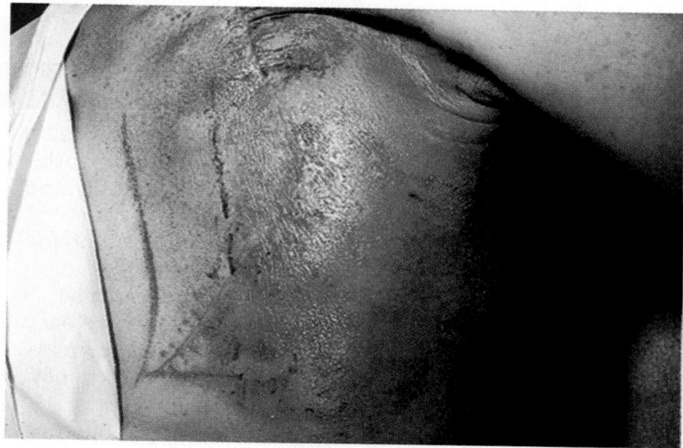

Fig. 14-17 Wet desquamation.

should be lubricated with a nonirritating lotion or solution that contains no metal, alcohol, perfume, or additives that irritate the skin. Wet reactions must be kept clean and protected from further damage. Prevention of infection and facilitation of wound healing are the therapeutic goals. Even in the patient who is immunosuppressed, the development of infections within the radiated field is extremely rare.

Irradiated skin should be protected from extremes of temperature to prevent trauma. Heating pads, ice packs, and hot water bottles cannot be used in the treatment field. Constricting garments, rubbing, harsh chemicals, and deodorants may also traumatize the skin and should be avoided. The use of corticosteroids and hydrogen peroxide remains controversial because of their interference with wound healing. Because protocols vary widely, the guidelines presented in Table 14-16 should be clarified with the department of radiotherapy before being instituted.

Oral, oropharynx, and esophageal reactions. The mucosal linings of the oral cavity, oropharynx, and esophagus are sensitive to the effects of radiation therapy. Mucosal epithelium in the buccal mucosa is lost by the twelfth day of treatment. Desquamation develops first on the soft palate followed by the hypopharynx, vallecula, floor of the mouth, cheeks, medial aspect of the mandible, laryngeal surface of the epiglottis, interarytenoid area, base of the tongue, vocal cords, and the dorsum of the tongue. Capillary engorgement, edema, and leukocyte infiltration characterize the acute reaction. These changes arise in both external beam and brachytherapy treatments. Salivary glands may swell acutely from interstitial edema and duct obstruction after the first treatment. A decrease in salivary flow with resultant xerostomia (dry mouth) occurs during therapy. Serous acini appear to be more severely damaged than mucous acini, leaving saliva thick and ropey. This thick saliva is less able to perform the functions of cleansing teeth and moistening food so that the taste receptors can be stimulated. Food must be dissolved in saliva to be tasted. Taste loss is progressive during therapy, and by the end of treatment patients often report that all food has lost its flavor. With radiation doses of 3000 cGy, the patient can barely detect a sucrose solution equivalent in sweetness to 25 teaspoons of sugar.[25]

Collaborative care of oral, oropharyngeal, and esophageal reactions. The oral cavity and esophageal effects of radiotherapy have the potential to compromise nutritional status. Oral assessment and meticulous intervention are essential to prevent infection and to facilitate nutritional intake. Difficulty swallowing, which characterizes esophageal reactions, further impedes eating. Patients report feeling that they have a "lump" as they swallow and that "foods get stuck." The individual with head and neck cancer often begins therapy in a compromised nutritional state related to poor eating habits associated with alcohol and tobacco abuse. All of these factors make the patient extremely vulnerable to malnutrition. Common side effects experienced by the individual with head and neck cancer include fatigue, loss of taste, anorexia, sore throat, cough, and changes in saliva.[25]

The patient should be taught to examine the oral cavity. The mucous membranes, characteristics of saliva, and ability to swallow must be assessed. Oral care includes pretreatment evaluation by a dentist to perform all necessary dental work before the initiation of treatment. The patient should also be taught how to perform oral care and be fitted with fluoride trays to use during treatment. Compliance to this protocol significantly reduces the risk of radiation caries, which develop as a result of loss of saliva. These dental caries are extremely damaging to the teeth, resulting in the need for extraction. Saliva substitutes are available and may be offered to patients, although many find that drinking large amounts of water has an equivalent effect. Oral care should be performed at least before and after each meal and at bedtime. A saline solution of 1 teaspoon of salt in 1 L of water is an effective cleansing agent. One teaspoon of sodium bicarbonate may be added to the oral care solution to decrease odor, alleviate pain, and dissolve mucin. Tooth brushing and flossing are critical unless contraindicated by decreased platelet counts. This is rarely seen when radiation is used alone, but it may be a concern with combined modality therapy.

Alleviation of mucositis or pain in the throat can be achieved by systemic analgesics and antibiotics, as well as coating agents, which include antacids and sucralfate suspension. Combinations of coating and analgesic compounds may be used. Antacids, diphenhydramine (Benadryl), and viscous Xylocaine have been mixed in equal proportions to use as a component of oral care. The solutions may be swallowed to alleviate esophagitis. Any coating solution must be cleansed and not allowed to build up on the mucosa where it could serve as a medium for infection.

PATIENT TEACHING GUIDE

Table 14-16 Radiation Skin Reactions

1. Gently cleanse the skin in the treatment field using a mild soap (Ivory, Dove), tepid water, a soft cloth, and a gentle patting motion. Rinse thoroughly and pat dry.
2. Apply nonmedicated, nonperfumed, moisturizing lotion or creams, such as baby lotion, oil, aloe gel, or cream to alleviate dry skin. This substance must be gently cleansed from the treatment field before each treatment and reapplied. (*NOTE:* Care differs from institution to institution.) Dusting with cornstarch may reduce itching.
3. Cleanse the area involved with half-strength hydrogen peroxide and normal saline solution if a level III reaction is present. The solution is best applied with an irrigating syringe to avoid friction. Rinse the area with saline solution. Expose the area to air as often as possible. If copious drainage is present, nonadhesive absorbent dressings are warranted, and they must be changed as soon as they become wet. Observe the area daily for signs of infection.
4. Instruct the patient to avoid wearing tight-fitting clothing such as brassieres, girdles, and belts over the treatment field.
5. Instruct the patient to avoid wearing harsh fabrics, such as wool and corduroy. A lightweight cotton garment is best. If possible, expose the treatment field to air.
6. Instruct the patient to use gentle detergents such as Dreft and Ivory Snow to wash clothing that will come in contact with the treatment field.
7. Instruct the patient to avoid direct exposure to the sun. If the treatment field is in an area that is exposed to the sun, protective clothing such as a wide-brimmed hat should be worn during exposure to the sun.
8. Avoid all sources of heat (hot water bottles, heating pads, and sun lamps) on the treatment field.
9. Avoid exposing the treatment field to cold temperatures (ice bags or cold weather).
10. Instruct the patient to avoid swimming in salt water or in chlorinated pools during the time of treatment.
11. Instruct the patient to avoid the use of all medication, deodorants, perfumes, powders, or cosmetics on the skin in the treatment field. Tape, dressings, and adhesive bandages should also be avoided unless permitted by the radiation therapist. Avoid shaving the hair in the treatment field.
12. Sensitive skin must continue to be protected after the treatment is completed. Teach the patient to do the following:
    a. Avoid direct exposure to the sun. A sunscreen agent and protective clothing must be worn if the potential of exposure to the sun is present.
    b. Use an electric razor if shaving is necessary in the treatment field.

Infection, particularly with *Candida*, can occur in individuals receiving head and neck radiation. The incidence increases dramatically in protocols using concomitant chemotherapy with agents such as bleomycin. Oral nystatin, ketoconazole, fluconazole, or clotrimazole may be prescribed to treat the infection.[25,26]

Feedings of soft, nonirritating high-protein and high-caloric foods should be offered frequently throughout the day. Extremes of temperature, as well as tobacco and alcohol, should be avoided. Nutritional supplements (e.g., Ensure) as an adjunct to meals and fluid intake must be encouraged. The patient should be weighed several times each week to ensure that excessive amounts of weight have not been lost. Families are an integral part of the health care team. As taste loss increases, the family's role in assisting the patient to eat becomes increasingly critical. If family members are not available, alternative avenues of support such as volunteers and home aides are indicated.[26]

Pulmonary effects. The effects of radiation on the lung include both acute and late reactions. Radiation doses in the lung are actually magnified because there is no reduction of the dose through tissue. Treatment planning limits the amount of radiation dose to the lung. When the lungs are irradiated, there is damage to the alveolar type II pneumocyte, which is the cell that produces surfactant. Surfactant is a phospholipid substance that decreases surface tension and prevents alveolar collapse. When exposed to radiation, type II pneumocytes initially secrete more surfactant in response to injury. Later, the gradual decrease in surfactant leads to a tendency toward alveolar collapse, which accentuates lung damage. Damage to the lung results in dyspnea and cough. Pneumonitis is the acute reaction related to blistering of capillary endothelial cells, platelet thrombi, and luminal obstruction. This reaction is often asymptomatic, although an increase in cough, fever, and night sweats may occur. Infiltrates that conform to the shape of the radiation field are evident on chest x-ray. The symptomatic individual may require corticosteroids to provide relief, but symptoms may reappear precipitously when these drugs are withdrawn abruptly. Furthermore, corticosteroids do not prevent the development of fibrosis. Bronchodilators, expectorants, bed rest, and oxygen are preferable to steroids.

One to three months after treatment, alveolar cells begin to slough with exudation and accumulation of fluid in interstitial spaces. Fibrosis develops 3 to 6 months after treatment with sclerosis of alveolar walls and loss of pulmonary function. With small radiation treatment doses the fibrosis that results is usually not clinically significant.

Collaborative care of pulmonary effects. The pulmonary effects of radiation are frightening to the patient because they may involve an exacerbation of the symptoms that precipitated the cancer diagnosis. Cough and dyspnea may increase. The cough becomes more productive as alveoli that had been blocked are opened as the tumor responds to treatment. As treatment continues, the cough becomes dry as the mucosa begins to be altered by the radiation. Cough suppressants may be indicated at night.

Oxygen, if prescribed for symptomatic pneumonitis, must be used judiciously if the patient has chronic obstructive pulmonary disease (see Chapter 27). The patient may mistakenly believe that increasing oxygen flow is an appropriate response to treat increasing dyspnea. Other symptoms reported by individuals receiving chest radiation include fatigue, skin irritation, anorexia, and sore throat. If the patient experiences dyspnea, anxiety may be pronounced. Lying flat on the treatment table and being alone in the room potentiate anxiety. Teaching must be reinforced frequently with the family present because the patient often forgets what has been told. Alleviation of obstruction reduces anxiety and dyspnea.

Gastrointestinal effects. The mucosa of the GI tract is highly proliferative with surface cells being replaced every 2 to 6 days. Radiation alters gastric secretion by direct injury to cells. Radiation gastritis is evident after the first week of therapy with hyperemia, microscopic hemorrhage, and exudation. The secretion of mucus, hydrochloric acid, and pepsin decreases with further treatment. The intestinal mucosa is one of the most radiosensitive tissues. Reepithelization occurs within 96 hours following destruction of the mucosa. Nausea, vomiting, and diarrhea result from radiation of the GI tissue. Malabsorption of protein, fats, and carbohydrates occurs. Excessive bile salts entering the intestine may also lead to diarrhea. Cholestyramine may be indicated as an antidiarrheal because it binds with bile salts.

Collaborative care of gastrointestinal effects. Nausea and vomiting are early reactions of radiation to the GI tract, occurring as soon as after the first treatment. The etiology of GI reactions may be related to the release of serotonin from the GI tract, which then stimulates the chemoreceptor trigger zone and the vomiting center in the brain. Further GI irritation is related to cellular death. Prophylactic administration of antiemetics 1 hour before treatment is recommended. The patient may find that eating a light meal of nonirritating food before treatment is also helpful. The development of *anticipatory nausea* and *vomiting* can occur in the patient receiving radiation. This conditioned response develops over time in the individual who has unrelieved nausea and vomiting. As the patient repeatedly experiences these symptoms, a framework of cues is created associated with nausea and vomiting to the point that encountering the cues even without receiving treatment may precipitate nausea and vomiting. In some individuals this response persists after treatment ends. This type of reaction does not develop in the patient who does not experience posttreatment vomiting, which underscores the necessity for prophylactic treatment.

The patient experiencing nausea and vomiting must be assessed for signs and symptoms of dehydration and alkalosis. Fluid intake is recorded to ensure that an adequate volume is being consumed and retained. Nausea and vomiting are usually successfully managed when conventional radiation doses and field sizes are used.

Diarrhea is a reaction of the bowel to radiation. The small bowel is extremely sensitive and does not tolerate significant radiation doses. Treating the patient with a full bladder may serve to move the small bowel out of the treatment field. The malabsorption of bile salts and the irritation of the bowel wall contribute to the development of diarrhea that occurs when abdominal and pelvic fields are radiated. Nonirritating diets and low-residue diets, as well as antidiarrheals and antispasmodics, are recommended. Lukewarm sitz baths may alleviate discomfort and cleanse the rectal area. The rectal area must be kept clean and dry to maintain mucosal integrity. The nurse should inspect the anal area. The patient should record the number, volume, consistency, and character of stools per day. Adequate food and fluid intake promote healing and mucosal integrity. Meticulous perianal care is essential. Systemic analgesia is warranted for the painful skin irritations that may develop.

Reproductive effects. The effects of radiation on the ovary and testes are determined by the dose delivered. The testes are very sensitive to radiation, and protection of the testicles is achieved whenever possible. Doses of 15 to 30 cGy temporarily decrease the sperm count with aspermia at 35 to 230 cGy. In some cases, 200 cGy may result in permanent aspermia. The patient receiving 300 to 600 cGy either recovers in 2 to 5 years or not at all. Pretreatment status may be a significant factor as a low sperm count and loss of motility are seen in individuals with testicular cancer and Hodgkin's disease before any therapy. Combined modality treatment or prior chemotherapy with alkylating agents enhances and prolongs the effects of radiation on the testes. When radiation is used alone with conventional doses and appropriate shielding, testicular recovery often occurs.[27]

Compromise of reproductive function in men may also result from erectile dysfunction following pelvic radiation and related vascular and neurologic effects. The incidence of erectile dysfunction with radiation is reportedly less than with non–nerve-sparing surgery. Brachytherapy for prostate cancer further decreases this risk.

The radiation dose necessary to induce ovarian failure changes with age. Permanent cessation of menses occurs in 95% of women less than 40 years of age at 500 to 1000 cGy and at 375 cGy in women more than 40 years of age. Unlike the testes, there is no avenue for repair of ovarian function. The ovaries are shielded whenever possible. If exploratory laparotomies are performed in women with Hodgkin's disease, the ovaries may be moved out of the radiation field.[28]

Other factors that influence reproductive or sexual functioning in women include reactions in the cervix and endometrium. These tissues withstand a high radiation dose with minimal sequelae, accounting for the ability to treat endometrial and cervical cancer with high external and brachytherapy doses. Acute reactions such as tenderness, irritation, and loss of lubrication compromise sexual activity. Late effects of combined internal and external therapy include vaginal shortening related to fibrosis and loss of elasticity and lubrication.

Collaborative care of reproductive effects. The patient and her or his partner require information about the expected effects of treatment relative to reproductive issues. Potential infertility can be a significant consequence for the individual, and counseling may be indicated. Pretreatment harvesting of sperm or ova may be considered. Specific suggestions to manage side effects that have an impact on sexual functioning include using a water-soluble vaginal lubricant and a vaginal dilator after pelvic radiation. The nurse must be able to encourage discussion of issues related to sexuality, offer specific suggestions, and make referrals for ongoing counseling when indicated.

Coping with Radiation Therapy. Assisting the patient to cope with the anxieties of receiving radiation is an essential component of the nursing role. The necessity of coming for treatment five times per week forces the individual to confront the cancer on an almost daily basis.[29] The demands on the patient and the family and the disruption of normal activities created by the treatment schedule are difficult to handle. In conjunction with the social worker, the nurse should assist with planning for transportation with available resources such as the American Cancer Society, churches, and community resources.

Anxiety is almost always present in the patient receiving therapy. The uncertainties regarding treatment and the fears of receiving radiation are most evident at the beginning of therapy. Anxiety continues to be a factor at the end of treatment

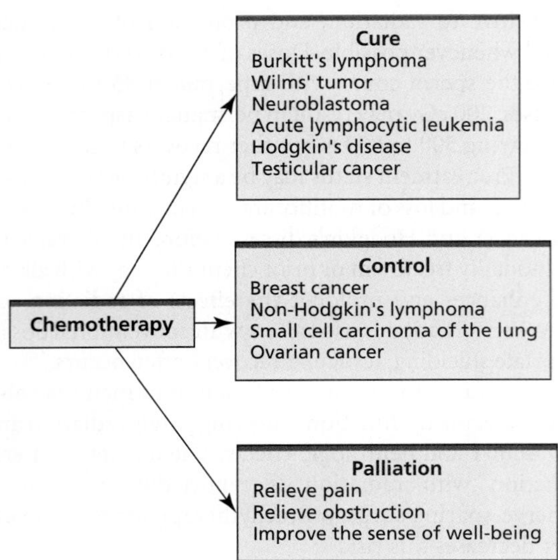

Fig. 14-18 Goals of chemotherapy.

when outcomes are still unknown. Anxiety may increase in some patients when treatment ends. The patient must realize that he or she will be followed and that support is ongoing. The impact of radiation on the quality of life of the patient undergoing therapy may be minimized with information and support. The patient may find that relaxation techniques and humor can be used to lessen anxiety. The nurse should encourage the appropriate use of humor. Research on the long-term effects, both physical and emotional, on the quality of life of the individual receiving radiation is needed.[30]

The nurse plays an important role in the management of the individual receiving radiation therapy. Patient education and symptom management allow the individual to cope with therapy while maintaining the highest possible quality of life.

Chemotherapy

Chemotherapy is the systemic treatment of cancer with chemicals (drugs). In the 1940s chemotherapy was in its infancy. Nitrogen mustard, a chemical warfare agent used in World Wars I and II, was used in the treatment of acute leukemia, and a folic acid antimetabolite (5-FU) was found to have antitumor activity. In the 1950s considerable experimentation with single-drug therapy began. In the 1960s the emphasis was on the development and use of combination chemotherapy. In the 1970s chemotherapy was established as an effective treatment modality for cancer. By the 1980s clinical studies looked at the effect of high doses of chemotherapy used in the treatment of cancers previously resistant to therapy. Chemotherapy is now used in the treatment of many solid tumors and is the primary therapy for leukemias and some lymphomas. Chemotherapy has gone from a palliative, "last-ditch effort" treatment modality to one that can cure certain cancers, control other cancers for long periods of time, and offer palliative relief of symptoms when cure or control no longer is possible[31] (Fig. 14-18).

Effect on Cells. The effect of chemotherapy is at the cellular level. All cells (cancer cells and normal cells) enter the cell cycle for replication and proliferation (see Fig. 14-1). The effects of the chemotherapeutic agents are described in relationship to the cell cycle. The two major categories of chemotherapeutic drugs are cell cycle–nonspecific and cell cycle phase–specific drugs.

Cell cycle–nonspecific chemotherapeutic drugs have their effect on the cells that are in the process of cellular replication and proliferation, as well as on the cells that are in the resting phase (G_0).

Cell cycle phase–specific chemotherapeutic drugs have their effect on cells that are in the process of cellular replication or proliferation (G_1, S_1, G_2, or M). These drugs exert their most significant effect during specific phases of the cell cycle.

Cell cycle phase–specific and cell cycle–nonspecific agents are often administered in combination with one another. The aim of this approach is to promote a better response using agents that function by differing mechanisms.[32]

The goal of chemotherapy is to reduce the number of cancer cells present in the primary tumor site(s) and metastatic tumor site(s). Several factors determine the response of cancer cells to chemotherapy:

1. Mitotic rate of the tissue from which the tumor arises. The more rapid the mitotic rate, the greater the response to chemotherapy. Chemotherapy is the treatment of choice for acute leukemia, choriocarcinoma of the placenta, Wilms' tumor (used in conjunction with surgery), and neuroblastoma. These cancer cells have a rapid rate of cellular proliferation.
2. Size of the tumor. The smaller the number of cancer cells, the greater the response to chemotherapy.
3. Age of the tumor. The younger the tumor, the greater the response to chemotherapy. Younger tumors have a greater percentage of proliferating cells.
4. Location of the tumor. Certain anatomic sites provide a protected environment from the effects of chemotherapy. For example, only a few drugs (nitrosoureas and bleomycin) cross the blood-brain barrier.
5. Presence of resistant tumor cells. Mutation of cancer cells within the tumor mass can result in variant cells that are resistant to chemotherapy. Resistance can also occur because of the biochemical inability of some cancer cells to convert the drug to its active form.
6. Physiologic and psychologic status of the host. A state of optimum health and a positive attitude will allow the patient to better withstand aggressive chemotherapy.

When the cancer first begins to grow, most of the cells are actively dividing. As the tumor increases in size, more and more cells become inactive and convert to a resting state (G_0). Since most chemotherapeutic agents are most effective against dividing cells, cells can escape death by staying in the G_0 phase. The main problem in cancer chemotherapy is the presence of drug-resistant resting and noncycling cells.

One method to prevent the existence of drug-resistant tumor cells is the use of high-dose chemotherapy. The aim of this approach is to maximize the effects of the drug at the cellular level before the problem of resistance occurs. An example of high-dose chemotherapy is the use of cytarabine (Ara-C) for the treatment of leukemia. The standard dose of this agent is 100 mg/m^2. However, the intensified regimen of this agent includes a dose of 3000 mg/m^2.[2,32]

Classification of Chemotherapeutic Drugs. Chemotherapeutic drugs are categorized or classified according to their structure and mechanisms of action (Table 14-17 and

Table 14-17 Classification of Chemotherapy Drugs

Mechanisms of Action	Examples
Alkylating Agents	
Cell Cycle–Nonspecific Drugs	
Damage DNA by causing breaks in the double-strand helix (similar to the effect of radiation therapy); if repair does not occur, cells will die immediately (cytocidal) or when they attempt to divide (cytostatic)	Mechlorethamine (nitrogen mustard), cyclophosphamide (Cytoxan), chlorambucil (Leukeran), melphalan (Alkeran), thiotepa, busulfan (Myleran), dacarbazine (DTIC), ifosfamide (Ifex), estramustine (Emcyt)
Heavy metal effect on DNA	Cisplatin (Platinol), carboplatin (Paraplatin)
Antimetabolites	
Cell Cycle Phase–Specific Drugs	
Interfere with synthesis of DNA by mimicking certain essential cellular metabolites that cell incorporates into synthesis of DNA; cells will die immediately (cytocidal)	Methotrexate (Amethopterin), cytarabine (Ara-C, Cytosar), 5-fluorouracil (5-FU), 6-mercaptopurine (6-TG), thioguanine (6-TG), floxuridine (FUDR), vidarabine (Vira-A), 5-azacytidine, hexamethylmelamine, pentostatin (Nipent), fludarabine (Fludara), hydroxyurea (Hydrea)
Antitumor Antibiotics	
Cell Cycle–Nonspecific Drugs	
Modify function of DNA and interfere with transcription of RNA; cells will die immediately (cytocidal) or when they attempt to divide (cytostatic)	Doxorubicin (Adriamycin), bleomycin (Blenoxane), mitomycin (Mutamycin), daunorubicin (Daunomycin), dactinomycin (Actinomycin D), idarubicin (Idamycin),
mithramycin	(Mithracin)
Plant Alkaloids (Mitotic Inhibitors)	
Cell Cycle Phase–Specific Drugs	
Interrupt cellular replication in mitosis at metaphase; cells will die immediately (cytocidal)	Vinblastine (Velban), vincristine (Oncovin), etoposide (VePesid), paclitaxel (Taxol), vinorelbine (Navelbine), taxotere (Docetaxel), vindesine (Eldisine), teniposide (Vumon)
Nitrosureas	
Cell Cycle–Nonspecific Drugs	
Have similar effect to alkylating agents and also block specific enzymes needed for the synthesis of purine; cells will die immediately (cytocidal) or when they attempt to divide (cytostatic)	Carmustine (BCNU), lomustine (CCNU), semustine (Methyl CCNU), streptozocin (Zanosar), chlorozotozin (DCNU)
Corticosteroids	
Cell Cycle–Nonspecific Drugs	
Disrupt the cell membrane and inhibit synthesis of protein; decrease circulating lymphocytes; inhibit mitosis, depress immune system; increase feeling of well-being	Cortisone, hydrocortisone, methylprednisone, methylprednisolone, prednisone, dexamethasone (Decadron)
Hormones	
Cell Cycle–Nonspecific Drugs	
Stimulate the process of cellular differentiation; metastatic lesions are less able to survive in unfavorable environment; decrease the process of cellular proliferation	Androgens (testosterone, fluoxymesterone [Halotestin]), estrogens (diethylstilbestrol [DES]), progestins (Provera, Delalutin, Megace)
Miscellaneous	
Destroys exogenous supply of L-asparagine, which is needed for cellular proliferation; normal cells can synthesize but cannot be synthesized by cancer cells	L-Asparaginase (Elspar)
Antiestrogens used in breast cancer	Tamoxifen (Nolvadex)
Antiadrenal drug blocks adrenal steroid production	Aminoglutethimide (Cytadren)
Produces single- and double-strand breaks in DNA	Amsacrine (m-AMSA)
Suppresses mitosis at interphase, appears to alter preformed DNA, RNA, and protein	Procarbazine (Matulane, Natulan)
Suppresses adrenocortical activity, modifies peripheral metabolism of steroids	Mitotane (Lysodren)
Inhibits DNA and RNA synthesis	Mitoxantrone (Novantrone)

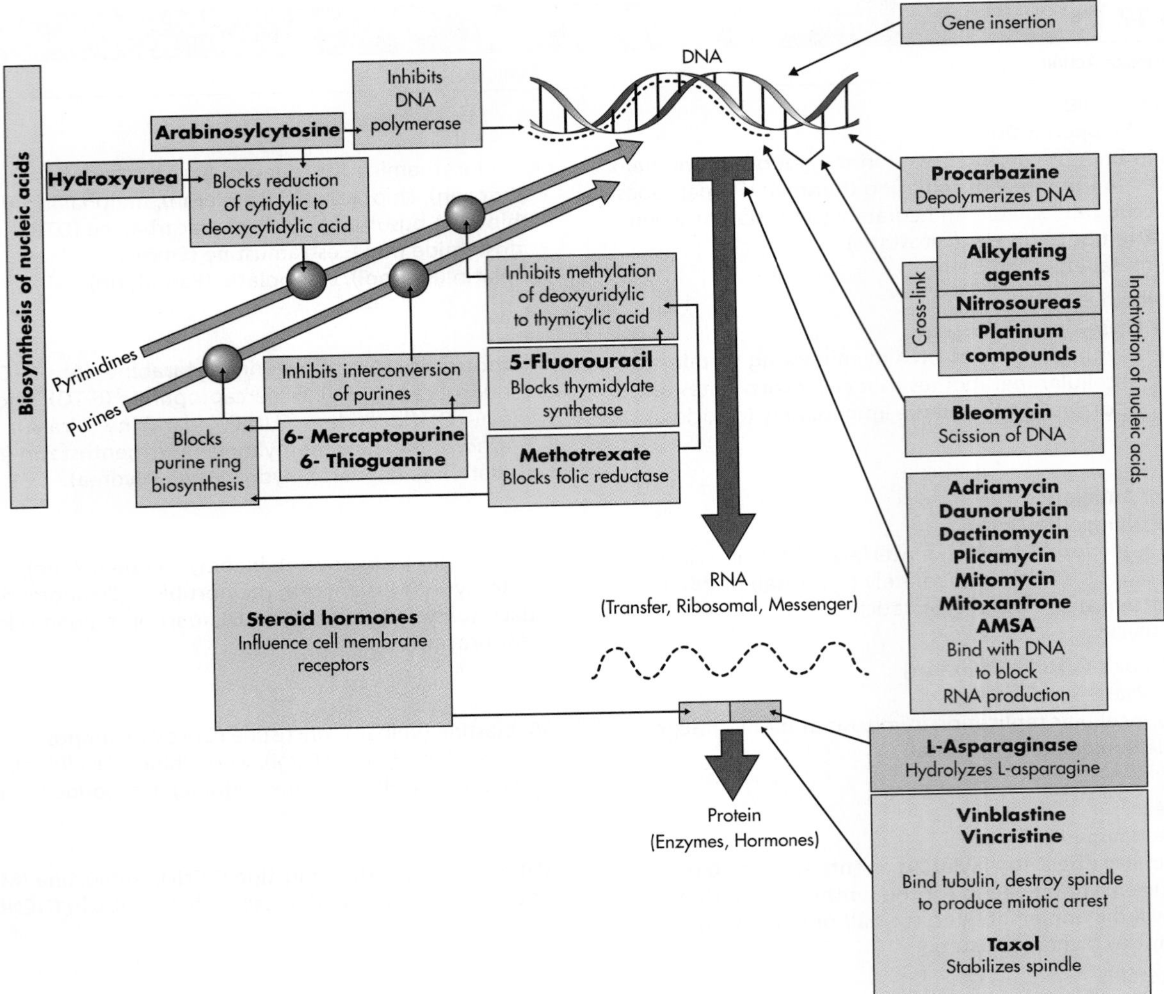

Fig. 14-19 Mechanisms of action of chemotherapeutic and biologic agents.

Fig. 14-19). Each drug in a particular classification has many similarities, but major differences in the drugs are also evident.

Methods of Administration. Chemotherapy can be administered by several routes (Table 14-18). The oral and intravenous (IV) routes are the most common. One of the major concerns with the IV administration of antineoplastic drugs is possible irritation of the vessel wall by the drug or, even worse, *extravasation* (infiltration of drugs into tissues surrounding the infusion site) causing local tissue damage. Many chemotherapeutic drugs are *vesicants*—agents that when accidentally infiltrated into the skin cause severe local tissue breakdown and necrosis. Some guidelines to promote safe use of the chemotherapeutic drugs by IV administration follow:

1. Know specifics about the safe administration of chemotherapy.
2. Start an IV infusion of normal saline solution or 5% dextrose in water or saline solution with a small-lumen short needle or catheter. Ensure that recent venipunctures have not been performed proximal to the IV site. Avoid using an arm that has poor lymphatic drainage or that has previously received radiation therapy.

Table 14-18 Methods of Chemotherapy Administration

Method	Examples
Oral	Cyclophosphamide
Intramuscular	Bleomycin
Intravenous	Doxorubicin, vincristine
Intracavitary (pleural, peritoneal)	Radioisotopes, alkylating agents, methotrexate
Intrathecal	Methotrexate, cytarabine
Intraarterial	DTIC, 5-FU, methotrexate, floxuridine
Perfusion	Alkylating agents
Continuous infusion	5-FU, methotrexate, cytarabine
Subcutaneous	Cytarabine
Topical	5-FU cream

3. Select a vein that is large enough to promote infusion without irritating the intima of the vein. When a vesicant is administered, avoid the veins in the hand, wrist, and antecubital area.
4. Instruct the patient to immediately report any changes in sensation, especially burning or stinging pain.
5. Check for a blood return before infusing the chemotherapeutic drug. However, a blood return does not always indicate an intact vein.
6. If more than one drug is to be administered, give the vesicant agents first, when the vein is at its optimum integrity. (NOTE: This method is controversial. Some believe that vesicants should be administered last or given between two nonvesicants.)
7. Slowly push those drugs that are to be given by the push or bolus method. Give in small increments (0.5 to 1.0 ml). Pause 30 to 60 seconds after each increment, and allow the IV infusion to flush the vein; check blood return, and again gently push 0.5 to 1.0 ml of the medication. Repeat until the medication has been given and allow the IV infusion to flush the vein for several minutes.
8. Avoid continuous peripheral IV infusions of vesicant agents. If given peripherally, the patient receiving the vesicant agent must be monitored directly for local tissue responses at all times.
9. Stop the IV infusion immediately if the patient complains of a burning or stinging pain or if an infiltration is suspected. If the drug is an irritant, check for blood return and, if present, continue to administer the drug. If it is a vesicant, stop the infusion and begin appropriate extravasation procedures.
10. Use transparent tape to secure needle placement and allow direct observation of area.
11. If extravasation occurs:
    a. Stop the IV infusion immediately; notify the physician, or use the standing written orders for treatment related to the specific vesicant agent.
    b. Remove the IV infusion tubing and aspirate any remaining drug with a new syringe.
    c. Inject the prescribed antidote (if one is available) in the infusion needle or in a "pin cushion" fashion in the skin surrounding the needle site.
    d. Apply a topical corticosteroid cream, if prescribed.
    e. Elevate the site.
    f. Apply cold compresses for the first 24 to 48 hours unless a plant alkaloid has been infiltrated; heat is applied following extravasation of plant alkaloids.
    g. Document the extravasation.
    h. Observe the site at designated intervals.
    i. A plastic surgeon may be consulted, depending on the extent of anticipated damage.[32]
    j. Provide the patient with written home care instructions.

Pain is the cardinal symptom of extravasation, although extravasation has been known to occur without causing pain. Swelling, redness, and the presence of vesicles on the skin are other signs of extravasation. After a few days, the tissue may begin to ulcerate and necrose. The process has the potential to progress to a deep, wide crater that often warrants closure with skin grafts. If infection occurs, this is a serious problem that may be life threatening.

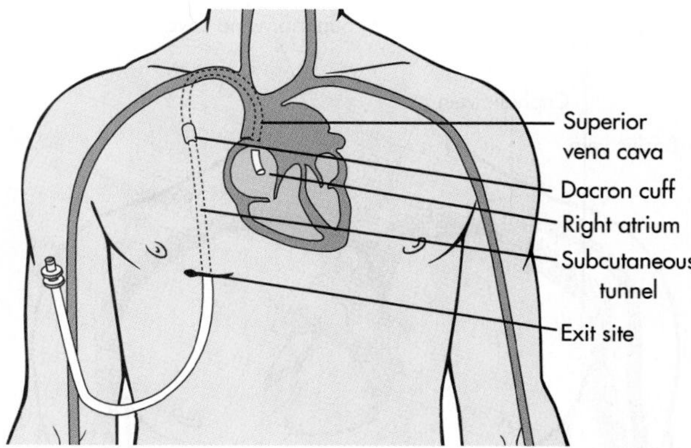

Fig. 14-20 Silastic right atrial catheter placement. Note tip of the catheter in the right atrium.

Chemotherapy can also be administered by means of a vascular access device. Vascular access devices are placed in large vessels (venous or arterial) and permit frequent, continuous, or intermittent administration of chemotherapy, biologic therapy, and other products, thus avoiding multiple punctures for vascular access. These devices are indicated in instances of limited vascular access, intensive chemotherapy, continuous infusion of vesicant agents, and projected long-term need for vascular access. In addition to their usefulness in administration of chemotherapeutic agents, vascular access devices can be used to administer additional fluids, such as blood products, parenteral nutrition, and other medications, and for venous blood sampling. The advantages of vascular access devices are that they provide for rapid dilution of chemotherapy, decreased incidence of extravasation, and reduced need for venipuncture. Three major types of vascular access devices are Silastic right atrial catheters, implanted infusion ports, and infusion (external and implanted) pumps.

Silastic right atrial catheters. Silastic right atrial catheters (Hickman, Broviac, Specialty Access Products, and Raaf) are single-, double-, or triple-lumen catheters approximately 90 cm in length with internal diameters ranging from 1 to 2 mm (Fig. 14-20). These catheters are inserted with the aid of local or general anesthesia through a central vein with the tip resting in the right atrium of the heart. The other end of the catheter is tunneled through subcutaneous tissue and exits through a separate incision on the chest or abdominal wall. A Dacron cuff on the catheter serves to stabilize the catheter and may also decrease the incidence of infection. Accurate placement must be verified by chest x-ray before the catheter can be used. Care requirements include cap change, cleansing, heparin flush, and dressing change. The exact frequency and procedures for these requirements vary from institution to institution. Reported complications with these catheters include occlusion, sepsis, bleeding, venous thrombosis, technical problems, and local infection at the exit site.[33]

The Groshong catheter is a distinct type of tunneled central venous catheter. The unique features of this catheter are the existence of a pressure-sensitive valve near the distal end, which precludes the need for heparin flushing and clamping, and its

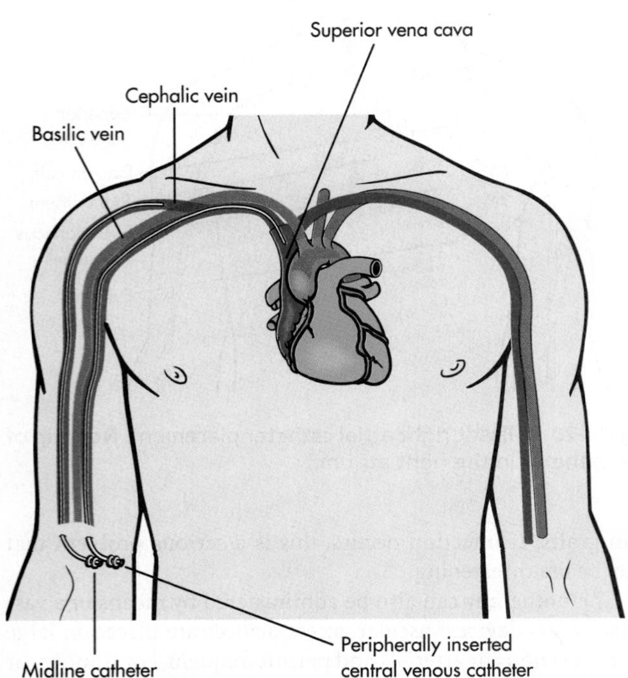

Fig. 14-21 Placement of peripherally inserted central venous catheters (PICC) and midline catheters (MLC).

placement 2 to 3 cm above the right atrium in the superior vena cava.

Peripherally inserted central venous catheters and midline catheters. Peripherally inserted central venous catheters (PICCs) (e.g., C-PICS, Per-Q-Cath, Intracath, L-Cath, Ven-A-Cath, Viggio Hydrocath, and Groshong PICC) and midline catheters (MLCs) (e.g., Landmark Midline Catheter and L-Cath) are single- or double-lumen, nontunneled, polymer catheters that are primarily used in cancer care for immediate central venous access or when the need for infusion therapy is beyond the capacity of the patient's existing, long-term venous access device[34] (Fig. 14-21). These catheters are used for short-term IV therapy, frequent administration of blood products, blood drawing, and intermittent or continuous drug infusions. These catheters are placed by a physician or a specially trained nurse.

PICC lines are inserted at or just above the antecubital fossa and advanced to a position with the tip ending in the distal one third of the superior vena cava. These lines are up to 60 cm in length with gauges ranging from 24 to 16. They can be in place for up to 6 months. The technique for placement of a PICC line involves insertion of the catheter through a needle with the use of a guide wire or forceps to advance the line.

MLC lines are catheters that are placed between the antecubital fossa and the head of the clavicle. These catheters are shorter than PICC lines (15 to 20 cm) with the tip resting in the larger vessels of the upper arm. PICC lines can be used for this purpose. However, specific MLCs have been developed (Landmark Midline Catheter and L-Cath). MLCs are made of an elastomeric hydrogel that becomes approximately 50 times softer approximately 2 hours following insertion because of contact with body fluids. As a result, the gauge of the catheter increases and the length of the line increases. The MLC can be placed

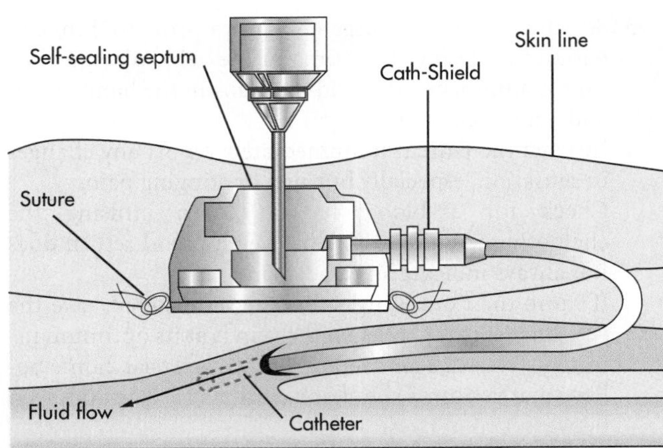

Fig. 14-22 Cross-section of implantable port displaying access of the port with the Huber needle. Note the deflected point of the Huber needle, which prevents coring of the port's septum.

above or below the antecubital fossa. Following venipuncture, the needle is withdrawn into a tube, and the catheter is advanced using a catheter advancement tab.

Complications of PICC and MLC lines include catheter occlusion and phlebitis. Urokinase can be used to lyse obstructions. If phlebitis occurs, it usually appears within 7 to 10 days following insertion. Signs of phlebitis include redness, edema, and tenderness along the track of the catheter line. The catheter should be removed, and the tip of the catheter must be cultured. The arm in which a PICC or MLC is in place should not be used for blood pressures or blood drawing.[34]

Implanted infusion ports. Implanted infusion ports (Hickman Port, Port-A-Cath, Infusaid MicroPort, Norport LS, Lifeport, and Groshong Port) consist of a central venous catheter connected to an implanted, single or double subcutaneous injection port (Fig. 14-22). The catheter is placed into the desired vein and the other end is connected to a port that is sutured to the chest wall muscle and surgically implanted in a subcutaneous pocket on the chest wall. The port consists of a metal sheath with a self-sealing silicone septum. It is accessed via the septum by means of a special Huber-point needle that has a deflected tip to prevent coring of the septum. Huber-point needles are also available with the tip at a 90° angle for longer infusions. Care requirements include dressing change, cleansing, and flushing. Complications attributed to implanted infusion ports include clotting, catheter migration, infection, bleeding, thrombosis, air embolism, and infection at the exit site or in the pocket. Formation of "sludge" (accumulation of clotted blood and drug precipitate) may also occur within the port septum. The risk of sludge formation is increased by "gouging" of the septal floor by the Huber-point needle. New implanted ports (Opti-Port) have been developed to reduce the risk of sludge formation.[35]

Infusion pumps. Infusion pumps are used in cancer treatment primarily for the continuous infusion of chemotherapy by IV, subcutaneous, intraarterial, and epidural routes. Infusion pumps can be worn externally or implanted surgically. The various types of external infusion pumps (Autosyringe, Cormed, Infumed 200, Deltec-Pharmacia, Pancreatec, Travenol Infusor)

Sideport
Bacterial filter
Needle stop
Inlet septum
Bellows
Outlet flow restrictor
A
Needle stop
Drug chamber
Silicone rubber coating
Charging fluid chamber
Outlet catheter
Suture loop

B

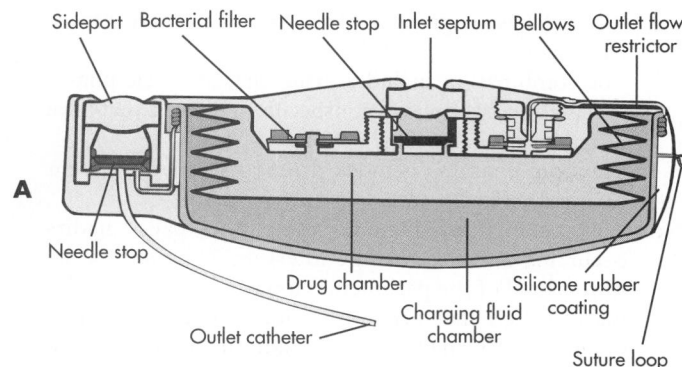

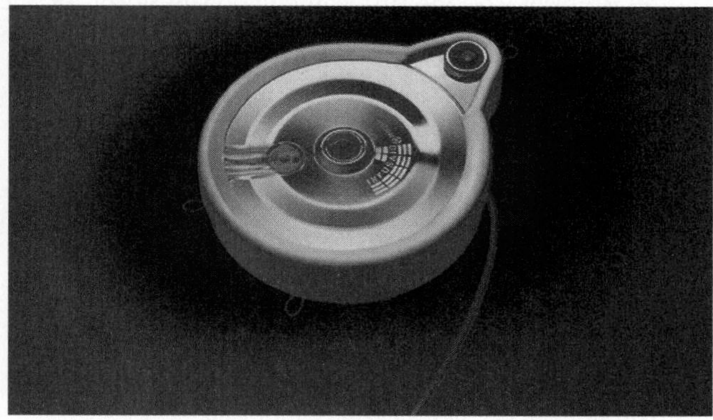

Fig. 14-23 **A,** Cross-section of the implantable pump displaying its two chambers: the drug chamber (inner) and the charging fluid chamber (outer). As the drug chamber is filled, the bellows expand, compressing the charging fluid in the outer chamber. The resulting increased pressure in the outer chamber forces the drug through a membrane filter and preset flow restrictor, thus ensuring a nearly constant flow. **B,** Infusaid pump.

differ in terms of their mechanisms of action, components, and capabilities.

Implanted infusion pumps (Infusaid and Medtronic) are used primarily for intraarterial administration of chemotherapy (Fig. 14-23). This approach permits continuous infusion of the chemotherapeutic agent directly to the area of the tumor while sparing the patient the systemic effects of the drug. Some implanted pumps have two silicone septums. The second septum can be used for bolus medication administration. The most common use of this method of chemotherapy administration has been hepatic artery infusion in the treatment of liver metastasis, usually from primary colon cancer.

Implanted pumps also consist of a catheter that is threaded into the designated artery. The catheter is attached to a pump apparatus that consists of two chambers: an inner chamber that serves as the drug reservoir and an outer chamber that contains vapor pressure providing a source of power for the pump. The pump is implanted surgically in a subcutaneous pocket. Access to the pump is via a silicone septum with a Huber-point needle. Flow rate of the pump can be affected by drug concentration, the length and diameter of the silastic catheter, and the patient's body temperature. Thus dose alterations may be required if the patient experiences a change in temperature or travels to higher altitudes. Complications that have been associated with implanted infusion pumps include infection, thrombosis, clotting of the catheter, and pump malfunction.[36]

Other access devices used in the treatment of the person with cancer include the Tenckhoff catheter used in the administration of intraperitoneal chemotherapy and the Ommaya reservoir, which delivers agents directly to the central nervous system (CNS).

Regional Chemotherapy Administration. Regional treatment with chemotherapy involves the delivery of the drug directly to the tumor site. The advantage of administering chemotherapy by this method is that higher concentrations of the drug can be delivered to the tumor with reduced systemic toxicity. Several regional delivery methods have been developed, including intraarterial, intraperitoneal, intrathecal or intraventricular, and intravesical bladder chemotherapy.[37]

Intraarterial chemotherapy. Intraarterial chemotherapy delivers the drug to the tumor via the arterial vessel supplying the tumor. This method has been used for the treatment of osteogenic sarcoma; cancer of the head and neck, bladder, brain, and cervix; melanoma; primary liver cancer; and metastatic liver disease. One method of intraarterial drug delivery involves the surgical placement of a catheter that is subsequently connected to an external infusion pump or an implanted infusion pump for infusion of the chemotherapeutic agent. Generally, intraarterial chemotherapy results in reduced systemic toxicity. The type of toxicity experienced by the patient is dependent on the site of the tumor being treated.[31]

Intraperitoneal chemotherapy. Intraperitoneal chemotherapy involves the delivery of chemotherapy to the peritoneal cavity for treatment of peritoneal metastases from primary colon and ovarian cancers, mesothelioma, and malignant ascites. Temporary silastic catheters (Tenckhoff, Hickman, and Groshong) are percutaneously or surgically placed into the peritoneal cavity for short-term administration of chemotherapy. Alternatively, an implanted port can be used to administer chemotherapy intraperitoneally. Chemotherapy is generally infused into the peritoneum in 1 to 2 L of fluid and allowed to "dwell" in the peritoneum for a period of 1 to 4 hours. Following the "dwell time," the fluid is usually drained from the peritoneum. Complications of peritoneal chemotherapy include abdominal pain; catheter occlusion, dislodgement, and migration; and infection.[36]

Intrathecal or intraventricular chemotherapy. Cancers that metastasize to the CNS, most commonly breast, lung, GI, leukemia, and lymphoma, are difficult to treat because the blood-brain barrier often prevents distribution of chemotherapy to this area. One method used to treat metastasis to the CNS is intrathecal chemotherapy. This method involves a lumbar puncture and injection of chemotherapy through the dura and arachnoid and into the subarachnoid space. However, this method has resulted in incomplete distribution of the drug in the CNS, particularly to the cisternal and ventricular areas.

To ensure more uniform distribution of chemotherapy to the cisternal and ventricular areas, an Ommaya reservoir is often inserted. An Ommaya reservoir is a silastic, dome-shaped disk with an extension catheter that is surgically implanted through the cranium into a lateral ventricle. In addition to more

Table 14-19 Cells with Rapid Rate of Proliferation

Cells and Generation Time	Effect of Cell Destruction
Bone marrow stem cell, 6-24 hr	Myelosuppression; infection, bleeding, anemia
Neutrophils, 12 hr	Leukopenia, infection
Epithelial cells lining the gastrointestinal tract, 12-24 hr	Anorexia, stomatitis, esophagitis, nausea and vomiting, diarrhea
Cells of the hair follicle, 24 hr	Alopecia
Ova or testes, 24-36 hr	Reproductive dysfunction

consistent drug distribution, the Ommaya reservoir precludes the use of repeated, painful lumbar punctures. Complications of intrathecal or intraventricular chemotherapy include headache, nausea, vomiting, fever, and nuchal rigidity.[36]

Intravesical bladder chemotherapy. The patient with superficial transitional cell cancer of the bladder often has recurrent disease following traditional surgical therapy. Instillation of chemotherapy into the bladder promotes destruction of cancer cells and reduces the incidence of recurrent disease. Additional benefits of this therapy include reduced urinary and sexual dysfunction. The chemotherapeutic agent is instilled into the bladder via a urinary catheter and retained for 1 to 3 hours. Complications of this therapy include dysuria, urinary frequency, hematuria, and bladder spasms.[36]

Effects of Chemotherapy on Normal Tissues. Chemotherapeutic agents cannot selectively distinguish between normal cells and cancer cells. When normal cells are destroyed, the patient experiences certain signs and symptoms that are the expected side effects or toxic effects of chemotherapy. Effects of chemotherapy are caused by destruction of cells with a rapid rate of cellular proliferation (Table 14-19); response of the body to the products of cellular destruction (cellular waste products in circulation may cause fatigue, anorexia, and taste alterations); and specific drug toxicities (Table 14-20).

The adverse effects of these drugs can be classified as acute, delayed, or chronic. Acute toxicity includes vomiting, allergic reactions, and arrhythmias. Delayed effects include mucositis, alopecia, and bone marrow depression. Mucositis can result in mouth sores, gastritis, and diarrhea. Chronic toxicities involve damage to organs such as the heart, liver, kidneys, and lungs.

Treatment Plan. When chemotherapy is used in the treatment of cancer, several drugs are usually given in combination. Today, single-drug chemotherapy is rarely chosen for a treatment plan. The drugs given are carefully selected to most effectively kill the cancer cells while allowing the normal cells to repair themselves and proliferate. The dose of each drug is carefully calculated according to the body weight or the body surface area of the patient being treated. The choice of the drugs selected to be given together to treat a particular cancer is based on the following principles of combination chemotherapy:

1. The drugs used in the treatment plan are effective against the cancer being treated.
2. When drugs are given in combination, a synergistic effect occurs.
3. The combination includes drugs that are cycle phase-specific and cycle phase-nonspecific and drugs that have different mechanisms of action.
4. The combination includes drugs that have different toxic side effects.
5. The combination includes drugs that cause nadirs occurring at different time intervals. The *nadir* is the lowest level of the peripheral blood cell counts (particularly WBC) that occurs secondary to bone marrow depression. The nadir following administration of most chemotherapy drugs occurs in 7 to 28 days.

The MOPP protocol, the first combination protocol for the treatment of Hodgkin's disease, is an example of a combination chemotherapy treatment regimen:

Nitrogen mustard (M)
Cycle phase-nonspecific
Alkylating agent
Toxic side effects: myelosuppression, nausea, vomiting, alopecia
Nadir: 7 to 14 days
Oncovin (O)
Cycle phase-specific
Plant alkaloid
Toxic side effects: neurotoxicity, alopecia
Nadir: unknown
Procarbazine (P)
Cycle phase-specific
Monoamine oxidase (MAO) inhibitor
Toxic side effects: myelosuppression, nausea, vomiting
Nadir: 2 to 8 weeks
Prednisone (P)
Toxic side effects: steroid effects
Nadir: unknown

The agents in this drug protocol differ in mechanisms of action, toxic side effects, and nadir, but the combination is synergistic in nature and effectively destroys the cancer cells present in the early stages of Hodgkin's disease.

The drugs are given according to a specific schedule that includes a time of drug administration and a time of rest from drug administration. The rest period is necessary to allow the normal body cells that have been destroyed to proliferate and repair the damaged tissue. The example in Table 14-21 (p. 305) describes a typical MOPP schedule. This drug schedule is repeated a specific number of times. Most chemotherapy treatment plans extend for 6 months or longer. The patient is evaluated before the administration of each course of chemotherapy to determine whether the normal cells have proliferated to a sufficient degree.

Often the most difficult decision to make is when to stop the administration of chemotherapy. The patient is evaluated according to the following criteria:

1. *Complete remission.* Complete absence of all evidence of cancer and a return to the usual performance status occur; the duration of a complete remission must exceed 1 month.

Table **14-20** Toxic Side Effects of Chemotherapy

Chemotherapeutic Agent	Myelosuppression	Mucositis	Nausea and Vomiting	Alopecia	Vesicant (V)/ Irritant (I)	Allergic Reaction	Other Specific Toxicities
Aminoglutethimide (Cytadren)	+	–	+	–	–	–	Skin rash; sensory alterations, including lethargy, visual blurring, vertigo, ataxia, and nystagmus; hyponatremia, hyperkalemia, cortisol insufficiency
Actinomycin D (Cosmegan)	+	+	+	+	+ (V)	0	Diarrhea
Amsacrine (m-AMSA)	+	0	+	0	+ (V)	0	Flulike syndrome, venoocclusive disease, hepatotoxicity
5-Azacytidine	+	+	+	0	0	0	Hepatotoxicity
Busulfan (Myleran)	+	0	±	0	0	0	Pulmonary fibrosis
Bleomycin (Blenoxane)	±	+	±	+	0	+	Pulmonary toxicity, skin rash
Camptothecin-11 (CPT-11)	+	–	+	+	–	–	Diarrhea, pulmonary toxicity
Carboplatin (Paraplatin)	+	0	+	0	0	0	Pigmentation at injection site, hepatotoxicity, neurotoxicity, renal toxicity, pulmonary toxicity
Carmustine (BCNU)	+	+	+	0	+ (I)	0	Hepatotoxicity
Chlorambucil (Leukeran)	+	0	±	0	0	0	
Chlorodeoxyadenosine	+	0	0	0	0	0	Neurotoxicity, renal toxicity
Cisplatin (Platinol)	+	0	+	0	0	+	Nephrotoxicity, peripheral neuropathy, ototoxicity
Cladribine (Leustatin)	+	–	+	–	–	–	Fever, rash, diarrhea, constipation, cough, shortness of breath, tachycardia, edema
Cortisone	+	–	–	–	–	–	Gastric irritation, hyperglycemia, sodium and water retention, hypokalemia, hypocalcemia, behavioral changes
Cyclophosphamide (Cytoxan)	+	0	+	+	0	0	Sterile hemorrhagic cystitis, heart failure
Cytarabine (Cytosar, Ara-C)	+	+	+	+	0	0	Hepatotoxicity
Dacarbazine (DTIC) (Daunomycin)	+	0	+	0	+ (I)	+	Hypotension
Diethylstilbestrol (DES)	0	0	+	0	0	0	Congestive heart failure
Doxorubicin (Adriamycin)	+	+	+	+	+ (V)	0	Cardiotoxicity, diarrhea
Estramustine (Emcyt)	+	–	+	–	+ (V)	0	Diarrhea, hepatotoxicity, hypocalcemia, hypophosphatemia, gynecomastia, congestive heart failure, thrombophlebitis, rash
Etoposide (VePesid)	+	0	+	+	+ (I)	±	Hepatotoxicity, neurotoxicity, hypotension
Floxuridine (FUDR)		+	+	+	0	0	Diarrhea, rash
Fludarabine (Fludara)	+	+	+	–	–	–	Pulmonary toxicity, pericardial effusion, neurotoxicity
5-Fluorouracil (5-FU)	+	+	±	±	0	0	Diarrhea, photosensitivity
Fluoxymesterone (Halotestin)	0	0	+	0	0	0	Masculinization
Gemcitabine (Gemzar)	+	–	+	–	–	–	Flulike symptoms

Continued

Table 14-20 Toxic Side Effects of Chemotherapy—cont'd

Chemotherapeutic Agent	Myelo-suppression	Mucositis	Nausea and Vomiting	Alopecia	Vesicant (V)/ Irritant (I)	Allergic Reaction	Other Specific Toxicities
Hexamethylmelamine	+	0	+	±	0	0	Peripheral neuropathy
Hydroxyurea (Hydrea)	+	+	+	+	0	0	
Idarubicin (Idamycin)	+	+	+	+	0	0	Cardiomyopathy
Ifosfamide (Ifex)	±	0	±	+	0	0	Hematuria, neurotoxicity, hemorrhagic cystitis
L-Asparaginase (Elspar)	0	0	+	0	0	+	Major organ failure
Lomustine (CCNU)	+	+	+	±	0	0	Hepatotoxicity
Megestrol acetate (Megace)	0	0	0	+	0	0	Fluid retention
Mechlorethamine (nitrogen mustard)	+	0	+	+	+ (V)	0	
Melphalan (Alkeran)	+	±	±	+	0	0	Rare pulmonary toxicity, secondary malignancy
6-Mercaptopurine (6-MP)	+	+	+	0	0	0	Hepatotoxicity
Methotrexate (MTX, Amethopterin)	+	+	±	±	0	0	Nephrotoxicity
Mithramycin (Mithracin)	+	+	+	0	+ (V)	0	Hemorrhagic tendency
Mitomycin (Mutamycin)	+	+	+	+	+ (V)	0	Nephrotoxicity, pulmonary toxicity
Mitotane (Lysodren)	−	−	+	−	−	−	Diarrhea, neurotoxicity, skin irritation or rash
Mitoxantrone (Novantrone)	+	+	+	+	0	0	Drug fever, diarrhea, increased liver enzymes
Oxaliplatin	+	−	+	−	−	−	Peripheral neuropathy
Oxymethalone (Anadrol-50)	0	0	+	0	0	0	Hepatotoxicity
Paclitaxel (Taxol)	+	0	+	±	0	±	Sensory neuropathy
Pentostatin (Nipent)	+	−	+	+	+ (V)	−	Nephrotoxicity, hepatotoxicity, mental status changes, pulmonary toxicity, severe conjunctivitis
Prednisolone	0	0	0	0	0	0	Steroid side effects
Prednisone	0	0	0	0	0	0	Steroid side effects
Procarbazine (Matulane)	+	±	+	0	0	0	Monoamine oxidase inhibitor
Semustine (Methyl CCNU)	+	+	+	0	0	0	
Streptozocin (Zanosar)	+	0	+	±	+ (I)	0	Nephrotoxicity
Tamoxifen (Nolvadex)	±	0	+	0	0	0	
Taxotere (Docetaxel)	+	−	−	+	−	+	Rash, fluid and electrolyte imbalance, peripheral edema, pleural effusion
Teniposide (Vumon)	+	−	+	+	+ (I)	+	Hypotension, hepatoxicity, cardiac arrhythmias, peripheral neuropathy
6-Thioguanine (6-TG)	+	+	+	0	0	0	Hepatotoxicity
Thiotepa	+	−	+	−	−	+	Sexual dysfunction, secondary malignancies, dizziness, headache, fever
Uracil mustard	+	0	+	±	0	0	
Vinblastine (Velban)	+	+	+	±	+ (V)	0	Neurotoxicity
Vincristine (Oncovin)	0	0	0	+	+ (V)	0	Neurotoxicity
Vindesine (Eldisine)	+	±	+	+	+ (V)	−	Peripheral neuropathy, constipation, rash, diarrhea
Vinorelbine (Navelbine)	+	+	+	+	+ (V)	−	Neurotoxicity, diarrhea, hepatotoxicity, injection site reaction, sexual/reproductive dysfunction

+, Common; ±, infrequent; 0, uncommon; −, no effect.

Table 14-21 MOPP Chemotherapeutic Drug Schedule

Drug	1	2	3	4	5	6	7	8	9	10	11	12	13	14	15-28
	Days														
Nitrogen mustard (intravenous administration)	↔							↔							
Oncovin (intravenous administration)	↔							↔							*
Procarbazine (oral administration)	←													→	
Prednisone (oral administration)	←													→	

*No drugs given.

2. *Partial remission.* Regression of 50% or more of the disease process without evidence of progression and with subjective improvement is noted. The duration of a partial remission is usually several months.
3. *Improvement.* Regression of 25% to 50% of the disease process with subjective improvement is noted.
4. *No response.* Regression of 25% or less of the disease with no subjective improvement is noted.
5. *Progression.* Progression of the disease process is noted.

With a complete remission that has extended for a time, the chemotherapy is usually discontinued, and the patient is evaluated at frequent intervals. When partial remission or improvement occurs, the same treatment plan or a revised treatment plan is followed over a long period (several years), and the patient is evaluated frequently. No response or progression of disease warrants a change in the treatment plan or a decision to use treatment for palliation.

Safe Preparation, Administration, and Disposal of Chemotherapeutic Agents. An important issue in cancer care is that working with antineoplastic agents may be hazardous for health professionals. It is suspected that the person preparing or giving chemotherapy may absorb the drug through inhalation of particles when reconstituting a powder in an open ampule and through skin contact. There may also be some risk in handling the vomitus and excreta of persons receiving chemotherapy.

The only well-known hazard associated with chemotherapy is that of cutaneous reactions following skin contact with certain drugs, including BCNU (Carmustine), mechlorethamine (nitrogen mustard), doxorubicin (Adriamycin), and other vesicants. The literature accompanying these drugs specifically cautions against skin and eye contact to prevent possible skin reactions and corneal damage.

Guidelines for the safe handling of chemotherapeutic agents have been developed by the Occupational Safety and Health Administration (OSHA) and the Oncology Nursing Society. These guidelines are summarized in Table 14-22.[36,37]

NURSING MANAGEMENT: CHEMOTHERAPY

The role of the nurse in cancer chemotherapy has greatly expanded during the past decade. Regardless of the health care agency setting, the nurse will meet the individual who is receiving or who has received chemotherapy. One of the most important responsibilities of the nurse is that of differentiating between toxic effects of the drug and progression of the malignant process. The nurse also must differentiate between tolerable side effects and acute toxic effects of chemotherapeutic agents. For example, nausea and vomiting are expected and controllable side effects of many drugs. However, if paresthesia occurs with the use of vincristine or signs of heart failure appear with the use of doxorubicin, these serious reactions must be reported to the physician so that drug dosages can be modified or discontinued. Some toxicities associated with chemotherapy may not be reversible. For example, ototoxicity may be an irreversible effect of cisplatin therapy, especially at higher doses. Periodic testing of hearing may be necessary to monitor for this toxicity. Specific nursing measures related to problems associated with chemotherapy are presented in NCP 14-1.

Nausea and vomiting are the most commonly observed GI side effects. Vomiting may occur within 1 hour of administration and may last for 24 hours or more. Several antiemetic drugs are available (see Chapter 39 and Table 39-5). Metoclopramide (Reglan), ondansetron (Zofran), granisetron (Kytril), and dexamethasone (Decadron) have also been used to decrease nausea and vomiting caused by chemotherapy. Nursing management related to nausea and vomiting is presented in the nursing care plan for the patient with cancer (NCP 14-1).

Results of laboratory studies of the patient who is receiving chemotherapy should be monitored. Particular attention should be given to the WBC (especially neutrophil count), platelet, and RBC counts. If the WBC count falls to less than 2000 per μl (2×10^9/L), the drug regimen may need to be modified or discontinued. Every possible measure should be taken to prevent infections in a patient with leukopenia (see nursing care plan on neutropenia in [NCP 29-3]). If the platelet count falls to less than 50,000 per μl (50×10^9/L), the patient must be assessed for any signs of bleeding, and measures should be taken to prevent bleeding (see the nursing care plan on thrombocytopenia in [NCP 29-2]). Platelet transfusions may be necessary. RBC transfusions may also be indicated for treatment of symptomatic anemia. However, anemia is an uncommon problem in the patient receiving chemotherapy.[38]

Uric acid and creatinine levels are usually monitored weekly. Optimum hydration is important to prevent uric acid crystals from causing obstructive uropathy. Allopurinol is often administered as a prophylactic measure if extensive cell breakdown is expected. Other diagnostic monitoring depends on the type of drug. For example, an electrocardiogram (ECG) is performed, and cardiac ejection fractions are measured to

Table 14-22 Guidelines for Safe Handling of Chemotherapeutic Agents

Preparation

- Prepare all chemotherapeutic agents in a central area and under a class II or III vertical laminar-flow biologic safety cabinet, vented to the outside.
- Agents should be prepared by a pharmacist, who should do the following:
  - Wear a disposable, protective gown with long sleeves and elastic cuffs and disposable, surgical, nonpowdered latex gloves
  - Place a disposable, plastic-backed liner on the work surface
  - Post hazardous warning signs in the mixing area
  - Use aseptic technique
  - Avoid puncturing gloves or inoculating self
  - Use Luer-Lok fittings where possible
  - Vent all vials
  - Wrap gauze around neck of ampule when opening
  - Prime tubing under safety cabinet before cytotoxic drug is added
  - Place all exposed waste in an approved disposable container

Administration and Exposure to Excreta and Vomitus During Administration

- Wear disposable, surgical, nonpowdered latex gloves.
- Wear disposable gown and mask.
- Use Luer-Lok fittings where possible.
- Never expel air from syringes, recap needles, or use venting tubing with IV bottles.

Disposal

- Wear disposable, surgical, nonpowdered latex gloves during disposal of all disposable items used in the preparation and administration of chemotherapeutic agents, body fluids, and linen.
- Place all disposable items (needles, syringes, vials, and ampules) coming in contact with antineoplastic agents in an approved, leak-proof container.
- Place a waterproof pad over the bedpan or toilet to avoid back-splashing of urine or stool while flushing.
- Discard waste containers in an approved incinerator.
- Place contaminated linen in labeled, double bags; wash linen separately.

Spills

- Wear disposable, surgical, nonpowdered latex gloves.
- Wear disposable gown with elastic cuffs.
- Use "spill kits" containing all materials necessary for proper handling.

Personnel Recommendations

- Teach all persons likely to be exposed to antineoplastic agents or excreta the necessary precautions.
- Prevent contact of pregnant or lactating women with chemotherapeutic agents.
- Distribute workload to minimize employee exposure to chemotherapeutic agents.
- Provide periodic health screening for exposed persons.
- Document patterns of exposure.

monitor the potential cardiotoxic effects of doxorubicin and daunorubicin.[39]

Patient Education

Education of the patient is an extremely important part of the nurse's role related to chemotherapy. To decrease the fear and anxiety often associated with chemotherapy, the patient must be told what to expect during a course of treatment. The patient's attitude toward treatment should be explored so that any misconception or fear can be discussed. The patient must be told of the possible side effects of chemotherapy that may be experienced during treatment. This may be a discouraging revelation. Therefore good nursing judgment is essential to determine the amount of information the patient can assimilate. The patient must be reassured that this is a temporary situation and that she or he should be feeling better within a few weeks after chemotherapy is discontinued. The patient should also be informed that supportive care (e.g., antiemetics and antidiarrheals) will be provided as needed.

Management of Hair Loss

Many emotions are experienced and expressed when hair loss occurs, including anger, grief, embarrassment, and fear. For some persons, the loss of hair is one of the most stressful events experienced during the course of the illness. Alopecia caused by the administration of chemotherapeutic agents is usually reversible. The degree and duration of hair loss depend on the type and dose of the chemotherapeutic agent, the duration of the treatment, and the nutritional status of the patient. Sometimes the hair begins to grow back while the patient is still receiving chemotherapeutic agents, but generally the hair cells do not grow back until the agents are discontinued. Often the new hair has a different color and texture than the hair that was lost.

Counseling Regarding Sexual and Reproductive Function

Sexual dysfunction may be manifested as temporary or permanent sterility, temporary or permanent disruption in the menstrual cycle, temporary or permanent impotence, or chromosomal damage leading to possible genetic mutation. The patient should be instructed to use an effective means of birth control during the time of chemotherapy or radiation therapy and for up to 2 years after treatment. This is necessary to avoid birth defects as a result of chromosomal damage, to allow the sperm count to return to normal, and to determine the expected prognosis of the patient. Sexual or genetic counseling is necessary before the conception of a child to determine the risk of chromosomal damage.

Sexual relations can be continued in the usual patterns during and after treatment if an effective method of birth control is used. It may be necessary to alter the time of day chosen for sexual relations if fatigue is a problem. Early morning may be the time the patient feels most rested.

Denuding of the epithelial lining of the vagina may result in inflammation, edema, and ulceration. Sexual intercourse should be avoided if mucositis or ulceration is present. Sitz baths or sitting in a tub of warm water will provide some degree of comfort. A steroid-based cream available by prescription

14-1 NURSING CARE PLAN PATIENT WITH CANCER*

Expected Patient Outcomes	Nursing Interventions and *Rationales*
NURSING DIAGNOSIS **Pain** *related to* effects of the disease or its treatment *as manifested by* facial mask, complaints of pain, guarding.	
▪ Reduction of pain to a tolerable and manageable level.	▪ Assess pain *to provide a baseline for treatment.* ▪ Confront and correct fears of addiction *to reduce the possibility of undertreating the patient's pain.* ▪ Use an "analgesic ladder" (Step 1: nonopioid, Step 2: weak opioid, Step 3: strong opioid) (see Fig. 14-24) *because the pain increases with disease progression and requires stronger treatment.* ▪ Teach patient complementary pain management techniques (imagery, relaxation, biofeedback, etc.) *to augment pain management strategies.*
NURSING DIAGNOSIS **Altered nutrition: less than body requirements** *related to* anorexia, nausea, and vomiting *as manifested by* fatigue, reported or observed inadequate food intake relative to minimum daily requirements with or without weight loss.	
▪ Maintenance of body weight and adequate energy for ADLs. ▪ Decreased episodes of nausea and vomiting.	▪ Avoid punitive or judgmental statements about food intake or weight loss *to avoid the nurse taking an adversarial role.* ▪ Administer antiemetic medication as prescribed *to minimize GI effects.* ▪ Maintain a pleasant, quiet, restful environment *to avoid triggering nausea or vomiting and to allow for maximum rest.* ▪ Modify diet to include bland, lukewarm, high-calorie, high-protein foods *to prevent triggering vomiting and provide additional calories.* ▪ Try small, frequent feedings every few hours rather than fewer large meals *to facilitate gastric emptying and prevent early satiety.* ▪ Teach patient to eat and drink slowly *to allow patient to enjoy the taste and to prevent bloating.* ▪ Ensure adequate fluid hydration with chemotherapy *to dilute drug levels and reduce stimulation of vomiting receptors.* ▪ Provide a well-balanced diet that includes all food groups with increased protein-calorie intake *to promote positive nitrogen balance.* ▪ Gently encourage patient to eat, but avoid nagging *to prevent establishing a negative meal environment.* ▪ Avoid foods that are gas forming, such as salads, cabbage, broccoli, fruits, and beer, *because they can promote nausea and a sense of fullness.* ▪ Serve all foods attractively and in a pleasant environment *to stimulate appetite.* ▪ Teach the patient to sip the nutritional supplement slowly between meals *to avoid bloating.* ▪ Teach the patient what to eat rather than stressing the fact that more food should be eaten. (Home-prepared items are often more appealing.)
NURSING DIAGNOSIS **Ineffective management of therapeutic regimen** *related to* lack of knowledge of long-term management of cancer *as manifested by* frequent questions by patient and/or caregiver regarding self-care, treatment, side effects; observed inability of patient and/or caregiver to manage technical aspects of long-term care.	
▪ Patient/caregiver express confidence in ability to manage long-term care. ▪ Adequate knowledge base to provide care.	▪ Determine knowledge and technical skills needed by patient/caregiver *to plan needed instruction.* ▪ Assess current level of knowledge and skill *to determine the abilities of the patient and caregiver to perform tasks correctly.* ▪ Teach required skills and provide information to patient and caregiver *to increase their knowledge level.* ▪ Provide opportunity for follow-up evaluation and teaching *to increase patient/caregiver confidence and ensure correct performance of tasks.*

Continued

14-1 NURSING CARE PLAN PATIENT WITH CANCER—continued

Expected Patient Outcomes	Nursing Interventions and *Rationales*
NURSING DIAGNOSIS	**Altered oral mucous membrane** *related to* chemotherapy or radiation *as manifested by* verbalization or signs of pain or discomfort in mouth, coated tongue, xerostomia (dry mouth), halitosis, swollen membranes; oral lesions; hemorrhagic gingivitis, leukoplakia, stomatitis, dysphagia.
■ No oral pain. ■ No infections in the oral mucosa. ■ No break in integrity of oral mucosa.	■ Assess oral mucosa daily. ■ Teach patient to inspect oral cavity *because stomatitis usually occurs 4 to 14 days after treatment begins.* ■ Remove dentures at night *to avoid further irritation.* ■ Observe for dryness, redness, and white or yellow membrane and the presence of any breaks in integrity of tissues. ■ Distinguish stomatitis from candidiasis and other oral problems, such as xerostomia and herpes, *so appropriate treatment is used.* ■ Use mouthwashes of baking soda, baking soda and saline, or normal saline solution every 2 hr *to provide comfort.* ■ Use soft-bristle toothbrushes, sponge-tipped applicators, or an irrigation syringe as cleansing agents *to prevent trauma.* ■ Avoid the use of lemon and glycerin swabs for mouth care *because they increase dryness and irritation.* ■ Apply topical anesthetics, such as viscous Xylocaine or oxethazaine, as ordered *to provide pain relief.* ■ Modify diet to avoid hot, spicy, acidic foods *to avoid irritation.* ■ Discourage use of irritants such as tobacco and alcohol. ■ Encourage drinking of water or other liquids at frequent intervals throughout the day or use of an artificial saliva *to keep mucous membranes moist.* ■ Apply a small amount of petroleum jelly, lip gloss, or moisturizer to the lips regularly *to promote comfort and prevent dryness.*
NURSING DIAGNOSIS	**Fatigue** *related to* the effects of cancer or treatment *as manifested by* verbal report of lack of energy and inability to maintain usual routines.
■ Satisfactory activity level relative to phase of disease or treatment.	■ Inform the patient that fatigue is an expected side effect of therapy and that it usually begins during the first week of therapy, reaches its peak in 2 weeks, continues, and then gradually disappears 2 to 4 weeks after treatment has ended. ■ Encourage patient to rest when fatigued, to maintain usual lifestyle patterns as closely as possible, and to pace activities in accordance with energy level *because rest periods are essential to conserve energy.*
NURSING DIAGNOSIS	**Ineffective individual coping** *related to* depression secondary to diagnosis and treatment, uncertain outcome, disruption in lifestyle, or financial burden of illness *as manifested by* verbalized or observed inability to manage affective component of diagnosis and resulting symptoms; threats or attempts to commit suicide; concerns over financial implications of disease
■ Appropriate response to problems. ■ Able to seek and/or accept support and assistance.	■ Have patient direct own care when possible *to encourage patient independence.* ■ Provide information *to allow patient to make informed choices regarding treatment regimen and plan of care.* ■ Facilitate communication between patient and family *to foster a supportive network.* ■ Assess and mobilize patient's support system. ■ Refer patient to social services for financial assistance if appropriate *to provide additional resources.* ■ Assess need for further counseling.

Continued

14-1 NURSING CARE PLAN PATIENT WITH CANCER—continued

Expected Patient Outcomes	Nursing Interventions and *Rationales*
NURSING DIAGNOSIS	**Body-image disturbance** *related to* hair loss, disfiguring surgery, and weight loss *as manifested by* expressions of concern with changes in body; refusal to interact with visitors; isolation; frequent crying; refusal to care for self or to look in mirror.
▪ Able to verbalize acceptance of changes in body appearance and function.	▪ Provide psychologic support and prepare patient for expected hair loss *to lessen shock of event when it occurs.* ▪ Encourage patient to select a wig and begin to wear it before hair loss begins and to wear a scarf or turban *to conceal hair loss.* ▪ Use a mild, protein-based shampoo, cream rinse, and hair conditioner every 4 to 7 days *to avoid drying remaining hair.* ▪ Avoid excessive shampooing, brushing, and combing of hair *to reduce hair loss.* ▪ Avoid use of electric hair dryers, curlers, curling rods, and hair spray *to minimize scalp irritation and decrease hair loss.* ▪ Help patient select clothing and colors that minimize weight loss or effects of disfiguring surgery. ▪ Assure patient that value as a person is not associated with external appearance. ▪ Discuss expected physical changes with family members and advise them of ways to assist patient with acceptance *to prepare the family and to foster family relationships.*
NURSING DIAGNOSIS	**Altered family processes** *related to* cancer diagnosis of family member *as manifested by* observed communication problems among family members; lack of family support related to physical, emotional, and/or spiritual needs of patient.
▪ Family members communicate about patient and cooperate in care of patient. ▪ Family will seek outside help when needed.	▪ Assess family structure and support system *to determine amount and quality of support available to patient.* Teach needed skills to family members. ▪ Provide opportunity for discussion of caregiving and emotional implications of role changes *to promote verbalization of feelings and shared understanding of problems.* ▪ Assist family members to set realistic expectations for patient and themselves. ▪ Provide guidance on course of disease and anticipated outcome *so planning can be accomplished.*
NURSING DIAGNOSIS	**Risk for infection** *related to* leukopenia, depressed immune system, and multiple exposure to microorganisms.‡

COLLABORATIVE PROBLEMS

Nursing Goals	Nursing Interventions and *Rationales*
POTENTIAL COMPLICATION	**Bleeding** *related to* thrombocytopenia.†
POTENTIAL COMPLICATION	**Hyperuricemia** *related to* chemotherapy.
▪ Monitor for signs of hyperuricemia. ▪ Report deviations from acceptable parameters. ▪ Carry out medical and nursing interventions.	▪ Monitor for high level of uric acid excretion in urine, high serum uric acid, obstructive uropathy, decreased urine output, nausea, vomiting, lethargy. ▪ Record intake and output *to determine fluid balance.* ▪ Encourage fluids *to prevent uric acid crystals from causing obstruction.* ▪ Evaluate blood urea nitrogen (BUN) and serum creatinine levels *to identify early changes in renal function.* ▪ Administer allopurinol (Zyloprim) as ordered *to reduce endogenous uric acid production.*

*Only nursing diagnoses that apply to all types of cancer are included in this nursing care plan.
†See NCP on thrombocytopenia (NCP 29-2).
‡See NCP on neutropenia (NCP 29-3).

may also provide comfort. A water-based lubricant may be used at the time of intercourse to increase vaginal lubrication, which is necessary to prevent trauma to the vaginal lining and to prevent discomfort or pain.

The patient should be encouraged to use other forms of physical contact to obtain sexual pleasure during the period of disruption in sexual functioning. Hugging, caressing, touching, and quiet talking can provide sexual pleasure when sexual intercourse is not possible. The patient's partner must be included in all teaching and counseling sessions to be fully informed of the temporary or permanent changes in the patient's sexual functioning. Both patient and partner must understand that adjustments in sexual functioning patterns will take time, patience, and understanding.

Late Effects of Radiation and Chemotherapy

Cancer survivors are achieving long-term remission and survival rates because of advancements in treatment modalities. However, these forms of therapy (especially radiation and chemotherapy) may produce long-term sequelae termed *physiologic late effects* that occur months to years after cessation of therapy. Every body system can be affected to some extent by chemotherapy and radiation therapy. The effects of radiation on the body's tissues are caused by cellular hypoplasia of stem cells and alterations in the fine vasculature and fibroconnective tissues. In addition to the acute toxicities, chemotherapy can have long-term effects related to the loss of cells' proliferative reserve capacity. The additive effects of multiagent chemotherapy before, during, or after a course of radiotherapy can significantly increase the resulting physiologic late effects. Some physiologic late effects of radiation and chemotherapy are summarized in Table 14-23.

Table 14-23 Possible Late Effects of Radiation and Chemotherapy

Body System	Effects
Cardiac	Chronic cardiomyopathy Myocardial fibrosis
Pulmonary	Diffuse alveolar damage Pneumonitis Fibrosis
Gastrointestinal	Hepatotoxicity Enteritis Esophagitis Fistula formation
Renal and urologic	Nephrotoxicity Nephritis Hemorrhagic cystitis Acute tubular necrosis
Neurologic	Neuropathy Autonomic nervous system disorders Hearing loss Myelopathy Necrotizing leukoencephalopathy
Endocrine	Gonadal impairment Ovarian destruction Infertility Disturbances in sexual functioning

The cancer survivor may also be at risk for leukemias and other secondary malignancies resulting from therapy for the primary cancer. However, the potential risk for developing a second malignancy does not contraindicate the use of cancer treatment; the overall risk of developing neoplastic complications is low, and the latency period may be long.

The cancer treatments most frequently implicated in causing secondary malignancy are the alkylating chemotherapeutic agents and high-dose radiation, which can induce cancers at the exposure site. The exact mechanism of oncogenesis of radiation and chemotherapy remains unclear. It could be related to interactions between immunosuppressive factors, direct cellular damage, and carcinogenic effects along with other environmental carcinogens.

Acute leukemias occurring as secondary malignancies have been most widely reported after treatment for Hodgkin's disease, but they also occur in survivors of ovarian, lung, and breast cancers. Secondary malignancies other than leukemias include multiple myeloma after radiation therapy for breast cancer; non-Hodgkin's lymphoma after treatment for Hodgkin's disease; and cancers of the bladder, kidney, and ureters after the use of cyclophosphamide. Radiation therapy for breast, lung, ovarian, uterine, and thyroid cancers, non-Hodgkin's lymphoma, and Hodgkin's disease has been linked to secondary osteosarcoma of the rib, scapula, clavicle, humerus, sternum, ilium, and pelvis. Fibrosarcomas have been reported several years after radiation therapy for astrocytoma, glioblastoma, and pituitary adenoma. Unfortunately, secondary malignancies are usually resistant to therapy.[39]

Biologic Therapy

Biologic therapy, now recognized as the fourth cancer treatment modality, can be effective alone or in association with surgery, radiotherapy, and chemotherapy. Biologic therapy or biologic response modifier therapy consists of agents that modify the relationship between the host and the tumor by altering the biologic response of the host to the tumor cells. Biologic agents may affect host-tumor response in three ways: (1) they have direct antitumor effects; (2) they restore, augment, or modulate host immune system mechanisms; and (3) they have other biologic effects, such as interfering with the cancer cells' ability to metastasize or differentiate.[40]

Since 1986 the Food and Drug Administration (FDA) has approved several biologic agents for cancer therapy, and many more are being investigated. Knowledge and experience with these agents are rapidly gaining with increased understanding of the immune system, advancements in molecular biology, development of monoclonal antibodies, and modern technologic equipment.

Interferons. Interferons are naturally occurring complex proteins of which there are three types: (1) α-interferon, produced by WBCs; (2) β-interferon, produced by fibroblasts and macrophages; and (3) γ-interferon, produced by T lymphocytes. Interferons are cytokines that have antiviral, antiproliferative, and immunomodulatory properties (see Table 12-4). The antiviral activity of interferons was first identified in 1957. Interferons protect cells infected by viruses from attack by other viruses, and they inhibit replication of viral

DNA (see Fig. 12-5). The antiproliferative effects of interferons are not completely understood. However, they have been shown to inhibit DNA and protein synthesis in tumor cells and to stimulate the expression of tumor-associated antigens on tumor cell surfaces, thus increasing the potential for an immune response against the tumor cell. Interferons modulate the immune response by their direct interaction with lymphocytes and monocytes or macrophages. They are also capable of mediating the function of other cytokines such as IL-2 and TNF and enhancing the antigenic expression in some tumor types. Interferons have also been shown to increase the cytotoxic activity and killing potential of NK cells.[40]

Because of the protein nature of interferons, they cannot be administered orally. Therefore they are administered IV, intramuscularly (IM), and subcutaneously. To date, the best dose, route, and frequency of administration have not been determined for many malignancies. In addition, α-interferon is made by different pharmaceutical companies such as interferon alfa-2a (Roferon-a) made by Roche and interferon alfa-2b (Intron-a) made by Schering. It is important to stress to the patient that these different brands of interferon are not interchangeable. If the patient begins to take one form of interferon, the brand of interferon being taken must not be changed unless recommended by the physician.

α-Interferon has been approved by the FDA for the treatment of hairy cell leukemia, Kaposi's sarcoma (KS), adjuvant treatment for melanoma, genital warts (caused by papillomavirus), and hepatitis B and C. α-Interferons have also demonstrated effectiveness in the treatment of renal cell carcinoma, chronic myelogenous leukemia, T cell lymphomas, multiple myeloma, ovarian carcinoma, and carcinoid tumors. Clinical trials continue to investigate the use of interferons to treat other malignancies.

Interleukins. Many ILs have been identified (see Table 12-4), although not all are undergoing clinical investigation. The ILs are a family of biologic agents that perform a variety of functions. Most ILs induce a multitude of biologic activities resulting in the activation of the immune system or alteration in the functional capacity of cancer cells. Currently, many of the ILs are in the clinical or preclinical research phases of development for potential use in the treatment of cancer and other diseases. In 1992 aldesleukin (Proleukin), a recombinant form of IL-2, was approved by the FDA for the treatment of renal cell carcinoma.

IL-2 is a cytokine produced by T lymphocytes that was first identified as an agent capable of stimulating proliferation of T lymphocytes. It was later found to activate NK cells and lymphokine-activated killer (LAK) cells. Activated NK cells make up part of a group of cytotoxic lymphocytes that mediate lymphokine-activated killing. IL-2 also stimulates the release of other cytokines, including γ-interferon, TNF, IL-1, and IL-6. IL-2 has been administered by IV bolus, continuous infusion, subcutaneous injection, and peritoneal infusion. The agent has been administered alone, in combination with chemotherapeutic agents, and with LAK cells.

Another approach to the use of IL-2 involves the isolation of lymphocytes from the tumor itself. These cells, known as tumor-infiltrating lymphocytes (TILs), are a subpopulation of lymphocytes that can be cultured with IL-2 and then reinfused into the patient. TIL cells have been found to be more tumoricidal than LAK cells.

Positive clinical responses with IL-2 and LAK cells have been reported in patients with metastatic renal cell cancer and malignant melanoma. In addition to its use with LAK and TIL cells, IL-2 has been administered alone or in conjunction with other lymphokines such as α-, β-, and γ-interferon. Research on uses of IL-2 in cancer therapy is continuing.[40]

Monoclonal Antibodies. Monoclonal antibodies are antibodies or immunoglobulins produced by B lymphocytes that are capable of binding to specific target cells, including tumor cells. A large number of monoclonal antibodies (MoAbs) are currently being investigated for diagnostic and treatment capabilities. (Hybridoma technology for the production of MoAbs is described in Chapter 12.) The diagnostic use of MoAbs is primarily for the imaging of tumors to locate areas of metastatic disease and for radioimmunoassays and enzyme-linked immunoassays in laboratory studies.

MoAbs can be conjugated or attached to other agents such as radioisotopes, toxins, chemotherapeutic agents, and other biologic agents. The goal of this approach is for the antibody to deliver the conjugated MoAb directly to the targeted cancer cells for their ultimate destruction.

MoAbs have demonstrated limited effectiveness in treating lymphomas; acute and chronic lymphocytic leukemias; T cell leukemia; and ovarian, gastric, and colon cancers. Two MoAbs have received FDA approval: muromonab-CD3 (Orthoclone OKT-3), a MoAb targeted to the CD3 receptor of human T cells, for the treatment of acute rejection in renal transplant patients; and satumomab pendetide (Onco Scint CR/OV) for the detection of colorectal and ovarian cancers.

MoAbs are administered by the infusion method. There is a risk, although rare, of anaphylaxis associated with the administration of MoAbs. This potential exists because most MoAbs are produced by mouse lymphocytes and thus represent a foreign protein to the human body. Onset of anaphylaxis can occur within 5 minutes of administration and can be a life-threatening event. Administration of the MoAb should be stopped immediately, an emergency code called, and 0.5 ml IV epinephrine 1:10,000 solution administered over 5 minutes.[41] (See Chapter 12 for a discussion of nursing management of anaphylaxis.)

Hematopoietic growth factors. Hematopoietic growth factors (HGFs), or colony-stimulating factors (CSFs), are a family of glycoproteins produced by various cells. HGFs stimulate production, maturation, regulation, and activation of cells of the hematologic system. After release, HGFs attach to receptors on the cell surface of peripheral blood cells and hematopoietic precursors (precursors of mature blood cells). HGFs then stimulate production, maturation, release from the bone marrow, and functional ability of blood cells.

Colony-stimulating factors. These include granulocyte colony–stimulating factor (G-CSF), granulocyte-macrophage colony–stimulating factor (GM-CSF), macrophage colony–stimulating factor (M-CSF or CSF-1), and multicolony stimulating factor (IL-3).

CSFs are naturally produced hormone-like proteins that regulate hematopoiesis and functions of mature WBC. There are a number of potential clinical uses of HGFs. They may hasten recovery from bone marrow depression after standard and high-dose chemotherapy and bone marrow transplantation or decrease bone marrow suppression associated with chemotherapy administration. HGFs may also reestablish bone marrow function in aplastic anemia, myelodysplastic syndrome, and leukemia and may be effective in the management of sepsis or parasitic infections. These functions are important because neutropenia is a major cause of morbidity and mortality associated with cancer and cancer treatment.[42]

G-CSF was approved for clinical use by the FDA in 1991 under the name of filgrastim (Neupogen) for the treatment of neutropenia. It stimulates the production and function of neutrophils. G-CSF can be administered subcutaneously or by IV infusion. The most commonly reported side effect of G-CSF therapy is medullary bone pain, which occurs most often in the lower back, pelvis, and sternum. This pain generally develops at the time the neutrophil count begins to recover and lasts for about 24 hours. The pain associated with G-CSF therapy is usually relieved with nonnarcotic analgesics.[42]

GM-CSF was approved by the FDA in 1991 under the name of sargramostim (Leukine, Prokine) for the management of neutropenia associated with bone marrow transplantation. Approval was expanded in 1994 to include the use of GM-CSF in the management of bone marrow transplant failure or delay in bone marrow engraftment and after chemotherapy in the treatment of acute myelogenous leukemia. GM-CSF stimulates the production and function of neutrophils, eosinophils, and monocytes. In addition, GM-CSF stimulates these cells to produce cytokines. GM-CSF can be administered either subcutaneously or by IV infusion. The most common side effects associated with GM-CSF administration include medullary bone pain, similar to the bone pain associated with G-CSF administration, and leukocytosis and eosinophilia.[42]

IL-3 is a multipotential stimulator of hematopoietic stem cells. IL-3 has been shown to stimulate the growth of neutrophils, monocytes, eosinophils, basophils, and platelet cell lines. IL-3 is being investigated for the treatment of bone marrow failure and for its ability to enhance myeloid recovery after chemotherapy, radiotherapy, and bone marrow transplantation. M-CSF is also undergoing investigation for its potential role in cancer treatment.

Erythropoietin. Erythropoietin (EPO) is an HGF responsible for stimulating growth of the erythroid precursor cells that ultimately mature into red blood cells. EPO is normally made by the kidneys. EPO was initially approved by the FDA in 1987 for the management of chronic anemia associated with end-stage renal disease. In 1993 FDA approval was expanded to include management of chemotherapy-related anemia. EPO is a well-tolerated HGF with only a rare occurrence of hypertension associated with administration.

Toxic and Side Effects of Biologic Agents. The administration of one biologic agent usually induces the endogenous release of other biologic agents. The release and action of these biologic agents results in systemic immune and inflammatory responses. The toxicities and side effects of biologic agents are related to dose and schedule. Table 14-24 summarizes the potential side effects associated with specific biologic agents. Common side effects include constitutional flulike symptoms, including headache, fever, chills, myalgias, fatigue, malaise, weakness, photosensitivity, anorexia, and nausea. With interferons the flulike symptoms almost invariably appear. However, the severity of the flulike symptoms associated with interferon therapy generally decreases over time. Acetaminophen administered every 4 hours, as prescribed, often reduces the severity of the flulike syndrome. The patient is commonly premedicated with acetaminophen in an attempt to prevent or decrease the intensity of these symptoms.[41] In addition, large amounts of fluids help decrease the symptoms.

Tachycardia and orthostatic hypotension are also commonly reported. IL-2 can cause capillary leak syndrome, which can result in pulmonary edema. Other toxic and side effects may involve the CNS, renal and hepatic systems, and cardiovascular system. These effects are found particularly with interferons and IL-2.

NURSING MANAGEMENT: BIOLOGIC THERAPY

Some problems experienced by the patient receiving biologic therapy are quite different from those observed with more traditional forms of cancer therapy. For example, capillary leak syndrome and pulmonary edema, observed with high doses of IL-2, are problems that require critical care nursing. These critical care requirements are new to many oncology nurses. Other problems, such as bone marrow depression and fatigue, are more familiar but exist at different levels of severity than those customarily associated with other forms of cancer therapy. Bone marrow depression occurring with biologic therapy administration is generally more transient and less severe than that observed with chemotherapy. Fatigue associated with biologic therapy can be so severe that it can constitute a dose-limiting toxicity.

Nursing interventions for flulike syndrome include the administration of acetaminophen before treatment and every 4 hours after treatment. Intravenous meperidine has been used to control the severe chills associated with some biologic agents. Other nursing measures include monitoring of vital signs and temperature, planning for periods of rest for the patient, and assisting with activities of daily living (ADLs).

A wide range of neurologic deficits have been observed with interferon and IL-2 therapy. The nature and extent of these problems have not been completely elucidated. However, these problems are understandably frightening to the patient and the family, who must be taught to observe for neurologic problems (e.g., confusion, memory loss, difficulty making decisions, insomnia), report their occurrence, and institute appropriate safety and support measures.[43]

Bone Marrow and Stem Cell Transplantation

Bone marrow transplantation (BMT) has become an effective, lifesaving procedure for a number of malignant and nonmalignant diseases (Table 14-25). BMT offers hope to many patients whose diseases are otherwise incurable.[44,45] BMT has become one of the most promising treatments for a number of cancers. In recent years there has been a dramatic increase in the number of BMT and transplant centers.

Whether the diagnosis is a malignant or nonmalignant disease, the goal of BMT is cure. Cure rates are still low, but are steadily increasing. Even if there is no cure, most transplants result in a period of remission. BMT is an intensive procedure with many risks, and some patients die from complications of the BMT or from relapse of the original disease. Because it is a

Table **14-24** Side Effects of Biologic Therapy

	Interferons	Interleukin-2 (IL-2)	Granulocyte Colony–Stimulating Factor (G-CSF)	Granulocyte-Macrophage–Colony Stimulating Factor (GM-CSF)
Flulike syndrome	Fever, chills, malaise, fatigue	Fever, chills, malaise, fatigue, myalgia	Fever, chills, myalgias, headache	Fever, chills, myalgias, headache, fatigue
Central nervous system	Impaired concentration and memory, confusion, lethargy, somnolence, seizures	Disorientation, impaired concentration and memory, somnolence, severe anxiety and agitation		
Renal/hepatic	Proteinuria, increased transaminase levels	Oliguria; anuria; azotemia; increased BUN, serum creatinine, serum bilirubin, and liver enzymes; hypoalbuminemia, hepatomegaly		
Gastrointestinal	Nausea, vomiting, diarrhea, anorexia	Nausea, vomiting, anorexia, diarrhea, stomatitis		
Hematologic	Leukopenia, thrombocytopenia, anemia	Anemia, thrombocytopenia, lymphopenia, eosinophilia		Leukocytosis, eosinophilia
Cardiovascular-pulmonary	Hypotension, tachycardia, arrhythmia, myocardial ischemia	Capillary leak syndrome, hypotension, tachycardia, arrhythmias, myocardial ischemia, rare myocardial infarction, pulmonary congestion		Dyspnea
Integumentary	Alopecia, irritation at injection site	Diffuse, pruritic, erythematous rash, dry desquamation, inflammatory reaction at injection site	Generalized rash	Facial flushing, generalized rash, inflammation at injection site
Endocrine		Hypothyroidism; increased ACTH, cortisol, prolactin, growth hormone, and acute phase proteins	Generalized rash	
Miscellaneous	Photophobia, impotence, decreased libido	Decreased libido, arthralgia	Bone pain	Bone pain, fluid retention

highly toxic therapy, the patient must weigh the significant risks of treatment-related death or treatment failure (relapse) with the hope of cure.

BMT allows for the safe use of very high doses of chemotherapy or radiation therapy to patients whose tumors have developed resistance or failed to respond to standard doses of chemotherapy and radiation.

Types of Bone Marrow Transplants. Bone marrow transplants can be allogeneic, autologous, or syngeneic. In *allogeneic marrow transplantation* the infused bone marrow is acquired from a donor who has been determined to be human leukocyte antigen (HLA) matched to the recipient in terms of tissue typing. HLA typing involves testing WBCs to identify genetically inherited antigens common to both donor and recipient that are important in compatibility of transplanted tissue.

Table **14-25** Uses for Bone Marrow Transplantation

Malignant Diseases	Nonmalignant Diseases
Acute and chronic myelogenous leukemia	Sickle cell disease
Acute lymphocytic leukemia	Thalassemia
Myelodysplastic syndrome	Aplastic anemia
Hodgkin's disease	Immunodeficiency diseases
Non-Hodgkin's lymphoma	Severe autoimmune diseases
Multiple myeloma	
Breast cancer	
Testicular cancer	
Ovarian cancer	

(HLA tissue typing is discussed in Chapters 12 and 44.) Often this is a family member but may be an unrelated donor found through a bone marrow registry. The goal of allogeneic transplantation is the engraftment and subsequent normal proliferation and differentiation of the donated marrow in the host. The most common indication for allogeneic transplant is leukemia.

In *autologous marrow transplantation* patients receive their own bone marrow. The aim of this approach is to enable patients to receive intensive chemotherapy or radiation while supporting them with their own bone marrow. In this type of BMT the patient's own marrow is removed, treated, stored, and reinfused.

Syngeneic marrow transplantation involves obtaining stem cells from one identical twin and infusing them into the other. Identical twins have identical HLA types and are a perfect match.

Harvest Procedures. Bone marrow can be "harvested" via a procedure conducted in the operating room using general or spinal anesthesia in which multiple bone marrow aspirations are carried out, usually from the iliac crest, but also from the sternum. The entire harvest procedure usually takes 1 to 2 hours, and the patient can be discharged following recovery. Following harvest the donor may experience pain at the collection site, which can be treated with mild analgesics. The donor's body will replace the bone marrow in a few weeks.

After harvest, autologous bone marrow may be treated (purged) to remove cancer cells. Many different pharmacologic, immunologic, physical, and chemical agents have been used for this purpose. The bone marrow is then frozen (cryopreserved) and stored until it is used for transplantation. In allogeneic transplants, the marrow can be harvested, processed, and infused into the recipient within a few hours of donation.

Preparative Regimens. In malignant diseases the goal of BMT is to rescue the marrow after the patient has received high doses of chemotherapy with or without radiation aimed at treating the underlying disease. Following harvesting of the marrow, the patient is given high-dose chemotherapy with or without radiation therapy. Total body radiation can be used for immunosuppression or to treat the disease.

After the therapy the marrow that was removed is thawed and given back to the patient through a needle in a vein to replace the destroyed marrow. The stem cells reconstitute, or "rescue," the recipient's hematopoeitic system. Usually 2 to 4 weeks are required for the transplanted marrow to start producing hematopoeitic blood cells. During this pancytopenic period it is critical for the patient to be in a protective isolation environment receiving supportive care. RBC and platelet transfusions usually are necessary to maintain circulating RBCs and platelets during this time.

Complications. Bacterial, viral, and fungal infections are common following BMT. Prophylactic antibiotic therapy may reduce their incidence. A potentially serious complication of allogeneic transplant is graft-versus-host disease. This occurs when the T lymphocytes from the donated marrow (graft) recognize the recipient (host) as foreign and begin to attack certain organs such as the skin, liver, and intestines. Graft-versus-host disease is discussed in Chapter 12.

Peripheral Stem Cell Transplantation. An emerging and promising alternative to BMT is peripheral stem cell transplant (PSCT).[46] This procedure is based on the fact that peripheral or circulating stem cells are capable of repopulating the bone marrow. PSCT is a type of transplant that differs from BMT primarily in the method of collection of stem cells. Because there are fewer stem cells in the blood than in the bone marrow, mobilization of stem cells from the bone marrow into the peripheral blood can be done using chemotherapy or hematopoietic growth factors. Common growth factors that are used are GM-CSF and G-CSF.

The donor's blood is collected via pheresis, in which the person is attached to a cell separator machine that removes peripheral stem cells and then returns the blood to the person. This procedure is called leukapheresis and usually takes 2 to 4 hours to complete. In autologous transplants the stem cells are purged to kill any cancer cells and then frozen and stored until used for transplantation. Although many of the same steps (harvesting, intensive chemotherapy, reinfusion) of BMT are used in PSCT, the hematologic recovery period in PSCT is shorter, and fewer, less severe complications are seen.

Cord Blood Stem Cells. Umbilical cord blood is rich in hematopoietic stem cells, and successful allogeneic transplants have been performed using this source. Cord blood can be HLA typed and cryopreserved. A disadvantage of cord blood is the possibility of insufficient numbers of stem cells to permit transplant to adults.

Gene Therapy

The use of gene therapy is currently being investigated for the treatment of cancer. Gene therapy is discussed in Chapter 12.

Nutritional Therapy

Nutritional problems that most frequently occur in the patient with cancer are malnutrition, anorexia, altered taste sensation, nausea, vomiting, diarrhea, stomatitis, and mucositis. These problems can be caused by a combination of many factors, including drug toxicity, effects of radiation therapy, tumor involvement, recent surgery, emotional distress, or difficulty with ingestion or digestion of food. If the patient is inadequately nourished, the normal cells will not be able to recover from the effects of therapy, and the immune system will be depressed because of depletion of protein stores.

Malnutrition. The patient with cancer usually experiences protein and calorie malnutrition characterized by fat and muscle depletion. (Assessment of the degree of malnutrition is discussed in Chapter 38.) Foods suggested for increasing the protein intake to facilitate repair and regeneration of cells are presented in Table 14-26. High-caloric foods that provide energy and minimize weight loss are presented in Table 14-27. A sample high-caloric, high-protein diet is presented in Table 38-13.

The nurse should suggest the need for a nutritional supplement to the physician as soon as a 5% weight loss is noted or if the patient has the potential for protein and caloric malnutrition. Albumin and prealbumin levels should be monitored. Once a 10 lb (4.5 kg) weight loss occurs, it is difficult to maintain the nutritional status. The patient can be taught to use nutritional supplements in place of milk when cooking or baking. Foods to which nutritional supplements can be easily added include scrambled eggs, pudding, custard, mashed potatoes, cereal, and cream sauces. Packages of Instant Breakfast can be

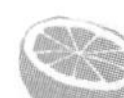

NUTRITIONAL THERAPY

Table 14-26 Protein Foods with High Biologic Value

Milk

Whole milk (1 cup) = 9 g protein

Double-strength milk—1 quart of whole milk plus 1 cup of dried skim milk blended and chilled: 1 cup = 14 g protein

Milk shake—1 cup of ice cream plus 1 cup of milk = 15 g protein, 416 calories

Use evaporated milk, double-strength milk, or half-and-half to make casseroles, hot cereals, sauces, gravies, puddings, milk shakes, and soups.

Yogurt (regular and frozen)—check labels and purchase brand with highest protein content: 1 cup = 10 g protein

Eggs

Egg = 6 g protein

Eggnog (1 cup) = 15.5 g protein

Add eggs to salads, casseroles, and sauces. Deviled eggs are especially well tolerated.

Desserts that contain eggs include angel food cake, sponge cake, custard, and cheesecake.

Cheese

Cottage	½ cup	15 g protein
American	1 slice	3 g protein
Cheddar	1 slice	6 g protein
Cream	1 tbsp	1 g protein

Use cheese in a sandwich or as a snack.

Add cheese to salads, casseroles, sauces, and baked potatoes.

Cheese spread with crackers is a wholesome snack that can be made and stored in the refrigerator for easy accessibility.

Meat, Poultry, Fish

Beef	3 oz	approx. 21 g protein
Pork	3 oz	approx. 19 g protein
Chicken	½ breast	approx. 26 g protein
Fish	3 oz	approx. 30 g protein
Tuna fish	6½ oz	approx. 44.5 g protein

Add meat, poultry, and fish to salads, casseroles, and sandwiches.

Add strained and junior baby meats to soups and casseroles.

Cocktail weiners or deviled ham on crackers are wholesome snacks. These snacks can be made and stored in the refrigerator for easy accessibility.

NUTRITIONAL THERAPY

Table 14-27 High-Caloric Foods

Mayonnaise	1 tbs	=	101 cal
Butter or margarine	1 tsp	=	35 cal
Sour cream	1 tbs	=	72 cal
Peanut butter	1 tbs	=	94 cal
Whipped cream	1 tbs	=	53 cal
Corn oil	1 tbs	=	119 cal
Jelly	1 tbs	=	49 cal
Ice cream	1 cup	=	256 cal
Honey	1 tbs	=	64 cal

used as indicated or sprinkled on cereals, desserts, and casseroles.

If the malnutrition cannot be treated with dietary intake, it may be necessary to use enteral or parenteral nutrition as an adjunct nutritional measure. (Enteral and parenteral nutrition are discussed in Chapter 38.)

Anorexia. It is important to realize that the anorexia experienced by the patient with cancer is a challenging problem. An intervention may be effective one day and ineffective the next. Continual assessment and intervention are necessary to successfully manage this problem. The nurse must develop the philosophy that something can be done to prevent or minimize anorexia, evaluate each intervention, and continue to use those interventions that have been successful in the past. Some suggestions are presented in NCP 14-1.

Altered Taste Sensation. It is theorized that cancer cells release substances that resemble amino acids and stimulate the bitter taste buds. The patient may also experience an alteration in the sweet taste sensation, as well as in the sour and salty taste sensations. Meat may also taste bitter to the patient. At this time the physiologic basis of these varied taste alterations is unknown. Other causes of altered taste sensation are presented in Table 14-15. The patient with an altered taste problem should be instructed to avoid foods that are disliked. Frequently the patient may feel compelled to eat certain foods because those foods are believed to be beneficial. The patient can be taught to experiment with spices and other seasoning agents in an attempt to mask the taste alterations that are occurring. Lemon juice, onion, mint, basil, and fruit juice marinades may improve the taste of certain meats and fish. Bacon bits, onion, and pieces of ham may enhance the taste of vegetables. An additional amount of a spice or seasoning agent is usually not an effective way to enhance the taste.

Unproven Methods of Cancer Treatment

Unproven methods of cancer treatment, sometimes referred to as *cancer quackery,* are as old as the disease itself. Cancer quackery is defined as the intentional misrepresentation or misapplication of measures that delay or impede the entry of the patient into the health care system for treatment. Today, cancer quackery is a multimillion-dollar business in North America. Fear appears to be the major factor that motivates a patient to seek "miracle cures." Other factors include an impatience with the progress of the present cancer treatment, the need to exercise control over daily life, the impersonal approach of health care workers, a need for hope when terminal illness is a reality, a lack of information on methods that are proven versus those that are not, and the suspicion that the health care system is not providing the most effective treatment plan available.[47]

The major hazard of cancer quackery is that it delays or prevents the patient from receiving proven methods of cancer diagnosis and treatment. This delay may make the difference between cure or control and terminal illness. The nurse can play a significant role in preventing or minimizing the use of cancer quackery by doing the following:

1. Provide the patient with accurate information concerning the benefits of the proven methods of cancer treatment.
2. Inform the American Cancer Society, the local medical association, the health department, and the local consumer protection office when it is learned that the patient is being approached by persons promoting unproven methods of cancer treatment.
3. Discuss the fallacies of the unproven methods of cancer treatment with the patient and the family.

The current methods of cancer quackery include chemicals and drugs, dietary alterations, occult techniques, and mechanical devices.

Chemicals and Drugs. Two drugs that have been associated with cancer quackery are krebiozen (the "wonder drug" of the 1950s and 1960s) and Laetrile (the wonder drug of the 1970s and 1980s). A National Cancer Institute study on a large number of patients who used krebiozen failed to demonstrate any anticancer effects of this drug. Chemical analysis revealed that the major ingredient of krebiozen is mineral oil with minute amounts of creatine and amyl alcohol.

Laetrile, also known as vitamin B_{17} and Cyto H-3, has been actively used as a treatment for cancer for the past 25 to 30 years. The active ingredient of Laetrile is hydrogen cyanide, and it is derived from apricot or peach pits. It is available in parenteral and tablet form; the parenteral form contains 30 to 40 times as much cyanide as the oral form. There is no evidence of an anticancer effect of this drug.

Because Laetrile is frequently used by the patient with cancer and until recently has been thought of as a harmless drug, the nurse must be aware of the possible toxic effects that may be experienced. The cyanide content of Laetrile is released in the presence of hydrolyzine β-glucosidase enzymes. These enzymes are present in raw fruits and vegetables, such as lettuce, mushrooms, green peppers, celery, and sweet almonds. When these foods are eaten after the ingestion of Laetrile, cyanide intoxication may occur. The bacteria of the intestinal tract are also thought to contain this enzyme. When the cyanide is released, it inhibits cellular respiration, and the resulting hypoxia produces symptoms such as dizziness, nausea or vomiting, hypotension, and shock. Because the drug is not controlled by the FDA, many impurities may exist that have the potential for causing systemic bacterial, viral, and fungal infections.

Dietary Alterations. Books that propose cures for cancer enumerate the foods to eat and to avoid, offer special recipes, and often recommend the use of an expensive blender to ensure the proper potency of the food mixture. Examples of nutritional alterations that have been used are eating raw foods; fasting for long periods of time; following the grape diet, the carrot juice diet, or the coffee and Coke diet; and using coffee, buttermilk, or yogurt enemas while on a special diet. None of these diets has been found effective in treating cancer. Nutritional alterations can have a profound effect on the patient with cancer. It is important that cancer patients have good nutritional intake to maintain weight and prevent a negative nitrogen balance.

Occult Techniques. The most commonly used occult form of cancer quackery is "psychic surgery." This surgery without an incision is performed by a healer. The patient comes to the healer with the problem, has the healing surgery, and leaves believing that the tumor has been removed. During the surgery the area where the problem exists is massaged and rubbed with animal blood. At some point the patient is shown a piece of animal tissue and is told that it is the diseased tissue or organ. This tissue is thrown away, the massage with blood continues, and the patient is told that the tumor is gone and the cancer is cured.

Mechanical Devices. The use of mechanical devices is an old form of cancer quackery that has recently lost its popularity. These devices are usually nothing more than light bulbs, vibrators, low-voltage generators, dials, and knobs. The patient is told to place the device on or in front of the area of cancer for a certain amount of time each day, and the device will destroy the cancer.

Supportive Care. One of the greatest assets of cancer quackery is the emotional support given to the patient and the patient's family. This factor should demonstrate to the nurse the need to provide psychologic support, caring, and active listening to the cancer patient and the family. The nurse should be available, listen, and counsel the patient during times when side effects are being experienced, when treatment is not effective, and when the patient is experiencing fear, anger, and depression.

If the patient chooses an unproven method of cancer treatment, the nurse should support the patient and assume a nonjudgmental attitude. The nurse should attempt to persuade the patient to continue the proven treatment plan and to maintain the nutritional status while using an unproven method of cancer treatment. Belief in the treatment may provide a placebo effect that may offer some benefits. It is important that all doors remain open to the patient so that a return to the health care system can be made without feelings of fear or guilt.

COMPLICATIONS RESULTING FROM CANCER

The patient may develop complications related to the continual growth of the malignancy or the side effects of treatment.

Infection

Infection is a frequent cause of death in the patient with cancer. The usual sites of infection include the lungs, GU system, mouth, rectum, peritoneal cavity, and blood (septicemia). Infection occurs as a result of the ulceration and necrosis caused by the tumor, compression by the tumor of vital organs, and the state of neutropenia caused by the disease process or the treatment of cancer. Fungi and gram-negative bacteria are the usual causative organisms.

Many patients are neutropenic when an infection develops. In these individuals, infection may cause significant morbidity and may be rapidly fatal if not treated promptly. The classic manifestations of infection are not often present in a patient with neutropenia and a depressed immune system. (Neutropenia is discussed in Chapter 29.)

Oncologic Emergencies

Oncologic emergencies are life-threatening emergencies that can occur as a result of cancer or cancer treatment. These emergencies can be obstructive, metabolic, or infiltrative.

Obstructive Emergencies. Obstructive emergencies are primarily caused by tumor obstruction of an organ or blood vessel. Obstructive emergencies include superior vena cava syndrome, spinal cord compression syndrome, third space syndrome, and intestinal obstruction.

Superior vena cava syndrome. Superior vena cava syndrome results from obstruction of the superior vena cava by a tumor. The clinical manifestations include facial edema, periorbital edema, distention of veins of the neck and chest, headache, and seizures. The presence of a mediastinal mass is often visible on chest x-ray. The most common causes are Hodgkin's disease, non-Hodgkin's lymphoma, and lung cancer. Superior vena cava syndrome is considered a serious medical problem, and management usually involves radiation therapy to the site of obstruction and treatment of the primary tumor. Chemotherapy may be administered concurrently with the radiation therapy.

Spinal cord compression. Spinal cord compression is the result of the presence of a malignant tumor in the epidural space of the spinal cord. The most common primary tumors that produce this problem are breast, lung, prostate, GI, melanoma, and renal tumors. Lymphomas also pose a risk if diseased lymph tissue invades the epidural space. The manifestations are back pain that is intense, localized, and persistent, accompanied by vertebral tenderness and aggravated by Valsalva's maneuver; motor weakness and dysfunction; sensory paresthesia and loss; and autonomic dysfunction. Radiation therapy is used for the patient with slowly progressive neurologic deficits and radiosensitive tumors. Surgery is usually recommended for the patient with rapidly progressive neurologic signs, especially if the tumors are relatively radioresistant.[48] Activity limitations and pain management are important nursing interventions.

Third space syndrome. Third space syndrome involves a shifting of fluid from the vascular space to the interstitial space that primarily occurs secondary to extensive surgical procedures, biologic therapy, or septic shock. Initially patients exhibit signs of hypovolemia, including hypotension, tachycardia, low central venous pressure, decreased urine output, and increased urine specific gravity. Treatment includes fluid, electrolyte, and plasma protein replacement. During recovery hypervolemia can occur, resulting in hypertension, elevated central venous pressure, weight gain, and shortness of breath. Treatment generally involves reduction in fluid administration and fluid balance monitoring.

Intestinal obstruction. Chapter 40 contains a complete discussion of intestinal obstruction.

Metabolic Emergencies. Metabolic emergencies are caused by the production of ectopic hormones directly from the tumor or secondary to cancer treatment. Ectopic hormones arise from tissues that do not normally release these hormones. Cancer cells become depressed and return to a more embryologic form, thus allowing the stored potential of the cells to become evident. Metabolic emergencies include hypercalcemia, syndrome of inappropriate antidiuretic hormone, septic shock, acute tumor lysis syndrome, and disseminated intravascular coagulation.

Syndrome of inappropriate antidiuretic hormone. Syndrome of inappropriate antidiuretic hormone (SIADH) results from abnormal or sustained production of antidiuretic hormone (ADH). (See Chapter 47). SIADH occurs most frequently in carcinoma of the lung and can also occur in cancer of the pancreas, duodenum, brain, esophagus, colon, ovary, prostate, bronchus, and nasopharynx; leukemia; mesothelioma; reticulum cell sarcoma; Hodgkin's disease; thymoma; and lymphosarcoma. Cancer cells in these tumors are actually able to manufacture, store, and release ADH. The chemotherapeutic agents vincristine and cyclophosphamide also stimulate the release of ADH from the pituitary or tumor cells. Symptoms of SIADH include weight gain, weakness, anorexia, nausea, vomiting, personality changes, seizures, and coma. Treatment of SIADH includes fluid restriction and, in severe cases, IV administration of 3% sodium chloride solution.

Hypercalcemia. Hypercalcemia can occur in the presence of cancer that involves the bone such as in metastatic disease of the bone or multiple myeloma, or when a parathyroid hormone–like substance is secreted by cancer cells in the absence of bony metastasis. Hypercalcemia resulting from malignancies that have metastasized occurs most frequently in patients with lung, breast, kidney, colon, ovarian, or thyroid cancer. Hypercalcemia resulting from secretion of parathyroid hormone–like substance occurs most frequently in hypernephromas; squamous cell carcinoma of the lung; head and neck, cervical, and esophageal cancer; lymphomas; and leukemia. Immobility and dehydration can contribute to or exacerbate hypercalcemia.

The primary manifestations of hypercalcemia include apathy, depression, fatigue, muscle weakness, electrocardiogram changes, polyuria and nocturia, anorexia, nausea, and vomiting. Serum levels of calcium in excess of 12 mg/dl (3 mmol/L) can be life threatening. Chronic hypercalcemia can result in nephrocalcinosis and irreversible renal failure. The long-term treatment of hypercalcemia is aimed at the primary disease. Acute hypercalcemia is treated by hydration (3 L/day), diuretic (particularly loop diuretics) administration, and plicamycin (Mithracin) (formerly mithramycin) if the patient has severe symptoms. Other pharmacologic interventions that may be used to inhibit bone resorption include etidronate disodium (Didronel), pamidronate (Aredia), calcitonin, and oral phosphates.[49]

Tumor lysis syndrome. Acute tumor lysis syndrome (TLS) is a metabolic complication that occurs in some patients with cancer and is frequently triggered by chemotherapy. It results from the rapid destruction of a large number of tumor cells, which can cause fatal biochemical changes. TLS is often associated with tumors that have high growth rates and are sensitive to the effects of chemotherapy. If not identified and treated quickly, TLS can result in acute renal failure.

The four hallmark signs of TLS are hyperuricemia, hyperphosphatemia, hyperkalemia, and hypocalcemia. TLS usually occurs within the first 24 to 48 hours after the initiation of chemotherapy and may persist for approximately 5 to 7 days. The primary goal of TLS management is preventing renal failure and severe electrolyte imbalances. The primary treatment includes increasing urine production using hydration therapy and decreasing uric acid concentrations using allopurinol.

Septic shock and disseminated intravascular coagulation. Septic shock is discussed in Chapter 61, and disseminated intravascular coagulation is discussed in Chapter 29.

Infiltrative Emergencies. Infiltrative emergencies occur when malignant tumors infiltrate major organs or secondary to cancer therapy. The most common infiltrative emergencies are cardiac tamponade and carotid artery rupture.

Cardiac tamponade. Cardiac tamponade results from fluid accumulation in the pericardial sac, constriction of the pericardium by tumor, or pericarditis secondary to radiation therapy to the chest. Manifestations include a heavy feeling over the chest, shortness of breath, tachycardia, cough, dysphagia, hiccups, hoarseness, nausea, vomiting, excessive perspiration, decreased level of consciousness, pulsus paradoxus, distant or muted heart sounds, and extreme anxiety. Emergency management is aimed at reduction of fluid around the heart and includes surgical establishment of a pericardial window or an indwelling pericardial catheter. Supportive therapy includes administration of oxygen therapy, intravenous hydration, and vasopressor therapy.

Carotid artery rupture. Rupture of the carotid artery occurs most frequently in patients with cancer of the head and neck secondary to invasion of the arterial wall by tumor or erosion following surgery or radiation therapy. Bleeding can manifest as minor oozing or spurting of blood in the case of a "blowout" of the artery. In the presence of a blowout, pressure should be applied to the site with a finger. Intravenous fluid and blood products are administered in an attempt to stabilize the patient for surgery. Surgical management involves ligation of the carotid artery above and below the rupture site and reduction of local tumor.

PSYCHOLOGIC SUPPORT

Psychologic support of the patient is an important aspect of cancer care. Because of the effectiveness of cancer treatment, many patients with cancer are cured or their disease is controlled for long periods of time. In light of this trend in cancer treatment, emphasis must be placed on maintaining an optimal quality of life after the diagnosis of cancer. A positive attitude of patient, family, and caregivers toward cancer and cancer treatment has a significant positive impact on the quality of life that the patient experiences. A positive attitude may also influence the prognosis of the patient with cancer.

The diagnosis of cancer is viewed by most persons as a crisis. The most common fears experienced by the patient with cancer include disfigurement, dependency, pain, emaciation, financial depletion, abandonment, and death.

To cope with these fears, the patient with cancer will use and experience different behavioral patterns: shock, anger, denial, bargaining, depression, helplessness, hopelessness, rationalization, acceptance, and intellectualization. These behavioral patterns may occur at any time during the process of cancer. However, some patterns appear to occur more frequently or at a greater intensity at certain specific stages of the disease process. The following factors may determine how the patient will cope with the diagnosis of cancer:

1. *Ability to cope with stressful events in the past* (e.g., loss of job, major disappointment). By simply asking how the patient has coped with stressful events, the nurse can gain an understanding of the patient's coping patterns, the effectiveness of the usual coping patterns, and the usual coping time framework.
2. *Availability of significant others.* The patient who has effective support systems tends to cope more effectively than the patient who does not have a meaningful, available support system.
3. *Ability to express feelings and concerns.* The patient who is able to express feelings and needs and who seeks and asks for help appears to cope more effectively than the patient who internalizes feelings and needs.
4. *Age at the time of diagnosis.* Age determines the coping strategies to a great degree. For example, a young mother with cancer may have concerns that differ from those of a 70-year-old woman with cancer.
5. *Extent of disease.* Cure or control of the disease process is usually easier to cope with than the reality of terminal illness.
6. *Disruption of body image.* Disruption of the body image (e.g., radical neck dissection, alopecia, mastectomy) may intensify the psychologic impact of cancer.
7. *Presence of symptoms.* Symptoms such as fatigue, nausea, diarrhea, and pain may intensify the psychologic impact of cancer.
8. *Past experience with cancer.* If past experiences with cancer have been negative, the patient will probably view the present status as negative.
9. *Attitude associated with the cancer.* A patient who feels in control and has a positive attitude about cancer and cancer treatment is better able to cope with the diagnosis and treatment of cancer than the patient who feels hopeless, helpless, and out of control.

To facilitate the development of a hopeful attitude about cancer and to support the patient and the family during the various stages of the process of cancer, the nurse should do the following:

1. Be available and continue to be available, especially during difficult times.
2. Exhibit a caring attitude.
3. Listen actively to fears and concerns.
4. Provide relief from distressing symptoms.
5. Provide essential information regarding cancer and cancer care.
6. Maintain a relationship based on trust and confidence; be open, honest, and caring in the approach.
7. Use touch to exhibit caring. A squeeze of the hand or a hug may at times be more effective than words.
8. Assist the patient in setting realistic, reachable short-term and long-term goals.
9. Assist the patient in maintaining usual lifestyle patterns.
10. Maintain hope, which is the key to effective cancer care. Hope varies, depending on the status of the patient—hope that the symptoms are not serious, hope that the treatment is curative, hope for independence, hope for relief of pain, hope for a longer life, or hope for a peaceful death. Hope provides control over what is

occurring and is the basis of a positive attitude toward cancer and cancer care.

Most patients with advanced cancer know that they are dying. Attempts at circumventing the truth are usually recognized by the patient and cause feelings of distrust and hostility toward the person who makes such attempts. Honesty and openness are the best approaches. Most patients will surprise caregivers by expressing relief at a willingness to discuss what is foremost in their minds, their imminent death.

Organizations and journals available as resources for the nurse are listed in the Resources section at the end of this chapter. In many cities, local units of the American Cancer Society provide a wide variety of services.

Management of Cancer Pain

Patients with cancer commonly experience pain, which can be caused by both the disease and its treatment. Undertreatment of cancer pain is common.

Because data such as vital signs and patient behaviors are not reliable indicators of pain, especially long-standing, chronic pain, it is *essential* that every patient with cancer be assessed for pain by first asking the question "Do you have pain?" If the patient's self-report is affirmative, further data are obtained and documented initially and at regular intervals on the location and intensity of the pain, what it feels like, and how it is relieved. Patterns of change also should be assessed. The patient report should *always* be believed and accepted as the primary source of assessment data. Table 14-28 presents assessment questions that may facilitate this data collection.

Table 14-28 Essential Components of Cancer Pain Assessment and Relevant Assessment Questions

Location	Where is the pain? (There may be more than one place.)
Intensity	How bad is the pain? (See Chapter 9 for rating scales.)
Quality	What does the pain feel like? (See Chapter 9 for descriptors.)
Pattern	Has the pain changed? What makes the pain better or worse?
Relief	What do you do to control your pain?
Measures	Are medications used? Does the relief measure help much? How much?

Modified from Agency for Health Care Policy and Research: *Patient guide, clinical practice guideline, managing cancer pain,* Rockville, Md, 1994, US Department of Health and Human Services.

Pharmaceutical interventions, including nonsteroidal anti-inflammatory drugs, opioids, and adjuvant pain medications, should be used following the World Health Organization Analgesic Ladder (Fig. 14-24). Analgesic medications should be given on a regular schedule, around the clock, with additional doses as needed for breakthrough pain.[50] Oral administration of the medication is preferred. It is important to remember that with opioid drugs such as morphine the appropriate dose is whatever is necessary to control the pain with the least side

CRITICAL THINKING EXERCISES

CASE STUDY

Cancer

Patient Profile

Ms. L. is a 32-year-old woman who is scheduled for radiation treatment following a lumpectomy (surgical removal of malignant tumor in her breast).

Subjective Data

- Expresses a great deal of fear and anxiety about radiation therapy
- Believes she should have had a mastectomy; therefore she would not have needed radiation
- States that no one has told her about what to expect related to radiation therapy
- Has two young children at home and is concerned about their care

Critical Thinking Questions

1. What are potential side effects of radiation therapy to the chest?
2. What are appropriate nursing interventions to control these side effects?
3. What should Ms. L. be taught about skin care in the treatment field?
4. How should she be helped to reduce her anxiety and fear about beginning radiation therapy?
5. Based on the assessment data provided, write one or more appropriate nursing diagnoses. Are there any collaborative problems?

NURSING RESEARCH ISSUES

1. Do patients who have been successfully treated for cancer with radiation or chemotherapy know about the late effects of treatment?
2. What is the quality of life for patients 5 or more years following successful radiation therapy?
3. What are the most challenging or difficult problems encountered by hospice nurses?
4. Is there a difference in quality of life between the patient receiving traditional chemotherapy as compared with the patient receiving biologic therapy?
5. Can relaxation strategies, such as guided imagery, decrease the side effects associated with chemotherapy?
6. Why do some individuals choose nontraditional methods of cancer treatment?

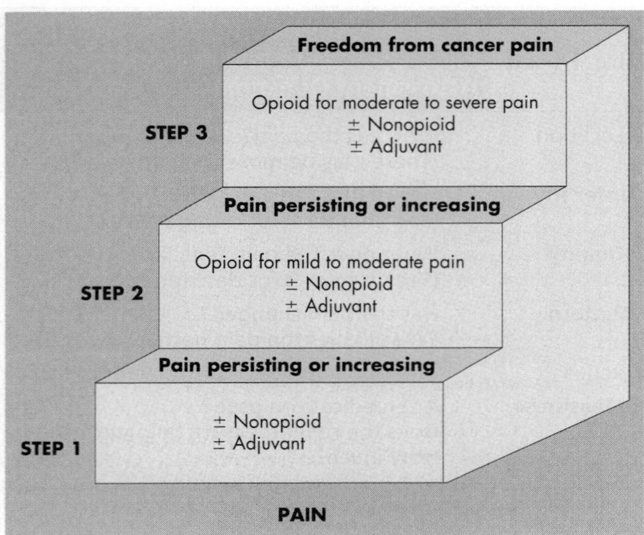

Fig. 14-24 The World Health Organization (WHO) three-step analgesic ladder.

effects. Principles of patient-controlled analgesia should also be followed. Fear of addiction is not warranted but must be addressed as part of patient education issues relevant to pain control, because fear of addiction is a significant barrier to appropriate pain management.

Nonpharmacologic interventions, including relaxation therapy and imagery, can be effectively used to manage pain.[51] Additional strategies to relieve pain are discussed in Chapter 9.

REVIEW QUESTIONS

The number of the question corresponds to the same-numbered objective at the beginning of the chapter.

1. Trends in the incidence and control of cancer include
   a. a decrease in cancer deaths in females with cancer of the lung.
   b. an increase in the number of individuals who are surviving cancer.
   c. an increase in cancer to the most common cause of death in the United States.
   d. a decrease in the overall incidence of cancer in both men and women.
2. Cancer is a name for a large group of diseases, all of which are characterized by
   a. increasing differentiation of cells.
   b. production of toxins that alter cells.
   c. rapid, explosive proliferation of cells.
   d. cell growth that escapes normal control.
3. A characteristic of the stage of progression in the development of cancer is
   a. oncogenic viral transformation of target cells.
   b. a reversible steady growth facilitated by carcinogens.
   c. a period of latency before clinical detection of cancer.
   d. proliferation of cancer cells in spite of host control mechanisms.
4. The primary protective role of the immune system related to malignant cells is
   a. surveillance for cells with tumor-associated antigens.
   b. binding with free antigen released by malignant cells.
   c. production of blocking factors that immobilize cancer cells.
   d. responding to a new set of antigenic determinants on cancer cells.
5. The primary difference between benign and malignant neoplasms is the
   a. rate of cell proliferation.
   b. site of malignant tumor.
   c. requirements for cellular nutrients.
   d. characteristic of tissue invasiveness.
6. Important nursing roles related to prevention and detection of cancer include
   a. instructing people to eat low-fiber, refined-carbohydrate diets.
   b. instructing persons on ways to increase capacity to cope with stress.
   c. teaching people to have annual screening tests for all detectable cancer sites.
   d. using people's natural fear of cancer to motivate changes in unhealthy lifestyles.
7. The goals of cancer treatment are based on the principle that
   a. initial treatment is always directed toward cure of the cancer.
   b. surgery is the single most effective treatment for solid tumors.
   c. a combination of treatment modalities is effective for controlling many cancers.
   d. although cancer cure is rare, quality of life can be increased with treatment modalities.
8. The nurse explains to a patient undergoing brachytherapy of the cervix that she
   a. must undergo simulation to locate the treatment area.
   b. requires the use of radioactive precautions during nursing care.
   c. may experience desquamation of the skin on the abdomen and upper legs.
   d. requires shielding of the ovaries during treatment to prevent ovarian damage.
9. When administering intravenous vesicant chemotherapeutic drugs the nurse should
   a. monitor the patient for symptoms of neurotoxicity.
   b. administer an antiemetic 30 minutes before the drug is started.
   c. initiate the IV with normal saline or a dextrose solution to ensure patency.
   d. expect the patient to complain of some burning and stinging as the medication is infused.
10. Stomatitis, a common side effect of chemotherapeutic agents, occurs because the
    a. site of the malignancy is near the oral cavity.
    b. general health of the patient with cancer is poor.
    c. chemotherapeutic drugs have an external, local, and irritating effect.
    d. rapidly dividing cells of the mucous membranes of the mouth are being destroyed.
11. The nurse teaches the patient receiving IL-2 about the drug based on the knowledge that this agent is administered primarily for the purpose of
    a. inhibiting DNA and protein synthesis in tumor cells.
    b. stimulating the production of tumoricidal lymphocytes.
    c. enhancing the antigenic expression of antigens on tumor cell surfaces.
    d. preventing bone marrow suppression associated with chemotherapy administration.

12. The nurse counsels the patient receiving radiation therapy or chemotherapy that
    a. if the treatment is successful a return to normal physiologic function can be expected.
    b. if nausea and vomiting during treatment becomes severe the treatment plan will be modified.
    c. effective birth control methods should be used during and for up to 2 years following treatment.
    d. the cycle of fatigue-depression-fatigue that may occur during treatment can be reduced by restricting activity.
13. An inappropriate nursing intervention to promote nutrition in the patient with cancer is
    a. stimulating taste sensation by the addition of spices and seasonings to food.
    b. providing increased protein for normal cell recovery and immune system function.
    c. reminding the patient to eat a high-calorie, high-protein snack every 1 to 2 hours to prevent weight loss.
    d. alerting the physician that nutritional supplements may be needed when the patient has a 10 lb weight loss.
14. If a patient decides to take Laetrile, the nurse should inform the patient that
    a. a pulmonary fungal infection will probably develop.
    b. chemotherapy and Laetrile should not be taken simultaneously.
    c. buttermilk should be drunk simultaneously to avoid toxic effects.
    d. foods with hydrolyzine β-glucosidase enzymes should be avoided.
15. Syndrome of inappropriate ADH (SIADH) that occurs in certain types of cancer is primarily due to
    a. autoimmune reaction.
    b. gram-negative septicemia.
    c. invasiveness of cancer cells.
    d. ectopic hormonal production.
16. A patient has recently been diagnosed with early stages of breast cancer. Which of the following is most appropriate for the nurse to focus on?
    a. maintaining patient's hope
    b. discussing child care for patient's children
    c. preparing a will and advance directives
    d. discussing the patient's past experiences with her grandmother's cancer

References

1. *Cancer Facts and Figures—1998,* Atlanta, 1998, American Cancer Society.
2. DeVita VT, Helman S, Rosenberg SA, editors: *Cancer: principles and practice of oncology,* Philadelphia, 1997, Lippincott-Raven.
3. LeMarbre PJ, Groenwald SL: Biology of cancer. In Groenwald SL and others, editors: *Cancer nursing: principles and practice,* ed 4, Boston, 1997, Jones & Bartlett.
4. Yarbro JW: Carcinogenesis. In Groenwald SL and others, editors: *Cancer nursing: principles and practice,* ed 4, Boston, 1997, Jones & Bartlett.
5. Marks R: Prevention and control of melanoma: the public health approach, *CA Cancer J Clin* 46:4, 1996.
6. Dudjak LA: Cancer metastasis, *Semin Oncol Nurs* 8:40, 1992.
7. Kim YS, Liotta LA, Kohn EC: Cancer invasion and metastasis, *Hosp Pract* 28:92, 1993.
8. Folkman J: Angiogenesis in cancer, vascular, rheumatoid and other diseases, *Nature Med* 1:27, 1995.
9. Hubbard SM, Liotta LA: The biology of metastases. In Baird SB, editor: *Cancer nursing: a comprehensive textbook,* ed 2, Philadelphia, 1996, Saunders.
10. Post-White J: The immune system, *Semin Oncol Nurs* 12:2, 1996.
11. Workman ML, Ellerhorst-Ryan J, Hargrave-Koertge V: *Nursing care of the immunocompromised patient,* Philadelphia, 1993, Saunders.
12. *Cancer-related checkups: If you're between 18 and 39: if you're 40 or over,* Atlanta, 1996, American Cancer Society.
13. Perez C, Brady L: Preface. In Perez C, Brady L, editors: *Principles and practice of radiation oncology,* ed 3, Philadelphia, 1998, Lippincott.
14. Kaplan H: Historic milestones in radiobiology and radiation therapy, *Semin Oncol* 4:479, 1979.
15. Stein J: Some observations of the history of irradiation therapy, *Endocur Hyperthermia Oncology* 1:59, 1985.
16. Withers HR: Biological basis of radiation therapy for cancer, *Lancet* 339:156, 1992.
17. Chapman J, Allalunis-Turner M: Cellular and molecular targets in normal tissue radiation injury. In Gutin P, Leibel SL, Sheline G, editors: *Radiation injury to the central nervous system,* New York, 1991, Raven Press.
18. Withers HR: Biologic basis of radiation therapy. In Perez C, Brady L, editors: *Principles and practice of radiation oncology,* ed 3, Philadelphia, 1998, Lippincott.
*19. Blackmar A: Radiation-induced skin alterations, *Medsurg Nurs* 6:172, 1997.
*20. Phillips T: Early and late effects of radiation on normal tissues. In Gutin P, Leibel S, Sheline G, editors: *Radiation injury to the central nervous system,* New York, 1991, Raven Press.
21. Hilderly L, Dow K: Radiation oncology. In Baird S, McCorkle R, Grant M, editors: *Cancer nursing: a comprehensive textbook,* ed 2, Philadelphia, 1996, Saunders.
22. Winningham M: Walking program for people with cancer: getting started, *Cancer Nurs* 4:270, 1991.
23. Mock V and others: Effects of exercise on fatigue, physical functioning and emotional distress during radiation for breast cancer, *Oncol Nurs Forum* 24: 991, 1997.
24. Chahbazian C: The skin. In Cox J: *Moss' radiation oncology: rationale, technique, results,* ed 7, St Louis, 1994, Mosby.
*25. Marcial V: The oral cavity and oropharynx. In Cox J: *Moss' radiation oncology: rationale, technique, results,* ed 7, St Louis, 1994, Mosby.
*26. Iwamoto R: Alterations in oral status. In Baird S, McCorkle R, Grant M, editors: *Cancer nursing: a comprehensive textbook,* ed 2, Philadelphia, 1996, Saunders.
27. Schover LR: *Sexuality and fertility after cancer,* New York, 1997, Wiley.
28. Dembo A: The ovary. In Cox J: *Moss' radiation oncology: rationale, techniques, results,* ed 7, St Louis, 1994, Mosby.
29. Oberst M and others: Self-care burden, stress appraisal, and mood among persons receiving radiotherapy, *Cancer Nurs* 14:71, 1991.
30. Christman N: Uncertainty and adjustment during radiotherapy, *Nurs Res* 39:17, 1990.
31. Krakoff IH: Systemic treatment of cancer, *CA Cancer J Clin* 46:134, 1996.
32. Bender CM: Nursing implications of antineoplastic therapy. In Itano J, Taoka K, editors: *The core curriculum for oncology nursing practice,* ed 3, Philadelphia, 1997, Saunders.
33. Baranowski L: Central venous access devices: current technologies, uses and management, *J Intravenous Nurs* 16:3, 1993.
34. Ryder MA: Peripherally inserted central venous catheters, *Nurs Clin North Am* 28:4, 1993.
35. Gullo SM: Implanted ports: technologic advances and nursing care issues, *Nurs Clin North Am* 28:4, 1993.
36. Barton-Burke M, Wilkes GM, Ingwersen K, editors: *Cancer chemotherapy: a nursing process approach,* Boston, 1996, Jones & Bartlett.
37. Oncology Nursing Society: *Cancer chemotherapy guidelines and recommendations for practice,* Pittsburgh, 1996, Oncology Nursing Society Press.
38. Wujcik D: Infection control in cancer patients, *Nurs Clin North Am* 28:639, 1993.
39. Wilkes GM: Potential toxicities and nursing management. In Barton-Burke M, Wilkes GM, Ingwersen K, editors: *Cancer chemotherapy: a nursing process approach,* Boston, 1996, Jones & Bartlett.
40. Aggarwal BB, Puri R, editors: *Human cytokines: their role in disease and therapy,* 1995, Blackwell Scientific.

41. Reiger PT: Biotherapy: the fourth modality. In Barton-Burke M, Wilkes GM, Ingersen K, editors: *Cancer chemotherapy: a nursing process approach,* Boston, 1996, Jones & Bartlett.
42. Farrell MM: Biotherapy and the oncology nurse, *Semin Oncol* 12:82, 1996.
43. Bender CM: Cognitive dysfunction associated with cancer and cancer therapy, *Medsurg Nurs* 4:5, 1995.
44. Bone marrow transplantation. In Groenwald SL and others, editors: *Cancer nursing: principles and practice,* ed 4, Boston, 1997, Jones & Bartlett.
45. Whedon MB, Wujcik D, editors: *Blood and marrow stem cell transplantation: principles, practice, and nursing insights,* ed 2, Sudbury, Mass, 1997, Jones & Bartlett.
46. Thomas ED: Stem cell transplantation: past, present and future, *Arch Immunol Ther Exp* 45:1, 1997.
47. Henke Yarbro C: Questionable methods of cancer therapy. In Groenwald SL and others, editors: *Cancer nursing: principles and practice,* ed 4, Boston, 1997, Jones & Bartlett.
48. Held JL, Peahota A: Nursing care of the patient with spinal cord compression, *Oncol Nurs Forum* 20, 1993.
49. Clayton K: Cancer-related hypercalcemia, *AJN* 97:42, 1997.
50. Agency for Health Care Policy and Research: *Clinical practice guidelines, management of cancer pain,* Rockville, Md, 1994, US Department of Health and Human Services.
51. Wallace KG: Analysis of recent literature concerning relaxation and imagery interventions for cancer pain, *Cancer Nurs* 20:79, 1997.

*Nursing research-based articles.

Resources

American Association for Cancer Education (AACE)
PO Box 601
Snellville, GA 30278-0601
http://rpci.med.buffalo.edu/departments/education/aace2.html

American Cancer Society
1599 Clifton Road NE
Atlanta, GA 30329
404-320-3333
http://www.cancer.org

American Institute for Cancer Research
1759 R Street NW
Washington, DC 20009
202-328-7744
800-843-8114
Fax: 202-328-7226
http://www.aicr.org

American Society of Clinical Oncology (ASCO)
435 North Michigan Avenue, Suite 1717
Chicago, IL 60611
312-644-0828

Association of Community Cancer Centers (ACCC)
11600 Nebel Street, Suite 201
Rockville, MD 20852
301-984-9496

Canadian Cancer Society
10 Alcorn Avenue, Suite 200
Toronto, Ontario M4V 1E4
Canada
416-961-7223
http://www.cancer.ca

Cancer Archives
http://cure.medinfo.org/lists/cancer/index.html

Cancer Care, Inc.
1180 Avenue of the Americas
New York, NY 10036
800-813-HOPE

Cancer Federation, Inc.
21250 Box Spring Road
Morena Valley, CA 92388
714-682-7989

Cancer Guide
http://cancerguide.org/

Cancer Hotline
800-525-3777
800-638-6070 (Alaska)
800-636-5700 (District of Columbia)
808-524-1234 (Hawaii, call collect)

Cancer Information Service (CIS)
NIH Building 31, Room 10A 24
Bethesda, MD 20892
1-800-4-CANCER
1-800-638-6070 (Alaska)
524-1234 (Hawaii; in Oahu, dial direct; call collect from neighboring islands)

Cancer News on the Net
http://www.cancernews.com

International Society of Nurses in Cancer Care
Mulberry House, The Royal Marsden Hospital
Fulham Road
London SW3 6JJ
England
071-252-8171, ext. 2123

International Union Against Cancer
3 rue du Conseil General
1205 Geneva
Switzerland
http://www.uicc.ch/

Memorial Sloan-Kettering Cancer Center
1275 York Avenue
New York, NY 10021
212-639-2000
http://www.mskcc.org/

National Cancer Institute—International Cancer Information Center (CancerNet and CancerFax)
Building 82, Room 123
Bethesda, MD 20892
800-4-CANCER
301-496-4907
Fax: 301-402-0212
http://www.nci.nih.gov/

National Coalition for Cancer Survivorship (NCCS)
1010 Wayne Avenue, 5th Floor
Silver Spring, MD 20910
301-650-8868
301-565-9670

National Foundation for Cancer Research
7315 Wisconsin Avenue, Suite 500-W
Bethesda, MD 20814
301-654-1250
Fax: 301-654-5824

OncoLink (cancer information site)
http://www.oncolink.upenn.edu

Oncology Nursing Society
501 Holiday Drive
Pittsburgh, PA 15220
412-921-7373
http://www.ons.org

Society of Gynecologic Oncologists
401 N. Michigan Avenue
Chicago, IL 60611
312-644-6610
http://www.sgo.org/

***For additional Internet resources, see the website for this book at* www.mosby.com/MERLIN/medsurg_lewis**

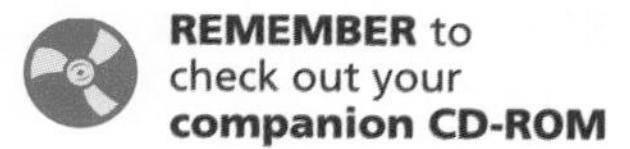

NURSING MANAGEMENT

15 Fluid, Electrolyte, and Acid-Base Imbalances

Mima M. Horne & Eleanor F. Bond

www.mosby.com/MERLIN/medsurg_lewis

LEARNING OBJECTIVES

1. Describe the composition of the major body fluid compartments.
2. Define the following processes involved in the regulation of movement of water and ions between the body fluid compartments: diffusion, osmosis, filtration, hydrostatic pressure, oncotic pressure, and osmotic pressure.
3. Describe the etiology, laboratory diagnostic findings, clinical manifestations, and nursing and collaborative management of the following disorders:
   a. Water excess and deficit
   b. Sodium and volume imbalances: hypernatremia and hyponatremia
   c. Potassium imbalance: hypokalemia and hyperkalemia
   d. Magnesium imbalance: hypomagnesemia and hypermagnesemia
   e. Calcium imbalance: hypocalemia and hypercalemia
   f. Phosphate imbalance: hypophosphatemia and hyperphosphatemia
   g. Acid-base imbalances: metabolic acidosis, metabolic alkalosis, respiratory acidosis, respiratory alkalosis
4. Describe the composition of common intravenous fluid solutions.

HOMEOSTASIS

The body is composed of a variety of fluid spaces. In the healthy person, the volume and composition of each space remains constant. Nutrients are delivered to body cells, wastes removed, and daily intake of water and electrolytes distributed to and removed from the various fluid spaces without disrupting the composition of the various body fluid compartments. The maintenance of this constant environment in the face of continual changes is termed *homeostasis.* This chapter describes the ways in which this dynamic equilibrium is maintained, the things that can happen in illness when homeostasis is disrupted, the signs and symptoms the patient will experience when homeostasis is disrupted, and actions the health care provider can take to prevent or treat alterations in fluid and electrolyte balance.

Stressors such as disease and injury commonly alter the normal regulatory processes that maintain the dynamic internal fluid and electrolyte balance. Fluid and electrolyte disorders are common in illness. Monitoring for, preventing, and treating such disorders are important parts of caring for patients.

WATER CONTENT OF THE BODY

Water is the primary component of the body, accounting for approximately 60% of the body weight in the adult. Water is the solvent in which body salts, nutrients, and wastes are dissolved and transported. The water content varies with gender, body mass, and age (Fig. 15-1). In men, the percentage of body weight that is composed of water is generally greater than in women because men tend to have more lean body mass than women. Adipose tissue contains less water than an equivalent volume of muscle tissue.[1] In the older adult body water content averages 45% to 55% of body weight. In the infant, water content is 70% to 80% of the body weight. Older adults have less fluid reserve and are at a greater risk for fluid-related problems than young adults.[2]

Body Fluid Compartments

The two major fluid compartments in the body are intracellular and extracellular (Fig. 15-2). Approximately two thirds of the body water is located within cells and is termed *intracellular fluid* (ICF); the ICF constitutes approximately 42% of body weight. The body of a 70 kg man would contain approximately 42 L of water, of which 30 L would be located within cells. *Extracellular fluid* (ECF) consists of the fluid spaces between cells (interstitial fluid and lymph) and the plasma space. The ECF consists of one third of the body water, or about 17% of the total weight; this would amount to about 11 L in a 70 kg man. About one third of the ECF is in the plasma space (3 L in our example), and two thirds is in the interstitium (8 L in our example).

A third small but important fluid compartment is the *transcellular space.* This usually consists of approximately 1 L. The fluid in the transcellular space is secreted and reabsorbed by epithelial cells. It includes fluid in the cerebrospinal space, gastrointestinal (GI) tract, and pleural, synovial, and peritoneal

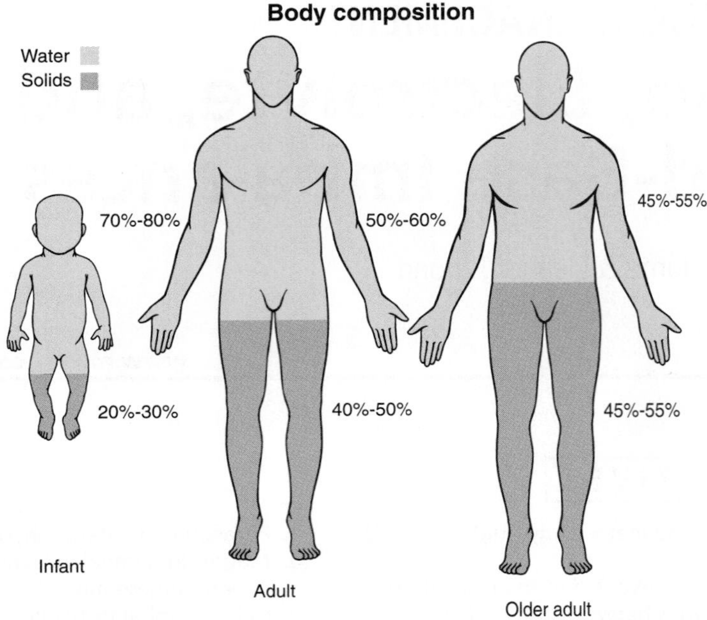

Fig. 15-1 Changes in body water content with age.

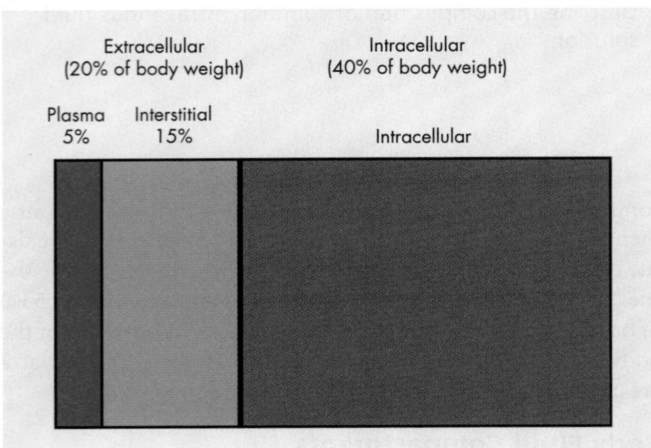

Fig. 15-2 Fluid compartments in the body.

fluid spaces. If the transcellular fluid is not reabsorbed, but instead is lost (e.g., vomiting), the loss of the transcellular fluid can produce serious fluid and electrolyte imbalances.

The term *effective circulating blood volume* (ECBV) is important in understanding fluid and electrolyte balance. It describes the plasma volume in addition to the blood cells circulating within the blood vessels. It is the volume perfusing the tissues and sensed by the volume receptors. Normally, the ECBV varies with ECF volume. In certain clinical conditions (e.g., ascites, burn injury, nephrosis), the balance between the ECBV and the interstitial volume shifts, with the ECBV diminished relative to the interstitial volume and relative to the overall ECF volume.

Fluid spacing is a term sometimes used to describe the distribution of body water. *First spacing* describes the normal distribution of fluid in the ICF and ECF compartments. *Second spacing* refers to an abnormal accumulation of interstitial fluid (i.e., edema). *Third spacing* occurs when fluid accumulates in areas that normally have no fluid or only a minimum amount of fluid. Examples of third spacing are ascites, sequestration of fluid in the abdominal cavity with peritonitis, and edema associated with burns.

Calculation of Fluid Gain or Loss

One liter of water weighs 2.2 lb (1 kg). If a patient drinks 240 ml (8 oz) of fluid, weight gain will be 0.5 lb (0.24 kg). A patient receiving diuretic therapy who loses 4.4 lb (2 kg) in 24 hours has experienced a fluid loss of approximately 2 L. An adult patient who is fasting might lose approximately 1 to 2 lb per day. A sudden weight loss exceeding this is likely due to loss of body fluid. A sudden weight gain similarly is suggestive of a gain of fluid. Body weight change is an excellent indicator of fluid volume loss or gain.

ELECTROLYTES

Electrolytes are substances whose molecules dissociate or split into ions when placed in water. *Ions* are electrically charged particles. *Cations* are positively charged ions. Examples include sodium (Na^+), potassium (K^+), calcium (Ca^{2+}), and magnesium (Mg^{2+}) ions. *Anions* are negatively charged ions. Examples include bicarbonate (HCO_3^-), chloride (Cl^-), and phosphate (PO_4^{3-}) ions. Most proteins bear a negative charge and are thus anions. The electrical charge of an ion is termed its *valence.* Cations and anions combine according to their valence. (Terminology related to body fluid chemistry is presented in Table 15-1.)

Measurement

The concentration of electrolytes can be expressed in milligrams per deciliter (mg/dl), millimoles per liter (mmol/L), or milliequivalents per liter (mEq/L). The international standard

Table 15-1 Terminology Related to Body Fluid Chemistry

Anion	Ion that carries a negative charge
Cation	Ion that carries a positive charge
Electrolyte	Substance that dissociates in solution into ions (charged particles); a molecule of sodium chloride (NaCl) in solution becomes Na^+ and Cl^-
Nonelectrolyte	Substance that does not dissociate into ions in solution; examples include glucose and urea
Osmolality	A measure of the total solute concentration per kilogram of solvent
Osmolarity	A measure of the total solute concentration per liter of solution
Solute	Substance that is dissolved in a solvent
Solution	Homogeneous mixture of solutes dissolved in a solvent
Solvent	Substance that is capable of dissolving a solute (liquid or gas)
Valence	The degree of combining power of an ion

for measuring electrolytes is mmol/L. The combining power of electrolytes is measured in mEq/L. For sodium ion (Na^+), 2.3 mg/dl (or 23 mg/L), 1 mmol/L, and 1 mEq/L all refer to the same concentration of sodium. Milliequivalents equal millimoles multiplied by the valence of the ion:

$$\text{mEq/L} = \text{mmol/L} \times \text{valence}$$

The weight of an electrolyte gives no direct information regarding the number of ions or the number of charges carried by an electrolyte. Because milliequivalents express the chemical combining power of an electrolyte, ions combine milliequivalent for milliequivalent and not millimole for millimole. For example, 1 mEq (1 mmol) of sodium combines with 1 mEq (1 mmol) of chloride, and 1 mEq (0.5 mmol) of calcium combines with 1 mEq (1 mmol) of chloride.

Electrolyte Composition of Fluid Compartments

Electrolyte composition varies between the ECF and ICF. The overall concentration of the electrolytes is approximately the same in the two compartments. However, concentrations of specific ions differ greatly (Fig. 15-3). In the ICF the most prevalent cation is potassium; there are small amounts of magnesium and sodium. The prevalent anion is phosphate, with some protein and a small amount of bicarbonate. In the ECF the main cation is sodium; there are small amounts of potassium, calcium, and magnesium. The primary ECF anion is chloride; there are small amounts of bicarbonate, sulfate, and phosphate anions. The plasma has substantial amounts of protein. However, the amount of protein in the plasma is less than in the ICF. There is a very small amount of protein in the interstitium.

MECHANISMS CONTROLLING FLUID AND ELECTROLYTE MOVEMENT

Many different processes are involved in the movement of electrolytes and water between the ICF and ECF. Electrolytes move according to their concentration and electrical gradients, toward the areas of lower concentration and toward areas with the opposite charge. Some of the processes include simple diffusion, facilitated diffusion, and active transport. Water moves as driven by two forces: hydrostatic pressure and osmotic pressure.

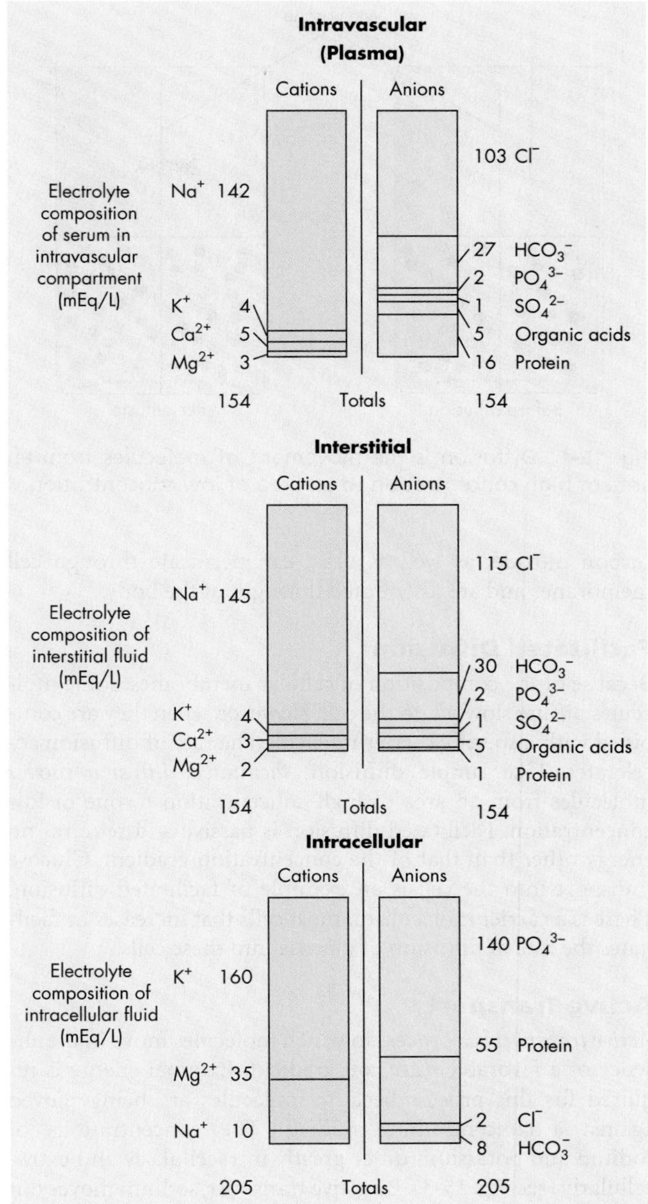

Fig. 15-3 Electrolyte content of fluid compartments.

Diffusion

Diffusion is the movement of molecules from an area of high concentration to one of low concentration (Fig. 15-4). It occurs in liquids, gases, and solids. Net movement of molecules stops when the concentrations are equal in both areas. The membrane separating the two areas must be permeable to the diffusing substance for the process to occur. Simple diffusion requires no external energy. Gases such as oxygen, nitrogen, and

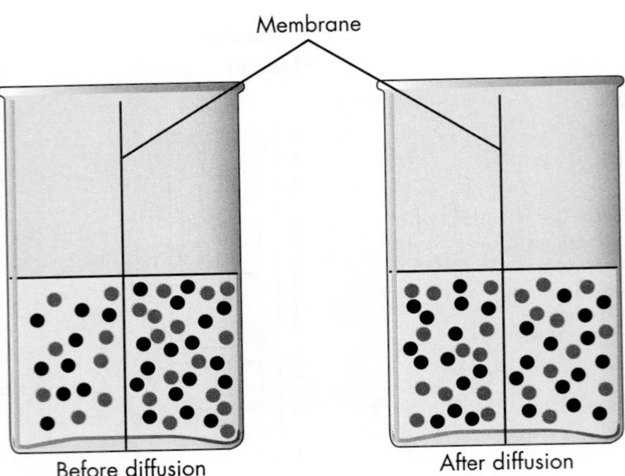

Fig. 15-4 Diffusion is the movement of molecules from an area of high concentration to an area of low concentration.

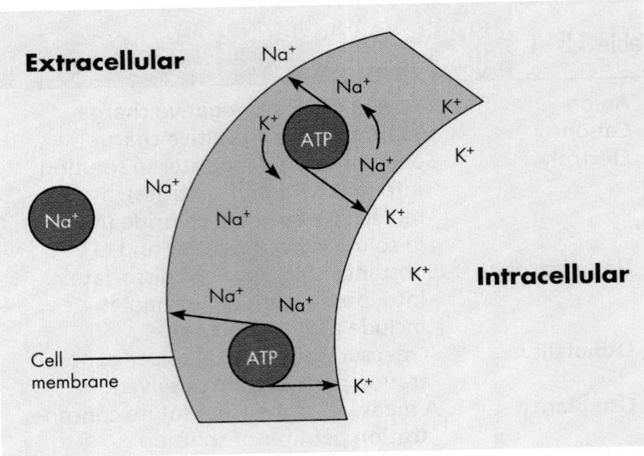

Fig. 15-5 Sodium-potassium pump. As sodium (Na^+) diffuses into the cell and potassium (K^+) diffuses out of the cell, an active transport system supplied with energy delivers sodium back to the extracellular compartment and potassium to the intracellular compartment. *ATP,* adenosine triphosphate.

carbon dioxide, as well as urea, can permeate through cell membranes and are distributed throughout the body.

Facilitated Diffusion

Because of the composition of cellular membranes, some molecules diffuse slowly into the cell. However, when they are combined with a specific carrier molecule, the rate of diffusion accelerates. Like simple diffusion, *facilitated diffusion* moves molecules from an area of high concentration to one of low concentration. Facilitated diffusion is passive and requires no energy other than that of the concentration gradient. Glucose transport into the cell is an example of facilitated diffusion. There is a carrier molecule on most cells that increases or facilitates the rate of diffusion of glucose into these cells.

Active Transport

Active transport is a process in which molecules move in the absence of a favorable diffusion gradient. External energy is required for this process because molecules are being moved against a concentration gradient. The concentrations of sodium and potassium differ greatly intracellularly and extracellularly (see Fig. 15-3). By active transport, sodium moves out of the cell and potassium moves into the cell to maintain this concentration difference (Fig. 15-5). The energy source for the sodium-potassium pump is adenosine triphosphate (ATP), which is produced in the mitochondria.

Osmosis

Osmosis is the movement of water between two compartments separated by a membrane permeable to water but not to a solute. Water moves through the membrane from an area of low solute concentration to an area of high solute concentration (Fig. 15-6); that is, water moves from the more dilute compartment (has more water) to the side that is more concentrated (has less water). The semipermeable membrane prevents movement of solute particles. Osmosis requires no outside energy sources and stops when the concentration differences disappear or when hydrostatic pressure builds and is sufficient to oppose any further movement of water. Diffusion and osmosis are important in maintaining the fluid volume of body cells.

Osmotic pressure can be understood in terms of imagining a chamber in which two compartments are separated by a membrane permeable to water and not to the solute (see Fig. 15-6). Water will move from the less concentrated side to the more concentrated side of the vessel. At some point the pressure generated by the height of the higher column of water will oppose the further movement of water. *Osmotic pressure* is the amount of pressure required to stop the osmotic flow of water.

Osmotic pressure is determined by the concentration of solutes in solution. It is measured in milliosmoles and may be expressed as either fluid osmolarity or fluid osmolality. Osmolality measures the osmotic force of solute per unit of weight of solvent (mOsm/kg or mmol/kg); osmolarity measures the total milliosmoles of solute per unit of total volume of solution (mOsm/L). For body fluids, which are dilute, the terms *osmolality* and *osmolarity* may be used interchangeably. Osmolality is the test typically performed to evaluate the concentration of plasma and urine.

Measurement of Osmolality. Osmolality is approximately the same in the various body fluid spaces. Determining osmolality is important because it indicates the water balance of the body. To assess the state of the body water balance, one can measure or estimate plasma osmolality. Normal plasma osmolality is between 275 and 295 mOsm/kg. A value greater than 295 mOsm/kg indicates that the concentration of particles is too great or that the water content is too little. This condition is termed *water deficit.* A value less than 275 mOsm/kg indicates too little solute for the amount of water or too much water for the amount of solute. This condition is termed *water excess.* Both conditions are clinically significant.

Plasma osmolality can be measured in most clinical laboratories. Because the major determinants of the plasma osmolality are sodium salts, glucose, and urea, one can calculate the effective plasma osmolality based on the concentrations of those compounds by using the following equation:

$$\text{Effective osmolality} = 2 \times [Na^+]p + [\text{glucose}]/18$$

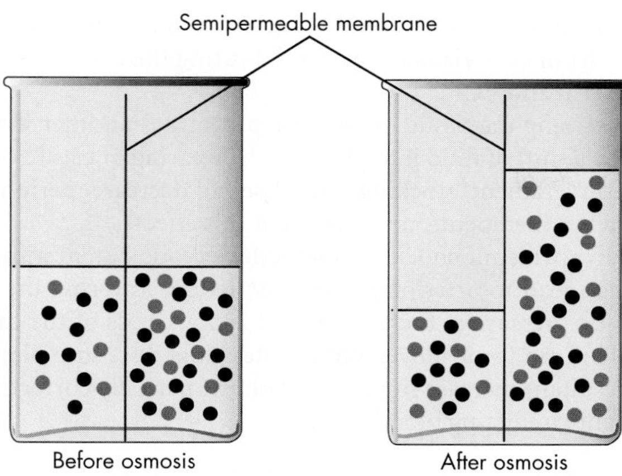

Fig. 15-6 Osmosis is the process of water movement through a semipermeable membrane from an area of low solute concentration to an area of high solute concentration.

where $[Na^+]p$ and [glucose] are the plasma concentrations of sodium and glucose in mEq/L and mg/dl, respectively. The sodium concentration is multiplied by 2 to account for the presence of an equivalent number of anions. Glucose concentration is divided by one tenth the molecular weight to calculate the number of osmotically active particles per liter.

It is sometimes recommended that the blood urea nitrogen (BUN) be included in the calculation of plasma osmolality. This is done by adding a third term to the above equation (+ BUN/2.8), with the BUN expressed in mg/dl. However, the urea moves freely between body fluid compartments; it has no lasting effect on water movement across cell boundaries and is sometimes dubbed an "ineffective osmole." Therefore one can estimate the actual osmolality more accurately by including the BUN. One can measure the effective plasma osmolality by eliminating the BUN term; the latter is the more physiologically meaningful estimate. Osmolality of urine can range from 100 to 1300 mOsm/kg, depending on the amount of antidiuretic hormone (ADH) and the renal response to it.

Water balance is maintained via the finely tuned balance of water intake and excretion. Water intake is controlled by thirst resulting in water consumption. Water excretion is controlled in the kidneys by the action of ADH. Both thirst and ADH release are regulated by the hypothalamus. As the body osmolality increases (water deficit), the person experiences thirst and will consume water if able. The water deficit is sensed in the hypothalamus, and more ADH is released from the posterior pituitary. When more ADH is present, more water is reabsorbed in the kidneys, and the water deficit tends to become corrected. The same mechanisms function when there is water excess. Thirst is inhibited, less ADH is released, and more water is excreted from the kidneys.[3]

Osmotic Movement of Fluids. Cells are affected by the osmolality of the fluid that surrounds them. Fluids with the same osmolality as the cell interior are termed *isotonic.* Solutions in which the solutes are less concentrated than the cells are termed *hypotonic* (hypo-osmolar). Those with solutes more concentrated than cells are termed *hypertonic* (hyperosmolar) (Table 15-2).

Normally, the ECF and ICF are isotonic to one another; hence no net movement of water occurs. In the metabolically active cell there is a constant exchange of substances between the compartments, but no net gain or loss of water occurs.

Table 15-2 Body Water (H_2O) Balance and Tonicity

Water Status	Osmolality	Effect on Cell Size
H_2O excess (hypotonic)	Less than 275 mOsm/kg (mmol/kg)	Swelling
Normal H_2O balance (isotonic)	275-295 mOsm/kg (mmol/kg)	None
H_2O deficit (hypertonic)	More than 300 mOsm/kg (mmol/kg)	Shrinking

If a cell is surrounded by hypotonic fluid, water moves into the cell, causing it to swell and possibly to burst. If a cell is surrounded by hypertonic fluid, water leaves the cell to dilute the ECF; the cell shrinks and may eventually die.

Hydrostatic Pressure

Hydrostatic pressure is the force within a fluid compartment. In the blood vessels hydrostatic pressure is related to the dynamic force added to the fluid by the pumping of the heart and to the height of the column of fluid within the vessel. Hydrostatic pressure in the vascular system gradually decreases as the blood moves through the arteries until it is about 40 mm Hg at the arterial end of a capillary. Because of the size of the capillary bed and fluid movement into the interstitium, the pressure decreases to about 10 mm Hg at the venous end of the capillary. Hydrostatic pressure is the major force that moves water out of the vascular system at the capillary level.

Oncotic Pressure

Oncotic pressure (colloidal osmotic pressure) is osmotic pressure exerted by colloids in solution. In plasma, protein molecules attract water and contribute to the total osmotic pressure in the vascular system. Unlike electrolytes, the large molecular size prevents proteins from leaving the vascular space through pores in capillary walls. Plasma oncotic pressure is approximately 25 mm Hg. Some proteins are found in the interstitial space; they exert an oncotic pressure of approximately 1 mm Hg.

FLUID MOVEMENT IN CAPILLARIES

There is normal movement of fluid between the capillary and the interstitium. The amount and direction of movement are determined by the interaction of (1) capillary hydrostatic pressure, (2) plasma oncotic pressure, (3) interstitial hydrostatic pressure, and (4) interstitial oncotic pressure.

Capillary hydrostatic pressure and interstitial oncotic pressure cause the movement of water *out* of the capillaries. Plasma oncotic pressure and interstitial hydrostatic pressure cause the movement of fluid *into* the capillary. At the arterial end of the capillary (Fig. 15-7), capillary hydrostatic pressure exceeds plasma oncotic pressure, and fluid is moved into the interstitium. At the venous end of the capillary, the capillary hydrostatic pressure is lower than plasma oncotic pressure, and fluid is drawn back into the capillary by the oncotic pressure created by plasma proteins.

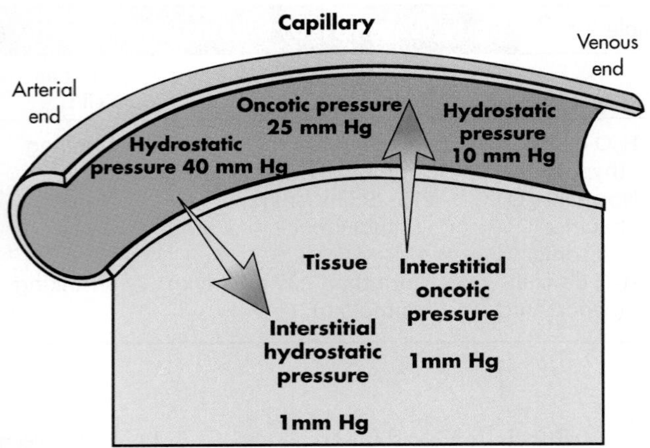

Fig. 15-7 Dynamics of fluid exchange between the capillary and the tissue. An equilibrium exists between forces filtering fluid out of the capillary and forces absorbing fluid back into the capillary. Note that the hydrostatic pressure is greater at the arterial end of the capillary than the venous end. The net effect of pressures at the arterial end of the capillary causes a movement of fluid into the tissue. At the venous end of the capillary there is net movement of fluid back into the capillary.

Fluid Shifts

If capillary or interstitial pressures are altered, fluid may abnormally shift from one compartment to another. Clinically, the two shifts of fluid seen most often are plasma-to-interstitial, seen in persons with edema, and interstitial-to-plasma, seen in persons with dehydration.[4]

Shifts of Plasma to Interstitial Fluid. Accumulation of fluid in the interstitium (edema) occurs if venous hydrostatic pressure rises, plasma oncotic pressure decreases, or interstitial oncotic pressure rises. Edema may also develop if there is an obstruction of lymphatic outflow that causes decreased removal of interstitial fluid.

Elevation of venous hydrostatic pressure. Increasing the pressure at the venous end of the capillary inhibits fluid movement back into the capillary. Causes of increased venous pressure include fluid overload, congestive heart failure, liver failure, obstruction of venous return to the heart (e.g., tourniquets, restrictive clothing, venous thrombosis), and venous insufficiency (e.g., varicose veins).

Decrease in plasma oncotic pressure. Fluid remains in the interstitium if the plasma oncotic pressure is too low to draw fluid back into the capillary. Decreased oncotic pressure is seen when the plasma protein content is low. This can result from excessive protein loss (nephrotic syndrome), deficient protein synthesis (liver disease), and deficient protein intake (malnutrition).

Elevation of interstitial oncotic pressure. Trauma, burns, and inflammation can damage capillary walls and allow plasma proteins to accumulate in the interstitium. The resultant increased interstitial oncotic pressure draws fluid into the interstitium and retains it there.

Shifts of Interstitial Fluid to Plasma. Fluid is drawn into the plasma space whenever there is an increase in the plasma osmotic-oncotic pressure. This could happen with administration of colloids, dextran, mannitol, or hypertonic solutions. Fluid is drawn from the interstitium. In turn, water is drawn from cells via osmosis, equilibrating the osmolality between ICF and ECF.

Increasing the tissue hydrostatic pressure is another way of causing a shift of fluid into plasma. The wearing of elastic compression gradient stockings or hose to decrease peripheral edema is a therapeutic application of this effect.

In hypovolemic shock, sympathetic nervous system stimulation can lead to arteriolar vasoconstriction, lowering the hydrostatic pressure at the arterial and venous ends of the capillary. This can favor movement of interstitial fluid into plasma. The resultant increase in vascular volume partially corrects the deficient circulating blood volume.

FLUID MOVEMENT BETWEEN EXTRACELLULAR FLUID AND INTRACELLULAR FLUID

Changes in the osmolality of the ECF alter the volume of cells. Increased ECF osmolality (water deficit) pulls water out of cells until the two compartments have a similar osmolality. Water deficit is associated with neurologic symptoms caused by altered central nervous system (CNS) function as brain cells shrink. Decreased ECF osmolality (water excess) develops as the result of gain or retention of excess water. In this case, cells swell. Again, the primary symptoms are neurologic as a result of brain cell swelling as water shifts into the cells.

REGULATION OF WATER BALANCE

Hypothalamic Regulation

Osmolar balance is regulated by the hypothalamus. Osmoreceptors in the hypothalamus detect a change in the osmolarity of as little as 1 mOsm/L. When the osmolality is increased (i.e., the concentration of solutes is increased), thirst is stimulated and ADH is released. (ADH is synthesized in the hypothalamus but stored and secreted by the posterior pituitary.) Thirst causes the patient to drink water. ADH acts in the distal and collecting tubules to cause water reabsorption in the kidneys. Together these factors result in increased free water in the body and decreased osmolality. If the osmolarity is diminished, the opposite occurs. Thirst and ADH release are suppressed. The collecting tubules become more permeable to water, and water is eliminated via the urine.

Water ingestion in the conscious patient is regulated by the thirst receptors located in the hypothalamus. The thirst mechanism is stimulated by hypotension and increased serum osmolality. An intact thirst mechanism is critical because it is the primary protection against the development of hyperosmolality. The patient who cannot recognize or act on the sensation of thirst is at risk for fluid deficit and hyperosmolality. The sensitivity of the thirst mechanism decreases in older adults.

The desire to consume fluids is also affected by social and psychologic factors not related to fluid balance. A dry mouth will cause the patient to drink, even when there is no measurable body water deficit. Water ingestion will equal water loss in the individual who has free access to water, a normal thirst and ADH mechanism, and normally functioning kidneys.

Pituitary Regulation

The posterior pituitary releases ADH, which regulates water retention by the kidneys. The distal tubules and collecting ducts in the kidneys respond to ADH by becoming more permeable to water so that water is reabsorbed into the blood and not ex-

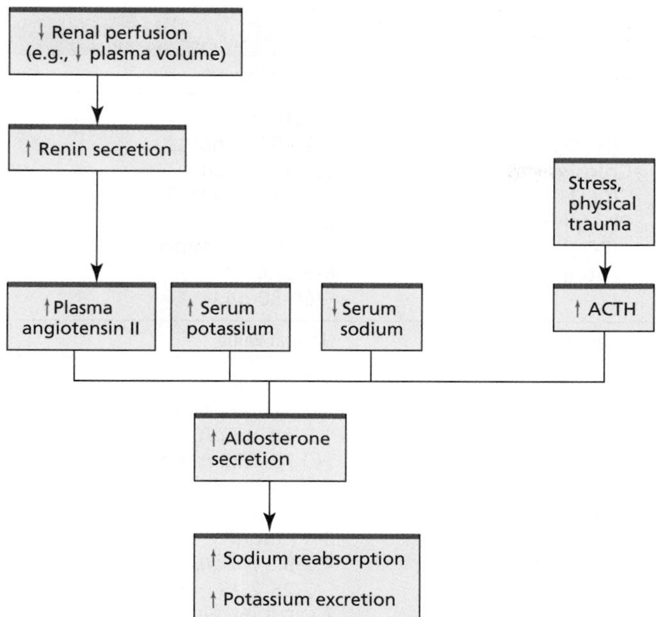

Fig. 15-8 Factors affecting aldosterone secretion.

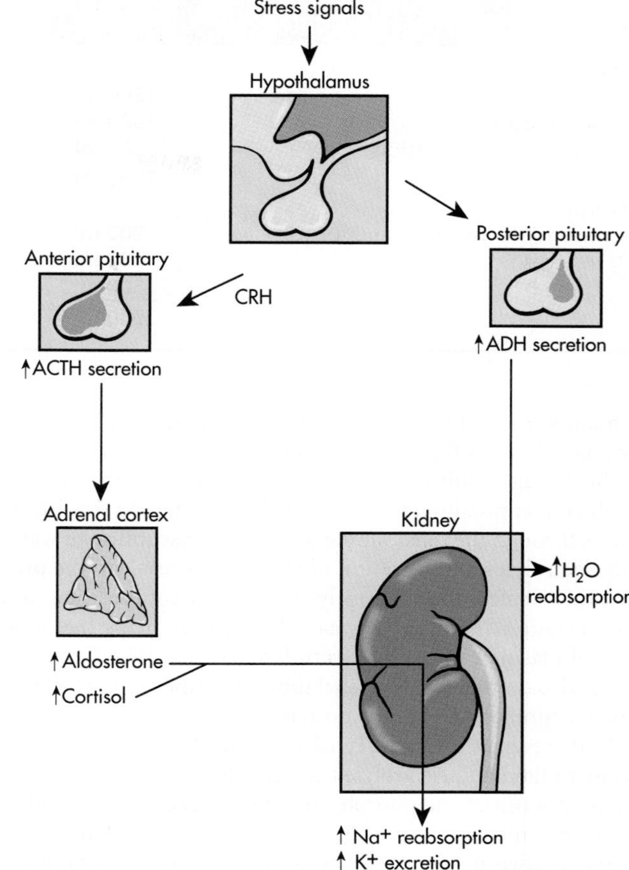

Fig. 15-9 Effects of stress on fluid and electrolyte balance.

creted in urine. An increase in plasma osmolality or a decrease in circulating volume will stimulate ADH secretion. Other factors that stimulate ADH release include stress, nausea, nicotine, and morphine. These factors usually result in shifts of osmolality within the range of normal values. It is common for the postoperative patient to have a lower serum osmolality after surgery, possibly because of the effects of stress and narcotic analgesia.

A pathologic condition seen occasionally is termed *syndrome of inappropriate antidiuretic hormone* (SIADH) (see Chapter 47). Causes of SIADH includes abnormal or ectopic ADH production in CNS disorders such as brain tumors or abscesses, brain injury, and pulmonary diseases such as pneumonia or tuberculosis. The inappropriate ADH causes water retention, which produces a decrease in plasma osmolality below the normal value and a relative increase in urine osmolality with a decrease in volume.

Reduction in the release or action of ADH produces diabetes insipidus (see Chapter 47). A copious amount of dilute urine is excreted because the renal tubules and collecting ducts do not appropriately reabsorb water. The patient with diabetes insipidus exhibits extreme polyuria and, if alert, polydipsia. Symptoms of dehydration and hypernatremia develop if the water losses are not adequately replaced.

Adrenal Cortical Regulation

ECF volume is maintained by a combination of hormonal influences. ADH affects only water reabsorption. Hormones released by the adrenal cortex help regulate both water and electrolytes. Two groups of hormones secreted by the adrenal cortex include glucocorticoids and mineralocorticoids. The glucocorticoids primarily have an antiinflammatory effect and increase serum glucose levels, whereas the mineralocorticoids (e.g., aldosterone) enhance sodium retention and potassium excretion (Fig. 15-8). When sodium is reabsorbed, water follows as a result of osmotic changes.

Cortisol is the most common example of a naturally occurring glucocorticoid. In large doses, cortisol has both glucocorticoid (glucose elevating and antiinflammatory) and mineralocorticoid (sodium-retention) properties. The adrenocortical hormone cortisol is secreted normally and whenever the body experiences stress. Many body systems, including fluid and electrolyte balance, are affected by stress (Fig. 15-9).

Aldosterone is the naturally occurring mineralocorticoid with potent sodium-retaining and potassium-excreting capability. The secretion of aldosterone may be stimulated by decreased renal perfusion or decreased sodium delivery to the distal portion of the renal tubule. The kidneys respond by secreting renin into the plasma. Angiotensinogen produced in the liver and normally found in blood is acted on by the renin to form angiotensin I, which converts to angiotensin II, which stimulates the adrenal cortex to secrete aldosterone. In addition to the renin-angiotensin mechanism, increased plasma potassium, decreased plasma sodium, and increased release of adrenocorticotropic hormone (ACTH) from the anterior pituitary all act directly on the adrenal cortex to stimulate the secretion of aldosterone (see Fig. 15-8).

Renal Regulation

The primary organs for regulating fluid and electrolyte balance are the kidneys (see Chapter 42). The kidneys regulate water balance through adjustments in urine volume. Similarly, urinary excretion of most electrolytes is adjusted so that a balance

Table 15-3 Normal Fluid Balance in the Adult

Intake	
Fluids	1200 ml
Solid food	1000 ml
Water from oxidation	300 ml
	2500 ml
Output	
Insensible loss (skin and lungs)	900 ml
In feces	100 ml
Urine	1500 ml
	2500 ml

is maintained between overall intake and output. The total plasma volume is filtered by the kidneys many times each day. In the average adult the kidney reabsorbs 99% of this filtrate, producing approximately 1.5 L of urine per day. As the filtrate moves through the renal tubule, selective reabsorption of water and electrolytes and secretion of electrolytes result in the production of urine that is greatly different in composition and concentration than the plasma. This process helps maintain normal plasma osmolality, electrolyte balance, blood volume, and acid-base balance. The renal tubules are the site for the hormonal action of ADH and aldosterone.

With severely impaired renal function, the kidneys cannot maintain fluid and electrolyte balance. This condition results in edema, potassium and phosphorus retention, acidosis, and other electrolyte imbalances (see Chapter 44). Renal function is typically decreased in the elderly person, placing the patient at increased risk for fluid and electrolyte imbalances. In particular, the ability to concentrate urine may be reduced in the older adult.

Cardiac Regulation

Atrial naturetic factor (ANF) is a hormone released by the cardiac atria in response to increased atrial pressure. ANF is increased in the presence of any condition that results in volume expansion or increased cardiac filling pressures (e.g., congestive heart failure). The primary actions of ANF are direct vasodilation and increased urinary excretion of sodium and water. The full physiologic role of ANF has yet to be identified.[4]

Gastrointestinal Regulation

Daily water intake and output are between 2000 and 3000 ml (Table 15-3). The gastrointestinal tract accounts for most of the water intake. Water intake includes fluids, water from food metabolism, and water present in solid foods. Lean meat is approximately 70% water, whereas the water content of many fruits and vegetables approaches 100%.

Most of the body water is excreted by the kidneys. A small amount of water is eliminated by the GI tract in feces.

Insensible Water Loss

Insensible water loss, which is unavoidable vaporization from the lungs and skin, assists in regulating body temperature. Normally, about 900 ml per day is lost. The amount of water loss is increased by accelerated body metabolism, which occurs with increased body temperature and exercise.

Water loss through the skin should not be confused with the vaporization of water excreted by sweat glands. Only water is lost by insensible perspiration. Excessive sweating (sensible perspiration) caused by fever or high environmental temperatures may lead to large losses of water and electrolytes.

Table 15-4 Normal Serum Electrolyte Values

Anions	Normal Value
Bicarbonate (HCO_3^-)	20-30 mEq/L (20-30 mmol/L)
Chloride (Cl^-)	96-106 mEq/L (96-106 mmol/L)
Phosphate (PO_4^{3-})	2.8-4.5 mg/dl (0.90-1.45 mmol/L)
Protein	6-8 g/dl (60-80 g/L)
Cations	**Normal Value**
Potassium (K^+)	3.5-5.5 mEq/L (3.5-5.5 mmol/L)
Magnesium (Mg^{2+})	1.5-2.5 mEq/L (0.75-1.25 mmol/L)
Sodium (Na^+)	135-145 mEq/L (135-145 mmol/L)
Calcium (Ca^{2+}) (Total)	9-11 mg/dl 4.5-5.5 mEq/L (2.25-2.75 mmol/L)
Calcium (Ionized)	4.5-5.5 mg/dl (1.13-1.38 mmol/L)

FLUID AND ELECTROLYTE IMBALANCES

Fluid and electrolyte imbalances occur to some degree in most patients with a major illness or injury because illness disrupts the normal homeostatic mechanism. Some fluid and electrolyte imbalances are directly caused by illness or disease (e.g., burns, congestive heart failure). At other times, therapeutic measures (e.g., intravenous fluid replacement, diuretics) cause or contribute to fluid and electrolyte imbalances.

The imbalances are commonly classified as deficits or excesses. Each imbalance is discussed separately. (For normal values, see Table 15-4.) In actual clinical situations, more than one imbalance found in the same patient is common. For example, a patient with prolonged nasogastric suction will lose Na^+, K^+, H^+, and Cl^-. These imbalances may result in a deficiency of both sodium and potassium, as well as metabolic alkalosis and fluid volume deficit.

SODIUM AND VOLUME IMBALANCES

Sodium plays a major role in maintaining the concentration and volume of the ECF. Sodium is the main cation of the ECF and the primary determinant of ECF osmolality. Sodium imbalances are typically associated with parallel changes in osmolality. Because of its impact on osmolality, sodium affects the water distribution between the ECF and the ICF. Sodium is also important in the generation and transmission of nerve impulses and the regulation of acid-base balance. Serum sodium is measured in milliequivalents per liter or millimoles per liter.

The GI tract absorbs sodium from foods. Typically, daily intake of sodium far exceeds the body's daily requirements. Sodium leaves the body through urine, sweat, and feces. The kidneys are the primary regulator of sodium balance. Urinary

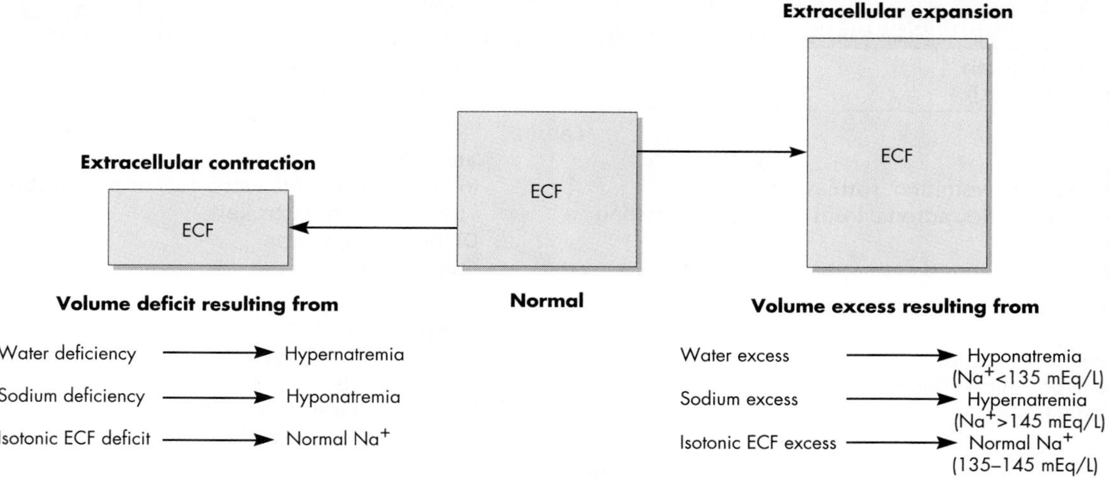

Fig. 15-10 Differential assessment of extracellular fluid (ECF) volume.

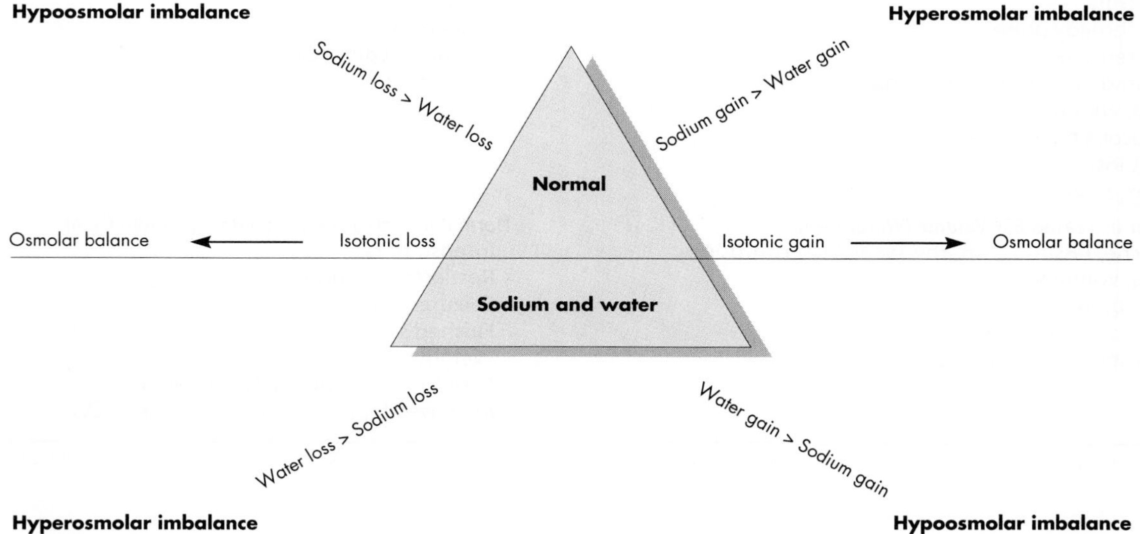

Fig. 15-11 Isotonic gains and losses affect mainly the extracellular fluid (ECF) compartment with little or no water movement into the cells. Hypertonic imbalances cause water to move from inside the cell into the ECF to dilute the concentrated sodium, causing cell shrinkage. Hypotonic imbalances cause water to move into the cell, causing cell swelling.

excretion of excess sodium is adjusted in part through the action of aldosterone. The kidneys regulate the ECF concentration of sodium by excreting or retaining water under the influence of ADH. The serum sodium level reflects the ratio of sodium to water, not necessarily the loss or gain of sodium. Thus changes in the serum sodium level may reflect either a primary water imbalance, a primary sodium imbalance, or a combination of the two. Sodium imbalances are typically associated with imbalances in ECF volume (Figs. 15-10 and 15-11).

HYPERNATREMIA

Common causes of hypernatremia are listed in Table 15-5. An elevated serum sodium may occur with water loss or sodium gain. Because sodium is the major determinant of the ECF osmolality, hypernatremia causes hyperosmolality. In turn, hyperosmolality causes a shift of water out of the cells, which leads to cellular dehydration.

As discussed earlier, the primary protection against the development of hyperosmolality is thirst. As the plasma osmolality increases, the thirst center in the hypothalamus is stimulated, and the individual seeks fluids. Although increased release of ADH is another important protective response to hypernatremia, thirst provides the ultimate defense.[1]

Hypernatremia is not a problem in an alert person who has access to water, is able to swallow, and can sense thirst. Hypernatremia secondary to water deficiency is often the result of an impaired level of consciousness or an inability to obtain fluids. The unconcious patient is at risk because of an inability to express thirst and act on it. Often the older adult, especially if ill, does not drink enough fluids because of a reduction in the sensitivity of the thirst center and decreased mobility.

Several clinical states can produce water loss and hypernatremia. A deficiency in the synthesis or a release of ADH from the posterior pituitary gland (central diabetes insipidus) or a

Table 15-5 Water and Sodium Imbalances: Causes and Clinical Manifestations

Water Excess/Hyponatremia (Na^+ <135 mEq/L [mmol/L])	Water Deficit/Hypernatremia (Na^+ >145 mEq/L [mmol/L])
Causes	
Sodium Loss	**Water Loss**
GI losses: Diarrhea, vomiting, fistulas, NG suction	Increased insensible water loss or perspiration (high fever, heatstroke)
Renal losses: Diuretics, adrenal insufficiency, Na^+ wasting renal disease	Diabetes insipidus
Skin losses: Burns, wound drainage	Osmotic diuresis
Water Gain	**Sodium Gain**
SIADH	IV hypertonic NaCl
Congestive heart failure	IV sodium bicarbonate
Excessive hypotonic IV fluids	IV excessive isotonic NaCl
Primary polydipsia	Primary hyperaldosteronism
	Saltwater near drowning
Clinical Manifestations	
Decreased ECF Volume (Sodium Loss)	**Decreased ECF Volume (Water Loss)**
Irritability, apprehension, confusion	Intense thirst, dry, swollen tongue
Postural hypotension	Restlessness, agitation, twitching
Tachycardia	Seizures, coma
Rapid, thready pulse	Weakness
Decreased CVP	Postural hypotension, decreased CVP
Decreased jugular venous filling	Weight loss
Nausea, vomiting	
Dry mucous membranes	
Weight loss	
Tremors, seizures, coma	
Normal or Increased ECF Volume (Water Gain)	**Normal or Increased ECF Volume (Sodium Gain)**
Headache, lassitude, apathy, weakness, confusion	Intense thirst
Nausea, vomiting	Restlessness, agitation, twitching
Weight gain	Seizures, coma
Increased blood pressure, increased CVP	Flushed skin
Muscle spasms, seizures, coma	Weight gain
	Peripheral and pulmonary edema
	Increased blood pressures, increased CVP

CVP, central venous pressure; *ECF,* extracellular fluid; *GI,* gastrointestinal; *IV,* intravenous; *NG,* nasogastric; *SIADH,* syndrome of inappropriate antidiuretic hormone.

decrease in kidney responsiveness to ADH (nephrogenic diabetes insipidus) can result in profound diuresis resulting in a water deficit and hypernatremia. More common causes include concentrated hyperosmolar tube feedings and osmotic diuresis, which occurs with hyperglycemia (uncontrolled diabetes mellitus) or after the administration of osmotic diuretics (mannitol). Other causes include insensible loss with high fever and severe diarrhea. Excessive sweating without water replacement also leads to hypernatremia.

Sodium intake in excess of water intake can also result in hypernatremia. Examples of sodium gain include intravenous administration of hypertonic saline or sodium bicarbonate, use of sodium-containing medications, excessive oral intake of sodium (ingestion of seawater), or primary aldosteronism caused by a tumor of the adrenal glands.

The clinical manifestations of hypernatremia are listed in Table 15-5. Symptoms are primarily the result of changes in the plasma osmolality that lead to changes in the volume of cellular water. Dehydration of neurons leads to neurologic manifestations such as intense thirst, lethargy, agitation, seizures, and even coma. Sodium excess also has a direct effect on the irritability and conduction of nerve cells, causing them to be more easily excited. Patients with hypernatremia will also exhibit the symptoms of any accompanying volume imbalance.

Collaborative Care

The goal of treatment in hypernatremia that is caused by either water loss or sodium gain is to treat the underlying cause. In primary water deficit the continued water loss must be prevented, and water replacement must be provided. If oral fluids cannot be ingested, intravenous solutions of 5% dextrose in water or hypotonic saline may be given initially. Serum sodium levels must be reduced gradually to prevent too rapid a shift of water back into the cells. Overly rapid correction of hypernatremia can result in cerebral edema. The risk is greatest in the patient who has developed hypernatremia over several days or longer.

Families caring for the incapacitated older adult or comatose person at home must be instructed in the need for adequate provision of water for these at-risk patients.[2] Iso-osmolar or hypo-osmolar liquid formulas do not provide adequate free water for patients with abnormal water losses.

The goal of treatment for sodium excess is to dilute the sodium concentration and to promote excretion of the excess sodium. Intravenous solutions of 5% dextrose in water are usually given in combination with diuretics. Sodium intake will also be restricted. (See Chapter 47 for specific treatment of diabetes insipidus.)

HYPONATREMIA

Hyponatremia may result from loss of sodium-containing fluids or from water excess. Hyponatremia causes hypo-osmolality with a shift of water into the cells.

Common causes of hyponatremia caused by water excess are inappropriate use of sodium-free or hypotonic intravenous (IV) fluids especially after surgery or major trauma, after unchecked fluid intake in patients with renal failure, or with psychiatric disorders associated with excessive water intake. SIADH will result in dilutional hyponatremia caused by abnormal retention of water. (See Chapter 47 for a discussion of the causes of SIADH.)

Losses of sodium-rich body fluids (caused by abnormal GI tract, kidney, or skin losses) alone will not result in hyponatremia because these are either isotonic or hypotonic fluids; that is, sodium is lost with an equal or greater proportion of water. However, the physiologic response to this volume loss (i.e., release of ADH and thirst) can lead to the development of hyponatremia as a result of retention of water.[5]

Clinical manifestations of water excess include rapid weight gain and increased central venous pressure (CVP). Neurologic symptoms develop with hyponatremia secondary to a reduction in the plasma osmolality with a shift of water into brain cells. The clinical manifestations of hyponatremia are listed in Table 15-5.

Collaborative Care

In hyponatremia that is caused by water excess, fluid restriction is often all that is needed to treat the problem. If severe symptoms (seizures) develop, small amounts of intravenous hypertonic saline solution (3% NaCl) are given to restore the serum sodium level while the body is returning to a normal water balance. Treatment of hyponatremia associated with abnormal fluid loss includes fluid replacement with sodium-containing solutions. Replacing losses with commercially available oral rehydration fluids containing electrolytes instead of pure water may help prevent the development of hyponatremia in the home setting. As with hypernatremia, chronic hyponatremia must be corrected slowly to prevent neurologic damage secondary to myelinolysis (destruction of myelin).[5]

EXTRACELLULAR FLUID VOLUME IMBALANCES

ECF volume deficit (hypovolemia) and ECF volume excess (hypervolemia) are commonly occurring clinical conditions (Table 15-6). ECF fluid volume imbalances are typically accompanied by one or more electrolyte imbalances. As previously discussed, volume imbalances are often associated with changes in the serum sodium level. Fluid volume deficit can occur with abnormal loss of body fluids (e.g., diarrhea, fistula drainage, hemorrhage, polyuria), decreased intake, or a plasma-to-interstitial fluid shift. Fluid volume excess may result from excessive intake of fluids, abnormal retention of fluids (e.g., congestive heart failure, renal failure), or interstitial-to-plasma fluid shift. Although shifts in fluid between the plasma and interstitium do not alter the overall volume of the ECF, these shifts do result in changes in the clinically important intravascular volume.

Table 15-6 Causes of ECF Volume Imbalances

ECF Volume Deficit	ECF Volume Excess
Increased Loss	**Increased Retention**
Vomiting	Congestive heart failure
Diarrhea	Cushing's syndrome
Fistula drainage	Chronic liver disease with portal hypertension
GI tract suction	Long-term use of corticosteroids
Excessive sweating	Renal failure
Third-space fluid shifts (e.g., burns, intestinal obstruction)	
Overuse of diuretics	
Hemorrhage	
Decreased Intake	**Increased Intake**
Nausea	Rare with adequate renal function
Anorexia	Excessive IV administration of fluids
Inability to drink	
Inability to obtain water	

Collaborative Care

The goal of treatment for fluid volume deficit is to correct the underlying cause and to replace both water and electrolytes. Balanced IV solutions, such as lactated Ringer's solution, are usually given. Isotonic sodium chloride is used when rapid volume replacement is indicated. Blood is administered when volume loss is due to blood loss.

The goal of treatment for fluid volume excess is removal of sodium and water without producing abnormal changes in the electrolyte composition or osmolality of ECF. The primary cause must be identified and treated. Intravenous therapy is usually not indicated for this type of fluid imbalance. Diuretics and fluid restriction are the primary forms of therapy. Restriction of sodium intake may also be indicated. If the fluid excess leads to ascites or pleural effusion, an abdominal paracentesis or thoracentesis may be necessary.

NURSING MANAGEMENT: SODIUM AND VOLUME IMBALANCES

■ Nursing Diagnoses

Nursing diagnoses and collaborative problems for the patient with various fluid and sodium imbalances include, but are not limited to, the following.

Extracellular fluid volume excess:

- Fluid volume excess *related to* increased sodium and water retention
- Risk for impaired skin integrity *related to* edema
- Body image disturbance *related to* altered body appearance secondary to edema
- Potential complications: pulmonary edema, ascites

Extracellular fluid volume deficit:

- Fluid volume deficit *related to* excessive ECF losses or decreased fluid intake
- Potential complication: hypovolemic shock

Hypernatremia:

- Risk for injury *related to* altered sensorium and seizures secondary to abnormal CNS function

Hyponatremia:

- Risk for injury *related to* altered sensorium and decreased level of consciousness secondary to abnormal CNS function

Nursing Implementation

Intake and Output. The use of 24-hour intake and output records gives valuable information regarding fluid and electrolyte problems. Sources of excessive intake or fluid losses can be identified on a properly recorded intake-and-output flowsheet. Intake should include oral, IV, and tube feedings and retained irrigants. Output includes urine, excess perspiration, wound or tube drainage, vomitus, and diarrhea. Fluid loss from wounds and perspiration should be estimated. Urine specific gravity measurements can be done. Readings of greater than 1.025 indicate a concentrated urine, whereas those of less than 1.010 indicate a dilute urine.

Vital Signs. Signs and symptoms of ECF volume excess and deficit are reflected in changes in blood pressure, heart rate, respiratory rate, CVP readings, and lung sounds. In fluid volume excess, tachycardia secondary to sympathetic nervous system stimulation occurs. The pulse is rapid and bounding. Because of the expanded intravascular volume, the pulse is not easily obliterated. The respiratory rate is increased. Blood pressure is usually elevated secondary to the increased volume, along with CVP. With pulmonary congestion and edema, the patient will experience shortness of breath, and moist crackles will be auscultated.

In mild to moderate fluid volume deficit, compensatory mechanisms include sympathetic nervous system stimulation of the heart and peripheral vasoconstriction. Stimulation of the heart increases heart rate and, combined with vasoconstriction, maintains blood pressure within normal limits. A change in position from lying to sitting or standing may elicit a further increase in heart rate or a decrease in blood pressure (orthostatic hypotension). If vasoconstriction and tachycardia provide inadequate compensation, hypotension occurs when the patient is recumbent. Severe fluid volume deficit can cause a weak, thready pulse that is easily obliterated. The decreased volume is also reflected in a significantly reduced CVP. The respiratory rate increases as a result of decreased tissue perfusion and hypoxia. Severe, untreated fluid deficit will result in shock.

Neurologic Changes. Changes in neurologic function may occur with sodium and water imbalances. With increased water volume and hyponatremia, water moves by osmosis into the brain cells. Alternatively, decreased water volume and hypernatremia cause water to shift out of the cerebral cells with resultant shrinkage. Profound volume depletion may cause an alteration in sensorium secondary to reduced cerebral tissue perfusion.

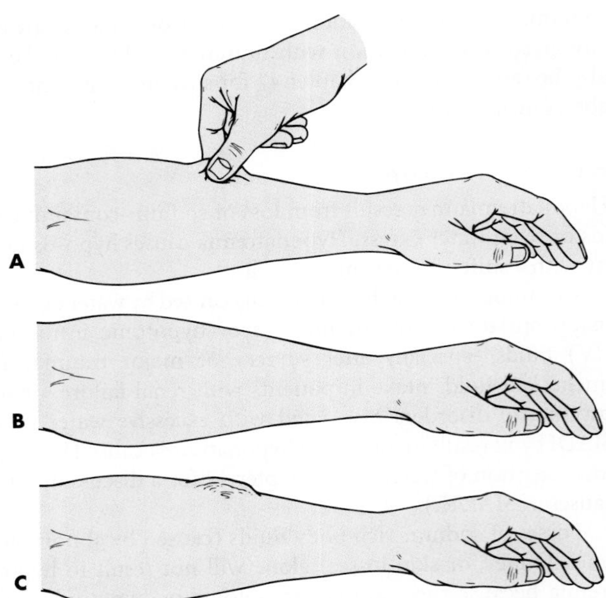

Fig. 15-12 Assessment of skin turgor. **A** and **B,** When normal skin is pinched, it resumes shape in seconds. **C,** If the skin remains wrinkled for 20 to 30 seconds, the patient has poor skin turgor.

Assessment of neurologic function includes evaluation of (1) the level of consciousness, which includes responses to verbal and painful stimuli and the determination of a person's orientation to time, place, and person; (2) pupillary response to light and equality of pupil size; and (3) voluntary movement of the extremities, degree of muscle strength, and reflexes.

Daily Weights. Accurate daily weights provide the best bedside measurement of volume status. An increase of 1 kg (2.2 lb) is equal to 1000 ml fluid retention (provided the person has maintained usual dietary intake or has not been on nothing-by-mouth [NPO] status). However, weight changes can be relied on only if obtained under standardized conditions. An accurate weight requires the patient to be weighed at the same time every day and on the same carefully calibrated scale. Excess clothing and bedding should be removed and all drainage bags should be emptied before the weighing. If bulky dressings or tubes are present, which may not necessarily be used every day, a notation regarding these variables should be recorded on the flowsheet or nursing notes.

Skin Assessment and Care. Clues to fluid volume deficit and excess can be detected by inspection of the skin. Skin should be examined for turgor and mobility. Normally a fold of skin, when pinched, will readily move and, on release, will rapidly return to its former position. Skin areas over the sternum, abdomen, and anterior forearm are the usual sites for evaluation of tissue turgor (Fig. 15-12).

In fluid volume deficit, skin turgor is diminished; there is a lag in the pinched skinfold's return to its original state. The skin may be cool and moist if there is sympathetic vasoconstriction to compensate for the decreased fluid volume. Mild hypovolemia usually does not stimulate this compensatory response; consequently, the skin will be warm and dry. Volume deficit may also cause the skin to appear dry and wrinkled. These signs may be difficult to evaluate in the older adult because the patient's skin may be normally dry, wrinkled, and nonelastic. Oral mucous membranes will be dry, the tongue may be furrowed, and the individual often complains of thirst. Routine oral care is critical to the comfort of the dehydrated patient and the patient who is fluid restricted for managment of fluid volume excess.

Skin that is edematous may feel cool because of fluid accumulation and a decrease in blood flow secondary to the pressure of the fluid. The fluid can also stretch the skin causing it to feel taut and hard. Edema is assessed by pressing with a thumb or forefinger over the edematous area. A grading scale is used to standardize the description if an indentation (ranging from 1+ [slight, 2 mm indentation] to 4+ [pitting, 8 mm indentation]) remains when pressure is released. The areas to be evaluated for edema are those where soft tissues overlie a bone. Skin areas over the tibia, fibula, and sacrum are the preferred sites.

Good skin care for the person with fluid volume excess or deficit is important. Edematous tissues must be protected from extremes of heat and cold, prolonged pressure, and trauma. Frequent skin care and changes in position will protect the patient from skin breakdown. Elevation of edematous extremities helps promote venous return and fluid reabsorption. Dehydrated skin needs frequent care without the use of soap. The application of moisturizing creams or oils will increase moisture retention and stimulate circulation.

Other Nursing Measures. The rates of infusion of intravenous fluid solutions should be carefully monitored. Attempts to "catch up" should be approached with extreme caution, particularly when large volumes of fluid or certain electrolytes are involved. This is especially true in patients with cardiac, renal, or neurologic problems. The nurse should encourage and often assist the older or debilitated patient to maintain an adequate oral intake. Patients receiving tube feedings need supplementary water added to their enteral formula.

The patient with nasogastric suction should not be allowed to drink water because it will increase the loss of electrolytes. Occasionally the patient may be given small amounts of ice chips to suck. A nasogastric tube should always be irrigated with isotonic saline solution and not with water. Water causes diffusion of electrolytes into the stomach; the electrolytes are then suctioned away.

POTASSIUM IMBALANCES

Potassium is the major ICF cation with 98% of the body potassium being intracellular. For example, potassium concentration within muscle cells is approximately 140 mEq/L; potassium concentration in the ECF is 3.5 to 5.5 mEq/L. The sodium-potassium pump in cell membranes maintains this concentration difference by pumping potassium into the cell and sodium out, a process fueled by the breakdown of ATP.

The small amount of potassium in the ECF is critically important because ECF potassium concentration is the primary factor setting resting membrane potential in most excitable cells. Changes in ECF potassium level alter the excitability of muscle, neurons, and many other tissues, including pancreatic islet cells, which release insulin. Because of its effects on cellular excitability, ECF potassium contributes to cardiac rate and rhythm, transmission and conduction of nerve impulses, skeletal muscle contraction, and function of smooth muscle and many endocrine tissues. ICF potassium has roles in cellular metabolism and functions in the regulation of protein and glycogen synthesis.[6]

Understanding a patient's potassium balance requires analysis of the intake and output of potassium and the movement of potassium between the ICF and ECF. The typical Western diet contains approximately 50 to 100 mEq of potassium daily, mainly from fruits, dried fruits, and vegetables. Many salt substitutes contain substantial potassium. Patients receive potassium from parenteral sources including IV fluids, stored blood, and potassium-penicillin.

About 90% of the daily potassium intake is eliminated by the kidneys; the remainder is lost in the stool and sweat. In the patient with good renal function, renal potassium loss is regulated by many factors, including ECF and ICF potassium, ECF sodium, and blood volume. There is an inverse relationship between sodium and potassium reabsorption in the kidneys. Factors that cause sodium retention (e.g., low blood volume, increased aldosterone level) cause potassium loss in the urine. Large urine volumes can be associated with excess loss of potassium in the urine. If kidney function is significantly impaired, toxic levels of potassium may be retained.

Disruptions in the dynamic equilibrium between ICF and ECF potassium often cause clinical problems. Clinicians use the mechanisms involved in this equilibrium to remedy hypokalemia and hyperkalemia. Among the factors causing potassium to move from the ECF to the ICF are the following: insulin, beta-adrenergic stimulation (as when epinephrine is released in stress, coronary ischemia, delerium tremens, or administered as in patients with asthma or premature labor), alkalosis, and rapid cell building (as when folic acid or cobalamin [Vitamin B_{12}] is administered to the patient with megaloblastic anemia, stimulating marked production of platelets and red blood cells). Factors that cause potassium to move from the ICF to the ECF include acidosis, trauma to cells (as in massive soft tissue damage or in tumor lysis), and exercise. Both digoxin-like drugs and beta-adrenergic blocking drugs (such as propanolol [Inderal]) can impair uptake of potassium into cells, resulting in the higher ECF potassium concentration. Causes of potassium imbalance are summarized in Table 15-7.

HYPERKALEMIA

Hyperkalemia may be caused by a massive intake of potassium, impaired renal excretion, shift of potassium from the ICF to the ECF, or a combination of these factors. The most common cause of hyperkalemia is renal failure. Hyperkalemia is also common in association with hyperglycemia in uncontrolled diabetes mellitus, in patients with massive cell destruction (e.g., burn or crush injury or tumor lysis), rapid transfusion of aged blood, and catabolic state (e.g., severe infections). Metabolic acidosis, particularly when the chloride is normal, is associated with a shift of potassium ion from the ICF to the ECF as hydrogen ions move into the cell. Adrenal insufficiency leads to retention of K^+ in the serum because of aldosterone deficiency. Certain medications, such as potassium-sparing diuretics and angiotensin-converting enzyme (ACE)

Table 15-7 Potassium Imbalances: Causes and Clinical Manifestations

Hypokalemia ($K^+ < 3.5$ mEq/L [mmol/L])	Hyperkalemia ($K^+ > 5.5$ mEq/L [mmol/L])
Causes	
Potassium Loss	**Excess Potassium Intake**
GI losses: Diarrhea, vomiting, fistulas, NG suction	Excessive or rapid parenteral administration
Renal losses: Diuretics, hyperaldosteronism, magnesium depletion	Potassium-containing drugs (e.g., potassium-penicillin)
Skin losses: Diaphoresis	Potassium-containing salt substitute
Dialysis	
Shift of Potassium into Cells	**Shift of Potassium Out of Cells**
Increased insulin (e.g., IV dextrose load)	Acidosis
Alkalosis	Tissue catabolism (e.g., fever, sepsis, burns)
Tissue repair	Crush injury
Increased epinephrine (e.g., stress)	Tumor lysis syndrome
Lack of Potassium Intake	**Failure to Eliminate Potassium**
Starvation	Renal disease
Diet low in potassium	Potassium-sparing diuretics
Failure to include potassium in parenteral fluids if NPO	Adrenal insufficiency
	ACE inhibitors
Clinical Manifestations	
Fatigue	Irritability
Muscle weakness	Anxiety
Leg cramps	Abdominal cramping, diarrhea
Nausea, vomiting, ileus	Weakness of lower extremities
Soft, flabby muscles	Paresthesias
Paresthesias, decreased reflexes	Irregular pulse
Weak, irregular pulse	Cardiac standstill if hyperkalemia sudden or severe
Polyuria	
Hyperglycemia	
Electrocardiograph Changes	**Electrocardiograph Changes**
ST segment depression	Tall, peaked T wave
Flattened T wave	Prolonged PR interval
Presence of U wave	ST depression
Ventricular arrhythmias (e.g., PVCs)	Loss of P wave
Bradycardia	Widening QRS
Enhanced digitalis effect	Ventricular fibrillation
	Ventricular standstill

ACE, angiotensin-converting enzyme; *NPO,* nothing by mouth; *PVC,* premature ventricular contraction.

inhibitors, may contribute to the development of hyperkalemia. Both of these types of medications reduce the kidneys's ability to secrete and therefore excrete excess potassium (see Table 15-7).

Clinical Manifestations

Hyperkalemia causes membrane depolarization, altering cell excitability. Skeletal muscles become weak or paralyzed. The patient may experience cramping leg pain. Leg muscles are affected initially; respiratory muscles are spared. Cardiac cells depolarize as well, leading to abnormal conduction and potentially fatal arrhythmias.[7] Ventricular fibrillation or cardiac standstill may occur. Cardiac depolarization is impaired, leading to flattening of the P wave and widening of the QRS wave. Repolarization occurs more rapidly, resulting in shortening of the Q-T interval and causing the T wave to be narrower and more peaked. Figure 15-13 illustrates the electrocardiographic (ECG) effects of hypokalemia and hyperkalemia. Other clinical manifestations are listed in Table 15-7.

NURSING AND COLLABORATIVE MANAGEMENT: HYPERKALEMIA

■ Nursing Diagnoses

Nursing diagnoses and collaborative problems for the patient with hyperkalemia include, but are not limited to, the following:

- Risk for injury *related to* lower extremity muscle weakness and seizures
- Potential complication: arrhythmias

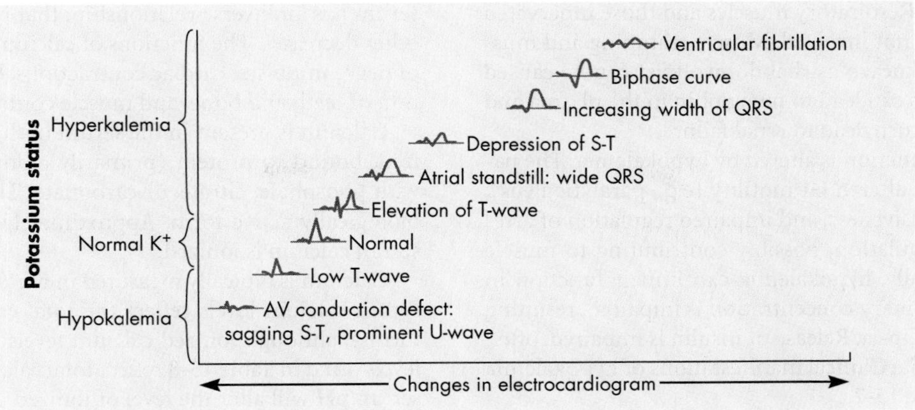

Fig. 15-13 Electrocardiogram changes associated with alterations in potassium status.

Nursing Implementation

Treatment of hyperkalemia consists of the following:

1. Eliminate oral and parenteral potassium intake (see Table 44-8).
2. Increase elimination of potassium. This is accomplished via diuretics, dialysis, and use of ion-exchange resins such as sodium polystyrene sulfonate (Kayexalate). Increased fluid intake can enhance renal potassium elimination.
3. Force potassium from the ECF to the ICF. This is accomplished by administration of intravenous insulin (along with glucose so the patient does not become hypoglycemic) or via administration of IV sodium bicarbonate. Rarely, a beta-adrenergic drug (e.g., epinephrine) is administered.
4. Reverse the membrane effects of the elevated ECF potassium. Calcium ion can immediately reverse the effect of the depolarization on cell excitability. Calcium gluconate is administered intravenously.

In cases where the elevation of potassium is mild and the kidneys are functioning, it may be sufficient to withhold potassium from the diet and intravenous sources and increase renal elimination by administering fluids and possibly diuretics. Kayexalate, which is administered via the GI tract, binds potassium in exchange for sodium, and the resin is excreted in feces (see Chapter 44). All patients with clinically significant hyperkalemia should be monitored electrocardiographically to detect arrhythmias and to monitor the effects of therapy. Patients with moderate hyperkalemia should additionally receive one of the treatments to force potassium into cells, usually insulin and glucose. The patient experiencing dangerous cardiac arrhythmias should receive calcium gluconate immediately to protect the patient while the potassium is being eliminated and forced into cells. Hemodialysis is an effective means of removing potassium from the body in the patient with renal failure.

HYPOKALEMIA

Hypokalemia (low serum potassium) can result from abnormal losses of potassium from a shift of potassium from ECF to ICF, or rarely from abnormally restricted potassium intake. The most common causes of hypokalemia are abnormal losses, either via the kidneys or GI tract. Abnormal losses occur when the patient is diuresing, particularly in the patient with an elevated aldosterone level. Aldosterone is released when the circulating blood volume is low; it causes sodium retention in the kidneys but loss of potassium in the urine. Magnesium deficiency may contribute to the development of potassium depletion resulting from increased urinary excretion. GI tract losses from diarrhea, vomiting, and ileostomy drainage can cause hypokalemia.

Metabolic alkalosis can cause a shift of potassium into cells, lowering the potassium in the ECF and causing symptomatic hypokalemia. Hypokalemia is sometimes associated with the treatment of diabetic ketoacidosis because of a combination of factors, including an increased urinary potassium loss and a shift of potassium into cells with the administration of insulin and correction of acidosis. A less common cause of hypokalemia is the sudden initiation of cell formation; for example, the formation of red blood cells (RBCs) as in treatment of anemia with cobalamin, folic acid, or erythropoeitin.

Clinical Manifestations

Hypokalemia alters resting membrane potential. It most commonly is associated with hyperpolarization, or increased negative charge within the cell. This causes excitability problems in many types of tissue. The most serious clinical problems are cardiac. The incidence of potentially lethal ventricular arrhythmias is increased in hypokalemia. Patients should be monitored with ECG for signs of hypokalemia. These changes include impaired repolarization, resulting in a flattening of the T wave and eventually in emergence of a U wave. The P wave amplitude may increase and may become peaked. Patients taking digoxin experience increased digoxin toxicity if their serum potassium is low. Skeletal muscle weakness and paralysis may occur with hypokalemia. As with hyperkalemia, symptoms are most often observed in the legs. Respiratory muscles and those innervated by cranial nerves are not involved. Muscle cramping and muscle cell breakdown (known as rhabdomyolysis) can be caused by hypokalemia. This can lead to myoglobin in the plasma and urine, which can, in turn, lead to renal failure.

Smooth muscle function is altered by hypokalemia. The patient may experience altered GI motility (e.g., paralytic ileus), altered airway responsiveness, and impaired regulation of arteriolar blood flow regulation, possibly contributing to muscle cell breakdown. Finally, hypokalemia can impair function in nonmuscle tissue. Urinary concentration is impaired, resulting in polyuria and polydipsia. Release of insulin is impaired, often causing hyperglycemia. Clinical manifestations of hypokalemia are presented in Table 15-7.

NURSING AND COLLABORATIVE MANAGEMENT: HYPOKALEMIA

Nursing Diagnoses

Nursing diagnoses and collaborative problems for the patient with hypokalemia include, but are not limited to, the following:

- Risk for injury *related to* muscle weakness and hyporeflexia
- Potential complication: arrhythmias

Nursing Implementation

Hypokalemia is treated by giving potassium chloride supplements and increasing dietary intake of potassium. Potassium chloride (KCl) supplements can be given orally or intravenously. Except in severe deficiencies, KCl is never given unless there is urine output of at least 0.5 ml/kg body weight per hour. KCl supplements added to IV solutions should never exceed 60 mEq/L. The preferred level is 40 mEq/L. The rate of IV administration of KCl should not exceed 10 to 20 mEq per hour to prevent hyperkalemia and cardiac arrest. When given intravenously, potassium may cause pain in the area of the vein where it is entering. Central IV lines should be used when rapid correction of hypokalemia is necessary. Potassium may also be replaced with potassium phosphate.

The patient who is taking diuretics (especially thiazide and loop diuretics) should be aware of the need to increase dietary potassium intake (see Table 44-8). It may be necessary for the patient to take oral KCl supplements or salt substitutes that contain potassium. The patient should be taught which foods are high in potassium. The patient should also be instructed to recognize the clinical manifestations of hypokalemia and to report them to the health care provider. If a patient is also taking digitalis preparations, the serum potassium level must be closely monitored because hypokalemia enhances the action of digitalis.

CALCIUM IMBALANCES

Calcium is obtained from ingested foods. However, only about 30% is absorbed in the GI tract. More than 99% of the body's calcium is combined with phosphorus and concentrated in the skeletal system. Bones serve as a readily available store of calcium. Thus wide variations in serum calcium levels are avoided by regulating the movement of calcium into or out of the bone. Usually the amount of calcium and phosphorus found in the serum has an inverse relationship; that is, as one increases, the other decreases. The functions of calcium include transmission of nerve impulses, cardiac contractions, blood clotting, formation of teeth and bone, and muscle contraction.

Calcium is present in the serum in three forms: free or ionized; bound to protein (primarily albumin); and complexed with phosphate, citrate, or carbonate. The ionized form is the biologically active form. Approximately one half of the total serum calcium is ionized.

Calcium is typically measured in mg/dl. As usually reported, serum calcium levels reflect the total calcium level (all three forms), although ionized calcium levels may be reported. The levels listed in Table 15-8 reflect total calcium levels. Changes in serum pH will alter the level of ionized calcium without altering the total calcium level. Acidosis decreases calcium binding to albumin, leading to more ionized calcium, and alkalosis increases calcium binding. Alterations in serum albumin levels affect interpretation of total calcium levels. Low albumin levels result in a drop in the total calcium level, although the level of ionized calcium does not change as much.

Calcium balance depends on the proper functioning of three hormones: vitamin D, parathyroid hormone (PTH), and calcitonin.[8] Vitamin D is formed through the action of ultraviolet (UV) rays on a precursor found in the skin or is ingested in the diet. Vitamin D is important for absorption of calcium from the gastrointestinal tract.

PTH is produced by the parathyroid gland. Its production and release are stimulated by low serum calcium levels. PTH increases bone resorption (movement of calcium out of bones), increases GI absorption of calcium, and increases renal tubule reabsorption of calcium.

Calcitonin is produced by the thyroid gland and is stimulated by high serum calcium levels. It opposes the action of PTH and thus lowers the serum calcium level by decreasing GI absorption, increasing bone mineralization, and promoting renal excretion. Causes of calcium imbalances are listed in Table 15-8.

HYPERCALCEMIA

Hypercalcemia is most commonly associated with malignancy, with or without skeletal metastasis, multiple myeloma, hyperparathyroidism, vitamin D overdose, and prolonged immobilization.[9] Hypercalcemia rarely occurs from increased calcium intake (e.g., ingestion of antacids containing calcium or excessive administration during cardiac arrest).

Clinical Manifestations

Excess serum calcium causes decreased memory span, confusion, disorientation, fatigue, muscle weakness, constipation, and cardiac arrhythmias (see Table 15-8).

NURSING AND COLLABORATIVE MANAGEMENT: HYPERCALCEMIA

Nursing Diagnoses

Nursing diagnoses and collaborative problems for the patient with hypercalcemia include, but are not limited to, the following:

- Risk for injury *related to* neuromuscular and sensorium changes
- Potential complication: arrhythmias

Table 15-8 Calcium Imbalances: Causes and Clinical Manifestations

Hypocalcemia (Ca^{2+} <9 mg/dl [2.25 mmol/L])	Hypercalcemia (Ca^{2+} >11 mg/dl [2.75 mmol/L])
Causes	
Decreased Total Calcium	**Increased Total Calcium**
Chronic renal failure	Multiple myeloma
Elevated phosphorus	Other malignancy
Primary hypoparathyroidism	Prolonged immobilization
Vitamin D deficiency	Hyperparathyroidism
Magnesium deficiency	Vitamin D overdose
Acute pancreatitis	Thiazide diuretics
Loop diuretics	Milk-alkali syndrome
Chronic alcoholism	
Diarrhea	
Decreased serum albumin (patient is usually asymptomatic due to normal ionized calcium level)	
Decreased Ionized Calcium	**Increased Ionized Calcium**
Alkalosis	Acidosis
Excess administration of citrated blood	
Clinical Manifestations	
Easy fatigability	Lethargy, weakness
Depression, anxiety, confusion	Depressed reflexes
Numbness and tingling in extremities and region around mouth	Decreased memory
Hyperreflexia, muscle cramps	Confusion, personality changes, psychosis
Chvostek's sign	Anorexia, nausea, vomiting
Trousseau's sign	Bone pain, fractures
Laryngeal spasm	Polyuria, dehydration
Tetany, seizures	Nephrolithiasis
	Stupor, coma
Electrocardiograph Changes	**Electrocardiograph Changes**
Elongation of ST segment	Shortened ST segment
Prolonged QT interval	Shortened QT interval
Ventricular tachycardia	Ventricular arrhythmias
	Increased digitalis effect

Nursing Implementation

The basic treatment of hypercalcemia is promotion of excretion of calcium in urine by administration of a loop diuretic (furosemide [Lasix] or ethacrynic acid [Edecrin]) and hydration of the patient with isotonic saline infusions. In hypercalcemia the patient must drink 3000 to 4000 ml of fluid daily to promote the renal excretion of calcium and to decrease the possibility of renal calculi formation.

Synthetic calcitonin can also be administered to lower serum calcium levels. Plicamycin (Mithracin) (formerly called mithramycin), a cytotoxic antibiotic, inhibits bone resorption and thus lowers the serum calcium level. A diet low in calcium may be prescribed. Mobilization with weight-bearing activity is encouraged to enhance bone mineralization. In hypercalcemia associated with malignancy the drug of choice is pamidronate (Aredia), which inhibits the activity of osteoclasts.

HYPOCALCEMIA

Any condition that causes a decrease in the production of PTH may result in the development of hypocalcemia. This may occur with surgical removal of a portion of or injury to the parathyroid glands during thyroid or neck surgery. Acute pancreatitis is another potential cause of hypocalcemia. The patient who receives multiple blood transfusions can become hypocalcemic because the citrate used to anticoagulate the blood binds with the calcium. Sudden alkalosis may also result in symptomatic hypocalcemia despite a normal total serum calcium level because of a reduction in the level of ionized calcium. Hypocalcemia can occur if the diet is low in calcium or if there is increased loss of calcium with laxative abuse and malabsorption syndromes. (See Table 15-8 for the clinical manifestations and etiologies of hypocalcemia.)

Clinical Manifestations

Because calcium is essential for conduction of nerve impulses and muscle contraction, procedures that evaluate neuromuscular irritability are useful for assessing a low serum calcium level. *Trousseau's sign* refers to carpal spasms induced by inflating a blood pressure cuff on the arm (Fig. 15-14). The blood pressure cuff is inflated above the systolic pressure. Carpal spasms become evident within 3 minutes if hypocalcemia is present. *Chvostek's sign* is contraction of facial muscles in response to a tap over the facial nerve in front of the ear (see Fig. 15-14), and it also indicates hypocalcemia with latent tetany.

Tetany refers to the increased neuroexcitability and sustained muscle contraction associated with hypocalcemia.

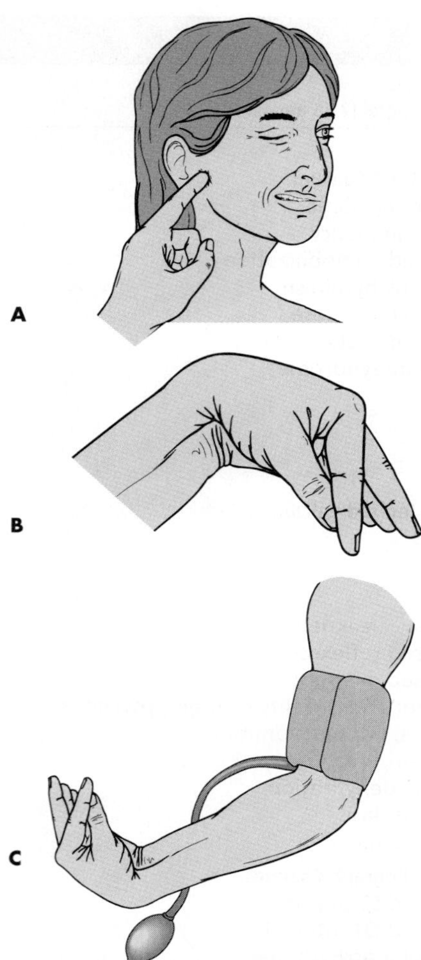

Fig. 15-14 Tests for hypocalcemia. **A,** Chvostek's sign is a contraction of facial muscles in response to a light tap over the facial nerve in front of the ear. **B,** Trousseau's sign is a carpal spasm induced by **C,** inflating a blood pressure cuff above the systolic pressure for a few minutes.

Manifestations of impending tetany include positive Chvostek's and Trousseau's signs (see Fig. 15-14), laryngeal stridor, dysphagia, and numbness and tingling around the mouth or in the extremities. Other clinical manifestations of hypocalcemia are listed in Table 15-8.

NURSING AND COLLABORATIVE MANAGEMENT: HYPOCALCEMIA

■ Nursing Diagnoses

Nursing diagnoses and collaborative problems for the patient with hypocalcemia include, but are not limited to, the following:

- Risk for injury *related to* tetany and seizures
- Potential complications: fracture, respiratory arrest

■ Nursing Implementation

The primary goal in treatment of hypocalcemia is aimed at treating the cause. Hypocalcemia can be treated with oral or IV calcium supplements. Calcium carbonate (oral) and calcium gluconate IV are commonly used as supplements. Hypocalcemia is managed as an emergency when tetany, seizues, hypotension, cardiac arrhythmias, or laryngeal spasms are present. Emergency treatment includes an inital IV dose of calcium followed by continuous calcium infusion.[10] Care must be taken because infiltration of IV calcium can cause sloughing of the tissue. Calcium is not given intramuscularly (IM) because it will precipitate in the muscle. A diet high in calcium-rich foods may be ordered along with vitamin D supplements for the patient with hypocalcemia. Synthetic PTH can also be given. Pain and anxiety must be adequately treated in the patient with suspected hypocalcemia because hyperventilation-induced respiratory alkalosis can precipitate hypocalcemic symptoms. Any patient who has had thyroid or neck surgery must be observed closely for manifestations of hypocalcemia because of the proximity of the surgery to the parathyroid glands.

PHOSPHATE IMBALANCES

Phosphorus is a primary anion in the ICF and is essential to the function of muscle, red blood cells, and the nervous system. It is deposited with calcium for bone and tooth structure. It is also involved in the acid-base buffering system, in the mitochondrial energy production of ATP, in cellular uptake and use of glucose, and as an intermediary in the metabolism of carbohydrates, proteins, and fats.

Maintenance of normal phosphate balance requires adequate renal functioning because the kidneys are the major route of phosphate excretion. A small amount is lost in the feces. A reciprocal relationship exists between phosphorus and calcium in that a high serum phosphate level tends to cause a low calcium concentration in the serum.

Hyperphosphatemia

The major condition that can lead to hyperphosphatemia is acute or chronic renal failure that results in an altered ability of the kidneys to excrete phosphate. Other causes include chemotherapy for certain malignancies (lymphomas), excessive ingestion of milk or phosphate-containing laxatives, and large intakes of vitamin D that increase GI absorption of phosphorus (Table 15-9).

Clinical manifestations of hyperphosphatemia (presented in Table 15-9) primarily relate to metastatic calcium-phosphate precipitates. Ordinarily, calcium and phosphate are deposited only in bone. However, an increased serum phosphate concentration along with calcium precipitates readily, and calcified deposits can occur in soft tissue such as joints, arteries, skin, kidneys, and cornea (see Chapter 44). Other manifestations of hyperphosphatemia are neuromuscular irritability and tetany, which are related to the low serum calcium levels often associated with high serum phosphate levels.

Management of hyperphosphatemia is aimed at identifying and treating the underlying cause. Ingestion of foods and fluids high in phosphorus (e.g., dairy products) should be restricted. Adequate hydration and correction of hypocalcemic conditions can enhance the renal excretion of phosphate. For the patient with renal failure, measures to reduce serum phosphate levels include calcium supplements, phosphate-

Table 15-9 Phosphate Imbalances: Causes and Clinical Manifestations

Hypophosphatemia (PO_4^{-3} <2.8 mg/dl [0.9 mmol/L])	Hyperphosphatemia (PO_4^{-3} >4.5 mg/dl [1.45 mmol/L])
Causes	
Malabsorption syndrome	Renal failure
Nutritional recovery syndrome	Chemotherapeutic agents
Glucose administration	Enemas containing phosphorus (e.g., Fleet Enema)
Total parenteral nutrition	Excessive ingestion (e.g., milk, phosphate-containing laxatives)
Alcohol withdrawal	Large vitamin D intake
Phosphate-binding antacids	Hypoparathyroidism
Recovery from diabetic ketoacidosis	
Respiratory alkalosis	
Clinical Manifestations	
Central nervous system dysfunction (confusion, coma)	Hypocalcemia
Rhabdomyolysis	Muscle problems; tetany
Renal tubular wasting of Mg^{+2}, Ca^{+2}, HCO_3^-	Deposition of calcium-phosphate precipitates in skin, soft tissue, cornea, viscera, blood vessels
Cardiac problems (arrhythmias, decreased stroke volume)	
Muscle weakness, including respiratory muscle weakness and difficulty weaning	
Osteomalacia	

binding agents or gels, and dietary phosphate restrictions (see Chapter 44).

Hypophosphatemia

Hypophosphatemia (low serum phosphate) is seen in the patient who is malnourished or has malabsorption syndromes. Other causes include alcohol withdrawal, parenteral nutrition with inadequate phosphorus replacement, use of phosphate-binding antacids, and nutritional recovery syndrome (refeeding after starvation). During the anabolic phase of metabolism, an influx of phosphorus into the cells occurs. Table 15-9 lists causes of phosphorus imbalances.

Most clinical manifestations of hypophosphatemia (presented in Table 15-9) relate to a deficiency of ATP or 2,3-diphosphoglycerate (2,3-DPG), an enzyme in RBCs. Both conditions result in impaired cellular energy resources and oxygen delivery to tissues. Hemolytic anemia may occur because of the fragility of the RBCs. Acute manifestations include CNS depression, confusion, and other mental changes. Other manifestations include muscle weakness and pain, arrhythmias, and cardiomyopathy.

Management of a mild phosphorus deficiency may involve oral supplementation (e.g., Neutra-Phos) and ingestion of foods high in phosphorus (e.g., dairy products). Severe hypophosphatemia can be serious and may require IV administration of sodium phosphate or potassium phosphate. Frequent monitoring of serum phosphate levels is necessary to guide intravenous therapy. Sudden symptomatic hypocalcemia, secondary to increased calcium phosphorus binding, is a potential complication of IV phosphorus administration.

MAGNESIUM IMBALANCES

Magnesium is the second most abundant intracellular cation. It functions as a coenzyme in the metabolism of carbohydrates and protein. It is also involved in metabolism of cellular nucleic acids and proteins. Regulation of magnesium is not well understood, but many of the factors that regulate calcium balance

Table 15-10 Causes of Magnesium Imbalances

Hypomagnesemia	Hypermagnesemia
Diarrhea	Renal failure (especially if patient is given magnesium products)
Vomiting	Excessive administration of magnesium for treatment of eclampsia
Chronic alcoholism	Adrenal insufficiency
Impaired gastrointestinal absorption	
Malabsorption syndrome	
Prolonged malnutrition	
Large urine output	
Nasogastric suction	
Poorly controlled diabetes mellitus	
Hyperaldosteronism	

(e.g., PTH, vitamin D) influence magnesium balance. About 50% to 60% of the body's magnesium is contained in bone. The kidneys are the primary route of magnesium excretion. Causes of magnesium imbalances are listed in Table 15-10. Neuromuscular excitability is profoundly affected by alterations in serum magnesium. Hypomagnesemia (a low serum magnesium level) produces neuromuscular and CNS hyperirritability. Additionally, diets low in magnesium are believed to be a risk factor for hypertension, cardiac arrhythmias, ischemic heart disease, and sudden cardiac death.[11] Decreased intracellular magnesium levels may contribute to the hypertension, abnormal glucose tolerance, and insulin resistance common in diabetes.[12] A high serum magnesium level (hypermagnesemia) depresses neuromuscular and CNS functions.

Hypermagnesemia

Hypermagnesemia usually occurs only with an increase in magnesium intake accompanied by renal insufficiency or failure. A patient with chronic renal failure who ingests products containing magnesium (e.g., Maalox, milk of magnesia) will have a problem with excess magnesium. Magnesium excess

Table 15-11 Causes of Protein Imbalances

Hypoproteinemia	Hyperproteinemia
Decreased food intake Starvation Diseased liver Massive burns Loss of albumin in renal disease Major infection	Dehydration Hemoconcentration

Table 15-12 Terms in Acid-Base Physiology

Acid	Donor of hydrogen ion (H^+); separation of an acid into H^+ and its accompanying anion in solution
Acidemia	Signifying an arterial blood pH of less than 7.35
Acidosis	Process that adds acid or eliminates base from body fluids
Alkalemia	Signifying an arterial blood pH of more than 7.45
Alkalosis	Process that adds base or eliminates acid from body fluids
Base	Acceptor of hydrogen ions; chemical combining of acid and base when hydrogen ions are added to a solution containing a base; bicarbonate (HCO_3^-) most abundant base in body fluids
Buffer	Substance that reacts with an acid or base to prevent a large change in pH
pH	Negative logarithm of the H^+ concentration

could develop in the pregnant woman who receives magnesium sulfate for the management of eclampsia.

Initial clinical manifestations of a mildly elevated serum magnesium concentration include lethargy, drowsiness, and nausea and vomiting. As the levels of serum magnesium increase, deep tendon reflexes are lost, followed by somnolence; then respiratory and, ultimately, cardiac arrest can occur.

Management of hypermagnesemia should focus on prevention. Persons with renal failure should not take magnesium-containing medication and must be cautioned to review all over-the-counter medication labels for magnesium content. The emergency treatment of hypermagnesemia is IV administration of calcium chloride or calcium gluconate to physiologically oppose the effects of the magnesium on cardiac muscle. Promoting urinary excretion with fluid will decrease serum magnesium. The patient with impaired renal function will require dialysis because the kidneys are the major route of excretion for magnesium.

Hypomagnesemia

Hypomagnesemia tends to develop gradually. Prolonged IV feeding without magnesium supplementation and excessive losses of fluids from the GI tract are potential causes. The most common causes are chronic alcoholism and uncontrolled diabetes mellitus. The significant clinical manifestations include confusion, hyperactive deep tendon reflexes, tremors, and seizures. Magnesium deficiency also predisposes to cardiac arrhythmias. Clinically, hypomagnesemia resembles hypocalcemia and may contribute to the development of hypocalcemia. Hypomagnesemia may also be associated with hypokalemia that does not respond well to potassium replacement. This occurs because intracellular magnesium is critical to normal function of the sodium-potassium pump.

Mild magnesium deficiencies can be treated with oral supplements and increased dietary intake of foods high in magnesium (e.g., green vegetables, nuts, bananas, oranges, peanut butter, chocolate). If the condition is severe, parenteral IV or IM magnesium (e.g., magnesium sulfate) should be administered. Too rapid administration of magnesium can lead to cardiac or respiratory arrest.

PROTEIN IMBALANCES

Plasma proteins, particularly albumin, are a significant determinant of plasma volume. Because of their large molecular size, they remain in the vascular space and contribute to the colloidal oncotic pressure. Causes of protein imbalances are listed in Table 15-11. Hypoproteinemia can occur over time. Causes related to intake are anorexia, malnutrition, starvation, fad dieting, and poorly balanced vegetarian diets. Poor absorption of protein can occur in certain GI malabsorptive diseases. Protein can shift out of the intravascular space with inflammation. Increased breakdown of proteins occurs with elevated basal metabolic rates and catabolic states, such as fever, infection, and certain malignancies. Increased use of protein occurs with cell growth and repair after surgical wounds or burns. Hemorrhage with loss of red blood cells can be a cause of protein deficit. The kidneys can lose large amounts of protein, especially albumin, in nephrotic syndrome.

Clinical manifestations of protein deficit include edema (from decreased oncotic pressure), slow healing, anorexia, fatigue, anemia, and muscle loss that results from the breakdown of body tissue to meet the body's need for protein. Ascites is an example of third-space shifting that may develop with hypoproteinemia.

Management of protein deficit includes providing a high-carbohydrate, high-protein diet and dietary protein supplements. If the patient cannot meet the needs for protein orally, enteral nutrition or total parenteral nutrition may be used. (Protein-calorie malnutrition is discussed in Chapter 38.)

Hyperproteinemia is rare, but it can occur with dehydration-induced hemoconcentration.

ACID-BASE IMBALANCES

Hydrogen Ion Concentration

The acidity or alkalinity of a solution depends on its hydrogen ion (H^+) concentration. An increase in H^+ concentration leads to acidity; a decrease leads to alkalinity. (Definitions related to acid-base balance are presented in Table 15-12.)

Despite the fact that acids are produced by the body daily, the hydrogen ion concentration of body fluids is small (0.0004 mEq/L). This tiny amount is maintained within a narrow range to ensure optimal cellular function. Hydrogen ion concentration is usually expressed as a negative logarithm (symbolized as

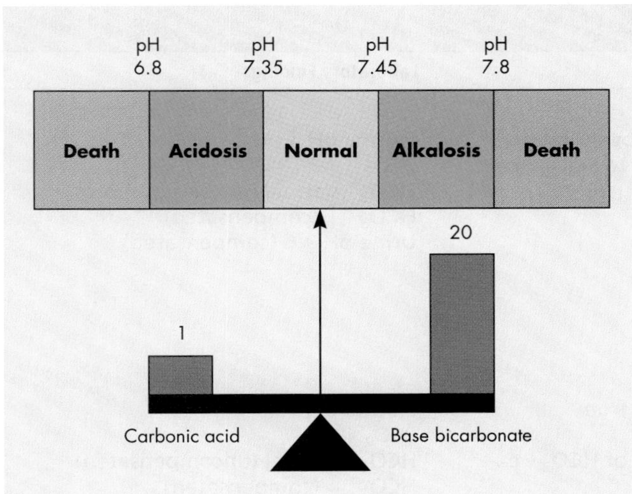

Fig. 15-15 The normal range of plasma pH is 7.35 to 7.45. A normal pH is maintained by a ratio of 1 part carbonic acid to 20 parts base bicarbonate.

pH) rather than in milliequivalents. The use of the negative logarithm means that the lower the pH, the higher the hydrogen ion concentration. In contrast to a pH of 7, a pH of 8 represents a tenfold decrease in hydrogen ion concentration.

The pH of a chemical solution may range from 1 to 14. A solution with a pH of 7 is considered neutral. An acid solution has a pH less than 7, and an alkaline solution has a pH greater than 7. Blood is slightly alkaline (pH 7.35 to 7.45); yet if it drops below 7.35, the person has *acidosis,* even though the blood may never become truly acidic. If the blood pH is greater than 7.45, the person has *alkalosis* (Fig. 15-15). The pH of blood is computed through the use of the Henderson-Hasselbalch equation (Table 15-13). This equation demonstrates that the pH level is determined by the ratio of base (bicarbonate) to acid (carbonic acid). A 20-to-1 relationship must exist to maintain the pH within a normal range.

Acid-Base Regulation

The body's metabolic processes constantly produce acids. These acids must be neutralized and excreted to maintain acid-base balance. Normally the body has three mechanisms by which it regulates acid-base balance to maintain the arterial pH between 7.35 and 7.45. These mechanisms are the buffer systems, the respiratory system, and the renal system.

The regulatory mechanisms react at different speeds. Buffers react immediately; the respiratory system responds in minutes and reaches maximum effectiveness in hours; the renal response takes 2 to 3 days to respond maximally, but the kidneys can maintain balance for a long period of time.

Buffer System. The buffer system is the fastest-acting system and the primary regulator of acid-base balance. Buffers act chemically to change strong acids into weaker acids or to bind acids to neutralize their effect. The buffers in the body include carbonic acid–bicarbonate, monohydrogen-dihydrogen phosphate, intracellular and plasma protein, and hemoglobin buffers.

A buffer consists of a weakly ionized acid or a base and its salt. The mechanisms of buffering function to minimize the effect of acids on blood pH until they can be excreted from the body. The carbonic acid (H_2CO_3)–bicarbonate (HCO_3^-) buffer system neutralizes hydrochloric acid (HCl) in the following manner:

Table 15-13 Henderson-Hasselbalch Equation

$$pH = pK\ (\text{constant}) + \log \frac{\text{base}}{\text{acid}}$$
$$= 6.1 + \log \frac{HCO_3^-\ (\text{renal})}{H_2CO_3\ (\text{lung})}$$
$$= 6.1 + \log \frac{25.4\ \text{mEq}}{1.27}$$
$$= 6.1 + \log \frac{20}{1}$$
$$= 6.1 + 1.3$$
$$= 7.4$$

$$\underset{\text{strong acid}}{H^+Cl^-} + \underset{\text{strong base}}{Na^+HCO_3^-} \rightarrow \underset{\text{salt}}{NaCl} + \underset{\text{weak acid}}{H_2CO_3}$$

In this way, HCl is prevented from making a large change in the solution's pH, and more H_2CO_3 is formed. The carbonic acid, in turn, is broken down to H_2O and CO_2. The CO_2 is excreted by the lungs. In this process the buffer system maintains the 20:1 ratio between bicarbonate and carbonic acid and the normal pH.

The phosphate buffer system is composed of sodium and other cations in combination with HPO_4^{2-} and $H_2PO_4^-$. This buffer system acts in the same manner as the bicarbonate system. Strong acids are neutralized to form a weak acid of sodium biphosphate, which can be excreted in the urine, and sodium chloride: $Na_2HPO_4 + HCl \rightarrow NaCl + NaH_2PO_4$. When a strong base is added to the system, it is neutralized to form a weak base and H_2O:

$$NaOH + NaH_2PO_4 \rightarrow Na_2HPO_4 + H_2O$$

Intracellular and extracellular proteins are an effective buffering system throughout the body. The protein buffering system acts like the bicarbonate system. Some of the amino acids of proteins contain free acid radicals, -COOH, which can dissociate into CO_2 and H. Other amino acids have basic radicals, $-NH_3OH$, which can dissociate into NH_3^+ and OH^-, which can combine with a H^+ to form H_2O.

Using the "chloride shift" mechanism, hemoglobin regulates pH by shifting chloride in and out of RBCs in exchange for bicarbonate. This shift is regulated by the level of oxygen in blood.

The cell can also act as a buffer by shifting hydrogen in and out of the cell. With an accumulation of H^+ in the ECF, the intracellular compartment can accept hydrogen in exchange for another cation (e.g., sodium or potassium).

The body buffers an acid load better than it neutralizes base excess. Buffers cannot maintain pH without the adequate functioning of the respiratory and renal systems.

Respiratory System. The lungs excrete carbon dioxide and water, which are by-products of cellular metabolism. When released into circulation, CO_2 enters red blood cells and combines with H_2O to form H_2CO_3. The carbonic acid dissociates

Table **15-14** Acid-Base Imbalances

Common Causes	Pathophysiology	Laboratory Findings
Respiratory Acidosis		
Chronic obstructive pulmonary disease Barbiturate or sedative overdose Chest wall abnormality (e.g., obesity) Severe pneumonia Atelectasis Respiratory muscle weakness (e.g., Guillain-Barré syndrome) Mechanical underventilation	CO_2 retention from hypoventilation Compensatory response to HCO_3^- retention by kidney	Plasma pH ↓ PCO_2 ↑ HCO_3^- normal (uncompensated) HCO_3^- ↑ (compensated) Urine pH <6 (compensated)
Respiratory Alkalosis		
Hyperventilation (caused by hypoxia, pulmonary emboli, anxiety, fear, pain, exercise, fever) Stimulated respiratory center caused by septicemia, encephalitis, brain injury, salicylate poisoning Mechanical overventilation	Increased CO_2 excretion from hyperventilation Compensatory response of HCO_3^- excretion by kidney	Plasma pH ↑ PCO_2 ↓ HCO_3^- normal (uncompensated) HCO_3^- ↓ (compensated) Urine pH >6 (compensated)
Metabolic Acidosis		
Diabetic ketoacidosis Lactic acidosis Starvation Severe diarrhea Renal tubular acidosis Renal failure Gastrointestinal fistulas Shock	Gain of fixed acid, inability to excrete acid or loss of base Compensatory response of CO_2 excretion by lungs	Plasma pH ↓ PCO_2 ↓ (compensated) HCO_3^- ↓ Urine pH <6 (compensated)
Metabolic Alkalosis		
Severe vomiting Excess gastric suctioning Diuretic therapy Potassium deficit Excess $NaHCO_3$ intake Excessive mineralocorticoids	Loss of strong acid or gain of base Compensatory response of CO_2 retention by lungs	Plasma pH ↑ PCO_2 ↑ (compensated) HCO_3^- ↑ Urine pH >6 (compensated)

into hydrogen ions and bicarbonate. The free hydrogen is buffered by hemoglobin molecules, and the bicarbonate diffuses into the plasma. In the pulmonary capillaries, this process is reversed, and CO_2 is formed and excreted by the lungs. The overall reversible reaction is expressed as the following:

$$CO_2 + H_2O \leftrightarrows H_2CO_3 \leftrightarrows H^+ + HCO_3^-$$

The amount of CO_2 in the blood directly relates to carbonic acid concentration and subsequently to hydrogen ion concentration. With increased respirations, less CO_2 remains in the blood. This leads to less carbonic acid and fewer H^+ ions. With decreased respirations, more CO_2 remains in the blood. This leads to increased carbonic acid and more hydrogen ions.

The rate of excretion of CO_2 is controlled by the respiratory center in the medulla of the brain. If increased amounts of CO_2 or hydrogen ions are present, the respiratory center stimulates an increased rate and depth of breathing. Respirations are inhibited if the center senses low H^+ or CO_2 levels.

As a compensatory mechanism the respiratory system acts on the $CO_2 + H_2O$ side of the reaction by altering the rate and depth of breathing to "blow off" or "retain" carbon dioxide. If a respiratory problem is the cause of an acid-base imbalance (e.g., respiratory failure), the respiratory system loses its ability to correct a pH alteration.

Renal System. Under normal conditions the kidneys reabsorb and conserve all of the bicarbonate they filter. The kidneys can generate additional bicarbonate and eliminate excess hydrogen ions as compensation for acidosis. The three mechanisms of acid elimination include (1) secretion of small amounts of free hydrogen into the renal tubule, (2) combination of hydrogen ions with ammonia (NH_3) to form ammonium (NH_4^+), and (3) excretion of weak acids.

The body depends on the kidneys to excrete a portion of the acid produced by cellular metabolism. Thus the kidneys normally excrete an acidic urine (average pH equals 6). They are able to act on the $H^+ + HCO_3^-$ side of the reaction. As a compensatory mechanism, the pH of the urine can decrease to 4 and increase to 8. If the renal system is the cause of an acid-base imbalance (e.g., renal failure), it loses its ability to correct a pH alteration. In the patient with renal failure, metabolic acidosis is the usual finding.

Alterations in Acid-Base Balance

An acid-base imbalance is produced when the ratio of 1:20 between acid and base content is altered (Table 15-14). A primary disease or process may alter one side of the ratio (e.g., CO_2 retention in pulmonary disease). The compensatory process attempts to maintain the other side of the ratio (e.g.,

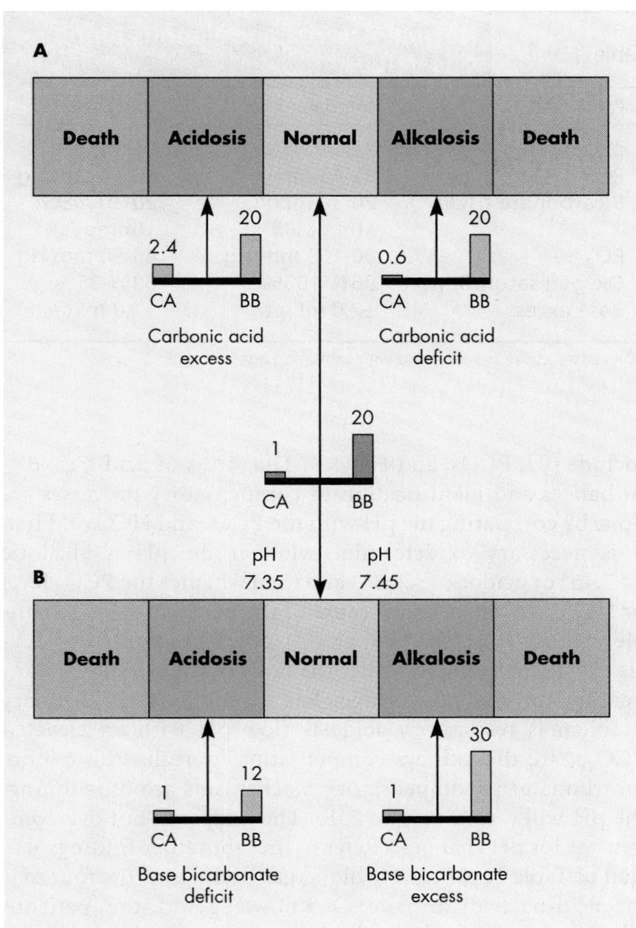

Fig. 15-16 Kinds of acid-base imbalances. **A,** Respiratory imbalances caused by carbonic acid (CA) excess and carbonic acid deficit. **B,** Metabolic imbalances caused by base bicarbonate (BB) deficit and base bicarbonate excess.

increased renal bicarbonate reabsorption). When the compensatory mechanism fails, an acid-base imbalance results. The compensatory process may be inadequate because either the pathophysiologic process is overwhelming or there is insufficient time for the compensatory process to function.

Acid-base imbalances are classified as respiratory or metabolic. Respiratory imbalances affect carbonic acid concentrations; metabolic imbalances affect the base bicarbonate. Therefore acidosis can be caused by an increase in carbonic acid (respiratory acidosis) or a decrease in bicarbonate (metabolic acidosis). Alkalosis can be caused by a decrease in carbonic acid (respiratory alkalosis) or an increase in bicarbonate (metabolic alkalosis). Imbalances may be further classified as acute or chronic. Chronic imbalances allow greater time for compensatory changes.

Respiratory Acidosis. Respiratory acidosis (carbonic acid excess) occurs whenever there is hypoventilation (see Table 15-14). Carbon dioxide and subsequently carbonic acid accumulate in the blood. Carbonic acid dissociates, liberating H^+, and there is a decrease in pH. If carbon dioxide is not eliminated from the blood, acidosis results from the accumulation of carbonic acid (Fig. 15-16, *A*).

Table 15-15 Clinical Manifestations of Acidosis

Respiratory ($\uparrow PCO_2$)	Metabolic ($\downarrow HCO_3^-$)
Appearance	
Drowsiness	Drowsiness
Coma	Coma
Behavior	
Disorientation	Confusion
Dizziness	
Cardiovascular	
Decreased blood pressure	Decreased blood pressure
Ventricular fibrillation	Arrhythmias
Peripheral vasodilation	Peripheral vasodilation
Gastrointestinal	
No significant findings	Nausea, vomiting, diarrhea, abdominal pain
Neuromuscular	
Headache	Headache
Seizures	
Respiratory	
Rapid, shallow breaths or hypoventilation with hypoxia	Deep, rapid respirations

The kidneys conserve bicarbonate and secrete increased concentrations of hydrogen ion into the urine. In acute respiratory acidosis the renal compensatory mechanisms begin to operate within 24 hours. Therefore a normal serum bicarbonate level usually can be found until the kidneys have compensated for the imbalance.

Respiratory Alkalosis. Respiratory alkalosis (carbonic acid deficit) occurs with hyperventilation (Table 15-15). Anxiety, CNS disease, sepsis, and mechanical overventilation all increase ventilation and decrease the PCO_2 level. This leads to decreased carbonic acid and alkalosis (Fig. 15-16, *A*).

Compensated respiratory alkalosis is uncommon unless the patient has been maintained on a ventilator or has a CNS problem. A decreased bicarbonate level differentiates compensated respiratory alkalosis from acute or uncompensated respiratory alkalosis.

Metabolic Acidosis. Metabolic acidosis (base bicarbonate deficit) occurs when an acid other than carbonic acid accumulates in the body or when bicarbonate is lost from body fluids (see Table 15-14 and Fig. 15-16, *B*). In both cases a bicarbonate deficit results. Keto acid accumulation in diabetic ketoacidosis and lactic acid accumulation with shock are examples of accumulation of acids. Severe diarrhea results in loss of bicarbonate. In renal disease the kidneys lose their ability to reabsorb bicarbonate and secrete hydrogen ions.

The compensatory response is to increase CO_2 excretion by the lungs. The patient often develops Kussmaul's respiration (deep, rapid breathing). In addition, the kidneys attempt to excrete additional acid.

Metabolic Alkalosis. Metabolic alkalosis (base bicarbonate excess) occurs when a loss of acid (prolonged vomiting or gastric suction) or a gain in bicarbonate (ingestion of

Table 15-16 Clinical Manifestations of Alkalosis

Respiratory ($\downarrow PCO_2$)	Metabolic ($\uparrow HCO_3^-$)
Appearance	
Lethargy	Dizziness
Behavior	
Light-headedness	Irritability
Confusion	Nervousness
	Confusion
Cardiovascular	
Tachycardia	Tachycardia
Arrhythmias	Arrhythmias
Gastrointestinal	
Nausea	Anorexia
Vomiting	Nausea
Epigastric pain	Vomiting
Neuromuscular	
Tetany	Tremors
Numbness	Hypertonic muscles
Tingling of extremities	Muscle cramps
Hyperreflexia	Tetany
Seizures	Tingling of fingers and toes
	Seizures
Respiratory	
Hyperventilation	Hypoventilation

baking soda) occurs (see Table 15-14 and Fig. 15-16, *B*). The compensatory mechanism is a decreased respiratory rate to increase CO_2. Renal excretion of bicarbonate also occurs.

Mixed Acid-Base Disorders. A mixed acid-base disorder occurs when two or more simple disorders are present at the same time. The pH will depend on the type, severity, and acuity of each of the simple disorders involved. Respiratory acidosis combined with metabolic alkalosis (e.g., chronic obstructive lung disease treated with diuretic therapy) may result in a near-normal pH, while respiratory acidosis combined with metabolic acidosis will cause a greater decrease in pH than either disorder alone. An example of a mixed acidosis appears in a patient in cardiopulmonary arrest. Hypoventilation elevates the carbon dioxide level, and anaerobic metabolism produces lactic acid. An example of a mixed alkalosis is the case of a patient who is hyperventilating because of postoperative pain and is also losing acid secondary to nasogastric suctioning.

Clinical Manifestations

Clinical manifestations of acidosis and alkalosis are summarized in Tables 15-15 and 15-16. Because a normal pH is vital to all cellular reactions, the clinical manifestations of acid-base imbalances are generalized and nonspecific. The actual compensatory mechanisms also produce some clinical manifestations. For example, the deep, rapid respirations of a patient with metabolic acidosis are an example of respiratory compensation. In alkalosis, hypocalcemia may concurrently be found and accounts for many of the clinical manifestations.

Blood Gas Values. Blood gas values provide essential information for evaluation of acid-base problems.[13] These

Table 15-17 Normal Arterial and Venous Blood Gas Values

Parameter	Arterial	Venous
pH	7.35-7.45	7.35-7.45
PCO_2	35-45 mm Hg	40-45 mm Hg
Bicarbonate (HCO_3^-)	20-30 mEq/L (mmol/L)	20-30 mEq/L (mmol/L)
PO_2*	80-100 mm Hg	40-50 mm Hg
Oxygen saturation	96%-100%	60%-85%
Base excess	±2.0 mEq/L	±2.0 mEq/L

*Decreases above sea level and with increasing age.

include pH, PCO_2, and HCO_3^-. Diagnosis of acid-base disturbances and identification of compensatory processes are done by correlating the pH with the PCO_2 and HCO_3^-. First, it is necessary to determine whether the pH is alkalotic (>7.45) or acidotic (<7.35) and then whether the PCO_2 level or HCO_3^- is the primary cause of the pH change. For example, acidosis is caused by high CO_2 levels or low HCO_3^- levels. Next, determine whether the body is attempting to compensate for the pH change. For example, if the primary problem is respiratory acidosis (low pH with an elevated PCO_2), are the kidneys compensating by reabsorbing more bicarbonate? If compensatory mechanisms are functioning, the pH will return toward 7.40. The body will not overcompensate for pH changes. (Refer to the laboratory findings section of Table 15-14 for the blood gas findings of the four major acid-base disturbances.) Knowledge of the patient's clinical situation and the physiologic extent of renal and respiratory compensation enables the clinician to identify mixed acid-base disorders.

Blood gas analysis will also show the PCO_2 and oxygen saturation. These values are used to identify hypoxemia. Arterial blood gases are usually obtained. The values of blood gases differ slightly between arterial and venous samples (Table 15-17). (Blood gases are discussed in Chapter 24).

ASSESSMENT OF FLUID, ELECTROLYTE, AND ACID-BASE IMBALANCES

Subjective Data

Important Health Information

Past health history. The patient should be questioned about any past health history of problems involving the kidneys, heart, GI system, or lungs that could affect the present fluid and electrolyte balance. Information about specific diseases such as diabetes mellitus, diabetes insipidus, chronic obstructive pulmonary disease, ulcerative colitis, and Crohn's disease should be obtained from the patient.

Medications. An assessment of the patient's current and past use of medications is important. The ingredients in many drugs, especially over-the-counter drugs, are often overlooked as sources of sodium, potassium, calcium, magnesium, and other electrolytes. Many prescription drugs can cause fluid and electrolyte problems, including diuretics, corticosteroids, and electrolyte supplements.

Surgery or other treatments. The patient should be asked about past or present renal dialysis, kidney surgery, and bowel

COMMON ASSESSMENT ABNORMALITIES

Table 15-18 Fluid and Electroyte Imbalances

Finding`	Possible Cause
Skin	
Poor skin turgor	Fluid volume deficit
Cold, clammy skin	Sodium deficit, shift of plasma to interstitial fluid
Pitting edema	Fluid volume excess
Flushed, dry skin	Sodium excess
Pulse	
Bounding pulse	Fluid volume excess, shift of interstitial fluid to plasma
Rapid, weak, thready pulse	Shift of plasma to interstitial fluid, sodium deficit, fluid volume deficit
Weak, irregular, rapid pulse	Severe potassium deficit
Weak, irregular, slow pulse	Severe potassium excess
Blood Pressure	
Hypotension	Fluid volume deficit, shift of plasma to interstitial fluid, sodium deficit
Hypertension	Fluid volume excess, shift of interstitial fluid to plasma
Respirations	
Deep, rapid breathing	Metabolic acidosis
Shallow, slow, irregular breathing	Metabolic alkalosis
Shortness of breath	Fluid volume excess
Moist crackles	Fluid volume excess, shift of interstitial fluid to plasma
Skeletal Muscle	
Cramping of exercised muscle	Calcium deficit, magnesium deficit, alkalosis
Carpal spasm (Trousseau's sign)	Calcium deficit, magnesium deficit, alkalosis
Flabby muscles	Potassium deficit
Positive Chvostek's sign	Calcium deficit, magnesium deficit, alkalosis
Behavior or Mental	
Picking at bedclothes	Potassium deficit, magnesium deficit
Indifference	Fluid volume deficit, sodium deficit
Apprehension	Shift of plasma to interstitial fluid
Extreme restlessness	Potassium excess, fluid volume deficit
Confusion and irritability	Potassium deficit, fluid volume excess, calcium excess, magnesium excess, H_2O excess
Decreased level of consciousness	H_20 excess

or kidney surgery resulting in a temporary or permanent external collecting system such as a colostomy or nephrostomy.

Functional Health Patterns

Health perception–health management pattern. If the patient is currently experiencing a problem related to fluid and electrolyte balance, a careful description of the illness including onset, course, and treatment should be obtained.

Nutritional-metabolic pattern. The patient should be questioned regarding diet, especially whether she or he has been on a special diet such as a reducing, low-sodium, or fad diet. If the patient is on a special diet, such as low sodium or high potassium, his or her ability to comply with the dietary prescription should be determined.

Elimination pattern. Note should be made of the patient's usual bowel and bladder habits. Any deviations from the expected elimination pattern such as diarrhea, nocturia, or polyuria should be carefully documented.

Activity-exercise pattern. The patient's exercise pattern is important to determine because excessive perspiration secondary to exercise could result in a fluid and electrolyte problem. Also, the patient's exposure to extremely high temperatures as a result of leisure or work activity should be determined. The patient should be asked what practices are followed to replace fluid and electrolytes lost through excessive perspiration.

Cognitive-perceptual pattern. The patient should be queried about any changes in sensations such as numbness, tingling, fasciculations, or muscle weakness that could indicate a fluid and electrolyte problem. Additionally, both the patient and the family should be asked if any changes in mentation or alertness have been noted such as confusion, memory impairment, or lethargy.

Objective Data

Physical Examination. There is no specific physical examination to assess fluid and electrolyte balance. Common abnormal assessment findings of major body systems offer clues to possible fluid and electrolyte imbalances (Table 15-18).

Laboratory Values. Normal serum electrolyte values are a good starting point for identifying fluid and electrolyte imbalance (see Table 15-4). However, they often provide only cursory information. Serum electrolyte values reflect the concentration of that electrolyte in the ECF. They do not necessarily provide information concerning the concentration of the electrolyte in the ICF. For example, the majority of the potassium in the body is found intracellularly. Changes in serum potassium values may be the result of a true deficit or excess of potassium or may reflect the movement of potassium into or out of the cell.

Table 15-19 Normal Daily Maintenance Requirements for Fluids and Electrolytes

Maintenance IVs	Volume	Na^+ and Cl^-	K^+	Glucose
5% dextrose and 0.45% normal saline with 20 mEq KCl/L	2000 ml	154 mEq	40 mEq	100 g (50 g/L)
10% dextrose in water ($D_{10}W$)	1000 ml			100 g (100 g/L)
	3000 ml	154 mEq	40 mEq	200 g

An abnormal serum sodium level may reflect a sodium problem or, more likely, a water problem. A reduced hematocrit value could indicate anemia, or it could be caused by fluid volume excess.

Other laboratory tests that are helpful in evaluating the presence of or risk for fluid and electrolyte imbalances include serum and urine osmolality, serum glucose, BUN, serum creatinine, urine specific gravity, and urine electrolytes. In the presence of fluid and electrolyte imbalances, urine values assist the clinician in determining whether the kidneys are helping to correct the imbalance or are contributing to the imbalance. The patient with hypokalemia will have a low urinary potassium level if the kidney is able to compensate for the deficiency. If the kidney is unable to compensate (e.g., because of diuretic therapy), the urine potassium will be high.

In addition to arterial and venous blood gases, serum electrolytes can provide important information concerning a patient's acid-base balance. Changes in the serum bicarbonate (often reported as total CO_2 or CO_2 content on an electrolyte panel) will indicate the presence of metabolic acidosis (low bicarbonate level) or alkalosis (high bicarbonate level). Calculation of the anion gap (serum sodium level minus chloride and bicarbonate levels) can help determine the source of metabolic acidosis. The anion gap is increased in metabolic acidosis associated with acid gain (e.g., lactic acidosis, diabetic ketoacidosis) but remains normal (10 to 14 mmol/L) in metabolic acidosis caused by bicarbonate loss (e.g., diarrhea).

ORAL FLUID AND ELECTROLYTE REPLACEMENT

In all cases of fluid, electrolyte, and acid-base imbalances the treatment is directed toward correction of the underlying cause. The specific diseases or disorders that cause these imbalances are discussed in various chapters throughout this text. Mild fluid and electrolyte deficits can be corrected using oral rehydration solutions containing water, electrolytes, and glucose. Glucose not only provides calories but also promotes sodium absorption in the small intestine. Commercial oral rehydration solutions are now available in markets and pharmacies for home use.

INTRAVENOUS FLUID AND ELECTROLYTE REPLACEMENT

IV fluid and electrolyte therapy are commonly used to treat many different fluid and electrolyte imbalances. Many patients need maintenance IV fluid therapy only while they cannot take oral fluids (e.g., during and after surgery). Other patients need corrective or replacement therapy for losses that have already occurred. The amount and type of solution are determined by the normal daily maintenance requirements and by imbalances identified by laboratory results. The normal daily requirement for fluids and electrolytes is as follows:

Electrolytes: Na^+—100 to 150 mEq; K^+— 40 to 60 mEq
Fluid: 1500 ml/m^2 body surface (2650 ml for a 70 kg adult with 1.76 m^2 body surface)

An example of normal daily maintenance IV therapy is presented in Table 15-19.

Solutions

Hypotonic. A hypotonic solution provides more water than electrolytes, diluting the ECF. Osmosis then produces a movement of water from the ECF to the ICF. After osmotic equilibrium has been achieved, the ICF and the ECF have the same osmolality, and both compartments have been expanded. Examples of hypotonic fluids are given in Table 15-20. Maintenance fluids are usually hypotonic solutions (e.g., 0.45% NaCl) because normal daily losses are hypotonic. Additional electrolytes (e.g., KCl) may be added to maintain those levels.

Although 5% dextrose in water is considered an isotonic solution, the dextrose is quickly metabolized, and the net result is the administration of free water (hypotonic) with proportionately equal expansion of the ECF and ICF. One liter of a 5% dextrose solution provides 50 g of dextrose or 170 calories. Although this amount of dextrose is not enough to meet caloric requirements, it helps prevent ketosis associated with starvation. Pure water cannot be administered IV because it would cause hemolysis of red blood cells.

Isotonic. Administration of an isotonic solution expands only the ECF. There is no net loss or gain from the ICF. An isotonic solution is the ideal fluid replacement for a patient with an ECF volume deficit. Examples of isotonic solutions include lactated Ringer's solution and 0.9% NaCl. Lactated Ringer's solution contains sodium, potassium, chloride, calcium, and lactate (the precursor of bicarbonate) in about the same concentrations as those of the ECF. It is contraindicated in the presence of lactic acidosis because of the body's decreased ability to convert lactate to bicarbonate.

Isotonic saline (0.9% NaCl) has a sodium concentration (154 mEq/L) somewhat higher than plasma (135 to 145 mEq/L) and a chloride concentration (154 mEq/L) significantly higher than the plasma chloride level (96 to 106 mEq/L). Thus excessive administration of isotonic NaCl can result in elevated sodium and chloride levels.

Hypertonic. A hypertonic solution initially raises the osmolality of ECF and expands it. Examples are listed in Table 15-20. In addition, the higher osmotic pressure draws water

Table 15-20 Composition and Use of Commonly Prescribed Crystalloid Solutions

Solution	Tonicity	mOsm/kg	Glucose (g/L)	Indications and Considerations
Dextrose in Water				
5%	Isotonic	278	50	■ Provides free water necessary for renal excretion of solutes ■ Used to replace water losses and treat hypernatremia ■ Provides 170 calories/L ■ Does not provide any electrolytes
10%	Hypertonic	556	100	■ Provides free water only, no electrolytes ■ Provides 340 calories/L
Saline				
0.45%	Hypotonic	154	0	■ Provides free water in addition to Na^+ and Cl^- ■ Used to replace hypotonic fluid losses ■ Used as maintenance solution although it does not replace daily losses of other electrolytes ■ Provides no calories
0.9%	Isotonic	308	0	■ Used to expand intravascular volume and replace extracellular fluid losses ■ Only solution that may be administered with blood products ■ Contains Na^+ and Cl^- in excess of plasma levels ■ Does not provide free water, calories, other electrolytes ■ May cause intravascular overload or hyperchloremic acidosis
3.0%	Hypertonic	1026	0	■ Used to treat symptomatic hyponatremia ■ Must be administered slowly and with extreme caution because it may cause dangerous intravascular volume overload and pulmonary edema
Dextrose in Saline				
5% in 0.225%	Isotonic	355	50	■ Provides Na^+, Cl^-, and free water ■ Used to replace hypotonic losses and treat hypernatremia ■ Provides 170 calories/L
5% in 0.45%	Hypertonic	432	50	■ Same as 0.45% NaCl except provides 170 calories/L
5% in 0.9%	Hypertonic	586	50	■ Same as 0.9% NaCl except provides 170 calories/L
Multiple Electrolyte Solutions				
Ringer's Solution	Isotonic	309	0	■ Similar in composition to plasma except that it has excess Cl^+, no Mg^{2+}, and no HCO_3^- ■ Does not provide free water or calories ■ Used to expand the intravascular volume and replace extracellular fluid losses
Lactated Ringer's (Hartmann's) Solution	Isotonic	274	0	■ Similar in composition to normal plasma except does not contain Mg^{2+} ■ Used to treat losses from burns and lower gastrointestinal tract ■ May be used to treat mild metabolic acidosis but should not be used to treat lactic acidosis ■ Does not provide free water or calories

Modified from Horne MM, Swearingen PL: *Pocket guide to fluid, electrolyte, and acid-base balance*, ed 3, St Louis, 1997, Mosby.

out of the cells into the ECF. Hypertonic solutions (e.g., 3% NaCl) require frequent monitoring of blood pressure, lung sounds, and serum sodium levels and should be used with caution because the risk of intravascular fluid volume excess.

Although concentrated dextrose and water solutions (10% dextrose or greater) are hypertonic solutions, once the dextrose is metabolized, the net result is the administration of water. The free water provided by these solutions will ultimately expand both the ECF and ICF. The primary use of these solutions is in the provision of calories. Concentrated dextrose solutions may be combined with amino acid solutions, electrolytes, vitamins, and trace elements to provide total parenteral nutrition (see Chapter 38). Solutions containing 10% dextrose or less may be administered through a peripheral IV line. Solutions with greater concentrations of dextrose must be administered through a central line.

Intravenous Additives. In addition to the basic solutions that provide water and a minimum amount of calories

CRITICAL THINKING EXERCISES

CASE STUDY

Fluid and Electrolyte Imbalance

Patient Profile

H.T., a 42-year-old man with type 1 diabetes mellitus and renal insufficiency, is homebound because of an infected ankle ulcer and osteomyelitis of the femur. The home health nurse provides daily dressing changes and IV vancomycin (Vancocin). Medications include enalapril (Vasotec) and insulin.

Subjective Data

- Complains of overall weakness, extreme muscle weakness in his legs, extreme thirst, and dizziness when he stands
- Has diarrhea and frequent urination
- States he omitted morning dose of insulin because of poor dietary intake

Objective Data

- Heart rate 95 and irregular
- Blood pressure 140/95
- Blood glucose >500 mg/dl (28 mmol/L) taken on home glucometer
- Dry oral mucous membranes

Critical Thinking Questions

1. Based on his clinical manifestations, what fluid imbalance does H.T. have?
2. What additional assessment data should the nurse obtain?
3. What are his risk factors for fluid and electrolyte imbalances?
4. The nurse draws blood for a serum chemistry evaluation. What potentially dangerous electrolyte imbalance does his history and symptoms suggest?
5. The home health nurse notifies the physician of H.T.'s situation and receives an immediate order for insulin. How will insulin help his fluid and electrolyte imbalances?

and electrolytes, there are additives to replace specific losses. These additives are mentioned previously during the discussion of the particular electrolyte deficiencies. KCl, calcium chloride, magnesium sulfate, and bicarbonate are common additives to the basic (IV) solutions.

Recommendations for giving potassium vary, but in general no more than 10 mEq per hour is considered safe for routine administration. Potassium can be safely diluted as 40 mEq/L of solution with a maximum of 60 mEq/L.

Plasma Expanders. Plasma expanders stay in the vascular space and increase the osmotic pressure. Plasma expanders include colloids, dextran, and hetastarch. Colloids are protein solutions such as plasma, albumin, and commercial plasmas (e.g., Plasmanate). Albumin is available in two concentrations: 5% and 25% solutions. The 5% solution has an albumin concentration similar to plasma and will expand the intravascular fluid milliliter for milliliter. In contrast, the 25% albumin solution is hypertonic and will draw additional fluid from the interstitium. Dextran is a complex synthetic sugar. Because dextran is metabolized slowly, it remains in the vascular system for a prolonged period but not as long as the colloids. It pulls additional fluid into the intravascular space. Hetastarch is a synthetic colloid that works similarly to dextran.

If the patient has lost blood, whole blood or packed red blood cells are necessary to restore hemoglobin. Packed red blood cells have the advantage of giving the patient primarily red blood cells; the blood bank can use the plasma for blood components. Whole blood with its additional fluid volume may cause circulatory overload. Although packed cells have a decreased plasma volume, they will increase the oncotic pressure and pull fluid into the intravascular space. Loop diuretics may be administered with blood to prevent symptoms of fluid volume excess in anemic patients who are not volume depleted.

REVIEW QUESTIONS

The number of the question corresponds to the same-numbered objective at the beginning of the chapter.

1. The primary cation in the fluid compartment that constitutes the greatest percentage of total body water is
   a. sodium.
   b. chloride.
   c. potassium.
   d. calcium.
2. If the blood plasma has a higher osmolality than the fluid within a red blood cell, the mechanism involved in equalizing the fluid concentration is
   a. osmosis.
   b. diffusion.
   c. active transport.
   d. facilitated diffusion.

3a. Conditions that result in decreased serum albumin will result in
   a. decreased hydrostatic pressure with plasma shifts from the interstitium to the vasculature.
   b. increased hydrostatic pressure with plasma shifts from the vasculature to the interstitium.
   c. increased oncotic pressure with plasma shifts from the interstitium to the vasculature.
   d. decreased oncotic pressure with plasma shifts from the vasculature to the interstitium.

3b. Implementation of nursing care for the patient with hypernatremia includes
   a. fluid restriction.
   b. administration of hypotonic IV fluids.
   c. administration of a cation exchange resin.
   d. increased water intake for patients on nasogastric suction.

3c. Weak, irregular pulse, poor muscle tone, confusion, and irritability are common assessment findings in the patient with
   a. sodium deficit.
   b. calcium deficit.
   c. potassium deficit.
   d. fluid volume deficit.

3d. Which of the following patients would be at greatest risk for the potential development of hypermagnesemia?
   a. 65-year-old woman with hypertension taking beta-adrenergic blockers
   b. 50-year-old man with benign prostate hyperplasia and a urinary tract infection
   c. 42-year-old woman with systemic lupus erythematosus and renal failure
   d. 83-year-old man with prostate cancer and hypertension

3e. Which of the following statements is accurate?
   a. Hypercalcemia rarely occurs from increased calcium intake.
   b. In patients with hypercalcemia it is important to restrict fluid intake.
   c. Any condition that causes decreased parathyroid hormone results in hypercalcemia.
   d. Patients who have had thyroid surgery must be closely monitored for hypercalcemia.

3f. Aldosterone regulates fluid and electrolyte balance by
   a. promoting sodium loss by the kidney when plasma osmolality is increased.
   b. stimulating the kidneys to retain water when plasma osmolality is increased.
   c. blocking reabsorption of sodium by the kidney when plasma osmolality is increased.
   d. promoting sodium reabsorption by the kidney when plasma osmolality is decreased.

3g. In respiratory acidosis, compensation would be accomplished by
   a. lungs retaining CO_2.
   b. lungs eliminating CO_2.
   c. kidneys retaining bicarbonate.
   d. kidneys eliminating bicarbonate.

4. The ideal fluid replacement for the patient with an ECF fluid volume deficit is
   a. isotonic.
   b. hypotonic.
   c. hypertonic.
   d. a plasma expander.

References

1. Horne MM, Heitz UE, Swearingen PL: *Pocket guide to fluids and electrolytes,* ed 3, St Louis, 1997, Mosby.
2. O'Donnell ME: Assessing fluid and electrolyte balance in elders, *AJN* 95:41, 1995.
3. Lee CAB, Barrett CA, Ignatavicius DD: *Fluids and electrolytes: a practical approach,* ed 4, Philadelphia, 1996, Davis.
4. Lee CAB and others: *Fluids and electrolytes: a practical approach,* ed 4, Philadelphia, 1996, FA Davis.
5. Laureno R, Karp BI: Myelinolysis after correction of hyponatremia, *Ann Intern Med* 126:57, 1997.
6. Halperin ML, Goldstein MB: *Fluid, electrolyte, and acid-base physiology—a problem based approach,* ed 2, Philadelphia, 1994, Saunders.
7. Fabius DB: How to recognize electrolyte imbalances on an ECG, *Hosp Nurs* 32:1, 1998.
8. Locker FG: Hormonal regulation of calcium homeostasis, *Nurs Clin North Am* 31:797, 1996.
9. Kaplan M: Hypercalcemia of malignancy: a review of advances in physiology, *Oncol Nurs Forum* 21:1039, 1994.
10. Reber PM, Heath H: Hypocalcemic emergencies, *Med Clin North Am* 79:93, 1995.
11. Toffaletti J: Physiology and regulation—ionized calcium, magnesium and lactate measurements in critical care settings, *Am J Clin Pathol* 104(4 suppl 1):88, 1995.
12. Tosiello L: Hypomagnesemia and diabetes mellitus, *Arch Intern Med* 156:1143, 1996.
13. Tasota FJ, Wesmiller SW: Balancing act: keeping blood pH in equilibrium, *Nursing* 28:34 1998.

Resources

Intravenous Nurses' Society (INS)
Fresh Pond Square
10 Fawcett Street
Cambridge, MA 02138
617-441-3008
Fax: 617-441-3009
http://www.ins1.org

***For additional Internet resources, see the website for this book at* www.mosby.com/MERLIN/medsurg_lewis**

SECTION

3

THE SURGICAL EXPERIENCE

SECTION OUTLINE

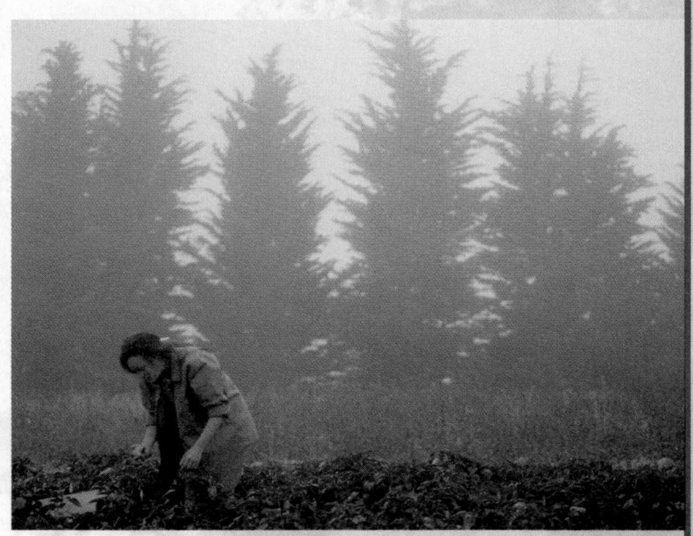

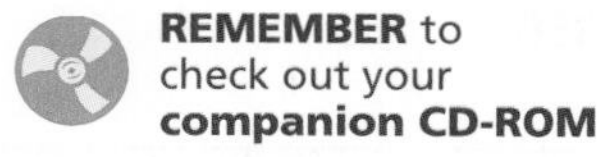

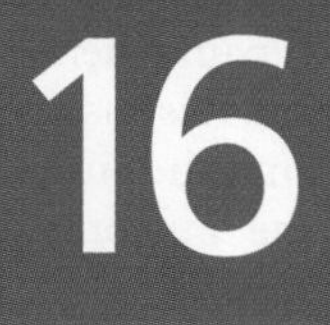

16 NURSING MANAGEMENT Preoperative Patient

Kim Litwack

www.mosby.com/MERLIN/medsurg_lewis

LEARNING OBJECTIVES

1. Identify the common purposes of surgery.
2. Describe the purpose and components of a preoperative assessment.
3. Interpret the significance of data related to the preoperative patient's health status and operative risk.
4. Explain the components and purpose of informed consent for surgery.
5. Describe the nursing role in the psychologic and educational preparation of the surgical patient.
6. Discuss the day-of-surgery preparation for the surgical patient.
7. Identify the purposes and types of preoperative medication.
8. Identify the special considerations of preoperative preparation for the older adult surgical patient.

Surgery can be defined as the art and science of treating diseases, injuries, and deformities by operation and instrumentation. The surgical procedure involves the interaction of the patient, the surgeon, and the nurse. Surgery may be performed for any of the following purposes:

1. Diagnosis: lymph node biopsy or bronchoscopy
2. Cure: removal of a ruptured appendix or benign ovarian cyst
3. Palliation: cutting a nerve root (rhizotomy) to remove symptoms of pain, or creating a colostomy to bypass an inoperable bowel obstruction
4. Cosmetic improvement: repairing a burn scar or changing breast shape (mammoplasty)
5. Prevention: removal of a mole before it becomes malignant or removal of the colon in familial polyposis to prevent cancer
6. Exploration: determination of the extent or nature of a disease (e.g., laparotomy).

Specific suffixes are commonly used in combination with identifying a body part or organ in naming surgical procedures (Table 16-1).

SURGICAL SETTINGS

Surgery may be a carefully planned and anticipated event in a person's life (elective surgery), or the need for surgery may sometimes arise with sudden and unanticipated urgency (emergency surgery). Both elective and emergency surgery may be performed in a variety of settings. The setting in which a surgical procedure may be safely and effectively performed is influenced by the extent of the surgery, the possible complications, and the general condition of the patient.

In the past the patient scheduled for a surgical procedure was admitted to the hospital the day before surgery to complete an appropriate preoperative assessment and laboratory testing. Surgery was usually performed in a hospital operating room (OR) and involved a hospital stay of several days. Today, because of increased interest in cost containment and advances in technology, the majority of surgical patients are admitted to the hospital on the day of surgery (same-day admission) or not admitted at all (outpatient).

An increasing number and type of surgical procedures are being performed as ambulatory procedures in emergency departments, doctor's offices, freestanding surgical clinics, and outpatient surgery units in hospitals. Ambulatory surgical procedures can be performed with the use of a general, regional, or local anesthetic, usually take less than 2 hours, require less than a 3-hour stay in the postanesthesia care unit (PACU), and do not require an overnight hospital stay.

The popularity of ambulatory surgery has steadily increased during the last decade. In some cases this concept has been mandated by third-party payers—private insurance companies, government insurers (Medicare and Medicaid), and health maintenance organizations (HMOs). Ambulatory surgery is generally preferred by patients, physicians, and third-party payers for several reasons. Patients like the convenience, physicians prefer the flexibility in scheduling, and the cost is usually less for both the patient and the insurer. Ambulatory surgery generally involves fewer laboratory tests, fewer preoperative and postoperative medications, less psychologic stress (especially in young children and older adults), and less susceptibility to hospital-acquired infections.

Regardless of where the surgery is performed, the nurse plays a significant role in preparing the patient for surgery, maintaining surveillance of the patient during surgery,

Reviewed by Virginia Printz-Feddersen, RNC, MSN, CNS, CNOR, CNRN, Clinical Nurse Specialist, Lovelace Health Systems, Albuquerque, NM; and Jill H. Pendarvis, RNC, MA, CNOR, Emeritus Associate Professor, Intercollegiate Center for Nursing Education, Spokane, Wash.

Table 16-1 Suffixes Describing Surgical Procedures

Suffix	Meaning	Example
-ectomy	Excision or removal of	Appendectomy
-lysis	Destruction of	Electrolysis
-orrhaphy	Repair or suture of	Herniorrhaphy
-oscopy	Looking into	Endoscopy
-ostomy	Creation of opening into	Colostomy
-otomy	Cutting into or incision of	Tracheotomy
-plasty	Repair or reconstruction of	Mammoplasty

preventing complications, and facilitating recovery following surgery. To perform this role effectively, the nurse must have certain basic information. First, the nurse must verify the nature of the disorder requiring surgery and any coexisting disease processes. Second, the nurse must know the individual patient's response to a stressful situation. Third, the nurse must assess the results of appropriate diagnostic tests done preoperatively. Finally, the nurse must consider the bodily alterations and possible risks and complications associated with the surgical procedure.

The preoperative nursing measures included in this chapter are those that are applicable to the preparation of any surgical patient. Specific measures in preparation for particular surgical procedures (e.g., abdominal, thoracic, or orthopedic surgery) are covered in other chapters of this text.

PSYCHOSOCIAL REACTIONS TO SURGERY

Even when planned well in advance, surgery is a psychologic and a physiologic experience that elicits the stress response. The stress response is a desirable mechanism that enables the body to adapt and heal in the postoperative period. If stressors or the response to the stressors are excessive, the stress response can be magnified and recovery can be affected. The nurse who is aware of a patient's perceived or actual stressors can provide support and the needed information during the preoperative period so that stress will not become distress. (See Chapter 7 for a discussion of stress.)

Emotional reactions to impending surgery and hospitalization often intensify in the older adult. Hospitalization may represent to the patient a physical decline and loss of health, mobility, and independence. The older adult may view a hospital as a place to die or as a stepping-stone to nursing home placement. The nurse can be instrumental in allaying anxieties and fears and maintaining and restoring the self-esteem of the older adult during the surgical experience (see section on gerontologic considerations on p. 373).

Common Fears

Fear of pain and discomfort is nearly universal. It includes concern about feeling pain during and after surgery. The nurse can reassure the patient that surgery will not begin before the anesthetic has taken effect and that adequate anesthesia will be maintained throughout the procedure. The nurse can encourage the patient to talk with the anesthesia care provider (ACP) for clarification. The nurse can help the patient who fears postoperative pain by emphasizing the availability of drugs for pain relief.

Fear of the unknown is also extremely common. It is based on lack of information about what to expect during the surgical experience and on the uncertainty about the outcome of surgery. The dread of cancer, so prevalent in society, often contributes to this fear, both when the surgery is for diagnostic purposes and when the diagnosis is known. The patient may have totally unrealistic expectations of what surgery will be like. This may be a result of past experiences or the vicarious experiences provided by friends' stories and the mass media, especially television. The nurse can relieve the patient's fear of the unknown by providing accurate, specific information about what to expect. The surgeon should be informed if the patient requires any additional information or if the fear seems excessive.

Fear of mutilation or alteration of body image may be a factor, not only when radical surgery or amputation is to be performed, but also when less extensive surgery is required. The prospect of blood being shed provokes anxiety in some persons. The presence of even a small scar on the body is abhorrent to others. A person's body image and the perception of a threat to it are unique. The nurse must listen to and assess the patient's concern about this aspect of surgery with an open, nonjudgmental attitude.

Fear of death may be greater when patients know that they have a malignancy or are a poor surgical risk. However, it may be experienced by others who are contemplating even minor procedures. Surgery may be postponed if the patient is convinced that it will lead to death. Attitude and emotional state influence the surgical outcome. The nurse should inform the surgeon if a patient expresses fear related to survival.

Fear of anesthesia may include concern about an unpleasant induction, hazards or complications (such as brain damage or paralysis), or loss of control while under its influence. The nurse can reassure the patient that anesthesia does not have the effect of "truth serum." The patient needs to know that it is not usual for persons to reveal their deepest secrets while under anesthesia. The ACP can provide detailed information about what the patient can expect to experience with the particular agents to be used.

Fear of disruption of life pattern may be present in varying degrees. It may range from fear of permanent disability to concern about not being able to play golf for a few weeks. Concerns about separation from family and about how spouse or children are managing are common. Financial concerns may be related either to an anticipated loss of income or to the costs of surgery.[1]

PATIENT INTERVIEW

Screening before surgery usually begins with a patient interview. The interview allows for the development of a relationship between the patient and the nurse. The interview is often the patient's first contact with the surgical facility and will frequently set the tone of the patient's opinion of the entire experience. The prescreening interview may occur in advance or on the day of surgery.

The primary purposes of the patient interview are to (1) obtain patient information, (2) provide information about surgery and anesthesia, and (3) get the patient's consent for surgery. The interview is also a time to (1) assess the patient's emotional state and readiness for surgery, (2) explore the patient's expectations about surgery and anesthesia, and

(3) reinforce and clarify these expectations as indicated. The interview provides an opportunity for the patient and family to ask questions about surgery, anesthesia, and postoperative care.

The preoperative interview also allows for assessment of the patient's and family's emotional response to surgery. The nurse who is aware of a patient's and family's perception of stressors can provide the support needed during the preoperative period so that stress will not become distress. Emotional reactions to surgery and anesthesia vary. The extent of a patient's and family's fears will be influenced by past surgical experiences, knowledge, hopes about the outcome of surgery, and personal coping mechanisms.

The nurse records preoperative data about the patient to be used as a basis for comparison during the intraoperative and postoperative periods, as well as to individualize postoperative care (Fig. 16-1).

ASSESSMENT OF THE PREOPERATIVE PATIENT

Although nursing assessment and intervention are discussed separately, both are simultaneously done in practice. The overall goal of preoperative assessment is patient safety and includes the following specific assessments:[2,3]

1. Determine the adequacy of the patient's health status to undergo the proposed surgery.
2. Identify and correct (if possible) any operative risk factors.
3. Determine whether surgery should be done as an inpatient, an outpatient, or a same-day admission.
4. Establish baseline data for comparison in the postoperative period.
5. Plan and institute preoperative care.
6. Select the anesthetic medication and technique best suited to the patient and type of surgery to be performed.

Subjective Data

Psychosocial Assessment. A psychosocial assessment of the preoperative patient should gather information about how the patient perceives the surgical experience (Table 16-2). This information can be gathered by the nurse during the admission nursing interview and throughout the ongoing nurse-patient relationship. The extremely anxious patient also needs additional consideration during the assessment process. The nurse must avoid introducing new concepts or terms that may increase the anxiety level and further impair thought processes and cognitive ability.

Past Health History. Initially, the nurse will explore the patient's understanding of the need for surgery and specific patient complaints that may have caused the patient to seek medical attention. For example, a patient scheduled for a total knee replacement may indicate problems with increasing pain and mobility limitations.

Women should be asked about menstrual and obstetric history. This includes obtaining the date of the patient's last menstrual period. The purpose for obtaining this information is to avoid possible maternal and fetal exposure to anesthetics during the first trimester of pregnancy. This type of questioning may be embarrassing for a teenager in the presence of parents or guardians. The nurse may elect to ask these questions with parents or guardians out of the room.

Obtaining information about the patient's family health history is also important, including any adverse reactions to or problems with anesthesia. Anesthesiologists were first made aware of a phenomenon, later to be known as malignant hyperthermia, when a young man in Australia reported that 10 of his family members died while undergoing anesthesia. The genetic predisposition for malignant hyperthermia is now well documented. (For further information on malignant hyperthermia, see Chapter 17.)

A family history of cardiac and endocrine disease should be investigated. A family history of sudden cardiac death, myocardial infarction, and coronary artery disease should alert the nurse to the possibility of similar diseases in the patient. A family history of diabetes should also be investigated because of the familial predisposition to both type 1 and type 2 diabetes mellitus.

The last component of the patient history is the systems review. Specific questions should be asked to confirm the presence or absence of disease. Systems alterations may influence the choice of anesthetic agents and techniques, intraoperative monitoring priorities, and the type of care administered postoperatively. If the patient is being evaluated before the day of surgery, the review of systems, combined with patient history data, will suggest the need for preoperative laboratory tests. Many physiologic stressors may put the patient at risk for surgical complications, whether the surgery is an elective or an emergency procedure. A physiologic assessment of the preoperative patient is presented in Table 16-3.

Cardiovascular system. The purpose of evaluating a patient's cardiovascular function is to determine the presence of preexisting disease or functional problems (e.g., mitral valve prolapse) that may increase perioperative risk. It is important to inquire about any history of cardiac problems, including hypertension, angina, arrhythmias, and myocardial infarction. The patient may respond or understand questions better if asked in lay terms about a history of high blood pressure, chest pain, palpitations, or heart attack. It is also important to inquire about any history of congestive heart failure and edema (e.g., swelling or fluid retention). The nurse should also inquire whether the patient has seen a cardiologist in the past, is using cardiac medications, or has ever undergone any cardiac surgical procedures, including catheterization, pacemaker insertion, or bypass surgery.[2-4]

Ideally, the patient who has had a myocardial infarction should wait at least 6 months for elective surgery to decrease the risk of reinfarction.[2,3] If the patient has a history of hypertension, medical approval by an internist is recommended.[4] If the patient has a history of congenital, rheumatic, or valvular heart disease, antibiotic prophylaxis before surgery may be used to decrease the risk of bacterial endocarditis[2] (see Chapter 35).

The patient will usually be monitored electrocardiographically during and after surgery. The patient who receives digitalis therapy will have serum potassium levels carefully monitored to avoid the adverse and toxic effects of anesthetic agents. Dehydration may require preoperative correction with fluid therapy. Although a preoperative fluid balance assessment should be completed for all patients, it is especially critical for the older adult because the reduced adaptive capacity leaves a narrow margin of safety between overhydration and underhydration.

Respiratory system. It is important to inquire about any history of dyspnea (at rest or with exertion), coughing (dry or productive), hemoptysis, and asthma. If a patient has a history of

Text continues on p. 362

Rush-Presbyterian-St. Luke's Medical Center
Chicago, Illinois

Patient Data Base-Nursing Assessment
___ Same Day Admission ___ General Admission

REASON FOR THIS HOSPITAL ADMISSION: ____________________

HOW DO YOU RATE YOUR HEALTH (PATIENT'S)? POOR ______ FAIR ______ GOOD ______ EXCELLENT ______
PLEASE EXPLAIN ____________________

ALLERGIES (FOOD, MEDICATION, OTHER) & TYPE OF REACTION: ____________________

MEDICATION HISTORY

PLEASE LIST ALL PRESCRIPTION AND NONPRESCRIPTION MEDICATIONS THAT YOU ARE CURRENTLY TAKING

NAME OF MEDICATION	DOSE OF MEDICATION	TIME OF DAY MEDICATION IS TAKEN	NAME OF MEDICATION	DOSE OF MEDICATION	TIME OF DAY MEDICATION IS TAKEN

DO YOU SMOKE? YES ______ NO ______ AMT ______ /DAY HAVE YOU SMOKED IN THE PAST? YES ______ NO ______
HOW MUCH ALCOHOL DO YOU DRINK? ____________________
DO YOU TAKE ANY OTHER ANY DRUGS? YES ______ NO ______ TYPE OF DRUG: ______

DISCHARGE PLANNING

MARITAL STATUS: MARRIED ______ SINGLE ______ DIVORCED ______ WIDOWED ______ CHILDREN: YES ______ # ______ NO ______
OCCUPATION: ______ NUMBER OF YEARS ______
NAME AND PHONE NUMBER OF IMMEDIATE FAMILY MEMBER OR FRIEND: ______
______ NONE: ______
LEVEL OF EDUCATION: GRADE SCHOOL ______ HIGH SCHOOL ______ COLLEGE ______
WHAT IS YOUR PRIMARY LANGUAGE? ______

HAVE YOU USED HOME HEALTH CARE SERVICES? YES ______ NO ______ IF YES, WHICH AGENCY: ______
WHERE WILL YOU GO AFTER BEING DISCHARGED FROM THE HOSPITAL: HOME ______ REHAB. FACILITY ______
NURSING HOME ______ UNCERTAIN ______ OTHER ______
WHAT TYPE OF ASSISTANCE DO YOU THINK YOU MIGHT NEED AFTER LEAVING THE HOSPITAL? ______
UNSURE AT THIS TIME: ______

Fig. 16-1 Adult surgical database.

NUTRITION

WHAT IS YOUR NORMAL DIET?
GENERAL ____ SPECIAL ____

ARE YOU HAVING:	YES	NO
CHANGES IN APPETITE?	___	___
CHANGES IN THIRST?	___	___
INTOLERANCE TO FOOD?	___	___
IF YES, TO WHAT TYPES OF FOOD:		
PROBLEMS CHEWING OR SWALLOWING?	___	___
DO YOU HAVE LOOSE TEETH?	___	___

SLEEP PATTERN

	YES	NO
DO YOU HAVE DIFFICULTY SLEEPING?	___	___
DO YOU USE SLEEPING PILLS OR SPECIAL ROUTINES TO HELP YOU SLEEP?	___	___

PLEASE SPECIFY: ____

ACTIVITY

	YES	NO
DO YOU EXERCISE REGULARLY?	___	___
DO YOU HAVE SUFFICIENT ENERGY FOR ACTIVITIES?	___	___
HAVE YOU HAD AN INCREASE IN FALLS OR STUMBLING?	___	___

DESCRIBE: ____

ELIMINATION

DO YOU:	YES	NO
MOVE YOUR BOWELS DAILY?	___	___
IF NO, HOW OFTEN:		
HAVE CONSTIPATION?	___	___
HAVE DIARRHEA?	___	___
USE A LAXATIVE? (TYPE):	___	___
HAVE AN INCREASE IN URINARY FREQUENCY?	___	___
LOSE CONTROL OF BLADDER?	___	___
USE ANY URINARY/OSTOMY APPLIANCE? (TYPE):	___	___

PERCEPTUAL PATTERN

DO YOU HAVE PROBLEMS WITH:	YES	NO
SENSATION?	___	___
VISION?	___	___
HEARING?	___	___
PAIN?	___	___

DESCRIBE ANY PAIN YOU CURRENTLY HAVE. INCLUDE THINGS THAT CAUSE IT AND RELIEVE IT: ____

COPING / STRESS

HAVE YOU EVER EXPERIENCED:	YES	NO
MOOD SWINGS?	___	___
DEPRESSION?	___	___
ANXIETY?	___	___
DO YOU HAVE ANY QUESTIONS OR CONCERNS REGARDING SEXUAL ACTIVITY?	___	___
HAVE THERE BEEN ANY MAJOR CHANGES IN YOUR LIFE WITHIN THE PAST YEAR?	___	___
DO YOU HAVE FINANCIAL CONCERNS RELATED TO YOUR HEALTH CARE OR HOSPITALIZATION?	___	___

COMMENTS: ____

SPIRITUAL

DO YOU HAVE ANY RELIGIOUS OR CULTURAL BELIEFS THAT WE SHOULD BE AWARE OF WHILE YOU ARE HOSPITALIZED? **YES** **NO**
IF YES, EXPLAIN: ____

RELATIONSHIP PATTERNS

DO YOU LIVE: ALONE ____ WITH OTHERS ____
APARTMENT ____ HOUSE ____ OTHER ____
ARE THERE STAIRS? YES ____ # ____ NO ____
DO YOU HAVE SOMEONE AVAILABLE TO ASSIST YOU AFTER YOU GO HOME? YES __ NO __
PLEASE SPECIFY WHO: ____

ACTIVITIES OF DAILY LIVING

PLEASE CHECK (✓) ANY AREAS WITH WHICH YOU NEED HELP:
EATING __ BATHING __ COMBING HAIR __
GETTING DRESSED: UPPER __ LOWER __
MOVING TO/FROM: BED __ WHEEL CHAIR __
TOILET __ TUB/SHOWER __
CAN YOU MOVE ALONE WHILE: SITTING __ STANDING __ IN BED __

DO YOU HAVE/USE:	YES	NO	BROUGHT TO HOSPITAL YES	BROUGHT TO HOSPITAL NO
DENTURES: FULL/UPPER	___	___	___	___
FULL/LOWER	___	___	___	___
PARTIAL/UPPER	___	___	___	___
PARTIAL/LOWER	___	___	___	___
GLASSES:	___	___	___	___
CONTACT LENSES:	___	___	___	___
HEARING AID:	___	___	___	___
WALKER:	___	___	___	___
CRUTCHES:	___	___	___	___
CANE:	___	___	___	___
WHEEL CHAIR:	___	___	___	___
PROSTHETIC DEVICE:	___	___	___	___

PLEASE SPECIFY: ____

Fig. 16-1 (continued)

PLEASE ANSWER THE FOLLOWING QUESTIONS ABOUT YOUR HEALTH HISTORY BY PLACING A CHECK(÷) IN THE APPROPRIATE COLUMN. YOU MAY USE THE SPACE UNDER "COMMENTS" TO ADD ANY ADDITIONAL INFORMATION ABOUT YOUR HEALTH HISTORY.

DO YOU HAVE OR HAVE YOU EVER HAD:	**YES**	**NO**	**COMMENTS:**
ARTHRITIS OR JOINT PROBLEMS?	____	____	
ASTHMA, BRONCHITIS, PNEUMONIA OR BREATHING DIFFICULTIES?	____	____	
BLEEDING DISORDERS OR PROBLEMS WITH BLOOD CLOTS?	____	____	
CIRCULATION PROBLEMS?	____	____	
DIABETES?	____	____	
DIZZINESS OR FAINTING?	____	____	
LIVER PROBLEMS?	____	____	
HEART PROBLEMS?	____	____	
HIGH BLOOD PRESSURE?	____	____	
INFECTIOUS DISEASE:			
HEPATITIS?	____	____	
TUBERCULOSIS?	____	____	
AIDS?	____	____	
OTHER: ____________			
KIDNEY, BLADDER OR PROSTATE PROBLEMS?	____	____	
RASHES, SORES OR REDDENED AREAS?	____	____	
IF YES, WHERE: ____________			
SEIZURES?			
STOMACH PROBLEMS?	____	____	
STROKE?	____	____	
OTHER HEALTH PROBLEMS: ____________			

HAVE ANY MEMBER(S) OF YOUR FAMILY (BLOOD RELATIONS) HAD ANY OF THE FOLLOWING PROBLEMS:

	YES	**NO**	**RELATIONSHIP**		**YES**	**NO**	**RELATIONSHIP**
HEART DISEASE?	____	____	____________	DIABETES?	____	____	____________
HIGH BLOOD PRESSURE?	____	____	____________	CANCER?	____	____	____________
STROKE?	____	____	____________	PROBLEMS WITH ANESTHESIA?	____	____	____________
OTHER HEALTH PROBLEMS?	____	____	____________				

LIST ANY PREVIOUS SURGERIES YOU HAVE HAD:

SURGERY: ____________ DATE: ____________

WHAT TYPE OF ANESTHESIA HAVE YOU HAD?

GENERAL ____ LOCAL ____ OTHER ____________

PLEASE DESCRIBE ANY PROBLEMS YOU HAD WITH PREVIOUS ANESTHESIA OR SURGERY (SUCH AS NAUSEA, DIFFICULTY WAKING UP, ALLERGIC REACTIONS, ETC.): ____________

FEMALE PATIENTS ONLY: WHAT WAS THE DATE OF YOUR LAST MENSTRUAL PERIOD? ____________

DO YOU HAVE ANY REASON TO BELIEVE YOU MIGHT BE PREGNANT? YES ____ NO ____

PATIENT / FAMILY SIGNATURE: ____________ DATE: ____________

INTERVIEWER / REVIEWER: ____________ DATE: ____________

UNABLE TO OBTAIN SUBJECTIVE INFORMATION DUE TO: ____________

Fig. 16-1 Adult surgical database. (continued)

DAY OF ADMISSION

DATE: ______________ TIME: ________ A.M./P.M. MODE OF ARRIVAL: W/C ____ CART ____ AMBULATORY ____

ACCOMPANIED BY: ______________ PATIENT SEX: M ____ F ____ AGE: ____

DISPOSITION OF VALUABLES: HOSPITAL VAULT ____ SENT HOME ____ NONE ____

DISPOSITION OF BELONGINGS / PROSTHESIS: FAMILY ______ STORAGE ______ WITH PATIENT ______

SPECIFY TYPE OF BELONGINGS / PROSTHESIS: ______________

COMPLETE THIS SECTION FOR ALL SAME DAY SURGICAL AND GENERAL ADMISSION PATIENTS:

GENERAL APPEARANCE:

PULSE: ________ RESP: ________ BP: ________ TEMP: ________ ALERT & ORIENTED x 3: ________

REG: ________ UNLABORED: ________ LYING: ________ WEIGHT: ________ HEIGHT: ________

IRREG: ________ BREATH SOUNDS: SITTING: ________

APICAL / RADIAL CLEAR & BILATERALLY: STANDING: ________

________ EQUAL: ________ RT. / LT. ARM ________

ADDITIONAL COMMENTS: ______________

____

RN SIGNATURE ______________ DATE: ________ TIME: ________

COMPLETE THIS SECTION FOR ALL GENERAL ADMISSION PATIENTS:

CIRCULATION/SKIN: Movement, circulation, & sensation intact in all extremities ______

Skin color: WNL ______ Other ______________

Skin lesions: Yes ______ No ______ Location/size ______________ Braden score: ________

Edema: Yes ______ No ______ Location/degree ______________

ABDOMEN: Soft, nontender, nondistended ______ Other: ______________

Bowel sounds: Normal ______ Other: ______________ Date of last bowel movement: ________

Stoma/Ostomy/Tubes: ______________

NEUROMUSCULAR: Gait: Steady ______ Unsteady ______ Muscle tone: Good ______ Fair ______ Poor ______

Joint swelling: Yes ______ No ______ Where ______________

ADDITIONAL COMMENTS: ______________

____

RN SIGNATURE ______________ DATE: ________ TIME: ________

ORIENTATION TO UNIT:	YES	NO	PT. UNABLE		YES	NO	PT. UNABLE
Tour of room complete	____	____	____	Safety precautions explained	____	____	____
Visiting policies explained	____	____	____	Identification/allergy band on	____	____	____
Demonstrates use of call light	____	____	____				

RN SIGNATURE ______________ DATE: ________ TIME: ________

Fig. 16-1 (continued)

Table 16-2 Psychosocial Assessment of the Preoperative Patient

Situational Changes
- Determine support systems, including family, significant others, group and institutional structure, and religious and spiritual orientation.
- Define current degree of personal control, decision making, and independence.
- Consider the impact of surgery and hospitalization and the possible effects on lifestyle.

Concerns with the Unknown
- Identify specific areas of concern.
- Identify expectations of surgery, changes in current health status, and effects on daily living.

Concerns with Body Image
- Identify current roles or relationships and view of self.
- Determine perceived or potential changes in role or relationships and their impact on body image.

Past Experiences
- Review previous surgical experiences, hospitalizations, and treatments.
- Determine responses to those experiences (positive and negative).
- Identify current perceptions of surgical procedure in relation to the above and information from others (e.g., a neighbor's view of a personal surgical experience).

Knowledge Deficit
- Identify understanding of the surgical procedure, including preparation, care, interventions, activities, restrictions, and expected outcomes.
- Identify the accuracy of information the patient has received from others, including health care team, family, friends, and neighbors.

Table 16-3 Physiologic Assessment of the Preoperative Patient

Cardiovascular Status
- Identify acute or chronic problems; focus on the presence of angina, hypertension, congestive heart failure, and recent history of myocardial infarction.
- Assess baseline pulses: apical, radial, and pedal for rate and characteristics (compare one side to the other).
- Assess for the presence of edema (including dependent areas), noting location and severity.
- Assess neck veins for distention.

Respiratory Status
- Identify acute or chronic problems; note the presence of infection or chronic obstructive lung disease.
- Note the history of smoking, including the time interval since the last cigarette and the number of pack-years. (Remember that although smoking should be discouraged preoperatively, it may be difficult for patients to stop during this time of anxiety.)
- Assess breath sounds for normal and adventitious sounds; determine baseline respiratory rate, pattern, and the use of accessory muscles of respiration.

Integumentary and Musculoskeletal Status
- Assess mucous membranes for dryness and intactness.
- Determine skin status; note drying, bruising, or breaks in integrity of surface.
- Note any limitations in range of motion, weakness, or impairments to ambulation.
- Identify any drug therapies that may affect coagulation (e.g., aspirin and nonsteroidal antiinflammatory agents).

Nutritional Status
- Weigh patient.
- Determine recent weight loss through a diet history (e.g., a negative nitrogen balance may lead to postoperative complications of delayed or impaired wound healing, fluid imbalances, and infection).
- Assess food and fluid intake patterns (older adults frequently have a preexisting nutritional deficit).
- Identify any drug therapies that may affect electrolyte balance. Consider prescribed and over-the-counter medications (e.g., potassium-depleting diuretics, excessive use of laxatives or antacids).
- Assess the presence of dentures and bridges (loose dentures or teeth may be dislodged during intubation).

See related body system chapters for more specific assessments and related laboratory studies.

asthma, the nurse should inquire about the patient's use of bronchodilators and the frequency and triggers of an asthma attack.

The patient should be asked about any recent or chronic upper respiratory infections. The presence of an upper airway infection normally results in the cancellation or postponement of elective surgery because the patient is at an increased risk of bronchospasm, laryngospasm, decreased oxygen saturation, and problems with secretions. The patient with a history of chronic obstructive pulmonary disease (COPD) and asthma is also at risk for postoperative pulmonary complications, including hypoxemia and atelectasis.[5,6]

The patient who smokes should be encouraged to abstain preoperatively but may find this difficult during a time of heightened anxiety. Any physical condition likely to influence or compromise respiratory function should also be noted. These include obesity and spinal, chest, and airway deformities. Depending on the patient's history and physical examination, baseline pulmonary function tests and arterial blood gases (ABGs) may be ordered preoperatively.

Nervous system. Preoperative evaluation of neurologic functioning includes assessing the patient's ability to respond to questions, to follow commands, and to maintain orderly thought patterns. Appropriateness of response and thought must be evaluated. This is particularly important for the patient who is expected to prepare for surgery and to complete preoperative preparation on an outpatient basis. If deficits are noted, careful assessment should determine its extent and if the problem can be corrected before surgery. If the problem cannot be corrected, it is important to determine whether there are appropriate resources and support to assist the patient.

It is also important to inquire about any history of cerebrovascular accidents (strokes), transient ischemic attacks, spinal cord injury, and diseases of the nervous system, such as cerebral palsy, myasthenia gravis, Parkinson's disease, and multiple sclerosis.[2]

Renal system. Because many people in the United States and Canada are affected by renal disease, it is important to include questions about preexisting renal disease.[2] Renal dysfunction is associated with a number of alterations, including fluid and electrolyte imbalances, coagulopathies, increased risk for infection, and impaired wound healing. Another important consideration is the recognition that many medications are metabolized and excreted by the kidney. A decrease in renal function may contribute to an altered response to medications and unpredictable drug elimination.

Hepatic system. The liver is involved in glucose homeostasis, fat metabolism, protein synthesis, drug and hormone metabolism, and bilirubin formation and excretion.[4] The liver detoxifies many anesthetics and adjunctive drugs. Therefore hepatic dysfunction will result in systemic effects. In addition, the patient with liver disease may have problems with glucose control, clotting abnormalities, and response to drug effects, all of which may increase perioperative risk.

Musculoskeletal system. It is important, particularly in the elderly, to inquire about a history of musculoskeletal problems.[7] If the patient has arthritis, all affected joints should be identified. Mobility restrictions may influence intraoperative and postoperative positioning and postoperative ambulation. If the neck is affected, intubation and airway management may be difficult. Any mobility aids such as a cane, walker, or crutches should be brought with the patient to the hospital on the day of surgery.

Nutritional status. Assessment of nutritional status includes recognition of two problems that can increase operative risk—obesity and nutritional deficiencies. Obesity stresses both the cardiac and pulmonary system. Obesity makes access to the surgical site more difficult and thus prolongs the surgery.[2] It predisposes the patient to wound dehiscence, wound infection, and incisional herniation because adipose tissue impairs approximation of the wound edges and is less vascular than other tissues. The inhalation anesthetic is absorbed and stored by adipose tissue and then released postoperatively. Therefore the obese patient requires more anesthetic and recovers more slowly from its effects.

Nutritional deficiencies of protein and vitamins A, C, and B complex are particularly significant because each of these substances is essential for wound healing. The older adult is often at risk for malnutrition and fluid volume deficits associated with poor eating habits and a lack of dentition, as well as economic restrictions. Nutritional deficiencies impair the ability to recover from surgery. Surgery may be postponed until the patient gains or loses weight and deficiencies are corrected. It is important to remember that the obese patient can also be protein and vitamin deficient. The nurse should also be alert for patients suffering from undernutrition related to eating disorders.

Endocrine system. Diabetes mellitus is a risk factor for both anesthesia and surgery. The diabetic patient is at risk for the development of hypoglycemia, ketosis, cardiovascular alterations, delayed wound healing, and infection.[2] It is important to clarify with the patient's surgeon or anesthesia provider whether the patient should take the usual dose of insulin on the day of surgery. Some practitioners prefer that the patient take only half of the usual dose; others ask that the patient take either the usual dose or take no insulin at all. If the insulin dose is held, the patient will be managed with periodic blood glucose checks and supplemented, if necessary, with regular (short-acting, rapid-onset) insulin.

Infection. Although the presence of an acute infection often results in the cancellation of elective surgery, patients with active chronic infections such as acquired immunodeficiency syndrome (AIDS) and tuberculosis may still have surgery. When preparing the patient for surgery, it should be remembered that infection control precautions must be taken with every patient. (Infection control guidelines are discussed in Chapter 11.)

Medications. The patient should be questioned about current medication use, including the use of over-the-counter medications. This is an important area to explore because these medications may interact with anesthetics, often increasing or decreasing potency and effectiveness. It is especially important to consider the effects of drugs used for heart disease, hypertension, immunosuppression, anticoagulation, and endocrine replacement.

In addition, knowledge about current medication usage can alert the nurse to obtain and evaluate laboratory tests. For example, if the patient is receiving warfarin (Coumadin) or aspirin, a coagulation profile should be obtained. A patient on diuretic therapy may need to have a potassium level obtained. If the patient is taking medications for arrhythmias, a preoperative electrocardiogram (ECG) should be obtained.[8] Insulin or antidiabetic agents used in the management of the patient with diabetes may require dose or agent adjustments during the perioperative period because of increased body metabolism, decreased caloric intake, stress, and anesthesia. Tranquilizers potentiate the effect of narcotics and barbiturates, which are agents used for anesthesia. Antihypertensive medication may predispose the patient to shock from the com-

HEALTH HISTORY

Table 16-4 Preoperative Patient

Health Perception–Health Management Pattern
- What has the doctor explained to you about your surgery?
- Have you had surgery before?*
- Have you or any family members ever experienced any problems with anesthesia?*
- Do you smoke?* If yes, how many packs daily? For how many years?
- Do you have any chronic illnesses?*
- Are you taking any medications?* Are you allergic to any medication?*
- What is your usual use of alcohol?

Nutritional-Metabolic Pattern
- What is your usual or present height and weight?
- Have you had a recent weight gain or loss?*
- Do you have any food preferences or dislikes?*
- Do you have any difficulty chewing or swallowing?*
- Do you take vitamins?*
- Do you have any problems healing?*
- Do you have a history of liver problems?*

Elimination Pattern
- Do you experience any problems with constipation?*
- Do you experience any problems with urinary elimination?*

Activity-Exercise Pattern
- Do you have a history of high blood pressure or cardiac disease?*
- Do you have any history of dyspnea, coughing, hemoptysis, COPD, or asthma?*
- Do you presently have an upper respiratory infection?*
- Do you have any musculoskeletal problems that might affect positioning during surgery or activity level after surgery?*
- Do you have any limitation in mobility of your neck?*
- Do you require any special equipment for ambulation?*

Sleep-Rest Pattern
- Describe any problems you have with sleeping.
- Do you use sleeping pills?*

Cognitive-Perceptual Pattern
- Do you wear glasses, contact lenses, or hearing aid?*
- How would you describe your pain tolerance?
- What methods have you found effective for pain relief?

Self-Perception–Self-Concept Pattern
- How do you feel about having this surgery?
- Have you experienced any changes in the way you feel about yourself or your body?*

Role-Relationship Pattern
- Will this surgery create any problems in your usual roles or relationships?*
- Will you have the support you feel you need following discharge?

Sexuality-Reproductive Pattern
- Do you expect this surgery to have any impact on your usual sexual activity?*

Coping–Stress Tolerance Pattern
- How do you feel about this surgery?
- Do you feel you will be able to cope following this surgery?

Value-Belief Pattern
- Do you have a conflict between your planned surgery and your value or belief system?*

*If yes, describe.
COPD, chronic obstructive pulmonary disease.

bined effect of the medication and the vasodilator effect of some anesthetic agents.

The nurse should also determine whether the patient is correctly taking currently prescribed medications. Is the patient taking the medication as ordered, or has the patient stopped taking the medication because of cost, side effects, or the feeling that ongoing therapy is no longer needed? Inquiry about medication use provides an ideal area for patient teaching and for referral of the patient to the physician who prescribed the medication.

When inquiring about medication use, it is important to ask about medication intolerance and drug allergies. Medication intolerance usually results in side effects that are uncomfortable or unpleasant for the patient but are not life threatening. These effects include nausea, constipation, diarrhea, and rash. A true drug allergy produces an anaphylactic or anaphylactoid reaction, causing cardiopulmonary compromise, including hypotension, tachycardia, bronchospasm, and possibly pulmonary edema. By being aware of medication intolerance and drug allergies, it will be possible to avoid the use of these drugs and ideally maintain patient comfort, safety, and stability. If a medication intolerance or drug allergy is noted, the patient's chart should be labeled accordingly, and an allergy wrist band should be put on the patient on the day of surgery.

It is also important to inquire about nondrug allergies, including allergies to foods, chemicals, and pollen. The patient with a history of allergic responsiveness has a greater potential for demonstrating hypersensitivity reactions to drugs administered during anesthesia.[2]

Patients should also be screened for possible latex allergies. The American College of Allergy, Asthma, and Immunology (ACAAI) recommends that patients be screened in the following five areas:[9]

1. Risk factors
2. Contact dermatitis
3. Contact urticaria (e.g., hives)
4. Aerosol reactions
5. History of reactions that suggest an allergy to latex

Risk factors include long-term, multiple exposures to latex products (e.g., health care personnel, rubber industry workers).

Table 16-5 Preoperative Rating of Patient's Physical Status

Rating	Examples
I. Healthy patient with no systemic disease	Patient with no significant past or present health history
II. Mild systemic disease without functional limitations	Patient with a history of asthma controlled with β-agonist inhaler
III. Severe systemic disease associated with definite functional limitations	Patient with history of chronic asthma controlled with β-agonist inhaler and inhaled steroids; not wheezing
IV. Severe systemic disease that is ongoing threat to life	Patient with a history of asthma, poorly controlled with β-agonist and oral steroids; PaO_2 50 mm Hg; wheezing; chest x-ray changes
V. Patient unlikely to survive for more than 24 hr with or without surgery	Patient in status asthmaticus, intubated, ventilated, IV corticosteroids, IV aminophylline

IV, intravenous.

Additional risk factors include a history of hay fever, asthma, and allergies to certain foods (e.g., avocados, kiwi, bananas, chestnuts, potatoes, peaches, apricots). (Latex allergies are discussed in Chapter 12.)

Although it may be difficult or embarrassing, the patient should be asked about possible drug use, abuse, and addiction. The categories of drugs most likely to be used and abused include tobacco, alcohol, opioids, marijuana, and cocaine. Questions should be asked matter-of-factly, and the patient should be encouraged to respond truthfully. Surprisingly, when patients become aware of the potential interactions of these drugs with anesthetic medications, most patients will respond honestly about their drug use. Specific to smoking, the patients should be encouraged to stop 6 weeks before surgery to decrease the risk of intraoperative and postoperative respiratory complications.[2] Alcohol, when used chronically, will place the surgical patient at risk (see Chapter 10). When liver function is decreased, metabolism of anesthetic agents is prolonged, nutritional status is altered, and the potential for postoperative complications is increased.

Surgery and Other Treatments. The patient should be questioned about previous surgical procedures and anesthetics. These answers will provide information about the patient's exposure to anesthetics and about any postoperative complications that may have occurred. For example, the patient may report having had an allergic reaction to a medication or may have developed pneumonia after a previous surgery.

Functional Health Patterns. It is important to review each functional health pattern of the patient before surgery. Questions to ask a preoperative patient are listed in Table 16-4.

Objective Data

Physical Examination. It is a requirement of the Joint Commission on Accreditation of Healthcare Organizations (JCAHO) that all patients admitted to the OR have a documented physical examination in the chart. This examination may be done in advance of surgery or on the day of surgery. It may be performed by an advanced practice nurse, a surgeon, an internist, or an anesthesiologist.

In consideration of the patient interview and physical examination, the ACP will assign the patient a physical status rating. This rating is designed to be an indicator of perioperative risk and overall outcome. Table 16-5 defines the current physical status classification rating scale.

Laboratory Testing. Ideally, preoperative laboratory tests should be ordered on the basis of the individual patient history and physical examination. However, many facilities have a written protocol for preoperative laboratory tests. Commonly ordered preoperative laboratory tests can be found in Table 16-6. It is often the responsibility of the nurse sending the patient to surgery to ensure that laboratory data are on the chart. In some institutions it is the nurse who screens the data for abnormalities, informing the surgeon and ACP as appropriate.

NURSING MANAGEMENT: PREOPERATIVE PATIENT

Preoperative Teaching

If the patient is an inpatient, most of the patient and family teaching should be done the evening before surgery. If the patient is an outpatient as is more common, the teaching is generally done in the surgeon's office or preadmission surgical clinic and reinforced on the morning of surgery. Some ambulatory surgical centers have the staff telephone the patients the evening before surgery to answer last minute questions and to reinforce teaching.

Preoperative teaching includes information about preoperative routines, such as the approximate time of surgery and postoperative recovery, and the purpose and goals of postanesthesia care and routines. The patient may receive instruction about deep breathing, use of incentive spirometry, and use of patient-controlled analgesia pumps. The patient will also receive surgery-specific information. For example, a patient having a total joint replacement will be instructed about the use of an immobilizer and possibly about the use of an epidural catheter for postoperative pain control. A patient having open heart surgery will be told about the intensive care unit and its routines.

Preoperative teaching also includes information about any preoperative preparation required before surgery. These preparations may include the need for a preoperative shower or

Table 16-6 Common Preoperative Laboratory Tests

Test	Area Assessed
Urinalysis	Renal status, hydration, urinary tract infection and disease
Chest x-ray	Pulmonary disorders, cardiac enlargement
Blood studies: RBC, Hb, Hct, WBC, WBC differential	Anemia, immune status, infection
Electrolytes	Metabolic status, renal function, diuretic side effects
ABGs, oximetry	Pulmonary and metabolic function
Prothrombin (INR) or partial thromboplastin time	Bleeding tendencies
Blood glucose	Metabolic status, diabetes mellitus
Creatinine	Renal function
Blood urea nitrogen	Renal function
Electrocardiogram	Cardiac disease, electrolyte abnormalities
Pulmonary function studies	Pulmonary status
Liver function tests	Liver function
Type and crossmatch	Blood availability for replacement (elective surgery patients may have own blood available)
Pregnancy	Reproductive status

ABGs, arterial blood gases; *Hb,* hemoglobin; *Hct,* hematocrit; *INR,* international normalized ratio; *RBC,* red blood cells; *WBC,* white blood cells.

PATIENT & FAMILY TEACHING GUIDE

Table 16-7 Preoperative Preparation

1. Instruct patient about preoperative procedures
   a. Time of surgery
   b. Food and fluid restrictions
   c. Informed consent
   d. Physical preparation required (e.g., bowel or skin preparation)
2. Instruct patient about intraoperative experiences
   a. Operating room environment
   b. Roles of anesthesia care provider, scrub nurse, circulating nurse
3. Instruct patient about postoperative procedures
   a. Awakening in recovery room
   b. Purpose of frequent vital signs assessment
   c. Pain control and other comfort measures
   d. Importance of turning, coughing, deep breathing
4. Encourage patient and family members to verbalize concerns
5. Assess patient's and family's areas of concern and respond appropriately

enema. Patients also must be instructed about preoperative food and fluid restrictions. The patient is usually instructed to have nothing by mouth (NPO), including food and fluids, after midnight on the evening before surgery. This protocol may vary if the patient is having local anesthesia. It will be important to verify the NPO protocol of a specific institution when instructing patients, because varying NPO protocols exist. Restriction of fluids and food is designed to minimize the potential risk of aspiration on induction of anesthesia and to decrease the risk of postoperative nausea and vomiting. The patient who has not followed this instruction may have surgery delayed or canceled. It is particularly important that the ambulatory surgical patient understands and adheres to these restrictions.[10]

The positive values of preoperative teaching include an increased satisfaction with nursing care by the patient and nurse, as well as a reduction in fear and anxiety, postoperative vomiting, postoperative pain and the use of pain medications, the number of complications, the duration of hospitalization, and the recovery time following discharge. In addition, the patient has a right to know what to expect and how to participate effectively during the surgical experience.

In preparing the patient psychologically for surgery, the nurse must strike a balance between telling so little that the patient is unprepared and telling so much that the patient is overwhelmed. The nurse who observes carefully and listens sensitively to the patient can usually determine how much information is enough in each instance.

The nurse should be particularly aware of the effect of anxiety on learning and should allow time for repetition, reinforcement, and verification of the patient's understanding. All teaching should be documented in the patient's medical record. A patient teaching guide is presented in Table 16-7. Additional information related to patient education may be found in Chapter 6.

Preoperative Teaching for Outpatients

The outpatient and family should also receive instruction about day-of-surgery events, including patient registration, parking, what to wear, what to bring, and the need to have a responsible adult present for transportation home after surgery.

In addition, the patient should be told the time to arrive and the time of surgery. Arrival time is often 1 to 2 hours before the scheduled time of surgery to allow for completion of preoperative paperwork and preparation and to ensure that all necessary laboratory results have been obtained.

Legal Preparation for Surgery

Before nonemergency surgery can be legally performed, the patient must sign a voluntary and informed consent in the presence of a witness. This document protects the patient, surgeon, and the hospital and its employees (Fig. 16-2). Informed

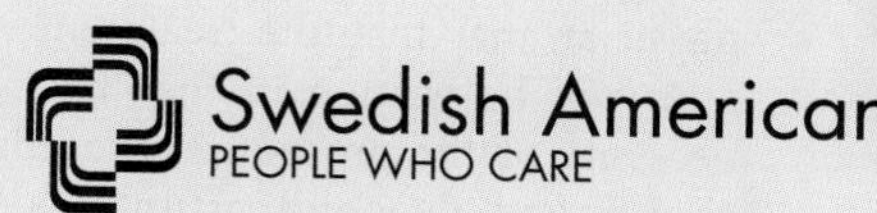

CONSENT TO OPERATION, ANESTHETICS, OBSTETRICAL PROCEDURES, AND OTHER MEDICAL SERVICES

Date ______________ Time ______________ AM PM

1) I authorize the performance on ______________
(Name of patient)
of the following operation ______________
to be performed under the direction of Dr. ______________

2) I consent to the performance of operations and procedures in addition to or different from those now contemplated whether or not arising from presently unforeseen conditions, which the above named doctor or associates or assistants may consider necessary or advisable in the course of the operation.

3) I consent to the administration of such anesthetics as may be considered necessary or advisable by the physician for this service with the exception of ______________
(State "None," "Spinal Anesthesia," etc.)

4) I consent to the photographing or televising of the operation or procedures to be performed, including appropriate portions of my body for medical, scientific, or educational purposes, provided my identity is not revealed by the pictures or by descriptive texts accompanying them.

5) For the purpose of advancing medical education, I consent to the admittance of observers to the operating room.

6) I consent to the disposal by hospital authorities of any tissues or parts that may be removed.

7) I am aware that sterility may result from this operation. I know that a sterile person is not capable of becoming a parent.

8) The nature and purpose of the operation, possible alternative methods of treatment, the risks involved, and the possibility of complications have been fully explained to me. No guarantee or assurance has been given by anyone as to the results that may be obtained.

____
(Signature of Patient or Authorized Person to Consent for Patient)

____
(Witness)

*Note: Cross out any paragraphs above that do not apply.

Fig. 16-2 Operative consent.

consent is an active, shared decision-making process between the provider and the recipient of care.

For consent to be valid, three conditions must be met. First, there must be *adequate disclosure* of the diagnosis; the nature and purpose of the proposed treatment; the risks and consequences of the proposed treatment; the probability of a successful outcome; the availability, benefits, and risks of alternative treatments; and the prognosis if treatment is not instituted. Second, the patient must demonstrate *sufficient comprehension* of the information being provided. Because preoperative medications may cloud a patient's comprehension, the operative consent must be signed before any preoperative medication is given. Third, the recipient of care must *give consent voluntarily.* The patient must not be persuaded or coerced in any way to undergo the procedure.[11]

Although the physician is ultimately responsible for obtaining the consent, the nurse may be responsible for obtaining and witnessing the patient's signature on the consent form. At this

ETHICAL DILEMMAS

Informed Consent

SITUATION

The nurse discusses a patient's impending surgery in the preoperative holding area. It becomes obvious that this competent adult patient was not fully informed of the alternatives to this surgery. She has signed the consent form but clearly was not fully informed about her options. What should the nurse do?

DISCUSSION

Informed consent requires that patients be fully informed about the need for surgery, the nature of the surgery, and the alternatives to surgery. If this patient was not fully counseled about her alternatives, she could not have given her informed consent to this surgery. No one should attempt to coerce a patient into signing a consent form or witness a form that has not been fully explained. The nurse should make sure that the patient discusses with her surgeon any and all questions and concerns she might have about the surgery before she is anesthetized. Her rights to full disclosure are of greater importance than maintaining the surgical schedule.

ETHICAL AND LEGAL PRINCIPLES

- Elements of informed consent include full disclosure of risks, benefits, and alternatives; competency of the patient to understand the information and make a decision; and voluntary (not coerced) agreement.
- A patient's autonomy and bodily integrity are best upheld and protected by full disclosure of risks, benefits, and alternatives.
- Medical paternalism would maintain the position that (1) medical professionals know what is best for patients, (2) patients can never fully understand enough to give fully informed consent, and (3) the contract with the patient implies consent to appropriate treatment. However, it is unethical and illegal to deny complete information on the grounds that full disclosure might be worse than withholding information or alternatives.

time the nurse can be a patient advocate, verifying that the patient (or family member) understands the consent form and its implications. The nurse has an important role as a patient advocate in ensuring that consent for surgery is truly voluntary and informed. The nurse will contact the surgeon and explain the need for additional information if the patient is unclear about operative plans. The patient must be aware that permission may be withdrawn at any time, including after the permit has been signed.

If the patient is a minor, is unconscious, or is mentally incompetent to sign the permit, the written permission may be signed by a responsible family member. Local hospital policies should be checked for further clarification on this matter.

A true medical emergency may override the need to obtain consent. When immediate medical treatment is needed to preserve life or to prevent serious impairment to life and the individual patient is incapable of giving consent, the next of kin may give consent. If reaching the next of kin is not possible, the physician may institute treatment without written consent. A note will be written in the chart documenting the medical necessity of the procedure. Procedures for obtaining consent vary among states and institutions. The nurse should be aware of the state's nurse practice act and the institutional or agency policies that apply to an individual situation.

Advance Directives. With advances in technology and pharmacology, new limits have been reached in the artificial support of patients through artificial ventilation, hydration, and nutrition. Ethical issues of withholding care and withdrawing care challenge all health care providers. The issue of withholding care is distinctly different from withdrawing life-sustaining treatment once it has been initiated. Health care providers have several options available related to withdrawing care, which may vary somewhat from state to state. These options include the following:

1. Obtain a court order to withdraw treatment.
2. Wait for death.
3. Follow advance directives, including a living will and durable power of attorney.
4. Follow verbal refusal of the patient for life support.
5. Follow directives of a surrogate decision maker.

Because these situations are often unexpected and occur suddenly, it is now required by law that before surgery inpatients be provided the opportunity to sign advance directives, including a living will and power of attorney. Figures 16-3 and 16-4 provide examples of these forms. Many centers offer the forms to outpatients as well. A living will recognizes the right of a person to make a written declaration instructing the person's physician to withhold or withdraw death-delaying procedures in the event that the person becomes terminally ill and is unable to express his or her wishes. It may be signed by any patient 18 years of age and older in the presence of two witnesses. A durable power of attorney for health care recognizes the right of an individual to delegate control over treatment decisions to another person in the event that the individual becomes incompetent.[12] It is often the nurse who is responsible for providing the forms to the patient, for answering questions, and for placing the signed forms in the chart.

Day of Surgery

Day-of-surgery preparation will vary a great deal depending on whether the patient is an inpatient or an outpatient. If the patient is an inpatient, it will be the responsibility of the hospital nurse to ensure that the patient is ready and appropriately prepared for surgery. If the patient is an outpatient, the patient or family member will share the responsibility for preoperative preparation. The nursing responsibility immediately before surgery includes final preparation of the patient, as well as checking to determine that all orders have been carried out and that records are complete and ready to accompany the patient to the OR.

The patient should be assisted as necessary in dressing for surgery. Most institutions require that a patient wear a hospital gown with no underclothes. Some surgery centers allow the patient to wear underwear, depending on the surgical procedure to be performed. It is recommended that the patient wear no cosmetics or nail polish, because observation of skin color

DURABLE POWER OF ATTORNEY FOR HEALTH CARE

POWER OF ATTORNEY made this ______ day of ______ 19 ______

1. I, the undersigned, hereby appoint (insert name and address of agent) ______

______

as agent to act for me and in my name to make any and all decisions for me concerning my personal care, medical treatment, hospitalization and health care and to require, withhold or withdraw any type of medical treatment or procedure, even though my death may ensue. My agent shall have the same access to my medical records that I have, including the right to disclose the contents to others. My agent shall also have full power to make disposition of any part or all of my body for medical purposes, authorize an autopsy and direct the disposition of my remains. (Neither the attending physician nor any other health care provider may act as your agent.)

2. The powers granted above shall be subject to the following rules or limitations (if none, leave blank):

______

______

(The subject of life-sustaining treatment is of particular importance. For your convenience in dealing with that subject, some general statements concerning the withholding or removal of life-sustaining treatment are set forth below. If you agree with one of these statements, you may initial that statement; but do not initial more than one.)

____ (I do not want my life prolonged nor do I want life-sustaining treatment to be provided or continued if my agent believes the burdens of the treatment outweigh the expected benefits. I want my agent to consider the relief of suffering, the expense involved and the quality as well as the possible extension of my life in making decisions concerning life-sustaining treatment.

____ (I want my life to be prolonged and I want life-sustaining treatment to be provided or continued unless I am in a coma which my attending physician believes to be irreversible, in accordance with reasonable medical standards at the time of reference. If and when I have suffered irreversible coma, I want life-sustaining treatment to be withheld or discontinued.

____ (I want my life to be prolonged to the greatest extent possible without regard to my condition, the chances I have for recovery or the cost of the procedures.

3. This power of attorney shall become effective on ______
4. This power of attorney shall terminate on ______
5. If any agent named by me shall die, become legally disabled, resign, refuse to act or be unavailable, I name the following (each to act alone and successively, in the order named) as successors to such agent:

______

______

6. If a guardian of my person is to be appointed, I nominate the following to serve as such guardian (If same as agent, leave blank):

______

7. I am fully informed as to all the contents of this form and understand the full import of this grant of power to my agent.

Signed ______
Principal

The principal has had an opportunity to read the above form and has signed the form or acknowledged his or her signature or mark on the form in my presence.

______ (Witness) Residing at ______

(You may, but are not required to, request your agent and successor agents to provide specimen signature below. If you include specimen signature in this Power of Attorney, you must complete the certification opposite the signatures of the agents.)

Specimen signatures of agent (and successors)	I certify that the signature of my agent (and successors) are correct.
______ (agent)	______ (principal)
______ (successor agent)	______ (principal)
______ (successor agent)	______ (principal)

Fig. 16-3 Durable power of attorney for health care.

will be important and equipment used to monitor oxygenation will be placed on the patient's fingertip (pulse oximeter). An identification band should be put on the patient and, if applicable, an allergy band. All patient valuables should be returned to a family member or locked up according to institutional protocol. If the patient prefers not to remove a wedding ring, the ring can be taped securely to the finger to prevent loss. All prostheses, including dentures, contact lenses, and glasses, are generally removed to prevent loss or damage to them. Hearing aids are usually left in place to allow the patient to better follow instructions. Consideration should be given to the privacy and self-esteem needs of the patient.

The patient should be encouraged to void before going into surgery. This should be done before the administration of any preoperative medication. Many preoperative medications have the potential to interfere with balance and judgment and could

LIVING WILL DECLARATION

This declaration is made this ________ day of ________________, 19 ____ (month, year). I, ______________________________, being of sound mind, willfully and voluntarily make known my desires that my moment of death shall not be artificially postponed.

If at any time I should have an incurable and irreversible injury, disease, or illness judged to be a terminal condition by my attending physician who has personally examined me, and has determined that my death is imminent except for death delaying procedures. I direct that such procedures which would only prolong the dying process be withheld or withdrawn, and that I be permitted to die naturally with only the administration of medication, sustenance, or the performance of any medical procedure deemed necessary by my attending physician to provide me with comfort care.

In the absence of my ability to give directions regarding the use of such death delaying procedures, it is my intention that this declaration shall be honored by my family and physician as the final expression of my legal right to refuse medical or surgical treatment and accept the consequences from such refusal.

Signed ______________________

City, County and State of Residence ______________________________

The declarant is personally known to me and I believe him or her to be of sound mind. I did not sign the declarant's signature above for or at the direction of the declarant. At the date of this instrument I am not entitled to any portion of the estate of the declarant according to the laws of intestate succession or to the best of my knowledge and belief, under any will of declarant or other instrument taking effect at declarant's death, or directly financially responsible for declarant's medical care.

Witness ______________________

Witness ______________________

Fig. 16-4 Living will.

result in a patient fall. Urination before surgery prevents involuntary elimination under anesthesia, lessens the chance of accidental nicking of the bladder during surgery, and reduces the possibility of urinary retention during early postoperative recovery.

The use of a preoperative checklist (Fig. 16-5) will help ensure that no detail has been omitted. The nurse should determine that all preoperative orders and procedures have been completed and that the chart and documentation is complete before giving any preoperative medications. It is especially important to verify the presence of a signed operative consent, laboratory data, a history and physical examination report, a record of any consultations, baseline vital signs, and nurses' notes complete to that point.

Preoperative Medications

Preoperative medications are used for a variety of reasons, as summarized in Table 16-8. A patient may receive a single drug

St. Joseph Hospital, Inc.
Albuquerque, New Mexico
☐ St. Joseph Hospital
☐ St. Joseph West Mesa Hospital

ADDRESSOGRAPH

PREOPERATIVE CHECK LIST

Name of Procedure ______
Date of Surgery ______

	INITIALS O.R.	UNIT
1. Operative Permit signed and on chart: (initial if completed)		
2. History and Physical in chart: (initial if present)		
3. New Progress and Doctor's order sheet on chart: (initial if present)		
4. Consultation: ______ NA ______		
5. Laboratory results: Hct: ______ Hgb: ______ K+ ______		
6. Miscellaneous Pre-Op Lab studies: SMAC ______ Chest X-Ray ______ ECG ______ Type & Cross Match ______ # of units ______		
7. Allergies: ______ NKA ______ Front of chart labelled ______ NPO ______		
8. Prosthetic removed: Contact lenses ______ glasses ______ limb ______ eyes ______ hearing aid ______ dentures ______ removable bridgework ______ capped teeth present ______ location ______ etc. ______		
9. Old chart to O.R. with patient: ______ Not requested ______ No old chart ______		
10. Preoperative Medication given: ______ TIME: ______ None ordered ______		
11. Vital Signs: (time taken) ______ B.P. ______ P ______ R ______ T ______		
12. Skin prep on unit: ______ wash ______ scrub ______ shower ______		
13. Wearing hospital gown: ______ other: ______		
14. Hairpins and/or wig removed: ______ NA ______		
15. Make-up, false eyelashes and nail polish removed: ______ NA ______		
16. Disposition of valuables: (money, credit cards) To business office ______ family ______ none ______ To O.R. with patient: Rings (taped) ______ religious articles ______ NONE ______		
17. Antiembolism stockings/bandages: Applied ______ with patient ______ NA ______		
18. Urinary status: voided ______ catheterized ______ indwelling cath ______		
19. Medications to O.R. with patient: ______ none ______		
20. Addressograph on chart ______		
21. Chart and transport slip checked ______		
Chart signed off ______		

Signature and Title	initials	Signature and Title	initials

Fig. 16-5 Preoperative checklist.

or a combination of drugs (Table 16-9). Benzodiazepines and barbiturates are used for their sedative and amnestic properties. Anticholinergics are given to reduce secretions. Narcotics may be given to decrease intraoperative anesthetic requirements and to decrease any pain associated with placement of IV catheters or other preoperative monitors. Antiemetics may be given to decrease nausea and vomiting.

Other medications that may be administered preoperatively include antibiotics, heparin, eyedrops, and routine prescription medications. Antibiotics may be ordered for a patient with a history of congenital or valvular heart disease to prevent the development of bacterial endocarditis. They may also be ordered for the patient undergoing surgery where wound contamination is either a potential risk (e.g., gastrointestinal surgery) or where wound infection could have serious postoperative consequences (e.g., cardiac and joint replacement surgery). Antibiotics are most commonly administered IV and may be started either preoperatively or in the OR.[13]

The use of low-dose heparin (5000 to 10,000 units subcutaneously) or enoxaparin (Lovenox) administered 6 to 12 hours preoperatively has been shown to reduce the rate of deep venous thrombosis and pulmonary embolism by 60%. Because most patients are not admitted to the hospital preoperatively, it has also been shown that heparin therapy may be started up to 2 days after surgery with similar outcomes.[13]

Eyedrops are commonly ordered and administered preoperatively for the patient undergoing cataract and other eye surgery. Many times the patient will require multiple sets of eyedrops, administered at 5-minute intervals. It is important to administer these drugs as ordered and on time to adequately prepare the eye for surgery.

Administering preoperative medications would be easier if two lists of medications were developed; the first would list the medications that are always given on the day of surgery, and the second would list those that are never given on the day of surgery. It would facilitate patient teaching and eliminate confusion. Unfortunately, such lists do not exist. Most patients will be advised to take routine cardiac, antihypertensive, and asthma medications on the day of surgery. It is important to carefully check written preoperative orders and to clarify which medications should be taken on the day of surgery. In the case of insulin it is important to clarify the dose.

Premedications may be administered orally, IV, subcutaneously, or IM. Oral medications should be given 60 to 90 minutes before the patient arrives in the OR. Because patients are fluid restricted before surgery, it is important for the patient to swallow these medications with only a minimal amount of water. Intramuscular and subcutaneous injections should be given 30 to 60 minutes before arrival (minimally 20 minutes).[13] Intravenous medications are usually administered to the patient after arrival to the preoperative holding area or OR. Once the medication is given, charting should be completed because the patient is now prepared for surgery and ready for transport to the OR. Premedication should be administered to the patient after all other preoperative preparation has been completed. The patient should be told that the medications will help with relaxation, and drowsiness may occur without loss of consciousness. If an anticholinergic drug is used, the patient needs to know that although the mouth will feel dry, no fluids should be taken.

Table 16-8 Purposes of Preoperative Medication

- Relieve apprehension and anxiety
- Promote sedation and amnesia
- Provide analgesia
- Facilitate induction of anesthesia
- Prevent nausea and vomiting
- Prevent autonomic reflex response
- Decrease anesthetic requirements
- Decrease respiratory and gastrointestinal secretions

Transportation to the Operating Room

If the patient is an inpatient, the OR staff sends transport personnel to the patient's room with a cart to transport the patient to surgery. The nurse assists the patient in transferring from the hospital bed to the OR cart, and the side rails of the cart are raised and secured. The nurse should ensure that the chart goes with the patient, as well as any ordered preoperative equipment, such as antiembolism devices or the patient's inhaler if the patient is an asthmatic. In many institutions the family may accompany the patient to the holding area.

If the patient is an outpatient, the patient may be transported to the OR by cart or wheelchair, or in the absence of premedication may even walk accompanied to the OR. In all cases it is important for the nurse to ensure patient safety in transport.

Because the patient is leaving the nursing unit or outpatient area for surgery, it will be important for the nurse to instruct the family where to wait for the patient during surgery. Many hospitals have a surgical waiting room where personnel communicate the status of the patient to the family. It is in this waiting room that the surgeon can locate the family after surgery and where families can be notified that the surgery is complete.

While the patient is in surgery the hospital nurse can prepare the patient's room in consideration of the patient's needs after surgery. The bed is remade, and, if necessary, disposable pads are placed for any anticipated drainage. Any additional necessary equipment, including IV poles, oxygen, suction, and additional pillows for positioning, should also be placed in the room. The

DRUG THERAPY

Table 16-9 Frequently Used Preoperative Medications

Class	Purpose and Effects	Drug
Benzodiazepines	Reduce anxiety Induce sedation Induce amnesia	Midazolam (Versed) Diazepam (Valium) Lorazepam (Ativan)
Narcotics	Relieve discomfort during preoperative procedures	Morphine Meperidine (Demerol) Fentanyl (Sublimaze)
H_2-receptor antagonists	Increase gastric pH Decrease gastric volume	Cimetidine (Tagamet) Famotidine (Pepcid) Ranitidine (Zantac)
Antacids	Increase gastric pH	Sodium citrate
Antiemetics	Increase gastric emptying Decrease nausea and vomiting	Metoclopramide (Reglan) Droperidol (Inapsine)
Anticholinergics	Decrease oral and respiratory secretions Prevent bradycardia	Atropine Glycopyrrolate

room should be organized to facilitate entry of the transport cart. By having these items readily available and the room ready, patient transfer from the PACU or the OR will be smooth.

GERONTOLOGIC CONSIDERATIONS

Preoperative Patient

Approximately 24% of all surgical procedures are performed on patients older than 65 years of age.[7] The most frequently performed procedures in the older adult are cataract extraction, prostatectomy, herniorraphy, cholecystectomy, and hip stabilization.[7]

The risks associated with anesthesia and surgery increase in the older patient. In general, the older the patient, the greater the risk of complications after surgery. The surgical risk in the older adult relates to normal physiologic aging changes that compromise organ function, reduce reserve capacity, and limit the body's ability to adapt to stress. (Physiologic changes associated with aging are presented in Table 4-1.) This decreased ability to cope with stress, compounded by the common additional burden of one or more chronic illnesses, anxiety, and the surgery itself, increases the risk of complications. The increased risks are not only a result of aging, but are caused by the increased prevalence of coexisting diseases and by a decline in basic bodily functioning. It is important to consider the physiologic status or condition of the patient in planning care and not simply the chronologic age.

When preparing the older adult for surgery, it is important to obtain a detailed history and complete physical examination. Often this patient will be referred to an internist for medical approval before surgery. Preoperative laboratory tests, including an ECG and a chest x-ray, will be important in planning the choice and technique of anesthesia. Inquiry about family support will also be important. With the increase in outpatient surgical procedures and shorter postoperative hospitalizations, family support is an important consideration in the continuity of care for the older patient.

The nurse must remember that the thought processes and cognitive abilities may be slowed or impaired in some older adults. In addition, vision and hearing may be diminished. Therefore the older patient may require increased time to complete preoperative testing, dress for surgery, understand preoperative instructions, and complete any needed preoperative preparation.

Adding to situational change and loss, the perceived threat or loss of health associated with surgery may be overwhelming to the older adult. This overwhelming loss, which can affect independence, lifestyle, and self-esteem, may result in ineffective coping. The nurse must be particularly alert when assessing and caring for the older adult surgical patient. An event that has little effect on a younger patient may be overwhelming to the older patient.

CRITICAL THINKING EXERCISES

CASE STUDY

Preoperative Patient

Patient Profile

Mrs. Frances D., an 82-year-old retired librarian, is admitted to the hospital with complaints of abdominal pain, alternating diarrhea and constipation, and blood in her stool.

Subjective Data

- Has history of hypertension for 40 years
- Takes hydrochlorothiazide
- Has history of diabetes mellitus, type 2, since age 60, diet controlled
- Has surgical history that includes a cesarean section at age 30 and appendectomy at age 19
- Has not eaten for 2 days and has had decreasing oral intake for the past 2 weeks
- Reports a 10 lb weight loss
- Sleeps poorly at night and is drowsy during the day
- Lives alone and has no immediate family

Objective Data

Physical Examination

Alert, well-oriented, slightly obese older woman with painful, palpable abdominal mass.

Diagnostic Studies

- Ultrasound—abdominal mass in area of transverse colon
- Hematocrit—27%
- Stool for guaiac—positive

Collaborative Care

Scheduled for exploratory laparotomy, colon resection, and possible colostomy.

Critical Thinking Questions

1. What factors may influence Mrs. D.'s response to hospitalization and surgery?
2. Given Mrs. D.'s history, what preoperative laboratory tests would you want to assess and why?
3. What potential perioperative complications might you expect for Mrs. D.?
4. What topics would you include in Mrs. D.'s preoperative teaching plan?
5. Based on the assessment data presented, write one or more appropriate nursing diagnoses. Are there any collaborative problems?

NURSING RESEARCH ISSUES

1. Can a patient assessment effectively predict the need for specific preoperative laboratory tests as opposed to using a predetermined list of required preoperative laboratory tests?
2. Does the preoperative administration of antiemetics to specific patient groups reduce the incidence of nausea and vomiting in the postoperative period?
3. Does the nurse use preoperative patient interview data in planning preoperative instruction?
4. Is there a difference in the accuracy of preoperative assessment data collected by a patient-completed form as compared with a nurse-completed questionnaire?

REVIEW QUESTIONS

The number of the question corresponds to the same-numbered objective at the beginning of the chapter.

1. Which of the following surgical procedures involves removal of a body organ?
   a. colostomy
   b. mammoplasty
   c. herniorrhaphy
   d. cholecystectomy
2. A patient reports having an allergy to penicillin. Which of the following questions would elicit the most useful information for the nurse?
   a. "When did the reaction occur?"
   b. "Did you notify your physician of the allergy?"
   c. "What type of allergic reaction did you have?"
   d. "What infection did you have that required penicillin?"
3. The patient who is at greatest risk for surgical and anesthetic complications is
   a. a 42-year-old scheduled for a breast biopsy.
   b. a 3-year-old boy scheduled for a hernia repair.
   c. an 80-year-old scheduled for an exploratory laparotomy.
   d. an 18-year-old scheduled for an emergency appendectomy.
4. The nurse's role in informed consent for surgery may include
   a. obtaining the patient's signature on the consent form.
   b. asking the patient for consent for the planned procedure.
   c. explaining the risks and consequences of the proposed surgery.
   d. informing the patient of the prognosis if the surgical procedure is refused.
5. A nursing intervention to assist a preoperative patient in coping with fear of pain would be to
   a. describe the degree of pain expected.
   b. explain the availability of pain medication.
   c. divert the patient when talking about pain.
   d. inform the patient of the frequency of pain medication.
6. The nursing measure that should be performed last on the morning of surgery is to
   a. ask patient to void in the bathroom.
   b. check chart for signed consent form.
   c. administer preanesthetic medication.
   d. remove jewelry and lock up securely.
7. The nurse administering preoperative medication recognizes that
   a. preoperative medications may help reduce anesthetic requirements.
   b. intravenous medications can be administered only by an anesthesiologist on the day of surgery.
   c. a preoperative diazepam (Valium) tablet should be administered within 15 minutes of scheduled surgery.
   d. an intramuscular injection of secobarbital should be administered 2 hours before the scheduled surgery.
8. A primary consideration in the instruction of the older preoperative patient is
   a. using large-print material.
   b. teaching early in the morning.
   c. standing very close to aid communication.
   d. recognizing that cognitive function may be decreased.

References

*1. Malone M: Top patient concerns: comfort and education, *Same Day Surg* 6:69, 1996.
2. Williams G: Preoperative assessment and health history interview, *Nurs Clin North Am* 32:395, 1997.
3. Pasternak L: Preanesthesia evaluation of the surgical patient, *ASA Refresher Courses in Anesthesiology* 16:205, 1996.
4. McGoldrick K: *Ambulatory anesthesiology,* Baltimore, 1995, Williams & Wilkins.
*5. Brooks-Brunn J: Minimizing pulmonary complications, *Heart Lung* 24:94, 1995.
6. Litwack K: *Postoperative pulmonary complications,* Sacramento, 1995, CME Resource.
7. Litwack K: *The elderly surgical patient,* Sacramento, 1995, CME Resource.
8. Litwack K: Care of the special needs patient, *Nurs Clin North Am* 32:457, 1997.
9. Guidelines for the management of latex allergies and safe use of latex in perioperative practice settings, *AORN J* 66:726, 1997.
10. Lancaster K: Patient teaching in ambulatory surgery, *Nurs Clin North Am* 32:417, 1997.
11. Ireland D: Legal issues in ambulatory surgery, *Nurs Clin North Am* 32:469, 1997.
12. Berrio M, Levesque M: Advance directives. Most patients don't have one. Do yours? *AJN* 96:25, 1996.
13. Litwack K: *Postanesthesia care nursing,* ed 2, St Louis, 1995, Mosby.

Resources

Resources for this chapter are listed after Chapter 18 on p. 413.

*Nursing research-based articles.

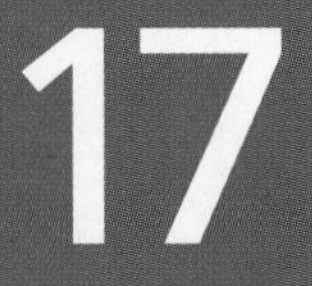

REMEMBER to check out your **companion CD-ROM**

17 NURSING MANAGEMENT Patient During Surgery

Patricia Robertson Hercules, Bettyann Hutchisson, Kim Litwack, & Chuck Biddle

www.mosby.com/MERLIN/medsurg_lewis

LEARNING OBJECTIVES

1. Describe the physical environment of the operating room and the holding area.
2. Describe the functions of the members of the surgical team.
3. Identify needs experienced by the patient undergoing surgical procedures.
4. Discuss the role of the perioperative nurse when managing the care of the patient undergoing surgery.
5. Describe basic principles of aseptic technique used in the operating room.
6. Differentiate between general and regional or local anesthesia, including advantages, disadvantages, and rationale for choice of the anesthetic technique.
7. Identify the basic techniques and drugs used to induce and maintain general anesthesia.
8. Discuss techniques for administering local and regional anesthesia.
9. Discuss the characteristics of adjunct agents used with general anesthesia.

Nursing care of the surgical patient requires an understanding of surgery and surgical interventions. This knowledge allows the nurse to monitor the patient's response to the stressors related to the surgical experience. Use of the nursing process during the operative phase of care is necessary as a framework for the delivery of care. The needs of the patient determine the type of nursing care delivered. These needs are based on the current health status of the patient and the type of surgical intervention anticipated.

Historically, surgical interventions have taken place in the traditional environment of the hospital operating room (OR) suite. The advancements in surgical technology, improvements in the administration of anesthesia, and the changes in health care have resulted in where and how surgery is performed. The number of surgical procedures being performed in the ambulatory surgery setting is rising, thereby lowering the number of cases being performed in the hospital environment. According to the SMG Marketing Group, hospitals are predicting a decrease of in-house surgical procedures and an increase in outpatient procedures (Table 17-1). Although all surgical specialties are represented in the ambulatory surgery setting, ophthalmology, gynecology, plastic surgery, and ear, nose, and throat (ENT) are the specialties with the highest patient loads.

The perioperative nurse must remember that the surgical procedure holds the same seriousness and potential for complications regardless of where it is being performed. The patient and family members still have the same needs and fears regardless of where the procedure is being performed. The nurse must still maintain asepsis in the surgical environment, keep current on the new technologies, and continue to be a patient advocate for safe practice.

Differences that are noted in the ambulatory surgery setting as compared with the traditional in-hospital surgery setting include healthier patient populations, shorter procedures, quicker turnovers, and less time available for perioperative teaching of the patient and family.

For the purposes of this chapter, the traditional OR suite and role and function of the perioperative nurse will be used to discuss the management of the patient during the surgical experience.

PHYSICAL ENVIRONMENT

Operating Room

The traditional surgical environment is a unique acute care setting removed from other hospital clinical units. It is controlled geographically, environmentally, and bacteriologically, and it is restricted in terms of the inflow and outflow of personnel (Fig. 17-1). It is preferable to have the physical location of the OR adjacent to the postanesthesia care unit (PACU) and the surgical intensive care unit for quick transportation of the surgical postoperative patient and close proximity to anesthesia personnel if complications arise. This allows for close collaboration for postanesthesia recovery and intensive care follow-up. Careful consideration of the design, location, and control of the physical environment assists with the prevention of infection and provides physical safety and comfort for the patient.

Several methods are used to prevent the transmission of infection. Filters and controlled airflow in the ventilating systems provide dust control. Positive air pressure in the rooms

Reviewed by Virginia Printz-Feddersen, RNC, MSN, CNS, CNOR, CNRN, Clinical Nurse Specialist, Lovelace Health Systems, Albuquerque, NM; and Jill H. Pendarvis, RNC, MA, CNOR, Emeritus Associate Professor, Intercollegiate Center for Nursing Education, Spokane, Wash.

Table 17-1 Inpatient vs. Outpatient Surgery Trends for Hospitals

	Total Inpatient Surgical Operations (× 1000)	Total Outpatient Surgical Operations (× 1000)
1990	10,903	11,020
1992	10,766	12,129
1994	10,326	12,691
1996	9,968	14,147
1998*	9,543	15,443

Source: SMG Marketing Group, Oct 1996.
*Projection.

prevents air from entering the OR from the halls and corridors. Dust-collecting surfaces such as open shelves, windows, and ledges are omitted. Materials that are resistant to the corroding effects of strong disinfectants are used. The functional design facilitates the practice of aseptic technique by the OR team.

Physical safety and comfort are aided by the use of OR furniture that is adjustable, easy to clean, and easy to move. All equipment is checked frequently to ensure electrical safety. The lighting is designed to provide a low- to high-intensity range for a precise view of the surgical site. A communication system provides a means for the delivery of routine and emergency messages.[1,2,3]

The temperature is controlled from 68° F to 75° F (20° C to 24° C), and the humidity is regulated at a minimum of 50% to facilitate patient comfort under the surgical drapes, team comfort during the procedure, and an environment that is unfavorable to bacterial incubation and growth.[1,3]

The privacy of the patient is achieved by restricting the influx of hospital personnel and visitors. Special permission must be obtained to enter the suite during the surgical procedure. The complexity of an ongoing operative procedure does not allow for the presence of extraneous personnel and visitors (Fig. 17-2).

Holding Area

The holding area, frequently called the preoperative holding area, is a special waiting area inside or outside the surgical suite. The size varies according to hospital design and can range from a centralized area to accommodate numerous patients to a small designated area immediately outside the actual room scheduled for the surgical procedure. In the holding area the perioperative nurse makes the final identification and assessment before the patient is transferred into the OR for surgery.[4,5] Many minor procedures can also be performed in the holding area, such as inserting intravenous (IV) catheters and arterial lines, removing casts, and medication administration.

In some settings another area for holding is identified as the admission, observation, and discharge (AOD) area. This area is designed to allow early-morning admissions for outpatient surgery, same-day admission, and inpatient holding before surgery. In this holding area the nurse can assess the patient for preoperative data, observe the patient both before and after surgery, and allow recovery for a sufficient length of time before discharge to either the home or an inpatient room. The AOD area significantly affects the patient's stay throughout outpatient surgery and prevents unnecessary overnight stays in the inpatient setting.[4,5]

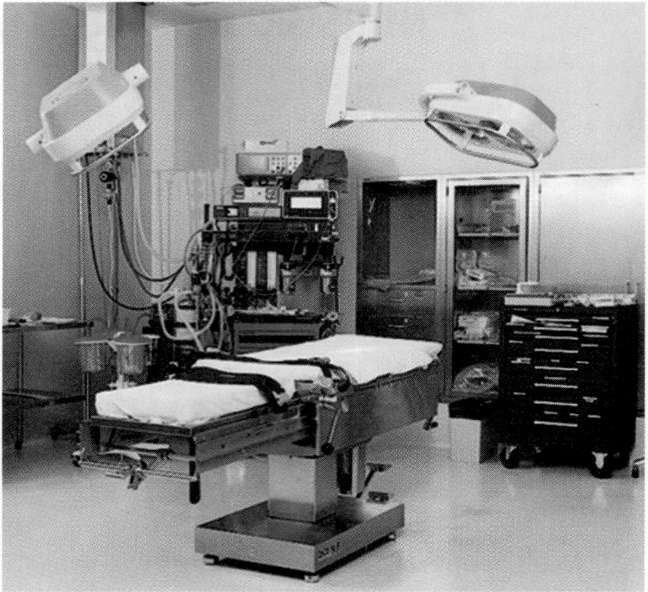

Fig. 17-1 Traditional operating room.

Some institutions permit the family or a friend to wait with the patient until it is time to be transferred to the OR. Separation from loved ones just before surgery can produce anxiety, and allowing them to stay with the patient alleviates stress.

SURGICAL TEAM

Registered Nurse

When the patient awaiting surgery arrives from home or is transported from the acute care inpatient area to the holding area, the nurse is usually the first member of the surgical team encountered. Along with the final assessment and necessary tasks before the surgery, the nurse provides physical comfort measures and assists through communication and touch in reducing the patient's anxiety.

The perioperative nurse is a registered nurse who implements patient care based on the nursing process. Different functions may be assumed by the perioperative nurse that involve either sterile or nonsterile activities. If the nurse is not scrubbed, gowned, and gloved and remains in the unsterile field, the function of *circulating* is implemented. If the nurse follows the designated scrub procedure, is gowned and gloved in sterile attire, and remains in the sterile field, the function of *scrubbing* is implemented. Some specific intraoperative activities of each function are outlined in Table 17-2.

The perioperative nurse is not limited to task-oriented duties and actively implements nursing care throughout the patient's surgical experience. Examples of nursing activities that characterize each phase surrounding the surgical experience are presented in Table 17-3.

Licensed Practical Nurse and Surgical Technician

In many institutions the scrubbed function is performed by a trained OR surgical technician or a licensed practical nurse.

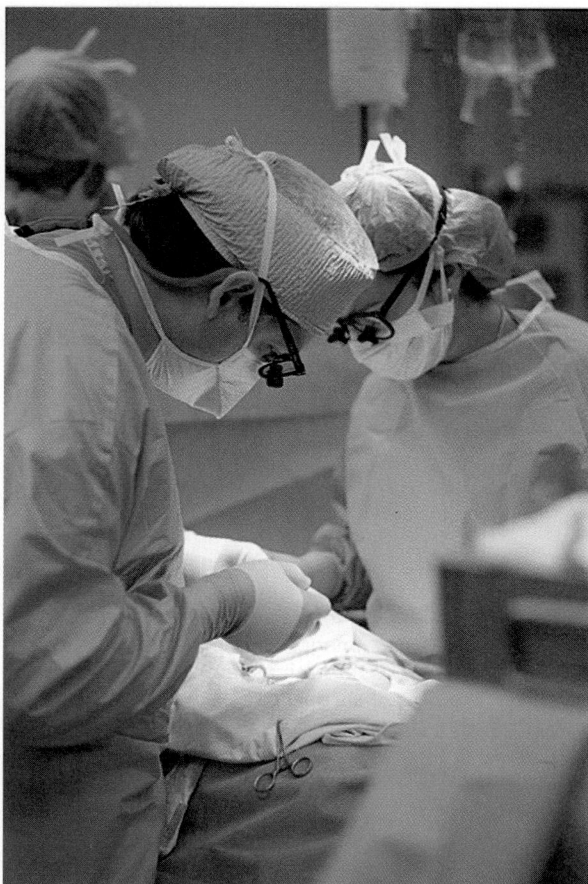

Fig. 17-2 The complexity of the operative procedure does not allow for the influx of extra personnel or visitors.

Table 17-2 Intraoperative Activities of the Perioperative Nurse

Circulating/Nonsterile Activities

- Reviews anatomy, physiology, and the surgical procedure
- Assists with preparing the room
  - Practices aseptic technique
  - Monitors the activities of others
  - Ensures that needed items are available and sterile (if required)
  - Checks mechanical and electrical equipment and environmental factors
  - Arranges the furniture in workable order
- Identifies and assesses the patient, then plans and coordinates the intraoperative nursing care
- Checks the chart and relates pertinent data
- Admits the patient to the operating room suite
- Assists with transferring the patient to the operating table
- Participates in insertion and application of monitoring devices
- Protects the patient during induction of anesthesia
- Positions the patient
- Prepares the patient's skin for the surgical procedure
- Monitors the draping procedure and all activities requiring asepsis
- Completes the intraoperative record
- Records, labels, and sends to proper locations tissue specimens and cultures
- Measures blood and fluid loss
- Records amount of drugs and medications used during local anesthesia
- Coordinates all activities in the room with team members and other health-related personnel and departments
- Counts sponges, needles, and instruments.
- Monitors practices of aseptic technique in self and others
- Accompanies the patient to the postanesthesia recovery area
- Reports pertinent information to the recovery area nurses

Scrub/Sterile Activities

- Reviews anatomy, physiology, and the surgical procedure
- Assists with preparation of the room
- Scrubs, gowns, and gloves self and other members of the surgical team
- Prepares the instrument table and organizes sterile equipment for functional use
- Assists with the draping procedure
- Passes instruments to the surgeon and assistants by anticipating their needs
- Counts sponges, needles, and instruments
- Monitors practices of aseptic technique in self and others
- Keeps track of irrigation solutions used for calculation of blood loss
- Reports amounts of local anesthesia and epinephrine solutions used by anesthesia care provider

The scrubbed, or assistive, person assists the surgeon by passing instruments and implementing other technical functions during the surgical procedure. This role is supervised by and can also be assumed by a registered nurse.

Surgeon and Assistant

The surgeon is the physician who performs the surgical procedure. The surgeon may be the patient's primary physician or one who was selected by the patient's physician or the patient. The surgeon is primarily responsible for the following:

1. Preoperative patient history and physical assessment, including need for surgical intervention, choice of surgical procedure, and management of preoperative workup
2. Patient safety and management in the OR
3. Postoperative management of the patient

The surgeon's assistant is usually a physician who functions in an assisting role during the surgical procedure. The assistant usually holds retractors to expose surgical areas and assists with hemostasis and suturing. In some instances, especially in educational settings, the assistant may perform some portions of the operative procedure under the direct supervision of the surgeon.

In some institutions the surgeon's assistant is a registered nurse or a nonphysician who functions in the role of the

Table 17-3 Examples of Nursing Activities Surrounding the Surgical Experience

Preoperative	Intraoperative	Postoperative
Assessment	**Implementation**	**Evaluation**
Home/Clinic/Holding Area Initiates initial preoperative assessment Plans teaching methods appropriate to patient's needs Involves family in interview	**Maintenance of Safety** Ensures that the sponge, needle, and instrument counts are correct Positions the patient Functional alignment Exposure of surgical site Maintenance of position throughout procedure Applies dispersive electrode to patient Provides physical support	**Postanesthesia/Discharge Area** Determines patient's immediate response to surgical intervention
Surgical Unit Completes preoperative assessment Coordinates patient teaching with other nursing staff Develops a plan of care	**Monitoring of Physical Status** Reports changes in patient's pulse, respirations, temperature, and blood pressure Distinguishes normal from abnormal cardiopulmonary data Monitors blood loss Monitors urine output as applicable	**Surgical Unit** Evaluates effectiveness of nursing care in the OR Determines patient's level of satisfaction with care given during perioperative period Evaluates products used on patient in the OR Determines patient's psychologic status Assists with discharge planning
Surgical Suite Verifies surgical site Assesses patient's level of consciousness, skin integrity, mobility, emotional status, and functional limitations Reviews chart Identifies patient	**Monitoring of Psychologic Status** Provides emotional support to patient Stands near or touches patient during procedures and induction Continues to assess patient's emotional status Communicates patient's emotional status to other appropriate members of the health care team	**Home/Clinic** Seeks patient's perception of surgery in terms of the effects of anesthetic agents, impact on body image, immobilization Determines family's perceptions of surgery
Planning Determines a plan of care	**Communication of Intraoperative Information** States patient's name States type of surgery performed Provides contributing intraoperative factors (e.g., drain, catheters, and blood loss) States physical limitations States impairments resulting from surgery Reports patient's preoperative level of consciousness Communicates necessary equipment needs	

OR, operating room.

assistant under the direct supervision of the physician. Hospital policies define this role and physician responsibility when the assistant's position is filled by a nonphysician.

Registered Nurse First Assistant

Nursing roles in the perioperative setting change and evolve as technology and health care change. One of these changes is the use of the registered nurse first assistant (RNFA). The RNFA works in collaboration with the surgeon to produce an optimal surgical outcome for the patient. The Association of Operating Room Nurses (AORN) revised position statement of RNFAs says this perioperative nurse must have formal education for this role and will assist the surgeon by handling tissue, using instruments, providing exposure to the surgical site, assisting with hemostasis, and suturing.[3,6]

Anesthesia Care Provider

The term *anesthesia care provider* (ACP) may be defined as "one who administers anesthesia" and can refer to an anesthesiologist or a nurse anesthetist. An anesthesiologist is a medical doctor who has completed a residency in the field of anesthesia and is credentialed by the American Board of Anesthesiology. A nurse anesthetist is a registered nurse who has passed a national certification examination to become a certified registered nurse anesthetist (CRNA). Both the anesthesiologist and the CRNA are qualified to administer anesthetics to the patient and

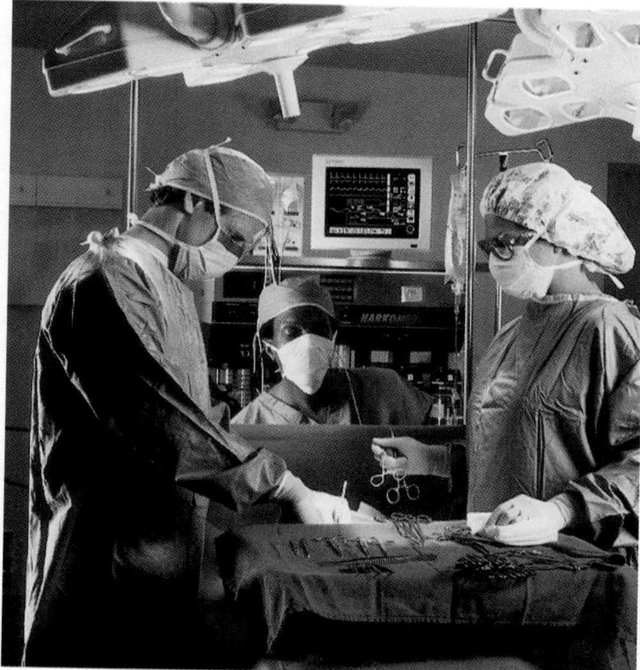

Fig. 17-3 Members of the surgical team collaborate on the care of the patient before, during, and after the surgical procedure.

assume responsibility for the maintenance of physiologic homeostasis throughout the intraoperative period.

Anesthesia may be provided by the anesthesiologist or CRNA, working alone or in combination. The latter is often termed the *anesthesia team approach.* When working in the team approach, the anesthesiologist assumes the responsibility of supervision of the CRNA while the CRNA administers the anesthesia. When the CRNA is practicing alone, the surgeon assumes the responsibility for medical supervision. The ACP is also governed by state practice acts and the policies of the hospital where the provider is practicing.

The following responsibilities are generally accepted by the ACP:

1. Assess the patient preoperatively to determine the safest anesthetic for the particular patient's needs and anticipated operative procedure.
2. Prescribe preoperative and adjunctive medications.
3. Monitor patient's cardiac status.
4. Monitor patient's vital signs throughout the procedure.
5. Administer the anesthetic during the surgical procedure, and inform the surgeon if difficulties arise during the patient's anesthetic course.
6. Administer fluids and electrolytes, medications, and blood products throughout the surgical procedure.
7. Supervise the postanesthesia recovery of the patient in the PACU, and document the patient's postanesthetic recovery in the first 24 hours.

In preparation for and carrying out the surgical procedure, members of the surgical team (circulating nurse, scrub assistant, surgeon, assistant, and ACP) collaborate to ensure that the patient is receiving the best possible care (Fig. 17-3).

NURSING MANAGEMENT: PATIENT BEFORE SURGERY

The preoperative assessment of the surgical patient establishes baseline data for intraoperative and postanesthesia care. Assessment data that are provided by the patient and family in the holding area and data from the inpatient nursing units are verified and important to ensure that a plan of care can be developed.

Psychosocial Assessment. The perioperative nurse who cares for the patient in the OR is knowledgeable about the ongoing activities that occur when a patient is transferred into the surgical suite. This knowledge allows for informative and reassuring explanations, especially to the anxious patient. General questions regarding surgery or anesthesia can usually be answered by the perioperative nurse. Examples of these questions include, "When will I go to sleep?" "Who will be in the room?" "When will my doctor arrive?" "How much of my body will be exposed and to whom?" "Will I be cold?" "When will I wake up?" Specific questions relating to details of the surgical procedure and anesthesia are referred to the surgeon or ACP.

It is especially important that the perioperative nurse has knowledge of the patient's spiritual and cultural habits and beliefs. Care must be taken that infringement on the patient's rights and privileges is not made without consent.

Physical Assessment. Physical assessment data that are specifically important to intraoperative nursing care include baseline data such as vital signs, height, weight, age, allergic reactions to both food and medication, condition and cleanliness of skin, skeletal and muscle impairments, perceptual difficulties, level of consciousness, nothing-by-mouth (NPO) status, and any sources of pain or discomfort. Vital signs are important as baseline data when drugs and anesthetics are administered. These data provide a means to evaluate the effects of intraoperative medications. Height and weight of the patient guide the nurse regarding the width and length of the operating table. Age may indicate the need for extra warmth because there are age-related decreases in body metabolism. Some allergic reactions may be avoided with such simple measures as a change in "prepping" solutions or the type of tape used with dressings. Catastrophic reactions can be eliminated if latex sensitivity is determined before the procedure begins. (See discussion of latex allergies on p. 388. Latex allergies are also discussed in Chapters 12 and 16.) The condition and cleanliness of the skin determine the amount and type of intraoperative skin preparation solutions and will alert the team to the potential for infection as a result of open or closed skin lesions. Knowledge of skeletal and muscle impairments helps prevent injury during positioning. Perceptual difficulty, such as a vision or hearing impairment, will guide the nurse in adapting communication techniques to individual needs. An altered level of consciousness necessitates increased safety and protection techniques. Communicating identified sources of pain to other health team members prevents subjecting the patient to unnecessary discomfort.

Chart Assessment. Required chart data vary with hospital policy, patient condition, and specific surgical procedures. Examples of data that are obtained during the preoperative assessment include the following:

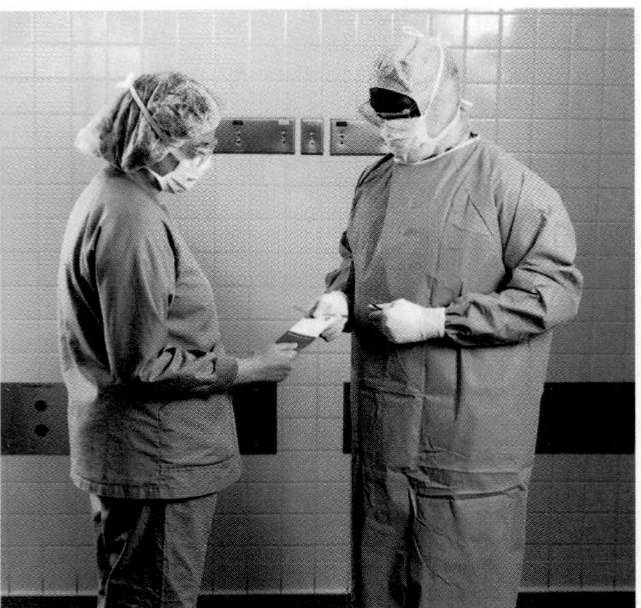

Fig. 17-4 Surgical attire is worn by all persons entering the operating room suite.

1. History and physical examination
2. Urinalysis
3. Complete blood cell count
4. Serum electrolyte values
5. Chest x-ray
6. Electrocardiogram
7. Other diagnostic tests (e.g., computed tomography [CT] scan)
8. Human immunodeficiency virus (HIV) status (in some situations)
9. Pregnancy testing (if applicable)
10. Surgical consent
11. Allergies
12. Type and crossmatch if applicable

A knowledge of these chart data will contribute to an understanding of past and present history, cardiopulmonary status, and potential for infection.

Admitting the Patient. Hospital policy designates the exact procedure that should be followed when admitting the patient to the holding area and OR suite. A general routine includes initial greeting, extension of human contact and warmth, and proper identification. The identification process includes asking the patient to state her or his name, the surgeon's name, and the operative procedure and location. In addition, the hospital identification numbers are compared with the patient's own identification band and chart. The patient is further identified by the surgeon before anesthesia induction. In some institutions identification may take place in the holding area and, in others, in the OR itself.

The admitting procedure is continued with reassessment of the patient and allowance of time for last-minute questions. The nurse continues to review the chart for the previously mentioned data and notes any abnormalities or changes. The patient is questioned concerning valuables, prostheses, and last intake of food and fluid. Validation is made that the correct preoperative medication was given, if ordered. A warm blanket, pillow, or position adjustment is provided if the patient is uncomfortable. Most hospitals require the patient's hair to be covered just before transfer to the OR suite to reduce potential shedding.

NURSING MANAGEMENT: PATIENT DURING SURGERY

Room Preparation. Before transferring the patient into the scheduled OR, the nurse spends significant time preparing the room to ensure privacy, safety, and prevention of infection. Surgical attire (pants and shirts, masks, protective eyewear, and caps or hoods) is worn by all persons entering the OR suite (Fig. 17-4). All electrical and mechanical equipment is checked for proper functioning. Aseptic technique is practiced as each surgical item is opened and placed systematically on the instrument table. Sponges, needles, and instruments are counted to ensure accurate retrieval at the close of the procedure.[4,7]

During this time and during the procedure the functions of the teams are delineated. The scrub person will scrub hands and arms, don sterile gown and gloves, and touch only those items in the sterile field. The circulating nurse remains in the unsterile field and implements those activities that permit touching all unsterile items and the patient.

Transferring the Patient. Once the patient has been properly identified and the OR has been adequately prepared, the patient is transported into the room for the surgery. Each time a patient is transferred from one bed to another, the wheels of the stretcher should be locked, and a sufficient number of personnel should be available to lift, guide, and prevent accidental falling. Once the patient is on the operating table, safety straps should be snugly placed across the patient's thighs. At this time the monitor leads (e.g., electrocardiograph leads) are usually applied and an IV catheter is inserted if it was not in place when the patient arrived from the holding area.

Scrubbing, Gowning, and Gloving. All sterile members of the surgical team (scrub assistant, surgeon, surgical technician, and assistant) are required to cleanse their hands and arms by scrubbing with a brush and detergent before entering the sterile field. This is done to eliminate dirt and skin oil to decrease the microbial count as much as possible. The surgical scrub helps prevent the growth of microbes beneath the surgical glove and gown. The detergent used should be a broad-spectrum microbiocidal agent. The procedure should involve a minimum of 2 minutes of mechanical friction with a specially designed sterile surgical brush. During the actual procedure of scrubbing, the team members' fingers and hands should be scrubbed first with progression to the arms and elbows. The hands should be held higher than the elbows at all times to prevent detergent suds and water from draining from the unclean (above elbows) to the clean and previously scrubbed areas (hands and fingers).[1,3,7]

Once the scrub procedure is completed, the team members enter the room to put on the surgical gowns and gloves. Because the gowns and gloves are sterile, it is permissible for the scrubbed people to manipulate and organize all sterile items for use during the procedure.

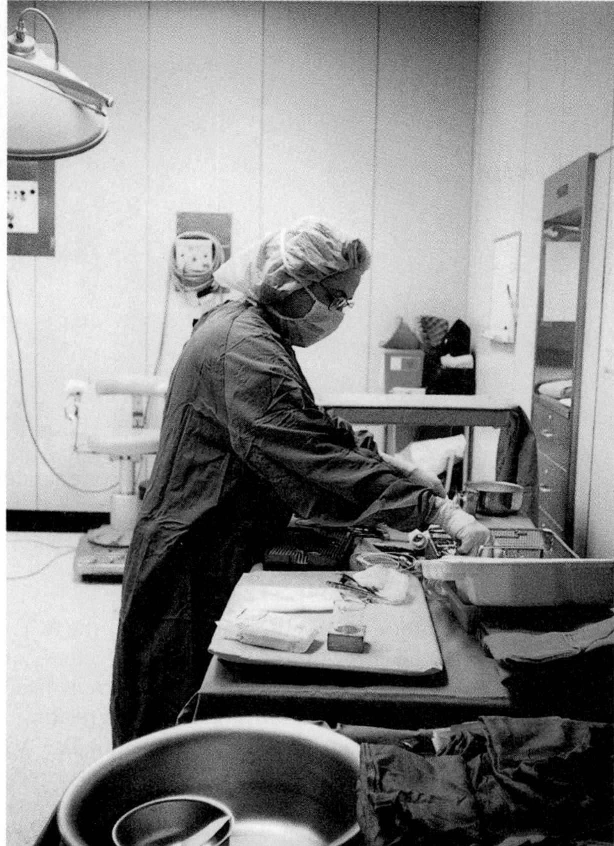

Fig. 17-5 A sterile field is created before surgery.

Table 17-4 Principles of Basic Aseptic Technique in the Operating Room

1. All materials that enter the sterile field must be sterile.
2. Sterilization is the only means by which an item can be considered sterile; if it comes in contact with an unsterile item, it becomes contaminated.
3. Contaminated items should be removed immediately from the sterile field.
4. Sterile team members must wear only sterile gowns; once dressed for the procedure, they should recognize that all parts of the gown are considered *unsterile* except the front from chest to table level and the sleeves to 2 inches above the elbow.
5. A wide margin of safety must be maintained between the sterile and unsterile field.
6. Team members' motions should be from sterile to sterile or from unsterile to unsterile.
7. Tables are considered sterile only at tabletop level, and items extending beneath this level are considered contaminated.
8. The edges of a sterile package are considered contaminated once the package has been opened.
9. Bacteria travel on airborne particles and will enter the sterile field with excessive air movements and currents.
10. Bacteria travel with moisture and liquids by capillary action from surface to surface and contamination occurs.
11. Bacteria harbor on the patient's and the team members' hair, skin, and respiratory tracts and must be confined by appropriate covers, masks, and scrubbing.

Basic Aseptic Technique. To prevent infections, aseptic technique is practiced in the OR to prevent the entrance of microorganisms into the surgical wound. This is implemented through the creation and maintenance of a sterile field (Fig. 17-5). The center of the sterile field is the site of the surgical incision. Inanimate items in the sterile field include surgical items and equipment that have been sterilized by appropriate sterilization methods.

There are specific principles that the team members should understand to practice aseptic technique. Unless these principles are followed, the safety of the patient is compromised, and the potential for postoperative infection is increased. Table 17-4 presents basic principles of aseptic technique.[1,3,7]

In addition to following the principles of aseptic technique, the surgical team is responsible for following the guidelines established by the U.S. Occupational Safety and Health Administration (OSHA) to protect the patient and the team from exposure to blood-borne pathogens. These guidelines emphasize universal precautions, engineering and work practice controls, and the use of personal protective equipment such as gloves, gowns, aprons, caps, face shields, masks, and protective eye wear (see Table 11-18). This is especially important in the OR environment because of the high potential for exposure to blood-borne pathogens.[8,9]

Assisting the Anesthesia Care Provider. While the perioperative nurse checks the OR to complete its preparation, the anesthesia care provider (ACP) prepares the patient for the administration of the anesthetic. The nurse must understand the mechanism of anesthetic administration and the pharmacologic effects of the agents. The nurse should know the location of all emergency drugs and equipment in the OR area.

The circulating nonsterile perioperative nurse may be involved in placing monitoring devices to be used during the surgical procedure (e.g., urinary catheter, electrocardiogram leads) and the electrical grounding pad. If the patient is to have a general anesthetic, the nurse remains at the patient's side to ensure safety and to assist the ACP. These responsibilities may include obtaining blood pressure measurements, starting an IV line, and protecting the patient from falling.

Positioning the Patient. Positioning the patient usually follows induction of a general anesthetic. If an alternative anesthetic technique (e.g., epidural or local anesthesia) is used, the ACP will indicate when to begin the positioning of the patient. When positioning for the surgical procedure, care must be used to (1) provide correct skeletal alignment; (2) prevent undue pressure on nerves, bony prominences, eyes, and skin; (3) provide for adequate thoracic excursion; (4) prevent occlusion of arteries and veins; (5) avoid stretching and compression of nerve tissue; (6) provide modesty in exposure; and (7) recognize and respect individual needs such as previously assessed aches, pains, or deformities. It is a nursing responsibility to secure the extremities, provide adequate padding and support, and obtain sufficient physical or mechanical help to avoid unnecessary straining of self or patient.

Various positions in which the patient may be placed include supine, prone, Trendelenburg's, lateral, kidney, lithotomy, jackknife, and sitting. The supine is the most common position used. It is suited for surgery involving the abdomen, heart, and breast. Following anesthesia, if only one arm is tucked at the patient's side the head will be turned toward the extended arm. The prone position allows easy access for back surgeries (e.g., laminectomies). The lithotomy position is used for some types of pelvic organ surgery (e.g., vaginal hysterectomy).

Preparing the Surgical Site. The purpose of skin preparation, or "prepping," is to reduce the number of organisms available to migrate to the surgical wound. The task of prepping is usually the responsibility of the circulating nurse.

The skin is prepared by mechanically scrubbing or cleansing around the surgical site with antimicrobial agents identified as being nonallergic to the patient. If the patient is very hairy or if the hair will interfere with the surgical procedure, the nurse will remove it using clippers. This will be done as close to incision time as possible. The area is then scrubbed in a circular motion. The principle of scrubbing from the clean area (site of the incision) to the dirty area (periphery) is observed at all times. A liberal area is cleansed to allow for added protection and unexpected occurrences during the procedure.

After preparation of the skin, the sterile members of the surgical team drape the area. Only the site to be incised is left exposed.

Safety Considerations. All surgical procedures, regardless of where they take place, can put the patient at risk for injury. These injuries can be infections, physical injury from positioning or equipment used, or the surgery itself. Lasers and new technologies in electrosurgical units can cause injury to the patient and surgical staff. The perioperative nurse must be familiar with fire safety issues to protect the patient and staff against burns. Smoke evacuators are being used in the OR on a more regular basis to decrease the amount of smoke plume in the perioperative setting (Fig. 17-6).

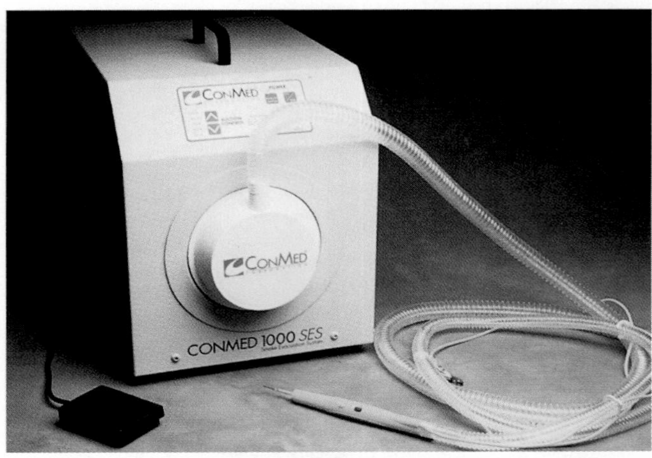

Fig. 17-6 The use of a smoke evacuator is recommended when using an electrosurgical unit.

Patient After Surgery

Through constant observation of the surgical progress, the ACP anticipates the end of the surgical procedure and uses appropriate types and doses of anesthetic agents so that their effects will be minimal at the end of the surgical procedure. This also allows greater physiologic control of the patient during the transfer to the PACU.

The ACP and the surgeon or another member of the surgical team accompany the patient to the PACU. A report of the patient's status and the procedure is communicated. The OR nurse evaluates the patient's response to nursing care based on outcome criteria established when the plan of care was developed (Table 17-5).[2,6,10]

CLASSIFICATION OF ANESTHESIA

The anesthetic technique and agents are selected by the ACP in collaboration with the surgeon and the patient. Factors contributing to the decision include the patient's current health status and history, emotional stability, and factors relating to the operative procedure (e.g., length, position, site). The ACP validates this information during the preoperative assessment, obtains anesthesia consent, writes orders for the preoperative medication, and assigns the patient an anesthesia classification. The anesthesia classification, an independent guideline for the ACP, is based on the physiologic status of the patient with no regard to the surgical procedure to be performed. A scale of 1 to 5 is used with 1 being a healthy patient and 5 being a moribund patient having surgery as a last resort or resuscitative effort. An intraoperative complication is more likely to develop with a higher classification number (see Table 16-5).

Anesthesia is classified according to the effect that it has on the patient's sensorium (central nervous system) and pain perception. *General anesthesia* is defined as a loss of sensation with loss of consciousness, skeletal muscle relaxation, analgesia, and elimination of the somatic, autonomic, and endocrine responses, including coughing, gagging, vomiting, and sympathetic responsiveness. *Local anesthesia* is defined as the loss of sensation without loss of consciousness. Local anesthesia may be induced topically or via infiltration intracutaneously or subcutaneously. *Conscious sedation* ("twilight sleep") is defined as a depressed level of consciousness following intravenous administration of a benzodiazepine, usually in combination with a narcotic. Conscious sedation retains the patient's ability to maintain her or his own airway and respond appropriately to verbal commands, yet achieves a level of emotional and physical acceptance of a painful procedure (e.g., colonoscopy). *Regional anesthesia* is defined as the loss of sensation to a region of the body when a specific nerve or group of nerves is blocked with the administration of a local anesthetic without loss of consciousness (e.g., spinal, epidural, or peripheral nerve block).

General Anesthesia

General anesthesia is usually the technique of choice for patients who (1) are having surgical procedures that require sig-

Table 17-5 Projected Outcomes for the Surgical Patient

- Demonstration of knowledge of the physiologic and psychologic responses to surgical intervention
- Absence of infection
- Maintenance of skin integrity
- Freedom from injury related to positioning, extraneous objects, or chemical, physical, and electrical hazards
- Maintenance of fluid and electrolyte balance
- Satisfaction with pain relief
- Participation in the rehabilitative process

nificant skeletal muscle relaxation, last for long periods of time, require awkward positions because of the location of the incisional site, or require control of respiration; (2) are extremely anxious; (3) refuse or have contraindications for local or regional anesthetic techniques; and (4) are uncooperative because of their emotional status, lack of maturity, intoxication, head injury, or pathophysiologic processes that do not permit them to remain immobile for any length of time. General anesthesia may be administered by an IV, inhalation, or rectal route (Table 17-6).

Intravenous Induction Agents. Virtually all routine adult general anesthetics begin with an IV induction agent. These agents induce a pleasant sleep, with a rapid onset of action that patients find desirable. A single dose lasts only a few minutes, long enough for an endotracheal tube to be placed and an inhalation agent to be started. Induction agents are classified as either barbiturates or nonbarbiturate hypnotics.

Barbiturates. In the past the IV agents used to induce general anesthesia have been the short-acting barbiturates. Of those available, the two most frequently used are thiopental (Pentothal) and methohexital (Brevital). Induction with both agents is rapid and only a small dose is required. In higher doses, these agents can cause cardiovascular alterations, hypotension, tachycardia, and respiratory depression. However, because the duration of action of these agents is extremely short (less than 5 minutes), the need for intervention to manage the side effects of these drugs is minimal. Rectal administration of short-acting barbiturates is rarely used today because acceptable pharmacologic alternatives are available.

Nonbarbiturate hypnotics. Etomidate (Amidate) and propofol (Diprivan) are nonbarbiturate hypnotic agents. Unlike the barbiturates, etomidate produces little change in cardiovascular dynamics, and therein lies its greatest benefit. Etomidate is useful for hemodynamically unstable patients who require emergency surgery. Etomidate is associated with adverse effects, including myoclonia (transient skeletal muscle movements), hiccoughs, nausea and vomiting, and inhibition of adrenocortical synthesis. Because of these side effects, etomidate is used only in situations where no other anesthetic alternative exists.

Propofol (Diprivan) is the newest induction agent. Classified as an intravenous hypnotic, propofol has a rapid onset of action with the added benefit that it can be used for the maintenance of anesthesia, as well as induction. As a nonbarbiturate, propofol is rapidly eliminated, making it the ideal agent for short outpatient procedures. Propofol also causes less nausea and vomiting than other induction agents, with some evidence suggesting that it may have direct antiemetic action.[11]

DRUG THERAPY

Table 17-6 General Anesthesia Drugs and Methods

Intravenous Agents
- Barbiturates
  - Thiopental (Pentothal)
  - Methohexital (Brevital)
- Nonbarbiturate hypnotics
  - Etomidate (Amidate)
  - Propofol (Diprivan)

Inhalation Agents
- Volatile liquids
  - Halothane (Fluothane)
  - Enflurane (Ethrane)
  - Isoflurane (Forane)
  - Desflurane (Suprane)
  - Sevoflurane (Ultane)
- Gaseous agents
  - Nitrous oxide

Anesthesia Adjuncts
- Narcotics
  - Fentanyl (Sublimaze)
  - Sufentanil (Sufenta)
  - Morphine sulfate
  - Meperidine (Demerol)
  - Alfentanil (Alfenta)
  - Remifentanil (Ultiva)
- Sedative-hypnotics
  - Midazolam (Versed)
  - Diazepam (Valium)
  - Lorazepam (Ativan)
- Muscle relaxants
  - Depolarizing agents
    - Succinylcholine (Anectine)
  - Nondepolarizing agents
    - Vecuronium (Norcuron)
    - Atracurium (Tracrium)
    - Pancuronium (Pavulon)
    - Tubocurarine (Curare)
    - Metocurarine (Metubine)
    - Gallamine (Flaxedil)
    - Pipecuronium (Arduan)
    - Doxacurium (Nuromax)
    - Rocuronium (Zemuron)
    - Mivacurium (Mivacron)
- Antiemetics
  - Droperidol (Inapsine)
  - Ondansetron (Zofran)
  - Metoclopramide (Reglan)
  - Prochlorperazine (Compazine)
  - Promethazine (Phenergan)

Dissociative Anesthetics
- Ketamine hydrochloride (Ketalar)

Inhalation Agents. Inhalation agents are the foundation of general anesthesia. The inhalation agents used for general anesthesia may be volatile liquids (liquid at room temperature) or gases (gas at room temperature). Volatile liquids are administered through a specially designed vaporizer after being mixed with oxygen as a carrier gas.

Inhalation agents enter the body through the alveoli in the lungs. They may be administered through a mask, an endotracheal tube, a laryngeal mask airway, or a tracheostomy. Ease of administration and rapid excretion by ventilation make them desirable agents. One undesirable characteristic is the irritating effect of inhalation agents on the respiratory tract. Complications that may arise are coughing, laryngospasm (muscular constriction of the larynx), bronchospasm, increased secretions, and respiratory depression.[12]

Inhalation agents are most commonly administered via an endotracheal tube placed into the trachea once the patient has been induced with an intravenous agent. The endotracheal tube permits control of ventilation and airway protection, both for patency and to prevent aspiration. Complications of endotracheal intubation include those primarily associated with its insertion and removal. These include damage to teeth and lips, laryngospasm, laryngeal edema, postoperative sore throat, and hoarseness caused by injury or irritation of the vocal cords or surrounding tissues.

Volatile liquids. There are currently five volatile liquid anesthetics being used today, including halothane (Fluothane), enflurane (Ethrane), isoflurane (Forane), desflurane (Suprane), and sevoflurane (Ultane). Although there are variations among the agents, all are bronchodilators, vasodilators, myocardial depressants, and muscle relaxants. The incidence of postoperative nausea and vomiting is relatively low with these agents. However, patient variability, procedure factors, and anesthetic adjuncts often result in patients experiencing postoperative nausea and vomiting. Because these agents are eliminated rapidly and there is little remaining analgesia, the patient must be assessed for the onset of pain.

Halothane is a potent bronchodilator, making the agent a useful one for patients with preexisting pulmonary disease, including asthma and chronic obstructive pulmonary disease. During its administration, cardiac depression and peripheral vasodilation resulting in hypotension may occur. Because of these hemodynamic effects, and because halothane can be hepatotoxic under certain circumstances, its use has decreased dramatically in favor of newer agents. Use of this agent is still common in inhalation inductions in children because its odor is relatively nonirritating and fairly acceptable to patients.

Enflurane is a potent vasodilator, dilating all major arterioles by direct smooth muscle relaxation. Cerebral blood flow increases, with a rise in intracranial pressure. Seizure activity has been seen during enflurane anesthesia at high concentrations. Enflurane's major weakness is its high degree of lipid solubility, resulting in a prolonged, unpredictable duration of action. It is rarely used.

Isoflurane is more rapid in its onset and duration than enflurane. It undergoes minimal metabolism and is essentially devoid of toxicity to any organs of the body. Isoflurane causes less cardiovascular depression than either halothane or enflurane and therefore may be better tolerated by patients.

Desflurane is structurally similar to isoflurane with one distinct chemical difference. It is this difference that causes its relative insolubility in blood and tissues, resulting in a rapid induction and rapid emergence from anesthesia. This may be a particularly useful benefit for patients having outpatient surgical procedures. Its cardiovascular effects are similar to those of isoflurane, and it does not appear to cause renal or hepatic toxicity. It is the most widely used volatile anesthetic agent today.

Sevoflurane is the most recently FDA-approved inhalation anesthetic. Like desflurane, it is highly insoluble, essentially nonmetabolized, and predictable in its effects on the cardiovascular and respiratory systems, and it allows for rapid induction and emergence from anesthesia. It is nonirritating to the respiratory tract.

Nitrous oxide. Nitrous oxide is the most widely used gaseous inhalation agent, primarily because of its adjunctive properties in potentiating the other volatile anesthetics. By potentiating the other agents, the ACP can use lesser concentrations of the volatile agents, thereby decreasing the negative side effects of these agents and increasing the speed of induction. Its primary disadvantage is that nitrous oxide is a relatively weak anesthetic, so it is rarely used alone. In addition to being administered with a volatile agent, nitrous oxide is also administered with oxygen to prevent hypoxemia.

Adjuncts to General Anesthesia. The administration of general anesthesia is rarely limited to one agent. Drugs added to an inhalation anesthetic (other than an IV induction agent) are termed *adjuncts.* These agents are added to the anesthetic regimen specifically to achieve unconsciousness, analgesia, amnesia, muscle relaxation, or autonomic nervous system control. Because no one agent can produce all of the desired outcomes of a general anesthetic, multiple medications are used to achieve the goals. Adjuncts include opiates, sedative-hypnotics (benzodiazepines), neuromuscular blocking agents (muscle relaxants), and antiemetics.

Opiates. Opiates are also termed *narcotics.* Narcotics are used preoperatively for sedation and analgesia (morphine), intraoperatively for induction and maintenance of anesthesia (fentanyl [Sublimaze], sufentanil [Sufenta], remifentanil [Ultiva], alfentanil [Alfenta]), and postoperatively for pain management (fentanyl, meperidine, morphine). The narcotics used intraoperatively are primarily morphine derivatives.

Narcotics are used to alter the perception of pain and the response to pain. Intraoperatively, narcotics are used to produce sufficient analgesia to reduce or abolish nervous system responses to surgical stimuli. When administered before the end of a surgical procedure, the residual analgesia often carries over into the PACU, allowing the patient to awaken relatively pain free.

All narcotics produce dose-related respiratory depression. Respiratory depression may be difficult to detect in the OR and therefore requires close observation and pulse oximetry monitoring. Respiratory depression can be reversed with naloxone (Narcan). However, its use is often associated with a reversal of the analgesic effects of the narcotics as well.

Cardiovascular side effects of narcotics are minimal in usual analgesic doses. In high doses, and when combined with other anesthetics, bradycardia and peripheral vasodilation are seen. Narcotics also have a direct stimulating effect on the vomiting center in the medulla. This may result in aspiration if the patient is too sedated to maintain his or her own airway.

Sedative-hypnotics (benzodiazepines). Sedative-hypnotics (benzodiazepines) are widely used for premedication before surgery for their amnestic effects, as agents for the induction and maintenance of anesthesia, for conscious sedation, as sup-

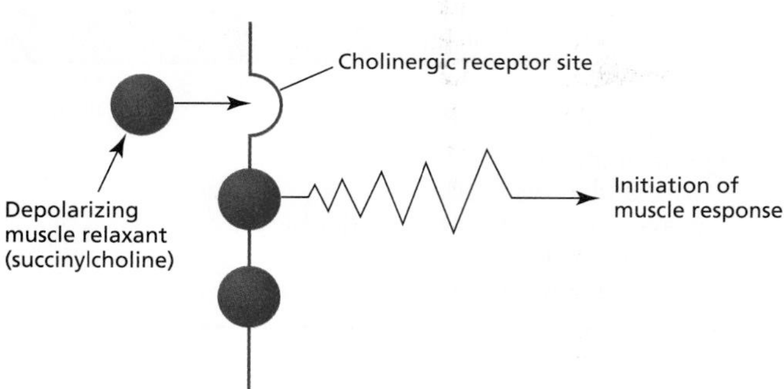

Fig. 17-7 Depolarization with succinylcholine.

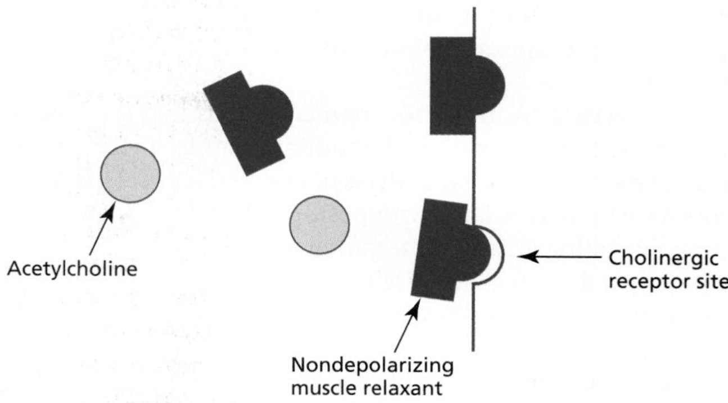

Fig. 17-8 Mode of action of nondepolarizing muscle relaxants.

plemental intravenous sedation during local and regional anesthesia, and for postoperative anxiety and agitation. Currently three benzodiazepines are used clinically: diazepam (Valium), midazolam (Versed), and lorazepam (Ativan). Because of its excellent amnestic property, shorter duration of action, and absence of pain on injection, midazolam is presently the most frequently used. It is most commonly administered intravenously or via intramuscular injection. It is the most common anesthesia adjunct in both ambulatory surgery settings and in conscious sedation. The other agents are limited in their usefulness because of their long duration of action. Benzodiazepines potentiate the effects of narcotics, increasing the potential for respiratory depression. Flumazenil (Romazicon) is a specific benzodiazepine antagonist in the event that reversal is required.

Neuromuscular blocking agents. Neuromuscular blocking agents (muscle relaxants) are used as adjuncts to general anesthesia to facilitate endotracheal intubation and to optimize surgical working conditions by providing relaxation (paralysis) of skeletal muscles. Neuromuscular blocking agents interrupt the transmission of nerve impulses at the neuromuscular junction.[13] Based on their mechanisms of action, neuromuscular blocking agents are classified as either depolarizing or nondepolarizing muscle relaxants.

Depolarizing muscle relaxants mimic the action of acetylcholine. Depolarizing agents bind to cholinergic receptor sites on muscle cells, causing depolarization of the cellular membrane (Fig. 17-7). As long as the cell remains depolarized, it is incapable of responding to further stimulation of acetylcholine, resulting in neuromuscular blockade. Succinylcholine (Anectine) is currently the only depolarizing muscle relaxant being used. Succinylcholine has a rapid onset of action (30 to 60 seconds) and a short duration of action (3 to 5 minutes), making it an ideal agent to use for intubation.

Nondepolarizing agents (see Table 17-6) compete with acetylcholine at the cholinergic receptor site. The high concentration of nondepolarizing muscle relaxant blocks the acetylcholine from reaching the motor end plate of the muscle cell. Neuromuscular transmission is inhibited, resulting in neuromuscular blockade (Fig. 17-8). The duration of action of the nondepolarizing agents ranges from short acting (10 to 20 minutes) to intermediate acting (20 to 40 minutes) to long acting (50 to 105 minutes). Selection of a nondepolarizing agent for a given patient depends on the duration of the procedure to be performed, the route of elimination of the drug (in consideration of the patient's renal and hepatic function), and potential adverse drug side effects and the patient's ability to tolerate them. The nondepolarizing muscle relaxants are reversible with anticholinesterase agents (e.g., neostigmine, pyridostigmine, edrophonium). Anticholinesterases restore neuromuscular function by binding to the enzyme acetylcholinesterase and inactivating it. As acetylcholinesterase is inactivated, levels of acetylcholine are allowed to rebuild. Acetylcholine ultimately displaces the nondepolarizing muscle relaxant, allowing for restoration of normal neuromuscular transmission (Fig. 17-9).

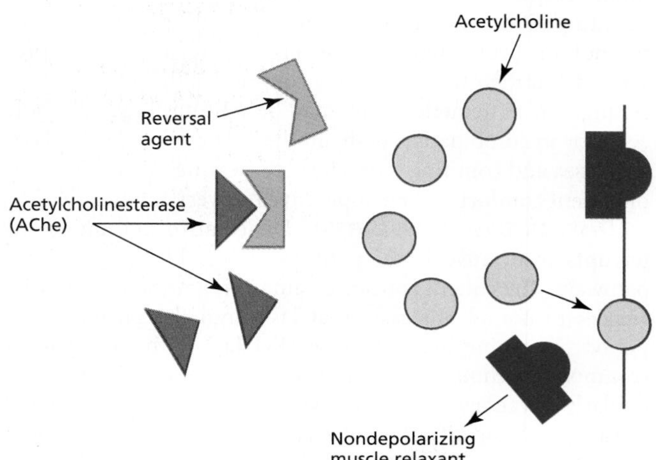

Fig. 17-9 Reversal of neuromuscular blockade.

Disadvantages involving the administration of muscle relaxants are of special concern to the ACP and postanesthesia nurse.[14] The duration of their action may be longer than the surgical procedure, or reversal agents may not be effective in completely eliminating the residual effects. The patient should be carefully observed for airway patency and adequacy of respiratory muscle movement. Lack of movement or poor return of reflexes and strength may indicate the need for an artificial airway and ventilator. If the patient is intubated, the endotracheal tube should not be removed without careful assessment of return of muscular strength, level of consciousness, and the minute volume (respiratory rate times tidal volume).

Antiemetics. Antiemetics are medications that are used to prevent and treat nausea and vomiting. Nausea and vomiting are the most common side effects of anesthesia. Numerous factors have been associated with postoperative nausea and vomiting, including anesthetic techniques, anesthetic agents, narcotics, gender (female), weight (obese), type of surgical procedure, pain, and a history of prior nausea and vomiting or motion sickness.

Although there are a number of antiemetics being used clinically, each has a different mechanism of action. Droperidol (Inapsine) antagonizes the emetic effects of narcotics. Metoclopramide (Reglan) increases gastric emptying and has direct antiemetic properties. Ondansetron (Zofran) is a selective serotonin receptor antagonist and is used to prevent nausea and vomiting. Other antiemetics such as prochlorperazine (Compazine) or promethazine (Phenergan) are sometimes prescribed, but their use is generally confined to the postoperative setting. An antiemetic agent may be administered as a sole agent or in combination with another antiemetic. Prophylaxis of nausea and vomiting is preferred to treatment, both in terms of patient comfort and postoperative recovery time.

Dissociative Anesthesia. Dissociative anesthesia interrupts associative brain pathways while blocking sensory pathways. The patient appears catatonic, is amnestic, and experiences profound analgesia that lasts into the postoperative period. Ketamine hydrochloride (Ketalar) is the agent most commonly administered as a dissociative anesthetic. It is particularly advantageous because ketamine can be administered intravenously or intramuscularly; it is a potent analgesic and amnestic.

This type of anesthetic is used for diagnostic or therapeutic procedures that do not require muscle relaxation, yet require profound analgesia and amnesia (e.g., burn scrubs and dressing changes). Because ketamine is a phencyclidine (PCP) derivative, the drug may cause hallucinations and nightmares, particularly in adult patients, greatly limiting its usefulness. Coadministration of a benzodiazepine decreases the potential for this adverse reaction.

Local Anesthesia

Local anesthetics block the initiation and transmission of electrical impulses along nerve fibers by preventing increases in cellular permeability to sodium ions. The decrease in sodium ion permeability slows the rate of cellular depolarization. A conduction blockade occurs because no action potential is generated. With progressive increases in local anesthetic concentration, the transmission of autonomic, then somatic sensory, and finally somatic motor impulses is blocked. This produces autonomic nervous system blockade, anesthesia, and skeletal muscle paralysis in the area of the affected nerve. If only autonomic and sensory blockade is desired, as with epidural anesthesia, a lower concentration of local anesthetic is used. Local anesthetics frequently administered include procaine (Novocain), tetracaine (Pontocaine), lidocaine (Xylocaine), mepivacaine (Carbocaine), bupivacaine (Marcaine), and ropivacaine (Naropin).

Table 17-7 Methods for Administering Local Anesthesia

- Topical application
- Local infiltration
- Regional injection
  - Peripheral nerve block
  - Intravenous regional block (Bier block)
  - Spinal anesthesia (block)
  - Epidural anesthesia (block)

Local anesthesia allows an operative procedure to be performed on a particular part of the body without loss of consciousness or sedation. Because there is little systemic absorption of the drug, recovery is rapid with little residual drug "hangover." The duration of action of the local anesthetic frequently carries over into the postoperative period, providing continued analgesia. In addition, the use of a local anesthetic in a regional technique provides an alternative to a general anesthetic in a physiologically compromised patient.

The disadvantages of local anesthetics include the technical difficulty and discomfort that may be associated with injecting them, inadvertent intravenous administration producing hypotension and potentially seizures, and the inability to precisely match the duration of action of the agents administered to the duration of the surgical procedure.

Methods of Administration. There are a variety of methods for administering local anesthetics (Table 17-7). *Topical application* is application of the agent directly to the skin, mucous membranes, or open surface. Eutectic mixture of local anesthetics (EMLA cream), a combination of lidocaine and prilocaine, can be applied to the skin to produce localized dermal anesthesia (see Chapter 9). EMLA has proven particularly useful in children when placing intravenous lines. *Local infiltration* is the injection of the agent into the tissues through which the surgical incision will pass.

Regional (peripheral) nerve block is achieved by the injection of a local anesthetic into or around a specific nerve or group of nerves. Nerve blocks may be used to provide intraoperative anesthesia and postoperative analgesia and for the diagnosis and treatment of chronic pain. Examples of common regional nerve blocks include brachial plexus, intercostal, and retrobulbar blocks. *Intravenous regional nerve block (Bier block)* is the intravenous injection of a local anesthetic into an extremity following mechanical exsanguination using a compression bandage and a tourniquet. This type of block provides not only analgesia, but the ability to work in a bloodless field. Spinal and epidural anesthesia are also types of regional anesthesia.

Spinal and epidural anesthesia. A spinal anesthetic involves the injection of a local anesthetic into the cerebrospinal fluid found in the subarachnoid space, usually below the level of L-2. The local anesthetic mixes with cerebrospinal fluid, and depending on the extent of its spread, various levels of anesthesia are achieved. Because the local anesthetic is administered directly into the cerebrospinal fluid, a spinal anesthetic produces an autonomic, sensory, and motor blockade. Patients experience vasodilation and may become hypotensive as a result of the autonomic block, feel no pain as a result of the

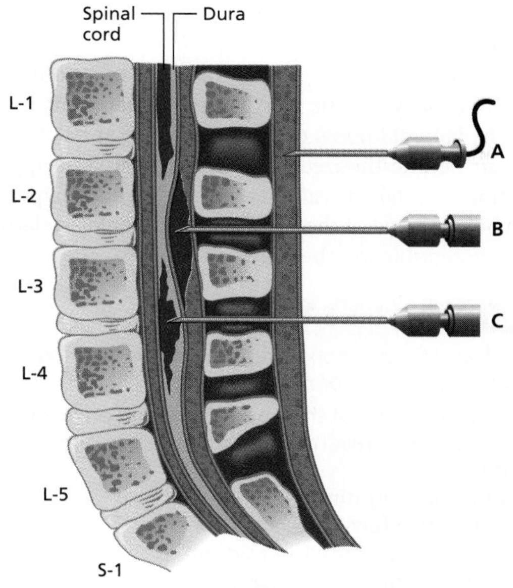

Fig. 17-10 Location of needle point and injected anesthetic relative to dura. **A,** Epidural catheter. **B,** Single-injection epidural. **C,** Spinal anesthesia. (Interspaces most commonly used are L4-5, L3-4, and L2-3.)

sensory block, and are unable to move as a result of the motor block. The duration of action of the spinal anesthetic depends on the agent selected and the dose administered. A spinal anesthetic may be used for procedures involving the groin, perineum, or lower extremity.

An epidural block involves injection of a local anesthetic into the epidural (extradural) space via either a thoracic or lumbar approach. Local anesthetics work by binding to nerve roots as they enter and exit the spinal cord. By using a low concentration of local anesthetic, sensory pathways are blocked, but motor fibers remain intact. In higher doses, both sensory and motor fibers are blocked (Fig. 17-10). Epidural anesthesia may be used as the sole anesthetic for a surgical procedure, or a catheter may be placed to allow for intraoperative use with continued use into the postoperative period for analgesia, using lower doses of epidurally administered local anesthetic, usually in combination with a narcotic. Epidural anesthesia is commonly used in labor and delivery, for vascular procedures involving the lower extremity, and for hip and knee replacement surgeries.

During the surgical procedure when spinal or epidural anesthesia is used, the patient can remain fully conscious or sedation can be achieved intravenously. The onset of spinal anesthesia is faster than that seen with an epidural, but the end results with either approach are usually similar. The patient must be closely observed for signs of autonomic nervous system blockade, including hypotension, bradycardia, nausea, and vomiting. Should "too high" a block be achieved, the patient may experience inadequate respiratory excursion and apnea. The level of the sensory and sympathetic block is controlled by the site of injection; the amount and strength of drug used; the speed of injection; the patient's height, weight, and body habitus; and the specific gravity of the solution used.

One advantage of epidural (extradural) injection over spinal (subarachnoid) injection is a decreased incidence of headache. The headache experienced after spinal anesthesia is thought to occur following leakage of spinal fluid at the site of injection. The incidence of headache is decreasing with the common use of smaller-gauge spinal needles (25 to 27 gauge) and the use of noncutting, "pencil-point" spinal needles. A headache following an epidural may occur when a 17- to 18-gauge needle is advanced too far and the dura is punctured, resulting in the leakage of cerebrospinal fluid.

Additional Anesthetic Considerations

Controlled hypotension is a technique used to decrease the amount of expected blood loss by lowering the blood pressure during the administration of anesthesia. *Hypothermia* is the deliberate lowering of body temperature to decrease metabolism, thus reducing both the demand for oxygen and anesthetic requirements. *Cyroanesthesia* involves cooling or freezing a localized area to block pain impulses of nerves. *Hypnoanesthesia* uses hypnosis to produce an alteration in pain consciousness. *Acupuncture* achieves loss of sensation by the use of intense local stimulation with fine-gauge needles at strategic points throughout the body.

GERONTOLOGIC CONSIDERATIONS

Patient During Surgery

Although anesthetic agents have become safer and more predictable, the elderly often demonstrate varying and unique responses to medications. Because of this, anesthetic drugs should be carefully titrated when given to older adults. Physiologic changes in aging may alter the patient's response not only to the anesthetic, but to blood and fluid loss and replacement, hypothermia, pain, and the tolerance of the surgical procedure and positioning. Advances in pharmacology, better understanding of the physiologic changes of aging, and improved technology allowing for careful monitoring of patient responses have made anesthesia and delivery safer than ever for older adults.[15] The older adult's response to all anesthetic agents must be carefully monitored and the postoperative recovery assessed before the patient is left without close supervision (e.g., transferred from the PACU to a surgical unit).[16]

Many older adults experience a decrease in their ability to communicate and follow directions as a result of alterations in vision or hearing. These factors pose a special need for clear and concise communication in the OR, especially when preoperative sedation is superimposed on the existing sensory deficit. Skin elasticity in the older adult is decreased because of loss of collagen. As a result, the skin is sensitive to injury from tape, electrodes, warming and cooling blankets, and certain types of dressing. In addition, the older adult often has fragile bones and osteoarthritis. These factors reinforce the need for careful transferring, lifting, and positioning techniques.

Catastrophic Events in the Operating Room

Unanticipated intraoperative events occasionally occur. Although some might be anticipated (e.g., cardiac arrest in an unstable patient, massive blood loss during trauma surgery), others may occur without warning, demanding immediate intervention by all members of the OR team. Two of these events are anaphylactic reactions and malignant hyperthermia.

Anaphylactic Reactions. Anaphylaxis is the most severe form of an allergic reaction, manifesting with life-threatening pulmonary and circulatory complications. Anesthesia providers administer an array of drugs to patients, such as anesthetics, antibiotics, blood products, and plasma expanders, and because any parenterally administered material can theoretically produce an allergic response, vigilance and rapid intervention is key. An anaphylactic reaction causes hypotension, tachycardia, bronchospasm, and possibly pulmonary edema. Antibiotics cause the greatest number of perioperative allergic reactions.[17] (Anaphylaxis is discussed in Chapter 12.)

Latex allergy has become a particular hazard in the perioperative setting, given the use of gloves, catheters, endotracheal tubes, and many other devices containing latex. Reactions to latex have ranged from urticaria to anaphylaxis with symptoms appearing immediately or at some time during the surgical procedure.[18] The patient must be treated at the onset of symptom identification. Latex allergy protocols should be set up in each institution so that a latex-safe environment can be provided in susceptible individuals, including health care workers, others with frequent latex exposure (e.g., patients who require frequent procedural or surgical intervention), and those with documented reactions (e.g., itching, rash) to latex-containing materials, such as balloons.

Latex allergic reactions can potentially be eliminated if properly assessed for in the preoperative period. Questions during the preoperative assessment may elicit undocumented sensitivity (e.g., "Do your lips feel numb when blowing up balloons?"). Currently a latex allergy protocol is available through the AORN. (Latex allergies are also discussed in Chapters 12 and 16.)

Malignant Hyperthermia. Malignant hyperthermia (MH) is a rare metabolic disease characterized by often fatal hyperthermia with rigidity of skeletal muscles. It occurs in affected people exposed to certain anesthetic agents. Succinylcholine, especially in conjunction with the volatile inhalation agents, appears to be the primary trigger of the disorder, although other factors, such as stress, trauma, and heat, have been implicated. When it does occur, it is usually during general anesthesia, but it may manifest in the recovery period as well. It is autosomal dominant in inheritance but is variable in its genetic penetrance, so predictions based on family history are important but inconsistent. The fundamental defect is hypermetabolism of skeletal muscle resulting from altered control of intracellular calcium, leading to muscle contracture, hyperthermia, hypoxemia, lactic acidosis, and hemodynamic and cardiac alterations.

Tachycardia, tachypnea, hypercarbia, and ventricular ectopy are generally seen but are nonspecific to MH. MH is generally diagnosed after all other causes are rapidly ruled out. The rise in body temperature is not an early sign of MH. Unless promptly detected with rapid initiation of appropriate intervention, malignant hyperthermia can result in cardiac arrest and death. The definitive treatment of MH is prompt administration of dantrolene sodium (Dantrium), which slows catabolism, along with symptomatic support to correct hemodynamic instability, acidosis, hypoxemia, and elevated temperature. A treatment protocol is available from the Malignant Hyperthermia Association of the United States and is usually displayed in the OR.[19]

To prevent MH it is important for the nurse to obtain a careful family history and be alert to its development perioperatively. The patient known or suspected to be at risk for this disorder can be anesthetized with minimal risks if appropriate precautions are taken. Patients with malignant hyperthermia should be informed of the condition so that close relatives who may be susceptible may be tested.

REVIEW QUESTIONS

The number of the question corresponds to the same-numbered objective at the beginning of the chapter.

1. The characteristic of the operating room environment that facilitates the prevention of infection in the surgical patient is
   a. adjustable lighting.
   b. conductive furniture.
   c. filters in the ventilating system.
   d. explosion-proof electrical plugs.
2. An activity that is carried out by nurses performing both sterile and nonsterile activities in the operating is
   a. checking electrical equipment.
   b. passing instruments to the surgeon and assistants.
   c. coordinating activities occurring in the operating room.
   d. assisting ACP with monitoring of patient during surgery.
3. Assessment of a patient with a musculoskeletal impairment on arrival to the operating room enables the nurse to meet the patient's needs during
   a. preparation of the skin.
   b. induction of anesthesia.
   c. positioning on the operating table.
   d. explanations about the surgical activities.
4. The perioperative nurse's primary responsibility for the care of the patient undergoing surgery is
   a. developing an individualized plan of nursing care for the patient.
   b. carrying out specific tasks related to surgical policies and procedures.
   c. ensuring that the patient has been assessed for safe administration of anesthesia.
   d. performing a preoperative history and physical assessment to identify patient needs.
5. When scrubbing at the scrub sink, the surgical team members should
   a. scrub from elbows to hands.
   b. scrub without mechanical friction.
   c. scrub for a minimum of 10 minutes.
   d. hold the hands higher than the elbows.
6. Mrs. Jones is scheduled for an abdominal hysterectomy. She is extremely anxious and has a tendency to hyperventilate when upset. The type of anesthetic that would probably be most appropriate for Mrs. Jones is
   a. a spinal block.
   b. an epidural block.
   c. a dissociative anesthethic.
   d. an inhalation general anesthetic.
7. Intravenous induction for general anesthesia is the method of choice for most patients because
   a. the patient is not intubated.
   b. they are nonexplosive agents.
   c. induction is rapid and pleasant.
   d. the odor of the agent is not offensive.

8. The injection of the local anesthetic into the tissues through which the surgical incision will pass is the technique of
   a. nerve block.
   b. local infiltration.
   c. topical application.
   d. regional application.
9. The anesthetic adjunct agent that is most likely to impair respiratory muscle movement following the completion of surgery is
   a. diazepam (Valium).
   b. fentanyl (Sublimaze).
   c. pancuronium (Pavulon).
   d. succinylcholine (Anectine).

References

1. Atkinson LJ: *Berry and Kohn's operating room techniques,* ed 8, St Louis, 1996, Mosby.
2. Groah L: *Operating room nursing,* ed 2, San Mateo, Calif, 1995, Appleton & Lange.
3. Meeker MH, Rothrock JC: *Alexander's care of the patient in surgery,* ed 11, St Louis, 1999, Mosby.
4. DeLong DL: Preoperative holding area, *AORN J* 55:563, 1992.
5. Longinow LT, Rzeszewski LB: The holding room, *AORN J* 57:914, 1993.
6. Association of Operating Room Nurses: Patient outcome standards. In *AORN standards and recommended practices,* Denver, 1997, Association of Operating Room Nurses.
7. Association of Operating Room Nurses: Recommended practices for maintaining a sterile field. In *AORN standards of practice,* Denver, 1997, Association of Operating Room Nurses.
8. Department of Labor, Occupational Safety and Health Administration, *Federal Register* 56(235):part 1920, 1991.
9. Fairchild SS: *Perioperative nursing,* ed 2, Boston, 1996, Jones & Bartlett.
10. Phippen ML, Wells MP: *Perioperative nursing practice,* Philadelphia, 1993, Saunders.
11. Siler JN, Fisher SM, Boon P: A comparative study of total intravenous anesthesia technique versus a standard anesthetic technique for outpatient surgical procedures, *Semin Anes* 11:14, 1992.
12. Walker JR: What is new with inhaled anesthetics: part 2, *J Perianesth Nurs* 11:404, 1996.
13. Walker JR: Neuromuscular relaxation and reversal: an update, *J Perianesth Nurs* 12:264, 1997.
14. Booth M: Clinical aspects of nurse anesthesia practice. Sedation and monitored anesthesia care, *Nurs Clin North Am* 31:667, 1996.
15. Dodds C: Anaesthetic drugs in the elderly, *Pharmacol Ther* 66:369, 1995.
16. Burney TL, Badlani GH: Anesthetic considerations in the geriatric patient, *Urol Clin North Am* 23:19, 1996.
17. White PF: *Ambulatory anesthesia and surgery,* London, 1997, Saunders.
18. American Association of Nurse Anesthetists: Latex allergy protocol, *AANA* 61:223, 1993.
19. Malignant Hyperthermia Association of the United States: *Suggested therapy for malignant hyperthermia emergency,* Darien, Conn, 1998, MHaus International.

Resources

Resources for this chapter are listed after Chapter 18 on p. 413.

REMEMBER to check out your companion CD-ROM

18 NURSING MANAGEMENT Postoperative Patient

Kim Litwack

www.mosby.com/MERLIN/medsurg_lewis

LEARNING OBJECTIVES

1. Identify the components of an initial postanesthesia assessment.
2. Identify the nursing responsibilities in admitting patients to the postanesthesia care unit (PACU).
3. Explain the etiology and nursing assessment and management of potential problems of patients in the PACU.
4. Describe the initial nursing assessment and management immediately after transfer from the PACU to the general care unit.
5. Explain the etiology and nursing assessment and management of potential problems during the postoperative period.
6. Identify the information needed by the postoperative patient in preparation for discharge.

The postoperative period begins immediately after surgery and continues until the patient is discharged from medical care. This chapter focuses on the common features of postoperative nursing care for the patient undergoing surgery. The problems and nursing care related to specific surgical procedures are discussed in the appropriate chapters of this text.

POSTOPERATIVE CARE IN THE POSTANESTHESIA CARE UNIT

The patient's immediate recovery period is supervised by a postanesthesia care nurse, an educated specialist working in a specially equipped environment. The postanesthesia care unit (PACU) is located adjacent to the operating room (OR) to minimize transportation of the patient immediately after surgery and to provide ready access to anesthesia and surgical personnel.

Postanesthesia Care Unit Admission

The initial admission of the patient to the PACU is a joint effort between the anesthesia care provider (ACP) and the PACU nurse. This collaborative effort fosters a smooth transfer of care. To ensure patient safety and continuity of care, the ACP gives a verbal report to the admitting PACU nurse. A complete report includes details of the surgical and anesthetic course, preoperative conditions warranting or influencing the surgical or anesthetic outcome, and PACU treatment plans.[1] Table 18-1 summarizes the components of a complete anesthesia report.

Reviewed by Virginia Printz-Feddersen, RNC, MSN, CNS, CNOR, CNRN, Clinical Nurse Specialist, Lovelace Health Systems, Albuquerque, NM; and Jill H. Pendarvis, RNC, MA, CNOR, Emeritus Associate Professor, Intercollegiate Center for Nursing Education, Spokane, Wash.

A priority in admitting a patient to the PACU is an assessment designed to

1. Determine the patient's physiologic status at the time of admission to the PACU
2. Allow periodic reevaluation of the patient so that physiologic trends become apparent
3. Establish the patient's baseline parameters
4. Assess the ongoing status of the surgical site
5. Assess recovery from anesthesia, noting residual effects
6. Allow comparison of current patient status with preoperative findings and discharge criteria[2]

A specific assessment priority is an evaluation of respiratory and circulatory adequacy.[3] Assessment will be made of the patient's airway patency and rate and quality of respirations. Breath sounds should be auscultated throughout all lung fields.

Oxygen therapy will be used if the patient has had general anesthesia or the ACP orders it. Oxygen therapy is given via nasal cannula or face mask. The use of oxygen aids in the elimination of anesthetic gases and helps meet the increased demand for oxygen needed in the immediate postoperative period. If the patient requires postoperative ventilation, a ventilator will be provided. Pulse oximetry monitoring will be initiated because it provides a noninvasive means of assessing the adequacy of oxygenation. (Pulse oximetry is discussed in Chapter 24.)

During this initial assessment, any signs of inadequate oxygenation and ventilation should be identified (Table 18-2). Any evidence of respiratory compromise requires prompt intervention. Commonly occurring respiratory problems for patients in the PACU are discussed on p. 391-396.

Electrocardiographic (ECG) monitoring will be initiated to determine cardiac rate and rhythm. Any deviation from preoperative findings should be noted and evaluated. Blood pressure

Table 18-1 Postanesthesia Admission Report

General Information
Patient name
Age
Anesthesia care provider
Surgeon
Surgical procedure
Intraoperative Management
Anesthetic medications
Other medications received preoperatively or intraoperatively
Blood loss
Fluid replacement totals, including blood transfusions
Urine output
Intraoperative Course
Unexpected anesthetic events or reactions
Unexpected surgical events
Vital signs and monitoring trends
Results of intraoperative laboratory tests
Patient History
Indication for surgery
Medical history, medications, allergies
Postanesthesia Care Unit Plan
Potential and expected problems (with plan for intervention)
Suggested PACU course
Acceptable parameters for laboratory test results
PACU discharge plan

PACU, postanesthesia care unit.

Table 18-2 Clinical Manifestations of Inadequate Oxygenation

Central Nervous System
Restlessness
Agitation
Muscle twitching
Seizures
Coma
Cardiovascular System
Hypertension
Hypotension
Tachycardia
Bradycardia
Arrhythmias
Integumentary System
Cyanosis
Poor capillary refill
Skin flushed and moist
Pulmonary System
Increased to absent respiratory effort
Use of accessory muscles
Abnormal breath sounds
Abnormal arterial blood gases
Renal System
Urine output <0.5 ml/kg/hr

should be measured and compared with baseline readings. Any invasive monitoring (e.g., arterial blood pressure monitoring) will be initiated. Body temperature and skin color and condition should also be assessed. Any evidence of inadequate circulatory status requires prompt intervention. Commonly occurring cardiovascular problems for patients in the PACU are discussed on p. 396-397.

The initial neurologic assessment will focus on level of consciousness; orientation; sensory and motor status; and size, equality, and reactivity of the pupils. The patient may be awake, drowsy but arousable, or asleep. Occasionally the patient may wake up agitated in what is referred to as *emergence delirium.* If the patient has had a regional anesthetic (e.g., spinal or epidural), sensory and motor blockade may still be present.

The assessment of the urinary system focuses on intake and output and electrolyte status. Intraoperative fluid totals will be communicated as part of the anesthesia report. The PACU nurse will note the presence of all intravenous (IV) lines, irrigation solutions and infusions, and all output devices, including catheters and wound drains. Intravenous infusions will be regulated according to postoperative orders.

The PACU nurse will also assess the surgical site, noting the condition of any dressings and the type and amount of any drainage. Postoperative orders related to site care will be instituted. All data obtained in the admission assessment are documented on a PACU record, a form specific to postanesthesia and postsurgical care (Fig. 18-1).

Even the patient who has been told what to expect after surgery may be frightened or confused on awakening in the strange environment. Because hearing is the first sense to return in the unconscious patient, the nurse should explain all activities from the moment of admission to the PACU. Orientation includes explaining to the patient that the surgery is completed, that the patient is in the recovery room, and that the family or significant other has been notified, and noting who is caring for the patient, what is being done, and what time it is.

After the initial assessment is completed, the PACU nurse will continue to apply the skills of ongoing assessment, diagnosis, and intervention. The patient's response to intervention is also noted. The goal of PACU care is to identify actual and potential patient problems that may occur as a result of anesthetic administration and surgical intervention and to intervene appropriately. The American Society of Perianesthesia Nursing (ASPAN) has defined Standards of Perianesthesia Nursing Practice (1995) to guide PACU care of adult, pediatric, and geriatric patients.[4]

Common postoperative problems include airway compromise (obstruction), respiratory insufficiency (hypoxemia and hypercarbia), cardiac compromise (hypotension, hypertension, and arrhythmias), neurologic compromise (emergence delirium and delayed awakening), hypothermia, pain, and nausea and vomiting (Fig. 18-2). Each of these problems and appropriate nursing interventions are discussed.

Potential Alterations in Respiratory Function

Etiology

In the immediate postanesthetic period the most common causes of airway compromise include obstruction, hypoxemia, and hypoventilation (Table 18-3). Patients at particular risk include those who have had general anesthesia, are older,

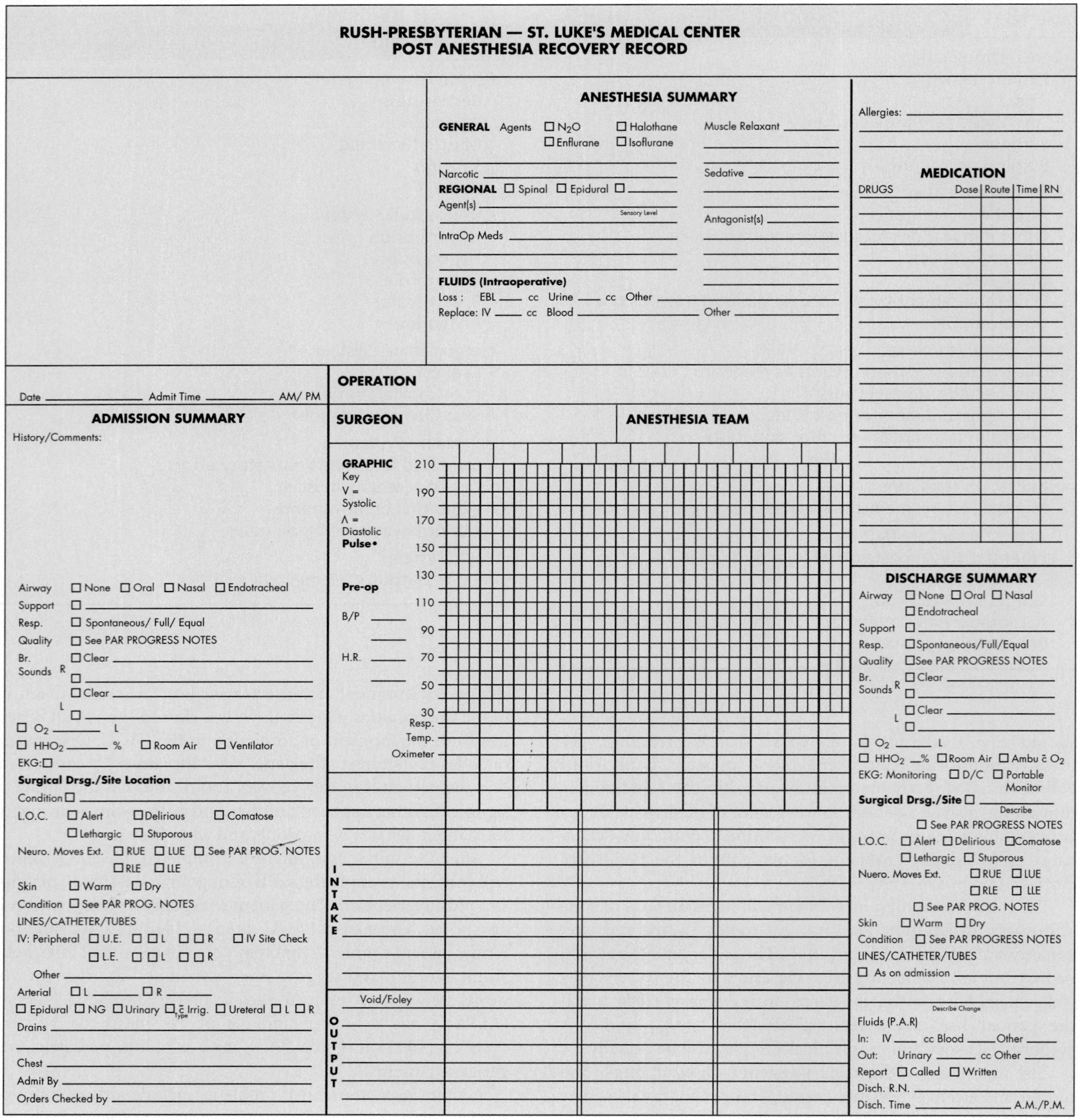

RUSH-PRESBYTERIAN — ST. LUKE'S MEDICAL CENTER
POST ANESTHESIA RECOVERY RECORD

ANESTHESIA SUMMARY

GENERAL Agents ☐ N_2O ☐ Halothane ☐ Enflurane ☐ Isoflurane Muscle Relaxant ______

Narcotic ______ Sedative ______

REGIONAL ☐ Spinal ☐ Epidural ☐ ______

Agent(s) ______ Sensory Level

Antagonist(s) ______

IntraOp Meds ______

FLUIDS (Intraoperative)

Loss: EBL ____ cc Urine ____ cc Other ______

Replace: IV ____ cc Blood ______ Other ______

Allergies: ______

MEDICATION

DRUGS	Dose	Route	Time	RN

Date ______ Admit Time ______ AM/ PM

ADMISSION SUMMARY

History/Comments:

Airway ☐ None ☐ Oral ☐ Nasal ☐ Endotracheal

Support ☐ ______

Resp. ☐ Spontaneous/ Full/ Equal

Quality ☐ See PAR PROGRESS NOTES

Br. Sounds R ☐ Clear ______ ☐ ______

L ☐ Clear ______ ☐ ______

☐ O_2 ______ L

☐ HHO_2 ______ % ☐ Room Air ☐ Ventilator

EKG:☐ ______

Surgical Drsg./Site Location ______

Condition ☐ ______

L.O.C. ☐ Alert ☐ Delirious ☐ Comatose ☐ Lethargic ☐ Stuporous

Neuro. Moves Ext. ☐ RUE ☐ LUE ☐ See PAR PROG. NOTES ☐ RLE ☐ LLE

Skin ☐ Warm ☐ Dry

Condition ☐ See PAR PROG. NOTES

LINES/CATHETER/TUBES

IV: Peripheral ☐ U.E. ☐ ☐ L ☐ ☐ R ☐ IV Site Check

☐ L.E. ☐ ☐ L ☐ ☐ R

Other ______

Arterial ☐ L ______ ☐ R ______

☐ Epidural ☐ NG ☐ Urinary ☐ Type c̄ Irrig. ☐ Ureteral ☐ L ☐ R

Drains ______

Chest ______

Admit By ______

Orders Checked by ______

OPERATION

SURGEON **ANESTHESIA TEAM**

GRAPHIC Key V = Systolic Λ = Diastolic **Pulse•**

210 190 170 150 130 110 90 70 50 30

Pre-op

B/P ______

H.R. ______

Resp.

Temp.

Oximeter

INTAKE

Void/Foley

OUTPUT

DISCHARGE SUMMARY

Airway ☐ None ☐ Oral ☐ Nasal ☐ Endotracheal

Support ☐ ______

Resp. ☐ Spontaneous/Full/Equal

Quality ☐ See PAR PROGRESS NOTES

Br. Sounds R ☐ Clear ______ ☐ ______

L ☐ Clear ______ ☐ ______

☐ O_2 ______ L

☐ HHO_2 __% ☐ Room Air ☐ Ambu c̄ O_2

EKG: Monitoring ☐ D/C ☐ Portable Monitor

Surgical Drsg./Site ☐ ______ Describe

☐ See PAR PROGRESS NOTES

L.O.C. ☐ Alert ☐ Delirious ☐ Comatose ☐ Lethargic ☐ Stuporous

Nuero. Moves Ext. ☐ RUE ☐ LUE ☐ RLE ☐ LLE

☐ See PAR PROG. NOTES

Skin ☐ Warm ☐ Dry

Condition ☐ See PAR PROGRESS NOTES

LINES/CATHETER/TUBES

☐ As on admission ______

Describe Change

Fluids (P.A.R)

In: IV ____ cc Blood ____ Other ____

Out: Urinary ____ cc Other ____

Report ☐ Called ☐ Written

Disch. R.N. ______

Disch. Time ______ A.M./P.M.

Fig. 18-1 PACU record.

smoke heavily, have lung disease, are obese, or have undergone airway, thoracic, or abdominal surgery. However, respiratory complications may occur with any patient who has been anesthetized.

Airway obstruction is most commonly caused by blockage of the airway by the patient's tongue (Fig. 18-3, p. 396). The base of the tongue falls backward against the soft palate and occludes the pharynx. It is most pronounced in the supine position and in the patient who is extremely somnolent after surgery. Less common causes of airway obstruction include laryngospasm, retained secretions, and laryngeal edema (croup).

Hypoxemia, specifically a PaO_2 of less than 60 mm Hg, is characterized by a variety of nonspecific clinical signs and symptoms, ranging from agitation to somnolence, hypertension to hypotension, and tachycardia to bradycardia. Pulse oximetry will indicate a low oxygen saturation (less than

		ARTERIAL GASES							ELECTROLYTES					Hb/Hct		INITIAL
Time	Parameters O_2 or Vent.	pH	pCO_2	pO_2	HCO_3	Total CO_2	BE	O_2 Sat %	Na	K	Cl	Ca	Glucose	Hb	Hct	

SIGNATURE & TITLE

TESTS/PROCEDURES		
TEST	TIME DONE/SENT	COMMENTS OR RESULTS
EKG		
MODEL S		
SMA_6		

X-RAY EXAMINATION	TIME DONE
☐ CXR	
☐ PELVIS	

P.A.R. PROGRESS NOTES

Fig. 18-1 (continued)

90%-92%). Arterial blood gas analysis should be used to confirm hypoxemia if the pulse oximetry indicates a low O_2 saturation.

The most common cause of postoperative hypoxemia is *atelectasis.* Atelectasis may be the result of bronchial obstruction caused by retained secretions or decreased respiratory excursion. Hypotension and low cardiac output states can also contribute to the development of atelectasis. Other causes of hypoxemia that may occur in the PACU include pulmonary edema, aspiration, and bronchospasm.

Pulmonary edema is caused by an accumulation of fluid in the alveoli and may be the result of fluid overload; left ventricular failure; or prolonged airway obstruction, sepsis, or aspiration. Pulmonary edema is characterized by hypoxemia, crackles on auscultation, decrease in pulmonary compliance, and the presence of infiltrates on chest x-ray.

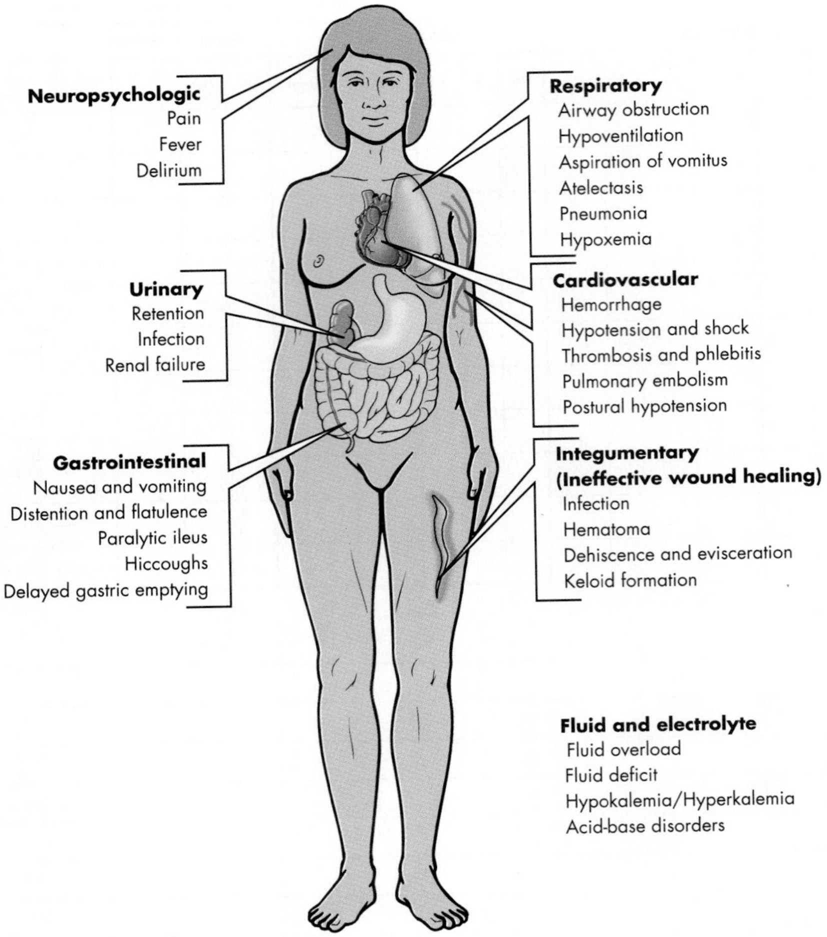

Fig. 18-2 Potential problems in the postoperative period.

Aspiration of gastric contents is a potentially serious airway emergency. Symptoms include bronchospasm, hypoxemia, atelectasis, interstitial edema, alveolar hemorrhage, and respiratory failure. Gastric aspiration may also cause laryngospasm, infection, and pulmonary edema. Because of the serious consequences of gastric aspiration, prevention, as opposed to treatment, is the goal. Patients identified as being at risk (obese, pregnant, history of hiatal hernia, gastroesophageal reflux disease [GERD], peptic ulcer, or trauma) may be premedicated with a histamine (H_2) blocker before induction of anesthesia. The anesthesia care provider will take special precautions to protect the airway during induction of and emergence from anesthesia.

Bronchospasm is the result of an increase in bronchial smooth muscle tone with resultant closure of small airways. Airway edema develops, causing secretions to build up in the airway. The patient will have wheezing, dyspnea, use of accessory muscles, hypoxemia, and tachypnea. Bronchospasm may be due to aspiration, endotrachael intubation, suctioning, histamine release from mast cells stimulated by medications, or an allergic response. It is seen in greater frequency in patients with asthma and chronic obstructive pulmonary disease (COPD).

Hypoventilation, a common complication in the PACU, is characterized by a decreased respiratory rate or effort, hypoxemia, and an increasing $PaCO_2$ (hypercapnia). Hypoventilation may occur as a result of depression of the central respiratory drive (secondary to anesthesia or pain medication), poor respiratory muscle tone (secondary to neuromuscular blockade or disease), or a combination of both.

NURSING MANAGEMENT: RESPIRATORY COMPLICATIONS

■ Nursing Assessment

For an adequate respiratory assessment, the nurse must evaluate airway patency, chest symmetry, and the depth, rate, and character of respirations. The nurse can place a cupped hand over the patient's nose and mouth to evaluate the forcefulness of exhaled air.

The chest wall should be observed for symmetry of movement with a hand placed lightly over the xiphoid process. It should also be determined whether abdominal or accessory muscles are being used for breathing. If the muscles are moving excessively, it may indicate respiratory distress.

Breath sounds should be auscultated anteriorly, laterally, and posteriorly. Decreased or absent breath sounds will be detected when airflow is diminished or obstructed. The presence of crackles or wheezes requires notification of the ACP.

Regular monitoring of vital signs and use of pulse oximetry permit the nurse to recognize early signs of respiratory distress. The presence of hypoxemia from any cause may be reflected by

Table 18-3 Common Immediate Postoperative Respiratory Complications

Complications and Causes	Mechanisms	Manifestations	Interventions
Airway Obstruction			
Tongue falling back	Muscular flaccidity associated with decreased consciousness and muscle relaxants	Use of accessory muscles Snoring respirations Decreased air movement	Stimulate patient Jaw thrust Chin lift Artificial airway
Retained thick secretions	Secretion stimulation by anesthetic agents Dehydration of secretions	Noisy respirations Rhonchi	Suctioning Deep breathing and coughing IV hydration IPPB with mucolytic agent Chest physical therapy
Laryngospasm	Irritation from endotracheal tube or anesthetic gases Most likely to occur after removal of endotracheal tube	Inspiratory stridor (crowing respiration) Sternal retraction Acute respiratory distress	Oxygen Positive-pressure ventilation IV muscle relaxant Lidocaine/corticosteroids
Laryngeal edema	Allergic drug reaction Mechanical irritation from intubation Fluid overload	Similar to laryngospasm	Oxygen Antihistamines or corticosteroids Sedatives Possible intubation
Hypoxemia			
Atelectasis	Bronchial obstruction caused by secretions or decreased lung volumes	↓ Breath sounds ↓ Oxygen saturation	Humidified oxygen Deep breathing Incentive spirometry Early mobilization
Pulmonary edema	↑ Hydrostatic pressure ↓ Interstitial pressure ↑ Capillary permeability	Crackles Infiltrates on chest x-ray Fluid overload ↓ Oxygen saturation	Oxygen therapy Diuretics Fluid restriction
Pulmonary embolism	Thrombus dislodged from periphery; lodged in pulmonary artery	Acute tachypnea Dyspnea Tachycardia Hypotension ↓ Oxygen saturation	Oxygen therapy Cardiopulmonary support Heparin therapy
Aspiration	Inhalation of gastric contents	Bronchospasm Atelectasis Crackles Respiratory distress ↓ Oxygen saturation	Oxygen therapy Cardiac support Antibiotics/corticosteroids
Bronchospasm	Increased smooth muscle tone with closure of small airways	Wheezing Dyspnea Tachypnea ↓ Oxygen saturation	Oxygen therapy Bronchodilators
Hypoventilation			
Depression of central respiratory drive	Medullary depression from anesthetics/narcotics/sedatives	Shallow respirations ↓ Respiratory rate/apnea ↓ PaO_2 ↑ $PaCO_2$	Stimulation Reversal of narcotics/ benzodiazepines Mechanical ventilation
Poor respiratory muscle tone	Neuromuscular blockade Neuromuscular disease	As above	Reversal of paralysis Mechanical ventilation
Mechanical restriction	Tight casts, dressings, positioning, and obesity prevent lung expansion	As above	Elevate head of bed Repositioning Loosen dressings
Pain	Shallow breathing to prevent incisional pain	As above Complaints of pain Guarding behavior	Analgesic therapy in reduced dose

IPPB, intermittent positive-pressure breathing.

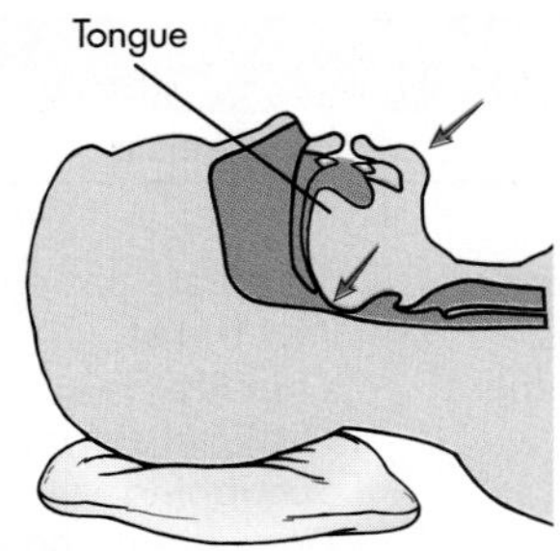

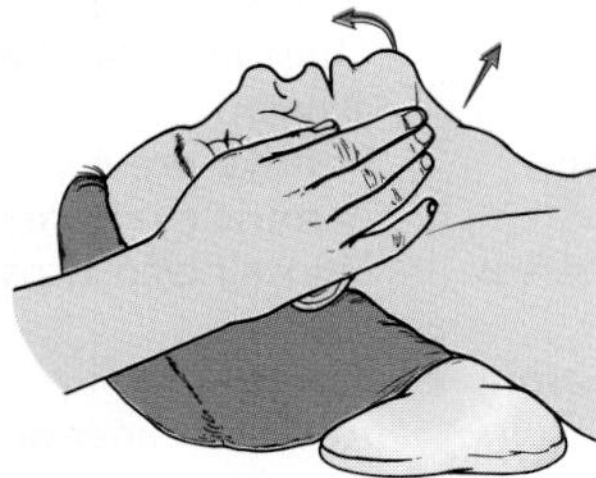

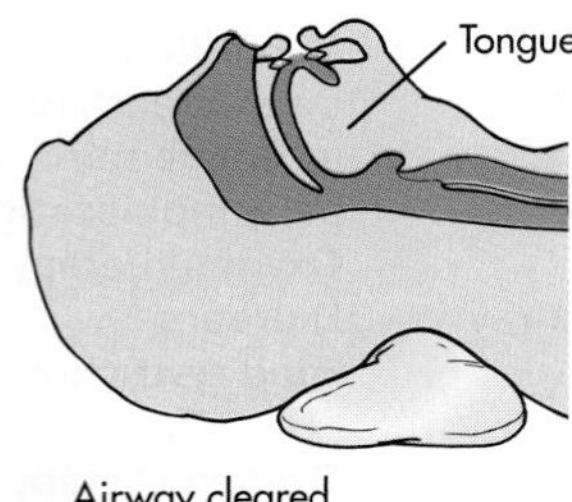

Fig. 18-3 Etiology and relief of airway obstruction due to patient's tongue.

rapid breathing, gasping, apprehension, restlessness, and a rapid or thready pulse. Impaired ventilation may initially be detected by the observation of slowed breathing or diminished chest and abdominal movement during the respiratory cycle.

The characteristics of sputum or mucus should be noted and recorded. Mucus from the trachea and throat is colorless and thin in consistency. Sputum from the lungs and bronchi is thick with a slight yellow tinge.

Nursing Diagnoses

Nursing diagnoses and collaborative problems related to potential respiratory complications for the patient in the PACU include, but are not limited to, the following:

- Ineffective airway clearance
- Ineffective breathing pattern
- Impaired gas exchange
- Risk for aspiration
- Potential complication: hypoxemia

Nursing Implementation

In the PACU, nursing interventions are designed to both prevent and treat respiratory problems. Proper positioning of the patient to facilitate respirations and protect the airway is essential. Unless contraindicated by the surgical procedure, the unconscious or semiconscious patient is positioned in a lateral position (Fig. 18-4). Once conscious, the patient is usually returned to a supine position with the head of the bed elevated. This position maximizes expansion of the thorax by decreasing the pressure of the abdominal contents on the diaphragm.

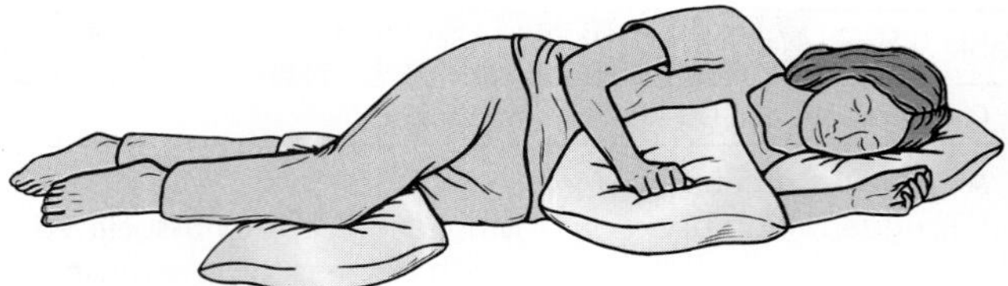

Fig. 18-4 Position of patient during recovery from general anesthesia.

Deep breathing is encouraged to facilitate gas exchange and to promote the return to consciousness. The patient should be taught to take in slow, deep breaths, ideally through the nose, to hold the breath, and to then slowly exhale. A patient can perform this type of breathing independently or with the aid of an incentive spirometer. This type of breathing is also useful as a relaxation strategy when the patient is anxious or in pain. Other nursing interventions will be specific to the cause of the respiratory complication, as detailed in Table 18-3.

Potential Alterations in Cardiovascular Function

Etiology

In the immediate postanesthetic period the most common cardiovascular complications include hypotension, hypertension, and arrhythmias. Patients at greatest risk for alterations in cardiovascular function include those with alterations in respiratory function, those with a cardiac history, the elderly, the debilitated, and the critically ill.

Hypotension is evidenced by signs of hypoperfusion to the vital organs, especially the brain, heart, and kidneys. Clinical signs of disorientation, loss of consciousness, chest pain, oliguria, and anuria reflect hypoxemia and the loss of physiologic compensation. Intervention must be timely to prevent the devastating complications of myocardial ischemia or infarction, cerebral ischemia, renal ischemia, and bowel infarction.

The most common cause of hypotension in the PACU is unreplaced fluid and blood loss. As a result, treatment will be directed toward restoring circulating volume. If there is no response to fluid administration, myocardial dysfunction should be considered to be the cause of hypotension.

Primary cardiac dysfunction, as may occur in the case of myocardial infarction, cardiac tamponade, or pulmonary embolism, results in an acute fall in cardiac output. Secondary myocardial dysfunction occurs as a result of the negative chronotrope (rate) and negative inotrope (force) effects of medications, such as beta blockers, digoxin, or narcotics.

Other causes of hypotension include decreased low systemic vascular resistance, arrhythmias, and measurement errors that may occur if a blood pressure cuff is incorrectly sized.

Hypertension is defined as a 20% to 30% increase above the resting blood pressure. Hypertension, a common finding in the PACU, is most frequently the result of sympathetic stimulation that may be the result of pain, anxiety, bladder distention, or respiratory compromise. Hypertension may also be the result of hypothermia and preexisting hypertension, and it may be seen after vascular and cardiac surgery as a result of revascularization.

Arrhythmias are most commonly the result of an identifiable cause as opposed to myocardial injury. The leading causes include hypokalemia, hypoxemia, hypercarbia, alterations in acid-base status, circulatory instability, and preexisting heart disease. Hypothermia, pain, surgical stress, and many anesthetic agents are also capable of causing arrhythmias.

NURSING MANAGEMENT: CARDIOVASCULAR COMPLICATIONS

■ Nursing Assessment

The most important aspect of the cardiovascular assessment is frequent monitoring of vital signs. They are usually monitored every 15 minutes, or more often until stabilized, and then at less frequent intervals. Postoperative vital signs should be compared with preoperative and intraoperative readings to determine when the signs are stabilizing at a normal level for the patient's situation. The ACP or surgeon should be notified if the following occur:

1. Systolic blood pressure is less than 90 mm Hg or greater than 160 mm Hg.
2. Pulse rate is less than 60 beats per minute or greater than 120 beats per minute.
3. Pulse pressure narrows.
4. Blood pressure gradually decreases during several consecutive readings.
5. An irregular cardiac rhythm develops.
6. There is a significant variation from preoperative readings.

Cardiac monitoring is recommended for patients who have a history of cardiac disease and for all older adult patients who have undergone major surgery, regardless of whether they have cardiac problems. An apical-radial pulse should be assessed carefully, and any irregularities should be reported.

Assessment of skin color, temperature, and moisture provides valuable information in detecting cardiovascular problems. Hypotension accompanied by a normal pulse and warm, dry, pink skin usually represents the residual vasodilating effects of anesthesia and suggests only a need for continued observation. Hypotension accompanied by a rapid pulse and cold, clammy, pale skin may be caused by impending hypovolemic shock and requires immediate treatment.

■ Nursing Diagnoses

Nursing diagnoses and collaborative problems related to potential cardiovascular complications for the patient in the PACU include, but are not limited to, the following:

- Decreased cardiac output
- Fluid volume deficit
- Altered tissue perfusion
- Potential complication: hypovolemic shock

■ Nursing Implementation

Nursing interventions in the PACU are designed to prevent and treat cardiovascular complications. Treatment of hypotension should always begin with oxygen therapy. Volume status should be assessed, and errors of blood pressure measurement should be ruled out. Because the most common cause of hypotension is fluid loss, IV fluid boluses will be given to normalize blood pressure. Primary cardiac dysfunction may require pharmacologic intervention. Secondary cardiac dysfunction may require discontinuation of causative medications. Peripheral vasodilation may require vasoconstrictive agents to normalize systemic vascular resistance.

Treatment of hypertension will center on addressing the cause of sympathetic stimulation and eliminating the precipitating cause. Treatment may include the use of analgesics, assistance in voiding, and correction of respiratory problems. Rewarming will correct hypothermia-induced hypertension. If the patient has preexisting hypertension or has undergone cardiac or vascular surgery, pharmacologic intervention designed to reduce blood pressure will usually be required.

Because the majority of arrhythmias seen in the PACU have identifiable causes, treatment is directed toward eliminating the cause. Correction of these physiologic alterations will, in most instances, correct the arrhythmias. In the event of life-threatening arrhythmias, protocols of advanced cardiac life support will be applied (see Chapter 34).

Potential Alterations in Neurologic Function

Etiology

Postoperatively, emergence delirium remains the neurologic alteration that causes the most concern to the practitioner. *Emergence delirium* is defined as a condition characterized by extreme alterations in arousal, orientation, perception, affect, and attention. The patient is frequently combative. Common causes of emergence delirium include hypoxemia, adverse reactions to anesthetic medications, chemical dependency, metabolic alterations, pain, bladder distention, and hypothermia.[5]

Delayed awakening may also be a problem postoperatively. Fortunately, the most common cause of delayed awakening is prolonged drug action, particularly of narcotics, sedatives, and inhalational anesthetics, as opposed to neurologic injury.

NURSING MANAGEMENT: NEUROLOGIC COMPLICATIONS

■ Nursing Assessment

The patient's level of consciousness, orientation, and ability to follow commands should be assessed. The size, reactivity, and equality of the pupils should be determined. The patient's sensory and motor status should also be assessed. If the neurologic status is altered, possible causes should be determined.

■ Nursing Diagnoses

Nursing diagnoses related to potential neurologic complications for the patient in the PACU include, but are not limited to, the following:

- Sensory-perceptual alterations
- Risk for injury
- Altered thought processes
- Impaired verbal communication

■ Nursing Implementation

The most common cause of postoperative agitation is hypoxemia. As a result, attention must be addressed toward evaluation of respiratory function. Once hypoxemia has been ruled out as the cause of postoperative delirium and all potentially known causes have been addressed, sedation may prove beneficial in controlling the agitation and for providing for patient and staff safety. Emergence delirium is time limited and will resolve before the patient is discharged from the PACU. Because the most common cause of delayed awakening is prolonged drug action, usually delays in awakening spontaneously resolve with time. If necessary, benzodiazepines and narcotics may be pharmacologically reversed with antagonists.

Until the patient is awake and able to communicate effectively, it will be the responsibility of the PACU nurse to act as a patient advocate and to maintain patient safety at all times. This includes having the side rails up, securing IV lines and artificial airways, verifying the presence of identification and allergy bands, and monitoring physiologic status.

Hypothermia

Etiology

Hypothermia, defined as a body temperature of less than 96° F (35.5° C), occurs when heat loss exceeds heat production.[1] Hypothermia may be the result of radiant heat loss (loss of heat from a warm body to a cold OR), convective heat loss (loss of heat from the body to ambient air), conductive heat loss (loss of heat from a warm body to a cold OR table), or evaporative loss (loss of heat from exposed viscera to the air).[1,3]

Although all patients are at risk for hypothermia, the older, debilitated, or intoxicated patient is at an increased risk. Long surgical procedures and prolonged anesthetic administration also place the patient at an increased risk for hypothermia.[3]

Hypothermia has the potential to compromise physiologic stability and increase perioperative risk. Metabolic processes slow down, decreasing metabolism and elimination of anesthetic agents. Renal function decreases, cardiac rate and rhythm disturbances may develop, and central nervous system (CNS) depression is accentuated. Systemic vascular resistance is increased as a result of peripheral vasoconstriction.[1]

NURSING MANAGEMENT: HYPOTHERMIA

■ Nursing Assessment

Vital signs, including temperature, should be determined. Temperature may be taken orally or via the tympanic membrane or axilla. Use of rectal temperature monitoring is rare; use of skin temperature monitoring is unreliable. The color and temperature of the skin should also be assessed.

■ Nursing Diagnoses

The nursing diagnosis for the patient with hypothermia includes, but is not limited to, risk for altered body temperature.

■ Nursing Implementation

Passive rewarming (i.e., shivering) raises basal heat metabolism. Active rewarming requires the application of external warming devices and may include warm blankets, heated aerosols, radiant warmers, forced air warmers, or heated water mattresses. When using any external warming device, body temperature should be monitored at 15-minute intervals, and care should be taken to prevent burns. In addition, oxygen therapy is used to treat the increased demand for oxygen accompanying the increase in body temperature.

Pain and Discomfort

Etiology

Despite the availability of analgesic medications and pain-relieving techniques, pain remains a common problem and a significant fear for the patient in the PACU and during the postoperative period. Pain may be the result of surgical manipulation, positioning, or the presence of internal devices such as an endotracheal tube or catheter, or it may occur as the patient begins to mobilize postoperatively. Other sources of physical and emotional discomfort include anxiety about the outcome of surgery, embarrassment from having removed dentures or other prostheses, shivering, and a full bladder.[1]

NURSING MANAGEMENT: PAIN

■ Nursing Assessment

The patient should be observed for indications of pain (e.g., restlessness). In addition, the patient should be questioned about the degree and characteristics of the pain.

■ Nursing Diagnoses

Nursing diagnoses for the patient experiencing pain and discomfort include, but are not limited to, the following:

- Pain
- Anxiety

■ Nursing Implementation

Interventions for pain include pharmacologic and behavioral therapy. Intravenous narcotics provide the most rapid relief. Medications are administered slowly and titrated to allow for optimal pain management with minimal to no adverse drug side effects. More sustained relief may be obtained through the use of epidural catheters, patient-controlled analgesia, or regional anesthetic blockade. Comfort measures, including touch, reuniting the patient and family, and rewarming, also contribute to patient comfort.

Pain management is most likely to be successful if the treatment plan is initiated with involvement of the patient, the ACP, and the PACU nurse. The goals should be to determine the most effective therapy, medication, and dose and to determine the best response to therapy. Once discharged from the PACU to an inpatient unit, the medical-surgical nurse will replace the PACU nurse as a member of the pain management team. For more information on nursing assessment and management of patients in pain, see Chapter 9.

Nausea and Vomiting

Etiology

Nausea and vomiting are significant problems in the immediate postoperative period. These problems are responsible for unanticipated hospital admission of day-surgery patients, increased patient discomfort, delays in discharge, and patient dissatisfaction with the surgical experience.[1,3]

Numerous factors have been identified as contributing to the development of nausea and vomiting, including anesthetic agents and techniques, gender (female), weight (obesity), type of surgery (eye, testicular, and gynecologic), and a history of nausea and vomiting after surgery or motion sickness.[1]

NURSING MANAGEMENT: NAUSEA AND VOMITING

■ Nursing Assessment

The patient should be questioned about feelings of nausea. If vomiting occurs, it is important to determine the quantity, characteristics, and color of the vomitus.

■ Nursing Diagnoses

Nursing diagnoses for the patient experiencing nausea and vomiting include, but are not limited to, the following:

- Nausea
- Risk for fluid volume deficit

■ Nursing Implementation

Intervention for nausea and vomiting is primarily the use of antiemetic or prokinetic drugs (see Chapter 39). In the PACU, oral fluids should be given only as indicated and tolerated. Intravenous fluids will provide hydration until the patient is able to tolerate oral fluids. Care should also be taken to prevent aspiration if the patient vomits while still sleepy from anesthesia. Having suction equipment readily available at the bedside and turning the patient's head to the side will help protect the patient from aspiration.

Surgical Care of the Patient in the Postanesthesia Care Unit

In addition to meeting the postanesthesia needs of the patient in the PACU, the PACU nurse will also attend to the surgery-specific (e.g., abdominal, thoracic) needs of the patient. The nursing assessment and management of the patient having a specific surgical procedure are discussed in the appropriate chapters of this text.

Table 18-4 Postanesthesia and Ambulatory Surgery Discharge Criteria

Postanesthesia Discharge Criteria
Patient awake (or baseline)
Vital signs stable
No excess bleeding or drainage
No respiratory depression
Oxygen saturation >90%
Report given
Ambulatory Surgery Discharge Criteria
All PACU discharge criteria met
No IV narcotics for last 30 minutes
Minimal nausea and vomiting
Voided (if appropriate to surgical procedure/orders)
Able to ambulate if age-appropriate and not contraindicated
Responsible adult present to accompany patient
Discharge instructions given and understood

Discharge from the Postanesthesia Care Unit

The patient leaving the PACU may be discharged to an intensive care unit, inpatient unit, an ambulatory care unit, or home. The choice of discharge site is based on patient acuity, access to follow-up care, and the potential for postoperative complications.

The decision to discharge the patient from the PACU is based on written discharge criteria. Discharge from an ambulatory care PACU requires that the patient meet additional criteria. Examples of discharge criteria are provided in Table 18-4.

Ambulatory Surgery Discharge. In an outpatient surgery setting the nurse must provide preoperative and postoperative care in a limited amount of time. This presents the nurse with numerous challenges. The nurse must assess the patient and resources, plan for postdischarge care, implement the plan, and evaluate the patient's and family's understanding of the information and their ability to provide for self-care at home, often in just a few hours.[6]

The patient leaving an ambulatory surgery setting must be able to provide a degree of self-care and will be discharged to home, and must therefore be mobile and alert. Postoperative pain and nausea and vomiting must be controlled. Overall, the patient must be stable and near the level of preoperative functioning for discharge from the unit. On discharge, instructions specific to the type of anesthesia received and the surgery are given to the patient verbally and reinforced with written directions. The type of information included in teaching is detailed later in this chapter. The patient may not drive and must be accompanied by a responsible adult at the time of discharge. A follow-up evaluation of the patient's status is made by telephone, and any specific questions and concerns are addressed.

Although ambulatory surgical procedures are minimally invasive, the nurse must carefully determine not only readiness for discharge, but home care needs of the individual. It is important to determine availability of assistive personnel (e.g., family, friends), access to a pharmacy for prescriptions, access to a phone in the event of an emergency, and access to follow-up care.

RESEARCH
IMPLICATIONS FOR NURSING PRACTICE

Outpatient Follow-up

Citation Twersky R, Fishman D, Homel P: What happens after discharge? Return hospital visits after ambulatory surgery, *Anesth Analg* 84:319, 1997.

Purpose To examine the frequency of return hospital visits after ambulatory surgery discharge and to identify any predictor variables for their occurrence.

Methods Retrospective review of hospital records for all patients returning to the same hospital within 30 days after ambulatory surgery was conducted. Data on the return hospital visits that resulted in rehospitalization (as an inpatient or to the ambulatory surgery unit [ASU]) or required treatment as an outpatient in the emergency department (ED) were recorded.

Results and Conclusions Of the 6243 patients who underwent an ambulatory surgical procedure, 187 (3%) returned to the same hospital; almost one half of the returns were for complications. Of all the returns, 54% returned to the ED; 46% were rehospitalized as inpatients or to ASU. Bleeding was the most common reason (41.5%) for all returns with 76.5% of these patients treated and discharged through the ED. Other common reasons for return included fever and infection (15%), pain (9.8%), swelling (7.3%), urinary retention (6.1%), and wound disruption (5.9%). Patients undergoing genitourinary surgery had the highest return rate. Patients under age 40 were more likely to be treated and released, while patients over age 65 were more likely to be readmitted.

Implications for Nursing Practice Patients with bleeding were most likely to return to the ED and be discharged to home, so more effective preprocedure and postprocedure patient education may reduce this occurrence. Better informing patients regarding the prognosis of bleeding, and advising them of treatment alternatives, could reduce inappropriate patient returns to the ED. Care should also be taken when providing discharge instructions about common postoperative complications such as bleeding and infection, especially to patients over age 65.

CARE OF THE POSTOPERATIVE PATIENT ON THE CLINICAL UNIT

Before discharging the patient from the PACU, the PACU nurse will provide a verbal report about the patient to the receiving nurse. The report will summarize the operative and postanesthetic period.

The nurse who receives the patient on the clinical unit will assist PACU transport personnel in transferring the patient from the PACU cart onto the bed. Care must be taken to protect IV lines, wound drains, dressings, and traction devices. The use of a draw sheet and sufficient personnel will facilitate transfer.

Vital signs should be obtained, and patient status should be compared with the report provided by the PACU. Documentation of the transfer is then completed, followed by a more in-depth assessment (Table 18-5). Postoperative orders and appropriate nursing care are then initiated.

Although many of the potential problems that may occur in the PACU are time limited to the immediate postoperative period, a number of potential complications may occur during the extended postoperative recovery period on the medical-surgical unit. Nursing assessment and management are based on awareness of the potential complications of surgery in general, as well as complications specific to the surgical procedure. A general nursing care plan (NCP 18-1) for the postoperative patient follows.

Early ambulation is the most significant general nursing measure to prevent postoperative complications. Since it was first advocated nearly 40 years ago, the value of early ambulation has been obvious. The exercise associated with walking (1) increases muscle tone; (2) improves gastrointestinal (GI) and urinary tract function; (3) stimulates circulation, which prevents venous stasis and speeds wound healing; and (4) increases vital capacity and maintains normal respiratory function.[7] Ambulation is especially important for the older adult patient because hazards of immobility develop earlier, last longer, and may have more lasting effects in the older adult.[8]

Table 18-5 Nursing Assessment and Care of Patient on Admission to Clinical Unit

- Record time of patient's return to unit
- Take baseline vital signs
  - Assess airway and breath sounds
- Assess neurologic status, including level of consciousness and movement of extremities
- Assess wound, dressing, drainage tubes
  - Note type and amount of drainage
  - Connect tubing to gravity or suction drainage
- Assess color and appearance of skin
- Assess urinary status
  - Note time of voiding
  - Note presence of catheter and total output
  - Check for bladder distention or urge to void
  - Note catheter patency
- Assess pain and discomfort
  - Note last dose and type of pain control
  - Note current pain intensity
- Position for airway maintenance, comfort, safety (bed in low position, side rails up)
- Check IV infusion
  - Note type of solution
  - Note amount of fluid remaining
  - Note flow rate
  - Check integrity of insertion site and size of catheter
- Attach call light within reach and reorient patient to use of call light
- Ensure that emesis basin and tissues are available
- Determine emotional condition and support
  - Check for presence of family member or significant other
- Check and carry out postoperative orders

18-1 NURSING CARE PLAN POSTOPERATIVE PATIENT*

Expected Patient Outcomes	Nursing Interventions and *Rationales*
NURSING DIAGNOSIS	**Pain** *related to* surgical incision and reflex muscle spasm *as manifested by* complaints of pain, tense and guarded body posture, facial grimacing, restlessness, irritability, moaning, diaphoresis, tachycardia.
▪ Satisfaction with pain relief ▪ No interference with postoperative recovery	▪ Assess pain for character, location, and effectiveness of relief measures *to plan appropriate interventions.* ▪ Position *to relieve pain.* ▪ Teach patient correct use of patient-controlled analgesia *to ensure effectiveness and control.* ▪ Use nonpharmacologic pain relievers (in addition to pharmacologic intervention) such as distraction, massage, and imagery *to reduce pain.*
NURSING DIAGNOSIS	**Nausea** *related to* gastrointestinal distention and medication or anesthesia effects *as manifested by* complaints of nausea, refusal to take fluids or solids, observed or reported vomiting.
▪ Reduced or no episodes of nausea and vomiting	▪ Assess precipitating factors and eliminate when possible (e.g., unpleasant smells, sights, pain) *to prevent initiating episode of nausea or vomiting.* ▪ Maintain patency of nasogastric tube if present *to prevent accumulation of gastric content and subsequent vomiting and aspiration.* ▪ *Assess bowel sounds* to determine presence, frequency, and characteristics of bowel sounds. ▪ Advance diet only as tolerated. ▪ Monitor gastrointestinal effects of medications, especially narcotics, *to determine if this is a possible source of the nausea.* ▪ Administer antiemetics as indicated.
NURSING DIAGNOSIS	**Risk for infection** *related to* surgical incision, inadequate nutrition and fluid intake, presence of environmental pathogens, invasive catheters, and immobility.
▪ No evidence of infection such as fever, pain or swelling at operative site, or purulent wound drainage	▪ Monitor for and report the following *to determine possible presence of infection:* elevated body temperature; red, swollen, warm area surrounding incision, invasive lines, or indwelling catheters; elevated white blood cell count; elevated pulse and respiratory rate; purulent drainage from wound. ▪ Use strict aseptic technique in providing wound care, including hand washing and sterile dressing technique, *to prevent wound contamination.* ▪ Administer antibiotics if ordered. ▪ Ensure a minimum of 2000 calories and 2500 ml fluid per day (greater if metabolic demands are increased) *to ensure adequate calories for tissue repair.* ▪ Weigh daily and notify physician if greater than 5% weight loss from baseline *to modify nutritional plan.* ▪ Minimize exposure to environmental pathogens by avoiding contact between patient and others with infection *to prevent cross-contamination.* ▪ Help patient turn, cough, and breathe deeply every 1 to 2 hours while awake *to prevent respiratory infection.*
NURSING DIAGNOSIS	**Ineffective airway clearance** *related to* ineffective cough and tenacious secretions *as manifested by* abnormal breath sounds, shallow respirations, nonproductive cough.
▪ Clear breath sounds ▪ Effective cough	▪ Provide for pain relief before having the patient cough and breathe deeply *to encourage cooperation and pain-free performance.* ▪ Provide a minimum of 2500 ml fluids per day unless contraindicated *to liquefy secretions for easier removal.* ▪ Assist patient with turning, coughing, and deep breathing every 1 to 2 hours while awake *to aid in removal of secretions and prevent formation of mucous plug.* ▪ Monitor use of incentive spirometer *to expand the lungs fully.* ▪ Discourage smoking. ▪ Suction if necessary *to remove secretions the patient is unable to remove unaided.* ▪ Monitor breath sounds and temperature *to detect early signs of infection.* ▪ Assist with early mobility *to increase respiratory excursion.*

Continued

18-1 NURSING CARE PLAN POSTOPERATIVE PATIENT*—continued

Expected Patient Outcomes	Nursing Interventions and *Rationales*
NURSING DIAGNOSIS	**Anxiety** *related to* lack of knowledge about follow-up care *as manifested by* frequent questioning about self-care at home, concern over difficulty in performing any part of self-care at home.
▪ Satisfaction with own knowledge and skill level or with plan made for home care.	▪ Teach patient and family about signs and symptoms of infection to observe and report, nutritional needs of patient, activity restrictions, wound care, and medication requirements *to decrease anxiety and increase sense of control.* ▪ Ensure patient's or family member's skills in performing self-care before discharge or arrange for referral for home care *to ensure continuity of care using appropriate technique.* ▪ Allow sufficient practice in technical skills such as dressing change for patient or family member *to become confident.* ▪ Together with patient, identify aspects of self-care with which assistance may be needed *so appropriate referrals can be made.* ▪ Assist patient to plan follow-up care with surgeon *to avoid delay in appropriate follow-up.*
NURSING DIAGNOSIS	**Constipation** *related to* inadequate intake, decreased physical activity, and medications that decrease bowel activity *as manifested by* hard, formed stool, straining at stool, or defecation less than 3 times per week.
▪ Usual bowel pattern.	▪ Assess bowel elimination *to determine need for intervention.* ▪ Maintain daily fluid intake of 2500 ml or more *to soften fecal mass.* ▪ Provide increased fiber in diet if appropriate *to increase fecal bulk and retention of fluid in fecal mass.* ▪ Increase activity as tolerated *to increase peristalsis.* ▪ Administer stool softeners as ordered *to soften fecal mass.*

COLLABORATIVE PROBLEMS

Nursing Goals	Nursing Interventions and *Rationales*
POTENTIAL COMPLICATION	**Hemorrhage** *related to* ineffective vascular closure or alterations in coagulation.
▪ Monitor operative site for signs of hemorrhage. ▪ Report deviations from acceptable parameters. ▪ Carry out appropriate medical and nursing interventions.	▪ Observe surgical site and dressings regularly (q hr for 4 hr, then q4hr) *to detect signs of bleeding, including dependent sites.* ▪ Monitor vital signs regularly from q15min to q2-4hr as indicated *to detect signs of hypovolemia.* ▪ Report abnormalities such as decreasing blood pressure; rapid pulse and respirations; cool, clammy skin; pallor; bright red blood on dressing. ▪ Monitor for changes in mental status, such as restlessness and sense of impending doom, *as indicators of inadequate cerebral perfusion.* ▪ Monitor hematocrit and hemoglobin levels *because decreases may indicate hemorrhage.* ▪ Monitor platelet levels *because decreases may indicate bleeding tendencies.* ▪ Monitor coagulation function tests *because elevations may indicate bleeding tendencies.*
POTENTIAL COMPLICATION	**Thromboembolism** *related to* dehydration, immobility, vascular manipulation, or injury.
▪ Monitor for signs of thromboembolism. ▪ Report deviation from acceptable parameters. ▪ Carry out appropriate medical and nursing interventions.	▪ Assess for signs of thromboembolism, such as redness, swelling, pain; increased warmth along path of vein; positive Homans' sign; edema or pain in extremity; chest pain; hemoptysis; tachypnea; dyspnea; restlessness. ▪ Administer subcutaneous heparin (if ordered) *to decrease clot formation.* ▪ Teach or perform range of motion to lower extremities and encourage early ambulation *to maintain muscle contractions and adequate vascular flow.* ▪ Avoid pressure under knees from bed or pillows *to avoid pressure on veins, constriction of circulation, or pooling and stasis of blood.* ▪ Apply antiembolism stockings and sequential compression device, if ordered. Remove for 1 hr every 8 to 10 hr *to allow for skin assessment.* ▪ Maintain adequate hydration *to prevent hypovolemia and subsequent sludging of cells.*

Continued

18-1 NURSING CARE PLAN POSTOPERATIVE PATIENT*—continued

Nursing Goals	Nursing Interventions and *Rationales*
POTENTIAL COMPLICATION	**Urinary retention** *related to* horizontal positioning, pain, fear, analgesic and anesthetic medications, or surgical procedure.
▪ Monitor for signs of urinary retention. ▪ Report deviation from acceptable parameters. ▪ Carry out appropriate medical and nursing interventions.	▪ Assess for bladder pain and distention, decreased or absent urinary output *to determine if a problem is present.* ▪ Monitor intake and output *to determine fluid balance.* ▪ Percuss bladder routinely for 48 hr postoperatively *to assess for distention.* ▪ Notify physician if no urine output within 6 hr after surgery. ▪ Position patient in as normal position as possible for voiding. ▪ Provide privacy. ▪ Use appropriate pain measures *to reduce anxiety so voiding will be easier.* ▪ Provide explanation and encouragement *to relieve patient's fears.* ▪ Monitor urinary effects of analgesic and anesthetic medications *because they could be a source of urinary retention.*
POTENTIAL COMPLICATION	**Paralytic ileus** *related to* bowel manipulation, immobility, pain medication, and anesthetics.
▪ Monitor for signs of paralytic ileus. ▪ Report deviation from acceptable parameters. ▪ Carry out appropriate medical and nursing interventions.	▪ Assess for abdominal distention, presence of flatus or stool, bowel sounds, or nausea and vomiting *to determine if paralytic ileus is present.* ▪ Maintain NPO status until peristalsis returns and ensure patency of nasogastric tube *to prevent vomiting.* ▪ Provide frequent oral hygiene for patient comfort.

*This is a general nursing care plan for the postoperative patient. It should be used in conjunction with a nursing care plan specific to the type of surgery being performed.

Potential Alterations in Respiratory Function

Etiology

Atelectasis and pneumonia can occur in the postoperative surgical patient and are particularly common after abdominal and thoracic surgery. *Atelectasis* (alveolar collapse) occurs when mucus blocks bronchioles or when the amount of alveolar surfactant (the substance that holds the alveoli open) is reduced (Fig. 18-5). As air becomes trapped beyond the plug and is eventually absorbed, the alveoli collapse. Atelectasis may affect a portion or an entire lobe of the lungs.

The postoperative development of mucous plugs and decreased surfactant production are directly related to hypoventilation, constant recumbent position, ineffective coughing, and smoking. Increased bronchial secretions occur when the respiratory passages are irritated by heavy smoking, acute or chronic pulmonary infection or disease, and the drying of mucous membranes that occurs with intubation, inhalation anesthesia, and dehydration. Without intervention, atelectasis can progress to pneumonia when microorganisms grow in the stagnant mucus and an infection develops.

NURSING MANAGEMENT: RESPIRATORY COMPLICATIONS

■ Nursing Assessment

Nursing assessment of the patient's respiratory rate, patterns, and breath sounds is essential to identify potential respiratory problems.

■ Nursing Diagnoses

Nursing diagnoses and collaborative problems related to potential respiratory complications for the postoperative patient include, but are not limited to, the following:

- Ineffective airway clearance
- Ineffective breathing pattern
- Impaired gas exchange
- Potential complication: pneumonia
- Potential complication: atelectasis

■ Nursing Implementation

Deep-breathing and coughing techniques help the patient prevent alveolar collapse and move respiratory secretions to larger airway passages for expectoration. The patient should be assisted to breathe deeply 10 times every hour. The use of an incentive spirometer is helpful in providing visual feedback of respiratory effort. Diaphragmatic or abdominal breathing is accomplished by inhaling slowly and deeply through the nose, holding the breath for a few seconds, and then exhaling slowly and completely through the mouth. The patient's hands should be placed lightly over the lower ribs and upper abdomen. This allows the patient to feel the abdomen rise during inspiration and fall during expiration.

Following four to six deep breaths, the patient should cough deeply from the lungs rather than the throat. If secretions are present in the respiratory passages, deep breathing often will move them up to stimulate the cough reflex without any voluntary effort by the patient, and they can then be expectorated.

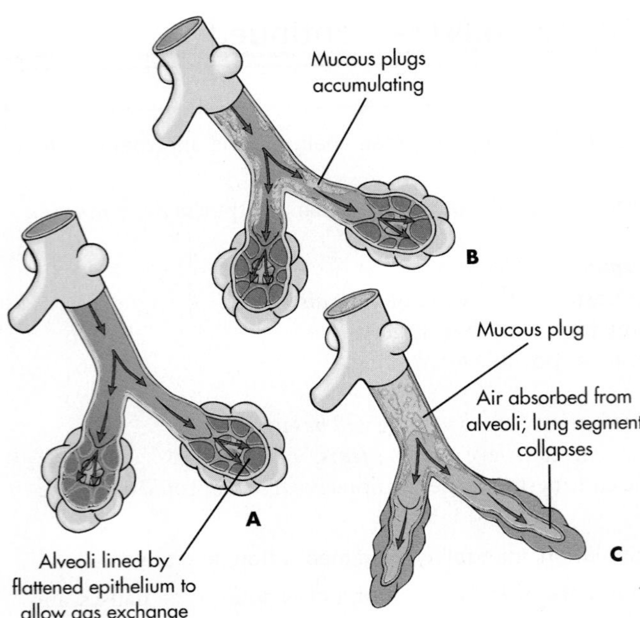

Fig. 18-5 Postoperative atelectasis. **A,** Normal bronchiole and alveoli. **B,** Mucous plug in bronchiole. **C,** Collapse of alveoli due to atelectasis following absorption of air.

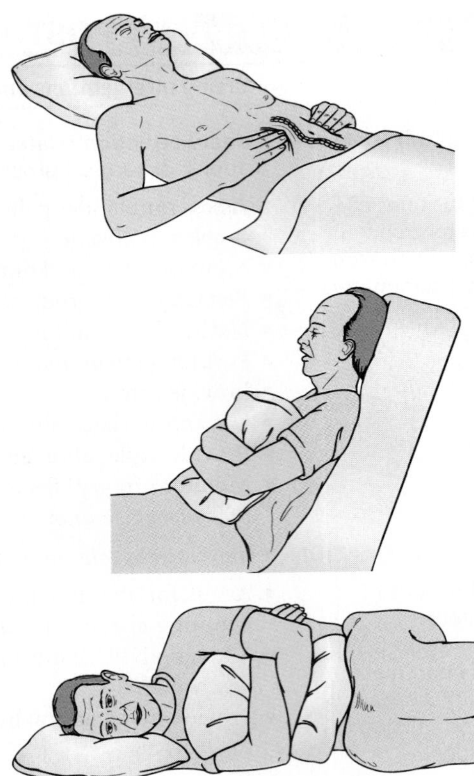

Fig. 18-6 Techniques for splinting wound when coughing.

Splinting the incision with a pillow or a rolled blanket provides support to weakened muscles and protection for abdominal incisions and also aids in coughing and expectoration of secretions (Fig. 18-6). Incentive spirometry can be used as an adjunct to traditional deep-breathing and coughing techniques.[9]

The patient's position should be changed every 1 to 2 hours to allow full chest expansion and increase perfusion of both lungs. Ambulation, not just sitting in a chair, should be aggressively carried out as soon as physician approval is given. Adequate and regular analgesic medication should be provided because incisional pain often is the greatest deterrent to patient participation in effective ventilation and ambulation. The patient should also be reassured that these activities will not cause the incision to separate. Adequate hydration, either parenteral or oral, is essential to maintain the integrity of mucous membranes and to keep secretions thin and loose for easy expectoration.

Potential Alterations in Cardiovascular Function

Etiology

Postoperative fluid and electrolyte imbalances are contributing factors to alterations in cardiovascular function. They may develop as a result of a combination of the body's normal response to the stress of surgery, excessive fluid losses, and improper IV fluid replacement. The body's fluid status directly affects cardiac output. Fluid retention during the first 2 to 5 postoperative days can be the result of the stress response (see Chapter 7). This body response serves to maintain both blood volume and blood pressure (see Fig. 7-6). Fluid retention results from the secretion and release of two hormones by the pituitary—adrenocorticotropic hormone (ACTH) and antidiuretic hormone (ADH). ACTH stimulates the adrenal cortex to secrete moderate amounts of aldosterone resulting in sodium and water retention, which increases blood volume. ADH release leads to increased H_2O reabsorption and decreased urinary output, which ultimately increases blood volume.

Fluid overload may occur during this period of fluid retention when IV fluids are administered too rapidly, when chronic (e.g., cardiac or renal) disease exists, or when the patient is an older adult. Conversely, fluid deficit may be related to slow or inadequate fluid replacement, which leads to decreases in cardiac output and tissue perfusion. Untreated preoperative dehydration or intraoperative or postoperative losses from vomiting, bleeding, wound drainage, or suctioning may be contributing factors to fluid deficits.

Hypokalemia can be a consequence of urinary and GI tract losses, and it results when potassium is not replaced in IV fluids. The loss of potassium directly affects the contractility of the heart and thus may also contribute to decreased cardiac output and overall body tissue perfusion. Adequate replacement of potassium is usually 40 mEq per day. However, it should not be given until adequate renal function has been established. A urine output of at least 0.5 ml/kg per hour is generally considered indicative of adequate renal function.

Cardiovascular status is also affected by the state of tissue perfusion or blood flow. The stress response contributes to an increase in clotting tendencies in the postoperative patient by increasing platelet production and circulating levels of corticosteroids. Deep vein thrombosis (DVT) may form in leg veins as a result of inactivity, body position, and pressure, all of which lead to venous stasis and decreased perfusion. Deep vein thrombosis, especially common in the older adult, obese individual, and immobilized patient, is a potentially life-threatening complication because it may lead to pulmonary embolism. Pulmonary embolism should be suspected in any patient complaining of tachypnea, dyspnea, and tachycardia, particularly when the patient is already receiving oxygen therapy. Symptoms may include chest pain, hypotension, hemoptysis, arrhythmias, and congestive heart failure. Definitive diagnosis requires pulmonary angiography. *Superficial thrombophlebitis* is an uncomfortable but less ominous complication that may develop in a leg vein as a result of venous stasis or in the arm veins as a result of irritation from IV catheters or solutions. If a piece of a clot becomes dislodged and travels to the lung, it can cause a pulmonary infarction of a size proportionate to the vessel in which it lodges.

Syncope (fainting) is another factor that reflects the cardiovascular status. It may indicate decreased cardiac output, fluid deficits, or defects in cerebral tissue perfusion. Syncope frequently occurs as a result of postural hypotension when the patient ambulates. It is more common in the older adult or in the patient who has been immobile for long periods of time. Normally when the patient quickly moves to a standing position, the arterial pressoreceptors respond to the accompanying fall in blood pressure with sympathetic nervous stimulation, which produces vasoconstriction. This sympathetic nervous system response causes an increase in, and therefore maintains, blood pressure. These sympathetic and vasomotor functions may be diminished in the older adult and the immobile or postanesthetic patient. Consequently, syncope develops when the patient sits up rapidly or during ambulation.

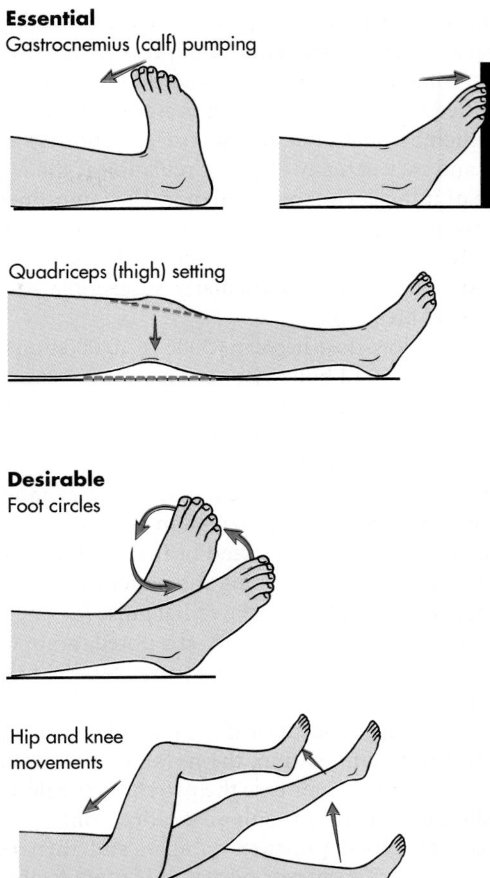

Fig. 18-7 Postoperative leg exercises.

NURSING MANAGEMENT: CARDIOVASCULAR COMPLICATIONS

■ Nursing Assessment

Specific assessment of cardiovascular function includes the regular monitoring of the patient's blood pressure, heart rate, pulses, and skin temperature and color. Results should be compared with preoperative status and the immediate postoperative and intraoperative findings.

■ Nursing Diagnoses

Nursing diagnoses and collaborative problems related to potential cardiovascular complications for the postoperative patient include, but are not limited to, the following:

- Decreased cardiac output
- Fluid volume deficit
- Fluid volume excess
- Altered tissue perfusion
- Activity intolerance
- Potential complication: thromboembolism

■ Nursing Implementation

An accurate intake and output record should be kept during the postoperative period, and laboratory findings (e.g., electrolytes, hematocrit) should be monitored. Nursing responsibilities relating to IV management are critical during this period. In particular the nurse should be alert for symptoms of too slow or too rapid a rate of fluid replacement. Assessment should also be made of the infusion site for discomfort and the hazards associated with the IV administration of potassium, such as pain in the area of the vein where it is entering and cardiac arrest. Thirst is one of the most annoying discomforts with which the postoperative patient must contend. This may be related to the drying effects of anticholinergic drugs, anesthetic gases, and fluid deficits. Adequate and regular mouth care is helpful while the patient cannot ingest food or drink by mouth.

Leg exercises (Fig. 18-7) should be encouraged 10 to 12 times every 1 to 2 hours. The muscular contraction produced by these exercises and by ambulation facilitates venous return from the lower extremities. The ambulating patient should pick up the feet rather than shuffling them so that muscular contraction is maximized. When confined to bed, the patient should alternately flex and extend the legs. When the patient is sitting in a chair or lying in bed, there should be no pressure to impede venous flow through the popliteal space. Crossed legs, pillows behind the knees, and elevation of the knee gatch must be avoided.

Some surgeons routinely prescribe elastic stockings or mechanical aids such as sequential compressive devices to stimulate and enhance the massaging and milking actions that are transmitted to the veins when leg muscles contract. The nurse must remember that these aids are useless if the legs are not exercised and may actually impair circulation if the legs remain inactive or if the devices are sized or applied improperly. When in use, elastic stockings must be removed and reapplied at least twice daily for skin care and inspection. The skin of the heels and post-tibial areas is particularly susceptible to increased pressure and breakdown.

The use of low-dose heparin (5000 to 10,000 units subcutaneously every 8 to 12 hours) or enoxaparin (Lovenox) is a prophylactic measure for venous thrombosis and embolism. Neither drug significantly increases the risk of bleeding during surgery or in the postoperative period.[7,10]

The nurse may prevent syncope by making changes slowly in the patient's position. Progression to ambulation can be achieved by first raising the head of the patient's bed for 1 to 2 minutes and then by assisting the patient to sit on the side of the bed while monitoring the radial pulse for rate and quality. If no changes or complaints are noted, ambulation can be started. If faintness occurs, the nurse can help the patient sit on the edge of the bed while continuing to monitor the pulse. If changes occur or if the patient complains of feeling faint during ambulation, the nurse should provide assistance to a nearby chair or ease the patient to the floor. The patient should remain in either location until recovery is evidenced by blood pressure stability, and then be helped back to the bed. If faintness occurs, it is often frightening for the patient and for the unprepared nurse, but syncope poses no real physiologic danger, although injury can result from a fall.

Potential Alterations in Urinary Function

Etiology

Low urine output (800 to 1500 ml) in the first 24 hours may be expected, regardless of fluid intake. This low output is caused by increased aldosterone and ADH secretion resulting from the stress of surgery, fluid restriction before surgery, and loss of fluids caused by evaporation during surgery, drainage, and diaphoresis. By the second or third day, the patient will begin to have increasing urinary output after fluid has been mobilized, and the immediate stress reaction subsides.

Acute urinary retention can occur in the postoperative period for a variety of reasons. Anesthesia depresses the nervous system, including the micturition reflex arc and the higher centers that influence it. This allows the bladder to fill more completely than normal before the urge to void is felt. Anesthesia also impedes voluntary micturition. Anticholinergic and narcotic drugs may also interfere with the ability to initiate voiding or to empty the bladder completely.

Retention is more likely to occur after lower abdominal or pelvic surgery because spasm or guarding of the abdominal and pelvic muscles interferes with their normal function in micturition. Pain may alter perception and interfere with the patient's awareness of the less intense sensation arising as the bladder fills. Voiding ability is probably impaired to the greatest extent by immobility and the recumbent position in bed. Lack of skeletal muscle activity decreases smooth muscle (bladder detrusor) tone, and the supine position reduces the ability to relax the perineal muscles and external sphincter.

Oliguria, the diminished output of urine, can be a manifestation of acute renal failure and is a less common although more serious problem after surgery. It may result from renal ischemia caused by inadequate renal perfusion or altered cardiovascular function.

NURSING MANAGEMENT: URINARY COMPLICATIONS

■ Nursing Assessment

The urine of the postoperative patient should be examined for both quantity and quality. The color, amount, consistency, and odor of the urine should be noted. Indwelling catheters should be assessed for patency, and urine output should be at least 0.5 ml/kg per hour. If a catheter is not present, the patient should be able to void approximately 200 ml of urine following surgery. Most people urinate within 6 to 8 hours after surgery. If no voiding occurs, the abdominal contour should be inspected and the bladder palpated and percussed for distention.

■ Nursing Diagnoses

Nursing diagnoses and collaborative problems related to potential urinary complications for the postoperative patient include, but are not limited to, the following:

- Altered urinary elimination
- Potential complication: acute urinary retention

■ Nursing Implementation

The nurse may facilitate voiding by normal positioning of the patient—sitting for women and standing for men. Providing reassurance to the patient regarding the ability to void and the use of techniques such as running water, drinking water, or pouring warm water over the perineum may also be of assistance. Ambulation, preferably to the bathroom, and the use of a bedside commode are additional helpful measures to assist in voiding.

The surgeon often leaves an order to catheterize the patient in 8 to 12 hours if voiding has not occurred. Because of the possibility of infection associated with catheterization, the nurse should first try other measures to induce voiding and validate that the bladder is actually full. If the bladder becomes overdistended, it is traumatized and more susceptible to infection if catheterization becomes necessary. In assessing the need for catheterization, the nurse should consider fluid intake during and after surgery and determine bladder fullness (e.g., palpable fullness above the symphysis pubis, discomfort when pressure is applied over the bladder, or the presence of the urge to void). Straight catheterization is preferred because of the possibility of infection associated with an indwelling catheter.

Potential Alterations in Gastrointestinal Function

Etiology

Slowed GI mobility and altered patterns of food intake may lead to the development of several distressing postoperative symptoms that are most pronounced after abdominal surgery. Nausea and vomiting may be caused by the action of anesthetics or narcotics, delayed gastric emptying, slowed peristalsis resulting from the handling of the bowel during surgery, and resumption of oral intake too soon after surgery.

Abdominal distention is another common problem caused by decreased peristalsis as a result of handling of the intestine during surgery and limited dietary intake before and after surgery. Motility of the large intestine may be reduced for 3 to 5 days, although motility in the small intestine resumes within 24 hours. Swallowed air and GI secretions may accumulate in the colon, producing flatulence and gas pains.

Hiccoughs (singultus) are intermittent spasms of the diaphragm caused by irritation of the phrenic nerve, which innervates the diaphragm. Postoperative sources of direct irritation of the phrenic nerve may be gastric distention, intestinal obstruction, intraabdominal bleeding, and a subphrenic abscess. Indirect irritation of the phrenic nerve may be produced by acid-base and electrolyte imbalances. Reflex irritation may come from drinking hot or cold liquids or from the presence of a nasogastric tube. Hiccoughs usually last a short time and subside spontaneously; occasionally they may be persistent but are rarely debilitating.

NURSING MANAGEMENT: GASTROINTESTINAL COMPLICATIONS

■ Nursing Assessment

The abdomen should be auscultated in all four quadrants to determine the presence, frequency, and characteristics of the bowel sounds. Bowel sounds are frequently absent or diminished in the immediate postoperative period when peristalsis is decreased. If vomiting occurs, the emesis should be evaluated for color, consistency, and amount.

■ Nursing Diagnoses

Nursing diagnoses and collaborative problems related to potential GI complications for the postoperative patient may include, but are not limited to, the following:

- Nausea
- Altered nutrition: less than body requirements
- Potential complication: paralytic ileus
- Potential complication: hiccoughs

■ Nursing Implementation

Depending on the nature of the surgery, the patient may resume oral intake as soon as the gag reflex returns. Sometimes the patient is kept on nothing by mouth (NPO) status for several days until bowel sounds are heard. Although the patient is receiving NPO, IV infusions are given to maintain fluid and electrolyte balance. A nasogastric tube may be used to decompress the stomach to prevent nausea, vomiting, and abdominal distention. When oral intake is allowed after the return of bowel sounds, clear liquids are begun, and the IV infusion is continued, usually at a reduced rate. If oral intake is well tolerated by the patient, the IV is discontinued, and the diet is advanced until a regular diet is tolerated.

While the patient is on NPO status, regular mouth care is essential for comfort and stimulation of salivary glands. Nausea and vomiting may be prevented or relieved by the administration of an antiemetic drug given IV, intramuscularly, or by rectal suppository. In some instances a nasogastric tube is inserted when symptoms persist.

Abdominal distention may be prevented or minimized by early and frequent ambulation and by resumption of a normal diet, both of which stimulate intestinal peristalsis. The nurse should assess the patient regularly to detect the resumption of normal intestinal peristalsis as evidenced by the return of bowel sounds and the passage of flatus. The nasogastric tube must be clamped or suction turned off when the abdomen is auscultated.

The patient may need to be encouraged to expel flatus and assured that expulsion is necessary and desirable. Gas pains, which tend to become pronounced on the second or third postoperative day, may be relieved by ambulation and frequent repositioning. Positioning the patient on the right side permits gas to rise along the transverse colon and facilitates its release. Bisacodyl (Dulcolax) suppositories may be ordered to stimulate peristalsis and expulsion of flatus.

The postoperative patient who is hiccoughing should first be assessed in an attempt to determine the cause. In many instances simple irrigation of the nasogastric tube to restore patency will solve the problem.

Potential Alterations of the Integument

Etiology

Surgery generally involves an incision through the skin and underlying tissues. An incision disrupts the protective skin barrier and needs wound healing, which is one of the major concerns during the postoperative period.

An adequate nutritional state is essential for wound healing. Amino acids are readily available for the healing process because of the catabolic effects of the stress-related hormones (e.g., cortisol, catecholamines). The patient who was well nourished preoperatively can tolerate the postoperative delay in nutritional intake. However, the patient with preexisting nutritional deficits, such as with chronic diseases (e.g., diabetes, ulcerative colitis, alcoholism), are more prone to problems of wound healing. Wound healing is also a concern for the older adult and is affected by multiple factors.

Wound infection may result from contamination of the wound from three major sources: (1) exogenous flora present in the environment and on the skin, (2) oral flora, and (3) intestinal flora. The incidence of wound sepsis is higher in patients who are malnourished, immunosuppressed, or older, or

Table 18-6 Expected Drainage from Tubes and Catheters

Substance	Daily Amount	Color	Odor	Consistency
Indwelling Catheter				
Urine	500-700 ml, 1-2 days postop; 1500-2500 ml thereafter	Clear, yellow	Ammonia	Watery
Gastrostomy Tube				
Gastric contents	Up to 1500 ml/day	Pale, yellow-green Bloody following GI surgery	Sour	Watery
Nasogastric Tube				
Gastric contents	Up to 1500 ml	Pale yellow-green Bloody following GI surgery	Sour	Watery
Hemovac				
Wound drainage	Variable with procedure	Variable with procedure Usually serosanguineous	Same as wound dressing	Variable
T-Tube				
Bile	500 ml	Bright yellow to dark green	Acid	Thick

GI, gastrointestinal.

who have had a prolonged hospital stay or a lengthy surgical procedure (lasting more than 3 hours). Patients undergoing bowel surgery, particularly following a traumatic injury, are at a particularly high risk. Infection may involve the entire incision and may extend downward through the deeper tissue layers. An abscess may form locally, or the infection may penetrate entire body cavities, as in peritonitis. Evidence of wound infection usually does not become apparent before the third to the fifth postoperative day. The signs include local manifestations of redness, swelling, and increasing pain and tenderness at the site. Systemic signs are fever and leukocytosis.

An accumulation of fluid in a wound may create pressure, impair circulation and wound healing, and predispose to infection. Because of these reasons the surgeon may place a drain in the incision or make a stab wound adjacent to the incision to allow for drainage. These drains may be made of soft rubber and drain into a dressing, or they may be firm catheters attached to a Hemovac or other source of gentle suction. Wound healing and complications are discussed in Chapter 11.

NURSING MANAGEMENT: SURGICAL WOUNDS

■ Nursing Assessment

Nursing assessment of the wound and dressing requires knowledge of the type of wound, drains inserted, and expected drainage related to the specific type of surgery. A small amount of serous drainage is common from any type of wound. If a drain is in place, a moderate to large amount of drainage may be expected. For example, an abdominal incision with accompanying drain is expected to have a moderate amount of serosanguineous drainage in the first 24 hours. In contrast, an inguinal herniorrhaphy should have only minimal serous drainage during the postoperative period.

In general, drainage is expected to change from sanguineous (red) to serosanguineous (pink) to serous (straw-colored) during a period of hours to days. Bloody drainage may be normal after certain types of surgery (e.g., chest surgery). A continuation of bleeding with no decrease in volume, or an increase in drainage after it has once subsided, often signals a problem.[11] Wound infection may be accompanied by purulent drainage. Wound dehiscence (separation and disruption of previously joined wound edges) may be preceded by a sudden discharge of brown, pink, or clear drainage.

■ Nursing Diagnoses

Nursing diagnoses related to surgical wounds of the postoperative patient include, but are not limited to, the following:

- Impaired tissue integrity
- Risk for infection

■ Nursing Implementation

When drainage occurs on the dressing, the type, amount, color, consistency, and odor of drainage should be noted and recorded. Expected drainage from tubes is outlined in Table 18-6. The effect of position changes on drainage should also be assessed. The surgeon should be notified of any excessive or abnormal drainage and significant changes in vital signs.

The incision may be initially covered with a dressing immediately after surgery. If there is no drainage after 24 to 48 hours, the incision may be opened to the air. Agency policy determines whether the nurse may change the initial operative dressing or simply reinforce it if the dressing is saturated.

When a dressing is changed, the number and type of drains present should be noted. Care should be taken to avoid dislodging drains during dressing removal. When the dressing is changed, the incision site should be examined carefully. The area around the sutures may be slightly reddened and swollen, which is an expected inflammatory response. However, the skin around the incision should be normal color and temperature. Abnormal findings include unusually warm skin around the incision, purple hard areas in the site (possibly from hemorrhage into the tissue), and other signs of infection.[12,13] The nurse should wear gloves when removing a dressing. Sterile technique should be used when any new dressing is applied. If healing is by primary intention, little or no drainage is present, and no drains are in place, a single-layer dressing is sufficient. When drains are in place, when moderate to heavy drainage is occurring, or when healing occurs other than by primary intention, a multiple-layer dressing is needed. Wound care and dressings are discussed in Chapter 11.

Potential Alterations in Neurologic Function

Etiology

Pain and fever are two clinical manifestations that may present problems for the postoperative patient. The assessment and management of the patient in pain are discussed in Chapter 9. Postoperative pain is caused by the interaction of a number of physiologic and psychologic factors. The skin and underlying tissues have been traumatized by the incision and retraction during surgery. In addition, there may be reflex muscle spasms around the incision. Anxiety and fear, sometimes related to the anticipation of pain, create tension and further increase muscle tone and spasm. The effort and movement associated with deep breathing, coughing, and changing position may aggravate pain by creating tension or pull on the incisional area.

When the internal viscera is cut, no pain is felt. However, pressure in the internal viscera elicits pain. Therefore deep visceral pain may signal the presence of a complication such as intestinal distention, bleeding, or abscess formation.

Postoperative pain is usually most severe within the first 48 hours and subsides thereafter. Variation is considerable, according to the procedure performed and the patient's individual pain tolerance or perception.

Temperature variation in the postoperative period provides valuable information about the patient's status. Hypothermia may be present in the immediate postoperative period while the patient is recovering from the effects of anesthesia and body heat loss during surgery. Fever may occur at any time during the postoperative period (Table 18-7). A mild elevation (up to 100.4° F [38° C]) during the first 48 hours usually reflects the surgical stress response. A moderate elevation (higher than 100.4° F [38° C]) is caused more frequently by respiratory congestion or atelectasis and less frequently by dehydration. After the first 48 hours a moderate to marked elevation (higher than 99.9° F [37.7° C]) is usually caused by infection.

Table 18-7 Significance of Postoperative Temperature Changes

Time After Surgery	Temperature	Possible Causes
Up to 12 hr	Hypothermia to 94° F (34.5° C)	Effects of anesthesia Body heat loss in surgical exposure
First 24-48 hr	Elevation to 100.4° F (38° C)	Inflammatory response to surgical stress
	Above 100.4° F (38° C)	Lung congestion, atelectasis Dehydration
Third day and later	Elevation above 100° F (37.7° C)	Wound infection Urinary infection Respiratory infection Phlebitis

Wound infection, particularly from aerobic organisms, is often accompanied by a fever that spikes in the afternoon or evening and returns to near-normal levels in the morning. The respiratory tract may be infected secondary to stasis of secretions in areas of atelectasis. The urinary tract may be infected secondary to catheterization. Superficial thrombophlebitis may occur at the IV site or in the leg veins. The latter may produce a temperature elevation between 7 and 10 days after surgery.

Intermittent high fever accompanied by shaking chills and diaphoresis suggests septicemia. This may occur at any time during the postoperative period because microorganisms may have been introduced into the bloodstream during surgery, especially in GI or genitourinary (GU) procedures, or picked up later from the site of a wound or a urinary or vein infection.

NURSING MANAGEMENT: NEUROLOGIC COMPLICATIONS

■ Nursing Assessment

The initial aspect of the neurologic assessment is a determination of the level of consciousness. The anesthetized patient resumes consciousness in a predictable pattern. By the time the patient returns to the clinical unit, she or he is usually awake or easily arousable. The nurse must be alert for possible deepening of anesthesia effects, especially when administering pain medication in the early postoperative period.

Pain assessment may be difficult in the early postoperative period. The patient may not be able to verbalize the presence or severity of pain. The nurse should observe for behavioral clues of pain such as a wrinkling face or brow, a clenched fist, moaning, diaphoresis, and an increased pulse rate.

Nursing Diagnoses

Nursing diagnoses related to potential neurologic complications for the postoperative patient may include, but are not limited to, the following:

- Sensory-perceptual alterations
- Pain
- Risk for altered body temperature

Nursing Implementation

Postoperative pain relief is a nursing responsibility because the surgeon's orders for analgesic medication and other comfort measures are usually written on an as-needed basis. During the first 48 hours or longer, narcotic analgesics (e.g., morphine) are required to relieve moderate-to-severe pain. After that time, nonnarcotic analgesics, such as nonsteroidal anti-inflammatory agents, may be sufficient as pain intensity decreases.

During the first 24 to 48 hours, the patient should be medicated freely every 3 to 4 hours if necessary because (1) the greatest relief is obtained when an analgesic is administered as pain is beginning rather than when it has become more severe and (2) relative freedom from pain is essential to gain the patient's cooperation in activities of deep breathing, coughing, turning, and ambulating.[14,15] When the patient does request pain medication, it should be given promptly because time perception is altered by pain and minutes can seem like hours.

Analgesic administration should be timed to ensure that it is in effect during activities that may be painful for the patient, such as ambulating. Although narcotic analgesics are often essential for the postoperative patient's comfort, there are undesirable side effects. Side effects such as constipation, nausea and vomiting, respiratory and cough depression, and hypotension are most common with the opiates.

Before administering any analgesic, the nurse should first assess the nature of the patient's pain, including location, quality, and intensity. If it is incisional pain, analgesic administration is appropriate. If it is chest or leg pain, medication may simply mask a complication that must be reported and documented. If it is gas pain, narcotic medication can aggravate it. The nurse should notify the physician and request a change in the order if the analgesic either fails to relieve the pain or makes the patient excessively lethargic or somnolent.

Patient-controlled analgesia (PCA) and epidural analgesia are two alternative approaches for pain control. The goals of PCA are to provide immediate analgesia and to maintain a constant, steady blood level of the analgesic agent. PCA involves self-administration of predetermined doses of analgesia by the patient. The route of delivery may be IV, oral, or epidural. (PCA is discussed in Chapter 9.)

Epidural analgesia is the infusion of pain-relieving medications through a catheter placed into the epidural space surrounding the spinal cord. The goal of epidural analgesia is delivery of medication directly to opiate receptors in the spinal cord. The administration may be intermittent or constant and is monitored by the nurse. The overall effectiveness and the technique of administration result in a constant circulating level and a total reduced dose of medication.

A number of other measures may be helpful in preventing or relieving postoperative pain. If abdominal surgery has been performed, the patient should be instructed to use the limbs rather than the abdominal muscles in turning and getting out of bed. Techniques of controlled breathing or relaxation may be used for pain relief. Both methods have a similar rationale, which includes anxiety reduction, attention distraction, muscle relaxation, and provision of a sense of control over the pain experience.[15]

The nurse's role with respect to postoperative fever may be preventive, diagnostic, and therapeutic. Meticulous asepsis is a preventive measure that should be maintained with regard to the wound and IV site, and frequent observation for early signs of inflammation.

The patient's temperature is usually measured every 4 hours for the first 48 hours postoperatively and then less frequently if no problems develop. If fever develops, chest x-rays may be taken and, depending on the suspected cause, cultures of the wound, urine, or blood are obtained. If infection is the source of the fever, antibiotics are started as soon as cultures have been obtained. If the fever is extreme (105.8° F [41° C]), antipyretic drugs and body-cooling measures will be employed.

Potential Alterations in Psychologic Function

Etiology

Anxiety and depression may occur in the postoperative patient. These states may be more pronounced in the patient who has had radical surgery (e.g., colostomy) or amputation or whose findings suggest a poor prognosis (e.g., inoperable tumor). A history of a neurotic or psychotic disorder should alert the nurse to the possibility of postoperative anxiety and depression. However, these responses may develop in any patient as part of the grief response to loss of a body organ or disturbance in body image and may be exacerbated by a lowered response to stress.

Confusion or delirium may arise from a variety of psychologic and physiologic sources, including fluid and electrolyte imbalances, hypoxemia, drug toxicity, sleep deprivation, and sensory alteration, deprivation, or overload. Delirium tremens caused by alcohol withdrawal may be responsible for as much as 25% of all postoperative delirium.[5] Delirium tremens is a reaction characterized by restlessness, insomnia and nightmares, tachycardia, apprehension, confusion and disorientation, irritability, and auditory or visual hallucinations. It may be treated by the administration of sedating agents and by patient restraint (see Chapter 10).

NURSING MANAGEMENT: PSYCHOLOGIC FUNCTION

Nursing Diagnoses

Nursing diagnoses related to potential alterations in psychologic function in the postoperative patient include, but are not limited to, the following:

- Anxiety
- Ineffective individual coping
- Body image disturbance

■ Nursing Implementation

The nurse attempts to prevent psychologic problems in the postoperative period by providing adequate support for the patient. Supportive measures include taking time to listen and talk with the patient, offering explanations and genuine reassurance, and encouraging the presence and assistance of significant others. The nurse must observe and evaluate the patient's behavior to distinguish a normal reaction to the stress situation from one that is becoming abnormal or excessive. The recognition of the alcohol withdrawal syndrome in a patient not previously known to be an alcoholic presents a particular challenge. Any unusual or disturbed behavior should be reported immediately so that diagnosis and treatment may be instituted.

Planning for Discharge and Follow-up Care

Preparation for the patient's discharge is an ongoing process throughout the surgical experience that begins during the preoperative period. The informed patient is therefore prepared as events unfold and gradually assumes greater responsibility for self-care during the postoperative period. As the day of discharge approaches, the nurse should be certain that the patient has the following information:

1. Care of wound site and any dressings, including bathing recommendations
2. Action and possible side effects of any medications; when and how to take them
3. Activities allowed and prohibited; when various physical activities can be resumed safely (e.g., driving a car, returning to work, sexual intercourse, leisure activities)
4. Dietary restrictions or modifications
5. Symptoms to be reported (e.g., development of incisional tenderness or increased drainage, discomfort in other parts of the body)
6. Where and when to return for follow-up care
7. Answers to any individual questions or concerns

If the physician has not provided information about particular diet or activity prescriptions or restrictions, the nurse should either obtain this information or encourage the patient to do so. Attention to complete discharge instruction may prevent needless distress for the patient. Written instructions are important for reinforcing verbal information. The nurse should specifically document in the record the discharge instructions provided to the patient and family. For the patient, the postoperative phase of care continues and extends into the recuperative period. Assessment and evaluation of the patient after discharge may be accomplished by a follow-up call or by a visit from a home health nurse.

Increasingly, patients are being discharged to home with many medical or surgical needs. It is expected that the patient, with assistance from family, friends, or home health care, will continue self-care in the home. This may include dressing changes, wound care, or catheter or drain care. Working through the discharge planner for the hospital unit, or the case manager, the nurse can facilitate the transition of care from hospital-based to home care, without jeopardizing the quality of care.

GERONTOLOGIC CONSIDERATIONS

Postoperative Patient

In general, older patients experience a more difficult and longer postoperative recovery.[16] The older adult has a decrease in respiratory function, including decreased ability to cough, decreased thoracic compliance, and decreased lung tissue. These alterations in pulmonary status lead to an increase in the work of ventilation and a decreased ability to readily eliminate pharmacologic agents. Reactions to anesthetic agents must be carefully monitored and their postoperative elimination assessed before the patient is left without close supervision. Pneumonia is a common postoperative complication in the elderly.[16]

Vascular function in the older adult is altered because of plaque formation and decreased elasticity in the blood vessels. Cardiac function is often compromised, and compensatory responses to changes in blood pressure and volume are limited. Circulating blood volume is decreased, and hypertension is common. Cardiovascular parameters must be closely monitored throughout surgery and the postoperative period.

Renal perfusion in the older adult normally decreases; the result is a reduction in the ability to eliminate drugs that are excreted by the kidney. This increases the patient's susceptibility to renal failure. Renal function must be carefully assessed in the postoperative phase of the patient's care.

Observing for changes in mental status is an important part of postoperative care in older adults. Postoperative delirium is common in the elderly in the postoperative period. Factors such as age, alcohol abuse, low baseline cognition, severe metabolic derangement, hypoxia, hypotension, and type of surgery appear to contribute to postoperative delirium. Anesthetics, notably anticholinergic drugs and benzodiazepines, increase the risk for delirium. Despite the above recommendations, postoperative delirium in the elderly is poorly understood.[17] One way that the nurse can differentiate delirium from dementia is to observe for alterations in the level of consciousness, since they may indicate a diagnosis of delirium rather than dementia.[16] In patients with an acute change in mental status, a potentially reversible cause should be considered, such as an infection or side effect of analgesic medication.

Postoperative pain tends to be undertreated in all patients, especially older patients.[15] Many older patients are hesitant to request pain medication. They may believe that pain is an inevitable consequence of surgery and they need to just tolerate it. Nurses may not appropriately assess pain in patients who do not report their pain. Some older patients are hesitant to learn how to use PCA machines. The nurse should know that the surgery will usually result in pain, and if untreated, could have a negative effect on recovery. The nurse should emphasize to the patient and family that appropriate pain relief can help promote recovery.

CRITICAL THINKING EXERCISES

CASE STUDY

Postoperative Patient

Patient Profile

Edward G., 74-year-old retired college professor, has just undergone a left hip pinning after a fall. The surgery, performed while the patient was under general anesthesia, was uneventful.

Subjective Data

- Was in excellent health before fall
- Played tennis three times each week
- Walked 20 to 30 miles per week
- Always had problems sleeping
- Difficulty hearing, wears hearing aid
- Upset with injury and its impact on activity
- Has no relatives or friends to assist with care

Objective Data

Admitted to PACU with abduction pillow between his legs, two peripheral IV catheters, a self-suction drain from the hip dressing, and an indwelling urinary catheter

Collaborative Care

Postoperative orders include the following:

- Vital signs per PACU routine
- Dextrose 5% in 0.45 normal saline at 100 ml/hr
- Morphine via patient-controlled analgesia 1 mg q 6 min (30 mg max in 4 hr) for pain
- Advance diet as tolerated
- Triflow spirometry q hr × 10

Critical Thinking Questions

1. What are the potential postanesthetic problems that the nurse might expect with Mr. G.?
2. What nursing interventions would be appropriate to prevent these complications from occurring?
3. What factors may predispose Mr. G. to the following problems: atelectasis, infection, pulmonary embolism, nausea and vomiting?
4. How should it be determined when Mr. G. is sufficiently recovered from general anesthesia to be discharged to the clinical unit?
5. What potential postoperative problems might the nurse on the clinical unit expect?
6. Based on the assessment data presented, write one or more appropriate nursing diagnoses. Are there any collaborative problems?

NURSING RESEARCH ISSUES

1. Does early mobilization of specific patient groups prevent the development of postoperative respiratory complications?
2. What are the unique differences in discharging a patient to home as opposed to a clinical unit?
3. Does the use of written discharge criteria accurately predict patient readiness for discharge?
4. Is patient-controlled intravenous delivery of narcotics more effective in controlling postoperative pain than intramuscular injections of narcotics?
5. Does an early phone call from a nurse during the first week of postoperative discharge reduce the occurrence of hospital readmission and postoperative complications?
6. Do antiembolism/compression stockings assist in the prevention of deep vein thromboses?

REVIEW QUESTIONS

The number of the question corresponds to the same-numbered objective at the beginning of the chapter.

1. As soon as the patient enters the PACU, the priority assessment by the nurse is
   a. urinary output.
   b. ECG monitoring.
   c. level of consciousness.
   d. airway patency and respiratory status.
2. Nursing interventions indicated during the patient's recovery from general anesthesia in the PACU include
   a. placing the patient in a supine position.
   b. encouraging deep breathing and coughing.
   c. restraining patients during episodes of emergence delirium.
   d. withholding analgesics until the patient is discharged from PACU.
3. Postoperative nausea and vomiting presents the greatest risk for
   a. a 14-year-old, 40 kg boy following an orchiopexy under general anesthesia.
   b. an 81-year-old, 55 kg woman following a cystoscopy under local anesthesia.
   c. a 45-year-old, 70 kg man following an arthroscopy under epidural anesthesia.
   d. a 23-year-old, 125 kg woman following a diagnostic laparoscopy under general anesthesia.
4. Following admission of the postoperative patient to the clinical unit, which of the following assessment data requires the most immediate attention?
   a. oxygen saturation of 85%
   b. respiratory rate of 13/min
   c. blood pressure of 90/60 mm Hg
   d. temperature of 94.3° F (34.6° C)
5. A urine output averaging 20 ml/hr for the first postoperative day
   a. is a normal expected finding.
   b. requires a return to the operating room.
   c. requires an evaluation of the patient's fluid status.
   d. is normal if the patient had genitourinary surgery.

6. In preparation for discharge after surgery the nurse should advise the patient regarding
   a. a time frame for when various physical activities can be resumed.
   b. the rationale for abstinence from sexual intercourse for 4 to 6 weeks.
   c. the need to call hospital clinical unit to report any abnormal signs or symptoms.
   d. the necessity of a referral to nutritional center for management of dietary restrictions.

References

1. Litwack K: *Post anesthesia care nursing,* ed 2, St Louis, 1995, Mosby.
2. Litwack K: Immediate postoperative care: a problem-oriented approach. In Vender J, Spiess B, editors: *Post anesthesia care,* Philadelphia, 1992, Saunders.
3. Litwack K: Postanesthesia assessment: what medical-surgical nurses need to know, *Medsurg Nurs* 2:294, 1993.
4. American Society of Perianesthesia Nurses: *Standards for perianesthesia nursing practice,* Richmond, 1998, The Society.
5. Cole MG, Primeau F, McCusker J: Effectiveness of interventions to prevent delirium in hospitalized patients: a systematic review, *Can Med Assoc J* 155:1263, 1996.
6. Dougherty J: Same-day surgery: the nurse's role, *Orthop Nurs* 15:15, 1996.
7. Verhaeghe R, Verstraete M: Prophylaxis of venous thromboembolism in surgery, *Acta Chir Belg* 97:106, 1997.
8. Litwack K: *The elderly surgical patient,* Sacramento, 1995, CME Resource.
9. Richardson J, Sabanathan S: Prevention of respiratory complications after abdominal surgery, *Thorax* 52(suppl 3):S35, 1997.
10. Bergquist D: New approaches to prevention of deep vein thrombosis, *Thrombos Haemost* 78:684, 1997.
11. Briggs M: Principles of closed surgical wound care, *J Wound Care* 6:288, 1997.
12. Hunt TK, Hopf HW: Wound healing and wound infection. What surgeons and anesthesiologists can do, *Surg Clin North Am* 77:587, 1997.
13. Kravitz M: Outpatient wound care, *Crit Care Nurs Clin North Am* 8:217, 1996.
14. McCaffery M: *Pain assessment and intervention in clinical practice,* ed 2, St Louis, 1999, Mosby.
15. Pasero CL, McCaffery M: Managing postoperative pain in the elderly, *AJN* 96:38, 1996.
16. Nusbaum NJ: How do geriatric patients recover from surgery? *South Med J* 89:950, 1996.
17. Parikh SS, Chung F: Postoperative delirium in the elderly, *Anesth Analg* 80:1223, 1995.

Resources

American Association of Nurse Anesthetists (AANA)
222 South Prospect Avenue
Park Ridge, IL 60068-4001
847-692-6968
fax: 847-692-6968
http://www.aana.com/

American College of Surgeons
633 N. St. Clair Street
Chicago, IL 60611-3211
312-202-5000
fax: 312-202-5001
http://www.facs.org/

American Society of Anesthesiologists
520 N. Northwest Highway
Park Ridge, IL 60068-2573
847-825-5586
fax: 847-825-1692
http://www.asahq.org/

American Society of PeriAnesthesia Nurses (ASPAN)
6900 Grove Road
Thorofare, NJ 08086
609-845-5557
fax: 609-848-1881
http://www.aspan.org/

Association of Operating Room Nurses (AORN)
2170 South Parker Road, Suite 300
Denver, CO 80231-5711
800-755-2676
http://www.aorn.org

Association of Surgical Technicians
7108-C South Alton Way, Suite 100
Englewood, CO 80112-2106
303-694-9130
fax: 303-694-9169

Canadian Anesthetists' Society
1 Eglinton Avenue East, Suite 208
Toronto, Ontario M4P 3A1 CANADA
416-480-0602
fax: 416-480-0320
http://www.cas.ca/

Michigan Association of Nurse Anesthetists (MANA)
http://www.rust.net/~orest/mana.htm

Operating Room Nurses' Association of Canada
http://www.ornac.ca/

For additional Internet resources, see the website for this book at **www.mosby.com/MERLIN/medsurg_lewis**

SECTION

4

PROBLEMS RELATED TO ALTERED SENSORY INPUT

SECTION OUTLINE

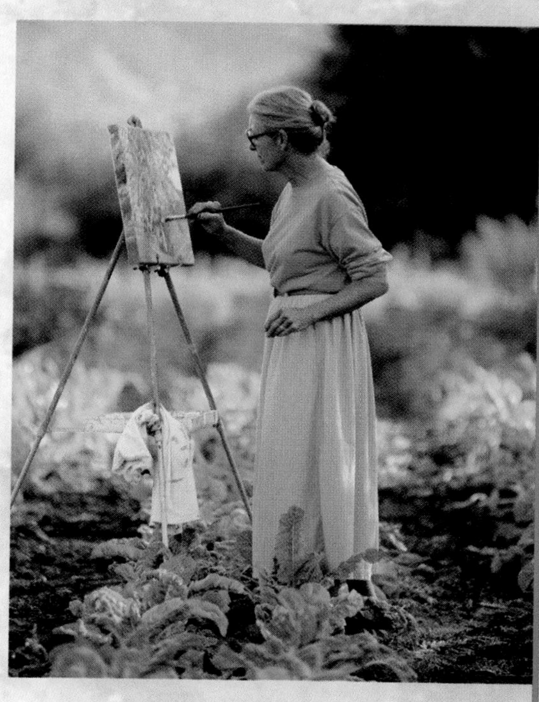

REMEMBER to check out your companion CD-ROM

19 NURSING ASSESSMENT Visual and Auditory Systems

Sarah C. Smith & Mary E. Wilbur

www.mosby.com/MERLIN/medsurg_lewis

LEARNING OBJECTIVES

1. Describe the structures and functions of the visual and auditory systems.
2. Describe the physiologic processes involved in normal vision and hearing.
3. Identify the significant subjective and objective assessment data related to the visual and auditory systems that should be obtained from the patient.
4. Describe the appropriate techniques used in the physical assessment of the visual and auditory systems.
5. Differentiate normal from common abnormal findings of a physical assessment of the visual and auditory systems.
6. Describe age-related changes in the visual and auditory systems and differences in assessment findings.
7. Describe the purpose, significance of results, and nursing responsibilities related to diagnostic studies of the visual and auditory systems.

STRUCTURES AND FUNCTIONS OF THE VISUAL SYSTEM

The visual system consists of the internal and external structures of the eyeball, the refractive media, and the visual pathways. The internal structures are the iris, lens, ciliary body, choroid, and retina. The external structures are the eyebrows, eyelids, eyelashes, lacrimal system, conjunctiva, cornea, sclera, and extraocular muscles. The entire visual system is important for visual function. Light reflected from an object in the field of vision passes through the transparent structures of the eye and, in doing so, is refracted (bent) so that a clear image can fall on the retina. From the retina, the visual stimuli travel through the visual pathway to the occipital cortex, where they are perceived as an image.

Visual and Structure Function

Eyeball. The eyeball, or globe, is composed of three layers (Fig. 19-1). The tough outer layer is composed of the sclera and the transparent cornea. The middle layer consists of the uveal tract (iris, choroid, and ciliary body) and the innermost layer is the retina. The anterior chamber lies between the iris and the posterior surface of the cornea, whereas the posterior chamber lies between the anterior surface of the lens and the posterior surface of the iris. These chambers are filled with aqueous humor secreted by the ciliary body (Fig. 19-2). The anatomic space between the posterior lens surface and the retina is filled with the vitreous gel.

Refractive Media. For light to reach the retina, it must pass through a number of structures: the cornea, aqueous humor, lens, and vitreous. Each structure has a different density and plays a role in helping the image fall focused on the retina.

Reviewed by Mary S. Merchant, RN, MSN, FNP, Continuum of Care Manager, Medical University of South Carolina, Charleston, SC.

The transparent cornea is the first structure through which light passes. It is responsible for the majority of light refraction necessary for clear vision.[1]

Aqueous humor, a clear watery fluid, fills the anterior and posterior chambers of the anterior cavity of the eye. Aqueous humor is produced by the ciliary process and passes through the pupil from the posterior chamber into the anterior chamber (see Fig. 19-2). It drains through the trabecular meshwork located in the angle formed by the cornea and iris and into the canal of Schlemm. This circular canal conveys fluid into scleral veins, which enter the circulation of the body. The aqueous humor bathes and nourishes the lens and the endothelium of the cornea. Excess production or decreased outflow can elevate intraocular pressure above the normal 10 to 21 mm Hg, a condition termed *glaucoma.*

The lens is a biconvex structure located behind the iris and supported in place by small fibers called *zonules.* The primary function of the lens is to bend light rays, allowing the rays to fall onto the retina. The lens shape is modified by action of the ciliary zonules as part of *accommodation,* a process that allows the patient to focus on near objects, such as in reading. Because light rays pass through the lens, the lens must remain clear. Anything altering the clarity of the lens affects light transmission.

Vitreous humor is located in the posterior cavity, the large area behind the lens and in front of the retina (see Fig. 19-1). Light passing through the vitreous may be blocked by any nontransparent substance within the vitreous. The effect on vision varies, depending on the amount, type, and location of the substance blocking the light. For example, in the case of hemorrhage into the vitreous, little light will reach the retina, and vision will be severely compromised. However, cellular debris that accumulates from normal cell metabolism will cause only a relatively small shadow on the retina (a "floater"). The vitreous becomes more liquid with aging.[2]

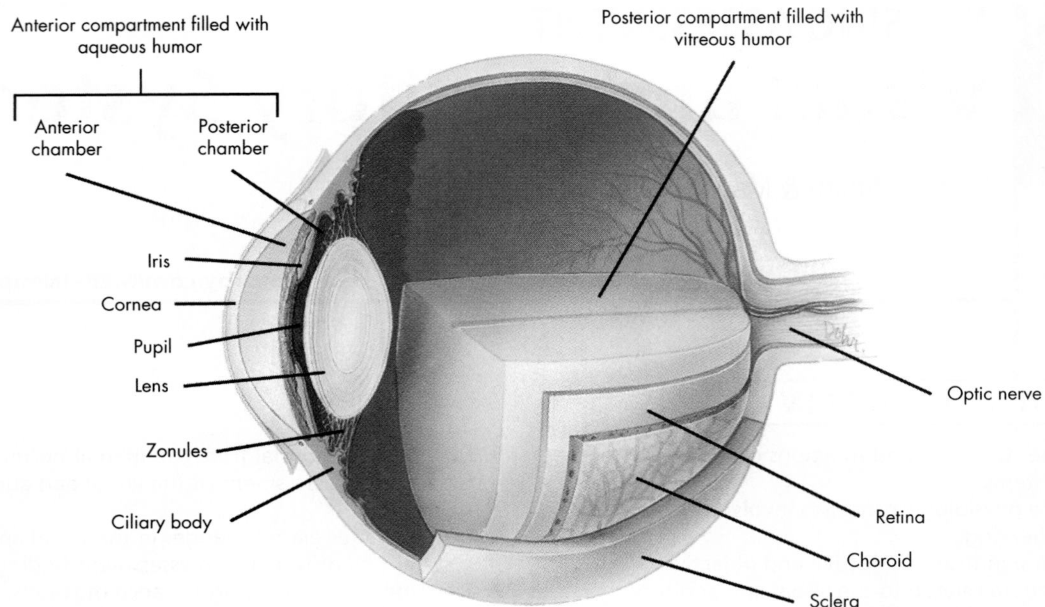

Fig. 19-1 The human eye.

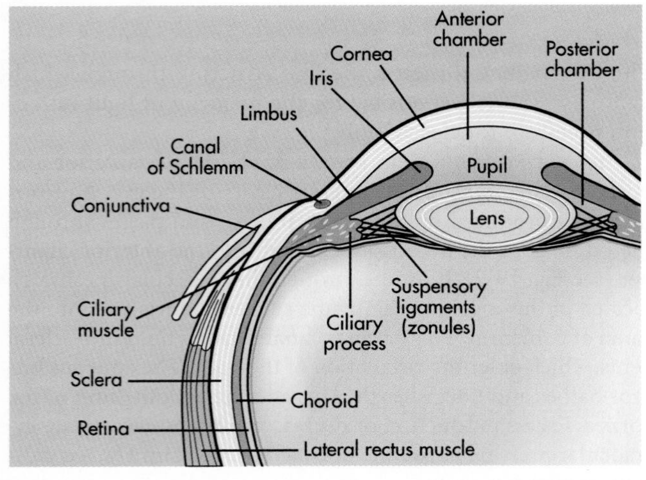

Fig. 19-2 Close-up view of ciliary body, zonules, lens, and anterior and posterior chambers. The aqueous humor flows from the ciliary process, over the anterior lens, and into the anterior chamber through the pupil, where it drains through the canal of Schlemm.

Refractive Errors. *Refraction* is the ability of the eye to bend light rays so that they fall on the retina. In the normal eye, parallel light rays are focused through the lens into a sharp image on the retina. This condition is termed *emmetropia* and means that light is focused exactly on the retina, not in front of it or behind it. When the light does not focus properly, it is called a *refractive error.*

The individual with *myopia* can see near objects clearly (nearsightedness), but objects in the distance are blurred. This condition occurs when an image is focused in front of the retina, either because the eye is too long or because there is excessive refracting power (Fig. 19-3, *A*). A concave lens is used to correct the light refraction so that objects seen in the distance are focused clearly on the retina (Fig. 19-3, *B*).

The individual with *hyperopia* can see distant objects clearly (farsightedness), but close objects are blurred. This condition occurs when an image is focused behind the retina, either because the eye is too short or because there is inadequate refracting power (Fig. 19-3, *C*). A convex lens is used to correct the refraction (Fig. 19-3, *D*).

Astigmatism is caused by an unevenness in the corneal or lenticular curvature, causing horizontal and vertical rays to be focused at two different points on the retina, which results in visual distortion. It can be myopic or hyperopic in nature in relation to where the image falls.

Presbyopia is a form of hyperopia, or farsightedness, that occurs as a normal process of aging, usually around age 40. As the lens ages and becomes less elastic, it loses refractive power, and the eye can no longer accommodate for near vision. As with hyperopia, convex lenses are used to correct the light refraction so that the presbyopic individual can see clearly to read and accomplish other near-vision tasks.

Visual Pathways. Once the image travels through the refractive media, it is focused on the retina, inverted, and reversed left to right (Fig. 19-4). For example, if the visualized object is in the upper part of the left temporal visual field, it will be focused in the lower part of the nasal retina, upside down, and as a mirror image. From the retina, the impulses travel through the optic nerve to the optic chiasm where the nasal fibers of each eye cross over to the other side. Fibers from the left field of both eyes form the left optic tract and travel to the left occipital cortex. The fibers from the right field of both eyes form the right optic tract and travel to the right occipital cortex. This arrangement of the nerve fibers in the visual pathways allows determination of the anatomic location of abnormalities in those nerve fibers by interpretation of the specific visual field defect (Fig. 19-4).

External Structures and Functions

Eyebrows, Eyelids, and Eyelashes. The eyebrows, eyelids, and eyelashes serve an important role in protecting

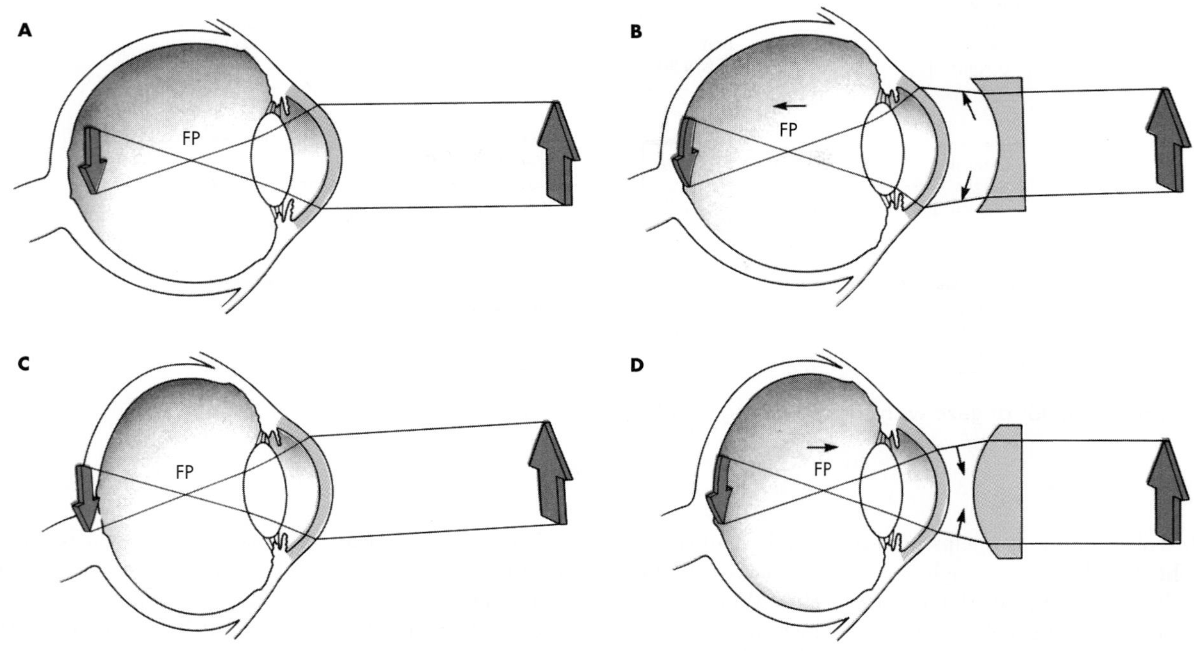

Fig. 19-3 Refraction disorders. **A** and **B,** Abnormal and corrected refraction observed in myopia and **C** and **D,** hyperopia. *FP,* focal point.

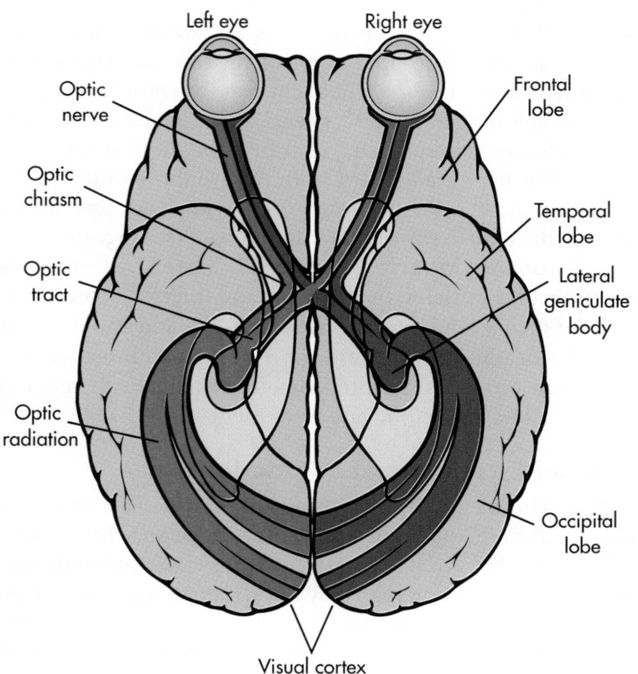

Fig. 19-4 The visual pathway. Fibers from the nasal portion of each retina cross over to the opposite side of the optic chiasma, terminating in the lateral geniculate body of the opposite side. Location of a lesion in the visual pathway determines the resulting visual defect.

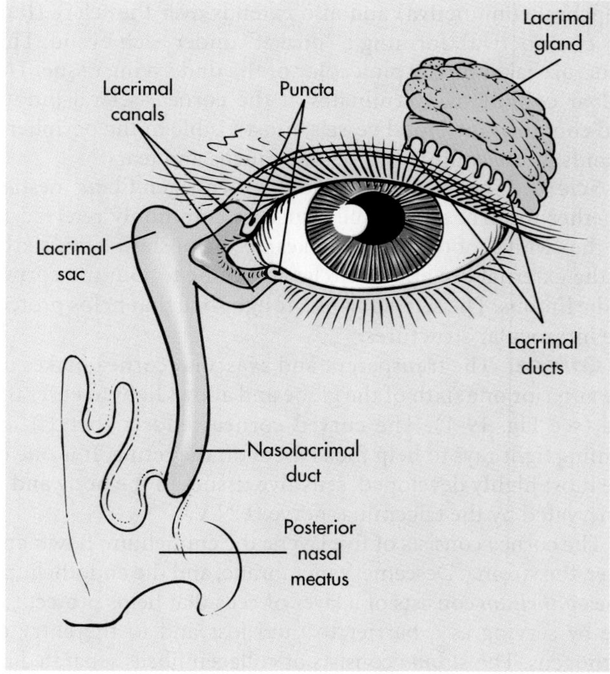

Fig. 19-5 External eye and lacrimal apparatus. Tears produced in the lacrimal gland pass over the surface of the eye and enter the lacrimal canal. From there the tears are carried through the nasolacrimal duct to the nasal cavity.

the eye. They provide a physical barrier to dust and foreign particles (Fig. 19-5). The eye is further protected by the surrounding bony orbit and by fat pads located below and behind the globe, or eyeball.

The upper and lower eyelids join at the medial and lateral canthi, forming the *palpebral fissure,* which normally measures 10 to 12 mm.[3] The upper eyelid blinks spontaneously approximately 15 times a minute. Blinking distributes tears over the anterior surface of the eyeball and helps control the amount of light entering the visual pathway.

The eyelids open and close through the action of muscles innervated by cranial nerve VII (CN VII), which is the facial

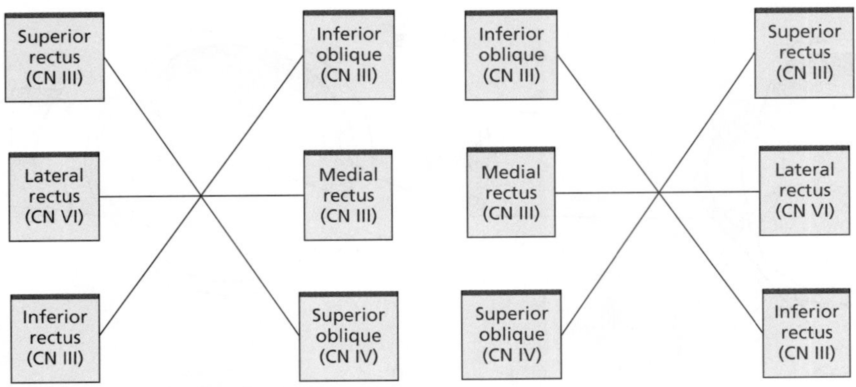

Fig. 19-6 Cardinal fields of gaze with corresponding muscles and nerves.

nerve. Muscular action also helps hold the eyelids against the eyeball. The *tarsal plate,* a tough sheet of connective tissue within the lids, maintains the shape of the eyelids. When open, the upper eyelid rests just below the *limbus* (the junction of the cornea and sclera). Sebaceous glands, located in the eyelids, help form the lipid layer of the tear film.

Conjunctiva. The conjunctiva is a transparent mucous membrane that covers the inner surfaces of the eyelids (the palpebral conjunctiva) and also extends over the sclera (bulbar conjunctiva), forming a "pocket" under each eyelid. This structure takes on the pink color of the underlying tissue. The bulbar conjunctiva terminates at the corneal-scleral limbus and contains tiny blood vessels, most visible in the periphery. Glands in the conjunctiva secrete mucus and tears.

Sclera. The sclera is composed of collagen fibers meshed together to form an opaque structure commonly referred to as the "white" of the eye. It makes up the posterior five sixths of the external eye and encircles the globe to join the cornea at the limbus. The sclera forms a tough shell that helps protect the intraocular structures.

Cornea. The transparent and avascular cornea makes up the anterior one sixth of the globe and allows light to enter the eye (see Fig. 19-1). The curved cornea refracts (bends) incoming light rays to help focus them on the retina. It is one of the most highly developed, sensitive tissues in the body and is innervated by the trigeminal nerve (CN V).

The cornea consists of five layers: the epithelium, Bowman's layer, the stroma, Descemet's membrane, and the endothelium. The *epithelium* consists of a layer of cells that helps protect the eye by serving as a barrier to fluid loss and to the entry of pathogens. The *stroma* consists of collagen fibrils separated by the ground substance, which has a unique ability to hold water. The stroma is relatively water free to maintain transparency. Any abnormality that disrupts the normal state of stromal hydration can result in stromal edema with a resulting loss of corneal clarity and a decrease in visual acuity. The corneal endothelium also consists of a single layer of cells, but unlike the cells of the epithelium, which regenerate if destroyed, the endothelial cells are limited in their regenerative ability. When these cells are damaged or destroyed, repair of an endothelial defect occurs primarily by the enlargement and spreading of the cells to fill in the defect.

The avascular cornea obtains oxygen primarily through absorption from the tear film layer that bathes the epithelium. A small amount of oxygen is obtained from the aqueous humor through the endothelial layer, which is also responsible for transporting other nutrients into the corneal tissues.

Lacrimal Apparatus. The lacrimal system consists of the lacrimal gland and ducts, the lacrimal canals and puncta, the lacrimal sac, and the nasolacrimal duct. In addition to the lacrimal gland, other glands provide secretions to make up the mucous, aqueous, and lipid layers of the tear film that covers the anterior surface of the globe. The tear film moistens the eye and provides oxygen to the cornea. Lid and globe movements are both involved in spreading tears over the anterior surface of the eye. The tears are drained from the eye through the upper and lower puncta, then through the lacrimal sac, and finally through the nasolacrimal duct into the nose (see Fig. 19-5).

Extraocular Muscles. Each eye is moved by three pairs of extraocular muscles: the superior and inferior rectus muscles, the medial and lateral rectus muscles, and the superior and inferior oblique muscles (Fig. 19-6). Neuromuscular coordination produces simultaneous movement of the eyes in the same direction (conjugate movement).

Internal Structures and Functions

Iris. The iris provides the color of the eye. This structure has a small round opening in its center, the *pupil,* which allows light to enter the eye. The pupil constricts via action of the iris sphincter muscle (innervated by CN III) and dilates via action of the iris dilator muscle (innervated by CN V) to control the amount of light that enters the eye. The constrictor muscle of the iris is stimulated by light falling on the retina and by accommodation. The autonomic nervous system also affects pupil size. Sympathetic stimulation results in contraction of the radial muscle and dilation of the pupil. Parasympathetic stimulation results in contraction of the circular muscle and constriction of the pupil.

Crystalline Lens. The crystalline lens is a biconvex, avascular, transparent structure located behind the iris. It is supported by the anterior and posterior ciliary zonules. The lens is composed of thick gelatinous material enclosed in a clear capsule. The primary function of the lens is to bend light rays so that they fall onto the retina. Accommodation occurs when the eye focuses on a near object and is facilitated by contraction of the ciliary body, which changes the shape of the lens.

Ciliary Body. The ciliary body consists of the ciliary muscles, which surround the lens and lie parallel to the sclera; the ciliary zonules, which attach to the lens capsule; and the ciliary processes, which constitute the terminal portion of the ciliary body. The ciliary processes lie behind the peripheral part of the iris and secrete aqueous humor.

Choroid. The choroid is a highly vascular structure that serves to nourish the ciliary body, the iris, and the outer portion of the retina. It lies inside and parallel to the sclera and extends from the area where the optic nerve enters the eye to the ciliary body (see Fig. 19-1).

Retina. The retina is the innermost layer of the eye that extends and forms the optic nerve. Neurons make up the major portion of the retina. Therefore retinal cells are unable to regenerate if destroyed. The retina lines the inside of the eyeball, extending from the area of optic nerve to the ciliary body (see Fig. 19-1). It is responsible for converting images into a form the brain can understand and process as vision. The retina is composed of two types of photoreceptor cells: rods and cones. Rods are stimulated in dim or darkened environments, and cones are receptive to colors in bright environments. There are approximately 130 million photoreceptors in each human retina, with rods outnumbering cones by approximately 13:1.[4] The center of the retina is the *fovea centralis,* a pinpoint depression composed only of densely packed cones. This area of the retina provides the sharpest visual acuity. Surrounding the fovea is the macula, an area less than 1 square millimeter, which has a high concentration of cones and is relatively free of blood vessels.[5] Nourishment to the macula comes from two sources: the choroid and the underlying pigment epithelium, which is the deepest layer of the retina.

With the exception of the macula, the retina is nourished by retinal arterioles and veins. This blood supply enters the eye through the optic disc, located nasally from the macula. The optic disc is the area where the optic nerve (CN II) exits the eyeball. Within the disc is the physiologic cup, a depression that can be visualized through the pupil with an ophthalmoscope. The retinal veins and arteries can also be visualized in this way and can provide information about the vascular system in general.

GERONTOLOGIC CONSIDERATIONS

Effects of Aging on the Visual System

Every structure of the visual system is subject to changes as the individual ages. Whereas many of these changes are relatively benign, others may result in severely compromised visual acuity in the older adult. The psychosocial impact of poor vision or blindness can be highly significant. Age-related changes in the visual system and differences in assessment findings are presented in Table 19-1.

ASSESSMENT OF THE VISUAL SYSTEM

Assessment of the visual system may be as simple as determining a patient's visual acuity or as complex as collecting complete subjective and objective data pertinent to the visual system. To do an appropriate ophthalmic evaluation, the nurse must determine which parts of the data collection are important for each particular patient.

Subjective Data

Important Health Information

Past health history. Information about the patient's past health history should include both ocular and nonocular history. The nurse should ask the patient specifically about systemic diseases, such as diabetes, hypertension, cancer, rheumatoid arthritis, syphilis and other sexually transmitted diseases (STDs), acquired immunodeficiency syndrome (AIDS), muscular dystrophy, myasthenia gravis, multiple sclerosis, inflammatory bowel disease, and hypothyroidism or hyperthyroidism, because many of these diseases have ocular manifestations. It is particularly important to determine if the patient has any history of cardiac or pulmonary disease because beta-adrenergic blocking agents are often used to treat glaucoma. These medications can slow heart rate, decrease blood pressure, and exacerbate asthma or emphysema.[6]

A history of tests for visual acuity should be obtained, including the date of the last examination and change in glasses or contact lenses. The nurse should specifically ask about a history of strabismus, amblyopia, cataracts, retinal detachment, or glaucoma. Any trauma to the eye, its treatment, and sequelae should be noted.

The patient's nonocular history can be significant in assessing or treating the ophthalmic condition. Specifically, the nurse should ask the patient about previous surgeries or treatments related to the head, as well as about previous trauma to the head.

Medications. If the patient takes medication, the nurse should obtain a complete list, including over-the-counter (OTC) medicines, eyedrops, and herbal or "natural" supplements or substances. Many patients do not think OTC drugs, eyedrops, or herbal agents are "real" medications and may not mention their use unless specifically questioned. However, many of these drugs have ocular effects. For example, many cold preparations contain a form of epinephrine that can dilate the pupil. The nurse should also note the use of any antihistamines or decongestants, because these drugs can cause ocular dryness. The nurse should specifically ask whether the patient uses any prescription drugs such as corticosteroids, thyroid medications, or agents such as oral hypoglycemics and insulin to lower blood glucose levels. Cortisone preparations can contribute to the development of glaucoma or cataracts. It is especially important to indicate whether the patient is taking any beta-adrenergic blocking medications, because these can be potentiated by the beta-blocking agents used to treat glaucoma.

Each drug the patient uses should correspond with a disease or disorder described in the patient's history. If a medication cannot be correlated with a disease or disorder, the nurse should ask the patient to explain why the drug is used. Finally, the nurse should determine whether the patient has allergies to medications or other substances.

Surgery or other treatments. Surgical procedures related to the eye or brain should be noted. Brain surgery and the subsequent swelling can cause pressure on the optic nerve or tract, resulting in visual alterations. Any laser procedures to the eye should also be documented. The effect of any eye surgery or

GERONTOLOGIC DIFFERENCES IN ASSESSMENT

Table 19-1 Visual System

Changes	Differences in Assessment Findings
Eyebrows and Eyelashes	
Loss of pigment in the hair	Graying of eyebrows, eyelashes
Eyelids	
Loss of orbital fat, decreased muscle tone	Entropion, ectropion, mild ptosis
Tissue atrophy, prolapse of fat into eyelid tissue	Blepharodermachalasis (excessive upper lid skin)
Conjunctiva	
Tissue damage related to chronic exposure to ultraviolet light or to other chronic environmental exposure	Pinguecula (small yellowish spot usually on the medial aspect of the conjunctiva)
Sclera	
Lipid deposition	Scleral color yellowish as opposed to bluish
Cornea	
Cholesterol deposits in peripheral cornea	Arcus senilis (milky or yellow ring encircling periphery of cornea)
Tissue damage related to chronic exposure	Pterygium (thickened, triangular bit of pale tissue that extends from the inner canthus of eye to the nasal border of the cornea)
Decrease in water content, atrophy of nerve fibers	Decreased corneal sensitivity
Epithelial changes	Loss of corneal luster
Accumulation of lipid deposits	Blurring of vision
Lacrimal Apparatus	
Decreased tear secretion	Dryness
Malposition of the eyelid resulting in tears overflowing the lid margins instead of draining through the puncta	Tearing, irritated eyes
Iris	
Increased rigidity of iris	Decreased pupil size
Dilator muscle atrophy or weakness	Slower recovery of pupil size after light stimulation
Loss of pigment	Change of iris color
Ciliary muscle becomes smaller, stiffer	Decrease in near vision and accommodation
Lens	
Biochemical changes in lens proteins, oxidative damage, chronic exposure to ultraviolet light	Cataracts
Increased rigidity of lens	Presbyopia
Opacities in the lens (may also be related to opacities in the cornea and vitreous)	Complaints of glare
Accumulation of yellow substances	Yellow color of lens
Retina	
Retinal vascular changes related to arteriosclerosis and hypertension	Narrowed, pale, straighter arterioles; acute branching
Decrease in cones	Changes in color perception
Loss of photoreceptor cells, retinal pigment, epithelial cells, and melanin	Decreased visual acuity
Age-related macular degeneration as a result of vascular changes	Loss of central vision
Vitreous	
Liquefaction and detachment of the vitreous	Increased complaints of "floaters"

laser treatment on visual acuity is important information for the nurse to obtain.

Functional Health Patterns. The ophthalmic patient may seek health care for a specific problem or for regular ophthalmic care. When the patient needs routine ophthalmic care, the nurse will focus the assessment of functional patterns on issues related to health promotion. When the patient has a recognized problem, the nurse will direct the assessment to identify those issues related to the patient's specific problem.

Ocular problems do not always affect the patient's visual acuity. For example, patients with blepharitis or diabetic retinopathy may not have any visual deficit. The nurse should be aware that many conditions can cause vision loss. The focus of the functional health pattern assessment depends on the pres-

HEALTH HISTORY

Table 19-2 Visual System

Health Perception–Health Management Pattern
- Describe the change in your vision. Describe how this affects your daily life.
- Do you wear protective eyewear (sunglasses or safety goggles)?*
- Do you wear contact lenses? If so, how do you take care of them?
- If you use eyedrops, how do you instill them?
- Do you have any allergies that cause eye symptoms?
- Do you have a family history of cataracts, glaucoma, or macular degeneration?

Nutritional-Metabolic Pattern
- Do you take any nutritional supplements?
- Does your visual problem affect your ability to obtain and prepare food?*

Elimination Pattern
- Do you have to strain to defecate?*

Activity-Exercise Pattern
- Are your activities limited in any way by your eye problem?*
- Do you participate in any leisure activities that have the potential for eye injury?*

Sleep-Rest Pattern
- Are your eyes affected by the amount of sleep you get?*

Cognitive-Perceptual Pattern
- Does your eye problem affect your ability to read?*
- Do you have any eye pain?* Do you have any eye itching, burning, or foreign body sensation?*

Self-Perception–Self-Concept Pattern
- How does your eye problem make you feel about yourself?

Role-Relationship Pattern
- Do you have any problems at work or home because of your eyes?*
- Have you made any changes in your social activities because of your eyes?

Sexuality-Reproductive Pattern
- Has your eye problem caused a change in your sex life?*
- For women—Are you pregnant? Do you use birth control?*

Coping–Stress Tolerance Pattern
- Do you feel able to cope with your eye problem?*
- Are you able to acknowledge the effects of your eye problem on your life?*

Value-Belief Pattern
- Do you have any conflicts about the treatment of your eye problem?*

*If yes, describe.

ence or absence of vision loss and whether the loss is permanent or temporary. Table 19-2 lists suggested health history questions to obtain data relating to the functional health patterns.

Health perception–health management pattern. The patient's age is pertinent in considering cataracts, macular problems, glaucoma, and other ophthalmic conditions. Men are more likely than women to have color blindness.[7] African-Americans and older individuals are at higher risk of damage to the optic nerve from glaucoma.[8]

The ophthalmic patient in a clinic or office setting is often seeking routine eye care or a change in the prescription of eyewear. However, there can be some underlying concern that the patient may not mention or even recognize. Even the hospitalized or surgical patient may not completely understand why he or she is receiving care. The nurse should obtain this information by asking, "Why are you here today?"

The patient's visual health can affect activities at home or at work. It is important to know how the patient perceives the current health problem. As outlined in Table 19-2, the nurse can guide the patient in defining the current problem and how it affects the patient's normal activities. The nurse should also assess the patient's ability to accomplish all necessary self-care, especially any eye care related to the patient's ophthalmic problem.

The nurse should assess the patient's ocular health care activities. The patient may not recognize the importance of eye safety practices such as wearing protective eyewear during potentially hazardous activities or avoiding noxious fumes and other eye irritants. Information about the use of sunglasses in bright lights should be obtained. Prolonged exposure to ultraviolet (UV) light can affect the retina. Night driving habits and any problems encountered should be noted. Today, millions of people wear contact lenses, but many do not care for them properly.[9] The type of contact lenses used and the patient's wearing and care habits may provide information for teaching.

Information about allergies should be obtained. Allergies often cause eye symptoms such as itching, burning, watering, drainage, and blurred vision.

Many hereditary systemic diseases (e.g., sickle cell anemia) can significantly affect ocular health. In addition, many refractive errors and other eye problems are hereditary. For these reasons the nurse should obtain a careful family history of both ocular and nonocular diseases. Specifically, the nurse should ask if the patient has a family history of diseases such as arteriosclerosis, diabetes, thyroid disease, hypertension, arthritis, or cancer. The nurse should also determine whether the patient has a family history of ocular problems such as cataracts, tumors, glaucoma, refractive errors (especially myopia and hyperopia), or retinal degenerative conditions (e.g., macular degeneration, retinal detachment, retinitis pigmentosa).

Nutritional-metabolic pattern. The patient's intake of antioxidant vitamins and trace minerals can be important to ocular health. Adequate intake of vitamins C and E may be beneficial in preventing or delaying retinal damage, and zinc deficiency is linked to erythematous scales in the periorbital area.[10,11]

Elimination pattern. Straining to defecate (Valsalva's maneuver) can raise the intraocular pressure. Although there is some evidence that elevating the intraocular pressure by normal activities is not detrimental to the surgical incision made during eye surgery, many surgeons do not want the patient straining. The nurse should assess the patient's usual pattern of elimination and determine whether there is the potential for constipation in the patient who has had ophthalmic surgical procedures.

Activity-exercise pattern. The patient's usual level of activity or exercise may be affected by reduced vision, by symptoms accompanying an ocular problem, or by activity restrictions following a surgical procedure. For example, a patient with *hyphema* (intraocular bleeding) may be on bed rest or have severely restricted activity. The diabetic patient with lower limb prostheses will have additional ambulation difficulties if diabetic retinopathy with vision loss is present.

The nurse should also inquire about leisure activities during which the patient may incur an ocular injury. For example, gardening, woodworking, and other craft activities can result in corneal or conjunctival foreign bodies or even penetrating injuries of the globe. Injuries to the globe or bony orbit can also occur after blows to the head or eye during sports activities such as racquetball, baseball, and tennis. Cross-country skiers may develop corneal fungal ulcers after an abrasion caused by low-hanging tree limbs. Other leisure activities such as needlepoint, fly tying, or birdwatching may have high-level visual demands and produce eye strain.

Sleep-rest pattern. In the otherwise healthy person, lack of sleep may cause ocular irritation, especially in the patient who wears contact lenses. Normal sleep patterns may be disrupted in the patient with painful eye problems such as corneal abrasions. The patient with alkali burns of the eye requires continuous irrigation of the ocular surface until the pH of the conjunctival sac returns to normal levels.[12] Normal sleep will be disrupted during this time.

Cognitive-perceptual pattern. The entire assessment of the ophthalmic patient focuses on the sense of sight, but it is important not to overlook other cognitive or perceptual problems. For example, the functional ability of a patient with a visual deficit will be further compromised if the patient also has hearing problems. The patient who cannot see to read has increased difficulty in following postoperative instructions if there is also trouble hearing or remembering verbal instructions. The patient who does not understand or read English may require written or verbal instructions and information in the native language.

Eye pain is always an important symptom to assess. Corneal abrasions, iritis, and acute glaucoma manifest with pain and are serious eye problems. Infections and foreign bodies can also cause less severe eye discomfort and are also potentially serious. If eye pain is present, the patient should be questioned about treatment and response.

Self-perception–self-concept pattern. The loss of independence that can follow a partial or complete loss of vision, even if the condition is temporary, can have devastating effects on the patient's self-concept. The nurse should carefully evaluate the potential effect of vision loss on the patient's self-image. For instance, disabling glare from a cataract may prevent nighttime driving or even limit daytime driving, resulting in a diminished self-image. In today's highly mobile society, loss of ability to drive can represent a significant loss of independence and self-esteem. The patient with severe ptosis or other disfiguring ophthalmic conditions may be embarrassed by her or his appearance and suffer from a poor self-image.

Role-relationship pattern. The patient's ability to maintain the necessary or desired roles and responsibilities in the home, work, and social environments can be negatively affected by ocular problems. For example, macular degeneration may decrease the patient's visual acuity to a level inadequate to function at work. Many occupations place workers in conditions in which eye injury may occur. For example, factory workers may be at risk from flying metal debris. Information should be obtained about eye-safety practices, such as the use of goggles or safety glasses. Workers can also be exposed to eye strain in the office from video display terminals, poor lighting, and glare.

The patient with diabetes may not be able to see well enough to self-administer insulin. This patient may resent the dependence on a family member who takes over this function. The patient with exophthalmos may be embarrassed by his or her appearance and avoid usual social activities. The nurse should sensitively inquire if the patient's preferred roles and responsibilities have been affected by the ocular problem.

Sexuality-reproductive pattern. The inactivity that may be associated with low vision, blindness, and certain eye problems and surgeries can negatively affect a patient's sexuality. The patient with severe vision loss may develop such a poor self-image that the ability to be sexually intimate is lost. The nurse can assure the patient that low vision or blindness does not affect a person's ability to be sexually expressive. For many sexually expressive acts, touch is more important than vision.

If a patient with low vision or blindness has a family, assistance with child-rearing tasks may be necessary. The nurse should determine the need and availability of help if this situation is present.

Coping–stress tolerance pattern. The patient with temporary or permanent visual problems will experience emotional stress. The nurse should assess the patient's coping level, coping mechanisms, and availability of social and personal support systems.

The patient with permanent visual loss experiences the usual stages of grief after the loss. The nurse should assess the potential need for psychosocial counseling and eventual vocational rehabilitation.

Value-belief pattern. The nurse must be sensitive to the individual values and spiritual beliefs of each patient, because the patient makes decisions regarding ophthalmic care based on those values and beliefs. It can be difficult to understand why a

Table 19-3 Normal Physical Assessment of the Visual System

- Visual acuity 20/20 OU; no diplopia
- External eye structures symmetric without lesions or deformities
- Lacrimal apparatus nontender without drainage
- Conjunctiva clear; sclera white
- PERRLA
- Lens clear
- EOMI
- Disc margins sharp
- Retinal vessels normal with no hemorrhages or spots

EOMI, extraocular movements intact; *OU,* both eyes; *PERRLA,* pupils equal, round, reactive to light and accommodation.

patient refuses treatment that has potential benefit or wants treatment that may have limited potential benefit. The nurse should assess the patient's value-belief pattern that serves as the basis for making those decisions.

Objective Data

Physical Examination. Physical examination of the visual system includes inspecting the ocular structures and determining the status of their respective functions. Physiologic functional assessment includes determining the patient's visual acuity, determining the patient's ability to judge closeness and distance, assessing extraocular muscle function, evaluating the visual fields, observing pupil function, and measuring the intraocular pressure. Assessment of ocular structures should include examining the ocular adnexa, external eye, and internal structures. Some structures, such as the retina and blood vessels, must be visualized with the aid of various ophthalmic observation equipment, such as the biomicroscope and the ophthalmoscope.

Assessment of the visual system may include all of the following components, or it may be as brief as measuring the patient's visual acuity. The nurse will assess what is appropriate and necessary for the specific patient. All of the following assessments are in the nurse's scope of practice, but some require special training. Normal physical assessment of the visual system is outlined in Table 19-3. Age-related visual changes and differences in assessment findings are listed in Table 19-1. Assessment techniques related to vision are summarized in Table 19-4, and common assessment abnormalities are listed in Table 19-5.

Table 19-4 Assessment Techniques: Visual System

Technique	Description	Purpose
▪ Visual acuity testing	Patient reads from Snellen chart at 20 ft (distance vision test) or Jaeger's chart at 14 in (near vision test); examiner notes smallest print patient can read on each chart.	To determine patient's distance and near visual acuity
▪ Extraocular muscle function testing	Examiner has patient follow a light source or other fixation object through a complete field of gaze; in the cover-uncover test, examiner covers patient's eye and then uncovers it to see if eye has deviated under the cover.	To determine if patient's extraocular muscles are functioning in a normal manner, with no underaction or overaction
▪ Confrontation visual field test	Patient faces examiner, covers one eye, fixates on examiner's face, and counts number of fingers that the examiner brings into patient's field of vision.	To determine if patient has a full field of vision, without obvious scotomas
▪ Pupil function testing	Examiner shines light into patient's pupil and observes pupillary response; each pupil is examined independently; examiner also checks for consensual and accommodative response.	To determine if patient has normal pupillary response
▪ Tonometry	Applanation tonometer is gently touched to the anesthetized corneal surface; examiner looks through ocular of slit-lamp microscope, adjusts pressure dial until mires are aligned, and notes intraocular pressure reading.	To measure intraocular pressure (normal pressure is 10-21 mm Hg)
▪ Slit-lamp microscopy	Patient is seated with chin placed in chin rest; slit beam illuminates ocular structures; examiner looks through magnifying ocular to assess various structures.	To provide magnified view of the conjunctiva, sclera, cornea, anterior chamber, iris, lens, and vitreous
▪ Ophthalmoscopy	Examiner holds ophthalmoscope close to patient's eye, shining light into back of eye and looking through aperture on ophthalmoscope; examiner adjusts dial to select one of the lenses in ophthalmoscope that produces the desired amount of magnification to inspect ocular fundus.	To provide magnified view of retina and optic nerve head
▪ Color vision testing	Patient identifies numbers or paths formed by pattern of dots in series of color plates.	To determine patient's ability to distinguish colors
▪ Stereopsis testing	From a series of plates, patient identifies geometric pattern or figure that appears closer to patient when viewed through special spectacles that provide a three-dimensional view.	To determine patient's ability to see objects in three dimensions; to test depth perception
▪ Keratometry	Examiner aligns the projection and notes the readings of corneal curvature.	To measure the corneal curvature; often done before fitting contact lenses, before doing refractive surgery, or after corneal transplantation

COMMON ASSESSMENT ABNORMALITIES

Table 19-5 Visual System

Finding	Description	Possible Etiology and Significance
Subjective Data		
▪ Pain	Foreign body sensation	Superficial corneal erosion or abrasion; can result from contact lens wear or trauma; conjunctival or corneal foreign body; usually lessened with lid closure
	Severe, deep, throbbing	Anterior uveitis, acute glaucoma, infection; acute glaucoma also associated with nausea, vomiting
▪ Photophobia	Persistent abnormal intolerance to light	Inflammation or infection of cornea or anterior uveal tract (iris and ciliary body)
▪ Blurred vision	Gradual or sudden inability to see clearly	Refractive errors, corneal opacities, cataracts, retinal changes (detachment, macular degeneration), optic neuritis or atrophy, central retinal vein or artery thrombosis, refractive changes related to fluctuations in serum glucose
▪ Scotoma	Blind or partially blind area in the visual field	Disorders of the optic chiasm, glaucoma, central serous chorioretinopathy, age-related macular degeneration, injury, migraine headache
▪ Spots, floaters	Patient describes seeing spots, "spider webs," "curtain," or floaters within the field of vision	Most common cause is vitreous liquefaction (benign phenomenon); other possible causes include hemorrhage into the vitreous humor, retinal holes or tears, impending retinal detachment, vitreous detachment, intraocular hemorrhage, chorioretinitis
▪ Dryness	Discomfort, sandy, gritty, irritation, or burning	Decreased tear formation or changes in tear composition because of aging or various systemic diseases
▪ Halo around lights	Presence of a halo around lights	Refractive changes, corneal edema as a result of a sudden rise in intraocular pressure in angle-closure glaucoma or secondary glaucoma
▪ Glare	Headache, ocular discomfort, reduced visual acuity	Related to corneal inflammation or to opacities in the cornea, lens, or vitreous that scatter the incoming light; can also result from light scatter around edges of an intraocular lens; worse at night when pupil dilated
▪ Diplopia	Double vision	Abnormalities of extraocular muscle action related to muscle or cranial nerve pathology
Objective Data		
Eyelids		
▪ Allergic reactions	Redness, excessive tearing, and itching of lid margins	Many possible allergens; associated eye trauma can occur from rubbing itchy eyelids
▪ Hordeolum (sty)	Small, superficial white nodule along lid margin	Infection of a sebaceous gland of eyelid; causative organism is usually bacterial (most commonly *Staphylococcus aureus*)
▪ Chalazion	Reddened, swollen area on eyelid; involves deeper tissues than hordeolum; can be inflamed and tender	Granuloma formed around a sebaceous gland; occurs as a foreign body reaction to sebum in the tissue; can develop from a hordeolum or from rupture of a sebaceous gland with resulting sebum in the tissue
▪ Blepharitis	Redness, swelling, and crusting along lid margins	Bacterial invasion of lid margins; often chronic
▪ Dacryocystitis	Redness, swelling, and tenderness of medial area of lower lid (in region of lacrimal sac)	Blockage of nasolacrimal duct and subsequent infection
▪ Xanthelasma	Raised, yellowish plaques on eyelids usually on nasal portion	Lipid disorders; may be normal finding
▪ Ptosis	Dropping of upper lid margin, unilateral or bilateral	Mechanical causes as a result of eyelid tumors or excess skin; myogenic causes attributable to condition involving the levator muscle or myoneural junction, such as myasthenia gravis; neurogenic causes affecting third cranial nerve that innervates the levator muscle
▪ Entropion	Inward turning of upper or lower lid margin, unilateral or bilateral	Congenital causes resulting in development abnormalities; involutional entropion related to horizontal eyelid laxity; can cause irritation and tearing

Continued

COMMON ASSESSMENT ABNORMALITIES

Table 19-5 Visual System—cont'd

Finding	Description	Possible Etiology and Significance
Objective Data		
Eyelids—cont'd		
▪ Ectropion	Outward turning of lower lid margin	Mechanical causes as a result of eyelid tumors, herniated orbital fat, or extravasation of fluid; paralytic ectropion occurs when orbicularis muscle function is disturbed as with Bell's palsy
▪ Lid lag	Slower or absent closing of one lid	Possible involvement of CN VII
▪ Blepharospasm	Increased blink rate; when severe spasms occur, inability to open eyelids	Inflammation; involvement of CNs V and VII; can occur as a response to bright lights
▪ Decreased blink	Decreased rate of eyelid closure	Decreased corneal sensation; possible involvement of CN VII; dry eye and corneal damage may result if blink rate significantly decreased
Conjunctiva		
▪ Conjunctivitis	Redness, swelling of conjunctiva; may be itchy	Bacterial or viral infection; may be allergic response or inflammatory response to chemical exposure
▪ Subconjunctival hemorrhage	Appearance of blood spot on sclera; may be small or can affect entire sclera	Conjunctival blood vessels rupture, leaking blood into the subconjunctival space; caused by coughing, sneezing, eye rubbing, or minor trauma; generally requires no treatment
▪ Pinguecula	Raised area (growth) on conjunctiva; horizontally oriented in medial area of bulbar conjunctiva	Degenerative lesion related to chronic ultraviolet light or other environmental exposure
▪ Jaundice	Yellowish color of entire sclera	Jaundice related to liver dysfunction; yellow color normal after diagnostic study requiring intravenous fluorescein injection
Cornea		
▪ Corneal abrasion	Localized painful disruption of the epithelial layer of cornea, can be visualized with fluorescein dye	Trauma; overwear or improper fit of contact lenses
▪ Corneal opacity	Whitish area of normally transplant cornea; may involve entire cornea	Scar tissue formation related to inflammation; infection, trauma; degree of visual acuity deficit depends on location and size of opacity
▪ Pterygium	Triangular, horizontally oriented thickening of bulbar conjunctiva that extends past cornea-scleral border onto cornea	Commonly thought to be an extension of a pinguecula; degenerative lesion related to chronic ultraviolet light or other environmental exposure; surgical removal necessary if progression to central cornea
Globe		
▪ Exophthalmos	Protrusion of globe beyond its normal position within bony orbit; sclera often visible above iris when eyelids are open	Intraocular or periorbital tumors; thyroid eye disease; swelling or tumors of the frontal sinus; dry eye and corneal damage may occur as a result of inability to close eye normally
Pupil		
▪ Mydriasis	Pupil is larger than normal (dilated)	Emotional influences, trauma, acute glaucoma (fixed, mid-dilated), systemic or local drugs, head injury
▪ Miosis	Pupil is smaller than normal	Iritis, morphine and similar drugs, glaucoma treated with miotic agents
▪ Anisocoria	Pupils are unequal (constricted)	Central nervous system disorders; slight difference in pupil size is normal in a small percentage of the population
▪ Dyscoria	Pupil is irregularly shaped	Congenital causes (e.g., iris coloboma); acquired causes (e.g., trauma, iris-fixated intraocular lens implant, posterior synechiae surgery on iris)
▪ Abnormal response to light or accommodation	Pupils respond asymmetrically or abnormally to light stimulus or accommodation	Central nervous system disorders, general anesthesia

Continued

COMMON ASSESSMENT ABNORMALITIES

Table 19-5 Visual System—cont'd

Finding	Description	Possible Etiology and Significance
Iris		
▪ Heterochromia	Irises are different colors	Congenital causes (Horner's syndrome); acquired causes (chronic iritis, metastatic carcinoma, diffuse iris nevus or melanoma)
▪ Iridokinesis	Iris appears to shake on movement of eye	Aphakia
Extraocular Muscles		
▪ Strabismus	Deviation of eye position in one or more directions	Overaction or underaction of one or more extraocular muscles; can be congenital or acquired; neuromuscular involvement; CN III, IV, or VI involved
Visual Field Defect		
▪ Peripheral	Partial or complete loss of peripheral vision	Glaucoma; complete or partial interruption of visual pathway; migraine headache
▪ Central	Loss of central vision	Macular disease
Lens		
▪ Cataract	Opacification of lens, pupil can appear cloudy or white when opacity is visible behind pupil opening	Aging, trauma, electrical shock, diabetes, chronic systemic corticosteroid therapy, congenital
▪ Subluxation or dislocation	Edge of lens may be seen through pupil; "setting sun" sign	Trauma, systemic disease (e.g., Marfan's syndrome)

CN, cranial nerve.

Initial observation. The initial observation of the patient can provide information that will help the nurse focus the assessment. When first encountering the patient, the nurse may observe that the patient is dressed in clothing with unusual color combinations. This may indicate a color-vision deficit. The nurse may also note an unusual head position. The patient with diplopia may hold the head in a skewed position in an attempt to see a single image. The patient with a corneal abrasion or photophobia will cover the eyes with the hands to try to block out room light. The nurse can make a crude estimate of depth perception by extending a hand for the patient to shake.

During the initial observation, the nurse should also observe the overall facial and ophthalmic appearance of the patient. The eyes should be symmetric and normally placed on the face. The globes should not have a bulging or sunken appearance.

Assessing functional status

Visual acuity. The nurse should always record the patient's visual acuity for medical and legal reasons. The nurse must document the patient's visual acuity before the patient receives any care.

The patient sits or stands 20 feet (6 meters) from the Snellen chart with the usual correction (glasses or contact lenses) left in place unless they are used solely for reading. The nurse asks the patient to cover the left eye and read the smallest line that the patient can read comfortably. If the patient reads that line with two or fewer errors, the examiner instructs the patient to read the next lower line. The nurse notes the smallest line the patient can read with two or fewer errors, and records the standard of 20 feet (6 meters) and then the distance in feet on the line of the Snellen chart the patient read successfully. The nurse records the visual acuities using the ophthalmic abbreviations for right eye (*OD*, or *oculus dexter*), left eye (*OS*, or *oculus sinister*), and both eyes (*OU*, or *oculus uterque*). For example, for the patient who reads to the 30 foot (9 meter) line with the right eye, the nurse records the acuity as 20/30 OD. A visual acuity of 20/30 means that from 20 feet (6 meters) away, the patient can read the same letters that the person with normal vision can read from 30 feet (9 meters) away. *Legal blindness* is defined as the best-corrected vision in the better eye of 20/200 or less.[6] The nurse then asks the patient to cover the right eye, and the process is repeated.

If the patient cannot read letters, the examiner can use an eye chart with pictures or numbers. A second option is an eye chart that presents the letter E in four different directions. The examiner asks the patient to point in the direction the E faces.

To evaluate visual acuity when the patient is unable to see the 20/400 letter, the nurse holds up a number of fingers 3 to 5 feet (0.9 to 1.5 meters) in front of the patient and asks the patient to count them. If the patient is unable to count the fingers, the nurse holds up a different number of fingers at successively closer distances up to 1 foot and again asks the patient to count them. The examiner tests the opposite eye in the same manner and records the acuities of each eye. If the patient can count the number of fingers at 2 feet (0.6 meters), the nurse records the acuity as *FC* or *CF* ("finger counting" or "counts fingers") at 2 feet (0.6 meters). If the patient cannot count fingers, the nurse asks the patient to indicate if moving the hand is seen in front of the face. This level of visual acuity is *HM* ("hand motion"). *LP* ("light projection") is the term for a patient's visual acuity if only light can be seen.

If the patient has a complaint of visual problems with near vision, and for all patients 40 years of age or older, the nurse tests the near visual acuity. The patient is instructed to hold a Jaeger chart 14 inches (35.6 cm) from the eyes. The nurse covers the patient's left eye with the occluder, asks the patient to read successively smaller lines of print from the chart, and records the visual acuity that corresponds to the smallest line of print the patient can read comfortably. The procedure is repeated while covering the right eye. A near acuity of Jaeger$_1$ (J_1) indicates that the patient can read 4-point type at 14 inches (35.6 cm) and is considered normal. A near acuity of J_{10} indicates that the smallest print the patient can read at 14 inches (35.6 cm) is 14-point type and is moderately impaired. Normal newspaper print is 8-point type.

If the nurse must assess visual acuity without access to an eye chart, an accurate assessment is still possible. Examples of other stimuli acceptable for use include newsprint or the label on a container. The examiner records the acuity as "reads newspaper headline at _____ inches."

Extraocular muscle functions. The nurse observes the corneal light reflex to evaluate for weakness or imbalance of the extraocular muscles. In a darkened room, the nurse asks the patient to look straight ahead while a penlight is shone directly on the cornea. The light reflection should be located in the center of both corneas as the patient faces the light source.

Pupil function. Pupil function is determined by inspecting the pupils and their reactions to light. The pupils should be equal in size, round, and react briskly to light. In a small percentage of the population the pupils are unequal in size (anisocoria). The pupils should react to light directly (the pupil constricts when a light shines into the same eye) and consensually (the pupil constricts when a light shines into the opposite eye). The nurse should also check the accommodative response by having the patient fixate on an object held 2 to 3 feet (0.6 to 0.9 m) away and then bringing the object closer to the patient until the patient is fixating on the object at 6 to 8 inches (15 to 20 cm) away. The pupils should constrict when the patient tries to focus on the near object.

Intraocular pressure. Intraocular pressure can be measured by using a Schiotz or Tono-pen tonometer, but the most accurate readings are obtained by applanation tonometry (Fig. 19-7). The surface of the anesthetized cornea is applanated by the tonometer, and the cornea is observed through the biomicroscope. The normal intraocular pressure ranges from 10 to 21 mm Hg.

Assessing structures. The structures that constitute the visual system are assessed primarily by inspection. The visual system is unique because the nurse can directly inspect not only the external structures but also many of the internal structures. The iris, lens, vitreous, retina, and optic nerve can all be visualized directly through the clear cornea and pupil opening.

This direct inspection requires the examiner to use special observation equipment such as the slit lamp biomicroscope and the ophthalmoscope. This equipment permits examination of the conjunctiva, sclera, cornea, anterior chamber, iris, lens, vitreous, and retina under magnification. With the slit lamp microscope, a narrow beam or slit of light is directed onto the eye to brightly illuminate a small section. The patient's chin is positioned in a chin rest to stabilize the head. The ophthalmoscope is a handheld instrument with a light source and magnifying lenses that is held close to the patient's eye to visualize the posterior part of the eye. There is no pain or discomfort associated with these examinations.

As with other skills, using this equipment requires some special training and practice. However, special equipment provides the means for a thorough ophthalmic assessment that gives the nurse information not only about the ocular structures themselves but also about the patient's systemic condition.

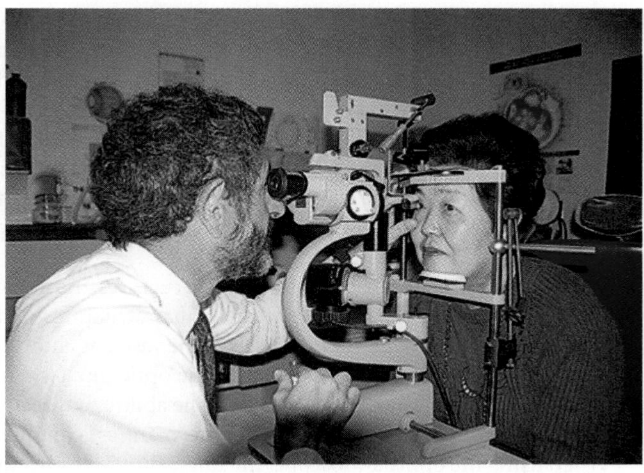

Fig. 19-7 Applanation tonometry.

Eyebrows, eyelashes, and eyelids. All structures should be present and symmetric, and without deformities, redness, or swelling. Eyelashes extend outward from the lid margins. The eyelids are positioned symmetrically with the upper and lower eyelids approximately at the corneal-scleral limbus and the lid margins against the globe. In normal closing, the upper and lower eyelid margins just touch. The lacrimal puncta should be open and positioned properly against the globe, with no swelling or redness around the lower puncta indicating lacrimal sac inflammation. If the sac is inflamed, pressure over the lacrimal sac may cause purulent material to ooze from the puncta.

Conjunctiva and sclera. The nurse can easily examine the conjunctiva and sclera at the same time. The examiner evaluates the color, smoothness, and presence of lesions. To examine the palpebral conjunctiva, the examiner places a forefinger over the cheekbone and gently pulls down. This maneuver exposes the palpebral conjunctiva of the lower lid for the nurse to assess color (normally pale pink), texture (normally smooth), and the presence of lesions or foreign bodies. The bulbar conjunctiva covering the sclera is normally clear, with fine blood vessels visible. These blood vessels are more common in the periphery.

The sclera is normally white, but it may take on a yellowish hue in the older individual because of lipid deposition. A pale blue cast caused by scleral thinning can also be normal in the older adult and in the infant (who have naturally thinner scleras). The blue cast is actually the vascular choroid showing through. A slight yellow cast may also be found in some dark-pigmented persons, such as African-Americans and Native-Americans.

Cornea. The cornea should be clear, transparent, and shiny. In an older patient, *arcus senilis,* which is a white ring at the limbus, is normal.

The nurse can use either a handheld oblique light or the slit lamp microscope to inspect the anterior chamber. The iris should appear flat and not bulging toward the cornea. The area between the cornea and the iris should be clear with no blood or purulent material visible in the anterior chamber. Because blood and purulent material have a viscosity greater than aqueous humor, they will settle to the lower portion of the chamber, if present.

Iris. Both irises should be of similar color and shape. However, a color difference between the irises occurs normally in a small portion of the population. The iris should be inspected with the upper lid raised. Any area of missing iris will be evident, because the absence of the colored iris tissue leaves what appears to be a dark, abnormally shaped "pupil." Round or notched areas of missing iris tissue are often the result of cataract or glaucoma surgery. The nurse should determine the cause of these areas and document the findings.

Retina and optic nerve. To assess these structures, the nurse uses an ophthalmoscope to magnify the ocular structures and bring them into crisp focus. Blood vessels in the vascular choroid are visible through the retinal tissues, as is the optic disc (where the optic nerve enters the back of the eye). The ability to directly view arteries, veins, and the optic nerve in this manner is unique.

When using the ophthalmoscope, the nurse directs the beam of light obliquely into the patient's pupil. The red reflex should be visible. This reflex results from the light reflecting off the pink color of the retina. Any dense areas in the lens, such as a cataract, will decrease the red reflex. The reflex is followed inward until the fundus, or back of the eye, comes into view. Both arterioles and veins can be seen. Arterioles are smaller, thinner, and lighter red and reflect light better than veins. The nurse should examine the areas where arterioles and veins cross for nicking or narrowing. These changes are associated with diabetes mellitus and hypertension.

The examiner follows a blood vessel toward the optic nerve. The optic nerve or disc is examined for size, color, and abnormalities. The disc is creamy yellow with distinct margins. A slight blurring of the nasal margin is common.

A central depression in the disc, called the physiologic cup, may be seen. This area is the exit site for the optic nerve. The cup should be less than one half the diameter of the disc. The nurse should document the presence of any unusual rings or crescents surrounding the disc.

There are normally no hemorrhages or exudates present in the fundus (retinal background). Careful inspection of the fundus can reveal the presence of retinal holes, tears, detachments, or lesions. Small hemorrhages can be associated with diabetes or hypertension and can appear in various shapes, such as dots or flames. Finally, the nurse examines the macula for shape and appearance. This area of high reflectivity is devoid of any blood vessels.

The nurse can obtain important information about the vascular system and the central nervous system (CNS) through direct visualization with an ophthalmoscope. Skilled use of this instrument requires practice, and it is not unusual for the nurse to be frustrated initially.

Special Assessment Techniques

Color vision. Testing the patient's ability to distinguish colors can be an important part of the overall assessment because some occupations may require accurate color discrimination. The Ishihara color test determines the patient's ability to distinguish a pattern of color in a series of color plates. In individuals of European ancestry, approximately 6% of males and 0.3% of females have a congenital color vision defect. The incidence of congenital color vision defects in individuals of non-European ancestry is lower.[7] Older adults have a loss of color discrimination at the blue end of the color spectrum and loss of sensitivity throughout the entire spectrum.

Stereopsis. Stereoscopic vision allows a patient to see objects in three dimensions. Any event that causes a patient to have monocular vision (e.g., enucleation, patching) results in the loss of stereoscopic vision. When stereopsis is not present, the individual's ability to judge distances is impaired. This disability can have serious consequences if the patient trips over a step when walking or follows too closely to another vehicle when driving.

DIAGNOSTIC STUDIES OF THE VISUAL SYSTEM

Diagnostic studies provide important information to the nurse in monitoring the patient's condition and planning appropriate interventions. These studies are considered objective data. Table 19-6 presents the most common basic diagnostic studies of the visual system.

STRUCTURES AND FUNCTIONS OF THE AUDITORY SYSTEM

The auditory system is composed of the peripheral auditory system and the central auditory system. The peripheral system includes the structures of the ear itself: the external, middle, and inner ear (Fig. 19-8). This system is concerned with the reception and perception of sound. The inner ear functions in hearing and balance. The central system (the brain and its pathways) integrates and assigns meaning to what is heard.

External Ear

The external ear consists of the auricle, or pinna, and the external auditory canal. The auricle is composed of cartilage and connective tissue covered with epithelium, which also lines the external auditory canal (see Fig. 19-8). The external auditory canal is a slightly S-shaped tube about 1 inch (2.5 cm) in length in the adult. The skin that lines the canal contains fine hairs and sebaceous glands. Wax-secreting glands are located deep within the canal. These glands secrete cerumen to keep the tympanum soft and waterproof.[14]

Hair is present in the outer half of the canal. This hair may be profuse and coarse, especially in the older male patient. The inner half of the ear canal is quite sensitive. The function of the external ear and canal is to collect and transmit sound waves to the tympanic membrane (eardrum). This shiny, translucent, pearl-gray membrane is composed of skin, connective tissue, and mucous membrane. It serves as a partition between the external auditory canal and the middle ear.

Middle Ear

Mucous membrane lines the middle ear and is continuous from the nasal pharynx via the eustachian tube. The middle ear cavity, which is located in the temporal bone, contains three tiny bones: malleus, incus, and stapes (called the ossicular chain). Vibrations of the tympanic membrane cause the ossicles to move and transmit sound waves to the oval window. This oval window vibration causes the fluid in the inner ear to move and stimulates the receptors of hearing. The round window covered with mucous membrane also opens into the inner ear and allows for dissipation of the fluid disturbances (round window reflex). The superior part of the middle ear is called the *epitympanum,* or the attic, and also communicates with air cells within

DIAGNOSTIC STUDIES

Table 19-6 Visual System

Study	Description and Purpose	Nursing Responsibilities*
▪ Retinoscopy	Objective (though inexact) measure of refractive error; handheld retinoscopy directs focused light into the eye, refractive error distorts the light, distortion is neutralized to determine refractive error; useful for patient unable to cooperate during process of subjective refraction (e.g., confused patients).	Procedure is painless; may need to help patient hold head still. Pupil dilation will make it difficult to focus on near objects; dilation may last from 3-4 hr.
▪ Refractometry	Subjective measure of refractive error; multiple lenses are mounted on rotating wheels; patient sits looking through apertures at Snellen acuity chart, lenses are changed; patient chooses lenses that make acuity sharpest; cycloplegic drugs used to paralyze accommodation during refraction process.	Same as retinoscopy.
▪ Visual field perimetry	Detailed mapping of the visual field; study uses semicircular, bowl-like instrument that presents patient with a light stimulus in various parts of the bowl; specific pattern of visual field loss used to diagnose glaucoma and certain neurologic deficits.	Procedure is painless but may be fatiguing; elderly or debilitated patient may need rest periods; patient must fixate on center target for accurate testing.
▪ Ultrasonography	A-scan probe is applanated against patient's anesthetized cornea; used primarily for axial length measurement for calculating power of intraocular lens implanted after cataract extraction; B-scan probe is applied to patient's closed lid; used more often than A-scan for diagnosis of ocular pathology such as intraocular foreign bodies or tumors, vitreous opacities, retinal detachments.	Procedure is painless (cornea is anesthetized for A-scan).
▪ Indirect ophthalmoscopy	Indirect ophthalmoscope is worn on examiner's head; light is projected through a handheld lens into patient's eye; stereoscopic view is larger and provides a better view of peripheral retina; always used when some retinal abnormality is suspected.	Light source is bright; patient may be uncomfortably photophobic, especially because pupil is dilated.
▪ Fluorescein angiography	Fluorescein (a nonradioactive, noniodine dye) is intravenously injected into antecubital or other peripheral vein, followed by serial photographs (over 10 min period) of the retina through dilated pupils; provides diagnostic information about flow of blood through pigment epithelial and retinal vessels; often used in diabetic patients to accurately locate areas of diabetic retinopathy before laser destruction of neovascularization.	If extravasation occurs, fluorescein is toxic to tissue; systemic allergic reactions are rare, but nurse should be familiar with emergency equipment and procedures; tell patient that dye can sometimes cause transient nausea or vomiting; yellow discoloration of urine and skin is normal and transient.
▪ Amsler grid test	Test is self-administered using a handheld card printed with a grid of lines (similar to graph paper); patient fixates on center dot and records any abnormalities of the grid lines, such as wavy, missing, or distorted areas; used to monitor macular problems.	Regular testing is necessary to identify any changes in macular function.
▪ Schirmer tear test	Study measures tear volume produced throughout fixed time period; one end of a strip of filter paper is placed in lower lid cul-de-sac; area of tear saturation is measured after 5 min; useful in diagnosing keratoconjunctivitis sicca.	Test may be done with closed or open eyes.

*Patient education regarding the purpose and method of testing is a nursing responsibility for all diagnostic procedures.

the mastoid bone. The air cells are lined with the same mucous membrane as the middle ear.

The middle ear cavity is filled with air, and equalization of atmospheric air pressure is accomplished by the eustachian tube. This tube is opened during yawning or swallowing. Blockage of the tube can occur with allergies, nasopharyngeal infections, and enlarged adenoids. The facial nerve (CN VII) traverses above the oval window of the middle ear. The thin, bony covering of the facial nerve (CN VII) can become damaged by chronic ear infection, skull fracture, or trauma during ear surgery, resulting in problems related to voluntary facial movements, eyelid closure, and taste discrimination.

The external and middle portions of the ear function to conduct and amplify sound waves from the environment. This portion of sound conduction is termed *air conduction.* Problems in these two parts of the ear may cause conductive hearing loss,

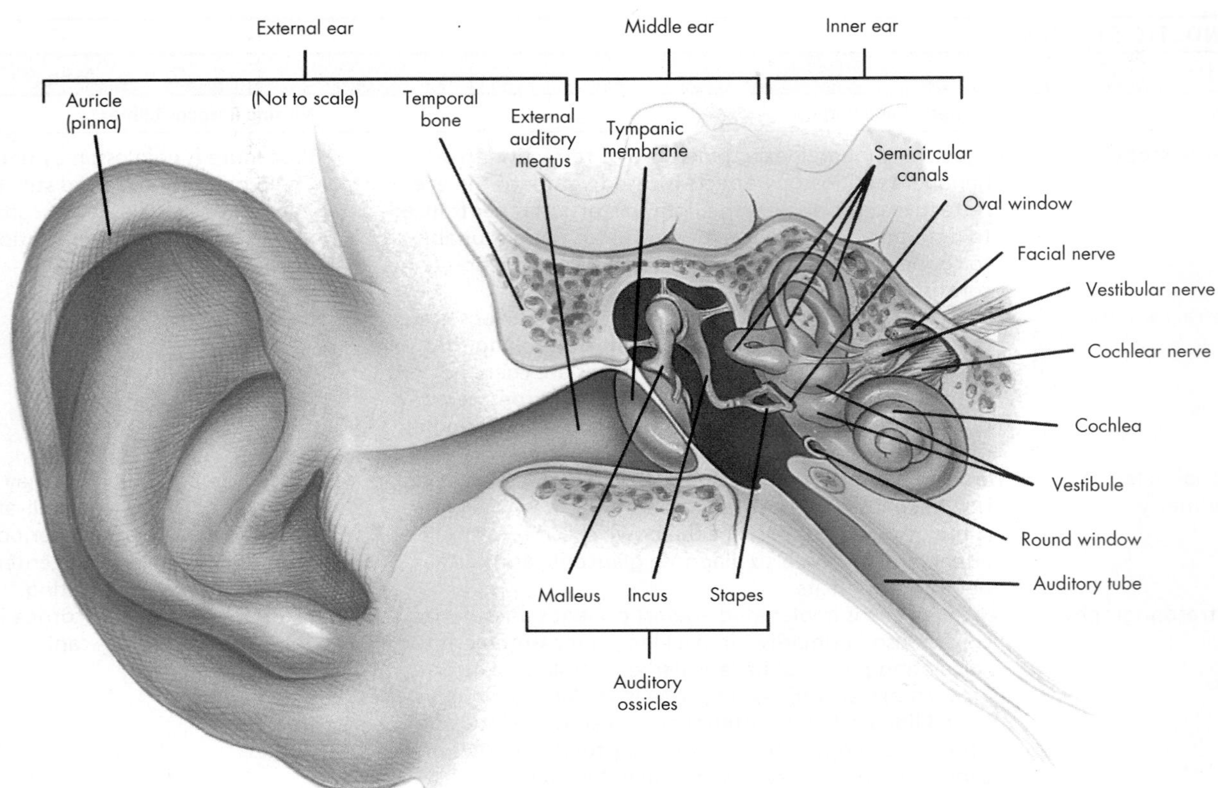

Fig. 19-8 External, middle, and inner ear.

resulting in an alteration in the patient's perception or sensitivity to sounds.

Inner Ear

The middle ear interfaces with the inner ear where the stapes meets the oval window. The inner ear is composed of the bony labyrinth and the membranous labyrinth and contains the functional organs for hearing and balance. The receptor organ for hearing is the cochlea, a coiled structure. It contains the organ of Corti, whose tiny hair cells respond to stimulation of selected portions of the basilar membrane according to pitch. This mechanical stimulus is converted into an electrochemical impulse and then transmitted by the acoustic portion of the vestibulocochlear nerve (CN VIII) to the brain to process and interpret sound.

Three semicircular canals and two sacs, the utricle and saccule, make up the organ of balance. These structures make up the membranous labyrinth, which is housed in a bony labyrinth. The membranous labyrinth is filled with endolymphatic fluid, and the bony labyrinth is filled with perilymphatic fluid. The perilymphatic fluid cushions these two sensitive organs and communicates with the brain and the subarachnoid spaces of the brain. The nervous stimuli are communicated by the vestibular portion of CN VIII.

Pathology of the inner ear or along the nerve pathway from the inner ear to the brain can result in *sensorineural hearing loss.* This may result in an alteration of the patient's perception or sensitivity to high-pitched tones. These may be experienced as a decrease in intensity, muffling of the intensity (increased sensitivity to loud sounds), or decrease in ability to understand spoken words (distortion). Problems within the central auditory system from the cochlear nuclei to the cortex cause *central hearing loss.* This type of hearing loss causes difficulty in understanding the meaning of the words heard. (Types of hearing loss are discussed in Chapter 20.)

Transmission of Sound. Sound waves are conducted by air and picked up by the auricles and auditory canal. The tympanic membrane is struck by the sound waves, causing it to vibrate. The central area of the tympanic membrane is connected to the malleus, which also starts to vibrate, transmitting the vibration to the incus, then the stapes. As the stapes moves back and forth, it pushes the membrane of the oval window in and out. Movement of the oval window produces waves in the perilymph.[15]

Once sound has been transmitted to the liquid medium of the inner ear, the vibration is picked up by the tiny sensory hair cells of the cochlea, which initiate nerve impulses. These impulses are carried by nerve fibers to the main branch of the acoustic portion of CN VIII and then to the brain.

GERONTOLOGIC CONSIDERATIONS

Effects of Aging on the Auditory System

Age-related changes of the auditory system can result in impaired hearing. *Presbycusis,* or hearing loss due to aging, has no clear-cut cause; however, several different variables in addition to aging are thought to be involved. The auditory system may encounter insults from a variety of sources, including noise exposure, vascular or systemic disease, nutrition, ototoxic drugs, and pollution during the life span. *Tinnitus,* or ringing in the

GERONTOLOGIC DIFFERENCES IN ASSESSMENT

Table 19-7 Auditory System

Changes	Differences in Assessment Findings
External Ear	
Increased production of and drier cerumen	Impacted earwax; potential hearing loss
Increased hair growth	Visible hair
Middle Ear	
Atrophic changes of tympanic membrane	Conductive hearing loss
Inner Ear	
Hair cell degeneration, neuron degeneration in auditory nerve and central pathways, reduced blood supply to cochlea	Presbycusis, diminished sensitivity to high-pitched sounds, impaired speech reception, tinnitus
Less effective vestibular apparatus in semicircular canals	Alterations in balance and body orientation

ears, may accompany the hearing loss that results from the aging process. Hearing loss, especially in the older adult, can have serious implications for the quality of life, including progressive physical and psychosocial dysfunction.[16] As the average life span increases, the number of people with progressive changes in the auditory system will also increase. Early identification of problems will ensure a more active and healthy patient population in their seventh and eighth decades.

Age-related changes in the auditory system and differences in assessment findings are presented in Table 19-7.

ASSESSMENT OF THE AUDITORY SYSTEM

Assessment of the auditory system includes assessment of the vestibular (balance) system because the two systems are so intimately related. It is often difficult to separate the symptomatology between the two systems. The nurse must help the patient describe symptoms and problems in order to differentiate the source of the problems. Health history questions to ask a patient with an auditory problem are listed in Table 19-8.

Initially the nurse should try to categorize symptoms related to dizziness and vertigo and separate them from symptoms related to hearing loss or tinnitus. The symptoms can be combined later in the assessment to help make the diagnosis and plan for the patient.

Subjective Data

Important Health Information

Past health history. Many problems related to the ear are sequelae of childhood illnesses or result from problems of adjacent organs. Consequently a careful assessment of past health problems is important.

The patient should be questioned about previous problems regarding the ears, especially problems experienced during childhood. The frequency of acute middle ear infections (otitis media); perforations of the eardrum; drainage; complications; and history of mumps, measles, or scarlet fever should be recorded. Congenital hearing loss can result from infectious diseases (rubella, influenza, or syphilis), teratogenic medications, or hypoxia in the first trimester of pregnancy. Pregnant women and young women of childbearing age should be questioned regarding whether they were vaccinated for rubella or have ever had rubella. If the patient is unsure about having had rubella, a blood test for this measles antibody can be performed.[17]

Symptoms such as dizziness, tinnitus, and hearing loss are recorded in the patient's words. It may be difficult for the patient to describe the dizziness. However, it is important that the patient describe the dizziness in detail using her or his own words. This careful description could help differentiate the cause.

Medications. Information about present or past medications that are ototoxic (cause damage to CN VIII) and can produce hearing loss, tinnitus, and vertigo should be obtained. The amount and frequency of aspirin use are important because tinnitus can result from high aspirin intake. Aminoglycosides, other antibiotics, salicylates, antimalarial agents, chemotherapeutic drugs, diuretics, and nonsteroidal antiinflammatory drugs (NSAIDs) are groups of drugs that are potentially ototoxic.[18] Careful monitoring is essential. Many drugs produce hearing loss that may be reversible with cessation of treatment.

Surgery or other treatments. Information regarding previous hospitalizations for ear surgery, as well as for tonsillectomy and adenoidectomy, should be obtained. Hospitalization or treatment for head injury should also be documented because a head injury may result in hearing loss. Use and satisfaction with a hearing aid should be documented. Problems with impacted cerumen should also be noted.

Functional Health Patterns. Hearing and balance problems can affect all aspects of a person's life. In order to assess the impact, health history questions can be asked based on a functional health pattern approach (see Table 19-8).

Health perception–health management pattern. The nurse should note the onset of hearing loss, whether sudden or gradual. It should be recorded who noted the onset, whether it be the patient, family, or significant others. Gradual hearing losses are most often noted by those who communicate with the patient. Sudden losses and those exacerbated by some other condition are most often reported by the patient.

Information about allergies is important because they can cause the eustachian tube to become edematous and prevent aeration of the middle ear. This occurs more frequently in children.

Information regarding family members with hearing loss and type of hearing loss is important. Some congenital hearing loss is hereditary. The age of onset of presbycusis also follows a familial pattern. Because prematurity can cause hearing problems, information about the patient's gestational age is also important. Premature infants may have been treated with an ototoxic drug. If knowledge of this event is important, it may be necessary to examine hospital records.

The patient should be questioned about personal practices used to preserve hearing. The use of protective ear covers or ear plugs is good practice for persons in high-noise environments. If the patient is a swimmer, the frequency and duration of swimming and use of ear protection should be documented.

HEALTH HISTORY

Table 19-8 Auditory System

Health Perception–Health Management Pattern

Hearing

- Have you had a change in your hearing?*
- If yes, how does this change affect your daily life?
- Do you use any devices to improve your hearing (e.g., hearing aid, special volume control, headphones for television or stereo)?*
- How do you protect your hearing?
- Do you have any allergies that result in ear problems?*

Balance

- Is your walking affected by dizziness or vertigo?*
- Does movement cause nausea or vomiting?
- Can you drive or walk alone? If no, elaborate.
- Are there any times of the day when your symptoms are worse?*

Tinnitus

- How long have you experienced ringing in your ears? Has it changed?
- When does it bother you the most?
- What things have you tried that help?

Nutritional-Metabolic Pattern

- Do you have any food allergies that affect your ears?*
- Do you notice any differences in symptoms with changes in diet?*

Elimination Pattern

- Does straining during a bowel movement cause you ear pain?*
- Does your ear problem cause nausea that interferes with your food intake?*
- Does chewing or swallowing cause you any ear discomfort?

Activity-Exercise Pattern

- Does your ear problem result in any change in your usual activity or exercise?*
- Do you need help with certain activities (lifting, bending, climbing stairs, driving, speaking) because of symptoms?*
- Do you have any limitations in activities of daily living because of your symptoms?*

Sleep-Rest Pattern

- Is your sleep disturbed by symptoms of tinnitus or dizziness?*

Cognitive-Perceptual Pattern

- Do you experience pain associated with your hearing or balance problem?* What relieves the pain? What makes it worse?
- Is your ability to communicate and understand affected by your symptoms?*

Self-Perception–Self-Concept Pattern

- Have changes in your hearing affected your self-esteem or feeling of independence?*

Role-Relationship Pattern

- What effect has your ear problem had on your work, family, or social life?
- Are you able to recognize the effects of your ear problems on your life?*
- Do you consider your ear problem a stressor?*

Sexuality-Reproductive Pattern

- Has your ear problem caused a change in your sex life?*

Coping–Stress Tolerance Pattern

- What coping mechanism do you use during time of exacerbation of symptoms?
- Do you feel able to cope with your hearing or balance problem? If no, describe.

Value-Belief Pattern

- Do you have a conflict between your planned treatment and your value-belief system?*

*If yes, describe.

Also, it is important to note the type of water in which the swimming takes place.

Nutritional-metabolic pattern. Both alcohol and sodium affect the amount of endolymph retained in the inner ear system. Patients with Meniere's disease generally notice some improvement in their symptoms with alcohol restriction and a low-sodium diet. Improvements and exacerbations associated with food intake should be noted. The patient should also be questioned about any ear pain or discomfort associated with chewing or swallowing that might decrease nutritional intake. This problem is often associated with a problem in the middle ear.

Elimination pattern. Elimination patterns and their association with ear problems are mainly of interest in the patient with perilymph fistula or the patient who is immediately postoperative. If the patient experiences frequent constipation or straining with bowel or bladder elimination, this may interfere with healing of a perilymph fistula or its repair. The post-stapedectomy patient especially needs to prevent the increased intracranial (and consequent inner ear) pressure associated with straining during bowel movements. Stool softeners may be ordered postoperatively for the patient who reports chronic problems with constipation.

Activity-exercise pattern. Activity-exercise review is most important when assessing the patient with vestibular problems. The patient should be questioned specifically about activities that relieve or exacerbate symptoms of dizziness or elicit nausea or vomiting. The patient with chronic vertigo syndrome (benign paroxysmal positional vertigo [BPPV]) notes that the symptoms improve throughout the day as adjustment to the visual and positional input from the environment occurs. If dizziness is a problem, the patient should be questioned about the onset, duration, frequency, and precipitating factors of this symptom.

Patients with Meniere's syndrome demonstrate increasing inability to compensate for environmental input as the day progresses. Symptoms are experienced particularly in the evening. The nurse and the patient should identify a list of activities and exercises that affect dizziness and vertigo. The patient may use habituation exercises to help control the symptoms. Habituation exercises involve frequent repetition of an activity that causes symptoms until the body adjusts and the activity is no longer a problem.

Sleep-rest pattern. The patient with chronic tinnitus should be questioned about sleep problems. Tinnitus can disturb sleep and activities conducted in a quiet environment. If a sleep problem is associated with tinnitus, the patient should be asked if any masking devices or techniques are used or have been tried to drown out the tinnitus.

Cognitive-perceptual pattern. Pain is associated with some ear problems, particularly those involving the middle ear. If pain is present, the patient should be asked to describe the pain and the treatments used for relief. The effect on the pain level when the auricle is moved should be noted.

Hearing loss is associated with many middle and inner ear problems. The nurse or family may report the patient's decreased hearing, or the patient may express concern about perceived hearing loss. If decreased hearing is noted, the patient and family should be questioned about the duration, severity, and circumstances associated with the decreased hearing.

Self-perception–self-concept pattern. The patient should be asked to describe how the ear problem has affected personal life and feelings about himself or herself. Hearing loss and chronic vertigo are particularly distressing for the patient. Hearing loss can result in embarrassing social situations that cause the patient to have a diminished self-concept. The nurse should sensitively question the patient about the occurrence of such situations.

The patient with chronic vertigo may at times be accused of alcohol intoxication. The patient should be asked if this has happened and how the situation was handled.

Role-relationship pattern. The patient should be questioned about the effect the ear problem has had on family life, work responsibilities, and social relationships. Hearing loss can result in strained family relations and misunderstandings. Failure to acknowledge hearing loss and failure to seek treatment can further hinder family relationships.

The patient should be questioned regarding employment or contact with environments that have excessive noise levels, such as work with jet engines and machinery, contact with the firing of firearms, and electronically amplified music. The use of preventive devices worn in noisy environments is important to document.

Many jobs rely on the ability to hear accurately and respond appropriately. If a hearing loss is present, the nurse should gather detailed information of the effect this has on the patient's job. The patient should be assisted to realistically evaluate the job situation.

Hearing loss often leaves the patient feeling isolated from valued social relationships. The nurse should gather information about social activities such as playing cards, going to movies, and attending church from before and since the hearing loss occurred. Comparison of the frequency and enjoyment of the events can indicate if a problem is present.

The unpredictability of vertigo attacks can have devastating effects on all aspects of a patient's life. Ordinary activities such as driving, child care, housework, climbing stairs, and cooking all have an element of danger. The patient should be asked to describe the effect of the vertigo on the many roles and responsibilities of life. Compensatory practices to avoid the development of dangerous situations should also be noted.

Table 19-9 Normal Physical Assessment of the Auditory System

Ears symmetric in location and shape
Auricles and tragus nontender, without lesions
Canal clear, tympanic membrane intact, landmarks and light reflex intact
Able to hear low whisper at 30 cm; Rinne test results AC > BC; Weber's test results, no lateralization

Sexuality-reproductive pattern. It should be determined if hearing loss or deafness has interfered with the establishment of a satisfactory sex life. Although intimacy does not depend on the ability to hear, it could interfere with establishing a relationship that could develop into a sexual relationship or maintaining a current relationship.

Coping–stress tolerance pattern. The patient should be asked to report the usual coping style, tolerance for stress, stress-reducing behaviors, and available support. This information enables the nurse to determine if the patient's resources are adequate to meet the demands imposed by the ear problem. If the nurse concludes that the patient seems unable to manage the situation produced by the ear problem, outside intervention may be required. Denial is a common response to a hearing problem and should be assessed.

Value-belief pattern. The patient should be questioned about any conflicts produced by the problem or treatment related to values or beliefs. Every effort should be made to resolve the problem so the patient does not experience additional stress.

Objective Data

Physical Examination. The nurse can collect valuable objective data regarding the patient's ability to hear during the health-history interview. Clues such as posturing of the head and appropriateness of responses should be noted. Does the patient ask to have certain words repeated? Does the patient intently watch the examiner but miss comments when not looking at the examiner? Such observations are significant and should be recorded. This is also important because the patient is often unaware of hearing loss or does not admit to changes in hearing until moderate losses have occurred. A normal assessment of the ear is listed in Table 19-9. Age-related changes of the auditory system and differences in assessment findings are listed in Table 19-7.

External ear. The external ear is inspected and palpated before examination of the external canal and tympanum. The auricle, preauricular area, and mastoid area are observed for equality of conformation of both ears, color of skin, nodules, swelling, redness, and lesions. The auricle and mastoid areas are then palpated for tenderness and nodules. Grasping the auricle may elicit pain, especially if inflammation of the external ear or canal is present.

External auditory canal and tympanum. Before inserting an otoscope, the nurse should inspect the canal opening for

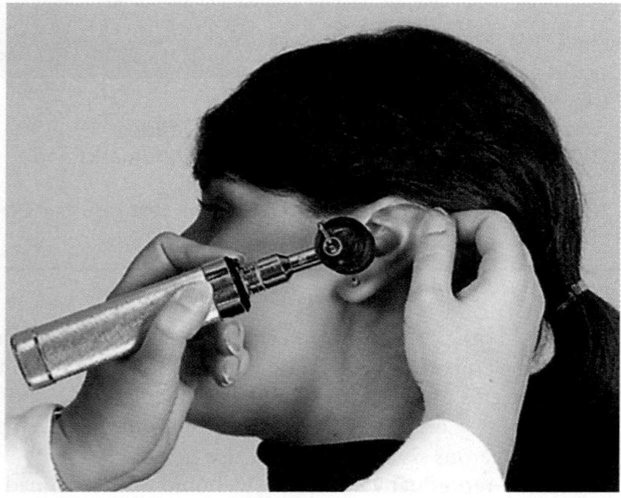

Fig. 19-9 Otoscopic examination of the adult ear. Auricle is pulled up and back. The hand holding the otoscope is braced against the face for stabilization.

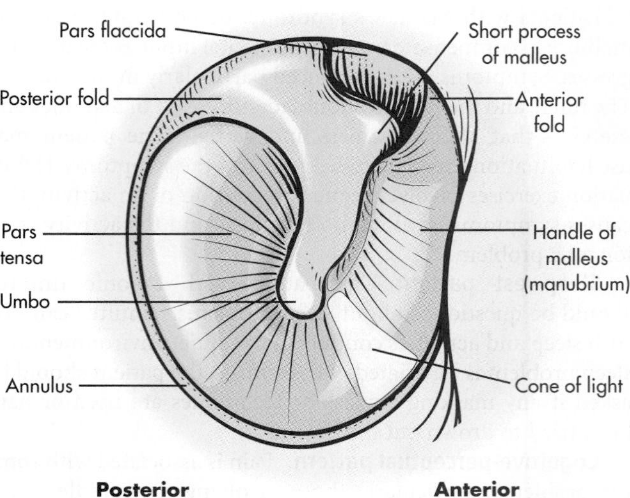

Fig. 19-10 Normal landmarks of the right tympanic membrane as seen through an otoscope.

patency, palpate the tragus, and move the ear about to check for discomfort. After inspecting the canal opening for patency, an otoscopic examination is performed. A speculum slightly smaller than the size of the ear canal is selected. The patient's head is tipped to the opposite shoulder. The top of the auricle is grasped and gently pulled up and back in adults and horizontally backward in children to straighten the canal. The otoscope, held in the examiner's right hand and stabilized on the patient's head by the fingers, is inserted slowly (Fig. 19-9). The canal is observed for size and shape and the color, amount, and type of cerumen. If a large amount of cerumen is present, the tympanum may not be visible. The tympanum is observed for color, landmarks, contour, and intactness (Fig. 19-10).

The tympanic membrane separates the external ear from the middle ear. It is pearl gray, white, or pink; shiny; and translucent. The anteroinferior quadrant is situated obliquely in the ear canal and is farthest from the examiner. The major landmarks are formed by the short process of the malleus superiorly, the handle or manubrium, and the umbo, the most depressed point of the concave tympanum. From the innermost part of the tympanum a light reflex or cone of light is formed with the point directed toward the umbo. The circumference of the tympanum is thickened into a dense, whitish, fibrous ring, or *annulus,* except in the superior area. The tympanum within the annulus is taut and is called the *pars tensa.* Superior to the short process of the malleus is the *pars flaccida,* the flaccid part of the tympanum. The malleolar folds are anterior and posterior to the short process of the malleus. The middle and inner ear cannot be examined with the otoscope because of the tympanic membrane. Table 19-10 summarizes common assessment abnormalities of the auditory system.

DIAGNOSTIC STUDIES OF THE AUDITORY SYSTEM

Table 19-11 describes diagnostic studies commonly used to assess the auditory system.

Tests for Hearing Acuity

Tests involving the whispered and spoken voice can provide gross screening information about the patient's ability to hear. Audiometric testing provides more detailed information that can be used for diagnosis and treatment.

In the whispered test the examiner stands 12 to 24 inches (30 to 61 cm) to the side of the patient and, after exhaling, speaks using a low whisper. A louder whisper is used if the patient does not respond correctly. Spoken voice, increasing in loudness, is similarly used. The patient is asked to repeat numbers or words or answer questions. Each ear is tested. The ear not being tested is masked with the patient occluding the ear or with the examiner moving a finger rapidly, close to the ear canal.

In another test a ticking watch is placed 0.5 to 2 inches (1.3 to 5 cm) from the ear being tested, and the opposite ear is masked. The patient with normal hearing should be able to hear the ticking. However, with the popularity of quartz movement watches, ticking watches are harder to find and the variation among watches makes this test a difficult one for assessing hearing acuity. The patient with sensorineural loss may not be able to hear the high-pitched tones of a ticking watch.

Tuning-Fork Tests. Tuning-fork tests aid in differentiating between conductive and sensorineural hearing loss. Tuning forks of 250, 500, and 1000 Hz are generally used for this examination. Both skill and experience are required to ensure accurate results. If a problem is suspected, further evaluation by pure-tone audiometry is essential. The most common tuning-fork tests are the Rinne test and Weber's test.

For the Rinne test the base of an activated tuning fork is held first against the mastoid bone and then in front of the ear canal (0.5 to 2 inches). The patient reports whether the sound is louder behind the ear (on the mastoid bone) or next to the ear canal. When the sound is no longer perceived behind the ear, the fork is moved next to the ear canal until the patient indicates that the sound is no longer heard. The Rinne test is positive when the patient reports that air conduction (AC) is heard longer than bone conduction (BC). This can indicate normal

COMMON ASSESSMENT ABNORMALITIES

Table 19-10 Auditory System

Finding	Description	Possible Etiology and Significance
External Ear and Canal		
▪ Sebaceous cyst behind ear	Usually within skin, possible presence of black dot (opening to sebaceous gland)	Removal or incision and drainage if painful
▪ Tophi	Hard nodules in the helix or antihelix consisting of uric acid crystals	Associated with gout, metabolic disorder; further diagnosis needed
▪ Impacted cerumen	Wax that has not normally been excreted from the ear; no visualization of eardrum	Decreased hearing possible, sensation of fullness in auditory canal, removal necessary before otoscopic examination
▪ Discharge in canal	Infection of external ear, usually painful	Swimmer's ear, infection of external ear; possibly caused by ruptured eardrum and otitis media
▪ Swelling of pinna, pain	Infection of glands of skin, hematoma caused by trauma	Aspiration (for hematoma)
▪ Scaling or lesions	Change in usual appearance of skin	Seborrheic dermatitis, squamous cell carcinoma, atrophic dermatitis
▪ Exostosis	Bony growth extending into canal causing narrowing of canal	Possible interference with visualization of tympanum, usually asymptomatic
Tympanum		
▪ Retracted eardrum	Appearance of shorter, more horizontal malleus; absent or bent cone of light	Absorption of air from middle ear, blockage of eustachian tube, negative pressure in middle ear
▪ Hairline fluid level, yellow-amber bubbles above fluid level	Caused by transudate of blood and serum, meniscus of fluid producing hairline appearance	Serous otitis media
▪ Bulging red or blue eardrum, lack of landmarks	Fluid-filled middle ear, pus, blood	Acute otitis media, perforation possible
▪ Perforation of eardrum (central or marginal)	Previous perforations of the eardrum that have failed to heal; thin, transparent layer of epithelium surrounding eardrum	Chronic otitis media
▪ Recruitment	Disproportionate loudness of sound from malfunction of inner ear	Hearing aid difficult to use

hearing or a sensorineural loss. If the patient hears the tuning fork better by bone conduction, the Rinne test is negative and indicates that a conductive hearing loss is present.

For Weber's test an activated tuning fork is placed on the midline of the skull, the forehead, or the teeth. The patient is asked to indicate where the sound is heard best. In normal auditory function the patient perceives a midline tone. If a patient has a conductive hearing loss in one ear, sound is heard louder (lateralizes) in that ear. If a sensorineural loss is present, sound is louder (lateralizes) in the unaffected ear.

Results of tuning fork tests are subjective. The patient with inconsistent test results or questionable results should be referred for more objective audiometric evaluation.

Audiometry. Audiometry is beneficial as a screening test for hearing acuity and as a diagnostic test for determining the degree and type of hearing loss. The audiometer produces pure tones at varying intensities to which the patient can respond. Sound is characterized by the number of vibrations or cycles that occur each second. Hertz (Hz) is the unit of measurement used to classify the frequency of a tone. The higher the frequency, the higher the pitch. Hearing loss can affect certain sound frequencies. The specific pattern produced on the audiogram by these losses can assist in the diagnosis of the type of hearing loss. The intensity or strength of a sound wave is expressed in terms of decibels (dB), ranging from 0 to 140 dB. The intensity of a sound required to make any frequency barely audible to the average normal ear is 0 dB. *Threshold* refers to the signal level at which pure tones are detected (pure tone thresholds) or the signal level at which the patient correctly hears 50% of the signals (speech detection thresholds).

Normal speech presented comfortably loud is approximately 40 to 65 dB; a soft whisper is 20 dB. Normally, a child and a young adult can hear frequencies from about 16 to 20,000 Hz, but hearing is most sensitive between 500 and 4000 Hz. This is similar to the frequencies contained in speech. A 40 to 45 dB

DIAGNOSTIC STUDIES

Table 19-11 Auditory System

Study	Description and Purpose	Nursing Responsibilities
Auditory		
▪ Pure-tone audiometry	Sounds are presented through earphones in soundproof room. Patient responds nonverbally when sound is heard. Response is recorded on an audiogram. Purpose is to determine hearing range of patient in terms of dB and Hz for diagnosing conductive and sensorineural hearing loss. Tinnitus can cause inconsistent results.	Nurse does not usually participate in examination.
▪ Bone conduction	Vibrator is placed on mastoid process, and hearing by bone conduction is recorded. Diagnoses conductive hearing loss.	
▪ One-syllable and two-syllable word lists	Words are presented and recorded at comfortable level of hearing to determine percentage correct and word understanding.	
▪ Auditory evoked potential (AEP)	Procedure is similar to electroencephalogram (See Table 53-9). Electrodes are attached to patient in a darkened room. Electrodes are placed typically at the vertex, mastoid process, or earlobes and forehead. A computer is used to isolate the auditory from other electrical activity of the brain.	Explain procedure to patient. Do not leave patient alone in the darkened room.
▪ Electrocochleography	Test is useful for uncooperative patient or patient who cannot volunteer useful information. Test records electrical activity in the cochlea and auditory nerve.	
▪ Auditory brainstem response (ABR)	Study measures electrical peaks along auditory pathway of inner ear to brain and provides diagnostic information related to acoustical neuromas, brainstem problems, and cerebrovascular accident (CVA).	
Vestibular		
▪ Caloric test stimulus	Endolymph of the semicircular canals is stimulated by irrigation of cold (68° F [20° C]) or warm (97° F [36° C]) solution into ear. Patient is seated or in supine position. Observation of type of nystagmus, nausea and vomiting, falling, or vertigo produced is helpful in diagnosing disease of labyrinth. Decreased function is indicated by decreased response and indicates disease of vestibular system. Other ear is tested similarly and results are compared.	Observe patient for vomiting, assist if necessary. Ensure patient safety.
▪ Electronystagmography (ENG)	Electrodes are placed near patient's eyes and movement of eyes (nystagmus) is recorded on graph during specific eye movements and when ear is irrigated. Study diagnoses diseases of vestibular system.	
▪ Posturography	Balance test that can isolate one semicircular canal from others to determine site of lesion.	Inform patient that test is time-consuming and uncomfortable; test can be discontinued at any time at patient's request.
▪ Rotatory chair testing	The patient is seated in a chair driven by a motor under computer control. Evaluates peripheral vestibular system.	

loss in these frequencies causes moderate difficulty in hearing normal speech. A hearing aid may be helpful because it amplifies sound. A patient with a loss primarily in the higher frequencies, such as 4000 through 8000 Hz, has difficulty distinguishing the high-pitched consonants. Words such as cat, hat, and fat may not be perceived accurately because the important information conveyed by the consonant is not heard. A hearing aid makes sound information louder but not clearer and so may not be helpful to the patient who has problems with *discrimination* of sounds or sound information because the consonants are still not heard enough to make speech understandable.

Screening audiometry. Screening audiometry is the testing of large numbers of persons with a fast, simple test to detect possible hearing problems. A pass-fail criterion is used to screen persons who will or will not be given additional diagnostic testing. Persons who fail the screening should be referred for threshold audiometry.

In screening audiometry, the audiometer is usually set at a hearing level of 10 to 20 dB. The patient wears earphones as the

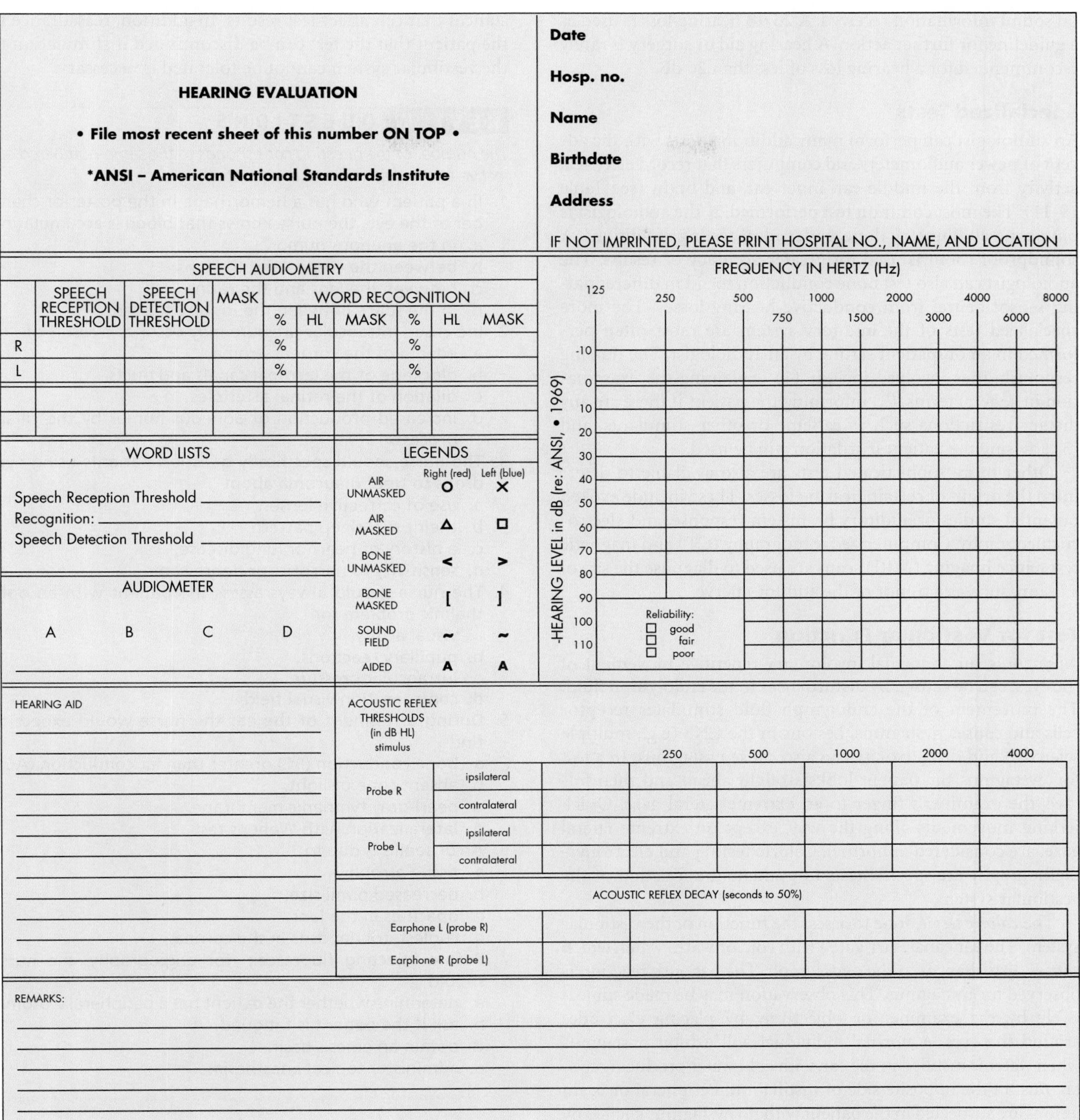

HEARING EVALUATION

• File most recent sheet of this number ON TOP •

*ANSI – American National Standards Institute

Date

Hosp. no.

Name

Birthdate

Address

IF NOT IMPRINTED, PLEASE PRINT HOSPITAL NO., NAME, AND LOCATION

SPEECH AUDIOMETRY

	SPEECH RECEPTION THRESHOLD	SPEECH DETECTION THRESHOLD	MASK	WORD RECOGNITION %	HL	MASK	%	HL	MASK
R				%			%		
L				%			%		

WORD LISTS

Speech Reception Threshold

Recognition:

Speech Detection Threshold

AUDIOMETER

A B C D

LEGENDS

	Right (red)	Left (blue)
AIR UNMASKED	O	X
AIR MASKED	Δ	□
BONE UNMASKED	<	>
BONE MASKED	[	]
SOUND FIELD	~	~
AIDED	A	A

FREQUENCY IN HERTZ (Hz)

125 250 500 1000 2000 4000 8000

750 1500 3000 6000

-HEARING LEVEL in dB (re: ANSI, • 1969)

-10 0 10 20 30 40 50 60 70 80 90 100 110

Reliability:
□ good
□ fair
□ poor

HEARING AID

ACOUSTIC REFLEX THRESHOLDS (in dB HL) stimulus

		250	500	1000	2000	4000
Probe R	ipsilateral					
	contralateral					
Probe L	ipsilateral					
	contralateral					

ACOUSTIC REFLEX DECAY (seconds to 50%)

Earphone L (probe R)					
Earphone R (probe L)					

REMARKS:

Fig. 19-11 The patient's hearing level is plotted on the audiogram.

tester sweeps across the available signal frequencies. The patient is directed to raise a hand when a sound is heard. Responses to air-conducted tones are checked at each frequency setting.

Pure-tone audiometry. A pure-tone audiometer produces pure tones at varied frequencies and intensities. Threshold audiometry generally determines thresholds for seven frequencies from 250 to 8000 Hz. The intensity is plotted against the frequency on an audiogram (Fig. 19-11). The right ear is represented by a red circle and the left ear by a blue X on the audiogram.

In a quiet setting a tone loud enough to be clearly heard by the patient is presented. The threshold level for frequency is then determined. A person with thresholds at 25 dB or higher will demonstrate problems in everyday communication. Usually the lower limit used for acceptable hearing for children is 15 to 20 dB because a child's ability to develop speech depends on sound information received. A 26 dB hearing loss is used as a guideline for further action. A hearing aid or surgery is rarely recommended for a hearing loss of less than 26 dB.[19]

Specialized Tests

An audiologist can perform many additional tests with the advent of newer audiometers and computers that record electrical activity from the middle ear, inner ear, and brain (see Table 19-11). The most common test performed by the audiologist is pure-tone audiometry done under ideal testing conditions. A soundproof room is used for greater accuracy of results. The audiologist can also test bone conduction to aid in differentiating sensorineural from conductive hearing losses. The more specialized tests of the auditory system are most often performed in an outpatient setting by an audiologist. The nursing responsibilities involved include (1) explaining the examination in general terms, (2) informing the patient if there are any dietary restrictions such as caffeine or other stimulants, and (3) advising the patient if sedation will be used.

Other more sophisticated tests are also available to determine the origin of certain hearing losses. These include evoked potential studies or auditory brainstem response, and electrocochleography. Computerized tomography (CT) and magnetic resonance imaging (MRI) scans are used to diagnose the site of a lesion, such as a tumor of the auditory nerve.

Test for Vestibular Function

Nystagmus, an abnormal involuntary repetitive movement of the eyes, can be caused by disturbances in the endolymph fluid. The movement of the endolymph fluid stimulates receptor cells and causes nystagmus. Lesions in the CNS (e.g., multiple sclerosis) and drug toxicity can also cause nystagmus. In a test for nystagmus the patient looks straight ahead and then follows the examiner's finger to an extreme lateral gaze. Quick jerking movements along the way, except on extreme lateral gaze, are considered abnormal. Caloric testing and electronystagmography are specific tests to evaluate the function of the vestibular system.

The *caloric test* is done to assess the function of the vestibular system. The ear canal is irrigated with cold or warm water, which causes disturbances in the endolymph. The patient's reaction is observed for nystagmus. This observation may be made subjectively by the examiner or objectively by placing electrodes around the eyes. A normal individual will exhibit nystagmus when water is instilled in the ear, with cold water producing nystagmus on the opposite side of instillation. Peripheral or brain lesions are suspected in the patient with no nystagmus elicited by caloric testing. Drugs that may alter the test results include alcohol, CNS depressants, and barbiturates. The patient's use of these substances should be known to the physician before testing.

Posturography. In the past few years, more sophisticated tests of the balance system have been developed, including platform posturography and rotational chair tests. These tests isolate one semicircular canal from the others to determine the site of a lesion causing vestibular disturbance. They can also provide data concerning the degree of disability caused by the disorder. These tests are time consuming, and in the vestibularly compromised patient can cause distress and discomfort, particularly nausea and vomiting. The patient will require pretest instructions regarding intake of substances that can affect test results. In addition, reassurance to the patient that the test can be discontinued if stimulation to the vestibular system cannot be tolerated is necessary.

REVIEW QUESTIONS

The number of the question corresponds to the same-numbered objective at the beginning of the chapter.

1. In a patient who has a hemorrhage in the posterior chamber of the eye, the nurse knows that blood is accumulating
   a. in the aqueous humor.
   b. between the cornea and the lens.
   c. between the lens and the retina.
   d. in the space between the iris and the lens.
2. Increased intraocular pressure may occur as a result of
   a. edema of the corneal stroma.
   b. blockage of the lacrimal canals and ducts.
   c. dilation of the retinal arterioles.
   d. increased production of aqueous humor by the ciliary process.
3. The nurse should specifically question patients using eyedrops to treat glaucoma about
   a. use of corrective lenses.
   b. their usual sleep pattern.
   c. a history of heart or lung disease.
   d. sensitivity to narcotics or depressants.
4. The nurse should always assess the patient with an ophthalmic problem for
   a. visual acuity.
   b. pupillary reactions.
   c. intraocular pressure.
   d. confrontation visual fields.
5. During assessment of the ear the nurse would expect to find
   a. bone conduction (BC) greater than air conduction (AC).
   b. absent cone of light.
   c. pearl-gray tympanic membrane.
   d. lateralization with Weber's test.
6. Arcus senilis is due to
   a. tissue atrophy.
   b. decreased pupil size.
   c. opacities in the lens.
   d. cholesterol deposits in the cornea.
7. Before injecting fluorescein for angiography, the nurse should
   a. determine whether the patient has a peripheral scotoma.
   b. ask if the patient is fatigued.
   c. obtain an emesis basin.
   d. administer topical anesthesia.

References

1. Talamo JH, Steinert RF: Keratorefractive surgery. In Albert DM, Jakobiec FA, editors: *Principles and practice of ophthalmology: clinical practice,* ed 2, vol 1, Philadelphia, 1999, Saunders.
2. Sahel JA, Brini A, Albert DM: Pathology of the retina and vitreous. In Albert DM, Jakobiec FA, editors: *Principles and practice of ophthalmology: clinical practice,* ed 2, vol 4, Philadelphia, 1999, Saunders.
3. Maus M: Basic eyelid anatomy. In Albert DM, Jakobiec FA, editors: *Principles and practice of ophthalmology: clinical practice,* ed 2, vol 3, Philadelphia, 1999, Saunders.
4. Berson EL: Hereditary retinal diseases: an overview. In Albert DM, Jakobiec FA, editors: *Principles and practice of ophthalmology: clinical practice,* ed 2, vol 2, Philadelphia, 1999, Saunders.
5. Newell FW: *Ophthalmology principles and concepts,* ed 8, St Louis, 1996, Mosby.

6. *Physicians' desk reference for ophthalmology,* ed 25, Montvale, NJ, 1997, Medical Economics Data Production Company.
7. Reichel E: Hereditary cone dysfunction syndromes. In Albert DM, Jakobiec FA, editors: *Principles and practice of ophthalmology: clinical practice,* ed 2, vol 2, Philadelphia, 1999, Saunders.
8. *Glaucoma panel quality of care committee: primary open-angle glaucoma suspect,* San Francisco, 1995, American Academy of Ophthalmology.
9. Okhravi N: *Manual of primary eye care,* Oxford, 1997, Butterworth-Heineman.
10. De La Paz MA, D'Amico DJ: Photic retinopathy. In Albert DM, Jakobiec FA, editors: *Principles and practice of ophthalmology: clinical practice,* ed 2, vol 2, Philadelphia, 1999, Saunders.
11. Bajart AM: Lid inflammations. In Albert DM, Jakobiec FA, editors: *Principles and practice of ophthalmology: clinical practice,* ed 2, vol 1, Philadelphia, 1999, Saunders.
12. Mead MD: Evaluation and initial management of patients with ocular and adnexal trauma. In Albert DM, Jakobiec FA, editors: *Principles and practice of ophthalmology: clinical practice,* ed 2, vol 5, Philadelphia, 1999, Saunders.
13. *Physicians' desk reference for ophthalmology,* ed 25, Montvale, NJ, 1997, Medical Economics Data Production Company.
14. Moore KL, Agur AMR: *Essential clinical anatomy,* Baltimore, 1996, Williams & Wilkins.
15. Van De Graaff K: *Human anatomy,* Dubuque, 1995, Wm C Brown.
16. Northern J: *Hearing disorders,* Boston, 1996, Allyn & Bacon.
17. Roland PS, Marple BFM : Disorders of inner ear, eighth nerve, and CNS. In Roland PS, Marple BF, Meryerhoff WL editors: *Hearing loss,* New York, 1997, Thieme.
18. Hughes G, Pensak M: *Clinical otology,* New York, 1997, Thieme.
19. Roeser RJ: *Roeser's audiology desk reference,* New York, 1996, Thieme.

Resources

Resources for this chapter are listed after Chapter 20 on p. 480.

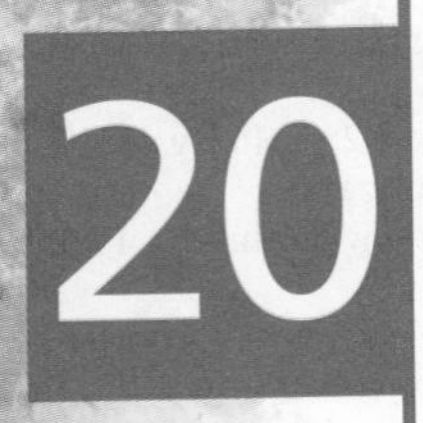

REMEMBER to check out your companion CD-ROM

20 NURSING MANAGEMENT Visual and Auditory Problems

Sarah C. Smith & Mary E. Wilbur

www.mosby.com/MERLIN/medsurg_lewis

LEARNING OBJECTIVES

1. Describe the types of refractive errors and appropriate corrections.
2. Describe the etiology and management of extraocular disorders.
3. Explain the pathophysiology, clinical manifestations, and nursing and collaborative management of the patient with selected intraocular disorders.
4. Describe the nursing measures that promote the health of the eyes and ears.
5. Explain the general preoperative and postoperative care of the patient undergoing surgery of the eye or ear.
6. Describe the action and uses of common pharmacologic agents used in treating problems of the eyes and ears.
7. Explain the pathophysiology, clinical manifestations, and nursing and collaborative management of common ear problems.
8. Compare the causes, management, and rehabilitative potential of conductive and sensorineural hearing loss.
9. Explain the use, care, and patient education related to assistive devices for eye and ear problems.
10. Describe the common causes and assistive measures for uncorrectable visual impairment and deafness.
11. Describe the measures used to assist the patient in adapting psychologically to decreased vision and hearing.

VISUAL PROBLEMS

Health Promotion

The nurse's role as a health educator with individuals, groups, and communities is extremely important in preventing health problems that have the potential for visual impairment. In addition to health education, the nurse can promote visual health by early recognition of conditions or situations that carry a high risk of visual impairment. The following is information about those adult conditions and situations amenable to nursing interventions.

1. Glaucoma is a significant cause of preventable visual impairment. Early recognition of glaucoma is extremely important in promoting visual health. The nurse can advocate and provide assistance for screening programs. In addition, the nurse should provide health information regarding the importance of regular ophthalmic examinations, especially to the patient at high risk for this disorder. The nurse can provide this information to an individual patient, groups of patients, or the general community.
2. Ocular trauma can lead to blindness or severe visual impairment. Many injuries can be prevented by identifying and correcting situations that may lead to eye injuries such as (1) failure to properly use eye protection during potentially hazardous work, hobby, or sports activities; (2) improper handling or storing of chemicals, especially strong alkalis or acids; (3) inappropriate response to ocular injuries, particularly failure to institute prompt, continuous ocular irrigation after exposure to a potentially toxic substance; and (4) failure to properly use seat belts or infant and child vehicle restraint devices. The nurse should take an active role in educating the patient about these potentially harmful situations.
3. As contact lens wear becomes increasingly common and contact lens companies continue to market directly to consumers, many people have become casual about wearing and caring for their lenses. Although contact lenses are generally safe and effective, they can be a significant potential source of ocular problems when the patient does not use or care for the lenses properly. The nurse should promote ocular health by teaching the patient correct wearing and cleaning techniques and recommending appropriate ophthalmic follow-up. Using incorrect solutions can be associated with severe ocular problems, and the nurse should stress using only approved contact lens solutions.
4. Women of childbearing age should be immunized against rubella, or German measles, to prevent congenital blindness in infants, which can result from rubella infection in the mother during the first trimester of pregnancy.[1] Persons who come in contact with this group of women, especially those who work in health care agencies, must be immunized as well.

Reviewed by Mary S. Merchant, RN, MSN, FNP, Continuum of Care Manager, Medical University of South Carolina, Charleston, SC.

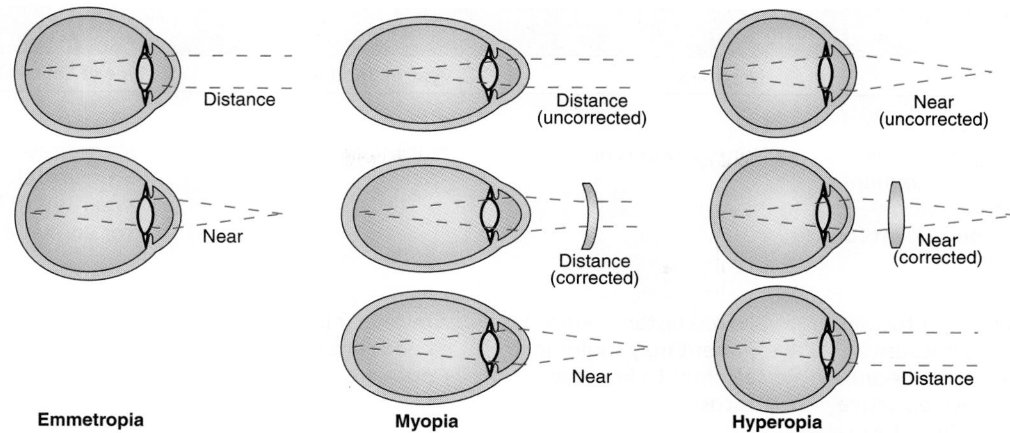

Fig. 20-1 Emmetropic, myopic, and hyperopic eyes with corrected and uncorrected vision.

5. Genetically transmitted syndromes and conditions often have ocular manifestations. The nurse working with the patient of childbearing age should be prepared to make referrals for genetic counseling when appropriate.

CORRECTABLE REFRACTIVE ERRORS

The most common visual problem is *refractive error*. This defect of the refracting media of the eye prevents light rays from converging into a single focus on the retina. Defects are a result of irregularities of the corneal curvature, the focusing power of the lens, or the length of the eye. The major symptom is blurred vision. In some cases the patient may also complain of ocular discomfort, eyestrain, or headaches. The patient with refractive errors uses corrective lenses to improve the focus of light rays on the retina (Fig. 20-1).

Myopia (nearsightedness) is the most common refractive error, with approximately 25% of Americans exhibiting this disorder. The prevalence of *hyperopia* (farsightedness) and *presbyopia* (farsightedness resulting from a decrease in the accommodative ability of the eye as a result of aging) is less common. However, approximately 80 million Americans wear some form of spectacle correction for refractive errors, approximately 25 million wear contact lenses, and several hundred thousand more have had keratorefractive surgery to correct refractive errors.[2] Table 20-1 summarizes the types of refractive errors and the appropriate corrections. Contrary to common belief, uncorrected refractive errors do not worsen the error, nor do they cause further pathology. However, refractive errors in young children should be corrected because children may develop *amblyopia* (reduced vision in the affected eye) if their refractive error is uncorrected.[2]

Myopia

Myopia (nearsightedness) causes light rays to be focused in front of the retina. Myopia may occur because of excessive light refraction by the cornea or lens or because of an abnormally long eye. Myopia may also occur because of lens swelling that occurs when blood glucose levels are elevated, as in uncontrolled diabetes. This type of myopia is transient and variable and fluctuates with the blood glucose level. During childhood, especially during adolescence when the child's growth rate increases, myopia may progress rapidly and require frequent changes in the patient's glasses. This excessive lengthening of the eye is often attributable to genetic factors.[3]

CULTURAL & ETHNIC CONSIDERATIONS

Hearing and Visual Problems

- Caucasians have a higher incidence of hearing impairment than African-Americans or Asian-Americans.
- Incidence and severity of glaucoma is increased among African-Americans when compared with Caucasians.
- Native Americans and African-Americans have a higher incidence of astigmatism than Caucasians.
- Native Americans have an increased incidence of otitis media when compared with Caucasians.
- Caucasians have a higher incidence of macular degeneration than Hispanic-Americans, African-Americans, or Asian-Americans.

Hyperopia

Hyperopia (farsightedness) causes the light rays to focus behind the retina and requires the patient to use accommodation to focus the light rays on the retina for near and far objects. This type of refractive error occurs when the cornea or lens do not have adequate focusing power or when the eyeball is too short.

Presbyopia

Presbyopia is the loss of accommodation because of age. As the eye ages, the crystalline lens becomes larger, firmer, and less elastic. These changes decrease the eye's accommodative ability. The accommodative ability continues to decline with each decade of life and, by approximately age 70 years, the accommodative power of the lens declines to zero.[4] When this occurs, the patient cannot focus on near objects without some form of visual aid.

Astigmatism

Astigmatism is caused by an unequal corneal curvature. This irregularity causes the incoming light rays to be bent unequally.

Table **20-1** Correction of Refractive Errors

Description	Symptoms	Type of Spectacles	Type of Contact Lenses*
Emmetropia			
Normal vision; light focuses on retina without accommodation for distance vision and with accommodation for near vision	None; vision is normal	Not indicated	Not indicated; some emmetropic patients wear tinted lenses for cosmetic reasons
Myopia			
Nearsightedness; light focuses in front of retina because eyeball is too long or because cornea or lens have excessive refractive power; light focuses on retina with accommodation for near vision	Blurred distance vision; patient may squint in an attempt to improve focus	Concave (minus); lens bends light rays outward	Rigid or soft; daily wear or extended wear
Hyperopia			
Farsightedness; light focuses behind retina because eyeball is too short or because cornea or lens have inadequate refractive power; light focuses on retina for distance vision	Blurred near vision; ocular fatigue from accommodative effort	Convex (plus); lens bends light rays inward	Rigid or soft; daily wear or extended wear
Astigmatism			
Light focuses at no clear point on the retina because corneal surface is irregularly curved; can occur with any of the above refractive errors	Blurred vision; ocular fatigue	Cylinder; lens bends light rays in different directions to align in a focused point	Rigid or soft toric; daily wear or extended wear
Presbyopia			
Light does not focus on retina for near vision because the aging crystalline lens can no longer accommodate	Blurred near vision; patient may attempt to obtain clear vision by holding objects further from the eyes	Convex for near vision; can be reading glasses or bifocals with reading correction in lower part of lens	Bifocal rigid or soft; monovision (one eye corrected for distance, one for near)
Aphakia			
Crystalline lens is absent because of congenital defect, trauma, or surgery (cataract extraction); eye loses approximately 30% of its refractive power	No near vision; if one eye is involved, the retinal image is one third larger than in the normal eye	Thick, convex; almost never used after cataract extraction today because of visual distortion, discomfort from heavy glasses, poor appearance, and superiority of IOL implant for aphakic correction	Rigid, soft; daily wear or extended wear; not used after cataract extraction in most cases today because of difficulty in handling lenses, complications related to wear, and superiority of IOL implant as aphakic correction

*See Table 20-2 for explanation of contact lens types.
IOL, intraocular lens.

Consequently, the light rays do not come to a single point of focus on the retina.

Aphakia

Aphakia is defined as the absence of the crystalline lens. The lens may be absent congenitally, or it may be removed during cataract surgery. A lens that is traumatically dislocated results in functional aphakia, although the lens remains in the eye. Because it accounts for approximately 30% of ocular refractive power, the absence of the lens results in a significant refractive error.[5] Without the focusing ability of the lens, images are projected behind the retina.

Nonsurgical Corrections

Glasses. Myopia, hyperopia, presbyopia, astigmatism, and aphakia can be modified by using the appropriate corrective lens (see Table 20-1). Myopia requires a minus corrective lens (concave), whereas hyperopia, presbyopia, and aphakia all require a plus corrective lens (convex). Glasses for presbyopia are often called reading glasses because they are usually worn for close work only. The presbyopic correction may also be combined with a correction for another refractive error, such as myopia or astigmatism. In these combined glasses the presbyopic correction is in the lower portion of bifocal or trifocal glasses. A newer type of correction for presbyopia, the "no-line" bifocal, is actually a multifocal lens that allows the patient to see clearly at any distance.

Aphakic glasses are very thick, making them heavy and unattractive to wear. The high degree of correction also causes images to be magnified about 25%. The glasses can provide good central vision but distort peripheral vision. This magnification and visual distortion is often unacceptable to the aphakic patient. With the modern surgical procedures prevalent today, patients seldom wear aphakic glasses for correction because of the associated visual problems. Astigmatism can occur in conjunction with any of the other refractive errors.

Contact Lenses. Contact lenses are another way to correct refractive errors. Contact lenses generally provide better vision than glasses because the patient has more normal peripheral vision without the distortion and obstruction of the glasses and their frames. Aphakic contact lenses magnify objects only approximately 7% and are visually superior to aphakic glasses.[6] However, many older patients have difficulty handling and caring for contact lenses. Table 20-2 describes the various types of contact lenses and the advantages and disadvantages of each.

Lenses may be either rigid or flexible (soft lenses). Rigid contact lenses ride on the tear film layer of the cornea and are held in place by surface tension. Blinking causes the tear film to move under and over the contact lens providing oxygen for the cornea. If the oxygen supply to the cornea is decreased, it becomes swollen, visual acuity decreases, and the patient experiences severe discomfort.

Because soft contact lenses do not ride on the corneal tear film layer, the cornea cannot receive oxygen from the tear film. Instead, the cornea receives oxygen through the soft contact lens, which is permeable to oxygen. Gas permeable rigid contact lenses also allow oxygen to reach the cornea through the lens itself.

Altered or decreased tear formation can make wearing contact lenses difficult. Tear production can be decreased by antihistamines, decongestants, diuretics, birth control pills, and the hormones produced during pregnancy. Allergic conjunctivitis with itching, tearing, and redness can also affect contact lens wear.

In general the nurse must know whether the patient wears contact lenses, the pattern of wear (daily versus extended), and care practices. The patient must remove daily wear lenses each night. The patient with extended wear lenses may generally wear the lenses as long as 1 week before removing them for cleaning, sterilizing, and an overnight period without lens wear. The nurse must be able to identify whether contact lenses are present and should know how to remove them in an emergency situation. Shining a light obliquely on the eyeball can help the nurse visualize a contact lens. If the patient can sit upright, the nurse can remove a rigid contact lens as follows: (1) wash hands with nonoily soap, rinse thoroughly, and dry with a lint-free towel; (2) stand at the patient's side (right side to remove right lens, left side to remove left lens); (3) place index finger of one hand near the lateral canthus; (4) hold the other hand beneath the patient's eye to catch the lens as it falls from the eye; (5) instruct the patient to blink; (6) as the patient blinks, use the index finger at the lateral canthus to gently pull the upper and lower lid tissue outward and slightly upward. The lens will fall into the nurse's hand and should be stored in a case filled with the appropriate solution and labeled with the patient's name. If the patient cannot sit upright or otherwise cooperate with the procedure, the nurse can remove a hard contact lens with a small suction cup designed for that purpose.

With the patient in any position, the nurse can remove a soft contact lens as follows: (1) wash hands with nonoily soap, rinse thoroughly, and dry with a lint-free towel; (2) stand at the patient's side (right side if the nurse is right-handed, left side if the nurse is left-handed); (3) place the middle finger of the dominant hand against the lower eyelid; (4) gently pull the lower eyelid down against the cheekbone; (5) with the thumb and index finger, slide the lens down off the cornea and onto the sclera; (6) bring the thumb and index finger together, gently pinching the lens off the eye. The nurse should store the lens in a case filled with normal saline solution and label the case with the patient's name.

The patient should know the signs and symptoms of contact lens problems that must be managed by the eye care professional. The patient may remember these symptoms better if the nurse uses the mnemonic device RSVP for *R*edness, *S*ensitivity, *V*ision problems, and *P*ain. The nurse must stress the importance of removing contact lenses *immediately* if any of these problems occur.

Surgical Therapy

Keratorefractive Surgery and Photorefractive Keratectomy. Keratorefractive surgery (surgery to alter the corneal curvature) is a new method of refractive correction. This surgical category includes a variety of procedures, including those in which the surgeon either makes cuts in the cornea or uses a laser and/or a special microsurgical knife to open and replace a flap of corneal tissue. Myopia is the refractive error most commonly corrected by refractive surgery. Currently it can be corrected by several methods.

Radial keratotomy (RK) is a technique in which the surgeon makes partial thickness, radial incisions in the patient's cornea, leaving an uncut optical zone in the center. The patient must evaluate the risk of serious complications, such as operative infection and corneal scarring, when considering this procedure.

Photorefractive keratectomy (PRK) is another procedure that uses an excimer laser to reshape the central corneal surface, primarily to correct myopia. There is evidence to suggest that final visual acuity is more predictable than with radial keratotomy, at least in the short term. *Laser-in-situ-keratomileusis (LASIK)* is a procedure where first a corneal flap is folded back, and then an excimer laser removes some of the internal layers of the cornea. Afterward, the flap is returned to normal position and allowed to heal in place. Early evidence supports claims that LASIK creates earlier visual stability in patients with a high degree of myopia than with PRK alone.[7] Unlike RK, both PRK and LASIK procedures affect the central zone of the cornea.

Intraocular Lens Implantation. The most common reason for aphakia is surgical removal of the lens during cataract extraction. In the past, the aphakic patient had to use either aphakic spectacles or, more recently, contact lenses for aphakic correction. However, the most common method of correction today is the surgical implantation of an *intraocular*

Table 20-2 Types of Contact Lenses

Type	Description	Advantages	Disadvantages	Wearing Schedule
Rigid Lenses				
■ Standard	Rigid plastic; smaller than cornea	Can be tinted for easier visibility out of the eye; longer lasting, least expensive to purchase; corrects all types of refractive errors	Requires separate care solutions for cleaning, storing, wetting; new patients (or those resuming wear after a period of nonwear) must gradually increase wearing time; initially uncomfortable, requires adaptation to obtain adequate comfort level	Daily wear; sleeping in lenses (either inadvertently or purposely) can cause corneal edema or severe pain from lack of oxygen to cornea
■ Gas permeable	Similar to standard rigid lenses, but plastic allows oxygen to pass through to cornea	Longer lasting than soft lenses; corrects all types of refractive errors; more comfortable initially than standard hard lenses; less adaptation time and fewer problems with corneal edema than standard hard lenses; flexible wearing schedule	Requires separate care solutions for cleaning, storing, wetting; more expensive to purchase than rigid standard contact lens	Daily wear
Soft Lenses				
■ Standard	Soft, flexible plastic; covers entire cornea and a small rim of sclera	Fits snugly on eye, allowing less invasion of foreign particles under the lens; initially more comfortable and less adaptation time than rigid lenses; can be worn intermittently	Less durable and more expensive than rigid lenses (cost may be similar to gas permeable rigid lenses); more susceptible to surface protein deposition that causes discomfort and vision problems; requires cleaning, sterilizing, and enzymatic removal of protein deposition, cannot correct for higher degrees of astigmatism	Daily wear only; sleeping in these lenses causes similar problems as sleeping in standard rigid lenses
■ High water content	Similar to standard soft lenses, but with a higher water content	Similar to standard soft lenses; allows more oxygen through lens so lens can be worn up to a week at a time without removal	Similar to standard soft lenses (with the exception that these can be extended wear); greater risk of complications related to contact lens wear than with standard soft lenses	Daily wear or extended wear
■ Toric	Similar to other standard soft lenses; special design to correct astigmatism	Similar to other soft lenses; can be custom ordered to correct patient's individual type of astigmatism	Similar to other soft lenses; more expensive than other types of lenses; can be more difficult to fit than nontoric soft lenses	Daily wear or extended wear
■ Disposable	Similar to other soft lenses but thinner	Similar to other soft lenses; frequent replacement decreases risk of complications related to contact lens wear	Similar to other soft lenses; cost may be greater (can be similar, depending on prevalent charges for replacement lenses)	Daily wear or extended wear; each lens can be worn as long as 2 weeks before disposal
■ Daily disposable	Similar to disposable	Similar to other soft lenses; daily disposal decreases risk of complications; good for patient who wear lenses only occasionally; no cleaning or disinfection necessary	Greater expense	Daily wear only; each lens is worn for 1 day and then discarded

Table 20-3 Definition of Legal Blindness in the United States

- Central visual acuity for distance of 20/200 or worse in the better eye (with correction)
- Visual field no greater than 20 degrees in its widest diameter or in the better eye

lens (IOL), usually at the time of the initial cataract extraction. The IOL is a small plastic lens that can be implanted either in the anterior or posterior chamber and provides very little optical distortion, especially compared with aphakic spectacles or even aphakic contact lenses. The type of IOL implanted depends on the cataract extraction technique and the surgeon's preference, but currently most IOLs are placed in the posterior chamber.

UNCORRECTABLE VISUAL IMPAIRMENT

The patient with correctable errors of vision is not functionally impaired. When no correction is possible, the patient's visual impairment may be moderate or profound. Approximately 4.8 million people in the United States have severe visual impairment, which is defined as the inability to read newsprint even with glasses. Of those individuals, only 9% have no useful vision, and the remaining 91% are considered partially sighted. The partially sighted individual may have significant visual abilities. It is important in working with the visually impaired patient to understand that a person classified as blind may have useful vision. Appropriate responses and interventions are dependent on the nurse's understanding of each patient's visual abilities.

Levels of Visual Impairment

The patient may be categorized by the level of visual loss.[8] *Total blindness* is defined as no light perception and no usable vision. *Functional blindness* is present when the patient has some light perception but no usable vision. The patient with either total or functional blindness is considered legally blind and may use vision substitutes such as guide dogs and canes for ambulation and Braille for reading. Vision enhancement techniques are not helpful.

The *legally blind* individual meets the criteria developed by the federal government to determine eligibility for federal and state assistance and income tax benefits (Table 20-3). The legally blind individual has some usable vision. The *partially sighted* individual who is not legally blind has a corrected visual acuity greater than 20/200 in the better eye and greater than 20 degrees of visual field, but the visual acuity is 20/50 or worse in the better eye. The patient who is partially sighted or legally blind can benefit greatly from vision enhancement techniques.

NURSING MANAGEMENT: SEVERE VISUAL IMPAIRMENT

■ Nursing Assessment

It is important to determine how long the patient has had a visual impairment because recent loss of vision has different implications for nursing care. The nurse should determine how the patient's visual impairment affects normal functioning. This may be done by questioning the patient about the level of difficulty encountered when doing certain tasks. For example, the nurse may ask how much difficulty the patient has when reading a newspaper, writing a check, moving from one room to the next, or viewing television. Other questions can help the nurse determine the personal meaning that the patient attaches to the visual impairment. The nurse can ask how the vision loss has affected specific aspects of the patient's life, whether the patient has lost a job, or what activities the patient does not engage in because of the visual impairment. The patient may attach many negative meanings to the impairment because of societal views of blindness. For example, the patient may view the impairment as punishment or view himself or herself as useless and burdensome. It is also important to determine the patient's primary coping strategies, emotional reactions, and the availability and strength of the patient's support systems.

■ Nursing Diagnoses

Nursing diagnoses depend on the degree of visual impairment and how long it has been present. Nursing diagnoses for the visually impaired patient include, but are not limited to, the following:

- Sensory-perceptual alterations *related to* visual deficit
- Risk for injury *related to* visual impairment and inability to see potential dangers
- Self-care deficits *related to* visual impairment
- Fear *related to* inability to see potential danger or accurately interpret environment
- Anticipatory grieving *related to* loss of functional vision
- Self-esteem disturbance *related to* loss of visual function and self-sufficiency
- Impaired social interaction *related to* visual deficits
- Diversional activity deficit *related to* inability to perform usual activities
- Social isolation *related to* increased difficulty in sustaining previous relationships

■ Planning

The overall goals are that the patient with recently impaired vision, or the patient with impaired adjustment to long-standing visual impairment, will (1) make a successful adjustment to the impairment, (2) verbalize feelings related to the loss, (3) identify personal strengths and external support systems, and (4) use appropriate coping strategies. If the patient has been functioning at an appropriate or acceptable level, the goal of the patient is to maintain the current level of function.

■ Nursing Implementation

Health Promotion. The nurse should encourage the partially sighted patient with preventable causes for further visual impairment to seek appropriate health care. For example, the patient with vision loss from glaucoma may prevent further visual impairment by complying with prescribed therapies and suggested ophthalmic evaluations. Other health promotion strategies were presented on p. 442 earlier in this chapter.

Acute Intervention. The nurse provides emotional support and direct care to the patient with recent visual

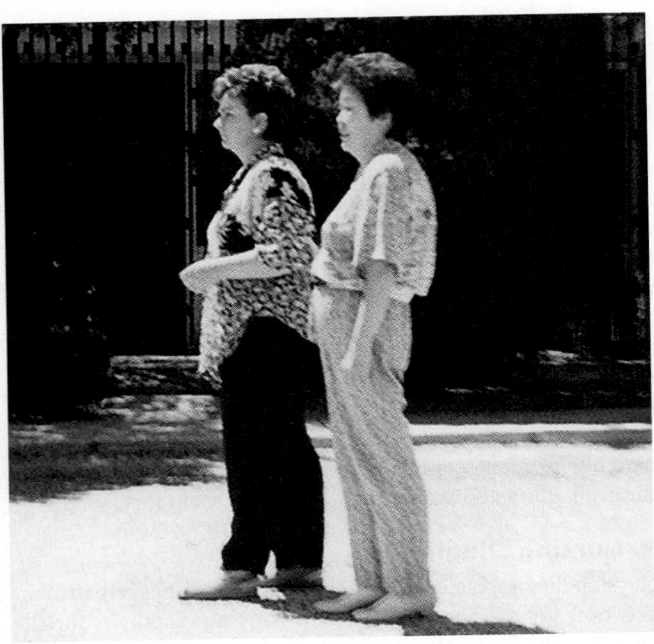

Fig. 20-2 Sighted-guide technique. The nurse serves as the sighted guide, walking slightly ahead of the patient with the patient holding the back of the nurse's arm.

impairment. Active listening and grief work facilitation are important components of nursing care for the recently visually impaired patient. The nurse should allow the patient to express anger and grief and should help the patient to identify fears and successful coping strategies. The family is intimately involved in the experiences that follow visual loss. With the patient's knowledge and permission, the nurse should include family members in discussions and encourage members to express their concerns.

Many people are uncomfortable around a blind or partially sighted individual because they are not sure what behaviors are appropriate. The nurse is responsible for knowing what is appropriate so that the patient does not become uncomfortable in the nurse's presence. Sensitivity to the patient's feelings without being overly solicitous or stifling the patient's independence is vital in creating a therapeutic nursing presence. The nurse should always communicate in a normal conversational tone and manner with the patient, and the nurse should address the patient, not a family member or friend that may be with the patient. Common courtesy dictates introducing oneself and any other persons who approach the blind or partially sighted patient and saying good-bye on leaving. Making eye contact with the partially sighted patient accomplishes several objectives. It ensures that the nurse speaks while facing the patient so the patient has no difficulty hearing the nurse. The nurse's head position validates that the nurse is attentive to the patient. Also, establishing eye contact ensures that the nurse will perceive the patient's facial or movement cues about reactions and responses.

The nurse should explain any activities or noises occurring in the patient's immediate surroundings. Orientation to the environment lessens the patient's anxiety or discomfort and facilitates independence. In orienting the partially sighted or blind patient to a new area, the nurse should identify one object as the focal point and describe the location of other objects in relation to it. For example the nurse may say, "The bed is straight ahead, approximately 10 steps. The chair is to the left, and the nightstand is to the right, near the head of the bed. The bathroom is to the left of the foot of the bed."

The nurse should assist the patient to each major object in the area, using the sighted-guide technique. When using this technique, the nurse stands slightly in front and to one side of the patient and offers an elbow for the patient to hold. The nurse serves as the sighted guide, walking slightly ahead of the patient with the patient holding the back of the nurse's arm (Fig. 20-2). When using this technique in any situation, the nurse should describe the environment to help orient the patient. For example the nurse may say, "We're going through an open doorway and approaching two steps down. There's an obstacle on the left." To assist the patient to sit, place one of his or her hands on the back of the chair.

When the partially sighted or blind patient places an object in a certain position, it should not be moved without the knowledge and consent of the patient. Objects on a table or food tray can be described in terms of the hours on a clock face. For example, the nurse may say, "Your book is at the 12 o'clock position, and your magnifier is at the 3 o'clock position," or "The eggs are at the 9 o'clock position, bacon at the 3 o'clock position, and toast at the 12 o'clock position." If the nurse is uncertain about providing help, it is perfectly appropriate to ask the patient if assistance is needed and, if so, how to provide it.

Ambulatory and Home Care. Rehabilitation after partial or total loss of vision can foster independence, self-esteem, and productivity. The nurse should know what services and devices are available for the partially sighted or blind patient and be prepared to make appropriate referrals for those services and devices. For the legally blind patient, the primary resource for services is the state agency for rehabilitation of the blind.[9] A list of agencies that serves the partially sighted or blind patient is available from the American Foundation for the Blind, 11 Penn Plaza, Suite 300, New York, NY 10001 (212-502-7600). Many of these agencies are listed in the resources section at the end of chapter.

Braille or audio books for reading and a cane or guide dog for ambulation are examples of vision substitution techniques. These are usually most appropriate for the patient with no functional vision. For most patients who have some remaining vision, vision enhancement techniques can provide enough help for many patients to learn to ambulate, read printed material, and accomplish activities of daily living (ADLs).

Optical devices for vision enhancement. Telescopic lenses for near or far vision and magnifiers of various types can often enhance the patient's remaining vision enough to allow the performance of many previously impossible tasks and activities. Most of these devices require some training and practice for successful use. Closed circuit television can provide magnification up to 60 times, allowing some patients to read, write, use computers, and do crafts. Although these systems are expensive and have limited portability, they are available in some public or university libraries.

Nonoptical methods for vision enhancement. *Approach magnification* is a simple but sometimes overlooked technique for enhancing the patient's residual vision. The nurse can recommend that the patient sit closer to the television or hold books closer to the eyes, which the patient may be reluctant to do unless encouraged. *Contrast enhancement* techniques include watching television in black and white, placing dark objects against a light background (e.g., a white plate on a black place mat), using a black felt-tip marker, and using contrasting colors (e.g., a red stripe at the edge of steps or curbs). Increased lighting can be provided by halogen lamps, direct sunlight, or gooseneck lamps that can be aimed directly at the reading material or other near objects. Large type is often helpful, especially in conjunction with other optical or nonoptical vision enhancements.

■ Evaluation

The overall expected outcomes are that the patient with severe visual impairment

- has no further progressive loss of vision
- is able to express adaptive coping strategies
- does not experience a decrease in self-esteem or social interactions
- functions safely within her or his own environment

GERONTOLOGIC CONSIDERATIONS

The elderly patient is at an increased risk for vision loss because cataracts, glaucoma, diabetic retinopathy, macular degeneration, and other potential causes of visual impairment are more common in the older patient. The older patient may have other deficits such as cognitive impairment or limited mobility, which further impact the ability to function in usual ways. Societal devaluation of the elderly may compound the self-esteem or isolation issues associated with the older patient's visual impairment. Financial resources may meet normal needs but can be inadequate in meeting increased demands of vision services or devices.

EYE TRAUMA

Although the eyes are well protected by the bony orbit and by fat pads, everyday activities can result in ocular trauma. Ocular injuries can involve the ocular adnexa, the superficial structures, or the deeper ocular structures. In the United States an estimated 1.3 million eye injuries occur each year. Of these injuries, 40,000 result in permanent visual impairment.[4] Table 20-4 outlines emergency management of the patient with an eye injury. Types of ocular trauma include blunt injuries, penetrating injuries, or chemical exposure injuries. Causes of ocular injuries include automobile accidents, accidental occurrences such as falls, sports and leisure activity injuries, assaults, or work-related situations.

Trauma is often a preventable cause of visual impairment. The nurse's role in individual and community education is extremely important in reducing the incidence of ocular trauma.

EXTRAOCULAR DISORDERS

INFLAMMATION AND INFECTION

One of the most common conditions encountered by the ophthalmologist is inflammation or infection of the external eye. Many external irritants or microorganisms affect the lids and conjunctiva and can involve the avascular cornea. It is a nursing responsibility to teach the patient appropriate interventions related to the specific disorder.

Hordeolum

A hordeolum (commonly called a sty) is an infection of the sebaceous glands in the lid margin. The most common bacterial infective agent is *Staphylococcus aureus.*[10] A red, swollen, circumscribed, and acutely tender area develops rapidly. The nurse should instruct the patient to apply warm, moist compresses at least four times a day until the abscess drains. This may be the only treatment necessary. If there is a tendency for recurrence, the patient should perform lid scrubs daily. In addition, appropriate antibiotic ointments or drops may be indicated.

Chalazion

A chalazion is an inflammation of a sebaceous gland in the lids. It may evolve from a hordeolum or may occur as a primary inflammatory response to the material released into the lid tissue when a blocked gland ruptures. The chalazion appears as a swollen, nonpainful, reddened area, usually on the upper lid. Initial treatment is similar to that for a hordeolum. If warm, moist compresses are ineffective in causing spontaneous drainage, the ophthalmologist may surgically remove the chronic lesion (this is normally an office procedure), or the ophthalmologist may inject the chronic lesion with corticosteroids.

Blepharitis

Blepharitis is a common chronic bilateral inflammation of the lid margins. The lids are red rimmed with many scales or crusts on the lid margins and lashes. The patient may primarily complain of itching but may also experience burning, irritation, and photophobia. Conjunctivitis may occur simultaneously.

If the blepharitis is caused by a staphylococcal infection, collaborative care includes the use of an appropriate ophthalmic antibiotic ointment. Seborrheic blepharitis, related to seborrhea of the scalp and eyebrows, is treated with an antiseborrheic shampoo for the scalp and eyebrows. Often blepharitis is caused by both staphylococcal and seborrheal microorganisms, and the treatment must be more vigorous to avoid hordeolum, keratitis (inflammation of the cornea), and other eye infections. Conscientious hygienic practices involving skin and scalp must be emphasized. Gentle cleansing of the lid margins with baby shampoo can effectively soften and remove crusting.

Conjunctivitis

Conjunctivitis is an infection or inflammation of the conjunctiva. Conjunctival infections may be caused by bacterial, viral, or chlamydial microorganisms. Conjunctival inflammation may result from exposure to allergens or chemical irritants (including cigarette smoke). The tarsal conjunctiva (lining the interior surface of the lids) may become inflamed as a result of a chronic foreign body in the eye, such as a contact lens or an ocular prosthesis.

Bacterial Infections. Acute bacterial conjunctivitis (pinkeye) is a common infection. Although it occurs in every age group, epidemics commonly occur in children because of their poor hygienic habits. In adults and children the most

✚EMERGENCY MANAGEMENT

Table 20-4 Eye Injury

Etiology	Assessment Findings	Intervention
Blunt Injury Fist Other blunt objects **Penetrating Injury** Fragments such as glass, metal, wood Knife, stick, or other large object **Chemical Injury** Alkaline Acid **Thermal Injury** Direct burn from curling iron or other hot surface Indirect burn from UV light (e.g., welding torch, sun lamp) **Foreign Bodies** Glass Metal Wood **Trauma** Blunt Penetrating **Burns** Chemical Thermal	▪ Pain ▪ Photophobia ▪ Redness—diffuse or localized ▪ Swelling ▪ Ecchymosis ▪ Tearing ▪ Blood in the anterior chamber ▪ Absent eye movements ▪ Fluid drainage from eye (e.g., blood, CSF, aqueous humor) ▪ Abnormal or decreased vision ▪ Visible foreign body ▪ Prolapsed globe ▪ Abnormal intraocular pressure	**Initial** ▪ Determine mechanism of injury. ▪ Ensure airway, breathing, circulation. ▪ Assess for other injuries. ▪ Assess visual acuity after irrigation for chemical exposure. ▪ Begin ocular irrigation *immediately* for chemical exposure. Use sterile saline or water if saline is unavailable. ▪ Do not put pressure on the eye. ▪ Begin ocular irrigation *immediately* in case of chemical exposure; do not stop until emergency personnel arrive to continue irrigation; sterile, pH-balanced, physiologic solution is best; if unavailable, use any nontoxic liquid. ▪ Do not attempt to treat the injury (except as noted above for chemical exposure). ▪ Stabilize foreign objects. ▪ Cover the eye(s) with dry, sterile patches and a protective shield. ▪ Do not give the patient food or fluids. ▪ Elevate head of bed 45 degrees. ▪ Do not put medication or solutions in the eye unless ordered by physician. ▪ Administer analgesia as appropriate. **Ongoing Monitoring** ▪ Reassure the patient. ▪ Monitor pain. ▪ Anticipate surgical repair for penetrating injury, globe rupture, or globe avulsion.

CSF, cerebrospinal fluid; *UV,* ultraviolet.

common causative microorganism is *S. aureus. Streptococcus pneumoniae* and *Haemophilus influenzae* are other common causative agents, but they are seen more often in children than adults. The patient with bacterial conjunctivitis may complain of irritation, tearing, redness, and a mucopurulent drainage. Although this typically occurs initially in one eye, it spreads rapidly to the unaffected eye. It is usually self-limiting, but treatment with antibiotic drops shortens the course of the disorder. Careful hand washing and using individual or disposable towels helps prevent spreading the condition.

Viral Infections. Conjunctival infections may be caused by many different viruses. The patient with *viral conjunctivitis* may complain of tearing, foreign body sensation, redness, and mild photophobia. Unless other ocular structures become involved, this condition is usually mild and self-limiting. However, it can be severe, with increased discomfort, subconjunctival hemorrhaging, or formation of *symblepharon* (adhesions between the bulbar and palpebral conjunctiva). Adenovirus conjunctivitis may be contracted in contaminated swimming pools and through direct contact with an infected patient.[11] Good hygiene practices decrease spread of the virus. Treatment is usually palliative. If the patient is severely symptomatic, topical corticosteroids provide temporary relief but have no benefit in the final outcome. Antiviral drops are ineffective and therefore not indicated.

Chlamydial Infections. Adult inclusion conjunctivitis (AIC) is caused by the oculogenital type of *Chlamydia trachomatis.* It is becoming more prevalent in the United States because of the increase in sexually transmitted chlamydial disease. The patient complains of a mucopurulent ocular discharge, irritation, redness, and lid swelling. Systemic symptoms may be present as well. For unknown reasons, this type of chlamydial infection does not carry the long-term consequences of *trachoma* (a sight-threatening keratoconjunctivitis caused by a different type of the *C. trachomatis* bacteria). It also differs from trachoma in that it is common in economically developed countries, whereas trachoma is rarely seen except in underdeveloped countries. The more benign nature of AIC may be related to lack of reexposure to the microorganism, the age of the patient at initial exposure, or a lower degree of pathogenicity of the oculogenital organism.[13]

Although topical treatment may be successful in the adult with chlamydial conjunctivitis, these patients have a high risk of concurrent chlamydial genital infection, as well as other sexually transmitted diseases. Consequently, all patients should be referred for further evaluation and systemic antibiotic therapy. The nurse's responsibility with the patient with chlamydial conjunctivitis includes education about the ocular condition, as well as the sexual implications of the condition.

Allergic Conjunctivitis. Conjunctivitis caused by exposure to some allergen can be mild and transitory, or it can be severe enough to cause significant swelling, sometimes ballooning the conjunctiva beyond the eyelids. The defining symptom of allergic conjunctivitis is itching. The patient may also complain of burning, redness, and tearing. Acutely, the patient may also have white or clear exudate. If the condition is chronic, the exudate is thicker and becomes mucopurulent. In addition to pollens, the patient may develop allergic conjunctivitis in response to animal dander, ocular solutions and medications, or even contact lenses. The nurse should instruct the patient to avoid the allergen if it is known. Artificial tears can be effective in diluting the allergen and washing it from the eye. Effective topical medications include antihistamines and corticosteroids.

Keratitis

Keratitis is an inflammation or infection of the cornea that can be caused by a variety of microorganisms or by other factors. The condition may involve the conjunctiva and the cornea. When it involves both, the disorder is *keratoconjunctivitis.*

Bacterial Infections. The intact cornea provides an effective defense against infection. However, when the epithelial layer is disrupted, the cornea can become infected by a variety of bacteria. The infected cornea can develop an ulcer with a mucopurulent exudate adherent to the ulcer. Topical antibiotics are generally effective, but eradicating the infection may require subconjunctival antibiotic injection or, in severe cases, intravenous (IV) antibiotics. Risk factors include mechanical or chemical corneal epithelial damage, soft contact lens wear (particularly with extended wear), debilitation, nutritional deficiencies, immunosuppressed states, and contaminated products (e.g., lens care solutions and cases, topical medications, cosmetics).[14]

Viral Infections. Herpes simplex virus (HSV) keratitis is the most frequently occurring infectious cause of corneal blindness in the Western hemisphere.[11] It is a growing problem, especially with immunosuppressed patients. It may be caused by HSV-1 or HSV-2 (genital herpes), although HSV-2 ocular infection is much less common. The resulting corneal ulcer has a characteristic dendritic (tree-branching) appearance, and it is often, although not always, preceded by infection of the conjunctiva or eyelids. Pain and photophobia are common. Up to 40% of patients with herpetic keratitis heal spontaneously. The spontaneous healing rate increases to 70% if the cornea is debrided to remove infected cells. Therapeutic management includes corneal debridement followed by topical therapy with idoxuridine drops or ointment (Stoxil, Herplex, IDU) for 2 to 3 weeks. Corticosteroids are contraindicated because they contribute to a longer course, possible deeper ulceration of the cornea, and systemic complications. If the ulcer is not responsive to idoxuridine within 1 to 2 weeks, vidarabine (Vira-A) or trifluridine (Viroptic) may be used topically. Pharmacologic therapy may also include acyclovir (Zovirax). Recurrent dendritic keratitis may be a problem.

The varicella-zoster virus (VZV) causes both chickenpox and *herpes zoster ophthalmicus (HZO)*. HZO may occur by reactivation of an endogenous infection that has persisted in latent form after an earlier attack of varicella or by direct or indirect contact with a patient with chickenpox or herpes zoster. It occurs most frequently in the older adult and in the immunosuppressed patient. Collaborative care of acute HZO may include narcotic or nonnarcotic analgesics for the pain, topical corticosteroids to reduce the inflammatory process, antiviral agents such as acyclovir (Zovirax) to reduce viral replication, mydriatic agents to dilate the pupil and relieve pain, and topical antibiotics to combat secondary infection. The patient may apply warm compresses and povidone-iodine gel to the affected skin (gel should not be applied near the eye).

Epidemic keratoconjunctivitis (EKC) is the most serious ocular adenoviral disease. EKC is spread by direct contact, including sexual activity. In the medical setting, contaminated hands and instruments can be the source of spread. The patient may complain of tearing, redness, photophobia, and foreign body sensation. In most patients, the disease involves only one eye. Treatment is primarily palliative and includes ice packs and dark glasses. In severe cases, therapy can include mild topical corticosteroids to temporarily relieve symptoms and topical antibiotic ointment to lubricate the cornea when membranes are present.[11] The nurse's most important role is to educate the patient and family members regarding good hygienic practices to avoid spreading the disease.

Chlamydial Infections. Trachoma is a severe keratoconjunctivitis caused by a variety of the *Chlamydia trachomatis* organism. It is the most common ocular disease in the world, affecting 500 million persons and often leading to blindness from corneal scarring.[12] Trachoma is especially prevalent in the Middle East, Africa, India, Southeast Asia, and South America, but also affects isolated groups in the Southwestern United States. Transmission of the disease is through contact with contaminated hands, bedding, linens, and eye-seeking flies. Treatment with topical and systemic antibiotics is effective but difficult to provide in the developing countries most afflicted with the disease. It is a preventable cause of blindness, requiring better sanitation and health delivery systems, as well as improved education.

Other Causes of Keratitis. Keratitis may also be caused by fungi (most commonly by the *Aspergillus, Candida,* and *Fusarium* species), especially in the case of ocular trauma in an outdoor setting where fungi are prevalent in the soil and moist organic matter. *Acanthamoeba* keratitis is caused by a parasite that is associated with contact lens wear, probably as a result of contaminated lens care solutions or cases. Homemade saline solution is particularly vulnerable to *Acanthamoeba* contamination. The nurse should instruct the patient who wears contact lenses about good lens care practices. Medical treatment of fungal and *Acanthamoeba* keratitis is difficult. Only one antifungal eye drop (natamycin) is approved by the Food and Drug Administration (FDA), and the *Acanthamoeba* organism is resistant to most drugs. If antimicrobial therapy fails, the patient may require a corneal transplant.

Exposure keratitis occurs when the patient cannot adequately close the eyelids. The patient with *exophthalmos* (protruding eyeball) from thyroid eye disease or masses posterior to the globe is susceptible to exposure keratitis.

NURSING MANAGEMENT: INFLAMMATION AND INFECTION OF THE EYES

■ Nursing Assessment

The nurse should assess ocular changes such as edema, redness, decreasing visual acuity, or discomfort, and document the findings in the patient's record. The nurse's assessment should also consider the psychosocial aspects of the patient's condition, especially when the patient has visual impairment associated with the condition.

Nursing Diagnoses

Nursing diagnoses for the patient with inflammation or infection of the external eye include, but are not limited to, the following:

- Pain *related to* irritation or infection of the external eye
- Anxiety *related to* uncertainty of cause of disease and outcome of treatment
- Sensory-perceptual alteration: visual *related to* diminished or absent vision

Planning

The overall goals are that the patient with inflammation or infection of the external eye will (1) maintain or improve visual acuity, (2) maintain an acceptable level of comfort and functioning during the course of the specific ocular problem, (3) avoid spread of infection, (4) promote appropriate health-seeking behaviors, and (5) comply with the prescribed therapy.

Nursing Implementation

Health Promotion. Careful asepsis and frequent, thorough hand washing are essential to prevent spreading organisms from one eye to the other, to other patients, to family members, and to the nurse. The nurse should dispose of any contaminated dressings in a proper waste container. The patient and family need information about avoiding sources of ocular irritation or infection and responding appropriately if an ocular problem occurs. The patient with infective disorders that may have a sexual mode of transmission or an associated sexually transmitted disease (STD) needs specific information about those disorders. The patient with contact lenses often does not comply with care regimens. The patient needs information about appropriate use and care of lenses and lens care products. The nurse should encourage the patient to follow the recommended regimens.

Acute Intervention. The nurse may apply warm or cool compresses if indicated for the patient's condition. Darkening the room and providing an appropriate analgesic are other comfort measures. If the patient's visual acuity is decreased, the nurse may need to modify the patient's environment or activities for safety.

The patient may require eye drops as frequently as every hour. If the patient receives two or more different drops, the nurse should stagger the eye drops to promote maximum absorption. For example, if two different eye drops are ordered hourly, the nurse should administer one drop on the hour and one drop on the half hour. This staggered schedule promotes maximum absorption.

The patient who needs frequent eye drop administration may experience sleep deprivation. Common symptoms include short attention span, irritability, confusion, and disorientation. Grouping necessary activities together and allowing periods of rest, in addition to providing a quiet environment, may be beneficial. The sleep-deprived patient may recognize abnormal behavior and be concerned or embarrassed. The nurse should reassure the patient that this behavior change is a normal consequence of lack of sleep.

Ambulatory and Home Care. The patient's primary need in the home environment is for information about required care and how to accomplish that care. The nurse should provide the patient and family with information about proper hygiene techniques to prevent contamination or limit the spread of inflammatory and infectious disorders. The patient and family also need information about proper techniques for medication administration. If the patient's vision is compromised, the nurse should provide suggestions for alternative ways to accomplish necessary daily activities and self-care. The patient who wears contact lenses and develops infections should discard all opened or used lens care products and cosmetics to decrease the risk of reinfection from contaminated products (a common problem and a probable source of infection for many patients).

Evaluation

The overall expected outcomes are that the patient with inflammation or infection of the external eye will

- cooperate with the treatment plan
- experience relief of ocular discomfort
- effectively cope with functional changes if decreased visual acuity is present
- obtain specific information to prevent recurrent disease

GERONTOLOGIC CONSIDERATIONS

The older patient may become confused or disoriented when visually compromised. The combination of decreased vision and confusion increases the risk of falls, which have potentially serious consequences for the older adult. Decreased vision may compromise the older patient's ability to function, causing concerns about maintaining independence and causing a decreased self-image. Decreased manual dexterity may make the instillation of prescribed eye drops difficult for some older adults.

DRY EYE DISORDERS

Complaints of dry eye are caused by a variety of ocular disorders characterized by decreased tear secretion or increased tear film evaporation. *Keratoconjunctivitis sicca* is caused by lacrimal gland dysfunction from an autoimmune mechanism. If the patient with keratoconjunctivitis sicca has associated dry mouth, the patient has primary Sjögren's syndrome. If the patient has associated rheumatoid arthritis, scleroderma, or systemic lupus erythematosus, the patient has secondary Sjögren's syndrome. The patient complains of a sandy or gritty sensation that typically worsens during the day and is better in the morning after eye closure with sleep. Treatment is directed at the underlying cause. With meibomian gland dysfunction, hot compresses and lid margin massage help express lipid into the tear film. With decreased tear secretion, the patient may use artificial tears or ointments but should avoid preserved products and use them sparingly because preservatives in the drops or overuse can cause further ocular irritation. In severe cases the ophthalmologist may temporarily or permanently surgically occlude the puncta, effectively providing the ocular surface with more available tears.

STRABISMUS

Strabismus is a condition in which the patient cannot consistently focus two eyes simultaneously on the same object. One eye may deviate in (*esotropia*), out (*exotropia*), up (*hypertropia*), or down (*hypotropia*). Strabismus in the adult may be caused by thyroid disease, neuromuscular problems of the eye muscles, entrapment of the extraocular muscles in orbital floor fractures, retinal detachment repair, or cerebral lesions. In the adult, the primary complaint with strabismus is double vision.

CORNEAL DISORDERS

Corneal Scars and Opacities

The cornea is an optically transparent tissue that allows light rays to enter the eye and focus on the retina, thus producing a visual image. Any corneal wound causes the stroma to become abnormally hydrated and decreases the normal transparency. A rigid contact lens can be effective in correcting the irregular astigmatism that results from corneal scars. In other situations the treatment for corneal scars or opacities is *penetrating keratoplasty* (corneal transplant). In penetrating keratoplasty the ophthalmic surgeon removes the full thickness of the patient's cornea and replaces it with a donor cornea or "button" that is sutured into place.[15] Although corneal problems leading to blindness are uncommon, a corneal transplant can restore vision that otherwise would be lost. Approximately 40,000 transplants are performed in the United States each year.

The time between the donor's death and the removal of the tissue should be as short as possible. Most surgeons prefer this interval to be 8 hours or less, but some eye banks provide donor eyes that have remained in the donor for as long as 18 hours.[16] The eye banks test donors for human immunodeficiency virus (HIV) and hepatitis B and C. The tissue is preserved in a special nutritive solution, and it can be kept for a week or longer in the storage media. Improved methods of tissue procurement and preservation, refined surgical techniques, postoperative topical corticosteroids, and careful follow-up have decreased graft rejection. The nurse plays an important role in promoting tissue donation through education of the individual, family, and the community, as well as by functioning in defined tissue procurement procedures.

Keratoconus

Keratoconus is a bilateral degenerative disease that is familial but has no exclusive inheritance pattern. It can be associated with Down syndrome, atopic dermatitis, Marfan syndrome, aniridia (congenital absence of the iris), and retinitis pigmentosa (hereditary disease characterized by bilateral primary degeneration of the retina beginning in childhood and progressing to blindness by middle age).

The anterior cornea thins and protrudes forward, taking on a cone shape. Keratoconus appears during adolescence and slowly progresses between the ages of 20 and 60 years. The only symptom is blurred vision caused by the variable astigmatism associated with the altered corneal shape. The astigmatism may be corrected with glasses or rigid contact lenses. The cornea can perforate as central corneal thinning progresses. Penetrating keratoplasty is indicated before perforation in advanced cases.

INTRAOCULAR DISORDERS

CATARACT

A *cataract* is an opacity within the crystalline lens. The patient may have a cataract in one or both eyes. If present in both eyes, one cataract may affect the patient's vision more than the other. Cataracts are the third leading cause of preventable blindness and the most common cause of self-declared visual disability in the United States. Approximately 50% of Americans between the ages of 65 and 74 years have some degree of cataract formation, and for those older than 75 years, the incidence increases to approximately 70%. Cataract removal is the most common surgical procedure for Americans older than 65 years. Congenital cataracts are relatively common, occurring in 1 of every 250 newborns (0.4%).[17]

Etiology and Pathophysiology

Although most cataracts are age-related (*senile cataracts*), they can be associated with other factors. These include blunt or penetrating trauma, congenital factors such as maternal rubella, radiation or ultraviolet (UV) light exposure, certain drugs such as systemic corticosteroids or long-term topical corticosteroids, and ocular inflammation. The patient with diabetes mellitus tends to develop cataracts at a younger age than does the patient without diabetes.

Cataract development is mediated by a number of factors. In senile cataract formation, it appears that altered metabolic processes within the lens cause an accumulation of water and alterations in the lens fiber structure. These changes affect lens transparency, causing vision changes.

Clinical Manifestations

The patient with cataracts may complain of a decrease in vision, abnormal color perception, and glare. Glare is due to light scatter caused by the lens opacities, and it may be significantly worse at night when the pupil dilates. The visual decline is gradual, but the rate of cataract development varies from patient to patient. Some patients may complain of a sudden loss of vision because they inadvertently cover their unaffected eye, and the decreased acuity of the eye with cataracts becomes "suddenly" apparent. Secondary glaucoma can also occur if the enlarging lens causes increased intraocular pressure (IOP).

Diagnostic Studies

Diagnosis is based on decreased visual acuity or other complaints of visual dysfunction. The opacity is directly observable by ophthalmoscopic or slit lamp microscopic examination. As noted earlier, a totally opaque lens creates the appearance of a white pupil. Table 20-5 outlines other diagnostic studies that may be helpful in evaluating the visual impact of a cataract.

Collaborative Care

The presence of a cataract does not necessarily indicate a need for surgery. For many patients the diagnosis is made long before they actually decide to have surgery. Nonsurgical therapy may postpone the need for surgery. Collaborative care for cataracts is presented in Table 20-5.

Nonsurgical Therapy. Currently, there is no available treatment to "cure" cataracts other than surgical removal. If the cataract is not removed, the patient's vision will continue

COLLABORATIVE CARE

Table 20-5 Cataract

Diagnostic
- Visual acuity measurement
- Ophthalmoscopy (direct and indirect)
- Slit lamp microscopy
- Glare testing, potential acuity testing in selected patients
- Keratometry and A-scan ultrasound (if surgery is planned)
- Other tests (e.g., visual field perimetry) may be indicated to differentiate visual loss of cataract from visual loss of other causes

Collaborative Therapy

Nonsurgical
- Change prescription of glasses
- Strong reading glasses or magnifiers
- Increased lighting
- Lifestyle adjustment
- Reassurance

Acute Care: Surgical Therapy

Preoperative
- Mydriatic, cycloplegic agents
- Nonsteroidal antiinflammatory drugs
- Topical antibiotics
- Antianxiety medications

Surgery
- Removal of lens
  - Phacoemulsification
  - Extracapsular extraction
- Correction of surgical aphakia
- Intraocular lens implantation (most frequent type of correction)
- Contact lens

Postoperative
- Topical antibiotic
- Topical corticosteroid or other antiinflammatory agent
- Mild analgesia if necessary
- Eye shield and activity as preferred by patient's surgeon

to deteriorate. However, palliative measures alone may help the patient. Often, changing the patient's glasses prescription can improve the level of visual acuity, at least temporarily. Other visual aids, such as strong reading glasses or magnifiers of some type, may help the patient with close vision. Increasing the amount of light to read or accomplish other near vision tasks is another useful measure. The patient may be willing to adjust lifestyle to accommodate for visual decline. For example, if glare makes it difficult to drive at night, a patient may elect to drive only during daylight hours or to have a family member drive at night. Sometimes informing and reassuring the patient about the disease process makes the patient comfortable about choosing nonsurgical measures, at least temporarily.

Surgical Therapy. When palliative measures no longer provide an acceptable level of visual function, the patient is an appropriate candidate for surgery. The patient's occupational needs and lifestyle changes are also factors affecting the decision to have surgery. In some instances, factors other than the patient's visual needs may influence the need for surgery. Lens-induced problems such as increased IOP may require

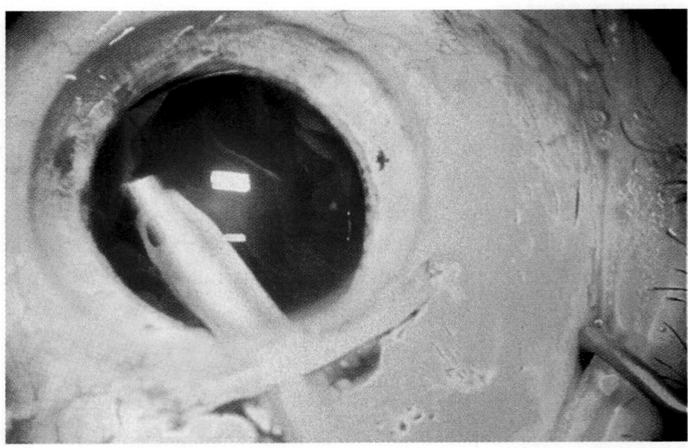

Fig. 20-3 Phacoemulsification of a cataractous lens through a self-sealing, scleral-tunnel incision. Note the circular opening in the anterior lens capsule.

lens removal. Opacities may prevent the ophthalmologist from obtaining a clear view of the retina in the patient with diabetic retinopathy or other sight-threatening pathology. In those cases the cataract may be removed to allow visualization of the retina and adequate management of the problem.

Preoperative phase. The patient's preoperative preparation should include an appropriate history and physical examination. Because almost all patients have local anesthesia, many physicians and surgical facilities do not require an extensive preoperative physical assessment. However, most cataract patients are older adults and may have several medical problems that should be evaluated and controlled before surgery. The surgeon may order preoperative antibiotic eye drops. The patient should not have food or fluids for approximately 6 to 8 hours before surgery. Almost all cataract patients are admitted to a surgical facility on an outpatient basis. The patient is normally admitted several hours before surgery to allow adequate time for necessary preoperative procedures.

The nurse will instill dilating drops and a nonsteroidal antiinflammatory eye drop to reduce inflammation and to help maintain pupil dilation. One type of drug used for dilation is a mydriatic, an α-adrenergic agonist that produces pupillary dilation by contraction of the iris dilator muscle. Mydriatics have little cycloplegic action (paralysis of accommodation). Another type is a cycloplegic, an anticholinergic agent that produces paralysis of accommodation (cycloplegia) by blocking the effect of acetylcholine on the ciliary body muscles. Cycloplegics produce pupillary dilation (mydriasis) by blocking the effect of acetylcholine on the iris sphincter muscle. Examples of mydriatics and cycloplegics are listed in Table 20-6, and nursing considerations are discussed on p. 456. The patient often receives preoperative antianxiety medication before the local anesthesia injection.

Intraoperative phase. Cataract extraction is an intraocular procedure. In *intracapsular extraction* the entire lens is removed with the capsule intact. In *extracapsular extraction* the anterior capsule is opened, and the lens nucleus and cortex are removed, leaving the remaining capsular bag intact. Although some surgeons still perform intracapsular extraction (and it may be necessary in instances of trauma), the intracapsular technique has been largely replaced by extracapsular extraction as the proce-

DRUG THERAPY

Table 20-6 **Topical Medications for Pupil Dilation**

Examples	Onset	Duration	Comments
Mydriatics			
Phenylephrine HCl (NeoSynephrine, Mydfrin)	45-60 min	4-6 hr	May cause tachycardia and elevated blood pressure, especially in elderly patient; can cause a reflexive decrease in heart rate when blood pressure rises; use punctal occlusion to limit systemic absorption
Hydroxyamphetamine-hydrobromide (Paredrine)	45-60 min	4-6 hr	Used diagnostically to differentiate postganglionic, central, or preganglionic Horner's syndrome
Cycloplegics			
Tropicamide (Mydriacyl, Tropicacyl)	20-40 min	4-6 hr	1% solution used in cycloplegic refraction; 0.5% solution used in fundus examination
Cyclopentolate HCl (AK-Pentolate, Cyclogyl, Ocu-Pentolate, Pentolair)	30-75 min	6-24 hr	Has been associated with psychotic reactions and behavioral disturbances, usually in children (especially in stronger concentrations); used in cycloplegic refraction, fundus examination, and uveitis
Homatropine hydrobromide (AK-Homatropine, Isopto Homatropine)	30-60 min	1-3 days	Used in cycloplegic refraction, uveitis; may be used for pupil dilation to allow patient to see around a central lens opacity
Scopolamine (Isopto Hyoscine)	20-60 min	3-7 days	Used in cycloplegic refraction, uveitis
Atropine (Atropisol, Atropair, Bufopto, Atropine, Isopto Atropine, Ocu-Tropine)	30-180 min	6-12 days	Used in cycloplegic refraction, uveitis

dure of choice in the United States. In extracapsular extraction, the surgeon can remove the lens nucleus by "scooping" it out with a lens loop, or by *phacoemulsification*, in which the nucleus is fragmented by ultrasonic vibration and aspirated from inside the capsular bag (Fig. 20-3). In either case, the remaining cortex is aspirated with an irrigation and aspiration instrument. The placement and type of incision varies among surgeons. Corneoscleral incisions require closure with sutures, while scleral tunnel incisions are self-sealing and require no closing suture. The incision required for phacoemulsification is considerably smaller than that required with intracapsular or standard extracapsular surgery.

Almost all patients now have an intraocular lens implanted at the time of cataract extraction surgery. Because most patients have an extracapsular procedure, the lens of choice is a posterior chamber lens that is implanted in the capsular bag behind the iris. At the end of the procedure, the patient receives injections of subconjunctival corticosteroid and antibiotic medications. Then an antibiotic and corticosteroid ointment is applied, and the patient's eye is covered with a patch and protective shield. The patch is usually worn overnight and removed during the first postoperative visit.

Postoperative phase. Unless complications occur, the patient is usually ready to go home within a few hours after the surgery as soon as the effects of sedative agents have dissipated. Postoperative medications usually include antibiotic and corticosteroid drops to prevent infection and decrease the postoperative inflammatory response. There is some evidence that postoperative activity restrictions and nighttime eye shielding are unnecessary. However, many ophthalmologists still prefer that the patient avoid activities that increase the IOP, such as bending or stooping, coughing, or lifting. Ophthalmologists may also recommend using an eye shield over the operative eye at night for protection.

The ophthalmologist will usually see the patient four to five times at increasing intervals throughout the 6 to 8 weeks following surgery. During each postoperative examination the surgeon will measure the patient's visual acuity, check anterior chamber depth, assess corneal clarity, and measure IOP. A flat anterior chamber may cause adhesions of the iris and cornea. The cornea may become hazy or cloudy from intraoperative trauma to the endothelium. Even on the first postoperative day the patient's uncorrected visual acuity in the operative eye may be good. However, it is not unusual or indicative of any problem if the patient's visual acuity is reduced immediately after surgery. The postoperative eye drops will be gradually reduced in frequency and finally discontinued when the eye has healed. When the eye is fully recovered, the patient will receive a final glasses prescription. Although the majority of the postoperative refractive error is corrected with the intraocular lens, the patient will still need glasses for near vision and for any residual refractive error.

NURSING MANAGEMENT: CATARACTS

■ Nursing Assessment

The nurse should assess the patient's distance and near visual acuity. If the patient is going to have surgery, the nurse should especially note the visual acuity in the patient's unoperated eye. With this information the nurse can determine how visually compromised the patient may be while the operative eye is patched and healing. In addition, the nurse should assess the psychosocial impact of the patient's visual disability and the patient's level of knowledge regarding the disease process and therapeutic options. Postoperatively it is important to assess the patient's level of comfort and ability to follow the postoperative regimen.

Nursing Diagnoses

Nursing diagnoses for the patient with a cataract include, but are not limited to, the following:

- Decisional conflict *related to* lack of knowledge about the condition and treatment options
- Self-care deficits *related to* visual deficit
- Anxiety *related to* lack of knowledge about the surgical and postoperative experience

Planning

Preoperatively the overall goals are that the patient with a cataract will (1) make informed decisions regarding therapeutic options and (2) experience minimal anxiety. Postoperatively the overall goals are that the patient with a cataract will (1) understand and comply with postoperative therapy, (2) maintain an acceptable level of physical and emotional comfort, and (3) remain free of infection or other complications.

Nursing Implementation

Health Promotion. There are no proven measures to prevent cataract development. However, it is probably wise (and certainly does no harm) to suggest that the patient wear sunglasses, avoid extraneous or unnecessary radiation, and maintain appropriate intake of antioxidant vitamins through good nutrition. The nurse can also provide information about vision enhancement techniques for the patient who chooses not to have surgery.

Acute Intervention. Preoperatively the patient with cataracts needs accurate information about the disease process and the treatment options, especially because cataract surgery is considered an elective procedure. For the patient who wants or needs to see better than is possible with medical interventions only, cataract surgery may not seem elective. However, in most cases there is no harm in not having surgery except that the patient has some degree of visual disability. The nurse should be available to give the patient and the family information to help them make an informed decision about appropriate treatment.

For the patient who elects to have surgery, the nurse is able to provide information, support, and reassurance about the surgical and postoperative experience that can reduce or alleviate the patient's anxiety.

When administering topical medications for pupil dilation before surgery (see Table 20-6 for examples), note that patients with dark irises may need a larger dose. Photophobia is common, and these patients need dark glasses. These medications produce transient stinging and burning and are contraindicated in patients with narrow-angle glaucoma because angle-closure glaucoma may be produced. Mydriatic agents can produce significant cardiovascular effects. When administering mydriatics, use punctal occlusion, especially in older and susceptible patients. When using cycloplegic agents for inflammatory disorders such as uveitis or iritis, the desired effect is to place the iris and ciliary body at rest, thus increasing patient comfort. This may help prevent posterior synechiae (adhesion of iris to cornea or lens).

PATIENT & FAMILY TEACHING GUIDE

Table 20-7 After Eye Surgery

- Teach patient and family proper hygiene and eye care techniques to ensure that medications, dressings, and/or surgical wound are not contaminated during necessary eye care.
- Teach patient and family about signs and symptoms of infection and when and how to report those to allow early recognition and treatment of possible infection.
- Instruct patient to comply with postoperative restrictions on head positioning, bending, coughing, and Valsalva's maneuver to optimize visual outcomes and prevent increased intraocular pressure.
- Instruct patient to instill eye medications using aseptic techniques and to comply with prescribed eye medication routine to prevent infection.
- Instruct patient to monitor pain and take prescribed medication for pain as directed and to report pain not relieved by prescribed medications.
- Instruct patient of the importance of continued follow-up as recommended to maximize potential visual outcomes.

Source: Goldblum K, editor: *Core curriculum for ophthalmic nursing,* American Society of Ophthalmic Registered Nurses, Dubuque, Ia, 1997, Kendall/Hunt Publishing.

Table 20-7 outlines patient and family teaching following eye surgery. The nurse should inform all patients that they will not have depth perception until their patch is removed (usually within 24 hours). This necessitates special considerations to avoid possible falls or other injuries. The patient with a significant visual impairment in the unoperated eye requires more assistance while the operative eye is patched. Once the patch is removed (usually within 24 hours) most patients with visual impairment in the unoperated eye will have adequate vision for necessary activities because the implanted IOL provides immediate visual rehabilitation in the operated eye. Occasionally the patient may require 1 or 2 weeks for the visual acuity in the operated eye to reach an adequate level for most of the visual needs. This patient will also need some special assistance until the vision improves. The postoperative cataract patient usually experiences little or no pain. There may be some scratchiness in the operative eye. Mild analgesics are usually sufficient to relieve these problems. If pain increases the patient should notify the surgeon because this may indicate hemorrhage, infection, or increased IOP. The nurse should also instruct the patient to notify the surgeon if there is increased or purulent drainage, increased redness, or any decrease in visual acuity. The following nursing care plan (NCP 20-1) outlines the nursing care for the patient following eye surgery.

Ambulatory and Home Care. For the cataract patient who has not had surgery, the nurse can suggest ways in which the patient may modify activities or lifestyle to accommodate the visual deficit produced by the cataract. The nurse should

20-1 NURSING CARE PLAN PATIENT AFTER EYE SURGERY

Expected Patient Outcomes	Nursing Interventions and *Rationales*
NURSING DIAGNOSIS	**Risk for injury** *related to* visual impairment or presence of eyepatch.
▪ No injury. ▪ Able to verbalize feelings of security about personal safety.	▪ Alter patient's environment *to reduce possibility of injuries resulting from unfamiliarity with the environment.* ▪ Assist with ambulation and activities of daily living to *reduce opportunities for injuries and provide verbal cueing.* ▪ Teach patient and family about possible sources of injury in the home environment *to allow them to identify and correct potentially harmful situations.*
NURSING DIAGNOSIS	**Pain** *related to* surgical manipulation of tissue *as manifested by* verbal complaint of pain and nonverbal cause of pain and pressure in the affected eye.
▪ Satisfaction with pain control.	▪ Apply warm or cold compresses *to reduce edema of eyelid and/or conjunctiva and provide soothing sensation.* ▪ Administer and teach patient to use analgesic as ordered *to relieve pain.* ▪ Teach patient to report increasing or unremitting pain *to allow early recognition and treatment of possible complications.*
NURSING DIAGNOSIS	**Anxiety** *related to* actual or potential permanent visual impairment *as manifested by* irritability and restlessness, frequent questions about outcome.
▪ Able to verbalize realistic understanding and acceptance of expected outcome. ▪ Hopeful attitude regarding best possible outcome.	▪ Use active listening techniques, encouraging patient to communicate *to allow patient to vent feelings and to validate patient's emotional responses.* ▪ Give careful explanations of all treatments and activities *to allow patient to feel a measure of control in the situation.* ▪ Include patient's family in planning and teaching *to foster their support of the patient.*
NURSING DIAGNOSIS	**Risk for self-care deficit** *related to* visual impairment and/or activity restrictions.
▪ Care needs met, with or without assistance.	▪ Assist patient with activities of daily living as needed or requested *to maintain health and self-esteem.* ▪ Help patient and family identify self-care deficits and alternative methods of accomplishing those activities, and refer to community support agencies if necessary *to assure availability of necessary assistance after discharge.*
NURSING DIAGNOSIS	**Risk for infection** *related to* disruption in normal body host defenses secondary to surgery.
▪ Free from infection.	▪ Teach patient to wash hands before instilling eye drops or cleansing around periorbital area *to prevent bacterial contamination of eye.* ▪ Teach patient not to touch tip of eye dropper to any surface *to prevent contamination.* ▪ Use prescribed medication appropriately to decrease risk of infection. ▪ Know signs and symptoms of infection and how to report *so early treatment can be initiated.*

COLLABORATIVE PROBLEM

Nursing Goals	Nursing Interventions and *Rationales*
POTENTIAL COMPLICATION:	**Increased intraocular pressure** *related to* surgery or postoperative activities.*
▪ Monitor for and report signs of increased intraocular pressure.	▪ Monitor for blurred or cloudy vision, halos around lights, severe and unrelieved eye pain, nausea and/or vomiting *to allow early recognition and treatment of possible increased intraocular pressure.*

*See Patient and Family Teaching Guide: After Eye Surgery (Table 20-7).

also provide the patient with accurate information about appropriate long-term eye care.

The trend toward outpatient surgery has clearly affected the patient with cataracts. Typically, the patient remains in the surgical facility for only a few hours instead of a few days. This shift in practice patterns has dramatically affected how the nurse provides the patient with postoperative care and teaching. The patient and the family are now responsible for almost all postoperative care, and the nurse should give them written and verbal instructions before discharge. These instructions should include information about postoperative eye care, activity restrictions, medications, follow-up visit schedule, and signs and symptoms of possible complications. The patient's family should be included in the instruction because some patients may have difficulty with self-care activities, especially if the vision in the unoperated eye is poor. The nurse should provide an opportunity for the patient and family to present return demonstrations of any necessary self-care activities.

Most patients experience little visual impairment following surgery. IOL implants provide immediate visual rehabilitation, and many patients achieve a usable level of visual acuity within a few days following surgery. Also, patients remain patched for only 24 hours, and many patients have good vision in their unoperated eye. A few patients may experience significant visual impairment postoperatively. These include patients who do not have an IOL implanted at the time of surgery, those who require several weeks to achieve a usable level of visual acuity following surgery, or those with poor vision in their unoperated eye. For those patients the time between surgery and receiving aphakic glasses or contacts can be a period of significant visual disability. The nurse can suggest ways in which the patient and the family can modify activities and the environment to maintain an adequate level of safe functioning. Suggestions may include getting assistance with steps, removing area rugs and other potential obstacles, preparing meals for freezing before surgery, or obtaining audio books for diversion until visual acuity improves.

■ Evaluation

Expected outcomes for the patient with a cataract after eye surgery are addressed in NCP 20-1 on p. 457.

GERONTOLOGIC CONSIDERATIONS

Most patients with cataracts are elderly. When the older patient is visually impaired, even temporarily, the patient may experience a loss of independence, lack of control over her or his life, and a significant change in self-perception. Societal devaluation of the older individual complicates these experiences. The older patient often needs emotional support and encouragement, as well as specific suggestions to allow a maximum level of independent function. The nurse can assure the older patient that cataract surgery can be accomplished safely and comfortably with minimal sedation. The change to outpatient surgery for cataract extraction is particularly beneficial for the older patient who may become confused or disoriented during hospitalization.

RETINAL DETACHMENT

A *retinal detachment* is a separation of the sensory retina and the underlying pigment epithelium, with fluid accumulation between the two layers. The incidence of nontraumatic retinal detachment is approximately 1 out of every 10,000 individuals each year. This number increases when aphakic individuals are included because retinal detachment is more likely to occur in aphakic patients. Including traumatic retinal detachments increases the incidence only slightly. In the patient with no other risk factors who has had a retinal detachment in one eye, the risk of detachment in the second eye is approximately 10%. Almost all patients with untreated, symptomatic retinal detachment become blind in the involved eye.

Etiology and Pathophysiology

There are many causes of retinal detachment. The most common cause is a retinal break. *Retinal breaks* are an interruption in the full thickness of the retinal tissue, and they can be classified as tears or holes. *Retinal holes* are atrophic retinal breaks that occur spontaneously. *Retinal tears* can occur as the vitreous humor shrinks during aging and pulls on the retina. The retina tears when the traction force exceeds the strength of the retina. Once there is a break in the retina, liquid vitreous can enter the subretinal space between the sensory layer and the retinal pigment epithelium layer, causing a *rhegmatogenous* retinal detachment. Less frequently, retinal detachment can occur when abnormal membranes mechanically pull on the retina. These are called *tractional* detachments. A third type of retinal detachment is the *secondary* or *exudative* detachment that occurs with conditions that allow fluid to accumulate in the subretinal space (e.g., choroidal tumors or intraocular inflammation). Risk factors for retinal detachment are listed in Table 20-8.

Clinical Manifestations

Patients with a detaching retina describe symptoms that include *photopsia* (light flashes), floaters, and a "cobweb," "hairnet," or ring in the field of vision. Once the retina has detached, the patient describes a painless loss of peripheral or central vision, "like a curtain" coming across the field of vision. The area of visual loss corresponds to the area of detachment. If the detachment is in the superior nasal retina, the visual field loss will be in the inferior temporal area. If the detachment is small or develops slowly in the periphery, the patient may not be aware of a visual problem.

Diagnostic Studies

Visual acuity measurements should be the first diagnostic procedure with any complaint of vision loss (Table 20-9). The ophthalmologist or nurse can directly visualize the retinal detachment using direct and indirect ophthalmoscopy or slit lamp microscopy in conjunction with a special lens to view the far periphery of the retina. Ultrasound may be useful to identify a retinal detachment if the retina cannot be directly visualized (e.g., when the cornea, lens, or vitreous is hazy or opaque).

Collaborative Care

The ophthalmologist will carefully evaluate the patient with retinal breaks to determine if prophylactic laser photocoagulation or cryopexy is necessary to avoid possible retinal detachment.

Table 20-8 Risk Factors for Retinal Detachment

High Myopia
Premature, accelerated rate of vitreous detachment; increased incidence of lattice degeneration

Aphakia
Retinal tears that presumably occur because of surgical disturbance of the vitreous

Proliferative Diabetic Retinopathy
Vitreous remains attached to areas of neovascularization as normal process of vitreal contraction occurs

Retinal Lattice Degeneration
Retinal holes common in lattice degeneration; vitreous remains attached to area of degeneration as the normal process of vitreal contraction occurs

Ocular Trauma
Retinal breaks after blunt or penetrating trauma allow fluid to accumulate in the subretinal space

Some retinal breaks are not likely to progress to detachment, and the ophthalmologist will simply watch the patient, giving precise information about the warning signs and symptoms of impending detachment and instructing the patient to seek immediate evaluation if any of those signs or symptoms are recognized. The general ophthalmologist will usually refer the patient with retinal detachments to a retinal specialist. Retinal detachment treatment has two objectives. The first is to seal any retinal breaks, and the second is to relieve inward traction on the retina. Several techniques are used to accomplish these objectives.

SURGICAL THERAPY

Laser Photocoagulation and Cryopexy

These techniques seal retinal breaks by creating an inflammatory reaction that causes a chorioretinal adhesion or scar. *Laser photocoagulation* involves using an intense, precisely focused light beam, such as the argon laser, to create an inflammatory reaction. The light is directed at the area of the retinal break. This produces a scar that seals the edges of the hole or tear and prevents fluid from collecting in the subretinal space and causing a detachment. The ophthalmologist may use photocoagulation alone if there is a single small tear with little or no detachment in the periphery and minimal subretinal fluid. For retinal breaks accompanied by significant detachment, the retinal surgeon may use photocoagulation intraoperatively in conjunction with scleral buckling. Tears or holes without accompanying retinal detachment may be treated prophylactically with laser photocoagulation if the ophthalmologist judges them to be at high risk of progressing to retinal detachment. When used alone, laser therapy is an outpatient procedure that usually requires only topical anesthetics, and the patient usually experiences minimal adverse symptoms during or following the procedure.

An alternate method used to seal retinal breaks is *cryopexy.* This procedure involves using extreme cold to create the inflammatory reaction that produces the sealing scar. The ophthalmologist applies the cryoprobe instrument to the external globe in the area over the tear. This is usually done on an outpatient basis and under local anesthesia. As with photocoagulation, cryotherapy may be used alone or during scleral buckling surgery. The patient may experience significant discomfort following cryopexy. The nurse should encourage the patient to take the prescribed pain medication following the procedure.

COLLABORATIVE CARE

Table 20-9 Retinal Detachment

Diagnostic
Visual acuity measurement
Ophthalmoscopy (direct and indirect)
Slit lamp microscopy
Ultrasound if cornea, lens, or vitreous are hazy or opaque

Collaborative Therapy

Preoperative
Mydriatic, cycloplegic
Photocoagulation of retinal break that has not progressed to detachment

Surgery to Seal Retinal Breaks and Relieve Traction on Retina
Photocoagulation
Cryoretinopexy
Scleral buckling procedure
Draining of subretinal fluid
Vitrectomy
Intravitreal bubble

Postoperative
Topical antibiotic
Topical corticosteroid
Analgesia
Mydriatics
Positioning and activity as preferred by patient's surgeon

Scleral Buckling

Scleral buckling is an extraocular surgical procedure that involves indenting the globe so that the pigment epithelium, choroid, and sclera move toward the detached retina. This not only helps seal retinal breaks, but also helps relieve inward traction on the retina. The retinal surgeon sutures a silicone implant against the sclera causing the sclera to buckle inward. The surgeon may place an encircling band over the implant if there are multiple retinal breaks, if the surgeon cannot locate suspected breaks, or if there is widespread inward traction on the retina (Fig. 20-4). If present, subretinal fluid may be drained by inserting a small-gauge needle to facilitate contact between the retina and the buckled sclera. Scleral buckling is usually accomplished under local anesthesia, and the patient may be discharged on the first postoperative day. Many surgeons now perform scleral buckling surgery as an outpatient procedure.

Intraocular Procedures

In addition to the extraocular procedures described, retinal surgeons may use one or more intraocular procedures in treating some retinal detachments. *Pneumatic retinopexy* is the intravitreal injection of special gases to form a temporary bubble in the vitreous that closes retinal breaks and provides appo-

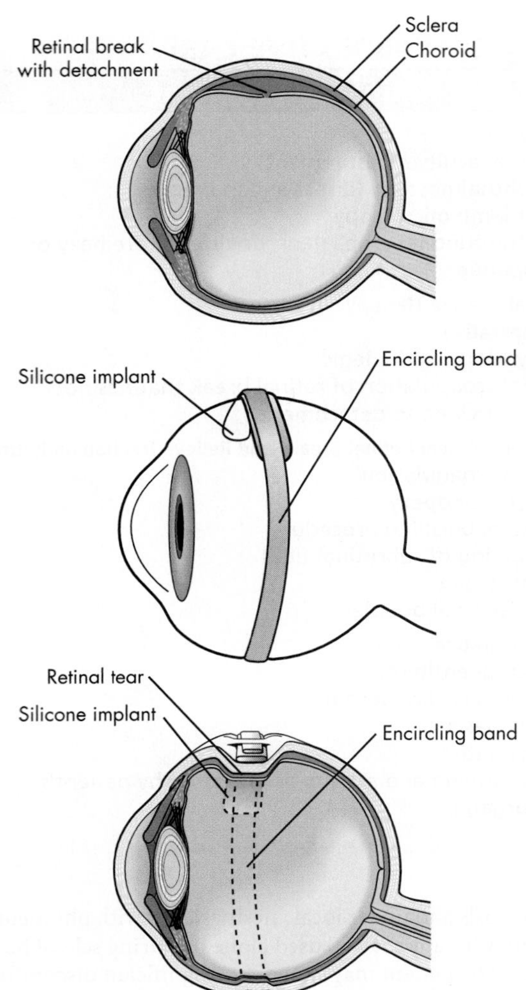

Fig. 20-4 Retinal break with detachment: surgical repair by scleral buckling technique.

sition of the separated retinal layers. Because the intravitreal bubble is temporary, this technique is combined with laser photocoagulation or cryotherapy. The patient with an intravitreal bubble must position the head so that the bubble is in contact with the retinal break. It may be necessary for the patient to maintain this position as much as possible for up to several weeks.[18]

Vitrectomy (surgical removal of the vitreous) may be used to relieve traction on the retina, especially when the traction results from proliferative diabetic retinopathy. Vitrectomy may be combined with scleral buckling to provide a dual effect in relieving traction. In *proliferative vitreoretinopathy* (PVR), membranes develop in the vitreous cavity and on the retinal surface, exerting traction that causes folds in the retina. Vitrectomy may be combined with membrane peeling to relieve traction in those cases.

Postoperative Considerations in Scleral Buckling and Intraocular Procedures

Reattachment is successful in 90% of retinal detachments. Visual prognosis varies, depending on the extent, length, and area of detachment. Postoperatively, the patient may be on bed rest and may require special positioning to maintain proper position of an intravitreal bubble. Length of hospitalization varies according to physician preference and third-party payer guidelines. The patient may use multiple topical medications, including antibiotics, antiinflammatory agents, or dilating agents. Activity recommendations vary according to physician preference, extent of the detachment, and the particular repair procedure.

NURSING MANAGEMENT: RETINAL DETACHMENT

Nursing Assessment

The nurse should elicit a careful description of the patient's visual symptoms and determine visual acuity. Confrontation visual fields may reveal a peripheral scotoma. If familiar with the techniques, the nurse may also visualize a detachment directly by ophthalmoscopy or slit lamp microscopy.

Nursing Diagnoses

Nursing diagnoses for the patient with retinal detachment include, but are not limited to, the following:

- Pain *related to* surgical correction and unusual positioning
- Fear *related to* possibility of permanent vision loss in affected eye
- Self-care deficits *related to* imposed activity restrictions and visual deficits

Planning

The overall goals are that the patient with retinal detachment will (1) experience minimal anxiety throughout the event, and (2) maintain an acceptable level of comfort postoperatively.

Nursing Implementation

The nurse should teach the patient at risk for retinal detachment the signs and symptoms of retinal detachment. The nurse can also promote use of proper protective eyewear to help avoid retinal detachments related to trauma.

In most cases retinal detachment is an urgent situation, and the patient is confronted suddenly with the need for surgery. The patient needs emotional support, especially during the immediate preoperative period when preparations for surgery produce additional anxiety. When the patient experiences postoperative pain, the nurse should administer prescribed pain medications and teach the patient to take the medication as necessary after being discharged. The patient may go home within a few hours of surgery or may remain in the hospital for several days, depending on the surgeon and the type of repair. Discharge planning and teaching is important, and the nurse should begin this process as early as possible because the patient may not remain hospitalized long. The nursing care plan on p. 457 outlines the nursing care for the patient following eye surgery. Patient and family teaching is discussed in Table 20-7.

The type and amount of activity restriction following retinal detachment surgeries varies greatly. The nurse should verify the prescribed level of activity with each patient's surgeon and help the patient plan for any necessary assistance related to activity restrictions. The nurse should teach the patient the signs and symptoms of retinal detachment because the risk of retinal detachment in the other eye is approximately 2% to 25%.

AGE-RELATED MACULAR DEGENERATION

Age-related macular degeneration (AMD) is an entity that is not precisely defined. However, for the purposes of this discussion, AMD is defined as a retinal degenerative process involving the macula and resulting in varying degrees of central vision loss. AMD is the most common cause of uncorrectable vision loss in adults over 52 years of age.

Etiology and Pathophysiology

Little is known about the etiology of AMD. Although it is clearly related to retinal aging, there is no explanation for the fact that not all aged retinas develop AMD and vision loss. The pathophysiologic mechanism may be an abnormal accumulation of waste material in the retinal pigment epithelium.[19] Cigarette smokers have a dose-related significantly higher risk of developing one form of AMD.[20]

Clinical Manifestations

The hallmark sign of AMD is the appearance of *drusen* in the fundus. Drusen appear as yellowish exudates beneath the retinal pigment epithelium and represent localized or diffuse deposits of extracellular debris. The patient may complain of blurred vision, the presence of scotomas, or *metamorphopsia* (distortion of vision).

Diagnostic Studies

In addition to visual acuity measurement, the primary diagnostic procedure is ophthalmoscopy. The examiner looks for drusen and other fundus changes associated with AMD. The Amsler grid test (see Table 19-6) may help define the involved area, and it provides a baseline for future comparison. Fundus photography and IV fluorescein angiography may be helpful in further defining the extent and type of degenerative disease.

Collaborative Care

There are no specific treatments for most patients with AMD. Laser treatment may help reduce visual loss in the patient with choroidal neovascularization. Laser treatment seals any leakage in the neovascular area, at least preventing progression of visual loss. However, in most cases of AMD, laser treatment is not helpful. Vitamin, mineral, and other nutritional supplements (e.g., zinc, selenium) are another possible treatment to slow or halt progression of visual loss. Unfortunately, this therapy is also of questionable value. When no treatment is possible, or when treatment fails, the patient with AMD can benefit from low-vision aids, such as magnifying lenses and amplification lamps.

The extent of this problem continues to grow as the number of individuals over 65 years of age increases. The permanent loss of central vision associated with AMD has significant psychosocial implications for nursing care. Nursing management of the patient with uncorrectable visual impairment is discussed on p. 447-449 and is appropriate for the patient with AMD. It is especially important when caring for the patient to avoid giving them the impression that "nothing can be done" about their problem. While it is true that therapy will not recover lost vision (and is not even appropriate in most cases) much can be done to augment the remaining vision. Just knowing that the ophthalmologist and nurse have not abandoned any attempt to help them can give these patients a more positive outlook.

RESEARCH

IMPLICATIONS FOR NURSING PRACTICE

Coping with Age-Related Macular Degeneration

Citation Duffy L: The experience of patients with age-related macular degeneration and the effectiveness of low-vision aids, *Ophthal Nurs* 1:14, 1997.

Purpose To determine how patients cope with their residual vision, to examine the effectiveness of low-vision aids, and to assess patient needs and resources for support.

Methods A case study design using qualitative and quantitative approaches with ten patients in Great Britain. Semistructured interviews were taped with nonparticipant observation in the patient's homes. Qualitative data analysis included memo writing, coding of data into categories, and thematic analysis. Thematic analysis is the search for themes or commonalities in the data.

Results and Conclusions Four main themes were qualitatively identified: physical effects of age-related macular degeneration (AMD), psychologic effects of AMD, coping strategies employed, and professional influences on rehabilitation. Observation revealed that although most (90%) patients used low-vision optical aids, only 40% did so without difficulty. Unmet rehabilitation needs in hospital and community included the provision of information, training in usage of optical aids, and ongoing support once the optical aid is obtained.

Implications for Nursing Practice Nurses should focus on careful assessment of patient needs related to AMD. Counseling may be needed for patients with anxiety or depression. Support from nurses is vital while the patient develops new coping skills. Patients cope better with visual impairment when education related to optical aids is ongoing and supported by nurses and other health care professionals.

GLAUCOMA

Glaucoma is not one disease but rather a group of disorders characterized by (1) increased IOP and the consequences of elevated pressure, (2) optic nerve atrophy, and (3) peripheral visual field loss. Glaucoma may occur congenitally, as a primary disease, or secondary to other ocular or systemic conditions. Intraocular pressure is regulated by the formation and reabsorption of aqueous humor; the presence of glaucoma is directly related to the balance or imbalance of this fluid. If elevated IOP is not recognized and treated, glaucomatous damage to the optic nerve and retinal cells result in atrophy and permanent vision loss. Glaucoma is the second leading cause of permanent blindness in the United States and the leading cause of blindness among African-Americans. At least 2 million persons have glaucoma, and, of these, more than 50% are unaware of their condition. Another 5 to 10 million persons have elevated IOP, placing them at increased risk of developing the disease. The incidence of glaucoma increases with age. One in 50 Caucasians are affected, however, 1 in 10 African-Americans develop glaucoma. Blindness from glaucoma is largely preventable with early detection and appropriate treatment.

Etiology and Pathophysiology

The etiology of glaucoma deals primarily with the consequences of elevated IOP. A proper balance between the rate of aqueous production (referred to as inflow) and the rate of aqueous reabsorption (referred to as outflow) is essential to maintain the IOP within normal limits. Intraocular pressure between 10 mm Hg and 21 mm Hg is considered normal intraocular tension. This range of IOP generally results in uniform ocular health and well-being. When the rate of inflow is greater than the rate of outflow, IOP can rise above the normal limits. If IOP remains elevated, permanent visual damage may begin.

Primary open-angle glaucoma (POAG) represents 90% of the cases of primary glaucoma. In POAG, the outflow of aqueous humor is decreased in the trabecular meshwork. In essence, the drainage channels become clogged, like a clogged kitchen sink.[21]

Primary angle-closure glaucoma (PACG) represents approximately 10% of the total number of glaucoma cases in the United States. As the name implies, the mechanism reducing the outflow of aqueous is angle closure. Usually, this is caused from the human lens bulging forward as a result of an age-related process. Angle closure may also occur as a result of pupil dilation in the patient with anatomically narrow angles. Dilation causes peripheral iris bulging with the same outcome of covering the trabecular meshwork and blocking the outflow channels. An acute attack may be precipitated by situations during which the pupil remains in a mid-dilated state long enough to cause an acute and significant rise in the IOP. This may occur because of drug-induced mydriasis, emotional excitement, or darkness. Drug-induced mydriasis may occur not only from topical ophthalmic preparations but also from many systemic medications (both prescription drugs and over-the-counter [OTC] drugs). The nurse should check drug documentation before administering medications to the patient with angle-closure glaucoma and should instruct the patient *not* to take any mydriatic-producing medications.

In *secondary glaucoma,* increased IOP results from other ocular or systemic conditions that may block the outflow channels in some way. Secondary glaucoma may be associated with various inflammatory processes that produce cells that can block the outflow channels. Inflammatory processes may also damage the trabecular meshwork. Trauma, intraocular or periorbital neoplasms, iris neovascularization, and other ocular or systemic disorders may also be associated with secondary glaucoma.

In *congenital glaucoma,* abnormal formation of the angle, iris, and trabecular channels results in poor aqueous drainage, which causes increased IOP. If the abnormalities are severe and occur early in the in utero stage, glaucomatous damage may already be significant at the time of birth.

Clinical Manifestations

POAG develops slowly and without symptoms. The patient with POAG reports no symptoms of pain or pressure. The patient usually does not notice the gradual visual field loss until peripheral vision has been severely compromised. Eventually the patient with untreated glaucoma has "tunnel vision" in which only a small center field can be seen, and all peripheral vision is absent.

Acute angle-closure glaucoma causes definite symptoms, including sudden, excruciating pain in or around the eye. This is often accompanied by nausea and vomiting. Visual symptoms include seeing colored halos around lights, blurred vision, and ocular redness. The acute rise in IOP may also cause corneal edema, giving the cornea a frosted appearance.

Manifestations of subacute or chronic angle closure glaucoma appear more gradually. The patient who has had a previous, unrecognized episode of subacute angle closure glaucoma may report a history of blurred vision, seeing colored halos around lights, ocular redness, or eye or brow pain.

Diagnostic Studies

IOP pressure is usually elevated in glaucoma. Normal IOP by applanation tonometry is 10 to 21 mm Hg. In the patient with elevated pressures, the ophthalmologist will usually repeat the measurements over a period of time to verify the elevation. In open-angle glaucoma, IOP is usually between 22 and 32 mm Hg. In acute angle-closure glaucoma, IOP may be 50 mm Hg or higher.

In open-angle glaucoma, slit lamp microscopy reveals a normal angle. In angle-closure glaucoma, the examiner may note a markedly narrow or flat anterior chamber angle, an edematous cornea, a fixed and moderately dilated pupil, and ciliary injection. Gonioscopy allows better visualization of the anterior chamber angle.

Measures of peripheral and central vision provide other diagnostic information. Whereas central acuity may remain 20/20 even in the presence of severe peripheral visual field loss, visual field perimetry may reveal subtle changes in the peripheral retina early in the disease process, long before actual scotomas develop. When visual field defects begin to appear, the initial scotoma is a small, football-shaped defect that gradually progresses to a nasal and superior field defect in chronic open-angle glaucoma. In acute angle-closure glaucoma, central visual acuity will be reduced if the patient has corneal edema, and the visual fields may be markedly decreased.

As glaucoma progresses, *optic disk cupping* occurs. This is visible with direct or indirect ophthalmoscopy. The optic disk becomes wider, deeper, and paler (light gray or white). Optic disk cupping may be one of the first signs of chronic open-angle glaucoma. Optic disk photographs are useful for comparison over time to demonstrate an increase in the cup-to-disk ratio and progressive blanching (Fig. 20-5).

Collaborative Care

The primary focus of glaucoma therapy is to keep the IOP low enough to prevent the patient from developing optic nerve damage. This damage is manifested by increasing visual field loss and progressive optic disk cupping. Specific therapies vary

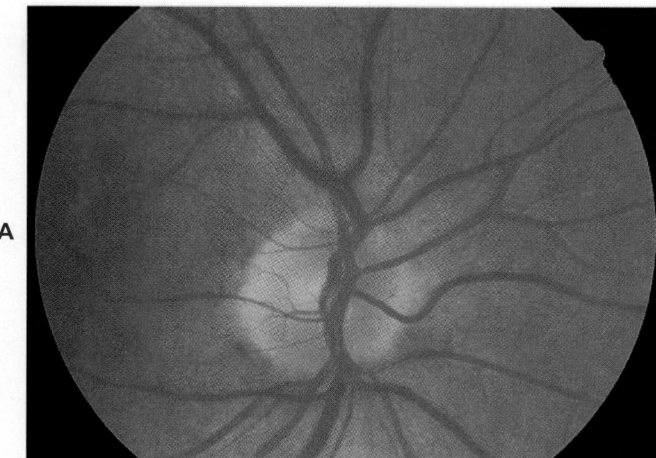

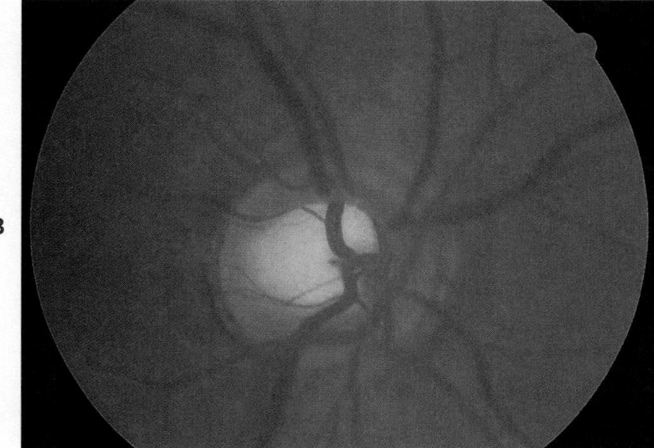

Fig. 20-5 **A,** In the normal eye, the optic cup is pink with little cupping. **B,** In the glaucomatous eye, the optic disk is bleached and optic cupping is present. (Note the appearance of the retinal vessels, which travel over the edge of the optic cup and appear to dip into it.)

with the type of glaucoma. The diagnostic and collaborative care of glaucoma is summarized in Table 20-10.

Chronic Open-Angle Glaucoma. Initial treatment in chronic open-angle glaucoma is with drugs (Table 20-11). With all drug therapy, the patient must understand that continued treatment and supervision are necessary because the medications control, but do not cure, the disease.

Argon laser trabeculoplasty (ALT) is a therapeutic option to lower IOP when medications are not successful or when occasionally the patient either cannot or will not use the drug therapy recommended. ALT is an outpatient procedure that requires only topical anesthetic. The topical drops anesthetize the cornea before the gonioscopy lens is applied, allowing visualization of the treatment area. Approximately 50 laser "spots" are evenly spaced around the superior or inferior 180 degrees of the trabecular meshwork. The laser stimulates scarring and contraction of the trabecular meshwork, opening the outflow channels. ALT reduces IOP approximately 75% of the time.[22] A second 180 degree area may be treated in a subsequent procedure. The patient uses topical corticosteroids for approximately

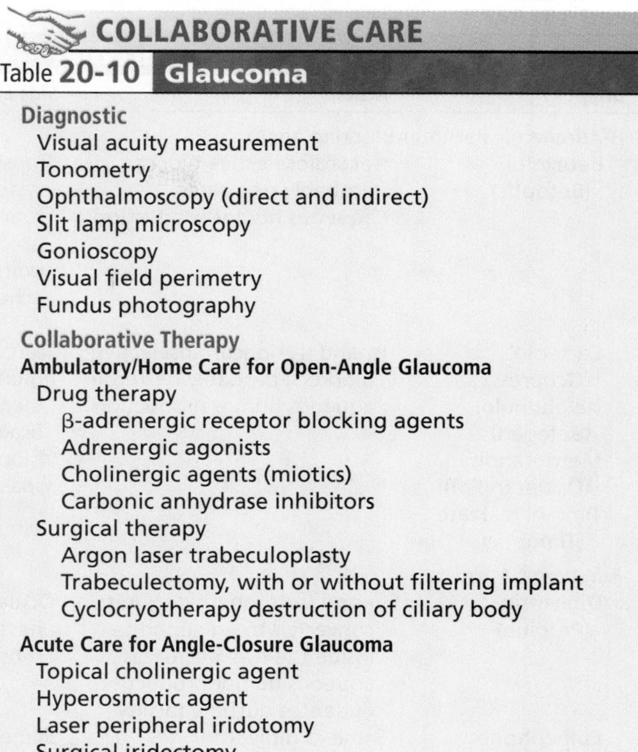

COLLABORATIVE CARE

Table 20-10 Glaucoma

Diagnostic
- Visual acuity measurement
- Tonometry
- Ophthalmoscopy (direct and indirect)
- Slit lamp microscopy
- Gonioscopy
- Visual field perimetry
- Fundus photography

Collaborative Therapy

Ambulatory/Home Care for Open-Angle Glaucoma
- Drug therapy
  - β-adrenergic receptor blocking agents
  - Adrenergic agonists
  - Cholinergic agents (miotics)
  - Carbonic anhydrase inhibitors
- Surgical therapy
  - Argon laser trabeculoplasty
  - Trabeculectomy, with or without filtering implant
  - Cyclocryotherapy destruction of ciliary body

Acute Care for Angle-Closure Glaucoma
- Topical cholinergic agent
- Hyperosmotic agent
- Laser peripheral iridotomy
- Surgical iridectomy

3 to 5 days following surgery. The most common complication is an acute postoperative IOP rise. Because the decrease in pressure is gradual, the patient continues taking the preoperative glaucoma medication. The ophthalmologist examines the patient 1 week after the procedure and again 4 to 6 weeks following surgery.

A *filtering procedure,* such as trabeculectomy, may be indicated if medical management and laser therapy are not successful. In this procedure the surgeon makes conjunctival and scleral flaps, removes part of the iris and trabecular meshwork, and closes the scleral flap loosely. Aqueous humor may now "percolate" out through the area of missing iris where it is trapped under the repaired conjunctiva and absorbed into the systemic circulation. The success rate of this filtering surgery is 75% to 85%. Mitomycin (Mutamycin) or 5-fluorouracil may increase the success rate by preventing scarring and subsequent closure of the opening created during surgery.

Cyclocryotherapy is another procedure that reduces IOP. The cryoprobe is touched to the sclera outside of the ciliary body. This freezes parts of the ciliary body, causing local destruction of the ciliary tissue and decreasing production of aqueous humor. The procedure may be repeated and can also be used in treating acute glaucoma.

An implant is another surgical option, usually reserved for the patient in whom filtration surgery has failed. It involves surgical placement of a small tube and reservoir to shunt aqueous humor from the anterior chamber to the implanted reservoir.

Acute Angle-Closure Glaucoma. Acute angle-closure glaucoma is an ocular emergency that requires immediate intervention. Miotics and oral or IV hyperosmotic agents are

DRUG THERAPY

Table 20-11 Acute and Chronic Glaucoma

Drug	Action	Side Effects	Nursing Considerations
β-Adrenergic Receptor Blocking Agents			
Betaxolol (Betoptic)	β_1 cardioselective blocker; probably decreases aqueous humor production	Transient discomfort; systemic reactions rarely reported but include bradycardia, heart block, pulmonary distress, headache, depression	Topical drops; minimal effect on pulmonary and cardiovascular parameters; contraindicated in patient with bradycardia, cardiogenic shock, or overt cardiac failure; systemic absorption can have additive effect with systemic β-blocking agents
Carteolol (Ocupress) Levobunolol (Betagan) Metripranolol (Optipranolol) Timolol maleate (Timoptic)	β_1 and β_2 noncardioselective blockers; probably decrease aqueous humor production	Transient ocular discomfort, blurred vision, photophobia, blepharoconjunctivitis, bradycardia, decreased blood pressure, bronchospasm, headache, depression	Topical drops; same as betaxolol; these noncardioselective β-blockers are also contraindicated in patients with asthma or severe COPD
Adrenergic Agonists			
Dipivefrin (Propine)	α- and β-Adrenergic agonist; converted to epinephrine inside the eye; decreases aqueous humor production, enhances outflow facility	Ocular discomfort and redness, tachycardia, hypertension	Topical drops; contraindicated in patient with narrow-angle glaucoma; teach punctal occlusion to patient at risk of systemic reactions
Epinephrine (Epifrin, Eppy, Claucon, Epitrate, Epinal, Eppy/N)	Same as dipivefrin	Same as dipivefrin, but can be more pronounced	Topical drops; same as dipivefrin
Apraclonidine (Lopidine) Bromonidine (Alphagan)	α-Adrenergic agonist; probably decrease aqueous humor production	Ocular redness; irregular heart rate	Topical drops; used to control or prevent acute postlaser IOP rise (used 1 hr before, and immediately after ALT and iridotomy, Nd: YAG laser capsulotomy); teach patient at risk of systemic reactions to occlude puncta
Latanoprost (Xalatan)	Prostaglandin F-Analog	Increased brown iris pigmentation, ocular discomfort and redness, dryness, itching, and foreign body sensation	Topical drops; teach patient to not exceed 1 drop per evening; have patient remove contact lens 15 min before instilling
Cholinergic Agents (Miotics)			
Carbachol (Isopto Carbachol)	Parasympathomimetic; stimulates iris sphincter contraction, causing miosis and opening of trabecular meshwork, facilitating aqueous outflow; also partially inhibits cholinesterase	Transient ocular discomfort, headache, browache, blurred vision, decreased dark adaptation, syncope, salivation, arrhythmias, vomiting, diarrhea, hypotension, retinal detachment in susceptible individual (rare)	Topical drops; caution patient about decreased visual acuity caused by miosis, particularly in dim light
Pilocarpine (Akarpine; Isopto Carpine, Pilocar, Pilopine, Piloptic, Pilostat)	Parasympathomimetic; stimulates iris sphincter contraction, causing miosis and opening of tabecular meshwork, facilitating aqueous humor outflow	Same as carbachol	Topical drops; same as carbachol
Carbonic Anhydrase Inhibitors			
Acetazolamide (Diamox) Dichlorphenamide (Daranide) Methazolamide (Neptazane)	Decreases aqueous humor production	Paresthesias, especially "tingling"in extremities; hearing dysfunction or tinnitus; loss of appetite; taste alteration; GI disturbances; drowsiness; confusion	Oral nonbacteriostatic sulfonamides; anaphylaxis and other sulfa-type allergic reactions may occur in patient allergic to sulfa; diuretic effect can lower electrolyte levels; ask patient about aspirin use; drug should not be given to patient on high-dose aspirin therapy

Continued

DRUG THERAPY

Table 20-11 Acute and Chronic Glaucoma—cont'd

Drug	Action	Side Effects	Nursing Considerations
Hyperosmolar Agents			
Glycerin liquid (Ophthalgan, Osmoglyn Oral)	Increases extracellular osmolarity so intracellular water moves to the extracellular and vascular spaces, reducing IOP	Nausea, vomiting, headache, confusion, disorientation, arrhythmia, severe dehydration	Oral liquid; used in acute glaucoma attacks or preoperatively when decreased IOP is desired; assess patient for susceptibility to pulmonary edema and CHF before administering hyperosmolar agents
Isosorbide solution (Ismotic)	Same as glycerin	Nausea, vomiting, headache, confusion, disorientation, syncope, lethargy, irritability	Oral liquid; same as glycerin
Mannitol solution (Osmitrol)	Same as glycerin	Nausea, vomiting, diarrhea, thrombophlebitis, hypertension, hypotension, tachycardia	IV solution; same as glycerin

ALT, argon laser trabeculoplasty; *CHF,* congestive heart failure; *COPD,* chronic obstructive pulmonary disease; *GI,* gastrointestinal; *IOP,* intraocular pressure; *IV,* intravenous.

usually successful in immediately lowering the IOP (see Table 20-10). A laser peripheral iridotomy or surgical iridectomy is necessary for long-term treatment and prevention of subsequent episodes. These procedures allow the aqueous humor to flow through a newly created opening in the iris and into normal outflow channels. One of these procedures may also be performed on the other eye as a precaution because many patients often experience an acute attack in the other eye.

Secondary Glaucoma. Secondary glaucoma is managed by treating the underlying problem and by using antiglaucoma drugs. If treatment fails, glaucoma can progress to absolute glaucoma, resulting in a hard, sightless, and usually painful eye requiring *enucleation* (surgical removal of the eye).

NURSING MANAGEMENT: GLAUCOMA

Glaucoma is a chronic condition that has long-term significant sight-threatening implications. Nursing management is focused on the chronicity of this disease and on the fact that visual impairment is preventable in most cases with proper therapeutic management.

■ Nursing Assessment

Because glaucoma is a chronic condition requiring long-term management, the nurse must carefully assess the patient's ability to understand and comply with the rationale and regimen of the prescribed therapy. In addition, the nurse should assess the patient's psychologic reaction to the diagnosis of a potentially sight-threatening chronic disorder. The nurse must include the patient's family in the assessment process because the chronic nature of this disorder impacts the family in many ways. Some families may become the primary providers of necessary care, such as eye drop administration or insulin injections, if the patient is unwilling or unable to accomplish these self-care activities. The nurse also assesses visual acuity, visual field, IOP, and fundus changes when appropriate.

■ Nursing Diagnoses

Nursing diagnoses for the patient with glaucoma include, but are not limited to, the following:

- Noncompliance *related to* the inconvenience and side effects of glaucoma medications
- Risk for injury *related to* visual acuity deficits
- Self-care deficits *related to* visual acuity deficits
- Pain *related to* pathophysiologic process and surgical correction

■ Planning

The overall goals are that the patient with glaucoma will (1) have no progression of visual impairment, (2) understand the disease process and rationale for therapy, (3) comply with all aspects of therapy (including medication administration and follow-up care), and (4) have no postoperative complications.

■ Nursing Implementation

Health Promotion. The nurse has an important role in educating the patient and family about the risk of glaucoma. In addition, the nurse should stress the importance of early detection and treatment in preventing visual impairment. This knowledge should encourage the patient to seek appropriate ophthalmic health care. The nurse may fulfill this teaching role by educating individual patients and families, groups of patients, or entire communities, depending on the nurse's practice setting. The patient should know that the incidence of glaucoma increases with age and that a comprehensive ophthalmic examination is invaluable in identifying persons with glaucoma or those at risk of developing glaucoma. The current recommendation is for an ophthalmologic examination every 2 to 4 years for persons between the ages of 40 and 64 years, and every 1 to 2 years for persons age 65 years or older. African-Americans in every age category should have examinations more often because of the increased incidence and more aggressive course of glaucoma in these individuals.

Acute Intervention. Acute nursing interventions are directed primarily toward the patient with acute angle-closure glaucoma and the surgical patient. The patient with acute angle-closure glaucoma requires immediate medication to lower the IOP, which the nurse must administer in a timely and appropriate manner according to the ophthalmologist's prescription. This patient may also be uncomfortable, and appropriate nursing comfort interventions may include darkening the environment, applying cool compresses to the patient's forehead, and providing a quiet and private space for the patient. Most surgical procedures for glaucoma are outpatient procedures. Acutely, the patient needs postoperative instructions and may require nursing comfort measures to relieve discomfort related to the procedure. The nursing care plan on p. 457 outlines the nursing care for the patient following eye surgery. Patient and family teaching is discussed in Table 20-7.

Ambulatory and Home Care. Because of the chronic nature of glaucoma the patient needs encouragement to follow the therapeutic regimen and follow-up recommendations prescribed by their ophthalmologist. The patient needs accurate information about the disease process and treatment options, including the rationale underlying each option. In addition, the patient needs information about the purpose, frequency, and technique for administration of prescribed antiglaucoma agents. In addition to verbal instructions, all patients should receive written instructions that contain the same information. This should be sufficiently detailed to provide all the necessary information without being so extensive that the patient becomes overwhelmed. The patient may be encouraged to comply with the medication regimen if the nurse promotes consideration of the sight-saving nature of the drops. The nurse can further encourage compliance by helping the patient identify the most convenient and appropriate times for medication administration or advocating a change in therapy if the patient reports unacceptable side effects.

■ Evaluation

The overall expected outcomes are that the patient with glaucoma will

- have no further loss of vision
- comply with recommended therapy
- safely function within own environment
- obtain relief from pain associated with the disease and surgery

GERONTOLOGIC CONSIDERATIONS

Many older patients with glaucoma have systemic illnesses or take systemic medications that may affect their therapy. In particular, the patient using a β-adrenergic blocking glaucoma agent may experience an additive effect if a systemic β-adrenergic blocking medication is also being taken. All β-adrenergic blocking glaucoma agents are contraindicated in the patient with bradycardia, greater than first degree heart block, cardiogenic shock, and overt cardiac failure. The noncardioselective β-adrenergic blocker glaucoma agents are also contraindicated in the patient with severe chronic obstructive pulmonary disease (COPD) or asthma. The hyperosmolar agents may precipitate congestive heart failure (CHF) or pulmonary edema in the susceptible patient. The older patient on high-dose aspirin therapy for rheumatoid arthritis should not take carbonic anhydrase inhibitors. The adrenergic agents can cause tachycardia or hypertension, which may have serious consequences in the older patient. The nurse should teach the older patient to occlude the puncta to limit the systemic absorption of glaucoma medications.

INTRAOCULAR INFLAMMATION AND INFECTION

The term *uveitis* is used to describe inflammation of the uveal tract, the retina, the vitreous body, or the optic nerve. This inflammation may be caused by bacteria, viruses, fungi, or parasites. *Cytomegalovirus retinitis* (CMV retinitis) is an opportunistic infection that occurs in patients with acquired immunodeficiency syndrome (AIDS) and in other immunosuppressed patients. The etiology of sterile intraocular inflammation includes autoimmune disorders, AIDS, malignancies, or those associated with systemic diseases such as juvenile rheumatoid arthritis and inflammatory bowel disease. Pain and photophobia are common symptoms.

Endophthalmitis is an extensive intraocular inflammation of the vitreous cavity. Bacteria, viruses, fungi, or parasites can all induce this serious inflammatory response. The mechanism of infection may be endogenous, in which the infecting agent arrives at the eye through the bloodstream, or exogenous, in which the infecting agent is introduced through a surgical wound or a penetrating injury. Although rare, most cases of endophthalmitis are a devastating complication of intraocular surgery or penetrating ocular injury and can lead to irreversible blindness within hours or days. Manifestations include ocular pain, photophobia, decreased visual acuity, headaches, upper lid edema, reddened and swollen conjunctiva, and corneal edema.

When all the layers of the eye (vitreous, retina, choroid, and sclera) are involved in the inflammatory response, the patient has *panophthalmitis*. In the final stages of extensive cases, the scleral coat may undergo bacterial or inflammatory dissolution. Subsequent rupture of the globe spreads the infection into the orbit or eyelids.

Treatment of intraocular inflammation is dependent on the underlying cause. Intraocular infections require antimicrobial agents, which may be delivered topically, subconjunctivally, intravitreally, systemically, or in some combination. Sterile inflammatory responses require antiinflammatory agents such as corticosteroids. The site and severity of the sterile inflammatory response determines whether topical, subconjunctival, or systemic corticosteroids are necessary.

The patient with intraocular inflammation is usually uncomfortable and may be noticeably anxious and frightened. The patient may fear sudden and total loss of vision. In some cases this fear is realistic, and the nurse should provide accurate information and emotional support to the patient and the family. In severe cases enucleation may be necessary. When the patient has lost visual function or even the entire eye, the patient will grieve the loss. The nurse's role includes helping the patient through the grieving process.

ENUCLEATION

Enucleation is the removal of the eye. The primary indication for enucleation is a blind, painful eye. This may result from absolute glaucoma, infection, or trauma. Enucleation may also be indicated in ocular malignancies, although many malignancies can be managed with cryotherapy, radiation, and chemotherapy. An extremely rare indication is *sympathetic ophthalmia,* in which the untraumatized eye develops an inflammatory response following the primary eye trauma. In this situation the traumatized eye is enucleated. The surgical procedure includes severing the extraocular muscles close to their insertion on the globe, inserting an implant to maintain the intraorbital anatomy, and suturing the ends of the extraocular muscles over the implant. The conjunctiva covers the joined muscles, and a clear conformer is placed over the conjunctiva until the permanent prosthesis is fitted. A pressure dressing helps prevent postoperative bleeding.

Postoperatively the nurse observes the patient for signs of complications including excessive bleeding or swelling, increased pain, displacement of the implant, or temperature elevation. Patient education should include the instillation of topical ointments or drops and wound cleansing. The nurse should also instruct the patient in the method of inserting the conformer into the socket in case it falls out. The patient is often devastated by the loss of an eye, even when enucleation occurs following a lengthy period of painful blindness. The nurse should recognize and validate the patient's emotional response and provide support to the patient and the family.

Approximately 6 weeks following surgery the wound is sufficiently healed for the permanent prosthesis. The prosthesis is fitted by an ocularist and designed to match the remaining eye. The patient should learn how to remove, cleanse, and insert the prosthesis. Special polishing is required periodically to remove dried protein secretions.

The nurse may need to remove the prosthesis when the patient is unable to do so. After thorough hand washing, the nurse pulls the patient's lower lid down and toward the cheekbone. The prosthesis will usually slip out (Fig. 20-6). A special small suction tip may be used if necessary. The prosthesis should be cleaned with a mild soap, rinsed well, and stored in a container lined with soft material to prevent damage. The patient's name should be clearly marked on the container. To reinsert the prosthesis, the nurse opens the upper lid by pressure on the upper bony orbit, places the top of the prosthesis under the upper lid, and pulls the lower lid down. The lower edge of the prosthesis will slip under the lower lid with a little pressure on the prosthesis (Fig. 20-7).

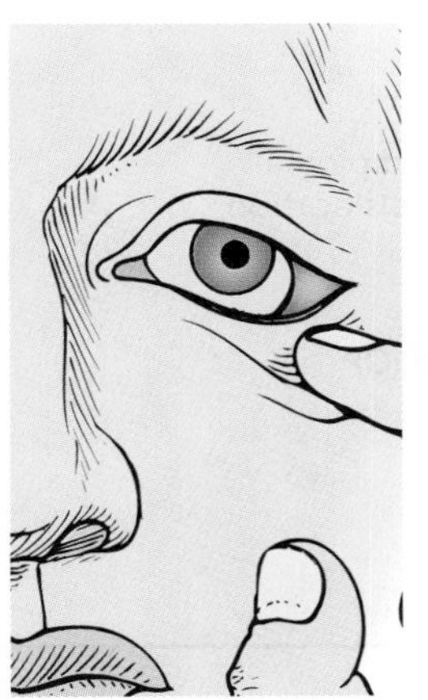
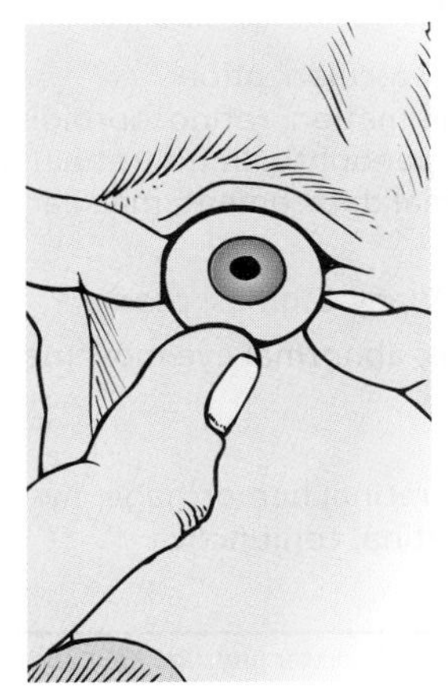

Fig. 20-6 Removal of ocular prosthesis.

OCULAR MANIFESTATIONS OF SYSTEMIC DISEASES

Many systemic diseases have significant ocular manifestations. Although it is not the purpose of this discussion to provide a full description of these disorders, it is important for the nurse to recognize that many systemic diseases have ocular symptoms. Conversely, ocular signs and symptoms may be the first finding or complaint in the patient with systemic diseases. One example is the patient with undiagnosed diabetes who seeks ophthalmic care for blurred vision. A careful health history and examination of the patient can reveal that the underlying cause of the blurred vision is lens swelling caused by uncontrolled hyperglycemia. Another example is the patient who seeks care for a conjunctival lesion. The ophthalmologist may be the first health care professional to make the diagnosis of AIDS based on the presence of a conjunctival Kaposi's sarcoma (KS). Table 20-12 lists some systemic diseases and the associated ophthalmic manifestations.

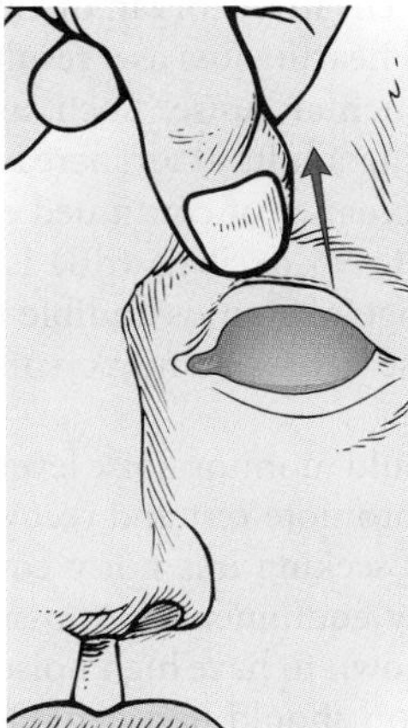
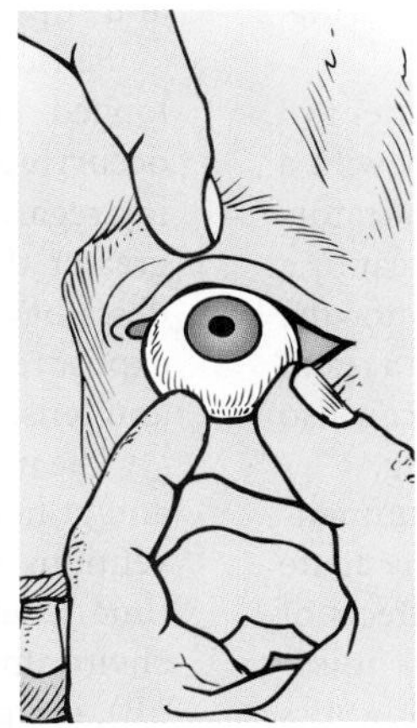
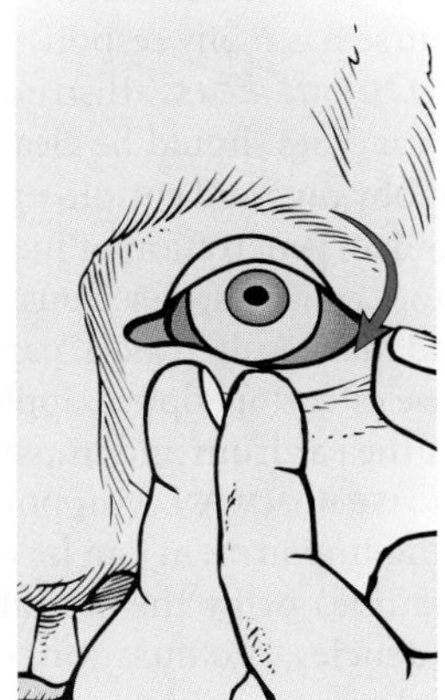

Fig. 20-7 Insertion of ocular prosthesis.

Table 20-12 Ocular Manifestations of Systemic Diseases or Syndromes

Systemic Entity	Ocular Manifestations
■ AIDS	Herpes zoster ophthalmicus, keratitis (bacterial and viral), CMV retinitis, endophthalmitis (bacterial and fungal), cotton-wool spots and microvasculopathy of the retina, KS of eyelids or conjunctiva
■ Albinism	Decreased visual acuity, photophobia, nystagmus, strabismus
■ Diabetes mellitus	Fluctuating refractive errors, diabetic retinopathy, macular edema, premature cataract development, increased incidence of glaucoma
■ Down syndrome	Myopia, cataracts, nystagmus, strabismus, keratoconus, upward and outward slant of palpebral fissures
■ Hypertension	Cotton-wool spots and hemorrhage of the retina, retinal lipid deposits
■ Systemic lupus erythematosus	Dry eye, retinal changes, uveitis, scleritis
■ Marfan's syndrome	Lens dislocation, high myopia, keratoconus, retinal detachment
■ Rheumatoid arthritis	Dry eye, keratitis, scleritis
■ Infections	
Botulism	Blurred vision, ptosis, diplopia, fixed, dilated pupil
Endocarditis	Subconjunctival or retinal petechiae
Tuberculosis	Conjunctivitis, keratitis, uveitis
Leprosy	Conjunctivitis, keratitis, uveitis, ptosis
Genital herpes	Herpes simplex keratitis
CMV infection	CMV retinitis
Measles	Conjunctivitis, keratitis, retinopathy
Congenital rubella	Cataracts, glaucoma
Histoplasmosis	Chorioretinal lesions, subretinal neovascularization
Toxoplasmosis	Necrotic retinal lesions, vitreal inflammation, retinochoroiditis
Lyme disease	Conjunctivitis, keratitis, episcleritis, panophthalmitis, retinal detachment, diplopia
Syphilis	Conjunctivitis, keratitis, uveitis, retinal detachment, macular edema, lens dislocation, glaucoma (congenital syphilis)
■ Temporal arteritis	Vision loss; palsies of CN III, IV, and VI; nystagmus; ptosis
■ Thyroid disease	Lid retraction, lid lag, exophthalmos, abnormal eye movement, increased IOP
■ Vitamin deficiencies	
A	Night blindness, corneal ulceration
B	Optic neuropathy, corneal changes, retinal hemorrhage, nystagmus
C	Hemorrhage in anterior chamber, retina, conjunctiva
D	Exophthalmos

AIDS, acquired immunodeficiency syndrome; *CMV,* cytomegalovirus; *CN,* cranial nerve; *IOP,* intraocular pressure, *KS,* Kaposi's sarcoma.

HEARING PROBLEMS

Health Promotion

The nurse has an important role in the preservation of hearing. To fulfill this role, the nurse has many responsibilities.

Keeping Objects Out of Ears. Instruct the patient to keep objects out of the ear. Ears should be cleaned only with a washcloth and finger. Bobby pins and cotton-tipped applicators should especially be avoided. Penetration of the middle ear by a cotton-tipped applicator can cause serious injury to the eardrum and ossicles and may result in facial paralysis as a result of nerve damage. The use of cotton-tipped applicators can also impact cerumen against the eardrum and impair hearing.

Environmental Noise Control. Support environmental noise control. Hearing impairment can be caused by acute loud noise (acoustic trauma) or by the cumulative effects of various intensities, frequencies, and durations of noise (noise-induced hearing loss). Acoustic trauma causes hearing loss from mechanical destruction of parts of the organ of Corti. Some recovery of function may occur in the first weeks after injury, but the remaining loss is permanent. Noise-induced hearing loss is probably caused by high-intensity stimulation of the cochlea resulting in mechanical damage of the hair cells and supporting cells in the organ of Corti.

Sensorineural hearing loss as a result of increased and prolonged environmental noise, such as amplified sound, is occurring in young adults at an increasing rate. Health teaching regarding avoidance of continued exposure to noise levels greater than 85 to 95 decibels (dB) is essential. Table 20-13 describes the range of sounds audible to humans. Continued exposure to noise causes some persons to be more irritable and tense.

The nurse should monitor noise levels in health care settings and at home to promote rest and recovery from illness. Interventions such as seeking less noisy equipment or a different time to use noisy equipment are possible solutions. In work environments known to have high noise levels (greater than 85 dB), ear protection should be worn. Occupational Safety and Health Administration (OSHA) standards require ear protection for workers in environments where the noise levels exceed

Table 20-13 Range of Sounds Audible to Human Ear

Typical	Example
Decibel	
0	Lowest sound audible to the human ear
30	Quiet library, soft whisper
40	Living room, quiet office, bedroom away from traffic
50	Light traffic at a distance, refrigerator, gentle breeze
60	Air conditioner at 20 ft, conversation, sewing machine
70	Busy traffic, noisy restaurant. At this decibel level, noise may begin to affect hearing if exposure is constant
Hazardous Zone for Hearing Loss	
80	Subway, heavy city traffic, alarm clock at two feet, factory noise. These noises are dangerous if exposure to them lasts for more than 8 hr
90	Truck traffic, noisy home appliances, shop tools, lawn mower. As loudness increases, the "safe" time exposure decreases; damage can occur in less than 8 hr
100	Chain saw, stereo headphones, pneumatic drill. Even 2 hr of exposure can be dangerous at this decibel level; with each 5 dB increase the safe time is cut in half
120	Rock band concert in front of speakers, sandblasting, thunderclap. The danger is immediate; exposure of 120 dB can injure ears
140	Gunshot blast, jet plane. Any length of exposure time is dangerous; noise at this level may cause actual pain in the ear
180	Rocket launching pad. Without ear protection, noise at this level causes irreversible damage; hearing loss is inevitable

From American Academy of Otolaryngology, 1993.

85 dB consistently. A variety of protectors is available that are worn over the ears or in the ears to prevent hearing loss. Periodic audiometric screening should be part of the health maintenance policies of industry. This provides baseline data on hearing to measure subsequent hearing loss.

The nurse should participate in hearing conservation programs in work environments. An industrial hearing conservation program should include noise exposure analysis, provision for control of noise exposure (hearing protectors), measurements of hearing, and employee-employer notification and education. Often a multidisciplinary team including an industrial hygienist, engineer, nurse, and audiometric technician is responsible for such a program.

Ear protection should be worn during skeet shooting and other recreational pursuits with high noise levels. Young adults should be encouraged to keep amplified music at a reasonable level and limit their exposure time. Hearing loss caused by noise is not reversible.

Immunizations. Promote childhood and adult immunizations, including the measles, mumps, and rubella (MMR) immunization. Various viruses can cause deafness as a result of fetal damage and malformations affecting the ear. Deafness occurs following exposure to rubella in the first trimester of pregnancy. The risk for congenital defects following exposure to rubella in the second and third trimester drops to 1%.[23] Women of childbearing age should be tested for immunity. A rubella antibody titer of 1:8 or greater shows the individual has immunity to rubella. If the titer is less, immunization with live vaccine should be given. The woman should avoid pregnancy for at least 3 months. Immunization is delayed if the woman is pregnant. Women who are susceptible to rubella can be vaccinated safely during the immediate puerperium.[24]

Ototoxic Drugs. Monitor the patient's reaction to drugs that are known to cause ototoxicity. Ototoxic drugs are capable of damaging one or both branches of the auditory nerve (CN VIII) and the inner ear. Signs and symptoms of cochlear toxicity are tinnitus and sensorineural hearing loss. Damage in the vestibule and semicircular canals can result in vertigo, horizontal nystagmus, nausea, and vomiting. Risk factors associated with ototoxicity include advanced age or extreme youth, renal or liver disease, a history of hearing loss, use of two or more potentially ototoxic drugs, dehydration, bacteremia, and a history of previous exposure to excessive noise or cranial irradiation.[25]

Drugs commonly associated with ototoxicity include aspirin, quinidine, quinine, loop diuretics, cisplatin, carboplatin, and aminoglycosides. The patient who is receiving these drugs should be assessed for development or exacerbation of signs and symptoms associated with ototoxicity. Ringing tinnitus may precede hearing loss. When these symptoms develop, immediate withdrawal of the drug may prevent further damage and may cause the symptoms to disappear. When withdrawal of the drug therapy is life threatening, the patient should be advised of the possibility of permanent hearing loss.

Risk for Hearing Loss. Identify the patient who has a potential for hearing loss. Children who are chronic mouth breathers need referral. Enlarged adenoids can block the nasal passages, as well as the eustachian tube, preventing aeration of the middle ear. This also predisposes the child to otitis media. Children who have acute otitis media frequently need to be observed for signs of chronic otitis media. It is important that children complete the full course of antibiotics prescribed for the acute episode.

Detection of Hearing Loss. Be observant of symptoms that indicate hearing loss at all ages. These symptoms include asking others to speak up, answering questions inappropriately, not responding when not looking at the speaker, straining to hear, cupping hands around ear, showing irritability with others who do not speak up, and increasing sensitivity to slight increases in noise level. Often the patient is unaware of minimal hearing loss or may compensate by using these mannerisms. Children will often be inattentive, bored, or uncooperative when they have decreased hearing caused by a middle ear infection (conductive type of loss) or an inner ear problem (sensorineural loss). Hearing loss in the older adult is often noticed first by family and friends of the patient who get tired of repeating or talking loudly.

EXTERNAL EAR AND CANAL

TRAUMA

Trauma to the external ear can cause injury to the subcutaneous tissue that may result in a hematoma. If the hematoma is not aspirated, inflammation of the membranes of the ear cartilage (perichondritis) can result. Antibiotics are given to prevent infection. Blows to the ear can also cause a conductive hearing loss if there is ossicular damage of the middle ear or if a perforation of the eardrum results. It is important to obtain a careful history of the accident and to assess the hearing of a patient who has had a blow to the ear or side of the head.

EXTERNAL OTITIS

The skin of the external ear and canal is subject to the same problems as skin anywhere on the body. *External otitis* involves inflammation or infection of the epithelium of the auricle and ear canal. Frequent swimming may alter the flora of the external canal to produce an infection often referred to as "swimmer's ear." Trauma caused by picking the ear or the use of sharp objects, such as hairpins, frequently causes the initial break in the skin.

Etiology

External otitis may be caused by infections, dermatitis, or both. Bacteria or fungi may be the cause. The bacteria most commonly cultured are *Pseudomonas aeruginosa, Proteus vulgaris, Escherichia coli,* and *S. aureus.* The most common fungi are *Candida albicans* and *Aspergillus* organisms. Fungi are often the causative agents of external otitis, especially in warm, moist climates. The warm, dark environment of the ear canal provides a good medium for the growth of microorganisms.

Clinical Manifestations and Complications

Pain (otalgia) is one of the first signs of external otitis. Even in mild cases, the patient may experience pain that is disproportionate to the infection. Pain is caused by the swelling of the bony ear canal as a result of the inflammatory process. Pain is especially noted on movement of the auricle or on application of pressure to the tragus (directly in front of the ear). Drainage from the ear may be serosanguineous or purulent. If it is the result of an infection caused by a *Pseudomonas* organism, the drainage will be green and have a musty smell. Temperature elevations occur when there is extensive involvement of the tissue. The swelling of the ear canal can block hearing and cause dizziness.

NURSING MANAGEMENT: EXTERNAL OTITIS

Diagnosis of external otitis is made by observation with the otoscope light using the largest speculum the ear will accommodate without causing the patient unnecessary discomfort. The eardrum may be normal if it can be seen. Culture and sensitivity studies of the drainage may be done. Aspirin or codeine will usually control the pain. After the ear canal is cleansed, a wick of cotton is placed in the canal to help deliver the antibiotic ear drops. Cotton wicks should be used with caution in young patients and confused or psychotic patients, who may push them farther into the ear. Topical antibiotics include polymyxin B, colistin, neomycin, and chloramphenicol (Chloromycetin). Nystatin is used for fungal infections. Corticosteroids may also be used unless the infection is fungal; corticosteroids are contraindicated in this case. If the surrounding tissue is involved, systemic antibiotics are prescribed. Warm, moist compresses or heat may be applied. Improvement should occur in 48 hours, but 7 to 14 days are required for complete resolution.

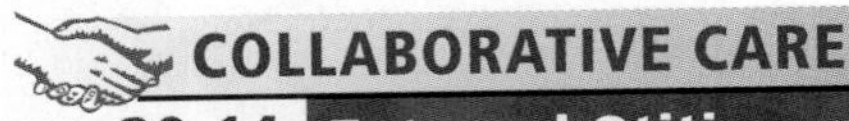
COLLABORATIVE CARE

Table 20-14 External Otitis

Diagnostic
- Otoscopic examination
- Culture and sensitivity

Collaborative Therapy
- Analgesics (depending on severity)
- Warm compresses
- Cleansing of canal
- Ear wick
- Antibiotic otic drops
- Systemic antibiotics

Careful handling and disposal of material saturated with drainage are important. Otic (ear) drops should be administered at room temperature because cold drops can cause dizziness in the patient by stimulation of the semicircular canals. The tip of the dropper should not touch the ear during administration to prevent contamination of the entire bottle of drops when the dropper is replaced in the bottle. The ear is positioned so that the drops can run down the canal. This position should be maintained for 2 minutes after ear drop administration to allow dispersion of drops. Collaborative care of external otitis is shown in Table 20-14.

CERUMEN AND FOREIGN BODIES IN THE EXTERNAL EAR CANAL

Impacted cerumen can cause discomfort and decreased hearing, which is often described as a hollow sensation. In the older person, the earwax becomes dense and drier. Tragal and external auditory canal hairs become thicker and coarser entrapping the hard dry cerumen in the canal.[26] Water that enters the canal during a shower or swimming may cause swelling of the cerumen, resulting in complete blockage of the canal. Symptoms of cerumen impaction are outlined in Table 20-15. Management involves irrigation of the canal with body-temperature solutions. Special syringes can be used and vary from the simple bulb syringe to special irrigating equipment used in the physician's office or clinic (Fig. 20-8). The patient is placed in a sitting position with an emesis basin under the ear. The auricle is pulled up and back, and the flow of solution is directed to the top of the canal. It is important that the ear canal not be completely occluded with the syringe tip. If irrigation does not remove the wax, a cerumen spoon can be used. Mild lubricant drops may be used (sometimes overnight) to soften the earwax, and irrigation may then be effective in removing the impacted cerumen. It may need to be removed by a physician using an operating microscope, suction, and microsurgical instruments.

The list of objects removed from the ear is extensive and includes animate, inanimate, vegetable, and mineral objects. Attempts to remove the object occasionally result in pushing it

Table 20-15 Clinical Manifestations of Cerumen Impaction

Hearing loss
Otalgia
Tinnitus
Vertigo
Cough
Cardiac depression (vagal stimulation)

further into the canal. Removal should be done by an otolaryngologist. Vegetable matter tends to swell and may create a secondary inflammation making removal more difficult.

Animate objects must be immobilized before removal. Mineral oil or lidocaine can be used to drown an insect.[27] The organism can then be removed with microscope guidance. If a wood tick has become attached to the tissue, it can be removed with ear forceps or it may be extracted under microscope guidance. Care should be taken to avoid crushing the wood tick, thereby leaving its head attached to the tissue, which may cause infection.

MALIGNANCY OF THE EXTERNAL EAR

Malignancies of the external ear (other than skin cancers) and canal are uncommon. The predominant signs include a chronic ulcer of the auricle and persistent drainage from the canal much like that seen with otitis externa. This drainage may be tinged with blood and does not diminish with treatment. Collaborative care includes biopsy and other diagnostic studies such as a computerized tomography (CT) scan to determine invasion of underlying tissue and bone. Treatment usually involves surgery. If the malignancy involves the ear canal and temporal bone, radical surgery of the middle and inner ear with resection of the facial nerve (CN VII), auditory nerve (CN VIII), and part of the temporal bone may be necessary.

Squamous cell carcinoma represents 55% of all skin cancers involving the ear. Cosmetic deformities are common and difficult to reconstruct. Basal cell carcinoma of the auricle accounts for approximately 1.5% of all basal cell carcinomas of the head and neck. It is usually seen in fair-skinned persons with long hours of sun exposure. These skin cancers can be excised surgically, or they may be serially excised using a special technique to microscopically examine the tissue to ensure that all residual cancer cells are resected. This procedure is known as Mohs' chemosurgery. These skin cancers are usually not life-threatening, and the cure rate after resection is greater than 90% in most cases. Melanoma may also occur on the external ear; treatment depends on the extent of the lesion. These lesions tend to metastasize either by lymphatics or the bloodstream.

MIDDLE EAR AND MASTOID

ACUTE OTITIS MEDIA

The most common problem of the middle ear is *acute otitis media*, usually a childhood disease associated with colds, sore throats, and blockage of the eustachian tube. The earlier the initial episode, the greater the risk of subsequent episodes. Risk

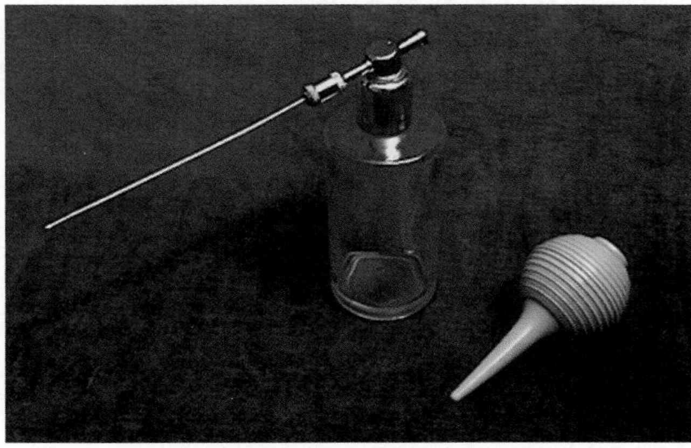

Fig. 20-8 Types of equipment used to irrigate the external ear canal. A bulb syringe (*right*) and an ear irrigation apparatus used in doctors' offices and clinics (*left*) are shown.

factors include young age, congenital abnormalities, immune deficiencies, passive smoke inhalation, eustachian tube damage from viral infections, family history of otitis media, recent upper respiratory infections, male gender, participation in day care, bottle feeding, and allergic rhinitis.[28] Although most patients have mixed infections, bacteria are the predominant etiologic agents. Pain, fever, malaise, headache, and reduced hearing are signs and symptoms of acute otitis media.

Collaborative care involves the use of antibiotics to eradicate the causative organism. Amoxicillin for 10 days is the current therapy of choice in the United States. Surgical intervention is generally reserved for the patient who does not respond to medical treatment. A *myringotomy* involves an incision in the tympanum to release the increased pressure and exudate in the ear. A tympanostomy tube may be placed for short- or long-term use. Prompt treatment of an episode of acute otitis media generally prevents spontaneous perforation of the tympanic membrane. In the adult patient for whom allergy may be an accompanying factor, antihistamines may also be prescribed. Otherwise, antihistamines have not proven effective.[29] Since the advent of treatment with antibiotics, the incidence of severe and prolonged infections of the middle ear and mastoid has been greatly reduced except in developing countries where health care is inadequate or people have limited access to health care.

CHRONIC OTITIS MEDIA AND MASTOIDITIS

Etiology and Pathophysiology

Untreated or repeated attacks of acute otitis media may lead to a chronic condition. Chronic infection of the middle ear is more common in persons who experience episodes of acute otitis media in early childhood. Organisms involved in chronic otitis media include *S. aureus, Streptococcus, Proteus mirabilis, P. aeruginosa*, and *E. coli*. Because the mucous membrane is continuous, both the middle ear and the air cells of the mastoid can be involved in the chronic infectious process.

Clinical Manifestations

Chronic otitis media is characterized by a purulent, mucoid, or serous discharge accompanied by hearing loss and occasionally

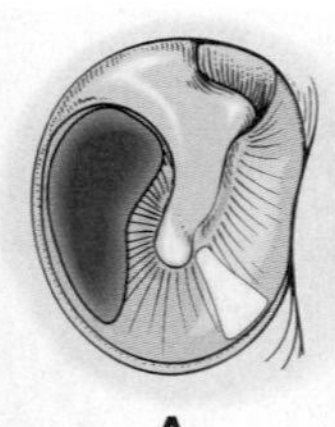

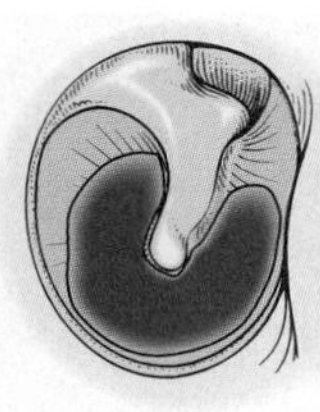

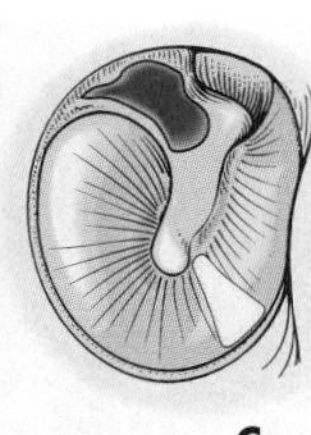

Fig. 20-9 Three common tympanic perforations. **A,** Small central perforation (hearing is usually good). **B,** Large central perforation around the handle of the malleus (hearing is usually poor). **C,** Marginal perforation of Shrapnell's membrane (hearing is usually good). Cholesteatomas commonly occur in patients with a marginal perforation and are always present with attic perforation.

by ear pain, nausea, and episodes of dizziness. The patient may complain of hearing loss that may be a result of destruction of the ossicles, a tympanic membrane perforation, or the accumulation of fluid in the middle ear space. Occasionally a facial palsy or an attack of vertigo may alert the patient to this condition. Chronic otitis media is usually painless, but if pain is present, it indicates fluid under pressure.

Complications

Untreated conditions can result in perforation of the eardrum and the formation of a cholesteatoma (an accumulation of keratinizing squamous epithelium in the middle ear). Its enlarging tumorlike behavior may destroy the adjacent bones, including the ossicles. Unless removed surgically a cholesteatoma can cause extensive damage to the structures of the middle ear, can erode the bony protection of the facial nerve, may create a labyrinthine fistula, or even invade the dura, threatening the brain. In addition to cholesteatoma, other complications of chronic otitis media include sensorineural hearing loss, facial nerve dysfunction, lateral sinus thrombosis, brain or subdural abscess, and meningitis.[27]

Diagnostic Studies

Otoscopic examination may reveal a marginal or central perforation of the eardrum (Fig. 20-9). Some eardrums may be healed but have an area that is more flaccid and thinner, indicating a previous perforation. Culture and sensitivity tests are necessary to identify the organisms involved so that the appropriate antibiotic can be prescribed. The audiogram may demonstrate no loss in hearing or a loss as great as 50 to 60 dB if the ossicles have been partially destroyed or disarticulated (separated). Sinus x-rays, magnetic resonance imaging (MRI), or a CT scan of the temporal bone may demonstrate bone destruction, absence of ossicles, or the presence of a mass, most likely a cholesteatoma.

Collaborative Care

The aim of treatment is to clear the middle ear of infection (Table 20-16). Systemic antibiotic therapy based on the culture and sensitivity results is initiated. In addition, the patient may need to undergo frequent evacuation of drainage and debris in an outpatient setting. Antibiotic ear drops and 2% acetic acid drops are also used to reduce infection. If there is a recurrence, the patient may need to be treated with parenteral antibiotics.

COLLABORATIVE CARE

Table 20-16 Chronic Otitis Media

Diagnostic
- Otoscopic examination
- Culture and sensitivity of middle ear drainage
- Mastoid x-ray

Collaborative Therapy
- Ear irrigations
- Acetic acid (equal amounts of white vinegar and warm water)
- Otic drops, powders
- Analgesics
- Antiemetics
- Systemic antibiotics
- Surgery
  - Tympanoplasty*
  - Mastoidectomy

*See Table 20-17.

Table 20-17 Surgical Therapy for Chronic Ear Infection

Myringoplasty
Surgical reconstruction limited to repair of a tympanic membrane perforation

Tympanoplasty without Mastoidectomy
An operation to eradicate disease in the middle ear and to reconstruct the hearing mechanism without mastoid surgery; with or without tympanic membrane grafting

Tympanoplasty with Mastoidectomy
An operation to eradicate disease in both the middle ear and the mastoid process and to reconstruct the middle ear conduction mechanism; with or without tympanic membrane grafting

In many cases of chronic otitis media, additional antimicrobial therapy is futile and its effectiveness is reduced as the number of treatments increases.

Surgical Therapy. Often chronic tympanic membrane perforations will not heal in response to conservative treatment, and surgery is necessary. Surgery involving reconstruction of the tympanic membrane and/or the ossicular chain is called a *tympanoplasty* (Table 20-17). Diseased tissue is removed, and the ossicles are examined and evaluated in reconstructing the conductive mechanism. This may be done with the use of partial or total ossicular prostheses in combination with a fascia graft to repair the perforation of the tympanic membrane. The incision may be endaural (incision within the ear canal) or postauricular (behind the auricle or ear), depending on the amount of involvement.

A *mastoidectomy* is often performed with tympanoplasty to remove diseased tissue and the source of infection. A modified mastoidectomy attempts to preserve functioning by removing as little structural tissue as possible. Removal of tissue stops at the middle ear structures that appear capable of functioning in the conduction of sound. A radical mastoidectomy, which involves complete removal of all middle ear structures, is required when disease is extensive or when complete exposure is necessary. No attempt is made to restore conductive hearing. The middle ear and mastoid become one large cavity. This surgery is rarely performed today, but it was not uncommon before antibiotics were available to treat ear infections. Patients seen today with a history of this type of surgery would have been children or young adults in the early 1940s or may have been raised in an area without adequate medical treatment.

NURSING MANAGEMENT: ACUTE OTITIS MEDIA

■ Following Tympanoplasty

Routine preoperative care is provided before tympanoplasty and includes teaching postoperative expectations. Postoperative concerns are the avoidance of complications such as disruption of the repair during the healing phase, facial nerve paralysis (rare), and increased pressure in the middle ear. The patient is instructed to avoid blowing the nose because this causes increased pressure in the eustachian tube and the middle ear cavity and could dislodge the tympanum graft. Coughing and sneezing can cause similar disruption and are to be avoided if possible. If the patient must cough or sneeze, leaving the mouth open will reduce the pressure. It is essential that the patient be helped when getting up the first time; because of dizziness and a loss of balance, a resulting fall may occur.

A cotton ball dressing is used for an endaural incision. If a postauricular incision is used and a drain is in place, a mastoid dressing is used. A 4 x 4-inch dressing is cut to fit behind the ear, and fluffs are applied over the ear to prevent the outer circular head dressing from placing pressure on the auricle. It is necessary to monitor the tightness of the dressing (to prevent tissue necrosis) and the amount and type of drainage postoperatively.

CHRONIC OTITIS MEDIA WITH EFFUSION

Chronic otitis media with effusion is an inflammation of the middle ear in which a collection of fluid is present in the middle ear space. The fluid may be thin, mucoid, or purulent. This condition is commonly called "glue ear," secretory otitis media, and serous otitis media. It may occur at any age but is more frequent in children. The fluid usually collects because of a malfunction of the eustachian tube, which commonly follows upper respiratory and chronic sinus infections, barotrauma (caused by pressure change), or otitis media. If the eustachian tube does not open and allow equalization of atmospheric pressure, negative pressure within the middle ear causes fluid transudation from the tissues. Allergic reaction of the mucosa creating edema can also cause blockage of the eustachian tube and cause fluid within the ear. Overgrowth of nasopharyngeal lymphoid tissue and chronic sinusitis are also factors that may contribute to middle ear effusion.

Complaints include a feeling of fullness of the ear, "plugged" feeling or popping, and decreased hearing. The patient does not experience pain, fever, or discharge from the ear. Otoscopic examination may reveal a normal tympanic membrane or minimal dullness and retraction. Tympanometry and pneumatoscopy may demonstrate limited tympanic membrane motion.

Decongestants, antihistamines, and corticosteroids, as well as antibiotics, have been used in the treatment of middle ear effusions. Exercises such as swallowing and gum chewing are used to open the eustachian tube. In addition, the patient may be taught Valsalva's maneuver (nose and mouth are closed off, forcing air into middle ear through the eustachian tube). If the effusion is not relieved after a period of time, a myringotomy is performed, usually under local or topical anesthesia with an operating microscope. A ventilating tube is frequently used for the person who has recurrent otitis media with effusion or dysfunction of the eustachian tube. The patient who has a ventilating tube in the eardrum must be instructed not to swim or get water in the ear. Despite efforts to correct inadequate middle ear aeration, eustachian tube dysfunction may persist, causing collapse of the eardrum, conductive hearing loss, and formation of a cholesteatoma. Adenoidectomy may also be done in conjunction with myringotomy to correct the underlying problem of middle ear aeration.

OTOSCLEROSIS

Otosclerosis, an autosomal dominant disease, is the fixation of the footplate of the stapes in the oval window. It is a common cause of conductive hearing loss in young adults, especially women, and may accelerate during pregnancy. It is a common finding in children who have a rare disease known as osteogenesis imperfecta. Otosclerosis is bilateral in 80% to 90% of patients. Spongy bone develops from the bony labyrinth, causing immobilization of the footplate of the stapes, which reduces the transmission of vibrations to the inner ear fluids. Although hearing loss is typically bilateral, one ear may show greater hearing loss progression. The patient is often unaware of the problem until the loss becomes so severe that communication is difficult. Loss of hearing usually becomes increasingly severe. Otosclerosis is more prevalent among Europeans and North Americans and half as common in African-Americans.

Otoscopic examination may reveal a reddish blush of the tympanum (Schwartz's sign) caused by the vascular and bony changes within the middle ear. Tuning fork tests help identify the conductive component of the hearing loss. On the Rinne test, bone conduction will be better than air conduction if hearing loss is greater that 25 dB. The Weber test lateralizes to the ear with the greater conductive hearing loss. An audiogram demonstrates good hearing by bone conduction, but poor hearing is demonstrated by air conduction or an air-bone gap audiogram. Usually at least a difference of 20 dB to 25 dB between air-conduction and bone-conduction levels of hearing is seen in otosclerosis.

Collaborative Care

A *stapedectomy* is the surgical treatment for otosclerosis and is usually performed under local anesthesia with sedation. The ear with poorer hearing is repaired first, and the other ear may be operated on 6 months to a year later. (Collaborative care of otosclerosis is shown in Table 20-18.)

In stapedectomy an endaural incision is made using the operating microscope for visualization. Generally the stapes superstructure is removed, and a small hole is made in the footplate with a drill or laser. A prosthesis made of stainless steel, Teflon, or other synthetic material completes the ossicular chain. Sound is then conducted with the prosthesis. The tympanum is rolled back into normal position, and Gelfoam is

COLLABORATIVE CARE

Table 20-18 Otosclerosis

Diagnostic
Otoscopic examination
Rinne test (512 Hz tuning fork)
Weber test
Audiometry
Tympanometry
Collaborative Therapy
Hearing aid
Surgery (stapedectomy)
Analgesics
Antiemetics
Antibiotics
Antimotion drugs

placed on the flap. A cotton ball is placed in the ear canal and a Band-Aid dressing is used to cover the ear. During surgery the patient will often report an immediate improvement in hearing in the operative ear. Because of the accumulation of blood and fluid in the middle ear, the hearing level decreases postoperatively but does return to near-normal levels. After stapedectomy, 90% of patients experience an improvement in hearing, in many instances near normal.[30]

A *perilymph fistula* (incomplete closure of the oval window) may occur with symptoms of fluctuating hearing levels, tinnitus, vertigo, and nystagmus. A small percentage of patients may develop a sensorineural hearing loss. Improved surgical techniques have dramatically lowered the incidence of perilymph fistula. An audiogram is repeated when the ear heals.

NURSING MANAGEMENT: OTOSCLEROSIS

Nursing management of the patient undergoing a stapedectomy is similar to that for the patient who has undergone a tympanoplasty. Postoperatively, the patient may experience dizziness, nausea, and vomiting as a result of stimulation of the labyrinth intraoperatively. Some patients demonstrate nystagmus on lateral gaze because of disturbance of the perilymph. Care should be taken to decrease sudden movements by the patient that may bring on or exacerbate dizziness. Actions (coughing, sneezing, lifting, bending, straining during bowel movements) should also be minimized.

INNER EAR PROBLEMS

Three symptoms that indicate disease of the inner ear are vertigo (whirling), sensorineural hearing loss, and tinnitus (ringing in the ear). Symptoms of vertigo arise from the vestibular labyrinth, whereas hearing loss and tinnitus arise from the auditory labyrinth. There is an overlap between manifestations of inner ear problems and CNS disorders.

MÉNIÈRE'S DISEASE

Ménière's disease (idiopathic endolymphatic hydrops) is characterized by symptoms caused by inner ear disease: episodic vertigo, tinnitus, fluctuating sensorineural hearing loss, and aural fullness. It causes significant disability for the patient because of sudden, severe attacks of vertigo with nausea and vomiting. Symptoms usually begin between 30 and 60 years of age. In 40% of patients with Ménière's disease, bilateral involvement is found.

The cause of the disease is unknown, but it results in an excessive accumulation of endolymph in the membranous labyrinth. The volume of endolymph increases until the membranous labyrinth ruptures, mixing high-potassium endolymph with low-potassium perilymph. These changes lead to degeneration of the delicate vestibular and cochlear hair cells. Attacks of vertigo are sudden with little or no warning. Attacks may be preceded by a sense of fullness in the ear, increasing tinnitus, and a decrease in hearing. The patient may experience the feeling of being pulled to the ground ("drop attacks"). Only 7% of patients with Ménière's report this symptom. Some patients report that they feel as if they are whirling in space. The duration of attacks may be hours or days, and may occur several times a year. Autonomic symptoms include pallor, sweating, nausea, and vomiting.

The clinical course of the disease is highly variable. Low-pitched tinnitus may be present continuously in the affected ear or it may be intensified during an attack. It is often described as a "roar," or "like the ocean." Hearing loss fluctuates, and with continued attacks, hearing recovery is often less complete with each episode, eventually leading to progressive permanent hearing loss.

NURSING AND COLLABORATIVE MANAGEMENT: MÉNIÈRE'S DIESEASE

Collaborative care of Ménière's disease (Table 20-19) includes diagnostic tests to rule out central nervous system disease. The audiogram demonstrates a mild low-frequency sensorineural hearing loss. Vestibular tests indicate decreased function.

A glycerol test may aid in the diagnosis of Ménière's disease. An oral dose of glycerol is given, and standard audiometry is tested before and approximately 2.5 hours after administration. Improvement in hearing or speech discrimination supports a diagnosis of Ménière's disease. The improvement is attributed to the osmotic effect of glycerol that pulls fluid from the inner ear. Although a positive test is diagnostic of Ménière's disease, a negative test does not rule out the condition.

During the acute attack, antihistamines, anticholinergics, and benzodiazepines can be used as suppressants of the labyrinth. Acute vertigo is treated symptomatically with bed rest, sedation, and antiemetics or drugs for motion sickness administered orally, rectally, or intravenously. The patient requires reassurance and counseling that the condition is not life threatening. Management between attacks may include vasodilation, diuretics, antihistamines, a low-sodium diet, and avoidance of caffeine and nicotine. Diazepam (Valium) and Antivert (Bonamine plus nicotinic acid) are commonly used to reduce the dizziness. Over a period of time, most patients respond to the prescribed medications but must learn to live with the unpredictability of the attacks. Approximately 75% to 85% of patients experience improvement with medical management and supportive therapy; the remainder of patients may, in time, require surgical intervention.[26]

Frequent and incapacitating attacks, reduced quality of life, and threatened unemployment are indications for surgical

COLLABORATIVE CARE

Table 20-19 Meniere's Disease

Diagnostic
- History
- Audiometric studies, including speech discrimination, tone decay
- Vestibular tests, including caloric test, positional test
- Electronystagmography
- Neurologic examination
- Glycerol test

Collaborative Therapy

Acute Care (one or more)
- Sedative (diazepam [Valium])
- Anticholinergic (atropine)
- Vasodilators
- Antihistamine (diphenhydramine [Benadryl])

Surgical Therapy

Conservative Surgical Intervention
- Endolymphatic shunt
- Vestibular nerve section

Destructive Surgical Intervention
- Labyrinthotomy
- Labyrinthectomy

Ambulatory/Home Care (one or more)
- Diuretics
- Antihistamines
- Vasodilators
- Neuroleptics
- Vitamins
- Diazepam (Valium)
- Low-salt diet
- Restriction of caffeine, nicotine, and alcohol intake

intervention. Surgical decompression of the endolymphatic sac is performed to reduce the pressure on the cochlear hair cells and to prevent further damage and hearing loss. If relief is not achieved with endolymphatic shunt surgery and hearing remains good, vestibular nerve resection may be performed to alleviate vertigo and preserve hearing. When involvement is unilateral, surgical ablation of the labyrinth, resulting in loss of the vestibular and hearing cochlear function, is performed. Careful therapeutic management can decrease the possibility of progressive sensorineural loss in many patients.

Nursing interventions are planned to minimize vertigo and provide for patient safety. During the acute attack the patient is kept in a quiet, darkened room in a comfortable position. Instruct the patient to avoid sudden head movements or position changes. Fluorescent or flickering lights or watching television may exacerbate symptoms and should be avoided. An emesis basin should be available because vomiting is common. To minimize the risk of falling the nurse should keep the siderails up and the bed low in position when the patient is in bed. The patient should be instructed to call for assistance when getting out of bed. Medications and fluids are administered parenterally, and intake and output are monitored. When the attack subsides, assist the patient with ambulation because unsteadiness may remain. Similar nursing care is provided after surgical ablation of the labyrinth. The patient will have severe tinnitus and vertigo, which decrease during a period of days or weeks as the brain adjusts to loss of vestibular input and postural stability is regained.

PRESBYCUSIS

Presbycusis, the hearing of old age, includes the loss of peripheral auditory sensitivity, a decline in word recognition ability, and associated psychologic and communication issues. Because consonants (high-frequency sounds) are the letters by which spoken words are recognized, the ability of the older person with presbycusis to understand the spoken word is greatly affected. Presbycusis usually reflects a gradual decline in hearing sensitivity. Vowels are heard, but some consonants fall into the high-frequency range and cannot be differentiated. This may lead to confusion and embarrassment because of the difference in what was said and what was heard.

The cause of presbycusis is related to degenerative changes in the inner ear such as loss of hair cells, reduction of blood supply, diminution of endolymph production, decreased basilar membrane flexibility, and loss of neurons in the cochlear nuclei. Noise exposure is thought to be a common factor related to presbycusis. Table 20-20 describes the classification of specific causes and associated hearing changes of presbycusis. Often, more than one type of presbycusis may be present in the same person. The prognosis for hearing depends on the cause of the presbycusis. Sound amplification with the appropriate device is often helpful in improving the understanding of speech. In other situations an audiologic rehabilitation program can be valuable.

The older adult is often reluctant to use a hearing aid for amplification. Reasons cited most often include cost, appearance, insufficient knowledge about hearing aids, amplification of competing noise, and unrealistic expectations. Most hearing aids and batteries are small, and neuromuscular changes such as stiff fingers, enlarged joints, and decreased sensory perception often make the care and handling of a hearing aid a difficult and frustrating experience for an older person. The elderly also tend to accept their losses as part of getting older and believe there is no need for improvement.

LABYRINTHITIS

Labyrinthitis is an inflammation of the inner ear affecting the cochlear or vestibular portion of the labyrinth or both. Infection can enter from the meninges, the middle ear, or the bloodstream. Symptoms include vertigo, tinnitus, and sensorineural hearing loss on the affected side. This condition is rare since the advent of antibiotics. *Nystagmus*, an abnormal rhythmic, jerking movement of the eyes, accompanies the vertigo and has a horizontal beat. Nystagmus is caused by abnormal currents in the endolymph fluid, causing the eyes to have a rhythmic jerking movement.

Suppurative labyrinthitis from infection causes severe vertigo with nausea and vomiting similar to that of an attack of Ménière's disease. Complete destruction of the cochlea and labyrinth occurs, causing permanent deafness. Loss of vestibular input causes extreme unsteadiness in the patient. The patient requires physical therapy to recondition the brain to interpret vestibular input. *Vestibular neuronitis* causes vertigo,

Table 20-20 Classification of Presbycusis

Type	Cause	Hearing Change and Prognosis
▪ Sensory	Atrophy of auditory nerve; loss of sensory hair cells	Loss of high-pitched sounds, little effect on speech understanding; good response to sound amplification
▪ Neural	Degenerative changes in cochlea and spinal ganglion	Loss of speech discrimination; amplification alone not sufficient
▪ Metabolic	Atrophy of blood vessels in wall of cochlea with interruption of essential nutrient supply	Uniform loss for all frequencies accompanied by recruitment*; good response to hearing aid
▪ Cochlear	Stiffening of basilar membrane, which interferes with sound transmission in the cochlea	Hearing loss increases from low to high frequencies; speech discrimination affected with higher frequency losses; helped by appropriate forms of amplification

*Abnormally rapid increase in loudness as sound intensity increases.

nausea, vomiting, and nystagmus. A viral infection may be the cause. The patient recovers after 7 to 10 days. Tinnitus is not present, and hearing loss does not occur. Toxic or serous labyrinthitis is associated with acute otitis media. It is caused by bacterial toxins diffusing through the round window membrane. High-frequency hearing loss and mild to moderate vertigo may occur.

ACOUSTIC NEUROMA

An *acoustic neuroma* (or vestibular schwannoma) is a benign tumor that occurs where the acoustic nerve (CN VIII) enters the internal auditory canal or the temporal bone from the brain. It is important that early diagnosis be made because the tumor can compress the facial nerve and arteries within the internal auditory canal. Once the tumor has expanded and become an intracranial neoplasm, more extensive surgery is necessary, reducing the chances of preserving hearing and normal facial nerve function. It can expand into the cerebellopontine angle and involve other cranial nerves and the brain by compression.

Early symptoms are associated with eighth cranial nerve compression and destruction. They include unilateral, progressive, sensorineural hearing loss, unilateral tinnitus, and mild intermittent vertigo. One of the earliest symptoms of an acoustic neuroma is reduced touch sensation in the posterior ear canal. Diagnostic tests include neurologic, audiometric, and vestibular tests, and CT scans and MRI with gadolinium enhancement.

Surgery to remove small tumors is performed through the middle cranial fossa or retrolabyrinthine approach, which preserves hearing and vestibular function. A translabyrinthine approach is usually used for medium-sized tumors and when hearing is minimal. Although hearing is destroyed by this approach, advantages include good access to the tumor and preservation of the facial nerve. Retrosigmoid (suboccipital) or transotic approaches are used for large tumors (larger than 3 cm). It is almost impossible to preserve hearing when the tumor is larger than 2 cm.

HEARING IMPAIRMENT AND DEAFNESS

Communication disorders are the primary handicapping disability in the United States. Twenty-eight million persons in the United States have impaired hearing in one or both ears. The majority of persons lost their hearing as adults. Hearing impairment is common among older adults. Nearly half of the persons who need assistance with hearing disorders are 65 years of age or older. Between 2% and 4% of children have a hearing loss, with 3 million school-age children affected.[31]

Types of Hearing Loss

Conductive Hearing Loss. *Conductive hearing loss* occurs in the outer and middle ear and impairs the sound being conducted from the outer to the inner ear. It is caused by conditions interfering with air conduction, such as impacted cerumen, middle ear disease, otosclerosis, and atresia or stenosis of the external auditory canal. The audiogram demonstrates an air-bone gap of at least 15 dB. The most common cause of conductive hearing loss is otitis media with effusion.

An air-bone gap occurs when hearing sensitivity by bone conduction is significantly better than by air conduction. The patient may speak softly because he or she hears his or her voice, which is conducted by bone, as being loud. This patient hears better in a noisy environment. A hearing aid is helpful for a patient with a 40 to 50 dB loss or more, although the device often is not necessary because of the excellent results of treatment of the underlying problem.

Sensorineural Hearing Loss. *Sensorineural hearing loss* is caused by impairment of function of the inner ear or its central connections. Congenital and hereditary factors, noise trauma during a period of time, aging (presbycusis), Ménière's disease, and ototoxicity can cause sensorineural hearing loss. Systemic diseases, such as tuberculosis, syphilis, Lyme disease, cytomegalovirus, HIV, and Paget's disease of the bone, can also cause sensorineural deafness. Immune diseases, diabetes, bacterial meningitis, and trauma are also causes of this type of hearing loss. The two main problems associated with sensorineural loss are the ability to hear sound but not to understand speech and lack of understanding of the problem by others. The ability to hear high-pitched sounds diminishes with sensorineural hearing loss. Consonants are high-pitched sounds that give intelligibility to speech. Words become difficult to distinguish, and sound becomes muffled. An audiogram demonstrates a loss in dB levels of the 4000 Hz range, which can progress to the 2000 Hz range. A hearing aid may help the patient who has a 30 dB loss or more by reducing the strain of trying to hear, but the sounds will still be muffled. *Presbycusis*, degenerative change of the inner ear, is a major cause of sensorineural hearing loss in the older adult. It is a progressive problem that results in many psychologic and communication issues. The control of inner ear diseases such as Ménière's disease can prevent further hearing loss. If using ototoxic drugs, hearing should be monitored frequently during treatment.

Mixed Hearing Loss. *Mixed hearing loss* is caused by a combination of conductive and sensorineural losses. Careful evaluation is needed before corrective surgery for conductive loss is planned because the sensorineural component of the hearing loss will still remain.

Central and Functional Hearing Loss. *Central hearing loss* is caused by problems in the CNS from the auditory nucleus to the cortex. The patient is unable to understand or to put meaning to the incoming sound. *Functional hearing loss* may be caused by an emotional or psychologic factor. The patient does not seem to hear or respond to pure-tone subjective hearing tests, but no organic cause can be identified. A careful history is helpful because there is usually a reference to deafness within the family. Psychologic counseling may help. Referral to qualified hearing and speech services is indicated.

Classification of Hearing Loss. Hearing loss can also be classified by the decibel (dB) level or loss as recorded on the audiogram. Normal hearing is in the 0 to 15 dB range. Slight hearing loss is in the 16 to 25 dB range. A mild impairment is present at the 26 to 40 dB hearing level. A moderate impairment is in the 41 to 55 dB range. A moderately severe impairment is in the 56 to 70 dB range. The severely impaired have a loss in the 71 to 90 dB range. The profoundly deaf have a loss greater than 91 dB. Many persons in this last group are congenitally deaf.

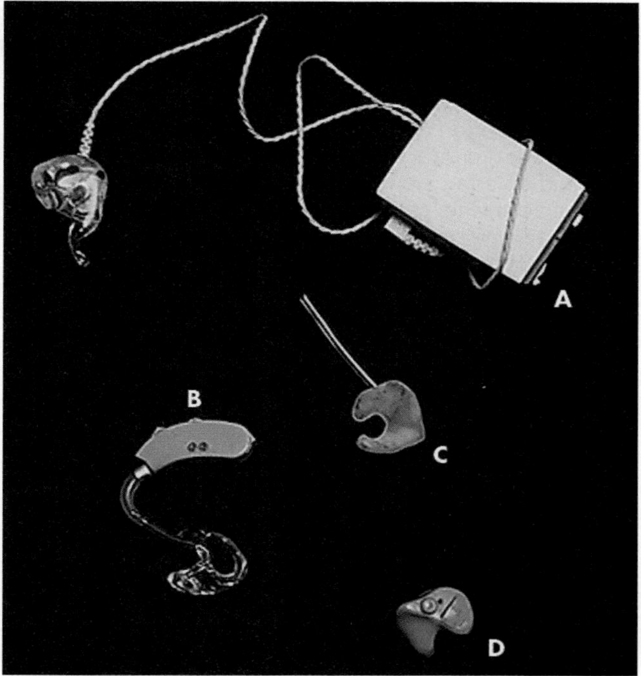

Fig. 20-10 Types of hearing aids and ear molds. **A,** Older aid worn on the body with a wire connected to the ear mold. **B,** Behind-the-ear aid with ear mold. **C,** Small ear mold. **D,** Smaller hearing aid worn in the ear canal.

Clinical Manifestations

If the hearing loss is congenital and significant, the young child will have significant speech and language problems. Rehabilitation must be started early.

Deafness is often called the "unseen handicap" because it is not until conversation is initiated with a deaf adult that the difficulty in communication is realized. It is important that the health professional be aware of the need for thorough validation of the deaf person's understanding of health teaching. Descriptive visual aids can be helpful. Because of the difficulty in communication, deaf persons often seek relationships with other deaf persons. The person who develops hearing loss later in life varies in the amount of loss and the reactions to it.

Interference in communication and interaction with others can be the source of many problems for the patient and family. Often the patient refuses to admit or may be unaware of impaired hearing. Irritability is common because of the concentration with which the patient must listen to understand speech. The loss of clarity of speech in the patient with sensorineural hearing loss is most frustrating. The patient may hear what is said but not understand it. Withdrawal, suspicion, loss of self-esteem, and insecurity are commonly associated with advancing hearing loss.

Collaborative Care: Patient with Impaired Hearing

Hearing Aids. It is important that the patient with a suspected hearing loss have a hearing assessment by a qualified audiologist, including examination and audiometric testing. If a hearing aid is indicated, it should be fitted by an audiologist or a speech and hearing specialist. There are many types of aids available each with advantages and disadvantages: the body-worn aid, the eyeglasses style, the behind-the-ear style, the in-the-ear style (Fig. 20-10), and the implantable hearing aid. The conventional hearing aid serves as a simple amplifier. For the patient with bilateral hearing impairment, binaural hearing aids provide the best sound lateralization and speech discrimination. Patients who are motivated and optimistic about using a hearing aid will be more successful users. The nurse must be prepared to give careful instruction on its use and maintenance and to assist the patient during the period of adjustment.

Initially, use of the hearing aid should be restricted to quiet situations in the home. The patient must first adjust to voices (including the patient's own) and household sounds. The patient should also experiment by increasing and decreasing the volume as situations require. As adjustment to the increase in sounds and background noise occurs, the patient will be ready to try a different listening environment, such as a small party where several people will be talking simultaneously. Next the environment can be expanded to the outdoors. After adapting to controlled situations, the patient will be ready to encounter environments such as the shopping mall or grocery store. Adjustment to different environments occurs gradually, depending on the individual patient.

When the hearing aid is not being worn, it should be placed in a dry cool area where it will not be inadvertently damaged or lost. The battery should be disconnected or removed. Battery life averages 1 week, and patients should be advised to purchase only a month's supply at a time. Earmolds should be cleaned weekly or as needed. Toothpicks or pipe cleaners may be used to clear a clogged eartip.

Speech Reading. Speech reading, commonly called lip reading, can be helpful in increasing communication. It allows for approximately 40% understanding of the spoken word. The patient is able to use visual cues associated with speech, such as gestures and facial expression, to help clarify

Table 20-21 Communication with the Patient with Impaired Hearing

Nonverbal Aids
- Draw attention with hand movements.
- Have speaker's face in good light.
- Avoid covering mouth or face with hands.
- Avoid chewing, eating, smoking while talking.
- Maintain eye contact.
- Avoid distracting environments.
- Avoid careless expression that the patient may misinterpret.
- Use touch.
- Move close to better ear.
- Avoid light behind speaker.

Verbal Aids
- Speak normally and slowly.
- Do not overexaggerate facial expressions.
- Do not overenunciate.
- Use simple sentences.
- Rephrase sentence; use different words.
- Write name or difficult words.
- Avoid shouting.
- Speak in normal voice directly into better ear.

the spoken message. In speech reading, many words will look alike to the patient (e.g., rabbit and woman). If the patient wears glasses, the glasses should be used to facilitate speech reading. The nurse can help the patient by using and teaching verbal and nonverbal communication techniques as described in Table 20-21. If a hearing aid is used, it should be readily available to the patient.

Cochlear Implant. The cochlear implant is being used as a hearing device for the profoundly deaf. The system consists of a surgically implanted induction coil beneath the skin behind the ear and an electrode wire placed in the cochlea. The implanted parts interface with an externally worn speech processor. The system stimulates auditory nerve fibers by an electric current so signals reach the brainstem's auditory nuclei and ultimately, the auditory cortex. The implant is intended for the patient whose sensorineural hearing loss is either congenital or acquired. The ideal candidate is one who has become deaf after acquiring speech and language. The adult who was born deaf or became deaf before learning to speak is generally not considered a candidate for a cochlear implant.[32]

The implant offers the profoundly deaf the ability to hear environmental sounds including speech at comfortable loudness levels. Multichannel cochlear implants also serve as aids to

CRITICAL THINKING EXERCISES

CASE STUDY

Argon Laser Trabeculoplasty

Patient Profile

Ms. R., an 83-year-old woman with rheumatoid arthritis, returns to the ambulatory clinic for follow-up care of primary open-angle glaucoma (POAG). Her current medical regimen includes topical Timoptic (Timolol maleate) 0.5% bid OU and Xalatan 0.005% q hs OU. Her intraocular pressures are stable on this regimen.

Subjective Data

- Reports stable vision.
- States she is not always successful in getting the eye drops instilled as her hands are gnarled and painful from rheumatoid arthritis.

Objective Data

- Distance and near visual acuity is stable at 20/40 OU.
- Goldmann visual field testing reveals a new scotoma in the right eye.

Collaborative Care

Argon laser trabeculoplasty (ALT) is performed in the right eye under topical anesthesia. One hour after the procedure, intraocular pressure measures 19 mm Hg and she is discharged home. Postoperative medication includes 1% Pred Forte (topical steroid) eye drops to be used qid for 3 days in the right eye. She is to continue her regular antiglaucomatous topical drops as before in both eyes. She will return in 2 weeks for an ALT in the left eye and a follow-up examination of the right eye.

Critical Thinking Questions

1. Explain the etiology of Ms. R's new scotoma.
2. Why might ALT be an appropriate therapy in this case?
3. What is the purpose of the topical corticosteroid drops after the laser procedure?
4. What topics should the nurse discuss in discharge teaching?
5. What is the therapeutic goal of ALT?
6. Based on the assessment data, write one or more appropriate nursing diagnoses. Are there any collaborative problems?

Nursing Research Issues

1. Do patients who receive keratorefractive surgery report greater well-being postoperatively as compared with preoperatively?
2. What are the main coping strategies of the patient with severe visual impairment? How can the nurse best support these strategies?
3. What strategies are most effective in educating patients about avoiding sources of ocular irritation?
4. What factors contribute to the decision-making process for the patient with a cataract who chooses surgery over continued palliative therapy?
5. Are the significant differences in elderly patient outcomes when postoperative care following eye surgery includes visits by a home health care nurse?
6. Compare the effectiveness of different interventions to decrease the vertigo associated with Ménière's disease.
7. Does family support significantly influence patient usage and adjustment to a hearing aid?
8. What motivates a patient following a tympanoplasty to comply with the therapeutic regimen?

speech production. Extensive training and rehabilitation are essential to receive maximum benefit from these implants. The positive aspects of a cochlear implant include providing sound to the person who heard none, improving lip reading, monitoring the loudness of the person's own speech, improving the sense of security, and decreasing feelings of isolation. With continued research the cochlear implant may offer the possibility of aural rehabilitation for a wider range of hearing impaired individuals.

Assisted Listening Devices. Numerous devices are now available to assist the hearing impaired person. Direct amplification devices, amplified telephone receivers, alerting systems that flash when activated by sound, an infrared system for amplifying the sound of the television, and a combination FM receiver and hearing aid are all aids that can be explored by the nurse based on individual patient's needs.

REVIEW QUESTIONS

The number of the question corresponds to the same-numbered objective at the beginning of the chapter.

1. Presbyopia occurs in older individuals because
   a. the retina degenerates.
   b. the crystalline lens becomes inflexible.
   c. the corneal curvature becomes irregular.
   d. it is associated with cataract development.
2. The most important nursing intervention in patients with epidemic keratoconjunctivitis is
   a. applying patches to the affected eyes.
   b. accurately measuring intraocular pressure.
   c. monitoring near visual acuity every 4 hours.
   d. teaching patient and family members good hygiene techniques.
3. Patients with an eye inflammation or infection should be taught
   a. to apply a cold washcloth with pressure to the inflamed area frequently.
   b. that acute conditions commonly lead to chronic problems.
   c. that regular careful hand washing may prevent the infection from spreading.
   d. to wear dark glasses to prevent irritation from UV light.
4. Rubella can cause hearing problems if
   a. exposure is after 20 weeks gestation.
   b. the mother had rubella before age 18 years.
   c. exposure is before 16 weeks gestation.
   d. the mother is vaccinated during the puerperium.
5. In preparing patients for retinal detachment surgery, the nurse should
   a. begin explaining how to care for an ocular prosthesis.
   b. assure patients that they can expect 20/20 vision following surgery.
   c. teach the family how to recognize when the patient is hallucinating.
   d. assess the patient's level of knowledge about retinal detachment and provide information appropriate to the situation.
6. The nurse should instruct patients with glaucoma that
   a. they should see their family practitioner or internist every 2 months.
   b. punctal occlusion will lessen systemic absorption of glaucoma eye drops.
   c. if they use their drops properly, they can expect full resolution of the glaucoma.
   d. the frequent pain caused by the increased intraocular pressure can be controlled with analgesics.
7. The nurse would suspect otosclerosis from assessment findings of hearing loss in
   a. a 26-year-old female who has 3 biologic children under the age of 5 years.
   b. a 42-year-old female African-American who has a history of serous otitis media.
   c. a 52-year-old male whose hearing loss is accompanied by vertigo and tinnitus.
   d. a 63-year-old male who can hear high-pitched sounds more effectively than low-pitched sounds.
8. The patient who has a sensorineural hearing loss
   a. has difficulty understanding speech.
   b. may have a reversal of damage caused by ototoxic drugs.
   c. hears low-pitched sounds better than high-pitched sounds.
   d. experiences clearer sounds with the use of a hearing aid.
9. The nurse teaches the patient with extended wear contact lenses that
   a. the lenses may be worn up to 1 week without removal.
   b. the lenses may be moistened with saliva if necessary.
   c. any saline solution may be used for moistening as long as it is hypertonic.
   d. they may continue lens wear if they experience only mild to moderate irritation or redness.
10. A nursing measure that is helpful in communicating with a hearing impaired patient is to
    a. overenunciate speech.
    b. use simple sentences.
    c. raise the voice to a higher pitch.
    d. write out all questions and responses.
11. Patients with permanent visual impairment
    a. feel most comfortable with other visually impaired persons.
    b. may experience the same grieving process that is associated with other losses.
    c. may feel threatened when others make eye contact during a conversation.
    d. usually need others to speak louder so they can communicate appropriately.

References

1. Thompson JM and others, editors: *Mosby's clinical nursing,* ed 4, St Louis, 1997, Mosby.
2. Guyton AC, Hall JE, editors: *Textbook of medical physiology,* ed 9, Philadelphia, 1996, Saunders.
3. Schull P, editor: *Mastering geriatric care,* Springhouse, Penn, 1997, Springhouse.
4. Browstein B, Bronner S, editors: *Functional movement in orthopaedic and sports physical therapy,* New York, 1997, Churchill Livingstone.
5. Mead MD, Sieck EA, Steinert RF: Optical rehabilitation of aphakia. In Albert DM, Jakobiec FA, editors: *Principles and practice of ophthalmology: clinical practice,* vol 2, Philadelphia, 1994, Saunders.
6. Tortora CM, Hersh PS, Blaker JW: Optics of intraocular lenses. In Albert DM, Jakobiec FA, editors: *Principles and practice of ophthalmology: clinical practice,* ed 2, vol 5, Philadelphia, 1999, Saunders.
7. McGhee et al: *Excimer in lasers in ophthalmology: principles and practice,* Oxford, 1997, Butterworth-Heinemann.
8. Kraut JA, McCabe CP: The problem of low vision: definition and common problems. In Albert DM, Jakobiec FA, editors: *Principles and practice of ophthalmology: clinical practice,* ed 2, vol 5, Philadelphia, 1999, Saunders.
9. Brandt JT, Nason FE: Community resources for the ophthalmic practice. In Albert DM, Jakobiec FA, editors: *Principles and practice of ophthalmology: clinical practice,* ed 2, vol 5, Philadelphia, 1999, Saunders.

10. Bajart AM: Lid inflammations. In Albert DM, Jakobiec FA, editors: *Principles and practice of ophthalmology: clinical practice,* ed 2, vol 5, Philadelphia, 1999, Saunders.
11. Pavan-Langston D: Viral disease of the cornea and external eye. In Albert DM, Jakobiec FA, editors: *Principles and practice of ophthalmology: clinical practice,* ed 2, vol 5, Philadelphia, 1999, Saunders.
12. Avery RK, Baker AS: Chlamydial disease. In Albert DM, Jakobiec FA, editors: *Principles and practice of ophthalmology: clinical practice,* vol 5, Philadelphia, 1994, Saunders.
13. Adamis AP, Schein OD: *Chlamydia* and *Acanthamoeba* infections of the eye. In Albert DM, Jakobiec FA, editors: *Principles and practice of ophthalmology: clinical practice,* vol 5, Philadelphia, 1994, Saunders.
14. Foulks GN: Bacterial infections of the conjunctiva and cornea. In Albert DM, Jakobiec FA, editors: *Principles and practice of ophthalmology: clinical practice,* vol 5, Philadelphia, 1994, Saunders.
15. Talamo JH, Steinert RF: Keratorefractive surgery. In Albert DM, Jakobiec FA, editors: *Principles and practice of ophthalmology: clinical practice,* vol 5, Philadelphia, 1994, Saunders.
16. Boruchoff SA: Penetrating keratoplasty. In Albert DM, Jakobiec FA, editors: *Principles and practice of ophthalmology: clinical practice,* ed 2, vol 5, Philadelphia, 1999, Saunders.
17. Streeten BW: Pathology of the lens. In Albert DM, Jakobiec FA, editors: *Principles and practice of ophthalmology: clinical practice,* vol 5, Philadelphia, 1994, Saunders.
18. Haynie GD, D'Amico DJ: Scleral buckling surgery. In Albert DM, Jakobiec FA, editors: *Principles and practice of ophthalmology: clinical practice,* vol 5, Philadelphia, 1994, Saunders.
19. Vingerling JR and others: Age-related macular degeneration and smoking, *Ach Ophthalmol* 114:1193, 1996.
20. Capone A, editor: Alternative therapies in macular degeneration, *Semin Ophthalmology,* 112:1997.
21. Thomas JV: Primary open-angle glaucoma. In Albert DM, Jakobiec FA, editors: *Principles and practice of ophthalmology: clinical practice,* vol 5, Philadelphia, 1994, Saunders.
22. Richter CU: Laser therapy of open-angle glaucoma. In Albert DM, Jakobiec FA, editors: *Principles and practice of ophthalmology: clinical practice,* ed 2, vol 5, Philadelphia, 1999, Saunders.
23. Neff C, Sprag M: *Maternal and child health nursing,* Philadelphia, 1996, Lippincott.
24. Novy M: The normal puerperium. In DeCherney A, Pernoll M, editors: *Current obstetric and gynecologic diagnosis and treatment,* ed 8, Norwalk, Conn, 1994, Appleton & Lange.
25. Northern J: *Hearing disorders,* Boston, 1996, Allyn & Bacon.
26. Roland PS, Marple BF: Disorders of inner ear, eighth nerve, and CNS. In Roland PS, Marple BF, Mererhoff WL, editors: *Hearing loss,* New York, 1997, Thieme.
27. Parisier SC, Kimmelman CP, Hanson MB: Diseases of the external auditory canal. In Hughes GB, Pensak ML, editors: *Clinical otology,* New York, 1997, Thieme.
28. Bluestone CD, Klein JO, *Otitis media in infants and children,* Philadelphia, 1995, Saunders.
29. Healy GB : Otitis media and middle ear effusions. In Ballenger JJ, Snow JB, editors: *Otorhinolaryngology,* ed 15, Baltimore, 1996, Williams & Wilkins.
30. Thompson J and others, editors: *Mosby's clinical nursing,* St Louis, 1997, Mosby.
31. Schuller DE, Schleuning AJ: *DeWeese and Saunders' Otolaryngology—head and neck surgery,* ed 8, St Louis, 1994, Mosby.
32. Telischi F, Hodges A, Balkany T: Cochlear implants for deafness, *Hosp Pract* 29:55, 1994.

Resources

Acoustic Neuroma Association
PO Box 12402
Atlanta, GA 30355
404-237-2704
http://anausa.org/

Alexander Graham Bell Association for the Deaf
3417 Volta Place NW
Washington, DC 20007-2778
202-337-5220 (voice/TTY)
http://www.agbell.org/

American Academy of Otolaryngology
One Prince Street
Alexandria, VA 22314-3357
703-836-4444
http://www.entnet.org/

American Deafness & Rehabilitation Association
PO Box 251554
Little Rock, AR 72225
501-868-8850
Fax: 501-868-8812

American Foundation for the Blind
11 Penn Plaza, Suite 300
New York, NY 10001
212-502-7600
Fax: 212-502-7777
http://www.igc.apc.org/afb/index.html

American Society of Cataract & Refractive Surgery
4000 Legato Road, Suite 850
Fairfax, VA 22033
703-591-2220
Fax: 703-591-0614
http://www.ascrs.org/

American Society of Ophthalmic Registered Nurses, Inc.
PO Box 193030
San Francisco, CA 94119
415-561-8513

American Speech-Language-Hearing Association
10801 Rockville Pike
Rockville, MD 20852
301-897-5700

Associated Services for the Blind
919 Walnut Street
Philadelphia, PA 19107

Association for Education & Rehabilitation of the Blind & Visually Impaired
206 N. Washington Street, Suite 320
Alexandria, VA 22314
703-548-1884
Fax: 703-683-2926

Association for Research in Vision & Opthamology
9650 Rockville Pike
Bethesda, MD 20814-3998
301-571-1844
Fax: 301-571-8311
http://www.faseb.org/arvo/

Better Hearing Institute
5021-B Backlick Road
Annandale, VA 22003
702-642-0580
800-EAR-WELL
Fax: 703-750-9302
http://www.betterhearing.org/

Canadian Hard of Hearing Association
2435 Holly Lane, Suite 205
Ottawa, ON, Canada K1V 7P2
800-263-8068
613-526-1584
613-526-2692 (TTY)
Fax: 613-526-4718
http://www.cyberus.ca/~chhanational/english.html

Canadian National Institute for the Blind
1929 Bayview Avenue
Toronto, ON, Canada M4G 3E8
416-486-2500
Fax: 416-480-7677
http://www.cnib.ca/

Deaf World Web
http://deafworldweb.org/

Ear Foundation
Baptist Hospital
Nashville, TN 37236
800-545-HEAR
http://www.theearfound.com/

Eye Bank Association of America
1001 Connecticut Avenue NW, Suite 601
Washington, DC 20036
202-775-4999
http://www.restoresight.org

EyeNet
American Academy of Ophthalmology
PO Box 7424
San Francisco, CA 94120-7424
415-561-8500
http://www.eyenet.org/

Fight for Sight
160 East 56th Street, Eighth floor
New York, NY 10022

Glaucoma Research Foundation
490 Post Street, Suite 830
San Francisco, CA 94102-9950
415-986-3162
Fax: 415-986-3763

Guide Dogs for the Blind, Inc.
P.O. Box 151200
San Rafael, CA 94915-1200
415-499-4000
Fax: 415-499-4035
800-295-4050
http://www.guidedogs.com/

Guide Dog Users, Inc.
57 Grandview Avenue
Watertown, MA 02172
617-926-9198

Guiding Eyes for the Blind
611 Granite Springs Road
Yorktown Heights, NY 10598
914-245-4024
800-942-0149
Fax: 914-245-1609
http://www.guiding-eyes.org/

International Hearing Dog, Inc.
5901 E. 89th Avenue
Henderson, CO 80640-8315
303-287-3277

International Hearing Society
20361 Middlebelt Road
Livonia, MI 48512
810-478-2610
800-521-5247

International Society of Refractive Surgery
1175 Springs Centre South Blvd, Suite 152
Altamonte Springs, FL 32714
407-786-7446
Fax: 407-786-7447
http://www.isrs.org/

National Association for Visually Handicapped
22 West 21st Street
New York, NY 10010
212-889-3141
Fax: 212-727-2931
http://www.navh.org/

National Association for the Deaf
814 Thayer Avenue
Silver Spring, MD 20910-4500
301-587-1788
301-587-1789 (TTY)
Fax: 301-587-1791
http://www.ececs.uc.edu/~jbelland/interests/sign/nad.html

National Braille Association
3 Townline Circle
Rochester, NY 14623-2513
716-427-8620
716-427-0263
http://members.aol.com/nbaoffice/index.htm

National Federation for the Blind
814 4th Avenue Suite 200
Grinnell, IA 50112
515-236-3366

National Information Center on Deafness
800 Florida Avenue NE
Washington, DC 20002-3695
202-651-5051
202-651-5052 (TTY)
Fax: 202-651-5054
http://www.gallaudet.edu/~nicd/

National Institute on Deafness & Other Communication Disorders
National Institutes of Health
Building 31, Room 3C35
9000 Rockville Pike
Bethesda, MD 20892
301-907-7653
http://www.nih.gov/nidcd/

Prevent Blindness America
800-331-2020
http://www.preventblindness.org

Prevention of Blindness Society
1775 Church Street NW
Washington, DC 20036
202-234-1010
202-234-1020

Recording for the Blind & Dyslexic, Inc.
20 Roszel Road
Princeton, NJ 08540
800-803-7201
http://www.rfbd.org/

Self-Help for Hard of Hearing People
7910 Woodmont Avenue, Suite 1200
Bethesda, MD 20814
301-657-2248
301-657-2249-TTY
Fax: 301-913-9413
http://www.shhh.org/

Talking Books: National Library Service for the Blind & Visually Handicapped
Library of Congress
Washington, DC 20540
http://lcweb.loc.gov/nls/nls.html

Telecommunications for the Deaf
8630 Fenton Street, # 604
Silver Spring, MD 20910
301-589-3006-TTY
301-589-3786-voice
Fax: 301-589-3797
http://www.tdi-online.org/

Vestibular Disorders Association (English & Spanish)
PO Box 4467
Portland, OR 97208-4467
503-229-7705
Fax: 503-229-8064
http://www.teleport.com/~veda/

***For additional Internet resources, see the website for this book at* www.mosby.com/MERLIN/medsurg_lewis**

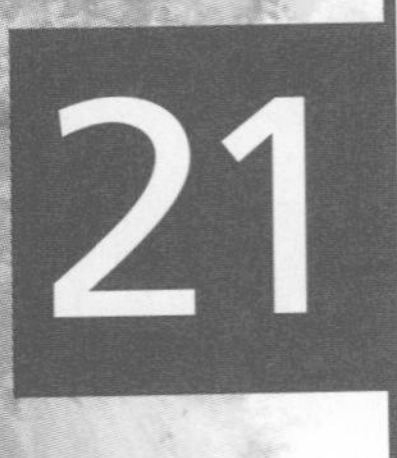

REMEMBER to check out your companion CD-ROM

21 NURSING ASSESSMENT Integumentary System

Shannon Ruff Dirksen

www.mosby.com/MERLIN/medsurg_lewis

LEARNING OBJECTIVES

1. Describe the structures and functions of the integumentary system.
2. Describe age-related changes in the integumentary system and differences in assessment findings.
3. Describe the significant subjective and objective data related to the integumentary system that should be obtained from a patient.
4. Describe specific assessments to be made during the physical examination of the skin and appendages.
5. Explain the critical components for describing a lesion.
6. Describe the appropriate techniques used in the physical assessment of the integumentary system.
7. Explain the structural and assessment differences in dark skin color.
8. Differentiate normal from common abnormal findings of a physical assessment of the integumentary system.
9. Describe the purpose, significance of results, and nursing responsibilities of diagnostic studies related to the integumentary system.

The integumentary system is the largest body organ and is composed of the skin, hair, nails, and glands. The skin is further divided into three layers: epidermis, dermis, and hypodermis (subcutaneous tissue) (Fig. 21-1).

STRUCTURES AND FUNCTIONS OF THE SKIN AND APPENDAGES

Structures

The epidermis is the outermost layer of the skin. The dermis, the second skin layer, contains a framework of highly vascular connective tissue. The hypodermis is composed primarily of subcutaneous fat and loose connective tissue.

Epidermis. The epidermis, the avascular superficial layer of the skin, is made up of an outer dead cornified portion that serves as a protective barrier and a deeper, living portion that folds into the dermis. Together these layers measure 0.05 mm to 0.1 mm in thickness. The epidermis is nourished by blood vessels in the dermis. The epidermis is replaced with new cells every 30 days. The two types of epidermal cells are the melanocytes (5%) and the keratinocytes (95%).

Melanocytes are scattered throughout the basal layer (*stratum germinativum*) of the epidermis. They secrete melanin, a pigment that gives color to the skin and hair and protects the body from damaging ultraviolet (UV) sunlight. Sunlight and hormones stimulate melanin production. All races have approximately the same number of melanocytes.[1] The wide range of skin and hair colors is caused by the amount of melanin produced; more melanin results in darker skin color.

Keratinocytes are synthesized from epidermal cells in the basal layer. Initially these cells are undifferentiated; as they mature (keratinize) they make their way to the surface where they flatten and die to form the outer skin layer (*stratum corneum*). Keratinocytes produce a specialized protein, *keratin*, which is vital to the protective barrier function of the skin. The upward movement of keratinocytes from the basement membrane to the stratum corneum takes approximately 4 weeks. If dead cells slough off too rapidly, the skin will appear thin and eroded. If new cells form faster than old cells are shed, the skin becomes scaly and thickened. Changes in this cell cycle account for many dermatologic problems.

Dermis. The dermis is the supportive connective tissue layer below the epidermis. Dermal thickness varies from 1 mm to 4 mm. The dermis is highly vascular and assists in body temperature and blood pressure regulation. Collagen forms the greatest part of the dermis and is responsible for the mechanical strength of the skin. Elastin fibers, nerves, lymphatic vessels, hair follicles, and sebaceous and sweat glands are also found in the dermis.

The dermis is divided into two layers, an upper *papillary* layer and a deeper, thicker *reticular* layer. The papillary layer is folded into ridges or papillae, which extend into the upper epidermal layer. These exposed surface ridges form congenital patterns called fingerprints and footprints. The reticular layer contains collagen and elastic and reticular fibers that give support to the skin.

Hypodermis (Subcutaneous Tissue). The hypodermis is not actually part of the skin. The hypodermis is

Reviewed by Sandra Somma, RN, BSN, Staff Nurse, Yale New Haven Hospital, New Haven, Conn.

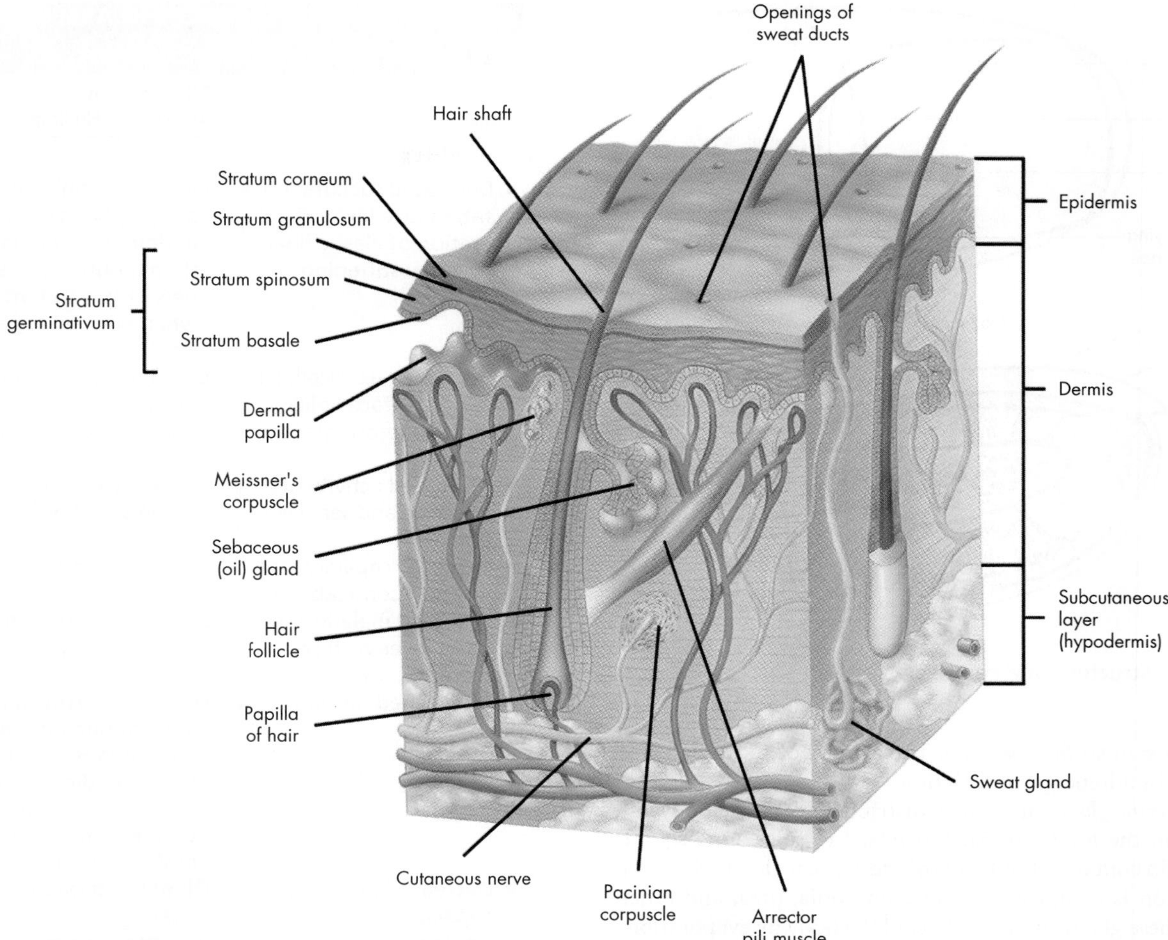

Fig. 21-1 Microscopic view of the skin in longitudinal section. The epidermis is shown raised at one corner to reveal the ridges in the dermis.

traditionally discussed with the skin because it attaches the skin to underlying tissues and organs; in addition, loose connective tissue and fat cells provide insulation. The anatomic distribution of subcutaneous tissue varies according to sex, heredity, age, and nutritional status. This layer also stores lipids, regulates temperature, and provides shock absorption.

Epidermal Appendages. Appendages of the skin include the hair, nails, and glands (sebaceous, apocrine, and eccrine). These structures develop from the epidermal layer and are located in both the epidermis and the dermis. They receive nutrients, electrolytes, and fluids from the dermis. Hair and nails form from specialized keratin that becomes hardened.

Hair grows on most of the body except for the lips, palms of the hand, the soles of the feet, and parts of the external reproductive organs. The color of the hair is a result of heredity and is determined by the type and amount of melanin in the hair shaft. Hair grows approximately 1 cm per month, 50 to 100 hairs are lost each day, and its rate of growth is not affected by cutting. Baldness results when lost hair is not replaced. This absence of hair may be disease or treatment related or due to heredity, particularly in males.[2]

Nails grow from the nail matrix, which is the white crescent-shaped area that extends beyond the proximal nail fold or *lunula* (Fig. 21-2). The *cuticle* is the part of the stratum corneum, which covers the nail root. Nails grow at a rate of 1 mm per week, with toenail growth somewhat slower. A lost fingernail usually regenerates in 3 to 6 months, whereas a lost toenail may require 12 months or more for regeneration. The viable part of a nail lies in the matrix behind the lunula. As long as the matrix remains intact, nail growth will occur. Nail growth may vary according to the person's age and health. Nail color ranges from pink to yellow or brown depending on skin color. Nails can be injured by direct trauma.

Sebaceous, apocrine, and eccrine glands all develop from the epidermal layer and are located in the dermis. The *sebaceous glands* secrete sebum, which is emptied into the hair shaft. Sebum is somewhat bacteriostatic and consists mainly of lipids. These glands depend on sex hormones, particularly testosterone, to regulate sebum secretion and production. Sebum secretion varies across the life span according to sex hormone levels. Sebaceous glands are present on all areas of the skin except the palms and soles, and are most numerous and largest on the face, scalp, upper chest, and back.

The *apocrine glands* are located primarily in the axillae, breast areolae, anogenital area, external ear, and eyelids. These sweat glands secrete a milky substance that becomes odoriferous when

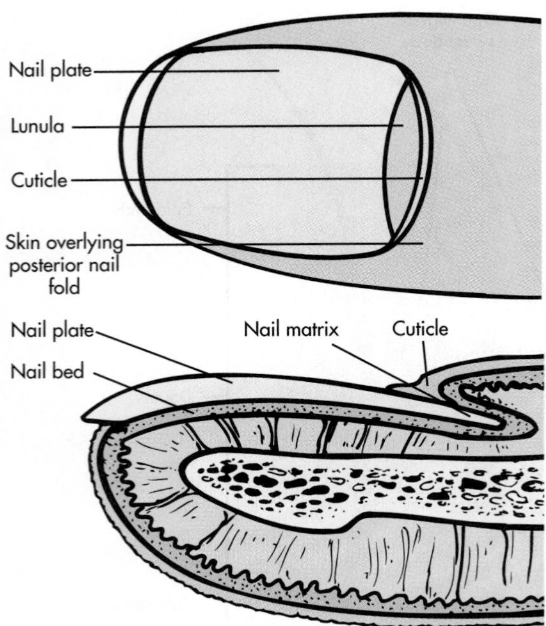

Fig. 21-2 Structure of a nail.

altered by skin surface bacteria. The activity of these glands is mediated by adrenergic innervation.

The *eccrine glands* are widely distributed over the body, especially on the forehead, back, palms, and soles. One square inch of skin contains about 3000 of these sweat glands. Sweat or perspiration is composed of salts, ammonia, urea, and other wastes. These glands function to cool the body by evaporation, to excrete waste products through the pores of the skin, and to moisturize surface cells.

Functions of the Integumentary System

The primary function of the skin is to protect the underlying tissues of the body by serving as a surface barrier to the external environment. The skin also acts as a barrier against invasion by bacteria and excessive loss of water.

The skin with its nerve endings and special receptors provides sensory perception for environmental stimuli. These highly specialized nerve endings supply information to the brain related to pain, heat and cold, touch, pressure, and vibration. The skin controls heat regulation by its ability to respond to changes in internal and external temperature by vasoconstriction and vasodilation. Related to heat regulation is the skin's function of excretion. Between 600 ml and 900 ml of water are lost daily through insensible perspiration. In addition, sebum and sweat are secreted by the skin and lubricate the skin surface. Endogenous synthesis of vitamin D, which is critical to calcium and phosphorus metabolism, occurs in the epidermis. Vitamin D is synthesized by the action of UV light on vitamin D precursors in epidermal cells.

The aesthetic functions of the skin include the mirroring of various emotions such as anger or embarrassment, as well as displaying the individual identity of a person. The role of absorption at the cutaneous level is a subject of active research and an increasing number of medications are effectively delivered via patches applied directly to the skin.

GERONTOLOGIC DIFFERENCES IN ASSESSMENT

Table 21-1 Integumentary System

Changes	Differences in Assessment Findings
Skin	
■ Decreased subcutaneous fat, muscle laxity, degeneration of elastic fibers, collagen stiffening	Increased wrinkling, sagging breasts and abdomen, redundant flesh around eyes, slowness of skin to flatten when pinched together (tenting)
■ Decreased extracellular water, surface lipids, and sebaceous gland activity	Dry, flaking skin with possible signs of excoriation caused by scratching
■ Decreased activity of apocrine and sebaceous glands	Dry skin with minimal to no perspiration
■ Increased capillary fragility and permeability	Evidence of bruising
■ Increased melanocytes in basal layer with pigment accumulation	Senile lentigines on face and back of hands
■ Diminished blood supply	Decrease in rosy appearance of skin and mucous membranes; skin is cool to touch; diminished awareness of pain, touch, temperature, and peripheral vibration
■ Decreased proliferative capacity	Diminished rate of wound healing
■ Decreased immunocompetence	Increase in neoplasms
Hair	
■ Decreased melanin and melanocytes	Graying hair
■ Decreased oil	Dry, coarse hair; scaly scalp
■ Decreased density of hair follicles	Thinning and loss of hair; loss of hair in outer half or outer third of eyebrow
■ Cumulative androgen effect; decreasing estrogen levels	Facial hirsutism; baldness
Nails	
■ Decreased peripheral blood supply	Thick, brittle nails with diminished growth
■ Increased keratin	Ridging
■ Decreased circulation	Prolonged return of blood to nails on blanching

GERONTOLOGIC CONSIDERATIONS

Effects of Aging on the Integumentary System

There are many changes in the skin of the aging person. Although many changes are not serious except for their cosmetic effect, others are more serious and need careful evaluation. Age-related changes of the integumentary system and differences in assessment findings are listed in Table 21-1.

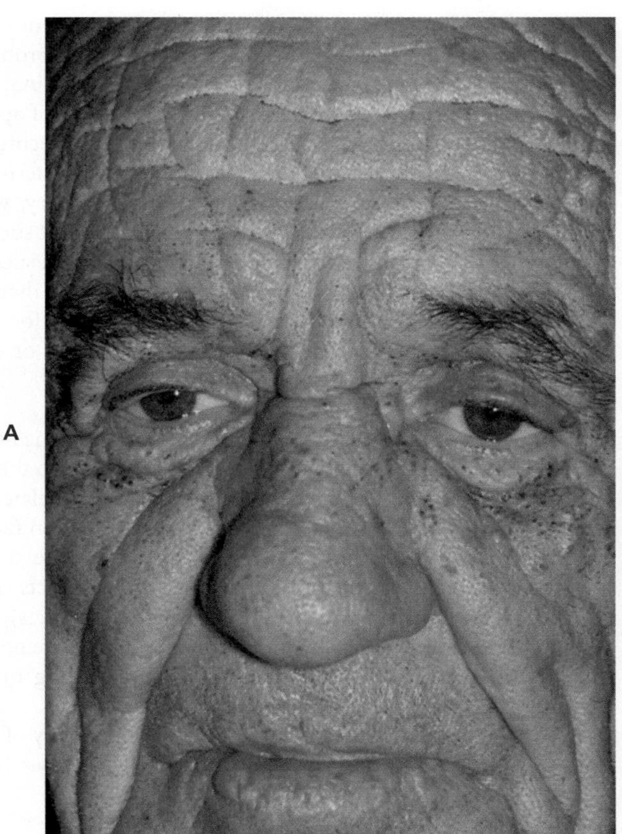

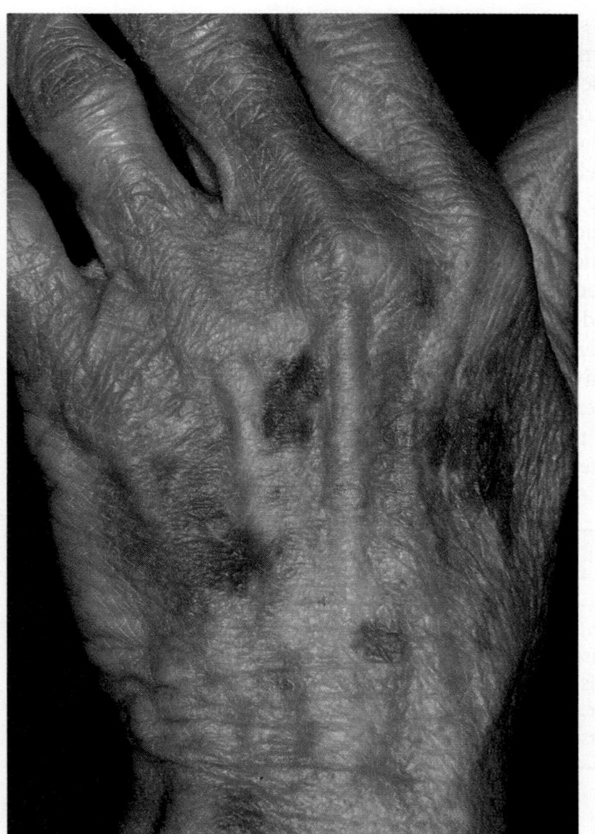

Fig. 21-3 **A,** Photoaging. Wrinkling resulting from chronic sun exposure. **B,** Photoaging. Bleeding occurs with minor injury to the sun-damaged surfaces of the hands.

The rate of age-related skin changes is influenced by heredity and a personal history of sun exposure, hygiene practices, nutrition, and general state of health. Skin changes that are related to aging include decreased firmness and flexibility, dryness, roughness, wrinkling, and benign neoplasms.[3]

The junction between the dermis and the epidermis becomes flattened and the epidermis contains fewer melanocytes. In addition, the dermis loses volume and has fewer blood vessels. Scalp, pubic, and axillary hair becomes depigmented and thinner. A loss of melanin results in gray hair. The nail-plate thins and nails become brittle, thicker, and prone to splitting and yellowing.

Chronic exposure to UV rays is the major contributor to the wrinkling of skin. Sun damage to the skin is cumulative. The wrinkling of sun-exposed areas such as the face is more marked than in sun-shielded areas such as the buttocks. Poor nutrition contributes to aging of the skin resulting from a decreased intake of protein, calories, and vitamins. With aging, collagen fibers stiffen, elastic fibers degenerate, and the amount of subcutaneous tissue decreases. These changes, with the added effects of gravity, lead to wrinkling (Fig. 21-3, *A* and *B*).

Benign neoplasms related to the aging process can occur on the skin. These growths include *seborrheic keratoses, cherry angiomas,* and *skin tags.* A common premalignant lesion is an *actinic keratosis,* which appears on areas of chronic sun exposure, especially in the person who has a fair complexion and light eyes (blue, green, or hazel). These cutaneous lesions place an individual at increased risk for squamous cell and basal cell carcinomas. The aging person is more susceptible to skin cancers because there is a decline in the capacity to repair cellular (DNA) damage caused by sun exposure.

Decreased subcutaneous fat leads to an increased risk of trauma injury, hypothermia, and skin shearing, which may lead to pressure ulcers. With aging, the eccrine and apocrine glands atrophy causing dry skin and decreasing body odor. The growth rate of the hair and nails decreases as a result of atrophy of the involved structures. Vitamin deficiencies can cause dry, thin hair that has a tendency to fall out.

ASSESSMENT OF THE INTEGUMENTARY SYSTEM

Assessment of the skin begins at the initial contact with the patient and continues throughout the examination. Specific areas of the skin are examined during examination of other areas of the body unless the chief complaint is that of a dermatologic nature. A general statement about the skin should be recorded (Table 21-2), and specific problems should be noted under the appropriate system. In addition, health history questions presented in Table 21-3 should be asked when a skin problem is noted.

Subjective Data

Important Health Information

Past health history. Past health history will indicate previous trauma, surgery, or prior disease that involves the skin. The nurse should determine if the patient has noticed any dermatologic manifestations of systemic problems such as jaundice (liver disease), delayed wound healing (diabetes mellitus), cyanosis (respiratory disorder), and pallor (anemia). Table 22-13 lists additional manifestations of systemic problems. Specific information related to food, pet, and drug allergies and skin reactions to insect bites and stings should also be obtained. A history of chronic or unprotected exposure to UV light, as well as radiation treatments, should be noted.

Medications. The patient should be questioned about skin-related problems that occurred as a result of taking prescription or over-the-counter (OTC) medications. A thorough medication history is important, especially in relation to vitamins, corticosteroids, hormones, antibiotics, and antimetabolites, because these medications may often cause side effects that are manifested in the skin.

Table 21-2 Normal Physical Assessment of the Integumentary System

Skin: even-toned and warm; good turgor; no petechiae, purpura, lesions, or excoriations.
Nails: pink, round, and mobile with 160-degree angle.
Hair: shiny and full; amount and distribution appropriate for age and sex; no flaking of scalp, forehead, or pinna.

The nurse should document the use of prescription or OTC medications used specifically to treat a primary skin problem such as acne or a secondary skin problem such as itching. If a preparation is used, the name, length of use, method of application, and effectiveness of the medication should be recorded.

Surgery or other treatments. It is important to determine if any surgical procedures, including cosmetic surgery, were performed on the skin. If a biopsy was done, the result should be recorded. Any treatments specific for a skin problem such as phototherapy or for a health problem such as radiation therapy should be noted. In addition, treatments undergone for primarily cosmetic purposes, such as tanning booth use or cosmetic "peels" should also be documented.

Functional Health Patterns

Health perception–health management pattern. The nurse should ask about the patient's health practices related to the integumentary system, such as the usual self-care habits related to daily hygiene. The frequency of use and sun protection factor (SPF) number of sun protection products should be documented. Assessment of the use of personal care products (e.g., shampoos, moisturizing agents, and cosmetic products), including brand name, quantity, and frequency, should be noted. A description of any current skin problem including onset, symptoms, course, and treatment should be recorded.

Information should be obtained about family history of any skin diseases, including congenital and familial diseases (e.g.,

HEALTH HISTORY

Table 21-3 Integumentary System

Health Perception–Health Management Pattern
- Describe your daily hygiene practices.
- What skin products are you currently using?
- Describe any current skin condition, including onset, course, and treatment (if any).
- Do you have any pets?

Nutritional-Metabolic Pattern
- Describe any changes in the condition of your skin, hair, nails, and mucous membranes.
- Are the conditions related to changes in your diet, including supplemental vitamins and minerals?*
- Have you noticed any changes in the way sores or lesions heal?*

Elimination Pattern
- Have you noticed changes in you skin related to excessive sweating, dryness, or swelling?

Activity-Exercise Pattern
- Do your leisure activities involve the use of any chemicals that are potentially toxic to the skin?*
- What is your sun protection program?

Sleep-Rest Pattern
- Does your skin condition keep you awake or awaken you after you have fallen asleep?

Cognitive-Perceptual Pattern
- Do you have any unusual sensations of heat, cold, or touch?*
- Do you have any pain associated with your skin condition?*
- Do you have any joint pain?*

Self-Perception–Self-Concept Pattern
- How does your skin condition make you feel about yourself?

Role-Relationship Pattern
- Has your skin condition changed your relationships with others?*
- Have you changed your lifestyle because of your skin condition?*
- Are there any environmental skin irritants at your current or previous work place or home?*

Sexuality-Reproductive Pattern
- Has your skin condition changed your intimate relationships with others?*
- Has your birth control method, if used, caused a skin problem?*

Coping–Stress Tolerance Pattern
- Are you aware of any situation or stressor that changes your skin condition?*
- Do you feel that stress plays a role in your skin condition?*
- How do you handle stress?

Value-Belief Pattern
- Are there any cultural beliefs that influence your thinking or feelings about your skin condition?*
- Are there any treatment options that you would be opposed to using?*

*If yes, describe.

alopecia and psoriasis) and systemic diseases with dermatologic manifestations (e.g., diabetes, thyroid disease, cardiovascular diseases, immune disorders). In addition, a family and personal history of skin cancer, particularly melanoma, should be noted.

Nutritional-metabolic pattern. The nurse should question the patient about any changes in the condition of skin, hair, nails, and mucous membranes and whether they are related to dietary changes. A diet history reveals the adequacy of nutrients essential to healthy skin such as vitamins A, D, E, and C; dietary fat; and protein. Food allergies that cause cutaneous reactions should also be noted. Obese patients should be asked if they have areas of chafing or maceration where moisture accumulates in overlapping skin areas. Changes in the time for wound healing to occur should be questioned and recorded.

Elimination pattern. The patient should be questioned about conditions of the skin such as dehydration, edema, and pruritus, which can indicate alterations in fluid balance. If incontinence is a problem, the condition of the skin in the anal and perineal areas should be determined.

Activity-exercise pattern. Information should be obtained about environmental hazards in relation to hobbies and recreation activities, including exposure to known cutaneous carcinogens, chemical irritants, and allergens. The patient should be asked if any changes occur in the skin during exercise or other activities.

Sleep-rest pattern. The patient should be questioned about disturbances in sleep patterns caused by a skin condition. For example, pruritus can be distressing and cause major alterations in normal sleep patterns. Also, poor sleep and resulting tiredness is often reflected in a patient's face by dark circles under the eyes and a decreased firmness in the facial skin.

Cognitive-perceptual pattern. The nurse should ascertain the patient's perception of the sensations of heat, cold, pain, and touch. Discomfort associated with a skin condition should be noted, especially when observed in intact skin. Joint pain related to the patient's skin condition should also be recorded.

Self-perception–self-concept pattern. Assessment should be made of the feelings related to sadness, anxiety, or despair in relation to the patient's skin condition. The patient should be observed for signs of decreased self-esteem and a poor or altered body image.

Role-relationship pattern. It is important to determine how the patient's skin condition affects relationships with family members, peers, and work associates. Assessment should be made of the changes in lifestyle that have occurred relative to the skin condition.

The patient should be questioned regarding the effect of environmental factors on the skin such as occupational exposure to irritants, sun, and unusually cold or unhygienic conditions. Contact dermatitis caused by allergies and irritants is a common skin problem associated with occupation.[4]

Sexuality-reproductive pattern. The nurse should tactfully question and assess the effect of the patient's skin condition on sexual activity. The nurse should also make note of the reproductive status of the female patient relative to possible therapeutic interventions. For example, isotretinoin (Accutane), which is used to treat acne, is a teratogenic drug that causes abnormal fetal development and, consequently, should not be used by a woman who could become pregnant.

Coping–stress tolerance pattern. It is important for the nurse to assess and question the patient about the role stress may play in creating or exacerbating the skin condition. The patient should be questioned as to what coping strategies are used to manage the skin condition.

Value-belief pattern. The patient should be questioned about cultural or religious beliefs that could influence the perception of self-image as related to the skin condition. Assessment should also be made of values and beliefs that might influence or limit the choice of treatment options.

Objective Data

Physical Examination. Characteristics of *primary (basic) skin lesions* are shown in Fig. 21-4. *Secondary skin lesions* are shown in Fig. 21-5. General principles when conducting an assessment of the skin are as follows:

1. Have a private examination room of moderate temperature with good lighting; a room with exposure to daylight is preferred.
2. Ensure that the patient is comfortable and in a dressing gown that allows easy access to all skin areas.
3. Be systematic, and proceed from head to toe.
4. Compare symmetrical parts.
5. Perform a general inspection and then a lesion-specific examination.
6. Use the metric system when taking measurements.
7. Use appropriate terminology and nomenclature when reporting or documenting.

Photographs are useful when accurate findings are needed.

Inspection. The skin is inspected for general color and pigmentation, vascularity or bruising, and the presence of lesions or discolorations. The critical factor in assessment of skin color is change. A skin color that is normal for a particular patient can be a sign of a pathologic condition in another patient. The color of the skin depends on the amount of melanin (brown), carotene (yellow), oxyhemoglobin (red), and reduced hemoglobin (bluish-red) present at a particular time. The most reliable areas in which to assess color are the areas of least pigmentation, such as the sclera, conjunctiva, nail beds, lips, and buccal mucosa. Activity, emotions, cigarette smoking, and edema as well as respiratory, renal cardiovascular, and hepatic disorders can all directly affect the color of the skin. Table 21-4 describes assessment variations in light- and dark-skinned individuals.

The skin is examined for possible problems related to vascularity, such as areas of bruising, and vascular and purpuric lesions, such as angioma, petechiae, or purpura. Reaction to direct pressure should be noted. If a lesion blanches on direct pressure and then refills, the redness is due to dilated blood vessels. If the discoloration remains, it is the result of subcutaneous or intradermal bleeding. Any pattern of bruising, for example, in the shape of the hand or fingers or bruises at different stages of resolution should be noted. These may be indications of other health problems or abuse and should be further investigated.

If lesions are found on the skin, the color, size, distribution, location, and shape should be recorded. Skin lesions are usually described by using words that describe the lesions' configuration (pattern in relation to other lesions, Table 21-5) and distribution (arrangement of lesions over an area of skin, Table 21-6).

During systematic inspection it is important to note any unusual odors. Colonized lesions and overgrowth of yeast in calluses or *intertriginous* (overlapping) areas are often associated with distinctive odors. Tattoos and needle-track marks should

Macule
A circumscribed, flat discoloration, which may be brown, blue, red, or hypopigmented

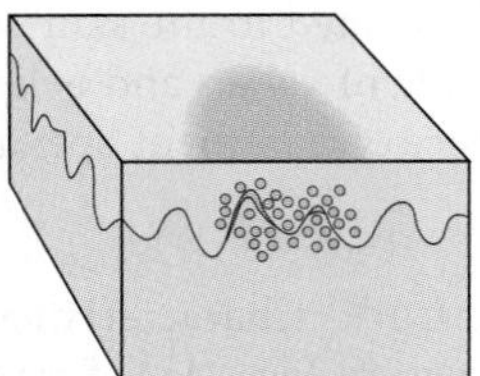

Vesicle
A circumscribed collection of free fluid up to 0.5 cm in diameter

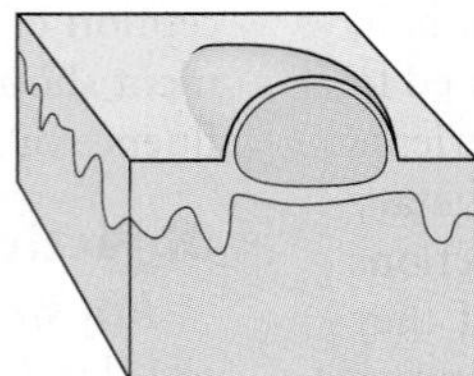

Plaque
A circumscribed, elevated, superficial, solid lesion more than 0.5 cm in diameter, often formed by the confluence of papules

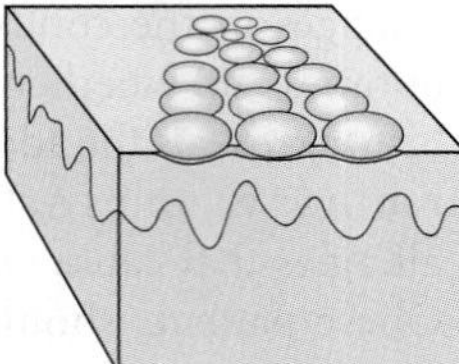

Nodule
A circumscribed, elevated, solid lesion more than 0.5 cm in diameter; a large nodule is referred to as a tumor

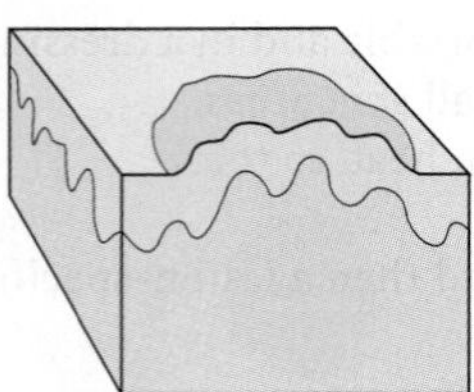

Papule
An elevated solid lesion up to 0.5 cm in diameter; color varies; papules may become confluent and form plaques

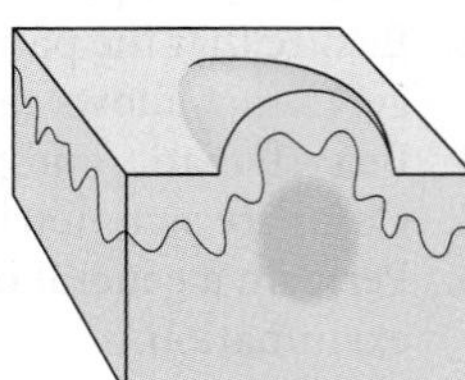

Pustule
A circumscribed collection of leukocytes and free fluid that varies in size

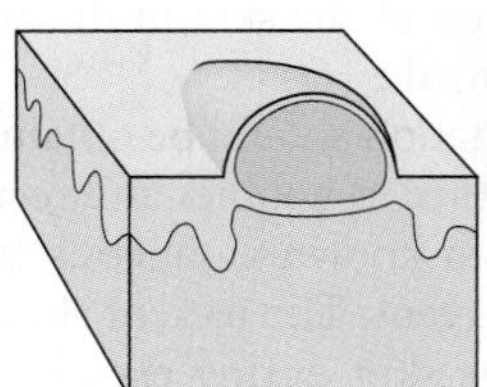

Wheal
A firm edematous plaque resulting from infiltration of the dermis with fluid; wheals are transient and may last only a few hours

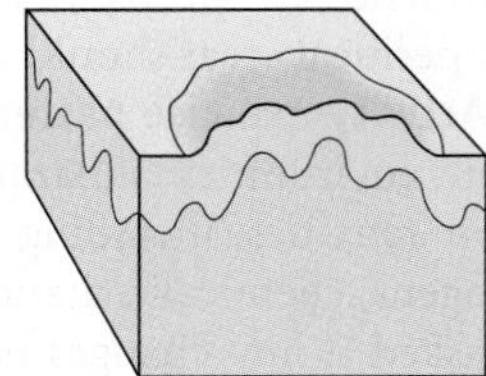

Fig. 21-4 Characteristics of primary skin lesions.

Scales
Excess dead epidermal cells that are produced by abnormal keratinization and shedding

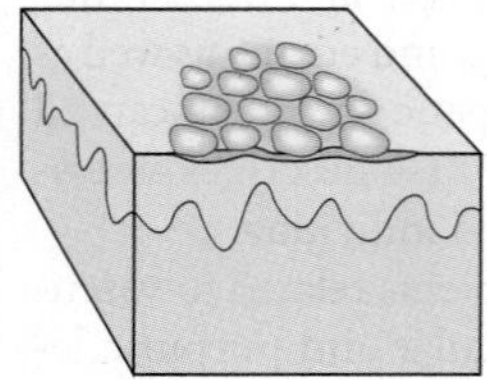

Scar
An abnormal formation of connective tissue implying dermal damage; after injury or surgery scars are initially thick and pink but become white and atrophic

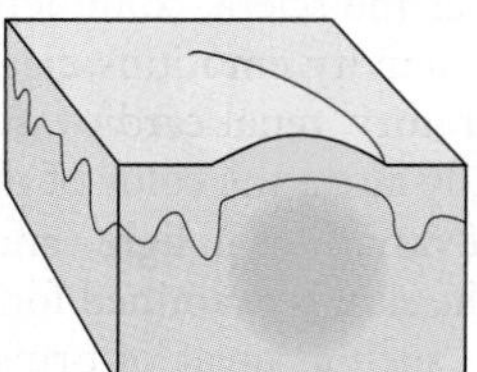

Erosions
A focal loss of epidermis; erosions do not penetrate below the dermoepidermal junction and therefore heal without scarring

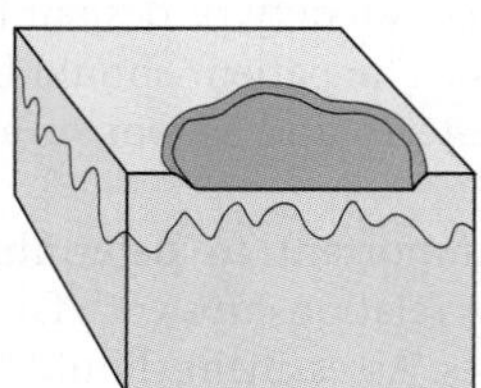

Ulcers
A focal loss of epidermis and dermis; ulcers heal with scarring

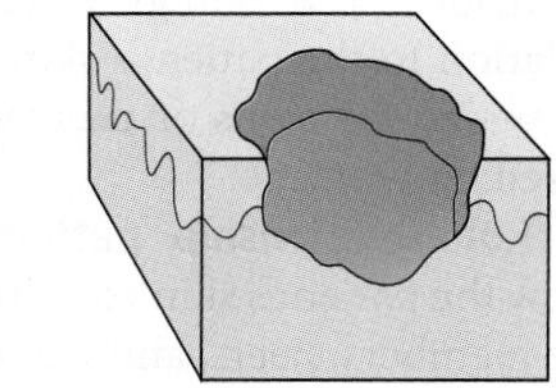

Fissure
A linear loss of epidermis and dermis with sharply defined, nearly vertical walls

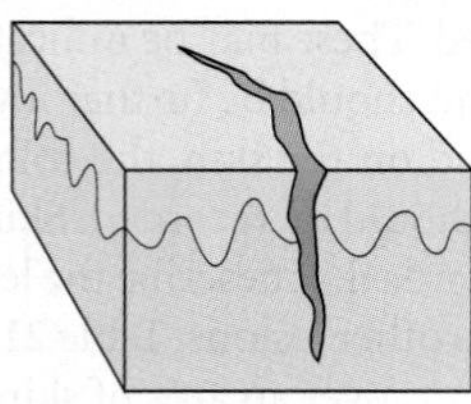

Atrophy
A depression in the skin resulting from thinning of the epidermis or dermis

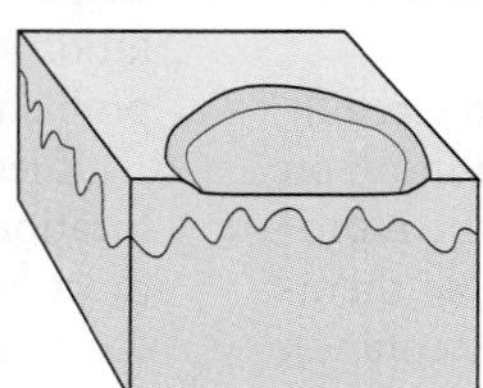

Crusts
A collection of dried serum and cellular debris; a scab

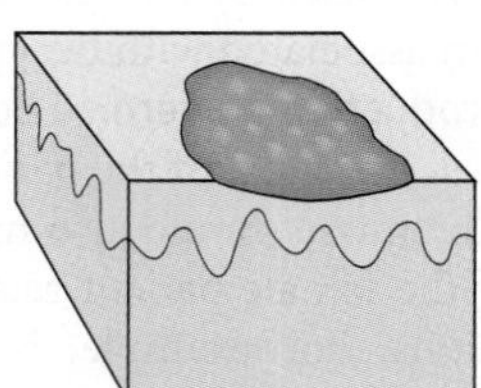

Fig. 21-5 Characteristics of secondary skin lesions.

Table 21-4 Assessment Variations in Light- and Dark-Skinned Individuals

Clinical Sign	Light Skin	Dark Skin
Cyanosis	Grayish-blue tone, especially in nail beds,ear lobes, lips, mucous membranes, and palms and soles of feet	Ashen or gray color most easily seen in the conjunctiva of the eye, oral mucous membranes, and nail beds
Ecchymosis (bruise)	Dark red, purple, yellow, or green color, depending on age of bruises	Deeper bluish or black tone; difficult to see unless occurring in an area of light pigmentation
Erythema	Reddish tone, possibly accompanied by increased skin temperature secondary to localized inflammation	Deeper brown or purple skin tone with evidence of increased skin temperature secondary to inflammation
Jaundice	Yellowish color of skin, sclera, fingernails, palms of hands, and oral mucosa	Yellowish-green color most obviously seen in sclera of eye (do not confuse with yellow eye pigmentation, which may be evident in dark-skinned patients), palms of hands, and soles of feet
Pallor	Pale skin color that may appear white or ashen, also evident on lips, nail beds, and mucous membranes	Underlying red tone in brown or black skin is absent. Light-skinned African-Americans may have yellowish brown skin; dark-skinned African-Americans may appear ashen or gray
Petechiae	Lesions appear as small, reddish-purple pinpoints, best observed on abdomen and buttocks	Difficult to see; may be evident in the buccal mucosa of the mouth or conjunctiva of the eye
Rash	May be visualized as well as felt with light palpation	Not easily visualized, but may be felt with light palpation
Scar	Generally heals, showing narrow scar line	Frequently has keloid development, resulting in a thickened, raised scar

Adapted from Thompson J, Wilson S: *Health assessment for nursing practice,* St Louis, 1996, Mosby.

Table 21-5 Lesion Configuration Terminology

Name	Appearance
Annular	Ring-shaped
Gyrate	Ring-spiral–shaped
Iris lesions	Concentric rings or "bull's eyes"
Linear	In a line
Nummular, discoid	Coinlike
Polymorphous	Occurring in several forms
Punctuate	Marked by points or dots
Serpiginous	Snakelike

Table 21-6 Lesion Distribution Terminology

Term	Description
Asymmetric	Unilateral distribution
Confluent	Merging together
Diffuse	Wide distribution
Discrete	Separate from other lesions
Generalized	Diffuse distribution
Grouped	Cluster of lesions
Localized	Limited areas of involvement that are clearly defined
Satellite	Single lesion in close proximity to a large grouping
Solitary	A single lesion
Symmetric	Bilateral distribution
Zosteriform	Bandlike distribution along a dermatome area

be examined and noted for location and the characteristics of the surrounding skin area.

Inspection of the hair should include an examination of all body hair. Note the distribution, texture, and quantity of hair. Changes in the normal distribution of body hair and growth may indicate an endocrine disorder. Inspection of the nails should include a careful examination of nail shape, thickness, curvature, and surface. Any grooves, pitting, or ridges should be noted. Changes in nail smoothness or thickness can occur with anemia, psoriasis, and decreased vascular circulation.

Palpation. The skin is palpated to provide information about temperature, turgor and mobility, moisture, and texture. *Temperature* of the skin is best assessed by using the backs of the hands. The skin should be warm without being hot. The temperature of the skin increases when blood flow to the dermis is increased. There will be a localized temperature increase with burns and local inflammation. A generalized increase in temperature will result from fever. A decreased body temperature may occur when shock, chilling, or emotional trauma is present.

Turgor and *mobility* refer to the elasticity of the skin. The nurse assesses turgor by gently pinching an area of skin under the clavicle. Skin with good turgor should move easily when lifted and should immediately return to its original position when released. There is a loss of turgor with dehydration and aging.

Moisture of the skin is the dampness or dryness of the skin. Moisture increases in intertriginous areas and with high humidity. The amount of moisture on the skin varies with environmental temperature, muscular activity, body weight, and body temperature. The skin should be intact with no flaking, scaling, or cracking. Skin generally becomes drier with increasing age.

Texture refers to the fineness or coarseness of the skin. The skin should feel smooth and firm with the surface evenly thin in most areas. Thickened callus areas are normal on the soles

COMMON ASSESSMENT ABNORMALITIES

Table 21-7 **Integumentary System**

Finding	Description	Possible Etiology and Significance
Alopecia	Loss of hair (localized or general)	Heredity, friction, rubbing, traction, trauma, stress, infection, inflammation, chemotherapy, pregnancy, emotional shock, tinea capitis, immunologic factors
Angioma	Tumor consisting of blood or lymph vessels	Normal increase with aging, liver disease, pregnancy, varicose veins
Carotenemia (Carotenosis)	Yellow discoloration of skin, no yellowing of sclerae, most noticeable on palms and soles	Vegetables containing carotene (e.g., carrots, squash), hypothyroidism
Comedo (blackheads and whiteheads)	Keratin, sebum microorganism, and epithelial debris within a dilated follicular opening	Acne vulgaris
Cyanosis	Slightly bluish-gray or dark purple discoloration of the skin and mucous membranes caused by presence of excessive amounts of reduced hemoglobin in capillaries	Cardiorespiratory problems; vasoconstriction, asphyxiation, anemia, leukemia, and malignancies
Cyst	Sac containing fluid or semisolid material	Obstruction of a duct or gland, parasitic infection
Depigmentation (vitiligo)	Congenital or acquired loss of melanin resulting in white, depigmented areas	Genetic, chemical and pharmacologic agents, nutritional and endocrine factors, burns and trauma, inflammation and infection
Ecchymosis	Large, bruiselike lesion caused by collection of extravascular blood in dermis and subcutaneous tissue	Trauma, bleeding disorders
Erythema	Redness occurring in patches of variable size and shape	Heat, certain drugs, alcohol, ultraviolet rays, any problem that causes dilation of blood vessels to the skin
Excoriation	Superficial excavations of epidermis	Pruritus, trauma
Hematoma	Extravasation of blood of sufficient size to cause visible swelling	Trauma, bleeding disorders
Hirsutism	Male distribution of hair in women	Abnormality of gonads or adrenal glands, decrease in estrogen level, familial trait
Intertrigo	Dermatitis of overlying surfaces of the skin	Moisture, obesity, *Monilia* infections
Jaundice	Yellow (in Caucasians) or yellowish-brown (in African-Americans) discoloration of the skin, best observed in the sclera secondary to increased bilirubin in the blood	Liver disease, red blood cell hemolysis; pancreatic cancer, common bile duct obstruction
Keloid	Hypertrophied scar beyond margin of incision or trauma	Predisposition more common in African-Americans
Lichenification	Thickening of the skin with accentuated skin markings	Repeated scratching, rubbing, and irritation
Mole (melanocytic nevus)	Benign overgrowth of melanocytes	Defects of development; excessive numbers and large, irregular moles; often familial
Petechiae	Pinpoint, discrete deposit of blood less than 1 mm to 2 mm in the extravascular tissues and visible through the skin or mucous membrane	Inflammation, marked dilation, blood vessel trauma, blood dyscrasia that results in bleeding tendencies (e.g., thrombocytopenia)
Telangiectasia	Visibly dilated, superficial, cutaneous small blood vessels, commonly found on face and thighs	Aging, acne, sun exposure, alcohol, liver failure, corticosteroid medication, radiation, certain systemic diseases, skin tumors; normal variant
Tenting	Failure of skin to return immediately to normal position after gentle pinching	Aging, dehydration, cachexia
Varicosity	Increased prominence of superficial veins	Interruption of venous return (e.g., from tumor, incompetent valves, inflammation)

and palms and relate to weight bearing. Increased thickness is often work-related and as a result of excessive pressure.

Common assessment abnormalities of the skin are described in Table 21-7.

Assessment of Dark Skin Color

Genetic factors determine the skin color of the individual. The darker skin tones result from the reflection of light as it strikes the underlying skin pigment. An increased amount of melanin pigment produced by the melanocytes results in the darker skin color. This increased melanin forms a natural sun shield for dark skin and results in a decreased incidence of skin cancer in these individuals.

The structures of dark skin are no different than those of lighter skin, but they are often more difficult to assess (Table 21-4). Assessment of color is more easily made in areas where

DIAGNOSTIC STUDIES

Table 21-8 Integumentary System

Study	Description and Purpose	Nursing Responsibility
Biopsy		
▪ Punch	Special punch biopsy instrument of appropriate size used. Instrument rotated to appropriate level to include dermis and some fat. Suturing may or may not be done.	Verify that consent form is signed (if needed). Assist with preparation of site, anesthesia, procedure, and hemostasis. Apply dressing, and give postprocedure instructions to patient. Properly identify specimen.
▪ Excisional	Useful when good cosmetic results and entire removal desired. Skin closed with subcutaneous and skin sutures.	Same as above
▪ Incisional	Elliptical incision made in lesion too large to excise. Adequate specimen obtained without causing an extensive cosmetic defect.	Same as above
▪ Shave (Subsection)	Single-edged razor blade used to shave off lesions. Performed on superficial lesions. Provides full-thickness specimen of stratum corneum.	Same as above
Microscopic Tests		
▪ Potassium hydroxide	Hair, scales, or nails examined for hyphae of fungal infection. Specimen is put on a glass slide and 10% to 40% concentration of potassium hydroxide added.	Instruct patient regarding purpose of test. Prepare slide.
▪ Tzanck test (Wright's and Giemsa's stain)	Fluid and cells from vesicles or bullae examined. Used to diagnose herpes virus. Specimen put on slide, stained, and examined microscopically.	Inform patient of purpose of test. Use sterile technique for collection of fluid.
▪ Culture	The test identifies fungal, bacterial, and viral organisms. For fungi, scraping performed if the fungus is systemic involving the skin. For bacteria, material obtained from intact pustules, bullae, or abscesses. For viruses, bullae scraped and exudate taken from center of lesion.	Instruct patient regarding purpose and specific procedure. Properly identify specimen. Follow instructions for storage of specimen if not sent to laboratory.
▪ Mineral oil slides	To check for infestations, scrapings are placed on slide with mineral oil.	Instruct patient of purpose of test. Prepare slide.
▪ Immunofluorescent studies	Some cutaneous diseases have specific, abnormal antibody proteins that can be identified by fluorescent studies. Both skin and serum can be examined.	Inform patient of purpose of test. Assist in obtaining specimen.
Miscellaneous		
▪ Wood's light	Examination of skin with long-wave ultraviolet light causes specific substances to fluoresce (e.g., *Pseudomonas* organisms, fungal infections, vitiligo)	Explain purpose of examination. Inform patient it is not painful.
▪ Diascopy	Examination of the skin using gentle pressure with a transparent object to check lesion vascularity.	Explain procedure to patient.
▪ Patch test	Used to determine whether patient is allergic to any testing material. Small amount of potentially allergenic material applied under occlusion, usually to skin on back.	Explain purpose and procedure to patient. Instruct patient to return in 48 hr for removal of allergens and evaluation. Inform patient if reevaluation is needed at 96 hr.

the epidermis is thin, such as the lips and mucous membranes. Rashes are often difficult to observe and may need to be palpated.

African-Americans are predisposed to certain skin conditions, including pseudofolliculitis, keloids, and mongolian spots. Because of the darkness of the skin of some individuals, color often cannot be used as an indicator of systemic conditions (e.g., flushed skin with fever). A bluish hue may be evident in the gums and skin of dark-skinned individuals.[5]

DIAGNOSTIC STUDIES OF THE INTEGUMENTARY SYSTEM

Diagnostic studies provide important information to the nurse in monitoring the patient's condition and planning appropriate interventions. These studies are considered to be objective data. Table 21-8 contains diagnostic studies common to the integumentary system.

The main diagnostic techniques related to skin problems are inspection of an individual lesion and a careful history related to the problem. If a definitive diagnosis cannot be made by these techniques, other tests may be indicated. The Wood's lamp (black light) is frequently used in the diagnosis of certain skin and hair diseases.[6]

Biopsy is one of the most common diagnostic tests used in the evaluation of a skin lesion. A biopsy is indicated in all conditions in which a malignancy is suspected or a specific diagnosis is questionable. Techniques include punch, incisional, excisional, and shave (subsection) biopsies. The method used is related to factors such as the site of the biopsy, cosmetic result desired, and the type of tissue to be obtained.

Other diagnostic procedures used include stains and cultures for fungal, bacterial, and viral infections. *Immunofluorescence* is a special technique used on biopsy specimens and may be indicated in certain conditions such as bullous diseases and systemic lupus erythematosus. *Patch testing* and *photopatch testing* may be used in the evaluation of contact, photoallergic, and photodistributed dermatitis.[7]

REVIEW QUESTIONS

The number of the question corresponds to the same-numbered objective at the beginning of the chapter.

1. Secretions that originate from the sebaceous glands are regulated by
   a. sympathetic nervous system stimulation.
   b. cool skin temperatures.
   c. androgens.
   d. parasympathetic nervous system stimulation.
2. Age-related changes in the skin of the aging person are
   a. thick, brittle nails.
   b. lighter skin tones, which burn easily.
   c. increased tenting of skin.
   d. oilier skin and hair.
3. When assessing the activity-exercise pattern in relation to the skin, the nurse questions the patient regarding
   a. the presence of superficial pain or itching.
   b. the presence of dark circles under the eyes.
   c. exposure to environmental allergens or irritants.
   d. daily hygiene and use of personal care products.
4. During physical examination of the patient's skin the nurse should
   a. provide a private, well-lighted room.
   b. wear gloves during palpation of the skin.
   c. focus initially on examination of specific lesions or problem areas.
   d. maintain the patient's privacy by undressing only areas that are abnormal.
5. While examining a patient the nurse notes small, raised, solid lesions that merge with one another on the patient's forearm. The nurse would describe this finding as
   a. diffuse pustular gyrate lesions.
   b. generalized pustules with confluence.
   c. punctuate, macular satellite lesions.
   d. confluent, annular papules forming plaque.
6. Palpation of the skin is the most appropriate technique to assess
   a. skin texture.
   b. the presence of lesions.
   c. the vascularity of the skin.
   d. presence of intertriginous areas.
7. During assessment of patients with dark skin color the nurse recognizes that
   a. the skin is thicker because of increased activity by melanocytes.
   b. dark skin is normally warmer and drier than light-colored skin.
   c. changes in skin color common in some systemic conditions may not be apparent.
   d. assessment of color changes is more easily made on the soles of the feet and palms of the hand.
8. On observing areas of excoriation on the patient's arms and legs, the nurse would question the patient regarding
   a. itching.
   b. sun exposure.
   c. excessive sweating.
   d. bleeding disorders.
9. If a more definitive diagnosis of a lesion is needed, the most common diagnostic tool used is
   a. biopsy.
   b. Tzanck test.
   c. Wood's light.
   d. potassium hydroxide.

References

1. Thibodeau G, Patton K: *Anatomy and physiology*, ed 4, St Louis, 1999, Mosby.
2. Sauer G, Hall J: *Manual of skin diseases*, ed 7, Philadelphia, 1996, Lippincott-Raven.
3. Sanders S: Integumentary system. In Lueckenotte A: *Textbook of gerontologic nursing*, St Louis, 1996, Mosby.
4. Diepgen T, Coenraads P: Inflammatory skin diseases, II: Contact dermatitis. In Williams H, Strachan D, editors: *The challenge of dermato-epidemiology*, Boca Raton, Fla, 1997, CRC Press.
5. Thompson J, Wilson S: *Health assessment for nursing practice*, St Louis, 1996, Mosby.
6. Fitzpatrick T and others, editors: *Color atlas and synopsis of clinical dermatology*, ed 2, New York, 1994, McGraw-Hill.
7. Goldsmith L, Lazarus G, Thorp M: *Adult and pediatric dermatology*, Philadelphia, 1997, FA Davis.

Resources

Resources for this chapter are listed after Chapter 22 on p. 522.

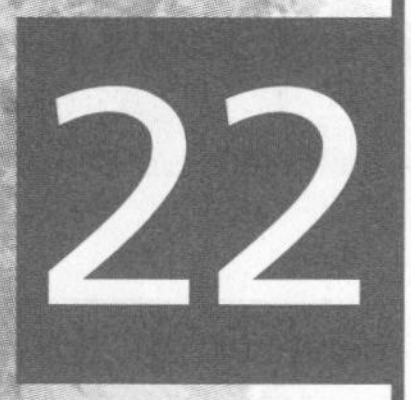

REMEMBER to check out your companion CD-ROM

22 NURSING MANAGEMENT Integumentary Problems

Noreen Heer Nicol & Anne Marie Ruszkowski

www.mosby.com/MERLIN/medsurg_lewis

LEARNING OBJECTIVES

1. Describe health promotion practices related to the skin.
2. Explain the etiology, clinical manifestations, and nursing and collaborative management of common acute dermatologic problems.
3. Describe the psychologic and physiologic effects of chronic dermatologic conditions.
4. Explain the etiology, clinical manifestations, and management of malignant dermatologic disorders.
5. Explain the etiology, clinical manifestations, and management of bacterial, viral, and fungal infections of the integument.
6. Explain the etiology, clinical manifestations, and management of infestations and bites.
7. Explain the etiology, clinical manifestations, and management of dermatologic disorders related to allergies.
8. Explain the etiology, clinical manifestations, and management related to benign dermatologic disorders.
9. Describe the dermatologic manifestations of common systemic diseases.
10. Explain the indications and nursing management related to plastic surgery and skin grafts.
11. Explain the etiology, clinical manifestations, and management of pressure sores.

Problems of the skin often present difficult management challenges. Clothing and cosmetics can disguise or cover some skin problems, but many problems cannot be hidden so easily. The emotional impact of skin problems often is more serious than the skin problem itself. For instance, acne is little more than a nuisance disease in relation to overall health. However, to the adolescent attempting to establish personal identity and self-esteem, it can be a barrier to acceptance in a peer group and pleasant social outlets. The actual seriousness of a skin problem and the emotional impact of the problem may often be two separate issues.

In this chapter, nursing and collaborative care of integumentary problems are presented before specific dermatologic problems are discussed. These common considerations apply to many different dermatologic problems.

INTEGUMENTARY PROBLEMS

Health Promotion

Health promotion practices related to problems of the skin often parallel practices appropriate for general good health. The skin reflects both physical and psychologic well-being. Specific health promotion activities appropriate to good skin health include avoidance of environmental hazards, adequate rest and exercise, proper hygiene and nutrition, and cautious use of self-treatment.

Environmental Hazards

Sun exposure. Many people are unaware that the effects of years of exposure to the sun are cumulative and damaging. The ultraviolet (UV) rays of the sun cause degenerative changes in the dermis, resulting in premature aging (i.e., loss of elasticity, thinning, wrinkling, and drying of the skin). Prolonged and repeated sun exposure is a major factor in precancerous and cancerous lesions. Actinic damage, actinic keratoses, basal cell epithelioma, squamous cell epithelioma, and malignant melanoma are dermatologic problems associated directly or indirectly with sun exposure.[1]

Nurses should be strong advocates of safe sun practices. Vitamin D_3 is produced in the skin and is necessary for vitamin D synthesis. However, only a few minutes of sun on small areas of the body are adequate to meet this need. Specific wavelengths of the sun (Table 22-1) have different effects on the skin. Ultraviolet B (UVB) appears to be the major factor in the development of skin cancer, while ultraviolet A (UVA) augments the carcinogenic effects of UVB. Tanning is the skin's response to injury by the sun and is caused by increased production of melanin. When sun exposure is excessive, the turnover time of the skin is shortened and results in peeling. Fair-skinned persons should be especially cautious about excessive sun exposure, since they have smaller amounts of the natural protection afforded by melanin.

Sunscreens can filter UVA and UVB wavelengths. There are two types of sunscreen—chemical and physical. *Chemical*

Reviewed by Sandra Somma, RN, BSN, Staff Nurse, Yale New Haven Hospital, New Haven, Conn.

CULTURAL & ETHNIC CONSIDERATIONS

Integumentary Problems

- African-Americans and Native-Americans have a lower incidence of skin cancer than Caucasians.
- Caucasians, especially those living in sunny climates, have a high incidence of skin cancer.
- Skin assessment may be difficult in individuals with darker skin. The oral mucous membranes and conjunctiva are areas where pallor, cyanosis, and jaundice are more readily detected. The palms of the hands and soles of feet can also be used for assessment of the skin of darker individuals.

Table 22-1 Wavelengths of the Sun and Effects on Skin

Wavelength	Nanometer Rating	Effect
Short (UVC)	Below 290	Does not reach earth; blocked by atmosphere
Middle (UVB)	280-320	Causes sunburn and cumulative effect of sun damage
Long (UVA)	320-400	Can produce elastic tissue damage and actinic skin damage; contributes to formation of skin cancer

sunscreens are designed to absorb or filter UV light, resulting in diminished UV light penetration into the epidermis. *Physical sunscreens* are thick, opaque, and reflect UV radiation. They block all UVA and UVB radiation, as well as all visible light.

The Food and Drug Administration (FDA) has rated popular sunscreen products according to their *sun protection factor (SPF)*. This is a method of measuring the effectiveness of a sunscreen in filtering and absorbing UVB radiation. There is no similar rating of products to screen UVA. Patients should be taught to look for the term "broad spectrum" on the packaging indicating a wide range of absorbance, particularly for UVB wavelengths.

Para-aminobenzoic acid (PABA) has been removed from many sunscreen products because it stains clothing and can cause allergic reactions, including contact dermatitis.

Consumers need to select the sunscreen most appropriate for their needs. PABA and PABA esters, cinnamates, salicylates, and methyl anthranilate block UVB rays. Parsol blocks UVA rays and is added to some sunscreens. The benzophenones block both UVA and UVB rays (Table 22-2).[2] Waterproof sunscreens should be used by swimmers and persons who perspire profusely. Directions accompanying specific products should be followed because application time before exposure varies according to the product.

The general recommendation is that everyone should use a sunscreen with a minimum SPF of 15 daily.[3] Sunscreens with an SPF of 15 or more filter 92% of the UVB responsible for erythema and make sunburn unlikely in most individuals when applied appropriately.

The nurse can also inform the patient about other means of protection from the damaging effects of the sun, such as wearing a large-brimmed hat and a long-sleeved shirt of a lightly woven fabric or carrying an umbrella. Patients need to know that the rays of the sun are most dangerous between 10 AM and 2 PM standard time or 11 AM and 3 PM daylight saving time, regardless of the latitude. Even on overcast days a serious sunburn can occur, since up to 80% of UV rays can penetrate through the clouds. Other factors that increase the possibility of sunburn include being at high altitudes, being in snow, which reflects 85% of the sun's rays, or being in or near water. Patients should be warned of the dangers of tanning booths and sun

Table 22-2 Sunscreen Ingredients and Ultraviolet Light Protection

Sunscreen Ingredients	Ultraviolet Light (UVL) Protection
Chemical	
Benzophenones	UVA and UVB
PABA and PABA esters	UVB
Cinnamates	UVB
Salicylates	UVB
Miscellaneous	
Methyl anthranilate	UVB
Parsol	UVA
Physical Sunscreens	
Titanium dioxide	UVA and UVB
Zinc oxide	UVA and UVB

UVA, long-wavelength of UVL; *UVB*, middle-wavelength of UVL.

lamps, which are predominantly UVA.[4] No presently available sunscreen blocks all UVA.

Certain topical and systemic medications potentiate the effect of the sun, even with brief exposure. Categories of drug therapy that may contain common photosensitizing medications are listed in Table 22-3. The nurse should be aware that many medications are included in these categories, and the photosensitivity of each individual drug should be examined. The chemicals in these medications absorb light and release energy that harms cells and tissues. The clinical symptoms of drug-induced photosensitivity are that of an exaggerated sunburn with swelling, erythema, papular, plaque-like lesions, and vesicles. Skin that is at risk for photosensitivity reactions can be protected by the use of sunscreen products. Nurses have a role in educating patients who are taking these medications about their photosensitizing effect.

Irritants and allergens. Patients can present to the nurse with irritant or allergic dermatitis, two types of contact dermatitis. *Irritant contact dermatitis* is produced by direct chemical injury to the skin and has a nonimmunologic etiology. *Allergic contact dermatitis* is an agent-specific, type IV delayed hypersensitivity response. This response requires sensitization

DRUG THERAPY

Table 22-3 Categories of Drugs That May Cause Photosensitivity

Categories	Examples
Anticancer drugs	Methotrexate, vinorelbine (Navelbine)
Antidepressants	Amitriptyline (Elavil), clomipramine (Anafranil), doxepin (Sinequan)
Antiarrhythmics	Quinidine, amiodarone (Cordarone)
Antihistamines	Diphenhydramine (Benadryl), chlorpheniramine, clemastine (Tavist)
Antimicrobials	Tetracycline, sulfamethoxazole, azithromycin, ciprofloxacin (Cipro)
Antifungals	Griseofulvin, ketoconazole (Nizoral)
Antipsychotics	Chlorpromazine (Thorazine), haloperidol (Haldol)
Diuretics	Furosemide (Lasix), hydrochlorothiazide (HydroDiuril)
Hypoglycemics	Tolbutamide (Orinase), glipizide (Glucotrol), chlorpropamide (Diabenese)
Nonsteroidal antiinflammatory drugs	Diclofenac (Voltaren), piroxicam (Feldene), sulindac (Clinoril)

and occurs only in individuals who are genetically predisposed to react to a particular antigen.[5] (See Chapter 12.)

The nurse should counsel his or her patients to avoid known irritants (e.g., ammonia, harsh detergents). Skin patch testing (application of allergens) is necessary to determine the most likely sensitizing agent.[6] Usually the nurse is the first health care provider to detect a contact allergy to various tapes, gloves (latex) and adhesives. The nurse must also be aware that prescribed and over-the-counter (OTC) topical and systemic medications used to treat a variety of conditions may cause dermatologic reactions.[7]

Radiation. Although most radiology departments are extremely cautious in protecting both themselves and their patients from the effects of excessive radiation, the nurse should help the patient make intelligent decisions about radiologic procedures. X-rays can be invaluable in both diagnosis and therapy, but indiscriminate use can cause serious side effects to the skin, as well as other body processes. In the past (30 years ago), cystic acne was treated with radiation. This information is important, since the patients who were thus treated have an increased incidence of basal cell carcinoma.

Rest and Sleep. Rest and sleep are important health-promotion considerations in relation to the skin. Although the exact effects of sleep are not known, it is thought to be restorative. Rest reduces the threshold of itching and the potential skin damage from the resultant scratching.

Exercise. Exercise increases circulation and dilates the blood vessels. In addition to the healthy glow produced by exercise, the psychologic effects can also improve one's appearance and mental outlook. However, caution must be used to avoid or protect the exerciser from overexposure to heat, cold, and sun during outdoor exercise.

Hygiene. Hygienic practices should match the skin type, lifestyle, and culture of the patient. The person with oily skin should cleanse the skin with a drying agent more often than the person with dry skin. Dry skin might benefit from superfatted soaps and measures to increase moisture, such as the application of moisturizers to the skin.

The normal acidity of the skin (pH 4.2 to 5.6) and perspiration protect against bacterial overgrowth. Most soaps are alkaline and cause a neutralization of the skin surface and loss of protection. The use of more neutral soaps, as well as avoiding hot water and vigorous rubbing, can noticeably decrease local irritation and inflammation.

In general, the skin and hair should be washed often enough to remove excess oil and excretions and to prevent odor. Older persons should avoid the use of harsh soaps and shampoos because of the increasing dryness of their skin. Moisturizers should be used after bath or shower, while the skin is still damp, to seal in this moisture.

Nutrition. A well-balanced diet adequate in all food groups can produce healthy skin, hair, and nails. Certain elements are particularly essential to good skin health. These elements include the following:

1. *Vitamin A*—essential for maintenance of normal cell structure, specifically epithelial cells. It is necessary for normal wound healing. The absence of vitamin A causes conjunctiva dryness and poor wound healing.
2. *Vitamin B complex*—essential to complex metabolic functions. Deficiencies of niacin and pyridoxine manifest as dermatologic symptoms such as erythema, bullae, and seborrhea-like lesions.
3. *Vitamin C (ascorbic acid)*—essential for connective tissue formation and normal wound healing. Absence of vitamin C causes symptoms of scurvy, including petechiae, bleeding gums, and purpura.
4. *Vitamin K* deficiency—interferes with normal prothrombin synthesis in the liver and can lead to cutaneous purpura.
5. *Protein*—necessary in amounts adequate for cell growth and maintenance. It is also necessary for normal wound healing.
6. *Unsaturated fatty acids*—necessary to maintain the function and integrity of cellular and subcellular membranes in tissue metabolism, especially linoleic and arachidonic acids.

Obesity has an adverse effect on the skin. This increase in subcutaneous fat can lead to stretching and overheating. Overheating secondary to the greater insulation provided by fat causes an increase in sweating, which has an adverse effect on normal or inflamed skin. Obesity also has an influence on the development of type 2 diabetes mellitus with its concomitant skin complications (see Chapter 46).

Self-treatment. The nurse needs to increase the patient's awareness of the dangers of self-diagnosis and treatment. The wide variety of OTC skin preparations can confuse the consumer. General instructions that the nurse can discuss with the patient would stress the duration of the treatment and the need to follow package directions closely. Skin problems are generally slow to produce symptoms and slow to resolve. If the package insert of an OTC drug says its use should not exceed 7 days, this warning should be heeded. If the directions say to apply twice daily, the urge to double the dose and hasten the cure must be avoided. If any systemic signs of inflammation or extension of the skin problem (e.g., an increased number of lesions or increased erythema or swelling) develop, self-care should be stopped and the help of a professional should be enlisted.

GENERAL MEASURES TO TREAT ACUTE DERMATOLOGIC PROBLEMS

Diagnostic Studies

A careful history is of prime importance in the diagnosis of skin problems. The clinician must be skilled at detecting any evidence that could lead to the cause of the extraordinary number of skin problems. After a careful history and physical examination, individual lesions are inspected. On the basis of the history, physical examination, and appropriate diagnostic tests, either medical, surgical, or combination therapy is planned.

Collaborative Care

Many different treatment methods are used in dermatology. Some are disease specific, whereas others work for unknown reasons. Advances in this field have brought relief to many previously chronic, untreatable conditions. Many of the specific therapeutic treatments require specialized equipment and are usually reserved for use by the dermatologist. Drug therapy is prescribed by many clinicians. The effectiveness of this therapy can often be related to the base (or vehicle) in which the medication is prepared. Table 22-4 summarizes the common agents used as bases for topical preparations and their therapeutic considerations.

DRUG THERAPY

Table 22-4 Common Bases for Topical Medications

Agent	Therapeutic Considerations
Powder	Promotion of dryness, increase in evaporation, absorbing of moisture possible, common base for antifungal preparations
Lotion	Suspension of insoluble powders in water; cooling and drying, with residual powder film after evaporation of water; useful in subacute pruritic eruptions
Cream	Emulsions of oil and water, most common base for topical medications, lubrication, and protection
Ointment	Oil with differing amounts of water added in suspension, lubrication and prevention of dehydration, petrolatum most common
Paste	Mixture of powder and ointment, used when drying effect necessary because moisture is absorbed

Phototherapy. Two types of ultraviolet light (UVL), or a combination of the two types (UVA, UVB), are used to treat many dermatologic conditions. Ultraviolet wavelengths cause erythema, desquamation, and pigmentation and may cause a temporary suppression of basal cell mitosis followed by a rebound increase in cell turnover.

Psoralen plus UVA light (PUVA) is a form of phototherapy. The photosensitizing drug psoralen is given to patients 90 minutes before exposure to UVA to enhance the effect of UVL in the UVA spectrum. Usually a moisturizing agent or a tar preparation is applied to the affected area in a thin layer before exposure to UVB. Conditions that are responsive to effective wavelengths with or without drugs include atopic dermatitis, cutaneous T-cell lymphoma, pruritus, psoriasis, and vitiligo.

UVL in the specific wavelengths can be produced artificially. Therapeutic doses of UVA and UVB can be measured and used to treat spectrum-specific diseases (Fig. 22-1). Frequent skin assessments must be performed on all patients receiving phototherapy. Inappropriate exposure to UVL can result in basal or squamous cell carcinoma, as well as severe erythema or burn to the skin. Patients should be cautioned about the potential hazards of using photosensitizing chemicals and further exposure to UV rays from sunlight or artificial UVL during the course of phototherapy. Protective eye wear that blocks 100% of ultraviolet light is prescribed for patients receiving PUVA, since psoralen is absorbed by the lens of the eye. The eye wear is used to prevent cataract formation. Patients are instructed to use the eye wear for 24 hours after taking the medication when outdoors or near a bright window because UVA penetrates glass. The recent evidence of immunosuppressive effects of PUVA requires careful ongoing monitoring of patients.

Radiation Therapy. The use of radiation for the treatment of cutaneous malignancies varies greatly according to local practice and availability. Even if radiotherapy is planned, a biopsy must first be performed to obtain a pathologic diagnosis.

Radiation to malignant cutaneous lesions is a painless treatment that is similar in cost to surgery. It produces minimal damage to surrounding tissue. It is a particularly effective treatment for the older adult or debilitated patient who cannot tolerate even a minor surgical procedure and for such areas as the nose, eyelids, and canthal areas, where preservation of the surrounding tissue is of prime consideration. Careful shielding is necessary to prevent ocular lens damage if the irradiated area is around the eyes.

Radiation therapy usually requires multiple visits. It is most effective on lesions above the neck. However, it produces permanent hair loss (alopecia) of the irradiated areas. Adverse effects include telangiectasia, atrophy, hyperpigmentation, depigmentation, ulceration, chronic radiodermatitis, and squamous cell carcinoma. Radiation therapy is discussed in Chapter 14.

Total-body skin irradiation (body is bombarded with high-energy electrons) may be the treatment of choice or adjunctive therapy for cutaneous T-cell lymphoma. Treatment follows a

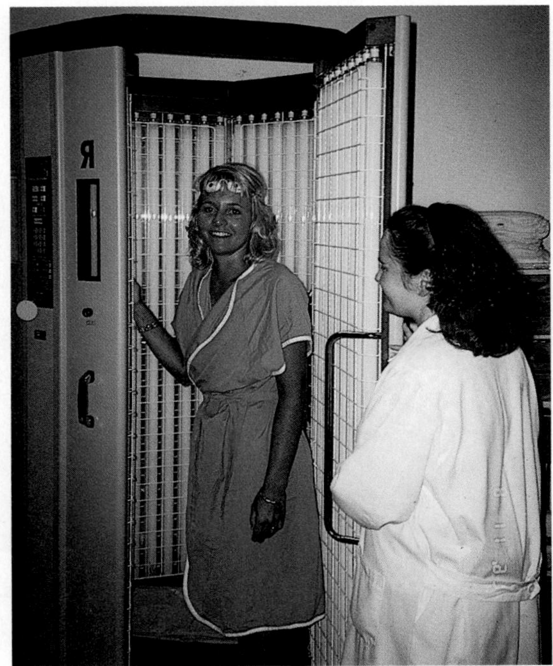

Fig. 22-1 Phototherapy is a method for treating spectrum-specific diseases. The patient's eyes must be protected during the phototherapy session. PUVA unit is illustrated in photo.

lengthy course, and toxicity to internal organs must be avoided. Patients experience varying degrees of hair loss and radiation dermatitis with transient loss of sweat gland function. This treatment ages the skin about 20 years.

Laser Technology. Laser treatment is expanding rapidly as an efficient surgical tool for many types of dermatologic problems. Lasers are able to produce measurable, repeatable, consistent zones of tissue damage. They can cut, coagulate, and vaporize tissue to some degree. The wavelength determines the type of delivery system used and the intensity of the energy delivered.

The surgical use of laser energy requires a focusing device to produce a small, high-density spot of energy that can be carefully focused on the surgical site and controllably directed to the operative site. Written policies and procedures should cover laser safety and be reviewed by all personnel working with laser equipment. Laser light does not accumulate in body cells and cannot cause cellular changes or damage.

There are several types of lasers generally available in most offices and hospitals. The CO_2 laser is the most common treatment. This laser has numerous applications as a vaporizing and cutting tool for most tissues. The argon laser emits light that is primarily absorbed by hemoglobin and helps in the treatment of vascular and other pigmented lesions. Other less common lasers include the use of copper and gold vapors, tunable dye and neodymium yttrium aluminum garnet (Nd:YAG). Dermatologic uses of the various lasers include coagulation of vascular lesions, removal of tattoos, and the treatment of basal cell carcinoma (BCC), condylomas, plantar warts, and keloids.

Drug Therapy

Antibiotics. Antibiotics are used both topically and systemically to treat dermatologic problems, and they are often used in combination. If used, topical antibiotics should be applied to clean skin. Common OTC topical antibiotics include bacitracin and polymyxin B. Prescription topical antibiotics include mupirocin (used for staphylococcus), gentamicin (used for *Staphylococcus* and most gram-negative organisms), and erythromycin (used for gram-positive cocci [staphylococci and streptococci] and gram-negative cocci and bacilli). Topical erythromycin and clindamycin (solutions or gels) are used in the treatment of acne vulgaris. Many of the more popular systemic antibiotics are not used topically because of the danger of allergic contact dermatitis.

If there are signs of systemic infection, a systemic antibiotic should be used. Systemic antibiotics are useful in the treatment of bacterial infections and acne vulgaris. The most frequently used are synthetic penicillin, erythromycin, and tetracycline. These drugs are particularly useful for erysipelas, cellulitis, carbuncles, and severe, infected eczema. Culture and sensitivity of the lesion can guide the choice of antibiotic. Patients require drug-specific instructions on the proper technique of taking or applying antibiotics. For instance, oral tetracycline must be taken on an empty stomach and should never be taken with a dairy product, which would interfere with absorption.

Corticosteroids. Corticosteroids are particularly effective in treating a wide variety of dermatologic conditions and can be used topically, intralesionally, or systemically. *Topical corticosteroids* are used for their local antiinflammatory action, as well as for their antipruritic effects. Attempts to diagnose a lesion should be made before a corticosteroid preparation is applied, since corticosteroids will mask the clinical manifestations. Corticosteroids are useful in the treatment of many dermatologic problems. Once a sufficient amount of medication is dispensed, limits should be set on the duration and frequency of application. The potency of a particular preparation is related to the concentration of active drug in the preparation. With prolonged use, the more potent corticosteroid formulations can cause adrenal suppression, especially if occlusive dressings are used. High-potency corticosteroids may produce side effects when their use is prolonged, including atrophy of the skin resulting from impaired cell mitosis and capillary fragility and susceptibility to bruising. In general, dermal and epidermal atrophy does not occur until a corticosteroid has been used 2 to 3 weeks. If drug use is discontinued at the first sign of atrophy, recovery usually occurs in several weeks. Rosacea eruptions, severe exacerbations of acne vulgaris, and dermatophyte infections may also occur. Rebound dermatitis is not uncommon when therapy is stopped, and this can be reduced by tapering potencies of topical corticosteroids with improvement.

Low-potency corticosteroids such as hydrocortisone act more slowly but can be used for a longer period of time without producing serious side effects. Low-potency corticosteroids are safe to use on the face and intertriginous (opposing skin surfaces) areas, such as the axillae. The potency of a particular preparation is related to the concentration of active drug in the preparation. The ointment form represents the most efficient delivery system. Creams and ointments should be applied in thin layers and slowly massaged into the site one to three times a day as prescribed. Accurate and adequate topical therapy is often the key to successful outcomes.

Intralesional corticosteroids are injected directly into or just beneath the lesion. This method provides a reservoir of medication with an effect lasting several weeks to months. Intralesional injection is commonly used in the treatment of psoriasis, *alopecia areata* (patchy hair loss), cystic acne, hypertrophic scars, and keloids. A 2.5 to 10 mg/ml suspension of triamcinolone acetonide (Kenalog) is the most common dose range for intralesional injection. A small amount is injected into the site of each lesion.

Systemic corticosteroids can have remarkable results in the treatment of dermatologic conditions. However, they often have undesirable systemic effects (see Chapter 47). Corticosteroids can be administered as short-term therapy for acute conditions such as contact dermatitis caused by poison ivy. Long-term corticosteroid therapy for dermatologic conditions is reserved for chronic bullous diseases, severe systemic effects of collagen and immunologic responses, and as a last resort when other therapies have failed.

The side effects of both topical and systemic long-term corticosteroid therapy must always be considered when such therapy is used to treat chronic skin conditions. The dangers of prolonged use of topical corticosteroids are discussed earlier in this section.

Antihistamines. Oral antihistamines are used to treat conditions that exhibit urticaria; angioedema; the pruritus associated with many dermatologic problems such as atopic dermatitis, psoriasis, and contact dermatitis; and other allergic cutaneous reactions. Antihistamines compete with histamine for the receptor site, thus preventing its effect. Antihistamines may have anticholinergic, antipruritic, and/or sedative effects. Several different antihistamines may have to be tried before the satisfactory therapeutic effect is achieved. Sedating antihistamines are often preferred, since the tranquilizing and sedative effect offer symptomatic relief. The patient should be warned about sedative effects, a particular problem when driving or operating heavy machinery. A new generation of antihistamines binds to peripheral histamine receptors, providing antihistamine action without sedation. Antihistamines should be used with particular caution in the older adult because of their long half-life and their anticholinergic effects.

Topical Fluorouracil. Fluorouracil (5-FU) is a topical cytotoxic agent with selective toxicity for sun-damaged cells. 5-FU is available in three strengths (1%, 2%, and 5%) and is used for the treatment of premalignant skin disease, especially actinic keratosis. Since systemic absorption of the drug is minimal, systemic side effects are virtually nonexistent. When a diagnosis of skin cancer has been established, 5-FU is generally not used.[8]

Patient compliance is the major problem with the use of 5-FU. The medication produces painful, eroded areas over the damaged skin within 4 days. Treatment must continue with applications one to two times a day for 2 to 4 weeks. Healing may take up to 3 weeks after medication is stopped. Since fluorouracil is a photosensitizing drug, the patient must be instructed to avoid sunlight during treatment. Patients should be educated about the effect of the medication and should be warned that they will look worse before they look better. 5-FU causes dermatitis, so patients should plan their social activities accordingly. After effective treatment, treated skin is smooth and free of actinic keratoses, although sometimes a second course is necessary.

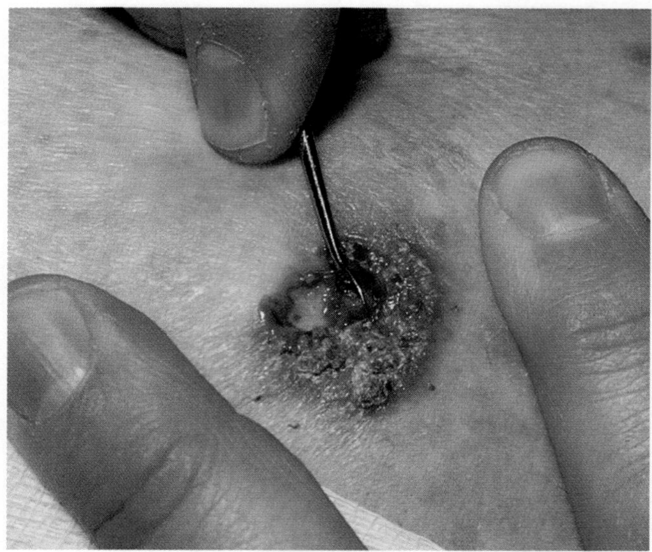

Fig. 22-2 Curettage of an inflamed seborrheic keratosis.

Diagnostic and Surgical Therapy

Skin Scraping. Scraping is done with a scalpel blade in order to obtain a sample of surface cells for microscopic inspection and diagnosis.

Electrodesiccation and Electrocoagulation. Electrical energy can be converted to heat by the tip of an electrode. This results in tissue being destroyed by burning. The major uses of this type of therapy are point coagulation of bleeding vessels to obtain hemostasis and destruction of small telangiectasias. *Electrodesiccation* usually involves more superficial destruction, and a monopolar electrode is used. *Electrocoagulation* has a deeper effect, with better hemostasis and an increased possibility of scarring. A dipolar electrode is used for electrocoagulation.

Curettage. *Curettage* is the removal of tissue using an instrument with a circular cutting edge attached to a handle (Fig. 22-2). The tissue is scooped away. Although the curette is not usually strong enough to cut normal skin, it is useful for removing many types of small skin tumors, such as warts, molluscum contagiosum, seborrheic keratoses, and small basal and squamous cell cancers. The area to be curetted is anesthetized before the procedure. Hemostasis is obtained by use of one of several methods, electrocoagulation, ferric subsulfate (Monsel's solution), gelatin foam, aluminum chloride, or a gauze pressure dressing. A small scar may form. The specimen may be sent for biopsy.

Punch Biopsy. *Punch biopsy* is a common dermatologic procedure used to obtain a tissue sample for histologic study or to remove small lesions (Fig. 22-3). Its use is generally reserved for lesions of less than 0.5 cm. Before anesthesia is used, the biopsy area is outlined so that landmarks will not be obscured by the anesthetizing agent. The biopsy punch cores out a small cylinder of skin when its sharp edge is twirled between the fingers. The core of skin is snipped from the subcu-

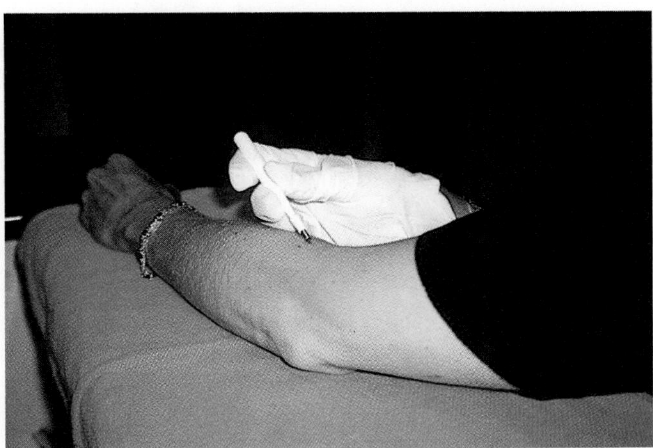

Fig. 22-3 Punch biopsy used to obtain tissue sample.

taneous fat and appropriately preserved for examination. Hemostasis is achieved by using methods as with curettage but sites of 3 mm or larger are often closed with sutures. Other types of biopsies are discussed in Table 21-8 and Chapter 21.

Cryosurgery. Some skin lesions can be destroyed by freezing. Topical liquid nitrogen is the agent most commonly used for cryosurgery. Although the exact mechanism is not clearly understood, the use of liquid nitrogen causes death or destruction of the treated skin.

Liquid nitrogen can be applied topically (directly onto the benign or precancerous lesion) with a cotton swab or with the appropriate container (Cry-AC) for several freeze-and-thaw cycles. Patients are informed that they will feel a cold sensation. The lesion will first become swollen and red, and it may blister. Next, a scab will form and fall off in 1 to 3 weeks. The skin lesion will be sloughed along with the scab. Growth of new skin follows. Cryosurgery is a useful treatment for common and genital warts, cutaneous tags, seborrheic keratoses, actinic keratoses, and many other less common skin conditions. Cryosurgery is inexpensive, rapid, and leaves minimal scarring. The major disadvantage of this treatment is lack of a tissue specimen, and potential for destruction of adjacent healthy tissue.

Excision. *Excision* should be considered if the lesion involves the dermis. Complete closure of the excised area usually results in a good cosmetic result.

Another type of excision is the *Mohs' micrographic surgery,* which is a microscopically controlled removal of a cutaneous malignancy. This procedure sections the surgical specimen horizontally, so that 100% of the surgical margin can be examined. Any residual tumor not removed by the first surgical excision can be removed in serial excisions performed the same day. The benefit of this treatment is preservation of normal tissue, producing the smallest possible wound. The procedure is done as an outpatient with a local anesthetic.

NURSING MANAGEMENT: DERMATOLOGIC PROBLEMS

Ambulatory and Home Care

Dermatologic conditions are not common reasons for hospitalization. Although it may not be the primary reason for hospitalization, many hospitalized patients will exhibit concurrent skin problems that warrant nursing intervention and patient education.

If the patient is in an acute-care setting, the nurse will be both administering and teaching the appropriate treatments. If the patient is in an outpatient setting, the nursing focus will be on patient education, with opportunities provided for demonstration and repeated demonstration. Subsequent visits provide the opportunity to evaluate patient understanding and treatment effectiveness.

Nursing interventions related to dermatologic conditions fall into broad categories. They are applicable to many skin problems in both inpatient and outpatient settings. The nursing care for a patient with chronic skin lesions is presented in NCP 22-1.

Wet dressings. The use of wet dressings is a common dermatologic procedure used to dry exudative lesions, relieve itching, suppress inflammation, and debride a wound. In addition, wet dressings increase penetration of topical medications, promote sleep by relieving discomfort, and enhance removal of scales, crusts, and exudate. Such materials as thin sheeting, gauze sponges, thermal underwear, or tube socks can be used for dressings. Ingenuity is sometimes required when odd-shaped parts of the body must be covered.

The prescribed dressing is put into fresh solution, held until it is no longer dripping, and applied to the affected area. The dressing should be left in place 15 to 30 minutes. The compress is then removed and replaced with a new one. This treatment may be used two to four times a day or continuously. If the skin appears macerated, the dressings should be discontinued for 2 to 3 hours. The patient should be protected from discomfort and chilling by using linens and bedclothes with pads or plastic.

Tap water, at room temperature, is the most common solution where water quality is adequate. Filtered or sterile water may be indicated in some locations. Potassium permanganate must be completely dissolved before use, since the crystals that do not dissolve may burn the skin. This solution must be freshly prepared to maintain its oxidative properties. If potassium permanganate solution turns brown, it should be discarded and fresh solution made. Boric acid is not recommended as a wet dressing solution because of potential systemic toxicity as a result of percutaneous absorption, especially on open skin. The best solution to use on the eyes is plain cool water.

Wet dressings do not need to be sterile. They should be cool when an antiinflammatory effect is desired and tepid when the purpose is to debride an infected, crusted lesion. These treatments are excellent ways to remove the scabs left by the collection of debris at a wound site.

Baths. Baths are appropriate when large body areas need to be treated. They also have sedative and antipruritic effects. Some medications, such as oilated oatmeal (Aveeno), potassium permanganate, and sodium bicarbonate, can be added directly to the bath water. One cup of the mixture can be added to 2 cups of water and then added to the bath water. The tub should be full enough to cover affected areas. Both the bath water and the prescribed solution should be at a temperature that is comfortable for the patient. The patient can soak for 15 to 20 minutes three to four times a day, depending on the

22-1 NURSING CARE PLAN PATIENT WITH CHRONIC SKIN LESIONS

Expected Patient Outcomes	Nursing Interventions and *Rationales*
NURSING DIAGNOSIS	**Altered comfort: pruritus*** *related to* presence of skin lesions *as manifested by* scratching, areas of excoriated skin, agitation, and anxiety over itching sensation.
▪ Satisfactory control of pruritus.	▪ Decrease environmental irritants (e.g., heat, scratchy coverings) *to reduce vasodilation and sensory stimulation.* ▪ Use appropriate topical and/or systemic corticosteroids *to reduce inflammation.* ▪ Provide a cool environment and cool soaks or wet dressings *to promote vasoconstriction.* ▪ Administer oral antihistamines as necessary *to reduce the itch sensation.* ▪ Provide diversional activities *to distract patient from discomfort or pruritus.*
NURSING DIAGNOSIS	**Risk for infection** *related to* open lesion and presence of environmental pathogens.
▪ No evidence of secondary infection such as redness, edema, or exudate.	▪ Monitor for open draining lesions; redness, swelling, and pain at lesion sites; lymphadenopathy and fever; indications of scratching *to detect presence of infection.* ▪ Practice and teach careful hand washing and bathing. Use proper disposal of dressings and contaminated linens *to prevent secondary infections.* ▪ Keep patient's nails trimmed short *to prevent skin excoriation from scratching.*
NURSING DIAGNOSIS	**Impaired skin integrity** *related to* dehydration, frequent wetting and drying of skin, dryness from treatment medications *as manifested by* destruction of skin layers.
▪ Moist, well-lubricated, intact skin.	▪ Provide adequate fluid (2000 to 3000 ml/day) intake *to maintain normal hydration status.* ▪ Avoid frequent wetting and drying of skin without proper use of topical lubricants. ▪ Encourage use of superfatted soap *to prevent drying of skin and encourage moisture retention.* ▪ Apply skin lotion/cream/ointments immediately after bathing *to trap moisture and reduce water loss.*
NURSING DIAGNOSIS	**Self-esteem disturbance** *related to* presence of unsightly lesions *as manifested by* verbalization of self-disgust and despair over appearance of lesions, isolation, reluctance to look at lesions or participate in self-care.
▪ Realistic hope for resolution of open lesions. ▪ Maintenance of normal social relationships.	▪ Discuss situation in open, accepting manner *to assist patient to express feelings.* ▪ Do not show shock or disgust at the sight of lesions *to prevent further decrease in self-esteem.* ▪ Provide counseling, if indicated, *to assist patient in accepting situation.*
NURSING DIAGNOSIS	**Altered health maintenance** *related to* lack of knowledge of disease process, management plan, prevention of scarring, and use of OTC medications *as manifested by* questions about self-care.
▪ Confidence in ability to care for self and explore surgical options. ▪ Understanding of disease process and management plan.	▪ Answer questions completely *to foster knowledge base of pertinent issues.* ▪ Teach patient about disease process, management plan, care of lesions *to foster independence and boost confidence in ability to manage self-care.* ▪ Discuss possible cosmetic surgery options *so patient can make informed decisions.* ▪ Advise patient to carefully follow guidelines for OTC medications *to prevent misuse or worsening of condition.*
NURSING DIAGNOSIS	**Social isolation** *related to* decreased activities secondary to poor self-image, fear of rejection, and lack of knowledge related to cover-up techniques *as manifested by* lack of social activities, verbalization of dissatisfaction with social life.
▪ Satisfaction with social life.	▪ Encourage socialization in patient's interest areas *to reduce sense of isolation and worthlessness.* ▪ Teach skillful use of cosmetics, cover-up agents, and clothing *to maximize personal appearance and encourage socialization.*

*This is not a currently accepted NANDA nursing diagnosis but is under consideration.
OTC, over-the-counter.

severity of the dermatitis and the patient's discomfort. It is important to stress to the patient that the skin not be rubbed dry with a towel but gently patted to prevent increasing irritation and inflammation. The addition of oils makes the bathtub extremely slippery and should be avoided. If oils are used in the tub, the utmost caution must be used in transferring patients to prevent accidents. To sustain the hydrating effect sealing moisturizers or medications should be applied to the skin directly after the bath. This helps to retain the moisture in the hydrated cells.

Topical medications. A thin layer of ointment, cream, or lotion should be applied to clean skin and spread evenly in a downward motion. An alternate method is to apply the medication directly onto the dressings. Pastes are designed to protect the affected area. They should be applied thickly with a tongue blade or a gloved hand. Draining lesions and lesions with greasy medication can be covered with a light dressing to prevent soiling clothes. Patients need specific directions on proper application technique of prescribed topical medications.

Control of pruritus. *Pruritus* (itching) can be caused by almost any physical or chemical stimulus to the skin, such as drugs, insects, and dry skin. The itch sensation is carried by the same nonmyelinated nerve fibers as pain.[9] If the epidermis is damaged or absent, the sensation will be felt as pain rather than an itch.

The itch-scratch cycle must be broken to prevent excoriation and eventual lichenification. Control of pruritus is also important because it is difficult to diagnose a lesion that is excoriated and inflamed.

Certain circumstances make itching worse. Anything that causes vasodilation, such as heat or rubbing, should be avoided. Dryness of the skin lowers the itch threshold and increases the itch sensation. Any internal or external factors that increase blood flow to an area increase itching.

The nurse can use or teach the patient various methods to break the itch cycle. A cool environment may cause vasoconstriction and decrease itching. The use of topical corticosteroids reduces inflammation and promote vasoconstriction, but should be reserved for use with appropriate dermatologic problems. Menthol, camphor, or phenol can be used to numb the itch receptors. Systemic antihistamines can be used if necessary to provide relief to a patient while the underlying cause of the pruritus is diagnosed and treated. The principle side effect of most antihistamines is sedation. This may, in fact, be desirable, since pruritus is often worse at night and interferes with sleep.

Wet dressings can be used effectively to relieve pruritus. Thin, cotton sheets or thermal underwear are placed in warm water, wrung out, and placed over the pruritic area. After 10 to 15 minutes the dressing is removed and the skin is patted dry and a lubricant or medication applied. This procedure can be repeated as necessary for comfort.

Prevention of spread. Although most skin problems are not contagious, universal precautions indicate the need for gloves with open or bleeding wounds. Procedures should be explained to the patient in order to avoid demoralizing an already sensitive patient. However, if in doubt, the nurse should wear gloves until a definite diagnosis has been established. The most common contagious lesions that the nurse should be cautious with include impetigo, staphylococcus, pyoderma, primary chancre and secondary syphilis lesions, scabies, and pediculosis. Careful hand washing and safe disposal of soiled dressings are the best means of preventing spread of skin problems.

Prevention of secondary infections. Open lesions on the skin are susceptible to invasion by other viral, bacterial, or fungal organisms. Meticulous hygiene, hand washing, and dressing changes are important to prevent secondary infections. Also, the patient should be warned about scratching lesions, which can cause excoriations and create a portal of entry for pathogens. The patient's nails should be trimmed short to minimize trauma from scratching.

Specific skin care. Nurses are often in a position to advise patients regarding care of the skin following simple dermatologic surgical procedures, such as skin biopsy, excision, and cryosurgery. Patient follow-up should be individualized. In general, instructions include dressing changes, use of topical antibiotics, and the signs and symptoms of infection. After a dermatologic procedure any oozing wound should be regularly cleansed with a saline solution. An antibiotic ointment may then be applied with a dressing that is both absorbent and nonadherent.

Wounds that are kept moist and covered heal more rapidly and with less scarring. Initially, a scab should be left alone to be a protective coating for the damaged skin beneath it. Scabs can be covered during the day for cosmetic purposes and should be protected at night from premature removal through rubbing against sheets. Scabs will separate naturally from healed epidermis.

A wound that required stitches can be covered with a variety of different dressings. Stitches will generally be removed in 4 to 10 days. Sometimes every other stitch is removed after the third day. Incision lines may require daily cleansing, usually with plain tap water. If necessary a topical antibiotic is applied and the wound is either covered with a dry sterile dressing or left open to air. The patient may experience some swelling and discomfort in the first 24 hours. Mild analgesics such as acetaminophen should control the discomfort. The patient needs to know the manifestations of inflammation such as redness, fever, or increased pain or swelling and signs of infection, such as purulent drainage. If these manifestations occur, they should be reported to the health care provider.

Psychologic effects of chronic dermatologic problems. Emotional stress can occur for persons who suffer from chronic skin problems such as psoriasis, atopic dermatitis, or severe acne. The sequelae of chronic skin problems could result in employment problems with subsequent financial implications, a frail and easily damaged body image, problems with sexuality, and increasing and progressive frustration. The usual lack of systemic overt illness coupled with the visibility of the skin lesions often presents a real problem to the patient.

The nurse must continue to be optimistic and help the patient comply with the prescribed regimen. The patient must be allowed to verbalize the "Why me?" question, even though there is no ready answer. Reinforcement of the prescribed hygiene and treatment measures is an important part of the nursing management. Dermatology patient support groups are listed with the American Academy of Dermatology (web site: www.aad.org). These groups are extremely useful for accurate patient support and education materials.

Many lesions can be camouflaged with the skillful use of cosmetics. Individual sensitivity to product ingredients must always be considered in the selection of a cosmetic product. Oil free, hypoallergenic cosmetics are available and could be beneficial to the allergic patient. Rehabilitative cosmetics are available to help camouflage and deemphasize such lesions as vitiligo or melasma (tan to brown patches on the face) or healed postoperative wound sites. These commercially available products are opaque, smudge resistant, and water resistant.

In addition to specific skin conditions that tend to chronicity, other factors affecting the outcome of long-term dermatologic problems include skin type, history of previous exacerbations, family history, complications, intolerance to therapy, environmental factors, lack of adherence to the prescribed regimen, endocrine factors, and psychologic factors. Lesions that follow a chronic pattern often are associated with lichenification and scarring.

Physiologic effects of chronic dermatologic problems. *Scarring* and *lichenification* are the result of chronic dermatologic problems. Scars occur when ulceration takes place and reflect the pattern of healing in the area. Scars are pink and vascular at first. As they age they become avascular and white with increasing strength. Different parts of the body scar differently, such as the face and neck, which heal fairly well because of a good blood supply.

The location of the scar is the determining factor with respect to its cosmetic implications. Facial scars are the most damaging psychologically, since they are so visible. Creative use of cosmetics can do much to mask the scarring of chronic skin conditions. The best treatment is prevention of scarring by control of the problem in the acute phase.

Lichenification is another consequence of chronic skin problems. It is the thickening of skin as a result of proliferation of keratinocytes with accentuation of the normal markings of the skin. Lichenification is caused by scratching or rubbing of the skin and is often associated with atopic dermatoses and pruritic conditions. Although any area of the body may be affected, the hands and forearms are common sites. Treatment of the cause of the itching is the key to prevention of lichenification. Excoriations are often evident in the thickened skin as a result of the pruritus.

DISORDERS OF THE INTEGUMENTARY SYSTEM

Malignant Conditions

Malignant neoplasms of the skin exhibit the characteristics of all malignant conditions (Chapter 14). However, skin malignancies generally grow slowly (Fig. 22-4). The presence of a persistent lesion that does not heal is highly suspicious of a malignancy and should be biopsied. Adequate and early treatment can often lead to complete cure. The fact that skin lesions are so visible increases the likelihood of early detection and diagnoses. Patients should be taught to self-examine their skin regularly.

Risk Factors. Risk factors for skin malignancies include having a fair skin type (blonde or red hair and blue or green eyes), history of chronic sun exposure, family history of skin cancer, outdoor occupation, and exposure to tar and systemic arsenicals. In addition, three severe sunburns before age 20 years greatly increase a person's subsequent risk of developing cutaneous melanoma.[10] Dark-skinned persons are less susceptible to skin cancer because of the naturally occurring increase in melanin, the most effective sunscreen. The incidence of skin cancer increases with proximity to the equator (latitude) and high altitude because of the increased intensity of UVB exposure.[11] Depletion of the stratosphere ozone layer has also been implicated in the increased incidence of skin cancer.[12]

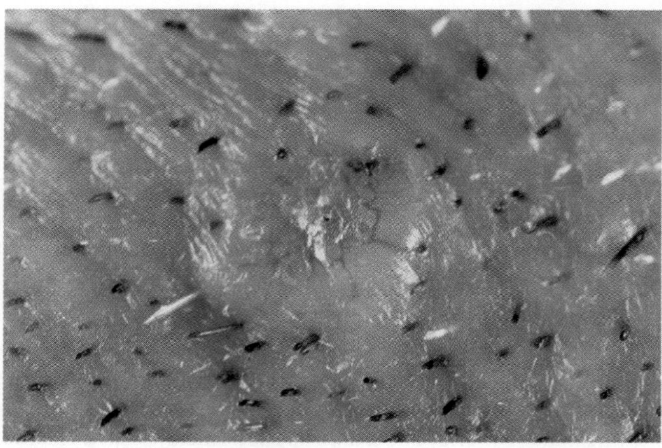

Fig. 22-4 Basal cell carcinoma. Magnification of early lesion found on upper lip after careful facial examination. Note the typical pearly border.

Nonmelanoma Skin Cancers. Nonmelanoma skin cancer is the most common form of neoplasm in countries with large numbers of Caucasian inhabitants and high exposure to UVL. In the United States and most countries throughout the world, there are greater than half a million new cases yearly.[13] The most common sites for development of nonmelanoma skin cancer are in sun-exposed areas and include the face, head, neck, back of the hands, and arms. A biopsy should be performed to confirm the diagnosis before specific treatment is started.

Although the number of deaths attributable to nonmelanoma skin cancer is small, the tumors have an inherent potential for severe local destruction, permanent disfigurement, and disability. The most common etiologic factor, chronic sun exposure, should be consciously avoided by the use of sunscreens and protective clothing.

Actinic keratosis. *Actinic keratosis* is a premalignant form of squamous cell carcinoma (SCC) that affects nearly all of the elderly white population. Actinic keratoses, also known as solar keratoses, are hyperkeratotic papules and plaques occurring on sun-exposed areas. The clinical appearance of actinic keratoses can be quite varied. The typical lesion is an irregularly shaped, flat, slightly erythematous macule or papule with indistinct borders and an overlying hard keratotic scale or horn. Many forms of treatment are used, including cryotherapy, 5-FU, surgical removal, tretinoin (Retin-A), and chemical peeling agents.

Basal cell carcinoma. *Basal cell carcinoma (BCC)* is a locally invasive malignancy arising from epidermal basal cells. The clinical manifestations are described in Table 22-5. Multiple treatment modalities are used, depending on the tumor location and histologic subtype, history of recurrence, and patient characteristics.[14] Treatment modalities include electrodesiccation and curettage, excision, cryosurgery, radiation therapy, Mohs' surgery, topical chemotherapy, and intralesional α-interferon.

Table 22-5 Premalignant and Malignant Conditions of the Skin

Etiology and Pathophysiology	Clinical Manifestations	Treatment and Prognosis
Actinic Keratoses		
Actinic (sun) damage (precursor of squamous cell carcinoma)	Flat or slightly elevated, dry, hyperkeratotic scaly papule; possibly flat, rough, or verrucous; adherent scale, which returns when removed; often multiple; rough scale on red base; often on erythematous sun-exposed areas; increase in number with age	Curettage, electrosurgery, cryosurgery, chemical caustics, topical application of 5-FU over entire area for 14-21 days; no effect on healthy skin and other lesions; recurrence possible even with adequate treatment; untreated lesions possibly leading to squamous cell carcinoma (1% incidence)
Dysplastic Nevus Syndrome		
Morphologically between common acquired nevi and melanoma; histogenetic precursor of cutaneous malignant melanoma	Often larger than 5 mm; irregular border, possibly notched; variegated color mixture of tan, brown, black, red, and pink with single mole; presence of at least one flat portion, often at edge of mole; frequently multiple; uncommon before puberty; most common site on back, but possible in uncommon mole sites such as scalp or buttocks	Marker of increased risk for melanoma; careful monitoring of persons suspected of familial tendency to melanoma or dysplastic nevus syndrome necessary to increase likelihood of early diagnosis of melanoma; indication for excisional biopsy for suspicious lesions
Basal Cell Carcinoma		
Change in basal cells; no maturation or normal keratinization; continuing division of basal cells and formation of enlarging mass; related to excessive sun exposure, genetic skin type, arsenicals, x-ray radiation, scars, and some types of nevi; basal cells possibly pigmented but absent in nevi	**Nodular and Ulcerative** Small, slowly enlarging papule; borders semitranslucent or "pearly," with overlying telangiectasia; erosion, ulceration, and depression of center; normal skin markings lost **Superficial** Erythematous, sharply defined, barely elevated multinodular plaques with varying scaling and crusting; similar to eczema but not pruritic	Excisional surgery, chemosurgery, electrosurgery, cryosurgery; 95% cure rate; slow-growing tumor that invades local tissue; metastasis rare
Squamous Cell Carcinoma		
Frequent occurrence on previously damaged skin (e.g., from sun, radiation, scar); malignant tumor of squamous (prickle) cell of epidermis; invasion of dermis, surrounding skin; metastasis possible	**Early** Firm nodules with indistinct borders with scaling and ulceration; opaque **Late** Covering of lesion with scale or horn from keratinization; most common on sun-exposed areas such as face and hands	Surgical removal, cryosurgery, radiation therapy, chemosurgery, Mohs' procedure or microscopically controlled excision, electrodesiccation, and curettage; untreated lesion possibly metastasizes to regional lymph nodes; high cure rate with early detection and treatment
Cutaneous T-Cell Lymphoma		
Origination in skin; chronic, slowly progressing disease with grave prognosis; possible etiologies of environmental toxins and chemical exposure	Prevalent in twice as many men as women in United States; classic presentation involving three stages—patch, plaque, and tumor; history of persistent macular eruption followed by gradual appearance of indurated plaques	Topical nitrogen mustard, radiation therapy, systemic chemotherapy, PUVA, and extracorporeal photopheresis; 5-yr life expectancy with only skin manifestations and no treatment; greatly decreased survival rate with generalized erythroderma with exfoliation and abnormal cells in bloodstream
Malignant Melanoma		
Neoplastic growth of melanocytes anywhere on skin, eyes, or mucous membranes; classification according to major histologic mode of spread; potential invasion and widespread metastases	Irregular color, irregular surface, irregular border; variegated color including red, white, blue, black, gray, brown; flat or elevated, eroded or ulcerated; often under 1 cm in size; most common sites in males and females on back; in females in chest and lower legs	Wide excision, full-thickness surgical removal; correlation of survival rate with depth of invasion; poor prognosis unless diagnosis and treatment early; spreading by local extension, regional lymphatic vessels, and bloodstream; adjuvant therapy after surgery may be necessary if lesion greater than 1.5 mm in depth

Continued

Table 22-5 Premalignant and Malignant Conditions of the Skin—cont'd

Etiology and Pathophysiology	Clinical Manifestations	Treatment and Prognosis
Kaposi's Sarcoma*		
Multicentric neoplasms that occur with increasing frequency in HIV-infected individuals; occurs predominantly in homosexual men; multiple vascular nodules appearing in the skin, mucous membranes, and viscera; severity ranges from minor to fulminant with extensive cutaneous and visceral involvement	Wide range of presentation; initially, small reddish, purple nodules on skin; lesions range in size from a few mm to several cm, can cause lymphedema and disfigurement particularly when confluent; systemic involvement has symptoms associated with organ (e.g., lungs and shortness of breath)	Diagnosis based upon biopsy of suspicious lesion; treatment dependent on severity of lesions and patient's immune status; attempt to avoid treatments to further suppress immune system; possible treatments include localized radiation, intralesional vinblastine, α-interferon, combination chemotherapy and cryotherapy

*Refer to Chapter 13 for more information.
HIV, human immunodeficiency virus; *PUVA,* psoralen ultraviolet A.

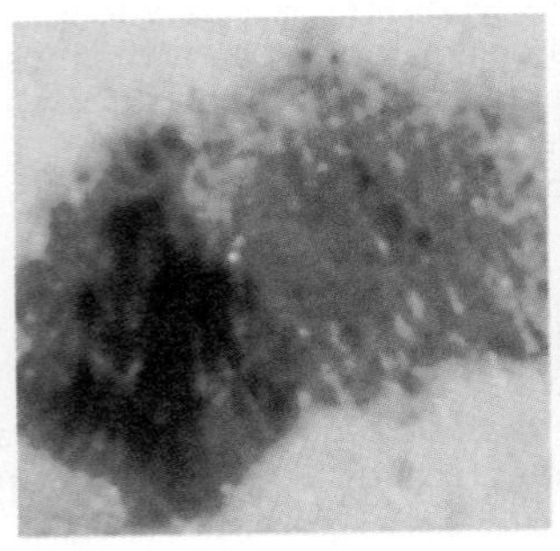
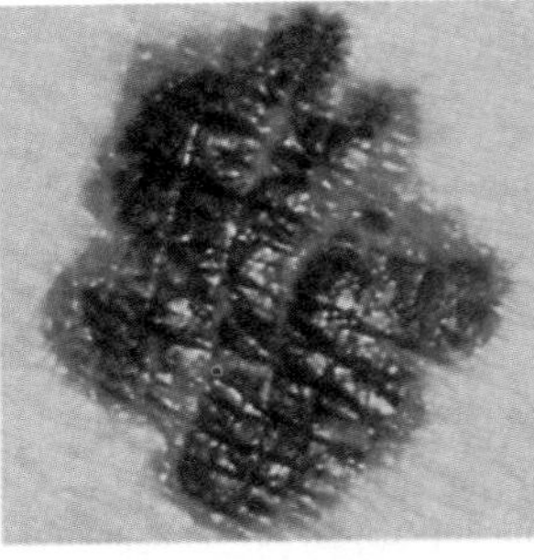
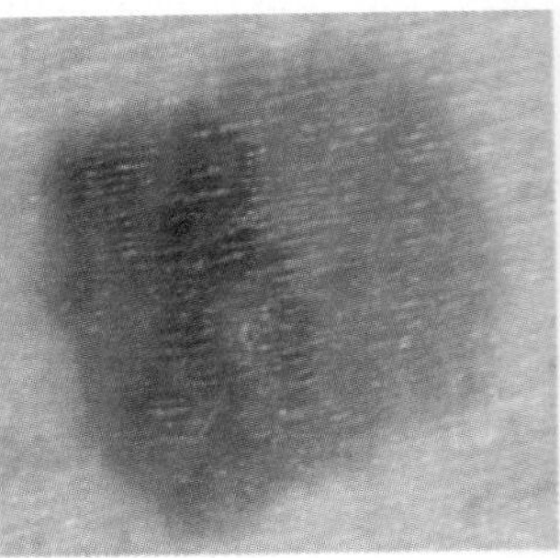
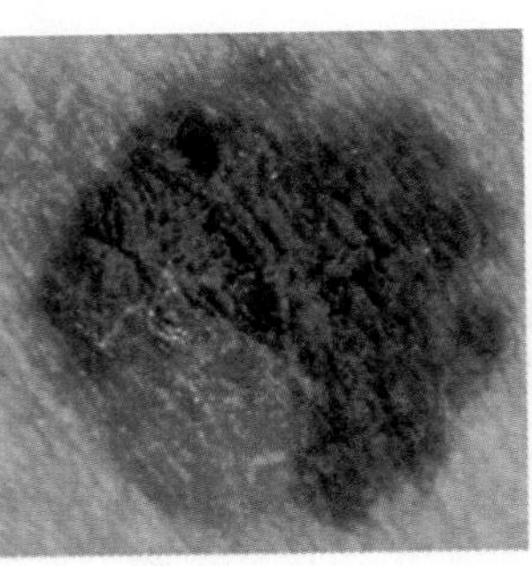

A, Asymmetry **B**, Border **C**, Color **D**, Diameter

Fig. 22-5 The ABCDs of melanoma. **A,** Asymmetry: one half unlike the other half. **B,** Border: irregular, scalloped, or poorly circumscribed border. **C,** Color: varied from one area to another; shades of tan and brown; black; sometimes white, red, or blue; change in shape, size, or color of mole. **D,** Diameter: larger than 6 mm as a rule (diameter of a pencil eraser)

Squamous cell carcinoma. SCC is a malignant neoplasm of keratinizing epidermal cells. It frequently occurs on skin previously damaged by such events as burns, scars, and irradiation. Unlike BCC, SCC has the potential to metastasize. The clinical manifestations are described in Table 22-5. Treatment consists of surgical excision, radiation, and Mohs' surgery. Cryosurgery and electrodesiccation and curettage have been used successfully in small primary tumors. There is a high cure rate with early detection and treatment.

Malignant Melanoma. *Malignant melanoma* is a tumor arising in cells producing melanin, usually the melanocytes of the skin. Melanoma has the ability to metastasize to any organ, including the brain and heart. This is the most deadly skin cancer and is increasing worldwide faster than any other cancer.[16] Risk factors that may contribute to this increase include UV radiation; skin sensitivity; genetic, hormonal, and immunologic factors; and recreational lifestyle changes that lead to greater sun exposure.[10] Cutaneous melanoma is nearly 100% curable by excision if diagnosed when the malignant cells are restricted to the epidermis. The most important prognostic factor is tumor thickness at the time of presentation. If spread to regional lymph nodes occurs, the patient has a 50% 5-year survival. If metastasis occurs, treatment is largely palliative.

The four types of cutaneous melanoma are *superficial spreading* (SSM), *lentigo maligna* (LMM), *acral-lentiginous* (ALM), and *nodular* (NM). SSM commonly occurs on chronically sun-exposed areas such as the legs and upper back. LMM usually is commonly located on the face. ALM appears on the soles, palms, mucous membranes, and terminal phalanges. ALM is more common in Asian and black people. NM occurs more often in males and can be located anywhere on the body. It is the most frequent misdiagnosed melanoma because it resembles a blood blister or polyp.[17] Patients should consult their physician immediately if their moles or lesions show any of the clinical signs (ABCDs) of melanoma. (Fig. 22-5).

The initial treatment of malignant melanoma is a wide surgical excision with a margin of normal skin. Subsequent treatment modalities such as chemotherapy, nonspecific immunotherapy, chemoimmunotherapy, and radiation may be planned, depending on the stage of the disease.[18] Gene therapy is currently being examined as another treatment option (see Chapter 12 for discussion of these therapies).

Dysplastic nevus syndrome. An abnormal mole pattern called *dysplastic nevus syndrome (DNS)* places a person at increased risk of melanoma.[15] There are two subtypes of DNS, familial and sporadic. The earliest clinically detectable abnormality associated with this syndrome is an increase in the number of morphologically normal-looking nevi at around the age of 2 to 6 years. Another proliferation occurs around adolescence, and new nevi appear throughout life. Obtaining a detailed family history related to melanoma and DNS is an important responsibility of the clinician.

Table **22-6** Common Bacterial Infections of the Skin

Etiology and Pathophysiology	Clinical Manifestations	Treatment and Prognosis
Impetigo		
Group A β-hemolytic streptococci, staphylococci, or combination of both; associated with poor hygiene and low socioeconomic status; primary or secondary infection; contagious	Vesiculopustular lesions that develop thick, honey-colored crust surrounded by erythema; pruritic; most common on face	**Systemic Antibiotics** Oral penicillin, benzathine penicillin IM, erythromycin **Local Treatment** Warm saline or aluminum acetate soaks followed by soap-and-water removal of crusts; topical antibiotic cream; with no treatment, glomerulonephritis possible when streptococcal strain nephritogenic; meticulous hygiene essential
Folliculitis		
Usually staphylococci; present in areas subjected to friction, moisture, oil, or grease	Small pustule at hair follicle opening with minimal erythema; development of crusting; most common on scalp, beard, extremities in men; tender to touch	Soap (e.g., Hibiclens) and water cleansing; topical antibiotics (e.g., Bactroban); warm compresses of water or aluminum acetate solution; healing usually without scarring; if lesions extensive and deep, possible scarring and loss of involved hair follicles
Furuncle		
Deep infection with staphylococci around hair follicle, often associated with severe acne or seborrheic dermatitis	Tender erythematous area around hair follicle; draining of pus and core of necrotic debris on rupture; most common on face, back of neck, axillae, breasts, buttocks, perineum, thighs; painful	Incision and drainage, occasionally antibiotics, meticulous care of involved skin, frequent application of warm, moist compresses
Furunculosis		
Increased incidence in patients who are obese, chronically ill, or regularly exposed to grease or oils or who have diabetes mellitus	Lesions as above; malaise, regional adenopathy, elevated temperature	Warm compresses; systemic antibiotic after culture and sensitivity study of drainage (usually semisynthetic, penicillinase-resistant, oral penicillin such as cloxacillin and oxacillin); measures to reduce surface staphylococci include antimicrobial cream to nares, armpits, and groin and antiseptic to entire skin; often recurrent with scarring; incision and drainage of soft lesions; prevention or correction of predisposing factors; meticulous personal hygiene
Carbuncle		
Multiple, interconnecting furuncles	Many pustules appearing in erythematous area, most common at nape of neck	Treatment same as furuncles; often recurrent despite production of antibodies; healing slow with scar formation

Continued

Infections

Bacterial Infections. The skin is covered with numerous microorganisms, especially bacteria. *Staphylococcus epidermidis* and diphtheroids are the most common bacteria present on the skin. The skin provides an ideal environment for bacterial growth, with abundant supplies of warmth, nutrients, and water.

Bacterial infection occurs when the balance between the host and the microorganisms is altered. This can occur as a primary infection following a break in the skin. It can also occur as a secondary infection to already damaged skin or as a sign of a systemic disease (Table 22-6).

Healthy persons can develop bacterial skin infections. Predisposing factors such as moisture, obesity, skin disease,

Table 22-6 Common Bacterial Infections of the Skin—cont'd

Etiology and Pathophysiology	Clinical Manifestations	Treatment and Prognosis
Cellulitis		
Inflammation of subcutaneous tissues; possibly secondary complication or primary infection; often following break in skin; *S. aureus* and streptococci usual causative agents; deep inflammation of subcutaneous tissue from enzymes produced by bacteria	Hot, tender, erythematous, and edematous area with diffuse borders; malaise and fever	Moist heat, immobilization and elevation, systemic antibiotic therapy, hospitalization if severe; progression to gangrene possible if untreated
Erysipelas		
Superficial cellulitis primarily involving the dermis; group A β-hemolytic streptococci	Red, hot, sharply demarcated plaque that is indurated and painful; bacteremia possible; most common on face and extremities; toxic signs, such as fever, elevated white blood cell count, headache, malaise	Systemic antibiotics—usually penicillin; hospitalization often required

IM, intramuscular.

✚ EMERGENCY MANAGEMENT

Table 22-7 Surface Skin Wound

Etiology	Assessment Findings	Interventions
Blunt Direct blow to skin (e.g., fist, baseball bat, rock) Indirect blow to skin (e.g., blast wave from gunshot) **Penetrating** Puncture or cutting of skin surface (e.g., knife, stick, glass)	▪ Contusion ▪ Laceration ▪ Avulsion ▪ Abrasion ▪ Bleeding ▪ Pain ▪ Neurovascular compromise	**Initial** ▪ Ensure airway, breathing, and circulation before management of surface injury. ▪ Identify and treat other more serious injuries. ▪ Control bleeding with direct pressure or pressure dressing. ▪ Assess for impaled objects, pieces of glass, or debris. ▪ Do not remove *impaled* object. Stabilize for removal under controlled environment. ▪ Cleanse wounds carefully with isotonic solution. Cover with moist saline gauze until wound is closed. ▪ Shave as small an area as possible with scalp wound. ▪ Never shave eyebrows. ▪ Fold avulsed skin flap into normal position, then control bleeding. Apply bulky sterile dressing to area and immobilize injured part. ▪ Determine tetanus immunization status. ▪ Use sticky side of a wide piece of tape to remove surface slivers of glass. **Ongoing** ▪ Monitor vital signs and neurovascular status of injured extremity.

systemic corticosteroids and antibiotics, chronic disease, and diabetes mellitus all increase the likelihood of infection. Good hygiene practices and general good health inhibit bacterial infections. If an infection is present, the resulting drainage is infectious. Meticulous skin hygiene and infection control practices are necessary to prevent spread of the infection.

Trauma is a common predisposing factor to skin infection. Table 22-7 outlines the emergency care of a patient with a surface skin wound.

Viral Infections. Viral infections of the skin are as difficult to treat as viral infections anywhere in the body. When a cell is infected by a virus, a lesion can result (Fig. 22-6). Lesions can also result from an inflammatory response to the viral infections. Herpes simplex, herpes zoster, and warts are the most common viral infections affecting the skin. (Table 22-8).

Fungal Infections. Because of the large number of identified fungi, it is almost impossible to avoid exposure to some pathologic varieties. Many fungi have valuable func-

Table 22-8 Common Viral Infections of the Skin

Etiology and Pathophysiology	Clinical Manifestations	Treatment and Prognosis
Herpes Simplex Virus Type 1*		
Generally oral infections; virus remaining in nerve root ganglion and possibly returning to skin to produce recurrence when exacerbated by sunlight, trauma, menses, stress, and systemic infection; contagious to those not previously infected; increase in severity with age, transmission by respiratory droplets or virus-containing fluid, such as saliva or cervical secretions; no protection against subsequent infection in other areas with episodes of infection in one area	**First Episode** Symptoms occurring 3-7 days or more after contact; painful local reaction; grouped vesicles on erythematous base; systemic symptoms, such as fever and malaise possible or asymptomatic presentation possible **Recurrent** Small; recurrence in similar spot; characteristic grouped vesicles on erythematous base	Symptomatic medication; soothing, moist compresses; petrolatum to lesions; scarring not usual result; antiviral agents such as acyclovir (Zovirax), famciclovir (Famvir), and valacyclovir (Valtrex)
Herpes Simplex Virus Type 2		
Generally genital infections; recurrence more frequent than oral-labial infections	Same as for herpes simplex virus type 1	Same as for herpes simplex virus type 1
Herpes Zoster		
Activation of the varicella-zoster virus; frequent occurrence in immunosuppressed patients; potentially contagious to anyone who has not had varicella or who is immunosuppressed	Linear patches along dermatome of grouped vesicles on erythematous base; usually unilateral and on trunk; burning, pain, and neuralgia preceding outbreak; mild to severe pain during outbreak	Symptomatic; antiviral agents such as acyclovir, famciclovir, and valacyclovir; wet compresses, white petrolatum to lesions; analgesia; mild sedation at bedtime; systemic corticosteroids to shorten course and decrease likelihood of postherpetic neuralgia (controversial); usual healing without complications but scarring possible; postherpetic neuralgia possible
Verruca Vulgaris		
Caused by human papillomavirus; spontaneous disappearance in 1-2 yr possible; mildly contagious by autoinoculation; specific response dependent on body part affected	Circumscribed, hypertrophic, flesh-colored papule limited to epidermis; painful on lateral compression	Multiple treatments, including surgery— scoop removal with scissors and currette; liquid nitrogen therapy; blistering agents—cantharidin; keratolytic agents—salicylic acid; CO_2 laser therapy, treatment can result in scarring
Plantar Warts		
Caused by human papillomavirus	Wart on bottom surface of foot, growing inward because of pressure of walking or standing; painful when pressure applied; interrupted skin markings; cone-shaped with black dots (thrombosed vessels) when pared	Usual treatment is liquid nitrogen or frequent paring followed by application of patches of impregnated chemicals to decrease regrowth; over-aggressive destruction possibly resulting in painful, hypertrophic scar

*Herpes simplex is also discussed in Chapter 50.

tions in food preparation (e.g., molds, cheese) and drug synthesis (e.g., penicillin). However, some fungi can cause serious infections. Common fungal infections of the skin are presented in Table 22-9.

Microscopic examination of the scraping of suspicious skin lesions in 10% to 20% potassium hydroxide is an easy, inexpensive diagnostic measure to determine the presence of fungus. The appearance of hyphae (threadlike structures) is indicative of a fungal infection.

Infestations and Insect Bites

The possibilities for exposure to insect bites and infestations are almost limitless. In many instances, an allergy to the venom plays a major role in the reaction. In other cases, the clinical

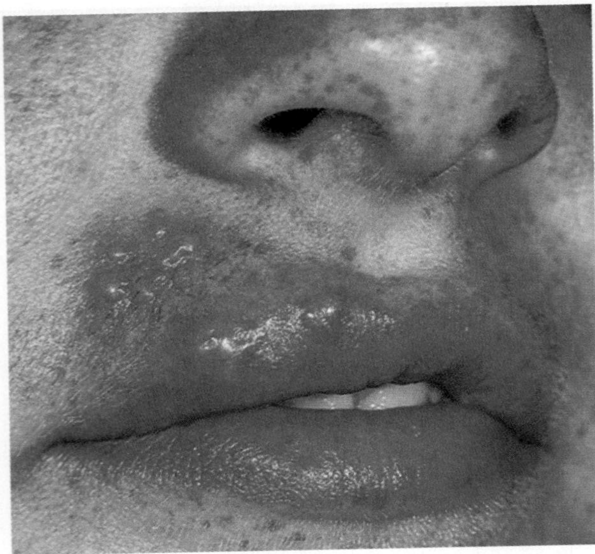

Fig. 22-6 Herpesvirus on the lips. Typical presentation with vesicles on the lips and extending on to the skin.

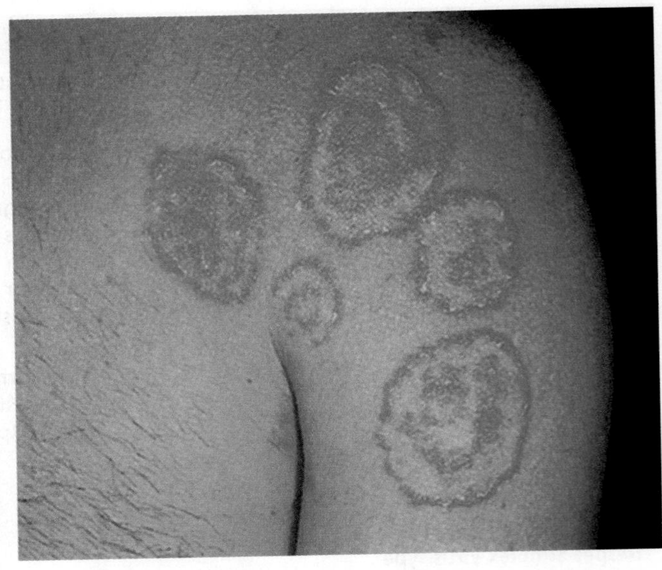

Fig. 22-7 Tinea corporis (ringworm). Typical presentation with an advancing red scaly border. Designation of "ring worm" is obvious.

Table 22-9 Common Fungal Infections of the Skin and Mucous Membranes

Etiology and Pathophysiology	Clinical Manifestations	Treatment and Prognosis
Candidiasis Caused by *Candida albicans;* also known as moniliasis; 50% of adults symptom-free carriers; presenting in warm, moist areas such as crural area, oral mucosa, and submammary folds; HIV infection, chemotherapy, radiation, and organ transplantation related to depression of cell-mediated immunity that allow yeast to become pathogenic; production of symptoms by imbalance between host and normal inhabitant of gastrointestinal tract, mouth, and vagina	**Mouth** White, cheeselike patches leaving erosions when removed **Vagina** Vaginitis, with red, edematous, painful vaginal wall, white patches; vaginal discharge; pruritus; pain on urination and intercourse **Skin** Diffuse papular erythematous rash with pinpoint satellite lesions around edges of affected area	Microscopic examination and culture; nystatin or other specific medication as vaginal suppository or oral lozenge; abstinence or use of condom; eradication of infection with appropriate medication; skin hygiene to keep it clean and dry; mycostatin powder effective on skin lesions; avoidance of lubricants
Tinea Corporis Various dermatophytes, commonly referred to as ringworm (Fig. 22-7)	Typical annular appearance, well-defined margins with fine cigarette paper scale; erythematous	Cool compresses; topical antifungals for isolated patches; creams or solutions of miconazole (Monistat) and clotrimazole (Lotrimin)
Tinea Cruris Various dermatophytes, commonly referred to as jock itch	Well-defined border in groin area	Topical antifungal cream or solution
Tinea Unguium Various dermatophytes	Only few nails on one hand affected; nails on toes possibly affected; fungal scale close to outer margin of lesion; brittle, thickened, broken nails with white or yellow discoloration	Topical antifungal cream or solution; griseofulvin moderately successful on fingernails; poor response on toenails; debridement of toenails to normal contour if problematic
Tinea Pedis Various dermatophytes, commonly referred to as athlete's foot	Interdigital scaling and maceration; erythema and blistering; pruritus; painful	Topical antifungal cream or solution

Table 22-10 Common Infestations and Insect Bites

Name	Etiology and Pathophysiology	Clinical Manifestations	Treatment and Prognosis
Bees and Wasps	*Hymenoptera*	Intense, burning, local pain; swelling and itching; severe hypersensitivity possibly leading to anaphylaxis	Cool compresses; local application of antipruritic lotion; antihistamines if indicated; usually uneventful recovery
Bedbugs	*Cimicidae;* feeding periodic, usually at night; present in furniture, walls during day	Wheal surrounded by vivid flare; firm urticaria transforming into persistent lesion; severe pruritis; often grouped in threes appearing on noncovered parts of body	Bedbug controlled by chlorocyclohexane; lesions usually requiring no treatment; severe itching possibly requiring use of antihistamines or topical steroids
Pediculosis Head lice Body lice Pubic lice	*Pediculus humanus* var. *capitis;* *Pediculus humanus* var. *corporis;* *Phthirius pubis;* obligate parasites that suck blood, leave excrement and eggs on skin, live in seams of clothing (if body lice) and in hair as nits; transmission of pubic lice often by sexual contact	Minute, red, noninflammatory; points flush with skin; progression to papular wheal-like lesions; pruritis; secondary excoriation, especially parallel linear excoriations in intrascapular region; firmly attached to hair shaft in head and body lice	γ-Benzene hexachloride or pyrethrins to treat various parts of body; application as directed; contact screening with bed partners, playmates, shared head gear
Scabies	*Sarcoptes scabiei;* penetration of stratum corneum; depositing of eggs; allergic reaction resulting from presence of eggs, feces, mite parts; transmission by direct physical contact, only occasionally by shared personal items	Severe itching, especially at night, usually not on face; presence of burrows, especially in interdigital webs, flexor surface of wrists, and anterior axillary folds; redness, swelling, vesiculation	10% crotamiton, γ-benzene hexachloride, benzyl benzoate 12-25%; complete eradication possible; recurrence possible; treatment of sexual partner in positively diagnosed scabies; antibiotics if dermatitis and secondary infections present
Ticks	*Borrelia burgdorferi* (spirochete transmitted by ticks in certain areas) causes Lyme disease; endemic areas that include Northeast, Mid-Atlantic states, parts of Midwest and West (see Chapter 60)	Spreading, ringlike rash 3-4 wk after bite; commonly in groin, buttocks, axillae, trunk, and upper arms and legs; warm, itchy, or painful rash; flulike symptoms; cardiac, arthritic, and neurologic manifestations possible; unreliable laboratory test; no acquired immunity	Oral antibiotics, such as doxycycline, tetracycline; intravenous antibiotics for arthritic, neurologic, and cardiac symptoms; rest and healthy diet

manifestations are a reaction to the eggs, feces, or body parts of the invading organism (see Fig. 22-9 later in this chapter). Certain persons react with a severe hypersensitivity (anaphylaxis), which can be life threatening.

Prevention of insect bites by avoidance or by the use of repellents is somewhat effective. Meticulous hygiene related to personal articles, clothing, bedding, examination and care of pets, as well as careful selection of sexual partners, can reduce the incidence of infestations. Routine inspection is necessary where there is a risk of tick bites and Lyme disease (Table 22-10).

Allergic Dermatologic Problems

Dermatologic problems associated with allergies and hypersensitivity reactions present a real challenge to the clinician (Table 22-11). The pathophysiology related to allergic and contact dermatitis is discussed in Chapter 12. A careful family history and discussion of exposure to possible offending agents provide valuable data. Patch testing involves the application of allergens to the patient's skin (usually on the back) for 48 hours, after which the test sites are examined for erythema, papules, vesicles, or all of these. Patch testing is used to determine possible causative agents. This information is valuable to the patient. The best treatment of allergic dermatitis is avoidance of causative agent. The extreme pruritus of contact dermatitis and its potential for chronicity make it a frustrating problem for the patient, the nurse, and the dermatologist.

Table 22-11 Common Allergic Conditions of the Skin

Etiology and Pathophysiology	Clinical Manifestations	Treatment and Prognosis
Contact Dermatitis		
Manifestation of delayed hypersensitivity, absorbed agent acting as antigen, sensitization after several exposures, appearance of lesions 2-7 days after contact with allergen	Red, hivelike papules and plaques; sharply circumscribed with occasional vesicles; exposed areas more common; usually pruritic; relation of area of dermatitis to causative agent (e.g., metal allergy and dermatitis on ring finger)	Topical corticosteroids, antihistamines; skin lubrication; elimination of contact allergen; avoidance of irritating affected area; systemic corticosteroids if sensitivity severe
Urticaria		
Usually allergic phenomena; presence of edema in upper dermis resulting from a local increase in permeability of capillaries, usually from histamine	Spontaneously occurring and rounded elevations, varying size, usually multiple	Removal of source; antihistamine therapy
Drug Reaction		
Any drug that acts as antigen and causes hypersensitivity reaction possible cause, certain drugs more prone to reactions (e.g., penicillin) mediated by circulating antibodies	Rash of any morphology; often red, macular and papular, semiconfluent, generalized rash with abrupt onset; appearance as late as 14 days after cessation of drug; possibly pruritic	Withdrawal of drug if possible; antihistamines, local or systemic corticosteroids possibly necessary
Atopic Dermatitis		
Exact cause unknown, often beginning in infancy and decreasing in incidence with age, association with allergic conditions, elevation of IgE levels common, genetically determined, often family history, decreased itch threshold, stress and increased water contact (e.g., frequent hand washing, thumb sucking), other possible agents	Scaly, red to red-brown, circumscribed lesions; accentuation of skin markings; pruritic; symmetric eruptions common in antecubital and popliteal space in adults	Topical corticosteroids, phototherapy, coal tar therapy, intralesional corticosteroids, lubrication of dry skin, systemic corticosteroids if severe, reduction of stress, antibiotics for secondary infection

IgE, immunoglobin E.

Benign Dermatologic Problems

Although the list of benign dermatoses is extensive, some of the most commonly seen and distressing problems are summarized in Table 22-12.

DERMATOLOGIC MANIFESTATIONS OF SYSTEMIC DISEASES

Dermatologic manifestations of systemic disease may be either specific or nonspecific. Specific conditions display the same pathophysiologic process in relation to the skin as the internal disease process. Nonspecific conditions do not resemble the internal problem but are helpful in establishing a diagnosis. The skilled clinician should always consider the possibility that a particular dermatosis is a clue to an internal, less obvious problem.

Certain life changes have recognized associated dermatoses. At puberty, male- or female-pattern hair growth will be evident as a secondary sex characteristic. Increased apocrine gland activity can lead to body odor. The increased sebaceous gland activity stimulated by androgens can result in seborrhea and acne.

Pregnancy is characterized by physiologic skin changes, including hyperpigmentation and increased perspiration. Menopause is often accompanied by hot flashes, increased perspiration, facial hair growth, and varying degrees of scalp hair loss. Skin problems related to aging include dryness, wrinkling, hyperpigmentation, and actinic changes. Dermatologic manifestations of systemic diseases are presented in Table 22-13.

PLASTIC SURGERY

Elective Cosmetic Surgery

The possible cosmetic changes that can be made surgically are almost limitless. Cosmetic surgery includes such techniques as breast enlargement; breast reduction; chemical, mechanical, and surgical face-lift; eyelid lift; hair transplant; nose corrections; removal of double chin; correction of receding or prominent chin; abdomen or thigh lift; buttocks reduction; correction of elephant ears; and liposuction of many body areas.

Table 22-12 Common Benign Conditions of the Skin

Etiology and Pathophysiology	Clinical Manifestations	Treatment and Prognosis
Acne		
Inflammatory disorder of sebaceous glands; more common in teenagers but possible development in adulthood; persistence into adulthood possible; secondary result of iodides, bromides, corticosteroids, androgen-dominant birth control pills	Noninflammatory lesions, including comedones (blackheads) and closed comedones (whiteheads); inflammatory lesions, including papules and pustules; most common on face, neck, and upper back	Mechanical removal of multiple lesions with comedo extractor after comedo opened with fine needle or blade; topical application of benzoyl peroxide as antibacterial and peeling agent; use of peeling and irritating agents such as retinoic acid; long-term antibiotic therapy—topical or systemic; phototherapy; aim of treatment to suppress new lesions; spontaneous remission possible; often improvement with exposure to sun Use of isotretinoin (Accutane) for severe cystic acne to possibly provide lasting remission; contraindicated in pregnant women or women intending to become pregnant while on drug; monitoring of liver function and pregnancy tests, cholesterol, and triglycerides essential
Moles		
Grouping of normal cells derived from melanocyte-like precursor cells; hereditary predisposition possible	Hyperpigmented areas that vary in form and color; flat, slightly elevated, haloid, verrucoid, polypoid, dome-shaped, sessile, or papillomatous; preservation of normal skin markings; hair growth possible	No treatment necessary except for cosmetic reasons; skin biopsy for diagnostic decisions
Psoriasis		
Chronic dermatitis, which involves excessively rapid turnover of epidermal cells; family predisposition	Sharply demarcated scaling plaques of the scalp, elbows, and knees; palms, soles, and fingernails possibly affected; localized or general, intermittent or continuous	Aim of retarding growth of epidermal cells; difficult to medicate; usually topical corticosteroids, tar, anthralin; intralesional injection of corticosteroids for chronic plaques; sunlight; ultraviolet light, alone or with topical or systemic potentiation; no cure; control possible; antimetabolites (especially methotrexate) for difficult cases
Seborrheic Keratoses		
Benign, genetically determined growths; found in increasing number with age; no association with sun exposure	Irregularly round or oval, flat-topped papules or plaques; surface often warty; appearance of being stuck on; increase in pigmentation with age of lesion; usually multiple and possibly itchy	Removal by curettage or cryosurgery for cosmetic reasons or to eliminate source of irritation; minimal scarring
Skin Tags		
Common after midlife; appearance on neck, axillae, and upper trunk	Small, skin-colored, soft, pedunculated papules	No treatment unless for cosmetic reasons or because of repeated trauma; surgical removal possible (if requested); usually just "clipping off" without anesthesia
Lipoma		
Benign tumor of adipose tissue, often encapsulated, most common in 40- to 60-year-old age group	Rubbery, compressible, round mass of adipose tissue; single or multiple; variable in size, possibly extremely large; most common on trunk, back of neck, and forearms	Usually no treatment, biopsy to differentiate from liposarcoma, excision usual treatment (when indicated)

Continued

Table 22-12 Common Benign Conditions of the Skin—cont'd

Etiology and Pathophysiology	Clinical Manifestations	Treatment and Prognosis
Vitiligo		
Unknown cause; genetically influenced, most noticeable in dark-skinned persons and those with summer tan; complete absence of melanocytes; noncontagious	Focal amelanosis (complete loss of pigment); macular; variation in size and location; usually symmetric and permanent	Attempts at repigmentation with exposure to UVA and psoralens; depigmentation of pigmented skin with extensive disease (>50% of body involved); cosmetics and stains for camouflage and to deemphasize vitiliginous areas
Lentigo		
Increased number of normal melanocytes in basal layer of epidermis; senile lentigos ("liver spots") related to aging and sun exposure	Hyperpigmented, brown to black, flat lesion; usually on sun-exposed areas	Treatment only for cosmetic purposes, liquid nitrogen; possible recurrence in 1-2 yr

The reasons for the surgery are as varied as the techniques. The most common reason that people suffer the discomfort and financial expense (most are not covered by insurance) of cosmetic surgery is to improve their body image. People project their personal image of themselves; if they feel better about themselves as a result of cosmetic surgery, they will often act more confident and self-assured. Often social position and economic considerations are part of the decision. Increased longevity provides a larger population to whom cosmetic surgery is especially appealing.

Regardless of the reason the patient elects to have cosmetic surgery, the nurse should maintain a supportive, nonjudgmental attitude. If the patient wishes to change a body feature perceived as unattractive, then it is a personal decision to undergo cosmetic surgery and the nurse should support this decision.

Chemical Face-lift or Peel. A chemical face peel uses a cauterant to the skin to cause a controlled burn. This results in superficial destruction of the upper layers of the skin and a tightening of the deep layers. The most common indications for a chemical peel include pigmentation problems, skin damage as a result of radiation, freckles, superficial acne scarring, and actinic and seborrheic keratoses.

A solution (buffered phenol, trichloroacetic acid, or other exfoliation acids) is applied to the skin with care taken to avoid the eyes. Posttreatment care is prescribed specifically by the physician. It may include refraining from activities, talking, and chewing, and it may involve the application of compresses and topical ointments. There may be moderate swelling and crusting for 1 week. Within 7 to 8 days new skin appears, and healing is complete by 10 days. Redness will persist for 6 to 8 weeks. A pink tone will be apparent for several months. Once healing is complete, the skin will have a more youthful appearance because of a new superficial layer of skin.

Since there is a reduction of melanin as a result of this procedure, the patient must be instructed to absolutely avoid the sun for 6 months to prevent unsightly hyperpigmentation. Chemical peeling is accepted as a treatment for wrinkles and certain types of hyperpigmentation.

Topical Tretinoin. Topical application of tretinoin (Retin-A) provides some reversal of photodamaged skin and normal aging changes.[19] Fine and coarse wrinkling improves. There is a reduction in the number of lentigines (age spots) and in the color of freckles. Actinic keratoses decrease in number. Deep wrinkles and expression lines are usually not affected by tretinoin. The main adverse effect is a cutaneous reaction characterized by erythema, swelling, and scaling, which generally improves when treated with emollients or when the frequency of tretinoin application is decreased to every other day or stopped altogether.

The response to tretinoin appears to be dose-related. The usual dose is 0.025%, 0.05%, or 0.1% in a cream or gel base. Gradual introduction to tretinoin begins with application every other day, aiming for nightly application as tolerated. Treatment is not usually stopped when inflammation occurs unless the inflammation is severe. Maximum response occurs after 8 to 12 months of treatment. Thereafter application three to four times a week should maintain improvement. A sunscreen must be used in combination with tretinoin to prevent further sun damage and to protect against the greater photosensitivity that patients experience during tretinoin therapy.

Alpha-Hydroxy Acids. Topical alpha-hydroxy acids are now in use for similar indications as topical tretinoin. Optimal dosages are still under investigation, but erythema appears to be less of a problem with the use of alpha-hydroxy acids.[20]

Dermabrasion. *Dermabrasion* is the removal of the epidermis and a portion of the superficial layer of the dermis with preservation of sufficient epidermal adnexa to allow for spontaneous reepithelialization of the abraded surface. Dermabrasion is used to treat acne scars, hypertrophic scars, and sun-damaged and wrinkled skin, and it is also used to correct pigmentary abnormalities, usually on the face.

In general, the instructions to patients who have dermabrasion are focused on prevention of drying. Emollients or antibiotic ointments and wet soaks are included in the instructions and are to be applied at varying times on particular postopera-

Table 22-13 **Dermatologic Manifestations of Systemic Problems***

Systemic Problem	Dermatologic Manifestations
Endocrine	
Hyperthyroidism	Increased sweating, warm skin with persistent flush, thin nails, vitiligo and alopecia, fine, soft hair
Hypothyroidism	Cold, dry, pale to yellow skin; slighly hyperkeratotic epidermis with follicular plugging; generalized nonpitting edema; dry, coarse, brittle hair; brittle, slow-growing nails
Glucocorticoid excess (Cushing's syndrome), induced endogenously or exogenously	Atrophy; striae; epidermal thinning; telangiectasia; acne, decreased subcutaneous fat over extremities; thin, loose dermis; impaired wound healing; increased vascular fragility; mild hirsutism; excessive collection of fat over clavicles, back of neck, abdomen, and face; increased incidence of pyodermas
Addison's disease	Loss of body hair (especially axillary), generalized hyperpigmentation (especially in folds)
Androgen excess	Enlarged facial pores, male sex characteristics, acne, acceleration of coarse hair growth
Androgen deficiency—postpuberty	Development of sparse hair; marked reduction in sebum production
Hypoparathyroidism	Opaque, brittle nails with transverse ridges; coarse, sparse hair with patchy alopecia; eczematous and exfoliative dermatitis; hyperkeratotic and maculopapular eruptions
Hyperpituitarism (acromegaly)	Coarsened skin, deepened lines; increased oiliness and sweating; acne; increased number of nevi, hyperpigmentation; hypertrichosis
Hypopituitarism (Froëlich's syndrome)	Smooth skin; scant hair growth; obesity; small, thin fingernails
Diabetes mellitus	Increased xanthomas and carotene, shin spots, necrobiosis lipoidica diabeticorum, delayed wound healing
Gastrointestinal	
Ulcerative colitis, Crohn's disease	Pyoderma gangrenosum, mouth ulcers
Liver disease and biliary tract obstruction	Jaundice, itching, pigmentary abnormalities, alterations in nails and hair, spider angiomas, telangiectasia
Deficiency of essential fatty acids	Scaly skin
Malabsorption syndrome	Acquired ichthyosis
Cystic fibrosis	Abnormal sweat gland function resulting in failure to converse sodium
Musculoskeletal and Connective Tissue	
Systemic lupus erythematosus	Maculopapular semiconfluent rash (butterfly rash)
Scleroderma	Leathery hardening and stiffness of skin
Dermatomyositis	Edema; purplish-red upper eyelids; butterfly rash; scaly, macular erythema over knuckles; linear telangiectasia of posterior nail fold
Metabolic	
Lipidoses	Xanthomas
Vitamin A deficiency	Generalized dry hyperkeratoses
Hypervitaminosis A	Hair loss, dry skin
Vitamin B_1 (thiamine) deficiency	Edema, redness of soles of feet
Vitamin B_2 (riboflavin) deficiency	Red fissures at corner of mouth, glossitis
Nicotinic acid (niacin) deficiency	Pellagra; redness of exposed areas of hand or foot; face or neck; infected dermatitis
Immune	
Drug sensitivity	Rash of any morphology
Serum sickness	Pruritus
Cancer of breast, stomach, lung, uterus, kidney, ovary, colon, bladder	Metastasis to skin
Hodgkin's disease	Pruritus and nonspecific erythemas
Lymphomas	Papules, nodules, plaques, pruritus
Cardiovascular	
Arteriosclerosis	Decreased oxygenation leading to gangrene
Rheumatic heart disease	Petechiae, urticaria, rheumatoid nodules, erythema nodosum and multiforme
Periarteritis nodosa	Periarteritis nodules
Thromboangiitis obliterans (Buerger's disease)	Superficial migrating thrombophlebitis, pallor or cyanosis, gangrene, ulceration

Continued

Table 22-13 Dermatologic Manifestations of Systemic Problems*—cont'd

Systemic Problem	Dermatologic Manifestations
Respiratory	
Inadequate oxygenation secondary to respiratory disease	Cyanosis
Hematologic	
Anemia	Pallor, hyperpigmentation, pale mucous membranes, hair loss, nail dystrophy
Clotting disorders	Purpura, petechiae, ecchymosis
Renal	
Chronic renal failure	Dry skin, pruritis, uremic frost, pallor, dry skin, bruises
Reproductive	
Primary syphilis	Chancre
Secondary syphilis	Generalized skin lesions
Late benign syphilis	Gummas
Paget's disease	Eczematous patch of nipple and areola
Neurologic	
Syringomyelia, chronic sensory polyneuropathies, spinal cord trauma	Trophic changes in skin resulting from sensory denervation, pressure ulcers, anesthesia, paresthesias

*Refer to the systemic disease for specific information.

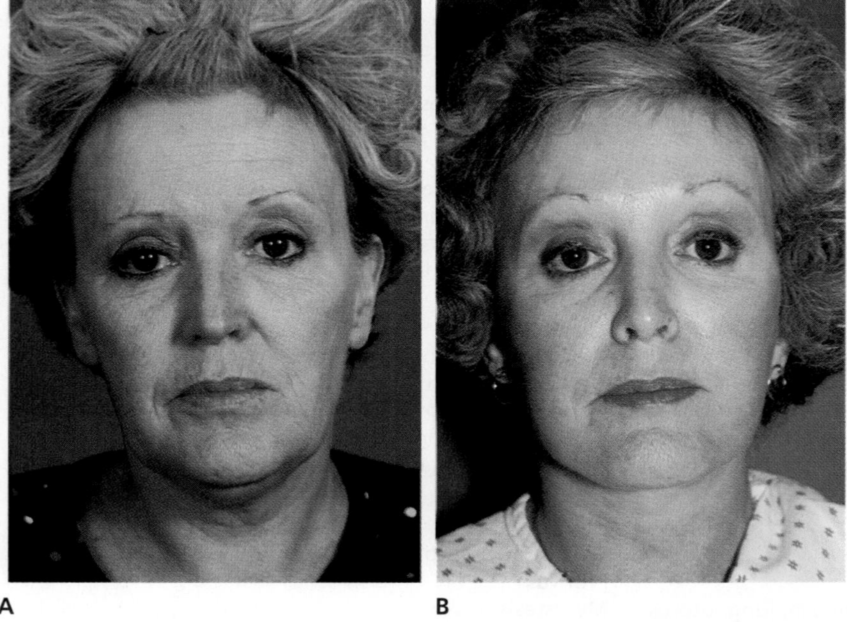

Fig. 22-8 Face-lift. **A,** Preoperative. **B,** Postoperative.

tive days. Patients are instructed to use a heavy layer of emollient when not using wet soaks. Instructions for postoperative wound care vary widely among practitioners. Specific care should be well understood by the patient. Sunscreens (SPF 30) should be used if the patient is outdoors. The most common complications include hyperpigmentation, hypopigmentation, keloids, herpes simplex, milia, persistent erythema, telangiectasia, and infection.

Face-lift. A *face-lift* (rhytidectomy) is the lifting and repositioning of the lower two thirds of the face and neck to improve appearance (Fig. 22-8). Indications for this procedure include the following:

1. Redundant soft tissue resulting from disease (e.g., smallpox or acne scarring)
2. Asymmetrical redundancy of soft tissues (e.g., facial palsy)
3. Redundant soft tissue resulting from trauma
4. Preauricular lesions

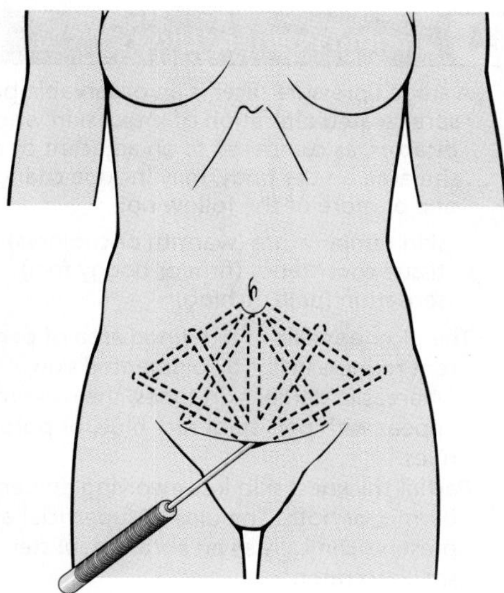

Fig. 22-9 Liposuction. Site of incision and tunneling pattern for abdominal liposuction procedure.

5. Redundant soft tissues resulting from solar elastosis (sagging of the skin as a result of sun damage), changes in body weight, and the effects of gravity
6. Restoration of body image

The surgical approach and lines of incisions vary according to the nature of the deformity and the position of the hairline. Prevention of hematoma formation is the most important postoperative consideration. A pressure dressing is usually used the first 24 to 48 hours to reduce the possibility of hematoma formation. Complications can occur if the person smokes or is involved in vigorous exercise. Once the dressing is removed, there is little pain. The sutures are removed sometime from the fifth to the tenth postoperative day. Antibiotics are used at the discretion of the surgeon. Infection is not a common problem.

Liposuction. *Liposuction* is a technique for removing subcutaneous fat to improve facial and body contours. Although not a substitute for diet and exercise, it can be successful in removing areas of fat from virtually any body area that is resistant to other techniques.

Although relatively free of complications, possible contraindications for the procedure include use of anticoagulants, history of inflammatory disease, uncontrolled hypertension, diabetes mellitus, and poor cardiovascular status. Persons under 40 years of age with good skin elasticity are the best candidates. However, patients ranging in age from 16 to 70 years can be treated successfully.[17]

The procedure is usually performed on an outpatient basis with the aid of local anesthesia. One or more sessions may be necessary, depending on the size of the area to be treated. A blunt-tipped cannula is inserted through a 1/2-inch incision and pushed into the fat to break it loose from the fibrous stroma. Multiple repeated thrusts disrupt the fat and create tunnels (Fig. 22-9). The loosened fat is removed with a very powerful suction. The area is taped. Firm bandaging helps to contour the skin and reduce the chance of postoperative bleeding and fluid accumulation. It may take several months for the final results to be evident.

NURSING MANAGEMENT: COSMETIC SURGERY

Many cosmetic surgical procedures are being performed in well-equipped day surgery units or in plastic surgeons' office surgery suites. There are several nursing interventions appropriate for the patient who has had cosmetic surgery, regardless of where the surgery was done.

Preoperative Management. A major consideration relates to informed consent and realistic expectations of what cosmetic surgery can accomplish. Although this information is usually provided by the surgeon, the nurse can and should reinforce this information and answer questions and concerns. For instance, a face-lift has little or no effect on deep wrinkling of the forehead and temples, deep nasolabial grooves, or vertical lip wrinkles. Before and after treatment photographs of similar cases are often useful in helping the patient to set realistic expectations.

The patient also needs to understand the time frame for healing. Complete results may not be evident until 1 year after the procedure. The oozing, crusting stage of the abrasive procedure must be explained so the patient can plan time off from work if this seems necessary. The final results of the cosmetic procedure are affected by the patient's age, general state of health, and skin type. If a health problem is present, efforts should be made to correct or control the problem before the procedure is performed.

Postoperative Phase. Most of the cosmetic procedures are not extremely painful. Usually mild analgesics are sufficient to keep the patient comfortable.

Although infection is not a common problem after cosmetic surgery, the nurse should assess the surgical sites for signs of infection. The patient should be aware of signs of infection and told to report any such signs and symptoms immediately so that appropriate antibiotic intervention can be started.

If the surgery involved alteration in the circulation to the skin, such as the undermining done in a face-lift, a careful monitoring of adequate circulation is necessary. Warm, pink skin that blanches on pressure indicates that adequate circulation is present in the surgical area.

Skin Grafts

Uses. Skin grafts may be necessary to provide protection to underlying structures or to reconstruct areas for cosmetic or functional purposes. Ideally, wounds heal by primary intention. However, large, surgically created wounds, trauma, and chronic wounds can cause extensive tissue destruction, making primary intention healing impossible. In these cases, skin grafting may be necessary. Improved surgical techniques make it possible to graft skin, bone, cartilage, fat, fascia, muscles, and nerves. For cosmetically pleasing results, the color, thickness, texture, and hair-bearing nature of skin used for grafting must be chosen to match the recipient site. (Skin grafting is discussed in Chapter 23.)

Types. The two types of skin grafts are free grafts and skin flaps. *Free grafts* are further classified according to the method of providing a blood supply to the grafted skin. One method is to transfer the graft (epidermis and part or all of the dermis) to the recipient site from the donor site. If the graft is an autograft (from the patient's own body) or an isograft (from an identical twin), it will revascularize and become fixed to the new site. Chapter 23 discusses full and split skin grafts in detail. Another method of free skin grafting is by reconstructive microsurgery. With the use of an operating microscope, circulation is immediately established in the free flap by anastomosis of the blood vessels from the skin flap to the vessels in the recipient site.

Skin flaps involve moving a section of skin and subcutaneous tissue from one part of the body to another without terminating the vascular attachment. The vascular attachment is called a *pedicle.* Skin flaps are used to cover wounds with a poor vascular bed, when padding is needed, and to cover wounds over cartilage and bone. There may be a need for intermediate flap placement if the recipient site is far removed from the donor site. For instance, a skin flap from the thigh to the head would require an intermediate graft. The flap is advanced to the recipient site when circulation is well established at the intermediate site. The type of flap and the route of transfer are determined according to the needs of the patient and the nature of the defect to be repaired.

Soft tissue expansion is a technique for providing skin for resurfacing a defect, such as a burn scar, for removing a disfiguring mark, such as a tattoo, or as a preliminary step in breast reconstruction. A subcutaneous tissue expander of an appropriate size and shape is placed under the skin, usually as an outpatient procedure. Weekly expansion with saline solution can be done in a health care setting or by the patient at home. This expansion procedure is repeated until the skin reaches the size needed for the repair. This may take from several weeks to 3 to 4 months. Once sufficient skin is available, the old incision is opened, the expander is removed, and the soft tissue is ready to be used as an advancement flap. The tissue expander next to a defect retains the primary tissue characteristics such as color and texture.

NURSING MANAGEMENT: SKIN GRAFTS

After a skin graft, several areas must be assessed. The most critical assessment is checking for adequate vascular supply to the grafted site. If the area is not covered by a dressing, it should be regularly assessed for color, warmth, capillary refill, and turgor. If the grafted area has a dressing, it is usually left in place until removed by the surgeon. Systemic signs of infection, such as fever and pain, must be monitored.

Although pain is not usually a major problem, the nurse should provide pain relief when necessary. Conversation, diversion, and massage to areas other than the surgical site, as well as medication, should be used to maintain patient comfort. The immobility enforced by certain grafting procedures presents the expected potential complications of pneumonia, pulmonary emboli, and pressure ulcers. Aggressive measures by nurses should be instituted to prevent such complications.

Skin grafting may involve long periods of hospitalization, with the constant threat of graft death. Since this is a particularly difficult time emotionally for the patient, the nurse must be supportive and understanding. Expectations of the results of the graft must be realistic if the patient is not to suffer depression as the result of unfulfilled expectations. The family and friends of the patient need consideration and explanation of procedures and restrictions imposed by the grafting procedures.

Table 22-14 Staging Pressure Ulcers

Stage I	A stage I pressure ulcer is an observable pressure-related alteration of intact skin whose indicators, as compared to an adjacent or opposite area on the body, may include changes in one or more of the following: skin temperature (warmth or coolness) tissue consistency (firm or boggy feel) sensation (pain, itching) The ulcer appears as a defined area of persistent redness in lightly pigmented skin, whereas in darker skin tones, the ulcer may appear with persistent red, blue, or purple hues.
Stage II	Partial-thickness skin loss involving epidermis, dermis, or both. The ulcer is superficial and presents clinically as an abrasion, blister, or shallow crater.
Stage III	Full-thickness skin loss involving damage to or necrosis of subcutaneous tissue that may extend down to, but not through, underlying fascia. The ulcer presents clinically as a deep crater with or without undermining of adjacent tissue.
Stage IV	Full-thickness skin loss with extensive destruction, tissue necrosis, or damage to muscle, bone, or supporting structures (e.g., tendon, joint capsule). Undermining and sinus tracts may also be associated with Stage IV pressure ulcers.

Source: Fifth National NPUAP Conference: *Task Force on Darkly Pigmented Skin and Stage I Pressure Ulcers,* Approved Feb 1998, and Bergstrom N and others: *Treatment of pressure ulcers,* Clinial Practice Guideline, no. 15. Rockville, Md: U.S. Department of Health and Human Services, Public Health Service, Agency for Health Care Policy and Research. AHCPR Publication no. 95-0652, Dec. 1994.

PRESSURE ULCERS*

Etiology and Pathophysiology

A pressure ulcer is a localized area of tissue necrosis caused by unrelieved pressure, tissue layers sliding over other tissue layers (shearing), and excessive moisture.[21] Factors that put a patient at risk for the development of pressure ulcers include impaired circulation, obesity, elevated body temperature, anemia, contractures, mental deterioration, physical dependence, immobility, incontinence, and old age. Systemic illnesses such as diabetes, collagen disease, vascular diseases, leprosy, and neurologic disorders that affect sensation also result in greater risk of ulcer formation. More than 95% of all pressure ulcers occur over a bony prominence, primarily the pelvic girdle.[22] Pressure ulcers are graded or staged according to their deepest level of tissue damage (Table 22-14).

Clinical Manifestations

The clinical manifestations of pressure ulcers depend on the stage of the ulcer. Figure 22-10 illustrates the four pressure ulcer stages. Identification of Stage I pressure ulcers (Fig. 22-11) may be difficult in patients with dark skin.[23] According to the National Pressure Ulcer Advisory Panel (NPUAP), when eschar is present, accurate staging of the pressure ulcer is not possible until the eschar is removed by debridement.[24] If the pressure ulcer be-

*This section was contributed by Elizabeth A. Ayello.

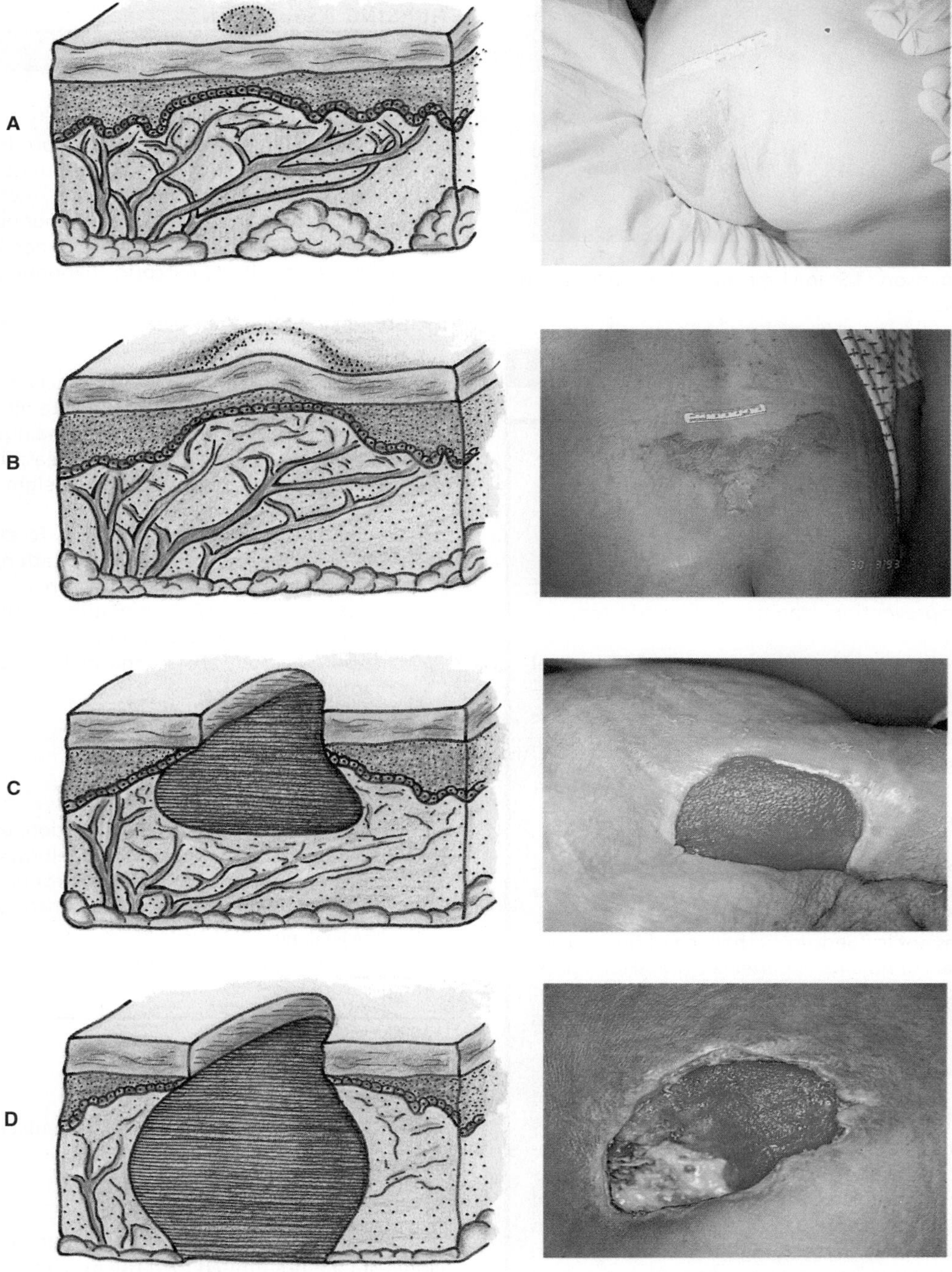

Fig. 22-10 Diagram of stages of pressure ulcers. **A,** Stage I pressure ulcer. **B,** Stage II pressure ulcer. **C,** Stage III pressure ulcer. **D,** Stage IV pressure ulcer.

comes infected, the patient may display signs of infection, such as leukocytosis and fever. In addition, the pressure ulcer may increase in size, odor, and drainage, have necrotic tissue, and be indurated, warm, and painful. The most common complication of a pressure ulcer is recurrence.

NURSING AND COLLABORATIVE MANAGEMENT: PRESSURE ULCERS

Care of a patient with a pressure ulcer requires local care of the wound and support measures such as adequate nutrition and pressure relief. The current trend is to keep a pressure sore slightly moist, rather than dry, to enhance reepithelialization. In addition to the nurse, other members of the health team, such as the plastic surgeon, the dietician, the physical therapist, and the occupational therapist, can provide valuable input into the complex treatment necessary to prevent and treat pressure ulcers. Both conservative and surgical strategies are used in the treatment of pressure ulcers, depending on the stage and condition of the ulcer. Therapeutic and nursing management will be discussed together, since the activities are interrelated.

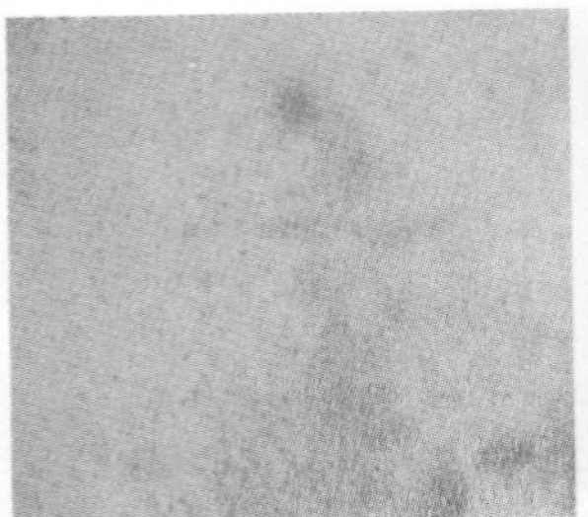

Fig. 22-11 Comparison of Stage I pressure ulcers in light- and dark-skinned patients.

RESEARCH
IMPLICATIONS FOR NURSING PRACTICE

Knowledge of Pressure Ulcer Prevention

Citation Pieper B, Mattern J: Critical care nurses' knowledge of pressure ulcer prevention, staging, and description, *Ostomy/Wound Management* 43:2, 1997.

Purpose To evaluate critical care nurses' knowledge of pressure ulcer prevention, staging, and description.

Methods Cross-sectional survey design using 75 critical care nurses. Nurses answered a pressure ulcer survey developed from Agency for Health Care Policy and Research (AHCPR) guideline on prediction and prevention. The survey content included pressure ulcer risk and prevention, staging, and wound description. This content was considered basic for nursing practice.

Results and Conclusions The percentage of total items answered correctly ranged from 15% to 83%. The highest area of incorrect answers was wound description. The total score was not influenced by the type of nursing education or years of nursing experience. The AHCPR pressure ulcer guideline had only been read by 12% of nurses. The knowledge deficit about pressure ulcers was significant.

Implications for Nursing Practice Lowering the incidence of pressure ulcers requires nurses to be knowledgeable about pressure ulcer prevention and development. Ongoing education of nurses about pressure ulcer prediction, prevention, and treatment strategies is essential for effective patient care. Pressure ulcer prevention in all patients, especially those at high risk and those who are critically ill, must be a primary goal of competent nursing care. A decrease in pressure ulcers results in cost savings and higher quality of care. Pressure ulcers are a national health concern and information about prevention must be shared among nurses and implemented in patient care.

■ Nursing Assessment

Patients should be assessed for pressure ulcer risk initially on admission and at periodic intervals. Risk assessment should be done using a validated assessment tool such as the Braden scale.[24] Subjective and objective data that should be obtained from a person with a pressure ulcer are presented in Table 22-15.

NURSING ASSESSMENT

Table 22-15 Pressure Ulcer

Subjective Data

Important Health Information

Past health history: Stroke, spinal cord injury; prolonged bed rest or immobility; circulatory impairment; poor nutrition; altered level of consciousness; prior history of pressure ulcer; immunologic abnormalities; advanced age; diabetes; anemia; trauma

Medications: Use of narcotics, hypnotics, systemic corticosteroids

Surgery or other treatments: Recent surgery

Functional Health Patterns

Nutritional-metabolic: Obesity, emaciation; decreased fluid, calorie, or protein intake; vitamin or mineral deficiencies; clinically significant malnutrition as indicated by low serum albumin, decreased total lymphocyte count, and decreased body weight (15% less than ideal body weight)

Elimination: Incontinence of urine, feces, or both

Activity-exercise: Weakness, debilitation, inability to turn and position body; contractures

Cognitive-perceptual: Pain or altered cutaneous sensation in pressure ulcer area; decreased awareness of pressure on body areas; capacity to follow treatment plan

Objective Data

General

Fever

Integumentary

Diaphoresis, edema, and discoloration, especially over bony areas such as sacrum, hips, elbows, heels, knees, ankles, shoulders, and ear rims, progressing to increased tissue damage characteristic of ulcer stages*

Possible Findings

Leukocytosis, positive cultures for microorganisms from pressure ulcer

*See Fig. 22-10.

■ Nursing Diagnoses

Nursing diagnoses for the patient with pressure ulcers may include, but are not limited to, those presented in NCP 22-2.

■ Planning

The overall goals are that the patient with a pressure ulcer will (1) have no deterioration of the ulcer stage, (2) reduce or eliminate the factors that lead to pressure ulcers, (3) not develop an infection in the pressure ulcer, and (4) have no recurrence.

■ Nursing Implementation

Health Promotion. A primary nursing responsibility is the identification of patients at risk for the development of pressure ulcers.

Prevention remains the best treatment for pressure ulcers. Devices, such as alternating pressure mattresses, foam mattresses

22-2 NURSING CARE PLAN PATIENT WITH A PRESSURE ULCER

Expected Patient Outcomes	Nursing Interventions and *Rationales*
NURSING DIAGNOSIS	**Impaired skin integrity** *related to* pressure and inadequate circulation *as manifested by* evidence of pressure ulcer.
▪ Intact skin. ▪ Healing of skin wounds without complications.	▪ Assess causative factors such as activity, mobility, presence or absence of sensory deficits, nutrition and hydration status, circulation and oxygenation, skin moisture status *to reduce or eliminate factors that contribute to development or progression of the pressure ulcer.* ▪ Assess and document wound on a regular basis in relation to location, length, width and depth of wound, amount of granulation tissue visible and/or epithelialization, necrotic tissue, local or systemic infection, presence and character of exudate, including volume, color, consistency, and odor *to provide baseline and ongoing data for monitoring pressure ulcer.* ▪ Stage the wound. ▪ Use pressure relief devices (e.g., foam boots, wheelchair cushions). ▪ Institute position change schedule q2hr *to avoid prolonged pressure in one area.* ▪ Keep heels off of bed. ▪ Keep head of bed at or below 30 degree angle and flat when not contraindicated *to avoid sacral and buttock pressure.* ▪ Use pillows or foam *to prevent direct contact between bony prominences such as knees or ankles.* ▪ Use assistive devices *to aid patient movement (e.g., trapeze, turning sheets, lifts).* ▪ Protect patient's skin from excess moisture *to prevent maceration.* ▪ Institute 2000 to 3000 calories/day (more if increased metabolic demands), 2000 ml/day of fluid *to provide calories, protein, and fluids necessary for tissue repair.* ▪ Offer *vitamin and mineral supplements* if there are deficiencies. ▪ Initiate prescribed local treatment based on pressure ulcer characteristics and in accordance with AHCPR Guidelines.* ▪ Educate patient and family relative to cause, prevention, and treatment of pressure ulcer *to prevent recurrence.* ▪ Reduce factors that contribute to deterioration of the pressure ulcer *such as malnutrition, unrelieved pressure, shear forces, and moisture.*

**Pressure ulcer treatment: Clinical practice guideline,* Agency for Health Care Policy and Research, US Department of Health and Human Services, No 95-0653, Dec 1994.

PATIENT & FAMILY HOME CARE GUIDE

Table 22-16 Pressure Ulcer

- Identify and explain risk factors and etiology of pressure ulcers to patient and family.
- Assess all at-risk patients at time of first hospital and/or home visit and thereafter at regular intervals.
- Teach family care techniques for incontinence. If incontinence occurs, cleanse skin at time of soiling, use topical moisture barriers, and use pads or briefs that are absorbent.
- Demonstrate correct positioning to decrease risk of skin breakdown. Instruct family to reposition bed-bound patient at least every 2 hours, chair-bound patient every hour (See *"Further Teaching Instructions" in NCP 22-2*).
- Assess resources (i.e., adequacy of caregiver availability and skill, finances, and equipment) of patients requiring pressure ulcer care at home. When selecting ulcer care dressing, consider cost and amount of caregiver time.
- Teach patient and/or caregiver to use clean dressings over sterile dressings using "no touch" technique when changing dressings. Instruct family on disposal of contaminated dressings.
- Teach patient and family to inspect skin daily. Assess and document pressure ulcer status at least weekly; may require help from patient and family.
- Evaluate program effectiveness in preventing and treating pressure ulcers.

Adapted from Potter P, Perry A: *Fundamentals of nursing,* ed 4, St Louis, 1997, Mosby, and AHCPR Panel for the Treatment of pressure ulcers, AHCPR Publication No 95-9652, Rockville, Md, Agency for Health Care Policy and Research, Public Health Service, US Department of Health and Human Services, Clinical Practice Guideline, No 15, 1994.

with adequate stiffness and thickness, wheelchair cushions, padded commode seats, foam boots, and lift sheets are useful in reducing pressure and shearing force. However, they are not adequate substitutes for frequent repositioning. Once a person has been identified as being at risk for pressure ulcer development, prevention strategies should be implemented. See patient and family home care in Table 22-16.

Acute Intervention. Once a pressure ulcer has developed, the nurse should initiate interventions based on the stage, size, and presence of infection. Careful documentation should be made of the size of the pressure ulcer. A plastic ruler or wound-measuring card can be used to note the ulcers' maximum length and width in centimeters. To find the depth of the ulcer, gently place a sterile cotton-tipped applicator into the deepest part of the ulcer. The length of the portion of the applicator that probed the ulcer can then be measured. To assess healing, pictures of the pressure ulcer may be taken initially and at regular intervals during the course of treatment.[25] Pressure ulcers should be reassessed at least weekly.

Local care of the pressure ulcer may involve debridement, wound cleaning, and the application of a dressing. A pressure ulcer that has necrotic tissue or eschar (except for dry stable necrotic heels) must have the tissue removed by either surgical/sharp, mechanical, enzymatic, or autolytic debridement methods.[24] Once the pressure ulcer has been successfully debrided and has a clean granulating base, the goal is to provide an appropriate wound environment that supports moist wound healing and prevents disruption of the newly formed granulation tissue. Reconstruction of the pressure ulcer site by operative repair including skin grafting, skin flaps, musculocutaneous flaps, or free flaps may be necessary.

Pressure ulcers should be cleaned with noncytotoxic solutions that do not kill or damage the cells such as fibroblasts. Solutions such as Dakin's solution (sodium hypochlorite solution), acetic acid, povidone iodine, and hydrogen peroxide are cytotoxic and therefore should not be used to clean pressure ulcers. It is also important to use enough irrigation pressure to adequately clean the pressure ulcer without causing trauma or damage to the wound.[26]

After the pressure ulcer has been cleansed, it should be covered with an appropriate dressing. Some factors to consider when selecting a dressing are maintenance of a moist environment, prevention of wound desiccation (drying out), ability to absorb the wound drainage, location of the wound, amount of caregiver time, cost of the dressing, presence of infection, clean versus sterile dressings, and care delivery setting.[24] A wet-to-dry dressing should never be used on a clean granulating pressure ulcer; this type of dressing should only be used for mechanical debridement of the wound. (Dressings are discussed in Chapter 11 and Table 11-17).

Stage II through IV pressure ulcers are considered to be contaminated or colonized with bacteria. It is important to re-

CRITICAL THINKING EXERCISES

CASE STUDY

Basal Cell Carcinoma

Patient Profile

Lee Smith, 61, is a fair-skinned, blue-eyed retired tennis instructor who enjoys gardening and swimming. She comes to the clinic for evaluation of a persistent lesion.

Subjective Data

- Has a 5-month history of a slowly enlarging papule on the posterior side of her right ear.
- States that a scab forms, falls off, and then reforms.
- Anxious that the lesion may be cancer and require extensive, disfiguring surgery.

Objective Data

Physical Examination

- Has a 6-mm ulcerating lesion with semitranslucent border
- Telangiectasia overlies the lesion

Diagnostic Studies

- Biopsy results: basal cell epithelioma

Critical Thinking Questions

1. What factors placed the patient at risk for this diagnosis?
2. What are the usual manifestations associated with basal cell carcinoma?
3. What treatment options are available for this patient?
4. What are some preoperative and postoperative considerations for this patient?
5. How would you address Mrs. Smith regarding her anxiety over surgery outcomes?
6. What would you include in a patient teaching plan to address future sun exposure?
7. Based on the assessment data presented, write one or more appropriate nursing diagnoses. Are there any collaborative problems?

NURSING RESEARCH ISSUES

1. What strategies are the most effective in educating patients about safe sun practices? How might these strategies vary based on the patient's age?
2. What factors influence the decision to undergo cosmetic surgery?
3. Do patients with dermatologic disorders who receive laser therapy significantly differ in their care needs as compared with those patients receiving phototherapy and radiation therapy?
4. Are there significant relationships between economic factors and caregiver support in preventing pressure ulcer development in high-risk patients receiving home health care?

member that in persons who have chronic wounds or who are immunocompromised, the clinical signs of infection (purulent exudate, odor, erythema, warmth, tenderness, edema, pain, fever, and elevated white cell count) may not be present even though the pressure ulcer is infected.

The maintenance of adequate nutrition is an important nursing responsibility for the patient with a pressure ulcer. Often, the patient is debilitated and has a poor appetite secondary to inactivity. The caloric intake needed to correct and maintain a nutritional balance may be as high as 4200 calories a day. Oral feedings should be high in calories and proteins and should be supplemented with vitamins and minerals. Nasogastric feedings can be used to supplement the oral feedings. If necessary, parenteral nutrition consisting of amino acid and glucose solutions is used when oral and nasogastric feedings are inadequate. NCP 22-2 on p. 519 outlines the care for the patient with a pressure ulcer.

Ambulatory and Home Care. Since the recurrence of pressure ulcers is common, the education of both the patient and the care provider in prevention techniques is extremely important (See Table 22-16). The care provider needs to know the etiology of pressure ulcers, prevention techniques, early signs, nutritional support, and care techniques for active pressure ulcers. Since the patient with a pressure ulcer often requires extensive care for other health problems, it is important that the nurse support the caregiver through the added responsibility of pressure ulcer treatment.

Evaluation

Expected outcomes for the patient with a pressure ulcer are addressed in NCP 22-2 on p. 519.

REVIEW QUESTIONS

The number of the question corresponds to the same-numbered objective at the beginning of the chapter.

1. The nurse advises a patient with photosensitivity to use a sunscreen that contains
   a. cinnamates.
   b. benzophenones.
   c. methyl anthranilate.
   d. PABA (para-aminobenzoic acid).
2. In teaching a patient who is using topical corticosteroids to treat an acute dermatitis, the nurse should tell the patient that
   a. topical corticosteroids usually do not cause systemic side effects.
   b. the cream form represents the most efficient system of delivery.
   c. abruptly discontinuing the use of topical corticosteroids will cause a reappearance of the dermatitis.
   d. creams and ointments should be applied with a glove in small amounts to prevent further infection.
3. A patient with psoriasis tells the nurse that she has quit her job as a receptionist because she feels her appearance is disgusting to customers. The nursing diagnosis that best describes this patient response is
   a. ineffective coping related to lack of social support.
   b. impaired skin integrity related to presence of lesions.
   c. anxiety related to lack of knowledge of the disease process.
   d. social isolation related to decreased activities secondary to fear of rejection.
4. In teaching a patient with malignant melanoma about this disorder, the nurse recognizes that the prognosis of the patient is most dependent on
   a. the thickness of the lesion.
   b. the degree of color change in the lesion.
   c. how much superficial spread the lesion has.
   d. the amount of ulceration present in the lesion.
5. The nurse identifies a nursing diagnosis of risk for infection transmission as a high priority for the patient with
   a. psoriasis on the palms and soles.
   b. candidiasis of the nails.
   c. tinea pedis.
   d. impetigo on the face.
6. A mother and her 2 children have been diagnosed with pediculosis corporis at a health center. An appropriate measure in treating this condition is
   a. topical application of griseofulvin.
   b. moist compresses applied frequently.
   c. administration of systemic antibiotics.
   d. washing the body with pyrethrins.
7. A common site for the lesions associated with atopic dermatitis is the
   a. buttocks.
   b. temporal area.
   c. antecubital space.
   d. palmar surface of the feet.
8. During assessment of a patient the nurse notes an area of red, sharply defined plaques covered with silvery scales that are mildly itchy on the patient's knee and elbow. The nurse recognizes this finding as
   a. lentigo.
   b. psoriasis.
   c. actinic keratoses.
   d. seborrheic keratoses.
9. Dermatologic symptoms of Cushing's syndrome would include
   a. generalized hyperpigmentation.
   b. increased sweating.
   c. thickened skin.
   d. telangiectasia.
10. Important patient instruction after a chemical peel includes
    a. avoidance of sun exposure.
    b. application of firm bandages.
    c. limitation of vigorous exercise.
    d. use of mild heat to prevent drying.
11. A patient is assessed to be at risk for the development of a pressure ulcer. Based on this information, the nurse should
    a. vigorously massage reddened bony prominences daily.
    b. keep head of bed elevated to 90° at all times.
    c. implement a q 2 hr turning schedule.
    d. have the patient maintain a high fat diet.

References

1. Marks R: An overview of skin cancers, *Cancer Suppl* 75:607, 1995.
2. Wentzell JM: Sunscreen: the ounce of prevention, *Am Fam Phys* 4:1713, 1996.
3. Taylor CR, Sober AS: Sun exposure and skin disease, *Ann Rev Med* 47:181, 1996.
4. Rhodes A: Public education and cancer of the skin, *Cancer* 75:613, 1995.
5. Marks JG, DeLeo VA: *Contact and occupational dermatology,* ed 2, St Louis, 1997, Mosby.

6. Memon A, Friedman P: Studies on the reproducibility of allergic contact dermatitis, *Br J Dermatol* 134:208, 1996.
7. Skidmore-Roth L: *Mosby's 1999 Nursing drug reference,* St Louis, 1999, Mosby.
8. Varricchio C, editor: *Cancer source book for nurses,* ed 7, Sudbury, Mass, 1997, Jones & Bartlett.
9. Teofoli P and others: Itch and pain, *Int J Dermatol* 35:159, 1996.
10. Schucter L and others: A prognostic model for predicting 10-year survival in patients with primary melanoma, *Ann Intern Med* 125:369, 1996.
11. Gallagher RD and others: Chemical exposure, medical history and risk of SCC and BCC, *Cancer Epidem* 5:419, 1996.
12. Markey A: Etiology and pathogenesis of squamous cell carcinoma, *Clin Dermatol* 13:537, 1995.
13. Landis S and others: Cancer statistics 1998, *CA Cancer J Clin* 48:6, 1998.
14. Fleming I and others: Principles of management of basal and squamous cell carcinoma of the skin, *Cancer* 75:699, 1995.
15. Sober AJ, Burstein JM: Precursors to skin cancer, *Cancer* 75:645, 1995.
16. Rigel D: Malignant melanoma: perspectives on incidence and its effects on awareness, diagnosis, and treatment, *CA Cancer J Clin* 46:195, 1996.
17. Habif TP: *Clinical dermatology: a color guide to diagnosis and therapy,* ed 3, St Louis, 1996, Mosby.
18. Gale D, Kiley K: Malignant melanoma and adjuvant alpha interferon-2b for patients at high risk of relapse, *Clin J Oncol Nurs* 2:5, 1998.
19. Noble S, Wagstaff AJ: Tretinoin: A review of its pharmacological properties and clinical efficiency in the topical treatment of photodamaged skin, *Drugs Aging* 6:479, 1995.
20. Ditre CM and others: Effects of alpha-hydroxy acids on photoaged skin: a pilot clinical, histological and ultrastructural study, *J Am Acad Derm* 34:187, 1996.
21. Maklebust J, Sieggreen M: *Pressure ulcers–guidelines for prevention and nursing management,* ed 2, Springhouse, Penn, 1996, Springhouse.
22. Barczak CA and others: Fourth national pressure ulcer prevalence survey, *Adv Wound Care* 10:18, 1997.
23. Henderson CT and others: Draft definition of stage I pressure ulcers: inclusion of persons with darkly pigmented skin, *Adv Wound Care* 10:16, 1997.
*24. Bergstrom N and others: Treatment of pressure ulcers, Clinical practice guidelines, no 15, Rockville, Md: US Department of Health and Human Services, Public Health Service, Agency for Health Care Policy and Research, AHCPR Publication No 95-0652, 1994.
25. Xakellis GC, Frantz RA: Pressure ulcer healing: what is it? what influences it? how is it measured? *Adv Wound Care* 10:20, 1997.
26. Barr JE: Principles of wound cleansing, *Ostomy/Wound Management* 41:155, 1995.

*Nursing research-based article.

Resources

AcneNet
http://www.derm-infonet.com/acnenet/toc.html

American Academy of Dermatology
930 North Meacham Rd.
Schaumburg, IL 60173
847-330-0230
888-462-DERM
http://www.aad.org/

American Society of Plastic & Reconstructive Surgical Nurses, Inc.
East Holly Avenue
Box 56
Pitman, NJ 08071-0056
609-256-2340
Fax: 609-589-7463
http://www.qicon.com/asprsn/

Dermatology Foundation
1560 Sherman Avenue
Evanston, IL 60201-4808
http://www.dermfnd.org/

National Eczema Association for Science & Education
1221 SW Yamhill, Suite 303
Portland, OR 97205
503-228-4430
503-273-8778
800-818-7546

National Pediculosis Association
P.O. Box 610189
Newton, MA 02161
781-449-NITS
http://www.headlice.org/

National Psoriasis Foundation
660 SW 92nd, Suite 300
Portland, OR 97223
503-244-7404
Fax: 503-245-0626
http://www.psoriasis.org/

Skin Cancer Foundation
245 Fifth Avenue, Suite 1403
New York, NY 10016
800-SKIN-490
212-725-5176
Fax: 212-725-5751
http://www.skincancer.org/

***For additional Internet resources, see the website for this book at* www.mosby.com/MERLIN/medsurg_lewis**

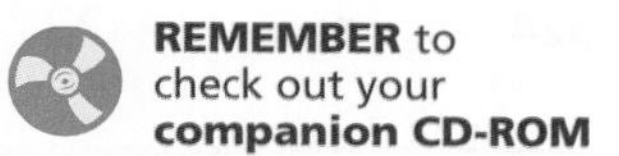

23 NURSING MANAGEMENT Patient with Burns

Kathleen C. Solotkin & Cindy J. Knipe

www.mosby.com/MERLIN/medsurg_lewis

LEARNING OBJECTIVES

1. Describe the causes and prevention of burn injuries.
2. Describe the burn injury classification system.
3. Describe the relationship between the involved structures and the clinical appearance of partial- and full-thickness burns.
4. Identify the parameters used to determine the severity of burns.
5. Describe the pathophysiology, clinical manifestations, complications, and nursing and collaborative management of each burn phase.
6. Explain fluid and electrolyte shifts during the emergent and acute burn phases.
7. Describe the nutritional needs of the burn patient during the three burn phases.
8. Explain the physiologic and psychosocial aspects of burn rehabilitation.
9. Describe the nursing management of the emotional needs of the burn patient and family.
10. Discuss the issues involved and rationale for preparing the burn patient to return home.
11. Describe the interventions that the nurse may use in the management of pain in the burn patient.

Burn wounds occur when there is contact between tissue and an energy source, such as heat, chemicals, electrical current, or radiation. The resulting effects are influenced by the intensity of the energy, the duration of exposure, and the type of tissue injured.

An estimated 2.5 million Americans seek medical care each year for burns. Approximately 100,000 are hospitalized, and 70,000 require intensive care services. An estimated 12,000 of these people die annually as a direct result of their burns. Approximately 1 million will sustain substantial or permanent disabilities resulting from their burn injury. Children (especially preschool-aged children) and older adults account for more than two thirds of all burn fatalities.[1]

The major cause of fires in the home is carelessness with cigarettes. Other causes of burns include hot water from water heaters set above 140° F (60° C), cooking accidents, space heaters, combustibles such as gasoline and charcoal lighter fluid, steam from radiators, and chemicals.

Most burn injuries can be prevented. The nurse as a citizen and health care provider is in a good position to conduct home safety assessments and to educate people about burn injuries before accidents occur. Home safety measures include the use of smoke alarms and fire extinguishers. Families should have fire drills, and each family member should know where to go and what to do in case of a fire. Local fire departments can inform the public of regional fire codes and perform home safety checks.

Reviewed by Judy Knighton, RN, MScN, Clinical Nurse Specialist—Burns, The Wellesley Central Hospital, Toronto, Ontario, Canada.

Knowledge of potential sources for burn injury allows problem solving for burn prevention (Tables 23-1 and 23-2). Teaching people proper use of appliances (e.g., space heaters), electrical cords, wiring, outlets, outdoor grills, and hot water heaters can prevent burn injury. The nurse can be instrumental in teaching home care of minor burns to the public. The industrial nurse should teach burn prevention in the work setting.

TYPES OF BURN INJURY

Thermal Burns

The most common type of burn is thermal injury, which can be caused by flame, flash, scald, or contact with hot objects (Table 23-2 and Fig. 23-1).

Chemical Burns

Chemical burns are the result of tissue injury and destruction from necrotizing substances. With chemical injuries, it is important to remove the person from the burning agent, or vice versa. The latter is accomplished by lavaging the affected area with copious amounts of water. Any clothing containing the chemical should be removed, because the burning process will continue as long as the chemical is in contact with the skin. Tissue destruction may continue for up to 72 hours after a chemical injury.

Chemicals can cause respiratory problems and other systemic manifestations, as well as skin or eye injuries. When chlorine is inhaled, the toxic gas produces respiratory distress. Byproducts of burning substances (e.g., carbon) are toxic to the sensitive respiratory mucosa.

Chemical burns are most commonly caused by acids. However, alkali burns also occur, and they are more difficult to man-

Table 23-1 Common Places and Causes of Burn Injury

Occupational Hazards	
Steam pipes	Electricity from power lines
Chemicals	Combustible fuels
Hot metals	
Tar	
Home and Recreational Hazards	
Hot water heaters set higher than 140° F (60° C)	Improper use of outdoor grills
Multiple extension cords per outlet	Improper use of flammables (e.g., starter fluid, gasoline, kerosene)
Frayed or defective wiring	Hot grease or liquids from cooking
Pressure cookers	Excessive exposure to sunlight
Microwaved food	Electrical storms
Radiators	
Open space heaters	
Carelessness with cigarettes or matches	

Table 23-2 Causes of Burn Injury

Cause	Examples
Flame	Clothing ignited with fire
Flash	Flame burn associated with explosion (combustible fuels)
Scald	Hot bath water
	Spilled hot beverages
	Hot grease or liquids from cooking
	Steam burns (pressure cookers, microwaved food, automobile radiators)
Contact	Hot metal (outdoor grill)
	Hot, sticky tar

age than acid burns. Alkaline substances are not neutralized by tissue fluids as readily as acid substances. Alkalis adhere to tissue, causing protein hydrolysis and liquefaction. This damage continues even when the alkali is neutralized. Examples of alkalis that cause burn injury are cleaning agents, drain cleaners, and lyes.

Smoke and Inhalation Injury

Inhalation of hot air or noxious chemicals can cause damage to the tissues of the respiratory tract. Although damage to the respiratory mucosa can occur, it seldom happens because the vocal cords and glottis close as a protective mechanism. Gases are cooled to body temperature before they reach the lung tissue. Smoke inhalation injuries are an important determinant of mortality in fire victims. Inhalation injuries are present in 20% to 30% of the patients admitted to burn centers and account for 60% to 70% of burn patient deaths.[2]

There are three types of smoke and inhalation injuries:

1. *Carbon monoxide poisoning.* Carbon monoxide (CO) poisoning and asphyxiation account for the majority of deaths at the fire scene. CO is produced by the incomplete combustion of burning materials. It is subsequently inhaled and displaces oxygen (O_2) on the hemoglobin molecule, causing hypoxia, carboxyhemoglobinemia, and ultimately death when the CO levels are high. Often the victims of fires, especially those who have been trapped in a closed space, will have elevated carboxyhemoglobin levels. If CO intoxication

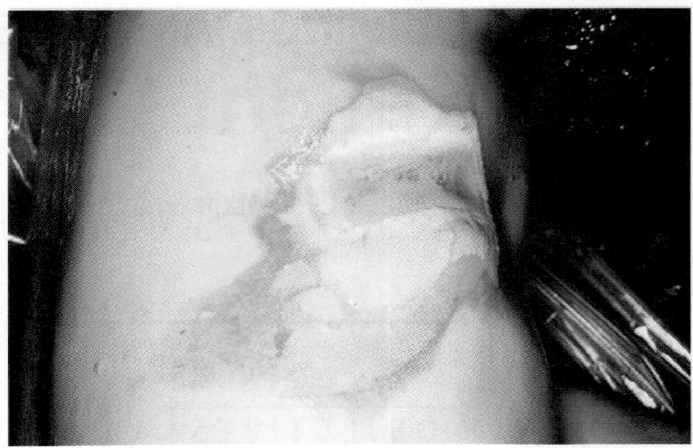
A

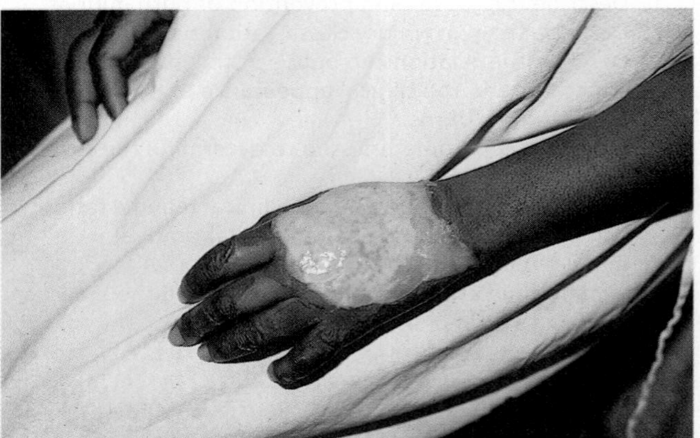
B

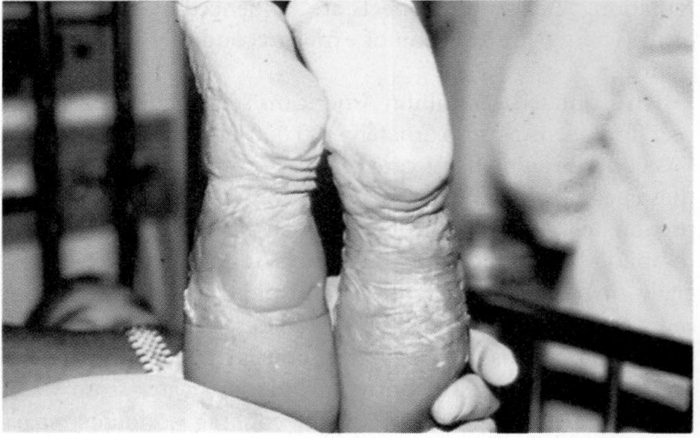
C

Fig. 23-1 Types of burn injury. **A,** Patient with full-thickness thermal burn. **B,** Partial-thickness burn to the hand. **C,** Partial-thickness burns secondary to immersion in hot water.

is suspected, the patient should be quickly treated with 100% humidified O_2 and the carboxyhemoglobin level should be measured when feasible. CO poisoning may occur in the absence of burn injury to the skin.

2. *Inhalation injury above the glottis.* This injury may be caused by the inhalation of hot air, steam, or smoke. Mucosal burns of the oropharynx and larynx are manifested by redness, blistering, and edema. Mechanical obstruction can occur quickly, presenting a true medical emergency. Often a reliable clue that this injury is likely is the presence of facial burns, singed nasal hair, hoarseness, painful swallowing, and darkened oral and nasal membranes.
3. *Inhalation injury below the glottis.* A general principle to remember is that inhalation injury above the glottis is thermally produced, and below the glottis it is usually chemically produced. The tissue injury to the lower respiratory tract is related to the length of exposure to smoke or toxic fumes. Clinical manifestations may not appear until 12 to 24 hours after the burn, and then they may manifest as acute respiratory distress syndrome (see Chapter 62).

These patients must be observed closely for signs of respiratory distress or compromise and must be treated quickly and efficiently if they are to survive. Respiratory tract complications from burn injury are discussed in detail later in this chapter.

Electrical Burns

Injury from electrical burns results from coagulation necrosis that is caused by intense heat generated from an electric current (Fig. 23-2). It can also result from direct damage to nerves and vessels causing tissue anoxia and death. The severity of the electrical injury depends on the amount of voltage, tissue resistance, current pathways, and surface area in contact with the current and on the length of time the current flow was sustained. Tissue densities offer various amounts of resistance to electric current. For example, fat and bone offer the most resistance, whereas nerves and blood vessels offer the least resistance. Current that passes through vital organs (e.g., brain, heart, kidneys) will produce more profound damage than current that passes through other tissue. In addition, electrical sparks may ignite the patient's clothing, causing a combination of thermal and electrical injury.

Nursing assessment of the patient with electrical injury should be thorough. Often the wounds of electrical current entry and exit are all that are visible, masking the possibility of extensive, underlying tissue damage. Noting the patient's position when the injury was sustained in conjunction with identifying the entry and exit wounds can help the nurse assess which underlying organ structures may have been affected. Contact with electrical current can cause tetanic muscle contractions strong enough to fracture the long bones and vertebrae. Another reason to suspect long bone or spinal fractures is a fall. Most electrical injuries occur when the victim is elevated above the ground (e.g., during the work of a utility pole lineperson) and comes in contact with a current source. For this reason, all patients with electrical burns should be considered at risk for a potential cervical spine injury. Cervical spine immobilization should be used during transport and subsequent spinal x-rays taken to rule out any injury.

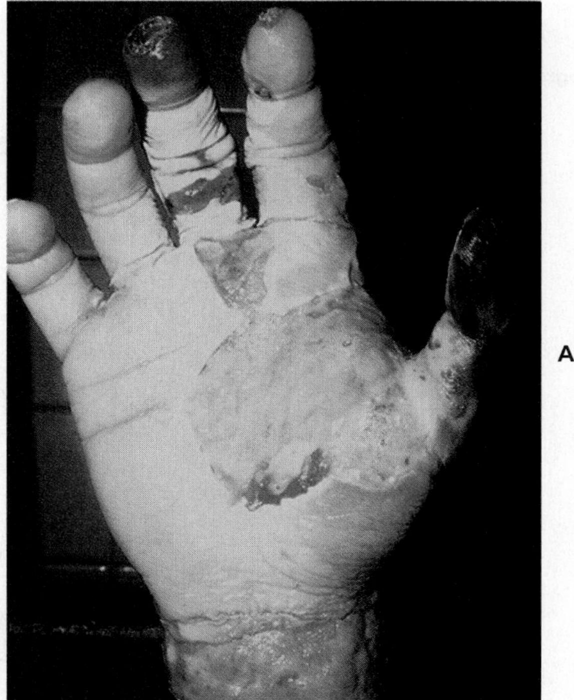

A

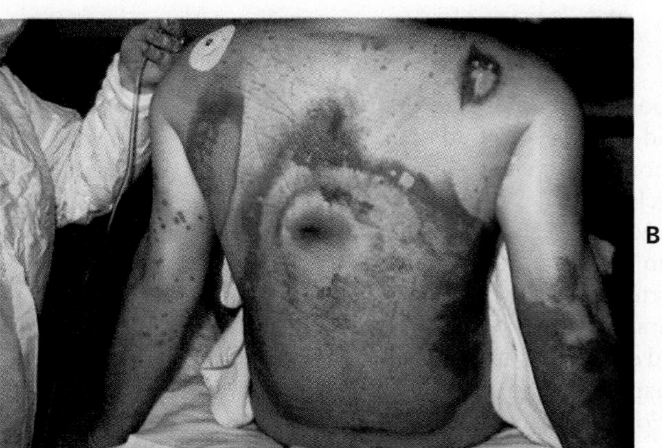

B

Fig. 23-2 Electrical injury produces heat coagulation of blood supply and contact area as electric current passes through the skin. **A,** Hand. **B,** Back.

Electrical injury puts the patient at risk for cardiac arrest or arrhythmias, severe metabolic acidosis, and myoglobinuria, which can lead to acute renal tubular necrosis (ATN). The electrical shock event can cause immediate cardiac standstill or fibrillation. If this occurs, cardiopulmonary resuscitation (CPR) should be initiated immediately. Delayed cardiac arrhythmias or arrest may also occur without warning during the first 24 to 48 hours after injury; therefore the patient should be monitored continuously. Because of extensive tissue destruction and cell rupture, severe metabolic acidosis develops within minutes after the injury, even in the absence of cardiac arrest. Arterial

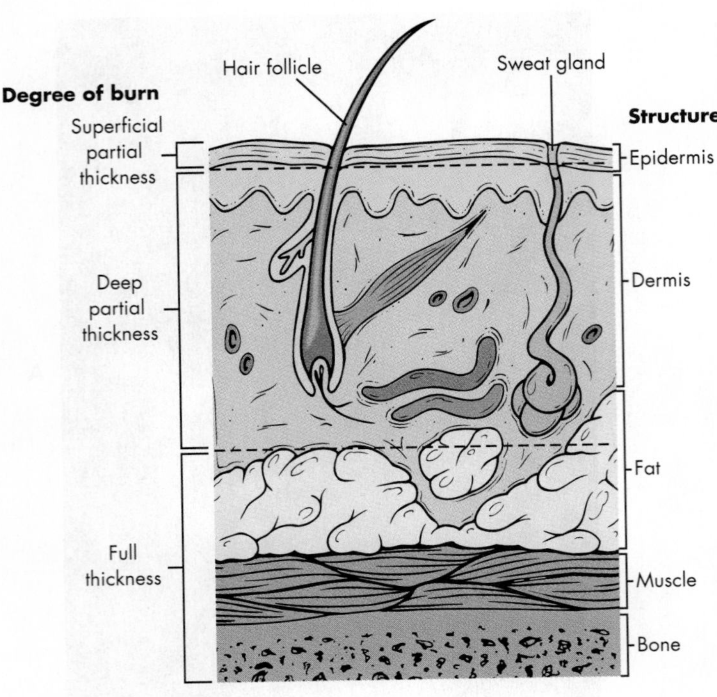

Fig. 23-3 Cross section of skin indicating the degree of burn and structures involved.

blood gas (ABG) analysis should be performed to assess the acid-base balance. Sodium bicarbonate may be administered in amounts sufficient to maintain the serum pH at near-normal levels.

Myoglobin is released from muscle tissue into the circulation whenever massive muscle damage occurs. It is then transported to the kidneys where it can mechanically block the renal tubules because of its large size. This process can result in ATN and eventual acute renal failure if not appropriately treated (see Chapter 44). Treatment consists of infusing Ringer's lactate solution at a rate sufficient to maintain urine output at 75 to 100 ml per hour until urine sample analyses indicate that the myoglobin has been flushed from the circulatory system. In addition, an osmotic diuretic (e.g., mannitol) may be given to maintain urine output.

Cold Thermal Injury

Cold thermal injury, or frostbite, is discussed in Chapter 64.

CLASSIFICATION OF BURN INJURY

The treatment of burns is related to the severity of the injury. Severity is determined by (1) depth of burn, (2) extent of burn calculated in percent of total body surface area (TBSA), (3) location of burn, and (4) patient risk factors.

Depth

Burn injury involves the destruction of the integumentary system. The skin is divided into three layers: the epidermis, dermis, and subcutaneous tissue (Fig. 23-3). The epidermis, or nonvascular outer layer of the skin, is approximately as thick as a sheet of paper. It is composed of many layers of nonliving epithelial cells that provide a protective barrier to the skin, hold in fluids and electrolytes, regulate heat, and keep harmful agents in the external environment from injuring or invading the body. The dermis, which lies below the epidermis, is approximately 30 to 45 times thicker than the epidermis. The dermis contains connective tissues with blood vessels and highly specialized structures consisting of hair follicles, nerve endings, sweat glands, and sebaceous glands. Under the dermis lies the subcutaneous tissue, which contains major vascular networks, fat, nerves, and lymphatics. The subcutaneous tissue acts as a shock absorber and heat insulator for the underlying structures, which include the muscles, tendons, bones, and internal organs.

In the past, burns were defined by degrees: first-degree, second-degree, and third-degree burns. The American Burn Association now advocates a more explicit definition categorizing the burn according to depth of skin destruction: partial-thickness and full-thickness burns. Table 23-3 reflects the comparison of the depth of injury.

Extent

Two commonly used guides for determining the extent of a burn wound are the Lund-Browder chart (Fig. 23-4, *A*) and the Rule of Nines (Fig. 23-4, *B*). (Only partial-thickness and full-thickness burns are included when calculating TBSA.) The Lund-Browder chart is considered more accurate because the patient's age in proportion to relative body-area size is taken into account. The Rule of Nines, which is easy to remember, is considered adequate for initial assessment of an adult burn patient. For irregular- or odd-shaped burns, the palmar surface of the patient's hand is considered to be approximately 1% of the TBSA. The extent of a burn is often revised after edema has subsided and demarcation of zones of injury has occurred.

Table 23-3 Classification of Burn Injury Depth

Classification	Clinical Appearance	Cause	Structure
Partial-thickness skin destruction			
▪ Superficial (First-degree)	Erythema, blanching on pressure, pain and mild swelling, no vesicles or blisters (although after 24 hr skin may blister and peel)	Superficial sunburn Quick heat flash	Only superficial devitalization with hyperemia is present. Tactile and pain sensation intact.
▪ Deep (Second-degree)	Fluid-filled vesicles that are red, shiny, wet (if vesicles have ruptured); severe pain caused by nerve injury; mild-to-moderate edema	Flame Flash Scald Contact burns Chemical tar	Epidermis and dermis involved to varying depth. Some skin elements, from which epithelial regeneration can occur, remain viable.
Full-thickness skin destruction ▪ (Third- and fourth-degree)	Dry, waxy white, leathery, or hard skin; visible thrombosed vessels; insensitivity to pain and pressure because of nerve destruction; possible involvement of muscles, tendons, and bones	Flame Scald Chemical Tar Electric current	All skin elements and nerve endings destroyed. Coagulation necrosis present.

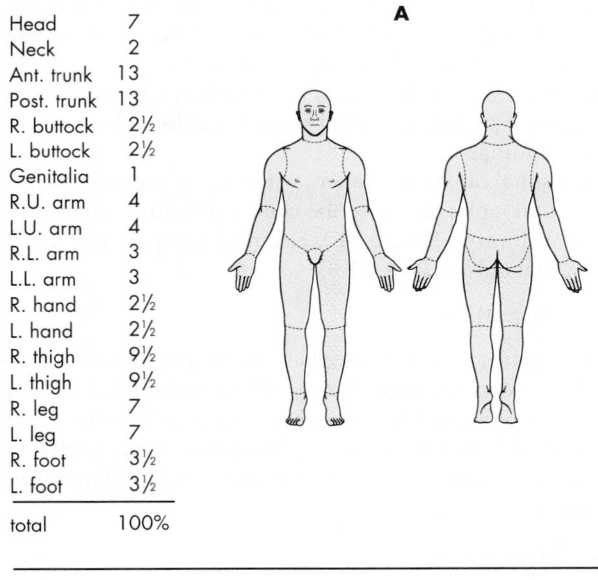

A
Head 7
Neck 2
Ant. trunk 13
Post. trunk 13
R. buttock 2½
L. buttock 2½
Genitalia 1
R.U. arm 4
L.U. arm 4
R.L. arm 3
L.L. arm 3
R. hand 2½
L. hand 2½
R. thigh 9½
L. thigh 9½
R. leg 7
L. leg 7
R. foot 3½
L. foot 3½
total 100%

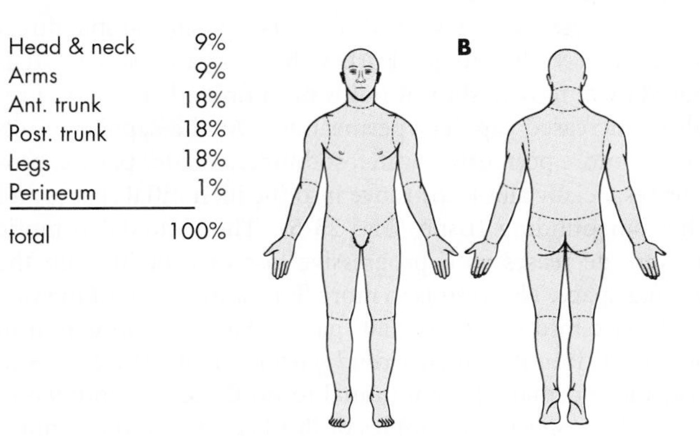

B
Head & neck 9%
Arms 9%
Ant. trunk 18%
Post. trunk 18%
Legs 18%
Perineum 1%
total 100%

Fig. 23-4 **A,** Lund and Browder chart. By convention, areas of partial-thickness injury are colored in blue and areas of full-thickness injury in red. Superficial partial-thickness burns are not calculated. **B,** Rule of Nines chart.

Location

The location of the burn wound has a direct relationship to the severity of the burn injury.[3] Burns of the face and neck and circumferential burns of the chest may inhibit respiratory function by virtue of mechanical obstruction secondary to edema or eschar formation. These injuries may also indicate the possibility of inhalation injury and respiratory mucosal damage.

Burns of the hands, feet, joints, and eyes are of concern because they make self-care impossible and jeopardize later function. Hands and feet are difficult to manage medically because of superficial vascular and nerve-supply systems.

The ears and nose, composed mainly of cartilage, are susceptible to infection because of poor blood supply to the cartilage. Burns of the buttocks or genitalia are highly susceptible to infection. Circumferential burns of the extremities can cause circulatory compromise distal to the burn with subsequent neurologic impairment of the affected extremity.

Patient Risk Factors

The older adult heals more slowly and has more difficulty with rehabilitation than a younger adult. Infection of the burn wound and pneumonia are common complications in the older patient.

Any patient with preexisting cardiovascular, pulmonary, or renal disease has a poorer prognosis for recovery because of the tremendous demands placed on the body by a burn injury. The patient with diabetes mellitus or peripheral vascular disease is at high risk for gangrene and poor healing, especially with foot and leg burns. General physical debilitation from any chronic disease, including alcoholism, drug abuse, and malnutrition, renders the patient less physiologically competent to deal with a burn injury. In addition, the patient who concurrently sustained fractures, head injuries, or other trauma has a poorer prognosis for recovery from the burn injury.

Major versus Minor Burns

The American Burn Association classifies burns into major, moderate uncomplicated, and minor injuries by depth, extent,

Table 23-4 American Burn Association Adult Burn Classification

Magnitude of Burn Injury	Partial Thickness* (Second-Degree)	Full Thickness* (Third-Degree)	Other Factors
Minor	<15%	<2%	Does not involve special care areas (eyes, ears, face, hands, feet, perineum); excludes electrical injury, inhalation injury, complicated injury (fractures), all high-risk patients (extremes of age, concomitant disease)
Moderate uncomplicated	15-25%	<10%	Excludes electrical injury, inhalation injury, complicated injury, all high-risk patients; does not involve special care areas
Major	>25%	>10%	Includes all burns involving hands, face, eyes, ears, feet, or perineum; includes inhalation injury, electrical injury, complicated burn injury, and all high-risk patients; patient should be transferred to a burn unit

*Figures indicate percentage of total body surface area involved.

location, and risk factors (Table 23-4). The American Burn Association recommends that major burn injuries be treated at burn centers or burn units that have optimal facilities and personnel for handling such severe trauma.

PHASES OF BURN MANAGEMENT

Burn management can be classified into three phases: emergent (resuscitative), acute, and rehabilitative. Prehospital care will also briefly be discussed.

Prehospital Care

The initial consideration in aiding the burn victim is to remove the person from the source of the burn and stop the burning process.[4] The caregiver must be protected from becoming part of the incident. In the case of electrical injuries, initial management involves removing the patient from contact with the source of current by a trained individual. Most chemical burns are best treated by brushing solid particles off the skin, followed by thorough lavage with water. (For handling specific agents, refer to a hazardous materials text.) Small thermal burns (10% or less TBSA) may be covered with a clean, cool, tap water–dampened towel for the patient's comfort and protection until definitive medical care is instituted. It is believed that cooling of the injured area (if small) within 1 minute minimizes the depth of injury. Tap water is acceptable for flushing. Time should not be wasted trying to find sterile water, saline solution, or antidotes.

If the thermal burn area is large, primary considerations are focused on airway, breathing, and circulation (the ABCs):

Airway: check for patency, soot around nares, or singed nasal hair.
Breathing: check for adequacy of ventilation.
Circulation: check for presence and regularity of pulses.

If the burn is large, it is not advisable to immerse the burned body part in cool water because doing so would lead to extensive heat loss. The burn should never be packed in ice. As much clothing as possible should be removed. The patient should be wrapped in a dry, clean sheet or blanket to prevent further contamination of the wound and to provide warmth.

The burn patient may also have sustained other injuries that take priority over the burn wound. It is important for the individual involved in the prehospital phase of burn care to adequately communicate the circumstances of the injury to the receiving hospital. This is especially important when the injury involves entrapment in a closed space, hazardous chemicals, or possible trauma.

Prehospital care of the patient with various types of burns is presented in tables that describe chemical burns (Table 23-5), inhalation injury (Table 23-6), electrical burns (Table 23-7), and thermal burns (Table 23-8).

Emergent Phase

The emergent (resuscitative) phase is the period of time required to resolve the immediate problems resulting from burn injury. This phase may last from burn onset to 5 or more days, but it usually lasts 24 to 48 hours. This phase begins with fluid loss and edema formation and continues until fluid mobilization and diuresis begin.

Pathophysiology

Fluid and Electrolyte Shifts. The greatest initial threat to a patient with a major burn is hypovolemic shock.[5] It is caused by a massive shift of fluids out of blood vessels as a result of increased capillary permeability. As the capillary walls become more permeable, water, sodium, and later plasma proteins (especially albumin) move into the interstitial spaces and other surrounding tissue (Fig. 23-5). The colloidal osmotic pressure decreases with progressive loss of protein from the vascular space. This results in more fluid shifting out of the vascular space into the interstitial spaces. (Fluid accumulation in the interstitium is termed *second spacing.*) Fluid also moves to areas that normally have minimal to no fluid, a phenomenon termed *third spacing.* Examples of third spacing in burn injury are exudate and blister formation.

The net result of the fluid shift is intravascular volume depletion. Edema, decreased blood pressure (BP), increased

EMERGENCY MANAGEMENT

Table 23-5 Chemical Burns

Etiology	Assessment Findings	Interventions
Acids Alkalis Corrosives Organophosphates	▪ Burning ▪ Redness, swelling of injured tissue ▪ Degeneration of exposed tissue ▪ Discoloration of injured skin ▪ Localized pain ▪ Edema of surrounding tissue ▪ Respiratory distress if chemical inhaled ▪ Decreased muscle coordination (if organophosphate) ▪ Paralysis	**Initial** ▪ Ensure patent airway. ▪ Assess airway, breathing, and circulation before decontamination procedures. ▪ Brush dry chemical from skin before irrigation. ▪ Flush chemical from wound and surrounding area with saline solution or water. ▪ Remove clothing, including shoes, watches, jewelry, and contact lenses if face exposed. ▪ Establish IV access with large-bore catheter needle if greater than 15% TBSA burn. ▪ Blot skin dry with clean towels. Do *not* rub dry. ▪ Cover burned areas with dry, sterile dressing or clean, dry sheet. ▪ Anticipate intubation if significant inhalation injury present. ▪ Contact poison control center for assistance. **Ongoing Monitoring** ▪ Monitor airway if airway exposed to chemicals.

TBSA, total body surface area.

EMERGENCY MANAGEMENT

Table 23-6 Inhalation Injury

Etiology	Assessment Findings	Interventions
Exposure of respiratory tract to intense heat or flames Inhalation of noxious chemicals, smoke, or carbon monoxide	▪ Rapid, shallow respirations ▪ Increasing hoarseness ▪ Coughing ▪ Singed nasal or facial hair ▪ Smoky breath ▪ Carbonaceous sputum ▪ Productive cough with black, gray, or bloody sputum ▪ Irritation of upper airways or burning pain in throat or chest ▪ Difficulty swallowing ▪ Restlessness, anxiety ▪ Altered mental status, including confusion, coma ▪ Decreased oxygen saturation ▪ Arrhythmias	**Initial** ▪ Ensure patent airway. ▪ Administer high-flow oxygen by non-rebreather mask. ▪ Remove patient's clothing. ▪ Establish IV access with large-bore catheter needle. ▪ Place in high Fowler's position unless spinal injury suspected. ▪ Assess for facial/neck burns or other trauma. ▪ Obtain arterial blood gas, carboxyhemoglobin levels, and chest radiograph. **Ongoing Monitoring** ▪ Monitor vital signs, level of consciousness, oxygen saturation, respiratory status, and cardiac rhythm. ▪ Anticipate need for cricothyrotomy or tracheostomy for significant laryngeal edema. ▪ Anticipate need for fiberoptic bronchoscopy or intubation if respiratory distress develops.

pulse, and other manifestations of hypovolemic shock are clinically detectable signs (see Chapter 61). If not corrected, these events can lead to irreversible shock and death.

Another source of fluid loss is insensible loss by evaporation from large, denuded body surfaces. The normal insensible loss of 30 to 50 ml per hour may increase to as much as 200 to 400 ml per hour in the severely burned patient.

The circulatory status is also impaired because of hemolysis of red blood cells (RBCs). The RBCs are hemolyzed by a circulating factor released at the time of the burn, as well as by the direct insult of the burn injury. Thrombosis in the capillaries of burned tissue causes an additional loss of circulating RBCs. An elevated hematocrit is commonly caused by hemoconcentration resulting from fluid loss. After fluid balance has been

✚ EMERGENCY MANAGEMENT

Table 23-7 **Electrical Burns**

Etiology	Assessment Findings	Interventions
Alternating Current Electric wires Utility wires **Direct Current** Lightning Defibrillator	▪ Leathery, white, or charred skin ▪ Burn odor ▪ Impaired touch sensation ▪ Minimal or absent pain ▪ Arrhythmias ▪ Cardiac arrest ▪ Entrance and exit wounds ▪ Diminished peripheral circulation in injured extremity ▪ Thermal burns if clothing ignites ▪ Fractures or dislocations from force of current ▪ Head injury if fall occurred ▪ Depth and extent of wound difficult to visualize; assume injury greater than what is seen ▪ Delayed effects include prolonged amnesia and cataracts	**Initial** ▪ Removal from current source must be done by trained personnel with special equipment to prevent injury to rescuer. ▪ Assess and treat patient *after* removal from source of current. ▪ Ensure patent airway. ▪ Stabilize cervical spine. ▪ Administer high-flow oxygen by non-rebreather mask. ▪ Establish IV access with large-bore catheter needle. ▪ Remove patient's clothing. ▪ Check pulses distal to burns. ▪ Cover burn sites with dry sterile dressing. ▪ Assess for any other injuries (e.g., fractures, head injury). **Ongoing Monitoring** ▪ Monitor cardiac rhythm, vital signs, level of consciousness, oxygen saturation, neurovascular status in injured limbs. ▪ Monitor urine output to ensure adequate volume. ▪ Monitor urine for development of myoglobinuria secondary to muscle breakdown. ▪ Anticipate administration of mannitol for myoglobinuria and hemoglobinuria.

✚ EMERGENCY MANAGEMENT

Table 23-8 **Thermal Burns**

Etiology	Assessment Findings	Interventions
Hot liquids or solids Flash flame Open flame Steam Hot surface Ultraviolet rays	**Partial-Thickness (Superficial)** ▪ Redness ▪ Pain ▪ Moderate to severe tenderness ▪ Minimal edema ▪ Blanching with pressure **Partial-Thickness (Deep)** ▪ Moist blebs, blisters ▪ Mottled white, pink to cherry red ▪ Hypersensitive to touch or air ▪ Moderate to severe pain ▪ Blanching with pressure **Full-Thickness** ▪ Dry, leathery eschar ▪ White, waxy, dark brown, or charred appearance ▪ Strong burn odor ▪ Impaired sensation when touched ▪ Absence of pain with severe pain in surrounding tissues ▪ Lack of blanching with pressure	**Initial** ▪ Ensure patent airway. ▪ Stop the burning process. ▪ Inspect face and neck for singed nasal hair, hoarseness of voice, stridor, soot in the sputum. ▪ Administer high-flow oxygen by non-rebreather mask. ▪ Establish IV access with large-bore catheter. ▪ Begin rapid fluid replacement. ▪ Remove clothing and jewelry. ▪ Identify and treat associated injuries (e.g., fractured ribs, pneumothorax). ▪ Determine depth, extent, and severity of burn. ▪ Administer IV analgesia. ▪ Cover large burns with dry, sterile dressing. ▪ Anticipate intubation with significant inhalation injury. ▪ Apply cool compresses or immerse in cool water for minor injuries only (less than 10% TBSA burn). ▪ Insert urinary catheter for severe burns. ▪ Prevent loss of body heat. ▪ Transport as soon as possible to a burn center. ▪ Do not debride burns or apply topical agents before transfer to a burn center. ▪ Administer tetanus prophylaxis as appropriate. **Ongoing Monitoring** ▪ Monitor vital signs, level of consciousness, oxygen saturation, cardiac rhythm, urine output. ▪ Monitor temperature. ▪ Monitor pain and medicate as needed.

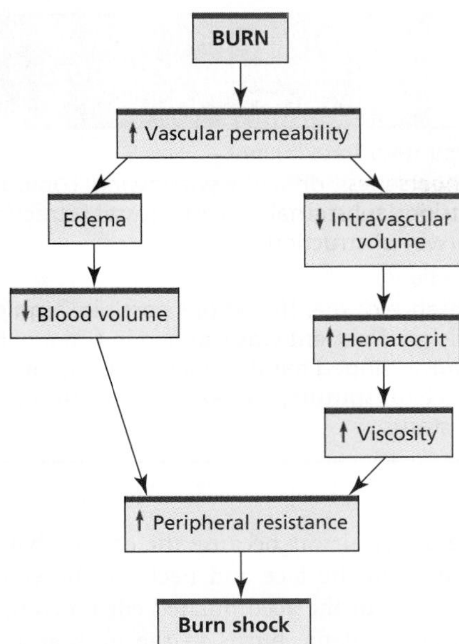

Fig. 23-5 At the time of major burn injury, there is increased capillary permeability. All fluid components of the blood begin to leak into the interstitium, causing edema and a decreased blood volume. The red blood cells and white blood cells do not leak. Therefore the hematocrit increases and the blood becomes viscous. The combination of decreased blood volume and increased viscosity produces increased peripheral resistance. Burn shock, a type of hypovolemic shock, rapidly ensues and continues for about 24 hours.

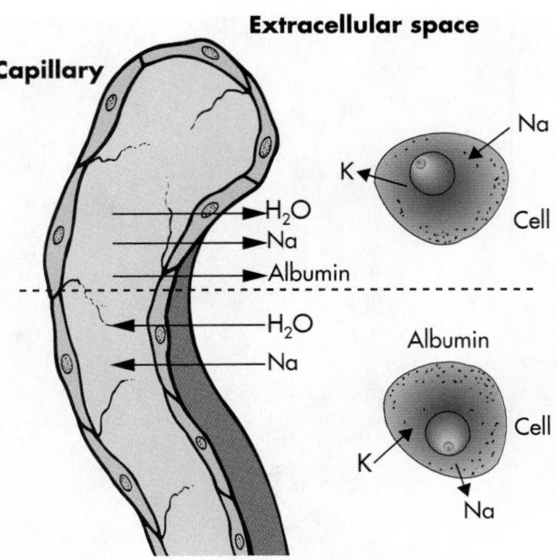

Fig. 23-6 The effects of burn shock during the first 24 hours are shown above the dotted line. As the capillary seal is lost, the interstitial edema fluid is formed. The cellular integrity is also altered, with sodium (Na) moving into the cell in abnormal amounts and potassium (K) leaving the cell. The shifts after the first 24 hours are shown below the dotted line. The water and sodium move back into the circulating volume through the capillary. The albumin remains in the interstitium. Potassium is transported into the cell and sodium is transported out as the cellular integrity returns.

restored, lowered hematocrit levels are found secondary to dilution, and an anemic state is more readily detectable.

Sodium and potassium are involved in electrolyte shifts. Sodium rapidly shifts to the interstitial spaces and remains there until edema formation ceases (Fig. 23-6). A potassium shift develops initially because injured cells and hemolyzed RBCs release potassium into the extracellular spaces.

Toward the end of the emergent phase, if fluid replacement is adequate, capillary membrane permeability will be restored. Fluid loss and edema formation cease. Interstitial fluid gradually returns to the vascular space (see Fig. 23-6). Clinically, diuresis is noted with low urine specific gravities. Serum potassium levels may be markedly elevated initially as fluid mobilization brings potassium from the interstitium to the vascular space. Hypokalemia may occur later as a result of the loss of potassium from diuresis and potassium movement back into cells. Serum sodium levels increase as sodium returns to the vascular space. Normal serum sodium values occur later with loss of sodium in urine.

Inflammation and Healing. Burn injury causes coagulation necrosis whereby tissues and vessels are damaged or destroyed. Polymorphonuclear leukocytes and monocytes accumulate at the site of injury. Fibroblasts and newly formed collagen fibrils appear and begin wound repair within the first 6 to 12 hours after injury. (The inflammatory response is discussed in Chapter 11.)

Immunologic Changes. Burn injury causes widespread impairment of the immune system.[6] The skin barrier to invading organisms is destroyed, circulating levels of immunoglobulins are decreased, and many changes in white blood cells (WBCs), both quantitative and qualitative, occur. Depression of neutrophil chemotactic, phagocytic, and bactericidal activity is found after burn injury. Burn size–related alterations of lymphocyte populations include decreased T-helper cells and increased T-suppressor cells. In addition, decreased levels of interleukin-1 (produced by macrophages) and interleukin-2 (produced by lymphocytes) are also found in some patients with burn injury. All of these changes in the immune system can make the burn patient more susceptible to infection.

Clinical Manifestations

The burn patient may be in shock from pain and hypovolemia. Frequently areas of full-thickness and deep partial-thickness burns are initially anesthetic because the nerve endings are destroyed. Superficial to moderate partial-thickness burns are painful. Blisters filled with fluid and protein may occur in partial-thickness burns. Fluid is not actually lost from the body as much as it is sequestered in the interstitial spaces and third spaces. It is hard to visualize severe dehydration in someone who is so obviously edematous. The patient may have signs of adynamic ileus as a result of the body's response to massive trauma and potassium shifts. Shivering may occur as a result of chilling that is caused by heat loss, anxiety, or pain.

The patient may have difficulty recalling the sequence of events that preceded the burn injury. Unconsciousness or altered mental status in a burn patient, however, is usually not a result of the burn. The most common reason is hypoxia associated with smoke inhalation. Other possibilities include head trauma and an overdose of sedative or pain medication.

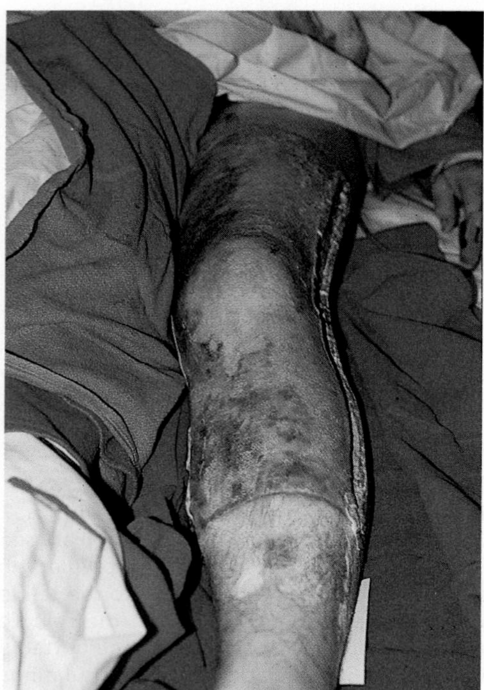

Fig. 23-7 Escharotomy of the lower extremity.

Complications

The three major organ systems most susceptible to complications during the emergent phase of burn injury are the cardiovascular, respiratory, and renal systems.

Cardiovascular System. Cardiovascular system complications include arrhythmias and hypovolemic shock, which may progress to irreversible shock. Circulation to the extremities can be severely impaired by circumferential burns and subsequent edema formation. These processes occlude the blood supply, causing ischemia, necrosis, and eventually gangrene. Escharotomies (incisions through the eschar) are frequently performed to restore circulation to compromised extremities (Fig. 23-7).

Initially there is an increase in blood viscosity with burn injuries because of the fluid loss that occurs in the emergent period. Microcirculation is impaired because of the damage to skin structures that contain small capillary systems. These two events result in a phenomenon termed *sludging*. Sludging can be corrected by adequate fluid replacement.

Respiratory System. The respiratory system is especially vulnerable to two types of injury: (1) upper airway burns that cause edema formation and obstruction of the airway and (2) inhalation injury (Table 23-9). Upper airway distress may occur with or without smoke inhalation, and airway injury at either level may occur in the absence of burn injury to the skin.

Upper respiratory tract injury. Upper respiratory tract injury results from direct heat injury or edema formation and can lead to mechanical airway obstruction and asphyxia. The edema associated with an upper respiratory tract burn injury can be massive and the onset insidious, and it occurs in most patients with major thermal burn injuries. Mechanical obstruction of the airway is not limited to the patient with flame burns of the upper airway because the edema that accompanies scald burns to the face and neck can be equally lethal when the pressure of the accumulated edema compresses the airway externally.[7] Flame burns to the neck and chest may contribute to respiratory difficulty because the inelastic eschar becomes tight and constricting from the underlying edema.

Table 23-9 Clinical Manifestations of Respiratory Injury Associated with Burns

Upper Respiratory Tract Injury

Edema, hoarseness, difficulty swallowing, copious secretions, stridor, substernal and intercostal retractions, total airway obstruction

Inhalation Injury

Initial absence of manifestations possible; high degree of suspicion if patient was trapped in fire and has facial burns, singed nasal or facial hair; dyspnea, carbonaceous sputum, wheezing, hoarseness, altered mental status

Inhalation injury. Inhalation injury refers to a direct insult at the alveolar level secondary to the inhalation of chemical fumes or smoke. The result is interstitial edema that prevents the diffusion of oxygen from the alveoli into the circulatory system. The patient with smoke inhalation frequently exhibits *no* physical manifestations of injury during the first 24 hours after sustaining a major burn. The only diagnostic indicator may be a history of prolonged exposure to smoke or fumes; therefore the nurse must be especially sensitive to signs of respiratory distress such as increased agitation or change in the rate or character of respirations. Sputum that contains carbon may be present. Generally there is no correlation between the extent of TBSA burn and severity of inhalation injury because inhalation injury is a factor of time exposure plus the type and density of the material inhaled. The initial chest x-ray may appear normal, and the ABG values may be within the normal range.

Impaired gas exchange related to CO poisoning often accompanies smoke inhalation. Inhalation of CO can produce significant hypoxemia. CO, produced by incomplete combustion of carbon-containing materials, has an affinity for hemoglobin 200 times that of oxygen. Carboxyhemoglobin concentration should be measured as soon as the patient reaches the hospital. The presence of increased concentrations of carboxyhemoglobin suggests that the patient has inhaled a significant amount of smoke. The characteristic cherry-red skin and mucous membranes associated with CO poisoning may not be present in the patient with burn shock because of the decrease in blood flow to the skin.

Other respiratory problems. The patient with preexisting respiratory problems (e.g., chronic obstructive pulmonary disease) is more predisposed to developing a respiratory infection. Pneumonia is a common complication of major burns (especially in the older adult) because of debilitation, abundant microbial flora, and the relative immobility of the patient. If fluid replacement is vigorous, the patient can develop pulmonary edema.

Renal System. The most common renal complication of a burn in the emergent phase is ATN. Because of the hypovolemic

COLLABORATIVE CARE

Table 23-10 Patient with Burns

Emergent Phase	Acute Phase	Rehabilitation Phase
Fluid therapy Assess fluid needs.* Begin IV fluid replacement. Insert indwelling urinary catheter. Monitor urine output. Wound care Start hydrotherapy or cleansing. Debride as necessary. Assess extent and depth of burns. Initiate topical antibiotic therapy. Administer tetanus toxoid or tetanus antitoxin.	Fluid therapy Replace fluids, depending on individual patient needs. Wound care Assess wound daily. Observe for complications. Continue hydrotherapy, cleansing. Continue debridement (if necessary). Early excision and grafting Provide homografts. Provide autografts. Care for donor site.	Counsel and teach patient and family. Encourage and assist patient in resuming self-care. Begin physical therapy for maintenance and rehabilitation of motion. Correct contractures and scarring (surgery, physical therapy, or splinting). Discuss possible cosmetic or reconstructive surgery.

*See Tables 23-11 and 23-12.
IV, intravenous; *RBCs,* red blood cells.

state, blood flow to the kidneys is decreased, causing renal ischemia. If this continues, acute renal failure may develop.

With full-thickness and electrical burns, myoglobin (from muscle cell breakdown) and hemoglobin (from RBC breakdown) are released into the bloodstream and occlude renal tubules. Adequate fluid replacement and diuretics can counteract myoglobin and hemoglobin obstruction of the tubules.

NURSING AND COLLABORATIVE MANAGEMENT: EMERGENT PHASE

In the emergent phase, patient survival depends on quick and thorough assessment and intervention.[8] It may be the nurse who makes the initial assessment of depth, degree, and percent of burn and who coordinates the actions of the burn team. From the onset of the burn event until the patient is stabilized, nursing and collaborative management predominantly consists of airway management, fluid therapy, and wound care (Table 23-10). See the accompanying nursing care plan (NCP 23-1).

Airway Management

Airway management involves early nasotracheal or endotracheal intubation before the airway is actually compromised. Early intubation eliminates the necessity for emergency tracheostomy after respiratory problems have become apparent. In general the patient with major injuries involving burns to the face and neck requires intubation within 1 to 2 hours after burn injury. (Nasotracheal and endotracheal intubations are discussed in Chapter 63.) After intubation, the patient may be placed on ventilatory assistance, and the delivered oxygen concentration is determined by assessing ABG values. Extubation may be indicated when the edema resolves, usually 3 to 6 days after burn injury, unless severe inhalation injury is involved. Escharotomies may be needed to relieve respiratory distress secondary to circumferential, full-thickness burns of the neck and trunk.

Within 6 to 12 hours after injury in which smoke inhalation is probable, the patient should have a fiberoptic bronchoscopy to assess the lower respiratory tract. Significant findings include the appearance of carbonaceous material, mucosal edema, vesicles, erythema, hemorrhage, and ulceration.

Treatment of inhalation injury includes administration of humidified air and 100% oxygen as required. The patient should be placed in a high Fowler's position (unless contraindicated by a possible spinal injury), encouraged to cough and deep breathe every hour, repositioned every 1 to 2 hours, given chest physiotherapy, and suctioned as necessary. If respiratory failure is impending, nasotracheal or endotracheal intubation should be performed and the patient should be supported with mechanical ventilation. Positive end-expiratory pressure (PEEP) may be used to prevent collapse of the alveoli and progressive respiratory failure (see Chapter 63). Bronchodilators may be administered intravenously to treat severe bronchospasm. CO poisoning is treated by administering 100% O_2 until the carboxyhemoglobin levels return to normal. Hyperbaric O_2 therapy may also be useful in accelerating the excretion of CO. However, patients may need to be transported to another part of the hospital for therapy or to another hospital entirely, and their important resuscitative treatment unnecessarily delayed.

Fluid Therapy

As soon as the patient arrives at a health care facility, at least one (and usually two) large-bore intravenous (IV) replacement line is secured, preferably by percutaneous puncture. If this is not feasible, a jugular or subclavian line is inserted through unburned or even burned tissue. A cutdown is a final measure but is rarely used because of the high incidence of infection and sepsis. It is critical to establish IV access that can accommodate large volumes of fluid.

The extent of an adult's burn wound should be assessed using the Rule of Nines (see Fig. 23-4). This will allow for estimation of fluid resuscitation requirements.

IV fluid therapy is usually instituted in the patient with burns greater than 20% TBSA.[9] The type of fluid replacement is determined by size and depth of burn, age of the patient, and individual considerations such as dehydration in the preburn state or preexisting chronic illness. Each burn center has a

23-1 NURSING CARE PLAN BURN PATIENT

Expected Patient Outcomes	Nursing Interventions and *Rationales* — Emergent Phase	Acute Phase	Rehabilitative Phase
NURSING DIAGNOSIS **Risk for fluid volume deficit** *related to* evaporative loss, plasma loss, and shift of fluid into interstitium secondary to burn injury.			
▪ Output >30 to 50 ml/hr. ▪ Stable vital signs. ▪ Clear sensorium. ▪ Sodium and potassium levels within acceptable range. ▪ Systolic blood pressure >90 mm Hg.	▪ Assess every 1-2 hr: pulses, blood pressure, circulation, and sensation to all extremities; mental status; intake and output; pulmonary function *to determine status of major body systems.* ▪ Monitor weight daily *to evaluate fluid/nutritional status.* ▪ Monitor serial laboratory tests *to determine fluid and electrolyte status.* ▪ Give fluids according to patient needs.	▪ Use emergent-phase interventions as necessary. ▪ Monitor electrolyte levels regularly. ▪ Provide oral fluids if patient is able to drink *to increase fluid intake and patient comfort.*	▪ No intervention is required.
NURSING DIAGNOSIS **Pain** *related to* burn injury and treatment *as manifested by* demonstration of discomfort and pain.			
▪ Satisfaction with level of pain control.	▪ Administer IV analgesia as needed *to manage pain.* ▪ Administer medication for pain 30 min before interventions. ▪ Evaluate effectiveness of medication. ▪ Provide emotional support. ▪ Reposition patient carefully using lifting sheet as necessary *to avoid further trauma to skin.*	▪ Plan adequate rest periods *to facilitate coping.* ▪ Administer medication before interventions. ▪ Teach relaxation techniques, guided imagery, distraction *to augment other pain relief measures.* ▪ Plan diversional activities *to distract patient from present situation.*	▪ Be aware that patient's pain may be replaced by itchiness. ▪ Keep skin lubricated with water-based moisturizers *to prevent drying.* ▪ Teach patient to watch for injuries to new skin.
NURSING DIAGNOSIS **Self-care deficits** *related to* pain, immobility, and perceived helplessness *as manifested by* inability or unwillingness to participate in self-care.			
▪ Optimal performance of self-care.	▪ Assess patient's ability to perform self-care activities. ▪ Assist or intervene as appropriate. ▪ Assist patient in remaining in emotional control *to reduce feelings of helplessness.*	▪ Increase patient's self-care activities as appropriate. ▪ Ensure that patient participates in planning care as able *to increase sense of control.*	▪ Assess and arrange for needed adaptations in living arrangements and lifestyle *to accommodate optimal self-care.*

Continued

23-1 NURSING CARE PLAN BURN PATIENT—continued

Expected Patient Outcomes	Nursing Interventions and *Rationales*		
	Emergent Phase	**Acute Phase**	**Rehabilitative Phase**
NURSING DIAGNOSIS	**Altered nutrition: less than body requirements** *related to* increased caloric demands and inability to ingest increased requirements *as manifested by* weight loss and negative nitrogen balance.		
▪ Positive nitrogen balance. ▪ Weight loss not >10% of body weight.	▪ Maintain patient NPO with NG tube to low intermittent suction *to allow for decompression of the stomach.* ▪ Assess return of bowel sounds *to determine when oral intake can be resumed.* ▪ Institute progressive diet *to meet nutritional needs when bowel sounds return.* ▪ Chart caloric intake *to monitor adequacy of diet.*	▪ Continue to monitor peristalsis. ▪ Titrate tube feedings to patient tolerance *to prevent diarrhea.* ▪ Offer high-protein, high-carbohydrate diet *to meet increased nutritional needs.* ▪ Assess patient food preferences and offer favored foods when patient is able to eat.	▪ Continue to meet nutritional needs. ▪ Once skin coverage is achieved, reduce calories *to prevent excess weight gain (if necessary).*
NURSING DIAGNOSIS	**Risk for infection** *related to* impaired skin integrity, endogenous flora, suppressed immune response.		
▪ Wound free of debris and loose necrotic tissue. ▪ Absence of wound infections.	▪ Use good hand-washing technique. ▪ Use sterile technique during topical antibiotic application and dressing changes *to prevent contaminating burn area.* ▪ Shave appropriate areas *to reduce possibility of contamination.* ▪ Evacuate blisters and remove devitalized tissue *to eliminate medium for bacterial growth.* ▪ Apply topical antibiotic or sterile dressings as indicated; start systemic IV antibiotics (if indicated) *to decrease probability of infection.* ▪ Give tetanus vaccine if necessary. ▪ Observe wound daily for separation of eschar; check wound margins for cellulitis. ▪ Monitor vital signs and temperature.	▪ Monitor burn wound margins *to detect signs of infection such as purulent drainage, edema, redness.* ▪ Note any change in behavior or sensorium. ▪ Perform hydrotherapy and debridement carefully *to remove wound debris and effectively cleanse wound.* ▪ Monitor body temperature, WBC count, and urine output *to detect signs of sepsis.* ▪ Monitor donor sites *to detect possible infection.*	▪ Instruct patient and family about signs and symptoms of infection *so early treatment can be initiated.* ▪ Teach family how to perform dressing changes *to ensure proper technique and increase their sense of control.*

Continued

23-1 NURSING CARE PLAN BURN PATIENT—continued

Expected Patient Outcomes	Nursing Interventions and *Rationales* Emergent Phase	Acute Phase	Rehabilitative Phase
NURSING DIAGNOSIS **Anxiety** *related to* pain, guilt associated with injury, lack of knowledge about treatment and outcome, financial needs, and appearance *as manifested by* questions about treatment and prognosis, withdrawn or overtly angry behavior, expression of concerns about scarring.			
▪ Reduction of anxiety. ▪ Body language indicating rest and comfort. ▪ Able to talk about changes in self-image.	▪ Administer and evaluate effectiveness of pain medication. ▪ Encourage family visits and participation in care *to increase feelings of support.* ▪ Be open to patient's expressions of feelings about burn event *so patient has opportunity to express emotions.* ▪ Describe burn process and clinical progress to patient and family. ▪ Explain therapeutic interventions, precautionary measures (e.g., gowning, hand washing) *to elicit cooperation and decrease anxiety.*	▪ Assist patient and family in setting realistic expectations for patient's progress. ▪ Consider psychiatric evaluation for patients and families who exhibit symptoms of posttraumatic stress disorder.	▪ Provide ways for patient and family to maintain contact with hospital personnel after discharge *to promote continuity of care and minimize anxiety.* ▪ Consider referral to support group. ▪ Plan counseling if needed.
NURSING DIAGNOSIS **Body image disturbance** *related to* disfigurement secondary to burn *as manifested by* verbalized negative comments about appearance, unwillingness to look at self or participate in self-care.			
▪ Realistic goals regarding future lifestyle. ▪ Acceptance of altered body image.	▪ Reassure patient and family that swelling will subside in 2 to 4 days *so patient realizes that it is not permanent.*	▪ Plan for family interaction *to foster feeling of support and reduce sense of isolation.* ▪ Explain expected appearance during treatments *to decrease misconceptions.* ▪ Be realistic and positive during interventions. ▪ Set goals within limitations *so patient can feel a sense of accomplishment.*	▪ Assess need for and provide means of professional counseling (psychologic and vocational) if appropriate *to reduce impact of the burn event on the patient's life.* ▪ Reassure patient that appearance of burn wounds will continue to improve even after healing has taken place.

NG, nasogastric; *NPO*, nothing by mouth; *WBC*, white blood cell.

preference for a replacement regimen. Fluid replacement is accomplished with either crystalloid solutions (physiologic saline, lactated Ringer's, or 5% dextrose and saline) or colloids (albumin, dextran, or other commercially prepared solutions).

Of the many formulas that are used for fluid replacement, the Brooke formula and the Parkland (Baxter) formula are the most commonly employed (Tables 23-11 and 23-12). All formulas are estimates. The Parkland formula has been widely used because it is easy to calculate and monitor and it provides a reliable method of fluid replacement for most patients.

As noted in Table 23-12, the Parkland formula gives fluid in the following manner: 4 ml lactated Ringer's solution per kilogram of body weight per percent TBSA burned. This quantity is calculated for the first 24 hours, with one half of the total quantity given in the first 8 hours after injury because it is during that period that fluid loss is greatest. (NOTE: This 24 hours is not calculated from time of arrival to hospital but from the time of injury.) One quarter of the total quantity is then given in the second 8-hour period, and the final quarter is given in the last 8-hour period.

The second 24 hours of fluid replacement consists of ensuring adequate dextrose in water replacement to maintain a serum sodium level below 140 mEq/L (140 mmol/L). Colloidal solutions (e.g., Plasmanate, albumin) are also routinely given. The amount is calculated with a formula and the patient's body weight, which predicts the replacement volume. Colloidal solu-

Table 23-11 Formulas for Estimating Fluid Replacement of an Adult Burn Patient

	First 24 Hours	Second 24 Hours	
Formula	Crystalloids	Colloids	Glucose in Water
Brooke (modified)	Lactated Ringer's solution: 2.0 ml/kg/% burn; ½ given during first 8 hr; ½ given during next 16 hr	0.3 to 0.5 ml/kg/% burn	Amount to replace estimated evaporative losses
Parkland (Baxter)	Lactated Ringer's solution: 4 ml/kg/% burn; ½ given first 8 hr; ¼ given each next 8 hr	20-60% of calculated plasma volume	Amount to replace estimated evaporative losses

Table 23-12 Fluid Resuscitation with the Parkland (Baxter) Formula*

Formula

4 ml lactated Ringer's solution
per
kg body weight
per
% TBSA burn
= total fluid requirement for first 24 hr after burn

Application

½ of total in first 8 hr
¼ of total in second 8 hr
¼ of total in third 8 hr

Example

For a 70 kg patient with a 50% TBSA burn:
4 ml × 70 kg × 50% TBSA burn = 14,000 ml
= 14 L in 24 hr
½ of total in first 8 hr = 7000 ml (875 ml/hr)
¼ of total in second 8 hr = 3500 ml (436 ml/hr)
¼ of total in third 8 hr = 3500 ml (436 ml/hr)

*Formulas are guidelines. Fluid is administered at a rate to produce 30 to 50 ml of urine output per hour.
TBSA, total body surface area.

tions are not usually given until the second 24 hours, when capillary permeability begins to return to normal, because premature infusion of colloid solutions could result in leakage out of the vascular space as a result of increased capillary permeability. After this time, the plasma remains in the vascular space and expands the circulating volume.

Assessment of the adequacy of fluid replacement is best made by use of more than one parameter. Urinary output is the most commonly used parameter. Assessment parameters include the following:

1. Urine output: 30 to 50 ml/hr in an adult.
2. Cardiopulmonary factors: BP (systolic >90 to 100 mm Hg), pulse rate (<100), respiration (16 to 20 breaths per minute). (BP is most appropriately measured by an arterial line. Peripheral measurement is often invalid because of vasoconstriction and edema.)
3. Sensorium: alert and oriented to time, place, and person.

Wound Care

Wound care should be delayed until a patent airway, adequate circulation, and adequate fluid replacement have been established. Full-thickness wounds will be dry and waxy white to dark brown and will have little to no sensation because nerve endings have been destroyed. Partial-thickness wounds are pink to cherry red and wet and shiny with serous exudate. These wounds may or may not have intact blisters and are painful when touched or exposed to air.

Cleansing and debridement can be done in a tank (Fig. 23-8), shower, or bed. Debridement may need to be done in the operating room (OR) (Fig. 23-9). During these procedures, loose, necrotic skin is removed. Large blisters may be opened to eliminate media for bacterial growth. All burned areas with hair (except eyebrows) should be shaved, including the head and perineum. Thereafter, daily shaving is required to minimize pathogen accumulation. Care should be taken to accomplish this procedure as quickly and deftly as possible. Immersion in a tank for longer than 20 to 30 minutes can cause electrolyte loss from open burned areas. Prolonged immersion can lead to chilling after the bath and cross-contamination of wounds from one area of the body to another. Because of these factors, some institutions do not submerge the patient. Instead the patient can be showered. The water does not need to be sterile, and tap water not exceeding 104° F (40° C) is acceptable. Because pathogenic organisms are present on the burn wound, a surgical detergent, disinfectant, or cleansing agent may be used. The patient may be bathed two times daily to limit the amount of bacterial growth. However, that degree of frequency may be too painful and psychologically demanding for many patients. A once-daily bath or shower followed by a dressing change in the patient's room is a popular alternative in many burn centers.

Infection is the most serious threat to further tissue injury and possible sepsis.[10] Survival is directly related to prevention of wound contamination. The source of infection in burn wounds is the patient's own flora, predominantly from the skin, respiratory tract, and gastrointestinal (GI) tract. The prevention of cross-contamination from one patient to another is a priority for nursing care.

Two methods of wound treatment used to control infection are the open method and the closed method. In the open method the patient's burn is covered with a topical antibiotic and has no dressing. The closed method uses sterile gauze

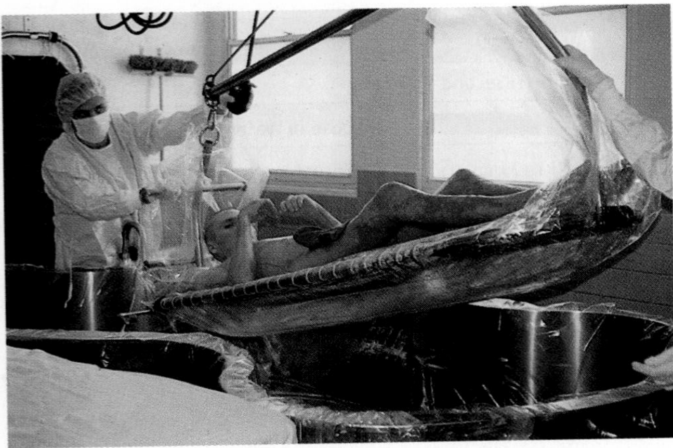

Fig. 23-8 Patient is being bathed in a tank. Bathing presents an opportunity for physical therapy as well as wound care.

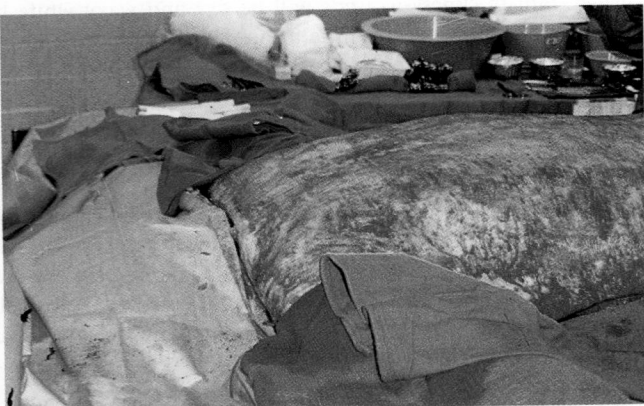

Fig. 23-9 Operative debridement of full-thickness burns is necessary to prepare the wound for grafting.

dressings impregnated with or laid over a topical antibiotic. These dressings may be changed two to three times every 24 hours.

When the patient's wounds are exposed, the staff must wear disposable hats, masks, gowns, and gloves. When removing dressings and washing the wound, the nurse should use nonsterile disposable gloves. Sterile gloves are used when applying ointments and sterile dressings. In addition, the room must be kept warm (approximately 85° F [29.4° C]). All attire is changed before the nurse treats another patient. Careful hand washing is also required to prevent cross-contamination. After the patient has been treated in the tub, the tank and agitators are disinfected with a chemical preparation.

Coverage is the primary goal for burn wounds.[11] Because there is rarely enough unburned skin in the major burn patient for immediate skin grafting, other temporary wound closure methods are used. Allograft or homograft skin (usually from cadavers) is commonly used for wound closure (Table 23-13). However, rejection eventually occurs because the host's immune system reacts against the foreign substance.

Table 23-13 Sources of Grafts

Source	Graft Name	Coverage
Porcine skin	Heterograft or xenograft (different species)	Temporary (3 days to 2 wk)
Cadaveric skin	Homograft or allograft (same species)	Temporary (3 days to 2 wk)
Patient's own skin	Autograft	Permanent
Patient's own skin and cell culture	Cultured epithelial autograft	Permanent

Other Care Measures

Care of special areas is initiated by the nurse. The face is vascular and subject to a greater amount of edema. Facial care is performed by the open method because facial dressings cause disorientation and confusion. Eye care for corneal burns or edema is done with slightly warmed physiologic saline rinses as often as every hour. Periorbital edema can prevent opening of the eyes. This can be frightening to the patient; the nurse must assure the patient that the swelling is not permanent and that vision will soon be restored. Instillation of methylcellulose drops or artificial tears into the eyes for moisture provides additional comfort and prevents corneal abrasions.

Hands and arms should be extended and elevated on pillows or in slings to minimize edema. Splints may need to be applied to burned hands and feet to maintain them in functional positions.

Ears should be kept free of pressure because of their poor vascularization and predisposition to infection. The patient with ear burns is not allowed to use pillows because of the danger of the burned ear sticking to the pillow case, thereby causing bleeding, pain, or infection of the ear cartilage. The patient with neck burns is not allowed to use pillows in order to prevent wound contraction.

The perineum must be kept clean and as dry as possible. In addition to providing hourly urine outputs, an indwelling catheter prevents urine contamination of the perineal area. Frequent perineal and catheter care is essential.

Routine lab tests are performed initially and serially to monitor electrolyte balance. Blood for measurement of ABGs may be drawn to determine adequacy of ventilation and perfusion.

Physical therapy is begun immediately, sometimes in the tank. Early range-of-motion (ROM) exercises are necessary to facilitate mobilization of the extravasated fluid back into the vascular bed. Exercise of body parts also maintains function and reassures the patient that movement is still possible.

Drug Therapy

Analgesics and Sedatives. Analgesics are ordered to promote patient comfort. Early in the postburn period, IV

DRUG THERAPY

Table 23-14 Drugs Commonly Used in Burn Treatment

Types and Names of Drugs	Purpose
Nutritional Support	
Vitamins A, C, E, and multivitamins	Promotes wound healing
Minerals: zinc, folate, iron (ferrous sulfate, ferrous gluconate)	Promotes cellular integrity and hemoglobin formation
Analgesia and Sedative	
Morphine	Diminishes pain perception
Meperidine (Demerol)	Diminishes pain perception
Fentanyl (Sublimaze)	Diminishes pain perception
Methadone	Relieves pain, elevates mood
Haloperidol (Haldol)	Produces antipsychotic and sedative effects, promotes sleep
Midazolam (Versed)	Has short-acting amnestic properties
Gastrointestinal Support	
Cimetidine (Tagamet)	Decreases incidence of Curling's ulcer
Nystatin (Mycostatin)	Prevents overgrowth of *Candida albicans* in oral mucosa
Mylanta, Maalox	Neutralizes stomach acid

pain medications should be given because (1) GI function is slowed or impaired because of shock or paralytic ileus, and (2) intramuscular (IM) injections will not be absorbed adequately in burned or edematous areas, causing pooling of medications in the tissues. When fluid mobilization begins, the patient could be inadvertently overdosed from the interstitial accumulation of previous IM medications.

Common narcotics used for pain control are listed in Table 23-14. The need for analgesia should be evaluated. The drug of choice for pain control is morphine, but meperidine and methadone may also be used. These drugs provide adequate pain control and a sedative effect. The patient may be in great pain with large burns (especially predominantly partial-thickness burns). Withholding pain medication in the early phases of burn injury is not only inhumane but also unethical.

Tetanus Immunization. Tetanus toxoid is given routinely to all burn patients because of the likelihood of anaerobic burn-wound contamination. In the absence of active immunization within 10 years before the burn injury, tetanus immunoglobulin should be administered.

Antimicrobial Agents. After the wound is cleansed, topical antibacterial agents are applied and may be covered with a light dressing or left open to air (Fig. 23-10). Systemic antibiotics are not usually used in controlling burn wound flora, especially after 48 hours, because there is little or no blood supply to the burn eschar, and consequently, there is little delivery of the antibiotic to the wound. Topical burn agents penetrate the eschar, thereby inhibiting bacterial invasion of the wound (Table 23-15). Silver sulfadiazine is commonly used because it is effective, and unlike mafenide (Sulfamylon), it is painless. Systemic sepsis remains a leading cause of death in the patient with major burns because resistant organisms develop with exposure of bacteria to topical agents over time. Most burn centers use one topical agent almost exclusively and change to another at the first sign of microorganism resistance. Systemic antibiotic therapy is initiated when the clinical diagnosis of invasive burn wound sepsis is made or when some other source of sepsis is identified (e.g., pneumonia).

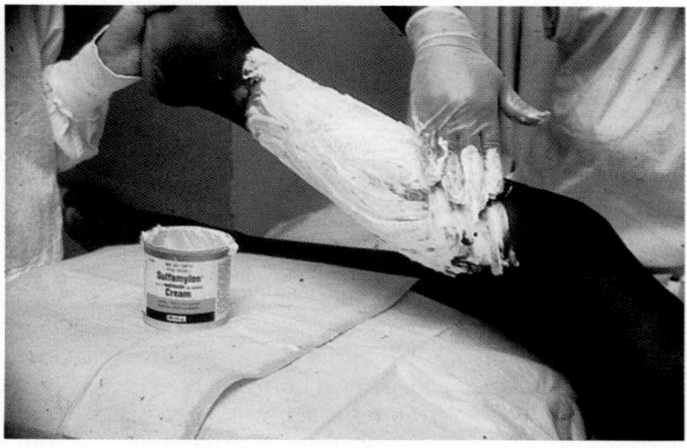

Fig. 23-10 Patient being treated with mafenide (Sulfamylon).

Frequently, superinfections develop in the patient's mucous membranes (mouth and genitalia) as a result of antibiotic therapy and low resistance in the host. The offending organism is usually *Candida albicans.* Oral infection is treated with nystatin (Mycostatin) mouthwash. When a normal diet is resumed, yogurt or *Lactobacillus* (Lactinex) may be given by mouth to reintroduce the normal intestinal flora that have been destroyed by antibiotic therapy.

Nutritional Therapy

Fluid replacement takes priority over nutritional needs in the initial emergent phase. The patient with large burns frequently develops paralytic ileus within a few hours as a result of the body's response to major trauma. A nasogastric tube is inserted and connected to low intermittent suction for decompression. When bowel sounds return at 48 to 72 hours after injury, alimentation can be initiated beginning with clear liquids and progressing to a diet high in protein and calories.

A hypermetabolic response proportional to the size of the wound is observed. Resting metabolic expenditure may be increased by 50% to 100% above normal for major burns. Core temperature is elevated. Plasma catecholamines, which stimulate heat production, and substrate mobilization are increased. Massive catabolism is characterized by protein breakdown and increased gluconeogenesis. Caloric needs are often in the 5000 kcal per day range. Failure to supply adequate calories and protein leads to malnutrition and delayed healing. The patient is not freely given water to drink. Rather,

DRUG THERAPY

Table 23-15 Topical Antibiotic Therapy

Topical	Indications	Advantages	Disadvantages
Silver sulfadiazine (Silvadene)	Gram-positive and gram-negative organisms, *Candida albicans*	Wide-spectrum antibacterial action No limit to motion Can use light or no dressings Fast, painless, easy to apply	Possible depression of granulocyte formation Possible allergic reaction to sulfa
Mafenide acetate (Sulfamylon)	Gram-positive and gram-negative organisms Most anaerobes Ear burns Electrical burns	Wide-spectrum antibacterial action Most effective topical antibiotic Penetrates eschar, cartilage Open treatment possible	Possible pain on application Acid-base disturbance because it is a carbonic anhydrase inhibitor Possible allergic reaction to sulfa
Bacitracin	Superficial burns Staphylococcal organisms Facial burns	Can be safely used on autografts and homografts Nonpainful Inexpensive Requires only 1-time-daily application	May cause itching, rash
Mupirocin (Bactroban)	Effective against many organisms resistant to silver sulfadiazine Use based on sensitivity results	Painless Safe for use on CEA Inhibits bacterial and protein synthesis	Possible itching, burning, rash Potential renal toxicity if used over large area

CEA, cultured epithelial autograft

calorie-containing liquids are given because of the great need for calories and the potential for water intoxication.

Major advances have been made in the area of liquid nutritional supplementation (see Chapter 38). A thin latex feeding tube can be advanced by fluoroscopic guidance into the duodenum, bypassing the stomach. This allows for quicker absorption of nutrients and a decrease in the nausea and vomiting associated with high-volume tube feedings into the stomach. This patient can be maintained on a more continuous feeding schedule, which does not have to be interrupted by surgical interventions (e.g., debridement, grafting). Because the liquid goes past the pyloric sphincter, the patient does not have to remain without food or water for extended periods as is required when the tube is in the stomach. Early and continuous enteral feeding promotes optimal conditions for wound healing and immunocompetence. Because of their direct effect on morbidity and mortality, early, continuous enteral feedings are recommended after burn injury.[12]

Supplemental vitamins and iron may be given as early as the emergent phase. However, the need for these supplements usually does not occur until the acute phase.

Acute Phase

The acute phase begins with the mobilization of extracellular fluid and subsequent diuresis. The acute phase is concluded when the burned area is completely covered or when the wounds are healed. This may take weeks or many months.

Pathophysiology

Burn injury involves pathophysiologic changes in many body systems. Diuresis from fluid mobilization occurs, and the patient is no longer grossly edematous. Areas that are full- or partial-thickness burns are more evident. Bowel sounds return. The patient is now aware of the enormity of body changes and the presence of pain. Healing begins when WBCs have surrounded the burn wound and phagocytosis begins. Necrotic tissue begins to slough. Fibroblasts lay down matrices of the collagen precursors that eventually form granulation tissue. Kept free from infection, a partial-thickness burn wound will heal from the edges and from below; however, full-thickness burn wounds, unless extremely small, must be covered by skin grafts. Often, healing time and length of hospitalization are decreased by early excision and grafting.

Clinical Manifestations

Full-thickness wounds will be dry and waxy white to dark brown and will have little to no sensation because nerve endings have been destroyed. Partial-thickness wounds are pink to cherry red and wet and shiny with serous exudate. These wounds may or may not have intact blisters and are painful when touched or exposed to air. With time, the margins of full-thickness eschar will begin to separate, allowing for debridement of the wound. Usually full-thickness wounds will require surgical debridement and skin grafting to speed the healing process.

Partial-thickness wounds will also form eschar but will not be as thick, so they will begin separating sooner and healing more quickly. Once partial-thickness eschar is removed, epithelialization begins at the wound margins and appears as red or pink scar tissue. The epithelial buds eventually close in the wound, and the wound heals spontaneously without surgical intervention. This is expected to occur in 10 to 14 days.

Laboratory Values

Because the body is attempting to reestablish fluid and electrolyte homeostasis in the initial acute phase, it is important to follow serum electrolyte levels closely.

Sodium. *Hyponatremia* can occur with silver nitrate topical antibiotic therapy as a result of sodium loss through the eschar. If hydrotherapy is too lengthy (usually longer than 20 to 30 minutes), the hypotonicity of the bath water pulls sodium from the open burn areas. Other causes of hyponatremia include excessive GI drainage, diarrhea, and excessive water intake. Symptoms of hyponatremia include weakness, dizziness, muscle cramps, fatigue, headache, tachycardia, and confusion. The burn patient may also develop a dilutional hyponatremia called *water intoxication.* To avoid this condition, the patient should drink fluids other than water, such as juice, soft drinks, or nutritional supplements.

Hypernatremia may be seen after successful fluid replacement if copious amounts of hypertonic solutions were required. Other causes of hypernatremia include improper tube feeding therapy or inappropriate fluid administration. Manifestations of hypernatremia include thirst; dried, furry tongue; lethargy; confusion; and possibly seizures.

Potassium. *Hyperkalemia* is noted if the patient has renal failure, adrenocortical insufficiency, or massive deep muscle injury with large amounts of potassium released from damaged cells. Cardiac arrhythmias and ventricular failure can occur with excessive elevations (potassium level >7 mEq/L [7 mmol/L]). Muscle weakness and electrocardiographic changes are observed clinically (see Chapter 15).

Hypokalemia is observed with silver nitrate therapy and lengthy hydrotherapy. Other causes of this deficit include vomiting, diarrhea, prolonged GI suction, and prolonged IV therapy without potassium supplementation. Constant potassium losses occur through the burn wound.

Complications

Infection. The body's first line of defense, the skin, has been destroyed by burn injury. Pathogens often proliferate before phagocytosis has adequately begun. If the bacterial density at the junction of the eschar with underlying viable tissue rises to greater than 10^5/g, the patient has a wound infection. In the presence of an infection, localized inflammation, induration, and suppuration can be seen at the burn wound margins.[10] Partial-thickness burns can convert to full-thickness burns in the presence of infection. A histologic examination of a burn-wound biopsy is the most reliable means of differentiating colonization of nonviable tissue from invasive infection of viable tissue. Invasive wound infections may be treated with systemic or topical antibiotics based on culture results.

Wound infection may progress to transient bacteremia from wound manipulation (e.g., after debridement and hydrotherapy). The patient may develop an invasive infection or sepsis. Manifestations of sepsis include an elevated temperature, increased pulse and respiratory rate, decreased BP, and decreased urine output. There may be mild confusion, chills, malaise, and loss of appetite. The WBC count will usually be between 10,000/μl (10×10^9/L) and 20,000/μl (20×10^9/L). There are functional defects in the WBCs, and the patient remains immunosuppressed for a period after the burn injury. The causative organisms of sepsis are usually gram-negative bacteria (e.g., *Pseudomonas, Proteus* organisms), putting the patient at further risk for septic shock.

When sepsis is suspected, cultures should be obtained immediately from all possible sources: urine, oropharynx, sputum, IV site, and wound. However, treatment should not be delayed pending results of the culture and sensitivity studies. Therapy will begin with antibiotics appropriate for the usual residual flora of the particular burn center. The topical antibiotic that is used may be continued or may be changed to another agent. At this stage, the patient's condition is critical, requiring close monitoring of vital signs.

Cardiovascular System. The same cardiovascular and respiratory system complications may be present in the acute phase as in the emergent phase.

Neurologic System. Neurologically, the patient usually has no physically based problems unless severe hypoxia from respiratory injuries or complications from electrical injuries occur. However, a poorly understood phenomenon is likely to be seen. The patient can become extremely disoriented, may withdraw or become combative, and have hallucinations and frequent nightmarelike episodes. Delirium is more acute at night and occurs more often in the older patient. This is a transient state lasting from a day or two to several weeks. Various causes have been considered, including electrolyte imbalance, stress, cerebral edema, sepsis, intensive care unit (ICU) psychosis syndrome, and the use of analgesics and antianxiety drugs.

Musculoskeletal System. The musculoskeletal system takes center stage for complications during the acute phase. As the burns begin to heal and scar tissue forms, the skin is less supple and pliant. ROM may be limited, and contractures can occur. Because of pain, the patient will prefer to assume a flexed position for comfort.

Gastrointestinal System. The GI system also exhibits complications during this phase. Adynamic ileus results from sepsis. However, diarrhea is more commonly present than ileus and can be caused by the use of supplemental feedings or antibiotics. Constipation can occur as a side effect of narcotic analgesics and decreased mobility. Curling's ulcer, a type of gastroduodenal ulcer characterized by diffuse superficial lesions, including mucosal erosion, is caused by a generalized stress response resulting in decreased production of mucus and increased gastric acid secretion. The best treatment of Curling's ulcer is prevention. The prophylactic use of antacids and H_2 histamine blockers (e.g., cimetidine [Tagamet]) inhibits histamine and stimulation of hydrochloric acid (HCl) secretion. Many major burn patients also have occult blood in their stools during the acute phase.

Endocrine System. Stress diabetes may be seen transiently because of stress-mediated cortisol and catecholamine release resulting in increased mobilization of glycogen stores, glycogenolysis, and subsequent production of glucose. There is also an increase in insulin production and release. However, insulin's effectiveness is decreased because of relative insulin insensitivity, leading to an elevated blood glucose level. Later, hyperglycemia can be caused by the supranormal caloric intake necessary to meet the metabolic requirements. When this

Table 23-16 Enzymatic Debriders Used in Burn Therapy

Topical	Indications	Advantages	Disadvantages
Collagenase (Santyl)	Aggressive debridement of necrotic tissue on deep partial-thickness wound	Does not harm healthy tissue Digests denatured collagen in devitalized tissue	Limited antimicrobial coverage Rare allergic sensitivity Expensive Effective only in narrow pH range of 6-8 Wound bed must be neutralized with Polysporin powder
Fibrinolysin/ desoxyribonuclease (Elase)	Debridement of devitalized tissue in partial-thickness wound	Attacks denatured DNA and fibrin in necrotic wounds Can be applied one time daily Compatible with other topicals	Possible burning Can harm healthy tissue Expensive
Accuzyme	Debridement of necrotic tissue on partial-thickness wound Liquefaction of purulent drainage	Derived from papaya—digests nonviable protein matter Will not harm healthy tissue Compatible with other topicals	Burning Stinging sensation Expensive

occurs, the treatment is supplemental insulin, not decreased feeding. Serum glucose is checked frequently and an appropriate amount of insulin is given if hyperglycemia is present. Glucometers may also be used to assess blood glucose; serum glucose samples are more accurate than capillary blood analysis by glucometer. As the patient's metabolic demands are met and less stress is placed on the entire system, this stress-induced condition is reversed.

NURSING AND COLLABORATIVE MANAGEMENT: ACUTE PHASE

The predominant therapeutic interventions in the acute phase are (1) fluid replacement, (2) physical therapy, (3) wound care, (4) early excision and grafting, and (5) pain management.

■ Fluid Replacement

Fluid replacement continues from the emergent phase into the acute phase on the basis of patient needs.[13] IV therapy is provided to replace fluid losses, administer medications, and administer transfusions. The type of fluid replacement depends on the patient's specific needs. Common types of replacement are normal saline solution, Ringer's lactate solution, and various concentrations of glucose in saline solution or water. Packed RBCs, fresh frozen plasma, and Plasmanate are also commonly given at this time.

■ Physical Therapy

Rigorous physical therapy is imperative to maintain optimal joint function. A good time for exercise is during and after hydrotherapy when the skin is softer and bulky dressings are removed. Passive and active ROM should be performed on all joints. The patient with neck burns should sleep without pillows or with the head hanging slightly over the top of the mattress to encourage hyperextension. Splints should be used to keep joints in functional positions and should be reexamined frequently to ensure an optimal fit.

■ Wound Care

Goals of wound care are to (1) cleanse and debride the area of necrotic tissue and debris that would promote bacterial growth, (2) minimize further destruction to viable skin, (3) promote wound reepithelialization or success of skin grafting, and (4) promote patient comfort.

Wound care consists of daily observation, assessment, cleansing, and debridement. Wound care begun in the emergent phase continues during the acute phase.

Debridement, dressing changes, topical antibiotic therapy, graft care, and donor site care may be performed two to three times daily.[14] Enzymatic debriders may be used for debridement of burn wounds (Table 23-16). Appropriate coverage of the graft (if it is not kept open to air) should include fine-mesh gauze in closest proximity to the graft before other dressings are applied. Xeroform dressing, a fine-mesh, absorbent gauze impregnated with 3% bismuth tribromophenate, may be used over grafted areas.[15] It has a petrolatum base that keeps the gauze from adhering to graft sites, and it also has mild antibacterial properties.

Sheet skin grafts must be free of serous collections or blebs. Blebs prevent the graft from interfacing and growing to the wound itself. Evacuation of blebs is done by aspiration with a tuberculin syringe or by pricking or cutting the peripheral margin of the bleb and rolling (with a sterile swab) the fluid from the center of the bleb to the exit site. The bleb should never be rolled to the edge of the graft. This serves only to separate adherent graft from the wound.

Donor site care methods have been controversial throughout the years.[16] Although the majority of burn centers continue to use heat lamp treatments with a Xeroform-covered donor site to facilitate drying, many new methods are being evaluated. The average healing time for a donor site is 10 to 14 days. Several of the newer methods potentially can decrease this healing time, which would facilitate earlier reharvesting of skin at the site. One new method of treatment promoting moist wound healing involves covering the Xeroform donor

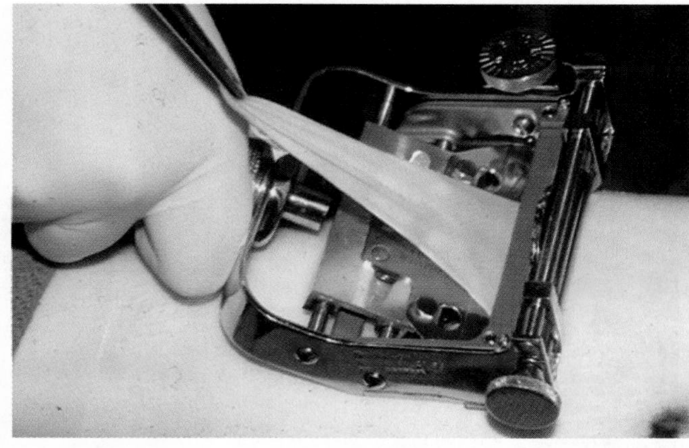
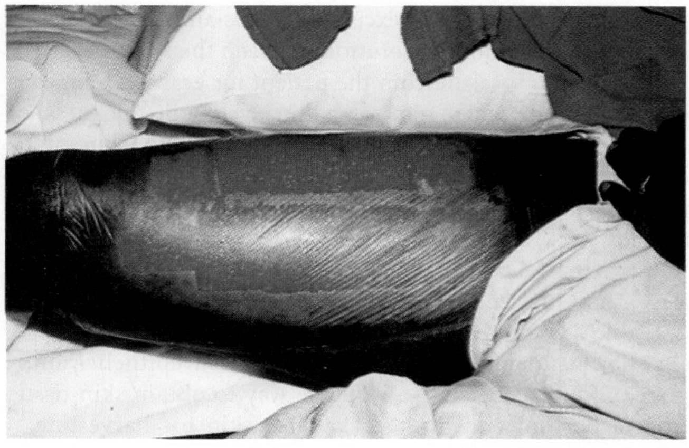
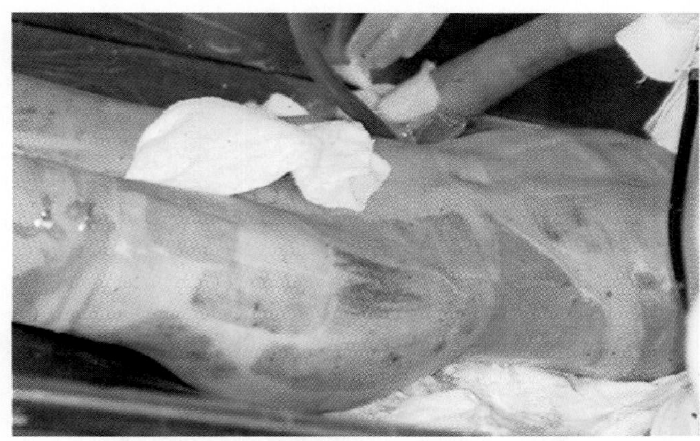
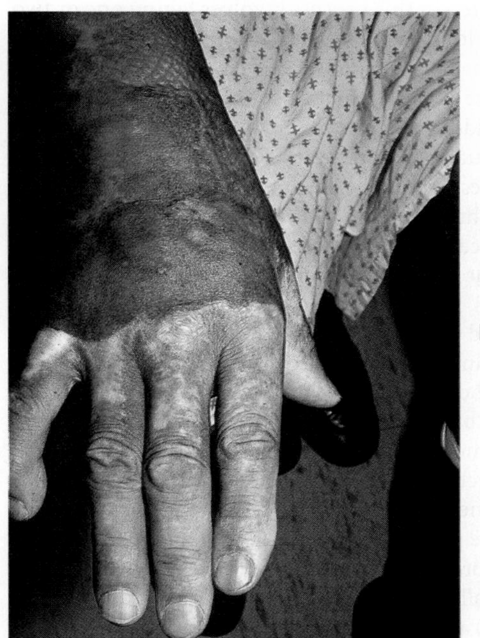

Fig. 23-11 **A,** The surgeon harvests skin from a patient's thigh using a dermatome. **B,** Appearance of donor site after harvesting split-thickness skin graft. Donor site is covered with a transparent occlusive dressing. **C,** Healed donor sites. **D,** Healed split-thickness skin graft to the hand.

site with bacitracin ointment 24 hours postoperatively. This is then covered with a bulky dressing that is changed twice daily, allowing for a moist environment with some topical antibiotic coverage.

Some centers use a transparent dressing that adheres to the periphery of the donor site. This permits an occlusive yet visible wound. Pigskin, silver sulfadiazene (Silvadene), and calcium alginate dressings are also being used with varying degrees of success. Each donor site dressing has specific nursing care aspects, and use varies among centers.

Excision and Grafting

Current therapeutic management of burn wounds involves early removal of the necrotic tissue followed by application of split-thickness autograft skin. This therapy has changed the management and mortality rate of burn patients. In the past, major burn patients had low rates of survival because healing and wound coverage took so long that the patient usually succumbed first to infection or malnutrition. Now, mortality rates can be greatly reduced and morbidity can be decreased by early intervention. Candidates for early excision and grafting are those with stable cardiovascular systems after initial fluid resuscitation.

During the procedure of excision and grafting, eschar is removed down to subcutaneous tissue or fascia, depending on the degree of injury. The graft must be placed on clean, viable tissue to achieve good adherence. Hemostasis is achieved by pressure and application of topical thrombin or epinephrine, after which the wound is covered with autograft skin (see Table 23-13). With early excision, function is restored and scar tissue formation is minimized. Because the dead tissue is planed off until viable tissue is reached, extensive bleeding is expected to occur, which may pose a problem when grafting is performed. Clots between the graft and the wound keep the graft from adhering to the wound. One method of managing the clotting problem is to excise the wound on one day and to graft it the next day. The excised wounds are soaked every 4 hours with an antibiotic solution between the surgeries.

Donor skin is taken from the patient for grafting by means of a dermatome, which removes a thin layer (split-thickness) of skin from an unburned site (Fig. 23-11). The donor skin can be meshed to allow for greater wound coverage, or it may be applied as a sheet graft for a better cosmetic result when grafting the face, neck, and hands.

Cultured Epithelial Autografts. In the patient with large body surface area burns, limited unburned skin may be available as a donor site for grafting, and available skin may also be unsuitable for harvesting. Cultured epithelial autograft (CEA) has become a valuable way to obtain skin tissue from a person with limited available skin for harvesting.[17] CEA is grown from biopsies obtained from the patient's own skin. The initial step in this process involves taking one or two small (2 to 3 cm long by 1 cm wide) biopsy specimens from unburned skin (usually the groin or axilla).

This procedure is performed as soon as possible after the patient has been identified as a candidate for this type of grafting, and it can usually be done at the bedside while the patient is under local anesthesia. The specimen is sent to a commercial laboratory where the skin biopsy specimens are disaggregated into single cells and are subsequently cultivated in a culture medium that contains epidermal growth factor. During the following 18 to 25 days the originally cultivated keratinocytes expand up to 10,000 times until they form confluent sheets that can be used as skin grafts. The cultured grafts are returned to the burn center where they are grafted on the patient's excised burn wounds. Because CEA grafts are only epidermal cells, meticulous care is required to prevent shearing injury or infection.

CEA grafts generate permanent skin coverage because they originate from the patient's own cells. CEA is applied surgically using the same procedure as with split-thickness autografts. CEA grafts generally form a seamless, smooth replacement skin tissue (Fig. 23-12) and have played an important role in the survival of the patient with major burns with limited skin for donor harvesting. In 24 days enough CEA can be generated to cover the entire body surface. However, problems related to CEA include the thin friable skin (resulting from lack of dermal cells) and contracture development.

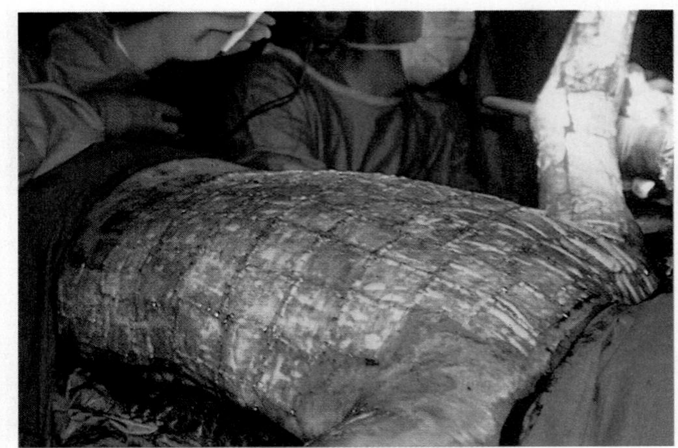

A

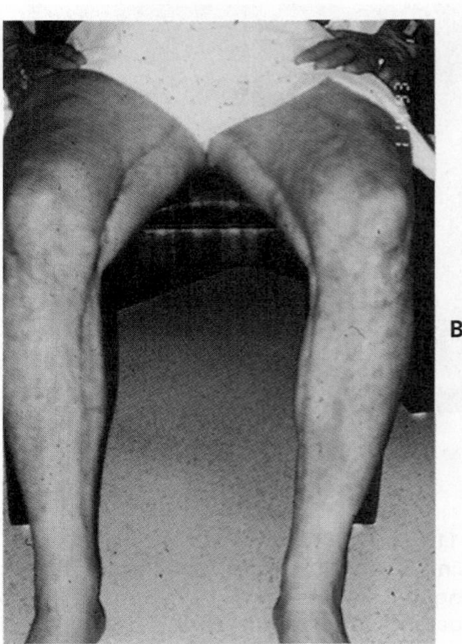

B

Fig. 23-12 Patient with cultured epithelial autograft. **A,** Intraoperative application of cultured epithelial autograft. **B,** Appearance of healed cultured epithelial autograft.

Artificial Skin. It has been recognized that any successful artificial skin must replace all functions of the skin and consist of a dermal and an epidermal portion. The Integra artificial skin dermal regeneration template is an example of the newest skin replacement system available in burn care.[18] It is indicated for use in postexcisional treatment of life-threatening full-thickness or deep partial-thickness burn wounds where conventional autograft is not available or advisable.

This artificial skin has a bilayer membrane composed of dermis and silicone. The wound is debrided, the bilayer membrane is placed dermal layer down first, and the wound is wrapped with dressings. The dermal layer functions as a biodegradable template that induces organized regeneration of new dermis by the body. The silicone layer remains intact as the dermal layer degrades. Final closure of the burn wound takes place several weeks later when thin epidermal autografts become available. The silicone is removed during surgery and replaced by the epidermal autografts.

Several other products are currently being investigated and evaluated in burn centers throughout North America, including Alloderm, a nonimmunogenic dermal transplant, and LifeSkin, a cultured composite autograft. Further evaluation must take place to determine the use and effectiveness of these products in burn wound management.

Pain Management

One of the most critical functions a nurse performs is pain assessment and management.[19] It becomes difficult in burn nursing to separate empathy from sympathy and to act appropriately when the patient is so vulnerable and ill. Almost every intervention that is performed for the patient causes pain. The patient may experience rare moments of relative comfort, but the patient knows that these moments will not last. The nurse must understand the physiologic as well as the psychologic bases of pain (see Chapter 9). Allowing the patient to ventilate feelings of anger, hostility, and frustration serves to assist the patient in expression of the pain. It is important to assess each patient's pain individually and consistently.

There are several interventions that the nurse may try to help the patient deal with pain. These interventions can also help the nurse cope with interventions that cause pain. First, it is helpful to get an order for a dosage range of a narcotic (e.g., morphine sulfate 5 to 10 mg IV) every 1 to 3 hours for pain. When the order is written this way, it allows the nurse some freedom to try medicating the patient according to responses to the medication. That is, the nurse may find that giving morphine 5 mg every hour works better than giving 10 mg every 3 hours. This method should include the patient's input if alert and also gives the patient some control over the pain. If the patient is unable to participate, the nurse will have to assess response to medication by physiologic parameters (i.e., heart rate, BP, and respiratory rate).

The second intervention is the use of several drugs in combination. This includes the use of morphine with haloperidol (Haldol), diazepam (Valium), or midazolam (Versed). The effect of midazolam is short-term amnesia, so if it is given 15 to 20 minutes before a dressing change, the patient will not necessarily recall the event. Midazolam lasts about 30 to 60 minutes after it is administered. Buprenorphine (Buprenex) is another drug that is useful. The mechanism of action is not entirely understood, but it is proposed that it exerts its analgesic effect via high-affinity binding to opiate receptors in the central nervous system. It is a narcotic antagonist so it cannot be used in combination with other narcotic analgesics. Buprenorphine may work well for the patient who does not obtain relief even with high doses of narcotics.

A third method of managing pain is an alternative manner in which the nurse and patient work together to find a way to cope with pain. It involves the use of relaxation tapes, visualization, guided imagery, biofeedback, and meditation. These techniques are used as adjuncts to traditional narcotic treatment of pain. They are not meant to be used exclusively to control pain in the burn patient.

The nurse works with the patient to identify the best strategy to manage the pain using one or more of these techniques. Visualization and guided imagery can be helpful to the nurse as well as the patient. These two techniques can take several forms, but the easiest method is for the nurse to ask questions about a favorite hobby or recent vacation. The nurse can then explore these areas further by asking questions that make the patient visualize and describe a favorite hobby or recent vacation. When using this method, both the nurse and the patient must focus on things besides the task at hand (e.g., a dressing change) to keep the conversation flowing. It is up to the nurse to maintain the exchange. Relaxation tapes can also be helpful, especially when played at night to help the patient fall asleep. The use of these techniques promotes a close nurse-patient relationship and can leave both with a sense of accomplishment.[20]

The most important point to remember about pain management is that the more control that the patient has in managing pain, the more successful it will be. There has been a recent trend toward the use of patient-controlled analgesia (PCA) pumps. An IV solution is made up to contain a certain dose of a narcotic per milliliter (e.g., morphine 2 mg/ml). The patient has a control that can be operated to deliver a preset dose of the IV narcotic. The machine is locked into this dose, so there is no possibility of the patient getting more than what is prescribed. (PCA is discussed in Chapters 9 and 18.)

Nutritional Therapy

The goals of nutritional management of the burn patient during the acute phase are to minimize energy demands and provide adequate calories and protein to promote healing. The burn patient is in a hypermetabolic and highly catabolic state as a result of the burn injury. Decreasing catecholamine release by minimizing pain, fear, anxiety, and cold can maximize patient comfort and conserve energy. Infection also increases the metabolic rate or expenditure.

Meeting daily caloric requirements is crucial. Estimated caloric needs for 24 hours for the adult with burns of greater than 20% TBSA can be calculated by the following formula:

$$(25 \text{ kcal} \times \text{kg of body weight}) + (40 \text{ kcal} \times \% \text{ TBSA burn})$$

Caloric needs are often 5000 kcal per day. By the end of the first week after burn injury, the patient's caloric and nutritional requirements should be met. The patient should be encourged to eat high-protein, high-carbohydrate foods to meet increased caloric needs. Ideally the patient should not lose more than 10% of preburn weight. Caloric requirements should be recalculated at least biweekly to prevent overfeeding and subsequent weight gain.

Optimally the patient should take a normal diet by mouth as soon as bowel function returns. If this is not possible, a feeding tube can be placed and a complete liquid diet administered. Diet supplements can be given by mouth or IV in the form of total parenteral nutrition (see Chapter 38).

If family members wish to bring in the patient's favorite foods, this should be encouraged. Appetite is usually diminished, and constant encouragement may be necessary to achieve adequate intake.

Rehabilitation Phase

The *rehabilitation phase* is defined as beginning when the patient's burn wound is covered with skin or healed and the patient is capable of assuming some self-care activity. This can occur as early as 2 weeks to as long as 2 or 3 months after the burn injury. Goals for this period are to assist the patient in resuming a functional role in society and to accomplish functional and cosmetic reconstruction.[21]

Pathophysiologic Changes and Clinical Manifestations

The burn wound heals either by primary intention or by grafting. Layers of epithelialization begin rebuilding the tissue structure destroyed by the burn injury. Collagen fibers present in the new scar tissue help healing and add strength to weakened areas. After healing, the new skin appears flat and pink. In

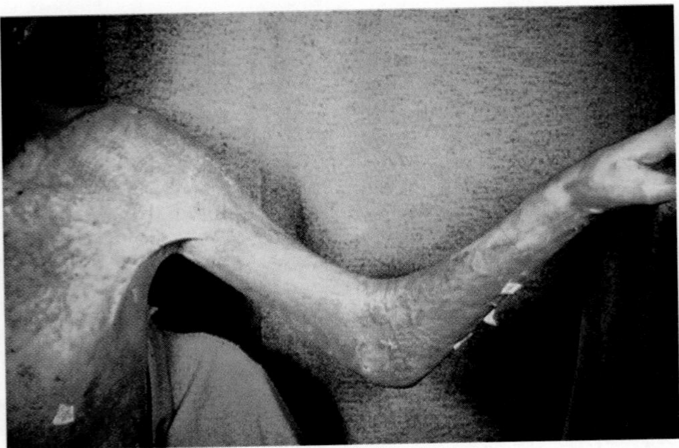

Fig. 23-13 Contracture of the axilla.

approximately 4 to 6 weeks the area becomes raised and hyperemic. If adequate ROM is not instituted, the new tissue will shorten, causing contracture. Mature healing is reached in 6 months to 2 years when suppleness has returned and the pink or red color has faded to a slightly lighter hue than the surrounding unburned tissue. It takes longer for more heavily pigmented skin to regain its dark color because many of the melanocytes are destroyed. Often skin never regains its original color.

Scarring has two components: discoloration and contour. The discoloration of scars fades with time. However, scar tissue tends to develop altered contours; that is, it is no longer flat or slightly raised but becomes elevated and enlarged above the original burn injury area. Pressure can help keep a scar flat. Gentle pressure is maintained on the healed burn with pressure garments. These garments are worn up to 24 hours a day for as long as 1 to 2 years after burn injury. They may be removed for short periods while bathing.

The patient will experience discomfort from itching where healing is occurring. Nivea or similar lotions and diphenhydramine (Benadryl) serve to ease the itching. As "old" epithelium is replaced by new cells, flaking will occur. The newly formed skin is extremely sensitive to trauma. Blisters are likely to form from slight pressure or friction. Additionally, these newly healed areas can be hypersensitive or hyposensitive to cold, heat, and touch. Grafted areas are more likely to be hyposensitive until peripheral nerve regeneration occurs. Healed burn areas must be protected from direct sunlight for 1 year to prevent hyperpigmentation and sunburn injury.

Complications

The most common complications of burn injury are skin and joint contractures and hypertrophic scarring (Fig. 23-13). Because of pain, the patient will prefer to assume a flexed position for comfort. This position predisposes the wounds to contracture formation. Positioning, splinting, and exercise should be instituted to minimize this complication. These procedures should be continued until the skin matures.

Areas that are most susceptible to contracture formation include the anterior and lateral neck areas, axillae, antecubital fossae, fingers, groin areas, popliteal fossae, and ankles. These areas encompass major joints. Not only does the skin over these areas develop contractures, but the underlying tissues such as the ligaments and tendons also have a tendency to shorten in the healing process. Therapy is aimed at extension of body parts because the flexors are stronger than the extensors. Legs should be wrapped before ambulation after grafting and donor site healing. This pressure prevents blister formation and promotes venous return. Once the skin is completely healed, pressure garments can replace leg wraps to grafted areas.

NURSING AND COLLABORATIVE MANAGEMENT: REHABILITATION PHASE

Members of the health care team share responsibility for assisting the patient to return to optimal function during the rehabilitation phase.[22] Because of the severe psychologic impact of burn injury, health care providers must be sensitive and attuned to the patient's feelings. They must assist patients to adjust emotionally by encouraging them to ventilate their fears regarding loss of function, deformity, disfigurement, and financial burdens. Care should also be taken to address individual spiritual and cultural needs. Having expressed these fears, patients can then be assisted in a realistic appraisal of the particular situations, emphasizing what they *can* do, not what *cannot* be done.

An individual's self-esteem is usually adversely affected by a burn injury. In some an overwhelming fear may be the loss of relationships because of perceived or actual physical disfigurement. In a society that values physical beauty, alterations in body image commonly result in psychologic distress. Allowing appropriate independence, return to preburn activities, and encouraging the patient to speak with other burn survivors will involve the patient in activities that may help restore self-esteem. Counseling continues after the patient goes home. Patients need reassurance that their feelings during this period of adjustment are normal and that frustration is to be expected as they attempt to resume normal lifestyles.

During the rehabilitation phase, both patient and family are actively learning how to care for the healing wounds. Because the patient may go home with unhealed open areas, instruction will be needed in dressing changes and wound care. An emollient water-based cream (e.g., Vaseline Intensive Care lotion for sensitive skin) should be used routinely on healed areas to keep the skin supple and to decrease itching and flaking. Diphenhydramine (Benadryl) may be used. The patient and family will need anticipatory guidance to know what to expect physiologically as well as psychologically during recovery.

Cosmetic or reconstructive surgery is often needed following major burns. It is important for the patient to understand the need for or possibility of reconstructive surgery before leaving the hospital.

The role of exercise and appropriate physical therapy cannot be overemphasized. The progression of physical therapy from hydrotherapy to passive ROM, active ROM, stretching, ambulation, and ultimate restoration of function is a lengthy and painful process that lasts for at least 1 year after burn injury. Constant encouragement and reassurance are necessary to maintain a patient's morale. The patient must regard physical therapy as an integral part of treatment.

Nutritional Therapy

By this time in the patient's recovery, the negative nitrogen balance should have been corrected. However, it is still important to maintain a high-calorie, high-protein diet. The problem with anorexia decreases at this time. As the oral intake increases, tube feedings are gradually tapered and discontinued. The patient with a functional problem associated with eating (especially burn injury to the hands) may need assistance from occupational therapy to obtain devices to correct or lessen the problem. Often all that is necessary is padding the handle of a fork or spoon with several layers of gauze so that a better grip is established. Toward the end of hospitalization, the patient occasionally needs assistance from a dietician. Because they have been encouraged to eat during the lengthy wound healing period, some patients may have difficulty controlling their appetite and avoiding unwanted weight gain as healing approaches completion.

Table 23-17 Emotional Responses of Burn Patients

Emotion	Possible Verbal Expression
Fear	Will I die? What will happen next? Will I be disfigured? Will my spouse or friends still love me?
Anxiety	I feel out of control. What's happening to me? When will it end?
Anger	Why did this happen to me? Those nurses enjoy hurting me.
Guilt	If only I'd been more careful. I was punished because I was bad.
Depression	It's no use going on like this. I don't care what happens to me. I wish people would leave me alone.

GERONTOLOGIC CONSIDERATIONS

The older patient presents many challenges for the burn team. Normal aging puts the patient at risk for injury because of the possibility of an unsteady gait, failing eyesight, and diminished hearing. Once injured the older adult has more complications in the emergent and acute phases of burn resuscitation because of preexisting medical conditions that may be present. For example, an older patient with diabetes, congestive heart failure, and chronic obstructive pulmonary disease will have morbidity and mortality rates exceeding a healthy younger patient. In the older patient, pneumonia is a frequent complication, wounds take longer to heal, and surgical procedures are less well tolerated. Because of all of these problems, strategies to prevent burn injuries are especially important in this population.

EMOTIONAL NEEDS OF THE PATIENT AND FAMILY

Because the nurse has the most prolonged contact with the patient and family, it is natural for the nurse to be seen as an important source of emotional support. The nurse is a valuable person in assisting the patient to maintain personal worth and reestablish a satisfactory body image. The nurse must have an almost unlimited supply of patience and understanding. Often the health care worker is the target for anger and hostility from the patient who has no other focus or method of expressing these feelings. Working with the family can be a challenge for the nurse.

Family members must understand and appreciate the importance of reestablishing the patient's independence. Family members will be confused by all the changes they see in the various burn phases and may benefit from repeated explanations of what to expect as the patient recovers. It may be helpful for some family members to view the burn wounds frequently so that they can see the progress of healing. The nurse should involve the family as team members during the patient's hospitalization.

The stress of the burn injury occasionally precipitates a psychiatric crisis. Treatment by a psychiatrist who can prescribe psychotropic drugs is indicated when this occurs. Early psychiatric intervention is also crucial if the patient has been previously treated for a psychiatric disorder or if the burn injury was the result of a suicide attempt.

The diagnosis of posttraumatic stress disorder is being made with increasing frequency in the burn patient population. Early intervention by appropriate professionals is associated with improved outcomes.

Because of the suddenness and severity of burn trauma, the patient and family are plunged into physical and emotional crises. The health care provider must be prepared to assess psychoemotional cues and provide appropriate intervention throughout the course of recovery.

The patient may experience thoughts and feelings that are frightening and disturbing, such as guilt about the burn accident, reliving the experience, fear of death, and concern about future therapy and the concomitant pain. Families may share any or all of these feelings. At times, family members will feel helpless when trying to assist their loved ones. During this period of adjustment, the nurse should provide time for the patient and the families to be alone. Family members may also be encouraged to assist with position changes and eating.

For the nurse to adequately manage the enormous range of emotional responses that the burn patient may exhibit, it is important to have an understanding of the circumstances of the burn, past family interactions, and past coping experiences with stressful stimuli. At any time the various emotional responses of fear, anxiety, anger, guilt, and depression may be experienced (Table 23-17).

A common emotional response is *regression*. The patient will revert to behavior that helped in coping with stressful situations in the past. Frank psychosis can also be observed. Unless the patient had a psychiatric condition before the burn injury, this psychosis is usually transient. Major emotional tasks confront patients and families. As more and more independence is expected from the patients, new fears must be confronted: "Can

I do it?" "Am I a desirable partner, parent?" Open communication among the patient, family members, friends, and burn team members is essential.

Therapeutic intervention for the patient at this point does not necessarily require the involvement of a psychiatrist. Nurses, physicians, social workers, or anyone else who has a rapport with the patient and a good understanding of personal feelings in such situations can be therapeutic. The patient can best convey some of these negative but normal emotions to a health care provider with whom he or she can communicate. Acknowledgment that the feelings are real and valid can do much to help the patient. The nurse should not belittle or scorn a patient's regression but should be firm and consistent in assisting the patient to cope.

The difficult issue of sexuality must be met with honesty. Physical appearance will be altered in the patient who has sustained a major burn. Acceptance of this alteration is difficult at first for the patient and significant other. The nature of skin injury in itself causes modifications in processing sexual stimuli. Touch is an important part of sexuality. Immature scar tissue may make the sensation of touch unpleasant or may dull it. This is usually transient, but the patient and family need to know that it is normal and receive anticipatory guidance from health care personnel to avoid undue emotional strain.

Family and patient support groups may be beneficial in meeting the patient's and family's emotional needs. Speaking with others who have experienced burn trauma can be beneficial, both in terms of reaffirming that the patient is feeling normal and in allowing for the sharing of helpful advice.

SPECIAL NEEDS OF THE NURSING STAFF

A logical extension of the emotional trauma experienced by the patient includes the emotional trauma for the nurse.[23] The nurse must deal with the patient who, at times, is unpleasant and hostile and with the fact that burn therapy is almost always painful. The nurse will sometimes see many hours of patient care suddenly destroyed by sepsis and death. Because of long hospitalizations and intense contact, relationships between the caregiver and the care receiver can result in strong bonds that can be healthy and healing or destructive and draining. The burn patient can develop demanding or punitive attitudes, which may cause the nurse to be reluctant to provide care. The nurse and patient can also develop warm, trusting, mutually satisfying relationships not only during hospitalization but also during long-term rehabilitation. Sometimes the bond can be so strong that the patient has difficulty separating from the hospital and staff. The frequency and intensity of family contact can also be rewarding as well as draining to the nurse. Newcomers to burn nursing often find it difficult to cope with not only the deformities caused by burn injury but also the odor, the unpleasant sight of the wound, and the reality of the pain that accompanies the burn.

Many nurses believe that the care they provide makes a critical difference in helping patients to survive and cope with a severe and multifaceted injury. It is this belief that keeps nurses caring for burn patients and their families.

RESEARCH
IMPLICATIONS FOR NURSING PRACTICE

Sexuality after Burn Injury

Citation Bianchi TL: Aspects of sexuality after burn injury. Outcomes in men, *Burn Care Rehabil* 18:183, 1997.

Purpose To study (1) the relationship between severity of burn injury and sexual-esteem, sexual-depression, and sexual-preoccupation in burn-injured men; and (2) the relationship between sociodemographic variables and sexual-esteem, sexual-depression, and sexual-preoccupation.

Methods Questionnaires were returned from a convenience sample ($n = 40$) of male burn survivors ages 19 to 39 years who were treated and discharged from a burn unit in the southeastern United States. Sociodemographic data were collected using the Instrument for Sociodemographic Data Collection. The Sexuality Scale, a 5-point-Likert design, 30-item questionnaire, was used to obtain information on three subscales: sexual-esteem, sexual-depression, and sexual-preoccupation.

Results and Conclusions Statistically significant positive relationships were demonstrated between sexual-preoccupation and sexual-esteem. Inverse relationships were demonstrated between age and sexual-preoccupation and also between sexual-esteem and sexual-depression. There was no relationship between severity of burn and sexual-esteem, sexual-depression, or sexual-preoccupation.

Implications for Nursing Practice With improvements in survival following burn injury, increased attention should be focused on quality of life. One of the most devastating consequences of burn injury is changes in body image and self-esteem, which can directly affect sexuality. Rehabilitation of burn patients should focus on issues related to sexuality. Nurses must recognize that even small burns may potentiate significant psychologic distress. The findings of this study reinforce the need for more research in the area of adjustment after burn injuries, particularly with regard to sexuality.

Support services for the burn nurse in the form of group meetings led by a psychiatrist, psychologist, psychiatric clinical nurse specialist, or social worker can be helpful. Peer support groups can serve a similar purpose of helping nursing staff to cope with difficult feelings that may be experienced when caring for the burn patient. The nurse may need the opportunity to ventilate feelings of anger and hostility to an impartial listener. This therapeutic communication process may make the difference between the nurse who can deliver effective nursing care and the nurse who provides mere custodial patient care.

CRITICAL THINKING EXERCISES

CASE STUDY

Severe Burn Patient

Patient Profile

Sylvia, a 24-year-old woman, was brought to the emergency department with extensive full-thickness burns to her upper body. Her gas stove exploded while she was manually lighting a burner.

Subjective Data

Complains of feeling very cold
Cannot remember the accident
Is hoarse and has difficulty talking
Expresses a great deal of fear

Objective Data

Physical Examination

- Is awake and oriented but in obvious distress
- Has dark brown, leathery burns involving the head, neck, chest, and upper extremities
- Has hair and eyebrows that are singed
- Nurse is unable to palpate peripheral pulses; apical pulse—140

Critical Thinking Questions

1. What are the first priorities in the prehospital environment? How should her airway be managed?
2. Why would Sylvia be considered at high risk for an inhalation injury?
3. What intervention should the nurse anticipate in a patient with full-thickness circumferential burns to the extremities?
4. Describe the rationale for Sylvia's lack of pain and her complaints of being cold. What medications might be considered to promote her comfort?
5. What fluid and electrolyte disturbances would be expected in the first 48 hours of Sylvia's hospitalization? Explain the physiologic bases for these changes.
6. What measures should be taken to support Sylvia's family?
7. Based on the assessment data presented, write one or more appropriate nursing diagnoses. Are there any collaborative problems?

NURSING RESEARCH ISSUES

1. What nursing interventions are most effective in preparing patients, families, and community nurses for the early discharge and post-hospitalization phase of burn care?
2. What nursing interventions are most effective in the management of burn pain?
3. What nutritional supplements are best tolerated in the emergent and acute phases of burn recovery?

REVIEW QUESTIONS

The number of the question corresponds to the same-numbered objective at the beginning of the chapter.

1. In presenting a program on fire and burn prevention for parents, the nurse focuses on the most common cause of household fires as
   a. unattended cooking.
   b. frayed or defective wiring.
   c. carelessness with cigarettes.
   d. improper use of inflammables.
2. The injury that is least likely to result in a full-thickness burn is
   a. sunburn.
   b. scald injury.
   c. chemical burn.
   d. electrical injury.
3. When assessing a partial-thickness burn the nurse would expect to find
   a. exposed fascia.
   b. dry, waxy appearance.
   c. red, shiny, wet appearance.
   d. absence of blanching with pressure.
4. The extent of burns is assessed by
   a. rating the location of burns at specific body sites.
   b. determining the presence of preexisting risk factors.
   c. estimating the ratio of full-thickness to partial-thickness burns.
   d. using guides to indicate burn location relative to total body surface.
5. An 82 kg patient has a 45% TBSA burn. Using 4 cc/kg/% TBSA during the first 12 hours after a burn injury, the nurse would anticipate a fluid replacement of
   a. 3690 ml.
   b. 7380 ml.
   c. 9225 ml.
   d. 14760 ml.
6. Fluid and electrolyte shifts that occur during the early emergent phase include
   a. adherence of albumin to vascular walls.
   b. movement of potassium into the vascular space.
   c. sequestering of sodium and water in interstitial fluid.
   d. hemolysis of red blood cells from large volumes of rapidly administered fluid.
7. To maintain a positive nitrogen balance in a major burn, the patient must
   a. eat a high-protein, low-fat, low-carbohydrate diet.
   b. increase normal adult caloric intake by about 3 times.
   c. eat at least 1500 calories per day in small frequent meals.
   d. eat rice and whole wheat for the chemical effect on nitrogen balance.

8. A therapeutic measure used to prevent hypertrophic scarring during the rehabilitative phase of burn recovery is
   a. applying pressure garments.
   b. performing active ROM at least every 4 hours.
   c. repositioning the patient every 2 hours.
   d. massaging the new tissue with water-based moisturizers.
9. It is important for the burn patient and family to
   a. see the burn wound three times per day.
   b. talk frequently with the nurse about the patient's progress.
   c. allow nurses to do total care for the patient to prevent infection.
   d. avoid discussion of the patient's progress to minimize false hope.
10. Discharge planning for the burn patient begins
    a. after grafting.
    b. on admission.
    c. after the emergent phase.
    d. at least 1 week before discharge.
11. Pain management for the burn patient is most effective when
    a. the nurse administers narcotics on a set schedule around the clock.
    b. the patient has as much control over the management of the pain as possible.
    c. the nurse has total freedom to administer narcotics within a dosage and frequency range.
    d. painful dressing changes and repositioning are delayed until the patient's pain is totally relieved.

References

1. American Burn Association, New York.
2. Monafo WW: Initial management of burns, *N Engl J Med* 335:1581, 1996.
3. Gordon M, Goodwin CW: Burn management. Initial assessment, management, and stabilization, *Nurs Clin North Am* 32:237, 1997.
4. Crawford ME, Rask H: Prehospital care of the burned patient, *Eur J Emerg Med* 3:247, 1996.
5. Staley M, Richard R: Management of the acute burn wound: an overview, *Adv Wound Care* 10:39, 1997.
6. Sparkes BG: Immunological responses to thermal injury, *Burns* 23:106, 1997.
7. Jordan BS, Harrington DT: Management of the burn wound, *Nurs Clin North Am* 32:251, 1997.
8. Shirani KZ and others: Update on current therapeutic approaches in burns, *Shock* 5:4, 1996.
9. Mann R, Heimbach D: Prognosis and treatment of burns, *West J Med* 165:215, 1996.
10. Greenfield E, McManus AT: Infectious complications: prevention and strategies for their control, *Nurs Clin North Am* 32:297, 1997.
11. Byers JF, Flynn MB: Acute burn injury: a trauma case report, *Crit Care Nurse* 16:55, 1996.
12. Mayes T: Enteral nutrition for the burn patient, *Nutr Clin Pract* 12(1 suppl):S43, 1997.
13. Rose JK and others: Advances in burn care, *Adv Surg* 30:71, 1996.
14. Wilson RE: Care of the burn patient, *Ostomy Wound Manage* 42:16, 1996.
15. Hansbrough W, Dore C, Hansbrough JF: Management of skin-grafted burn wounds with Xeroform and layers of dry coarse-mesh gauze dressing results in excellent graft take and minimal nursing time, *J Burn Care Rehabil* 16:531, 1995.
16. Hansbrough W: Nursing care of donor site wounds, *J Burn Care Rehabil* 16:337, 1995.
17. Raghunath M, Meuli M: Cultured epithelial autografts: diving from surgery into matrix biology, *Pediatric Surgery International* 12:478, 1997.
18. Cameron S: Changes in burn patient care, *Br J Theatre Nurs* 7:5, 1997.
19. Latarjet J, Choinere M: Pain in burn patients, *Burns* 21:344, 1995.
20. Davis ST, Sheely-Adolphson P: Burn management. Psychosocial interventions: pharmacologic and psychologic modalities, *Nurs Clin North Am* 32:331, 1997.
21. Pessina MA, Ellis SM: Burn management. Rehabilitation, *Nurs Clin North Am* 32:365, 1997.
22. Richard RL, Staley MJ: *Burn care and rehabilitation: principles and practice,* Philadelphia, 1994, Davis.
23. Steeves RH and others: Tasks of bereavement for burn center staffs, *J Burn Care Rehabil* 14:386, 1993.

Resources

American Academy of Facial Plastic and Reconstructive Surgery
310 South Henry Street
Alexandria, VA 22314
703-299-9291
800-332-FACE
http://www.aafprs.org/

American Burn Association
625 N. Michigan Avenue, Suite 1530
Chicago, IL 60611
800-548-BURN
http://www.ameriburn/org/home.htm

American Society of Plastic and Reconstructive Surgical Nurses
East Holly Avenue, Box 56
Pitman, NJ 08071
609-256-2340
Fax: 609-589-7463
http://asprsn.inurse.com/

Burn Foundation
1128 Walnut Street
Philadelphia, PA 19107
215-629-9200
http://www.ot.com/burn_prevention/

Canadian Association of Burn Nurses
The Wellesley Hospital
160 Wellesley Street East
Toronto, Ontario, Canada M4Y 1J3

International Society for Burn Injuries
2005 Franklin Street, #660
Denver, CO 80205

The Phoenix Society for Burn Survivors, Inc.
11 Rust Hill Road
Levitttown, PA 19056-2311
215-946-BURN
800-888-BURN
Fax: 215-946-4788
http://www.nvoad.org/phoenix.htm

***For additional Internet resources, see the website for this book at* www.mosby.com/MERLIN/medsurg_lewis**

SECTION

5

PROBLEMS OF OXYGENATION: VENTILATION

SECTION OUTLINE

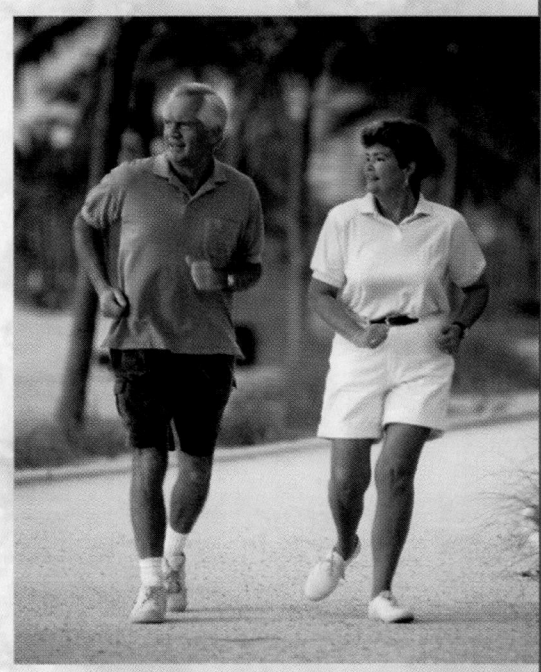

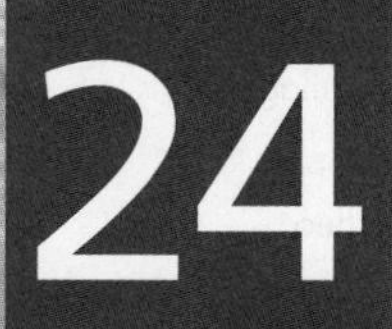

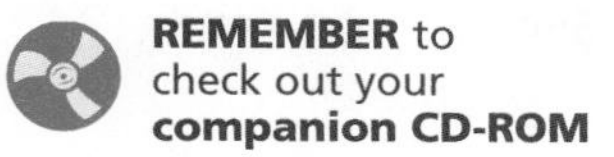

24 NURSING ASSESSMENT Respiratory System

Lynn F. Reinke & Leslie A. Hoffman

www.mosby.com/MERLIN/medsurg_lewis

LEARNING OBJECTIVES

1. Describe the structures and functions of the upper respiratory tract, the lower respiratory tract, and the chest wall.
2. Describe the process that initiates and controls inspiration and expiration.
3. Describe the process of gaseous diffusion within the lungs.
4. Identify the functions of the respiratory defense mechanisms.
5. Describe the significance of arterial blood gas values and the oxyhemoglobin dissociation curve in relation to respiratory function.
6. Identify the signs and symptoms of inadequate oxygenation and the implications of these findings.
7. Describe age-related changes in the respiratory system and differences in assessment findings.
8. Identify the significant subjective and objective assessment data that should be obtained from a patient.
9. Describe the techniques used in physical assessment of the respiratory system.
10. Differentiate normal from common abnormal findings of a physical assessment of the respiratory system.
11. Describe the purpose, nursing responsibilities, and significance of the results related to diagnostic studies of the respiratory system.

STRUCTURES AND FUNCTIONS OF THE RESPIRATORY SYSTEM

The primary purpose of the respiratory system is gas exchange, which involves the transfer of oxygen and carbon dioxide between the atmosphere and the blood. The respiratory system is divided into two parts: the upper respiratory tract and the lower respiratory tract (Fig. 24-1). The upper respiratory tract includes the nose, pharynx, adenoids, tonsils, epiglottis, larynx, and trachea. The lower respiratory tract consists of the bronchi, bronchioles, alveolar ducts, and alveoli. With the exception of the right and left main-stem bronchi, all lower airway structures are contained within the lungs. The right lung is divided into three lobes (upper, middle, and lower) and the left lung into two lobes (upper and lower) (Fig. 24-2). The structures of the chest wall (ribs, pleura, muscles of respiration) are also essential to respiration.

Upper Respiratory Tract

The nose is made of bone and cartilage. Internally, the nose is divided into two passages, or nares, by the septum. The interior of the nose is shaped into rolling projections called turbinates that increase the surface area for warming and moistening air.

Reviewed by Michele Geiger-Bronsky, RN, MSN, CS, FAACVPR, Nurse Practitioner/Respiratory Clinical Nurse Specialist, Maritime Health Works, Manitowec, Wisc.

The internal nose opens directly into the sinuses. The nasal cavity connects with the pharynx, a tubular passageway that is subdivided from above downward into three parts: the nasopharynx, the oropharynx, and the laryngopharynx.

The nose, like the rest of the respiratory tract, is lined with mucous membrane. As air enters the nose, it is warmed, moistened, and filtered by very small hairs. These actions serve a protective function. Inhaled particles that are larger than 10 μm (e.g., dust, bacteria) are trapped by nasal hairs or strike mucous membranes, thereby preventing them from reaching the lower airways. By the time air enters the alveoli, it should be 100% saturated with water vapor. Most of this humidification occurs in the nose. When humidifying air, the body loses approximately 250 ml of water per day, a process termed *insensible loss.*[1-4]

The olfactory nerve endings (receptors for the sense of smell) are located in the roof of the nose. The adenoids and tonsils, which are small masses of lymphatic tissue, are found in the nasopharynx and the oropharynx, respectively. Air can enter the oropharynx through the nose or the mouth. However, the mouth breather loses the filtering and humidifying functions of the nose.

The epiglottis is a small flap of tissue at the base of the tongue. During swallowing, the epiglottis covers the larynx, preventing solids and liquids from entering the lungs. If the epiglottis does not perform this protective function, food or liquids could be aspirated into the lungs. Any condition that alters the mental status or swallowing ability may impair the

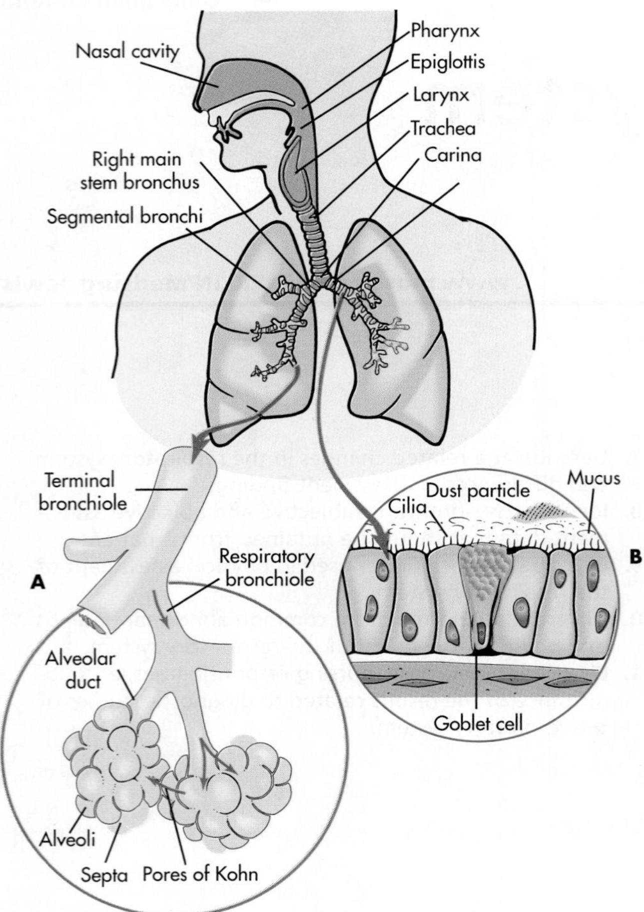

Fig. 24-1 Structures of the respiratory tract. **A,** Pulmonary functional unit. **B,** Ciliated mucous membrane.

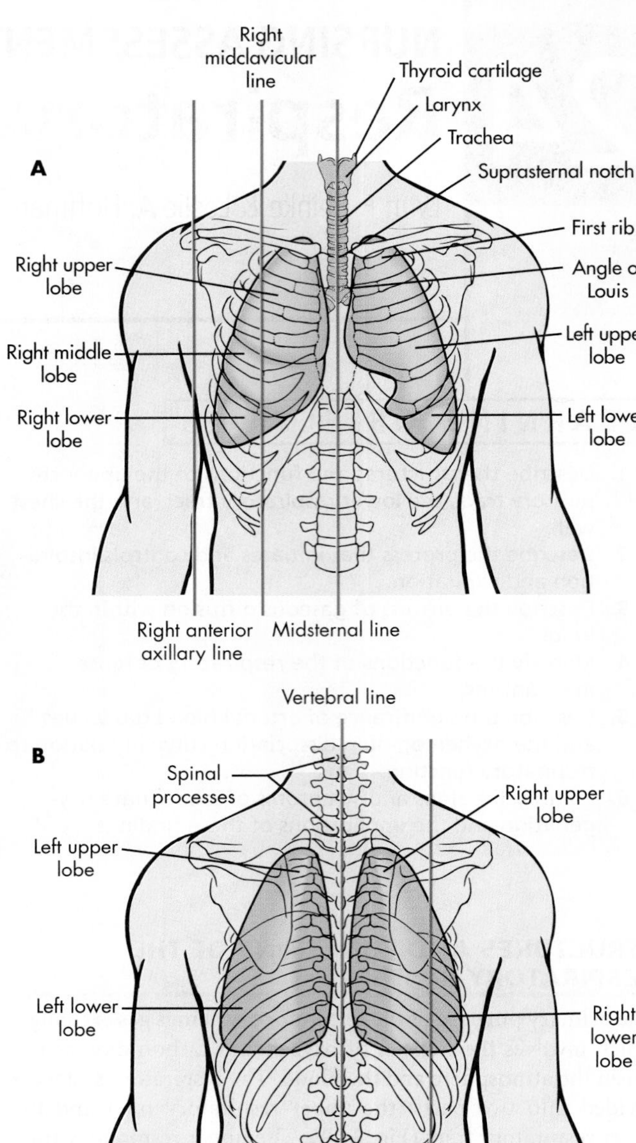

Fig. 24-2 Landmarks and structures of chest wall. **A,** Anterior view. **B,** Posterior view.

function of the epiglottis and hence predispose to aspiration. Examples include a decreased level of consciousness, a cerebrovascular accident, or the presence of a tracheostomy tube (see Chapter 25).[2,5]

After passing through the oropharynx, air moves through the laryngopharynx and the larynx, where the vocal cords are located, and then down into the trachea. The trachea is a cylindric tube about 5 inches (10 to 12 cm) long and 1 inch (1.5 to 2.5 cm) in diameter.[2] It is supported by U-shaped cartilages, which keep the trachea from collapsing. On the posterior surface, the cartilages of the trachea are bridged by connective tissue and smooth muscle. This design allows the esophagus to expand when a bolus of food is swallowed. The trachea bifurcates into the right and left main-stem bronchi at a point called the carina. The carina is located at the level of the manubriosternal junction. The manubriosternal junction is sometimes called the angle of Louis. The carina is highly sensitive, and touching it, as might occur during insertion of a suction catheter, can elicit vigorous coughing.[1-4]

Lower Respiratory Tract

Once air passes the carina, it is in the lower respiratory tract. The main-stem bronchi, pulmonary vessels, and nerves enter the lungs through a slit called the hilus. The right main-stem bronchus is shorter, wider, and straighter than the left main-stem bronchus. For this reason, aspiration is more likely in the right lung than in the left lung.

The main-stem bronchi subdivide several times to form the lobar, segmental, and subsegmental bronchi. Further divisions form the bronchioles. The most distant bronchioles are called the respiratory bronchioles. Beyond these lie the alveolar ducts and alveolar sacs (Fig. 24-3). The bronchioles are encircled by smooth muscles that constrict and dilate in response to various stimuli. The terms *bronchoconstriction* and *bronchodilation* are used to refer to a decrease or increase in the diameter of the airways caused by contraction of these muscles.

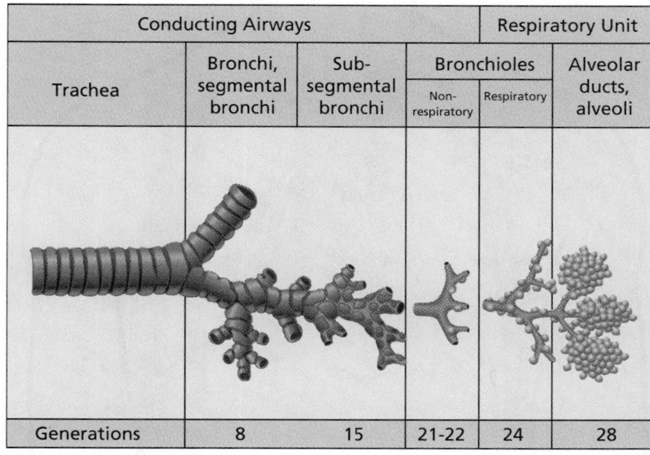

Conducting Airways
Respiratory Unit
Trachea
Bronchi, segmental bronchi
Sub-segmental bronchi
Bronchioles
Non-respiratory
Respiratory
Alveolar ducts, alveoli
Generations
8
15
21-22
24
28

Fig. 24-3 Structures of lower airways.

No exchange of oxygen or carbon dioxide takes place until air enters the respiratory bronchioles. The area of the respiratory tract from the nose to the respiratory bronchioles serves only as a conducting pathway and is therefore termed the *anatomic dead space* (VD) or *conducting zone.* This space must be filled with every breath, but the air that fills it is not available for gas exchange. In adults, a normal tidal volume (VT), or volume of air exchanged with each breath, is about 500 ml. Of each 500 ml inhaled, about 150 ml remains in the VD.[1-4]

After moving through the conducting zone, air reaches the respiratory bronchioles and alveoli (Fig. 24-4). Alveoli are small sacs that form the functional unit of the lungs. The alveoli are interconnected by pores of Kohn, which allow movement of air from alveolus to alveolus (see Fig. 24-1). Bacteria can also move through these pores, resulting in an extension of respiratory infection to previously noninfected areas. The 300 million alveoli in the adult have a total volume of about 2500 ml and a surface area for gas exchange that is about the size of a tennis court. The alveoli are separated from the capillaries by the interstitial layer or space (Fig. 24-5). The alveolar-capillary membrane is very thin (less than 1/5000 of an inch, or 1 μm) and is the site of gas exchange. In conditions such as pulmonary edema, excess fluid fills the interstitial space and alveoli, markedly impairing gas exchange.[1-4]

Surfactant. The lung can be conceptualized as a collection of 300 million bubbles (alveoli), each 0.3 mm in diameter.[1] Such a structure is inherently unstable and, as a consequence, the alveoli have a natural tendency to collapse. The alveolar surface is composed of two kinds of cells: type I and type II. Type I cells provide structure and type II cells secrete surfactant (see Fig. 24-5). Surfactant lowers surface tension in the alveoli, thereby reducing the amount of pressure needed to inflate the alveoli and decreasing the tendency of the alveoli to collapse.[3] Normally, each person takes a slightly larger breath, termed a *sigh,* after every five to six breaths. This sigh stretches the alveoli and causes surfactant to be secreted by type II cells.

Normal lung function depends on the continuous production and secretion of surfactant. When insufficient surfactant is present, the alveoli collapse. The term *atelectasis* refers to collapsed, airless alveoli (see Fig. 24-4). The postoperative patient is at risk for atelectasis because of the tendency to resist taking deeper, sigh breaths because of pain (see Chapter 18). In acute respiratory distress syndrome (ARDS), fluid enters the alveoli as a result of damage to the alveolar-capillary membrane. This results in inactivation or destruction of surfactant and subsequent widespread atelectasis (see Chapter 62).

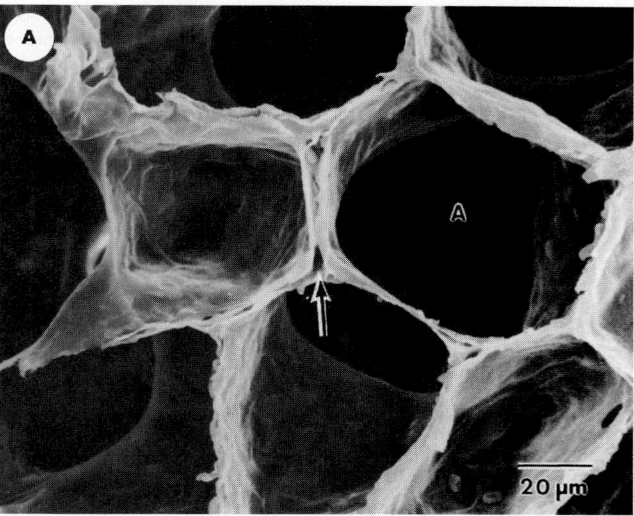

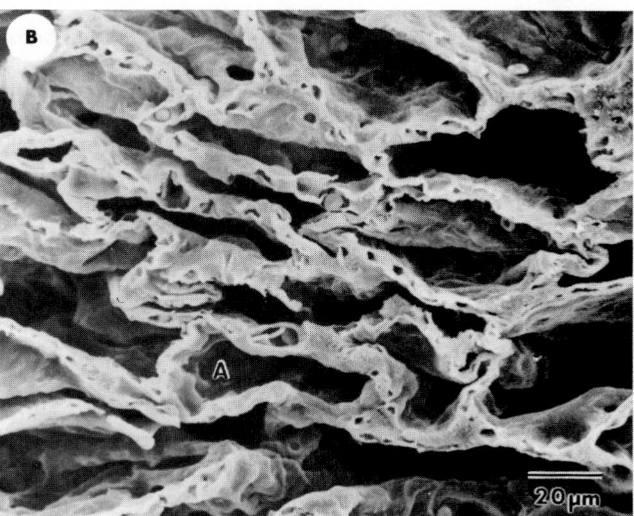

Fig. 24-4 Scanning electron micrograph of lung parenchyma. **A,** Alveoli *(A)* and alveolar capillary *(arrow)*. **B,** Effects of atelectasis. Alveoli (*A*) are partially or totally collapsed.

Blood Supply. The lungs have two different types of circulation: pulmonary and bronchial. The pulmonary circulation provides the lungs with blood for gas exchange. The pulmonary artery receives deoxygenated blood from the right ventricle of the heart and branches so that each pulmonary capillary is directly connected with many alveoli. Oxygen-carbon dioxide exchange occurs at this point. The pulmonary veins return oxygenated blood to the left atrium of the heart.

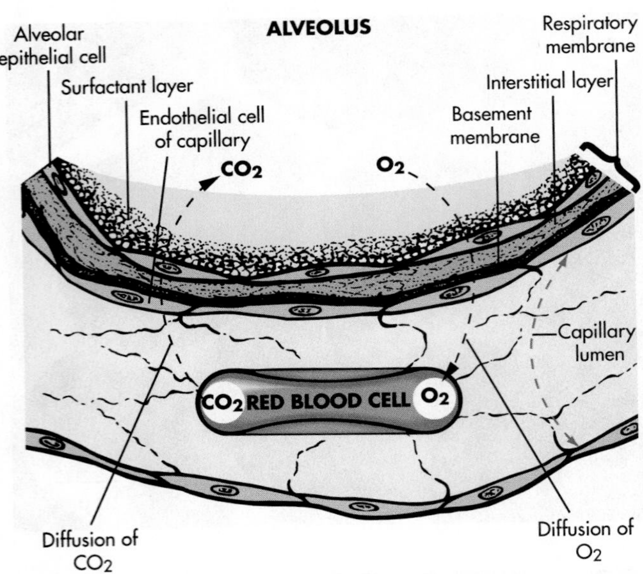

Fig. 24-5 A small portion of the respiratory membrane greatly magnified. An extremely thin interstitial layer of tissue separates the endothelial cell and basement membrane on the capillary side from the epithelial cell and surfactant layer on the alveolar side of the respiratory membrane. The total thickness of the respiratory membrane is less than 1/5000 of an inch.

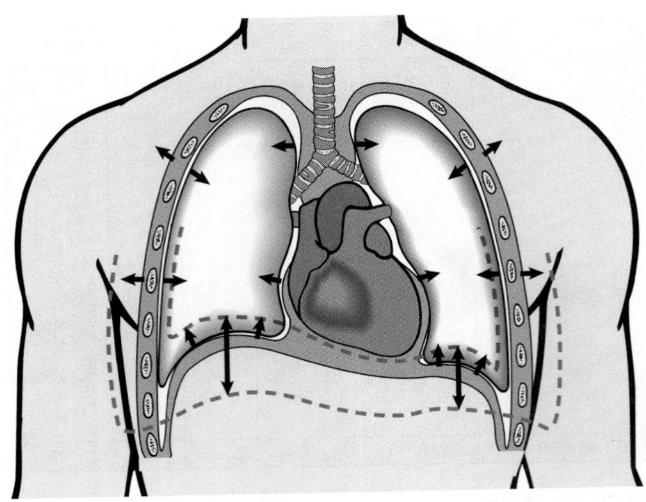

Fig. 24-6 Frontal section of chest showing movement of the lungs and chest wall during inspiration and expiration. During inspiration, the inspiratory muscles contract and the chest expands. Alveolar pressure becomes subatmospheric with respect to pressure at the airway opening and air flows into the lungs. During expiration, the inspiratory muscles relax. Recoil of the lung causes alveolar pressure to exceed pressure at the airway opening and air to flow out of the lungs. *Single arrows* show excursion of the lungs and chest wall. *Double arrows* show movement of the lung bases.

The bronchial circulation starts with the bronchial arteries, which arise from the thoracic aorta. The bronchial circulation provides oxygen to the bronchi and other pulmonary tissues. Blood returns from the bronchial circulation through the azygos vein into the left atrium. In the lung transplant recipient, the bronchial circulation is not reconnected when the donor lung is implanted. Therefore the donor bronchus depends on collateral circulation for viability until local tissue revascularization occurs (see Chapter 26).[6]

Chest Wall

The chest wall is shaped, supported, and protected by 24 ribs (12 on each side). The ribs and the sternum protect the lungs and heart from injury and are sometimes called the thoracic cage. The structures of the chest wall include the rib cage, pleura, and respiratory muscles.

The chest cavity is lined with a membrane called the parietal pleura, and the lungs are lined with a membrane called the visceral pleura. The parietal and visceral pleura are joined and form a closed, double-walled sac. The space between the pleural layers, termed the *intrapleural space,* is a potential space. In the normal adult, this space is filled with a thin film of fluid, which serves two purposes: it provides lubrication, allowing the layers of pleura to slide over each other during breathing; and it increases cohesion between the pleural layers, thereby facilitating expansion of the pleura and lung during inspiration. Fluid is drained from the pleural space by the lymphatic circulation.

Normally, the pleural space contains 20 to 25 ml of fluid. Several pathologic conditions may cause the accumulation of greater amounts of fluid, termed a *pleural effusion.* Pleural fluid may accumulate because malignant cells block lymphatic drainage or because there is an imbalance between intravascular and oncotic fluid pressures, such as occurs in congestive heart failure. Bacterial infection that extends to the pleura may also cause fluid accumulation. The term *empyema* is used to designate the presence of purulent pleural fluid. Pleuritic pain is a symptom of conditions involving the pleura. Pleuritic pain is caused when the parietal pleura is involved; the visceral pleura does not contain pain receptors.[7]

The diaphragm is the major muscle of respiration. During inspiration, the diaphragm contracts, pushing the abdominal contents downward. At the same time, the external intercostal muscles and parasternal muscles contract, increasing the lateral and anteroposterior dimension of the chest.[1] This causes the size of the thoracic cavity to increase (Fig. 24-6). As a consequence, intrathoracic pressure decreases, causing air to enter the lungs.

The diaphragm is made up of two hemidiaphragms, each innervated by the right and left phrenic nerves. The phrenic nerves arise from the spinal cord between C3 and C5, the third and fifth cervical vertebrae. If the phrenic nerve is injured, diaphragm function will be impaired. Causes of phrenic nerve injury include blunt, penetrating, or surgical trauma. Injury to the phrenic nerve results in hemidiaphragm paralysis with paralysis on the side of the injury.[1] Spinal cord injuries above the level of C3 result in total diaphragm paralysis. The patient with such an injury cannot breathe a normal V_T without assistance of a mechanical ventilator, since only a V_T of 50 to 100 ml (normal 500 ml) can be achieved. If the spinal cord injury is incomplete or below this level, the patient typically retains sufficient phrenic and diaphragmatic function to breathe without a mechanical ventilator.

Physiology of Respiration

Ventilation. Ventilation involves inspiration (movement of air into the lungs) and expiration (movement of air

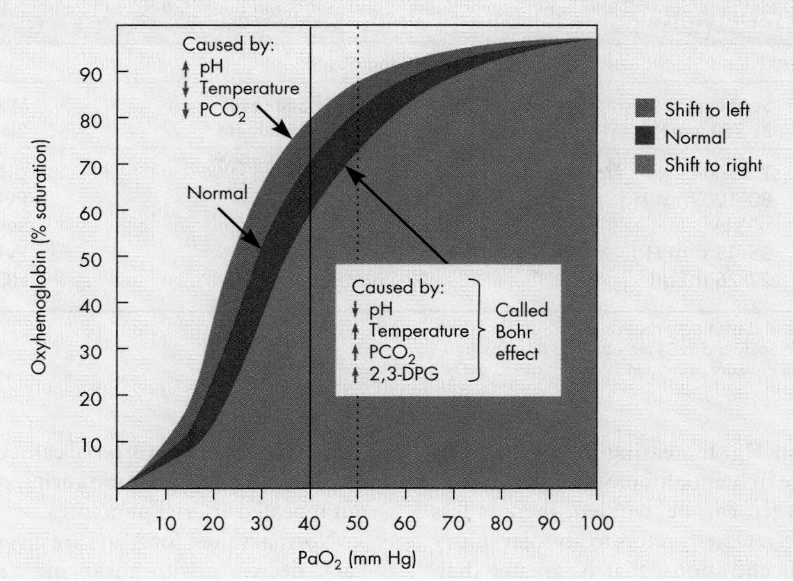

Fig. 24-7 Oxygen-hemoglobin dissociation curve. The effects of acidity and temperature changes are shown.

out of the lungs). Air moves in and out of the lungs because intrathoracic pressure changes in relation to pressure at the airway opening. Contraction of the diaphragm and intercostal and scalene muscles increases chest dimensions, thereby decreasing intrathoracic pressure. Gas flows from an area of higher pressure (atmospheric) to one of lower pressure (intrathoracic) (see Fig. 24-6). Some conditions (e.g., phrenic nerve paralysis, rib fractures, neuromuscular disease) may limit diaphragm or chest wall movement and cause the patient to breathe with smaller tidal volumes. As a result, the lungs do not fully inflate, and gas exchange is impaired. Interventions used to reverse this problem include mechanical phrenic nerve stimulation, nerve blocks to relieve pain from rib fractures, and mechanical ventilation.

In contrast to inspiration, expiration is passive. The elastic recoil of the chest wall and lungs allows the chest to passively return to its normal position. Intrathoracic pressure rises, causing air to move out of the lungs. Some conditions cause expiration to become an active process. For example, this may occur during an asthmatic exacerbation or when a patient with emphysema has severe dyspnea (see Chapter 27). During active or "labored" respirations, the scalene muscles and sternocleidomastoid muscles assist with expiration.

Elastic Recoil and Compliance. Elastic recoil is the tendency for the lungs to recoil after being stretched or expanded. The elasticity of lung tissue is due to the elastin fibers found in the alveolar walls and surrounding the bronchioles and capillaries.

Compliance (distensibility) is a measure of the elasticity of the lungs and thorax. When compliance is decreased, the lungs are more difficult to inflate. Examples include conditions that increase fluid in the lungs (e.g., pulmonary edema and ARDS); conditions that make lung tissue less elastic (e.g., pulmonary fibrosis or sarcoidosis); and conditions that restrict lung movement (e.g., pleural effusion). Compliance is increased as a result of aging and when there is destruction of alveolar walls and loss of tissue elasticity, as in emphysema.

Diffusion. Oxygen and carbon dioxide move back and forth across the alveolar capillary membrane by *diffusion*. The overall direction of movement is from the area of higher concentration to the area of lower concentration. Thus oxygen moves from alveolar gas (atmospheric air) into the arterial blood and carbon dioxide from the arterial blood into the alveolar gas. Diffusion continues until equilibrium is reached (see Fig. 24-5).[3]

The ability of the lungs to oxygenate arterial blood adequately is determined by examination of the arterial oxygen tension (PaO_2) and arterial oxygen saturation (SaO_2). Oxygen is carried in the blood in two forms: dissolved oxygen and oxygen in chemical combination with hemoglobin. The PaO_2 represents the amount of oxygen dissolved in the plasma and is expressed in millimeters of mercury (mm Hg). The SaO_2 is the amount of oxygen bound to hemoglobin in comparison with the amount of oxygen the hemoglobin can carry. The SaO_2 is expressed as a percentage. For example, if the SaO_2 is 90%, then 90% of the hemoglobin attachments for oxygen have oxygen bound to them.

Oxygen-Hemoglobin Dissociation Curve. The affinity of hemoglobin for oxygen is described by the oxygen-hemoglobin dissociation curve (Fig. 24-7). Oxygen delivery to the tissues depends on the amount of oxygen transported to the tissues and the ease with which hemoglobin gives up oxygen once it reaches the tissues. In the upper flat portion of the curve, fairly large changes in the PaO_2 cause a small change in hemoglobin saturation. For this reason, if the PaO_2 drops from 100 to 60 mm Hg, the saturation of hemoglobin changes only 7% (from the normal 97% to 90%). Thus the hemoglobin remains 90% saturated despite a 40 mm Hg drop in the PaO_2. This portion of the curve also explains the reason the patient is considered adequately oxygenated when the

Table 24-1 Normal Arterial and Venous Blood Gas Values*

Arterial Blood Gases			Mixed Venous Blood Gases	
Laboratory Value	Sea Level BP 760 mm Hg	1 Mile Above Sea Level (5280 ft) BP 629 mm Hg		
pH	7.35-7.45	7.35-7.45	pH	7.34-7.37
PaO_2	80-100 mm Hg	65-75 mm Hg	PvO_2	38-42 mm Hg
SaO_2	>95%†	>95%†	SvO_2	60%-80%†
$PaCO_2$	35-45 mm Hg	35-45 mm Hg	$PvCO_2$	44-46 mm Hg
HCO_3^-	22-26 mEq/L	22-26 mEq/L	HCO_3^-	24-30 mEq/L

*Assumes patient is ≤60 years of age and breathing room air.
†The same normal values apply when SpO_2 and SvO_2 are obtained by oximetry.
BP, barometric pressure; *PvO_2*, partial pressure of oxygen in venous blood; *SvO_2*, venous oxygen saturation.

PaO_2 is greater than 60 mm Hg. Increasing the PaO_2 above this level causes little change in hemoglobin saturation, and if high concentrations of oxygen can be avoided, there is less risk of oxygen toxicity. *Oxygen toxicity* refers to alveolar injury caused by high oxygen concentrations, that is, greater than 40% to 60%.[8]

The lower portion of the oxyhemoglobin dissociation curve indicates a different type of phenomenon. As the hemoglobin becomes further desaturated, larger amounts of oxygen are released for tissue use. This is an important method of maintaining the pressure gradient between the blood and the tissues. It also ensures an adequate oxygen supply to peripheral tissues, even if oxygen delivery is compromised.[8]

Many factors alter the affinity of hemoglobin for oxygen. When the oxygen dissociation curve shifts to the left, blood picks up oxygen more readily in the lungs but delivers oxygen less readily to the tissues. This is seen in alkalosis, in hypothermia, and with a decrease in arterial carbon dioxide tension ($PaCO_2$) (see Fig. 24-7). The patient with a condition that causes a leftward shift of the curve, such as with hypothermia that follows open heart surgery, may be given higher concentrations of oxygen until the body temperature normalizes. This helps compensate for decreased oxygen unloading in the tissues. When the curve shifts to the right, the opposite occurs. Blood picks up oxygen less rapidly in the lungs but delivers oxygen more readily to the tissues. This is seen in acidosis, hyperthermia, and when the $PaCO_2$ is increased.[8,9]

Two methods are used to assess the efficiency of gas transfer in the lung: analysis of arterial blood gases (ABGs) and oximetry. These measures are usually adequate if the patient is stable and not critically ill. The critically ill patient often has a condition that impairs tissue oxygen delivery. In this patient, cardiac output, oxygen consumption (VO_2), mixed venous oxygen tension (PvO_2), and venous oxygen saturation (SvO_2) may also be assessed (see Chapter 62).

Arterial Blood Gases. ABGs are measured to determine oxygenation status and acid-base balance. ABG analysis includes measurement of the PaO_2, $PaCO_2$, acidity (pH), and bicarbonate (HCO_3^-) in arterial blood. The SaO_2 is also calculated during this analysis.[8,9]

Blood for ABG analysis can be obtained by arterial puncture or from an arterial catheter that is typically placed in the radial or femoral artery. Both techniques are invasive and allow only intermittent analysis. Continuous intraarterial blood gas monitoring is also possible via a fiberoptic sensor or an oxygen electrode inserted into an arterial catheter.[8] An arterial catheter and continuous blood gas monitoring permit ABG sampling without repeated arterial punctures.

Normal values for ABGs are given in Table 24-1. The normal PaO_2 decreases with advancing age.[8] The normal PaO_2 also varies in relation to the distance above sea level. At higher altitudes, the barometric pressure is lower, resulting in a lower inspired oxygen pressure and a lower PaO_2 (see Table 24-1). Most airplanes are pressurized to approximate an altitude of 8000 feet above sea level. A normal person can expect a 16 to 32 mm Hg fall in PaO_2 at this altitude.[10] The patient who is already receiving oxygen therapy or the patient with a PaO_2 less than 72 mm Hg while breathing room air needs careful evaluation before air travel. Supplemental oxygen or a change in liter flow may be required during the flight. If oxygen is required, the airline should be contacted several weeks in advance to determine the procedures regarding air travel with oxygen.[10,11]

Mixed Venous Blood Gases. For the patient with a normal or near-normal cardiac status, an assessment of PaO_2 or SaO_2 is usually sufficient to determine adequate oxygenation. This is often not true for the patient with impaired cardiac output or who is hemodynamically unstable. Such a patient may have inadequate tissue oxygen delivery or abnormal oxygen consumption. The amount of oxygen delivered to the tissues and the amount of oxygen consumed can be calculated. The PvO_2 and SvO_2 can also be analyzed to determine if the tissues are receiving enough oxygen.

A catheter positioned in the pulmonary artery, termed a *pulmonary artery (PA) catheter,* is used for mixed venous sampling (see Chapter 63). Blood drawn from a PA catheter is termed a *mixed venous sample* because it consists of venous blood that has returned to the heart from all tissue beds and "mixed" in the right ventricle. Normal mixed venous values are given in Table 24-1. When tissue oxygen delivery is inadequate or when inadequate oxygen is transported to the tissues by the hemoglobin, the PvO_2 and SvO_2 fall. The value of mixed venous blood in the assessment of hypoxemia results from information provided about the pulmonary and cardiovascular system. The PaO_2 provides information about tissue oxygen supply to the tissues and the PvO_2 about tissue oxygen demand. A lower than normal PvO_2 suggests an inadequate oxygen supply to meet oxygen demand.[8]

Oximetry. ABG values provide accurate information about oxygenation and acid-base balance. However, they are invasive, require laboratory analysis, and expose the patient to the risk of bleeding from an arterial puncture. Arterial oxygen

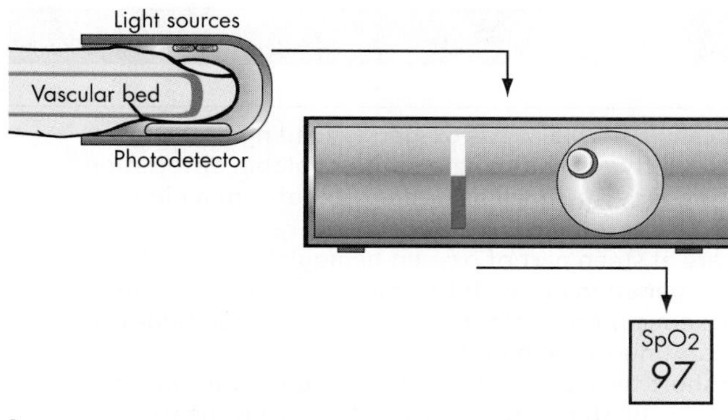

A

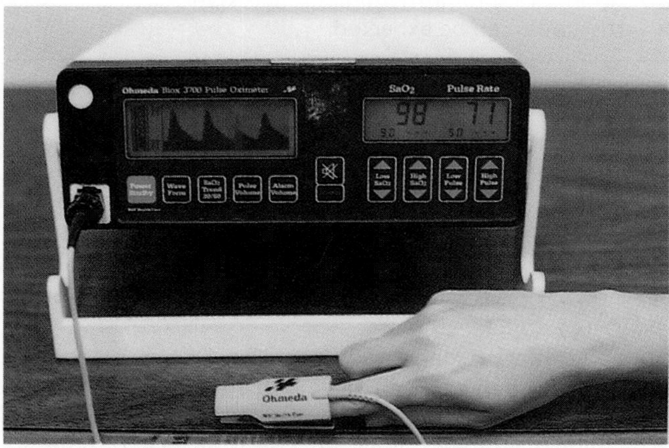

B

Fig. 24-8 **A,** A pulse oximeter passes light from a light-emitting diode through a vascular bed to a photodetector. The oximeter compares the amount of light emitted and absorbed and calculates the SpO_2. The oximeter displays SpO_2 as a digital reading. **B,** Portable pulse oximeter displays oxygen saturation and pulse rate.

saturation can be monitored continuously and noninvasively (i.e., without a blood sample) using pulse oximetry. The technique involves attaching a probe to the ear, finger, toe, forehead, or bridge of the nose (Fig. 24-8).

A pulse oximeter emits two wavelengths of light, one red and one infrared, which pass from a light-emitting diode (positioned on one side of the probe) to a photodetector (positioned on the opposite side). Well-oxygenated blood absorbs light differently than deoxygenated blood does. The oximeter determines the amount of light absorbed by the vascular bed and uses this information to calculate the saturation. Since arterial oxygen saturation can be determined from ABGs or by oximetry, SpO_2 is used to indicate the value obtained by pulse oximetry. SpO_2 and heart rate are displayed on the monitor as a digital reading (see Fig. 24-8, *B*). The normal SpO_2 is greater than 95%.[8]

Pulse oximetry is particularly valuable in intensive care units (ICUs), during exercise testing, and when determining oxygen flow rates for the patient on long-term oxygen therapy. Changes in SpO_2 can be quickly detected and modifications made in the plan of care (Table 24-2).[9] Pulse oximetry does not provide any information about ventilation status (pH, $PaCO_2$). Thus the use of pulse oximetry does not eliminate the need for ABGs.[8,9]

Values obtained by pulse oximetry become less accurate if the SpO_2 is less than 70%. At this level, the oximeter may display a value that is ±4% of the actual value; for example, if the SpO_2 is 70%, the actual value can range from 66% to 74%. Pulse oximetry is also inaccurate if there are hemoglobin variants, such as carboxyhemoglobin or methemoglobin, present. Other factors that can alter accuracy of pulse oximetry include motion, low perfusion, anemia, bright fluorescent lights, intravascular dyes, thick acrylic nails, and dark skin color. If there is doubt about the accuracy of the SpO_2 reading, an ABG analysis should be obtained to verify accuracy.

The technique of oximetry can also be used to monitor SvO_2.[8] With SvO_2 monitoring, the light-emitting probe is placed in one lumen of the PA catheter. A decrease in SvO_2 suggests that less oxygen is being delivered to the tissues or that more oxygen is being consumed. Changes in SvO_2 provide an early warning of a change in cardiac output and tissue oxygen delivery. Normal SvO_2 is 60% to 80%.

Oxygen Delivery. Information from ABGs or oximetry is used to assess adequacy of oxygenation. Several questions must be asked to determine if oxygenation is adequate:

1. What is the patient's SpO_2 or PaO_2 compared with expected normal values? (Normal values are given in Table 24-1.)
2. What is the degree of hypoxemia and what is the trend? Has there been a rapid decline in SpO_2 or PaO_2? A sudden drop in blood oxygen level can be life threatening. A gradual decline is tolerated with fewer symptoms. Critical values for SpO_2 and PaO_2 are given in Table 24-2.
3. Are there signs or symptoms of inadequate oxygenation? Changes in respiratory, cardiovascular, central nervous system, and renal function are seen when tissue oxygen delivery is inadequate (Table 24-3). Because the brain is very sensitive to a decrease in tissue oxygen delivery, the very first evidence of hypoxemia may be apprehension, restlessness, or irritability. If these signs or symptoms are observed, a change in the management plan is needed.
4. What is the oxygenation status with activity or exercise? Pulse oximetry is used to monitor SpO_2 levels during a standardized 6 minute walk distance test or with activities of daily living to assess for desaturation with activity. An SpO_2 ≤88% during exertion indicates the need for supplemental oxygen.

Control of Respiration

The respiratory center is composed of cell clusters in the medulla on the brainstem. These cells respond to chemical and mechanical signals from the body. Impulses are sent from the medulla to the respiratory muscles through the spinal cord and phrenic nerves. Respiration is controlled by chemoreceptors and mechanical sensors.

Chemoreceptors. A chemoreceptor is a receptor that responds to a change in the chemical composition ($PaCO_2$ and pH) of the fluid around it. Central chemoreceptors are located in the medulla and respond to changes in the hydrogen ion (H^+) concentration. An increase in the H^+ concentration (acidosis) causes the medulla to increase the respiratory rate and V_T. A decrease in H^+ concentration (alkalosis) has the

Table 24-2 Critical Values for PaO_2 and SpO_2*

PaO_2 (%)	SpO_2 (%)	Considerations
≥70	≥94	Adequate unless patient is hemodynamically unstable or has oxygen-unloading problem. With a low cardiac output, arrhythmias, a leftward shift of the oxyhemoglobin dissociation curve, or carbon monoxide inhalation, higher values may be desired. Benefits of a higher blood oxygen value need to be balanced against the risk of oxygen toxicity.
60	90	Adequate in almost all patients. Values are at steep part of oxygen-hemoglobin dissociation curve. Provides adequate oxygenation but with less margin of error than above.
55	88	Adequate for patients with chronic hypoxemia if no cardiac problems occur. These values are also used as criteria for prescription of continuous oxygen therapy.
40	75	Inadequate but may be acceptable on a short-term basis if the patient also has carbon dioxide retention. In this situation, respirations may be stimulated by a low PaO_2. Thus the PaO_2 cannot be raised rapidly. The nurse may use oxygen therapy by mask at a low concentration (24-28%) to gradually increase the PaO_2. Monitoring for arrhythmias is necessary.
<40	<75	Inadequate. Tissue hypoxia and cardiac arrhythmias can be expected.

*The same critical values apply for SpO_2 and SaO_2. Values pertain to rest or exertion.

Table 24-3 Signs and Symptoms of Inadequate Oxygenation

Signs and Symptoms	Onset
Respiratory	
Tachypnea	Early
Dyspnea on exertion	Early
Dyspnea at rest	Late
Use of accessory muscles	Late
Retraction of interspaces on inspiration	Late
Pause for breath between sentences, words	Late
Cardiovascular	
Tachycardia	Early
Mild hypertension	Early
Arrhythmias (e.g., premature ventricular contractions)	Early or late
Hypotension	Late
Cyanosis	Late
Cool, clammy skin	Late
Central Nervous System	
Unexplained apprehension	Early
Unexplained restlessness or irritability	Early
Unexplained confusion or lethargy	Early or late
Combativeness	Late
Coma	Late
Other	
Diaphoresis	Early or late
Decreased urinary output	Early or late
Unexplained fatigue	Early or late

opposite effect. Changes in $PaCO_2$ regulate ventilation primarily by their effect on the pH of the cerebrospinal fluid. When the $PaCO_2$ level is increased, more CO_2 is available to combine with H_2O and form carbonic acid (H_2CO_3). This lowers the cerebrospinal fluid pH and stimulates an increase in respiratory rate. The opposite process occurs with a decrease in $PaCO_2$ level.

Peripheral chemoreceptors are located in the carotid bodies at the bifurcation of the common carotid arteries and in the aortic bodies above and below the aortic arch. The peripheral chemoreceptors respond to decreases in PaO_2 and pH and to increases in $PaCO_2$. These changes also cause stimulation of the respiratory center.

In a healthy person an increase in $PaCO_2$ or a decrease in pH causes an immediate increase in the respiratory rate. The process is extremely precise. The $PaCO_2$ does not vary more than about 3 mm Hg if lung function is normal. Conditions such as chronic obstructive pulmonary disease (COPD) alter lung function and may result in chronically elevated $PaCO_2$ levels. In these instances, the patient will be relatively insensitive to further increases in $PaCO_2$ as a stimulus to breathe and may be maintaining ventilation largely because of a hypoxic drive from the peripheral chemoreceptors (see Chapter 27).[2,12]

Mechanical Receptors. Mechanical receptors (juxtacapillary and irritant) are located in the lungs, upper airways, chest wall, and diaphragm. They are stimulated by a variety of physiologic factors, such as irritants, muscle stretching, and alveolar wall distortion. Signals from the stretch receptors aid in the control of respiration. As the lungs inflate, pulmonary stretch receptors activate the inspiratory center to inhibit further lung expansion. This is termed the *Hering-Breuer reflex* and it prevents overdistention of the lungs. Impulses from the mechanical sensors are sent through the vagus nerve to the brain. Juxtacapillary (J) receptors are believed to cause the rapid respiration (tachypnea) seen in pulmonary edema. These receptors are stimulated by fluid entering the pulmonary interstitial space.

Respiratory Defense Mechanisms

Respiratory defense mechanisms are efficient in protecting the lungs from inhaled particles, microorganisms, and toxic gases. The defense mechanisms include filtration of air, the mucociliary clearance system, the cough reflex, reflex bronchoconstriction, and alveolar macrophages.

Filtration of Air. Nasal hairs filter the inspired air. In addition, the abrupt changes in direction of airflow that occur as air moves through the nasopharynx and larynx increase air turbulence. This causes particles and bacteria to come in contact on the mucosa lining these structures. Most large particles (greater than 5 μm in diameter) are removed in this manner.

The velocity of airflow slows greatly after it passes the larynx, facilitating the deposition of smaller particles (1 to 5 μm in size). They settle out similar to sand in a river, a process termed *sedimentation.* Particles less than 1 μm in size are too small to settle in this manner and are deposited in the alveoli. One example of small particles that can build up is coal dust, which can lead to pneumoconiosis. Particle size is important. Particles greater than 5 μm in size are less dangerous because they are removed in the nasopharynx or bronchi and do not reach the alveoli.[2]

Mucociliary Clearance System. Below the larynx, movement of mucus is accomplished by the mucociliary clearance system, commonly referred to as the *mucociliary escalator.* This term is used to indicate the interrelationship between the secretion of mucus and the ciliary activity. Mucus is continually secreted at a rate of about 100 ml per day by goblet cells and submucosal glands. It forms a mucous blanket that contains the impacted particles and debris from distal lung areas (see Fig. 24-1). The small amount of mucus normally secreted is swallowed without being noticed. Secretory immunoglobulin A (IgA) in the mucus contributes to protection against bacteria and viruses.

Cilia cover the airways from the level of the trachea to the respiratory bronchioles (see Fig. 24-1). Each ciliated cell contains approximately 200 cilia, which beat rhythmically about 1000 times per minute in the large airways, moving mucus toward the mouth. The ciliary beat is slower further down the tracheobronchial tree. As a consequence, particles that penetrate more deeply into the airways are removed less rapidly. Ciliary action is impaired by dehydration, smoking, inhalation of high oxygen concentrations, infection, and ingestion of drugs such as atropine, alcohol, anesthetics, and recreational drugs such as cocaine or crack. Patients with chronic bronchitis and cystic fibrosis have repeated upper respiratory infections. Cilia are often destroyed during these infections, resulting in impaired secretion clearance, a chronic productive cough, and frequent respiratory infections.[13]

Cough Reflex. The cough is a protective reflex action that clears the airway by a high-pressure, high-velocity flow of air. It is a backup for mucociliary clearance, especially when this clearance mechanism is overwhelmed or ineffective. Coughing is only effective in removing secretions above the subsegmental level (large or main airways). Secretions below this level must be moved upward by the mucociliary mechanism or by interventions such as postural drainage before they can be removed by coughing.

Reflex Bronchoconstriction. Another defense mechanism is reflex bronchoconstriction. In response to the inhalation of large amounts of irritating substances (e.g., dusts, aerosols), the bronchi constrict in an effort to prevent entry of the irritants. A person with hyperreactive airways, such as a person with asthma, experiences bronchoconstriction after inhalation of cold air, perfume, or other strong odors.

Alveolar Macrophages. Since ciliated cells are not found below the level of the respiratory bronchioles, the primary defense mechanism at the alveolar level is alveolar macrophages. Alveolar macrophages rapidly phagocytize inhaled foreign particles such as bacteria. The debris is moved to the level of the bronchioles for removal by the cilia or removed from the lungs by the lymphatic system. Particles that cannot be adequately phagocytized tend to remain in the lungs for indefinite periods and can stimulate inflammatory or fibrogenic responses. Coal dust and silica can stimulate a fibrous reaction (see Chapter 26). Because alveolar macrophage activity is impaired by cigarette smoke, the smoker who is employed in an occupation with heavy dust exposure (e.g., mining, foundries), is at an especially high risk for lung disease.

GERONTOLOGIC CONSIDERATIONS

Effects of Aging on the Respiratory System

Age-related changes in the respiratory system can be divided into alterations in structure, defense mechanisms, and respiratory control.[14] Structural alterations include a decrease in elastic recoil of the lung and a decrease in chest wall compliance. The anteroposterior diameter of the thoracic cage increases. Within the lung there is a decrease in the number of functional alveoli. Small airways in the lung bases close earlier in expiration. As a consequence, more inspired air is distributed to the lung apices and ventilation is less well matched to perfusion, causing a lowering of the PaO_2.[14] The PaO_2 associated with a given age can be calculated by means of the following equation:[14]

$$PaO_2\ (\text{mm Hg}) = 103.5 - 0.42 \times \text{Age in years}$$

For example, the normal PaO_2 for a patient 80 years of age is 70 mm Hg [103.5 - (0.42 × 80) = 70 mm Hg] as compared with a PaO_2 of 93 mm Hg for a 25-year-old person.

Respiratory defense mechanisms are less effective because of a decline in cell-mediated immunity and formation of antibodies. The alveolar macrophages are less effective at phagocytosis. An elderly patient has a less forceful cough and fewer and less functional cilia. Formation of secretory IgA, an important mechanism in neutralizing the effect of viruses, is diminished.[14]

Respiratory control is altered, resulting in a more gradual response to changes in blood oxygen or carbon dioxide level. The PaO_2 drops to a lower level and the $PaCO_2$ rises to a higher level before the respiratory rate changes.

There is much variability in the extent of these changes in persons of the same age. The elderly patient who has a significant smoking history, is obese, and is diagnosed with a chronic illness is at greatest risk of adverse outcomes.

Age-related changes in the respiratory system and differences in assessment findings are presented in Table 24-4.

ASSESSMENT OF THE RESPIRATORY SYSTEM

Correct diagnosis depends on an accurate health history and a thorough physical examination. A respiratory assessment can be done as part of a comprehensive physical examination or as an examination in itself. Judgment must be used in determining whether all or part of the history and physical examination will be completed based on problems presented by the patient and the degree of respiratory distress. If respiratory distress is severe, only pertinent information should be obtained and a thorough assessment should be deferred until the patient's condition stabilizes.

GERONTOLOGIC DIFFERENCES IN ASSESSMENT

Table 24-4 Respiratory System

Changes	Differences in Assessment Findings
Structure	
↓ Elastic recoil ↓ Chest wall compliance ↑ Anteroposterior diameter ↓ Functioning alveoli	Barrel chest appearance; ↓ chest wall movement; ↓ respiratory excursion; ↓ vital capacity; ↑ functional residual capacity; diminished breath sounds particularly at lung bases; ↓ PaO_2 and SaO_2; normal pH and $PaCO_2$
Defense Mechanisms	
↓ Cell-mediated immunity ↓ Specific antibodies ↓ Cilia function ↓ Cough force ↓ Alveolar macrophage function	↓ Cough effectiveness; ↓ secretion clearance; ↑ risk of upper respiratory infection, influenza, pneumonia. Respiratory infections may be more severe and last longer
Respiratory Control	
↓ Response to hypoxemia ↓ Response to hypercapnia	Greater ↓ in PaO_2 and ↑ in $PaCO_2$ before respiratory rate changes. Significant hypoxemia or hypercapnia may develop from relatively small incidents. Retained secretions, excessive sedation, or positioning that impairs chest expansion may substantially alter PaO_2 or SpO_2 values.

Subjective Data

Important Health Information

Past health history. The nurse should determine the frequency of upper respiratory problems (e.g., colds, sore throats, sinus problems, allergies) and if weather changes affect these problems. The patient with allergies should be questioned about possible precipitating factors such as medications, pollen, smoke, or pet exposure. Characteristics of the allergic reaction, such as runny nose, wheezing, scratchy throat, or tightness in the chest, and severity should be documented. The frequency of asthma exacerbations and cause, if known, should also be determined. Prior use of a peak expiratory flow rate (PEFR) meter and personal best values can be helpful information in determining the patient's current asthma status.

A history of lower respiratory problems, such as asthma, COPD, pneumonia, and tuberculosis, should also be elicited. Respiratory symptoms are often manifestations of problems that involve other body systems. Therefore the patient should be asked if there is a history of other health problems in addition to those involving the respiratory system. For example, the patient with cardiac dysfunction may experience dyspnea as a consequence of congestive heart failure. The patient with human immunodeficiency virus (HIV) infection may experience frequent respiratory infections because immune function is compromised.

Medications. The patient should be questioned carefully about prescription and over-the-counter drugs used to manage respiratory problems, such as antihistamines, bronchodilators, corticosteroids, cough suppressants, and antibiotics. Information about the reason for taking the medication, its name, the dose and frequency, length of time taken, its effect, and any side effects should be obtained.

If the patient is using oxygen to ease a breathing problem, the amount, method of administration, and effectiveness of the therapy should be documented. Safety practices related to using oxygen should also be assessed.

Surgery or other treatments. The nurse should determine if the patient has been hospitalized for a respiratory problem. If so, the dates, therapy (including surgery), and current status of the problem should be recorded.

The nurse should ask about the use of respiratory treatments such as nebulizer, humidifier, and airway clearance modalities, including a Flutter valve, high-frequency chest oscillation, postural drainage, and percussion. The frequency of these treatments and the results obtained are important for the nurse to know.

Functional Health Patterns. Health history questions to ask a patient with a respiratory problem are presented in Table 24-5.

Health perception–health management pattern. The patient should be asked if there has been a perceived change in health status within the last several days, months, or years. In COPD, lung function declines slowly over many years. The patient may not notice this decline because activity is altered to accommodate reduced exercise tolerance. If an upper respiratory infection is superimposed on a chronic problem, dyspnea and decreased exercise tolerance may occur very quickly. In asthma, symptoms may occur or worsen in the presence of exercise, animals, or change in temperature, causing the patient to avoid these activities.

Common cues that should alert the nurse to the possibility of respiratory problems should be explored and documented (Table 24-6). The course of the patient's illness, including when it began, the type of symptoms, and factors that alleviate or aggravate these symptoms, should be described. Because of the chronic nature of respiratory problems, the patient may relate a change in symptoms rather than the onset of new symptoms when describing the present illness. Such changes should be carefully documented because they often suggest the cause of illness. For example, a change in the volume, tenacity (thickness), or color of sputum suggests the onset of a lower respiratory tract infection.[4,15]

HEALTH HISTORY

Table 24-5 **Respiratory System**

Health Perception–Health Management Pattern

- Describe your daily activities. Has there been a change in activities you can perform in the last several days? Months? Years? If changed, was this because of your health?
- How do your breathing problems affect your self-care abilities?
- Have you ever smoked? Do you smoke now? If yes, how many cigarettes each day and for how long? Did you stop or cut back on your smoking because of your health?*
- Have you had a Pneumovax vaccination? When was your last flu shot?
- What types of alcoholic beverages do you drink? How often? How much?
- Do you ever use drugs to get high?* How often?
- What equipment helps you manage your respiratory problems? How often do you use it? Does it help? Cause problems?

Nutritional-Metabolic Pattern

- Have you recently lost weight because of difficulty eating secondary to a respiratory problem? How much? Voluntarily?
- Do any particular foods affect your sputum production or breathing?*

Elimination Pattern

- Does your respiratory problem make it difficult for you to get to the toilet?*
- Are you inactive because of dyspnea to the point where it causes constipation?

Activity-Exercise Pattern

- Are you ever short of breath during exercise?* At rest?*
- Do you get too short of breath to do the things you want to do?*
- Is your home one story? Two stories? How many steps from the street to your door?
- Are you able to maintain your typical activity pattern? If not, explain.
- What do you do when you get short of breath?

Sleep-Rest Pattern

- Do breathing problems cause you to awaken during the night?*
- Can you lie flat at night? If not, how many pillows do you use? Do you need to sleep upright in a chair?
- Are you or your sleep partner aware of any snoring?

Cognitive-Perceptual Pattern

- Do you have any pain associated with breathing?*
- Do you ever feel restless, irritable, or confused without a reason?*
- Do you have difficulty remembering things?*

Self-Perception–Self-Concept Pattern

- Describe how your respiratory problems have changed your life.
- Do you ever go out without using your oxygen? When and why?

Role-Relationship Pattern

- Has your respiratory problem caused any difficulties in your work, family, or social relationships?*

Sexuality-Reproductive Pattern

- Has your respiratory problem caused a change in your sexual activity?*
- Do you want to discuss ways to decrease dyspnea during sexual activity?

Coping–Stress Tolerance Pattern

- How often do you leave your home?
- Would you want to join a support group? Pulmonary rehabilitation program?
- Does stress have an effect on your breathing?*
- What effect does your respiratory problem have on your emotions?

Value-Belief Pattern

- How often do you miss taking your medications? Why?
- Do you think the things you have been told to do for your respiratory problems really help? If not, why?

*If yes, describe.

Table 24-6 **Cues to Respiratory Problems**

Manifestation	Description
Shortness of breath (dyspnea)	Distressful sensation of uncomfortable breathing. Most common complaint of people with respiratory problems. Person may become accustomed to sensation and not recognize its presence. Difficult to evaluate because it is a subjective experience.
Wheezing	May or may not be heard by patient. May be described as chest tightness.
Pleuritic chest pain	Described on a continuum from discomfort during inspiration to intense, sharp pain at the end of inspiration. Pain is usually aggravated by deep breathing and coughing.
Cough	Characteristics of cough are important diagnostic cues.
Sputum production	Material coughed up from lungs. Contains mucus, cellular debris, or microorganisms, and may contain blood or pus. Amount, color, and constituents of sputum are important diagnostic information.
Hemoptysis	Coughing up of blood; either gross, frankly bloody sputum, or blood-tinged sputum. Precipitating events should be investigated.
Voice change	Hoarseness, stridor (whistling sound during inspiration), muffling, or a barking cough may indicate abnormalities of upper airway, vocal cord dysfunction, or gastroesophageal reflux disease.

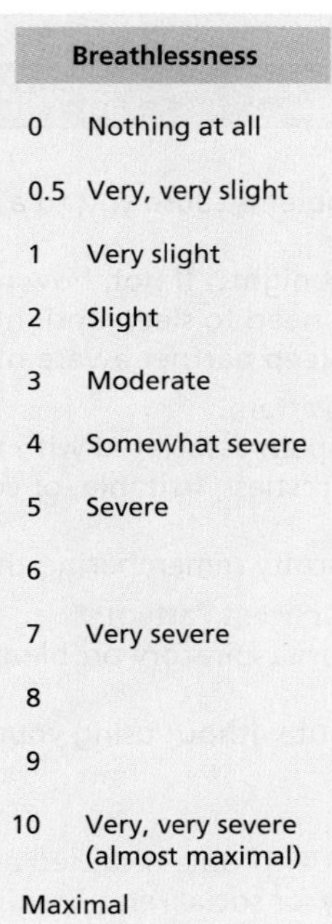

Breathlessness	
0	Nothing at all
0.5	Very, very slight
1	Very slight
2	Slight
3	Moderate
4	Somewhat severe
5	Severe
6	
7	Very severe
8	
9	
10	Very, very severe (almost maximal)
Maximal	

Fig. 24-9 Borg category-ratio scale. Using this scale from 0 to 10, how much shortness of breath do you have right now?

If dyspnea is present, the nurse should determine if it occurs at rest or with physical exertion. To determine the intensity of dyspnea, the use of a Borg scale or visual analog scale may be helpful (Fig. 24-9).

If a cough is present, the nurse should evaluate the quality of the cough. For example, a loose-sounding cough indicates the presence of secretions; a dry, hacking cough indicates airway irritation or obstruction; a harsh, barky cough suggests upper airway obstruction from inhibited vocal cord movement related to subglottic edema. The nurse should assess whether the cough is weak or strong, and productive or unproductive of secretions. Determining the onset and chronicity of a cough is helpful in the differential diagnosis process.

If the patient has a productive cough, the following characteristics of sputum should be evaluated: amount, color, consistency, and odor. The amount should be quantified in teaspoons, tablespoons, or cups per day. The nurse should note any recent increases or decreases in the amount. The normal color is clear or slightly whitish. If a patient is a cigarette smoker, the sputum is usually clear to gray with occasional specks of brown. The patient with COPD may exhibit clear, whitish, or slightly yellow sputum, especially in the morning on rising. If the patient reports any change from baseline to yellow, pink, red, brown, or green sputum, pulmonary complications should be suspected. Changes in consistency of sputum to thick, thin, or frothy should be noted. These changes may indicate dehydration, postnasal drip or sinus drainage, or possible pulmonary edema. Normally sputum should be odorless. A foul odor suggests an infectious process.

The patient should be questioned about a family history of respiratory problems that may be genetic or familial tendencies, such as asthma, emphysema resulting from alpha$_1$-antitrypsin deficiency, or cystic fibrosis. A history of family exposure to tuberculosis bacilli should be noted.

The nurse should ask where the patient has lived and traveled. Risk factors for tuberculosis include prior residence in Asia, Africa, or Latin America. Risk factors for fungal infections of the lung include living or traveling in the Southwest (coccidioidomycosis) and the Mississippi River Valley (histoplasmosis).[2]

The nurse should also ask about current and past smoking habits and quantify exposure in pack-years. This is done by multiplying the number of packs smoked per day by the number of years smoked. For example, a person who smoked 1 pack per day for 15 years has a 15 pack-year history. The risk of lung cancer rises in direct proportion to the number of cigarettes smoked. Smoking increases the risk of COPD and exacerbates symptoms of asthma and chronic bronchitis.

The nurse should ask if the patient received immunization for influenza (flu) and pneumococcal pneumonia (Pneumovax). Influenza vaccine should be administered yearly in the fall. Pneumovax is recommended for persons 65 years or older or those individuals with chronic cardiovascular disease, chronic pulmonary disease, or diabetes mellitus. Revaccination is currently advised only if the patient received the vaccine more than 5 years previously and was less than 65 years old at the time of vaccination. In persons with functional or anatomic asplenia or immunocompromised persons (e.g., transplant recipient), an initial vaccine is recommended and a single revaccination should be administered every 5 years after the initial dose.[16]

The patient should be asked about the use of equipment to manage respiratory symptoms (e.g., home oxygen therapy equipment, metered-dose inhaler [MDI] or nebulizer for medication administration, a positive airway pressure device for relief of sleep apnea). The patient should be questioned about the type of equipment used, frequency of use, its effect, and any side effects. The patient should be asked to demonstrate use of the MDI. Many patients do not know how to correctly use MDI devices (see Chapter 27).[10] Use of spacer devices with MDIs should be determined.

Nutritional-metabolic pattern. Weight loss is a symptom of many respiratory diseases. The nurse should determine if weight loss was intentional and, if not, if food intake is altered by anorexia (from medications), fatigue (from hypoxemia, increased work of breathing), early satiety (from lung hyperinflation), or social isolation. Anorexia and weight loss are common symptoms in patients with COPD, acquired immunodeficiency syndrome (AIDS), lung cancer, and tuberculosis. Fluid intake should also be noted. Dehydration can result in thickened mucus, which can cause airway obstruction.

Weight gain indicates possible fluid retention from cardiovascular dysfunction. Excessive weight interferes with normal ventilation and may cause sleep apnea (see Chapter 25).

Elimination pattern. Healthy elimination habits depend on the ability to reach a toilet when necessary. Activity intolerance secondary to dyspnea could result in urinary incontinence. Dyspnea (shortness of breath) can also be the cause of limited mobility, which can cause constipation. The patient with dyspnea should be questioned about both of these possibilities.

Activity-exercise pattern. The nurse should determine if the patient's activity is limited by dyspnea at rest or during exercise. The nurse should also note whether the patient's housing (e.g., number of steps, levels) poses a problem that increases social isolation.

The nurse should also inquire if the patient is able to carry out activities of daily living without dyspnea or other respiratory symptoms. If unable, the amount and type of care needed should be documented. Self-care strategies to minimize dyspnea should be reinforced. Immobility and sedentary habits can be risk factors for hypoventilation leading to atelectasis or pneumonia.

Sleep-rest pattern. The nurse should ask if the patient can sleep throughout the night. The patient with asthma or COPD may awaken at night with chest tightness, wheezing, or coughing. This suggests a need for a longer-acting bronchodilator or other medication change. The patient with cardiovascular disease (e.g., congestive heart failure) may sleep with the head elevated on several pillows. The patient with sleep apnea may complain of snoring, insomnia, and daytime drowsiness. The occurrence of night sweats should be documented because this can be a manifestation of tuberculosis.

Cognitive-perceptual pattern. Because hypoxia can cause neurologic symptoms, the nurse should ask about apprehension, restlessness, and irritability, which can indicate inadequate cerebral oxygenation (see Table 24-3). Hypoxemia interferes with the ability to learn and retain information.[17] For this reason, teaching may be more effective if another person is present during the teaching session to provide reinforcement at a later date.

The patient's ability to cooperate with the treatment plan should be assessed. Cognitive impairment may cause noncompliance or resistance to therapy. Failure to participate in needed therapy can result in exacerbation of respiratory problems.

The nurse should inquire about any discomfort or pain with breathing. A complaint of chest pain must be explored carefully to rule out cardiac involvement. Respiratory system problems such as pleurisy, fractured ribs, and costochondritis cause chest pain. Pleuritic pain is described as a sharp, stabbing pain associated with movement or deep breathing. Fractured ribs cause localized sharp pain associated with breathing. The pain of costochondritis is along the borders of the sternum and is associated with breathing.

Self-perception–self-concept pattern. Dyspnea limits activity, impairs ability to fulfill normal developmental role functions, and often alters self-esteem. Concern about a highly visible nasal cannula may cause the patient to resist using oxygen in public. The nurse should ask how the patient views body image in relation to that of others. Referral to a support group or pulmonary rehabilitation program may be beneficial in developing a support system and coping strategies.[18]

Role-relationship pattern. Acute or chronic respiratory problems can seriously affect performance in work or other related activities. The nurse should ask about the impact of activity, medications, oxygen, and special routines (e.g., pulmonary hygiene for cystic fibrosis) on the patient's family, job, and social life.

Progression of chronic respiratory problems that severely limit activity may have a negative impact on the patient's roles and responsibilities at home or on the job. The patient should be asked if any problems in these areas are present.

The nurse should document the nature of the patient's work and the frequency and intensity of exposure to fumes, toxins, asbestos, coal, or silica. Patient-specific allergens such as dust or fumes, which could be present in the work environment, should be investigated. Hobbies such as woodworking (sawdust) or pottery (silica) and exposure to animals (allergies) may also cause respiratory problems. Because of hyperreactive airways, exposure to fumes, smoke, and other chemicals may trigger wheezing in the asthmatic patient.

Sexuality-reproductive pattern. Most patients can continue to have good sexual relationships despite marked physical limitations. In a tactful manner, the nurse should determine whether breathing difficulties have caused alterations in sexual activity. If so, teaching can be provided about positions that decrease dyspnea during sexual activity and alternative strategies for sexual fulfillment.

Coping–stress tolerance pattern. Dyspnea causes anxiety and anxiety exacerbates dyspnea. The result is a vicious cycle—the patient avoids activities that cause dyspnea, becoming more deconditioned and more dyspneic. The outcome is often physical and social isolation. The nurse should ask how often the patient leaves home and interacts with others. Referral to a support group or pulmonary rehabilitation program may be beneficial.[18]

The chronic nature of many respiratory problems such as COPD and asthma can cause prolonged stress. Inquiry should be made into the patient's coping strategies to manage this stress.

Value-belief pattern. The nurse should determine the patient's adherence to the management regimen. If suboptimal, reasons for lack of adherence should be explored, including culturally specific beliefs, financial constraints (costs of prescriptions), failure to note benefit, or other reasons.

Objective Data

Physical Examination. Vital signs, including temperature, pulse, respirations, and blood pressure, are important data to collect before examination of the respiratory system.

Nose. The nose is inspected for inflammation, deformities, and symmetry. The nurse tilts the patient's head backward and pushes the tip of the nose upward gently. With a nasal speculum and a good light, the interior of the nose is inspected. The mucous membrane should be pink and moist, with no evidence of edema (bogginess), exudate, or bleeding. The nasal septum should be observed for deviation, perforations, and bleeding. Some nasal deviation is normal in an adult. The turbinates should be observed for polyps, which are abnormal, fingerlike projections of swollen nasal mucosa. Polyps may result from long-term irritation of the mucosa, as from allergies.

Mouth and pharynx. Using a good light source, the nurse inspects the interior of the mouth for color, lesions, masses, gum retraction, bleeding, and poor dentition. The tongue is inspected for symmetry and presence of lesions. The nurse observes the pharynx by pressing a tongue blade against the middle of the back of the tongue. The pharynx should be smooth and moist, with no evidence of exudate, ulcerations, or swelling. The color, symmetry, and any enlargement of the tonsils are noted. The nurse stimulates the gag reflex by placing a tongue blade on the back of the pharynx. A normal response (gagging) indicates that the cranial nerves IX and X are intact and that the airway is protected.

Neck. The nurse inspects the neck for symmetry and presence of tender or swollen areas. The lymph nodes are palpated while the patient is sitting erect with the neck slightly flexed. Progression is front to back from the nodes around the ears, to the nodes at the base of the skull, and then to those located under the angles of the mandible to the midline. The patient may have small, mobile, nontender nodes (shotty nodes), which are not a sign of a pathologic condition. Tender, hard, or fixed nodes indicate disease. The location and characteristics of any nodes that are palpated are described.[3,4]

Thorax and lungs. Imaginary lines can be pictured on the chest to help in identifying abnormalities (see Fig. 24-2). Abnormalities can be described in relation to their location to these lines (e.g., 2 cm from the right midclavicular line).

Chest examination is best performed in a well-lighted, warm room with measures taken to ensure the patient's privacy. Depending on the clinician's preference, either the anterior or the posterior chest may be examined first.

Inspection. The patient's anterior side of the chest should be exposed. If able, the patient should sit upright or lean on the bedside table. First, the nurse observes the patient's appearance and notes any evidence of respiratory distress, such as tachypnea, inability to lie flat, or use of accessory muscles. Next, the nurse determines the shape and symmetry of the chest. Chest movement should be equal on both sides, and the anteroposterior (AP) diameter should be equal to the side-to-side diameter. Normal AP diameter is 1:2 and is less than the transverse diameter, which is 5:7. An increase in AP diameter (e.g., barrel chest) may be a normal aging change or result from lung hyperinflation. The nurse observes for abnormalities in the sternum (e.g., pectus carinatum, a prominent protrusion of the sternum, and pectus excavatum, an indentation of the lower sternum above the xiphoid process).[4,19]

Next the respiratory rate, depth, and rhythm should be observed. The normal rate is 12 to 20 breaths per minute; in the elderly, it is 16 to 25 breaths per minute. Inspiration (I) should take half as long as expiration (E) (e.g., I:E = 1:2). The nurse should observe for abnormal breathing patterns, such as Kussmaul's (rapid, deep breathing), Cheyne-Stokes (a rhythmic increase and decrease in rate separated by periods of apnea), or Biot's (irregular breathing with apnea every 4 to 5 cycles) respirations.

Skin color provides clues to respiratory status. Cyanosis is best observed in a dark-skinned patient in the conjunctivae, lips, palms, and soles of the feet. Causes of cyanosis include hypoxemia or decreased cardiac output. The fingers should be inspected for evidence of clubbing (an increase in the angle between the base of the nail and the fingernail to 180 degrees or more, usually accompanied by an increase in the depth, bulk, and sponginess of the end of the finger).[2]

When the nurse is inspecting the posterior part of the chest, the patient should be asked to lean forward with arms folded. This position moves the scapula away from the spine, so there is more exposure of the area to be examined. The same sequence of observations that were done on the anterior part of the chest is performed on the posterior part. In addition, any spinal curvature is noted. Spinal curvatures that affect breathing include kyphosis, scoliosis, and kyphoscoliosis.

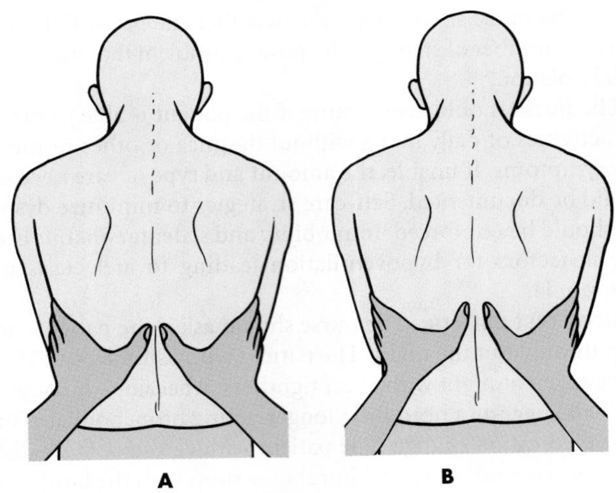

Fig. 24-10 Estimation of thoracic expansion. **A,** Exhalation. **B,** Maximal inhalation.

Palpation. The nurse determines tracheal position by gently placing the index fingers on either side of the trachea just above the suprasternal notch and gently pressing backward. Normal tracheal position is midline; deviation to the left or right is abnormal. Tracheal deviation occurs with a tension pneumothorax (toward the side contralateral to the pneumothorax), pneumonectomy (toward the surgical side), and lobar atelectasis (toward the collapsed lobe).[7,20]

The nurse determines symmetry of chest expansion and extent of movement at the level of the diaphragm. The nurse places the hands over the lower anterior chest wall along the costal margin and moves them inward until the thumbs meet at midline. The patient is asked to breathe deeply, and the nurse observes the movement of the thumbs away from each other. Normal expansion is 1 inch (2.5 cm). On the posterior side of the chest, the nurse places the hands at the level of the tenth rib and moves the thumbs until they meet over the spine (Fig. 24-10).

Normal chest movement is equal. Unequal expansion occurs when air entry is limited by conditions involving the lung (e.g., atelectasis, pneumothorax), the chest wall (e.g., incisional pain), or the pleura (e.g., pleural effusion). Equal but diminished expansion occurs in conditions that produce a hyperinflated or barrel chest or in neuromuscular disease (e.g., amyotrophic lateral sclerosis, spinal cord lesions). Movement may be absent or unequal over a pleural effusion, an atelectasis, or a pneumothorax.

Tactile fremitus (or vocal fremitus) is vibration of the chest wall produced by vocalization. To elicit this, the nurse places the palms of the hands against the patient's chest and asks the patient to repeat a phrase such as "ninety-nine." The nurse moves the hands from side to side and from top to bottom on the patient's chest (Fig. 24-11). All areas of the chest should be palpated and vibrations compared from similar areas. Tactile fremitus is most intense in the first and second interspace lateral to the sternum and between the scapulae because these areas are closest to the major bronchi. Fremitus is less intense farther away from these areas.[3,4,19]

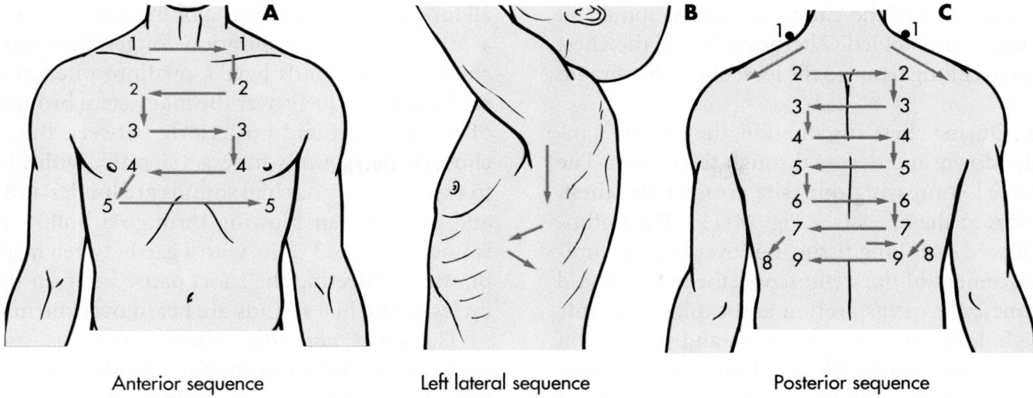

Fig. 24-11 Sequence for examination of the chest. **A,** Anterior sequence. **B,** Lateral sequence. **C,** Posterior sequence. For palpation, place the palms of the hands in the position designated as "1" on the right and left sides of the chest. Compare the intensity of vibrations. Continue for all positions in each sequence. For percussion, tap the chest at each designated position, moving downward from side to side, while comparing percussion notes. For auscultation, place the stethoscope at each position and listen to at least one complete inspiratory and expiratory cycle.

Table 24-7 Percussion Sounds

Sound	Description
Resonance	Low-pitched sound heard over normal lungs
Hyperresonance	Loud, lower-pitched sound than normal resonance heard over hyperinflated lungs, such as in chronic obstructive lung disease and acute asthma
Tympany	Drumlike, loud, empty quality heard over gas-filled stomach or intestine, or pneumothorax
Dull	Medium-intensity pitch and duration heard over areas of "mixed" solid and lung tissue, such as over the top area of the liver, partially consolidated lung tissue (pneumonia), or fluid-filled pleural space
Flat	Soft, high-pitched sound of short duration heard over very dense tissue where air is not present

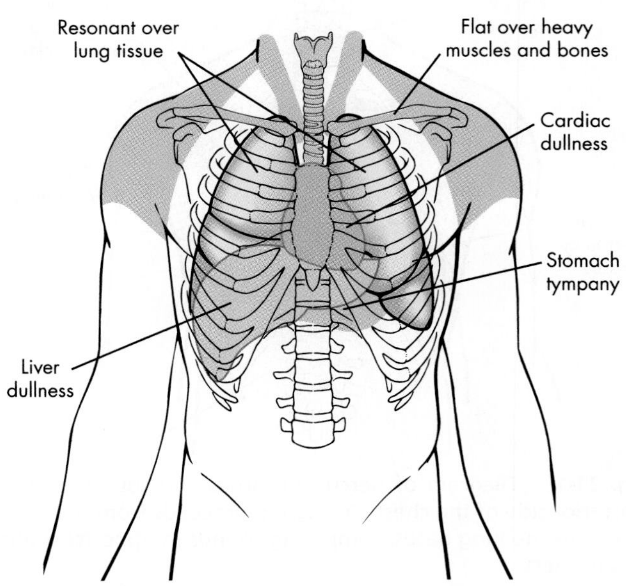

Fig. 24-12 Diagram of percussion areas and sounds in the anterior side of the chest.

Increase, decrease, or absence of fremitus should be noted. Increased fremitus occurs when the lung becomes filled with fluid or more dense. This is noted in pneumonia, in lung tumors, and above a pleural effusion (the lung is compressed upward). Fremitus is decreased if the hand is farther from the lung (e.g., pleural effusion) or the lung is hyperinflated (e.g., barrel chest). Absent fremitus may be noted with pneumothorax or atelectasis. The anterior of the chest is more difficult to palpate for fremitus because of the presence of large muscles and breast tissue.

Rhonchal fremitus is a palpable vibration caused by air traveling past thick bronchial mucus. It can be felt with the hand on the chest while the patient takes a deep inspiration, and may change or clear with coughing. Rhonchal fremitus is an abnormal finding.

Percussion. Percussion is done to assess density or aeration of the lungs. Percussion sounds are described in Table 24-7. (The technique for percussion is described in Chapter 5.)

The anterior of the chest is usually percussed with the patient in a semisitting or supine position. Starting below the clavicles, the nurse percusses downward, interspace by interspace (see Fig. 24-11). The area over lung tissue should be resonant, with the exception of the area of cardiac dullness (Fig. 24-12). For percussion of the posterior of the chest, the patient should sit leaning forward with arms folded. The posterior of the chest should be resonant over lung tissue to the level of the diaphragm (Fig. 24-13).

Auscultation. During chest auscultation, the patient is instructed to breathe slowly and deeply through the mouth. The nurse should proceed comparing opposite areas of the chest, from the lung apices to the bases (see Fig. 24-11). The stethoscope should be placed over lung tissue, not over bony prominences. At each placement of the stethoscope, the nurse should listen to at least one cycle of inspiration and expiration. Note the pitch (e.g., high, low), duration of sound, and presence of adventitious or abnormal sounds. The location of normal auscultatory sounds is more easily understood by visualization of a lung model (Fig. 24-14).

There are three normal breath sounds: vesicular, bronchovesicular, and bronchial. Vesicular sounds are relatively soft, low-pitched, gentle, rustling sounds. They are heard over all lung areas except the major bronchi. Vesicular sounds have a 3:1 ratio, with inspiration longer than expiration. Bronchovesicular sounds have a medium pitch and intensity and are heard anteriorly over the main-stem bronchi on either side of the sternum and posteriorly between the scapulae. Bronchovesicular sounds have a 1:1 ratio, with inspiration equal to expiration. Bronchial sounds are louder and higher pitched and resemble air blowing through a hollow pipe. Bronchial sounds have a 2:3 ratio, with a gap between inspiration and expiration, reflecting the short pause between these respiratory cycles. Bronchial sounds are heard over the manubrium.[4,19]

The term *abnormal breath sounds* is used to describe bronchial or bronchovesicular sounds heard in the peripheral lung fields. Adventitious sounds include crackles, rhonchi, wheezes, and pleural friction rubs.

A record of the normal physical assessment of the respiratory system is shown in Table 24-8. Common assessment abnormalities of the thorax and lungs are presented in Table

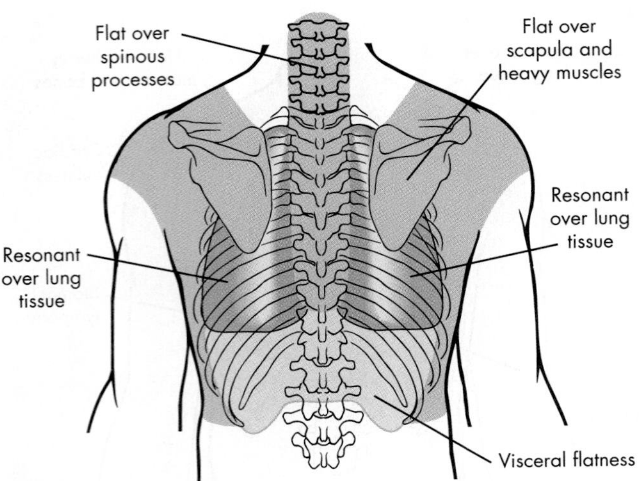

Fig. 24-13 Diagram of percussion areas and sounds in the posterior side of the chest. Percussion proceeds from the lung apices to the lung bases, comparing sounds in opposite areas of the chest.

Table 24-8 Normal Physical Assessment of the Respiratory System

- Nose is symmetric with no deformities. Nasal mucosa is pink and moist with no edema, exudate, or blood. Nasal septum is straight, without perforations. No polyps are evident.
- Oral mucosa is light pink and moist, with no exudate or ulcerations.
- Tonsils are present and not inflamed or enlarged.
- Pharynx is smooth, moist, and pink.
- Neck is symmetric and trachea is in the midline. No nodes are palpable.
- Chest has a normal configuration, with no evidence of injury. Respirations are normal, at the rate of 14/min. Excursion is equal bilaterally, with no increase in tactile fremitus. Percussion is resonant throughout. Breath sounds are normal throughout, without crackles, rhonchi, or wheezes. No axillary nodes are palpable.

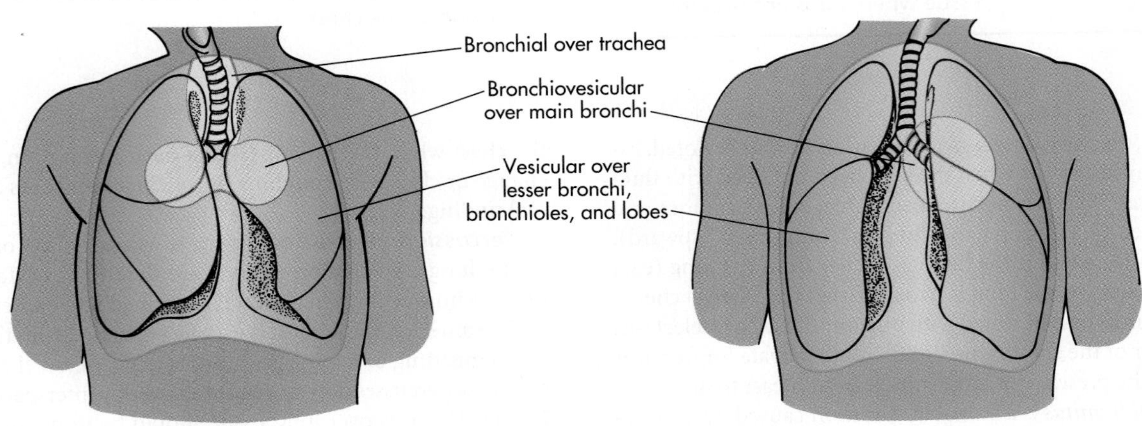

Fig. 24-14 Normal auscultatory sounds.

24-9. Chest examination findings in common pulmonary problems are presented in Table 24-10. Age-related changes in the respiratory system and assessment findings are presented in Table 24-4.

DIAGNOSTIC STUDIES OF THE RESPIRATORY SYSTEM

Blood Studies

Common blood studies used to assess the respiratory system are the hemoglobin (Hb), hematocrit (Hct), and ABG determinations (see Table 24-11). Table 24-11 also describes nursing responsibilities associated with these tests.

Oximetry

Oximetry is used to noninvasively monitor SpO_2 and SvO_2 (see Tables 24-1 and 24-2). Nursing care associated with oximetry is discussed in Table 24-11.

Sputum Studies

Sputum samples can be obtained by expectoration or bronchoscopy, a technique in which a flexible scope is inserted into

COMMON ASSESSMENT ABNORMALITIES

Table 24-9 Thorax and Lungs

Finding	Description	Possible Etiology and Significance*
Inspection		
■ Pursed-lip breathing	Exhalation through mouth with lips pursed together to slow exhalation.	COPD, asthma. Suggests ↑ breathlessness. Strategy taught to slow expiration, ↓ dyspnea.
■ Tripod position; inability to lie flat	Leaning forward with arms and elbows supported on overbed table.	COPD, asthma in exacerbation, pulmonary edema. Indicates moderate to severe respiratory distress.
■ Accessory muscle use; intercostal retractions	Neck and shoulder muscles used to assist breathing. Muscles between ribs pull in during inspiration.	COPD, asthma in exacerbation, secretion retention. Indicates severe respiratory distress, hypoxemia.
■ Splinting	Voluntary ↓ in tidal volume to ↓ pain on chest expansion.	Thoracic or abdominal incision. Chest trauma, pleurisy.
■ ↑ AP diameter	AP chest diameter equal to lateral. Slope of ribs more horizontal (90°) to spine.	COPD, asthma, cystic fibrosis. Lung hyperinflation. Advanced age.
■ Tachypnea	Rate >20 breaths/min; >25 breaths/min in elderly.	Fever, anxiety, hypoxemia, restrictive lung disease. Magnitude of ↑ above normal rate reflects increased work of breathing.
■ Kussmaul's respirations	Regular, rapid, and deep respirations.	Metabolic acidosis. ↑ in rate aids body in ↑ CO_2 excretion.
■ Cyanosis	Bluish color of skin best seen in earlobes, under the eyelids, or nail beds.	↓ Oxygen transfer in lungs, ↓ cardiac output. Nonspecific, unreliable indicator.
■ Clubbing of fingers	↑ Depth, bulk, sponginess of distal digit of finger.	Chronic hypoxemia. Cystic fibrosis, lung cancer, bronchiectasis.
■ Abdominal paradox	Inward (rather than normal outward) movement of abdomen during inspiration.	Inefficient and ineffective breathing pattern. Nonspecific indicator of severe respiratory distress.
Palpation		
■ Tracheal deviation	Leftward or rightward movement of trachea from normal midline position.	Nonspecific indicator of change in position of mediastinal structures. Medical emergency if caused by tension pneumothorax.
■ Altered tactile fremitus	Increase or decrease in vibrations.	↑ in pneumonia, pulmonary edema; ↓ in pleural effusion, atelectatic area, lung hyperinflation; absent in pneumothorax, large atelectasis.
■ Altered chest movement	Unequal or equal but diminished movement of two sides of chest with inspiration.	Unequal movement caused by atelectasis, pneumothorax, pleural effusion, splinting; equal but diminished movement caused by barrel chest, restrictive disease, neuromuscular disease.
Percussion		
■ Hyperresonance	Loud, lower-pitched sound over areas that normally produce a resonant sound.	Lung hyperinflation (COPD), lung collapse (pneumothorax), air trapping (asthma).
■ Dullness	Medium-pitched sound over areas that normally produce a resonant sound.	↑ Density (pneumonia, large atelectasis), ↑ fluid pleural space (pleural effusion).

Continued

COMMON ASSESSMENT ABNORMALITIES

Table 24-9 Thorax and Lungs—cont'd

Finding	Description	Possible Etiology and Significance*
Auscultation		
▪ Fine crackles	Series of short, explosive, high-pitched sounds heard just before the end of inspiration; result of rapid equalization of gas pressure when collapsed alveoli or terminal bronchioles suddenly snap open; similar sound to that made by rolling hair between fingers just behind ear	Interstitial fibrosis (asbestosis), interstitial edema (early pulmonary edema), alveolar filling (pneumonia), loss of lung volume (atelectasis), early phase of congestive heart failure
▪ Coarse crackles	Series of short, low-pitched sounds caused by air passing through airway intermittently occluded by mucus, unstable bronchial wall, or fold of mucosa; evident on inspiration and, at times, expiration; similar sound to blowing through straw under water; increase in bubbling quality with more fluid	Congestive heart failure, pulmonary edema, pneumonia with severe congestion, COPD
▪ Rhonchi	Continuous rumbling, snoring, or rattling sounds from obstruction of large airways with secretions; most prominent on expiration; change often evident after coughing or suctioning	COPD, cystic fibrosis, pneumonia, bronchiectasis
▪ Wheezes	Continuous high-pitched squeaking sound caused by rapid vibration of bronchial walls; first evident on expiration but possibly evident on inspiration as obstruction of airway increases; possibly audible without stethoscope	Bronchospasm (caused by asthma), airway obstruction (caused by foreign body, tumor), COPD
▪ Stridor	Continuous musical sound of constant pitch; result of partial obstruction of larynx or trachea	Croup, epiglottitis, vocal cord edema after extubation, foreign body
▪ Absent breath sounds	No sound evident over entire lung or area of lung	Pleural effusion, main-stem bronchi obstruction, large atelectasis, pneumonectomy, lobectomy
▪ Pleural friction rub	Creaking or grating sound from roughened, inflamed surfaces of the pleura rubbing together; evident during inspiration, expiration, or both and no change with coughing; usually uncomfortable, especially on deep inspiration	Pleurisy, pneumonia, pulmonary infarct
▪ Bronchophony, whispered pectoriloquy	Spoken or whispered syllable more distinct than normal on auscultation	Pneumonia
▪ Egophony	Spoken "e" similar to "a" on auscultation because of altered transmission of voice sounds	Pneumonia, pleural effusion

*Limited to common etiologic factors. (Further discussion of conditions listed may be found in Chapters 25 through 27.)
AP, anteroposterior; *COPD*, chronic obstructive pulmonary disease.

the airways. The specimens may be examined for culture and sensitivity to identify an infecting organism (e.g., *Mycobacterium, Pneumocystis carinii*) or to confirm a diagnosis (e.g., malignant cells). Nursing responsibilities for specimen collection are given in Table 24-11. Regardless of whether specimen tests are ordered, it is important to observe the sputum for color, blood, volume, and viscosity.

Skin Tests

Skin tests may be performed to test for allergic reactions or exposure to tuberculous bacilli or fungi. Skin tests involve the intradermal injection of an antigen. A positive result indicates that the patient has been exposed to the antigen. It does not indicate that disease is currently present. A negative result indicates that there has been no exposure or there is depression of cell-mediated immunity such as occurs in HIV infection.[21]

Nursing responsibilities are similar for all skin tests. First, to prevent a false-negative reaction, the nurse should be certain that the injection is intradermal and not subcutaneous. After the injection, the sites should be circled and the patient instructed not to remove the marks. When charting adminis-

Table 24-10 Chest Examination Findings in Common Pulmonary Problems

Problem	Inspection	Palpation	Percussion	Auscultation
Chronic bronchitis	Barrel chest; cyanosis	↓ Movement ↑ Fremitus	Hyperresonant or dull if consolidation	Crackles; rhonchi; wheezes
Emphysema	Barrel chest; tripod position; use of accessory muscles	↓ Movement	Hyperresonant or dull if consolidation	Crackles; rhonchi; diminished if no exacerbation
Asthma				
In exacerbation	Prolonged expiration; tripod position; pursed lips	↓ Movement ↓ Fremitus if hyperinflation	Hyperresonance	Wheezes; ↓ breath sounds ominous sign if no improvement (severely diminished air movement)
Not in exacerbation	Normal	Normal	Normal	Normal
Pneumonia	Tachypnea; use of accessory muscles; duskiness or cyanosis	Unequal movement if lobar involvement; ↑ fremitus over affected area	Dull over affected areas	Early: Bronchial sounds Later: Crackles; rhonchi
Atelectasis	No change unless involves entire segment, lobe	If small, no change. If large, ↓ movement; ↑ fremitus	Dull over affected areas	Crackles (may disappear with deep breaths); absent sounds if large
Pulmonary edema	Tachypnea; labored respirations; cyanosis	↓ Movement or normal movement	Dull or normal depending on amount of fluid	Fine or coarse crackles
Pleural effusion	Tachypnea; use of accessory muscles	↓ Movement ↑ Fremitus above effusion; absent fremitus over effusion	Dull	Diminished or absent over effusion; egophony over effusion
Pulmonary fibrosis	Tachypnea	↓ Movement	Normal	Crackles

tration of the antigen, the nurse should draw a diagram of the forearm and hand and label the injection sites. The diagram is especially helpful when more than one test is administered.

When reading test results, the nurse should use a good light. If induration is present, a marking pen should be brought in from the periphery on all four sides of the induration. As the pen touches the raised area, a mark should be made. The nurse then determines the diameter of the induration in millimeters. Reddened, flat areas are not measured.[22,23] See Table 24-12 for a description of reactions that indicate a positive tuberculosis skin test.

Radiographic Studies

Chest X-ray. A chest x-ray is the most commonly used test for respiratory diagnosis. It is also used to assess progression of disease and response to treatment. The most common views used are the posteroanterior and lateral. (See Table 24-11 for nursing responsibilities related to chest x-rays.)

Computed Tomography. A computed tomography (CT) scan may be used to examine cross sections of the entire body. CT scans are used to evaluate areas that are difficult to assess by conventional x-ray, such as the mediastinum, hilum, and pleura. With the addition of a contrast-enhanced medium- or high-resolution technique, all structures of the thorax can be inspected for evidence of disease.[24]

Magnetic Resonance Imaging. While in a strong magnetic field, the alignment of spinning nuclei can be changed with a superimposed radio frequency and the rate at which they return to alignment with the field can be measured. Magnetic resonance imaging (MRI) uses this technique to produce images of body structures. MRI has limited indications. It is most useful when evaluating images near the lung apex or spine and for distinguishing vascular from nonvascular structures.[24]

Ventilation-Perfusion Scan. A ventilation-perfusion ($\dot{V}/\dot{P}$) scan is used primarily to check for the presence of a pulmonary embolus. There is no specific preparation or aftercare. An intravenous (IV) radioisotope is given for the perfusion portion of the test, and the pulmonary vasculature is outlined and photographed. For the ventilation portion, the patient inhales a radioactive gas, which outlines the alveoli, and another photograph is taken. Normal scans show homogeneous radioactivity. Diminished or absent radioactivity suggests lack of perfusion or airflow.

Pulmonary Angiography. Pulmonary angiography is used to confirm the diagnosis of an embolus if findings of the lung scan are inconclusive. A series of x-rays is taken after radiopaque dye is injected into the pulmonary artery. This test also detects congenital and acquired lesions of the pulmonary vessels.

Positron Emission Tomography. Positron emission tomography (PET) scans involve the use of radionuclides with short half-lives. PET scans are used to distinguish benign and malignant solitary pulmonary nodules. Because malignant lung cells have an increased uptake of glucose, the PET scan, which uses an IV glucose preparation, can demonstrate increased uptake of glucose in malignant lung cells.

DIAGNOSTIC STUDIES

Table 24-11 Respiratory System

Study	Description and Purpose	Nursing Responsibility
Blood Studies		
▪ Hemoglobin	Test reflects amount of hemoglobin available for combination with oxygen. Venous blood is used. *Normal level* for adult man is 13.5-18 g/dl (135-180 g/L); *normal level* for adult woman is 12-16 g/dl (120-160 g/L).	Explain procedure and its purpose.
▪ Hematocrit	Test reflects ratio of red blood cells to plasma. Increased hematocrit (polycythemia) found in chronic hypoxemia. Venous blood is used. *Normal* for adult man is 40-54% (0.40-0.54); *normal* for adult woman is 38-47% (0.38-0.47).	Explain procedure and its purpose.
▪ ABGs	Arterial blood is obtained through puncture of radial or femoral artery or through arterial catheter. ABGs are performed to assess acid-base balance,ventilation status, need for oxygen therapy, change in oxygen therapy, or change in ventilator settings.* Continuous ABG monitoring is also possible via a sensor or electrode inserted into the arterial catheter.	Indicate whether patient is using oxygen (percentage, L/min). Avoid change in oxygen therapy or interventions (e.g., suctioning, position change) for 20 min before obtaining sample. Assist with positioning (e.g., palm up, wrist slightly hyperextended if radial artery is used). Collect blood into heparinized syringe. To ensure accurate results, expel all air bubbles, and place sample in ice, unless it will be analyzed in less than 1 min. Apply pressure to artery for 5 min after specimen is obtained to prevent hematoma at the arterial puncture site.
▪ Oximetry	Test monitors arterial or venous oxygen saturation. Device attaches to the earlobe, finger, or nose for SpO_2 monitoring or is contained in a pulmonary artery catheter for SvO_2 monitoring. Oximetry is used for continuous monitoring in ICUs, inpatient and outpatient settings, and exercise testing.†	Apply probe to finger, forehead, earlobe, or bridge of nose. When interpreting SpO_2 and SvO_2 values, first assess patient status and presence of factors that can alter accuracy of pulse oximeter reading. For SpO_2, these include motion, low perfusion, bright lights, use of intravascular dyes, acrylic nails, dark skin color. For SvO_2, these include change in O_2 delivery or O_2 consumption. For SpO_2, notify physician of ±4% change from baseline or ↓ to <90%. For SvO_2, notify physician of ±10% change from baseline or ↓ to <60%.
Sputum Studies		
▪ Culture and sensitivity	Single sputum specimen is collected in a sterile container. Purpose is to diagnose bacterial infection, select antibiotic, and evaluate treatment.	Instruct patient on how to produce a good specimen (see Gram's stain). If patient cannot produce specimen, bronchoscopy may be used (see Fig. 24-15).
▪ Gram's stain	Staining of sputum permits classification of bacteria into gram-negative and gram-positive types. Results guide therapy until culture and sensitivity results are obtained.	Instruct patient to expectorate sputum into the container after coughing deeply. Obtain sputum (mucoidlike), not saliva. Obtain specimen in early morning because secretions collect during night. If unsuccessful, try increasing oral fluid intake unless fluids are restricted. Collect sputum in sterile container (sputum trap) during suctioning or by aspirating secretions from the trachea. Send specimen to laboratory promptly.
▪ Acid-fast smear and culture	Test is performed to collect sputum for acid-fast bacilli (tuberculosis). A series of 3 early morning specimens is used.	Instruct patient on how to produce a good specimen (see Gram's stain). Cover specimen and send to laboratory for analysis.
▪ Cytology	Single sputum specimen is collected in special container with fixative solution. Purpose is to determine presence of abnormal cells that may indicate malignant condition.	Send specimen to laboratory promptly. Instruct patient on how to produce a good specimen (see Gram's stain). If patient cannot produce specimen, bronchoscopy may be used (see Fig. 24-15).
Radiology		
▪ Chest x-ray	Test is used to screen, diagnose, and evaluate change. Most common views are posteroanterior and lateral.	Instruct patient to undress to waist, put on gown, and remove any metal between neck and waist.

Continued

DIAGNOSTIC STUDIES

Table 24-11 Respiratory System—cont'd

Study	Description and Purpose	Nursing Responsibility
▪ Computed tomography (CT)	Test is performed for diagnosis of lesions difficult to assess by conventional x-ray studies, such as those in the hilum, mediastinum, and pleura. Images show structures in cross section.	Same as for chest x-ray.
▪ Magnetic resonance imaging (MRI)	Test is used for diagnosis of lesions difficult to assess by CT scan (e.g., lung apex near the spine).	Same as for chest x-ray. Instruct the patient to remove all metal (e.g., jewelry, watch) before test.
▪ Ventilation-perfusion ($\dot{V}/\dot{Q}$)	Test is used to identify areas of the lung not receiving airflow (ventilation) or blood flow (perfusion). It involves injection of radioisotope and inhalation of small amount of radioactive gas (xenon). A gamma-detecting device is used to record radioactivity. Ventilation without perfusion suggests pulmonary embolus.	Same as for chest x-ray. Also check for dye allergy. No precautions needed afterward because the gas and isotope transmit radioactivity for only a brief interval.
▪ Pulmonary angiogram	Study is used to visualize pulmonary vasculature and locate obstruction or pathologic conditions such as pulmonary embolus. A radiopaque dye is injected, usually through a catheter, into the pulmonary artery or right side of the heart.	Same as for chest x-ray. Know that dye injection may cause flushing, warm sensation, and coughing. Check pressure dressing site after procedure. Monitor blood pressure, pulse rate, and circulation distal to injection site. Report and record significant changes.
▪ Positron emission tomography (PET)	Test is used to distinguish benign and malignant lung nodules. It involves IV injection of a radioisotope with short half-life.	Same as for chest x-ray study. No precautions needed afterward because isotope only transmits radioactivity for brief interval.
Endoscopic Examinations		
▪ Bronchoscopy	Study is typically performed in outpatient procedure room. Flexible fiberoptic scope is used for diagnosis, biopsy, specimen collection, or assessment of changes. It may also be done to suction mucous plugs or to remove foreign objects.	Instruct patient to be on NPO status for 6-12 hr. Obtain signed permit. Give diazepam (Valium) if ordered by physician before procedure to aid relaxation. After procedure, keep patient NPO until gag reflex returns and monitor for laryngeal edema. If biopsy was done, monitor for hemorrhage and pneumothorax.
▪ Mediastinoscopy	Test is used for inspection and biopsy of lymph nodes in mediastinal area.	Prepare patient for surgical intervention. Obtain signed permit. Afterward, monitor as for bronchoscopy.
Biopsy		
▪ Lung biopsy	Specimens may be obtained by transbronchial or open-lung biopsy. This test is used to obtain specimens for laboratory analysis.	Same as bronchoscopy if procedure done with bronchoscope, and same as thoracotomy if open-lung biopsy done. Obtain signed permit.
Other		
▪ Thoracentesis	Test is used to obtain specimen of pleural fluid for diagnosis, to remove pleural fluid, or to instill medication. The physician inserts a large-bore needle through the chest wall into pleural space. Chest x-ray is always obtained after procedure to check for pneumothorax.	Explain procedure to patient and obtain signed permit before procedure. Position patient upright, instruct not to talk or cough, and assist during procedure. Observe for signs of inadequate oxygenation after procedure. If large volume of fluid is removed, monitor for decrease in shortness of breath. Send labeled specimens to laboratory.
▪ Pulmonary function test	Test is used to evaluate lung function. It involves use of a spirometer to diagram air movement as patient performs prescribed respiratory maneuvers.†	Avoid scheduling immediately after mealtime. Avoid administration of inhaled bronchodilator for 6 hr before procedure. Explain procedure to patient. Provide rest after the procedure.

*For normal values, see Tables 24-1 and 24-2.
†For normal values see Tables 24-12 and 24-13.
ABGs, arterial blood gases; *ICUs,* intensive care units; *IV,* intravenous; *NPO,* nothing by mouth.

Table 24-12 Interpreting Skin Reactions to Tuberculosis Testing

Size of Induration	Consider Positive in the Following Groups
5 mm or greater	▪ Recent close contact with person diagnosed with infectious TB. ▪ Chest x-ray with fibrotic lesions likely to be healed TB. ▪ Known or suspected HIV infection.
10 mm or greater	▪ Other medical risk factors known to substantially ↑ risk of TB once infection has occurred (e.g., diabetes mellitus, immunosuppressive therapy, end-stage renal disease, cancer of oropharynx or upper GI tract). ▪ Foreign-born from high-prevalence areas (e.g., Southeast Asia, Africa, Latin America). ▪ Medically underserved groups, homeless. ▪ Residents of long-term care facilities, prisons. ▪ IV drug users.
15 mm or greater	▪ All other persons.
False-negative reactions may occur in persons who were infected with TB many years ago and persons with an active current infection.	Causes include the following: ▪ Immunosuppression, overwhelming TB infection. ▪ Testing too soon after exposure to TB (up to 10 wk may be required to develop immune response). ▪ Aging (may result in decrease in delayed-type hypersensitivity). ▪ Long time since TB infection. Sensitivity to tuberculin may wane over the years, resulting in a negative reaction. However, the tuberculin test may stimulate (boost) ability to react to tuberculin, causing a positive reaction to future tests.
10-25% of persons with TB have a negative reaction if tested with tuberculin.	*Two-step testing* is therefore recommended for individuals likely to be tested often (i.e., health care providers and individuals who may have decrease in delayed hypersensitivity). Interpret as follows: ▪ 1st test positive, consider the person infected. ▪ 1st test negative, repeat 1-3 wk later. ▪ 2nd test positive, consider active or prior infection (depending on risk factors) and care for accordingly. ▪ 2nd test negative, consider uninfected. Interpret future positive test as a new infection.

GI, gastrointestinal; *HIV*, human immunodeficiency virus; *TB*, tuberculosis.

Endoscopic Examinations

Bronchoscopy. Bronchoscopy is a procedure in which the bronchi are visualized through a fiberoptic tube. Bronchoscopy may be used to obtain biopsy specimens, assess changes resulting from treatment, and remove mucous plugs or foreign bodies. Small amounts (30 ml) of sterile saline may be injected through the scope and withdrawn and examined for cells, a technique termed *bronchoalveolar lavage* (BAL). BAL is used to diagnose *Pneumocystis carinii* pneumonia (Fig. 24-15).[25]

Bronchoscopy can be performed in an outpatient procedure room, surgical suite, or at the bedside in ICU or on a medical-surgical floor, with the patient lying down or seated. After the nasal pharynx and oral pharynx are anesthetized with local anesthetic, the bronchoscope is coated with lidocaine (Xylocaine) and inserted, usually through the nose, and threaded down into the airways. Bronchoscopy can be done on mechanically ventilated patients. The scope is inserted through the endotracheal tube. The nursing care for this procedure is described in Table 24-11.

Mediastinoscopy. For mediastinoscopy, a scope is inserted through a small incision in the suprasternal notch and advanced into the mediastinum to inspect and biopsy lymph nodes. The test is used to diagnose carcinoma, granulomatous infections, and sarcoidosis. The procedure is performed in the operating room and the patient is given a general anesthetic.[25]

Lung Biopsy

Lung biopsy may be done transbronchially or as an open-lung biopsy. The purpose is to obtain tissue, cells, or secretions for evaluation. Transbronchial lung biopsy involves passing a forceps or needle through the bronchoscope. A specimen is obtained with forceps or aspirated through a needle (Fig. 24-16). Specimens can be cultured or examined for malignant cells. A combination of transbronchial lung biopsy and BAL is used to differentiate infection and rejection in lung transplant recipients. Nursing care is the same as for fiberoptic bronchoscopy. Open-lung biopsy is used when pulmonary disease cannot be diagnosed by other procedures. The patient is anesthetized, the chest is opened with a thoracotomy incision, and a biopsy specimen is obtained. Nursing care for the procedure is the same as for any patient who has a thoracotomy (see Chapter 26).

Thoracentesis

Thoracentesis is the insertion of a needle through the chest wall into the pleural space to obtain specimens for diagnostic evaluation, remove pleural fluid, and instill medication into the pleural space (Fig. 24-17). The patient is positioned sitting up-

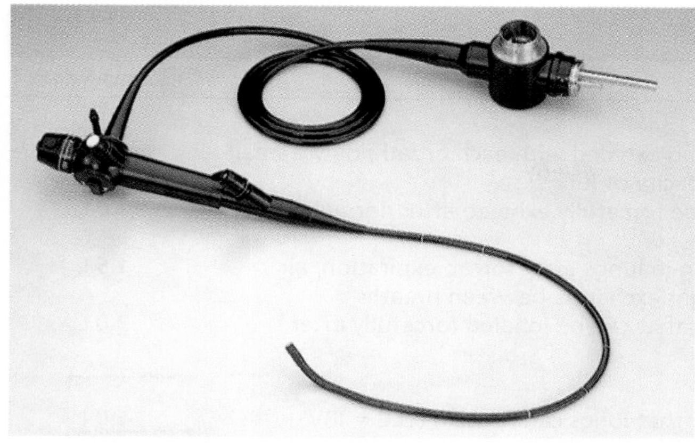

A

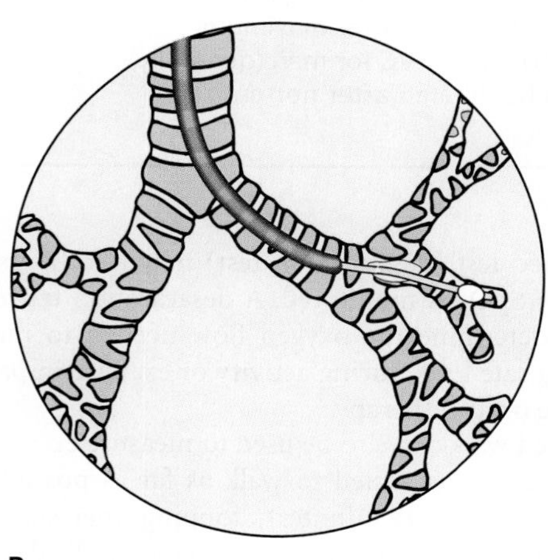

B

Fig. 24-15 Fiberoptic bronchoscope. **A,** The transbronchoscopic balloon-tipped catheter and the flexible fiberoptic bronchoscope. **B,** The catheter is introduced into a small airway and the balloon inflated with 1.5 to 2 ml air to occlude the airway. Bronchial alveolar lavage is performed by injecting and withdrawing 30 ml aliquots of sterile saline solution, gently aspirating after each instillation. Specimens are sent to the laboratory for analysis.

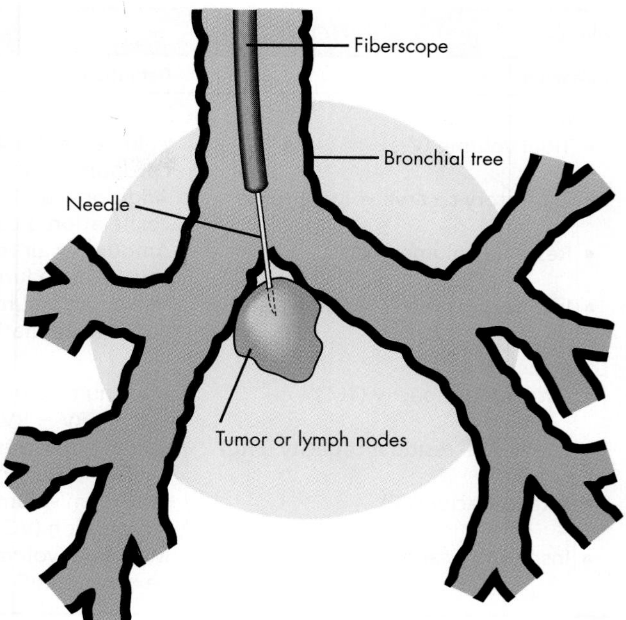

Fig. 24-16 Transbronchial needle biopsy. The diagram shows a transbronchial biopsy needle penetrating the bronchial wall and entering a mass of subcarinal lymph nodes or tumor.

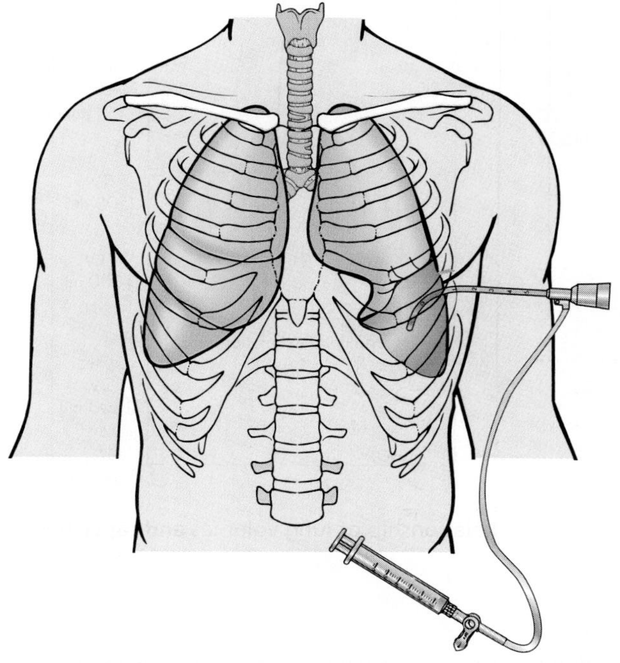

Fig. 24-17 Thoracentesis. The needle has penetrated the fluid-filled pleural space to remove fluid.

right with elbows on an overbed table. Feet and legs should be well supported. The skin is cleansed and a local anesthetic (Xylocaine) is instilled subcutaneously. A chest tube may be inserted to permit further drainage of fluid.[25] (Nursing care is described in Table 24-11.)

Pulmonary Function Tests

Pulmonary function tests (PFTs) measure lung volumes and airflow. The results of PFTs are used to diagnose pulmonary disease, monitor disease progression, evaluate disability, and evaluate response to bronchodilators. PFTs are performed with the use of a spirometer. The patient's age, sex, height, and weight are first obtained. This information is entered into the PFT computer and used to calculate the predicted value for each test. The patient inserts a mouthpiece, takes as deep a breath as possible, and exhales as hard, fast, and long as possible. Verbal coaching is given to ensure that the patient continues blowing out until exhalation is complete. The computer determines the actual value, predicted (normal) value, and percentage of the predicted value for each test. A normal value is 80% to 120% of the predicted value. Normal values for PFTs are shown in Tables 24-13 and 24-14 and Fig. 24-18.

Table 24-13 Lung Volumes and Capacities

Parameter	Definition	Normal Values
Volumes		
▪ Tidal volume (VT)	Volume of air inhaled and exhaled with each breath; only a small proportion of total capacity of lungs	0.5 L
▪ Expiratory reserve volume (ERV)	Additional air that can be forcefully exhaled after normal exhalation is complete	1.0 L
▪ Residual volume (RV)	Amount of air remaining in lungs after forced expiration; air available in lungs for gas exchange between breaths	1.5 L
▪ Inspiratory reserve volume (IRV)	Maximum volume of air that can be inhaled forcefully after normal inhalation	3.0 L
Capacities		
▪ Total lung capacity (TLC)X	Maximum volume of air that lungs can contain (TLC = IRV + VT + ERV + RV)	6.0 L
▪ Functional residual capacity (FRC)	Volume of air remaining in lungs at end of normal exhalation (FRC = ERV + RV); increase or decrease possible with lung disease	2.5 L
▪ Vital capacity (VC)	Maximum volume of air that can be exhaled after maximum inspiration (VC = IRV + VT + ERV); higher VC for men (generally)	4.5 L
▪ Inspiratory capacity (IC)	Maximum volume of air that can be inhaled after normal expiration (IC = VT + IRV)	3.5 L

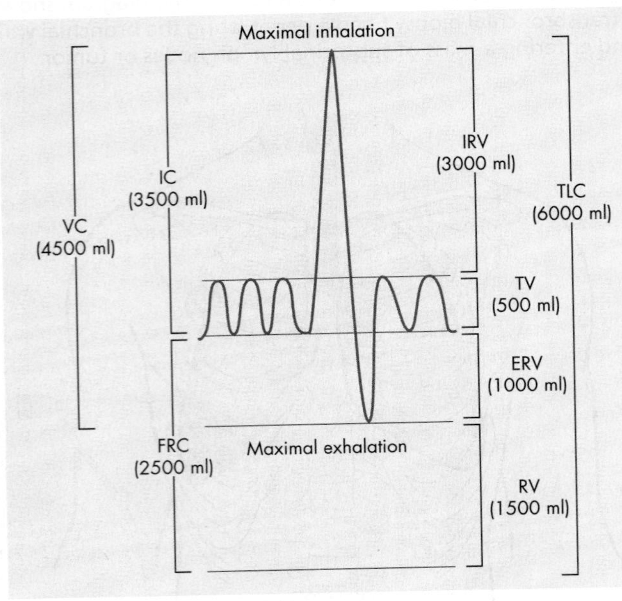

Fig. 24-18 Relationship of lung volumes and capacities.

Pulmonary function parameters can also be used to determine the need for mechanical ventilation or the readiness to be weaned from ventilatory support. Measurements of vital capacity, maximum inspiratory pressure, and minute ventilation are used to make this determination (see Table 24-13).[26]

Exercise Testing

Exercise testing is used in diagnosis, in determining exercise capacity, and for disability evaluation. A complete exercise test involves walking on a treadmill while expired oxygen and carbon dioxide, respiratory rate, heart rate, and rhythm are monitored.

A modified test (desaturation test) may also be used. In this case, only SpO_2 is monitored. A desaturation test can also be used to determine the oxygen flow needed to maintain the SpO_2 at a safe level during activity or exercise in patients who use home oxygen therapy.

A timed walk can also be used to measure exercise capacity. The patient is instructed to walk as far as possible during a timed period (6 or 12 minutes), stopping when short of breath, and continuing when able. The distance walked is measured and used to monitor progression of disease or improvement after rehabilitation.[27]

REVIEW QUESTIONS

The number of the question corresponds to the same-numbered objective at the beginning of the chapter.

1. The mechanism that stimulates the release of surfactant is
   a. deep breathing that stretches the alveoli.
   b. collapse of the alveoli that activates type I cells.
   c. activation of type II cells by fluid accumulation in the alveoli.
   d. movement of air from alveolus to alveolus through the pores of Kohn.
2. During inspiration, air enters the thoracic cavity as a result of
   a. stimulation of the respiratory muscles by the chemoreceptors.
   b. an increase in carbon dioxide and decrease in oxygen in the blood.
   c. decrease in intrathoracic pressure relative to pressure at the airway.
   d. an increase in intrathoracic pressure relative to pressure at the airway.
3. The ability of the lungs to adequately oxygenate the arterial blood is determined by examination of the
   a. arterial oxygen tension.
   b. carboxyhemoglobin level.
   c. arterial carbon dioxide tension.
   d. venous carbon dioxide tension.

Table 24-14 Common Measures of Pulmonary Function

Measure	Description	Normal Value*
▪ Forced vital capacity (FVC)	Amount of air that can be quickly and forcefully exhaled after maximum inspiration	Over 80% of predicted
▪ Forced expiratory volume in first second of expiration (FEV_1)	Amount of air exhaled in first second of FVC; valuable clue to severity of airway obstruction	Over 80% of predicted
▪ FEV_1/FVC	Dividing of value for FEV_1 by value for FVC; useful in differentiating obstructive and restrictive pulmonary dysfunction	Over 80% of predicted
▪ Forced midexpiratory flow rate ($FEF_{25\text{-}75\%}$)	Measurement of airflow rate in middle half of forced expiration; early indicator of disease of small airways	Over 80% of predicted
▪ Maximal voluntary ventilation (MVV)	Deep breathing as rapidly as possible for specified period; test for airflow, muscle strength, coordination, airway resistance; important factor in exercise tolerance	About 170 L/min
▪ Peak expiratory flow rate (PEFR)	Maximum airflow rate during forced expiration; aid in monitoring bronchoconstriction in asthma	Up to 600 L/min
▪ Maximum inspiratory pressure (MIP) or negative inspiratory force (NIF)	Amount of negative pressure generated on inspiration; indication of ability to breathe deeply and cough	<-80 cm H_2O

*Normal values vary with height, weight, age, and sex of patient.

4. The most important respiratory defense mechanism distal to the respiratory bronchioles is the
   a. impaction of particles.
   b. alveolar macrophage.
   c. reflex bronchoconstriction.
   d. mucociliary clearance mechanism.
5. A rightward shift of the oxygen-hemoglobin dissociation curve
   a. is caused by metabolic alkalosis.
   b. facilitates release of oxygen at the tissue level.
   c. interferes with release of oxygen at the tissue level.
   d. causes oxygen to have a greater affinity for hemoglobin.
6. Very early signs or symptoms of inadequate oxygenation include
   a. dyspnea and hypotension.
   b. cyanosis and cool clammy skin.
   c. unexplained apprehension and restlessness.
   d. increased urine output and diaphoresis.
7. During the respiratory assessment of the older adult the nurse would expect to find
   a. decreased pH and increased $PaCO_2$ levels.
   b. increased breath sounds in the lung apices.
   c. an increase in the anterior-posterior chest diameter.
   d. an early rise in respiratory rate in response to hypercapnia.
8. When assessing activity-exercise patterns related to respiratory health, the nurse inquires about
   a. dyspnea during rest or exercise.
   b. recent weight loss or weight gain.
   c. willingness to wear oxygen in public.
   d. ability to sleep through the entire night.
9. When percussing the chest, the nurse should compare sounds heard
   a. at the lung base and apex.
   b. on the anterior and posterior chest.
   c. over the scapulae and manubrium.
   d. on the left and right anterior and posterior chest in the same areas.
10. Normal assessment findings of the respiratory system include
    a. inspiratory chest expansion of 1 inch.
    b. percussion dullness over the lung bases.
    c. bronchovesicular sounds heard over the manubrium.
    d. presence of fremitus greater in the lower lobes than between the scapulae.
11. A diagnostic study that is most likely to be normal in a patient with pneumonia is
    a. oximetry.
    b. chest x-ray.
    c. sputum C & S.
    d. pulmonary angiogram.

References

1. Nai-San W: Anatomy. In Dail DH, Hammer SP, editors: *Pulmonary pathology,* ed 2, New York, 1994, Springer-Verlag.
2. Light RW: Mechanics of respiration. In George RB and others, editors: *Chest medicine: essentials of pulmonary and critical care medicine,* ed 3, Baltimore, 1995, Williams & Wilkins.
3. Dettemeier PA: *Pulmonary nursing care,* St Louis, 1992, Mosby.
4. Kersten LD: *Comprehensive respiratory nursing: a decision-making approach,* Philadelphia, 1989, Saunders.
5. Elpern EH and others: Pulmonary aspiration in mechanically ventilated patients with tracheostomies, *Chest* 105:563, 1994.
6. Peters JI, Levine SM: Lung transplantation. In George RB and others, editors: *Chest medicine: essentials of pulmonary and critical care medicine,* ed 3, Baltimore, 1995, Williams & Wilkins.
7. Light RW: Diseases of the pleura, mediastinum, chest wall, and diaphragm. In George RB and others, editors: *Chest medicine: essentials of pulmonary and critical care medicine,* ed 3, Baltimore, 1995, Williams & Wilkins.
8. Shoemaker WC, Parsa MH: Invasive and noninvasive physiologic monitoring. In Shoemaker WC and others, editors: *Textbook of critical care,* ed 3, Philadelphia, 1995, Saunders.

*9. Noll ML, Byers JF: Usefulness of measures of SvO_2, SpO_2, vital signs and derived dual oximetry parameters as indicators of arterial blood variables during weaning of cardiac surgery patients from mechanical ventilation, *Heart Lung* 24:220, 1995.

10. Schapira RM, Reinke LF: The outpatient diagnosis and management of chronic obstructive pulmonary disease: pharmacotherapy, administration of supplemental oxygen, and smoking cessation techniques, *J Gen Intern Med* 10:40, 1995.
11. Gong H: Air travel and oxygen therapy in cardiopulmonary patients, *Chest* 101:1104, 1992.
12. Pfister SM: Home oxygen therapy: indications, administration, recertification, and patient education, *Nurse Pract* 20:44, 1995.
13. Wanner A, Salathe M, O'Riordan T: Mucociliary clearance in the airways, *Am J Respir Crit Care Med* 154:1868, 1996.
14. Cotes JE: Physiology in the aging lung. In Crystal RG, West JB, Weibel ER, Barnes PJ, editors: *The lung: scientific foundations,* ed 2, Philadelphia, 1997, Lippincott-Raven.
15. Goroll AH, May LA, Mulley AG: *Primary care medicine, office evaluation and management of the adult patient,* ed 3, Philadelphia,1995, Lippincott.
16. Centers for Disease Control and Prevention: Prevention of pneumococcal disease: recommendations of the advisory committee on immunization practices, Atlanta, *MMWR,* Department of Health and Human Services 46, 1997.
17. Incalzi RA and others: Chronic obstructive pulmonary disease: an original model of cognitive decline, *Am Rev Respir Dis* 148:418, 1993.
18. Ries AL and others: Effects of pulmonary rehabilitation on physiologic and psychosocial outcomes in patients with chronic obstructive pulmonary disease, *Ann Intern Med* 122:823, 1995.
19. Bates B: *A visual guide to physical examination, thorax and lungs,* ed 3 (23 minute videocassette), Philadelphia, 1995, Lippincott.
20. Repasky TM: Tension pneumothorax, *AJN* 94:47, 1994.
21. Sasse S, Kramer F: Infectious and noninfectious pulmonary complications in patients infected with the human immunodeficiency virus. In George RB and others, editors: *Chest medicine: essentials of pulmonary and critical care medicine,* ed 3, Baltimore, 1995, Williams & Wilkins.
22. Sibilano H: TB or not TB: the tuberculosis index of suspicion nursing assessment tool, *Perspect Respir Nurs* 7:1, 1996.
23. Centers for Disease Control and Prevention: *Core curriculum on tuberculosis,* ed 3, Atlanta, 1994, Department of Health and Human Services.
24. Sostman HD, Matthay RA: Chest imaging. In George RB and others, editors: *Chest medicine: essentials of pulmonary and critical care medicine,* ed 3, Baltimore, 1995, Williams & Wilkins.
25. Anderson WM, Light RW: Invasive diagnostic procedures. In George RB, Light RW, Matthay MA, Matthay RA, editors: *Chest medicine: essentials of pulmonary and critical care medicine,* ed 3, Baltimore, 1995, Williams & Wilkins.
26. American Thoracic Society: Standardization of spirometry, 1994 update, *Am J Respir Crit Care Med* 152:1107, 1995.
27. Steele B: Timed walking tests of exercise capacity in chronic cardiopulmonary illness, *J Cardiopulm Rehabil* 16:25, 1996.

*

Resources

Resources for this chapter are listed after Chapter 27 on p. 715.

*Nursing research-based articles.

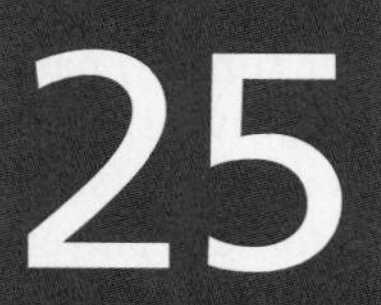

REMEMBER to check out your companion CD-ROM

25 NURSING MANAGEMENT Upper Respiratory Problems

Margaret M. Hickey & Leslie A. Hoffman

www.mosby.com/MERLIN/medsurg_lewis

LEARNING OBJECTIVES

1. Describe the clinical manifestations and nursing management of problems of the nose.
2. Describe the clinical manifestations and nursing management of problems of the paranasal sinuses.
3. Describe the clinical manifestations and nursing management of problems of the pharynx and larynx.
4. Discuss the nursing management of the patient who requires a tracheostomy.
5. Identify the steps involved in performing tracheostomy care and suctioning an airway.
6. Describe the risk factors and warning symptoms associated with head and neck cancer.
7. Discuss the nursing management of the patient with a laryngectomy.
8. Describe the methods used in voice restoration for the patient with temporary or permanent loss of speech.

The structures that make up the upper respiratory tract are the nose, paranasal sinuses, pharynx, larynx, and trachea. As a person breathes these structures are subjected to repeated exposure to microorganisms, fumes, gases, and carcinogens. For this reason, disorders that involve the upper respiratory tract are common.

STRUCTURAL AND TRAUMATIC DISORDERS OF THE NOSE

DEVIATED SEPTUM

Deviated septum is a deflection of the normally straight nasal septum. It is most commonly caused by trauma to the nose or congenital disproportion, a condition in which the size of the septum is not proportional to the size of the nose. On inspection, the septum is bent to one side, altering the air passage. Symptoms are variable. The patient may experience obstruction to nasal breathing, nasal edema, or dryness of the nasal mucosa with crusting and bleeding (epistaxis). A severely deviated septum may block drainage of mucus from the sinus cavities, resulting in infection (sinusitis). Nasal breathing is subjective, and only the patient can gauge the degree of obstruction and amount of discomfort it causes.[1]

Health promotion is aimed at prevention of precipitating factors, such as accidental falls in childhood. Medical management of deviated septum includes the use of decongestants or a nasal corticosteroid spray to reduce nasal edema (Fig. 25-1). Surgery is an option for patients with severe symptoms. A nasal septoplasty is performed to reconstruct and properly align the deviated septum. Nasal septoplasty can be performed alone or with a rhinoplasty. Complications are rare.

NASAL FRACTURE

Nasal fracture is most often caused by trauma of substantial force to the middle of the face. Complications of the fracture include airway obstruction, epistaxis, and cosmetic deformity. Nasal fractures are classified as unilateral, bilateral, or complex. A unilateral fracture typically produces little or no displacement. Bilateral fractures, the most common fractures, give the nose a flattened look. Powerful frontal blows cause complex fractures, which may also shatter frontal bones. Diagnosis is based on the health history, direct observation, and x-ray findings.

On inspection, the nurse should assess the patient's ability to breathe through each side of the nose and note the presence of edema, bleeding, or hematoma. There may be ecchymosis under one or both eyes. Ecchymosis involving both eyes is often termed *raccoon eyes.* The nose is inspected internally for evidence of septal deviation, hemorrhage, or clear drainage, which suggests leakage of cerebrospinal fluid (CSF). If clear drainage is observed, a specimen may be sent to the laboratory to determine if it is CSF. Injury of sufficient force to fracture nasal bones results in considerable swelling of soft tissues. With extensive swelling, it may be difficult to verify the extent of deformity or to repair the fracture until several days later when edema is subsiding.

The goals of nursing management are to reduce edema, prevent complications, educate the patient, and provide emotional support. Ice may be applied to the face and nose to reduce edema and bleeding. When a fracture is confirmed, the goal of management is to realign the fracture using closed or open

Reviewed by Michele Geiger-Bronsky, RN, MSN, CS, FAACVPR, Nurse Practitioner/Respiratory Clinical Nurse Specialist, Maritime Health Works, Manitowoc, Wisc.

Before using the inhaler, gently blow your nose, making sure your nostrils are clear.

Then follow these steps:

1. Remove the protective cap from the nasal inhaler.
2. Shake the canister well.
3. Hold the inhaler between the thumb and forefinger.
4. Tilt the head back slightly and insert the end of the inhaler into one nostril, pointing it slightly toward the outside nostril wall. Hold the other nostril closed with one finger.
5. Press down on the canister to release one dose and, at the same time, inhale gently.
6. Hold your breath for a few seconds, then breathe out slowly through the mouth.
7. Withdraw the inhaler from the nostril and repeat the process for the other nostril. If more than one puff is prescribed per nostril, repeat steps 4-6.
8. Replace the protective cap on the inhaler.

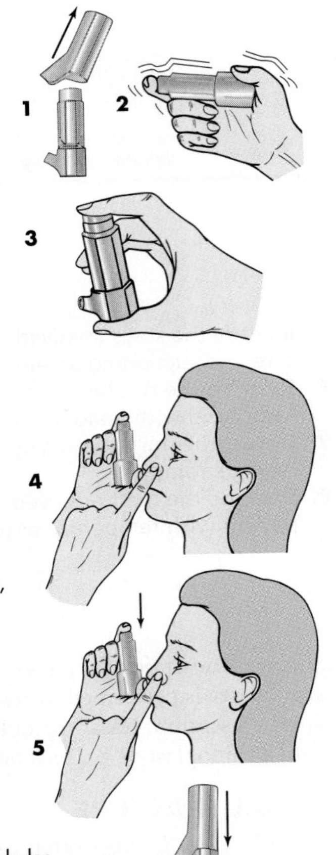

Fig. 25-1 Method for using an intranasal inhaler.

reduction (septoplasty, rhinoplasty). These procedures reestablish cosmetic appearance and proper function of the nose and provide an adequate airway.

RHINOPLASTY

Rhinoplasty, the surgical reconstruction of the nose, is performed for cosmetic reasons or to improve airway function when trauma or developmental deformities result in nasal obstruction. Assessment of the patient's expectations is a critical aspect of preparation for rhinoplasty. Any actual or perceived alteration in body image (e.g., a deformed or enlarged nose) can affect self-esteem and interactions with others. The patient's expectations concerning surgical results should be assessed with regard to the expected change. Photographs made to life-size measurements can be used to simulate appearance after the surgery and may help the patient decide whether to undergo rhinoplasty. Expected results of surgery should be explained frankly and truthfully to avoid disappointment.

Collaborative Care

Rhinoplasty is performed as an outpatient procedure using regional anesthesia. Nasal tissue may be added or removed, and the nose may be lengthened or shortened. Plastic implants are sometimes used to reshape the nose. After surgery, nasal packing may be inserted to apply pressure and prevent bleeding or septal hematoma formation. Nasal septal splints (small pieces of plastic or Silastic) may be inserted to help prevent scar tissue formation between the surgical site and lateral nasal wall. An external plastic splint is molded to the new shape of the nose and placed on the nose. Steri-Strips are placed to hold the skin against the septal cartilage. Typically, nasal packing is removed the day after surgery, and the splint is removed in 3 to 5 days.

NURSING MANAGEMENT: NASAL SURGERY

Examples of nasal surgery include rhinoplasty, septoplasty, and nasal fracture reductions. Before surgery, the patient should be instructed to not take aspirin-containing drugs for 2 weeks to reduce the risk of bleeding. Nursing interventions during the immediate postoperative period include assessment of respiratory status, pain management, and observation of the surgical site for hemorrhage and edema. Health teaching is important because these procedures involve a short hospital stay and the patient must be able to detect early and late complications. The final outcome is often pleasing to the patient. There is an interim period while edema and ecchymosis resolve before the final effect can be appreciated. Nursing diagnoses for the patient undergoing nasal surgery include, but are not limited to, those presented in NCP 25-1.

EPISTAXIS

Epistaxis (nosebleed) occurs in all age-groups, especially in children and the elderly. Epistaxis may be caused by trauma, foreign bodies, nasal spray abuse, illicit drug abuse, anatomic malformation, allergic rhinitis, or tumors. Any condition that prolongs bleeding time or alters platelet counts will also predispose the patient to epistaxis. Bleeding time may also be prolonged if the patient takes aspirin or nonsteroidal antiinflammatory drugs (NSAIDs). Conditions such as hypertension increase the risk of epistaxis if the blood pressure is elevated.

Children and young adults have a tendency to develop anterior nasal bleeding, whereas older adults more commonly have posterior nasal bleeding. Anterior bleeding occurs most frequently in Little's area on the anterior nasal septum, where several arteries join together. Within Little's area is Kiesselbach's plexus, a rich venous network vulnerable to trauma. Posterior bleeding usually occurs high on the nasal septum. A common area of bleeding is Woodruff's plexus, an area under the posterior portion of the inferior turbinate. Anterior bleeding usually stops spontaneously or can be self-treated, but posterior bleeding may require medical care.[1-3]

NURSING AND COLLABORATIVE MANAGEMENT: EPISTAXIS

Simple first aid measures should be used first to control epistaxis. The nurse should (1) keep the patient quiet; (2) place the patient in a sitting position, leaning forward, or if not possible,

25-1 NURSING CARE PLAN PATIENT WITH NASAL SURGERY (RHINOPLASTY, SEPTOPLASTY, NASAL FRACTURE REDUCTION)

Expected Patient Outcomes	Nursing Interventions and *Rationales*
NURSING DIAGNOSIS	**Altered health maintenance** *related to* lack of knowledge of postoperative course, pain management, and prevention of complications *as manifested by* questioning about care, anxiety.
▪ Able to verbalize correct information about expected routine and self-care.	▪ Explain surgical procedure, expected postoperative course, and required self-care *to decrease anxiety and increase patient cooperation.* ▪ Answer questions as needed. ▪ Assess patient perceptions about body image and expectation of surgery *to obtain information to use in patient care.*
NURSING DIAGNOSIS	**Ineffective breathing pattern** *related to* presence of packing, nasal edema, or intranasal splints *as manifested by* complaint of shortness of breath, alteration in respiratory rate, rhythm, or depth.
▪ Normal respiratory rate, rhythm, and depth. ▪ Pulse oximetry >90% (if ordered). ▪ Minimal to no swelling or bruising.	▪ Assess for respiratory distress. ▪ Elevate head of bed. ▪ Provide supplemental oxygen, if prescribed. ▪ Instruct patient not to blow nose; open mouth when sneezing and coughing *to maintain correct position of packing.* ▪ Apply cold compresses to incisional area *to promote vasoconstriction and reduce edema.* ▪ Instruct patient to call (if discharged) or inform the nurse (if hospitalized) if there is increased difficulty breathing or packing becomes dislodged *to allow early intervention to prevent respiratory distress.*
NURSING DIAGNOSIS	**Pain** *related to* edema from the surgical procedure *as manifested by* report of pain.
▪ Minimal or no pain.	▪ Teach patient correct analgesic schedule *to foster appropriate use of medications to prevent pain.* ▪ Describe to patient the amount of pain expected *to decrease anxiety and foster report of excessive pain, which could indicate a complication.* ▪ Teach patient nonpharmacologic measures (e.g., elevation of the head of the bed and application of cold compresses) *to minimize facial swelling and pain from edema.* ▪ Provide frequent mouth care and lubricate lips *to promote moist mucous membranes.* ▪ Teach patient to avoid use of aspirin and nonsteroidal antiinflammatory medications *because these drugs prolong bleeding time.* ▪ Teach patient gentle cleaning techniques, such as use of cotton swabs with hydrogen peroxide to clean crusting, and application of water-soluble jelly to lubricate when packing has been removed *to promote cleanliness and comfort and to decrease risk of infection.* ▪ Promote use of bedside humidifier *to decrease drying of mucosa and promote comfort.*
NURSING DIAGNOSIS	**Body image disturbance** *related to* postoperative edema and changed facial appearance *as manifested by* verbalization of concern about appearance.
▪ Expression of optimistic feelings about positive surgical outcome.	▪ Inform patient that most facial edema and bruising subsides gradually over several weeks *to decrease anxiety.* (It may take up to 8 months for all edema to subside.) ▪ Help patient to remain realistic regarding surgical results *to avoid disappointment.*

COLLABORATIVE PROBLEMS

Nursing Goals	Nursing Interventions and *Rationales*
POTENTIAL COMPLICATION	**Nasal hemorrhage** *related to* inadequate hemostasis and high vascularity of operative site.
▪ Monitor for signs of bleeding. ▪ Report deviation from acceptable parameter. ▪ Carry out appropriate medical and nursing interventions.	▪ Teach patient to report continued drainage of serosanguineous fluid from operative site after 24 hr and not to take aspirin or nonsteroidal antiinflammatory medications *because aspirin products increase the potential for bleeding.* ▪ Report to physician any fresh bleeding or displacement of the packing *so early treatment of hemorrhage is initiated.*

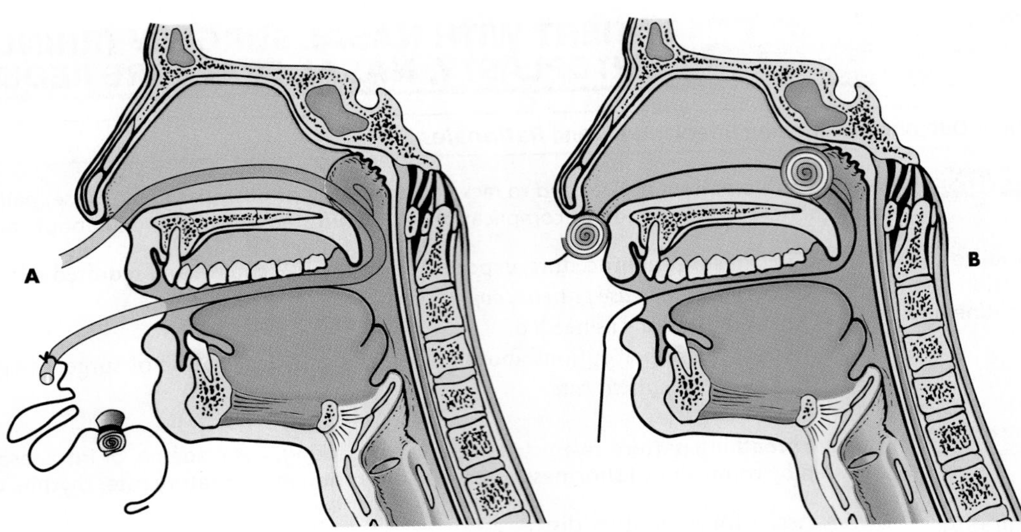

Fig. 25-2 Method for placing posterior nasal pack. **A,** Catheter is passed through the bleeding side of the nose and pulled out through the mouth with a hemostat. Strings are tied to the catheter and the pack is pulled up behind the soft palate and into the nasopharynx. **B,** Nasal pack in position in the posterior nasopharynx. Dental roll at the nose helps maintain correct position.

in a reclining position with head and shoulders elevated; (3) apply direct pressure by pinching the entire soft lower portion of the nose for 10 to 15 minutes; (4) apply ice compresses to the nose, and have the patient suck on ice; (5) partially insert a small gauze pad into the bleeding nostril, and apply digital pressure if bleeding continues; and (6) obtain medical assistance if bleeding does not stop.[2]

If first aid is not effective, management involves localization of the bleeding site and application of a vasoconstrictive agent, cauterization, or anterior packing. Anterior packing may consist of ribbon gauze impregnated with antibiotic ointment that is wedged firmly in the desired location and remains in place for 48 to 72 hours.[2] If posterior packing is required, the patient should be hospitalized. Inflatable balloons may be used as the nasal pack or gauze rolls may be inserted (Fig. 25-2).[3] Strings attached to the packing are brought to the outside and taped to the cheek for ease of removal. A nasal sling (a folded 2 × 2–inch gauze pad) should be taped over the nares to absorb drainage.

Posterior packing may alter consciousness and respiratory status, especially in the elderly. Some patients experience hypoventilation (increase in $PaCO_2$) and hypoxemia (decrease in PaO_2) sufficient to lead to cardiac arrhythmias or respiratory arrest.[3] The nurse should closely monitor respiratory rate, heart rate and rhythm, oxygen saturation using pulse oximetry (SpO_2), and level of consciousness and observe for signs of aspiration and infection. Because of the risk of complications, the patient may be admitted to a monitored unit to permit closer observation.

Packing is painful because sufficient pressure must be applied to stop the bleeding.[2] Nasal packing predisposes to infection from bacteria (e.g., *Staphylococcus aureus*) present in the nasal cavity.[2] The patient should receive a mild narcotic analgesic for pain (e.g., acetaminophen with codeine) and an antibiotic effective against staphylococci to protect against infection.

Posterior packs are left in place for a minimum of 3 days.[3] Before removal, the patient should be medicated for pain, because this procedure is very uncomfortable. After removal, the nares may be gently cleaned and lubricated with petroleum jelly.

Failure of posterior packing to control epistaxis indicates the need for surgery. The most common procedure involves ligation of the internal maxillary artery performed through a Caldwell-Luc incision under the upper lip to gain access to the artery. Ligation of other arteries may also be performed, if indicated.[3]

The patient can be discharged after being taught about home care. The patient should be instructed to avoid vigorous nose blowing, strenuous activity, lifting, and straining for 4 to 6 weeks. The patient should be taught to sneeze with the mouth open and to avoid the use of aspirin-containing products or NSAIDs.

INFLAMMATION AND INFECTION OF THE NOSE AND PARANASAL SINUSES

ALLERGIC RHINITIS

Allergic rhinitis is the reaction of the nasal mucosa to a specific antigen (allergen). Attacks of seasonal rhinitis usually occur in the spring and fall and are caused by allergy to pollens from trees, flowers, or grasses. The typical attack lasts for several weeks during times when pollen counts are high, disappears, and recurs at the same time the following year.[4,5] Perennial rhinitis is present intermittently or constantly. Symptoms are usually caused by specific environmental triggers such as pet dander, dust mites, molds, or particular foods.[4,5] Because symptoms of perennial rhinitis resemble the common cold, the patient may believe the condition is a continuous or repeated cold.

Clinical Manifestations

Manifestations of allergic rhinitis are nasal congestion; sneezing; watery, itchy eyes and nose; altered sense of smell; and thin watery nasal discharge.[4] The nasal turbinates appear pale, boggy, and swollen. The turbinates may fill the air space and

PATIENT & FAMILY HOME CARE GUIDE

Table 25-1 How to Reduce Symptoms of Allergic Rhinitis

1. **Avoidance is the best treatment.**
2. **Avoid house dust.** Use the approach "less is best." Focus on the bedroom. Remove carpeting. Limit furniture. Enclose the pillows, mattress, and springs in air-tight, vinyl encasements. Limit clothing in the bedroom to items used frequently. Place clothing in air-tight, zipper-sealed, vinyl clothes bags. Install an air filter. Close the air-conditioning vent into the room.
3. **Avoid house dust mites.** Wash bedding in hot water (130° F [54° C]) weekly. Wear a mask when vacuuming. Double-bag the vacuum cleaner. Install a filter on the outlet port of the vacuum cleaner. Avoid sleeping or lying on upholstered furniture. Remove carpets that are laid on concrete. If possible, have someone else clean the house.
4. **Avoid mold spores.** The three *D*s that promote growth of mold spores are darkness, dampness, and drafts. Avoid places where humidity is high (e.g., basements, camps on the lake, clothes hampers, greenhouses, stables, barns). Dehumidifiers are rarely helpful. Ventilate closed rooms, open doors, and install fans. Consider adding windows to dark rooms. Consider keeping a small light on in closets. A basement light with a timer that provides light several hours a day may decrease mold growth.
5. **Avoid pollens.** Stay inside with closed doors and windows during high-pollen season. Avoid the use of fans. Install an air conditioner with a good air filter. Wash filters weekly during high pollen season. Put the car air conditioner on "recirculate" when driving. Get someone else to tend to your yard.
6. **Avoid pet allergens.** Remove pets from the interior of the home. Clean the living area thoroughly. Do not expect instant relief. Symptoms usually do not improve significantly for 2 months following pet removal.
7. **Avoid smoke.** The presence of a smoker will sabotage the best of all possible symptom reduction programs.

Adapted from Boggs P: *Sneezing your head off? How to live with your allergic nose,* 1994, Boggs, pp. 125-137.

press against the nasal septum. The posterior ends of the turbinates can become so enlarged that they obstruct sinus aeration or drainage and result in sinusitis. With chronic exposure to allergens, the patient's responses include headache, congestion, pressure, and postnasal drip. The patient may complain of cough, hoarseness, or the recurrent need to clear the throat. Congestion may be sufficient to cause snoring. Nasal polyps may be present if the allergy has persisted for a long time.[4]

NURSING AND COLLABORATIVE MANAGEMENT: ALLERGIC RHINITIS

Several steps are used in managing allergic rhinitis. The most important step involves identifying triggers of allergic reactions (Table 25-1).[5] Drug therapy involves the use of antihistamines, decongestants, and nasal sprays (Table 25-2). An oral antihistamine or oral decongestant is typically used first. If this therapy is not effective, a nasal corticosteroid spray may be used to decrease inflammation. Corticosteroids administered by a nasal spray are poorly absorbed in the systemic circulation. Therefore systemic side effects are rare. Another alternative, a nasal anticholinergic spray, may also be effective in reducing rhinorrhea. Nasal decongestant sprays are not recommended because of the rebound effect from prolonged use.[5] Immunotherapy may be used if medications are not well tolerated, or are ineffective, and a specific allergen can be identified and cannot be avoided. Immunotherapy involves controlled exposure to small amounts of a known antigen through weekly injections with the goal to decrease sensitivity.[5] (Immunotherapy is discussed in Chapter 12.)

The patient should be instructed to keep a diary of times when the allergic reaction occurred and the activities that precipitated the reaction. Steps can then be taken to avoid these triggers. Avoidance is the best therapy (see Table 25-1). The patient receiving drug therapy needs careful instructions about proper use (see Table 25-2). The patient who is using classic antihistamines should be warned about sedative side effects. Nonsedating antihistamines eliminate or reduce drowsiness but are more costly. Intranasal corticosteroid or cromolyn sprays are effective for seasonal and perennial rhinitis. The best relief is often obtained by combining a nasal corticosteroid spray and a nonsedating antihistamine.[4,5]

ACUTE VIRAL RHINITIS

Acute viral rhinitis (common cold or acute coryza) is caused by viruses that invade the upper respiratory tract. It is the most prevalent infectious disease and is spread by airborne droplet sprays emitted by the infected person while breathing, talking, sneezing, or coughing or by direct hand contact. Frequency increases in the winter months, when people stay indoors and overcrowding is more common. Other factors, such as chilling, fatigue, physical and emotional stress, and the patient's compromised immune status, may increase susceptibility. The patient with acute viral rhinitis typically first experiences tickling, irritation, sneezing, or dryness of the nose or nasopharynx, followed by copious nasal secretions, some nasal obstruction, watery eyes, elevated temperature, general malaise, and headache. After the early profuse secretions, the nose becomes more obstructed, and the discharge is thicker. Within a few days the general symptoms improve, nasal passages reopen, and normal breathing is established.[6]

NURSING AND COLLABORATIVE MANAGEMENT: ACUTE VIRAL RHINITIS

Rest, fluids, proper diet, antipyretics, and analgesics are recommended. Complications of acute viral rhinitis include pharyngitis, sinusitis, otitis media, tonsillitis, and chest infections. Unless symptoms of complications are present, antibiotic therapy is not indicated. Antibiotics have no effect on viruses and, if taken injudiciously, may produce resistant organisms.

During the cold season, the patient with a chronic illness or a compromised immune status should be advised to avoid

DRUG THERAPY

Table 25-2 Allergic Rhinitis and Sinusitis

Preparation*	Mechanism of Action	Side Effects	Nursing Actions
Antihistamines **First-Generation Agents** **Ethanolamines** Carbinoxamine (Clistin) Clemastine (Tavist) Diphenhydramine (Benadryl) **Ethylenediamines** Pryilamine (Nisaval) Tripelennamine (PBZ) **Alkylamines** Brompheniramine (Dimetane) Chlorpheniramine (Chlor-Trimeton) Dexchlorpheniramine (Polaramine) Triprolidine (Actidil) **Piperazines** Hydroxyzine (Atarax, Vistaril) Cyclizine (Marezine) **Piperidine** Azatadine (Optimime) **Phenothiazines** Phenothiazine (Phenergan) **Second-Generation Agents** Astemizole (Hismanal)† Loratadine (Claritin)† Cetirizine (Zyrtec)† Fexofenadine (Allegra)† Mizolastine (Mizollen)†	Bind with H_1 receptors on target cells, blocking histamine binding. Relieve acute symptoms of allergic response (itching, sneezing, excessive secretions, mild congestion).	**First-generation agents** cross blood-brain barrier, bind to H_1 receptors in brain. Cause *sedation* (diminished alertness, slow reaction time, somnolence) and *stimulation* (restless, nervous, insomnia). Some drugs (e.g., ethanolamines) are more likely to cause sedation. Patients vary in their sensitivity to these side effects. The next most common side effects involve the GI system and include loss of appetite, epigastric distress, constipation, or diarrhea. May cause palpitations, tachycardia, urinary retention or frequency. Second-generation agents have limited affinity for brain H_1 receptors. Cause minimal sedation, few effects on psychomotor activities, bladder function.	**First generation agents:** ■ Warn patient that operating machinery and driving may be dangerous because of sedative effect. Drowsiness usually passes after 2 weeks of treatment. ■ Teach patient to report palpitations, change in heart rate, change in bowel, bladder habits. ■ Instruct patient not to use alcohol with antihistamines because of additive depressant effect. **Second generation agents:** ■ Teach patient to expect few, if any, side effects. ■ More expensive than classic antihistamines. ■ Rapid onset of action, no drug tolerance with prolonged use. **General interactions:** ■ Do not take with alcohol or any form of tranquilizer or sedative. ■ Do not take with any monamine oxidase inhibitor.
Decongestants **Oral** Pseudoephedrine (Sudafed) Phenylpropanolamine (Dura-Vent) **Topical (Nasal Spray)** Oxymetazoline (Dristan) Phenylephrine (Neo-Synephrine)	Stimulate adrenergic receptors on blood vessels, promote vasoconstriction and reduce nasal edema and rhinorrhea. Same as above.	CNS stimulation, causing insomnia, excitation, headache, irritability, increased blood and ocular pressure, dysuria, palpitations, tachycardia. Same as above, plus rhinitis medicamentosa (rebound nasal congestion).	■ Advise patient of adverse reactions. ■ Advise that some preparations are contraindicated for patients with cardiovascular disease, hypertension, diabetes, glaucoma, prostate hyperplasia, hepatic and renal disease. ■ Teach patient that these drugs should not be used for >3 days or more than 3-4 times a day. Longer use increases risk of rhinitis medicamentosa.
Corticosteroids **Nasal spray** Beclomethasone (Vancenase) Budesonide (Rhinocort) Flunisolide (Nasalide) Fluticasone (Flonase) Triamcinolone (Nasacort)	Inhibits inflammatory response. At recommended dose, systemic side effects are unlikely because of low systemic absorption. Systemic effects may occur with greater than recommended doses.	Mild transient nasal burning and stinging. In rare instances, localized fungal infection with *Candida albicans.*	■ Teach patient correct use (see Fig. 25-1). ■ Instruct patient to use on regular basis and not prn. ■ Reinforce that spray acts to decrease inflammation and effect is not immediate, as with decongestant sprays. ■ Discontinue use if nasal infection develops.

Continued

DRUG THERAPY

Table 25-2 **Allergic Rhinitis and Sinusitis—cont'd**

Preparation*	Mechanism of Action	Side Effects	Nursing Actions
Mast Cell Stabilizer **Nasal spray** Cromolyn spray (Nasalcrom) Nedocromil spray (Tilade)	Inhibits degranulation of sensitized mast cells which occurs after exposure to specific antigens.	Minimal side effects. Occasional burning or nasal irritation.	▪ Teach patient correct use (see Fig. 25-1). ▪ Reinforce that spray prevents symptoms. ▪ Begin 2 weeks before pollen season starts and use throughout pollen season. ▪ If isolated allergy, such as cat, use prophylactically (i.e., 10-15 min before exposure to allergen).
Anticholinergic **Nasal spray** Ipratropium bromide (Atrovent)	Blocks hypersecretory effects by competing for binding sites on the cell. Reduces rhinorrhea in the common cold, allergic and nonallergic rhinitis.	Dryness of the mouth and nose may occur. Does not cause systemic side effects.	▪ Teach patient correct use (see Fig. 25-1). ▪ Reinforce that spray prevents symptoms with onset of action within 1 hr of use. ▪ May reduce the need for other rhinitis medications.

Sources: Hardman JG, Limbird LE, editors: *Goodman & Gilman's the pharmacological basis of therapeutics,* ed 9, New York, 1996, McGraw-Hill. Rang HP and others: *Pharmacology,* New York, 1995, Churchill Livingstone.

*Partial listing of available medications.

†Second-generation antihistamines, generally less sedating.

crowded, close situations and other persons who have obvious cold symptoms. The nurse should recommend that the patient get adequate rest. If the patient cannot avoid such contacts, frequent hand washing and avoiding hand-to-face contact may help prevent direct spread.

Nursing diagnoses for the patient with an upper respiratory infection include, but are not limited to, those presented in NCP 25-2. Interventions are directed toward relieving annoying symptoms. The patient should be encouraged to drink increased amounts of fluids to liquefy secretions. Antihistamine or decongestant therapy reduces postnasal drip and significantly decreases severity of cough, nasal obstruction, and nasal discharge. The patient should also be taught to recognize the symptoms of secondary bacterial infection, such as a temperature higher than 100.4° F (38° C); exudate on the tonsils; tender, swollen glands; and a sore, red throat. In the patient with pulmonary disease, signs of infection include a change in consistency, color, or volume of the sputum. Because infection can progress rapidly, the patient with chronic respiratory disease may be taught to inspect the sputum and to begin antibiotics if these changes occur.[7]

INFLUENZA

Each year influenza (flu) causes significant morbidity and mortality rates. Estimates of influenza-related deaths range from 20,000 in years with low activity to 40,000 in years with severe epidemics. Most deaths occur in persons over 60 years of age with underlying heart or lung disease.[8,9] Influenza is preventable, yet only 50% of persons over 65 and 10% to 15% of those younger than 65 who are at high risk receive vaccination (Table 25-3).

Influenza virus has a remarkable ability to change over time, which accounts for the ability to cause widespread disease. There are three types of virus: A, B, and C. In some years, influenza A virus undergoes an antigenic drift (minor change), whereas in other years it undergoes an antigenic shift (major change). Fewer cases of influenza result when a minor change occurs because most persons have partial immunity. Influenza B virus tends to cause localized outbreaks. Infection with influenza C virus is common but unlikely to cause symptoms. Subtypes are named by the strain, site of isolation, and year (e.g., A/Beijing/184/93-like).[9]

Clinical Manifestations

The onset of flu is typically abrupt with systemic symptoms of headache, fever, chills, and myalgia accompanied by a cough and sore throat. Milder symptoms, similar to the common cold, may also occur. Physical findings are usually minimal with normal assessment on chest auscultation. Dyspnea and diffuse crackles are signs of pulmonary complications. In uncomplicated cases, symptoms subside within 7 days.[9] Some patients, particularly older adults, experience weakness or lassitude that persists for weeks. The convalescent phase may be marked by hyperactive airways and a chronic cough. Important diagnostic factors include the patient's health history, clinical findings, and the presence of other cases of influenza in the community.

The most common complication of influenza is pneumonia. Primary viral influenzal pneumonia is the least common but most serious complication. The patient develops symptoms of

25-2 NURSING CARE PLAN PATIENT WITH UPPER RESPIRATORY INFECTION

Expected Patient Outcomes	Nursing Interventions and *Rationales*
NURSING DIAGNOSIS	**Ineffective airway clearance** *related to* mucosal edema *as manifested by* cough, increased nasal and respiratory secretions, inability to tolerate breathing of cold air.
▪ Decreased or absent cough. ▪ Normal secretion production.	▪ Humidify air as needed *to assist in moisturizing respiratory mucosa.* ▪ Encourage intake of fluids *to assist in liquefying secretions.* ▪ Administer antihistamine-decongestant prn *to reduce postnasal drip and cough.* ▪ Administer throat lozenges or antitussive prn *to provide throat and cough relief.* ▪ Instruct patient to place a scarf or mask over the nose and mouth when breathing cold air *to prevent drying and irritation of oral and respiratory mucosa.*
NURSING DIAGNOSIS	**Risk for ineffective thermoregulation** *related to* infection.
▪ Temperature less than or equal to 100.4° F (38° C). ▪ Absence of chills and diaphoresis. ▪ Adequate state of hydration.	▪ Assess for temperature greater than 100.4° F (38° C), diaphoresis *so early intervention can be initiated.* ▪ Check temperature *to provide ongoing assessment of temperature and response to treatment.* ▪ Give antipyretic medications prn *to reduce temperature.* ▪ Use cooling sponge bath prn *to assist in temperature reduction by heat dissipation.* ▪ Keep patient dry and lightly covered *to avoid chilling* and a subsequent rise in temperature secondary to shivering. ▪ Encourage increased fluid intake *to replace fluid lost through perspiration and to ensure adequate circulating volume to promote positive renal function.*

COLLABORATIVE PROBLEMS

Nursing Goals	Nursing Interventions and *Rationales*
POTENTIAL COMPLICATION	**Viral/bacterial pneumonitis** *related to* secondary infection.
▪ Monitor for signs of pneumonitis. ▪ Report positive signs. ▪ Carry out appropriate medical and nursing interventions.	▪ Instruct patient about proper diet, rest, and activity *to avoid progression of illness.* ▪ Teach patient to report symptoms that do not resolve, such as increase in fever, dyspnea, or secretion production or change in volume, color, or consistency of secretions; tender glands; tonsil exudate *to promote early detection of any complications.* ▪ Administer antibiotics as prescribed if bacterial infection develops.

influenza that become more severe, rather than resolving, and may be fatal. The sputum, if produced, has no predominant organisms. Treatment is largely supportive. The patient who develops secondary bacterial pneumonia experiences gradual improvement of symptoms for 2 to 3 days and then cough and purulent sputum. Treatment with antibiotics is usually effective, if started early. Mixed viral and bacterial pneumonia involves symptoms of both types of pneumonia.[9]

Table 25-3 Target Groups for Influenza Immunization

Groups at High Risk
- Anyone ≥65 years old
- Adults of any age with chronic cardiac or pulmonary disease
- Adults who had regular medical follow-up or were hospitalized during the preceding year
- Residents of chronic care facilities
- Immunocompromised adults

Groups That Can Transmit Influenza to High Risk Persons
- Health care workers
- Providers of home care to high risk persons
- Household members of high risk persons

Modified from Centers for Disease Control and Prevention: Prevention and control of influenza. Recommendations of the Advisory Committee on Immunization Practices, *MMWR* 45(RR-5): 1, 1996.

NURSING AND COLLABORATIVE MANAGEMENT: INFLUENZA

The nurse should advocate influenza vaccination in patients at high risk during routine office visits or, if hospitalized, at the time of discharge (see Table 25-3). The vaccine is 70% to 90% effective in preventing influenza in adults. To be effective, the vaccine must be given in the fall (mid-October) before exposure occurs. Influenza vaccination is an indispensable part of the care of persons 65 years of age or older.[10] High priority

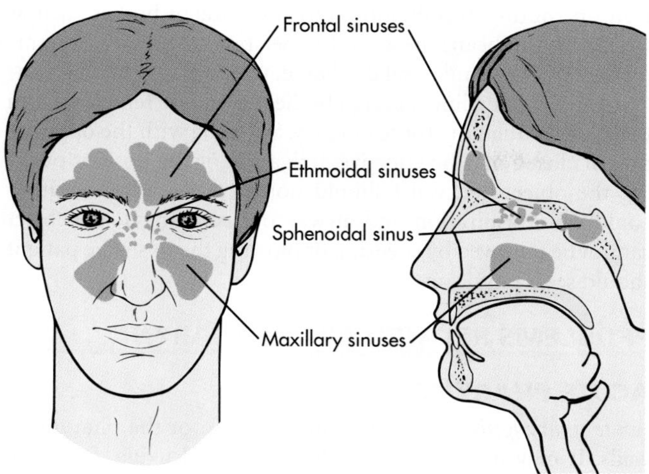

Fig. 25-3 Location of the sinuses.

should also be given to groups that can transmit influenza to high risk persons, such as health care workers. By being vaccinated, the nurse can decrease the risk of transmitting influenza to those who have less ability to cope with the effects of this illness.[10] Despite obvious benefits, many persons are reluctant to be vaccinated, especially among ethnic minority groups. Current vaccines are highly purified, and reactions are extremely uncommon. Soreness at the injection site is usually the only side effect. The only contraindication is hypersensitivity to eggs, since the vaccine is produced in eggs.

The primary goals in nursing management are supportive measures directed toward relief of symptoms and prevention of secondary infection (see NCP 25-2). Unless at high risk, the patient with influenza usually requires only symptomatic therapy unless complications develop. Older adults and those with a chronic illness may require hospitalization. Antibiotics are not indicated unless secondary bacterial infection occurs. Drug therapy with oral amantadine (Symmetrel) may be given to prevent or decrease symptoms of influenza A in high risk patients exposed to the flu but not vaccinated. This drug has a high incidence of side effects (e.g., stomach problems and hallucinations) and is poorly tolerated. Zanamivir (Relenza), a new agent that can be given by nasal spray or inhaled, is effective against both influenza A and B and has been shown to reduce symptom duration by 20%.[11]

SINUSITIS

Sinusitis develops when the ostia (exit) from the sinuses is narrowed or blocked by inflammation or hypertrophy (swelling) of the mucosa (Fig. 25-3). The secretions that accumulate behind the obstruction provide a rich medium for growth of bacteria, viruses, and fungi, all of which may cause infection.[12] Bacterial sinusitis is most commonly caused by *Streptococcus pneumoniae, Haemophilus influenzae,* or *Moraxella catarrhalis.* Viral sinusitis follows an upper respiratory infection in which the virus penetrates the mucous membrane and decreases ciliary transport. Fungal sinusitis is uncommon and is usually found in patients who are debilitated or immunocompromised.[13]

Acute sinusitis usually results from an upper respiratory infection, allergic rhinitis, swimming, or dental manipulation, all of which can cause inflammatory changes and retention of secretions. Chronic sinusitis is a persistent infection usually associated with allergies and nasal polyps. Chronic sinusitis generally results from repeated episodes of acute sinusitis that result in irreversible loss of the normal ciliated epithelium lining the sinus cavity.

Clinical Manifestations

Acute sinusitis causes significant pain over the affected sinus, purulent nasal drainage, nasal obstruction, congestion, fever, and malaise. The patient looks and feels sick. Assessment involves inspection of the nasal mucosa and palpation of the sinus points for pain. Findings that indicate acute sinusitis include a hyperemic and edematous mucosa, enlarged turbinates, and tenderness over the involved sinuses. Pain is caused by the accumulation of pus and absorption of air behind a blocked ostium. The patient may also experience recurrent headaches that change in intensity with position or when secretions drain.[14]

Chronic sinusitis is difficult to diagnose because symptoms may be nonspecific. The patient is rarely febrile. Although there may be facial pain, nasal congestion, and increased drainage, severe pain and purulent drainage are often absent. Symptoms may mimic those seen with allergies. X-rays of the sinuses or a sinus computed tomography (CT) scan may be performed to confirm the diagnosis. CT scans may show the sinuses to be filled with fluid or the mucous membrane to be thickened. Nasal endoscopy may be used to examine the sinuses and obtain drainage for culture. This test involves insertion of a flexible scope that allows extensive examination of the nasal cavity.[13]

Many patients with asthma have sinusitis. The link between these diseases is unclear. Sinusitis may trigger asthma by stimulating reflex bronchospasm. Alternatively, sinusitis and asthma may represent the same underlying disease in different parts of the respiratory tract.[12,13] Recognition of this problem is important because appropriate treatment of sinusitis often causes a reduction in asthma symptoms.

NURSING AND COLLABORATIVE MANAGEMENT: SINUSITIS

Therapy for acute sinusitis includes antibiotics to treat the infection, decongestants or expectorants to reduce tissue edema, nasal corticosteroids to decrease inflammation, and measures to promote mucous flow (Table 25-4). Classic antihistamines increase the viscosity of mucus and promote continued symptoms. Therefore their use should be avoided. Nonsedating antihistamines do not cause this problem. Antibiotic therapy is usually continued for 10 to 14 days for acute sinusitis. If symptoms do not resolve, the antibiotic should be changed to a broader-spectrum agent. With chronic sinusitis, mixed bacterial flora are often present and infections are difficult to eliminate. Broad-spectrum antibiotics are used for 4 to 6 weeks.

The patient with persistent or recurrent sinus complaints not alleviated by medical therapy may require nasal endoscopic surgery to relieve blockage caused by hypertrophy or septal deviation. This is an outpatient procedure usually performed

PATIENT TEACHING GUIDE

Table 25-4 Acute or Chronic Sinusitis

1. Keep well hydrated by drinking six to eight glasses of water to liquefy secretions.
2. Take hot showers twice daily; use a steam inhaler (15-minute vaporization of boiled water), bedside humidifier, or nasal saline spray to promote secretion drainage.
3. Report temperature of 100.4° F (38° C), which may indicate infection.
4. Follow prescribed medication regimen:
   - Take analgesics to relieve pain.
   - Take decongestants/expectorants to relieve swelling and improve breathing.
   - Take antibiotics, as prescribed, for infection. Be sure to take entire prescription and report continued symptoms or a change in symptoms.
   - Administer nasal sprays correctly.
5. Do not smoke, and avoid exposure to smoke. Smoke is an irritant and may worsen symptoms.
6. If allergies predispose to sinusitis, follow instructions regarding environmental control, drug therapy, and immunotherapy to reduce the inflammation and prevent sinus infection.

under local anesthesia. Discomfort is minimal, and more than 80% of those who have the procedure report substantial symptomatic improvement. The patient can return to work in 5 days but should limit strenuous activity for 3 to 4 weeks.[13]

Nursing diagnoses for the patient with acute sinusitis include, but are not limited to, those presented in NCP 25-3. Additional nursing measures for the treatment of sinusitis are presented in NCP 25-3.

OBSTRUCTION OF THE NOSE AND PARANASAL SINUSES

POLYPS

Nasal polyps are benign projections of edematous mucous membrane that form slowly in response to repeated inflammation of the sinus or nasal mucosa. Once nasal polyps are present, they enlarge, partly by growing and partly by swelling from increased edema, until they protrude into the airway or occlude the nose. Polyps may be multiple and can exceed the size of a grape. The patient may be anxious, fearing they are malignant. Clinical manifestations include nasal obstruction, nasal discharge (usually clear mucus), and speech distortion. Nasal polyps can be removed with endoscopic or laser surgery, but recurrence is common.

FOREIGN BODIES

A variety of foreign bodies may lodge in the upper respiratory tract. Inorganic foreign bodies such as buttons and beads may cause no symptoms, lie undetected, and be accidentally discovered on routine examination. Organic foreign bodies such as wood, cotton, beans, peas, and paper produce a local inflammatory reaction and nasal discharge, which may become purulent and foul smelling. Foreign bodies should be removed from the nose through the route of entry. Sneezing with the opposite nostril closed may be effective. Irrigation of the nose or pushing the object backward should not be done, because either could cause aspiration and airway obstruction. If the object cannot be removed by sneezing or blowing the nose, the patient should see a physician.

PROBLEMS RELATED TO THE PHARYNX

ACUTE PHARYNGITIS

Acute pharyngitis is an acute inflammation of the pharyngeal walls. It may include the tonsils, palate, and uvula. It can be caused by a viral, bacterial, or fungal infection. Viral pharyngitis accounts for approximately 70% of cases. Acute follicular pharyngitis ("strep throat") results from beta-hemolytic streptococcal invasion and accounts for an additional 15% to 20% of episodes. *Neisseria gonorrhoeae* and *Corynebacterium diphtheriae* are other bacterial organisms that infect the pharynx. Fungal pharyngitis, especially candidiasis, can develop with prolonged use of antibiotics or inhaled corticosteroids or in immunosuppressed patients, especially those with human immunodeficiency virus (HIV). (Management of the patient with HIV is discussed in Chapter 13.)

Clinical Manifestations

Symptoms of acute pharyngitis range in severity from complaints of a "scratchy throat" to pain so severe that swallowing is difficult. White, irregular patches suggest infection with *Candida albicans.* In viral infections, the throat may appear mildly red with some congestion of blood vessels. In strep throat, the throat is typically an intense red-purple with patchy yellow exudate and hypertrophy of lymphoid tissue. In diphtheria, a gray-white false membrane, termed a *pseudomembrane,* is seen covering the oropharynx, nasopharynx, and laryngopharynx and sometimes extends to the trachea. Appearance is not always diagnostic. Cultures are done to establish the cause and direct appropriate management. Even with severe infection, cultures may be negative.

NURSING AND COLLABORATIVE MANAGEMENT: ACUTE PHARYNGITIS

The goals of nursing management are infection control, symptomatic relief, and prevention of secondary complications. Because cultures can be negative even when infection is present, the patient suspected of having strep throat is often treated with antibiotics. *Candida* infections are treated with nystatin, an antifungal antibiotic. The preparation should be held in the mouth as long as possible before it is swallowed, and treatment should continue until symptoms are gone. The patient should be encouraged to increase fluid intake. Cool, bland liquids and gelatin will not irritate the pharynx; citrus juices should be avoided because they irritate the mucous membranes.

25-3 NURSING CARE PLAN PATIENT WITH ACUTE OR CHRONIC SINUSITIS

Expected Patient Outcomes	Nursing Interventions and *Rationales*
NURSING DIAGNOSIS	**Pain** *related to* decreased sinus drainage, inflammation or infection, and inadequate comfort measures *as manifested by* pain over involved sinuses, infected nasal drainage, facial pain, or complaints of congestion.
▪ No pain when pressure applied over involved sinus. ▪ No drainage of secretions. ▪ Correct technique used with vasoconstrictors. ▪ Normal temperature.	▪ Explain need to continue antibiotics for prescribed time *to decrease risk of recurrent infection.* ▪ Encourage increased fluid intake (6-8 glasses of water daily), hot shower in A.M. and P.M. followed by blowing the nose thoroughly *to promote cleansing of nasal passages and secretion drainage.* Alternative interventions include irrigating the nose with salt water (¼ to ½ tsp per quart of water) or steam inhalations (15 min vaporization of boiled water). ▪ Instruct patient in correct use of nasal inhalers (see Fig. 25-1) and other medications for predisposing illnesses (e.g., asthma, allergies). Reinforce need to adhere to medication regimen *to decrease risk of recurrent symptoms.* ▪ Instruct patient to elevate head of bed *to promote secretion drainage.* ▪ Teach patient correct analgesic schedule and use of decongestants/expectorants *to foster correct use of medications to relieve pain and swelling.* ▪ Teach patient to avoid use of antihistamines *because these drugs increase viscosity of mucus and promote continued symptoms.*
NURSING DIAGNOSIS	**Altered health maintenance** *related to* lack of knowledge of self-care, pain management, and prevention of chronic sinusitis *as manifested by* anxiety, questioning about care, continued purulent nasal discharge, sinus pain, cough.
▪ No nasal discharge, cough, sinus pressure. ▪ Accurate description of self-care requirements related to hydration, infection control, pain management.	▪ Instruct patient on use of pain, expectorant, decongestant, and antibiotic medications, nasal cleansing techniques, and nutrition and hydration issues *to increase the patient's knowledge of self-care.* ▪ Answer questions completely about self-care responsibilities *to promote health through knowledgeable self-care.* ▪ Instruct patient to follow interventions for acute sinusitis *to provide for early treatment and avoid chronic condition.* ▪ Teach patient to avoid factors that predispose to exacerbations, such as swimming and diving. ▪ If allergy is cause, follow instructions regarding environmental control, drug therapy, and immunotherapy *to reduce the sinus inflammation and prevent sinus infection.*
NURSING DIAGNOSIS	**Risk for infection** *related to* impaired mucosal integrity.
▪ No inflammation. ▪ Normal temperature and white blood cell count.	▪ Report a temperature of 100.4° F (38° C), *which may indicate infection.* ▪ Instruct patient to take medications as prescribed and report continued symptoms or a change in symptoms to health care provider *because these symptoms may indicate need for change in antibiotic regimen.* ▪ Report any signs of infection to health care provider.

PERITONSILLAR ABSCESS

Peritonsillar abscess typically occurs as a complication of acute pharyngitis or acute tonsillitis if bacterial infection results in invasion of one or both tonsils. The tonsils may enlarge sufficiently to threaten airway patency. The patient will experience a high fever, leukocytosis, and chills. Early detection and treatment with intravenous (IV) antibiotic therapy may clear the infection and prevent abscess development. If an abscess develops, incision and drainage are required. An emergency tonsillectomy may be performed or an elective tonsillectomy may be scheduled after the infection has subsided.

OBSTRUCTIVE SLEEP APNEA

Obstructive sleep apnea is a condition characterized by repetitive cessation of airflow during sleep. Airflow obstruction occurs when the tongue and the soft palate fall backward and partially or completely obstruct the pharynx (Fig. 25-4). The obstruction may last from 15 to 90 seconds. During the apneic period, the patient experiences severe hypoxemia (decreased PaO_2) and hypercapnia (increased $PaCO_2$). These changes are ventilatory stimulants and cause the patient to partially awaken. The patient has a generalized startle response, snorts, and gasps, which causes the tongue and soft palate to move forward

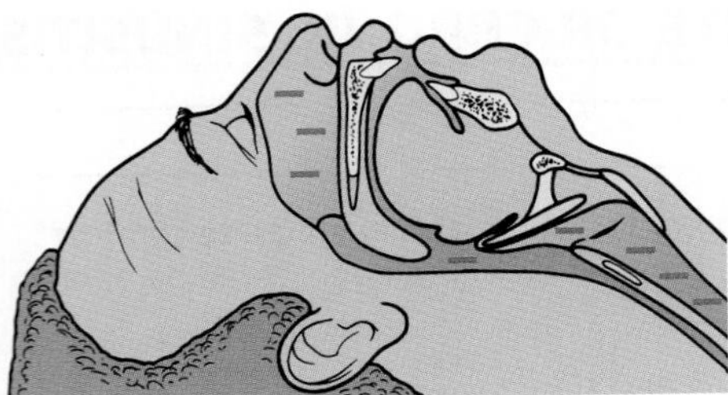

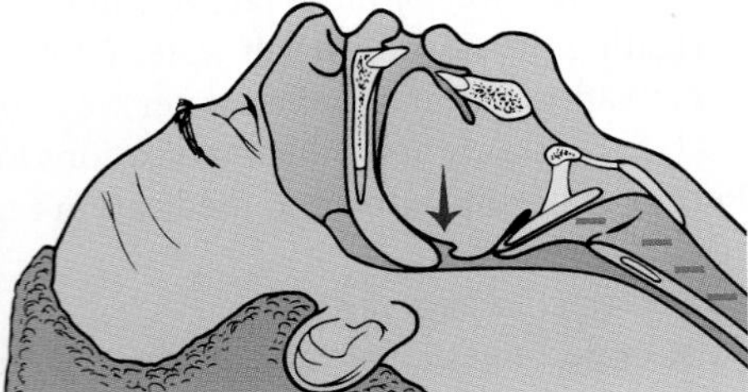

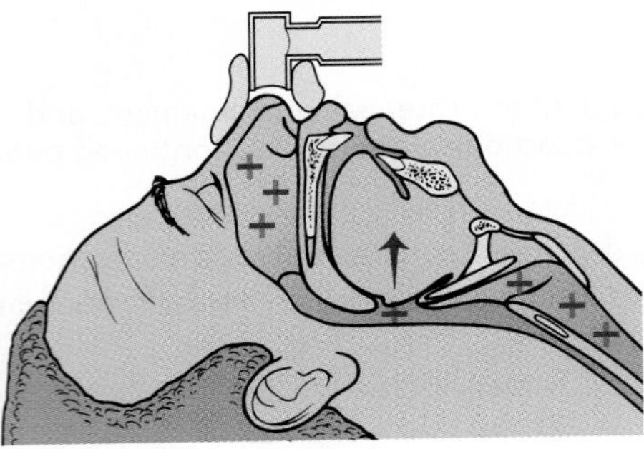

Fig. 25-4 How sleep apnea occurs. **A,** The patient predisposed to obstructive sleep apnea (OSA) has a small pharyngeal airway. **B,** During sleep, the pharyngeal muscles relax, allowing the airway to close. Lack of airflow results in repeated apneic episodes. **C,** With nasal CPAP, positive pressure splints the airway open, preventing airflow obstruction.

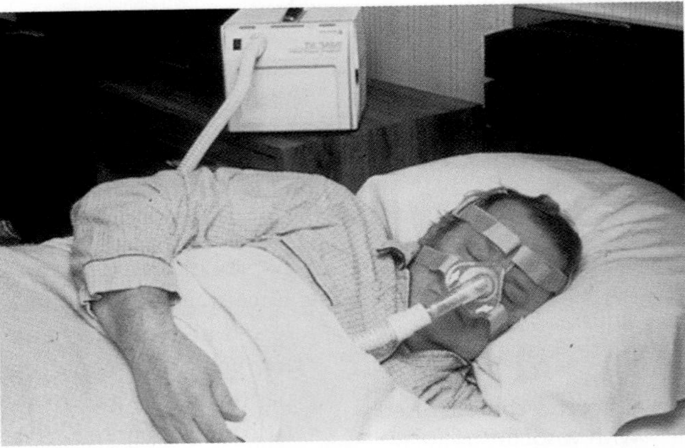

Fig. 25-5 Management of sleep apnea often involves sleeping with a nasal mask in place. The pressure supplied by air coming from the compressor opens the oropharynx and nasopharynx.

and the airway to open. Apnea and arousal cycles occur repeatedly, as many as 200 to 400 times during 6 to 8 hours of sleep.[15]

The cause of sleep apnea is not definitely known. However, three factors appear to be involved: (1) an anatomically small pharyngeal airway, (2) altered neural control of the respiratory muscles, and (3) hormonal imbalance. Sleep apnea occurs in 1% to 4% of otherwise healthy men. The disorder is 7 to 10 times more common in men than women.[15]

Clinical Manifestations and Diagnostic Studies

Clinical manifestations of sleep apnea include frequent awakening at night, insomnia, and excessive daytime sleepiness. The patient's bed partner may complain about loud snoring. The snoring may be so loud that both persons cannot sleep in the same room. Other symptoms include morning headaches (from hypercapnia, which causes vasodilation of cerebral blood vessels), personality changes, and irritability. Symptoms of sleep apnea alter many aspects of the patient's lifestyle. Chronic sleep loss predisposes to diminished ability to concentrate, impaired memory, failure to accomplish daily tasks, and interpersonal difficulties. The male patient may experience impotence. Driving accidents are more common in the patient with sleep apnea. Family life and the patient's ability to maintain employment are also often compromised. As a result, the patient may experience severe depression. The patient should be assessed to determine psychologic adjustment, and appropriate referral should be made, if problems are identified.

Diagnosis of sleep apnea is made during sleep with the use of polysomnography. The patient's chest and abdominal movement, oral airflow, nasal airflow, SpO_2, ocular movement, and heart rate and rhythm are monitored, and time in each sleep stage is determined. A diagnosis of sleep apnea requires documentation of multiple episodes of apnea (no airflow with respiratory effort) or hypopnea (airflow diminished 30% to 50% with respiratory effort).

NURSING AND COLLABORATIVE MANAGEMENT: SLEEP APNEA

Mild sleep apnea may respond to simple measures. The patient should be instructed to avoid sedatives and alcoholic beverages for 3 to 4 hours before sleep. Referral to a weight loss program may be beneficial, because excessive weight exacerbates symptoms. Symptoms may resolve with use of an oral appliance worn during the night. The appliance advances the mandible during sleep, preventing airflow obstruction.[16] Some individuals find a support group beneficial where concerns and feelings can be expressed and strategies discussed for resolving problems.[17]

In patients with more severe symptoms, nasal continuous positive airway pressure (nCPAP) may be used (Fig. 25-5). With nCPAP, the patient applies a nasal mask to the face that is attached to a high-flow blower.[15] The blower is adjusted to maintain sufficient positive pressure (5 to 15 cm H_2O) in the airway during inspiration and expiration to prevent airway collapse. Some patients cannot adjust to exhaling against the high pressure. A technologically more sophisticated therapy, bilevel positive airway pressure (BiPAP), capable of delivering a higher pressure during inspiration (when the airway is most likely to be occluded) and a lower pressure during expiration (when the airway is least likely to be occluded), may be helpful and is better tolerated. Although nCPAP is highly effective, compliance is poor, even if symptoms of sleep apnea are relieved.[18]

25-4 NURSING CARE PLAN PATIENT WITH SLEEP APNEA

Expected Patient Outcomes	Nursing Interventions and *Rationales*
NURSING DIAGNOSIS	**Sleep pattern disturbance** *related to* inability to sleep normally because of airflow obstruction during sleep *as manifested by* snoring, restlessness during sleep, morning headache, excessive daytime sleepiness.
▪ Recognition of relationship between sleep and breathing problem.	▪ Assist patient to recognize that breathing problems may be a cause of symptoms *to encourage compliance with therapy.* ▪ Assess severity of symptoms *to determine their effect on the patient's life and urgency for treatment.* ▪ Instruct patient not to use alcohol or sedatives for 3 to 4 hours before sleep *to promote more restful sleep.* ▪ Suggest that patient try sleeping on side *to minimize potential for airflow obstruction in supine position.* ▪ Teach need to avoid driving until management is effective *because daytime sleepiness may result in falling asleep while driving.*
NURSING DIAGNOSIS	**Self-esteem disturbance** *related to* changes in body image, role performance, and personal identity *as manifested by* unwillingness to discuss symptoms, refusal to take part in own care, withdrawal from social contacts.
▪ Attendance at support groups. ▪ Expression of positive feelings about self.	▪ Assess patient's ability to understand and cope with symptoms experienced *to determine effectiveness of coping.* ▪ Inform patient and bed partner about support groups *to share concerns and feelings with other patients with sleep apnea and to discuss strategies to deal with the problem.* ▪ Assess patient for symptoms of depression *because this is a common occurrence in sleep apnea.*
NURSING DIAGNOSIS	**Altered nutrition: greater than body requirements** *related to* increased appetite and inadequate exercise *as manifested by* inability to regulate caloric intake to reduce or maintain normal weight.
▪ Initiation of a weight-loss program. ▪ Achievement of weight goal.	▪ Assist patient to recognize that obesity is contributing to present illness *because this is a common predisposing factor.* ▪ Educate patient about weight-loss methods *to provide encouragement by knowledge of a variety of methods.*
NURSING DIAGNOSIS	**Altered health maintenance** *related to* lack of knowledge regarding use of equipment to modify breathing pattern *as manifested by* agitation; questioning about care; noncompliance with use of oral appliance or nCPAP; complaints of nasal dryness, burning, congestion; presence of epistaxis, conjunctivitis.
▪ Able to state purpose and demonstrate proper use of oral appliance or mask. ▪ Adherence to plan of care. ▪ Resolution of conjunctivitis and epistaxis. ▪ Correct fit of mask.	▪ Teach patient how to insert oral appliance *to ensure proper placement.* ▪ Ensure that oral appliance fits properly in mouth without excessive pressure on teeth or gums *to ensure maximum benefit and prevent pain.* ▪ Teach patient how to apply nCPAP mask and use device *to ensure maximum benefit.* ▪ Instruct patient that device will create a positive pressure, *which will help hold airway open during sleep.* ▪ Teach patient that conjunctivitis and epistaxis result from dry air flowing into eyes and nose. ▪ Instruct patient to use room humidifier or humidifier incorporated into airway circuit *because airflow is drying to nasal mucosa.* For traveling, humidifier can be replaced by chin strap. ▪ Teach patient that a corticosteroid or saline nasal spray may also be used *to reduce inflammation of or moisturize nasal mucosa.*

nCPAP, nasal continuous positive airway pressure.

If other measures fail, sleep apnea may be managed surgically. The two most common procedures are uvulopalatopharyngoplasty (UPPP or UP_3) and genioglossal advancement and hyoid myotomy (GAHM). UPPP involves excision of the tonsillar pillars, uvula, and posterior soft palate with the goal of removing the obstructing tissue. UPPP is often successful in relieving some, but not all, symptoms. GAHM involves advancing the attachment of the muscular part of the tongue on the mandible. This procedure limits airway obstruction by the tongue during sleep, and symptoms are relieved in up to 67% of patients.[19]

Nursing diagnoses for the patient with sleep apnea include, but are not limited to, those presented in NCP 25-4. Nursing management is important in assisting the patient to adopt a regimen that promotes adherence with this therapy (see NCP 25-4).

PROBLEMS RELATED TO THE TRACHEA AND LARYNX

AIRWAY OBSTRUCTION

Airway obstruction may be complete or partial. Complete airway obstruction is a medical emergency. Partial airway obstruction may occur as a result of aspiration of food or a foreign body. In addition, partial airway obstruction may result from laryngeal edema following extubation, laryngeal or tracheal stenosis, and neurologic depression. Symptoms include stridor, use of accessory muscles, suprasternal and intercostal retractions, wheezing, restlessness, tachycardia, and cyanosis. Prompt assessment and treatment are essential because partial obstruction may quickly progress to complete obstruction. Interventions to maintain a patent airway include use of the obstructed airway (Heimlich) maneuver, cricothyroidotomy, endotracheal intubation, and tracheostomy. The patient may have few symptoms if the obstruction is minor. Unexplained or recurrent symptoms indicate the need for additional tests, such as a chest x-ray, pulmonary function tests, and bronchoscopy.

TRACHEOSTOMY

A *tracheotomy* is a surgical incision into the trachea for the purpose of establishing an airway. A *tracheostomy* is the stoma (opening) that results from the tracheotomy. Indications for a tracheostomy are to (1) bypass an upper airway obstruction, (2) facilitate removal of secretions, (3) permit long-term mechanical ventilation, and (4) permit oral intake and speech in the patient who requires long-term mechanical ventilation.[20] Most patients who require mechanical ventilation are initially managed with an endotracheal tube, which can be quickly inserted in an emergency. (Care of the patient with an endotracheal tube is discussed in Chapter 63.) A tracheostomy requires surgical dissection and is therefore not typically an emergency procedure.

Several advantages make a tracheostomy the better option for long-term care. With a tracheostomy, there is less risk of long-term damage to the airway. Patient comfort may be increased because no tube is present in the mouth. The patient can eat with a tracheostomy because the tube enters lower in the airway (Fig. 25-6). If the tracheostomy cuff can be deflated or a speaking tube is used, the patient can also speak with a tracheostomy. Because the tracheostomy tube is more secure, mobility may be increased.[20,21]

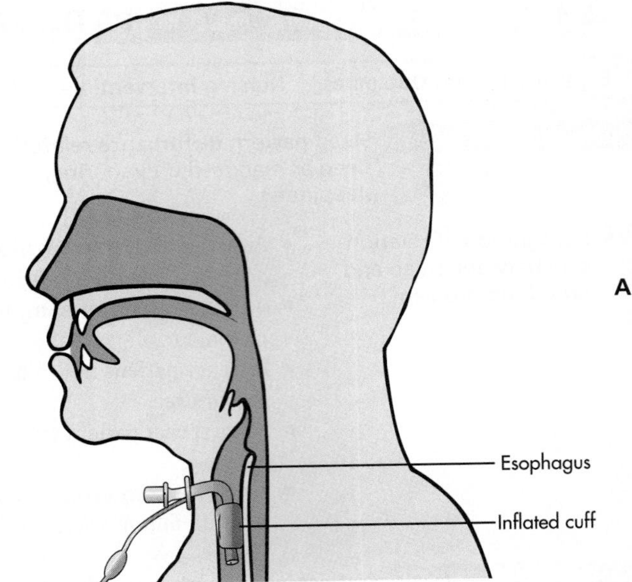

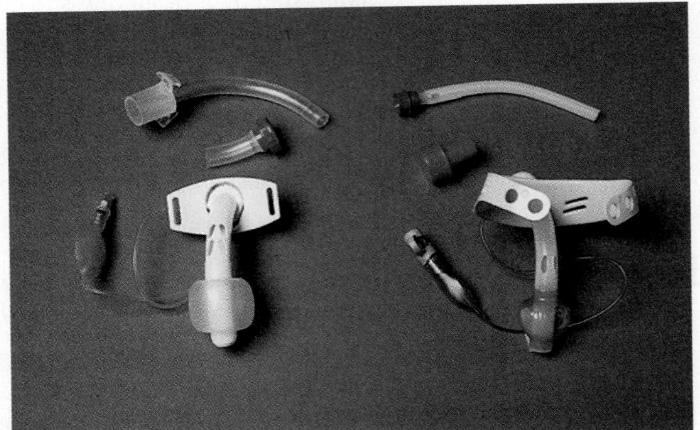

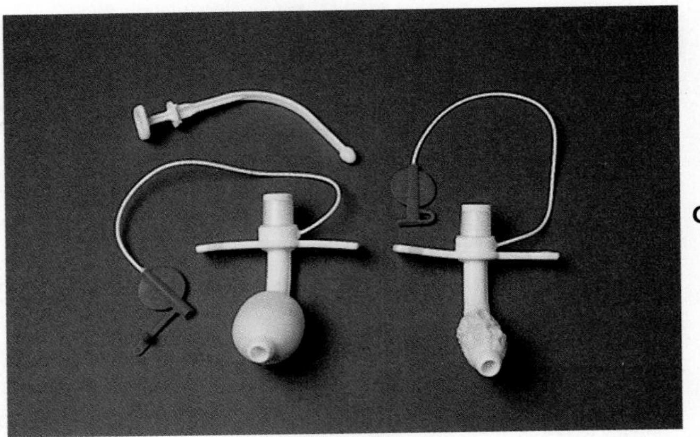

Fig. 25-6 Types of tracheostomy tubes. **A,** Tracheostomy tube inserted in airway with inflated cuff. **B,** Shiley and Portex fenestrated tracheostomy tube with cuff, inner cannula, decannulation plug, and pilot balloon. **C,** Bivona (Fome) tracheostomy tube with foam cuff and obturator (one cuff is deflated on tracheostomy tube). (See Tables 25-5 and NCP 25-5 for related nursing management.)

Table 25-5 Characteristics and Nursing Management of Tracheostomies

Tube	Characteristics	Nursing Management
Tracheostomy tube with cuff and pilot balloon (see Fig. 25-6, *A* and *B*)	When properly inflated, low-pressure, high-volume cuff distributes cuff pressure over large area, minimizing pressure on tracheal wall.	**Procedure for cuff inflation** ▪ Mechanically ventilated patient: Inflate the cuff to *minimal occlusion pressure* by slowly injecting air into the cuff until no leak (sound) is heard at peak inspiratory pressure (end of ventilator inspiration) when a stethoscope is placed over the trachea. Use cuff pressure monitor to determine cuff inflation pressure. An alternative approach, termed *minimal leak technique* (MLT), involves inflating the cuff to minimal occlusion pressure and withdrawing 0.1 ml of air. ▪ Spontaneously breathing patient: Inflate cuff to minimal occlusion pressure by slowly injecting air into the cuff until no sound is heard after deep breath or during inhalation with manual resuscitation bag. If using MLT, remove 0.1 ml of air while maintaining seal. MLT should not be used if there is risk of aspiration. ▪ Immediately after cuff inflation (both groups): Verify pressure is within accepted range ($\leq$20 mm Hg or $\leq$25 cm H_2O) with a manometer. Record cuff pressure and volume of air used for cuff inflation in chart. **Care of patients with an inflated cuff** ▪ Monitor and record cuff pressure q8hr. Cuff pressure should be $\leq$20 mm Hg or $\leq$25 cm H_2O to allow adequate tracheal capillary perfusion. If needed, remove or add air to the pilot tubing using a syringe and stopcock. Afterward, verify cuff pressure is within accepted range with manometer. ▪ Report inability to keep the cuff inflated or need to use progressively larger volumes of air to keep cuff inflated. Potential causes include tracheal dilation at the cuff site or a crack or slow leak in the housing of the one-way inflation valve. If the leak is due to tracheal dilation, the physician may intubate the patient with a larger tube. Cracks in the inflation valve may be temporarily managed by clamping the small-bore tubing with a hemostat. The tube should be changed within 24 hours.
Fenestrated tracheostomy tube (Shiley, Portex) with cuff,inner cannula, and decannulation plug (see Fig. 25-6, *B;* Fig. 25-9, *A*)	When inner cannula is removed, cuff deflated, and decannulation plug inserted, air flows around tube, through fenestration in outer cannula, and up over vocal chords. Patient can then speak	▪ Assess risk of aspiration before removing inner cannula. Deflate cuff. Note coughing. Have patient swallow a small amount of clear liquid (grape juice) or 30 ml of water with a few drops of blue food coloring. Observe secretions after patient coughs or when suctioned for presence of colored secretions. If no aspiration is noted, a fenestrated tube may be used. ▪ Never insert decannulation plug in tracheostomy tube until cuff is deflated and inner cannula removed. Prior insertion will prevent patient from breathing (no air inflow). This may precipitate a respiratory arrest. ▪ Assess for signs of respiratory distress when a fenestrated cannula is first used. If this occurs, the cap should be removed, the inner cannula replaced, and the cuff reinflated. ▪ Cuff management as described above.

Continued

NURSING MANAGEMENT: TRACHEOSTOMY

■ Providing Tracheostomy Care

Before the tracheotomy procedure, the nurse should explain to the patient and the family the purpose of the procedure and inform them that the patient will not be able to speak if an inflated cuff is used. The patient and the family should be told that normal speech will be possible as soon as the cuff can be deflated.

A variety of tubes are available to meet individual patient needs (Table 25-5). All tracheostomy tubes contain a faceplate or flange, which rests on the neck between the clavicles and outer cannula. In addition, all tubes have an obturator, which is used when inserting the tube (see Fig. 25-6, *C*). During insertion of the tube, the obturator is placed inside the outer cannula with its rounded tip protruding from the end of the tube to ease insertion. After insertion, the obturator must be immediately removed so air can flow through the tube. The obturator should be kept in an easily accessible place at the bedside (e.g., taped to the wall) so that it can be used quickly in case of accidental decannulation.[21]

Table 25-5 Characteristics and Nursing Management of Tracheostomies—cont'd

Tube	Characteristics	Nursing Management
Speaking tracheostomy tube (Portex, National) with cuff, two external tubings (see Fig. 25-9, *B*)	Has two tubings, one leading to cuff and second to opening above the cuff. When port is connected to air source, air flows out of opening and up over the vocal cords, allowing speech with cuff inflated.	■ Once tube is inserted, wait 2 days before use so that the stoma can close around the tube and prevent leaks. ■ When patient desires to speak, connect port to compressed air (or oxygen). Be certain to identify correct tubing. If gas enters the cuff, it will overinflate and rupture, requiring an emergency tube change. Use lowest flow (typically 4-6 L/min) that results in speech. High flows dehydrate mucosa. ■ Cover port adaptor. This will cause the air to flow upward. Instruct patient to speak in short sentences because voice becomes a whisper with long sentences. ■ Disconnect flow when patient does not want to speak to prevent mucosal dehydration. ■ Cuff management as described above.
Tracheostomy tube (Bivona Fome-Cuf) foam-filled cuff (see Fig. 25-6, *C*)	Cuff is filled with plastic foam. Before insertion, cuff is deflated. After insertion, cuff is allowed to fill passively with air. Pilot tubing is not capped, and no cuff pressure monitoring is required.	■ Before insertion, withdraw all air from the cuff using a 20 ml syringe. Cap pilot balloon tubing to prevent reentry of air. After tracheostomy is inserted, remove cap from pilot tubing allowing cuff to passively reinflate. ■ Do not inject air into tubing or cap pilot balloon tubing while in patient. Air will flow in and out in response to pressure changes (head turning). Place tag on tubing alerting staff not to cap or inflate cuff. ■ Deflate cuff daily via pilot balloon to evaluate integrity of cuff. Also assess ability to easily deflate cuff. Difficulty deflating cuff indicates a need for tube change. If aspirate returns with air, the cuff is no longer intact. ■ Tube can be used for up to 1 month in patients on home mechanical ventilation. Good choice for patients who require inflated cuff at home since teaching about cuff pressure is simplified.

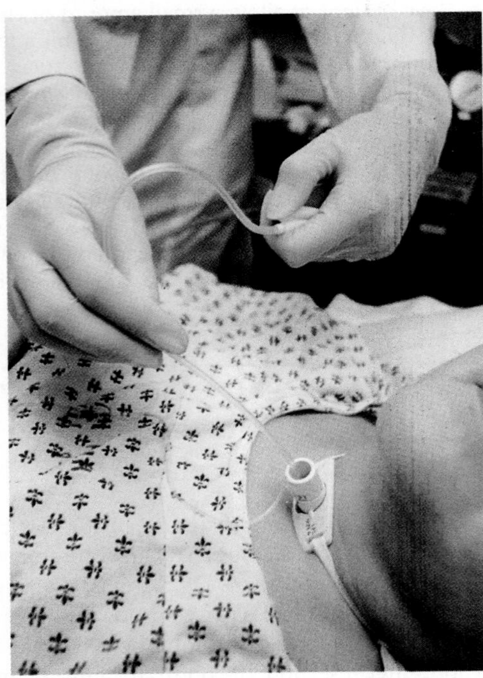

Fig. 25-7 Suctioning a tracheostomy. Using sterile technique, the suction catheter is being withdrawn from the airway while suction is applied. The pilot balloon tubing may be seen lying on the patient's chest.

Some tracheostomy tubes also have an inner cannula, which can be removed for cleaning (see Fig. 25-6, *B*). The cleaning procedure removes mucus from the inside of the tube. If humidification is adequate, mucus may not accumulate and a tube without an inner cannula can be used. Care of the patient with a tracheostomy involves suctioning the airway to remove secretions (Fig. 25-7 and Table 25-6). In addition, tracheostomy care includes changing tracheostomy ties (Fig. 25-8 and Table 25-7). If a disposable or nondisposable inner cannula is used, tracheostomy care also involves inner cannula care (see Table 25-7).

Both cuffed and uncuffed tracheostomy tubes are available. A tracheostomy tube with an inflated cuff is used if the patient is at risk of aspiration or needs mechanical ventilation. Because an inflated cuff exerts pressure on tracheal mucosa, it is important to inflate the cuff with the minimum volume of air required to obtain an airway seal. Cuff inflation pressure should not exceed 20 mm Hg or 25 cm H_2O because higher pressures may compress tracheal capillaries, limit blood flow, and predispose to tracheal necrosis. An alternative approach, termed the *minimal leak technique* (MLT), involves inflating the cuff with the minimum amount of air to obtain a seal and then withdrawing 0.1 ml air. A disadvantage of MLT is risk of aspiration from secretions leaking around the cuff. MLT should not be used when the tracheostomy was placed to bypass an upper airway obstruction, such as with head and neck surgical patients.[21,22]

Table 25-6 Procedure for Suctioning a Tracheostomy Tube

1. Assess the need for suctioning q2hr. Indications include coarse crackles or rhonchi over large airways, moist cough, increase in peak inspiratory pressure on mechanical ventilator, and restlessness or agitation if accompanied by decrease in SpO_2 or PaO_2. Do not suction routinely or if patient is able to clear secretions with cough.
2. If suctioning is indicated, explain procedure to patient.
3. Collect necessary sterile equipment: suction catheter (no larger than half the lumen of the tracheostomy tube), gloves, water, cup, and drape. If a closed tracheal suction system is used, the catheter is enclosed in a plastic sleeve and reused for 24 hours. No additional equipment is needed.
4. Check suction source and regulator. Adjust suction pressure until the dial reads −120 to −150 mm Hg pressure with tubing occluded.
5. Wash hands. Put on goggles and gloves.
6. Use sterile technique to open package, fill cup with water, put on gloves, and connect catheter to suction. Designate one hand as contaminated for disconnecting, bagging, and operating the suction control. Suction water through the catheter to test the system.
7. Assess SpO_2, heart rate, and rhythm to provide baseline for detecting change during suctioning.
8. Provide preoxygenation by (1) adjusting ventilator to deliver 100% O_2; (2) using a reservoir-equipped manual resuscitation bag (MRB) connected to 100% oxygen; or (3) asking the patient to take 3-4 deep breaths while administering oxygen. The method chosen will depend on the patient's underlying disease and acuity of illness. The patient who has had a tracheostomy for an extended period of time and is not acutely ill may be able to tolerate suctioning without use of an MRB or the ventilator.
9. Gently insert catheter *without suction* to minimize the amount of oxygen removed from the lungs. Insert the catheter approximately 5-6 inches. Stop if an obstruction is met.
10. Withdraw the catheter 1-2 cm and apply suction intermittently, while withdrawing catheter in a rotating manner. If secretion volume is large, apply suction continuously.
11. If the patient develops mucous plugs or thick secretions, a 3-5 ml bolus of normal saline may be instilled into the airway to loosen secretions sufficiently to clear the airway either through coughing or suctioning.
12. *Limit suction time to 10 seconds.* Discontinue suctioning if heart rate decreases from baseline by 20 beats, increases from baseline by 40 beats per minute, an arrhythmia occurs, or SpO_2 decreases to less than 90%.
13. After each suction pass, oxygenate with 3-4 breaths by ventilator, MRB, or deep breaths with oxygen.
14. Rinse catheter with sterile water.
15. Repeat procedure until airway is clear. Limit insertions of suction catheter to three passes.
16. Return oxygen concentration to prior setting.
17. Rinse catheter and suction the oropharynx or use mouth suction.
18. Dispose of catheter by wrapping it around fingers of gloved hand and pulling glove over catheter. Discard equipment in proper waste container.
19. Auscultate to assess changes in lung sounds. Record time, amount, and character of secretions and response to suctioning.

In some patients, cuff deflation is performed to remove secretions that accumulate above the cuff. Before deflation, the patient should cough up secretions, if possible, and the tracheostomy tube and mouth should be suctioned (see Fig. 25-7 and Table 25-6). This step is important to prevent secretions from being aspirated during deflation. The cuff is deflated during exhalation because the exhaled gas helps propel secretions into the mouth. The patient should also cough or be suctioned after cuff deflation. The cuff should be reinflated during inspiration. The volume of air required to inflate the cuff should be monitored daily because this volume may increase if there is tracheal dilation from cuff pressure. The nurse should assess the ability of the patient to protect the airway from aspiration and remain with the patient when the cuff is initially deflated unless the patient can protect the airway from aspiration and breathe without respiratory distress. When the patient can protect the airway from aspiration and does not require mechanical ventilation, a cuffless tracheostomy tube should be used.

Retention sutures are often placed in the tracheal cartilage when the tracheostomy is performed. The free ends should be taped to the skin in a place and manner that leaves them accessible if the tube is dislodged. Care should be taken not to dislodge the tracheostomy tube during the first few days when the stoma is not mature (healed). Because tube replacement can be difficult, several precautions are required: (1) a replacement tube of equal or smaller size is kept at the bedside, readily available for emergency reinsertion; (2) tracheostomy tapes are not changed for at least 24 hours after the insertion procedure; and (3) the first tube change is performed by a physician usually no sooner than 7 days after the tracheostomy.

If the tube is accidentally dislodged, the nurse should immediately attempt to replace it. The retention sutures are grasped and the opening is spread. The obturator is inserted in the replacement tube, a water-soluble lubricant is applied to the tip, and the tube is inserted in the stoma at a 45-degree angle to the neck. If insertion is successful, the obturator is removed immediately so that air can flow through the tube. Another method is to insert a suction catheter to allow passage of air and to serve as a guide for insertion. The tracheostomy tube should be threaded over the catheter and the suction catheter removed. If the tube cannot be replaced, assess the level of respiratory distress. Minor dyspnea may be alleviated by use of semi-Fowler's position until assistance

Table 25-7 Tracheostomy Care

1. Explain procedure to patient.
2. Collect necessary sterile equipment (e.g., suction catheter, gloves, water, basin, drape, tracheostomy ties, tube brush or pipe cleaners, 4 × 4s, hydrogen peroxide [3%], sterile water, and tracheostomy dressing [optional]). Note: Clean rather than sterile technique is used at home.
3. Position patient in semi-Fowler's position.
4. Assemble needed materials on bedside table next to patient.
5. Wash hands. Put on goggles and gloves.
6. Auscultate chest sounds. If rhonchi or coarse crackles are present, suction the patient if unable to cough up secretions (see Table 25-6).
7. Unlock and remove inner cannula, if present. Many tracheostomy tubes do not have inner cannulas. Care for these tubes includes all steps except for inner cannula care.
8. If disposable inner cannula is used, replace with new cannula. If a nondisposable cannula is used:
   a. Immerse inner cannula in 3% hydrogen peroxide and clean inside and outside of cannula using tube brush or pipe cleaners.
   b. Drain hydrogen peroxide from cannula. Immerse cannula in sterile water. Remove from sterile water and shake to dry.
   c. Insert inner cannula into outer cannula with the curved part downward and lock in place.
9. Remove dried secretions from stoma using 4 × 4 soaked in hydrogen peroxide. Rinse with another 4 × 4 soaked in sterile water. Gently pat area around the stoma dry. Be sure to clean under the tracheostomy face plate, using cotton swabs to reach this area.
10. Maintain position of tracheal retention sutures, if present, by taping above and below the stoma.
11. Change tracheostomy ties. Tie tracheostomy ties securely with room for one finger between ties and skin (see Fig 25-8). To prevent accidental tube removal, secure the tracheostomy tube by gently applying pressure to flange of the tube during the tie changes. *Do not change tracheostomy ties for 24 hr after the tracheotomy procedure.*
12. As an alternative, some patients prefer tracheostomy ties made of Velcro, which are easier to adjust. Other patients use plastic IV tubing because it is easily cleaned and dries without the need to replace the ties.
13. Unless excessive amounts of exudate are present, avoid using a tracheostomy dressing since this keeps the site moist and may predispose to infection.
14. If drainage is excessive, place dressing around tube (see Fig. 25-8). A tracheostomy dressing or unlined gauze should be used. Do not cut the gauze because threads may be inhaled or wrap around the tracheostomy tube. Change the dressing frequently. Wet dressings promote infection and stoma irritation.
15. Repeat care three times a day and as needed.

arrives. Severe dyspnea may progress to respiratory arrest. If this situation occurs, the stoma should be covered with a sterile dressing, and the patient should be ventilated with bag-mask ventilation until help arrives.

After the first tube change, the tube should be changed approximately once a month. When a tracheostomy has been in place for several months, the tract will be well formed. The patient can then be taught to change the tube using a clean technique at home (Fig. 25-10).[23] Teaching will vary, depending on the illness of the patient and the device selected.

Nursing diagnoses for the patient with a tracheostomy include, but are not limited to, those presented in NCP 25-5.

Swallowing Dysfunction

The patient who cannot protect the airway from aspiration requires an inflated cuff. However, an inflated cuff may promote swallowing dysfunction because the cuff interferes with the normal function of muscles used to swallow. For this reason, it is important to evaluate the risk for aspiration with the cuff deflated. The patient may be able to swallow without aspirating when the cuff is deflated but not when it is inflated. The cuff may then be left deflated or a cuffless tube substituted (see Fig. 25-9).

To evaluate aspiration risk, the cuff is deflated and the patient is instructed to swallow a small amount of clear liquid such as grape juice or 30 ml of water that has blue food coloring added. Any coughing and secretions are noted. If needed, the trachea is suctioned to check for the presence of blue-colored secretions. If there is no indication of aspiration, the patient is judged to have adequate epiglottic function without risk for aspiration.

Speech with a Tracheostomy Tube

A number of techniques promote speech in the patient with a tracheostomy. The spontaneously breathing patient may be able to talk by deflating the cuff, which allows exhaled air to flow upward over the vocal cords. This can be enhanced by the patient occluding the tube. Frequently, a small cuffless tube is inserted so exhaled air can pass freely around the tube. If the patient is on mechanical ventilation, speech may be possible by allowing a constant air leak around the cuff. In addition, tracheostomy tubes and valves have been designed to facilitate speech. The nurse can be an advocate in promoting use of these specialized devices. Their use can provide great psychologic benefit and facilitate self-care for the patient with a tracheostomy.

A fenestrated tube has openings on the surface of the outer cannula that permit air from the lungs to flow over the vocal cords (see Fig. 25-6, *B*, and Fig. 25-9, *A*). A fenestrated tube allows the patient to breathe spontaneously through the larynx, speak, and cough up secretions while the tracheostomy tube

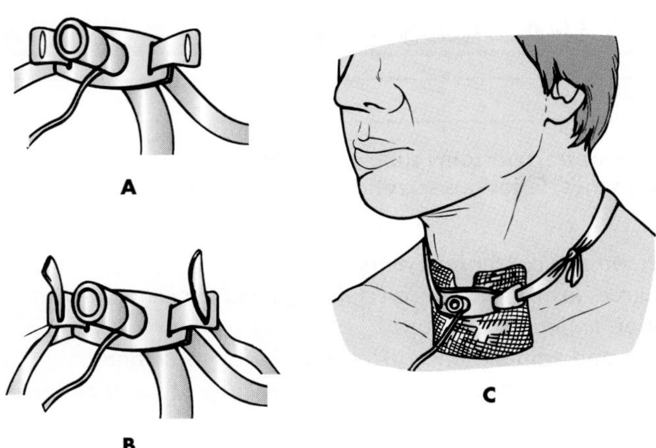

Fig 25-8 Changing tracheostomy ties. **A,** A slit is cut about 1 inch (2.5 cm) from the end. The slit end is put into the opening of the cannula. **B,** A loop is made with the other end of the tape. **C,** The tapes are tied together with a double knot on the side of the neck.

remains in place. It can be used by the patient who can swallow without risk of aspiration but requires suctioning for secretion removal. It may also be used by the patient who requires mechanical ventilation for fewer than 24 hours a day (e.g., during sleep).

Before this device is used, the patient's ability to swallow without aspiration is determined (see Table 25-5 and NCP 25-5). If there is no aspiration, (1) the inner cannula is removed, (2) the cuff is deflated, and (3) the decannulation cap is placed in the tube (see Fig. 25-9, *A*). It is important to perform the steps in order because severe respiratory distress may result if the tube is capped before the inner cannula is removed and the cuff deflated. When a fenestrated cannula is first used, the nurse should frequently assess the patient for signs of respiratory distress. If the patient is not able to tolerate the procedure, the cap should be removed, the inner cannula replaced, and the cuff reinflated. A disadvantage of fenestrated tubes is the potential for development of tracheal polyps from tracheal tissue granulating into the fenestrated openings.

A speaking tracheostomy tube has two pigtail tubings. One tubing connects to the cuff and is used for cuff inflation, and the second connects to an opening just above the cuff (see Fig. 25-9, *B*). When the second tubing is connected to a low-flow (4 to 6 L/min) air source, sufficient air moves up over the vocal cords to permit speech. The patient can then speak, although the cuff is inflated.

When a speaking tracheostomy valve is used, a cuffless tube must be in place or the cuff deflated to allow exhalation (Fig. 25-11). Ability to tolerate cuff deflation without aspiration or respiratory distress must also be evaluated in patients using this device. If there is no aspiration, the cuff is deflated and the valve is placed over the tracheostomy tube opening. The speaking valve contains a thin plastic diaphragm that opens on inspiration and closes on expiration. During inspiration, air flows in through the valve. During expiration, the diaphragm prevents exhalation and air flows upward over the vocal cords and into the mouth.[24-26]

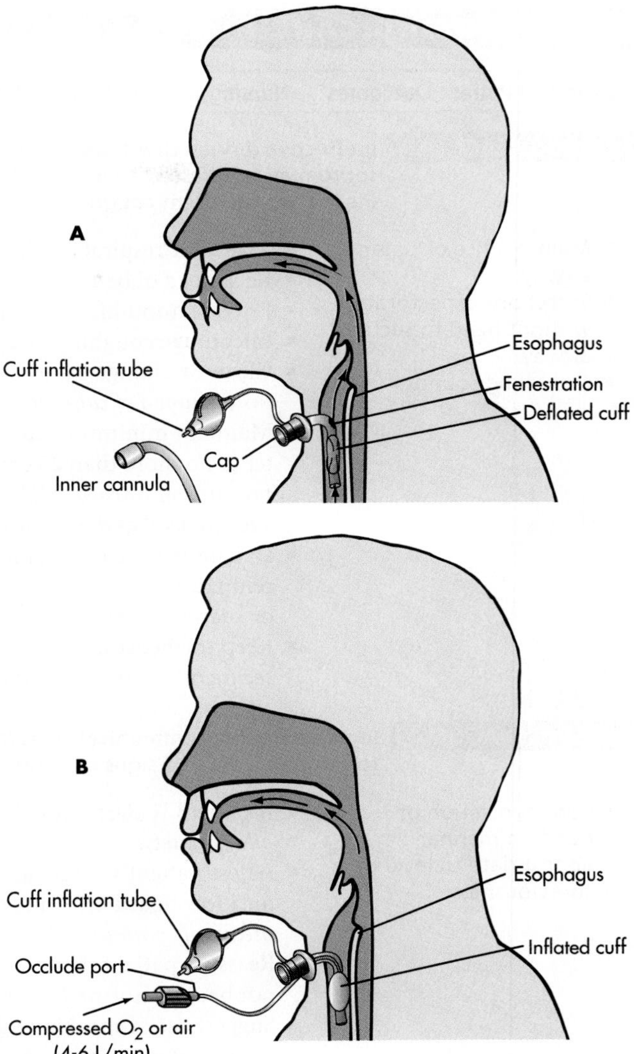

Fig. 25-9 Speaking tracheostomy tubes. **A,** Fenestrated tracheostomy tube with cuff deflated, inner cannula removed, and tracheostomy tube capped to allow air to pass over the vocal cords. **B,** Speaking tracheostomy tube. One tubing is used for cuff inflation. The second tubing is connected to a source of compressed air or oxygen. When the port on the second tubing is occluded, air flows up over the vocal cords, allowing speech with an inflated cuff. (See Tables 25-5 and NCP 25-5 for related nursing management.)

Decannulation

When the patient can adequately exchange air and expectorate secretions, the tracheostomy tube can be removed. The stoma is closed with tape strips and covered with an occlusive dressing. The dressing must be changed if it gets soiled or wet. The patient should be instructed to splint the stoma with the fingers when coughing, swallowing, or speaking. Epithelial tissue begins to form in 24 to 48 hours, and the opening will close in several days. Surgical intervention to close the tracheostomy is not required.

25-5 NURSING CARE PLAN PATIENT WITH A TRACHEOSTOMY

Expected Patient Outcomes	Nursing Interventions and *Rationales*
NURSING DIAGNOSIS	**Ineffective airway clearance** *related to* presence of tracheostomy tube and difficulty expectorating sputum *as manifested by* adventitious breath sounds, tenacious secretions, increase in restlessness, ineffective or absent cough.
▪ Maintenance of patent airway. ▪ Secretions expectorated without need to suction airway. ▪ Clear lung sounds.	▪ Assess for respiratory distress *to determine need for interventions.* ▪ Keep head of bed elevated 30-40 degrees *to allow a more forceful cough and to relieve dyspnea.* ▪ Provide humidification and hydration *to liquefy secretions.* ▪ Encourage coughing, deep breathing, and ambulation *to assist in mobilizing secretions.* ▪ Clean or change inner cannula, if present, as needed *to minimize buildup of secretions on inside lumen of cannula.* ▪ Maintain minimum cuff pressure while obtaining airway seal by measuring with manometer at no more than 25 cm H_2O pressure or with minimal leak technique (MLT) *to minimize pressure on trachea. MLT cannot be used if tracheostomy is to bypass upper airway obstruction such as head and neck surgery.* ▪ Deflate cuff at least daily *to remove accumulated secretions;* deflate during exhalation and reinflate during inhalation. Clear mouth and trachea before and after deflation by coughing or suctioning *to minimize aspiration.* ▪ Keep tracheostomy tube tied securely, allowing room for one finger between ties and skin *to secure tube from accidentally dislodging.*
NURSING DIAGNOSIS	**Impaired verbal communication** *related to* use of artificial airway and cuff *as manifested by* inability to communicate and signs of frustration.
▪ Communication of needs in manner appropriate to level of consciousness.	▪ If patient is alert, provide call bell within easy reach and respond immediately in person *to allay anxiety.* ▪ Assess patient's ability to read and write; provide with magic slate, pad and pencil, communication board with illustrations of requests, electrolarynx (Cooper-Rand) *as alternative means of communication.* ▪ Reassure patient that speech will return when cuff can be deflated (if total laryngectomy has not been performed) *to allay fear that situation is permanent.* ▪ Suggest use of speaking tubes (small, cuffless tube, fenestrated tube, speaking valve, speaking tracheostomy tube) *to permit speech.* ▪ Encourage gesturing *to communicate needs and desires.*
NURSING DIAGNOSIS	**Risk for infection** *related to* bypass of airway defense mechanisms and impaired skin integrity.
▪ Normal white blood cell count. ▪ Normal temperature. ▪ Clear mucus. ▪ No erythema or purulent secretions from stoma site.	▪ Monitor and report elevated white blood cell count and temperature, change in color of secretions, purulent drainage *to identify signs of infection and permit early medical intervention.* ▪ Use strict aseptic technique for suctioning and tracheostomy care during hospitalization *to reduce occurrence of infection.* ▪ Change oxygen-delivery equipment q48hr *to prevent contaminated tubing from being a source of infection.* ▪ Keep stoma clean and dry with frequent tracheostomy care.
NURSING DIAGNOSIS	**Altered nutrition: less than body requirements** *related to* decreased oral intake, altered taste sensation, and swallowing difficulty *as manifested by* inadequate caloric intake, weight loss.
▪ Usual appetite. ▪ Maintenance of normal body weight.	▪ Provide ongoing assessment of oral intake and caloric count if required *to assess adequacy of diet.* ▪ Monitor weight *to provide information for evaluation.* ▪ Provide high-calorie, high-protein food and beverages *to maximize nutritional intake.* ▪ Thicken foods and beverages if needed *to ease swallowing and minimize aspiration.* ▪ Assess for swallowing dysfunction *to determine if presence of inflated cuff is predisposing to aspiration.* ▪ Initiate enteral feedings if patient is unable to take in adequate oral intake *to maintain nutritional intake.* ▪ Perform mouth care q8hr and prn *to promote patient comfort and appetite.*

Continued

25-5 NURSING CARE PLAN PATIENT WITH A TRACHEOSTOMY—continued

Expected Patient Outcomes	Nursing Interventions and *Rationales*

NURSING DIAGNOSIS **Impaired swallowing** *related to* mechanical obstruction secondary to tracheostomy tube *as manifested by* inability to swallow without aspiration.

▪ Normal swallowing function. ▪ No aspiration.	▪ Assess swallow and gag reflexes by deflating cuff; note coughing *is an indicator of aspiration.* ▪ If patient tolerates cuff deflated, have patient swallow clear liquid (grape juice) or water with blue food coloring *to determine presence of aspiration.* If patient does not cough or no colored secretions are suctioned, the patient may tolerate eating with cuff deflated.

NURSING DIAGNOSIS **Ineffective management of therapeutic regimen** *related to* lack of knowledge about care of tracheostomy at home *as manifested by* questioning about care (patient or family), agitation, and restlessness when planning for discharge.

▪ Demonstration of techniques by patient and significant others for tracheostomy care. ▪ Able to verbalize expected outcomes and when to contact health care professionals if problems arise.	▪ Assess ability of patient and significant other to provide care at home, including tracheostomy tube care, stoma care, airway care, and ability to respond appropriately to emergencies *to determine if home care is feasible.* ▪ Teach good hand-washing technique *to minimize risk for infection.* ▪ Teach clean tracheostomy tube care and home preparation of sterile saline solution *so patient can care for self at home.* ▪ Teach clean suctioning, if needed, and use of one catheter for 24 hr *so patient can care for self at home.* ▪ Teach patient and significant other the signs and symptoms to report to health care professionals such as changes in secretions (yellow, green, or blood tinged) or elevated temperature *because these may be early signs of respiratory infection.* ▪ Make referral to home health nurse *to provide ongoing assistance and support.*

COLLABORATIVE PROBLEMS

Nursing Goals	Nursing Interventions and *Rationales*

POTENTIAL COMPLICATION **Hypoxemia** *related to* misplaced or improperly functioning tube, accumulated secretions.

▪ Monitor for signs of hypoxemia. ▪ Report deviations from acceptable parameters. ▪ Carry out appropriate medical and nursing interventions.	▪ Assess patient for restlessness, agitation, confusion, tachycardia, bradycardia, arrhythmias; SpO_2 less than 90%; accidental expulsion of tube from airway *to determine if tube is placed properly.* ▪ Elevate head of bed if tolerated. ▪ Auscultate chest *to determine need for suctioning.* If coarse crackles or rhonchi are present and patient cannot cough and clear secretions, suction airway. ▪ If unable to pass suction catheter, *tube is dislodged* and emergency measures must be implemented. ▪ If tube is dislodged or misplaced, grasp the retention sutures (if present) and spread opening. Lubricate tube and insert with obturator in place at 45 degree angle to neck. If successful, remove obturator immediately. ▪ Another method is to insert a suction catheter to allow the passage of air and to serve as a guide for insertion. Thread the tracheostomy tube over catheter and remove the suction catheter. ▪ If tube cannot be reinserted, assess the level of respiratory distress *to determine whether patient can breathe without tube for a short interval.* ▪ Notify physician. If distress is severe, ventilate with bag-mask ventilator until assistance arrives *to ensure adequate ventilation.*

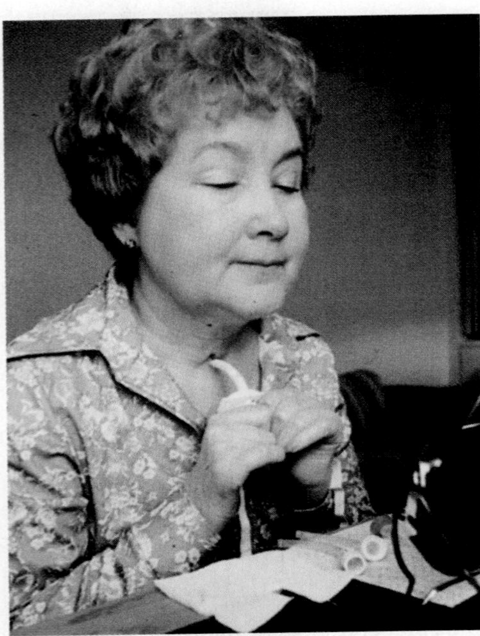

Fig. 25-10 Changing the tracheostomy tube at home. When a tracheostomy has been in place for several months, the tract will be well formed. The patient can then be taught to change the tube using a clean technique at home.

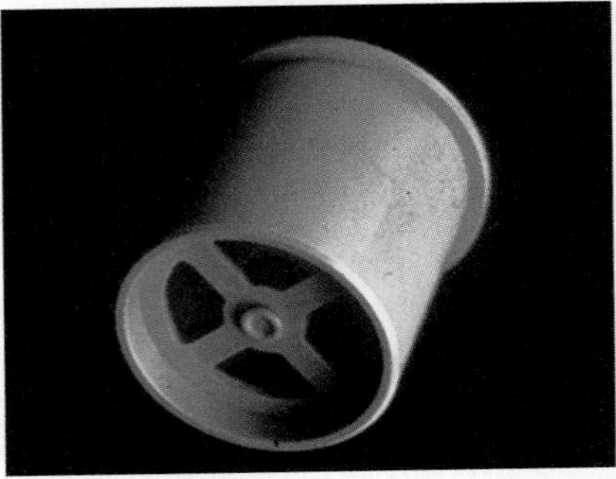

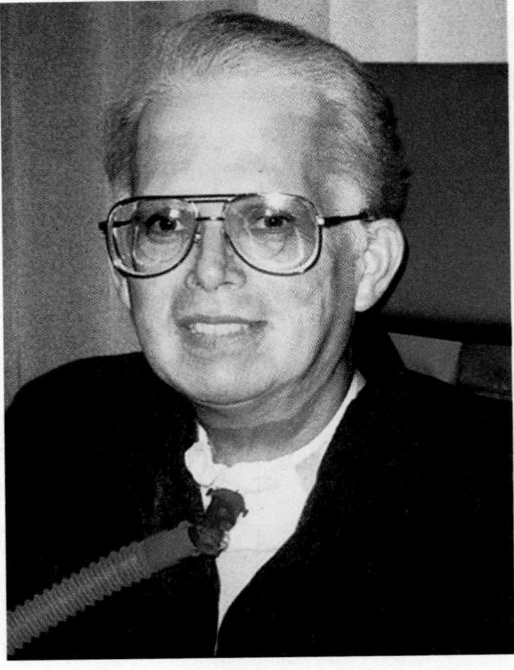

Fig. 25-11 Passy-Muir speaking tracheostomy valve. The valve is placed over the hub of the tracheostomy tube after the cuff is deflated. Two options are available: a white valve for non-ventilated patients and an aqua valve (shown) for ventilated patients. The valve contains a one-way valve that allows air to enter the lungs during inspiration and redirects air upward over the vocal cords into the mouth during expiration.

LARYNGEAL POLYPS

Laryngeal polyps may develop on the vocal cords from vocal abuse (e.g., excessive talking, singing) or irritation (e.g., intubation, cigarette smoking). The most common symptom is hoarseness. Polyps may be treated conservatively with voice rest. Surgical removal may be indicated for large polyps, which may cause dyspnea and stridor. Polyps are usually benign but may be removed because they may later become malignant.

CANCER OF THE HEAD AND NECK

In 1998 there were an estimated 55,000 new cases of head and neck cancer diagnosed in the United States with nearly 13,000 deaths. The male-to-female ratio is nearly 3:1. The incidence of this cancer is increasing in women, most likely because of rising tobacco and alcohol consumption. The usual age at diagnosis is 50 years or older. Although this disorder represents only about 5% of cancer cases, disability is great because of the potential loss of voice, disfigurement, and social consequences. Although specific causes are not known, there are well-known risk factors. Most (90%) head and neck cancers arise after prolonged use of tobacco and alcohol. Exposure to various noxious fumes and chemicals may also predispose to head and neck cancer. A viral etiology has been implicated in up to 15% of the cases. An association between the Epstein-Barr virus (EBV) and nasopharyngeal carcinomas has been suggested by the high incidence of elevated EBV titers in patients with nasopharyngeal carcinoma. Genetic research has shown that mutation in a tumor suppressor gene on human chromosome 17 is linked to head and neck cancer.[27-29]

Clinical Manifestations

The nurse is in a key position to detect early signs of head and neck cancer. Early detection is critical. If found early, the cure rate is high. However, early symptoms are often not reported because the patient does not know their significance or fears the consequences.[28,29]

Early signs and symptoms of upper airway cancer vary with tumor location. Cancer of the oral cavity may be a painless growth in the mouth, an ulcer that does not heal, or a change in fit of dentures. Pain is a late symptom that may be aggravated by acidic food. Cancers of the oropharynx, hypopharynx, and supraglottic larynx rarely produce early symptoms and are usually diagnosed in late stages. The patient may complain of persistent unilateral sore throat or otalgia (ear pain).

Hoarseness may be a symptom of early laryngeal cancer. If a lump in the neck or hoarseness lasts longer than 2 weeks, a medical evaluation is indicated. Some patients experience what feels like a lump in the throat or a change in voice quality. Late stages of head and neck cancers have easily detectable signs and symptoms including pain, dysphagia, decreased mobility of the tongue, airway obstruction, and cranial nerve neuropathies.[28]

The nurse should thoroughly examine the oral cavity, including the area under the tongue and dentures. The floor of the mouth, tongue, and lymph nodes in the neck should be bimanually palpated. There may be thickening of the normally soft and pliable oral mucosa. Leukoplakia (white patch) or erythroplakia (red patch) may be seen and should be noted for later biopsy. Both leukoplakia and carcinoma in situ (localized to a defined area) may precede invasive carcinoma by many years.[27,28]

Diagnostic Studies

If lesions are suspected, the upper airways may be examined using indirect laryngoscopy that involves using a laryngeal mirror to visualize the laryngeal area, or a flexible nasopharyngoscope may be used. The larynx and vocal cords are visually inspected for lesions and tissue mobility. A CT scan or magnetic resonance imaging (MRI) may be performed to detect local and regional spread. Neoplastic tissue is identifiable because it contains tissue of greater density or because it distorts, displaces, or destroys normal anatomic structures. Typically, multiple biopsy specimens are obtained to determine the extent of the disease.

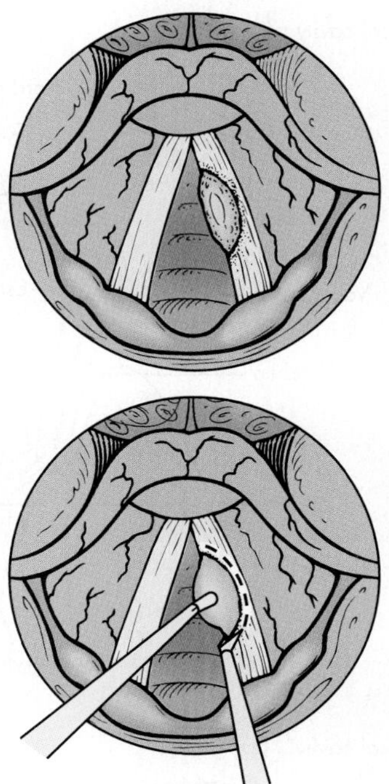

Fig. 25-12 Excision of laryngeal cancer. This cancer of the right vocal cord meets criteria for resection by transoral cordectomy. The cord is fully mobile and the lesion can be fully exposed. It does not approach or cross the anterior commissure.

Collaborative Care

Using the information obtained, a decision will be made about the stage of the disease based on tumor size (T), number and location of involved nodes (N), and extent of metastasis (M). TNM staging classifies disease as stage I to stage IV and guides treatment. Approximately one third of patients with head and neck cancers have highly confined lesions that are stage I or II at diagnosis. Such patients can undergo radiation therapy or surgery with the goal of cure. This goal is achieved in approximately 80% of patients with stage I disease and in 60% of patients with stage II disease. In stage III or IV disease, fewer than 30% of patients are cured.[28] Choice of treatment is based on medical history, extent of disease, cosmetic considerations, urgency of treatment, and patient choice.

Radiation therapy may be effective in curing early vocal cord lesions. This therapy is usually successful in eliminating the tumor while preserving the quality of the voice. If radiation therapy is not successful or the lesion is too advanced for this therapy, surgery may be performed. A cordectomy is used when there is a superficial tumor involving one cord. A cordectomy is a smaller version of a hemilaryngectomy (Fig. 25-12). A hemilaryngectomy involves removal of one vocal cord or part of a cord and requires a temporary tracheostomy. A supraglottic laryngectomy involves removing structures above the true cords–the false vocal cords and epiglottis. The patient is left at high risk of aspiration following surgery and requires a temporary tracheostomy. Both a hemilaryngectomy and supraglottic laryngectomy allow the voice to be preserved, but quality is breathy and hoarse.

Advanced lesions are treated by a total laryngectomy in which the entire larynx and preepiglottic region is removed and a permanent tracheostomy performed. Airflow patterns before and after total laryngectomy are shown in Fig. 25-13. Radical neck dissection frequently accompanies total laryngectomy to decrease the risk of lymphatic spread. Depending on the extent of involvement, extensive dissection and reconstruction may be performed. This procedure involves wide excision of the lymph nodes and their lymphatic channels (Fig. 25-14). Depending on the primary lesion and its extensiveness, the following structures may also be removed or transected: the sternocleidomastoid muscle and other closely associated muscles, internal jugular vein, mandible, submaxillary gland, part of the thyroid and parathyroid glands, and the spinal accessory nerve.

A modified neck dissection is performed whenever possible as an alternative to a radical neck dissection. The dissection is modified by sparing as many structures as possible to limit disfigurement and functional loss. A modified neck dissection usually involves dissection of the major cervical lymphatic vessels and lateral cervical space with preservation of nerves and vessels, including the sympathetic and vagus nerves, spinal accessory nerves, and internal jugular vein. Neck dissection with vocal cord cancer usually involves one side of the neck. However, if the lesion is midline, a bilateral neck dissection may be performed. When a bilateral neck dissection is performed, it

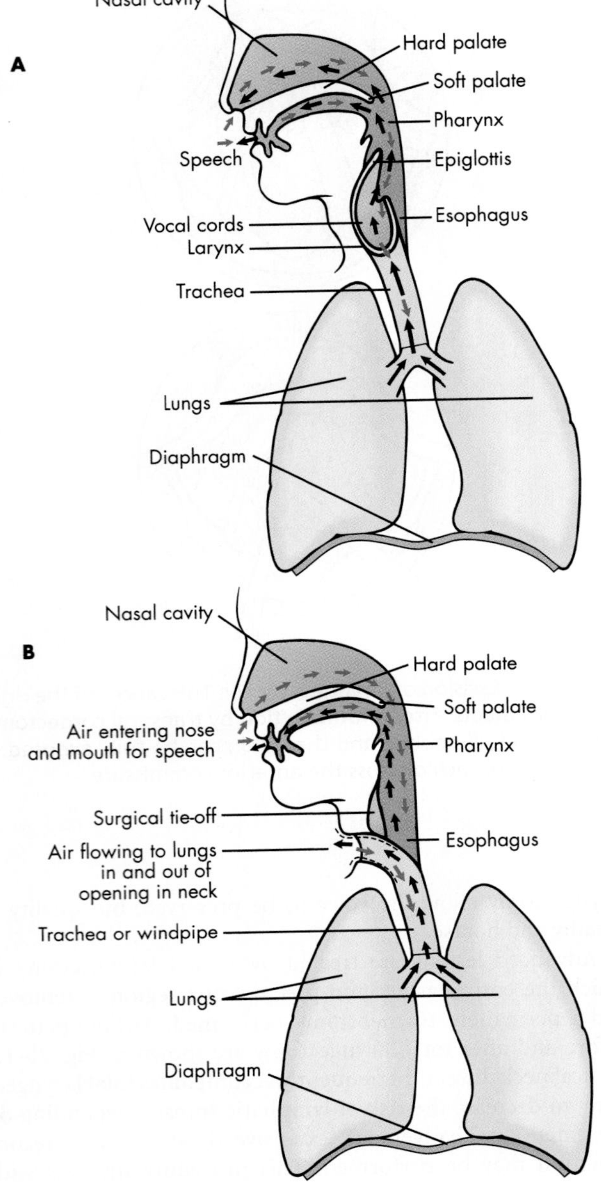

Fig. 25-13 **A,** Normal airflow in and out of the lungs. **B,** Airflow in and out of the lungs after total laryngectomy. Patients using esophageal speech trap air in the esophagus and release it to create sound.

is always modified on at least one side to minimize structural and functional deficits.

The patient may refuse surgical intervention for advanced lesions because of the extent of the procedure or may be judged to be at too great a medical risk to undergo the procedure. In this situation, external radiation therapy may be used as the sole treatment or a combination of chemotherapy and radiation therapy.

In addition, brachytherapy, a concentrated and localized method of delivering radiation that involves placing a radioactive source into or near the tumor, may be used to treat head and neck cancer. The goal is to deliver high doses of radiation to the target area while limiting exposure of surrounding tissues. Thin hollow plastic needles are inserted into the tumor area and a radioactive source, iridium seeds, is placed in the needles. The seeds emit continuous radiation. Brachytherapy can be used alone or combined with external radiation or surgical intervention. (Radiation therapy and brachytherapy are discussed in Chapter 14.)

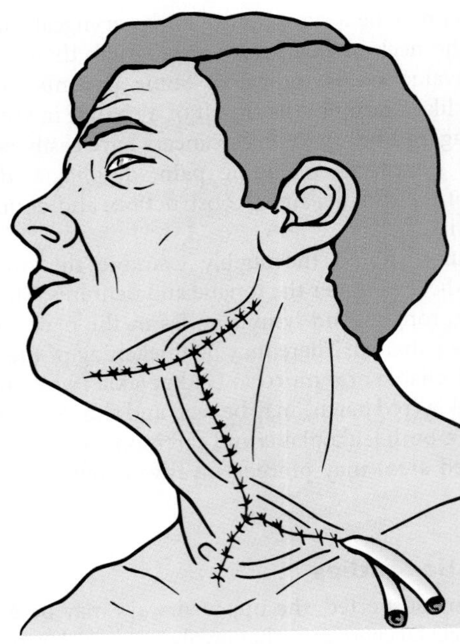

Fig. 25-14 Radical neck incision with suction tubing in place.

Nutritional Therapy. After radical neck surgery, the patient may be unable to take in nutrients through the normal route of ingestion because of swelling, the location of sutures, or difficulty with swallowing. Parenteral fluids will be given for the first 24 to 48 hours. After this time, tube feedings are usually given via a nasogastric or nasointestinal tube that was placed during surgery. Sometimes a temporary feeding gastrostomy may be used. (Nasogastric and gastrostomy feedings are described in Chapter 38.) Cervical esophagostomy and pharyngostomy have also been used. The nurse must observe for tolerance of the feedings and adjust the amount, time, and formula if nausea, vomiting, diarrhea, or distention occurs. The patient is usually instructed about the tube feedings. When the patient can swallow, small amounts of water are given. Close observation for choking is essential. Suctioning may be necessary to prevent aspiration.

Swallowing problems should be anticipated when the patient resumes eating. The type and degree of difficulty vary, depending on the procedure. When a supraglottic laryngectomy is performed, the surgeon excises the upper portion of the larynx, including the epiglottis and false vocal cords. The patient can speak because the true vocal cords remain intact. However, a new technique, the supraglottic swallow, must be learned to compensate for removal of the epiglottis and minimize risk of aspiration (Table 25-8). When learning this technique, it may be helpful to start with carbonated beverages because the effervescence provides cues about the liquid's position. With this exception, thin, watery fluids should be avoided

PATIENT TEACHING GUIDE

Table 25-8 Steps for Performing the Supraglottic Swallow

1. Take a deep breath to aerate lungs.
2. Perform Valsalva's maneuver to approximate cords.
3. Place food in mouth and swallow. Some food will enter airway and remain on top of closed vocal cords.
4. Cough to remove food from top of vocal cords.
5. Swallow so food is moved from top of vocal cords.
6. Breathe after cough-swallow sequence to prevent aspiration of food collected on top of vocal cords.

Adapted from Sigler BA, Schuring LT: *Ear, nose, and throat disorders,* St Louis, 1994, Mosby, p 240.

since they are difficult to swallow and increase the risk of aspiration. A better choice is nonpourable pureed foods, which are thicker and allow more control during swallowing.[1]

Good nutrition is important during radiation therapy because calories and protein are needed for tissue repair. Antiemetics or analgesics may be given before meals to reduce nausea and mouth pain. Bland foods may be better tolerated. Caloric intake may be increased by adding dry milk to foods during preparation, selecting foods high in calories, and using oral supplements. It is helpful to add sauces and gravies to food, which adds calories and moistens food so it is more easily swallowed. If an adequate intake cannot be maintained, enteral feedings may be used.

NURSING MANAGEMENT: CANCER OF THE HEAD AND NECK

Nursing Assessment

Subjective and objective data that should be obtained from a person with head and neck cancer are presented in Table 25-9.

NURSING ASSESSMENT

Table 25-9 Cancer of the Head and Neck

Subjective Data

Important Health Information

Past health history: Positive family history; prolonged tobacco use (cigarettes, pipes, cigars, chewing tobacco, smokeless tobacco); prolonged, heavy alcohol use; exposure to radiation or occupational exposures to heavy metals and fumes; history of viral infections (e.g., Epstein-Barr); poor oral hygiene

Medications: Prolonged use of over-the-counter medication for sore throat, decongestants

Functional Health Patterns

Health perception–health management: Does not value preventive health measures, long history of alcohol and tobacco use

Nutritional-metabolic: Mouth ulcer that does not heal, change in fit of dentures, change in appetite, weight loss, swallowing difficulty (e.g., sensation of lump in throat, pain with swallowing, aspiration when swallowing)

Activity-exercise: Fatigue with minimal exertion

Cognitive-perceptual: Sore throat, pain on swallowing, referred ear pain

Objective Data

Respiratory

Hoarseness, change in voice quality, chronic laryngitis, nasal voice, palpable neck mass and lymph nodes (tender, hard, fixed), tracheal deviation; dyspnea, stridor (late sign)

Gastrointestinal

White (leukoplakia) or red (erythoplakia) patches inside mouth, ulceration of mucosa, asymmetric tongue, exudate in mouth or pharynx, mass or thickening of mucosa

Possible Findings

Mass on direct or indirect laryngoscopy; tumor on soft tissue x-ray, computed tomography (CT) scan, or magnetic resonance imaging (MRI); positive biopsy

Nursing Diagnoses

Nursing diagnoses for the patient with head and neck cancer include, but are not limited to, those presented in NCP 25-6.

Planning

The overall goals are that the patient will have (1) a patent airway, (2) no spread of cancer, (3) no complications related to therapy, (4) adequate nutritional intake, (5) minimal to no pain, (6) the ability to communicate, and (7) an acceptable body image.

Nursing Implementation

Health Promotion. Development of head and neck cancer is closely related to personal habits, primarily tobacco use, including the use of cigarettes, cigars, chewing tobacco, and snuff. Snuff dipping, or the placement and retention of tobacco in the cheek, is becoming more common among U.S. youth. Another popular fad is cigar smoking. Long-term snuff users and cigar smokers are at increased risk of oral cancer. Prolonged alcohol use has been implicated as a potentiating factor in head and neck cancer.

The nurse should include information about risk factors in health teaching. If cancer has been diagnosed, tobacco cessation is still important. The patient with head and neck cancer who continues to smoke during radiation therapy has a lower rate of response and survival than the patient who does not smoke during radiation therapy.[27] Additionally, risk of a secondary primary cancer is significantly increased in patients who continue to smoke.

Acute Intervention. The patient and the family must be taught about the type of therapy to be performed and care required. Assessment of concerns is integral to the plan of care. The patient and family must deal with the psychologic impact of the diagnosis of cancer, alteration of physical appearance, and possible need for altered methods of communication. The care plan should include assessment of the patient's support system. The patient may not have someone to provide assistance after

25-6 NURSING CARE PLAN PATIENT WITH TOTAL LARYNGECTOMY OR RADICAL NECK SURGERY

Expected Patient Outcomes	Nursing Interventions and *Rationales*
NURSING DIAGNOSIS **Anxiety** *related to* lack of knowledge regarding surgical procedure, pain management, and prevention of complications *as manifested by* questioning about impending surgery, agitation, restlessness.	
■ Decrease in anxiety about surgery and a calm appearance. ■ Verbalization of confidence regarding surgical procedure.	■ Assess knowledge desired by patient *to allay fears and answer questions.* ■ Facilitate discussion of expected alterations in physical appearance and function; encourage sharing of feelings and concerns *to begin adjustment and acceptance.* ■ Provide information about what to expect after surgery (tracheostomy tube, stoma, incisions, alternative communication methods, nasogastric tube, drainage tubes, pain management) *to reduce patient's sense of helplessness and increase sense of control.*
NURSING DIAGNOSIS **Ineffective airway clearance** *related to* alteration in upper airway, tracheal stoma, presence of tracheostomy tube, difficulty expectorating sputum *as manifested by* ineffective or absent cough; rhonchi or coarse crackles on auscultation; abnormal rate, pattern of breathing.	
■ Patent airway. ■ Normal respiratory rate and pattern.	■ Auscultate chest and monitor respiratory rate, pattern, SpO_2, and level of consciousness q4hr for 24 hr postoperatively *to determine adequacy of respirations.* ■ Encourage coughing, deep breathing, and ambulating *to assist in mobilizing secretions.* ■ Suction tracheostomy tube/stoma as needed *to clear secretions.* ■ Administer humidified air or oxygen as prescribed into tracheostomy/stoma *to help keep secretions moist.* ■ Clean inner cannula of tracheostomy/laryngectomy tube three times daily and as needed *to prevent mucus from crusting, which may occlude the lumen.*
NURSING DIAGNOSIS **Altered tissue perfusion** *related to* tissue edema and disruption of vascular and lymphatic drainage *as manifested by* swollen and tense skin, serous drainage from wound drainage tubes.	
■ Decrease in tissue edema. ■ Minimal to no drainage from tubes. ■ Stable vital signs. ■ Healing of incision lines.	■ Maintain head of bed at 30 to 40 degrees *to decrease tissue edema.* ■ Monitor heart rate, blood pressure, hemoglobin, and hematocrit *to detect excessive bleeding.* ■ Monitor patency of drainage tubes, amount, color of drainage *to determine if drainage is excessive.* ■ Clean incision as prescribed *to prevent infection.*
NURSING DIAGNOSIS **Altered nutrition: less than body requirements** *related to* surgical procedure, edema, dysphagia, presence of a nasogastric tube *as manifested by* absence of oral intake.	
■ Normal oral intake. ■ Able to swallow. ■ Maintenance of body weight.	■ Provide frequent oral hygiene with saline rinses or dilute hydrogen peroxide *to promote comfort and remove drainage.* ■ Administer enteral feedings as ordered *to provide adequate nutrients while wound heals.* ■ When oral feedings begin, give clear liquids and advance as tolerated *to allow patient time to adjust to initiation of oral intake.* ■ Monitor caloric intake and weight to evaluate response.
NURSING DIAGNOSIS **Impaired verbal communication** *related to* removal of vocal cords *as manifested by* inability to speak.	
■ Able to communicate clearly using method of choice.	■ Evaluate the patient's ability to read and write. ■ Instruct in alternate methods of communication (magic slate, communication board, electrolarynx). ■ Encourage use of communication tools and allow adequate time for communication. ■ Consult with speech therapist *to learn use of voice prosthesis, electrolarynx, or esophageal speech.*

Continued

25-6 NURSING CARE PLAN PATIENT WITH TOTAL LARYNGECTOMY OR RADICAL NECK SURGERY—continued

Expected Patient Outcomes	Nursing Interventions and *Rationales*
NURSING DIAGNOSIS	**Body image disturbance** *related to* disfiguring surgery and loss of oral communication *as manifested by* withdrawal, depression, isolation, unwillingness to look at self or assist with care, refusal to see visitors.
▪ Acknowledgement of change in body structure and function. ▪ Able to communicate feelings about surgical changes. ▪ Participation in self-care.	▪ Assess patient's body image concept *to identify patients at risk for unsuccessful adjustment.* ▪ Provide privacy *to respect patient's request while adjusting to change in body function and appearance.* ▪ Encourage attention to personal hygiene *because improved appearance can boost self-esteem.* ▪ Encourage socialization with family and friends *because acceptance by significant others is a critical factor in patient's own acceptance.* ▪ Provide information about measures to help improve appearance such as wearing clothes with high collars and wearing accessories *to aid in successful adjustment.* ▪ Answer questions honestly about changes in body image *to convey acceptance and to provide accurate information.* ▪ Involve patient in self-care *because participation in self-care is a sign of successful adjustment.* ▪ Assure patient of self-worth *to increase acceptance of altered physical appearance.*
NURSING DIAGNOSIS	**Pain** *related to* surgical procedure *as manifested by* report of discomfort, facial mask of pain, changes in blood pressure, pulse, respiratory rate.
▪ Satisfactory pain control.	▪ Assess patient's manifestations of pain (e.g., facial expression, reluctance to cough or move) *to plan appropriate interventions.* ▪ Administer pain medication as prescribed and assess effectiveness *to reduce pain and prevent respiratory depression.* ▪ Logroll head and chest *to prevent strain on sutures.* ▪ Keep head of bed elevated 30 to 40 degrees at all times *to limit edema.* ▪ Refer patient to physical therapy for exercises to be used *to maintain strength and mobility of shoulder, which is compromised by radical neck dissection.*
NURSING DIAGNOSIS	**Ineffective management of therapeutic regimen** *related to* lack of knowledge about home care after discharge *as manifested by* verbalized concern about ability to manage self-care at home.
▪ Demonstration of steps to be used in carrying out self-care.	▪ Provide written instructions for patient and significant other *because an accurate reference reduces error.* ▪ Teach patient and significant other laryngectomy tube and stoma care allowing them to perform repeatedly in hospital *to ensure correct performance of technique.* ▪ Teach patient to cover stoma before performing activities such as shaving, application of makeup *to avoid inhalation of foreign materials.* ▪ Teach patient to report changes, such as stoma narrowing, difficulty swallowing, lump in the throat *to detect possible recurrence of tumor or tracheal stenosis.* ▪ Teach patient to provide adequate humidity at home using a bedside humidifier, sitting in a steamy bathroom, instillation of 3-5 ml sterile normal saline into laryngectomy tube/stoma. ▪ Teach patient to report changes in mucus production such as color changes (yellow or green) or blood-tinged secretions *because these may be signs of infection or tracheal irritation.* ▪ Make referral for home health care visit *to evaluate self-care.*

discharge, may not be employed, or may be employed in a job that cannot be continued. It may be helpful to consult a social worker to assist with discharge planning.

Radiation therapy. The nurse can suggest interventions to reduce side effects of radiation therapy.[1] Dry mouth (xerostomia), the most frequent and annoying problem, typically begins within a few weeks of treatment. The patient's saliva decreases in volume and becomes thick. The change may be temporary or permanent. Pilocarpine hydrochloride (Salagen) can be effective in increasing saliva production and should be started before the initiation of radiation therapy and continued for 90 days. Symptom relief can also be obtained by carrying a squirt or water bottle, increasing fluid intake, chewing sugarless gum or sugarless candy, using nonalcoholic mouth rinses (baking soda or glycerin solutions), and artificial saliva.

The patient may also complain of stomatitis, especially if the oral cavity is in the field of therapy. Irritation, ulceration, and pain are common complaints. Rinses of water and hydrogen peroxide (3:1 ratio) or baking soda and water (1 tsp baking soda to 8 oz water) can be used to clean and soothe irritated tissues.

Commercial mouthwashes and hot or spicy foods should be avoided because they are irritating. If the problem is severe, a mixture of equal parts of antacid, diphenhydramine (Benadryl), and topical lidocaine can be used. Skin over the radiated area often becomes reddened and sensitive to touch. All exposure to the sun should be avoided to reduce discomfort.

Surgical therapy. Preoperative care for the patient who is to have a radical neck dissection involves consideration of the patient's physical and psychosocial needs. Physical preparation is the same as for any major surgery, with special emphasis on oral hygiene. Explanations and emotional support are of special significance and should include postoperative measures relating to communication and feeding. The surgical procedure should be explained to the patient, and the nurse should make sure that the information is understood by the patient.

Teaching must be tailored to the planned surgical procedure. For surgeries that involve a laryngectomy, teaching should include information about expected changes in speech. The nurse or speech pathologist should demonstrate means of communicating other than speaking that can be used temporarily or permanently.

After surgery, maintenance of a patent airway is a priority. The inflammation in the surgical area may compress the trachea. The patient will be placed in a semi-Fowler's position to decrease edema and limit tension on the suture lines. Vital signs should be monitored frequently because of the risk of hemorrhage and respiratory compromise. Pressure dressings, packing, or drainage tubes (Hemovac, Jackson Pratt) may be used for wound management, depending on the type of surgical procedure. When a radical neck dissection is performed, wound suction using a portable system, such as a Hemovac, is usually used. If skin flaps are employed, dressings are typically not used. This allows better visualization of the incision and avoids excessive pressure on tissue. The drainage should be serosanguineous and gradually decrease in volume over 24 hours. Patency of drainage tubes should be monitored every 4 hours to ensure that they are properly removing serous drainage and for the amount and character of drainage. If the

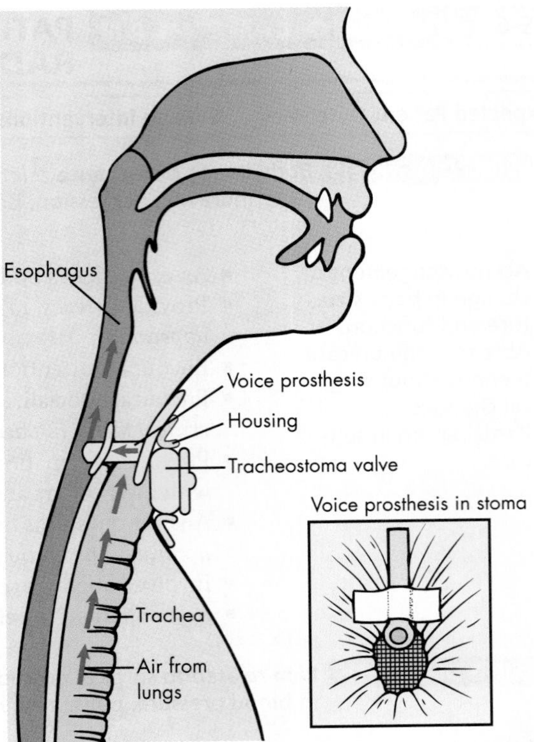

Fig. 25-15 Blom-Singer voice prosthesis and tracheostoma valve. With this prosthesis and valve, patients with a laryngectomy can speak normally. Inserts show laryngectomy stoma and voice prosthesis with tracheostoma valve removed.

tubing becomes obstructed, fluid will accumulate under the skin flap and predispose to impaired wound healing and infection. After drainage tubes are removed, the area should be closely monitored to detect any swelling. If fluid continues to accumulate, aspiration may be necessary.

Immediately after surgery, the patient with a laryngectomy requires frequent suctioning via the laryngectomy tube. Secretions typically change in amount and consistency over time. The patient may initially have copious blood-tinged secretions that diminish and thicken. If the patient develops mucous plugs or thick secretions, a 3 to 5 ml bolus of normal saline may be instilled into the airway to loosen secretions enough to clear the airway either through coughing or suctioning. With teaching, the patient can learn to use the bolus technique at home to assist in providing moisture and mobilizing secretions. The patient will also benefit from the use of a humidifier while hospitalized and at home.

Following a neck dissection, an exercise program should be instituted to maintain strength and movement in the affected shoulder and neck. This is especially important when the spinal accessory nerve and sternocleidomastoid muscles are sacrificed or damaged. Without exercise, the patient will be left with a frozen shoulder and limited range of neck motion. This exercise program should be continued following discharge to prevent future functional disabilities.

Voice rehabilitation. A speech therapist should meet with the patient following a total laryngectomy to discuss voice

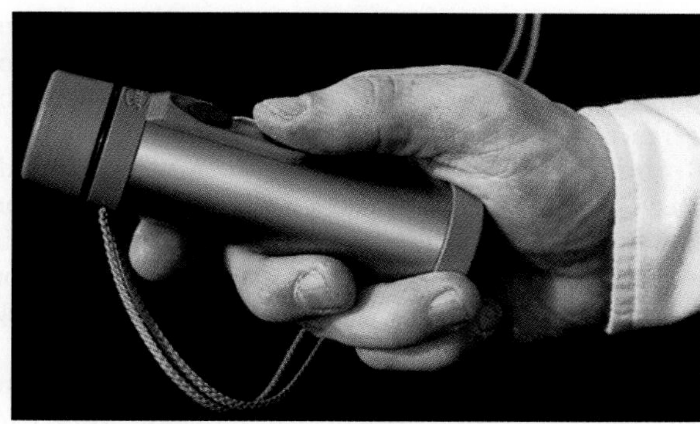

Fig. 25-16 Artificial larynx. Battery-powered electronic artificial larynx for patient who has total laryngectomy.

restoration options. The International Association of Laryngectomies, an association of laryngectomy patients, focuses on assisting patients to reestablish speech. Local groups, called Lost Cord Clubs, often provide member volunteers to visit the patient, preferably preoperatively. Several options are available to restore speech. These include use of a voice prosthesis, esophageal speech, and an electrolarynx.

The most commonly used voice prosthesis is the Blom-Singer prosthesis (Fig. 25-15).[30] This soft plastic device is inserted into a fistula made between the esophagus and the trachea. The puncture may be created at the time of surgery or afterward, depending on the preference of the surgeon. A red rubber catheter is placed in the tracheoesophageal puncture and must remain intact until a tract is formed. Once the tract is formed, the speech prosthesis is inserted. This prosthesis allows air from the lungs to enter the esophagus by way of the tracheal stoma. A one-way valve prevents aspiration of food or saliva from the esophagus into the tracheostomy. To speak, the patient manually blocks the stoma with the finger. Air moves from the lungs, through the prosthesis, into the esophagus, and out the mouth. Speech is produced by the air vibrating against the esophagus and is formed into words by moving the tongue and lips. A valve may also be used with this device. When the valve is in place, the stoma does not need to be closed with the finger to speak. The prosthesis must be cleaned regularly and replaced when it becomes blocked with mucus.

An electrolarynx is a handheld, battery-powered device that creates speech with the use of sound waves. One device, the Cooper-Rand, uses a plastic tube placed in the corner of the roof of the mouth to create vibrations. To create the most normal sound when using this device, the patient should (1) avoid trying to use the tongue to hold the tube in place; (2) compress the tone generator for short intervals and speak in phrases, rather than full sentences; (3) speak using large movements of the lips, tongue, and jaw, rather than keeping the mouth partially closed; (4) talk face-to-face with the listener; and (5) practice because development of skill takes time.

An artificial larynx is placed against the neck rather than in the mouth. This device is used after surgical healing is complete and there is no edema remaining (Fig. 25-16). With experience the patient can learn to move the lips in ways that create normal-sounding speech. With both devices, voice pitch is low, and the sound resembles that of a robot or machine.

TOTAL NECK BREATHER

(Front of Card)

EMERGENCY!

I am a Total Neck Breather
(Laryngectomee–No Vocal Cords)

I breathe ONLY through an opening in my neck, NOT through my nose or mouth.

If I have stopped breathing:
1. Expose my entire neck.
2. Give me **mouth to neck breathing only.**
3. Keep my head straight—chin up.
4. Keep neck opening clear with clean CLOTH (not tissue).
5. Use oxygen supply to neck opening ONLY, when I start to breathe again.

BE PROMPT–SECONDS COUNT I NEED AIR NOW!

(Back of All Cards)

Medical Problems
☐ Epilepsy ☐ Glaucoma
☐ Diabetes ☐ Peptic Ulcer
☐ Other ______

Medicines Taken Regularly
☐ Anticoagulants ☐ Cortisone or ACTH
☐ Heart drugs (Name and dose)
☐ Other ______

Dangerous Allergies
☐ Drugs (Name)
☐ Penicillin
☐ Other ______

Other Information
☐ Hard of hearing
☐ Speaks No English (Other)
☐ Wearing Contact Lenses
☐ Other ______
NAME ______
ADDRESS ______

PLEASE NOTIFY:
NAME ______
PHONE ______
ADDRESS ______
CITY ______

OR
NAME ______
PHONE ______
ADDRESS ______

INTERNATIONAL ASSOCIATION OF LARYNGECTOMEES

Fig. 25-17 Emergency identification of a neck breather.

Esophageal speech is a method of swallowing air, trapping it in the esophagus, and releasing it to create sound. The air causes vibration of the pharyngoesophageal segment and sound (which initially is similar to a belch). With practice 50% of patients develop some speech skills, but only 10% develop fluent speech.

Stoma care. Before discharge, the patient should be instructed in the care of the laryngectomy stoma.[29] The area around the stoma should be washed daily with a moist cloth. If a laryngectomy tube is in place, the entire tube must be removed at least daily and cleaned in the same manner as a tracheostomy tube. The inner cannula may need to be removed and cleaned more frequently. A scarf, a loose shirt, or a crocheted shield can be used to shield the stoma. The patient should cover the stoma when coughing, because mucus may be expectorated, and during any activity (e.g., shaving, applying makeup) that might lead to inhalation of foreign materials. Because water can easily enter the stoma, the patient should wear a plastic collar when taking a shower. Swimming is contraindicated. Initially, humidification will be administered via a tracheostomy mask. After discharge, a bedside humidifier can be substituted along with the instillation of 3 to 5 ml of sterile saline solution. Saline boluses provide humidification and stimulate coughing. A high oral fluid intake must be maintained, especially in dry weather. The patient should be told the importance of wearing a Medic Alert bracelet or other identification that alerts others in an emergency situation of the use of neck breathing (Fig. 25-17).

Since the patient no longer breathes through the nose, the ability to smell smoke and food may be lost. Advise the patient to install smoke and carbon monoxide detectors in the home. It is important for food to be colorful, attractively prepared, and nutritious, because taste may also be diminished secondary to the loss of smell, as well as radiation therapy.

Depression. Depression is common in the patient who has had a radical neck dissection. The patient may not be able to speak because of the tracheostomy and cannot control saliva. The neck and shoulders may be numb because of the transected nerves. The facial appearance may be significantly altered with swelling, edema, and deformities. The patient must understand that many of the physical changes are reversible as the edema subsides and the tracheostomy tube is removed. Depression may also be related to concern about the prognosis. The nurse can help the patient through the depression by allowing verbalization of feelings, conveying acceptance, and helping the patient regain an acceptable self-concept. Sometimes it is appropriate to obtain a psychiatric referral for the patient who is experiencing prolonged or severe depression.

Sexuality. The patient may feel less desirable sexually and may also feel inadequate. The nurse can assist the patient by allowing discussions regarding sexuality and encouraging the patient to discuss this problem with the sexual partner. It may be difficult for the patient to orally discuss sexual problems because of the alteration in communication. The nurse can allow the patient to plan how to communicate with the sexual partner and offer support and guidance to the sexual partner. Helping the patient see that sexuality involves much more than appearance may relieve some anxiety.

Ambulatory and Home Care. The patient is often discharged with a tracheostomy and a nasogastric or gastrostomy feeding tube. Home health care may need to be provided initially to evaluate the family's or the patient's ability to perform self-care activities. The patient and the family must be taught how to manage tubes and who to call if there are problems.

The patient can resume exercise, recreation, and sexual activity when able. Most patients can return to work 1 to 2 months after surgery. However, as many as 50% never return to full-time employment. The changes that follow a total laryngectomy can be upsetting. Loss of speech, loss of the ability to taste and smell, inability to produce audible sounds (including laughing and weeping), and the presence of a permanent tracheal stoma that produces undesirable mucus are often overwhelming to the patient. Although changes are discussed before surgery, the patient may not be prepared for the extent of these changes. If the patient has a significant other, the reaction of this person to the patient's altered appearance is important. Acceptance by another person can promote an improved self-image. Encouraging the patient to participate in self-care is another important part of rehabilitation.

CRITICAL THINKING EXERCISES

CASE STUDY

Cancer of the Larynx

Patient Profile

Mr. C., a 60-year-old man, was admitted for evaluation of mild pain on swallowing and a persistent sore throat over the past year.

Subjective Data

- States that his symptoms worsened in the last 2 months
- Has used various cold remedies to relieve symptoms without relief
- Has lost weight because of decrease in appetite and difficulty swallowing
- Has smoked 3 packs of cigarettes a day for 40 years
- Consumes 6 cans of beer a day

Objective Data

Laryngoscopy

- Enlarged cervical nodes

CT Scan

- Subglottic lesion with lymph node involvement

Collaborative Care

- Total laryngectomy with tracheostomy with inflated cuff
- Nasogastric tube

Critical Thinking Questions

1. What information in the assessment suggests that Mr. C. might be at risk for cancer of the larynx?
2. What diagnostic tests are typically performed to evaluate the extent of this problem?
3. What teaching should the nurse plan for Mr. C. before and after laryngectomy?
4. Discuss methods used to restore the voice after laryngectomy. How do these methods differ in regard to the techniques used to produce speech after removal of the vocal cords?
5. What teaching is required to assist this patient to assume self-care after his surgery? What precautions should the patient take because of his stoma?
6. Based on the assessment data presented, write one or more nursing diagnoses. Are there any collaborative problems?

NURSING RESEARCH ISSUES

1. In what ways does sleep apnea affect a patient's quality of life?
2. After a laryngectomy, what methods of voice restoration provide the most satisfaction for the patient?
3. What are the most effective ways for a patient with a tracheostomy to communicate?
4. What is the quality of life of patients following a radical neck dissection?
5. What factors are most likely to promote compliance with CPAP therapy?

Facial disfigurement and other mutilating aspects of radical head and neck surgery may have a major long-term impact on the patient's body image and lifestyle. Many of these surgical procedures leave a deformity, both functionally and cosmetically. It may be difficult for the patient to eat and speak, and the altered physical appearance may be embarrassing and depressing. The patient may need information about prosthetic devices, speech therapy, and further reconstructive surgery.

Reconstructive surgery may be performed at the time of the initial surgery or soon after the tumor is removed. Various types of flaps and grafts are used. It may be necessary to rebuild the nose or the mandible or to close oral cutaneous openings. Prosthetic materials, such as Silastic and Plastigel (which is soft), are often used to reconstruct various deformities.

Despite the use of surgical interventions and radiation therapy, the cure rate is disappointingly low for advanced head and neck cancer. Metastatic cancer is often painful, leaving the affected person in a severely debilitated state. If pain is a problem, a pain control regimen should be identified to provide comfort, and referral should be made to a hospice, if indicated.

Evaluation

Expected outcomes for the patient with head and neck cancer who is treated surgically are addressed in NCP 25-6.

REVIEW QUESTIONS

The number of the question corresponds to the same-numbered objective at the beginning of the chapter.

1. A patient was seen in clinic for an episode of epistaxis, which was controlled by placement of anterior nasal packing. During discharge teaching the nurse instructs the patient to
   a. avoid vigorous nose blowing and strenuous activity.
   b. use aspirin or aspirin-containing compounds for pain relief.
   c. apply ice compresses to the nose every 4 hours for the first 48 hours.
   d. leave the packing in place for 7 to 10 days until it is removed by the physician.
2. A patient with allergic rhinitis reports severe nasal congestion, sneezing, and watery, itchy eyes and nose most of the year. To teach the patient to control these symptoms, the nurse advises the patient to
   a. limit the duration of use of nasal decongestant spray to 10 days.
   b. keep a diary of when the allergic reaction occurs and what precipitates it.
   c. use oral decongestants at bedtime to prevent symptoms during the night.
   d. never use an intranasal spray and nonsedating antihistamine at the same time.
3. A patient with sleep apnea would like to avoid using a nasal CPAP device, if possible. To help him reach this goal the nurse suggests that he
   a. use an oral appliance at night.
   b. take a nap during the day so he is not so tired.
   c. place golf balls in a pocket sewn in the back of his pajamas.
   d. use mild sedatives or alcohol at bedtime to promote deeper sleep stages.
4. The patient with a tracheostomy can speak using all of the following devices except
   a. a cuffless tracheostomy tube.
   b. a fenestrated tracheostomy tube.
   c. a tube with an inflated foam cuff.
   d. a cuffed tube with the cuff deflated.
5. To prevent excessive pressure on tracheal capillaries, pressure in the cuff on a tracheostomy tube should be
   a. monitored every 2 to 3 days.
   b. less than 20 mm Hg or 25 cm H_2O.
   c. less than 30 mm Hg or 35 cm H_2O.
   d. sufficient to fill the pilot balloon until it is tense.
6. Which of the following is not an early symptom of cancer of the head and neck?
   a. hoarseness
   b. mouth ulcers that do not heal
   c. change in fit of dentures
   d. decreased mobility of the tongue
7. Nursing management of the patient immediately after a total laryngectomy includes all of the following except
   a. changing the surgical dressing.
   b. ensuring that the nasogastric tube is patent.
   c. placing the patient in semi-Fowler's position.
   d. monitoring function of the drainage tubes.
8. When using a voice prosthesis, the patient
   a. swallows air using Valsalva's maneuver.
   b. places a vibrating device in the mouth or on the neck.
   c. places a speaking valve over the laryngectomy stoma.
   d. blocks the stoma entrance with the finger, causing air to travel up over the vocal cords.

References

1. Sigler BA, Schuring LT: *Ear, nose, and throat disorders,* St Louis, 1993, Mosby.
2. Pulli RS, Hengerer AS: Epistaxis: evaluating and managing a common problem, *J Respir Dis* 17:764, 1996.
3. Pulli RS, Hengerer AS. Epistaxis: options for managing posterior bleeding, *J Respir Dis* 17:841, 1996.
4. Philip G, Togias AG: Allergic rhinitis: clues to the differential, *J Respir Dis* 16:359, 1995.
5. Philip G, Togias AG: Allergic rhinitis: today's approach to treatment, *J Respir Dis* 16:367, 1995.
6. Colman BH: *Hall and Colman's diseases of the nose, throat, ear, and head and neck: a handbook for students and practitioners,* New York, 1992, Churchill Livingstone.
7. Murray JE, Petty TL: *Frontline treatment for COPD,* Hackettstown, NJ, 1996, Snowdrift Pulmonary Foundation.
8. Fishman NO: Viral pneumonias. In Fishman AP, editor: *Pulmonary diseases and disorders companion handbook,* ed 2, New York, 1994, McGraw Hill.
9. Glezen WP: Influenza: time to prepare for the '96-97 season, *J Respir Dis* 17:643, 1996.
10. Gross PA, Hermongenes AW, Sacks HS, and others: The efficacy of influenza vaccine in elderly persons: a meta-analysis and review of the literature, *Ann Intern Med* 123:518, 1995.
11. Hayden FG and others: Efficacy and safety of the neuraminidase inhibitor zanamivir in the treatment of influenza virus infections, *N Engl J Med* 337:874, 1997.
12. Einarsson O, Wirth JA: Sinopulmonary syndromes, *Clin Pulm Med* 3:199, 1996.
13. Lockey RF: Management of chronic sinusitis, *Hosp Pract* 31:141, 1996.
14. Douville L: Pharmacologic highlights: management of acute sinusitis, *J Am Acad Nurse Pract* 7:407, 1995.
15. Schwab RJ: Sleep-disordered breathing. In Fishman AP, editor: *Pulmonary diseases and disorders companion handbook,* ed 2, New York, 1994, McGraw Hill.

16. Ferguson KA and others: A randomized crossover study of an oral appliance vs nasal-continuous positive airway pressure in the treatment of mild-moderate obstructive sleep apnea, *Chest* 109:1269, 1996.
17. Likar LL and others: Group education sessions and compliance with nasal CPAP therapy, *Chest* 111:1273, 1997.
18. Engleman HM and others: Self-reported use of CPAP and benefits of CPAP therapy, *Chest* 109:1470, 1996.
19. Atwood CW, Sanders MH, Strollo PJ: Palatal and nonpalatal surgery for sleep apnea hypopnea syndrome, *Clin Pulm Med* 4:205, 1997.
20. Hoffman LA: Timing of tracheostomy, *Respir Care* 39:378, 1994.
21. Weilitz PB, Dettenmeier PA: Test your knowledge of tracheostomy tubes, *AJN* 94:46, 1994.
22. Dettenmeier PA: *Pulmonary nursing care*, St Louis, 1992, Mosby.
23. Harlid R and others: Respiratory tract colonization and infection in patients with chronic tracheostomy: a one-year study in patients living at home, *Am J Respir Crit Care Med* 154:124, 1997.
24. Bell SD: Use of Passy-Muir tracheostomy speaking valve in mechanically ventilated patients, *Crit Care Nurse* 16:63, 1996.
25. Kaut K, Turcott JC, Lavery M: Passy-Muir speaking valve, *DCCN* 15:298, 1996.
26. Manzano JL and others: Verbal communication of ventilator-dependent patients, *Crit Care Med* 21:512, 1993.
27. Vokes EE and others: Head and neck cancer, *N Engl J Med* 328:184, 1993.
28. Lore JM: Early diagnosis and treatment of head and neck cancer, *CA Cancer J Clin* 45:325, 1995.
29. Haynes VL: Caring for the laryngectomy patient, *AJN* 96:16B, 1996.
30. Lochart JS, Bryce J: Restoring speech with tracheoesophageal puncture, *Nursing* 23:59, 1993.

Resources

International Association of Laryngectomees
7440 N. Shadeland Avenue, Suite 100
Indianapolis, IN 46250
317-570-4568
fax: 317-570-4570
http://www.larynxlink.com

For additional Internet resources, see the website for this book at **www.mosby.com/MERLIN/medsurg_lewis**

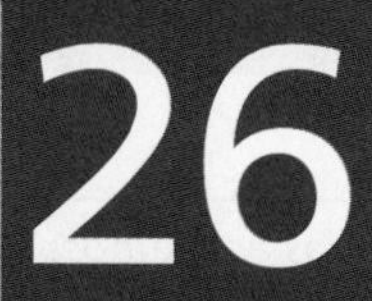

REMEMBER to check out your companion CD-ROM

26 NURSING MANAGEMENT Lower Respiratory Problems

Sharon Mantik Lewis

www.mosby.com/MERLIN/medsurg_lewis

LEARNING OBJECTIVES

1. Describe the pathophysiology, types, clinical manifestations, and collaborative care of pneumonia.
2. Explain the nursing management of the patient with pneumonia.
3. Describe the pathogenesis, classification, clinical manifestations, complications, diagnostic abnormalities, and nursing and collaborative management of tuberculosis.
4. Identify the causes, clinical manifestations, and nursing and collaborative management of pulmonary fungal infections.
5. Explain the pathophysiology, clinical manifestations, and nursing and collaborative management of bronchiectasis and lung abscess.
6. Identify the causative factors, clinical features, and management of occupational lung diseases.
7. Describe the causes, risk factors, pathogenesis, clinical manifestations, and nursing and collaborative management of lung cancer.
8. Describe the risks associated with cigarette smoking, various methods of smoking cessation, and the role of the nurse in assisting the patient to stop smoking.
9. Identify the mechanisms involved and the clinical manifestations of pneumothorax, fractured ribs, and flail chest.
10. Describe the purpose, methods, and nursing responsibilities related to chest tubes.
11. Explain the types of chest surgery and appropriate preoperative and postoperative care.
12. Compare and contrast extrapulmonary and intrapulmonary restrictive lung disorders in terms of causes, clinical manifestations, and collaborative management.
13. Describe the pathophysiology, clinical manifestations, and management of pulmonary hypertension and cor pulmonale.
14. Discuss the use of lung transplantation as a treatment for pulmonary disorders.

A wide variety of problems affect the lower respiratory system. Lung diseases that are characterized primarily by an obstructive disorder, such as asthma, emphysema, chronic bronchitis, and cystic fibrosis, are discussed in Chapter 27. All other lower respiratory problems are discussed in this chapter.

Pulmonary infections annually rank among the top 10 causes of death in the United States. Bacterial pneumonia remains the leading infectious cause of death despite the availability of antimicrobial agents. Tuberculosis, although potentially curable and preventable, still is a significant public health problem in the United States, Canada, and the rest of the world.

ACUTE BRONCHITIS

Acute bronchitis is an inflammation of the lower respiratory tract that is usually due to infection and occurs most frequently in patients with chronic respiratory disease. It also occurs in other individuals, usually as a sequela to an upper respiratory tract infection. Chronic bronchitis is a persistent inflammation of the lower respiratory tract without infection and is a type of chronic obstructive pulmonary disease (COPD is discussed in Chapter 27). Acute exacerbations of chronic bronchitis represent acute infection superimposed on chronic bronchitis (discussed in Chapter 27). Acute bronchitis is a self-limiting disease. However, acute exacerbation of chronic bronchitis is a potentially lethal condition.[1]

The cause of most cases of acute bronchitis is viral. However, bacterial causes (*Streptococcus pneumoniae* or *Haemophilus influenzae*) are also common in both smokers and nonsmokers.

In acute bronchitis, persistent cough following an acute upper airway infection (e.g., rhinitis, pharyngitis) is the most common symptom. Cough is often accompanied by production of clear, mucoid sputum, although some patients produce purulent sputum. Associated symptoms include fever, headache, and malaise. Physical examination may reveal mildly elevated temperature, pulse, and respiratory rate with normal breath sounds. Chest x-ray differentiates acute bronchitis from pneumonia because there is usually no evidence of consolidation or infiltrates with bronchitis.

Treatment of acute bronchitis is generally supportive, including fluids, rest, and cough suppressants if cough interferes

Reviewed by Sheena Ferguson, RN, MSN, CCRN, Pulmonary Clinical Nurse Specialist, University of New Mexico Hospital, Albuquerque, NM, and Barbara S. Levine, RN, PhD, CRNP, CS, Clinical Director, Gerontological Nursing Services, University of Pennsylvania Health System; Assistant Professor, Gerontological Nursing, University of Pennsylvania School of Nursing, Philadelphia, Penn.

Table 26-1 Risk Factors Predisposing to Pneumonia

Smoking
Air pollution
Altered consciousness: alcoholism, head injury, seizures, anesthesia, drug overdose
Tracheal intubation (endotracheal intubation, tracheostomy)
Upper respiratory tract infection
Chronic diseases: chronic lung disease, diabetes mellitus, heart disease, uremia, cancer
Immunosuppression
- Drugs (corticosteroids, cancer chemotherapy, immunosuppressive therapy after organ transplant)
- HIV

Malnutrition
Inhalation or aspiration of noxious substances
Debilitating illness
Bed rest and prolonged immobility
Altered oropharyngeal flora

HIV, human immunodeficiency virus.

Table 26-2 Causes of Pneumonia

Community-Acquired Pneumonia	Hospital-Acquired Pneumonia
*Streptococcus pneumoniae**	*Pseudomonas aeruginosa*
Mycoplasma pneumoniae	*Enterobacter*
Haemophilus influenzae†	*Escherichia coli*
Respiratory viruses	*Proteus*
Chlamydia pneumoniae	*Klebsiella*
Legionella pneumophila	*Staphylococcus aureus*
Oral anaerobes	*Streptococcus pneumoniae*
Moraxella catarrhalis	Oral anaerobes
Staphylococcus aureus	
Nocardia	
Enteric aerobic gram-negative bacteria (e.g., *Klebsiella*)	
Fungi	
Mycobacterium tuberculosis	

*Most common cause of community-acquired pneumonia (CAP).
†Second most common cause of CAP.

with sleep. Antibiotics are not usually prescribed unless the person is a smoker or has COPD.[2]

The patient with COPD who has symptoms of acute bronchitis is usually treated empirically with broad-spectrum antibiotics, and modifications in therapy are made if they prove ineffective. Often the patient with COPD is taught to recognize symptoms of acute bronchitis and to begin a course of antibiotics when symptoms occur. Many clinicians believe that a more severe infection often results if the patient delays taking antibiotics until after an examination by a physician. This delay may cause serious consequences for the patient with severe chronic lung disease.

PNEUMONIA

Pneumonia, or *pneumonitis,* is an acute inflammation of the lung parenchyma. Until 1936 pneumonia was the leading cause of death in the United States. Then sulfa drugs and penicillin were discovered and used to treat pneumonia. However, despite antibiotics, pneumonia is still common, and some types of the disease have a high mortality rate. Approximately 1% of the American population will have pneumonia at some time in their lives. Pneumonia is the sixth leading cause of death in the United States.[3]

Etiology

Normal Defense Mechanisms. Normally, the airway distal to the larynx is sterile because of protective defense mechanisms. These mechanisms include the following (see Chapter 24):

1. filtration of air
2. warming and humidification of inspired air
3. epiglottis closure over the trachea
4. cough reflex
5. mucociliary escalator mechanism
6. secretion of immunoglobulin A
7. alveolar macrophages

Factors Predisposing to Pneumonia. Pneumonia is more likely to result when defense mechanisms become incompetent or are overwhelmed by the virulence or quantity of infectious agents. Decreased consciousness depresses the cough and epiglottal reflexes, which may allow aspiration of oropharyngeal contents into the lungs. Tracheal intubation interferes with the normal cough reflex and the mucociliary escalator mechanism. It also bypasses the upper airways in which filtration and humidification of air normally take place. The mucociliary escalator mechanism is impaired by air pollution, cigarette smoking, viral upper respiratory infections (URIs), and normal changes of aging. In cases of malnutrition the formation and function of lymphocytes and polymorphonuclear leukocytes are altered. Certain diseases such as leukemia, alcoholism, and diabetes mellitus are associated with an increased frequency of gram-negative bacilli in the oropharynx.[4] (Gram-negative bacilli are not normal flora in the respiratory tract.) Altered oropharyngeal flora can also occur secondary to antibiotic therapy given for an infection elsewhere in the body. The risk factors predisposing to pneumonia are listed in Table 26-1.

Acquisition of Organisms. Organisms that cause pneumonia reach the lung by three methods:

1. Aspiration from the nasopharynx or oropharynx. Many of the organisms that cause pneumonia are normal inhabitants of the pharynx in healthy adults.
2. Inhalation of microbes present in the air. Examples include *Mycoplasma pneumoniae* and fungal pneumonias.
3. Hematogenous spread from a primary infection elsewhere in the body. An example is *Staphylococcus aureus.*

Types of Pneumonia

Pneumonia can be caused by bacteria, viruses, *Mycoplasma,* fungi, parasites, and chemicals. Although pneumonia can be classified according to the causative organism, a clinically more effective way is to classify pneumonia as *community-acquired pneumonia (CAP)* or *hospital-acquired pneumonia (HAP).*

Classifying pneumonia into CAP or HAP based on clinical situations is important because of differences in the likely causative organisms and the selection of appropriate antibiotics (Table 26-2).

Table 26-3 Patient Categories and Treatment for Community-Acquired Pneumonia According to ATS Guidelines

	Severity of Illness			
	Category 1: Mild to Moderate	Category 2: Mild to Moderate	Category 3: Moderately Severe	Category 4: Severe
Need for Hospitalization	No	No	Yes, not ICU	Yes, usually ICU
Age (yr)	≤60	<60 >60	All ages	All ages
Comorbidity	No	Yes Yes or no	Yes or no	Yes or no
Antibiotic therapy	▪ Macrolide:* consider a newer macrolide in a smoker or in the patient intolerant to erythromycin ▪ Tetracycline: but not always reliable against *S. pneumoniae* ▪ Quinolones**	▪ Second-generation cephalosporin† or trimethoprim/ sulfamethoxazole (Bactrim) or beta-lactam/beta-lactamase inhibitor§ ▪ May add erythromycin or other macrolide if *Legionella* is a concern ▪ Quinolones**	▪ Second- or third-generation cephalosporin‡ or beta-lactam/beta lactamase inhibitor§ ▪ May add erythromycin or other macrolide if *Legionella* is a concern (add rifampin if infection with *Legionella* is documented)	▪ Macrolide (add rifampin if *Legionella* is documented) ▪ Add third-generation cephalosporin with antipseudomonal activity (e.g., ceftazidime [Fortaz]) or other antipseudomonal agents (e.g., ciprofloxacin [Cipro])

Source: American Thoracic Society (ATS).
*Macrolides: azithromycin (Zithromax), clarithromycin (Biaxin), erythromycin.
†Second-generation cephalosporins: cefaclor (Ceclor), cefprozil (Cefzil).
‡Third-generation cephalosporins: ceftazidime (Fortaz); cefocerazone (Cefobid).
§Beta-lactam/beta-lactamase inhibitors: amoxicillin-clavulanate (Augmentin), ampicillin-sulbactam (Unasyn).
**Quinolones: ciprofloxacin (Cipro), ofloxacin (Floxin), levofloxacin (Levaquin), moxifloxacin (Avolox)
ICU, intensive care unit.

Community-Acquired Pneumonia. CAP is defined as a lower respiratory tract infection of the lung parenchyma with onset in the community or the first 2 days of hospitalization. The incidence in the United States is approximately 12 per 1000 adults. Hospitalizations occur in about 600,000 cases annually. The causative organism in CAP is identified only 50% of the time. Organisms that are commonly implicated in CAP include *Streptococcus pneumoniae, Haemophilus influenzae,* and atypical organisms (*Legionella, Mycoplasma, Chlamydia,* viral) (see Table 26-2). The American Thoracic Society guidelines classify patients with CAP into four categories based on severity of infection, need for hospitalization, older age (>60 years), and comorbidity (Table 26-3).[5]

Hospital-Acquired Pneumonia. HAP is pneumonia occurring 48 hours or longer after admission and not incubating at the time of hospitalization.[6] HAP is estimated to occur at a rate of 5 to 10 cases per 1000 hospital admissions, with the rate increasing by 6 to 20 times in patients requiring mechanical ventilation. Pneumonia has the highest morbidity and mortality rate of any nosocomial infection.[6] The microorganisms responsible for HAP are different than those organisms implicated in CAP (see Table 26-2). Bacteria are responsible for the majority of HAP infections, including *Pseudomonas* and *Enterobacter, Staphylococcus aureus,* and *Streptococcus pneumoniae.* Many of the organisms causing HAP enter the lungs after aspiration of particles from the patient's own pharynx. Immunosuppressive therapy, general debility, and endotracheal intubation may be predisposing factors. Respiratory therapy equipment that is not cleaned regularly is another source of infection. Patients with HAP are classified into three groups based on (1) severity of the patient's illness, (2) whether specific host or therapeutic factors predisposing to specific pathogens are present, and (3) whether the pneumonia is of early (<5 days after admission) or late (>5 days after admission) onset. The three groups are as follows (Table 26-4):

- Group 1: Patients without unusual risk factors who have mild to moderate HAP with onset at any time during hospitalization or severe HAP of early onset
- Group 2: Patients with specific risk factors who have mild to moderate HAP occurring any time during hospitalization
- Group 3: Patients with severe HAP either of early onset with specific risk factors or of late onset

Fungal Pneumonia. Fungi may also be a cause of pneumonia (see section on pulmonary fungal infections).

Aspiration Pneumonia. Aspiration pneumonia is frequently called *necrotizing pneumonia* because of the pathologic changes in the lungs. It usually follows aspiration of material in the mouth into the trachea and subsequently the lungs. The person who has aspiration pneumonia usually has a history of loss of consciousness (e.g., as a result of seizure, anesthesia, head injury, alcohol intake). With loss of consciousness the gag and cough reflexes are depressed, and aspiration is more likely to occur. The dependent portions of the lung are most often affected, primarily the superior segments of the lower lobes, which are dependent in the supine position.

The aspirated material, either food, water, or vomitus, is the triggering mechanism for the pathology of this type of pneumonia. If the aspirated material is an inert substance (e.g., bar-

Table 26-4 Organisms Associated with Hospital-Acquired Pneumonia and Recommended Antibiotics

Risk Factors	Core Organisms	Core Antibiotics
Group 1: Mild to moderate HAP, no unusual risk factors, onset at any time; or severe HAP with early onset		
	Core Organisms	**Core Antibiotics**
	▪ Enteric gram-negative bacilli (nonpseudomonal, e.g., *Enterobacter, Escherichia coli, Proteus, Klebsiella, Serratia marcescens, Haemophilus influenzae*) ▪ Methicillin-sensitive *Staphylococcus aureus* ▪ *Streptococcus pneumoniae*	Cephalosporin (second generation or nonantipseudomonal third generation) *or* Beta-lactam/beta-lactamase inhibitor *or* If allergic to penicillin, a fluoroquinolone* or clindamycin + aztreonam
Group 2: Mild to moderate HAP with risk factors associated with additional specific organisms, onset at any time		
Risk Factors	**Core *Plus* Specific At-Risk Organisms**	**Core Antibiotics *Plus* Additional Specific Coverage**
Abdominal surgery, aspiration	▪ Anaerobes	Clindamycin or beta-lactam/beta-lactamase inhibitor
Coma, head trauma, diabetes mellitus, renal failure	▪ *S. aureus*	+/− vancomycin (until MRSA ruled out)
High-dose corticosteroids	▪ *Legionella*	Erythromycin +/− rifampin
Prolonged ICU stay, corticosteroids, antibiotics, lung disease	▪ *Pseudomonas aeruginosa*	Treat as severe HAP (group 3)
Group 3: Severe HAP with risk factors, early onset; or severe HAP, late onset		
	Core Organisms *Plus*	**Antibiotics**
	▪ *P. aeruginosa* ▪ *Acinetobacter* species	Aminoglycoside or ciprofloxacin, *plus* One of the following: antipseudomonal penicillin, beta-lactam/beta-lactamase inhibitor, ceftazidime or cefoperazone (Cefobid), imipenem (Primaxin), aztreonam (Azactam) *and*
	▪ Consider MRSA	+/− vancomycin (if MRSA is a concern)

Adapted from American Thoracic Society: Hospital-acquired pneumonia in adults: diagnosis, assessment of severity, initial antimicrobial therapy: a consensus statement, *Am J Respir Crit Care Med* 153:1711, 1996.
*If *S. pneumoniae* not a concern.
MRSA, methicillin-resistant *S. aureus.*

ium or stomach contents), the initial manifestation is usually caused by obstruction of airways. When the aspirated materials contain gastric juice, there is chemical injury to the lung parenchyma with infection as a secondary event usually 48 to 72 hours later. The infecting organism is usually one of the normal oropharyngeal flora, and multiple organisms, including both aerobes and anaerobes, are isolated from the sputum of the patient with aspiration pneumonia. Antibiotic therapy should be based on an assessment of the severity of illness, where the infection was acquired (community versus hospital), and type of organisms present.[7]

Opportunistic Pneumonia. Certain patients with altered immune response are highly susceptible to respiratory infections. Individuals considered at risk include those who have severe protein-calorie malnutrition, immune deficiencies, transplants, and patients who are being treated with radiation therapy, chemotherapy drugs, and corticosteroids (especially for a prolonged period). The individual has a variety of altered conditions, including altered B and T lymphocyte function, depressed bone marrow function, and decreased levels or function of neutrophils and macrophages. In addition to the causative agents (especially gram-negative bacteria), other agents that cause pneumonia in the immunocompromised patient are *Pneumocystis carinii,* cytomegalovirus (CMV), and fungi.

Pneumocystis carinii is an opportunistic pathogen whose natural habitat is the lung. Although its classification has been historically considered to be a protozoa, it is now considered a fungus. This organism rarely causes pneumonia in the healthy individual. *Pneumocystis carinii* pneumonia (PCP) affects 70% of HIV-infected individuals and is the most common opportunistic infection in patients with acquired immunodeficiency syndrome (AIDS). In this type of pneumonia the chest x-ray usually shows a diffuse bilateral alveolar pattern of infiltration. In widespread disease the lungs are massively consolidated. However, chest x-ray interpretation may be nondiagnostic in many cases. Clinical manifestations are insidious and include fever, tachypnea, tachycardia, dyspnea, nonproductive cough, and hypoxemia. Breath sounds may be normal. Pulmonary physical findings are minimal in proportion to the serious nature of the disease. Treatment consists of a 21-day course of trimethoprim-sulfamethoxazole (Bactrim) as the primary agent and parenteral pentamidine (Nebupent). In populations at risk for development of *P. carinii* pneumonitis (e.g., patients with hematologic malignancies or AIDS), prophylaxis with trimethoprim-sulfamethoxazole may be advocated. Aerosolized pentamidine (Nebupent) is used as a prophylactic measure. (PCP is discussed in Chapter 13).

CMV, also called *cytomegalic inclusion virus,* is a cause of viral pneumonia in the immunocompromised patient, particularly in transplant recipients. CMV, a type of herpes virus, gives rise to latent infections and reactivation with shedding of infectious virus. This type of interstitial pneumonia can be a mild disease, or it can be fulminant and produce pulmonary insufficiency and death. Often, CMV coexists with other opportunistic bacterial or fungal agents in causing pneumonia. Treatment of CMV pneumonia includes IV ganciclovir (Cytovene) and foscarnet (Foscavir).

Pathophysiology

Pneumococcal pneumonia is the most common cause of bacterial pneumonia, and the pathophysiology related to this type of pneumonia will be discussed. There are four characteristic stages of the disease process:

1. *Congestion.* After the pneumococcus organisms reach the alveoli via droplets or saliva, there is an outpouring of fluid into the alveoli. The organisms multiply in the serous fluid, and the infection is spread. The pneumococci damage the host by their overwhelming growth and interference with lung function.
2. *Red hepatization.* There is massive dilation of the capillaries, and alveoli are filled with organisms, neutrophils, RBCs, and fibrin (Fig. 26-1). The lung appears red and granular, or liverlike, which is why the process is called *hepatization.*
3. *Gray hepatization.* Blood flow decreases, and leukocytes and fibrin consolidate in the affected part of the lung.
4. *Resolution.* Complete resolution and healing occur if there are no complications. The exudate becomes lysed and is processed by the macrophages. The normal lung tissue is restored, and the person's gas-exchange ability returns to normal.

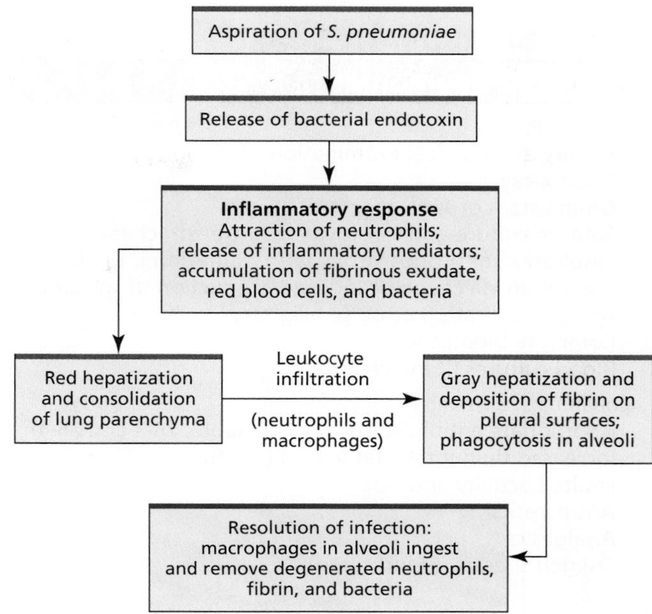

Fig. 26-1 Pathophysiologic course of pneumococcal pneumonia.

Clinical Manifestations

CAP has been traditionally thought to present as two syndromes: typical and atypical, although the distinctions are not clear. *Typical* pneumonia syndrome is characterized by sudden onset of fever, chills, cough productive of purulent sputum, and pleuritic chest pain (in some cases). On physical examination signs of pulmonary consolidation, such as dullness to percussion, increased fremitus, bronchial breath sounds, and crackles, may be found. In the elderly or debilitated patient, confusion or stupor may be the predominant finding. The typical pneumonia syndrome is usually caused by the most common pathogen in CAP, which is *S. pneumoniae.* but can also be due to other bacterial pathogens, such as *H. influenzae.*

The *atypical* syndrome is characterized by a more gradual onset, a dry cough, and extrapulmonary manifestations such as headache, myalgias, fatigue, sore throat, nausea, vomiting, and diarrhea. On physical examination crackles are often heard. Atypical pneumonia is classically produced by *Mycoplasma pneumoniae* but can also be caused by *Legionella* and *Chlamydia pneumoniae.*

Although the initial manifestations of viral pneumonia are highly variable, viruses also cause pneumonia that is usually characterized by an atypical presentation with chills, fever, dry nonproductive cough, and extrapulmonary symptoms. Primary viral pneumonia can be caused by influenza virus infection. Viral pneumonia is also found in association with systemic viral diseases such as measles, varicella-zoster, and herpes simplex.

Patients with hematogenous *S. aureus* pneumonia may have only dyspnea and fever. Necrotizing infection causes destruction of lung tissue. These patients are usually very sick.

Complications

Most cases of pneumonia generally run an uncomplicated course. However, complications can occur, and they develop more frequently in individuals with underlying chronic diseases and other risk factors. Complications may include the following:

1. *Pleurisy* (inflammation of the pleura) is a relatively common accompanying problem of pneumonia.
2. *Pleural effusion* can occur, and usually the effusion is sterile and is reabsorbed in 1 to 2 weeks. Occasionally, it requires aspiration by means of thoracentesis.
3. *Atelectasis* (collapsed, airless alveoli) of one or part of one lobe may occur. These areas usually clear with effective coughing and deep breathing.
4. *Delayed resolution* results from persistent infection and is seen on x-ray as residual consolidation. Usually, the physical findings return to normal within 2 to 4 weeks. Delayed resolution occurs most frequently in the pa-

COLLABORATIVE CARE

Table 26-5 Pneumonia

Diagnostic
- History and physical examination
- Chest x-ray
- Gram's stain of sputum
- Sputum culture and sensitivity test (transtracheal aspiration or bronchoscopy with aspiration if unable to obtain via cough or induced production of sputum)
- ABGs (if indicated) or pulse oximetry
- Complete blood count
- Blood cultures (if indicated)

Collaborative Therapy
- Appropriate antibiotic therapy (see Tables 26-3 and 26-4)
- Increased fluid intake (at least 3 L q24hr)
- Limited activity and rest
- Antipyretics
- Analgesics
- Oxygen therapy (if indicated)

ABGs, arterial blood gases.

tient who is older, is malnourished, is alcoholic, or has COPD.

5. *Lung abscess* is *not* a common complication of pneumonia. It is seen with pneumonia caused by *S. aureus* and gram-negative pneumonias (see section on lung abscess, later in this chapter).
6. *Empyema* (accumulation of purulent exudate in the pleural cavity) is relatively infrequent but requires antibiotic therapy and drainage of the exudate by a chest tube or open surgical drainage.
7. *Pericarditis* results from spread of the infecting organism from an infected pleura or via a hematogenous route to the pericardium (the fibroserous sac around the heart).
8. *Arthritis* results from systemic spread of the organism. The affected joints are swollen, red, and painful, and a purulent exudate can be aspirated.
9. *Meningitis* can be caused by *S. pneumoniae.* The patient with pneumonia who is disoriented, confused, or somnolent should have a lumbar puncture to evaluate the possibility of meningitis.
10. *Endocarditis* can develop when the organisms attack the endocardium and the valves of the heart. The clinical manifestations are similar to those of acute bacterial endocarditis (see Chapter 35).

Diagnostic Studies

The common diagnostic measures for pneumonia are presented in Table 26-5. History, physical examination, and chest x-ray often provide enough information to make management decisions without costly laboratory tests.

Chest x-ray often shows a typical pattern characteristic of the infecting organism and is an invaluable adjunct in the diagnosis of pneumonia. Lobar or segmental consolidation suggests a bacterial cause, usually *S. pneumoniae* or *Klebsiella.* Diffuse pulmonary infiltrates are most commonly caused by infection with viruses, *Legionella,* or opportunistic pathogens such as *Pneumocystis carinii.* Cavitary shadows suggest the presence of a necrotizing infection with destruction of lung tissue commonly caused by *S. aureus,* gram-negative bacteria, and *Mycobacterium tuberculosis.* Pleural effusions, which can occur in a variety of respiratory infections, can also be seen on x-ray.

A Gram's stain of the sputum provides information on the predominant causative organism. If the patient cannot voluntarily produce a sputum specimen, procedures such as transtracheal aspiration and fiberoptic bronchoscopy may be used. Transtracheal aspiration involves inserting a catheter into the trachea through the cricothyroid membrane and withdrawing secretions for testing. Blood and sputum cultures (if indicated) may take 24 to 72 hours.

Arterial blood gases (ABGs), if obtained, usually reveal hypoxemia. Leukocytosis is found in the majority of patients with bacterial pneumonia, usually with a white blood cell (WBC) count greater than 15,000/μl (15×10^9/L) with a shift to the left.

Collaborative Care

Prompt treatment with the appropriate antibiotic almost always cures bacterial and mycoplasmal pneumonia. In uncomplicated cases, the patient responds to drug therapy within 48 to 72 hours. Indications of improvement include decreased temperature, improved breathing, and reduced chest pain. Abnormal physical findings can last for more than 7 days.

In addition to antibiotic therapy, supportive measures may be used, including oxygen therapy to treat hypoxemia, analgesics to relieve the chest pain for patient comfort, and antipyretics such as aspirin or acetaminophen for significantly elevated temperature. During the acute febrile phase, the patient's activity should be restricted, and rest should be encouraged and planned.

Most individuals with mild to moderate illness who have no other underlying disease process can be treated on an outpatient basis. If there is a serious underlying disease or if the pneumonia is accompanied by severe dyspnea, hypoxemia, or other complications, the patient should be hospitalized. Guidelines for hospitalization for CAP are presented in Table 26-3.

Currently, there is no definitive treatment for viral pneumonia. Two antiviral drugs, amantadine (Symadine) and rimantadine (Flumadine), are approved for oral use in the treatment of influenza pneumonia. Amantadine acts by preventing the penetration of the virus into the host cell. Vaccines against adenovirus and influenza are currently available. Because adenovirus pneumonia is not common in the general population, the use of adenovirus vaccine has been limited to high-risk groups, such as military recruits. Influenza vaccine is considered a mainstay of prevention and is recommended annually for use in the individual considered to be at risk for serious influenza.

A clinical pathway for care of the patient with pneumonia follows.

Pneumococcal Vaccine. Pneumococcal vaccine is indicated primarily for the individual considered at risk who (1) has chronic illnesses such as lung and heart disease and diabetes mellitus, (2) is recovering from a severe illness, (3) is 65 years of age or older, or (4) is in a nursing home or other long-term care facility. This is particularly important because the rate of drug-resistant *S. pneumoniae* infections is increasing.[8]

The current recommendation is that pneumococcal vaccine is good for the person's lifetime. However, in the immunosup-

CLINICAL PATHWAY Pneumonia

Admit Date **DRG: 89** **LOS: 4–4.5 days** **Discharge Date: ________**

Pathway	ER- Day 1	Day 2	Day 3	Day 4–4.5
Critical Path Implemented				
Diagnostic Studies	■ BMP ■ CBC ■ Sputum C&S, gram stain ■ Chest X-ray ■ Pulse Ox Q___H & PRN ■ ECG ■ ABGs if O_2sat <90%	■ Pulse Ox qid	■ Pulse Ox Q shift	
Treatments	■ O_2____L/min via NC/Mask ■ HHN/CPT treatments q___hr & prn ■ Suction prn; RC to induce sputum for C&S/Gram stain if necessary	■ O_2____L/min via NC/Mask ■ HHN/CPT Rx q___hr & prn	■ Start weaning from O_2 ■ O_2____L/min prn ■ Suction prn	■ D/C O_2 ■ Obtain D/C orders for Resp. Rx
IV/Meds	■ IV __________ @ ___cc/hr ■ Antibiotics ■ Bronchodilators ■ Antipyretics analgesics ■ Steroids	■ See MAR	■ See MAR	■ Obtain D/C medication orders
Consults	■ Pulmonary Rehab (if Hx of COPD)			
Team Directives	Monitor & assess respiratory status with each VS check for: rate, depth exertion, breath sounds, fatigue and relief. Prevent fatigue with frequent rest periods, Use Shortness of Breath Scale to evaluate SOB and level of respiratory distress. VS q4hr with temp ×48hr, the q8hr with temp ×24hr, then q shift & prn with temp if stable. Physical assessment q shift. Trend respiratory assessment with pulse Ox readings, lab values, and respiratory treatments. Evaluate LOC and risk for aspiration q8hr & prn until stable. I & O; monitor and trend fluid balance status. Provide skin care and assist with ADLs to prevent fatigue. Provide emotional support and assist with reducing Pt/family anxiety. (sign/date/time)			
Diet	■ As specified on order sheet			
Activity & Safety	Bedrest with bedside commode Elevate HOB 30 degrees Turn, cough & deep breathe q2hr	Rest periods between activities Sit at bedside before standing	Frequent rest periods Increase activity level as tolerated	
Teaching Patient & Family	Orient Pt./family to unit Instruct to call staff for assist to BSC Instruct to call staff for episodes of dyspnea Teach re: Isolation precautions & good hand washing Explain diet, meds, activity level Explain all tests and procedures Explain the pathway plan of care & obtain signature denoting pt./family agreement & understanding	Teach effective cough technique (take several deep breaths, give 3-4 coughs on same exhalation to expel most of air) Teach pursed lip breathing technique Implement Pneumonia Teaching Plan (sign/date/time)		
Discharge Planning	Risk Screening Referrals from Database Assessment initiated Advance Directives reviewed Referral to Pulmonary Rehab initiated (if Pt. has history of COPD)	Facilitate Physician/Family discussion to plan for post-hospitalization care needs Assess need for follow up care Consults and confer with physician for orders		

Author: Molly Metzler, RN, BSN for Nanticoke Health Services. Licensed by the Center for Case Management, South Natick, Mass. Nanticoke Health Services.

Continued

Service

CM - Care Management
ET - Ostomy/Skin Care
RC - Respiratory Care
N - Nurse
PT - Physical Therapy
NS - Nutrition Services
RX - Pharmacist
SL - Speech/Language
CCC - Primary RN Clinical Care Coord.
SW - Social Work
OT - Occupational Therapy
HC - Home Care
DR - Physician
Card - Cardiology
Rad - Radiology
Rehab - Cardiac, Respiratory

CLINICAL PATHWAY Pneumonia—continued

DRG: 89 LOS: 4.5 days

Meets Expected Outcomes (initial)	ER-Day 1	MET	NOT	Day 2	MET	NOT	Day 3	MET	NOT	Day 4–4.5	MET	NOT
Impaired Gas Exchange: Altered O_2 supply due to decreased alveolar ventilation from narrowed airways. ■ $PaO_2 < 80$ mmHg ■ $PaCO_2 < 35$ mmHg ■ pH > 7.45 (Resp. Alk.) **OR:** pH <7.35 with PaO_2 > 45 & RR >20/min ■ Hypoventilation, crackles, cyanosis & altered LOC	■ Patient airway maintained ___/RC or N ■ Pt./Family able to express anxiety appropriately about severe illness and hospitalization___/N ■ $PaO_2 > 90$mmHg & $PaCO_2$ 35-45 mmHg, with pH 7.35-.45 & RR 12-24 after initiating O_2 & treatments ___/RC or N ■ Improved LOC, color pinker after O_2 & Rx ___/RC or N			■ Pt.'s color returning to baseline ___/N ■ Pulse Ox ≥90% ___/RC or N ■ Pt. alert & oriented at baseline level___/N ■ Breath sounds improving with decreased crackles and rales upon auscultation ___/RC or N ■ Productive cough ___/RC or N ■ RR 16-24/min ___/RC or N ■ Pt./Family anxiety level decreasing ___/N ■ Metabolically stable___/N			■ Color pink and O_2 saturation ≥ 90% during the weaning process from O_2 ___/RC or N ■ Alert and oriented at baseline level ___/N ■ Breath sounds with occasional crackles and rales upon auscultation ___/RC or N ■ RR 12-24/min, cough effective ___/RC or N ■ Family coping ___/N			■ Lungs clear, chest xray (if done before D/C) shows improvement___/RC or N ■ O_2 sat ≥ 90% off O_2 ___/RC or N ■ RR 12-20/min with effective cough ___/RC or N ■ Family support system in place and ready to take Pt. home ___/N		
Ineffective Airway Clearance: ■ Presence of tracheobronchial secretions from increased mucus production. ■ Audible wheezing ■ Congested cough with thick, tenacious mucus	■ Suctions easily (if indicated) after therapies initiated ___/RC or N ■ Mucus production decreasing after initiation of IV therapy and respiratory treatments___/RC or N ■ Pt. demonstrates effective cough technique ___/RC or N			■ Pt. able to cough productively to clear airway ___/RC or N ■ Lungs clearing, wheezing decreased ___/RC or N ■ Secretions thinner ___/RC or N			■ Productive cough, able to maintain clear airway___/RC or N ■ Minimal mucus production ___/RC or N ■ Lungs clear, few adventitious breath sounds___/RC or N ■ Clear, odorless secretions ___/RC or N ■ Minimal coughing ___/RC or N			■ Pt. able to breathe deeply without cough ___/RC or N ■ Pt. breathes easily; eupnia___/RC or N ■ Free of excessive cough ___/RC or N		
Activity Intolerance: Imbalance between O_2 supply and demand; decreased alveolar oxygen supply combined with greater metabolic demands from increased work of breathing. ■ Pt. complaint of fatigue ■ Dyspnea on exertion ■ Diaphoresis ■ Possible altered LOC	■ Rests between activities ___/N ■ Rest relieves pt.'s fatigue ___/N ■ Starts to use relaxation techniques to reduce stress ___/N ■ Pt. able to describe shortness of breath on SOB scale ___/N			■ Pt. verbalizes decreased fatigue and dyspnea after initiation of treatment ___/N ■ Pt. able to gradually increase activity with minimal dyspnea ___/N ■ Relaxation techniques are effective in reducing pt.'s stress and anxiety ___/N			■ Pt. able to perform ADLs (with assist from staff) with minimal dyspnea___/N ■ Pt. tolerating increased activity level___/N ■ Pt. able to pace activities to avoid becoming overly tired___/N			■ Pt. able to complete ADLs without fatigue or dyspnea ___/N		
Knowledge Deficit: ■ Bronchospasms, exposure to allergens ■ Importance in seeking early medical treatment ■ Importance of completing prescribed medication regimen ■ Questions regarding disease process	■ Pt./Family verbalize understanding of treatment plan and equipment use___/RC or N ■ Pt. able to demonstrate effective cough technique___/RC or N ■ Pt. cooperative with nebulizer/metered dose inhaler instructions___/RC or N			■ Pt./Family able to identify precipitating factors leading to respiratory infection (smoke, air pollution, persistent respiratory infection...) ___/RC or N ■ Pt. able to use MDI appropriately ___/RC or N ■ Pt. understands the importance of proper nutrition and hydration in prevention of illness ___/N			■ Pt. can state the signs and symptoms of early pulmonary infection (increased cough, increased sputum production with change in color from white to yellow-green) ___/RC or N ■ Pt. understands the importance of seeking early medical treatment when S/S present ___/RC or N			■ Pt. able to discuss medications; route, purpose, dosage, side effects, and precautions ___/Rx or N ■ Pt./Family know when and how to contact physician and access EMS if necessary ___/N ■ Pt. knows to ask the PCP about the Pneumonia vaccine after discharge from hospital ___/N		
Unmet Outcomes: (CCC Initials Required)	7-3 pm Resolved Planned /RN			7-3 pm Resolved Planned /RN			7-3 pm Resolved Planned /RN			7-3 pm Resolved Planned /RN		
	3-7 pm Resolved Planned /RN			3-7 pm Resolved Planned /RN			3-7 pm Resolved Planned /RN			3-7 pm Resolved Planned /RN		
	7-11 pm Resolved Planned /RN			7-11 pm Resolved Planned /RN			7-11 pm Resolved Planned /RN			7-11 pm Resolved Planned /RN		
	11-7 am Resolved Planned /RN			11-7 am Resolved Planned /RN			11-7 am Resolved Planned /RN			11-7 am Resolved Planned /RN		

pressed individual at risk for development of fatal pneumococcal infection (e.g., asplenic patient; patient with nephrotic syndrome, renal failure, or AIDS; or transplant recipient), it is thought that revaccination should be considered every 5 years.

Drug Therapy. The introduction of sulfonamides in the 1930s and penicillin in the 1940s revolutionized the treatment of pneumonia. The main problems with the use of antibiotics in pneumonia are the development of resistant strains of organisms and the patient's hypersensitivity or allergic reaction to certain antibiotics.

Most cases of community-acquired pneumonia in otherwise healthy adults do not require hospitalization. The oral antibiotic therapy administered is frequently empirical treatment with broad-spectrum antibiotics. (Empirical treatment is based on observation and experience without always knowing the exact cause.) Once the patient is categorized (see Table 26-3), empiric therapy can be based on the likely infecting organism.[5] For example, in the category 1 patients, these include *S. pneumoniae, M. pneumoniae,* respiratory viruses, *C. pneumoniae,* and *H. influenza.* Macrolides are the recommended therapy: either erythromycin or a newer macrolide if the patient is a smoker or is intolerant to erythromycin. Tetracycline is recommended for the patient who is allergic to macrolides, but this antibiotic is not reliably active against pneumococcus.[9]

For hospital-acquired pneumoniae, the American Thoracic Society recommends that empiric antibiotic therapy be based on the likely pathogens in the various patient groups (see Table 26-4).[6] Even with extensive diagnostic testing an etiologic agent is often not identified.

When using empiric therapy, it is important to recognize the nonresponding patient. Therapy may require modification based on the patient's culture results or clinical response. Clinical response is evaluated by factors such as a change in fever, sputum purulence, leukocytosis, oxygenation, x-ray patterns, and resolution of organ failure. Improvement is often not apparent for the first 48 to 72 hours, and empiric therapy need not be altered during this period unless deterioration is noted or culture results dictate otherwise.[6]

Patients with ventilator-associated pneumonia may experience rapid deterioration. Patients who deteriorate or fail to respond to therapy will require aggressive evaluation to assess noninfectious etiologies, complications, other coexisting infectious processes, or pneumonia caused by a resistant pathogen. It may be necessary to broaden antimicrobial coverage while awaiting results of cultures and other studies, such as computed tomograhy (CT) scan, ultrasound, or lung scans.[6]

Nutritional Therapy. Fluid intake of at least 3 L per day is important in the supportive treatment of pneumonia. If the patient has heart failure, fluid intake must be individualized. If oral intake cannot be maintained, IV administration of fluids and electrolytes may be necessary for the acutely ill patient. An intake of at least 1500 calories per day should be maintained to provide energy for the increased metabolic processes in the patient. Small, frequent meals are better tolerated by the dyspneic patient.

NURSING MANAGEMENT: PNEUMONIA

Nursing Assessment

Subjective and objective data that should be obtained from a patient with pneumonia are presented in Table 26-6.

Nursing Diagnoses

Nursing diagnoses for the patient with pneumonia may include, but are not limited to, those presented in NCP 26-1.

NURSING ASSESSMENT

Table 26-6 Pneumonia

Subjective Data	Objective Data
Important Health Information	**General**
Past health history: Lung cancer, COPD, diabetes, chronic debilitating disease, malnutrition, altered consciousness, AIDS, exposure to chemical toxins, dust, or allergens	Fever, restlessness or lethargy; splinting of affected area
Medications: Use of antibiotics; corticosteroids, chemotherapy, or any other immunosuppressants	**Respiratory**
Surgeries or other treatment: Recent abdominal or thoracic surgery, splenectomy, endotracheal intubation, or any surgery with general anesthesia	Tachypnea; pharyngitis; asymmetric chest movements or retraction; decreased excursion; nasal flaring; use of accessory muscles (neck, abdomen); grunting; crackles, friction rub on auscultation; dullness on percussion over consolidated areas, increased tactile fremitus on palpation; pink, rusty, purulent, green, yellow, or white sputum (amount may be scant to copious)
Functional Health Patterns	**Cardiovascular**
Health perception–health management: Cigarette smoking, alcoholism; recent upper respiratory tract infection, malaise	Tachycardia
Nutritional-metabolic: Anorexia, nausea, vomiting; chills	**Neurologic**
Activity-exercise: Prolonged bed rest or immobility; fatigue, weakness; dyspnea, cough (productive or nonproductive); nasal congestion	Changes in mental status, ranging from confusion to delirium
Cognitive-perceptual: Pain with breathing, chest pain, sore throat, headache, abdominal pain, muscle aches	**Possible Findings**
	Leukocytosis; abnormal ABGs with decreased or normal PaO_2, decreased $PaCO_2$, and increased pH initially, and later decreased PaO_2, increased $PaCO_2$, and decreased pH; positive sputum Gram's stain and culture; patchy or diffuse infiltrates, abscesses, pleural effusion, or pneumothorax on chest x-ray

AIDS, acquired immunodeficiency syndrome; *COPD,* chronic obstructive pulmonary disease.

26-1 NURSING CARE PLAN PATIENT WITH PNEUMONIA

Expected Patient Outcomes	Nursing Interventions and *Rationales*
NURSING DIAGNOSIS	**Ineffective breathing pattern** *related to* pneumonia and pain *as manifested by* rapid respirations, dyspnea, tachypnea, nasal flaring, altered chest excursion.
▪ Respiratory rate of 12-18 breaths/min. ▪ Feeling of comfort.	▪ Monitor vital signs and auscultate lungs every 2-4 hr *to provide ongoing data on patient's response to therapy.* ▪ Monitor arterial blood gases if ordered *to assess oxygenation status.* ▪ Administer oxygen as indicated *to maintain optimal oxygen level and increase patient comfort.* ▪ Position patient in semi-Fowler's or other comfortable position for breathing (may use reclining chairs) *to maximize lung expansion.*
NURSING DIAGNOSIS	**Ineffective airway clearance** *related to* pain, positioning, fatigue, and thick secretions *as manifested by* ineffective cough or thick, tenacious sputum; abnormal breath sounds; dyspnea.
▪ Clear breath sounds. ▪ Effective cough with expectoration of sputum. ▪ Normal chest x-ray or evidence of resolution.	▪ Assist patient to cough by splinting chest and teach patient how to cough effectively (inhale slowly through nose, exhale and cough) *to clear airways by bringing secretions to the mouth.* ▪ Give expectorants *to increase bronchial fluid production and promote expectoration* and cough suppressants *to relieve nonproductive cough* as ordered. ▪ Provide humidification of inhaled air *to maintain moisture of nasal/oral mucosa.* ▪ Maintain fluid intake of 3 L daily *to liquefy secretions.* ▪ Use chest physiotherapy or other airway clearance technique, if indicated, *to mobilize secretions.* ▪ Suction prn *to maintain patient airway.*
NURSING DIAGNOSIS	**Pain** *related to* pleuritis and ineffective pain management and/or comfort measures *as manifested by* pleuritic chest pain, pleural friction rub, shallow respirations, decreased breath sounds.
▪ Decreased or absent pain. ▪ Full lung excursion. ▪ Satisfaction with pain control.	▪ Assess pain level and location *to provide information on need for analgesia and other types of pain relief.* ▪ Administer analgesics as ordered *to relieve pain by interrupting CNS pathways.* ▪ Assist with intercostal nerve block if necessary *to treat pleuritic pain unresponsive to analgesics.* ▪ Observe for possible complications (e.g., pleural effusion, empyema) if pain persists *so appropriate treatment can be initiated.* ▪ Perform nonpharmacologic pain interventions such as back rubs, distraction, and relaxation technique *to relieve pain and reduce the need for analgesia.*
NURSING DIAGNOSIS	**Risk for altered health maintenance** *related to* lack of knowledge regarding treatment regimen after discharge.
▪ Adherence to treatment regimen, including medications, fluid therapy, activity schedule.	▪ Assess ability to continue self-care at home *to identify patient's knowledge about self-care and ability to manage self-care.* ▪ Encourage patient to continue on full course of antibiotic therapy *to prevent a relapse of pneumonia and the development of resistant strains of the organism.* ▪ Instruct patient on the importance of rest and limited activity *to maintain progress toward recovery and to prevent a relapse.* ▪ Encourage patient to obtain adequate rest, good nutrition, and fresh air *to assist the healing process.* ▪ If indicated, encourage patient to stop or decrease cigarette smoking *to improve the mucociliary clearance mechanism.* ▪ Teach patient to continue coughing and deep-breathing exercises *to remove secretions and improve ventilation.* ▪ Teach patient the importance of follow-up care and the need to seek medical attention for symptoms related to respiratory infections *to prevent relapse.* ▪ Encourage patients who have chronic illness (e.g., heart, lung, diabetes mellitus), are recovering from severe illness, are age 65 or older, or are in nursing homes or other long-term care facilities to obtain vaccinations (pneumococcal and influenza) *because these persons are at risk for pneumonia.*

Continued

26-1 NURSING CARE PLAN PATIENT WITH PNEUMONIA—continued

Expected Patient Outcomes	Nursing Interventions and *Rationales*
NURSING DIAGNOSIS	**Altered nutrition: less than body requirements** *related to* increased metabolism, fatigue, anorexia, nausea, and vomiting *as manifested by* weight loss.
▪ Maintenance of normal body weight. ▪ Adequate strength to perform activities of daily living.	▪ Assist with meals *to conserve energy.* ▪ Determine patient's food preferences and provide them when possible *to promote ingestion of adequate nutrients.* ▪ Provide means of oral hygiene before meals *to remove foul tastes related to sputum or medications.* ▪ Provide frequent small meals *to prevent pressure on diaphragm and minimize energy expenditure.* ▪ Monitor patient's weight and caloric intake *to assess need to adjust diet.*
NURSING DIAGNOSIS	**Hyperthermia** *related to* effects of illness *as manifested by* elevated temperature, diaphoresis, chills, flushing, thirst, headache, malaise.
▪ Normal body temperature. ▪ Increased comfort as fever subsides.	▪ Administer antibiotics as prescribed *to treat the infection.* ▪ Administer antipyretics as ordered *to reduce fever and increase patient's comfort.* ▪ Take temperature every 2-4 hr. ▪ Observe for continuing or recurring fever and report finding to physician *because this may indicate worsening of the illness.* ▪ Provide fluid intake (at least 3 L/day) *to replace fluid loss due to fever and diaphoresis.* ▪ Provide frequent clothing and linen changes if diaphoresis occurs *to keep patient comfortable and dry and to prevent chilling.*
NURSING DIAGNOSIS	**Activity intolerance** *related to* interrupted sleep-wake cycle, hypoxia, and weakness *as manifested by* fatigue, unwillingness or inability to exert self, dyspnea, increased pulse and respiration, dizziness on exertion.
▪ Verbalization of feeling of being rested. ▪ Able to perform activities of daily living without fatigue or dyspnea.	▪ Provide bed rest and limited physical activity *to conserve oxygen.* ▪ Assess response to activity *to evaluate patient's hypoxemia* and plan changes accordingly. ▪ Limit visitors and long conversations. ▪ Plan nursing care in blocks *to ensure periods of uninterrupted rest.* ▪ Place needed items (e.g., tissues, call bell) within easy reach *to conserve energy while facilitating independence.*

COLLABORATIVE PROBLEMS

Nursing Goals	Nursing Interventions and *Rationales*
POTENTIAL COMPLICATION	**Hypoxemia** *related to* impaired gas exchange in lungs.
▪ Monitor for signs of hypoxemia. ▪ Report deviations from acceptable parameters. ▪ Carry out appropriate medical and nursing interventions.	▪ Administer oxygen and antibiotics as ordered *to treat hypoxemia and infection.* ▪ Monitor vital signs as indicated. ▪ Assess and monitor mental status, such as restlessness, anxiety, confusion, and combative reactions, and respiratory status, such as cyanosis and changes in respiratory rate. ▪ Report changes from baseline values *to provide early treatment.*

CNS, central nervous system.

■ Planning

The overall goals are that the patient with pneumonia will have (1) clear breath sounds, (2) normal breathing patterns, (3) normal chest x-ray, and (4) no complications related to pneumonia.

■ Nursing Implementation

Health Promotion. There are many nursing interventions to help prevent the occurrence of, as well as the morbidity associated with, pneumonia. Teaching the individual to practice good health habits, such as proper diet and hygiene, adequate rest, and regular exercise, can maintain the natural resistance to infecting organisms. If possible, exposure to URIs should be avoided. If a URI occurs, it should be treated promptly with supportive measures (e.g., rest, fluids). If symptoms persist for more than 7 days, the person should obtain medical care. The individual at risk for pneumonia (e.g., the chronically ill and older adult) should be encouraged to obtain both influenza and pneumococcal vaccines.

In the hospital, the nursing role involves identifying the patient at risk (see Table 26-1) and taking measures to prevent the development of pneumonia. The patient with altered consciousness should be placed in positions (e.g., side-lying, upright) that will prevent or minimize the risk of aspiration. The patient should be turned and repositioned at least every 2 hours to facilitate adequate lung expansion and to discourage pooling of secretions.

The patient who has a feeding tube generally requires attention to measures to prevent aspiration (see Chapter 38). Although the distal end of the feeding tube is small, an interruption in the integrity of the lower esophageal sphincter still exists, which can allow reflux of gastric and intestinal contents.

The patient who has difficulty swallowing (e.g., stroke patient) needs assistance in eating, drinking, and taking medication to prevent aspiration. The patient who has recently had surgery and others who are immobile need assistance with turning and deep-breathing measures at frequent intervals (see Chapter 18). The nurse must be careful to avoid overmedication with narcotics or sedatives, which can cause a depressed cough reflex and accumulation of fluid in the lungs. The gag reflex should be present in the individual who has had local anesthesia to the throat before the administration of fluids or food.

Strict medical asepsis and adherence to infection control guidelines should be practiced by the nurse to reduce the incidence of nosocomial infections.[10] The patient with an infection should not be placed in the same room with a patient who is recovering from surgery or a patient with chronic lung disease. Respiratory therapy equipment should be properly cleaned and changed, and disposable equipment should be used as much as possible. Strict sterile aseptic technique should be used when suctioning a patient.

Acute Intervention. Although many patients with pneumonia are treated on an outpatient basis, the nursing care plan for a patient with pneumonia (see NCP 26-1) is applicable to both these individuals and in-hospital patients. It is important for the nurse to remember that pneumonia is an acute, infectious disease. Although most cases of pneumonia are potentially completely curable, complications can result. The nurse must be aware of these complications and their manifestations.

ETHICAL DILEMMAS

Guardianship

SITUATION

A 32-year-old man, institutionalized almost all of his life for profound developmental disabilities, is hospitalized for his fourth aspiration-related pneumonia in the last year. His physician believes that a feeding tube would solve the problem of aspiration and wants the family to agree to the procedure. The family believes his life span should not be extended by artificial means and refuses to give consent. The hospital is considering seeking a court-appointed guardian because the family is not acting in the best interest of the patient.

DISCUSSION

Disagreeing with the physician is not necessarily grounds for the family to be considered inappropriate guardians. In cases of profound developmental disabilities, it is difficult to distinguish who has the patient's *best interests* at heart; the family, the institution paid to attend to the patient, specialists who focus on a specific medical condition, or disability advocates. This patient has a medical condition that could probably be alleviated by the surgical placement of a feeding tube. However, there has yet to be a discussion about how the patient will adapt to the tube, what pleasures of taste he would lose, or how this would affect his ongoing care. The institution should also investigate the current feeding tube procedure to see if poor technique is a causative factor in his pneumonia. If so, appropriate teaching and training of the staff could correct the problem. Seeking a guardian hearing before these considerations would be premature.

ETHICAL AND LEGAL PRINCIPLES

- The state's position in favor of treating incompetent patients in order to preserve their life can be in direct opposition to the long-held assumption that parents have the right to make decisions for their incompetent adult children.
- Substituted judgment, basing the decision on what the patient himself would have decided, is difficult and may not be possible in cases of never-competent patients. However, best interest judgment can be based on the experience of the patient and extrapolation of the value, meaning, and pleasure he receives from life.
- Usually any person can petition the court for protection of an incompetent person. Courts are reluctant to intervene if the parents are functioning in a reasonable fashion. The law should be the last resort for treatment decisions.

Ambulatory and Home Care. The patient needs to be reassured that complete recovery from pneumonia is possible. It is extremely important to emphasize the need to take all of the prescribed medication and to return for follow-up medical care and evaluation. Adequate rest is needed to maintain progress toward recovery and to prevent a relapse. The patient should be told that it may be weeks before the usual vigor and sense of well-being are felt. A prolonged period of convalescence may be necessary for the older adult or chronically ill patient.

The patient considered to be at risk for pneumonia should be told about available vaccines and should discuss them with the health care provider. Deep-breathing exercises should be practiced for 6 to 8 weeks after the patient is discharged from the hospital.

Evaluation

The expected outcomes for the patient with pneumonia are presented in NCP 26-1.

TUBERCULOSIS

Tuberculosis (TB) is an infectious disease caused by *Mycobacterium tuberculosis.* It usually involves the lungs, but it also occurs in the kidneys, bones, adrenal glands, lymph nodes, and meninges and can be disseminated throughout the body.

With the introduction of chemotherapy in the late 1940s and early 1950s, there was a dramatic decrease in the prevalence of TB. Today 10 to 15 million people are infected with or harbor the tubercle bacillus. The majority of these individuals have healed or dormant TB. There have been approximately 29,000 cases per year of new active TB. Approximately 10% of these cases are relapses. These statistics indicate that TB, despite being potentially curable and preventable, is still a major public health problem in the United States. The major factors that have contributed to the resurgence of TB have been (1) the emergence of multidrug-resistant strains of *M. tuberculosis* and (2) epidemic proportions of TB among patients with human immunodeficiency virus (HIV) infections. HIV infection is the most important risk factor for the development of TB.[11]

Multidrug-resistant strains of TB have developed because TB patients' compliance with drug therapy was not monitored and therefore faltered, leading to treatment failure and development of resistant strains. Patients were lost to follow-up treatment or placed on drug regimens to which their infections were no longer susceptible. In general there was decreased vigilance in treating patients diagnosed with TB.[12]

Individuals at risk for TB include homeless persons, residents of inner-city neighborhoods, foreign-born persons (especially from Haiti and Southeast Asia), older adults, those in institutions (nursing homes, prisons), and the socioeconomically disadvantaged and medically underserved of all races. Immunosuppression from any etiology (e.g., HIV infection, malignancy) increases the risk of TB infection. The prevalence of TB is high in a few areas of the United States where there is a large population of Native-Americans, such as Arizona and New Mexico, and in counties near the Mexican border.

Etiology and Pathophysiology

M. tuberculosis, a gram-positive, acid-fast bacillus, is usually spread via airborne droplets, which are produced when the infected individual coughs, sneezes, or speaks. Once released into a room, the organisms are dispersed and can be inhaled. Brief exposure to a few tubercle bacilli rarely causes an infection. Rather, it is more commonly spread to the individual who has had repeated close contact with an infected person. TB is not highly infectious, and transmission usually requires close, frequent, or prolonged exposure. The disease cannot be spread by hands, books, glasses, dishes, or other fomites.

When the bacilli are inhaled, they pass down the bronchial system and implant themselves on the respiratory bronchioles or alveoli. The lower parts of the lungs are usually the site of initial bacterial implantation. After implantation, the bacilli multiply with no initial resistance from the host. The organisms are engulfed by phagocytes (initially neutrophils and later macrophages) and may continue to multiply within the phagocytes.

While a cellular immune response is being activated, the bacilli can be spread through the lymphatic channels to regional lymph nodes and via the thoracic duct to the circulating blood. Thus organisms may be spread throughout the body before sufficient activation of the cell-mediated immune response is available to bring the infection under control. The organisms find favorable environments for growth primarily in the upper lobes of the lungs, kidneys, epiphyses of the bone, cerebral cortex, and adrenal glands.

Eventually the acquired cellular immunity limits further multiplication and spread of the infection. A characteristic tissue reaction called an *epithelioid cell granuloma* results after the cellular immune system is activated. This granuloma (also called an *epithelioid cell tubercle*) is a result of fusion of the infiltrating macrophages. The granuloma is surrounded by lymphocytes. This reaction usually takes 10 to 20 days.

The central portion of the lesion (called a *Ghon tubercle*) undergoes necrosis characterized by a cheesy appearance and hence is named *caseous necrosis.* The lesion may also undergo liquefactive necrosis in which the liquid sloughs into connecting bronchi and produces a cavity. Tubercular material may enter the tracheobronchial system, allowing airborne transmission of infectious particles.

Healing of the primary lesion usually takes place by resolution, fibrosis, and calcification. The granulation tissue surrounding the lesion may become more fibrous and form a collagenous scar around the tubercle. A *Ghon complex* is formed, consisting of the Ghon tubercle and regional lymph nodes. Calcified Ghon complexes may be seen on chest x-ray.

CULTURAL & ETHNIC CONSIDERATIONS

Tuberculosis

- TB in the United States and Canada tends to be a disease of the older population, urban poor, minority groups, and patients with AIDS.
- At all ages the incidence of TB among non-Caucasians is at least twice that of Caucasians.
- Ethnic groups that have a high incidence of TB include foreign-born people from Asia, Africa, and Latin America. Native-Americans, Alaskan Natives, African-Americans, and Asian-Americans are also ethnic groups with a high incidence of TB.
- Southeastern Asian, Haitian, and Hispanic immigrants have incidence rates of TB similar to those of the countries from which they came.

Table 26-7 Classification of Tuberculosis (TB)

Class 0
No TB exposure, not infected (no history of exposure, negative tuberculin skin test)

Class 1
TB exposure, no evidence of infection (history of exposure, negative tuberculin skin test)

Class 2
TB infection without disease (significant reaction to tuberculin skin test, negative bacteriologic studies, no x-ray findings compatible with TB, no clinical evidence of TB)

Class 3
TB infection with clinically active disease (positive bacteriologic studies or both a significant reaction to tuberculin skin test and clinical or x-ray evidence of current disease)

Class 4
No current disease (history of previous episode of TB or abnormal, stable x-ray findings in a person with a significant reaction to tuberculin skin test; negative bacteriologic studies if done; no clinical or x-ray evidence of current disease)

Class 5
TB suspect (diagnosis pending); person should not be in this classification for more than 3 mo

Source: American Thoracic Society.

When a tuberculous lesion regresses and heals, the infection enters a latent period in which it may persist without producing a clinical illness. The infection may develop into clinical disease if the persisting organisms begin to multiply rapidly, or it may remain dormant.

If the initial immune response is not adequate, control of the organisms is not maintained and clinical disease results. Certain individuals are at a higher risk for clinical disease, including those who are immunosuppressed for any reason (e.g., patients with HIV infection, those receiving cancer chemotherapy or long-term corticosteroid therapy) or have diabetes mellitus.

Dormant but viable organisms persist for years. Reactivation of TB can occur if the host's defense mechanisms become impaired. The reasons for reactivation are not well understood, but they are related to decreased resistance found in older adults, individuals with concomitant diseases, and those who receive immunosuppressive therapy.

Classification

The American Thoracic Association and American Lung Association adopted a classification system that covers the entire population (Table 26-7).

Clinical Manifestations

In the early stages of TB the person is usually free of symptoms. Many cases are found incidentally when routine chest x-rays are taken, especially in older adults.

Systemic manifestations may initially consist of fatigue, malaise, anorexia, weight loss, low-grade fevers (especially in the late afternoon), and night sweats. The weight loss may not be excessive until late in the disease and is often attributed to overwork or other factors. Irregular menses may also be present in premenopausal women.

A characteristic pulmonary manifestation is a cough that becomes frequent and produces mucoid or mucopurulent sputum. Chest pain characterized as dull or tight may also be present. Hemoptysis is not a common finding and is usually associated with more advanced cases. Sometimes TB has more acute, sudden manifestations; the patient has high fever, chills, generalized flu-like symptoms, pleuritic pain, and a productive cough.

The HIV-infected patient with TB often has atypical physical examinations and chest x-ray findings. Classical signs such as fever, cough, and weight loss may be attributed to *Pneumocystis carinii* (PCP) or other HIV-associated opportunistic diseases. Clinical manifestations of respiratory problems must be carefully investigated to determine the cause.

Complications

Miliary TB. If a necrotic Ghon complex erodes through a blood vessel, large numbers of organisms invade the bloodstream and spread to all body organs. This is called *miliary* or *hematogenous TB.* The patient may be either acutely ill with fever, dyspnea, and cyanosis or chronically ill with systemic manifestations of weight loss, fever, and GI disturbance. Hepatomegaly, splenomegaly, and generalized lymphadenopathy may be present.

Pleural Effusion. A pleural effusion is caused by the release of caseous material into the pleural space. The bacteria-containing material triggers an inflammatory reaction and a pleural exudate of protein-rich fluid. A form of pleurisy called *dry pleurisy* may result from a superficial tuberculous lesion involving the pleura. It appears as localized pleuritic pain on deep inspiration.

Tuberculous Pneumonia. Acute pneumonia may result when large amounts of tubercle bacilli are discharged from the liquefied necrotic lesion into the lung or lymph nodes. The clinical manifestations are similar to those of bacterial pneumonia, including chills, fever, productive cough, pleuritic pain, and leukocytosis.

Other Organ Involvement. Although the lungs are the primary site of TB, other body organs may also be involved. The meninges may become infected. Bone and joint tissue may be involved in the infectious disease process. The kidneys, adrenal glands, lymph nodes, and both female and male genital tracts may also be infected.

Diagnostic Studies

Tuberculin Skin Testing. The body's immune response can be demonstrated by hypersensitivity to a tuberculin skin test. A positive reaction occurs 3 to 10 weeks after the initial infection, corresponding to the time needed to mount an immune response.

Purified protein derivative (PPD) of tuberculin is used primarily to detect the delayed hypersensitivity response. (The procedure for performing the tuberculin skin test is described in Chapter 24.) Once acquired, sensitivity to tuberculin tends to persist throughout life. A positive reaction indicates the pres-

COLLABORATIVE CARE

Table 26-8 Tuberculosis

Diagnostic
- Health history and physical examination
- Tuberculin skin test
- Chest x-ray
- Bacteriologic studies
  - Sputum smear
  - Sputum culture

Collaborative Therapy
- Long-term treatment with antimicrobial drugs*
- Follow-up bacteriologic studies

*See Tables 26-9 and 26-10.

ence of a tuberculous infection, but it does not show whether the infection is dormant or active, causing a clinical illness.

Because the response to TB skin testing may be decreased in the immunocompromised patient, induration reactions less than 10 mm may be considered positive. See Table 24-12 for the guidelines in interpreting TB skin tests.

Chest X-ray. Although the findings on chest x-ray examination are important, it is not possible to make a diagnosis of TB solely on the basis of this examination. This is because other diseases can mimic the x-ray appearance of TB. The abnormality most commonly found in TB is multinodular lymph node involvement with cavitation in the upper lobes of the lungs. This is often referred to as the *parenchymal lymph node complex.* Calcification of the lung lesions generally occurs within several years of the infection.

Bacteriologic Studies. The demonstration of tubercle bacilli bacteriologically is essential for establishing a diagnosis. Microscopic examination of stained sputum smears for acid-fast bacilli is usually the first bacteriologic evidence of the presence of tubercle bacilli. This is a quick, easy examination that provides valuable information. A major disadvantage is that more than 10,000 bacteria per milliliter of specimen are required to produce a positive smear. In addition to sputum, material for examination can be obtained from gastric washings, cerebrospinal fluid (CSF), or pus from an abscess.

The most accurate means of diagnosis is a culture technique. The major disadvantage of this method is that it may take 6 to 8 weeks for the mycobacterium to grow. The advantage is that it can detect small quantities (as few as 10 bacteria per milliliter of specimen).

Serologic diagnosis of TB using enzyme-linked immunosorbent assay (ELISA) methodology to measure IgG antibody against mycobacterial antigens is a new and promising technique. DNA fingerprinting uses the polymerase chain reaction technique to identify individual strains of *M. tuberculosis.*

Collaborative Care

Hospitalization for initial treatment of TB is not necessary in most patients. Most patients are treated on an outpatient basis (Table 26-8), and many can continue to work and maintain their lifestyles with few changes. Hospitalization may be used for diagnostic evaluation, for the severely ill or debilitated, and for those who experience adverse drug reactions or treatment failures.

The mainstay of TB treatment is drug therapy. Drug therapy is used to treat an individual with clinical disease and to prevent disease in an infected person.

Drug Therapy

Active disease. In view of the growing prevalence of multidrug-resistant TB, the patient with active TB should be managed aggressively. Standard therapy has been revised because of the increase in prevalence of drug-resistant TB. Treatment of TB usually consists of a combination of at least four drugs. The reason for combination therapy is to increase the therapeutic effectiveness and decrease the development of resistant strains of *M. tuberculosis.* It has been shown that single-drug therapy can result in rapid development of resistant strains.

The five primary drugs used are isoniazid, rifampin, pyrazinamide, streptomycin, and ethambutol (Table 26-9). Fixed-dose combination antituberculous drugs may enhance adherence to treatment recommendations. Combinations of isoniazid and rifampin (Rifamate) and of isoniazid, rifampin, and pyrazinamide (Rifater) are available to simplify therapy. Other drugs are primarily used for treatment of resistant strains or if the patient develops toxicity to the primary drugs. Many second-line drugs carry a greater risk of toxicity and require closer monitoring. Newer drugs for the treatment of TB that have not been placed in categories of first- or second-line drugs include the quinolones, especially ciprofloxacin (Cipro), ofloxacin (Floxin), and sparfloxacin (Zagam). Rifapentine (Priftin), a new drug to treat TB, can be used in combination with other TB drugs.

A problem with antituberculous therapy is the length of time medication must be taken. In the past, 18 to 26 months was the usual period of time required for individuals to adhere to the medical regimen. Shorter courses of therapy (6 to 9 months) have been shown to be effective. Three options for a treatment regimen are available (Table 26-10).

Treatment in areas where drug resistance is known to be a problem may consist of initial addition of drugs not in the resistance pattern for that area. Drug regimens should be adapted to the resistance pattern evident from sputum culture. In follow-up care for patients on long-term therapy, it is important to monitor the effectiveness of drugs and the development of toxic side effects. Usually sputum specimens are initially obtained weekly and then monthly to assess the effectiveness of the medication. The regimen is considered to be effective if the patient converts to a negative TB sputum status.

Although TB tends to have a rapidly progressive course in the patient coinfected with HIV, it responds well to standard medication. The coinfected patient should receive antituberculosis treatment for at least 6 months beyond the conversion of sputum cultures to negative status.

An important reason for follow-up care in the patient with TB is to ensure adherence to the treatment regimen. Noncompliance is a major factor in the emergence of multidrug resistance and treatment failures. Many individuals do not adhere to the treatment program in spite of understanding the disease process and the value of treatment. As a result, directly observed therapy (DOT) is usually prescribed for patients known to be at risk for noncompliance with therapy. DOT is an

DRUG THERAPY

Table 26-9 Tuberculosis (TB)

Drug	Mechanisms of Action	Side Effects	Comments
First-Line Drugs			
▪ Isoniazid (INH)	Interferes with DNA metabolism of tubercle bacillus	Peripheral neuritis, hepatotoxicity, hypersensitivity (skin rash, arthralgia, fever), optic neuritis, vitamin B_6 neuritis	Metabolism primarily by liver and excretion by kidneys, pyridoxine (vitamin B_6) administration during high-dose therapy as prophylactic measure, use as single prophylactic agent for active TB in individuals whose PPD converts to positive, ability to cross blood-brain barrier
▪ Rifampin (Rifadin)	Has broad-spectrum effects, inhibits RNA polymerase of tubercle bacillus	Hepatitis, febrile reaction, GI disturbance, peripheral neuropathy, hypersensitivity	Most common use with isoniazid, low incidence of side effects, suppression of effect of birth control pills, possible orange urine
▪ Ethambutol (Myambutol)	Inhibits RNA synthesis and is bacteriostatic for the tubercle bacillus	Skin rash, GI disturbance, malaise, peripheral neuritis, optic neuritis	Side effects uncommon and reversible with discontinuation of drug, most common use as substitute drug when toxicity occurs with isoniazid or rifampin
▪ Streptomycin	Inhibits protein synthesis and is bactericidal	Ototoxicity (eighth cranial nerve), nephrotoxicity, hypersensitivity	Cautious use in older adults, those with renal disease, and pregnant women; must be given parenterally
▪ Pyrazinamide	Bactericidal effect (exact mechanism is unknown)	Fever, skin rash, hyperuricemia, jaundice (rare)	High rate of effectiveness when used with streptomycin or capreomycin
Second-Line Drugs			
▪ Ethionamide (Trecator)	Inhibits protein synthesis	GI disturbance, hepatotoxicity, hypersensitivity	Valuable for treatment of resistant organisms Contraindication in pregnancy
▪ Capreomycin (Capastat)	Inhibits protein synthesis and is bactericidal	Ototoxicity, nephrotoxicity	Cautious use in older adults
▪ Kanamycin (Kantrex) and amikacin	Interferes with protein synthesis	Ototoxicity, nephrotoxicity	Use in selected cases for treatment of resistant strains
▪ Para-aminosalicylic acid (PAS)	Interferes with metabolism of tubercle bacillus	GI disturbance (frequent), hypersensitivity, hepatotoxicity	Interference with absorption of rifampin, infrequent use
▪ Cycloserine (Seromycin)	Inhibits cell-wall synthesis	Personality changes, psychosis, rash	Contraindication in individuals with a history of psychosis, use in treatment of resistant strains

DNA, deoxyribonucleic acid; *GI,* gastrointestinal; *PPD,* purified protein derivative; *RNA,* ribonucleic acid.

expensive but essential public health issue. The patient needs to have follow-up visits for 12 months after completion of therapy to check for the presence of resistant strains. Patients infected with *M. tuberculosis* but without active disease harbor small numbers of organisms.

The major side effect of isoniazid, rifampin, and pyrazinamide is hepatitis. Liver function tests should be monitored, especially in individuals over 35 years of age.[13] Elevation of liver transaminase enzymes up to three times normal without symptoms does not constitute an indication to stop therapy.

Prophylactic treatment. Drug therapy can be used to prevent a TB infection from developing into a clinical disease. The indications for preventive therapy (chemoprophylaxis) are presented in Table 26-11. Close contacts of individuals with infectious clinical TB should be examined with tuberculin skin tests.

Some individuals carry dormant TB infections that may develop into active disease in some situations. Examples include positive reactors who (1) demonstrate some degree of immunosuppression (e.g., person who is on prolonged corticosteroid therapy or has HIV infection), (2) have a malignant

DRUG THERAPY

Table 26-10 Regimen Options for the Initial Treatment of Tuberculosis

TB without HIV Infection

Option 1

Four-drug regimen consisting of isoniazid, rifampin, pyrazinamide, and either ethambutol or streptomycin. Therapy may be given daily or 2-3 times weekly if DOT. Ethambutol or streptomycin may be discontinued if susceptibility to isoniazid or rifampin is documented. Pyrazinamide should be discontinued after 8 wk. The total duration of therapy should be at least 6 mo and at least 3 mo after sputum cultures convert to negative. Fixed-dose combinations of rifampin and isoniazid (Rifamate) and rifampin, isoniazid, and pyrazinamide (Rifater) are available to simplify therapy.

Option 2

Daily isoniazid, rifampin, pyrazinamide, and streptomycin or ethambutol for 2 wk, followed by DOT twice-weekly administration of the same drugs for 6 wk, followed by DOT twice-weekly administrations of isoniazid and rifampin for 16 wk.

Option 3

DOT 3 times/wk administration of isoniazid, rifampin, pyrazinamide, and ethambutol or streptomycin for 6 mo.

TB with HIV Infection

Option 1, 2, or 3 can be used, but treatment regimens should continue for a total of 9 mo and at least 6 mo beyond culture conversion.

Source: Centers for Disease Control.
Note: The CDC advises consultation with a TB medical expert if the patient is symptomatic or smear or culture is positive after 3 months.
DOT, directly observed therapy.

condition such as Hodgkin's disease, or (3) have diabetes mellitus. The individual with any of these characteristics will benefit from prophylactic treatment for TB.

The drug generally used in prophylactic chemotherapy is isoniazid. It is effective and inexpensive and can be administered orally. Isoniazid is usually administered once daily for 6 months in an uncomplicated case or for 12 months for the individual with abnormal chest x-rays or who is HIV positive.

Vaccine. A number of live tuberculosis vaccines are available and are known collectively as BCG after the original strain of bacterium used in the vaccines (bacille Calmette-Guérin [BCG]).[13] BCG vaccination should be considered only if isoniazid chemoprophylaxis cannot be used. It is recommended for the person who has a negative tuberculin skin test but who is repeatedly exposed to pulmonary tuberculosis (e.g., person assigned to work in countries with a high prevalence rate). Vaccines should also be considered for communities or groups in which a high rate of new infections occurs despite aggressive treatment and surveillance programs.

NURSING MANAGEMENT: TUBERCULOSIS

■ Nursing Assessment

It is important to determine whether the patient was ever exposed to a person with TB. The patient should be assessed for productive cough, night sweats, afternoon temperature elevation, weight loss, pleuritic chest pain, and crackles over the apices of the lungs. If the patient has a productive cough, an early morning sputum specimen will be required for an acid-fast bacillus (AFB) smear to detect the presence of mycobacteria.

Table 26-11 Indications for Preventive TB Therapy

- Newly infected patient
- Person with known or suspected HIV infection and positive skin test
- Exposure of household members and other close associates to newly diagnosed patient
- Significant tuberculin skin test reactors with abnormal chest x-ray
- Significant tuberculin skin test reactors in special clinical situations (person takes corticosteroids; has diabetes mellitus, silicosis, gastrectomy, or end-stage renal disease)
- Other significant tuberculin skin test converters (≥10 mm increase within a 2 yr period for those less than 35 yr old; ≥15 mm increase for those greater than 35 yr old; all children less than 2 yr old with a >10 mm skin test)
- Other significant tuberculin skin test reactors in person less than 35 yr old (persons born outside of United States from high-prevalence countries; medically underserved low-income populations including high-risk racial or ethnic populations, such as African-Americans, Hispanic, and Native-Americans; residents in long-term care facilities)

Source: American Thoracic Society.

■ Nursing Diagnoses

Nursing diagnoses for the patient with TB may include, but are not limited to, the following:

- Ineffective breathing pattern *related to* decreased lung capacity
- Altered nutrition: less than body requirements *related to* chronic poor appetite, fatigue, and productive cough
- Noncompliance *related to* lack of knowledge of disease process, lack of motivation, and long-term nature of treatment
- Altered health maintenance *related to* lack of knowledge about the disease process and therapeutic regimen
- Activity intolerance *related to* fatigue, decreased nutritional status, and chronic febrile episodes

■ Planning

The overall goals are that the patient with TB will (1) comply with therapeutic regimen, (2) have no recurrence of disease, (3) have normal pulmonary function, and (4) take appropriate measures to prevent the spread of the disease.

■ Nursing Implementation

Health Promotion. The ultimate goal related to TB in the United States is eradication. The public health nurse and clinical nurse have especially important responsibilities. Selective screening programs in known risk groups are of value in detecting individuals with TB. The person with a positive

ETHICAL DILEMMAS

Patient Compliance

SITUATION

The health clinic for the homeless discovers that a patient with TB has not been complying with taking his medication. He tells the nurse that it is hard for him to get to the clinic to obtain the medication, much less to keep on a schedule. The nurse is concerned not only about this patient, but also about the risks for the other people at the shelter, in the park, and at the meal sites.

DISCUSSION

TB is a public health concern, as well as this individual's problem. Homelessness does not lend itself toward good compliance with medical treatment unless the patient is highly motivated and able to cope both with daily living issues and with his medical condition. If the TB is not treated appropriately, the patient may not only infect others, but his disease may develop a resistance to the medication, possibly leading to an even more resistant strain of the TB bacillus. There are two patients in this case: this particular patient and the public. To effectively help this person with his treatment program, social services must be involved. It might be possible to place him in a halfway house or group home until his treatment is completed. In any case, if he is unable or unwilling to cooperate, public health officials must be involved so that the public is protected.

ETHICAL AND LEGAL PRINCIPLES

- Compliance with a medical treatment plan helps to ensure the goals of treatment. If a patient cannot comply, the medical goals of treatment are compromised.
- Patient autonomy may be overridden by concerns about protecting the health of the public.
- Public health interests may be included in state statutes allowing medical personnel to detain and treat patients with infectious diseases.

tuberculin skin test should have a chest x-ray to assess for the presence of TB. Another important measure is to identify the contacts of the individual who has TB. These contacts should be assessed for the possibility of infection and the need for chemoprophylactic treatment.

When an individual has respiratory symptoms such as cough, dyspnea, or sputum production, especially if accompanied by a history of night sweats or unexplained weight loss, the nurse should assess for exposure to persons with TB. Even if the suspected respiratory problem is something else, such as emphysema, pneumonia, or lung cancer, it is possible that the patient may also have TB.

Acute Intervention. Acute in-hospital care is seldom required for the patient with TB. If hospitalization is needed, it is usually for a brief period. Respiratory isolation is indicated until the patient has been on adequate drug therapy for at least 2 weeks and has shown a clinical response to therapy. It is recommended that isolation be maintained on the patient with drug-resistant TB until smears are negative on 3 consecutive days. The patient who is unlikely to transmit tubercle bacilli (i.e., patient without a cough) does not necessarily need to be placed in respiratory isolation. Masks are of limited value unless they are made of fabric designed to filter out droplet nuclei. High-efficiency particulate air (HEPA) masks may be indicated because they can remove almost 100% of particles greater than 3 μm in diameter. Any mask used needs to be molded to fit tightly around the nose and mouth.

The patient should be taught to cover the nose and mouth with paper tissue every time he or she coughs, sneezes, or produces sputum. The tissues should be thrown into a paper bag and disposed of with the trash, burned, or flushed down the toilet. Masks are necessary only during face-to-face contacts. It is preferable that the patient wears the mask. The patient should also be taught careful hand-washing techniques after handling sputum and soiled tissues. Special precautions should be taken during high risk procedures such as sputum induction, bronchoscopy, or endoscopy.

Ambulatory and Home Care. Most treatment failures occur because the patient neglects to take the medication, discontinues it prematurely, or takes it irregularly. It is important for the nurse to develop a therapeutic, consistent relationship with each patient. The nurse must understand the patient's lifestyle and provide flexibility in planning a program that facilitates the patient's participation in and completion of therapy. The nurse should educate the patient so that the need for dedication to the prescribed regimen is fully understood by the patient. Ongoing reassurance helps the patient understand that adherence can mean cure. If the patient cannot or will not adhere to a self-administered medication regimen, medication may have to be given by a responsible person on a daily or intermittent basis. Notification of the public health department is essential if drug compliance is questionable so that follow-up of close contacts can be accomplished. In some cases the public health nurse will be responsible for DOT. In other situations, a spouse, grown child, other relative living with the patient, or co-worker may be asked to supervise drug taking.

Some patients may feel that there is a social stigma attached to TB. These feelings should be discussed, and the patient should be reassured that an individual with TB can be cured if the prescribed regimen is followed. Many people still remember when TB patients were sent away to TB sanitariums and isolated from society. The health care worker's attitude toward individuals with TB should be no different from the attitude toward those with pneumonia. Both diseases are infectious and potentially curable. The American Lung Association provides excellent literature for teaching about the disease, as well as providing emotional support to the patient and family.

When the chemotherapy regimen has been completed, most individuals can be considered adequately treated. Follow-up care may be indicated during the subsequent 12 months, including bacteriologic studies and chest x-ray. Because approximately 5% of individuals experience relapses, the patient should be taught to recognize the symptoms that indicate recurrence of TB. If these symptoms occur, immediate medical attention should be sought.

The patient needs to be instructed about certain factors that could reactivate TB, such as immunosuppressive therapy, ma-

Table 26-12 Fungal Infections of the Lung

Organism	Characteristics
Histoplasmosis *Histoplasma capsulatum*	Indigenous to soil of North American river valleys, inhalation of mycelia into lungs, infected individual often free of symptoms, generally self-limiting, chronic disease similar to TB
Coccidioidomycosis *Coccidioides immitis*	Indigenous to semiarid regions of southwestern United States, inhalation of arthrospores into lungs, suppurative and granulomatous reaction in lungs, symptomatic infection in one third of individuals
Blastomycosis *Blastomyces dermatitidis*	Indigenous to southeastern and midwestern United States, inhalation of fungus into lungs, progression of disease often insidious, possible involvement of skin
Cryptococcosis *Cryptococcus neoformans*	True yeast, indigenous worldwide in soil and pigeon excreta, inhalation of fungus into lungs, possible meningitis
Aspergillosis *Aspergillus niger* or *Aspergillus fumigatus*	True mold inhabiting mouth, widely distributed, invasion of lung tissue resulting in possible necrotizing pneumonia: in individual with asthma, allergic bronchopulmonary aspergillosis may require corticosteroid therapy
Candidiasis *Candida albicans*	Leading cause of mycotic infections in hospitalized and immunocompromised hosts, ubiquitous and frequent colonization of upper respiratory and GI tracts, infections often following broad-spectrum antibiotic therapy (systemic or inhaled), possible development of localized pulmonary infiltrate to widespread bilateral consolidation with hypoxemia
Actinomycosis *Actinomyces israeli*	Not a true fungus, pseudohyphae present; anaerobic, gram-positive, higher bacteria with branching hyphae; presence of necrotizing pneumonia after aspiration; pneumonitis, commonly in lower lobes with abscess or empyema formation
Nocardiosis *Nocardia asteroides*	Not a true fungus; aerobic, higher bacteria with branching hyphae; soil saprophyte widely distributed in nature; acquisition of infection from nature; rarely present in sputum without accompanying disease

lignancy, and prolonged debilitating illness. If the patient experiences any of these events, the health care provider must to be told so that reactivation of TB can be closely monitored. In some situations it may be necessary to put the patient on anti-TB chemotherapy.

■ Evaluation

The expected outcomes are that the patient with TB will have

- complete resolution of the disease
- normal pulmonary function
- absence of any complications

ATYPICAL MYCOBACTERIA

Pulmonary disease that closely resembles TB may be caused by atypical acid-fast mycobacteria. This type of pulmonary disease is indistinguishable from TB clinically and radiologically but can be differentiated by bacteriologic culture. These organisms are not believed to be airborne and thus are not transmitted by droplet nuclei.

Atypical mycobacteria that affect the lung include *M. kansasii, M. scrofulaceum, M. intracellularis,* and *M. xenopi.* These bacteria (especially *M. avium-intracellulare* and *M. scrofulaceum*) may also invade the cervical lymph nodes, causing lymphadenitis. This type of pulmonary disease typically occurs in white men with a history of COPD, cystic fibrosis, or silicosis. *Mycobacterium avium-intracellulare* is a common cause of opportunistic infections in the patient with HIV infection (see Chapter 13).

Treatment depends on identification of the causative agent and determination of drug sensitivity. Many of the drugs used in treating TB are used in combating infections from atypical mycobacteria.

PULMONARY FUNGAL INFECTIONS

Pulmonary fungal infections are increasing in incidence. They are found most frequently in seriously ill patients being treated with corticosteroids, antineoplastic and immunosuppressive drugs, or multiple antibiotics; they are also found in patients with AIDS and cystic fibrosis. Types of fungal infections are presented in Table 26-12. These infections are not transmitted from person to person, and the patient does not have to be placed in isolation. The clinical manifestations are similar to those of bacterial pneumonia. Skin and serology tests are available to assist in identifying the infecting organism. However, identification of the organism in a sputum specimen or in other body fluids is the best diagnostic indicator.

Collaborative Care

Amphotericin B is the drug most widely used in treating serious systemic fungal infections. It must be given intravenously to achieve adequate blood and tissue levels because it is poorly absorbed from the GI tract. Amphotericin B is considered a toxic drug with many possible side effects, including hypersensitivity reactions, fever, chills, malaise, nausea and vomiting, thrombophlebitis at the injection site, and abnormal renal function. Many of the side effects during infusion can be avoided by using aspirin or diphenhydramine (Benadryl) 1 hour before the infusion. Inclusion of a small amount of hydrocortisone in the infusion helps decrease the irritation of the veins. Monitoring of renal function is essential while a person is receiving this drug. Renal changes are at least partially reversible. Amphotericin infusions are incompatible with most other drugs. Amphotericin is frequently administered every other day after an initial period of several weeks of daily therapy. Total treatment with the drug may range from 4 to 10 weeks.

Oral imidazole and triazole compounds with antifungal activity such as ketoconazole (Nizoral), fluconazole (Diflucan), or itraconazole (Sporanox) have been successful in the treatment of fungal infections. Their effectiveness in treatment allows an alternative to the use of amphotericin B in many cases. Effectiveness of therapy can be monitored with fungal serology titers.

Flucytosine (Ancobon) has also been used in selected types of pulmonary fungal infections. It is given orally and becomes widely distributed in the body. Adverse reactions include abdominal discomfort, diarrhea, hepatotoxicity, and bone marrow suppression.

BRONCHIECTASIS

Etiology and Pathophysiology

Bronchiectasis is a disorder characterized by permanent, abnormal dilation of one or more large bronchi. The pathophysiologic change that results in dilation is destruction of the elastic and muscular structures of the bronchial wall. There are two pathologic types of bronchiectasis: saccular and cylindrical (Fig. 26-2). *Saccular bronchiectasis* occurs mainly in large bronchi and is characterized by cavity-like dilations. The affected bronchi end in large sacs. *Cylindrical bronchiectasis* involves medium-sized bronchi that are mildly to moderately dilated. *Fusiform bronchiectasis,* a subtype of cylindrical, tends to involve more "pouching" of the bronchi as opposed to dilation seen with cylindrical bronchiectasis.

Almost all forms of bronchiectasis are associated with bacterial infections. A wide variety of infectious agents can initiate bronchiectasis, including adenovirus, influenza virus, *Staphylococcus aureus, Klebsiella,* and anaerobes. Infections cause the bronchial walls to weaken, and pockets of infection begin to form. When the walls of the bronchial system are injured, the mucociliary mechanism is damaged, allowing bacteria and mucus to accumulate within the pockets. The infection becomes worse and results in bronchiectasis.

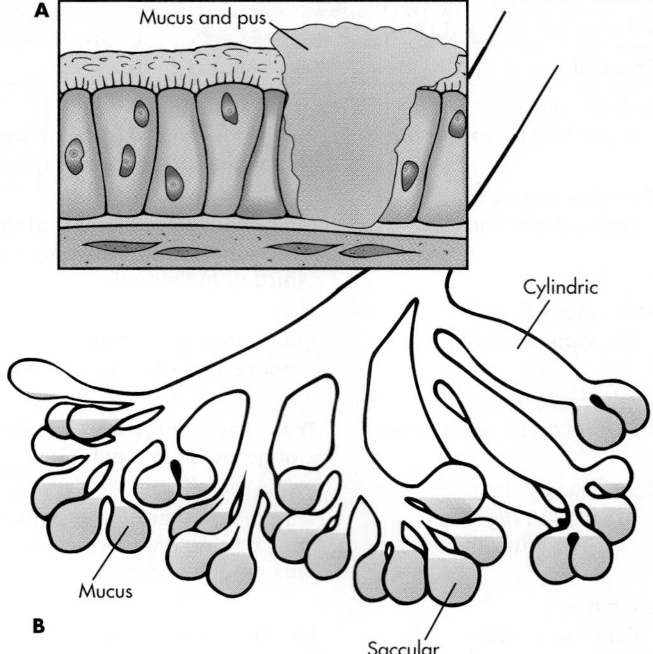

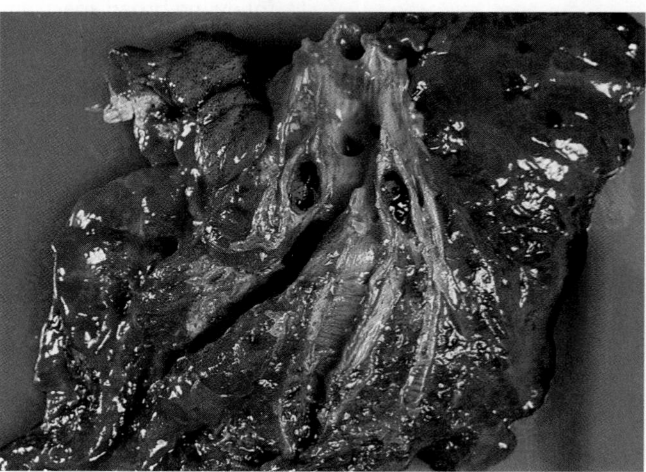

Fig. 26-2 Pathologic changes in bronchiectasis. **A,** Longitudinal section of bronchial wall where chronic infection has caused damage. **B,** Collection of purulent material in dilated bronchioles, leading to persistent infection. **C,** Cylindrical bronchiectasis. The dilated bronchi (**A**) and bronchioles (**B**) can be dissected almost to the pleural surface.

Bronchiectasis can be designated as *localized* or *generalized* based on the underlying cause. *Localized bronchiectasis* results from necrotizing or lobar pneumonia whose bronchiectatic sequelae are limited to one area of the lung or from focal airway obstructions. Obstructive processes of any kind can predispose an individual to bronchiectasis. Examples include lung tumors, tumor masses in the chest cavity, aspirated foreign objects, and thick, tenacious secretions such as those found in chronic bronchitis and cystic fibrosis. The obstruction causes the bronchi and bronchioles to distend and balloon out below the level of obstruction. This provides a good place for organisms to proliferate.

The most common cause of *generalized bronchiectasis* is multifocal necrotizing bacterial infection, but other conditions such as congenital factors, recurrent gastric aspiration, and toxic inhalations can predispose persons to the development of bronchiectasis. Congenital factors include altered bronchial structures such as cysts and cul-de-sacs, which lead to pooling of secretion. A defect in cilia, causing them to be immobile, is also associated with the development of bronchiectasis. In cystic fibrosis, there is retention and thickening of mucus that may plug the airways. A variety of immunodeficiency diseases are associated with recurrent bacterial pneumonias. Some inhalation exposures, particularly to irritant gases such as oxides of sulfur and nitrogen, have been noted as causes of bronchiectasis.

The disease process is often believed to start in childhood as an acquired disorder, beginning with respiratory complications secondary to influenza, measles, or whooping cough. Recurring lower respiratory tract infections are another pattern of disease in childhood that may predispose an individual to bronchiectasis. This pattern is typically seen in the individual who has cystic fibrosis, asthma, α_1-antitrypsin deficiency, or immunodeficiency diseases.

Clinical Manifestations

The primary manifestations of bronchiectasis vary considerably, depending on the extent and location of the disease process. They include chronic cough with production of mucopurulent sputum, hemoptysis, and recurrent pneumonia. The cough is paroxysmal and is often stimulated with position changes. Other manifestations include exertional dyspnea, fatigue, weight loss, anorexia, and fetid breath. On auscultation of the lungs, any combination of crackles, rhonchi, and wheezing may be heard. Sinusitis frequently accompanies diffuse bronchiectasis. The manifestations of advanced, widespread bronchiectasis are generalized wheezing, digital clubbing, and cor pulmonale.

Diagnostic Studies

An individual with a chronic productive cough with copious sputum (which may be blood streaked) should be suspected of having bronchiectasis. Characteristic findings in the health history, such as childhood diseases complicated by respiratory infections or chronic bronchitis, are significant. Chest x-rays are usually done and may show streaky infiltrates. Bronchography involves instilling liquid radiopaque material into the bronchial system via a catheter or bronchoscope, and in the past it was useful in evaluating individuals with moderate to severe cases of bronchiectasis. With the availability of CT scanning, the sensitivity for detecting bronchiectasis has improved. Bronchoscopy may be useful in identifying the source of secretions or sites of hemoptysis in the individual with a chronic productive cough.

Collecting sputum to evaluate its quantity, characteristics, and microbial content may provide additional information regarding the severity of impairment and the presence of active infection. Pulmonary function studies may be abnormal in advanced bronchiectasis, showing a decrease in vital capacity, expiratory flow, and maximum voluntary ventilation and an increase in ventilation-perfusion mismatching with resultant hypoxemia. A complete blood count may be normal or show evidence of leukocytosis or anemia from chronic infection within the thorax.

Collaborative Care

Bronchiectasis is difficult to treat. Antibiotics are the major form of treatment and should be given on the basis of sputum culture results. Other forms of drug therapy may include bronchodilators, mucolytic agents, and expectorants. Maintaining good hydration is important to liquefy secretions. Chest physical therapy and other airway clearance techniques are important to facilitate expectoration of sputum. (These techniques are discussed in Chapter 27.) The individual should reduce exposure to excessive air pollutants and irritants, avoid cigarette smoking, and obtain pneumococcal and influenza vaccinations.

Surgical resection of parts of the lungs, although not used as often as previously, may be done if more conservative treatment is not effective. Surgical resection of an affected lobe or segment may be indicated for the patient with repeated bouts of pneumonia, hemoptysis, and disabling complications. Surgery is not advisable when there is diffuse or widespread involvement. For selected patients who are disabled in spite of maximal therapy, lung transplantation is an option. (Lung transplantation is discussed later in this chapter.)

NURSING MANAGEMENT: BRONCHIECTASIS

The incidence of bronchiectasis has shown a decline in recent years. This is partially because of the administration of measles and pertussis vaccines, which decreases the incidence of bronchiectasis caused by these diseases. Early detection and treatment of lower respiratory tract infections prevent them from developing into complications such as bronchiectasis. Any obstructing lesion or foreign body should be removed promptly. Other measures to decrease the occurrence or progression of bronchiectasis include avoiding cigarette smoking and decreasing exposure to pollution. Children with persistent coughs should receive evaluations to determine the source of the problem.

An important nursing goal is to promote drainage and removal of bronchial mucus. Various airway clearance techniques can be effectively used to facilitate secretion removal. The patient should be taught effective deep-breathing exercises and effective ways to cough (see Table 27-20). Chest physical therapy with postural drainage should be done on affected parts of the lung (see Fig. 27-15). Some individuals require elevation of the foot of the bed by 4 to 6 inches to facilitate drainage. Pillows may be used in the hospital and at home to help the patient assume postural drainage positions. A Flutter mucus clearance device is a handheld device that provides airway vibration during the expiratory phase of breathing. Two to four 15-minute sessions daily by a patient who has been properly trained can provide satisfactory mucus clearance. Positive expiratory pressure (PEP) therapy is a breathing maneuver against an expiratory resistance often used in conjunction with nebulized medications. (Respiratory therapy procedures are explained in Chapter 27.)

Administration of the prescribed antibiotics, bronchodilators, or expectorants is important. The patient needs to understand the importance of taking the prescribed regimen of drugs to obtain maximum effectiveness. The patient should be aware of possible side effects or adverse effects that must be reported to the physician.

Rest is important to prevent overexertion. Bed rest may be indicated during the acute phase of the illness. Chilling and excess fatigue should be avoided.

Good nutrition is important and may be difficult to maintain because the patient is often anorexic. Oral hygiene to cleanse the mouth and remove dried sputum crusts may improve the patient's appetite. Offering foods that are appealing may also increase the desire to eat. Adequate hydration to help liquefy secretions and thus make it easier to remove them is extremely important. Unless there are contraindications such as concomitant congestive heart failure or renal disease, the patient should be instructed to drink at least 3 L of fluid daily. To accomplish this, the patient should be advised to increase fluid consumption from the baseline by increasing intake by one glass per day until the goal is reached. Generally the patient should be counseled to use low-sodium fluids to avoid systemic fluid retention.

Direct hydration of the respiratory system may also prove beneficial in the expectoration of secretions. Usually a bland aerosol with normal saline solution delivered by a jet-type nebulizer is used. The patient with bronchiectasis should avoid ultrasonic nebulizers because they often induce bronchospasm. At home a steamy shower can prove effective; expensive equipment that requires frequent cleaning is usually unnecessary. It is important that the patient medicate with an inhaled bronchodilator 10 to 15 minutes before using a bland aerosol to prevent bronchoconstriction.

The patient and family should be taught to recognize significant clinical manifestations to be reported to the health care provider. These manifestations include increased sputum production, grossly bloody sputum, increasing dyspnea, fever, chills, and chest pain.

LUNG ABSCESS

Etiology and Pathophysiology

Lung abscess is a pus-containing lesion of the lung parenchyma that gives rise to a cavity. The cavity is formed by necrosis of the lung tissue. In many cases the causes and pathogenesis of lung abscess are similar to those of pneumonia. The most common contributing factor to a lung abscess is aspiration of material into the lungs.[14] Risk factors for aspiration include alcoholism, seizure disorders, drug overdose, general anesthesia, and cerebrovascular accidents. Most lung abscesses are caused by infectious agents. In addition to producing infection, the organisms involved cause necrosis of the lung tissue. Examples include enteric gram-negative organisms (e.g., *Klebsiella*), *S. aureus,* and anaerobic bacilli (e.g., *Bacteroides, Actinomyces*). Lung abscess can also result from hematogenously spread lung infarct secondary to pulmonary embolus, malignant growth, TB, and various parasitic and fungal diseases of the lung.

The areas of the lung most commonly affected are the apical segments of the lower lobes and the posterior segments of the upper lobes. Fibrous tissue usually forms around the abscess in an attempt to wall it off. The abscess may erode into the bronchial system, causing the production of foul-smelling sputum. It may grow toward the pleura and cause pleuritic pain. Multiple small abscesses can occur within the lung.

Clinical Manifestations and Complications

The onset of a lung abscess is usually insidious, especially if anaerobic organisms are the primary cause. A more acute onset occurs with aerobic organisms. The most common manifestation is cough-producing purulent sputum (often dark brown) that is foul smelling and foul tasting. Hemoptysis is common, especially at the time that an abscess ruptures into a bronchus. Other common manifestations are fever, chills, prostration, pleuritic pain, dyspnea, cough, and weight loss. The history may reveal a predisposing condition such as alcoholism, pneumonia, or oral infection.

Physical examination of the lungs indicates dullness to percussion and decreased breath sounds on auscultation over the segment of lung involved. There may be transmission of bronchial breath sounds to the periphery if the communicating bronchus becomes patent and drainage of the segment begins. Crackles may also be present in the later stages as the abscess drains. Oral examination often reveals dental caries, gingivitis, and periodontal infection.

Complications that can occur include chronic pulmonary abscess, hemorrhage from abscess erosion into blood vessels, brain abscess as a result of the hematogenous spread of infection, bronchopleural fistula, and empyema from abscess perforation into the pleural cavity.

Diagnostic Studies

A chest x-ray taken before drainage of the abscess will reveal a solitary cavitary lesion with an air fluid level.[14] After the abscess is drained, a chest x-ray will show an area of consolidation with a wall around a lucent zone. Sputum culture and Gram's stain are necessary to identify the infecting organism. Sputum specimens may be obtained by transtracheal or transthoracic methods to avoid oral contamination. Bronchoscopy may be used in cases of abscess in which drainage is delayed or in which there are factors that suggest an underlying malignancy. Leukocytosis is usually present.

NURSING AND COLLABORATIVE MANAGEMENT: LUNG ABSCESS

Antibiotics given for a prolonged period (up to 6 to 8 weeks) are usually the primary method of treatment. Penicillin has historically been the drug of choice because of the frequent presence of anaerobic organisms. However, recent studies suggesting the presence of β-lactamase production by the anaerobic bacteria involved in abscesses of the lung indicate that drugs such as clindamycin (Cleocin) or metronidazole (Flagyl) in combination with penicillin should be used as primary therapy. Clindamycin is definitely the drug of choice for infections involving foul-smelling abscesses with large cavities or for the patient who has severe systemic toxicity.

Because of the need for prolonged antibiotic therapy, the patient must be aware of the importance of continuing the medication for the prescribed period. The patient needs to know about untoward side effects to be reported to the health care provider. Sometimes the patient is asked to return periodically during the course of antibiotic therapy for repeat cultures and sensitivity tests to ensure that the infecting organism is not becoming resistant to the antibiotic. When antibiotic therapy is completed, the patient is reevaluated.

The patient should be taught how to cough effectively (see Table 27-20). Chest physiotherapy and postural drainage are sometimes used to drain abscesses located in the lower or posterior portions of the lung. Postural drainage according to the lung area involved will aid the removal of secretions (see Fig. 27-15).

Frequent (every 2 to 3 hours) mouth care is needed to relieve the foul-smelling odor and taste from the sputum. Diluted hydrogen peroxide and mouthwash are often effective.

Rest, good nutrition, and adequate fluid intake are all supportive measures to facilitate recovery. If dentition is poor and dental hygiene is not adequate, the patient should be encouraged to obtain dental care (see Chapter 39).

Surgery is rarely indicated but occasionally may be necessary when reinfection of a large cavitary lesion occurs or to establish a diagnosis when there is evidence of an underlying neoplasm or chronic associated disease. The use of bronchoscopy for drainage of an abscess is controversial. Some clinicians believe that this procedure may spread the infection to other parts of the lung. If used, bronchoscopy should not be performed until after 24 to 48 hours of antimicrobial therapy.

ENVIRONMENTAL LUNG DISEASES

Environmental or occupational lung diseases result from inhaled dust or chemicals. The duration of exposure and the amount of inhalant have a major influence on whether the exposed individual will have lung damage. Another factor is the susceptibility of the host.

Pneumoconiosis is a general term for lung diseases caused by inhalation and retention of dust particles. The literal meaning of pneumoconiosis is "dust in the lungs." Examples of this condition are silicosis, asbestosis, and berylliosis. The classic response to the inhaled substance is diffuse parenchymal infiltration with phagocytic cells. This eventually results in *diffuse pulmonary fibrosis* (excess connective tissue). Fibrosis is the result of tissue repair after inflammation. Pneumoconiosis and other environmental lung diseases are presented in Table 26-13.

Chemical pneumonitis results from exposures to toxic chemical fumes. Acutely there is diffuse parenchymal injury characterized as pulmonary edema. Chronically the clinical picture is that of bronchiolitis obliterans, which is usually associated with a normal chest radiograph or shows hyperinflation. An example is silo filler's disease.

Hypersensitivity pneumonitis or extrinsic allergic alveolitis is the response seen when antigens are inhaled to which an individual is allergic. Examples include bird fancier's lung and farmer's lung.

Lung cancer, either squamous cell carcinoma or adenocarcinoma, is the most frequent cancer associated with asbestos exposure. People with more exposure are at a greater risk of disease. There is a minimum lapse of 15 to 19 years between first exposure and development of lung cancer. Mesotheliomas, both pleural and peritoneal, are also associated with asbestos exposure.

Clinical Manifestations

Acute symptoms of pulmonary edema may be seen following early exposures to chemical fumes. However, symptoms of many environmental lung diseases may not occur until at least 10 to 15 years after the initial exposure to the inhaled irritant. Dyspnea and cough are often the earliest manifestations. Chest pain and cough with sputum production usually occur later. Complications that often result are pneumonia, chronic bronchitis, emphysema, and lung cancer. Cor pulmonale is a late complication, especially in conditions characterized by diffuse pulmonary fibrosis. Manifestations of these complications can be the reason the patient seeks health care.

Pulmonary function studies often show reduced vital capacity. A chest x-ray will often reveal lung involvement specific to the primary problem. CT scans have been shown to be useful in detecting early lung involvement.

Occupational asthma refers to the development of symptoms of shortness of breath, wheezing, cough, and chest tightness as a result of exposure to fumes or dust that trigger an allergic response. The obstruction may initially be reversible or intermittent, but continued exposure results in permanent obstructive changes. The best-known causative agent in occupational asthma is toluene diisocyanate (TDI), which is used in the production of rigid polyurethane foam.

Collaborative Care

The best approach to management is to try to prevent or decrease environmental and occupational risks. Well-designed, effective ventilation systems can reduce exposure to irritants. Wearing masks is appropriate in some occupations. Periodic inspections and monitoring of workplaces by agencies such as the Occupational Safety and Health Agency (OSHA) and the National Institute for Occupational Safety and Health (NIOSH) reinforce the obligations of employers to provide a safe work environment.

Cigarette smoking adds increased insult to the lungs, and the person at risk for occupational lung disease should not smoke. Additionally, secondhand smoke is an important source of occupational exposure with increased risk for development of lung cancer. This has led to regulations requiring a smoke-free workspace for all employees.

Early diagnosis is essential if the disease process is to be halted. The best treatment is to decrease or stop exposure to the harmful agent. Some places of employment at which there is a known risk of lung disease may require periodic chest x-rays and pulmonary function studies for exposed employees. These measures can detect pulmonary changes before symptoms develop.

There is no specific treatment for most environmental lung diseases. Treatment is directed toward providing symptomatic relief. If there are coexisting problems, such as pneumonia, chronic bronchitis, emphysema, or asthma, they are treated.

LUNG CANCER

Lung cancer is the leading cause of death in men and women who have malignant disease in the United States. In 1998 an estimated 160,100 deaths occurred, accounting for 28% of all cancer deaths.[15] Until recently, many more cases of lung cancer were found in men than in women. That situation is changing, probably because cigarette smoking has become socially acceptable for women since the 1930s and 1940s. Beginning in 1987, deaths from lung cancer in women exceeded deaths from all other cancers. An estimated 171,500 new cases of lung cancer were diagnosed in 1998. The overall 5-year survival rate is only 14%, which is the poorest prognosis for any cancer other than cancers of the pancreas, liver, and esophagus.[15]

Lung cancer most commonly occurs in individuals more than 50 years of age who have a long history of cigarette smoking. The disease is found most frequently in persons 40 to 75 years of age, with peak incidence between 55 and 65 years of age.

Etiology and Risk Factors

Cigarette smoking as a chronic respiratory irritant is by far the major risk factor in the development of lung cancer. Smoking is

Table **26-13** Environmental Lung Diseases

Disease	Agents/Industries	Description	Complications
▪ Asbestosis	Asbestos fibers present in insulation, construction material (roof tiling, cement products), shipyards, textiles (for fireproofing), automobile clutch and brake linings	Disease appears 15-35 yr after first exposure. Interstitial fibrosis develops. Pleural plaques, which are calcified lesions, develop on pleura. Dyspnea, basal crackles, and decreased vital capacity are early manifestations.	Diffuse interstitial pulmonary fibrosis. Lung cancer, especially in cigarette smokers; mesothelioma (rare type of cancer affecting pleura and peritoneal membrane)
▪ Berylliosis	Beryllium dust present in aircraft manufacturing, metallurgy, rocket fuels	Noncaseating granulomas form. Acute pneumonitis occurs after heavy exposure. Interstitial fibrosis can also occur.	Progress of disease possible after removal of stimulating inhalant
▪ Bird fancier's, breeder's, or handler's lung	Bird droppings or feathers	Hypersensitivity pneumonitis is present.	Progressive fibrosis of lung
▪ Byssinosis	Cotton, flax, and hemp dust (textile industry)	Airway obstruction is caused by contraction of smooth muscles. Chronic disease results from severe airway obstruction and decreased elastic recoil.	Progression of chronic disease after cessation of dust exposure
▪ Coal worker's pneumoconiosis (black lung)	Coal dust	Incidence is high (20-30%) in coal workers. Deposits of carbon dust cause lesions to develop along respiratory bronchioles. Bronchioles dilate because of loss of wall structure. Chronic airway obstruction and bronchitis develop. Dyspnea and cough are common early symptoms.	Progressive, massive lung fibrosis; increased risk of chronic bronchitis and emphysema with smoking
▪ Farmer's lung	Inhalation of airborne material from moldy hay or similar matter	Hypersensitivity pneumonitis occurs. *Acute* form is similar to pneumonia, with manifestations of chills, fever, and malaise. *Chronic,* insidious form is type of pulmonary fibrosis.	Progressive fibrosis of lung
▪ Siderosis	Iron oxide present in welding materials, foundries, iron ore mining	Dust deposits are found in lung.	
▪ Silicosis	Silica dust present in quartz rock in mining of gold, copper, tin, coal, lead; also present in sandblasting, foundries, quarries, pottery making, masonry	In *chronic* disease, dust is engulfed by macrophages and may be destroyed, resulting in fibrotic nodules. *Acute* disease results from intense exposure in short time period. Within 5 yr, it progresses to severe disability from lung fibrosis.	Increased susceptibility to tuberculosis; progressive, massive fibrosis; high incidence of chronic bronchitis
▪ Silo filler's disease	Nitrogen oxides from fermentation of vegetation in freshly filled silo	Chemical pneumonitis occurs.	Progressive bronchiolitis obliterans

responsible for approximately 80% to 90% of all lung cancers. About 1 of every 10 heavy smokers eventually develops lung cancer.[15] Cigarette smoking causes a change in the bronchial epithelium, which usually returns to normal when smoking is discontinued. The risk of lung cancer is gradually lowered when smoking ceases and continues to decline with time. It is estimated that it takes approximately 15 years for the risk for lung cancer of a former smoker to equal that of a nonsmoker.

The risk of developing lung cancer is directly related to total exposure to cigarette smoke measured by total number of cigarettes smoked in a lifetime, depth of inhalation, and tar and nicotine content of the cigarettes smoked. The *Report of the*

CULTURAL & ETHNIC CONSIDERATIONS

Lung Cancer

- Lung cancer occurs more frequently and has a higher mortality rate among non-Caucasians.
- Lung cancer is the most commonly newly diagnosed cancer among African-Americans.
- Prevalence of cigarette smoking is higher among African-Americans and Hispanics than Caucasians.

Surgeon General presented data that showed that sidestream smoke is qualitatively similar to mainstream smoke and concluded that involuntary (secondhand) smoking poses a risk for the development of lung cancer in nonsmokers.[16]

Heredity may play a role in both the tendency to smoke and the predisposition to develop lung cancer. Because only a few persons (1 of 10) at risk actually develop lung cancer, there is probably a difference in the host's ability to deal with the repeated insult of smoking. Individuals with an early onset of lung cancer are most likely to have genetic susceptibility. A number of genes potentially determine susceptibility to lung cancer, including (1) protooncogenes and tumor suppressor genes, (2) genes encoding enzymes that metabolize procarcinogens to active carcinogens, and (3) enzymes that detoxify carcinogens.[17]

Those who smoke pipes and cigars have also been shown to have an increased risk of developing lung cancer, which is slightly higher than that of nonsmokers. Cigar smokers are at higher rate for lung cancer than are pipe smokers. However, heavy smoking of cigars and inhalation of smoke from small cigars have been shown to correlate with the rates of lung cancer observed in cigarette smokers.

Another major risk factor for lung cancer is inhaled carcinogens. These include asbestos, radon, nickel, iron and iron oxides, uranium, polycyclic aromatic hydrocarbons, chromates, arsenic, and air pollution. Exposure to these substances is common for employees of industries involved in mining, smelting, or chemical or petroleum manufacturing. The cigarette smoker who is also exposed to one or more of these chemicals or to high amounts of air pollution is at significantly higher risk for lung cancer.

Lung cancer does occur in individuals who have never smoked or worked with carcinogens. The reasons for this are not known, but heredity may play a part. The host's response to environmental insults is important in determining who develops lung cancer.

Another possible risk factor is preexisting pulmonary diseases such as TB, pulmonary fibrosis, bronchiectasis, and COPD. Chronic inflammatory conditions often precede cancer. The incidence of lung cancer correlates with the degree of urbanization and population density. One reason for this may be increased exposure to irritants and pollutants.

Pathophysiology

The pathogenesis of primary lung cancer is not well understood. More than 90% of cancers originate from the epithelium of the bronchus (bronchogenic). They grow slowly, and it takes 8 to 10 years for a tumor to reach 1 cm in size, which is the smallest detectable lesion on an x-ray. Lung cancers occur primarily in the segmental bronchi or beyond and have a preference for the upper lobes of the lungs (Fig. 26-3). Pathologic changes in the bronchial system show nonspecific inflammatory changes with hypersecretion of mucus, desquamation of cells, reactive hyperplasia of the basal cells, and metaplasia of normal respiratory epithelium to stratified squamous cells. (Pathologic types of lung cancer are presented in Fig. 26-4.)

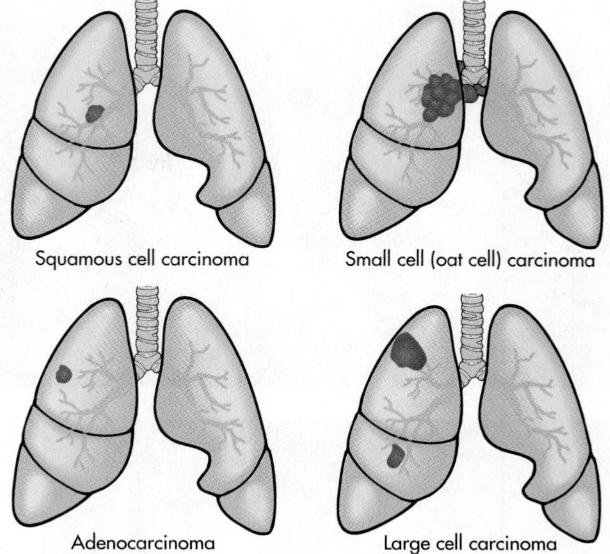

Fig. 26-3 Predominant sites of types of lung cancer.

Primary lung cancers are often categorized into two broad subtypes (Table 26-14), including non–small cell lung cancer and small cell lung cancer. Lung cancers metastasize primarily by direct extension and via the blood circulation and the lymph system. The common sites for metastatic growth are the liver, brain, bones, scalene lymph nodes, and adrenal glands.

Paraneoplastic syndrome. Certain lung cancers cause the *paraneoplastic syndrome,* which is characterized by various manifestations caused by certain substances (e.g., hormones, enzymes, antigens) produced by the tumor cells. Small cell lung cancers are most commonly associated with the paraneoplastic syndrome. The systemic manifestations are as follows:

1. *Hormonal* (Table 26-15)
2. *Dermatologic,* including dermatomyositis and acanthosis nigricans
3. *Neuromuscular,* including peripheral neuropathy, cortical cerebellar degeneration, and a syndrome similar to myasthenia gravis
4. *Vascular* and *hematologic,* including thrombocytopenic purpura, anemia, leukemia-like reaction, thrombophlebitis, and nonbacterial endocarditis
5. *Connective tissue,* including nonspecific arthralgias, hypertrophic pulmonary osteoarthropathy, and digital clubbing.

Clinical Manifestations

Lung cancer is clinically silent for most individuals for the majority of its course. The clinical manifestations of lung cancer are usually nonspecific and appear late in the disease process.

A

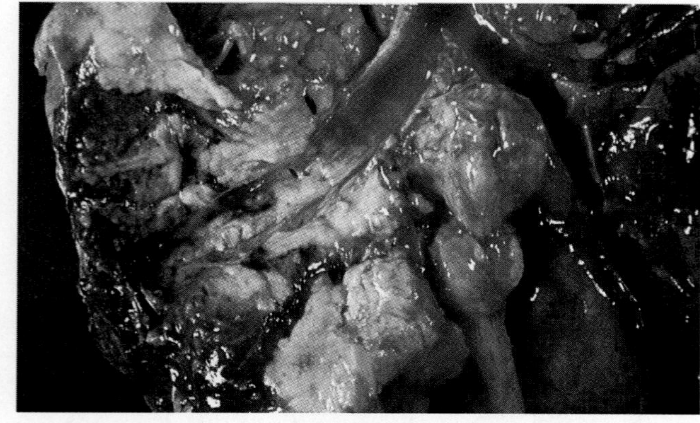

B

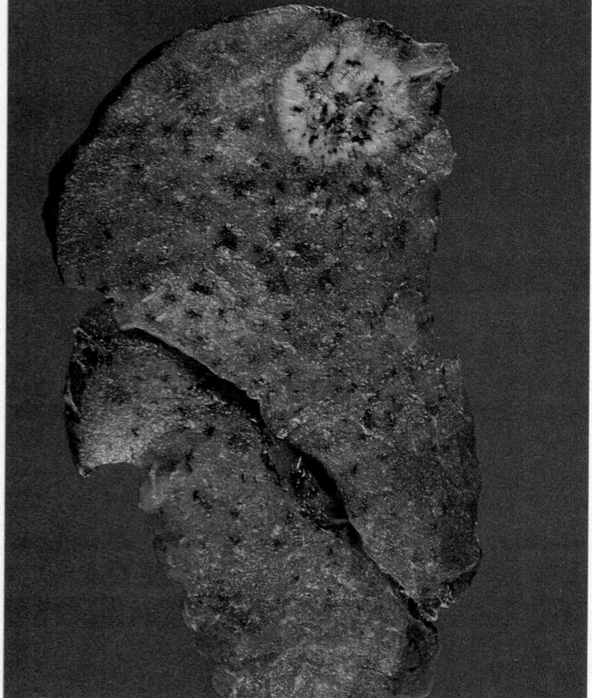

C

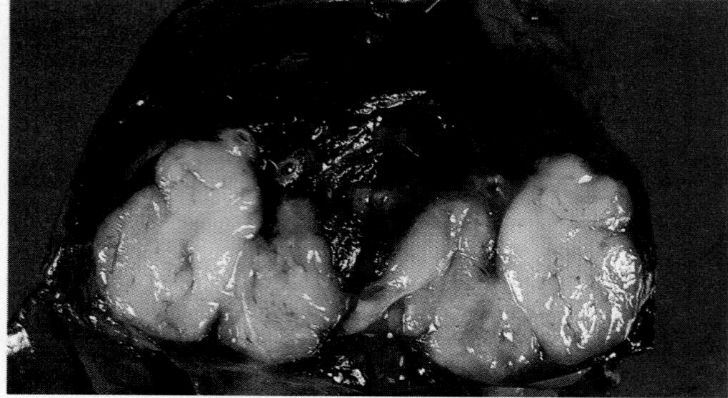

Fig. 26-4 Lung cancer. **A,** Squamous cell carcinoma. This hilar tumor originates from the main bronchus. **B,** Peripheral adenocarcinoma. The tumor shows prominent black pigmentation, suggestive of having evolved in an anthracotic scar. **C,** Small cell carcinoma. The tumor forms confluent nodules. On cross sectioning, the nodules have an encephalid appearance.

Manifestations depend on the type of primary lung cancer. Often there is extensive metastasis before symptoms become apparent. Persistent pneumonitis that is a result of obstructed bronchi may be one of the earliest manifestations, causing fever, chills, and cough.

One of the most significant symptoms, and often the one reported first, is a persistent cough that may be productive of sputum. Blood-tinged sputum may be produced because of bleeding caused by malignancy, but hemoptysis is not a common early presenting symptom. Chest pain may be present and localized or unilateral, ranging from mild to severe. Dyspnea and an auscultatory wheeze may be present if there is bronchial obstruction.

Later manifestations may include nonspecific systemic symptoms such as anorexia, fatigue, weight loss, and nausea and vomiting. Hoarseness may be present as a result of involvement of the recurrent laryngeal nerve. Unilateral paralysis of the diaphragm, dysphagia, and superior vena cava obstruction may occur because of intrathoracic spread of the malignancy. There may be palpable lymph nodes in the neck or axilla. Mediastinal involvement may lead to pericardial effusion, cardiac tamponade, and arrhythmias.

Diagnostic Studies

Chest x-rays are widely used in the diagnosis of lung cancer. Anyone who has had a cough or a change in a cough for more than 2 to 3 weeks should be evaluated by chest x-ray.[18] The findings may show the presence of the tumor or abnormalities related to the obstructive features of the tumor such as atelectasis and pneumonitis. The x-ray can also show evidence of metastasis to the ribs or vertebrae and the presence of pleural effusion.

CT scans are also used in the diagnosis of lung cancer. With CT scans, the location and extent of masses in the chest can be identified, as well as any mediastinal involvement or lymph node enlargement. Magnetic resonance imaging (MRI) may be used in combination with or instead of CT scans. Positron emission tomography (PET) promises to be a useful diagnostic tool in early detection of cancers and in staging and monitoring the effects of treatment. PET allows measurement of differential metabolic activity in normal and diseased tissues.

A definitive diagnosis of lung cancer is made by identifying malignant cells. Sputum specimens are usually obtained for cytologic studies and may identify tumors that involve the bronchial wall. An early-morning specimen that has been obtained by having the patient cough deeply provides the most accurate results. However, malignant cells may not be obtained even in the presence of a lung cancer.

The use of the fiberoptic bronchoscope is important in the diagnosis of lung cancer, particularly when the lesions are endobronchial or are in close proximity to an airway. It provides direct visualization and allows biopsy specimens to be obtained. A biopsy is usually the best method for establishing the presence of a malignant tumor.

Mediastinoscopy involves the insertion of a scope via a small anterior chest incision into the mediastinum. This is done to examine for metastasis in the anterior mediastinum or hilum or in the chest extrapleurally. It is also used to determine the stage of the lung cancer, which is important in determining the treatment plan.

Table 26-14 Comparison of the Types of Primary Lung Cancer

Cell Type	Risk Factors	Characteristics	Response to Therapy
Non–Small Cell Lung Cancer			
▪ Squamous cell (epidermoid) carcinoma	Almost always associated with cigarette smoking; is associated with exposure to environmental carcinogens (e.g., uranium, asbestos)	Accounts for 30-35% of lung cancers; is more common in men; arises from the bronchial epithelium, produces earlier symptoms because of bronchial obstructive characteristics; does not have a strong tendency to metastasize, metastasizes locally by direct extension, causes cavitating pulmonary lesions	Surgical resection is often attempted; life expectancy is better than for small cell lung cancer
▪ Adenocarcinoma	Has been associated with lung scarring and chronic interstitial fibrosis; is not related to cigarette smoking	Accounts for approximately 35-45% of lung cancers; is more common in women; often has no clinical manifestations until widespread metastasis is present; metastasizes via bloodstream; is most commonly located in peripheral portions of lungs*	Surgical resection is often attempted; cancer does not respond well to chemotherapy
▪ Large cell undifferentiated carcinoma	High correlation with cigarette smoking and exposure to environmental carcinogens	Accounts for 5-10% of lung cancers; commonly causes cavitation; is highly metastatic via lymphatics and blood; commonly peripheral rather than central	Surgery is not usually attempted because of high rate of metastases; tumor may be radiosensitive but often recurs
Small Cell Lung Cancer			
▪ Small cell anaplastic undifferentiated (includes oat cell)	Associated with cigarette smoking, exposure to environmental carcinogens	Accounts for 15-25% of lung cancers; is most malignant form; tends to spread early via lymphatics and bloodstream; is frequently associated with endocrine disturbances; predominantly central and can cause bronchial obstruction and pneumonia	Cancer has poorest prognosis; however, recent chemotherapy gains have been substantial; radiation is used as adjuvant therapy, as well as palliative measure; average median survival is 12-18 mo

*See Fig. 26-3.

Table 26-15 Ectopic Hormone Syndromes of Lung Cancer

Syndrome	Ectopic Hormone	Most Common Cell Type
Cushing's syndrome	Adrenocorticotropic hormone	Small cell
Syndrome of inappropriate antidiuretic hormone	Antidiuretic hormone	Small cell
Hypercalcemia	Parathyroid hormone	Squamous cell
Gynecomastia	Follicle-stimulating hormone	Large cell
Carcinoid syndrome	5-hydroxyindoleacetic acid (5-HIAA) from serotonin breakdown	Small cell

Pulmonary angiography and lung scans may be performed to assess overall pulmonary status. Fine-needle aspiration (FNA) may be used to obtain a tissue sample to determine tumor histology. FNA is most useful in cases involving a peripheral lesion near the chest wall, and it is usually attempted in an effort to avoid a thoracotomy. If a thoracentesis is performed to relieve a pleural effusion, the fluid should be analyzed for malignant cells. (Table 26-16 summarizes the diagnostic management of lung cancer.)

Staging

Staging of non–small cell lung cancer (NSCLC) is performed according to the TNM staging system in a manner similar to that for other tumors (Table 26-17). Assessment criteria are *T,*

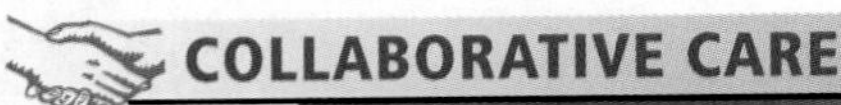

Table 26-16 Lung Cancer

Diagnostic
Health history and physical examination
Chest x-ray
Sputum for cytologic study
Bronchoscopy
CT scan
MRI
Spirometry (preoperative)
Mediastinoscopy
Pulmonary angiography
Lung scan
Fine-needle aspiration
Collaborative Therapy
Surgery
Radiation therapy
Chemotherapy
Phototherapy (Nd:YAG laser)
Biologic therapies

CT, computed tomography; *MRI*, magnetic resonance imaging; *Nd:YAG*, neodymium: yttrium-aluminum-garnet.

which denotes tumor size, location, and degree of invasion; *N*, which indicates regional lymph node involvement; and *M*, which represents the presence or absence of distant metastases. Depending on the TNM designation, the tumor is then staged, which assists in estimating prognosis and appropriate therapy.

Staging of small cell lung cancer (SCLC) has not been useful because the cancer has usually metastasized by the time a diagnosis is made. Instead, SCLC is determined to be *limited* (confined to one hemothorax and to regional lymph nodes) or *extensive* (any disease exceeding those boundaries).

Collaborative Care

Surgical Therapy. Surgical resection is usually the only hope for cure in lung cancer. Unfortunately, detection is often so late that the tumor is no longer localized and is not amenable to resection. Resectability of the tumor is a major consideration in planning the surgical intervention. Small cell carcinomas usually have widespread metastasis at the time of diagnosis. Therefore surgery is usually contraindicated. In contrast, squamous cell carcinomas are more likely to be treated with surgery because they remain localized, or if they metastasize they primarily do so by local spread.

Table 26-17 Lung Cancer TNM Classifications

Tumor Definitions

- T_x Tumor proved by cytologic studies but not visualized by radiograph or bronchoscope
- T_0 No evidence of tumor
- T_{is} Carcinoma in situ
- T_1 Tumor 3 cm or less in greatest dimension
- T_2 Tumor greater than 3 cm in diameter or invading visceral pleura or with atelectasis or obstructive pneumonitis extending to the hilum
- T_3 Tumor with direct extension into chest wall, diaphragm, mediastinal pleura, or pericardium without involvement of mediastinal viscera; tumor within 2 cm of carina but not involving carina
- T_4 Tumor invading mediastinum or carina or with malignant pleural effusion

Nodal Involvement

- N_0 No nodal metastasis
- N_1 Metastasis to peribronchial or ipsilateral hilar lymph nodes
- N_2 Metastasis to ipsilateral mediastinal or subcarinal lymph nodes
- N_3 Metastasis to contralateral mediastinal or hilar lymph nodes or any scalene or supraclavicular node

Distant Metastases

- M_0 No known metastasis
- M_1 Presence of distant metastasis

Stage Grouping

Occult Carcinoma	T_x	N_0	M_0
Stage 0	T_{is}	Carcinoma in situ	M_0
Stage I	T_1	N_0	M_0
	T_2	N_0	M_0
Stage II	T_1	N_1	M_0
	T_2	N_1	M_0
Stage IIIA	T_3	N_0	M_0
	T_3	N_1	M_0
	T_{1-3}	N_2	M_0
Stage IIIB	Any T	N_3	M_0
	T_4	Any N	M_0
Stage IV	Any T	Any N	M_1

TNM, tumor, node, metastases.

When the tumor is considered operable with a potential for cure, the patient's cardiopulmonary status must be evaluated to determine the ability to withstand surgery. This is done by clinical studies of pulmonary function, ABGs, and others, as indicated by the individual's status. Contraindications for thoracotomy include hypercapnia, pulmonary hypertension, cor pulmonale, and markedly reduced lung function. Coexisting conditions such as cardiac, renal, and liver disease are also contraindications for surgery.

A tumor may be potentially resectable, but if it is located in a critical area, such as the trachea or too close to the heart, it may be considered inoperable. The type of surgery performed is usually a *lobectomy* (removal of one or more lobes of the lung) and less often a *pneumonectomy* (removal of one entire lung).

Radiation Therapy. Radiation therapy is used as a curative approach in the individual who has a resectable tumor but who is considered a poor surgical risk. Adenocarcinomas are the most radioresistant type of cancer cell. Although small cell carcinomas are radiosensitive, radiation (even when used in combination with chemotherapy) does not significantly improve the mortality rate because of the early metastases of this type of cancer.

Radiation therapy is also done as a palliative procedure to reduce distressing symptoms such as cough, hemoptysis, bronchial obstruction, and superior vena cava syndrome. It can be used to treat pain that is caused by metastatic bone lesions or cerebral metastasis. Radiation used as a preoperative or postoperative adjuvant measure has not been found to significantly increase survival in the patient with lung cancer.

Chemotherapy. Chemotherapy may be used in the treatment of nonresectable tumors or as adjuvant therapy to surgery in non–small cell lung cancer with distant metastases. A variety of chemotherapy drugs and multidrug regimens (i.e., protocols) including combination chemotherapy have been used.[19,20] These drugs include etoposide (VePesid), carboplatin (Paraplatin), cisplatin (Platinol), paclitaxel (Taxol), vinorelbine (Navelbine), vindesine (Eldisine), cyclophosphamide (Cytoxan), ifosfamide (Ifex), docetaxel (Taxotere), gemcitabine (Gemzar), topotecan (Hycamtin), and irinotecan (Camptosar).

Chemotherapy has produced only modest survival benefits in patients with advanced non–small cell lung cancer. Chemotherapy has made a stronger impact in small cell lung cancer, but the majority of patients still die from the disease.[21]

Biologic Therapies. Biologic therapy as adjuvant therapy has been used in individuals with cancer, including malignant lung tumors. (Biologic therapy is discussed in Chapter 14.)

Phototherapy. Laser surgery, with the use of the neodymium: yttrium-aluminum-garnet (Nd:YAG) laser via a fiberoptic bronchoscope, makes it possible to remove obstructing bronchial lesions as large as 2 cm in depth. It is a complicated procedure that often requires general anesthesia to control the patient's cough reflex. Relief of the symptoms from airway obstruction as a result of thermal necrosis and shrinkage of the tumor can be dramatic. However, it is not a curative therapy for cancer.

Porfimer (Photofrin) has recently been approved for treatment of late-stage lung cancer. It is injected IV, selectively concentrates in tumor cells, and can be activated by laser light, producing a toxic form of oxygen that destroys tumor cells. Necrotic tissue is removed through a bronchoscope.

NURSING MANAGEMENT: LUNG CANCER

■ Nursing Assessment

It is important to determine the understanding of the patient and the family concerning the diagnostic tests (those completed as well as those planned), the diagnosis or potential diagnosis, the treatment options, and the prognosis. At the same time the nurse can assess the level of anxiety experienced by the patient and the support provided and needed by the patient's significant others. Subjective and objective data that should be obtained from a patient with lung cancer are presented in Table 26-18.

■ Nursing Diagnoses

Nursing diagnoses for the patient with lung cancer may include, but are not limited to, the following:

- Ineffective airway clearance *related to* increased tracheobronchial secretions
- Anxiety *related to* lack of knowledge of diagnosis or unknown prognosis and treatments
- Pain *related to* pressure of tumor on surrounding structures and erosion of tissues
- Altered nutrition: less than body requirements *related to* increased metabolic demands, increased secretions, weakness, and anorexia
- Altered health maintenance *related to* lack of knowledge about the disease process and therapeutic regimen
- Ineffective breathing pattern *related to* decreased lung capacity

■ Planning

The overall goals are that the patient with lung cancer will have (1) effective breathing patterns, (2) adequate airway clearance, (3) adequate oxygenation of tissues, (4) minimal to no pain, and (5) a realistic attitude toward treatment and prognosis.

■ Nursing Implementation

Health Promotion. The best way to halt the epidemic of lung cancer is for people to stop smoking. Important nursing activities to assist in the progress toward this goal include promoting smoking cessation programs and actively supporting education and policy changes deterring social, economic, and political patterns that have, in the past, encouraged smoking. Some recent important changes that have occurred as the result of nonsmokers' assertions that sidestream smoke is a health hazard are laws requiring designation of nonsmoking areas in most public places or prohibiting smoking and a ban on smoking on most airline flights. Other actions aimed at controlling tobacco use include restrictions on tobacco advertising on television and warning label requirements for cigarette packaging. These are examples of beginning steps toward the goal of a smokeless society. Other strategies may be to ban cigarettes and other tobacco products or to tax them heavily to prevent many people, such as adolescents, from taking up the habit or continuing it. Despite the small advances being made, tobacco-producing states and tobacco companies still have strong political influences.

For the individual who does have a smoking habit, efforts should be made to assist the smoker to stop smoking (Table 26-19). Nicotine's addictive properties make quitting a difficult task that requires much support. Nicotine replacement

NURSING ASSESSMENT

Table 26-18 Lung Cancer

Subjective Data	Objective Data
Important Health Information *Past health history:* Exposure to secondhand smoke; airborne carcinogens (e.g., asbestos, uranium, chromates, hydrocarbons, arsenic) or other pollutants; urban living environment; chronic lung disease, including TB, COPD, bronchiectasis *Medications:* Use of cough medicines or other respiratory medications **Functional Health Patterns** *Health perception–health management:* Smoking history; family history of lung cancer; frequent respiratory infections *Nutritional-metabolic:* Anorexia, nausea, vomiting, dysphagia (late); weight loss; chills *Activity-exercise:* Fatigue; persistent cough (productive or nonproductive); dyspnea, hemoptysis (late symptom) *Cognitive-perceptual:* Chest pain or tightness, shoulder and arm pain, headache, bone pain (late symptom)	**General** Fever, neck and axillary lymphadenopathy, paraneoplastic syndromes (syndrome of inappropriate ADH; ACTH secretion; hypercalcemia; vascular, neuromuscular, dermatologic, and connective tissue disorders) **Integumentary** Jaundice (liver metastasis); edema of neck and face (superior vena cava syndrome), digital clubbing **Respiratory** Wheezing, hoarseness, stridor, unilateral diaphragm paralysis, pleural effusions (late signs) **Cardiovascular** Pericardial effusion, cardiac tamponade, arrhythmias (late signs) **Neurologic** Unsteady gait (brain metastasis) **Musculoskeletal** Pathologic fractures, muscle wasting (late) **Possible Findings** Low serum sodium and hypercalcemia (paraneoplastic syndrome); observance of lesion on chest x-ray, CT scan, or lung scan; positive sputum or bronchial washings for cytologic studies; positive fiberoptic bronchoscopy and biopsy findings

ACTH, adrenocorticotropic hormone; *ADH,* antidiuretic hormone.

significantly lessens the urge to smoke and increases the percentage of smokers who successfully quit smoking. Nicotine patches are available in different strengths. A gradual taper in patch strength is used to wean the patient off of nicotine. Stop-smoking aids are listed in Table 26-19.

Research into smoking behaviors and successful strategies to promote smoking cessation is ongoing. However, many factors are recognized as being important in the initiation and continuation of smoking, such as peer pressure, rebelliousness, curiosity, self-image, environmental cues, and psychologic needs. Programs designed to assist the individual to stop smoking use strategies such as education, environmental control, social support, and slow nicotine withdrawal with varying degrees of success. Other methods offered in smoking cessation programs may involve hypnosis, acupuncture, behavioral interventions, and aversion therapy. The most successful programs combine a behavior modification approach with pharmacologic intervention to decrease nicotine dependence. Group support programs, individual therapy, and self-help options are also available.

The advice and motivation of health care professionals can be a powerful force in smoking cessation. However, many health care workers become cynical with regard to counseling their patients to abstain from tobacco use. Fewer than 5% of smokers are successful on their first attempt at quitting, and the average smoker requires multiple attempts before being successful. Support for the smoker includes education that smoking a few cigarettes during a cessation attempt (a slip) is much different than resuming the full smoking habit (a relapse). Despite the slip, smokers should be encouraged to continue the attempt at cessation without viewing the effort as a failure. Measures to assist an individual in quitting should be directed toward the meaning that smoking has to that individual. The nurse needs to be aware of resources in the community to assist the individual who is interested in quitting. Local chapters of the American Lung Association and the American Cancer Society have information on available programs.

An important part of concentrated efforts to prevent smoking-related health problems is recognizing what influences people, particularly children and adolescents, to begin smoking. Programs developed to help children explore the external influences (e.g., peer pressure) that may cause one to start smoking and that help them identify alternative behaviors make it less likely for these children to start smoking. An emphasis on the health hazards of smoking, as well as on those of other addictive behaviors, should be part of the total curriculum beginning in elementary schools.

The nurse who smokes is in a difficult position to help the patient change smoking habits. The nurse as a role model can do much to facilitate or harm educational attempts with persons in the community, as well as in the hospital. Therefore if the nurse smokes, the nurse must try to stop before serving as a role model for the patient. A smoker turned nonsmoker may be in a good position to suggest strategies for success.

When a nurse is obtaining a health history from a patient (even a patient with nonrespiratory problems), it is important to get information related to respiratory carcinogens. The

PATIENT TEACHING GUIDE

Table 26-19 Smoking Cessation

The following categories are methods that work for quitting smoking. Patients have the best chance of quitting if they use more than one method.

Stop-Smoking Methods

Nicotine Patch*

- Trade names for the nicotine patch include Nicoderm, Nicotrol, Habitrol, and Prostep. Nicoderm and Nicotrol are available as over-the-counter agents.
- Patches should be replaced every day (preferably in morning) and placed on the body between the neck and waist.
- Most smokers should start using a full-strength patch (15-22 mg of nicotine) daily for 4 wk and then use a weaker patch for another 4 wk (5-14 mg of nicotine).
- Side effects may include minor skin irritation, which is why it is important to apply the patch in a different place every day.

Nicotine Gum

- Nicotine gum (marketed as Nicorette) is sold over the counter in 2 mg and 4 mg strengths.
- One piece of 2 mg gum has the same amount of nicotine as one cigarette.
- Gum should be chewed until a "peppery" taste comes out and then placed between the cheek and gum.
- Each piece of gum should be used for about 30 min.

Nicotine Nasal Spray

- Nicotine in a nasal spray (marketed as Nicotrol NS) is sprayed directly into each nostril.
- Should be used in anticipation of or at the beginning of urge to smoke.
- Side effects include watery eyes and nose, burning sensation in nose, throat irritation, and sneezing or coughing.

Nicotine Inhaler

- Available in cartridge with small amount of nicotine (marketed as Nicotrol inhaler).
- Delivers one third the nicotine of one cigarette.
- Puffing on inhaler releases nicotine vapor into mouth.

Non-Nicotine Therapy

- Bupropion (Zyban), available by prescription, increases dopamine and epinephrine levels in the brain.
- These brain chemicals are also stimulated by nicotine and give a person energy and sense of well-being.
- Side effects include headache, dry mouth, difficulty sleeping, and drowsiness.

Dealing with Urges to Smoke and Stress

- Be aware of things that may cause you to want to smoke. For example, being around other smokers, being under time pressure, getting into an argument, feeling sad or frustrated, and drinking alcohol.
- Avoid difficult situations while you are trying to quit. Try to lower your stress level. Take time to do things you enjoy. Exercise, such as walking, jogging, or bicycling, can also help.
- Distract yourself from thoughts of smoking and the urge to smoke by talking to someone, getting busy with a task, or reading a book.

Support and Encouragement

- Counseling can help you learn how to live life as a nonsmoker. You may want to join a quit-smoking program.
- If you get the urge for a cigarette, call someone to help talk you out of it—preferably an ex-smoker.
- Do not be afraid to talk about how you feel—fears of not being able to quit or problems with family or friends. Your family, friends, or health care provider can offer encouragement and support. Self-help materials and hotlines are also available:
  - American Lung Association: 800-586-4872
  - American Cancer Society: 800-227-2345
  - Cancer Information Service: 800-422-6237
  - Smoking Cessation Consumer Tool Kit: 800-358-9295

Avoiding Relapse

Most relapses occur within the first 3 months after quitting. Do not be discouraged if you start smoking again. Remember, most people try several times before they finally quit. Explore different ways to break habits. You may have to deal with some of the following triggers that may cause relapse.

- *Change your environment.* Get rid of cigarettes and ashtrays in your home, car, and place of work. Get rid of the smell of cigarettes in your car and home. Avoid other tobacco products, such as cigars, pipes, and chewing tobacco.
- *Alcohol.* Consider limiting or stopping alcohol use while you are quitting smoking.
- *Other smokers at home.* Try to get your spouse or housemates to quit with you. Work out a plan to cope with others who smoke, and avoid being around them.
- *Weight gain.* Tackle one problem at a time. Work on quitting smoking first. Consider using nicotine gum to delay weight gain. (You will not necessarily gain weight.)
- *Negative mood or depression.* If these symptoms persist, talk to your health care provider. You may need treatment for depression.
- *Severe withdrawal symptoms.* Your body will go through many changes when you quit smoking. You may have a dry mouth, cough, or scratchy throat, and feel on edge. The patch or gum may help with cravings.
- *Thoughts.* Get your mind off cigarettes. Exercise and do things you enjoy.
- *Keep a list.* Keep a list of "slips" and near-slips, what caused them, and what you can learn from them.

Sources: You Can Quit Smoking. Consumer Version, Clinical Practice Guidelines, No. 18. AHCPR Publication No. 96-0695, Apr 1996. Agency for Health Care Policy and Research, Rockville, Md. http://www.ahcpr.gov/consumer/ch_quits.htm; *Mayo Clinic Health Letter,* Nov 1997.

*Do not use nicotine replacement aids while smoking cigarettes.

RESEARCH

IMPLICATIONS FOR NURSING PRACTICE

Nurse-Managed Smoking Cessation Intervention

Citation Wewers ME, Jenkins L, Mignery T: A nurse-managed smoking cessation intervention during diagnostic testing for lung cancer, *Oncol Nurs Forum* 24:1419, 1997.

Purpose To determine the effectiveness of a nurse-managed smoking cessation intervention.

Methods Fifteen adult male and female smokers with a suspected diagnosis of lung cancer who were admitted to an inpatient thoracic surgery unit for diagnostic testing were included in the study. They received a nurse-managed smoking cessation intervention during hospitalization with subsequent verification of smoking status at a clinic visit 6 weeks after intervention.

Results and Conclusions Eighty-seven percent of subjects reported an intent to quit smoking within a month. At 6 weeks after intervention 93% of the subjects reported at least one cessation attempt, and 40% were confirmed via saliva cotinine (major metabolite of nicotine) analysis as abstinent from smoking during the prior week.

Implications for Nursing Practice A nurse-managed smoking cessation intervention was successful in achieving short-term cessation. Hospitalization for diagnostic testing for lung cancer may represent an opportunity for nurses to encourage patients to stop smoking. Even after a person has been diagnosed with lung cancer, smoking cessation is important, because continued smoking in patients with lung cancer who are treated with chemotherapy or radiation have poorer outcomes.

patient should be asked about occupational exposure to asbestos, uranium, arsenic, nickel, iron and iron oxides, and excessive exposure to air pollution. In addition, a detailed history of cigarette smoking should be obtained. This information should be used to evaluate the patient's risk of developing lung cancer and also to teach the patient about early recognition of symptoms. Anyone with a history of exposure to respiratory carcinogens who has pneumonia that persists for longer than 2 weeks in spite of antibiotic therapy should be evaluated for the possibility of lung cancer.

The individual with a chronic cough or a change in the character of a cough should be encouraged to obtain care. In addition, the person with chronic or recurring respiratory infections should be carefully evaluated, especially if the person smokes cigarettes.

Acute Intervention. Care of the patient with lung cancer will initially involve support and reassurance during the diagnostic evaluation. (Specific nursing measures related to the diagnostic studies are outlined in Chapter 24.)

Another major responsibility of the nurse is to help the patient and the family deal with the diagnosis of lung cancer. The patient may feel guilty about cigarette smoking having caused the cancer and need to discuss this feeling with someone who has a nonjudgmental attitude. Questions regarding each patient's condition should be answered honestly. Additional counseling from a social worker, psychologist, or member of the clergy may be needed.

Specific care of the patient will depend on the treatment plan. Postoperative care for the patient having surgery is discussed later in this chapter. Care of the patient undergoing radiation therapy and chemotherapy is discussed in Chapter 14. The nurse has a major role in providing patient comfort, teaching methods to reduce pain, and assessing indications for hospitalization (see Chapter 14).

Ambulatory and Home Care. The patient who has had a surgical resection with intent to cure should be followed up carefully for manifestations of metastasis. The patient and family should be told to contact the physician if symptoms such as hemoptysis, dysphagia, chest pain, and hoarseness develop.

For many individuals who have lung cancer, little can be done to significantly prolong their lives. Radiation therapy and chemotherapy can be used to provide palliative relief from distressing symptoms. Constant pain becomes a major problem. (Measures used to relieve pain are discussed in Chapter 9. Care of the patient with cancer is discussed in Chapter 14.)

Evaluation

The expected outcomes are that the patient with lung cancer will have

- adequate breathing patterns
- minimal to no pain
- realistic attitude about prognosis

OTHER TYPES OF LUNG TUMORS

Other types of primary lung tumors include sarcomas, lymphomas, and bronchial adenomas. Bronchial adenomas are small tumors that arise from the lower trachea or major bronchi and are considered malignant because they are locally invasive and frequently metastasize. Clinical manifestations of bronchial adenomas include hemoptysis, persistent cough, localized obstructive wheezing, and purulent bronchitis. There may be secondary bronchiectasis in long-standing cases. Bronchial adenomas frequently cause endocrine paraneoplastic manifestations. They can usually be treated successfully with surgical resection.

The lungs are a common site for secondary metastases and are more often affected by metastatic growth than by primary lung tumors. The pulmonary capillaries, with their extensive network, are ideal sites for tumor emboli. In addition, the lungs have an extensive lymphatic network. The primary malignancies that spread to the lungs often originate in the gastrointestinal (GI) or genitourinary (GU) tracts and in the breast. General symptoms of lung metastases are chest pain and nonproductive cough.

Benign tumors of the lung are generally classified as *mesenchymal.* Their occurrence is rare, and they have the potential to become malignant. The most common mesenchymal tumors are chondromas, which arise in the bronchial cartilage, and leiomyomas, which are myomas of smooth, nonstriated muscle fibers.

Table 26-20 Common Traumatic Chest Injuries and Mechanisms of Injury

Mechanism of Injury	Common Related Injury
Blunt Trauma	
Blunt steering-wheel injury to chest	Rib fractures, flail chest, pneumothorax, hemopneumothorax, cardiac contusion, pulmonary contusion, cardiac tamponade, great vessel tears
Shoulder-harness seat belt injury	Fractured clavicle, dislocated shoulder, rib fractures, pulmonary contusion, pericardial contusion, cardiac tamponade
Crush injury (e.g., heavy equipment, crushing thorax)	Pneumothorax and hemopneumothorax, flail chest, great vessel tears and rupture, decreased blood return to heart with decreased cardiac output
Penetrating Trauma	
Gunshot or stab wound to chest	Open pneumothorax, tension pneumothorax, hemopneumothorax, cardiac tamponade, esophageal damage, tracheal tear, great vessel tears

Hamartomas of the lung are mixtures of fibrous tissue, fat, and blood vessels. They are congenital malformations of the connective tissue of the bronchiolar walls.

CHEST TRAUMA AND THORACIC INJURIES

Traumatic injuries fall into two major categories: (1) blunt trauma and (2) penetrating trauma. *Blunt trauma* occurs when the body is struck by a blunt object, such as a steering wheel. The external injury may appear minor, but the impact may cause severe, life-threatening internal injuries, such as a ruptured spleen. *Contrecoup trauma,* a type of blunt trauma, is caused by the impact of parts of the body against other objects. This type of injury differs from blunt trauma primarily in the velocity of the impact. Internal organs are rapidly forced back and forth within the bony structures that surround them so that internal injury is sustained not only on the side of the impact but also on the opposite side, where the organ or organs hit bony structures. If the velocity of impact is great enough, organs and blood vessels can literally be torn from their points of origin. Many head injuries are caused by contrecoup trauma.

Penetrating trauma occurs when a foreign body impales or passes through the body tissues (e.g., gunshot wounds, stabbings). Table 26-20 describes selective traumatic injuries as they relate to the categories of trauma and the mechanism of injury. Emergency care of the patient with a chest injury is presented in Table 26-21.

Thoracic injuries range from simple rib fractures to life-threatening tears of the aorta, vena cava, and other major vessels. The most common thoracic emergencies and their management are described in Table 26-22.

PNEUMOTHORAX

A *pneumothorax* is a complete or partial collapse of a lung as a result of an accumulation of air in the pleural space. This condition should be suspected after any blunt trauma to the chest wall. Pneumothorax may be closed or open. Pneumothorax associated with trauma may be accompanied by hemothorax, a condition called *hemopneumothorax.*

Closed Pneumothorax

Closed pneumothorax has no associated external wound. The most common form is a *spontaneous pneumothorax,* which is caused by rupture of small blebs on the visceral pleural space. The cause of the blebs is unknown. This condition occurs most commonly in male cigarette smokers between 20 and 40 years of age. There is a tendency for this condition to recur.

Other causes of closed pneumothorax include the following:

1. Injury to the lungs from mechanical ventilation
2. Injury to the lungs from insertion of a subclavian catheter
3. Perforation of the esophagus
4. Injury to the lungs from broken ribs
5. Ruptured blebs or bullae in a patient with COPD

Open Pneumothorax

Open pneumothorax occurs when air enters the pleural space through an opening in the chest wall (Fig. 26-5, *B*). Examples include stab or gunshot wounds and surgical thoracotomies. A penetrating chest wound is often referred to as a *sucking chest wound.*

An open pneumothorax should be covered with a vented dressing. (A vented dressing is one secured on three sides with the fourth side left untaped.) This allows air to escape from the vent and decreases the likelihood of tension pneumothorax developing. If the object that caused the open chest wound is still in place, it should not be removed until a physician is present. The impaled object should be stabilized with a bulky dressing.

Tension Pneumothorax

Tension pneumothorax may result from either an open or a closed pneumothorax (Fig. 26-6). In an open chest wound, a flap may act as a one-way valve; thus air can enter on inspiration but cannot escape. Intrathoracic pressure increases, the lung collapses, and the mediastinum shifts toward the unaffected side, which is subsequently compressed. As the intrathoracic pressure increases, cardiac output is altered because there is decreased venous return and compression of the great vessels. Tension pneumothorax can occur from mechanical ventilation and resuscitative efforts. Tension pneumothorax may also occur if chest tubes are clamped or become blocked in a patient after insertion for treatment of pneumothorax. Unclamping the tube or relief of the obstruction will remedy this situation.

EMERGENCY MANAGEMENT

Table **26-21** Chest Trauma

Etiology	Assessment Findings	Interventions
Blunt Motor vehicle accident Pedestrian accident Fall Assault with blunt object Crush injury Explosion **Penetrating** Knife Gunshot Stick Arrow Other missiles	**Respiratory** ▪ Dyspnea, respiratory distress ▪ Cough with or without hemoptysis ▪ Cyanosis of mouth, face, nail beds, mucous membranes ▪ Tracheal deviation ▪ Audible air escaping from chest wound ▪ Decreased breath sounds on side of injury ▪ Decreased O_2 saturation ▪ Frothy secretions **Cardiovascular** ▪ Rapid, thready pulse ▪ Decreased blood pressure ▪ Narrowed pulse pressure ▪ Asymmetric blood pressure values in arms ▪ Distended neck veins ▪ Muffled heart sounds ▪ Chest pain ▪ Crunching sound synchronous with heart sounds ▪ Arrhythmias **Surface Findings** ▪ Bruising ▪ Abrasions ▪ Open chest wound ▪ Asymmetric chest movement ▪ Subcutaneous emphysema	**Initial** ▪ Ensure patient airway. ▪ Administer high-flow O_2 with nonrebreather mask. ▪ Establish IV access with two large-bore catheters. Begin fluid resuscitation as appropriate. ▪ Remove clothing to assess injury. ▪ Cover sucking chest wound with nonporous dressing taped on three sides ▪ Stabilize impaled objects with bulky dressings. *Do not remove.* ▪ Assess for other significant injuries and treat appropriately. ▪ Stabilize flail rib segment with hand followed by application of large pieces of tape horizontal across the flail segment. ▪ Place patient in a semi-Fowler's position or position patient on the injured side if breathing is easier *after* cervical spine injury has been ruled out. **Ongoing Monitoring** ▪ Monitor vital signs, level of consciousness, oxygen saturation, cardiac rhythm, respiratory status, and urinary output. ▪ Anticipate intubation for respiratory distress. ▪ Release dressing if tension pneumothorax develops after sucking chest wound is covered.

Tension pneumothorax is a medical emergency because both the respiratory and circulatory systems are affected. If the tension in the pleural space is not relieved, the patient is likely to die from inadequate cardiac output or marked hypoxemia.[22] Nurses and paramedics are now being trained to insert large-bore needles and chest tubes into the chest wall to release the trapped air. Tension pneumothorax usually occurs during mechanical ventilation or resuscitative efforts.

Hemothorax

Hemothorax is an accumulation of blood in the intrapleural space. It is frequently found in association with open pneumothorax and is then called a hemopneumothorax. Causes of hemothorax include chest trauma, lung malignancy, complication of anticoagulant therapy, pulmonary embolus, and tearing of pleural adhesions.

Clinical Manifestations

If the pneumothorax is small, mild tachycardia and dyspnea may be the only manifestations. If the pneumothorax is large, respiratory distress may be present, including shallow, rapid respirations, dyspnea, and air hunger. Chest pain and a cough with or without hemoptysis may be present. On auscultation there are no breath sounds over the affected area, and hyperresonance may be present. A chest x-ray shows the presence of pneumothorax.

If a tension pneumothorax develops, severe respiratory distress, tachycardia, and hypotension occur. Mediastinal displacement occurs, and the trachea shifts to the unaffected side.

Collaborative Care

Treatment depends on the severity of the pneumothorax and the nature of the underlying disease. If the patient is stable, and the amount of air and fluid accumulated in the intrapleural space is minimal, no treatment may be needed as the pneumothorax resolves spontaneously. If the amount of air or fluid is minimal, the pleural space can be aspirated with a large-bore needle. As a lifesaving measure, needle venting (using a large bore needle) of the pleural space may be used. A Heimlich valve may also be used to evacuate air from the pleural space (see p. 647). The most definitive and common form of treatment of pneumothorax and hemothorax is to insert a chest tube and connect it to water-seal drainage (see p. 646).

Repeated spontaneous pneumothorax may need to be treated surgically by a partial pleurectomy, stapling, or laser pleurodesis to promote adherence of the pleurae to one another. The injection of doxycycline (Doryx), an irritating agent, can be used for pleurodesis.

FRACTURED RIBS

Rib fractures are the most common type of chest injury resulting from trauma. Ribs 4 through 9 are most commonly frac-

EMERGENCY MANAGEMENT

Table 26-22 Thoracic Injuries

Injury	Definition	Clinical Manifestations	Emergency Management
Pneumothorax	Air in pleural space (see Fig. 26-5).	Dyspnea, decreased movement of involved chest wall, diminished or absent breath sounds on the affected side, hyperresonance to percussion	Chest tube insertion with suction or vented drainage
Hemothorax	Blood in the pleural space, usually occurs in conjunction with pneumothorax.	Dyspnea, diminished or absent breath sounds, dullness to percussion, shock	Chest insertion, autotransfusion of collected blood, treatment of hypovolemia as necessary
Tension pneumothorax	Air in pleural space that does not escape. Continued increase in amount of air shifts intrathoracic organs and increases intrathoracic pressure (see Fig. 26-6).	Cyanosis, air hunger, violent agitation, tracheal deviation away from affected side, subcutaneous emphysema, neck vein distention, hyperresonance to percussion	Needle decompression followed by chest tube insertion
Flail chest	Fracture of two or more adjacent ribs in two or more places with loss of chest wall stability (see Fig. 26-7).	Paradoxic movement of chest wall, respiratory distress, associated hemothorax, pneumothorax, pulmonary contusion	Stabilize flail segment with intubation in some patients; taping in others; oxygen therapy; treat associated injuries; analgesia
Cardiac tamponade	Blood rapidly collects in pericardial sac, compresses myocardium because the pericardium does not stretch, and prevents heart from pumping effectively.	Muffled, distant heart sounds, hypotension, neck vein distention, increased central venous pressure	Pericardiocentesis with surgical repair as appropriate

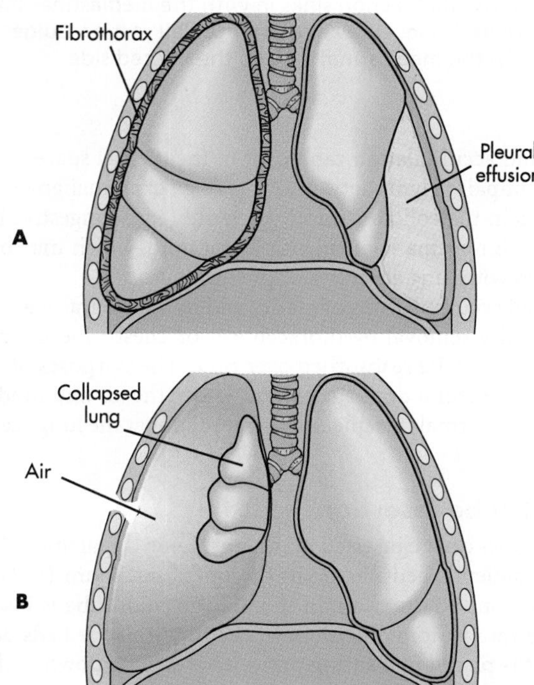

Fig. 26-5 Disorders of the pleura. **A,** Fibrothorax resulting from an organization of inflammatory exudate and pleural effusion. **B,** Open pneumothorax resulting from collapse of lung due to disruption of chest wall and outside air entering.

tured because they are least protected by chest muscles. If the fractured rib is splintered or displaced, it may damage the pleura and lungs.

Clinical manifestations of fractured ribs include pain (especially on inspiration) at the site of injury. The individual splints the affected area and takes shallow breaths to try to decrease the pain. Because the individual is reluctant to take deep breaths, atelectasis may develop because of decreased ventilation.

The main goal in treatment is to decrease pain so that the patient can breathe adequately to promote good chest expansion. Intercostal nerve blocks with local anesthesia may be used to provide pain relief. The nerves of the affected ribs and the two intercostal nerves above and below the injured rib are also blocked. The effect of the anesthesia lasts for a period of hours to days. It needs to be repeated as necessary to provide pain relief. Strapping the chest with tape or using a binder is not common practice. Most physicians believe that these measures should be avoided because they reduce lung expansion and predispose the individual to atelectasis. Narcotic drug therapy must be individualized and used with caution because these drugs can depress respirations.

FLAIL CHEST

Flail chest results from multiple rib fractures, causing instability of the chest wall (Fig. 26-7). The chest wall cannot provide the bony structure necessary to maintain bellows action and ventilation. The affected (flail) area will move paradoxically to

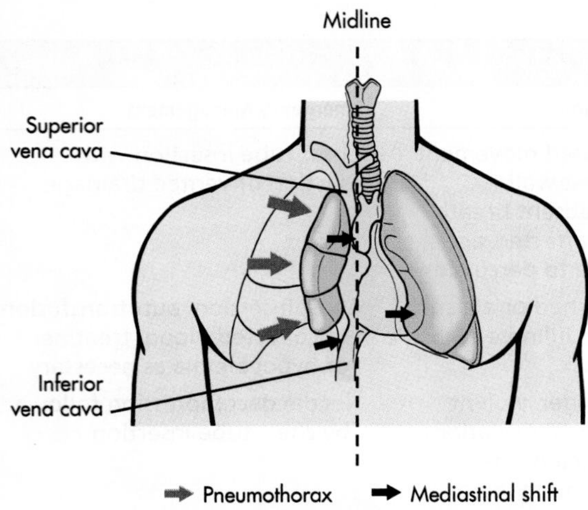

Fig. 26-6 Tension pneumothorax. As pleural pressure on the affected side increases, mediastinal displacement ensues with resultant respiratory and cardiovascular compromise.

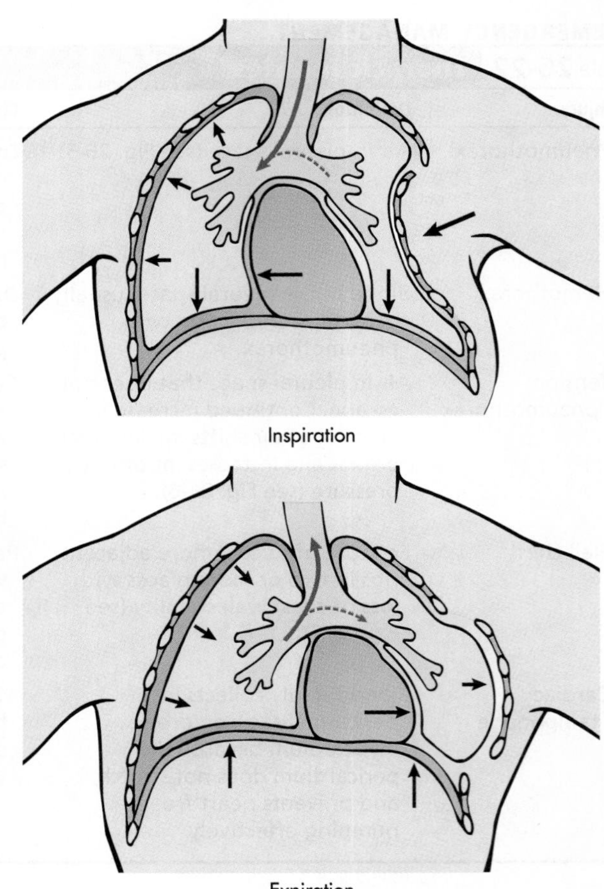

Fig. 26-7 Flail chest produces paradoxic respiration. On inspiration the flail section sinks in with the mediastinal shift to the uninjured side. On expiration the flail section bulges outward with the mediastinal shift to the injured side.

the intact portion of the chest during respiration. During inspiration the affected portion is sucked in, and during expiration it bulges out. This paradoxical chest movement prevents adequate ventilation of the lung in the injured area. The underlying lung may or may not have a serious injury. Associated pain and any lung injury, giving rise to loss of compliance, will contribute to an alteration in breathing patterns and lead to hypoxemia.

A flail chest is usually apparent on visual examination of the unconscious patient. The patient manifests rapid, shallow respirations and tachycardia. A flail chest may not be initially apparent in the conscious patient as a result of splinting of the chest wall. The patient moves air poorly, and movement of the thorax is asymmetric and uncoordinated. Palpation of abnormal respiratory movements, crepitus of the rib, chest x-ray, and ABGs assist in the diagnosis.

Initial therapy consists of adequate ventilation, humidified O_2, and careful administration of crystalloid IV solutions. The definitive therapy is to reexpand the lung and ensure adequate oxygenation. Although many patients can be managed without the use of mechanical ventilation, a short period of intubation and ventilation may be necessary until the diagnosis of the lung injury is complete.

Positive end-expiratory pressure (PEEP) used with mechanical ventilation to improve oxygenation will maintain positive pressure in the lungs throughout the respiratory cycle. Mechanical ventilation is discussed in Chapter 63. The lung parenchyma and fractured ribs will heal with time.

CHEST TUBES AND PLEURAL DRAINAGE

Under normal conditions, intrapleural pressure is below atmospheric pressure (approximately 4 to 5 cm H_2O below atmospheric pressure during expiration and approximately 8 to 10 cm H_2O below atmospheric pressure during inspiration). (Intrapleural pressure and the intrapleural space are described in Chapter 24.) If intrapleural pressure becomes equal to atmospheric pressure, the lungs will collapse (pneumothorax). Air can enter the intrapleural space by a variety of mechanisms, including traumatic chest injury (e.g., gunshot wound, fractured rib), thoracotomy, and spontaneous pneumothorax. Excess fluid accumulation can occur in the pleural space as a result of impaired lymphatic drainage (e.g., from malignancy) or changes in the colloid osmotic pressure (e.g., congestive heart failure). Empyema is purulent pleural fluid, which may be associated with lung abscesses or pneumonia.

Small accumulations of air or fluid in the pleural space may not require removal by thoracentesis or chest-tube insertion. Instead it may be reabsorbed over time. The purposes of chest tubes and pleural drainage are to remove the air and fluid and to restore normal intrapleural pressure so that the lungs can reexpand.

Chest Tube Insertion

Chest tubes can be inserted in the emergency department (ED), at the patient's bedside, or in the operating room (OR), depending on the situation. In the OR the chest tube is inserted via the thoracotomy incision. In the ED or at the bedside the patient is placed in a sitting position or is lying down with the affected side elevated. The area is prepared with antiseptic solution, and the site is infiltrated with a local anesthetic agent. After a small incision is made, one or two chest tubes are inserted into the pleural space. One catheter is placed anteriorly through the second intercostal space to remove air (Fig. 26-8).

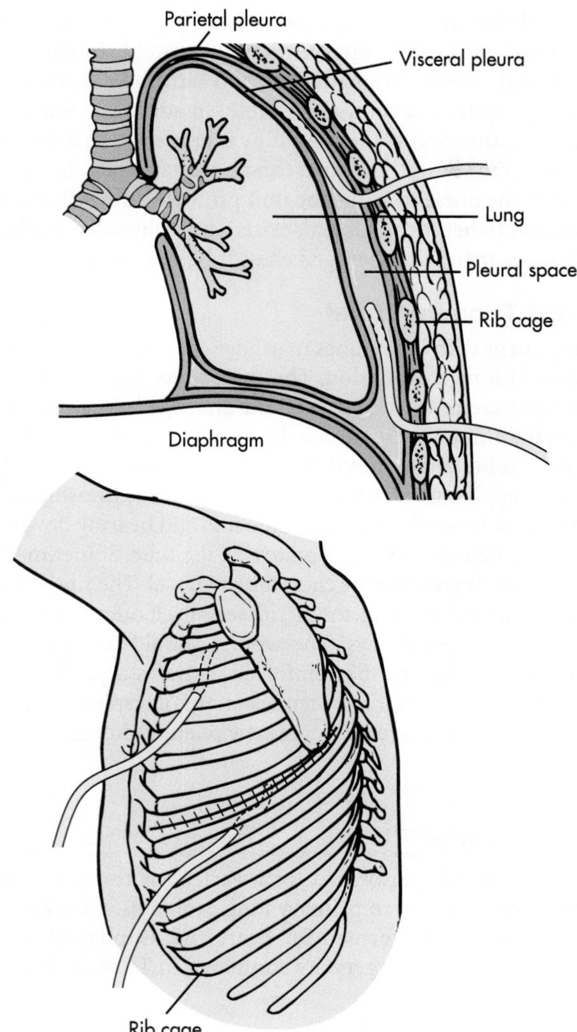

Fig. 26-8 Placement of chest tubes.

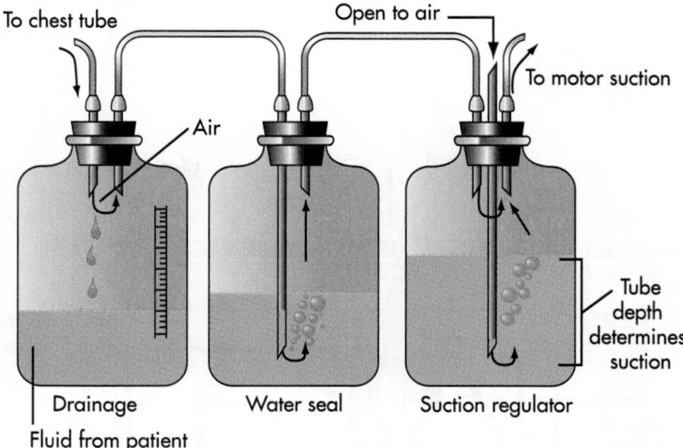

Fig. 26-9 Three-bottle water seal suction. *Bottle I* is the drainage bottle. A vertical piece of tape should be applied to the outer surface of the drainage bottle. The time and the fluid level should be marked hourly on the tape. *Bottle II* is the water-seal bottle. *Bottle III* is the suction control bottle. The length of glass tube below the water surface determines the amount of suction.

The other is placed posteriorly through the eighth or ninth intercostal space to drain fluid and blood.[23] The tubes are sutured to the chest wall, and the puncture wound is covered with an airtight dressing. During insertion, the tubes are kept clamped. After the tubes are in place in the pleural space, they are connected to drainage tubing and pleural drainage and the clamp is removed. Each tube may be connected to a separate drainage system and suction. More commonly, a Y-connector is used to attach both chest tubes to the same drainage system.

Pleural Drainage

Most pleural drainage systems have three basic compartments, each with its own separate function. The three compartments were bottles in early drainage systems and were known as the *three-bottle system* (Fig. 26-9).

The first compartment, or *collection chamber,* receives fluid and air from the chest cavity. The air in the chamber is vented to the second compartment, called the *water-seal chamber,* which acts as a one-way valve. Air enters from the collection chamber via a connector that enters under water in the second compartment. The air bubbles up through the water, and no air can reenter the collection chamber because of the water seal.

A third compartment, which is used to apply controlled suction to the system, is called the *suction control chamber.* The suction control chamber uses tubing submerged in a column of water, which is also vented to the atmosphere (see Fig. 26-9). Suction is applied to the chamber through a separate opening. The amount of suction applied is regulated by the depth of the tubing in the water, not by the amount of suction applied to the system. An increase in suction does not result in an increase in negative pressure applied to the system. Instead, excess suction merely draws in air through the vented tubing.[24]

The removal of air from the pleural space is facilitated during periods when the patient's intrathoracic pressure is increased, such as during exhalation, coughing, or sneezing. As a result, more air bubbles are noted in the water-seal chamber during these activities. A lack of bubbling during exhalation or coughing may indicate a blockage in the chest tube (e.g., kinking, clotting) or expansion of the lung with no further air in the pleural space.

A variety of commercial disposable plastic chest drainage systems are available. Most operate on the same principles as the three-bottle system. One popular system is the Pleur-evac shown in Fig. 26-10. (Note the correspondence of the chambers to the bottles shown in the three-bottle system in Fig. 26-9.) The manufacturer's suggestions for use are included with the equipment. The plastic units allow the patient mobility and decrease the risk of breaking or spilling the drainage system.

Heimlich Valves. Another device that may be used to evacuate air from the pleural space is the Heimlich valve. This valve is a collapsible rubber tube that is attached to the external end of the chest tube. The valve opens whenever the pressure is greater than atmospheric pressure and closes when the reverse occurs. The Heimlich valve functions like a water seal and is usually used for emergency transport or in special home care situations.

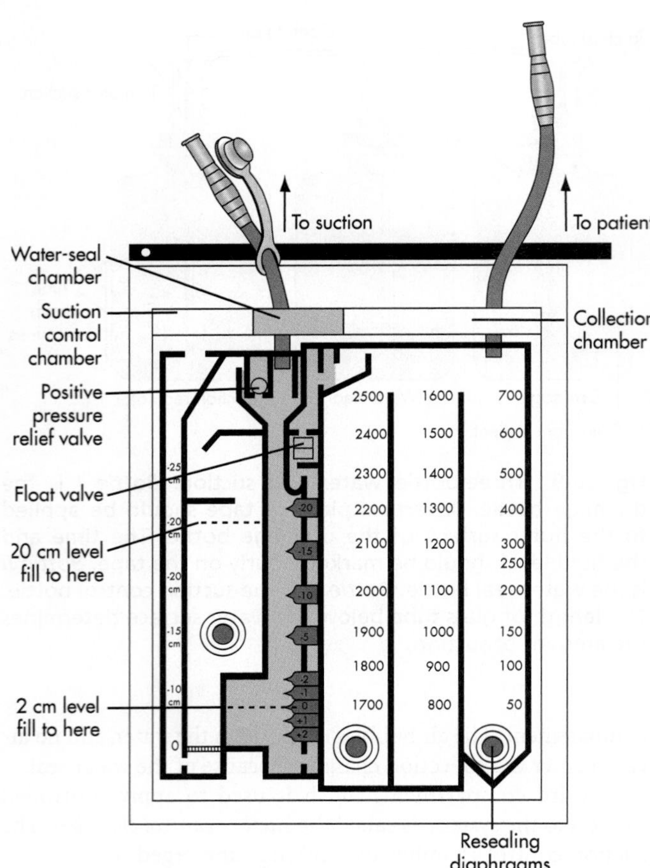

Fig. 26-10 Pleur-evac disposable chest suction system.

NURSING MANAGEMENT: CHEST TUBES

Some general guidelines for nursing care of the patient with chest tubes and water-seal drainage systems are presented in Table 26-23.

Milking and stripping of chest tubes may briefly increase the amount of negative pressure applied to the pleural space. The increased negative pressure should enhance the evacuation of fluid in chest tubes and prevent the development of clots and obstruction from the stagnation of fluids. Although further study is still needed to evaluate the effects of routine stripping of pleural and mediastinal tubes on the lung and mediastinal tissue, present practice advocates the use of these procedures when there is bloody drainage or when the fluid in the collection bottle tends to clot. When chest tubes are used for air collection alone, stripping and milking is not usually performed. Each clinical situation should be evaluated individually, and unit protocol and physician preferences should be ascertained before initiation of stripping and milking. The nurse should keep in mind that these procedures can cause the patient to experience pain and that dislodgement of the tube may occur if the tube is not stabilized above the area that is being stripped.

Clamping of chest tubes is no longer advocated as routine clinical practice unless they become disconnected. The danger of a rapid accumulation of air in the pleural space causing tension pneumothorax is far greater than that of a small amount of atmospheric air entering the pleural space. Chest tubes may be momentarily clamped to change the drainage apparatus or to check for air leaks.[23] If a chest tube becomes disconnected the most important intervention is reestablishment of the water-seal system immediately and attachment of a new drainage system as soon as possible. In some hospitals, when disconnection occurs the chest tube is immersed in sterile water (about 2 cm) until the system can be reestablished. It is important for the nurse to know the unit protocol, individual clinical situation (whether an air leak exists), and physician preference before resorting to prolonged chest tube clamping.

Chest Tube Removal

The patient with chest tubes may have chest x-rays to follow the course of lung reexpansion. The chest tubes are removed when the lungs are reexpanded and fluid drainage has ceased. Sometimes the amount of suction is decreased for a period of time before the tubes are removed. The tube is removed by cutting the sutures, applying a sterile petroleum jelly gauze dressing, having the patient take a deep breath, exhaling, and bearing down (Valsalva's maneuver), and then removing the tube. Sometimes pain medication is given before chest tube removal. The site is covered with an airtight dressing, the pleura seals itself off, and the wound is healed in several days. The wound should be observed for drainage and should be reinforced if necessary. The patient should be observed for any manifestations of respiratory distress, which may signify a recurrent or new pneumothorax.

CHEST SURGERY

Chest surgery is performed for a variety of reasons, some of which are unrelated to primary lung problems. For example, a thoracotomy is performed for heart and esophageal surgery. The types of chest surgery are compared in Table 26-24.

Preoperative Care

Before chest surgery, baseline data are obtained on the respiratory and cardiovascular systems. Diagnostic studies performed are pulmonary function studies, chest x-rays, electrocardiograph (ECG), ABGs, blood urea nitrogen (BUN), serum creatinine, blood glucose, serum electrolytes, and complete blood count. Additional studies of cardiac function such as cardiac catheterization may be done for the patient who is to undergo a pneumonectomy. A careful physical assessment of the lungs, including percussion and auscultation, should be done. This will allow the nurse to compare preoperative and postoperative findings.

The patient should be encouraged to stop smoking before surgery to decrease secretions and increase O_2 saturation. In the anxious period before surgery this is not an easy thing for the habitual smoker to do. Chest physiotherapy may be indicated to help drain the lungs of accumulated secretions. This is especially indicated for the patient with a lung abscess or bronchiectasis.

Preoperative teaching should include exercises for effective deep breathing and incentive spirometry. If the patient practices these techniques before surgery, the techniques will be easier to perform postoperatively. The patient should be told that adequate medication will be given to reduce the pain, and the patient is helped to splint the incision with a pillow to facilitate deep breathing.

Table 26-23 Guidelines for Care of Patient with Chest Tubes and Water-Seal Drainage

1. Keep all tubing as straight as possible and coiled loosely below chest level. Do not let the patient lie on it.
2. Keep all connections between chest tubes, drainage tubing, and the drainage collector tight. Taping at connections and at the top of the bottle helps prevent air leaks.
3. Keep the water seal and suction control chamber at the appropriate water levels by adding sterile water as needed, because water loss by evaporation may occur.
4. Mark the time of measurement and the fluid level on the drainage bottle according to the prescribed orders. Marking intervals may range from once per hour to every 8 hours. Any change in the quantity or characteristics of drainage (e.g., clear yellow to bloody) should be reported to the physician and recorded.
5. Observe for air bubbles in the water-seal chamber and fluctuations in the glass tube or chest tubes. Air should be bubbling out from the glass tube. If no fluctuations are observed (rising with inspiration and falling with expiration in the spontaneously breathing patient; the opposite occurs during positive-pressure mechanical ventilation), the drainage system is blocked or the lungs are reexpanded. If bubbling increases, there may be an air leak.
6. Check for bubbling in the water seal. Normally, this is intermittent. When bubbling is continuous and constant, the source of the air leak may be determined by momentarily clamping the tubing at successively distal points away from the patient until the bubbling ceases. Retaping tubing connections or replacing the drainage apparatus may be necessary to correct the air leak.
7. Monitor the patient's clinical status. Vital signs should be taken frequently, lungs auscultated, and the chest wall observed for any abnormal chest movements.
8. Never elevate the drainage system to the level of the patient's chest because this will cause fluid to drain back into the lungs. Secure the bottles to the metal drainage stand or racks. The drainage bottles should not be emptied unless they are in danger of overflowing.
9. Encourage the patient to breathe deeply periodically to facilitate lung expansion.
10. Check the position of the bottle. If the bottle is overturned and the water seal is disrupted, return the bottle to an upright position and encourage the patient to take a few deep breaths, followed by forced exhalations and cough maneuvers.

For most types of chest surgery, chest tubes are inserted and connected to water-sealed drainage systems. The purpose of these tubes should be explained to the patient. In addition, O_2 is frequently given the first 24 hours after surgery. Range-of-motion exercises on the surgical side similar to those for the mastectomy patient should be taught (see Chapter 49).

The thought of losing part of a vital organ is frequently frightening. The patient should be reassured that the lungs have a large degree of functional reserve. Even after the removal of one lung there is enough lung tissue to maintain adequate oxygenation.

The nurse should be available to deal with the questions asked by the patient and the family. Questions should be answered honestly. The nurse should try to facilitate the expression of concerns, feelings, and questions. (General preoperative care and teaching are discussed in Chapter 16.)

Surgical Therapy

Thoracotomy surgery is considered major surgery because the incision is large, cutting into bone, muscle, and cartilage. The two types of thoracic incisions are *median sternotomy*, performed by splitting the sternum, and *lateral thoracotomy*. The median sternotomy is primarily used for surgery involving the heart. The two types of lateral thoracotomy are posterolateral and anterolateral. The posterolateral thoracotomy is used for most surgeries involving the lung. The incision is made from the anterior axillary line below the nipple level posteriorly at the fourth, fifth, or sixth intercostal space. It is rarely necessary to remove the ribs. Strong mechanical retractors are used to gain access to the lung. The anterolateral incision is made in the fourth or fifth intercostal space from the sternal border to the midaxillary line. This procedure is commonly used for surgery or trauma victims, mediastinal operations, and wedge resections of the upper and middle lobes of the lung.

The extensiveness of the thoracotomy incision often results in severe pain for the patient after surgery. Because muscles have been severed, the patient is reluctant to move the shoulder and arm on the surgical side. Chest tubes are placed in the pleural space except in pneumonectomy surgery. In a pneumonectomy the space from which the lung was removed gradually fills with serosanguineous fluid.

Thorascopic Surgery. Thorascopic surgery (endoscopic thoracotomy) is a procedure that in many cases can avoid the impact of a full thoracotomy.[25] The procedure involves three to four 1-inch incisions made on the chest that allow the thorascope (a special fiberoptic camera) and instruments to be inserted and manipulated. *Video-assisted thorascopes* improve visualization because the surgeon can view the thoracic cavity from the video monitor. The thorascope is equipped with a camera that magnifies the image on the monitor. Thorascopy can be used to diagnose and treat a variety of conditions of the lung, pleura, and mediastinum.

The candidate for this type of procedure should not have a prior history of conventional thoracic surgery because the probability of adhesion formation would make access more difficult. The patient whose lesions are in the lung periphery or the mediastinum is a better candidate because of better accessibility. The patient considered for thorascopy should have sufficient pulmonary function preoperatively to allow the surgeon to perform conventional thoracotomy if complications occur (e.g., heavy bleeding). Other complications that may occur are diaphragmatic perforation, air emboli, persistent pleural air leaks, and tension pneumothorax.[25]

There are many benefits of thorascopic surgery when compared with a conventional thoracotomy procedure. These

Table 26-24 Chest Surgeries

Type	Description	Indication	Comments
■ Lobectomy	Removal of one lobe of lung	Lung cancer, bronchiectasis, TB, emphysematous bullae, benign lung tumors, fungal infections	Most common lung surgery, postoperative insertion of two chest tubes, expansion of remaining lung tissue to fill up space
■ Pneumonectomy	Removal of entire lung	Lung cancer (most common), extensive TB, bronchiectasis, lung abscess	Done only when lobectomy or segmental resection will not remove all diseased lung, no drainage tubes (generally), fluid gradually filling space where lung has been removed, turning of patient with unaffected side dependent contraindicated, position of patient on back or operative side with head elevated
■ Segmental resection	Removal of one or more lung segments	Bronchiectasis, TB	Technically difficult, done to remove lung segment, insertion of chest tubes, expansion of remaining lung tissue to fill space
■ Wedge resection	Removal of small, localized lesion that occupies only part of a segment	Lung biopsy, excision of small nodules	Need for chest tubes postoperatively
■ Decortication	Removal or stripping of thick, fibrous membrane from visceral pleura	Empyema	Use of chest tubes and drainage postoperatively
■ Exploratory thoracotomy	Incision into thorax to look for injured or bleeding tissues	Chest trauma	Use of chest tubes and drainage postoperatively
■ Thoracotomy not involving lungs*	Incision into thorax for surgery on other organs	Hiatal hernia repair, open heart surgery, esophageal surgery, tracheal resection, aortic aneurysm repair	—
■ Thoracoplasty	Removal of ribs without entering pleura	Reduction of size of chest cavity	Historical importance in treating TB, possible use to decrease lung size in area of chronic empyema, use before resectional surgery (rarely)
■ Thorascopy (endoscopic thoracotomy)	One to four 1-in incisions through which a special fiberoptic camera is introduced as well as other instruments and suction	Patient without prior thoracotomy; peripheral or mediastinal lesions; lung function must be sufficient to undergo conventional thoracotomy	Possible complications include heavy bleeding, diaphragmatic perforation, air emboli, tension pneumothorax; chest tube is inserted through one of the incisions; incisions may be sutured or closed with adhesive wound-approximating strips

*For comments on thoracotomy not involving the lungs, see discussion of individual diseases in text.

26-2 NURSING CARE PLAN PATIENT AFTER THORACOTOMY

Expected Patient Outcomes	Nursing Interventions and *Rationales*
NURSING DIAGNOSIS	**Ineffective airway clearance** *related to* inability to cough secondary to pain from surgical procedure and positioning *as manifested by* rhonchi, wheezes, inability to cough or deep breathe.
▪ Lungs clear to auscultation. ▪ Able to clear secretions.	▪ Place patient in semi-Fowler's position *to improve cardiac output and to maximize lung excursion.* ▪ Assist patient to turn, deep breathe, and cough every 1-2 hr initially *to help move or drain the lungs of accumulated secretions.* ▪ Splint chest incision *to facilitate breathing exercises and coughing.* ▪ Plan coughing and deep breathing after pain relief is obtained *to mobilize secretions, open closed airways, and achieve maximum lung inflation.* ▪ Auscultate lungs before and after deep-breathing and coughing regimens *to evaluate effectiveness of intervention.* ▪ Humidify air *to liquefy secretions for easier expectoration.* ▪ Perform suctioning if necessary *to assist in removing secretions from airway.*
NURSING DIAGNOSIS	**Impaired gas exchange** *related to* air and fluid collection in lungs and pleural space *as manifested by* tachycardia, abnormal respirations, abnormal ABGs.
▪ Full expansion of lungs. ▪ Normal breath sounds bilaterally. ▪ Normal ABGs.	▪ Monitor chest drainage system (see text) *to ensure adequate ventilation and to detect hemorrhage.* ▪ Monitor respiratory rate and pattern and ABG results *to allow early recognition of significant changes in respiratory function.* ▪ Administer low-flow oxygen (1-4 L/min) via nasal prongs or cannula *to treat hypoxemia.* ▪ Assist with position changes *to increase patient's comfort and to facilitate aeration of the lungs.*
NURSING DIAGNOSIS	**Ineffective breathing pattern** *related to* pain, position, and possible complication on affected side *as manifested by* shortness of breath, shallow respirations, use of accessory muscles.
▪ Respiratory rate 12-18 breaths/min. ▪ Ease of respiration.	▪ Auscultate lungs every 2-3 hr *to evaluate the rate, quality, and depth of patient's respirations and the need for tracheal aspiration.* ▪ Observe for manifestations of complications such as pneumothorax or hemothorax with symptoms of acute shortness of breath; shallow, rapid respirations; dyspnea; cough, and air hunger. ▪ Assist patient with deep breathing *to provide encouragement and improve results.* ▪ Position patient for comfort and ease of breathing *to increase compliance with respiratory treatments.* ▪ Encourage use of incentive spirometer every 2-3 hr *to provide visual feedback to the patient on effectiveness of respirations.*
NURSING DIAGNOSIS	**Anxiety** *related to* feelings of dyspnea and pain *as manifested by* anxious facial expression, inability to cooperate with instructions to breathe slowly.
▪ Relief from anxiety or able to manage level of anxiety.	▪ Stay with patient during procedures *to provide encouragement and explanations.* ▪ Assess patency of and drainage from chest tubes *to validate proper functioning.* ▪ Provide feedback from effective breathing *to provide encouragement and reduce anxiety.* ▪ Administer pain medication as ordered or implement nonpharmacologic measures such as distraction and relaxation *because pain increases anxiety and decreases compliance with necessary treatments.*

Table 26-25 Relationship of Lung Volumes to Type of Ventilatory Impairment

Interpretation	FVC	FEV_1	FEV_1/FVC	RV	TLC
Normal	Normal	Normal	Normal	Normal	Normal
Airway obstruction	Normal or low	Low	Low	High	High
Lung restriction	Low	Normal or low	Normal or high	Normal or low	Low
Obstruction and restriction	Low	Low	Low	Variable	Variable

FEV1, forced expiratory volume in 1 second; *FVC*, functional vital capacity; *RV*, residual volume; *TLC*, total lung capacity.

include less adhesion formation, minimal blood loss, less time under anesthesia, no ICU confinement in most cases, shorter hospitalization and faster recovery, less pain, and no need for postoperative rehabilitation therapy because of minimal disruption of thoracic structures. Patients who are not candidates for thoracotomy surgery can undergo thoracscopic surgery.

Chest tubes are placed at the end of the procedure through one of the incisions. The incisions are closed with sutures or a wound-approximating adhesive bandage. Nursing assessment and care postoperatively include monitoring respiratory status and lung reexpansion with the chest tubes and checking the incisions for drainage or dehiscence. The most common complication is prolonged air leak. A return to prior activities should be encouraged as quickly as possible. The hospital stay averages from 1 to 5 days, depending on the type of surgery.

Postoperative Care

Specific measures related to the care after a thoracotomy are presented in NCP 26-2. The specific follow-up care depends on the type of surgical procedure. General postoperative care is discussed in Chapter 18.

RESTRICTIVE RESPIRATORY DISORDERS

Restrictive respiratory disorders are characterized by decreased compliance of the lungs or chest wall or both. This is in contrast to obstructive disorders, which are characterized by increased resistance to airflow. Pulmonary function tests are the best means to use in differentiating between restrictive and obstructive respiratory disorders (Table 26-25). Restrictive disorders are characterized by reduced vital capacity (VC) and reduced total lung capacity (TLC), with a normal or reduced functional residual capacity (FRC) and residual volume (RV). Obstructive disorders are characterized by normal or decreased VC, increased TLC, reduced ratio of forced air expiration volume in the first second of expiration (FEV_1) to functional vital capacity (FVC), increased FRC, and increased RV. Mixed obstructive and restrictive disorders are often manifested. For example, a patient may have both chronic bronchitis (an obstructive problem) and pulmonary fibrosis (a restrictive problem).

Restrictive problems are generally categorized into extrapulmonary and intrapulmonary disorders. Extrapulmonary causes of restrictive lung disease include disorders involving the central nervous system (CNS), neuromuscular system, and chest wall (Table 26-26). In these disorders the lung tissue is normal. Intrapulmonary causes of restrictive lung disease involve the pleura or the lung tissue (Table 26-27).

Pleural Effusion

Types. The pleural space lies between the lung and chest wall and normally contains a very thin layer of fluid. Pleural effusion is a collection of fluid in the pleural space (Fig. 26-5, *A*). It is not a disease but rather a sign of a serious disease. It is frequently classified as *transudative* or *exudative* according to whether the protein content of the effusion is low or high, respectively. A transudate occurs primarily in noninflammatory conditions and is an accumulation of protein-poor, cell-poor fluid. Transudative pleural effusions (also called *hydrothorax*) are caused by (1) increased hydrostatic pressure found in congestive heart failure, which is the most common cause of pleural effusion, or (2) decreased oncotic pressure (from hypoalbuminemia) found in chronic liver or renal disease. In these situations, fluid movement is facilitated out of the capillaries and into the pleural space.

An exudate is an accumulation of fluid and cells in an area of inflammation. An exudative pleural effusion results from increased capillary permeability characteristic of the inflammatory reaction. This type of effusion occurs secondary to conditions such as pulmonary malignancies, pulmonary infections, pulmonary embolization, and GI disease (e.g., pancreatic disease, esophageal perforation).

The type of pleural effusion can be determined by a sample of pleural fluid obtained via thoracentesis (a procedure done to remove fluid from the pleural space). Exudates have a specific gravity above 1.015 and a high protein content, and the fluid is dark yellow or amber. Transudates have a lower specific gravity and low to no protein content, and the fluid is clear or pale yellow. The fluid can also be analyzed for red and white blood cells, malignant cells, bacteria, glucose, pH, and lactic dehydrogenase.

An *empyema* is a pleural effusion that contains pus. It is caused by conditions such as pneumonia, TB, and lung abscess. A complication of empyema is *fibrothorax,* in which there is fibrous fusion of the visceral and parietal pleurae (Fig. 26-5, *A*).

Clinical Manifestations

Common clinical manifestations of pleural effusion are progressive dyspnea and decreased movement of the chest wall on the affected side. There may be pleuritic pain from the underlying disease. Physical examination of the chest will indicate dullness to percussion and absent or decreased breath sounds over the affected area. The chest x-ray will indicate an abnormality if the effusion is greater than 250 ml. Manifestations of empyema include the manifestations of pleural effusion, as well as fever, night sweats, cough, and weight loss. A thoracentesis reveals an exudate containing thick, purulent material.

Table 26-26 Extrapulmonary Causes of Restrictive Lung Disease

Disease or Alteration	Description	Comments
Central Nervous System		
■ Head injury, CNS lesion (e.g., tumor, cerebrovascular accident)	Injury to or impingement on respiratory center, causing hypoventilation or hyperventilation; relationship of manifestations to increased intracranial pressure (see Chapter 54)	Management is directed toward treating the underlying cause, maintaining the airway, using mechanical ventilation for supportive care, and assessing for manifestations of increased intracranial pressure.
■ Narcotic and barbiturate use	Depression of respiratory center, respiratory rate of <12 breaths/min	Respiratory depression is caused by drug overdose or inadvertent administration of drugs to a person with respiratory difficulty. These drugs should not be administered to a person with a respiratory rate of <12 breaths/min.
Neuromuscular System		
■ Guillain-Barré syndrome	Acute inflammation of peripheral nerves and ganglia; paralysis of intercostal nerves leading to diaphragmatic breathing; paralysis of vagal preganglionic and postganglionic fibers leading to reduced ability of bronchioles to constrict, dilate, and respond to irritants	Patient often has to be put on mechanical ventilation for supportive care (see Chapter 57).
■ Amyotrophic lateral sclerosis	Progressive degenerative disorder of the motor neurons in the spinal cord, brain stem, and motor cortex; respiratory system involvement as a result of interruption of nerve transmission to respiratory muscles, especially diaphragm	See Chapter 57 for clinical manifestations and management.
■ Myasthenia gravis	Defect in neuromuscular junction, respiratory system involvement as a result of interruption of nerve transmission to respiratory muscles	See Chapter 57 for clinical manifestations and management.
■ Muscular dystrophy	Hereditary disease; eventual involvement of all skeletal muscles; paralysis of respiratory muscles, including intercostals, diaphragm, and accessory muscles	Pulmonary problems develop late in disease process.
Chest Wall		
■ Chest-wall trauma (e.g., flail chest, fractured rib)	Rib fracture causing inspiratory pain; voluntary splinting of chest, resulting in shallow, rapid breathing; impaired ventilatory ability caused by paradoxical breathing. See p. 643.	—
■ Pickwickian syndrome (extreme obesity)	Excess adipose tissue interfering with chest-wall and diaphragmatic excursion, somnolence from hypoxemia and CO_2 retention, polycythemia from chronic hypoxia	Weight loss generally causes reversal of symptoms. Prevention and prompt treatment of respiratory infections are important. Condition is worsened in supine position.
■ Kyphoscoliosis	Posterior and lateral angulation of the spine; restriction of ventilation as a result of alteration in thoracic excursion; increase in work of breathing; pattern of rapid, shallow breathing; reduction of lung volume; compression of alveoli and blood vessels	Only small number of persons with condition develop severe respiratory problems.

Thoracentesis

If the cause of the pleural effusion is not known, a diagnostic thoracentesis is needed to obtain pleural fluid for analysis (see Fig. 24-17). If the degree of pleural effusion is severe enough to impair breathing, a therapeutic thoracentesis is done to remove fluid.

A thoracentesis is performed by having the patient sit on the edge of a bed and lean forward over a bedside table. The puncture site is determined by chest x-ray, and percussion of the chest is used to assess the maximum degree of dullness. The skin is cleaned with an antiseptic solution and anesthetized locally. The thoracentesis needle is inserted into the intercostal

Table 26-27 Intrapulmonary Causes of Restrictive Lung Disease

Disease or Alteration	Description
Pleural Disorders	
▪ Pleural effusion	Accumulation of fluid in pleural space secondary to altered hydrostatic or oncotic pressure, fluid collection >250 ml, showing up on chest x-ray
▪ Pleurisy	Inflammation of pleura, classification as fibrinous (dry) or serofibrinous (wet), wet pleurisy accompanied by an increase in pleural fluid and possibly resulting in pleural effusion
▪ Pneumothorax	Accumulation of air in pleural space with accompanying lung collapse
Parenchymal Disorders	
▪ Atelectasis	Condition of lung characterized by collapsed, airless alveoli; possibly acute (e.g., in postoperative patient) or chronic (e.g., in patient with malignant tumor)
▪ Pneumonia	Acute inflammation of lung tissue caused by bacteria, viruses, fungi, chemicals, dusts, and other factors
▪ Pulmonary fibrosis	Excessive connective tissue in the lungs resulting from healing and tissue repair after inflammation, possible localized fibrosis (e.g., from lung abscess, TB, pneumonia) or diffuse (e.g., from pneumoconiosis, sarcoidosis, cystic fibrosis, Hamman-Rich syndrome), progressive dyspnea on exertion as a result of decreased compliance of lungs and increased work of breathing. Diffuse pulmonary fibrosis is progressively disabling and frequently fatal.
▪ ARDS*	Atelectasis, pulmonary edema, congestion, and hyaline membrane lining the alveolar wall; result of variety of conditions, including shock lung, O_2 toxicity, gram-negative sepsis, cardiopulmonary bypass, and aspiration pneumonia.

*See Chapter 62 for clinical manifestations and management.
ARDS, acute respiratory distress syndrome.

space. Fluid can be aspirated with a syringe, or tubing can be connected to allow fluid to drain into a sterile collecting bottle. After the fluid is removed, the needle is withdrawn, and a bandage is applied over the insertion site.

Usually only 1000 to 1200 ml of pleural fluid are removed at one time to prevent mediastinal shift and compromised venous return. A follow-up chest x-ray should be done to detect a possible pneumothorax that could have been induced by perforation of the visceral pleura. During and after the procedure the patient should be observed for any manifestations of respiratory distress.

Collaborative Care

The main goal of management of pleural effusions is to treat the underlying cause. For example, adequate treatment of CHF with diuretics and sodium restriction will result in decreased pleural effusions. The treatment of pleural effusions secondary to malignant disease represents a more difficult problem. These types of pleural effusions are frequently recurrent and accumulate quickly after thoracentesis. Infusions of cancer chemotherapeutic agents directly into the pleural space may be used to decrease the number of recurrent effusions.

Treatment of empyema is directed at drainage of the pleural space via thoracentesis or a closed thoracotomy tube. Appropriate antibiotic therapy is also needed to eradicate the causative organism. If a fibrothorax results from the empyema and causes severe pulmonary restriction, a decortication surgical procedure is done in which the pleural membranes are separated.

PLEURISY

Pleurisy (also called *pleuritis*) is an inflammation of the pleura. The most common causes are pneumonia, TB, chest trauma, pulmonary infarctions, and neoplasms. The inflammation usually subsides with adequate treatment of the primary disease. Pleurisy can be classified as *fibrinous* (dry), with fibrinous deposits on the pleural surface, or *serofibrinous* (wet), with increased production of pleural fluid that may result in pleural effusion.

The pain of pleurisy is typically abrupt and sharp in onset and is aggravated by inspiration. The patient's breathing is shallow and rapid to avoid unnecessary movement of the pleura and chest wall. A pleural friction rub may occur, which is the sound over areas where inflamed visceral and parietal pleura rub over one another during inspiration. This sound is usually loudest at peak inspiration but can be heard during exhalation as well.

Treatment of pleurisy is aimed at treating the underlying disease and providing pain relief. Taking analgesics and lying on or splinting the affected side may provide some relief. The patient should be taught to splint the rib cage when coughing. Intercostal nerve blocks may be done if the pain is severe.

ATELECTASIS

Atelectasis is a condition of the lungs characterized by collapsed, airless alveoli. The most common cause of atelectasis is airway obstruction that is resulting from retained exudates and secretions. This is frequently observed in the postoperative patient. Normally the pores of Kohn provide for collateral passage of air from one alveolus to another. Deep inspiration is necessary to open the pores effectively. For this reason, deep-breathing exercises are important in preventing atelectasis in the high-risk patient (e.g., postoperative, immobilized patient). Pulmonary fibrosis can occur as a complication of chronic atelectasis. (The prevention and treatment of atelectasis are discussed in Chapter 18.)

PULMONARY FIBROSIS

A common cause of diffuse pulmonary fibrosis is environmental or occupational inhalation of organic and inorganic substances (see section earlier in this chapter). Other causes of diffuse pulmonary fibrosis include the Hamman-Rich syndrome (an unusual form of interstitial pneumonia) and sarcoidosis.

Table 26-28 Causes of Pulmonary Edema

Congestive heart failure
Overhydration with intravenous fluids
Hypoalbuminemia: nephrotic syndrome, hepatic disease, nutritional disorders
Altered capillary permeability of lungs: inhaled toxins, inflammation (e.g., pneumonia), severe hypoxia, near-drowning
Mechanical ventilation
Malignancies of the lymph system
Respiratory distress syndrome (e.g., O_2 toxicity)
Unknown causes: neurogenic condition, narcotic overdose, high altitude

Sarcoidosis is a systemic disease of unknown cause characterized by the presence of granulomatous inflammation of the lungs in about 90% of the patients. The disease may be systemic and involve the skin, eyes, liver, kidney, or heart. The disease is most common in African-Americans between the ages of 20 and 35. The clinical course of the disease varies from self-limiting to progressive, widespread granulomatous inflammation and fibrosis. Marked pulmonary fibrosis can be present with severe restrictive lung disease. Cor pulmonale can develop in the advanced stages. There is no specific treatment for sarcoidosis. Often the disease is self-limiting, and the patient gets well without treatment. Corticosteroids have been used to relieve symptoms and suppress the acute inflammation.

VASCULAR LUNG DISORDERS

PULMONARY EDEMA

Pulmonary edema is an abnormal accumulation of fluid in the alveoli and interstitial spaces of the lungs. It is a complication of various heart and lung diseases (Table 26-28). It is considered a medical emergency and may be life threatening.

Normally, there is a balance between the hydrostatic and oncotic pressures in the pulmonary capillaries. If the hydrostatic pressure increases or the colloid oncotic pressure decreases, the net effect will be fluid leaving the pulmonary capillaries and entering the interstitial space. This stage is referred to as *interstitial edema.* At this stage the lymphatics can usually drain away the excess fluid. If fluid continues to leak from the pulmonary capillaries it will enter the alveoli. This stage is referred to as *alveolar edema.* Pulmonary edema interferes with gas exchange by causing an alteration in the diffusing pathway between the alveoli and the pulmonary capillaries.

The most common cause of pulmonary edema is left-sided congestive heart failure (CHF). (The clinical manifestations and management of pulmonary edema are described in Chapter 33.) Chronic forms of pulmonary edema are not common. This condition can be asymptomatic for a long period of time while structural changes such as pulmonary fibrosis result. An early manifestation of this condition may be paroxysmal nocturnal dyspnea as a result of increased hydrostatic pressure in the lungs in the recumbent position.

PULMONARY EMBOLISM

Pulmonary emboli arise from thrombi in the venous circulation or right side of the heart (thromboembolism) and from other sources, such as amniotic fluid, air, fat, bone marrow, and foreign IV material. The most common source of the thrombus is the deep veins of the legs. The thrombus breaks loose and travels as an embolus until it lodges in the pulmonary vasculature.

The result of the thromboembolic occlusion is complete or partial occlusion of the pulmonary arterial blood flow to parts of the lung. Thus the lung tissue distal to the embolus is ventilated but not perfused. As the pressure increases in the pulmonary vasculature, pulmonary hypertension may result. (Pulmonary embolism is described in detail in Chapter 36.)

PULMONARY HYPERTENSION

Pulmonary hypertension compromises a variety of disorders occurring as a primary disease (primary pulmonary hypertension) or as a complication of a large number of respiratory and cardiac disorders. Pulmonary hypertension is elevated pulmonary pressure resulting from an increase in pulmonary vascular resistance to blood flow through small arteries and arterioles. A 60% to 70% reduction in the pulmonary vascular bed is required before pulmonary hypertension develops.

Etiology and Pathophysiology

Normally the pulmonary circulation is characterized by low resistance and low pressure. Cardiac output can increase significantly with no increase in the pressure in the pulmonary vasculature. In pulmonary hypertension the increase in vascular resistance may be anatomic or vasomotor related in origin. The reasons for an anatomic increase in vascular resistance include (1) loss of capillaries as a result of alveolar wall damage, as found in COPD; (2) stiffening of the pulmonary vasculature, as found in pulmonary fibrosis; and (3) obstruction of blood flow, as found with pulmonary emboli.

Vasomotor increase in pulmonary vascular resistance is found in conditions characterized by alveolar hypoxia and hypercapnia. These conditions cause localized vasoconstriction and shunting of blood away from poorly ventilated alveoli. Alveolar hypoxia and hypercapnia can be caused by a wide variety of conditions, including the pickwickian syndrome, kyphoscoliosis, neuromuscular diseases, and other conditions characterized by alveolar hypoventilation with normal lungs.

It is possible to have a combination of anatomic restriction and vasomotor constriction. This is found in the patient with long-standing chronic bronchitis who has chronic hypoxia in addition to loss of lung tissue.

Primary Pulmonary Hypertension. *Primary pulmonary hypertension* is not associated with either pulmonary or cardiac disease. The person with this disorder is typically a woman between the ages of 20 and 40. The basic cause of the problem is unknown, although it is thought that there is an abnormality of the endothelial cells of the pulmonary arterial system. There also appears to be a genetic basis for its occurrence. No definitive therapy is available, and the course is often continual downhill progression often occurring within several years of onset of symptoms.

Clinical Manifestations

The most common manifestations of pulmonary hypertension are dyspnea, fatigue, chest pain, and occasionally syncope with exercise. These symptoms initially occur only when there is an increased cardiac output (e.g., during exercise or with fever) or during hypoxemia (e.g., with pulmonary infection). Eventually the condition occurs even during rest. Pulmonary hypertension increases the workload of the right ventricle and causes right ventricular hypertrophy (a condition called cor pulmonale) and eventually heart failure. A chest x-ray generally shows enlarged central pulmonary arteries and clear lung fields. An enlarged right heart may be seen. Echocardiogram usually reveals right ventricular hypertrophy.

Collaborative Care

Treatment of pulmonary hypertension caused primarily by pulmonary or cardiac disorders consists mainly of treating the underlying disorder, such as COPD or pulmonary emboli. Early recognition of pulmonary hypertension is essential to interrupt the self-perpetuation cycle responsible for the progression of this problem (Fig. 26-11).

Many patients with primary pulmonary hypertension can be effectively managed with calcium channel blocker therapy, such as nifedipine (Adalat) and diltiazem (Cardizem), and epoprostenol (Flolan) therapy. Epoprostenol, a prostacyclin that promotes pulmonary vasodilation, reduces pulmonary vascular resistance but has little effect on the systemic vascular resistance.[26] Its administration requires the placement of an indwelling catheter and continuous infusion pump. The major problems have been infections related to vascular access. Intravenous adenosine (Adenocard) and inhaled nitric oxide have also been used to decrease pulmonary vascular resistance.

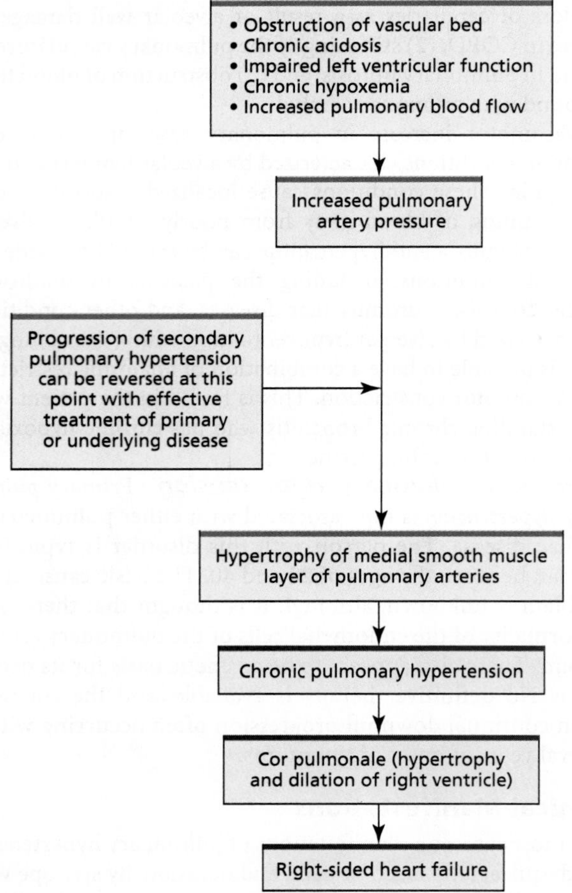

Fig. 26-11 Pathogenesis of pulmonary hypertension and cor pulmonale.

Diuretic therapy relieves dyspnea and peripheral edema and may be useful in reducing right ventricular volume overload. Anticoagulant therapy has also been used based on evidence that thrombosis in situ is common. Lung transplantation is recommended for those patients who do not respond to epoprostenol and progress to severe right-sided heart failure. Recurrence of the disease has not been reported in individuals who have undergone transplantation.

COR PULMONALE

Cor pulmonale is enlargement of the right ventricle secondary to diseases of the lung, thorax, or pulmonary circulation. Pulmonary hypertension is usually a preexisting condition in the individual with cor pulmonale. Cor pulmonale may be present with or without overt cardiac failure. The most common cause of acute cor pulmonale is a massive pulmonary embolism. However, cor pulmonale is usually chronic, resulting from alveolar hypoxia in COPD. Almost any disorder that affects the respiratory system can cause cor pulmonale. The etiology and pathogenesis of pulmonary hypertension and cor pulmonale are outlined in Fig. 26-11.

Clinical Manifestations

Clinical manifestations of cor pulmonale include dyspnea, chronic productive cough, wheezing respirations, retrosternal

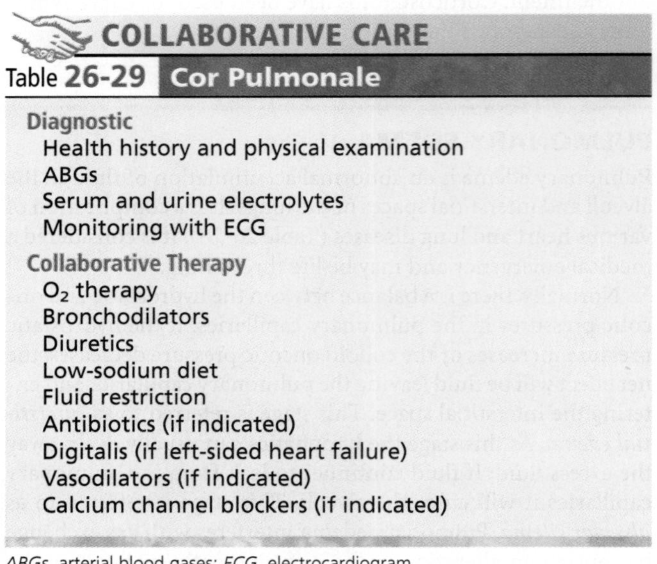
COLLABORATIVE CARE

Table 26-29 Cor Pulmonale

Diagnostic
- Health history and physical examination
- ABGs
- Serum and urine electrolytes
- Monitoring with ECG

Collaborative Therapy
- O_2 therapy
- Bronchodilators
- Diuretics
- Low-sodium diet
- Fluid restriction
- Antibiotics (if indicated)
- Digitalis (if left-sided heart failure)
- Vasodilators (if indicated)
- Calcium channel blockers (if indicated)

ABGs, arterial blood gases; *ECG*, electrocardiogram.

Table 26-30 Indications for Lung Transplant

- Emphysema
- α_1-Antitrypsin deficiency
- Idiopathic pulmonary fibrosis
- Primary pulmonary hypertension
- Interstitial lung disease
- Cystic fibrosis
- Bronchiectasis
- Pulmonary fibrosis secondary to other diseases (e.g., sarcoidosis)
- Congenital heart disease with Eisenmenger's complex

or substernal pain, and fatigue. Chronic hypoxemia leads to polycythemia and increased total blood volume and viscosity of the blood. (Polycythemia is often present in cor pulmonale secondary to COPD.) Compensatory mechanisms that are secondary to hypoxemia can aggravate the pulmonary hypertension. Episodes of cor pulmonale in a person with underlying chronic respiratory problems are frequently triggered by an acute respiratory tract infection.

If heart failure accompanies cor pulmonale, additional manifestations such as peripheral edema; weight gain; distended neck veins; full, bounding pulse; and enlarged liver will also be found. (Heart failure is discussed in Chapter 33.) A chest x-ray will show an enlarged right ventricle and pulmonary artery.

Collaborative Care

The primary management of cor pulmonale is directed at treating the underlying pulmonary problem that precipitated the heart problem (Table 26-29). Low-flow O_2 therapy is used to correct the hypoxemia and reduce vasoconstriction in chronic states of respiratory disorders. In acute states (e.g., those caused by pulmonary emboli), higher concentrations of O_2 may be required. If fluid, electrolyte, and acid-base imbalances are present, they must be corrected. Diuretics and a low-sodium diet will help decrease the plasma volume and the load on the heart. Bronchodilator therapy is indicated if the underlying respiratory problem is due to an obstructive disorder. Antibiotic therapy is indicated if the cor pulmonale was precipitated by an infection. Digitalis may be used if there is left-sided heart failure. Phlebotomies may be needed in the patient with hematocrit level above 60 g/dl (600 g/L) to reduce the hematocrit and blood volume.

Chronic management of cor pulmonale resulting from COPD is similar to that described for COPD (see Chapter 27). Continuous low-flow O_2 during sleep; exercise; and small, frequent meals may allow the patient to feel better and be more active. Other treatments include those for pulmonary hypertension and include vasodilator therapy, calcium channel blockers, and anticoagulants. When medical treatment fails, lung transplantation is an option for some patients.

LUNG TRANSPLANTATION

Lung transplantation has evolved as a viable therapy for patients with end-stage lung disease. Improved selection criteria, technical advances, and better methods of immunosuppression have resulted in improved survival rates. A variety of

CRITICAL THINKING EXERCISES

CASE STUDY

Tuberculosis

Patient Profile

Mr. G., a 56-year-old Hispanic male, was admitted to the hospital with symptoms of right-sided chest pain and coughing up blood.

Subjective Data

- Has been homeless and living on the street for the past 6 months
- Has had increasingly severe pain in the right side during the past 2 weeks
- Describes the pain as "like a knife stabbing him" and is almost unable to breathe when it hits
- Thinks he has lost weight because he needs a rope to hold up his pants
- Describes frequent episodes of awakening in the night soaking wet

Objective Data

Physical Examination

- Thin, disheveled man appearing older than stated age.
- Chest auscultation revealed diffuse rhonchi.

Diagnostic Studies

- Serum albumin 2.8 g/dl (28 g/L)
- WBC 20,000/µl (20×10^9/L)
- Induced sputum specimen gray with red streaking
- Stain of sputum revealed many acid-fast bacilli

Chest X-ray

- Diffuse alveolar infiltrates in lower right lobe accompanied by small pleural effusion

Critical Thinking Questions

1. What types of infectious disease precautions should be taken related to his hospitalization?
2. What clinical manifestations of TB did Mr. G. exhibit? Explain their pathophysiologic bases.
3. With a new diagnosis of TB, what drugs will probably be given to Mr. G.?
4. What will the nurse need to consider in planning discharge arrangements for Mr. G.?
5. Based on the assessment data presented, write one or more appropriate nursing diagnoses. Are there any collaborative problems?

NURSING RESEARCH ISSUES

1. What are effective measures that a nurse can institute to increase patient compliance with long-term antituberculosis medication?
2. Compare the effectiveness of various smoking cassation methods (e.g., hypnosis, aversion therapy, nicotine weaning).
3. What position should a patient assume following lung surgery for comfort and maximum oxygenation?
4. Does an aggressive nurse-managed community program related to TB therapy increase patient compliance with therapy?
5. Is there a significant improvement in the quality of life of the patient following lung transplantation?

pulmonary disorders are potentially treatable with some type of lung transplantation (Table 26-30). Various transplant options are available, including single lung transplant, bilateral lung transplant, heart-lung transplant, and living related lobe transplant.[27]

Because donor lungs are the scarcest of the common solid organs transplanted, patients with end-stage lung disease undergo extensive evaluation. The candidate for lung transplantation should not have any significant psychiatric disorders or systemic diseases, should not be an active smoker, and should not have a malignancy or recent history of malignancy or renal or liver insufficiency. The candidate and the family undergo thorough psychologic screening to determine the ability to cope with a postoperative regimen that requires strict adherence to immunosuppressive therapy, continuous monitoring for early signs of infection, and prompt reporting of manifestations of infection for medical evaluation. Additionally, they must have the financial ability, either through medical insurance or private funds, to afford the procedure, postoperative immunosuppressive drugs, and medical follow-up care.

Immunosuppressive therapy usually includes cyclosporine, azathioprine (Imuran), and prednisone. Immunosuppressive drugs are discussed in Chapter 44 and Table 44-12.

Infection is an early pulmonary postoperative complication of lung transplantation. Initially, patients experience a shallow breathing pattern and difficulty in clearing secretions secondary to denervation of the lung below the trachea, with a resultant decrease in mucociliary clearance and lymphatic drainage. Infection in the transplant recipient is the most significant cause of morbidity and death. The immunosuppression necessary to prevent rejection makes the recipient susceptible to many pathogens, including bacterial, fungal, viral, and protozoal organisms. Infections are primarily pulmonary and are usually either nosocomial or opportunistic in nature. Aggressive pulmonary clearance measures, including aerosolized bronchodilators, chest physiotherapy, and deep-breathing and coughing techniques, are mandatory to minimize potential complications.

Acute rejection of lung transplants is commonly seen within the first 3 months after transplantation, and symptoms include dyspnea, low grade fever, tachypnea, and chest x-ray findings ranging from infiltrates to consolidation. Treatment of rejection consists of administration of high-dose IV methylprednisolone. (Treatment of rejection is discussed in Chapter 44.)

Bronchiolitis obliterans (obstructive defect that affects the airways, causing progressive occlusion) is the primary manifestation of chronic rejection in lung transplant patients.[28] The onset, usually at least 6 months after transplant, is often subacute, with gradual onset of progressive obstructive airflow defect, including cough, dyspnea, and recurrent lower respiratory tract infection. There is no effective therapy for bronchiolitis obliterans.

Patients are discharged with portable spirometry devices to monitor their own pulmonary function. As lung transplantation continues to evolve, hope for a prolonged life with improved quality is realistic for some individuals with end-stage lung disease.

REVIEW QUESTIONS

The number of the question corresponds to the same-numbered objective at the beginning of the chapter.

1. In assessing a patient with pneumococcal pneumonia, the nurse recognizes that clinical manifestations of this condition include
   a. fever, chills, and a productive cough with rust-colored sputum.
   b. a nonproductive cough and night sweats that are usually self-limiting.
   c. a gradual onset of nasal stuffiness, sore throat, and purulent productive cough.
   d. an abrupt onset of fever, nonproductive cough, and formation of lung abscesses.
2. An appropriate nursing intervention for a pneumonia patient with the nursing diagnosis of ineffective airway clearance related to thick secretions and fatigue would be to
   a. perform postural drainage every hour.
   b. provide analgesics as ordered to promote patient comfort.
   c. administer oxygen as prescribed to maintain optimal oxygen levels.
   d. teach the patient how to cough effectively to bring secretions to the mouth.
3. A patient with tuberculosis has a nursing diagnosis of noncompliance. The nurse recognizes that the most common etiologic factor for this diagnosis in patients with TB is
   a. fatigue and lack of energy to manage self-care.
   b. lack of knowledge about how the disease is transmitted.
   c. little or no motivation to adhere to a long-term drug regimen.
   d. feelings of shame and the response to the social stigma associated with TB.
4. A patient has been receiving high-dose corticosteroids and broad-spectrum antibiotics for treatment of serious trauma and infection. The nurse plans care for the patient knowing that the patient is most susceptible to
   a. candidiasis.
   b. aspergillosis.
   c. histoplasmosis.
   d. coccidioidomycosis.
5. The primary goal for the patient with bronchiectasis is that the patient will
   a. have no recurrence of disease.
   b. have normal pulmonary function.
   c. maintain removal of bronchial secretions.
   d. avoid environmental agents that precipitate inflammation.
6. A common pathophysiologic characteristic of many types of pneumoconiosis is
   a. liquefactive necrosis.
   b. benign tumor growth.
   c. diffuse airway obstruction.
   d. diffuse pulmonary fibrosis.
7. The type of lung cancer generally associated with the best prognosis because it is potentially surgically resectable is
   a. adenocarcinoma.
   b. small cell carcinoma.
   c. squamous cell carcinoma.
   d. undifferentiated large cell carcinoma.

8. A patient who smokes tells the nurse that she wants to quit smoking. The best response by the nurse is to tell the patient that
   a. if she is really committed to stopping, that is all that is needed to quit.
   b. to overcome the nicotine addiction it is almost always necessary to join a group support program.
   c. setting a date to stop and then quitting "cold turkey" is the most difficult but is associated with fewer relapses.
   d. the use of nicotine replacement aids with behavioral interventions is the most successful method of stopping.
9. The nurse identifies a flail chest in a trauma patient when
   a. multiple rib fractures are determined by x-ray.
   b. a tracheal deviation to the unaffected side is present.
   c. paradoxic chest movement occurs during respiration.
   d. there is decreased movement of the involved chest wall.
10. The nurse notes fluctuation of the water level in the tube submerged in the water-seal chamber in a patient with closed chest-tube drainage. The nurse should
    a. continue to monitor this normal finding.
    b. check all connections for a leak in the system.
    c. lower the drainage collector further from the chest.
    d. clamp the tubing at progressively distal points away from the patient until the fluctuations stop.
11. A nursing measure that should be instituted after a pneumonectomy includes
    a. monitoring chest-tube drainage and functioning.
    b. positioning the patient on the unaffected side or back.
    c. range-of-motion exercises on the affected upper extremity.
    d. ascultating frequently for lung sounds on the affected side.
12. Guillain-Barré syndrome causes respiratory problems primarily by
    a. depressing the CNS.
    b. deforming chest-wall muscles.
    c. paralyzing the diaphragm secondary to trauma.
    d. interrupting nerve transmission to respiratory muscles.
13. A patient with COPD asks why the heart is affected by the respiratory disease. The nurse's response to the patient is based on the knowledge that cor pulmonale is characterized by
    a. pulmonary congestion secondary to left ventricular failure.
    b. excess serous fluid collection in the alveoli caused by retained respiratory secretions.
    c. right ventricular hypertrophy secondary to increased pulmonary vascular resistance.
    d. right ventricular failure secondary to compression of the heart by hyperinflated lungs.
14. In responding to a patient with emphysema who asks about the possibility of a lung transplant, the nurse knows that lung transplantation is contraindicated in patients
    a. with cor pulmonale.
    b. who currently smoke.
    c. with end-stage lung disease.
    d. older than 50 years of age.

References

1. Levine BS: Pulmonary conditions. In Meredith PV, Horan NJ, editors: *Adult primary care, a handbook for nurse practitioners,* Philadelphia, Saunders (in press).
2. Esposito AL, Dempsey CJ, Doyle JM: Acute bronchitis. In Rakel RE, editors: *Conn's current therapy,* Philadelphia, 1997, Saunders.
3. Fine MJ and others: A prediction rule to identify low-risk patients with community-acquired pneumonia, *N Engl J Med* 336:243, 1997.
4. Levinson ME: Pneumonia including necrotizing pulmonary infections (lung abscess). In Fauci AS and others; editors: *Harrison's principles of internal medicine,* ed 14, New York, 1998, McGraw-Hill.
5. Gotfried M: Appropriate use of antibiotics in treatment of community-acquired pneumonia, *Infect Med* 13(suppl A):15, 1996.
6. Mayer J, Campbell GD: ATS recommendations for treatment of adults with hospital-acquired pneumonia, *Infect Med* 13:1027, 1996.
7. Cassiere HA: Aspiration pneumonia: current concepts and approach to management, *Medscape Resp Care* 2, 1998.
8. Herman CM, Chen GJ, High KP: Pneumococcal penicillin resistance and the cost-effectiveness of pneumococcal vaccine, *Infect Med* 15:233, 1998.
9. Rodvold KA: A treatment algorithm for CAP based on the ATS guidelines, *Infect Med* 13(suppl A):22, 1996.
10. Calianno C: Pneumonia—repelling a deadly invader, *Nursing* 26:33, 1996.
11. Carter M: TB prevention and treatment, *Infect Med* 15:32, 1998.
12. Bradford WZ, Daley CL: Multiple drug-resistant tuberculosis, *Infect Dis Clin North Am* 12:157, 1998.
13. Jordan TJ, Mangura BT, Reichman LB: Management after exposure to tuberculosis, *Hosp Pract* 32:73, 1997.
14. Cassiere HA, Fein AM: Lung abscess: diagnosis and treatment, *Medscape Resp Care 1,* 1997.
15. American Cancer Society: *Cancer facts and figures,* 1998.
16. Report of the Surgeon General: The health consequences of involuntary smoking, Washington, DC, US Department of Health and Human Services.
17. Minna JD: Neoplasms of the lung. In Fauci AS and others, editors: *Harrison's principles of internal medicine,* ed 14, New York, 1998, McGraw-Hill.
18. Chiramannil A: Lung cancer, *AJN* 98:46, 1998.
19. Chiappori A, DeVore RF, Johnson DH: New agents in the management of non–small-cell lung cancer, Cancer Control: *JMCC* 4:317, 1997.
20. Bonomi P: Eastern Cooperative Oncology Group experience with chemotherapy in advanced non–small cell lung cancer, *Chest* 113 (suppl 1):13S, 1998.
21. Lilenbaum RC: Recent advances in chemotherapy for lung cancer, *Curr Opin Pulm Med* 2:285, 1996.
22. Laskowski-Jones L: Meeting the challenge of chest trauma, *AJN* 95:23, 1995.
23. O'Hanlon-Nichols T: Commonly asked questions about chest tubes, *AJN* 96:60, 1996.
24. Pettinicchi TA: Trouble shooting chest tubes, *Nursing* 28:58, 1998.
25. Shawgo T: Thoracoscopic surgery: a new approach to pulmonary disease, *Crit Care Nurse* 16:76, 1996.
26. Gaine SP, Rubin LJ: Medical and surgical treatment options for pulmonary hypertension, *Am J Med Sci* 315:179, 1998.
27. Wood DE and others: Lung transplantation part I: indications and operative management, *West J Med* 165:355, 1996.
28. Edelman JD, Kotloff RM: Lung transplantation: a disease-specific approach, *Clin in Chest Med* 18:627, 1997.

Resources

Resources for this chapter are listed after Chapter 27 on p. 715.

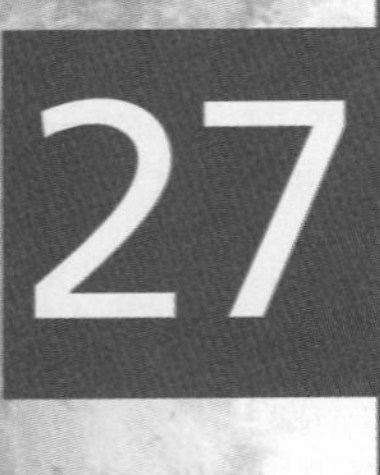
 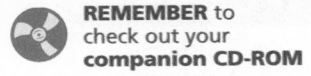

REMEMBER to check out your companion CD-ROM

27 NURSING MANAGEMENT Obstructive Pulmonary Diseases

Kathleen Oare Lindell & Trisch Van Sciver

www.mosby.com/MERLIN/medsurg_lewis

LEARNING OBJECTIVES

1. Describe the etiology, pathophysiology, clinical manifestations, and collaborative care of asthma.
2. Describe the nursing management of the patient with asthma.
3. Differentiate among the etiology, pathophysiology, clinical manifestations, and collaborative care of the patient with chronic bronchitis and emphysema.
4. Describe the effects of cigarette smoking on the lungs.
5. Explain the nursing management of the patient with chronic bronchitis and emphysema.
6. Identify the indications for oxygen therapy, methods of delivery, and complications of oxygen administration.
7. Describe the pathophysiology, clinical manifestations, collaborative care, and nursing management of the patient with cystic fibrosis.

Obstructive pulmonary diseases include those diseases characterized by increased resistance to airflow as a result of airway obstruction or airway narrowing. Airway obstruction may result from accumulated secretions, edema, and swelling of the inner lumen, bronchospasm, or destruction of lung tissue. Asthma, a reactive airway disease, is a chronic inflammatory lung disease that results in airflow obstruction, but is reversible. Emphysema and chronic bronchitis are also forms of chronic obstructive pulmonary disease (COPD), and most often are irreversible in nature. The patient with asthma has variations in airflow over time, whereas the limitation in expiratory airflow in the patient with emphysema or chronic bronchitis is generally more constant. The patient with a diagnosis of obstructive lung disease may have distinguishing features of two or all three of these diseases.[1] Cystic fibrosis, another form of obstructive lung disease, is a genetic disorder that produces airway obstruction because of changes in glandular secretions.

ASTHMA

Asthma is defined as a chronic inflammatory disorder of the airways in which inflammation causes varying degrees of obstruction in the airways.[2] This inflammation causes recurrent episodes of wheezing, breathlessness, chest tightness, and cough, particularly at night and in the early morning. The airway obstruction may reverse spontaneously or with treatment. The hyperresponsiveness of the airways is variable, producing spontaneous fluctuations in the severity of obstruction. The clinical course of asthma is unpredictable, ranging from paroxysms of dyspnea and wheezing to unremitting symptoms such as in status asthmaticus.[2]

Asthma affects an estimated 1 in 20 Americans with 14 to 15 million people affected. The incidence of asthma has increased 60% since the 1980s.[2] It is not really known why the incidence has increased. The morbidity associated with asthma is dramatic. It affects school attendance, occupational choices, physical activity, and many other aspects of life. Only 5000 people die of asthma annually. However, asthma hospitalization rates have markedly increased. The highest hospitalization rates are among African-Americans and children, and death rates for asthma are consistently highest among African-Americans aged 15 to 24 years. Underdiagnosis and inappropriate therapy are the major contributors to asthma morbidity and mortality. The high morbidity rates related to asthma may be attributed to limited access to health care, an inaccurate assessment of disease severity, a delay in seeking help, inadequate medical treatment, nonadherence to prescribed therapy, and an increase of allergens in the environment.[2,3]

Triggers of Asthma Attacks (Table 27-1)

Allergens. In some persons with asthma, an exaggerated IgE response to certain allergens (e.g., dust, pollen, grasses, animal danders) occurs. These allergens attach to IgE receptors on mast cells (Fig. 27-1). The IgE-mast cell complexes re-

Reviewed by Janet T. Crimlisk, RN, MS, NP, CS, Pulmonary Clinical Nurse Specialist and Adult Nurse Practitioner, Boston Medical Center, Boston, Mass; and Alicia M. Horkan, RN, MSN, CEN, Director, Emergency Services, Colquitt Regional Medical Center, Moultrie, Ga.

Table 27-1 Triggers of Acute Asthma Attacks

- Allergen inhalation
  - Animal danders
  - House dust mite
  - Pollens
  - Molds
- Air pollutants
  - Exhaust fumes
  - Perfumes
  - Oxidants
  - Sulfur dioxides
  - Cigarette smoke
  - Aerosol sprays
- Viral upper respiratory infection
- Sinusitis
- Exercise and cold, dry air
- Drugs
  - Aspirin
  - Nonsteroidal antiinflammatory drugs
  - β-adrenergic blockers
- Occupational exposure
  - Metal salts
  - Wood and vegetable dusts
  - Industrial chemicals and plastics
  - Pharmaceutical agents
- Food additives
  - Sulfites (bisulfites and metabisulfites)
  - Tartrazine
- Hormones/menses
- Gastroesophageal reflux

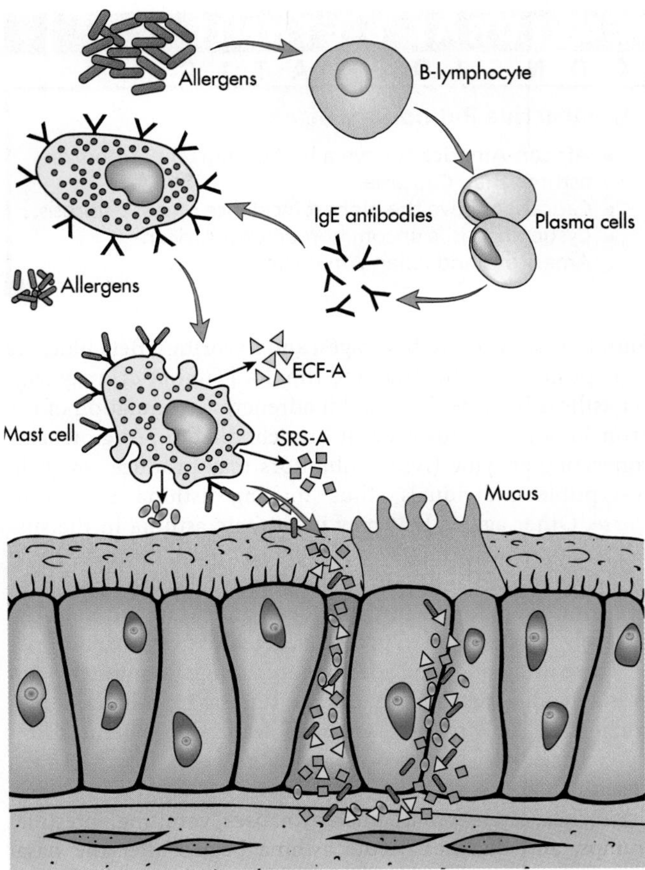

Fig. 27-1 The early phase response in asthma is triggered when an allergen or irritant cross-links IgE receptors on mast cells, which are then activated to release histamine and other inflammatory mediators.

main for a long time so that a second exposure to the allergen triggers mast cell degranulation even years after the initial exposure to the antigen. (Allergic reactions are discussed in Chapter 12.)

Respiratory Infections. Respiratory infections (especially viral infections) are one of the most common precipitating factors of an acute asthma attack. Bacterial respiratory infections, with the exception of sinusitis, rarely play a major role in exacerbations of asthma. Infections cause inflammatory changes in the tracheobronchial system and alter the mucociliary mechanism. Therefore they increase the hyperresponsiveness of the bronchial system. Increased airway responsiveness can last from 2 to 8 weeks after the infection in both normal and asthmatic persons. A respiratory infection may trigger airway inflammation and cause asthma that subsides in 2 to 3 weeks, or it may trigger asthma that continues for several months and then subsides spontaneously or after medical intervention. The patient with asthma should avoid people with colds or flu, get yearly influenza vaccinations, and avoid taking over-the-counter (OTC) cold remedies unless approved by the health care provider.

Nose and Sinus Problems. Approximately 30% of asthmatics have chronic sinus problems and more have nasal problems.[4] These problems include allergic rhinitis, which can be seasonal or perennial, and nasal polyps. Sinus problems are usually related to inflammation of the mucous membranes, most commonly from noninfectious causes such as allergies. However, bacterial sinusitis may also occur. Sinusitis must be treated and large nasal polyps removed for the asthma patient to have good control. (Sinusitis is discussed in Chapter 25.)

Exercise. Asthma that is induced or exacerbated during physical exertion is called exercise-induced asthma (EIA). Typically, EIA occurs after several minutes of vigorous exercise (e.g., jogging, aerobics, walking briskly, climbing stairs) and is characterized by bronchospasm, shortness of breath, cough, and wheezing. Cromolyn (Intal), β_2-agonists*, and nedocromil (Tilade) have successfully maintained bronchodilation during exercise when they were inhaled 10 to 20 minutes before exercise. Long-acting β_2-agonists (e.g., salmeterol [Serevent]) may also be of value. The patient should perform a brief warm-up of stretching for 2 to 3 minutes before exercise. When exercising in cold or dry climate conditions, breathing through a scarf or mask may decrease the likelihood of symptoms.

Drugs and Food Additives. Sensitivity to drugs may occur in some asthmatic persons, especially those with nasal polyps. Approximately 12% to 25% of people with asthma have what is termed the *asthma triad*—nasal polyps, asthma, and sensitivity to aspirin and nonsteroidal antiinflammatory drugs (NSAIDs). Salicylic acid can be found in many OTC drugs and some foods, beverages, and flavorings. In some asthmatics who ingest aspirin or NSAIDs (e.g., ibuprofen, indomethacin), wheezing will develop in approximately 2 hours. Some patients are also sensitive to salicylates, which are

*The terms β-adrenergic agonists, β-agonists, and β-adrenergics are used interchangeably in this textbook.

CULTURAL & ETHNIC CONSIDERATIONS

Obstructive Pulmonary Diseases

- African-Americans have a higher mortality rate from asthma than Caucasians.
- Caucasians have the highest incidence of cystic fibrosis.
- Cystic fibrosis is uncommon among African-Americans and Asian-Americans.

found in many foods, beverages, and flavorings. Beta blockers (e.g., propanolol [Inderal] and timolol [Timoptic]) may trigger asthma because they inhibit adrenergic stimulation of the bronchioles and thus prevent bronchodilation. Angiotensin-converting enzyme (ACE) inhibitors may produce cough in susceptible individuals, thus making asthma symptoms worse. Other agents that may precipitate asthma in the susceptible patient are tartrazine (yellow dye no. 5 found in many foods), vitamins, and sodium metabisulfite (a food preservative commonly found in fruits, beer, and wine and used extensively in salad bars to protect vegetables from oxidation).

These drugs and food additives are thought to interfere with prostaglandin metabolic pathways, leading to enhanced production of leukotrienes, some of which are potent bronchoconstrictors. The onset of a typical reaction occurs 15 minutes to 3 hours after ingestion and is marked by profuse rhinorrhea, often accompanied by nausea, vomiting, intestinal cramps, and diarrhea. Acute asthma begins after the nasal symptoms appear. Pretreatment with corticosteroids or cromolyn does not prevent the reaction. Epinephrine, given shortly after the onset, usually controls the symptoms.

Although sensitivity to salicylates persists for many years, the nature and severity of the reaction can change over time. Dietary restrictions of tartrazine (if applicable) and avoidance of aspirin and NSAIDs are required.

Food allergies may cause asthma symptoms. Avoidance diets may be needed to prevent asthma. However, food allergies triggering asthma in adults are rare but are more common in children.

Gastroesophageal Reflux Disease. The exact mechanism by which gastroesophageal reflux disease (GERD) causes asthma is unknown. It is postulated that reflux of stomach acid into the esophagus can be aspirated into the lungs and cause reflex bronchoconstriction. Although GERD is primarily involved in nocturnal asthma, it can trigger daytime asthma as well. Patients with hiatal hernia, excessive stress, and a prior history of reflux or ulcer disease may have acid reflux as an asthma trigger. (GERD is discussed in Chapter 39.)

Emotional Stress. Another factor often discussed in relationship to the etiology of asthma is psychologic or emotional stress. Asthma is not a psychosomatic disease. Psychologic factors can interact with the asthmatic response to worsen or ameliorate the disease process. An asthma attack caused by any trigger can produce panic and anxiety, which are not unexpected emotions during this experience. The extent to which psychologic factors contribute to the induction and continuation of any given acute exacerbation is unknown, but it probably varies from patient to patient and in the same patient from episode to episode.

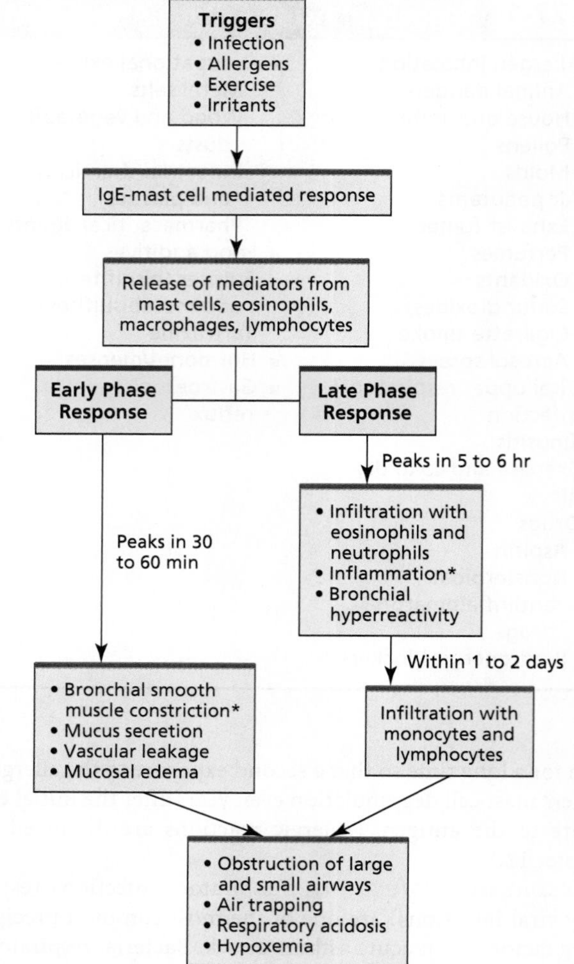

Fig. 27-2 Early and late phase responses of asthma. Items with an *asterisk* are primary processes.

Pathophysiology

The hallmarks of asthma are airway inflammation and nonspecific hyperirritability or hyperresponsiveness of the tracheobronchial tree. The mechanisms that induce asthma remain unknown. The airway hyperresponsiveness seen in asthma is caused by bronchoconstriction in response to physical, chemical, and pharmacologic agents. Traditionally asthma has been considered a disease characterized by bronchospasm. However, the pathophysiologic changes associated with asthma are also due to inflammation in the airways.

The early-phase response in asthma is characterized by bronchospasm, which induces the inflammatory sequelae of the late-phase response (Fig. 27-2). The early-phase response is triggered when an allergen or irritant cross-links IgE receptors on mast cells found beneath the basement membrane of the bronchial wall (see Fig. 27-1). The mast cells become activated with subsequent release of granules (see Table 11-11) and disruption of the phospholipid cell membrane. Both processes result in the release of histamine, bradykinin, leukotrienes, prostaglandins, platelet-activating factor, and chemotactic factors.[5] A similar process can occur in a susceptible patient after exercise. These mediators cause intense inflammation associated with the classic immediate reaction of asthma, which consists of bronchial smooth muscle constriction, increased vasodilation and permeability, and epithelial damage. Clinically the effects are bronchospasm, increased mucus secretion, edema formation, and increased amounts of tenacious sputum (see Fig. 27-2). This immediate response peaks within 30 to 60 minutes of exposure to the trigger (e.g., allergen, irritant) and subsides in another 30 to 90 minutes. Clinically the patient has wheezing, chest tightness, dyspnea, and cough.

The late-phase response in asthma peaks 5 to 6 hours after exposure and may last for several hours or days. It is characterized primarily by inflammation. Eosinophils and neutrophils infiltrate the airways. These cells can subsequently release mediators that cause mast cells to release histamine and other mediators that eventually set up a self-sustaining cycle. In addition, lymphocytes and monocytes influx into the area.

These events, which define the late-phase response, increase airway reactivity that may worsen the symptoms of future asthma attacks. The person becomes hyperresponsive to specific allergens and nonspecific stimuli such as air pollution, cold air, and dust. Identifying the original trigger may be difficult at this point, and less stimulation is required to produce a reaction. The airway hyperreactivity may be related to the exposure of sensory nerve endings as a result of epithelial injury caused by the repeated late-phase responses. Increased airway resistance leads to air trapping in the alveoli and hyperinflation of the lungs.[6-8]

The prominent pathophysiologic features of asthma are a reduction in airway diameter and an increase in airway resistance related to mucosal inflammation, constriction of bronchial smooth muscle, and excess production of mucus (Fig. 27-3). Accompanying these changes are bronchial smooth muscle hypertrophy, basement membrane thickening, mucous gland hypertrophy, thick and tenacious sputum, hyperinflation, and air trapping in the alveoli leading to an increased work of breathing. As a consequence of these events, alterations in respiratory muscle function, abnormal distribution of both ventilation and perfusion, and altered arterial blood gases (ABGs) occur. Although asthma is considered a disease of the airways, eventually all aspects of pulmonary function are compromised during an asthma attack. If airway inflammation is not treated or does not resolve, it may eventually cause progressive, irreversible lung damage.

In addition to the inflammatory aspects of asthma, alterations in the neural control of the airways have been postulated. It is possible, however, that these defects are secondary to the inflammatory process. The autonomic nervous system, consisting of the parasympathetic and sympathetic systems, innervates the bronchi. Airway smooth muscle tone is regulated by the parasympathetic nervous system via the vagus nerve. Afferent and efferent impulses are conducted through the vagus nerve to the medulla and back to the lungs. When airway nerve endings are stimulated by mechanical or chemical stimuli (e.g., air pollution, cold air, dust, allergens), increased release of acetylcholine causes bronchoconstriction.

Both α- and β-adrenergic receptors of the sympathetic nervous system are located in the bronchi. When the α-adrenergic receptors are stimulated, bronchoconstriction occurs. When the β-adrenergic receptors (β_2-adrenergic receptors are primarily located in the bronchi) are stimulated, bronchodilation

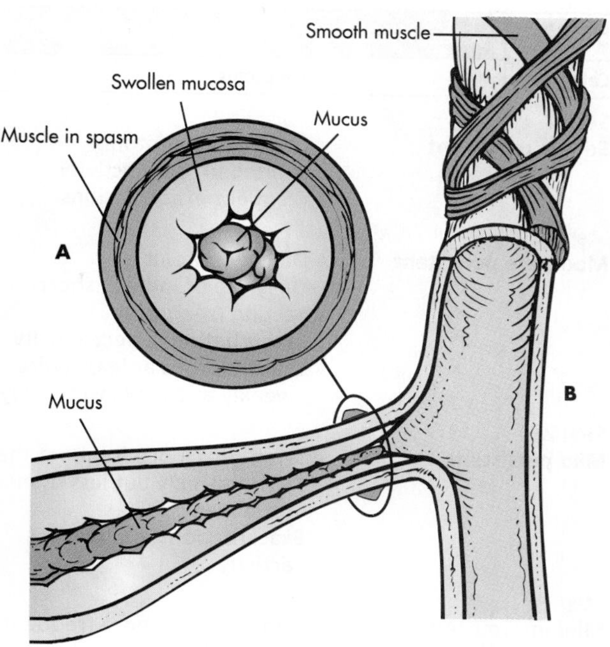

Fig. 27-3 Factors causing expiratory obstruction in asthma. **A,** Cross-section of a bronchiole occluded by muscle spasm, swollen mucosa, and mucus in the lumen. **B,** Longitudinal section of a bronchiole.

occurs. Epinephrine acts on both α- and β-adrenergic receptors, and β_2-adrenergic drugs act primarily on β-adrenergic receptors.

Clinical Manifestations

Asthma is characterized by an unpredictable and variable course. It causes recurrent episodes of wheezing, breathlessness, chest tightness, and cough, particularly at night and in the early morning. An attack of asthma may have an abrupt onset or may be more gradual. Attacks often occur at night and may last for a few minutes to several hours. Between attacks the patient may be asymptomatic with normal and abnormal pulmonary function. However, in some persons, compromised pulmonary function may result in a state of continuous asthma and chronic debilitation characterized by irreversible airway disease.

The characteristic clinical manifestations of asthma are wheezing, cough, dyspnea, and chest tightness after exposure to a precipitating factor or trigger. Expiration may be prolonged. Instead of a normal inspiratory-expiratory ratio of 1:2, it may be prolonged to 1:3 or 1:4. Normally the bronchioles constrict during expiration. However, as a result of bronchospasm, edema, and mucus in the bronchioles, the airways become narrower than usual. Thus it takes longer for the air to move out of the bronchioles. This produces the characteristic wheezing, air trapping, and hyperinflation.

Wheezing is an unreliable sign to gauge the severity of an attack. Many patients with minor attacks wheeze loudly, whereas others with severe attacks do not wheeze. The patient with severe asthmatic attacks may have no audible wheezing because of the marked reduction in airflow. For wheezing to

Table 27-2 Classification of Asthma Severity: Clinical Features Before Treatment

Category	Symptoms	Nocturnal Symptoms	Pulmonary Function*
Step 4 **Severe persistent**	Continual symptoms Limited physical activity Frequent exacerbations	Frequent	FEV_1/PEFR is no greater than 60% of predicted. PEFR variability exceeds 30%.
Step 3 **Moderate persistent**	Daily symptoms Daily use of inhaled short-acting β_2-agonist Exacerbations affect activity Exacerbations at least twice weekly and may last for days	More frequent than once weekly	FEV_1/PEFR exceeds 60% but is less than 80% of predicted. PEFR variability exceeds 30%.
Step 2 **Mild persistent**	Symptoms more frequent than twice weekly but less than once a day Exacerbations may affect activity	More frequent than twice monthly	FEV_1/PEFR is at least 80% of predicted. PEFR variability is between 20% and 30%.
Step 1 **Mild intermittent**	Symptoms no more frequent than twice weekly Asymptomatic and with normal PEFR between exacerbations Exacerbations brief (hours to days) Intensity of exacerbations varies	No more frequent than twice monthly	FEV_1/PEFR is at least 80% of predicted. PEFR variability is less than 20%.

Source: *Practical guide for the diagnosis and management of asthma, based on Expert panel report 2: guidelines for the diagnosis and management of asthma,* Washington, DC, 1997, National Institutes of Health.

*Percent predicted values for forced expiratory volume in 1 second (FEV_1) and percent of personal best for peak expiratory flow rate (PEFR).

NOTES:

- Patients should be assigned to the most severe step in which *any* feature occurs. Clinical features for individual patients may overlap across steps.
- An individual's classification may change over time.
- Patients at any level of severity of chronic asthma can have mild, moderate, or severe exacerbations of asthma. Some patients with intermittent asthma experience severe and life-threatening exacerbations separated by long periods of normal lung function and no symptoms.
- Patients with two or more asthma exacerbations per week (i.e., progressively worsening symptoms that may last hours or days) tend to have moderate to severe persistent asthma.

occur, the patient must be able to move enough air to produce the sound. Wheezing usually occurs first on exhalation. As asthma progresses the patient may wheeze during inspiration and expiration. Severely diminished breath sounds are an ominous sign, indicating severe obstruction and impending respiratory failure.

In some patients with asthma, cough is the only symptom. The bronchospasm may not be severe enough to cause airflow obstruction, but it can increase bronchial tone and cause irritation and stimulation of the cough receptors. The cough may be nonproductive. Mobilizing secretions may be difficult. Secretions may be thick, tenacious, white, gelatinous mucus.

The person with asthma has difficulty with air movement in and out of the lungs, which creates a feeling of suffocation. Therefore during an acute attack, the person with asthma usually sits upright or slightly bent forward using the accessory muscles of respiration to try to get enough air. The more difficult the breathing becomes, the more anxious the patient feels.

Examination of the patient during an acute attack usually reveals signs of hypoxemia, which may include restlessness, increased anxiety, inappropriate behavior, increased pulse and blood pressure, and pulsus paradoxus greater than 12 mm Hg. The respiratory rate is significantly increased (usually greater than 30 breaths per minute) with the use of accessory muscles. Percussion of the lungs indicates hyperresonance, and auscultation indicates the presence of inspiratory or expiratory wheezing. Diminished or absent breath sounds may indicate a significant decrease in air movement resulting from exhaustion and an inability to generate enough muscle force to ventilate. Diminished or absent breath sounds may also indicate atelectasis or pneumothorax.

Classification of Asthma

Asthma can be classified as mild intermittent, mild persistent, moderate persistent, or severe persistent (Table 27-2). Patients may progress up or down in the level of asthma severity over the course of their disease. Good asthma control correlates with minimal symptoms, ability to sleep through the night, and ability to participate in sports, exercise, and strenuous activity.

Complications

Severe acute asthma can result in complications such as rib fractures, pneumothorax, pneumomediastinum, atelectasis, pneumonia, and status asthmaticus.

Table 27-3 Arterial Blood Gas Results Correlated with Clinical Manifestations During an Acute Asthmatic Attack

Time Frame	pH	$PaCO_2$	PaO_2	Physiologic Event	Clinical Manifestations
Early in attack	↑	↓	↓	Alveolar hyperventilation → hypocarbia Hypoxemia secondary to ventilation-perfusion mismatch Adequate alveolar ventilation CO_2 not being eliminated as well	Use of all accessory muscles of ventilation to overcome increased airway resistance Increased heart rate, diaphoresis, chest tightness, cough, wheezing
Progressive attack	N	N	↓	Decrease in effective alveolar ventilation Hypercarbia indicating that ventilation is no longer adequate	Tiring of patient and difficulty with increased work of breathing
Prolonged attack, status asthmaticus	↓	↑	↓	Alveolar hypoventilation → respiratory acidosis Worsening hypoxemia as result of hypoventilation and ventilation-perfusion mismatch	Exhaustion, diminished breath sounds, intubation and mechanical ventilation necessary

Status Asthmaticus. Status asthmaticus is a severe, life-threatening asthma attack that is refractory to usual treatment and places the patient at risk for developing respiratory failure. An axiom describes status asthmaticus: "The longer it lasts, the worse it gets, and the worse it gets, the longer it lasts." Acute asthmatic attacks account for nearly 1 million emergency department (ED) visits a year in the United States, with hundreds of thousands of hospital admissions each year. Of the persons with asthma admitted to the hospital, approximately 10% require intensive care unit (ICU) monitoring or ventilatory assistance for status asthmaticus.[9]

Causes of status asthmaticus include viral illnesses, ingestion of aspirin or other NSAIDs, emotional stress, increases in environmental pollutants or other allergen exposure, abrupt discontinuation of drug therapy (especially corticosteroids and theophylline), abuse of aerosol medication, and ingestion of β-adrenergic blocking agents.[9] Usually the patient reports a history of poorly controlled asthma progressing over days or weeks.

The clinical manifestations of status asthmaticus result from increased airway resistance as a consequence of edema, mucus plugging, and bronchospasm with subsequent air trapping and hyperinflation. The patient has clinical manifestations similar to those of asthma, but they are more severe and more prolonged. Extreme anxiety, fear of suffocation, severely increased work of breathing, and diaphoresis are common. Absence of diaphoresis may indicate significant dehydration. Sternocleidomastoid, intercostal, and supraclavicular muscle retractions reflect increased work of breathing. If obtainable, the peak expiratory flow rate (PEFR) is usually less than 100 to 150 L per minute.

Although wheezing is often audible without a stethoscope, auscultation may not always be reliable because the airflow obstruction may be so severe in some patients that audible wheezing or other abnormal lung sounds may not be produced because of insufficient airflow, also referred to as "quiet chest." The chest appears fixed in a hyperinflated position and is often described as "tight," indicating severely decreased movement of air through the constricted bronchial airways.

Forced exhalation with the use of the abdominal musculature can result in increased intrathoracic pressure transmitted to the great vessels and heart. Neck vein distention and a pulsus paradoxus of 40 mm Hg or higher may result. Usually it is difficult to auscultate pulsus paradoxus secondary to a noisy chest or increased work of breathing. (Pulsus paradoxus is described in Chapter 35.) Hypertension, sinus tachycardia, and ventricular arrhythmias may occur. These three conditions are related to hypoxemia, catecholamines from an endogenous response to hypoxia, and underlying coronary artery disease in the older adult population. Electrocardiogram (ECG) results may show sinus tachycardia or signs of strain on the right side of the heart secondary to pulmonary vasoconstriction, which may be seen as P pulmonale and a right axis deviation.

Hypoxemia with hypocapnia usually occurs initially as the patient attempts to hyperventilate and maintain adequate oxygenation and ventilation. As the severity of the attack increases, the work of breathing increases, making it more difficult for the patient to overcome the increased resistance to breathing. The patient becomes fatigued, causing more carbon dioxide (CO_2) retention. ABGs deteriorate to normocapnia (normal arterial CO_2 pressure) and then ultimately to hypercapnia and hypoxemia (Table 27-3). A moderate elevation in $PaCO_2$ may be tolerated without intubation and mechanical ventilation if the patient remains alert and cooperative and continues to improve during the first 2 to 3 hours of treatment.

Complications of status asthmaticus include pneumothorax, pneumomediastinum, acute cor pulmonale with right ventricular failure, and severe respiratory muscle fatigue leading to respiratory arrest. Death from status asthmaticus is usually the result of respiratory arrest or cardiac failure.

Diagnostic Studies

Wheezing and respiratory distress characterize a variety of disorders, including asthma, chronic bronchitis, emphysema, cystic fibrosis, pulmonary edema, upper airway and bronchial obstruction, tracheobronchitis, bronchiolitis, aspiration, and pulmonary embolism. Therefore certain diagnostic studies

COLLABORATIVE CARE

Table 27-4 Asthma

Diagnostic
Health history and physical examination
Pulmonary function studies including response to bronchodilator therapy
Peak expiratory flow monitoring
Chest x-ray
Measurement of ABGs or oximetry
Allergy skin testing (if indicated)
Blood level of eosinophils and IgE (if indicated)
Collaborative Therapy
Mild or Persistent Asthma
Identification and avoidance/elimination of triggers
Desensitization (immunotherapy) if indicated
Patient and family education
Drug therapy (see Table 27-5)
Asthma management plan (see Table 27-10)
Status Asthmaticus
Inhaled β_2-adrenergic drugs or anticholinergic agents
IV aminophylline (if indicated)
O_2 by mask or nasal prongs
IV corticosteroids
IV fluids
IV magnesium
Intubation and assisted ventilation (if indicated)
Heliox therapy

ABGs, arterial blood gases; *IgE,* immunoglobulin E.

must be performed to determine whether these symptoms are caused primarily by asthma (Table 27-4). The severity of the clinical manifestations of asthma determines the appropriate diagnostic studies.

In the patient who is not in distress, a detailed history may indicate previous attacks of a similar nature, often precipitated by a known cause. Seasonal attacks may indicate pollen triggers. Attacks that occur at night may be caused by sleeping with a cat, sleep apnea, gastroesophageal reflux, or mattress dust mites. It is important to determine whether the patient can sleep through the night or participate in an aerobic exercise program. This information helps identify asthma triggers.

Pulmonary function tests are usually within normal limits between attacks if the patient has no other underlying pulmonary disease. Pulmonary function tests are frequently used to diagnose and manage asthma and are an essential objective measurement of airflow obstruction. The patient with asthma usually has a decrease in forced expiratory volume in 1 second (FEV_1), PEFR, FEV_1 to forced vital capacity (FVC) ratio (FEV_1/FVC), and forced expiratory flow rate measured during the middle of FVC ($FEF_{25\%-75\%}$), with the degree of obstruction depending on the values obtained. (The normal values for pulmonary function tests are discussed in Chapter 24.) PEFR correlates with FEV_1 and is a helpful tool for the patient's clinician to diagnose and manage asthma.

These parameters decrease from their baseline levels during an exacerbation, and some patients may be within normal limits during a remission. Rarely do clinicians require confirmation of the diagnosis by inducing bronchospasm with bronchial provocation testing with known quantities of bronchial irritants such as histamine and methacholine. An increase of 12% to 15% or more in the FEV_1 in response to a bronchodilator when the patient is not experiencing an exacerbation is another diagnostic indicator of asthma.

Eosinophils in the sputum and serum eosinophilia (greater than or equal to 5% of the total white blood cell [WBC]) and elevated serum IgE levels are highly suggestive of asthma in a symptomatic patient. A chest x-ray in an asymptomatic patient with asthma is usually normal. During an acute attack the chest x-ray shows hyperinflation. In a mild asthma attack, ABGs (if obtained) would indicate respiratory alkalosis with an arterial oxygen pressure (PaO_2) near normal. Hypercapnia and respiratory and metabolic acidosis indicate severe disease. In mild asthma pulse oximetry monitoring is sufficient to determine oxygenation status.

Allergy skin testing may be of some value to determine sensitivity to specific allergens (antigens). However, a positive skin test does not necessarily mean that the allergen (antigen) is causing the asthma attack. On the other hand, a negative allergy test does not mean that the asthma is not allergy related. A radioallergosorbent test (RAST) is sometimes used to identify allergic causes in certain patients who show negative skin tests and in those who should not be tested (e.g., patients with severe eczema).

If the patient has wheezing and acute distress, it is not feasible to obtain a detailed health history (although a family member may supply some pertinent information). During an acute attack of asthma, bedside spirometry (specifically FEV_1 or FVC, but usually PEFR) may be used to monitor pulmonary function test results. Serial spirometric parameters, oximetry, and measurement of ABGs help provide information about the severity of the attack and the response to therapy. A complete blood cell count (CBC) and serum electrolytes are also obtained to help direct the course of therapy.

A sputum specimen for Gram's stain and culture may be obtained to rule out the presence of bacterial infection, especially if the patient has purulent sputum, a history of upper respiratory tract infection, a fever, or an elevated WBC count. A chest x-ray obtained during an acute attack usually shows hyperinflation. Occasionally the chest x-ray reveals complications of asthma such as mucoid impaction, pneumothorax, atelectasis, or pneumomediastinum.

Collaborative Care

Mild Intermittent and Persistent Asthma. To help health care professionals bridge the gap between current knowledge and practice, the National Heart, Lung, and Blood Institute's (NHLBI) National Asthma Education and Prevention Program (NAEPP) has convened two expert panels to prepare guidelines for the diagnosis and management of asthma. The charge of the first panel was to develop a report that would provide a general approach to diagnosing and managing asthma based on current science.[2] The second expert panel report (EPR-2) critically reviewed and expanded on the first. The goal of the expert panel is to serve as a comprehensive guide to diagnosing and managing asthma. Implementation of EPR-2 recommendations is likely to increase

Table 27-5 Stepwise Approach for Managing Asthma in Adults

Step	Daily Medication for Long-Term Control	Medication for Quick Relief
Step 4 **Severe persistent**	**Two daily medications** Antiinflammatory agent (high-dose inhaled corticosteroid) ***and*** Long-acting bronchodilator (inhaled or oral β_2-agonist or theophylline) ***and*** Oral corticosteroid	Short-acting inhaled β_2-agonist Daily use or increasing use indicates need for additional long-term therapy
Step 3 **Moderate persistent**	**One or two daily medications** Antiinflammatory agent (medium-dose inhaled corticosteroid) ***and/or*** Medium-dose inhaled corticosteroid plus long-acting bronchodilator	Short-acting inhaled β_2-agonist Daily use or increasing use indicates need for additional long-term therapy
Step 2 **Mild persistent**	**One daily medication** Antiinflammatory agent (low-dose inhaled corticosteroid, cromolyn, or nedocromil) ***or*** Sustained-release theophylline **Note:** Leukotriene modifiers may be considered	Short-acting inhaled β_2-agonist Daily use or increasing use indicates need for additional long-term therapy
Step 1 **Mild intermittent**	**No daily medication**	Short-acting inhaled β_2-agonist Use more than twice weekly may indicate need to initiate long-term therapy

Action Key

Step up if control is not maintained. First, review the patient's medication technique, compliance, and control of environmental triggers.

Step down gradually if review of status at 1- to 6-month intervals suggests reduction in treatment is possible.

Note: Stepped therapy is a guide to assist clinical decision making, not a specific prescription. As a general rule, use the highest appropriate step to gain control quickly. A rescue course of systemic corticosteroids may be needed at any time. Patient education is necessary for environmental control, recognition of warning signals, and medication and monitoring technique assessment and reinforcement at all steps.

Source: *Practical guide for the diagnosis and management of asthma, based on Expert panel report 2: guidelines for the diagnosis and management of asthma,* Washington, DC, 1997, National Institutes of Health.

some costs of asthma care by increasing the initial care and use of medications, but asthma diagnosis and management are expected to improve, which should reduce the numbers of lost school and work days, hospitalizations, emergency department (ED) visits, and deaths caused by asthma.[2,10]

Education for an active partnership with patients remains the cornerstone of asthma management and should be carried out by health care providers delivering asthma care. Education should start at the time of asthma diagnosis and be integrated into every step of clinical asthma care. Asthma self-management should be tailored to the needs of each patient, maintaining a sensitivity to cultural beliefs and practices. Emphasis should be placed on evaluating outcomes in terms of the patient's perceptions of improvement, especially quality of life and the ability to engage in usual activities.

The patient who has persistent airflow obstruction and frequent attacks of asthma should be taught to avoid triggers of acute attacks and to premedicate before exercising. The choice of drug therapy depends on the severity of symptoms (Table 27-5). The patient with mild intermittent asthma or EIA should use inhaled β_2-adrenergic agents, cromolyn (Intal), or nedocromil (Tilade) before exercising or when anticipating exposure to allergens known to cause asthma. Persistent asthma requires regular or maintenance use of inhaled antiinflammatory medication. These include inhaled corticosteroids (used at lowest possible dose to manage symptoms), cromolyn (Intal), and nedocromil (Tilade). In mild persistent asthma cromolyn and nedocromil can be used in place of inhaled corticosteroids. For severe persistent asthma, inhaled or oral corticosteroids, inhaled or oral β_2-agonists, and theophylline may be used to alleviate symptoms. Some persons require continuous oral corticosteroids, which should be maintained at as low a dosage as possible and administered on alternate days (if possible) to reduce systemic side effects.

A patient frequently comes to the ED or a physician's office in acute respiratory distress. The choice of treatment of acute asthma depends on the severity of the attack and response to initial therapy. Severity can be measured objectively by measuring FEV_1 or PEFR. Assessing the degree or amount of change from the patient's personal best PEFR (if known) and the patient's baseline pulse oximetry results can help determine the severity of the attack. Oxygen (O_2) therapy should be started immediately, and its administration should be monitored by pulse oximetry and in more severe cases by measurement of ABGs. Initial therapy should include inhaled β_2-adrenergic agonists administered by metered-dose inhaler (MDI) using spacer devices or nebulizer. Generally, aerosolized medications by nebulizer therapy or by MDI used correctly with a spacer are given every 20 minutes to 4 hours as necessary.[2]

Corticosteroids are indicated if the initial response is insufficient (e.g., no response within 30 to 60 minutes), if the patient has had several recent asthma attacks, or if the patient is receiving oral corticosteroid therapy. The choice of oral or IV administration of corticosteroids depends on the severity of the attack. Therapy should be continued until the patient is breathing comfortably, wheezing has disappeared, and pulmonary function study results are near baseline values.[3] Although the value of administering aminophylline in the treatment of acute asthma has been questioned, intravenous (IV) aminophylline may be considered if the asthma attack is severe or there is minimal or no response to inhaled β_2-agonists.

Status Asthmaticus. Management of the patient with status asthmaticus focuses on correcting hypoxemia and improving ventilation. Most of the therapeutic measures are the same as for acute asthma. It may be necessary, however, to increase the frequency and dose of inhaled bronchodilators. When an MDI is used, the typical dose is two to six puffs every 5 to 20 minutes, depending on the medication selected. Continuous β-agonist nebulizer therapy may be given. Therapy with inhaled agents is usually initiated despite prior home use, because drug delivery at home may have been submaximal and higher doses given under supervision may be beneficial.

Continuous monitoring of the patient is critical. Obtaining even a PEFR during a severe asthma attack is usually not possible. IV aminophylline administration may be added to the treatment regimen if the patient does not respond to β-adrenergic agonists. IV corticosteroids are administered, although their peak effect is not apparent for 6 to 12 hours. IV methylprednisolone is administered every 4 to 6 hours. Sometimes IV magnesium sulfate is given to act as a bronchodilator. Although it is no longer listed in the guidelines for asthma management, subcutaneous epinephrine is occasionally administered. If administered, patients need their BP and ECG monitored closely.

Supplemental O_2 is given by mask or nasal prongs to achieve a PaO_2 of at least 60 mm Hg or an O_2 saturation of greater than or equal to 90%. An arterial catheter may be inserted to facilitate frequent ABG monitoring. Because the patient's insensible loss of fluids is increased and the metabolic rate is increased, IV fluids are given to provide optimal hydration. Sodium bicarbonate administration is usually limited to treatment of severe metabolic or respiratory acidosis (pH less than 7.29), because effective bronchodilation by adrenergic agents is not possible if the patient has extreme acidosis. Bronchoscopy, although rarely performed during an acute attack, may be necessary to remove thick mucous plugs.

Occasionally, asthma attacks are so severe that the patient requires mechanical ventilation if there is no response to treatment. Indications for mechanical ventilation are persistent or progressive CO_2 retention and respiratory acidosis, clinical deterioration indicated by fatigue, hypersomnolence, metabolic acidosis, and cardiopulmonary arrest. In status asthmaticus the goals of initiating mechanical ventilation are to achieve a PaO_2 greater than or equal to 60 mm Hg, O_2 saturation greater than or equal to 90%, and a normal pH. Heliox therapy, which is a mixture of oxygen and helium, is sometimes used during mechanical ventilation or with continuous nebulization to decrease airway resistance and improve ventilation.

Louder wheezing may actually occur in the airways that are responding to the therapy as airflow in the airways increases. As improvement continues and airflow increases, breath sounds increase and wheezing decreases. As the patient begins to respond to therapy and symptoms begin to subside, it is important to remember that despite the disappearance of most of the bronchospasm, the edema and cellular infiltration of the airway mucosa and the viscous mucous plugs may take several days to improve. Thus intensive therapy must be continued even after clinical improvement has occurred. IV corticosteroids are usually tapered rapidly, and the patient is placed on oral corticosteroids, which are tapered over several weeks. Inhaled corticosteroids are usually added when the oral dose is tapered. IV aminophylline (if used), frequent airway care with aerosolized medications, and chest physiotherapy (if indicated) are continued for several days after clinical improvement is noted. The patient's cough often becomes productive of mucous plugs, and breath sounds improve. If the patient is asked to perform a forced expiratory maneuver, a faint wheeze may still be heard. Finally, the patient can be switched to oral bronchodilators and can use a β-adrenergic MDI before discharge.[9]

Drug Therapy (Table 27-6). The NAEPP recommends a stepwise approach to drug therapy with the type and amount of medication dictated by asthma severity (see Table 27-5). The NAEPP emphasizes that persistent asthma requires daily long-term therapy in addition to appropriate medications to manage acute asthma exacerbations.[10] To clarify this concept, the NAEPP now categorizes medications into two general classifications: (1) long-term–control medications to achieve and maintain control of persistent asthma and (2) quick-relief medications to treat symptoms and exacerbations.[2] Because inflammation is considered an early and persistent component of asthma, therapy for persistent asthma must be directed toward long-term suppression of the inflammation.

Antiinflammatory drugs. Because chronic inflammation is a primary component of asthma, corticosteroids, which suppress the inflammatory response, are the most potent and effective antiinflammatory medication currently available.

Table 27-6 Drugs Used in the Treatment of Asthma and Chronic Obstructive Pulmonary Disease

Drug	Route of Administration	Mechanisms of Action	Side Effects	Comments
β-Adrenergic Agonists				
Metaproterenol (Alupent, Metaprel)	Nebulizer, oral tablets, elixir, MDI	Stimulates β-adrenergic receptors, producing bronchodilation. Increases mucociliary clearance.	Tachycardia, BP changes, nervousness, palpitations, muscle tremors, nausea, vomiting, vertigo, insomnia, dry mouth, headache, hypokalemia.	Should not be used in patient with angina or other cardiac disorders. Has fairly rapid onset of action (5-10 min). Duration of action is 3-4 hr. Oral lasts up to 8 hr.
Albuterol (Proventil, Ventolin, Proventil HFA)	Nebulizer, MDI, oral tablets, rotahaler	Selectively stimulates β_2 receptors, producing bronchodilation.	Same as above but cardiac effects are less.	Has rapid onset of action (1-3 min). Duration of action is 4-8 hr.
Pirbuterol (Maxair)	MDI	Same as above.	Same as metaproterenol but cardiac effects are less.	
Terbutaline (Bicanyl, Brethine, Brethair)	Oral tablets, nebulizer, subcutaneous, MDI	Same as above.	Same as above.	Has slow onset of action (except nebulized and subcutaneous route). Duration of action is 4-6 hr.
Bitolterol (Tornalate)	MDI	Same as above.	Same as above.	Duration of action is 4-8 hr.
Epinephrine (Adrenalin)	Subcutaneous, MDI, nebulizer	Stimulates α, β_1, and β_2 receptors, producing bronchodilation.	Headache, dizziness, palpitations, tremors, restlessness, hypertension, arrhythmias, tachycardia.	Used primarily to treat severe bronchial asthma attacks. Should not be used in patient with arrhythmias or hypertension. Instruct patient regarding self-administration of inhalants.
Salmeterol (Serevent)	MDI, DPI	Long acting.	Headache, sore throat, diarrhea, upper respiratory tract infection.	Not to exceed 2 puffs every 12 hours. Not to be used for acute exacerbations.
Antiinflammatory Agents				
Hydrocortisone (Solu-Cortef) Methylprednisolone (Medrol) (Solu-Medrol) Prednisone	IV Oral IV Oral	Have antiinflammatory and immunosuppressive effects. Decrease edema in bronchial airways. Act synergistically with β_2-agonists. Decrease mucus secretion. Effective in late-phase reaction of asthma.	Cushingoid appearance, skin changes (acne, striae, bruising), osteoporosis, increased appetite, obesity; peptic ulcer, hypertension, hypokalemia, cataracts, menstrual irregularities, muscle weakness, immunosuppression, catabolism, dysphonia, growth retardation.	Alternate-day therapy minimizes side effects. Oral dose should be taken in morning with food or milk. When given in high doses, patient must be observed for epigastric distress. H_2 blockers (ranitidine, cimetidine) and antacids may help minimize GI effects. The patient taking long-term corticosteroids may be given vitamin D and calcium to prevent osteoporosis. Should never be abruptly discontinued but tapered gradually over time to prevent adrenal insufficiency. If during tapering patient has recurrence of symptoms, physician should be notified. May be used concomitantly with bronchodilator.

Continued

DRUG THERAPY

Table 27-6 **Drugs Used in the Treatment of Asthma and Chronic Obstructive Pulmonary Disease—cont'd**

Drug	Route of Administration	Mechanisms of Action	Side Effects	Comments
Beclomethasone (Vanceril, Beclovent, Vanceril DS)	MDI, nasal spray	Same as above. Acts locally in respiratory tract with relatively little systemic absorption.	Oral thrush infections, hoarseness, irritated throat, dry mouth, cough, few systemic effects.	Not recommended for acute asthma attack. Rinse mouth with water or mouthwash after use to prevent oral fungal infections. Use of space device with MDI may decrease incidence of thrush. Use after MDI bronchodilator. MDI steroids may be discontinued during acute asthma attack. Nasal spray is used for allergic rhinitis.
Triamcinolone (Azmacort)	MDI	Same as above.	Same as above.	Same as above. Advantage is that it has a built-in spacer device.
Flunisolide (AeroBid, AeroBid-M)	MDI	Same as above.	Same as above.	AeroBid-M contains menthol.
Fluticasone (Flovent)	MDI, DPI	Same as above but with higher potency.	High incidence of yeast infections.	Same as beclomethasone.
Budesonide (Pulmicort)	MDI, DPI	Same as above.	Same as above.	
Cromolyn (Intal)	Nebulizer, MDI, nasal spray	Inhibits release of histamine and SRS-A by acting directly on mast cell. May act by interference with calcium ion influx across cell membrane. Exact mechanism unknown.	Irritation of throat, relatively nontoxic effects, bronchospasm.	Used for asthma (e.g., before exercise) prophylactically if allergen is causative agent. Instruct patient in correct use of inhaler. May follow treatment with glass of water to reduce pharyngeal irritation. May take 4-6 wk before clinical response occurs. Nasal spray (Nasalcrom) used for allergic rhinitis.
Nedocromil (Tilade)	MDI	Similar to cromolyn but with broad-spectrum effects.	Same as above. Transient unpleasant taste, rhinitis.	
Anticholinergics				
Ipratropium (Atrovent)	Nebulizer, MDI	Blocks action of acetylcholine, resulting in bronchodilation.	Drying of oral mucosa, cough, flushing of skin, bad taste.	Alternating schedules of β-adrenergic agonists and atropine administration may be helpful in some patients. Temporary blurred vision will occur if sprayed in eyes.
Ipratropium and albuterol (Combivent)	MDI	Combination of anticholinergic and β-agonist		Patients must be careful not to overuse and take as prescribed.

Methylxanthine Derivatives				
IV agent: aminophylline Oral: Aerolate Choledyl SA Elixophyllin Quibron Slo-Bid Slo-Phyllin Theo-Dur Theolair Theo 24 Uni-Dur Uniphyl	Oral tablets, IV, elixir	Major effects are relaxation of bronchial smooth muscles and improved contractility of fatigued diaphragm. Other effects are mild diuresis, increased gastric acid secretion, stimulation of mucociliary clearance, stimulation of CNS and respiration, pulmonary vasodilation, improved exercise tolerance.	Tachycardia, BP changes, arrhythmias, anorexia, nausea, vomiting, nervousness, irritability, headache, muscle twitching, flushing, epigastric pain, diarrhea, insomnia, palpitations.	Wide variety of response to drug metabolism exists. Half-life is decreased by smoking and is increased by heart failure and liver disease. Cimetidine, ciprofloxacin, erythromycin, and several other drugs may rapidly increase theophylline levels. Gastrointestinal side effects may be alleviated by taking drug with food or antacids. Patient should be instructed to lie down if dizziness is experienced. Patient must be encouraged to take drugs even when feeling well. Extra doses should not be taken when symptoms are present unless prescribed. Side effects should be reported but medication not stopped unless symptoms are severe.
Mucolytics				
Acetylcysteine (Mucomyst) (10% and 20%)	Nebulizer	Enzyme breaks down mucoproteins. Decreases viscosity of mucus and enhances mobilization of secretions.	Bronchospasm, hemoptysis, nausea, vomiting.	After administration of mucolytics, secretions may become profuse. Use of mucolytic agents may not be necessary if patient is kept well hydrated and humidified. Usually combined with bronchodilator when administered.
Guaifenesin (Humibid)	Oral tablets	Expectorant that helps loosen phlegm.	No serious side effects.	
Leukotriene Modifiers				
Leukotriene Receptor Antagonist				
Zafirlukast (Accolate) Montelukast (Singulair)	Oral tablets	Blocks the action of leukotrienes once they are formed. Has both bronchodilators and antiinflammatory effects.	Headache, dizziness; nausea, vomiting, diarrhea, fatigue, abdominal pain	Take at least 1 hour before or 2 hours after meals. Affects metabolism of erythromycin and theophylline. Not to be used to treat acute asthma episodes.
Leukotriene Inhibitors				
Zileuton (Zyflo)	Oral tablets	Inhibits the synthesis of leukotrienes. Has both bronchodilator and antiinflammatory effects.	Elevated liver enzymes; dizziness, insomnia, dyspepsia, abdominal pain	Monitor liver enzymes. May interfere with metabolism of Coumadin and theophylline. Not to be used to treat acute asthma episodes.

BP, blood pressure; *CNS*, central nervous system; *DPI*, dry powder inhaler; *GI*, gastrointestinal; *IV*, intravenous; *MDI*, metered-dose inhaler; *SRS-A*, slow-reacting substance of anaphylaxis.

The inhaled form is used in the long-term control of asthma. Systemic corticosteroids are used in long-term therapy to gain prompt control of asthma in exacerbation and also to manage severe persistent asthma that is not controlled with maximal inhaled therapy.[2]

Corticosteroids. Corticosteroids are remarkably effective in suppressing the inflammation induced by asthma, but are still greatly underused.[11] Corticosteroids do not block the classic immediate response to irritants, allergens, or exercise, but they do block the late-phase response and subsequent bronchial hyperresponsiveness.[12] The onset of action of corticosteroids occurs approximately 3 to 6 hours after oral administration. They act by inhibiting the release of mediators from macrophages and eosinophils, reducing the microvascular leakage in the airways, inhibiting the influx of inflammatory cells into the reactive site, and decreasing peripheral blood eosinophilia.

Usually inhaled corticosteroids must be administered for at least 4 to 5 days before a therapeutic effect can be seen. Newer inhaled corticosteroids (e.g., fluticasone [Flovent], budesonide [Pulmicort]) begin to have a therapeutic effect in 48 to 72 hours. Corticosteroids given by inhalation are active topically and can usually control the disease without systemic side effects. When administered in the aerosol form as MDIs, little systemic absorption occurs, thus eliminating the side effects that result from adrenal suppression seen with oral or IV corticosteroids.

Oropharyngeal candidiasis, hoarseness, and dry cough are local adverse effects caused by inhalation of corticosteroids. These problems can be reduced or prevented by using a spacer with the MDI and by gargling the mouth with water after each use. Using a spacer or holding device for inhalation of inhaled corticosteroids can be helpful in getting more medication into the lungs and less into the stomach, thus decreasing systemic side effects.

Short courses of orally administered corticosteroids are indicated for acute exacerbations of asthma. Side effects associated with short-term therapy include insomnia, heartburn, mood swings, blurry vision, headache, increased appetite, and weight gain. Maintenance doses of oral corticosteroids may be necessary to control asthma in a minority of patients with severe chronic asthma when long-term therapy is required. A single dose in the morning to coincide with endogenous cortisol production and alternate-day dosing are associated with fewer side effects. Side effects of long-term corticosteroid therapy are discussed in Chapter 47.

Postmenopausal women with asthma who use corticosteroids should take adequate amounts of calcium and vitamin D and participate in regular weight-bearing exercise. (Osteoporosis is discussed in Chapter 59.)

Cromolyn and nedocromil. Cromolyn (Intal) is often classified as a mast cell stabilizer. However, its exact mechanism of action is unknown. It inhibits the immediate response from exercise and allergens and prevents the late-phase response. Long-term administration can reduce bronchial hyperreactivity and prevent the increased bronchial hyperreactivity associated with pollens in susceptible asthmatics. It is the antiinflammatory drug of choice in children, but it can also be used successfully in adults for seasonal asthma. It is particularly effective in exercise-induced asthma when used 10 to 20 minutes before exercise. Patient education should emphasize the rationale for use and the correct method of administration of cromolyn.

Nedocromil (Tilade) is a bronchial antiinflammatory agent that has a broad spectrum of effects. It is similar to cromolyn and inhibits both the immediate and late phases of asthmatic response, as well as reduces bronchial hyperreactivity. It can be used as a pretreatment therapy before exposure to environmental irritants, cold air, allergens, or exercise. It is most effective in mild intermittent or mild persistent asthma where frequent bronchodilator therapy is required. The usual dosage is two puffs four times a day, but twice-a-day dosages are usually prescribed. The most common side effects are a transient, mild, unpleasant taste and rhinitis.

Leukotriene modifiers. Two new groups of drugs, leukotriene receptor antagonists (zafirlukast [Accolate], montelukast [Singulair]) and leukotriene synthesis inhibitors (zileuton [Zyflo]), are currently being used for the treatment of asthma. These types of drugs interfere with the synthesis or block the action of leukotrienes. Leukotrienes are produced from arachidonic acid metabolism (see Fig. 11-7). Leukotrienes are potent bronchoconstrictors, and some also cause airway edema and inflammation, thus contributing to the symptoms of asthma.[12] A broad range of patients, from those with mild symptoms to those with more severe asthma, can benefit from taking leukotriene modifiers. They are not indicated for use in the reversal of bronchospasm in acute asthma attacks. It is also recommended that these drugs not be used as the only therapy for treatment of persistent asthma. A major advantage of these drugs is that they have both bronchodilator and antiinflammatory effects.[13]

Bronchodilators. Three classes of bronchodilator drugs currently used in asthma therapy are β-adrenergic agonists, methylxanthine derivatives, and anticholinergics.

β-Adrenergic agonist drugs. Inhaled β_2-agonists such as albuterol (Proventil, Proventil HFA, and Ventolin), metaproterenol (Alupent), bitolterol (Tornalate), and pirbuterol (Maxair) have an onset of action within minutes and are effective for 4 to 8 hours. Inhaled β-agonists are indicated for the short-term relief of bronchoconstriction and are the treatment of choice for acute exacerbations of asthma. β_2-Agonists are also useful in preventing bronchospasm precipitated by exercise and other stimuli because they prevent mediator release from mast cells. They do not inhibit the late-phase response. If used frequently, inhaled β_2-agonists may produce tremors, anxiety, tachycardia, palpitations, and nausea.

Longer-acting (8 to 12 hour) inhaled β_2-agonists include salmeterol (Serevent). These drugs are useful for nocturnal asthma. Patient education should stress that these drugs are used only every 12 hours and are not used as reserve therapy to obtain quick relief from bronchospasm like the shorter-acting β-agonists.

Orally administered β-agonists are less useful because of the increased incidence of side effects. The most common side effects of inhaled β-agonists are tremor, tachycardia, and palpitations. Some of these side effects can be decreased by teaching the patient to avoid contact between the medication and the tongue. Because the tongue has many blood vessels, rapid absorption of these drugs can occur. Excessive use of β-agonists may cause hypokalemia. Therefore their use should be monitored carefully in patients on long-term diuretic or corticosteroid therapy.

Methylxanthines. Methylxanthine (theophylline) preparations are less effective bronchodilators than inhaled β-agonists.[10] The trend is now toward introducing theophylline as an additional bronchodilator later in the therapeutic regimen. Theophylline may have a synergistic effect with β-agonists. It is not effective as an inhalant and must be given orally or IV as aminophylline. Sustained-release theophylline preparations are preferable for maintenance therapy.

Although the exact mechanism of action is unknown, the main therapeutic action of methylxanthine derivatives is bronchodilation, which is useful in the early-phase response. Only minimal bronchodilation occurs at therapeutic theophylline concentrations.

Theophylline alleviates the early phase of asthma attacks and the bronchoconstrictive portion of the late-phase asthmatic response. However, it has no effect on bronchial hyperresponsiveness. Long-acting theophylline products administered at bedtime may be used to treat the patient with nocturnal asthma. The main problem with theophylline is the relatively high incidence of side effects, which include nausea, headache, gastrointestinal distress, tachycardia, arrhythmias, and seizures.

Theophylline administration requires monitoring of its serum concentrations for safe and effective use. Many foods, drugs, and pathophysiologic conditions can alter the metabolism of theophylline. The end result can be subtherapeutic or toxic concentrations with previously appropriate doses. Drugs that inhibit the metabolism of theophylline, thus causing elevated levels of theophylline in the blood, include cimetidine (Tagamet), erythromycin, ciprofloxacin (Cipro), diltiazem (Cardizem), verapamil (Calan, Isoptin), and allopurinol.

Anticholinergic drugs. Airway diameter is predominantly controlled by the parasympathetic division of the autonomic nervous system. The effects of acetylcholine on the airways are increased mucus secretion and smooth muscle contraction, resulting in bronchoconstriction. Anticholinergic agents (e.g., ipratropium [Atrovent]) inhibit only the component of bronchoconstriction related to the parasympathetic nervous system. Thus these drugs are less effective than β_2-agonists and are usually used in combination with other bronchodilators. Anticholinergic agents produce most of their bronchodilation in larger airways, in contrast to β_2-agonists, which act primarily in smaller airways. Anticholinergics are not useful in routine asthma management but may be used as alternative bronchodilators for patients with severe adverse effects from β_2-agonist inhalers. They may also provide additive effects used in combination with β_2-agonists (e.g., Combivent).

The onset of action of anticholinergics is slower than β_2-agonists, peaking at 1 hour and lasting longer, usually up to 4 to 6 hours. Systemic side effects of inhaled anticholinergics are uncommon because they are poorly absorbed.

Patient teaching related to drug therapy. Information about medications should include the name, dosage, method of administration, and schedule, taking into consideration meal times and other activities of daily living (ADLs), purpose, side effects, appropriate action if side effects occur, consequences of improper use, and the importance of refilling the prescription before the medication runs out.

One of the major factors in asthma management is the correct administration of medications.[14] The majority of asthma medications are administered only or preferably by inhalation. Inhalation of drugs is often preferred to oral administration because a lower dose is needed and systemic side effects are reduced. In addition, the onset of action of bronchodilators is faster. Inhalation devices include nebulizers and MDIs. Nebulizers, which generally deliver a larger dose of medication, are usually used for severe asthma. MDIs are usually effective, but some persons, particularly older adults, may have problems with the coordination needed to activate the MDI and inhale the medication. Poor coordination can be solved by the use of spacer devices (Aerochamber, Inspirease) (Fig. 27-4) or the use of a breath-activated MDI (Maxair Autoinhaler). If the patient is still unable to receive adequate medication, a nebulizer may be used.

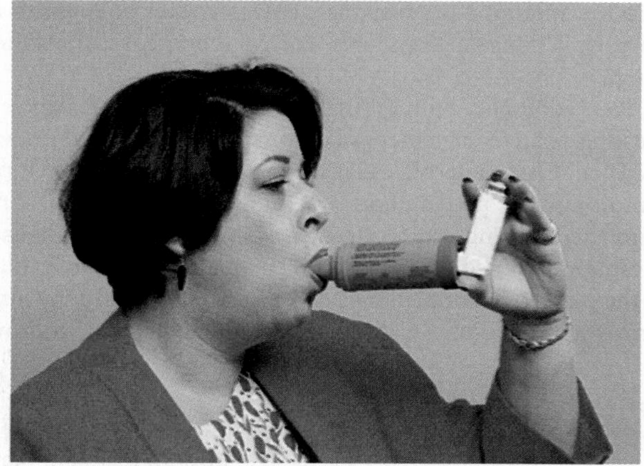

Fig. 27-4 Example of an AeroChamber spacer used with a metered-dose inhaler.

The patient should be given instructions on the use of MDIs (Fig. 27-5). Many patients using MDI are performing the technique incorrectly. Because at best only 10% to 15% of the inhaled medication reaches the lung, correct use of MDI technique is imperative. Problems commonly observed with MDI use are presented in Table 27-7. It is helpful to observe the patient from the side and evaluate each step in the MDI process. Even experienced asthmatic inhaler users frequently make errors in technique. Videos (available from pharmaceutical companies) on correct inhaler technique can be helpful.

The inhaler should be cleaned by removing the dust cap and rinsing it in warm water (see Fig. 27-5). The patient who needs to use several MDIs is often unclear about the order in which to take the medications. As a general rule, β_2-agonists should be used first to open the airway if needed at that time. Corticosteroid inhalers should be used last because they require gargling after use to prevent oral candidiasis. Numbering the inhalers in order of use and marking the number of puffs in large, indelible markers on the inhaler has proved valuable for some patients.

One of the major problems with metered-dose drugs is the potential for overuse (i.e., using them much more frequently than prescribed rather than seeking needed medical care), especially β-agonist MDIs. As a patient develops additional asthmatic symptoms, she or he may use the β-agonist MDI repeatedly. β-Agonists help by relieving bronchospasm; they do not treat the inflammatory response. Therefore the patient must receive explicit instructions in the correct therapeutic use of these drugs.

Poor adherence with asthma therapy is a major challenge in the long-term management of chronic asthma. The patient will use β-agonist inhalers because they provide immediate relief of symptoms. The patient, however, often does not take the long-term therapy (inhaled corticosteroids or cromolyn) regularly because no immediate benefit is seen. It is important to explain to the patient the importance and purpose of taking the long-term therapy regularly, emphasizing that maximal improvement may take more than 1 week. It is important to emphasize that without regular use the swelling in the airways may progress and the asthma will likely worsen over time.

Nonprescription combination drugs. Several nonprescription combination drugs are available over the counter. They are usually combinations of a bronchodilator, an expectorant, and a sedative (Table 27-8). These agents are advertised as drugs to relieve bronchospasm. In general they should be avoided. Many persons consider these drugs safe because they can be obtained without a prescription. Some of the dangers of these drugs are as follows:

How To Use Your Metered-Dose Inhaler the Right Way

Using an inhaler seems simple, but most patients do not use it the right way. When you use your inhaler the wrong way, less medicine gets to your lungs. (Your doctor may give you other types of inhalers.)

For the next 2 weeks, read these steps aloud as you do them or ask someone to read them to you. Ask your doctor or nurse to check how well you are using your inhaler.

Use your inhaler in one of the three ways pictured below (**A** or **B** are best, but **C** can be used if you have trouble with **A** and **B**).

Steps for Using Your Inhaler

Getting ready

1. Take off the cap and shake the inhaler.
2. Breathe out all the way.
3. Hold your inhaler the way your doctor said (A, B, or C below).

Breathe in slowly

4. As you start breathing in **slowly** through your mouth, press down on the inhaler **one** time. (If you use a holding chamber, first press down on the inhaler. Within 5 sec, begin to breathe in slowly.)
5. Keep breathing in **slowly**, as deeply as you can.

Hold your breath

6. Hold your breath as you count to 10 slowly, if you can.
7. For inhaled quick-relief medicine (β_2-agonists), wait about 1 min between puffs. There is no need to wait between puffs for other medicines.

A. Hold inhaler 1 to 2 in in front of your mouth (about the width of two fingers).

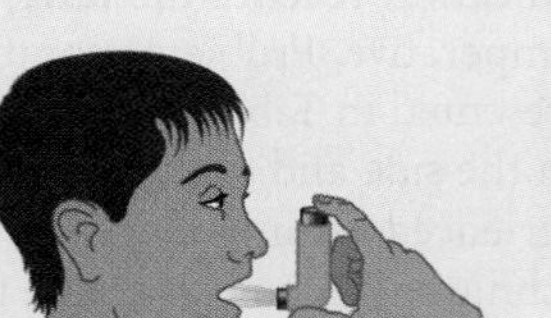

B. Use a spacer/holding chamber. These come in many shapes and can be useful to any patient.

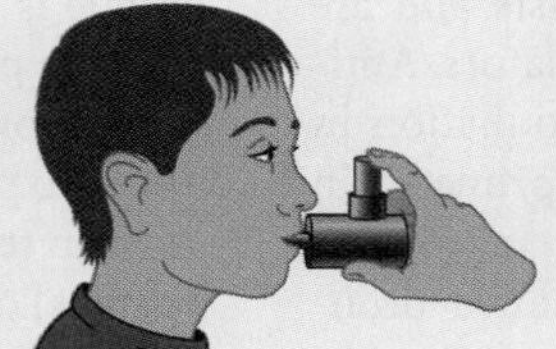

C. Put the inhaler in your mouth. Do not use for steroids.

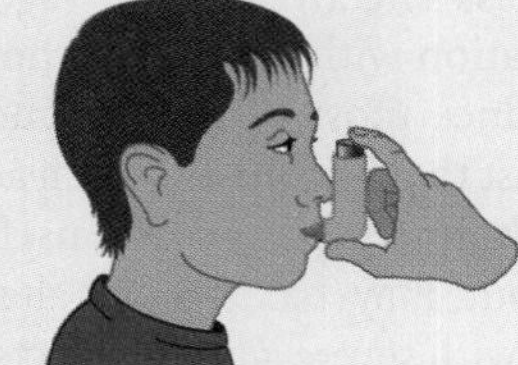

Clean Your Inhaler as Needed

Look at the hole where the medicine sprays out from your inhaler. If you see "powder" in or around the hole, clean the inhaler. Remove the metal canister from the L-shaped plastic mouthpiece. Rinse only the mouthpiece and cap in warm water. Let them dry overnight. In the morning, put the canister back inside. Put the cap on.

Know When to Replace Your Inhaler

For medicines you take each day (an example): Say your new canister has 200 puffs (number of puffs is listed on canister) and you are told to take 8 puffs per day.

8 puffs per day) 200 puffs in canister = 25 days

So this canister will last 25 days. If you started using this inhaler on May 1, replace it on or before May 25.

You can write the date on your canister.

For quick-relief medicine take as needed and count each puff.

Do not put your canister in water to see if it is empty. This does not work.

Fig. 27-5 How to use your metered-dose inhaler the right way.

1. Epinephrine, found in Primatene spray, acts only for a short time and may increase the patient's heart rate and blood pressure.
2. Theophylline, taken with other xanthines including caffeine, has an additive effect. Side effects include central nervous system (CNS) and cardiovascular effects, vomiting, nausea, and anorexia.
3. A combination of ephedrine (found in many OTC decongestants) and theophylline causes synergistic stimulation of the central nervous and cardiovascular systems. Side effects include nervousness, heart palpitations and arrhythmias, tremors, and insomnia.

An important teaching responsibility of the health professional is to warn the patient about the dangers associated with nonprescription combination drugs. These drugs are especially dangerous to a patient with underlying cardiac problems. The patient who persists in taking one of these medications should be cautioned to read and follow the accompanying directions on the label. Another way of discouraging the use of these drugs is to carefully monitor and reevaluate the effectiveness of the prescribed drug therapy. The drug regimen may have to be adjusted to help the patient obtain maximum relief from bronchospasm. An attitude of understanding and caring will often reassure the patient that the health care worker is concerned. This may prevent the patient from attempting to find relief at the local drugstore.

Table 27-7 Problems Encountered with Metered-Dose Inhaler Use

1. Failing to coordinate activation with inspiration
2. Activating MDI in the mouth while breathing through nose
3. Inspiring too rapidly
4. Not holding the breath for 10 sec (or as close to 10 sec as possible)
5. Holding MDI upside down or sideways
6. Inhaling more than 1 puff with each inspiration
7. Not shaking MDI before use
8. Not waiting a sufficient amount of time between each puff
9. Not opening mouth wide enough, causing medication to bounce off teeth, tongue, or palate
10. Not having adequate strength to activate MDI
11. Unable to understand and incorporate directions

NURSING MANAGEMENT: ASTHMA

Nursing Assessment

If a patient can speak and is not in acute distress, a detailed health history, including identification of any precipitating factors and what has helped alleviate attacks in the past, can be taken. Subjective and objective data that should be obtained from a patient with asthma are presented in Table 27-9.

Nursing Diagnoses

Nursing diagnoses for the patient with asthma may include, but are not limited to, those presented in NCP 27-1.

Planning

The overall goals are that the patient with asthma will have (1) normal or near-normal pulmonary function, (2) normal activity levels (including exercise and other physical activity), (3) no recurrent exacerbations of asthma or decreased incidence of asthma attacks, and (4) adequate knowledge to participate in and carry out management.

Nursing Implementation

Health Promotion. The nursing role in preventing asthma attacks or decreasing their severity focuses primarily on teaching the patient and family. The patient should be taught to identify and avoid known personal triggers for asthma (e.g., cigarette smoke, pet dander) and irritants (e.g., cold air, aspirin, foods, cats, indoor air pollution). If cold air cannot be avoided, dressing properly with scarves or using a mask helps reduce the risk of an asthma attack. Aspirin and NSAIDs should be avoided if they are known to precipitate an attack. Many OTC drugs contain aspirin, and the patient should be instructed to read the labels carefully. β-Adrenergic receptor blocking agents (e.g., propranolol [Inderal]) are contraindicated because they inhibit bronchodilation. Desensitization (immunotherapy) may be partially effective in decreasing the patient's sensitivity to known allergens (see Chapter 12).

Table 27-8 Nonprescription Combination Asthma Drugs

	Ingredients		
Drug Product	**Sympathomimetic**	**Xanthine**	**Other**
Amodrine	Ephedrine	Aminophylline	Phenobarbital
Asthma Nefrin inhalant	Epinephrine	—	Chlorobutanol
Bronkaid tablets	Ephedrine	Theophylline	Guaifenesin
Bronkaid mist	Epinephrine	—	Ascorbic acid, alcohol
Bronkotabs	Ephedrine	Theophylline	Guaifenesin, phenobarbital
Primatene M tablets	Ephedrine	Theophylline	Pyrilamine
Primatene P tablets	Ephedrine	Theophylline	Phenobarbital
Primatene Mist	Epinephrine	—	Ascorbic acid, alcohol
Tedral	Ephedrine	Theophylline	Phenobarbital
Vaponefrin inhalant	Epinephrine	—	Chlorobutanol
Verquad	Ephedrine	Theophylline	Guaifenesin, phenobarbital

NURSING ASSESSMENT

Table 27-9 Asthma

Subjective Data	Objective Data
Important Health Information *Past health history:* Allergic rhinitis or sinusitis; previous asthma attack; exposure to pollen, danders, feathers, mold, dust, inhaled irritants, weather changes, exercise, smoke; sinus infections; gastroesophageal reflux *Medications:* Use of and compliance with corticosteroids, bronchodilators, cromolyn sodium, anticholinergics, antibiotics; medications that may precipitate an attack in susceptible asthmatics such as aspirin, nonsteroidal antiinflammatory drugs, beta-blockers **Functional Health Patterns** *Health perception–health management:* Family history of allergies or asthma; recent upper respiratory infection or sinus infection *Activity-exercise:* Fatigue, decreased or absent exercise tolerance; dyspnea, cough, productive cough with yellow or green sputum; chest tightness, feelings of suffocation, air hunger *Sleep-rest:* Interrupted sleep, insomnia *Coping–stress tolerance:* Fear, anxiety, emotional distress, stress in work environment or in the home	**General** Restlessness or exhaustion, confusion, upright or forward-leaning body position **Integumentary** Diaphoresis, cyanosis (circumoral, nailbed) **Respiratory** Wheezing, crackles, diminished or absent breath sounds, and rhonchi on auscultation; hyperresonance on percussion; sputum (thick, white, tenacious), increased work of breathing with use of accessory muscles; intercostal and supraclavicular retractions; tachypnea with hyperventilation; prolonged expiration **Cardiovascular** Tachycardia, pulsus paradoxus, jugular venous distention, hypertension or hypotension, premature ventricular contractions **Possible Findings** Abnormal ABGs during attacks, decreased O_2 saturation, serum and sputum eosinophilia, elevated serum IgE, positive skin tests for allergens, chest x-ray demonstrating hyperinflation with attacks, abnormal pulmonary function tests showing decreased flow rates; FVC, FEV_1, PEFR, and FEV_1/FVC ratio that improve between attacks and with bronchodilators

FEV_1, forced expiratory volume at 1 second; *FVC,* forced vital capacity, *PEFR,* peak expiratory flow rate.

Prompt diagnosis and treatment of upper respiratory tract infections and sinusitis may prevent an exacerbation of asthma. If occupational irritants are involved as etiologic factors, the patient may need to consider changing jobs. The patient should be encouraged to maintain a fluid intake of 2 to 3 L per day, good nutrition, and adequate rest. If exercise is planned, administering a β-agonist, cromolyn, or nedocromil 10 to 20 minutes before the activity should prevent bronchospasm.

Acute Intervention. During an acute attack of asthma, it is important to monitor the patient's respiratory and cardiovascular systems. This includes auscultating lung sounds; taking the pulse rate, respiratory rate, and BP; and monitoring ABGs, pulse oximetry, and FEV_1 and PEFR. The patient's work of breathing (i.e., use of accessory muscles, degree of fatigue) and response to therapy should also be evaluated. If the patient's condition deteriorates, the physician must be notified immediately to initiate prompt medical intervention. Nursing interventions include administering O_2, bronchodilators, chest physical therapy, and medications (as ordered) and ongoing patient monitoring, including the effectiveness of these interventions.

An important nursing goal during an acute attack is to decrease the patient's sense of panic. A calm, quiet, reassuring attitude may help the patient relax. The patient should be positioned comfortably (usually sitting) to maximize chest expansion. Staying with the patient and being available provide additional comfort. Encouraging slow breathing using pursed lips for prolonged exhalation can be helpful.

When the acute attack subsides, the nurse should provide rest and a quiet, calm environment for the patient. When the patient has recovered from exhaustion, the nurse should attempt to obtain information about the patient's health history and pattern of asthma. If family members are present, they may be able to provide information about the patient's health history. A thorough physical assessment should be completed (see Table 27-9). This information is important in planning an individualized nursing care plan for the patient. Well-thought-out written plans involving the patient and significant others increase the patient's knowledge and control of the situation and may help improve confidence and compliance.

Ambulatory and Home Care. It is important to remember that asthma is potentially controllable and that every effort should be made to keep the patient free of symptoms. The patient with asthma usually takes several medications with different routes of administration and time frames for dosage (e.g., tapering corticosteroid schedules, using several different inhalers with different indications). The drug regimen itself can be confusing and complex. The patient with asthma must learn about the numerous medications and develop self-management strategies. The patient and the health professional need to monitor the patient's responsiveness to medication. It is easy to undermedicate or overmedicate a patient with asthma unless careful monitoring is ongoing. Some

27-1 NURSING CARE PLAN PATIENT WITH ASTHMA

Expected Patient Outcomes	Nursing Interventions and *Rationales*
NURSING DIAGNOSIS	**Ineffective breathing pattern** *related to* increased airway resistance caused by bronchospasm, mucosal edema, and mucus production *as manifested by* dyspnea, wheezing, rapid respiratory rate, use of accessory muscles.
▪ Absence of wheezing and chest tightness. ▪ Return of appropriate breath sounds indicating better airflow. ▪ Respiratory rate of 12-24/min. ▪ ABGs/oximetry and pulmonary function tests within normal limits or returned to baseline.	▪ Assess heart rate, respiratory rate, lung sounds, decreased airflow, accessory muscle use, and color of mucous membranes and lips *to identify acute dyspnea.* ▪ Provide comfortable position (e.g., bed rest in high Fowler's position or recliner chair) *to maximize chest expansion and promote prolonged expiratory phase to reduce trapped air.* ▪ Administer bronchodilators as ordered *to treat bronchospasm.* ▪ Administer O_2 as ordered *to increase oxygen saturation.* ▪ Auscultate breath sounds *to monitor effectiveness of treatment and patient status.* ▪ Monitor ABGs or pulse oximetry *to monitor oxygen saturation,* PaO_2*, and* $PaCO_2$. ▪ Premedicate with bronchodilators before deep-breathing and coughing exercises or chest physiotherapy *to open airways for more efficient movement of sputum toward mouth.* ▪ Evaluate effectiveness of nebulizer treatments by assessing lung sounds, secretion clearance, PEFR, and oximetry *to assess need for increase or decrease in frequency of treatments.* ▪ Teach patient to breathe deeply through the nose and exhale 2-3 times as long as inspiration through pursed lips *to increase vital capacity and increase* PaO_2 *and decrease respiratory rate.*
NURSING DIAGNOSIS	**Ineffective airway clearance** *related to* bronchospasm, ineffective cough, excessive mucus production, tenacious secretions, and fatigue *as manifested by* ineffective cough, inability to raise secretions, adventitious breath sounds.
▪ Breath sounds indicating good air movement. ▪ Effective or productive cough of clear or white secretions.	▪ Monitor and control environment for possible allergens (e.g., dust, smoke, flowers) *to reduce exacerbating asthma attack.* ▪ Teach effective coughing techniques *so patient can clear airways by propelling secretions toward mouth for expectoration.* ▪ If patient is unable to cough or expectorate secretions, evaluate possible causes (e.g., respiratory muscle fatigue, pain, thick secretions, severe bronchospasm, decreased level of consciousness) *so appropriate intervention can be initiated.* ▪ As ordered, assist in and evaluate administration of bronchodilator drugs, mucolytic drugs (e.g., guaifenesin), corticosteroid therapy, chest physiotherapy *to improve respiratory status.* ▪ Observe and note character and quantity of coughed or suctioned sputum and secretions *to determine presence of infection.* ▪ If ordered, send sputum for Gram's stain and culture and sensitivity.
NURSING DIAGNOSIS	**Anxiety** *related to* difficulty breathing, perceived or actual loss of control, and fear of suffocation *as manifested by* restlessness, elevated pulse and blood pressure.
▪ Calm feeling. ▪ Less anxiety over asthma.	▪ Give simple, concise explanations demonstrating and repeating (as necessary) *to increase understanding and foster cooperation.* ▪ Stay with the patient *to provide reassurance and reduce anxiety.* ▪ Anticipate patient's needs. ▪ Provide anticipatory guidance for patient to prevent exacerbations. ▪ Promptly treat any exacerbations of an attack *to prevent development of status asthmaticus.* ▪ Place in room near nurses' station *to provide reassurance to patient that help is nearby and to allow for frequent observation.* ▪ Teach relaxation techniques *to reduce anxiety.* ▪ Explain that some medications (e.g., frequent β_2-agonists, corticosteroids, theophylline) may further increase anxiety and irritability.

Continued

27-1 NURSING CARE PLAN PATIENT WITH ASTHMA—continued

Expected Patient Outcomes	Nursing Interventions and *Rationales*
NURSING DIAGNOSIS **Risk for infection** *related to* decreased pulmonary function, ineffective airway clearance, and possible corticosteroid therapy.	
■ No sputum or clear to white sputum. ■ Normal temperature. ■ Clear chest x-ray.	■ Assess for manifestations of a respiratory infection such as elevated temperature, pulse, and respiration; increased coughing; change in color, consistency, or amount of sputum; adventitious breath sounds. ■ If sputum is mucopurulent, obtain sputum Gram's stain and culture and sensitivity *to determine infecting organism.* ■ Administer antibiotic as ordered *to treat the infection.* ■ Monitor temperature q4hr and prn, sputum character and quantity *to assess for signs of infection.* ■ Monitor for localized decrease in breath sounds, decreased PaO_2, inability to raise secretions *to determine a worsening of condition.* ■ Provide deep-breathing and coughing exercises (if needed) *to improve breathing and raise secretions.*
NURSING DIAGNOSIS **Ineffective management of therapeutic regimen** *related to* lack of knowledge about asthma and its treatment *as manifested by* frequent questioning regarding all aspects of long-term management (refer to patient and family teaching guide [Table 27-12]).	

PEFR, peak expiratory flow rate.

patients may benefit from keeping a diary to record medication use, the presence of wheezing or coughing, PEFR, the drug's side effects, and the activity level. This information will be valuable in helping the health care provider adjust the medication. The patient must understand the importance of continuing the medication even when symptoms are not present. If worsening bronchospasm or severe side effects of the drugs occur, the patient should seek medical attention.

Good nutrition is important. Physical exercise (e.g., swimming, walking, stationary cycling) within the patient's limit of tolerance is also beneficial. If dyspnea occurs on exertion, it can often be prevented with the use of a β-agonist MDI, cromolyn, or nedocromil. Adequate rest and uninterrupted (from asthma symptoms) sleep are important.

A written asthma management plan (Table 27-10) should be developed together with the patient and family. Most plans are developed based on the patient's asthma symptoms and peak flow readings. A management plan can be established when the patient's best peak flow is established and the patient has good asthma control (e.g., not waking up at night with asthma symptoms, able to perform some type of aerobic exercise or strenuous activity, not having frequent daily symptoms).

To follow the management plan, the patient must measure his or her peak flow at least daily. Patients with asthma frequently do not perceive changes in their breathing. The longer a person has asthma, the more the person becomes used to breathing at lower lung capacities. Therefore peak flow monitoring when done correctly can be a good objective measurement of asthma (Table 27-11). Using PEFR is similar to using BP monitoring in a person with hypertension.

If a patient's PEFR is within the green zone (usually 80% to 100% of the person's personal best), the patient should remain on her or his usual medications.[15] Patients who get a cold or sinus infection, which may trigger asthma, can usually increase the dose of the corticosteroid inhaler one third to one half, depending on the asthma management plan. The dose can be decreased once the cold subsides.

If the PEFR is within the yellow zone (usually 50% to 80% of personal best), it indicates caution. Something is triggering the patient's asthma. Different strategies may be employed by the patient based on the asthma management plan. For example, the patient could use the β_2-agonist inhaler more frequently.

If the PEFR is in the red zone (50% or less of personal best), it indicates a serious problem. Definitive action must be taken. In addition to increasing the use of β_2-agonist inhalers, oral corticosteroids may be indicated. The patient may also need to contact or be seen by the health care provider.

It is important to emphasize to the patient the need to monitor PEFR daily because most people get in trouble with their asthma over time. Although it may occur, it is unusual for a patient's PEFR to drop from the green zone to the red zone quickly. Usually the patient has time to make changes in medications, avoid triggers, and notify the health care provider.

When developing a management plan, it is important to involve the patient's family. Often the family member feels frustrated and does not know how to help. The family member or significant other should be taught what can be done to help the patient during an asthmatic attack. This person should know where the patient's inhalers, oral medications, and emergency phone numbers are located. The significant other can also be instructed on how to decrease the patient's anxiety if an asthma attack occurs. When the patient is stabilized or controlled, the significant other can gently remind the patient about doing daily PEFR by asking questions such as, "What zone are you in? How's your peak flow today?"

Table 27-10 Asthma Management Plan

Name: **Personal Best Peak Flow:** **Date:**

Green—GO

- Breathing is good
- No coughing, wheezing, chest tightness, or shortness of breath
- No problems talking or walking

Peak Flow Number:
_________ to _________
(80-100% of Best)

PLAN A: Continue regular medicines. Use **preventer** medicines all the time.
Brochodilator Inhaler **(Quick Reliever):** __________
Steroid Inhaler **(Preventer/Controller):** __________
Other Inhaler/Nebs: __________
Additional Instructions:

- At the first sign of a cold, you may double the dose of the steroid inhaler until the cold subsides. Then resume usual dose.
- Monitor your peak flows daily. When exposed to triggers or when you have a cold, monitor your peak flows at least 2 times/day or more.
- Use quick reliever medicine 10 minutes before exercise if you have exercise-induced asthma.

Yellow—CAUTION

- Mild to moderate symptoms
- Coughing, wheezing, chest tightness, or shortness of breath
- No problems talking or walking but may feel anxious
- Unable to sleep because of asthma symptoms

Peak Flow Number:
_________ to _________
(50-80% of Best)

PLAN B: Continue Plan A and add quick reliever medicine.

❶ Immediately take 2-4 puffs of quick reliever __________ or by nebulizer treatment.
❷ Wait 20 minutes.
- If peak flow returns to Green Zone or asthma symptoms subside, follow Green Zone plan.
- If peak flow remains in the Yellow Zone and/or symptoms do not improve, repeat ❶ and ❷. You may repeat this a third time if still not improved.

❸ If still in the Yellow Zone after ______ hours and/or symptoms do not improve, __________ or begin prednisone (Deltasone) or Medrol on the following schedule: __________

WARNING: If at any time you progress to the Red Zone, proceed to Plan C.

Red—STOP—Danger

Severe Symptoms

- Continuous coughing, wheezing, chest tightness, or shortness of breath
- Able to speak in short sentences only but feel very anxious
- Lips and nails still pink color

Peak Flow Number:
_________ to _________
(0-50% of Best)

PLAN C: This is the **DANGER ZONE!** Act immediately.

❶ Immediately take 2-6 puffs of quick reliever or nebulizer treatment __________
❷ If you are still in the Red Zone in 10-20 minutes, begin prednisone (Deltasone) or Medrol on the following schedule, if instructed to do so: __________
❸ Repeat ❶ and ❷ for a total of three times in 1 hour if asthma symptoms persist.
❹ Call your health care provider if you do not have instructions to begin prednisone (Deltasone) or Medrol or if your symptoms do not improve.

Very Severe Symptoms ➡

- Severe chest tightness, struggling to breathe, hunching over, chest pulled or sucked in with each breath
- Having trouble walking and talking
- Must stop activity you are doing and cannot start again
- Lips and nails may be blue

STOP

PLAN D: Call 911 immediately to be taken to the emergency room.

- Take 6 puffs of beta bronchodilator (quick reliever) inhaler every 5-10 minutes OR take a continuous nebulizer treatment while waiting or in route.
- If you have prednisone, take 40 mg immediately.

Any time you are having an asthma episode **STAY CALM.** Breathe out slowly through pursed lips. If possible, identify the specific trigger for this episode and try to avoid it. If you need help, call your health care provider.

____________________ ____________________
Provider Signature *Patient Signature*

Source: Lovelace Health Systems Adult Asthma Program, Albuquerque, NM.

PATIENT TEACHING GUIDE

Table 27-11 **How to Use Your Peak Flow Meter**

A peak flow meter helps you check how well your asthma is controlled. Peak flow meters are most helpful for people with moderate or severe asthma.

This guide will tell you (1) how to find your personal best peak flow number, (2) how to use your personal best number to set your peak flow zones, (3) how to take your peak flow, and (4) when to take your peak flow to check your asthma each day.

Starting Out: Find Your Personal Best Peak Flow Number

To find your personal best peak flow number, take your peak flow each day for 2 to 3 weeks. Your asthma should be under good control during this time. Take your peak flow as close to the times listed below as you can. (These times for taking your peak flow are *only* for finding your personal best peak flow. To check your asthma each day, you will take your peak flow in the morning.

- Between noon and 2:00 PM each day.
- Each time you take your quick-relief medicine to relieve symptoms. (Measure your peak flow *after* you take your medicine.)
- Any other time your doctor suggests.

Write down the number you get for each peak flow reading. The highest peak flow number you had during the 2 to 3 weeks is your personal best.

Your personal best can change over time. Ask your doctor when to check for a new personal best.

Your Peak Flow Zones

Your peak flow zones are based on your personal best peak flow number. The zones will help you check your asthma and take the right actions to keep it controlled. The colors used with each zone come from the traffic light.

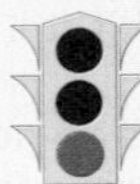

Green Zone (80 - 100% of your personal best) signals **good control.** Take your usual daily long-term–control medicines, if you take any. Keep taking these medicines even when you are in the yellow or red zones.

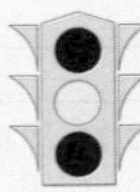

Yellow Zone (50 - 79% of your personal best) signals **caution: your asthma is getting worse.** Add quick-relief medicines. You might need to increase other asthma medicines as directed by your doctor.

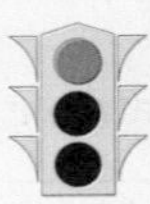

Red Zone (below 50% of your personal best) signals **medical alert!** Add or increase quick-relief medicines and call your doctor ***now.***

Ask your doctor to write an action plan for you that tells you:

- The peak flow numbers for *your* green, yellow, and red zones. Mark the zones on your peak flow meter with colored tape or a marker.
- The medicines you should take while in each peak flow zone.

How to Take Your Peak Flow

1. Move the marker to the bottom of the numbered scale.
2. Stand up or sit up straight.
3. Take a deep breath. Fill your lungs all the way.
4. Hold your breath while you place the mouthpiece in your mouth, between your teeth. Close your lips around it. Do **not** put your tongue inside the hole.
5. Blow out as hard and fast as you can. Your peak flow meter will measure how fast you can blow out air.
6. Write down the number you get. But if you cough or make a mistake, do not write down the number. Do it over again.
7. Repeat steps 1 through 6 two more times. Write down the highest of the three numbers. This is your peak flow number.
8. Check to see which peak flow *zone* your peak flow number is in. Do the actions your doctor told you to do while in that zone.

Your doctor may ask you to write down your peak flow numbers each day. You can do this on a calendar or other paper. This will help you and your doctor see how your asthma is doing over time.

Checking Your Asthma: When to Use Your Peak Flow Meter

- **Every morning** when you wake up, *before* you take medicine. Make this part of your daily routine.
- **When you are having asthma symptoms or an attack.** And after taking medicine for the attack. This can tell you how bad your asthma attack is and whether your medicine is working.
- Any other time your doctor suggests.

If you use more than one peak flow meter (such as at home and at school), be sure that both meters are the same brand.

Bring to Each of Your Doctor's Visits

- Your peak flow meter.
- Your peak flow numbers if you have written them down each day.

Also, ask your doctor or nurse to check how you use your peak flow meter—just to be sure you are doing it right.

Source: *Practical guide for the diagnosis and management of asthma, based on Expert panel report 2: guidelines for the diagnosis and management of asthma,* Washington, DC, 1997, National Institutes of Health.

PATIENT & FAMILY TEACHING GUIDE

Table 27-12 **Asthma**

Goal: To assist patient in improving quality of life through education, increased understanding, and promotion of lifestyle practices that support successful living with asthma.

Teaching Topic	Resources
What Is Asthma? ▪ Basic anatomy and physiology of lung ▪ Pathophysiology of asthma ▪ Relationship of pathophysiology to signs and symptoms ▪ Measurement and correlation of pulmonary function tests and peak expiratory flow rate	*Teach Your Patient about Asthma: A Clinician's Guide* (Publication 92-2737, National Institutes of Health) *The Asthma Handbook* (American Lung Association)
What Is Good Asthma Control?	Discussion with patient on personal ideas of good control. Videotape—*Essence of Life* (Glaxo—sponsored by Allen and Hansbury's Respiratory Institute)
Hindrances to Asthma Treatment and Control ▪ Intermittent nature of symptoms ▪ Role of denial ▪ Poor perception of asthma severity by patient	Discussion with patient and family about possible hindrances
Environmental/Trigger Control ▪ Identifications of possible triggers and possible preventive measures ▪ Avoidance of allergens and other triggers ▪ Need to maintain good hydration	Trigger diary kept by patient Handouts from National Asthma Education and Prevention Program (NIH Publication 97-4053)
Medications ▪ Types (include mechanism of action) β_2-agonists Cromolyn/nedocromil Corticosteroids Methylxanthines Leukotriene modifiers	*Understanding Lung Medications: How They Work—How to Use Them* (American Lung Association)
▪ Establishing medication schedule ▪ Use of preventive/maintenance agents (e.g., antiinflammatory agents) ▪ Regular use	Asthma Management Plan (see Table 27-10) Write out medication list and schedule
Correct Use of Meter-Dose Inhaler, Spacer, and Nebulizer	Videotape—*Managing Your Asthma* (Glaxo) (Fig. 27-5)
Breathing Techniques ▪ Pursed-lip breathing ▪ Diaphragmatic breathing	Demonstration–return demonstration
Correct Use of Peak Flow Meter	Table 27-11 Videotape—*Managing Your Asthma* (Glaxo) *Facts about Peak Flow Meters* (American Lung Association)
Asthma Management Plan ▪ Peak flow zones ▪ Individualize plan ▪ Early recognition of infection	Table 27-10 Living with Asthma and the Asthma Handbook (American Lung Association) Patient completes plan and discusses it with health care provider

Counseling may be indicated to help the patient and the family resolve personal, family, social, and occupational problems that have resulted from asthma. Relaxation therapies (e.g., yoga, meditation, relaxation techniques, breathing techniques) may be of value in helping a patient relax respiratory muscles and decrease the respiratory rate. A healthy emotional outlook can also be important in preventing future asthma attacks. One resource that can be used when teaching the patient about asthma is the American Lung Association, which has educational materials about asthma, including *The Asthma Handbook.* Table 27-12 is a patient and family teaching guide for the patient with asthma.

■ Evaluation

The expected outcomes for the patient with asthma are presented in NCP 27-1.

Table 27-13 Effects of Tobacco Smoke on the Respiratory System

Area of Defect	Acute Effects	Long-Term Effects
Respiratory mucosa		
Nasopharyngeal	↓ Sense of smell	Cancer
Tongue	↓ Sense of taste	Cancer
Vocal cords	Hoarseness	Chronic cough, cancer
Bronchus and bronchioles	Bronchospasm, cough	Chronic bronchitis, asthma, cancer
Cilia	Paralysis, sputum accumulation, cough	Chronic bronchitis, cancer
Mucous glands	↑ Secretions, ↑ cough	Hyperplasia and hypertrophy of glands, chronic bronchitis
Alveolar macrophages	↓ Function	Increased incidence of infection
Elastin and collagen fibers	↑ Destruction by proteases, ↓ function of antiproteases (α_1-antitrypsin), ↓ synthesis and repair of elastin	Emphysema

EMPHYSEMA AND CHRONIC BRONCHITIS

Chronic obstructive pulmonary disease (COPD) is defined as a disease state characterized by the presence of airflow obstruction caused by chronic bronchitis or emphysema. The airflow obstruction is generally progressive, may be accompanied by airway hyperreactivity, and may be partially reversible. In the past, asthma was generally defined along with COPD. Now, inflammation is considered the distinguishing feature of asthma, and therefore asthma has now been defined separately. Patients with COPD may have asthma, and some patients with asthma may go on to develop fixed or irreversible airflow obstruction. *Chronic bronchitis* is defined as the presence of chronic productive cough for 3 months in each of 2 successive years in a patient in whom other causes of chronic cough have been excluded. *Emphysema* is defined as abnormal permanent enlargement of the airspaces distal to the terminal bronchioles, accompanied by destruction of their walls and without obvious fibrosis. Although the preferred terms are *emphysema* and *chronic bronchitis,* there is usually some overlap between them.[1]

More than 15 million persons in the United States suffer from emphysema and chronic bronchitis. The estimated number of those with COPD has doubled in the last 25 years. The number of women with COPD is on the rise because of the increased number of women smoking cigarettes. COPD is the fourth-leading cause of death in the United States. More than one half of COPD patients die within 10 years of diagnosis. Observed increases in morbidity and mortality rates appear to be related to past trends in cigarette smoking. Since smoking frequency has decreased over the past 30 years, there should be a decrease in COPD mortality rates in the future.[1,16]

Etiology

Exposure to tobacco smoke is the primary cause of COPD in the United States.[17,18]

Cigarette Smoking. The major risk factor for developing COPD is cigarette smoking. Although the prevalence of cigarette smoking in the United States has decreased since 1964, it is still a major public health concern among young people. Nearly all first use of tobacco occurs before high school graduation, and each day 3000 teenagers start to smoke. In spite of an overall decline in the number of smokers in the United States and much of the developed world, the prevalence of cigarette smoking continues to increase in many developing countries.[17]

Clinically significant airway obstruction develops in 15% of smokers, and 80% to 90% of COPD deaths in the United States are related to tobacco smoking. For most Americans who die of lung diseases related to cigarette smoking, death is preceded by a long period of debilitating morbidity characterized by frequent hospitalizations and loss of many years of productivity. Cigarette smoking is extremely costly to both the individual and society. More than one out of every five deaths in the United States is the result of smoking. Cigarette smoking remains the most preventable cause of premature death in the United States. In addition to being linked with emphysema, chronic bronchitis, and lung cancer, cigarette smoking has also been implicated as a factor in cancers of the mouth, pharynx, larynx, esophagus, pancreas, kidney, stomach, cervix, and bladder. Cigarette smoking is responsible for approximately 87% of deaths from lung cancer.[17,18]

When cigarettes are smoked, approximately 4000 chemicals and gases are inhaled into the lungs. Many carcinogens have been isolated from cigarette smoke; 3,4-benzpyrene is the most dangerous. At least 43 other components have been identified as carcinogens, co-carcinogens, tumor promoters, tumor initiators, and mutagens. Nicotine is probably not a carcinogen, but it has other deleterious effects. It acts by stimulating the sympathetic nervous system, resulting in increased heart rate (HR), increased peripheral vasoconstriction, increased BP, and increased cardiac workload. These effects of nicotine compound the problems in a person with coronary artery disease (CAD).[17]

Cigarette smoke has several direct effects on the respiratory tract (Table 27-13). The irritating effect of the smoke causes hyperplasia of cells, including goblet cells, which subsequently results in increased production of mucus. Hyperplasia reduces airway diameter and increases the difficulty in clearing secretions. Smoking reduces the ciliary activity and may cause actual loss of ciliated cells. Smoking also produces abnormal dilation of the distal air space with destruction of alveolar walls. Many cells develop large, atypical nuclei, which is considered a precancerous condition.[17]

After only 1 year of smoking, changes in small airway function can develop. In the early stages these changes are mostly inflammatory with mucosal edema and an influx of inflammatory cells. In later stages, however, peribronchiolar fibrosis is present. These inflammatory changes in small airways can be reversed with smoking cessation, at least in the younger person.

Carbon monoxide (CO), a component of tobacco smoke, is also present in similar concentrations in automobile exhaust. CO has a high affinity for hemoglobin and combines with it more readily than does O_2, thereby reducing the smoker's O_2-carrying capacity. The smoker inhales a lower percentage of O_2 than normal, resulting in less O_2 available at the alveolar level. The heart's need for O_2 is increased because of the stimulatory effect of nicotine on the sympathetic nervous system. Because the blood's O_2-carrying capacity is reduced, the heart must pump more rapidly to adequately supply tissues with O_2. CO also seems to impair psychomotor performance and judgment and may cause anxiety.

Passive smoking is the exposure of nonsmokers to cigarette smoke, also known as environmental tobacco smoke (ETS) or secondhand smoke. Children whose parents smoke have a higher prevalence of respiratory symptoms and respiratory disease and appear to have small but measurable deficiencies in tests of pulmonary function when compared with children of nonsmokers. In adults, involuntary smoke exposure is associated with decreased pulmonary function, increased risk for lung cancer, and increased mortality rates from ischemic heart disease.[1]

Infection. Recurring respiratory tract infections are a major contributing factor to the aggravation and progression of COPD. Recurring infections impair normal defense mechanisms, making the bronchioles and alveoli more susceptible to injury. In addition, the person with COPD is more prone to respiratory infections, which subsequently intensify the pathologic destruction of lung tissue and the progression of COPD. The most common causative organisms are *Haemophilus influenzae, Streptococcus pneumoniae,* and *Moraxella catarrhalis.* Retained secretions provide a good medium for their proliferation.

Ambient Air Pollution. High levels of urban air pollution are demonstrably harmful to persons with heart or lung disease, but the role of environmental air pollution in the etiology of COPD in the United States is unclear; its role appears to be small when compared with that of cigarette smoking.

Heredity. α_1-Antitrypsin (AAT) is the only known genetic abnormality that leads to COPD. AAT deficiency accounts for less than 1% of COPD in the United States. Also known as α_1-protease inhibitor, AAT is a serum protein produced by the liver and normally found in the lungs. Severe AAT deficiency leads to premature emphysema, often with chronic bronchitis and occasionally with bronchiectasis. Emphysema results when lysis of lung tissues by proteolytic enzymes from neutrophils and macrophages occurs because of the AAT deficiency. Normally AAT inhibits the action of these enzymes. Therefore lower levels of AAT result in insufficient inactivation and subsequent destruction of lung tissue. Smoking greatly exacerbates the disease process in these patients.

The level of AAT is controlled by a pair of autosomal codominant genes. Low levels of AAT are related to homozygosity for the deficiency gene (ZZ), intermediate levels to heterozygosity (MZ), and normal values to homozygosity for the normal gene (MM). The incidence of ZZ homozygous individuals ranges from 1 out of 3500 persons to 1 out of 1670 persons, and 5% to 10% of persons are heterozygous. In the recessive gene homozygous group, onset of symptoms often occurs by the age of 40, and the disease is found as frequently in women as in men. The people with this type of emphysema are primarily of Northern European origin.[19]

IV or nebulizer-administered AAT (Prolastin) augmentation therapy has recently been approved for persons with AAT deficiency. The infusions are administered weekly.[19] Its effectiveness in slowing the progression of the disease continues to be evaluated.

Aging. Some degree of emphysema is common in the lungs of the older person, even a nonsmoker. Aging results in changes in the lung structure, the thoracic cage, and the respiratory muscles. Clinically significant emphysema, however, is usually not caused by aging alone.

As people age there is gradual loss of the elastic recoil of the lung. The lungs become more rounded and smaller. The number of functional alveoli decreases as a result of the loss of the alveolar supporting structures and loss of the intraalveolar septum. These changes are similar to those seen in the patient with emphysema. Thinner alveolar walls contribute to loss of alveolar septal tissue and alveolar capillaries. With fewer capillaries available for gas exchange, arterial oxygen levels decrease. The PaO_2 falls at a rate of 4 mm Hg for each decade of life, beginning after 20 years of age. The surface area available for gas exchange decreases from 80 m^2 at 20 years of age to 65 to 70 m^2 by 70 years of age.

Thoracic cage changes result from osteoporosis and calcification of the costal cartilages. The thoracic cage becomes stiff and rigid, and the ribs are less mobile. The shape of the rib cage gradually changes because of the increased functional residual capacity (FRC), causing it to expand and become rounded. These changes result in a decreased compliance of the chest wall and an increase in the work of breathing.

Pathophysiology

It is common clinically to find a combination of emphysema and chronic bronchitis in the same person, often with one condition predominating (Fig. 27-6).

Emphysema. Emphysema is a condition of the lungs characterized by abnormal, permanent enlargement of the air spaces distal to the terminal bronchioles, accompanied by destruction of their walls, and without obvious fibrosis. Structural changes include (1) hyperinflation of alveoli; (2) destruction of alveolar walls; (3) destruction of alveolar capillary walls; (4) narrowed, tortuous, small airways; and (5) loss of lung elasticity.

There are two major types of emphysema: centrilobular and panlobular (Fig. 27-7). In centrilobular emphysema the primary area of involvement is the central part of the lobule. Respiratory bronchioles enlarge, the walls are destroyed, and the bronchioles become confluent. Chronic bronchitis is often associated with centrilobular emphysema, which is more common than panlobular emphysema.

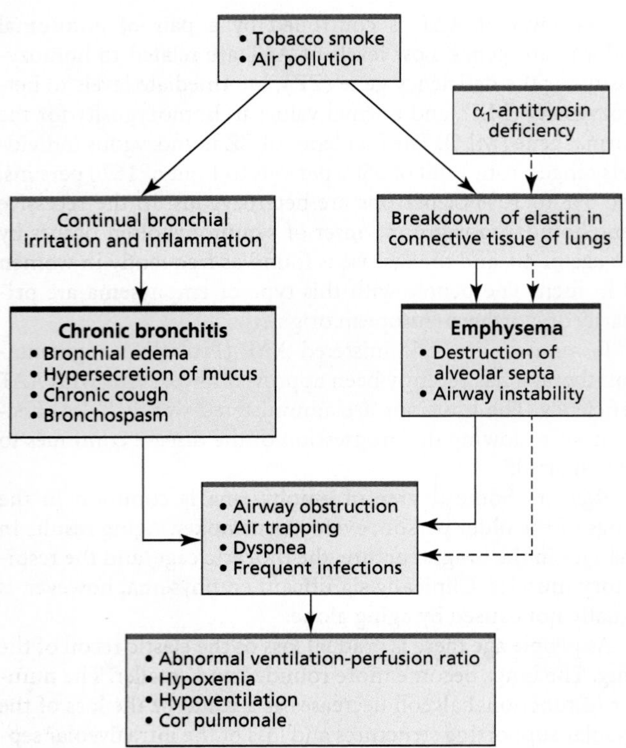

Fig. 27-6 Pathophysiology of chronic bronchitis and emphysema. *Dashed arrows,* role of α_1-antitrypsin deficiency, if present.

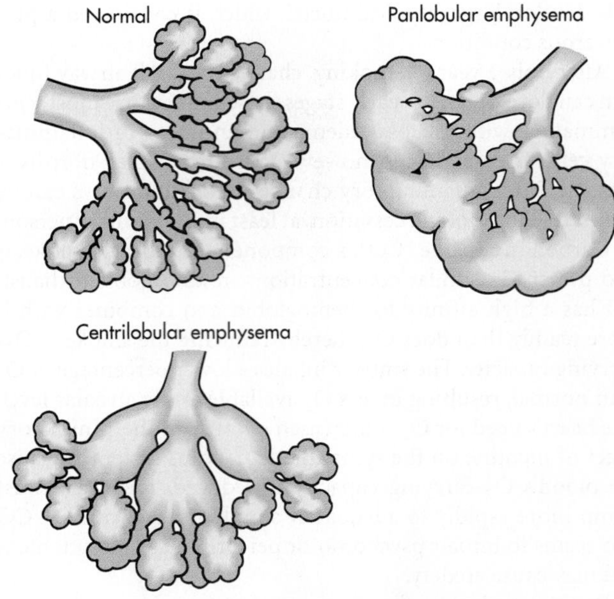

Fig. 27-7 Morphologic types of emphysema. In panlobular emphysema the entire primary lobule is involved, with destruction and distention distal to the respiratory bronchioles. In centrilobular emphysema, destruction is central, involving primarily the respiratory bronchioles.

In contrast, panlobular emphysema involves distention and destruction of the whole lobule. Respiratory bronchioles, alveolar ducts and sacs, and alveoli are all affected. There is progressive loss of lung tissue and a decreased alveolar-capillary surface area. Severe panlobular emphysema is usually found in persons with AAT deficiency. In some patients with emphysema, bullae (large cystic areas) develop. When emphysema is severe, it is difficult to distinguish the two types, which may coexist in the same lung.

The pathophysiologic mechanisms involved in emphysema are not totally understood. Small bronchioles become obstructed as a result of mucus, smooth muscle spasm, the inflammatory process, and collapse of bronchiolar walls. Recurrent infectious processes lead to increased production and stimulation of neutrophils and macrophages. These cells release proteolytic enzymes that can destroy alveolar tissue. This process results in more inflammation, more edema, and exudate formation.

In a healthy person there is a balance between elastases and proteases and antiproteases in the lungs. In smokers the numbers of neutrophils and macrophages are increased. Release of their elastases and proteases may overwhelm the normal antiprotease defense. In addition, smoking inactivates AAT. In AAT-related emphysema, AAT activity is greatly diminished and may be overwhelmed by normal protease activity.

In emphysema, elastin and collagen, the supporting structures of the lung, are destroyed. As a result there is no pull or traction on the walls of the bronchioles. Like air being blown into a paper bag, air goes into the lungs easily but is unable to come out on its own and remains in the lung. Thus the bronchioles tend to collapse (especially on expiration) and air is trapped in the distal alveoli, resulting in hyperinflation and overdistention of the alveoli. This trapped air in the lungs gives the patient the typical barrel-chested appearance. In emphysema the lungs can be inflated easily but can deflate only partially. As more alveoli are destroyed and alveoli coalesce, larger air spaces called blebs (in the visceral pleura) and bullae (in the lung parenchyma) may develop (Fig. 27-8).

Because of the loss of alveolar walls and the capillaries surrounding them, the amount of surface area that is available for diffusion of O_2 in the blood decreases. The patient with emphysema compensates for this problem by increasing the respiratory rate to increase alveolar ventilation. Typically the patient with pure emphysema does not have difficulty with hypoxemia at rest until late in the disease. However, hypoxemia may develop during exercise, and the patient may benefit from supplemental O_2. Hypercapnia and respiratory acidosis do not develop until late in the disease process.

Chronic Bronchitis. Chronic bronchitis is excessive production of mucus in the bronchi accompanied by a recurrent cough that persists for at least 3 months of the year during at least 2 successive years. Pathologic changes in the lung consist of (1) hyperplasia of mucous-secreting glands in the trachea and bronchi, (2) increase in goblet cells, (3) disappearance of cilia, (4) chronic inflammatory changes and narrowing of small airways, and (5) altered function of alveolar macrophages, leading to increased bronchial infections. Fre-

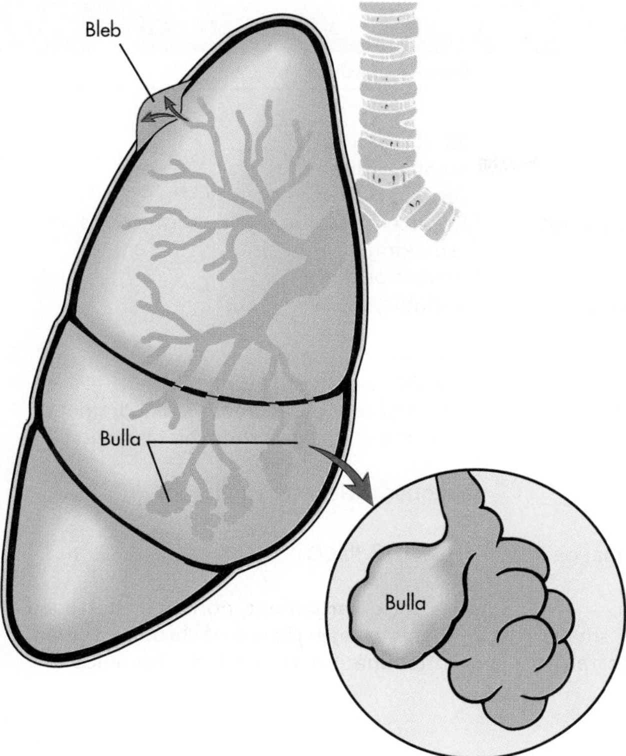

Fig. 27-8 Pulmonary blebs and bullae.

quently the airways are colonized with microorganisms. Infections can occur when the organisms increase. Excess amounts of mucus are found in the airways and sometimes may occlude small bronchioles. Eventually, scarring of the bronchial walls may occur. In contrast to emphysema, the alveolar structure and capillaries are normal.

Chronic inflammation is the primary pathologic mechanism involved in causing the changes characteristic of chronic bronchitis. The inflammatory response causes vasodilation, congestion, and mucosal edema. The mucous glands are stimulated to become hyperplastic. This hyperplasia, inflammatory swelling, and excess, thick mucus cause narrowing of the airway lumen and result in diminished airflow. Greater resistance to airflow increases the work of breathing. Hypoxemia and hypercapnia develop more frequently in chronic bronchitis than in emphysema. Because the constricted bronchioles are clogged with mucus, there is a physical barrier to ventilation. In addition, there is a diminished respiratory drive, with a tendency to hypoventilate and retain CO_2. As a result, many areas of the lung are not ventilated, and O_2 diffusion cannot occur. Frequently the patient with chronic bronchitis requires O_2 both at rest and during exercise as the disease progresses. Peribronchial fibrosis may also result from the healing process secondary to inflammatory changes.

Coughing is stimulated by retained mucus that cannot adequately be removed as a result of decreased cilia and mucociliary activity. The cough is often ineffective to remove secretions adequately because the person cannot inspire deeply enough to cause air to flow distal to retained secretions. Frequently, bronchospasm develops in the patient with chronic bronchitis. Bronchospasm is usually more common in the patient with a history of cigarette smoking or asthma. The bronchospasm adds to the already increased airway resistance, resulting in further increased work of breathing and impaired gas exchange.

Clinical Manifestations

The clinical manifestations of COPD vary from those of pure emphysema to those of pure chronic bronchitis. Most patients with COPD have features of both (Table 27-14).

Emphysema. An early symptom of emphysema is dyspnea, which becomes progressively more severe. The patient will first complain of dyspnea on exertion that progresses to interfering with ADLs to dyspnea at rest. Minimal coughing is present, with no sputum or small amounts of mucoid sputum. As more alveoli become overdistended, increasing amounts of air are trapped. This causes a flattened diaphragm and an increased anteroposterior diameter of the chest, forming the typical barrel chest. Effective abdominal breathing is decreased because of the flattened diaphragm from the overdistended lungs. The person becomes more of a chest breather, relying on the intercostal and accessory muscles. This type of breathing, however, is not that effective because the ribs become fixed in an inspiratory position.

Hypoxemia (especially during exercise) may be present, but hypercapnia does not develop until late in the disease. The person is characteristically thin and underweight, but the exact cause for this is not well understood. One possibility is that the patient is in a hypermetabolic state with increased energy requirements that are partly due to the increased work of breathing. Even when the patient has adequate calorie intake, weight loss is still experienced. The patient with emphysema has protein-calorie malnutrition with loss of lean muscle mass and subcutaneous fat. (Malnutrition is discussed in Chapter 38.)

Later in the course of the disease, secondary chronic bronchitis may develop. In advanced stages, finger clubbing may be present in both emphysema and chronic bronchitis. Other characteristics are presented in Table 27-15.

Chronic Bronchitis. The earliest symptom in chronic bronchitis is usually a frequent, productive cough during most winter months. It is often exacerbated by respiratory irritants and cold, damp air. Bronchospasm can occur at the end of paroxysms of coughing. Frequent respiratory infections are another common manifestation. Somewhat later, dyspnea on exertion may develop. A history of cigarette smoking for many years is almost always present. Unfortunately, a patient often attributes chronic cough to smoking rather than lung disease, thus delaying initiation of treatment. In addition, the patient may not be aware of the cough because she or he becomes accustomed to it.

Hypoxemia and hypercapnia result from hypoventilation caused by increased airway resistance. The bluish-red color of the skin results from polycythemia and cyanosis. Polycythemia develops as a result of increased production of red blood cells secondary to the body's attempt to compensate for chronic

Table 27-14 Comparison of Emphysema and Chronic Bronchitis*

	Emphysema	Chronic Bronchitis
Clinical Features		
Age	30-40 yr (onset) 60-70 yr (disabling)	20-30 yr (onset) 40-50 yr (disabling)
Body build	Thin	Tendency toward obesity
Health history	Generally healthy, occasional insidious dyspnea, smoking	Recurrent respiratory tract infections, smoking
Weight loss	Often marked	Absent or slight
Dyspnea	Slowly progressive and eventually disabling	Variable, relatively late
Sputum	Scanty, mucoid	Copious, mucopurulent
Cough	Negligible	Considerable
Chest examination	Marked increase in AP diameter, quiet or diminished breath sounds, limited diaphragmatic excursion	Slight to marked increase in AP diameter, scattered crackles, rhonchi, wheezing
Cor pulmonale	Rare except terminally	Frequent with many episodes
Diagnostic Study Results		
ABGs	Near normal, mild ↓ PaO_2, normal or ↓ $PaCO_2$	↓ PaO_2, ↑ $PaCO_2$
Chest x-ray	Hyperinflation, flat diaphragm, attenuated peripheral vessels, small or normal heart, widened intercostal margins	Cardiac enlargement, normal or flattened diaphragm, evidence of chronic inflammation, congested lung fields
Lung volumes		
Total lung capacity	Increased	Normal or slightly increased
Residual volume	Increased	Increased
Vital capacity	Decreased	Decreased
FEV_1	Decreased	Decreased
FEV_1/FVC	Decreased (<70%)	Decreased (<70%)
Hematocrit and hemoglobin	Normal until late in disease	Increased
Pathology	Panlobular emphysema	Centrilobular emphysema

*Most persons with COPD have features of both pulmonary emphysema and chronic bronchitis.
AP, anteroposterior; *FEV_1*, forced expiratory volume in 1 second; *FVC*, forced vital capacity.

Table 27-15 Correlation of FEV_1 with Probable Clinical Manifestations

Approximate FEV_1 (ml)	Probable Clinical Manifestation
1500	Shortness of breath just beginning to be noticed
1000	Shortness of breath with activity
500	Shortness of breath at rest

hypoxemia. Hemoglobin concentrations may reach 20 g/dl (200 g/L) or more. Cyanosis develops when there is at least 5 g/dl (50 g/L) or more of circulating unoxygenated hemoglobin.

A person with chronic bronchitis is usually of normal weight or heavyset, with a robust appearance. Emphysema of the centrilobular type frequently develops.

Complications

Cor Pulmonale. *Cor pulmonale* is hypertrophy of the right side of the heart, with or without heart failure, resulting from pulmonary hypertension. In COPD, pulmonary hypertension is caused primarily by constriction of the pulmonary vessels in response to alveolar hypoxia, with acidosis further potentiating the vasoconstriction (Fig. 27-9). Chronic alveolar hypoxia also causes pulmonary arteriolar muscle hypertrophy. Chronic hypoxia also stimulates erythropoiesis, which causes polycythemia and increases the viscosity of the blood.

Normally the right ventricle and pulmonary circulatory system are low-pressure systems compared with the left ventricle and systemic circulation. When pulmonary hypertension develops, the pressures on the right side of the heart must increase to push blood into the lungs. Eventually, right-sided heart failure develops.

The clinical manifestations of cor pulmonale are related to dilation and failure of the right ventricle with subsequent intravascular volume expansion and systemic venous congestion. Heart sound changes include accentuation of the pul-

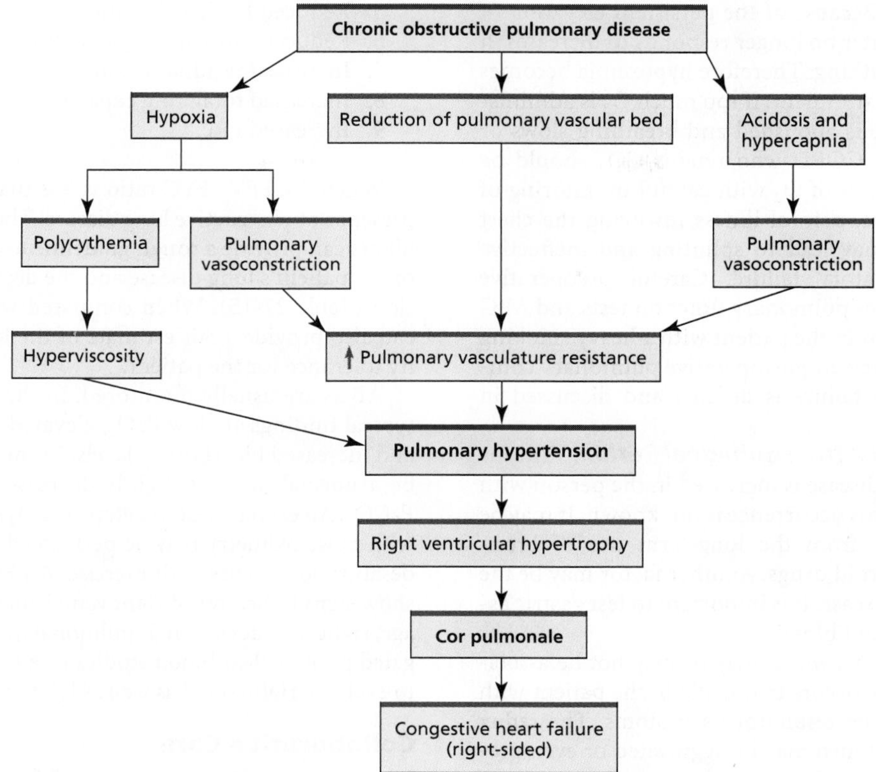

Fig. 27-9 Mechanisms involved in the pathophysiology of cor pulmonale secondary to chronic obstructive pulmonary disease.

monic component of the second heart sound, right-sided ventricular diastolic S_3 gallop, and early systolic ejection click along the left sternal border. ECG changes include increased P wave amplitude (P pulmonale) in leads II, III, and aVF; a tendency for right axis deviation; and incomplete right bundle branch block. Overt manifestations of right-sided heart failure may develop, which include distended neck veins (jugular venous distention), hepatomegaly with right upper quadrant tenderness, ascites, epigastric distress, peripheral edema, and weight gain.

Management of cor pulmonale is continuous low-flow O_2. Long-term O_2 therapy can reverse the progression of pulmonary hypertension in the patient with COPD.[16,20] Although use of digitalis is not indicated for right-sided heart failure, it is used when a left-sided heart failure is present. Dietary salt restriction is sometimes recommended, especially if overt congestive heart failure (CHF) is present. Although diuretics are generally used, they are prescribed with caution because of their tendency to deplete potassium and chloride and reduce intravascular volume and cardiac output. (Cor pulmonale is discussed further in Chapter 26.)

Acute Exacerbations of Chronic Bronchitis. The airways of patients with stable chronic COPD are colonized with *Streptococcus pneumoniae* and *Haemophilus influenzae* that are relatively nonpathogenic in these patients. Factors that impair the normal function of the mucociliary system and thus slow or prevent the removal of particulate matter may result in the potential for acute infection. The most common organisms causing acute bronchitis are *H. influenzae, M. catarrhalis,* and *S. pneumoniae.* As COPD becomes more severe, *Pseudomonas, Klebsiella pneumoniae,* and *E. coli* are frequent causes.[21]

Clinical manifestations of an acute exacerbation include worsened cough, hemoptysis, wheezing, increased shortness of breath, and changes in the amount, color, consistency, or viscosity of the sputum. Patients are treated with antibiotics, as well as increases in bronchodilator usage, possibly corticosteroids, humidification, and postural drainage.

Acute Respiratory Failure. The most common event leading to acute respiratory failure in COPD is acute respiratory tract infection (usually viral) or acute bronchitis. Frequently COPD patients wait too long to contact their health care provider when they develop fever, increased cough and dyspnea, or other symptoms suggestive of exacerbations of COPD. An exacerbation of cor pulmonale occurring either alone or simultaneously with other etiologic causes of acute respiratory failure may lead to acute respiratory failure. Discontinuing bronchodilator or corticosteroid medication may also precipitate respiratory failure. The use of β-blocker medications (e.g., propranolol [Inderal]) may also exacerbate acute respiratory failure in the patient with an asthmatic component to the COPD.

The indiscriminate use of sedatives and narcotics, especially in the preoperative or postoperative patient who retains CO_2, may suppress ventilatory drive and lead to respiratory failure. Hypercapnia presents a serious problem when O_2

therapy is being given. Because of the persistent elevation of CO_2, the respiratory center no longer responds to increases in CO_2 by stimulating breathing. Therefore hypoxemia becomes the primary respiratory stimulant. If too much O_2 is administered, the hypoxic drive is abolished and breathing slows or stops. The person with COPD who retains CO_2 should be treated with low flow rates of O_2 with careful monitoring of ABGs. Surgery or severe, painful illness involving the chest or abdominal organs may lead to splinting and ineffective ventilation and respiratory failure. Careful preoperative screening, which includes pulmonary function tests and ABG monitoring, is important in the patient with a heavy smoking history and COPD to prevent postoperative pulmonary complications. (Respiratory failure is defined and discussed in Chapter 62.)

Peptic Ulcer and Gastroesophageal Reflux. The incidence of peptic ulcer disease is increased in the person with COPD. The reason for this occurrence is not known. It may be because of side effects from the long-term use of bronchodilator or corticosteroid drugs. Another factor may be the stressful nature of the disease. It is important to test gastric aspirates and feces for occult blood.

Gastroesophageal reflux, which may or may not be associated with a hiatal hernia, occurs frequently in the patient with COPD and may aggravate respiratory symptoms. The reflux and accompanying heartburn may be aggravated or even precipitated by theophylline or β-adrenergic drugs. As a result of esophageal irritation or aspiration into the tracheobronchial tree, reflux airway constriction and obstruction may occur. (Treatment of hiatal hernia and gastroesophageal reflux is discussed in Chapter 39.)

Pneumonia. Pneumonia is a frequent complication of COPD. The most common causative agents are *S. pneumoniae, H. influenzae,* and viruses. The most common manifestation is purulent sputum. Systemic manifestations such as fever, chills, and leukocytosis may not be present. (Treatment of pneumonia is discussed in Chapter 26.)

Diagnostic Studies

An important goal of the diagnostic workup is to determine the major disease component of COPD, the severity of the disease, and impact of disease on the patient's quality of life. These factors enable the health care provider to design an individualized treatment plan. Chest x-rays taken early in the disease may not show abnormalities. Later in the disease the findings presented in Table 27-14 may be present.

A history and physical examination are extremely important in a diagnostic workup of the patient.[20] Pulmonary function studies are useful in diagnosing and assessing the severity of COPD. Usually spirometry before and after bronchodilation is ordered. The most significant findings are related to increased resistance to expiratory airflow. Typical findings are as follows:

1. Reduced FEV_1
2. Reduced $FEF_{25\%-75\%}$
3. Reduced maximum voluntary ventilation (MVV)
4. Reduced vital capacity (VC)
5. Reduced FEV_1/FVC ratio
6. Reduced diffusing capacity for carbon monoxide
7. Increased residual volume
8. Increased total lung capacity
9. Increased FRC

When the FEV_1/FVC ratio is less than 70%, it suggests the presence of obstructive lung disease. The value of FEV_1 in milliliters can provide a rough guideline to determine the severity of the patient's lung disease and the degree of disease progression (Table 27-15). When compared with previous values, it can also provide a fair estimate of the level of expected activity tolerance for the patient.

ABGs are usually monitored. In the later stages of COPD, typical findings are low PaO_2, elevated $PaCO_2$, decreased pH, and increased bicarbonate levels. In the early stages there may be a normal or only slightly decreased PaO_2 and a normal $PaCO_2$. An exercise test to determine O_2 saturation in the blood with pulse oximetry may be performed to evaluate how much desaturation occurs with exercise. An ECG may be normal or show signs indicative of right ventricular failure (e.g., low voltage, right-axis deviation, P pulmonale). An echocardiogram or gated pool nuclear blood studies (see Chapter 30) can be used to evaluate right-sided as well as left ventricular function.

Collaborative Care

In general, COPD is an irreversible process. The reversible components are airway size and secretions. Certain patients with COPD have emphysema that may be described as fixed airway disease; that is, there is no reversibility. The primary goals of care for the COPD patient are to (1) improve ventilation, (2) promote secretion removal, (3) prevent complications and progression of symptoms, (4) promote patient comfort and participation in care, and (5) improve quality of life as much as possible (Table 27-16). The majority of these patients are treated as outpatients. They are hospitalized for acute exacerbations and complications such as respiratory failure, pneumonia, and CHF.

A clinical pathway for care of the patient with exacerbation of COPD is provided on p. 690.

Smoking Cessation. Cessation of cigarette smoking in the early stages is probably the most significant factor in slowing the progression of the disease.[17] After discontinuation of smoking, the accelerated decline in pulmonary function slows and pulmonary function usually improves. Thus the sooner the smoker stops, the less pulmonary function is lost and the sooner the symptoms decrease, particularly cough and sputum production. The health care provider has a responsibility to do the following:

1. *Ask.* Systematically identify each tobacco user at every visit.
2. *Advise.* Strongly urge all smokers to quit, and identify smokers willing to make a quit attempt.
3. *Assist.* If the patient expresses an interest in quitting, assist by helping the patient with a quit plan, encouraging nicotine replacement therapy (except in special circumstances), giving key advice on successful quitting, and providing supplementary materials.

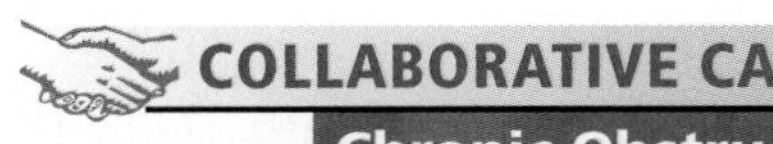

Table 27-16 Chronic Obstructive Pulmonary Disease

Diagnostic
- Health history and physical examination
- Chest x-ray
- Pulmonary function tests
- Sputum specimen for Gram's stain and culture (if indicated)
- ABG
- ECG
- Exercise testing with oximetry (if indicated)
- Echocardiogram or cardiac nuclear scans (if indicated)

Collaborative Therapy
- Treatment of respiratory infections
- Bronchodilator therapy
  - β-adrenergic agonists
  - Anticholinergic agents (ipratropium)
  - Long-acting theophylline preparations
- Corticosteroids
- PEFR monitoring (if indicated)
- Chest physiotherapy and postural drainage (if indicated)
- Breathing exercises and retraining
- Hydration of 3 L/day (if not contraindicated)
- Cessation of cigarette smoking
- Appropriate rest periods
- Patient and family education
- Influenza immunization yearly
- Pneumovax immunization
- Low flow rate O_2 (if indicated)
- Progressive plan of exercise
- Pulmonary rehabilitation program

ECG, electrocardiogram.

4. *Arrange.* Schedule follow-up contact either in person or via telephone.[18] The use of nicotine replacement therapy and the newer, non-nicotine medication bupropion (Zyban) may be helpful in minimizing the effects of nicotine withdrawal.[22,23] These adjunctive therapies should be combined with other modalities such as support groups, education materials, and behavior modification programs. Hypnosis and acupuncture have also been helpful. Regardless of the methods used to stop smoking, the most important factor is that the person is committed to stopping.[18] (Smoking cessation techniques are discussed in Chapter 26 in the section on lung cancer and in Table 26-19.)

Other environmental or occupational irritants should be evaluated for their possible negative effect, and ways to control or avoid them should be determined. For example, aerosol hair sprays and smoke-filled rooms should be avoided. The patient with COPD should have a vaccination with influenza virus vaccine yearly and with pneumococcal vaccine. Pneumococcal revaccination is recommended every 5 years for the patient with COPD. The patient with COPD is extremely susceptible to pulmonary infections.

Respiratory infections should be treated as soon as possible. Often the best indication of the presence of a respiratory infection is the increasing quantity, viscosity, or purulence of sputum. Some patients are given a 7- to 10-day supply of antibiotics and are instructed to begin taking them at the first signs of change in sputum. The most common antibiotics given are amoxicillin, amoxicillin with clavulanate (Augmentin), ciprofloxacin (Cipro), erythromycin, and trimethoprim-sulfamethoxazole (Bactrim, Septra).[24]

Drug Therapy. Bronchodilator drug therapy is often helpful in relieving symptoms. Although patients with COPD do not respond as dramatically as those with asthma to bronchodilator therapy, a reduction in dyspnea and an increase in FEV_1 are usually achieved. Most physicians believe that bronchodilator therapy is best given as maintenance therapy rather than as a treatment for acute symptoms. However, the routine use of bronchodilator therapy in all patients with COPD is controversial, especially in people with pure emphysema.

β-Adrenergic agonists are routinely used as bronchodilators in the treatment of COPD. The preferred route of administration is by MDI or nebulizer. Anticholinergic agents, especially ipratropium (Atrovent) by inhaler, are even more effective bronchodilators than β-agonists in the patient with emphysematous COPD. Inhaled anticholinergics are the preferred route of delivery, and they have minimal side effects. These medications are also available in combination (Combivent [albuterol and ipratropium]) via MDI and aerosol therapy. These drugs are best taken on a regular basis. The use of long-acting theophylline in the treatment of COPD is controversial. Although it has some action as a mild bronchodilator in the patient with partial reversibility of airflow obstruction, its main value may be to improve contractility of the diaphragm and decrease diaphragmatic fatigue.

The use of corticosteroid therapy in COPD also is controversial. The person most likely to benefit from these drugs has a history of childhood asthma, has bronchospasm, has a relatively short duration of disease, or has frequent exacerbations that do not respond to therapy with β-agonists and theophylline.[1]

Oxygen Therapy. Oxygen therapy is frequently used in the treatment of COPD and other problems associated with hypoxemia. Oxygen is a colorless, odorless, tasteless gas that constitutes 20.95% of the atmosphere. Administering supplemental O_2 raises the partial pressure of oxygen (PO_2) in inspired air. Used clinically it is considered a drug, but for reimbursement purposes, it is considered durable medical equipment.

Indications for use. Oxygen is usually administered to treat hypoxemia caused by (1) respiratory disorders such as COPD, cor pulmonale, pneumonia, atelectasis, lung cancer, and pulmonary emboli; (2) cardiovascular disorders such as myocardial infarction, arrhythmias, angina pectoris, and cardiogenic shock; and (3) CNS disorders such as overdose of narcotics, head injury, and disordered sleep (sleep apnea).[25,26]

Methods of administration. The goal of O_2 administration is to supply the patient with adequate O_2 to maximize the

CLINICAL PATHWAY Exacerbation of COPD

Admit Date:	DRG: 88		LOS: 4 days	Discharge Date: ____
Pathway	**ER-Day 1**	**Day 2**	**Day 3**	**Day 4**
Critical Path Implemented				
Diagnostic Studies	■ BMP ■ CBC ■ Theophylline level ■ Pulse Ox ____ ■ Chest x-ray	■ Pulse OX	■ Schedule O.P. PFTs ■ Chest x-ray ■ Pulse Ox at rest and with activity ■ CBC, Theo level, lytes	■ Pulse OX
Treatments	■ O_2 ____ L/min via NC ■ Nebulizer Rx ____ ■ Peak flow before and after first treatment, then qd prn	■ O_2 ____ L/min via NC	■ O_2 ____ L/min via NC	■ O_2 ____ L/min via NC
IV/Meds	■ IV fluids ____ @ ___cc/hr ■ Aminophylline ■ IV steroids ■ Bronchodilator	■ See MAR ➜	➜	➜
Consults	■ Pulmonary Rehab	■ Nutrition Services	■ Home Health Care	
Team Directives	( ) Monitor respirations for rate, depth, exertion, ease. Use Shortness of Breath Scale to evaluation and document patient's SOB rating. ( ) VS q2hr x 4hr, then q4hr with temperature ( ) Physical assessment (especially breath sounds) q12hr and prn with changes in condition ( ) Monitor and trend lab values, pulse Ox readings, sputum production and characteristics ( ) Provide skin care and assist with ADLs ( ) Implement measures to prevent fatigue, promote rest, and reduce anxiety ( ) Provide emotional support to pt/family through frequent patient checks (q2hr with VS) (sign/date/time) ____/____/____, ____/____/____, ____/____/____, ____/____/____			
Diet	■ Regular diet, no added salt, encourage fluids. Provide supplements if indicated.			
Activity and Safety	■ Bed rest with bedside commode ■ Routine safety measures ■ Elevate HOB ____/____/____	( ) Rests periods after activity ( ) Sit on side of bed, assist with ADLs ( ) Progress as tolerated ____/____/____		( ) OOB, ambulate in room and hall as tolerated ____/____/____
Teaching Patient and Family	( ) Orient to unit ( ) Instruct to call nurse with dyspnea and for assistance to commode ( ) Teach pursed-lip breathing technique ( ) Teach effective cough technique ( ) Explain diet, meds, and activity level ( ) Explain tests, procedures, and treatments ____/____/____, ____/____/____	( ) Encourage fluids ( ) Explain nebulizer treatments ( ) Teach use of Metered-Dose Inhaler and Peak flow measurement ( ) Teach about meds; dosages, frequency, precautions, potential side effects ____/____/____, ____/____/____		( ) Reinforce importance of taking all of prescribed antibiotics ( ) Teach signs and symptoms of respiratory infection and importance of notifying physician ( ) Review family's EMS plan ____/____/____, ____/____/____
Discharge Planning	( ) Initial assessment of risk indicators completed and referrals made ( ) Advance Directives reviewed ____/____/____	( ) Need for home O_2 evaluated and provider notified ( ) Need for Home Health Care reviewed with family and provider notified of expected discharge date ( ) Follow-up appointment(s) with physician(s), and O.P. PFTs arranged ____/____/____, ____/____/____		

Author: Molly Metzler, RN, BSN, for Nanticoke Health Services. Licensed by the Center for Case Management, South Natick, Mass, Nanticoke Health Services.

CLINICAL PATHWAY Exacerbation of COPD—continued

DRG: 88 **LOS: 4 days**

Meets Expected Outcomes (initial)	ER- Day 1	MET	NOT	Day 2	MET	NOT	Day 3	MET	NOT	Day 4	MET	NOT
Impaired Gas Exchange: Altered O_2 supply 2° to decreased alveolar ventilation and perfusion due to fluid in alveoli. ■ $PaO_2 < 60$ mm Hg ■ pH < 7.35 ■ RR > 20/min ■ Crackles, wheezes, cyanosis, altered LOC	■ Pt.'s airway maintained ___/RC or N ■ Pt. using pursed-lip breathing technique ___/RC or N ■ Air exchange improving within 2 hours of initial HHN, CPT, IV fluids, and Meds ___/RC or N ■ Pulse Ox ≥ 88% on O_2 ___/RC or N ■ Pt with improved LOC after initial Rx ___/N			■ Lungs clearing, with decreased crackles and wheezes, on auscultation ___/RC or N ■ LOC WNL for pt's baseline ___/N ■ Pulse Ox ≥ 90% on O_2 ___/RC or N ■ RR 20/min (± 5) ___/RC or N			■ Air exchange improving on auscultation ___/RC or N ■ Pulse Ox stabilized at >90% as pt is weaned from O_2 ___/RC or N ■ RR stabilized WNL for pt baseline ___/RC or N			■ Pulse Ox ≥90% of O_2 ___/RC or N ■ Air exchange WNL for pt's baseline ___/RC or N		
Ineffective Airway Clearance: Presence of tracheobronchial secretions 2° to increased fluid in lungs. ■ Wheezing ■ Coughing (ineffective) ■ Pink, frothy mucus	■ Using effective diaphragmatic breathing to help maintain airway ___/RC or N ■ Decreased mucus viscosity after initial IV fluid load ___/RC or N ■ Pt using effective cough technique (takes several deep breaths, then gives 3–4 coughs on same exhalation to expel most of air) ___/RC or N			■ Able to cough productively to clear airway ___/RC or N ■ Secretions thinner ___/RC or N ■ Mucus production controlled ___/RC or N			■ Pt. has clear, odorless secretions ___/RC or N ■ Pt. able to breathe deeply without coughing ___/RC or N ■ Pt. able to breathe easily, eupnea ___/RC or N ■ Pt. free of excessive cough ___/RC or N			■ No evidence of respiratory distress ___/RC or N		
Activity Intolerance: Imbalance between O_2 supply and demand 2° to decreased alveolar oxygen supply and greater metabolic demands due to increased work of breathing. Pt c/o: ■ Fatigue ■ Diaphoresis ■ Dyspnea on exertion ■ Altered LOC	■ Rests between activities ___/N ■ Able to describe SOB on Shortness of Breath Scale ___/N ■ Relaxation techniques are effective in reducing Pt/family stress and anxiety ___/N ■ LOC improved ___/N			■ Verbalizes decrease in fatigue with increasing activity level ___/N ■ Gradually increases activity level without increasing SOB ___/N ■ Able to use relaxation and breathing techniques to reduce SOB ___/N			■ Able to complete ADLs with minimal fatigue or dyspnea ___/N ■ Incorporating relaxation and breathing techniques into daily routines ___/N			■ No dyspnea on exertion ___/N ■ Able to use relaxation and breathing techniques to control SOB and fatigue ___/N		
UNMET OUTCOMES: (CCC Initials Required)	7-3p ( ) Resolved ( ) Planned /RN			7-3p ( ) Resolved ( ) Planned /RN			7-3p ( ) Resolved ( ) Planned /RN			7-3p ( ) Resolved ( ) Planned /RN		
	3-7p ( ) Resolved ( ) Planned /RN			3-7p ( ) Resolved ( ) Planned /RN			3-7p ( ) Resolved ( ) Planned /RN			3-7p ( ) Resolved ( ) Planned /RN		
	7-11p ( ) Resolved ( ) Planned /RN			7-11p ( ) Resolved ( ) Planned /RN			7-11p ( ) Resolved ( ) Planned /RN			7-11p ( ) Resolved ( ) Planned /RN		
	11-7a ( ) Resolved ( ) Planned /RN			11-7a ( ) Resolved ( ) Planned /RN			11-7a ( ) Resolved ( ) Planned /RN			11-7a ( ) Resolved ( ) Planned /RN		

Continued

Service

CM - Care Management
ET - Ostomy/Skin Care
RC - Respiratory Care
N - Nurse
PT - Physical Therapy
NS - Nutrition Services
RX - Pharmacist
SL - Speech/Language
CCC - Primary RN Clinical Care Coord.
SW - Social Work
OT - Occupational Therapy
HC - Home Care
DR - Physician
Card - Cardiology
Rad - Radiology
Rehab - Cardiac, Respiratory

Patient informed of plan:

Health care provider signature, date, time

CLINICAL PATHWAY Exacerbation of COPD—continued

DRG: 88 LOS: 4 days

Meets Expected Outcomes (initial)	ER- Day 1	MET	NOT	Day 2	MET	NOT	Day 3	MET	NOT	Day 4	MET	NOT
Potential Fluid Volume Excess: Compromised regulatory mechanism ■ Weight gain > 5 lb ■ Electrolyte imbalance ■ Peripheral edema ■ Jugular vein distension	■ Hourly UO > 30 cc ___/N ■ Peripheral edema and JVD decreasing after initiation of Rx ___/N ■ K^+ between 3.5–5 mEq/L ___/N ■ Na^+ between 147–160 mEq/L ___/N			■ Heart rate range ~ 60-100 BPM___/N ■ UO volume increased; reflecting in weight loss___/N (1 L fluid = 1 kg) ■ Minimal peripheral edema and JVD ___/N			■ VS stable ___/N ■ Fluid balance maintained ___/N ■ Electrolytes stable ___/N ■ Weight stabilizing ___/N			■ Fluid balance stable ___/N		
Knowledge Deficit: ■ S/S respiratory infection; impending exacerbation of disease ■ Breathing and relaxation techniques ■ Effective cough ■ Meds and Treatment ■ Pulmonary Rehab and follow-up medical care	■ Pt/family verbalizes understanding of treatment regimen and equipment ___/N ■ Pt/family understand the purpose of and can demonstrate pursed-lip breathing and relaxation techniques ___/N ■ Pt can demonstrate effective cough___/N			■ Pt. can demonstrate appropriate use of metered-dose inhaler ___/RC or N ■ Pt/family have an opportunity to talk to Pulmonary Rehab staff for follow up ___/Rehab or N ■ Pt/family understand home medication regimen ___/Rx or N ■ Community resources reviewed and discussed with pt/family ___/N,NCM or SWCM			■ Home care follow-up plans confirmed ___/N,NCM or SWCM ■ Patient can state the importance of adequate hydration ___/N ■ Pt/family can state the signs and symptoms of impending pulmonary infection (increased cough, sputum production, change in sputum color from white to yellow-greenish) ___/RC or N			■ Pt/family can list medications, route, purpose, dosage, precautions, and side effects ___/N or RX ■ Pt. can state the importance of consulting with the physician before taking OTC remedies ___/N or RX ■ Pt/family know when and how to contact EMS in case of emergency ___/N		
UNMET OUTCOMES: (CCC Initials Required)	7-3p ( ) Resolved ( ) Planned /RN			7-3p ( ) Resolved ( ) Planned /RN			7-3p ( ) Resolved ( ) Planned /RN			7-3p ( ) Resolved ( ) Planned /RN		
	3-7p ( ) Resolved ( ) Planned /RN			3-7p ( ) Resolved ( ) Planned /RN			3-7p ( ) Resolved ( ) Planned /RN			3-7p ( ) Resolved ( ) Planned /RN		
	7-11p ( ) Resolved ( ) Planned /RN			7-11p ( ) Resolved ( ) Planned /RN			7-11p ( ) Resolved ( ) Planned /RN			7-11p ( ) Resolved ( ) Planned /RN		
	11-7a ( ) Resolved ( ) Planned /RN			11-7a ( ) Resolved ( ) Planned /RN			11-7a ( ) Resolved ( ) Planned /RN			11-7a ( ) Resolved ( ) Planned /RN		

Table 27-17 Methods of Oxygen Administration

Advantages	Disadvantages	Nursing Interventions
Low Flow Delivery Devices		
Nasal Cannula		
Cannula may be used by a restless patient. It is a safe and simple method that is relatively comfortable and acceptable. It is useful for a patient requiring low O_2 concentrations (e.g., those with chronic CO_2 retention). It allows patient to move about in bed. Patient can eat, talk, or cough while wearing device.	Cannula is difficult to maintain in position and can be easily dislodged. Patient must be alert and cooperative to keep cannula in proper place. High flow rates (>5 L/min) dry nasal membranes and may cause pain in frontal sinuses.	Nasal cannula should be stabilized when caring for a restless patient. A flow rate of 2 L/min gives an O_2 concentration of approximately 28%. Amount of O_2 inhaled depends on room air and patient's breathing pattern. Most patients with COPD can tolerate 2 L/min via cannula.
Simple Face Mask		
O_2 can be given quickly for short periods. O_2 concentrations of 35-50% can be achieved with flow rates of 6-12 L/min. Mask provides adequate humidification of inspired air.	Lack of patient tolerance results in inadequate therapy. Mask may be uncomfortable because tight seal must be maintained between face and mask. Mask may produce pressure necrosis of the skin and confines heat radiating from the face about nose and mouth. It must be removed to eat or drink.	Wash and dry under mask q2hr. Mask must fit snugly. Nasal cannula may be provided while patient is eating. Watch for pressure necrosis at the top of ears from elastic straps. (Gauze or other padding may be used to alleviate this problem.) Method requires at least 5 L/min flow to prevent accumulation of expired air in the mask.
Nasal Catheter		
Catheter allows continuous uninterrupted O_2 therapy. Patient receives O_2 even if a mouth breather. Catheter does not interfere with patient care. It is rarely used except for short-term procedures (e.g., bronchoscopy).	Catheter must be inserted into nasopharynx through a nostril and can produce excoriation of the nares. High flow rates (>6 L/min) can cause drying of nasal membranes. Inadvertent gas flow distends the stomach. Cannula does not permit a high degree of humidification and must be taped to patient's face.	Catheter should be changed q8hr, alternate the nostrils. Distance that catheter is to be inserted is measured from distance between tip of nose and earlobe. A flow rate of 5-6 L/min gives an O_2 concentration of approximately 30%. Method is best used for short-term therapy.
Partial Rebreathing Mask		
Mask is lightweight and easy to use. Reservoir bag conserves O_2. Concentrations of 40-60% can be achieved using flow rates of 6-10 L/min.	Mask cannot be used with a high degree of humidity.	Method is useful when blood O_2 concentrations must be raised. It is not recommended for patient with COPD and should never be used with a nebulizer. Bag should not be allowed to deflate during inspiration.
Non-Rebreathing Mask		
High concentrations of O_2 can be delivered accurately. O_2 flows into bag and mask during inhalation. Valve prevents expired air from flowing back into bag. Concentrations of 60-90% can be achieved.	Mask cannot be used with a high degree of humidity.	Mask should fit snugly. Flow rate must be sufficient to keep bag from collapsing during inspiration. Bag should not be allowed to deflate during inspiration.

Continued

O_2-carrying ability of the blood. There are various methods of O_2 administration (Table 27-17 and Figs. 27-10 and 27-11). The method selected depends on factors such as the fraction of inspired oxygen (FIO_2) and humidification required, patient cooperation, comfort, cost, and available financial resources.

Oxygen delivery systems are classified as low- or high-flow systems based on whether the system provides the entire inspired atmosphere to a patient in a fixed oxygen concentration. Most methods of O_2 administration are low-flow devices that deliver O_2 in concentrations that vary with the person's respiratory pattern. In contrast, the Venturi mask is a high-flow device that delivers fixed concentrations of O_2 independent of the patient's respiratory pattern. With the Venturi mask, O_2 is delivered to a small jet (Venturi device) in the center of a wide-based cone (Fig. 27-10, *C*). Air is entrained (pulled through) openings in the cone as O_2 flows through the small jet. The mask has large vents through which exhaled air can escape. The degree of restriction or narrowness of the jet determines the amount of entrainment and dilution of pure O_2 with room air and thus the concentration of O_2.[26,27] Mechanical ventilators are another example of a high-flow O_2 delivery system.

Table 27-17 Methods of Oxygen Administration—cont'd

Advantages	Disadvantages	Nursing Interventions
Oxygen-Conserving Cannula		
Cannula has a built-in reservoir that increases O_2 concentration delivered and allows patient to use lower flow, usually 30-50%, which increases comfort and lowers cost. It is reportedly more comfortable than standard cannulas.	Cannula cannot be cleaned: manufacturer recommends changing cannula every week. It is more expensive than standard cannulas and requires evaluation with ABGs and oximetry to determine correct flow for patient. Cannula is highly visible. Cannula heavy on ears.	Method is generally indicated for patient requiring long-term O_2 therapy at home versus during hospitalization. It may be "moustache" or "pendant" type. May cause necroses over the tops of the ears; can be padded.
Transtracheal Catheter†		
Catheter is less visible. Flow requirement may be reduced 60-80%, which greatly increases amount of time available from portable source of O_2. Less nasal irritation occurs.	Patient and family must learn entire program of care for tracheostoma and how to replace catheter. Procedure is invasive. Procedure and replacement adds costs to O_2 therapy.	Method may not be appropriate for patient with excessive mucus production from mucus plugging.
Face Tent		
Tent is ideal for providing moderate- to high-density aerosol. O_2 concentration administered varies with O_2 flow rate.	Face tent is less reliable than face mask for maintaining high inspiration of O_2 concentration.	Open plastic mask fits under chin. Temperature of aerosol must be checked to maintain at or near body temperature. It is rarely used.
Tracheostomy Collar		
Collar can deliver high humidity and O_2 via tracheostomy.	Condensed fluid in tubing may drain into tracheostomy. Water traps are usually put in. Secretions collect inside collar and around tracheostomy. O_2 concentration is lost into atmosphere because collar does not fit tightly.	Collar attaches to neck with elastic strap and should be removed and cleaned at least q4hr to prevent aspiration of fluid and infection.
Tracheostomy T Bar		
Tight fit allows better O_2 and humidity delivery than tracheostomy collar.	Condensed fluid in tubing may drain into tracheostomy. Water traps are usually put in.	T bar must be removed for suctioning. Mörch swivel may be used to eliminate the need for removal. It should be emptied as necessary.
Tent or Incubator		
Tent or incubator has ability to control temperature and humidity.	Tent or incubator has limited usefulness. It is difficult to maintain adequate concentrations of O_2. Method isolates patient from environment.	Tent should be flushed with O_2 every time it is opened. Nurse should assess for leaks around canopy.
High Flow Delivery Devices		
Venturi Mask*		
Mask can deliver precise, high flow rates of O_2. Lightweight plastic, cone-shaped device is fitted to face. Masks are available for delivery of 24%, 28%, 31%, 35%, 40%, and 50% O_2. Adaptors can be applied to increase humidification.	Mask is uncomfortable and must be removed when patient eats. Patient can talk but voice may be muffled. Other disadvantages are the same as those discussed for the simple face mask.	Entrainment device on mask must be changed to deliver higher concentrations of O_2. Method is especially helpful for administering low, constant O_2 concentrations to patients with COPD. Air entrainment ports must not be occluded.

*See Fig. 27-10, *C*.
†See Fig. 27-11.

Humidification and nebulizers. Oxygen obtained from cylinders or wall systems is dry. Dry oxygen has an irritating effect on mucous membranes and dries secretions. Therefore it is important that O_2 be humidified when administered, either by humidification or nebulization. A common device used for humidification when the patient has a catheter, cannula, or low-flow mask is a bubble-through humidifier. It is a small plastic jar filled with sterile distilled water that is attached to the O_2 source by means of a flowmeter. O_2 passes into the jar, bubbles through the water, and then goes through tubing to the patient's catheter, cannula, or mask. The purpose of the bubble-through humidifier is to restore the humidity conditions of room air. However, the need for bubble-through humidifiers at flow rates between 1 and 4 L per minute is controversial when humidity in the environment is adequate.[27]

Another means of administering humidified O_2 is via a nebulizer. It delivers particulate water mist (aerosols) with nearly 100% humidity. The humidity can be raised by heating the

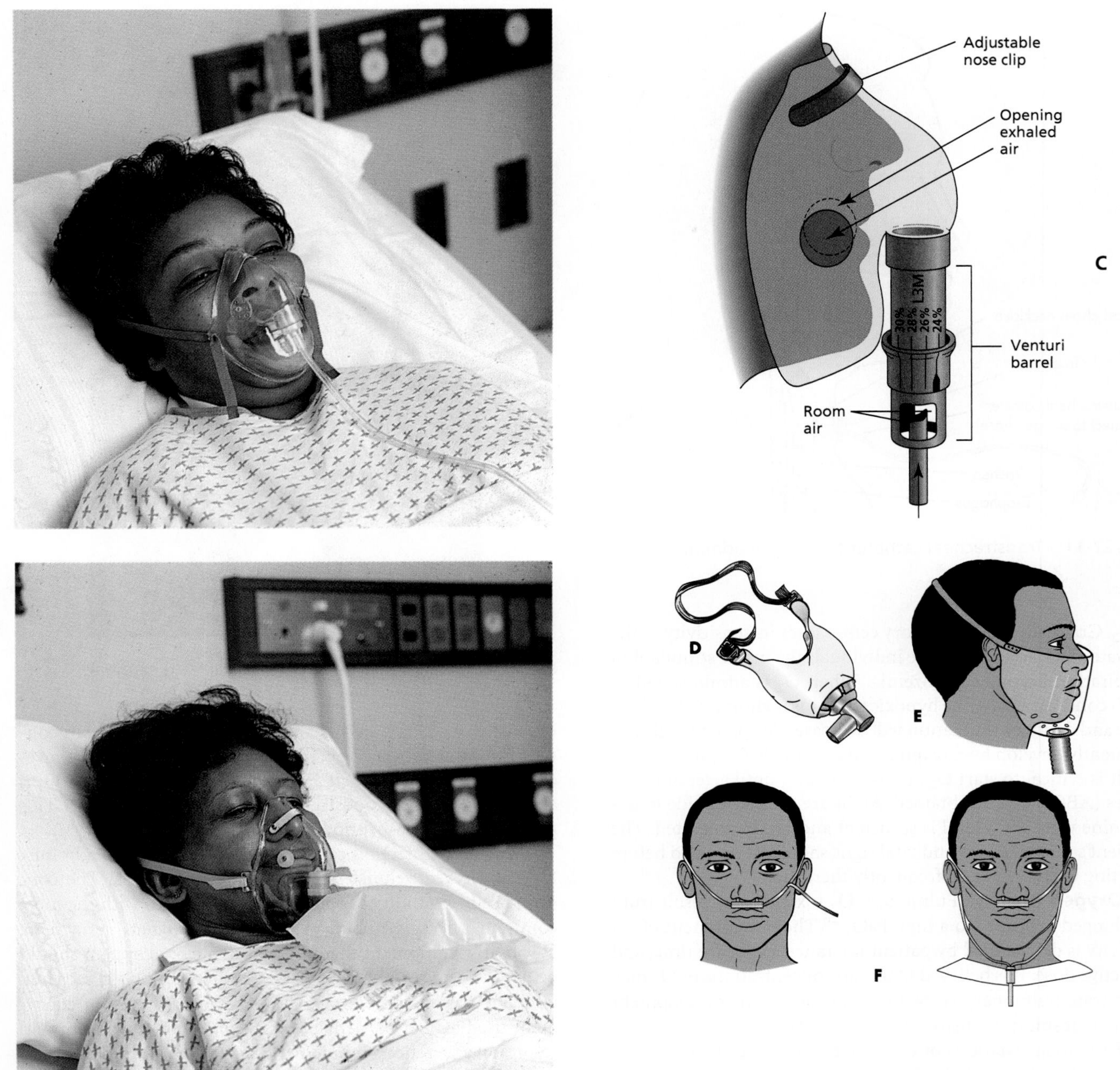

Fig. 27-10 Methods of oxygen administration. Shown are **A,** Simple face mask. **B,** Plastic face mask with reservoir bag. **C,** Venturi mask. **D,** Tracheostomy mask. **E,** Face tent. **F,** Standard nasal cannulas.

water, which increases the ability of the gas to hold moisture. Heated (98.6° F [37° C]) and humidified (100%) gas is required when the upper airway is bypassed. When nebulizers are used, large-size tubing should be employed to connect the device to a face mask or T bar. If small-size tubing is used, condensation can occlude the flow of O_2.

Complications

Combustion. Oxygen supports combustion and increases the rate of burning. This is why it is important that smoking be prohibited in the area in which O_2 is being used. A "No Smoking" sign should be prominently displayed on the patient's door. The patient should also be cautioned against smoking cigarettes with O_2 prongs or a catheter in place.

Carbon dioxide narcosis. In some cases of respiratory distress, increasing the O_2 flow rate may be harmful. Normally, carbon dioxide (CO_2) accumulation is a major stimulant of the respiratory center. However, the individual with a long-standing history of COPD (i.e., one who may be a CO_2 retainer and confirmed with arterial blood gases) or the patient who is heavily sedated may have a tendency to hypoventilate and to retain

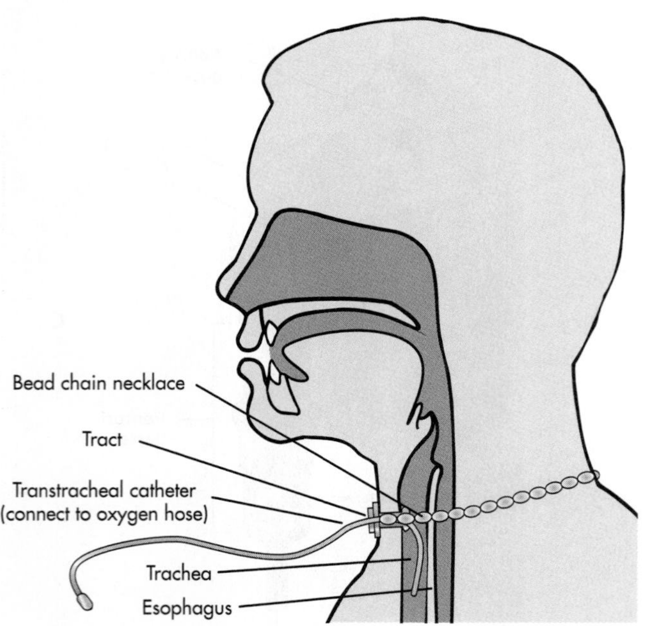

Fig. 27-11 Transtracheal catheter for oxygen administration.

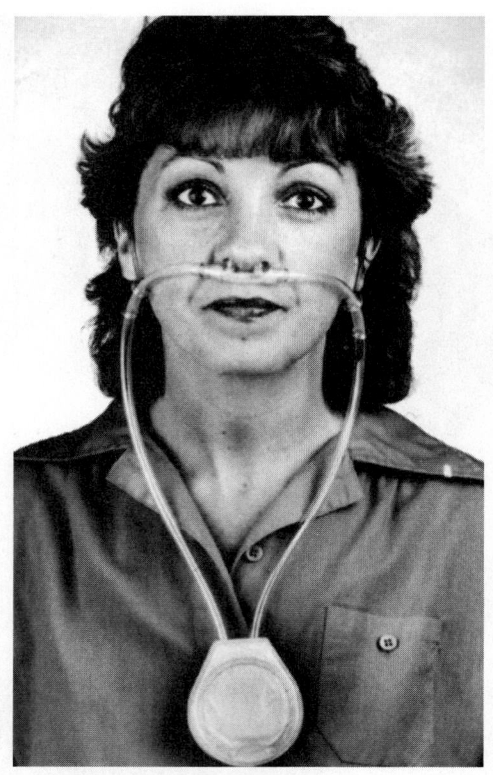

Fig. 27-12 Pendant-type oxygen-conserving cannula.

CO_2. Gradually, the respiratory center loses its sensitivity to the elevated CO_2 level. For these individuals the major stimulant of respiration becomes hypoxemia. When O_2 is administered in high concentrations, the hypoxic stimulus is eliminated and the rate and depth of ventilation will decrease. The patient will subsequently develop hypercapnia and eventually CO_2 narcosis.

It is critical to start O_2 at low flow rates until arterial blood gases (ABGs) can be obtained. ABGs are used as a guide to determine what FIO_2 level is sufficient and can be tolerated. The patient's mental status and vital signs should be assessed before starting O_2 therapy and frequently thereafter.

Oxygen toxicity. Pulmonary O_2 toxicity may result from prolonged exposure to a high PaO_2.[26] The development of O_2 toxicity is determined by patient tolerance, exposure time, and effective dose. It is believed that high concentrations of O_2 may inactivate pulmonary surfactant and lead to the development of acute respiratory distress syndrome (ARDS).

Early manifestations of O_2 toxicity are reduced vital capacity, cough, substernal chest pain, nausea and vomiting, paresthesia, nasal stuffiness, sore throat, and malaise. The later stages of O_2 toxicity affect the alveolar-capillary gas exchange unit, causing edema and production of copious sputum. The end stage of O_2 toxicity is progressive fibrosis of the lungs. Prevention of O_2 toxicity is important for the patient who is receiving O_2. The amount of O_2 administered should be just enough to maintain the PaO_2 within a normal or acceptable range for the patient. ABGs should be monitored frequently to evaluate the effectiveness of therapy and to guide the tapering of supplemental O_2. A safe limit of O_2 concentrations has not yet been established. All levels above 50% and used for longer than 24 hours should be considered potentially toxic. Levels of 40% and below may be regarded as relatively nontoxic and may not result in development of significant O_2 toxicity if the exposure period is short.

Absorption atelectasis. Normally nitrogen, which constitutes 79% of the air that is breathed, is not absorbed into the bloodstream. This prevents alveolar collapse. When high concentrations of O_2 are given, nitrogen is washed out of the alveoli and replaced with O_2. If airway obstruction occurs, the O_2 is absorbed into the bloodstream and the alveoli collapse. This process is called absorption atelectasis.

Infection. Infection can be a major hazard of O_2 administration. Heated nebulizers present the highest risk. The constant use of humidity supports bacterial growth with the most common infecting organism being *Pseudomonas aeruginosa.* Disposable equipment that operates as a closed system should be used. There should be a hospital policy stating the required frequency of equipment changes based on the type of equipment used at that particular institution. Both equipment and respiratory secretions should be stained using Gram's stain and cultured frequently.

Chronic oxygen therapy at home. Improved prognosis and quality of life has been noted in patients with COPD who receive nocturnal or continuous O_2 to treat hypoxemia.[28] This improved prognosis results from preventing progression of the disease and subsequent cor pulmonale. The benefits of long-term continuous oxygen therapy include improved neuropsychologic function, increased exercise tolerance, decreased hematocrit, and reduced pulmonary hypertension. It also improves sleep and may reduce nocturnal arrhythmias.[29]

The potential benefit of long-term O_2 therapy should be evaluated when the patient's condition has stabilized. There should be an accurate, current diagnosis and an optimal medical regimen prescribed by a physician knowledgeable in the treatment of respiratory disease. Short-term home O_2 therapy (1 to 30 days) may be indicated for the patient in whom hypoxemia persists after discharge from the hospital. For example, the patient with underlying COPD who develops a serious respira-

Table 27-18 Home Oxygen Delivery Systems

System	Advantages	Disadvantages	Comments
▪ Liquid oxygen	Portable unit* can be refilled by patient from reservoir. Portable unit holds 6-8 hr supply at 2 L/min; reservoir will last approximately 7-10 days at 2 L/min continuously.	Liquid system slightly more expensive, depending on location; not available everywhere; generally limited to urban areas.	As liquid warms to gas, some is vented from the system. In summer, evaporation is accelerated and may decrease reservoir duration to <1 wk.
▪ Compressed tank O_2 (H or J tank/E or A cylinder)	Good availability in most areas. Portability possible with cart. Aluminum E or A cylinders available that are markedly lighter than steel and easier to maneuver.	Duration of H or J tank at 2 L/min flow about 50 hr; storage of 4-5 large cylinders in the home necessary to have 1 wk to 10-day supply; portable cylinder on cart is cumbersome and heavy. Duration of E cylinder at 2 L/min approximately 4-5 hr; A cylinder at 2 L/min will last approximately 8-10 hr.	Some smaller tanks (D or M) may be used; these can be refilled from large cylinders and weigh about 10 lb. Tank can be carried on shoulder strap, backpack, or fanny pack or placed on portable cart.
▪ Concentrator or extractor (E or A cylinder)	On wheels, movable from room to room; weekly delivery of supply not necessary, because unit delivers oxygen continuously; compact, excellent system for rural or homebound patient.	Older models can be noisy; increase in electricity bill by \$20-\$30 a month (not reimbursable by insurance); >3 L flow resulting in significant decrease in concentration. Patient will need backup O_2 tank in case electricity fails.	Concentrator should be kept in room other than bedroom; extension tubing should be used if noise disturbs sleep.
▪ Pulse or demand delivery system	Simple to use; delivery rate changes with respiratory rate, (i.e., the faster the patient's rate, the higher the rate of delivery).	Mechanically complex; only safe use with portable system when patient is awake unless there is an alarm to detect disconnection of patient. Oxygenation possibly less efficient with exertion.	System may be a separate unit that can be used with liquid or cylinder, or can be "built in" to portable liquid oxygen unit. Less drying, rarely needs humidification.

*Portable usually refers to units weighing more than 10 lb (4.5 kg) and ambulatory units weigh less than 10 lb.

tory infection may continue to have clearing of the infection after completion of antibiotic therapy and discharge from the hospital. This patient may demonstrate continued hypoxemia for 4 to 6 weeks after discharge. It is important to measure the patient's oxygenation status 2 to 3 months after an acute episode to determine if the oxygen is still warranted.[25,29]

Patients whose disease is stable with a PaO_2 of 55 mm Hg or less (corresponding to an SaO_2 of 88% or less) should receive long-term oxygen therapy. A patient whose PaO_2 is between 55 and 59 mm Hg (SaO_2 89%) and who exhibits signs of tissue hypoxia, such as cor pulmonale, erythrocytosis, edema from right-sided heart failure, or impaired mental status, should also receive long-term O_2 therapy. Desaturation only during exercise or sleep suggests consideration of oxygen therapy specifically under those conditions. These guidelines are generally accepted and have been adopted by Medicare as reimbursement criteria. Patients may receive oxygen only during exercise or sleep or at both times. The need for oxygen during these periods should be evaluated with oximetry. (Pulse oximetry is discussed in Chapter 24.)

Periodic reevaluations are necessary for the patient who is using chronic supplemental O_2. Generally the recommendation is that the patient should be reevaluated every 30 to 90 days during the first year of therapy and annually after that, as long as the patient remains stable. This frequency of reevaluation is used by Medicare and other third-party payers for reimbursement determinations.[25,29]

Nasal cannulas, either regular or the O_2-conserving type (Table 27-17 and Fig. 27-12) are usually used to deliver O_2 from a central source in the home. The source may be a liquid O_2 storage system, compressed O_2 in tanks, or an O_2 concentrator or extractor, depending on the patient's home environment, activity level, and proximity to an O_2 supply company (Table 27-18). The patient can use extension tubing (up to 50 feet) without adversely affecting the O_2 flow delivery to increase mobility in the home, provided that the flowmeter is the back pressure–compensated type. Small portable systems may be provided for the patient who remains active outside the home (Fig. 27-13).

Reservoir cannulas operate on the principle of storing O_2 in a small reservoir during exhalation. The O_2 is then delivered to the patient during the subsequent inhalation, similar to a bolus effect. The reservoir cannulas can reduce flow requirements by approximately 50%. There is a pendant type (see Fig. 27-12). Another type that fits onto the frame of eyeglasses is also available and is less visible on the face.

Other delivery devices for chronic O_2 therapy include transtracheal O_2 delivery and intermittent-demand O_2 delivery systems. Transtracheal O_2 delivery requires a surgical procedure to insert the small O_2 catheter into the patient's trachea (see Fig. 27-11). Nursing care involves teaching the patient and

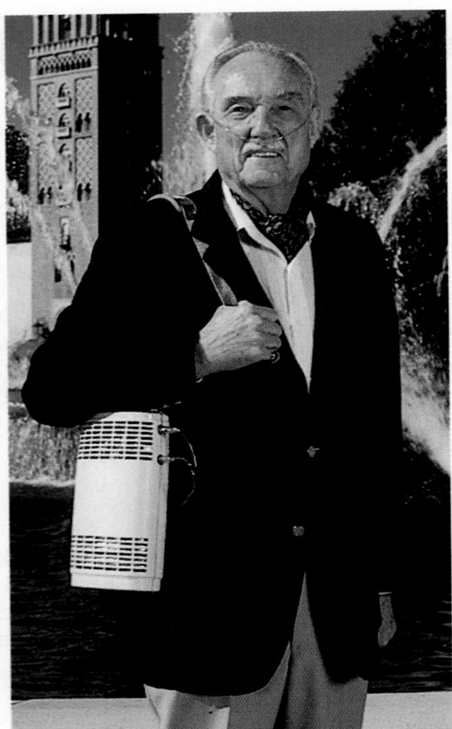

Fig. 27-13 Ambulatory liquid oxygen system.

family how to care for supplemental O_2 transtracheally. The transtracheal catheter is less visible than nasal cannulas and there is no nasal irritation. It also reduces the O_2 flow requirement by 30% to 50%.

Intermittent-demand delivery systems are mechanically complex devices. They deliver "pulses" of O_2 to the patient, usually during inspiration, and thus eliminate wasted flow during exhalation as is experienced during continuous flow. There are intermittent-demand units that operate independently of a particular system and units that are built into the delivery device itself.

Home O_2 systems are usually rented from a company that sends a respiratory therapist or pulmonary nurse specialist to the patient's home. The therapist teaches the patient how to use the O_2 system, how to care for it, and how to recognize when the supply is running low and needs to be reordered. Home care guides for teaching the patient and family about use of O_2 at home are presented in Table 27-19.

The patient who uses home O_2 should be encouraged to remain active and to travel normally. If travel is by automobile, arrangements can be made for O_2 to be available at the destination point. O_2 supply companies can often assist in these arrangements. If a patient wishes to travel by bus, train, or airplane, these parties require notification when reservations are made of the need for O_2 during the travel. A high altitude simulation test (HAST) may be performed in a hospital pulmonary function laboratory to determine the oxygen prescription required for the altitude at which the patient will be flying. Because airplane cabins are pressurized to an elevation of 7000 or 8000 feet, the patient who uses supplemental O_2 should have O_2 provided during flight. The plane's O_2 system must be used. Patients may not use their own O_2 system during flight because it is not properly pressurized. Airlines allow patients to bring their oxygen system to be carried in the baggage compartment for use at the point of destination, but the reservoirs (liquid or tank) must be empty and the valves left open. Some patients may need to avoid prolonged exposure to high elevations during travel unless they are instructed by their physician regarding adjustments in their O_2 flow to attempt to compensate for altitude.[25]

PATIENT & FAMILY HOME CARE GUIDE

Table 27-19 Home Oxygen Use

Mask/Cannula
- Ensure that the straps are not too tight
- Remove 2-3 times/day to wash and dry skin where straps are and stimulate skin
- Pad any pressure points
- Observe tops of ears for skin breakdown from pressure points

Oral and Nasal Mucous Membranes
- Assess oral and nasal mucous membranes 2-3 times/day
- Use water-based gel on lips and nasal mucosa
- Provide frequent oral hygiene
- Provide humidification via humidifier or nebulizing device

Decreasing Risk for Infection
- Remove mask or collar and cleanse with water 2-3 times/day
- Cleanse skin carefully at this time and observe for cuts, scratches, and bruises
- Change disposable equipment frequently
- Remove secretions that are coughed out

Decreasing Risk of Fire Injuries
- Post "No Smoking" warning signs in home where they can be seen
- Do not use electric razors, portable radios, open flames, wool blankets, or mineral oils in the area where oxygen is in use
- Do not allow smoking in the home

NOTE: A good resource for patients is *About Oxygen Therapy at Home,* a booklet published by the American Lung Association.

Surgical Therapy for Chronic Obstructive Pulmonary Disease. Three different surgical procedures have been used in severe COPD. One of the oldest is bullectomy (removal of bullae). Bullae are abnormally dilated air spaces within the lungs (see Fig. 27-8). These large bullae compress normal and abnormal lung tissue. Some large bullae may cause repeated pneumothorax or hemoptysis. This operation is rarely performed because only a small percentage of COPD patients have large bullae.

Another type of surgery that is currently being used is lung volume reduction surgery (LVRS).[30,31] The rationale for this type of surgery is that by reducing the size of the hyperinflated emphysematous lungs, there is decreased airway obstruction and increased room for normal alveoli. The procedure reduces lung volume and improves lung and chest wall mechanics. There are different types of LVRS. In one approach a median sternotomy is performed and parts of each lung are removed and tissue reattached using a stapling device. Another approach is a video-assisted thoracoscopy that can be performed unilaterally or bilaterally. In this approach either a stapling or laser procedure can be done, or they can be done together.[31] The most common postoperative complication is pneumonia. The National Institutes of Health is currently funding a large multicenter study to evaluate the effectiveness of LVRS.

The third surgical procedure is lung transplantation. COPD patients are the largest group of patients on waiting lists for lung transplantation. Although single-lung transplant is the most commonly used technique, bilateral transplantation can be performed. In appropriately selected patients with COPD, lung transplantation prolongs life, improves functional capacity, and enhances quality of life. However, rejection and effects of immunosuppressive therapy remain an obstacle.[32] Lung transplantation does not offer a cure but rather an exchange of one set of medical problems for another. (Lung transplantation is discussed in Chapter 26.)

Respiratory Care. Respiratory care is usually a collaborative effort involving respiratory therapists and nurses. Respiratory care includes breathing retraining, effective cough techniques, chest physiotherapy, and aerosol-nebulization therapy.

Breathing retraining. The patient with COPD develops an increased respiratory rate with a prolonged expiration to compensate for dyspnea. In addition, the accessory muscles of breathing in the neck and upper part of the chest are used excessively to promote chest wall movement. These muscles are not designed for long-term use and as a result the patient experiences increased fatigue. Breathing exercises can assist the patient during rest and activity (e.g., lifting, walking, stair climbing). The main types of breathing exercises are (1) pursed-lip breathing and (2) diaphragmatic breathing.

The purpose of using pursed-lip breathing is to prolong exhalation and thereby prevent bronchiolar collapse and air trapping. The patient is taught to inhale slowly through the nose and then to exhale slowly through pursed lips, almost as if whistling. Exhalation should be at least three times as long as inhalation. It is helpful to have the nurse demonstrate the breathing exercises so the patient can imitate the action. The following techniques can be used to teach pursed-lip breathing:

1. Blow through a straw in a glass of water with the intent of forming small bubbles.
2. Blow at a lit candle enough to bend the flame without blowing it out.
3. Steadily blow a table-tennis ball across a table.

Diaphragmatic (abdominal) breathing focuses on using the diaphragm instead of the accessory muscles to achieve maximum inhalation and to slow the respiratory rate. The patient should be made aware of the difference between chest breathing and abdominal breathing. This can be achieved by having the patient lie down or assume a semi-Fowler's position and by placing one hand on the chest and the other on the abdomen. The patient should observe which hand moves during inspiration. The abdomen should protrude on inhalation with diaphragmatic breathing and contract on exhalation as the diaphragm pushes the air out of the lungs. The nurse should emphasize the value of diaphragmatic movement in increasing lung expansion.

PATIENT TEACHING GUIDE

Table 27-20 Guidelines for Effective Coughing

1. Patient assumes a sitting position with head slightly flexed, shoulders relaxed, knees flexed, and forearms supported by pillow, and if possible, with feet on the floor.
2. Patient then drops head and bends forward while using slow, pursed-lip breathing to exhale.
3. Sitting up again, patient uses diaphragmatic breathing to inhale slowly and deeply.
4. Patient repeats steps 2 and 3 three to four times to facilitate mobilization of secretions.
5. Before initiating a cough, patient should take a deep abdominal breath, bend slightly forward, and then huff cough (cough three to four times on exhalation). Patient may need to support or splint thorax or abdomen to achieve a maximum cough.

To practice diaphragmatic breathing, the patient should keep the hand on the abdomen and concentrate on filling up the abdomen by inhaling slowly through the nose. Another technique is to wrap a towel gently around the abdomen and to pull it tight during exhalation. The patient then attempts to stretch the towel with slow inhalation by diaphragmatic breathing. On exhalation the patient uses pursed-lip breathing and draws the towel tighter to promote effective expiration.

Another technique to assist in diaphragmatic breathing is to place a small pillow, magazine, book, or small bag of beans on the abdomen. This approach provides tactile stimulation and visual feedback. If the object rises on inspiration, the patient is given positive feedback that diaphragmatic breathing is taking place.

Pursed-lip breathing and diaphragmatic breathing should be practiced together for 8 to 10 repetitions three or four times a day. These techniques give the patient more control over breathing, especially during exercise and periods of dyspnea.

In the setting of extreme acute dyspnea when the patient is hospitalized for infection or heart failure, it is more important to focus on helping the patient slow the respiratory rate by using the principles of pursed-lip breathing. Diaphragmatic (abdominal) breathing requires more energy and thus should be taught only when the patient has achieved a stable rehabilitative state such as before discharge or in a home care rehabilitation program.

Effective coughing. Many patients with COPD have developed ineffective coughing patterns that do not adequately clear their airways of sputum. In addition, they fear they may develop spastic coughing, resulting in dyspnea. Guidelines for effective coughing are presented in Table 27-20. Huff coughing is an effective technique that the patient can be easily taught. The main goals of effective coughing are to conserve energy, reduce fatigue, and facilitate removal of secretions.

Chest physiotherapy. Chest physiotherapy (CPT) is indicated in the patient with (1) excessive bronchial secretions who has difficulty clearing secretions with expectorated sputum production greater than 25 to 30 ml a day, (2) evidence or suggestion of retained secretions in the presence of an artificial airway, or (3) lobar atelectasis caused by or suspected of being caused by mucous plugging.

Table 27-21 Steps in Chest Physiotherapy

1. Perform procedure 1 hr before meals or 1-3 hr after meals.
2. Administer bronchodilator (if nebulized or MDI is ordered) approximately 15 min before procedure.
3. Collect needed equipment such as tissues, emesis basin, paper bag, and pillows.
4. Help patient assume correct position for postural drainage based on findings from x-ray, auscultation, palpation, and percussion of chest. Position should be maintained for 5-15 min to mobilize secretions via gravity.
5. Observe patient during treatment to assess tolerance. Particularly observe breathing and color changes, especially duskiness in face.
6. Have patient take several deep abdominal breaths.
7. Percuss appropriate area for 1-2 min.
8. Vibrate the same area while the patient exhales 4-5 deep breaths.*
9. Assist patient to cough while assuming same position. Splinting with towel or hands may be necessary to aid in effective coughing. Patient may have to assume sitting position to generate enough airflow to expel secretions. (Coughing productively may be a long waiting process that may occur 30 min after procedure.) Suction may be necessary if coughing is not effective.
10. Repeat percussion, vibration, and coughing until patient no longer expectorates mucus.
11. Repeat same procedure in all necessary positions.
12. After procedure, help patient assume a comfortable position, assist with oral hygiene, and discard used tissues.
13. Monitor for hypoxemia if patient having any respiratory difficulty during the procedure.
14. Evaluate and chart effectiveness of treatment by amount of sputum produced and the results of auscultation. Also chart patient tolerance.

*If using an electronic vibrator, use for periods of 5-20 min in each position according to the patient's tolerance.
MDI, metered dose inhaler.

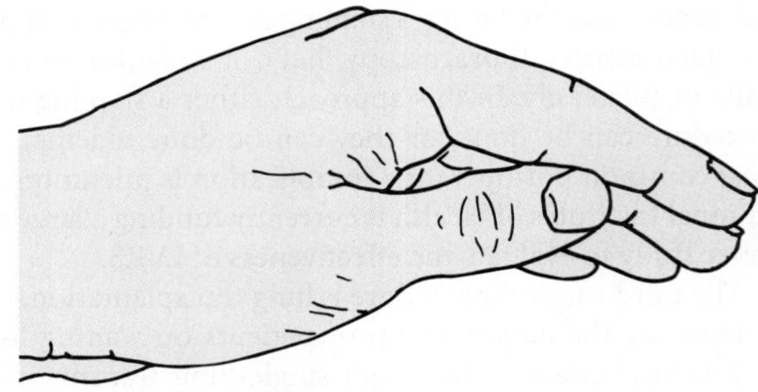

Fig. 27-14 Cupped-hand position for percussion. The hand should be cupped as though scooping up water.

Chest physiotherapy consists of percussion, vibration, and postural drainage (Table 27-21). Percussion and vibration are manual or mechanical techniques used to augment postural drainage. Postural drainage uses the principle of gravity to assist in bronchial drainage. Percussion and vibration are used after the patient has assumed a postural drainage position to assist in loosening the mobilized secretions. Percussion, vibration, and postural drainage may assist in bringing secretions into larger, more central airways. Effective coughing is then necessary to help raise these secretions. After each drainage position change, the patient should be given time to cough and deep breathe. These techniques are individualized based on the patient's pulmonary condition and response to the initial treatment. Sometimes it takes several hours after CPT for secretions to be expectorated. It is important to evaluate CPT for both its effectiveness and relief of the patient's symptoms. CPT should be performed by an individual who has been properly trained. Complications associated with improperly performed CPT include fractured ribs, bruising, hypoxemia, and discomfort to the patient. CPT may not be beneficial and may be stressful for some patients. Some patients may develop hypoxemia and bronchospasms with CPT.

Percussion. Percussion is performed in the appropriate postural drainage position with the hands in a cuplike position (Fig. 27-14). The hands are cupped, and the fingers and thumbs are closed. The cupped hand should create an air pocket between the patient's chest and the hand. Both hands are cupped and used in an alternating rhythmic fashion. Percussion is accomplished with flexion and extension of the wrists. If it is performed correctly, a hollow sound should be heard. The air-cushion impact facilitates the movement of thick mucus. A thin towel should be placed over the area to be percussed, or the patient may choose to wear a T-shirt or hospital gown. Percussion should not be performed over the kidneys, sternum, spinal cord, or any tender or painful area. Other contraindications to percussion include hemoptysis, carcinoma, and induced bronchospasm.

Vibration. Vibration is accomplished by tensing the hand and arm muscles repeatedly and pressing mildly with the flat of the hand on the affected area while the patient slowly exhales a deep breath. The vibrations facilitate movement of secretions to larger airways. Mild vibration is tolerated better than percussion and can be used in situations where percussion may be contraindicated. Commercial vibrators are available for hospital and home use.

Postural drainage. The lungs are divided into five lobes, with three on the right side and two on the left side. There are 18 segments in the lungs, which can be drained by 18 positions. Figure 27-15 shows the modified postural drainage positions most often used in clinical practice. The purpose of various positions in postural drainage is to drain each segment toward the larger airways. The postural drainage positions are determined by the areas of involved lung, which are assessed by chest x-rays, percussion, palpation, and auscultation. Aerosolized bronchodilators and hydration therapy are frequently administered before postural drainage. The chosen postural drainage position is maintained for 5 to 15 minutes. The degree of slope can be obtained with pillows, blocks, books, or a tilt board.

The frequency and choice of postural drainage positions depend on the location of retained secretions and patient tolerance to dependent positions. A common order is two to four times a day. In acute situations, postural drainage may be performed as frequently as every 1 to 2 hours. The procedure should be planned to occur and be completed at least 1 hour before meals or 3 hours after meals.

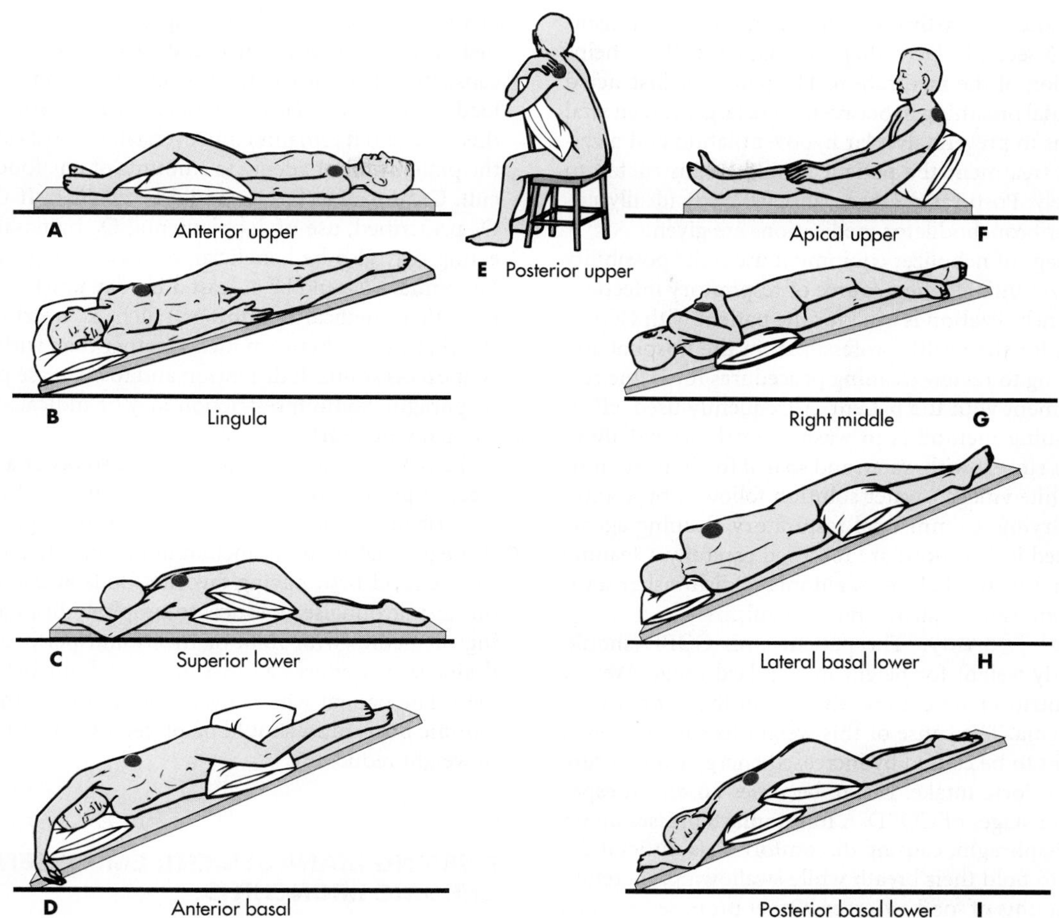

Fig. 27-15 Representative positions for postural drainage. *Shaded areas* in each drawing indicate the segment of the lung in which drainage is promoted.

If a patient has difficulty in assuming various positions, adaptations will need to be made by reducing the angle or length of time of the procedure. A side-lying position can be used for the patient who cannot tolerate a head-down position. Some positions for postural drainage (e.g., Trendelenburg's) should not be performed on the patient with chest trauma, hemoptysis, heart disease, or head injury, and in other situations where the patient's condition is not stable.

Flutter mucus clearance device. The Flutter mucus clearance device is a handheld device that provides positive expiratory pressure (PEP) treatment for patients with mucus-producing conditions. The Flutter valve works by (1) vibrating the airways (which loosens mucus from airway walls), (2) intermittently increasing the endobronchial pressure (which helps maintain the patency of the airway), and (3) accelerating expiratory airflow. It helps move mucus up through the airways to the mouth where the mucus can be expectorated.

The Flutter valve has been used in place of CPT in some patients in whom chest physiotherapy cannot be used (e.g., patients with pneumothorax or right-sided heart failure). Although the Flutter valve is mostly used in patients with cystic fibrosis, it has been effectively used in patients with chronic bronchitis and bronchiectasis.

Aerosol-nebulization therapy. Medications for COPD patients are most often delivered via metered-dose inhalers. This is the preferred delivery route, although devices that deliver a suspension of fine particles of liquid in a gas may also be used to deliver medications to the COPD patient. Nebulizers are usually powered by a compressed air or O_2 generator. At home the patient may have an air-powered compressor; in the hospital, wall O_2 or compressed air is used to power the nebulizer.

Aerosolized medication orders must include the medication, dose, diluent, and whether it is to be nebulized with O_2 or compressed air. If O_2 is inadvertently used, a patient could become apneic if hypoxia was the primary respiratory stimulant. Medication is nebulized or reduced to a fine spray, and depending on several factors, including droplet size, it can be inhaled into the patient's tracheobronchial tree. The advantage to aerosol-nebulization therapy is a rapid-acting form of administration with few systemic effects. Medications that are routinely nebulized include albuterol and ipratropium. Other medications infrequently used that can be administered by nebulization include antibiotics, pentamidine, and DNase (Pulmozyme).

The patient is placed in an upright position that allows for most efficient breathing to ensure adequate penetration and deposition of the aerosolized medication. The patient must breathe slowly and deeply through the mouth and hold inspiration for 2 to 3 seconds. Deep diaphragmatic breathing helps ensure deposition of the medication. The patient is instructed to do normal tidal breathing in between these larger forced vital capacity breaths to prevent alveolar hypoventilation and dizziness. After the treatment the patient should be instructed to cough effectively. Postural drainage and CPT are ideally administered after bronchodilator medications are given.

A disadvantage of nebulizer equipment use is the possibility that the nebulizer unit will be a source of respiratory infection. Because home nebulization is used for the patient with COPD, it is important for the health professional in the hospital and home care setting to review cleaning procedures for home respiratory equipment with the patient. A frequently used, effective home-cleaning method is to wash the nebulizer daily in soap and water, rinse it with water, and soak it for 20 to 30 minutes in a 1:1 white vinegar–water solution followed by a water rinse and air drying. Commercial respiratory cleaning agents may also be used if directions are followed carefully. Cleaning the nebulizer in the top shelf of an automatic dishwasher saves time, and the hot water destroys most organisms.

Nutritional Therapy. The patient with COPD should try to keep body weight for height in standard range. Weight loss and malnutrition are commonly seen in the patient with severe emphysema. The cause of this weight loss is unknown, but it is thought to be caused by increased energy expenditure or inadequate caloric intake. Eating becomes an effort, especially in the later stages of COPD. A full stomach presses up on the flattened diaphragm, causing discomfort. It is difficult for some patients to hold their breath while swallowing; therefore inadequate amounts of food are eaten. Other proposed reasons for malnutrition include loss of appetite related to a decreased sense of taste and smell and gastrointestinal disturbances.

To decrease dyspnea and conserve energy, the patient should rest at least 30 minutes before eating and should select foods that can be prepared in advance. The patient should eat five to six small, frequent meals to avoid feelings of bloating and early satiety when eating. Exercises and treatments should be avoided at least 1 hour before and after eating. The exertion involved in the preparation and eating of food is often fatiguing. The use of a microwave oven may help conserve patient energy in food preparation.

Many patients with COPD have feelings of bloating and early satiety when eating. This sensation can be attributed to swallowing air while eating, side effects of medication (especially corticosteroids and theophylline), and the abnormal position of the diaphragm relative to the stomach in association with hyperinflation. A full stomach puts pressure on the diaphragm and decreases lung movement. Liquid, blenderized, or commercial diets may be helpful. Foods that require a great deal of chewing should be avoided or served in another manner (e.g., grated, pureed). Cold foods may give less of a sense of fullness than hot foods.

The patient with emphysema has a greater than normal nutritional requirement for protein and calories. A high-calorie, high-protein diet is recommended and can be divided into five to six small meals a day. High-protein, high-calorie nutritional supplements can be offered between meals. Ice cream added to these supplements can help increase calories. (Nutritional supplements are discussed in Chapter 38.) A high-carbohydrate diet may need to be avoided in the patient who retains CO_2 because carbohydrates metabolize into CO_2 and increase the CO_2 load of the patient. However, research is currently being done in this area, and it remains controversial. In most cases just getting the patients to eat adequate amounts of any foods can be difficult. Gas-forming foods should be avoided. If the patient has O_2 prescribed, use of supplemental O_2 by nasal prongs while eating may also be beneficial, because eating expends energy. Fluid intake should be at least 3 L a day unless contraindicated for other medical conditions, such as heart failure. Fluids should be taken between meals (rather than with them) to prevent excess stomach distention and to decrease pressure on the diaphragm. Sodium restriction may be indicated if there is accompanying heart failure.

Loss of appetite and nausea may also occur as a result of increased production of mucus and as an effect of some of the prescribed medications. If anorexia is a problem, various strategies can be used, including having the patient eat high-calorie food first; having favorite foods available; and adding butter, mayonnaise, or sauces to supply additional calories. Taking medicines with milk or meals and performing bronchial drainage procedures approximately 1 hour before meals may help. The patient who is overweight, more commonly seen in chronic bronchitis, should be placed on a low-fat diet to assist in weight reduction.

NURSING MANAGEMENT: EMPHYSEMA AND CHRONIC BRONCHITIS

■ Nursing Assessment

Subjective and objective data that should be obtained from a person with emphysema or chronic bronchitis are presented in Table 27-22.

■ Nursing Diagnoses

The nursing diagnoses for the patient with emphysema and chronic bronchitis may include, but are not limited to, those presented in NCP 27-2.

■ Planning

The overall goals are that the patient with COPD will have (1) return of baseline respiratory function, (2) ability to perform ADLs, (3) relief from dyspnea, (4) no complications related to COPD, (5) knowledge and ability to implement a long-term treatment regimen, and (6) overall improved quality of life.

■ Nursing Implementation

Health Promotion. The incidence of COPD would decrease if more people would not begin smoking or would stop smoking. Avoiding or controlling exposure to occupational and environmental pollutants and irritants is another preventive measure to maintain healthy lungs. (These factors are discussed in the section on nursing management of lung cancer in Chapter 26.)

Early detection of small-airway disease is important. The person who has smoked for only a few years may have early evidence of obstructive airway disease. These changes often can-

NURSING ASSESSMENT

Table 27-22 Emphysema or Chronic Bronchitis

Subjective Data

Important Health Information

Past health history: Long-term exposure to chemical pollution, respiratory irritants, occupational fumes, dust; recurrent respiratory infections; previous hospitalizations

Medications: Use and duration of use of O_2, bronchodilators, corticosteroids, antibiotics, anticholinergics, OTC drugs, herbs

Functional Health Patterns

Health perception–health management: Smoking (pack-years, including passive smoking); family history of respiratory disease

Nutritional-metabolic: Anorexia, weight loss or gain

Activity-exercise: Fatigue, inability to perform ADLs; palpitations, swelling of feet; progressive dyspnea, especially on exertion; wheezing; recurrent cough; sputum production with changes in color, odor, viscosity, amount; orthopnea

Elimination: Constipation, gas, bloating

Sleep-rest: Insomnia; sitting up position for sleeping, paroxysmal nocturnal dyspnea

Cognitive-perceptual: Chest and abdominal soreness, headache

Objective Data

General

Debilitation, anxiety, depression, restlessness, assumption of upright position

Integumentary

Cyanosis (bronchitis), pallor or ruddy color, poor skin turgor, thin skin, digital clubbing, easy bruising; peripheral edema (cor pulmonale)

Respiratory

Rapid, shallow breathing; inability to speak; prolonged expiratory phase; pursed-lip breathing; wheezing; rhonchi, crackles, diminished or bronchial breath sounds; decreased chest excursion and diaphragm movement; use of accessory muscles; hyperresonant or dull chest sounds on percussion

Cardiovascular

Tachycardia; arrhythmias, jugular vein distention, distant heart tones, right-sided S_3 (cor pulmonale), edema (especially in feet)

Gastrointestinal

Ascites, hepatomegaly (cor pulmonale)

Musculoskeletal

Muscle atrophy, increased anteroposterior diameter (barrel-chest)

Possible Findings

Abnormal ABGs, polycythemia, pulmonary function tests showing expiratory airflow obstruction (e.g., low FEV_1, low FEV_1/VC, large RV, low PEFR compared with baseline, decreased expiratory flow rate), chest x-ray showing flattened diaphragm and hyperinflation or infiltrates, ECG showing arrhythmias

ADLs, activities of daily living; *OTC,* over-the-counter; *RV,* residual volume; *VC,* vital capacity.

not be detected from pulmonary function studies until extensive damage is present. It is extremely important for the person to stop smoking and avoid inhaling irritants while the disease is still reversible. Failure to follow this advice will inevitably lead to irreversible COPD.

As health care professionals, nurses who smoke should reevaluate the smoking behavior and its relationship to their health. It is also important for nurses to counsel patients and peers regarding the harmful effects of smoking and to encourage them to quit. Referring patients and peers to self-help groups in the community may be especially valuable. These groups are sponsored by organizations such as the American Lung Association, American Cancer Society, and American Heart Association. These groups also have literature available that provides helpful guidelines, encouragement, and support. Nurses should participate actively in developing policies establishing smoke-free working environments for themselves and others, controlling smoking in public places, requiring self-extinguishing cigarettes to prevent fire deaths and injuries, prohibiting advertising and tobacco promotions, and mandating health warning labels on cigarette packages. Nurses, physicians, and respiratory therapists who smoke and smell of cigarette smoke should be aware that the odor of their clothes can be offensive to patients.

Early diagnosis and treatment of respiratory tract infections are other ways to decrease the incidence of COPD. Avoiding exposure to large crowds in the peak periods for influenza may be necessary, especially for the older adult and the person with a history of respiratory problems. Influenza and pneumococcal pneumonia vaccines are recommended for the patient with COPD.

Families with a history of AAT deficiency should be aware of the genetic nature of the disease. Genetic counseling may be appropriate for the patient who is planning to have children.

Acute Intervention. The patient with COPD will require acute intervention for complications such as pneumonia, cor pulmonale, and acute respiratory failure. (The nursing care for these conditions is discussed in Chapters 26 and 62.) Once the crisis in these situations has been resolved, the nurse can assess the degree and severity of the underlying respiratory problem. (The section on assessment in Chapter 24 provides a beginning basis to use in obtaining information from the patient.) The information obtained will help plan the nursing care.

27-2 NURSING CARE PLAN PATIENT WITH CHRONIC OBSTRUCTIVE PULMONARY DISEASE

Expected Patient Outcomes	Nursing Interventions and *Rationales*
NURSING DIAGNOSIS **Ineffective airway clearance** *related to* expiratory airflow obstruction, ineffective cough, decreased airway humidity, and infection in airways *as manifested by* dyspnea, ineffective or absent cough, presence of abnormal breath sounds, or diminished breath sounds.	
■ Normal breath sounds for patient. ■ Effective coughing.	■ Facilitate deep breathing by elevating head or sitting patient up *to maximize ventilation and prolong expiratory phase, which reduces trapped air.* ■ Position in semi-Fowler's position *to facilitate cough and prevent aspiration.* ■ Ensure hydration (oral intake approximately 2-3 L/day, humidified ambient air) *to liquefy secretions for easier expectoration.* ■ Teach effective cough techniques *to minimize airway collapse and aid in proper coughing.* ■ Provide chest physiotherapy (positioning, percussion, and vibration) when indicated *to use effect of gravity in removing secretions.* ■ Coordinate inhaled bronchodilator administration *to facilitate clearance of retained secretions.* ■ Teach alternative cough techniques (e.g., quad, huff), signs and symptoms of infection, and airway clearance techniques *to prepare patient for self-care at home.*
NURSING DIAGNOSIS **Impaired gas exchange: hypercapnia** *related to* alveolar hypoventilation *as manifested by* headache on awakening, $PaCO_2 \geq 45$ mm Hg and abnormal for patient's baseline.	
■ $PaCO_2$ of 35-40 mm Hg or usual compensated baseline value. ■ Demonstration of correct techniques to normalize $PaCO_2$ (e.g., secretion clearance and bronchodilator therapies). ■ Improved mental status.	■ Provide frequent stimulation (e.g., talking, turning, and positioning) *to keep patient moving and to mobilize secretions.* ■ Teach pursed-lip breathing *to prolong expiratory phase and slow respiratory rate.* ■ Assist patient to assume position of comfort (e.g., tripod position, elevated backrest, supported upper extremities to fix shoulder girdle) *to maximize respiratory excursion.* ■ Avoid use of respiratory depressants *to ensure adequate alveolar ventilation.* ■ Administer and teach appropriate use of bronchodilators *to treat bronchospasm and narrowing of bronchi.* ■ Teach potential hazard of excessive levels of inspired O_2 to patients with blunted CO_2 drive *because excess O_2 will depress respiratory drive.* ■ Teach signs, symptoms, and consequences of hypercapnia (e.g., confusion, somnolence, headache, irritability, decrease in mental acuity, increase in respiration, facial flush, diaphoresis) *so problem can be recognized early and treatment initiated.* ■ Teach avoidance of central nervous system depressants, *which further depress respirations.*
NURSING DIAGNOSIS **Impaired gas exchange: hypoxemia** *related to* alveolar hypoventilation, low ventilation/perfusion ratio, diffusion impairment, decreased ambient O_2, and decreased barometric pressure (high altitude) *as manifested by* $PaO_2 < 60$ mm Hg or $SaO_2 < 90\%$ at rest, confusion.	
■ Return of PaO_2 to normal range for patient. ■ Increased independence in activities of daily living. ■ Improved mental status.	■ Administer O_2 if appropriate *to increase O_2 saturation without depressing respiratory drive.* ■ Select O_2 supply systems and devices (e.g., nasal cannulas, mask) that are appropriate to patient's activities of daily living (rest, sleep, exercise) *to minimize impact on preferred lifestyle.* ■ Avoid unnecessary activity and provide assistance with activities of daily living *to reduce CO_2 retention.* ■ Teach and encourage deep breathing and pursed-lip breathing *to clear airways by propelling secretions toward mouth and to minimize air trapping.* ■ Implement airway clearance techniques, if appropriate. ■ Teach patient and family early signs and symptoms of impaired gas exchange (e.g., increased respiratory rate, irritability, anxiety, restlessness, dyspnea) *so interventions can be initiated promptly.* ■ Administer and teach appropriate use of bronchodilator. ■ Counsel patient about management of hypoxemia associated with air travel or increased altitude.

Continued

27-2 NURSING CARE PLAN PATIENT WITH CHRONIC OBSTRUCTIVE PULMONARY DISEASE—continued

Expected Patient Outcomes	Nursing Interventions and *Rationales*
NURSING DIAGNOSIS	**Self-care deficits** *related to* lowered energy level, hypoxemia, and depression *as manifested by* inability to perform activities of daily living without assistance.
▪ Able to perform activities of daily living by self or with assistance.	▪ Assess type of self-care deficits *to have baseline data for planning care.* ▪ Teach measures such as lifting on exhalation, using assistive devices for work activities, transferring techniques, pacing activities, and planning periods of rest *to conserve energy.* ▪ Refer to occupational therapy when appropriate *for analysis of energy-conserving aids and activities.* ▪ Administer O_2 if appropriate. ▪ Teach appropriate physical conditioning exercises *to increase strength and endurance.* ▪ Investigate need for personal assistance in home and refer to agencies that provide necessary assistance *to ensure that basic needs are met.*
NURSING DIAGNOSIS	**Altered nutrition: less than body requirements** *related to* poor appetite, lowered energy level, shortness of breath, gastric distention, sputum production, and depression *as manifested by* weight loss >10% of ideal body weight, serum albumin level below normal laboratory values, lack of interest in food.
▪ Maintenance of body weight within normal range for height and age. ▪ Normal serum protein and albumin levels.	▪ Monitor daily caloric intake, weight, and serum albumin *to determine adequacy of intake.* ▪ Provide menu suggestions for high-protein, high-calorie foods. ▪ Give patient high-protein, high-calorie liquid supplements if necessary *to provide adequate calories and protein to prevent weight loss and muscle wasting.* ▪ Plan periods of rest after food intake *to compensate for blood flow diversion to the GI tract for digestion.* ▪ Provide O_2 supplement during meals as required and prescribed. ▪ Refer to agency for financial or nutritional assistance as necessary (e.g., Meals-on-Wheels, food stamps) *to ensure nutritional adequacy after discharge.* ▪ Be aware that patient may benefit from six small meals throughout the day *because this reduces bloating.*
NURSING DIAGNOSIS	**Sleep pattern disturbance** *related to* anxiety, dyspnea, depression, hypoxemia or hypercapnia, and shortness of breath *as manifested by* insomnia, lethargy, fatigue, restlessness, irritability; orthopnea, paroxysmal nocturnal dyspnea.
▪ Feeling of being rested. ▪ Improvement in sleep pattern. ▪ Rested feeling on awakening.	▪ Identify usual sleep habits *to provide baseline data.* ▪ Ask patient why she or he is having difficulty sleeping, and identify causes of discomfort and wakefulness. ▪ Observe for signs and symptoms of sleep apnea syndrome such as frequent awakening at night, insomnia, and excessive daytime sleepiness *so appropriate interventions can be initiated.* ▪ Identify patient-specific methods of relaxation, and teach patient relaxation methods *to foster sleep.* ▪ Encourage exercise and activity during daylight hours *because this will improve sleep at night.* ▪ Instruct patient regarding position for easier breathing. ▪ Administer O_2 (if appropriate) *to increase* PaO_2. ▪ Instruct patient in maintaining an environment conducive to rest (e.g., clothing, temperature, position, noise level). ▪ Teach avoidance of alcoholic beverages, caffeine products, or other stimulants before bedtime *to reduce interference with sleep.*

Continued

27-2 NURSING CARE PLAN PATIENT WITH CHRONIC OBSTRUCTIVE PULMONARY DISEASE—continued

Expected Patient Outcomes	Nursing Interventions and *Rationales*
NURSING DIAGNOSIS	**Sexual dysfunction** *related to* dyspnea, effect of medications, and psychologic factors *as manifested by* decrease in desire for or interest in sex; decrease in social interactions with actual or potential sexual partners.
▪ Satisfaction with sexual functioning.	▪ Determine basis for dysfunction (physical or psychologic) *to plan appropriate interventions.* ▪ Teach use of O_2 during sexual activities and use of β-agonist metered-dose inhaler 10 minutes before sexual activities, if appropriate, *to reduce dyspnea secondary to hypoxemia.* ▪ Provide opportunity for patient and significant other to discuss feelings regarding problem *to foster sharing and mutual problem solving.* ▪ Help partner to understand change *so guilt and blame do not enter relationship.* ▪ Encourage patient and partner to explore other means of sexual expression and planning of sexual activity in terms of energy levels during the day *so means of sexual expression is maintained.* ▪ Counsel patient and partner on sexual positions *to conserve energy.* ▪ Refer for counseling, if indicated.
NURSING DIAGNOSIS	**Body image disturbance** *related to* changes in body appearance, function, illness, treatment *as manifested by* verbalization of decreased ability to function.
▪ Maintenance of social contacts. ▪ Expression of positive feelings about self.	▪ Assess patient for carelessness in dress and grooming; expression of depression or anxiety; difficulty in decision making; withdrawal from social situations, family interactions, and work-related responsibilities; ineffectual social interactions; verbal and nonverbal expression of decrease in self-worth; increase in dependent behaviors *to determine if there is a self-esteem problem.* ▪ Help patient identify and optimize physical and psychologic strengths. ▪ Help patient maintain social interactions by participation in family and social activities *to increase sources of pleasure and maintain self-esteem.* ▪ Help family or significant others to understand patient's limitations and need for acceptance *so they will continue to provide support to the patient.* ▪ Help family understand patient's need for independence and feeling of significant worth *to prevent family from treating patient as an invalid.* ▪ Refer for psychologic intervention or to support groups as needed.
NURSING DIAGNOSIS	**Risk for infection** *related to* decreased pulmonary function, possible corticosteroid therapy, ineffective airway clearance, and lack of knowledge regarding signs and symptoms of infection and preventive measures.
▪ Use of behaviors designed to minimize risk of infection. ▪ Aware of need to seek medical attention for appropriate treatment. ▪ No infection.	▪ Assess for change in color, quantity, odor, and viscosity of sputum; difficulty in mobilizing secretions; foul oral odor; increase in cough; increase in dyspnea; fever; chills; diaphoresis; increase in respiratory rate; abnormal breath sounds (gurgles, wheezing); hypoxemia or hypercapnia; excessive fatigue *to determine if an infection is present.* ▪ Teach patient to use good hand-washing techniques and avoid contact (whenever possible) with persons with respiratory infections *to minimize source of infection.* ▪ Encourage patient to obtain vaccines for influenza and pneumococcal pneumonia *to decrease occurrence or severity of influenza or pneumonia.* ▪ Teach proper care and cleaning of home respiratory equipment *to eliminate this source of infection.* ▪ Instruct patient to seek medical attention for manifestations of early infection *so treatment can be started promptly.* ▪ Teach patient to initiate plan of care previously discussed with physician when infections occur (e.g., increase fluid intake, begin antibiotics, increase corticosteroid dosage) *so appropriate self-care is initiated promptly.*

ETHICAL DILEMMAS

Living Will

SITUATION

A 79-year-old man with emphysema is admitted to the hospital in respiratory failure. His living will was executed 5 years ago and a copy was given to his wife and physician at that time. The wife brings the document to the intensive care unit and tells the nurse that the hospital must stop treating her husband and allow him to die as he requested. However, the oldest son is threatening the hospital with a lawsuit if its staff does not provide full care to his father.

DISCUSSION

A legally executed living will is binding in most states. If the patient is not mentally competent or physically able to explain his wishes regarding continuation of medical treatment, this advance directive is designed to speak for him. The son has no legal right to object to this directive if the document was duly executed by the patient when he was competent. Under the Patient Self-Determination Act, the hospital would have asked a competent, adult patient about his advance directives at the time of admission. His physician is obligated to follow the patient's directives if (1) the physician agrees that he is terminally ill and another physician concurs with that diagnosis and (2) it does not conflict with the physician's beliefs. If this physician is unable to follow the directives, the physician must transfer the care of this patient to another physician who will honor them. Professional counseling should be sought for the son and the wife as they face the impending death of the patient.

ETHICAL AND LEGAL PRINCIPLES

- The Patient Self-Determination Act was enacted in 1990. All health care facilities and agencies that receive Medicaid or Medicare reimbursements are covered under the act. It requires that on admission or enrollment in a health plan, information must be given to patients regarding their rights to make medical decisions for themselves and to execute advance directives (living wills and durable powers of attorney for health care decisions.)
- Living wills are a patient's advance directives regarding terminal illness condition and, in some states, persistent vegetative state. They specifically request that certain life-sustaining treatments be withheld or withdrawn, and they may also indicate the refusal of such maintenance medical care as artificial hydration and nutrition. Not all states have these statutes, and the laws vary in definition and content.
- A legally executed living will is the expression of a patient's wishes and should hold the same weight as the verbal expression of a currently competent patient. The son's wishes do not outweigh his father's wishes.

Ambulatory and Home Care. By far the most important aspect in the long-term care of the patient with COPD is education (Table 27-23). Because COPD is a chronic, debilitating disease, the patient will benefit by being able to exert some control over the disease. Because each COPD patient has different learning expectations, motivations, and needs, teaching must be adapted individually. Therefore it is important to assess the patient's level of knowledge, motivations, and goals before beginning to teach or develop a teaching plan. The nurse should help the patient understand that it is possible to plan treatment aimed at preserving lung function and slowing the progression of the disease. Patient and family participation in the treatment plan is essential. Respiratory care, as well as other related approaches, will be ongoing.

The health professional usually finds that it is not realistic to teach everything at one time. For example, if the patient has been hospitalized recently for acute respiratory failure resulting from a respiratory infection, the focus of teaching may be on helping the patient identify the signs and symptoms of a respiratory infection (e.g., fever, increased dyspnea, purulent sputum, increased use of inhalers or nebulizer treatments without relief) and writing a plan with input from the patient that may be used if these symptoms recur. The plan may include the following: notify the physician, increase fluid intake, increase nebulizer treatments (e.g., from twice a day to four times a day) with the physician's order, begin taking prescribed antibiotics, monitor for decrease or increase in symptoms, and notify the physician of the effects of these interventions.

Pulmonary rehabilitation. Pulmonary rehabilitation should be considered for all patients with symptomatic COPD. According to the American Thoracic Society, the objectives of pulmonary rehabilitation are to (1) control and alleviate as much as possible the symptoms and pathophysiologic complications of respiratory impairment and (2) teach the patient how to achieve optimal capability for carrying out ADLs. The overall goal is to increase the quality of life. The components of pulmonary rehabilitation include physical therapy (e.g., bronchial hygiene, exercise conditioning, breathing retraining, energy conservation), nutrition, and education and other topics such as smoking cessation, environmental factors, health promotion, psychologic counseling, and vocational rehabilitation. Although much of this intervention should be routinely included in the comprehensive approach to the patient with COPD, the referral of the patient to a structured pulmonary rehabilitation program should also be considered for the patient with moderate to severe COPD.[33,34]

Activity considerations. Energy conservation is another important component in COPD rehabilitation. This patient is typically an upper thoracic and neck breather who uses accessory muscles rather than the diaphragm. Thus the patient has difficulty performing upper-extremity activities, particularly those activities that require arm elevation above the head.[33] Exercise training of the upper extremities may improve function and reduce dyspnea. Frequently the patient has already adapted alternative energy-saving practices for ADLs. Alternative methods of hair care, shaving, showering, and reaching may need to be explored. An occupational therapist may help with ideas in these areas. Assuming a tripod posture (elbows supported on a table, chest in fixed position) and a mirror placed on the table during use of an electric razor or hair dryer conserves much more energy than when the patient stands in front of a mirror to shave or blow-dry hair. If the patient uses home oxygen therapy, it is essential that the patient wear the oxygen during activities of hygiene, because these are energy consuming. The patient should be encouraged to make a schedule and plan daily and weekly activities so as to leave plenty of time for rest

PATIENT & FAMILY TEACHING GUIDE

Table 27-23 Chronic Obstructive Pulmonary Disease

Goal: To assist patient and family in improving quality of life through education and promotion of lifestyle practices that support successful living with COPD.

Teaching Topic	Resources
What is COPD?	
■ Basic anatomy and physiology of lung ■ Basic pathophysiology of COPD ■ Signs and symptoms of COPD, respiratory infection, heart failure	*Help Yourself to Better Breathing* (American Lung Association) Videos (American Lung Association)
Breathing Retraining	
■ Pursed-lip breathing ■ Abdominal (diaphragm) breathing	Demonstration and return demonstration
Energy Conservation Techniques	
■ Pacing and pursing (pacing activity and using pursed-lip breathing with activities)	*Around the Clock with COPD: Helpful Hints for Respiratory Patients* (American Lung Association)
Medications	
■ Types (include mechanism of action) Methylxanthines β_2-agonists Corticosteroids Anticholinergics Antibiotics ■ Establishing medication schedule	*Understanding Lung Medications: How They Work—How to Use Them* (American Lung Association) Write out medication list and schedule
Correct Use of Metered-Dose Inhaler, Spacer, and Nebulizer	Fig. 27-5
Home Oxygen	
■ Explanation of rationale for use ■ Guide for home O_2 use	*About Oxygen Therapy at Home* (American Lung Association) Table 27-19
Psychosocial Emotional Issues	
■ Concerns about interpersonal relationships Dependency Intimacy ■ Problems with emotions Depression Anxiety Panic ■ Effects of medications ■ Support and rehabilitation groups	*Intimacy and Lung Disease* (American Lung Association) Open discussion (sharing with patient, significant other, and family)
COPD Management Plan	
■ Focusing on self-management ■ Knowing usual signs/symptoms ■ Need to report changes ■ Cause of flare-ups ■ Recognition of signs and symptoms of respiration infection, heart failure ■ Yearly follow-up	Nurse and patient develop and write up COPD management plan that meets individual needs
Healthy Nutrition	
■ Strategies to lose weight (if overweight) ■ Strategies to gain weight (if underweight)	Consultation with dietitian

RESEARCH
IMPLICATIONS FOR NURSING PRACTICE

Impact of Pulmonary Rehabilitation on Self-Efficacy

Citation Scherer YK, Schmieder LE: The effect of a pulmonary rehabilitation program on self-efficacy, perception of dyspnea, and physical endurance, *Heart Lung* 26:15, 1997.

Purpose To determine the effect of participation in an outpatient pulmonary rehabilitation (OPR) program on changes in self-efficacy, perception of dyspnea, and exercise endurance in patients with chronic obstructive pulmonary disease (COPD).

Methods The study was designed to measure preprogram and postprogram scores of 60 patients with a diagnosis of COPD (age range 35 to 82) participating in an OPR consisting of an educational and exercise training. In addition, methods to increase self-efficacy were integrated into the OPR. Preprogram and postprogram measurements were obtained on the COPD Self-Efficacy Scale (CSES), Dyspnea Scale, and distance walked on a 12-minute walking-distance test.

Results and Conclusions There was a significant difference between preprogram and postprogram scores on all three measures. The results indicated that higher self-efficacy scores on the CSES were correlated with lower perception of dyspnea and greater distances walked in 12 minutes. An OPR can improve self-efficacy or confidence in patients' ability to manage or avoid breathing difficulty.

Implications for Nursing Practice Improvement in self-efficacy may be a factor in decreased perception of dyspnea and increased exercise tolerance. Methods to increase self-efficacy expectations with education and exercise training provide an approach to assist patients with COPD to manage their breathing difficulty more effectively.

periods. The patient should also try to sit as much as possible when performing activities. Another energy-saving tip is to exhale when pushing, pulling, or exerting effort during an activity.

Walking is by far the best physical exercise for the COPD patient. Coordinated walking with slow, pursed-lip breathing without breath holding is a difficult task that requires conscious effort and frequent reinforcement. During coordinated walking and breathing, the patient is taught to breathe through the nose while taking one step, then to breathe out through pursed lips while taking two to four steps (the number depends on the patient's tolerance). Walking should occur at a slow pace with rest periods when necessary so the patient can sit or lean against an object such as a tree or post. The patient may need to ambulate using O_2. Once the patient is able to successfully perform coordinated walking with pursed-lip breathing, diaphragmatic breathing may also be incorporated if the patient has practiced and mastered this technique at rest. The nurse should walk with the patient, giving verbal reminders when necessary regarding breathing (inhalation and exhalation) and steps. Walking with the patient helps decrease anxiety and helps maintain a slow pace. It also enables the nurse to observe the patient's actions and physiologic responses to the activity. Many patients with moderate or severe COPD are anxious and fearful of walking or performing exercise. These patients and their families require much support while they build the confidence they need to walk or to perform daily exercises.

The patient should be encouraged to walk 15 to 20 minutes a day with gradual increases. Severely disabled patients can begin at a slow pace by walking for 2 to 5 minutes three times a day and slowly building up to 20 minutes a day, if possible. Adequate rest periods should be allowed. Some patients benefit from using their β-agonist MDI approximately 10 minutes before exercise. Parameters that may be monitored in the patient with mild COPD are resting pulse and pulse rate after walking. Pulse rate after walking should not exceed 75% to 80% of the maximum heart rate (maximum heart rate is age in years subtracted from 220). In the patient with other than mild COPD and without significant heart disease, it is usually dyspnea and the limitation in breathing rather than increased heart rate that limits the exercise. Thus it is better to use the patient's perceived sense of dyspnea as an indication of exercise tolerance. The Borg scale (see Fig. 24-9) can be used to have the patient determine the intensity of dyspnea.

The patient should be told that shortness of breath will probably increase during exercise (as it does for a healthy individual) but that the activity is not being overdone if this increased shortness of breath returns to baseline within 5 minutes after the cessation of exercise. The patient should be told to wait 5 minutes after completion of exercise before using the β-agonist MDI to allow a chance to recover. During this time, slow, pursed-lip breathing should be used. If it takes longer than 5 minutes to return to baseline, the patient most likely has overdone it and should proceed at a slower pace during the next exercise period. The patient may benefit from keeping a diary or log of the exercise program. The diary can help provide a realistic evaluation of the patient's progress. In addition, the diary can help motivate the patient and add to the patient's sense of accomplishment. Stationary cycling can also be used either alone or with walking. Cycles and treadmills are particularly valuable when weather prevents walking outside.

Sexual activity. Modifying but not abstaining from sexual activity can also contribute to a healthy psychologic well-being. Using an inhaled bronchodilator before sexual activity can help ventilation. The patient with COPD will also use less energy if these guidelines are followed: (1) plan sexual activity during the part of the day when breathing is best, (2) use slow pursed-lip breathing, (3) refrain from sexual activity after eating or other strenuous activity, (4) do not assume a dominant position, and (5) do not prolong foreplay. These aspects of sexual activity require open communication between partners regarding their needs and expectations.

Sleep. Adequate sleep is extremely important. Getting adequate amounts of sleep can be difficult for the COPD patient. Medications may cause restlessness and insomnia. Many patients with COPD have postnasal drip or nasal congestion that may cause coughing and wheezing at night. Nasal saline sprays before sleep and in the morning may help. The health care

ETHICAL DILEMMAS

Advance Directives

SITUATION

A 50-year-old woman is being treated for complications from her COPD. She is currently on a respirator and not coherent because of the drugs she is receiving. Her life partner, another woman, has been with her throughout this hospitalization. The patient had executed a valid durable power of attorney for health care decisions before this admission and had named her partner as her primary agent. However, the patient's parents and siblings have arrived and demand to be in charge of her treatment decisions. They do not accept the partner or the patient's appointment of this woman to make decisions for her.

DISCUSSION

One of the reasons people execute a durable power of attorney for health care decisions is to avoid the bickering over who should be making those decisions. This patient seems to have been competent when she determined who knew her wishes well enough to make decisions based on them. It was her right to name anyone as her agent, even a non–family member and a person who has no legal relationship to her. The family members can make demands, but they have no legal rights in this situation unless they have evidence that the partner is not basing decisions on the values of the patient.

ETHICAL AND LEGAL PRINCIPLES

- Most states do not have statutes that allow a "significant other" to be automatically considered a legal surrogate decision maker in cases where a patient has not named an agent. Those that do, however, give significant others the same priority as spouses. They have priority over parents, siblings, and grown children.
- Whatever a person's relationship is to his or her designated agent, there is no legal right for family members to override that designation unless there is proof that the agent is not making decisions based on substituted judgment (deciding as the patient himself or herself would).
- It is crucial to know the law regarding surrogate decision makers and agents in the state in which one practices.

provider may also prescribe a nasal decongestant or nasal steroid inhaler that may be used at bedtime. Long-acting theophylline preparations frequently aid in promoting sleep by decreasing bronchospasm and airway obstruction. If the patient is a restless sleeper, snores, stops breathing while asleep, and has a tendency to fall asleep during the day, sleep apnea may be present (see Chapter 25).

Psychosocial considerations. Healthy psychologic coping is often the most difficult task to accomplish. People with COPD frequently have to deal with many lifestyle changes that may involve decreased ability to care for themselves, decreased energy for social activities, and loss of a job.

When a patient with COPD is first diagnosed or when a patient has complications that require hospitalization, the nurse should expect a variety of emotional responses from the person ranging from denial and guilt to depression. Guilt may result from the knowledge that the disease was caused largely by cigarette smoking. Depression may be experienced as the severity and chronicity of the disease are realized. Denial may result if the disease is not yet severe enough to cause much physical limitation. The nurse should convey a sense of understanding and caring to the patient.

Emotions frequently encountered include depression, anxiety, social isolation, denial, and dependence. One study suggests that 45% of patients with moderate to severe COPD suffer from depression.[35] Recognizing the manifestations of depression is important but can be difficult in COPD. Paying close attention to the presence of a depressed appearance, social withdrawal, self-pity, and pessimistic attitude can be important clues to depression.

Expression of these emotions becomes complicated because of the relationship of emotional expression to breathing. For example, anxiety normally produces an increase in respiratory rate, and depression usually goes along with inactivity, which in the COPD patient can translate into decreased exercise tolerance, increased dyspnea, increased dependence, and, ultimately, worsening of depression. A vicious cycle of emotional entrapment can occur. Learning new ways to express emotions with the use of relaxation techniques involving breathing can be helpful. Slowing the pace with frequent rest periods, open and honest communication with supportive significant others, and avoidance of anxiety-producing situations (if necessary) may need to be learned.

The patient with COPD may benefit from several relaxation techniques. One is the use of a progressive relaxation technique in which the patient listens either to a tape or to the patient's own or another voice and gradually begins to tighten and relax muscle groups. Relaxation may begin in the head and neck area and end in the legs. Self-hypnosis, biofeedback, meditation, and massage (self-massage or massage from others) are other alternative relaxation therapies. Support groups at local American Lung Associations, hospitals, and clinics can also be helpful.

The patient frequently asks whether moving to a warmer or drier climate will help. In general, such a move is not significantly beneficial. Moving to places with an elevation of 4000 feet or more should be discouraged because of the lower partial pressure of O_2 found in the air at higher elevations. A disadvantage of moving may be that a person leaves an occupation, friends, and familiar environment, which could be psychologically stressful. Any advantage gained from a different climate may be outweighed by the psychologic effects of the move.

■ Evaluation

The expected outcomes for the patient with COPD are presented in NCP 27-2. 

CYSTIC FIBROSIS

Cystic fibrosis (CF) is an autosomal recessive, multisystem disease characterized by altered function of the exocrine glands involving primarily the lungs, pancreas, and sweat glands. Abnormally thick, abundant secretions from mucous glands can lead to a chronic, diffuse, obstructive pulmonary disorder in almost all patients. Exocrine pancreatic insufficiency is associated with 85% to 90% of cases of CF. Sweat glands excrete increased amounts of sodium and chloride.

Cystic fibrosis affects approximately 30,000 persons in the United States. The disease occurs primarily in Caucasians, with a frequency of 1 in 3000 births among Caucasians and 1 in 17,000 births among African-Americans. Both sexes are equally affected. Approximately 4% to 5% (1 in 20) of the general population are carriers of the gene transmitting CF, with 20% of these being young adults.[36] The first signs and symptoms typically occur in children, but some patients are not diagnosed until they are adults.

CF was once exclusively a pediatric disease. However, because of improvements in therapy, approximately 34% of patients reach adulthood and nearly 10% live past the age of 30. The average life span is 28 years.[36] Each person has an individual spectrum of the disease and time course of deterioration.

Etiology and Pathophysiology

CF is an autosomal recessive disease resulting from mutations in a gene located on chromosome 7. The most common mutation in the CF gene is known as the CF transmembrane regulator (CFTR). The primary defect in CF is abnormally regulated chloride channel activity. This defect alters ionic transport of sodium and chloride across epithelial surfaces. The high concentrations of sodium and chloride in the sweat of the patient with CF result from decreased chloride reabsorption in the sweat duct. The basic pathophysiologic mechanism is obstruction of exocrine gland ducts with thick, viscous secretions that adhere to the lumen of the ducts. The glands distal to the duct eventually undergo fibrosis.

In the respiratory system, both upper and lower respiratory tracts can be affected. Upper respiratory tract manifestations may be present and include chronic sinusitis and nasal polyposis. The hallmark of respiratory involvement in CF is its effect on the airways. The disease progresses from being a disease of the small airways (chronic bronchiolitis) to an entity that eventually involves the larger airways and finally causes destruction of lung parenchyma. Thick secretions obstruct bronchioles and lead to air trapping and hyperinflation of the lungs. The stasis of mucus provides an excellent growth medium for bacteria. CF is characterized by chronic airway infection. The most common organisms cultured from the sputum of a patient with CF are *S. aureus, H. influenzae,* and *P. aeruginosa.*

Lung disorders that can result include pneumonia, bronchiolitis, bronchitis, bronchiectasis, atelectasis, and emphysema. There is progressive loss of lung tissue from inflammation and scarring, and the resultant chronic hypoxia leads to pulmonary hypertension and cor pulmonale. Blebs and large cysts in the lung are also severe manifestations of lung destruction. Other pulmonary complications include hemoptysis, which can sometimes be fatal, and pneumothorax. Hemoptysis may range from scant streaking to major bleeding.

Initially, CF is an obstructive lung disease caused by the overall obstruction of the airways with mucus. Later, CF also progresses to a restrictive lung disease because of the fibrosis, lung destruction, and thoracic wall changes. Death usually results from loss of pulmonary function. Cor pulmonale is a common late complication caused by extensive loss of lung tissue and chronic hypoxia.

Pancreatic insufficiency is caused primarily by mucus plugging the pancreatic duct and its branches, which results in fibrosis of the acinar glands of the pancreas. The exocrine function of the pancreas is altered and may be lost completely. Pancreatic enzymes such as trypsinogen, lipase, and amylase do not reach the intestine to digest ingested nutrients. There is malabsorption of fat, protein, and fat-soluble vitamins (vitamins A, D, E, K). Fat malabsorption results in steatorrhea, and protein malabsorption results in failure to grow and gain weight. In advanced pancreatic insufficiency, endocrine function may also be affected.

Diabetes mellitus may occur if the islets of Langerhans become fibrotic. Cystic fibrosis–related diabetes mellitus affects approximately 15% of all patients with CF. It differs from type 1 diabetes in that some insulin is secreted, it is nonketotic, and it is slow in onset. It differs from type 2 diabetes in that individuals are underweight (as opposed to being obese), the onset is in a younger age population, and the individual is hypoinsulinemic. Routine screening is indicated by following serum glucose values. Depending on the response to the glucose challenge, the individual may require insulin.

The sweat glands of the CF patient secrete normal volumes of sweat but are unable to absorb sodium chloride from sweat as it moves through the sweat duct. Therefore they excrete four times the normal amount of sodium and chloride in sweat. This abnormality does not seem to affect the general health of the person, but it is useful as a diagnostic indicator.

Individuals with CF often have gastrointestinal problems. Many health care professionals are aware of the intestinal obstruction seen in the newborn period (meconium ileus). However, gastroesophageal reflux disease (GERD), distal intestinal obstructive syndrome (DIOS), and constipation are common. GERD is a major problem in individuals with CF, particularly in those with pulmonary disease. The relationship between reflux and exacerbation of respiratory disease is not known, but it is known that these two entities enhance each other.

DIOS is a syndrome that results from intermittent obstruction in the ileal-cecal area in patients with pancreatic insufficiency. The degree to which the bowel is obstructed may vary with each episode, and a partial obstruction may progress to a complete obstruction. While complete obstruction requires gastric decompression and a surgical consultation, partial and uncomplicated episodes of DIOS are treated with ingestion of a balanced polyethylene glycol electrolyte solution. Constipation develops in the sigmoid colon and progresses proximally, while DIOS develops in the ileal-cecal area and progresses distally. Careful monitoring of bowel habits and patterns are essential.

The liver may become involved. Biliary cirrhosis may not be recognized until late in the disease. Hepatobiliary disease is common in the older patient. Chronic cholestasis, inflammation, fibrosis, and portal hypertension can occur. Intestinal obstructions can also occur. Once resolved, they recur in almost one half of patients.

Clinical Manifestations

The clinical manifestations of CF vary depending on the severity of the disease. An initial finding of meconium ileus in the newborn infant is present in 10% to 15% of persons with CF. Early manifestations in childhood are failure to grow, clubbing, persistent cough with mucus production, tachypnea, and large, frequent bowel movements. A large, protuberant abdomen may develop with an emaciated appearance of the extremities.

The first symptom of CF in the adult is frequently cough. With time the cough becomes persistent and produces viscous, purulent, often greenish-colored sputum. Other respiratory problems that may be indicative of CF are recurring lung infections such as bronchiolitis, bronchitis, and pneumonia. As the disease progresses, periods of clinical stability are interrupted by exacerbations characterized by increased cough, weight loss, increased sputum, and decreases in pulmonary function. Over time the exacerbations become more frequent and the recovery of lost lung function less complete, ultimately leading to respiratory failure.[37]

Distal intestinal obstruction causes right lower quadrant pain, loss of appetite, emesis, and often a palpable mass. Insufficient pancreatic enzyme release causes the typical pattern of protein and fat malabsorption with frequent, bulky, foul-smelling stools.

The function of the reproductive system is altered. This finding is important because more persons with CF are living to adulthood. The male adult is usually sterile (although not impotent) as a result of structural changes in the vas deferens, seminal vesicles, and epididymis. The female adult usually has delayed menarche. During exacerbations, menstrual irregularities and secondary amenorrhea are fairly common for the woman. She may be unable to become pregnant because of the increased viscosity of the cervical mucus. Women with CF do become pregnant, but the fertility rate is lower than in healthy women. The baby is heterozygous (and hence a carrier) for CF if the father is not a carrier. If the father is a carrier, there is a 50% chance that the baby will have CF.

The severity and progression of the disease vary from person to person. In the last decade, it has been shown that with early diagnosis and immediate institution of intensive care, the prognosis can be significantly improved.

Complications

Pneumothorax is common (greater than 10% of patients) in patients with cystic fibrosis. The presence of small amounts of blood in sputum is common in the CF patient with lung infection. Massive hemoptysis is life threatening. With advanced lung disease, digital clubbing becomes evident in almost all patients with CF. Respiratory failure and cor pulmonale are late complications of CF.

Diagnostic Studies

The main diagnostic test for CF is the sweat chloride test with the pilocarpine iontophoresis method. Pilocarpine carried by a small electric current is used to stimulate sweat production. The sweat is collected on filter paper or gauze and then analyzed for sodium and chloride concentrations. The test takes approximately 40 minutes. Values greater than 65 mEq/L for both sodium and chloride are suggestive of CF, especially in a person who has other clinical features of the disease. The degree of sodium and chloride elevation does not necessarily correlate with the severity of the disease. Fetal diagnosis can now be made by analyzing gene markers from the chorionic villus tissue. Other diagnostic studies include chest x-ray, pulmonary function tests, fecal analysis for fat, and duodenoscopy for quantitative determination of pancreatic enzymes.

Because of the large number of CF mutations, DNA analysis is not used for primary diagnosis. It is likely that DNA analysis will be performed increasingly in CF patients to corroborate the diagnosis.

Collaborative Care

The major objectives of therapy in CF are to (1) promote clearance of secretions, (2) control infection in the lungs, and (3) provide adequate nutrition.

Management of pulmonary problems in CF aims at relieving airway obstruction and controlling infection. Drainage of thick bronchial mucus is assisted by aerosol and nebulization treatments of medications used to liquefy mucus and to facilitate coughing. The abnormal viscoelastic properties of CF secretions are primarily caused by mucus glycoproteins and DNA from degenerated neutrophils. Agents that degrade the high concentrations of DNA in CF sputum (e.g., DNase [Pulmozyme]) decrease sputum viscosity and increase airflow. Bronchodilators (e.g., β_2-agonists, theophylline) and mucolytics may be used.

Airway clearance techniques are critical in reducing mucus. These techniques include CPT, postural drainage, and expiratory pressure breathing. Flutter mucus clearance devices are also effective in promoting mucus removal. Individuals with CF may have a preference for a certain technique that works well for them in a daily routine. (These airway clearance techniques are discussed in the section on respiratory therapy for COPD earlier in this chapter.)

Aerobic exercise seems to be effective in clearing the airways. Important needs to consider when planning an aerobic exercise program for the patient with CF are (1) frequent rest periods interspersed throughout the exercise regimen, (2) meeting increased nutritional demands of exercise, (3) observing for manifestations of hyperthermia, and (4) drinking large amounts of fluid and replacing salt losses.

More than 95% of CF patients die of complications resulting from lung infection. Antimicrobial treatment is initiated for the treatment of infection. The use of antibiotics should be carefully guided by sputum culture results. Early intervention with antibiotics is useful, and long courses of antibiotics are the usual treatment. Prolonged high-dose therapy may be necessary because many drugs are abnormally metabolized and rapidly excreted in the patient with CF. Pharmacokinetic and kidney function studies therefore should be monitored closely. Oral agents commonly used are trimethoprim-sulfamethoxazole, tetracycline, chloramphenicol, cephalosporins, antistaphylococcal penicillins, and oral quinolones, especially ciprofloxacin. Although oral and aerosolized antimicrobial therapy is usually adequate 20% to 80% of the time, some patients require a 2- to 4-week course of IV antimicrobial therapy. If home facilities are adequate, the CF patient and the family may choose to continue parenteral therapy at home. The usual treatment for acute infectious exacerbation is an aminoglycoside combined with penicillin, or a third-generation cephalosporin. Aerosolized bronchodilators and antiinflammatory agents (e.g., cromolyn) are used in selected patients, particularly before CPT (see Table 27-21). The patient with cor pulmonale or hypoxemia may require home O_2 therapy (O_2 therapy is discussed earlier in this chapter). Sclerosing of the pleural space or partial pleural stripping and pleural abrasion performed surgically are usually indicated for recurrent episodes of pneumothorax.

CF has become a leading indication for either heart-lung or lung transplantation. (Lung transplants are discussed in Chapter 26.) Lung transplantations for the patient with CF have resulted in significant improvement of pulmonary function.

The management of pancreatic insufficiency includes pancreatic enzyme replacement of lipase, protease, and amylase (e.g., Cotazym, Creon, Ultrase, Viokase, Zymase) administered before each meal and snack. A high-calorie, high-protein diet and multivitamins are recommended. Fat restriction usually is not necessary. Fat-soluble vitamins (vitamins A, D, E, and K) must be supplemented. Use of caloric supplements improves nutritional status. Added dietary salt is indicated whenever sweating is excessive, such as during hot weather, in the presence of fever, or from intense physical activity.

Gene therapy has been used as an experimental therapy for treating CF.[38] (Gene therapy is discussed in Chapter 12.)

NURSING MANAGEMENT: CYSTIC FIBROSIS

■ Nursing Assessment

Subjective and objective data that should be obtained from the patient with cystic fibrosis are presented in Table 27-24.

■ Nursing Diagnoses

Nursing diagnoses for the patient with CF may include, but are not limited to, the following:

- Ineffective airway clearance *related to* abundant, thick bronchial mucus, weakness, and fatigue
- Ineffective breathing pattern *related to* bronchoconstriction, anxiety, airway obstruction
- Impaired gas exchange *related to* recurring lung infections
- Altered nutrition: less than body requirements *related to* dietary intolerances, intestinal gas, and altered pancreatic enzyme production

■ Planning

The overall goals are that the patient with CF will have (1) adequate airway clearance, (2) reduced risk factors associated with respiratory infections, (3) ability to perform ADLs, (4) no complications related to CF, and (5) active participation in planning and implementing a therapeutic regimen.

■ Nursing Implementation

The nurse and other health professionals can assist young adults to gain independence by helping them assume responsibility for their care and for their vocational or school goals. An important issue that should be discussed is sexuality. Delayed or irregular menstruation is not uncommon. There may be delayed development of secondary sex characteristics such as breasts in girls. The person may use the illness to avoid certain events or relationships. The healthy person may hesitate to make friends with someone who is sick. Other crises and life transitions that must be dealt with in the young adult include building confidence and self-respect on the basis of achievements, persevering with employment goals, developing motivation to achieve, learning to cope with the treatment program, and adjusting to the need for dependence if health fails.

The issue of marrying and having children is difficult. Genetic counseling may be an appropriate suggestion for the couple considering having children. Many men with CF are sterile. Women with the disease may have difficulty becoming pregnant. In addition, any children produced will either be a carrier of CF or have the disease. Another concern is the shortened life span of the parent with CF, and the parent's ability to care for the child must be taken into consideration.

NURSING ASSESSMENT

Table 27-24 Cystic Fibrosis

Subjective Data

Important Health Information

Past health history: Recurrent respiratory and sinus infections, persistent cough with excessive sputum production

Medications: Use of and compliance with corticosteroids, bronchodilators, antibiotics, herbs

Functional Health Patterns

Health perception–health maintenance: Family history of cystic fibrosis; diagnosis of cystic fibrosis in childhood

Nutritional-metabolic: Dietary intolerances, voracious appetite, weight loss

Elimination: Intestinal gas; large, frequent bowel movements

Activity-rest: Fatigue, decreased exercise tolerance; dyspnea, cough, excessive mucus or sputum production

Cognitive-perception: Abdominal pain

Sexuality-reproductive: Delayed menarche, menstrual irregularities, and secondary amenorrhea; decreased fertility in men and women

Objective Data

General

Anxiety, depression, restlessness; failure to thrive

Integumentary

Cyanosis (circumoral, nailbed), digital clubbing; salty skin

Respiratory

Persistent runny nose, diminished breath sounds, sputum (thick, white, tenacious), hemoptysis, increased work of breathing, use of accessory muscles of respiration, barrel chest

Cardiovascular

Tachycardia

Gastrointestinal

Protuberant abdomen; abdominal distention; foul, fatty stools

Possible Findings

Abnormal ABGs and pulmonary function tests; abnormal sweat chloride test, chest x-ray, fecal fat analysis

CRITICAL THINKING EXERCISES

CASE STUDY

Asthma

Patient Profile

Mrs. S., age 30, comes to the emergency department (ED) with severe wheezing, dyspnea, and anxiety. She was in the ED only 6 hours ago with an acute asthma attack.

Subjective Data

- Treated in the ED previously with nebulized albuterol and responded quickly
- Can speak only one- to three-word sentences
- Is allergic to cigarette smoke
- Began to experience increased shortness of breath and tightness in her chest when she returned home
- Used albuterol MDI repeatedly at home without relief

Objective Data

Physical Examination

- Uses accessory muscles to breathe
- Has audible wheezing
- Respiratory rate 34/min
- Auscultation reveals no air movement in lower lobes
- Heart rate 126 beats/min

Diagnostic Studies

ABGs: PaO_2 80 mm Hg, $PaCO_2$ 35 mm Hg, pH 7.46
PEFR: 150 L/min (personal best: 400 L/min)

Critical Thinking Questions

1. Why did Mrs. S. return to the ED? Explain the pathophysiology of this exacerbation of asthma.
2. What are the nursing care priorities for Mrs. S.?
3. What are the complications the nurse must be ready for based on her assessment?
4. What should be included in her discharge plan of care?
5. Based on the assessment data presented, write one or more nursing diagnoses. Are there any collaborative problems?

NURSING RESEARCH ISSUES

1. What effect does a planned exercise program have on respiratory function in the patient with COPD?
2. Can the use of relaxation techniques reduce dyspnea in the patient with asthma or COPD?
3. What types of breathing retraining techniques result in the greatest improvement in oxygenation?
4. What are the most common patient care problems with an adult who has CF?
5. What are the most effective nursing care measures to promote airway clearance?
6. What are the most effective measures to improve upper arm strength and endurance and reduce dyspnea in the patient with COPD?

Acute intervention for the patient with CF includes relief of bronchoconstriction, airway obstruction, and airflow limitation. Interventions include aggressive CPT, antibiotics, oxygen therapy, and corticosteroids in severe disease. Good nutrition is important to support the immune system. Advances in long-term vascular access (e.g., implanted ports) have made IV access and administration of medication much easier. This has also eased the transition for IV treatment at home.

CPT is the mainstay of intervention for ineffective airway clearance for these patients. Home management of cystic fibrosis includes an aggressive plan of postural drainage with percussion and vibration, aerosol-nebulization therapy, and breathing retraining. The patient is taught controlled coughing techniques, deep breathing exercises, and progressive exercise conditioning such as a bicycling program or arm ergometry.

The family and the person with CF have a great financial and emotional burden. The cost of drugs, special equipment, and health care is often a financial hardship. As CF patients are living to childbearing age, family planning and genetic counseling are important. The burden of living with a chronic disease at a young age can be emotionally overwhelming. Community resources are often available to help the family. In addition, the Cystic Fibrosis Foundation can be of assistance. As the person continues toward and into adulthood, the nurse and other skilled health professionals should be available to help the patient and family cope with complications resulting from the disease.

REVIEW QUESTIONS

The number of the question corresponds to the same-numbered objective at the beginning of the chapter.

1. Asthma is best characterized as
   a. an inflammatory disease.
   b. a steady progression of bronchoconstriction.
   c. an obstructive disease with loss of alveolar walls.
   d. a chronic obstructive disorder characterized by mucus production.
2. In evaluating the asthmatic patient's knowledge of self-care, the nurse recognizes that additional instruction is needed when the patient says,
   a. "I use my corticosteroid inhaler when I feel short of breath."
   b. "I get a flu shot every year and see my doctor if I have an upper respiratory infection."
   c. "I use my bronchodilator inhaler before I visit my aunt who has a cat, but I only visit for a few minutes because of my allergies."
   d. "I walk 30 minutes every day but sometimes I have to use my bronchodilator inhaler before walking to prevent me from getting short of breath."
3. A plan of care for the patient with COPD would include
   a. chronic corticosteroid therapy.
   b. reduction of risk factors for infection.
   c. high flow rate oxygen administration.
   d. lung exercises that involve inhaling longer than exhaling.

4. The effects of cigarette smoking on the respiratory system include
   a. increased proliferation of ciliated cells.
   b. hypertrophy of the alveolar membrane.
   c. destruction of all alveolar macrophages.
   d. hyperplasia of goblet cells and increased production of mucus.
5. One of the most important things a nurse can teach a patient with emphysema is to
   a. move to a hot, dry climate.
   b. perform chest physical therapy.
   c. know the early signs of respiratory infection.
   d. obtain adequate rest in the supine position.
6. The major advantage of a Venturi mask is that it can
   a. deliver up to 80% O_2.
   b. provide continuous 100% humidity.
   c. deliver a precise concentration of O_2.
   d. be used while a patient eats and sleeps.
7. Diagnostic studies that the nurse would expect to be abnormal in a person with CF are
   a. insulin tolerance and blood sugars.
   b. pancreatic enzymes and hormones.
   c. sweat test and vitamin B tolerance test.
   d. pulmonary function study and sweat test.

References

1. American Thoracic Society: Standards for the diagnosis and care of patients with chronic obstructive pulmonary disease, *Am J Respir Crit Care Med (Suppl)* 152:5, 1995.
2. National Institutes of Health: *Highlights of The Expert Panel Report 2: Guidelines for the diagnosis and management of asthma,* pub no 97-4051A, 1997, US Department of Health and Human Services.
3. Fish J and others: Asthma care: new treatment strategies, new expectations, *Patient Care* 31:16, 1997.
4. Einarsson O, Wirth JA: Sinopulmonary syndromes, *Clin Pulm Med* 3:199, 1996.
5. Krishna MT, Chauhan AJ, Holgate ST: Molecular mediators of asthma: current insights, *Hosp Pract* 31:115, 1996.
6. Middleton A: Managing asthma: it takes teamwork, *AJN* 97:39, 1997.
7. Canales MA: Asthma management: putting your patient on the team, *Nursing* 27:33, 1997.
8. Fishman A and others: *Fishman's pulmonary diseases and disorders,* New York, 1997, McGraw-Hill.
9. Levy BD, Kitch B, Fanta CH: Medical and ventilatory management of status asthmaticus, *Intensive Care Med* 24:105, 1998.
10. Richman E: Asthma diagnosis and management: new severity classifications and therapy alternatives, *Clinician Reviews* 7:76, 1997.
11. Rachelefsky G: Helping patients live with asthma, *Hosp Pract* 30:51, 1995.
12. Drazen JM: New directions in asthma drug therapy, *Hosp Pract* 33:25, 1998.
13. O'Byrne PM, Israel E, Drazen JM: Antileukotrienes in the treatment of asthma, *Ann Intern Med* 127:472, 1997.
14. Canales MAP: Asthma management: putting your patient on the team, *Nursing* 27:33, 1997.
15. Mathews PJ: Monitoring the air waves using a peak flowmeter, *Nursing* 27:57, 1997.
16. Schapira R, Reinke L: The outpatient diagnosis and management of chronic obstructive pulmonary disease: pharmacotherapy, administration of supplemental oxygen, and smoking cessation techniques, *J Gen Intern Med* 10:40, 1995.
17. American Thoracic Society: Cigarette smoking and health, *Am J Respir Crit Care Med* 153:861, 1996.
18. The Agency for Health Care Policy and Research: Smoking cessation clinical practice guideline, *JAMA* 275:1270, 1996.
19. Barker AF and others: Replacement therapy for hereditary alpha$_1$-antitrypsin deficiency. A program for long-term administration, *Chest* 105:1046, 1994.
20. Ferguson GT: Screening and early intervention for COPD, *Hosp Pract* 33:67, 1998.
21. Grossman RF: Acute exacerbations of chronic bronchitis, *Hosp Pract* 32:85, 1997.
22. Wood A, Henningfield J: Nicotine medications for smoking cessation, *N Engl J Med* 333:1196, 1995.
23. Hurt RD and others: A comparison of sustained-release bupropion and placebo for smoking cessation, *N Engl J Med* 337:1195, 1997.
24. Hanson MJ: Caring for a patient with COPD: how to help him breathe easier once the damage is done, *Nursing* 27:39, 1997.
25. Tarpy SP, Celli B: Long-term oxygen therapy, *N Engl J Med* 333:710, 1995.
26. Calianno C and others: Oxygen therapy: giving your patient breathing room, *Nursing* 25:33, 1995.
27. Somerson SJ and others: Mastering emergency airway management, *AJN* 96:24, 1996.
28. O'Donohue WJ: Home oxygen therapy, *Med Clin North Am* 80:611, 1996.
29. Petty TL, O'Donohue WJ: Further recommendations for prescribing, reimbursement, technology development, and research in long-term oxygen therapy, *Am J Respir Crit Care Med* 150:875, 1994.
30. MacGregor RJ, Schakenbach LH: Lung volume reduction surgery: a new breath of life for emphysema patients, *Medsurg Nurs* 5:245, 1996.
31. Newsome EA, Ott BB: Lung volume reduction: surgical treatment for emphysema, *Am J Crit Care* 6:423, 1997.
32. Trulock EP: Lung transplantation for COPD, *Chest* 113(4 suppl):269S, 1998.
*33. Breslin EH: Respiratory muscle function in patients with chronic obstructive pulmonary disease, *Heart Lung* 25:271, 1996.
*34. Scherer YK, Schmieder LE: The effect of a pulmonary rehabilitation program on self-efficacy, perception of dyspnea, and physical endurance, *Heart Lung* 26:15, 1997.
35. Wingate BJ, Hansen-Flaschen J: Anxiety and depression in advanced lung disease, *Clin Chest Med* 18:495, 1997.
36. Rosenstein BJ, Zeitlin PL: Cystic fibrosis, *Lancet* 351:277, 1998.
37. Ruzal-Shapiro C: Cystic fibrosis: an overview, *Radiol Clin North Am* 36:143, 1998.
38. Alton EW and others: Towards gene therapy for cystic fibrosis: a clinical progress report, *Gene Therapy* 5:291, 1998.

*Nursing research-based articles.

Resources

American Thoracic Society
1740 Broadway
New York, NY 10019
212-315-8700
http://www.thoracic.org

Division of Tuberculosis Elimination
Centers for Disease Control
1600 Clifton Road NE
Atlanta, GA 30333
404-639-8120
http://www.cdc.gov/nchstp/tb/default.htm

National Heart, Lung, and Blood Institute
National Institutes of Health
4733 Bethesda Avenue, Suite 530
Bethesda, MD 20814
301-951-3260
http://www.nhlbi.nih.gov/nhlbi/nhlbi.htm

***For additional Internet resources, see the website for this book at* www.mosby.com/MERLIN/medsurg_lewis**

SECTION

6

PROBLEMS OF OXYGENATION: TRANSPORT

SECTION OUTLINE

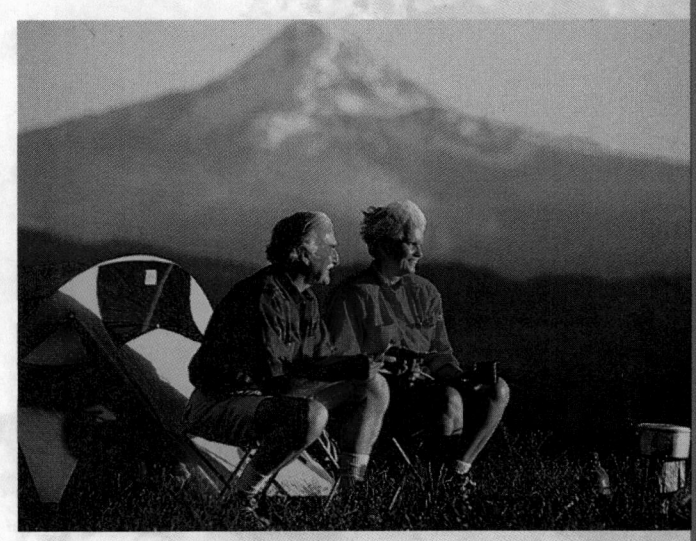

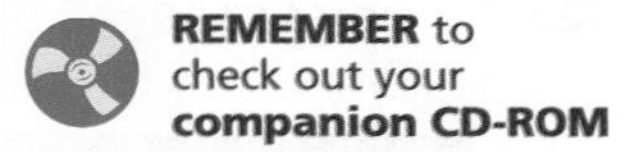
REMEMBER to check out your companion CD-ROM

28 NURSING ASSESSMENT Hematologic System

Ann M. O'Mara & Marie Bakitas Whedon

www.mosby.com/MERLIN/medsurg_lewis

LEARNING OBJECTIVES

1. Describe the structures and functions of the hematologic system.
2. Differentiate among the different types of blood cells and their functions.
3. Explain the process of hemostasis.
4. Describe the age-related changes in the hematologic system and differences in hematologic studies.
5. Identify the significant subjective and objective assessment data related to the hematologic system that should be obtained from a patient.
6. Describe the appropriate techniques used in the physical assessment of the hematologic system.
7. Differentiate normal from common abnormal findings of a physical assessment of the hematologic system.
8. Describe the purpose, significance of results, and nursing responsibilities related to diagnostic studies of the hematologic system.

Hematology is the study of blood and blood-forming tissues. This includes the blood cells, the bone marrow, the spleen, and the lymph system. A basic knowledge of hematology is useful in clinical settings to evaluate the patient's ability to transport oxygen and carbon dioxide, coagulate blood, and combat infections. Another important homeostatic function of the blood cells is removing old and dead cells. This function is accomplished by the mononuclear phagocyte system (MPS). The MPS, formerly known as the reticuloendothelial system, is composed of monocytes and macrophages. The role of the MPS in phagocytosis and the immune response is described in Chapters 11 and 12.

STRUCTURES AND FUNCTIONS OF THE HEMATOLOGIC SYSTEM

Bone Marrow

Bone marrow is the soft material that fills the central core of bones. It is the blood-forming tissue that produces the three major cell components of the blood: erythrocytes (red blood cells [RBCs])(Fig. 28-1), leukocytes (white blood cells [WBCs]), and platelets. The blood components develop from a common stem cell, but as they mature and differentiate several distinct cell types evolve (Fig. 28-2). An understanding of the function of particular blood cell types enhances the nurse's ability to interpret laboratory data.

Reviewed by Suzanne Shaffer, MN, RN, AOCN, Director of Nursing Practice, Department of Nursing, University of Kansas Medical Center and Hospital, Kansas City, Kans.

In the fetus, most of the bone marrow actively produces blood cells. However, in the adult, active production of marrow is generally limited to the ends of long bones, vertebrae, flat cranial bones, sternum, ribs, scapulae, clavicles, pelvis, and sacrum.

Blood Cells

Erythrocytes. *Erythropoiesis,* which is the production of erythrocytes (see Fig. 28-1), or RBCs, is largely regulated by cellular oxygen requirements and general metabolic activity. The process of erythropoiesis is stimulated by hypoxia and controlled hormonally by erythropoietin, a hormone synthesized and released by the kidney. Erythropoietin stimulates the bone marrow to increase erythrocyte production. Erythropoiesis is also influenced by the availability of nutrients. The essential nutrients for erythropoiesis include iron, cobalamin (vitamin B_{12}), and folic acid.[1]

Several distinct cell types evolve during erythrocyte maturation (Fig. 28-2). The *reticulocyte* is an immature erythrocyte. The reticulocyte count measures the rate at which new RBCs appear in the circulation. Reticulocytes are capable of maturing to mature erythrocytes within 48 hours of release into circulation. Therefore assessing the number of reticulocytes is a useful means of evaluating the rate and adequacy of erythrocyte production. The functions of erythrocytes include transport of gases (both oxygen and carbon dioxide) and assistance in maintaining the acid-base balance through the buffering capability of hemoglobin.

Hemoglobin, the major component of erythrocytes, gives RBCs their characteristic red color when combined with oxygen. Iron and protein form the molecular structure of hemoglobin. The function of hemoglobin is to transport oxygen. Therefore, although adequate oxygen may be inspired into the

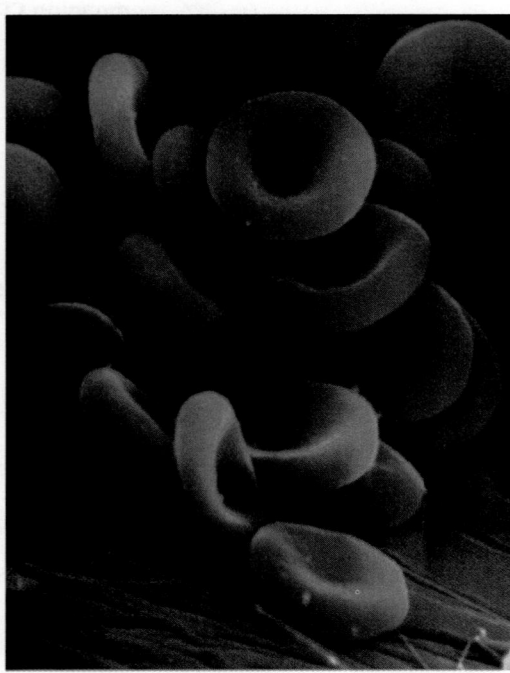

Fig. 28-1 Mature erythrocytes. Scanning electron micrograph of mature erythrocytes.

lungs, it may not reach the tissues unless there is an adequate amount of hemoglobin to carry it. Consequently the significance of any type of anemia, a state of reduced RBCs or hemoglobin, is its effect on tissue oxygenation.

Hemolysis (destruction of erythrocytes) by macrophages removes abnormal, defective, damaged, and old RBCs from circulation. Hemolysis occurs in the bone marrow, liver, and spleen, and it increases bilirubin production. The normal life span of an erythrocyte is 120 days.

Leukocytes. Leukocytes (WBCs) also develop in a series of cell types that vary in maturity (see Fig. 28-2). The three general classes of mature circulating leukocytes are granulocytes, monocytes, and lymphocytes (Fig. 28-3). The main function of the granulocytes and monocytes is phagocytosis of bacteria and foreign particles that invade the body. *Phagocytosis* is a process by which WBCs ingest or engulf any unwanted organism and then digest and kill it. The main function of lymphocytes is related to the immune response (see Chapter 12).

Granulocytes. Granulocytes, which contain granules in their cytoplasm, consist of neutrophils, eosinophils, and basophils. They are also known as polymorphonuclear leukocytes (PMNs).

The maturation cycle of neutrophils is shown in Fig. 28-2. Following the metamyelocyte stage (see Fig. 28-2), the neutrophil matures into a band or stab, followed by a mature PMN. The band or stab stage is similar to the metamyelocyte except that the nucleus has become horseshoe shaped. Although band cells are sometimes found in the peripheral circulation of normal persons and are capable of phagocytosis, the mature neutrophil is much more effective at phagocytosis. The nucleus of the neutrophil is segmented into two to five lobes connected by thin chromatin strands, hence the nickname "segs" for these mature neutrophils.

Neutrophils have strong phagocytic activity. They are the primary phagocytic cells involved in acute inflammatory responses. Eosinophils have a similar but reduced ability for phagocytosis. One of their primary functions is to engulf antigen-antibody complexes formed during an allergic response. They also are able to defend against parasitic infections. Basophils have a limited role in phagocytosis. Their granules in the cytoplasm contain heparin, serotonin, and histamine. If a basophil is stimulated by an antigen or by tissue injury, it will respond by releasing its granules. This is part of the response seen in allergic and inflammatory reactions.

Monocytes. Monocytes are produced in the bone marrow and circulate briefly in the blood. They are large, slow-moving, potent phagocytic cells that can ingest small or large masses of matter, such as bacteria, dead cells, tissue debris, and old or defective RBCs. Monocytes are the second type of WBCs to arrive at the scene of an injury (neutrophils are the first). When monocytes leave the blood and enter and remain in the tissues, they differentiate into macrophages. Macrophages are very effective phagocytic cells.

In tissues, resident macrophages are given special names (e.g., Kupffer cells in the liver, osteoclasts in the bone, and alveolar macrophages in the lung). They protect the body from pathogens at these entry points and are more phagocytic than monocytes. Macrophages also interact with lymphocytes to facilitate the humoral and cellular immune responses.

Lymphocytes. Lymphocytes are produced in the bone marrow and form the basis of the cellular and humoral immune responses. Two lymphocyte subtypes are B cells and T cells. B cells mediate the humoral immune response. When B cells are stimulated by antigens, they are activated to form specialized antibody factories, called plasma cells. Plasma cells produce antibodies, termed *immunoglobulins,* that mediate humoral immunity.

T cell precursors originate in the bone marrow and then migrate to the thymus gland for further differentiation. The T cells mediate cellular immunity, and they are involved in the cellular immune response against intracellular viruses, tuberculosis, contact irritants (e.g., poison ivy), cancer, parasites, fungi, and transplant antigens that provoke rejection of organs. Various subtypes of T cells have been identified. Among these are the T-helper cells and the T-suppressor cells. Human immunodeficiency virus (HIV) infections cause decreases and alterations of T-helper cells, leaving the individual vulnerable to the previously mentioned pathogens, as well as malignancies. (The details of lymphocyte function are presented in Chapter 12, and HIV infections are discussed in Chapter 13.)

Platelets. Platelets, or thrombocytes, are derived from megakaryocytes (see Fig. 28-2). The primary function of platelets is to aid in blood clotting. Platelet performance depends on both quantitative and qualitative features.[2] Platelets must be available in sufficient numbers (quantitatively sufficient) and must be structurally and metabolically sound to work properly (qualitatively adequate). Platelets are also involved in homeostasis by maintaining capillary integrity by working as "plugs" to close any openings in the capillary wall. At the site of any damage, platelet activation is initiated. Increasing numbers of platelets accumulate to form a platelet plug. Platelets are also important in the process of clot shrinkage and retraction.

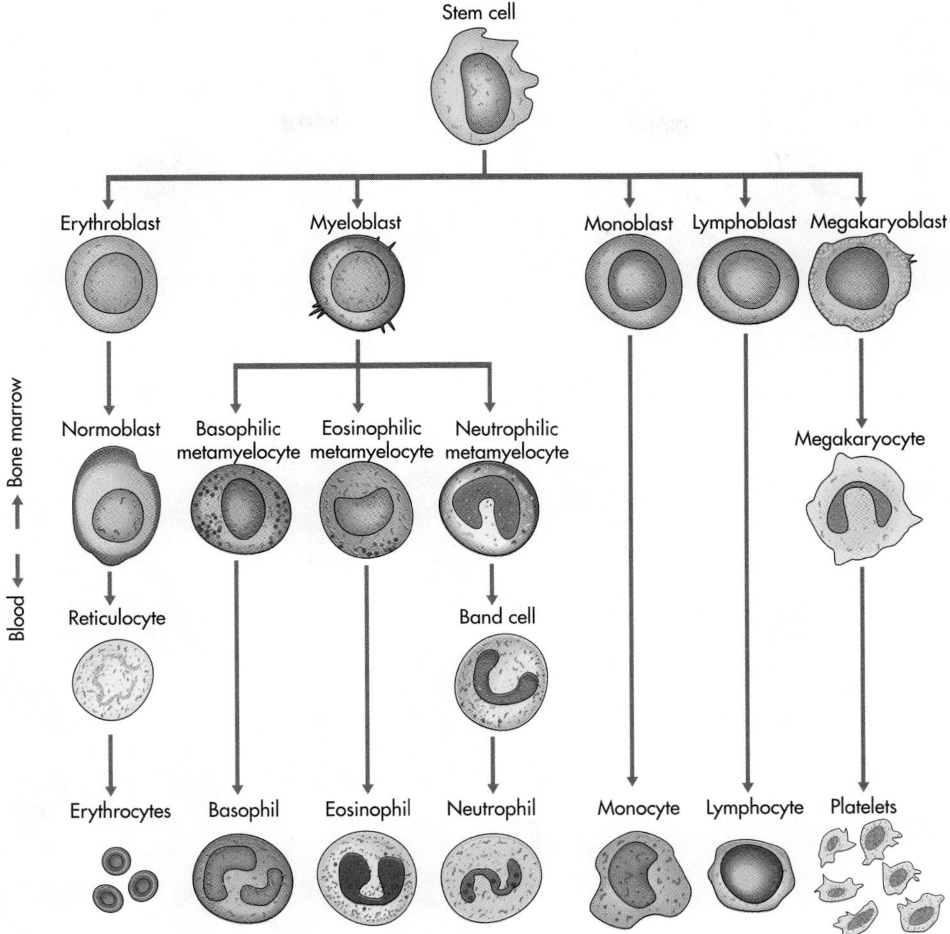

Fig. 28-2 Development of blood cells.

Spleen

Another component of the hematologic system is the spleen, which is located in the upper left quadrant of the abdomen. The functions of the spleen can be classified into four general groups:

1. *Hematopoietic function.* The spleen produces RBCs during fetal development.
2. *Filter function.* The splenic structure provides an ideal filter mechanism. For example, the spleen removes old and defective erythrocytes from the circulation by the MPS. Another example of filtering involves the reuse of iron. The spleen is able to catabolize hemoglobin released by hemolysis and return the iron component of the hemoglobin to the bone marrow for reuse.
3. *Immune function.* The spleen contains a rich supply of lymphocytes and monocytes.
4. *Storage function.* Approximately 30% of the platelet mass is stored in the spleen.

Lymph System

The lymph system, consisting of lymphatic capillaries, ducts, and lymph nodes, carries fluid from the interstitial spaces to the blood. It is by means of the lymph that proteins, fat from the gastrointestinal (GI) tract, and certain hormones are able to return to the blood. The lymph system also returns excess interstitial fluid to the blood, which is important in preventing the development of edema.

Lymph fluid is pale yellow interstitial fluid that has diffused through lymphatic capillary walls. It circulates through a special vasculature, much as blood moves through blood vessels. The formation of lymph fluid increases when interstitial fluid pressure rises, thereby forcing more fluid into the lymph system. When too much interstitial pressure develops or when something interferes with the reabsorption of lymph, lymphedema develops. The lymphedema that may occur as a complication of a radical mastectomy is often caused by the obstruction of lymph flow resulting from the removal of lymph nodes.

The lymphatic capillaries are thin-walled, endothelium-lined vessels that have an irregular diameter. They are somewhat larger than blood capillaries and do not contain valves. Lymphatic capillaries unite to form lymphatic vessels that carry all lymph to either the right lymphatic duct or the thoracic duct. These large lymphatic ducts drain into subclavian veins in the neck.

The lymph nodes are also a part of the lymphatic system. Structurally the nodes are small, round to bean-shaped organs of varying sizes. A primary function of lymph nodes is filtration of bacteria and foreign particles carried by lymph. Lymph nodes are distributed throughout the body along lymph vessels. They are situated both superficially and deep. The superficial

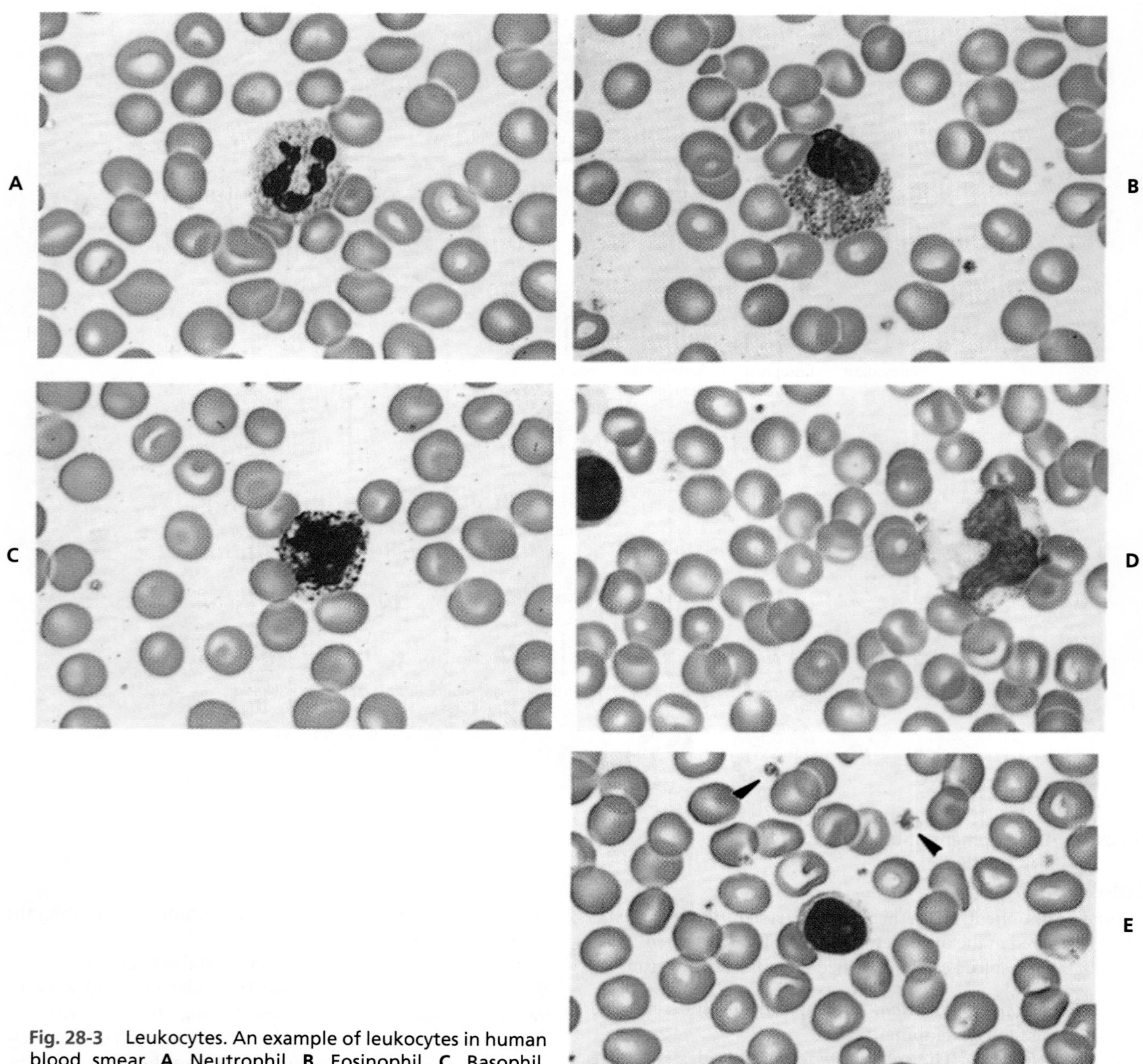

Fig. 28-3 Leukocytes. An example of leukocytes in human blood smear. **A,** Neutrophil. **B,** Eosinophil. **C,** Basophil. **D,** Monocyte. **E,** Lymphocyte.

nodes can be palpated, but the deep nodes must be visualized radiographically.

Liver

The liver functions as a filter but also produces all the procoagulants that are essential to hemostasis and blood coagulation. Other functions of the liver are described in Chapter 41.

Normal Clotting Mechanisms

Hemostasis is a normal homeostatic process of blood clotting and blood lysing. Blood clotting minimizes blood loss when various body structures are injured. Three components contribute to normal clotting: vascular response, platelet response, and plasma clotting factors.

Vascular Response. When a blood vessel is injured, an immediate local vasoconstrictive response occurs. Vasoconstriction reduces the leakage of blood from the vessel not only by restricting the vessel size but also by pressing the endothelial surfaces together. The latter reaction enhances vessel wall stickiness and maintains closure of the vessel even after the vasoconstriction subsides. Vascular spasm may last for 20 to 30 minutes, thus allowing time for the platelet response and plasma clotting factors to be activated.

Platelet Response. Platelets are activated when they are exposed to interstitial collagen from an injured blood vessel.

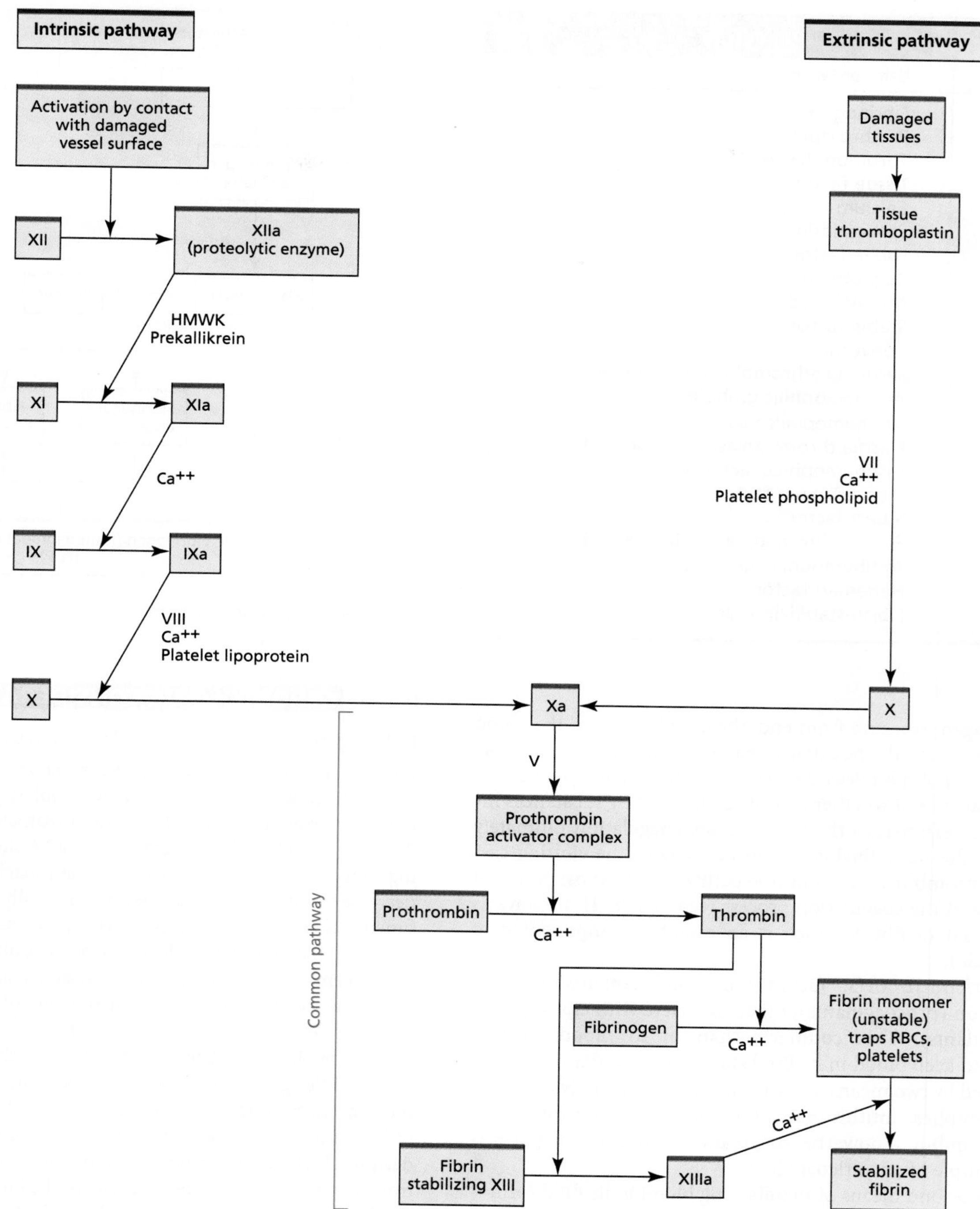

Fig. 28-4 Coagulation mechanism showing steps in the intrinsic pathway and extrinsic pathway as it would occur in the test tube. *HMWK,* high molecular weight kininogen. *RBCs,* red blood cells.

Platelets stick to one another and form clumps. The stickiness is termed *adhesiveness,* and the formation of clumps is termed *aggregation* or *agglutination.* When a blood vessel is injured, the circulating platelets are exposed to the collagen from the inner lining of the vessel. This interaction causes the platelets to release substances such as platelet factor 3 (PF3) and serotonin, which facilitate coagulation. At the same time, platelets release adenosine diphosphate (ADP), which increases platelet adhesiveness and aggregation, thereby enhancing the formation of a platelet plug.

In addition to their independent contribution to clotting, platelets also facilitate the reactions of the plasma clotting factors. As Fig. 28-4 shows, platelet lipoproteins stimulate necessary conversions in the clotting process.

Plasma Clotting Factors. The plasma clotting factors are labeled with both names and Roman numerals (Table 28-1). Plasma proteins circulate in inactive forms until stimulated to initiate clotting through one of two pathways, intrinsic or extrinsic. These two pathways have undergone only in vitro observations and analyses.[3] The intrinsic pathway is activated

Table 28-1 Coagulation Factors

Factor	Name or Synonym
I	Fibrinogen
II	Prothrombin
III	Thromboplastin Tissue factor
IV	Calcium
V	Proaccelerin Labile factor Ac globulin
VI	Not assigned
VII	Stable factor Convertin Serum prothrombin conversion accelerator
VIII	Antihemophilic globulin Antihemophilic factor
IX	Plasma thromboplastin component Antihemophilic factor B
X	Stuart-Prower factor Stuart factor
XI	Plasma thromboplastin antecedent Antihemophilic factor C
XII	Hageman factor
XIII	Fibrin-stabilizing factor

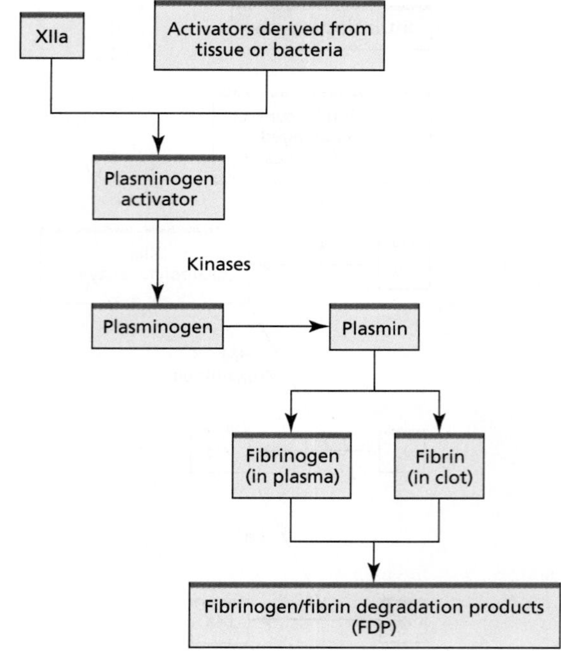

Fig. 28-5 Fibrinolytic system.

by collagen exposure from endothelial injury when the blood vessel is damaged. The extrinsic pathway is initiated when tissue thromboplastin is released extravascularly from injured tissues.

Regardless of whether clotting is initiated by substances internal or external to the blood vessel, coagulation ultimately follows the same final common pathway of the clotting cascade. Thrombin, in the common pathway, is the most powerful enzyme in the coagulation process (see Fig. 28-4). It converts fibrinogen to fibrin, which is an essential component of a blood clot.

Anticoagulants. Just as some blood elements foster coagulation (procoagulants), others interfere with clotting (anticoagulants). This countermechanism to blood clotting serves to keep blood in its fluid state. Anticoagulation may be achieved by two means, antithrombins and fibrinolysis. As the name implies, antithrombins keep blood fluid by antagonizing thrombin, a powerful coagulant. Endogenous heparin is an example of an anticoagulant.

The second means of maintaining blood in its fluid form is fibrinolysis. The fibrinolytic system is initiated when plasminogen is activated to plasmin (Fig. 28-5). Thrombin is one of the substances that can activate the conversion of plasminogen to plasmin, thereby propagating fibrinolysis. The plasmin attacks either fibrin or fibrinogen by splitting the molecules into smaller elements known as fibrin split products (FSPs) or fibrin degradation products (FDPs). (More information about FSPs can be found in Table 28-7 and in the discussion of disseminated intravascular coagulation in Chapter 29.)

If fibrinolysis is excessive, the patient will be predisposed to bleeding. In such a situation, bleeding results from the destruction of fibrin in platelet plugs or from the anticoagulation effects of increased FSPs, which include impaired platelet aggregation, reduced prothrombin, and an inability to stabilize fibrin.

GERONTOLOGIC CONSIDERATIONS

Effects of Aging on the Hematologic System

Physiologic aging is a gradual process that involves cell loss and organ atrophy. After age 30, marrow cellularity (stem cells) decreases from approximately 80% to approximately 50% at age 65. After age 65, cellularity decreases to 30%.[4] Although the remaining stem cells maintain their functional capacity to divide, they decrease in number because they are gradually replaced by nonfunctional fat cells. In the bone marrow, decreased cellularity and decreased marrow reserves leave the older adult more vulnerable to problems with clotting, oxygen transport, and fighting infection. This will result in a diminished ability of an older adult to compensate for an acute or a chronic illness.[4]

Hemoglobin levels begin to decrease in both men and women after middle age, with the lowest levels seen in older people. Estimates of the prevalence of anemia in the elderly range from a low of 2% among upper socioeconomic class, independent living elderly to a high of 40% among institutionalized elderly.[5] Although iron deficiency is usually responsible for the low hemoglobin levels, the cause of anemia in many older patients has no known etiology. Iron absorption is not impaired in the older patient, but nutritional intake of iron-rich foods is decreased and the use of iron supplements may be decreased. It is essential to assess for indications of disease processes such as GI bleeding before concluding that decreased hemoglobin levels are caused solely by aging. The osmotic fragility of RBCs is increased in the older person, and this may account for the increased mean corpuscular volume (MCV) and the decreased mean corpuscular hemoglobin concentration (MCHC) of RBCs of the older person.

The total WBC count and differential are generally not affected by aging.[4] Leukocyte function is also well preserved. However, during an infection, the older adult may have only a minimal elevation in the total WBC count. These laboratory

GERONTOLOGIC DIFFERENCES IN ASSESSMENT

Table 28-2 **Effects of Aging on Hematologic Studies**

Study	Changes
CBC Studies	
Hb	Decreased
MCV	Increased
MCHC	Decreased
WBC count	Diminished response to infection
Platelets	Unchanged
Clotting Studies	
Partial thromboplastin time	Reduced
Fibrinogen	May be elevated
Factors V, VII, VIII, IX	May be elevated
ESR	Increased significantly
Iron Studies	
Serum iron	Reduced
Total iron-binding capacity	Reduced

CBC, complete blood count; *ESR,* erythrocyte sedimentation rate; *Hb,* hemoglobin; *MCHC,* mean corpuscular hemoglobin concentration; *MCV,* mean corpuscular volume; *WBC,* white blood cell.

findings suggest a diminished marrow granulocyte reserve in older adults. Platelets are unaffected by the aging process. However, changes in vascular integrity from aging can manifest as easy bruising.

The effects of aging on hematologic studies are presented in Table 28-2. Immune changes related to aging are presented in Chapter 12.

ASSESSMENT OF THE HEMATOLOGIC SYSTEM

Much of the evaluation of the hematologic system is based on a thorough health history. Consequently, the nurse must be knowledgeable about what to include in the health history so that questions may be phrased in a manner eliciting the most information related to the hematologic problem. Key questions to ask a patient with a hematologic problem are presented in Table 28-3.

Subjective Data

Important Health Information

Past health history. It is important to learn whether the patient has had prior hematologic problems. A previous laboratory determination of anemia must be explored, as should diagnoses of mononucleosis, malabsorption, liver disorders (e.g., hepatitis, cirrhosis), thrombophlebitis or thrombosis, and spleen disorders. Diseases of the blood, such as leukemia, should be documented.

Medications. Many drugs may interfere with normal hematologic function (Table 28-4). Antineoplastic agents used to treat malignant disorders may cause depression of the bone marrow (see Chapter 14). A complete drug history of both prescription and over-the-counter medications is an important component of a hematologic assessment. Further use of vitamins or herbal substances should be explored. Many patients will not volunteer the use of alternative medicine practices in which they engage.

Surgery or other treatments. Specific past surgical procedures to ask the patient about include splenectomy, tumor removal, prosthetic heart valve placement, surgical excision of the duodenum (where iron absorption occurs), partial or total gastrectomy (which removes parietal cells, thus reducing intrinsic factor and the absorption of cobalamin), and ileal resection (where cobalamin absorption takes place). The nurse should also ascertain how wound healing progressed postoperatively and if and when any bleeding problems occurred in relation to the surgery. Wound healing and bleeding should be discussed as responses to past injuries (including minor trauma) and to dental extractions. The nurse should also ask the patient about any recurring infections and problems with blood clotting.

Functional Health Patterns

Health perception–health management pattern. The nurse should ask the patient to describe the usual and present state of health. To assist the patient in maintaining optimal health, it is important to identify the health perceptions, health practices, and preventive practices.

Complete biographic data are needed, including age, sex, race, and ethnic background. There is a known genetic influence in certain hematologic conditions, as well as in other blood diseases that follow familial patterns. For example, sickle cell disease occurs primarily in African-Americans, and pernicious anemia occurs most commonly in persons of Northern European descent.

When a family health history is taken, the following health problems should be explored: jaundice, anemia, malignancies, RBC dyscrasias such as sickle cell disease, and bleeding disorders such as hemophilia. The number of previous blood transfusions and possible complications during administration should be determined. Known allergies and allergic reactions, including anaphylaxis, should be documented.

Risk factors such as alcohol and cigarette use that might disrupt the hematologic system must be assessed. Alcohol use must be tactfully explored. Alcohol is a caustic agent to GI mucosa, and damage to the GI tract secondary to alcohol can cause local bleeding. Hematemesis (bright red, brown, or black vomitus) can be a symptom of this problem and should be investigated. Chronic alcohol abusers frequently have vitamin deficiencies. Alcohol also exerts a damaging effect on platelet function and the liver, where several clotting factors are produced. Consequently, bleeding problems can develop and should be anticipated in cases of known alcohol abuse.

Nutritional-metabolic pattern. During the patient interview and assessment, the nurse should obtain the patient's weight and determine if the patient has experienced any recent changes associated with anorexia, nausea, vomiting, or oral discomfort. A dietary history may provide clues about the cause of erythrocyte deficiencies. Iron, cobalamin, and folic acid are necessary for the development of RBCs. Iron and folic acid deficiencies are associated with inadequate intake of foods such as liver, meat, eggs, whole-grain and enriched breads and cereals, potatoes, leafy green vegetables, dried fruits, legumes, and citrus fruits. Folic acid deficiencies may be offset by a diet including foods that are also high in iron.

Any changes in the skin's texture or color should be explored. The patient should be asked about any bleeding of gum tissue. Any petechiae or ecchymotic areas on the skin should be noted. If present, the frequency, size, and cause should be documented. Petechiae pinpoint an accumulation of blood in the skin or mucous membranes. Small vessels leak under pressure,

HEALTH HISTORY

Table 28-3 Hematologic System

Health Perception–Health Management Pattern
- Do you have any difficulty performing daily activities because of a lack of energy?*
- Do you smoke or drink alcohol?*
- Have you ever received a blood transfusion?*
- Is there any family history of anemia, cancer, bleeding, or clotting problems?*
- List the medications you are taking.

Nutritional-Metabolic Pattern
- Do you have any difficulties with eating, chewing, or swallowing?*
- How has your appetite been?
- Do you take any vitamins, nutritional supplements, or iron?*
- Is nausea and vomiting a problem for you?*
- Have you had any unusual bleeding or bruising?*
- Have there been recent changes in the condition of your skin?*
- Have you experienced night sweats or cold intolerance?*
- Have you noticed any swelling in your armpits, neck, or groin?*

Elimination Pattern
- Have you had black or tarry stools?*
- Have you noticed any blood in your urine?*
- Have you had any decrease in urinary output?*
- Do you ever have diarrhea?*

Activity-Exercise Pattern
- Have you experienced excessive fatigue recently?*
- Do you have any shortness of breath at rest? With activity?*
- Do you have any limitations in joint motion?*
- Do you have a problem with unsteady gait?*
- After activity do you ever notice bleeding or bruising?*

Sleep-Rest Pattern
- Do you feel fatigued? Are you more fatigued than usual?*
- Do you feel rested upon awakening? If no, explain.

Cognitive-Perceptual Pattern
- Have you experienced any numbness or tingling?*
- Have you had any problems with your vision, hearing, or taste?*
- Have you noticed any changes in your mental functions?*
- Do you have any pain such as bone, joint, or abdominal pain, or abdominal fullness?*
- Do you have pain when moving your joints?*
- Have your muscles been sore or achy recently?*

Self-Perception–Self-Concept Pattern
- Does your health problem make you feel differently about yourself?*
- Do you have any physical changes that cause you distress?*

Role-Relationship Pattern
- Does your occupation bring you into contact with hazardous substances?*
- Has your present illness caused a change in your roles and relationships?*

Sexuality-Reproductive Pattern
- Has your hematologic problem caused any sexual problems that concern you?*
- Women: When was your last menses? Did you consider your cycle normal? How long does your bleeding usually last? Have you had any increase in cramping or clotting?*
- Men: Do you experience impotence?*

Coping–Stress Tolerance Pattern
- Do you have a support system to assist you when needed?
- What coping strategies do you use during exacerbation of symptoms?

Value-Belief Pattern
- How do you feel about blood transfusions?
- Do you have any conflicts between your planned therapy and your value-belief system?*

*If yes, describe.

and the platelet numbers are insufficient to stop the bleeding. Petechiae are more likely to occur where clothing constricts the circulation.

The patient should also be questioned about any swelling in the neck, armpits, or groin. A careful description of the swelling should be made and should include size, texture, movability, and tenderness. Primary lymph tumors are usually not painful. A nontender swollen lymph node may be a sign of Hodgkin's disease or non-Hodgkin's lymphoma.

Any incidents of fever should be explored thoroughly. It should be determined if the patient currently has a fever, recurring fevers, chills, or night sweats.

Elimination pattern. The patient should be asked if blood has been noted in the urine or stool or if black, tarry stools have occurred. Also, any decrease in urinary output or diarrhea should be documented.

Activity-exercise pattern. Because fatigue is a prominent symptom in many hematologic disorders, the patient should be asked about feelings of tiredness. Weakness and complaints of heavy extremities should also be determined. Symptoms of apathy, malaise, dyspnea, or palpitations should be documented. Any change in the patient's ability to perform activities of daily living (ADLs) should be noted.

Sleep-rest pattern. The patient's feeling of being rested after a night's sleep should be determined. Fatigue secondary to a hematologic problem often will not be resolved following sleep.

Cognitive-perceptual pattern. Pain may also be caused by a hematologic problem and should be assessed. Arthralgia (joint pain) may indicate an autoimmune disorder or may be caused by gout secondary to increased uric acid production as a result of a hematologic malignancy or hemolytic anemia. Aching bones may result from pressure of expanding bone marrow. Hemarthrosis (blood in a joint) occurs in the patient with bleeding disorders and can be painful.

Paresthesias, numbness, and tingling may be related to a hematologic disorder and should be noted. Any changes in

Table 28-4 **Drugs Affecting Hematologic Function and Laboratory Values***

Drug	Clinical Use	Hematologic Effect
Aminosalicylic acid (Pamisyl, PAS)	Antituberculin	Leukocytosis secondary to hypersensitivity
Amphotericin B (Fungizone)	Antifungal	Anemia
Acetylsalicylic acid (aspirin) and aspirin-containing compounds (e.g., Empirin, Percodan)	Analgesic, antipyretic, antiinflammatory	Reduced platelet aggregation, prolonged bleeding time
Azathioprine (Imuran)	Immunosuppression	Anemia, leukopenia
Carbamazepine (Tegretol)	Antiseizure agent	Anemia, leukopenia, thrombocytopenia
Chloramphenicol (Chloromycetin)	Antibiotic	Anemia, neutropenia, thrombocytopenia
Chlorothiazide (Diuril)	Diuretic	Thrombocytopenia (occasional)
Oral contraceptives and diethylstilbestrol	Birth control, menopausal symptoms, functional uterine bleeding, cancer of prostate	Increase in factors II, V, VII, VIII, IX, X; increase in fibrinogen; increase in thrombin; decrease in prothrombin and partial thromboplastin times; increase in coagulation and thromboemboli formation (overall)
Diphenylhydantoin (Dilantin)	Antiseizure agent, antiarrhythmic	Anemia
Epinephrine (Adrenalin)	Sympathomimetic	Leukocytosis
Glucocorticoids (Prednisone)	Antiinflammatory	Lymphopenia, neutrophilia
Isoniazid (INH)	Antituberculin	Neutropenia
Methyldopa (Aldomet)	Antihypertensive	Hemolytic anemia
Phenacetin (APC, Empirin compound)	Analgesic, antipyretic	Anemia
Phenylbutazone (Butazolidin)	Antiinflammatory	Anemia, leukopenia, neutropenia, thrombocytopenia
Procainamide hydrochloride (Pronestyl)	Antiarrhythmic	Agranulocytosis
Quinidine sulfate	Antiarrhythmic	Agranulocytosis, anemia, thrombocytopenia
Trimethoprim-sulfamethoxazole (Bactrim, Septra)	Antibacterial	Anemia, leukopenia, neutropenia, thrombocytopenia
Antineoplastic agents	Immunosuppression, malignancies	Anemia, leukopenia, thrombocytopenia
Nonsteroidal antiinflammatory drugs	Antiinflammatory, analgesic, antipyretic	Inhibition of platelet aggregation

*This represents only a partial listing of drugs affecting the hematologic system.

vision, hearing, taste, or mental status should also be carefully assessed.

Self-perception–self-concept pattern. The effect of the health problem on the patient's perception of self and personal abilities should be determined. The effect of certain problems, such as bruising, petechiae, and lymph node swelling, on the patient's personal appearance should also be assessed.

Role-relationship pattern. The patient should be questioned about any past or present occupational or household exposures to radiation or chemicals. If such exposure has occurred, the type, amount, and duration of the exposure should be determined.

It is known that a person who has been exposed to radiation, as a treatment modality or by accident, has a higher incidence of certain hematologic problems. The same is true of a person who has been exposed to chemicals (e.g., benzene, lead, naphthalene, and phenylbutazone). These chemicals are commonly used by potters, dry cleaners, or individuals involved with occupations that use adhesives. The patient should also be questioned about a history in the military. Many Vietnam War veterans were exposed to dioxin-containing defoliant (Agent Orange), which has been linked with leukemia and lymphoma. The nurse also should assess the impact of the present illness on the patient's usual roles and responsibilities.

Sexuality-reproductive pattern. A careful menstrual history should be obtained from women, including the age at which menarche and menopause began, duration and amount of bleeding, incidence of clotting and cramping, and any associated problems. Any intrapartum or postpartum bleeding problems should also be documented. Men should be asked if they have any problems related to impotence because this is not uncommon in men with hematologic problems.

Coping–stress tolerance pattern. The patient with a hematologic problem often needs assistance with ADLs. The patient should be asked if adequate support is available to meet daily needs. The patient's usual methods of handling stress should also be determined. In the patient with platelet disorders or hemophilia, the potential for hemorrhage can be so frightening that usual life patterns may be drastically curtailed, affecting the person's quality of life. The nurse should explore the accuracy of the patient's understanding of the problem.

Value-belief pattern. Often the person with hematologic problems needs a blood transfusion or bone marrow transplant. The nurse should determine if these types of treatments are problematic for the patient. In addition, the nurse should determine if the planned therapy causes any conflicts with the patient's value-belief system. The nurse should be cognizant of cultural differences related to blood and blood transfusions.

Objective Data

Physical Examination. A complete physical examination is necessary to accurately examine all systems that affect or are affected by the hematologic system (see Chapter 5). For example, a decreasing level of consciousness may be caused by an intracranial hemorrhage, and this indicates the need for a neurologic examination. Increasing abdominal girth may be related to an enlarged spleen, an enlarged liver, or abdominal bleeding. This finding warrants the need for a complete GI examination. The nurse must be aware that signs and symptoms can be caused by hematologic problems, even though these are not the obvious cause[6] (Table 28-5).

Lymph nodes are distributed throughout the body. The superficial nodes can be evaluated by light palpation (Fig. 28-6). Deep nodes are examined radiographically. Lymph nodes should be assessed symmetrically with regard to location, size (in centimeters), degree of fixation (e.g., movable, fixed), tenderness, and texture.

The examiner should lightly palpate lymph nodes over the appropriate areas. The pads of the index and third fingers are most often used when assessing the lymph nodes. The examiner should gently roll the skin over the area and concentrate on feeling for possible lymph node enlargement. When not specifically examined for their status, lymph nodes are usually palpated during the examination of the region where the nodes are located. For example, the axillary lymph nodes are examined at the completion of a breast examination.

It is important to develop a sequence when examining the lymph nodes. The lymph nodes of the head and neck drain areas of the mouth, throat, breast, thorax, and arms. A convenient sequence for examination is preauricular, posterior auricular, occipital, tonsillar, submaxillary, submental, superficial cervical, posterior cervical chain, deep cervical chain, and supraclavicular (see Fig. 28-6).

The axillary lymph nodes drain lymph from the chest wall, breasts, arms, and hands. The pectoral, subscapular, and lateral groups of nodes are palpated next. The epitrochlear nodes, located in the antecubital fossa between the biceps and triceps muscles, are then examined. These nodes drain specific areas of the forearm and hand. The inguinal lymph nodes, which drain the lower extremities, are palpated last.

Lymph nodes are generally not palpable unless there is residual enlargement from a previous or current infection. It may be normal to find small (0.5 to 1.0 cm), mobile, discrete, firm, nontender nodes, termed *shotty nodes.* Tender nodes are usually a result of inflammation, whereas hard or fixed nodes suggest malignancy.

Additional hematologic data can also be acquired from other body systems. It is important to include careful inspection of the skin (see Chapter 21) and palpation of the liver and spleen (see Chapter 37) in a hematologic assessment. The most direct means of evaluating the hematologic system is through laboratory analysis and other diagnostic studies.

DIAGNOSTIC STUDIES OF THE HEMATOLOGIC SYSTEM

The nurse should recognize the need to thoroughly explain any diagnostic procedures to the patient. It is common for a patient to be anxious when faced with illness. Therefore instructions must be simple, clear, and repeated when necessary to decrease anxiety and ensure the patient's compliance with preparatory protocols. Whether studies are performed on an outpatient or an inpatient basis, written instructions regarding the procedures facilitate compliance. If a diverse ethnic population is served, it is helpful to have instructions translated into the patients' dominant language.

The repeated acquisition of blood specimens may be distressing for the patient. Some patients and staff members become concerned that the amount of blood withdrawn for tests could lead to adverse effects. Although multiple blood studies may be uncomfortable, it is only in rare situations that diagnostic blood withdrawal predisposes the patient to significant volume loss.

The nurse must capitalize on all appropriate opportunities to use independent nursing assessment and clinical judgment. For example, when there is a suspicion of bleeding, it is important to perform guaiac tests of the stool, nasogastric secretions, or emesis and a Hematest of the urine.

Laboratory Studies

Complete Blood Count. The complete blood count (CBC) involves several laboratory tests (Table 28-6), each of which serves to assess the three major blood cells formed in the bone marrow. Although the status of each cell type is important, the entire system may be disrupted by diseases, as well as by treatment of diseases. When the entire CBC is suppressed, a condition termed *pancytopenia* exists. In such cases the patient needs care directed toward the management of anemia, infection, and hemorrhage (see Chapter 29). The effects of aging on hematologic studies are presented in Table 28-2.

Red blood cells. Normal values of some RBC tests are reported separately for men and for women because normal values are based on body mass and men usually have a larger body mass than women.

The hemoglobin (Hb) value is reduced in cases of anemia, hemorrhage, and states of hemodilution, such as those that occur when the fluid volume is excessive. Increases in hemoglobin are found in polycythemia or in states of hemoconcentration, which can develop from volume depletion.

The hematocrit (Hct) value is determined by spinning blood in a centrifuge, which causes erythrocytes and plasma to separate. The erythrocytes, being the heavier elements, settle to the bottom. The hematocrit value represents the percentage of RBC as compared to the total blood volume. Reductions and elevations of hematocrit value are seen in the same conditions that raise and lower the hemoglobin value. The hematocrit value generally equals three times the hemoglobin value.

COMMON ASSESSMENT ABNORMALITIES

Table 28-5 Hematologic System

Finding	Possible Etiology and Significance
Skin	
Pallor of skin or nail beds	Decrease in quantity of hemoglobin (anemia)
Flushing	Increase in hemoglobin (polycythemia)
Jaundice	Accumulation of bile pigment caused by rapid or excessive hemolysis
Purpura, petechiae, ecchymoses, hematoma	Hemostatic deficiency of platelets or clotting factors resulting in hemorrhage into the skin
Excoriation and pruritus	Scratching from intense pruritus secondary to disorders such as Hodgkin's disease, increased bilirubin
Leg ulcers	Common in sickle cell disease, especially prominent on the malleoli on the ankles
Brownish discoloration	Hemosiderin and melanin from the breakdown of erythrocytes, iron deposits secondary to transfusional iron overload
Cyanosis	Reduced hemoglobin
Telangiectasis	Hyperemic spot caused by capillary or small artery dilation; small angioma with a tendency to hemorrhage
Angioma	A benign tumor consisting primarily of blood or lymph vessels
Spider nevus	Branched growth of dilated capillaries resembling a spider; associated with liver disease, elevated estrogen levels as in pregnancy
Nails	
Rigid longitudinally, flattened, concave	Chronic, severe iron-deficiency anemia
Eyes	
Jaundiced sclera	Accumulation of bile pigment because of rapid or excessive hemolysis
Conjunctival pallor	Reduction in quantity of hemoglobin (anemia)
Retinal hemorrhages	More frequent in concurrent states of thrombocytopenia and anemia than with thrombocytopenia alone
Dilation of the veins	Polycythemia
Mouth	
Pallor	Reduction in quantity of hemoglobin (anemia)
Gingival and mucosal ulceration	Neutropenia, severe anemia
Gingival infiltration (swelling, reddening, bleeding)	Leukemia caused by impeded movement of granulocytes and monocytes through gingiva-tooth attachment into mucous membrane or by inability of impaired leukocytes to combat oral infections
Gingival or mucosal bleeding	Hemorrhagic diseases, thrombocytopenia
Smooth tongue texture	Pernicious and iron-deficiency anemia
Lymph Nodes	
Lymphadenopathy, tenderness	Normal response to infection in infants and children; cancerous invasion causative factor in adults; enlargement caused by infection, foreign infiltrates, or metabolic disturbances, especially with lipids
Chest	
Widened mediastinum	Enlarged lymph nodes
Generalized sternal tenderness	Leukemia resulting from increased bone marrow cellularity, causing increase in pressure and bone erosion
Localized sternal tenderness	Multiple myeloma as a result of stretching of periosteum
Tachycardia	Compensatory mechanism in anemia to increase cardiac output
Widened pulse pressure	Compensatory mechanism in anemia to increase cardiac output by increasing stroke volume
Murmurs	Usually systolic murmur in anemia caused by increased quantity and speed of low-viscosity blood going through pulmonic valve
Bruits (especially carotid bruits)	Anemia caused by increased flow of low-viscosity blood swirling through blood vessels
Angina pectoris	Anemia
Abdomen	
Hepatomegaly	Leukemia, cirrhosis, or fibrosis secondary to iron overload from sickle cell or thalassemia
Splenomegaly	Leukemia, lymphomas, mononucleosis
Splenic bruits and rubs	Splenic infarction

Continued

COMMON ASSESSMENT ABNORMALITIES

Table 28-5 Hematologic System—cont'd

Finding	Possible Etiology and Significance
Nervous System	
Pain and touch, position and vibratory sensation, tendon reflexes	Impaired nervous system function because of cobalamin deficiency or compression of nerves by masses
Back and Extremities	
Back pain	Acute hemolytic reaction from flank pain because of renal involvement with hemolysis; multiple myeloma from enlarged tumors that stretch periosteum or weaken supportive tissue, causing ligament strain and muscle spasm, sickle cell disease
Arthralgia	Leukemia as a result of aching in bones that contain marrow, sickle cell disease from hemarthrosis
Bone pain	Bone invasion by leukemia cells, bone demineralization resulting from various hematopoietic and solid malignancies enhancing possibility of pathologic fractures, sickle cell disease

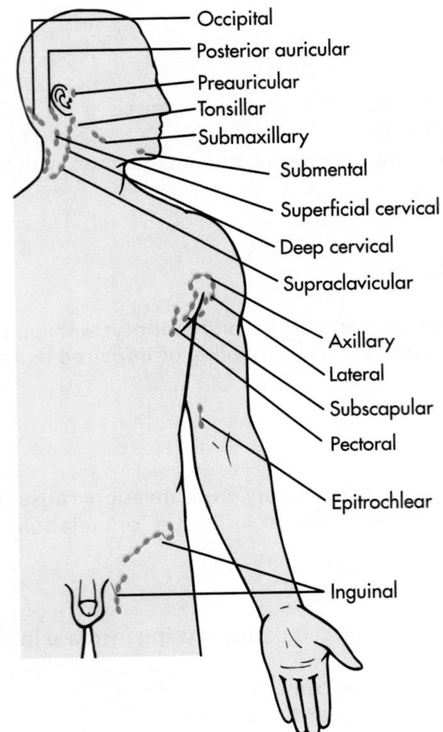

Fig. 28-6 Palpable superficial lymph nodes.

The total RBC count is reported as RBC × $10^6/\mu l$. However, total RBC count is not always reliable in determining the adequacy of RBC function. Consequently, other data, such as hemoglobin, hematocrit, and RBC indices, must also be evaluated. The RBC count is altered by the same conditions that raise and lower the hemoglobin and hematocrit values.

RBC indices are special indicators that reflect RBC volume, color, and hemoglobin saturation (see Table 28-6). These parameters may provide insight into the cause of anemia. (The significance of these parameters is discussed further in Chapter 29.)

White blood cells. The WBC differential is of considerable significance because it is possible for the total WBC count to remain essentially normal despite a marked change in one type of leukocyte. For example, a patient may have a normal WBC count of 8800/μl while the differential count may show a relative proportion of lymphocytes to be reduced to 10%. This is an abnormal finding that warrants further investigation.

An important concept related to neutrophil counts is the shift to the left. When infections are severe, more granulocytes are released from the bone marrow as a compensatory mechanism. To meet the increased demand, many young, immature polymorphonuclear neutrophils or bands are released into circulation. The usual laboratory procedure is to report the WBCs in order of maturity (see Fig. 28-2), with the less mature forms on the left side of the written report. Consequently the existence of many immature cells is termed a *shift to the left.*

Platelet count. Bleeding may occur when the platelet count is depressed, which is a condition termed *thrombocytopenia.* If platelets are functioning properly, most hematologists believe that a patient can undergo necessary surgery with platelet counts as low as 50,000/μl (normal count is 150,000 to 400,000/μl). Once platelet counts drop to between 20,000 and 30,000/μl, spontaneous hemorrhage is probable. When platelets are depressed to 10,000/μl, the possibility of intracerebral hemorrhage is significantly increased.[7] Clotting studies are presented in Table 28-7.

Erythrocyte Sedimentation Rate. Erythrocyte sedimentation rate (ESR, or sed rate) measures the sedimentation or settling of RBCs and is used as a nonspecific measure of many diseases, especially inflammatory conditions. Increased ESRs are common during acute and chronic inflammatory reactions when cell destruction is increased. They are also found in persons with malignancy, myocardial infarction, and end-stage renal disease. Although the ESR is a nonspecific test, it is often used as a routine screening procedure.

Table 28-6 Complete Blood Count Studies

Study	Description and Purpose	Normal Values
Hb	Measurement of gas-carrying capacity of RBC	Women: 12-16 g/dl (120-160 g/L) Men: 13.5-18 g/dl (135-180 g/L)
Hct	Measure of packed cell volume of RBC expressed as a percentage of the total blood volume	Women: 38-47% (.38-.47) Men: 40-54% (.40-.54)
Total RBC count	Count of number of circulating RBCs	Women: 4.0-5.0 × 10^6/μl (4.0-5.0 × 10^{12}/L) Men: 4.5-6.0 × 10^6/μl (4.5-6.0 × 10^{12}/L)
Red cell indices		
$MCV = \frac{Hct \times 10}{RBC \times 10^6}$	Determination of relative size of RBC; low MCV reflection of microcytosis, high MCV reflection of macrocytosis	82-98 fl
$MCH = \frac{Hb \times 10}{RBC \times 10^6}$	Measurement of average weight of Hb/RBC; low MCH indication of microcytosis or hypochromia, high MCHC indication of macrocytosis	27-33 pg
$MCHC = \frac{Hb}{Hct} \times 100$	Evaluation of RBC saturation with Hb; low MCHC indication of hypochromia, high MCHC evident in spherocytosis	32-36% (.32-.36)
WBC count	Measurement of total number of leukocytes	4000-11,000 /μl (4-11 × 10^9/L)
WBC differential	Determination of whether each kind of WBC is present in proper proportion, determination of absolute value by multiplying percentage of cell type by total WBC count and dividing by 100	Neutrophils: 50-70% (.50-.70) Eosinophils: 2-4% (.02-.04) Basophils: 0-2% (0-.02) Lymphocytes: 20-40% (.20-.40) Monocytes: 4-8% (.04-.08)
Platelet count	Measurement of number of platelets available to maintain platelet clotting functions (not measurement of quality of platelet function)	150,000-400,000 /μl (150-400 × 10^9/L)

Hb, hemoglobin; *Hct*, hematocrit; *MCH*, mean corpuscular hemoglobin; *MCHC*, mean corpuscular hemoglobin concentration; *MCV*, mean corpuscular volume.

Blood Typing and Rh Factor. Blood group antigens (A and B) are found only on RBC membranes and form the basis for the ABO blood typing system. The presence or absence of one or both of the two inherited antigens is the basis for the four blood groups: A, B, AB, and O. Blood group A has A antigens, group B has B antigens, group AB has both antigens, and group O has neither A nor B antigens. Each person has antibodies in the serum termed anti-A and anti-B that react with A or B antigens. These antibodies are found when the corresponding antigen is absent from the RBC surface. For example, B antibodies are found in persons with blood group A (Table 28-8).

Blood reactions based on ABO incompatibilities result from intravascular hemolysis of the RBCs. Erythrocytes agglutinate when a serum antibody is present to react with the antigens on the RBC membrane. For example, agglutination would occur in the blood of a person with type A blood when blood is transfused from a person with B antigens (i.e., type B or AB) into the person with type A blood. The anti-B antibodies in the type A blood would react with the B antigens, thus initiating the process that results in RBC hemolysis.

The Rh system is based on a third antigen, D, which is also found on the RBC membrane. Rh-positive persons have the D antigen, whereas Rh-negative persons do not. Approximately 85% of the Caucasian population is Rh positive and 15% is Rh negative; in the African-American population, the distribution is slightly higher (90% and 10%, respectively).[7] As a result of transfusion therapy or during childbirth, an Rh-negative person may be exposed to Rh-positive blood. Such exposure results in formation of an antibody, anti-D, which acts against Rh antigens. (Rh-positive persons normally have no anti-D.) The person is then sensitized to Rh-positive blood, and a second exposure to Rh-positive blood will cause a severe hemolytic reaction. A Coombs' test can be used to evaluate the person's Rh status (Table 28-9).

Lymphangiography

Lymphangiography is radiologic visualization of the lymph system after the injection of dye. The purpose of this procedure is to assess deep lymph nodes. Although its use has decreased, it continues to have a role in staging Hodgkin's and non-Hodgkin's lymphomas. This test may be used in conjunction with other tests such as computerized tomography (CT) scans or gallium scans to fully identify lymph nodes involved with cancer. Allergies to shellfish and iodine, and previous reactions to dyes, should be ascertained before doing a lymphangiogram.

The procedure begins with the intracutaneous injection of a blue dye into the webs of the toes. (It is less commonly done through the hands.) The dye is absorbed by the lymph vessels, making them visible through the skin on the dorsum of the foot. Once visible the dorsum of each foot is injected with a

Table 28-7 Clotting Studies

Study	Description and Purpose	Normal Values
Platelet count	Count of number of circulating platelets	150,000-400,000/μl
Prothrombin time (PT)	Assessment of extrinsic coagulation by measurement of factors I, II, V, VII, X	12-15 sec
International normalized ratio (INR)	Standardized system of reporting PT based on a reference calibration model and calculated by comparing the patient's PT with a control value.	2.0-3.0*
Activated partial thromboplastin time (APTT)	Assessment of intrinsic coagulation by measuring factors I, II, V, VIII, IX, X, XI, XII; longer with use of heparin	30-45 sec
Automated coagulation time (ACT)	Evaluation of intrinsic coagulation status; more accurate than APTT; used during dialysis, coronary artery bypass procedure, arteriograms	150-180
Thromboplastin generation test (TGT)	Reflection of generation of thromboplastin; if abnormal, second stage done to identify missing coagulation factor	< 12 sec (100%)
Bleeding time	Measurement of time small skin incision bleeds; reflection of ability of small blood vessels to constrict	1-6 min
Thrombin time	Reflection of adequacy of thrombin; prolonged thrombin time indication that coagulation is inadequate secondary to decreased thrombin activity	8-12 sec
Fibrinogen	Reflection of level of fibrinogen; increase in fibrinogen possible indication of enhancement of fibrin formation, making patient hypercoagulable; decrease in fibrinogen indicates that patient possibly predisposed to bleeding	200-400 mg/dl (2.0-4.0 g/L)
Fibrin split products†	Reflection of degree of fibrinolysis; reflection of excessive fibrinolysis and predisposition to bleed (if present); possible indication of disseminated intravascular coagulation	< 10 mg/L
Clot retraction	Reflection of clot shrinkage or retraction from sides of test tube after 24 hours; used to confirm a platelet problem	50-100% in 24 hr
Capillary fragility test (Tourniquet test, Rumpel-Leede test)	Reflection of capillary integrity when positive or negative pressure is applied to various areas of the body; positive test indication of thrombocytopenia, toxic vascular reactions	No petechiae or negative
Protamine sulfate tests	Reflection of presence of fibrin monomer (portion of fibrin remaining after elements that polymerize and stabilize clot detach); positive test indication of predisposition to bleed and possible presence of disseminated intravascular coagulation	Negative

*Desired level for anticoagulation regimens.
†Also called fibrin degradation products (FDP)

Table 28-8 ABO Blood Group Names and Compatibilities*

Blood Group	Red Blood Cell Agglutinogen(s)	Serum Agglutinin(s)	Compatible Donor Blood Groups	Incompatible Donor Blood Groups
A	A	Anti-B	A and O	B and AB
B	B	Anti-A	B and O	A and AB
AB	A and B	Neither	A, B, AB, and O	None
O	Neither (universal donor)	Anti-A and anti-B	O	A, B, and AB

*ABO blood groups are named for the antigen found on the RBCs. Compatibility is based on the antibodies present in the serum.

local anesthetic agent, and a small superficial incision is made over the lymph vessels. The lymph vessel is then cannulated with a small needle. Once the needle is inserted it is important that the patient not move the feet to avoid the possibility of dislodging the needle. When the lymph vessels are cannulated, a radiopaque oil is injected slowly by means of an automated pump. The usual dose of oil for an adult is 7 ml in each foot administered for a duration of 45 to 60 minutes. Fluoroscopy may be used during the injection to watch the filling of the lymph vessels. Immediately after the dye has been injected several x-rays will be taken from various angles. A second set of x-rays will be taken the next day when the lymph channels are emptied. The incisions on the feet are sutured closed when the procedure is complete.

The lymph nodes can also be seen by means of isotopic (technetium 99m) lymphangiography. Compared with radi-

Table 28-9 Miscellaneous Laboratory Blood Studies

Study	Description and Purpose	Normal Values
ESR	Measurement of sedimentation or settling of RBCs in 1 hr. Inflammatory processes cause an alteration in plasma proteins, resulting in aggregation of RBC and making them heavier. The faster the sedimentation rate, the higher the ESR.	Women: 1-20 mm in 1 hr Men: 1-15 mm in 1 hr
Reticulocyte count	Measurement of immature RBCs; reflection of bone marrow activity in producing RBCs	0.5-1.5% of RBC count (0.005-0.015 of RBC count)
Bilirubin	Measurement of degree of RBC hemolysis or liver's inability to excrete normal quantities of bilirubin; increase in indirect bilirubin with hemolytic problems	Total: 0.2-1.3 mg/dl (3.4-22 μmol/L) Direct: 0.1-0.3 mg/dl (1.7-5.1 μmol/L) Indirect: 0.1-1.0 mg/dl (1.7-17 μmol/L)
Iron Serum iron	Reflection of amount of iron combined with proteins in serum; accurate indication of status of iron storage and use	50-150 μg/dl (9.0-26.9 μmol/L)
Total iron-binding capacity	Measurement of percentage of saturation of transferrin, a protein that binds iron; evaluation of amount of extra iron that can be carried	250-410 μg/dl (45-73 μmol/L)
Coombs' test	Differentiation among types of hemolytic anemias; detection of immune antibodies	
Direct	Detection of antibodies that are attached to RBCs	Negative
Indirect	Detection of antibodies in serum	Negative

ESR, erythrocyte sedimentation rate.

ographic lymphangiography, isotopic lymphangiography is less invasive and does not require dye injection. However, the isotope's short life prevents serial studies.

Nursing responsibilities related to lymphangiography and other common studies of the hematologic system are presented in Table 28-10.

Biopsies

Biopsy procedures specific to hematologic assessment are bone marrow examination and lymph node biopsy. In general, these procedures are done when a diagnosis cannot be established from a peripheral blood smear or when more information about the possible hematologic problem is needed.

Bone Marrow Examination. Bone marrow examination is important in the evaluation of many hematologic disorders. It involves the aspiration or biopsy of bone marrow with a syringe and needle. The aspirate is made into smears that are useful for cytologic diagnosis.

The site of bone marrow aspiration is determined by the age of the patient and the skill of the physician or specially credentialed nurse. In adults, the sites most easily aspirated are the anterior and posterior iliac crests. The tibia may provide an additional site in young children. Although hazards of bone marrow aspiration are minimal, there is a possibility of penetrating the bone and damaging underlying structures.

The skin over the puncture site is cleansed with a bactericidal agent. The skin, subcutaneous tissue, and periosteum are infiltrated with a local anesthetic agent. In addition, systemic analgesics or tranquilizers are often administered before the procedure to minimize pain and decrease anxiety. The patient may be uncomfortable when the periosteum is penetrated. Once the area is anesthetized, the special marrow needle is inserted through the cortex of the bone. The stylet of the needle is then removed, the hub is attached to a 10 ml syringe, and 0.2 to 0.5 ml of the fluid marrow is aspirated. The aspiration is experienced by the patient as a suction pain, which may be quite uncomfortable although it lasts for only a few seconds.

After the marrow aspiration, the needle is removed. Pressure is applied over the aspiration site to ensure hemostasis. If the patient is thrombocytopenic, pressure may be required for 5 to 10 minutes or longer.

If a bone biopsy is required, the preparatory procedure remains the same, but a different needle is used. The needle has a cutting blade that allows a specimen of the bone to be removed. When either a marrow aspirate or a biopsy specimen is acquired, a glass slide is carefully prepared with a thin film of the marrow.

Lymph Node Biopsy. Lymph node biopsy involves obtaining lymph tissue for histologic examination to determine the diagnosis and therapy. This may be accomplished by either an open biopsy or a closed (needle) biopsy. In the open biopsy procedure, an incision is made, and the lymph node and surrounding tissue are dissected whenever possible. Care must be taken because neoplastic cells can be disseminated during the biopsy procedure if the scalpel passes through tissues containing cancerous cells. An open biopsy is performed in the operating room using either local or general anesthesia.

A closed (needle) biopsy may also be performed to analyze lymph tissue. This bedside or outpatient technique is performed by a skilled physician. Sterile technique is essential throughout the procedure. Nursing personnel must recognize the possibility of insidious bleeding, and direct pressure should be applied to the area after the biopsy procedure to achieve hemostasis. Frequent observations of the site for bleeding and monitoring of vital signs should be done, especially if the platelet count is low. The sterile dressing should be changed as ordered, and the wound should be inspected for healing and infection. It is important to recognize that if a needle biopsy is negative, it may signify only that the cancer cells were not a part of the tissue in the biopsy specimen. However, a positive finding is sufficient evidence for confirming a diagnosis.

DIAGNOSTIC STUDIES

Table 28-10 Hematologic System

Study	Description and Purpose	Nursing Responsibility
Urine Studies		
■ Bence Jones protein	An electrophoretic measurement is used to detect the presence of the Bence Jones protein, which is found in most cases of multiple myeloma. Negative finding indicates that patient is normal.	Acquire random urine specimen.
Radioisotope Studies		
■ Liver/spleen scan	Radioactive isotope is injected intravenously. Images from the radioactive emissions are used to evaluate the structure of the spleen and liver. Patient is not a source of radio-activity.	No specific nursing responsibilities
■ Bone scan	Same procedure as for the spleen scan except used for the purpose of evaluating the structure of the bones.	No specific nursing responsibilities
■ Isotopic lymphangiography	Radionuclide study is used to assess lymph nodes and lymph system. Technetium 99m is used. Technique is less invasive than radiographic lymphangiography.	No specific nursing responsibilities
Radiologic Studies		
■ Lymphangiography	Purpose is to evaluate deep lymph nodes. Radiopaque oil-based dye is infused slowly into the lymph vessels via small needles in the dorsum of each foot. Radiographs are taken immediately and on next day.	Inform the patient about what to anticipate. Obtain consent form. Assess for iodine sensitivity. Give preoperative sedation, if indicated. Instruct patient that urine will be blue from the dye excretion for 1-2 days. Inform patient that transient fever, general malaise, and diffuse muscle aches may be experienced for 12-24 hr. Watch for signs of oil embolus to lungs (hacking cough, dyspnea, pleuritic pain, and hemoptysis).
■ Computed tomography (CT)	Noninvasive radiologic examination using computer-assisted x-ray evaluates the spleen, liver, or lymph nodes.	No specific nursing responsibilities
■ Magnetic resonance imaging (MRI)	Noninvasive procedure produces sensitive images of soft tissue without using contrast dyes. No ionizing radiation is required. Technique is used to evaluate spleen, liver, and lymph nodes.	Instruct patient to remove all metal objects and ask about any history of surgical insertion of staples, plates, or other metal appliances. Inform patient of need to lie still in small chamber.
Biopsies		
■ Bone marrow	Technique involves removal of bone marrow through a locally anesthetized site to evaluate the status of the blood-forming tissue. It is used to diagnose multiple myeloma, all types of leukemia, and some lymphomas and to stage some solid tumors (e.g., breast cancer). It is also done to assess efficacy of leukemic therapy.*	Explain procedure to patient. Obtain signed consent form. Consider preprocedure analgesic administration to enhance patient comfort and cooperation. Apply pressure dressing after procedure. Assess biopsy site for bleeding.
■ Lymph node biopsy	Purpose is to obtain lymph tissue for histologic examination to determine diagnosis and therapy.	Explain procedure to patient. Obtain signed consent form. Use sterile technique in dressing changes after procedure. Carefully evaluate wound for healing. Assess patient for complications, especially bleeding and edema.
Open	Test is performed in operating room with direct visualization of the area.	
Closed (needle)	Test is performed at bedside or in office.	
Blood Studies†		

*See Chapter 29.
†See Tables 28-6, 28-7, and 28-9.

REVIEW QUESTIONS

The number of the question corresponds to the same-numbered objective at the beginning of the chapter.

1. An individual who lives at a high altitude may normally have an increased RBC because
   a. high altitudes cause vascular fluid loss leading to hemoconcentration.
   b. hypoxia caused by decreased atmospheric oxygen stimulates erythropoiesis.
   c. the function of the spleen in removing old erythrocytes is impaired at high altitudes.
   d. impaired production of leukocytes and platelets leads to proportionally higher red cell counts.
2. Disorders such as myeloblastic leukemia that arise from myeloblast cells in the bone marrow will have the primary effect of causing
   a. increased incidence of cancer.
   b. decreased production of antibodies.
   c. decreased phagocytosis of bacteria.
   d. increased allergic and inflammatory reactions.
3. An anticoagulant such as warfarin that interferes with the production of prothrombin will alter the clotting mechanism during
   a. platelet aggregation.
   b. activation of thrombin.
   c. the release of tissue thromboplastin.
   d. stimulation of factor activation complex.
4. When reviewing laboratory results of an 83-year-old patient with an infection, the nurse would expect to find
   a. minimal leukocytosis.
   b. decreased platelet count.
   c. increased hemoglobin and hematocrit levels.
   b. decreased erythrocyte sedimentation rate (ESR).
5. Significant information obtained from the patient's health history that relates to the hematologic system includes
   a. jaundice.
   b. bladder surgery.
   c. early menopause.
   d. multiple pregnancies.
6. While assessing the lymph nodes the nurse
   a. applies gentle, firm pressure to deep lymph nodes.
   b. palpates the deep cervical and supraclavicular nodes last.
   c. lightly palpates superficial lymph nodes with the index and third fingers.
   d. uses the tips of the second, third, and fourth fingers to apply deep palpation.
7. A normal finding of the lymph node examination is
   a. shotty nodes.
   b. hard, fixed nodes.
   c. firm, tender nodes.
   d. mobile, hard nodes.
8. Immediately following a bone marrow biopsy and aspiration the nurse should instruct the patient to
   a. expect to receive a blood transfusion.
   b. lie still with a sterile pressure dressing intact.
   c. lie with knees slightly bent and head elevated.
   d. cleanse the site immediately with povidone-iodine.

References

1. Erickson JMM: Anemia, *Semin Oncol Nurs* 12:1, 1996.
2. George JN, Shattil SJ: The clinical importance of acquired abnormalities of platelet function, *N Engl J Med* 324:27, 1991.
3. Mann KG, Gaffney D, Bovill EG: Molecular biology, biochemistry, and lifespan of plasma coagulation factors. In Beutler E, editor: *Williams hematology textbook,* ed 5, New York, 1995, McGraw-Hill.
4. Lipschitz DA: Aging of the hematopoietic system. In *Principles of geriatric medicine and gerontology,* ed 3, New York, 1994, McGraw-Hill
5. Walsh JR: Hematologic problems. In Cassel CK, editor: *Geriatric medicine,* ed 3, New York, 1997, Springer.
6. Williams WJ: Approach to the patient. In Beutler E, editor: *Williams hematology textbook,* ed 5, New York, 1995, McGraw-Hill.
7. Fischbach F: *A manual of laboratory and diagnostic tests,* ed 5, Philadelphia, 1996, Lippincott.

Resources

Resources for this chapter are listed after Chapter 29 on p. 789.

REMEMBER to check out your companion CD-ROM

29 NURSING MANAGEMENT Hematologic Problems

Ann M. O'Mara & Marie Bakitas Whedon

www.mosby.com/MERLIN/medsurg_lewis

LEARNING OBJECTIVES

1. Describe the general clinical manifestations and complications of anemia.
2. Differentiate between the etiologic and morphologic classifications of anemia.
3. Describe the etiologies, specific clinical manifestations, diagnostic findings, and nursing and collaborative management of iron-deficiency, megaloblastic, and aplastic anemias and anemia of chronic disease.
4. Explain the nursing management of anemia secondary to blood loss.
5. Describe the pathophysiology, clinical manifestations, and nursing and collaborative management of anemia caused by increased erythrocyte destruction, including sickle cell disease and acquired hemolytic anemias.
6. Describe the pathophysiology and nursing and collaborative management of polycythemia.
7. Explain the pathophysiology, clinical manifestations, and nursing and collaborative management of various types of thrombocytopenia.
8. Describe the types, clinical manifestations, diagnostic findings, and nursing and collaborative management of hemophilia and von Willebrand disease.
9. Explain the pathophysiology, diagnostic findings, and nursing and collaborative management of disseminated intravascular coagulation.
10. Describe the etiology, clinical manifestations, and nursing and collaborative management of neutropenia.
11. Describe the pathophysiology, clinical manifestations, and nursing and collaborative management of myelodysplastic syndromes.
12. Compare and contrast the major types of leukemia regarding age at onset and distinguishing clinical and laboratory findings.
13. Explain the nursing and collaborative management of acute and chronic leukemias.
14. Compare Hodgkin's disease and non-Hodgkin's lymphomas in terms of clinical manifestations, staging, and nursing and collaborative management.
15. Describe the pathophysiology, clinical manifestations, and nursing and collaborative management of multiple myeloma.
16. Describe the spleen disorders and related collaborative care.
17. Describe the nursing management of the patient receiving transfusions of blood and blood components.

ANEMIA

Definition and Classification

Anemia is a reduction below normal in the number of erythrocytes, the quantity of hemoglobin, and the volume of packed red cells (hematocrit) caused by rapid blood loss, impaired production of erythrocytes, or increased destruction of erythrocytes. Because red blood cells (RBCs) transport oxygen (O_2), erythrocyte disorders can lead to tissue hypoxia. This hypoxia accounts for many of the clinical manifestations of anemia. Anemia is not a specific disease; it is a manifestation of a pathologic process. Anemia is identified and classified by laboratory evaluation. Once anemia is identified, further investigation must be done to determine its cause.[1]

Anemia can result from primary hematologic problems or can develop as a secondary consequence of defects in other body systems. The many kinds of anemia can be grouped according to either a *morphologic* or an *etiologic* classification. Morphologic classification is based on descriptive, objective laboratory information about erythrocyte size and color. (The terms used in this classification system are explained in Chapter 28.) Etiologic classification is related to the clinical conditions causing the anemia, such as decreased erythrocyte production, blood loss, or increased erythrocyte destruction (Table 29-1). Although the morphologic system is the most accurate means of classifying anemias, it is easier to discuss patient care by focusing on the etiologic problem. Table 29-2 relates morphologic classifications to various etiologies.

Mechanisms to Compensate for Hypoxia

Regardless of the type of anemia, a decrease in erythrocytes reduces the blood's O_2-carrying capacity, which leads to tissue hypoxia. The physiologic effects of anemia are caused by tissue hypoxia and activation of compensatory mechanisms that attempt to meet cellular O_2 needs. The four major compensatory responses to anemia are as follows:

Reviewed by Judy Kaye, RN, CNRN, CCRN, ANP, GNP, CS, PhDc, Critical Care/Neuroscience Clinical Specialist, Adult and Gerontology Nurse Practitioner, University Hospital, Augusta, Ga.

Table 29-1 Etiologic Classification of Anemia

Decreased Erythrocyte Production
- Decreased hemoglobin synthesis
  - Iron deficiency
  - Thalassemias (decreased globin synthesis)
  - Sideroblastic anemia (decreased porphyrin)
- Defective DNA synthesis
  - Cobalamin (vitamin B_{12}) deficiency
  - Folic acid deficiency
- Decreased number of erythrocyte precursors
  - Aplastic anemia
  - Anemia of leukemia and myelodysplasia
  - Chronic diseases or disorders

Blood Loss
- Acute
  - Trauma
  - Blood vessel rupture
- Chronic
  - Gastritis
  - Menstrual flow
  - Hemorrhoids

Increased Erythrocyte Destruction*
- Intrinsic
  - Abnormal hemoglobin (HbS—sickle cell anemia)
  - Enzyme deficiency (G6PD)
  - Membrane abnormalities (paroxysmal nocturnal hemoglobinuria)
- Extrinsic
  - Physical trauma (prosthetic heart valves, extracorporeal circulation)
  - Antibodies (isoimmune and autoimmune)
  - Infectious agents and toxins (malaria)

*Hemolytic anemias.
DNA, deoxyribonucleic acid; *G6PD*, glucose-6-phosphate dehydrogenase; *HbS*, hemoglobin S.

Table 29-2 Relationship of Morphologic Classification and Etiologies of Anemia

Morphology	Etiology
Normocytic, normochromic	Acute blood loss, hemolysis, chronic renal disease, chronic disease, cancers, sideroblastic anemia, refractory anemia, diseases of endocrine dysfunction, aplastic anemia, pregnancy
Macrocytic, normochromic	Cobalamin (vitamin B_{12}) deficiency, folic acid deficiency, liver disease (including effects of alcohol abuse), postsplenectomy
Microcytic, hypochromic	Iron-deficiency anemia, thalassemia, lead poisoning

1. A shift of the oxygen-hemoglobin dissociation curve to the right, thereby facilitating removal of more O_2 by the tissues at the same partial pressure of O_2 (Fig. 29-1)
2. Redistribution of blood from tissues that have a low O_2 requirement (e.g., skin) to tissues that have higher O_2 needs (e.g., brain, muscle, myocardium)

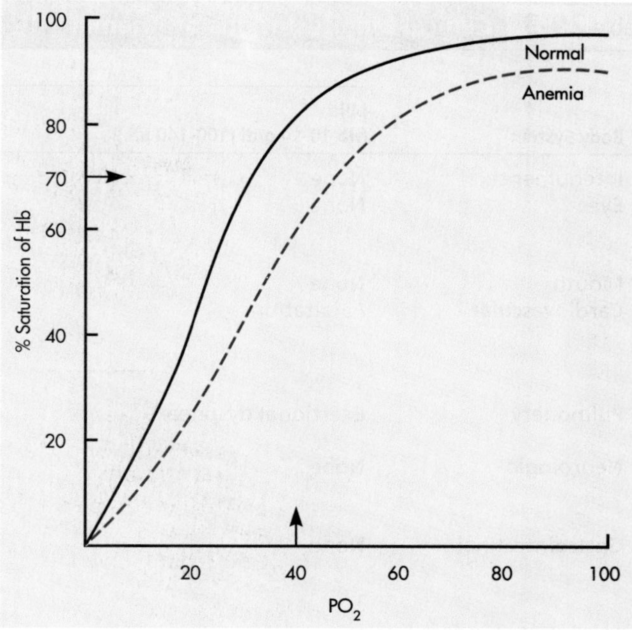

Fig. 29-1 Oxygen-hemoglobin dissociation curve. The oxygen-hemoglobin curve of a normal person (*solid line*) with hemoglobin of 15 g/dl compared to that of a person with anemia (*dashed line*) with hemoglobin of 6 g/dl. The shift to the right seen with the anemic person is a compensatory mechanism. While the O_2 transport capability of hemoglobin is decreased with the shift to the right, hemoglobin release of O_2 to the tissues is facilitated; that is, hemoglobin gives up O_2 more readily when the curve shifts to the right.

3. Increased cardiac output (CO) achieved by increased heart rate (HR) or increased stroke volume (SV) to meet O_2 demands of the tissues
4. Increased rate of RBC production (within 4 to 5 days) after erythropoietin synthesis (by the kidneys) has increased in response to tissue hypoxia

Clinical Manifestations

The clinical manifestations of anemia are primarily caused by the body's response to tissue hypoxia. The intensity of the manifestations varies depending on the severity of the anemia and the presence of coexisting diseases. The severity of anemia can be determined by the hemoglobin (Hb) levels. Mild states of anemia (Hb 10 to 14 g/dl [100 to 140 g/L]) may exist without causing symptoms. If symptoms develop, they are usually caused by an underlying disease or a compensatory response to heavy exercise. These symptoms include palpitations, dyspnea, and diaphoresis. In cases of moderate anemia (Hb 6 to 10 g/dl [60 to 100 g/L]), the cardiopulmonary symptoms may be increased and may be associated with rest as well as activity. The patient with severe anemia (Hb less than 6 g/dl [60 g/L]) displays many clinical manifestations involving multiple body systems (Table 29-3).

Integumentary Changes. Integumentary changes include pallor, jaundice, and pruritus. The pallor results from reduced amounts of hemoglobin and reduced blood flow to the skin. Jaundice occurs when there is an increased concentration of serum bilirubin, which increases when hemolysis of RBCs occurs. Pruritus occurs because of increased serum and

Table 29-3 Clinical Manifestations of Anemia

Body System	Severity of Anemia: Mild (Hb 10-14 g/dl [100-140 g/L])	Moderate (Hb 6-10 g/dl [60-100 g/L])	Severe (Hb <6 g/dl [<60 g/L])
Integument	None	None	Pallor, jaundice,* pruritus*
Eyes	None	None	Icteric conjunctiva and sclera,* retinal hemorrhage, blurred vision
Mouth	None	None	Glossitis, smooth tongue
Cardiovascular	Palpitations	Increased palpitations	Tachycardia, increased pulse pressure, systolic murmurs, intermittent claudication, angina, CHF, MI
Pulmonary	Exertional dyspnea	Dyspnea	Tachypnea, orthopnea, dyspnea at rest
Neurologic	None	None	Headache, vertigo, irritability, depression, impaired thought processes
Gastrointestinal	None	None	Anorexia, hepatomegaly, splenomegaly, difficulty swallowing, sore mouth
Musculoskeletal	None	None	Bone pain
General	None	Fatigue	Sensitivity to cold, weight loss, lethargy

*Caused by hemolysis.
CHF, congestive heart failure; *Hb,* hemoglobin; *MI,* myocardial infarction.

CULTURAL & ETHNIC CONSIDERATIONS

Hematologic Problems

- Sickle cell disease has a high incidence among African-Americans.
- Thalassemia has a high incidence among African-Americans and people of Mediterranean origin.
- Tay-Sachs disease has the highest incidence in families of Eastern European Jewish origin, especially the Ashkenazic Jews.
- Pernicious anemia has a high incidence among Scandinavians and African-Americans.

skin bile salt concentrations. In addition to the skin, the sclera of the eyes and mucous membranes should be evaluated for jaundice because they reflect the integumentary changes more accurately, especially in a dark-skinned individual.

Cardiopulmonary Manifestations. Cardiopulmonary manifestations of severe anemia result from additional attempts by the heart and lungs to provide adequate amounts of oxygen to the tissues. CO is maintained by increasing the heart rate. The low viscosity of the blood contributes to the development of systolic murmurs and bruits. In extreme cases or when concomitant heart disease is present, angina pectoris and myocardial infarction (MI) may occur if myocardial O_2 needs cannot be met. Congestive heart failure (CHF), cardiomegaly, pulmonary and systemic congestion, ascites, and peripheral edema may develop if the heart is overworked for an extended period of time.

NURSING MANAGEMENT: ANEMIA

This section will discuss general nursing management of anemia. Specific care related to various types of anemia is discussed later in this chapter.

■ Nursing Assessment

Subjective and objective data that should be obtained from an individual with anemia are presented in Table 29-4.

■ Nursing Diagnoses

Nursing diagnoses for the patient with anemia include, but are not limited to, those presented in NCP 29-1.

■ Planning

The overall goals are that the patient with anemia will (1) assume normal activities of daily living, (2) maintain adequate nutrition, and (3) develop no complications related to anemia.

■ Nursing Implementation

The numerous causes of anemia necessitate different nursing interventions specific to the needs of the patient. Nevertheless, there are certain general components of care for all patients with anemia that are presented in NCP 29-1.

Dietary and lifestyle changes (described with specific types of anemia) can reverse some anemias so that the patient can return to the former state of health. Acute interventions include blood transfusions, drug therapy (e.g., erythropoietin, vitamin supplements), and oxygen therapy. However, correcting the etiology of the anemia is ultimately the goal of therapy. Ongoing

NURSING ASSESSMENT

Table 29-4 Anemia

Subjective Data	Objective Data
Important Health Information *Past health history:* Recent blood loss or trauma; chronic liver, endocrine, or renal disease (including dialysis); GI disease (malabsorption syndrome, ulcers, gastritis, or hemorrhoids); inflammatory disorders; exposure to radiation or chemical toxins (arsenic, lead, benzenes, copper) *Medications:* Use of vitamin and iron supplements; aspirin, anticoagulants, oral contraceptives, phenobarbital, penicillins, NSAIDs, phenacetin, quinine, quinidine, phenytoin (Dilantin), methyldopa (Aldomet), sulfonamides *Surgery and other treatments:* Recent surgery, small bowel resection, gastrectomy, prosthetic heart valves **Functional Health Patterns** *Health perception–health management:* Family history of anemia; malaise *Nutritional-metabolic:* Nausea, vomiting, anorexia, weight loss; dysphagia, dyspepsia, heartburn, night sweats, cold intolerance *Elimination:* Hematuria, decreased urinary output; diarrhea, constipation, flatulence, tarry stools, bloody stools *Activity-exercise:* Fatigue, muscle weakness, and decreased strength; dyspnea, orthopnea, cough, hemoptysis; palpitations *Cognitive-perceptual:* Headache; abdominal, chest, and bone pain; painful tongue; paresthesias of feet and hands; pruritis; disturbances in vision, taste, or hearing; vertigo; hypersensitivity to cold *Sexuality-reproductive:* Menorrhagia, metrorrhagia; recent or current pregnancy; male impotence	**General** Lethargy, apathy, general lymphadenopathy, fever **Integumentary** Pale skin and mucous membranes; blue, pale white, or icteric sclera; cheilitis; poor skin turgor; brittle, spoon-shaped fingernails; jaundice; petechiae; ecchymoses; nose or gingival bleeding; poor healing; dry, brittle, thinning hair **Respiratory** Tachypnea **Cardiovascular** Tachycardia, systolic murmur, arrhythmias; postural hypotension, widened pulse pressure, bruits (especially carotid); intermittent claudication, ankle edema **Gastrointestinal** Hepatosplenomegaly; glossitis; beefy, red tongue; stomatitis; abdominal distention; anorexia **Neurologic** Confusion, impaired judgment, irritability, ataxia, unsteady gait, paralysis **Possible Findings** ↓ RBC; ↓ Hb; ↓ Hct; ↓ serum iron, ferritin, folate, or cobalamin (vitamin B_{12}); heme (guaiac)–positive stools; ↓ serum erythropoietin level

GI, gastrointestinal; *Hct,* hematocrit; *NSAIDs,* nonsteroidal antiinflammatory drugs; *RBC,* red blood cells.

assessment of the patient's knowledge regarding adequate nutritional intake and compliance to drug therapies should be included in the plan of care.[2]

GERONTOLOGIC CONSIDERATIONS

Anemia

Anemia is common in older adults because of their poor nutritional intake and decreased intestinal absorption of iron. Women more than 60 years of age have a prevalence of anemia as high as women in childbearing years.[3] Nutritional deficiencies account for the majority of anemia seen in older adults. Physical debilitation and depression among older adults can interfere with their ability to maintain adequate nutrition (Table 29-5).[4] Signs and symptoms of anemia may go unrecognized in the older adult or are mistaken as normal aging changes. These symptoms include confusion, ataxia, fatigue, worsening angina, and CHF. Multiple comorbid conditions in older adults increase the likelihood of occurrence of many types of anemia. However, these same conditions and the bias about what constitutes "normal aging" also contribute to the difficulty in diagnosing reversible causes of anemia. For example, an easily reversible iron-deficiency anemia presenting as ataxia may go unrecognized and untreated in an older patient. The nurse can play a major role in providing appropriate health assessment and related interventions for the older adult.

ANEMIA CAUSED BY DECREASED ERYTHROCYTE PRODUCTION

Normally RBC production (erythropoiesis) is in equilibrium with RBC destruction and loss. This balance ensures that an adequate number of erythrocytes are available at all times. RBCs must be replenished on a regular basis because they are viable for only 120 days. Three significant alterations in erythropoiesis may occur that decrease RBC production: (1) decreased hemoglobin synthesis may lead to iron-deficiency anemia, thalassemia, and sideroblastic anemia; (2) defective DNA synthesis in RBCs (e.g., cobalamin [vitamin B_{12}] deficiency, folic acid deficiency) may lead to megaloblastic anemias; and (3) diminished availability of erythrocyte precursors may result in aplastic anemia and anemia of chronic disease (see Table 29-1).

29-1 NURSING CARE PLAN PATIENT WITH ANEMIA

Expected Patient Outcomes	Nursing Interventions and *Rationales*
NURSING DIAGNOSIS	**Activity intolerance** *related to* weakness and malaise *as manifested by* difficulty in tolerating increased activity (e.g., increased pulse, respiration).
▪ Participation in activities of daily living (e.g., bathing, dressing, grooming, feeding) to greatest extent possible. ▪ Vital signs within acceptable range.	▪ Plan care to alternate periods of rest and activity *to provide activity without tiring the patient.* ▪ Strive for a 1:3 rest/activity ratio; assist patient with activities of daily living as needed. ▪ Place objects within patient's reach *to conserve strength.* ▪ Limit visitors, phone calls, noise, and interruptions by hospital staff *to reduce demands placed on patient.* ▪ Monitor vital signs *to evaluate activity tolerance.* ▪ Monitor hematocrit and hemoglobin *as a guide to planning activities.*
NURSING DIAGNOSIS	**Altered nutrition: less than body requirements** *related to* anorexia and treatment *as manifested by* weight loss, low serum albumin, decreased iron levels, vitamin deficiencies, below usual body weight.
▪ Maintenance of body weight, then gradually increase within range of ideal.	▪ Teach patient about high-protein, high-calorie foods *to increase intake of essential nutrients needed for hematopoiesis.* ▪ With input from patient, establish range of optimal weight outcomes, as well as dietary plan *to involve patient and increase compliance.* ▪ Teach and monitor use of a food diary *to increase patient's awareness of actual intake and increase intake.* ▪ Suggest eating small, frequent meals with snacks throughout the day.
NURSING DIAGNOSIS	**Ineffective management of therapeutic regimen** *related to* lack of knowledge about lifestyle adjustments, appropriate nutrition, and medication regimen *as manifested by* questioning about lifestyle adjustments, diet, medication prescriptions.
▪ Knowledge about lifestyle changes, nutrition, and medication regimen.	▪ Review and teach patient about lifestyle changes and nutrition and medication information *to promote compliance.* ▪ Teach about and monitor response to supplemental drugs that aid in RBC production *since it is difficult to correct severe anemia by diet alone.* ▪ Suggest follow-up resources to help patient maintain gains and adjustments throughout recovery.

COLLABORATIVE PROBLEMS

Nursing Goals	Nursing Interventions and *Rationales*
POTENTIAL COMPLICATION	**Hypoxemia** *related to* decreased hemoglobin.
▪ Monitor for signs of hypoxemia. ▪ Report deviations from acceptable parameter. ▪ Carry out appropriate medical and nursing interventions.	▪ Assess for manifestations of hypoxemia such as dyspnea, decrease in O_2 saturation, increase $PaCO_2$, cyanosis *to initiate early intervention.* ▪ Administer O_2 as ordered *to saturate all available hemoglobin.* ▪ Transfuse with blood products as ordered *to increase hemoglobin.* ▪ Change patient's position slowly; evaluate dizziness *as sign of cerebral hypoxia.* ▪ Monitor hemoglobin *to determine severity of anemia and response to treatment.* ▪ Position patient *to promote maximum thoracic excursion.* ▪ Teach effective breathing exercises and relaxation techniques *to relieve dyspnea.*

NUTRITIONAL THERAPY

Table 29-5 Nutrients Needed for Erythropoiesis

Nutrient	Role in Erythropoiesis	Food Sources
Cobalamin (vitamin B_{12})	RBC maturation	Red meats, especially liver
Folic acid	RBC maturation	Green leafy vegetables, liver, meat, fish, legumes, whole grains
Iron	Hemoglobin synthesis	Liver and muscle meats, eggs, dried fruits, legumes, dark green leafy vegetables, whole-grain and enriched bread and cereals, potatoes
Vitamin B_6	Hemoglobin synthesis	Meats (especially pork and liver), wheat germ, legumes, potatoes, cornmeal, bananas
Amino acids	Synthesis of nucleoproteins	Eggs, meat, milk and milk products (cheese, ice cream), poultry, fish, legumes, nuts
Vitamin C	Conversion of folic acid to its active forms, aids in iron absorption	Citrus fruits, leafy green vegetables, strawberries, cantaloupe

IRON-DEFICIENCY ANEMIA

Iron-deficiency anemia, one of the most common chronic hematologic disorders, is found in 30% of the world's population. In the United States, those most susceptible to iron-deficiency anemia are the very young, those on poor diets, and healthy women in their reproductive age.[5]

Iron is present in all RBCs as heme in hemoglobin and in a stored form. The heme in hemoglobin accounts for two thirds of the body's iron. The other one third of iron is stored as ferritin and hemosiderin in macrophages in the bone marrow, spleen, and liver. Normally, 1 mg of iron is lost daily through the gastrointestinal (GI) tract, sweat, and urine. When the stored iron is not replaced, hemoglobin production is reduced.

Etiology

Iron deficiency may develop from inadequate dietary intake, malabsorption, blood loss, or hemolysis. Iron is obtained from dietary intake. Approximately 1 mg of every 10 to 20 mg of iron ingested is absorbed in the duodenum. Therefore only approximately 5% to 10% of ingested iron is absorbed. This amount of dietary iron is adequate to meet the needs of men and older women, but it may be inadequate for those individuals who have higher iron needs (e.g., children, pregnant women). Table 29-5 lists nutrients needed for erythropoiesis.

Malabsorption of iron may occur after certain types of GI surgery and in malabsorption syndromes. Iron absorption primarily occurs in the duodenum. Surgical procedures for gastric ulcers may involve removal or bypass of the duodenum (see Chapter 39). Malabsorption syndromes may involve disease of the duodenum, where iron is normally absorbed. The absorption of iron is impeded in malabsorption states because the disease has altered or destroyed the absorptive surface.

Blood loss is a major cause of iron deficiency in adults. Two milliliters of whole blood contain 1 mg of iron. The major sources of chronic blood loss are from the GI and genitourinary (GU) systems. GI bleeding is often not apparent and therefore may exist for a considerable time before the problem is identified. Loss of 50 to 75 ml of blood from the upper GI tract is required for stools to appear as black or *melena.* The black color results from the iron in the RBCs. Common causes of GI blood loss in the adult are peptic ulcer, gastritis, esophagitis, diverticuli, hemorrhoids, and neoplasia. GU blood loss occurs primarily from menstrual bleeding. The average monthly menstrual blood loss is about 45 ml and causes the loss of about 22 mg of iron. Postmenopausal bleeding is rarely significant but also can contribute to anemia in a susceptible older woman.

Pregnancy contributes to iron deficiency because of the diversion of iron to the fetus for erythropoiesis, blood loss at delivery, and lactation. In addition to anemia of chronic renal failure, dialysis treatment may induce iron-deficiency anemia because of the blood lost in the dialysis equipment and frequent blood sampling.

Clinical Manifestations

In the early course of iron-deficiency anemia, the patient may be free of symptoms. As the disease becomes chronic, any of the general manifestations of anemia may develop (see Table 29-3). In addition, specific clinical symptoms may occur related to iron-deficiency anemia. Pallor is the most common finding, and *glossitis* (inflammation of the tongue) is the second most common; another finding is *cheilitis* (inflammation of the lips). In addition, the patient may report headache, paresthesias, and a burning sensation of the tongue, all of which are caused by lack of iron in the tissues.

Diagnostic Studies

Laboratory abnormalities characteristic of iron-deficiency anemia are presented in Table 29-6. Other diagnostic studies are done to determine the cause of the iron deficiency. For example, endoscopy and colonoscopy may be used to detect GI bleeding.

Collaborative Care

The main goal of collaborative care of iron-deficiency anemia is to treat the underlying disease that is causing reduced intake (e.g., malnutrition, alcoholism) or absorption of iron. In addition, efforts are directed toward replacing iron (Table 29-7).

Table 29-6 Laboratory Study Findings in Anemias

	Iron Deficiency	Thalassemia Major	Cobalamin (Vitamin B_{12}) Deficiency	Folic Acid Deficiency	Aplastic Anemia	Chronic Disease	Acute Blood Loss	Chronic Blood Loss	Sickle Cell Anemia	Hemolytic Anemia
Hb/Hct	↓	↓	↓	↓	↓	↓	↓	↓	↓	↓
MCV	↓	N	↑	↑	N	N	N	↓	N	N
MCH	↓	N	N or slight ↓	N or slight ↓	N	N	N	↓	N	N
MCHC	↓	N	↑	↑	N	N	N	↓	N	N
Reticulocytes	N or ↓	↑	↓	N	↓	N	N	N or ↑	↑	↑
Serum iron	↓	↑	N	N	±N	↓	N	↓	N to ↑	↑
TIBC	↑	↑	N	N	±N	↓	N	↓	N to ↓	↓
Bilirubin	N to ↓	↑	N	N	N	±N	N	N to ↓	↑	N to ↑
Platelets	N or ↑	—	↓	—	↓	↑	—	↑	↑	—
Other findings	—	—	↓cobalamin, positive Schilling test, achlorhydria	↓ folate	↓ WBC	—	—	—	See Table 29-11	—

MCH, mean corpuscular hemoglobin; *MCHC*, mean corpuscular hemoglobin concentration; *MCV*, mean corpuscular volume; *N*, normal; *TIBC*, total iron-binding capacity; *WBC*, white blood cell.

COLLABORATIVE CARE

Table 29-7 Iron-Deficiency Anemia

Diagnostic
- History and physical examination
- Hct and Hb levels
- RBC count, including morphology
- Reticulocyte count
- Serum iron
- Serum ferritin
- Total iron-binding capacity
- Fecal examination for occult blood

Collaborative Therapy
- Identification and treatment of underlying cause
- Administration of ferrous sulfate or ferrous gluconate
- Administration of iron dextran IM or IV
- Diet rich in foods containing iron
- Nutritional education
- Transfusion of packed RBCs (symptomatic patient only)

IM, intramuscular; *IV*, intravenous; *RBCs*, red blood cells.

This may be done through increasing the intake of iron. The patient should be taught which foods are good sources of iron (see Table 29-5). If nutrition is already adequate, increasing iron intake by dietary means may not be reasonable because it is difficult for nutritional intake to exceed 7 mg of iron per 1000 kcal without the use of dietary supplements (e.g., an 8 oz steak supplies 8 mg of iron). Consequently, oral or occasionally parenteral iron supplements are used. If the iron deficiency is from significant acute blood loss, transfusion of packed RBCs may be required.

Drug Therapy. Oral iron should be used whenever possible because it is inexpensive and convenient. Many iron preparations are available. Four factors should be considered in the administration of iron:

1. The dosage should provide 150 to 200 mg elemental iron daily. This can be ingested in three or four daily doses, with each tablet or capsule of the iron preparation containing between 50 and 100 mg of iron (e.g., a 325 mg tablet of ferrous sulfate contains 50 mg of elemental iron).
2. Iron is best absorbed in an acidic environment. For this reason and to avoid binding the iron with food, iron should be taken about an hour before meals, when the duodenal mucosa is most acidic. Taking iron with vitamin C (ascorbic acid) or orange juice, which contains ascorbic acid, also enhances iron absorption. Gastric side effects, however, may necessitate ingesting iron with meals. Enteric-coated iron may be ineffective because the iron may not be released in an area of the intestine that facilitates absorption.
3. Undiluted liquid iron may stain the patient's teeth; therefore it should be diluted and ingested through a straw.
4. GI side effects of iron administration may occur, including pyrosis (heartburn), constipation, and diarrhea. If side effects develop, the dose and type of iron supplement may be adjusted. For example, many individuals who need supplemental iron cannot tolerate ferrous sulfate because of the effects of the sulfate base. However, ferrous gluconate may be an acceptable substitute. All patients should know that the use of iron preparations will cause their stools to become black because excess iron is excreted by the GI tract. Constipation is common, and the patient should be told about this side effect because constipation may be a reason for decreased patient compliance.

In some situations, it may be necessary to administer iron parenterally. Parenteral use of iron is indicated for malabsorption, intolerance of oral iron, a need for iron beyond oral limits, and poor patient compliance in taking the oral preparations of iron. Parenteral iron can be given intramuscularly (IM) or intravenously (IV).

Because IM iron solutions may stain the skin, separate needles should be used for withdrawing the solution and for injecting the medication. Approximately 0.5 ml of air should be left in the syringe to clear the iron completely from the syringe. Iron should be given deep IM in the upper outer quadrant of the buttocks, with a 2 inch to 3 inch needle with a 19 to 20 gauge. Preferably, no more than 2 ml of iron is given in a single injection. A Z-track technique should be used for injection to prevent leakage of the iron solution to the subcutaneous (SC) tissue. The site should not be massaged after the injection is given. IV administration of iron dextran should not be mixed with other medications or added to parenteral nutrition solutions. It should be given undiluted and at a rate of no more than 1 ml/min. The IV line should be flushed with normal saline.

NURSING MANAGEMENT: IRON-DEFICIENCY ANEMIA

It is important to recognize groups of individuals who are at an increased risk for the development of iron-deficiency anemia. These include infants, teenage girls, premenopausal and pregnant women, persons from low socioeconomic backgrounds, older adults, and individuals experiencing blood loss. Diet teaching, with an emphasis on foods high in iron, is important for these groups. Supplemental iron is especially important for the pregnant woman. Appropriate nursing measures are presented in NCP 29-1. If anemia is present, it is important to discuss with the patient the need for diagnostic studies to identify the cause. The Hb level and RBC count should be reassessed to evaluate the response to therapy. Compliance with dietary and drug therapy should be emphasized. To replenish the body's iron stores, the patient should take iron therapy for 2 to 3 months after the Hb level returns to normal. An older adult patient may require lifelong iron supplementation. If the Hb level remains low, the patient must be reevaluated for the cause of anemia.

THALASSEMIA

Another cause of decreased erythrocyte production is termed *thalassemia*. As in iron deficiency, it is a disease of inadequate production of normal hemoglobin. Hemolysis also occurs in thalassemia, but insufficient production of normal hemoglobin

Table 29-8 Classification of Megaloblastic Anemias

Cobalamin (Vitamin B_{12}) Deficiency
Dietary deficiency
Deficiency of gastric intrinsic factor
Pernicious anemia
Gastrectomy
Intestinal malabsorption
Increased requirement
Folic Acid Deficiency
Dietary deficiency
Impaired absorption
Increased requirement
Drug-Induced Suppression of DNA Synthesis
Folate antagonists
Metabolic inhibitors
Alkylating agents
Nitrous oxide
Inborn Errors
Hereditary orotic aciduria
Defective folate metabolism
Lesch-Nyhan syndrome
Defective transport of cobalamin
Erythroleukemia

is the predominant problem. In contrast to iron-deficiency anemia, in which heme synthesis is the problem, thalassemia involves a problem with the globin protein. Therefore the basic defect of thalassemia is abnormal hemoglobin synthesis.

Etiology

Thalassemias are a group of autosomal recessive genetic disorders commonly found in members of ethnic groups whose origins are near the Mediterranean Sea. An individual with thalassemia may have a heterozygous or homozygous form of the disease. A person who is heterozygous has one thalassemic gene and one normal gene and is said to have *thalassemia minor* or *thalassemic trait,* which is a mild form of the disease. A homozygous person has two thalassemic genes, causing a severe condition known as *thalassemia major.*

Clinical Manifestations

The patient with thalassemia minor is frequently asymptomatic because the patient adjusts to the gradually acquired chronic state of anemia. Occasionally, splenomegaly may develop in this patient, and mild jaundice may occur if malformed erythrocytes are rapidly hemolyzed. The person who has thalassemia major is pale and displays other general symptoms of anemia (see Table 29-3). In addition, the person has pronounced splenomegaly and hepatomegaly. Jaundice from RBC hemolysis is prominent. Chronic bone marrow hyperplasia leads to expansion of the marrow space. This may cause thickening of the cranium and maxillary cavity, leading to an appearance resembling Down syndrome. Thalassemia major is a life-threatening disease in which growth, both physical and mental, is often retarded.

Collaborative Care

The laboratory abnormalities of thalassemia major are summarized in Table 29-6. Thalassemia minor requires no treatment because the body adapts to the reduction of normal hemoglobin. Thalassemia major is usually treated with blood transfusions and chelation therapy (therapy to reduce the iron overloading that sometimes occurs with chronic transfusion therapy). No specific drug or diet therapies are effective in treating thalassemia. Transfusions are administered to keep the Hb level at approximately 10 g/dl (100 g/L). This level is low enough to foster the patient's own erythropoiesis without enlarging the spleen. Because RBCs are sequestered in the enlarged spleen, thalassemia may be treated by splenectomy. However, even with therapy, the person with thalassemia major will experience growth failure, hemochromatosis, and cardiac failure that are often fatal.[6]

MEGALOBLASTIC ANEMIAS

Megaloblastic anemias are disorders caused by impaired DNA synthesis and characterized by the presence of large RBCs. When DNA synthesis is impaired, defective RBC maturation results. The RBCs are large (macrocytic) and abnormal and are referred to as *megaloblasts.* Macrocytic RBCs are easily destroyed because of their fragile membranes. Although the overwhelming majority of megaloblastic anemias result from cobalamin (vitamin B_{12}) and folate deficiencies, this type of red blood cell deformity can also occur from suppression of DNA synthesis by drugs, from inborn errors of cobalamin and folic acid metabolism, and from erythroleukemia (malignant blood disorder characterized by a proliferation of erythropoietic cells in bone marrow) (Table 29-8). Common forms of megaloblastic anemia are cobalamin deficiency (e.g., pernicious anemia) and folic acid deficiency.

Cobalamin Deficiency

Normally, a protein termed *intrinsic factor* (IF) is secreted by the parietal cells of the gastric mucosa. IF is required for cobalamin (extrinsic factor) absorption. Therefore if IF is not secreted, cobalamin cannot be absorbed. (Cobalamin is normally absorbed in the distal ileum.) In pernicious anemia, gastric secretion of IF is defective. Although once fatal, pernicious anemia is now treatable. The term *pernicious anemia* has been used inappropriately to describe any cobalamin deficiency. However, pernicious anemia is only one cause of cobalamin deficiency, and the term should be used only to describe the situations in which the gastric mucosa is not secreting IF or when there is inadequate secretion of IF because of gastric resection (see Table 29-8).

Etiology

Pernicious anemia is a disease of insidious onset that generally begins in middle age or later (usually after age 40). In this condition, IF secretion fails because of gastric mucosal atrophy. Pernicious anemia is an autoimmune disease; the gastric atrophy of pernicious anemia probably results from destruction of the parietal cells.

Pernicious anemia occurs frequently in persons of Northern European ancestry, particularly Scandinavians, and African-Americans. In African-Americans, the disease tends to begin early, occurs with high frequency in women, and is often severe.

Cobalamin deficiency can occur in a patient who has a gastrectomy, in a patient who has a small bowel resection involving the ileum, or in Crohn's disease. Cobalamin deficiency results from the loss of IF-secreting gastric mucosal surface or impaired absorption of cobalamin in the distal ileum.

Clinical Manifestations

General symptoms of anemia related to cobalamin deficiency develop because of tissue hypoxia (see Table 29-3). GI manifestations include a sore tongue, anorexia, nausea, vomiting, and abdominal pain. Typical neuromuscular manifestations include weakness, paresthesias of the feet and hands, reduced vibratory and position senses, ataxia, muscle weakness, and impaired thought processes ranging from confusion to dementia. Because cobalamin deficiency-related anemia has an insidious onset, it may take several months for these manifestations to develop.

Diagnostic Studies

Laboratory data reflective of cobalamin deficiency anemia are presented in Table 29-6. The erythrocytes appear large (macrocytic) and have abnormal shapes. This structure contributes to erythrocyte destruction because the cell membrane is fragile. Additional studies may need to be performed. Serum cobalamin levels will be reduced. A gastric analysis is done to ascertain the cause of the cobalamin deficiency. A nasogastric (NG) tube is inserted, pentagastrin is injected to stimulate gastric juice secretion, and the gastric juice is aspirated via the NG tube for a period of time. If analysis of the gastric juice reveals *achlorhydria* (the absence of free HCl in a pH never lower than 3.5), depressed parietal cell function can be determined. A gastroscopy and biopsy of the gastric mucosa may also be done.

Another means of assessing parietal cell function is by a Schilling test. After radioactive cobalamin is administered to the patient, the amount of cobalamin excreted in the urine is measured. An individual who cannot absorb cobalamin excretes only a small amount of this radioactive form. The same procedure may be followed with the addition of IF parenterally. Absorption of cobalamin when IF is added is diagnostic of pernicious anemia.

Collaborative Care

Regardless of how much cobalamin is ingested, the patient is not able to absorb it if IF is lacking or there is impaired absorption in the ileum, so dietary management is not a reasonable approach for cobalamin replacement. However, the patient should be instructed on adequate dietary intake to maintain good nutrition (see Table 29-6). Parenteral administration of cobalamin (cyanocobalamin or hydroxocobalamin) is the treatment of choice. Without cobalamin administration, these individuals will die in 1 to 3 years. The efficacy of cobalamin injections in altering the otherwise fatal course cannot be overemphasized. The dosage and frequency of cobalamin administration may vary. A typical treatment schedule consists of 1000 μg cobalamin IM daily for 2 weeks, then weekly until the Hct is normal, then monthly for life. An intranasal form of cyanocobalamin (Nascobal) is now available. It is a nasal gel that is self-administered once weekly.

As long as supplemental cobalamin is used, the anemia can be controlled. Hematologic manifestations can be completely reversed. However, most long-standing neuromuscular complications will not be reversed by this therapy.

NURSING MANAGEMENT: PERNICIOUS ANEMIA

Because of the familial predisposition involved, patients who have a positive family history of pernicious anemia should be evaluated for symptoms. Although disease development cannot be prevented, early detection and treatment can lead to reversal of symptoms.

The nursing measures presented in the nursing care plan for the patient with anemia (see NCP 29-1) are appropriate for the patient with cobalamin deficiency anemia. In addition to these measures, the nurse should ensure that injuries are not sustained because of the diminished sensations to heat and pain resulting from the neurologic impairment. The patient must be protected from burns and trauma. If heat therapy is required, the patient's skin must be evaluated at frequent intervals to detect redness. Irritation from NG tubes and restrictive clothing may not be perceived by the patient because of reduced pain sensations.

Ongoing care is primarily related to ensuring good patient compliance in returning for monthly cobalamin injections. There must also be careful follow-up to assess for neurologic difficulties that were not fully corrected by adequate cobalamin replacement therapy. Because the potential for gastric carcinoma is increased in pernicious anemia, the patient should have frequent and careful evaluation for this problem.

Folic Acid Deficiency

Folic acid deficiency also causes megaloblastic anemia. Folic acid is required for DNA synthesis leading to RBC formation and maturation. Common causes of folic acid deficiency include the following:

1. Poor nutrition, especially a lack of leafy green vegetables, liver, citrus fruits, yeast, dried beans, nuts, and grains
2. Malabsorption syndromes, particularly small bowel disorders
3. Drugs that impede the absorption and use of folic acid (e.g., methotrexate, oral contraceptives), as well as antiseizure agents (e.g., phenobarbital, diphenylhydantoin)
4. Alcohol abuse and anorexia
5. Hemodialysis patients, because folic acid is dialyzable

The clinical manifestations of folic acid deficiency are similar to those of cobalamin deficiency. The disease develops insidiously, and the patient's symptoms may be attributed to other coexisting problems such as cirrhosis or esophageal varices. GI disturbances include dyspepsia and a smooth, beefy red tongue. The absence of neurologic problems is an important diagnostic finding. This lack of neurologic involvement differentiates folic acid deficiency from cobalamin deficiency.

The diagnostic findings for folic acid deficiency are presented in Table 29-6. In addition, the serum folate level is low (normal is 3 to 25 ng/ml [7 to 57 mol/L]), the serum cobalamin level is normal, and the gastric analysis is positive for hydrochloric acid.

Folic acid deficiency is treated by replacement therapy. The usual dose is 1 mg per day by mouth. In malabsorption states, up to 5 mg per day may be required. The duration of treatment depends on the reason for the deficiency. The patient should be encouraged to eat foods containing large amounts of folic acid (see Table 29-5).

ANEMIA OF CHRONIC DISEASE

Hypoproliferative anemias (decreased erythrocyte precursors) may develop in several chronic conditions. One specific cause is end-stage renal disease. There is a relationship between the degree of anemia and the severity of uremia. Although several mechanisms may be involved in the development of anemia with renal disease, the primary factor is decreased erythropoietin, a hormone made in the kidneys that is necessary for erythropoiesis. With impaired renal function, decreased levels of erythropoietin are produced (see Chapter 44).

Other chronic, inflammatory, or malignant diseases can lead to the *anemia of chronic disease.* Chronic liver disease may also contribute to the development of anemia. Anemia may result from the folic acid deficiencies caused by inadequate nutrition in abusers of alcohol or from blood loss caused by chronic gastritis. The use of alcohol itself may reduce erythropoiesis. Anemia may also result from splenomegaly, which is commonly found in advanced stages of cirrhosis (see Chapter 41).

Chronic inflammation and malignant tumors are other conditions in which anemia may be present. The mechanisms involved include increased RBC destruction accompanied by a failure to augment erythropoiesis to compensate for the rise in destruction. Chemotherapy with heavy metals (e.g., cisplatin, carboplatin) for malignant diseases is a common cause of anemia in neoplastic disease.[7] Anemia related to human immunodeficiency virus (HIV) and its treatment are other causes of anemia.

Chronic endocrine diseases may also lead to anemia. Hypopituitary and hypothyroid states both lead to reduced tissue metabolism; therefore tissue oxygen needs are diminished, leading to a reduced production of erythropoietin by the kidneys. Adrenal dysfunction caused by either adrenalectomy or Addison's disease also results in anemia.

Anemia of chronic disease must first be recognized and differentiated from anemias of other etiologies. Findings of elevated serum ferritin and increased iron stores will distinguish it from iron-deficiency anemia. Effective treatment for anemia of chronic disease begins with specific therapy of the underlying etiology. The anemia of chronic disease is not responsive to iron, folic acid, or cobalamin. Because the anemia is rarely severe, blood transfusions are rarely indicated. Anemia related to end-stage renal disease does respond to erythropoietin therapy (see Chapter 44).

APLASTIC ANEMIA

One of the most severe forms of anemia related to reduced erythrocyte production is a group of disorders termed *aplastic, hypoplastic,* or *pancytopenic* anemias. These anemias are life-threatening stem cell disorders characterized by hypoplastic, fatty bone marrow and that result in pancytopenia. Aplastic anemia is somewhat of a misnomer because in most cases all marrow elements—erythrocytes, leukocytes, and platelets—are quantitatively decreased, although they are qualitatively normal.

Table 29-9 Causes of Aplastic Anemia

Congenital
Fanconi's syndrome
Dyskeratosis congenita
Schwachman-Diamond syndrome
Acquired
Radiation
Chemical agents and toxins
Drugs
Viral and bacterial infections
Pregnancy
Idiopathic

Etiology

The incidence of aplastic anemia is low, affecting approximately 4 persons per 1 million. There are various etiologic classifications for aplastic anemia, but they can be divided into two major groups: congenital (or idiopathic) or acquired (Table 29-9).

1. Congenital origin caused by chromosomal alterations (approximately 30% of the aplastic anemias that appear in childhood are inherited).
2. Acquired as a result of exposure to ionizing radiation, chemical agents (e.g., benzene, insecticides, arsenic, alcohol), viral and bacterial infections (e.g., hepatitis, parvovirus, miliary tuberculosis), and prescribed medications (e.g., alkylating agents, antiseizure agents, antimetabolites, antimicrobials, gold). The causes of 70% of acquired cases of aplastic anemia are idiopathic.[8]

Clinical Manifestations

Aplastic anemia usually develops insidiously. Clinically the patient may have symptoms caused by suppression of any or all bone marrow elements. General manifestations of anemia such as fatigue and dyspnea, as well as cardiovascular and cerebral responses, may be seen (see Table 29-3). The patient with granulocytopenia is susceptible to infection and generally has a fever. Thrombocytopenia is manifested by a predisposition to bleeding (e.g., petechiae, ecchymoses, epistaxis).

Diagnostic Studies

The diagnosis is confirmed by laboratory studies. Because all marrow elements are affected, hemoglobin, white blood cell (WBC), and platelet values are often decreased in aplastic anemia (see Table 29-6). However, the RBC indices are normal. The condition is therefore classified as a normocytic, normochromic anemia. The reticulocyte count is low. Bleeding time is prolonged.

Aplastic anemia can be further evaluated by assessing various iron studies. The serum iron and total iron-binding capacity (TIBC) are elevated as initial signs of erythroid suppression. Bone marrow examination may be done for any anemic state. However, the findings are especially important in aplastic anemia because the marrow is hypocellular, with increased yellow marrow (fat content), a finding termed *dry tap.*

NURSING AND COLLABORATIVE MANAGEMENT: APLASTIC ANEMIA

Management of aplastic anemia is based on identifying and removing the causative agent (when possible) and providing supportive care until the pancytopenia reverses. Nursing interventions appropriate for the patient with pancytopenia from aplastic anemia are presented in the nursing care plan for the patient with anemia (NCP 29-1) earlier in this chapter and the nursing care plans for thrombocytopenia (NCP 29-2) and neutropenia (NCP 29-3) later in this chapter. Nursing actions are directed at preventing complications from infection and hemorrhage.

The prognosis of untreated aplastic anemia is poor (approximately 75% fatal). However, advances in medical management, including bone marrow transplantation and immunosuppressive therapy with antithymocyte globulin (ATG) and cyclosporine, have improved outcomes significantly. ATG is a horse serum, containing polyclonal antibodies against human T cells. The rationale for this therapy is that aplastic anemia is an immune-mediated disease.[8] (ATG and cyclosporine are discussed in Chapter 44.)

The treatment of choice for adults less than 45 years of age who have a human leukocyte antigen (HLA)–matched donor is allogeneic bone marrow transplantation. The best results occur in a younger patient who has not had previous blood transfusions. Prior transfusions increase the risk of graft rejection. (Bone marrow transplants are discussed in Chapter 14.)

For the older adult or the patient without HLA-matched siblings, the treatment of choice is immunosuppression with ATG or cyclosporine. Response to this therapy may be only partial, but transfusions usually can be avoided.

ANEMIA CAUSED BY BLOOD LOSS

Anemia resulting from blood loss may be caused by either acute or chronic problems.

ACUTE BLOOD LOSS

Acute blood loss occurs as a result of sudden hemorrhage. Causes of acute blood loss include trauma, complications of surgery, and diseases that disrupt vascular integrity. There are two clinical concerns in such situations. First, there is a sudden reduction in the total blood volume that can lead to hypovolemic shock. Second, if the acute loss is more gradual, the body maintains its blood volume by slowly increasing the plasma volume. Consequently, the circulating fluid volume is preserved, but the number of erythrocytes available to carry O_2 is significantly diminished.

Clinical Manifestations

The clinical manifestations of anemia from acute blood loss are caused by the body's attempts to maintain an adequate blood volume and meet O_2 requirements. Table 29-10 summarizes the clinical manifestations of patients with varying degrees of blood volume loss. It is essential to understand that clinical signs and symptoms are valuable indicators of the degree of blood loss because laboratory data may not accurately reflect the severity of hemorrhage for 2 to 3 days.

Table 29-10 Clinical Manifestations of Acute Blood Loss

Volume Lost (%)	Clinical Manifestations
10	None
20	No detectable signs or symptoms at rest, tachycardia with exercise and slight postural hypotension
30	Normal supine blood pressure and pulse at rest, postural hypotension and tachycardia with exercise
40	Blood pressure, central venous pressure, and cardiac output below normal at rest; rapid, thready pulse and cold, clammy skin
50	Shock and potential death

The nurse should be alert to the patient's expression (verbal or nonverbal) of pain. Internal hemorrhage may cause pain because of tissue distention, organ displacement, and nerve compression. Pain may be localized or referred. In the case of retroperitoneal bleeding, the patient may not experience abdominal pain. Instead, the patient may have numbness and pain in a lower extremity secondary to compression of the lateral cutaneous nerve, which is located in the region of the first to third lumbar vertebrae. The major complication of acute blood loss is shock (see Chapter 61).

Diagnostic Studies

When blood volume loss is sudden, the body reacts by vasoconstriction. Because plasma volume has not yet had a chance to increase, the loss of RBC mass is not reflected in laboratory data, and the values may seem normal or high for 2 to 3 days. However, once the plasma is replaced by endogenous and exogenous means, the RBC mass is less concentrated. At this time, erythrocytes, Hb, and Hct levels are usually low and reflect the blood loss.

Collaborative Care

Collaborative care is initially concerned with (1) replacing blood volume to prevent shock and (2) identifying the source of the hemorrhage and stopping the blood loss. IV fluids used in emergencies include dextran, Hetastarch, albumin, or crystalloid electrolyte solutions such as lactated Ringer's. The amount of infusion varies with the solution used. (Management of shock is discussed in Chapter 61.)

Once volume replacement is established, attention can be directed to correcting RBC loss. The body needs 2 to 5 days to manufacture more RBCs in response to increased erythropoietin. Consequently, blood transfusions (packed RBCs) may be needed if the blood loss is significant.

The patient may also need supplemental iron because the availability of iron affects the marrow production of erythrocytes. When anemia exists after acute blood loss, dietary sources of iron will probably not be adequate to maintain iron pools. For every 2 ml of blood lost, 1 mg of iron is also lost. Therefore oral or parenteral iron preparations are administered.

NURSING MANAGEMENT: ACUTE BLOOD LOSS

In the case of trauma, it may be impossible to prevent the situation leading to the blood loss. For the postoperative patient, careful evaluation of blood loss from various drainage tubes and dressings facilitates early assessment of the source of bleeding and related appropriate treatment. The nursing care plan for the patient with anemia is relevant to the anemia resulting from acute blood loss. In this situation, blood product replacement (described at the end of this chapter) is almost certainly necessary.

Once the source of hemorrhage is identified, blood loss is controlled, and fluid and blood volume are replaced, the anemia should begin to correct itself. There should be no need for long-term treatment of this type of anemia.

CHRONIC BLOOD LOSS

The sources of chronic blood loss are similar to those of iron-deficiency anemia (e.g., bleeding ulcer, hemorrhoids, menstrual and postmenopausal blood loss). The effects of chronic blood loss are usually related to the depletion of iron stores and are usually considered as iron-deficiency anemia. Management of chronic blood loss anemia involves identifying the source and stopping the bleeding. Supplemental iron may be required. The nursing measures presented in NCP 29-1 are relevant to anemia of chronic blood loss.

ANEMIA CAUSED BY INCREASED ERYTHROCYTE DESTRUCTION

The third major cause of anemia is the destruction, or hemolysis, of RBCs at a rate that exceeds production. Hemolysis can occur because of problems intrinsic or extrinsic to the RBCs. Intrinsic hemolytic anemias result from defects in the RBCs themselves caused by abnormal hemoglobin (e.g., sickle cells), enzyme deficiencies that alter glycolysis (glucose-6-phosphate dehydrogenase [G6PD] deficiency), or RBC membrane abnormalities. Intrinsic hemolytic anemias are usually hereditary. More common are the extrinsic hemolytic anemias, which are acquired. The patient's RBCs are normal, but damage is caused by external factors such as trapping of cells within the sinuses of the liver or spleen, antibody-mediated destruction, toxins, or mechanical injury (e.g., prosthetic heart valves).

The two sites of hemolysis are classified as intravascular or extravascular. Intravascular destruction occurs within the circulation; extravascular hemolysis takes place in the macrophages of the spleen, liver, and bone marrow. The spleen is the primary site of the destruction of RBCs that are old, defective, or moderately damaged. Figure 29-2 indicates the sequence of events involved in extravascular hemolysis.

The patient with hemolytic anemia manifests the general symptoms of anemia (see Table 29-3) and clinical manifestations specific to this type of anemia. Jaundice is likely because the increased destruction of RBCs causes an elevation in biliru-

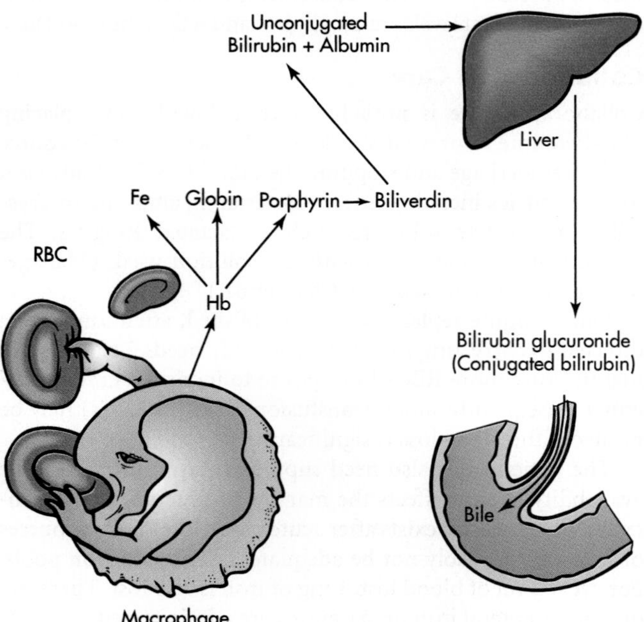

Fig. 29-2 Sequence of events in extravascular hemolysis.

ETHICAL DILEMMAS

Genetic Testing and Truth Telling

SITUATION

A couple who have a child with sickle cell disease have come in for genetic testing. They are considering whether or not to have another child, and want to know the risk for sickle cell. The results have come back and must be communicated to the couple. The tests prove that the husband could not be the biologic father of the child with sickle cell anemia. What should the nurse do?

DISCUSSION

Paternity is an issue that should be discussed with a couple before they have genetic testing. This couple may already know that he is not the child's biologic father, but are concerned about the risks for a subsequent child. Only the mother may know that this man is not the child's father, or maybe neither of them knows. It would be advisable to attempt to reach the mother directly and give her the information. If this is not possible, it will take great tact to explain the reasons why a subsequent child is not at risk because this man has no recessive gene for sickle cell. The couple contracted for the testing and counseling, so it is not acceptable to withhold the truth from one of them. The decisions about the marriage and the future children they might produce are not the responsibility of the nurse.

ETHICAL AND LEGAL PRINCIPLES

- Although knowledge is, itself, neutral, its effects may be devastating.
- When a contractual agreement has been made for the provision of information, it is not ethical to withhold that information from one of the parties.
- There is no ethical obligation to give the information about genetic risks to the biologic father of the child since he did not contract with the provider for testing and counseling. It could be offered, however, if the mother were willing to tell the nurse how to contact him.

bin levels. The spleen and liver may enlarge because of their hyperactivity, which is related to macrophage phagocytosis of the defective erythrocytes.

In all causes of hemolysis a major focus of treatment is to maintain renal function. When an RBC is hemolyzed, the hemoglobin molecule is released and filtered by the kidneys. The accumulation of hemoglobin molecules can obstruct the renal tubule and lead to acute tubular necrosis (see Chapter 44).

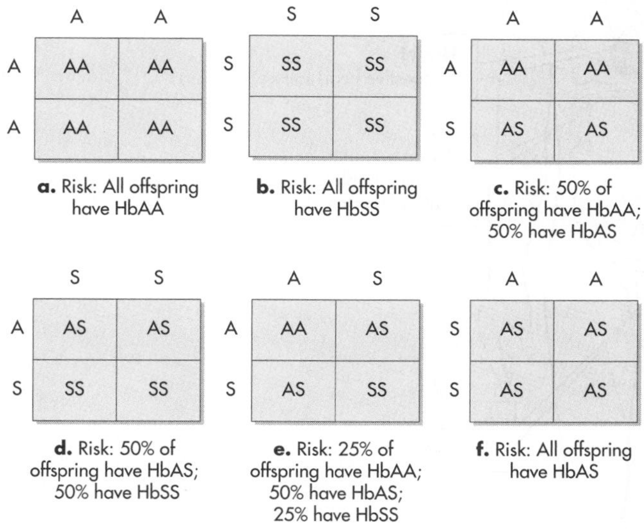

Fig. 29-3 Inheritance patterns of sickle cell disease. The boxes represent the possible genetic makeup of children from parents with various genotypes.

SICKLE CELL DISEASE

Sickle cell disease (SCD) is a family of genetic disorders caused by the abnormal properties conveyed to sickle cell RBC by mutant sickle cell hemoglobin (HbS). SCD affects more than 50,000 Americans and is predominant in African-Americans, occurring in an estimated prevalence of 1 in 375 live births. It can also affect people of Mediterranean, Caribbean, South and Central American, Arabian, or East Indian ancestry. It is an incurable disease that is often fatal by middle age.[9]

Etiology and Pathophysiology

Sickle cell anemia, one type of SCD, is an autosomal recessive genetic disorder in which the person is homozygous for HbS. Some persons may have sickle cell trait, a mild condition that may be asymptomatic. A person with sickle cell trait is heterozygous, with approximately one fourth of the hemoglobin in the abnormal S form and three fourths in the normal A form (Fig. 29-3). If two parents have sickle cell trait, there is a 25% chance with each pregnancy that the child will have sickle cell anemia. The mutation that causes HbS to develop involves one amino acid. One valine amino acid is substituted for a glutamic acid. This substitution leads to an abnormal linking reaction that causes the development of deformed crescent-shaped cells when O_2 tension is lowered (Fig. 29-4).

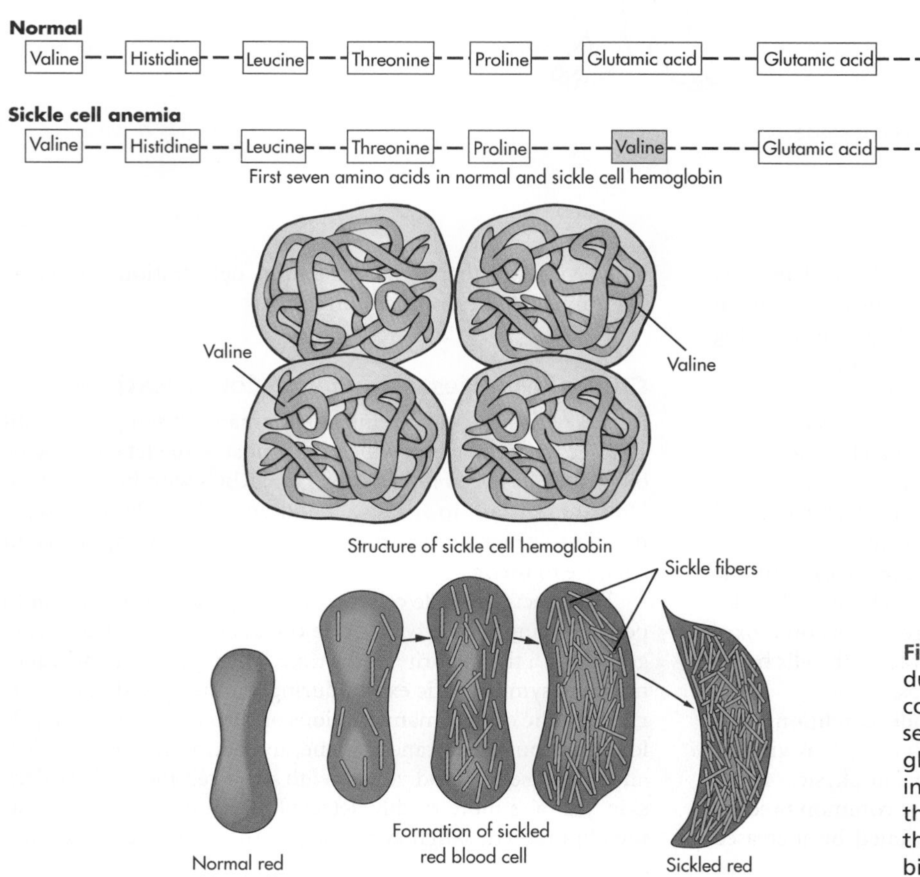

Fig. 29-4 Sickle cell hemoglobin is produced by a recessive allele of the gene encoding the chain of hemoglobin. It represents a single amino acid change from glutamic acid to valine at the sixth position in the chain. In the folded-chain molecule the sixth position contacts the chain, and the amino acid change causes the hemoglobins to aggregate into long chains, altering the shape of the cell.

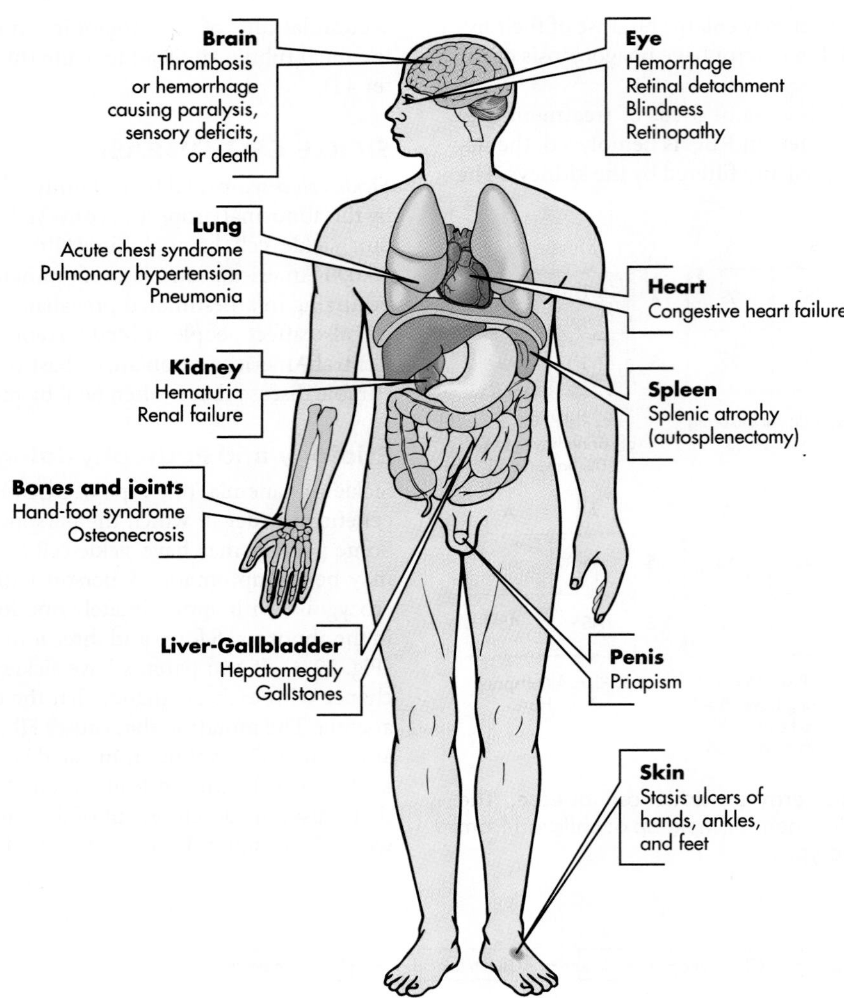

Fig. 29-5 Clinical manifestations of sickle cell disease.

When hypoxia occurs in a patient with sickle cell anemia, the RBC containing HbS changes from a biconcave disk to an elongated, crescent or sickle cell. These sickling cells may clog the small capillaries. The resulting hemostasis promotes a self-perpetuating cycle of local hypoxia, deoxygenation of more erythrocytes, and more sickling. As blood vessels become occluded, thrombosis occurs. This can ultimately lead to ischemia and necrosis of the infarcted tissue from lack of O_2. With repeated infarction there is gradual involvement of all body systems, especially the spleen, lungs, kidneys, and brain. The abnormal shape of the hemoglobin is recognized by the body, and the cell is hemolyzed. Sickled cells are also destroyed randomly. Initially the sickling is reversible on reoxygenation but eventually becomes irreversible, with cells being hemolyzed, and hemolytic anemia develops.

Precipitating factors for sickling include conditions that cause hypoxia or deoxygenation of the RBCs, such as viral or bacterial infections, high altitudes, emotional or physical stress, surgery, and blood loss. Infection is the most common precipitating factor.[9] Sickling can also be precipitated by increased blood viscosity that may result from dehydration caused by vomiting, diarrhea, or diaphoresis.

Clinical Manifestations and Complications

Infants with sickle cell anemia do not manifest symptoms until 10 to 12 weeks of age, at which time most of the fetal hemoglobin (HbF) has been replaced by HbS. RBCs with high levels of HbF are resistant to sickling. Children with sickle cell disease manifest a general impairment of growth and development and a failure to thrive.

The effects of sickle cell disease vary greatly from person to person. Many people with sickle cell anemia are in reasonably good health the majority of the time. The typical patient is anemic but asymptomatic except during painful episodes. Patients manifest the clinical manifestations of chronic anemia with pallor of mucous membranes, fatigue, and decreased exercise tolerance. Because most individuals with sickle cell anemia have dark skin, pallor is more readily detected by examining the mucous membranes. The skin may have a grayish cast. Because of the he-

Table 29-11 Laboratory Assessment of Sickle Cell Trait and Sickle Cell Anemia

Study	Description	Sickle Cell Trait	Sickle Cell Anemia
Peripheral smear	Small amount of peripheral blood specimen is smeared on a slide.	Normal	Partially or completely sickled cells
Sickle cell preparation	Blood specimen reaction is observed in hypoxic setting.	Sickle cells	Sickle cells
Sickledex	Blood is mixed with a solution that deoxygenates HbS; this becomes insoluble and causes turbidity. Development of cloudiness is positive for presence of HbS.	Positive	Positive
Hemoglobin electrophoresis	Blood specimen is exposed to electric field and types of hemoglobin are separated.	HbS and HbA	HbS

molysis, jaundice is common and patients are prone to gallstones (cholelithiasis).

Organs that have a high need for O_2 are most often affected and form the basis for many of the complications of sickle cell disease (Fig. 29-5). The heart may become ischemic and enlarged, leading to congestive heart failure. *Acute chest syndrome* is characterized by fever, chest pain, cough, pulmonary infiltrates, and dyspnea. In most instances, the etiology is unknown. Pulmonary infarctions may cause pulmonary hypertension, heart failure, and ultimately cor pulmonale. Retinal vessel obstruction may result in hemorrhage, scarring, retinal detachment, and blindness. The kidneys may be injured from the increased blood viscosity and the lack of O_2. The spleen becomes small because of repeated scarring, a phenomenon termed *autosplenectomy.* Hepatomegaly is a frequent finding. Stroke can result from thrombosis and infarction of cerebral blood vessels. Bone changes may include osteoporosis and osteosclerosis after infarction. Chronic leg ulcers can result from the hypoxia and are especially prevalent around the ankles.

Priapism (condition of prolonged or constant penile erection) is a potentially serious problem and can last from several hours to several days. Aching in the joints, especially those of the hands and feet, is a common complaint. The painful bone infarction of the *hand-foot syndrome* (painful swelling of hands and feet) is often the first symptom of SCD. The pain associated with these attacks is often described as deep gnawing and throbbing.[10] The patient with SCD is particularly prone to infection. One reason for this is the failure of the spleen to phagocytize foreign substances because of impairment of splenic function. Pneumonia is the most common infection and often is of pneumococcal origin. Infections must be treated vigorously with antibiotics.

In addition to these chronic manifestations of sickle cell disease, an acute episode or *sickle cell crisis* (exacerbations of sickling) may occur. The most common type of crisis results from vaso-occlusion (occlusion of blood vessels from sickled cells). Tissue hypoxia occurs and ultimately leads to tissue death and pain. This type of crisis may appear suddenly and affect various parts of the body, especially the chest, back, extremities, and abdomen. A crisis may persist for days to weeks. The pain experienced with an acute painful crisis typically is severe. Crises may have a sudden onset and occasionally fatal outcome. Crisis may occur frequently and then may not recur for months or years. Some vaso-occlusive crises are triggered by stress, cold water exposure, dehydration, hypoxia, and infection, but most occur without an obvious cause.

Shock is a possible development in sickle cell crisis. Capillary hypoxia may result in changes in membrane permeability, leading to plasma loss, hemoconcentration, and further circulatory stagnation, causing a reduction of the circulating fluid volume.

Current median survival of individuals with sickle cell disease is approximately 40 to 50 years. The major causes of mortality are renal and pulmonary failure.

Diagnostic Studies

Screening tests to identify sickle cell disease or trait are available (Table 29-11). A person with sickle cell anemia has a severe form of hemolytic anemia. The Hb level usually ranges from 5 to 11 g/dl (50 to 110 g/L). The mean RBC survival time is 15 days. As a result of the accelerated RBC breakdown, the patient has characteristic clinical findings of hemolysis (jaundice, elevated serum bilirubin levels) and abnormal laboratory test results (see Table 29-6). Skeletal x-rays will demonstrate bone and joint deformities and flattening. Magnetic resonance imaging may be used to diagnose a cerebrovascular accident caused by blocked cerebral vessels from sickled cells.

NURSING AND COLLABORATIVE MANAGEMENT: SICKLE CELL DISEASE

Collaborative care for a patient with sickle cell anemia is essentially supportive. There is no specific treatment for the disease. Patients with sickle cell disease should be taught to avoid high altitudes, maintain adequate fluid intake, and treat infections promptly. Pneumovax and *Haemophilus influenzae* vaccines should be administered. Therapy is usually directed toward alleviating the symptoms from complications of the disease. For example, chronic leg ulcers may be treated with bed rest, antibiotics, warm saline soaks, mechanical or enzyme debridement, and grafting if necessary. Priapism is managed with pain medication and nifedipine (Procardia).

Sickle cell crises may require hospitalization. O_2 may be administered to treat hypoxia and control sickling. Rest is instituted to reduce metabolic requirements, and fluids and electrolytes are administered to reduce blood viscosity and maintain renal function. Transfusion therapy is indicated when an aplastic crisis occurs.

Acute painful episodes caused by sickling are the most common cause for sickle cell patients to seek medical care. Pain management poses a number of challenges to the health care provider. Undertreatment of sickle cell pain is a major problem.[10] Large doses of continuous (not prn) narcotic analgesics are the mainstay of pain management during the acute phase. Patients with sickle cell disease metabolize narcotics more rapidly than normal. Patient-controlled analgesia (PCA) may be used during an acute crisis. (PCA is discussed in Chapter 9.) After discharge patients will often continue on oral narcotic analgesics. Health care personnel must overcome their fears of narcotic addiction to treat pain optimally and to avoid prolonging the duration of pain.

Patients with acute chest syndrome are treated with broad-spectrum antibiotics, O_2 therapy, and adequate fluid therapy. Because these patients have an increased need for folic acid, it is important for them to obtain daily supplementation. Blood transfusions should be used judiciously to treat a crisis. They have little if any role in the treatment between crises. In general, iron therapy is not indicated.

Although many antisickling agents have been tried, hydroxyurea (Droxia) is the only one that has been shown to be clinically beneficial.[11] The drug interferes with normal erythropoiesis and results in increased levels of HbF, which lessens the sickling process and decreases the incidence of crises. The effects of hydroxyurea are enhanced with concomitant use of erythropoietin.

Allogeneic bone marrow transplantation is the only available treatment that can cure sickle cell disease. However, its use remains uncommon. (Bone marrow transplants are discussed in Chapter 14.) Recent advances in gene therapy technology provide promise for the future treatment of SCD. (Gene therapy is discussed in Chapter 12.)

Patient education is important in the long-term care for the patient. The patient and family must understand the basis of the disease and the reasons for supportive care. The patient must be taught ways to avoid crises, which include taking steps to reduce the chance of developing hypoxia, such as avoiding high altitudes, and seeking medical attention quickly to counteract problems such as upper respiratory tract infections. Education on pain control is also needed because the pain during a crisis may be severe and often requires considerable analgesia.

GLUCOSE-6-PHOSPHATE DEHYDROGENASE DEFICIENCY

Glucose-6-phosphate dehydrogenase (G6PD) is an RBC enzyme that acts as the initial catalyst in glycolysis. G6PD deficiency is a sex-linked disorder and directly affects the erythrocyte's ability to resist oxidative damage. Consequently, when G6PD is reduced, there is a decrease in glucose use by the RBCs. If erythrocytes are exposed to oxidative foods and drugs, the metabolic needs of RBCs increase. However, the G6PD deficiency interferes with glucose metabolism and leads to damage of older RBCs, which are then destroyed by hemolysis.

G6PD deficiency is relatively common, especially in African-Americans and in persons of Mediterranean or Jewish heritage. Hemolytic episodes are triggered by viral and bacterial infections. Drugs and toxins also cause hemolysis in persons deficient in G6PD. Drugs that may cause oxidative problems include antimalarial drugs, sulfonamides, nitrofurantoins, analgesics (e.g., phenacetin), and chloramphenicol.

Managing the hemolysis seen in G6PD deficiency is relatively easy. Because only older RBCs are destroyed by the oxidative agent, the younger cells survive. The cause of the hemolytic reaction must be removed. During the period of acute hemolysis, the patient will require rest, adequate hydration, and assessment of kidney function. Attention should be focused on preventing the hemolytic disorders by treating infections promptly and screening high risk individuals for G6PD deficiency before giving an oxidative drug.

ACQUIRED HEMOLYTIC ANEMIA

Extrinsic causes of hemolysis can be separated into three categories: (1) physical factors, (2) immune reactions, and (3) infectious agents and toxins. Physical destruction of RBCs results from the exertion of extreme force on the cells. Traumatic events causing disruption of the RBC membrane include hemodialysis, extracorporeal circulation used in heart-lung bypass, and prosthetic heart valves. In addition, the force needed to push blood through abnormal vessels, such as those that have been burned or affected by angiopathic disease (e.g., diabetes mellitus), may also physically damage RBCs.

Antibodies may destroy RBCs by the mechanisms involved in antigen-antibody reactions. The reactions may be of an isoimmune or autoimmune type. Isoimmune reactions occur when antibodies develop against antigens from another person of the same species. Blood transfusion reactions typify this response, especially when donor cells are hemolyzed by the recipient's antibodies because of an ABO mismatch. Another isoimmune reaction is termed *hemolytic disease of the newborn* (HDN). In the past this disorder was termed *erythroblastosis fetalis.* In this situation, maternal antibodies that have been previously sensitized either through previous pregnancy or transfusion destroy the RBCs of the fetus, resulting in a hemolytic anemia.

Autoimmune reactions result when individuals develop antibodies against their own erythrocytes. Autoimmune hemolytic reactions may be idiopathic, developing with no prior hemolytic history as a result of the immunoglobulin IgG covering the RBCs, or secondary to other autoimmune diseases (e.g., systemic lupus erythematosus), leukemia, lymphoma, or drugs (penicillin, indomethacin, phenylbutazone, phenacetin, quinidine, quinine, and methyldopa).

The third category of acquired hemolytic disorders is caused by infectious agents and toxins. Infectious agents can foster hemolysis in four ways: (1) by invading the RBC and destroying its contents (e.g., parasites such as in malaria); (2) by releasing hemolytic substances (e.g., *Clostridium perfringens*); (3) by generating an antigen-antibody reaction; and (4) by contributing to splenomegaly as a means of increasing the removal of damaged erythrocytes from the circulation.

Various agents may be toxic to RBCs and cause hemolysis. These hemolytic toxins involve chemicals such as oxidative drugs, arsenic, lead, copper, and snake venom.

Laboratory findings in hemolytic anemia are presented in Table 29-6. Treatment and management of acquired hemolytic anemias involve general supportive care until the causative agent can be eliminated or at least rendered less injurious to the erythrocytes. Supportive care may include administering corticosteroids and blood products or removing the spleen.

HEMACHROMATOSIS

Hemachromatosis (HH) is an autosomal recessive disease characterized by increased intestinal iron absorption and consequent increased tissue iron deposition. It is the most common genetic disorder among Caucasians, with an incidence of 1 in 300. Total body iron concentration in normal individuals is 2 to 6 g. Individuals with HH accumulate iron at a rate of 0.5 to 1.0 g each year and may exceed total iron concentrations of 50 g. Symptoms of HH usually develop between 40 and 60 years of age. In addition to the primary genetic defect, HH occurs secondary to diseases such as thalassemia and sideroblastosis. It may also be caused by multiple blood transfusions.

Initially the excess iron accumulates in the liver and causes liver enlargement and eventually cirrhosis. Then other organs become affected resulting in diabetes mellitus, skin pigment changes (bronzing), cardiac changes (e.g., cardiomyopathy), arthritis, and testicular atrophy. Physical examination reveals an enlarged liver and spleen and pigmentation changes in the skin. Laboratory values demonstrate an elevated serum iron, TIBC, and serum ferritin. A liver biopsy can quantify the amount of iron and is the definitive way to establish the diagnosis.

The goal of treatment is to remove excess iron from the body and give supportive treatment. Iron removal is achieved by removing 500 ml of blood each week for 2 to 3 years until the iron stores in the body are depleted. Then less frequent removal of blood is needed to maintain iron levels within normal limits. Management of organ involvement (e.g., diabetes mellitus, heart failure) is the same as conventional treatment for these problems. The most common causes of death are cirrhosis, liver failure, hepatic carcinoma, and cardiac failure. With early diagnosis and treatment, life expectancy is normal. However, many cases go undetected and untreated.

POLYCYTHEMIA

Polycythemia is the production and presence of increased numbers of RBCs. The increase in erythrocytes can be so great that blood circulation is impaired as a result of the increased blood viscosity (hyperviscosity) and volume (hypervolemia).

Etiology and Pathophysiology

The two types of polycythemia are primary polycythemia, or polycythemia vera, and secondary polycythemia (Fig. 29-6). Their etiologies and pathogenesis differ, although their complications and clinical manifestations are similar. Polycythemia vera is considered a myeloproliferative disorder arising from a chromosomal mutation in a single pluripotent stem cell. Therefore not only are erythrocytes involved but also granulocytes and platelets, leading to increased production of each of these blood cells. The disease develops insidiously and follows a chronic, vacillating course. It usually develops in patients more than 50 years of age. With this myeloproliferative disorder the patient has enhanced blood viscosity and blood volume and congestion of organs and tissues with blood. Splenomegaly is common.

Secondary polycythemia is caused by hypoxia rather than a defect in the development of the RBC. Hypoxia stimulates erythropoietin production in the kidney, which in turn stimulates erythrocyte production. The need for O_2 may be due to high altitude, pulmonary disease, cardiovascular disease, alveolar hypoventilation, defective O_2 transport, or tissue hypoxia. Consequently, secondary polycythemia is a physiologic response in which the body tries to compensate for a problem rather than a pathologic response. (Secondary polycythemia is discussed in the section on COPD in Chapter 27.)

Clinical Manifestations and Complications

Circulatory manifestations of polycythemia vera occur because of the hypertension caused by hypervolemia and hyperviscosity. They are often the first symptoms and include subjective complaints of headache, vertigo, dizziness, tinnitus, and visual disturbances. In addition, the patient may experience angina, CHF, intermittent claudication, and thrombophlebitis, which may be complicated by embolization. These manifestations are caused by blood vessel distention, impaired blood flow, circulatory stasis, thrombosis, and tissue hypoxia caused by the hypervolemia and hyperviscosity. The most common

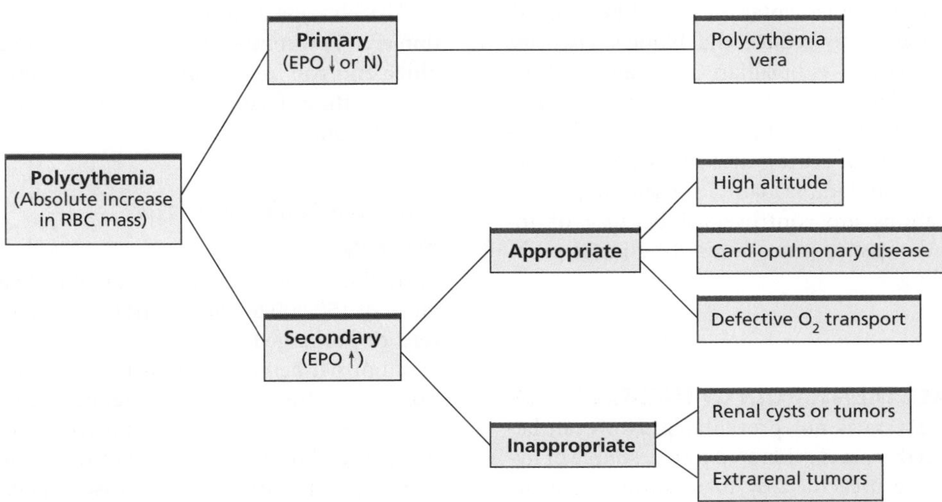

Fig. 29-6 Differentiating between primary and secondary polycythemia. *EPO*, erythropoietin; *N*, normal.

serious complication is cerebrovascular accident secondary to thrombosis. Generalized pruritus may be a striking symptom and is related to histamine release from an increased number of basophils and mast cells.

Hemorrhagic phenomena caused by either vessel rupture from overdistention or inadequate platelet function may result in petechiae, ecchymoses, epistaxis, or GI bleeding. Hemorrhage can be acute and catastrophic.

Hepatomegaly and splenomegaly from organ engorgement may contribute to patient complaints of satiety and fullness. The patient may also experience pain from peptic ulcer caused by either increased gastric secretions or liver and spleen engorgement. Plethora (ruddy complexion) may also be present.

Hyperuricemia is caused by the increase in RBC destruction that accompanies the excessive RBC production. Uric acid is one of the products of cell destruction. As RBC destruction increases, uric acid production also increases, thus leading to hyperuricemia. This problem may cause a secondary form of gout (a form of arthritis).

Diagnostic Studies

The following laboratory manifestations are seen in a patient with polycythemia vera: (1) elevated hemoglobin and RBC count; (2) elevated WBC count with basophilia; (3) elevated platelets (thrombocytosis) and platelet dysfunction; (4) elevated leukocyte alkaline phosphatase, uric acid, and cobalamin levels; and (5) elevated histamine levels.

Bone marrow examination in polycythemia vera shows hypercellularity of RBCs, WBCs, and platelets. Splenomegaly is found in 90% of patients with primary polycythemia but does not accompany secondary polycythemia.

Collaborative Care

Once the diagnosis of polycythemia vera is made, treatment is directed toward reducing blood volume and viscosity and bone marrow activity. Phlebotomy may be done to diminish blood volume until the desired Hct level is achieved. The aim of phlebotomy is to reduce and keep the Hct less than 45% to 48%. Generally, at the time of diagnosis 300 to 500 ml of blood may be removed every other day until the Hct is reduced to normal levels. An individual managed with repeated phlebotomies eventually becomes deficient in iron, although this effect is rarely symptomatic. Iron supplementation should be avoided. Hydration therapy is used to reduce the blood's viscosity. Myelosuppressive agents such as busulfan (Myleran), hydroxyurea (Hydrea), melphalan (Alkeran), and radioactive phosphorus may be given to inhibit bone marrow activity. Allopurinol may reduce the number of acute gouty attacks. Antiplatelet agents, such as aspirin and dipyridamole, used to prevent thrombotic complications are controversial because of increased irritation of the gastric mucosa resulting in GI problems, including bleeding.

NURSING MANAGEMENT: POLYCYTHEMIA VERA

Primary polycythemia vera is not preventable. However, because secondary polycythemia is generated by any source of hypoxia, problems may be prevented by maintaining adequate oxygenation. Therefore controlling chronic pulmonary disease and avoiding high altitudes may be important.

When acute exacerbations of polycythemia vera develop, the nurse has several responsibilities. Depending on the institution's policies, the nurse may either assist with or perform the phlebotomy. Fluid intake and output must be evaluated during hydration therapy to avoid fluid overload (which further complicates the circulatory congestion) and underhydration (which can cause the blood to become even more viscous). If myelosuppressive agents are used, the nurse must administer the drugs as ordered, observe the patient, and teach the patient about medication side effects.

Assessment of the patient's nutritional status in collaboration with the dietitian may be necessary to offset the inadequate food intake that can result from GI symptoms of fullness, pain, and dyspepsia. Activities must be instituted to decrease thrombus formation. The relative immobility normally imposed by hospitalization puts the patient at risk for thrombus formation. Active or passive leg exercises, and ambulation when possible, should be initiated.

Because of its chronic nature, polycythemia vera requires ongoing evaluation. Phlebotomy may need to be done every 2 to 3 months, reducing the blood volume by about 500 ml each time. The nurse must evaluate the patient for the development of complications.

Although the incidence is small, leukemia and lymphomas develop in some patients with polycythemia vera. These occurrences may be caused by the chemotherapeutic drugs used to treat the disease, or they may be secondary to a disorder in the stem cells that progresses to erythroleukemia. The major cause of morbidity and mortality from polycythemia vera is related to thrombosis (e.g., CVA).

PROBLEMS OF HEMOSTASIS

The hemostatic process involves the vascular endothelium, platelets, and coagulation factors, which normally function in concert to arrest hemorrhage and repair vascular injury. (These mechanisms are described in Chapter 28.) Disruption in any of these components may result in bleeding or thrombotic disorders.

Three major disorders of hemostasis discussed in this section are (1) thrombocytopenia (low platelet count), (2) hemophilia and von Willebrand disease (inherited disorders of specific clotting factors), and (3) disseminated intravascular coagulation.

THROMBOCYTOPENIA

Etiology

Thrombocytopenia is a reduction of platelets below the normal range of 150,000 to 400,000/μl (150 to 400 $\times 10^9$/L). Acute, severe, or prolonged decreases from this normal range can result in abnormal hemostasis that manifests as prolonged bleeding from minor trauma to spontaneous bleeding without injury.

Platelet disorders can be inherited (e.g., Wiskott-Aldrich syndrome), but the vast majority are acquired. Acquired disorders can occur because of decreased platelet production or in-

Table 29-12 Causes of Thrombocytopenia

Decreased Platelet Production
- Inherited
  - Fanconi's syndrome (pancytopenia)
  - Hereditary thrombocytopenia
- Acquired
  - Aplastic anemia
  - Hematologic malignant disorders
  - Myelosuppressive drugs
  - Chronic alcoholism
  - Exposure to ionizing radiation
  - Viral infections
  - Deficiencies of cobalamin, folic acid

Increased Platelet Destruction
- Nonimmune
  - Thrombotic thrombocytopenic purpura
  - Pregnancy
  - Infection
  - Drug induced
  - Severe burns
- Immune
  - Immune thrombocytopenic purpura
  - Human immunodeficiency virus infection
  - Drug induced
- Splenomegaly

Table 29-13 Drugs, Spices, and Vitamins That Can Cause Abnormalities of Platelet Function

Suppression of Platelet Production
- Thiazide diuretics, alcohol, estrogen, chemotherapeutic drugs

Abnormal Platelet Aggregation
- Nonsteroidal antiinflammatory drugs: ibuprofen (Advil, Motrin), indomethacin (Indocin), naproxen (Naprosyn, Aleve)
- Antibiotics: penicillins, cephalosporins
- Analgesics: aspirin and aspirin-containing drugs (see Table 29-15)
- Spices: ginger, cumin, tumeric, cloves, garlic
- Vitamins: vitamin C, vitamin E
- Heparin

creased platelet destruction (Table 29-12). Many of these abnormalities of platelet number occur following ingestion of some foods and medications (Table 29-13). Aspirin doses as low as 60 mg (a baby aspirin) can alter the function of circulating platelets. Normal function is restored with the generation of newly formed platelets. It is important for the nurse to be aware of the numerous conditions that may affect platelet production and destruction.[12]

Immune Thrombocytopenic Purpura. The most common acquired thrombocytopenia is a syndrome of abnormal destruction of circulating platelets termed *immune thrombocytopenic purpura* (ITP). It was originally termed *idiopathic thrombocytopenic purpura* because its cause was unknown; however, it is now believed that ITP is an autoimmune disease. In ITP, platelets are coated with antibodies. Although these platelets function normally, when they reach the spleen, the antibody-coated platelets are recognized as foreign and are destroyed by macrophages.

Platelets normally survive 8 to 10 days, but in ITP, survival is only 1 to 3 days. Acute ITP is seen predominantly in children following a viral illness. Chronic ITP occurs most commonly in women between 20 and 40 years of age. Chronic ITP has a gradual onset, and transient remissions occur.

Thrombotic Thrombocytopenic Purpura. Thrombotic thrombocytopenic purpura (TTP) is an uncommon syndrome characterized by microangiopathic hemolytic anemia, thrombocytopenia, neurologic abnormalities, fever (in the absence of infection), and renal abnormalities. The disease is associated with enhanced agglutination of platelets, which form microthrombi that deposit in arterioles and capillaries. The cause of the platelet agglutination is unknown. TTP is seen primarily in adults between 20 and 50 years of age, with a slight female predominance. The syndrome is occasionally precipitated by the use of estrogen or by pregnancy. TTP is a medical emergency because bleeding and clotting occur simultaneously.

Heparin-Induced Thrombocytopenia and Thrombosis Syndrome. One of the risks associated with the broad and increasing use of heparin is the development of the life-threatening condition called heparin-induced thrombocytopenia and thrombosis syndrome (HITTS), also called white clot syndrome. Platelet destruction and vascular endothelial injury are the two major responses to what is believed to be an immune-mediated mechanism.[13] The immune response promotes platelet aggregation leading to decreased circulating platelets and ultimately thrombocytopenia. In addition, platelet-fibrin thrombi are formed. Platelet aggregation also induces heparin to be neutralized, thus more heparin is required to maintain therapeutic activated partial thromboplastin times. HITTS can be mild (type I) or severe (type II), and estimates vary from 5% to as high as 25% incidence rate. A lower incidence is seen in patients receiving porcine preparations of heparin.[13]

Clinical Manifestations

Despite different etiologies, clinical manifestations of thrombocytopenia are similar. Thrombocytopenia is most commonly manifested by the appearance of small, flat, pinpoint red or reddish brown microhemorrhages termed *petechiae.* When the platelet count is low, RBCs may leak out of the blood vessels and into the skin to cause petechiae. When petechiae are numerous, the resulting reddish skin bruise is termed *purpura.* Larger purplish lesions caused by hemorrhage are termed *ecchymoses* (Fig. 29-7). Ecchymoses may be flat or raised; pain and tenderness sometimes are present.

Prolonged bleeding after routine procedures such as venipuncture or IM injection may also indicate thrombocytopenia. Because the bleeding may be internal, the nurse must also be aware of manifestations that reflect this type of blood loss, including weakness, fainting, dizziness, tachycardia, abdominal pain, and hypotension.

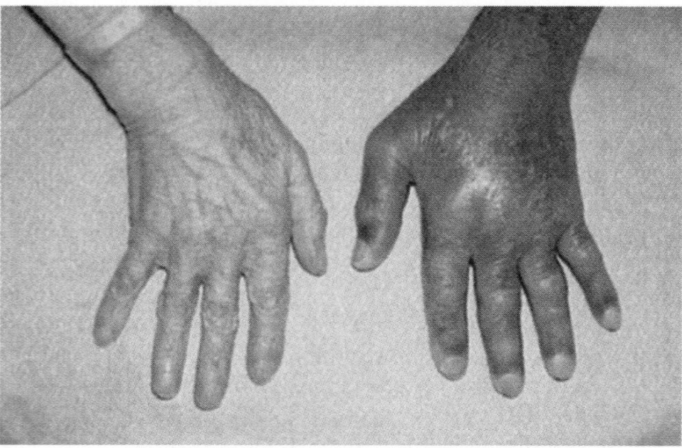

Fig. 29-7 Example of ecchymoses.

The major complication of thrombocytopenia is hemorrhage. The hemorrhage may be insidious or acute and internal or external. It may occur in any area of the body, including the joints, retina, and brain. Cerebral hemorrhage may be fatal in persons with ITP. Insidious hemorrhage may first be detected by discovering the anemia that accompanies blood loss.

Diagnostic Studies

The platelet count is decreased in cases of thrombocytopenia. Any reduction below 150,000/μl (150 × 10^9/L) may be termed *thrombocytopenia.* However, prolonged bleeding from trauma or injury does not usually occur until platelet counts are less than 50,000/μl (50 × 10^9/L). When the count drops below 20,000/μl (20 × 10^9/L), spontaneous, life-threatening hemorrhages (e.g., intracranial bleeding) can occur. Platelet transfusions are generally not recommended until the count is below 20,000/μl (20 × 10^9/L) unless the patient is actively bleeding.

The bleeding time is a test of primary hemostasis and will be prolonged in any disorder of platelet function. Laboratory tests that assess secondary hemostasis or coagulation, such as the prothrombin time (PT) and activated partial thromboplastin time (APTT), can be normal even in severe thrombocytopenia. When destruction of circulating platelets is the etiology, bone marrow analysis shows megakaryocytes (precursors of platelets) to be normal or increased, even though circulating platelets are reduced. Additionally, special blood analyses using flow cytometry and other techniques can detect antiplatelet antibodies as the source of destruction. Bone marrow examination is done to rule out production problems as the cause of thrombocytopenia (e.g., leukemia, aplastic anemia, and other myeloproliferative disorders).

Anemia is present in proportion to the amount of blood lost. Therefore it is important to monitor Hb and Hct values and to observe the patient for cardiopulmonary distress and other manifestations of anemia. When thrombocytopenia occurs with anemia characterized by altered RBC morphology, including spherocytes, fragmented cells (schistocytes), and pronounced reticulocytosis, a diagnosis of TTP should be suspected. These findings are partially as a result of intravascular fibrin deposition causing a "slicing" of RBCs. In TTP, thrombocytopenia may be severe, but coagulation studies are normal.

COLLABORATIVE CARE

Table 29-14 Thrombocytopenia

Diagnostic
- History and physical examination
- Platelet count
- Bleeding time
- Bone marrow aspiration and biopsy
- Hematocrit and hemoglobin levels

Collaborative Therapy

Immune thrombocytopenic purpura
- Corticosteroids
- Platelet transfusions
- Intravenous immunoglobulin
- Danazol
- Immunosuppressives (cyclophosphamide, azathioprine)
- Splenectomy

Thrombotic thrombocytopenic purpura
- Plasma infusion
- Plasmapheresis and plasma exchange
- High-dose prednisone
- Splenectomy

Decreased production problem
- Identification and treatment of cause
- Corticosteroids
- Platelet transfusions
- Thrombopoietin (investigational)

Collaborative Care

Collaborative care of thrombocytopenia differs based on the etiology of the thrombocytopenia. Discussion of management strategies for these different etiologies follows.

Immune Thrombocytopenic Purpura. Multiple therapies are used to manage the patient with ITP (Table 29-14). Corticosteroids are used to treat ITP because of their ability to suppress the phagocytic response of splenic macrophages. This alters the spleen's recognition of platelets and increases the platelets' life spans. In addition, corticosteroids depress autoimmune antibody formation. Initial treatment is with prednisone, which reduces the binding of antibody to the platelet surface. Corticosteroids also reduce capillary fragility and bleeding time. The mechanism of action for this response is poorly understood.

Treatment may also include high doses of IV immunoglobulin in the patient who is unresponsive to corticosteroids or splenectomy. The immunoglobulin works by competing with the antiplatelet antibodies for macrophage receptors. IV immunoglobulin effectively raises the platelet count, but the beneficial effects are temporary.

Danazol, an androgen, has been used with success in some patients. Immunosuppressive therapy used in refractory cases includes vincristine (Oncovin), vinblastine (Velban), azathioprine (Imuran), and cyclophosphamide (Cytoxan).

Splenectomy is indicated if the patient does not respond to prednisone initially or requires unacceptably high doses to maintain an adequate platelet count. Approximately 80% of patients benefit from splenectomy, resulting in a complete or partial remission. The effectiveness of splenectomy is based on four factors. First, the spleen contains an abundance of the macrophages that sequester and destroy platelets. Second, structural features of the spleen enhance antibody-coated platelets and macrophage interaction. Third, some antibody synthesis occurs in the spleen; thus antiplatelet antibodies decrease after splenectomy. Fourth, the spleen normally sequesters approximately one third of the platelets, so its removal increases the number in circulation.

Platelet transfusions may be used to increase platelet counts in cases of life-threatening hemorrhage. Platelets should not be administered prophylactically because of the possibility of antibody formation. ABO compatibility is not a necessary prerequisite for platelet transfusions. However, after multiple platelet transfusions, a patient may develop anti-HLA antibodies to the transfused platelets. Therefore by using lymphocyte typing to match HLA types of the donor and the recipient, multiple platelet transfusions can be given with fewer complications. In addition, the patient may be premedicated with an antihistamine (e.g., diphenhydramine [Benadryl]) and hydrocortisone to decrease the possibility of reacting to platelet transfusions. Sometimes meperidine (Demerol) is used for symptomatic treatment of platelet transfusion reactions in combination with an antihistamine and a corticosteroid. The mechanism of action of meperidine in controlling this reaction is not well understood, but it is believed to reset the temperature-regulating center in the hypothalamus. Aspirin and aspirin-containing compounds should be avoided in the patient with thrombocytopenia (Table 29-15).

Thrombotic Thrombocytopenic Purpura. TTP is treated with emergency plasma infusion or plasmapheresis. The mechanism for the therapeutic response is not fully understood. Treatment should be continued daily until the patient is in complete remission. Splenectomy, corticosteroids, dextran (antiplatelet agent), and vincristine or vinblastine have also been used with success.[14]

Heparin-Induced Thrombocytopenia and Thrombosis Syndrome. Heparin must be discontinued when HITTS is first recognized.[13] The most commonly used treatment modalities are plasmapheresis to clear the platelet-aggregating IgG from the blood, protamine sulfate to interrupt the circulating heparin, thrombolytic agents to treat the thromboembolic events, and surgery to remove white clots. Lepirudin (Refludan), an inhibitor of thrombin, has recently been approved to treat HITTS. It is important to note that platelet transfusions are not effective because they may enhance thromboembolic events.

Acquired Thrombocytopenia from Decreased Platelet Production. The management of acquired thrombocytopenia is based on identifying the cause and treating the disease or removing the causative agent. If the precipitating factor is unknown and being investigated, the patient may receive corticosteroids to enhance capillary integrity. Platelet transfusions are given if life-threatening hemorrhage develops. Splenectomy is not used because the spleen is not contributing to the thrombocytopenia.

Often, acquired thrombocytopenia is caused by another underlying condition (e.g., aplastic anemia, leukemia) or therapy used to treat another problem. For example, in acute leukemia all blood cell types may be depressed. Additionally, the patient may receive chemotherapeutic drugs that cause bone marrow suppression. If the patient can be adequately supported throughout the course of chemotherapy-induced thrombocytopenia, the disease-related thrombocytopenia will also resolve.

Oprelvekin (Neumega), a platelet growth factor that is a recombinant form of interleukin-11, stimulates the bone marrow to produce platelets.[15] It is being used to treat chemotherapy-induced thrombocytopenia.

Table 29-15 Products Containing Aspirin and Aspirin-like Compounds

Nonprescription	Prescription
Alka-Seltzer Antacid/Pain Reliever Effervescent Tablets	Darvon Compound-65
Alka-Seltzer Plus Cold Medicine Tablets	Disalcid Capsules/Tablets
Anacin Caplets/Tablets	Easprin Tablets
Anacin Maximum Strength Tablets	Empirin with Codeine Tablets
Arthritis Pain Formula Tablets	Equagesic Tablets
Arthritis Strength Bufferin Tablets	Fiorinal Capsules/Tablets
Ascriptin Caplets/Tablets	Fiorinal with Codeine Capsules/Tablets
Ascriptin A/D Caplets	Lortab ASA Tablets
Aspergum	Magsal Tablets
Bayer Aspirin Caplets/Tablets	Mono-Gesic Tablets
Bayer Children's Chewable Tablets	Norgesic and Norgesic Forte Tablets
Bayer Plus Tablets	Percodan and Percodan-Demi Tablets
Maximum Bayer Caplets/Tablets	Robaxisal Tablets
8-Hour Bayer Extended-Release Tablets	Salflex Tablets
BC Powder	Soma Compound Tablets
BC Cold Powder	Soma Compound with Codeine Tablets
Buffaprin Caplets/Tablets	Synalgos-DC Capsules
Bufferin Arthritis Strength Caplets	Talwin Compound Tablets
Bufferin Caplets/Tablets	Trilisate Tablets/Liquid
Cama Arthritis Pain Reliever Tablets	
Doan's Pills Caplets	
Ecotrin Caplets/Tablets	
Empirin Tablets	
Excedrin Extra-Strength Caplets/Tablets	
Midol Caplets	
Mobigesic Analgesic Tablets	
Norwich Tablets	
P-A-C Analgesic Tablets	
Sine-Off Tablets, Aspirin Formula	
St. Joseph Adult Chewable Aspirin	
Therapy Bayer Caplets	
Trigesic	
Ursinus Inlay-Tabs	
Vanquish Analgesic Caplets	

NURSING ASSESSMENT

Table 29-16 Thrombocytopenia

Subjective Data

Important Health Information

Past health history: Recent hemorrhage, excessive bleeding, or viral illness; HIV infection; cancer (especially leukemia or lymphoma); aplastic anemia; systemic lupus erythematosus; cirrhosis; exposure to radiation or toxic chemicals; disseminated intravascular coagulation

Medications: Use of thiazide diuretics, furosemide (Lasix), aspirin, acetaminophen, estrogens, gold salts, nonsteroidal antiinflammatory drugs, phenylbutazone (Butazolidin), penicillins, cephalothin, streptomycin, sulfonamides, quinidine, quinine, phenobarbital, methyldopa (Aldomet), phenytoin (Dilantin), chlorpropamide (Diabenese), meprobamate (Equanil), chemotherapy drugs, drugs listed in Tables 29-13 and 29-15

Functional Health Patterns

Health perception–health management: Family history of bleeding problems; malaise

Nutritional-metabolic: Bleeding gingiva; coffee-ground or bloody vomitus; easy bruising

Elimination: Hematuria, dark or bloody stools

Activity-exercise: Fatigue, weakness, fainting; epistaxis, hemoptysis; dyspnea

Cognitive-perceptual: Pain and tenderness in bleeding areas (e.g., abdomen, head, extremities); headache

Sexuality-reproductive: Menorrhagia, metrorrhagia

Objective Data

General

Fever, lethargy

Integumentary

Petechiae, ecchymoses, purpura

Gastrointestinal

Splenomegaly, abdominal distention; guaiac-positive stools

Possible Findings

Platelet count $<150,000/\mu l$ ($150 \times 10^9/L$), prolonged bleeding time, decreased hemoglobin and hematocrit; normal or increased megakaryocytes in bone marrow examination

NURSING MANAGEMENT: THROMBOCYTOPENIA

Nursing Assessment

Subjective and objective data that should be obtained from a patient with thrombocytopenia are presented in Table 29-16.

Nursing Diagnoses

Nursing diagnoses for the patient with thrombocytopenia may include, but are not limited to, those presented in NCP 29-2.

Planning

The overall goals are that the patient with thrombocytopenia will (1) have no gross or occult bleeding, (2) maintain vascular integrity, and (3) manage home care to prevent any complications related to an increased risk for bleeding.

Nursing Implementation

Health Promotion. It is important for the nurse to discourage excessive use of over-the-counter (OTC) medications known to be possible causes of acquired thrombocytopenia. Many medications contain aspirin as an ingredient (see Table 29-15). Aspirin reduces platelet adhesiveness, thus potentially contributing to thrombocytopenia.

It is also important for the nurse to encourage persons to have a complete medical evaluation if manifestations of bleeding tendencies (e.g., prolonged epistaxis, petechiae) develop. In addition, the nurse must observe for early signs of thrombocytopenia in the patient receiving cancer chemotherapy drugs.

Acute Intervention. The goal during acute episodes of thrombocytopenia is to prevent or control hemorrhage (see NCP 29-2). In the patient with thrombocytopenia, bleeding is usually from superficial sites; deep bleeding (into muscles, joints, abdomen) usually occurs only when clotting factors are diminished. It is important to emphasize that a seemingly minor nosebleed may lead to hemorrhage in a patient with severe thrombocytopenia. Bleeding from the posterior nasopharynx may be difficult to detect because the blood may be swallowed. If an IM or SC injection is unavoidable, the use of a small-gauge needle and application of direct pressure for at least 5 to 10 minutes after injection is indicated.

In a woman with thrombocytopenia, menstrual blood loss may exceed the usual amount and duration. Counting sanitary napkins used during menses is another important intervention to detect excess blood loss. Fifty milliliters of blood will completely soak a sanitary napkin. Suppression of menses with hormonal agents may be indicated during predictable periods of thrombocytopenia to reduce blood loss from menses (e.g., during chemotherapy and bone marrow transplantation).

The proper administration of platelet transfusions is an important nursing responsibility. Platelet concentrates, derived from fresh whole blood, can increase the platelet level effectively. One unit of platelets, a yellow liquid that is usually 30 to 50 ml in volume, can be derived by centrifuging 500 ml of whole blood. Platelet concentrates from multiple units of blood (usually from six to eight different donors) can be pooled together for a single administration. The degree of increase or increment from a pooled platelet product varies widely and is usually measured by performing a platelet count within 1 hour following the transfusion.

Platelet transfusions can also be prepared by pheresing single donors. This may be indicated when HLA-matched platelets

29-2 NURSING CARE PLAN PATIENT WITH THROMBOCYTOPENIA

Expected Patient Outcomes	Nursing Interventions and *Rationales*
NURSING DIAGNOSIS	**Risk for altered oral mucous membrane** *related to* treatment, disease, or blood-filled bullae.
▪ Pink, moist, lesion-free oral mucosa, tongue, and lips.	▪ Assess oral mucosa daily for presence of blood-filled bullae in mouth; bleeding; tender gingivae and lips *to provide information for planning interventions.* ▪ Remove dentures daily and assess oral cavity *to assess underlying gums and mouth for bullae or bleeding areas.* ▪ Provide oral hygiene with minimal friction: use soft-bristle toothbrush, cotton swabs, mild mouthwash, or irrigating syringe *to gently cleanse mouth without trauma.* ▪ Evaluate integrity of nares, especially if nasogastric tube, endotracheal tube, or nasal O_2 is in use *to determine need for prophylactic or treatment interventions.*
NURSING DIAGNOSIS	**Risk for injury** *related to* interventions and tissue sensitivity to trauma.
▪ Maintenance of tissue integrity. ▪ No evidence of petechiae, ecchymoses, purpura, hematoma.	▪ Initiate IV therapy judiciously; consider use of alternative venous access devices *to reduce number of venipunctures.* ▪ Avoid IM and SC injections; if used, apply local pressure with dry, sterile 2 × 2 inch gauze for 5-10 min after needle is removed *to prevent bleeding into tissue surrounding puncture site.* ▪ Use electric razor for shaving *to reduce potential for skin nicks.* ▪ Reduce frequency of cuff blood pressures and alternate extremities used for readings; pad rails and other firm surfaces, especially if patient is combative or at risk for seizures; be very gentle when turning patient or changing dressings *to reduce tissue trauma and subsequent bleeding into tissue.*
NURSING DIAGNOSIS	**Ineffective management of therapeutic regimen** *related to* lack of knowledge of disease process, activity, nutrition, and medication *as manifested by* frequent questioning about disease management, anxiety, restlessness.
▪ Verbalization or demonstration by patient or family of required knowledge and skills to manage home care.	▪ Assess learning needs related to disease management *to plan appropriate interventions.* ▪ Teach patient about disease process, medication, and activity and dietary recommendations *to decrease anxiety and prevent complications.* ▪ Discuss complications and signs that should be reported such as trauma prevention, need for high fluid intake, medication management, and need for periods of rest and exercise *so patient will be knowledgeable and able to manage own care or direct others in care.* ▪ Provide opportunities for patient to verbalize concerns *because discussing these with a supportive other decreases anxiety.*

COLLABORATIVE PROBLEMS

Nursing Goals	Nursing Interventions and *Rationales*
POTENTIAL COMPLICATION	**Hemorrhage** *related to* acute blood loss.
▪ Monitor for signs of hemorrhage. ▪ Report deviations from acceptable parameters. ▪ Carry out appropriate medical and nursing interventions.	▪ Evaluate mucous membranes and skin each shift or more often *to detect presence of epistaxis, petechiae, ecchymoses, hematomas.* ▪ Test excretions regularly for occult blood and observe for blood in emesis, sputum, feces, urine, nasogastric secretions, wound secretions *to detect potential presence of bleeding.* ▪ Assess CBC and platelet count daily or more often if warranted *to monitor for bleeding.* ▪ Do not administer aspirin or aspirin-containing products *because of their effects on platelet adhesiveness.* ▪ Teach patient to avoid over-the-counter medications that contain aspirin (see Table 29-15). ▪ Use ice, packing, or direct pressure *to control active bleeding.* ▪ Teach patient to avoid Valsalva's maneuver (e.g., straining at stool); administer stool softeners as ordered; avoid rectal temperatures, suppositories, and enemas; teach patient to cough, sneeze, and blow nose gently; administer medications to suppress vomiting and coughing *to avoid activities that could cause hemorrhage.* ▪ Administer platelets or other blood components as ordered *to treat bleeding or replace blood loss from hemorrhage.*

Table 29-17 Comparison of Hemophilic States

Disorder	Deficiency	Inheritance Pattern
Hemophilia A	Factor VIII	Recessive sex-linked (transmitted by female carriers, displayed almost exclusively in men)
Hemophilia B	Factor IX	Recessive sex-linked (transmitted by female carriers, displayed almost exclusively in men)
von Willebrand disease	vWf and platelet dysfunction	Autosomal dominant, seen in both sexes Recessive (in severe forms of the disease)

vWF, von Willebrand factor.

are needed, especially for patients requiring multiple platelet transfusions. In this procedure, blood is removed from the donor, the platelets are removed, and the rest of the blood is reinfused into the donor. This procedure results in 200 to 400 ml of platelets and plasma.

Once acquired from a donor, platelets can be stored at room temperature for 1 to 5 days. Gentle agitation of the bag is useful to prevent the platelets from adhering to the plastic. The actual transfusion procedure (described later in this chapter) may vary among institutions but may involve the use of specialized leukocyte reduction filters. In a severely immunocompromised patient these products are also radiated to further ensure WBC removal and prevent the complication of graft-versus-host disease (see Chapter 12).

Ambulatory and Home Care. The patient with ITP who is receiving corticosteroids should be monitored frequently for the response to therapy. If the ITP is reversed by splenectomy, there is usually no recurrence. The person with acquired thrombocytopenia must be taught to avoid causative agents when possible (see Table 29-13). If the causative agents cannot be avoided (e.g., chemotherapy), the patient should learn to avoid injury or trauma during these periods and to detect the clinical signs and symptoms of bleeding caused by thrombocytopenia. The patient with either ITP or acquired thrombocytopenia should have planned periodic medical evaluations to assess the patient's status and to intercede in situations in which exacerbations and bleeding are likely to occur.

Evaluation

The expected outcomes for the patient with thrombocytopenia are presented in NCP 29-2.

HEMOPHILIA AND VON WILLEBRAND DISEASE

Hemophilia is a hereditary bleeding disorder caused by defective or deficient coagulation factors. The two major forms of hemophilia, which can occur in mild to severe forms, are hemophilia A (classic hemophilia, factor VIII deficiency) and hemophilia B (Christmas disease, factor IX deficiency). The disorder termed *von Willebrand disease* is a related disorder involving a congenitally acquired deficiency of the von Willebrand coagulation protein. Factor VIII is synthesized in the liver and circulates complexed to von Willebrand protein (vWF).

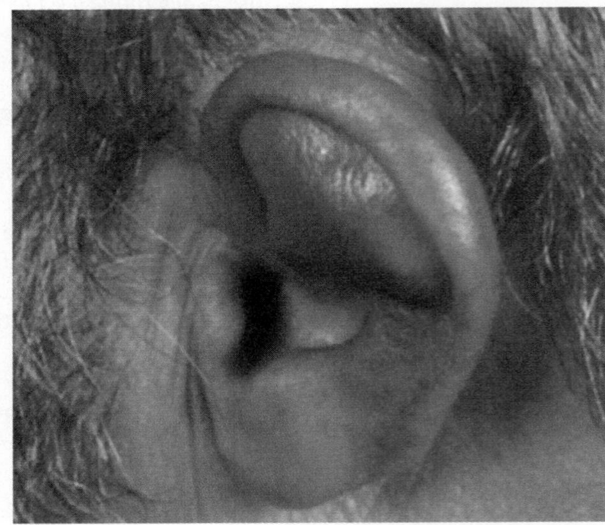

Fig. 29-8 Hematoma that developed in a person with hemophilia after trauma to the ear.

Hemophilia A is the most common form of hemophilia; it makes up approximately 80% of all cases. The incidence of hemophilia A is approximately 1 in 10,000 males; hemophilia B is seen in 1 in 100,000 males. von Willebrand disease is considered the most common congenital bleeding disorder in humans, with estimates as high as 1 in 100. However, because this disease can also exist in mild to severe forms, life-threatening hemorrhage in patients is rare (1 in 1 million).[16] The deficiency and inheritance patterns of these three forms of inherited coagulopathies are compared in Table 29-17.

Clinical Manifestations and Complications

Clinical manifestations and complications related to hemophilia include (1) slow, persistent, prolonged bleeding from minor trauma and small cuts (Fig. 29-8); (2) delayed bleeding after minor injuries (the delay may be several hours or days); (3) uncontrollable hemorrhage after dental extractions or irritation of the gingiva with a hard-bristle toothbrush; (4) epistaxis, especially after a blow to the face; (5) GI bleeding from ulcers and gastritis; (6) hematuria from GU trauma and splenic rupture resulting from falls or abdominal trauma; (7) ecchymoses and subcutaneous hematomas (common); (8) neurologic signs, such as pain, anesthesia, and paralysis, which may develop from nerve compression caused by hematoma forma-

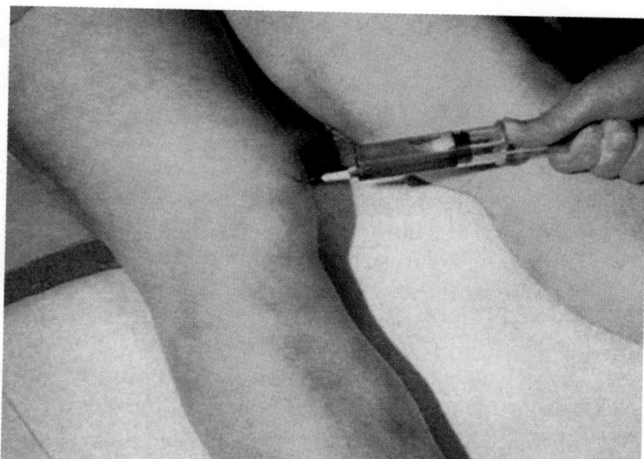

Fig. 29-9 Acute hemarthrosis of right knee in a patient with severe hemophilia. Blood from the synovial cavity is being aspirated with a needle and syringe.

tion; and (9) hemarthrosis (bleeding into the joints) (Fig. 29-9), which may lead to joint deformity severe enough to cause unresolvable crippling (most commonly in the knees, elbows, shoulders, hips, and ankles).

These manifestations are especially important when seen in children because the disease may not yet be diagnosed. In adults, these developments may be the first sign of a newly diagnosed mild form of the disease that escaped detection through a childhood free of major injuries, dental procedures, or surgeries. However, these manifestations can also suggest that the hemophilia is poorly controlled. All clinical manifestations relate to bleeding, and any bleeding episode in persons with hemophilia may result in death from hemorrhage.

Hemophilia had been considered primarily a disease of childhood because of early death from complications. At the beginning of the century the median life expectancy was 11 years. By the 1970s advances in its treatment enabled persons with hemophilia to have a median life expectancy of 68 years. Unfortunately, the AIDS epidemic and the contamination of blood products reduced this figure to 49 years in the late 1980s. Presently, about 90% of older persons severely affected with hemophilia are seropositive for HIV infection, which was transmitted via cryoprecipitates and factor concentrates. Before 1986 donated blood and blood products were not tested for HIV antibody. Longer-term survival is now being observed because of improved preparation of factor VIII concentrates, improved screening techniques of donor populations, and heat-treatment of the product to further reduce the likelihood of transmission of both HIV and hepatitis B and C viruses.[17] The development of hepatitis C in hemophilia patients was also common for many years because of lack of an available test to detect it and the use of pooled blood products. Hepatitis C antibody screening is now routinely done on all donated blood and blood products.

Diagnostic Studies

Laboratory studies are used to determine the type of hemophilia present. Any factor deficiency within the intrinsic system (factors VIII, vWF, IX, XI, or XII) will yield the laboratory results presented in Table 29-18.

Table 29-18 Laboratory Results in Hemophilia

Test	Comments
Prothrombin time	No involvement of extrinsic system
Thrombin time	No impairment of thrombin-fibrinogen reaction
Platelet count	Adequate platelet production
Partial thromboplastin time	Prolonged because of deficiency in any intrinsic clotting system factor
Bleeding time	Prolonged in von Willebrand disease because of structurally defective platelets, normal in hemophilia A and B because platelets not affected
Factor assays	Reduction of factor VIII in hemophilia A, vWF in von Willebrand disease, reduction of factor IX in hemophilia B

DRUG THERAPY

Table 29-19 Concentrate Factors Used in Treating Hemophilia

Factor VIII	
Plasma-Derived Products	**Recombinant Products***
Monoclate	Recombinate
Hemofil	Kogenate
Profilate	
Koate	
Humate	
Factor IX	
Plasma-Derived Products	
Alpha-Nine	Bebulin
Mononine	Autoplex
Konyne	FEIBA
Profilnine	Hyate

*Produced by hamster cell lines transfected with a gene for factor VIII.

Collaborative Care

The goals of collaborative care are to prevent and treat bleeding. The therapeutic regimens for persons with hemophilia or von Willebrand disease focus on maintaining adequate blood levels of the deficient clotting factors. This goal is achieved by assessing clinical manifestations, determining blood levels of the involved factors, and administering the necessary factors.

Replacement of deficient clotting factors is the primary means of supporting a patient with hemophilia. In addition to treating acute crises, replacement therapy may be given before surgery and dental care as a prophylactic measure. The standard therapeutic products are described in Table 29-19. Fresh frozen plasma, once commonly used for replacement therapy, is rarely used today. Cryoprecipitate, which primarily contains factor VIII and fibrinogen, is prepared from plasma, frozen rapidly, and kept frozen until used. Before administration, the cryoprecipitate is thawed slowly.

Most patients with hemophilia A use factor VIII concentrate, which is prepared from multiple donors and supplied as a lyophilized powder. A number of processes have increased the safety of factor VIII therapy. First, heat-treating the concentrate in solution or after lyophilization inactivates HIV. Second, treating the concentrate with chemicals, including solvent-detergent mixtures, can specifically inactivate viruses. Highly purified factor VIII can be produced by adsorbing and eluding factor VIII from monoclonal antibody columns. The discovery of the factor VIII gene in 1984 and recombinant DNA techniques have allowed for the production of factor VIII by recombinant DNA technology (see Chapter 12). This product appears to be equivalent to its plasma-derived counterpart; because donors are not involved, it should prevent infectious complications.

Factor IX deficiency is treated with factor IX concentrate, which is available as a lyophilized concentrate and contains prothrombin and factors VII and X. Monoclonally purified or recombinant factor IX preparations are undergoing clinical trials.

For certain subtypes of von Willebrand disease, desmopressin acetate (also known as DDAVP), a synthetic analog of vasopressin, may be used to stimulate an increase in factor VIII and von Willebrand factor. This drug acts on endothelial cells to cause the release of von Willebrand factor, which subsequently binds with factor VIII, thus increasing their concentration. Beneficial effects (e.g., decreased bleeding time) of DDAVP, when administered IV, are seen within 30 minutes and can last for more than 12 hours. Because the effect of DDAVP is relatively short-lived, the patient must be closely monitored and repeated doses may be necessary. It is an appropriate therapy for procedures such as dental extractions or care. An intranasal form has been developed and may be indicated for home therapy for some patients with mild to moderate forms of the disease.[16]

Complications of treatment of hemophilia include development of inhibitors to factors VIII or IX, transfusion-transmitted infectious disorders, allergic reactions (more commonly seen with the use of cryoprecipitate), and thrombotic complications with the use of factor IX because it contains activated coagulation factors. Because of the improved viral-depleting processes and donor screening practices, the risk of HIV and hepatitis transmission is greatly reduced from the pre-1986 incidence.

The most common difficulties with acute management are starting factor replacement therapy too late and stopping it too soon. Generally, minor bleeding episodes should be treated for at least 72 hours. Surgery and traumatic injuries may dictate support for 10 to 14 days. Because of the short half-life of the factors, regular intermittent or continuous infusions have been used to manage bleeding episodes or expected traumatic procedures. Chronically, development of inhibitors to the factor products has occurred and requires individualized expert patient management.

NURSING MANAGEMENT: HEMOPHILIA

■ Nursing Implementation

Health Promotion. Because of the hereditary nature of hemophilia, referral for genetic counseling is essential when considering preventive measures. This is especially important because persons with hemophilia are living longer and reaching an age when reproduction is possible.

Acute Intervention. Nursing interventions are related primarily to controlling bleeding and include the following:

1. Stop the topical bleeding as quickly as possible by applying direct pressure or ice, packing the area with Gelfoam or fibrin foam, and applying topical hemostatic agents such as thrombin.
2. Administer the specific coagulation factor concentrate ordered to raise the patient's level of the deficient coagulation factor.
3. When joint bleeding occurs, it is important to totally rest the involved joint, in addition to administering antihemophilic factors to help prevent crippling deformities from hemarthrosis. The joint may be packed in ice. Analgesics are given to reduce severe pain. However, aspirin and aspirin-containing compounds should *never* be used. As soon as bleeding ceases, it is important to encourage mobilization of the affected area through range-of-motion exercises and physical therapy. Actual weight bearing is avoided until all swelling has resolved and muscle strength has returned.
4. Manage any life-threatening complication that may develop as a result of hemorrhage. Examples include nursing interventions to prevent or treat airway obstruction from hemorrhage into the neck and pharynx, as well as early assessment and treatment of intracranial bleeding.

Ambulatory and Home Care. Home management is a primary consideration for the patient with hemophilia because the disease follows a progressive, chronic course. The quality and the length of life may be significantly affected by the patient's knowledge of the illness and how to live with it. The patient and family can be referred to a local chapter of the National Hemophilia Society to encourage associations with other individuals who are dealing with the problems of hemophilia. The nurse must provide ongoing assessment of the patient's adaptation to the illness. Psychosocial support and assistance should be readily available as needed.

Most of the long-term care measures are related to patient education. The patient with hemophilia must be taught to recognize disease-related problems and to learn which problems can be resolved at home and which require hospitalization. Immediate medical attention is required for severe pain or swelling of a muscle or joint that restricts movement or inhibits sleep and for a head injury, a swelling in the neck or mouth, abdominal pain, hematuria, melena, and skin wounds in need of suturing.

Daily oral hygiene must be performed without causing trauma. Understanding how to prevent injuries is another consideration. This is no easy task; there are many potential sources of trauma. The patient can learn to participate in noncontact sports (e.g., golf) and wear gloves when doing household chores to prevent cuts or abrasions from knives, hammers, and other tools. The patient should wear a Medic Alert tag to ensure that health care providers know about the hemophilia in case of an accident.

The patient needs information about routine follow-up care, and the compliance with scheduled visits must be assessed. A reliable person can be taught to self-administer some of the factor replacement therapies at home.

■ Evaluation

The overall expected outcomes are similar to those for the patient with thrombocytopenia and are presented in NCP 29-2.

DISSEMINATED INTRAVASCULAR COAGULATION

Disseminated intravascular coagulation (DIC) is a serious bleeding disorder resulting from abnormally initiated and accelerated clotting. Subsequent decreases in clotting factors and platelets ensue, which may lead to uncontrollable hemorrhage. The term *DIC* can be misleading because it suggests that blood is clotting. However, the paradox of this condition is characterized by the profuse bleeding that results from the depletion of platelets and clotting factors. DIC is always caused by an underlying disease. The underlying disease must be treated for the DIC to resolve.

Etiology and Pathophysiology

DIC is not a disease; it is an abnormal response of the normal clotting cascade stimulated by another disease process or disorder. The diseases and disorders known to predispose a patient to DIC are listed in Table 29-20. DIC can occur as an acute, catastrophic condition, or it may exist at a subacute or chronic level. Each condition may have one or multiple triggering mechanisms to start the cascade. For example, tumors and traumatized or necrotic tissue release tissue factor into circulation. Endotoxin from gram-negative bacteria activates several steps in the coagulation cascade.

Initially in DIC, the normal coagulation mechanisms are enhanced. Abundant intravascular thrombin, the most powerful coagulant, is produced (Fig. 29-10). It catalyzes the conversion of fibrinogen to fibrin and enhances platelet aggregation. There is widespread fibrin and platelet deposition in capillaries and arterioles, resulting in thrombosis. Excessive clotting activates the fibrinolytic system, which in turn lyses the newly formed clots, creating fibrin-split (fibrin-degradation) products. These products have anticoagulant properties and inhibit normal blood clotting. Ultimately with fibrin split products accumulating and clotting factors being depleted, the blood loses its ability to clot. Therefore a stable clot cannot be formed at injury sites. This situation predisposes the patient to hemorrhage.

Chronic DIC is most commonly seen in patients with longstanding illnesses such as malignant disorders or autoimmune diseases. The incidence of DIC associated with malignancy ranges from 10% to 75%, depending on the malignancy studied.[18] Occasionally these patients have subclinical disease manifested only by laboratory abnormalities. However, the clinical spectrum ranges from easy bruising to hemorrhage and from hypercoagulability to thrombosis.

Clinical Manifestations

There is no well-defined sequence of events in acute DIC. Bleeding in a person with no previous history or obvious cause should be questioned because it may be one of the first manifestations of acute DIC. Other nonspecific manifestations can include weakness, malaise, and fever.

There are both bleeding and thrombotic manifestations in DIC. Bleeding manifestations of DIC are multifactorial (see Fig. 29-10) and result from consumption and depletion of platelets and coagulation factors, as well as clot lysis and formation of fibrin split products that have anticoagulant properties. Bleeding manifestations include integumentary problems, such as pallor, petechiae, oozing blood, venipuncture site bleeding, hematomas, and occult hemorrhage; respiratory problems, such as tachypnea, hemoptysis, and orthopnea; cardiovascular problems, such as tachycardia and hypotension; GI changes, such as upper and lower GI bleeding, abdominal distention, and bloody stools; urinary problems, such as hematuria; neurologic changes, such as vision changes, dizziness, headache, changes in mental status, and irritability; and musculoskeletal changes, such as bone and joint pain.

Table 29-20 Predisposing Conditions to Development of Disseminated Intravascular Coagulation

Acute DIC
- Shock
  - Hemorrhagic
  - Cardiogenic
  - Anaphylactic
- Septicemia
- Hemolytic processes
  - Transfusion of mismatched blood
  - Acute hemolysis from infection or immunologic disorders
- Obstetric conditions
  - Abruptio placenta
  - Amniotic fluid embolism
  - Septic abortion
- Tissue damage
  - Extensive burns and trauma
  - Heat stroke
  - Severe head injury
  - Transplant rejections
  - Postoperative damage, especially after extracorporeal membrane oxygenation
  - Fat and pulmonary emboli
  - Snakebites
  - Glomerulonephritis
  - Acute anoxia (e.g., after cardiac arrest)
  - Prosthetic devices

Subacute DIC
- Malignant disease
  - Acute leukemias
  - Metastatic cancer
- Obstetric
  - Retained dead fetus

Chronic DIC
- Liver disease
- Systemic lupus erythematosus
- Localized malignancy

DIC, disseminated intravascular coagulation.

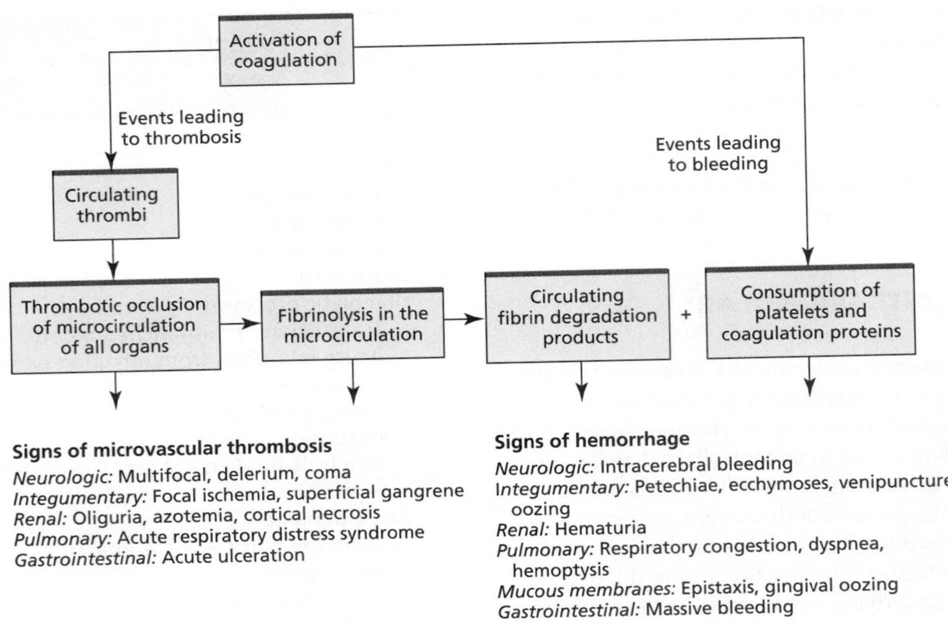

Fig. 29-10 The sequence of events that occur during disseminated intravascular coagulation (DIC), leading to the clinical appearance of thrombotic and hemorrhagic phenomena.

Thrombotic manifestations are a result of fibrin or platelet deposition in the microvasculature (see Fig. 29-10) and include integumentary changes, such as acral cyanosis, ischemic tissue necrosis (e.g., gangrene), and hemorrhagic necrosis; respiratory changes, such as tachypnea, dyspnea, pulmonary emboli, and acute respiratory distress syndrome; cardiovascular changes, such as ECG changes and venous distention; GI changes, such as abdominal pain and paralytic ileus; and urinary changes, such as oliguria.

Diagnostic Studies

Tests used to diagnose acute DIC and their findings are listed in Table 29-21. As more clots are made in the body, more breakdown products from fibrinogen and fibrin are also formed. These are termed *fibrin split products* (FSPs) or *fibrin degradation products* (FDPs), and they work in three ways to interfere with blood coagulation. First, they coat the platelets and interfere with platelet function. Second, they interfere with thrombin and thereby disrupt coagulation. Third, the FSPs attach to fibrinogen, which interferes with the polymerization process necessary to form a stable clot. A much more specific test that is replacing measurement of FSP is the D-Dimer assay. D-Dimer, a specific polymer resulting from the breakdown of fibrin (and not fibrinogen), is a much more specific marker of the degree of fibrinolysis. In general, tests that measure *raw materials* needed for coagulation (e.g., platelets and fibrinogen) are reduced, and values that measure *times to clot* are prolonged. Fragmented erythrocytes (schistocytes), indicative of partial occlusion of small vessels by fibrin thrombi, may be found on blood smears.

Table 29-21 Laboratory Abnormalities of Acute Disseminated Intravascular Coagulation

Test	Finding (Incidence)
Screening Tests	
Prothrombin time	Prolonged (75%) Normal or shortened (25%)
Partial thromboplastin time	Prolonged (50-60%)
Activated partial thromboplastin time	Prolonged
Thrombin time	Prolonged
Fibrinogen	Reduced
Platelets	Reduced to below 100,000/μl (100×10^9/L) to 5000/μl (5×10^9/L) in some
Special Tests	
Fibrin split products (FSP)*	Elevated (75-100%)
Factor assays (for factors V, VII, VIII, X, XIII)	Reduced
D-Dimers (cross-linked fibrin fragments)	Elevated (more reliable than FSP)
Antithrombin III	Reduced (90%)

*Fibrin degradation products (FDP).

Collaborative Care

It is important to diagnose DIC quickly, institute therapy that will resolve the underlying causative disease or problem, and provide supportive care for the manifestations resulting from the pathology of DIC itself. The treatment of DIC remains controversial and under investigation as researchers attempt to determine the most suitable means of managing this dangerous syndrome. Consequently it is imperative that the nurse maintain an ongoing awareness of current modes of therapy. Regardless of the etiology, treating the primary disease process is essential to the resolution of DIC.

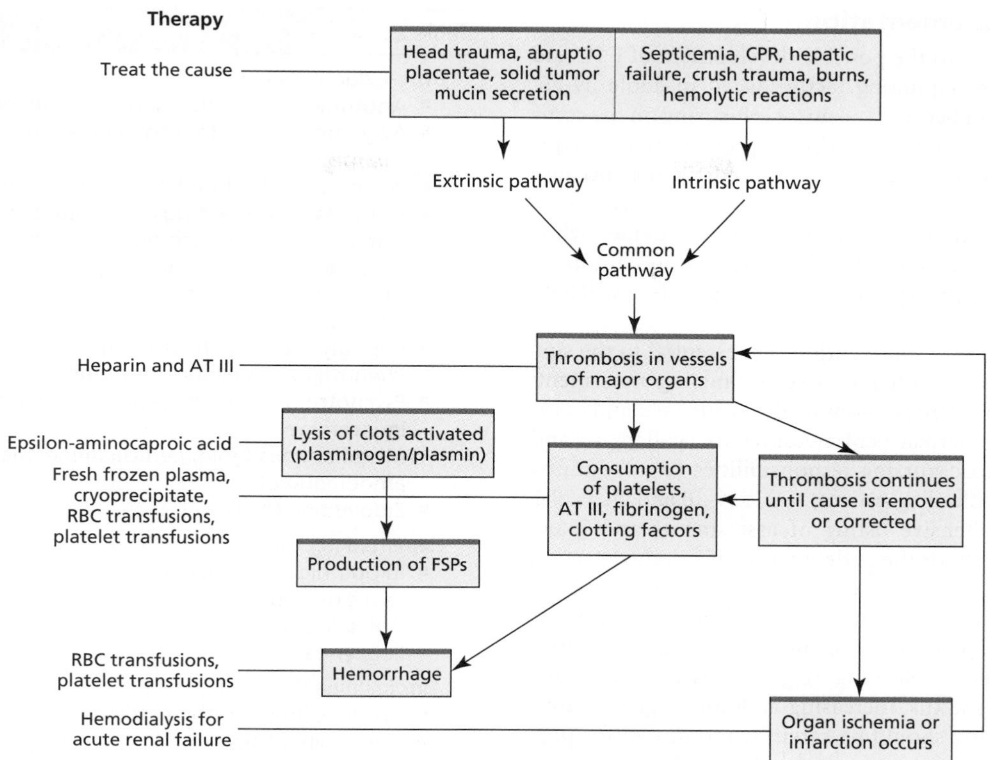

Fig. 29-11 Intended sites of action for therapies in disseminated intravascular coagulation. *CPR*, cardiopulmonary resuscitation; *FSP*, fibrin split products.

Depending on its severity, a variety of different methods are used to provide supportive and symptomatic management of DIC (Fig. 29-11). First, if chronic DIC is diagnosed in a patient who is not bleeding, no therapy for DIC is necessary. Treatment of the underlying disease may be sufficient to reverse the DIC (e.g., antineoplastic therapy when DIC is caused by malignancy). Second, when the patient with DIC is bleeding, therapy is directed toward providing support with necessary blood products while treating the primary disorder. The blood products are administered on the basis of specific component deficiencies. Platelets are given to correct thrombocytopenia, cryoprecipitate replaces factor VIII and fibrinogen, and fresh frozen plasma (FFP) replaces all clotting factors except platelets and provides a source of antithrombin.

A patient with manifestations of thrombosis is often treated by anticoagulation with heparin. However, the use of heparin in the treatment of DIC remains controversial. Antithrombin III (AT III), a cofactor of heparin that becomes depleted during DIC, has been used alone or in conjunction with heparin when levels of this factor are low. Hirudin, a thrombin inhibitor and neutralizer, is also being studied as a blocker of the abnormal coagulation process.[18] Another treatment that has been used is epsilon aminocaproic acid (EACA, Amicar) because of its ability to inhibit fibrinolysis. The use of EACA is controversial because it can enhance thrombosis. Generally it is used only as adjunctive therapy to heparin. Blood product support with platelets, cryoprecipitate, and FFP is usually reserved for a patient with life-threatening hemorrhage. The concern is that one is adding "fuel to the fire" of already activated coagulation. However, it may be the only method to avoid fatal hemorrhage in some patients. Therapy will stabilize a patient, prevent exsanguination or massive thrombosis, and permit institution of definitive therapy to treat the underlying cause.

Chronic DIC does not respond to oral anticoagulants, but it can be controlled with long-term use of heparin. Some patients with indolent (inactive and slowly developing) tumors and severe, chronic DIC may need continuous infusion of heparin with portable pumps.

NURSING MANAGEMENT: DISSEMINATED INTRAVASCULAR COAGULATION

Nursing Diagnoses

Nursing diagnoses for patient with DIC may include, but are not limited to, the following:

- Altered cerebral, cardiopulmonary, renal, GI, and peripheral tissue perfusion *related to* bleeding and sluggish or diminished blood flow secondary to thrombosis
- Pain *related to* bleeding into tissues and diagnostic procedures
- Decreased cardiac output *related to* fluid volume deficit and hypotension
- Anxiety *related to* fear of the unknown, disease process, diagnostic procedures, and therapy

Nursing Implementation

Nurses must be alert to the possible development of DIC and especially to the precipitating factors listed in Table 29-20. This may be difficult because the nurse is focusing on the complex care often required by the primary problem that precipitated the DIC. The nurse must also remember that because DIC is secondary to an underlying disease, appropriate care for managing the causative problem must be provided while providing supportive care related to the manifestations of DIC. Correcting the primary disease (when possible) will help resolve the DIC.

Appropriate nursing interventions are essential to the survival of a patient with acute DIC. Astute, ongoing assessment; active attention to manifestations of the syndrome; and institution of appropriate treatment measures are challenging and sometimes paradoxic nursing responsibilities (e.g., administering heparin to a bleeding patient). Table 29-16 and NCP 29-2 provide a comprehensive listing of assessments and interventions appropriate for the patient with DIC. Early detection of bleeding, both occult and overt, must be a primary goal. The patient should be thoroughly assessed for signs of external bleeding (e.g., petechiae, oozing at IV or injection sites) and signs of internal bleeding (e.g., increased heart rate, changes in mental status, increasing abdominal girth, pain). Any sites of bleeding should be carefully monitored for progression or response to supportive therapies. Tissue damage should be minimized and the patient protected from additional foci of bleeding.

An additional nursing responsibility is to administer blood products properly if they are ordered. Infusing cryoprecipitate or FFP is similar to giving any other blood product (see Table 29-36). Cryoprecipitate comes in bags of 10 to 20 ml each. When it is used to treat DIC, multiple bags of cryoprecipitate may be required to support the patient. A unit of FFP that contains 200 to 280 ml takes about 20 minutes to thaw.

Table 29-22 Causes of Neutropenia

Drug-Induced Causes
- Antitumor antibiotics (daunorubicin, doxorubicin)
- Alkylating agents (nitrogen mustards, busulfan, chlorambucil)
- Antimetabolites (methotrexate, 6-mercaptopurine)
- Antiinflammatory drugs (phenylbutazone)
- Antibacterial drugs (chloramphenicol, trimethoprim-sulfamethoxazole, penicillins)*
- Antiseizure drugs (phenytoin)*
- Antithyroids*
- Hypoglycemics (tolbutamide)*
- Phenothiazines (chlorpromazine)*
- Psychotropics and antidepressants (clozapine, imipramine)
- Miscellaneous (gold, penicillamine, mepacrine, amodiaquine)
- Zidovudine (AZT)

Hematologic Disorders
- Idiopathic neutropenia
- Cyclic neutropenia
- Aplastic anemia
- Leukemia

Autoimmune Disorders
- Systemic lupus erythematosus
- Felty's syndrome
- Rheumatoid arthritis

Infections
- Viral (e.g., hepatitis, influenza, HIV, measles)
- Fulminant bacterial infection (e.g., typhoid fever, miliary tuberculosis)

Miscellaneous
- Severe sepsis
- Bone marrow infiltration (e.g., carcinoma, tuberculosis, lymphoma)
- Hypersplenism (e.g., portal hypertension, Felty's syndrome, storage diseases [e.g., Gaucher's disease])
- Nutritional deficiencies (cobalamin, folic acid)

*Infrequent causes of neutropenia.

NEUTROPENIA

Leukopenia refers to a decrease in the total WBC count (granulocytes, monocytes, and lymphocytes). *Granulocytopenia* is a deficiency of granulocytes, which include neutrophils, eosinophils, and basophils. The neutrophilic granulocytes, which play a major role in phagocytizing pathogenic microbes, are closely monitored in clinical practice as an indicator of a patient's risk for infection. A reduction in neutrophils is termed *neutropenia.* (Some clinicians use the terms *granulocytopenia* and *neutropenia* interchangeably because the largest constituency of the granulocyte family is the neutrophils.) The absolute neutrophil count is determined by multiplying the total WBC count by the percentage of neutrophils. For example, a person with a total WBC of 9800/μl (9.8×10^9/L) and a neutrophil percentage of 72% would have a total of neutrophil count of 7056/μl (7.1×10^9/L). *Neutropenia* is defined as a neutrophil count of less than 1000 to 1500/μl (1 to 1.5×10^9/L).[19] However, in considering the clinical significance of neutropenia it is important to know the rapidity of the decrease in the neutrophil count (gradual or rapid), degree of neutropenia, and duration. The faster the drop, the more profound the bone marrow suppression and the greater the likelihood of developing infection.

Neutropenia is not a disease; it is a syndrome that occurs with a variety of conditions or diseases (Table 29-22). It can also be an expected effect, side effect, or unintentional effect of taking certain medications. The most common cause of neutropenia is iatrogenic, resulting from widespread use of cytotoxic and immunosuppressive therapy used in the treatment of malignancies and autoimmune diseases. A brief overview of the clinical, diagnostic, and therapeutic implications of neutropenia is provided as a foundation for considering the effect of neutropenia in other diseases of WBCs that follow in this chapter.

Clinical Manifestations

The patient with neutropenia is predisposed to infection with nonpathogenic organisms that normally constitute normal body flora, as well as opportunistic pathogens. When the WBC count is depressed or immature WBCs are present, normal

COLLABORATIVE CARE

Table 29-23 Neutropenia

Diagnostic
- History and physical examination
- WBC count with differential count
- WBC morphology
- Hct and Hb values
- Reticulocyte and platelet count
- Bone marrow aspiration or biopsy
- Cultures of nose, throat, sputum, urine, stool, obvious lesions, blood (as indicated)
- Chest x-ray

Collaborative Therapy
- Identification and removal of cause of neutropenia (if possible)
- Identification of site of infection (if present) and causative organism
- Antibiotic therapy
- Hematopoietic growth factors (G-CSF, GM-CSF)
- Protective (reverse) isolation
- High-efficiency particulate air (HEPA) filtration
- Laminar airflow isolation

G-CSF, granulocyte colony–stimulating factor; *GM-CSF,* granulocyte-macrophage colony–stimulating factor.

phagocytic mechanisms are impaired. Because of the diminished phagocytic response, the classic signs of inflammation—redness, heat, and swelling—may not occur. WBCs are the major component of pus; therefore, in the patient with neutropenia, pus formation (e.g., as a visible skin lesion or as pulmonary infiltrates on a chest x-ray) is also absent. Therefore the presence of fever is of great significance in recognizing the presence of infection in a neutropenic patient.[20]

When fever occurs in a neutropenic patient, it is generally assumed to be caused by infection and requires immediate attention because the immunocompromised, neutropenic patient lacks normal protective mechanisms. A neutropenic condition can lead to a rapid and sometimes fatal progression of minor infections to sepsis. The mucous membranes of the throat and mouth, the skin, the perianal area, and the pulmonary system are common entry points for pathogenic organisms in susceptible hosts. Clinical manifestations related to infection at these sites include complaints of sore throat and dysphagia, appearance of ulcerative lesions of the pharyngeal and buccal mucosa, diarrhea, rectal tenderness, vaginal itching or discharge, shortness of breath, and nonproductive cough. These seemingly minor complaints can progress to fever, chills, sepsis, and septic shock if not recognized and treated in early stages.

Systemic infections caused by bacterial, fungal, and viral organisms are common in patients with neutropenia. The patient's own flora (normally nonpathogenic) have been identified as contributing significantly to life-threatening infections such as pneumonia. Organisms that are known to be common sources of infection include gram-positive *Staphylococcus aureus* and aerobic gram-negative organisms. *Pneumocystis carinii* is an especially serious cause of pneumonia. Fungi that are involved include *Candida* (usually *C. albicans*) and *Aspergillus.* Viral infections caused by reactivation of herpes simplex and zoster are common following prolonged periods of neutropenia.[20]

Diagnostic Studies

The primary diagnostic tests for assessing neutropenia are the peripheral WBC count and bone marrow aspiration and biopsy (Table 29-23). A total WBC count of less than 5000/μl (5×10^9/L) reflects leukopenia. However, only a differential count can confirm the presence of neutropenia (neutrophil count <1000 to 1500/μl [1 to 1.5×10^9/L]). If the differential WBC count reflects an absolute neutropenia of 500 to 1000/μl (0.5 to 1.0×10^9/L), the patient is at moderate risk for a bacterial infection; an absolute neutropenia of less than 500/μl (0.5×10^9/L) places the patient at severe risk.

A peripheral blood smear is used to assess for immature forms of WBCs. The Hct level, reticulocyte count, and platelet count are done to evaluate general bone marrow function. Bone marrow aspirations and biopsies are done to examine cellularity and cell morphology. Additional studies may be done as indicated to assess spleen and liver function.

NURSING AND COLLABORATIVE MANAGEMENT: NEUTROPENIA

The factors involved in the nursing and collaborative care of neutropenia include (1) determining the cause of the neutropenia; (2) identifying the offending organisms if an infection has developed; (3) instituting prophylactic, empiric, or therapeutic antibiotic therapy; (4) administering hematopoietic growth factors (e.g., granulocyte colony–stimulating factor [G-CSF] and granulocyte-macrophage colony–stimulating factor [GM-CSF]); and (5) instituting protective isolation practices, such as strict hand washing, visitor restrictions, private room, high-efficiency particulate air (HEPA) filtration, or laminar airflow (LAF) environment (see Table 29-23).

Occasionally the cause of the neutropenia can be easily removed (e.g., by termination of phenothiazines). However, neutropenia can also be a side effect that must be tolerated as a necessary step in therapy (e.g., chemotherapy or radiation therapy). In some situations the neutropenia resolves when the primary disease is treated (e.g., tuberculosis).

One aspect of vigilant monitoring of the neutropenic patient is constantly evaluating for signs and symptoms of infection. Early identification of a potentially infective organism depends on acquiring cultures from various sites. Serial blood cultures (at least two) and cultures of sputum, throat, lesions, wounds, urine, and feces are essential in the surveillance of the patient. It may also be necessary to do a tracheal aspiration, bronchoscopy with bronchial brushings, or lung biopsy to diagnose the cause of pneumonic infiltrates. Despite these many tests, the causative organism is usually identified only in approximately one half of patients.[20]

When a febrile episode occurs in a neutropenic patient, antibiotic therapy must be initiated immediately. The life-threatening nature of infection in a neutropenic host necessitates the institution of broad-spectrum antibiotics before the determination of a specific causative organism by culture. Administration of antibiotics is usually by the IV route because of the rapidly lethal effects of infection. However, some oral antibiotics are highly effective and routinely used for prophylaxis against infection in some neutropenic patients. Antibiotics are often used in combinations because of their synergistic effects. Combinations of antibiotics are also used in the event that multiple organisms are responsible for the infectious symptoms. Usually an aminoglycoside is used with an antipseudomonal penicillin or cephalosporin. Regardless of the combination, the nurse must observe for side effects of antimicrobial agents. Side effects common to aminoglycosides include nephrotoxicity and ototoxicity; side effects common to cephalosporins include rashes, fever, and pruritus.

G-CSF (filgrastim [Neupogen]) and GM-CSF (sargramostim [Leukine, Prokine]) can be used to treat a neutropenic patient. These factors are especially beneficial in enhancing granulocyte recovery after chemotherapy and shorten the period of vulnerability to fatal infections. These CSFs also have the potential benefit of enhancing the phagocytic and cytotoxic activities of neutrophils. In addition to growth factors, monocyte-CSF, interferon-gamma, and interleukin-1 (IL-1), IL-3, and IL-6 may show potential usefulness in treating neutropenic patients.[20] (These factors are discussed in Chapter 12.)

An important consideration in the care of a neutropenic patient is the determination of the best means to protect the patient whose own defenses against infection are compromised. The principles to keep in mind to accomplish this goal are (1) the patient's normal flora is the most common source of microbial colonization and infection; (2) transmission of organisms from humans most commonly occurs by direct contact with the hands; (3) air, food, water, and equipment provide additional opportunities for infection transmission; and (4) health care providers with transmittable illnesses and other patients with infections can also be sources of infection transmission under certain conditions.

Strict hand washing by all persons coming in contact with the compromised patient is the major method to prevent transmission of harmful pathogens. The Centers for Disease Control and Prevention (CDC) advocates hand washing before, during, and after care. This seemingly routine technique has a significant effect in reducing infection. It must be emphasized and enforced despite its seeming simplicity.

The CDC also encourages separating immunocompromised patients from those who are infected or who have conditions that increase the probability of transmitting infections (e.g., poor hygiene caused by lack of understanding or cognitive dysfunction). Private rooms are useful whenever possible. HEPA filtration is an air-handling method with a high-flow filtering system that can reduce or eliminate the number of aerosolized pathogens in the environment. Although it is expensive to install, it is often used for a patient with severe prolonged neutropenia. Care routines in an HEPA environment are essentially the same as care in any other private room.

For severely immunocompromised patients (e.g., bone marrow transplants, high-dose chemotherapy) routine protective isolation techniques may be warranted. These include LAF rooms, nonabsorbable prophylactic antibiotics, and avoidance of fresh fruit and vegetables. Although LAF rooms can reduce the incidence of hospital-acquired infections in severely neutropenic patients, long-term survival has not been increased in most of these patients. Cost, lack of sufficient improvement in long-term survival, and the psychologic effects to a patient isolated in an LAF room have contributed to the declining construction of new LAF rooms.[21] The nursing measures presented in NCP 29-3 are important in the treatment of the patient with neutropenia.

The value of effective nursing care in reducing the development of infection or limiting its extent cannot be overemphasized. Regular assessment and early detection of infectious sources are key roles for the nurse in reducing morbidity and mortality from infection.

MYELODYSPLASTIC SYNDROME

Myelodysplastic syndrome (MDS) is any of a group of related hematologic disorders characterized by a change in the quantity and quality of bone marrow elements. Other terms used to describe this hematologic disorder include preleukemia, hematopoietic dysplasia, refractory anemia with excessive myeloblasts, subacute myeloid leukemia, oligoplastic leukemia, and smoldering leukemia.[22]

Etiology and Pathophysiology

The etiology of MDS is unknown. Its manifestations result from neoplastic transformation of the pluripotent hematopoietic stem cells within the bone marrow. MDS is referred to as a clonal disorder because some bone marrow stem cells continue to function normally while others (a specific clone) do not. Occasionally one type of MDS transforms into another. In approximately 30% of cases, MDS will progress to acute myelogenous leukemia. Typically, life-threatening anemia, thrombocytopenia, and neutropenia will occur during the advanced stage of MDS.

The abnormal clone of the stem cells is usually found in the bone marrow but eventually may be found in circulation. In contrast to acute myelogenous leukemia (AML), in which the leukemic cells show little normal maturation, the clonal cells in MDS always display some degree of maturity. Disease progression is slower than in AML. However, eventually the bone marrow is replaced partly or wholly by the abnormal cells.

Clinical Manifestations

MDS is found more often in the elderly and is most often discovered as a result of testing for complications of anemia, thrombocytopenia, or neutropenia. However, there are other cases in which there are no symptoms and diagnosis results from a routine complete blood count (CBC).

Infection and bleeding are common and result from either inadequate numbers of or poorly functioning circulating cells or platelets. Neutropenia usually precedes infection. Some patients may have normal numbers of granulocytes but become infected as a result of the ineffective functioning of these circulating granulocytes.

Diagnostic Studies

Bone marrow aspiration and biopsies are essential for both the diagnosis and the classification of the specific types of myelodysplasia. In MDS the bone marrow is normocellular, hypocellular, or hypercellular in the presence of peripheral cy-

29-3 NURSING CARE PLAN PATIENT WITH NEUTROPENIA

Expected Patient Outcomes	Nursing Interventions and *Rationales*
NURSING DIAGNOSIS	**Risk for infection** *related to* decreased neutrophils and altered response to microbial invasion and presence of environmental pathogens.
▪ Free from signs and symptoms of infection. ▪ Minimal exposure to environmental pathogens.	▪ Monitor for fever and absolute neutrophil count *to identify signs of and potential for infection.* ▪ Evaluate for presence of chills and malaise and determine temperature q4hr *because fever may be the only indication of infection.* ▪ Report temperature elevations >100.4° F (38° C) to physician immediately *in order to promptly initiate antibiotic therapy because of the rapidly lethal effects of infection.* ▪ Be aware of chills, complaints of being cold when environment is warm, sore throat, persistent cough, chest pain, burning on urination, rectal pain, confusion *because these may be local and systemic signs of infection.* ▪ Use proper skin preparation techniques for initiating and maintaining IVs, caring for venous access devices, or obtaining blood culture specimens *to reduce the risk of introducing infection through the skin.* ▪ Establish antibiotic administration schedule *to maximize pharmacologic effects and minimize side effects of drugs.* ▪ Assess for superinfections *because these may develop with extended use of antibiotics.* ▪ Institute good hand-washing technique with antiseptic solution for all persons in contact with patient; place patient in private room; limit or screen visitors and hospital staff members with colds or potentially communicable illnesses *to prevent the transmission of harmful pathogens to patient.* ▪ Teach patient necessary personal hygiene techniques (e.g., hand washing, pulmonary hygiene). ▪ Routinely culture common sources of contamination (e.g., bathtubs or shower heads, respiratory therapy equipment) *to determine possible environmental sources of harmful pathogens.* ▪ Avoid invasive procedures to the greatest extent possible (e.g., venipunctures, urinary catheters, enemas, rectal suppositories). Provide meticulous perianal care *to prevent perirectal abscess.* ▪ Administer hematopoietic growth factors as ordered (e.g., G-CSF, GM-CSF) *to increase patient's WBC count and reduce infection risk during periods of neutropenia.*

G-CSF, granulocyte colony-stimulating factor; *Gm-CSF*, granulocyte-monocyte colony-stimulating factor.

topenias. MDS is staged according to clinical and laboratory findings. The relationship between the number of circulating blast cells and the number of blast cells in the bone marrow serves as the main indicator of prognosis in this disease.

NURSING AND COLLABORATIVE MANAGEMENT: MYELODYSPLASTIC SYNDROME

Supportive treatment of MDS is based on the premise that the aggressiveness of treatment should match the aggressiveness of the disease. Supportive treatment consists of simple hematologic monitoring (serial bone marrow and peripheral blood examinations), antibiotic therapy, or transfusions with blood products. Side effects and toxicities from supportive treatment include anemia, thrombocytopenia, and blood transfusion reactions.

Differentiation-inducing agents can correct the defective maturation of the hematopoietic stem cell clone in the marrow in about 25% to 35% of patients. Some agents have been shown to transform nonfunctional immature blasts and promyelocytes into functional mature granulocytes.[22] These agents include retinoic acid (Tretinoin) and cytarabine (Ara-C). Response rates have ranged from no response to improvement in survival in some patients. Side effects and toxicities from retinoic acid include dry skin, dry lips, myalgias, lethargy, and hypercalcemia. Bone marrow transplantation, biologic therapy, and colony-stimulating factors have also been used in an attempt to treat bone marrow dysfunction of MDS. However, because of the aggressiveness of these treatments, they are not often tolerated by older patients.

Nursing care of a patient with MDS is similar to that of a patient with manifestations of anemia (see nursing care plan for the patient with anemia [NCP 29-1]), thrombocytopenia (see nursing care plan for the patient with thrombocytopenia [NCP 29-2]), and neutropenia (see nursing care plan for the patient with neutropenia [NCP 29-3]). The nurse must educate the patient about the risks of infection, bleeding, and fatigue.

Table 29-24 Types of Leukemia

Type/Incidence*	Age of Onset	Clinical Manifestations	Diagnostic Findings
Acute myelogenous leukemia—33%	Increase in incidence with advancing age, peak incidence between 60-70 yr of age	Fatigue and weakness, headache, mouth sores, minimal hepatosplenomegaly and lymphadenopathy, anemia, bleeding, fever, infection, sternal tenderness	Low RBC count, Hb, Hct; low platelet count; low to high WBC count with myeloblasts; greatly hypercellular bone marrow with myeloblasts
Acute lymphocytic leukemia—11%	Before 14 yr of age, peak incidence between 2-9 yr of age and in older adults	Fever; pallor; bleeding; anorexia; fatigue and weakness; bone, joint, and abdominal pain; generalized lymphadenopathy; infections; weight loss; hepatosplenomegaly; headache; mouth sores; neurologic manifestations, including CNS involvement, increased intracranial pressure, secondary to meningeal infiltration	Low RBC count, Hb, Hct; low platelet count; low, normal, or high WBC count; transverse lines of rarefaction at ends of metaphysis of long bones on x-ray; hypercellular bone marrow with lymphoblasts; lymphoblasts also possible in cerebrospinal fluid
Chronic myelogenous leukemia—15%	25-60 yr of age, peak incidence around 45 yr of age	No symptoms early in disease, fatigue and weakness, fever, sternal tenderness, weight loss, joint pain, bone pain, massive splenomegaly, increase in sweating	Low RBC count, Hb, Hct; high platelet count early, lower count later; increase in polymorphonuclear neutrophils, normal number of lymphocytes, and normal or low number of monocytes in WBC differential; low leukocyte alkaline phosphatase; presence of Philadelphia chromosome in 90% of patients
Chronic lymphocytic leukemia—25%	50-70 yr of age, rare below 30 yr of age, predominance in men	No symptoms usually, detection of disease often during examination for unrelated condition, chronic fatigue, anorexia, splenomegaly and lymphadenopathy, hepatomegaly	Mild anemia and thrombocytopenia with disease progression; increase in peripheral lymphocytes; increase in presence of lymphocytes in bone marrow

*This is the incidence based on all types of leukemia; the number does not add up to 100% because approximately 16% are unclassifiable.

LEUKEMIA

Leukemia is the general term used to describe a group of malignant disorders affecting the blood and blood-forming tissues of the bone marrow, lymph system, and spleen. Leukemia occurs in all age-groups. It results in an accumulation of dysfunctional cells because of a loss of regulation in cell division. It follows a progressive course that is eventually fatal if untreated. An estimated 28,700 new cases were diagnosed in 1998.[23] Table 29-24 summarizes the relative incidences of the different subtypes and their hallmark features. Although often thought of as a disease of children, the number of adults affected with leukemia is 10 times that of children.

Etiology and Pathophysiology

Regardless of the specific type of leukemia, there is generally no single causative agent in the development of leukemia. Most leukemias result from a combination of factors, including genetic and environmental influences. Chromosomal changes, first recognized in chronic myelogenous leukemia (which involves Philadelphia chromosome), have led to discoveries of how normal genes, once transformed, can result in abnormal genes (oncogenes) capable of causing many types of cancers, including leukemias (see Chapter 14). Chemical agents (e.g., benzene), chemotherapeutic agents (e.g., alkylating agents), viruses, radiation, and immunologic deficiencies have all been associated with the development of leukemia in susceptible hosts. There is an increased incidence of leukemia in radiologists, persons who lived near nuclear bomb test sites or nuclear reactor accidents (e.g., Chernobyl), survivors of the bombing of Nagasaki and Hiroshima, and persons previously treated with radiotherapy or chemotherapy. Although RNA retroviruses cause a number of leukemias in animals, a viral cause for a human leukemia has been established only for some patients with adult T cell leukemia, which is caused by the human T cell leukemia virus type I (HTLV-1). This form of leukemia is endemic in southwestern Japan and parts of the Caribbean and central Africa.

The two major categories of leukemia are acute and chronic. Acute leukemia is characterized by the clonal proliferation of

Table 29-25 The French-American-British (FAB) Classification of Acute Myelogenous Leukemias

Classification	Category	Abbreviation	Percent of Cases
AML M1	Myeloblastic leukemia	AML	19%
AML M2	Myeloblastic leukemia with maturation	AML	29%
AML M3	Promyelocytic leukemia	APL	9%
AML M4	Myelomonocytic leukemia	AMML	19%
AML M5	Monocytic leukemia	AMoL	15%
AML M6	Erythroleukemia	AEL	4%
AML M7	Megakaryoblastic leukemia	AMegL	4%
AML M0	Undifferentiated leukemia		1%

immature hematopoietic cells. The leukemia arises following malignant transformation of a single hematopoietic progenitor, followed by cellular replication and expansion of the transformed clone. The most prominent characteristic of the neoplastic cell in acute leukemia is a defect in maturation beyond the myeloblast or promyelocyte level in acute myelogenous leukemia and the lymphoblast level in acute lymphocytic leukemia (see Fig. 28-1).

Chronic lymphocytic leukemia (CLL) is a neoplasm of activated B lymphocytes. The CLL cells, which morphologically resemble mature, small lymphocytes of the peripheral blood, accumulate in the bone marrow, blood, lymph nodes, and spleen in large numbers.

Chronic myelogenous leukemia (CML) is a clonal stem cell disorder characterized by greatly increased myelopoiesis and the presence of the Philadelphia chromosome. The chromosomal abnormality found in 90% of individuals with CML is the translocation of genetic material from chromosome 22 to chromosome 9. The resulting chromosome 22 is termed the *Philadelphia chromosome.* Although no specific etiologic agent has been identified, an increased incidence of CML was observed in survivors of the atomic bombs in Japan. The incidence of CML in these individuals was dose related.

Clinical Manifestations

The clinical manifestations of leukemia are varied (see Table 29-24). Essentially they relate to problems caused by bone marrow failure and the formation of masses composed of leukemic infiltrates. Bone marrow failure results from (1) bone marrow crowding by abnormal cells and (2) inadequate production of normal marrow elements. The patient is predisposed to anemia, thrombocytopenia, and decreased number and function of WBCs.

As leukemia progresses, fewer normal blood cells are produced. Abnormal WBCs continue to accumulate because they do not go through the normal cell life cycle to death. The increased numbers of WBCs can lead to infiltration and damage to the bone marrow, lymph nodes, spleen, and other organs, including the central nervous system (CNS). Leukemic infiltration leads to problems such as splenomegaly, hepatomegaly, lymphadenopathy, bone pain, meningeal irritation, and oral lesions. Solid masses resulting from collections of leukemic cells, called *chloromas,* can also occur.

Diagnostic Studies and Classification

The goal of diagnostic studies is to define the subclass or specific type of leukemia so that the appropriate treatment and prognosis can be determined. Peripheral blood evaluation and bone marrow examination are the primary methods of diagnosing and classifying the subtypes of leukemia. (See Tables 29-25 and 29-26 for these classifications.) Morphologic, histochemical, immunologic, and cytogenetic methods are all used to identify cell subtypes and the stage of development of leukemic cell populations. Further studies such as lumbar puncture and computed tomography (CT) scan can determine the presence of leukemic cells outside of the blood and bone marrow.

Table 29-26 French-American-British (FAB) Classification of Acute Lymphocytic Leukemias

L1	Common childhood leukemia
L2	Adult acute lymphocytic leukemia
L3	Rare subtype, blasts resembling those in Burkitt's lymphoma

In the past, the designations of acute and chronic leukemia had significant prognostic implications related to the duration of the illness. However, current therapeutic measures have increased the survival of patients with certain forms of acute leukemia beyond that of patients with certain forms of chronic leukemia. Although the terms *acute* and *chronic* are still used, they refer primarily to cell maturity and the nature of the disease onset. In acute leukemia, the bone marrow is infiltrated with young, undifferentiated, immature cells, often termed *blasts.* The disease has a rapid onset and requires immediate and aggressive intervention. The bone marrow in an individual with chronic leukemia consists primarily of differentiated mature WBCs, and the disease onset is more gradual.

Additional classification of leukemia is done by identifying the type of leukocyte involved, whether of myelogenous origin (granulocyte, monocyte, erythrocyte, megakaryocyte) or of lymphocytic origin. By combining the acute and chronic categories with the cell type involved, specific types of leukemia can be identified. Four major types of leukemia are acute lymphocytic leukemia (ALL), acute myelogenous leukemia (AML) (also called acute nonlymphoblastic leukemia [ANLL]), chronic myelogenous (granulocytic) leukemia (CML), and chronic lymphocytic leukemia (CLL). Other defining features of these leukemic subtypes are presented in Table 29-24.

Leukemias are also classified using the French-American-British (FAB) classification system. The FAB system divides acute myelogenous leukemia into seven subtypes (see Table 29-25) according to the direction of differentiation along one or more cell lines and the degree of cellular maturation. Three types of acute lymphocytic leukemia (see Table 29-26) are distinguished by certain cytologic features and the degree of heterogeneity of the leukemic cell population. The traditional AML (ANLL) and ALL labels are used in conjunction with the FAB nomenclature. Additional work is being done using monoclonal antibodies, molecular cell markers, and genetic probes to more accurately distinguish among the many types of leukemic WBCs and their precursors to facilitate diagnosis, classification, and treatment of leukemia.

Acute Myelogenous Leukemia. AML is also referred to as ANLL, as previously mentioned. Although only one fourth of all leukemias are of this subtype, it makes up approximately 85% of the acute leukemias in adults. Its onset is often abrupt and dramatic. A patient may have serious infections and abnormal bleeding.

AML is characterized by uncontrolled proliferation of myeloblasts, the precursors of granulocytes (see Fig. 28-1). There is hyperplasia of the bone marrow and spleen. The clinical manifestations are usually related to replacement of normal hematopoietic cells in the marrow by leukemic cells and, to a lesser extent, to infiltration of other organs (see Table 29-24).

Acute Lymphocytic Leukemia. ALL is most common in children and accounts for 15% of acute leukemia in adults. In ALL, immature lymphocytes proliferate in the bone marrow. Fever is present in the majority of patients at the time of diagnosis. Signs and symptoms may appear abruptly with bleeding or fever, or they may be insidious with progressive weakness, fatigue, and bleeding tendencies. CNS manifestations are especially common in ALL and represent a serious problem. Leukemic meningitis caused by arachnoid infiltration occurs in many patients with ALL.

Chronic Myelogenous Leukemia. CML is also termed *chronic granulocytic leukemia* (CGL). CML is caused by excessive development of neoplastic granulocytes in the bone marrow. The excess neoplastic granulocytes move into the peripheral blood in massive numbers and ultimately infiltrate the liver and spleen. Immature and mature granulocytes are found in the bone marrow and peripheral blood, but mature cells are dominant peripherally.

Complications of CML are related to a blast crisis in which chronic leukemia transforms to acute disease (infiltration of more immature cells). In a blastic crisis increased numbers of myeloblasts are found in both the bone marrow and blood. The chronic phase of CML can persist for 2 to 4 years and can usually be well controlled with treatment. Without treatment the chronic phase of the disease will ultimately progress to a more symptomatic accelerated phase, ending in a brief blastic phase in which the disease resembles its acute counterpart. Once CML transforms to an accelerated or blastic phase, it is often refractory to therapy and the patient may live for only a few months.

Chronic Lymphocytic Leukemia. CLL is characterized by the production and accumulation of functionally inactive but long-lived, mature-appearing lymphocytes. The type of lymphocyte involved is usually the B cell. The lymphocytes infiltrate the bone marrow, spleen, and liver. Lymph node enlargement throughout the body is commonly present. There is an increased incidence of infection. Complications from CLL are uncommon initially but may develop as the disease advances. Pressure on nerves from enlarged lymph nodes can cause pain and even paralysis. Mediastinal node enlargement can lead to pulmonary symptoms. Because CLL is a disease of older adults, treatment decisions must be made by considering the progression of the disease and the side effects of treatment. Many individuals in the early stages of CLL require no treatment.

Hairy Cell Leukemia. Hairy cell leukemia accounts for approximately 2% of all adult leukemias. It is a chronic disease of lymphoproliferation predominantly involving B lymphocytes that infiltrate the bone marrow and spleen. Cells have a "hairy" appearance under the microscope. The spleen sequesters increasing numbers of normal hematopoietic cells, making splenomegaly a common finding. Hairy cell leukemia is usually seen in male patients over 40 years of age. A patient with hairy cell leukemia usually has symptoms from splenomegaly, pancytopenia, infection caused by impaired host defense, or vasculitis. Many asymptomatic patients are detected on routine CBC. α-Interferon, pentostatin (Nipent), and cladribine (Leustatin) are effective agents in the treatment of this type of leukemia.

Unclassified Leukemias. Occasionally the subtype of leukemia cannot be identified. The malignant leukemic cells may have lymphoid, myeloid, or mixed characteristics. Often these patients do not respond to treatment. Typically a patient with undifferentiated leukemia has a poorer prognosis. Response to treatment will help identify if a correct diagnosis has been made.

Collaborative Care

Once a diagnosis of leukemia has been made, collaborative care includes remission induction with chemotherapeutic drugs and, sometimes, radiation therapy. Other considerations include regular examination of patients on an ongoing basis to evaluate their progress and supportive interventions to prevent complications of the disease and the therapy (e.g., hemorrhage, infection). The nurse must understand the principles of cancer chemotherapy, including cellular kinetics, the use of multiple drugs rather than single agents, and the cell cycle. (See the section on chemotherapy in Chapter 14.)

Attaining remission is the initial goal of treatment for leukemia. Although not all forms of leukemia are considered curable at this time, attaining an initial remission or disease control is currently a realistic option for the majority of patients. In complete remission there is no evidence of overt disease on physical examination, and the bone marrow and peripheral blood appear normal. A lesser state of control is known as partial remission. Partial remission is characterized by no overt clinical disease and a normal peripheral blood smear, but there is still evidence of disease in the bone marrow. The survival period after diagnosis is increasing as a result of attaining and maintaining remissions. Each time there is a relapse, the succeeding remission may be more difficult to achieve and shorter in duration (Figs. 29-12 and 29-13). With each subsequent therapy a patient needs to consider the likelihood of attaining remission versus experiencing potentially life-threatening side effects.

The chemotherapeutic treatment of acute leukemia is divided into stages. The first stage, *induction therapy*, is the attempt to induce or bring about a remission. Induction is aggressive treatment that seeks to destroy leukemic cells in the

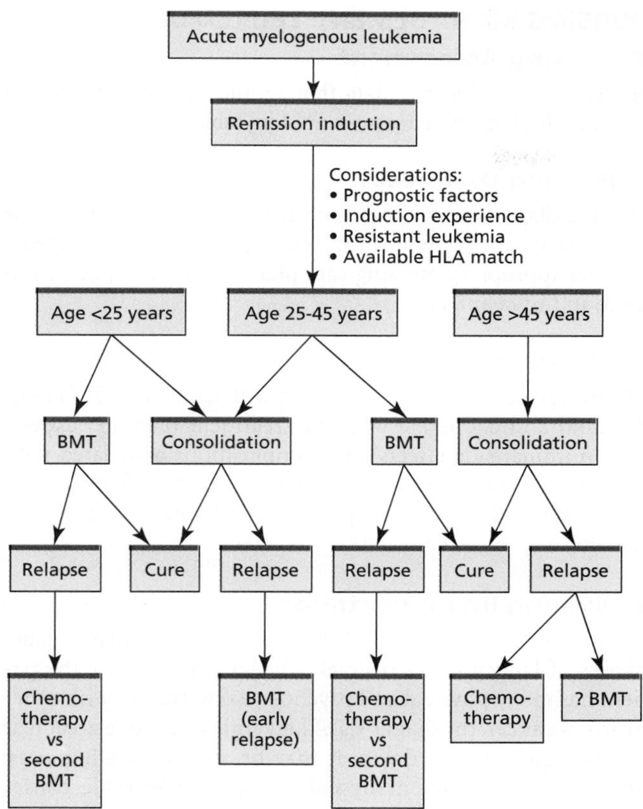

Fig. 29-12 Treatment considerations and options for patients with acute myelogenous leukemia. *BMT,* bone marrow transplant. *HLA,* human leukocyte antigen.

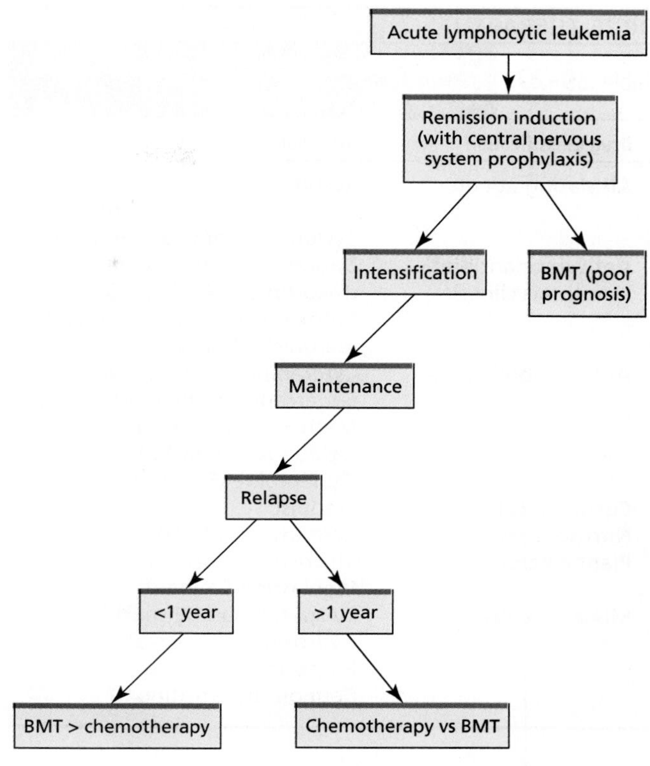

Fig. 29-13 Treatment considerations and options for patients with acute lymphocytic leukemia. *BMT,* bone marrow transplant.

tissues, peripheral blood, and bone marrow. During induction therapy a patient may become devastatingly ill and predisposed to complications because the bone marrow is severely depressed by the drugs. Throughout induction, therapeutic and nursing interventions focused on anemia, thrombocytopenia, and neutropenia may significantly affect the patient's survival. Common chemotherapy for induction of acute myelogenous leukemia includes cytarabine (cytosine arabinoside), an antimetabolite, given for 7 days, and 3 days of antitumor antibiotics (anthracyclines) including daunorubicin, doxorubicin, idarubicin, amsacrine, or mitoxantrone. After one course of induction therapy, approximately 70% of newly diagnosed patients will achieve complete remission.[24,25]

Terms used to describe postremission chemotherapy include intensification, consolidation, and maintenance. *Intensification,* or high-dose therapy, may be given immediately after induction therapy for several months. This therapy may use the same drugs as those used in induction but at higher dosages. Other drugs that target the cell in a different way than those used for induction may also be added. *Consolidation therapy* is started after a remission is achieved. It may consist of one or two additional courses of the same drugs used during induction or involve high-dose therapy (intensive consolidation). The purpose of consolidation therapy is to eliminate remaining leukemic cells.

Maintenance therapy is treatment with lower doses of the same drugs used in induction or other drugs given every 3 to 4 weeks for a prolonged period, usually years. Usually there are few complications and this therapy is well tolerated. The goal is to maintain the remission once it is achieved, thereby keeping the body free of leukemic cells. Each leukemia requires differing lengths of time on maintenance therapy. In AML maintenance therapy is rarely effective and therefore rarely administered.[25]

In addition to chemotherapy, corticosteroids and radiation therapy can also have a role in the complex therapeutic plans for the patient with leukemia. Total body radiation may be used to prepare a patient for bone marrow transplantation, or it may be restricted to certain areas (fields) such as the liver and spleen or other organs affected by infiltrates. In acute lymphocytic leukemia, prophylactic intrathecal methotrexate is given to decrease the chance of CNS involvement, which is common in this particular type of leukemia. When CNS leukemia does occur, cranial radiation is given. Although the incidence of infectious complications has been reduced with the use of biologic therapy, the overall mortality rate has not been affected. This, coupled with its high cost, limits the routine use of biologic therapy. (Biologic therapy is discussed in Chapter 14.)

Chemotherapy Regimens. The chemotherapeutic agents used to treat leukemia vary. The choice of drugs and the sequence of therapy depend on the preference of the oncologist and on current research findings. Table 29-27 lists chemotherapeutic agents used to treat leukemia. Table 29-28 gives examples of treatment regimens used in various types of leukemia.

Combination chemotherapy is the mainstay of treatment for leukemia. The three purposes for using multiple drugs are

DRUG THERAPY

Table 29-27 Chemotherapeutic Agents Used to Treat Leukemia

Drug Classification	Drug Name
Alkylating agents	Busulfan (Myleran)
	Chlorambucil (Leukeran)
	Cyclophosphamide (Cytoxan)
Antitumor antibiotics (Anthracyclines)	Daunorubicin (Cerubidine)
	Doxorubicin (Adriamycin)
	Mitoxantrone (Novantrone)
	Idarubicin (Idamycin)
Antimetabolites	Cytarabine (Cytosar, Ara-C)
	6-mercaptopurine (Purinethol)
	Methotrexate (Folex)
	6-thioguanine (6-TG)
	Fludarabine (Fludara)
Corticosteroid	Prednisone
Nitrosoureas	Carmustine (BCNU)
Plant alkaloid	Vincristine (Oncovin)
	Vinblastine (Velban)
Miscellaneous	L-Asparaginase (Elspar)
	Hydroxyurea (Hydrea)
	Etoposide (VePesid)
	Retinoic acid (tretinoin)

to (1) decrease drug resistance, (2) minimize the toxicity of high doses of single agents by using multiple drugs with varying toxicities, and (3) interrupt cell growth at multiple points in the cell cycle.

Acronyms made from the letters of the drugs used in combination chemotherapy may be used to identify the regimen. For example, *COAP* stands for *c*yclophosphamide, *O*ncovin, *a*rabinoside, and *p*rednisone. This combination of drugs is used to treat acute leukemia.

Bone Marrow and Stem Cell Transplantation. Bone marrow and stem cell transplantation are other forms of therapy used for patients with different forms of leukemia, including ALL, AML, and CML. In leukemia, the goal of transplant is to totally eliminate leukemic cells from the body using combinations of chemotherapy with or without total body irradiation. This treatment also eradicates the patient's hematopoietic stem cells, which are then replaced with those of an HLA-matched sibling or volunteer donor (allogeneic), with those of an identical twin (syngeneic), or with the patient's own (autologous) stem cells that were removed (harvested) before the intensive therapy. (Bone marrow and peripheral stem cell transplantation is discussed in Chapter 14.)

The primary complications of patients with allogeneic BMT are graft-versus-host disease (GVHD), relapse of leukemia (especially ALL), and infection (especially interstitial pneumonia). GVHD is discussed in Chapter 12. Relapse of the underlying disease is also a difficult problem to solve because of the inability for even intensive therapy to eliminate every leukemic cell. Because transplantation has serious associated risks, the patient must weigh the significant risks of treatment-related death or treatment failure (relapse) with the hope of cure.[26,27]

NURSING MANAGEMENT: LEUKEMIA

Nursing Assessment

Subjective and objective data that should be obtained from a patient with leukemia are presented in Table 29-29.

Nursing Diagnoses

Nursing diagnoses for the patient with leukemia include those appropriate for anemia, thrombocytopenia, and neutropenia (see the appropriate nursing care plans [NCPs 29-1, 29-2, and 29-3] in this chapter).

Planning

The overall goals are that the patient with leukemia will (1) understand and cooperate with the treatment plan, (2) experience minimal side effects and complications associated with both the disease and its treatment, and (3) feel hopeful and supported during the periods of treatment, relapse, or remission.

Nursing Implementation

Acute Intervention. The nursing role during acute phases of leukemia is extremely challenging because the patient has many physical and psychosocial needs. As with other forms of cancer, the diagnosis of leukemia can evoke great fear and be equated with death. It may be viewed as a hopeless, horrible disease with many painful and undesirable consequences. The diagnosis of leukemia elicits many emotional responses based on the realization that life is finite. The nurse has a special responsibility in helping the patient and family deal with these feelings. The nurse must help the patient realize that although the future may be uncertain, one can have a meaningful quality of life while in remission or with disease control. The family also needs help in adjusting to the stress of this abrupt onset of serious illness (e.g., dependence, withdrawal, changes in role responsibilities, and alterations in body image) and the losses imposed by the sick role. The diagnosis of leukemia often brings with it the need to make difficult decisions at a time of profound stress for the patient and family.

The nurse is an important advocate in helping the patient and family understand the complexities of treatment decisions and expected side effects and toxicities. A patient empowered by knowledge of the disease and treatment can have a more positive outlook and improved quality of life. A patient may require isolation or may need to temporarily relocate to an appropriate treatment center. These situations can lead a patient to feel deserted and isolated at the time when the most support is needed. The nurse has contact with a patient 24 hours a day, and can help reverse feelings of abandonment and loneliness by balancing the demanding technical needs with a humanistic, caring approach. Therefore a nurse faces a special challenge in learning how to meet the intense psychosocial needs of a patient with leukemia while continuing to offer the complex physical care that is usually required. Consulting with other health professionals (e.g., psychiatric clinical specialists, oncology clinical specialists, social workers) may help the nurse develop the skills required to meet the many needs of a patient with leukemia.

DRUG THERAPY

Table 29-28 Treatments Used in Leukemia

Drug Therapy	Other Therapy
Acute Myelogenous Leukemia	
Daunorubicin, cytarabine, doxorubicin, idarubicin, 6-thioguanine, mitoxantrone, combination chemotherapy of antitumor antibiotic and cytosine arabinoside or antitumor antibiotic and cytosine arabinoside and thioguanine	Bone marrow and stem cell transplant (see Chapter 14)
Acute Lymphocytic Leukemia	
Daunorubicin, doxorubicin, vincristine, prednisone, L-asparaginase, cyclophosphamide, methotrexate, 6-mercaptopurine, cytarabine, combination chemotherapy of cyclophosphamide and vincristine and prednisone and antitumor antibiotic and L-asparaginase, combination chemotherapy of daunorubicin and cytarabine and 6-mercaptopurine and vincristine and prednisone	Cranial radiation therapy, intrathecal methotrexate
Chronic Myelogenous Leukemia	
Busulfan (Myleran); hydroxyurea (Hydrea); combination chemotherapy including any of the following: cytarabine, thioguanine, daunorubicin, methotrexate, prednisone, vincristine, L-asparaginase, carmustine, 6-mercaptopurine	Radiation (total body or spleen), bone marrow and stem cell transplant, α-interferon, leukapheresis
Chronic Lymphocytic Leukemia	
Chorambucil (Leukeran), cyclophosphamide (Cytoxan), prednisone (CVP protocol (cyclophosphamide, vincristine, and prednisone), fludarabine	Radiation (total body, lymph nodes, or spleen), splenectomy, colony-stimulating factors, α-interferon

NURSING ASSESSMENT

Table 29-29 Leukemia

Subjective Data

Important Health Information

Past health history: Exposure to chemical toxins (e.g., benzene, arsenic), radiation, or viruses (Epstein-Barr, HTLV-1); chromosome abnormalities (Down syndrome, Klinefelter's syndrome, Fanconi's syndrome), immunologic deficiencies; organ transplantation; frequent infections; bleeding tendencies

Medications: Use of phenylbutazone (Butazolidin), chloramphenicol, chemotherapy

Surgery and other treatments: Radiation exposure; prior radiation and chemotherapy for cancer

Functional Health Patterns

Health perception–health management: Family history of leukemia; malaise

Nutritional-metabolic: Mouth sores, weight loss; chills, night sweats; nausea, vomiting, anorexia, dysphagia, early satiety; easy bruising

Elimination: Hematuria, decreased urine output; diarrhea, dark or bloody stools

Activity-exercise: Fatigue with progressive weakness; dyspnea, epistaxis, cough

Cognitive-perceptual: Headache; muscle cramps; sore throat; generalized sternal tenderness, bone, joint, abdominal pain; paresthesias, numbness, tingling, visual disturbances

Sexuality-reproductive: Prolonged menses, menorrhagia, impotence

Objective Data

General

Fever, generalized lymphadenopathy, lethargy

Integumentary

Pallor or jaundice; petechiae, ecchymoses, purpura, reddish-brown to purple cutaneous infiltrates, macules, and papules

Cardiovascular

Tachycardia, systolic murmurs

Gastrointestinal

Gingival bleeding and hyperplasia; oral ulcerations, herpes and *Candida* infections; perirectal irritation and infection; hepatosplenomegaly

Neurologic

Seizures, disorientation, confusion, decreased coordination, cranial nerve palsies, papilledema

Musculoskeletal

Muscle wasting

Possible Findings

Low, normal, or high WBC count with shift to the left (↑ blast cells); anemia, decreased hematocrit and hemoglobin, thrombocytopenia, Philadelphia chromosome; hypercellular bone marrow aspirate or biopsy with myeloblasts, lymphoblasts, and markedly reduced normal cells

HTLV-1, human T cell leukemia virus, type 1.

RESEARCH
IMPLICATIONS FOR NURSING PRACTICE

Hope in Cancer Patients

Citation Koopmeiners L and others: How healthcare professionals contribute to hope in patients with cancer, *Oncol Nurs Forum* 24:1501, 1997.

Purpose To explore whether health care professionals influence the level of hope in patients with cancer and, if so, how they influence patients' hope.

Methods Descriptive, qualitative design was used to study 32 male and female patients in an adult hematology/oncology unit. Semistructured interviews were conducted in the patients' rooms. The interviews were analyzed by content analysis, and themes and subthemes were identified that described the roles of health care professionals.

Results and Conclusions Health care professionals can positively and negatively influence hope. Hope was facilitated by being present, giving information, and demonstrating caring behaviors. Negative influences in hope primarily concerned the way in which health care professionals gave information. The conclusions were that health care professionals do influence patients' perceptions of their hope. Although most nursing interventions enhance hope, nurses can reduce a patient's sense of hope if information provided or attitude toward the patient is insensitive or disrespectful.

Implications for Nursing Practice Hope is one of the most essential elements in the lives of patients with cancer. Nurses can increase patients' hope by being present, taking time to talk, and being helpful. They should provide information and answer questions in a compassionate, positive, honest, and respectful manner. Caring behaviors such as thoughtful gestures, showing warmth and genuineness, and being friendly and polite also increase patients' hope. Caring behaviors may play a major role in influencing patients' level of hope, increasing their quality of life, and possibly even increasing their survival.

From a physical care perspective, the nurse is challenged to make astute assessments and plan care to help the patient survive the severe side effects of chemotherapy. The life-threatening results of bone marrow suppression (anemia, thrombocytopenia, neutropenia) require aggressive nursing interventions (see NCPs 29-1, 29-2, and 29-3). Additional complications of chemotherapy may affect the patient's GI tract, nutritional status, skin and mucosa, cardiopulmonary status, liver, kidneys, and neurologic system. (Nursing interventions related to chemotherapy are discussed in Chapter 14.)

The nurse must be knowledgeable about all drugs being administered. This includes the mechanism of action, purpose, routes of administration, usual doses, potential side effects, safe-handling considerations, and toxic effects of the drugs. In addition, the nurse must know how to assess laboratory data reflecting the effects of the drugs. Patient survival and comfort during aggressive chemotherapy are significantly affected by the quality of nursing care.

Ambulatory and Home Care. Ongoing care for the patient with leukemia is necessary to monitor for signs and symptoms of disease control or relapse. For a patient requiring long-term or maintenance chemotherapy, the fatigue of long-term chronic disease management can become arduous and discouraging. Therefore a patient and the significant other must be educated to understand the importance of the continued diligence in disease management and the need for follow-up care. At a minimum the patient and significant other must be taught about the drugs and when to seek medical attention.

The goals of rehabilitation for long-term survivors of childhood and adult leukemia are to manage the physical, psychologic, social, and spiritual consequences and delayed effects from the disease and its treatment. (Delayed effects are discussed in Chapter 14.) Assistance may be needed to reestablish the various relationships that are a part of the patient's life. Friends and family may not know how to interact with the patient. The patient and family must learn to regain attitudes of health and life while facing the real fear of relapse of disease. Involving the patient in survivor networks, support groups, or services such as Can Surmount and Make Today Count may help the patient adapt to living after a life-threatening illness. Exploring resources in the community (e.g., American Cancer Society, Leukemia Society, Meals-on-Wheels, wheelchair taxis) may reduce the financial burden and the feelings of dependence. Spiritual support may give the patient inner strength and peace.

The patient will need support in adapting to any physical limitations or changes imposed by the illness. Vigilant follow-up care by providers who are aware of the unique needs of a cancer survivor is of the utmost importance for early recognition and treatment of long-term or delayed physical, psychologic, and social effects. The nurse may involve other health care providers in meeting the patient's needs. However, often these needs will require the initiation of a referral or consultation. For example, physical therapy personnel may be asked to develop an exercise program to prevent posttreatment deficits caused by drug-induced peripheral neuropathy. These needs can also include other concerns such as growth and development concerns for childhood survivors, vocational retraining, and reproductive concerns for a patient of childbearing age.[26,27] The long-term recovery following treatment for leukemia affects the quality of the patient's life.

Evaluation

The expected outcomes are that the patient with leukemia will

- cope effectively with diagnosis, treatment regimen, and prognosis
- attain and maintain adequate nutrition
- experience no complications related to disease or treatment
- feel comfortable and supported throughout treatment

Table 29-30 Comparison of Hodgkin's Disease and Non-Hodgkin's Lymphoma

	Hodgkin's	Non-Hodgkin's
Cellular origin	Unknown	B lymphocytes (90%) T lymphocytes (10%)
Spread at presentation	Localized to regional	Disseminated
B symptoms*	Common	Uncommon
Histopathologic classification	Singular	Many different classifications (see Table 29-33)
Curability	>75%	30-40%

*B symptoms include fever, night sweats, and weight loss.

LYMPHOMAS

Lymphomas are malignant neoplasms originating in the bone marrow and lymphatic structures resulting in the proliferation of lymphocytes. The cause for the currently rising incidence is not entirely understood, although AIDS-related lymphoma is certainly a factor. Lymphomas are the fifth most common type of cancer in the United States.[23] Two major types of lymphoma—Hodgkin's disease and non-Hodgkin's lymphoma (NHL)—are discussed in this chapter. A comparison of these two types of lymphoma is presented in Table 29-30.

HODGKIN'S DISEASE

Hodgkin's disease, which makes up 15% of all lymphomas, is a malignant condition characterized by proliferation of abnormal giant, multinucleated cells, called *Reed-Sternberg cells,* which are located in lymph nodes. The disease has a bimodal age-specific incidence, occurring most frequently in persons from 15 to 35 years of age and above 50 years of age. In adults, it is twice as prevalent in men as in women.

Etiology and Pathophysiology

Although the cause of Hodgkin's disease remains unknown, several key factors are thought to play a role in its development. The main interacting factors include infection with Epstein-Barr virus (EBV), genetic predisposition, and exposure to occupational toxins.

Normally, the lymph nodes are composed of connective tissues that surround a fine mesh of reticular fibers and cells. In Hodgkin's disease the normal structure of lymph nodes is destroyed by hyperplasia of monocytes and macrophages. The main diagnostic feature of Hodgkin's disease is the presence of Reed-Sternberg cells in lymph node biopsy specimens. The disease is believed to arise in a single location (it originates in lymph nodes in 90% of patients) and then spreads along adjacent lymphatics. It eventually infiltrates other organs, especially the lungs, spleen, and liver. In approximately two thirds of patients the cervical lymph nodes are the first to be affected. When the disease begins above the diaphragm, it remains confined to lymph nodes for a variable period of time. Disease originating below the diaphragm frequently spreads to extralymphoid sites such as the liver.

Clinical Manifestations

The onset of symptoms in Hodgkin's disease is usually insidious. The initial development is most often enlargement of cervical, axillary, or inguinal lymph nodes. This lymphadenopathy affects discrete nodes that remain movable and nontender. The enlarged nodes are not painful unless pressure is exerted on adjacent nerves.

The patient may notice weight loss, fatigue, weakness, fever, chills, tachycardia, or night sweats. A group of initial findings including fever, night sweats, and weight loss (termed *B symptoms*) correlates with a worse prognosis. After the ingestion of even small amounts of alcohol, individuals with Hodgkin's disease may complain of a rapid onset of pain at the site of disease. The cause for the alcohol-induced pain is unknown. Generalized pruritus without skin lesions may develop. Cough, dyspnea, stridor, and dysphagia may all reflect mediastinal node involvement.

In more advanced disease there is hepatomegaly and splenomegaly. Anemia results from increased destruction and decreased production of erythrocytes. Other physical signs vary depending on where the disease has spread. For example, intrathoracic involvement may lead to superior vena cava syndrome, enlarged retroperitoneal nodes may cause palpable abdominal masses or interfere with renal function, jaundice may occur from liver involvement, and spinal cord compression leading to paraplegia may occur with extradural involvement. Bone pain occurs as a result of bone involvement.

Diagnostic and Staging Studies

Peripheral blood analysis, lymph node biopsy, bone marrow examination, and radiologic evaluation are important means of evaluating Hodgkin's disease. Peripheral blood analysis often reveals a microcytic hypochromic anemia, neutrophilic leukocytosis (15,000 to 28,000/μl [15 to 28 $\times$ 10^9/L]), which may be associated with lymphopenia, and an increased platelet count. Leukopenia and thrombocytopenia may develop, but they are usually a consequence of treatment, advanced disease, or superimposed hypersplenism. Other blood studies may show hypoferremia caused by excessive iron uptake by the liver and spleen, elevated leukocyte alkaline phosphatase from liver and bone involvement, hypercalcemia from bone involvement, and hypoalbuminemia from liver involvement.

Excisional lymph node biopsy offers a definitive means of diagnosis. If removed, an enlarged peripheral lymph node can be examined histologically for the presence of the diagnostic Reed-Sternberg cells.

Bone marrow biopsy is performed as an important aspect of staging. In Hodgkin's disease there may be indications of granulocytic and megakaryocytic hyperplasia, but these findings are not unique to Hodgkin's disease. Reed-Sternberg cells may also be found in the bone marrow of patients with advanced disease.

Radiologic evaluation can help define all sites of the disease. Chest x-rays, radioisotope studies, and CT scans may show mediastinal lymphadenopathy, renal displacement caused by retroperitoneal node enlargement, abdominal lymph node enlargement, and liver, spleen, bone, and brain infiltration. Some clinicians also use lymphangiography, a radiographic dye study that uses blue dye injected into the lymphatic system to assess the lymph nodes and lymph vessels. This test can also visualize the sometimes difficult to see retroperitoneal structures.

Diagnostic studies are conducted to assess the stage of Hodgkin's disease. However, there also is a need to demonstrate the actual extent of disease involvement. In the past, a surgical procedure (called a staging laparotomy including splenectomy) was performed to visualize the actual extent of disease involvement. Technologic advances in CT scanning and magnetic resonance imaging (MRI) have augmented the array of techniques available for noninvasive evaluation. Although controversial, many institutions continue to use surgical staging to ensure accurate identification of all sites of disease involvement.

NURSING AND COLLABORATIVE MANAGEMENT: HODGKIN'S DISEASE

Using all of the information from the various diagnostic studies, a stage of disease is determined (Fig. 29-14). Treatment decisions are made based on the stage of disease. Staging involves determining the extent and involvement of the disease. This is important because Hodgkin's disease may be localized or diffuse. Treatment depends on the nature and extent of the disease. The nomenclature used in staging involves an A or B classification, depending on whether symptoms are present when the disease is found, and a Roman numeral (I to IV) that reflects the location and extent of the disease.

Once the stage of Hodgkin's disease is established, management focuses on selecting a treatment plan (Table 29-31). Treatment for Hodgkin's disease has improved considerably and is aimed at cure. The least amount of treatment is used to achieve cure yet minimize the short-term and long-term complications. Radiation therapy given to affected areas over 4 to 6 weeks can cure 95% of patients with stage I or stage II disease. Combination chemotherapy is used in some early stages in patients believed to have resistant disease or be at high risk for relapse. Stage IIIA disease is treated with both radiotherapy and chemotherapy. The role of radiation as a supplement to chemotherapy in stages III and IV varies depending on sites of disease. Advances in treatment now enable some stage IIIB and stage IV diseases to be cured with high-dose chemotherapy and bone marrow or peripheral stem cell transplantation (see Chapter 14).

Intensive chemotherapy with or without the use of bone marrow and peripheral stem cell transplantation and hematopoietic growth factors is the treatment of choice for advanced Hodgkin's disease (stages IIIB and IV). Transplantation has allowed patients to receive higher, potentially curative doses of chemotherapy while reducing life-threatening leukopenia. Combination chemotherapy works well because, as in leukemia, drugs are used that have an additive antitumor effect without increasing side effects. As with leukemia, therapy must be aggressive; therefore potentially life-threatening problems are encountered in an attempt to achieve a remission.[28]

Two chemotherapy regimens termed *MOPP* and *ABVD* have been used alone and in combination to induce remissions in 80% of patients. The acronyms are described in Table 29-32. About 60% to 70% of these patients will be cured.

Maintenance chemotherapy does not contribute to increased survival once a complete remission is achieved. Occasionally, single drugs may be administered palliatively to patients who cannot tolerate intensive combination therapy. A serious consequence of the treatment for Hodgkin's disease is the later development of secondary malignancies (see Chapter 14).

The nursing care for Hodgkin's disease is largely based on managing pancytopenia and other side effects of therapy. Because the survival of patients with Hodgkin's disease depends on their response to treatment, supporting the patient through the immunosuppressive state is extremely important.

The patient undergoing radiotherapy will need special nursing consideration. The skin in the radiation field requires special attention. Also, the nurse must understand the concepts related to administration of radiotherapy (see Chapter 14).

Psychosocial considerations are just as important as they are with leukemia. Although the prognosis for Hodgkin's disease is better than that for many forms of cancer or leukemia, patients must still be helped to deal with all of the physical, psychologic, social, and spiritual consequences of their disease. Evaluation of patients for long-term effects of therapy is important because delayed consequences of disease and treatment may not be apparent for many years.[29] (Secondary malignancies and delayed effects are discussed in Chapter 14.)

NON-HODGKIN'S LYMPHOMA

Non-Hodgkin's lymphomas (NHLs) are a heterogeneous group of malignant neoplasms of the immune system affecting all ages. They are classified according to different cellular and lymph node characteristics (Table 29-33). As more information about the cell types is discovered, evolving schemas have been used to describe different subtypes. A variety of clinical presentations and courses are recognized, from indolent (slowly developing) to rapidly progressive disease. Common names for different types of NHLs include Burkitt's lymphoma, reticulum cell sarcoma, and lymphosarcoma. There is no hallmark feature in NHLs that parallels the Reed-Sternberg cell of Hodgkin's disease. However, all NHLs involve lymphocytes arrested in various stages of development.

NHLs can originate outside the lymph nodes, the method of spread can be unpredictable, and the majority of patients have widely disseminated disease at the time of diagnosis. The primary clinical manifestation is painless lymph node enlargement. Because the disease is usually disseminated when it is diagnosed, other symptoms will be present depending on where the disease has spread (e.g., hepatomegaly with liver involvement).

Patients with high-grade lymphomas may have lymphadenopathy and constitutional ("B") symptoms such as fever, night sweats, and weight loss. The peripheral blood is usually normal, but some lymphomas manifest in a "leukemic" phase.

Diagnostic studies used for NHL resemble those used for Hodgkin's disease. Lymph node biopsy establishes the cell type

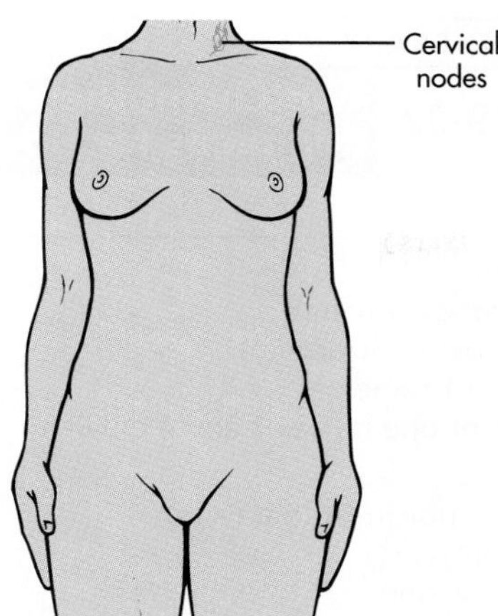

Stage I
Involvement of a single lymph node or a single extranodal site

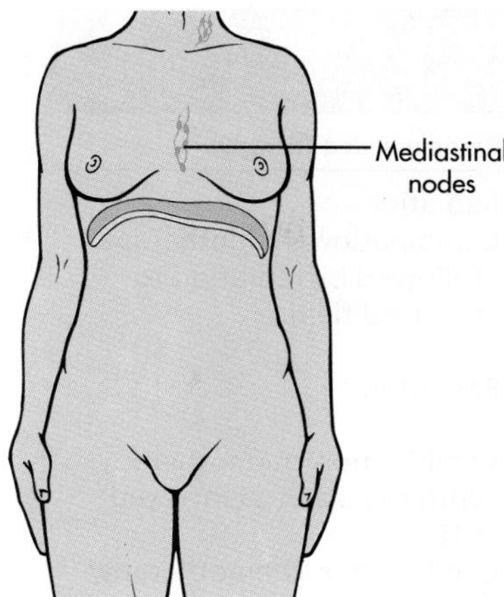

Stage II
Involvement of two or more lymph node regions on the same side of the diaphragm or localized involvement of an extranodal site and one or more lymph node regions of the same side of diaphragm

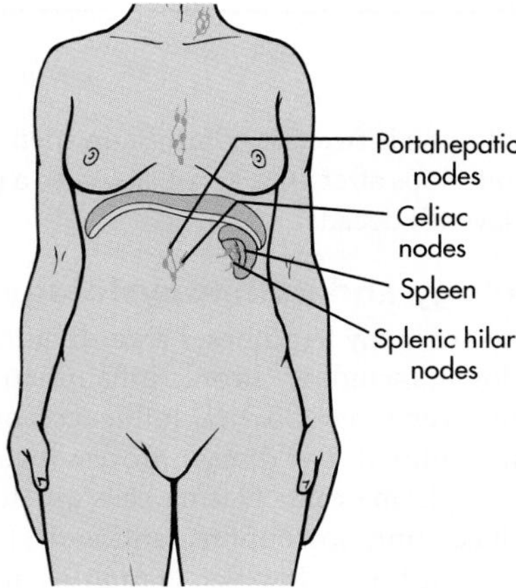

Stage III
Involvement of lymph node regions on both sides of the diaphragm. May include a single extranodal site, the spleen, or both; now subdivided into lymphatic involvement of the upper abdomen in the spleen (splenic, celiac, and portal nodes) (*Stage* III_1) and the lower abdominal nodes in the periaortic, mesenteric, and iliac regions (*Stage* III_2)

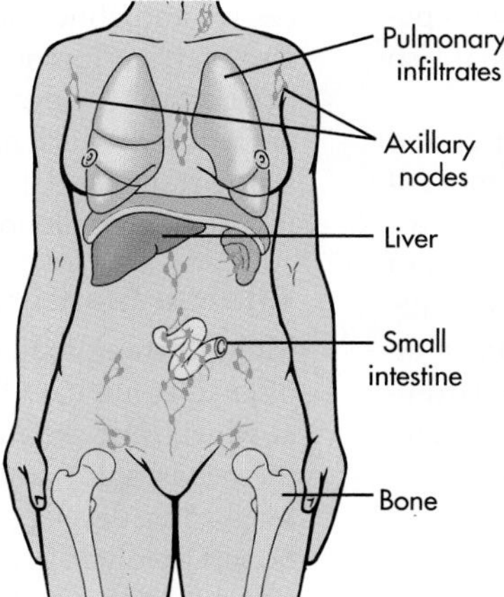

Stage IV
Diffuse or disseminated disease of one or more extralymphatic organs or tissues with or without associated lymph node involvement; the extranodal site is identified as *H*, hepatic; *L*, lung; *P*, pleura; *M*, marrow; *D*, dermal; *O*, osseous

Fig. 29-14 Staging system for Hodgkin's disease and non-Hodgkin's lymphoma.

Table 29-31 Guidelines for Treatment of Hodgkin's Disease

Stage	Recommended Therapy
I, II (A or B)	Radiation
I, II (A or B, with mediastinal mass >⅓ diameter of the chest)	Combination chemotherapy* followed by radiation to involved field
IIIA$_1$ (minimal abdominal disease)	Radiation
IIIA$_2$ (extensive abdominal disease)	Combination chemotherapy* with radiation to involved sites
IIIB	Combination chemotherapy*
IV (A or B)	Combination chemotherapy*

*Combination chemotherapy may be used in conjunction with stem cell transplant (see Chapter 14).

DRUG THERAPY

Table 29-32 Two Chemotherapeutic Regimens for Hodgkin's Disease

Drug	Schedule
MOPP	
Nitrogen ***M***ustard	Days 1 and 8
Vincristine (***O***ncovin)	Days 1 and 8
Procarbazine	Days 1-14
Prednisone (cycles 1 and 4 only)	Days 1-14
ABVD	
Doxorubicin (***A***driamycin)	Days 1 and 15
Bleomycin	Days 1 and 15
Vinblastine	Days 1 and 15
Dacarbazine (DTIC)	Days 1 and 15

Repeat cycle every 28 days for a minimum of six cycles. Complete remission must be documented before discontinuing therapy. Therapy may continue for two cycles after remission.

and pattern. Staging, as described for Hodgkin's disease, is used to guide therapy (see Fig. 29-14). The prognosis for NHL is generally not as good as that for Hodgkin's disease.

Treatment for NHL involves radiotherapy and chemotherapy (Table 29-34). Ironically, more aggressive lymphomas are more responsive to treatment and more likely to be cured. In contrast, indolent lymphomas have a naturally long course but are difficult to effectively treat. Radiotherapy alone may be effective for treatment of stage I disease, but combination radiation therapy and chemotherapy is used for other stages. Initial chemotherapy uses alkylating agents such as cyclophosphamide and chlorambucil. However, numerous combinations have been used to try to overcome the resistant nature of this disease. The most common chemotherapeutic regimen is CHOP (cyclophosphamide, doxorubicin [Adriamycin], vincristine [Oncovin], prednisone). Other combination therapies include cyclophosphamide, vincristine, prednisone (CVP) and cyclophosphamide, vincristine [Oncovin], procarbazine, and prednisone (COPP). Furthermore, high-dose therapy with peripheral blood stem cell or bone marrow transplantation is also commonly employed.

Biologic therapy, such as α-interferon, interleukin-2, and tumor necrosis factor, is also being investigated for treatment of NHL. α-interferon (Intron A) is used in conjunction with anthracycline chemotherapeutic drugs for the initial treatment of clinically aggressive NHL. Rituximab (Rituxan), a genetically engineered monoclinal antibody against the CD20 antigen on the suface of normal and malignant B lymphocytes, is used to treat NHL. Once bound to the cells, rituximab causes lysis and cell death. (Biologic therapy is discussed in Chapter 14.)

MALIGNANCIES OF PLASMA CELLS

MULTIPLE MYELOMA

Multiple myeloma, or plasma cell myeloma, is a condition in which neoplastic plasma cells infiltrate the bone marrow and destroy bone. A patient usually lives for approximately 2 years after diagnosis if untreated. The incidence of multiple myeloma is approximately 2 to 3 per 100,000 people, which is similar to that of Hodgkin's disease or chronic lymphocytic leukemia. The disease is twice as common in men as in women and usually develops after 40 years of age, with a peak incidence around the seventh decade.

Etiology and Pathophysiology

There are many hypotheses regarding the etiology of multiple myeloma, including chronic inflammation, chronic hypersensitivity reactions, and viral influences, but no actual cause has been identified. The disease process involves excessive production of plasma cells. Plasma cells are activated B cells, which produce immunoglobulins (antibodies) that normally serve to protect the body. However, in multiple myeloma the malignant plasma cells infiltrate the bone marrow and produce abnormal and excessive amounts of immunoglobulin (usually IgG, IgA, IgD, or IgE). This abnormal immunoglobulin is termed a *myeloma protein.* Furthermore, plasma cell production of excessive and abnormal amounts of cytokines (IL-4, IL-5, IL-6) also plays an important role in the pathologic process of bone destruction. As myeloma protein increases, normal plasma cells are reduced, which further compromises the body's normal immune response. Ultimately, the plasma cells destroy bone and invade the lymph nodes, liver, spleen, and kidneys.

Clinical Manifestations

Multiple myeloma develops slowly and insidiously. The patient often does not manifest symptoms until the disease is advanced, at which time skeletal pain is the major manifestation. Pain in the pelvis, spine, and ribs is particularly common. Diffuse osteoporosis develops as the myeloma protein destroys more bone. Osteolytic lesions are seen in the skull, vertebrae, and ribs. Vertebral destruction can lead to collapse of vertebrae with ensuing compression of the spinal cord, requiring emergency measures to prevent paraplegia (e.g., radiation, surgery, chemotherapy). Loss of bone integrity can lead to the development of pathologic fractures. Bony degeneration also causes calcium to be lost from bones, eventually causing hypercalcemia.

Hypercalcemia may cause renal, GI, or neurologic changes such as polyuria, anorexia, and confusion. In addition, cell de-

Table 29-33 Classification of Non-Hodgkin's Lymphomas

Low Grade
- Small lymphocytic
- Follicular, small cleaved cell
- Follicular, mixed small cleaved and large cell

Intermediate Grade
- Follicular, large cell
- Diffuse, small cleaved cell
- Diffuse, mixed; small and large
- Diffuse, large cell

High Grade
- Large cell, immunoblastic
- Lymphoblastic
- Small noncleaved cell

Table 29-34 Guidelines for Treatment of Non-Hodgkin's Lymphoma

	Recommended Therapy	
Grade	**Stage I, II_1***	**Stages II_2,† III, IV**
Low	Localized irradiation	Observation until disease progression, then palliative irradiation or single-agent or combination chemotherapy
Intermediate	Combination chemotherapy with localized radiation	Combination chemotherapy
High	Combination chemotherapy (high dose) with localized radiation	Combination chemotherapy (high dose)

*Stage II_1 = nonbulky disease.
†Stage II_2 = bulky disease >10 cm or ⅓ diameter of chest.

struction contributes to the development of hyperuricemia. Along with the high protein levels caused by the presence of the myeloma protein, hyperuricemia can result in renal failure from renal tubular obstruction and interstitial nephritis from the uric acid precipitates. The patient may display symptoms of anemia, thrombocytopenia, and granulocytopenia, all of which are related to the replacement of normal bone marrow elements with plasma cells.

Diagnostic Studies

Evaluating multiple myeloma involves laboratory, radiologic, and bone marrow examination. High serum protein may be present as evidenced by an "M" spike on serum electrophoresis. Pancytopenia, hyperuricemia, hypercalcemia, and elevated creatinine may also be found. In addition, an abnormal globulin termed *Bence Jones protein* is found in the urine of a patient with multiple myeloma.

Radiologic studies, including bone scans, are done to establish the degree of bone involvement. These studies document the presence of diffuse bony lesions, demineralization, and osteoporosis in affected areas of the skeleton.

Bone marrow analysis shows significantly increased numbers of plasma cells in the bone marrow. Other components of the marrow, particularly megakaryocytes, may be normal.

Collaborative Care

The therapeutic approach involves managing both the disease and its symptoms because with treatment the chronic phase of multiple myeloma may last for more than 10 years. Ambulation and adequate hydration are used to treat hypercalcemia, hyperuricemia, and dehydration. Weight bearing helps the bones reabsorb some calcium, and fluids dilute calcium and prevent protein precipitates from causing renal tubular obstruction. Control of pain is another goal of management. Analgesics, orthopedic supports, and localized radiation help reduce the skeletal pain. Pamidronate disodium (Aredia) is used for the treatment of skeletal pain and instability. It inhibits bone resorption without inhibiting bone formation and mineralization. It is given concurrently with initial chemotherapy to reduce bone destruction and skeletal fractures.

Chemotherapy is used to reduce the number of plasma cells. The agents most frequently used are the alkylating drugs, including melphalan (Alkeran), cyclophosphamide (Cytoxan), chlorambucil (Leukeran), and carmustine (BCNU). Corticosteroids may be added because they exert an antitumor effect in some patients. The VAD regimen (vincristine, doxorubicin [Adriamycin], and dexamethasone) can be used for patients who do not respond to alkylating agents. Radiotherapy is another important component of treatment, primarily because of its palliative effect on localized lesions. Bone marrow and peripheral blood stem cell transplantation is curative in some patients with multiple myeloma. Transplant and α-interferon are being investigated in the treatment of multiple myeloma.

Drugs may be used to treat complications of multiple myeloma. For example, allopurinol (Zyloprim) may be given to reduce hyperuricemia, and IV furosemide (Lasix) promotes renal excretion of calcium. Calcitonin and pamidronate may be used to treat moderate to severe hypercalcemia.

NURSING MANAGEMENT: MULTIPLE MYELOMA

The focus of care for the neuromuscular system has to do with the bony involvement and sequelae from bone breakdown. Administering pamidronate and maintaining adequate hydration are primary nursing considerations to minimize problems from hypercalcemia. Fluids are administered to attain a urinary output of 1.5 to 2 L per day. This may require an intake of 3 to 4 L. In addition, weight bearing helps bones reabsorb some of the circulating calcium, and corticosteroids may augment the excretion of calcium. Once chemotherapy is initiated, the uric acid levels rise because of the increased cell destruction. Hyperuricemia must be resolved by ensuring adequate hydration and using allopurinol.

Because of the potential for pathologic fractures, the nurse must be careful when moving and ambulating the patient. A slight twist or strain in the wrong area (e.g., a weak area in the patient's bones) may be sufficient to cause a fracture.

Pain management requires innovative and knowledgeable nursing interventions. If radiotherapy is used to diminish pain from localized myeloma lesions, appropriate skin care techniques must be used. Analgesics, such as nonsteroidal antiinflammatory drugs, acetaminophen, or an acetaminophen/opioid combination, may be more effective than opioids alone in diminishing bone pain. Braces, especially for the spine, may also help control pain. As in any pain management situation, the nurse is responsible for assessing the patient and for implementing necessary nursing measures to alleviate the pain (see Chapter 9).

The patient's psychosocial needs require sensitive, skilled management. As with leukemia, it is important to help the patient and significant others adapt to changes fostered by chronic sickness, deal with reality, and adjust to the losses related to the disease process. The symptoms of multiple myeloma remit and exacerbate. Consequently acute care is needed at various times during the course of the illness. The final, acute phase is unresponsive to treatment and usually short in duration. The way in which patients and families deal with confronting death may be affected by the manner in which they learned to accept and live with the chronic nature of the disease.

Table 29-35 Causes of Splenomegaly

- Hereditary hemolytic anemias
  - Sickle cell disease
  - Thalassemia
- Autoimmune cytopenias
  - Acquired hemolytic anemia
  - Immune thrombocytopenia
- Infections and inflammations
  - Bacterial endocarditis
  - Infectious mononucleosis
  - Systemic lupus erythematosus
  - Sarcoidosis
  - Human immunodeficiency virus infection
  - Viral hepatitis
- Infiltrative diseases
  - Acute and chronic leukemia
  - Lymphomas
  - Polycythemia vera
- Congestion
  - Cirrhosis of the liver
  - Congestive heart failure

DISORDERS OF THE SPLEEN

The spleen performs many functions and is affected by many illnesses. There are many different causes of splenomegaly (Table 29-35). The term *hypersplenism* refers to the occurrence of splenomegaly and peripheral cytopenias (anemia, leukopenia, thrombocytopenia). The degree of splenic enlargement varies with the disease. For example, massive splenic enlargement occurs with chronic myelocytic leukemia, hairy cell leukemia, and thalassemia major. Mild splenic enlargement occurs with congestive heart failure and systemic lupus erythematosus.

When the spleen enlarges, its normal filtering and sequestering capacity increases. Consequently there is often a reduction in the number of circulating blood cells. A slight to moderate enlargement of the spleen is usually asymptomatic and found during a routine examination of the abdomen. Even massive splenomegaly can be well tolerated, but the patient may complain of abdominal discomfort and early satiety. Other techniques to assess the size of the spleen include ^{99}Tc-colloid liver-spleen scan, CT scan, and ultrasound scan.

Occasionally laparotomy and splenectomy are indicated in the evaluation or treatment of splenomegaly. Splenectomy can have a dramatic effect in increasing peripheral RBC, WBC, and platelet counts. Another major indication for splenectomy is splenic rupture. The spleen may rupture from trauma, inadvertent tearing during other surgical procedures, and diseases such as mononucleosis.

Nursing responsibilities for the patient with spleen disorders vary depending on the nature of the problem. Splenomegaly may be painful and may require analgesic administration; care in moving, turning, and positioning; and evaluation of lung expansion because spleen enlargement may impair diaphragmatic excursion. If anemia, thrombocytopenia, or leukopenia develops from splenic enlargement, nursing measures must be instituted to support the patient and prevent life-threatening complications. If splenectomy is performed, the nurse must provide the meticulous care warranted after any surgery. In addition, there must be special observation for hemorrhage, which could lead to shock, fever, and abdominal distention.

After splenectomy, immunologic deficiencies may develop. IgM levels are reduced, and IgG and IgA values remain within normal limits. Postsplenectomy patients are especially vulnerable to infection. A younger patient is at significantly greater risk than an older patient, but the risk is present for all ages. This patient is highly susceptible to infection from encapsulated organisms such as pneumococcus. This complication is prevented by immunization with polyvalent pneumococcal vaccine (e.g., Pneumovax).

BLOOD COMPONENT THERAPY

Blood component therapy is frequently used in managing hematologic diseases. Many therapeutic and surgical procedures depend on blood product support. However, blood component therapy only temporarily supports the patient until the underlying problem is resolved. Because transfusions are not free from hazards, they should be used only if necessary. Nurses must be careful to avoid developing a complacent attitude about this common but potentially dangerous therapy.

Traditionally, the term *blood transfusion* meant the administration of whole blood. Blood transfusion now has a broader meaning because of the ability to administer specific components of blood such as platelets, RBCs, or plasma (Table 29-36).

Administration Procedure

Blood components can be administered safely through a 19-gauge or larger needle into a free-flowing IV line. Larger size needles (e.g., 19 gauge) may be preferred if rapid transfusions are given. Smaller-size needles can be used for platelets, albumin, and cryoprecipitates. Peripherally inserted central catheters (PICCs) are not recommended because of increased incidence of clogged lines due to slow blood flow.[30] The blood administration tubing with a filter should have a stopcock or other means to develop a closed system, with blood open to

ETHICAL DILEMMAS

Religious Issues

SITUATION

An elderly woman is transferred from a nursing home because of gastrointestinal bleeding from an unknown cause. Some of her family members tell the nurse that she is a Jehovah's Witness and must not receive blood products. If she does not have exploratory surgery and transfusions, the physicians believe that she will die.

DISCUSSION

Competent adults have the right to make medical decisions based on their religious beliefs. If the patient is not able to communicate her wishes and has no advance directives, a determination must be made about her religious beliefs before treatment decisions are made. Appropriate methods to make this determination include consulting with the local church officials, inquiring about a wallet card identifying her religious affiliation and beliefs, and discussing her religious beliefs and involvement with her family. Jehovah's Witnesses believe that if they receive blood products, there are eternal consequences. If there is doubt about the patient's involvement in this church or commitment to the tenets of this faith, potentially lifesaving surgery and transfusion would be acceptable.

ETHICAL AND LEGAL PRINCIPLES

- Competent adult patients have the right to refuse medical treatment whether or not the refusal is based on their religious beliefs.
- If a patient is not competent and has no advance directives, health care providers must protect the patient by determining whether it is the *patient's* belief, not the family's, that is the basis for refusing treatment.
- In two cases involving Jehovah's Witnesses in the 1960s, judges' decisions were based on the competency of the patient. A competent patient's wish to refuse treatment was upheld; an incompetent patient's wishes were not clear and the transfusion was ordered.

one port and isotonic saline solution infusing through the other. Dextrose solutions or lactated Ringer's should not be used because they induce RBC hemolysis. No other additives (including medications) should be given via the same tubing as the blood unless the tubing is cleared with saline solution.

When the blood or blood components have been obtained from the blood bank, positive identification of the donor blood and recipient must be made. Improper product-to-patient identification causes 90% of transfusion reactions, thus placing a great responsibility on nursing personnel to carry out the identification procedure appropriately. The nurse should follow the policy and procedures at the place of employment. The blood bank is responsible for typing and crossmatching the donor's blood with the recipient's blood.

The blood should be administered as soon as it is brought to the patient. It should not be refrigerated on the nursing unit. If the blood is not used right away, it should be returned to the blood bank.

During the first 15 minutes or 50 ml of blood infusion, the nurse should stay with the patient. If there are any untoward reactions, they are most likely to occur at this time. The rate of infusion during this period should be no more than 2 ml/min. Blood should not be infused quickly unless an emergency exists. Rapid infusion of cold blood may cause the patient to become chilled. If rapid replacement of large amounts of blood is necessary, a blood-warming device may be used.

After the first 15 minutes, the rate of infusion is governed by the clinical condition of the patient and the product being infused. Most patients not in danger of fluid overload can tolerate the infusion of 1 unit of packed red blood cells over 2 hours. The transfusion should not take more than 4 hours to administer. Blood remaining after 4 hours should not be infused because of the length of time it has been removed from refrigeration.

Blood Transfusion Reactions

If a transfusion reaction occurs, the following steps should be taken: (1) stop the transfusion; (2) maintain a patent IV line with saline solution; (3) notify the blood bank and the physician immediately; (4) recheck identifying tags and numbers; (5) monitor vital signs and urine output; (6) treat symptoms per physician order; (7) save the blood bag and tubing and send them to the blood bank for examination; (8) complete transfusion reaction reports; (9) collect required blood and urine specimens at intervals stipulated by hospital policy to evaluate for hemolysis; and (10) document on transfusion reaction form and patient chart. The blood bank and laboratory are responsible for identifying the type of reaction.

The complications of transfusion therapy may be significant and necessitate judicious evaluation of the patient. Blood transfusion reactions can be classified as acute or delayed (Tables 29-37 and 29-38).

Acute Reactions

Acute hemolytic reactions. The most common cause of hemolytic reactions is transfusion of ABO-incompatible blood (see Table 28-8). This is an example of a type II cytotoxic hypersensitivity reaction (see Chapter 12). Severe hemolytic reactions are rare. Most mistakes are caused by mislabeling specimens and administering blood to the wrong individual.

When an acute hemolytic reaction occurs, antibodies in the recipient's serum react with antigens on the donor's RBCs. This results in agglutination of cells, which can obstruct capillaries and block blood flow. Hemolysis of the RBCs releases free hemoglobin into the plasma. The hemoglobin is filtered by the kidney and may be found in the urine (hemoglobinuria). Hemoglobin may obstruct the renal tubules, leading to acute renal failure (see Chapter 44).

The clinical manifestations of an acute hemolytic reaction may be mild or severe and usually develop within the first 15 minutes of transfusion. Free hemoglobin in blood and urine specimens obtained at the onset of the reaction will provide evidence of an acute hemolytic reaction. Delayed transfusion reactions may occur 2 to 14 days after the administration of blood. (The clinical manifestations and nursing management

Table 29-36 Blood Products*

Description	Special Considerations	Indications for Use
Packed RBC		
Packed RBCs are prepared from whole blood by sedimentation or centrifugation. One unit contains 250-350 ml.	Use of RBCs for treatment allows remaining components of blood (e.g., platelets, albumin, plasma) to be used for other purposes. There is less danger of fluid overload. Packed RBCs are preferred RBC source because they are more component specific.	Severe or symptomatic anemia, acute blood loss.
Frozen RBC		
Frozen RBCs are prepared from RBCs using glycerol for protection and frozen. They can be stored for 3 yr at −188.6° F (−87° C).	They must be used within 24 hr of thawing. Successive washings with saline solution remove majority of WBCs and plasma proteins.	Autotransfusion, patient with previous febrile reactions to transfusions. Infrequently used because filters remove most WBCs.
Platelets		
Platelets are prepared from fresh whole blood within 4 hr after collection. One unit contains 30-60 ml of platelet concentrate.	Multiple units of platelets can be obtained from one donor by plateletpheresis. They can be kept at room temperature for 1-5 days depending on type of collection and storage bag used. Bag should be agitated periodically. Expected increase is 10,000/μl/U. Failure to have a rise may be due to fever, sepsis, splenomegaly, or DIC.	Bleeding caused by thrombocytopenia, platelet levels <10,000-20,000/μl (10-20 × 10^9/L)
Fresh Frozen Plasma		
Liquid portion of whole blood is separated from cells and frozen. One unit contains 200-250 ml. Plasma is rich in clotting factors but contains no platelets. It may be stored for 1 yr. It must be used within 2 hr after thawing.	Use of plasma in treating hypovolemic shock is being replaced by pure preparations such as albumin plasma expanders.	Bleeding caused by deficiency in clotting factors (e.g., DIC, hemorrhage, massive transfusion)
Albumin		
Albumin is prepared from plasma. It can be stored for 5 yr. It is available in 5% or 25% solution.	Albumin 25 g/100 ml is osmotically equal to 500 ml of plasma. Hyperosmolar solution acts by moving water from extravascular to intravascular space.	Hypovolemic shock, hypoalbuminemia
Cryoprecipitates and Commercial Concentrates		
Cryoprecipitate is prepared from fresh frozen plasma, with 10-20 ml/bag. It can be stored for 1 yr. Once thawed, must be used.	See Table 29-20.	Replacement of clotting factors, especially factor VIII and fibrinogen.

*Component therapy has replaced the use of whole blood, which accounts for less than 10% of all transfusions.
DIC, disseminated intravascular coagulation.

for the patient with a hemolytic reaction are presented in Table 29-37.)

Febrile reactions. Febrile reactions are most commonly caused by leukocyte incompatibility. Many individuals who receive five or more transfusions develop circulating antibodies to WBCs. Febrile reactions can often be prevented by using filters to leukocyte deplete RBCs and platelets. Leukocyte-poor blood products (filtered, washed, or frozen) can also be used to prevent febrile reactions.

Mild allergic reactions. Allergic reactions result from the recipient's sensitivity to plasma proteins of the donor's blood. These reactions are more common in an individual with a history of allergies. Antihistamines may be used to prevent allergic reactions. Epinephrine or corticosteroids may be used to treat a severe reaction.

Circulatory overload. An individual with cardiac or renal insufficiency is at risk for developing circulatory overload. This is especially true if a large quantity of blood is infused in a short

Table 29-37 Acute Transfusion Reactions

Reaction	Cause	Clinical Manifestations	Management	Prevention
Acute hemolytic	Infusion of ABO-incompatible whole blood, RBCs or components containing 10 ml or more of RBCs. Antibodies in the recipient's plasma attach to antigens on transfused red blood cells causing RBC destruction.	Chills, fever, low back pain, flushing, tachycardia, tachypnea, hypotension, vascular collapse, hemoglobinuria, acute jaundice, dark urine, bleeding, acute renal failure, shock, cardiac arrest, death.	Treat shock if present. Draw blood samples for serologic testing slowly to avoid hemolysis from the procedure. Send urine specimen to the laboratory. Maintain BP with IV colloid solutions. Give diuretics as prescribed to maintain urine flow. Insert indwelling urinary catheter or measure voided amounts to monitor hourly urine output. Dialysis may be required if renal failure occurs. Do not transfuse additional RBC-containing components until blood bank has provided newly crossmatched units.	Meticulously verify and document patient identification from sample collection to component infusion.
Febrile, nonhemolytic (most common)	Sensitization to donor WBCs, platelets, or plasma proteins.	Sudden chills and fever (rise in temperature of >1° C), headache, flushing, anxiety, muscle pain.	Give antipyretics as prescribed—avoid aspirin in thrombocytopenic patients. *Do not restart transfusion* unless physican orders.	Consider leukocyte-poor blood products (filtered, washed, or frozen) for patients with a history of two or more such reactions.
Mild allergic	Sensitivity to foreign plasma proteins.	Flushing, itching, urticaria (hives).	Give antihistamine as directed. If symptoms are mild and transient, transfusion may be restarted slowly. Do not restart transfusion if fever or pulmonary symptoms develop.	Treat prophylactically with antihistamines. Consider washed RBCs and platelets.
Anaphylactic and severe allergic	Sensitivity to donor plasma proteins. Infusion of IgA proteins to IgA-deficient recipient who has developed IgA antibody.	Anxiety, urticaria, wheezing, progressing to cyanosis, shock, and possible cardiac arrest.	Initiate CPR, if indicated. Have epinephrine ready for injection (0.4 ml of a 1:1000 solution SC or 0.1 ml of 1:1000 solution diluted to 10 ml with saline for IV use). *Do not restart transfusion.*	Transfuse extensively washed RBC products, from which all plasma has been removed. Use blood from IgA-deficient donor. Use autologous components.
Circulatory overload	Fluid administered faster than the circulation can accommodate.	Cough, dyspnea, pulmonary congestion, headache, hypertension, tachycardia, distended neck veins.	Place patient upright with feet in dependent position. Administer prescribed diuretics, oxygen, morphine. Phlebotomy may be indicated.	Adjust transfusion volume and flow rate based on patient size and clinical status. Have blood bank divide unit into smaller aliquots for better spacing of fluid input.
Sepsis	Transfusion of bacterially infected blood components.	Rapid onset of chills, high fever, vomiting, diarrhea, marked hypotension, or shock.	Obtain culture of patient's blood and send bag with remaining blood and tubing to blood bank for further study. Treat septicemia as directed—antibiotics, IV fluids, vasopressors.	Collect, process, store, and transfuse blood products according to blood banking standards and infuse within 4 hr of starting time.

Modified from Transfusion Therapy Guidelines for Nurses, National Blood Resources Education Program, US Department Health and Human Services.
CPR, cardiopulmonary resuscitation.

period of time. When blood is needed, it should be infused as slowly as possible, and the patient can be monitored with central venous pressure readings. Central venous pressure readings above 15 cm H_2O usually indicate circulatory overload. If a pulmonary artery catheter is in place, pulmonary artery wedge pressure readings above 18 mm Hg indicate elevated left atrial pressure and impending heart failure.

Sepsis. Blood products can become infected from improper handling and storage. Bacterial contamination of blood products can result in bacteremia, sepsis, or septic shock. However, with careful handling, bacterial contamination and growth rarely occur.

Massive blood transfusion reaction. An acute complication of transfusing large volumes of blood products is termed *massive blood transfusion reaction.* Massive blood transfusion reactions can occur when replacement of RBCs or blood exceeds the total blood volume within 24 hours. In this situation, an imbalance of normal blood elements can result because clotting factors, albumin, and platelets are not found in RBC transfusions.

Additional problems such as hypothermia, citrate toxicity, hypocalcemia, and hyperkalemia may occur when massive blood transfusions are given. Hypothermia with cardiac arrhythmias can result from rapid infusion of large quantities of cold blood. Blood-warming equipment can prevent this problem. Citrate toxicity and hypocalcemia can occur from the use of large quantities of blood products, which usually have citrate as part of the storage solution; calcium binds to the citrate. Citrate toxicity is likely to develop when blood is transfused at a rate of 1 unit in 10 minutes (or 8 to 10 units of RBCs within a few hours). Symptoms such as muscle tremors and ECG changes may be observed with hypocalcemia but can be prevented or reversed by the infusion of 10% calcium gluconate (10 ml with every liter of citrated blood).[31] Hyperkalemia results when potassium leaks from RBCs in stored blood. Mild to severe signs and symptoms can occur, including nausea, muscle weakness, diarrhea, paresthesias, flaccid paralysis of the cardiac or respiratory muscles, and cardiac arrest. Electrolyte monitoring is an important aspect of care when massive transfusions are necessary.

Delayed Transfusion Reactions

Delayed transfusion reactions include delayed hemolytic reactions (discussed previously), infections, iron overload, and graft-versus-host disease (see Table 29-38).

Infection. Infectious agents transmitted by blood transfusion include hepatitis B and C viruses, HIV, human herpesvirus type 6 (HSV-6), Epstein-Barr virus (EBV), human T cell leukemia (HTLV-1), cytomegalovirus (CMV), and malaria. Hepatitis is the most common viral infection transmitted, although its incidence has been decreasing. Hepatitis B virus can be detected in the blood by the presence of hepatitis B surface antigen (HBsAg). A test for hepatitis C antibodies in donor blood is used to exclude the use of any donated blood testing positive for hepatitis C. Therefore the risk of transmission of hepatitis C has been reduced.

In the past, HIV was transmitted by contaminated blood and blood products. This posed a serious problem for an individual who received infected transfusions. Patients with hemophilia who received antihemophiliac factors, which had been prepared from pooled plasma of a large number of donors of

Table 29-38 Delayed Transfusion Reactions

Reaction	Clinical Manifestations
Delayed hemolytic	Fever, mild jaundice, decreased hematocrit. Occurs as early as 3 days or as late as several months, but usually 7-14 days posttransfusion as the result of destruction of transfused RBC by alloantibodies not detected during crossmatch. Generally, no acute treatment is required, but hemolysis may be severe enough to warrant further transfusions.
Hepatitis B	Elevated liver enzymes (AST and ALT), anorexia, malaise, nausea and vomiting, fever, dark urine, jaundice. Usually resolves spontaneously within 4-6 wk. Chronic carrier state can develop and can result in permanent liver damage. Treat symptomatically. (See Chapter 41.)
Hepatitis C	Similar to hepatitis B, but symptoms are usually less severe. Chronic liver disease and cirrhosis may develop. Before introduction of anti-HCV test, accounted for 90-95% of all posttransfusion hepatitis. Treat symptomatically. (See Chapter 41.)
Human immunodeficiency virus (HIV)	Can be asymptomatic for up to several years or may develop flulike symptoms within 2-4 wk. Later signs and symptoms include weight loss, diarrhea, fever, lymphadenopathy, thrush, pneumocystis pneumonia.
Iron overload	Excess iron is deposited in the heart, liver, pancreas, and joints, causing dysfunction. Congestive heart failure, arrhythmias, impaired thyroid and gonadal function, diabetes, arthritis, cirrhosis. Commonly occurs in patients receiving >100 units for chronic anemia over a period of time. Treat symptomatically. Deferoxamine (Desferal), which chelates and removes accumulated iron via the kidneys, may be administered IV or SC.
Graft-versus-host disease	Fever, rash, diarrhea, hepatitis. Result of replication of donor lymphocytes (graft) in the transfusion recipient (host). No effective therapy available. To prevent, irradiate blood products intended for immunocompromised patients. Some believe that irradiated blood products are indicated for first-degree family members' donations also. (See Chapter 12.)
Other	Other infectious diseases and agents may be transmitted via transfusion, including cytomegalovirus, HTLV-I, and those causing malaria.

Modified from Transfusion Therapy Guidelines for Nurses, National Blood Resources Education Program, US Department Health and Human Services.
ALT, alanine aminotransferase; *AST,* aspartate aminotransferase; *HTLV-1,* human T cell leukemia virus, type 1.

which some donors were infected, have a high rate of HIV infection from transfusion sources. Presently, the use of recombinant antihemophilic factors (see Table 29-19), donor education, donor screening, and HIV-antibody testing have greatly reduced the transmission of HIV by blood transfusion or factor replacement therapy.

AUTOTRANSFUSION

Autotransfusion, or autologous transfusion, consists of removing whole blood from a person and transfusing that blood into the same person. The problems of incompatibility, allergic reactions, and transmission of disease can be avoided. Methods of autotransfusion include the following:

1. *Autologous donation* or *elective phlebotomy (predeposit transfusion).* A person donates blood before a planned surgical procedure. The blood can be frozen and stored for up to 3 years. Usually the blood is stored without being frozen and is given to the person within a few weeks of donation. This technique is especially beneficial to the patient with a rare blood type or for any patient that might be expected to require limited blood product support during a major surgical procedure (e.g., elective joint surgery).
2. *Autotransfusion.* A newer method for replacing blood volume involves safely and aseptically collecting, filtering, and returning the patient's own blood lost during a major surgical procedure or from a traumatic injury. This system was originally developed in response to patients' concerns about the safety of blood from blood products. However, today it provides an important way to safely replace volume and stabilize bleeding patients.[32] Collection devices can be attached to drains following chest or orthopedic procedures. Sometimes the collection device is a component of the drainage system. Some systems allow blood to be automatically and continuously reinfused; others require collection for a period of time (usually no longer than 2 to 4 hours) and then are reinfused. Drainage after the first 24 hours or drainage that is suspected to contain pathogens should not be reinfused. Anticoagulants may or may not be added before reinfusion. Development of clots after blood is filtered through the collection system can sometimes prevent reinfusion of the blood. Sometimes blood that has been collected has become depleted of its normal coagulation factors; therefore monitoring coagulation studies in the patient receiving an autotransfusion is important.[33]

CRITICAL THINKING EXERCISES

CASE STUDY

Leukemia

Patient Profile

J., a 35-year-old man, went to the emergency department because of severe bruising caused by a fall while hiking.

Subjective Data

- Complains of oral pain and white patches covering his tongue
- Has had a 2-month history of fatigue, malaise, and flu symptoms
- Has taken numerous prescribed antibiotics and increased rest and sleep in the past 2 months without relief of symptoms

Objective Data

Physical Examination

- Has bruises and ecchymoses from fall
- Gingiva has petechiae and patchy white spots
- Temperature 102.2° F (39° C)
- Has splenomegaly

Laboratory Results

- Hct 30%
- WBC 120,000/μl (120×10^9/L)
- Platelet count 25,000/μl (25×10^9/L)

Bone Marrow Biopsy

- Multiple myeloblasts (>50%)

Critical Thinking Questions

1. What components of the laboratory test results suggest acute leukemia?
2. How is acute myelogenous leukemia treated?
3. What is the prognosis for J.?
4. What are the main priorities for patient teaching with a newly diagnosed young adult with leukemia?
5. Based on the assessment data presented, write one or more nursing diagnoses. Are there any collaborative problems?

NURSING RESEARCH ISSUES

1. What nursing interventions can assist the patient to manage fatigue from anemia?
2. How effective are different types of isolation procedures in the prevention of infection in an immunocompromised patient?
3. What is the quality of life for a patient following bone marrow transplantation?
4. What is the impact on the family when one of its members is receiving chemotherapy for leukemia?
5. What are the most effective ways to train a nurse to administer blood and blood products?
6. How does leukemia affect the lifestyle of an affected individual?
7. What is the quality of life for a patient with recurrent sickle cell crises?
8. What strategies are effective for pain management in patients with sickle cell crises?

REVIEW QUESTIONS

The number of the question corresponds to the same-numbered objective at the beginning of the chapter.

1. In a severely anemic patient the nurse would expect to find
   a. dyspnea and tachycardia.
   b. cyanosis and pulmonary edema.
   c. cardiomegaly and pulmonary fibrosis.
   d. ventricular arrhythmias and wheezing.
2. When obtaining assessment data from a patient with a microcytic, normochromic anemia the nurse would question the patient about
   a. folic acid intake.
   b. dietary intake of iron.
   c. a history of gastric surgery.
   d. a history of sickle cell anemia.
3. A nursing intervention for a patient with the severe anemia of chronic renal disease includes
   a. monitoring stools for guaiac.
   b. instructions in high-iron diet.
   c. monitoring urine intake and output.
   d. teaching self-injection of erythropoietin.
4. A patient with anemia secondary to heavy menstrual blood loss describes her dietary intake to the nurse. For breakfast the nurse recommends that whole grain cereal be substituted for
   a. scrambled eggs.
   b. sausage and toast.
   c. fresh fruit and yogurt.
   d. granola bar with raisins.
5. The nursing management of a patient in sickle cell crisis includes
   a. bed rest and heparin therapy.
   b. blood transfusions and iron replacement.
   c. aggressive analgesic and oxygen therapy.
   d. platelet administration and monitoring of CBC.
6. A complication of the hyperviscosity of polycythemia is
   a. thrombosis.
   b. cardiomyopathy.
   c. pulmonary edema.
   d. disseminated intravascular coagulation (DIC).
7. When providing care for a patient with thrombocytopenia, the nurse must avoid administering aspirin or aspirin-containing products because they
   a. interfere with platelet aggregation.
   b. may contribute to the destruction of thrombocytes.
   c. may mask the fever that occurs with thrombocytopenia.
   d. alter blood flow to the homeostatic mechanisms in the brain.
8. The nurse would anticipate that a patient with von Willebrand's disease undergoing surgery would be treated with administration of vWF and
   a. factor VI.
   b. factor VII.
   c. factor VIII.
   d. thrombin.
9. DIC is a disorder in which
   a. the coagulation pathway is genetically altered leading to thrombus formation in all major blood vessels.
   b. an underlying disease depletes hemolytic factors in the blood leading to diffuse thrombotic episodes and infarcts.
   c. a disease process stimulates coagulation processes with resultant depletion of clotting factors leading to diffuse hemorrhage.
   d. an inherited predisposition causes a deficiency of clotting factors that leads to overstimulation of coagulation processes in the vasculature.
10. Appropriate nursing actions when caring for a hospitalized patient with severe neutropenia include
    a. perirectal care and platelet administration.
    b. oral care and red blood cell administration.
    c. monitoring lung sounds and invasive blood pressures.
    d. strict hand washing and frequent temperature assessment.
11. Because myelodysplastic syndromes arise from the pluripotent hematopoietic stem cell in the bone marrow, laboratory results the nurse would expect to find include
    a. an excess of platelets.
    b. an excess of T cells.
    c. a deficiency of granulocytes.
    d. a deficiency of all cellular blood components.
12. A type of leukemia that is common but rarely fatal in older adults includes
    a. acute myelocytic leukemia.
    b. acute lymphocytic leukemia.
    c. chronic lymphocytic leukemia.
    d. chronic granulocytic leukemia.
13. Multiple drugs are primarily used in combinations to treat leukemia and lymphoma because
    a. there are fewer toxic and side effects.
    b. the chance that one drug will be effective is increased.
    c. they can interrupt cell growth at multiple points in the cell cycle.
    d. they are more effective without having exacerbating side effects.
14. The nurse is aware that a major difference between Hodgkin's disease and non-Hodgkin's lymphoma is that
    a. Hodgkin's disease is considered potentially curable.
    b. Hodgkin's disease occurs only in young adults.
    c. non-Hodgkin's lymphoma requires a staging laparotomy.
    d. non-Hodgkin's lymphoma is treated only with radiation therapy.
15. A patient with multiple myeloma becomes confused and lethargic. The nurse would expect that these clinical manifestations may be explained by diagnostic results that indicate
    a. hyperkalemia.
    b. hyperuricemia.
    c. hypercalcemia.
    d. CNS myeloma.
16. When reviewing the patient's hematologic laboratory values after a splenectomy the nurse would expect to find
    a. leukopenia.
    b. RBC abnormalities.
    c. decreased hemoglobin.
    d. increased platelet count.
17. Complications of transfusions that can be decreased by the use of leukocyte reduction filters for red blood cells and platelets are
    a. chills and back pain.
    b. leukostasis and neutrophilia.
    c. fluid overload and pulmonary edema.
    d. transmission of cytomegalovirus and alloimmunization.

References

1. Thibodeau GA, Patton KT: *Anatomy and physiology,* ed 3, St Louis, 1996, Mosby.
2. Van Fleet Wilens N: The geriatric patient. In Rice R, editor: *Home health nursing practice: concepts and application,* ed 2, St Louis, 1996, Mosby.
3. Beard JL, Ashraf R, Smiciklas-Wright H: Iron nutrition in the elderly. In Watson RR, editor: *Handbook of nutrition in the aged,* ed 2, Boca Raton, Fla, 1994, CRC Press.
4. Lipschitz DA: Anemia. In Hazzard WR and others, editors: *Principles of geriatric medicine and gerontology,* ed 3, New York, 1994, McGraw-Hill.
5. Fairbanks VF, Beutler E: Iron deficiency. In Beutler E and others, editors: *Williams hematology,* ed 5, New York, 1995, McGraw-Hill.
6. Weatherall DJ: The thalassemias. In Beutler E and others, editors: *Williams hematology,* ed 5, New York, 1995, McGraw-Hill.
7. Nissenblatt MJ: *Managing cancer-related anemia,* New Jersey, 1994, Ortho Biotech (monograph).
8. Paquette RL and others: Long-term outcome of aplastic anemia in adults treated with antithymocyte globulin: comparison with bone marrow transplantation, *Blood* 85:283, 1995.
9. Bunn HF: Pathogenesis and treatment of sickle cell disease, *N Engl J Med* 337:762, 1997.
10. Davies SC, Oni L: Management of patients with sickle cell disease, *BMJ* 315:656, 1997.
11. Howard LW, Kennedy LD: Hydroxyurea in the treatment of sickle-cell anemia, *Ann Pharmacother* 31:1393, 1997.
12. Shuey KM: Platelet-associated bleeding disorders, *Semin Oncol Nurs* 12:15, 1996.
13. Broughton S: Heparin has its risks, *Can Nurse* 91:25, 1995.
14. Kajis-Wyllie M: Thrombotic thrombocytopenia purpura, *Crit Care Nurse* 15:44, 1995.
15. Rust DM: FDA approves first biologic drug to promote platelet production, *Oncology Nurs Forum* 251:608, 1998.
16. Kleinert D and others: von Willebrand's disease: a nursing perspective, *J Obstet Gynecol Neonatal Nurs* 26: 271, 1997.
17. Roberts H, Hoffman M: Hemophilia and related conditions—inherited deficiencies of prothrombin (factor II), factor V, and factors VII to XII. In Beutler E and others, editors: *Williams hematology,* ed 5, New York, 1995, McGraw-Hill.
18. Wheeler A, Rubenstein EB: Current management of disseminated intravascular coagulation, *Oncology* 8:69, 1994.
19. Van Der Meer JWM: Defects in host defense mechanisms. In Rubin RR, Young LS, editors: *Clinical approach to infection in the compromised host,* ed 3, New York, 1994, Plenum Medical.
20. Noskin GA, Phair JP, Murphy RL: Diagnosis and management of infections in the immunocompromised host. In Shulman ST and others, editors: *The biologic and clinical basis of infectious diseases,* ed 5, Philadelphia, 1997, Saunders.
21. Buchsel PC: Allogenic bone marrow transplantation. In Groenwald SL and others, editors: *Cancer nursing: principles and practice,* ed 4, Boston, 1997, Jones & Bartlett.
22. Utley SM: Myelodysplastic syndromes, *Semin Oncol Nurs* 12:51, 1996.
23. *Cancer facts and figures, 1998,* American Cancer Society.
24. Wujcik D: Leukemia. In Groenwald SL and others, editors: *Cancer nursing: principles and practice,* ed 4, Boston, 1997, Jones & Bartlett.
25. Wiernik PH: Diagnosis and treatment of adult acute myelogenous leukemia. In Wiernik PH and others, editors: *Neoplastic diseases of the blood,* ed 4, New York, 1996, Churchill Livingstone.
26. O'Connell SA, Schmit-Pokorny K: Blood and marrow stem cell transplantation: indications, procedure, process. In Whedon MB, Wvjcik D, editors: *Blood and marrow stem cell transplantation,* ed 2, Boston, 1997, Jones & Bartlett.
27. DeMeyer E, Whedon MB, Ferrell B: Quality of life after transplantation. In Whedon MB, Wvjcik D, editors: *Blood and marrow stem cell transplantation,* ed 2, Boston, 1997, Jones & Bartlett.
28. McFadden ME: Malignant lymphomas. In Groenwald SL and others, editors: *Cancer nursing: principles and practice,* ed 4, Boston, 1997, Jones & Bartlett.
29. Yellen SB, Cella DF, Bonomi A: Quality of life in people with Hodgkin's disease, *Oncology* 7:41, 1993.
30. Fitzpatrick L, Fitzpatrick T: Blood transfusion. Keeping your patient safe, *Nursing* 27:34, 1997.
31. Gloe D: Common reactions to transfusions, *Heart Lung* 20:506, 1991.
32. Gobel BH: Bleeding disorders. In Groenwald SL and others, editors: *Cancer nursing principles and practice,* ed 4, Boston, 1997, Jones & Bartlett.
33. Smith RN and others: Autotransfusion, *Nursing* 25:52, 1995.

Resources

American Sickle Cell Anemia
P.O. Box 1971
10300 Carnegie Avenue
Cleveland, OH 44106
216-229-4500
Fax: 216-229-4500

Cooley's Anemia Foundation
129-09 26th Avenue #203
Flushing, NY 11354
800-522-7222
718-321-CURE (2873)
Fax: 718-321-3340
http://www.thalassemia.org/

Hemochromatosis Foundation
PO Box 8569
Albany, NY 12208-0596
518-489-0972
http://laran.waisman.wisc.edu/fv/www/lib_hemo.htm

International Myeloma Foundation
2129 Stanley Hills Drive
Los Angeles, CA 90046
213-654-3023
800-452-2873
Fax: 213-656-1182
http://www.myeloma.org/

Leukemia Society of America
600 Third Avenue
New York, NY 10017
212-573-8484
http://www.leukemia.org/

National Association for Sickle Cell Disease, Inc.
3345 Wilshire Boulevard
Los Angeles, CA 90010-1880
800-421-8453
Fax: 213-736-5211

National Heart, Lung, and Blood Institute
National Institutes of Health
4733 Bethesda Avenue, Suite 530
Bethesda, MD 20814
301-951-3260
http://www.nhlbi.nih.gov/nhlbi/nhlbi.htm

National Hemophilia Foundation
110 Green Street, Room 303
New York, NY 10012
212-219-8180

Sickle Cell Disease Association of America, Inc.
200 Corporate Point, #495
Culver City, CA 90230-7633
310-216-6363
800-421-8453
Fax: 310-215-3722
http://www.sickle.qpg.com/

Triad Sickle Cell Anemia Foundation
1102 East Market Street
Greensboro, NC 27420-0964
919-274-1507
Fax: 919-275-7984

For additional Internet resources, see the website for this book at **www.mosby.com/MERLIN/medsurg_lewis**

SECTION

7

PROBLEMS OF OXYGENATION: PERFUSION

SECTION OUTLINE

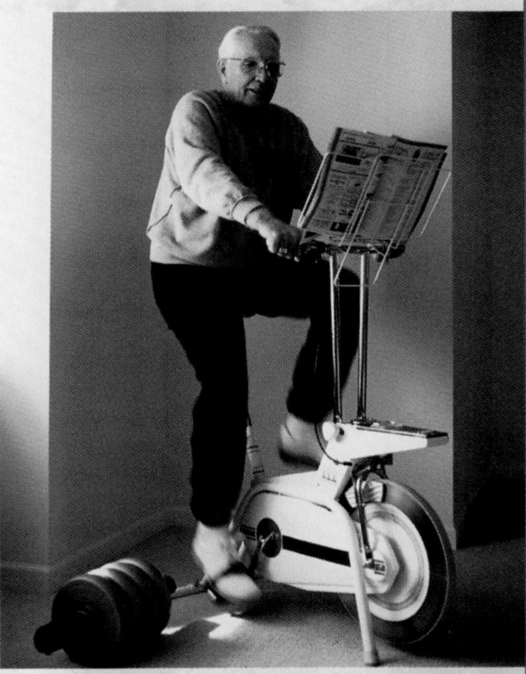

30 NURSING ASSESSMENT Cardiovascular System

Anita M. Ralstin

LEARNING OBJECTIVES

1. Describe the anatomic location and function of the following cardiac structures: pericardial layers, atria, ventricles, semilunar valves, and atrioventricular valves.
2. Describe coronary circulation and the areas of heart muscle supplied by each blood vessel.
3. Explain the normal sequence of events involved in the conduction pathway of the heart.
4. Describe the structure and function of arteries, capillaries, and veins.
5. Define blood pressure and the mechanisms involved in its regulation.
6. Identify the significant subjective and objective assessment data related to the cardiovascular system that should be obtained from a patient.
7. Describe the appropriate techniques used in the physical assessment of the cardiovascular system.
8. Differentiate normal from common abnormal findings of a physical assessment of the cardiovascular system.
9. Describe the age-related changes of the cardiovascular system and differences in assessment findings.
10. Describe the purpose, significance of results, and nursing responsibilities of invasive and noninvasive diagnostic studies of the cardiovascular system.
11. Identify waveforms of a normal electrocardiogram and components of the normal sinus rhythm.

STRUCTURES AND FUNCTIONS OF THE CARDIOVASCULAR SYSTEM

Heart

Structure. The heart is a four-chambered hollow muscular organ approximately the size of a fist. It is the pump of the cardiovascular system. The heart lies within the thorax between the lungs in the mediastinal space. Its beating is often palpable at the fifth intercostal space approximately 2 inches left of the midline (Fig. 30-1). This pulsation, arising at the apex of the heart, is termed the *point of maximum impulse* (PMI).

The heart wall is composed of three layers. The endocardium is the thin inner lining, the myocardium is the middle muscular layer, and the epicardium is the outer serous membrane. The pericardium (pericardial sac) surrounds the heart, enclosing it the way a glove encloses a fist. This sac consists of a visceral (inner) layer and a parietal (outer) layer. The visceral layer is in contact with the epicardium. Between the visceral and parietal layers is the pericardial space. A small amount of fluid in this space acts as a lubricant and reduces the friction caused by the movement of the layers with each contraction.

The heart's four chambers are separated by a septum, with two chambers on the right side and two chambers on the left side. The upper chambers on each side are the atria, and the lower chambers are the ventricles. The atrial myocardium is thinner than that of the ventricles. The left ventricular wall is much thicker than the right ventricular wall. Its added thickness provides the force for the left ventricle to pump blood into the systemic circulation. The thinner-walled right ventricle pumps against a lower pressure into the lungs.

Blood Flow Through the Heart

Cardiac valves. The right atrium receives venous blood from the inferior and superior venae cavae and the coronary sinus. The blood then passes through the tricuspid valve into the right ventricle. With each contraction, the right ventricle pumps blood into the pulmonary artery. At the entrance to the pulmonary artery is the pulmonic valve.

Blood from the lungs flows into the left atrium by way of the pulmonary veins. It then passes through the mitral valve and into the left ventricle. As the heart contracts, blood is ejected through the aortic valve into the aorta and thus enters the systemic circulation (Fig. 30-2).

The four valves of the heart serve to keep blood flowing in one direction. The atrioventricular (AV) valves (tricuspid and mitral) prevent backflow of blood into the atria during ventricular contraction. The cusps of the valves are twice the size of the orifice and are attached to thin strands of fibrous tissue termed *chordae tendineae* (Fig. 30-3). Chordae are anchored in the papillary muscles of the ventricles. The support of the valves by the chordae tendineae prevents the eversion of the leaflets into the atria during ventricular contraction. The pulmonic and aortic valves prevent blood from regurgitating into the ventricles at the end of each ventricular contraction. These valves, also known as semilunar valves, have three cusps. No additional support structures are necessary for the semilunar valves.

Blood Supply to the Myocardium. The myocardium has its own coronary circulation. Immediately above the cusps of the aortic valve are the sinuses of Valsalva, with openings to

Reviewed by Kathleen C. Ashton, RN, CS, PhD, Clinical Assistant Professor, Department of Nursing, Rutgers, the State University of New Jersey, Camden, NJ.

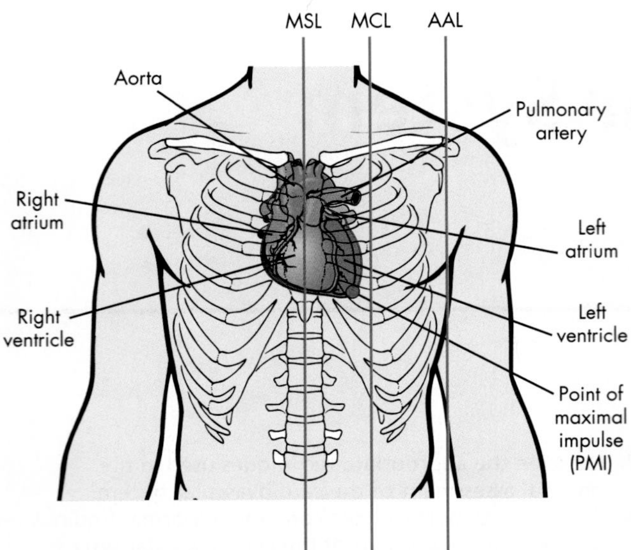

Fig. 30-1 Orientation of the heart within the thorax. Red lines indicate the midsternal line (MSL), midclavicular line (MCL), and anterior axillary line (AAL).

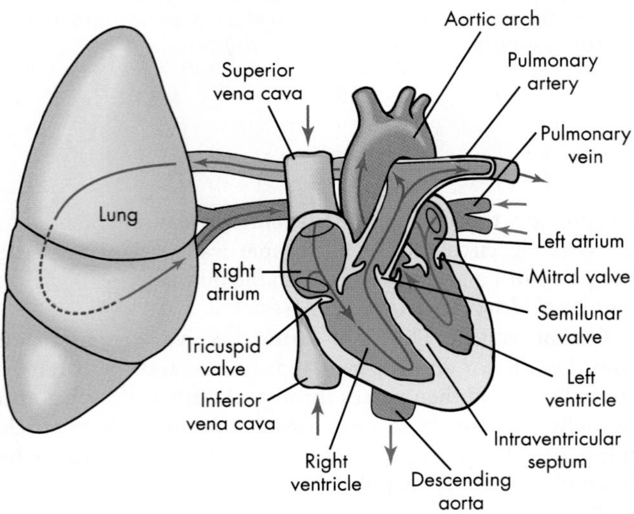

Fig. 30-2 Schematic representation of blood flow through the heart. Arrows indicate direction of flow.

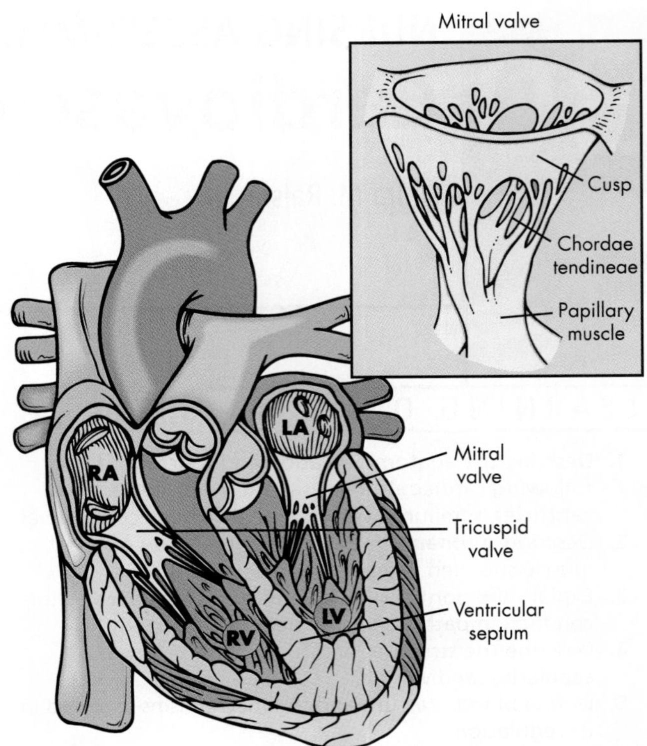

Fig. 30-3 Anatomic structures of the atrioventricular (AV) valves. *LA,* Left atrium; *LV,* left ventricle; *RA,* right atrium; *RV,* right ventricle.

the right and left coronary arteries. Blood flow into the coronary arteries occurs primarily during diastole. The branches of the coronary arteries carry blood to different areas of the myocardium (Fig. 30-4). The right coronary artery and its branches usually supply the right atrium, the right ventricle, and a portion of the posterior wall of the left ventricle. The left coronary artery and its branches (left anterior descending artery and left circumflex artery) supply the left atrium and the left ventricle. In 90% of all persons, the AV node, part of the cardiac conduction system, receives its blood supply from the right coronary artery. For this reason, obstruction of this artery often causes serious defects in cardiac conduction.

If blood flow through any part of the coronary arterial system is reduced, an imbalance between oxygen supply and demand occurs. *Ischemia,* which is a reversible cellular injury, produces tissue hypoxia, a decreased energy supply, and a buildup of toxic metabolic wastes. This may reduce the mechanical and electrical activity of the heart. Myocardial hibernation is the decreased mechanical functioning as a result of decreased persistent and significant blood flow to the myocardium.[1]

Infarction is the permanent loss of blood flow to the myocardium and results in cell death. The overall effect of ischemia or infarction depends on the size of the area deprived of oxygen (O_2). If blood flow is reduced over months or years, alternate routes may develop in enough time to nourish the endangered myocardium. These alternate routes are termed *collateral circulation.*

The divisions of coronary veins parallel the coronary arteries. Most of the blood from the coronary system drains into the coronary sinus, which empties into the right atrium near the entrance to the inferior vena cava (see Fig. 30-4).

Conduction System. In the heart wall there is specialized nerve tissue responsible for creating and transporting the electrical impulse. The final result is myocardial contraction. This electrical impulse is created by the sinoatrial (SA) node by the rapid influx of sodium ions into the cells and the outflux of potassium ions. This shift in electrolytes reduces the polarized condition that exists when node cells are at rest (i.e., electrically negative inside, positive outside), and the cell membranes become depolarized. This change in polarity is termed an *action potential.* The action potential created at that instant moves in concentric waves throughout the atria. The SA node is a tiny knob of tissue in the wall of the right atrium, near the entrance of the superior vena cava (Fig. 30-5). The

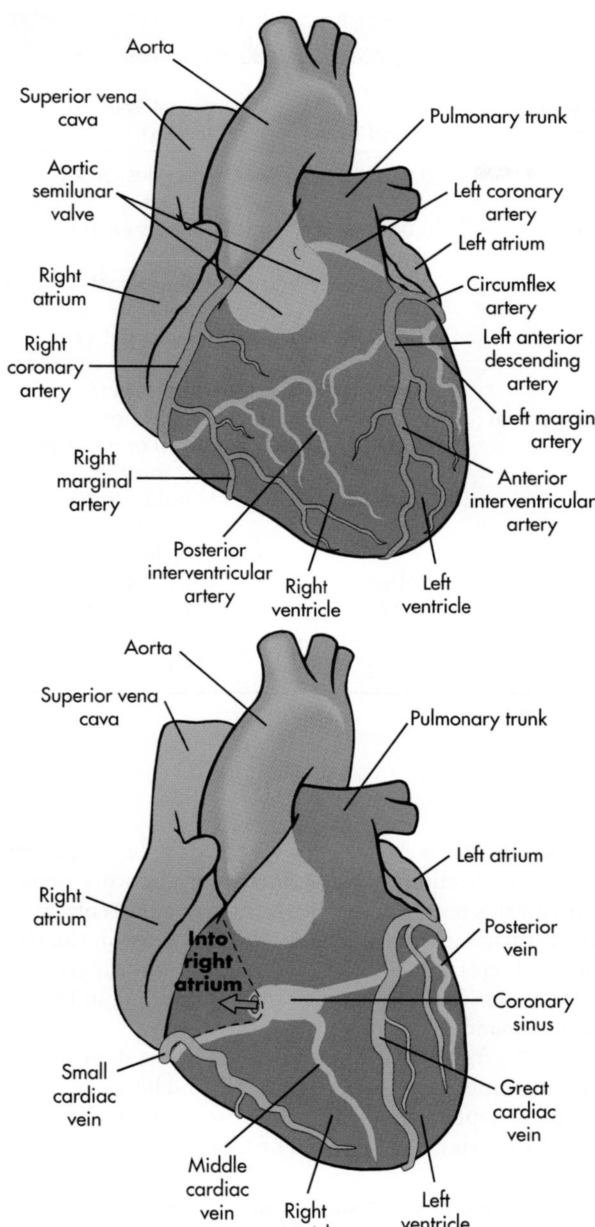

Fig. 30-4 Coronary arteries and veins.

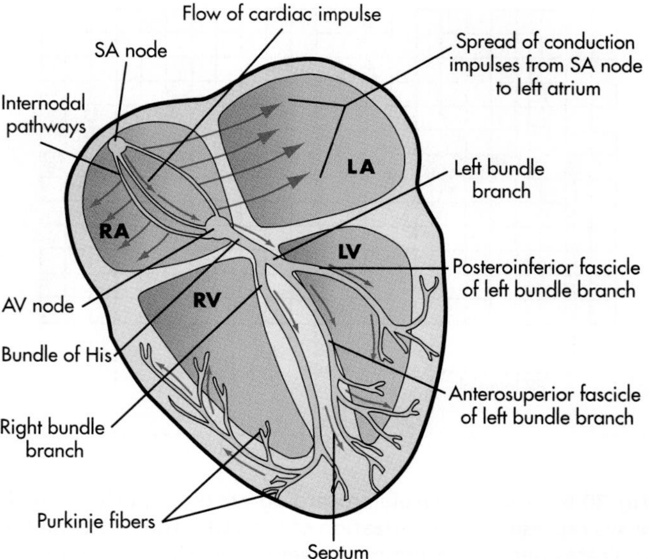

Fig. 30-5 Conduction system of the heart. *AV,* atrioventricular; *SA,* sinoatrial.

SA node is called the pacemaker of the heart. Each impulse generated at the SA node travels swiftly through the atrial muscle fibers of both atria by internodal pathways and cell-to-cell conduction.

Mechanical contraction of the heart muscle follows the depolarization of the cells. Contraction occurs when the actin and myosin filaments of the contractile units of the heart move together. Calcium, which flows into the cell after depolarization, initiates this contraction. The uniform and quick delivery of the electrical impulse allows the atria to contract as one unit.

The electrical impulse travels from the atria to the AV node located in the base of the right atrium near the septum. The electrical impulse pauses briefly in the AV node, which allows contraction and emptying of the atria before contraction of the ventricles begins. The excitation then moves through the bundle of His and along the interventricular septum by way of the left and right bundle branches. The left bundle branch has two fascicles, an anterior and a posterior. From there the action potential diffuses widely through the walls of both ventricles by means of Purkinje fibers. The efficient ventricular conduction system delivers the impulse within 0.12 seconds. This triggers a uniform myocardial contraction.

The cardiac cycle starts with depolarization of the SA node. Its climax is ejection of blood into the pulmonary and systemic circulations. It ends with repolarization when the contractile fiber cells and the conduction pathway cells regain their resting polarized condition. Cardiac muscle cells have a compensatory mechanism that makes them unresponsive or refractory to restimulation during the action potential. During systole there is an absolute refractory period during which cardiac muscle does not respond to any stimuli. After this period, cardiac muscle gradually recovers its excitability and a relative refractory period occurs by early diastole.

Electrocardiogram. The electrical activity of the heart can be detected on the body surface and is recorded as an electrocardiogram (ECG). The letters *P, QRS, T,* and *U* are used to identify the separate waveforms (Fig. 30-6). The first wave, P, begins with the firing of the SA node and represents depolarization of the fibers of the atria. The QRS wave represents depolarization from the AV node throughout the ventricles. There is a delay of impulse transmission through the AV node that accounts for the time sequence between the end of the P wave and the beginning of the QRS wave. The T wave represents repolarization of the ventricles. The U wave, if seen, represents delayed ventricular repolarization and may be associated with hypokalemia.

Intervals between these waves reflect the length of time it takes for the impulse to travel from one area of the heart to

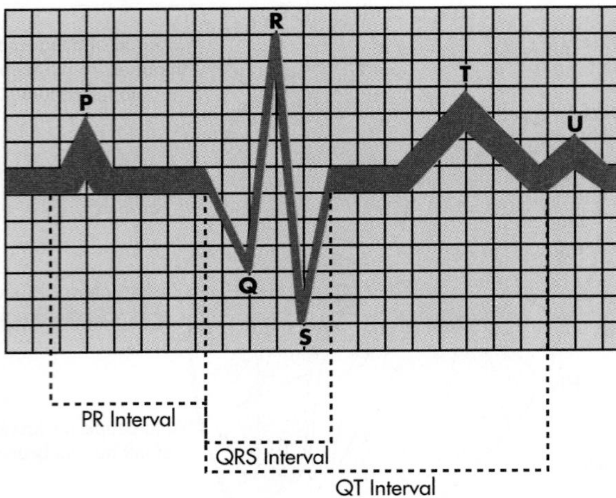

Fig. 30-6 The normal electrocardiogram (ECG) pattern. The P wave represents depolarization of the atria. The QRS complex indicates depolarization of the ventricles. The T wave represents repolarization of the ventricles. The U wave, if present, may indicate hypokalemia or repolarization abnormalities. The PR interval is a measure of the time required for the impulse to spread from the sinoatrial node to the ventricles.

Table 30-1 Electrocardiogram Waves

Normal Waveforms and Intervals	Normal Timing	Normal Sinus Rhythm*
P	0.06-0.12 sec	Precedes QRS-T waves
QRS	0.04-0.12 sec wave	Follows each P
T	0.16 sec	Follows each QRS wave
PR interval	0.12-0.20 sec	Should not vary from one complex to another
QT interval	Varies with pulse rate (0.31-0.38 sec at heart rate of 72 beats/min)	Should not vary from one complex to another Should not be more than half the RR interval
RR interval	Varies with pulse rate	Should be equidistant, with slight variations on respiration

*At 60-100 beats/min.

another. These time intervals can be measured (Table 30-1), and deviations from these time references often indicate pathology.

Mechanical System. The electrical system triggers mechanical activity. Contraction of myocardium results in ejection of blood from the cardiac chamber and is termed *systole.* Relaxation of the muscle is termed *diastole.* Cardiac output (CO) is the measurement of mechanical efficiency. CO is the amount of blood pumped by each ventricle in 1 minute. It is calculated by multiplying the amount of blood ejected from one ventricle with one heart beat, the stroke volume (SV), by the heart rate (HR) per minute:

$$CO = SV \times HR$$

For the normal adult at rest, CO is maintained in the range of 4 to 8 L per minute.[2] Cardiac index (CI) is the CO divided by the body mass index (BMI). The CI adjusts the CO to the body size. The normal CI is 2.8 to 4.2 L per minute per meter squared ($L/min/m^2$).[2]

Factors affecting cardiac output. Numerous factors can affect either the HR or the SV and thus the CO. The HR is regulated primarily by the autonomic nervous system. The factors affecting the SV are preload, contractility, and afterload.[1]

Starling's law states that, to a point, the more the fibers are stretched, the greater their force of contraction. The volume of blood in the ventricles at the end of diastole, before the next contraction, is called preload. Preload determines the amount of stretch placed on myocardial fibers.

Contractility can be increased by norepinephrine released by the sympathetic nervous system, as well as by epinephrine, whether produced endogenously by the adrenal medulla or administered as a drug. Increasing contractility raises the SV by increasing ventricular emptying.

Afterload is the peripheral resistance against which the left ventricle must pump. Afterload is affected by the size of the ventricle, wall tension, and arterial blood pressure. If the arterial blood pressure is elevated, the ventricles will meet increased resistance to ejection of blood, increasing the work demand. Eventually this results in ventricular hypertrophy (enlargement of the cardiac muscle tissue without an increase in the size of cavities). Increasing preload, contractility, and afterload increase the workload of the myocardium resulting in increased oxygen demand.

Cardiac Reserve. The cardiovascular system must respond to numerous situations in health and illness (e.g., exercise, stress, hypovolemia). The ability to respond to these demands by altering CO threefold or fourfold is termed *cardiac reserve.*

The increase in CO results from an increase in HR or SV. The HR can increase to as high as 180 beats per minute for short periods without deleterious effects. The SV can be increased by increasing either preload or contractility.

Vascular System

Blood Vessels. The three major types of blood vessels in the vascular system are the arteries, veins, and capillaries. Arteries travel away from the heart and, except for the pulmonary artery, carry oxygenated blood. Veins travel toward the heart and, except for the pulmonary veins, carry deoxygenated blood. Small arteries are called arterioles, and small veins are called venules. Blood circulates from the heart into arteries, arterioles, capillaries, venules, veins, and back to the heart.

Arteries and arterioles. The arterial system differs from the venous system by the amount and type of tissue that makes up arterial walls (Fig. 30-7). The large arteries have thick walls that are composed mainly of elastic tissue. This elastic property cushions the impact of the force from systemic blood pressure and provides a recoil that propels blood

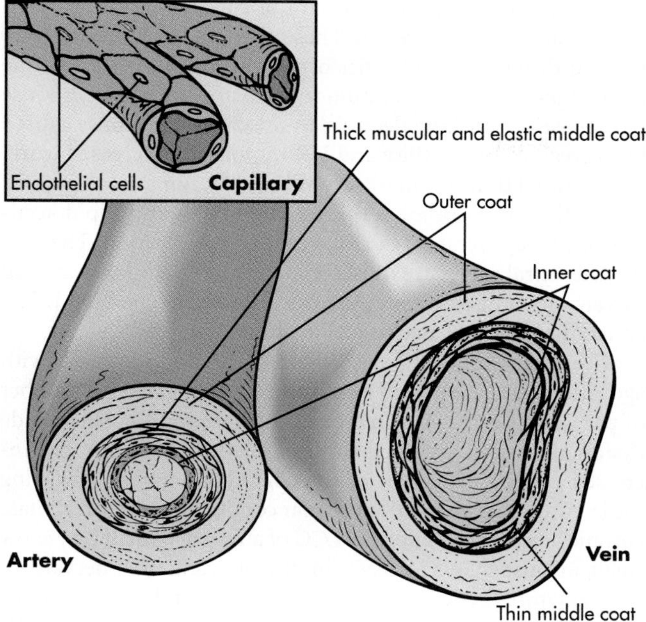

Fig. 30-7 Comparative thickness of layers of the artery, vein, and capillary.

forward into the circulation. Large arteries also contain some smooth muscle. Examples of large arteries are the aorta and the pulmonary artery.

Arterioles have relatively little elastic tissue but a lot of smooth muscle. They respond readily to local conditions such as low O_2, increasing levels of CO_2, and other wastes by dilating or constricting. The amount of blood flow to each organ and various tissues is directly related to the degree of constriction of the arteriole lumen. Arterioles serve as the major control of arterial blood pressure and distribution of blood flow.

Capillaries. The thin capillary wall is made up of endothelial cells, with no elastic or muscle tissue present (see Fig. 30-7). There are many miles of capillaries in an adult. The exchange of cellular nutrients and metabolic end products takes place through these many thin-walled vessels.

Veins and venules. Veins are large-diameter, thin-walled vessels that return blood to the right atrium (see Fig. 30-7). The venous system is a low-pressure, high-volume system. The larger veins contain semilunar valves at intervals to maintain the blood flow toward the heart and to prevent backward flow. The amount of blood in the venous system is affected by a number of factors, including arterial flow, compression of veins by skeletal muscles, alterations in thoracic and abdominal pressures, and right atrial pressure.

The largest veins are the superior vena cava, which returns blood to the heart from the head, neck, and arms, and the inferior vena cava, which returns blood to the heart from the lower part of the body. These large-diameter vessels are affected by the pressure in the right side of the heart. Elevated right atrial pressure can cause distended neck veins or liver engorgement as a result of resistance to blood flow.

Venules are relatively small tubules made up of a small amount of muscle and connective tissue. Venules collect blood from various capillary beds and channel it to the larger veins.

Regulation of the Cardiovascular System

Autonomic Nervous System. The autonomic nervous system consists of the sympathetic nervous system and the parasympathetic nervous system.

Effect on the heart. Stimulation of the sympathetic nervous system increases the HR, the speed of impulse conduction through the AV node, and the force of atrial and ventricular contractions. This effect is mediated by specific sites in the heart called β-adrenergic receptors that are receptors for norepinephrine and epinephrine.

In contrast, stimulation of the parasympathetic system (mediated by the vagus nerve) causes a decrease in HR by the action on the SA node and slows conduction through the AV node.

Effect on the blood vessels. The source of neural control of blood vessels is the sympathetic nervous system. The α-adrenergic receptors are located in the vascular smooth muscle. Stimulation of the α-adrenergic receptors results in vasoconstriction. Decreased stimulation to the α-adrenergic receptors causes vasodilation.

The parasympathetic nerves have selective distribution in the blood vessels. Stimulation of the parasympathetic nerves to each organ results in a specialized response. Blood vessels to skeletal muscle do not receive parasympathetic input.[1]

Baroreceptors. Baroreceptors in the aortic arch and carotid sinus (at the origin of the internal carotid artery) are sensitive to stretch or pressure within the arterial system. Stimulation of these receptors sends information to the vasomotor center in the brainstem. This results in inhibition of the sympathetic nervous system and enhancement of the parasympathetic influence, causing a decreased HR and peripheral vasodilation.

Decreased arterial pressure causes the opposite effect. Baroreceptors influence only temporary changes in blood pressure and heart rate.

Chemoreceptors. Chemoreceptors are located in the aortic arch and carotid body. They are capable of initiating changes in HR and arterial pressure in response to chemical stimulation. They are stimulated by decreased arterial O_2 pressure (PO_2), increased arterial carbon dioxide pressure (PCO_2), and decreased plasma pH. When the chemoreceptor reflexes are stimulated, they subsequently stimulate the vasomotor center to increase cardiac activity.

Blood Pressure

The arterial blood pressure (BP) is a measure of the pressure exerted by blood against the walls of the arterial system. The systolic blood pressure (SBP) is the peak pressure exerted against the arteries when the heart contracts. The diastolic blood pressure (DBP) is the residual pressure of the arterial system during ventricular relaxation. BP is usually expressed as the ratio of systolic to diastolic pressure.

The two main factors influencing BP are CO and systemic vascular resistance (SVR):

$$BP = CO \times SVR$$

SVR is the force opposing the movement of blood. This force is created primarily in small arteries and arterioles.

Measurement of Arterial Blood Pressure. BP can be measured by invasive and noninvasive techniques. The invasive technique consists of catheter insertion into an artery.

The catheter is attached to a recording device, and the pressure is measured directly (see Chapter 63).

However, the easiest technique is the noninvasive, indirect measurement of BP with a sphygmomanometer and a stethoscope. The sphygmomanometer consists of an inflatable cuff and a pressure gauge. The BP is measured externally by listening for sounds of turbulent blood flow through a compressed artery (Korotkoff sounds). The brachial artery is the usual site for taking BP.

After placing the appropriate size cuff on the extremity, the cuff is inflated to a pressure in excess of the systolic pressure. This causes blood flow in the artery to cease. As the pressure in the cuff is lowered, the artery is auscultated for Korotkoff sounds. There are five phases of Korotkoff sounds. The first phase is a tapping sound caused by the spurt of blood into the constricted artery as the pressure in the cuff is gradually deflated. This sound is considered the SBP. The fifth phase occurs when the sound disappears and is known as the DBP.[3] Clinically the blood pressure is recorded as 120/80. Occasionally an auscultatory gap is heard. An auscultatory gap is a loss of sound between the SBP and the DBP. The BP could be measured incorrectly if the cuff is not inflated to exceed the true SBP.

In addition to the manual technique, another noninvasive way to measure BP indirectly is to use an automatic cycling device. These automated BP monitors have been found to correlate closely with the results obtained by auscultating BP.

Ambulatory BP monitoring may be used to diagnose hypertension more accurately in some patients (see Chapter 31).The monitor consists of a BP cuff and a lightweight microprocessing unit. This method records a patient's BP at preset intervals during routine activities. At the end of the monitoring period (usually 24 hours), the data that are recorded and stored in the microprocessing unit are transferred to a printer. The printed results are then interpreted.

Pulse Pressure and Mean Arterial Pressure. Pulse pressure is the difference between the systolic and diastolic pressures. It is normally about one third of the systolic pressure. If the BP is 120/80, the pulse pressure is 40. An increased pulse pressure may occur during exercise or in individuals with arteriosclerosis of the larger arteries. A decreased pulse pressure may be found in cardiac failure or hypovolemia.

Another measurement related to BP is mean arterial pressure (MAP). It is not the average of the diastolic and systolic pressures because the duration of diastole exceeds that of systole at normal HRs. MAP is calculated by adding the diastolic pressure to one third of the pulse pressure:

$$\text{MAP} = \text{DBP} + {}^{1}/_{3}\ \text{pulse pressure}$$

A person with a BP of 120/60 has a MAP of 80.

GERONTOLOGIC CONSIDERATIONS

Effects of Aging on the Cardiovascular System

Cardiovascular disease is the most common cause of hospitalization and death in older adults in North America. The most common cardiovascular problem is coronary arteriosclerosis. It is difficult to separate normal aging changes from the pathophysiologic changes of atherosclerosis. Current research suggests that some of the normal changes of aging promote arteriosclerosis, hypertension, and cardiac failure.[4]

With increased age, the amount of collagen in the heart increases and elastin decreases. These changes affect the contractile and distensible properties of the myocardium. One of the major age-associated alterations in the cardiovascular response to exercise is a striking decrease in the cardiac response caused by decreased contractility and HR response to increased work. The resting HR is not markedly affected by aging.

Cardiac valves become thicker and stiffer from lipid accumulation, degeneration of collagen, and calcification. The aortic and mitral valves are most frequently affected. This can lead to valve incompetence or stenosis. The turbulent blood flow across the affected valve results in a murmur.[5]

The number of pacemaker cells in the SA node decreases with age. An elderly person may have only 10% of the normal number of pacemaker cells.[5] This increases the likelihood of sinus node dysfunction with sustained sinus bradycardia. Fibrosis and increased microcalcification of the conduction system involving the left bundle branch in ventricular conduction may precipitate chronic heart block. A normal ECG of an aging patient may show small, inconspicuous increases in PR, QRS, and QT intervals.

The sympathetic nervous system control of the cardiovascular system decreases with aging. The number and function of β-adrenergic receptors in the heart decrease with age. Therefore the older adult has a decreased response to physical and emotional stress and is less sensitive to β-adrenergic agonist drugs.

Arterial blood vessels thicken and become less elastic with age. Arteries increase their sensitivity to vasopressin (antidiuretic hormone).[4] Both of these changes contribute to an increase in blood pressure with age. An increase in systolic pressure and a lower rate of increase in the diastolic pressure cause a widening of the pulse pressure. Despite the changes associated with aging, the heart is able to function adequately under normal circumstances, and hypertension should not be considered a normal consequence of aging.

Age-related changes in the cardiovascular system and differences in assessment findings are presented in Table 30-2.

ASSESSMENT OF THE CARDIOVASCULAR SYSTEM

Subjective Data

A careful health history and physical examination should aid the nurse in differentiating symptoms that reflect a cardiovascular problem from problems of other body systems. For instance, it is important to determine if weight gain is because of overeating or a manifestation of fluid retention. Is shortness of breath caused by congestive heart failure (CHF) or chronic obstructive pulmonary disease (COPD)? Common chief cues that should alert the nurse to the possibility of underlying cardiovascular problems should be explored and documented (Table 30-3).

Important Health Information

Past health history. Many illnesses affect the cardiovascular system directly or indirectly. The patient should be questioned about a history of chest pain, shortness of breath, alcoholism or excessive drinking, anemia, rheumatic fever, streptococcal sore throat, congenital heart disease, stroke, syncope, hypertension, thrombophlebitis, intermittent claudication, varicosities, and edema.

Medications. An assessment of the patient's current and past use of medication should be made. This includes both

GERONTOLOGIC DIFFERENCES IN ASSESSMENT

Table 30-2 Cardiovascular System

Changes	Differences in Assessment Findings
Chest Wall	
Senile kyphosis	Altered chest landmarks for palpation, percussion, and auscultation; distant heart sounds
Heart	
Myocardial hypertrophy, increase in collagen and scarring, decrease in elasticity	Decrease in cardiac reserve, slight decrease in HR
Downward displacement	Difficulty in isolating apical pulse
Decrease in CO, HR, SV in response to exercise or stress	Slowed, decreased response to stress; slowed recovery from activity
Cellular aging changes and fibrosis of conduction system	Decrease in amplitude of QRS complex and lengthening of PR, QRS, and QT intervals; left axis deviation; irregular cardiac rhythms
Valvular rigidity from calcification, sclerosis, or fibrosis, impeding complete closure of valves	Systolic murmur (aortic or mitral) possible without being indication of cardiovascular pathology
Blood Vessels	
Arterial stiffening caused by loss of elastin in arterial walls, thickening of intima of arteries and progressive fibrosis of media	Elevation in systolic and possibly diastolic BP (e.g., 160/90); possible widened pulse pressures; more pronounced arterial pulses; pedal pulses diminished

BP, blood pressure; *CO,* cardiac output; *HR,* heart rate; *SV,* stroke volume.

over-the-counter (OTC) drugs and prescription drugs. For example, aspirin, which prolongs the blood clotting time, is contained in many drugs used to alleviate cold symptoms.

A medication assessment should list the name of the drug and the patient's understanding of its purpose and side effects. Drugs that may adversely affect the cardiovascular system also should be assessed. Some of these, and examples of their effect on the cardiovascular system, are as follows:

Tricyclic antidepressants—arrhythmias
Phenothiazines—arrhythmias and hypotension
Oral contraceptives—thrombophlebitis
Doxorubicin (Adriamycin)—cardiomyopathy
Lithium—arrhythmias
Corticosteroids—sodium and fluid retention
Theophylline preparations—tachycardia and arrhythmias
Recreational or abused drugs—tachycardia and arrhythmias

Surgery or other treatments. The patient should also be asked about specific treatments, past surgeries, or hospital admissions related to cardiovascular problems. Any hospitalizations for diagnostic workups or cardiovascular symptoms should be explored. It should be noted whether an ECG or a chest x-ray was taken for baseline data.

Functional Health Patterns. The strong correlation between components of a patient's lifestyle and cardiovascular health supports the need to review each functional health pattern. Key questions to ask a person with a cardiovascular problem are listed in Table 30-4.

Health perception–health management pattern. The nurse should ask the patient about the presence of cardiovascular risk factors. Major risk factors include elevated serum lipids, hypertension, cigarette smoking, sedentary lifestyle, and

Table 30-3 Cues to Cardiovascular Problems

Manifestation	Description
Fatigue	No energy, need more rest than usual, normal activities result in tiring
Fluid retention	Weight gain, bloated feeling; swelling; tightening of clothing; shoes no longer fitting comfortably; marks or indentations left from constricting garments
Irregular heartbeat	Sensation of heart in throat or skipped beats, racing heart; dizziness
Dyspnea	Air hunger, especially after exertion; pillows or upright chair necessary for sleep
Pain	Indigestion, burning, numbness, tightness, or pressure in midchest; epigastric or substernal pain, radiating to shoulder, neck, arms
Tenderness in calf of leg	Inability to bear weight; swelling of the involved extremity; inflamed, warm skin over vein
	Distended, discolored, tortuous veins in calves of legs; ache in lower extremities after standing for short periods
Dizzy, light-headed	Dizzy with change of position; woozy, unstable, weak

HEALTH HISTORY

Table 30-4 Cardiovascular System

Health Perception–Health Management Pattern
- Have you noticed an increase in cardiovascular symptoms such as chest pain or dyspnea?*
- Do you practice any preventive measures to decrease cardiac risk factors?*
- Do you foresee any potential self-care problems because of your cardiovascular problem?*

Nutritional-Metabolic Pattern
- Describe your usual daily dietary intake, including fat, sodium, and fluid.
- What is your present weight? What was your weight one year ago? If different, explain.
- Does eating cause fatigue or shortness of breath?*

Elimination Pattern
- Do your feet or ankles ever swell?*
- Have you ever taken medication to help you get rid of excess fluid?*

Activity-Exercise Pattern
- Are your activities or exercise limited because of your cardiovascular problem?*
- Are your activities of daily living restricted because of your cardiovascular problem?*
- Do you experience any discomfort or side effects as a result of exercise or activity?*

Sleep-Rest Pattern
- How many pillows do you sleep on at night?
- How many times a night do you awaken to urinate?
- Do you ever wake up suddenly and feel as if you cannot catch your breath?*

Cognitive-Perceptual Pattern
- Have you noticed any changes in your memory or level of awareness?*
- Do you ever experience dizziness?*
- Do you find it difficult to verbally express yourself?*
- Do you experience any pain (e.g., chest pain, leg pain with activity) as a result of your cardiovascular problem?*

Self-Perception–Self-Concept Pattern
- Have your perceptions of yourself changed since you were diagnosed with a cardiovascular disease?*
- How has your cardiovascular disease affected your life and your self-esteem?

Role-Relationship Pattern
- Describe how this illness has affected the roles that you play in your daily life.
- Describe how this illness has affected your relationships.
- How have your significant others been affected by your disease?

Sexuality-Reproductive Pattern
- Has your sexual behavior changed?*
- Do you experience any cardiac-related symptoms during intercourse?*
- Do any of your medications affect your ability to participate in sexual activities?*

Coping–Stress Tolerance Pattern
- Do you practice any stress reduction techniques?*
- Describe your normal coping mechanisms for stress.
- Who or where would you turn to during a time of stress? Are these people or services helping you now?*
- Do you feel capable of handling your present health situation? Explain.
- Do you experience any cardiovascular symptoms such as chest pain or palpitations during times of stress?*

Values-Belief Pattern
- What influence has your value-belief system had during your illness?
- Do you feel any conflicts between your value-belief system and your planned therapy?*
- Describe any cultural or religious beliefs that may influence the treatment of your cardiovascular problem.

*If yes, describe.

obesity. Stressful lifestyle and diabetes mellitus should also be investigated.

If the patient smokes, the number of pack years of smoking (number of packs smoked per day multiplied by the number of years the patient has smoked) should be estimated. The patient's attitude about smoking, as well as attempts to stop, should be documented. Alcohol use should also be recorded. This information should include type of beverage, amount, frequency, and any changes in the reaction to it. The use of habit-forming drugs, including recreational drugs, also should be noted. Finally, of importance for teaching and discharge planning, is knowledge of the patient's perception of how this illness may affect the future level of wellness and ability for self-care.

A question about the patient's allergies is appropriate. The nurse should determine whether a drug reaction or allergic reaction was ever experienced. If the patient has been treated for allergies, understanding of this therapy should be ascertained. The patient should also be asked whether an anaphylactic reaction has ever been experienced.

Confirmed illnesses of blood relatives can highlight any hereditary or familial tendencies toward coronary artery disease, peripheral vascular disease, hypertension, bleeding, cardiac disorders, diabetes mellitus, atherosclerosis, and stroke. In addition, disorders affecting the vascular system, such as intermittent claudication and varicosities, may be familial. Finally, a family health history of noncardiac conditions such as asthma, renal disease, and obesity should be assessed because they can affect the cardiovascular system.

Nutritional-metabolic pattern. Being underweight or overweight may indicate potential cardiovascular problems. Thus it is important to assess the patient's weight history in relation to height and build. A typical day's diet should be examined for its adequacy in relation to the patient's lifestyle. The amount of salt, saturated fats, and triglycerides in the patient's diet should be determined. In addition to actual food habits, which are influenced greatly by ethnicity, the patient's attitudes and plans in relation to diet should be investigated. Food intake and exercise patterns should be complementary.

Elimination pattern. Skin color, temperature, integrity, and turgor may provide valuable information about circulatory problems. Atherosclerosis may produce cool, cyanotic extremities, and edema may indicate heart failure. The patient on diuretics may report increased urinary elimination. Problems with constipation should be investigated and documented. Straining at stool (Valsalva maneuver) should be avoided in a patient with cardiovascular problems.

Cardiovascular problems may impair the patient's ability to get to a toilet as quickly as necessary. The patient should be questioned about this if incontinence or constipation are problematic.

Activity-exercise pattern. The benefit of exercise to cardiovascular health is indisputable, with sustained aerobic exercise being most beneficial. The nurse should carefully inquire about the types of exercise done, the duration and frequency of each, and the occurrence of any unwanted effects. The length of time the exercise program has been practiced should be recorded, along with participation in individual or group sports. Any symptoms indicative of cardiovascular problems such as lightheadedness, chest pain, shortness of breath, or claudication during exercise should be noted.

The patient should also be questioned about any limitations in activities of daily living (ADLs) as a result of a cardiovascular problem. Such problems are often associated with fatigue and depression, which are common symptoms of cardiac disease. The nurse should also gather information about the patient's leisure and recreational activities. Any decrease in previous abilities should be noted.

Sleep-rest pattern. Although there are many possible causes, cardiovascular problems are often the cause for interrupted sleep. Paroxysmal nocturnal dyspnea (attacks of shortness of breath especially at night that awaken the patient) are associated with advanced heart failure. Many patients with heart failure may need to sleep with their head elevated on pillows. The nurse should note the number of pillows needed for comfort. Nocturia, a common finding with cardiovascular patients, interrupts normal sleep patterns.

Cognitive-perceptual pattern. It is important that the nurse asks both the patient and significant others about cognitive-perceptual problems. Any pain associated with the cardiovascular system such as chest pain and claudication should be reported. Cardiovascular problems such as arrhythmias, hypertension, and stroke may cause problems with vertigo, language, and memory.

Self-perception–self-concept pattern. If a cardiovascular event has been of acute origin, the patient's self-perception is often affected. Invasive diagnostic and palliative procedures often lead to body image concerns for the patient. When the cardiovascular disease is chronic in nature, the patient may not be able to identify the cause but can often describe the inability to "keep up" previous levels of activity or accomplishments. This too may affect the patient's self-esteem. Therefore it is essential to inquire about the effects of the illness on the patient.

Role-relationship pattern. The patient's sex, race, and age are all related to cardiovascular health and are therefore important basic information. In addition, discussing the patient's marital status, role in the household, number of children and their ages, living environment, and significant others assist the nurse in identifying strengths and support systems in the patient's life. The nurse must assess the patient's level of satisfaction or dissatisfaction in each assigned role, which may alert the clinician to possible areas of stress or conflict.

Sexuality-reproductive pattern. The patient should be asked about the effect of the cardiovascular problem on sexual patterns and satisfaction. It is common for the patient to have a fear of sudden death during sexual intercourse, causing a major alteration in sexual behavior. Fatigue or shortness of breath may also curtail sexual activity. Impotence may be a symptom of peripheral vascular disease and is a side effect of some medications used in treating cardiovascular problems (e.g., β-adrenergic blockers, diuretics).

Many medications used to treat cardiovascular problems, particularly those used to treat hypertension, can result in impotence (see Table 31-8). This side effect may result in noncompliance with medical treatment. Counseling of both the patient and partner may be indicated.

Coping–stress tolerance pattern. The patient should be asked to identify areas that cause stress or anxiety. Potentially stressful areas include marital relationships, family, occupation, church, friends, finances, and housing. Although many persons enjoy certain activities, these activities can be stressful at the same time that they are rewarding. The usual methods of coping with stress should be investigated.

Behaviors such as explosive, rapid speech and emotions such as anger and hostility have been associated with a risk of cardiac disease. Further research has made a strong link between hostility and heart disease.[6] The patient and the family should be asked about the frequency of these types of behavior.

Information about support systems such as family, extended family and friends, psychologists, or religious groups may provide excellent resources for developing a plan of care.

Values-belief pattern. Individual values and beliefs, which are greatly affected by culture, may play a significant role in the level of conflict a patient faces when dealing with a diagnosis of cardiovascular disease. Some patients may attribute their illness to punishment from God; others may feel that a "higher power" may assist them. Knowledge of a patient's values and beliefs will give the nurse and allied professionals excellent information to intervene during periods of crisis. It is also important to determine if the proposed plan of care causes any conflict with the patient's value system.

Objective Data

Physical Examination

Vital signs. After the patient's general appearance has been observed, vital signs, including BP, heart and respiratory rate, and temperature, are taken. The BP should be measured while the patient is sitting, lying, and standing. An appropriate cuff size should be used for accurate readings. Normally there is a reduction of up to 15 mm Hg in the systolic blood pressure and 3 to 5 mm Hg in the diastolic blood pressure in the standing position. BP measurements should be taken in both arms. These readings may vary from 5 to 15 mm Hg. A greater variance indicates pathology. BP in the lower extremities is expected to be 10 mm Hg higher than in the upper extremities.

Peripheral vascular system

Inspection. Inspection of the skin color, hair distribution, and venous blood flow provides information about arterial blood flow and venous return. The extremities should be inspected for conditions such as edema, thrombophlebitis, varicose veins, and lesions such as stasis ulcers. Edema in the extremities can be caused by gravity, interruption of venous return, or elevation of right atrial pressure.

A measure used for assessing arterial flow to the extremities is the capillary filling time. The patient's nail beds are squeezed to produce blanching and observed for the return of color. With normal arterial capillary perfusion, the color will return within 3 seconds.

The large veins in the neck (internal and external jugular) should be inspected while the patient is gradually elevated to an upright position. Distention and prominent pulsations of these neck veins can be caused by right atrial pressure elevation.

Palpation. Palpation of the pulses in the neck and extremities also provides information on arterial blood flow. The pulses should be palpated to assess the volume and pressure within each vessel. Characteristics of the arteries on the right and left sides of the body should be compared. It is important to palpate each carotid pulse separately to avoid vagal stimulation and subsequent arrhythmias.

When palpating the arteries identified in Fig. 30-8, the assessor should note the pressure of the pulse wave or how far the vessel wall distends when the pulse occurs. This judgment of the pulsation volume is recorded as normal, bounding, thready, or absent. A scale may be used to document pulse volume or amplitude:[3]

0—Absent
1+—Weak, thready
2+—Normal
3+—Full, bounding

The rigidity (hardness) of the vessel should also be noted. The normal pulse will feel like a tap, whereas a vessel wall that is narrowed or bulging will vibrate. A term for a palpable vibration is *thrill.*

Auscultation. An artery that has a narrowed or bulging wall may also create an abnormal buzzing or humming termed a *bruit.* It can be heard through a stethoscope placed over the vessel. Auscultation of major arteries such as the carotids, abdominal aorta, and femoral should be part of the initial cardiovascular assessment. Abnormalities of the cardiovascular system are described in Table 30-5.

Thorax

Inspection and palpation. An overall inspection of the bony structures of the thorax, including the sternoclavicular joints, the manubrium, and the upper part of the sternum, is the initial step in the examination. Pulsations of the aortic arch or the innominate arteries may be observed or palpated in this area in some normal persons. Thrills caused by abnormalities of these vessels may also be detected.

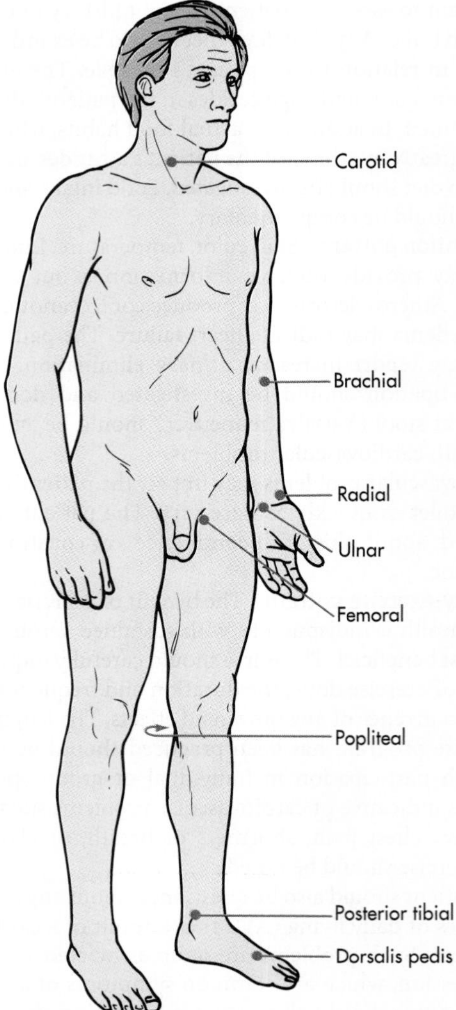

Fig. 30-8 Common sites for palpating arteries.

Next, inspect and palpate the areas where the cardiac valves project their sounds by identifying the intercostal spaces (ICSs). The raised notch, angle of Louis, that is created where the manubrium and the body of the sternum are joined is readily palpable in the midline of the sternum. The angle of Louis is at the level of the second rib and can therefore be used to count ICSs and locate specific auscultatory areas.

The following auscultatory areas can be located (Fig. 30-9): the aortic area in the second ICS to the right of the sternum, the pulmonic area in the second ICS to the left of the sternum, the tricuspid area in the fifth left ICS close to the sternum, and the mitral area in the left midclavicular line at the level of the fifth ICS. A fifth auscultatory area is Erb's point, located at the third left ICS near the sternum.

Normally, no pulsations are felt in these areas unless the patient has a thin chest wall. Valvular disorder may be suspected if abnormal pulsations or thrills are felt. Next, the epigastric area, which lies on either side of the midline just below the xyphoid process, is inspected and palpated. The pulsation of the abdominal aorta may be visible and can normally be palpated here. Next, the precordium, which is located between the apex

COMMON ASSESSMENT ABNORMALITIES

Table 30-5 Cardiovascular System

Findings	Description	Possible Etiology and Significance
Pulse		
Pulse volume		
Bounding	Sharp, brisk, rapidly rising pulse	Bradycardia, anemia, aortic valve incompetence
Thready	Weak, slowly rising pulse	Blood loss, mitral valve stenosis
Absent	Lack of pulse	Atherosclerosis, thrombus, trauma
Thrill	Vibration of vessel or chest wall	Aneurysm, aortic regurgitation
Rigidity	Stiffness or inflexibility of vessel wall	Hardening or thickening of wall, atherosclerosis
Bruit	Humming heard through stethoscope placed over vessel	Narrowing of vessel, atherosclerosis, or aneurysm
Tachycardia	Heart rate greater than 100 beats/min	Exercise, anxiety, shock, need for increased cardiac output
Bradycardia	Heart rate less than 60 beats/min	Rest, SA node (pacemaker) damage, athletic conditioning, side effect of drugs (e.g., β-adrenergic blockers)
Arrhythmia	Irregular heart rate, skipped heart beats	Damage to cardiac conduction pathway, ischemia, side effect of drugs
Venous Abnormalities		
Distended neck veins	Vertical distance between intersection of angle of Louis and level of jugular distention greater than 3 cm with patient sitting at 45° angle	Elevated right atrial pressure
Pitting edema of lower extremities or sacral area	Visible finger indentation after application of firm pressure	Interruption of venous return to heart, fluid in tissues
Thrombophlebitis	Inflammation of vein associated with red, warm, tender, hard vein; edema, pain, tenderness of extremity	Venous stasis, damage to endothelial layer of vein, hypercoagulability of blood
Positive Homans' sign	Presence of calf pain during sharp dorsiflexion of foot	Thrombophlebitis
Skin		
Unusually warm hands or feet	Warmer than normal	Possible thyrotoxicosis and severe anemia
Cold hands or feet	Cold to touch, external covering necessary for comfort	Intermittent claudication, peripheral arterial obstruction, low cardiac output
Central cyanosis	Bluish or purplish tinge in central areas such as tongue, conjunctivae, inner surface of lips	Incomplete O_2 saturation of arterial blood due to pulmonary or cardiac disorders (e.g., congenital defects)
Peripheral cyanosis	Bluish or purplish tinge in extremities or in nose and ears	Reduced blood flow because of heart failure, vasoconstriction, cold environment
Color changes in extremities with postural change	Pallor, cyanosis, mottling of skin after limb elevation; glossy skin	Chronic decreased arterial perfusion
Stasis ulcers	Darkly pigmented, edematous areas of skin; open or oozing fluid	Poor venous return, varicose veins, incompetent venous valves
Extremities		
Clubbing of nail beds	Obliteration of normal angle between base of nail and skin	Endocarditis, congenital defects, prolonged O_2 deficiency
Splinter hemorrhages	Small red to black streaks under fingernails	Infective endocarditis (infection of endocardium, usually in area of cardiac valves)

Continued

COMMON ASSESSMENT ABNORMALITIES

Table 30-5 Cardiovascular System—cont'd

Findings	Description	Possible Etiology and Significance
Extremities—cont'd		
Abnormal capillary filling time	Blanching of nail bed for more than 3 sec after release of pressure	Reduced arterial capillary perfusion, anemia
Varicose veins	Visible dilated, tortuous vessels in lower extremities	Incompetent valves in vein
Asymmetry in limb circumference	Measurable swelling of involved limb	Thrombophlebitis, varicose veins
Arterial bruit	Turbulent flow sound in peripheral artery	Arterial obstruction or aneurysm
Cardiac Auscultatory Abnormalities		
Third heart sound (S_3)	Extra heart sound, low pitched, ending in early diastole, similar to sound of a gallop	Left ventricular failure; mitral valve regurgitation, volume overload, hypertension (possible)
Fourth heart sound (S_4)	Extra heart sound, low pitched, ending in late diastole, similar to sound of a gallop	Forceful atrial contraction from resistance to ventricular filling (e.g., in left ventricular hypertrophy, pulmonary stenosis, hypertension, coronary artery disease, aortic stenosis)
Cardiac murmurs	Turbulent sounds occurring between normal heart sounds; characterized by loudness, pitch, shape, quality, duration, timing	Cardiac valve disorder, abnormal blood flow patterns

SA, sinoatrial.

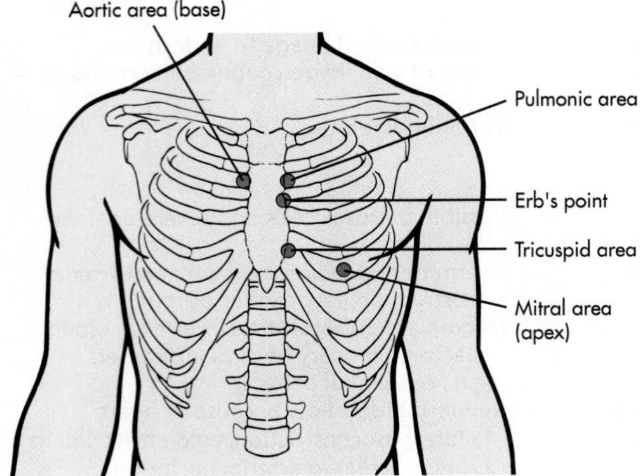

Fig. 30-9 Cardiac auscultatory areas.

and the sternum, is inspected for heaves. *Heaves* are sustained lifts of the chest wall in the precordial area that can be seen or palpated. They may be caused by left ventricular enlargement. Normally no pulsations are seen or felt here.

The mitral valve area is inspected for the PMI while the patient is recumbent. This pulsation or ventricular thrust normally has a short duration and lies within the midclavicular line in the fifth ICS (apex). If the PMI is not visible, the area should be palpated by placing the palm of the right hand in the apical area and feeling for the thrust. If the PMI is palpable, its position is recorded in relation to the midclavicular line and ICSs. When the PMI is left of the midclavicular line, the heart may be enlarged.

Percussion. The borders of the right and left sides of the heart can be estimated by percussion. The nurse stands to the right of the recumbent patient and percusses along the curve of the rib in the fourth and fifth ICSs, starting at the midaxillary line. The percussion note over the heart is dull in comparison with the resonance over the lung and is recorded in relation to the midclavicular line.

Auscultation. The movement of the cardiac valves creates some turbulence in the blood flow. The vibration of the blood causes normal heart sounds (Fig. 30-10). These sounds can be heard through a stethoscope placed on the chest wall. The first heart sound (S_1), which is associated with the closure of the tricuspid and mitral (AV) valves, has a soft *lubb* sound. The second heart sound (S_2), which is associated with the closure of the aortic and pulmonic (semilunar) valves, has a sharp *dupp* sound. S_1 signals the beginning of systole. S_2 signals the beginning of diastole (Fig. 30-11). The nurse should listen to the auscultatory areas in sequence with both the diaphragm and bell of the stethoscope.

The first and second heart sounds are heard best with the diaphragm of the stethoscope because they are high pitched. Extra heart sounds (S_3 or S_4), if present, are heard best with the bell of the stethoscope because they are low pitched. Leaning forward while sitting accentuates sounds from the second ICSs (aortic and pulmonic areas). The left lateral decubitus position accentuates sounds produced at the mitral area.

The nurse listens at the apical area with the diaphragm of the stethoscope while simultaneously palpating the radial pulse. If fewer radial than apical pulses are counted, a pulse deficit is present. A patient with a pulse deficit should have the apical and radial pulse taken often to monitor this abnormality. A judgment about the rhythm (regular or irregular) is also made when listening at the apex.

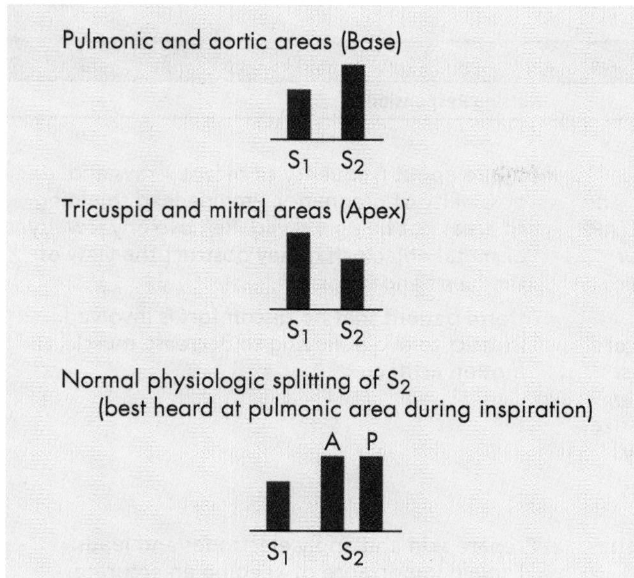

Fig. 30-10 Heart sounds. *A*, aortic; *P*, pulmonic.

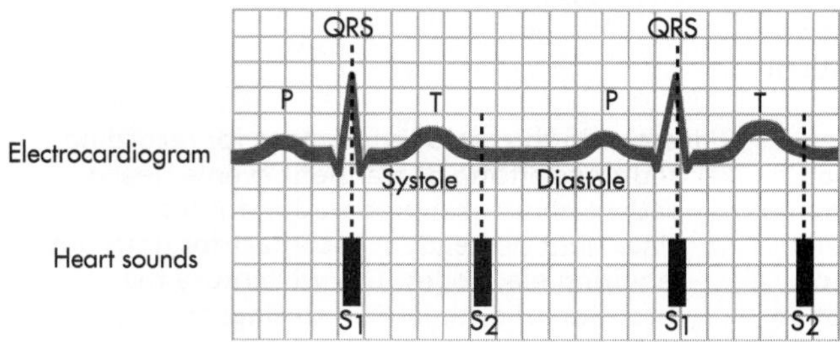

Fig. 30-11 Relationship of electrocardiogram, cardiac cycle, and heart sounds.

Palpating one carotid artery while auscultating is also important because it allows differentiation of S_1 from S_2 and systole from diastole. Because S_1 (lubb) occurs almost simultaneously with ventricular ejection, it is heard when the carotid pulse is felt. When listening at the other valvular areas, the nurse should always concentrate on the periods of systole and diastole as well as on the first and second heart sounds.

Normally no sound is heard between S_1 and S_2 during the periods of systole and diastole. Sounds that are heard during these periods probably represent abnormalities and should be described. An exception to this is a normal splitting of S_2, which is best heard at the pulmonic area during inspiration. Splitting of this heart sound can be abnormal if it is heard during expiration or if it is constant (fixed) during the respiratory cycle.

The S_3 heart sound is a low-intensity vibration of the ventricular walls usually associated with ventricular filling. An S_3 heart sound may occur in patients with left ventricular failure or mitral valve regurgitation. It is heard closely after S_2 and is known as a ventricular gallop. The S_4 heart sound is a low-frequency vibration caused by atrial contraction. It closely precedes S_1 of the next cycle and is known as an atrial gallop. An S_4 heart sound may occur in patients with coronary artery disease, left ventricular hypertrophy, or aortic stenosis.

Table 30-6 Normal Physical Assessment of the Cardiovascular System

Inspection	Normal skin color with capillary refill <3 sec; thorax symmetric with no visible PMI; no JVD with patient at 45° angle
Palpation	PMI palpable in fifth ICS at MCL; no forceful pulsations, thrills, or heaves; slight palpable pulsations of abdominal aorta in epigastric area; carotid and extremity pulses 2+ and equal bilaterally; no evidence of impaired arterial flow or venous return in lower extremities
Percussion	Unable to distinguish right-sided heart border
Auscultation	S_1 and S_2 heard; HR 72 and regular; no murmurs or extra heart sounds

ICS, intercostal space; *JVD*, jugular venous distention; *MCL*, midclavicular line; *PMI*, point of maximum impulse.

Murmurs are sounds produced by turbulent blood flow through the heart or the walls of large arteries. Most murmurs are the result of cardiac abnormalities, but some occur in normal cardiac structures. Murmurs are graded on a six-point scale of loudness and recorded as a Roman numeral ratio; the numerator is the intensity of the murmur and the denominator is always VI, which indicates that the six-point scale is being used. Number I indicates a soft, faint murmur; number VI indicates a murmur that can be heard without a stethoscope.[3]

If an abnormal sound is heard, it should be documented. This description should include the timing (during systole or diastole), location (the site on the chest where it is heard the loudest), pitch (heard best with the diaphragm or the bell of the stethoscope), position (heard best when patient is recumbent, sitting and leaning forward, or in the left lateral decubitus position), characteristic (harsh, musical, soft, short, long), and any other abnormal findings (irregular cardiac rhythms or palpable chest wall heaves) associated with the sound.

The abnormal sounds occurring during systole and diastole are classified as either murmurs or extra sounds. The most common abnormal sounds and abnormal assessment findings are described in Table 30-5. A method of recording data from the cardiovascular assessment is presented in Table 30-6.

DIAGNOSTIC STUDIES OF THE CARDIOVASCULAR SYSTEM

Numerous diagnostic procedures add to the information obtained from the history and physical examination of the cardiovascular system. These procedures are usually classified as noninvasive or invasive. If only needle insertion for withdrawal of blood or injection of dye is used, these studies are usually considered noninvasive. Catheter insertion for angiography is considered an invasive procedure. The most common studies used to assess the cardiovascular system are presented in Table 30-7. Certain responsibilities of the nurse remain the same regardless of whether the patient is to undergo an invasive or a

Text continues on p. 810.

DIAGNOSTIC STUDIES

Table 30-7 Cardiovascular System

Study	Description and Purpose	Nursing Responsibility
	Noninvasive	
Chest X-ray	Patient is placed in two upright positions to examine the lung fields and size of the heart. The two common positions are anterior/posterior (AP) and left lateral. Normal heart size and contour for the individual's age, sex, and size are noted.	Inquire about frequency of recent x-rays and possibility of pregnancy. Provide lead shielding to areas not being viewed. Remove any jewelry or metal objects that may obstruct the view of the heart and lungs.
ECG	Electrodes are placed on the chest and extremities, allowing the ECG machine to record cardiac electrical activity from different views. Can detect rhythm of heart, site of pacemaker, conduction abnormalities, position of heart, size of atria and ventricles, and presence of injury.	Inform patient that no discomfort is involved. Instruct to avoid moving to decrease muscle motion artifact.
Ambulatory ECG Monitoring		
▪ Holter monitoring	Recording of ECG rhythm for 24-48 hr and then correlating rhythm changes with symptoms recorded in diary. Normal patient activity is encouraged to simulate conditions that produce symptoms. Electrodes are placed on chest and a recorder is used to store information until it is recalled, printed, and analyzed for any rhythm disturbance. It can be performed on an inpatient or outpatient basis.	Prepare skin and apply electrodes and leads. Explain importance of keeping an accurate diary of activities and symptoms. Tell patient that no bath or shower can be taken during monitoring. Skin irritation may develop from electrodes.
▪ Transtelephonic event recorders	It allows more freedom than a regular Holter monitor. It records rhythm disturbances that are not frequent enough to be recorded in one 24 hr period. Some units have electrodes that are attached to the chest and have a loop of memory that captures the onset and end of an event. Other types are placed directly on patient's wrist, chest, or fingers and have no loop of memory, but record the patient's ECG in real time. Recordings are transmitted over the phone to a receiving unit, and the recordings are printed out for review. Tracings can then be erased and the unit can be reused.	Instruct in the use of equipment for recording and transmitting of transient events. Teach patient about skin preparation for lead placement or steady skin contact for units not requiring electrodes. This will ensure the reception of optimal ECG tracings for analysis.
Exercise Treadmill Test	Various protocols are used to evaluate the effect of exercise tolerance on myocardial function. A common protocol uses 3 min stages at set speeds and elevation of the treadmill belt. Continual monitoring of vital signs and ECG rhythms or ischemic changes are important in the diagnosis of left ventricular function and coronary artery disease. An exercise bike may be used if the patient is unable to walk on the treadmill.	Instruct patient to wear comfortable clothes and shoes that can be used for walking and running. Instruct patient about procedure and application of lead placement. Monitor vital signs and obtain 12-lead ECG before exercise, during each stage of exercise, and after exercise until all vital signs and ECG changes have returned to normal. Monitor patient's symptoms throughout procedure.
Echocardiogram ▪ M-mode ▪ Two-dimensional ▪ Cardiac Doppler ▪ Color flow imaging	Transducer that emits and receives ultrasound waves is placed in four positions on the chest above the heart. Transducer records sound waves that are bounced off the heart. Also records direction and flow of blood through the heart and transforms it to audio and graphic data that measure valvular abnormalities, congenital cardiac defects, and cardiac function.	Place patient in a supine position on left side facing equipment. Instruct family and patient about procedure and sensations (pressure and mechanical movement from head of transducer). No contraindications to procedure exist.

Continued

DIAGNOSTIC STUDIES

Table 30-7 Cardiovascular System—cont'd

Study	Description and Purpose	Nursing Responsibility
▪ Stress echocardiogram	Combination of exercise treadmill test and echocardiogram. Resting images of the heart are taken with ultrasound and then the patient exercises. Post-exercise images are taken immediately after exercise (within 1 min of stopping exercise). Differences in left ventricular wall motion and thickening before and after exercise are evaluated.	Instruct and prepare patient for exercise treadmill. Inform patient that ultrasound is not harmful and the importance of speed in returning to examination table for imaging after exercise. Contraindications include any patient unable to reach peak exercise.
▪ Dobutamine echocardiogram	Used as a substitute for the exercise stress test in individuals unable to walk on a treadmill. Dobutamine (a positive inotropic agent) is infused IV and dosage is increased in 5 min intervals while echocardiogram is performed to detect wall motion abnormalities at each stage.	Start IV infusion. Administer dobutamine. Monitor vital signs before, during, and after test until baseline achieved. Monitor patient for signs and symptoms of distress during procedure.
▪ Transesophageal echocardiogram	A probe with an ultrasound transducer at the tip is swallowed. The physician controls angle and depth. As it passes down the esophagus, it sends back clear images of heart size, wall motion, valvular abnormalities, and possible source of thrombi without interference from lungs or chest ribs. A contrast medium may be injected IV for evaluating direction of blood flow if an atrial or ventricular septal defect is suspected. Doppler ultrasound and color flow imaging can also be used concurrently.	Instruct patient to be NPO for at least 6 hr before test. A tranquilizer will be given and throat locally anesthetized, so if done as an outpatient, a designated driver is needed. Monitor vital signs and oxygen saturation levels and perform suctioning continually during procedure. Explain to patient the proper procedure for easy passage of transducer. Assist patient to relax. Patient may not eat or drink until gag reflex returns.
Nuclear Cardiology	Study involves IV injection of radioactive isotopes. Radioactive uptake is counted over the heart by scintillation camera. It supplies information about myocardial contractility, myocardial perfusion, and acute cell injury.	Explain procedure to patient. Establish IV line for injection of isotopes. Explain that radioactive isotope used is a small, diagnostic amount and will lose most of its radioactivity in a few hours. Inform the patient that he or she will be lying down on back with arms extended over head for a period of time. Repeat scans are performed within a few minutes to hours after the injection.
▪ Thallium 201 scan	Thallium 201 is injected IV and used to evaluate blood flow in different parts of heart. Cold spots correlate with areas of infarction. For stress testing, IV thallium is given 1 min before the patient reaches maximum heart rate on bicycle or treadmill. Patient is then required to continue exercise for 1 min to circulate the radioactive isotope. Actual scanning must be done within 5-10 min after exercise. A second resting scan is performed 2-4 hr later and compared to post-exercise scan.	Explain procedure to patient. Instruct patient to eat only a light meal between scans.
▪ Dipyridamole thallium scan	As with a thallium exercise test, dipyridamole (Persantine) is also injected. Dipyridamole acts as a powerful vasodilator and will increase blood flow to well-perfused coronary arteries. Scanning procedure is same as with thallium scan.	Explain procedure to patient. Instruct patient to hold all caffeine products for 12 hr before procedure.
▪ Technetium 99m Sestamibi scan	Technetium 99m Sestamibi is injected IV and taken up in area of MI, producing hot spots. Maximum results are produced when performed 1-6 days after suspected MI. Waiting period after injection is $1\frac{1}{2}$-2 hr.	Explain procedure to patient.

Continued

DIAGNOSTIC STUDIES

Table 30-7 Cardiovascular System—cont'd

Study	Description and Purpose	Nursing Responsibility
▪ Blood pool imaging	Technetium 99m pertechnetate is injected intravenously. Single injection allows sequential evaluation of heart for several hours. Study is indicated for patients with recent MI or congestive heart failure, especially if not recovering well. It can be used to measure effectiveness of various cardiac medications and can be done at patient's bedside.	Explain procedure to patient. Inform patient that procedure involves little or no risk.
▪ Positron emission tomography (PET)	Uses two radionuclides. Nitrogen-13-ammonia is injected intravenously first and scanned to evaluate myocardial perfusion. A second radioactive isotope, fluoro-18-deoxyglucose, is then injected and scanned to show myocardial metabolic function. In the normal heart, both scans will match, but in an ischemic or damaged heart, they will differ. The patient may or may not be stressed. A baseline resting scan is usually obtained for comparison.	Instruct patient on procedure. Explain that patient will be scanned by a machine and will need to stay still for a period of time. Patient's glucose level must be between 60 and 140 mg/dl (3.3-7.8 μmol/L) for accurate glucose metabolic activity. If exercise is included as part of testing, patient will need to be NPO and refrain from tobacco and caffeine for 24 hr before test.
Magnetic Resonance Imaging (MRI)	Noninvasive imaging technique obtains information about cardiac tissue integrity, aneurysms, ejection fractions, cardiac output, and patency of proximal coronary arteries. It does not involve ionizing radiation and is an extremely safe procedure. It provides images in multiple planes with uniformly good resolution. It has limited use in critical care patients because of access and equipment problems. It cannot be used in persons with any implanted metallic devices.	Explain procedure to patient. Inform patient that the small diameter of the cylinder, along with loud noise of the procedure, may cause panic or anxiety. Antianxiety medications and music may be recommended.
Blood Studies		
▪ Creatine kinase (CK)	CK enzymes are present in heart, skeletal muscle, and brain. Within 4-6 hr of MI, CK is elevated. It returns to normal within 3-4 days. *Normal:* <160 U/ml (2.67 μkat/L) (men) <130 U/ml (2.17 μkat/L) (women)	Avoid CK elevation created by IM injections that damage muscle cells.
▪ CK-MB fraction	Immunochemical process using monoclonal antibodies that measures this cardiospecific enzyme within 10-30 min. Concentrations > 7.5 ng/ml are highly indicative of MI. Begin to rise 4-6 hr after MI.	Serial sampling should be done in conjunction with ECG.
▪ AST (SGOT)	Within 6-8 hr after MI, AST rises. It peaks within 24-48 hr and returns to normal in 4-8 days. It is not specific to cardiac muscle damage. *Normal:* 7-40 U/ml (0.12-0.67 μkat/L)	Because AST can be elevated by other disorders such as liver damage, thorough history is important.
▪ Myoglobin	Low molecular protein that is 99-100% sensitive for myocardial injury. Serum concentrations rise 1-4 hr after MI and peak in 6-9 hr. *Normal:* <92 ng/ml (men) <76 ng/ml (women)	Cleared from the circulation rapidly and therefore must be measured within first 18 hr of onset of chest pain.
▪ Troponin	Contractile proteins that are released following an MI. Both troponin T and troponin I are highly specific to cardiac tissue. *Normal:* Troponin T: <0.1 ng/ml Troponin I: <0.1-3.1 ng/ml	Rapid bedside assays are available.

Continued

DIAGNOSTIC STUDIES

Table 30-7 Cardiovascular System—cont'd

Study	Description and Purpose	Nursing Responsibility
■ **Blood Studies—cont'd**		
■ Lactic dehydrogenase (LDH)	LDH has five different isoenzymes. Pattern of elevation is similar to that of AST after MI except that LDH remains elevated for 5-7 days. *Normal:* <100 U/L (<1.67 μkat/L)	When drawing blood, make certain it is not hemolyzed because this will falsely raise LDH level.
■ LDH_1 and LDH_2	LDH isoenzyme subgroups are contained in heart muscle. Test determines LDH_1/LDH_2 ratio. If $LDH_1/LDH_2 > 1$, it is indicative of MI.	
Serum Lipids		
■ Cholesterol	Cholesterol is a blood lipid. Elevated cholesterol is considered a risk factor for atherosclerotic heart disease. Level can be measured at any time of the day in a nonfasting state. *Normal:* 140-200 mg/dl (3.62-5.17 mmol/L) (varies with age and sex)	Explain procedure to patient. Cholesterol levels can be obtained in a nonfasting state, but for triglyceride levels and lipoproteins, fasting state for at least 12 hr (except for water) is necessary, and no alcohol intake is allowed for 24 hr before testing.
■ Triglycerides	Triglycerides are mixtures of fatty acids. Elevations are associated with cardiovascular disease. *Normal:* 40-190 mg/dl (0.45-2.15 mmol/L) (varies with age)	
■ Lipoproteins	Electrophoresis is done to separate lipoproteins into HDL, LDL, and VLDL and chylomicrons. There are marked day-to-day fluctuations in serum lipid levels. More than one determination is needed for accurate diagnosis and treatment. *Normal:* varies with age. Desirable LDL is <130 mg/dl (3.4 mmol/L). Desirable HDL is 37-70 mg/dl (0.97-1.83 mmol/L) for men; 40-88 mg/dl (1.05-2.30 mmol/L) for women.	Cardiac risk factors are assessed by dividing the total cholesterol level by the HDL level. *Risk* / *Men* / *Women* Low 3.43 3.27 Average 4.97 4.44 Moderate 9.55 7.95 High 25.99 11.04
Drug Levels	Blood tests done to determine therapeutic and toxic levels of drugs in body.	Ensure appropriate timing of test with medication schedule.
■ Digoxin	Therapeutic level is 1-2 ng/ml; toxic level is >3 ng/ml.	
■ Quinidine	Therapeutic level is 2.5-5 μg/ml; toxic level is >5 μg/ml.	
■ Propranolol (Inderal)	Therapeutic level is 20-85 ng/ml; toxic level is >150 ng/ml.	
	Invasive	
Cardiac Catheterization	Study involves insertion of catheter into heart. Information can be obtained about O_2 saturation and pressure readings within chambers. Dye can be injected to assist in examining structure and motion of heart. Procedure is done by insertion of catheter into a vein (for right side of heart) or an artery (for left side of heart) (see text).	Before procedure, obtain written permission. Withhold food and fluids for 6-18 hr before procedure. Give sedative, if ordered. Inform patient about use of local anesthesia, insertion of catheter, and feeling of warmth and fluttering sensation of heart as catheter is passed. Note that patient may be instructed to cough or take a deep breath when catheter is inserted and that patient is monitored by ECG throughout procedure. After procedure, assess circulation to extremity used for catheter insertion. Check peripheral pulses, color, and sensation of extremity every 15 min for 1 hr and then with decreasing frequency. Observe injection site for swelling and bleeding. Place sandbag over arterial site, if indicated. Monitor vital signs. Assess for abnormal HR, arrhythmias, and signs of pulmonary emboli (respiratory difficulty).

Continued

DIAGNOSTIC STUDIES

Table 30-7 Cardiovascular System—cont'd

Study	Description and Purpose	Nursing Responsibility
Coronary Angiography	Study involves injection of radiopaque dye directly into coronary arteries by same procedure as for cardiac catheterization. It is used to evaluate patency of coronary arteries and collateral circulation.	Same as for cardiac catheterization.
Intracoronary Ultrasound (ICUS)	Invasive study used to provide ultrasound information about the coronary arteries. A very small ultrasound probe is introduced into the coronary artery, similar to coronary angiography. Information obtained is used to asses size and consistency of plaque, arterial walls, and effectiveness of intracoronary artery treatment.	Same as for cardiac catheterization.
Hemodynamic Monitoring	Hemodynamic monitoring of arterial blood pressures, pulmonary artery pressure, pulmonary artery wedge pressure, and cardiac output are discussed in Chapter 63.	
Electrophysiology Study (EPS)	Invasive study used to record intracardiac electrical activity using catheters (with multiple electrodes) inserted via the femoral vein into the right side of heart. The catheter electrodes record the electrical activity in different cardiac structures. In addition, arrhythmias can be induced.	Obtain written consent. Antiarrhythmic medications may be discontinued several days before study. Keep patient NPO 6-8 hr before test. Give premedication to promote relaxation and throughout the procedure if ordered. Place the patient on cardiac monitor after the procedure.
Peripheral Arteriography and Venography*	Study involves injection of radiopaque dye into either arteries or veins. Serial x-rays taken to detect and visualize any atherosclerotic plaques, occlusion, aneurysms, or traumatic injury.	Carefully explain procedure to patient. Give mild sedative, if ordered. Check extremity with puncture site for pulsation, warmth, color, and motion after procedure. Inspect insertion site for bleeding or swelling. Observe patient for allergic reactions to dye.
Digital Subtraction Angiography	Type of arteriography that involves IV injection of contrast media. Catheter is threaded into superior vena cava. When contrast media circulate through arteries, computerized subtraction technique "subtracts" structures that block clear view of arteries. Most portions of cardiovascular system (except coronary arteries) can be studied by this technique. It can be performed on an outpatient basis and has fewer complications than arteriography. Fluoroscopy is used to help position catheter.	Keep patient NPO 2 hr before test. Inform patient that slight feeling of warmth may be experienced as contrast medium is injected and that ECG monitoring is done throughout procedure. Explain to patient that test takes about 1 hr.

*Additional peripheral vascular diagnostic studies are found in Table 36-9.
AST, aspartate aminotransferase; *BP,* blood pressure; *CHF,* congestive heart failure; *CO,* cardiac output; *ECG,* electrocardiogram; *HDL,* high-density lipoproteins; *HR,* heart rate; *LDL,* low-density lipoproteins; *MI,* myocardial infarction; *SGOT,* serum glutamic-oxaloacetic transaminase; *VLDL,* very-low density lipoproteins.

noninvasive procedure. First, the nurse must see that the procedure is scheduled and that any necessary preliminaries (e.g., special diets or changes in medication) are completed. Appropriate safety measures, such as the use of bedside rails after administration of preprocedure medications or identification of patient allergies, should be instituted. Comfort measures, such as oral care before the procedure, are important. The nurse must also check to see that the patient's permission for the procedure has been obtained if it is required. It is important that the patient understand the procedure. The patient may have inaccurate information that causes unnecessary anxiety regarding the diagnostic study.

Noninvasive Studies

Chest X-Ray. A radiographic picture can depict cardiac contours, heart size and configuration, and anatomic changes in individual chambers (Fig. 30-12). The radiographic image records any displacement or enlargement of the heart, and it is more accurate than percussion in determining the size of the heart. In addition to cardiac abnormalities, the presence of

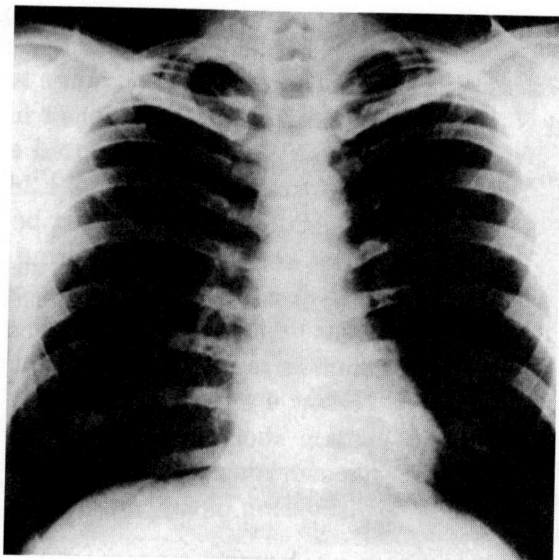

Fig. 30-12 Chest x-ray showing outline of the heart.

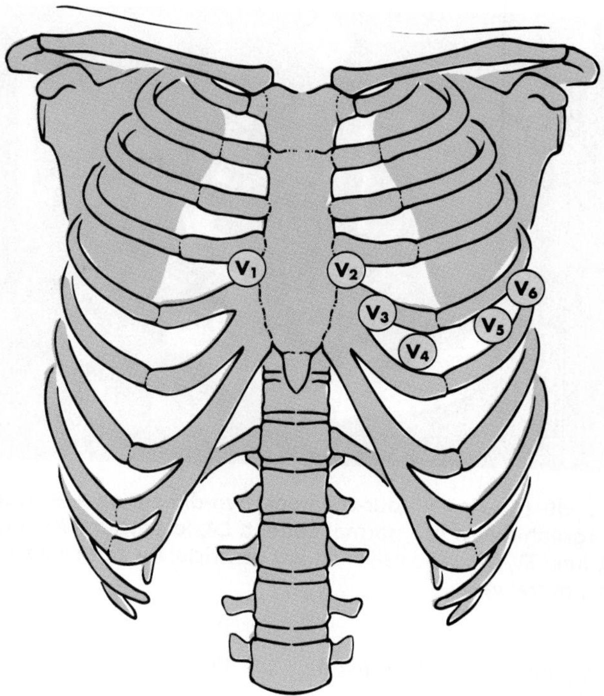

Fig. 30-13 Placement of chest leads (V leads) for a 12-lead electrocardiogram.

extra fluid around the heart may be detected by these radiographic images.

Electrocardiogram. The basic P, QRS, T waveforms (see Table 30-1) are used to assess cardiac function. Deviations from the normal sinus rhythm can indicate abnormalities in heart function. There are many types of electrocardiographic monitoring, including resting, exercise or stress testing, and continuous ambulatory monitoring.

A resting ECG helps identify at one point in time primary conduction abnormalities, cardiac arrhythmias, cardiac hypertrophy, pericarditis, myocardial ischemia, site and extent of myocardial infarction (MI), pacemaker performance, and effectiveness of drug therapy. It is used to monitor recovery from an MI.

In an exercise or stress ECG, the person pedals a stationary bicycle or walks on a treadmill while ECG and BP measurements are taken to evaluate the heart's response to physical stress. This test is valuable in assessing asymptomatic cardiac disease and helping to define limits for exercise programs.

Continuous ambulatory ECG can provide more diagnostic information than a standard resting ECG, which records less than 1 minute of the heart's activity. In this test, a portable Holter monitor is attached to the patient, and the ECG is recorded during a 24- to 48-hour period while the person performs usual activities. The person records these activities in a log book so that cardiac responses to level of activity can be studied (see Table 30-7).

Electrocardiogram leads. Recording of an ECG involves the use of multiple electrodes. An electrode is placed on each of the four limbs. The right-leg electrode is used as an inactive ground electrode. Six electrodes are placed on the precordium.

Electrical impulses generated by the heart are picked up by the electrodes, magnified by an amplifier, and recorded. The recording is done by machines that produce a direct tracing by a stylus on graph paper. An ECG records only those events occurring during the few seconds of the recording.

Each combination of electrodes used in standard electrocardiography is called a *lead*. Each lead gives a continuous recording of changes in potential (or voltage) during the cardiac cycle between any two of the electrodes or between one electrode and a combination of others.

Like a camera taking a picture from different angles, ECG leads take pictures of the myocardium. In a standard 12-lead ECG, the electrodes attached to the arms, legs, and chest measure current, or take pictures, from 12 different views or leads. The three limb leads are I, II, and III. Lead I records the direction of electric current and voltage detected between the right- and left-arm electrodes. Lead II is a right-arm and left-leg combination. Lead III records the electrical activity using the left-arm and left-leg electrodes. The unipolar augmented limb leads (aVR, aVF, and aVL) measure electrical potential between one augmented limb lead and the electrical midpoint of the remaining two leads. The chest electrodes are placed in various locations, starting at the right sternal border in the fourth ICS (V_1) and moving across the chest (V_1 through V_6), as indicated in Fig. 30-13. These are known as chest or V leads.

Unfortunately, the 12-lead ECG has limitations, with some areas of the myocardium left completely invisible to "the camera's vision." Because of lead placement, invisible areas of the myocardium include the portions of the right ventricle and the posterior wall of the left ventricle. If a more definitive diagnosis is needed for a posterior wall or right ventricular infarct, six V leads of the right chest may be obtained. Similar to the 12-lead ECG, the additional six leads are obtained by placing electrodes across the right side of the chest in the mirror image of the left chest leads.

Ambulatory Electrocardiogram Monitoring

Holter monitoring. In Holter monitoring a recorder is worn by the patient for 24 to 48 hours, and the resulting ECG information is then stored until it is played back for printing and evaluation. Holter monitoring gives the patient freedom to perform those activities that are associated with the cardiovascular

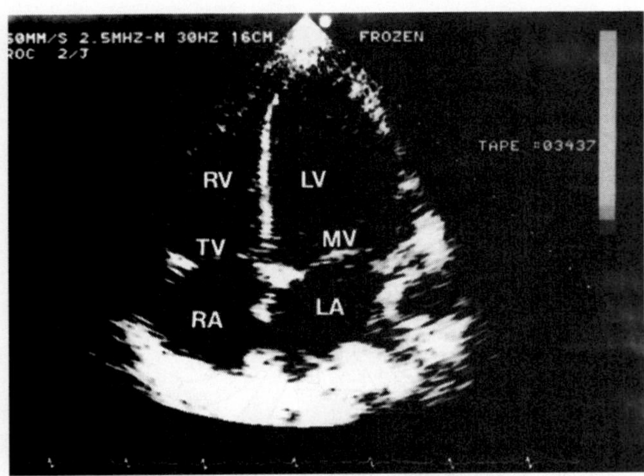

Fig. 30-14 Apical four-chamber two-dimensional echocardiographic view in a normal patient. *LA,* left atrium; *RA,* right atrium; *TV,* tricuspid valve; *LV,* left ventricle; *RV,* right ventricle; *MV,* mitral valve.

symptoms while documenting any ECG changes associated with these activities.

Transtelephonic event recorders. This type of recorder is helpful for monitoring less frequent ECG events. The monitor is a portable unit using electrodes to transmit a limited ECG over the phone to a receiving device. A disadvantage of this type of monitoring is that if the event occurs for only a short duration, the symptoms may be over before the patient puts on the device and calls the assigned number.

Exercise Testing. Cardiac symptoms frequently occur only with activity. Exercise testing is a method used to evaluate the ECG, BP, and symptoms with activity. Specific protocols for the exercise are followed. The placement of electrodes is similar to a regular 12-lead placement for the chest leads V_1 through V_6. Limb leads are placed on upper and lower chest walls to alleviate muscle interference during exercise. Resting blood pressures and ECGs are performed in the supine position, while standing, and after hyperventilation to provide a baseline for comparison of any changes during exercise.

As the patient exercises on a treadmill or stationary bicycle, the blood pressure, ECG, and often the oxygen saturation level are measured and monitored. The patient exercises to either peak HR (calculated by subtracting the person's age from 220) or to peak exercise tolerance, at which time the test is terminated and the treadmill is slowed while the patient continues walking. The test is also terminated for moderate to severe chest discomfort or significant ST segment depression indicating ischemic changes associated with coronary artery disease. After the treadmill belt is stopped, the patient lies down to rest. The ECG is monitored after exercise for rhythm disturbances or, if ECG changes did occur with exercise, for return to baseline.

Patient selection for exercise testing is appropriate for individuals free of limitations of walking or using the bicycle and those without abnormal ECGs that limit diagnostic interpretation (e.g., pacemakers, left bundle branch block).

Echocardiogram. The echocardiogram uses ultrasound waves to record the movement of the structures of the heart. In the normal heart, ultrasonic sound waves directed at the heart are reflected back in typical configurations (Fig. 30-14). The echocardiogram provides information about abnormalities of (1) valvular structure and motion, (2) cardiac chamber size and contents, (3) ventricular muscle and septal motion and thickness, (4) the pericardial sac, and (5) the ascending aorta.

Two commonly used types are the M-mode (motion-mode) and the two-dimensional (2-D, real-time, cross-sectional) echocardiogram. In the M-mode, a single ultrasound beam is directed toward the heart, recording the motion of the intracardiac structures, as well as detecting wall thickness and chamber size. The 2-D echocardiogram sweeps the ultrasound beam through an arc, producing a cross-sectional view, and shows correct spatial relationships among the structures.

Newer developments in echocardiography include Doppler technology and color flow imaging. Doppler technology allows for sound evaluation of the flow or motion of the scanned object (heart valves, ventricular walls, blood flow). Color flow imaging (duplex) is the combination of 2-D echocardiography and Doppler technology. It uses color changes to demonstrate the velocity and direction of blood flow.[7] Detection of pathologic conditions, such as valvular leaks and congenital defects, can be diagnosed with much greater ease.

Stress echocardiography, a combination of treadmill test and ultrasound images, evaluates segmental wall motion abnormalities. By using a digital computer system to compare images before and after exercise, wall motion and segmental function can be clearly seen. This diagnostic test provides the information of an exercise stress test with the information gained from an echocardiogram.[8]

For those individuals unable to exercise, infusion of dobutamine causes a pharmacologic stress on the heart while the patient is resting. The same ultrasound technology is used.

Transesophageal echocardiography (TEE) is used when posterior structures of the heart require more precise echocardiography than 2-D echocardiography can provide. The TEE uses a modified, flexible endoscope probe with an ultrasound transducer in the tip for imaging of the heart and great vessels. This probe is attached to the regular ultrasound machine so that M-mode, 2-D images, pulsed Doppler, and color flow imaging can be used. The TEE provides information on left ventricular function and wall motion. In addition, it can evaluate valvular prosthetic dysfunction, bacterial endocarditis, congenital heart disease, aortic dissection, mitral valve dysfunction, aortic aneurysm, and atrial thrombi.[9]

This technique can be used in more than one setting. It has proven helpful in intraoperative procedures because it does not interfere with the operative field and provides continuous monitoring of heart function. Knowledge regarding the adequacy of valve repair, valve replacement, and septal closures can be obtained before removal of cardiopulmonary bypass.

Outpatient TEE procedures are also performed with topical anesthesia and intravenous sedation. The patient must have taken no food or liquids for 6 to 8 hours before the procedure. The probe is introduced into the esophagus until the transducer tip is positioned at the level of the heart. The procedure lasts approximately 15 minutes. After the examination the patient may not drink or eat until the gag reflex returns.

The risks of TEE are minimal. However, complications may include perforation of the esophagus, hemorrhage, arrhythmias, vasovagal reactions, and transient hypoxemia. TEE is contraindicated if the patient has a history of esophageal disorders, dysphagia, or radiation therapy to the chest wall.

Nuclear Cardiology. Single photon emission computed tomography (SPECT) is growing in use for the evaluation of the myocardium at risk of infarction and to determine infarction size.[10] Small amounts of radioactive isotope are injected intravenously, and recordings are made of the radioactivity emitted over a specific area of the body. The total radiation exposure is minimal. The circulation of this tagged material can be used to detect coronary artery blood flow, intracardiac shunts, motion of ventricles, and size of the heart chambers. The most commonly used nuclear imaging tests include thallium imaging, technetium-99m Sestimibi scanning, and blood pool imaging. The use of new isotopes is in development. Technetium-99m Sestimibi scanning is the currently favored SPECT technique. This is due to the improvements in routine isotope scanning and lower cost than positron emission tomography (PET) scanning.[11] PET scanning uses two isotopes (see Table 30-7). PET scans are highly sensitive in distinguishing between viable and nonviable myocardial tissue. Cost limits the widespread use of PET scanning.[12]

Perfusion imaging is also used with exercise testing to determine whether the coronary blood flow changes with increased activity. Stress exercising imaging may show an abnormality even when a resting image is normal. This procedure is indicated to diagnose coronary artery disease, determine the prognosis in already diagnosed coronary disease, assess the physiologic significance of a known coronary lesion, and assess the effectiveness of various therapeutic modalities such as bypass surgery or angioplasty.

If a patient is unable to tolerate exercise, an IV infusion of dipyridamole (Persantine) is given to dilate the coronary arteries and therefore simulate the effect of exercise. After the dipyridamole takes effect, the isotope is injected and the procedure proceeds. The patient is required to lie flat for 40 minutes while the pictures are taken. The patient must have nothing by mouth until the imaging is complete. All caffeine and theophylline products must be held 12 hours before the study.

Magnetic Resonance Imaging. Although not widely used because of equipment size and access, magnetic resonance imaging (MRI) allows detection and localization of MI areas. An MRI is comparable to other established imaging modalities in assessing infarct size and location.[12] Further research is needed to determine if this imaging technique will become more commonly used in diagnosing cardiac problems.

Blood Studies. Numerous blood studies contribute information about the cardiovascular system. For example, studies of the blood itself reflect the oxygen-carrying capacity (red blood cell count and hemoglobin) and coagulation properties (clotting times). (See Chapter 28 for hematology studies.)

Diagnostic tests for myocardial infarction. When cells are injured, they release their cell contents, including enzymes, into the circulation. The enzymes characteristic of cardiac injury are creatine kinase (CK), lactic dehydrogenase (LDH), and serum aspartate aminotransferase (AST), formerly called serum glutamic-oxaloacetic transaminase (SGOT). Because these enzymes are found in a variety of body tissues, they can be elevated as a result of injury to the muscles, liver, brain, and other organs. For this reason, isoenzymes, multiple forms of an enzyme, can be identified by electrophoresis and are organ specific. Their determination is a better indicator of cardiac injury than assessment of the total enzymes. In addition to enzymes, cell contents measured are the cell proteins troponin and myoglobin.

CK is present in heart muscle, skeletal muscle, and brain tissue. CK-MM is found primarily in skeletal muscle, and CK-BB is found in the brain and nervous tissue. CK-MB elevation is specific for myocardial tissue injury, and a rise may be detected within 4 to 6 hours after an MI. CK-MB has been the "gold standard" in measuring the extent of myocardial damage. However, the traditional methodology (electrophoresis) to perform this test may take a few hours, thereby decreasing the crucial "time to treatment" for the patient with acute chest pain. A rapid quantitative CK-MB_{mass} has now been developed and takes 30 to 45 minutes to perform.[13] This test allows more rapid diagnosis of acute MI.

There are five isoenzymes of LDH, with LDH_1 and LDH_2 primarily found in the heart, red blood cells, and kidneys; LDH_3 found in the lungs; and LDH_4 and LDH_5 found in the liver and skeletal muscle. Usually LDH_1 and LDH_2 levels rise 8 to 12 hours after an acute MI. An elevated LDH level in which LDH_1 levels exceed LDH_2 levels (the reversal of their normal pattern) is a reliable indication of acute MI.

AST is present in the heart, liver, skeletal muscles, kidneys, pancreas, and red blood cells (RBCs). Although a high correlation exists between an MI and elevated AST levels, no heart-specific isoenzymes exist to assist in identifying the specific organ damaged. Therefore testing for AST in assessment of myocardial injury is often considered superfluous.

Troponin is a myocardial muscle protein released into circulation after injury. There are two subtypes, troponin T and troponin I, and they are specific to myocardial tissue. Normally there is no circulating troponin, so a rise in its level is diagnostic of myocardial damage.[13] Troponin T reaches peak levels within 12 hours and has a high specificity at 3 to 6 hours following onset of symptoms. This blood test is becoming more popular and valuable in the diagnosis of MI because results can be obtained within 20 minutes of drawing the specimen.

Myoglobin is another protein marker of acute MI that is providing new information for diagnosis. Myoglobin elevation is a sensitive indicator of myocardial injury, and serum elevations occur within 1 to 2 hours after injury but decline rapidly after 7 hours. Results can be available within 20 minutes.

Rapid bedside assays are becoming more readily available for many of the diagnostic serum markers. These will decrease the time required for laboratory results. The nurse must consider the time frame for these markers to appear in the serum and the adjunctive data (patient symptoms and ECG changes) that complete the diagnostic picture for myocardial infarction.

Blood lipids. Blood lipids consist of triglycerides, cholesterol, and phospholipids. They circulate in the blood bound to protein. Thus they are often referred to as lipoproteins.

Triglycerides are the main storage form of lipids and constitute approximately 95% of fatty tissue. Cholesterol, a structural component of cell membranes and plasma lipoproteins, is a precursor of glucocorticoids, sex hormones, and bile salts. In addition to being absorbed from food in the GI tract, cholesterol can also be synthesized in the liver. Phospholipids contain glycerol, fatty acids, phosphates, and a nitrogenous compound. Although formed in most cells, phospholipids usually enter the circulation as lipoproteins synthesized by the liver. Apoproteins are water-soluble proteins that combine with most lipids to form lipoproteins.

Different classes of lipoproteins contain varying amounts of the naturally occurring lipids. Electrophoresis is done to separate lipoproteins into the following groups:

1. Chylomicrons: primarily exogenous triglycerides from dietary fat
2. Very-low-density lipoproteins (VLDLs): primarily endogenous triglycerides with moderate amounts of phospholipids and cholesterol
3. Low-density lipoproteins (LDLs): mostly cholesterol with moderate amounts of phospholipids
4. High-density lipoproteins (HDLs): about one-half protein and one-half phospholipids and cholesterol

An elevation in LDL has a strong and direct association with coronary artery disease (CAD); increased HDL has been inversely associated with the risk of CAD. High levels of HDL serve a protective role by mobilizing cholesterol from tissues. Although the association between elevated serum cholesterol levels and CAD exists, determination of total cholesterol level is not sufficient for the assessment of coronary risk. It is important to determine whether elevated cholesterol levels are related to increased LDL or HDL.

Triglyceride elevations have had a questionable role in CAD etiology until recently. It has now been shown that high triglyceride levels are linked to the progression of CAD.[14]

A lipid profile serum test usually consists of cholesterol, triglycerides, LDL, and HDL measurements. Frequently a risk assessment for CAD is given by comparing the total cholesterol to HDL ratio.[15] An increase in the ratio indicates increased risk. This combination provides more information than either value alone (see Table 30-7). The patient must fast for 12 to 14 hours before the blood draw to eliminate the effects of a recent meal.

Evidence indicates that levels of plasma apolipoprotein A-1 (the major HDL protein) and apolipoprotein B (the major LDL protein) are better predictors of CAD than HDL or LDL. Therefore measurements of these lipoproteins may replace cholesterol-lipoprotein determinations in assessing the risk of CAD.

Lipoprotein A [Lp(a)] is a newly recognized lipoprotein being assessed for its role in CAD. Increased levels of Lp(a), especially with increased levels of LDH, are strongly associated with the progression in arteriosclerosis. In addition, Lp(a) is found to have thrombogenic properties that increase the risk of clot formation at the site of intravascular lesions.[16]

Invasive Studies

Invasive studies are performed if definitive information is required. These include cardiac catheterization, coronary angiography, electrophysiology, and intracoronary ultrasound.

Cardiac Catheterization. Cardiac catheterization is a common outpatient procedure. It provides a means of obtaining information about CAD, congenital heart disease, valvular heart disease, and ventricular function. Cardiac catheterization can be used to measure intracardiac pressures and O_2 levels in various parts of the heart, as well as CO. With injection of dye and x-ray visualization, the chambers of the heart can be outlined and wall motion observed.

Cardiac catheterization is performed by insertion of a radiopaque catheter into the right or left side of the heart. For the right side of the heart, a catheter is inserted through an arm vein (basilic or cephalic) or a leg vein (femoral). The catheter is advanced into the vena cava, the right atrium, and the right ventricle. The catheter is further inserted into the pulmonary artery, and pressures are recorded. The catheter is then advanced until it is wedged or lodged in position. This position is called the pulmonary artery wedge position. The pulmonary artery wedge position (wedge pressure) obstructs the flow and pressure from the right side of the heart and looks forward through the pulmonary capillary bed to the pressure in the left side of the heart. The wedge pressure is used to determine the function of the left side of the heart.

The left-sided approach is performed by insertion of a catheter into the femoral artery. The brachial artery can be used if necessary. The catheter is passed in a retrograde manner up the aorta, across the aortic valve, and into the left ventricle.

With right and left heart catheterization, blood is taken from various chambers and analyzed for its O_2 content. Pressures in the various chambers are recorded. With the use of dye injections, the structures of the heart can be visualized, and the size and function of the chambers can be determined. Patients frequently feel a temporary hot and flushed sensation with the dye injection.

Complications of cardiac catheterization include looping, kinking, or breaking off of the catheter; blood loss; allergic reaction to the dye; infection, thrombus formation; air or blood embolism; arrhythmias; MI; cerebrovascular accident; puncture of the ventricles, cardiac septum, lung tissue; and rarely, death.

The nurse has preprocedure and postprocedure responsibilities for the patient undergoing cardiac catheterization. The patient should be told how long the catheterization procedure will take (2 to 3 hours) and where it will take place. Most hospitals have a cardiac catheterization laboratory specifically designed for the procedure. (See Table 30-7 for the nursing responsibilities related to cardiac catheterization.)

Coronary Angiography. When coronary anatomic or diagnostic information is required, coronary angiography (arteriography) is performed in conjunction with a cardiac catheterization. The approach is modified so that the catheters are inserted up the aorta and into the opening of the coronary arteries. Dye is injected and x-rays are taken. The procedure is repeated for the other coronary artery. The patient should be informed that a flush may be felt when the dye is injected.

The nursing responsibilities for this procedure are the same as for a patient with cardiac catheterization.

Electrophysiology Study. Electrophysiology study (EPS) is the direct study and manipulation of the electrical activity of the heart using electrodes placed inside the cardiac chambers. It provides information on SA node function, AV node conduction, and ventricular conduction. It is particularly helpful in diagnosing the tissue source for arrhythmias. Patients with a history of symptomatic supraventricular or ventricular tachycardias may obtain an accurate diagnosis and treatment with this technique.

Catheters are inserted in a similar method as for right and left heart catheterization. These catheters are placed at specific anatomic sites within the heart to record electrical activity. Nursing care for patients after EPS include close ECG monitoring, puncture site assessment, vital signs, and other responsibilities related to care following a cardiac catheterization.

Intracoronary Ultrasound. Intracoronary ultrasound (ICUS), also known as intravascular ultrasound (IVUS), is an invasive procedure performed in the catheterization laboratory. The two- or three-dimensional ultrasound images provide a cross-sectional view of the arterial walls of the coronary arteries.[17]

A miniature transducer attached to a small catheter is introduced through a peripheral artery and advanced to the artery to be studied. Once in the artery, ultrasound images are obtained. The health of the arterial layers is assessed, as is the composition, location, and thickness of plaque.

ICUS is currently used in conjunction with coronary angiography to diagnose severity of coronary artery disease. It is increasingly being used to evaluate the vessel response to treatments such as stent placement and athrectomy.[18]

Because the patient will most often have ICUS in addition to angiography or an invasive treatment, nursing care of the patient following ICUS is similar to that following cardiac catheterization (see Table 30-7).

Blood Flow and Pressure Measurements

Peripheral vessel blood flow. Duplex imaging is useful in the diagnoses of occlusive disease in the peripheral blood vessels and for the diagnosis of thrombophlebitis. Peripheral vessel blood flow can be assessed by injection of radiopaque material into the appropriate arteries or veins (arteriography and venography). With these tests, arterial occlusions and venous abnormalities can be located. (Additional studies of peripheral blood vessels are discussed in Chapter 36 and Table 36-9.)

Hemodynamic monitoring. Hemodynamic bedside monitoring of pressures of the cardiovascular system are frequently used to assess cardiovascular status. Invasive hemodynamic monitoring using intraarterial and pulmonary artery catheters can be used to monitor arterial BP, intracardiac pressures, and CO (see Chapter 63). Central venous pressure (CVP) monitoring is indicated when a patient has a significant alteration in fluid volume. The CVP reflects the pressure in the right atrium and is a measurement of preload. The CVP can be used as a guide in fluid volume management of overhydration or dehydration.

CVP can be measured with a pulmonary artery catheter (see Chapter 63) or a central venous line threaded through the jugular or subclavian vein into the superior vena cava. Two different methods to take CVP measurements include a mercury (mm Hg) system or a water (cm H_2O) manometer system. The end of the catheter is connected to a three-way stopcock, a fluid system, and a water manometer or to a pressure transducer. The normal CVP is 2 to 9 mm Hg (3 to 12 cm H_2O).

For an accurate reading, the base of the manometer should be at the level of the right atrium (the phlebostatic axis). The pressure readings directly reflect the right ventricular filling and diastolic pressure. The CVP reading is influenced by the function of the left side of the heart, pressures in the pulmonary vessels, venous return to the heart, and the position of the patient when the reading is taken. The last factor must be kept in mind to obtain an accurate reading. CVP monitoring has been augmented with the use of pulmonary artery monitoring.

REVIEW QUESTIONS

The number of the question corresponds to the same-numbered objective at the beginning of the chapter.

1. A patient with a tricuspid valve disorder will have impaired blood flow between the
   a. vena cava and right atrium.
   b. left atrium and left ventricle.
   c. right atrium and right ventricle.
   d. right ventricle and pulmonary artery.
2. A patient with an MI of the anterior wall of the left ventricle most likely has an occlusion of the
   a. left circumflex artery.
   b. right marginal artery.
   c. left anterior descending artery.
   d. right anterior descending artery.
3. If the Purkinje system is damaged, conduction of the electrical impulse is impaired through the
   a. atria.
   b. AV node.
   c. bundle of His.
   d. ventricles.
4. Prolonged pressure on the skin causes reddened areas at the point of contact due to
   a. arterial vasodilation from smooth muscle relaxation.
   b. compression of veins resulting in venous engorgement.
   c. occlusion of major arteries causing infarction of the tissue.
   d. tissue damage and inflammation resulting from impaired capillary blood flow.
5. When a person's blood pressure rises, the homeostatic mechanism to compensate for an elevation involves stimulation of
   a. chemoreceptors that inhibit sympathetic nervous system causing vasodilation.
   b. baroreceptors that inhibit the sympathetic nervous system causing a decreased heart rate.
   c. chemoreceptors that stimulate the sympathetic nervous system causing an increased heart rate.
   d. baroreceptors that inhibit the parasympathetic nervous system causing vasodilation.
6. When checking the capillary filling time of a patient the color returns in 10 seconds. The nurse recognizes this finding as indicative of
   a. a normal response.
   b. thrombus formation in the veins.
   c. lymphatic obstruction of venous return.
   d. impaired arterial flow to the extremities.
7. The auscultatory area in the left midclavicular line at the level of the fifth ICS is the
   a. mitral area.
   b. aortic area.
   c. tricuspid area.
   d pulmonic area.
8. When assessing the patient the nurse notes a palpable precordial thrill. This finding may be caused by
   a. gallop rhythms.
   b. heart murmurs.
   c. pulmonary edema.
   d. right ventricular hypertrophy.
9. When assessing the cardiovascular system of a 79-year-old patient the nurse expects to find
   a. a narrowed pulse pressure.
   b. diminished carotid artery pulses.
   c. difficulty in isolating the apical pulse.
   d. an increased heart rate in response to stress.
10. An important nursing responsibility for a patient having an invasive cardiovascular diagnostic study includes
   a. checking the peripheral pulses and percutaneous site.
   b. instructing the patient about radioactive isotope injection.
   c. informing the patient that general anesthesia will be given.
   d. assisting the patient to do a surgical scrub of the insertion site.

11. A P wave on an ECG represents an impulse
    a. arising at the SA node and repolarizing the atria
    b. arising at the SA node and depolarizing the atria
    c. arising at the AV node and depolarizing the atria
    d. arising at the AV node and spreading to the bundle of His

References

1. Berne RM, Levy MN: *Cardiovascular physiology,* ed 7, St Louis, 1997, Mosby.
2. Woods SL and others: *Cardiac nursing,* ed 3, Philadelphia, 1995, Lippincott.
3. Kinney MR, Packa DR: *Andreoli's comprehensive cardiac care,* ed 8, St Louis, 1996, Mosby.
4. Frolkis VV, Bezrukov VV, Kulchitshy OK: *The aging cardiovascular system: physiology and pathology,* New York, 1996, Springer.
5. Matteson MA: *Gerontological nursing: concepts and practice,* ed 2, Philadelphia, 1997, Saunders.
6. Delonas LR: Beyond type A: hostility and coronary artery disease—implication for research, *Rehabil Nurs* 21:4, 1996.
7. Hartnell GC: Developments in echocardiography, *Radiol Clin North Am* 32:3, 1994.
8. Johns PJ, Abraham SA, Eagle KA: Dipyridamole-thallium versus dobutamine echocardiographic stress testing: a clinician's viewpoint, *Am Heart J* 130:5, 1995.
9. Ansari A: Transesophageal two dimensional echocardiography: current perspectives, *Prog Cardiovasc Dis* 35:5, 1993.
10. O'Keefe JH, Barnhart CS, Bateman TM: Comparison of stress echocardiography and stress myocardial perfusion scintigraphy for diagnosing coronary artery disease and assessing its severity, *Am J Cardiol* 75:25D, 1995.
11. Merz CNB, Berman DS: Imaging techniques for coronary artery disease: current status and future direction, *Clin Cardiol* 20:526, 1997.
12. Brown KA: Prognostic value of cardiac imaging in patients with known or suspected coronary artery disease: comparison of myocardial perfusion imaging, stress echocardiography, and positron emission tomography, *Am J Cardiol* 75:35D, 1995.
13. Cheesbro MJ: Using serum markers in the early diagnosis of myocardial infarction, *Am Fam Physician* 55:8, 1997.
14. Assmann G, Schulte H, von Eckardstein A: Hypertriglyceridemia and elevated lipoprotein (a) are risk factors for major coronary events in middle-aged men, *Am J Cardiol* 77:1179, 1996.
15. Fishbach FT: *A manual of laboratory and diagnostic tests,* Philadelphia, 1996, Lippincott.
16. Blackman MC, Busby-Whitehead MJ: Clinical implications of abnormal lipoprotein metabolism. In Barker LR and others, eds: *Principles of ambulatory medicine,* ed 3, Baltimore, 1995, Williams & Wilkins.
17. Foster GP and others: Variability in the measurement of intracoronary ultrasound images: implication for the identification of atherosclerotic plaque regression, *Clin Cardiol* 20:11, 1997.
18. Tenaglia A: Intravascular ultrasound and balloon percutaneous transluminal coronary angioplasty, *Cardiol Clin* 15:1, 1997.

Resources

Resources for this chapter are listed after Chapter 36 on p. 1009.

REMEMBER to check out your companion CD-ROM

31 NURSING MANAGEMENT Hypertension

Barbara S. Levine

www.mosby.com/MERLIN/medsurg_lewis

LEARNING OBJECTIVES

1. Describe the mechanisms involved in the regulation of blood pressure.
2. Identify the pathophysiologic mechanisms associated with primary hypertension.
3. Describe the clinical manifestations and complications of hypertension.
4. Describe strategies for the prevention of primary hypertension.
5. Describe the collaborative care for hypertension, including drug and nutritional therapy.
6. Discuss the management of the older adult patient with hypertension.
7. Describe the nursing management of the patient with hypertension, emphasizing patient education.
8. Describe the clinical manifestations and management of hypertensive crisis.

NORMAL REGULATION OF BLOOD PRESSURE

Blood pressure (BP) is the force exerted by the blood against the walls of the blood vessel and must be adequate to maintain tissue perfusion during activity and rest. The maintenance of normal BP and tissue perfusion requires the integration of both systemic factors and local peripheral vascular effects. Arterial BP is primarily a function of cardiac output and systemic vascular resistance. The relationship is summarized by the following equation:

$$\text{Arterial blood pressure} = \text{Cardiac output} \times \text{Systemic vascular resistance}$$

Cardiac output (CO) is the total blood flow through the systemic or pulmonary circulation per minute. CO can be described as the stroke volume (amount of blood pumped out of the left ventricle per beat [approximately 70 ml]) multiplied by the heart rate (HR) for 1 minute. *Systemic vascular resistance* (SVR) is the force opposing the movement of blood within the blood vessels. Radius of the small arteries and arterioles is the principal factor determining vascular resistance. A small change in the radius of the arterioles creates a major change in the SVR. If SVR is increased and CO remains constant or increases, arterial BP will increase.

The mechanisms that regulate BP can affect either CO or SVR, or both. Regulation of BP is a complex process involving nervous, cardiovascular, renal, and endocrine functions (Fig. 31-1). BP is regulated by both short-term (seconds to hours) and long-term (days to weeks) mechanisms. Short-term mechanisms, including the autonomic nervous system and vascular endothelium, are active within a few seconds. Long-term mechanisms include renal and hormonal processes that regulate arteriolar resistance and blood volume.

Sympathetic Nervous System

The nervous system, which reacts within seconds after a decrease in arterial pressure, increases BP primarily by activation of the sympathetic nervous system (SNS). Increased SNS activity increases HR and cardiac contractility, produces widespread vasoconstriction in the peripheral arterioles, and promotes the release of renin from the kidney. The net effect of SNS activation is to increase arterial pressure by increasing both CO and SVR.

Change in BP is sensed by specialized nerve cells (baroreceptors) and transmitted to the vasomotor centers in the brainstem. Information received in the brainstem is relayed throughout the brain by complex networks of interneurons exciting or inhibiting efferent nerves, thereby influencing cardiovascular function. Sympathetic efferent nerves innervate cardiac and vascular smooth muscle cells. Under normal conditions, a low level of continuous sympathetic activity maintains tonic vasoconstriction. BP may be reduced by withdrawal of tonic SNS activity or by stimulation of the parasympathetic nervous system, which decreases the HR (via the vagus nerve) and thereby decreases CO.

The neurotransmitter norepinephrine (NE) is released from sympathetic nerve endings. NE activates receptors located in the sinoatrial node, myocardium, and vascular smooth muscle. The response to NE depends on the type and density of receptors present. Sympathetic nervous system receptors are classified as α_1, α_2, β_1, and β_2. β_1-Receptors in the heart respond to NE with increased HR (chronotropic), increased force of contraction (inotropic), and increased speed of conduction. Diminished responsiveness of cardiovascular cells to sympathetic stimulation is one of the most significant cardiovascular effects of aging. α_1-Receptors located in peripheral vasculature cause vasoconstriction when activated. The smooth muscle of the blood vessels have both α_1 and β_2-receptors (Table 31-1).

Reviewed by Elizabeth Chapman, RN, MS, CCRN, ICU Staff Nurse, Columbia Garden Park; Nursing Faculty, MGCCC-Jefferson Davis Campus, Long Beach, Miss.

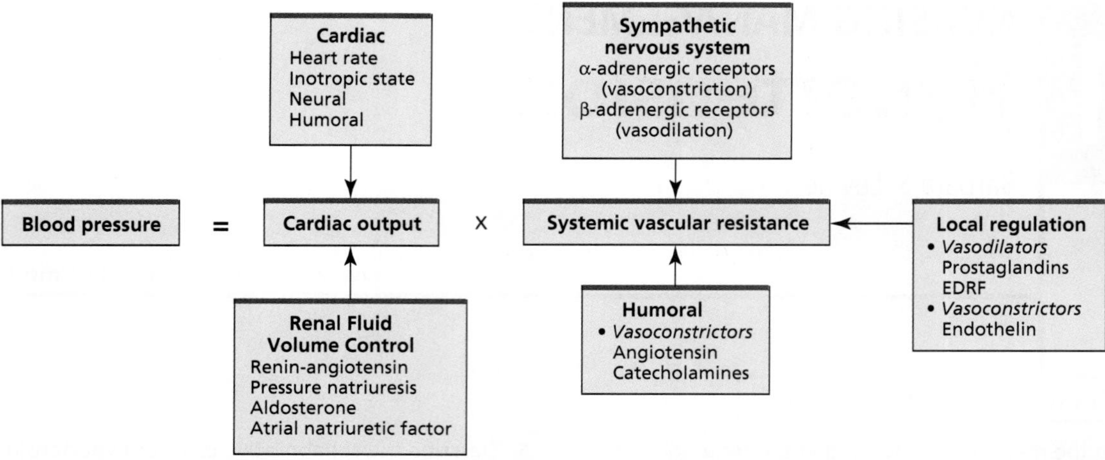

Fig. 31-1 Factors influencing blood pressure. *EDRF,* endothelium-derived relaxing factor.

Table 31-1 Sympathetic Nervous System Receptors Influencing Blood Pressure

Receptor	Location	Response When Activated
α_1	Vascular smooth muscle	Vasoconstriction
	Heart	Increased contractility
α_2	Presynaptic membrane	Inhibition of norepinephrine release
	Vascular smooth muscle	Vasoconstriction
β_1	Heart	Increased contractility (positive inotropic effect)
		Increased heart rate (positive chronotropic effect)
		Increased conduction (positive dromotropic effect)
	Juxtaglomerular cells	Increased renin secretion
β_2	Smooth muscle of peripheral blood vessels in skeletal muscle and coronary arteries	Vasodilation
Dopaminergic receptors	Primarily renal and mesenteric blood vessels	Vasodilation

β_2-Receptors are activated primarily by epinephrine released from the adrenal medulla and cause vasodilation.

The sympathetic vasomotor center, located in the medulla, interacts with many areas of the brain to maintain normal BP under various conditions. During exercise the motor area of the cortex is stimulated, activating the vasomotor center and the SNS through neuronal connections. This causes an appropriate increase in BP to accommodate the increased oxygen demand of the exercising muscles. During postural change from lying to standing, there is a transient decrease in BP. The vasomotor center is stimulated and activates the SNS, causing peripheral vasoconstriction and increased venous return to the heart. If this response did not occur, there would be inadequate blood flow to the brain, resulting in dizziness. Cerebral cortical perceptions such as pain and stress activate the vasomotor centers through the neuronal connections.

Baroreceptors. *Baroreceptors* (pressoreceptors) are specialized nerve cells located in the carotid arteries and arch of the aorta. They are sensitive to stretching and, when stimulated by an increase in BP, send inhibitory impulses to the sympathetic vasomotor center in the brainstem. Inhibition of sympathetic activity results in decreased heart rate, decreased force of contraction, and vasodilation in peripheral arterioles. Increased parasympathetic activity (vagus nerve) reduces HR further.

A fall in BP, sensed by the baroreceptors, leads to activation of the SNS. The result is constriction of the peripheral arterioles, increased HR, and increased contractility of the heart. The baroreceptors have an important role in the maintenance of BP stability during normal activities. In the presence of long-standing hypertension, the baroreceptors become adjusted to elevated levels of BP and recognize this level as "normal." The baroreceptor reflex is less responsive in some older adults.

Vascular Endothelium

The vascular endothelium is a single cell layer that lines the blood vessels. Previously considered inert, it has the ability to produce vasoactive substances and growth factors. Nitric oxide, an endothelium-derived relaxing factor (EDRF), helps maintain low arterial tone at rest, inhibits growth of the smooth muscle layer, and inhibits platelet aggregation. Other substances released by the vascular endothelium with local vasodilator effects include prostacyclin and endothelium-derived hyperpolarizing factor.

Endothelin (ET) is an extremely potent vasoconstrictor. There are three subclasses of endothelins (ET-1, ET-2, and ET-3).

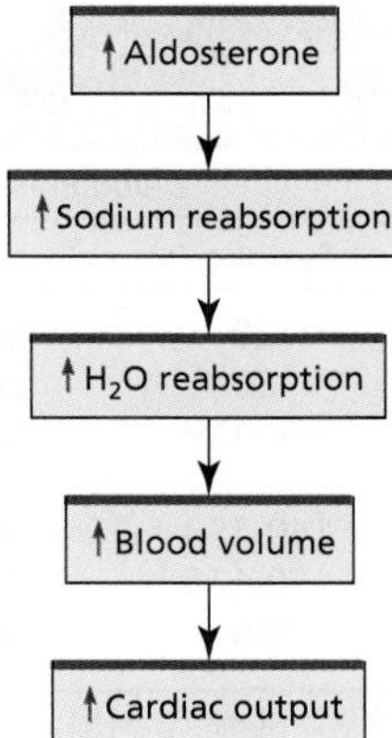

Fig. 31-2 Mechanisms of action of aldosterone.

ET-1 is the most important endothelin for the maintenance of vasomotor tone. ET-1 also causes adhesion and aggregation of neutrophils and stimulates smooth muscle growth. Endothelial function and dysfunction is an area of active investigation. There is some evidence that vascular endothelial dysfunction may contribute to atherosclerosis and primary hypertension. The prevention or reversal of endothelial dysfunction may become important therapeutic areas in the future.

Renal System

The kidneys contribute to BP regulation by controlling sodium excretion and extracellular fluid (ECF) volume (see Chapter 42). Sodium retention results in water retention, which causes an increased ECF volume. This increases the venous return to the heart, increasing the stroke volume, which elevates the BP through an increase in CO.

The renin-angiotensin-aldosterone system also plays an important role in BP regulation. In response to sympathetic stimulation, decreased blood flow through the kidneys, or decreased serum sodium concentration, renin is secreted from the juxtaglomerular apparatus in the kidney. Renin is an enzyme that converts angiotensinogen to angiotensin I. Angiotensin-converting enzyme (ACE) converts angiotensin I into angiotensin II (A-II), which can increase BP by two different mechanisms (see Fig. 42-6). First, A-II is a potent vasoconstrictor and increases vascular resistance, resulting in an immediate increase in BP. Second, over a period of hours or days, A-II increases BP indirectly by stimulating the adrenal cortex to secrete aldosterone, which causes sodium and water retention by the kidneys resulting in increased blood volume and increased CO (Fig. 31-2).

Angiotensin II also functions at a local level within the heart and blood vessels. Recent evidence suggests that local vasoactive effects of A-II (vasoconstriction and growth promotion) may contribute to atherosclerosis and primary hypertension.[1]

Prostaglandins (PGE_2 and PGI_2) secreted by the renal medulla have a vasodilator effect on the systemic circulation. This results in decreased systemic vascular resistance and lowering of BP. (Prostaglandins are discussed in Chapter 11.)

Endocrine System

Stimulation of the SNS results in release of epinephrine along with a small fraction of norepinephrine by the adrenal medulla. Epinephrine increases CO by increasing HR and myocardial contractility. Epinephrine activates β_2-receptors in peripheral arterioles of skeletal muscle, causing vasodilation. In peripheral arterioles with only α_1-receptors (skin and kidneys), epinephrine causes vasoconstriction.

The adrenal cortex is stimulated by A-II to release aldosterone. (Release of aldosterone is also regulated by other factors, such as low sodium levels [see Chapters 45 and 47].) Aldosterone stimulates the kidneys to retain sodium and therefore water. This increases BP by increasing CO (see Fig. 31-2).

An increased blood sodium osmolarity level stimulates the release of antidiuretic hormone (ADH) from the posterior pituitary gland. ADH increases the ECF volume by promoting the reabsorption of water in the distal and collecting tubules of the kidneys. The resulting increase in blood volume can cause an elevation in BP.

In the healthy person, these regulatory mechanisms function in response to the demands of the body. When hypertension develops, one or more of the BP-regulating mechanisms are defective. Collaborative care and nursing management are directed toward normalizing BP and preventing target organ disease.

HYPERTENSION

Definition

Hypertension is sustained elevation of BP. In adults, hypertension exists when systolic blood pressure (SBP) is equal to or greater than 140 mm Hg or diastolic blood pressure (DBP) is equal to or greater than 90 mm Hg for extended periods of time. The diagnosis of hypertension requires that elevated readings be present on at least three occasions during several weeks.

Significance

High BP means that the heart is working harder than normal, putting both the heart and the blood vessels under strain. High BP may contribute to myocardial infarctions, cerebrovascular accident (CVA), renal failure, and atherosclerosis. Approximately 2.2 million Americans age 15 and older have disabilities resulting from high BP.[2]

The status of hypertension control has improved considerably over the past 20 years. Large-scale education programs provided by various organizations have increased awareness of hypertension. The percentage of patients with hypertension on medication who have their BP controlled has also improved substantially. Until 1993 cardiovascular mortality and stroke had decreased among all adult population groups in the United States. Because high BP is one of the major risk factors for coronary artery disease (CAD) and the most important risk factor for CVA, it is inferred that progress in detection, treatment, and control of hypertension contributed to the decline in the mortality rates of these diseases.[3] However, these dramatic improvements have slowed. Since 1993 the rate of CAD appears to be stable. However, CVA rates have increased slightly, and the incidence of end-stage renal disease and the prevalence of heart failure are increasing.[3]

Hypertension causes no symptoms to motivate a person to seek treatment. When symptoms do occur, they signify either secondary causes of hypertension or effects of sustained elevation of BP on target organs (coronary artery disease, left

CULTURAL & ETHNIC CONSIDERATIONS

Hypertension

- African-Americans, Puerto Ricans, Cubans, and Mexican-Americans have a higher incidence of hypertension than do Caucasians.
- African-Americans have the highest incidence of hypertension.
- African-American women have a particularly high incidence of hypertension.
- African-Americans have a higher mortality rate related to hypertension than Caucasians.
- African-Americans and Caucasians living in the southeastern United States have a higher incidence of hypertension than similar ethnic groups living in other parts of the United States.

ventricular hypertrophy, cerebrovascular disease, peripheral vascular disease, or renal insufficiency).

In the United States, 50 million people either have elevated BP (SBP of 140 mm Hg or greater or DBP of 90 mm Hg or greater) or are taking antihypertensive medication.[2] The prevalence of hypertension increases with age and is higher in African-Americans than in Caucasians. In comparison to Caucasians, African-Americans develop high BP at an earlier age, and it is more severe at any decade. As a result, African-Americans have a higher prevalence of stroke, heart disease, and end-stage renal disease when compared with Caucasians. In addition, African-Americans have a higher mortality rate at every level of BP elevation than do Caucasians. In both races, the prevalence is higher in less educated as compared with more educated people. Hypertension is more prevalent in men than in women until the age of 55. From age 55 to 75 the prevalence is about equal for men and women, and after age 75 it is more prevalent in women than men.[2]

Classification of Hypertension

Table 31-2 describes the BP classification for people 18 years of age and older. The Joint Commission classifies hypertension according to stages (1 through 3) with the addition of a *high normal* category.[3] These experts consider the person with BP in the high normal category to be at higher risk for the development of definite hypertension and recommend more frequent monitoring than the person with lower BP.[3] The risk of progression from high normal to definite hypertension is controversial. Other experts caution that use of this category risks labeling a very large number of people.[4] The etiology of hypertension can be classified as either primary (essential) or secondary.

Primary Hypertension. Primary hypertension accounts for 95% of all cases of hypertension, with the onset usually between the ages of 30 and 50 years. Although the exact cause of primary hypertension is unknown, several contributing factors, including increased SNS activity, overproduction of sodium-retaining hormones and vasoconstrictors, increased sodium-intake, greater than ideal body weight, diabetes mellitus, and excessive alcohol intake, have been identified.[5,6] Primary hypertension is the focus of this chapter because of its prevalence in clinical practice.

Table 31-2 Classification of Blood Pressure for Adults Aged 18 Years and Older*

Category	Blood Pressure, mm Hg Systolic		Diastolic
Optimal†	<120	and	<80
Normal	<130	and	<85
High normal	130-139	or	85-89
Hypertension‡			
Stage 1	140-159	or	90-99
Stage 2	160-179	or	100-109
Stage 3	≥180	or	≥110

From US Department of Health and Human Services: *The Sixth Report of the Joint National Committee on Detection, Evaluation, and Treatment of High Blood Pressure (JNC-VI),* Washington, DC, 1997, National Institutes of Health.
*Not taking antihypertensive drugs and not acutely ill.
†Optimal blood pressure with respect to cardiovascular risk is less than 120/80 mm Hg. However, unusually low readings should be evaluated for clinical significance.
‡Based on the average of two or more readings taken at each of two or more visits after an initial screening. When systolic and diastolic blood pressures fall into different categories, the higher category should be selected to classify the individual's blood pressure status. For example, 160/92 should be classified as stage 2 hypertension, and 174/120 should be classified as stage 3 hypertension. Isolated systolic hypertension is defined as systolic blood pressure 140 mm Hg or greater and diastolic blood pressure less than 90 mm Hg and staged appropriately (e.g., 170/82 mm Hg is defined as stage 2 isolated systolic hypertension).
NOTE: In addition to classifying stages of hypertension based on average blood pressure levels, the clinician should specify presence or absence of target organ disease and additional risk factors. This specificity is important for risk classification and treatment.

Secondary Hypertension. Secondary hypertension is elevated BP with a specific cause that often can be identified and corrected. This type of hypertension accounts for less than 5% of hypertension in adults but more than 80% of hypertension in children. If a person below age 20 or over age 50 suddenly develops hypertension, especially if it is severe, a secondary cause should be suspected. Clinical findings that suggest secondary hypertension include unprovoked hypokalemia, abdominal bruit, variable pressures with history of tachycardia, sweating and tremor, or a family history of renal disease. Causes of secondary hypertension include the following: (1) coarctation or congenital narrowing of the aorta; (2) renal disease such as renal artery stenosis and parenchymal disease (see Chapter 43); (3) endocrine disorders such as pheochromocytoma, Cushing's syndrome, and hyperaldosteronism (see Chapter 47); (4) neurologic disorders such as brain tumors, quadriplegia, and head injury; (5) sleep apnea; (6) medications such as sympathetic stimulants (including cocaine), monoamine oxidase inhibitors taken with tyramine-containing foods, estrogen replacement therapy, oral contraceptive pills, and nonsteroidal antiinflammatory drugs (NSAIDs); and (7) pregnancy-induced hypertension. Treatment of secondary hypertension is directed at eliminating the underlying cause. Secondary hypertension contributes to hypertensive crisis. (See section at end of this chapter.)

Pathophysiology of Primary Hypertension

For arterial pressure to rise, there must be an increase in either CO or SVR. Increased CO is sometimes found in the early and borderline hypertensive person. Later in the course of hypertension, SVR rises and the CO returns to normal. The hemodynamic hallmark of hypertension is persistently increased SVR. This persistent elevation in SVR may come about in various ways. Factors that are known to be related to the development

Table 31-3 Risk Factors in Primary Hypertension

Age	BP rises progressively with increasing age. Elevated BP is present in approximately 50% of people over 65 years of age.
Sex	Hypertension is more prevalent in men in young adulthood and early middle age. After age 55, hypertension is more prevalent in women.
Race	Incidence of hypertension is twice as great in African-Americans as in Caucasians.
Family history	Level of BP is strongly familial. Risk of hypertension increases for those with a close relative having hypertension.
Obesity	Weight gain is associated with increased frequency of hypertension. The risk is greatest with central abdominal obesity.
Cigarette smoking	Smoking greatly increases the risk of cardiovascular disease. Hypertensives who smoke are at even greater risk.
Excess dietary sodium	High sodium intake can contribute to hypertension in some patients and can decrease the efficacy of certain antihypertensive medications.
Elevated serum lipids	Elevated levels of cholesterol and triglycerides are primary risk factors in atherosclerosis. Hyperlipidemia is more common in hypertensives.
Alcohol	Excessive alcohol intake is strongly associated with hypertension. Hypertensive patients should limit their daily intake of ethanol to 1 oz.
Sedentary lifestyle	Regular physical activity can help control weight and reduce cardiovascular risk. Physical activity may decrease blood pressure.
Diabetes mellitus	Hypertension is more common in diabetics. When hypertension and diabetes coexist, complications are more severe.
Socioeconomic status	Hypertension is more prevalent in lower socioeconomic groups and among the less educated.
Stress	People exposed to repeated stress may develop hypertension more frequently than others. People who become hypertensive may respond differently to stress than those who do not become hypertensive.

of primary hypertension or contribute to its consequences are presented in Table 31-3.

Heredity. The level of BP is strongly familial, although it is not known exactly what is inherited that leads to high BP. Studies of BP correlation within families indicate that the heritability of both systolic and diastolic blood pressure is approximately 20% to 40%. Heritability estimates based on twin studies tend to be higher (60%) but may reflect greater environmental similarity.[7] Genetic observations to date suggest that primary hypertension is polygenic and that alteration in renal function with resultant salt and water retention is the final common pathway.[7] In most cases, primary hypertension results from the interaction of genetic, environmental, and demographic factors.

Water and Sodium Retention. Excessive sodium intake is considered responsible for initiation of hypertension in some people. Studies on populations with a low sodium intake (usually primitive hunter-gatherer societies) show little or no hypertension and no progressive increase in BP with age as is found in industrialized societies. In addition, when people from these societies adopt industrialized lifestyles, the prevalence of hypertension increases. When sodium is restricted in many hypertensive people, their BP falls. A high sodium intake may activate a number of pressor mechanisms and cause water retention. Although almost everyone in Western countries consumes a high-sodium diet, only about 20% will develop hypertension. This indicates that some degree of sodium sensitivity must be present for high sodium intake to trigger the development of hypertension.[6]

Altered Renin-Angiotensin Mechanism. In normotensive people, increased BP (e.g., associated with exercise) inhibits renin secretion by the kidney. Thus primary hypertension might be expected to be associated with low levels of plasma renin activity (PRA). About 31% of people with primary hypertension have low PRA, 50% have normal PRA, and 20% have high PRA. High PRA results in the increased conversion of angiotensinogen to angiotensin (see Fig. 42-6). Angiotensin II causes direct arteriolar constriction, promotes vascular hypertrophy, and induces aldosterone secretion. Thus altered renin-angiotensin mechanisms may contribute to the development and maintenance of hypertension.[1,8]

Stress and Increased Sympathetic Nervous System Activity. It has long been recognized that arterial pressure is influenced by factors such as anger, fear, and pain. Physiologic responses to stress, which are normally protective, may persist to a pathologic degree, resulting in prolonged increase in SNS activity. Increased sympathetic stimulation produces increased vasoconstriction, increased HR, and increased renin release. Increased renin activates the angiotensin mechanism and increases aldosterone secretion, both leading to elevated BP. Studies have shown that people exposed to high levels of repeated psychologic stress develop hypertension to a greater extent than those who do not experience as much stress. As stress is a part of everyday life, it may be that those who develop hypertension respond differently to stress.[6]

Insulin Resistance and Hyperinsulinemia. Abnormalities of glucose, insulin, and lipoprotein metabolism are common in primary hypertension. They are not present in secondary hypertension and do not improve when hypertension is treated. Therefore these abnormalities may contribute to the development of primary hypertension and to its complications. Evidence suggests that high insulin concentration in the blood stimulates SNS activity and impairs nitric oxide–mediated vasodilation. Additional pressor effects of insulin include vascular hypertrophy and increased renal sodium reabsorption.[9]

Endothelial Cell Dysfunction. Vascular endothelial cells are known to be the source of multiple vasoactive substances. Some hypertensive people have a reduced vasodilator response to nitric oxide. Endothelin produces pronounced and prolonged vasoconstriction. The role of endothelial dysfunction in the pathogenesis and treatment of hypertension is an area of active investigation.[10]

GERONTOLOGIC CONSIDERATIONS

Hypertension

More than 50% of the U.S. population 65 years of age and older has elevated SBP or DBP, increasing the risk of cardiovascular disease and stroke.[2] The following age-related physical changes play a role in the pathophysiology of hypertension in the older adult: (1) loss of tissue elasticity; (2) increased collagen content and stiffness of the myocardium; (3) increased peripheral vascular resistance; (4) decreased β-adrenergic receptor sensitivity; (5) blunting of baroreceptor reflexes; (6) decreased renal function; and (7) decreased renin response to sodium and water depletion.

In the older adult taking antihypertensive medication, absorption of some drugs may be altered as a result of decreased splanchnic blood flow. Metabolism and excretion of drugs may also be prolonged.

Careful technique is important in assessing BP in older adults. In some older people, there is a wide gap between the first Korotkoff sound and subsequent beats. This is called the auscultatory gap. Failure to inflate the cuff enough may result in seriously underestimating the SBP. This problem can be avoided by palpating the brachial or radial artery while inflating the cuff to a level above the disappearance of the pulse.

Isolated Systolic Hypertension. *Isolated systolic hypertension* (ISH) is defined as a sustained elevation in SBP equal to or greater than 160 mm Hg with a DBP less than 90 mm Hg. (A one-time isolated reading of increased SBP is not classified as ISH.) SBP in the range of 140 to 159 mm Hg with DBP less than 90 mm Hg constitutes borderline ISH.[11] Although ISH does occur in the young, it is much more common in the elderly and more prevalent in women and African-Americans. Older adults often have ISH caused by loss of elasticity in large arteries from atherosclerosis.

In the past, ISH was not treated because of the belief that excessive lowering of the DBP would occur, leading to greater problems. Side effects of medication were also a concern. The results of several studies have shown that it is both safe and beneficial to treat ISH in the elderly, and that to do so decreases the incidence of stroke and cardiovascular morbidity and mortality.[11,12]

As with primary hypertension, treatment of ISH begins with lifestyle modifications, particularly if the BP is not severely elevated. If measures such as sodium and alcohol restriction, weight reduction for the overweight, and regular physical activity are not sufficient to lower the SBP below 160 mm Hg, drug therapy is indicated.

Because of varying degrees of impaired baroreceptor reflex mechanisms, postural or orthostatic hypotension occurs often in older adults, especially in those with ISH. Postural hypotension in this age-group is often associated with volume depletion or chronic disease states, such as decreased renal and hepatic function or electrolyte imbalance.[13] To reduce the likelihood of postural hypotension, antihypertensive drugs should be started at low doses and increased cautiously. BP and pulse should be measured in the reclining and standing positions at every visit.

Pseudohypertension. Pseudohypertension, or false hypertension, can occur with sclerosis of the large arteries. Sclerotic arteries do not collapse under the cuff, presenting much higher cuff pressures than are actually present within the vessels. Pseudohypertension is suspected if arteries feel rigid or when few retinal or cardiac signs are found relative to the pressures obtained by cuff. Osler's maneuver may help detect pseudohypertension. This maneuver is performed by inflating the BP cuff to a level above the measured SBP and then palpating the radial artery. If a pulseless radial artery is palpable, pseudohypertension is a possibility. (Normally, arteries collapse and are not palpable when they are not filled with blood.) The only way to accurately measure BP in pseudohypertension is through the use of an intraarterial catheter.

Clinical Manifestations

Hypertension is often called the "silent killer" because it is frequently asymptomatic until it becomes severe and target organ disease has occurred. A patient with severe hypertension may experience a variety of symptoms secondary to effects on blood vessels in the various organs and tissues or to the increased workload of the heart. These secondary symptoms include fatigue, reduced activity tolerance, dizziness, palpitations, angina, and dyspnea. In the past, symptoms of hypertension were thought to include headache, nosebleeds, and dizziness. However, these symptoms are not more frequent in people with hypertension than in the general population.[6]

Complications

The most common complications of hypertension are target organ disease (Table 31-4) occurring in the heart (hypertensive heart disease), brain (cerebrovascular disease), peripheral vasculature (peripheral vascular disease), kidney (nephrosclerosis), and eyes (retinal damage).

Hypertensive Heart Disease

Coronary artery disease. Hypertension is a major risk factor for coronary artery disease. The mechanisms by which hypertension contributes to the development of atherosclerosis are not fully defined. The "response-to-injury" hypothesis of atherogenesis purports that hypertension disrupts the coronary artery endothelium thus exposing the intimal layer to activated white blood cells and platelets. Growth factors released by the vascular endothelium and platelets may induce smooth muscle proliferation within the lesion.[14] These arteriolar changes may account for a high incidence of coronary artery disease and the resulting problems of angina and MI.

Left ventricular hypertrophy. Sustained high blood pressure increases cardiac work and produces left ventricular hypertrophy (LVH) (Fig. 31-3). Initially, LVH is an adaptive or compensatory mechanism that strengthens cardiac contraction and increases cardiac output. However, increased contractility increases myocardial work and oxygen consumption. When the heart can no longer meet the demands for myocardial oxygen, heart failure develops. Progressive LVH, especially in association with coronary artery disease, is associated with the development of heart failure.

Heart failure. Heart failure occurs when the heart's compensatory adaptations are overwhelmed and the heart can no longer pump enough blood to meet the metabolic needs of the body (see Chapter 33). Contractility is depressed, and stroke volume and cardiac output are decreased. The patient may

Table 31-4 Manifestations of Target Organ Disease

Organ System	Manifestations
Cardiac	Clinical, electrocardiographic, or radiologic evidence of coronary artery disease Left ventricular hypertrophy or "strain" by electrocardiography or left ventricular hypertrophy by echocardiography Left ventricular dysfunction or cardiac failure
Cerebrovascular	Transient ischemic attack or stroke
Peripheral vascular	Absence of one or more major pulses in the extremities (except for dorsalis pedis) with or without intermittent claudication; aneurysm
Renal	Serum creatinine ≥1.5 mg/dl (130 μmol/L) Proteinuria (1+ or greater) Microalbuminuria
Retinopathy	Hemorrhages or exudates, with or without papilledema

From US Department of Health and Human Services: *The Sixth Report of the Joint National Committee on Detection, Evaluation, and Treatment of High Blood Pressure (JNC-VI),* Washington, DC, 1997, National Institutes of Health.

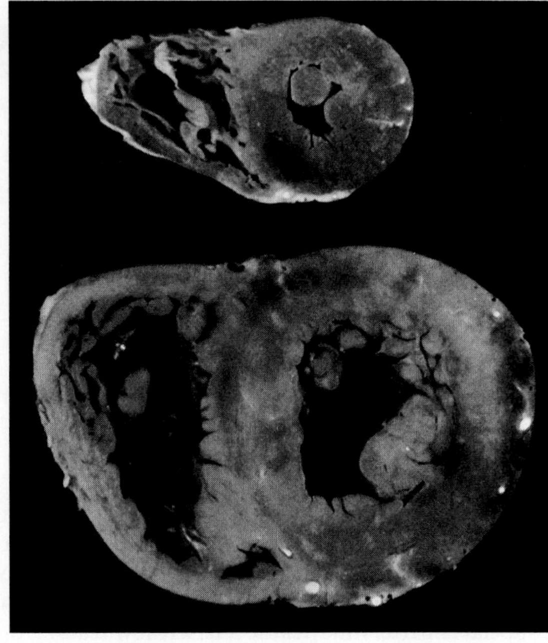

Fig. 31-3 Massively enlarged heart caused by hypertrophy of both ventricles. The normal heart weighs 325 g. The heart with biventricular hypertrophy weighs 1100 g. The patient had suffered from severe systemic hypertension.

complain of shortness of breath on exertion, paroxysmal nocturnal dyspnea, and fatigue. Signs of an enlarged heart may be present on physical examination, and an electrocardiogram (ECG) may show electrical changes indicative of LVH.

Cerebrovascular Disease. Atherosclerosis is the most common cause of cerebrovascular disease. Hypertension is a major risk factor for atherosclerosis and stroke. Even in mildly hypertensive people, the risk of stroke is four times higher than in normotensive people. Adequate control of BP effectively diminishes the risk of stroke.

Atherosclerotic plaques are commonly distributed at the bifurcation of the common carotid artery into the internal and external carotid arteries. Portions of the atherosclerotic plaque, or the blood clot that forms on the plaque, may break off and travel to intracerebral vessels, producing a thromboembolism. The patient may experience transient ischemic attacks or a stroke. (These conditions are discussed in Chapter 55.)

Hypertensive encephalopathy may occur after a marked rise in BP if the cerebral blood flow is not decreased by autoregulation. *Autoregulation* is a physiologic process that maintains constant cerebral blood flow despite fluctuations in arterial blood pressure. Normally as pressure in the cerebral blood vessels rises, the vessels constrict to maintain constant flow. When arterial blood pressure exceeds the body's ability to autoregulate, the cerebral vessels suddenly dilate and cerebral edema develops, producing a rise in intracranial pressure. If left untreated, patients die quickly from brain damage. (Cerebral blood flow and autoregulation are discussed in Chapter 54.)

Peripheral Vascular Disease. As it does with other vessels, hypertension speeds up the process of atherosclerosis in the peripheral blood vessels, leading to the development of aortic aneurysm, aortic dissection, and peripheral vascular disease (see Chapter 36). Intermittent claudication (ischemic muscle pain precipitated by activity and relieved with rest) is a classic symptom of peripheral vascular disease. Abdominal aortic aneurysm may be felt as a pulsating mass on physical examination.

Nephrosclerosis. Hypertension is one of the leading risk factors for end-stage renal disease, especially among African-Americans. Some degree of renal dysfunction is usually present in the hypertensive patient, even one with a minimally elevated BP.[6] Renal dysfunction is the direct result of ischemia caused by the narrowed lumen of the intrarenal blood vessels. Gradual narrowing of the arteries and arterioles leads to atrophy of the tubules, destruction of the glomeruli, and eventual death of nephrons. Initially intact nephrons can compensate, but these changes may eventually lead to renal failure. Common laboratory indications of renal dysfunction are microalbuminuria, proteinuria, elevated blood urea nitrogen (BUN) and serum creatinine levels, and microscopic hematuria. The earliest symptom of renal dysfunction is usually nocturia.

Retinal Damage. An ophthalmoscope is used to visualize the blood vessels of the eye. The appearance of the retina provides important information about the severity of the hypertensive process. The retina is the only place in the body where the blood vessels can be directly visualized. Therefore damage to retinal vessels provides an indication of vessel damage in the heart, brain, and kidney. Manifestations of severe retinal damage include blurring of vision, retinal hemorrhage, and loss of vision.

Retinal changes are graded according to the severity of damage. The Keith-Wagener classification of retinal changes is presented in Table 31-5. Grade I and II changes may be seen with

Table 31-5 Keith-Wagener Classification of Retinal Changes

Grade I	Vascular spasm and arteriolar narrowing in terminal branches of vessels
Grade II	Definite arteriovenous nicking (arterioles cross vein and compress it)
Grade III	Flame-shaped hemorrhages and fluffy cotton-wool exudates
Grade IV	Any of the above and papilledema (swelling of optic disc)

stage 1 or 2 hypertension. Grade III and IV hypertensive retinopathy indicate stage 3 hypertension.

Diagnostic Studies

Measurements should be taken in both arms when initially evaluating a patient's BP. If there is a difference between arms, the arm with the higher reading should be used for all subsequent measurements. This is because atherosclerotic narrowing of the subclavian artery may cause a falsely low reading on the side in which the narrowing occurs. The average of at least two BP measurements (taken 2 to 5 minutes apart while the patient is sitting) should be used to determine if the patient should return for further evaluation. If the first two readings differ by more than 5 mm Hg, additional readings should be obtained.[3] Postural changes in BP and pulse should be measured in older adults, people taking antihypertensive drugs, and when orthostatic hypotension is suspected.

There is some controversy as to how extensive a diagnostic workup should be performed in the initial evaluation of a person with hypertension. Because most hypertension is classified as primary hypertension, testing for secondary causes is not routinely done. Basic laboratory studies are performed to evaluate target organ disease, determine overall cardiovascular risk, or establish baseline levels before initiating therapy.

Table 31-6 lists basic laboratory studies that are performed in a person with sustained hypertension. Routine urinalysis, BUN, and serum creatinine levels are used to screen for renal involvement. Measurement of serum electrolytes, especially potassium levels, is important to detect hyperaldosteronism. Blood glucose level should be assessed. Serum cholesterol and triglyceride levels provide information about additional risk factors that predispose to atherosclerosis. Uric acid levels are determined to establish a baseline, since the levels often rise with diuretic therapy. An electrocardiogram provides baseline information regarding the cardiac status. Because of the prognostic importance of LVH, echocardiography is performed frequently. If the patient's age, history, physical examination findings, or severity of hypertension point to a secondary cause, further diagnostic tests may be indicated.

Ambulatory Blood Pressure Monitoring. Some patients have elevated BP readings in a clinical setting and normal readings when BP is measured elsewhere. This phenomenon is referred to as "white coat" hypertension. When white coat hypertension is suspected, blood pressure measurement at home or in the community may be helpful. Many fire stations and hospital auxiliaries provide BP measurement as a community service. Alternatively, a fully automated system that measures BP at preset intervals over a 24-hour period may be used. The equipment includes a BP cuff and a small microprocessing unit that fits into a pouch worn on a shoulder strap or belt. Patients are asked to maintain a diary of activities that may have affected BP. This procedure may be helpful in patients with suspected white coat hypertension, apparent drug resistance, hypotensive symptoms with hypertensive medications, episodic hypertension, and autonomic dysfunction.[3] The usual fee for this procedure is $150 to $310, and it is not recommended for routine evaluation of patients with primary hypertension.

As with most physiologic phenomena, BP demonstrates diurnal variability expressed as sleep-wakefulness difference. For day-active people, BP is highest in the early morning, decreases during the day, and is lowest at night. Some patients with hypertension do not show a normal, nocturnal fall in BP. The absence of diurnal variability has been associated with more target organ damage. The presence or absence of diurnal variability can be determined by continuous ambulatory BP monitoring.

COLLABORATIVE CARE

Table 31-6 Hypertension

Diagnostic
- History and physical examination
- Routine urinalysis
- Serum electrolytes and uric acid
- BUN and serum creatinine
- Blood glucose (fasting, if possible)
- Complete blood count
- Serum lipid profile, cholesterol, and triglycerides
- Electrocardiogram

Collaborative Therapy
- Periodic monitoring of BP
  - Every 3-6 months once BP is stabilized
- Assignment of risk level (see Table 31-7)
- Diet
  - Restrict sodium
  - Reduce weight (if indicated)
  - Restrict cholesterol and saturated fats
  - Maintain adequate intake of potassium
  - Maintain adequate intake of calcium and magnesium
- Physical activity
- Cessation of smoking
- Modification of alcohol intake
- Antihypertensive drugs (see Table 31-8)

Collaborative Care

Clinical guidelines for the therapeutic management of hypertension have been published by several groups.[3,4,15] Consensus among the guidelines exists in the following areas: (1) BP elevation should usually be assessed carefully over several months before initiating treatment; (2) the decision to treat hypertension should be made in the context of overall cardiovascular risk; (3) isolated systolic hypertension should be treated; (4) lifestyle modifications should provide the foundation for treatment; (5) primary and systolic hypertension should be treated in older adults up to 85 years; and (6) there are five categories of first-line drugs.

Table 31-7 Risk Stratification and Treatment of Hypertension

Blood Pressure Stages (mm Hg)	Risk Group A (No Risk Factors; No TOD/CCD)	Risk Group B (At Least One Risk Factor, Not Including Diabetes; No TOD/CCD)	Risk Group C (TOD/CCD, Diabetes, or Both, with or without Other Risk Factors)
High normal (130-135/85-89)	Lifestyle modification	Lifestyle modification	Drug therapy
Stage 1 (140-159/90-99)	Lifestyle modification (up to 12 months)	Lifestyle modification* (up to 6 months)	Drug therapy
Stages 2 and 3 (≥160/≥100)	Drug therapy	Drug therapy	Drug therapy

From US Department of Health and Human Services: *The Sixth Report of the Joint National Committee on Detection, Evaluation, and Treatment of High Blood Pressure (JNC-VI),* Washington, DC, 1997, National Institutes of Health.

*For patients with multiple risk factors, clinicians should consider drugs as initial therapy plus lifestyle modifications.

NOTE: For example, a patient with diabetes mellitus and a BP of 142/94 mm Hg plus left ventricular hypertrophy (LVH) should be classified as having stage 1 hypertension with target organ disease (LVH) and another risk factor (diabetes mellitus). This patient would be categorized as "stage 1, risk group C," and recommended for immediate initiation of drug therapy. Lifestyle modification should be adjunctive therapy for all patients recommended for drug therapy.

For patients with multiple risk factors, the clinician should consider drugs as initial therapy plus lifestyle modifications. For patients with heart failure, renal insufficiency, or diabetes, the clinician should consider drugs as initial therapy plus lifestyle modifications.

TOD/CCD indicates target organ disease/clinical cardiovascular disease.

Risk Stratification

The risk of cardiovascular disease in people with hypertension is determined by the level of BP, the presence of target organ disease, and other risk factors. These factors independently modify the risk for cardiovascular disease. The Joint National Committee on Detection, Evaluation, and Treatment of High Blood Pressure (JNC-VI) guidelines (1997) for the management of hypertension assign patients to risk groups based on these factors.[3,4] Risk group A includes patients with high normal BP or stage 1, 2, or 3 hypertension who do not have clinical cardiovascular disease, target organ disease, or other risk factors. Risk group B includes patients with hypertension who do not have clinical cardiovascular disease or target organ disease, have one or more cardiovascular risk factors, but do not have diabetes. Risk group C includes patients with hypertension who have clinical cardiovascular disease or target organ damage. The JNC-VI recommends that patients with high normal BP as well as renal insufficiency, heart failure, or diabetes be placed in risk group C.[3] The goal in treating a hypertensive patient is to reduce overall cardiovascular risk and to control BP by the least intrusive means possible. Treatment recommendations by risk group are summarized in Table 31-7.

Follow-up monitoring of the BP is very important. The frequency of monitoring varies initially with the level of BP. After the BP has stabilized, follow-up visits should be scheduled every 3 to 6 months to ensure continued control of BP, provide support for lifestyle changes, detect side or adverse effects of medications, and assess for target organ damage.

Lifestyle Modifications

Lifestyle modifications should be used in all hypertensive patients either as definitive or adjunctive therapy. These modifications are directed toward reducing BP and overall cardiovascular risk. Modifications include (1) dietary changes, (2) limitation of alcohol intake, (3) regular physical activity, and (4) avoidance of tobacco use (smoking and chewing). Based on assigned risk group (see Table 31-7), lifestyle modifications are usually continued for up to 1 year before drug therapy is used (Fig. 31-4). Factors that may prompt a decision for early drug therapy include stage 2 or 3 hypertension, the presence of risk factors, target organ disease, clinical cardiovascular or cerebrovascular disease, and diabetes.

Nutritional Therapy. Dietary management of hypertension consists of restriction of sodium; maintenance of dietary potassium, calcium, and magnesium intake; and calorie restriction if the patient is overweight. Two recent dietary intervention trials demonstrated reductions in BP comparable to those usually seen with single-drug therapy for mild hypertension.[16,17] Epidemiologic observations and clinical trials have shown an association between sodium intake and BP. Short-term studies have shown an average decrease of 4.9 mm Hg in SBP and 2.6 mm Hg in DBP with moderate reduction in sodium intake.[3]

The average American intake of salt totals 15 g per day. The JNC-VI recommends restricting salt intake to less than 6 g of salt (NaCl) (less than 2.3 g of sodium) per day. This involves not adding salt in the preparation of foods or at meals and avoiding foods known to be high in sodium (see Table 33-11).

This level of sodium restriction may be enough to control BP in some patients with stage 1 hypertension. If drug therapy is needed, a lower dose may be effective if the patient also restricts sodium intake.[3] Furthermore, moderate sodium restriction lessens the risk of hypokalemia associated with diuretic therapy. However, people with hypertension respond differently to salt restriction. This heterogeneity of response has led to attempts to define subgroups of people with hypertension as "salt sensitive" or "salt resistant." Patients with low renin activity, such as African-Americans and older adults, are more likely to respond to salt restriction with a reduction in BP.[5]

The significance of other dietary elements for the control of hypertension is not certain. There is evidence that greater levels of dietary potassium, calcium, and vitamin D are associated with lower BP in the general population and in those with hypertension.[17] Based on available data, it is recommended that people with hypertension maintain adequate potassium (>100 mEq/day) and calcium (>1 g/day) intake from food sources.[3,5] Although it is important to maintain an adequate intake of calcium for general health, calcium supplements are not recommended to lower BP. Caffeine may raise BP acutely, but there is no long-term relationship between caffeine intake and elevated BP. Caffeine restriction is not recommended to lower BP.

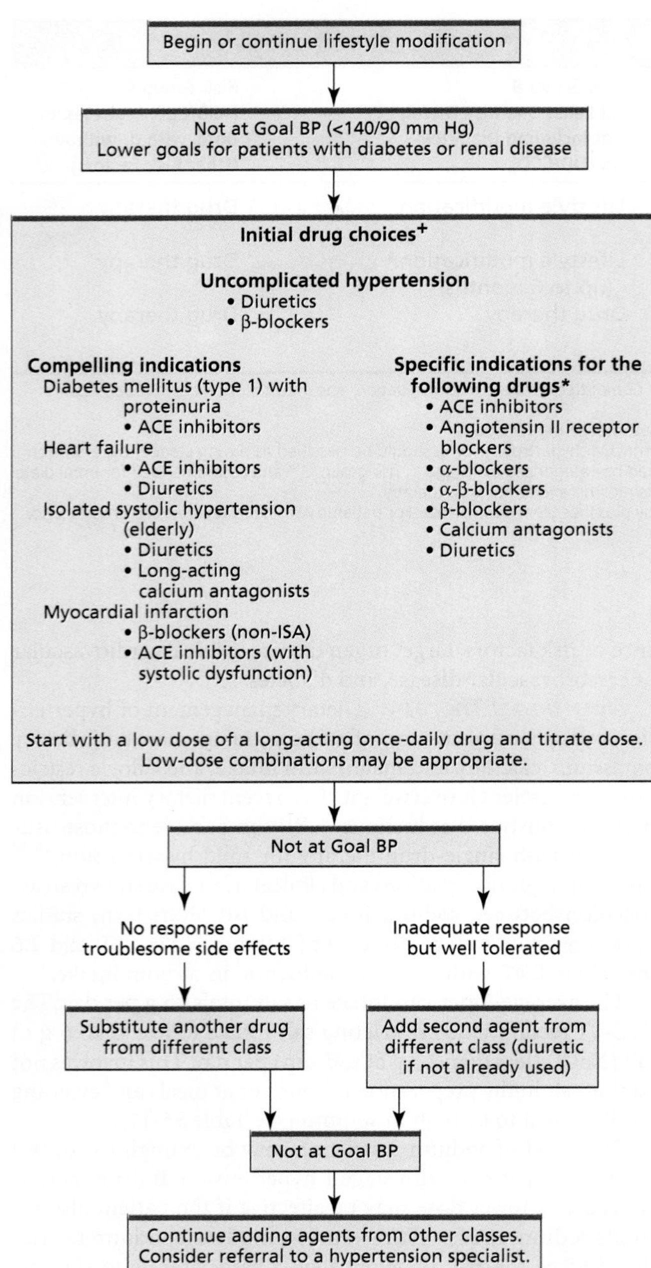

Fig. 31-4 Treatment algorithm for hypertension. *ACE,* angiotension- converting enzyme; *ISA,* intrinsic sympathetic activity.

Overweight individuals have an increased incidence of hypertension and increased cardiovascular risk. Weight reduction has a significant effect on lowering BP in many people, and the effect is seen with even moderate weight loss. When a person decreases caloric intake, sodium and fat intake may also be reduced. Although reducing the fat content of the diet has not been shown to produce sustained benefits in BP control, it may slow the progress of atherosclerosis and reduce overall cardiovascular risk (see Chapter 32). Weight reduction through a combination of dietary calorie restriction and physical activity is recommended for overweight hypertensive patients.

Modification in Alcohol Consumption. Excessive alcohol consumption is strongly associated with hypertension, and available studies suggest that the consumption of three or more alcoholic drinks daily is a risk factor for heart disease and stroke. Hypertensive patients who drink alcohol should be advised to limit their alcohol intake to 1 ounce per day (the amount of alcohol in 2 oz of 100-proof whiskey, 8 oz of wine, or 24 oz of beer).[3] Because women absorb more ethanol than men and lighter-weight people are more susceptible to the effects of alcohol than heavier-weight people, women and lighter-weight men should further restrict alcohol to 0.5 ounce per day.[3] Excessive alcohol consumption is the most frequent cause of secondary hypertension in the United States.

Physical Activity. To promote cardiovascular health, it is recommended that all adults accumulate 30 minutes or more of moderate-intensity physical activity on most, or preferably all, days of the week.[18] Moderately intense activity such as brisk walking, jogging, and swimming can lower BP, promote relaxation, and decrease or control body weight. Regular activity of this type can reduce SBP in the hypertensive patient by approximately 10 mm Hg.[3] Sedentary people should be advised to increase activity levels gradually. People with heart disease or other serious health problems need a thorough examination, possibly including a stress test, before beginning an exercise program.[3]

Avoidance of Tobacco Products. Nicotine contained in tobacco causes vasoconstriction and increases BP in hypertensive people. In addition, smoking tobacco is a major risk factor for cardiovascular disease. The cardiovascular benefits of discontinuing tobacco use can be seen within 1 year in all age-groups. Everyone, especially a hypertensive patient, should be strongly advised to avoid tobacco use. The lower amounts of nicotine contained in smoking cessation aids usually will not raise BP and may be used as indicated. People who continue to use tobacco products should be advised to monitor their BP during use.

Stress Management. Although stress can raise BP on a short-term basis and has been implicated in the development of hypertension, controversy exists as to the benefit of stress management in the prevention and treatment of hypertension. Some studies of relaxation techniques and biofeedback have shown short- and long-term BP-lowering effects. Consequently, some clinicians recommend stress management techniques as routine management of hypertension.[19] Other studies have found little effect of stress management in the treatment of hypertension.[20,21] The JNC-VI does not recommend the use of relaxation techniques for the prevention or definitive treatment of hypertension.[3]

Drug Therapy. The general goals of drug therapy are to achieve BP less than 131/85 in young adults with mild hypertension. In older adults with elevation of both systolic and diastolic BP, lowering BP to less than 140/90 mm Hg is desirable. For older adults with isolated systolic hypertension the goal of treatment should be to achieve a systolic BP less than 140 mm Hg if tolerated.[3]

The drugs currently available for treating hypertension have two main actions: reduction of SVR and volume of circulating blood (Table 31-8). The drugs used in the treatment

Text continues on p. 831

DRUG THERAPY

Table 31-8 Hypertension

Agent	Mechanism of Action	Side Effects and Adverse Effects	Nursing Considerations
Diuretics			
Thiazide and Related Diuretics			
Bendroflumethiazide (Naturetin) Benzthiazide (Aquatag, Exna) Chlorothiazide (Diuril) Hydrochlorothiazide (Esidrix, HydroDiuril, Oretic) Hydroflumethiazide (Saluron) Indapamide (Lozol) Metolazone (Zaroxolyn) Methyclothiazide (Enduron) Polythiazide (Renese) Quinethazone (Hydromax) Trichlormethiazide (Metahydrin, Naqua)	Inhibit NaCl reabsorption in the distal convoluted tubule; increase excretion of Na^+ and Cl^-. Initial decrease in ECF; sustained decrease in SVR. Lowers BP moderately in 2 to 4 weeks.	Fluid and electrolyte imbalances (volume depletion, hypokalemia, hyponatremia, hypochloremia, hypomagnesemia, hypercalcemia, hyperuricemia, metabolic alkalosis); CNS effects (vertigo, headache, weakness); GI effects (anorexia, nausea, vomiting, diarrhea, constipation, pancreatitis); sexual problems (impotence and decreased libido); blood dyscrasias; and dermatologic (photosensitivity, skin rash) effects. Decreased glucose tolerance.	Monitor for orthostatic hypotension, hypokalemia, and alkalosis. Thiazides may potentiate cardiotoxicity of digoxin by producing hypokalemia. Dietary sodium restriction reduces the risk of hypokalemia. NSAIDs can decrease diuretic and antihypertensive effect of thiazide diuretics. Advise patient to supplement with potassium-rich foods. Current doses are lower than previously recommended.
Loop Diuretics			
Bumetanide (Bumex) Ethacrynic acid (Edecrin) Furosemide (Lasix) Torsemide (Demadex)	Inhibits NaCl reabsorption in the thick ascending limb of the loop of Henle. Profoundly increased excretion of Na^+ and Cl^-. More potent diuretic effect than thiazides, but shorter duration of action, less effective for hypertension.	Fluid and electrolyte imbalance as with thiazides except not hypercalcemia. Ototoxicity (hearing impairment, deafness, vertigo) that is usually reversible. Metabolic effects including hyperuricemia, hyperglycemia, increased LDL cholesterol and triglycerides with decreased HDL cholesterol.	Monitor for orthostasis and electrolyte abnormalities as with thiazide diuretics. Loop diuretics remain effective despite renal insufficiency. Diuretic effect of drug increases at higher doses.
Potassium-Sparing Diuretics			
Amiloride (Midamor) Triamterine (Dyrenium)	Reduce K^+ and Na^+ exchange in the distal and collecting tubules. Reduce the excretion of K^+, H^+, Ca^{2+}, and Mg^{2+}.	Hyperkalemia, nausea, vomiting, diarrhea, headache, leg cramps, and dizziness.	Monitor for orthostatic hypotension and hyperkalemia. Potassium-sparing diuretics are contraindicated in renal failure and used with caution in patients on ACE inhibitors or angiotensin II blockers. Avoid potassium supplements.
Spironolactone (Aldactone)	Inhibits the Na^+-retaining and K^+-excreting effects of aldosterone in the distal and collecting tubules.	Same as amiloride and triamterine; may cause gynecomastia, impotence, decreased libido, and menstrual irregularities.	
Adrenergic Inhibitors			
Central-Acting Adrenergic Antagonists			
Clonidine (Catapres)	Reduces sympathetic outflow from CNS. Reduces peripheral sympathetic tone, produces vasodilation; decreases SVR and BP.	Dry mouth, sedation, impotence, nausea, dizziness, sleep disturbance, nightmares, restlessness, and depression. Symptomatic bradycardia in patients with conduction disorder.	Sudden discontinuation may cause withdrawal syndrome including rebound hypertension, tachycardia, headache, tremors, apprehension, and sweating. Chewing gum or hard candy may relieve dry mouth. Alcohol and sedatives increase sedation. May be given transdermally with fewer side effects and better compliance.

Continued

DRUG THERAPY

Table 31-8 Hypertension—cont'd

Agent	Mechanism of Action	Side Effects and Adverse Effects	Nursing Considerations
Adrenergic Inhibitors (continued)			
Central-Acting Adrenergic Antagonists (continued)			
Guanabenz (Wytensin)	Same as clonidine.	Same as clonidine.	Same as clonidine, but not available in transdermal.
Guanfacine (Tenex)	Same as clonidine.	Same as clonidine.	Same as clonidine, but not available in transdermal.
Methyldopa (Aldomet)	Same as clonidine.	Sedation, fatigue, orthostatic hypotension, decreased libido, impotence, dry mouth, hemolytic anemia, hepatotoxicity, sodium and water retention, depression.	Instruct patient about daytime sedation and avoidance of hazardous activities. Administration of a single daily dose at bedtime minimizes sedative effect.
Peripheral-Acting Adrenergic Antagonists			
Guanethidine (Ismelin)	Prevents peripheral release of norepinephrine, resulting in vasodilation; lowers CO and reduces SBP more than DBP.	Marked orthostatic hypotension, diarrhea, cramps, bradycardia, retrograde or delayed ejaculation, sodium and water retention.	May cause severe postural hypotension; not recommended for use with cerebrovascular or coronary insufficiency or in older adults; advise to rise slowly and wear support stockings. Hypotensive effect is delayed for 2-3 days and lasts 7-10 days after withdrawal. Once-daily dosing.
Guanadrel sulfate (Hylorel)	Same as guanethidine.	Similar to guanethidine.	Must be given twice daily.
Reserpine (Serpasil)	Depletes central and peripheral stores of norepinephrine; results in peripheral vasodilation (decreases SVR and BP).	Sedation and inability to concentrate; depression; nasal stuffiness.	Contraindicated with history of depression. Monitor mood and mental status regularly. Advise patient to avoid barbiturates, alcohol, and narcotics.
α_1-Adrenergic Blockers			
Doxazosin (Cardura) Prazosin (Minipress) Terazosin (Hytrin)	Blocks α_1 effects producing peripheral dilation (decreases SVR and BP).	Variable amount of postural hypotension depending on the plasma volume. May see profound orthostatic hypotension with syncope within 90 minutes after initial dose. Retention of salt and water.	Prazosin reduces resistance to the outflow of urine and symptoms of prostatism. Taking drug at bedtime reduces risks associated with orthostatic hypotension. Beneficial effects on lipid profile.
Phentolamine (Regitine)	Blocks α-adrenergic receptors, resulting in peripheral vascular dilation (decreases SVR and BP).	Acute, prolonged hypotension, cardiac arrhythmias, tachycardia, weakness, flushing. Abdominal pain, nausea, and exacerbation of peptic ulcer.	Used in short-term management of pheochromocytoma. Also used locally to prevent necrosis of skin and subcutaneous tissue after extravasation of an α-adrenergic agent.

Continued

DRUG THERAPY

Table 31-8 Hypertension—cont'd

Agent	Mechanism of Action	Side Effects and Adverse Effects	Nursing Considerations
Adrenergic Inhibitors (continued)			
β-Adrenergic Blockers			
Acebutolol (Sectral) Atenolol (Tenormin) Betaxolol (Kerlone) Bisoprolol (Zebeta) Carteolol (Cartrol) Carvedilol (Coreg) Metoprolol (Lopressor) Nadolol (Corgard) Penbutolol (Levatol) Pindolol (Visken) Propranolol (Inderal) Timolol (Blocadren)	Reduce BP by antagonizing β-adrenergic effects. Decrease CO and reduce sympathetic vasoconstrictor tone. Decrease renin secretion by kidney.	Bronchospasm, atrioventricular conduction block, impaired peripheral circulation, nightmares, depression, weakness, reduced exercise capacity. May induce or exacerbate heart failure in susceptible patients. Sudden withdrawal of β-blockers may cause rebound hypertension and exacerbate symptoms of ischemic heart disease.	β-Adrenergic blockers vary in lipid solubility, selectivity, and sympathomimetic effect, which explains different therapeutic and side effect profiles of specific agents. Monitor HR regularly. Use with caution in patients with diabetes mellitus (as may mask signs of hypoglycemia) and asthma.
Esmolol (Brevibloc)	Reduces BP by antagonizing β_1-adrenergic effects.		IV administration; rapid onset and very short duration of action.
Combined α- and β-Adrenergic Blocker			
Labetalol (Normodyne, Trandate)	α_1-, β_1-, and β_2-blocking properties producing peripheral vascular dilation and decreased heart rate. Reduces CO, SVR, and BP.	Dizziness, fatigue, nausea, vomiting, dyspepsia, paresthesia, nasal stuffiness, impotence, edema. Hepatic toxicity.	Same as β-blockers. IV form available for hypertensive crisis in hospitalized patients. Patients must be kept supine during IV administration. Assess patient tolerance of upright position (severe postural hypotension) before allowing upright activities (e.g., commode).
Direct Vasodilators			
Diazoxide (Hyperstat)	Direct arterial vasodilation reduces SVR and BP.	Reflex sympathetic activation producing increased HR, CO, and salt and water retention. Hyperglycemia, especially in type 2 diabetes.	IV use only for hypertensive crisis in hospitalized patients. Administer only into peripheral vein.
Hydralazine (Apresoline)	Direct arterial vasodilation reduces SVR and BP.	Headache, nausea, flushing, palpitations, tachycardia, dizziness, and angina. Hemolytic anemia, vasculitis, and rapidly progressive glomerulonephritis.	IV use for hypertensive crisis in hospitalized patients. Twice-daily oral dosage. Not used as monotherapy because of side effects. Contraindicated with coronary heart disease; used with caution in patients over 40 years of age.
Minoxidil (Loniten)	Direct arterial vasodilation reduces SVR and BP.	Reflex tachycardia, marked sodium and fluid retention (may require loop diuretics for control), and hirsutism. May cause ECG changes (flattened and inverted T waves) not related to ischemia.	Reserved for treatment of severe hypertension associated with renal failure and resistant to other therapy. Once- or twice-daily dosage.
Nitroglycerin (Tridil)	Relaxes arterial and venous smooth muscle reducing preload and SVR. At low dose, venous dilation predominates; at higher dose, arterial dilation is present.	Hypotension, headache, vomiting, flushing.	IV use for hypertensive crisis in hospitalized patients with myocardial ischemia. Administered by continuous IV infusion with pump or control device.

Continued

DRUG THERAPY

Table 31-8 Hypertension—cont'd

Agent	Mechanism of Action	Side Effects and Adverse Effects	Nursing Considerations
Direct Vasodilators (continued)			
Sodium nitroprusside (Nipride)	Direct arterial vasodilation reduces SVR and BP.	Acute hypotension, nausea, vomiting, muscle twitching. Signs of thiocyanate toxicity include anorexia, nausea, fatigue, and disorientation.	IV use for hypertensive crisis in hospitalized patients. Administered by continuous IV infusion with pump or control device. Use intraarterial monitoring of BP. Light-resistant bags, bottles, and administration sets must be used; stable for 24 hr. Monitor thiocyanate levels with prolonged (≥24 to 48 hr) use.
Ganglionic Blockers			
Trimethaphan (Arfonad)	Interrupts adrenergic control of arteries, results in vasodilation, and reduces SVR and BP.	Visual disturbance, dilated pupils, dry mouth, urinary hesitancy, subjective chilliness.	IV use for initial control of BP in patient with dissecting aortic aneurysm. Administered by continuous IV infusion with pump or control device.
Angiotensin Inhibitors			
Angiotensin-Converting Enzyme Inhibitors			
Benazepril (Lotensin) Captopril (Capoten) Cilazapril (Inhibace) Enalapril (Vasotec) Fosinopril (Monopril) Lisinopril (Prinivil, Zestril) Moexipril (Univasc) Perindopril (Aceon) Ramipril (Altace) Quinapril (Accupril) Trandolapril (Mavik)	Inhibit angiotensin-converting enzyme; reduces conversion of angiotensin I to angiotensin II (A-II); prevents A-II–mediated vasoconstriction.	Hypotension, loss of taste, cough, hyperkalemia, acute renal failure, skin rash, angioneurotic edema.	Aspirin and NSAIDs may reduce drug effectiveness. Addition of diuretic enhances drug effect. Should not be used with potassium-sparing diuretics. Can cause fetal morbidity or mortality. Captopril may be given orally for hypertensive crisis.
Enalaprilat (Vasotec Injection)	Inhibit angiotensin-converting enzyme when oral agents not appropriate.	Same as oral forms.	Given IV over 5 minutes; may be given every 6 hours.
Angiotensin II Receptor Blockers			
Candesartan (Atacand) Eprosartan (Teveten Irbesartan (Avapro) Losartan (Cozaar) Tasosartan (Verdia) Valsartan (Diovan)	Prevent action of angiotensin II and produce vasodilation and increasing salt and water excretion.	Hyperkalemia, decreased renal function.	Full effect on BP may not be seen for 3-6 weeks.
Calcium Channel Blockers			
Amlodipine (Norvasc) Diltiazem (Cardizem) Felodipine (Plendil) Isradipine (Dynacirc) Mibefradil (Posicor) Nicardipine (Cardene) Nifedipine (Procardia) Nisoldipine (Sular) Verapamil (Isoptin) Verapamil SR	Blocks movement of extracellular calcium into cells causing peripheral vasodilation and decreased SVR.	Nausea, headache, dizziness, peripheral edema. Reflex tachycardia. Reflex decrease in HR (with diltiazem); constipation (with verapamil).	Use with caution in patients with heart failure. Contraindicated with second- or third-degree heart block. IV nicardipine available for hypertensive crisis in hospitalized patients.

ACE, angiotensin-converting enzyme; *CO*, cardiac output; *DBP*, diastolic blood pressure; *ECF*, extracellular fluid; *HDL*, high-density lipoprotein; *LDL*, low-density lipoprotein; *NSAID*, nonsteroidal antiinflammatory drug; *SBP*, systolic blood pressure; *SVR*, systemic vascular resistance.

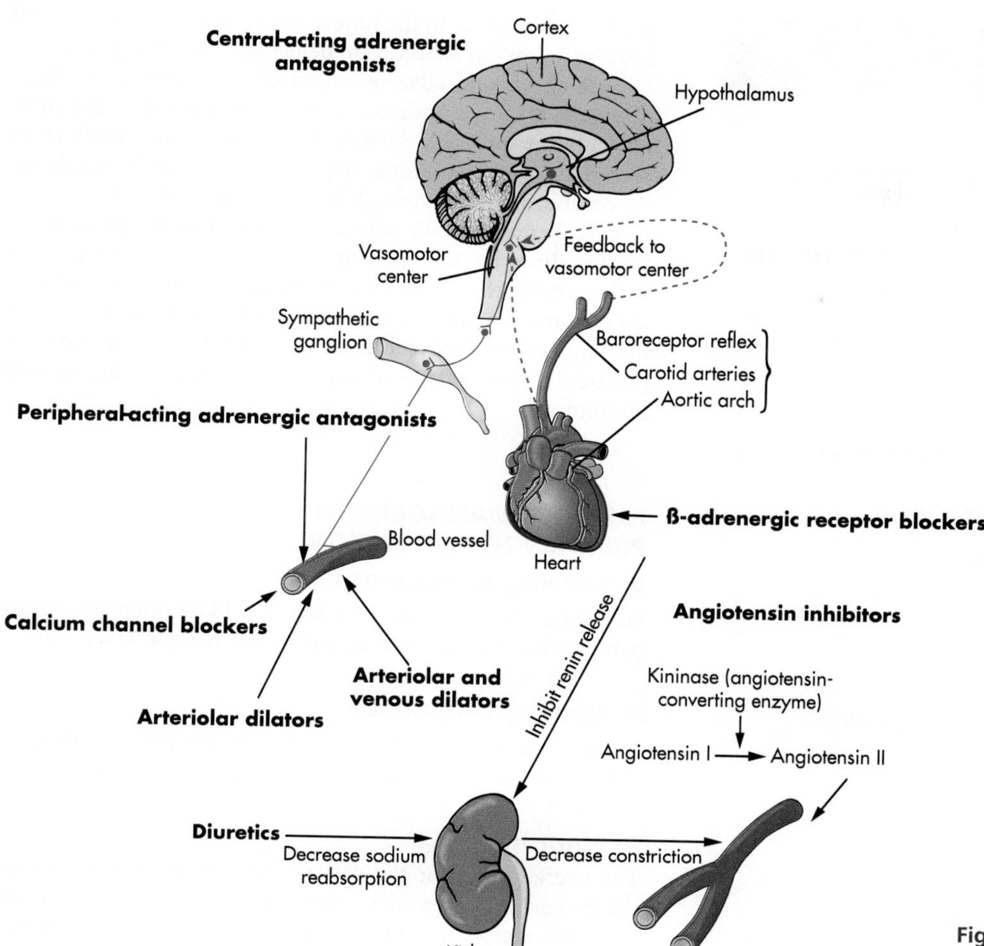

Fig. 31-5 Site and method of action of various antihypertensive drugs.

of hypertension include diuretics, adrenergic (sympathetic) inhibitors, vasodilators, angiotensin inhibitors, and calcium channel blockers. The various sites and methods of action are presented in Fig. 31-5.

Although the precise action of diuretics in the reduction of BP is unclear, it is known that they promote sodium and water excretion, reduce plasma volume, decrease sodium in the arteriolar walls, and reduce the vascular response to catecholamines. Adrenergic-inhibiting agents act by diminishing the sympathetic effects that increase BP. Adrenergic inhibitors include drugs that act centrally on the vasomotor center and peripherally at the neuroeffector junction to inhibit norepinephrine release or to block the adrenergic receptors on blood vessels. Direct vasodilators decrease the BP by relaxing vascular smooth muscle and reducing SVR. Angiotensin inhibitors reduce angiotensin II (A-II)–mediated vasoconstriction and salt and water conservation. ACE inhibitors reduce A-II concentration, and A-II receptor blockers prevent angiotension from binding to its receptors in the walls of the blood vessels. Calcium channel blockers increase sodium excretion and cause arteriolar vasodilation by preventing the movement of extracellular calcium into cells (see Chapter 32).

Drug therapy is recommended for all patients with stage 2 or 3 hypertension that is not controlled by lifestyle measures. Because of the higher risk of hypertensive complications, drug therapy is also recommended for all hypertensive patients with diabetes, clinical cardiovascular or cerebrovascular disease, and target organ disease.[3] Based on studies that have shown decreased cardiovascular morbidity and mortality rates associated with the use of diuretics and β-blockers, these agents are recommended for the initial drug therapy of uncomplicated hypertension.[3,4] Angiotensin inhibitors, adrenergic receptor blockers, and calcium channel blockers are also effective in lowering BP and may be used as first-line drugs. Direct-acting vasodilators, the α_2-adrenergic agonists, and the peripheral-acting adrenergic antagonists are not recommended for single-drug therapy because of their side effects.

The selection of a first-line drug is influenced by cost, the presence of other medical conditions, patient characteristics, and side effects. The initial drug is started at a low dose for several weeks. If, after 1 to 3 months, the BP is not controlled, the dose of the first-line drug can be increased, a second drug from a different class can be substituted, or a second drug from a different class can be added. If the addition of the second drug controls the BP, the clinician may try withdrawing the first drug. Many times, the patient with mild to moderate hypertension can be controlled with only one drug.[3] Before proceeding with the addition or substitution of medication, con-

Table 31-9 Causes for Lack of Responsiveness to Therapy

Nonadherence to Therapy
- Cost of medication
- Instructions not clear or not given to the patient in writing
- Inadequate or no patient education
- Lack of involvement of the patient in the treatment plan
- Side effects of medication
- Organic brain syndrome (e.g., memory deficit)
- Inconvenient dosing

Drug-related Causes
- Doses too low
- Inappropriate combinations (e.g., two centrally acting adrenergic inhibitors)
- Rapid inactivation (e.g., hydralazine)
- Drug interactions
  - Nonsteroidal antiinflammatory drugs
  - Oral contraceptives
  - Sympathomimetics
  - Antidepressants
  - Adrenal steroids
  - Nasal decongestants
  - Licorice-containing substances (e.g., chewing tobacco)
  - Cocaine
  - Cyclosporine
  - Erythropoietin

Associated Conditions
- Increasing obesity
- Alcohol intake more than 1 oz/day

Secondary Hypertension
- Renal insufficiency
- Renovascular hypertension
- Pheochromocytoma
- Primary aldosteronism

Volume Overload
- Inadequate diuretic therapy
- Excess sodium intake
- Fluid retention from reduction of blood pressure
- Progressive renal damage

Pseudohypertension

From US Department of Health and Human Services: *The Sixth Report of the Joint National Committee on Detection, Evaluation, and Treatment of High Blood Pressure (JNC-VI)*, Washington, DC, 1997, National Institutes of Health.

sideration should be given to possible reasons for the lack of response to drug therapy (Table 31-9).

For stage 3 hypertension, the plan is essentially the same, but the interval between medication changes may be shortened, and therapy may need to be started with more than one drug. The addition of a third or fourth drug, including the centrally and peripherally acting adrenergic antagonists and direct vasodilators, may be necessary.

After one year of good BP control, step-down therapy may be tried. The number of medications and their dosages are gradually decreased to the lowest amount that controls the BP. Regular follow-up is needed to detect any elevation of BP.[3]

Side effects and adverse effects of antihypertensive drugs may be so severe or undesirable that the patient does not comply with therapy. Table 31-8 describes the major side effects of each drug. Hyperuricemia, hyperglycemia, and hypokalemia are common side effects with both thiazide and loop diuretics. Hyperkalemia can be a serious side effect of the potassium-sparing diuretics and ACE inhibitors. Impotence may occur with many of the diuretics. Orthostatic hypotension and sexual dysfunction are two undesirable effects of adrenergic-inhibiting agents. Tachycardia and orthostatic hypotension are potential adverse effects of both vasodilators and angiotensin inhibitors.

NURSING MANAGEMENT: PRIMARY HYPERTENSION

■ Nursing Assessment

Subjective and objective data that should be obtained from a patient with hypertension are presented in Table 31-10.

■ Nursing Diagnoses

Nursing diagnoses for the patient with hypertension include, but are not limited to, those presented in Table 31-11.

■ Planning

The overall goals for the patient with hypertension are that the patient will (1) achieve and maintain desired BP; (2) understand, accept, and implement the therapeutic plan; (3) experience minimal or no unpleasant side effects of therapy; and (4) be confident of ability to manage and cope with this condition.

■ Nursing Implementation

Health Promotion. Primary prevention of hypertension provides an attractive alternative to the costly cycle of managing hypertension and its complications. Current recommendations for primary prevention are based on lifestyle modifications that have been shown to prevent or delay the expected rise in BP in susceptible people.[3] A diet rich in fruits, vegetables, and low-fat dairy foods, with reduced saturated and total fats, significantly lowers BP.[17] This diet has been recommended for primary prevention in the general population. Dietary modifications that do not require active participation of the individual, such as a reduction in the amount of sodium chloride added to processed foods, may be even more effective.[3]

Individual patient evaluation. The majority of cases of hypertension are identified through routine screening procedures such as insurance, preemployment, and military physical examinations. The nurse in these settings, as well as in most other practice settings, is in an ideal position to assess for the presence of hypertension, identify the risk factors for hypertension and coronary artery disease, and educate the patient regarding these conditions. In addition to BP determination, a complete health

NURSING ASSESSMENT

Table **31-10** **Hypertension**

Subjective Data	Objective Data
Important Health Information *Past health history:* Known duration and past workup of high BP; cardiovascular, cerebrovascular, renal, or thyroid disease; diabetes mellitus; pituitary disorders; obesity; dyslipidemia; menopause or hormone replacement status *Medications:* Use of any prescription or over-the-counter, illicit, or herbal medications; previous use of antihypertensive drug therapy **Functional Health Patterns** *Health perception–health management:* Family history of hypertension or cardiovascular disease; smoking or other tobacco use, alcohol use; sedentary lifestyle *Nutritional-metabolic:* Usual salt and fat intake; weight gain or loss *Elimination:* Nocturia *Activity-exercise:* Fatigue; dyspnea on exertion, palpitations on exertion, anginal chest pain; intermittent claudication, muscle cramps *Cognitive-perceptual:* Dizziness; blurred vision, paresthesias *Sexual-reproductive:* Impotence *Coping–stress tolerance:* Stressful life events	**Cardiovascular** BP consistently above 140 mm Hg systolic or 90 mm Hg diastolic, orthostatic change in BP and pulse; retinal vessel changes, abnormal heart sounds; laterally displaced, sustained, forceful, apical pulse; diminished or absent peripheral pulses; carotid, renal, ischial, or femoral bruits; presence of edema **Musculoskeletal** Truncal obesity; abnormal waist-hip ratio **Neurologic** Mental status changes; localized edema **Possible Findings** **Serum Chemistries** Abnormal serum electrolytes (especially potassium); elevated BUN, creatinine, glucose, cholesterol, and tryglyceride levels; proteinuria, microalbuminuria; evidence of ischemic heart disease and left ventricular hypertrophy on EEG; evidence of structural heart disease and left ventricular hypertrophy on echocardiogram

MI, myocardial infarction.

assessment should include such factors as age, sex, race, diet history (including sodium and alcohol intake), weight patterns, and family history of heart disease, stroke, renal disease, and diabetes mellitus. Medications taken, both prescribed and over-the-counter, should be noted. The patient should be asked about any previous history of high BP and the results of treatment (if any) (see Table 31-10).

Initially, the BP is taken two or three times, at least 2 minutes apart, with the average pressure recorded as the value for that visit. Waiting for at least 2 minutes between readings allows the venous blood to drain from the arm and prevents inaccurate readings. Size and placement of BP cuff are important considerations for accurate measurement. The width of the inflatable bladder should be 40% and length should be 80% of the arm circumference. Use of a cuff that is too small or too large will result in readings that are falsely high or low, respectively.

BP measurements of both arms should be performed initially to detect any differences between arms. Atherosclerotic narrowing of the subclavian artery can cause a falsely low reading on the side where the narrowing occurs. Therefore the arm with the higher reading should be used for all subsequent BP measurements. The patient's arm is uncovered and placed at the level of the heart. The cuff should be inflated until no pulse is felt in the brachial artery located in the antecubital fossa of the arm being used. The cuff is then inflated an additional 10 to 20 mm Hg to ensure vascular occlusion. The pressure is released at 2 mm Hg per second. Releasing any slower or faster may create inaccurate readings. Both SBP and DBP should be recorded, with the DBP recorded as the disappearance of sound (Table 31-12).

The BP and pulse are initially measured with the patient in either the supine or the sitting position after at least 5 minutes of rest. BP and pulse should be measured again after 2 minutes in the standing position. Usually the SBP decreases on standing, whereas the DBP and pulse increase. A decrease of more than 10 mm Hg in SBP or any decrease in DBP when standing is abnormal and should prompt further investigation. Common causes of abnormal postural BP values include intravascular volume loss (such as with diuretic therapy) and inadequate vasoconstrictor mechanisms related to disease or medications.

Screening programs. The nurse involved in a screening program should be aware of general guidelines for BP detection and evaluation (Table 31-13). At the time of the BP measurement, each person should be informed in writing of the numeric value of the reading and, if necessary, why further evaluation is important. Effort and resources should be focused on controlling BP in the person already identified as having hypertension; identifying and controlling BP in high risk groups such as African-Americans, obese people, and blood relatives of people with hypertension; and screening those with limited access to the health care system.[22]

Table 31-11 Nursing Diagnoses and Collaborative Problems Associated with Hypertension

Nursing Diagnoses

Altered health maintenance *related to* lack of knowledge of pathology, complications, and management of hypertension

Anxiety *related to* complexity of management regimen, possible complications, and lifestyle changes associated with hypertension

Sexuality dysfunction *related to* effects of antihypertensive medication

Ineffective management of therapeutic regimen *related to* (specify)
- lack of knowledge
- unpleasant side effects of medication
- return of BP to normal while on medication
- high cost of some medications
- inconvenient schedule for taking medications
- lack of trusting relationship with health care provider

Body image disturbance *related to* diagnosis of hypertension

Collaborative Problems

Potential complication: adverse effects from antihypertensive therapy

Potential complication: hypertensive crisis

Potential complication: cerebrovascular accident

Table 31-12 Appropriate Technique for Measuring Blood Pressure

1. Patient should be seated with the arm bared, supported, and positioned at heart level. The patient should not have smoked or ingested caffeine within 30 minutes before measurement.
2. Blood pressure should be taken in both arms initially.
3. Measurement should not begin until patient has had 5 minutes of quiet rest.
4. The appropriate cuff size must be used to ensure an accurate measurement. The rubber bladder should nearly (at least 80%) or completely encircle the arm. Cuff width should be at least 40% of the arm circumference. Several sizes of cuffs (e.g., child, adult, and large adult) should be available.
5. Measurements should be taken with a mercury sphygmomanometer, a recently calibrated aneroid manometer, or a calibrated electronic device.
6. Both systolic and diastolic pressures should be recorded. The disappearance of sound should be used for the diastolic reading.
7. Two or more readings (taken at least 2 minutes apart) should be averaged. If the first two readings differ by more than 5 mm Hg, additional readings should be obtained.
8. The patient should be informed of the reading and advised of the need for periodic remeasurement.

From US Department of Health and Human Services: *The Sixth Report of the Joint National Committee on Detection, Evaluation, and Treatment of High Blood Pressure (JNC-VI),* Washington, DC, 1997, National Institutes of Health.

Cardiovascular risk factor modification. Education regarding cardiovascular risk factors is appropriate for individual and targeted screening programs. Modifiable cardiovascular risk factors include hypertension, obesity, diabetes mellitus, elevated serum lipids, tobacco use, and physical inactivity. Risk factors can easily be identified and modification discussed with the patient. (Health-promoting behaviors for cardiovascular risk factors are discussed in Table 32-4.)

Ambulatory and Home Care. The primary nursing responsibilities for long-term management of hypertension are to assist the patient in reducing BP and complying with the treatment plan. Nursing actions include patient and family education, detection and reporting of adverse treatment effects, compliance assessment and enhancement, and evaluation of therapeutic effectiveness (Table 31-14). Patient education includes the following: (1) diet therapy; (2) drug therapy; (3) physical activity; (4) home monitoring of BP (if appropriate); and (5) tobacco cessation (if applicable).

Nutritional therapy. The patient and family, especially the member who prepares the meals, should be educated about sodium-restricted diets. They should be instructed on reading labels of over-the-counter drugs, packaged foods, and health products (e.g., baking soda–containing toothpaste) to identify hidden sources of sodium. It is helpful to review the patient's normal diet and to identify foods high in sodium. Analysis of a 3-day diet history will help identify foods high in sodium in the patient's usual diet. (Weight-reduction diets are discussed in Chapter 38, and diets low in cholesterol and saturated fats are discussed in Chapter 32.)

Drug therapy. Patient and family education related to drug therapy is needed to identify and minimize side effects and to cope with therapeutic effects. Side effects of antihypertensive drug therapy are common. Side effects may be an initial response to a drug and may decrease with continued use of the drug. Informing the patient about side effects that lessen with time may enable the individual to continue taking the medicine. The number or severity of side effects may be related to the dosage, and it may be necessary to change the drug or decrease the dosage. In this case, the patient should be advised to report the side effects to the person who prescribed the medication.

A common side effect of several of these drugs is orthostatic hypotension. This condition is caused by an alteration of the autonomic nervous system's mechanisms for regulating pressure, which are required for position changes. Consequently, the patient may feel dizzy, weak, and faint when assuming an upright position after sitting or lying down. Specific measures to control or decrease orthostatic hypotension are presented in Table 31-14.

Sexual dysfunction may occur with many of the antihypertensive drugs (see Table 31-8) and can be a major reason that a patient does not adhere to the treatment plan. Rather than discussing a sexual problem with a health professional, the patient may decide to discontinue using the drug. Often the nurse must approach the patient on this sensitive subject and encourage discussion of any sexual dysfunction that may be experienced.

Table 31-13 **Recommendations for Follow-Up Based on Initial Set of Blood Pressure Measurements for Adults Age 18 and Older**

Initial Screening Blood Pressure (mm Hg)*		
Systolic	**Diastolic**	**Follow-Up Recommended**†
<130	<85	Recheck in 2 years
130-139	85-89	Recheck in 1 year‡
140-159	90-99	Confirm within 2 months‡
160-179	100-109	Evaluate or refer to source of care within 1 month
≥180	≥110	Evaluate or refer to source of care immediately or within 1 week depending on clinical situation

*If systolic and diastolic categories are different, follow recommendations for shorter follow-up (e.g., 160/86 mm Hg should be evaluated or referred to source of care within 1 month).
†Modify the scheduling of follow-up according to reliable information about past blood pressure measurements, other cardiovascular risk factors, or target organ disease.
‡Provide advice about lifestyle modifications.

PATIENT & FAMILY TEACHING GUIDE

Table 31-14 **Hypertension**

When presenting information to the patient or family, the nurse should do the following:

1. Provide the numerical value of the patient's BP and explain that it exceeds normal limits.
2. Inform the patient that hypertension is usually asymptomatic and symptoms do not reliably indicate BP levels.
3. Explain that hypertension means elevated BP and does not relate to a "hyper" personality.
4. Explain that long-term follow-up and therapy are necessary.
5. Explain that therapy will not cure but should control hypertension.
6. Tell the patient that controlled hypertension is usually compatible with an excellent prognosis and a normal lifestyle.
7. Explain the potential dangers of uncontrolled hypertension.
8. Be specific about the names, actions, dosages, and side effects of prescribed medications.
9. Tell the patient to plan regular and convenient times for taking medications.
10. Tell the patient not to discontinue drugs abruptly because withdrawal may cause a severe hypertensive reaction.
11. Tell the patient not to double up on doses when a dose is missed.
12. Inform the patient that if BP increases, not to take an increased medication dosage before consulting with the health care provider.
13. Tell the patient not to take a medication belonging to someone else.
14. Inform the patient that side effects of medication often diminish with time.
15. Tell the patient to consult with the health care provider about changing drugs or dosages if impotence or other sexual problems develop.
16. Tell the patient to supplement diet with foods high in potassium (e.g., citrus fruits and green leafy vegetables) if taking potassium-losing diuretics.
17. Tell the patient to avoid hot baths, excessive amounts of alcohol, and strenuous exercise within 3 hr of taking medications that promote vasodilation.
18. Explain that to decrease orthostatic hypotension, the patient should arise slowly from bed, sit on side of bed for a few minutes, stand slowly, not stand still for prolonged periods of time, do leg exercises to increase venous return, sleep with head of bed raised or on pillows, and lie or sit down when dizziness occurs.

The sexual problems may be easier for the patient to discuss and handle once it has been explained that the drug may be the source of the problem and the side effects can be decreased or eliminated by changing to another antihypertensive drug. The patient should be encouraged to discuss side effects with the health professional who prescribed the medication. There are so many options now in treating hypertension that a plan that is acceptable to the patient should be achievable.

Some unpleasant effects of drugs result from their therapeutic effect, but the impact can be minimized. For example, dry mouth and frequent voiding are unpleasant effects of diuretics. Sugarless gum or candy may relieve the dry mouth. The nurse can assist the patient to develop a medication schedule to minimize unpleasant effects. When frequent urination interrupts sleep, taking the diuretic earlier in the day may be beneficial. Side effects of vasodilators and adrenergic inhibitors decrease if the drugs are given in the evening. It should be remembered that BP is lowest during the night and highest shortly after awakening. Therefore medicines with 24-hour duration of action should be taken as early in

RESEARCH
IMPLICATIONS FOR NURSING PRACTICE

Accuracy of Home BP Measurement

Citation Merrick RD, Olive KE, Hamdy RC, and others: Factors influencing the accuracy of home blood pressure measurement, *South Med J* 90:1110, 1997.

Purpose To determine the accuracy of BP measurements obtained by patients using their own blood pressure monitoring device (BPMD) and to ascertain factors that affect the accuracy of patient measurements.

Methods Ninety-one volunteers participated in a study in which they brought their own BPMD and then had their BP checked by a trained technician. They also completed a 30-item questionnaire regarding demographic variables, their BPMDs, and knowledge of hypertension. Patient BP measurements were defined as accurate if the systolic and diastolic BP readings were each within 10 mm Hg of the systolic and diastolic measurements done by the technician.

Results and Conclusions Of 91 patients, 31 (34%) obtained inaccurate readings. The inaccuracy could not be attributed to the type of the instrument, the cost of the instrument, the educational level of the user, or the age of the instrument. Fifty-three percent of the volunteers had never received instructions on the use of their instrument. This study shows that a significant number of inaccurate readings are obtained by patients using BPMDs. Supervision of their use should be incorporated into patient teaching to ensure that there is a reasonable correlation between values obtained using the mercury sphygmomanometer and the BPMD.

Implications for Nursing Practice Over the past few years BPMDs have become available for individuals to measure their BP in the convenience of their home. Health care providers should ask the patients to bring their BPMDs to the clinic or office for comparison readings on each visit. More effort by manufacturers and the medical and nursing community should be expended to teach patients how to more accurately use their BPMDs.

the morning as possible (e.g., 4 or 5 AM if the patient awakens to void).

Physical activity. Physical activity is bodily movement produced by skeletal muscles that requires energy expenditure.[18] Health benefits from physical activity can be achieved with moderate-intensity activities. The goal for all adults is to accumulate 30 minutes of moderate-intensity activity daily. Generally physical activity is more likely to be sustained if it is safe and enjoyable, fits easily into the daily schedule, and does not generate financial or social costs. Shopping malls in many communities are open early in the morning (before shopping hours) and provide a warm, safe, flat area for walking. In some communities, health clubs offer special "off-peak" rates to encourage physical activity among older adults. Cardiac rehabilitation programs offer supervised exercise with education about reduction of cardiovascular risk factors. Nurses can assist people with hypertension to increase their physical activity by identifying and communicating the need for increased activity, explaining the difference between physical activity and exercise, assisting in initiating activity, and following up appropriately.

Home blood pressure monitoring. Some patients benefit from regularly monitoring their BP at home. Home BP measurement may give a more valid indication of the BP because the patient is more relaxed. It is important to emphasize to the patient that a single reading is not as important as a series of readings over a period of time. The patient should be instructed to take BP readings weekly (unless otherwise instructed) once the BP has stabilized. A log of the BP measurements should be maintained by the patient and brought to office visits.

Home BP readings may help achieve patient compliance by reinforcing the need to remain on therapy. A patient may become excessively concerned with the BP readings when using home monitoring. Generally, however, this practice should reassure the patient that the treatment is effective.

Patient compliance. A major problem in the long-term management of the patient with hypertension is poor compliance with the prescribed treatment plan.[23] The reasons are many and include inadequate patient instruction, unpleasant side effects of drugs, return of BP to normal range while on medication, lack of motivation, high cost of drugs, and lack of a trusting relationship between the patient and the health care provider. In addition to using BP determinations as an indicator of compliance, the nurse should also assess the patient's diet, activity level, and lifestyle.

Individual assessment to determine the reasons the patient is not complying with the treatment plan and the development of an individualized plan with the patient's assistance are essential. The plan should be compatible with the patient's personality, habits, and lifestyle. Active patient participation increases the likelihood of adherence to the treatment plan. Measures such as involving the patient in scheduling medication convenient to a daily routine, helping the patient link pill taking with another daily activity, and involving family members (if necessary) help increase patient compliance. Substituting combination tablets for multiple drugs once the BP is stabilized may also facilitate compliance, since the patient has to take fewer drugs each day and the cost may be less. It is important to help the patient and the family understand that hypertension is a chronic condition that cannot be cured but can be controlled with drug therapy, diet therapy, physical activity, periodic evaluation, and other relevant lifestyle changes.

■ Evaluation

The overall expected outcomes are that the patient with hypertension will

- achieve and maintain desired BP
- understand, accept, and implement the therapeutic plan
- experience minimal or no unpleasant side effects of therapy

Table 31-15 Causes of Hypertensive Crisis

Exacerbation of chronic hypertension
Renovascular hypertension
Preeclampsia, eclampsia
Pheochromocytoma
Drugs (cocaine, amphetamines, oral contraceptive pills)
Monoamine oxidase inhibitors taken with tyramine-containing foods
Rebound hypertension (from abrupt withdrawal of clonidine or β-adrenergic blockers)
Necrotizing vasculitis
Head injury
Acute aortic dissection

HYPERTENSIVE CRISIS

Hypertensive crisis is a severe and abrupt elevation in BP, arbitrarily defined as a diastolic BP of 120 to 130 mm Hg. The rate of rise of BP is more important than the absolute value in determining the need for emergency treatment. Patients with chronic hypertension can tolerate much higher BP than previously normotensive people. Prompt recognition and management of hypertensive crisis is essential to decrease the threat to organ function and life.

Hypertensive crisis occurs most commonly in patients with a history of hypertension who have failed to comply with their prescribed medications or who have been under medicated. In this setting, rising BP is thought to trigger endothelial damage and the release of vasoconstrictor substances. A vicious cycle of BP elevation ensues leading to life-threatening damage to target organs. Hypertensive crisis related to cocaine or crack use is becoming a more frequent problem. Other drugs such as amphetamines, phencyclidine (PCP), and lysergic acid diethylamide (LSD) may also precipitate hypertensive crisis that may be complicated by drug-induced seizures, stroke, myocardial infarction, or encephalopathy.[5,6] Table 31-15 lists causes of hypertensive crisis.

Hypertensive crisis is classified by the degree of organ damage and the rapidity with which the BP must be lowered. *Hypertensive emergency,* which develops over hours to days, is a situation in which a patient's BP is severely elevated with evidence of acute target organ damage, especially damage to the central nervous system. Hypertensive emergencies include hypertensive encephalopathy, intracranial or subarachnoid hemorrhage, acute left ventricular failure with pulmonary edema, myocardial infarction, renal failure, and dissecting aortic aneurysm. *Hypertensive urgency,* which develops over days to weeks, is a situation in which a patient's BP is severely elevated but there is no clinical evidence of target organ damage.

Clinical Manifestations

A hypertensive emergency may be manifested as hypertensive encephalopathy, a syndrome in which a sudden rise in arterial pressure is associated with headache, nausea, vomiting, seizures, confusion, stupor, and coma. Other common manifestations are blurred vision and transient blindness. The manifestations of encephalopathy are probably the results of cerebral edema and spasms of cerebral vessels.

Renal insufficiency ranging from minor impairment to complete renal shutdown may occur. Rapid cardiac decompensation ranging from unstable angina to infarction and pulmonary edema is also possible with chest pain and dyspnea. Aortic dissection causes excruciating chest and back pain often accompanied by diaphoresis, and the loss of pulses in an extremity.

Patient assessment is extremely important, especially monitoring for signs of neurologic dysfunction, retinal damage, heart failure, pulmonary edema, and renal failure. The neurologic manifestations are often similar to the presentation of a CVA. However, a hypertensive crisis does not show focal or lateralizing signs often seen with a CVA.

NURSING AND COLLABORATIVE MANAGEMENT: HYPERTENSIVE CRISIS

BP level alone is a poor indicator of the seriousness of the patient's condition and is not the major factor in deciding the treatment for a hypertensive crisis. The association between elevated BP and signs of new or progressive end-organ damage (e.g., cerebrovascular, cardiac, retinal, or renal involvement) determines the seriousness of the situation.

When treating hypertensive emergencies, the mean arterial pressure (MAP) is often used instead of systolic and diastolic readings to guide and evaluate therapy. MAP is calculated as DBP plus pulse pressure (SBP minus DBP):

$$\text{MAP} = \text{DBP} + \frac{1}{3}\ \text{Pulse pressure}$$

Hypertensive emergencies require hospitalization, parenteral administration of antihypertensive drugs, and intensive care monitoring. Generally, the initial treatment goal is to decrease MAP 10% to 20% in the first 1 to 2 hours with further gradual reduction over the next 24 hours. Lowering the BP too far or too fast may decrease cerebral perfusion and could precipitate a stroke. A patient who has aortic dissection, unstable angina, or signs of myocardial infarction must have the SBP lowered to 100 to 120 mm Hg as quickly as possible.[6]

The intravenous (IV) drugs used for hypertensive emergencies include vasodilators (such as sodium nitroprusside, nitroglycerin, diazoxide [Hyperstat], and hydralazine [Apresoline]), adrenergic inhibitors (such as phentolamine [Regitine], labetalol [Normodyne], esmolol [Brevibloc]), and the ACE inhibitor enalaprilat (Vasotec). Sodium nitroprusside is the most effective parenteral drug for the treatment of hypertensive emergencies. Fenoldopam (Corlopam), a new IV drug for the treatment of hypertensive emergencies, selectively activates dopamine receptors, resulting in renal and systemic vasodilation. Oral agents may be administered in addition to the parenteral drugs to help make an earlier transition to long-term therapy. The mechanisms of action and the adverse effects of these drugs are presented in Table 31-8.

Administered intravenously the drugs have a rapid (within seconds to minutes) onset of action. The patient's BP and pulse should be taken every 2 to 3 minutes during the initial administration of these drugs. The use of an intraarterial line (see Chapter 63) or an automated BP monitoring machine (e.g., Dynamap) to monitor the BP is ideal. The rate of drug administration is titrated according to the level of BP. It is important to prevent hypotension and its effects in a person whose body has adjusted to hypertension. An excessive reduction in BP may cause stroke, MI, or visual changes. Continual ECG monitoring is frequently done to observe for cardiac arrhythmias. Extreme caution is needed in treating the patient with coronary artery disease or cerebral vascular insufficiency. Hourly urinary output should be measured to assess renal perfusion. Careful monitoring of vital signs and urinary output provides information regarding the effectiveness of these drugs and the patient's response to therapy. Patients receiving IV antihypertensive drugs may be restricted to bed; getting up (e.g., to use the commode) may cause severe cerebral ischemia and fainting.

Regular, ongoing assessment is essential to evaluate the patient with severe hypertension. Frequent neurologic checks, including level of consciousness, pupillary size and reaction, movement of extremities, and reactions to stimuli, help detect any changes in the patient's condition. Cardiac, pulmonary, and renal systems should be monitored for decompensation caused by the severe elevation in BP (e.g., pulmonary edema, CHF, angina, and renal failure).

Hypertensive urgencies usually do not require IV medications but can be managed with oral agents. The patient with a hypertensive urgency may not need hospitalization, but requires frequent follow-up.[6] The oral drugs most frequently used for hypertensive urgencies are captopril (Capoten) and clonidine (Catapres) (see Table 31-8). Sublingual or oral nifedipine was previously used for hypertensive urgencies, but it is no longer recommended. The disadvantage of oral medications is the inability to regulate the dosage moment to moment, as can be done with IV medications.

A patient with severe elevation of BP but without target organ damage (hypertensive urgency) may not require emergent drug therapy or hospitalization. Allowing the patient to sit for 20 or 30 minutes in a quiet environment may significantly reduce BP. Oral drugs may then be instituted or adjusted. Additional nursing interventions include encouraging the patient to verbalize fears, answering questions concerning the hypertension, and eliminating excess noise in the patient's environment. If a patient with a hypertensive urgency is not hospitalized, outpatient follow-up should be arranged within 24 hours.

Once the hypertensive crisis is resolved, it is important to determine the cause. The patient will need appropriate management and extensive education to avoid future crisis.

CRITICAL THINKING EXERCISES

CASE STUDY

Primary Hypertension

Patient Profile

Mr. R. is a 45-year-old African-American man with no previous history of hypertension. At a screening clinic, his BP was found to be 180/120 mm Hg.

Subjective Data

- Father died of stroke at age 60
- Mother is alive but has hypertension
- States that he feels fine and is not a "hyper" person
- Smokes one pack of cigarettes daily
- Drinks a six-pack of beer on Friday and Saturday nights
- Believes that BP medication interferes with his love life

Objective Data

Physical Examination

- Grade I/IV Keith-Wagener retinopathy
- Sustained apical impulse palpable in the fourth intercostal space just lateral to the midclavicular line

Diagnostic Studies

- ECG: left ventricular hypertrophy
- Urinalysis: protein 31 mg/dl (0.3 g/L)
- Serum creatinine level: 1.6 mg/dl (141 μmol/L)

Collaborative Care

- Low-sodium diet
- Hydrochlorothiazide 12.5 mg/day

Critical Thinking Questions

1. What risk factors for hypertension are present?
2. What evidence of target organ damage is present?
3. What misconceptions about hypertension should be corrected?
4. What areas would you focus on in teaching this patient about his illness?
5. Based on the assessment data presented, write one or more appropriate nursing diagnoses. Are there any collaborative problems?

NURSING RESEARCH ISSUES

1. Does a person believe that if the personal risk factors for hypertension are reduced, chances of developing hypertension will be reduced?
2. What are the perceptions and attitudes of the nurse toward the efficacy of hypertension screening?
3. Do the perceptions of daily stress in the hypertensive patient differ from the perceptions of daily stress in the normotensive patient?
4. Do the patient and family members who are taught BP measurement by videotaped instruction measure BP as accurately as those who are taught by personal instruction?
5. Does home monitoring of BP increase the patient's compliance with antihypertensive therapy?

REVIEW QUESTIONS

The number of the question corresponds to the same-numbered objective at the beginning of the chapter.

1. If a patient has decreased cardiac output caused by fluid volume deficit and marked vasodilation, the regulatory mechanism that will increase the blood pressure by improving both of these is
   a. release of antidiuretic hormone (ADH).
   b. secretion of prostaglandins PGE_2 and PGI_2.
   c. stimulation of the sympathetic nervous system.
   d. activation of the renin-angiotensin-aldosterone system.
2. While obtaining subjective assessment data from a patient with hypertension, the nurse recognizes that a modifiable risk factor for the development of hypertension is
   a. hyperlipidemia.
   b. excessive alcohol intake.
   c. a family history of hypertension.
   d. consumption of a high-carbohydrate, high calcium-diet.
3. Target organ damage that can occur from hypertension includes
   a. headache and dizziness.
   b. retinopathy and diabetes.
   c. hypercholesterolemia and renal dysfunction.
   d. renal dysfunction and left ventricular hypertrophy.
4. A high risk population that should be targeted in the primary prevention of hypertension is
   a. smokers.
   b. African-Americans.
   c. business executives.
   d. middle-aged women.
5. In teaching a patient with hypertension about controlling the condition, the nurse recognizes that
   a. all patients with elevated BP require medication.
   b. it is not necessary to limit salt in the diet if taking a diuretic.
   c. obese persons must achieve a normal weight in order to lower BP.
   d. lifestyle modifications are indicated for all persons with elevated BP.
6. A major consideration in the management of the older adult with hypertension is to
   a. prevent pseudohypertension from converting to true hypertension.
   b. recognize that the older adult is less likely to comply with the drug therapy than a younger adult.
   c. ensure that the patient receives larger initial doses of antihypertensive drugs because of impaired absorption.
   d. use careful technique in assessing the BP of the patient because of the possible presence of an auscultatory gap.
7. A patient with newly diagnosed hypertension has a blood pressure of 158/98 after 12 months of exercise and diet modifications. The nurse advises the patient that
   a. medication may be required because the BP is still not within the normal range.
   b. continued monitoring of the BP every 3 to 6 months is all that will be necessary for treatment.
   c. since lifestyle modifications were not effective they do not need to be continued and drugs will be used.
   d. he will have to make more vigorous changes in his lifestyle if he wants to stay off medication for his hypertension.
8. A patient is admitted to the hospital in hypertensive crisis. The nurse recognizes that the hypertensive urgency differs from hypertensive emergency in that
   a. the BP is always higher in a hypertensive emergency.
   b. hypertensive emergencies are associated with evidence of target organ damage.
   c. hypertensive urgency is treated with rest and tranquilizers to lower the BP.
   d. hypertensive emergencies require intraarterial catheter measurement of the BP.

References

1. Vaughan DE: The renin-angiotensin system and fibrinolysis, *Am J Cardiol* 79:12, 1997.
2. American Heart Association: *Heart stroke facts,* Dallas, 1996.
3. Sixth Report of the Joint National Committee on Detection, Evaluation, and Treatment of High Blood Pressure (JNC-VI), *Arch Intern Med* 157:2413, 1997.
4. 1993 guidelines for the management of mild hypertension: memorandum from a World Health Organization/International Society of Hypertension meeting, *J Hypertens* 11:905, 1993.
5. Oparil S, McCarron DA: High blood pressure. In Dale DC, Federman DD, editors: *Scientific American medicine,* New York, 1997, Scientific American.
6. Kaplan NM: Systemic hypertension: mechanisms and diagnosis. In Braunwald E, editor: *Heart disease: a textbook of cardiovascular medicine,* ed 5, Philadelphia, 1997, Saunders.
7. Jorde LB, Carey JC, White RL: *Medical genetics,* ed 2, St Louis, 1999, Mosby.
8. Cody RJ: The integrated effects of angiotensin II, *Am J Cardiol* 79:9, 1997.
9. Reaven GM, Lithell H, Lansberg L: Hypertension and associated metabolic abnormalities—the role of insulin resistance and the sympathoadrenal system, *N Engl J Med* 334:374, 1996.
10. Vanhouette PM: Endothelial dysfunction in hypertension, *J Hypertens* 14(suppl):S83, 1996.
11. SHEP Cooperative Research Group: prevention of stroke by antihypertensive drug treatment in older persons with isolated systolic hypertension, *JAMA* 265:3255, 1991.
12. Dahlof B and others: Morbidity and mortality in the Swedish Trial in old patients with hypertension (STOP-hypertension), *Lancet* 338:1281, 1991.
13. Kochar MS: Hypertension in elderly patients: the special concerns in this growing population, *Postgrad Med* 91: 393, 1992.
14. Ross R: Mechanisms of atherosclerosis: a perspective for the 1990s, *Nature* 362:801, 1993.
15. Ogilvie RI and others: Report of the Canadian Hypertension Society Consensus Conference: 3. Pharmacologic treatment of essential hypertension, *Can Med Assoc J* 149:875. 1993.
16. McCarron DA and others: Nutritional management of cardiovascular risk factors: a randomized clinical trial, *Arch Intern Med* 157:169, 1997.
17. Appel LJ and others: The effect of dietary patterns on blood pressure: results from the Dietary Approaches to Stop Hypertension (DASH) clinical trial, *N Engl J Med* 336:1117, 1997.
18. NIH Consensus Development Panel on Physical Activity and Cardiovascular Health: Physical activity and cardiovascular health, *JAMA* 276:241, 1996.
19. Johnston DW: Stress management in the treatment of mild primary hypertension, *Hypertension* 17:III-63, 1991.
20. Montfrans G and others: Relaxation therapy and continuous ambulatory blood pressure in mild hypertension: a controlled study, *BMJ* 310:1368, 1990.
21. The Trials of Hypertension Prevention Collaborative Research Group: The effects of nonpharmacologic interventions on blood pressure of persons with high normal levels: results of the trials of hypertension prevention, phase 1, *JAMA* 267:1213, 1992.

22. National High Blood Pressure Education Program Working Group Report on Primary Prevention of Hypertension, *Arch Intern Med* 153:186, 1993.
23. Eaton LE, Buck EA, Catanzaro JE: The nurse's role in facilitating compliance in clients with hypertension, *Medsurg Nurs* 5:339, 1996.

Resources

High Blood Pressure Information Center
National Heart, Lung and Blood Institute
4733 Bethesda Avenue, Suite 530
Bethesda, MD 20814
301-951-3260
http://www.nhlbi.nih.gov/nhlbi/nhlbi.htm

Hypertension Information Center
http://pharminfo.com/disease/cardio/HT_info.html

***For additional Internet resources, see the website for this book at* www.mosby.com/MERLIN/medsurg_lewis**

REMEMBER to check out your companion CD-ROM

32 NURSING MANAGEMENT Coronary Artery Disease

Linda Griego Martinez & Mary Ann House-Fancher

www.mosby.com/MERLIN/medsurg_lewis

LEARNING OBJECTIVES

1. Describe the etiology and pathophysiology of coronary artery disease.
2. Explain the nursing role in health promotion related to risk factors for coronary artery disease.
3. Describe the precipitating factors, types, clinical manifestations, and collaborative care, including drug therapy, of stable and unstable angina pectoris.
4. Explain the nursing management of the patient with stable and unstable angina pectoris.
5. Describe the pathophysiology of myocardial infarction from the onset of injury through the healing process.
6. Describe the clinical manifestations, complications, diagnostic study results, and collaborative care of myocardial infarction.
7. Describe the nursing management of the patient following a myocardial infarction.
8. Identify the emotional and behavioral reactions to myocardial infarction.
9. Describe the precipitating factors, types, clinical presentation, and collaborative care of the patient with or at risk for sudden cardiac death.

CORONARY ARTERY DISEASE

Coronary artery disease (CAD) is a type of blood vessel disorder that is included in the general category of atherosclerosis. The term *atherosclerosis* is derived from two Greek words: *athere,* meaning "fatty mush," and *skleros,* meaning "hard." This word combination indicates that atherosclerosis begins as soft deposits of fat that harden with age. Atherosclerosis is often referred to as "hardening of the arteries." Although this condition can occur in any artery in the body, the atheromas (fatty deposits) have a preference for the coronary arteries. Arteriosclerotic heart disease (ASHD), cardiovascular heart disease (CVHD), ischemic heart disease (IHD), coronary heart disease (CHD), and CAD are synonymous terms used to describe this disease process. Other terms used to describe the disease mechanisms involved in CAD are plaque formation, atheromatous deposits, and coronary occlusions.

Significance

Cardiovascular diseases are the major cause of death in the United States (Fig. 32-1). The American Heart Association (AHA) reports that almost 490,000 persons die each year of heart attacks. Although the death rate has decreased by 28.7% between 1985 and 1995, heart attacks, or myocardial infarctions (MIs), are still the leading cause of all cardiovascular disease deaths and deaths in general. An estimated 58,200,000 persons have one or more types of cardiovascular disease.[1,2] The estimated prevalence of CAD by age is presented in Fig. 32-2.

Reviewed by Deborah K. Drummonds, RN, MN, CCRN, CEN, Assistant Professor, Adult and Gerontological Health, Georgia College and State University School of Health Science, Milledgeville, Ga.; and Deborah L. Roush, RN, MSN, Assistant Professor, College of Nursing, Valdosta State University, Valdosta, Ga.

Etiology and Pathophysiology

Atherosclerosis is the major cause of CAD. It is characterized by a focal deposit of cholesterol and lipids, primarily within the intimal wall of the artery. The genesis of plaque formation is the result of complex interactions between the components of the blood and the elements forming the vascular wall.[1] The concept of endothelial injury is central to current theories of atherogenesis. Table 32-1 summarizes theories of atherogenesis, with endothelial injury being the leading theory for the cause of atherosclerotic disease.

Intact normal endothelium is nonreactive to platelets and leukocytes as well as coagulation, fibrinolytic, and complement factors. However, the endothelial lining can be altered as a result of chemical injuries, such as hyperlipidemia (nondenuding), or high-shear stress, such as hypertension (denuding). With either type of endothelial alteration, platelets are activated, and they release a growth factor that stimulates smooth muscle proliferation. The smooth muscle cell proliferation entraps lipids, which are calcified over time and form an irritant to the endothelium on which platelets adhere and aggregate. Thrombin is generated, and fibrin formation and thrombi occur (Fig. 32-3). Endothelial replication is normally slow in adults, but in the presence of hypertension and hyperlipidemia, increased cell turnover leads to transient repeated denuding of the endothelium.

Development Stages. CAD takes many years to develop. When it becomes symptomatic, the disease process is usually well advanced. The stages of development in atherosclerosis are (1) fatty streak, (2) raised fibrous plaque resulting from smooth muscle cell proliferation, and (3) complicated lesion (Fig. 32-4).

Fatty streak. Fatty streaks, the earliest lesions of atherosclerosis, are characterized by lipid-filled smooth muscle cells.[2] As streaks of fat develop within the smooth muscle cells, a yellow

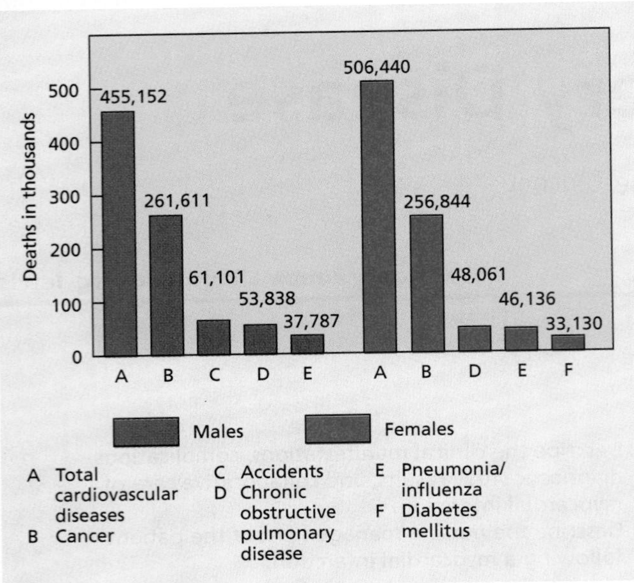

Fig. 32-1 Leading causes of death for all males and females.

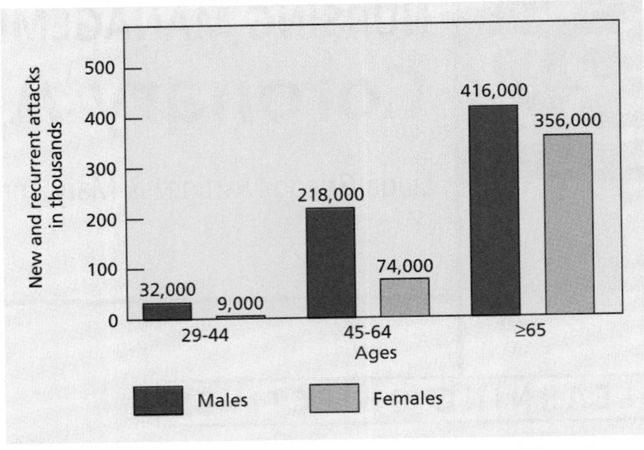

Fig. 32-2 Estimated annual number of Americans experiencing heart attack by age and sex.

tinge appears. Fatty streaks are usually observed in the coronary arteries by age 15 and involve an increasing amount of surface area as the patient ages. It is generally believed that they are reversible.

Raised fibrous plaque. The raised fibrous plaque stage is the beginning of progressive changes in the arterial wall. These changes appear in the coronary arteries by the age of 30 and increase with age. The arterial wall changes are initiated by chronic endothelial injury that results from many factors, including elevated blood pressure (BP), high blood cholesterol, heredity, carbon monoxide produced by smoking, immune reactions, and possibly toxic substances within the blood.

Normally the endothelium repairs itself immediately, but in the person with CAD the endothelium is *not* rapidly replaced, allowing low-density lipoproteins and growth factors from platelets to stimulate smooth muscle proliferation and thickening of the arterial wall. Once endothelial injury has occurred, lipoproteins (the carrier substances within the bloodstream) transport cholesterol and other lipids into the arterial intima (see Fig. 32-4). Lipids may cause smooth muscle damage and contribute to plaque thickening and instability.[2] As these lipids and other substances pass through the vessels, they adhere to the roughened, damaged wall, thereby causing the lesion buildup or structural abnormality. Collagen tissue, elastic fibers, and smooth muscle cells filled with fat cover the lesion. The fibrous plaque appears grayish or whitish. These plaques can form on one portion of the artery or in a circular fashion involving the entire lumen. The borders can be smooth or irregular with rough, jagged edges.[2]

Platelets also play a part in the hypertrophy of smooth muscle cells. Once the artery's inner wall has become damaged, platelets may accumulate in large numbers, leading to a thrombus. The thrombus may adhere to the wall of the artery, leading to narrowing or total occlusion of the artery.

Complicated lesion. The final stage in the development of the atherosclerotic lesion is the most dangerous. The plaque consists of a core of lipid materials (mainly cholesterol) within an area of dead tissue. With the incorporation of lipids, thrombi, damaged tissue, and accumulation of calcium, the growing lesion becomes complex. As the lesion continues to grow and become complex, necrotic tissue that is dark and hardened appears within the arteries, causing rigidity and hardening. This complicated lesion may totally or partially occlude the artery.

Collateral Circulation. Normally some arterial branching, termed *collateral circulation,* exists within the coronary circulation. The growth of collateral circulation is attributed to two factors: (1) the inherited predisposition to develop new blood vessels and (2) the presence of chronic ischemia. When an atherosclerotic plaque occludes the normal flow of blood through a coronary artery and ischemia is chronic, increased collateral circulation develops (Fig. 32-5). When occlusion of the coronary arteries occurs slowly over a long period, there is a greater chance of adequate collateral circulation developing, and the myocardium may still receive an adequate amount of oxygen. However, with rapid-onset CAD or coronary spasm, the time is inadequate for collateral development, and a diminished arterial flow results in a more severe ischemia or infarction. Clinically the younger person is frequently seen to have a more severe myocardial infarction as a result of inadequate collateral formation.

Risk Factors for Coronary Artery Disease

Risk factors are characteristics or conditions that are statistically associated with a high incidence of a disease. Many risk factors have been associated with CAD. These associations are derived from studies of large populations. Risk factors in different populations may vary. For example, major risk factors for CAD in the United States, such as high serum cholesterol and hypertension, are less prevalent in Japanese and Puerto Rican populations.[3]

Risk factors can be categorized as unmodifiable and modifiable (Table 32-2). Unmodifiable risk factors are age, gender, race, and genetic inheritance. Modifiable risk factors include elevated serum lipids, hypertension, smoking, obesity, physical inactivity, and stress in daily living. Although control of

Table **32-1** Theories of Atherogenesis

Endothelial Injury
Endothelium is "injured" by hyperlipidemia, hypertension, or other chemical irritants. Factors are released into the subendothelium and induce the migration of smooth muscle cells into the intima. Smooth muscle cells initiate synthesis of collagen, elastic fiber proteins, and proteoglycans (a substance that tends to provide a nonthrombogenic surface). Intracellular and extracellular lipids begin to accumulate, as well as platelets and other clotting factors, and a lesion-associated superimposed thrombus is formed.

Lipid Infiltration
Lipids from the circulation enter the endothelium and accumulate in smooth muscle in response to mechanical or inflammatory trauma. Lipoproteins become trapped, and damage occurs. Endothelial permeability is altered.

Aging
Atherosclerotic changes occur in everyone and become more evident as aging progresses.

Thrombogenic
Red blood cells, platelets, and lipids accumulate along the intima of arteries. Microthrombi form. Platelets aggregate, releasing substances that alter endothelial permeability. The thrombus extends and reactivates the cycle.

Vascular Dynamics
Mechanical factors (e.g., hypertension) increase intraluminal pressure, which leads to altered membrane permeability, resulting in increased lipid infiltration.

Capillary Hemorrhage
Lipids accumulate in plaques as a result of capillary hemorrhage.

Lipid Metabolic
Low-density lipoproteins migrate into the arterial wall, accumulating in the intimal and medial layers of the artery. Cholesterol is deposited by the low-density lipoproteins.

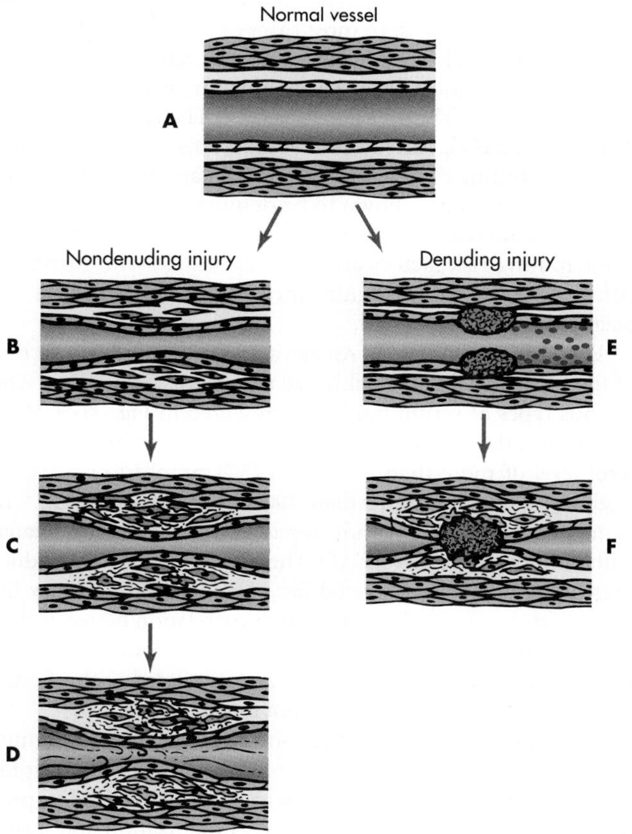

Fig. 32-3 Response to endothelial injury. **A,** Normal vessel, endothelium intact. **B,** Nondenuding injury (e.g., hyperlipidemia) with smooth muscle proliferation. **C,** Addition of collagen and fibroelastic tissues that narrow lumen. **D,** Narrowed lumen with calcification and irregular blood flow. **E,** Denuding injury with platelet adherence and aggregation or frank clot formation. **F,** Eventual thrombosis leading to infarction.

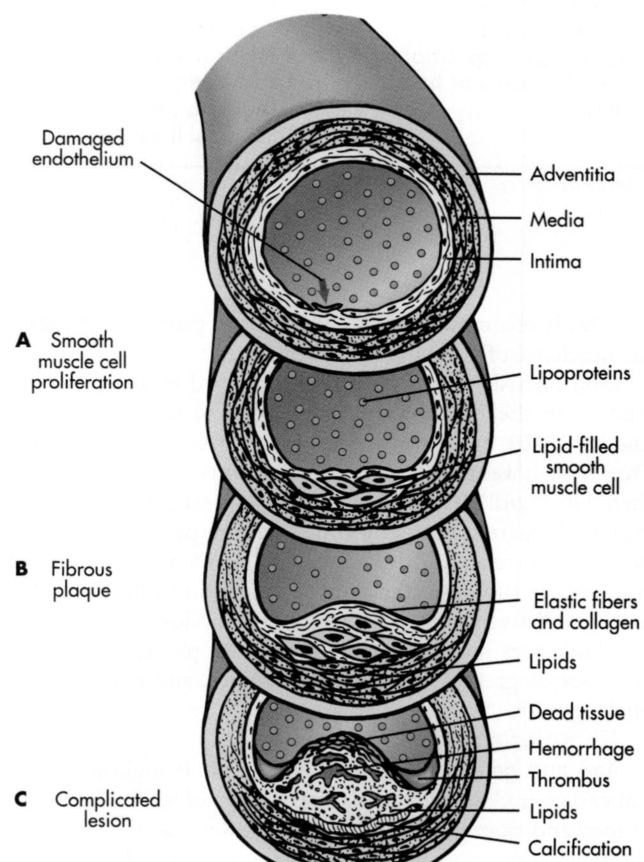

Fig. 32-4 The stages of development in the progression of atherosclerosis include **A,** smooth muscle cell proliferation, which creates **B,** a raised fibrous plaque and **C,** a complicated lesion.

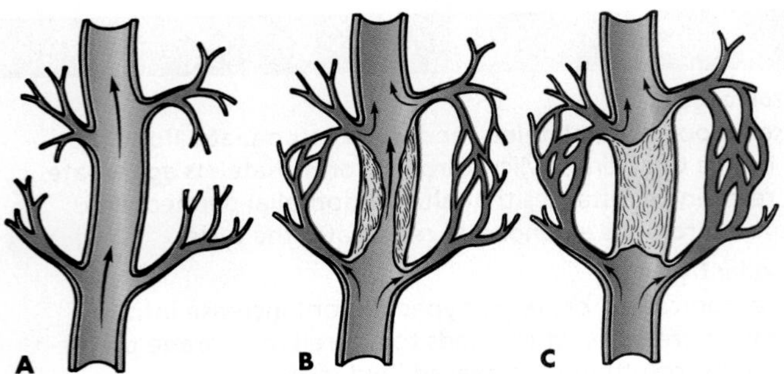

Fig. 32-5 Vessel occlusion with collateral circulation. **A,** Open, functioning coronary artery. **B,** Partial coronary artery closure with collateral circulation being established. **C,** Total coronary artery occlusion with collateral circulation bypassing the occlusion to supply the myocardium.

Table 32-2 Risk Factors for Coronary Artery Disease

Unmodifiable	Modifiable
Age	**Major**
Gender (men > women until 60 yr of age)	Elevated serum lipids
Race (African-Americans < Caucasians)	Hypertension
Genetic predisposition and family history of heart disease	Cigarette smoking
	Obesity
	Physical inactivity
	Contributing
	Diabetes mellitus*
	Stressful lifestyle

*May be hereditary.

CULTURAL & ETHNIC CONSIDERATIONS

Coronary Artery Disease

- Caucasian, middle-aged men have the highest incidence of coronary artery disease.
- African-Americans have an early age of onset of coronary artery disease.
- African-American women have a higher incidence of coronary artery disease than Caucasian women.
- African-Americans have more severe coronary artery disease than Caucasians.
- Native-Americans less than 35 years of age have heart disease mortality rates twice as high as other Americans.
- Hispanics have lower death rates from heart disease than non-Hispanics.
- Major modifiable cardiovascular risk factors for Native-Americans are obesity and diabetes mellitus.

diabetes is recommended, it has not been proven to decrease the incidence of CAD in the United States.

Data on risk factors have been obtained in several major studies. In the Framingham study (one of the most widely known), 5209 men and women were observed for 20 years. Over time, it was noted that elevated serum cholesterol (greater than 240 mg/dl), elevated systolic BP (greater than 160 mm Hg), and cigarette smoking (one or more packs a day) were positively correlated with an increased incidence of CAD. The younger the subject at the time of induction to the study, the more predictive were the values. Other implicated risk factors and indicators included diabetes mellitus, physical inactivity, electrocardiographic (ECG) abnormalities, and reduced lung vital capacity.

Unmodifiable Risk Factors

Age and gender. The incidence of MI is highest for the Caucasian, middle-aged man. After the age of 65, the incidence in men and women equalizes, although there is early evidence suggesting that more women are being seen with CAD earlier because of increased stress, increased cigarette smoking, presence of hypertension, and use of birth control pills.

Family history and heredity. Genetic predisposition is an important factor in the occurrence of CAD, although the exact mechanism of inheritance is not fully understood. Some congenital defects in coronary artery walls predispose the person to the formation of plaques. Familial hyperlipoproteinemia, an autosomal dominant trait, has been strongly associated with CAD at early ages. In most cases of angina or MI, the patient can name a close family member who has died either suddenly of an unknown cause or of a documented heart attack.

Modifiable Major Risk Factors. The American Heart Association has classified the modifiable risk factors as major and contributing risk factors. Major risk factors are those that medical research has shown to be definitely associated with a significant increase in the risk of the development of CAD. Contributing risk factors are those associated with increased risk of CAD, but their significance and prevalence have not been precisely determined.[3]

Elevated serum lipids. An elevated serum lipid level is one of the four most firmly established risk factors for CAD.[2-5] The various types of serum lipids are presented in Fig. 32-6. More specifically, the risk of CAD is associated with a serum cholesterol level of more than 200 mg/dl (5.2 mmol/L) or a fasting triglyceride level of more than 200 mg/dl (1.7 mmol/L).[5] In women elevated triglyceride levels are especially associated with an increased risk of CAD. The liver is capable of producing cholesterol from saturated fats, even when the dietary intake of fats is severely limited. A high correlation between cholesterol and triglyceride levels has been found. Elevated triglyceride and cholesterol levels are correlated with obesity, physical inactivity, and high alcohol intake.

For lipids to be used and transported by the body, they must become soluble in blood by combining with proteins. Lipids combine with protein to form macromolecules called lipoproteins. Lipoproteins are vehicles for fat mobilization and transport. The different types of lipoprotein vary in composition and are classified as high-density lipoproteins (HDLs), low-density lipoproteins (LDLs), and very-low-density lipoproteins (VLDLs) (see Fig. 32-6).

HDLs contain more protein by weight and less lipid than any other lipoprotein. HDLs carry lipids away from arteries and to the liver for metabolism (Fig. 32-7). Therefore high serum HDL

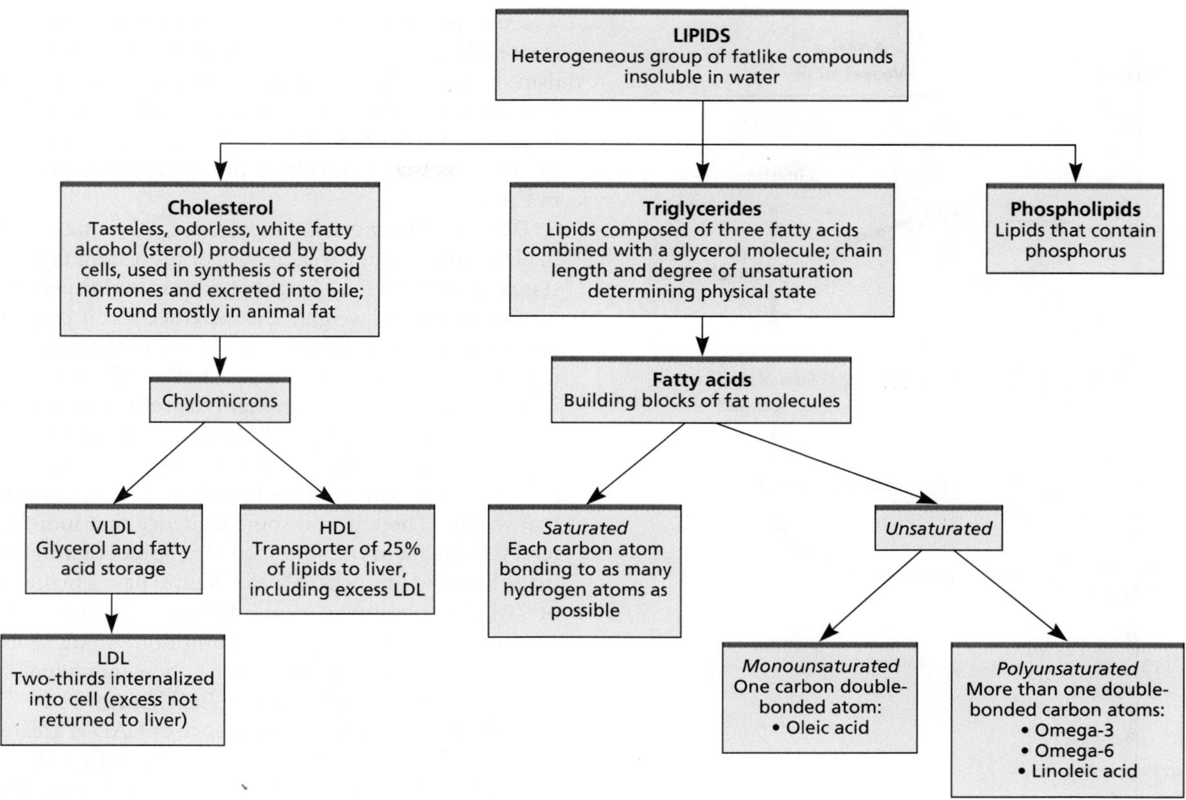

Fig. 32-6 Types of serum lipids. *HDL,* high-density lipoprotein; *LDL,* low-density lipoprotein; *VLDL,* very-low-density lipoprotein.

levels are desirable. This process of HDL transport prevents lipid accumulation within the arterial walls. The higher the HDL levels in the blood, the lower the risk of CAD. HDL levels are generally higher in women than in men and are increased by physical activity and estrogen. The person who has had an MI has lower concentrations of HDL than matched controls. In general, HDL levels are high in children and women, decrease with age, and are low in persons with CAD. Current research on drug and dietary therapy is concentrating on ways to increase HDL levels.

HDLs are broken down into HDL_2 and HDL_3. HDL_2 seems to protect the arteries from developing atherosclerosis. Exercise significantly raises HDL_2, which helps clear out the fat load from the blood plasma. Premenopausal women have HDL_2 levels approximately three times greater than men. After menopause, their HDL_2 levels quickly approximate those of men.

LDLs contain more cholesterol than any of the other lipoproteins and have an affinity for arterial walls.[6] Elevated LDL levels correlate most closely with an increased incidence of atherosclerosis. Therefore low serum LDL levels are desirable.

VLDLs contain most of the triglycerides. The direct correlation of VLDLs with heart disease is uncertain. High VLDL concentrations may increase the risk of premature atherosclerosis when associated with other factors such as diabetes, hypertension, and cigarette smoking.

Hypertension. The second major risk factor in CAD is hypertension, which is defined as a BP greater than or equal to 140/90 mm Hg. In the Framingham study, a threefold increase in the incidence of CAD was reported for middle-aged men with arterial pressures exceeding 160/95 mm Hg compared with those with BP of 140/90 mm Hg or less.[3] The cause of hypertension in 90% of those affected is unknown, but it is usually controllable with diet or medication.

The stress of a constantly elevated BP increases the rate of atherosclerotic development. This is related to the shearing stress, causing denuding injury of the endothelial lining. Atherosclerosis, in turn, causes narrowed, thickened arterial walls and decreases the distensibility and elasticity of vessels. More force is required to pump blood through diseased arterial vasculature, and this increased force is reflected in a higher BP. This increased workload is also manifested by left ventricular hypertrophy and a loss of efficiency and stroke volume with each contraction. Salt intake is positively correlated with elevated BP because of fluid retention, adding volume and increasing systemic vascular resistance (SVR) to the cardiac workload.

Smoking. A third major risk factor in CAD is cigarette smoking. The risk of developing CAD is two to six times higher in cigarette smokers than in nonsmokers. Two large studies have shown strong evidence that chronic exposure to environmental tobacco smoke also increases the risk of CAD.[7,8] Risk is proportional to the number of cigarettes smoked. Changing to lower-nicotine or filtered cigarettes does not affect risk. Cessation of smoking has been shown to reduce the risk to nonsmoker levels within 3 years.[5] Pipe and cigar smokers have not been found to have an increased risk of CAD.

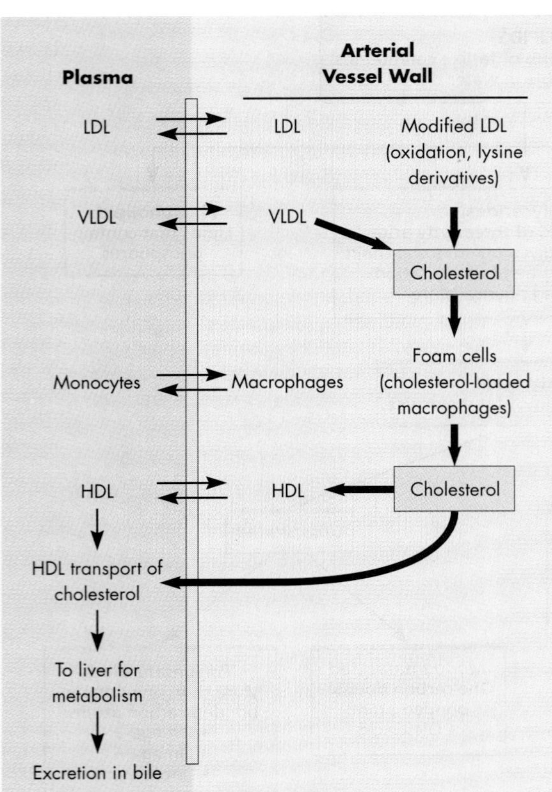

Fig. 32-7 Specific types of plasma lipoproteins (*LDL* and *VLDL*) deliver cholesterol to cells of the blood vessel wall, mostly to macrophages that become cholesterol foam cells. These are predominant early features of atherosclerotic lesions. *HDL* is an important cholesterol-transporting carrier, delivering cholesterol to the liver to be excreted in the bile.

Nicotine in cigarette smoke causes catecholamine (epinephrine, norepinephrine) release. These hormones cause an increased heart rate (HR), peripheral vasoconstriction, and increased BP. These changes increase the cardiac workload, necessitating greater myocardial oxygen consumption.

Carbon monoxide, a by-product of combustion, affects the oxygen-carrying capacity of hemoglobin by reducing the sites available for oxygen transport. Thus the effects of an increased cardiac workload, combined with the oxygen-depleting effect of carbon monoxide from smoking, significantly decrease the oxygen available to the myocardium. There is also some indication that carbon monoxide may be a chemical irritant as well, thus causing nondenuding injury to the endothelium.

Physical inactivity. Physical inactivity is a fourth major modifiable risk factor. Physical inactivity implies a lack of adequate physical exercise on a regular basis. Some practitioners define regular physical exercise as exercise that occurs at least three times a week for at least 30 minutes, causing perspiration and an increase in HR by 30 to 50 beats per minute.

The mechanism by which physical inactivity predisposes to CAD is still unknown. Physically active people have increased HDL levels, and exercise enhances fibrinolytic activity, thus reducing the risk of clot formation. It is also believed that exercise encourages the development of collateral circulation.

Exercise training for those who are physically inactive decreases the risk of CAD through more efficient lipid metabolism, increased HDL_2 production, and more efficient oxygen extraction from the working muscle groups, thereby decreasing the cardiac workload. It may be observed that physically active persons are seldom obese, thus eliminating two risk factors in CAD.[5]

Obesity. The mortality rate from CAD is statistically higher in obese (defined as a weight 30% or more than that considered standard for a person's height and body build) persons than in persons of normal weight. The increased risk is proportional to the degree of obesity. However, obesity in the absence of other risk factors probably subjects a person to only a modest increase in risk. Obese persons are thought to produce increased levels of LDL, which are strongly implicated in atherosclerosis. Obesity is often associated with hypertension, which is three times more likely to develop in an obese person than in a person with normal weight. There is also some evidence that individuals who tend to store fat in the abdomen (an "apple" figure) rather than in the hips and buttocks (a "pear" figure) have a higher incidence of CAD.[5] As obesity increases, the heart size grows, causing increased myocardial oxygen consumption. In addition, there is an increase in type 2 diabetes in the obese individual.

Modifiable Contributing Risk Factors

Diabetes mellitus. The incidence of CAD is greater among persons who have diabetes, even those with well-controlled blood glucose levels, than the general population. The patient with diabetes manifests CAD not only more frequently but also at an earlier age. There is no age difference between diabetic men and women for the onset of manifestations of CAD. Diabetes virtually eliminates the lower incidence of CAD in women. Latent diabetes is frequently diagnosed at the time of infarction. Because the person with diabetes has an increased tendency toward connective tissue degeneration, it is thought that this condition may account for the tendency toward atheroma development seen in the diabetic population. Diabetic patients also have alterations in lipid metabolism and tend to have high cholesterol and triglyceride levels.[5]

Stress and behavior patterns. Several behavior patterns have been correlated with CAD. However, the study of these behaviors remains controversial and complex. The Framingham study provided evidence that certain behaviors and lifestyles are conducive to the development of CAD.[4,5,9,10] Type A and type B behaviors were described by Friedman and Rosenman in the 1960s and were further elaborated in the 1970s by Jenkins and Zyzanski.[9] Type A behaviors include perfectionism and a hard-working, driving personality. The type A person suppresses anger and hostility, has a sense of time urgency, is impatient, and creates stress and tension, often when a situation does not warrant it (Table 32-3). This person is more prone to heart attacks than a type B person, who is more easygoing, takes upsets in stride, knows personal limitations, takes time to relax, is not an overachiever, and is able to keep priorities in perspective. Although not all characteristics are present in one person all the time, people tend to be either type A or type B. Meta-analysis of the type A personality studies done in the 1980s has shown that the studies that demonstrated a positive correlation between type A personality and CAD were equal in number to the studies that failed to show a correlation with CAD.[9]

Table 32-3 Type A Personality Characteristics

Perfectionistic
Competitive
Aggressive
Constantly time-oriented
Has hurry sickness
Never says "no"
Compulsive
Impatient
Always tense
Unduly irritable
Obsessed with number of sales made, articles written, patients seen, forms completed
Holds in feelings
Never has leisure time
Rarely takes a relaxing vacation or day off

Source: Friedman M, Roseman RH: *Type A behavior and your heart,* Greenwich, Conn, 1974, Fawcett.

Studies now are focusing on specific components of the type A personality. Specifically, hostility and anger have both been linked with CAD, especially in men.[5,9,10] Researchers studying spousal combinations of type A husbands married to highly educated wives have found a positive correlation with this spousal combination and the men's risk for CAD.[11] Continued research is needed in the field of personality, behavior, and risk for CAD.

Stress has also been correlated with the development of CAD. Sympathetic nervous system (SNS) stimulation and its effect on the heart is generally considered to be the physiologic mechanism by which stress predisposes to the development of CAD. SNS stimulation causes an increased release of epinephrine and norepinephrine. This stimulation influences the heart by increasing the HR and intensifying the force of myocardial contraction. Therefore the demand for oxygen consumption greatly increases. Also, stress-induced mechanisms can cause elevated lipid levels and alterations in blood coagulation, which can lead to increased atherogenesis.[12]

Homocysteine. High blood levels of homocysteine have been linked to an increased risk for CAD and other cardiovascular diseases.[13] Homocysteine, a sulfur-containing amino acid, is produced by the breakdown of the essential amino acid methionine, which is found in dietary protein.

High homocysteine levels possibly contribute to atherosclerosis by (1) damaging the inner lining of blood vessels, (2) promoting plaque buildup, and (3) altering the clotting mechanism to make clots more likely to occur.

Research is ongoing to determine if a decline in homocysteine can reduce the risk of heart disease. Currently a general recommendation for a screening test has not yet been developed. B-complex vitamins—B_6, B_{12}, and folic acid—have been shown to work together to lower blood levels of homocysteine.

Health Promotion. The appropriate management of risk factors in CAD may prevent, modify, or retard the progression of the disease. In the United States during the past 20 to 30 years there has been a gradual and persistent decline in coronary deaths. The decline can be attributed to the efforts of consumers to become generally healthier and individual initiatives to alter unhealthy and hazardous lifestyles. Emphasis on prevention and early treatment of heart disease must be ongoing.

Identification of high risk persons. In both the acute care setting and the community, the nurse should identify the person at risk for CAD. Risk screening involves obtaining personal and family health histories. The patient should be questioned about a family history of heart disease in parents, grandparents, or siblings. The presence of any cardiovascular symptoms should be noted. Environmental factors, such as eating habits, type of diet, and level of exercise, are assessed to elicit lifestyle patterns. A psychosocial history is included to determine smoking habits, alcohol ingestion, type A behaviors, recent life-stressing events, sleeping habits, and the presence of anxiety or depression. The place of work and the type of work can provide important information on the kind of activity performed; exposure to pollutants, allergens, or noxious chemicals; and the degree of emotional stress associated with employment.

The nurse should identify the patient's attitudes and beliefs about health and illness. This information can give some indication of how disease and lifestyle changes may affect the patient and can reveal possible misconceptions about heart disease. Knowledge of the patient's educational background is frequently helpful in deciding at what level to begin teaching. If the patient is taking medications, it is important to know what they are, when they are taken, and what the patient's attitude is regarding the taking of medications.

Management of high risk persons. Once a high risk person is identified, preventive measures can be taken. Risk factors such as age, gender, and genetic inheritance cannot be modified. However, the person with any of these risk factors can modify the risk of CAD by controlling or changing the additive effects of modifiable risk factors. For example, a young man with a family history of heart disease can decrease the risk of an MI by maintaining an ideal weight, getting adequate physical exercise, reducing intake of saturated fats, and not smoking.

The person who has modifiable risk factors should be encouraged and motivated to make changes in lifestyle to reduce the risk of heart disease. The nurse can play a major role in teaching health-promoting behaviors to the person at risk for CAD (Table 32-4). For highly motivated persons, knowing how to reduce this risk may be the only information needed to get them to make changes.

For the person who is less motivated to assume responsibility for health, the idea of risk factor reduction may be so remote that the person is unable to perceive a threat of CAD in his or her life. Especially in the absence of symptoms, few persons desire to make lifestyle changes. The nurse should first assist this person in clarifying personal values. Then by explaining the risk factors and having the person identify the personal vulnerability to various risks, the nurse may help the person recognize the susceptibility to CAD. The nurse may also help the person set realistic goals and allow the person to choose which risk factor to change first. Some persons are reluctant to change until they begin to manifest overt symptoms or actually suffer an infarction. Others, having suffered a heart attack, may find the idea of changing lifelong habits totally unacceptable. The nurse must be able to identify such attitudes and respect them as human rights.

PATIENT TEACHING GUIDE

Table 32-4 Behaviors to Decrease Risk Factors for Coronary Artery Disease

Risk Factor	Health-Promoting Behaviors
Hypertension	▪ Have regular BP checkups ▪ Take prescribed medications for BP control ▪ Reduce salt intake ▪ Stop smoking ▪ Control or reduce weight ▪ Exercise regularly
Elevated serum lipids	▪ Reduce animal (saturated) fat intake ▪ Reduce total fat intake ▪ Adjust total caloric intake to achieve and maintain ideal body weight ▪ Engage in regular exercise program ▪ Increase amount of complex carbohydrates and vegetable proteins in diet
Smoking	▪ Enroll in structured program to stop smoking if support system is needed ▪ Change daily routines associated with smoking to reduce desire to smoke ▪ Substitute other activities for smoking ▪ Ask family members to support efforts to stop smoking
Physical inactivity	▪ Develop and maintain routine for physical activity that is done at least three times a week ▪ Increase activities to a fitness level
Stressful lifestyle	▪ Increase awareness of behaviors that are detrimental to health ▪ Alter patterns that are conducive to stress and rushing (e.g., get up 30 min earlier so breakfast is not eaten on way to work; take 20 min/day to meditate) ▪ Set realistic goals for self ▪ Reassess priorities in light of health needs ▪ Learn to cope with unavoidable stress ▪ Avoid excessive and prolonged stress ▪ Plan time for adequate rest and sleep
Obesity	▪ Change eating patterns and habits ▪ Reduce caloric intake ▪ Exercise regularly to increase caloric expenditure ▪ Avoid fad and crash diets, which are not effective in the long run ▪ Avoid large, heavy meals
Diabetes mellitus*	▪ Follow the recommended diet ▪ Reduce weight and control diet ▪ Monitor blood glucose levels regularly

*See Chapter 46 for additional health-promoting behaviors.

Physical fitness. The last two decades have seen a surge of interest in attaining and maintaining health. Physical fitness has become a field of major importance. Communities are developing exercise programs for persons of all ages and with all health needs, ranging from aerobic exercise classes to cardiac walking-jogging programs. Local YMCAs often sponsor exercise classes, jogging courses, bicycling courses, and related offerings. Many shopping malls open their doors in the early morning to allow people to walk indoors. The American Heart Association takes pride in its annual "Heart Walk," as well as other events dramatizing the need for physical activity to promote health. Many large corporations provide gymnasiums where their employees can exercise. For many people, running may be inadvisable; these people should be encouraged to pursue walking, swimming, or whatever exercise will accommodate their individual physical abilities.

Health education in schools. The recent awareness of the body and physical health is also seen in school systems. The school nurse has an important role in teaching good health practices. Besides teaching physical fitness topics, the school nurse can inform students on how the body functions and responds to daily living. Lifestyle habits can be positively influenced at early ages to decrease the need for drastic changes later in life that confront the students' parents. The school nurse should take advantage of the social climate that promotes health and health practices and find innovative ways to present these values to a receptive, youthful audience before the habits of that audience become inflexible. Health awareness programs have been initiated as early as preschool to try to establish health patterns for life. Follow-up on the effectiveness of early childhood health education will not yield data on cardiac risk for many years to come, yet the energy and effort to change lifestyle patterns cannot be left until adulthood, when habits are set. The nurse can provide valuable consultation to schools and the educational process at all levels. In many areas of the country, school nurses have several schools to oversee, making it difficult to do classes. The American Heart Association has established school programs such as "Heart Power," which provides the teaching materials for teachers to incorporate into their curriculum. Volunteers from the association are also available to help teachers educate children in their schools about healthy habits for better cardiac health.

Nutritional Therapy. The patient with elevated serum cholesterol and triglyceride levels should first achieve a normal weight, if overweight. Then the patient should be maintained on a diet that emphasizes a decreased intake of saturated fat and cholesterol, such as the step 1 diet recommended by the American Heart Association.[6] Red meats, eggs, and milk products are major sources of saturated fat and cholesterol. If the serum triglyceride level is elevated, alcohol intake and simple sugars should be reduced or eliminated. If within 6 months there is no trend toward lower blood cholesterol, the patient should be placed on the step 2 diet of the American Heart Association, which further restricts intake of saturated fats and cholesterol (Table 32-5).[6]

The average reduction in total serum cholesterol levels with diet is 10% to 15%.[6] The highly motivated individual who adheres stringently to a low-fat diet may reduce total cholesterol more dramatically. Several studies have demonstrated regression in coronary atherosclerosis and reduction in coronary events by lifestyle changes, including a low-saturated-fat diet, smoking cessation, and increase in physical activity.[5,6,14] Many of these studies also included drug therapy as well.[6,14] These studies demonstrate the importance of lowering cholesterol in the individual at risk for CAD.

Drug Therapy. The person with serum cholesterol levels of more than 200 mg/dl (5.2 mmol/L) is at high risk for CAD and should be treated. Treatment usually begins with dietary caloric restriction, decreased dietary fat content, lower cholesterol intake, and exercise instruction. Serum cholesterol levels are reassessed after 6 months of diet therapy. If they remain elevated, drug therapy may be started (Table 32-6). Various drugs are available to treat hyperlipidemia[15] (Table 32-7).

Drugs that increase lipoprotein removal. The major route of elimination of cholesterol is via conversion to bile acids in the liver. Two bile acid–sequestering agents are currently available. These resins primarily lower LDL cholesterol and also cause an increase in HDL. The resins are nonabsorbable compounds that interfere with the enterohepatic circulation of bile acids. There is increased conversion of cholesterol to bile acids and decreased hepatic cholesterol content.

The two resins that are available are cholestyramine (Questran) and colestipol (Colestid). A preparation of cholestyramine (Colybar) containing 4 g of cholestyramine in a bar form is also available. Administration of these drugs can be associated with complaints related to palatability and with a variety of upper and lower gastrointestinal (GI) symptoms, including constipation, abdominal pain, belching, heartburn, and nausea. The resins have been known to interfere with absorption of other drugs, such as warfarin, thiazides, thyroid hormones, and β-adrenergic blockers. Separating the time of administration of the resins from that of other drugs may decrease this adverse effect.

Drugs that restrict lipoprotein production. Nicotinic acid (niacin) is a B vitamin that has been used in conjunction with diet therapy. Nicotinic acid is highly effective in lowering cholesterol and triglyceride levels by interfering with their synthesis. Adverse effects of this drug may include severe flushing, pruritus, and GI distress.

Clofibrate (Atromid) is effective primarily in lowering serum triglyceride levels and has some cholesterol-lowering activity as well. It appears to act by decreasing the synthesis of lipids. Adverse effects include malaise, nausea, diarrhea, and occasional increases in liver enzymes.

Gemfibrozil (Lopid) is primarily effective in lowering VLDL levels and triglycerides, and it also increases HDL cholesterol. Although most patients tolerate the drug well, complaints may include GI irritability. Fenofibrate (Tricor) is particularly effective in treating patients with very high serum triglyceride levels. This drug should not be taken with statin medications.

Lovastatin (Mevacor), pravastatin (Pravachol), simvastatin (Zocor), fluvastatin (Lescol), atorvastatin (Lipitor), and cerivastatin (Baycol) are all competitive inhibitors of the biosynthesis of cholesterol. The statin drugs reduce the synthesis of cholesterol in the liver by blocking HMG-CoA reductase, a key enzyme in cholesterol synthesis. Adverse effects of these drugs include rash, gas, stomach cramps or pain, elevated liver enzymes, nausea, constipation or diarrhea, headaches, and opacities of eye lenses. A baseline eye examination may be required before administration of these drugs is started. Liver enzymes must be monitored during therapy.

Drug therapy for hyperlipidemia is likely to be prolonged, perhaps continuing for a lifetime. It is essential that diet modification be used to minimize the need for drug therapy. The patient must fully understand the rationale and goals of treatment, as well as the safety and side effects of drugs.[15]

CLINICAL MANIFESTATIONS OF CORONARY ARTERY DISEASE

There are three major clinical manifestations of CAD: angina pectoris, acute MI, and sudden cardiac death.

ANGINA PECTORIS

Angina pectoris is literally translated as pain (angina) in the chest (pectoris). Myocardial ischemia is expressed symptomatically as angina. More specifically, angina pectoris is transient chest pain caused by myocardial ischemia. It usually lasts for only a few minutes (3 to 5 minutes) and commonly subsides when the precipitating factor (usually exertion) is relieved. Typical exertional angina should not persist longer than 20 minutes after rest and administration of nitroglycerin.

Pathophysiology

Myocardial ischemia develops when the demand for myocardial oxygen exceeds the ability of the coronary arteries to supply it (Table 32-8). The primary reason for insufficient blood flow is narrowing of coronary arteries by atherosclerosis. Although skeletal muscles extract only 20% of available oxygen and maintain a reserve, the myocardium (at rest) extracts 60% to 85% of the available oxygen. If myocardial oxygen needs are not met from this near-maximum extraction, coronary blood flow is increased through vasodilation and increased rate of flow.

In the person with CAD the coronary arteries are unable to dilate to meet increased metabolic needs because they are already chronically dilated beyond the obstructed area. For ischemia secondary to atherosclerosis to occur, the artery is usually 75% or more stenosed. In addition, the diseased heart has difficulty increasing the rate of blood flow. This creates an oxygen deficit. In addition to atherosclerotic stenosis, oxygen deficit is caused by coronary artery spasm and coronary thrombosis. In coronary artery spasm the constriction is transient and reversible and causes either subtotal or total narrowing of

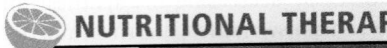

NUTRITIONAL THERAPY

Table 32-5 Coronary Artery Disease

Comparison of Step 1 Low-Fat Diet and Step 2 Low-Fat Diet

Principles of Step 1 Diet

Visible fat (e.g., butter, cream, margarine, salad dressing, cooking oil) is restricted to 1 tsp/meal. Unsaturated vegetable oils should be used.

Only lean meats, skim milk or 1% milk, and no more than three egg yolks per week are used.

Food high in fat content (e.g., avocados, fat, meat, olives, nuts) are avoided.

Cooking methods such as steaming, baking, broiling, grilling, or stir-frying in small amounts of fat are recommended.

Principles of Step 2 Diet

Only leanest cuts of meats allowed.

Organ meats and shrimp are restricted because they are high in cholesterol although low in total fat.

Only one egg yolk per week is used because egg yolk is high in cholesterol. Egg white or egg substitutes may be used as desired.

Vegetable oils are used in cooking and food preparation. Coconut and palm oils are not allowed because of their high content of saturated fats. Choose margarine that contains 2 g or less of saturated fat per tablespoon.

Skim milk is highly recommended. Low-fat yogurt and low-fat cheeses may be used. Low-fat ice milk, frozen yogurt, or sherbet may be used.

Sample Menus

	Step 1			Step 2		
Breakfast 1 fruit 1 starch 3 eggs/wk 1 fat 1 skim milk	½ cup orange juice ¾ cup dry cereal 1 poached egg 1 slice toast with 1 tsp butter or margarine 1 cup skim milk Coffee with sugar	1 banana 1/2 cup oatmeal 1 flour tortilla 1 cup skim milk Coffee with 1 tsp cream	¼ cantaloupe ½ cup corn meal mush 1 scrambled egg 1 slice toast with 1 tsp butter or margarine 1 cup skim milk Coffee with sugar	½ cup orange juice ¾ cup dry cereal Low-cholesterol egg 1 slice toast with 1 tsp special vegetable oil margarine 1 cup skim milk Coffee with sugar	1 banana ½ cup oatmeal 1 corn tortilla with 1 tsp special vegetable oil margarine 1 cup skim milk Coffee with sugar	¼ cantaloupe ½ cup corn meal mush 1 slice toast with 1 tsp special vegetable oil margarine 1 cup skim milk Coffee with sugar
Lunch 2 meat 2 starch 1 vegetable 1 starch 1 fat 1 dessert	2 oz baked chicken Mashed potato Tossed salad with vinegar, lemon juice Bread with 1 tsp margarine or butter Angel food cake Iced tea with sugar and lemon	3 oz lean hamburger Hamburger bun Lettuce, tomato, pickle, 1 tsp mustard Sherbet Carbonated beverage	2 oz baked fish Baked potato Zucchini Bread with 1 tsp butter or margarine Gelatin dessert Lemonade	3 oz baked chicken (skinless) Mashed potato with 1 tsp special vegetable oil margarine Tossed salad with vinegar, vegetable oil Angel food cake Iced tea with sugar and lemon	¾ cup dry cottage cheese with peach slices Saltine crackers Cucumber and tomato slices 1 tsp special vegetable oil Sherbet Carbonated beverage	4 oz baked fish Fried potatoes (cooked with allowed oils) Zucchini Cornbread (made with allowed oils) Gelatin dessert Lemonade

Continued

NUTRITIONAL THERAPY

Table 32-5 Coronary Artery Disease—cont'd

	Step 1			Step 2		
Dinner 2 meat 2 starch 1 vegetable 1 fat 1 fruit 1 skim milk	2 oz lean roast beef Rice Green beans Dinner roll with 1 tsp butter or margarine Canned peach 1 cup skim milk	Green chili stew (made with 2 oz lean beef cubes, potato slices, tomato, chili) 1 flour tortilla Pudding (made from skim milk and egg whites) Fruit punch	2 oz lean pork chop Corn on the cob Okra Bread with 1 tsp margarine or butter Watermelon slice Buttermilk	2 oz lean roast beef Rice with 1 tsp special vegetable oil margarine Green beans Dinner roll with 1 tsp special vegetable oil margarine Canned peach 1 cup skim milk	2 oz green chili stew (made with lean beef cubes, potato slices, tomato, chili) 1 corn tortilla with 1 tsp special vegetable oil margarine Pudding (made from skim milk and egg whites) Fruit punch	3 oz breaded lean pork chop Corn on the cob with 1 tsp special vegetable oil margarine Okra Biscuit (made with allowed oils) Watermelon slice Buttermilk

Table 32-6 Treatment Decisions for High Blood Cholesterol Based on Low-Density Lipoprotein Cholesterol Levels

Patient Category	Initiation Level	LDL Goal
Dietary Therapy		
Without CAD and with fewer than two risk factors	≥160 mg/dl (4.1 mmol/L)	≤160 mg/dl (4.1 mmol/L)
Without CAD and with two or more risk factors	≥130 mg/dl (3.4 mmol/L)	≤130 mg/dl (3.4 mmol/L)
With CAD	>100 mg/dl (2.6 mmol/L)	≤100 mg/dl (2.6 mmol/L)
Drug Treatment		
Without CAD and with fewer than two risk factors	≥190 mg/dl (4.9 mmol/L)	≤130 mg/dl (4.1 mmol/L)
Without CAD and with two or more risk factors	≥160 mg/dl (4.1 mmol/L)	≤130 mg/dl (3.4 mmol/L)
With CAD	≥130 mg/dl (3.4 mmol/L)	≤100 mg/dl (2.6 mmol/L)

From Summary of the Second Report of the National Cholesterol Education Program (NCEP) Expert Panel on Detection, Evaluation, and Treatment of High Cholesterol in Adults (Adult Treatment Panel II), *Circulation* 89:1330, 1996.
CAD, coronary artery disease; *LDL,* low-density lipoprotein.

the coronary artery. The coronary artery spasm is usually associated with an underlying atherosclerotic plaque, although spasms do occur in arteries without significant stenosis. The duration of the spasm determines whether the myocardium will sustain ischemia (not resulting in cell death) or actual infarction (resulting in cell death).

Other factors responsible for a discrepancy between myocardial oxygen needs and oxygen supply include low BP, low blood volume, drugs causing vasoconstriction, valvular disorders, stenosis of the coronary ostia (either congenital or secondary to syphilis), and aortic stenosis. Excessive catecholamine stimulation (e.g., from cocaine intoxication or overdose, chronic congestive heart failure), anemia, oxygen-hemoglobin disorders, and chronic lung disease may also contribute to myocardial ischemia.

The left ventricle (LV) is most susceptible to ischemia and injury because of its higher myocardial oxygen demand, larger mass, higher wall tension, and higher systemic pressures. Ischemia causes transient LV dysfunction resulting in an increased LV diastolic pressure. Ischemia also causes elevated pulmonary artery wedge pressure (PAWP) and elevated right-sided heart pressure. Arrhythmias may occur in the presence of myocardial ischemia because of cellular irritability. Arrhythmias decrease the efficiency of the cardiac pump and thereby increase the need for myocardial oxygen while decreasing the available supply.

Up to 80% of patients with myocardial ischemia are asymptomatic.[16] This type of ischemia is termed *silent ischemia.* This creates an iceberg phenomenon in which the angina is merely the tip of the iceberg. Ischemia with pain (angina) or without pain has the same prognosis. Diabetes mellitus and hypertension are associated with an increased prevalence of silent ischemia. This phenomenon occurs in patients with and without diabetes mellitus–related neuropathy. It is important to remember that the myocardium is at risk when ischemia is present, regardless of whether it is asymptomatic or manifests as angina.

DRUG THERAPY

Table 32-7 **Hyperlipidemia**

Name	Mechanisms of Action	Side Effects	Nursing Considerations
Cholestyramine (Questran, Colybar)	Bile acid–binding resin, increases production of LDL receptors in liver Increases synthesis of cholesterol for use by liver as bile acids	Unpleasant gritty quality to taste GI disturbances (e.g., nausea, dyspepsia, constipation) Skin rash	Be aware that drug is effective and safe for long-term use, that side effects diminish with time, and that drug interferes with absorption of digoxin, thiazides, β-blockers, fat-soluble vitamins, folic acid.
Colestipol (Colestid)	Same as cholestyramine	Same as cholestyramine	Same as cholestyramine.
Nicotinic acid (niacin, Nicobid, Niac, Nicospan)	Inhibits synthesis and secretion of VLDL and LDL from liver Increases HDL levels	Hot flashes and pruritus in upper torso and face GI disturbances (e.g., nausea and vomiting, dyspepsia, diarrhea)	Be aware that most side effects subside with time and that decreased liver function and arrhythmias may occur with high doses. Have patient take aspirin 1/2 hr before drug to prevent flushing and take drug with meal.
Clofibrate (Atromid)	Promotes lipolysis of VLDL and reduces hepatic VLDL synthesis Reduces triglyceride levels	Nausea, diarrhea, weight gain Elevated liver enzymes	Monitor liver function tests. Increased incidence of gallbladder disease
Gemfibrozil (Lopid) Fenofibrate (Tricor)	Reduces hepatic VLDL synthesis and inhibits VLDL secretion Reduces triglyceride levels	Mild GI disturbances (e.g., nausea and diarrhea)	Be aware that drug is generally well tolerated.
Lovastatin (Mevacor) Pravastatin (Pravachol) Simvastatin (Zocor) Fluvastatin (Lescol) Atorvastatin (Lipitor) Cerivastatin (Baycol)	Increases liver rate of LDL removal from plasma Decreases liver synthesis of LDL	Rash, mild GI disturbances, insomnia, elevated liver enzymes (lens opacities, rhabdomyolysis [specifically lovastatin])	Be aware that drug is well tolerated with few side effects. Monitor patient with liver function tests and eye examinations.

ECG, electrocardiogram; *GI*, gastrointestinal; *HDL*, high-density lipoprotein; *LDL*, low-density lipoprotein; *VLDL*, very-low-density lipoprotein.

On the cellular level, the myocardium becomes cyanotic within the first 10 seconds of coronary occlusion, and ECG changes appear. With total occlusion of the coronary arteries, contractility ceases after several minutes, depriving the myocardial cells of glucose for aerobic metabolism. Anaerobic metabolism begins and lactic acid accumulates. Myocardial nerve fibers are irritated by the increased lactic acid and transmit a pain message to the cardiac nerves and upper thoracic posterior roots (the reason for referred cardiac pain to the left shoulder and arm). In ischemic conditions cardiac cells are viable for approximately 20 minutes. With restoration of blood flow, aerobic metabolism resumes and contractility is restored. Cellular repair also begins.

Precipitating Factors. Extracardiac factors may precipitate myocardial ischemia and anginal pain. These include the following:[17]

1. *Physical exertion* increases the HR. Increasing the HR decreases the time the heart spends in diastole, which is the time of greatest coronary blood flow. Walking outdoors is the most common form of exertion that produces an attack. Isometric exertion of the arms, as in raking leaves, painting, or lifting heavy objects, also causes exertional angina.
2. *Strong emotions* stimulate the sympathetic nervous system and increase the work of the heart. This results in an increase in HR, BP, and myocardial contractility.
3. *Consumption of a heavy meal* (especially if the person exerts afterward) can increase the work of the heart. During the digestive process, blood is diverted to the GI system, causing a low flow rate in the coronary arteries.
4. *Temperature extremes,* either hot or cold, increase the workload of the heart (blood vessels constrict in response to a cold stimulus; blood vessels dilate and blood pools in the skin in response to a hot stimulus). Cold weather also causes increased metabolism to maintain internal temperature regulation.
5. *Cigarette smoking* causes vasoconstriction and an increased HR because of nicotine's stimulation of catecholamine release. It also diminishes available oxygen by increasing the level of carbon monoxide.
6. *Sexual activity* increases the cardiac workload and sympathetic stimulation. In a person with severe CAD, the resulting extra workload of the heart may precipitate angina.
7. *Stimulants,* such as cocaine, cause increased HR and subsequent myocardial oxygen demand. Stimulation of catecholamine release is the precipitating factor.

Table 32-8 Factors Determining Myocardial Oxygen Needs

Decreased Oxygen Supply	Increased Oxygen Demand or Consumption
↓ Hematocrit	↑ HR
↓ Hemoglobin-binding capacity	↑ Contractility
↓ Coronary blood flow	↑ Left ventricular wall tension
↑ Diastolic pressure	↑ Systolic BP
↑ Coronary vascular resistance	↑ Ventricular volume
Coronary spasm	↑ Myocardial wall thickness
↓ Blood volume	

8. *Circadian rhythm patterns* have been related to the occurrence of stable angina, Prinzmetal's angina, MI, and sudden cardiac death. These manifestations of CAD tend to occur in the early morning after awakening.

Types of Angina

Stable Angina. Stable angina (classic) refers to chest pain occurring intermittently over a long period with the same pattern of onset, duration, and intensity of symptoms. Stable angina is usually exercise induced. Pain at rest is unusual. An ECG usually reveals ST segment depression, indicating subendocardial ischemia. The discomfort may be mild or severe and disabling, but it is usually infrequent. Stable angina can be controlled with medications on an outpatient basis. Because stable angina is often predictable, medications can be timed to provide peak effects during the time of day when angina is likely to occur. For example, if angina occurs when rising, the patient can take medication as soon as awakening and wait 30 minutes to 1 hour before engaging in activity.

Unstable Angina. Unstable angina (progressive, crescendo, or preinfarction angina) is different from stable angina. Unlike stable angina, it is unpredictable. The patient with stable angina may develop unstable angina, or unstable angina may be the first clinical manifestation of CAD. The patient with previously diagnosed stable angina will describe a significant change in the pattern of angina. It will occur with increasing frequency and is easily provoked by minimal or no exercise, during sleep, or even at total rest. The patient without previously diagnosed angina will describe anginal pain that has progressed rapidly in the last few weeks to days, often culminating in pain at rest.[18]

Recent findings associate unstable angina with deterioration of a once stable atherosclerotic plaque. In the majority of cases, the once stable plaque has ruptured, exposing the intima to blood and stimulating platelet aggregation and local vasoconstriction with thrombus formation.[19,20] This unstable lesion is at increased risk of complete thrombosis of the lumen with progression to MI. This is why these patients require immediate hospitalization with ECG monitoring and bed rest. The unstable lesion can progress to an MI, or it can return to a stable lesion (Fig. 32-8). Aspirin and systemic anticoagulation are the treatments of choice for unstable angina. If the patient is not already on antianginal agents, nitrates or β-blockers are the first line of treatment.[18] Calcium channel blockers can be added if the patient is already on adequate doses of nitrates or β-blockers or if the patient cannot tolerate the other two drugs or has variant angina.[18]

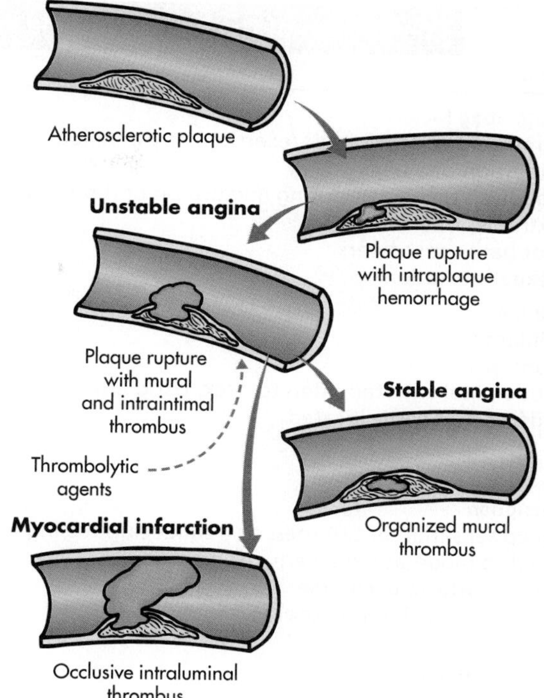

Fig. 32-8 Coronary thrombogenesis secondary to atherosclerotic plaque progression.

Prinzmetal's Angina. Prinzmetal's angina (variant angina) often occurs at rest, usually in response to spasm of a major coronary artery. It is a rare form of angina and is frequently seen in patients with a history of migraine headaches and Raynaud's phenomenon. The spasm may occur in the absence of CAD, as well as with documented disease. Prinzmetal's angina is not usually precipitated by increased physical demand. Coronary spasm can be described as a strong contraction of smooth muscle in the coronary artery caused by an increase in intracellular calcium ions. Factors that may precipitate coronary artery spasm include increased myocardial oxygen demand and increased levels of a variety of substances (e.g., histamine, angiotensin, epinephrine, norepinephrine, prostaglandins). When spasm occurs, the patient experiences pain and marked, transient ST segment elevation. The pain may occur during rapid eye movement (REM) sleep when myocardial oxygen consumption increases; it may be relieved by some form of exercise or it may disappear spontaneously. Cyclical, short bursts of pain at a usual time each day may also occur with this type of angina.

Nocturnal Angina and Angina Decubitus. Nocturnal angina occurs only at night but not necessarily when the person is in the recumbent position or during sleep. Angina decubitus is chest pain that occurs only while the person is lying down and is usually relieved by standing or sitting.

Clinical Manifestations

The most common initial symptom of a patient with angina is chest pain or discomfort (Table 32-9). The exact cause of the pain is unknown, but neurogenic pain at the site of

Table 32-9 Comparison of the Pain of Angina Pectoris and Myocardial Infarction

Angina	Myocardial Infarction
Precipitating Factors	
Stress, either physiologic (exertion) or psychologic	Exertion or at rest
Digestion of a heavy meal	Physical or emotional stress
Valsalva's maneuver during micturition or defecation	Often no precipitating factors or any factor associated with angina
Extremes of weather	
Hot baths or showers	
Sexual excitation	
Location	
Midanterior chest	Midanterior chest
Substernal	Substernal
Abdominal with radiation to neck, back, arms, fingers	Subscapular, midscapular
Diffuse, not easily located	Diffuse
	Radiation to neck and jaw or down left arm or both arms to fingers
Description	
Deep sensation of tightness or a squeezing feeling	Severe pressure, squeezing, or heaviness with a crushing, oppressive quality
Mild to moderate in severity or pressure	Report of such severe pain that patient would rather die than experience pain again
Similar attacks each time	Residual "soreness" for several days following MI
Twinges or dullness in thoracic area	
Onset and Duration	
Gradual or sudden onset	Sudden onset
Usual duration of 15 min or less (usually no more than 30 min)	Duration of 30 min to 2 hr
Relief from nitroglycerin	No relief from rest or nitroglycerin
Associated Clinical Manifestations	
Apprehension	Apprehension
Dyspnea	Nausea and vomiting
Diaphoresis	Dyspnea
Nausea	Diaphoresis
Desire to void	Extreme fatigue
Belching	Dizziness or faintness (after abatement of pain)

MI, myocardial infarction.

ischemia is most likely. On direct questioning, some patients may deny feeling pain but will refer to a vague sensation, a strange feeling, pressure, or ache in the chest. It is an unpleasant feeling, often described as a constrictive, squeezing, heavy, choking, or suffocating sensation. Many persons complain of severe indigestion or burning. Although most of the discomfort experienced by persons with angina appears substernally, the sensation may occur in the neck or radiate to various locations, including the jaw, shoulders, and down the arms (Fig. 32-9). Often people will complain of pain between the shoulder blades and dismiss it as not being heart pain. Depending on the severity of the anginal attack, the person may remain motionless or may clench a fist over the sternal area. The person experiencing angina often refers to a feeling of anxiety and impending doom. Associated symptoms may include shortness of breath, cold sweat, weakness, or paresthesias of one or both arms. Relief of classic angina pectoris is usually obtained with rest or cessation of activity. Prinzmetal's angina differs from stable or unstable angina in that it is longer in duration and may wake the patient from sleep.

Complications

Arrhythmias, such as premature contractions or fibrillation, may occur in a person with angina. The cells deprived of oxygen and nutrients may become irritable and develop into sites for ectopic pacemaker cells. Decreased myocardial contractility also occurs in the person experiencing angina.

Because some anginal pains may be vague, the patient may not perceive the discomfort as important and dismiss its occurrence. When chest pain is reported to a health care provider, the diagnosis of angina may not be the first consideration because many problems can mimic midthoracic discomfort. Exertional discomfort in any of the areas shown in Fig. 32-9 should be evaluated to rule out angina.

Diagnostic Studies

When a patient has a history indicating CAD, the physician may order several diagnostic studies (Table 32-10). After a detailed health history and physical examination, a chest x-ray is usually taken to look for cardiac enlargement, cardiac calcifications, and pulmonary congestion. Laboratory tests may be done to ascertain serum lipid and cardiac enzyme values.

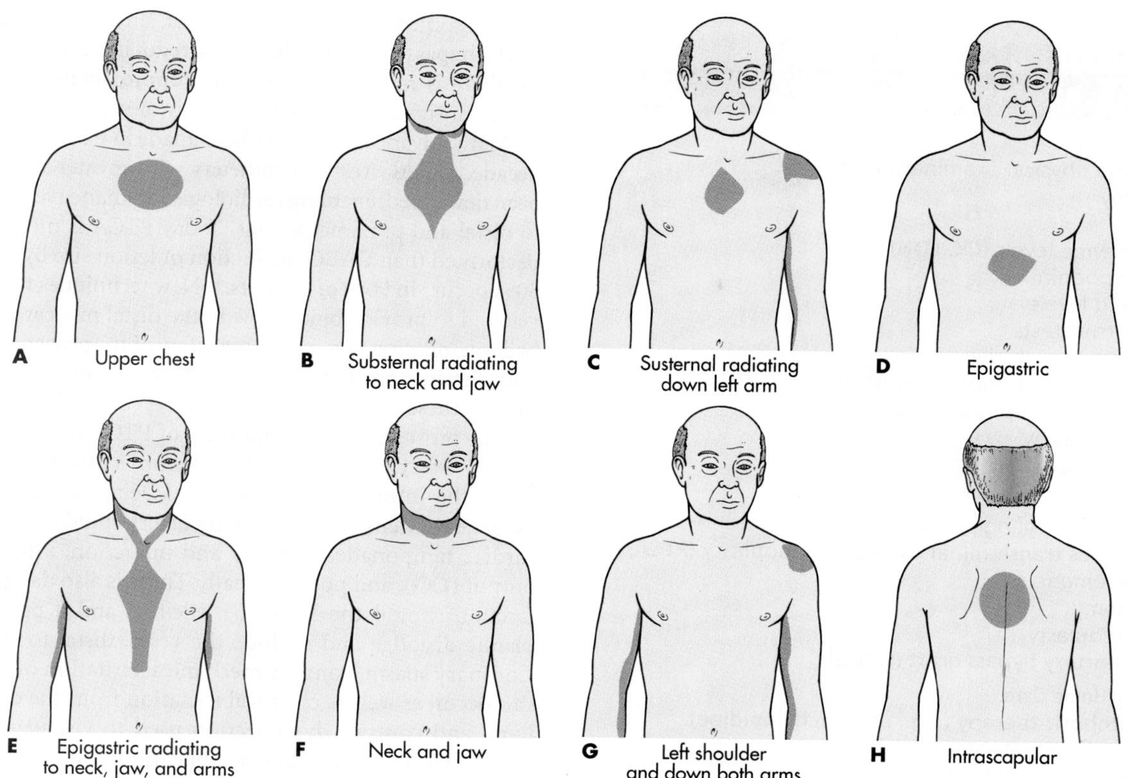

Fig. 32-9 Location of chest pain during angina or MI. **A,** Upper chest. **B,** Substernal, radiating to neck and jaw. **C,** Substernal, radiating down left arm. **D,** Epigastric. **E,** Epigastric, radiating to neck, jaw, and arms. **F,** Neck and jaw. **G,** Left shoulder and down both arms. **H,** Intrascapular.

Serum lipid levels are assessed to screen for positive risk factors, and enzyme levels are checked to rule out the occurrence of an infarction. An ECG is obtained and compared with an earlier tracing when possible.

Frequently, treadmill exercise testing is done for the patient with stable angina to examine ST segment changes during exercise as an indirect assessment of coronary artery perfusion. (Unstable angina is a contraindication for using the treadmill.) Severely abnormal ECGs on exercise testing, indicating gross disease processes, may show the need for angiography. Unfortunately, the ECG stress test is not always conclusive for CAD. A false-positive reaction may be found (especially in women), and a false-negative reaction may be seen if the patient is exercised submaximally or if only one coronary artery is involved. Ambulatory 24- to 48-hour ECG monitoring with patient-recorded activity may be effective in identifying silent ischemia. It is also helpful in differentiating Prinzmetal's angina because the incidence of spasm occurs more commonly in early hours (5 to 6 AM).

Nuclear imaging is being widely used as a noninvasive measurement of myocardial perfusion. Thallium 201 and Sestimibi are the isotopes of choice to detect ischemia, and technetium 99m pyrophosphate is used to detect the "hot spots" of actual infarcted tissue.[21] Thallium or Sestimibi stress tests are also frequently performed. The patient is injected with the isotope and proceeds with exercise on a treadmill, with scanning done at peak exercise and 2 to 4 hours after exercise. For the patient unable to exercise, a dipyridamole (Persantine) and radioisotope test may be done. The patient is injected with both dipyridamole and a radioisotope and then scanned. Dipyridamole will cause vasodilation in healthy arteries, and the radioisotope will "light up" the areas of the heart that are well perfused. Regions of the heart that are not well perfused will show up on the scan as "cold spots." A repeat scan is done 2 to 4 hours later to see if the cold spots have reversed after the dipyridamole has worn off.

Positron emission tomography (PET), a noninvasive technique, is also useful in identifying and quantifying ischemia and infarction (see Chapter 30 and Table 30-7).

The physician may propose coronary angiography. This study allows visualization of the coronary arteries for obstruction and helps determine the treatment and prognosis. The patient with unstable angina should undergo coronary angiography to evaluate the extent of the disease and to determine the most appropriate therapeutic modality. Coronary angiography is the only way to confirm the diagnosis of Prinzmetal's angina.

Other new techniques for diagnosing coronary artery stenosis include the use of echocardiography with exercise. Stress echocardiograms may be used when a patient has an abnormal baseline ECG. The patient has a baseline echocardiogram before exercise stress testing and then proceeds with the treadmill exercise test. Immediately after the conclusion of the test, another echocardiogram is performed to detect any new regional abnormal wall motion. This increases the sensitivity of the treadmill test.

Another technique using an echocardiogram can be used for the patient who is unable to exercise. In this patient, a dobutamine stress echocardiogram can be performed. Echocardiography is done during a stepwise infusion of dobutamine, which causes a progressive increase in HR just as occurs with exercise; that is, the heart is being exercised chemically.

COLLABORATIVE CARE

Table 32-10 Angina Pectoris

Diagnostic
History and physical examination
Chest x-ray
ECG
Serum enzyme levels (CK, LDH)
Cardiac troponin
Serum lipid levels
Exercise stress tests
Nuclear imaging studies
Position emission tomography (PET)
Coronary angiography studies
Echocardiography
Collaborative Therapy
Acute Care
Nitroglycerin (sublingual, IV)
Percutaneous transluminal coronary angioplasty (PTCA)
Stent placement
Atherectomy
Laser angioplasty
Coronary artery bypass graft (CABG)
Ambulatory/Home Care
Antithrombotic therapy (e.g., aspirin, ticlopidine)
Nitroglycerin ointment (e.g., Nitrol)
Transdermal controlled-release nitrates
Long-acting nitrates (e.g., Isordil, Sorbitrate, Imdur)
β-Adrenergic blocking agents
Calcium-blocking agents
Management of risk factors for coronary artery disease (see Table 32-4)

CK, creatine kinase; *LDH,* lactic dehydrogenase.

Again, abnormality of the regional wall motion is determined. The test is stopped if a wall motion abnormality or angina develops or the patient reaches the target HR or the peak dobutamine dose. Atropine IV may also be used to help reach target HR.

Collaborative Care

The most common initial therapeutic intervention for angina is the use of nitrate therapy to enhance coronary blood flow (see Table 32-10). Emergency care of the patient with chest pain is presented in Table 32-11. The treatment of CAD may include percutaneous transluminal coronary angioplasty (PTCA), stent placement, atherectomy, laser angioplasty, and coronary artery bypass surgery.

Percutaneous Transluminal Coronary Angioplasty. A common intervention for angina is PTCA.[18,22] In a catheterization laboratory a catheter equipped with an inflatable balloon tip is inserted into the appropriate coronary artery. When the lesion is located, the catheter is passed through and just past the lesion, the balloon is inflated, and the atherosclerotic plaque is compressed, resulting in vessel dilation.

The advantages of PTCA are that (1) it provides an alternative to surgical intervention; (2) it is performed with local anesthesia; (3) it eliminates the recovery from sternotomy required for bypass surgery and its complications; (4) the patient is ambulatory 24 hours after the procedure; (5) the length of hospital stay is approximately 1 to 3 days compared with the 4- to 6-day stay of someone having open heart surgery with a coronary artery bypass graft (CABG), thus reducing hospital costs; and (6) there is rapid return to work (approximately 1 week after PTCA) instead of a 2- to 8-week convalescence after CABG.

Many advancements have been made in PTCA during the last decade. Guidewires and catheters with greater flexibility have been developed, enabling cardiologists to maneuver the catheters to distal and proximal lesions. Today PTCA is more frequently performed than CABG. Reduction of lesion size by greater than 50% occurs in 90% of patients.[22] New techniques have been developed to provide blood flow to the distal myocardium during balloon inflation, increasing the safety of the procedure. Dilation may also be done for stenotic grafts from a previous CABG, although these vessels usually require repeated dilation.

The most serious complication of PTCA is dissection of the dilated artery where the intimal lesion is pushed farther up or down the intimal lining instead of being compressed. If the damage is extensive, the coronary artery could rupture, causing cardiac tamponade, ischemia and infarction, a fall in cardiac output (CO), and possible death. There is also danger from infarction should the lesion be calcified and a portion of the plaque dislodge and occlude the vessel distal to the catheter. Coronary spasm from the mechanical irritation of the catheter can occur, as well as chemical irritation from the catheter, balloon, and contrast dye injection used to visualize the artery. Abrupt closure is another complication that can occur in the first 24 hours after PTCA. Factors related to abrupt closure include a diffuse, complicated lesion, severe stenosis (greater than 90%), presence of thrombus before dilation, and lesions in vessels supplying collateral circulation.[23] The risk of restenosis after PTCA is approximately 30% in the first 3 to 6 months.[22] Restenosis occurs more commonly in smokers, diabetics, and patients with hypercholesterolemia.[24]

Stent Placement. Stents are used to treat abrupt or threatened abrupt closure and restenosis following PTCA. Stents are expandable meshlike structures designed to maintain vessel patency by compressing the arterial walls and resisting vasoconstriction (Fig. 32-10).[23,25] Stents are carefully placed over the angioplasty site to hold the vessel open. Because stents are thrombogenic, the patient is usually treated with antiplatelet agents such as aspirin, ticlopidine (Ticlid), or clopidogrel (Plavix). If the procedure was difficult or less than ideal, or placement of the stent is detected by intracoronary ultrasound, an IV infusion of abciximab (ReoPro), a platelet aggregation inhibitor, can be used.[26,27] Abciximab helps to prevent the abrupt closure of treated coronary arteries. It prevents clot formation by preventing fibrinogen and other adhesive molecules from binding to platelets. Occasionally a patient might be placed on warfarin (Coumadin) for 1 to 3 months.[26,27] The primary complications from stent placement are hemorrhage and vascular injury. Less common complications are stent thrombosis, acute MI, emergency CABG, stent embolization, and coronary spasm.[23] The possibility of arrhythmias is always present.

Atherectomy. Atherectomy is another technique used to treat CAD. With atherectomy the plaque is shaved off using a type of rotational blade (Fig. 32-11). Atherectomy decreases the incidence of abrupt closure as compared with PTCA. However, it is limited to use in proximal and middle portions of a vessel greater than 3 mm in diameter, less than 15 mm long, and not heavily calcified. It is superior to PTCA in lesions lo-

✚EMERGENCY MANAGEMENT

Table **32-11** **Chest Pain**

Etiology	Assessment Findings	Interventions
Cardiovascular Angina Myocardial infarction Arrhythmia Pericarditis Aortic aneurysm **Pulmonary** Pleurisy Pneumonia Spontaneous pneumothorax Pulmonary edema Pulmonary embolus **Chest Trauma** Rib/sternal fracture Flail chest Cardiac tamponade Pneumothorax Hemothorax Pulmonary contusion Aortic injury Great vessel injury **Others** Costochondritis Stress Strenuous exercise Drugs Shock Hiatal hernia	▪ Pain in chest, neck, arm, or shoulder ▪ Cold, clammy skin ▪ Diaphoresis ▪ Nausea and vomiting ▪ Abdominal pain ▪ Heartburn ▪ Dyspnea ▪ Weakness ▪ Anxiety ▪ Feeling of impending doom ▪ Tachycardia ▪ Irregular HR ▪ Palpitations ▪ Arrhythmias ▪ Decreased BP ▪ Narrowed pulse pressure ▪ Unequal BP readings in upper extremities ▪ Syncope, loss of consciousness ▪ Decreased oxygen saturation ▪ Decreased or absent breath sounds ▪ Pericardial friction rub	**Initial** ▪ Ensure patent airway. ▪ Administer oxygen by nasal cannula or nonrebreather mask. ▪ Insert two IV catheters. ▪ Obtain 12-lead ECG. ▪ Determine location of pain. Assess severity using pain scale (0-10). ▪ Medicate for pain as ordered (e.g., morphine, nitroglycerin). ▪ Identify underlying rhythm. ▪ Obtain cardiac enzymes levels. ▪ Assess need for thrombolytic therapy as appropriate. ▪ Administer aspirin and β-adrenergic blockers for cardiac-related chest pain unless contraindicated. **Ongoing Monitoring** ▪ Monitor vital signs, level of consciousness, cardiac rhythm, and oxygen saturation. ▪ Monitor pain and remedicate as needed. ▪ Reassure patient. ▪ Anticipate need for intubation if respiratory distress is evident. ▪ Prepare for CPR, defibrillation, transcutaneous pacing, or cardioversion.

CPR, cardiopulmonary resuscitation.

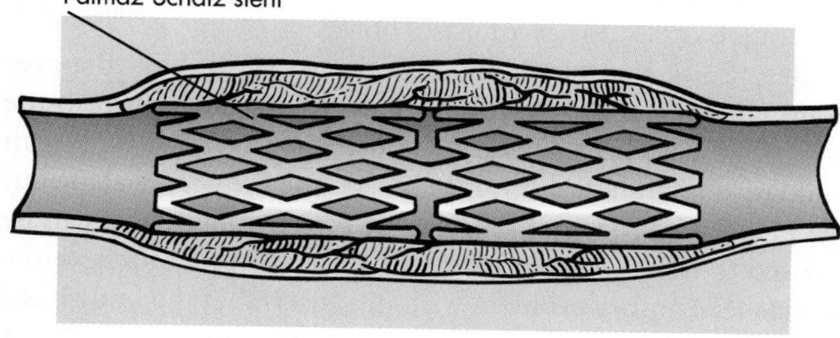

Fig. 32-10 Palmaz-Schatz stent, an articulated stainless steel mesh deployed by balloon inflation.

cated in branches or attachment sites of a bypass graft but carries the same risk for thrombosis and restenosis rate as conventional PTCA.[28,29]

Laser Angioplasty. In laser angioplasty a catheter is introduced through a peripheral artery into the diseased coronary artery. A small laser on the tip of the catheter vaporizes the plaqued areas of the artery, thereby facilitating blood flow. A disadvantage of this procedure is that the technique needs refinement so that the proper laser strength for a given thickness of atherosclerotic plaque will be known. Research has found laser angioplasty useful in relieving stenosis that develops in stents, in extracting pacemaker leads, and in vein graft occlusions.[28]

Coronary Artery Bypass Surgery. Generally, CABG is recommended if the patient has (1) significant left main coronary artery obstruction, (2) triple-vessel disease, or (3) two-vessel disease unresponsive to medical therapy. Bypass surgery is usually recommended for the person with unstable angina who demonstrates a poor response to therapy, requiring repeat angioplasty. The success of such treatment varies. (Coronary artery bypass surgery is discussed in Chapter 33.)

Drug Therapy

Antiplatelet aggregation therapy. Antiplatelet aggregation therapy is the first line of pharmacologic intervention in the treatment of angina. Aspirin is the drug of choice. Recent studies indicate that up to a 50% reduction in unstable angina progression to MI occurs with the use of aspirin.[18,30] As little as one baby aspirin daily may be effective in inhibiting platelet aggregation. For patients unable to tolerate aspirin or in patients with recent gastrointestinal bleeding, ticlopidine or clopidogrel may be given.[18]

Nitrates. Nitrates, which are commonly classified as vasodilators, are the next step in the treatment of angina. Nitrates produce their principal effects by the following:

1. *Dilating peripheral blood vessels.* This results in decreased SVR, venous pooling, and decreased venous

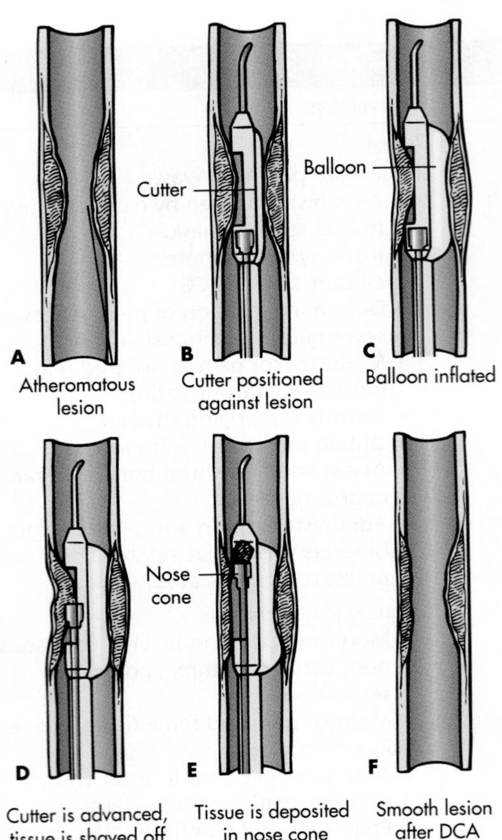

Fig. 32-11 Directional coronary atherectomy (DCA). **A,** Atheromatous lesion. **B,** DCA cutter is introduced over a guidewire into the coronary artery and positioned with the window against lesion. **C,** Balloon is inflated to maintain cutting position against the lesion. **D,** As the rotating cutter is advanced across the lesion, atheromatous tissue is shaved off. **E,** Tissue is deposited in the nose cone. **F,** Smooth lesion after DCA.

blood return to the heart. Therefore myocardial oxygen requirements are lessened because of the reduced cardiac workload.

2. *Dilating coronary arteries and collateral vessels.* This may increase blood flow to the ischemic areas of the heart. However, when the coronary arteries are severely atherosclerotic, coronary dilation is difficult to achieve.[30,31]

Nitroglycerin. Nitroglycerin given sublingually will usually relieve pain in approximately 3 minutes and has a duration of approximately 20 to 45 minutes. The usual recommended dose is one tablet taken sublingually, which can be followed at 5-minute intervals with two more doses. If nitroglycerin tablets have been necessary and relief from anginal pain has not been obtained after three tablets and 15 minutes, the patient should be instructed to seek immediate medical attention.

Nitroglycerin can be used prophylactically before undertaking an activity that the patient knows may precipitate an anginal attack. In these instances the patient can take a tablet 5 to 10 minutes before beginning the activity. Any changes in the usual pattern of pain, especially increasing frequency or nocturnal angina, should be reported to the physician.

Nitroglycerin tablets are marketed in light-resistant bottles closed with metal caps. Because they tend to lose potency, the patient should be advised to purchase a new supply every 6 to 9 months.

Nitroglycerin ointment. Nitroglycerin (Nitrol and Nitropaste) is a 2% nitroglycerin topical ointment dosed by the inch. It is placed on the skin where it is absorbed, producing anginal prophylaxis for 3 to 6 hours. It has been found to be especially useful for nocturnal and unstable angina because it acts for a longer period of time than sublingual (SL) nitroglycerin. Its disadvantages include its messiness and its rapid absorption, necessitating repeated application.[30]

Transdermal controlled-release nitrates. Currently two systems are available for transdermal drug administration: reservoir and matrix. Transderm-Nitro is the reservoir system, in which the drug migrates to the absorption site through a rate-controlled permeable membrane. Nitro-Dur and Nitro-Disc are the matrix system, in which the drug is slowly dispersed through a polymer matrix to the skin absorption site. Both reservoir and matrix delivery systems offer the advantages of steady plasma levels within the therapeutic range during 24 hours, thus making only one application a day necessary. The reservoir system has the disadvantage of dose dumping if the reservoir seal is punctured or broken. An advantage of the matrix system is that there can be no dose dumping. Both systems achieve plasma drug level steady states by 2 hours.

Long-acting nitrates. Long-acting nitrates such as isosorbide dinitrate and isosorbide mononitrate (Isordil, Sorbitrate, Imdur) are longer acting than SL nitroglycerin and, when used in adequate doses, are effective in reducing the incidence of anginal attacks. Their mechanisms of action and side effects are similar to those of nitroglycerin. The effects of oral isosorbide dinitrate may last for as long as 8 hours.

Because of the vasodilating properties of nitrates, the predominant side effect of all nitrate drugs is headache from the dilation of cerebral blood vessels. Sometimes the body can build up a tolerance to the drug so that the headaches abate but the principal antianginal effect is still present. Patients can be advised to take acetaminophen with their nitrate to relieve the headache. Another problem with nitrates is that the body has a tendency to develop a tolerance to the effects of nitrates.[30,31] A strategy found effective to combat this tolerance is providing a nitrate-free period of at least 8 hours within each 24-hour period. This nitrate-free period should be at night unless the patient experiences nocturnal angina. Other complications of the vasodilator drugs are orthostatic hypotension (nitrate syncope) and an aggravation of cerebral vascular insufficiency.

Intravenous nitroglycerin. Intravenous (IV) nitroglycerin (Nitrol IV, Nitrostat IV, Nitro-Bid IV, Tridil) has been used in treating the hospitalized patient with unstable angina. It has an immediate onset of action and can be titrated to prevent, treat, and stop acute attacks of angina. The goal of therapy should aim at stopping anginal pain and reducing systolic BP by 15% or mean arterial pressure (MAP) by 10%.[30,31] IV nitroglycerin has also been used in treatment of MI. The rationale for use in MI has been to increase the collateral blood flow to the ischemic area and reduce myocardial oxygen demand

NURSING ASSESSMENT

Table 32-12 Angina Pectoris

Subjective Data

Important Health Information

Past health history: Previous history of MI, angina, aortic stenosis, or cardiomyopathy; hypertension, diabetes mellitus, anemia, lung disease; hyperlipidemia

Medications: Use of nitrates, calcium channel blockers, β-adrenergic blockers, antihypertensive drugs, lipid-lowering agents

Functional Health Patterns

Health perception–health management: Family history of heart disease; sedentary lifestyle; smoking

Nutritional-metabolic: Usual fat and sodium intake; indigestion, heartburn, nausea, belching

Elimination: Desire to void

Activity-exercise: Palpitations; dyspnea; dizziness, weakness

Cognitive-perceptual: Diffuse substernal chest pain or pressure (squeezing, constricting, aching, sharp, tingling) lasting <20 min; referral to arms (especially left), jaw, neck, shoulders, back and usually associated with a precipitating factor; relief with rest or nitroglycerin; paresthesia of arms

Coping–stress tolerance: Stressful lifestyle; apprehension, anxiety; feeling of impending doom

Objective Data

General

Anxiety

Integumentary

Cool, clammy, pale skin

Cardiovascular

Tachycardia, pulsus alterans, arrhythmias (especially ventricular), ventricular gallop, atrial gallop

Possible Findings

Negative cardiac enzymes, elevated serum lipids; positive exercise stress test and thallium scans; demonstration of ST and T wave abnormalities on ECG; cardiac enlargement or calcifications, pulmonary congestion on chest x-ray; abnormal wall motion with stress echocardiogram; positive coronary angiography

because of decreasing preload and afterload. Tolerance is also a side effect of IV nitrate therapy. An effective strategy for this phenomenon is titrating down the dose at night during sleep and titrating the dose up during the day.

Beta-adrenergic blockers. β-adrenergic blocking agents are the one class of drugs that have been shown to decrease morbidity and mortality rates in patients with CAD, especially following acute MI. However, β-adrenergic blocking agents have many side effects and are sometimes poorly tolerated.[18,30] β-adrenergic blocking agents available for the prophylaxis of angina are propranolol (Inderal), metoprolol (Lopressor), nadolol (Corgard), atenolol (Tenormin), oxyprendol (Trasicor), pindolol (Visken), and timolol (Blocadren) (See Table 31-8). These drugs produce a direct decrease in myocardial contractility, HR, SVR, and BP, all of which reduce the myocardial oxygen demand. Side effects of β-adrenergic blockers may include bradycardia, hypotension, wheezing, and GI complaints. Many patients also complain of weight gain, depression, and sexual dysfunction. β-adrenergic blockers should not be discontinued abruptly without medical supervision.

Calcium channel blocking agents. Calcium channel blocking agents such as nifedipine (Procardia), verapamil (Calan, Isoptin), diltiazem (Cardizem), and nicardipine (Cardene) are the next step in the management of angina. Most of these agents have sustained-release versions for longer action with the hope of increased patient adherence. The three primary effects of calcium channel blockers are (1) systemic vasodilation with decreased SVR, (2) decreased myocardial contractility, and (3) coronary vasodilation. Each drug manifests these effects to a different degree. Calcium channel blockers have a depressant effect on the sinoatrial (SA) node rate of discharge, and the conduction velocity through the atrioventricular (AV) node is decreased, thus slowing the HR. (See Table 31-8 for a list of calcium channel blockers).

Cardiac muscle and vascular smooth muscle cells are more dependent on extracellular calcium than skeletal muscles and are therefore more sensitive to calcium channel blocking agents. The effect of calcium channel blockers on smooth muscle of both coronary and systemic arteries is to cause relaxation and relative vasodilation, thus increasing blood flow. Verapamil and diltiazem have antiarrhythmic properties (see Chapter 34). Myocardial perfusion is enhanced with calcium channel blockers by increased coronary blood flow through vasodilation and reduction in myocardial oxygen demand mediated through a decrease in HR and afterload. Calcium channel blocking agents have also been effective in controlling angina from either "fixed" atherosclerotic lesions or vasospasm. Verapamil, nifedipine, and diltiazem have also been shown to consistently decrease systemic BP in the hypertensive patient.

Calcium channel blockers potentiate the action of digoxin by increasing serum digoxin levels during the first week of therapy. Therefore serum digoxin levels should be closely monitored on institution of this therapy, and the patient should be taught the signs and symptoms of digoxin toxicity.

NURSING MANAGEMENT: ANGINA

■ Nursing Assessment

Subjective and objective data that should be obtained from a patient with angina are presented in Table 32-12.

■ Nursing Diagnoses

Nursing diagnoses for the patient with angina may include, but are not limited to, the following:

- Pain (chest pain or discomfort) *related to* ischemic myocardium
- Anxiety *related to* diagnosis and awareness of having heart disease, pain and limited activity tolerance, uncertainties about the future, diagnostic tests, and pending surgery
- Decreased CO *related to* myocardial ischemia affecting contractility
- Activity intolerance *related to* myocardial ischemia

■ Planning

The overall goals are that the patient with angina will (1) experience pain relief, (2) have reduced anxiety, (3) have adequate knowledge of the problem and prescribed treatment, and (4) modify risk factors.

■ Nursing Implementation

Health Promotion. Behaviors to reduce risk factors for CAD are presented in Table 32-4 and discussed on p. 847-848.

Acute Intervention. Some of the main nursing objectives for the patient with angina are pain assessment, evaluation of treatment, and reinforcement of appropriate therapy. Because chest pain can be caused by many factors other than ischemia (e.g., pericarditis, valvular disease, pulmonary artery stenosis, MI, congestive cardiomyopathy), it is important to have a clear understanding of the patient's chest pain. The questions a nurse asks may elicit a history of anginal pain. The nurse should determine whether breathing in or out or changing positions makes the patient's chest pain better or worse. Anginal pain does not vary with body position or respirations. In contrast, the pain of pericarditis does. It should be ascertained whether the pain is deep or superficial, mild or intense. Cardiac pain is usually described as deep and intense, but occasionally it may be characterized as a dull ache. Few persons can successfully ignore cardiac pain.

The patient should be asked whether the pain is diffuse or well localized. Cardiac pain is usually diffuse. The patient may rub the entire chest to explain where the pain is occurring. The nurse should instruct the patient to quantify each pain experience by rating the pain on a scale from 1 to 10, with 10 being excruciating pain and 1 being barely noticeable pain. By doing this, the nurse can assess the effectiveness of treatment during a pain experience and discriminate between subsequent pain experiences.

If a nurse is present during an anginal attack, the following measures should be instituted: (1) administration of oxygen, (2) determination of vital signs, (3) 12-lead ECG, (4) prompt pain relief first with a nitrate followed by a narcotic analgesic if needed, (5) physical assessment of the chest, and (6) comfortable positioning of the patient. The patient will most likely appear distressed and have pale, cool, clammy skin. The BP and heart rate will probably be elevated, and an atrial gallop (S_4) sound may be heard. If a ventricular gallop (S_3) is heard, it may indicate LV decompensation. A murmur may be heard during an anginal attack secondary to ischemia of a papillary muscle. The murmur is likely to be transient and abates with the cessation of symptoms. Supportive and realistic assurance and a calm, soothing manner help reduce the patient's anxiety.

The patient must be instructed in the proper use of SL nitroglycerin. It should be easily accessible to the patient at all times. However, patients should be taught not to carry nitroglycerin in their pockets because heat from the body can cause loss of potency of the tablets. For protection from degradation, it should be kept in a tightly closed dark glass bottle. The patient should be instructed to place a nitroglycerin tablet beneath the tongue and allow it to dissolve. This should cause a fizzing or slightly warm feeling locally. The patient should be warned that HR may increase and a pounding headache, dizziness, or flushing may occur. The patient should be cautioned against quickly rising to a standing position because postural hypotension may occur after nitroglycerin ingestion. If the pain has not been relieved after 5 minutes, the patient should be told to take another nitroglycerin tablet. This procedure may be repeated for pain relief every 5 minutes, not to exceed the ingestion of three tablets. If pain persists after three doses, the patient should seek immediate medical attention.

Ambulatory and Home Care. The patient should be reassured that a long, productive life is possible, even with angina. Prevention of angina is preferable to its treatment, and this is where instruction is important. The patient should be educated regarding CAD and angina, precipitating factors, risk factors, and medications.

Patient teaching can be handled in a variety of ways. One-to-one contact between the nurse and the patient is often the most effective procedure. The time spent in providing daily care is often an ideal teaching period. Teaching tools, such as pamphlets, videotapes, a heart model, and especially written information, are necessary components of patient and family education.

The patient should be assisted in identifying factors that precipitate angina (see Table 32-9). The patient should be given instruction on how to avoid or control precipitating factors. For example, the patient should be cautioned to avoid exposures to extremes of weather and taught not to eat large, heavy meals. If a heavy meal is ingested, adequate rest should be planned for 1 to 2 hours after eating because blood is shunted to the GI tract to aid digestion.

The patient should be assisted in identifying personal risk factors in CAD. Once these risk factors are known, various methods of decreasing them should be discussed (see Table 32-4).

Educating the patient and the family about diets that are low in sodium and reduced in saturated fats may be appropriate. Maintaining ideal body weight is important in controlling angina because weight above this level increases the myocardial workload and may cause pain. Eating large meals also contributes to angina, and the patient may need to eat several small meals in place of three moderate to large meals each day.

Adhering to a regular, individualized exercise program that conditions the heart rather than overstresses the myocardium is important. Most patients can be advised to walk briskly on a flat surface 30 minutes a day at least 3 days a week. For more individualized instruction, the nurse should consult with a physician or a physical therapist in instructing the patient regarding an exercise program.

It is important to educate the patient and the family in the use of nitroglycerin. Nitroglycerin tablets or ointments may be used prophylactically before an emotionally stressful situation, sexual intercourse, or physical exertion (e.g., climbing a long flight of stairs).

Counseling should be provided to assess the psychologic adjustment of the patient and the family to the diagnosis of CAD and the resulting angina pectoris. Many patients feel a threat to their identity and self-esteem and are unable to fill their roles in society. These emotions are normal and real.

■ Evaluation

The expected outcomes are that the patient with angina will

- experience pain relief and have no further episodes of anginal pain.
- take actions to modify risk factors for CAD.
- adhere to drug and diet therapies.
- be knowledgeable of disease process.
- experience no complications

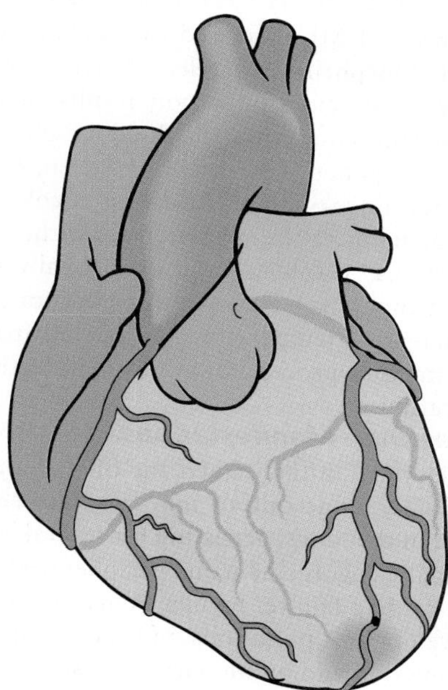

Fig. 32-12 Occlusion of coronary artery, resulting in a myocardial infarction.

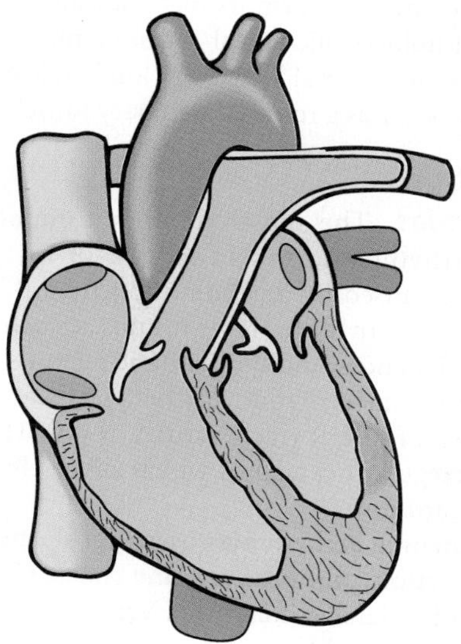

Fig. 32-13 Transmural myocardial infarction involving the thickness of the total wall.

MYOCARDIAL INFARCTION

An MI occurs when ischemic intracellular changes become irreversible and necrosis results. Angina as a result of ischemia causes reversible cellular injury, and infarction is the result of sustained ischemia, causing irreversible cellular death (Fig. 32-12).

The prehospital mortality rate among patients with acute MI is approximately 30% to 50%. The mortality rate among patients who reach the hospital is approximately 5%. Most of these deaths occur within the first 3 to 4 days.[32]

Pathophysiology

Cardiac cells can withstand ischemic conditions for approximately 20 minutes before cellular death (necrosis) begins. Contractile function of the heart stops in the areas of myocardial necrosis. The degree of altered function depends on the area of the heart involved and the size of the infarct. Most infarcts involve the LV. A *transmural MI* occurs when the entire thickness of the myocardium in a region is involved (Fig. 32-13). A *subendocardial MI* (nontransmural) exists when the damage has not penetrated through the entire thickness of the myocardial wall.

Infarctions are described by the area of occurrence as anterior, inferior, lateral, or posterior wall infarctions (Fig. 32-14). Common combinations of areas are the anterolateral or anteroseptal MI. An inferior MI is also called a diaphragmatic MI.

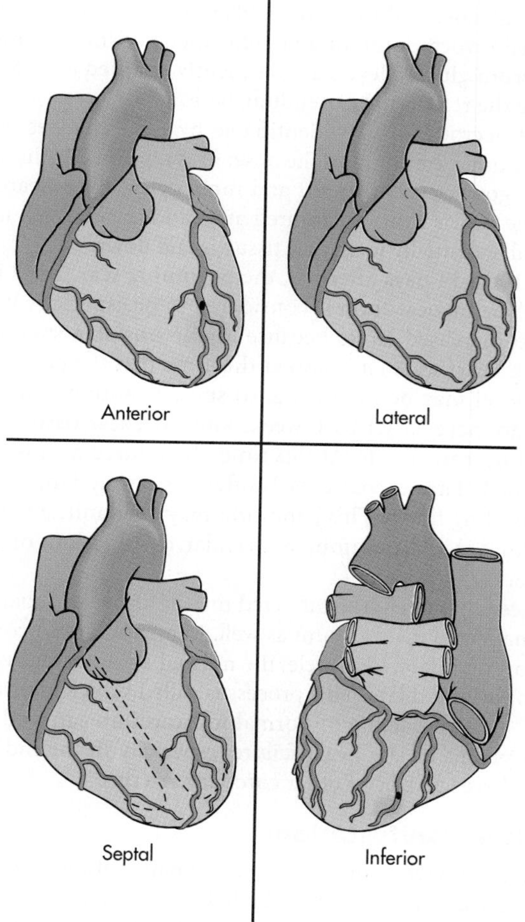

Fig. 32-14 Four common locations where myocardial infarction occurs.

The location and area of the infarct correlate with the part of the coronary circulation involved. For example, inferior wall infarctions are usually the result of right coronary artery lesions. Anterior wall infarctions are usually caused by lesions in the left anterior descending artery. Lesions in the left circumflex artery usually cause posterior or inferior MIs.

The degree of preestablished collateral circulation also determines the severity of infarction. In an individual with a history of heart disease, adequate collateral channels may have been established that provide the area surrounding the infarction site with a blood supply and oxygen. This is one explanation why the younger person who has a severe MI is often more likely to have a more serious impairment than an older person with the same degree of occlusion.

Healing Process. The body's response to cell death is the inflammatory process (see Chapter 11.) Within 24 hours, leukocytes infiltrate the area. Enzymes are released from the dead cardiac cells and are important diagnostic indicators of MI. (See section on serum cardiac markers later in this chapter.) The proteolytic enzymes of the neutrophils and macrophages remove all necrotic tissue by the second or third day. During this time, the necrotic muscle wall is thin. The development of collateral circulation improves areas of poor perfusion and may limit the zones of injury and infarction. Once infarction takes place, catecholamine-mediated lipolysis and glycogenolysis occur. These processes allow the increased plasma glucose and free fatty acids to be used by the oxygen-depleted myocardium for anaerobic metabolism. For this reason, serum glucose levels are frequently elevated after MI and may be the reason for a pseudodiabetic state.

The necrotic zone is identifiable by ECG changes and by technetium scanning after the onset of symptoms. At this point, the phagocytes (neutrophils and monocytes) have cleared the necrotic debris from the injured area, and the collagen matrix that will eventually form scar tissue is laid down.

At 10 to 14 days after MI, the beginning scar tissue is still weak. The myocardium is considered to be especially vulnerable to increased stress because of the unstable state of the healing heart wall. (It is also at this time that the patient's activity level may be increasing, so special caution and assessment are necessary.) By 6 weeks after MI, scar tissue has replaced necrotic tissue. At this time, the injured area is said to be healed. The scarred area is often less compliant than the surrounding fibers. This condition may be manifested by uncoordinated wall motion, ventricular dysfunction, or pump failure.

These changes in the infarcted muscle also cause changes in the unaffected myocardium as well. In an attempt to compensate for the infarcted muscle, the normal myocardium will hypertrophy and dilate. This process is called ventricular remodeling.[32,33] Remodeling of normal myocardium can lead to the development of late heart failure, especially in the individual with atherosclerosis of other coronary arteries.

Clinical Manifestations

Pain. Severe, immobilizing chest pain not relieved by rest or nitrate administration is the hallmark of an MI (see Table 32-9). The pain is caused by the inadequate oxygen supply to the myocardium. Persistent and unlike any other pain, it is usually described as a heaviness, tightness, or constriction. Common locations are substernal or retrosternal, radiating to the neck, jaw, and arms or to the back. It may occur while the patient is active or at rest, asleep or awake, and it commonly occurs in the early morning hours. It usually lasts for 20 minutes or more and is described as more severe than anginal pain. The pain may be located atypically in the epigastric area. The patient may have taken antacids without relief. Some patients may not experience pain but may have "discomfort," weakness, or shortness of breath.

Nausea and Vomiting. The patient may be nauseated and vomit. Nausea and vomiting can result from reflex stimulation of the vomiting center by the severe pain. These symptoms can also result from vasovagal reflexes initiated from the area of the infarcted myocardium.

Sympathetic Nervous System Stimulation. During the initial phases of MI, increased catecholamines (norepinephrine and epinephrine) are released. The increased sympathetic nervous system stimulation results in diaphoresis and vasoconstriction of peripheral blood vessels. On physical examination, the patient's skin will be ashen, clammy, and cool. This condition is often referred to as a "cold sweat."

Fever. The temperature may increase within the first 24 hours up to 100.4° F (38° C) and occasionally to 102.2° F (39° C). The temperature elevation may last for as long as 1 week. This increase in temperature is a systemic manifestation of the inflammatory process caused by cell death in the infarcted myocardium.

Cardiovascular Manifestations. The BP and heart rate may be elevated initially. Later the BP may drop because of decreased CO. Urine output may be decreased. Crackles may be noted in the lungs, persisting for several hours to several days. Hepatic engorgement and peripheral edema may indicate overt cardiac failure. Jugular veins may be distended and may have obvious pulsations, indicating early right ventricular dysfunction and pulmonary congestion.

Cardiac examination may reveal abnormal precordial movements suggestive of ventricular aneurysm. Heart sounds may seem distant, but close auscultation may reveal splitting of heart sounds, indicating LV dysfunction. Other abnormal sounds suggesting ventricular dysfunction are S_3 and S_4. In addition, the presence of murmurs may indicate valve incompetency. A loud holosystolic apical murmur may indicate valve incompetency or a septal defect. A loud holosystolic apical murmur may occur as a result of papillary muscle rupture.

Complications

Arrhythmias. The most common complications after an MI are arrhythmias, present in 80% of MI patients. Arrhythmias are caused by any condition that affects the myocardial cell's sensitivity to nerve impulses, such as ischemia, electrolyte imbalances, and sympathetic nervous system stimulation. The intrinsic rhythm of the heartbeat is disrupted, causing either a fast HR (tachycardia), a slow HR (bradycardia), or an irregular beat, all of which adversely affect the ischemic myocardium.

Life-threatening arrhythmias occur most often with anterior wall infarction, pump failure, and shock. Complete heart block is seen in massive infarction. Ventricular fibrillation, a common cause of sudden death, is a lethal arrhythmia that most often occurs within the first 4 hours after the onset of pain. Premature ventricular contractions (PVCs) may precede ventricular tachycardia and fibrillation. Ventricular arrhythmias must be treated immediately. (See Chapter 34 for a detailed description of arrhythmias and their management.)

Congestive Heart Failure. Congestive heart failure (CHF) is a complication that occurs when the pumping power of the heart has diminished. In the patient with an acute MI it is common to see some degree of LV dysfunction in the first 24 hours. Depending on the severity and extent of the injury, CHF occurs initially with subtle signs such as slight dyspnea, restlessness, agitation, or slight tachycardia. Jugular vein distention from right-sided heart failure, crackles heard in the lungs, distention of upper lobe veins on an upright chest x-ray, and the presence of an S_3 or S_4 heart sound may indicate the onset of heart failure. (The treatment of acute CHF is discussed in Chapter 33.)

Cardiogenic Shock. Cardiogenic shock occurs when inadequate oxygen and nutrients are supplied to the tissues because of severe LV failure. It occurs when there is loss of function of at least 40% of the LV because of infarction. Cardiogenic shock occurs less often since the advent of thrombolytic therapy and acute coronary intervention, but when it occurs, it carries a high mortality rate. It often requires aggressive management, including control of arrhythmias, intraaortic balloon pump therapy, and support of contractility with the use of vasoactive drugs. The goal of therapy is to maximize oxygen delivery and prevent complications such as acute renal failure.

Papillary Muscle Dysfunction. Papillary muscle dysfunction may occur if the infarcted area includes or is adjacent to these structures. Papillary muscle dysfunction causes mitral valve regurgitation, which increases the volume of blood in the left atrium. This condition aggravates an already compromised LV. It is detected by a systolic murmur at the cardiac apex radiating toward the axilla. Papillary muscle rupture is a severe complication causing massive mitral valve regurgitation, which results in dyspnea, gross pulmonary edema, and decreased CO. Treatment consists of rapid afterload reduction with nitroprusside or intraaortic balloon pumping and immediate open heart surgery with mitral valve replacement.

Ventricular Aneurysm. Ventricular aneurysm results when the infarcted myocardial wall becomes thinned and bulges out during contraction (Fig. 32-15). In the acute stage after MI this is termed an *ischemic bulge.* If the aneurysm still exists after scar tissue is laid down, it is termed a *ventricular aneurysm.* Ventricular aneurysms are identified by palpation of ectopic impulses; bulges seen on x-ray, echocardiogram, or fluoroscopy; or persistent, long-term ST segment changes on an ECG. Ventricular angiography can definitively diagnose ventricular aneurysm.

The patient with a ventricular aneurysm may experience intractable CHF, arrhythmias, and angina. Besides ventricular rupture, which is fatal, ventricular aneurysms harbor thrombi, cause arrhythmias, and promote LV dysfunction. Surgical excision is the treatment for ventricular aneurysms severe enough to cause dysfunction.

Pericarditis. Acute pericarditis, an inflammation of the visceral or parietal pericardium, or both, may result in cardiac compression, decreased ventricular filling and emptying, and cardiac failure.[34] It may occur 2 to 3 days after an acute MI as a common complication of the infarction. Chest pain, which may vary from mild to severe, is aggravated by inspiration, coughing, and movement of the upper body and usually accompanies acute pericarditis. The pain may radiate to the back and down to the left arm, making it difficult to differentiate from an acute MI. The pain may be relieved by sitting in a forward position.

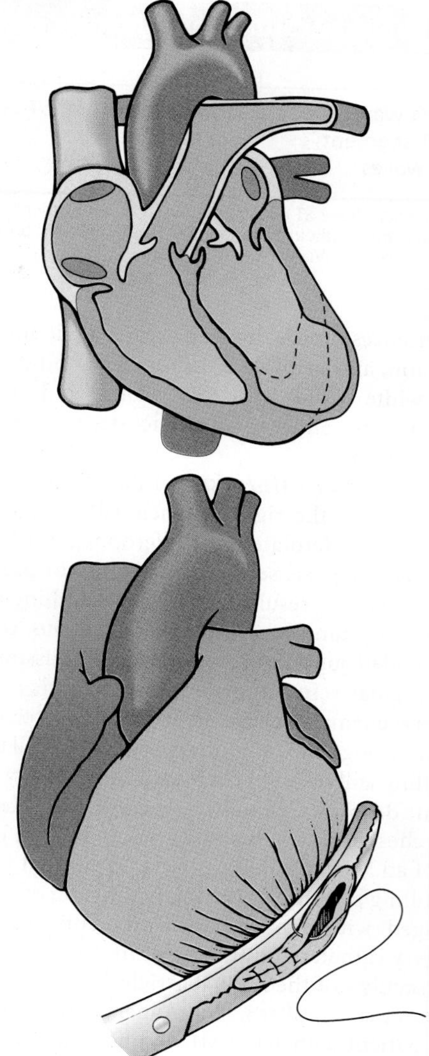

Fig. 32-15 Ventricular aneurysm and surgical repair.

Assessment of the patient with pericarditis may reveal a friction rub over the pericardium. The sound may be best heard with the diaphragm of the stethoscope at the mid to lower sternal border. It may be persistent or intermittent. Fever may also be present.

Diagnosis of pericarditis can be made with serial 12-lead ECGs. ECG changes reflect the inflammation and may produce characteristic ST-T segment elevations that are persistent. Treatment may include pain relief by aspirin, corticosteroids, or nonsteroidal antiinflammatory drugs.

Dressler's Syndrome. Dressler's syndrome (post-MI syndrome) is characterized by pericarditis with effusion and fever that develops 1 to 4 weeks after MI. It may also occur after open heart surgery. It is thought to be caused by an antigen-antibody reaction to the necrotic myocardium. The

Table 32-13 Electrocardiogram Changes with Myocardial Infarction*

Phase I	Phase II	Phase III	Phase IV
Abnormal Q waves Elevated ST segment Inverted T waves	Gradual return of ST segment to baseline	Return of T waves to normal or near-normal configuration	Remnant Q wave

*Inferior wall infarction shows ST elevation, T inversion, and pathophysiologic Q wave in leads II, III, and aVF; inferolateral and posterolateral wall infarction shows reduced R and T inversion, with or without ST elevation in V_5, V_6, and aVL; posterior wall infarction shows mirror image of normal ECG; anterior wall infarction shows typical infarction pattern in leads I, aVL, V_2-V_6.

patient experiences pericardial pain, fever, a friction rub, left pleural effusion, and arthralgia. Laboratory findings include an elevated white blood cell (WBC) count and an elevated sedimentation rate. Short-term corticosteroids are used to treat this condition.

Right Ventricular Infarction. Infarctions that primarily cause damage to the right ventricle (RV) are often seen with large inferior, inferolateral, or inferoposterior MIs. These RV infarctions can cause severe compromise of perfusion to the pulmonary system resulting in decreased filling of the LV. The patient will manifest symptoms of venous congestion such as distended jugular veins often with Kussmaul's sign (bulging of jugular veins on inspiration), hepatic congestion, and peripheral edema. Because the RV is unable to adequately pump blood through the pulmonary system and fill the LV, reduced LV filling will result in decreased contractility of the LV, hypotension, drop in CO, and tachycardia. ST elevation of right-sided chest leads (V_3 R and V_4 R) can be seen in the first few hours of an MI causing RV infarct. Treatment is aimed at increasing filling pressure of the LV by infusion of fluids carefully managed with pressure measurements using a pulmonary artery catheter and the use of inotropic agents to increase contractility of the right ventricle.[35]

Pulmonary Embolism. Pulmonary embolism may be seen in the patient with acute MI who has had bouts of CHF or arrhythmias or has been extremely immobile because of prolonged bed rest. The source of the thrombus may be the roughened endocardium or leg veins. Early detection of emboli is accomplished by observing for pallor or cyanosis, heart failure unresponsive to treatment, and an unexplained pleural effusion. Acute massive pulmonary embolism causes sudden, severe dyspnea and is usually fatal. (Pulmonary emboli are discussed in more detail in Chapter 36.)

Diagnostic Studies

Common diagnostic parameters used to determine whether a person has sustained an acute MI include (1) the patient's history of pain, risk factors, and health history; (2) 12-lead ECG consistent with acute MI (ST-T wave elevations of greater than 1 mm or more in two contiguous leads); and (3) serial measurement of myocardial serum enzymes and troponin.

Clinical Presentation. The patient's clinical presentation is important. However, many patients do not have the classic unrelenting chest pain characteristic of acute MI. The patient may complain of a feeling of weakness, severe indigestion, shortness of breath, or chest discomfort. Risk factor analysis may indicate the patient's propensity for an acute event. Any patient's presentation that is suggestive of an acute MI should be treated as quickly as possible to rule out an infarction.

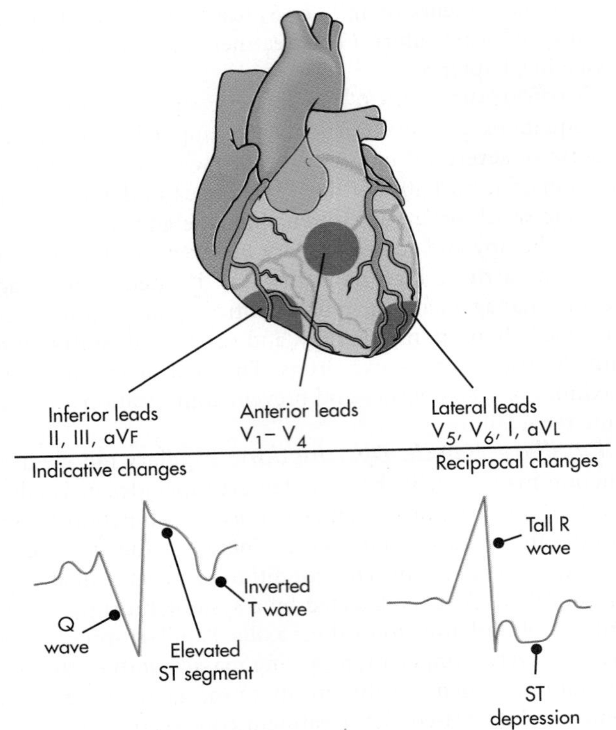

Fig. 32-16 Indicative changes occur in leads that examine the area of infarction. Reciprocal changes occur in leads opposite the area of infarction.

Electrocardiogram Findings. Serial ECGs are approximately 80% specific for diagnosing an acute MI and represent a leading diagnostic criterion. Areas of ischemia or infarction may be noted on the ECG. Changes in rate and rhythm of the heart may also be diagnostic for abnormalities. Because the acute infarction is a dynamic process that occurs with time, the ECG may reveal the time sequence of ischemia, injury, infarction, and resolution of the infarction (Table 32-13).

The 12-lead ECG may be normal when the patient comes to the emergency department (ED) with a complaint of pain typical of ischemic chest pain, but within a few hours it may have changed to show the infarction process. These changes take place when cellular damage has occurred, interrupting the normal electrical depolarization. Because many patients with an acute MI have nondiagnostic ECGs on admission to an ED, it is important to do repeat ECGs on patients every 30 minutes to 2 hours while in the ED.

Figure 32-16 correlates the anatomy with areas of infarction and with changes that occur on the 12-lead ECG. Changes that are present in the leads that examine infarcted areas of the heart

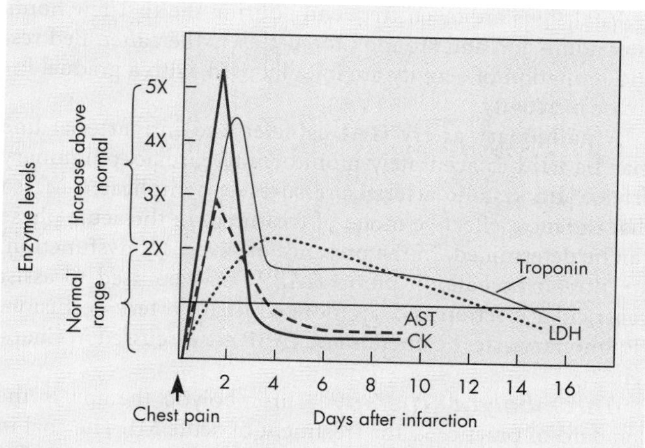

Fig. 32-17 Serum cardiac markers in the blood after myocardial infarction. *AST,* aspartate aminotransferase; *CK,* creatine kinase; *LDH,* lactic dehydrogenase.

are called *indicative changes* (i.e., they are indicative of infarction). Changes in the leads opposite infarcted areas are called *reciprocal changes.*

In general the area of infarction correlates more closely with side effects and complications than with mortality rates. With inferior wall damage, AV blocks are commonly seen because the right coronary artery perfuses the SA and AV node tissue in 80% to 90% of people. CHF, LV aneurysms, cardiogenic shock, and complete heart block are more frequently seen with anterior MI because the front surface of the LV and part of the septum are damaged. An inferior wall MI may also cause CHF, arrhythmias, and cardiogenic shock.

Serum Cardiac Markers. Certain proteins, called serum cardiac markers, are released into the blood in large quantities from necrotic heart muscle after an MI. These markers, specifically cardiac serum enzymes and troponin, are important diagnostic criteria for an acute MI. The cardiac enzymes are creatine kinase (CK), lactic dehydrogenase (LDH), and aspartate aminotransferase (AST). When cardiac cells die, their cellular enzymes are released into circulation. The increase in serum enzymes that occurs after cellular death can demonstrate whether cardiac damage is present and the approximate extent of the damage. Because there are no cardiac muscle–specific enzymes for AST, its use in diagnosing an MI has decreased. (Figure 32-17 indicates the peak level and duration of these markers in the presence of MI.) Other causes of increased serum enzymes may make the differential diagnosis more difficult. These include pulmonary embolism, intramuscular damage, seizure activity, cardiopulmonary resuscitation, and other muscle-damaging events.

CK levels begin to rise approximately 4 to 6 hours after an acute MI and return to normal within 3 to 4 days. The CK enzymes may be fractionated into bands, including the MB band. The MB band is specific to the myocardial cell and may more specifically quantify myocardial damage. Depending on the individual laboratory, MB bands greater than 3% indicate MI.

Troponin is a myocardial muscle protein released into circulation after an injury. In the heart there are two subtypes: troponin T and troponin I. Cardiac-specific troponin T (cTnT) and cardiac-specific troponin I (cTnI) have different amino acid sequences than skeletal muscle forms of these proteins. Therefore these markers are highly specific indicators of MI.

Troponin rises as quickly as CK and remains elevated for 2 weeks. It is usually used in conjunction with total CK and the MB fraction, but has replaced LDH in many institutions.[36]

Although the traditional cardiac enzymes are excellent diagnostic indicators of an acute MI, they are not immediately available to the physician or nurse because the laboratory needs time to analyze the results. Now there are rapid whole blood bedside assays for serum cardiac markers. They facilitate management decisions, especially in patients with nondiagnostic ECGs. These markers aid in the rapid diagnosis of acute MI. All of these tests are not yet available in every clinical facility. (Cardiac enzyme studies and troponin are also discussed in Chapter 30.)

Myoglobin is released into circulation within only a few hours after an MI. Although it is one of the first serum cardiac markers that increases after an MI, it lacks cardiac specificity. In addition, it is rapidly excreted in urine so that blood levels return to normal range within 24 hours after an MI.

Other Measures. For the assessment of cardiac size and pulmonary congestion, an initial chest x-ray is helpful but not diagnostic of an acute MI. The appearance of distended upper lobe veins may indicate early LV dysfunction. The WBC count may rise to 12,000 to 14,000/μl (12 to 14 $\times 10^9$/L) or higher. Increases in fasting blood glucose levels to 300 mg/dl (16.7 mmol/L) may also occur secondary to the body's stress response to injury.

Nuclear imaging has become increasingly important in establishing the diagnosis of MI. It is considered an extremely sensitive indicator of myocardial damage. Myocardial nuclear scans, done by injecting IV radioactive isotopes, can help establish the diagnosis of acute MI when other data are inconclusive. After an IV injection of thallium, the amount of thallium present in each myocardial region is determined by two factors: the amount of coronary blood flow to that region and the degree of viable myocardium. Ischemia or infarcted myocardial regions receiving little or no coronary blood flow accumulate little or no thallium. Such regions appear as cold spots on the scan and thus indicate an area of ischemia or infarct. However, this technique does not differentiate old from new infarcts.

Technetium pyrophosphate scanning can be used to localize areas of acute necrosis. When given intravenously to the patient, technetium complexes with calcium in necrotic myocardial tissue. An area of infarct is visualized as a zone of increased radionuclide uptake and thus derives the name *hot spot.* Optimum time for imaging after an acute MI is 24 to 48 hours, but the scan may remain positive for as long as 10 days. (Nuclear imaging is also described in Chapter 30 and Table 30-7.)

Collaborative Care

Initial management of the patient with MI is best accomplished in a cardiac care unit (CCU), where constant monitoring is available. Arrhythmias may be detected by the nurse trained in continuous ECG monitoring techniques, and appropriate treatment can be instituted. An IV route is established to provide an accessible means for emergency drug therapy. Morphine sulfate or meperidine may be given intravenously for relief of pain. Oxygen is usually administered by nasal cannula at a rate of 2 to 4 L per minute. The collaborative care management of MI is presented in Table 32-14,

COLLABORATIVE CARE

Table 32-14 Myocardial Infarction

Diagnostic
- History and physical examination
- Serum enzyme levels (e.g., CK, LDH)
- Cardiac troponin
- 12-lead ECG
- Chest x-ray
- CBC, thyroid profile
- Nuclear imaging studies
- Echocardiography
- Cardiac catheterization

Collaborative Therapy

Acute Care
- IV therapy
- Continual ECG monitoring
- Morphine sulfate IV 2-4 mg every 5 min or as needed (meperidine if patient is allergic to morphine)
- Nitroglycerin IV
- Oxygen therapy
- Monitoring of vital signs every 1-4 hr
- Lidocaine IV drip infusion (if ordered)
- Thrombolytic therapy (if indicated)
- Anticoagulant therapy (e.g., heparin IV)
- Inotropic drugs
- β-Adrenergic blockers
- ACE inhibitors
- Antithrombotic therapy (e.g., ASA)
- Antiarrhythmic drugs
- Bed rest with progressive activity
- Recording of intake and output
- Percutaneous transluminal coronary angioplasty (PTCA)
- Coronary artery bypass graft (CABG)

Ambulatory/Home Care
- ASA 80-325 mg per day
- Patient education (see Table 32-22)
- Progressive rehabilitation program (see Tables 32-21 and 32-23)
- Dietary restrictions, if necessary (see Table 32-5)
- Management of risk factors for CAD (see Table 32-4)

ACE, angiotensin-converting enzyme; *ASA*, acetylsalicylic acid; *CAD*, coronary artery disease; *CBC*, complete blood count; *CK*, creatine kinase; *LDH*, lactic dehydrogenase.

and typical admission orders containing diagnosis and treatment orders are shown in Table 32-15. A clinical pathway for care of the patient with acute myocardial infarction is provided on p. 868.

A continuous IV infusion of lidocaine may be given to the patient who has frequent PVCs which may precede ventricular fibrillation. The use of prophylactic lidocaine is not currently recommended by the American College of Cardiology (ACC)/AHA Practice Guidelines for the treatment of acute MI unless the patient has sustained ventricular tachycardia or ventricular fibrillation.[37]

Vital signs are taken frequently during the first few hours after admission and are monitored closely thereafter. Bed rest and limitation of activity are initially used, with a gradual increase in activity.

A pulmonary artery (PA) catheter and intraarterial line may be used to accurately monitor intracardiac, pulmonary artery, and systolic arterial pressures in complicated MI so that the most effective mode of treatment in the acute phase can be determined. In the presence of severe LV dysfunction, an intraaortic balloon pump (IABP) may be used to assist ventricular ejection and promote coronary artery perfusion. (Pulmonary artery catheters and IABP are discussed in Chapter 63.)

Thrombolytic Therapy. Thrombolytic therapy is the standard of practice in the treatment of acute MI. The goal in the treatment of acute MI is to salvage as much myocardial muscle as possible. Historically, treatment of acute MI had been directed only at the patient's signs and symptoms (i.e., arrhythmia and CHF), and nothing was done for the acute process of infarction. This treatment modality decreased mortality rates from 30% to approximately 15% in the 1970s. With the advent of thrombolytic therapy, treatment has progressed to actually stopping the infarction process instead of just treating symptoms. In the 1990s mortality rates have decreased to 2.5% to 5% with thrombolytic treatment.[37,38]

It is now known that 80% to 90% of all acute MIs are secondary to thrombus formation.[34,37,38,39] Perfusion to the myocardium distal to the occlusion is halted, causing progressive ischemia, cell death, necrosis, and acute MI. The acute MI process takes time. The earliest tissue to become ischemic is the subendocardium (the innermost layer of tissue in the cardiac muscle). Necrosis spreads toward the epicardium in a phenomenon termed the *wave front of necrosis*.[37] Myocardial cells do not die instantly. It takes approximately 4 to 6 hours for the entire thickness of the muscle to become necrosed in the majority of patients; this is termed a *transmural infarction.*

Treatment of the acute MI is geared to quickly dissolve the thrombus in the coronary artery and reperfuse the myocardium before cellular death occurs. To be of most benefit, thrombolytics must be given as soon as possible, preferably within that first 6 hours after the onset of pain. If reperfusion occurs within that time, a 25% reduction in mortality rate has been shown.[38]

Indications and contraindications. The commonly used thrombolytics (Table 32-16) can be given by the intracoronary or IV route. IV thrombolytic therapy is preferred because it can be given quickly, with excellent results in opening the artery. Although these drugs have different mechanisms of action and different pharmacokinetics, they all produce an open artery by lysis of the thrombus in the coronary artery.

Because all the thrombolytics produce lysis of the pathologic clot, they may also lyse homeostatic clots (such as in the stomach or over a postoperative site). Therefore patient selection is important because persons receiving thrombolytic therapy may have a minor or major bleeding episode as a consequence of therapy. Not all patients who have an acute MI are candidates for thrombolytic therapy (Table 32-17). Inclusion criteria to receive an IV thrombolytic agent are (1) chest pain typical of acute MI less than or equal to 6 hours in duration

Table 32-15 Cardiac Care Unit Admission Orders

Admission

Continuous monitor, rhythm strips, and arrhythmia analysis
Vital signs q2hr for first 8 hr, then q4hr from 6 AM to midnight or as needed
Intake and output hourly
IV infusion of 500 ml 5% dextrose and water to keep vein open
Diet: Determined by condition of patient _clear liquids and advance as tolerated_
Daily weight ✓
(Must be checked if wish to have done)
Oxygen 3 L/min by cannula or 5-8 L/min by mask
Absolute bed rest with bathroom privileges for 24 hr

CPR*

Defibrillation with 200 joules for ventricular fibrillation
Type of resuscitation:
DNR ______ EPS (treatment of arrhythmias and defibrillation only—no CPR to be done) ______ Full ACLS ✓

Arrhythmias

Lidocaine 75-100 mg bolus, then IV drip (500 ml 5% dextrose in water with 2 g lidocaine) of 2-4 mg/min for PVCs more than 6/min, R-on-T, multifocal or sequential PVCs at a rate >110
Atropine 0.5-1.0 mg IV for ventricular rate <50 with BP <90 and/or symptoms of poor cerebral perfusion

Medication

Pain
Severe _Morphine Sulfate 2-4 mg IV every 5 min. until relief_
Mild _Acetaminophen 650 mg PO every 3-4 hr._
Hypnotic _Restoril 15 mg po hs MR x 1_
Laxative _MOM 30 cc q hs prn_ Stool softener _Colace 100 mg PO bid_
Antiemetic —
Antithrombotic _ASA i po q am_
Anticoagulant _(5% dextrose in water) Heparin 25,000 U/500 ml to run at 1000 U/hr; titrate to maintain PTT 1 1/2 - 2X baseline per unit protocol_

Laboratory

Cardiac profile on admittance and q8hr x 3
ECG Dates _4/5, 4/6, 4/7_
Serum K^+ every other day while in CCU, PTT every am while on heparin
Routine lab UA, CBC, serum electrolytes, PTT
Other _Chest x-ray on admittance (if not done in ED)_

*By certified personnel only.
ACLS, Advanced cardiac life support; *ASA,* acetylsalicyclic acid; *CCU,* cardiac care unit; *DNR,* do not resuscitate; *EPS,* electrophysiology study; *ED,* emergency department; *PO,* by mouth; *PRN,* as required; *PTT,* partial thromboplastin time; *PVC,* premature ventricular contraction; *UA,* urinary analysis.

(some centers extend the time limit to 12 hours); (2) chest pain for more than 6 hours if intermittent with ongoing ischemia; (3) 12-lead ECG findings consistent with acute MI, irrespective of location; and (4) no condition that may cause a predisposition to hemorrhage.[37]

Procedure. Once the patient has been assessed in the ED for risk factors of possible side effects of the therapy and is considered a candidate, IV thrombolysis can begin. An agent is selected according to the patient's profile and the physician's preference. Each hospital has a protocol to follow for administration of thrombolytic agents. However, there are several common factors. Blood is drawn, three lines for IV therapy are started, and all other invasive procedures are done before the thrombolytic agent is given, reducing the possibility of bleeding in the patient.

The time therapy begins is noted, and the patient is monitored frequently during the dose and maintenance protocol. ECG, vital signs, and heart and lung assessments are completed as often as every 5 minutes to evaluate the patient's response to therapy. When reperfusion occurs (i.e., the coronary artery that was occluded is patent, and blood flow is reestablished to the myocardium), several clinical markers may occur. These include chest pain resolution; return of ST segment to baseline on the ECG; the presence of reperfusion arrhythmias; and marked, rapid rise of the CK enzyme within 3 hours of therapy, peaking within 12 hours. The CK levels increase as the dead myocardial cells release CK enzymes into the circulation after perfusion has been restored to the area.

The nurse must closely monitor the patient for signs of reperfusion arrhythmias, including an increase in premature ventricular contractions, ventricular tachycardia, ventricular fibrillation, and accelerated idioventricular rhythm. Sometimes bradycardia, AV blocks, and asystole can occur, depending on the location of the infarction. Unfortunately, these clinical markers do not always occur when the artery opens. If they do occur, the nurse should document their presence and have another ECG done.

CLINICAL PATHWAY Acute Myocardial Infarction

Admit Date:	DRG: 122	LOS: 4 days	Discharge Date: ____

Pathway				
Critical Path Implemented	**ER-ICU Day 1**	**ICU Day 2**	**PCU Day 3**	**PCU Day 4**
Diagnostic Studies	▪ CMP ▪ Mg ▪ Myoglobin ▪ Troponin ▪ PT/PTT ▪ Chest x-ray ▪ Pulse ox stat; consider ABGs ▪ ECG ▪ LDH, AST,CK q8hx2 after initial labs	▪ ECHO ▪ Consider cardiac enzymes (LDH, AST, CK) 24 hr after initial series	▪ Holter ▪ Consider SAECG (if low EF or significant V. ectopy on Holter)	▪ Consider modified ETT, and discharge if negative ▪ Consider OP Card. Cath if modified ETT is positive
Treatments	▪ Initiate thrombolytic therapy protocol within 30-60 min of arrival to ER on appropriate candidates, then transfer to ICU. ▪ Oxygen ____ L/min continuous via NC ▪ Cardiac monitoring ▪ Pulse ox continuous ▪ If Pt. experiences chest pain, obtain ECG and give SL NTG, notify physician			
IV/Meds	▪ IV ______ @ ___cc/Hr ▪ NTG drip ▪ Heparin ▪ MS IVP ▪ Antidysrhythmics ▪ SL NTG ▪ ASA ▪ Stool softener ▪ Beta blocker ▪ Consider nitrates		▪ Initiate weaning from drips	▪ Order discharge medications
Consults	▪ Cardiology	▪ Cardiac Rehab ▪ Nutrition Services		▪ Consider Home Health Care visits
Team Directives	( ) Evaluate ECG strips q shift and prn for rhythm, ST segment analysis, ectopy. ( ) Monitor Pt.'s response to thrombolytics; assess hourly for bleeding while on thrombolytics and anticoagulation Rx. ( ) VS per ICU/PCU routine. Daily weights. Strict I & O. ( ) Monitor CP for site, duration, quality, radiation and assess for pain relief using 0-5 pain scale. Notify physician of increasing CP, ST elevations, or changes in cardiac rhythm. ( ) Physical assessment per ICU/PCU routine. Cardiopulmonary assessment q2h and prn. ( ) Monitor and trend lab values. (sign/date/time)____/____/____, ____/____/____ ( ) Monitor and trend hemodynamic status ____/____/____, ____/____/____ ( ) Provide emotional support and assist in reducing Pt./family anxiety by allowing visitation and providing information.			
Diet	▪ NPO/Clear Liquid Diet. Advance as tolerated to 2/gm Na, low cholesterol, no caffeine.			
Activity & Safety	( ) Routine safety measures ( ) Bed rest with beside commode ( ) Initiate cardiac step levels ( ) Active & passive ROM	( ) Frequent rest periods (sign/date/time) ____/____/____ ____/____/____	( ) Cardiac step level ____ ____/____/____	( ) Cardiac step level ____ ____/____/____
Teaching Patient & Family	( ) Orient to unit ( ) Provide updated information to Pt./family routinely and frequently to enable them to make informed care decisions and to assist in their coping process. ( ) Explain the 0-5 pain scale to describe chest pain/discomfort ( ) Explain cardiac step levels ( ) Explain the MI pathway ____/____/____, ____/____/____		( ) Explain all tests and procedures ( ) Initiate the Acute MI teaching plan ( ) Teach Pt./family how to take a pulse ( ) Diet education initiated (sign/date/time) ____/____/____, ____/____/____	
Discharge Planning	( ) Risk screening referrals from Database initiated ( ) SW and Nursing Case Management initiated discharge planning ( ) Advance Directives reviewed ( ) Referral to Cardiac rehab initiated ____/____/____, ____/____/____ (sign/date/time)		( ) Facilitate physician/family discussion to plan for post-hospitalization care needs ( ) Assess need for follow-up care consults/ referrals and confer with physician for orders ____/____/____, ____/____/____	

Continued

Author: Molly Metzler, RN, BSN for Nanticoke Health Services. Licensed by the Center for Case Management, South Natick, MA Nanticoke Health Services.

CLINICAL PATHWAY Acute Myocardial Infarction—continued

Expected Outcomes DRG: 122 LOS: 4 days

Meets Expected Outcomes (initial)	ER-ICU Day 1	MET	NOT	ICU Day 2	MET	NOT	PCU Day 3	MET	NOT	PCU Day 4	MET	NOT
Chest Pain: Related to myocardial ischemic process. ▪ Pt. describes chest pain as crushing, tightness in sternal area, pain extending down arm ▪ Dyspnea ▪ Cyanosis ▪ Altered muscle tone ▪ Diaphoresis ▪ BP & pulse changes ▪ Abnormal cardiac enzymes	▪ Pt. is pain free within 30 min of arrival to ER ___/N ▪ Thrombolytics initiated within 30 min of arrival to ER___/N ▪ Pt. able to describe pain using 0-5 pain scale___/N ▪ Respiratory symptoms improved after O_2___/RC or N ▪ VS stabilizing ___/N ▪ Color improved after O_2___/N			▪ Pain is managed with medications and comfort measures___/N ▪ Pulse ox ≥93% on O_2/RC or N ▪ VS continue to stabilize___/N ▪ Pt./Family aware of factors that intensify pain and modifies behavior accordingly___/N ▪ No dyspnea, cyanosis, or diaphoresis___/N ▪ Muscle tone relaxing___/N ▪ Lab values normalizing___/N			▪ No new episodes of chest pain ___/N ▪ Pulse ox ≥93% on prn O_2___/RC or N ▪ VS stable___/N ▪ Pt. is comfortable ___/N ▪ No dyspnea___/N ▪ Color pink___/N ▪ No diaphoresis ___/N ▪ Pt. is able to relax ___/N ▪ Labs stabilizing ___/N			▪ Pt./Family know how to manage pain with medication and nonpharmaceutical measures once discharged ___/N ▪ Pt./Family know when and how to access EMS if chest pain returns ___/N		
Altered CO: Related to ischemic myocardial muscle damage and risk of bleeding from treatment. ▪ BP <90 systolic ▪ HR >100/min with rhythm changes ▪ RR >20/min ▪ UO <30 cc/hour ▪ Bleeding/ Hemorrhage from thrombolytics or heparin ▪ Bruising from heparin Rx	▪ BP ≥90 systolic ___/N ▪ HR ≤90/min ___/N ▪ Rhythm stabilizing with medications ___/N ▪ RR ≤20/min and stabilizing on O_2___/RC or N ▪ UO ≥30 cc/hr___/N ▪ Safety precautions to minimize/prevent bleeding implemented ___/N			▪ Hemodynamic stabilization achieved within 24 hrs of admission___/N ▪ VS stabilizing___/N ▪ ECG evolving with ST segment returning to baseline___/N ▪ UO >30/cc/Hr___/N ▪ No bleeding/bruising evident___/N			▪ Pt. remains hemodynamically stable___/N ▪ VS stable___/N ▪ ECG evolving with ST segment returning to baseline___/N ▪ No bleeding/ bruising___/N			▪ Pt.'s CO stable___/N ▪ Pt. is fluid-volume stable___/N ▪ Pt. knows signs and symptoms of bleeding and to report bleeding/ excess bruising to PCP and/or cardiologist ___/N		
Anxiety: Related to a life-threatening illness: ▪ Inability to focus and cope ▪ Chest pain, rapid pulse, hyperventilation, nausea, sweating, constipation or diarrhea ▪ Insomnia, restlessness ▪ Feelings of fear, denial, uncertainty, regret, apprehension	▪ Pt./Family are provided with up-to-date information for care decisions and to help reduce fear___/N ▪ Pt./Family follow simple instructions ___/N ▪ Pt./Family express that they are anxious ___/N			▪ Pt./Family able to state the cause of their anxiety___/N ▪ Pt./Family perform stress reduction techniques to reduce anxiety___/N ▪ Pt./Family identify support systems to assist with coping___/N			▪ Pt. effectively performing relaxation techniques to reduce stress and anxiety___/N ▪ Pt./Family involved in care decisions and demonstrate the development of coping skills___/N			▪ Pt. demonstrates a decrease in physical manifestations of anxiety___/N ▪ Support systems to enable effective coping in place for discharge ___/N		

Continued

Another major concern with therapy is reocclusion of the artery. In this situation the patient seems to have a reperfused artery and is stable. However, because the area around the thrombus is unstable, another clot may form or spasm of the artery may occur. Because of this possibility, most physicians begin heparin therapy. An IV bolus is given, followed by a heparin drip to maintain the patient's partial thromboplastin time (PTT) at one to two times normal. This prevents another clot from forming in the coronary artery. If another clot develops, the patient has similar complaints of chest pain, ECG changes, and hemodynamic compromise. The physician is notified and further action is taken to determine the cause of the reocclusion. The patient may go to the cardiac catheterization laboratory for further invasive diagnostic procedures or PTCA. Sometimes the patient will again receive thrombolytic therapy.

The major complication with thrombolytic therapy is bleeding. The patient is receiving an agent that causes clot dissolution, and this may cause the patient to bleed. Prevention of bleeding is essential, and proper patient selection and

CLINICAL PATHWAY Acute Myocardial Infarction—continued

Expected Outcomes	DRG: 122						LOS: 4 days					
Meets Expected Outcomes (initial)	**ER-ICU Day 1**	MET	NOT	**ICU Day 2**	MET	NOT	**PCU Day 3**	MET	NOT	**PCU Day 4**	MET	NOT
Activity Intolerance: Imbalance of O_2 supply and demand from decreased cardiac output. ■ Dyspnea on exertion ■ Easily fatigued ■ Chest pain/discomfort ■ ECG changes reflecting ischemia ■ VS changes with increased activity	■ Pt./Family understand the importanct of rest in recovery from an acute MI___/N ■ Pt. able to identify activities that precipitate CP___/N ■ Pt. modifies activities accordingly with frequent rest periods___/N			■ No dyspnea on exertion noted___/N ■ ECG stabilizing with minimal activity level ___/N ■ Pt. able to tolerate OOB to BSC/chair without dyspnea___/N ■ VS remain stable with increased activity ___/N			■ Progressing through cardiac step levels without dyspnea, or ECG changes___/N ■ RR ≤24/min with increases in activity ___/N ■ HR ≤110 min/or within 20/min of resting HR with increases in activity ___/N ■ Cardiac rehab program reviewed with Pt./family ___/Cardiac Rehab or N			■ Pt./Family understand activity limits and restrictions for discharge___/N ■ Cardiac rehab in place post-discharge___/N ■ VS stable with ADLs___/N ■ NSR on monitor___/N		
Knowledge Deficit: Acute MI and implications for lifestyle changes. ■ Diet ■ Exercise/Activity ■ Smoking cessation ■ Possible changes in alcohol consumption ■ Medications ■ Disease process ■ Risk factors ■ Stress reduction ■ Importance of medical follow up and compliance with treatment regimen ■ When and how to access EMS	■ Pt. understands importance of notifying nurse of chest pain/discomfort ___/N ■ Pt. understands 0-5 pain scale and is able to describe pain in terms of quality, intensity, duration, radiation, and relief ___/N ■ Pt./Family understand activity restrictions___/N ■ Pt./Family understand the diagnosis of Acute MI___/N			■ Pt./Family understand the cardiac step level progression___/N ■ Dietary modifications discussed with Nutrition Services___/NS or N ■ Pt./Family verbalize activities that promote relaxation and reduce stress___/N ■ Pt./Family demonstrate readiness to learn about MI disease process___/N			■ Pt./Family identify risk factors for MI___/N ■ Pt./Family verbalize understanding of relationship between angina, CVD, and MI___/N ■ Pt./Family verbalize understanding of basis dietary parameters for CVD___/NS or N ■ Pt./Family have discussed med regimen with PCP/RX or cardiologist and verbalize understanding of regimen___/Rx or N ■ Pt./Family member able to take own pulse ___/N			■ Pt./Family verbalize understanding of med regimen___/Rx or N ■ Pt./Family have completed initial MI teaching process and are scheduled for rehab___/CardRehab or N ■ Pt./Family have discussed potential for OP cardiac cath with PCP/Cardiologist and procedure is scheduled ___/CardRehab or N ■ Pt./Family understand importance of follow-up medical care___/N ■ Pt./Family verbalize understanding of discharge instructions ___/N		
UNMET OUTCOMES: (CCC Initials Required)	7-3p ( ) Resolved ( ) Planned /RN			7-3p ( ) Resolved ( ) Planned /RN			7-3p ( ) Resolved ( ) Planned /RN			7-3p ( ) Resolved ( ) Planned /RN		
	3-7p ( ) Resolved ( ) Planned /RN			3-7p ( ) Resolved ( ) Planned /RN			3-7p ( ) Resolved ( ) Planned /RN			3-7p ( ) Resolved ( ) Planned /RN		
	7-11p ( ) Resolved ( ) Planned /RN			7-11p ( ) Resolved ( ) Planned /RN			7-11p ( ) Resolved ( ) Planned /RN			7-11p ( ) Resolved ( ) Planned /RN		
	11-7a ( ) Resolved ( ) Planned /RN			11-7a ( ) Resolved ( ) Planned /RN			11-7a ( ) Resolved ( ) Planned /RN			11-7a ( ) Resolved ( ) Planned /RN		

Service

CM - Care Management	RX - Pharmacist	HC - Home Care
ET - Ostomy/Skin Care	SL - Speech/Language	DR - Physician
RC - Respiratory Care	CCC - Primary RN Clinical Care Coord.	Card - Cardiology
N - Nurse	SW - Social Work	Rad - Radiology
PT - Physical Therapy	OT - Occupational Therapy	Rehab - Cardiac, Respiratory
NS - Nutrition Services		

Patient informed of plan: ____________________

Health care provider signature, date, time:

screening are imperative. Ongoing nursing assessment is also essential. Minor bleeding is expected. If minor bleeding does occur (such as surface bleeding from IV sites or gingival bleeding), it can be controlled by pressure dressing or ice packs, and thrombolytic therapy should not be stopped. If, however, there is a major bleeding episode, the physician should be notified and the thrombolytic therapy should be stopped. The nurse must pay particular attention to signs and symptoms of bleeding such as a drop in BP, an increase in HR, blood in the NG aspirate or stool, hematuria, a sudden decrease in the patient's level of consciousness, and oozing of blood from IV or catheter sites. If any of these manifestations develop, the physician should be notified and thrombolytic therapy may be discontinued.

DRUG THERAPY

Table 32-16 Thrombolytic Agents Used to Treat Myocardial Infarction

Aniosoylated plasminogen–streptokinase activator complex (APSAC, anistreplace [Eminase])
Recombinant plasminogen activator (rPA, reteplase [Retavase])
Tissue plasminogen activator (tPA, alteplase [Activase])
Streptokinase (Streptase)
Urokinase (Abbokinase)

DRUG THERAPY

Table 32-17 Contraindications for Thrombolytic Therapy

Absolute Contraindications
- History of hemorrhagic stroke
- Uncontrolled hypertension
  - Systolic BP >180 mm Hg
  - Diastolic BP >120 mm Hg
- Recent surgery or trauma (within 3 mo)
- Active internal bleeding
- Known bleeding disorder
- Suspected aortic dissection
- Pregnancy

Relative Contraindications
- History of ischemic stroke
- Poorly controlled hypertension (BP >165/95)
- Recent, prolonged, traumatic CPR
- Acute pericarditis
- Active peptic ulcer
- Diabetic hemorrhagic retinopathy
- Atrial fibrillation
- History of recent GI bleeding
- Cardiogenic shock

Cardiac Catheterization. Although the treatment for acute MI is to lyse the thrombus and reperfuse the myocardium, some patients may not be candidates for thrombolytic therapy or may have a complicated course necessitating an emergent cardiac catheterization. The patient with acute MI may have a catheterization early in the treatment phase to locate the exact lesion (or lesions) and to assess the severity, the presence of collateral circulation, and LV function.

With actual visualization of the coronary artery system and LV function, the physician can prescribe a treatment modality most beneficial to the patient. Possible therapies include direct intracoronary thrombolytic therapy, PTCA, IABP insertion, or CABG.

Percutaneous Transluminal Coronary Angioplasty. PTCA may be performed as first-line treatment instead of thrombolytics, especially in the patient exhibiting signs of cardiogenic shock or in the patient in whom thrombolytic therapy was unsuccessful. PTCA is a nonoperative alternative to surgery for the patient who has coronary artery narrowing. Transluminal dilation can increase the diameter of the artery with the use of percutaneous, fluoroscopically guided catheters to relieve stenotic or occlusive lesions.

The technique is similar to cardiac catheterization. A double-lumen polyvinyl balloon catheter is guided into the coronary artery to the site of the occlusion. The balloon is inflated at the site of stenosis, thereby directly increasing the diameter of the artery. After PTCA, regional coronary blood flow is increased and myocardial metabolism is restored. PTCA is therefore indicated for the relief of myocardial ischemia in the patient with noncalcified, occlusive, compressible coronary artery lesions. Emergent PTCA following MI has a slightly higher rate of abrupt closure than elective PTCA.[38] Therefore the use of stents in the setting of acute MI has increased. (Elective PTCA is described earlier in this chapter.)

Coronary Artery Bypass Graft Surgery. CABG surgery may be a treatment choice in a select group of patients with acute MI. Other revascularization procedures include minimal invasive coronary artery bypass surgery and transmyocardial laser revascularization. (Surgical procedures are discussed in Chapter 33.)

Drug Therapy

IV nitroglycerin. IV nitroglycerin (Tridil) may be used in the initial therapeutic treatment of the patient with an acute MI. Nitroglycerin given intravenously may reduce pain and decrease preload and afterload while increasing the myocardial oxygen supply. Its action may also increase collateral circulation to the ischemic areas of the myocardium. The dose of nitroglycerin is titrated to a dose that decreases the patient's pain while maintaining an adequate BP (no lower than 90 to 100 systolic). The major side effect of IV nitroglycerin is headache or hypotension accompanied by diaphoresis, nausea, vomiting, and occasionally arrhythmias (e.g., tachycardia).

Antiarrhythmic drugs. Arrhythmias are the most common complications after an MI. (The drugs used in the treatment of arrhythmias are discussed in Chapter 34.)

Morphine. Morphine sulfate is given for acute chest pain relief because it reduces anxiety and fear and decreases the cardiac workload by lowering myocardial oxygen consumption, reducing contractility, lowering BP, and slowing the HR. Morphine is given intravenously because (1) after infarction there may be poor peripheral perfusion, which may cause pooling of medication, rendering the medication ineffective until the circulation is restored and at which time a drug overdose may occur; (2) serum enzymes are affected by an intramuscular (IM) injection; and (3) bleeding may occur at the site of the injection if the patient has received thrombolytic therapy or is on heparin.

Meperidine (Demerol) may be given, but it is used less frequently than morphine. Both drugs can depress respirations, which may cause hypoxia, a condition to be avoided in myocardial ischemia and infarction.

Positive inotropic drugs. Positive inotropic drugs that increase the heart's contractility may be used in the patient with acute MI. However, caution should be used. This group of drugs increases the heart's demand for oxygen (increased myocardial oxygen consumption [MVO_2]) at a time when therapy is used to decrease the demand and increase the heart's supply of oxygen (increased flow). Digitalis, amrinone (Inocor), and dobutamine (Dobutrex) are examples of drugs that increase the heart's pumping action (contractility). Their use is indicated when LV failure is present. Nursing interventions during the use of inotropic therapy should include frequent vital signs and heart and lung assessment for evidence of further LV failure or ischemia.

Beta-adrenergic blockers. The use of β-adrenergic blockers early in the acute phase of the MI and during a 1-year follow-up regimen can decrease morbidity. The patient who uses β-adrenergic blockers in the treatment of an acute MI and for 1 year following the infarction has a decreased chance of reinfarction and increased survival.[37,39]

Drug choice and dose depend on the physician. Nursing interventions during the use of β-adrenergic blockers in acute MI should include frequent vital signs and heart and lung assessment. Bradycardia, heart block, and hypotension may result.

Calcium channel blockers. Calcium channel blockers (e.g., verapamil [Cardizem]) may also be used in the treatment of acute MI but have not been shown to be beneficial in reducing morbidity and mortality rates. They may be used in the treatment of MI where the patient also underwent PTCA to restore perfusion. In this setting, calcium channel blockers may be used to prevent coronary spasm. They may also be used for patients in whom β-adrenergic blockers are contraindicated.[39]

Angiotensin-converting enzyme inhibitors. Angiotensin-converting enzyme (ACE) inhibitors (e.g., captopril [Capoten], enalapril [Vasotec]) may be used following MIs. The use of ACE inhibitors can help prevent ventricular remodeling and prevent or slow the progression of heart failure. (See Chapter 31 and Table 31-8 for a discussion on ACE inhibitors.)

Stool softeners. After an MI the patient is predisposed to constipation as a result of bed rest and narcotic administration. Stool softeners such as dioctyl sodium sulfosuccinate (Colace) are given to facilitate and promote the comfort of bowel evacuation. This prevents straining and the resultant vagal stimulation from the Valsalva's maneuver. Vagal stimulation produces bradycardia and can provoke arrhythmias. Another real danger of straining is that when the action is stopped, venous return to the heart is suddenly increased. This may result in overloading of a weakened heart.

Nutritional Therapy. Diet is restricted in saturated fats and cholesterol (see Table 32-5) and is sometimes low in sodium to prevent fluid retention. The patient may have a clear liquid diet the first day when there may still be nausea.

NURSING ASSESSMENT

Table 32-18 Myocardial Infarction

Subjective Data

Important Health Information

Past health history: Previous angina or MI, hypertension, diabetes mellitus

Medications: Use of nitrates, calcium channel blockers, antihypertensive medications, lipid-lowering agents

Functional Health Patterns

Health perception–health management: Family history of heart disease; sedentary lifestyle; smoking

Nutritional-metabolic: Nausea, vomiting, indigestion, heartburn

Activity-exercise: Profound weakness, dyspnea, palpitations, syncope

Elimination: Urinary output, straining at stool

Cognitive-perceptual: Severe substernal or precordial pain, described as heavy or crushing, lasting more than 30 minutes and not relieved by rest or nitrates; radiation to jaw, neck, back, or arms possible

Coping–stress tolerance: Recurrent or persistent stress; apprehension, feeling of impending doom

Objective Data

General

Fever, anxiety, restlessness

Integumentary

Cold, clammy, pale skin

Respiratory

Tachypnea, crackles

Cardiovascular

Tachycardia or bradycardia; arrhythmias (especially ventricular); elevated BP (initially); S_4, possible S_3; murmur and rub and diminished heart tones

Urinary

Decreased urinary output

Possible Findings

Positive serum cardiac markers, leukocytosis; normal chest x-ray or signs of pulmonary congestion, cardiomegaly; abnormal Q waves, ST-T wave elevations, inverted T waves on ECG; positive radionuclide scan, coronary arteriography

NURSING MANAGEMENT: MYOCARDIAL INFARCTION

Nursing Assessment

Subjective and objective data that should be obtained from a patient with an MI are presented in Table 32-18.

Nursing Diagnoses

Nursing diagnoses for the patient with an MI may include, but are not limited to, those presented in NCP 32-1.

Planning

The overall goals are that the patient with a myocardial infarction will (1) experience relief of pain, (2) have no progression of MI, (3) receive immediate and appropriate treatment, (4) cope effectively with associated anxiety, (5) cooperate with rehabilitation plan, and (6) modify or alter risk factors.

Nursing Implementation

Acute Intervention. Acute nursing interventions for the patient with MI are best done in a specialized care unit such as a CCU. Since the advent of CCUs in the early 1960s, medical and nursing care has improved dramatically, and countless lives have been saved.

Acute nursing intervention includes the initial CCU stay (1 to 2 days) and the rest of hospitalization (4 to 6 days). Priorities for nursing interventions in the initial phase of recovery after MI include pain assessment and relief, physiologic monitoring, promotion of rest and comfort, alleviation of stress and anxiety,

32-1 NURSING CARE PLAN PATIENT WITH MYOCARDIAL INFARCTION

Expected Patient Outcomes	Nursing Interventions and *Rationales*
NURSING DIAGNOSIS	**Pain** *related to* lactic acid production from myocardial ischemia and decreased myocardial oxygen supply *as manifested by* severe chest pain, tightness, or constriction, radiation of pain to neck, arms, or back.
▪ Verbalization that chest pain or referred pain is relieved.	▪ Administer O_2 through nasal cannula *to increase oxygenation of myocardial tissue and prevent further tissue ischemia.* ▪ Administer morphine sulfate IV as needed *to decrease anxiety and decrease the cardiac workload by lowering myocardial oxygen consumption, reducing contractility, lowering BP, and slowing the heart rate.* ▪ Administer antianginal agents as ordered *to increase blood flow to myocardium, decrease workload, and reduce pain.* ▪ Monitor vital signs q1-2hr *to provide ongoing assessment of patient's response to treatment.* ▪ Continue to evaluate patient's level of comfort *as an evaluation of myocardial ischemia and response to treatment.* ▪ Explain the importance of early reporting of pain to *provide treatment and prevent further ischemia.* ▪ *Obtain 12-lead ECG during pain episode to help differentiate angina from extension of MI or pericarditis.*
NURSING DIAGNOSIS	**Altered cardiac tissue perfusion** *related to* myocardial damage, inadequate cardiac output, and potential pulmonary congestion *as manifested by* decrease in BP, oliguria, crackles, hepatic engorgement, peripheral edema, splitting of heart sounds, presence of S_4 and S_3.
▪ BP and pulse rate within normal limits for individual. ▪ Respiratory rate of 12-18/min. ▪ Urine output >30 cc/hr.	▪ Assess BP, pulse rate, heart sounds, and respiratory rate every hour initially and then prn. ▪ Monitor intake and output every hour *to assess adequacy of renal perfusion and renal function.* ▪ Minimize cardiac workload during healing *to decrease the oxygen needs of the myocardium.* ▪ Explain necessity of bed rest and decreased activity *to promote patient cooperation.* ▪ Allow rest periods between concentrated nursing care times *to reduce fatigue and O_2 requirements of myocardium.* ▪ Monitor O_2 administration *to ensure adequacy of O_2 supply to the myocardium.* ▪ Assess comfort level (try to keep patient free of pain) *because pain is an indication of myocardial ischemia and can produce anxiety, which increases O_2 needs.*
NURSING DIAGNOSIS	**Anxiety** *related to* perceived threat of death, pain, possible lifestyle changes *as manifested by* restlessness, agitation, verbalization of concern over many health-related aspects such as lifestyle changes and prognosis.
▪ Physical and emotional comfort. ▪ Expression of sense of well-being.	▪ Monitor anxiety level *as anxiety increases the need for O_2.* ▪ Determine patient's past coping mechanisms and effectiveness *to encourage their use or assist in modifying if needed.* ▪ Encourage use of relaxation techniques *to enhance self-control.* ▪ If patient needs information, provide it simply and clearly *so it can be understood.* ▪ Assess support systems and incorporate into plan of care if effective *because family may be most effective in reducing patient's stress.*
NURSING DIAGNOSIS	**Activity intolerance** *related to* fatigue secondary to decreased cardiac output and poor lung and tissue perfusion *as manifested by* fatigue with minimal activity, inability to care for self without dyspnea, and increase in pulse rate.
▪ Absence of dyspnea and fatigue on exertion.	▪ Assess level of fatigue, weakness, and potential for activity progression to provide baseline data for developing a care plan. ▪ Encourage patient to maintain bed rest until instructed otherwise *to reduce cardiac workload.*

Continued

32-1 NURSING CARE PLAN PATIENT WITH MYOCARDIAL INFARCTION —continued

Expected Patient Outcomes	Nursing Interventions and *Rationales*
NURSING DIAGNOSIS Cont'd	
▪ Stable vital signs with progressive increase in activity.	▪ Have articles patient may want or need within easy reach *to minimize activity, conserve energy, and foster independence.* ▪ Monitor BP, HR, respiration, and skin color *to monitor patient's response to activity and adjust as necessary.* ▪ Administer O_2 prn during activity *to increase O_2 availability for cardiac and other organ perfusion.* ▪ Plan gradual activity progression *to increase activity tolerance without rapidly increasing cardiac workload.*
NURSING DIAGNOSIS **Self-esteem disturbance** *related to* lack of control, illness event, and perceived or actual role changes *as manifested by* expression of feelings of helplessness and low self-esteem, minimal participation in self-care.	
▪ Understanding of importance of limiting activity at this time.	▪ Allow patient as much autonomy as possible by giving necessary information to decrease anxiety and *promote autonomy.* ▪ Allow patient to assist in planning care *to reinforce patient's value as a person and to maintain his or her independence.*
NURSING DIAGNOSIS **Sleep pattern disturbance** *related to* complex treatment regimen, pain, anxiety, stressful environment, and frequent interruptions *as manifested by* report of feeling tired on awakening, frequent napping, fitful sleep with frequent interruptions.	
▪ Feeling of being rested. ▪ Minimal interruptions during sleep.	▪ Assess sleep patterns and patient's perception of quality of sleep. ▪ Monitor flow of people into patient's room *to reduce noise and confusion and prevent sensory overload.* ▪ Plan nursing care to provide optimal rest *to encourage myocardial healing.* ▪ Provide calm, restful environment *to reduce stimuli and promote sleep.* ▪ Attempt to maintain patient's sleep-wake cycle *because lack of sleep impedes healing and may produce confusion.* ▪ If patient's condition is stable, do not awaken for vital signs *so that patient may have an uninterrupted sleep cycle.*
NURSING DIAGNOSIS **Ineffective management of therapeutic regimen** *related to* lack of knowledge of disease process, rehabilitation, home activities, diet, and medications *as manifested by* frequent questioning about illness, management, and aftercare.	
▪ Able to describe appropriate responses for future symptoms, recommended lifestyle changes, immediate plan of care, appropriate expectations after discharge, and activity and diet guidelines.	▪ Assess patient's understanding of therapeutic regimen *to obtain information on patient's education needs.* ▪ Teach at patient's level of understanding *so that the information is understood* and *to increase likelihood of behavior change.* ▪ Provide guidelines with rationale for recommended actions to be taken *so patient has a clear understanding of why he or she is being asked to change specific behaviors.* ▪ Make recommendations to patient in a realistic manner *so that patient can see self carrying them out.* ▪ Include family when information is given, especially regarding discharge, *to get the cooperation of the patient's most significant support system.* ▪ Be specific when giving discharge instructions; write them down for patient to take home *to be available for reference.*

Continued

32-1 NURSING CARE PLAN PATIENT WITH MYOCARDIAL INFARCTION —continued

Expected Patient Outcomes	Nursing Interventions and *Rationales*
NURSING DIAGNOSIS	**Anticipatory grieving** *related to* actual or perceived losses secondary to cardiac condition *as manifested by* possible losses, such as occupation, role, status, and previous lifestyle.
▪ Resolution of grief over losses and changes.	▪ Assess potential losses and changes that patient will need to make *to evaluate patient's perception of losses and changes and alter if unrealistic or unnecessary.* ▪ Encourage discussion of ways to alter lifestyle to patient's satisfaction *to minimize impact of changes.* ▪ Assure patient of self-worth *to strengthen his or her self-image.* ▪ Assist patient to plan realistic lifestyle adjustments *to increase the probability of compliance and avoid unnecessary changes.*

and understanding of the patient's emotional and behavioral reactions. Proper management of these priorities decreases the oxygen needs of a compromised myocardium. In addition, the nurse should institute measures to avoid the hazards of immobility while encouraging rest.

Pain. Morphine should be given as needed to eliminate or reduce chest pain. The nurse should instruct the patient to rate the pain on a scale of 1 to 10 to assist in the assessment and treatment of pain. Because a patient does not always verbalize pain, the nurse must be attuned to other manifestations of pain, such as restlessness, elevated heart rate or BP, clutching of the bedclothes, or other nonverbal cues. IV nitroglycerin, if given, should be titrated. Once pain is relieved, the nurse may have to deal with denial in a patient who interprets the absence of pain as an absence of cardiac damage. After the pain medication has been administered, the efficacy of the drug and the patient's response should be assessed and documented.

Monitoring. A patient has continuous ECG monitoring while in the CCU and usually after transfer to a step-down or general unit. The nurse should be trained in ECG interpretation so that arrhythmias causing further deterioration of the cardiovascular status can be identified and treated. During the initial period after MI, ventricular fibrillation is the most common lethal arrhythmia. In many patients, this arrhythmia is preceded by PVCs or ventricular tachycardia (VT).

In addition to frequent vital signs, intake and output should be evaluated at least once a shift, and physical assessment should be carried out to detect deviations from the patient's baseline parameters. Included is an assessment of lung sounds and heart sounds and inspection for evidence of fluid retention (e.g., distended neck veins, hepatic engorgement, presacral or anterior tibial edema). Because a patient is frequently on strict bed rest initially, dorsiflexion of the feet (Homans' sign) to elicit deep calf pain should also be done to evaluate the presence of deep-vein thrombosis.

Assessment of the patient's oxygenation status is helpful, especially if the patient is receiving oxygen. Also, the nares should be checked for irritation or dryness, which can cause considerable discomfort if the nasal route is used for oxygen administration.

Table 32-19 Phases of Rehabilitation

Phase I—*Time when patient is in the CCU:* Activity level depends on severity of MI; patient may rest in bed or chair; attention focuses on management of pain, anxiety, arrhythmias, and cardiogenic shock
Phase II—*Time from transfer from the CCU to discharge from hospital:* Resumption of activities begins to the point of self-care at the time of discharge; information giving and teaching are appropriate at this time
Phase III—*Time of convalescence at home:* Patient and family examine and possibly restructure lifestyles and roles; exercise program begins, commonly a walking program, which progresses daily during first week and then weekly; patient undergoes exercise treadmill test at about 8 wk to determine workload of recovering myocardium
Phase IV—*Time of recovery and maintenance:* Involvement with the community rehabilitation program for physical training and fitness continues

Rest and comfort. With a severe insult to the myocardium, as in the case of infarction, it is important for the nurse to promote rest and comfort. Bed rest may be ordered for the first 2 to 3 days in a severe MI. A patient with an uncomplicated MI may rest in a chair.

When sleeping or resting, the body requires less work from the heart than it does when active. It is important to plan nursing and therapeutic actions to ensure adequate rest periods free from interruption. Comfort measures that can promote rest are smooth bedclothes, frequent oral care, adequate warmth, dim lighting, a quiet atmosphere, and assurance that personnel are nearby and responsive to the patient's needs.

It is important that the patient understand the reasons why activity is limited. However, in spite of this limitation the patient is not completely restricted. Gradually the cardiac workload is increased through more demanding physical tasks so that the patient can achieve a discharge activity level adequate for home care. Phases of rehabilitation are outlined in Table 32-19.

Anxiety. Anxiety is present in all patients in various degrees. The nurse's role is to identify the source of anxiety and assist the patient in reducing it. If the patient is afraid of being alone, a family member should be allowed to sit quietly by the bedside or to check in with the patient frequently. If a source of anxiety is fear of the unknown, the nurse should explore these concerns with the patient and help with appropriate reality testing.

If anxiety is caused by lack of information, the nurse should provide teaching appropriate to the patient's stated need and level. The nurse should answer the patient's questions with clear, simple explanations sufficient to reduce the patient's anxiety.

It is important to start teaching at the patient's level rather than to present a prepackaged protocol. Frequently the patient is not yet ready to hear about the pathogenesis of heart disease. The earliest questions usually relate to how the disease affects perceived control and independence. These questions include the following:

When will I leave the CCU?
When can I be out of bed?
When will I be discharged?
When can I return to work?
How much change will I have to make in my life?
Will this happen again?

The nurse should advise that a more complete teaching program begins once the patient is feeling stronger. Frequently the patient may not be able to consciously examine the most pervasive concern of MI patients: Am I going to die? Even if a patient denies this concern, it is helpful for the nurse to initiate conversation by remarking that fear of dying is a common concern reported by most patients who have suffered an MI. This gives the patient "permission" to talk about an uncomfortable and fearful topic.

Emotional and behavioral reactions. The emotional and behavioral reactions of a patient are varied and frequently follow a predictable response pattern (Table 32-20). The role of the nurse in intervention is to understand what the patient is currently experiencing, to assist the patient in testing reality, and to support the use of constructive coping styles. Denial may be a positive coping style in the early phase of recovery from MI.

The nurse has an obligation to maximize and enhance the patient's social support systems. This entails assessing the support structure of the patient and family and allowing it to function. Often the patient is separated from the most significant support system at the time of hospitalization. The nurse's role can include talking with the family, informing them of the patient's progress, allowing the patient and the family to interact as necessary, and supporting the family members who will be able to provide the necessary support to the patient. Open visitation is helpful in decreasing anxiety and increasing support for the patient with an MI. Social isolation has been associated with negative outcomes following MI in both men and women.[40,41] It is important for the nurse to help the patient identify support systems that can help the patient after discharge.

Ambulatory and Home Care. *Rehabilitation* may be defined as the process of helping the patient adjust to a disability by teaching integration of all resources and concentrating more on existing abilities than on permanent disabilities. Cardiac rehabilitation is the restoration of a person to an optimal state of function in six areas: physiologic, psychologic, mental, spiritual, economic, and vocational. Many persons recover from an MI physically, yet they may never attain psychologic well-being because of misconceptions about the illness or a need to practice illness behaviors. Returning to work and resuming all activities have long been outcome measures of cardiac rehabilitation and are important in terms of the cost-effectiveness of cardiac care and rehabilitation. A sample rehabilitation program is presented in Table 32-21.

In considering rehabilitation, the nurse and patient must recognize that CAD is a chronic disease. It will not be cured, nor will it disappear by itself. Therefore basic changes in lifestyle must be made to promote recovery and health. These changes must frequently be made at a time when a person is middle-aged and is already dealing with aging and all its associated stresses. The patient must also realize that recovery takes time. Resumption of physical activity after MI is slow

Table 32-20 Emotional and Behavioral Responses to Acute Myocardial Infarction

Denial
- May have history of ignoring symptoms related to heart disease
- Minimizes severity of medical condition
- Ignores activity restrictions
- Avoids discussing MI or its significance

Anger
- Is commonly expressed as, "Why did this happen to me?"
- May be directed at family, staff, or medical regimen

Anxiety and Fear
- Fears death and long-term disability
- Overtly manifests apprehension, restlessness, insomnia, tachycardia
- Less overtly manifests increased verbalization, projection of feelings to others, hypochondriasis
- Fears activity, recurrent heart attacks, and sudden death

Dependency
- Is totally reliant on staff
- Is unwilling to perform tasks or activities unless approved by physician
- Wants to be monitored by ECG at all times
- Is hesitant to leave CCU or hospital

Depression
- Experiences mourning period concerning loss of health, altered body function, and changes in lifestyle
- Realizes seriousness of situation
- Begins to worry about future implications of health problem
- Shows manifestations of withdrawal, crying, anorexia, apathy
- May be more evident after discharge

Realistic Acceptance
- Focuses on optimum rehabilitation
- Plans changes compatible with altered cardiac function

Table 32-21 **Inpatient Rehabilitation: Five-Step Myocardial Infarction Program (Revised 1996: Grady Memorial Hospital/Emory University School of Medicine)**

Step	Date	M.D. Initials	Nurse/ Exercise Specialist Notes	Supervised Exercise	CCU/Step-Down Unit Activity	Educational Activity
				CCU		
1	____			Active and passive ROM all extremities in bed Teach patient ankle plantar and dorsiflexion—repeat hourly when awake	Partial self-care Feed self Dangle legs on side of bed Use bedside commode Sit in chair 15 min, 1-2 times/day	Orientation to CCU Personal emergencies, social service aid as needed Bedside teaching (CCU staff)
2	____			Active ROM all extremities, sitting on side of bed or bedside chair	Sit in chair 15-30 min, 2-3 times/day Complete self-care	Orientation to rehabilitation team, program Smoking cessation Educational literature if requested Planning transfer from CCU
				Step-Down Unit		
3	____			Warm-up exercises, 2-2.5 METs: Stretching ROM Calisthenics Walk in hall 50-70 ft and back at slow pace	Sit in chair ad lib Walk in room Walk to class with supervision OOB as tolerated	Normal cardiac anatomy and function Development of atherosclerosis What happens when myocardial infarction occurs Coronary risk factors and their control Diet
4	____			Teach pulse counting, Borg Scale ROM and calisthenics, 3 METs Practice walking few stair steps Walk 300-500 ft bid Instruct on home exercise	Tepid shower or tub bath, with supervision Walk in corridor prn	Heart attack management: Medications Exercise Surgery Response to symptoms Family, community adjustments on return home Work simplification techniques (as needed)
5	____			Continue above activities Check pulse counting Walk up flight of steps Walk 500 ft bid Continue home exercise instruction; present information regarding outpatient exercise program	Continue all previous activities Predischarge exercise test (as appropriate)	Discharge planning Medications, diet, activity Return appointments Schedules tests Return to work Community resources Educational literature Medication cards

Modified from Wegner N: Rehabilitation of the patient with coronary heart disease. In Alexander RW and others: *Hurst's the heart,* ed 9, New York, 1998, McGraw-Hill.
MET, metabolic equivalent; *OOB,* out of bed; *OT,* occupational therapy, *ROM,* range of motion.

and gradual. However, with appropriate and adequate supportive care, recovery is more likely to occur. (See Research Box, p. 878.)

Patient education. Once the acute stage of MI has passed, the patient is transferred to a progressive care or regular hospital unit. The goals of nursing care are ongoing. In addition, an important nursing goal is patient and family education. This teaching begins with the CCU nurse and progresses through the staff nurse to the community health nurse. The purpose of education is to give the patient and family the tools they need to make informed decisions about attainment of health. For teaching to be meaningful, the patient must be aware of the need to learn. Careful assessment of the patient's learning needs helps the nurse set goals and objectives that are realistic.

The timing of the teaching is important. When patients or families are in crisis (either physiologic or psychologic), they may not be very interested in patient education issues. It is important to remember that early questions should be

RESEARCH
IMPLICATIONS FOR NURSING PRACTICE

Nursing Care of MI Patients

Citation Riegel B, Thomason T, Carlson B: Nursing care of patients with acute myocardial infarction, *Crit Care Nurse* 17:23, 1997.

Purpose A national survey was done to determine the treatment strategies and knowledge base of bedside clinical nurses caring for acute myocardial infarction patients. In particular, the goal was to determine if nursing practice was congruent with the current body of published research findings.

Methods A survey called the Assessment and Treatment of Patients with Acute Myocardial Infarction Tool was completed by 882 randomly selected nurses across the United States who were caring for acute myocardial infarction patients. This tool obtained information on the following areas: pain assessment and management, activity management, treatment strategies, and practices for teaching patients.

Results and Conclusions Patients with acute myocardial infarctions are being managed by nurses with varied educational backgrounds. Although much of the care provided is consistent with the current state of knowledge, some of the reported practices (e.g., use of bedpan instead of letting the patient use a bedside commode, factors to consider when allowing a patient to ambulate) are not research based. Some nurses found that lack of time and poor support from administration were the factors that most discouraged the use of research findings in practice. Another explanation for the variable use of research findings is that nurses are not yet convinced by the results and therefore do not use published research findings in practice.

Implications for Nursing Practice There is a need for the development and use of standards of care, clinical pathways, and other tools that provide nurses with research-based guidance in the care of patients. Nurses need to establish their practice on research findings rather than tradition, which may be erroneous and outdated. When adequate research is available, nursing policies and procedures should reflect current research findings. When available research is insufficient, additional research is needed.

answered initially in simple, brief terms, without detailed elaboration, and that the answers to these questions require repetition and follow-up (elaboration). When the shock and disbelief accompanying a crisis subside, the patient and family are better able to focus on new information.

In addition to teaching the patient and the family what they wish to know, several types of information are considered necessary in achieving optimal health. A teaching guide for the patient with MI is presented in Table 32-22.

Some nurses have found that an algorithm sheet that lists these patient teaching categories and who taught the information is helpful in documenting information given to the patient and family.

PATIENT TEACHING GUIDE
Table 32-22 Myocardial Infarction

- Anatomy and physiology of the heart and vessels
- Cause and effect of atherosclerosis
- Definition of terms (e.g., CAD, angina, MI, sudden death, CHF)
- Signs and symptoms of angina and MI and reasons they occur
- Healing after infarction
- Identification of risk factors (see Table 32-4)
- Rationale for tests and treatments, including ECG, blood tests, and angiography as well as monitoring, rest, diet, and medications
- Appropriate expectations about recovery and rehabilitation (anticipatory guidance)
- Measures to take to promote recovery and health
- Importance of the gradual, progressive resumption of activity

When medical terminology is used, its meaning should be explained in lay terms. For example, it can be explained that the heart, a four-chambered pump, is a muscle that needs oxygen like all other muscles, and when vessels become narrowed by atherosclerosis, the process is similar to a buildup of mineral deposits inside water pipes, which causes less water to flow through at a higher pressure. It is a good idea for the nurse to have a model of the heart or to use a pad and pencil to sketch what is being explained. Literature written for a nonmedical audience is available through the American Heart Association. Videotapes are also helpful tools that can be used to teach patients.

Anticipatory guidance involves preparing the patient and the family for what to expect in the course of recovery and rehabilitation. By learning what to expect during treatment and recovery, the patient gains a sense of control over life. This sense of perceived control allows the patient to consciously consider stressors and thus possibly to promote recovery.

The idea of perceived control is operationalized as the process by which the patient exercises choice and makes decisions by cutting back. Cutting back is one way of minimizing the psychologic and physiologic losses after MI (or any other life-changing event). The patient considers what must be cut back (changed), weighs this against what should be cut back, and finally determines what will be cut back. For example, a middle-aged man who smokes two packs of cigarettes a day, is 20 pounds overweight, and gets no physical exercise has a seemingly overwhelming task. He may decide that he *can* live with a weight-reduction diet and will get more exercise (although perhaps not daily) but that it is not possible for him to quit smoking. He reasons that because he is modifying two of the three risk factors, he will be safe if he cuts back on smoking. Ideally the smoking risk factors should be a priority for this patient, but if information regarding risks and effects of smoking is not accepted, the nurse must respect the patient's need for control.

Physical exercise. Exercise is an integral part of the rehabilitation program. It is necessary for optimal physiologic functioning and psychologic well-being. It has a direct, positive effect on maximal oxygen uptake, increasing CO, decreasing blood lipids, decreasing BP, increasing blood flow through the coronary arteries, increasing muscle mass and flexibility, improving the psychologic state, and assisting in weight loss and control. A regular schedule of moderate exercise, even after many years of sedentary living, is beneficial.

One method used to identify levels of physical activities is through metabolic equivalent (MET) units: 1 MET is the amount of oxygen needed by the body at rest: 3.5 ml of oxygen per kilogram per minute or 1.4 cal/kg of body weight per minute. The MET is used to determine the energy costs of various exercises (Table 32-23).

In the hospital, the activity level is gradually increased so that by the time of discharge the patient can tolerate moderate-energy activities of 3 to 5 MET. Many patients with an uncomplicated MI are in the hospital approximately 5 days. By day 4 or 5, the patient can ambulate in the hallway. Many physicians order low-level treadmill tests before discharge to assess readiness for discharge, accurate HR for an exercise prescription, and potential for reinfarction. If tests are positive (i.e., ischemia at a low level of energy expenditure), the patient is evaluated for cardiac catheterization before discharge and possible bypass grafting. If the test is negative, a catheterization may be suggested for 1 month after discharge. Because of the short hospitalization, it is critical to give the patient specific guidelines for activity and exercise so that overexertion will not occur. It is helpful to stress that when the patient "listens to what the body is saying"—the most important facet of recovery—uncomplicated recovery should proceed.

Teaching the patient to check the pulse rate is a nursing responsibility. The patient should be taught the parameters within which to exercise. The patient should be told the maximum HR that should be present at any point. If the HR exceeds this level or does not return to the rate of the resting pulse, within a few minutes the patient should stop. The patient should be instructed to stop exercising if pain or dyspnea occurs.

In a normal, healthy person the minimum threshold for improving cardiorespiratory fitness is 60% of the age-predicted maximum HR (which is calculated by subtracting the person's age from 220). The ideal training target HR is 80% of maximum HR. The patient who has been physically inactive and is just beginning an exercise program should do so under supervision whenever possible. The more important factor is the patient's response to exercise in terms of symptoms rather than absolute HR. This is a point that cannot be overstressed in teaching of the MI patient. In addition, a cardiac patient on medications (especially β-adrenergic blockers) may not be able to increase HR to any degree and should have a treadmill test to determine an individual target HR. Basic guidelines for cardiac conditioning are presented in Table 32-24.

The basic categories of exercise are static (isometric) and dynamic (isotonic). Most daily activities are a mixture of the two. Static exercise involves the development of tension during muscular contraction but produces little or no change in muscle length or joint movement. Lifting, carrying, and pushing heavy objects are primarily isometric activities. Since the HR and BP increase rapidly during isometric work, exercise programs involving isometric exercises should be limited.

Table 32-23 Energy Expenditure in Metabolic Equivalents

Low-Energy Activities (Less Than 3 METs or Less Than 3 cal/min)	**Calories Burned**
Activities in Hospital	
Resting supine	1.0
Sitting	1.2
Eating	1.4
Conversing	1.4
Washing hands, face	2.5
Activities Outside Hospital	
Sewing by hand	1.4
Sweeping floor	1.7
Painting, sitting	2.5
Driving car	2.8
Assembling radio	2.7
Sewing by machine	2.9
Moderate-Energy Activities (3-6 METs or 3-5 cal/min)	
Activities in Hospital	
Sitting on bedside commode	3.6
Walking at 2.5 mph	3.6
Showering	4.2
Using bedpan	4.7
Walking at 3.75 mph	5.6
Activities Outside Hospital	
Bricklaying	4.0
Tractor plowing	4.2
Ironing, standing	4.2
Mopping	4.2
Bowling	4.4
Cycling at 5.5 mph on level ground	4.5
Golfing	5.0
Dancing	5.5
High-Energy Activities (6-8 METs or 6-8 cal/min)	
Ambulating with braces and crutches	8.0
Performing carpentry	6.8
Mowing lawn by hand	7.7
Playing singles tennis	7.1
Riding on trotting horse	8.0
Walking at 5 mph	6.5
Ascending stairs	7.0
Very High-Energy Activities (8-10 METs or 8-10 cal/min)	
Skiing	9.9
Jogging at 5 mph	8.0
Shoveling snow	8.5
Ascending stairs with a 17 lb load	9.0
Extremely High-Energy Activities (more than 10 METs or more than 11 cal/min)	
Playing handball	
Cycling at 13 mph	
Ascending stairs with a 22 lb load	

MET, metabolic equivalent unit.

PATIENT TEACHING GUIDE

Table 32-24 Exercise Guidelines After an MI

Type of Exercise
Exercise should be regular, rhythmic, and repetitive, using large muscles to build up endurance (e.g., walking, cycling, swimming, rowing).

Intensity
Exercise intensity should be determined by the patient's HR. If a treadmill test has not been performed, the person recovering from MI should not exceed 20 beats per minute over the resting pulse rate.

Duration
Exercise can be from 20 to 30 minutes. It is important to begin slowly at personal tolerance (perhaps only 5 to 10 minutes) and build up to 30 minutes.

Frequency
The patient should exercise three times a week. If done at low duration (5 to 10 minutes), exercise can be done daily but is best done on nonconsecutive days.

Warm-up/Cooldown
Mild stretching for 3 to 5 minutes before the exercise activity and 5 minutes after the activity is important. Activity should not be started or stopped abruptly.

PATIENT TEACHING GUIDE

Table 32-25 Sexual Activity After Myocardial Infarction

- Planning of resumption of sexual activity should correspond to sexual activity before the heart attack.
- Physical training (exercise) seems to improve the physiologic response to coitus; therefore daily exercise during recovery should be encouraged.
- Consumption of food and alcohol should be reduced before intercourse is anticipated (e.g., waiting 3-4 hr after ingesting a large meal before engaging in sexual activity).
- Familiar surroundings and a familiar partner reduce anxiety.
- Masturbation may be a useful sexual outlet and may reassure the patient that sexual activity is still possible.
- Temperature should be comfortable, not extreme. Hot or cold showers should be avoided just before and just after intercourse.
- Foreplay is desirable because it allows a gradual increase in heart rate before orgasm.
- Positions during intercourse are a matter of individual choice.
- Orogenital sex places no undue strain on the heart. This form of sexual expression depends entirely on the individuals involved.
- A relaxed atmosphere free of fatigue is optimal.
- Prophylactic use of nitrates is effective in decreasing angina during sexual activity.
- Anal intercourse may cause undue cardiac stress because of the possibility of inducing a vasovagal response.

Isotonic exercises involve changes in muscle length and joint movement with rhythmic contractions at relatively low muscular tension. Walking, jogging, swimming, bicycling, and jumping rope are examples of activities that are predominantly isotonic. Isotonic exercise can put a safe, steady load on the heart and lungs and may also improve the circulation in many organs.

Resumption of sexual activity. It is important to include sexual counseling for cardiac patients and their partners. This often-neglected area of discussion may be difficult for both patients and health care providers to approach. However, the cardiac patient's concern about resumption of sexual activity after MI often produces more stress than the physiologic act itself. About one third of men and women do not resume sexual activity or have a decrease in sexual activity after MI.[41] The majority of these patients changed their sexual behavior not because of physical problems, but because they were concerned about sexual inadequacy, death during coitus, and impotence. The misconceptions held by these persons could have been clarified with specific counseling by a concerned and knowledgeable health care provider.

Before the nurse provides guidelines on resumption of sexual activity, it is important to know the physiologic status of the patient, the physiologic effects of sexual activity, and the psychologic effects of having a heart attack. Sexual activity for middle-aged men with their usual partners is no more strenuous than climbing two flights of stairs.

Many nurses are unsure of how and when to begin counseling about resumption of sex. It is helpful to consider sex as a physical activity and to discuss or explore feelings in this area when other physical activities are discussed. One helpful approach is, "Many people who have had a heart attack wonder when they will be able to resume sexual activity. Has this been of concern to you?" Another is, "If this has been of concern to you, this information should be helpful." This type of nonthreatening statement brings up the topic, allows the patient to explore personal feelings, and gives the patient an opportunity to raise questions with the nurse or another health care provider. Common guidelines are presented in Table 32-25.

The patient needs to know that the inability to perform sexually after MI is common and that impotence usually disappears after several attempts. The nurse should reinforce the idea that patience and understanding usually solve the problem.

It is not uncommon for a patient who experiences chest pain on physical exertion to have some angina during sexual stimulation or intercourse. The patient should be instructed to take nitroglycerin prophylactically. It is also helpful to have the patient avoid sex soon after a heavy meal or after excessive ingestion of alcohol, when extremely tired or stressed, or with unfamiliar partners. Anal intercourse is to be avoided because of the likelihood of eliciting a vasovagal response.

The patient should be counseled that resumption of sex depends on the patient and his or her partner's emotional readiness and on the physician's assessment of the extent of recovery. It is usually recommended that a patient refrain from sex until

4 to 8 weeks after MI. Some physicians believe that the patient should decide when ready to resume sex. Others say that a patient must be able to climb two flights of stairs briskly without dyspnea or angina before sexual activity can be resumed.

Reading material on resumption of sexual activity may be presented to the patient to facilitate discussion. The nurse should return to clarify and explain as necessary. Calmly and matter-of-factly introducing the subject of resumption of sexual activity during teaching about physical activity has positive effects of eliciting questions and concerns that might not have otherwise surfaced. For example, the nurse might begin, "Sexual activity is like other forms of activity and should be gradually resumed after MI. If your ability to perform sexually is concerning you, the energy expenditure has been found to be no more than walking briskly or climbing two flights of stairs." This forms a factual basis for the patient to begin to seek information and explore personal feelings about resuming sex.

■ Evaluation

The expected outcomes for the patient with an MI are presented in NCP 32-1.

SUDDEN CARDIAC DEATH

Sudden cardiac death (SCD) is unexpected death from cardiac causes. In SCD there is a disruption in cardiac function, producing an abrupt loss of cerebral blood flow. Death occurs within 1 hour of the onset of acute symptoms. It occurs secondary to natural (not accidental or traumatic) causes. The affected person may or may not have a documented prior history of cardiovascular disease. In 25% of patients who die of CAD, sudden cardiac death may be the first sign of trouble.[3]

Sudden cardiac death accounts for approximately 350,000 deaths a year in the United States.[42] Only 20% of SCD survivors are discharged from the hospital without neurologic impairment. CAD is the most common cause of SCD, accounting for 80% of all SCDs. Fifty-six percent occur out of the hospital or in the ED. It is difficult to predict who is at risk for SCD. However, poor left ventricular function ejection fraction (less than 40%) has been found to be the strongest predictor.[42,43] Although increased sympathetic nervous system activity has been linked with the development of cardiac arrhythmias, continued research is needed.[43]

Etiology

Victims of SCD usually have multivessel coronary atherosclerosis. However, many of these persons have no known history of cardiovascular disease. Less commonly, SCD may occur as a result of a primary LV outflow obstruction. These obstructions may be secondary to such diseases as aortic stenosis, hypertrophic cardiomyopathy, and coarctation of the aorta.

Persons who experience SCD as a result of CAD fall into two groups: (1) those who had an acute MI and (2) those who did not have an acute MI. The latter group accounts for the majority of cases of SCD.[3] In this instance, victims usually have no warning signs or no known precedent symptoms. Typically, death is a result of arrhythmias, usually ventricular tachycardia, ventricular fibrillation, or both. The patient is at risk for recurrent sudden death, probably because of continued electrical instability of the myocardium that caused the initial event to occur.

The second, smaller group of patients includes those who have had an acute MI and have suffered sudden cardiac death. In these cases the patients usually do have prodromal symptoms, such as chest pain and dyspnea, and they have less chance of recurrent sudden cardiac death than those who have not had MI.

Risk Factors

Persons at increased risk for sudden cardiac death include those with the following risk factors:

1. Male gender (especially African-American men)
2. Family history of premature atherosclerosis
3. Cigarette smoking
4. Diabetes mellitus
5. Hypercholesterolemia
6. Hypertension
7. Cardiomegaly
8. Ejection fraction less than 40%
9. History of ventricular arrhythmias

NURSING AND COLLABORATIVE MANAGEMENT: SUDDEN CARDIAC DEATH

Survivors of SCD generally require a diagnostic workup to determine whether they have had an acute MI. Thus serial cardiac enzymes and ECGs must be obtained, and the patient must be treated accordingly. (See section on collaborative care of MI.) In addition, because most persons with SCD have CAD secondary to multivessel coronary atherosclerosis, cardiac catheterization is indicated to determine the possible location and extent of coronary artery occlusion. Percutaneous transluminal coronary angioplasty or CABG bypass graft surgery may be indicated (see Chapter 33).

Most SCD patients have a lethal arrhythmia (usually ventricular arrhythmia) that is associated with a high incidence of recurrence. Thus it is useful to know when those persons are most likely to have a recurrence and what drug therapy is the most effective treatment. Assessment of arrhythmias in these patients includes 24-hour Holter monitoring, exercise stress testing, and electrophysiology study (EPS). EPS is performed under fluoroscopy; pacing electrodes are placed in selected intracardiac areas, and stimuli are selectively used to attempt to evoke arrhythmias. The patient's response to various antiarrhythmic medications can be determined and monitored in a controlled environment. (EPS is discussed in Chapter 30.)

Most commonly, a patient who has experienced SCD can be treated with antiarrhythmic medications such as procainamide (Pronestyl), quinidine, and amiodarone (Cordarone). However, some selected patients are refractory to drug therapy and may require implantation of a ventricular defibrillator (see Chapter 34).

The nurse caring for a survivor of SCD should be attuned to the patient's psychosocial adaptation to this sudden "brush with death." Many of these patients develop a "time bomb" mentality. They fear the recurrence of cardiopulmonary arrest and may become anxious, angry, and depressed. Their families are likely to experience the same feelings. Wives of male survivors of SCD often experience a great deal of anxiety and fear of recurrence. The wives often feel responsible for the prevention of another event.[44] The grief response varies among persons and families. The nurse should be attuned to the specific needs of the patient and the family and educate them accordingly while providing appropriate emotional support.

GERONTOLOGIC CONSIDERATIONS

Coronary Artery Disease

The incidence of cardiac disease is greatly increased in older adults and is the leading cause of death in older persons. Angina can be disabling in this population, and affected persons increasingly rely on health care services to remain independent.[45]

The nurse caring for the older adult with CAD must be aware of the physiologic changes that occur in the cardiovascular system. Structural changes in the myocardium include increased collagen and fat deposition, myofibrillar degeneration, and endocardial thickening resulting in abnormalities in diastolic filling of the ventricles.[45] Calcification of the heart valves and degeneration of the conduction system can also occur. The majority of pacemakers are placed in persons more than 65 years of age. In addition, resting HR decreases with age, and maximum HR with exercise decreases with age.

In the older adult, loss of elastic fibers and increased collagen in the arterial media diminish elasticity and distensibility of arteries.[45,46] These changes cause an increased systolic BP and SVR, which can result in accelerated atherosclerosis. These combined changes lead to a decrease in CO by 1% a year. This decrease in CO is probably secondary to decreased contractility of the myocardium and increased afterload caused by the increase in SVR. In addition, decreased arterial wall elasticity blunts the responsiveness to baroreceptors in the aortic arch and carotid arteries.[45] Circulating norepinephrine levels also increase with age. However, β-adrenergic receptors may be less responsive to catecholamines.

The nurse must be aware of the changes in an older adult and must keep in mind the effect that nursing care may have on these patients. Because older adults have decreased responsiveness to catecholamines, their response to stress may be blunted; HR may not rise as quickly in response to pain or to declining CO. They often have atypical symptoms when experiencing an acute MI. Sudden shortness of breath may be more common than classic substernal chest pain. Associated diaphoresis may not be a predominant manifestation of an MI. The sudden occurrence of symptoms such as profound weakness and dyspnea should be investigated.

Many of the antianginal agents that cause postural hypotension and decrease preload may not be well tolerated in the older patient secondary to the decreased responsiveness of the baroreceptors and impaired diastolic filling of the ventricles.[45,46] The patient who has been on bed rest should sit for 3 to 5 minutes before ambulating. Also, antianginal agents that can slow HR must be used with caution in the patient who may have degeneration of the conduction system. The patient may be at increased risk of drug toxicity because of declining hepatic and renal function.

The older patient should be included in a cardiac rehabilitation program. Activity performance, endurance, and ability to tolerate stress can be improved in the older adult with physical training. Positive psychologic benefits can be derived from a planned exercise program and can include increased self-esteem and emotional well-being and improved body image.[47]

When planning an exercise program for the older adult, the nurse should remember the following: (1) longer warm-up periods are needed, (2) longer periods of low-level activity or longer rest periods between sessions are advisable, and (3) heat intolerance may be caused by decreased ability to sweat efficiently. The patient should be taught to avoid exercising in extremes of temperature and to maintain a moderate pace. Target HR for an older adult is 60% to 75% of the maximum HR. The older adult should exercise a minimum of 30 to 40 minutes three or four times a week.

Studies have shown that aggressive treatment of hypertension and hyperlipidemia will stabilize plaques in the coronary arteries of older adults, and cessation of cigarette smoking helps decrease the risk of MI at any age.[46] Encouraging the older patient to adopt a healthy lifestyle may increase quality of life and reduce the risks of CAD.

Older adults have a greater incidence of unstable angina as well as more complications from an acute MI than younger patients.[46] Complications commonly found in an older patient with an acute MI include an increased incidence of atrial fibrillation, atrial flutter, complete heart block, CHF, myocardial rupture, and cardiogenic shock. Given this greater risk, aggressive management with thrombolytic therapy or direct PTCA in the older adult patient with an acute MI is recommended.[48]

β-adrenergic blocker therapy has also been shown to greatly benefit the older population, but side effects such as CHF and heart block are more common. PTCA is another aggressive treatment used for controlling CAD in the older patient. However, in patients more than 70 years of age there is a significantly increased incidence of complications with this procedure.

Elective CABG is generally well tolerated in the older patient. However, the incidence of postoperative complications is high, including arrhythmias, stroke, and infection. The nurse caring for older adults must be aware that, although the benefits of treatment may outweigh risks in this population, complications are higher than in younger individuals. The nurse must be alert to early signs and symptoms of complications and aggressively try to prevent and treat them. Nursing research has shown that despite increased early postoperative complications, once these individuals are home their time of recovery is similar to patients younger than age 70.[45]

WOMEN AND CORONARY ARTERY DISEASE

Traditionally CAD has been viewed as an affliction of middle-aged men, when in fact CAD is the number one killer of American women. Approximately 500,000 deaths occur from cardiovascular disease in women per year.[49] Only recently has there been research focusing on the manifestations and course of CAD in women. Women tend to manifest CAD 10 years later in life than men, and most women have symptoms of angina rather than MI.[49,50] The exercise treadmill test has a low sensi-

RESEARCH
IMPLICATIONS FOR NURSING PRACTICE

Women and Coronary Artery Disease

Citation Women and coronary disease: relationship between descriptors of signs and symptoms and diagnostic and treatment course, *Am J Crit Care* 7:175, 1998.

Purpose To explore the relationship between descriptors of signs and symptoms of coronary artery disease and follow-up care and to investigate any differences between male and female patients.

Methods Structured interviews with patients and chart audits were used to assess initial signs and symptoms, associated cardiac-related signs and symptoms, and the diagnostic tests and interventions used for treatment. The sample consisted of 98 patients (51 women and 47 men) who were admitted with a medical diagnosis of myocardial infarction.

Results and Conclusions Chest pain was the most common sign or symptom reported by both men and women. The four most common associated signs and symptoms were identical in men and women: fatigue, rest pain, shortness of breath, and weakness. However, significantly more women than men reported loss of appetite, paroxysmal nocturnal dyspnea, and back pain. Women were also less likely than men to have angiography and to receive IV nitroglycerin, heparin, and thrombolytic agents as part of the acute management of myocardial infarction.

Implications for Nursing Practice Nurses should learn to anticipate nonspecific signs and symptoms, such as back pain, anorexia, and light-headedness, in women with myocardial infarction. Nurses also should recognize that chest pain may not be the initial symptom in women and that women may have more vague complaints of pain than men do that warrant further investigation. Nurses have a key role in advocating for female patients to ensure that the patients receive appropriate diagnostic and treatment options. In addition, nurses and other health care providers can educate the public about the risk that heart disease will develop in one of three women and about ways to modify cardiovascular risk factors to decrease individual risk.

tivity and specificity in women, and 30% to 40% of women have false-positive results.[49] This may be because women have lower hematocrits, higher pulmonary and systolic BP responses to exercise, and ST segment depression from circulating estrogen. Exercise echocardiography is the most accurate test for the detection of CAD in women.[49]

Women also have a much higher mortality rate within 1 year following MI than men.[49,50] Women are also more likely to have reinfarction within 1 year.[49,50] This increased mortality rate was thought to be as a result of women developing CAD at a later age in life when they are more likely to have other illnesses such as diabetes, hypertension, and heart failure. However, even when these comorbidities have been taken into consideration, women still have a higher mortality rate following MI than men.

Women who have CABG surgery have a higher mortality rate and more complications after surgery than men. This is because women have smaller arteries, are older, and are referred more frequently for CABG with severe or unstable angina requiring urgent or emergent surgery.[49,50] Long-term survival rates are similar for men and women following CABG, but women report less relief from angina, poorer health, and more symptoms than men. Women also have higher rates of coronary dissection and hospital mortality than men following PTCA, but men have a higher incidence of restenosis.[50] However, women have a decreased incidence of sudden cardiac death compared with men.

Although risk factors of CAD for men and women are similar, the significance of these risk factors may be different. Diabetes mellitus has been found to be the most single powerful predictor of CAD in women. Women with diabetes have five to seven times the risk for developing CAD than nondiabetic women.[50] Studies have shown that estrogen replacement in postmenopausal women reduces their risk for CAD by 50%. Furthermore, estrogen replacement lowers LDL and raises HDL cholesterol in postmenopausal women. Smoking, a major risk factor for both men and women, may also carry specific problems for women. Smoking has been linked to a decrease in estrogen levels and hence early menopause. Cigarette smoking has been identified as the most powerful contributor to CAD in women younger than age 50.[51] Hypertension is a risk factor for CAD in women. In postmenopausal women, hypertension is associated with a higher incidence of CAD than men, and in premenopausal women, it increases the risk of death from CAD tenfold.[49]

Implications for Nursing

Because CAD in women more often manifests with angina and women have a poorer prognosis following acute MI, aggressive education about the reduction of risk factors and counseling about lifestyle modification should be implemented after diagnosis of disease in an attempt to prevent an acute MI. The nurse must recognize that women have significant post-MI and post-CABG morbidity and mortality rates. Women should be assessed for the presence of other diseases such as diabetes mellitus and hypertension that can affect their recovery after an MI. The nurse should closely assess for early complications following MI, PTCA, and CABG.

Because women generally develop CAD at a later age than men, they often are widowed. The nurse should assess the patient's social support systems and refer to agencies that can assist in recovery where indicated. Cardiac rehabilitation programs are just as beneficial for women as men. Specific instruction should be given for activities that can be performed following recovery from MI or CABG. Studies of psychosocial outcomes following CABG are conflicting. Some studies report that women suffer many psychosocial difficulties after cardiac surgery; others report that women actually have less depression and anxiety.[52] Preoperative assessment of anxiety, depression, and social support should be done to facilitate optimal recovery from CABG.[52]

CRITICAL THINKING EXERCISES

CASE STUDY

Myocardial Infarction

Patient Profile

M.T., a 46-year-old successful businessman, was rushed to the hospital by a rescue squad after experiencing crushing substernal pain radiating down his left arm. He also complained of dizziness and nausea.

Subjective Data

- Has a history of angina pectoris and hypertension
- Is overweight but recently lost 10 pounds
- Bowls occasionally
- Has three teenage children who are causing "problems"
- Recently experienced loss of best friend and business partner, who died from cancer

Objective Data

Physical Examination

- Diaphoretic, short of breath
- BP 165/100, pulse 120, respiratory rate 26/min

Diagnostic Studies

- Cholesterol 350 mg/dl (9.1 mmol/L)
- CK 730 U/L (12.17 μkat/L)
- ECG shows premature ventricular contractions
- Inferolateral wall MI

Collaborative Care

- Streptokinase 1.5 million units IVPB over 40 to 60 min
- Morphine 2 to 4 mg IV q5min prn for chest pain
- Oxygen 2 L/min
- ASA 80 to 325 mg per day
- Bed rest
- Vital signs every hour

Critical Thinking Questions

1. Which coronary artery was most likely occluded in M.T.'s coronary circulation?
2. Explain the pathogenesis of CAD. What risk factors may contribute to its development? What risk factors were present in M.T.'s life?
3. What is angina pectoris? How does angina differ from MI?
4. List the clinical manifestations that M.T. exhibited and explain their pathophysiologic bases.
5. Explain the significance of the results of the laboratory tests and ECG findings.
6. For each treatment measure M.T. received, explain the physiologic reason for its use.
7. Based on the assessment data presented, write one or more appropriate nursing diagnoses. Are there any collaborative problems?

NURSING RESEARCH ISSUES

1. Are patients with CABG more likely to make lifestyle changes than patients who are treated with PTCA?
2. Do the activities that precipitate angina differ between those who are older than 65 years as compared with younger people?
3. Is there a gender bias in the treatment of patients with CAD?
4. Does estrogen replacement delay the onset of symptomatic CAD in women?
5. Is a nurse-monitored rehabilitation program more effective than a self-monitored program?
6. What risk factors for CAD are most significant for women?

REVIEW QUESTIONS

The number of the question corresponds to the same-numbered objective at the beginning of the chapter.

1. In teaching a patient about coronary artery disease, the nurse explains that the changes that occur in this disorder involve
   a. diffuse involvement of plaque formation in coronary veins.
   b. formation of fibrous tissue around coronary artery orifices.
   c. accumulation of lipid and fibrous tissue within the coronary arteries.
   d. chronic vasoconstriction of coronary arteries leading to permanent vasospasm.
2. After teaching about ways to decrease risk factors for CAD, the nurse recognizes that additional instruction is needed when the patient says,
   a. "I would like to add weight lifting to my exercise program."
   b. "I can't keep my blood pressure normal without medication."
   c. "I can change my diet to decrease my intake of saturated fats."
   d. "I will change my lifestyle to reduce activities that increase my stress."
3. A hospitalized patient with angina pectoris tells the nurse that she is having chest pain. The nurse bases his actions on the knowledge that anginal pain
   a. will be relieved by rest, nitroglycerin, or both.
   b. is less severe than pain of a myocardial infarction.
   c. indicates that irreversible cellular damage is occurring.
   d. is frequently associated with vomiting and extreme fatigue.
4. In planning education for the patient with angina, the nurse includes information related to
   a. symptoms of digitalis toxicity.
   b. prophylactic use of nitroglycerin.
   c. behavior modification to prevent recurrent MI.
   d. knowledge of foods that are high in potassium.
5. In planning activity for the patient recovering from an MI, the nurse recognizes that the healing heart wall is most vulnerable to stress
   a. 3 weeks after the infarction.
   b. 4 to 6 days after the infarction.

c. 10 to 14 days after the infarction.
d. when healing is complete at 6 to 8 weeks.

6. A patient is admitted to the CCU with chest pain of 24 hours' duration, ECG findings consistent with an acute MI, and occasional ventricular arrhythmias. The nurse plans care for the patient based on the expectation that the patient will be managed with
   a. subcutaneous nitroglycerin.
   b. endotracheal intubation.
   c. continuous ECG monitoring.
   d. thrombolytic therapy with tissue plasminogen activator.
7. A patient 5 days after MI is restless and apprehensive. The nurse can help by
   a. providing all care by doing everything for the patient.
   b. structuring the environment and routine so that the patient can rest.
   c. allowing the patient to participate in planning and carrying out activities.
   d. encouraging the family to provide for the patient's physical care and emotional support.
8. Three days after MI a patient states that he does not understand what the alarm is about because his problem is just bad indigestion. His reaction is an example of
   a. anger.
   b. denial.
   c. projection.
   d. depression.
9. The most common pathologic finding in individuals with sudden cardiac death is
   a. cardiomyopathies.
   b. mitral valve disease.
   c. atherosclerotic heart disease.
   d. left ventricular hypertrophy.

References

1. American Heart Association: *1998 heart and stroke facts statistics,* Dallas, 1997, American Heart Association.
2. Berliner JA and others: Atherosclerosis: basic mechanisms oxidation, inflammation, and genetics, *Circulation* 91:2488, 1995.
3. American Heart Association: *Heart and stroke facts,* Dallas, 1997, American Heart Association.
4. Kannel WB: CHD risk factors: a Framingham study update, *Hosp Pract* 25:119, 1990.
5. Froelicher ES and others: Risk factor screening, *J Cardiovasc Nurs* 10:30, 1995.
6. National Cholesterol Education Program: Second report of the expert panel on detection, evaluation and treatment of high blood cholesterol in adults (Adult Treatment Panel II), *Circulation* 89:1330, 1994.
7. Steenland K, Than M, Lally C, Heath C: Environmental tobacco smoke and coronary heart disease in the American Cancer Society CPS II Cohort, *Circulation* 94:622, 1996.
8. Kawachi I and others: A prospective study of passive smoking and coronary heart disease, *Circulation* 95:2374, 1997.
9. Delunas LR: Beyond type A: hostility and coronary heart disease—implications for research and practice, *Rehabil Nurs* 21:196, 1996.
10. Kawachi I and others: A prospective study of anger and coronary heart disease, *Circulation* 94:2090, 1996.
11. Frankish CJ, Linden W: Spouse-pair risk factors and cardiovascular reactivity, *J Psychosom Res* 40:37, 1996.
12. Engler MB, Engler MM: Assessment of the cardiovascular effects of stress, *J Cardiovasc Nurs* 10:51, 1995.
13. Nygard O and others: The role of homocysteine in arteriosclerosis, *N Engl J Med* 337:230, 1997.
14. Haskell WL and others: Effects of intensive atherosclerosis and clinical cardiac events in men and women with coronary artery disease, *Circulation* 89:975, 1994.
15. Talbert RL: Hyperlipidemia. In Dipiro JT and others, editors: *Pharmacotherapy: a pathophysiologic approach,* ed 3, Stamford, Conn, 1997, Appleton & Lange.
16. Weiner DA and others: Significance of silent myocardial ischemia during exercise testing in women: report from the coronary artery surgery study, *Am Heart J* 129:465, 1995.
17. Thelan LA and others: *Critical care nursing,* ed 3, St Louis, 1998, Mosby.
18. Braunwald E and others: *Diagnosing and managing unstable angina,* PHS, AHCPR, NHLBI 94-0603, Rockville, Md, 1994, US Department of Health and Human Services.
19. Shah PK: New insights into the pathogenesis and prevention of acute coronary syndromes, *Am J Cardiol* 79:17, 1997.
20. Servi S and others: Correlation between clinical and morphologic findings in unstable angina, *Am J Cardiol* 77:128, 1996.
21. Berman D and others: Risk stratification in coronary artery disease: implications for stabilization and prevention, *Am J Cardiol* 79:10, 1997.
22. Bachinsky WB, Barnathan ES: Angioplasty in multivessel coronary artery disease, *Hosp Pract* 29:27, 1994.
23. Strimike CL: Caring for a patient with an intracoronary stent, *AJN* 95:40, 1995.
*24. Juran NB and others: Survey of current practice patterns for percutaneous transluminal coronary angioplasty, *Am J Crit Care* 5:442, 1996.
25. Gardner E and others: Intracoronary stent update: focus on patient education, *Crit Care Nurse* 16:65, 1996.
26. Moussa I and others: Subacute stent thrombosis and the anticoagulation controversy: changes in drug therapy, operator technique, and the impact of intravascular ultrasound, *Am J Cardiol* 78:13, 1996.
27. Brezina K, Murphy M, Stonner T: Care of the patient receiving ReoPro following angioplasty, *J Invasive Cardiol* 6(A):38A, 1994.
28. Coodley EL: CHD: when medical therapy fails, *Hosp Pract* 31:13, 1996.
29. Perra BM: Managing coronary atherectomy patients in a special procedure unit, *Crit Care Nurse* 15:57, 1995.
30. Talbert RL: Ischemic heart disease. In Dipiro JT and others, editors: *Pharmacotherapy: a pathophysiologic approach,* ed 3, Stamford, Conn, 1997, Appleton & Lange.
31. Abrams J: Beneficial actions of nitrates in cardiovascular disease, *Am J Cardiol* 77:31-C, 1997.
32. Pasternak RC, Braunwald E: Acute myocardial infarction. In Isselbacher KJ and others, editors: *Harrison's principles of internal medicine,* ed 14, New York, 1997, McGraw-Hill.
33. Connors KF, Gervasio AL: Postmyocardial infarction patients: experience from the SAVE trial, *Am J Crit Care* 4:23, 1995.
34. O'Donnell L: Complications of MI: beyond the acute stage, *AJN* 96:25, 1996.
35. Sewart S, Kucia A, Poropat S: Early detection and management of right ventricular infarction: the role of the critical care nurse, *DCCN* 14:282, 1995.
36. Futterman LG, Lemberg L: SGPT, LDH, HBCK, CPK, CPK-MB, MB^1, MB^2, CTCT, CTNC, CTNI, *Am J Crit Care* 6:333, 1997.
37. Ryan RJ and others: ACC/AHA guidelines for the management of patients with acute myocardial infarction, *J Am Coll Cardiol* 34:890, 1999.
38. Ryan TJ: Angioplasty in acute myocardial infarction, *Hosp Pract* 30:33, 1995.
39. Flapah AD: Management after a first myocardial infarction, *Hosp Pract* 31:133, 1996.
*40. McCauley KM: Assessing social support in patients with cardiac disease, *J Cardiovasc Nurs* 10:73, 1995.
41. Brezinka V, Kittel F: Psychosocial factors of coronary heart disease in women: a review, *Soc Sci Med* 42:1351, 1995.
42. Chang D, Goldstein S: Sudden cardiac death in ischemic heart disease, *Compr Ther* 23:95, 1997.
43. Barron HV, Lesh MD: Autonomic nervous system and sudden cardiac death, *J Am Coll Cardiol* 27:1053, 1996.
*44. Doolittle ND, Sauve MJ: Impact of aborted sudden cardiac death on survivors and their spouses: the phenomenon of different reference points, *Am J Crit Care* 4:389, 1995.

45. Rossi MS: The octogenarian cardiac surgery patient, *J Cardiovasc Nurs* 9:75, 1995.
46. Kannel WB: Cardiovascular risk factors in the older adult, *Hosp Pract* 31:135, 1996.
47. Lavie CJ, Milani RV: Effects of cardiac rehabilitation programs on exercise capacity, coronary risk factors, behavioral characteristics, and quality of life in a large elderly cohort, *Am J Cardiol* 76:177, 1995.
48. Laster SB and others: Results of direct percutaneous transluminal coronary angioplasty in octogenarians, *Am J Cardiol* 76:10, 1996.
49. Jensen L, King KM: Women and heart disease: the issues, *Crit Care Nurs* 17:45, 1997.
50. Moser DK: Correcting misconceptions about women and heart disease, *AJN* 97:26, 1997.
*51. Cronin SN, Logsdon C, Miracle V: Psychosocial and functional outcomes in women after coronary artery bypass surgery, *Crit Care Nurs* 17:19, 1997.
*52. Sauve J, Frotin F: Factors related to recovery of women following coronary artery surgery, *Cardiovasc Nurs* 32:1, 1996.

*Nursing research-based articles.

Resources

Resources for this chapter are listed after Chapter 33 on p. 917.

REMEMBER to check out your companion CD-ROM

33 NURSING MANAGEMENT Congestive Heart Failure and Cardiac Surgery

Mary Ann House-Fancher & Linda Griego Martinez

www.mosby.com/MERLIN/medsurg_lewis

LEARNING OBJECTIVES

1. Compare the pathophysiology of systolic and diastolic ventricular failure.
2. Discuss the compensatory mechanisms involved in congestive heart failure.
3. Describe the nursing and collaborative management, including diet and nutritional therapy, of the patient with chronic congestive heart failure.
4. Describe the nursing and collaborative management of the patient with acute congestive heart failure and pulmonary edema.
5. Compare the different types of cardiomyopathy regarding pathophysiology, clinical manifestations, and nursing and collaborative management.
6. Describe the indications for cardiac transplantation and the nursing management of cardiac transplant recipients.
7. Describe the preoperative and postoperative management of the patient who has cardiac surgery.

CONGESTIVE HEART FAILURE

Congestive heart failure (CHF) is a cardiovascular condition in which the heart is unable to pump an adequate amount of blood to meet the metabolic needs of the body's tissues. CHF is not a disease; it is a syndrome caused by a variety of pathophysiologic processes (Table 33-1). CHF is characterized by left ventricular dysfunction, reduced exercise tolerance, diminished quality of life, and shortened life expectancy.

Significance

CHF is associated with numerous types of heart disease, particularly with long-standing hypertension and coronary artery disease (CAD). More than one half of the deaths from heart disease are attributable to end-stage CHF. Currently about 4.9 million people in the United States have CHF. The American Heart Association (AHA) estimates that 400,000 new cases of CHF occur each year. The 5-year mortality rate for heart failure is about 50%. In the past 15 years deaths from CHF have increased 116%. The rate of sudden cardiac death (SCD) in a patient with CHF is 6 to 9 times higher than the rate for the general population. About 20% of individuals who have a heart attack will be disabled with heart failure within 6 years.[1]

The patient with CHF has an impaired quality of life, restrictions in functional capacity, and numerous symptoms. CHF is the single most frequent cause of hospitalization for people age 65 and older.[2,3] Currently, CHF continues to have a poor prognosis and is likely to remain a major clinical and health care problem.

Etiology and Pathophysiology

Risk Factors. Although CAD and advancing age are the primary risk factors for CHF, there are also other factors, including hypertension, diabetes, cigarette smoking, obesity, high cholesterol levels, and proteinuria.[3] Hypertension is a major contributing factor, increasing the risk of CHF approximately threefold. The risk of CHF increases progressively with the severity of hypertension, and systolic and diastolic hypertension equally predict risk. Diabetes mellitus predisposes an individual to CHF regardless of the presence of concomitant CAD or hypertension. Diabetes is more likely to predispose to CHF in women than in men.[4] The presence of these risk factors should alert health care providers to the possibility of the development of CHF.

Etiology. CHF may be caused by any interference with the normal mechanisms regulating cardiac output (CO). CO depends on (1) preload, (2) afterload, (3) myocardial contractility, (4) heart rate (HR), and (5) metabolic state of the individual. Any alteration in these factors can lead to decreased ventricular function and the resultant manifestations of CHF. The major causes of CHF may be divided into two subgroups: (1) underlying cardiac diseases (see Table 33-1) and (2) precipitating causes (Table 33-2). Underlying cardiac diseases that cause CHF may be congenital or acquired. Precipitating causes often increase the workload of the ventricles, causing a

Reviewed by Carmella Moran, RN, MSN, Senior Department Chair, St. Joseph College of Nursing, Naperville, Ill.

Table 33-1 Common Causes of Congestive Heart Failure

Chronic	Acute
Coronary artery disease	Acute myocardial infarction
Hypertensive heart disease	Arrhythmias
Rheumatic heart disease	Pulmonary emboli
Congenital heart disease	Thyrotoxicosis
Cor pulmonale	Hypertensive crises
Cardiomyopathy	Rupture of papillary muscle
Anemia	Ventricular septal defect
Bacterial endocarditis	

decompensated condition that leads to decreased myocardial function. Precipitating causes are generally more amenable to treatment than cardiac diseases.

Pathology of Ventricular Failure. Ventricular failure can be described as (1) a defect in systolic function that results in impaired ventricular emptying or (2) a defect in diastolic function that causes an impairment in ventricular filling. It is now recognized that patients with heart failure actually comprise three distinct groups: (1) those with failure of systolic ejection, (2) those with abnormal resistance to diastolic filling, and (3) those with mixed systolic and diastolic dysfunction.[5]

Systolic failure. Systolic failure is the most common cause of CHF. It is a defect in the ability of the cardiac myofibrils to shorten, which decreases the muscles' ability to contract (pump). This causes the left ventricle to lose its ability to generate enough pressure to eject blood forward through the high-pressure aorta. Inability to move blood forward through the aorta results in (1) a decreased left ventricular ejection fraction (LVEF), (2) an acute increase in left ventricular end-diastolic pressure (LVEDP), (3) an increase in pulmonary artery wedge pressure (PAWP), and (4) an increase in fluid accumulation in the pulmonary vascular bed (pulmonary congestion). Systolic failure is caused by impaired contractile function (e.g., myocardial infarction), increased afterload (e.g., hypertension), or mechanical abnormalities (e.g., valvular heart disease). Therefore systolic failure is characterized by low forward blood flow.

Diastolic failure. In contrast, diastolic failure is not a disorder of contractility, but of relaxation and ventricular filling. In fact, there is normal or hyperdynamic systolic function. Diastolic failure is characterized by high filling pressures and the resultant venous engorgement in both the pulmonary and systemic systems. The diagnosis of diastolic failure is made on the basis of the presence of pulmonary congestion and pulmonary hypertension in the setting of a normal ejection fraction.

Diastolic failure is usually the result of left ventricular hypertrophy from chronic systemic hypertension, aortic stenosis, or infiltrative and hypertrophic cardiomyopathy. Diastolic failure is commonly seen in older adults as a result of myocardial fibrosis and hypertension, which are common in this population.[6]

Mixed systolic and diastolic failure. Systolic and diastolic failure of mixed origin is seen in disease states such as dilated cardiomyopathy (DCM), a condition in which poor systolic function (weakened muscle function) is further compromised by dilated left ventricular walls that are unable to relax. This patient often has extremely poor ejection fractions, high pulmonary pressures, and biventricular failure (both ventricles may be dilated and have poor filling and emptying capacity).

The patient with ventricular failure of any type has low systemic arterial blood pressure, low CO, and poor renal perfusion. Poor exercise tolerance and ventricular arrhythmias are also common. When pulmonary congestion and edema are present, the diagnosis of CHF may be made. Whether a patient arrives at this point acutely from a myocardial infarction (MI) or chronically from worsening cardiomyopathy or hypertension, the body's response to this low CO is to mobilize its compensatory mechanisms to maintain CO and blood pressure (BP).

Compensatory Mechanisms. CHF can have an abrupt onset as with acute MI, or it can be an insidious process resulting from slow, progressive changes. The overloaded heart resorts to certain compensatory mechanisms to try to maintain adequate CO.[7] The main compensatory mechanisms include (1) ventricular dilation, (2) ventricular hypertrophy, (3) increased sympathetic nervous system stimulation, and (4) hormonal response.

Dilation. Dilation is an enlargement of the chambers of the heart. It occurs when pressure in the heart chambers (usually the left ventricle) is elevated over time. The muscle fibers of the heart stretch and thereby increase their contractile force. Initially this increased contraction leads to increased CO and maintenance of arterial blood pressure and perfusion. Therefore dilation is an adaptive mechanism to cope with increasing blood volume. Eventually this mechanism becomes inadequate because the elastic elements of the muscle fibers are overstretched and overstrained.

Hypertrophy. In chronic CHF, hypertrophy is an increase in the muscle mass and cardiac wall thickness in response to overwork and strain. It occurs slowly because it takes time for this increased muscle tissue to develop. Hypertrophy generally follows persistent or chronic dilation and thus further increases the contractile power of the muscle fibers. This will lead to an increase in CO and maintenance of tissue perfusion. However, hypertrophic heart muscle has poor contractility.

Sympathetic nervous system activation. Sympathetic nervous system stimulation is often the first mechanism triggered in low CO states. However, it is the least effective compensatory mechanism. Because there is inadequate stroke volume and CO, there is increased sympathetic nervous system activation, resulting in the increased release of epinephrine and norepinephrine. This results in an increased heart rate, myocardial contractility, and peripheral vascular constriction. Initially this increase in HR and contractility improves CO. However, over time these factors act in a detrimental fashion by increasing the myocardium's need for oxygen and the workload of the already failing heart. The vasoconstriction causes an immediate increase in preload, which may initially increase CO. However, an increase in venous return to the heart, which is already volume overloaded, actually worsens ventricular performance.

Hormonal response. As the CO falls, blood flow to the kidneys decreases, causing decreased glomerular blood flow. This is interpreted by the juxtaglomerular apparatus in the kidneys as decreased volume. In response, the kidneys release renin, which converts angiotensinogen to angiotensin (see Chapter 42 and Fig. 42-6). Angiotensin causes (1) the adrenal cortex to release aldosterone, which causes sodium retention, and (2) in-

Table 33-2 **Precipitating Causes of Congestive Heart Failure**

Cause	Mechanism
Anemia	Decreases O_2-carrying capacity of the blood, stimulating ↑ in CO to meet tissue demands
Infection	Increases O_2 demand of tissues, stimulating ↑ CO
Thyrotoxicosis	Increases the tissue metabolic rate, accelerating HR and workload of the heart
Hypothyroidism	Indirectly predisposes to ↑ atherosclerosis; severe hypothyroidism decreases myocardial contractility
Arrhythmias	May decrease CO and increase workload and O_2 requirements of the myocardial tissue
Bacterial endocarditis	Infection: increases metabolic demands and O_2 requirements Valvular dysfunction: causes stenosis and regurgitation
Pulmonary embolism	Increases pulmonary pressure and exerts a pressure load on the RV, leading to RV hypertrophy and failure
Pulmonary disease	Increases pulmonary pressure and exerts a pressure load on the RV, leading to RV hypertrophy and failure
Paget's disease	Increases workload of the heart by ↑ the vascular bed in skeletal muscle
Nutritional deficiencies	May decrease cardiac function by ↓ myocardial muscle mass and contractility
Hypervolemia	Increases preload and causes volume load on the RV

CO, Cardiac output; *HR,* heart rate; *RV,* right ventricle.

creased peripheral vasoconstriction, which increases the arterial pressure.

The posterior pituitary senses the increased osmotic pressure and it secretes antidiuretic hormone (ADH). ADH increases water reabsorption in the renal tubules, causing water retention and therefore increased blood volume. Therefore the blood volume is increased in a person who is already volume overloaded.

Cardiac compensation occurs when compensatory mechanisms succeed in maintaining adequate CO for tissue perfusion. Cardiac decompensation occurs when these mechanisms can no longer maintain adequate CO and clinical signs and symptoms appear as a consequence of inadequate tissue perfusion. Without treatment, this state is fatal. Even with treatment, the prognosis is poor.

Types of Congestive Heart Failure

CHF is usually manifested by biventricular failure, although one ventricle may precede the other in dysfunction.[6] Normally the pumping actions of the left and right sides of the heart complement each other, producing a continuous flow of blood. However, as a result of pathologic conditions, one side may fail while the other side continues to function normally for a period of time. Because of the prolonged strain, the functioning side of the heart will eventually fail, resulting in biventricular failure.

The most common form of initial heart failure is left-sided failure (Fig. 33-1). LV failure will usually lead to and be the main cause of right-sided failure. Right-sided failure can occur without preceding LV failure as a result of right ventricular MI or cor pulmonale (see Fig. 26-11).

Left-Sided Failure. Left-sided failure results from LV dysfunction, which causes blood to back up through the left atrium and into the pulmonary veins. The increased pulmonary pressure causes fluid extravasation from the pulmonary capillary bed into the interstitium and then the alveoli, which is manifested as pulmonary congestion and edema. The most common causes of left-sided failure are diseases of the coronary arteries, hypertension, cardiomyopathy, and rheumatic heart disease.

When an MI occurs, myocardial tissue is damaged and, with time, replaced by scar tissue. The ischemic tissue and the scar tissue are less elastic and have less contractility than undamaged myocardium. The loss of myocardial mass increases the workload on the remaining functional tissue. If the functioning myocardium cannot compensate for this loss, the volume of blood ejected from the ventricle is decreased and heart failure results. This failure may have a rapid onset (acute CHF) or a more insidious onset (chronic CHF).

When hypertension is present, the heart must pump blood against high arterial pressure. Eventually this can lead to LV hypertrophy. Hypertrophic muscle has poor contractility and will result in failure with time. Cardiomyopathy (discussed later in this chapter) is the third leading cause of CHF. There are different types of cardiomyopathy, but the end result is loss of the left ventricle's ability to maintain adequate CO, resulting in CHF.

Right-Sided Failure. Right-sided failure from a diseased right ventricle (RV) causes backward flow to the right atrium and venous circulation. Venous congestion in the systemic circulation results in peripheral edema, hepatomegaly, splenomegaly, vascular congestion of the gastrointestinal (GI) tract, and jugular venous distention. The primary cause of right-sided failure is left-sided failure. In this situation, left-sided failure results in pulmonary congestion and increased pressure in the blood vessels of the lung (pulmonary hypertension). Eventually, chronic pulmonary hypertension results in right-sided hypertrophy and failure. Cor pulmonale (right ventricular dilation and hypertrophy caused by pulmonary pathology) can also cause right-sided failure. Causes of cor pulmonale include chronic obstructive pulmonary disease (COPD) and pulmonary emboli. Right ventricular infarction may also cause RV failure. (Cor pulmonale is discussed in Chapter 26.)

Clinical Manifestations of Acute Congestive Heart Failure

Regardless of etiology, acute heart failure typically manifests as *pulmonary edema,* a term used to refer to an acute, life-threatening situation in which the lung alveoli become filled with

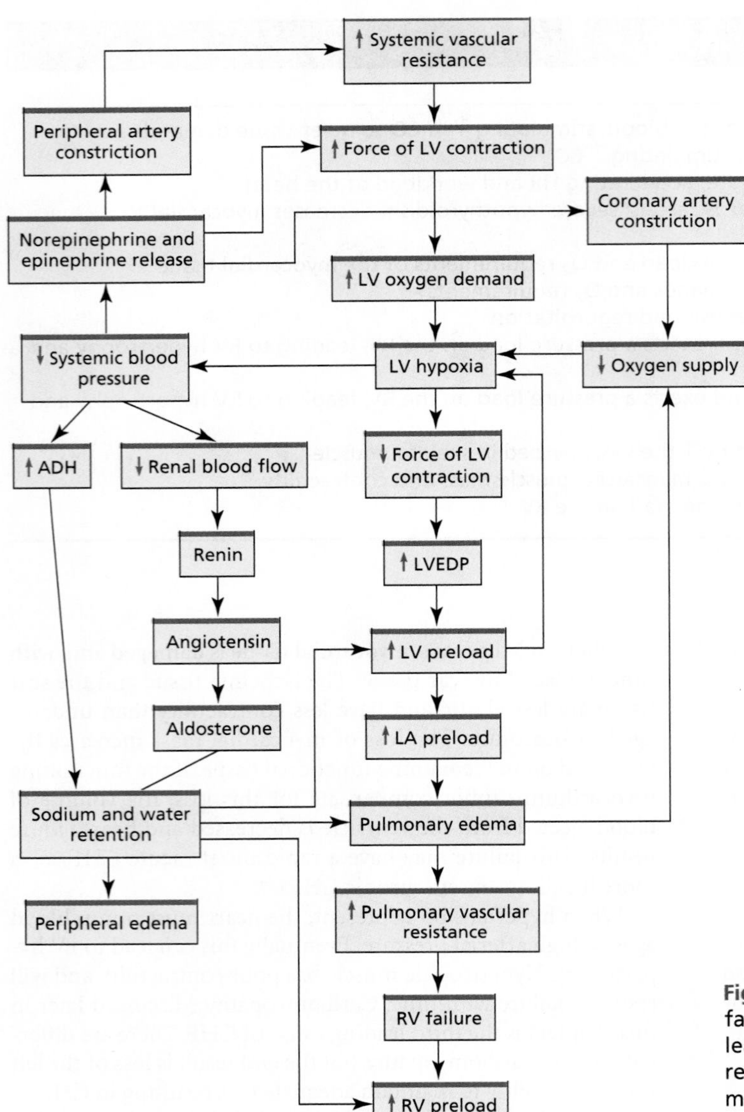

Fig. 33-1 Left ventricular (LV) heart failure (congestive heart failure) from elevated systemic vascular resistance. LV failure leads to right ventricular (RV) heart failure. Systemic vascular resistance and preload are exacerbated by renal and adrenal mechanisms. *ADH,* antidiuretic hormone; *LA,* left atrial; *LVEDP,* left ventricular end-diastolic pressure.

serous or serosanguineous fluid (Fig. 33-2). The most common factor in the onset of pulmonary edema is LV failure caused by CAD. (Other etiologic factors for pulmonary edema are listed in Table 26-28.)

In most cases of acute heart failure, there is an increase in the pulmonary venous pressure caused by decreased efficiency of the LV. This results in engorgement of the pulmonary vascular system. As a result, the lungs become less compliant, and there is increased resistance in the small airways. In addition, the lymphatic system increases its flow to help maintain a constant volume of the pulmonary extravascular fluid. This early stage is clinically associated with a mild increase in the respiratory rate and a decrease in arterial PaO_2.

If pulmonary venous pressure continues to increase, the increase in intravascular pressure causes more fluid to move into the interstitial space than the lymphatics can drain. There is *interstitial edema* at this point. There is more severe tachypnea, and x-ray changes can be noted. If the pulmonary venous pressure increases further, the tight alveoli lining cells are disrupted and a fluid containing red blood cells (RBCs) moves into the alveoli (alveolar edema). As the disruption becomes worse from further increases in the pulmonary venous pressure, the alveoli and airways are flooded with fluid (see Fig. 33-2). This is accompanied by a worsening of the blood gases (i.e., lower PaO_2 and possible increased $PaCO_2$ and progressive acidemia).

Clinical manifestations of pulmonary edema are unmistakable. The patient may be agitated, pale, and possibly cyanotic. The skin is clammy and cold from vasoconstriction caused by stimulation of the sympathetic nervous system. The patient has severe dyspnea, as evidenced by the obvious use of accessory muscles of respiration, a respiratory rate greater than 30 per minute, and orthopnea. There may be wheezing and coughing with the production of frothy, blood-tinged sputum. Auscultation of the lungs may reveal bubbling crackles, wheezes, and rhonchi throughout the lungs. The patient's HR is rapid, and BP may be elevated or decreased depending on the severity of the edema.

Clinical Manifestations of Chronic Congestive Heart Failure

The clinical manifestations of chronic CHF depend on the patient's age, the underlying type and extent of heart disease,

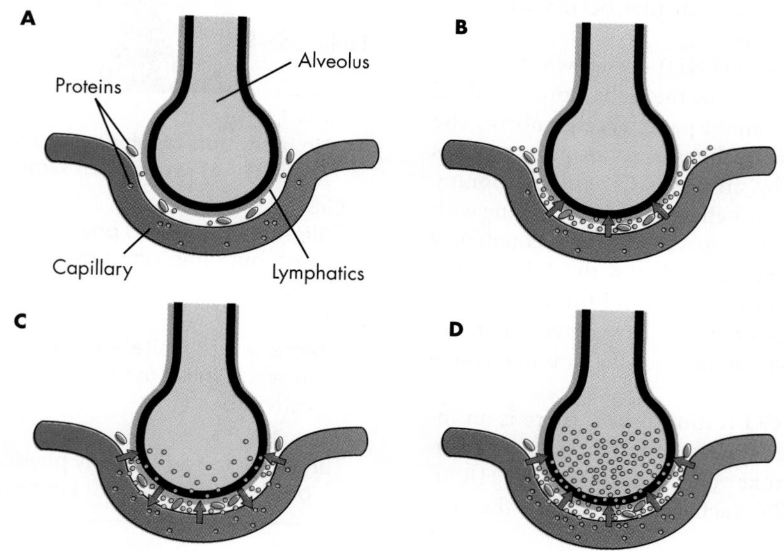

Fig. 33-2 As pulmonary edema progresses, it inhibits oxygen and carbon dioxide exchange at the alveolar capillary interface. **A,** Normal relationship. **B,** Increased pulmonary capillary hydrostatic pressure causes fluid to move from the vascular space into the pulmonary interstitial space. **C,** Lymphatic flow increases in an attempt to pull fluid back into the vascular or lymphatic space. **D,** Failure of lymphatic flow and worsening of left ventricular heart failure result in further movement of fluid into the interstitial space and into the alveoli.

Table 33-3 Clinical Manifestations of Heart Failure

Right-Sided Heart Failure	Left-Sided Heart Failure
Signs	**Signs**
RV heaves	LV heaves
Murmurs	Cheyne-Stokes respirations
Peripheral edema	Pulsus alternans (alternating pulses: strong, weak)
Weight gain	Increased HR
Edema of dependent body parts (sacrum, anterior tibias, pedal edema)	PMI displaced inferiorly and posteriorly (LV hypertrophy)
Ascites	↓ PaO_2, slight ↑ $PaCO_2$ (poor oxygen exchange)
Anasarca (massive generalized body edema)	Crackles (pulmonary edema)
Jugular venous distention	S_3 and S_4 heart sounds
Hepatomegaly (liver engorgement)	
Right-sided pleural effusion	
Symptoms	**Symptoms**
Fatigue	Fatigue
Dependent edema	Dyspnea (shallow respirations up to 32-40/min)
Right upper quadrant pain	Orthopnea (shortness of breath in recumbent position)
Anorexia and GI bloating	Dry, hacking cough
Nausea	Pulmonary edema
	Nocturia
	Paroxysmal noctural dyspnea

PMI, point of maximal impulse.

and which ventricle is failing to pump effectively. Table 33-3 lists the manifestations of LV and RV failure. The patient with chronic CHF will probably have manifestations of biventricular failure.

Fatigue. Fatigue is one of the earliest symptoms of chronic CHF. The patient notices fatigue after activities that normally are not tiring. The fatigue is caused by decreased CO, impaired circulation, and decreased oxygenation of the tissues. It is sometimes described as "sick fatigue" because of the decreased amounts of blood reaching the musculoskeletal system.

Dyspnea. Dyspnea is a common sign of chronic CHF. It is caused by increased pulmonary pressures secondary to interstitial and alveolar edema. This results in poor gas exchange because of fluid in the alveoli. The shortness of breath makes the patient conscious of air hunger that prompts rapid, shallow respirations. Dyspnea can occur with mild exertion or at rest. *Orthopnea* is shortness of breath that occurs when the patient is in a recumbent position.

Paroxysmal nocturnal dyspnea (PND) occurs when the patient is asleep. It is probably caused by the reabsorption of fluid from dependent body areas when the patient is recumbent. The patient awakens in a panic, has feelings of suffocation, and has a strong desire to seek relief by sitting up. Careful questioning of patients often reveals adaptive behavior such as sleeping with two or more pillows to aid breathing. A dry, hacking cough may be the first clinical symptom for the patient with CHF. Because there are increased pulmonary pressures and fluid accumulation in the lung tissues, the patient may have a persistent, dry cough, unrelieved with position or over-the-counter cough suppressants.

Tachycardia. Because CO is diminished, there is an increased sympathetic nervous system stimulation to compensate for low output. If the stroke volume decreases, the HR increases to maintain the CO. Tachycardia may be the first clinical sign of CHF.

Edema. Edema is a common sign of CHF. It may occur in the legs (peripheral edema), liver (hepatomegaly), abdominal cavity (ascites), lungs (pulmonary edema and pleural effusion), and other parts of the body. If the patient is in bed, sacral edema may develop. Pressing the edematous skin with the finger may leave a transient indentation (*pitting edema*). The development of dependent edema or a sudden weight gain of 5 pounds (2.3 kg) or more is often indicative of exacerbated CHF.

Nocturia. A person with chronic CHF will have decreased CO, impaired renal perfusion, and decreased urinary output during the day. However, when the person lies down at night, fluid movement from interstitial spaces back into the circulatory system is enhanced. This causes increased renal blood flow and diuresis. The patient may complain of having to void six or seven times during the night.

Skin Changes. Because tissue capillary oxygen extraction is increased in a person with chronic CHF, the skin may appear dusky. It is also cool and may be cool to the touch from diaphoresis. Often the lower extremities are shiny and swollen, with diminished or absent hair growth. Chronic swelling may result in pigment changes causing the skin to appear brown in areas covering the ankles and lower legs. The peripheral vasoconstriction that occurs to shunt blood to vital organs is a minor compensatory mechanism in chronic CHF.

Behavioral Changes. Cerebral circulation may be impaired with chronic CHF, especially in the presence of more widespread atherosclerosis. The patient or family may report unusual behavior, including restlessness, confusion, and decreased attention span or memory.

Chest Pain. In the presence of atherosclerosis, CHF can precipitate chest pain because of decreased coronary perfusion from decreased CO and increased myocardial work. Anginal-type pain may accompany either acute or chronic CHF.

Weight Changes. Many factors contribute to weight changes. Initially there may be a progressive weight gain from fluid retention. The patient with CHF has an increased metabolic rate. At the same time, decreased oxygen and nutrients are transported to the tissues. Often the patient is too sick to eat. Abdominal fullness from ascites and hepatomegaly frequently causes anorexia and nausea. In many cases the muscle and fat loss is masked by the patient's edematous condition. The actual weight loss may not be apparent until after the edema subsides.

Table 33-4 New York Heart Association Functional Classification of Persons with Congestive Heart Failure

Class 1
No limitation on physical activity; ordinary physical activity not resulting in symptoms

Class 2
Slight limitation on physical activity; no symptoms at rest, but symptoms possible with ordinary physical activity

Class 3
More severe limitations; patient usually comfortable at rest; clinical manifestations with usual physical activities

Class 4
Inability to carry on any physical activity without producing symptoms; symptoms possible at rest

Complications of Congestive Heart Failure

Pleural Effusion. Pleural effusion results from increasing pressure in the pleural capillaries. A transudation of fluid occurs from these capillaries into the pleural space. The pleural effusion usually develops in the right lower lobe initially. (Pleural effusion is discussed in Chapter 26.)

Arrhythmias. Patients with CHF have a high risk of fatal arrhythmias. Nearly one half experience sudden cardiac death, usually because of ventricular tachyarrhythmias. (Sudden cardiac death is discussed in Chapter 32.)

Left Ventricular Thrombus. With acute or chronic CHF, the enlarged LV and poor CO combine to increase the chance of thrombus formation in the LV. Current guidelines by the American College of Cardiology and AHA recommend anticoagulation in patients with CHF and atrial fibrillation or very poor left ventricular function (e.g., ejection fraction less than 20%). Once a thrombus has formed, it may also decrease LV contractility, decrease CO, and further worsen the patient's perfusion. The development of emboli from the thrombus is also a possibility and can result in a cerebrovascular accident (CVA).

Hepatomegaly. CHF can lead to severe hepatomegaly. The liver lobules become congested with venous blood. The hepatic congestion leads to impaired liver function. Eventually liver cells die, fibrosis occurs, and cirrhosis can develop (see Chapter 41).

Classification of Congestive Heart Failure

The New York Heart Association has developed functional guidelines for classifying people with CHF. The classification is based on the person's tolerance to physical activity (Table 33-4).

Diagnostic Studies

The primary goal in diagnosis is to determine the underlying etiology of heart failure. Diagnostic measures to assess the

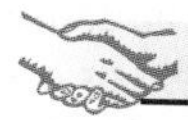

COLLABORATIVE CARE

Table 33-5 Acute Congestive Heart Failure and Pulmonary Edema

Diagnostic
- History and physical examination
- ABGs, serum chemistries, liver profile
- Chest x-ray
- Hemodynamic monitoring
- Twelve-lead ECG and monitor
- Echocardiogram
- Nuclear imaging studies
- Cardiac catheterization

Collaborative Therapy
- Maintenance of patient in high Fowler's position
- Oxygen by mask or nasal catheter
- Morphine IV
- Diuretics IV
  - Furosemide (Lasix)
  - Bumetanide (Bumex)
- Nitroglycerin IV
- Nitroprusside IV
- Inotropic therapy (see Table 33-7)
- BP, HR, RR, PAWP, urinary output at least q1hr
- Daily weights
- Possible cardioversion
- Endotracheal intubation and mechanical ventilation
- Treatment of underlying cause

ABGs, arterial blood gases; *PAWP,* pulmonary artery wedge pressure; *RR,* respiratory rate.

COLLABORATIVE CARE

Table 33-6 Chronic Congestive Heart Failure

Diagnostic
- History and physical examination
- Determination of underlying cause
- Serum chemistries, renal profile, liver profile
- Chest x-ray
- ECG
- Exercise-stress testing
- Nuclear imaging studies
- Echocardiography
- Hemodynamic monitoring
- Cardiac catheterization

Collaborative Therapy
- Treatment of underlying cause
- Oxygen therapy at 2-6 L/min
- Rest
- Digitalis preparations
- Diuretics (see Table 33-9)
- Vasodilator drugs
  - ACE inhibitors
  - Nitrates
- Inotropic drugs
  - Amrinone (Inocor)
  - Milrinone (Primacor)
  - Dopamine (Intropin)
  - Dobutamine (Dobutrex)
- Antiarrhythmic drugs
- β-adrenergic blocking drugs
  - Carvedilol (Coreg)
- Daily weights
- Sodium-restricted diet
- Intraaortic balloon pump
- Ventricular assist device
- Cardiac transplant

ACE, angiotensin-converting enzyme.

cause and degree of heart failure include physical examination, chest x-ray, electrocardiogram (ECG), hemodynamic assessment, echocardiogram, and cardiac catheterization. Diagnostic studies used for the patient with acute CHF are presented in Table 33-5 and those for the patient with chronic CHF are presented in Table 33-6.

NURSING AND COLLABORATIVE MANAGEMENT: ACUTE CONGESTIVE HEART FAILURE AND PULMONARY EDEMA

The goal of therapy is to improve left ventricular function by decreasing intravascular volume, decreasing venous return (preload), decreasing afterload, improving gas exchange and oxygenation, increasing CO, and reducing anxiety. Table 33-5 lists the major components of the therapeutic approach. Many of the measures may be done simultaneously.

■ Decreasing Intravascular Volume

Decreasing intravascular volume with the use of diuretics improves LV function by reducing venous return to the failing LV. A loop diuretic (e.g., furosemide [Lasix], bumetanide [Bumex]) is the drug of choice for decreasing volume because it may be administered quickly by IV push and its action within the kidney occurs rapidly.

By decreasing venous return to the LV and thereby reducing preload, the overfilled LV contracts more efficiently and CO improves. This measure increases LV function, decreases pulmonary vascular pressures, and improves gas exchange.

IV nitroglycerin (NTG) is a vasodilator used in the treatment of acute and chronic CHF. NTG reduces circulating volume by decreasing preload and also increases coronary artery circulation by dilating the coronary arteries. Therefore NTG reduces preload, slightly reduces afterload (in high doses), and increases myocardial oxygen supply.

■ Decreasing Venous Return

Decreasing venous return (preload) reduces the amount of volume returned to the LV during diastole. This can be accomplished by placing the patient in a high Fowler's position with the feet horizontal in the bed or dangling at the bedside. This position helps decrease venous return because of the pooling of blood in the extremities. This position also increases the thoracic capacity, allowing for improved ventilation.

Decreasing Afterload

Afterload is the amount of wall tension the LV must develop during systole to eject blood into the aorta; that is, it is the amount of work the LV has to produce to eject blood into the systemic circulation. Systemic vascular resistance (SVR) is a determinant of afterload, as is LV filling. If afterload is reduced, the CO of the LV improves and thereby decreases pulmonary congestion.

IV nitroprusside (Nipride) is a potent vasodilator that reduces preload and afterload. Because of its potent effects on the vascular system, it is the drug of choice for the patient with pulmonary edema. By reducing both preload and afterload (by arteriolar and venous dilation), myocardial contraction improves, increasing CO and reducing pulmonary congestion. Complications of IV nitroprusside include (1) hypotension, which may require the use of dobutamine (Dobutrex) IV to maintain a mean arterial BP greater than or equal to 60 mm Hg, and (2) thiocyanate toxicity that can develop after 48 hours of use. Morphine also reduces preload and afterload. It dilates both the pulmonary and systemic blood vessels, a goal in decreasing pulmonary pressures and improving the exchange of gases. It also reduces anxiety.

Improving Gas Exchange and Oxygenation

Gas exchange may be improved by several measures. IV morphine decreases oxygen demands, which may be raised as a result of anxiety and subsequent increased musculoskeletal and respiratory activity. Administration of oxygen helps increase the percentage of oxygen in inspired air. (Oxygen therapy is discussed in Chapter 27.) In severe pulmonary edema the patient may need to be intubated and placed on a mechanical ventilator.

Improving Cardiac Function

Digitalis improves LV function by its positive inotropic action. Digitalis increases contractility but also increases myocardial oxygen consumption. Newer inotropic drugs (e.g., dobutamine [Dobutrex], amrinone [Inocor], milrinone [Primacor]) that increase myocardial contractility without increasing oxygen consumption are more effective. Dobutamine, amrinone, and milrinone also cause increased peripheral vasodilation. Whatever increase in maximal oxygen consumption (MVO_2) is induced by these agents is counteracted by subsequent vasodilation. However, these drugs are potent vasoactive substances requiring close observation and monitoring of the patient.

Hemodynamic monitoring may become necessary if rapid resolution of symptoms does not occur with diuretics, morphine, and NTG or if the patient becomes hypotensive. (Hemodynamic monitoring is discussed in Chapter 63.) Once a pulmonary artery catheter is in position, accurate measurement of PAWP may be made and effective therapy instituted to maximize CO. A PAWP of 14 to 18 mm Hg will generally achieve the goal of increasing CO. BP control can also be maintained with other drugs if needed (see Chapter 31).

Reducing Anxiety

Reduction of anxiety is facilitated by the sedative action of morphine administered IV. When morphine is used, the patient must be watched closely for respiratory depression. In addition, a calm approach in providing care helps reduce anxiety.

Once the patient is more stable, determination of the cause of pulmonary edema is important. Diagnosis of systolic or diastolic failure will then determine further management protocols. Aggressive drug therapy may continue with IV forms of inotropic drugs, vasodilators, and angiotensin-converting enzyme (ACE) inhibitors. Nursing care focuses on continual physical assessment, hemodynamic monitoring, and monitoring the patient's response to treatment.

Collaborative Care: Chronic Congestive Heart Failure (see Table 33-6)

One of the most important goals in the treatment of CHF is to treat the underlying cause. If arrhythmias have precipitated the failure, they should be treated accordingly[8] (see Chapter 34). If the underlying cause is hypertension, antihypertensives should be used in treatment (see Chapter 31). Valvular defects can be treated with surgery. If the cardiac dysfunction is a result of ischemic heart disease, specific interventions such as thrombolytic therapy and percutaneous transluminal coronary angiography or coronary artery bypass surgery may be needed. For those who survive ventricular tachyarrhythmias, the use of an implantable cardioverter-defibrillator (ICD) has become a standard practice. (ICDs are discussed in Chapter 34.)

Several mechanical options are available to sustain deteriorating CHF patients, especially those awaiting cardiac transplantation. The intraaortic balloon pump (IABP) is widely used as a short-term bridge to cardiac surgery, including transplantation. However, the limitations of bed rest, infection, and vascular complications preclude long-term use. (IABPs are discussed in Chapter 63.) Ventricular assist devices (VADs) provide highly effective long-term support for up to 2 years and have become standard care in most U.S. heart transplant centers.[9] (VADs are discussed in Chapter 63.)

Although therapeutic advances have had a favorable impact on the long-term prognosis for many CHF patients, for the majority the clinical course is characterized by repeated hospitalizations, progressive deterioration, and risk of sudden death. Given the generally grim prognosis, cardiac transplantation is often the treatment of choice. However, the lack of donor hearts and the challenges of postoperative care make it an option for only a small number of patients with CHF. Stringent criteria are necessary to select the few patients with advanced CHF who can even hope to receive a transplanted heart.[9] (Heart transplants are discussed later in this chapter.)

In a person with CHF, oxygen saturation of the blood is reduced because the blood is not adequately oxygenated in the lungs. Administration of oxygen improves saturation and assists greatly in meeting tissue oxygen needs. Thus oxygen therapy helps relieve dyspnea and fatigue. Optimally either arterial blood gases (ABGs) or pulse oximetry is used to monitor the effectiveness of oxygen therapy (see Chapter 27).

Physical and emotional rest allows the patient to conserve energy and decreases the need for additional oxygen. The degree of rest recommended depends on the severity of heart failure. A patient with severe CHF must be on bed rest with limited activity. A patient with mild to moderate CHF can be ambulatory with a restriction of strenuous activity. The patient should

DRUG THERAPY

Table 33-7 Positive Inotropic Agents Used to Treat Congestive Heart Failure

Sodium-potassium-ATPase inhibitors
- Digitalis (Lanoxin)

β-Adrenergic agonists
- Dopamine (Intropin)
- Dobutamine (Dobutrex)

Phosphodiesterase inhibitors
- Amrinone (Inocor)
- Milrinone (Primacor)

be instructed to participate in limited activities with adequate recovery periods in between.

Drug Therapy: Chronic Congestive Heart Failure. General therapeutic objectives for drug management of CHF include (1) the identification of the type of CHF and underlying causes, (2) the correction of sodium and water retention and volume overload, (3) the reduction of cardiac workload, (4) the improvement of myocardial contractility, and (5) the control of precipitating and complicating factors.[10] Because CHF is a complex syndrome, it is unlikely that any single pharmacologic agent would be successful alone. A combination of drugs that meet the preceding objectives has been most successful in treating the patient with CHF.

Positive inotropic drugs. The use of positive inotropic drugs in the patient with CHF is directed at improving cardiac contractility to increase CO, decrease LV diastolic pressure, and decrease systemic vascular resistance. The types of positive inotropic agents are listed in Table 33-7.

Digitalis preparations. Digitalis preparations (cardiac glycosides) have been the mainstay in the treatment of CHF and have been used for more than 200 years. Currently, digitalis is the only oral inotropic agent approved by the Food and Drug Administration (FDA) for use in the treatment of CHF. However, the use of digitalis preparations has recently become controversial because they have never been shown to reduce mortality rates, but they do seem to offer some benefit in moderate to severe CHF by reducing hospitalizations. They are particularly useful in the treatment of heart failure accompanied by atrial flutter, fibrillation, and a rapid ventricular rate. Digitalis preparations increase the force or strength of cardiac contraction (inotropic action). They also decrease the conduction speed within the myocardium and slow the HR (chronotropic action). This action allows for more complete emptying of the ventricles, thus diminishing the volume remaining in the ventricles during diastole. CO increases because of an increased stroke volume (SV) from improved contractility.

An individual receiving digitalis preparations is subject to digitalis toxicity (Table 33-8). Some of the earliest symptoms of toxicity are anorexia, nausea, and vomiting. Visual disturbances, such as "yellow" vision can occur with digitalis toxicity. Arrhythmias are a common indication of digitalis toxicity. Although almost any arrhythmia can occur, the types most frequently found are premature beats, atrial fibrillation, and first-degree heart block.

Hypokalemia is one of the most common causes of digitalis toxicity resulting in arrhythmias because low serum potassium

DRUG THERAPY

Table 33-8 Manifestations of Digitalis Toxicity

Cardiovascular System
Bradycardia; tachycardia; pulse deficit; arrhythmias, including premature ventricular contractions, first-degree atrioventricular blocks, atrial fibrillation

Gastrointestinal System
Anorexia, nausea, vomiting, diarrhea, abdominal pain

Neurologic System
Headache, drowsiness, confusion, insomnia, muscle weakness

Visual System
Double vision, blurred vision, colored vision (usually green or yellow), visual halos

levels enhance ectopic pacemaker activity. Monitoring the serum potassium levels of patients receiving both digitalis preparations and potassium-losing diuretics (e.g., thiazides, loop diuretics) is essential. Other electrolyte imbalances, such as hyperkalemia, hypercalcemia, and hypomagnesemia, can also precipitate toxicity.

Diseases of the kidney and liver increase the susceptibility to digitalis toxicity because most of the preparations are metabolized and eliminated by these organs. An older adult is especially prone to digitalis toxicity because digitalis accumulation occurs sooner with decreased liver and kidney function and slowed body metabolism, which occur with aging.

The usual treatment of toxicity consists of withholding the drug until the symptoms subside. In the case of life-threatening toxicity, digoxin immune Fab (ovine [Digibind]) is an antidote that can be given. The treatment of life-threatening arrhythmias is instituted as needed (see Chapter 34).

Beta-adrenergic agonists. β-Adrenergic agonists include dopamine (Intropin), dobutamine (Dobutrex), epinephrine, and norepinephrine (Levophed). Stimulation of β-adrenergic receptors results in an increase in cyclic adenosine monophosphate (cAMP) within the myocardial cells and an increase in contractility. The β-adrenergic agents are typically used as a short-term treatment of acute exacerbations of CHF in the intensive care unit (ICU). Their role in long-term therapy of CHF is controversial. Potential problems related to long-term treatment with β-adrenergic agonists include tolerance, increased ventricular irritability, and increased need for oxygen by the myocardium.

Dopamine (Intropin) is an adrenergic agonist used for therapy of severe heart failure and cardiogenic shock. In addition to increasing myocardial contractility, as above, it also has the valuable property in severe CHF or shock of specifically increasing blood flow to the renal, mesenteric, coronary, and cerebral vascular beds. Thereby, its use can lead to increased urine output, as well as help perfuse other vascular beds. The action of dopamine is highly effective in the CHF patient since it increases cardiac output (contractility), as well as urine output (decreases preload).

Phosphodiesterase inhibitors. Inhibition of phosphodiesterase increases cAMP, which enhances calcium entry into

DRUG THERAPY

Table 33-9 **Diuretic Therapy Used in Congestive Heart Failure***

Drugs	Mechanism of Action	Side Effects and Adverse Effects
Thiazides		
Chlorothiazide (Diuril) Hydrochlorothiazide (HydroDiuril, Oretic, Esidrix) Chlorthelidone (Hygroton) Indapamide (Lozol) Metolazone (Zaroxolyn)	Increase in sodium, chloride, and water excretion by inhibiting reabsorption of sodium and chloride in the distal tubule; excretion of potassium in conjunction with sodium	Hypokalemia, hyperuricemia, hypercalcemia, hyperglycemia, dermatologic reactions
Loop Diuretics		
Furosemide (Lasix) Ethacrynic acid (Edecrin) Bumetanide (Bumex) Torsemide (Demadex)	Potent diuretics that increase urine output by preventing sodium, chloride, and water reabsorption in the loop of Henle and distal tubule	Hypokalemia, hyperglycemia, hyperuricemia
Potassium-sparing Agents		
Spironolactone (Aldactone)	Inhibition of action of aldosterone in distal tubule; increased sodium excretion and potassium retention	Hyperkalemia, gynecomastia, amenorrhea, GI disturbances
Triamterene (Dyrenium)	Unknown mechanism of action; action on distal tubule to cause sodium excretion and potassium retention	Hyperkalemia, nausea and vomiting, leg cramps
Combination Agents		
Aldactazide (spironolactone and hydrochlorothiazide)	More potent diuretic effect than single agents alone	GI disturbances, dizziness, dry mouth, avoidance of hypokalemia possible
Dyazide (triamterene and hydrochlorothiazide)	Potassium-sparing effects	Same as above

*For more information on diuretic therapy, see Table 31-8.

the cell and improves myocardial contractility. Phosphodiesterase inhibitors are also potent vasodilators. They increase CO and reduce arterial pressure (decreased afterload). These drugs are not currently available in oral form; therefore they are limited to short-term use in the critical care setting.[11]

Amrinone (Inocor) increases myocardial contraction, increases CO, promotes peripheral vasodilation, and decreases SVR, thus augmenting performance of the LV. Adverse reactions include arrhythmias, thrombocytopenia, and GI effects. Because of amrinone's strong vasodilatory effect, hypotension may occur.

Milrinone (Primacor) is a newer phosphodiesterase inhibitor and appears to be more potent than amrinone (Inocor), better tolerated, and with fewer side effects (especially thrombocytopenia). Although milrinone has a direct positive inotropic effect, the improvement in cardiac function is probably a result of a combination of beneficial changes in preload and afterload, as well as inotropic effects.[10,11]

In summary, inotropic agents are clearly beneficial when used in the short term. However, controversy exists about their long-term role in the treatment of CHF. Although inotropic agents improve hemodynamic function and exercise tolerance, other effects may be harmful. Considerations to be weighed in the treatment of CHF patients include the potential to increase MVO_2, which can induce myocardial ischemia, exacerbate or stimulate arrhythmias, and cause more rapid deterioration of muscle function.

Diuretics. Diuretics are used in heart failure to mobilize edematous fluid, reduce pulmonary venous pressure, and reduce preload (Table 33-9). If excess extracellular fluid is excreted, blood volume returning to the heart can be reduced and cardiac function improved.

Diuretics act on the kidney by promoting excretion of sodium and water. Many varieties of diuretics are available, and some have specific indications for use. Thiazide diuretics are usually the first choice in chronic CHF because of their convenience, safety, low cost, and effectiveness. They are particularly useful in treating edema secondary to CHF and in controlling hypertension. The thiazides inhibit sodium reabsorption in the distal tubule, thus promoting excretion of sodium and water.

Four potent diuretics, all classified as loop diuretics, are furosemide (Lasix), ethacrynic acid (Edecrin), bumetanide (Bumex), and torsemide (Demadex). These drugs act on the ascending loop of Henle to promote sodium, chloride, and water excretion. Furosemide is more commonly used in acute CHF and pulmonary edema because it is slightly more predictable in its response. Bumetanide is a short-acting diuretic with a rapid onset and a half-life of 1 to 1.5 hours. It is used when furosemide has not produced diuresis or when a patient is allergic to furosemide. Problems in using bumetanide include reduction in serum potassium levels, ototoxicity, and possible allergic reaction in the patient who is sensitive to sulfa-type drugs.

Spironolactone (Aldactone) and triamterene (Dyrenium) are potassium-sparing diuretics that promote sodium and water excretion but block potassium excretion. A combination of diuretics may be administered for maximum potential (see Table 33-9).

Because there are numerous effective diuretic agents available, the choice is usually based on whether the CHF is chronic or acute, on the degree or severity of symptoms, or on special needs caused by renal insufficiency or electrolyte abnormalities.

Vasodilator drugs. Vasodilator drugs are the only class of drugs clearly shown to improve survival in overt heart failure. The goals of vasodilator therapy in the treatment of CHF include (1) increasing venous capacity, (2) improving ejection fraction through improved ventricular contraction, (3) slowing the process of ventricular dysfunction, (4) decreasing heart size, and (5) avoiding stimulation of the neurohormonal responses initiated by the compensatory mechanisms of CHF.[11]

Sodium nitroprusside. Nitroprusside is the most commonly used IV vasodilator in the management of acute CHF and pulmonary edema (see earlier in this chapter).

Nitrates. Nitrates cause vasodilation by acting directly on the smooth muscle of the vessel wall. Their effects primarily involve increasing venous capacitance, dilating the pulmonary vasculature, and improving arterial compliance. Therefore the major hemodynamic effect of nitrates is to decrease preload. Nitrates are of particular benefit in the management of myocardial ischemia related to CHF because they promote vasodilation of the coronary arteries. One specific deterrent to the use of nitrates in CHF is nitrate tolerance. Frequent dosing with drug-free periods may help reduce this effect.

Angiotensin-converting enzyme inhibitors. ACE inhibitors have become the vasodilator of choice in the patient with mild to severe CHF. The conversion of angiotensin I to the potent vasoconstrictor angiotensin II requires the presence of ACE. ACE inhibitors such as captopril (Capoten), enalapril (Vasotec), and lisinopril (Prinivil, Zestril) exert their effects through blocking ACE, resulting in decreased levels of angiotensin II (see Table 31-8). Plasma aldosterone levels are also reduced.[10,11]

Because CO is dependent on afterload in chronic CHF, the reduction in SVR seen with the use of ACE inhibitors produces a significant increase in CO. Furthermore, with the use of ACE inhibitors, although BP may be decreased, tissue perfusion is maintained or is increased as a result of improvement of CO and redistribution of regional blood flow. Other hemodynamic changes include a reduction in (1) pulmonary artery pressure, (2) right arterial pressure, and (3) left ventricular filling pressure.[11]

Activation of the sympathetic nervous system is augmented by the renin-angiotensin system, so treatment of CHF with an ACE inhibitor reduces norepinephrine levels and the effects of this potent catecholamine. Beneficial consequences of this decrease in sympathetic activity include (1) a reduction in ventricular wall stress (decreased afterload and workload of the LV), (2) decrease in ventricular arrhythmias, and (3) increased vagal tone (decreased HR).[10,11]

The differences between the three major ACE inhibitors—captopril, enalapril, and lisinopril—are related to onset and duration of action. Side effects of ACE inhibitors include symptomatic hypotension, chronic cough, and renal insufficiency (in high doses). Aging and baseline renal insufficiency slow the metabolism of ACE inhibitors and may therefore lead to increased serum drug levels.[7] It is recommended that these drugs be started at the lowest dose and that BP and renal function be monitored at regular intervals. Overall, ACE inhibitors are well tolerated by patients.[12,13] In patients who are unable to tolerate the ACE inhibitors (e.g., those with chronic cough), an angiotensin II blocker such as losartan (Cozaar) or valsartan (Diovan) may be used (see Table 31-8).

Beta-adrenergic blocking agents. Another agent recently approved for use in CHF is carvedilol (Coreg). Carvedilol is the only β-blocker to be specifically approved for treating CHF. However, its use is restricted to mild to moderate CHF. It directly blocks the sympathetic nervous system's negative effects on the failing heart. It is used in combination with ACE inhibitors, digitalis, and diuretics. Carvedilol must be started gradually, increasing the dosage slowly every 2 weeks as tolerated by the patient.

Nutritional Therapy: Chronic Congestive Heart Failure. Diet education and weight management are critical to the patient's control of chronic CHF. The nurse or dietitian should obtain a detailed diet history, determining not only what foods the patient eats and when but also the sociocultural value of food. The nurse can use this database to assist the patient in solving problems and developing an individual diet plan. The patient should be taught what foods are low and high in sodium and ways to enhance food flavors without the use of salt (e.g., substituting lemon juice and various spices).

The edema of chronic CHF is often treated by dietary restriction of sodium. The degree of sodium restriction depends on the severity of the heart failure and the effectiveness of diuretic therapy. Diets that are severely restricted in sodium are rarely prescribed because they are unpalatable and patient compliance is poor.

The normal daily dietary intake of sodium ranges from 3 to 7 g. A commonly prescribed diet for a patient with mild CHF is a 2 g sodium diet (Table 33-10). All foods high in sodium should be eliminated (Table 33-11). For more severe CHF, sodium intake is restricted to 500 to 1000 mg. On this diet, milk, cheese, bread, cereals, canned soups, and some canned vegetables must be eliminated. The patient and family must be instructed on how to read labels to look for sodium as an ingredient.

Fluid restrictions are not commonly prescribed for the patient with mild to moderate CHF. Diuretic therapy and digitalis preparations act as effective diuretics to promote fluid excretion. However, in moderate to severe CHF, fluid restrictions are usually implemented.

Instructing patients to weigh themselves daily is important for monitoring fluid retention, as well as weight reduction. Patients should be instructed to weigh themselves at the same time each day, preferably before breakfast, while wearing the same type of clothing. This helps ensure valid comparisons from day to day and helps identify early signs of fluid retention. If a patient experiences a weight gain of 3 lb (1.4 kg) over 2 to 5 days, the primary care provider should be called.

NUTRITIONAL THERAPY

Table 33-10 Low-Sodium Diets

General Principles

Do not add salt or seasonings containing sodium when preparing foods.
Do not use salt at the table.
Avoid high-sodium foods.*
Limit milk products to 2 cups daily.

Sample Menu Plans for 2 g Sodium Diet*

Breakfast		
1 cup low-fat or skim milk ¾ cup puffed wheat Sugar Toast 1 tsp. margarine Scrambled egg substitute Coffee	½ cup low-fat or skim milk ½ cup cream of wheat Sugar Tortilla Coffee	½ cup low-fat or skim milk ½ cup grits Boiled egg 1 tsp butter 1 biscuit made with low-sodium baking powder Coffee
Lunch		
½ cup chicken salad sandwich with 1 tsp mayonnaise Fresh fruit 1 cup low-fat or skim milk Iced tea	½ cup pinto beans ½ cup chili with meat Tossed salad with oil and vinegar Tortilla ½ cup gelatin dessert Coffee	2 oz baked fish Carrots Roll and 1 tsp butter Canned fruit Coffee
Dinner		
3 oz roast beef 1 baked potato 2 tsp sour cream 1 tsp margarine ½ cup green beans 1 dinner roll ½ cup sherbet Coffee	3 oz broiled fish ½ cup fried potatoes ½ cup zucchini or corn 1 cup chocolate pudding Bread and 1 tsp margarine Coffee	3 oz baked chicken ½ cup boiled potatoes ½ cup greens cooked without salt pork 1 cup ice cream Sugar cookies Coffee

Modifications for Other Low-Sodium Diets

500 mg Sodium Diet

Restrict milk products to 1 cup daily.
Limit meat to 4 oz daily.
Use salt-free butter, bread, vegetables, and starches.

1000 mg Sodium Diet

Restrict milk products to 1 cup daily.
Use salt-free butter and vegetables.

4 g Sodium Diet

Allow cooking with small amounts of salt.
Allow 3 cups milk products daily.

*See Table 33-11.

NURSING MANAGEMENT: CHRONIC CONGESTIVE HEART FAILURE

■ Nursing Assessment

Subjective and objective data that should be obtained from a patient with CHF include those presented in Table 33-12.

■ Nursing Diagnoses

Nursing diagnoses for the patient with CHF include, but are not limited to, those presented in NCP 33-1.

■ Planning

The overall goals are that the patient with CHF will have (1) decreased peripheral edema, (2) decreased shortness of breath, (3) increased exercise tolerance, (4) compliance with medications prescribed, and (5) no complications related to CHF.

■ Nursing Implementation

Health Promotion. An important measure used to prevent heart failure is the treatment or control of the underlying heart disease.[3] For example, in rheumatic valvular disease, valve replacement should be planned before lung congestion develops. Another important preventive measure concerns early and continued treatment of hypertension. Hyperlipidemic states in persons with CAD should be managed with diet, exercise, and medication. The use of antiarrhythmic agents or pacemakers is indicated for people with serious arrhythmias or conduction disturbances. When a patient is diagnosed with CHF, preventive care should focus on slowing the progression of the disease. Knowledge of the importance of following the medication, diet, and exercise regimens is essential. The in-hospital nurse may request home nursing care

NUTRITIONAL THERAPY

Table 33-11 High-Sodium Diets

Beverages	Mineral water, club soda, Dutch-processed cocoa
Breads	Saltines, baking powder biscuits, muffins, Bisquick, pretzels, salted snack crackers and chips; quick breads such as cornbread, nut bread; pancakes, waffles (including mixes)
Cereals	Instant cooked cereal, processed bran cereal, commercial granola
Dairy	Commercial buttermilk, regular cheese
Desserts	Commercial baked products, baked products and puddings made from mixes
Fats	Bacon fat, salted nuts or seeds, commercial dips (e.g., containing sour cream), regular salad dressings, mayonnaise
Juices	Tomato juice, V-8 juice, Clamato, Bloody Mary mixes
Meat	Smoked or cured products: bacon, ham, sausage, salt pork, hot dogs, lunch meat, corned or chipped beef, organ meats, shellfish, sardines, herring, anchovies, caviar, kosher meats, canned tuna fish and salmon, mackerel
Potato or substitute	Salted potato chips, salted french fries, instant potatoes, rice, noodle mixes
Seasonings	Salt, excessive amounts of baking powder, baking soda; celery, onion, and garlic salt and other seasoned salt and peppers; meat tenderizers, Accent, MSG, worcestershire, soy sauce, mustard, catsup, horseradish, chili sauce, tomato sauce, barbeque sauce, steak sauce
Soup	Commercial soups, bouillon cubes, powdered dehydrated soups
Vegetables	Sauerkraut, tomato juice, V-8 juice, vegetables in creamed or seasoned sauces, frozen vegetables processed with salt or sodium
Miscellaneous	Olives; pickles; salted popcorn; commercially prepared, frozen, or canned entrees (e.g., pot pies, TV dinners); Mexican, Italian, Oriental dishes as ordinarily prepared

MSG, monosodium glutamate.

NURSING ASSESSMENT

Table 33-12 Congestive Heart Failure

Subjective Data

Important Health Information

Past health history: CAD (including recent MI), hypertension, cardiomyopathy, valvular or congenital heart disease, diabetes mellitus, thyroid or lung disease, rapid or irregular heartbeat

Medications: Use of and compliance with any cardiac medications; use of diuretics, estrogens, corticosteroids, phenylbutazone, nonsteroidal antiinflammatory drugs

Functional Health Patterns

Health perception–health management: Fatigue

Nutritional-metabolic: Usual sodium intake; nausea, vomiting, anorexia, stomach bloating; weight gain

Elimination: Nocturia, decreased daytime urinary output, constipation

Activity-exercise: Dyspnea, orthopnea, cough; palpitations; dizziness, fainting

Sleep-rest: Number of pillows used for sleeping; paroxysmal nocturnal dyspnea

Cognitive-perceptual: Chest pain or heaviness; RUQ pain, abdominal discomfort; behavioral changes

Objective Data

Integumentary

Cool, diaphoretic skin; cyanosis or pallor, peripheral edema (right-sided heart failure)

Respiratory

Tachypnea, crackles, rhonchi, wheezes; frothy, blood-tinged sputum

Cardiovascular

Tachycardia, S_3, S_4, murmurs; pulsus alternans, PMI displaced inferiorly and posteriorly, jugular vein distention

Gastrointestinal

Abdominal distention, hepatosplenomegaly, ascites

Neurologic

Restlessness, confusion, decreased attention or memory

Possible Findings

Altered serum electrolytes (especially Na^+ and K^+), elevated BUN, creatinine, or liver function tests; chest x-ray demonstrating cardiomegaly, pulmonary congestion, and interstitial pulmonary edema; echocardiogram showing increased chamber size and decreased wall motion; atrial and ventricular enlargement on ECG; ↑ PAP, ↑ PAWP, ↓ CO, ↓ CI, ↓ O_2 saturation, ↑ SVR on hemodynamic monitoring

BUN, blood urea nitrogen; *CAD,* coronary artery disease; *CI,* cardiac index; *ECG,* electrocardiogram; *MI,* myocardial infarction; *NSAIDs,* nonsteroidal antiinflammatory drugs; *PAP,* pulmonary artery pressure; *PAWP,* pulmonary artery wedge pressure; *RUQ,* right upper quadrant; *SVR,* systemic vascular resistance.

33-1 NURSING CARE PLAN PATIENT WITH CONGESTIVE HEART FAILURE

Expected Patient Outcomes	Nursing Interventions and *Rationales*
NURSING DIAGNOSIS	**Activity intolerance** *related to* fatigue secondary to cardiac insufficiency, pulmonary congestion, and inadequate nutrition *as manifested by* dyspnea, shortness of breath, increase/decrease in pulse on exertion.
▪ Able to tolerate activity. ▪ Needs met to satisfaction.	▪ Assess patient daily for dyspnea, fatigue, and pulse rate *to determine level of activity that can be performed.* ▪ Provide emotional and physical rest *to reduce oxygen consumption and to relieve dyspnea and fatigue.* ▪ Provide frequent small feedings instead of three large meals per day *because increased cardiac output is needed for digestion.* ▪ Teach patient about expenditure of energy with various activities *to promote self-monitoring of appropriate activities.**
NURSING DIAGNOSIS	**Sleep pattern disturbance** *related to* nocturnal dyspnea, inability to assume favored sleep position, and nocturia *as manifested by* inability to sleep through night.
▪ Rested feeling after sleep.	▪ Explain etiology of nocturnal dyspnea *to reduce fear caused by waking up in acute dyspneic state.* ▪ Explore with patient alternative positions of comfort such as sleeping with two or more pillows *to relieve dyspnea.* ▪ Have patient take diuretics early in the day *to decrease urination during the night.*
NURSING DIAGNOSIS	**Fluid volume excess** *related to* pump failure and fluid retention *as manifested by* edema, dyspnea on exertion.
▪ Reduced or absence of edema.	▪ Evaluate degree of peripheral edema and measure abdominal girth daily *to provide data on patient's response to treatment.* ▪ Administer digitalis agents *to improve cardiac output by improving contractility* and diuretics *to mobilize edematous fluid.* ▪ Assess intake and output every shift *to monitor fluid balance.* ▪ Weigh patient daily *to monitor fluid retention and weight reduction.* ▪ Observe manifestations of hypokalemia *since hypokalemia sensitizes the myocardium to digitalis.* ▪ Provide sodium-restricted diet as ordered *to minimize further fluid retention.*
NURSING DIAGNOSIS	**Risk for impaired skin integrity** *related to* edema or immobility.
▪ No breakdown of skin at edematous areas.	▪ Monitor for signs of edema such as taut, shiny skin, sacral edema, pitting edema, or dependent edema *to identify location and severity of edema.* ▪ Assess edematous areas for skin breakdown *because these areas have increased susceptibility to breakdown.* ▪ Perform passive range of motion to extremities q4hr *to facilitate venous return of the fluid.* ▪ Handle edematous skin gently because *tissue is painful and fragile.* ▪ Turn and reposition q2hr *to prevent skin breakdown.* ▪ Pad bony prominences *to reduce pressure and subsequent skin breakdown.*
NURSING DIAGNOSIS	**Impaired gas exchange** *related to* increased preload, mechanical failure, or immobility *as manifested by* increased respiratory rate, shortness of breath, dyspnea on exertion.
▪ Respiratory rate of 12-18/min.	▪ Elevate head of bed to Fowler's position *to improve ventilation by decreasing venous return to the heart and increasing thoracic capacity.* ▪ Support patient's arms with pillows *to move arms off and away from chest to facilitate breathing.* ▪ Encourage active range of motion of feet and legs *to improve circulation through muscle contraction.* ▪ Administer oxygen by nasal cannula *to improve oxygen saturation, assist in meeting tissue oxygen needs, and relieve dyspnea and fatigue.* ▪ Auscultate for lung and heart sounds q4hr *to evaluate patient's response to treatments.* ▪ Use pulse oximetry *to monitor oxygenation status.*

Continued

33-1 NURSING CARE PLAN PATIENT WITH CONGESTIVE HEART FAILURE —continued

Expected Patient Outcomes	Nursing Interventions and *Rationales*
NURSING DIAGNOSIS	**Anxiety** *related to* dyspnea or perceived threat of death *as manifested by* restlessness, irritability, expression of feelings of life threat.
▪ Feeling less apprehensive about condition and prognosis.	▪ Assess facial expression and behavior for feeling of apprehension *to allow for early identification and treatment of anxiety.* ▪ Allow patient to ask questions *to relieve some anxiety by having accurate information.* ▪ Answer call light promptly and explain all procedures *to promote sense of security.* ▪ Demonstrate calm behavior with patient *to increase confidence in caregiver and relieve anxiety.* ▪ Use measures to decrease dyspnea (e.g., rest, elevation of head of bed) *to reduce anxiety and improve breathing.*
NURSING DIAGNOSIS	**Ineffective management of therapeutic regimen** *related to* lack of knowledge regarding signs and symptoms of CHF, proper diet, and medications *as manifested by* lack of adherence to low-sodium diet and questioning about disease, diet, and medications.
▪ Expression of knowledge of disease process and dietary and medication regimen. ▪ Adherence to therapeutic regimen.	▪ Teach patient manifestations to report, including shortness of breath at rest; swelling of ankles, feet, or abdomen; loss of appetite, nausea, or vomiting; weight gain of 2-3 lb (0.9-1.4 kg) in a 2-day period; frequent urination; persistent cough; changes in HR ±20 beats different from usual *so patient will know signs and symptoms of worsening CHF.* ▪ Instruct patient on dietary restrictions (e.g., low-sodium diet, possible weight reduction) and medication regimen *to ensure that an adequate nutritional intake and correct medications are taken.*

*See Table 33-13.

for the patient and family to provide for follow-up of care and to monitor the patient's response to treatment. Early detection of signs and symptoms of worsening failure may help modify care and prevent an acute episode requiring further hospitalization.

Acute Intervention. Many persons with CHF do not experience an acute episode. If they do, they are usually initially managed in a critical care unit and later transferred to a general unit when their condition has stabilized. The nursing care plan for the patient with CHF (see NCP 33-1) applies to the patient with stabilized acute or chronic CHF.

Ambulatory and Home Care. CHF is a chronic illness for most persons. Important nursing responsibilities are (1) educating the patient about the physiologic changes that have occurred and (2) assisting the patient to adapt to both the physiologic and psychologic changes. It must be emphasized to the patient that it is possible to live productively with this health problem. Home health care is a vital factor in preventing future hospitalization for this patient. Home nursing care will follow up with ongoing clinical assessments, monitoring vital signs, and response to therapies. Managing these patients out of the hospital is a priority of care. A patient and family teaching guide for the patient with CHF is presented in Table 33-13.

Patients with CHF are usually required to take medication for the rest of their lives. This often becomes difficult because a patient may be asymptomatic when CHF is under control. It must be stressed that the disease is chronic and that medication must be continued to keep the heart failure under control.

The patient should evaluate the action of the prescribed medication. The patient should be taught to recognize the manifestations of digitalis toxicity (see Table 33-8). The patient should also be taught how to take the pulse rate and to know under what circumstances drugs, especially digitalis preparations, should be withheld and a physician consulted. The pulse rate should always be taken for 1 full minute. A pulse rate lower than 50 to 60 beats per minute may be a contraindication to taking a digitalis preparation unless specified otherwise by the health care provider. A slow pulse rate may indicate a need to alter the digitalis therapy. However, in the absence of primary heart block or the development of ventricular ectopy, a pulse rate of 60 beats per minute or less is not a contraindication to taking digitalis. A pulse rate of 50 beats per minute (especially in a patient who is also taking β-blocking drugs) may be acceptable.

The patient should also be taught the symptoms of hypokalemia if diuretics that cause potassium excretion are being taken. (Manifestations of hypokalemia are discussed in Chapter 15.) Hypokalemia sensitizes the myocardium to digitalis. Consequently, toxicity may develop from an ordinary dose of digitalis. Frequently the patient who is taking thiazide or loop diuretics is given supplemental potassium.

The nurse, physical therapist, or occupational therapist can instruct the patient in energy-saving and energy-efficient behaviors after an evaluation of daily activities has been done. For example, once the nurse understands the patient's daily routine, suggestions can be made for simplification of work or modification of an activity. Frequently the patient needs a

PATIENT & FAMILY TEACHING GUIDE

Table 33-13 Congestive Heart Failure

Rest
1. Have a regular daily rest and activity program.
2. After exertion, such as exercise and ADLs, plan a rest period.
3. Shorten working hours or schedule rest period during working hours.
4. Avoid emotional upsets.

Drug Therapy
1. Take each medication as prescribed daily.
2. Develop a check-off system (e.g., daily chart) to ensure medications have been taken.
3. Take pulse rate each day before taking medications. Know the parameters that your health care provider wants for your heart rate.
4. Learn to take own BP at determined intervals. Know your acceptable BP limits.
5. Know signs and symptoms of orthostatic hypotension and how to prevent them.
6. Know the signs and symptoms of potassium depletion.
7. Know signs and symptoms of internal bleeding; bleeding gums, increased bruises, blood in stool or urine, and what to do.
8. Know own INR if taking Coumadin, and how often to have blood monitored.

Dietary Therapy
1. Consult the written diet plan and list of permitted and restricted foods.
2. Examine labels to determine sodium content. Also over-the-counter medicines such as laxatives, cough medicines, antacids.
3. Avoid using salt.
4. Weigh at same time daily.
5. Report weight gain of more than 2-3 lb (0.9-1.4 kg) in a few days.
6. Eat small, frequent meals.

Activity Program
1. Increase walking and other activities gradually, provided they do not cause fatigue and dyspnea.
2. Avoid extremes of heat and cold.
3. Keep regular appointments with health care provider.

Ongoing Monitoring
1. Know the signs and symptoms of recurring or progressing heart failure.
2. Recall the symptoms experienced when illness began; reappearance of previous symptoms may indicate a reoccurrence.
3. Report immediately to health care provider any of the following:
   a. Gain in weight
   b. Loss of appetite
   c. Shortness of breath during activity
   d. Shortness of breath at rest
   e. Swelling of ankles, feet, or abdomen
   f. Persistent cough
   g. Frequent urination at night
   h. Waking breathless in the night

INR, international normalized ratio.

prescription for rest after an activity. Many hard-driving persons need that "permission" to not feel "lazy." Sometimes an activity that the patient enjoys may need to be eliminated. In such situations the patient should be helped to explore alternative activities that cause less physical and cardiac stress. The physical environment may require modification in situations in which there is an increased cardiac workload demand (e.g., frequent climbing of stairs). The nurse can help the patient identify areas where outside assistance can be obtained.

The home health nurse is essential in the care of the CHF patient and family. Frequent physical assessments, including vital signs and weight, are extremely important. Home health nurses frequently work within protocols set up with the patient's physician and health care team. The protocols may enable the nurse and patient to identify problems, such as an increase in weight and HR as evidence of worsening failure, and institute interventions to prevent hospitalization. This may include altering medications and fluid restrictions. Home health nursing care of CHF patients is paramount in reducing the number of hospitalizations, increasing functional capacity, and increasing quality of life.[14,15]

Evaluation

The expected outcomes for the patient with CHF are presented in NCP 33-1.

RESEARCH
IMPLICATIONS FOR NURSING PRACTICE

Social Support in Older Women with Heart Failure

Citation Friedman MM: Social support sources among older women with heart failure: continuity versus loss over time, *Res Nurs Health* 20:319, 1997.

Purpose To examine whether older women with heart failure experience continuity or loss of their emotional and tangible support sources over a period of 18 months during the course of their illness.

Methods In-home interviews were conducted with 57 older (55 yr) women following a hospital admission for heart failure. Two interviews 18 months apart were done. The questionnaires obtained data on demographic information, perceived social support, social support sources, psychologic well-being, and satisfaction with life.

Results and Conclusions Over the 18-month period both emotional and tangible support sources were quite stable. These findings suggest that most older women in this study are embedded in an informal network made up of family and friends who provide continuous emotional and tangible support. The older women who did lose primary support sources frequently replaced them with others from their informal support network. Women who did experience more loss of their tangible support services were more likely to report feelings of depressed affect.

Implications for Nursing Practice Heart failure is a major cause of disability in older women that is marked by activity intolerance and inability to perform activities of daily living. Ongoing assistance from support sources is essential to patients with heart failure residing in the community. Home nursing services may be useful in assessing support services and psychologic well-being of patients with heart failure. This assessment could identify vulnerable individuals in need of intervention.

CARDIOMYOPATHY

Cardiomyopathy (CMP) is a term used to describe a group of heart muscle diseases of unknown etiology that primarily affect the structural or functional ability of the myocardium. Diagnosis of CMP is made by the patient's clinical manifestations and noninvasive and invasive cardiac procedures to rule out other causes of dysfunction. This patient is a particular challenge to the nurse and often has unique management and care needs.

CMPs can be classified as primary or secondary. Primary CMPs are those conditions in which the etiology of the heart disease is unknown. The heart muscle in this instance is the only portion of the heart involved, and other cardiac structures are unaffected. In secondary CMP the cause of the myocardial disease is known and is secondary to another disease process. Common causes of secondary CMP are ischemia, viral infections, alcohol intake, drug abuse, and pregnancy (Table 33-14).

Table 33-14 Causes of Secondary Cardiomyopathy

Dilated	Hypertrophic	Restrictive
Ischemic	Genetic	Amyloid
Valvular	Hypertension	Endomycardial fibrosis
Infectious	Obstructive valvular disease	Löffler's disease
Pregnancy	Thyroid disease	Sarcoidosis
Metabolic	Glycogen storage disease	Neoplastic tumor
Hypertension	Friedreich's ataxia	Ventricular thrombus
Cardiotoxic	Infants of diabetics	
Alcohol		
Adriamycin		
Cobalt		
Cocaine		

The World Health Organization has classified CMP conditions into three general types: dilated (congestive), hypertrophic, and restrictive (Table 33-15).[16] Each of these types has its own pathogenesis, clinical presentation, and treatment protocols. All these types of CMP can lead to cardiomegaly and CHF.

DILATED CARDIOMYOPATHY

Etiology and Pathophysiology

Dilated (congestive) cardiomyopathy is the most common type of CMP, accounting for greater than 90% of all cases, and is characterized by cardiomegaly with ventricular dilation, impairment of systolic function, atrial enlargement, and stasis of blood in the LV. Cardiomegaly is the result of primarily ventricular dilation (Fig. 33-3). Clinical sequence of this impaired systolic function closely resembles the situation in CHF. Because the ejection fraction falls and there is a lower CO, stasis of blood occurs. What differentiates this disorder from chronic CHF is that the walls of the ventricle do not become hypertrophic (Fig. 33-4). This is thought to be caused by the rapid destruction of cells, leaving the ventricles with little time to hypertrophy. Deterioration is rapid after the development of symptoms, and as many as 20% to 50% of patients are expected to die within 1 year.[16]

No specific cause has been identified, although dilated CMP often follows an infectious myocarditis. Thyrotoxicosis, diabetes mellitus, toxins (especially alcohol and cocaine), chemotherapeutic agents, nutritional deficiencies, pregnancy, and drugs causing a hypersensitivity reaction have all been associated with the development of dilated CMP. Regardless of the initial cause, it results in a diffuse inflammation and rapid degeneration of myocardial fibers that decrease contractile function.

Clinical Manifestations

The signs and symptoms of dilated CMP develop insidiously. The patient may have signs and symptoms of CHF. These symptoms can include a change in exercise tolerance, fatigue, dry cough, dyspnea, paroxysmal nocturnal dyspnea, orthopnea, palpitations, and anorexia. Signs can include S_3, S_4, tachycardia, pulmonary crackles, edema, weak peripheral pulses, pallor, hepatomegaly, and jugular venous distention. The patient may also have arrhythmias or systemic embolization.

Table 33-15 Characteristics of Cardiomyopathies

Dilated	Hypertrophic	Restrictive
Etiology		
Idiopathic condition, alcoholism, pregnancy, myocarditis, nutritional deficiency (vitamin B_1), exposure to toxins and drugs, genetic disease	Inherited disorder (autosomal dominant), possible chronic hypertension	Amyloidosis, postradiation, post–open heart surgery, diabetes mellitus
Major Manifestations		
Fatigue, weakness, palpitations, dyspnea, dry cough	Exertional dyspnea, fatigue, angina, syncope, palpitations	Dyspnea, fatigue, palpitations
Cardiomegaly		
Moderate to marked	Mild	Mild to moderate
Contractility		
Decreased	Increased or decreased	Normal or decreased
Valvular Incompetence		
Atrioventricular valves, particularly mitral	Mitral valve	Mitral valve
Arrhythmias		
Sinoatrial tachycardia, atrial and ventricular arrhythmias	Tachyarrhythmias	Atrial and ventricular arrhythmias
Cardiac Output		
Decreased	Decreased	Normal or decreased
Stroke Volume		
Decreased	Normal or increased	Decreased
Ejection Fraction		
Decreased	Increased	Normal or decreased
Outflow Tract Obstruction		
None	Increased	None

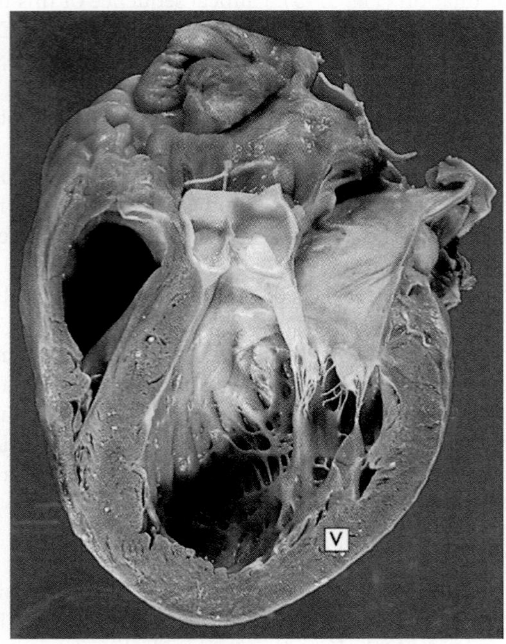

Fig. 33-3 Dilated cardiomyopathy. The dilated left ventricle has a thin wall (V).

Diagnostic Studies

The diagnosis of dilated CMP is made on the basis of the patient's history and by ruling out other conditions that cause CHF. The chest x-ray shows cardiomegaly. Signs of pulmonary venous hypertension may be present, as well as pleural effusion. The ECG may reveal tachycardia and arrhythmias. Conduction disturbances may also be present because of the stretching of the ventricular septum. Echocardiography is useful in distinguishing dilated CMP from other structural abnormalities. The size of the ventricular chamber can be assessed, the thickness of the heart muscle can be measured, and the valves can be evaluated.

Cardiac catheterization and coronary angiography are used in evaluating the manifestations of dilated CMP. The coronary arteries are usually normal. Left ventriculogram may reveal abnormal wall motion caused by the dilation, a thin wall, and dilated ventricles. Endomyocardial biopsy may be done at the time of the right heart catheterization. This rarely provides information significant for treatment, but it may rule out other diagnoses.

NURSING AND COLLABORATIVE MANAGEMENT: DILATED CARDIOMYOPATHY

Interventions focus on controlling CHF by enhancing myocardial contractility and decreasing afterload, similar to the treatment of chronic CHF (Table 33-16). Thus treatment is more palliative than curative. Digitalis is used in the presence of atrial

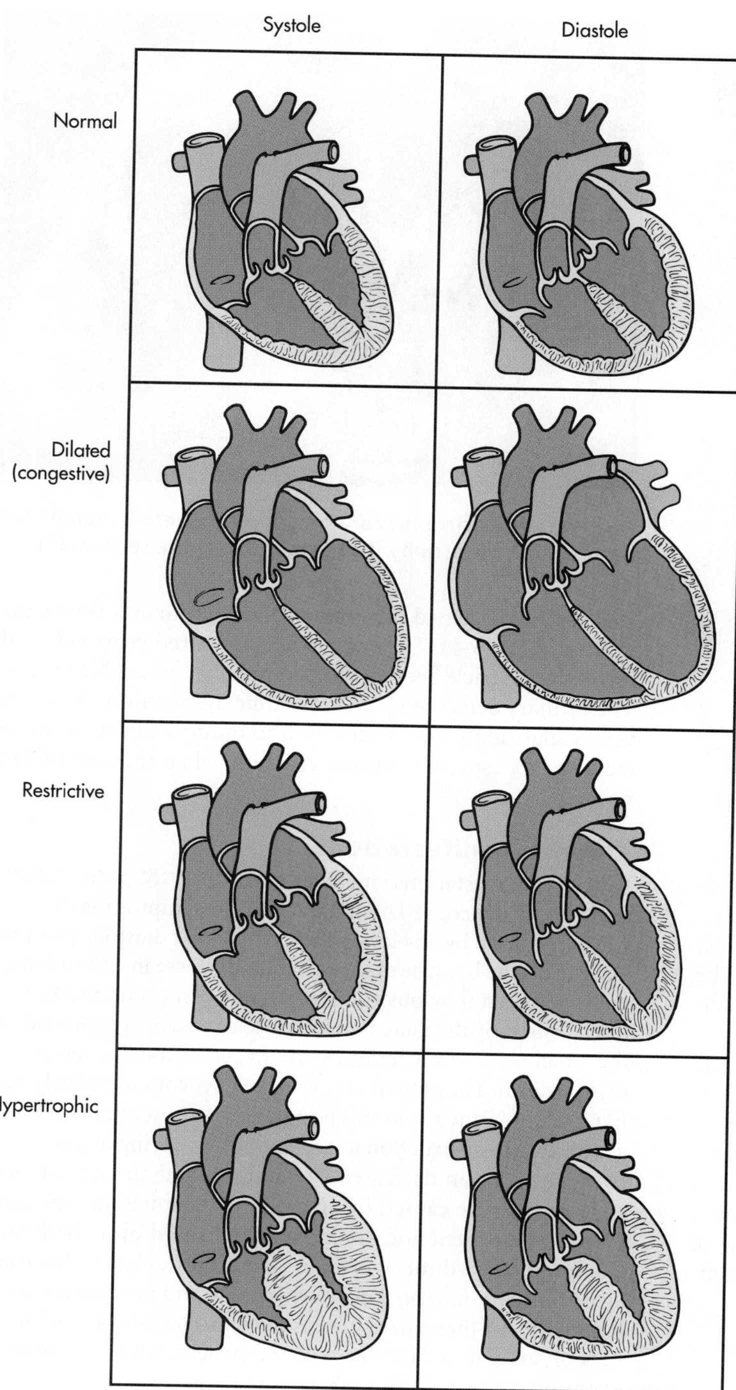

Fig. 33-4 Types of cardiomyopathies and the differences in ventricular diameter during systole and diastole, compared with a normal heart.

fibrillation, diuretics are used to decrease preload, and vasodilators such as the ACE inhibitors are used to reduce afterload. Drug therapy, nutritional therapy, and cardiac rehabilitation may help alleviate symptoms of CHF and improve CO. A patient with secondary dilated CMP must be treated for the underlying disease process. For example, the patient with alcohol-induced dilated CMP must abstain from all alcohol intake.

Unfortunately, dilated CMP does not respond well to therapy. Intermittent dobutamine (Dobutrex) or milrinone (Primacor) infusions are a therapy used in the treatment of dilated cardiomyopathy. The patient is admitted to the hospital for a 72-hour infusion of dobutamine or milrinone. Sometimes these infusions are done for an 8-hour period as an outpatient treatment or in the home. After infusion, many patients experience an improvement in symptoms that lasts several weeks after therapy.

The patient with terminal end-stage CMP may require cardiac transplantation. Currently approximately 50% of heart transplants are performed for treatment of cardiomyopathic conditions. Cardiac transplant recipients have a good prognosis for survival. However, donor hearts are difficult to obtain, and the surgical procedure is expensive. Many patients with dilated CMP die while awaiting heart transplantation.

COLLABORATIVE CARE

Table 33-16 Cardiomyopathies

Diagnostic
- History and physical examination
- ECG
- Chest x-ray
- Echocardiogram
- Nuclear imaging studies
- Cardiac catheterization
- Endocardial biopsy

Collaborative Therapy
- Treatment of underlying cause
- Digitalis (except in hypertrophic CMP in normal sinus rhythm)
- Diuretics
- ACE inhibitors
- Bed rest (if indicated)
- Anticoagulants (if indicated)
- Antiarrhythmics (if indicated)
- β-Adrenergic blocking agents (for hypertrophic CMP)
- Intermittent infusions of dobutamine (Dobutrex) or milronone (Primacor)
- Heart transplant
- Surgical correction

ACE, angiotensin-converting enzyme; *CMP*, cardiomyopathy.

Patients with dilated cardiomyopathy are very ill people with a grave prognosis who need expert nursing care. The patient's family must learn cardiopulmonary resuscitation (CPR) and how to access emergency care in their neighborhood. The nurse should include family members and other support systems when planning a patient's care.

Home health care nursing can provide the patient and the family with the continuous assessments and therapeutic interventions that are required to maximize and maintain the functional status. Observing for signs and symptoms of worsening failure, arrhythmias, and embolic formation are paramount in this patient, as well as monitoring drug responsiveness. Because the goal of therapy is to keep the patient functional and out of the hospital, home health nurses play a critical role in accomplishing these goals.

HYPERTROPHIC CARDIOMYOPATHY

Pathophysiology

Hypertrophic cardiomyopathy (HCM) produces asymmetric myocardial hypertrophy without ventricular dilation (Fig. 33-5). It seems to have an autosomal dominant genetic basis. HCM occurs less commonly than dilated CMP and is more common in men than in women.[16] It is usually diagnosed in young adulthood and is often seen in active, athletic individuals. Another name for this disorder is idiopathic hypertrophic subaortic stenosis (IHSS).

The four main characteristics of HCM are (1) massive ventricular hypertrophy; (2) rapid, forceful contraction of the LV; (3) impaired relaxation; and (4) obstruction to aortic outflow (not present in all patients). Ventricular hypertrophy is associated with a thickened intraventricular septum and ventricular wall (see Fig. 33-4). The end result is impaired ventricular filling as the ventricle becomes noncompliant and unable to relax. The primary defect of HCM is diastolic dysfunction. Decreased ventricular filling and obstruction to outflow can result in decreased CO, especially during exertion, when increased CO is needed.

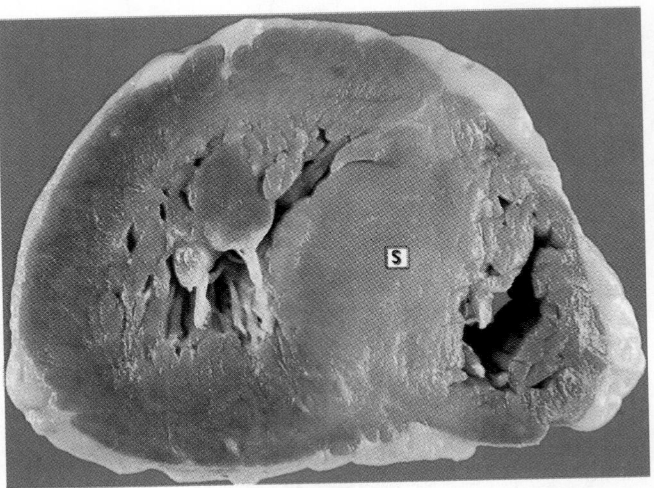

Fig. 33-5 Hypertrophic cardiomyopathy. There is marked left ventricular hypertrophy. This often affects the septum (*S*).

Clinical Manifestations

Patient manifestations include exertional dyspnea, fatigue, angina, and syncope. The most common symptom is dyspnea, which is caused by an elevated left ventricular diastolic pressure. Fatigue occurs because of the resultant decrease in CO and in exercise-induced flow obstruction. Angina can occur and is most often caused by the increased LV muscle mass or compression of the small coronary arteries by the hypercontractile ventricular myocardium. The patient may also have syncope, especially during exertion. Syncope in this population is most often caused by an increase in obstruction to aortic outflow during increased activity, resulting in decreased CO and cerebral circulation. Syncope can also be caused by arrhythmias. Palpitations are common in the patient and are most often caused by arrhythmias. Common arrhythmias include supraventricular tachycardia, atrial fibrillation, ventricular tachycardia, and ventricular fibrillation. Any of these arrhythmias may lead to loss of consciousness or sudden cardiac death of the patient, which is the most common cause of death in this population.

Diagnostic Studies

The chest x-ray is usually normal except in a patient with severe disease causing an increased cardiac silhouette. Increased voltage and duration of the QRS complex are the most common abnormalities on the ECG. These findings usually indicate ventricular hypertrophy. Ventricular arrhythmias are also frequently seen, with ventricular tachycardia the most common.

The echocardiogram is the primary diagnostic tool revealing the classic feature of HCM, which is LV hypertrophy. The echocardiogram may also demonstrate wall motion abnormalities and diastolic dysfunction. Cardiac catheterization may also be helpful in the diagnosis of HCM.

NURSING AND COLLABORATIVE MANAGEMENT: HYPERTROPHIC CARDIOMYOPATHY

Goals of intervention are to improve ventricular filling by reducing ventricular contractility and relieving LV outflow obstruction. These can be accomplished with the use of β-blockers or calcium channel blockers. Digitalis preparations are contraindicated in the patient unless they are used to treat atrial fibrillation. CHF may also be present in varying degrees but is usually not present until later stages. Antiarrhythmics are also used to control arrhythmias; however, their use has not been proven to prevent sudden death in this group. An alternative treatment for ventricular arrhythmias may be an implantable defibrillator (see Chapter 34). It has been found that ventricular or atrioventricular pacing can be beneficial for patients with HCM and outflow obstruction. By pacing the ventricles from the apex of the right ventricle, septal depolarization occurs first, allowing the septum to move away from the left ventricular wall and reducing the degree of obstruction of the outflow tract.

Some patients may be candidates for surgical treatment of their hypertrophied septum. The indications for surgery include severe symptoms refractory to therapy with marked obstruction to aortic outflow. The surgery is termed a *ventriculomyotomy and myectomy.* It involves incision of the hypertrophied septal muscle and resection of some of the hypertrophied muscle. Most patients have good symptomatic improvement after surgery and improved exercise tolerance.

Nursing interventions focus on relieving symptoms, observing for and preventing complications, and providing emotional and psychologic support. Education should focus on teaching patients to adjust lifestyle to avoid strenuous activity and dehydration. Any activity or procedure that causes an increase in systemic vascular resistance (thus increasing the obstruction to forward flow) is dangerous for this group of patients and should be avoided. The patient should be taught to space activities and allow for rest periods.

RESTRICTIVE CARDIOMYOPATHY

Etiology and Pathophysiology

Restrictive cardiomyopathy is the least common of the cardiomyopathic conditions. It is a disease of the heart muscle that impairs diastolic volume and stretch (see Fig. 33-4). Systolic function remains unaffected.

Although the specific etiology of restrictive CMP is unknown, a number of pathologic processes may be involved in its development. Myocardial fibrosis, hypertrophy, and infiltration produce stiffness of the ventricular wall. Secondary causes of restrictive CMP include amyloidosis, endocardial fibrosis, glycogen deposition, hemochromatosis, sarcoidosis, fibrosis of different etiology, and radiation to the thorax.

The principal characteristic of restrictive CMP is cardiac muscle stiffness. It is characterized by loss of ventricular compliance. The ventricles are resistant to filling and therefore demand high diastolic filling pressures to maintain CO.

Clinical Manifestations

Angina, syncope, fatigue, and dyspnea on exertion are common signs. The most common symptom is that of exercise intolerance because the myocardium cannot increase CO by producing a tachycardia without further compromising the ventricular filling.

Signs and symptoms include those similar to CHF. The patient may have signs of both left-sided and right-sided heart failure, including dyspnea, peripheral edema, ascites, and hepatic dysfunction. Kussmaul's sign (bulging of the internal jugular neck veins on inspiration) may also be present.

Diagnostic Studies

The chest x-ray may be normal, or it may show cardiomegaly. Pleural effusions and pulmonary congestion may be evident in the patient with progression to CHF. The ECG may reveal a tachycardia at rest. The most common arrhythmias are atrial fibrillation and complex ventricular arrhythmias. Echocardiogram may reveal the thickened ventricular wall of restrictive CMP, small ventricular cavities, and a dilated atria. Endomyocardial biopsy, computed tomography (CT) scan, and nuclear imaging may be helpful in a definitive diagnosis.

NURSING AND COLLABORATIVE MANAGEMENT: RESTRICTIVE CARDIOMYOPATHY

Currently no specific treatment for restrictive CMP exists. Interventions are aimed at improving diastolic filling and the underlying disease process. Treatment includes conventional therapy for CHF and arrhythmias. Heart transplant may also be a consideration. Nursing care is similar to the care of a patient with CHF. As in the treatment of patients with HCM, the patient should be taught to avoid situations that impair ventricular filling, such as strenuous activity, dehydration, and increases in SVR.

"CRACK" HEART

CMP caused by cocaine abuse is seen more frequently than ever before. Cocaine causes intense vasoconstriction of the coronary arteries and peripheral vasoconstriction, resulting in hypertension. This can result in increased myocardial oxygen needs and decreased oxygen supply to the myocardium and can cause ischemia and infarction. This may lead to an acute MI or ischemic CMP. Cocaine also causes high circulating levels of catecholamines. This may lead to further injury to myocardial cells and cause cell damage leading to ischemic or dilated CMP. The CMP produced is difficult to treat. Interventions deal mainly with the CHF that ensues. The patient has a poor prognosis and is not usually considered a candidate for heart transplantation.

CARDIAC SURGERY

Since the introduction of cardiopulmonary bypass in 1953 and the open heart surgery technique of Favaloro in 1967, there have been many modifications and technical improvements in the operating room and in perioperative patient care. Coronary artery bypass graft (CABG) procedures, heart valve repair and replacement, and heart transplantation have become routine

Table 33-17 Indications for Cardiac Surgery

Aneurysm of sinus of Valsalva
Constrictive pericarditis
Congenital heart defects
Coronary artery disease
Dissecting aortic aneurysm
Valvular insufficiency or stenosis
Ventricular aneurysm
Ventricular septal defect
Ventricular arrhythmias

surgical procedures (Table 33-17). Cardiac surgery today provides pain relief, improvement in lifestyle, and improved survival for the patient undergoing open heart surgical treatment.

The nurse who cares for this patient has been challenged to keep pace with rapid technologic advances in patient care, as well as caring for a patient who 10 to 20 years ago would not have been a surgical candidate. Patients today are older, have worse LV function (patients with ejection fractions below 35%), have progressive disease, have had previous sternotomies, have other systemic diseases that increase the risk of operation (e.g., diabetes mellitus, severe hypertension, renal disease), and require emergency operations secondary to failed angioplasty or acute MI. These groups of patients require specialized nursing care.

Myocardial Revascularization

Myocardial revascularization, or CABG, is the main surgical treatment for CAD. Indications for surgery have changed during the last decade, especially with the advent of percutaneous transluminal coronary angioplasty. The patient with CAD who has failed medical management or who has advanced disease is considered a candidate for surgical revascularization. A growing body of research indicates that surgical treatment, when compared with medical therapy, reduces angina, decreases overall costs, and improves patient survival.[17,18]

Surgical Procedures

CABG procedure. The CABG operation consists of the construction of new conduits (vessels to transport blood) between the aorta, or other major arteries, beyond the obstructed coronary artery (or arteries) (Fig. 33-6). This procedure provides blood flow beyond the stenosis so that the myocardium distal to the obstruction continues to receive blood flow. The coronary artery is considered stenotic if its diameter is narrowed by more than 75% to 80%.

This procedure usually involves a graft from the saphenous vein or the internal mammary artery for aortocoronary bypass. In the former procedure, the saphenous vein from one of the legs of the patient is removed and reversed (so that the valves will not obstruct the blood flow). Saphenous veins are used as free grafts and anastomosed proximally to the ascending aorta and distally to one (or more) coronary artery. Approximately 10% of vessel occlusions occur within the first several weeks after surgery and are caused by technical problems or thrombosis at the distal graft anastomosis. Saphenous veins used as grafts develop diffuse intimal hyperplasia, which contributes to ultimate stenosis and occlusions of the graft. Patency rates of these grafts are lower when the anastomosis is to a small coronary artery and to arteries supplying areas with scar tissue (infarction areas). The use of aspirin (80-325 mg PO daily) improves vein graft patency and is used postoperatively. Overall vein graft patency is estimated at 5 to 10 years.

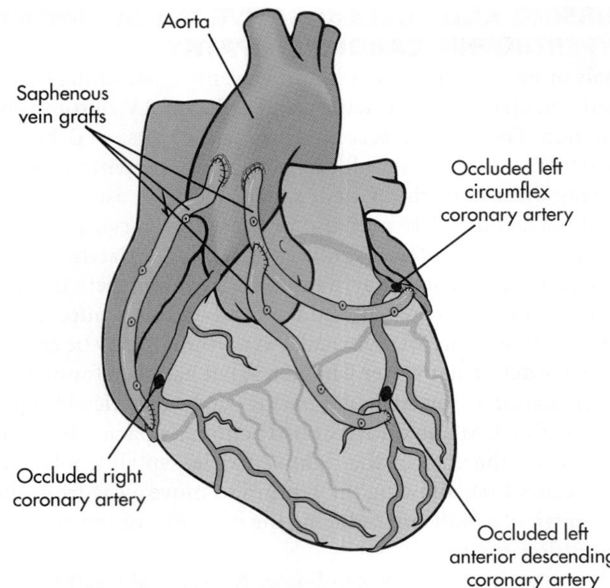

Fig. 33-6 Saphenous aortocoronary artery bypass or revascularization involves taking a piece of saphenous vein from the leg and creating a conduit for blood from the aorta to the area below the blockage in the coronary artery. A triple bypass is illustrated.

The use of the internal mammary artery (IMA) as a conduit was introduced in 1968. Patency rates of the IMA are 85% to 95% at 10 years.[17] Because the patency rate of the IMA is higher than that of saphenous veins, the IMA may prove to be a better conduit for improving long-term prognosis. Use of the left IMA, which is left attached to its origin from the left subclavian artery, is mobilized from the chest wall and anastomosed to the coronary artery distal to the stenosis. The right IMA may also be used in a similar fashion. The use of the left IMA and saphenous vein conduits together for patients with three-, four-, five-, or six-vessel bypass procedures is common.

If a patient has had previous CABG using saphenous vein grafts or IMA and at the time of reoperation has no conduits to harvest, the gastroepiploic artery or inferior epigastric artery may be used. These arteries are excellent conduits. However, use of these arteries creates the additional need for a laparotomy. This increases the length of surgery, and wound complications at the harvest site are not uncommon, especially in an obese or diabetic patient. Other arterial graft conduits, such as the splenic and radial arteries, have been used, but with slightly less successful patency rates than the IMA. Arm veins are more difficult to dissect and harvest, are thin and delicate, and may have been traumatized by previous intravenous injections. Because of the number of patients requiring reoperation, the use of alternative arteries and veins will become increasingly more common.

Revascularization surgery has an overall mortality rate of approximately 1% to 2%, with an 85% rate of functional improvement (85% of patients have their anginal pain completely eliminated).[17] CABG remains a palliative treatment for CAD and not a cure. It provides the patient with improved outcomes, quality of life, and survival.

Cardiovascular disease is the primary cause of morbidity and mortality for people more than 65 years of age. The number of older adults who are candidates for CABG has increased, and they have become a subpopulation of patients who have specialized needs before and after surgery.

The results of coronary revascularization are less favorable for women than men. CAD is the leading cause of death among women. The severity of the clinical variables in women, including a more severe angina and poorer CHF score (despite a better ejection fraction) and the smaller mean diameter of the coronary vessels, are all considered possible causes of their increased risk of CABG. The mortality rate of women undergoing CABG is often double that of men the same age.

Nursing care for the patient with a CABG involves caring for two surgical sites: the chest and the leg. The care of the leg wound is similar to the postoperative care after the stripping of varicose veins (see Chapter 36). The management of the chest wound, which involves a sternotomy, is similar to that of other chest surgeries (see Chapter 26).

MIDCABG procedure. With recent efforts to reduce cost, length of hospital stay, and morbidity a new approach to CABG surgery has been developed. Minimally invasive direct coronary artery bypass grafting (MIDCABG) has been introduced as an alternative to traditional CABG. This newer technique offers the patient with either left anterior descending (LAD) or right coronary artery (RCA) single-vessel disease, in whom medical management is not effective, an approach to surgical treatment other than sternotomy.[19,20]

With a thoracotomy surgical approach, a thoracoscope is used to mobilize the left IMA (LIMA). The heart is slowed using an IV infusion of β-adrenergic or calcium channel blockers. The LIMA is then anastomosed to the distal LAD (or RCA utilizing the right IMA). Before closure, the IV infusion of β-adrenergic or calcium channel blockers is stopped. A chest tube is placed in the left lateral chest and a mediastinal tube is also placed.[20]

Postoperative nursing care of the patient with a MIDCABG procedure is similar to routine cardiac surgery patients. Intravenous nitroglycerin is used to minimize ischemia and coronary artery spasm. Pain management in these patients is essential since a thoracotomy incision has a higher incidence of pain than a sternotomy.[21] Many of these patients may be managed with an epidural anesthesia. The recovery time is somewhat shorter and patients may resume their routine activities in a shorter time than patients who have a CABG procedure.[22]

The success of MIDCABG and its lowered hospital cost, stay, and morbidity and its future application for patients will depend on further research. Additional clinical experience, cost studies, and longer follow-up will be necessary to delineate the role of this procedure.

Transmyocardial laser revascularization. Transmyocardial laser revascularization (TMLR) is an indirect revascularization procedure that uses laser to create channels between the left ventricular cavity and the coronary microcirculation (ventriculocoronary anastomoses). The channels allow blood to flow into ischemic areas. The procedure is performed through a thoracotomy incision. A high-energy laser, triggered electrocardiographically, is focused through the wall of the ventricle, and usually as many as 40 transmural connections are established in the ischemic myocardium. The laser perforations are completed in 15 to 45 minutes. Currently treatment is limited to patients with advanced CAD who are not candidates for traditional bypass surgery.

Complications following TMLR include murmur, extra heart sounds (S_3, S_4), arrhythmias, and low cardiac output. Angina pain may continue, and the same antianginal medications should be continued after surgery. Cardiac rehabilitation is not begun until nuclear scans and physical examination confirm that the surgery was successful.

Valvular Surgeries

Successful replacement of diseased cardiac valves with valvular prostheses became a reality more than 30 years ago with the development of the Hacher and Starr caged ball prosthesis.[23] Since then, rapid technologic advances have occurred, and today there are a variety of protheses available for patients.

Heart valve prostheses can be broadly grouped into mechanical valve and biologic (tissue) valve categories (see Table 35-20). Both types of prostheses are associated with different valve-related complications, and the clinical superiority of one over the other has not been established. Before deciding which valve to use, factors in valve design, technical considerations, and long-term anticoagulation therapy should be considered.

Mechanical Valves. Currently available mechanical valves are long lasting and characterized by excellent durability. The durability of valves today usually exceeds the life expectancy of the patient requiring valvular replacement. Commonly used mechanical valves include the tilting disk valve and bileaflet valves, such as the St. Jude Medical, Bjork-Shiley, Medtronic-Hall, and Carbomedics valve.

Biologic Valves. Biologic valves are characterized by a low incidence of thromboembolism and valve thrombosis, and thus do not require long-term anticoagulation. The main concern with biologic valves is their shortened long-term durability and the potential risks, including reoperation, associated with tissue degeneration and failure. Biologic cardiac valve substitutes currently available include the porcine aortic valve, the bovine pericardial valve, and human aortic valves (also known as a homograft). The type of valve used depends on individual patient needs such as cardiac anatomic structure, age, past health history, contraindications to anticoagulation use, and lifestyle.

Both mitral and aortic valve disease may require valvular replacement when medical management is no longer effective in the presence of increasing heart failure. Almost all cardiac valvular surgeries require cardiopulmonary bypass. A closed mitral commissurotomy (valvulotomy) is the only possible exception. It involves incising the fused leaflets of the mitral valves if there is no significant calcification of the valve. (Chapter 35 describes the causes, collaborative care, and surgical intervention of valvular diseases.)

Ventricular Surgeries

Ventricular Septal Defects. Occasionally an adult may be diagnosed as having a ventricular septal defect (VSD) that is congenital in nature but had not been diagnosed early in life or progressed in size to cause oxygenation and exercise

Table 33-18 Indications and Contraindications for Cardiac Transplantation

Indications
Suitable physiologic/chronologic age
End-stage heart disease refractory to medical therapy
Functional class III or IV status (NYHA)
Vigorous and healthy individual (except for end-stage cardiac disease) who would benefit from procedure
Compliance with medical regimens
Demonstrated emotional stability and social support system
Financial resources available
Contraindications*
Systemic disease with poor prognosis
Active infection
Active or recent malignancy
Diabetes mellitus, type 1, with end-organ damage
Recent or unresolved pulmonary infarction
Severe pulmonary hypertension unrelieved with medication
Severe cerebrovascular or peripheral vascular disease
Irreversible renal or hepatic dysfunction
Active peptic ulcer disease
Severe osteoporosis
Severe obesity
History of drug or alcohol abuse or mental illness

*Contraindications may vary at different cardiac transplant centers.
NYHA, New York Heart Association.

tolerance problems. A VSD repair involves a primary closure (suturing) or a patch repair (pericardial patch, or grafted with a Gore-Tex or Dacron patch).

Ventricular septal rupture occasionally occurs as a complication of acute MI. Because this defect has a high mortality rate with medical treatment alone, surgical repair is indicated and may be performed on an emergency basis. The septal defect may be sutured or patched depending on the size of the rupture.

Ventricular Aneurysmectomy. Ventricular aneurysms located on the anterolateral or apical part of the LV may also be excised. These noncontracting areas interfere significantly with adequate cardiac contraction and CO. They are often a site for the development of mural thrombi within the ventricle. The ventricle is opened and allowed to collapse so that the thinned scar tissue is cut away and any thrombotic material removed before the ventricle is closed (see Fig. 32-15).

Septal Myotomy and Myectomy. Surgical intervention for HCM is indicated when the patient is symptomatic on optimal medical therapy and left ventricular outflow tract obstruction (LVOTO) is present. The goals of surgical therapy are to decrease LVOTO and improve quality of life. The most common operative procedure is left ventricular septal myotomy and myectomy. In this procedure, a portion of the hypertrophied septum is removed. A mitral valve replacement may be necessary to eliminate mitral insufficiency and decrease LVOTO. The outcomes for these patients are favorable. Postoperative complications include arrhythmias such as heart block or tachyarrhythmias. Another complication is VSD from septal perforation. During surgery a transesophageal echocardiogram is performed to detect a possible VSD before anastomosing the surgical incision.

Cardiomyoplasty

Cardiomyoplasty, a surgical method of augmenting cardiac function, usually involves the use of skeletal muscle such as the latissimus dorsi. The muscle is wrapped around the heart or the aorta, or it may be fashioned into a separate pumping chamber. The muscle is then stimulated with specialized burst pacing, which results in contraction and provides circulatory support. If clinical trials continue to produce favorable results, this procedure may become an important bridge to transplant. With the scarcity of donor hearts, the implications for skeletal muscle wrapping as a long-term alternative to transplant are promising.

Cardiac Transplantation

The first heart transplant was performed in 1967. Since that time, heart transplantation has become the treatment of choice for patients with end-stage heart disease who are unlikely to survive the next 6 to 12 months. Patients with CMP account for more than 50% of the cardiac transplant recipients. Dilated CMP is the most common type of CMP requiring transplantation. Inoperable CAD is the second most common indication for transplantation, accounting for 40% of candidates (Table 33-18).

Once an individual meets the criteria for cardiac transplantation, the goal of the evaluation process is to identify patients who would most benefit from a new heart.[24] In addition to the physical examination, psychologic assessment of candidates is valuable. A complete history of coping abilities, family support system, and motivation to follow through with the transplant and the rigorous transplantation regimen is essential. The complexity of the transplant process may be overwhelming to a patient with inadequate support systems and a poor understanding of the lifestyle changes required after transplant.

Once potential recipients are placed on the transplant list, they may wait at home and receive ongoing medical care if their medical condition is stable. If their condition is not stable, they may require hospitalization for more intensive therapy. Unfortunately, the overall waiting period for a transplant is long, and many patients die while waiting for a transplant.

Donor and recipient matching is based on body and heart size and ABO type. Tissue crossmatching between donor and recipient is generally not done because of difficulty in obtaining good matches and lack of correlation between match and outcome. Negative lymphocyte crossmatch (explained in Chapter 44) and avoidance of a transplantation from a cytomegalovirus (CMV)–positive donor to a CMV-negative recipient are important.

Most donor hearts are obtained at sites distant from the institution performing the transplant. The maximum acceptable ischemic time for cardiac transplant is 4 to 6 hours.

The recipient is prepared for surgery, and cardiopulmonary bypass is used. The usual surgical procedure involves removing the recipient's heart, except for the posterior right and left atrial walls and their venous connections. The recipient's heart is then replaced with the donor heart, which has been trimmed to match. Care is taken to preserve the integrity of the donor sinoatrial (SA) node so that a sinus rhythm may be achieved postoperatively.

Immunosuppressive therapy usually begins while the recipient is in the operating room. Regimens vary but they usually include azathioprine (Imuran), corticosteroids, and cyclosporine. (The mechanisms of action and side effects of these and other immunosuppressants are discussed in Chapter 44 and Table 44-12.) Cyclosporine was first used in heart transplantation in 1980. Currently it is used with corticosteroids for maintenance immunosuppression. Its use has resulted not only in reduced rejection, but also in slowing the rejection process so that early treatment can be instituted.

The postoperative care is similar to that of other open heart surgeries (see next section). Endomyocardial biopsies via the right internal jugular vein are performed at repeated intervals to detect rejection. In addition, peripheral blood T-lymphocyte monitoring is done to assess the recipient's immune status.

Because the patient is immunosuppressed, nursing management should involve prevention of infection, which is the leading cause of death in this population. Many deaths from infection occur during augmented immunosuppressive therapy for acute rejection episodes. Nursing care involves a great deal of emotional support and teaching of both the patient and the family, because transplantation is a last resort. In addition, often the patient is a long distance from home and significant others.

Advances in surgical technique and postoperative care have improved early survival rates after cardiac transplantation. Attention is directed toward improvements in immunosuppression and management of long-term complications. Nursing management continues to focus on promoting patient adaptation to the transplant process, monitoring, managing lifestyle changes, and ongoing education of the patient and family. Ongoing data collection and research continues in regard to quality of life, functional level, and rehabilitation of the cardiac transplant recipient.

Table 33-19 Complications of Cardiac Surgery

Complications of Cardiac Surgery
Early Postoperative Period
Low CO syndrome caused by hypovolemia, acidosis, acute MI, CHF, drugs such as propranolol, mediastinal tamponade, pulmonary embolism, or incomplete or faulty surgical repair
Acute MI, especially with aortocoronary bypass surgery
Cardiac arrhythmias
Hemorrhage
Pulmonary embolism, especially with saphenous vein aortocoronary bypass
Fever
Depression
Wound infection
Electrolyte disturbances
Systemic arterial hypertension
Cerebral infarcts caused by air or thrombus emboli
Confusion, agitation, and disorientation
Disseminated intravascular coagulation
Acute respiratory distress syndrome
Renal failure
Late Postoperative Period
Wound infection
Hepatitis
Pancreatitis (early or late)
Postpericardiotomy syndrome
Systemic arterial emboli and infective endocarditis, with valvular surgeries
Occlusion of graft

CHF, congestive heart failure.

Postoperative Complications Following Cardiac Surgery

The possible complications resulting from cardiac surgery are summarized in Table 33-19.

Low Cardiac Output Syndrome. The most common complication in the early postoperative period is low CO syndrome. Regardless of the surgical procedure, most patients after open heart surgery are in a controlled state of shock caused by fluid shifts and varying vascular tone. Low CO may be caused by relative hypovolemia secondary to blood loss and vascular dilation, or it may be caused by poor left ventricular function. It is evidenced by hypotension, oliguria, and cool extremities. If low CO is due to hypovolemia, the central venous pressure (CVP), left atrial pressure (LAP), and PAWP will be low.

The treatment for hypovolemia includes intravascular volume augmentation, calcium administration, and close observation for blood loss. Volume can be replaced by lactated Ringer's solution, colloids, or blood replacement in the form of packed RBCs (see Chapter 29). Careful recording of all intake and output (e.g., IV fluids, chest drainage, GI drainage, blood, urine, and medications) is essential to monitor fluid balance.

If the low CO is secondary to poor LV function, there may be a high LAP, low BP, decreased urine output, and high CVP and PAWP. Drug therapy is needed and may include diuretics, inotropic agents, or vasopressor agents.

Cardiac Tamponade. Mediastinal or cardiac tamponade may be a cause of low cardiac output syndrome. Cardiac tamponade is pressure on the heart caused by the accumulation of fluid, such as blood, in the pericardium. Clinical manifestations include a decrease in chest tube drainage, decrease in the precordial pulsation, and quiet heart sounds. A chest x-ray shows an enlarged heart and a widened mediastinum. The ECG may show a decrease in amplitude. The PAWP, LAP, and CVP are increased. Pulsus paradoxus, an abnormal (more than 10 mm Hg) fall in systolic BP on inspiration, may be present. It can be determined by taking the BP with a cuff. As the cuff is deflated, it is stopped at the first Korotkoff sound while the patient is breathing normally. If the Korotkoff sound is heard during both inspiration and expiration, no pulsus paradoxus exists. However, if the sound is heard only on expiration, the cuff is deflated slowly until the first Korotkoff sound is heard on both inspiration and expiration. If the difference in pressure between inspiration and expiration is greater than 10 mm Hg, the patient has significant pulsus paradoxus.

After open heart surgery the patient already has a mediastinal tube in place. Therefore the medical treatment for cardiac tamponade is one of the following:

1. Disconnect other chest tubes and clean out the mediastinal tube with a sterile catheter.
2. Remove the tube, break up the clot by inserting a gloved finger into the stoma, and then reinsert a new chest tube.
3. Return the patient to the operating room, where bleeding can be further assessed and treated.

The other treatment for cardiac tamponade in the patient who does not have mediastinal tubes in place is pericardiocentesis.

This procedure involves the insertion of a needle into the pericardium to remove fluid (see Fig. 35-6).

Arrhythmias. Arrhythmias are common postoperatively. A common cause of arrhythmias is serum potassium imbalance (i.e., hyperkalemia or hypokalemia), necessitating frequent evaluation of serum potassium levels. Frequent PVCs and ventricular tachycardia may be seen early in the postoperative period. Potassium replacement is essential in the care of this patient. The nurse must also look to other causes of ventricular arrhythmias (e.g., catheter placement, pH, ischemia, hypothermia) that must be evaluated and treated if necessary. Atrial flutter or fibrillation may occur as early as a few hours postoperatively, in the first 36 hours after aortocoronary bypass, or approximately 6 or 7 days postoperatively. Atrial arrhythmias are treated prophylactically with drugs such as digoxin or metoprolol (Lopressor). (See Chapter 34 for treatment of arrhythmias.) Initial treatment of rapid atrial fibrillation or flutter may also include IV diltiazem (Cardizem) to slow the ventricular response or ibutilide (Covert) to convert the rhythm back to a normal sinus rhythm. Atrial arrhythmias are common with mitral and aortic valve replacements. The patient who has aortic valve replacement for aortic stenosis is at high risk for arrhythmias. If PVCs are noted postoperatively, they are treated quickly with lidocaine. Pacing wires are inserted during surgery so that tachyarrhythmias can be paced in an overdrive method or bradyarrhythmias can be paced at a rate that will maximize CO.

Emboli. The cardiac patient is at risk for pulmonary embolism, which occurs most commonly after the third postoperative day. It is common in the patient with saphenous aortocoronary bypass surgery. Because the clinical manifestations of pulmonary emboli are not always overt, the nurse should report to the physician any patient who has transient weakness, dyspnea, or faintness. Lung scans are often used in the diagnosis. Anticoagulation is the usual method of treatment. (The prevention and treatment of pulmonary emboli are discussed in Chapter 36.)

Arterial embolism may occur after aortic or mitral valve surgery. The patient is frequently placed on long-term anticoagulant therapy. The patient must be observed for evidence of a cerebral embolism, such as a sudden change in level of consciousness, slurring of speech, or one-sided weakness. Extremities should be assessed for evidence of embolization, including pain, pulselessness, pallor, paresthesia, and paralysis.

Fever. Fever is a common complication of cardiac surgery. Causes of a fever include atelectasis, urinary tract infection, pneumonia, thrombophlebitis, drug reaction, transfusion reaction, and wound infection. An elevated temperature increases the workload of the heart because it increases metabolism. The nurse is involved in preventing potential problems that cause fever and assisting in collecting information to assess the cause. The patient's body temperature is taken at least every 4 hours. Treatment is directed toward treating the cause and reducing the fever.

Another possible cause of fever is endocarditis. It rarely occurs in the first weeks postoperatively, probably because of the widespread use of prophylactic antibiotics. However, it can occur early with valvular replacements. (Endocarditis is discussed in Chapter 35.)

Intraoperative Myocardial Infarction. Of primary importance in all cardiovascular surgery, especially in bypass grafts, is the preservation of myocardial tissue. The incidence of intraoperative and perioperative MI may be as high as 25%. Several methods of preserving myocardial tissue during surgery have been developed, primarily the use of hypothermia (cold cardioplegia).

During the immediate postoperative period, serial ECGs are taken and cardiac enzymes are assessed to detect intraoperative infarction. It is sometimes difficult to assess if an intraoperative MI has occurred. Cardiac enzymes may be elevated because of the surgical procedure itself, and an ECG may be difficult to evaluate (as with complete left bundle branch block). Nursing and medical interventions are aimed at preserving myocardial function at all times postoperatively. Monitoring SvO_2 and O_2 saturation gives the nurse a great deal of information about CO and O_2 utilization in this group of patients. If an infarct has occurred, the prognosis is worsened and the hospital stay is lengthened.

NURSING AND COLLABORATIVE MANAGEMENT: CARDIAC SURGERY

Preoperative Management

The preoperative period may vary from a few hours to a month or more depending on the patient's physical condition. Some conditions, such as a stab wound to the heart, require immediate surgical intervention. With other conditions, such as heart failure associated with mitral stenosis or regurgitation, the patient must be stabilized and prepared for surgery. It is desirable that the patient's cardiac and physical condition be stabilized before surgery. For example, arrhythmias should be controlled, CHF treated, BP and CO maximized, and anginal pain relieved.

Most patients have a cardiac catheterization to measure changes in pressure and blood gases in cardiac chambers and across valves. This is performed to look for structural abnormalities or to confirm the diagnosis and to assess LV function. Coronary arteriography is also done to observe the coronary perfusion of the myocardium. Other diagnostic studies include echocardiograms, stress testing, nuclear imaging, ABGs, and Doppler studies to evaluate peripheral perfusion.

In addition, baseline data are obtained just before surgery. These include a chest x-ray, ECG, coagulation studies (e.g., clotting time, prothrombin time, fibrinogen, and platelets), complete blood count (CBC), urinalysis, serum electrolytes, BUN and serum creatinine levels, and cardiac enzymes. Some patients also have thyroid studies and liver function studies. Pulmonary function studies may be performed on patients with pulmonary disease or a history of smoking. ABGs may be done preoperatively as a baseline for postoperative care. The patient also is blood typed and crossmatched.

Blood transfusions have become a major concern to many patients and their families. Preoperative teaching should include information regarding autotransfusion and autologous blood donation. If the surgery is planned, a patient may donate 1 unit of blood per week up to 3 units (3 weeks) and have fresh blood at the time of surgery (no freezing is required). A patient may also have the family donate blood (directed donor blood, which, when cross-typed, is given to the patient). Surgical procedures have improved with the use of blood cell savers and

PATIENT TEACHING GUIDE

Table 33-20 Preoperative Teaching List for Cardiac Surgery

Operating room	Provide trip to operating room to see area and meet staff (if desired) Provide trip to waiting room for family Inform patient that conversations and events from the operating room experience may be remembered
CCU or ICU	Provide trip to see area and meet staff (if desired)
Early postoperative period in CCU or ICU	Explain that patient may lose track of time and place and may have hallucinations (visual, auditory, taste) Explain ECG monitoring leads Discuss location and purpose of tubes and when they will be removed Discuss endotracheal tube; because patient cannot talk, devise method of calling a nurse Explain nasogastric tube Explain that arterial lines and monitors are used for pressure measurements Explain that venous lines and monitors are used for fluid or medication administration Explain that bloody red drainage will occur from the chest tubes and that a pulling sensation is felt when the tubes are removed Explain that retention catheter is used for input and output and ease of urine elimination Inform patient that thirst may be experienced Discuss noise level, sounds, alarms
Postoperative routine	Explain mechanical ventilation Explain suctioning Explain the importance of coughing, deep breathing, and turning Discuss frequent monitoring of vital signs and continuous cardiac monitoring
Pain medications	Explain that patient can ask for pain medication to be comfortable Inform patient that the body will be achy and sore for the first week postoperatively
Nebulizer treatment	Provide demonstration of incentive spirometer
Post-CCU or post-ICU routines	Provide overview of discharge regimens
General care unit	Discuss emotional reaction Explain that depression is common and should be short-lived Explain discharge plans, home health care

CCU, coronary care unit; *ICU*, intensive care unit.

subsequent autotransfusion of blood from the surgical field, to the point where many patients require no blood after surgery. The patient may return home with lower hemoglobin and hematocrit levels but can be treated successfully with iron replacement therapy and nutritional support.

Other baseline data obtained shortly before surgery include an accurate body weight to aid in fluid management and vital signs, including temperature, because an elevated temperature is an indication for postponement of surgery.

To improve the respiratory status, the patient who smokes must stop smoking at least 1 week and preferably 1 month or more before surgery. This helps decrease the amount of bronchial secretions and thus reduces the postoperative risk of atelectasis and pneumonia. However, it may be difficult for many patients to stop smoking because of their anxiety about the surgery.

It may be necessary to modify the patient's medications to prevent adverse reactions. Propranolol (Inderal) may be tapered 24 hours to 2 weeks before surgery if the patient tolerates weaning (i.e., has no anginal or hypertensive episodes). However, a patient who requires propranolol may be given positive inotropic agents in the early postoperative period to counteract the effects of propranolol. If possible, aspirin or warfarin (Coumadin) should be stopped 7 days before surgery. This may require the patient to be admitted preoperatively and started on IV heparin for anticoagulation. Although tapering or stopping these drugs may appear to be beneficial, many patients who undergo emergency surgeries do not discontinue these medications and do well postoperatively.

Patients receiving long-acting insulins will be switched to regular insulin on a sliding-scale basis during the perioperative period. They remain on the sliding scale into the postoperative period. Other drugs that may need modification include corticosteroids, antihypertensives, and phenothiazines. The nurse should check with the physician concerning changes in any drug that is questionable.

To prevent incisional infections, the patient should be instructed to shower several times using a bacteriostatic soap (e.g., Betadine, hexachlorophene). In addition, the patient is usually started on parenteral antibiotics within 12 hours of surgery. The physician discusses at length with the patient and significant others the nature of the surgery, including the procedures, expected outcomes, possible complications, and postsurgical care.

Nursing management in the preoperative period is primarily focused on teaching. Extensive preoperative teaching is a major responsibility of the nurse. It deals with general postoperative concerns (see Chapter 18), in addition to the specialized concerns related to cardiovascular surgery. The purpose of teaching is to help reduce anxiety. Table 33-20 outlines the topics that should be included. The patient should be encouraged to ask questions and discuss concerns. It is essential that the nurse report significant concerns to the physician so that a coordinated approach can be developed to deal with the patient's anxiety.

Family members should also be involved in the preoperative teaching. This will help alleviate their anxiety so that they can support the patient more effectively during this period. Many patients do not come to the hospital until the morning of surgery. In this situation, preoperative teaching should occur before this time, as an outpatient or in the physician's office.

Intraoperative Management

Many cardiovascular surgeries are being performed with the patient on a heart-lung machine or cardiopulmonary bypass. This allows the surgeon to work on a heart that has been put into asystole or a slowly contracting state. The heart-lung machine serves as a pump to circulate and oxygenate blood. The machine receives blood from catheters in the venae cavae or right atrium, oxygenates it, and returns the blood to the patient through a catheter in the aorta. This is usually done in conjunction with hypothermia (approximately 77° to 82° F [25° to 28° C] for bypass and valvular surgeries). The time on the heart-lung machine is closely monitored and kept to a minimum because the longer the patient is on it, the more complications may develop. In addition, careful anesthesia and precise monitoring of the cardiac rhythm, vital signs, blood gases, electrolytes, and coagulation status are components of the procedure.

At the end of the procedure, depending on the patient's condition (ventricular function) when coming off bypass, the surgeon may place monitoring lines for hemodynamic monitoring and management postoperatively. An intraaortic balloon pump (IABP) may also need to be inserted in the operating room in cases of poor left ventricular function. (Hemodynamic monitoring and intraaortic balloon pumps are discussed in Chapter 63.)

Postoperative Management

Complications that may occur as a result of cardiac surgery are outlined in Table 33-19. Much of the postoperative management is directed toward the prevention or early detection of these complications. Postoperative assessment is outlined in Table 33-21. The physician and nurses work closely during this time with much overlapping of functions, depending on the policies of the institution.

On completion of cardiac surgery, the patient is transferred immediately to a coronary care unit (CCU) or ICU. (Some hospitals have separate heart recovery rooms because the CCU and the operating room are not always in close proximity.) The nursing staff should have been notified of the patient's estimated time of arrival and status so that all the equipment is ready to provide care.

On arrival the patient should already be lying on the postoperative bed. Usually a team of two nurses admits the patient on arrival to the unit. This is a crucial time for the patient because complications may occur early and during transport. When the patient arrives, the nurse team will connect the monitoring devices (e.g., ECG, arterial lines, O_2 saturation monitor) and suction equipment (e.g., chest tubes, nasogastric tubes) so that the patient's hemodynamic parameters can be assessed immediately. The endotracheal tube is checked, and the patient is attached to a preset mechanical ventilator. As soon as the equipment is properly connected and calibrated, the nurse should assess the patient's neurologic, respiratory, and cardiac status to determine the level of anesthesia and the ventilation and perfusion status. Reports from the anesthesiologist and surgeon are often given during this initial assessment period. Baseline laboratory data are collected, including ABGs, serum electrolytes, CBC, clotting profile, lactate level, and cardiac enzymes. A chest x-ray is also taken immediately on arrival to the ICU.

The nurse also collects baseline data on the cardiovascular status by checking the arterial blood pressure, PAP, PAWP, LAP (if a line was inserted during surgery), heart sounds, cardiac rhythm, and peripheral pulses and O_2 saturations. If the patient has an Oximetrics pulmonary artery catheter, venous O_2 saturation (SvO_2) can be monitored continuously. The patient's monitoring devices (e.g., pulmonary artery catheter, left atrial line, Oximetrics SvO_2 monitoring) depend on the patient's preoperative condition, the intraoperative procedures and find-

Table 33-21 Postoperative Assessment after Cardiac Surgery

Nervous System
- Pupil size and reaction
- Orientation and level of consciousness
- Motor functioning

Respiratory System
- Placement of endotracheal tube
- Settings on mechanical ventilator
- Character of respirations
- Breath sounds and secretions
- Arterial blood gases

Cardiovascular and Hematologic Systems
- Cardiac rhythm
- Peripheral pulses
- Blood pressure
- Venous or pulmonary artery pressures
- Temperature
- Fluid status
- Chest tubes
- Coagulation status
- Cardiac output

Renal System
- Urinary output
- Urine character, color, specific gravity
- Electrolytes

Gastrointestinal System
- Nasogastric secretions
- Bowel sounds

Integumentary System
- Skin breakdown
- Incisional healing and drainage

Pain
- Quality or intensity
- Location

ings, the surgeon's preference, and the unit's protocol. Many patients return from surgery with only a CVP line; others may require a pulmonary artery catheter and an atrial and ventricular pacing wire, and they may be on an IABP. These variations are of primary importance in preparing for the patient and in planning for care.

Once the initial assessment is made, the patient is placed on frequent vital signs (e.g., BP and HR continuously and then every 15 minutes for the first 4 hours, then every 30 minutes for 4 hours, and later every hour). After the patient has had the initial assessment, CO, cardiac index, and SVR measurements may be done to assess LV function. Other indicators may be measured at least every hour, such as urinary output, PAWP or PAP, temperature, breath sounds, and other respiratory parameters. In addition, the wave patterns for the arterial pressure, pulmonary artery catheter, O_2 saturation, SvO_2, and ECG are constantly monitored for significant changes. Peripheral pulses and warmth of extremities also are checked every 1 to 2 hours.

Care of the patient's chest tubes is indicated by the surgeon's preference and the unit's protocol. Chest tubes must be kept patent so that blood from the mediastinum and pericardium can drain adequately. Plugging or clotting in the chest tube may obstruct the drainage and severely compromise the patient. Chest tube drainage (amount and character) is also assessed and recorded frequently (every 15 minutes for the first few hours postoperatively). (The nursing care of the patient with chest tubes is presented in Chapter 26.)

The patient also needs care to prevent problems associated with immobility. This includes turning from side to side. The head of the bed may be elevated 30 degrees when vital signs are stable. The patient may have antiembolic stockings in place. While on the ventilator, the patient must be suctioned (see Chapter 63). When the endotracheal tube is removed, the

CRITICAL THINKING EXERCISES

CASE STUDY

Congestive Heart Failure

Patient Profile

Mrs. E., a 62-year-old Hispanic woman, was admitted to the medical unit with complaints of increasing dyspnea on exertion.

Subjective Data

- Had a severe MI at 58 years of age
- Has experienced increasing dyspnea of exertion during the last 2 years
- Had a respiratory tract infection, frequent cough, and edema in legs 2 weeks ago
- Cannot walk two blocks without getting short of breath
- Has to sleep with head elevated on three pillows
- Does not always remember to take medication

Objective Data

Physical Examination

- Elderly woman in respiratory distress
- Heart murmur
- Moist crackles in both lungs
- Cyanotic lips and extremities

Diagnostic Studies

- Chest x-ray results: cardiomegaly with right and left ventricular hypertrophy; fluid in lower lobes of lungs

Collaborative Care

- Digoxin 0.25 mg qd
- Furosemide (Lasix) 40 mg bid
- Potassium 40 mEq PO bid
- Enalapril (Vasotec) 5 mg PO qd
- 2 g sodium diet
- Oxygen 6 L/min
- Daily weights

Critical Thinking Questions

1. Explain the pathophysiology of Mrs. E.'s heart disease.
2. What clinical manifestations of heart failure did Mrs. E. exhibit?
3. What is the significance of the findings of the chest x-ray?
4. Explain the rationale for each of the medical orders prescribed for Mrs. E.
5. What are appropriate nursing interventions for Mrs. E.?
6. What teaching measures should be instituted to prevent recurrence of an acute episode of heart failure?
7. Based on the assessment data presented, write one or more appropriate nursing diagnoses. Are there any collaborative problems?

NURSING RESEARCH ISSUES

1. What nursing measures are most effective in relieving shortness of breath in a patient with CHF?
2. What are effective ways of promoting optimum sleep-rest patterns in a patient with end-stage CHF?
3. What preoperative teaching methods are most effective in assisting the patient to prepare for a second open heart surgical procedure?
4. What are the psychoemotional needs of a spouse of an open heart surgical patient preoperatively and 2 months postoperatively?
5. What stressors are present for the family of a patient who is on a waiting list for a cardiac transplant?

patient should cough and deep breathe. The patient can also sit in a chair, usually by the end of the first day postoperatively. Progressive ambulation is then encouraged.

Most tubes and lines are removed within 1 to 3 days of surgery. Because rest periods are important, care must be planned to allow for uninterrupted sleep, especially during the early period of intensive care. Pain medications are also important because they allow the patient to be active and to participate in coughing and deep-breathing exercises. The patient and the family need many explanations and much support. They should be allowed to spend as much time together as the patient's condition allows.

After a short period in the ICU, the patient is moved to a step-down unit if further ECG monitoring or care is necessary; if the patient's condition is stable, the patient may be moved to a general surgical unit. After transfer, the patient's activity levels are gradually increased and nutritional patterns are resumed. Medication regimens are adjusted. Wound care is initiated according to physician preference or unit protocol. The patient is prepared for discharge, and referrals are made to appropriate community resources. Home regimens, including wound care, activity, and medications, are discussed, and the patient should be given written instructions. Wound care, diet, and activity levels should be discussed in specific terms with the patient and the family. Evaluation should be made of their level of knowledge and of the need for further teaching before discharge. Return appointments to the surgeon and referring physician are made before discharge so that the patient and family are aware of all follow-up procedures.

Home health nursing is critical when planning for the patient's discharge. Patients are now being discharged as early as the third postoperative day and may require daily home nursing care. Agencies that specialize in home care of the cardiovascular surgical patient can provide monitoring and assessment of activity levels, nutritional intake, bowel function, vital signs, daily weights, and adjustment of medications. Answering questions and providing assistance with bathing and activities of daily living are essential. These coordinated activities between the surgeon's office and the home health agency may prevent rehospitalization from complications identified and treated early and in the home.

REVIEW QUESTIONS

The number of the question corresponds to the same-numbered objective at the beginning of the chapter.

1. The nurse recognizes that primary manifestations of systolic ventricular failure include
   a. ↓ afterload and ↓ LVEDP.
   b. ↓ ejection fraction and ↑ PAWP.
   c. ↓ PAWP and ↑ left ventricular ejection fraction.
   d. ↑ pulmonary hypertension associated with normal ejection fraction.
2. The compensatory mechanism involved in congestive heart failure that leads to inappropriate fluid retention and additional workload of the heart is
   a. ventricular dilation.
   b. the hormonal response.
   c. ventricular hypertrophy.
   d. sympathetic nervous system activation.
3. A patient with chronic congestive heart failure and atrial fibrillation is treated with a digitalis preparation and a thiazide diuretic. To prevent possible complications of the combination of drugs the nurse
   a. monitors serum potassium levels.
   b. keeps an accurate measure of intake and output.
   c. teaches the patient about dietary restriction of potassium.
   d. withholds the digitalis and notifies the physician if the heart rate is irregular.
4. The medication used in the management of a patient with acute pulmonary edema that will decrease both preload and afterload and provide relief of anxiety is
   a. morphine.
   b. amrinone (Inocor).
   c. dobutamine (Dobutrex).
   d. aminophylline.
5. The nurse plans care for the patient with primary dilated cardiomyopathy based on the knowledge that
   a. family members may be at risk because of the genetic basis of the disease.
   b. the prognosis of the patient is poor and emotional support is a high priority of care.
   c. the condition may be successfully treated with surgical ventriculomyotomy and myectomy.
   d. medical management of the disorder focuses on treatment of the underlying cause.
6. Aware of the leading cause of death in patients with heart transplants, the nurse places high priority on nursing interventions that
   a. detect signs of rejection.
   b. prevent and detect infection.
   c. promote mobility and activity.
   d. prevent postoperative arrhythmias.
7. While caring for a cardiac surgery patient immediately postoperatively the nurse recognizes that the patient has low cardiac output secondary to poor left ventricular function based on the findings of
   a. ↑ PAWP and ↓ urinary output.
   b. pulsus paradoxus and ↑ PAWP.
   c. ↓ PAWP, ↓ CVP, and ↓ left atrial pressure.
   d. premature ventricular contractions and ↑ CVP.

References

1. American Heart Association website: www.americanheart.org.
2. Kannel WB, Belanger AJ: Epidemiology of heart failure, *Am Heart J* 121:951, 1991.
3. Funk M, Krumholz HM: Epidemiologic and economic impact of advanced heart failure, *J Cardiovasc Nurs* 10:1, 1996.
4. Guerra-Garcia H, Taffet G, Protas EJ: Considerations related to disability and exercise in elderly women with congestive heart failure, *J Cardiovasc Nurs* 11:60, 1997.
5. Ahrens SG: Managing heart failure: a blue print of success, *Nursing* 25:26, 1995.
6. Dracup K, Dunbar SB, Baker DW: Rethinking heart failure, *AJN* 95:23, 1995.
7. Oka RK: Physiologic changes in heart failure: what's new, *J Cardiovasc Nurs* 10:11, 1996.
8. Singh SN: Congestive heart failure and arrhythmias: therapeutic modalities, *J Cardiovasc Electrophysiol* 8:89, 1997.
9. Fisher ML, Balke CW, Freudenberger R: Therapeutic options in advanced heart failure, *Hosp Pract* 32:97, 1997.
10. Wright JM: Pharmacological management of congestive heart failure, *Crit Care Nurs Q* 18:22, 1995.
11. Moser DK: Maximizing therapy in the advanced heart failure patient, *J Cardiovasc Nurs* 10:29, 1996.
12. Pratt NG: Pathophysiology of heart failure: neuroendocrine response, *Crit Care Nurs Q* 18:22, 1995.

13. Meyer MS: Congestive heart failure: meet the challenge, *Medsurg Nurs* 4:341, 1995.
14. Jaarsma T, and others: Maintaining the balance: nursing care of patients with chronic heart failure, *Int J Nurs Stud* 34:213, 1997.
15. Sherman A: Critical care management of the heart failure patient in the home, *Crit Care Nurs Q* 18:77, 1995.
16. Bashore TM, Harrison JK, Davidson CT: Special diagnostic and therapeutic procedures in cardiac surgery. In Sabiston DC, Spencer FC, editors: *Surgery of the chest,* vol II, Philadelphia, 1995, Saunders.
17. Spencer FC, Galloway AC, Colvin SB: Surgical management of coronary artery disease. In Sabiston DC, Spencer FC, editors: *Surgery of the chest,* vol II, Philadelphia, 1995, Saunders.
18. Coodley EL: CHD: when medical therapy fails, *Hosp Pract* 31:13, 1996.
19. Vac KJ, Daake CJ, Lambrechts DS: Nursing care of patients undergoing thoracoscopic minimally invasive bypass grafting, *Am J Crit Care* 6:281, 1997.
20. Mizell JL, Maglish BL, Matheny RG: Minimally invasive direct coronary artery bypass graft surgery: introduction for critical care nurses, *Crit Care Nurse* 17:46, 1997.
21. Cohen AJ, and others: Effect of internal mammary harvest on postoperative pain and pulmonary function, *Ann Thorac Surg* 56:1107, 1993.
22. Shawgo T: Thoracoscopic surgery: a new approach to pulmonary disease, *Crit Care Nurse* 16:76, 1996.
23. Starr A, Edwards MC: Mitral replacement: clinical experience with a ball-valve prosthesis, *Ann Surg* 154:726, 1961.
24. Grady KL: When to transplant: recipient selection for heart transplantation, *J Cardiovasc Nurs* 10:58, 1996.
25. Hicks GL: Cardiac surgery, *J Am Coll Surg* 186:129, 1998.

Resources

American Association of Cardiovascular and Pulmonary Rehabilitation
7611 Elmwood Avenue, Suite 201
Middleton, WI 53562
608-831-6989
Fax: 608-831-5122
http://www.aacvpr.org

American College of Cardiology
http://www.acc.org

American Heart Association
7320 Greenville Avenue
Dallas, TX 75231
214-373-6300
http://www.amhrt.org

Council on Cardiovascular Nursing
American Heart Association
7320 Greenville Avenue
Dallas, TX 75231
214-373-6300
http://www.amhrt.org/Scientific/council/cvn/index.html

The Mended Hearts
7272 Greenville Avenue
Dallas, TX 75231
214-706-1442
http://www.mendedhearts.org

National Heart, Lung, and Blood Institute
National Institutes of Health
4733 Bethesda Avenue, Suite 530
Bethesda, MD 20814
301-951-3260
http://www.nhlbi.nih.gov/nhlbi/nhlbi.htm

National Heart Savers Association
9140 West Dodge Road
Omaha, NE 68114
402-398-1993
http://heartsavers.org/

For additional Internet resources, see the website for this book at **www.mosby.com/MERLIN/medsurg_lewis**

REMEMBER to check out your companion CD-ROM

34 NURSING MANAGEMENT Arrhythmias

Carolyn I. Johns

www.mosby.com/MERLIN/medsurg_lewis

LEARNING OBJECTIVES

1. Identify the clinical characteristics and electrocardiographic patterns of common arrhythmias.
2. Describe the nursing and collaborative management of common arrhythmias.
3. Differentiate between defibrillation and cardioversion, identifying indications for use and physiologic effects.
4. Describe the management of patients with temporary and permanent pacemakers.
5. Describe the management of a patient with an implantable cardioverter-defibrillator.
6. Explain the management of a patient undergoing electrophysiologic testing and radiofrequency catheter ablation therapy.
7. Explain the essential elements of basic cardiac life support.
8. Explain the essential elements of advanced cardiac life support.

ARRHYTHMIA IDENTIFICATION AND TREATMENT

The ability to recognize *arrhythmias,* which are abnormal cardiac rhythms, is an essential skill for the nurse. Cardiac monitoring is now used in a wide range of hospital and clinic settings.[1] Prompt assessment of an abnormal cardiac rhythm and the patient's response to the rhythm is critical. This chapter describes basic principles of common arrhythmias. For more information on arrhythmias, the reader should refer to detailed texts on electrocardiograph (ECG) interpretation.[1-4]

Conduction System: A Brief Review

Four properties of cardiac tissue enable the conduction system to initiate an electrical impulse, which is transmitted through the cardiac tissue stimulating muscle contraction (Table 34-1). The conduction system of the heart is made up of specialized neuromuscular tissue located throughout the heart (see Fig. 30-5). A normal cardiac impulse begins in the sinoatrial (SA) node in the upper right atrium. It is transmitted over the atrial myocardium via Bachmann's bundle and internodal pathways to the atrioventricular (AV) node. From the AV node, the impulse spreads through the bundle of His and down the left and right bundle branches, emerging in the Purkinje's fibers, which transmit the impulse to the ventricles.

Conduction to the point just before the impulse leaves the Purkinje's fibers takes place within the time of the PR interval of the ECG. When the impulse emerges from the Purkinje fibers, ventricular depolarization occurs, producing mechanical contraction of the ventricles and the QRS complex on the ECG. The electrical activity of the heart is illustrated in Fig. 30-6.

Nervous Control of the Heart

The autonomic nervous system plays an important role in the rate of impulse formation, the speed of conduction, and the strength of cardiac contraction. The components of the autonomic nervous system that affect the heart are the right and left vagus nerve fibers of the parasympathetic nervous system and fibers of the sympathetic nervous system.

Stimulation of the vagus nerve causes a decreased rate of firing of the SA node, slowed impulse conduction of the AV node, and decreased force of cardiac muscle contraction. Stimulation of the sympathetic nerves that supply the heart has essentially the opposite effect on the heart.[2]

Electrocardiogram Monitoring

The ECG is a graphic tracing of the electrical impulses produced in the heart. The wave forms on the ECG are produced by the movement of charged ions across the membranes of myocardial cells, representing depolarization and repolarization.

Table 34-1 Properties of Cardiac Tissue

Automaticity	Ability to initiate an impulse spontaneously and continuously
Contractility	Ability to respond mechanically to an impulse
Conductivity	Ability to transmit an impulse along a membrane in an orderly manner
Excitability	Ability to be electrically stimulated

Reviewed by Elizabeth Chapman, RN, MS, CCRN, ICU Staff Nurse, Columbia Garden Park; Nursing Faculty, MGCCC-Jefferson Davis Campus, Long Beach, Miss.

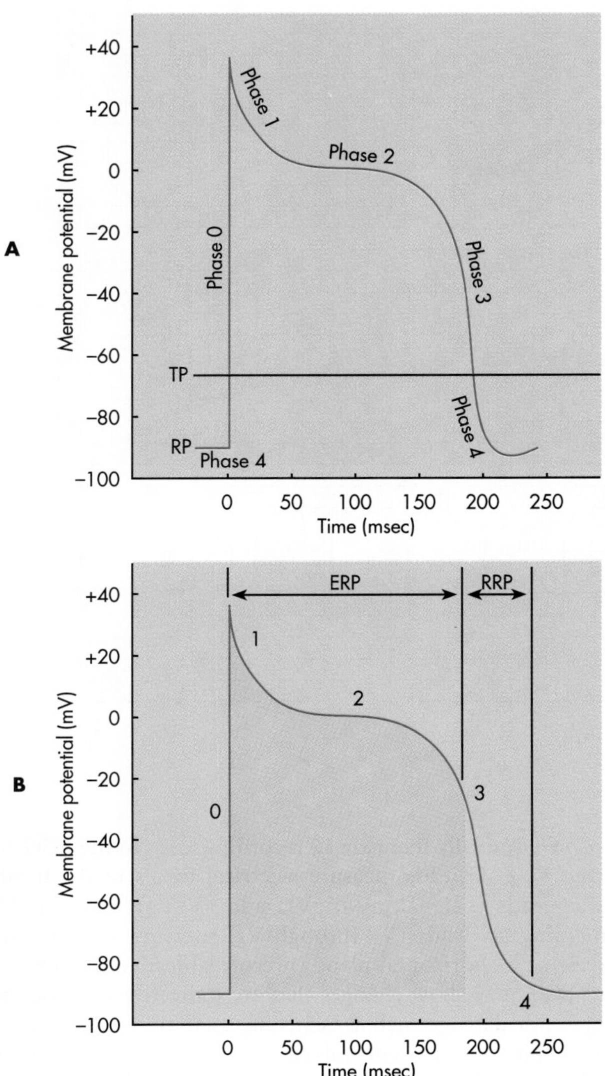

Fig. 34-1 **A,** Phases of the cardiac action potential. The electrical potential, measured in millivolts *(mV),* is indicated along the vertical axis of the graph. Time, measured in milliseconds *(msec),* is indicated along the horizontal axis. The action potential consists of three to five phases, labeled as phase *0* through phase *4.* Each phase represents a particular electrical event or combination of electrical events. The events, the duration of the events and action potential, and the transmembrane potential vary with the type of cardiac cell being measured. **B,** Two parts of the refractory period. The effective refractory period (*ERP*) extends from phase 0 to approximately −60 mV in phase 3. The remainder of the action potential is the relative refractory period (*RRP*).

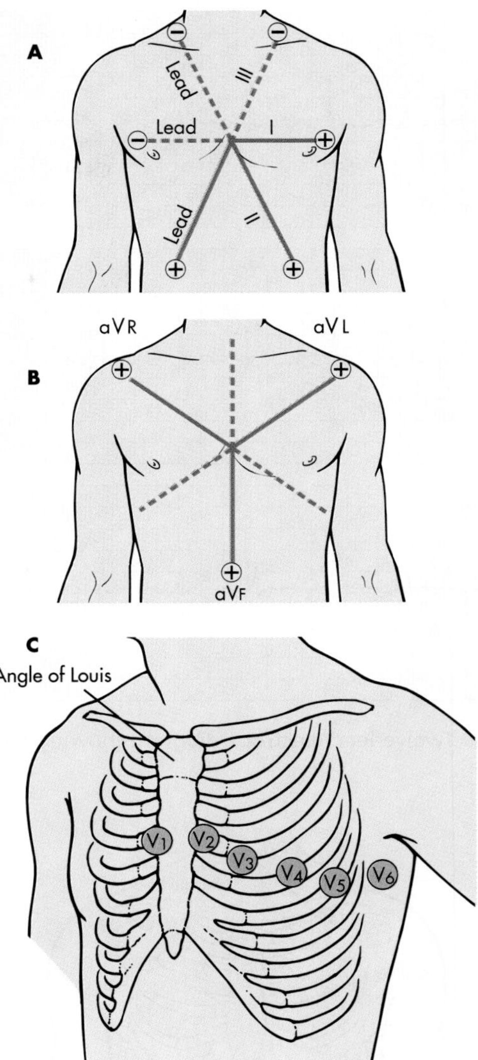

Fig. 34-2 **A,** Limb leads I, II, and III. Leads are located on the extremities. Illustrated are the angles from which these leads view the heart. **B,** Lead placement for augmented limb leads aVR, aVL, and aVF. These unipolar leads use the calculated center of the heart as their negative electrode. **C,** Lead placement for the chest electrodes: V_1, fourth intercostal space at the right sternal border; V_2, fourth intercostal space at the left sternal border; V_3, equidistant between V_2 and V_4; V_4, fifth intercostal space at the left midclavicular line; V_5, anterior axillary line and same horizontal level as V_4; V_6, midaxillary line and same horizontal level as V_4.

The membrane of a cardiac cell is semipermeable, allowing it to maintain a high concentration of potassium and a low concentration of sodium inside the cell. A high concentration of sodium and a low concentration of potassium are maintained outside the cell. The inside of the cell, when at rest, or in the *polarized* state, is negative compared with the outside. When a cell or groups of cells are stimulated, each cell membrane changes its permeability and allows sodium to migrate rapidly into the cell, making the cell positive compared with the outside (*depolarization*). A slower movement of ions across the membrane restores the cell to the polarized state, which is called *repolarization.* In Fig. 34-1 the phases are as follows: phase 4 is a polarized state; phase 0 is the upstroke of rapid depolarization; and phases 1, 2, and 3 represent repolarization.[3] Antiarrhythmic drugs have a direct effect on the action potential.[4] When antiarrhythmic drugs are used in a clinical setting, a nurse's understanding of the ionic shifts in the cardiac cell and the action potential mechanism is important.

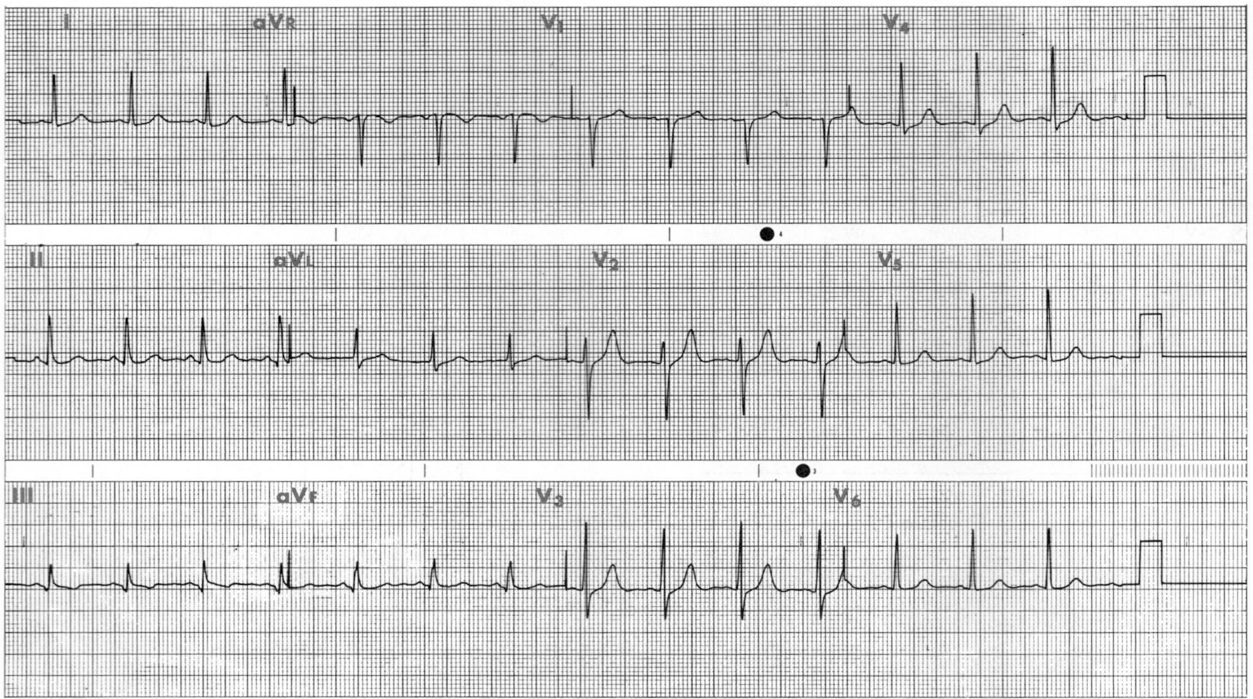

Fig. 34-3 Twelve-lead electrocardiogram showing a normal sinus rhythm.

A

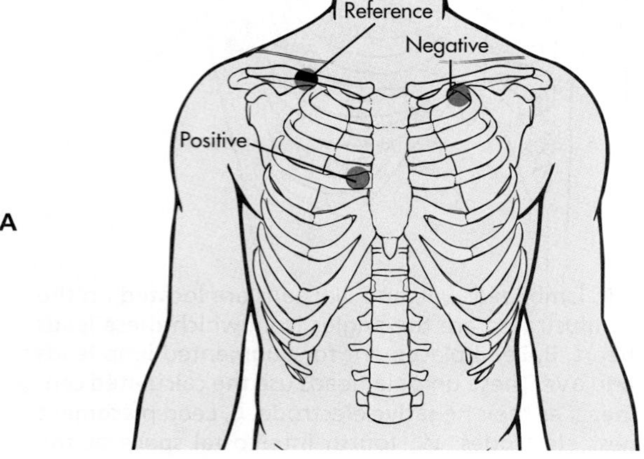

B

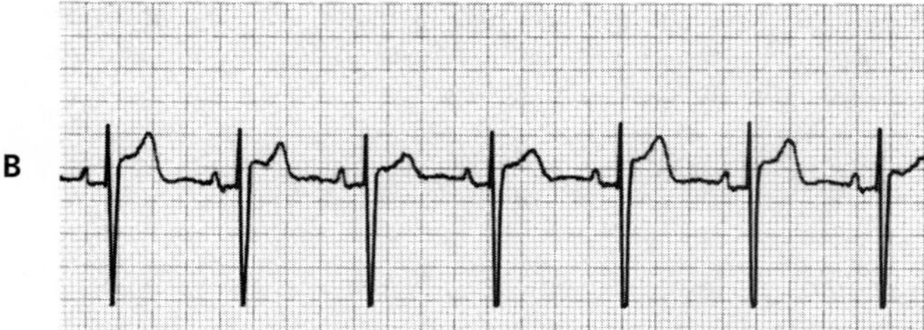

Fig. 34-4 **A,** Lead placement for MCL_1. **B,** Typical electrocardiogram tracing in lead MCL_1.

Conventionally there are 12 recording leads in the ECG. Six of the 12 ECG leads measure electrical forces in the frontal plane (leads I, II, III, aVR, aVL, and aVF) (Fig. 34-2). The remaining six leads (V_1 through V_6) measure the electrical forces in the horizontal plane (precordial lead sites). The 12-lead ECG may show changes that are indicative of structural changes or damage such as ischemia, infarction, enlarged cardiac chambers, electrolyte imbalance, or drug toxicity.[3] Obtaining 12 views of the heart is also helpful in the assessment of arrhythmias. An example of a normal 12-lead ECG appears in Fig. 34-3.

When a patient's ECG is being continuously monitored, 1 to 12 ECG leads are used. The most common leads used are lead II and lead MCL_1, which corresponds to V_1 in the standard 12-lead ECG (Fig. 34-4). These leads most clearly demonstrate the P wave and QRS complexes.[5]

The ECG can be visualized continuously on a monitor oscilloscope. A recording of the ECG "strip" is done on ECG paper attached to the monitor. This provides documentation of the patient's rhythms. It is a way to thoroughly assess an arrhythmia and measure complexes and intervals.

It is essential to know how to measure time and voltage on the ECG paper to correctly interpret an ECG. ECG paper consists of large (heavy lines) and small (light lines) squares (Fig. 34-5). Each large square incorporates 25 smaller squares (five horizontal and five vertical). Each small square represents 0.04 second horizontally and 0.1 mV vertically. This means that the large square equals 0.20 second and that 300 large squares equal 1.0 minute. Vertically, one large square is equal to 0.5 mV. These squares are used to calculate the heart rate (HR) and intervals between different ECG complexes.[5]

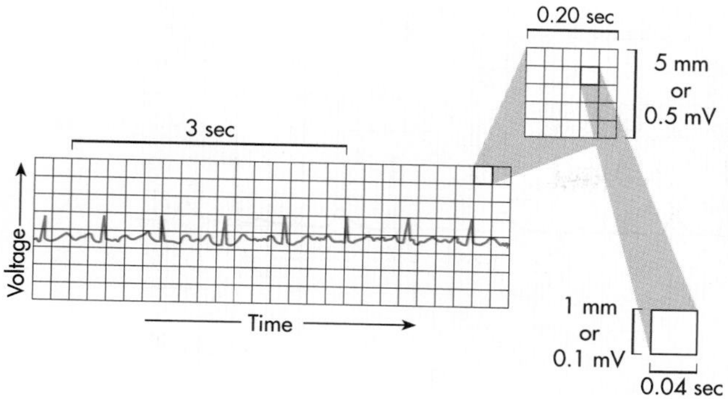

Fig. 34-5 Time and voltage on the electrocardiogram.

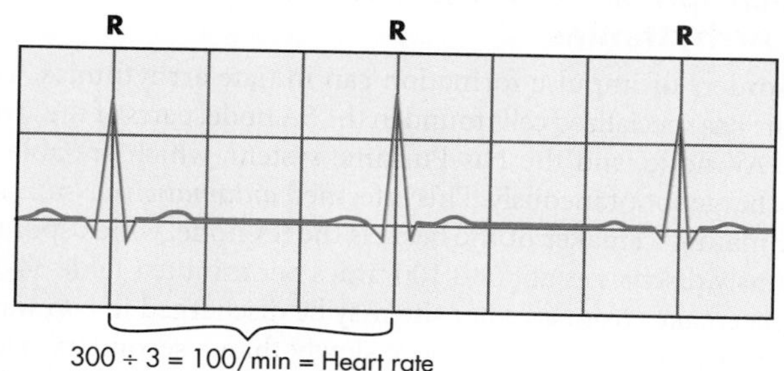

Fig. 34-6 When the rhythm is regular, heart rate can be determined at a glance.

A variety of methods can be used to calculate the HR from an ECG. Probably the most accurate way is to count the number of QRS complexes in 1 minute; however, this method is time-consuming. If the rhythm is regular, a simpler process can be used. Every 3 seconds a marker appears on the ECG paper. The nurse can count the number of QRS complexes in 6 seconds and multiply that number by 10. This will yield the number of complexes or beats per minute.

Another rapid method for calculating the HR when a regular rhythm is present is to count the number of small squares between two QRS complexes (R-R interval). An R wave is the first upward deflection of the QRS complex. The nurse divides 1500 by the number of small squares to get the precise HR. This method is accurate only if the rhythm is regular.[7]

The nurse can also count the number of large squares between two R waves and divide into 300 (Fig. 34-6). This method is also only accurate if the rhythm is regular.

An additional way to measure distances on the ECG grid is to use calipers. Calipers are used for fine measurements, especially for points of a specific wave. Many times a P or R wave will not fall directly on a light or heavy line. The fine points of the calipers can be placed exactly on the components to be measured and then moved to another part of the grid for time measurement, which is accurate to 0.04 second.

ECG leads are attached to the patient's chest wall via an electrode pad fixed with electrical conductive paste. For best contact, hair on the chest wall should be shaved and skin should be prepared with acetone to remove excess oil and debris. In the case of a diaphoretic patient, benzoin may be applied to the skin before electrode placement. If leads and electrodes are not firmly placed, or if there is muscle activity or electrical interference from an outside source, an artifact may be seen on the monitor. An *artifact* is a distortion of the baseline and waveforms seen on the ECG (Fig. 34-7). Accurate interpretation of cardiac rhythm is difficult when an artifact is present.

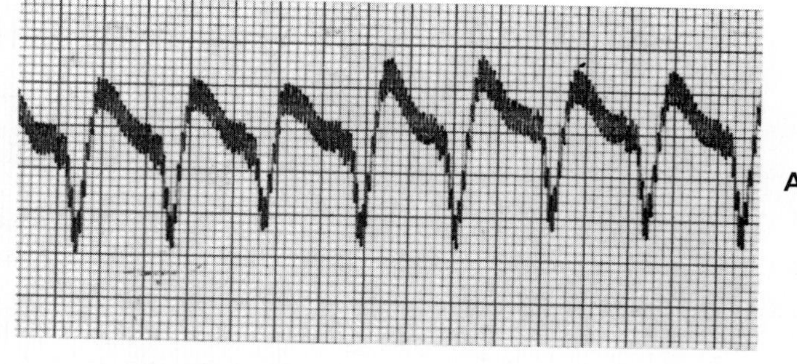

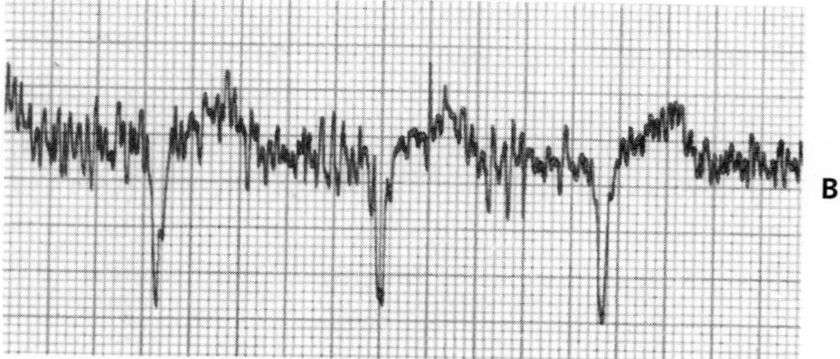

Fig. 34-7 **A,** Artifact—60-cycle interference. **B,** Artifact—muscular movement.

Telemetry Monitoring

Telemetry monitoring is the observation of a patient's heart rate and rhythm that is used for the diagnosis of arrhythmias.[6] Two types of systems are used for detecting arrhythmias by telemetry. The first type, a centralized monitoring system, requires a nurse or telemetry technician to constantly be observing all patients' rhythms at a central location. The second and most updated system of telemetry monitoring does not require constant nurse or technician surveillance. These systems have the capability of detecting and storing data on the type and frequency of arrhythmias. Sophisticated alarm systems provide different levels of detection of arrhythmias, depending on the severity of the arrhythmia. However, computerized monitoring systems are not fail-proof. Frequent nursing assessment is important when caring for monitored patients.

Assessment of Cardiac Rhythm

When assessing the cardiac rhythm the nurse must make an accurate interpretation of an arrhythmia and immediately proceed to evaluate the consequences of that arrhythmia for the individual patient. Assessment of the patient's hemodynamic response to an arrhythmia provides guidance in therapeutic intervention. If possible, a determination of the cause of the arrhythmia should be made. Tachycardias may cause a decrease in

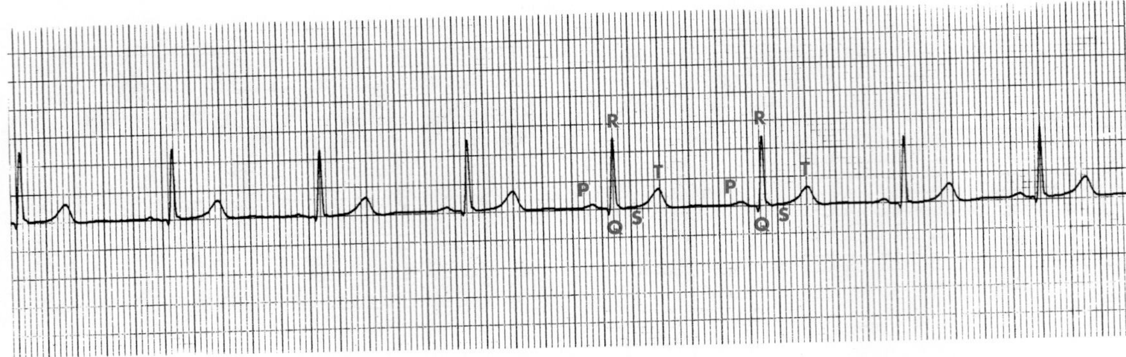

Fig. 34-8 Normal sinus rhythm in lead II.

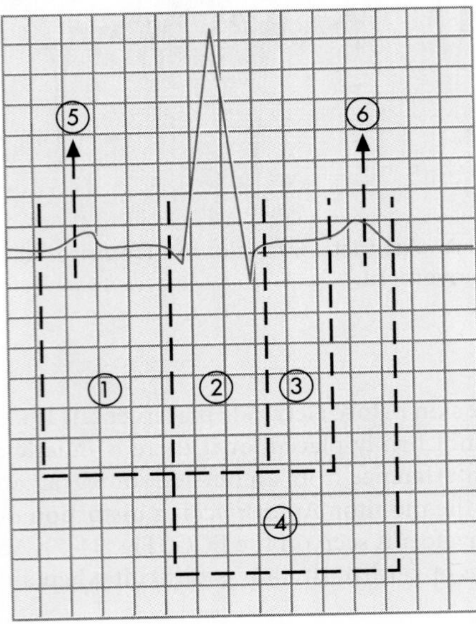

Fig. 34-9 The electrocardiogram complex as seen in a normal sinus rhythm. *1,* PR interval (normal is 0.12 to 0.20 second); *2,* QRS complex (normal is 0.04 to 0.12 second); *3,* ST segment (normal is 0.12 second); *4,* QT interval (normal is 0.34 to 0.43 second); *5,* P wave (normal is 0.06 to 0.12 second); *6,* T wave (normal is 0.16 second).

cardiac output (CO) and possible hypotension. Certain arrhythmias may bring about more life-threatening arrhythmias.[6] The patient, not just the arrhythmia, must be treated.

Normal sinus rhythm refers to the normal conduction pattern of the cardiac cycle, which originates in the SA node (Fig. 34-8). Figure 34-9 shows the normal electrical pattern of the cardiac cycle. Table 34-2 provides a description of ECG intervals and the significance of disturbances. The P wave represents the depolarization of the atrium (passage of an electrical impulse through the atrial muscle), causing atrial contraction. The QRS complex represents depolarization of the ventricles, causing ventricular contraction. The T wave represents repolarization of the ventricles. The PR interval represents the period when the impulse spreads through the atria, AV node, bundle of His, and Purkinje's fibers. The QRS interval represents the time it takes for depolarization of both ventricles. The QT interval represents the time it takes for complete depolarization and repolarization of the ventricles.

Electrophysiologic Mechanisms of Arrhythmias

Disorders of impulse formation can initiate arrhythmias. The heart has specialized cells found in the SA node, parts of the atria, the AV node, and the His-Purkinje system, which are able to discharge spontaneously. This is termed *automaticity.* Normally the main pacemaker of the heart is the SA node, which spontaneously discharges at 60 to 100 times per minute (Table 34-3). A pacemaker from another site may be discharged in two ways. If the SA node discharges more slowly than a secondary pacemaker, the electrical discharges from the secondary pacemaker may passively "escape." The secondary pacemaker will then discharge automatically at its intrinsic rate. These secondary pacemakers may originate from the AV node or the His-Purkinje system at rates of 40 to 60 times per minute and 30 to 40 times per minute, respectively. Another way that secondary pacemakers can originate is when they discharge more rapidly than the normal pacemaker of the SA node. Triggered beats (early or late) may come from an ectopic focus in the atria, ventricles, or AV nodal area. This may begin a "run" of an arrhythmia, which replaces the normal sinus rhythm.

The impulse started by a pacemaker focus must be conducted to the entire heart chamber. The property of myocardial tissue that allows it to be depolarized by a stimulus is called *excitability.* This is an important part of the transmission of the impulse from one fiber to another. The level of excitability is determined by the length of time after depolarization that the tissues can be restimulated. The recovery period after stimulation is called the *refractory phase* or *period.* The *absolute refractory phase* or *period* occurs when excitability is zero and heart tissue cannot be stimulated. The *relative refractory period* occurs slightly later in the cycle, and excitability is more likely. In states of full excitability, the heart is completely recovered. Figure 34-10 shows the relationship between the refractory period and the ECG.[2]

If conduction is depressed and if some areas of the heart are blocked, the unblocked areas are activated earlier than the blocked areas. When the block is unidirectional, this uneven conduction may allow the initial impulse to *reenter* areas that were previously not excitable but have recovered. The reentering impulse may be able to depolarize the atria and ventricles, causing a premature beat. If the *reentrant excitation* continues, tachycardia occurs.[4]

Arrhythmias occur as the result of various abnormalities and disease states.[3] The cause of an arrhythmia influences the

Table 34-2 Definition and Significance of Electrocardiogram Intervals*

Description	Duration (sec)	Significance of Disturbance
PR interval: From beginning of P wave to beginning of QRS complex; represents time taken for impulse to spread through the atria, AV node and bundle of His, the bundle branches, and Purkinje's fibers, to a point immediately preceding ventricular activation	0.12-0.20	Disturbance in conduction usually in AV node, bundle of His, or bundle branches but can be in atria as well
QRS interval: From beginning to end of QRS complex; represents time taken for depolarization of both ventricles	0.04-0.12	Disturbance in conduction in bundle branches or in ventricles
QT interval: From beginning of QRS to end of T wave; represents time taken for entire electrical depolarization and repolarization of the ventricles	0.34-0.43	Disturbances usually affecting repolarization more than depolarization such as drug effects, electrolyte disturbances, and rate changes

*HR influences the duration of these intervals, especially those of the PR and QT intervals.

Table 34-3 Rates of the Conduction System

SA node	60-100 times/min
AV junction	40-60 times/min
Purkinje's fibers	20-40 times/min

AV, atrioventricular; *SA*, sinoatrial.

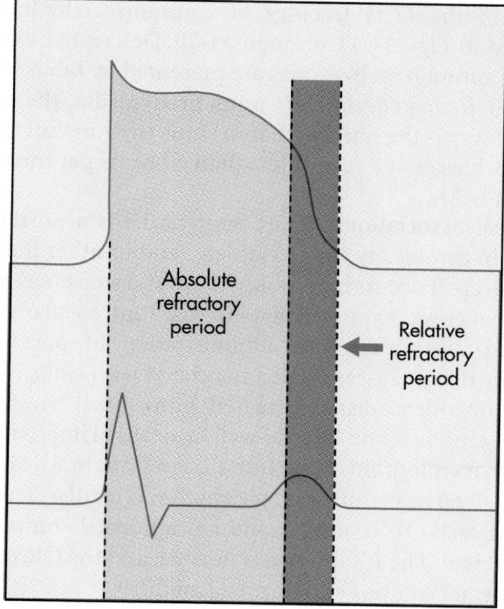

Fig. 34-10 Absolute and relative refractory periods correlated with the cardiac muscle's action potential and with an ECG tracing.

treatment of the patient. Common causes of arrhythmias are presented in Table 34-4.

Arrhythmias occurring in out-of-hospital settings present problems of management. Determination of the rhythm by cardiac monitoring is a high priority. Emergency care of the patient with an arrhythmia is outlined in Table 34-5. If indicated, the emergency medical system (EMS) is activated after the patient has been assessed.

Table 34-4 Common Causes of Arrhythmias

Drug effects or toxicity	Coffee, tea, tobacco
Myocardial cell degeneration	Electrolyte imbalances
Hypertrophy of cardiac muscle	Cellular hypoxia
Emotional crisis	Edema
Connective tissue disorders	Acid-base imbalances
Alcohol	Myocardial ischemia
Metabolic conditions (e.g., thyroid dysfunction)	Degeneration of the conduction system

Evaluation of Arrhythmias

In addition to continuous ECG monitoring during hospitalization, several other methods are used to evaluate cardiac arrhythmias and the effectiveness of antiarrhythmic drug therapy. An electrophysiology test (an invasive method) and Holter monitoring, event recorder monitoring, exercise treadmill testing, and signal-averaged ECG (all noninvasive methods) can be performed on both an inpatient and an outpatient basis.

Electrophysiologic (EPS) testing is performed to identify different mechanisms of tachyarrhythmias, as well as heart blocks, bradyarrhythmias, and arrhythmic causes of syncope. It can also be used to identify locations of accessory pathways and to determine the effectiveness of antiarrhythmic drugs. It involves introducing several electrode catheters transvenously to the right side of the heart with fluoroscopic guidance. Electrical stimulation to various areas of the atrium and ventricle is performed, and the inducibility of arrhythmias is determined.[2] During the procedure, the patient is sedated but conscious, since serious arrhythmias can be provoked, requiring immediate cardioversion or defibrillation. Preprocedure anxiety is common for the patient undergoing EPS. Emotional support from the nurse for these patients is important. Nursing care before and after the procedure is similar to that for cardiac catheterization. (EPS testing is also discussed in Chapter 30.)

The Holter monitor is a device that records the ECG while the patient is ambulatory.[4] The device can record heart rhythm for 24 to 48 hours while the patient performs daily activities.

EMERGENCY MANAGEMENT

Table 34-5 Arrhythmias

Etiology	Assessment Findings	Interventions
Hypoxia, shock Poisoning, drug ingestion Myocardial infarction, congestive heart failure, conduction defects Pulmonary disorders, near-drowning Electrolyte imbalances, metabolic imbalances Electric shock	▪ Irregular rate and rhythm, palpitations ▪ Chest, neck, shoulder, or arm pain ▪ Dizziness, syncope ▪ Dyspnea ▪ Extreme restlessness ▪ Decreased level of consciousness ▪ Feeling of impending doom ▪ Numbness, tingling of arms ▪ Weakness and fatigue ▪ Cold, clammy skin ▪ Diaphoresis ▪ Pallor ▪ Nausea and vomiting ▪ Decreased blood pressure ▪ Decreased O_2 saturation	**Initial** ▪ Ensure patent airway ▪ Administer O_2 via nasal cannula or non-rebreather mask ▪ Establish IV access ▪ Apply cardiac electrodes ▪ Identify underlying rhythm ▪ Identify ectopic beats **Ongoing Monitoring** ▪ Monitor vital signs, level of consciousness, O_2 saturation, and cardiac rhythm ▪ Anticipate need for intubation if respiratory distress evident ▪ Prepare to initiate CPR, defibrillation, or both

CPR, cardiopulmonary resuscitation.

The patient maintains a diary in which activities and any symptoms are recorded. Events in the diary can later be correlated with any arrhythmias observed on the recording. The monitor is generally a useful device for detecting significant arrhythmias and evaluating the effects of drugs during a patient's normal activities. It can also be used for detecting ischemia by analyzing ST segments. A limitation of the device is that the patient who has frequent ventricular arrhythmias, some of which may be lethal, may not have these arrhythmias during the monitored time.

The recent use of event monitors has greatly improved the evaluation of outpatient arrhythmias. Event monitors are recorders that are activated by the patient and can be used only at the time of the patient's symptoms related to the arrhythmia. The recorder is placed over the patient's chest during symptoms. The patient then transmits the rhythm to a central monitoring company via telephone. This is an easier method of documenting an arrhythmia than the 24-hour monitor, if symptoms are not occurring daily. (Ambulatory ECG monitoring is discussed in Chapter 30.)

The signal-averaged ECG (SAECG) is a high-resolution electrocardiogram used to identify the patient at risk for developing complex ventricular arrhythmias. A computerized program and ECG machine are used for the test. The identification of electrical activity called *late potentials* on the SAECG strongly suggests that the patient is at risk for developing serious ventricular arrhythmias.[4]

Exercise treadmill testing is used for evaluation of cardiac rhythm response to exercise. Exercise-induced arrhythmias can be reproduced and analyzed, and drug therapy can be evaluated. These tests are performed with routine treadmill testing protocols.

Types of Arrhythmias

When assessing a cardiac rhythm, a systematic approach must be used. The recommended approach is to note the rate, rhythm, P wave, QRS complex, relationship of P wave to QRS complex, PR interval, QRS interval, and QT interval. Questions to consider include the following: Are premature ventricular complexes present? Are escape beats present? What is the dominant rhythm? What is the clinical significance of the arrhythmia? What is the treatment for the particular arrhythmia? Examples of the ECG tracings of common arrhythmias are presented in Figs. 34-11 through 34-20. Descriptive characteristics of common arrhythmias are presented in Table 34-6.

Sinus Bradycardia. In sinus bradycardia, the conduction pathway is the same as that in sinus rhythm, but the sinus node discharges at a rate of less than 60 beats per minute (see Fig. 34-11, *A*).

Clinical associations. Sinus bradycardia is a normal sinus rhythm in aerobically trained athletes and in other individuals during sleep. It occurs in response to carotid sinus massage, Valsalva's maneuver, hypothermia, increased intraocular pressure, increased vagal tone, and administration of parasympathomimetic drugs. Disease states associated with sinus bradycardia are hypothyroidism, increased intracranial pressure, obstructive jaundice, and inferior wall myocardial infarction (MI).

Electrocardiogram characteristics. In sinus bradycardia, HR is less than 60 beats/min, and the rhythm is regular. The P wave precedes each QRS complex and has a normal contour and a fixed interval. The PR interval is normal, and the QRS complex has a normal contour and normal length.

Significance. The clinical significance of sinus bradycardia depends on how the patient tolerates it hemodynamically. Hypotension with decreased CO may occur in some circumstances. An acute MI may predispose the heart to escape arrhythmias and premature beats.

Treatment. Treatment consists of administration of atropine (an anticholinergic drug) for the patient with symptoms. Pacemaker therapy may be required.

Sinus Tachycardia. The conduction pathway is the same in sinus tachycardia as that in normal sinus rhythm. The discharge rate from the sinus node is increased as a result of vagal inhibition or sympathetic stimulation. The sinus rate is greater than 100 beats/min (see Fig. 34-11, *B*).

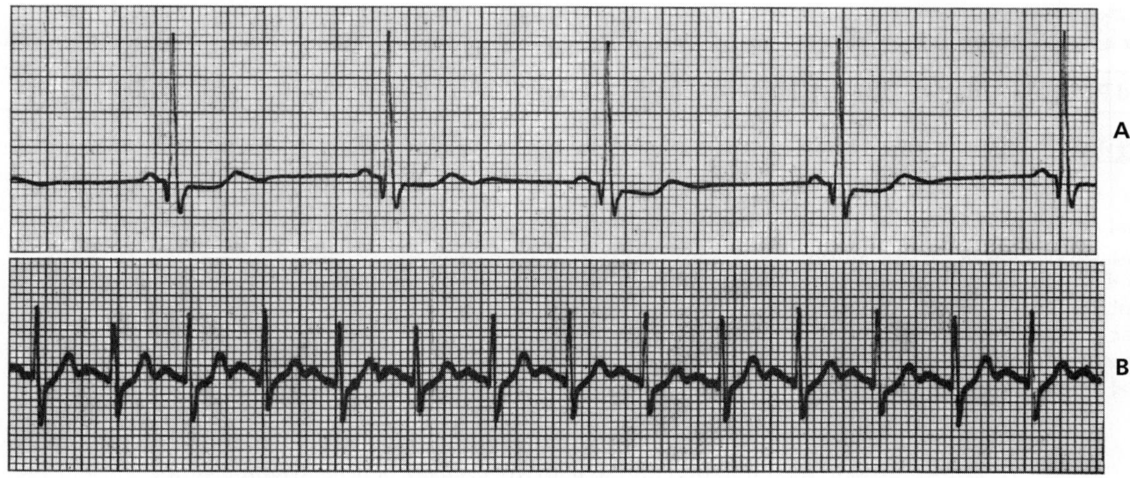

Fig. 34-11 **A,** Sinus bradycardia of 50 beats/min. **B,** Sinus tachycardia of 140 beats/min.

Table 34-6 Characteristics of Common Arrhythmias

Pattern	Rate and Rhythm	P Wave	PR Interval	QRS Complex
NSR	60-100 beats/min and regular	Normal	Normal	Normal
Sinus bradycardia	<60 beats/min and regular	Normal	Normal	Normal
Sinus tachycardia	>100 beats/min and regular	Normal	Normal	Normal
PAC	Usually 60-100 beats/min and irregular	Abnormal shape	Normal or variable	Normal (usually)
PSVT	100-300 beats/min and regular	Abnormal shape, may be hidden	Variable	Normal (usually)
Atrial flutter	*Atrial:* 250-350 beats/min and regular *Ventricular:* >100 beats/min and irregular	Sawtooth	Variable	Normal (usually)
Atrial fibrillation	*Atrial:* 350-600 beats/min and irregular *Ventricular:* >100 beats/min and irregular or possibly any rate	Chaotic	Not measurable	Normal (usually)
Junctional rhythms	40-140 beats/min and regular	Abnormal (may be hidden)	Variable	Normal (usually)
First-degree heart block	Normal and regular	Normal	>0.20 sec	Normal
Second-degree heart block				
Type I (Mobitz I, Wenckebach)	*Atrial:* Normal and regular *Ventricular:* Slower and irregular	Normal	Progressively lengthened	Normal QRS width, with pattern of one nonconducted QRS
Type II (Mobitz II)	*Atrial:* Usually normal and regular or irregular *Ventricular:* Slower and regular or irregular	P wave occurs in multiples	Normal or prolonged	Widened QRS, preceded by two or more P waves
Third-degree heart block	Ventricular rate 20-40 beats/min and regular	Normal, but no connection with QRS complex	Variable	Normal or widened, no connection with P waves
PVC	60-100 beats/min and irregular	Not usually present	Not measurable	Wide and distorted
Ventricular tachycardia	100-250 beats/min and regular or irregular	Not usually present	Not measurable	Wide and distorted
Ventricular fibrillation	Not measurable and irregular	Absent	Not measurable	Not measurable

NSR, normal sinus rhythm; *PAC,* premature atrial contraction; *PSVT,* paroxysmal supraventricular tachycardia; *PVC,* premature ventricular contraction.

34-1 NURSING CARE PLAN PATIENT WITH ARRHYTHMIAS

Expected Patient Outcomes	Nursing Interventions and *Rationales*
NURSING DIAGNOSIS	**Decreased cardiac output** *related to* arrhythmias *as manifested by* sudden drop in blood pressure, atrial or ventricular rate >100/min or <40/min, mental confusion, chest pain, dyspnea, oliguria.
▪ Arterial pressure >70 mm Hg, cardiac index >2 L/min, urine output >30 mL/hr. ▪ Cardiac rate and rhythm within normal limits. ▪ Normal mentation.	▪ Assess ECG continuously for rhythm; rate; PR, QRS, and QT intervals *to monitor cardiac status.* ▪ Monitor vital signs. ▪ Assess and document excessive fatigue, activity intolerance, dyspnea, orthopnea, palpitations, chest pain, light-headedness, dizziness, and nausea *as subjective evidence of hemodynamic status.* ▪ Assess and document pulse rate and regularity, BP status, respiratory status (crackles, rhonchi, wheezing), heart sounds (murmurs, gallops), edema of extremities and sacrum, skin (diaphoretic, cool) *as objective evidence of hemodynamic status.* ▪ Use IV drugs, CPR, etc. per unit protocol *to treat arrhythmias and sustain adequate cardiac output.* ▪ Maintain at least one patent IV site *as vascular access for IV medications.* ▪ Provide supplemental O_2 prn *to maintain adequate tissue* O_2 *saturation.* ▪ Monitor serum electrolytes including potassium and magnesium *because high or low levels may exacerbate arrhythmias.*
NURSING DIAGNOSIS	**Activity intolerance** *related to* inadequate cardiac output *as manifested by* vertigo or syncope on position change, dyspnea on exertion, standing blood pressure decreases >20 mm Hg, heart rate increases >20/min with positional change.
▪ Maintenance of optimal activity level. ▪ No ischemic pain on activity.	▪ Assess respiratory and cardiac status before activity *to determine advisability of planned activity and provide baseline data for comparison with postactivity status.* ▪ Observe and document response to activity *to evaluate patient progress and plan future activity.* ▪ Assess for medication side effects that affect activity such as fatigue, dizziness, decreased myocardial contractility, and exacerbation of arrhythmias *so medication or activity can be adjusted appropriately.*
NURSING DIAGNOSIS	**Fear** *related to* development of life-threatening cardiac arrhythmias *as manifested by* refusal to move or participate in care, need for constant attention, asking many or no questions, intent focus on cardiac monitoring.
▪ Participation in plan of treatment. ▪ Increase in psychologic and physiologic comfort.	▪ Assess patient's coping ability and strategies *to identify resources or problems.* ▪ Encourage verbalization of feelings *so patient can discuss reasons for fear.* ▪ Clarify and answer questions in regard to cardiovascular pathology, symptomatology, activity and diet restrictions, medications, and procedures *because accurate knowledge often reduces fear.*

COLLABORATIVE PROBLEMS

POTENTIAL COMPLICATION **Cardiac arrest** *related to* inadequate cardiac output.

Nursing Goals	Nursing Interventions and *Rationales*
▪ Monitor for signs of significant cardiac arrhythmias. ▪ Report deviations from acceptable parameters. ▪ Carry out appropriate medical and nursing interventions.	▪ Assess for and recognize immediately cardiac arrhythmias that can result in cardiac arrest. ▪ Initiate advanced cardiac life support procedures according to unit protocol.

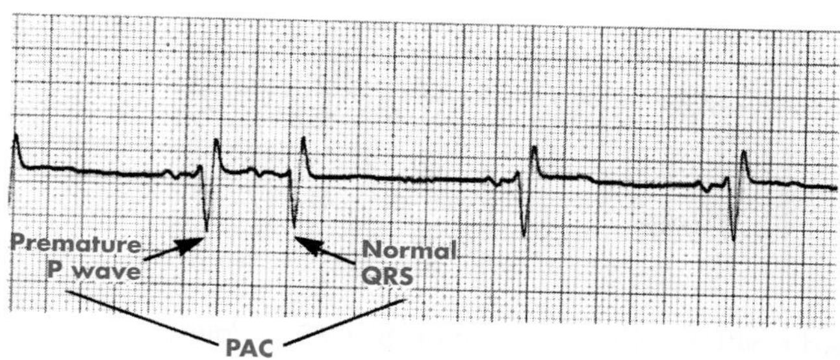

Fig. 34-12 Normally conducted premature atrial contraction (*PAC*). The early P wave is indicated by the *arrows,* and the QRS complex that follows is of normal shape and duration.

Clinical associations. Sinus tachycardia is associated with physiologic stressors such as exercise, fever, pain, hypotension, hypovolemia, anxiety, anemia, hypoxia, hypoglycemia, myocardial ischemia, congestive heart failure (CHF), and hyperthyroidism. It can also be an effect of drugs such as epinephrine, norepinephrine, caffeine, atropine, theophylline, nifedipine (Procardia), or hydralazine (Apresoline).

Electrocardiogram characteristics. In sinus tachycardia, HR is greater than 100 beats/min, and the rhythm is regular. The P wave is normal, precedes each QRS complex, and has a normal contour and fixed interval. The PR interval is normal, and the QRS complex has a normal contour.

Significance. The clinical significance of sinus tachycardia depends on the patient's tolerance of the increased HR. The patient may have symptoms of dizziness, and hypotension may occur. Increased myocardial oxygen consumption is associated with an increased HR. Angina or an increase in infarct size may accompany persistent sinus tachycardia in the patient with an acute MI.

Treatment. Treatment is determined by underlying causes. In certain settings, β-blocker therapy (e.g., propranolol [Inderal]) is used to reduce HR and decrease myocardial oxygen consumption.

Premature Atrial Contraction. A premature atrial contraction (PAC) is a contraction originating from an ectopic focus in the atrium in a location other than the sinus node. It originates in the left or right atrium and travels across the atria by an abnormal pathway, creating a distorted P wave (Fig. 34-12). At the AV node, it is stopped (nonconducted PAC), delayed (lengthened PR interval), or conducted normally. It moves through the AV node, and in most cases it is conducted normally through the ventricles.[5]

Clinical associations. In a normal heart, a PAC can result from emotional stress or the use of caffeine, tobacco, or alcohol. A PAC can also result from disease states such as infection, inflammation, hyperthyroidism, chronic obstructive pulmonary disease (COPD), heart disease (including atherosclerotic heart disease), valvular disease, and other diseases. A PAC can also be caused by an enlarged atrium.

Electrocardiogram characteristics. HR varies with the underlying rate and frequency of the PAC, and the rhythm is irregular. The P wave has a different contour from that of a normal P wave. It may be notched or have negative deflection, or it may be hidden in the preceding T wave. The PR interval may be shorter or longer than a normal PR interval originating from the sinus node, but it is within normal limits. The QRS complex is usually normal. If the QRS interval is 0.12 second or longer, abnormal conduction through the ventricles is present.

Significance. A PAC may be a prelude to supraventricular tachycardias.

Treatment. Treatment depends on the patient's symptoms. Withdrawal of sources of stimulation such as caffeine may be warranted. Drugs such as digoxin, quinidine, procainamide (Pronestyl), flecainide (Tambocor), and β-blockers can be used.

Paroxysmal Supraventricular Tachycardia. Paroxysmal supraventricular tachycardia (PSVT) is an arrhythmia originating in an ectopic focus anywhere above the bifurcation of the bundle of His (Fig. 34-13). Identification of the ectopic focus is sometimes difficult with a 12-lead ECG. It occurs with the reentrant phenomenon (reexcitation of the atria when there is a one-way block). A run of repeated premature beats is initiated and is usually heralded by a PAC. *Paroxysmal* refers to an abrupt onset and termination. Termination is sometimes followed by a brief period of asystole. Some degree of AV block may be present. PSVT occurring via an accessory pathway is designated as *orthodromic* or *antidromic* tachycardia. *Orthodromic* refers to anterograde, or forward conduction through the AV node and retrograde, or backward conduction, through the accessory pathway. *Antidromic* refers to the opposite: anterograde conduction through the accessory pathway and retrograde conduction through the AV node.[2]

Clinical associations. In the normal heart, PSVT is associated with overexertion, emotional stress, changes of position, deep inspiration, and stimulants such as caffeine and tobacco. PSVT is associated with rheumatic heart disease, Wolff-Parkinson-White (WPW) syndrome (conduction via accessory pathways), digitalis intoxication, coronary artery disease (CAD), or cor pulmonale.

Electrocardiogram characteristics. In PSVT, HR is 100 to 300 beats/min, and rhythm is regular. The P wave is often hidden in the preceding T wave and has an abnormal contour. The PR interval may be prolonged, shortened, or normal, and the QRS complex may have a normal or abnormal contour.

Significance. The clinical significance of PSVT depends on symptoms and HR. A prolonged episode and HR greater than 180 beats/min may precipitate a decreased CO with hypotension and myocardial ischemia.

Treatment. Treatment includes vagal stimulation and drug therapy. Vagal stimulation induced by carotid massage or Valsalva's maneuver may be used to treat PSVT. Adenosine (Adenocard) IV is most commonly used to convert PSVT to a normal sinus rhythm. This drug has a short half-life (10 seconds) and is well-tolerated by most patients.[8,9] Intravenous verapamil (Calan, Isoptin), diltiazem (Cardizem), digitalis, and propranolol (Inderal) can also be used. However, digitalis and calcium channel blockers can cause hemodynamic collapse in WPW syndrome. Persistent, recurring PSVT in WPW may ultimately be treated with radiofrequency catheter ablation of the accessory pathway.[10]

Atrial Flutter. Atrial flutter is an atrial tachyarrhythmia identified by recurring, regular, sawtooth-shaped flutter waves (Fig. 34-14, *A*) and is best visualized in leads II, III, aVF, and V_1 on the 12-lead ECG. It is usually associated with a slower ventricular response. Because of the refractory characteristic of the AV node, there is usually some AV block in a fixed ratio of flutter waves to QRS complexes (e.g., 2:1, 3:1).

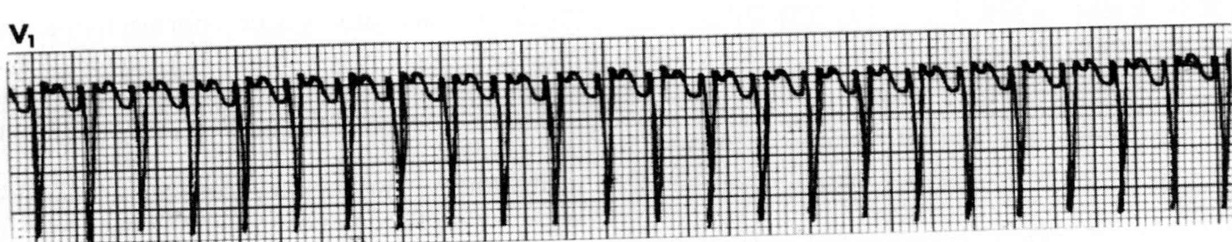

Fig. 34-13 AV nodal reentrant paroxysmal supraventricular tachycardia with P wave at the end of the QRS complex.

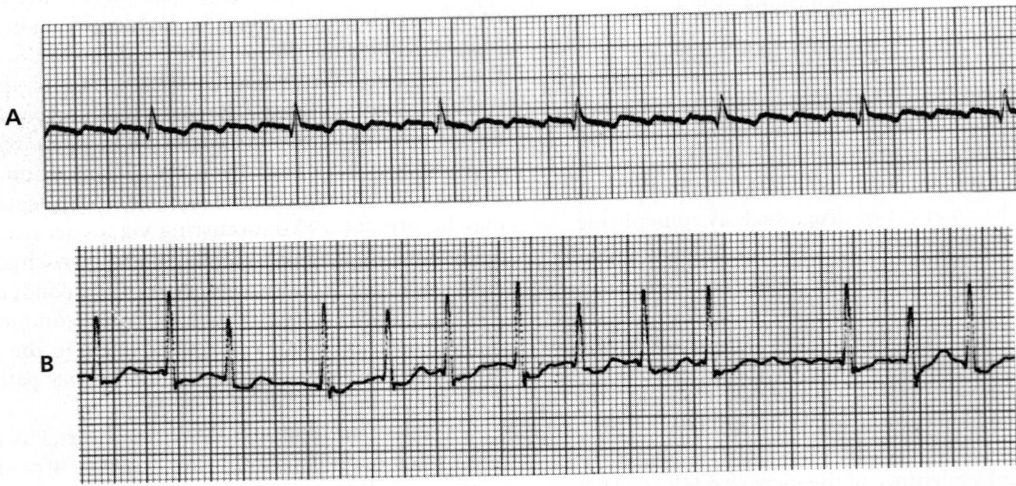

Fig. 34-14 **A,** Atrial flutter with a 4:1 conduction. **B,** Atrial fibrillation. Note the jagged, irregular baseline between the QRS complexes.

Clinical associations. Atrial flutter rarely occurs in a normal heart. In disease states, it is associated with CAD, hypertension, mitral valve disorders, pulmonary embolus, cor pulmonale, cardiomyopathy, hyperthyroidism, and the use of drugs such as digitalis, quinidine, and epinephrine.

Electrocardiogram characteristics. Atrial rate is 250 to 350 beats/min. The ventricular rate varies according to the conduction ratio. In 2:1 conduction, the ventricular rate is typically found to be approximately 150 beats/min. Atrial rhythm is regular, and ventricular rhythm is usually regular. The P wave is represented by sawtooth waves, the PR interval is variable, and the QRS complex is normal in contour.

Significance. High ventricular rates associated with atrial flutter can decrease CO and cause serious consequences such as heart failure, especially in the patient with underlying heart disease.[11]

Treatment. The primary goal in treatment of atrial flutter is to slow the ventricular response by increasing AV block. Electrical cardioversion may be used to convert the atrial flutter to sinus rhythm in an emergency situation. Drugs used include verapamil (Calan, Isoptin), diltiazem (Cardizem), digoxin, sotalol (Betapace), propafenone (Rythmol), quinidine, procainamide (Pronestyl), and β-blockers.

Ibutilide (Corvert) is effective at terminating atrial flutter in a closely monitored situation and is used intravenously.[12,13] Radiofrequency catheter ablation is increasingly being used as curative therapy of atrial flutter.

Atrial Fibrillation. Atrial fibrillation is characterized by a total disorganization of atrial electrical activity without effective atrial contraction (Fig. 34-14, *B*). The ECG demonstrates baseline fibrillatory waves or undulations of variable contour at a rate of 300 to 600 per minute. Ventricular response is irregular, and if the patient is untreated, the ventricular rate will be 100 to 160 beats/min. The arrhythmia may be chronic or intermittent.

Clinical associations. Atrial fibrillation usually occurs in the patient with underlying heart disease, such as rheumatic heart disease, cardiomyopathy, hypertensive heart disease, CHF, pericarditis, and CAD. It is also associated with thyrotoxicosis, alcoholism, infection, gastroenteritis, and stress. The term *lone atrial fibrillation* is used when no detectable cause is found for atrial fibrillation.[14]

Electrocardiogram characteristics. During atrial fibrillation, atrial rate may be as high as 350 to 600 beats/min. Ventricular rate can vary from as low as 50 beats/min to as high as 180 beats/min. Atrial rhythm is chaotic, and ventricular rhythm is usually irregular. Ventricular rhythm may be regular if there is complete AV block (ventricular escape rhythm). The P wave shows fibrillatory waves, but no definite P wave can be observed. The PR interval is not measurable, and the QRS complex usually has a normal contour.

Significance. Atrial fibrillation can often result in a decrease in CO because of ineffective atrial contractions and a rapid ventricular response. Thrombi may form in the atria as a

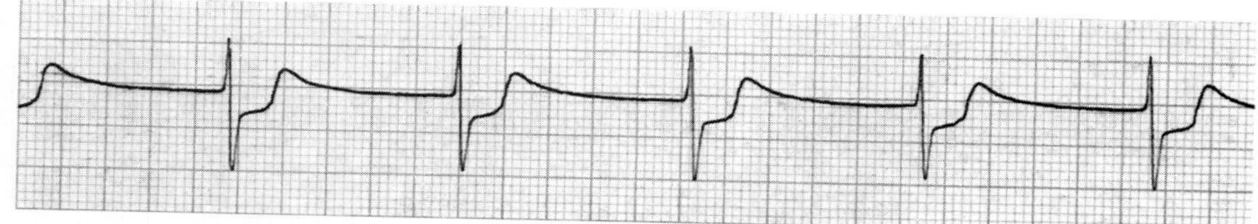

Fig. 34-15 Junctional rhythm of 57 beats per minute.

result of ineffective atrial contraction. An embolized clot may pass to the brain, causing a stroke. Risk of stroke increases fivefold with atrial fibrillation. Risk of stroke is even higher in patients with structural heart disease, hypertension, and at an age over 65 years. Anticoagulation with warfarin (Coumadin) is used to prevent stroke in atrial fibrillation.[15,16]

Treatment. The goal of treatment is a decrease in ventricular response. In emergency situations, cardioversion may be used to convert atrial fibrillation to a normal sinus rhythm. Medications used for pharmaceutical cardioversion or a decrease in ventricular response include digoxin, verapamil (Calan, Isoptin), diltiazem (Cardizem), quinidine, β-blockers, flecainide (Tambocor), propafenone (Rythmol), and sotalol (Betapace).[17] Low-dose amiodarone (Cordarone) is being increasingly used as antiarrhythmic therapy for atrial fibrillation.[18] Intravenous ibutilide is also being used for conversion of atrial fibrillation in the acute care setting.[12,13] If a patient has been in atrial fibrillation for more than 48 hours, anticoagulation therapy with warfarin (Coumadin) is recommended for 3 to 4 weeks before any attempt at conversion to sinus rhythm.[15,16]

Junctional Arrhythmia. Junctional rhythm refers to an arrhythmia that originates in the area of the AV node. The impulse may move in a retrograde fashion that produces an abnormal P wave occurring just before or after the QRS complex or that is hidden in the QRS complex. The impulse usually moves normally through the ventricles. Junctional premature beats may occur, and they are treated in a manner similar to that for PACs. Other junctional arrhythmias include junctional escape rhythm (Fig. 34-15), accelerated junctional rhythm, and junctional tachycardia. These arrhythmias are treated according to the patient's tolerance of the rhythm and the patient's clinical condition.

Clinical associations. Junctional escape rhythm is often associated with the aerobically trained individual who has sinus bradycardia. It may occur with acute MI, especially inferior MI, and dysfunction of the SA node. Accelerated junctional rhythm and junctional tachycardia are observed with acute inferior MI, digitalis toxicity, and acute rheumatic fever and during open heart surgery.

Electrocardiogram characteristics. In junctional escape rhythm, the HR is 40 to 60 beats/min, in accelerated junctional rhythm it is 60 to 100 beats/min, and in junctional tachycardia it is 100 to 140 beats/min. Rhythm is regular. The P wave is abnormal in contour and inverted, or it may be hidden in the QRS complex (see Fig. 34-15). The PR interval is less than 0.12 second when the P wave precedes the QRS complex. The QRS complex is usually normal.

Significance. Junctional escape rhythm serves as a safety mechanism occurring when the primary pacemaker has not been activated. Escape rhythms such as this should not be suppressed. Accelerated junctional rhythm and junctional tachycardia indicate a problem with the sinus node. If these rhythms are rapid, they may result in a reduction of CO and possible heart failure.

Treatment. Treatment varies according to the type of junctional arrhythmia. If a patient has symptoms with an escape junctional rhythm, atropine can be used. In accelerated junctional rhythm and junctional tachycardia caused by digoxin toxicity, the digoxin is withheld. In the absence of digitalis toxicity, propranolol (Inderal), phenytoin (Dilantin), or verapamil (Cardizem) may be used.

First-Degree AV Block. First-degree AV block is a type of AV block in which every impulse is conducted to the ventricles but the duration of AV conduction is prolonged (Fig. 34-16). This is manifested by a PR interval greater than 0.20 second. After the impulse moves through the AV node, it is usually conducted normally through the ventricles.

Clinical associations. First-degree AV block is associated with MI, chronic ischemic heart disease, rheumatic fever, hyperthyroidism, vagal stimulation, and drugs such as digitalis, β-blockers, flecainide (Tambocor), and IV verapamil (Cardizem).

Electrocardiogram characteristics. In first-degree AV block, HR is normal, and rhythm is regular. The P wave is normal, the PR interval is prolonged for more than 0.20 second, and the QRS complex usually has a normal contour.

Significance. First-degree AV block may be a precursor of higher degrees of AV block.

Treatment. There is no treatment for first-degree AV block.

Second-Degree AV Block, Type I. Type I AV block (Mobitz I, Wenckebach phenomenon) includes a gradual lengthening of the PR interval, which occurs because of the AV conduction time that is prolonged until an atrial impulse is nonconducted and a QRS complex is dropped (see Fig. 34-16). Once a ventricular beat is dropped, the cycle repeats itself with progressive lengthening of the PR intervals until another QRS complex is dropped. The rhythm appears on the ECG in a pattern of grouped beats. The duration of the QRS complex is normal or prolonged. Type I AV block most commonly occurs in the AV node, but it can also occur in the His-Purkinje system.

Clinical associations. Type I AV block may result from use of drugs such as digoxin or β-blockers. It may also be associated with ischemic cardiac disease and other diseases that can slow AV conduction.

Atrial rate is normal, but ventricular rate may be slower as a result of dropped QRS complexes. Ventricular rhythm is irregular. The PR interval progressively lengthens before the nonconducted P wave occurs. The P wave has a normal contour. The PR interval lengthens progressively until a P wave is nonconducted and a QRS complex is dropped. The QRS complex has a normal contour.

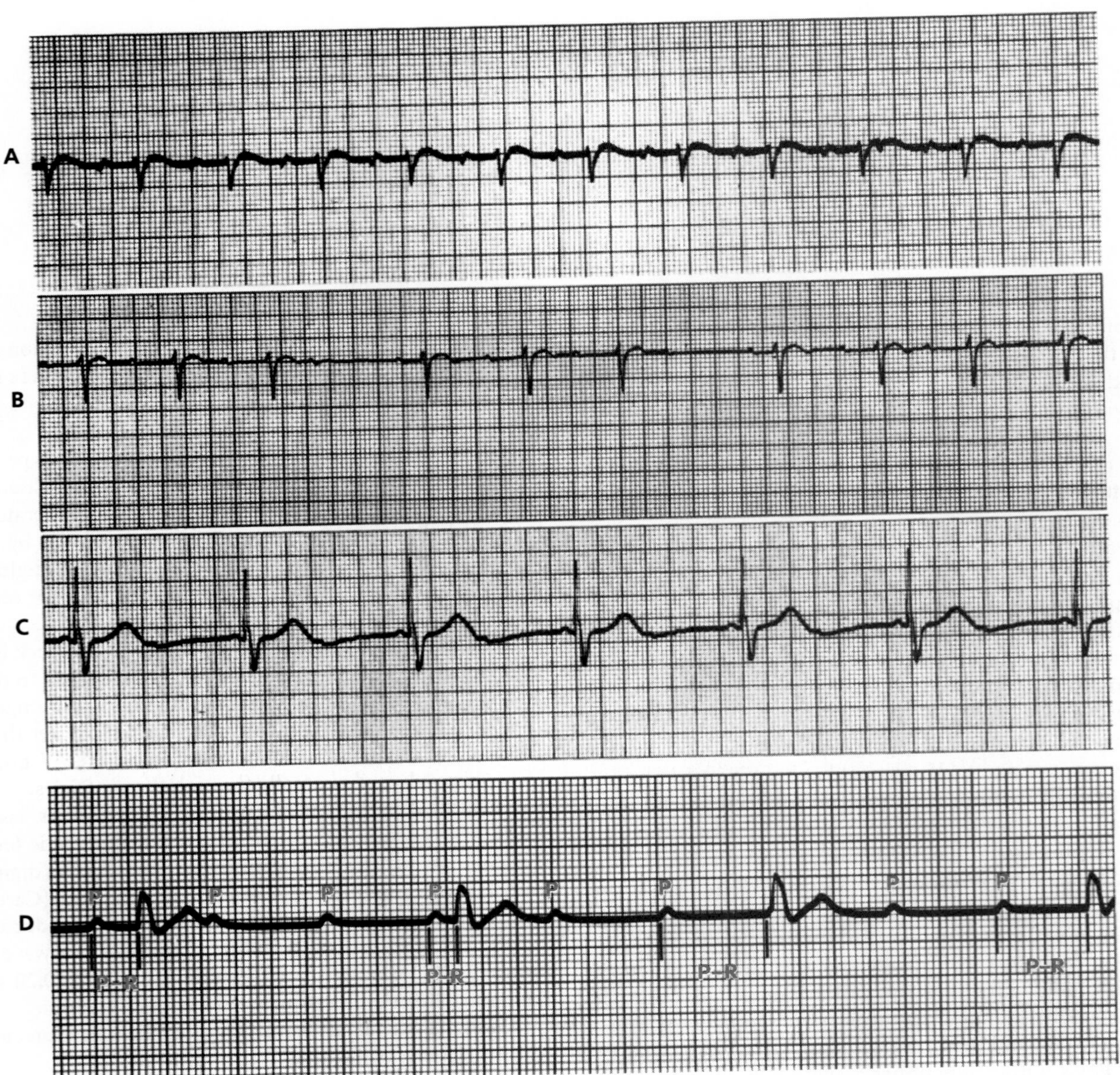

Fig. 34-16 Heart block. **A,** First-degree heart block. Note the delayed PR interval. **B,** Second-degree heart block, type I (Mobitz I, Wenckebach). **C,** Second-degree heart block, type II (Mobitz II). **D,** Complete heart block (third degree). The irregular PR intervals indicate the presence of a complete heart block.

Significance. Type I AV block is usually a result of myocardial ischemia in an inferior MI. It is almost always transient and is usually well tolerated. However, it may be a warning signal of an impending significant AV conduction disturbance.

Treatment. If the patient is symptomatic, atropine is used to increase HR, or a temporary pacemaker may be needed, especially if the patient has an acute MI.

Second-Degree Heart Block, Type II. In type II second-degree AV block (Mobitz II) a P wave is nonconducted without progressive antecedent PR lengthening, and this almost always occurs when a bundle branch block is present (see Fig. 34-16). On conducted beats, the PR interval is constant. Second-degree heart block is a more serious type of block in which a certain number of impulses from the sinus node are not conducted to the ventricles. This occurs in ratios of 2:1, 3:1, and so on when there are two P waves to one QRS complex, three P waves to one QRS complex, and so on. It may occur with varying ratios. Type II AV block almost always occurs in the His-Purkinje system.

Clinical associations. Type II AV block is associated with rheumatic and atherosclerotic heart disease, acute anterior MI, and digitalis toxicity.

Electrocardiogram characteristics. Atrial rate is usually normal. Ventricular rate depends on the intrinsic rate and the degree of AV block. Sinus rhythm is regular, but ventricular rhythm may be irregular. The P wave has a normal contour. The PR interval may be normal or prolonged but remains fixed on conducted beats. The QRS complex widens to more than 0.12 second because of bundle branch block.

Significance. Type II AV block often progresses to third-degree AV block and is associated with a poor prognosis. The reduced HR may result in decreased CO with subsequent hypotension and myocardial ischemia. Type II AV block is an indication for therapy with a permanent pacemaker.

Treatment. Temporary treatment before the insertion of a permanent pacemaker involves the use of a temporary pacemaker. Drugs such as atropine, epinephrine, or dopamine (Intropin) can be tried as temporary measures to increase HR until pacemaker therapy is available.

Third-Degree AV Heart Block. Third-degree AV heart block, which is complete heart block, constitutes one form of AV dissociation in which no impulses from the atria are conducted to the ventricles (see Fig. 34-16). The atria are stimulated and contract independently of the ventricles. The ventricular rhythm is an escape rhythm, and the focus may be above or below the bifurcation of the His bundle.

Clinical associations. Third-degree heart block is associated with fibrosis or calcification of the cardiac conduction system, CAD, myocarditis, cardiomyopathy, open heart surgery, and some systemic diseases such as amyloidosis and scleroderma.

Electrocardiogram characteristics. The atrial rate is usually a sinus rate of 60 to 100 beats/min. The ventricular rate depends on the site of the block. If it is in the AV node, the rate is 40 to 60 beats/min, and if it is in the Purkinje system, it is 20 to 40 beats/min. Atrial and ventricular rhythms are regular but asynchronous. The P wave has a normal contour. The PR interval is variable, and there is no time relationship between the P wave and the QRS complex. The QRS complex is normal if escape rhythm is initiated in the bundle of His or above. It is widened if escape rhythm is initiated below the bundle of His.

Significance. Third-degree AV block almost always results in reduced CO with subsequent ischemia and heart failure. Syncope from third degree AV block may result from severe bradycardia or even periods of asystole.

Treatment. A temporary pacemaker may be inserted or an external pacemaker applied on an emergency basis in a patient with acute MI. The use of drugs such as atropine, epinephrine, and dopamine (Intropin) are temporary treatments to increase HR and support BP before pacemaker insertion.

Premature Ventricular Contractions. A premature ventricular contraction (PVC) is a contraction originating in an ectopic focus in the ventricles. It is the premature occurrence of a QRS complex, which is wide and distorted in shape, compared with a QRS complex initiated from the supraventricular tissue (Fig. 34-17). The QRS complex is usually wider than 0.12 second, and the T wave is generally large and opposite in direction to the major deflection of the QRS complex. Retrograde conduction may occur, and the P wave may be seen following the ectopic beat. PVCs that are initiated from different foci appear different in contour from each other and are called *multifocal PVCs.* When every other beat is a PVC, it is called *ventricular bigeminy.* When every third beat is a PVC, it is called *ventricular trigeminy.* Two consecutive PVCs are called *couplets.* Three consecutive PVCs are called *triplets. Ventricular tachycardia* occurs when there are three or more consecutive PVCs. When a PVC falls on the T wave of a preceding beat, the *R on T phenomenon* occurs and is considered to be dangerous because it may precipitate ventricular tachycardia or ventricular fibrillation.

Clinical associations. PVCs are associated with stimulants such as caffeine, alcohol, aminophylline, epinephrine, isoproterenol (Isuprel), and digoxin. They are also associated with hypokalemia, hypoxia, fever, exercise, and emotional stress. Disease states associated with PVCs include MI, mitral valve prolapse (MVP), CHF, and CAD.

Electrocardiogram characteristics. HR varies according to intrinsic rate and number of PVCs. Rhythm is irregular because of premature beats. A retrograde P wave is possible; the P wave is rarely visible and is usually lost in the QRS complex of PVC. The PR interval is not measurable. The QRS complex is wide and distorted in shape, more than 0.12 second.

Significance. PVCs are usually a benign finding in the patient with a normal heart. In heart disease, depending on frequency, PVCs may reduce the CO and precipitate angina and heart failure. PVCs in ischemic heart disease or acute MI represent ventricular irritability. They may also occur as *reperfusion arrhythmias* after lysis of a coronary artery clot with thrombolytic therapy in acute MI, or following plaque reduction from a percutaneous transluminal coronary angioplasty (PTCA).

Treatment. Indications for treatment in an appropriate clinical setting include (1) six or more PVCs occurring per minute, (2) ventricular couplets and triplets, (3) multifocal PVCs, and (4) R on T phenomenon. If treatment is not initiated, ventricular tachycardia or ventricular fibrillation may occur. For treating PVCs, lidocaine is the drug of choice, with an initial IV bolus of 1 to 1.5 mg/kg followed by a second bolus of 0.5 to 1.5 mg/kg and continuous lidocaine infusion of 2 to 4 mg/min. Procainamide (Pronestyl) is the second drug of choice if lidocaine is ineffective.[11] Assessment of the patient's hemodynamic status is important to determine if treatment with drug therapy is indicated.

Ventricular Tachycardia. The ECG diagnosis of ventricular tachycardia is made when a run of three or more PVCs occurs. The QRS complex is distorted in appearance, with a duration exceeding 0.12 second and with the ST-T direction pointing opposite to the major QRS deflection (Fig. 34-18). It occurs when an ectopic focus or foci fire repetitively and the ventricle takes control as the pacemaker. The ventricular rate is 110 to 250 beats/min, and the R-R interval may be irregular or regular. AV dissociation may be present, with P waves occurring independently of the QRS complex. The atria may also be depolarized by the ventricles in a retrograde fashion.

Ventricular tachycardia may be sustained (lasting longer than 30 seconds) or nonsustained (lasting 30 seconds or less). Torsades de pointes (Fig. 34-19), or polymorphic ventricular tachycardia, is a type of ventricular tachycardia characterized by a QRS contour that gradually changes its polarity over a series of beats. It usually occurs when QT prolongation is present.

The appearance of ventricular tachycardia is an ominous sign because it usually indicates the presence of cardiac disease. It is considered to be a life-threatening arrhythmia because of decreased CO and the possibility of deterioration of ventricular tachycardia to ventricular fibrillation, which is a lethal arrhythmia.

Clinical associations. Ventricular tachycardia is associated with acute MI, CAD, significant electrolyte imbalances (e.g., potassium), cardiomyopathy, mitral valve prolapse, long QT syndrome, and coronary reperfusion after thrombolytic therapy. The arrhythmia has also been observed in the patient who has no evidence of cardiac disease.

Electrocardiogram characteristics. Ventricular rate is 110 to 250 beats/min. Rhythm may be regular or irregular. The

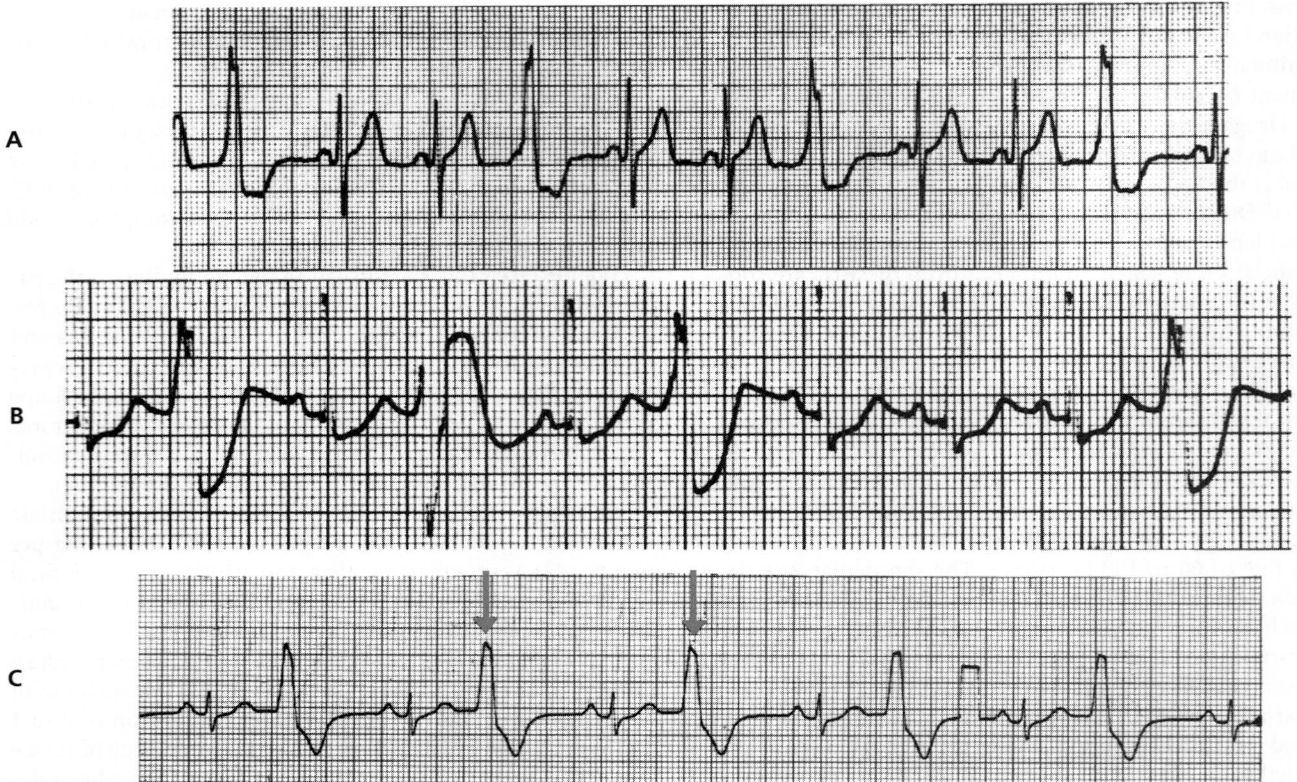

Fig. 34-17 Premature ventricular contractions (PVCs). **A,** Ventricular trigeminy. **B,** Multifocal PVC. **C,** Ventricular bigeminy.

P wave may be noted to "march through" the ventricular rhythm in AV dissociation, or it may occur after the QRS complex in a regular pattern of retrograde conduction. The PR interval is not measurable. The QRS interval is prolonged for more than 0.12 second, and the QRS complex contour is distorted.

Significance. Ventricular tachycardia may cause a severe decrease in CO as a result of decreased ventricular diastolic filling times and loss of atrial contraction. The result may be pulmonary edema, shock, and decreased blood flow to the brain. The arrhythmia must be treated quickly, even if it occurs only briefly and stops abruptly. Episodes may recur if prophylactic treatment is not begun. Ventricular fibrillation may also develop.

Treatment. If the patient is hemodynamically stable, treatment consists of administration of a lidocaine bolus with subsequent boluses. If this abolishes the tachycardia, a continuous lidocaine infusion of 2 to 4 mg/min should be started. If lidocaine is ineffective, IV procainamide (Pronestyl) may be tried. It may be given in an infusion of 20 mg/min until the arrhythmia is suppressed, hypotension occurs, the QRS complex is widened by 50% of its original width, or a total of 17 mg/kg of the drug has been injected. If this treatment is successful, a continuous procainamide infusion of 2 to 4 mg/min should be started. A third drug of choice is bretylium (Bretylol), given IV at a dose of 5 mg/kg for several minutes and increased to 10 mg/kg at 15 to 30 minutes (not to exceed 30 to 35 mg/kg). A continuous infusion of bretylium (1 to 2 mg/min) may be started.[11]

The acute treatment of torsades de pointes can be quite different than that of more common ventricular tachycardias. Magnesium sulfate infusion is the therapy of choice. Other therapies indicated for torsades de pointes include isoproterenol (Isuprel) or lidocaine infusions. Overdrive pacing is also used to suppress this arrhythmia.[9,19,20]

If a patient is unconscious or hemodynamically unstable, immediate cardioversion, starting initially with 50 joules, is the recommended treatment. A defibrillator is used in the synchronized mode for cardioversion. The machine is timed to discharge on an R wave in order to effectively convert the ventricular tachycardia to a sinus rhythm. If a patient is awake before cardioversion, a sedative may be given before delivery of the electrical discharge.[11]

Ventricular Fibrillation. Ventricular fibrillation is a severe derangement of the heart rhythm characterized on the ECG by irregular undulations of varying contour and amplitude (Fig. 34-20). This represents the firing of multiple ectopic foci in the ventricle. Mechanically the ventricle is simply "quivering," and no effective contraction or CO occurs.

Clinical associations. Ventricular fibrillation occurs in acute MI and myocardial ischemia and in chronic diseases such as CAD and cardiomyopathy. It may occur during cardiac pacing or cardiac catheterization procedures as a result of catheter stimulation of the ventricle. It may also occur with coronary reperfusion after thrombolytic therapy. Other clini-

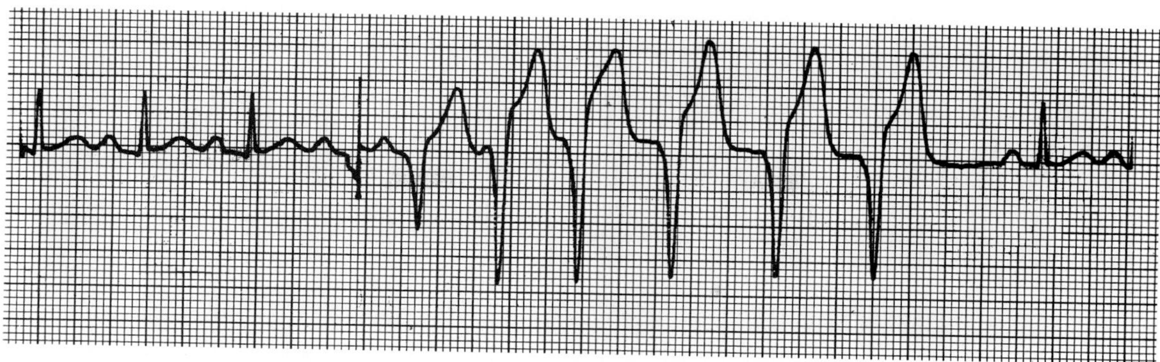

Fig. 34-18 Ventricular tachycardia.

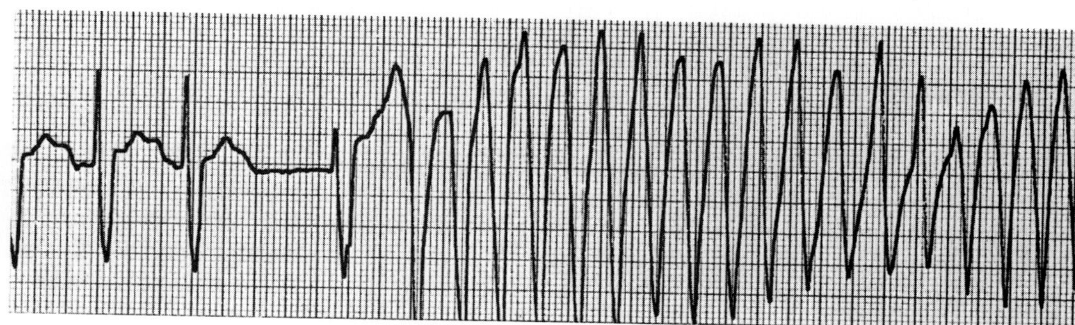

Fig. 34-19 Torsades de pointes.

cal associations are accidental electrical shock, hyperkalemia, and hypoxemia.

Electrocardiogram characteristics. HR is not measurable. Rhythm is irregular and chaotic. The P wave is not visible, and the PR interval and the QRS interval are not measurable.

Significance. Ventricular fibrillation results in unconsciousness, absence of pulse, apnea, and seizures. If left untreated, the patient with this condition will die.

Treatment. Treatment consists of immediate initiation of cardiopulmonary resuscitation (CPR) and initiation of advanced cardiac life support (ACLS) measures with the use of defibrillation and definitive drug therapy. If a defibrillator is immediately available, there should be no delay in using it.[11]

Asystole. Asystole represents the total absence of ventricular electrical activity. Occasionally, P waves can be seen. No ventricular contraction occurs because depolarization does not occur. This is a lethal arrhythmia that requires immediate treatment. Ventricular fibrillation may masquerade as asystole; thus the rhythm should be assessed in more than one lead. The prognosis of a patient with asystole is poor.

Clinical associations. Asystole is usually a result of advanced cardiac disease, a severe cardiac conduction system disturbance, or end-stage CHF.

Significance. Generally the patient with asystole has end-stage cardiac function or has a prolonged arrest and cannot be resuscitated.

Treatment. Treatment consists of CPR with initiation of ACLS measures, which include intubation and IV therapy with epinephrine and atropine.[11]

Pulseless Electrical Activity. *Pulseless electrical activity (PEA)*, a new term replacing *electromechanical dissociation*, describes a situation in which electrical activity can be observed on the ECG, but there is no mechanical activity of the ventricles and the patient has no pulse. Prognosis is poor unless the underlying cause can be identified and corrected. The most common correctable causes of PEA are hypovolemia, cardiac tamponade, tension pneumothorax, hypoxemia, hypothermia, and acidosis. Other less correctable causes of PEA include massive myocardial damage from infarction, prolonged ischemia during resuscitation, and pulmonary embolism. Treatment begins with CPR followed by intubation and IV therapy with epinephrine. Treatment is directed toward correction of the underlying cause.[11]

Sudden Cardiac Death. The term *sudden cardiac death (SCD)* or *sudden death* refer to cardiac death by an arrhythmia such as ventricular fibrillation. However, some electrophysiologists believe the terms can refer to death that is sudden by any cause. These causes may include ventricular arrhythmias, PEA, and aortic rupture. SCD is responsible for over 300,000 deaths per year in the United States.[21,22] (SCD is discussed in Chapter 32).

Proarrhythmia. Antiarrhythmic drugs may cause life-threatening arrhythmias similar to those for which they are administered. This concept is termed *proarrhythmia.* The patient who has severe left ventricular dysfunction is the most susceptible to a proarrhythmia. Class IA and IC drugs (Table 34-7), digoxin, and type III drugs can cause a proarrhythmic response. The first several days of drug therapy is the vulnerable period for

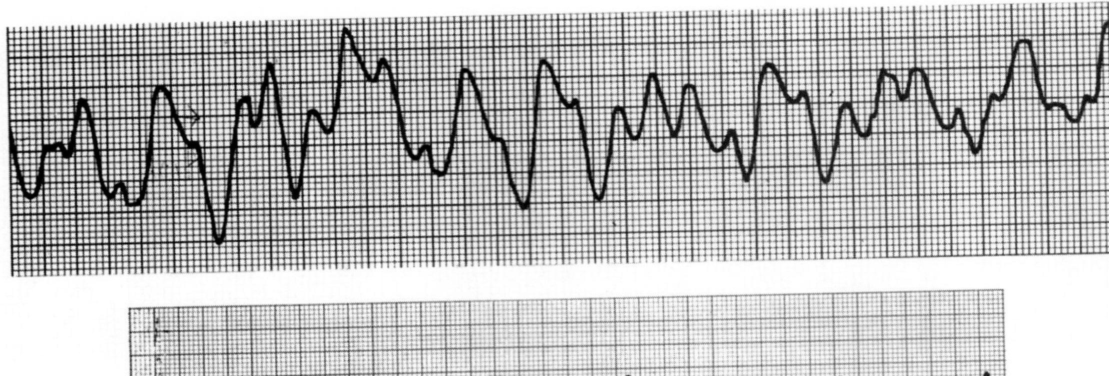

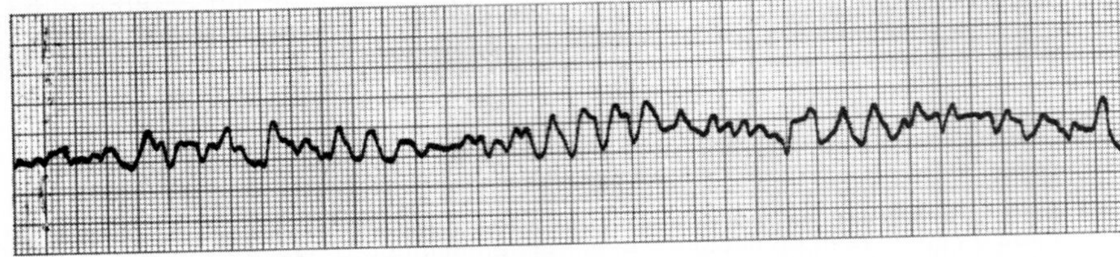

Fig. 34-20 Ventricular fibrillation.

developing proarrhythmias. For this reason, the beginning of most oral antiarrhythmic drug regimens using these classes of drugs should be done in a monitored hospital setting.[9]

Antiarrhythmic Drugs

An increasing number of antiarrhythmic drugs have become available.[9,10] Table 34-7 categorizes major drug classifications by primary effects on the cardiac intracellular action potential. Another arrhythmia drug classification system, originating in Europe, is being increasingly used. It classifies drugs according to their effect on ion channels and pumps and cardiac receptors.[23]

Defibrillation

Defibrillation is the most effective method of terminating ventricular fibrillation. It is most effective when the myocardial cells are not anoxic or acidotic. Therefore defibrillation should ideally be performed within 15 to 20 seconds of the onset of the arrhythmia. Defibrillation is accomplished by the passage of a direct current (DC) electrical shock through the heart that is sufficient to depolarize the cells of the myocardium. The intent is that subsequent repolarization of myocardial cells will allow the SA node to resume the role of pacemaker.[11] The output of a defibrillator is quantified in joules, or watts per second. The recommended energy for initial shock in defibrillation is 200 joules with a second shock of 200 to 300 joules as needed and a third shock of 360 joules if defibrillation is unsuccessful. High doses of electricity during defibrillation have been found to cause myocardial damage; thus the lowest effective electrical output is the one with which to start.

A defibrillator is one part of standard emergency equipment available (Fig. 34-21). There are many different models of defibrillators. The nurse should be familiar with the operation of the type of defibrillator that is used in the clinical setting. Proficiency verification in use of the defibrillator is recommended annually for nursing staff members who use it.

The following steps are to be taken for defibrillation: (1) CPR should be in progress if the defibrillator is not immediately available; (2) the defibrillator should be turned on, and the proper energy level should be selected; and (3) someone should

DRUG THERAPY

Table 34-7 Major Classifications of Antiarrhythmic Drugs

Classification I: Drugs That Depress Upstroke of Action Potential

A. Prolong Repolarization
- Quinidine
- Procainamide (Pronestyl)
- Disopyramide (Norpace)
- Moricizine* (Ethmozine)

B. Accelerate Repolarization
- Lidocaine
- Tocainide (Tonocard)
- Mexiletine (Mexitil)

C. Have Little or No Effect on Repolarization
- Flecainide (Tambocar)
- Propafenone (Rythmol)
- Moricizine* (Ethmozine)

Classification II: β-Adrenergic Blockers
- Propanolol (Inderal)
- Nadolol (Corgard)
- Timolol (Blocadren)
- Atenolol (Tenormin)
- Acebutolol (Sectral)
- Esmolol (Brevibloc)
- Metoprolol (Lopressor)
- Sotalol† (Betapace)
- Labetalol (Normodyne)

Classification III: Drugs That Prolong Repolarization
- Bretylium (Bretylate)
- Amiodarone (Cordarone)
- Sotalol† (Betapace)
- Ibutilide (Corvert)

Classification IV: Calcium Channel Blockers
- Diltiazem (Cardizem)
- Verapamil (Calan, Isoptin)

Potassium Channel Opener
- Adenosine (Adenocard)

Digitalis Preparations

*Moricizine has both class IA and IC properties.
†Sotalol has both class II and class III properties.

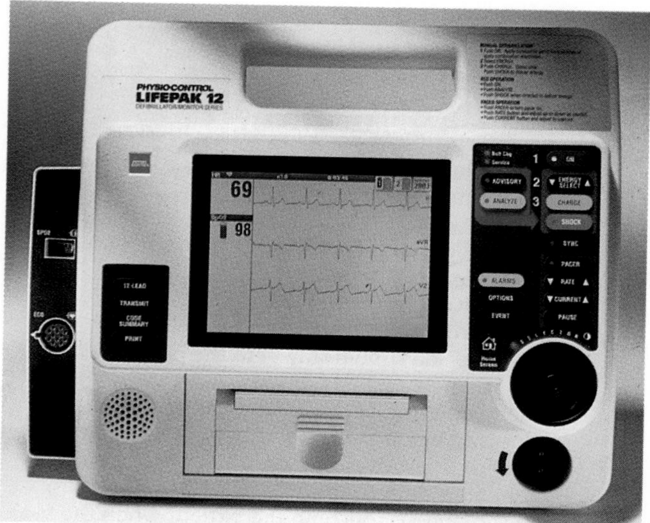

Fig. 34-21 Life-Pak: contains a monitor, defibrillator, and transcutaneous pacemaker.

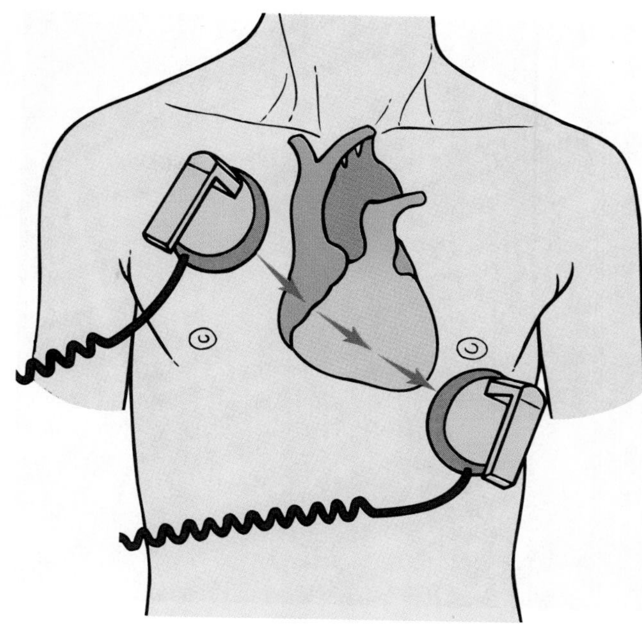

Fig. 34-22 Paddle placement and current flow in defibrillation.

make sure that the synchronizer switch is turned off. Conductive materials in the form of saline pads, electrode gel, or defibrillator gel pads are applied to the chest where defibrillator paddles will be placed. This decreases electrical impedance and helps prevent burns. The paddles are charged by a button on the defibrillator or a button on the paddles themselves. The paddles are placed on the chest wall (Fig. 34-22); one is placed to the right of the sternum just below the clavicle, and the other is placed to the left of the precordium. The operator applies 20 to 25 pounds of pressure to the paddles. The operator calls "all clear" to ensure that personnel are not touching the patient or the bed at the time of discharge. The defibrillator is then discharged by depressing buttons on both paddles simultaneously.

Electrical cardioversion is the therapy of choice for hemodynamically unstable ventricular or supraventricular tachyarrhythmias. A synchronized circuit in the defibrillator is used to deliver a countershock that is programmed to occur during the QRS complex of the ECG.

The procedure for cardioversion is the same as for defibrillation with the following exceptions: If synchronized cardioversion is done on a nonemergency basis when the patient is awake and hemodynamically stable, the patient may be sedated with diazepam (Valium) or midazolam (Versed) before the procedure. Strict attention to maintenance of a patent airway is important in this situation. When a patient with supraventricular tachycardia or ventricular tachycardia is hemodynamically unstable, cardioversion is performed as quickly as possible.

Implantable Cardioverter-Defibrillator. In the past 10 years the implantable cardioverter-defibrillator (ICD) has been developed as an acceptable treatment for the patient who has life-threatening ventricular arrhythmias. Indications for implantation of an ICD include cardiac arrest survivors, recurrent sustained VT, and prophylactically in patients who are at risk for SCD. Use of the ICD appears to significantly decrease cardiac mortality rates and has added a new dimension to the management of life-threatening arrhythmias and the prevention of SCD.[24,25]

The ICD consists of a lead system placed via a subclavian vein to the endocardium. A battery-powered pulse generator is implanted, usually subcutaneously, over the pectoral muscle. The pulse generator is similar to a pacemaker box but is somewhat larger. The newest systems are single-lead systems instead of previous multilead or patch systems[24] (Fig. 34-23). The ICD sensing system monitors the HR and rhythm and identifies ventricular tachycardia or ventricular fibrillation. Approximately 25 seconds after the sensing system detects a lethal arrhythmia, the defibrillating mechanism delivers a 25-joule or less shock to the patient's heart muscle. If the first shock is unsuccessful, the generator recycles and can continue to deliver shocks.[25]

Surgical risk and hospital length-of-stay have been greatly reduced with the use of the transvenous approach for implantation of the ICD. Previous approaches required thoracotomy or sternotomy. The transvenous approach decreases morbidity and medical costs related to surgical complications. In some centers, the implantation of an ICD is an outpatient procedure.[25] Occasionally an ICD is implanted during open heart surgery, which results in a different risk and complication profile.

In addition to defibrillation capabilities, the newest ICDs, or third-generation ICDs, are equipped with antitachycardia and antibradycardia pacemakers. These sophisticated devices use arrhythmia algorithms that detect arrhythmias and determine the appropriate programmed response. These devices initiate overdrive pacing of supraventricular and ventricular tachycardias, sparing the patient painful shocks from the defibrillator device. They also provide backup pacing for bradyarrhythmias occurring after defibrillation discharges.[24,25]

Education of the patient who is receiving an ICD is of extreme importance.[26,27] The patient experiences a variety of emotions, including fear of body image change, fear of recurrent arrhythmias, expectation of pain with ICD discharge (described as a feeling of a blow to the chest), and anxiety about going home. Table 34-8 describes the home care guidelines for the patient with an ICD and the patient's family. Participation in an ICD support group should be encouraged.[24]

A

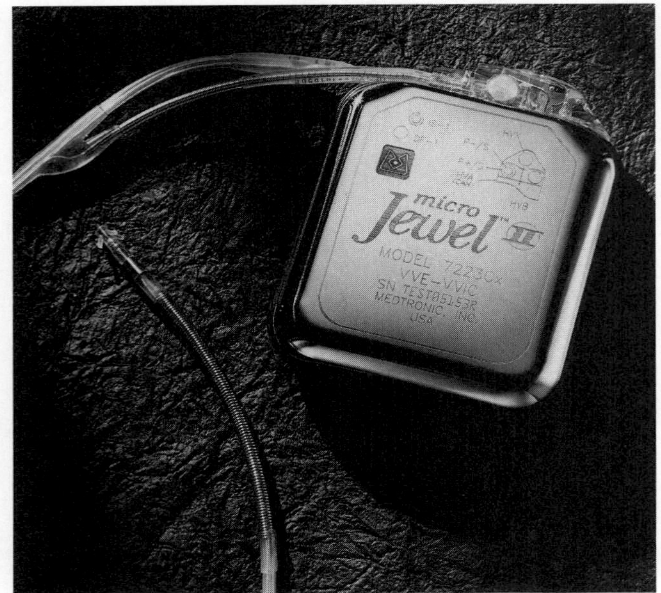

B

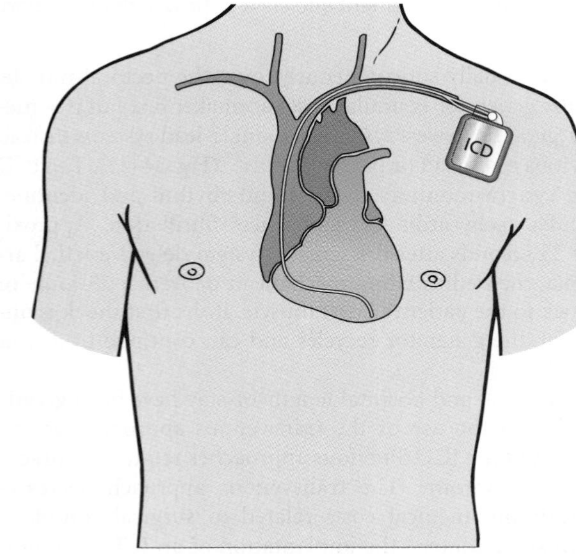

Fig. 34-23 **A,** The implantable cardioverter-defibrillator (ICD) pulse generator from Medtronics, Inc. **B,** The ICD is placed in a subcutaneous pocket over the pectoralis muscle. A single-lead system is placed transvenously from the pulse generator to the endocardium. The single lead detects arrhythmias and delivers an electrical shock to the heart muscle.

PATIENT & FAMILY HOME CARE GUIDE

Table 34-8 Implantable Cardioverter-Defibrillator (ICD)

1. Maintain close follow-up with physician for testing of ICD function and for inspection of ICD insertion site.
2. Watch for signs of infection at incision site (e.g., redness, swelling, drainage).
3. When the ICD fires:
   - The patient should lie down.
   - One person should stay with the patient while another contacts the physician.
   - Someone should call an ambulance if patient loses consciousness. CPR should be delayed until device fires unsuccessfully 4-7 times or fails to fire after 30 seconds.
   - If someone is touching the patient when the ICD fires, that person may feel a slight but harmless shock.
   - If alone, the patient should call an ambulance immediately and then lie down.
4. The ICD battery must be checked every 2 months.
5. A Medic Alert bracelet should be worn at all times.
6. An information card about the ICD should be easily accessible in the patient's wallet.
7. The manual for patients provided by the ICD manufacturer should be read.
8. Family members should learn CPR.
9. The nurse should assist patient with the development of positive coping strategies to reduce stress.
10. Avoid large electromagnetic and vibratory forces, which may turn off the device.
11. Generally, patients should be told that they should not drive until they have had a 6-month discharge-free period. This is the law in some states.

Pacemakers

The artificial cardiac pacemaker is an electronic device used in place of the SA node, the natural cardiac pacemaker of the heart. Implantable pacemakers were first developed in the 1950s. The artificial cardiac pacemaker is an electrical circuit in which the battery provides electricity that travels through a conducting wire to the myocardium, and the myocardium stimulates the heart to beat (i.e., it "captures" the heart).

Recent advances in technology have been applied extensively to pacemakers. This has resulted in sophisticated, noninvasive, programmable single- and dual-chambered pacemakers with specialized circuits that weigh only 40 to 50 g. Pacemakers have been developed that are more physiologically accurate, pacing both the atrium and the ventricle, as well as increasing HR when appropriate.[28,29]

Permanent pacemakers are those that are implanted totally within the body (Fig. 34-24), and temporary pacemakers are those with the power source outside the body (Fig. 34-25). The permanent pacemaker power source is implanted subcutaneously in the chest (see Fig. 34-24, *B*) or abdomen and is attached to pacer electrodes, which are threaded transvenously to the right ventricle or the right atrium. Indications for insertion of permanent pacemaker are listed in Table 34-9. Newer and experimental indications for pacing include vasovagal syncope, hypertrophic cardiomyopathy, long QT syndrome, and prevention of atrial fibrillation.[28,29]

Temporary pacemakers are usually used with a lead or wire threaded transvenously to the right ventricle and with a wire attached to a power source externally (Fig. 34-26). They are inserted in cardiac care units in emergency situations. Indications for temporary pacing are listed in Table 34-10.

Pacemaker malfunction is manifested by a failure to sense or a failure to capture. Failure to sense occurs when the pacemaker

A

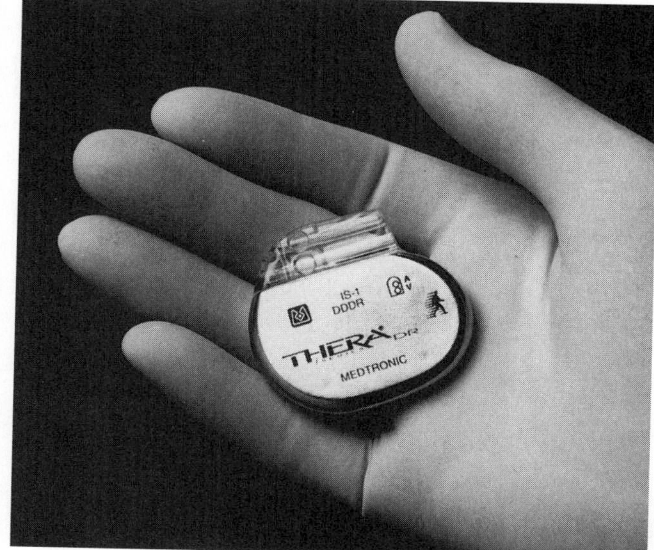

B

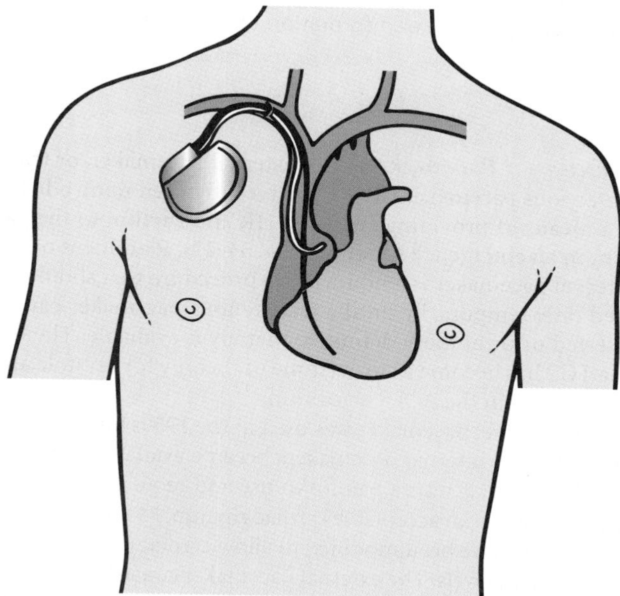

Fig. 34-24 **A,** A dual-chamber, rate-responsive pacemaker (shown here actual size) from Medtronic, Inc., is designed to detect body movement and automatically increase or decrease paced heart rates based on the level of physical activity. **B,** Cardiac leads in both the atrium and ventricle enable a dual-chamber pacemaker to sense and pace in both heart chambers.

fails to recognize spontaneous atrial or ventricular activity, and it fires inappropriately. Failure to sense may be caused by pacer lead fracture, battery failure, or movement of electrode. Failure to capture occurs when the electrical charge to the myocardium is insufficient to produce atrial or ventricular contraction. Failure to capture may be caused by pacer lead fracture, battery failure, electrode movement, or fibrosis at the electrode tip.

Complications of invasive temporary or permanent pacemaker insertion include infection and hematoma formation at the site of insertion of the pacemaker power source, pneumothorax, failure to sense or capture with possible bradycardia and significant symptoms, perforation of the atrial or ventricular septum by the pacing wire, and appearance of "end-of-life" battery parameters on testing the pacemaker. A decrease in CO may also be seen when a ventricular demand–ventricular inhibited mode pacer is inserted because of loss of atrial contractions (atrial "kick").

Measures taken to prevent and assess complications include prophylactic IV antibiotic therapy before and after insertion, assessment of chest x-ray after insertion to check lead placement and to rule out the presence of a pneumothorax, careful observation of insertion site, and continuous ECG monitoring of the patient's rhythm. After pacemaker insertion, the patient is maintained on bed rest for 12 hours, and minimal arm and shoulder activity is allowed to prevent dislodgement of the newly implanted pacemaker leads. The nurse should observe for signs of infection by assessing the incision for redness, swelling, or discharge. Temperature elevation should also be noted. Careful monitoring of the patient's rhythm is used to detect problems with sensing or capturing.

The nurse must provide patient education in addition to observation for complications after pacemaker insertion. The patient with a newly implanted pacemaker has many questions

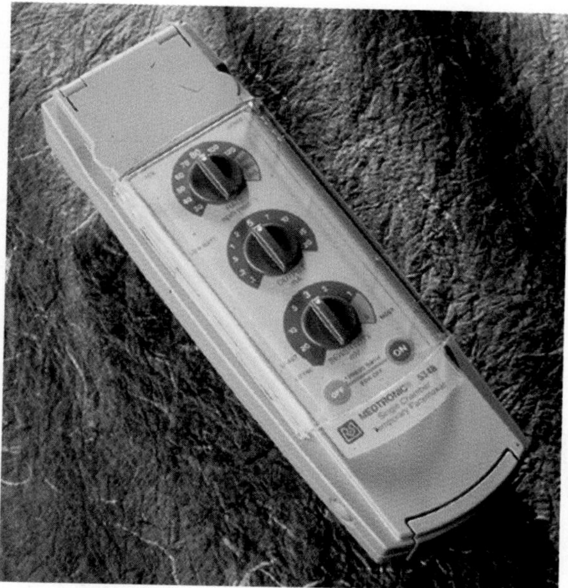

Fig. 34-25 Temporary external demand pacemaker.

Table 34-9 Indications for Permanent Pacemaker Therapy

Indications
Sinus node dysfunction
Third-degree AV block
Fibrosis or sclerotic changes of cardiac conduction system
Sick sinus syndrome
Mobitz II second-degree AV block
Hypersensitive carotid sinus syndrome
Chronic atrial fibrillation with slow ventricular response
Tachyarrhythmias
Bifascicular block

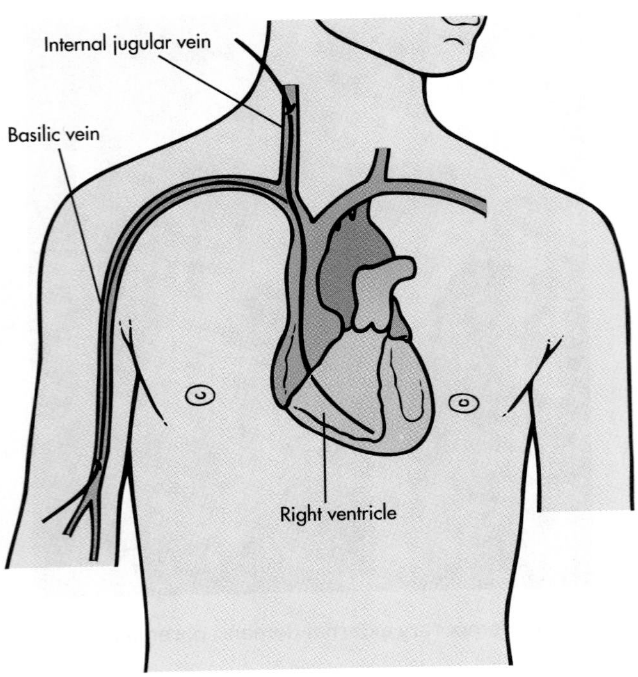

Fig. 34-26 Temporary pacemaker catheter insertion.

Table 34-10 Indications for Temporary Pacing

- Maintenance of adequate HR and rhythm during special circumstances such as surgery and postoperative recovery, cardiac catheterization or coronary angioplasty, during drug therapy that may cause bradycardia, and before implantation of a permanent pacemaker
- As prophylaxis after open heart surgery
- Acute anterior MI with second-degree or third-degree AV block or bundle branch block
- Acute inferior MI with symptomatic bradycardia and AV block
- Termination of AV nodal reentry or reciprocating tachycardia associated with WPW syndrome, atrial flutter, or ventricular tachycardia
- Suppression of ectopic atrial or ventricular rhythm
- Electrophysiologic studies to evaluate patient with bradyarrhythmias and tachyarrhythmias

WPW, Wolff-Parkinson-White.

about activity restrictions and fears concerning body image and becoming a "cardiac cripple" after the procedure. The goal of pacemaker therapy should be to enhance physiologic functioning and the quality of life. This should be emphasized to the patient, and the nurse should give concrete advice on activity restrictions. Patient and family education for the patient with a pacemaker is outlined in Table 34-11.

Pacemaker function can be checked by magnet placement during ECG assessment in the pacemaker clinic, or it can be done from the home using telephone transmitter devices. The patient is sometimes given devices to place on the fingers or directly over the pacemaker battery generator with an attachment to the telephone. In this way, the heart rhythm can be transmitted to the pacemaker clinic.

PATIENT & FAMILY TEACHING GUIDE

Table 34-11 Pacemaker

1. Maintain follow-up care with a physician to check the pacemaker site and begin regular pacemaker function checks with magnet and ECG evaluation.
2. Watch for signs of infection at incision site—redness, swelling, drainage.
3. Keep incision dry for 1 week after implantation.
4. Avoid lifting operative-side arm above shoulder level for 1 week.
5. Avoid direct blows to generator site.
6. Avoid close proximity to high-output electrical generators or to large magnets such as an MRI scanner. These devices can reprogram a pacemaker.
7. Microwave ovens are safe to use and do not threaten pacemaker function.
8. Travel without restrictions is allowed. The small metal case of an implanted pacemaker rarely sets off an airport security alarm.
9. The patient should be taught how to take the pulse.
10. Carry pacemaker information card at all times.

External Pacemaker. The external pacemaker, or transcutaneous pacemaker (TCP), has recently been reintroduced as a means of providing adequate HR and rhythm to the patient in an emergency situation (Fig. 34-27). Placement of the external pacemaker is a noninvasive procedure that should be used only temporarily until a transvenous pacemaker can be inserted or until more definitive therapy is available. The use of a TCP has become a cornerstone of therapy for asystole and bradycardia in the ACLS algorithms.[11]

The external pacemaker was used in the 1950s but lost favor in 1959 when internal pacemakers became available. Early external pacemakers were painful to use and required high voltage to maintain an acceptable cardiac rhythm. Modern external pacemakers have been modified to allow cardiac stimulation at lower voltage levels. The external pacemaker consists of a power source and a rate- and voltage-control device that is attached to two large electrode pads. One pad is positioned on the anterior part of the chest, usually on the V_2 or V_5 lead position, and the other pad is placed on the back between the spine and the left scapula at the level of the heart.[11]

Before initiating external pacemaker therapy, it is important to tell the patient what to expect. The uncomfortable muscle contractions that the pacemaker creates when the current passes through the chest wall should be explained. The patient should be reassured that the therapy is temporary and that every effort will be made to adjust the voltage settings of the pacemaker to improve comfort level. Mild analgesia may also be given.

Catheter Ablation Therapy

Catheter ablation therapy is a revolutionary development in the area of antiarrhythmic therapy. In 1981 transcatheter ablation of the AV node was introduced as a treatment for supraventricular arrhythmias. Radiofrequency energy (produced by high-frequency alternating current) has been most recently used to "burn" or ablate areas of the conduction system as definitive treatment of tachyarrhythmias.[8]

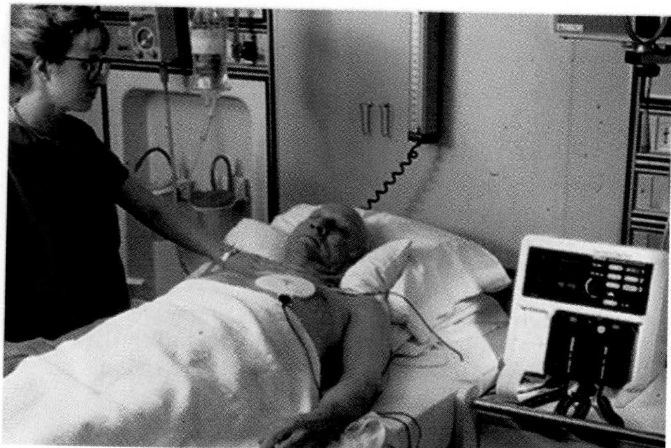

Fig. 34-27 Transcutaneous pacemaker.

The procedure is done following EPS that is used to map the source of the arrhythmia. An electrode-tipped ablation catheter is used to "burn" or ablate accessory pathways or ectopic sites in the atria, AV node, and ventricles. Catheter ablation is considered the nonpharmacologic treatment of choice for AV nodal reentrant tachycardia, for reentrant tachycardia related to accessory bypass tracts, and to control the ventricular response of certain tachyarrhythmias. The procedure is also used for atrial flutter. In some cases of uncontrolled ventricular response in atrial fibrillation or flutter that is unresponsive to medical therapy, complete ablation of the AV node or bundle of His is performed.

The ablation procedure is a highly successful therapy with a low complication rate. Care of the patient following ablation therapy is similar to that of a patient undergoing cardiac catheterization.

CARDIOPULMONARY RESUSCITATION

All health care workers should be skilled in CPR because *cardiac arrest,* the sudden cessation of breathing and adequate circulation of blood by the heart, may occur at any time or in any setting. CPR is the process of externally supporting the circulation and respiration of a person who has a cardiac arrest.[30] Resuscitation measures are divided into two components: basic life support (BLS) and ACLS. The American Heart Association establishes the standards for CPR and is actively involved in teaching BLS and ACLS to health professionals. The American Heart Association recommends that nurses and physicians working with patients be certified in BLS and ACLS. Certification involves attending formal classes and passing cognitive and motor skill tests.

CPR alone is not enough to save lives in most cardiac arrests. It is a vital link in the chain of survival that supports the victim until more advanced help is available. The chain of survival is composed of the following sequence: early activation of the EMS system, early CPR, early defibrillation, and early advanced care.[11]

Basic Life Support

BLS involves the external support of circulation and ventilation for a patient with cardiac or respiratory arrest through CPR.[30] Artificial respiration (mouth-to-mouth, mouth-to-mask, mouth-to-nose, mouth-to-stoma) and external chest compression substitute for spontaneous breathing and circulation. The major objective of performing CPR is to provide oxygen to the brain, heart, and other vital organs until appropriate therapeutic management and resuscitation efforts involving advanced life support methods can be initiated or until resuscitation efforts are ordered to be stopped.

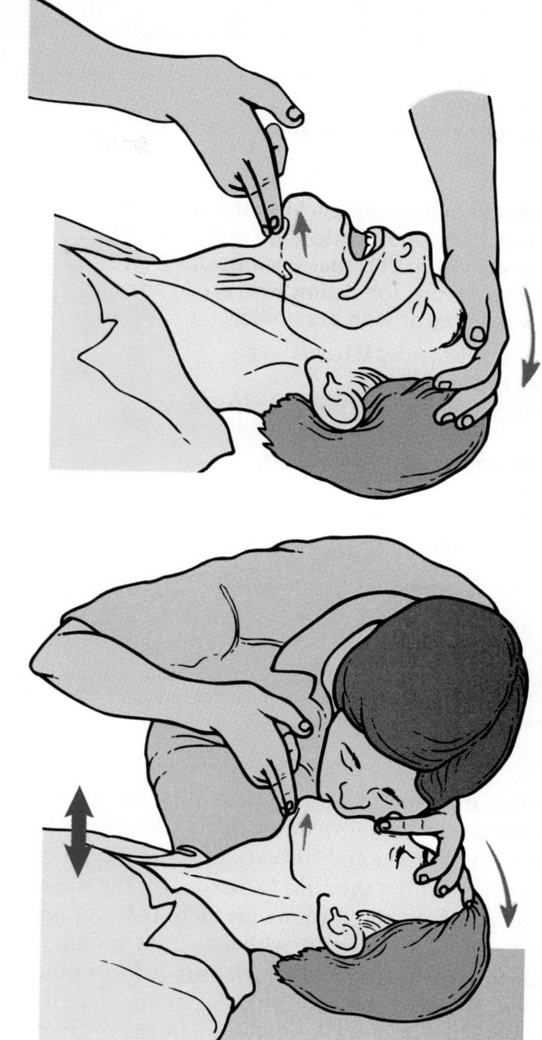

Fig. 34-28 The head tilt–chin lift maneuver is used to open the victim's airway to give mouth-to-mouth resuscitation. This procedure is carried out by placing one hand on the victim's forehead and applying firm, backward pressure with the palm to tilt the head back. The chin is lifted and brought forward with the fingers of the other hand.

Rapid intervention is the key to success and is critical in preventing biologic death or the death of brain cells. CPR must be initiated within 4 to 6 minutes of cardiac or pulmonary arrest. Brain cells begin to die (brain death) within 6 minutes of anoxia. It is critical that oxygenated blood be circulated during CPR. Unfortunately, even when CPR is performed with perfect technique, only 25% to 30% of the normal CO is achieved. National standards for knowledge and technique must be met for personnel to be certified to deliver CPR. Assessment of the victim must be stressed in teaching CPR. Each of the broad areas—airway, breathing, and circulation (the ABCs of CPR)—should be reviewed.

Airway and Breathing. The first steps in administering BLS are to confirm the absence of breathing and to establish a patent airway. Figure 34-28 demonstrates opening the airway

Table 34-12 Management of Foreign Body Airway Obstruction

Action	Helpful Hints
Conscious Adult	
1. Determine if victim is able to speak or cough.	Rescuer can ask, "Are you choking?" Victim may be using the universal distress signal of choking: clutching the neck between thumb and index finger
2. Abdominal thrust: perform the Heimlich maneuver until the foreign body is expelled or the victim becomes unconscious (Fig. 34-29).	Stand behind victim and wrap arms around victim's waist. Press fist into abdomen with quick inward and upward thrusts.
3. Chest thrust: for victims who are in advanced pregnancy or who are obese.	Chest thrusts: stand behind victim and place arms under victim's armpits to encircle the chest. Press with quick backward thrusts.
Victim Is or Becomes Unconscious	
1. Activate EMS.	Call 911.
2. Check for foreign body obstruction.	Sweep deeply into mouth with hooked finger to remove foreign body.
3. Attempt rescue breathing.	Open airway. Try to give two breaths. If needed, reposition the head and try again (Fig. 34-30).
4. If airway is obstructed, perform Heimlich maneuver.	Kneel astride the victim's thighs. Place the heel of one hand on the victim's abdomen, in the midline slightly above the navel and well below the tip of the xyphoid. Place the second hand on top of the first. Press into the abdomen with quick upward thrusts.
5. Repeat sequence until successful.	Alternate these maneuvers in rapid sequence: finger sweep, rescue breathing attempt, and abdominal thrusts.

Source: *Textbook of basic life support for healthcare providers,* Dallas, 1997, American Heart Association.
EMS, emergency medical services.

and performing mouth-to-mouth ventilation. An adult's airway is opened by hyperextending the head. The head tilt–chin lift maneuver is used and involves tilting the head back with one hand and lifting the chin forward with the fingers of the other hand. If no respirations are detected, the rescuer attempts to ventilate the victim with mouth-to-mouth resuscitation. Breaths are given with the victim's nostrils pinched and the rescuer's mouth placed around the victim's mouth to make a tight seal. Two slow breaths are given by the rescuer (1.5 to 2 seconds per breath). The volume of air of each ventilation should be approximately 800 ml, which can be determined by noting a rise of 1 to 2 inches in the victim's chest. When the victim has a tracheostomy, ventilation should be given through the stoma.[11,30]

If airflow is obstructed, the rescuer should reposition the head and repeat the attempt to provide ventilation. If the victim cannot be ventilated after repositioning the head, the rescuer should proceed with maneuvers to remove foreign bodies that may be obstructing the airway (Table 34-12).

In those rare instances when airway obstruction is not relieved by methods described in Table 34-12, additional procedures are necessary. These include transtracheal catheter ventilation and cricothyroidotomy, which must be attempted only by health care professionals experienced in these procedures.[11]

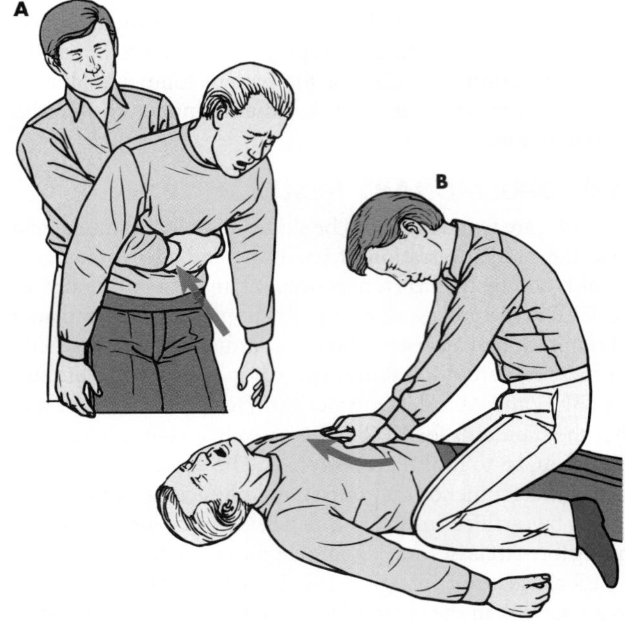

Fig. 34-29 **A,** Heimlich maneuver administered to a conscious (standing) victim of foreign body airway obstruction. **B,** Heimlich maneuver administered to an unconscious (lying) victim of foreign body airway obstruction—astride position.

External Cardiac Compressions. Cardiac arrest is characterized by the absence of a pulse in the large arteries of an unconscious victim who is not breathing. The carotid artery is used to determine the absence of a pulse. After an airway has been established and two ventilations have been delivered, the rescuer checks the pulse. While maintaining the head-tilt position with one hand on the forehead, the rescuer locates the victim's trachea with two or three fingers of the other hand. The rescuer then slides these fingers into the groove between the trachea and the muscles of the side of the neck where the carotid pulse can be felt. The technique is more easily performed on the side nearest the rescuer. If no pulse is palpated, chest compressions should be initiated.[30]

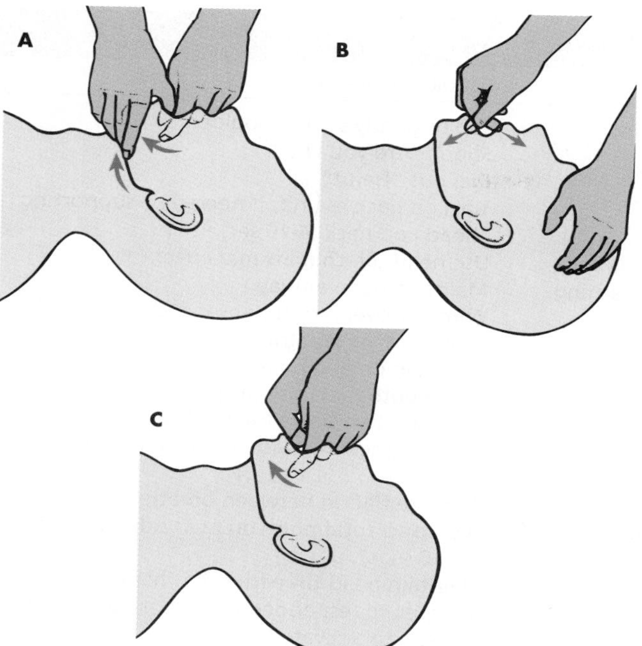

Fig. 34-30 **A,** Finger-sweep maneuver administered to an unconscious victim of foreign body airway obstruction. With the victim's head up, the rescuer opens the victim's mouth by grasping both the tongue and the lower jaw between the thumb and fingers and lifting (tongue-jaw lift). This action draws the tongue from the back of the throat and away from the foreign body. The obstruction may be partially relieved by this maneuver. **B,** Crossed-finger technique for opening the airway. If the rescuer is unable to open the mouth with tongue-jaw lift, the crossed-finger technique may be used. The rescuer opens the mouth by crossing index finger and thumb and pushing the teeth apart. **C,** The index finger of the rescuer's available hand is inserted along inside of the cheek and deeply into the throat to the base of the tongue. A hooking motion is used to dislodge the foreign body and maneuver it into the mouth for removal.

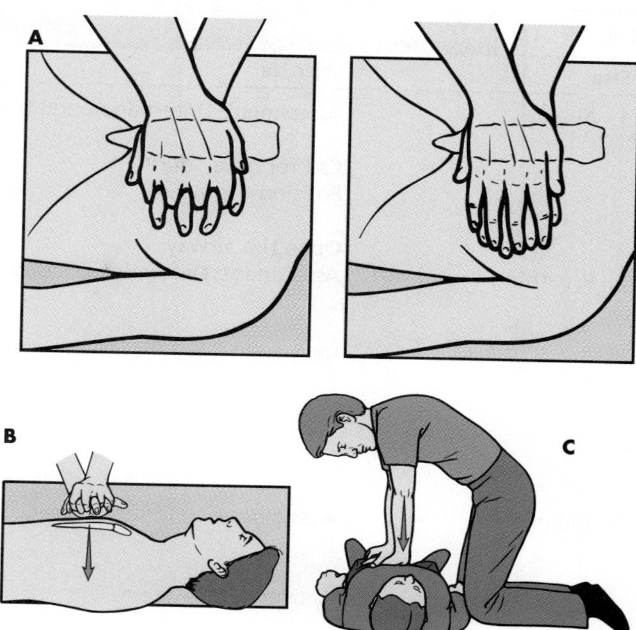

Fig. 34-31 Cardiopulmonary resuscitation. **A,** Position of the hands during application of external cardiac massage. **B,** When pressure is applied, the lower portion of the sternum is displaced posteriorly with the palm of the hand. **C,** To apply maximum downward pressure, the resuscitator leans forward so that both arms are at right angles to the patient's sternum and the elbows are locked.

The proper technique for administering chest compressions is shown in Fig. 34-31. External chest compression technique consists of serial, rhythmic applications of pressure on the lower half of the sternum. The victim must be in the horizontal supine position when the compressions are performed. The victim must be lying on a flat, hard surface, such as a CPR board (specially manufactured for use in CPR), a headboard from a cardiac care unit bed, or, if necessary, the floor. The rescuer should be positioned close to the side of the victim's chest.[30]

The following guidelines have been established for proper hand placement[30] (see Fig. 34-31, *A*):

1. With the middle and index fingers of the hand nearest the victim's legs, the rescuer locates the lower margin of the victim's rib cage on the side next to the rescuer.
2. The fingers are moved up the rib cage to the notch where the ribs meet the sternum.
3. The middle finger is placed on this notch, and the index finger is placed next to it on the lower end of the sternum. (This allows proper placement above the xiphoid process and prevents possible laceration of the liver by the xiphoid process during compressions.)
4. The heel of the hand nearest the victim's head is placed on the lower half of the sternum, close to the index finger of the other hand. The long axis of the heel of the rescuer's hand should be placed on the long axis of the sternum.
5. The first hand is removed from the notch and placed on top of the hand on the sternum so that both hands are parallel to each other.
6. The fingers are extended or interlaced and must be kept off the chest.[30]

The following guidelines have been established for proper compression technique[30] (see Fig. 34-31, *C*):

1. The elbows are locked into position, the arms are straightened, and the shoulders are positioned directly over the hands so that the thrust for each chest compression is straight down on the sternum.
2. The sternum must be depressed 1.5 to 2 inches (3.8 to 5.1 cm) for the normal-sized adult. The heart is compressed between the sternum and spine.
3. The external chest compression pressure is released to allow blood to flow into the chest and the heart. The pressure must be released and the chest allowed to return to its normal position after each compression. Arterial pressure during chest compression is maximal when the duration of compression is 50% of the compression-release cycle.[30]

Table 34-13 Adult One-Rescuer CPR

Step	Objective	Critical Performance
1. Airway	Assessment: Determine unresponsiveness.	Tap or gently shake shoulder. Shout "Are you OK?"
	Call for help.	Call out "Help!"
	Position the victim.	Turn on back as unit, if necessary, supporting head and neck (4-10 sec).
	Open the airway.	Use head tilt–chin lift maneuver.
2. Breathing	Assessment: Determine cessation of breathing.	Maintain open airway. With ear over mouth, observe chest: look, listen, feel for breathing (3-5 sec).
	Ventilate twice.	Maintain open airway. Seal mouth and nose properly. Ventilate two times for 1.5-2 sec/inflation. Observe chest rise (adequate ventilation volume). Allow deflation between breaths.
3. Circulation	Assessment: Determine absence of pulse.	Feel for carotid pulse on near side of victim (5-10 sec). Maintain head-tilt with other hand.
	Activate EMS system.	If someone responded to call for help, send person to activate EMS system. Total time, step 1—Activate EMS system: 15-35 sec.
	Begin chest compressions.	Kneel by victim's shoulders. Make landmark check before hands are placed. Maintain proper hand position throughout. Keep shoulders over victim's sternum. Maintain equal compression and relaxation. Compress 1.5-2 in. Keep hands on sternum during upstroke. Wait for complete chest relaxation on upstroke. Say any helpful mnemonic (e.g., one-and-two-and-three-and . . .). Remember that compression rate is 80-100/min (15/9-11 sec).
4. Compression-ventilation cycles	Do four cycles of 15 compressions and two ventilations.	Maintain proper compression-ventilation ratio of 15 compressions to two ventilations per cycle. Observe chest rise: 1.5-2 sec/inflation; four cycles/52-73 sec.
5. Reassessment	Determine absence of pulse.	Feel for carotid pulse (5 sec). If there is no pulse, go to step 6.
6. Continuation of CPR	Ventilate twice.	Ventilate two times. 1.5-2 sec Observe chest rise: 1-1.5 sec/inflation.
	Resume compression-ventilation cycles.	Feel for carotid pulse every few minutes.

Source: *Textbook of basic life support for healthcare providers,* Dallas, 1997, American Heart Association.

4. The hands should not be lifted from the chest or the position changed in any way so that correct hand position is maintained.

Rescue breathing and chest compressions are combined for an effective resuscitation effort of the victim of cardiopulmonary arrest. When there is one rescuer, the rate of compression should be 80 to 100 compressions per minute with a compression-ventilation ratio of 15 compressions to 2 ventilations (Table 34-13). The compression rate for two-rescuer CPR is 80 to 100 per minute, with a compression-ventilation ratio of 5:1 (Table 34-14).

It is preferable to have two persons performing CPR (see Table 34-14). One person, positioned at the victim's side, performs chest compressions while the other rescuer, positioned at the victim's head, maintains an open airway and performs

Table 34-14 Adult Two-Rescuer CPR

Step	Objective	Critical Performance
1. Airway	*One rescuer (ventilator):*	
	Assessment: Determine unresponsiveness.	Tap or gently shake shoulder.
	Position the victim.	Shout "Are you OK?"
	Open the airway.	Turn on back if necessary (4-10 sec).
		Use a proper technique to open airway.
2. Breathing	Assessment: Determine cessation of breathing.	Look, listen, and feel for breath (3-5 sec).
	Ventilate twice.	Observe chest rise: 1.5-2 sec/inflation.
3. Circulation	Assessment: Determine absence of pulse.	Feel for carotid pulse (5-10 sec).
	State assessment results.	Say "No pulse."
	Other rescuer (compressor):	When another rescuer comes, first rescuer asks if EMS has been activated.
	Get into position for compressions.	Put hands, shoulders in correct position.
	Locate landmark notch.	Check landmark.
4. Compression-ventilation cycles	*Compressor:* Begin chest compressions.	Correct ratio compressions-ventilations is 5:1.
		Compression rate is 80-100/min (5 compressions/3-4 sec).
		Say any helpful mnemonic.
		Stop compressing for each ventilation.
	Ventilator: Ventilate after every fifth compression and check compression effectiveness.	Ventilate once (1.5-2 sec/inflation).
		Check pulse occasionally to assess compressions.
	(Minimum of 10 cycles)	(Time for 10 cycles: 40-53 sec)
5. Calling for switch	*Compressor:* Call for switch when tired.	Give clear signal to change roles.
		Compressor completes fifth compression.
		Ventilator completes ventilation after fifth compression.
6. Switching	Simultaneously switch:	
	Ventilator: Move to chest.	Become compressor.
		Get into position for compressions.
		Locate landmark notch.
	Compressor: Move to head.	Become ventilator.
		Check carotid pulse (5 sec).
		Say "No pulse."
		Ventilate once (1.5-2 sec/inflation).
7. Continuation of CPR	Resume compression-ventilation cycles.	Repeat step 4.

Source: *Textbook of basic life support for healthcare providers,* Dallas, 1997, American Heart Association.

ventilations. When the person doing chest compressions becomes fatigued, the two rescuers should exchange positions as quickly as possible.[30]

The victim's condition must be assessed during CPR to determine the effectiveness of compressions and to determine whether the victim has resumed spontaneous circulation and breathing. The pulse should be checked by the ventilating rescuer during the compressions to assess the effectiveness of compressions in two-rescuer CPR. Chest compressions are stopped for 5 seconds at the end of the first minute and every few minutes thereafter to determine whether the victim has resumed spontaneous breathing and circulation. The goal of CPR is the return of spontaneous breathing and circulation, but it is rarely achieved without more definitive therapy with ACLS.

Advanced Cardiac Life Support

ACLS involves a systematic approach to treatment of cardiac emergencies with knowledge and skills necessary to provide early treatment. ACLS includes (1) basic life support (BLS); (2) the use of adjunctive equipment and special techniques for establishing and maintaining effective ventilation and circulation; (3) ECG monitoring and arrhythmia recognition; (4) establishment and maintenance of IV access; (5) therapies for emergency treatment of patients with cardiac or respiratory arrest (including stabilization in the postarrest phase); and (6) treatment of patient with suspected acute MI.[11]

The principle of early defibrillation has been emphasized in national emergency medical care organizations. With the invention of the automated external defibrillator (AED), which is simple to use and available throughout communities, more trained rescuers are available to provide early defibrillation. The importance of early, effective BLS and defibrillation before entrance into the ACLS system cannot be overemphasized.[11] Drugs used in ACLS are listed in Table 34-15.

Medical professionals trained in ACLS are taught treatment algorithms that are guidelines for treatment of specific cardiac

DRUG THERAPY

Table 34-15 Drugs Used in Advanced Cardiac Life Support

First-Line Drugs	Second-Line Drugs
Oxygen	**Inotropic Vasoactive Agents**
Epinephrine	Norepinephrine
Atropine	Dopamine (Intropin)
Antiarrhythmic Agents	Dobutamine (Dobutrex)
Lidocaine	Isoproterenol (Isuprel)
Procainamide (Pronestyl)	Amrinone (Inocor)
Bretylium (Bretylol)	Digitalis
Verapamil (Calan, Isoptin)	**Vasodilators/Antihypertensives**
Diltiazem (Cardizem)	Sodium nitroprusside
Adenosine (Adenocard)	Nitroglycerin
Miscellaneous	**Beta-Adrenergic Blockers**
Magnesium	Propanolol (Inderal)
Sodium bicarbonate	Metoprolol (Lopressor)
Morphine	Atenolol (Tenormin)
Calcium chloride	Esmolol (Brevibloc)
	Diuretics
	Furosemide (Lasix)
	Thrombolytic Agents
	Anisoylated plasminogen-streptokinase activator complex (APSAC, anistreplase [Eminase])
	Streptokinase (Streptase)
	Tissue plasminogen activator (tPA, alteplase [Activase])
	Recombinant plasminogen activator (rPA, reteplase [Retavase])

CRITICAL THINKING EXERCISES

CASE STUDY

Arryhthmia

Patient Profile

J.M., a 68-year-old retired postal worker, is admitted to the cardiac care unit following cardiac arrest. After defibrillation is performed by paramedics, J.M. is awake and lethargic but responding appropriately.

Subjective Data

- Has had two MIs and a history of CHF
- Has shortness of breath, even in a sitting position

Objective Data

Physical Examination

- Appears anxious
- BP 92/60, pulse 98/min, respirations 28/min
- Lungs: bilateral coarse crackles
- Heart: S_3 gallop at apex

Diagnostic Studies

- ECG: frequent PVCs
- Echocardiogram: severe left ventricular dysfunction with ejection fraction of 20%
- Serum potassium 2.9 mEq/L (2.9 mmol/L)

Collaborative Care

- Lidocaine infusion 2 mg/min
- Scheduled for electrophysiology study (EPS)

Critical Thinking Questions

1. Why is J.M. at risk for sudden cardiac death (ventricular fibrillation)?
2. Explain the rationale for using lidocaine after ventricular fibrillation.
3. What methods may be used to assess the effectiveness of the antiarrhythmic drugs?
4. Would J.M. be a candidate for an ICD?
5. If J.M. had ventricular fibrillation again while on a lidocaine infusion, what other IV medications would be tried?
6. Explain the significance of the serum potassium value.
7. Based on the assessment data provided, write one or more appropriate nursing diagnoses. Are there any collaborative problems?

emergencies. The algorithm can be adjusted to fit the needs of a particular patient or situation. Emphasis is placed on maintaining the basics of airway, breathing, and circulation and making judgments for effective treatment based on overall patient assessment.[11]

Nursing Role During a Code

There is potential for a "code," or cardiopulmonary arrest situation, in all hospital settings. The nurse should be well prepared to participate in resuscitation of a patient. The nurse must be familiar with code protocols, be familiar with emergency equipment in the crash cart, and keep current with BLS and ACLS skills.

It is important for the nurse to be familiar with the crash cart location and contents on the hospital unit. Most crash carts contain all necessary emergency supplies. Ideally, all crash carts in an individual hospital are organized in the same fashion.

REVIEW QUESTIONS

The number of the question corresponds to the same-numbered objective at the beginning of the chapter.

1. A patient with a stable blood pressure and no symptoms has the following electrocardiogram characteristics:
   Atrial rate—74 and regular
   Ventricular rate—62 and irregular
   P wave—normal contour
   PR interval—lengthens progressively until a P wave is not conducted
   QRS—normal contour

   The nurse would expect that treatment would involve
   a. epinephrine 1 mg IV push.
   b. isoproterenol IV continuous drip.
   c. immediate insertion of a temporary pacemaker.
   d. careful observation for symptoms of hypotension.
2. The cardiac monitor of a patient in the cardiac care unit following an acute MI indicates ventricular bigeminy. The nurse anticipates
   a. performing defibrillation.
   b. treatment with IV lidocaine.
   c. insertion of a temporary pacemaker.
   d. continuing monitoring without other treatment.
3. The nurse prepares a patient for electrical cardioversion knowing that cardioversion differs from defibrillation in that
   a. defibrillation requires a greater dose of electrical current.
   b. defibrillation is synchronized to countershock during the QRS complex.
   c. cardioversion is indicated only for treatment of atrial tachyarrhythmias.
   d. cardioversion may be done on a nonemergency basis with sedation of the patient.
4. When providing discharge instructions to a patient with a new permanent pacemaker the nurse teaches the patient to
   a. take and record a daily pulse rate.
   b. request special hand scanning at airport and other security gates.
   c. immobilize the arm and shoulder on the side of the pacemaker insertion for 6 weeks.
   d. avoid microwave ovens because they emit radio waves that alter pacemaker function.
5. The nurse plans care for the patient with an implantable cardioverter-defibrillator based on the knowledge that
   a. all members of the patient's family should learn CPR.
   b. antiarrhythmia drugs can be discontinued.
   c. the patient should not drive until 1 month after the ICD has been implanted.
   d. the patient is usually relieved to have the device implanted to prevent arrhythmias.
6. Important teaching for the patient who will be undergoing electrophysiologic monitoring includes explaining that
   a. a catheter will be placed in each of the femoral arteries to allow double catheter use.
   b. the patient will be given a general anesthetic to prevent the awareness of "near-death" experiences.
   c. ventricular tachycardia and ventricular fibrillation may be induced and treated during the procedure.
   d. the procedure is used to "burn" or ablate areas of the conduction system that are causing tachyarrhythmias.
7. The proper sequence for care of the obstructed airway victim who becomes unconscious is
   a. abdominal thrusts; finger sweep into mouth; call for second rescuer; attempt rescue breathing.
   b. call 911; finger sweep into mouth; attempt rescue breathing; abdominal thrusts if still obstructed.
   c. finger sweep into mouth; attempt rescue breathing; call 911; abdominal thrust if still obstructed.
   d. attempt rescue breathing; abdominal thrusts if still obstructed; finger sweep into mouth; call 911.
8. A procedure that is common to both BLS and ACLS is
   a. use of ECG monitoring.
   b. adminstration of emergency cardiac drugs.
   c. establishment and maintenance of IV access.
   d. establishment and maintenance of a patent airway.

References

1. Scrima DE: Foundations of arrhythmia interpretation, *Medsurg Nurs* 6:4, 1997.
2. Podrid PJ, Kowey PR: *Handbook of cardiac arrhythmia,* Baltimore, 1996, Williams & Wilkins.
3. Goldberger AL, Goldberger E: *Clinical electrocardiography: a simplified approach,* ed 5, St Louis, 1994, Mosby.
4. Vlay SC: *A practical approach to cardiac arrhythmias,* ed 2, Boston, 1996, Little, Brown.
5. Marriott HJL: *Marriott's manual of electrocardiography,* Orlando, 1995, The Trinity Press.
6. Walraven G: *Basic arrhythmias,* New Jersey, 1995, Brady-Prentice-Hall.
7. Ehrat KS: *The art of EKG interpretation—a self instructional text,* ed 4, Dubuque, Ia, 1997, Kendall/Hunt.
8. Messerli FH: *Cardiovascular drug therapy,* ed 2, Philadelphia, 1996, Saunders.
9. Fogoros RN: *Antiarrhythmic drugs—a practical approach,* Malden, Mass, 1997, Blackwell Science.
10. Futterman LG, Lemberg L: Radiofrequency catheter ablation for supraventricular tachycardias: part II, *Am J Crit Care* 3:77, 1994.
11. Cummins RO, editor: *Advanced cardiac life support,* Dallas, 1997, American Heart Association.
12. Roden DM: Ibutilide and the treatment of atrial arrhythmias, *Circulation* 94:1499, 1996.
13. Pill MW: Ibutilide: a new antiarrhythmic agent for the critical care environment, *Crit Care Nurse* 17:19, 1997.
14. Futterman LG, Lemberg L: Atrial fibrillation; an increasingly common and provocative arrhythmia, *Am J Crit Care* 5:379, 1996.
15. Prystowsky EN and others: Management of patients with atrial fibrillation, *Circulation* 93:1262, 1996.
16. Atrial Fibrillation Investigators: Risk factors for stroke and efficacy of antithrombotic therapy in atrial fibrillation, *Arch Intern Med* 154:1449, 1994.
17. Riley RD, Pritchett ELC: Pharmacologic management of atrial fibrillation, *J Cardiovasc Electrophysiol* 8:818, 1997.
18. Futterman LG, Lemberg L: Amiodarone: a late comer, *Am J Crit Care* 6:233, 1997.

19. Roden DM: A practical approach to torsades de pointes, *Clin Cardiol* 20:285, 1997.
20. Futterman LG, Lemberg L: The long QT syndrome: when syncope is common in the young and the elderly, *Am J Crit Care* 4:405, 1995.
21. Califf RM, Mark DB, Wagner GS: *Acute coronary care,* ed 2, St Louis, 1995, Mosby.
22. Myerburg RJ, Castellanos A: Cardiac arrest and sudden cardiac death. In Braunwald E, editor: *Heart disease,* ed 5, Philadelphia, 1997, Saunders.
23. Task Force of the Working Group on Arrhythmias of the European Society of Cardiology: The Sicilian Gambit. A new approach to the classification of antiarrhythmic drugs based on their actions on arrhythmogenic mechanisms, *Circulation* 84:1831, 1991.
24. Knight L and others: Caring for patients with third-generation implantable cardioverter-defibrillators, *Crit Care Nurse* 17:46, 1997.
25. Raviele A: Implantable cardioverter-defibrillator (ICD) indications in 1996: have they changed? *Am J Cardiol* 78(suppl 5A):21, 1996.
26. Fetter JG and others: Electromagnetic interference from welding and motors on implantable cardioverter defibrillators as tested in the electrically hostile work site, *J Am Coll Cardiol* 28:423, 1996.
27. Gallager RD: The impact of the implantable cardioverter defibrillator on quality of life, *Am J Crit Care* 6:16, 1997.
28. Horwood L and others: Antitachycardia pacing: an overview, *Am J Crit Care* 4:397, 1995.
29. Kusumoto FM, Goldschlager N: Cardiac pacing, *N Engl J Med* 334:89, 1996.
30. *Basic life support for health care providers,* Dallas, 1997, American Heart Association.

Resources

Resources for this chapter are listed after Chapter 33 on p. 917.

REMEMBER to check out your **companion CD-ROM**

35 NURSING MANAGEMENT Inflammatory and Valvular Heart Diseases

Nancy Stoetzner Kupper & Ellen Stoetzner Duke

www.mosby.com/MERLIN/medsurg_lewis

LEARNING OBJECTIVES

1. Describe the etiology, pathophysiology, and clinical manifestations of infective endocarditis and pericarditis.
2. Discuss the nursing and collaborative management of infective endocarditis and pericarditis.
3. Explain the importance of prophylactic antibiotic therapy in infective endocarditis.
4. Explain the etiology, clinical manifestations, and collaborative care of myocarditis.
5. Describe the etiology, pathophysiology, and clinical manifestations of rheumatic fever and rheumatic heart disease.
6. Discuss the nursing and collaborative management of the patient with rheumatic fever and rheumatic heart disease.
7. Identify the etiologies of congenital and acquired valvular heart diseases.
8. Discuss the pathophysiology, clinical manifestations, and diagnostic studies for the various types of valvular heart problems.
9. Describe the nursing and collaborative management of valvular heart disease.
10. Describe surgical interventions used in management of the patient with valvular heart problems.

INFLAMMATORY DISORDERS OF THE HEART

INFECTIVE ENDOCARDITIS

Infective endocarditis, previously known as bacterial endocarditis, is an infection of the endocardial surface with microorganisms present in the lesion.[1] The endocardium, the inner layer of the heart (Fig. 35-1), is contiguous with the valves of the heart. Therefore inflammation from infective endocarditis usually affects the cardiac valves.

Before the era of antibiotics, infective endocarditis was almost always fatal. The advent of penicillin therapy changed the prognosis dramatically, and mortality rates decreased appreciably. For example, the mortality rate of infective endocarditis from viridans streptococci is now less than 10%. In spite of the relatively uncommon nature of the disease, an estimated 5000 to 8000 new cases of endocarditis are diagnosed in the United States each year.[2] Infective endocarditis continues to pose a significant clinical challenge.

Classification

Two forms of infective endocarditis, subacute and acute, have been described. The subacute form has a longer clinical course of more insidious onset with less toxicity, and the causative organism is usually of low virulence (most often viridans streptococci). In contrast, the acute form has a shorter clinical course with a more rapid onset, increased toxicity, and a more pathogenic causative organism (usually *Staphylococcus aureus*).[1] Although this classification system has been used historically and may be conceptually useful, clinicians prefer to classify infective endocarditis based on the etiologic agent.

Etiology and Pathophysiology

The most common causative agents are bacterial, especially *S. aureus, Streptococcus pyogenes,* and *Streptococcus pneumoniae* (Table 35-1). Other possible pathogens include fungi, chlamydiae, rickettsiae, and viruses.

Infective endocarditis occurs when blood flow turbulence within the heart allows the causative organism to infect previously damaged valves or other endothelial surfaces. The damage may occur in individuals with underlying cardiac conditions (Table 35-2). A variety of invasive procedures (e.g., surgical interventions, intravenous injection, and diagnostic procedures) can allow large numbers of organisms to enter the bloodstream and trigger the infectious process (see Tables 35-2 and 35-5).

Conditions predisposing to infective endocarditis have changed because of decreasing incidence of rheumatic heart disease, increased recognition and treatment of mitral valve prolapse, the aging population with degenerative heart disease, and IV drug abuse.[3] With the increasing use of valve replacement, prosthetic valve endocarditis has continued to rise. Left-sided endocarditis is more common in patients with bacterial infections and underlying heart disease. The primary cause of

Reviewed by Linda Schakenbach, RN, MSN, CS, CCRN, CETN, Clinical Nurse Specialist, Surgical Nursing, Inova Fairfax Hospital, Annandale, Va.

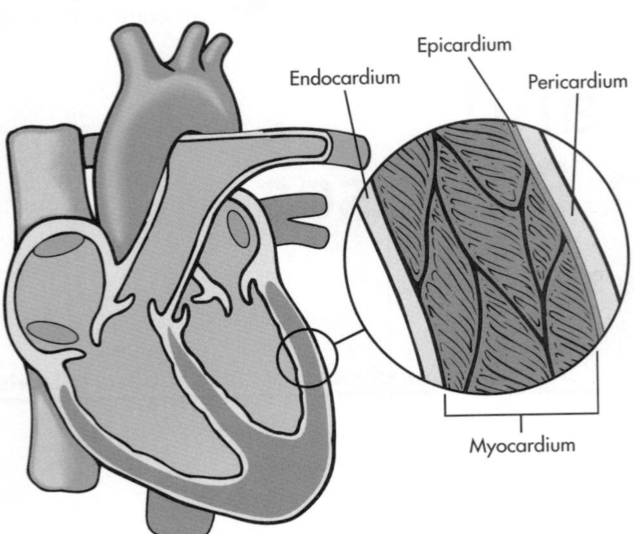

Fig. 35-1 Layers of the heart.

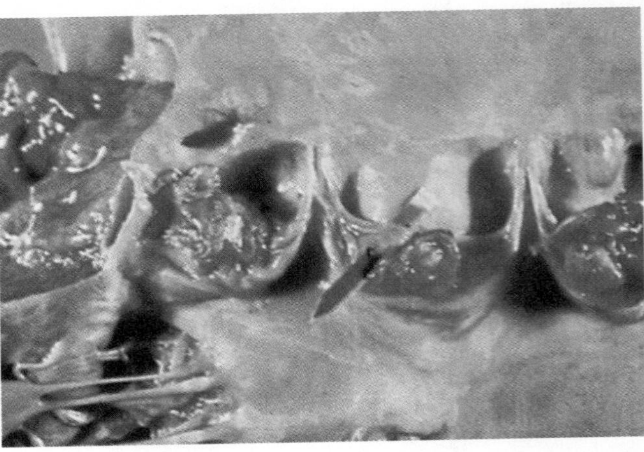

Fig. 35-2 Bacterial endocarditis of the mitral valve (caused by streptococci).

Table 35-1 Etiologic Organisms Associated with Infective Endocarditis

Streptococci
α-Hemolytic streptococci
Enterococci
Streptococcus bovis
Streptococcus pneumoniae
Staphylococci
Staphylococcus aureus
Staphylococcus epidermidis
Gram-negative Bacteria
Escherichia coli
Klebsiella
Pseudomonas
Polymicrobic Endocarditis
Staphylococcus agalactiae and methicillin susceptible *S. aureus*
Pseudomonas aeruginosa, α-hemolytic streptococci, and *Micrococcus*
Haemophilus, Actinobacillus, Cardiobacterium, Eikenella, and Kingella

Table 35-2 Predisposing Conditions to the Development of Infective Endocarditis

Cardiac Conditions
Rheumatic heart disease
Aortic valve leaflet abnormalities
Mitral valve prolapse with murmur
Cyanotic congenital heart disease
Prosthetic valves
Degenerative valvular lesions
Prior endocarditis
Marfan's syndrome
Asymmetric septal hypertrophy
Idiopathic hypertrophic subaortic stenosis
Noncardiac Diseases
Intravenous illicit drug use
Nosocomial bacteremia
Procedure-Associated Risks
Intravascular devices (leading to nosocomial bacteremia)
Procedures listed in Table 35-5

right-sided (tricuspid) lesions is IV drug abuse, especially cocaine abuse. Staphylococcal infections frequently occur in this patient population, although gram-negative bacilli, yeasts, or fungi may be the infecting organisms.

Vegetation, the primary lesions of infective endocarditis, consist of fibrin, leukocytes, platelets, and microbes that adhere to the valve surface or endocardium (Fig. 35-2). The loss of portions of these friable types of vegetation into the circulation results in embolization. Systemic embolization occurs from left-sided heart vegetation, progressing to organ (particularly the brain, kidneys, and spleen) and limb infarction. Right-sided heart lesions embolize to the lungs.

The infection may spread locally to cause damage to the valves or to their supporting structures. The resulting valvular incompetence and eventual invasion of the myocardium in the infectious disease result in congestive heart failure (CHF), generalized myocardial dysfunction, and sepsis (Fig. 35-3).

Clinical Manifestations

The findings in infective endocarditis are nonspecific and can involve multiple organ systems. Fever occurs in more than 90% of patients with endocarditis. Other nonspecific manifestations that may accompany fever include chills, weakness, malaise, fatigue, and anorexia. Arthralgias, myalgias, back pain, abdominal discomfort, weight loss, headache, and clubbing of fingers may occur in subacute forms of endocarditis.

Vascular manifestations of infective endocarditis include splinter hemorrhages (black longitudinal streaks) that may occur in the nailbeds. Petechiae may occur as a result of fragmentation and microembolization of vegetative lesions and are common in the conjunctivae, the lips, the buccal mucosa, the palate, and over the ankles, the feet, and the antecubital and

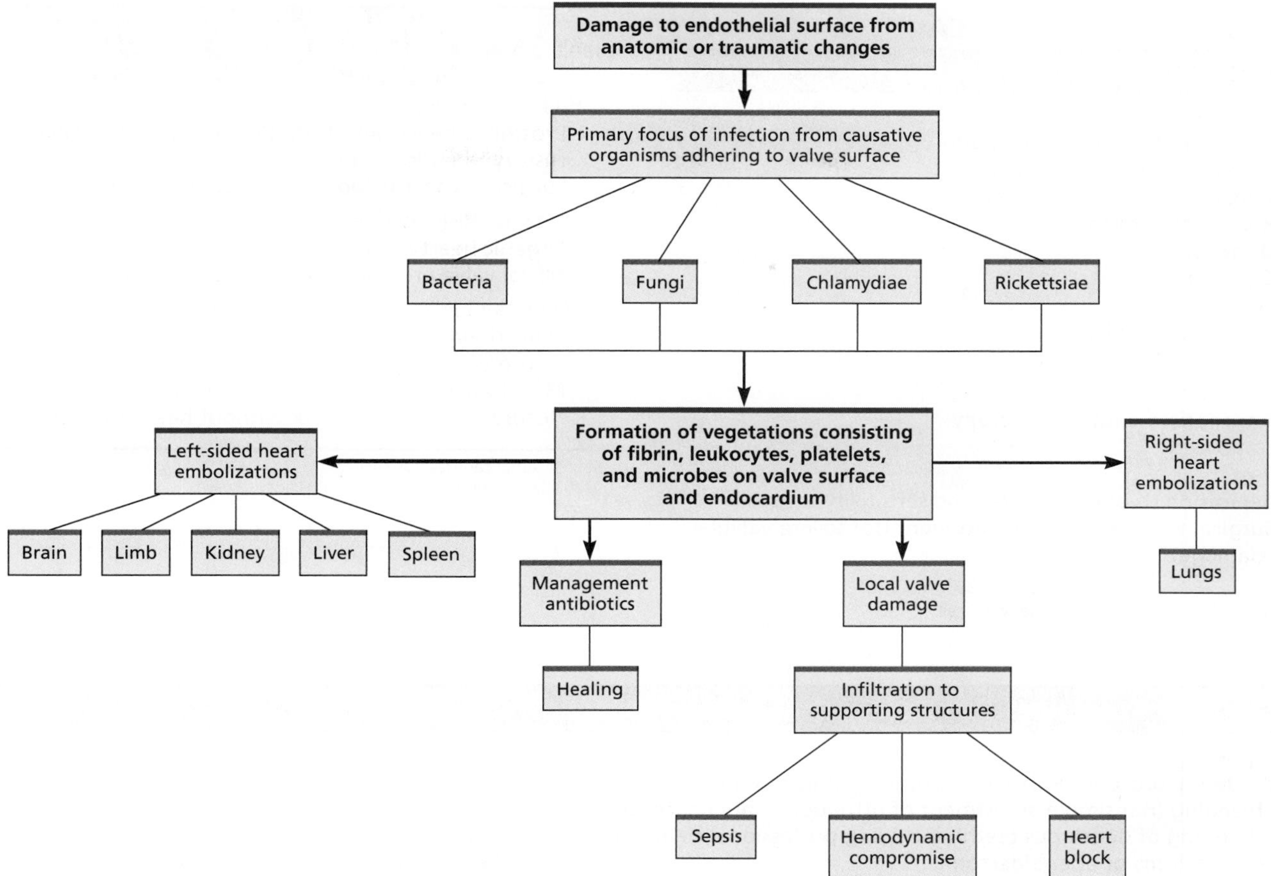

Fig. 35-3 Sequence of events in infective endocarditis.

popliteal areas. Osler's nodes (painful, tender, red or purple, pea-size lesions) may be found on the fingertips or toes. Janeway's lesions (flat, painless, small, red spots) may be found on the palms and soles. Funduscopic examination may reveal hemorrhagic retinal lesions called Roth's spots.

The onset of a new murmur is frequently noted with infective endocarditis, with the aortic and mitral valves most commonly affected. The mitral murmur of endocarditis is generally a mid-to-late systolic regurgitant type. The aortic murmur may be early diastolic. Murmurs are often absent in tricuspid endocarditis because right-sided heart pressures are too low to hear. CHF occurs in up to 80% of patients with aortic valve endocarditis and in approximately 50% of patients with mitral valve endocarditis.[1]

Clinical manifestations secondary to embolization in various body organs may also be present. Embolization to the spleen may result in sharp, left upper quadrant pain and splenomegaly. Local tenderness and abdominal rigidity may be present. Embolization to the kidneys may cause pain in the flank, hematuria, and azotemia. Emboli may lodge in small peripheral blood vessels of arms and legs and may cause gangrene. Embolization to the brain may cause neurologic problems such as hemiplegia, ataxia, aphasia, visual changes, and change in the level of consciousness. Pulmonary emboli may occur in right-sided endocarditis.

Diagnostic Studies

Obtaining the patient's recent health history is important in assessing infective endocarditis. Inquiry should be made regarding any recent (within the past 3 to 6 months) dental, urologic, surgical, or gynecologic procedures, including normal or abnormal obstetric delivery. Previous history of heart disease; recent cardiac catheterization; and skin, respiratory, or urinary tract infections should be documented.

Laboratory data, especially blood cultures, should also be assessed (Table 35-3). Blood cultures are the primary diagnostic tool for the evaluation of infective endocarditis. Positive blood cultures are found in 90% to 95% of patients with infective endocarditis. Two or three sets of blood cultures (a set consists of one aerobic and one anaerobic culture from one site) should be performed over a 24-hour period. Negative cultures should be kept for 3 weeks if the clinical diagnosis remains endocarditis, because of the possibility of a slow-growing, causative organism. The blood cultures may be obtained at 20-minute intervals if immediate antibiotic therapy is deemed necessary. Blood-culture bottles containing a resin to bind the antibiotic should be used if the patient is already receiving antibiotics. Culture-negative endocarditis may occur in those patients who have had previous antibiotic therapy, in patients with causative organisms that cannot be grown from blood using routine media (e.g., *Mycobacterium tuberculosis*), or in patients with right-sided infection of the heart.

A mild leukocytosis with average white blood cell (WBC) counts ranging from 10,000 − 11,000/μl ($10 - 11 \times 10^9$/L) and erythrocyte sedimentation rates (ESRs) greater than 30 mm per hour are often detectable. Proteinuria and positive rheumatoid factor may also be present in some patients with endocarditis.

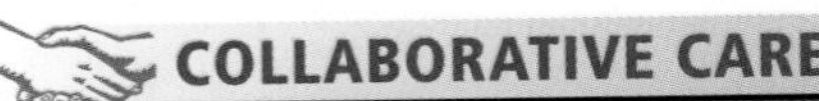

Table 35-3 Infective Endocarditis

Diagnostic
- History and physical examination
- Blood culture and sensitivity
- WBC count with differential
- Rheumatoid factor
- Urinalysis
- Chest x-ray
- ECG
- Echocardiography
- Cardiac catheterization

Collaborative Therapy
- Appropriate antibiotic therapy
- Antipyretics
- Rest
- Repetition of blood cultures and sensitivity tests
- Surgical valve repair or replacement (for severe valvular damage)

ECG, electrocardiogram; *WBC*, white blood cell.

Table 35-4 Antibiotic Prophylaxis to Prevent Endocarditis in Cardiac Conditions*

High-Risk Conditions
- Prosthetic heart valve (including biosynthetic valve)
- History of endocarditis
- Surgically constructed systemic-pulmonary shunts

Moderate-Risk Conditions
- Organic heart murmur
- Mitral valve prolapse with valvular regurgitation

Low-Risk Conditions (no prophylaxis)
- "Functional," "physiologic," or "innocent" heart murmur
- Mitral valve prolapse without valvular regurgitation
- History of rheumatic fever without heart murmur

Source: American Heart Association.
*Table lists common conditions, but is not inclusive.

Table 35-5 Procedures That Require Endocarditis Antibiotic Prophylaxis*

Oropharyngeal
- All dental procedures likely to produce gingival or mucosal bleeding (not simple adjustment of orthodontic appliances or shedding of deciduous teeth), including professional cleaning
- Tonsillectomy or adenoidectomy

Respiratory
- Surgical procedures or biopsy involving respiratory mucosa
- Bronchoscopy, especially with a rigid bronchoscope

Gastrointestinal
- Gallbladder surgery
- Colonic surgery
- Esophageal dilation
- Sclerotherapy of esophageal varices
- Colonoscopy

Genitourinary
- Cystoscopy
- Prostatic surgery
- Urethral catheterization (in presence of infection)
- Urinary tract surgery (in presence of infection)
- Vaginal hysterectomy
- Vaginal delivery in presence of infection

Cardiac
- Placement of prosthetic heart valves
- Surgically constructed systemic pulmonary shunts

Other
- Incision and drainage of infected tissue
- Surgery involving infected soft tissue

Modified from Dajani AS and others: Prevention of bacterial endocarditis: recommendations by the American Heart Association, *JAMA* 277:1796,1997.
*This table has selected procedures and is not all inclusive.

Echocardiography is valuable in the diagnostic workup for a patient with infective endocarditis when the blood cultures are negative, or for the patient who is a surgical candidate and has an active infection. Transesophageal echocardiograms and digital imaging using two-dimensional transthoracic echocardiograms can detect vegetation and abscesses on valves.

A chest x-ray examination is done to detect the presence of CHF. An electrocardiogram may reveal changes during endocarditis because the cardiac valves lie in proximity to cardiac conductive tissue, especially the atrioventricular (AV) node. Cardiac catheterization may be used when surgical intervention is being considered for patients with infective endocarditis.

Prophylactic Treatment

Cardiac lesions, prosthetic valves, acquired valvular disease, mitral valve prolapse, prior endocarditis, and noncardiac diseases are the principal risk factors for infective endocarditis.[2] Procedure-associated risks, including intravenous injection of recreational drugs and specific dental, medical, or surgical procedures, must also be considered.[3,4] Antibiotic prophylaxis is recommended for patients with specific cardiac conditions before they undergo certain dental or surgical procedures (Table 35-4). Procedures that require endocarditis prophylaxis are summarized in Table 35-5. Specific antibiotic regimens are recommended for dental, respiratory tract, gastrointestinal (GI), and genitourinary (GU) procedures.[5] Antibiotic prophylaxis should also be instituted in high risk patients who (1) are to undergo removal or drainage of infected tissue, (2) have indwelling cardiac pacemakers, (3) undergo renal dialysis, and (4) have ventriculoatrial shunts for management of hydrocephalus.[5-8]

Collaborative Care

Accurate identification of the infecting organism is the key to successful treatment. The appropriate antibiotic (usually given intravenously) is chosen on the basis of sensitivity studies.

DRUG THERAPY

Table 35-6 Treatment of Infective Endocarditis with Outpatient Antibiotic Therapy

Etiologic Agent or Clinical Situation	Antibiotic Regimen Options
Streptococcal endocarditis	IV/IM ceftriaxone*; IV/IM ceftriaxone* plus IV/IM gentamicin;† IV/IM ceftriaxone* followed by oral amoxicillin
Enterococcal endocarditis without renal failure	IV ampicillin plus IV/IM gentamicin†
Enterococcal endocarditis with renal failure	IV vancomycin‡
Staphylococcal endocarditis	IV nafcillin; IV vancomycin‡
Right-sided staphylococcal endocarditis in IV drug abusers	IV nafcillin plus tobramycin

Source: Dajani AS and others: Prevention of bacterial endocarditis. Recommendations of the American Heart Association, *Circulation* 96:358, 1997.
*Endocarditis is not an FDA-approved indication for ceftriaxone therapy.
†Serum concentrations should be monitored.
‡Establish dose according to renal function and serum drug level

NURSING ASSESSMENT

Table 35-7 Infective Endocarditis

Subjective Data	Objective Data
Important Health Information *Past health history:* Valvular, congenital, or syphilitic cardiac disease (including valve repair or replacement); previous endocarditis, childbirth, staphylococcal or streptococcal infections, nosocomial bacteremia *Medications:* Immunosuppressive therapy *Surgery and other treatments:* Recent obstetric or gynecologic procedures; invasive techniques including catheterization, cystoscopy, intravascular procedures; recent dental or surgical procedure **Functional Health Patterns** *Health perception–health management:* IV drug abuse, alcohol abuse; malaise *Nutritional-metabolic:* Weight gain or loss; anorexia; chills, diaphoresis *Elimination:* Bloody urine *Activity-exercise:* Exercise intolerance, generalized weakness, fatigue; cough, dyspnea on exertion, orthopnea; palpitations *Sleep-rest:* Night sweats *Cognitive-perceptual:* Chest, back, or abdominal pain; headache; joint tenderness, muscle tenderness	**General** Fever **Integumentary** Olser's nodes on extremities; splinter hemorrhages under nailbeds; Janeway's lesions on palms and soles; petechiae of skin, mucous membranes, or conjunctivae; purpura; peripheral edema, finger clubbing **Respiratory** Tachypnea, crackles **Cardiovascular** Arrhythmias, tachycardia, new or enhanced murmurs, S_3, S_4, retinal hemorrhages **Possible Findings** Leukocytosis, anemia, elevated ESR and cardiac enzymes; positive blood cultures; microscopic hematuria; echocardiogram showing chamber enlargement, valvular dysfunction, and vegetations; chest x-ray showing cardiomegaly and pulmonary infiltrates; ECG demonstrating ischemia and conduction defects

ESR, erythrocyte sedimentation rate.

Complete eradication of the organism generally takes weeks to achieve, and relapses are common. Traditionally this has meant a prolonged hospitalization for most patients with infective endocarditis. Currently, with the use of newer, more versatile antibiotics and in light of economic concerns, treatment of patients with infective endocarditis on an outpatient basis is becoming more common.[3] Table 35-6 outlines specific regimens for outpatient therapy of patients with endocarditis. Some patients require changes in antibiotics because of allergic reactions or other drug-related side effects.

The patient's antibiotic serum levels should be monitored periodically. Subsequent blood cultures may be performed to evaluate the effectiveness of antibiotic therapy. Blood cultures that remain positive indicate inadequate or inappropriate antibiotic administration, aortic root or myocardial abscess, or the wrong diagnosis (e.g., an infection elsewhere). Fever may persist for several days after treatment has been started and can be treated with aspirin, acetaminophen, fluids, and rest. Complete bed rest is usually not indicated unless the temperature remains elevated or there are signs of heart failure.

The results of drug therapy alone are generally poor in patients with fungal endocarditis and prosthetic valve endocarditis. Early valve replacement followed by prolonged drug therapy is recommended in these situations. Valve replacement has become an important adjunct procedure in the management of endocarditis, with it being used in greater than 25% of cases.

NURSING MANAGEMENT: INFECTIVE ENDOCARDITIS

■ Nursing Assessment

Subjective and objective data that should be obtained from a patient with infective endocarditis are presented in Table 35-7. Heart sounds should be assessed together with vital signs to

35-1 NURSING CARE PLAN PATIENT WITH INFECTIVE ENDOCARDITIS

Expected Patient Outcomes	Nursing Interventions and *Rationales*
NURSING DIAGNOSIS **Hyperthermia** *related to* infection of cardiac tissue *as manifested by* temperature elevation, diaphoresis, chills, headache, malaise, tachycardia, tachypnea.	
■ Normal temperature. ■ Normal pulse (60-100) beats/min. ■ Normal respirations (12-20 breaths/min). ■ Absence of chills, diaphoresis, headache.	■ Monitor temperature *to determine effectiveness of therapy.* ■ Administer antipyretics or sedatives as ordered *to reduce fever and assist in sleep.* ■ Reduce physical activity *to decrease cardiac workload.* ■ Administer antibiotics *to treat the causative agent.* ■ Monitor blood cultures and WBC count *to evaluate patient's response to treatment.* ■ Cover patient with light blankets *to prevent shivering and subsequent additional temperature elevation from increased muscular activity.*
NURSING DIAGNOSIS **Decreased cardiac output** *related to* valvular insufficiency and fluid overload *as manifested by* heart murmur, S_3, tachycardia, capillary refill time greater than 3 sec, diminished peripheral pulses, adventitious breath sounds, decreased urine output, restlessness, confusion.	
■ Sufficient cardiac output to maintain mean arterial BP $\geq$ 60 mm Hg and urine output greater than 0.5 ml/kg/hr.	■ Auscultate heart sounds, rate, and rhythm *to detect a change in the character of the cardiac murmur and the presence of extradiastolic sounds.* ■ Assess for peripheral and sacral edema *as indicators of ineffective circulation or fluid overload.* ■ Assess breath sounds *to identify pulmonary involvement, congestion, and fluid overload.* ■ Provide O_2 therapy *to increase O_2 to the myocardium and to promote comfort by relieving hypoxemia.* ■ Administer diuretics, inotropic therapy, and other medications as ordered *to promote diuresis and strengthen myocardial contractility.* ■ Plan rest periods *to reduce cardiac workload.* ■ Assess urine output *to monitor renal function and evaluate fluid status.* ■ Assess for changes in level of consciousness *to rule out embolization to the brain.*
NURSING DIAGNOSIS **Activity intolerance** *related to* generalized weakness and alteration in oxygen transport secondary to valvular dysfunction *as manifested by* fatigue, malaise, weakness, dyspnea, shortness of breath, pallor, cyanosis, confusion, vertigo, increased pulse, increased or decreased respiratory rate and BP.	
■ Completion of activities of daily living with no to minimal fatigue or physiologic distress.	■ Monitor vital signs during activity *to evaluate cardiac response.* ■ Monitor for signs of activity intolerance (e.g., tachycardia, hypertension, diaphoresis, shortness of breath) *to plan or alter activities.* ■ Reduce activity if systolic BP goes down 10 mm Hg *because this may indicate impaired ability of the heart to respond appropriately to increased activity.* ■ Teach patient to check pulse rate. ■ Instruct patient to reduce activity if pulse increases >20 beats/min and to not increase activity if resting pulse >100 beats/min, *since these signs indicate excessive cardiac effort.* ■ Plan rest periods between activities *to reduce cardiac workload.*
NURSING DIAGNOSIS **Anxiety** *related to* critical illness and hospitalization *as manifested by* restlessness, apprehension, withdrawal.	
■ Reduction in anxiety. ■ Increase in psychologic and physiologic comfort.	■ Observe for verbal and physiologic signs of anxiety *to diagnose anxiety and initiate a plan of care.* ■ Allow time for verbalization of fears related to illness, *since discussing fears openly is helpful in allaying anxiety.* ■ Encourage patient to discuss feelings and concerns about illness and hospitalization *to assess depth of feelings and accuracy of knowledge for planning interventions.* ■ Explain how all procedures and activities relate to patient's treatment plan *to give patient information that may reduce anxiety.* ■ Teach patient relaxation techniques such as imagery, muscle relaxation *to reduce anxiety by eliciting the relaxation response.*

Continued

35-1 NURSING CARE PLAN PATIENT WITH INFECTIVE ENDOCARDITIS —continued

Expected Patient Outcomes	Nursing Interventions and *Rationales*
NURSING DIAGNOSIS	**Altered health maintenance** *related to* lack of knowledge about disease and treatment process *as manifested by* nonperformance of desired prescribed health behaviors, verbalization of misconceptions about desired or prescribed health behaviors, requests for information.
▪ Increased understanding of disease process and self-care management.	▪ Assess patient's knowledge about disease and treatment process *to identify teaching needs.* ▪ Discuss symptoms of recurrent infection (e.g., fatigue, malaise, chills, elevated temperature, anorexia) *so physician can be notified and treatment initiated promptly.* ▪ Explain need to avoid persons with infections. ▪ Encourage early treatment of common infections such as cold and flu *to reduce the risk of recurrent infective endocarditis.* ▪ Explain need to report endocarditis history to the physician performing invasive procedures such as dental or gingival therapy, diagnostic tests, or medical and surgical procedures *so prophylactic antibiotic therapy can be initiated to prevent the possibility of infection.* ▪ Discuss names of prescribed medications, dosages, times of administration, purpose, and side effects *to promote safe drug therapy.*

COLLABORATIVE PROBLEMS

Nursing Goals	Nursing Interventions and *Rationales*
POTENTIAL COMPLICATION	**Emboli** *related to* dislodging of vegetations and immobility-related thrombophlebitis.
▪ Monitor for emboli to all organs. ▪ Report deviations from expected parameters. ▪ Carry out medical and nursing interventions.	▪ Perform pulmonary assessment, *since pulmonary emboli may produce decreased breath sounds, increased respiratory rate, dyspnea, and use of accessory muscles.* ▪ Monitor color of urine and specific gravity *to evaluate renal function for decreased output and hematuria.* ▪ Assess for abdominal pain, *since splenic emboli result in abdominal pain and splenomegaly.* ▪ Perform neurologic assessment *to detect signs of brain emboli.* ▪ Check temperature and pulses in extremities *since emboli may lodge in small peripheral blood vessels and cause gangrene.* ▪ Observe skin, eyes, mucous membranes for petechiae, *which occur as a result of fragmentation and microembolization of vegetative lesions.* ▪ Check fingernails for splinter hemorrhages; fingers, toes, palms, and soles of feet for Osler nodes; and skin surface for lesions *because these signs are indicative of emboli to the respective areas.* ▪ Observe for swelling, redness, calf tenderness *to identify possible signs of thrombophlebitis.* ▪ Apply elastic compression gradient stockings *to provide venous support to legs.* ▪ Teach patient leg exercises *to promote venous return and decrease the occurrence of thrombophlebitis.*

detect a change in the character of the cardiac murmur and the presence of extradiastolic sounds. Arthralgia is common and may involve multiple joints and may be accompanied by myalgias. The patient should be assessed for joint tenderness, decreased range of motion (ROM), and muscle tenderness. The oral mucosa, conjunctivae, upper chest, and lower extremities should be examined for petechiae. A general systems assessment should be completed to facilitate recognition of hemodynamic and embolic complications.

Nursing Diagnoses

Nursing diagnoses for the patient with infective endocarditis may include, but are not limited to, those presented in NCP 35-1.

Planning

The overall goals are that the patient with infective endocarditis will (1) have normal cardiac function, (2) have no residual cardiac damage, (3) perform activities of daily living (ADLs) without fatigue, and (4) understand the therapeutic regimen to prevent recurrence of endocarditis.

Nursing Implementation

Health Promotion. The incidence of infective endocarditis can be decreased by identifying individuals who are at risk for the development of endocarditis (see Tables 35-2 and 35-4). Assessment of the patient's history and an understanding of the disease process are crucial for planning and implementing appropriate health promotion strategies.

Education of the patient who is at risk or has had infective endocarditis helps reduce the incidence and recurrence of the disease. Education is crucial for the patient's understanding of and adherence to the planned treatment regimen. The patient should understand the need to avoid persons with infection, especially upper respiratory, and to report cold, flu, and cough symptoms. The importance of avoiding excessive fatigue and the need to plan rest periods before and after activity should be carefully explained to the patient. Good oral hygiene, including daily care and regular dental visits, is also important. The patient must inform all health care providers performing dental, medical, or surgical procedures of the history of heart disease. The patient should understand the significance of the prescribed prophylactic antibiotic therapy before any invasive procedure.

Acute Intervention. A patient with infective endocarditis has many problems that require astute nursing management (see NCP 35-1). Infective endocarditis generally requires treatment with antibiotics for 4 to 6 weeks. The patient requires in-hospital treatment and then may be a candidate for outpatient parenteral antibiotic therapy.

Physical assessment findings are nonspecific (see Table 35-7) but can help confirm the diagnosis and aid the treatment plans. Fever, chronic or intermittent, is a common early sign. Frequent assessment of body temperature is important because persistent, prolonged temperature elevations may mean that the drug therapy is ineffective.

The patient needs adequate periods of physical and emotional rest. Bed rest may be necessary when fever is present or when there are complications (e.g., heart damage). Otherwise the patient may ambulate and perform moderate activity.

Laboratory data should be monitored to determine the effectiveness of the long-term, high-dose antibiotic therapy received by the patient. IV lines should be monitored for patency, and antibiotics should be given when scheduled. The patient should be monitored continuously for undesirable reactions to drugs. To prevent problems because of immobility, the patient should wear elastic compression gradient stockings, perform ROM exercises, and turn, cough, and deep breathe every 2 hours.

The patient may experience anxiety and fear associated with the illness. The nurse must recognize this problem and implement strategies to help reduce the patient's fears and anxieties.

Ambulatory and Home Care. Patients who receive outpatient antibiotics will require vigilant home nursing care. Patients with active endocarditis are at risk for life-threatening complications, such as cerebral emboli and pulmonary edema. The adequacy of the home environment in terms of in-home companions and hospital access must be determined for successful management. After therapy is completed in either the home or the hospital setting, management will focus on educating the patient about the nature of the disease and on reducing the risk of reinfection. The patient should be instructed about symptoms that may indicate recurrent infection, such as fever, fatigue, malaise, and chills. If any of these symptoms occur, the patient should be aware of the importance of notifying the physician. The patient must be instructed about the need for prophylactic antibiotic therapy before any invasive procedure is performed (see Table 35-5). The nurse must explain to the patient the relationship of follow-up care, good nutrition, and early treatment of common infections (e.g., colds) to maintain good health.

Evaluation

Expected outcomes for the patient with infective endocarditis are presented in NCP 35-1.

ACUTE PERICARDITIS

Pericarditis is a condition caused by inflammation of the pericardial sac (the pericardium), which may occur on an acute basis. The pericardium is composed of the inner serous membrane (visceral pericardium) that closely adheres to the epicardial surface of the heart and the outer fibrous (parietal) layer (see Fig. 35-1). The pericardial space is the cavity between these two layers, and in the normal state it contains less than 50 ml of serous fluid. Although the pericardium may be congenitally absent or surgically removed, it serves a useful anchoring function, provides lubrication to decrease friction during systolic and diastolic heart movements, and assists in preventing excessive dilation of the heart during diastole.

Etiology and Pathophysiology

The common causes of acute pericarditis are listed in Table 35-8. Acute pericarditis in the adult patient is most often idiopathic, with a variety of suspected viral causes. The coxsackievirus B group is the most commonly identified virus and tends to elicit

Table 35-8 Etiologies of Pericarditis

Etiologies of Pericarditis
Infectious
Viral causes, including coxsackievirus B, coxsackievirus A, echovirus, adenovirus, mumps, Epstein-Barr, varicella zoster, hepatitis B
Bacterial causes, including pneumococci, staphylococci, streptococci, septicemia from gram-negative organisms
Tuberculosis
Fungal causes, including histoplasma, *Candida* species
Infections such as toxoplasmosis, Lyme disease
Noninfectious
Uremia
Acute myocardial infarction
Neoplasms, such as lung cancer, breast cancer, leukemia, Hodgkin's disease, lymphoma
Trauma after thoracic surgery, pacemaker insertion, cardiac diagnostic procedures
Radiation
Dissecting aortic aneurysm
Myxedema
Hypersensitive or Autoimmune
Delayed postmyocardial-pericardial injury
Post–myocardial infarction (Dressler's) syndrome
Postpericardiotomy syndrome
Rheumatic fever
Drug reactions (e.g., from procainamide [Pronestyl], hydralazine [Apresoline])
Rheumatologic diseases, including rheumatoid arthritis, systemic lupus erythematosus, scleroderma, ankylosing spondylitis

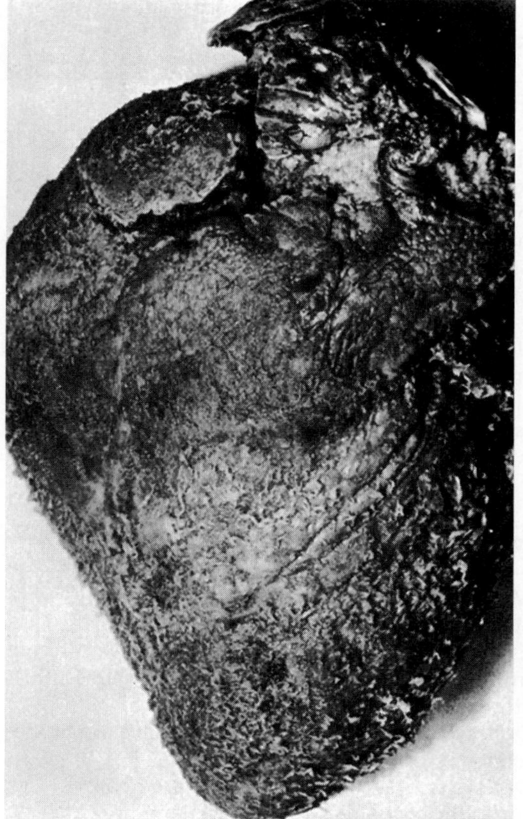

Fig. 35-4 Acute fibrinous pericarditis. There is a shaggy coat of fibrin covering the surface of the heart.

pleuropericarditis in adults (Bornholm disease) and myopericarditis in children. In addition to idiopathic or viral pericarditis, other causes of this syndrome include uremia, bacterial infection, acute myocardial infarction (MI), tuberculosis, neoplasm, and trauma.[9] Pericarditis in the acute MI patient may be described as two distinct syndromes.[10] Acute pericarditis immediately follows myocardial damage within the initial 48 to 72 hours. Dressler's syndrome (late pericarditis) appears 2 to 4 weeks after infarction.

An inflammatory response is the characteristic pathologic finding in acute pericarditis. There is an influx of neutrophils, increased pericardial vascularity, and eventually fibrin deposition on the visceral pericardium (Fig. 35-4).

Clinical Manifestations

Characteristic clinical manifestations found in acute pericarditis include chest pain, dyspnea, and a pericardial friction rub. The intense, pleuritic chest pain is generally sharpest over the left precordium or retrosternally but may radiate to the trapezius ridge and neck (mimicking angina), or sometimes to the epigastrium or abdomen (mimicking abdominal or other noncardiac pathologic conditions). The pain is aggravated by lying supine, deep breathing, coughing, swallowing, and moving the trunk and is eased by sitting up and leaning forward. The dyspnea accompanying acute pericarditis is related to the patient's need to breathe in rapid, shallow breaths to avoid chest pain and may be aggravated by fever and anxiety.

The hallmark finding in acute pericarditis is the pericardial friction rub. The rub is a scratching, grating, high-pitched sound believed to arise from friction between the roughened pericardial and epicardial surfaces.[10] It is best heard with the stethoscope diaphragm firmly placed at the lower left sternal border of the chest. The pericardial friction rub does not radiate widely or vary in timing from the heartbeat, but it may require frequent auscultation to identify because it may be elusive and transient. Timing the pericardial friction rub with the pulse (and not respirations) will help distinguish it from pleural rub.

Complications

Two major complications that may result from acute pericarditis are pericardial effusion and cardiac tamponade. Pericardial effusion is generally a rapid accumulation of excess pericardial fluid that occurs in chest trauma. However, a slowly developing effusion may result, as in tuberculous pericarditis. Large effusions may compress adjoining structures. Pulmonary tissue compression can cause cough, dyspnea, and tachypnea. Phrenic nerve compression can induce hiccups,

Table 35-9 Clinical Manifestations of Cardiac Tamponade

Decrease in systolic BP
Narrowing pulse pressure
Pulsus paradoxus (>10 mm Hg)
Increase in venous pressure, distention of neck veins
Tachycardia
Tachypnea
Possible friction rub
Muffled heart sounds
Low-voltage ECG
Rapid enlargement of cardiac silhouette on chest x-ray
Peripheral cyanosis
Anxiety
Chest pain

Table 35-10 Measurement of Pulsus Paradoxus

1. Make determination during quiet breathing with stable rhythm.
2. Establish systolic pressure.
3. Inflate BP cuff until no sounds are heard with stethoscope.
4. Deflate cuff slowly until systolic sounds are heard on expiration and note the pressure.
5. Deflate cuff until systolic sounds are heard throughout the respiratory cycle and note the pressure.
6. Determine the difference between (4) and (5). This will equal the amount of paradox:

Sounds heard in expiration at	110 mm Hg
Sounds heard throughout cycle at	82 mm Hg
Amount of paradox	28 mm Hg

The difference is usually less than 10 mm Hg. If the difference is greater than 10 mm Hg, cardiac tamponade may be present.

COLLABORATIVE CARE

Table 35-11 Acute Pericarditis

Diagnostic
- History and physical examination
- Auscultation of chest
- ECG
- Chest x-ray
- Echocardiography
- Pericardiocentesis
- Pericardial biopsy
- CT scan
- Nuclear scan of heart

Collaborative Therapy
- Treatment of underlying disease
- Bed rest
- Aspirin
- Nonsteroidal antiinflammatory agents
- Corticosteroids
- Pericardiocentesis (for large pericardial effusion or tamponade)

and compression of the recurrent laryngeal nerve may result in hoarseness. Heart sounds are generally distant and muffled, although blood pressure (BP) is usually maintained by compensatory mechanisms.

Cardiac tamponade develops as the pericardial effusion increases in size. Compensatory mechanisms ultimately fail to adjust to the decreased cardiac output. The patient with pericardial tamponade is often confused, agitated, and restless and has tachycardia and tachypnea with a low-output state (Table 35-9). The neck veins are usually markedly distended because of jugular venous pressure elevation, and a significant pulsus paradoxus is present. Pulsus paradoxus, an inspiratory drop in systolic BP greater than 10 mm Hg, results because the normal inspiratory decline in systolic BP of less than 10 mm Hg is exaggerated in cardiac tamponade. The technique for measurement of pulsus paradoxus is outlined in Table 35-10.

Diagnostic Studies

ECG changes in acute pericarditis are key diagnostic clues and evolve over a period of hours to days or weeks (Table 35-11). Four stages of ECG changes have been described: (1) initial diffuse ST segment elevations that concave upward and are present in all leads except aVR and V_1; (2) return of ST segments to baseline with T wave flattening several days later; (3) T wave inversion without the appearance of significant Q waves seen in acute MI; and (4) reversion of T wave changes to normal that may occur weeks or months later.[10] PR segment depression may also be present in the early stages of ST segment changes. The changes are believed to be caused by superficial myocardial inflammation or epicardial injury. Arrhythmias can accompany these ECG changes but are generally rare occurrences. When encountered, they are usually atrial arrhythmias in patients who also have myocardial or valvular pathologic conditions.

The chest x-ray findings are generally normal or nonspecific in acute pericarditis unless the patient has a large pericardial effusion (Fig. 35-5). Echocardiographic findings are much more useful in determining the presence of a pericardial effusion or cardiac tamponade. Additional diagnostic studies such as gallium radionuclide heart scans may be performed, although their sensitivity in diagnosing pericarditis has not yet been determined.

Laboratory testing focuses on the possible etiology of the pericarditis. For example, elevated blood urea nitrogen (BUN) levels and serum creatinine levels may indicate uremic pericarditis, or a positive tuberculin skin test may suggest tuberculous pericarditis. The fluid obtained during pericardiocentesis (Fig. 35-6) or the tissue from a pericardial biopsy may also be analyzed to determine the cause of the pericarditis.

Collaborative Care

Management of acute pericarditis is directed toward identification and treatment of the underlying problem (see Table 35-11). Antibiotics should be used to treat bacterial pericarditis. Corticosteroids are generally reserved for patients with pericarditis secondary to systemic lupus erythematosus, patients already

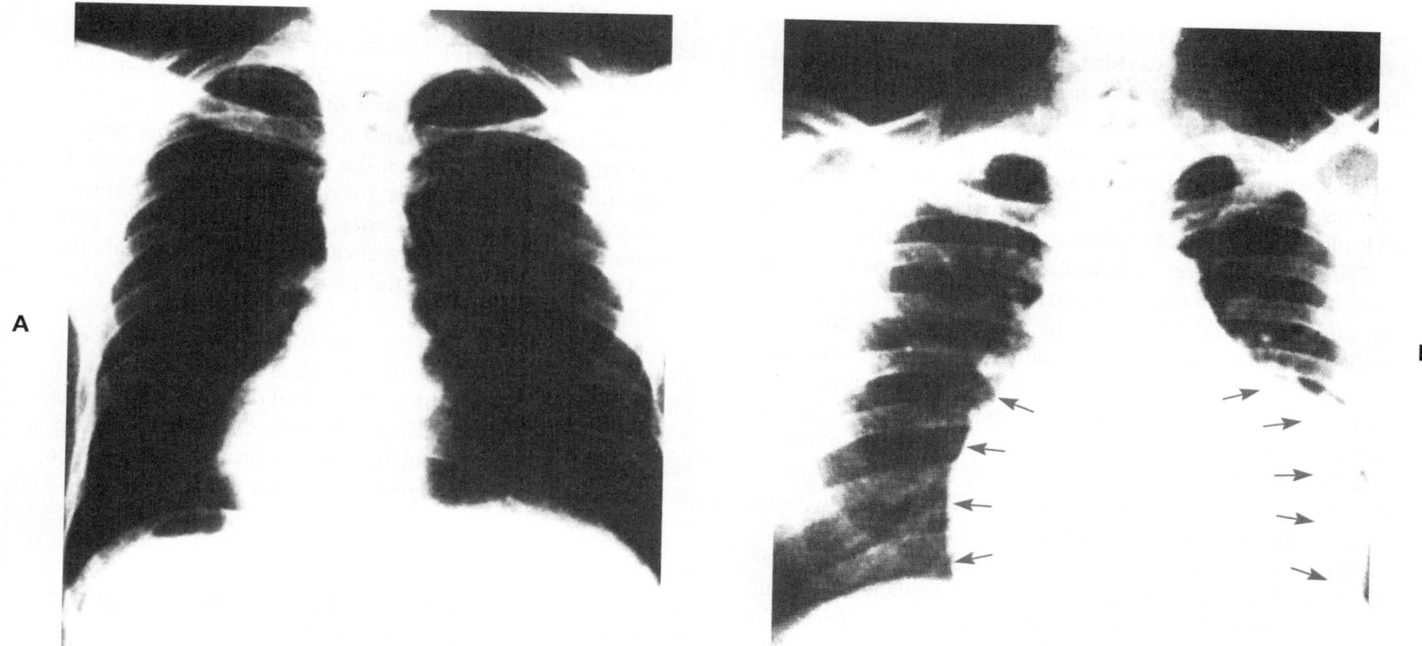

Fig. 35-5 **A,** X-ray of a normal chest. **B,** Pericardial effusion is present and the cardiac silhouette is enlarged with a globular shape *(arrows).*

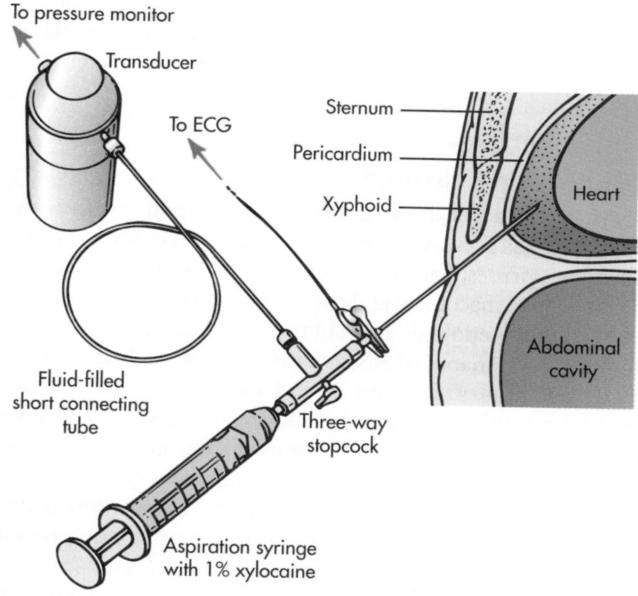

Fig. 35-6 Pericardiocentesis performed under sterile conditions in conjunction with electrocardiogram (ECG) and hemodynamic measurements.

taking corticosteroids for a rheumatologic or other immune system condition, or patients who do not respond to nonsteroidal antiinflammatory drugs (NSAIDs). When necessary, prednisone is usually given according to a tapering dosage schedule (see Chapter 47). Discriminate and careful administration of corticosteroids is advised because of their numerous side effects, such as peptic ulcer disease, sodium retention, hyperglycemia, hypokalemia, and Cushing's syndrome (see Chapter 47).

The pain and inflammation of acute pericarditis are usually treated with NSAIDs. High-dose salicylates (300 to 900 mg orally four times a day) or NSAIDs, such as indomethacin (Indocin), are commonly used.

Pericardiocentesis (see Fig. 35-6) is usually performed when acute cardiac tamponade has reduced the patient's systolic BP 30 mm Hg or more from baseline. Hemodynamic support for the patient being prepared for the pericardiocentesis may include administration of volume expanders and inotropic agents. The procedure is usually performed in the cardiac care unit or cardiac catheterization laboratory under sterile conditions and in conjunction with ECG, echocardiogram, and hemodynamic measurements. A 16- to 18-gauge needle is inserted into the pericardial space to remove fluid for analysis and to relieve cardiac pressure. Complications from pericardiocentesis include arrhythmias, pneumomediastinum, pneumothorax, myocardial laceration, cardiac tamponade, coronary artery laceration, and gastric fistula.

NURSING MANAGEMENT: ACUTE PERICARDITIS

The management of the patient's pain and anxiety during acute pericarditis are primary nursing considerations. Assessment of the amount, quality, and location of the pain is important, particularly in distinguishing the pain of acute MI (or reinfarction) from the pain of pericarditis. Careful nursing observations should be made regarding ischemic chest pain, which is generally located retrosternal in the left shoulder and arm with a pressure-like, burning quality and is unaffected by posture. In contrast, pericarditic pain is usually located in the precordium, left trapezius ridge and has a sharp, pleuritic quality that changes with respirations. Relief from this pain is often obtained by leaning forward, and the pain is worsened by recumbency. The ECG also aids in distinguishing these types of pain because acute MI usually involves localized ST segment changes, as compared with the ST segment changes present in all leads except aVR and V_1 during acute pericarditis.

Pain relief measures include maintaining the patient on bed rest with the head of the bed elevated to 45 degrees and providing a padded overbed table for the patient. Antiinflammatory medications help alleviate the patient's pain. However, because of the potential for GI problems with the use of high doses of these medications, nursing interventions should be directed toward management of this potential problem. Specific interventions include the administration of these drugs with food or milk and instruction of the patient to avoid any alcoholic beverages while taking the medications.

Anxiety-reducing measures for the patient with acute pericarditis include providing simple, complete explanations of all procedures performed. These explanations are particularly important for the patient whose diagnosis of acute pericarditis is being established and for the patient who has already experienced an acute MI and has pericarditis (Dressler's syndrome).

The real potential for decreased cardiac output (CO) also exists for the patient with acute pericarditis because of the possibility of cardiac tamponade. Monitoring for the signs and symptoms of tamponade (see Table 35-9) and making preparations for possible pericardiocentesis are important nursing responsibilities.

CHRONIC CONSTRICTIVE PERICARDITIS

Etiology and Pathophysiology

Constrictive pericarditis usually begins with an initial episode of acute pericarditis (often secondary to neoplasia, radiation, previous surgery, or idiopathic causes) and is characterized by fibrin deposition with a clinically undetected pericardial effusion. Organization and resorption of the effusion slowly follows with progression toward the chronic stage of fibrous scarring, thickening of the pericardium from calcium deposition, and eventual obliteration of the pericardial space. The fibrotic, thickened, and adherent pericardium encases the heart, thereby impairing the ability of the atria and ventricles to stretch adequately during diastolic filling.

Clinical Manifestations

Manifestations of chronic constrictive pericarditis occur over an extended time period and mimic those of CHF and cor pulmonale. They include dyspnea on exertion, lower extremity edema, ascites, fatigue, anorexia, and weight loss. The most prominent finding at the physical examination is elevated jugular venous pressure. Unlike cardiac tamponade, the presence of significant pulsus paradoxus is uncommon. Auscultatory findings include a pericardial knock, which is a loud early diastolic sound often heard along the left sternal border.

Diagnostic Studies

ECG changes may be nonspecific in chronic constrictive pericarditis but usually consist of low QRS voltage, generalized T wave inversion or flattening, and either P mitrale or atrial fibrillation. The cardiac silhouette on the chest x-ray may be normal or enlarged depending on the degree of pericardial thickening and the presence of a coexisting pericardial effusion. Echocardiographic findings may reveal a thickened pericardium, but without the presence of a large pericardial effusion. Distinctions between the myocardium and epicardium are difficult to ascertain.

Cardiac catheterization pressure tracings are more specific diagnostic tools in constrictive pericarditis. Abnormalities include elevation of the right and left atrial pressures with equilibration of these pressures during diastole. Other valuable diagnostic tools used to evaluate this condition are computed tomography (CT) and magnetic resonance imaging (MRI).

NURSING AND COLLABORATIVE MANAGEMENT: CHRONIC CONSTRICTIVE PERICARDITIS

Unless the patient is free of symptoms or the condition is inoperable, the treatment of choice for chronic constrictive pericarditis is a pericardiectomy. The pericardiectomy usually involves complete resection of the pericardium through a median sternotomy with the use of cardiopulmonary bypass. The postoperative prognosis is improved when the surgery is performed before the development of severe clinical disability. Postoperative nursing care after a pericardiectomy is similar to that of other open heart surgical procedures (see Chapter 33).

MYOCARDITIS

Etiology and Pathophysiology

Myocarditis, a focal or diffuse inflammation of the myocardium, has been associated with a variety of etiologic agents, including viruses, bacteria, rickettsiae, fungi, parasites, radiation, and pharmacologic and chemical factors.[11] Viruses are the most common etiologic agent in the United States and Canada, with a predominance of RNA viruses (coxsackievirus A and B, echovirus, influenza A and B, and mumps virus).[11] Certain medical conditions such as metabolic disorders and collagen-vascular diseases (e.g., systemic lupus erythematosus) may also precipitate myocarditis. Myocarditis may also occur when no causative agent or factor can be identified. Myocarditis is frequently associated with acute pericarditis, particularly when it is caused by coxsackievirus B strains or echoviruses.

The pathophysiologic mechanisms of myocarditis are poorly understood because there is usually a period of several weeks after the initial infection before the development of manifestations of myocarditis. Immunologic mechanisms may play a role in the development of myocarditis. The majority of infections are benign, self-limiting, and subclinical, although viral myocarditis in infants and pregnant women may be virulent.

Clinical Manifestations

The clinical features for patients with myocarditis are variable, ranging from a benign course without any overt manifestations to severe heart involvement or sudden death. Fever, fatigue, malaise, myalgias, pharyngitis, dyspnea, lymphadenopathy, and GI symptoms are early systemic manifestations of the viral illness.

Early cardiac manifestations appear 7 to 10 days after viral infection and include pericardial chest pain with an associated friction rub because pericarditis often accompanies myocarditis. Cardiac signs (S_3, crackles, jugular venous distention, and peripheral edema) may progress to CHF, including pericardial effusion, syncope, and possibly ischemic pain.

Diagnostic Studies

The ECG changes for a patient with myocarditis are often nonspecific and reflect associated pericardial involvement, including diffuse ST segment abnormalities. Arrhythmias and conduction disturbances may be present. Laboratory findings are also often inconclusive, with the presence of mild to moderate leukocytosis and atypical lymphocytes, elevated viral titers (virus is generally only present in tissue and fluid samples during the initial 8 to 10 days of illness), increased ESR, and elevated levels of myocardial enzymes such as aspartate aminotransferase (AST), creatine kinase (CK), and lactic dehydrogenase (LDH).

Histologic confirmation of myocarditis is possible through endomyocardial biopsy (EMB), a technique in which several small pieces of myocardial tissue are percutaneously removed from the right ventricle with a special instrument called a bioptome and microscopically examined. A biopsy done during the initial 6 weeks of acute illness is most diagnostic because this is the period in which lymphocytic infiltration and myocyte damage indicative of myocarditis are present. Special myocardial imaging techniques may also be used in the diagnostic evaluation of myocarditis.

Collaborative Care

The specific treatment for myocarditis has yet to be established and usually consists of managing associated cardiac decompensation. Digoxin is often used to treat ventricular failure because it improves myocardial contractility and reduces ventricular rate. Digoxin should be used cautiously in patients with myocarditis, because of the increased sensitivity of the heart to the adverse effects of this drug and the potential toxicity with minimal doses. Oxygen therapy, bed rest, restricted activity, and maintenance of standby emergency equipment are general supportive measures used for management of myocarditis.

Immunosuppression with agents such as prednisone, azathioprine (Imuran), and cyclosporine has been used in a limited number of patients with myocarditis to reduce myocardial inflammation and to prevent irreversible myocardial damage.[15] Administration of immunosuppressive agents is recommended only during the postinfectious stage of the disease, approximately 10 days after the onset of initial symptoms. If used early in the course of viral myocarditis, these drugs can actually increase tissue necrosis.[11] The use of corticosteroids for the treatment of myocarditis remains controversial because of the associated serious side effects and the lack of clear documentation of their efficacy.

NURSING MANAGEMENT: MYOCARDITIS

Decreased cardiac output is an ongoing nursing diagnosis in the care of the patient with myocarditis. Interventions focus on assessment for the signs and symptoms of CHF and institution of measures to decrease cardiac workload, such as the use of semi-Fowler's position, spacing of activity and rest periods, and provisions for a quiet environment. Prescribed medications that increase the heart's contractility and decrease the preload, afterload, or both are administered. Careful monitoring and evaluation of the patient taking these medications are necessary.

The patient may be anxious about the diagnosis of myocarditis, recovery from myocarditis, and therapy. Nursing measures include assessing the level of anxiety, instituting measures to decrease anxiety, and keeping the patient and family informed about therapeutic measures.

The patient who receives immunosuppressive therapy has additional problems of alterations in the immune response with the potential for infection and complications related to the therapy. Guidelines for care include monitoring for complications and providing the patient with a clean, safe environment by following proper infection control procedures.

The majority of individuals with myocarditis recover spontaneously. Occasionally, acute myocarditis progresses to chronic dilated cardiomyopathy (see Chapter 33).

RHEUMATIC FEVER AND HEART DISEASE

Rheumatic fever is an inflammatory disease of the heart potentially involving all layers (endocardium, myocardium, and pericardium). The resulting damage to the heart from rheumatic fever is termed *rheumatic heart disease,* a chronic condition characterized by scarring and deformity of the heart valves.

Acute rheumatic fever (ARF) is a complication of up to 3% of sporadic upper respiratory infections caused by group A β-hemolytic streptococci.[12] Initial and recurrent episodes of ARF are most common from ages 6 through 15. Most recurrences occur within 2 years of the initial episode.[12] Recurrent attacks of rheumatic fever are twice as common between the ages of 11 and 22 as they are after the age of 22. The frequency of recurrence of rheumatic fever after streptococcal infection is greater in those patients with rheumatic heart disease than in those who have not had cardiac injury during previous attacks.[13] Attacks do occur in adulthood and are probably more common than previously believed. However, the sequelae of rheumatic heart disease are found primarily in young adults.

A spectacular decline in the incidence of rheumatic fever was observed in the 1960s and 1970s. By the 1980s rheumatic fever had almost disappeared in developed countries such as the United States. However, it remained frequent and severe in most developing countries. Antibiotics, especially penicillin, are responsible for the decline in rheumatic fever. Antibiotics given within 9 days of the appearance of streptococcal sore throat, before the immune system completely responds, can prevent rheumatic complications.[14] A decrease in the prevalence of bacterial strains with the natural ability to trigger rheumatic complications has also contributed to the decline.

Etiology

Rheumatic fever almost always occurs as a delayed sequela (usually after 2 to 3 weeks) of a group A β-hemolytic streptococcal infection of the upper respiratory system, usually a pharyngeal infection. Streptococcal infections of the skin are not associated with ARF, and some strains of group A β-hemolytic streptococci do not cause rheumatic fever. Although all attacks of rheumatic fever follow a streptococcal infection, only a few streptococcal infections are followed by rheumatic fever.

In addition to the infecting organisms, socioeconomic factors, familial factors, and the presence of an altered immune response have a predisposing role in the development of rheumatic fever. The incidence of rheumatic fever is higher in low socioeconomic groups and remains a major public health problem in the poorer developing countries. Crowded living conditions may be the major factor contributing to this finding. Neglect, inadequate treatment, poor nutrition, and a lowered state of health may be other reasons why lower socioeconomic groups in the United States and Canada and persons in developing countries are more commonly affected. Rheumatic fever is more likely to develop in people living in urban areas than in rural communities. There also seems to be a familial tendency toward rheumatic fever, which may be genetically determined, possibly leading to an altered immune response.[15]

A great deal of interest has been generated by a number of well-documented "mini-epidemics" of acute rheumatic fever in the United States during the last decade. Typically these outbreaks have involved 10 to 75 cases during a circumscribed time period in a single region. Often these have involved only one strain of streptococcus at each location. These may be isolated cases, but there is a question of whether these outbreaks indicate a general upswing in acute rheumatic fever across the country.[16] In searching for the cause of the reappearance, researchers have focused their efforts on isolating strains of group A streptococci. Researchers have isolated highly virulent mucoid strains of the same M protein serotypes that were prevalent in epidemic rheumatic fever more than 30 years ago. Another finding under consideration is the role of hyaluronate (a principal constituent of the group A streptococcal capsule) in the pathogenesis of the disease. Streptococcal hyaluronate, previously thought to be nonantigenic, induces the production of antibodies in animals. It is theorized that the body may have an allergic response to the streptococcus, or the host has an autoimmune response in which antibodies to the streptococci attack host tissue.[15] In the majority of new patients, a sore throat was never noted or reported. The infection that set off the immune system was so mild that the patient did not seek medical care. These reemergent strains of streptococci are capable of causing rheumatic fever, while producing such mild sore throats that no treatment is sought until it is too late to prevent complications.

Pathophysiology

The correlation of streptococcal pharyngitis with rheumatic fever is conclusive, but the pathogenic mechanisms by which the streptococcal infection causes inflammation of the heart and other tissues are not well defined. The organism is not demonstrable in the lesions when rheumatic fever appears several days or weeks after the acute streptococcal infection. Normally, antibodies are produced in response to infections with

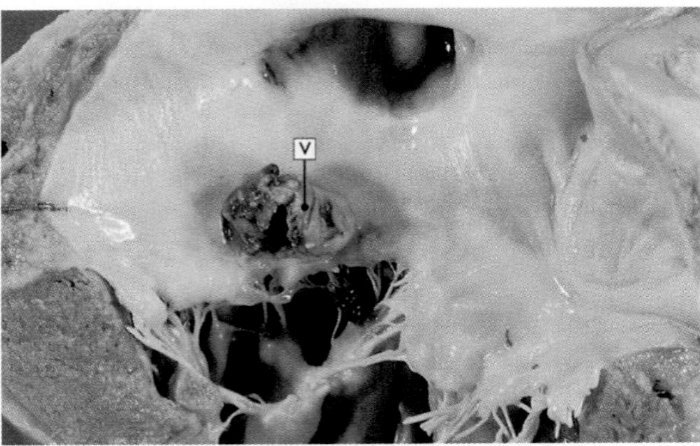

Fig. 35-7 Mitral stenosis and clumps of vegetation *(V)* containing platelets and fibrin. Mitral leaflets are thickened and fused and have clumps of vegetation containing platelets and fibrin.

streptococcal organisms. Episodes of primary and recurrent ARF have been associated with a greater antibody response than those found with uncomplicated streptococcal sore throats.

Manifestations of ARF appear to be related (in susceptible individuals) to an abnormal immunologic response to an upper respiratory infection with group A β-hemolytic streptococci. ARF probably affects the heart, joints, central nervous system (CNS), and skin because of an abnormal humoral and cell-mediated immune response to group A hemolytic streptococcal cell membrane antigens. It is possible that these antigens cross-react with other tissues and bind to receptors on heart, muscle, joint, and brain cells triggering immune and inflammatory responses.[17] However, the direct relationship of this cross-reactive phenomenon to pathology is unproven, and streptococcus-induced autoimmunity as a mechanism to explain the rheumatic process remains a popular but unestablished pathogenetic concept.

Cardiac Lesions and Valvular Deformities. About 40% of ARF episodes are marked by carditis, and all layers of the heart (endocardium, myocardium, and pericardium) may be involved. This generalized involvement gives rise to the term *rheumatic pancarditis.*

Rheumatic endocarditis is found primarily in the valves, with swelling and erosion of the valve leaflets. Vegetations form from deposits of fibrin and blood cells in areas of erosion (Fig. 35-7). The lesions initially create fibrous thickening of the valve leaflets, fusion of commissures and chordae tendineae, and fibrosis of the papillary muscle. Valve leaflets may fuse and become thickened or even calcified, resulting in stenosis. Reduction in the mobility of valve leaflets may occur with failure of the leaflets to appose, resulting in regurgitation. The mitral and aortic valves are most commonly affected; less commonly involved are the tricuspid valve and, rarely, the pulmonic valve.

Myocardial involvement is characterized by Aschoff's bodies, which are nodules formed by a reaction to inflammation with accompanying swelling and fragmentation of collagen fibers. As Aschoff's bodies age, they become more fibrous, and

Table 35-12 Modified Jones Criteria for Acute Rheumatic Fever

Major Criteria	Minor Criteria
Carditis	Fever
Polyarthritis	Previous occurrence of rheumatic fever or rheumatic heart disease
Chorea	Arthralgia
Erythema marginatum	Prolonged PR interval
Subcutaneous nodules	Laboratory findings*

Source: American Heart Association.
*See Table 35-13.

Table 35-13 Laboratory Test Abnormalities in Acute Rheumatic Fever

Antistreptolysin O titer	>250 IU/ml
Erythrocyte sedimentation rate	>15 mm/hr in men, >20 mm/hr in women
C-reactive protein	Positive
Throat culture	Positive for streptococci (usually negative)
WBC count	Elevated
Red blood cell parameters (Hct, Hb, RBCs)	Mild to moderate degree of normocytic, normochromic anemia

Hb, hemoglobin; *Hct,* hematocrit; *RBC,* red blood cell; *WBC,* white blood cell.

scar tissue is formed in the myocardium. In addition to Aschoff's bodies, a diffuse cellular infiltrate is present in interstitial tissues. This interstitial myocarditis may be more important than nodular Aschoff's bodies in producing heart failure.

Rheumatic pericarditis affects both layers of the pericardium, which become thickened and covered with a fibrinous exudate, and a serosanguineous pericardial fluid may be present. When healing occurs, fibrosis and adhesions develop that partially or completely obliterate the pericardial sac, but constrictive pericarditis does not occur.

These pathophysiologic changes in the heart may occur as a result of an initial attack of rheumatic fever. However, recurrent infections may cause further structural damage.

Extracardiac Lesions. The lesions of rheumatic fever are systemic, especially involving the connective tissue. The joints (polyarthritis), skin (subcutaneous nodules), CNS (chorea), and lungs (fibrinous pleurisy and rheumatic pneumonitis) can be involved in rheumatic fever.

Clinical Manifestations

The diagnosis of ARF is suggested by a clustering of signs and symptoms as well as from laboratory findings. When not observed in its most severe form, the disease may be difficult to differentiate from many illnesses with similar clinical manifestations. Criteria were established by T.D. Jones in 1944, revised by the American Heart Association in 1965, and updated in 1992 to provide a logical basis for diagnosis (Table 35-12). The presence of two major criteria or one major and two minor criteria indicates a high probability of ARF. Either combination must have evidence of an existing streptococcal infection.

Major Criteria. Carditis is the most important manifestation of ARF (see Table 35-12), with three signs including (1) an organic heart murmur or murmurs of mitral or aortic regurgitation, or mitral stenosis; (2) cardiac enlargement and CHF occurring secondary to myocarditis; and (3) pericarditis resulting in distant heart sounds, chest pain, a pericardial friction rub, or signs of effusion. Large effusions are rare but can lead to cardiac tamponade.

Polyarthritis, which is not a cause of permanent disability, is the most common finding in rheumatic fever. The inflammatory process affects the synovial membranes of the joints causing swelling, heat, redness, tenderness, and limitation of motion. The arthritis is migratory, affecting one joint and then moving to another. The larger joints are most frequently affected, particularly the knees, ankles, elbows, and wrists. The pain may prevent the patient from being able to walk.

Chorea (Sydenham's chorea) is the major CNS manifestation. It is characterized by weakness, ataxia, and choreic movement that is spontaneous, rapid, and purposeless, which tends to intensify with voluntary activity. Females under 18 years of age are primarily affected.

Erythema marginatum lesions are a less common feature of ARF. The bright-pink maplike macular lesions occur mainly on the trunk or inner aspects of the upper arm and thigh but never on the face. The rash is nonpruritic and nonpainful and is neither indurated nor raised. It is usually transitory (lasting for a few hours), may recur intermittently for months, and is exacerbated by heat (e.g., a warm bath).

Subcutaneous nodules are firm, small, hard, painless swellings found most commonly over bony prominences (e.g., knees, elbows, spine, scapulae). They frequently are not noticed by the person because the skin overlying the nodules moves freely and is not inflamed.

The presence of the major criteria of ARF vary among children and adults. In contrast to children, polyarthritis is the dominant clinical feature in adults, whereas carditis and subsequent valvular lesions are less prominent. In adults, two other major criteria, chorea and subcutaneous nodules, are usually not seen, and erythema marginatum occurs infrequently.

Minor Criteria. Minor clinical manifestations (see Table 35-12) are frequently present and are helpful in recognizing the disease. These criteria are too nonspecific to make a definitive diagnosis because they frequently occur in other diseases. The minor criteria are used as supplemental data to confirm the presence of rheumatic fever. Laboratory test abnormalities in rheumatic fever are presented in Table 35-13.

Complications

The course of rheumatic fever cannot be predicted at the onset of the disease, but generalizations can be made. Within 6 weeks, 75% of the symptoms associated with ARF attacks abate, and 90% abate within 3 months. Less than 5% of the symptoms last for more than 6 months.[17] Once all evidence of rheumatic inflammation has abated, rheumatic fever does not recur in the absence of a new streptococcal infection. If the initial episode is not associated with carditis, there is little likelihood of subsequent cardiac damage if repeated attacks do occur.

COLLABORATIVE CARE

Table 35-14 Rheumatic Fever

Diagnostic
- History and physical examination
- ASO titer
- Throat culture
- ESR
- C-reactive protein
- WBC count
- Chest x-ray
- Echocardiography
- ECG

Collaborative Therapy
- Bed rest (modified)
- Benzathine penicillin (1.2 million units IM) or procaine penicillin (600,000 units IM) qd for 10 days
- Acetylsalicylic acid
- Corticosteroids

ASO, antistreptolysin O; *ESR*, erythrocyte sedimentation rate.

A complication that can result from ARF is chronic rheumatic carditis. It results from changes in valvular structure that may occur months to years after an episode of ARF. Rheumatic endocarditis can result in fibrous tissue growth in valve leaflets and chordae tendineae with scarring and contractures. The mitral valve is most frequently involved. Other valves that may be affected are the aortic and tricuspid valves.

Diagnostic Studies

No single diagnostic test exists for rheumatic fever, but the results of combinations of laboratory studies suggest the presence of the disease (see Table 35-13). Throat cultures are usually negative at the onset of the disease because of the relatively long latent period of 10 days to several weeks after the precipitating infection. The most specific diagnostic test to confirm a recent group A streptococcal infection is measurement of the antistreptolysin O (ASO) titer. The ESR and measurement of C-reactive protein (CRP) are nonspecific tests indicative of a systemic inflammatory response.

An echocardiogram may show valvular insufficiency and pericardial fluid or thickening. A chest x-ray may show an enlarged heart if CHF is present. The most consistent electrocardiographic change is delayed AV conduction as evidenced in prolongation of the PR interval. Other ECG changes are frequent but nondiagnostic.

Collaborative Care

No specific treatment will cure rheumatic fever. Treatment consists of drug therapy and supportive measures (Table 35-14). Antibiotic therapy does not modify the course of the acute disease or the development of carditis. Penicillin eliminates residual group A β-hemolytic streptococci remaining in the tonsils and pharynx and prevents the spread of organisms to close contacts. Salicylates and corticosteroids are the two antiinflammatory agents most widely used in the management of ARF. Both are effective in controlling the fever and joint manifestations. Salicylates are used when arthritis is the main manifestation and corticosteroids are used if severe carditis is present.

Prolonged periods of bed rest have previously been recommended, but now the patient without carditis may be ambulatory as soon as acute symptoms have subsided and may return to normal activity when the antiinflammatory therapy has been discontinued. When carditis is present, ambulation is postponed until CHF has been controlled with treatment. Full activities should not be resumed until antiinflammatory therapy has been discontinued.

NURSING MANAGEMENT: RHEUMATIC FEVER AND HEART DISEASE

■ Nursing Assessment

Subjective and objective data that should be obtained from a patient with rheumatic fever and heart disease are presented in Table 35-15. Rheumatic fever is five times more likely to occur in a person with a previous history of rheumatic fever than in the general population. A higher incidence of ARF occurs in lower socioeconomic groups and in crowded living conditions. This may be related to poor treatment of streptococcal infections.

The skin of the patient should be assessed for subcutaneous nodules and erythema marginatum. The procedure involves palpation for subcutaneous nodules over all bony surfaces and along extensor tendons of the hands and feet. The nodules range in size from 1 to 4 cm and are hard, painless, and freely movable. Erythema marginatum can occur on the trunk and inner aspects of the upper arm and thigh. The erythematous maplike macules do not itch and are not raised. The possible presence of these bright pink macules should be assessed in good light because the rash is difficult to observe.

■ Nursing Diagnoses

Nursing diagnoses for the patient with rheumatic fever and heart disease may include, but are not limited to, those presented in NCP 35-2.

■ Planning

The overall goals are that the patient with rheumatic fever will (1) have no residual cardiac disease, (2) resume daily activities without joint pain, and (3) verbalize the ability to manage the disease.

■ Nursing Implementation

Health Promotion. Rheumatic fever is one of the few cardiovascular diseases that is preventable. Prevention is frequently classified as primary and secondary. Primary prevention involves early detection and immediate treatment of group A β-hemolytic streptococcal pharyngitis. Adequate treatment of streptococcal pharyngitis prevents initial attacks of rheumatic fever. Treatment consists of a single intramuscular (IM) injection of 0.6 to 1.2 million units of benzathine penicillin G or 10 days of oral penicillin G. If the patient is allergic to penicillin, clindamycin (Cleocin), vancomycin, or gentamicin may be substituted. Oral therapy requires faithful adherence to the full 10-day course of treatment. The nurse's

NURSING ASSESSMENT

Table 35-15 Rheumatic Fever

Subjective Data

Important Health Information

Past health history: Recent β-hemolytic streptococcal infection, previous rheumatic fever or rheumatic heart disease

Functional Health Patterns

Health perception–health management: Family history of rheumatic fever; malaise

Nutritional-metabolic: Anorexia, weight loss

Activity-exercise: Palpitations; generalized weakness, fatigue; ataxia

Cognitive-perceptual: Chest pain, abdominal pain; migratory joint pain and tenderness (especially large joints)

Objective Data

General

Low-grade fever

Integumentary

Subcutaneous nodules and erythema marginatum

Cardiovascular

Tachycardia, pericardial friction rub, distant heart sounds; gallop rhythm, diastolic and systolic murmurs, peripheral edema

Neurologic

Chorea (involuntary, purposeless, rapid motions; facial grimaces)

Musculoskeletal

Signs of polyarthritis including swelling, heat, redness, limitation of motion (especially of knees, ankles, elbows, shoulders, and wrists)

Possible Findings

Cardiomegaly on chest x-ray; delayed AV conduction on ECG; valve abnormalities, chamber dilation, and pericardial effusion on echocardiogram; elevated ASO titer, increased ESR, positive C-reactive protein, leukocytosis, decreased RBC, hemoglobin, and hematocrit

ASO, antistreptolysin O; *ESR,* erythrocyte sedimentation rate.

role is to educate people in the community to seek medical attention for symptoms of streptococcal pharyngitis and to emphasize the need for adequate treatment of a streptococcal sore throat.

Secondary prevention focuses on the use of prophylactic antibiotics to prevent recurrent rheumatic fever. A person who has had rheumatic fever is more susceptible to a second attack after a streptococcal infection. The best prevention is monthly injections of benzathine penicillin G.[13] Alternative treatment is administration of oral penicillin, sulfonamide, erythromycin, or gentamicin one or two times a day. Prophylactic treatment should continue for life in individuals who had rheumatic carditis as children. Rheumatic fever without carditis after the age of 18 may require only 5 years of prophylactic antibiotic therapy, or therapy may continue indefinitely in patients with frequent exposure to group A streptococcus.

Acute Intervention. The primary goals of managing a patient with ARF are to control and eradicate the infecting organism; prevent cardiac complications; relieve joint pain, fever, and other symptoms; and support the patient psychologically and emotionally. The nurse should administer antibiotics as ordered to treat the streptococcal infection and teach the patient that oral antibiotic therapy requires faithful adherence to the full 10 day course of therapy. Precautions with respiratory secretions should be maintained for 24 hours after the initiation of antibiotic therapy. Antipyretics should be administered as prescribed. Oral fluids should be encouraged if the patient is able to swallow; IV fluids should be administered as prescribed.

Promotion of optimal rest is essential to reduce the cardiac workload and to diminish the metabolic needs of the body. After the acute symptoms have subsided, the patient without carditis should ambulate. The patient may resume normal activity after the antiinflammatory therapy is discontinued. If the patient has carditis with CHF, bed rest restrictions should be applied. Again, full activity should not be allowed until antiinflammatory therapy is discontinued. Nonstrenuous activities should be encouraged once recovery has begun.

Relief of joint pain is an important nursing goal. Painful joints should be positioned for comfort and proper alignment. Removal of covers from painful joints can be done with a bed cradle. Heat may be applied, and salicylates may be administered to relieve joint pain.

Psychologic and emotional care can be more important than physical care, especially since the heart is often viewed as the center of life. Any alteration in cardiac function may be perceived as a threat to the person's body image.

Ambulatory and Home Care. Secondary prevention aims at preventing the recurrence of rheumatic fever. The patient with a previous history of rheumatic fever should be taught about the disease process, possible sequelae, and the continual need for prophylactic antibiotics. The patient must be made aware of the high risk of recurrence if a streptococcal infection develops and should be informed about the risk of exposure to streptococcal infections from contact with school-age children, individuals in military service, and people in health care positions. Ongoing patient education should encourage good nutrition and hygienic practices and reinforce the importance of receiving adequate rest.

The patient should be instructed in the use of prophylactic antibiotic therapy. The dosage of antibiotics used in maintenance prophylaxis of rheumatic fever is not adequate to prevent infective endocarditis when invasive procedures are performed. Additional prophylaxis is necessary if a patient with known rheumatic heart disease has dental or surgical procedures involving the upper respiratory, GI, or GU tract. The

35-2 NURSING CARE PLAN PATIENT WITH RHEUMATIC FEVER AND HEART DISEASE

Expected Patient Outcomes	Nursing Interventions and *Rationales*
NURSING DIAGNOSIS	**Activity intolerance** *related to* arthralgia secondary to joint pain and congestive heart failure *as manifested by* malaise, fatigue, weakness, dyspnea, shortness of breath, confusion, vertigo, increased pulse, increased or decreased respiratory rate and BP.
▪ Able to perform activities of daily living with minimal or no fatigue or physiologic distress.	▪ Assess patient's response to activity *to determine extent of problem and plan appropriate interventions.* ▪ Monitor heart rate/rhythm, BP, and respiratory rate before, during, and after activity *to determine degree of cardiac and pulmonary function.* ▪ Maintain bed rest during febrile periods *to promote resolution of inflammatory process and reduce cardiac workload.* ▪ Plan rest periods between activities *to balance demands that activity places on heart and to promote healing process.* ▪ Teach progressive exercise program after antiinflammatory therapy is discontinued noting patient responses to activity *so that activity is increased to patient's ability.* ▪ Treat arthralgia with rest and medication for pain *to promote healing and enable limited activity.*
NURSING DIAGNOSIS	**Ineffective management of therapeutic regimen** *related to* lack of knowledge concerning the need for long-term prophylactic antibiotic therapy and possible disease sequelae, lack of compliance, lack of resources *as manifested by* complications of rheumatic heart disease.
▪ Adherence to treatment regimen. ▪ Expression of confidence in managing disease. ▪ Able to describe signs and symptoms of valvular heart disease.	▪ Assess patient's knowledge, confidence, and resources for self-care *to initiate appropriate interventions.* ▪ Teach patient about the disease process, possible sequelae, and continued need for prophylactic antibiotics *to increase patient's control of disease and reduce the possibility of recurrence.* ▪ Inform patient of ways to reduce exposure to streptococcal infections *to reduce possibility of recurrence.* ▪ Teach patient the signs of valvular heart disease such as excessive fatigue, dizziness, palpitations, or dyspnea on exertion *because this is the most serious complication of rheumatic fever.*

nurse must explain the difference between these two prophylactic programs.

The patient should also be cautioned about the possibility of development of valvular heart disease. The nurse should teach the patient to seek medical attention if symptoms such as excessive fatigue, dizziness, palpitations, or exertional dyspnea develop.

Evaluation

The expected outcomes for a patient with rheumatic fever and heart disease are presented in NCP 35-2.

VALVULAR HEART DISEASE

The heart contains two atrioventricular valves, the mitral and the tricuspid, and two semilunar valves, the aortic and the pulmonic, which are located in four strategic locations to control unidirectional blood flow (Fig. 35-8). Types of valvular heart disease are defined according to the valve or valves affected and the two types of functional alterations, stenosis and regurgitation (Fig. 35-9).

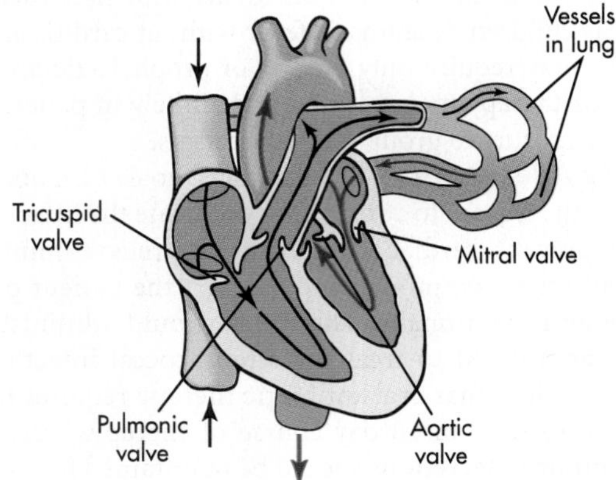

Fig. 35-8 Cross section of valves of the heart.

The pressure on either side of an open valve is normally equal. However, in a stenotic valve the valve orifice is restricted, impeding the forward flow of blood and creating a pressure gradient difference across an open valve.[18] The degree of stenosis is reflected in the pressure gradient differences (i.e., the higher the

Table 35-16 Congenital Heart Lesions

Lesion	Description
Ventricular septal defect	Hole in septum between two ventricles
Atrial septal defect	Hole in septum between two atria
Patent ductus arteriosus	Persistence of opening between aorta and pulmonary artery, which normally closes shortly after birth
Pulmonic stenosis	Narrowing of pulmonic valve
Coarctation of aorta	Stricture and narrowing of aorta caused by infolding of wall of aorta
Aortic stenosis	Narrowing of aortic valve
Tetralogy of Fallot	Ventricular septal defect, pulmonic stenosis, aorta overriding two ventricles, and right ventricular hypertrophy
Transposition of great vessels	Reversal of position of aorta and pulmonary artery; origination of aorta from right ventricle, origination of pulmonary artery from left ventricle
Persistent truncus arteriosus	Single vessel exiting the heart to supply blood to pulmonary and systemic circulations
Tricuspid atresia	Absence of communication between right atrium and right ventricle

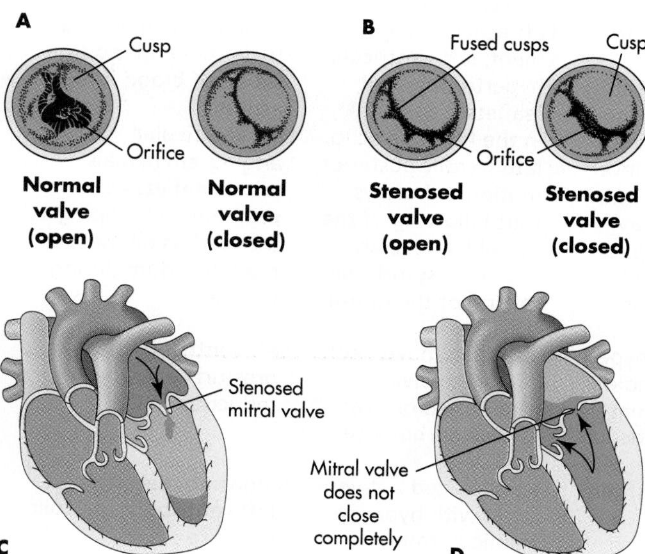

Fig. 35-9 Valvular stenosis and regurgitation. **A,** Normal position of the valve leaflets, or cusps, when the valve is open and closed. **B,** Open position of a stenosed valve *(left)* and open position of a closed regurgitant valve *(right).* **C,** Hemodynamic effect of mitral stenosis. The stenosed valve is unable to open sufficiently during left atrial systole, inhibiting left ventricular filling. **D,** Hemodynamic effect of mitral regurgitation. The mitral valve does not close completely during left ventricular systole, permitting blood to reenter the left atrium.

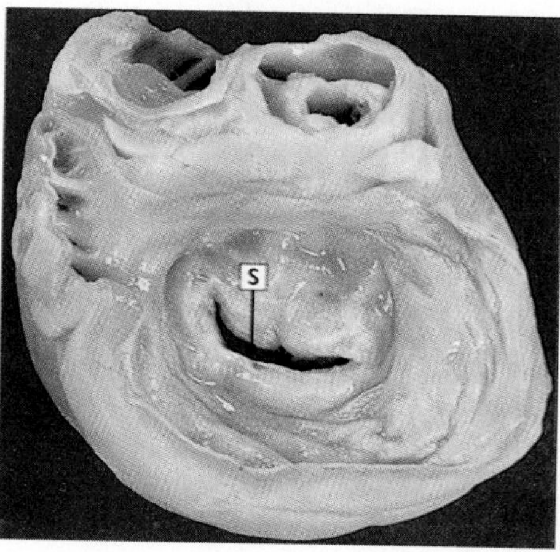

Fig. 35-10 Mitral stenosis with classic "fish mouth" orifice.

gradient, the greater the stenosis). In regurgitation (also called valvular incompetence or insufficiency) incomplete closure of the valve leaflets results in the backward flow of blood.

Valvular disorders occur in children and adolescents primarily from congenital conditions such as tricuspid atresia, pulmonary stenosis, and aortic stenosis (Table 35-16). The incidence of congenital heart disease in the United States is 1 out of every 100 newborns, of which 15% to 20% have some type of congenital valvular heart defect.[19] Rheumatic heart disease is a common cause of adult valvular disease.

Fenfluramine (Pondimin) and phentermine (Fastin, Adipex), used in combination to treat obesity, were associated with valvular heart disease. Fenfluramine was withdrawn from the market in 1997.

MITRAL STENOSIS

Etiology and Pathophysiology

The majority of adult cases of mitral stenosis result from rheumatic heart disease. Less common causes include congenital mitral stenosis, rheumatoid arthritis, and systemic lupus erythematosus. Rheumatic endocarditis causes scarring of the valve leaflets and the chordae tendineae. Contractures develop with adhesions between the commissures (the junctional areas) of the two leaflets (Fig. 35-10).[20] The stenotic mitral valve assumes a funnel shape because of the thickening and shortening of the structures composing the mitral valve. Obstruction to flow through the mitral valve results from these structural deformities and creates a pressure gradient difference between the left atrium and the left ventricle during diastole. The flow obstruction increases left atrial pressure and volume resulting in increased pressure in the pulmonary vasculature. Hypertrophy of the pulmonary vessels occurs in cases of chronic left

Table 35-17 Clinical Manifestations and Diagnostic Findings of Valvular Heart Diseases

	Clinical Manifestations	Electrocardiogram	Echocardiogram	Cardiac Catheterization
Mitral valve stenosis	Dyspnea, hemoptysis; fatigue; palpitations; loud, accentuated S_1; opening snap; low-pitched, rumbling diastolic murmur	Right axis deviation, left atrial enlargement, right ventricular hypertrophy, P "mitrale" (wide, M-shaped P wave), atrial flutter or fibrillation	Restricted movement of mitral valve leaflets; decreased size of orifice; diastolic turbulence	Left atrial pressure increased at end of diastole, reduction in CO
Mitral valve regurgitation	*Acute*—generally poorly tolerated with fulminating pulmonary edema and shock developing rapidly; systolic murmur	Left atrial enlargment, atrial fibrillation	Hyperdynamic left ventricular contraction in association with shock; allows visualization of regurgitant jets and flail chordae/leaflets	Dye injection in left ventricle showing regurgitation of blood into left atrium
	Chronic—weakness, fatigue, exertional dyspnea, palpitations; an S_3 gallop, holosystolic or pansystolic murmur	P mitrale, left ventricular hypertrophy, atrial flutter or fibrillation	Left atrial enlargement; left ventricular hypertrophy; flail leaflets	Dye injection in left ventricle showing regurgitation of blood into left atrium
Mitral valve prolapse	Palpitations, dyspnea, chest pain, activity intolerance, syncope; mobile midsystolic nonejection click and a late or holosystolic murmur	Usually normal; occasionally T wave inversion or biplasticity in leads II, III, and aVF are noted; complications of PVCs and tachyarrhythmias reported	On the M-mode echo, late systolic posterior motion or holosystolic billowing of the mitral leaflets; on 2-D echo, systolic billowing of the mitral leaflets	Left ventricular angiogram reveals mitral leaflets with prominent scalloping as the leaflets billow into the left atrium during systole
Aortic valve stenosis	Angina pectoris, syncope, heart failure, normal or soft S_1, prominent S_4, crescendo-decrescendo murmur	Left ventricular hypertrophy, left bundle branch block, complete atrioventricular heart block	Restricted movement of aortic valve; diminished orifice; systolic turbulence	Left ventricular systolic pressure increased, reduction in CO
Aortic valve regurgitation	*Acute*—abrupt onset of profound dyspnea, transient chest pain, progression to shock	Left ventricular strain	Normal-sized left ventricle with hyperdynamic systolic contraction; aortic dissection can be seen, if cause of acute process	Significant elevation of left ventricular diastolic pressure
	Chronic—fatigue, exertional dyspnea; Corrigan's pulse; heaving precordial impulse; diastolic high-pitched soft decrescendo diastolic murmur, characteristic Austin Flint murmur at diastolic rumble, systolic ejection click	Left ventricular hypertrophy	Enlarged left ventricle and dilated aortic root	Increase in left ventricular diastolic pressure, aortic root dye injection demonstrating regurgitation of blood into left ventricle
Tricuspid stenosis and regurgitation	Peripheral edema, ascites, hepatomegaly; diastolic low-pitched, decrescendo murmur with increased intensity during inspiration (stenosis), pansystolic murmur with increased intensity at inspiration (regurgitation)	Tall, peaked P waves; atrial fibrillation	Right ventricular dilation and paradoxic septal motion, usually poor visualization of tricuspid valve itself	Pressure gradient across tricuspid valve and increased right atrial pressure (stenosis), reflux of contrast medium into right atrium (regurgitation)

PVCs, premature ventricular contractions.

atrial pressure elevations. In chronic mitral stenosis, pressure overload occurs on the left atrium, the pulmonary vasculature, and the right ventricle.

Clinical Manifestations

Dyspnea, sometimes accompanied by hemoptysis, is the primary symptom of mitral stenosis because of reduced lung compliance (Table 35-17). Palpitations from atrial fibrillation and fatigue may also be present. Auscultatory findings generally include a loud or accentuated first heart sound, an opening snap (best heard at the apex with the stethoscope diaphragm), and a low-pitched, rumbling diastolic murmur (best heard at the apex with the stethoscope bell). Less frequently, patients with mitral stenosis may have hoarseness (from atrial enlargement), chest pain (from decreased CO), seizures (from emboli), or a cerebrovascular accident (from emboli) (see Table 35-17).

MITRAL REGURGITATION

Etiology and Pathophysiology

Mitral valve patency depends on the integrity of the mitral leaflets, the mitral annulus, the chordae tendineae, the papillary muscles, the left atrium, and the left ventricle. An anatomic or functional abnormality of any of these structures can result in regurgitation. Causes of chronic and acute mitral regurgitation are numerous and may be inflammatory, degenerative, infective, structural, or congenital in nature. The majority of cases may be attributed to chronic rheumatic heart disease, isolated rupture of chordae tendineae, mitral valve prolapse, ischemic papillary muscle dysfunction, and infectious endocarditis.

The regurgitant mitral orifice is parallel with the aortic valve, so the burden imposed on the left ventricle and the left atrium are determined by the etiology, severity, and duration of the mitral regurgitation. In chronic mitral regurgitation, volume overload on the left ventricle, the left atrium, and the pulmonary bed is created by the backward flow of blood from the left ventricle into the left atrium during ventricular systole, resulting in varying degrees of left atrial enlargement and left ventricular dilation. Acute mitral regurgitation does not result in dilation of the left atrium or left ventricle. Without dilation to accommodate the regurgitant volume, pulmonary vascular pressures rise, ultimately causing pulmonary edema.

Clinical Manifestations

The clinical course of mitral regurgitation is determined by the nature of its onset (see Table 35-17). The left atrium is relatively noncompliant, and when the atrium is abruptly distended, as occurs in papillary muscle rupture following a myocardial infarction, the sudden increases of volume and pressure are transmitted directly to the pulmonary vasculature. The resultant clinical picture in acute mitral regurgitation is that of pulmonary edema and shock. Patients will have thready, peripheral pulses and cool, clammy extremities. Auscultatory findings of a new systolic murmur may be obscured by a low CO state.

Patients with chronic mitral regurgitation may remain asymptomatic for many years until the development of some degree of left ventricular failure. Initial symptoms include weakness, fatigue, and dyspnea that gradually progress to orthopnea, paroxysmal nocturnal dyspnea, and peripheral edema. Patients with chronic mitral regurgitation have brisk carotid pulses. Auscultatory findings reflect accentuated left ventricular filling leading to an audible third heart sound (S_3) even in the absence of left ventricular dysfunction. The murmur is a loud pansystolic or holosystolic murmur at the apex radiating to the left axilla.

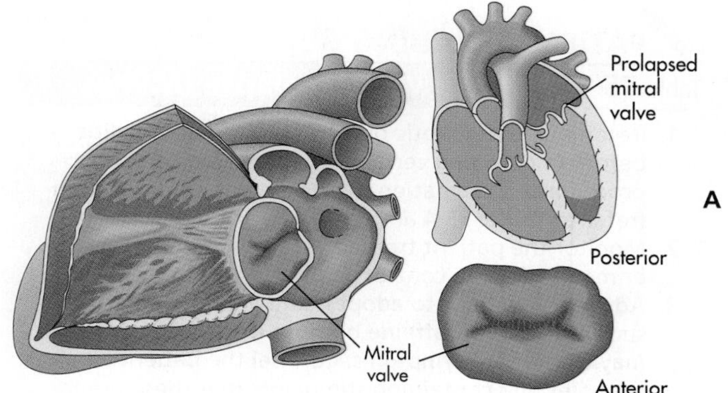

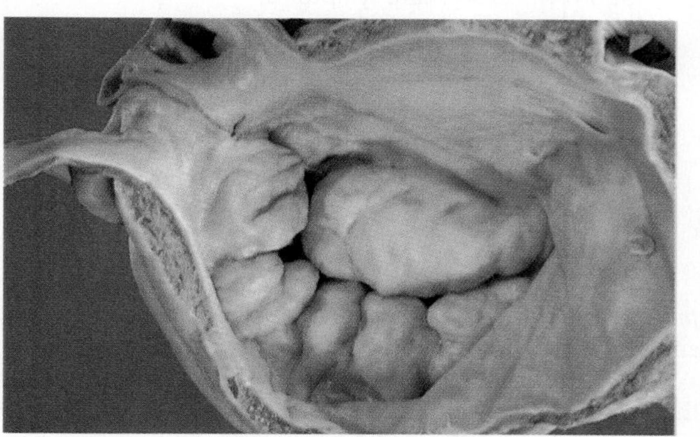

Fig. 35-11 Mitral valve prolapse. **A,** Normal mitral valve *(lower right)* and prolapsed mitral valve *(right).* Prolapse permits the valve leaflets to billow back into the atrium during left ventricular systole. The billowing causes the leaflets to part slightly, permitting regurgitation into the atrium. **B,** Looking down on the mitral valve, the ballooning of the leaflets is seen.

MITRAL VALVE PROLAPSE

Etiology and Pathophysiology

Mitral valve prolapse (MVP) is a failure of one or both leaflets to fit together resulting in displacement of an involved leaflet edge toward the atrium during systole (Fig. 35-11).[21] The etiology of MVP is unknown but is related to diverse pathogenic mechanisms of the mitral valve apparatus. MVP can occur in the presence of redundant mitral valve leaflets, elongated chordae tendineae, enlarged mitral annulus, and abnormally contracting left ventricular wall segments. The use of the term

PATIENT TEACHING GUIDE

Table 35-18 Mitral Valve Prolapse (MVP)

1. Recommend antibiotic prophylaxis for endocarditis before undergoing certain dental or surgical procedures if the patient has MVP with regurgitation (refer to Tables 35-4 and 35-6).
2. Monitor the patient treated with β-adrenergic blocker medications to control palpitations.
3. Advise the patient to adopt healthy eating patterns, such as avoiding caffeine because it is a stimulant and may exacerbate symptoms. Counsel the patient who uses diet pills containing stimulants that these preparations will exacerbate symptoms.
4. Instruct the patient to take over-the-counter drugs with caution and to check common ingredients, including caffeine, ephedrine, and pseudoephedrine.
5. Develop a planned aerobic exercise program and help the patient implement it.

prolapse is unfortunate because it is used even when the valve anomaly is functionally normal.

MVP is the most common form of valvular heart disease in the United States with prevalence ranging from 4% to 7% and reaching as high as 17% with detection by echocardiography alone. MVP is eight times as common among women as among men. It is reported most often in young women ages 14 to 30. It is usually benign, but serious complications can occur, including mitral regurgitation, infective endocarditis, sudden death, and cerebral ischemia.[21] There is an increased familial incidence in some patients with MVP resulting from a connective tissue defect affecting only the valve, or occuring as part of Marfan's syndrome or other hereditary conditions that influence the structure of collagen in the body. In many patients the abnormality detected by echocardiography is not accompanied by any other clinical manifestations of cardiac disease, and the significance of the finding is uncertain.[22]

Clinical Manifestations

MVP encompasses a broad spectrum of severity. Most patients are asymptomatic and remain so for their entire lives. Although severe mitral regurgitation is an uncommon complication of MVP, the latter has become the most common cause of isolated severe mitral regurgitation. A characteristic of MVP is a murmur from insufficiency that gets more intense through systole. This could be a late or holosystolic murmur. Another major sign is one or more clicks usually heard in midsystole to late systole, between the first heart sound (S_1) and second heart sound (S_2), and less frequently in early systole. The clicks may be constant or vary from beat to beat. MVP does not alter S_1 or S_2. M-mode echocardiography confirms MVP by demonstrating late-systolic prolapse, and two-dimensional echocardiography reveals leaflet billowing into the left atrium.

Arrhythmias, most commonly ventricular premature contractions, paroxysmal supraventricular tachycardia, and ventricular tachycardia, may cause palpitations, light-headedness, and dizziness. Infective endocarditis may occur in patients with mitral regurgitation associated with MVP.

Patients may or may not have chest pain. If episodes of chest pain occur, the episodes tend to occur in clusters, especially during periods of emotional stress. The chest pain may occasionally be accompanied by dyspnea, palpitations, and syncope. This chest pain does not respond to antianginal treatment (e.g., nitrates).

Patients with MVP generally have a benign, manageable course unless some severe problems associated with mitral regurgitation are present.[22] A teaching plan for patients with MVP is presented in Table 35-18.

AORTIC STENOSIS

Etiology and Pathophysiology

Congenitally abnormal stenotic aortic valves are generally discovered in childhood, adolescence, or young adulthood. A patient seen later in life usually has aortic stenosis as a result of rheumatic fever or senile fibrocalcific degeneration of a normal valve. In rheumatic valvular disease, fusion of the commissures and secondary calcification cause the valve leaflets to stiffen and retract, resulting in regurgitation. If it does occur secondary to rheumatic heart disease, mitral valve disease accompanies aortic stenosis. In contrast to mitral stenosis, isolated aortic valve stenosis is almost always nonrheumatic in origin. Although the incidence of rheumatic aortic valvular disease has been decreasing, senile or degenerative stenosis is expected to increase as the population ages.

Aortic stenosis results in obstruction of flow from the left ventricle to the aorta during systole. The effect is concentric left-ventricular hypertrophy and increased myocardial oxygen consumption because of the increased myocardial mass. As the disease course progresses and compensatory mechanisms fail, reduced CO leads to pulmonary hypertension.

Clinical Manifestations

Symptoms of aortic stenosis (see Table 35-17) generally develop when the valve orifice becomes approximately one third its normal size and classically include angina pectoris, syncope, and heart failure. The prognosis is poor for a patient with symptoms and whose valve obstruction is not relieved. Auscultatory findings of aortic stenosis typically reveal a normal or soft first heart sound (S_1), a diminished or absent second heart sound (S_2), a systolic, crescendo-decrescendo murmur that ends before the second heart sound (S_2), and a prominent fourth heart sound (S_4).

AORTIC REGURGITATION

Etiology and Pathophysiology

Aortic regurgitation may be the result of a primary disease of the aortic valve leaflets, the aortic root, or both. Acute aortic regurgitation is caused by bacterial endocarditis, trauma, or aortic dissection and constitutes a life-threatening emergency. Chronic aortic regurgitation is generally the result of rheumatic heart disease, a congenital bicuspid aortic valve, syphilis, or chronic rheumatic conditions such as ankylosing spondylitis or Reiter's syndrome.

The basic physiologic consequence of aortic regurgitation is retrograde blood flow from the ascending aorta into the left ventricle resulting in volume overload. The left ventricle initially compensates for chronic aortic regurgitation by dilation and hypertrophy. Myocardial contractility eventually declines and blood volumes increase in the left atrium and pulmonary vasculature. Ultimately, pulmonary hypertension and right ventricular failure develop.

Clinical Manifestations

Patients with acute aortic regurgitation have sudden clinical manifestations of cardiovascular collapse (see Table 35-17). The left ventricle is exposed to aortic pressure during diastole. The patient develops weakness, severe dyspnea, and hypotension that generally constitutes a medical emergency. Patients with chronic, severe aortic regurgitation have pulses that are of the "water-hammer" or collapsing type with abrupt distention during systole and quick collapse during diastole (Corrigan's pulse). Auscultatory findings may include a soft or absent S_1, presence of S_3 or S_4, and a soft, decrescendo high-pitched diastolic murmur. A systolic ejection murmur may also be heard, and the Austin-Flint murmur, a low-frequency diastolic rumble similar to that of mitral stenosis, may be auscultated.

The patient with chronic aortic regurgitation generally remains asymptomatic for years and is seen with exertional dyspnea, orthopnea, and paroxysmal nocturnal dyspnea only after considerable myocardial dysfunction has occurred (see Table 35-17). Angina pectoris occurs less frequently in aortic regurgitation than in aortic stenosis. However, a nocturnal angina accompanied by diaphoresis and abdominal discomfort may be present.

TRICUSPID VALVE DISEASE

Etiology and Pathophysiology

Tricuspid stenosis is extremely uncommon and occurs almost exclusively in patients with rheumatic mitral stenosis. It is also seen in IV drug users. In tricuspid stenosis, right atrial outflow is obstructed, resulting in right atrial enlargement and elevated systemic venous pressures. Tricuspid regurgitation is usually the result of pulmonary hypertension or right ventricular dysfunction. Volume overload of the right atrium and ventricle occurs in tricuspid regurgitation.

Clinical Manifestations

Both tricuspid stenosis and tricuspid regurgitation result in the backward flow of blood into the systemic circulation. Common manifestations are peripheral edema, ascites, and hepatomegaly. The murmur of stenosis is presystolic (sinus rhythm) or midsystolic (atrial fibrillation), and a pansystolic murmur may be heard in regurgitation. Both types of murmurs dramatically increase in intensity with inspiration.

PULMONIC VALVE DISEASE

Pulmonic valve disease is an uncommon entity and, in the case of pulmonary stenosis, is almost always congenital. Pulmonary regurgitation as an isolated abnormality has a benign course but is generally associated with disease of other valves.

COLLABORATIVE CARE

Table 35-19 Valvular Heart Disease

Diagnostic
- History and physical examination
- Chest x-ray
- ECG
- Echocardiography
- Cardiac catheterization

Collaborative Therapy

Nonsurgical
- Prophylactic antibiotic therapy
  - Rheumatic fever
  - Infective endocarditis*
- Digitalis
- Diuretics†
- Sodium restriction
- Anticoagulant agents
  - Warfarin (Coumadin)
  - Dipyramidole (Persantine)
  - Aspirin
- Antiarrhythmic drugs (see Table 34-7)
- Oral nitrates
- β-Adrenergic blockers (see Table 31-8)
- Percutaneous transluminal balloon valvuloplasty

Surgical
- Valvuloplasty
- Closed commissurotomy (valvulotomy)
- Open commissurotomy (valvulotomy)
- Annuloplasty
- Valve replacement

*See Tables 35-4 and 35-5.
†See Tables 33-9 and 31-8.

Diagnostic Studies for Valvular Heart Disease

Diagnosis of valvular heart disease is generally based on the results of a history, a physical examination, an echocardiogram, and a cardiac catheterization (if surgery is considered) (Table 35-19). Chest x-ray results, electrocardiogram (ECG) findings, and the clinical manifestations exhibited by the patient also aid in establishing the correct diagnosis.

An echocardiogram provides information on the structure and function of the valves and on enlargement of the chambers. Transesophageal echocardiography and Doppler color-flow imaging are particularly valuable in diagnosing and monitoring the progression of valvular heart disease. Cardiac catheterization detects pressure changes in the cardiac chambers, as well as pressure gradients across the valves. It also quantifies the size of the valve area. An ECG shows variation in the heart rate and rhythm and provides information about possible ischemia or chamber enlargement. Chest x-ray reveals the heart size, alterations in pulmonary circulation, and calcification of valves.

Collaborative Care of Valvular Heart Disease

Conservative Therapy. An important aspect of conservative management of valvular heart disease (see Table 35-19) is prevention of recurrent rheumatic fever and infective endocarditis. Treatment of valvular heart disease depends on the

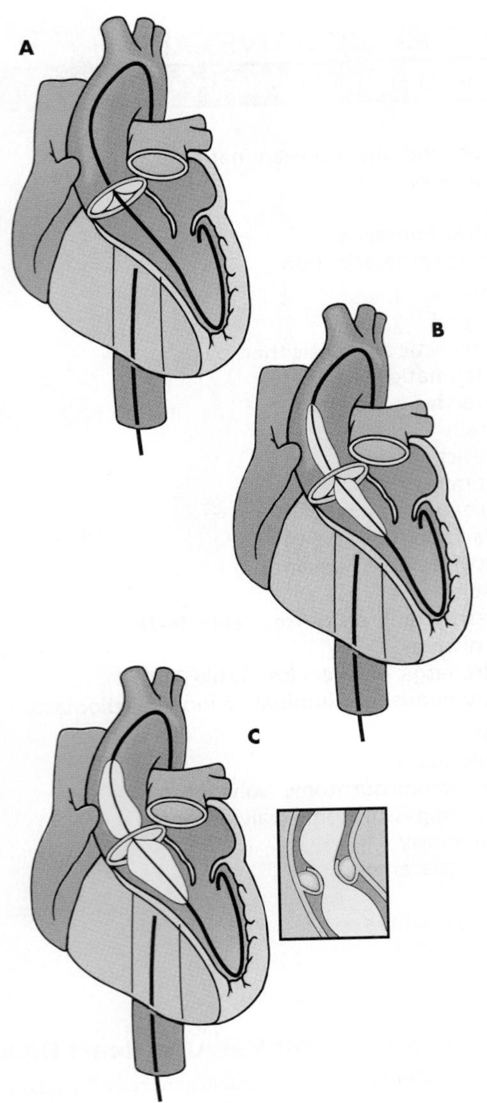

Fig. 35-12 Percutaneous transluminal balloon valvuloplasty (PTBV) procedure in a stenotic, calcific aortic valve. **A,** The loop of a wire guide, passed from the right femoral artery retrograde across the aortic valve, is seen nestling at the apex of the left ventricle. This positioning helps prevent perforation of the ventricular wall and minimizes ventricular ectopy. **B,** A 20 mm dilating balloon catheter, having been passed over the guide wire, is partially inflated; the indentation is caused by the stenosed valve. **C,** Full inflation of the balloon *(inset)* opens the aortic valve orifice.

valve involved and the severity of the disease. It focuses on preventing exacerbations of heart failure, acute pulmonary edema, thromboembolism, and recurrent endocarditis. If manifestations of CHF develop, digitalis, diuretics, and a low-sodium diet are recommended (see Chapter 33). Anticoagulant therapy is used to prevent and treat systemic or pulmonary embolization, and it is also used as a prophylactic measure in patients with atrial fibrillation. Arrhythmias, especially atrial arrhythmias, are common with valvular heart disease and are treated with digitalis, antiarrhythmic drugs, or

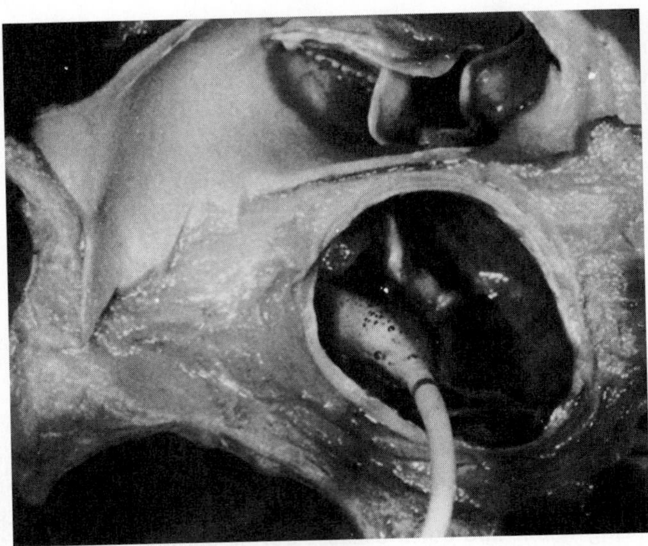

Fig. 35-13 Single balloon inflated through aortic valve orifice in the heart of a 73-year-old man with severe calcific aortic stenosis. Note that balloon does not occupy entire aortic valve opening, thereby allowing the patient to maintain perfusion throughout balloon inflation.

electrical cardioversion. β-adrenergic blocking drugs may be used to slow the ventricular rate in patients with atrial fibrillation. (Arrhythmias are discussed in Chapter 34.)

Oral nitrates may be prescribed for patients with aortic valvular disease. These drugs cause peripheral vasodilation, which reduces the blood volume returning to the heart and subsequently decreases the pressure gradient between the aorta and the left ventricle, allowing the ventricle to pump more effectively. In addition, nitrates improve coronary artery perfusion and reduce myocardial oxygen consumption.

Percutaneous transluminal balloon valvuloplasty. An alternative treatment for some patients with valvular heart disease is the percutaneous transluminal balloon valvuloplasty (PTBV) procedure (Fig. 35-12). Balloon valvuloplasty has been used for pulmonic, aortic, and mitral stenosis.[22] The procedure, performed in the cardiac catheterization laboratory, involves threading a balloon-tipped catheter from the femoral artery or from the femoral vein with transatrial septal puncture to the stenotic valve so that the balloon may be inflated in an attempt to separate the valve leaflets. A single- or double-balloon technique may be used for the PTBV procedure. A typical single balloon (the largest balloons available have a maximum inflation diameter of 30 mm) is shown inserted through the aortic valve orifice in Fig. 35-13. The double-balloon technique uses combinations of 10, 12, or 15 mm balloons inserted through each femoral artery to allow two balloons to be placed side by side into the valvular orifice, thus permitting a smaller arterial puncture and laceration.[23]

The PTBV procedure is generally indicated for older adult patients and for patients who are poor candidates for surgery. Complications are fewer for those undergoing PTBV as compared with those undergoing valve replacement. The long-term

ETHICAL DILEMMAS

Do Not Resuscitate

SITUATION

A 68-year-old man has been admitted for a second mitral valve surgery and possible coronary artery bypass. He was not compliant following his original surgery 5 years ago. The nurse worried about his future compliance with medication to reduce blood clotting, appropriate diet, and exercise. His kidneys are failing and he is on dialysis, but not tolerating it well. Both the patient and family want complete therapeutic treatment and refuse to discuss do not resuscitate (DNR) orders.

DISCUSSION

Lack of compliance in the past is not necessarily indicative of failure to comply in the future. As long as he can be maintained on medication, support, and dialysis, and no other organs fail, he has a good chance of survival. If, during periods of competency, he tells the nurses that he wants to keep fighting and he wants their help, the nurses have been told the wishes of a competent adult about his treatment. His family agrees and seems to be supportive. A DNR order is a *physician's* order, not a patient's advance directive or expressed wish. It would reasonably follow from certain advance directives and conversations with competent patients that a physician would place a DNR order in the chart, but that is the physician's decision. Legal problems could result if a DNR order were written against the expressed wishes of a patient and family, if the transfer of care was not attempted, or if a non–terminally ill patient died as a result of not being resuscitated.

ETHICAL AND LEGAL PRINCIPLES

- DNR orders should be discussed with the patient or the patient's family.
- DNR orders should be reviewed periodically during a hospitalization or institutionalization, and should be reassessed if there are subsequent admissions.
- DNR orders should be detailed enough to cover a full range of emergency support treatments (e.g., intubation, drugs).

results of PTBV seem promising. A recent study of patients undergoing PTBV indicated valve patency 1 year after the procedure, and 60% to 70% required no further surgical intervention after 5 years.[23]

Surgical Therapy. The decision for surgical intervention is based on the clinical state of the patient as generally appraised through use of the New York Heart Association classification system for functional disability (see Table 33-4). The type of surgery used for a particular patient depends on the valves involved, the valvular pathology, the severity of the disease, and the patient's clinical condition. All types of valve surgery are palliative, not curative, and patients will require lifelong health care.

Valve repair is becoming the surgical procedure of choice. Reparative or reconstructive procedures are often used in mitral or tricuspid valvular heart disease. Repair of these valves has a lower operative mortality rate than does replacement. Mitral commissurotomy (valvulotomy) is the procedure of choice for patients with pure mitral stenosis. The less precise closed (without cardiopulmonary bypass) method of commissurotomy has generally been replaced by the open method in the United States, Canada, and Western Europe.[20] The closed mitral commissurotomy is generally performed in developing nations where there is a higher number of younger patients with juvenile mitral stenosis. Cost considerations are a significant factor.[20] The closed procedure is usually performed with the aid of a transventricular dilator inserted through the apex of the left ventricle into the ostium of the mitral valve (versus the previous use of a simple transatrial finger fracture). In contrast, the direct vision or open procedure entails the establishment of cardiopulmonary bypass, removal of thrombi from the atrium and its appendage, commissure incision, and as indicated, separation of fused chordae, splitting of underlying papillary muscle, and debriding the valve of calcification.

Open surgical valvuloplasty involves repair of the valve by suturing the torn leaflets, chordae tendinae, or papillary muscles. It is primarily performed to treat mitral regurgitation or tricuspid regurgitation. The main advantage of a reparative procedure is that it avoids the risks associated with valve replacement. The disadvantage is that it may not be possible to establish total valve competence.

Further repair or reconstruction of the valve may be necessary and can be achieved by annuloplasty, a procedure also used in cases of mitral or tricuspid regurgitation. Annuloplasty entails reconstruction of the annulus, with or without the aid of prosthetic rings (e.g., a Carpentier ring).

Prosthetic valves. Valvular replacement may be required for mitral, aortic, tricuspid, and occasionally pulmonic valvular disease. The surgical treatment of choice for combined aortic stenosis and aortic regurgitation is valvular replacement (Fig. 35-14, Table 35-20).

Prosthetic valves have improved since the first caged-ball valve was introduced in 1952. Early valves disintegrated, stuck, became incompetent, changed the structure of cardiac chambers, caused emboli, and traumatized blood cells. Newer valves and improved surgical techniques have made valve replacement safer and long-term valvular functioning more effective. A wide variety of valves have been introduced in an attempt to find the most sound, nonthrombogenic, durable valve, and one that creates the least amount of stenosis.

The two categories of prosthetic valves are mechanical and biologic (tissue) valves. Mechanical valves are made of combinations of metal alloys, pyrolite carbon, and Dacron. Biologic valves are constructed from bovine, porcine, and human cardiac tissue. Within the past few years, major innovations in freezing and thawing techniques have enabled human grafts to be preserved for extensive periods without losing viability. Mechanical prosthetic valves are more durable and last longer than biologic tissue valves but have an increased risk of thromboembolism, which necessitates the use of long-term anticoagulant therapy. Biologic valves offer the patient freedom from anticoagulant therapy as a result of their low thrombogenicity. However, their durability is limited by the tendency for early calcification, tissue degeneration, and stiffening of the leaflets. Other

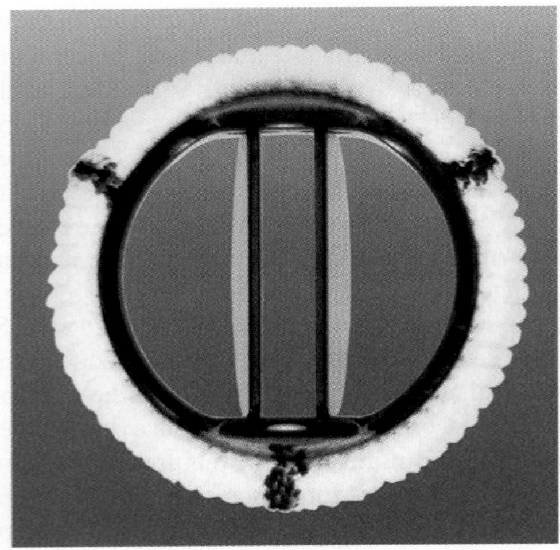

A

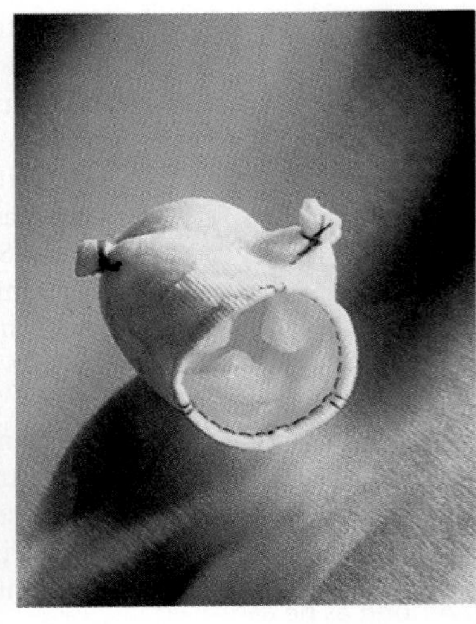

B

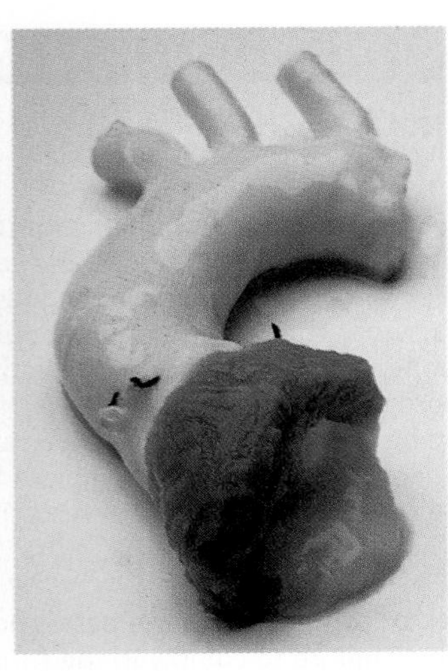

C

Fig. 35-14 Types of prosthetic and tissue valves. **A,** St. Jude Medical mechanical heart valve SJM Masters Series. **B,** Medtronic porcine heterograft valve. **C,** Baxter Healthcare aortic allograft valve.

Table 35-20 Types of Cardiac Prosthetic and Tissue Valves

Type	Description	Advantages	Disadvantages
Mechanical			
Caged-Ball Valve Starr-Edwards Smeloff-Cutter Magovern-Cromie	Metal cage with several struts mounted on a circular ring; hollow metal or plastic ball *(poppett)* inside of cage	High durability (up to 20 yr)	Possibility of blood clots forming on or around valve (thrombogenic) with risk of embolism Need for long-term anticoagulation therapy Very large size
Tilting-Disk Valve Bjork-Shiley Lillehei-Kaster Medtronic Hall	Mobile, lens-shaped disk attached to a circular sewing ring by two offset transverse struts; pyrolytic carbon composition	Hemodynamic efficiency High durability	Tendency toward thrombogenicity and embolism Need for long-term anticoagulation therapy
Bileaflet Valve St. Jude Medical Duromedics	Two pivoting semicircular disks that open centrally, mounted directly onto a sewing ring	Compact size; successful use in children and patients with small aortic roots	Possibility of thrombogenicity and embolism Need for long-term anticoagulation therapy
Biologic			
Porcine Heterograft Hancock Carpentier-Edwards Medtronic	Harvested aortic valve of pig that is preserved in glutaraldehyde and mounted on a specially designed sewing ring	Low thrombogenicity Need for anticoagulation therapy for only 3 mo after placement	Limited durability (failure rate increases sharply after 5-7 yr) Cumbersome structural design
Pericardial Heterograph Ionescu-Shiley Carpentier-Edwards	Three leaflets composed of pericardium from 16- to 18-month-old calves that are preserved in glutaraldehyde and mounted on a Dacron-covered frame	Low thrombogenicity Need for only short-term anticoagulation therapy Less resistance to blood flow; useful in patients with small aortic roots	Limited durability
Homograft Cadaver Valve	Harvested aortic valve from human cadaver that is initially frozen until needed for valve replacement; then thawed, trimmed, and sewn into place with special mounting material	Excellent hemodynamics No hemolysis/low risk for embolism Only rare need for anticoagulation therapy	Limited durability Not useful for mitral or tricuspid valve replacement

problems associated with prosthetic valves include paravalvular leaks and endocarditis.

Long-term anticoagulation is recommended for all patients with mechanical prostheses and for patients with biologic tissue valves who are in atrial fibrillation. Some patients with biologic tissue valves or annuloplasty with prosthetic rings may require anticoagulation during the first few months after surgery.

The choice of a valvular prosthesis depends on many factors. For example, if a patient cannot take anticoagulant therapy (e.g., women of childbearing age), a biologic valve may be considered. A mechanical valve may be considered for a younger patient because it is more durable and lasts longer. For patients over age 65 the importance of durability is less of an issue, but the risks of noncompliance or hemorrhage from anticoagulants may be greater. (The care of the patient requiring cardiac surgery is discussed in Chapter 33.)

NURSING MANAGEMENT: VALVULAR DISORDERS

Nursing Assessment

Subjective and objective data should be obtained from an individual with valvular disease and are presented in Table 35-21.

Nursing Diagnoses

Nursing diagnoses for the patient with valvular disease may include, but are not limited to, those presented in NCP 35-3.

Planning

The overall goals are that the patient with valvular heart disease will have (1) normal cardiac function, (2) improved activity tolerance, and (3) an understanding of the disease process and preventive measures.

Nursing Implementation

Health Promotion. Prevention of acquired rheumatic valvular disease is achieved by diagnosing and treating streptococcal infection and providing prophylactic antibiotics for patients with a history of rheumatic fever. The patient at risk for endocarditis and any patient with valvular heart disease must also be treated with prophylactic antibiotics (see Tables 35-4 and 35-5).

The patient must adhere to recommended therapies. The individual with a history of rheumatic fever, endocarditis, and congenital heart disease should know the symptoms suggestive of valvular heart disease so that early medical treatment may be obtained.

Acute Intervention and Ambulatory and Home Care. A patient with progressive valvular heart disease may require hospitalization or outpatient care for management of CHF, endocarditis, embolic disease, or arrhythmias. CHF is the most common reason for ongoing medical care.

The role of the nurse is to implement and evaluate the effectiveness of therapeutic management. Activity should be designed after considering the patient's limitations. An appropriate exercise plan can increase cardiac tolerance. However, activities that regularly produce fatigue and dyspnea should be restricted, and an explanation should be provided to the patient. Smoking should be discouraged. Strenuous physical exercise should be avoided because damaged valves may not be able to handle the required increase in CO. The patient should be assisted in planning the activities of daily living, with an emphasis on conserving energy, setting priorities, and taking planned rest periods.

NURSING ASSESSMENT

Table 35-21 Valvular Heart Disease

Subjective Data

Important Health Information

Past health history: Rheumatic fever, endocarditis, congenital defects, myocardial infarction, chest trauma, cardiomyopathy, syphilis, Marfan's syndrome, staphylococcal or streptococcal infections

Functional Health Patterns

Health perception–health management: IV drug abuse; fatigue

Activity-exercise: Palpitations; generalized weakness, activity intolerance; dizziness, fainting; dyspnea on exertion, cough, hemoptysis, orthopnea

Sleep-rest: Paroxysmal nocturnal dyspnea

Cognitive-perceptual: Anginal or atypical chest pain

Objective Data

General

Fever

Integumentary

Diaphoresis, flushing, cyanosis, clubbing; peripheral edema

Respiratory

Crackles, wheezes, hoarseness

Cardiovascular

Abnormal heart sounds, including opening snaps, clicks, thrills, systolic and diastolic murmurs, S_3, and S_4; arrhythmias, including premature atrial contraction, atrial fibrillation; tachycardia; increase or decrease in pulse pressure; hypotension, water-hammer or thready peripheral pulses, brisk carotid pulses

Gastrointestinal

Ascites, hepatomegaly

Possible Findings

Cardiomegaly, valve calcification, pulmonary congestion on chest x-ray; decrease in excursion, calcification or vegetation of leaflets or prolapse, chamber enlargement, turbulence on echocardiogram; abnormal chamber pressures and flow patterns on cardiac catheterization; atrial and ventricular hypertrophy, arrhythmias, conduction defects on ECG

S_3 and S_4, third and fourth heart sounds.

35-3 NURSING CARE PLAN PATIENT WITH VALVULAR HEART DISEASE

Expected Patient Outcomes	Nursing Interventions and *Rationales*
NURSING DIAGNOSIS	**Activity intolerance** *related to* insufficient oxygenation secondary to decreased cardiac output and pulmonary congestion *as manifested by* weakness, fatigue, shortness of breath, increase or decrease in heart rate, BP changes.
▪ Demonstration of cardiac tolerance to increased activity (e.g., stable heart rate, respirations, and BP).	▪ Assess and monitor patient responses to activity (e.g., heart rate, respirations, BP) *to plan appropriate interventions.* ▪ Plan rest periods between activities *to conserve energy and decrease cardiac demands.* ▪ Organize care *to minimize unnecessary disturbance.* ▪ Assist patient with personal care as necessary *to minimize fatigue and dyspnea and ensure patient needs are met.* ▪ Progressively increase activity *to increase cardiac tolerance.*
NURSING DIAGNOSIS	**Ineffective management of therapeutic regimen** *related to* lack of knowledge about disease process and prevention and treatment strategies *as manifested by* lack of compliance with therapeutic regimen.
▪ Knowledge of signs and symptoms that indicate a need to seek health care. ▪ Knowledge of need and when to use prophylactic antibiotics. ▪ Adherent to therapeutic regimen.	▪ Explain nature and cause of disease process *to ensure patient has adequate knowledge base on which to make decisions.* ▪ Teach signs and symptoms of heart failure and infective endocarditis *to ensure early reporting and treatment of complications.* ▪ Teach the need to avoid all invasive surgical or diagnostic procedures that may predispose to bacteremia until prophylactic antibiotics are given. ▪ Explain the importance of notifying the dentist, urologist, and gynecologist of valvular disease *so prophylactic antibiotic treatment can be initiated* (see Tables 35-4 and 35-5). ▪ Explain need for good oral hygiene and avoidance of fatigue *to minimize the opportunity for infection.* ▪ Discourage smoking *to prevent an increased cardiac workload and the oxygen-depleting effect of carbon monoxide from decreasing the* O_2 *available to all tissues.* ▪ Discuss the name of prescribed medication, dosage, purpose, and side effects *to promote safe and accurate self-medication.* ▪ Instruct patient to wear a Medic Alert bracelet.
NURSING DIAGNOSIS	**Sleep pattern disturbance** *related to* pulmonary congestion *as manifested by* fatigue and paroxysmal nocturnal dyspnea.
▪ Rested feeling on awakening.	▪ Elevate head of bed 30 to 40 degrees *to decrease venous return, reduce* O_2 *demand, and maximize respiratory excursion.* ▪ Administer oxygen as ordered *to increase* O_2 *saturation.* ▪ Reassure and remain with patient until respirations stabilize *to decrease anxiety and cardiac workload.* ▪ Eliminate environmental noise *to promote a restful environment conducive to sleep.*
NURSING DIAGNOSIS	**Fluid volume excess** *related to* cardiac failure *as manifested by* edema, dyspnea on exertion, shortness of breath.
▪ Reduced or absent edema.	▪ Monitor for manifestations of hypervolemia such as peripheral edema; taut, shiny skin; adventitious breath sounds *to detect hypervolemia.* ▪ Assess vital signs, auscultate breath sounds, assess jugular distention, measure intake and output, palpate for edema, and assess for weight gain (>2 lb [0.9 kg]/day or >5 lb [2.3 kg]/wk) *to monitor indicators of fluid balance.* ▪ Restrict sodium as ordered *to prevent fluid retention.* ▪ Monitor laboratory findings including electrolytes, hematocrit, BUN, and urinalysis *because specific changes can indicate hypervolemia.*

Continued

35-3 NURSING CARE PLAN PATIENT WITH VALVULAR HEART DISEASE —continued

Expected Patient Outcomes	Nursing Interventions and *Rationales*

COLLABORATIVE PROBLEMS

Nursing Goals	Nursing Interventions and *Rationales*
POTENTIAL COMPLICATION	**Decreased cardiac output** *related to* heart valve dysfunction.
▪ Monitor for signs of decreased cardiac output. ▪ Report deviations from acceptable parameters. ▪ Carry out medical and nursing interventions.	▪ Monitor BP, apical pulse, respirations, and breath and heart sounds *to assess for signs of decreased cardiac output* such as fatigue, malaise, shortness of breath, dyspnea on exertion, paroxysmal nocturnal dyspnea, palpitations, angina, vertigo, cardiac murmur, widened pulse pressure. ▪ Assess hemodynamic parameters (e.g., pulmonary artery pressure, pulmonary artery wedge pressure, cardiac output, central venous pressure) as ordered *as indicators of patient status.* ▪ Maintain bed rest as ordered *to decrease cardiac workload and O_2 demands.* ▪ Elevate head of bed 30 to 40 degrees *to reduce venous return, reduce O_2 demand, and maximize chest excursion.* ▪ Administer O_2 as ordered *to improve O_2 saturation.* ▪ Monitor cardiac rhythm *to detect changes from baseline.* ▪ Administer parenteral therapy as ordered and measure intake and output *to assess fluid balance.* ▪ Administer inotropic medication as ordered *to increase myocardial contractility.*
POTENTIAL COMPLICATION	**Systemic and pulmonary emboli** *related to* dislodgment of vegetations from heart valves.
▪ Monitor for signs of systemic or pulmonary emboli. ▪ Report deviations from acceptable parameters. ▪ Carry out medical and nursing interventions.	▪ Monitor for confusion, dyspnea, hemoptysis, pain, diminished or absent peripheral pulses, urine output, changes in skin color and temperature *to detect systemic and pulmonary emboli.* ▪ Auscultate breath sounds *to determine signs of pulmonary emboli such as crackles.* ▪ Administer anticoagulants and oxygen as ordered. ▪ Assess peripheral pulses and lower extremities for color, warmth, and edema *because changes in status can indicate peripheral embolization.* ▪ Perform range of motion (active or passive) to extremities, and apply elastic compression gradient stockings *to promote venous return and prevent venous stasis.*

Referral to a vocational counselor may be necessary if the patient has a physically or emotionally demanding job.

Auscultatory assessment of the heart should be performed to monitor the effectiveness of digitalis, β-adrenergic blocking agents, and antiarrhythmic drugs. Patients should be instructed to wear a Medic Alert bracelet. The patient must understand the importance of prophylactic antibiotic therapy to prevent endocarditis (see Tables 35-4 and 35-5). If the valve disease was caused by rheumatic fever, prophylaxis to prevent recurrence is necessary.

Urinary output and daily weight should be monitored when diuretics are prescribed. The patient's diet should be well-balanced nutritionally, with sodium restriction to prevent fluid retention.

The nurse should help the patient with a valvular disorder achieve and maintain an optimal level of health. Teaching regarding the actions and side effects of drugs is important to achieve compliance. When valvular heart disease can no longer be managed medically, surgical intervention is necessary. The patient who is on anticoagulation therapy after surgery for valve replacement must have the international normalized ratio (INR) checked regularly (usually monthly) to assess the adequacy of therapy. The INR is a standardized system of reporting prothrombin time.

Teaching instructions related to anticoagulant therapy are listed in Table 36-15. The patient must realize that valve surgery is not a cure, and that regular follow-up examinations by the health care provider will be required. The nurse also must teach the patient about when to seek medical care. Any manifestations of infection, congestive heart failure, signs of bleeding, and any planned invasive or dental procedures require the patient to notify the health care provider.

CRITICAL THINKING EXERCISES

CASE STUDY

Valvular Heart Disease

Patient Profile

Mrs. S., a 54-year-old woman, is admitted to the hospital for valvular heart disease.

Subjective Data

- Was told she had streptococcal throat infection as a child
- Was diagnosed 10 years ago with rheumatic heart disease
- Has shortness of breath at rest; cannot get out of bed without becoming dyspneic
- Takes digoxin (0.25 mg once a day)

Objective Data

Physical Examination

- Ankle edema
- Irregular pulse
- Crackles at lung bases
- Murmurs of mitral stenosis, mitral insufficiency, and aortic insufficiency

Diagnostic Studies

- Chest x-ray and ECG indicate enlarged left atrium

Critical Thinking Questions

1. Explain the cause of Mrs. S.'s valvular heart disease. What valves are most likely to become involved with rheumatic heart disease?
2. Differentiate between the characteristics of mitral stenosis and mitral regurgitation.
3. What other conservative treatment measures might be initiated for this patient in addition to digoxin?
4. What are important nursing measures for Mrs. S.?
5. On the basis of the assessment data provided, write one or more nursing diagnoses. Are there any collaborative problems?

NURSING RESEARCH ISSUES

1. What are effective nursing measures to facilitate patient compliance with prophylactic antibiotic therapy for endocarditis?
2. How does the quality of life of a patient having valvular heart surgery differ preoperatively as compared with postoperatively?
3. Does a planned aerobic exercise program decrease symptoms associated with mitral valve prolapse?
4. What health problems are observed most frequently by the nurse caring for a patient with rheumatic heart disease?

REVIEW QUESTIONS

The number of the question corresponds to the same-numbered objective at the beginning of the chapter.

1. A patient with a history of IV cocaine use has acute infective endocarditis. The nurse closely assesses the patient for signs and symptoms of
   a. pulmonary emboli.
   b. mitral valve regurgitation.
   c. streptococcal bacteremia.
   d. increased cardiac output.
2. The nurse suspects cardiac tamponade in a patient with acute pericarditis based on the finding of
   a. chest pain.
   b. pulsus paradoxus.
   c. mitral valve murmur.
   d. pericardial friction rub.
3. Prophylactic antibiotics are indicated to prevent infective endocarditis for at-risk individuals who
   a. are undergoing any dental procedure.
   b. are entering the third trimester of pregnancy.
   c. have acquired a viral respiratory tract infection.
   d. are exposed to human immunodeficiency virus.
4. The most common cause of myocarditis is
   a. viruses.
   b. radiation.
   c. endocarditis.
   d. myocardial infarction.
5. Teaching the patient with rheumatic fever about the disease, the nurse explains that rheumatic fever is
   a. a *Streptococcus viridans* infection.
   b. a viral infection of endocardium and valves.
   c. a sequela of β-hemolytic streptococcal infection.
   d. frequently triggered by immunosuppressive therapy.
6. Penicillin therapy for the patient with rheumatic fever is indicated to
   a. prevent chronic rheumatic carditis.
   b. relieve arthralgia and inflamed joints.
   c. prevent reinfection and recurrent rheumatic fever.
   d. destroy the infective microorganism and cure the disease.
7. The most common cause of adult valvular heart disease is
   a. myocarditis.
   b. rheumatic heart disease.
   c. congenital heart disease.
   d. subacute infective endocarditis.
8. Which of the following findings is indicative of accentuated left ventricular filling in a patient with chronic mitral regurgitation?
   a. A midsystolic click followed by an early systolic murmur.
   b. An audible third heart sound and a late diastolic murmur.
   c. An audible third heart sound and a pansystolic or holosystolic murmur.
   d. An audible third heart sound and a middiastolic click with a late diastolic murmur.

9. A patient hospitalized with aortic stenosis has a nursing diagnosis of activity intolerance related to insufficient oxygen secondary to decreased cardiac output. An appropriate nursing intervention for this patient is to
   a. monitor ECG to assess cardiac output.
   b. maintain on bed rest to reduce tissue oxygen demands.
   c. progressively increase activity to increase cardiac tolerance.
   d. use a semi-Fowler's position to decrease venous return and increase respiratory excursion.
10. The nurse caring for a patient scheduled for a percutaneous transluminal balloon valvuloplasty understands that this procedure
   a. is the treatment of choice for combined aortic stenosis and aortic regurgitation.
   b. is recommended for patients who are poor candidates for more extensive valvular surgery.
   c. involves the insertion of a transventricular dilator inserted into the opening of the valve.
   d. is a last resort treatment when other valvular repair procedures have not been effective.

References

1. Berbari EF, Cockerill FR, Steckelberg JM: Infective endocarditis due to unusual or fastidious microorganisms, *Mayo Clin Proc* 72:532, 1997.
2. Bansal RC: Infective endocarditis, *Med Clin North Am* 79:1205, 1995.
3. Aranki SF, Adams DH, Rizzo RJ: Determinants of early mortality and late survival in mitral valve endocarditis, *Circulation* 92(suppl II):143, 1995.
4. Wahl MJ: Myths of dental-induced endocarditis, *Arch Intern Med* 154:137, 1994.
5. Dajani AS and others: Prevention of bacterial endocarditis: recommendation by the American Heart Association, *JAMA* 277:1794, 1997.
6. Cetta F, Warnes C: Adults with congenital heart disease: patient knowledge of endocarditis prophylaxis, *Mayo Clin Proc* 70:50, 1995.
7. Oakley CM: The medical treatment of culture-negative infective endocarditis, *Eur Heart J* 16(suppl B):90, 1995.
8. Aragon T, Sande M: Infective endocarditis. In Stein JH, editor: *Internal medicine,* ed 5, St Louis, 1998, Mosby.
9. Dugan KJ: Caring for patients with pericarditis, *Nursing* 28:50, 1998.
10. Pericarditis: another cause of chest pain, *Harvard Heart Letter* 5:4, 1995.
11. Zayas R, Anguita M, Torres FL: Incidence of specific etiology and role of methods for specific etiologic diagnosis of primary acute pericarditis, *Am J Cardiol* 75:378, 1995.
12. Feldman T: Rheumatic heart disease, *Curr Opin Cardiol* 11:126, 1996.
13. Burge DJ, DeHoratius RJ: Acute rheumatic fever, *Cardiovasc Clin* 23:3, 1993.
14. Fraser EF: A review of the epidemiology and prevention of rheumatic heart disease: part I, *Cardiovascular Reviews and Reports* 17:3, 1996.
15. Carlquist JF and others: Immune response factors in rheumatic heart disease: meta-analysis of HLA-DR association and evaluation of additional class II alleles, *J Am Coll Cardiol* 26:452, 1995.
16. Fraser EF: A review of the epidemiology and prevention of rheumatic heart disease: part II, *Cardiovascular Reviews and Reports* 17:4, 1996.
17. Kaplan EL: Acute rheumatic fever. In Schlant RE, Alexander RW, editors: *Hurst's the heart,* ed 9, New York, 1998, McGraw-Hill.
18. Soovsky B, Dehner S: Patient education after valve surgery, *Crit Care Nurse* 14:117, 1994.
19. Rose AG: Etiology of valvular heart disease, *Curr Opin Cardiol* 11:98, 1996.
20. Citrin BS, Mensah GA, Byrd BF: Functional mitral stenosis resulting from large mitral valve prosthesis vegetation, *South Med J* 90:231, 1997.
21. Devereux RB: Recent developments in the diagnosis and management of mitral valve prolapse, *Curr Opin Cardiol* 10:107, 1995.
22. Hayes DD: Mitral valve prolapse revisited, *Nursing* 27:35, 1997.
23. Holloway S, Feldman T: An alternative to valvular surgery in the treatment of mitral stenosis: balloon mitral valvotomy, *Crit Care Nurse* 17:27, 1997.

Resources

Resources for this chapter are listed after Chapter 33 on p. 917.

REMEMBER to check out your **companion CD-ROM**

36 NURSING MANAGEMENT Vascular Disorders

Jennie Daugherty

www.mosby.com/MERLIN/medsurg_lewis

LEARNING OBJECTIVES

1. Describe the pathophysiology, clinical manifestations, and surgical management of aortic aneurysms.
2. Discuss the perioperative nursing care of a patient having an aortic aneurysm repair.
3. Describe the pathophysiology, clinical manifestations, and collaborative care of aortic dissection.
4. Identify the risk factors associated with atherosclerosis.
5. Describe the pathophysiology, clinical manifestations, and collaborative care of peripheral arterial occlusive disease.
6. Discuss the nursing management of the patient with acute arterial insufficiency affecting the lower extremities.
7. Identify three risk factors predisposing to the development of thrombophlebitis.
8. Differentiate between the clinical characteristics of superficial and deep vein thrombophlebitis.
9. Describe the nursing management of the patient with deep vein thrombophlebitis.
10. Explain the purpose and actions of commonly used anticoagulants and the nursing implications for patients receiving them.
11. Describe the pathophysiology, clinical manifestations, and nursing and collaborative management of pulmonary emboli.
12. Describe the pathophysiology and nursing management of venous stasis ulcers.

Problems of the vascular system include disorders of the aorta, arteries, veins, and lymphatic vessels. *Peripheral vascular disease* is a term used to describe a wide variety of conditions affecting these vessels in the neck, abdomen, and extremities.

DISORDERS OF THE AORTA

ANEURYSMS

Aneurysms are outpouchings or dilations of the arterial wall and are a common problem involving the aorta. Aneurysms of peripheral arteries can also occur but are far less common. Aneurysms occur in men more often than in women, and their incidence increases with age. Abdominal aortic aneurysms occur in 5% to 7% of people over age 60 in the United States. Half of all aneurysms greater than 6 cm in diameter rupture within 1 year.[1,2]

Etiology and Pathophysiology

Most aneurysms are found in the abdominal aorta below the level of the renal arteries. The aortic wall weakens and dilates with the turbulent blood flow. The growth rate of aneurysms is unpredictable, but the larger the aneurysm, the greater the risk of rupture. Thrombi are deposited on the aortic wall and can embolize.

Three fourths of true aortic aneurysms occur in the abdomen (Fig. 36-1) and one fourth in the thoracic aorta. Popliteal artery aneurysms rank third in frequency.

Although the cause of aneurysms is unknown, several risk factors are associated with the development of aneurysms, including hypertension, smoking, and atherosclerosis. A cause of aortic aneurysm is atherosclerosis with plaques composed of lipids, cholesterol, fibrin, and other debris deposited beneath the intima or lining of the artery. This plaque formation causes degenerative changes in the media (middle layer of the arterial wall), leading to loss of elasticity, weakening, and eventual dilation of the aorta.[2,3]

Several studies have shown a strong genetic component in the development of abdominal aortic aneurysms. Although the familial tendency to develop abdominal aortic aneurysms is primarily a genetic defect, no formal genetic analysis of family data has been performed. Less common causes of aneurysm formation include trauma, acute or chronic infections (e.g., tuberculosis, syphilis), and anastomotic disruptions.[4]

Classification

Aneurysms are generally divided into two basic classifications: true and false aneurysms (Fig. 36-2). A true aneurysm is one in which the wall of the artery forms the aneurysm, with at least one vessel layer still intact.

True aneurysms can be further subdivided into fusiform and saccular dilations. A fusiform aneurysm is circumferential and relatively uniform in shape. A saccular aneurysm is pouchlike with a narrow neck connecting the bulge to one side of the arterial wall.

Reviewed by Eileen Walsh, RN, MSN, CVN, Vascular Clinical Nurse Specialist, Jobst Vascular Center, The Toledo Hospital, Toledo, Ohio.

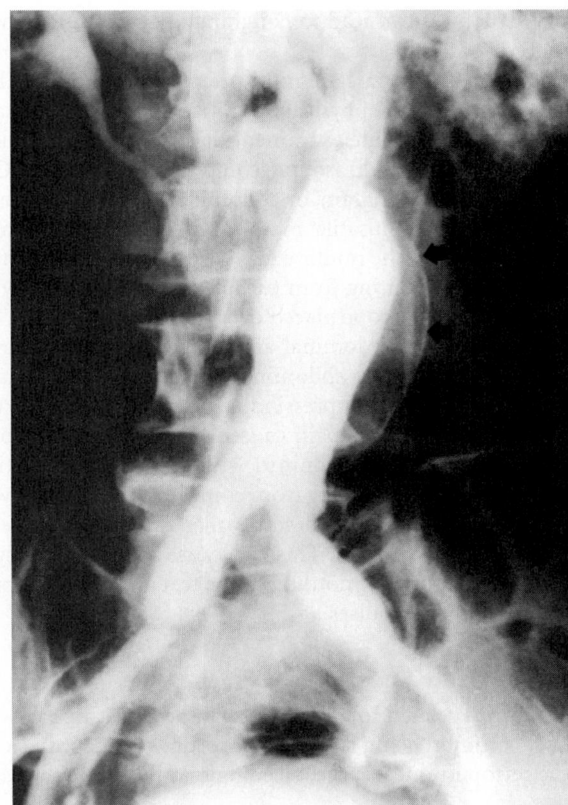

Fig. 36-1 Aortogram demonstrating fusiform abdominal aortic aneurysm. Note calcification of the aortic wall *(arrows)* and extension of the aneurysm into the common iliac arteries.

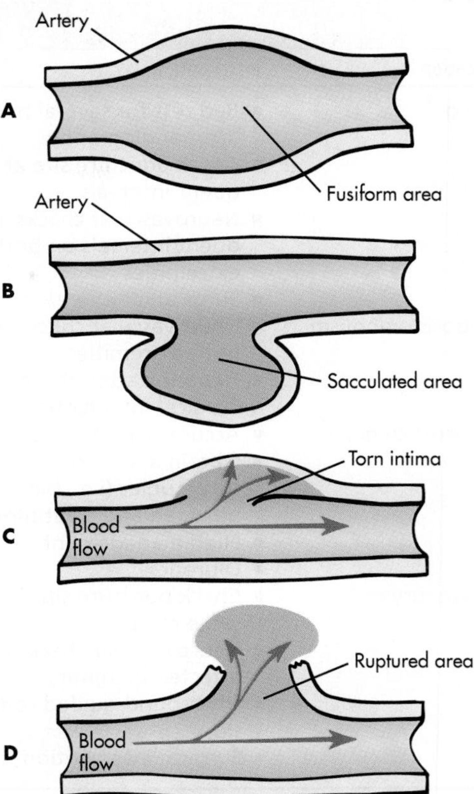

Fig. 36-2 **A,** True fusiform abdominal aortic aneurysm. **B,** True saccular aortic aneurysm. **C,** Dissecting aneurysm. **D,** False aneurysm, or pseudoaneurysm (pulsatile hematoma).

A false aneurysm, or pseudoaneurysm, is not an aneurysm but a disruption of all layers of the arterial wall resulting in bleeding that is contained or tamponaded by surrounding structures. False aneurysms may result from trauma, infection, or disruption of an arterial suture line after surgery. They may also result from arterial leakage after removal of cannulae such as upper or lower extremity arterial catheters and intraaortic balloon pump devices.

Aortic dissection is often misnamed "dissecting aneurysm" and occurs when there is a tear of the internal lining of the arterial wall that allows blood to enter between the intima and media, creating a false lumen (Fig. 36-3). With arterial pulsations, the blood may continue to dissect down the artery, involving branch arteries along the way. This process may be acute and life threatening or self-limiting, resulting in a chronic and stable process for a period of time.[5] (Aortic dissection is discussed later in this chapter.)

Clinical Manifestations

Thoracic aorta aneurysms are usually asymptomatic. When manifestations are present, they are varied. The most common manifestation is deep, diffuse chest pain. Aneurysms located in the ascending aorta and the aortic arch can produce hoarseness in the patient as a result of pressure on the recurrent laryngeal nerve. Pressure on the esophagus can cause dysphagia. If the aneurysm presses on the superior vena cava, it can cause decreased venous drainage resulting in distended neck veins and edema of the head and arms. Pressure of the aneurysm on pul-

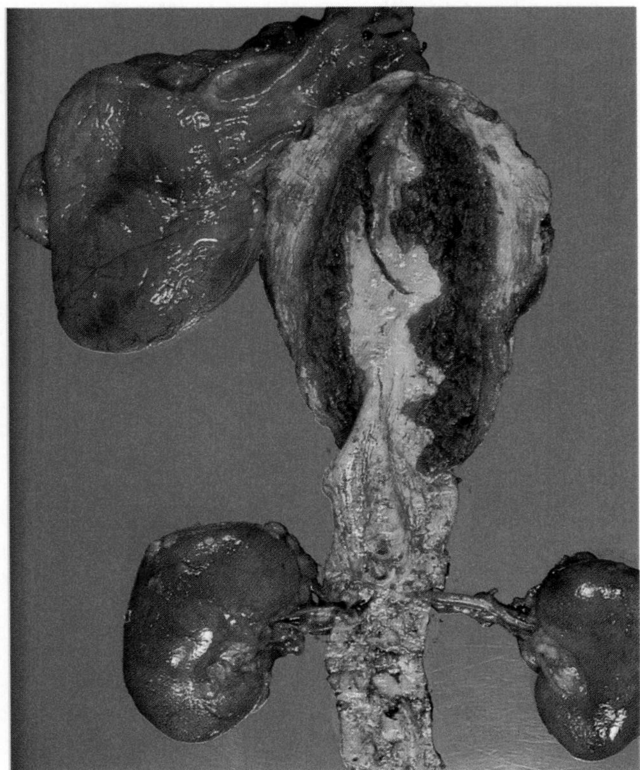

Fig. 36-3 Dissecting aneurysm of thoracic aorta.

Table 36-1 Complications of Angiography

Complication	Intervention
Bleeding	▪ Bed rest for several hours after angiography ▪ Check puncture site at frequent intervals ▪ Neurovascular checks at frequent intervals on both extremities ▪ Surgical intervention
Thrombosis/embolism	▪ Neurovascular checks of both extremities ▪ Heparinization/thrombolysis ▪ Surgical intervention
Renal insufficiency	▪ Accurate intake and output ▪ Obtain appropriate laboratory studies (i.e., blood urea nitrogen and creatinine) ▪ Fluid management ▪ Diuretics
Pseudoaneurysm	▪ Check puncture site for pulsatile mass ▪ Neurovascular checks of affected extremity ▪ Ultrasound-guided compression ▪ Surgical intervention

monary structures can lead to coughing, dyspnea, and airway obstruction.[6]

Abdominal aneurysms are most often asymptomatic. They are detected on routine physical examination or coincidentally when the patient is being examined for an unrelated problem (e.g., abdominal x-ray, ultrasound, computed tomography (CT) scan, intravenous pyelogram, or abdominal surgery). On physical examination a pulsatile mass in the periumbilical area slightly to the left of the midline may be detected. Bruits (murmur-like sounds resulting from turbulent blood flow) may be audible with a stethoscope placed over the aneurysm.

Symptoms of an abdominal aortic aneurysm may mimic pain associated with any abdominal or back disorder. Symptoms may result from compression of nearby anatomic structures. These include back pain caused by lumbar nerve compression and epigastric discomfort with or without alteration in bowel elimination resulting from compression on the bowel. Occasionally aneurysms, even small ones, spontaneously embolize plaque and thrombi. This can cause the "blue toe syndrome," in which patchy mottling of the feet and toes occurs in the presence of pedal pulses.

Complications

Complications related to aneurysms can be catastrophic, with the most common being rupture. If rupture occurs posteriorly into the retroperitoneal space, bleeding may be tamponaded by

Table 36-2 Types of Aortic Aneurysm Repair

Location of Aneurysm	Incision Site	Use of Bypass or Hypothermia	Nursing Considerations
▪ Ascending aorta with aortic valve insufficiency	Median sternotomy	Cardiopulmonary bypass and hypothermia are used.	If aortic valvular insufficiency is severe, prosthetic valve replacement is performed.
▪ Aortic arch	Median sternotomy	Cardiopulmonary bypass and hypothermia are used. If transverse aorta containing brachiocephalic vessels is involved, extracorporeal perfusion of brain is necessary.	Cold predisposes patient to arrhythmias. Watch neurologic signs.
▪ Descending thoracic aorta	Posterolateral at fourth intercostal space	Hypothermia is used. Cardiopulmonary bypass may be used.	Carlen's tube (double-cuffed endotracheal tube) deflates either lung and causes pulmonary stress and atelectasis. Good pulmonary care is important and ischemia to spinal cord is common.
▪ Abdominal aortic aneurysm	Xiphoid process to pubis	Bypass and hypothermia are not used. Arterial blood flow to lower extremities can be interrupted for time needed for surgical procedure.	Graft is placed within artery walls; this technique prevents graft from eroding into surrounding structures such as bowel.
	Retroperitoneal (left flank, similar to nephrectomy incision)	Bypass and hypothermia are not used.	Because abdominal cavity is not entered, the patient often has fewer problems with gastrointestinal and pulmonary dysfunction and less pain.

surrounding structures, preventing exsanguination. In this case the patient often has severe back pain and may or may not have back or flank ecchymosis (Turner's sign).

If rupture occurs anteriorly into the abdominal cavity, death from massive hemorrhage is likely. If the patient does reach the hospital, signs are manifestations of shock such as tachycardia, hypotension, pale clammy skin, decreased urine output, altered sensorium, and abdominal tenderness on palpation. (Shock is discussed in Chapter 61.)

Diagnostic Studies

Most aneurysms are found on routine physical or x-ray examination. Chest x-rays are useful in demonstrating the mediastinal silhouette and any abnormal widening of the thoracic aorta. A plain x-ray of the abdomen may show calcification within the wall of an abdominal aortic aneurysm.

When an electrocardiogram (ECG) is performed, it is used to rule out evidence of myocardial infarction (MI) because some persons may have symptoms suggestive of angina. Echocardiography assists in the diagnosis of aortic insufficiency related to ascending aortic dilation. Ultrasonography is useful for screening. A CT scan is the most accurate test to determine the anterior-to-posterior and cross-sectional diameter of the aneurysm and to identify the presence of thrombus in the aneurysm. Magnetic resonance imaging (MRI) may also be used to diagnose and assess the severity of aneurysms.

Aortography, anatomic mapping of the aortic system by contrast imaging, is not a reliable method of determining the diameter or length of an aneurysm. It may, however, be helpful in providing the surgeon with accurate information about the visceral, renal, or distal vessels. It is also useful if a suprarenal or thoracoabdominal aneurysm is suspected. Aortography is done with the use of a local anesthetic. A large needle with a stylet is inserted into the femoral artery, although a subclavian, axillary, brachial, or translumbar approach (through the back directly into the aorta) may also be used. A catheter is inserted and threaded through the needle into the artery. Contrast medium is then injected, and x-rays are taken with fluoroscopy. When all x-rays have been taken, the catheter is removed. Pressure is applied on the puncture site for several minutes or until the bleeding has stopped. Nursing implications following angiography (aortography is a type of angiography) are presented in Table 36-1.

Collaborative Care

The goal of management is to prevent rupture of the aneurysm. Therefore early detection and prompt treatment of the patient are imperative. Once an aneurysm is suspected, studies are performed to determine its exact size and location. A careful review of all body systems is necessary to identify any coexisting disorders, especially of the lungs, heart, or kidney, because they may influence the patient's risk for surgery. The carotid and coronary arteries should be assessed for significant atherosclerotic disease. If obstructions in these vessels are present, they may need to be corrected before the aneurysm is repaired. Generally, if coexisting problems are not severe, surgery is the treatment of choice. The type of surgery depends on the location of the aneurysm (Table 36-2).

Surgical Therapy. The only effective treatment of an aortic aneurysm is surgery. Surgery is needed for aneurysms of any size that are expanding rapidly in a patient who is symptomatic. For asymptomatic aneurysms, surgery is indicated if the diameter is greater than 6.5 cm. Surgery may be recommended in patients with aneurysm diameters of 4 to 5 cm.

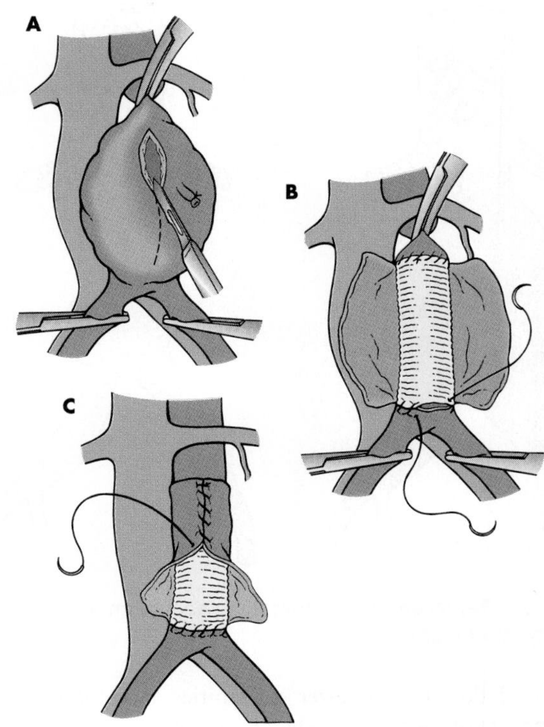

Fig. 36-4 Surgical repair of an abdominal aortic aneurysm. **A,** Incising the aneurysmal sac. **B,** Insertion of synthetic graft. **C,** Suturing native aortic wall over synthetic graft.

The surgical technique involves (1) incising the diseased segment of the aorta; (2) removing intraluminal thrombus or plaque; (3) inserting a synthetic arterial graft (Dacron or polytetrafluoroethylene), which is sutured to the normal aorta proximal and distal to the aneurysm; and (4) suturing the native aortic wall around the graft so that it will act as a protective cover (Fig. 36-4). If the iliac arteries are also aneurysmal, the entire diseased segment is replaced with a bifurcation graft (Fig. 36-5).

Before surgery, every effort is made to bring the patient into the best possible state of hydration and electrolyte balance. Any abnormalities in coagulation and blood cell count are corrected. The patient may receive antibiotics and baths with antiseptics before surgery. However, if the aneurysm has ruptured, immediate surgical intervention is required. Even with prompt care, the mortality rate is high (about 50%) after rupture and increases with the age of the patient. Aneurysms repaired electively have a surgical risk of 1% to 5%.[7]

All aneurysm resections require cross-clamping of the aorta proximal and distal to the aneurysm. When aneurysms are repaired electively, the patient is systemically anticoagulated with intravenous (IV) heparin before cross-clamping the aorta. This prevents clotting of pooled blood distal to the aneurysm. If surgery is performed emergently (as in the case of rupture), no anticoagulation is indicated. Most resections can be completed in 30 to 45 minutes, after which time the clamps are removed

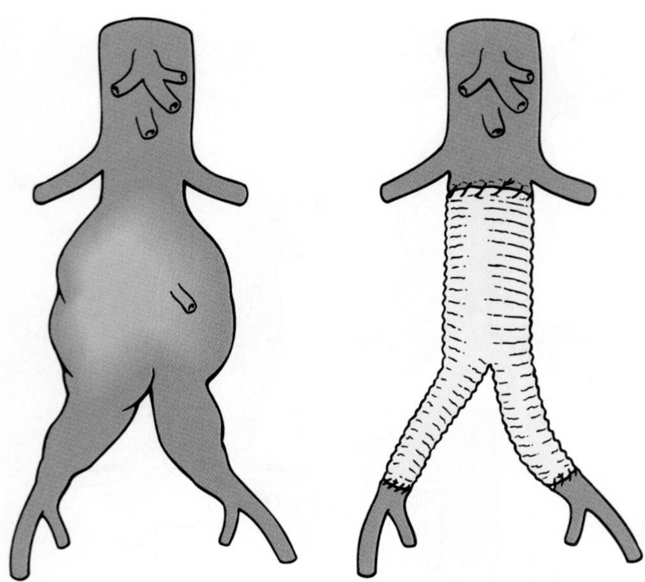

Fig. 36-5 Replacement of aortoiliac aneurysm with a bifurcated synthetic graft.

and blood flow to the lower extremities is restored. Use of autotransfusion, which recycles the patient's own blood, has markedly reduced the need for blood transfusions. (Autotransfusions are discussed in Chapter 29.)

Fortunately most abdominal aortic aneurysms originate below the origin of the renal arteries. However, if the aneurysm extends above the renal arteries or if the cross clamp must be applied above the renal arteries, adequate renal perfusion after removal of the clamp should be ascertained before closure of the abdominal incision. The risk of postoperative renal complications is significantly increased in patients who have surgical repair of aneurysms above the renal arteries.

With saccular aneurysms, it may be possible to excise only the bulbous lesion, repairing the artery by primary closure (suturing the artery together) or by application of an autogenous or synthetic patch graft over the arterial defect.

All patients undergoing aneurysmectomy should be placed in an intensive care unit (ICU) with appropriate support services and equipment postoperatively. When the patient arrives in the ICU, an endotracheal tube, an arterial line, a central venous pressure or pulmonary artery catheter, peripheral IV lines, an indwelling urinary catheter, and a nasogastric tube will likely be in place. If the thorax is entered during surgery, chest tubes will also be in place. Anesthesia may be done using a combination of general and epidural, with the epidural catheter left in place for epidural pain management.[8]

Endovascular graft procedure. The newest alternative to conventional surgical repair of an abdominal aortic aneurysm is the endovascular procedure.[9] The endovascular technique involves the transluminal placement of a sutureless aortic graft prosthesis across the aneurysm using the femoral artery. The graft is constructed from a Dacron cylinder, and the surface of the graft is supported with multiple rings of extraflexible wire. After the compactly folded graft is delivered through the sheath to the predetermined point, the graft is deployed and then pressed against the vessel by balloon inflation.

Patients must meet strict eligibility criteria to be a potential candidate for use of the devices. Some of the devices are custom made for each patient using data from CT scans, angiography, and ultrasound. In other institutions, the surgeons use knitted Dacron grafts combined with balloon expandable stents.

The benefits of endovascular repair include shortened length of hospital stay, small femoral incisions as opposed to a large abdominal incision, decreased morbidity and mortality rates, quicker recovery, and reduction in overall costs. Potential complications include bleeding, aortic dissection, graft thrombosis, embolization, graft leaks, and infection.

Currently, clinical trials are being conducted on several different devices. The endovascular graft technique offers many benefits for patients with abdominal aortic aneurysms.[10]

NURSING MANAGEMENT: ANEURYSMS

■ Nursing Assessment

The patient with an aneurysm may be symptomatic or may be totally free of symptoms. Therefore the nurse must use assessment skills to focus on early detection and treatment.

A thorough nursing history and assessment should be performed. Because most aneurysms are atherosclerotic and atherosclerosis is a systemic disease process, it is likely that the disease process is present throughout the body. Therefore it is important for the nurse to watch for signs of cardiac, pulmonary, cerebral, and peripheral vascular problems. The patient should be monitored for indications of rupture of the aneurysm, such as paleness; weakness; tachycardia; hypotension; abdominal, back, or groin pain; changes in sensorium; or a pulsating abdominal mass.

Establishing baseline data is important for later postoperative assessment and intervention. In addition to gathering data, the nurse should observe the patient closely for subtle abnormalities. Special attention should be paid to the character and quality of the peripheral pulses and the neurologic status. Arterial pulse sites and skin lesions in the lower extremities should be marked and documented before surgery.

■ Planning

The overall goals for a patient with an aneurysm include (1) normal tissue perfusion, (2) intact motor and neurologic function, and (3) no complications related to surgical repair such as thrombosis or infection.

■ Nursing Implementation

Health Promotion. The nurse must be aware of cardiovascular disease risk factors and be alert for opportunities to teach health measures to patients in the hospital and the community (see Chapter 32). Special attention should be given to the patient with a strong family history of aneurysm or any evidence of other cardiovascular disease. A trauma victim with abdominal or back pain should be urged to seek medical attention.

The patient should be encouraged to reduce risk factors known to be associated with atherosclerosis (see Table 32-4). These should include controlling hypertension, stopping smoking, and following a diet low in fats and cholesterol. These measures are also done to ensure continued graft patency following surgical repair.

Acute Intervention. The nursing role during the preoperative period should include teaching, providing support for the patient and family, and carefully assessing all body systems. It is imperative that problems be identified early and proper intervention instituted.

In addition to maintaining adequate respiratory function, fluid and electrolyte balance, and pain control in the postoperative period, the nurse must monitor graft patency and renal perfusion. The nurse can also assist in preventing ventricular arrhythmias, infections, and neurologic complications. Care of the patient with an aneurysm repair is described in NCP 36-1.

Graft patency. It is important to maintain adequate systemic blood pressure (BP) to promote graft patency. Prolonged hypotension may result in thrombosis of the graft as a result of decreased blood flow. Administration of IV fluids and blood components (as indicated) is essential to maintaining adequate blood flow to the graft. Central venous pressure readings or pulmonary artery pressures should be monitored hourly to help assess the patient's state of hydration.

Severe hypertension may cause undue stress on the proximal and distal arterial anastomoses, resulting in leakage of blood or rupture at the suture line. Drug therapy with diuretics or antihypertensive agents may be indicated if severe hypertension persists.

Ventricular arrhythmias. Ventricular arrhythmias are usually caused by hypoxia, hypothermia, or electrolyte imbalances. A patient with coexisting coronary artery disease is prone to arrhythmias. Nursing interventions include ECG monitoring, frequent electrolyte studies, and arterial blood gas (ABG) determinations. The patient who returns from surgery with hypothermia should be warmed with hyperthermia blankets.

Infection. The development of a prosthetic vascular graft infection can be a life-threatening complication. Nursing intervention to prevent infection should include ensuring that the patient receives a broad-spectrum antibiotic as prescribed to maintain adequate blood levels of the drug. It is important to assess body temperature regularly and to report any elevations. Laboratory data should be monitored for elevated white blood cell (WBC) count, which may be the first indication of an infection. In addition, the nurse should ensure adequate nutrition and observe the wound for evidence of poor healing, signs of infection, or any unusual drainage.

All IV, arterial, and central venous catheter insertion sites should be cared for carefully with the use of sterile technique because they are frequently a portal of entry for bacteria. Meticulous perineal care for the patient with an indwelling urinary catheter is also essential to minimize the risk of urinary tract infection. Surgical incisions should be kept clean and dry.

Gastrointestinal status. After conventional abdominal aneurysm resection, a paralytic ileus may develop as a result of anesthesia and the manual manipulation and displacement of the bowel for long periods during surgery. The intestines may become swollen and bruised, and peristalsis ceases for variable intervals. A retroperitoneal approach can be used to avoid bowel complications.

A nasogastric tube is inserted during surgery and connected to low, intermittent suction. This decompresses the stomach and duodenum, prevents aspiration of stomach contents, and decreases pressure on suture lines. The nasogastric tube should be irrigated with normal saline solution as needed, and the amount and character of the drainage should be recorded. The nurse should auscultate for the return of bowel sounds. The passing of flatus is a key sign of returning bowel function and should be noted.

It is unusual for paralytic ileus to persist beyond the fourth postoperative day. While the patient is receiving nothing by mouth (NPO), meticulous mouth care should be given every few hours. In some situations ice chips or lozenges may be given to the patient to soothe an irritated throat.

If the arterial blood supply to the bowel is disrupted during surgery, ischemia or death of intestinal tissue may result. This is evidenced by lack of bowel sounds, fever, abdominal distention, diarrhea, and bloody stools. Fortunately, this serious complication is uncommon.

Neurologic status. Neurologic complications can occur after surgical procedures on the aorta, especially when the ascending aorta and aortic arch are involved. Nursing intervention should include assessment of neurologic signs (hourly initially after surgery and less frequently thereafter), including level of consciousness, pupil size and response to light, ability to move all extremities, and quality of hand grasps (see Chapter 53). These should be recorded in detail with a careful description of the patient's response. Any alteration from the baseline assessment should be reported to the physician immediately.

Circulatory status. The anatomic location of the aneurysm indicates the areas of major concern related to circulatory status. All peripheral pulses should be checked regularly and recorded. This should be done every hour for several hours, depending on the nursing policy and routinely thereafter at frequent intervals. Pulses to be assessed may include the femoral, popliteal, posterior tibial, and dorsalis pedis (see Fig. 30-8).

When checking the pulses, the nurse should mark the location lightly with a ballpoint or felt-tip pen so that others can locate them easily. It is also important to note the temperature, color, and movement of the extremities.

Occasionally pulses in the lower extremities may be absent for a short time following surgery. This is usually due to vasospasm and hypothermia. A decreased or absent pulse in conjunction with a cool, pale, mottled, or painful extremity may indicate embolization of aneurysmal thrombus or plaque or occlusion of the graft. These findings should be reported to the surgeon immediately. In some patients the pulses may have been absent preoperatively because of coexistent arterial occlusive disease. Comparison with the preoperative status is essential to determine the etiology of a decreased or absent pulse and the proper treatment.

Renal perfusion. One of the causes of decreased renal perfusion is embolization of a fragment of thrombus or plaque from the aorta that subsequently lodges in a renal artery. This can cause obstruction and ischemia of one or both kidneys. Hypotension, dehydration, prolonged aortic clamping, or blood loss can also lead to decreased renal perfusion.

The patient returns from surgery with an indwelling urinary catheter in place. An accurate record of fluid intake and urinary

36-1 NURSING CARE PLAN PATIENT AFTER AORTIC ANEURYSM REPAIR

Expected Patient Outcomes	Nursing Interventions and *Rationales*
NURSING DIAGNOSIS **Risk for infection** *related to* presence of a prosthetic vascular graft and invasive lines.	
▪ Normal body temperature. ▪ No signs of infection.	▪ Monitor for signs of infection such as elevated body temperature; elevated WBC, HR, and respiratory rate; purulent drainage from incisions, as well as sites of invasive lines. ▪ Administer broad-spectrum antibiotic as ordered *to maintain adequate blood levels of the drug.* ▪ Monitor WBC count *because a rising count may be the first sign of infection.* ▪ Use aseptic technique in caring for incision and any indwelling IV line, tubing, or catheter *because these sites are potential portals of entry for infection.* ▪ Ensure adequate nutrition *to promote healing.*
NURSING DIAGNOSIS **Risk for altered peripheral tissue perfusion** *related to* graft thrombosis, embolism, or distal occlusion.	
▪ Patent arterial graft with adequate distal perfusion.	▪ Assess for diminished or absent peripheral pulses in lower extremities; color or temperature changes in legs; increased pain level *because these are indicators of altered peripheral perfusion.* ▪ Compare extremities for warmth and color *because differences may indicate impaired blood flow.* ▪ Administer IV fluids at prescribed rates *to ensure adequate hydration and renal perfusion.*

COLLABORATIVE PROBLEMS

Nursing Goals	Nursing Interventions and *Rationales*
POTENTIAL COMPLICATION **Cardiac arrhythmia** *related to* hypothermia, electrolyte imbalance, or coexisting coronary artery disease.	
▪ Monitor for signs of cardiac arrhythmias. ▪ Report deviation from acceptable parameters. ▪ Carry out medical and nursing interventions.	▪ Maintain temperature at about 37° C *to prevent arrhythmias resulting from hypothermia.* ▪ Administer O_2 as ordered by ventilator or mask *to reduce hypoxia.* ▪ Monitor the results of ABGs and serum electrolytes *to prevent imbalance from initiating an arrhythmia.* ▪ Keep lidocaine 100 mg IV bolus at bedside and administer as needed *to treat PVCs.*
POTENTIAL COMPLICATION **Hypovolemia** *secondary to* hemorrhage, extravascular fluid redistribution, or prolonged diuresis.	
▪ Monitor for signs of hypovolemia. ▪ Report deviation from acceptable parameters. ▪ Carry out medical and nursing interventions.	▪ Administer packed RBCs (as ordered) *to use as replacement if hemorrhage should occur.* ▪ Monitor BP and heart rate *to detect changes indicating hypovolemia such as decreased BP and increased heart rate.* ▪ Check hemoglobin and hematocrit q4-6hr and as needed. ▪ Observe abdomen and record girth *to assess for hemorrhage or extravascular fluid displacement.* ▪ Monitor pulmonary artery pressures and cardiac output *to assess for hypovolemia.*
POTENTIAL COMPLICATION **Altered renal perfusion** *related to* renal artery embolism, prolonged hypotension, or prolonged aortic cross-clamping intraoperatively.	
▪ Monitor for signs of altered renal perfusion. ▪ Report deviations from acceptable parameters. ▪ Carry out medical and nursing interventions.	▪ Monitor urinary output, daily weights, BUN, and serum creatinine *to detect signs of altered renal perfusion and renal failure.* ▪ Administer IV fluids and medications as ordered *to maintain adequate hydration, perfusion, and BP.* ▪ Monitor daily intake and output *to assess for dehydration or volume overload.* ▪ Assess BP *to ensure adequate systemic BP and perfusion.*
POTENTIAL COMPLICATION **Paralytic ileus** *related to* bowel manipulation, pain medication, and immobility.	
▪ Monitor for signs of paralytic ileus. ▪ Report deviations from acceptable parameters. ▪ Carry out medical and nursing interventions.	▪ Assess for absence of bowel sounds and flatus, abdominal distention, nausea, and vomiting *to detect signs of paralytic ileus.* ▪ Attach nasogastric tube to low suction *to decompress stomach and prevent aspiration.* ▪ Irrigate nasogastric tube with normal saline as needed *to ensure patency of the tube.* ▪ Give frequent oral care while patient is receiving nothing orally *to stimulate salivary glands and provide for patient comfort.* ▪ Encourage early ambulation (when possible) and turning q2hr while patient is awake *to foster return of peristalsis.*

BUN, blood urea nitrogen; *PVCs,* premature ventricular contractions.

output should be kept until the patient resumes the preoperative diet. Daily weights should be obtained. Central venous pressure readings and pulmonary artery pressures also provide important information regarding hydration status. Daily BUN and serum creatinine studies are performed to evaluate renal function.[11]

Ambulatory and Home Care. The patient may be apprehensive about returning home after major surgery involving the aorta. The nurse should encourage the patient to express any concerns and reassure the patient that normal activities of daily living can be resumed. The patient should be instructed to gradually increase activities. Fatigue, poor appetite, and irregular bowel habits are to be expected. Heavy lifting is avoided for at least 4 to 6 weeks following surgery. Observation of incisions for signs and symptoms of infection should be encouraged. Any redness, increased pain, or drainage from incisions should be reported to the physician. In addition, a fever greater than 100° F (37.8° C) should also be reported.

Sexual dysfunction in male patients is not uncommon after aneurysm repair surgery. This may occur because the internal hypogastric artery is disrupted, leading to altered blood flow to the penis. The patient should also be taught to observe for changes in color or warmth of the extremities. Select patients may be taught to palpate peripheral pulses and to assess changes in their quality. The patient who has received a synthetic graft should be aware that prophylactic antibiotics may be required before future invasive procedures, including any dental procedures.

There are situations in which operative repair is not performed. Examples of this are the presence of a very small aneurysm, a patient who is not a surgical candidate (e.g., severe lung or cardiac disease), or patient or family refusal to undergo repair. The patient who does not undergo surgical repair should be urged to receive regular routine physical examinations and should be reminded that any symptom, no matter how minor, must be investigated if it persists.

■ Evaluation

Expected outcomes for the patient who undergoes aortic aneurysm repair are addressed in NCP 36-1.

AORTIC DISSECTION

Aortic dissection, occurring most commonly in the thoracic aorta, is a longitudinal splitting of the medial layer of the artery by a column of blood (see Fig. 36-3). Aortic dissection affects men more often than women and occurs most frequently between the fourth and seventh decades of life. If not treated, aortic dissection has a 90% mortality rate.[5]

Etiology and Pathophysiology

Aortic dissection results from a small tear in the intimal lining of the artery, allowing blood to "track" between the intima and media and creating a false lumen of blood flow. As the heart contracts, each systolic pulsation causes increased pressure on the damaged area, which further increases the dissection. As it extends proximally or distally, it may occlude major branches of the aorta, cutting off blood supply to areas such as the brain, abdominal organs, kidneys, spinal cord, and extremities. Occasionally a small tear develops distally and the blood flow reenters the true vessel lumen.

Aortic dissection differs from an aortic aneurysm in that a false lumen is formed by separation of the intima from the media in dissection. In contrast, a true aneurysm involves dilation of the entire aortic wall.

The exact cause of dissection is uncertain, although many authorities attribute the cause to the destruction of the medial layer elastic fibers (cystic medial necrosis). Most people with dissection problems have hypertension. Persons with Marfan's syndrome (a disease of the connective tissue) have a high incidence of dissection. Pregnancy also promotes vascular stress as a result of increased blood volume. Areas that seem to undergo the greatest amount of stress and are thus most prone to dissection are the ascending aorta, the aortic arch, and the descending aorta beyond the origin of the left subclavian artery.

Classification

Aortic dissections are usually classified as type I, II, or III. Type I involves the ascending aorta and descending thoracic aorta. Type II involves only the ascending aorta, and type III involves the aorta distal to the subclavian artery.[6]

Clinical Manifestations

The patient with acute aortic dissection usually has sudden, severe pain in the back, chest, or abdomen. The pain is described as "tearing" or "ripping." The severe pain may mimic that of an MI. As the dissection progresses, pain may be located both above and below the diaphragm. Dyspnea may also be present.

If the arch of the aorta is involved, the patient may exhibit neurologic deficiencies, including an altered level of consciousness, dizziness, and weakened or absent carotid and temporal pulses. An ascending aortic dissection usually produces some degree of aortic valvular insufficiency, and a murmur is audible on auscultation. Severe insufficiency may produce left ventricular failure with the development of dyspnea and orthopnea caused by pulmonary edema. When either subclavian artery is involved, pulse quality and BP readings may vary between the left and right arms. As the dissection progresses down the aorta, the abdominal organs and lower extremities may begin to demonstrate evidence of altered tissue perfusion and ischemia.

Complications

A severe complication of dissection of the ascending aortic arch is cardiac tamponade, which occurs when blood escapes from the dissection into the pericardial sac. Clinical manifestations of cardiac tamponade include narrowed pulse pressure, distended neck veins, muffled heart sounds, and pulsus paradoxus (see Chapter 35).

Because the aorta is weakened by the medial dissection, it may rupture. Hemorrhage may occur into the mediastinal, pleural, or abdominal cavities.

Dissection can lead to occlusion of the arterial supply to many vital organs, such as the spinal cord, kidneys, and abdominal organs. Ischemia of the spinal cord produces symptoms varying from weakness to paralysis in the lower extremities and decreased pain sensation. Renal ischemia is usually manifested by low urinary output. Signs of abdominal ischemia

COLLABORATIVE CARE

Table 36-3 Aortic Dissection

Diagnostic
- History and physical examination
- ECG
- Chest x-ray
- CT scan
- Transesophageal echocardiography
- Magnetic resonance imaging (MRI)
- Aortography

Collaborative Therapy
- Bed rest
- Pain relief with narcotics
- Control of blood pressure
  - Trimethaphan (Arfonad)
  - Sodium nitroprusside (Nipride)
- Propranolol (Inderal)
- Labetalol (Normodyne)
- Aortic resection and repair

include abdominal pain, decreased bowel sounds, and altered bowel elimination.

Diagnostic Studies

The diagnostic studies used to assess dissection of the aorta are similar to those performed for aneurysms (Table 36-3). An ECG is done to rule out the possibility of an MI. Left ventricular hypertrophy is a common finding on an echocardiogram and is possibly related to changes caused by systemic hypertension. A chest x-ray may show a widening of the mediastinal silhouette, and left pleural effusion is not uncommon. A CT scan or MRI provides valuable information on the presence and severity of the dissection. After the patient's condition has stabilized, aortography is necessary to assess the extent of the dissection.

Collaborative Care

The goal of therapy for aortic dissection without complications is to lower the BP and myocardial contractility to diminish the pulsatile forces within the aorta (see Table 36-3). The use of trimethaphan (Arfonad) and nitroprusside (Nipride) IV rapidly reduces the BP. Intravenous β-blockers may also be used, such as propranolol (Inderal), or α-blockers and β-blockers such as labetalol (Normodyne). Propranolol is used to decrease the force of myocardial contractility.

Conservative Therapy. The patient with dissection without complications can be treated conservatively for an extended period. Supportive treatment is directed toward pain relief, blood transfusion (if required), and management of heart failure (if indicated). If the dissection is limited to the descending aorta, conservative therapy is usually adequate to treat the problem. Success of the treatment is judged by relief of pain, which is an indication of stabilization of the dissection. If the dissection involves the ascending aorta, surgery is usually indicated.

Surgical Therapy. Surgery is indicated when drug therapy is ineffective or when complications of aortic dissection (e.g., heart failure, leaking dissection, occlusion of an artery) are present. The aorta is fragile following surgery. Therefore surgery is delayed for as long as possible to allow time for edema in the area of dissection to decrease, to permit clotting of the blood in the false lumen, and to allow the healing process to begin.

Surgery for aortic dissection involves resection of the aortic segment containing the intimal tear and replacement with synthetic graft material. The extent of aortic replacement depends on the extent of the dissection.

NURSING MANAGEMENT: AORTIC DISSECTION

Nursing management related to an aortic dissection includes keeping the patient in bed in a semi-Fowler's position and maintaining a quiet environment. These measures assist in keeping the systolic BP at the lowest possible level. Narcotics and tranquilizers should be administered as ordered. Pain and anxiety must be managed for patient comfort, especially since they may cause elevations in the systolic BP.

Continuous IV administration of antihypertensive agents requires close nursing supervision. An ECG monitoring device is used, and an intraarterial pressure line is usually inserted (see Chapter 63). The nurse should observe for changes in the quality of peripheral pulses and for signs of increasing pain, restlessness, and anxiety. Vital signs are taken frequently, sometimes as often as every 2 to 3 minutes. A widening pulse pressure may indicate increasing aortic valvular insufficiency. If the blood vessels branching off the aortic arch are involved, decreased cerebral blood flow may alter the sensorium and level of consciousness. Postoperative care after surgery to correct the dissection is similar to that after aneurysmectomy (see the section on nursing management of aneurysms).

In preparation for discharge, the nurse should focus on patient and family teaching. The therapeutic regimen includes antihypertensive drugs, which are usually taken orally. The patient needs to understand that these drugs must be taken to control BP. Propranolol can be taken orally to continue to decrease myocardial contractility. It is important that the patient understand the drug regimen. The nurse should instruct the patient that if the pain returns or other symptoms progress, the patient must seek immediate help at the nearest health care facility.

ACUTE ARTERIAL OCCLUSIVE DISORDERS

Etiology and Pathophysiology

Acute arterial occlusion occurs suddenly, without warning signs. It can be caused by embolism, thrombosis of an already narrowed artery, or trauma. Embolization of a thrombus from the heart or an atherosclerotic aneurysm is the most frequent cause of acute arterial occlusion. Heart conditions in which thrombi are prone to develop include infective endocarditis, MI, mitral valve disease, chronic atrial fibrillation, cardiomyopathies, and prosthetic heart valves. The thrombi become dislodged and may travel to the lungs if they originate in the right side of the heart or to anywhere in the systemic circulation if they originate in the left side of the heart.

Arterial emboli tend to lodge at sites of arterial branching or in areas of atherosclerotic narrowing. An acute arterial occlusion causes the blood supply distal to the embolus to decrease. The degree and extent of symptoms depend on the size and location of the obstruction, the occurrence of clot fragmentation with embolism to smaller vessels, and the degree of peripheral vascular disease already present.

Sudden local thrombosis may occur at the location of an atherosclerotic plaque. Traumatic injury to the extremity itself may produce partial or total occlusion of a vessel from compression, shearing, or laceration. Acute arterial occlusion may also develop as a result of arterial dissection in the carotid artery or aorta or as a result of iatrogenic arterial injury (e.g., after arteriography).

Clinical Manifestations

Signs and symptoms of an acute arterial occlusion usually have an abrupt onset. The exception is when a sudden occlusion is superimposed on preexisting chronic arterial insufficiency. In this case the symptoms may be insidious because collateral circulation is well developed.

Clinical manifestations of acute arterial occlusion include the "six *Ps*:" pain, pallor, pulselessness, paresthesia, paralysis, and poikilothermia (adaptation of the ischemic limb to its environmental temperature, most often cool). Without immediate intervention, ischemia may progress to tissue necrosis and gangrene within hours. It should be noted that paralysis is a very late sign of acute arterial ischemia and signals the actual death of nerves supplying the extremity. Because nerve tissue is extremely sensitive to lack of oxygen, limb paralysis or ischemic neuropathy may persist after revascularization and may be permanent.

Collaborative Care

With acute arterial occlusion in the absence of adequate collateral circulation, early treatment is essential to keep the affected limb viable. Anticoagulant therapy is initiated immediately to prevent further enlargement of the thrombus and inhibit embolization. Continuous IV heparin is the agent of choice. The thrombus should be removed as soon as possible by embolectomy or thrombectomy. Balloon catheters can be used and are passed distal and proximal to the site to remove the clot material. Direct arteriotomy to perform an embolectomy or thromboendarterectomy may be necessary.

If the limb is stable using heparin, recently formed emboli may be effectively treated with an intraarterial infusion of a thrombolytic agent such as recombinant tissue plasminogen activator (r-tPA), streptokinase, or urokinase. These drugs work by directly dissolving the clot over a period of 24 to 48 hours. A percutaneous catheter is inserted into the femoral artery and threaded to the site of the clot. Bed rest is maintained and periodic angiograms are performed to monitor the resolution of the clot. This procedure can be effective and still have bleeding complications. Therefore patients are carefully selected and monitored by experienced critical care providers.

If the patient remains at risk for further embolization from a persistent source such as chronic atrial fibrillation, long-term treatment includes oral anticoagulation to prevent further acute episodes.

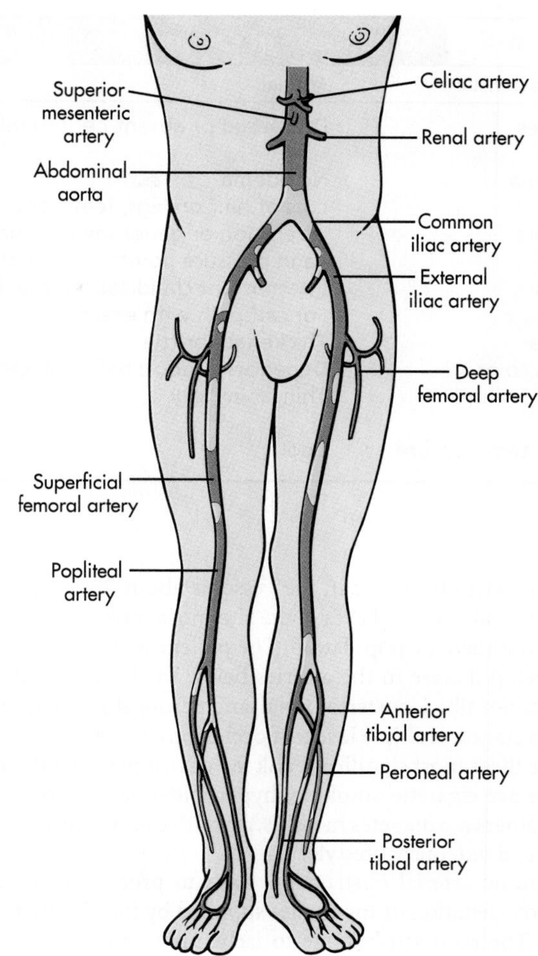

Fig. 36-6 Common anatomic locations of atherosclerotic lesions of the abdominal aorta and lower extremities.

CHRONIC ARTERIAL OCCLUSIVE DISEASE

LOWER EXTREMITY DISEASE

Chronic peripheral arterial occlusive disease involves progressive narrowing and degeneration and eventual obstruction of the arteries to the extremities, occurring predominantly in the legs. It may affect the aortoiliac, femoral, popliteal, tibial, peroneal vessels, or any combination of these areas (Fig. 36-6). Chronic arterial occlusion is a slowly progressive, insidious disease primarily attributed to the atherosclerotic process; hence the term *arteriosclerosis obliterans* is often used. It usually occurs in the sixth through eighth decades of life, primarily affects men, and has a familial tendency.[12] It occurs at an earlier age in patients with diabetes mellitus. Although the process may be slowed or arrested through risk factor modification, there is no cure. All treatments are palliative.

Etiology and Pathophysiology

The leading cause of chronic arterial occlusion is atherosclerosis, a gradual thickening of the intima and media, which leads to narrowing of the vessel lumen. Atherosclerosis primarily affects larger arteries. The involvement is generally segmental, with normal segments interspersed between involved ones. By

Table 36-4 Comparison of Chronic Arterial and Venous Insufficiency of the Lower Extremities

Characteristic	Arterial	Venous
Pulses	Decreased or absent peripheral pulses	Presence of peripheral pulses; may be difficult to palpate with edema
Edema	No edema	Edema around ankles and lower leg
Hair	Loss of hair on legs, feet, toes	Hair present
Ulcers	Ulceration or gangrene over bony prominences and pressure points on toes and feet	Ulceration around ankle, above or below medial malleoli; gangrene rare
Pain	Intermittent claudication (hip, buttock, thigh, or calf pain with exercise)	Dull ache or heaviness in calf or thigh
Nails	Thickened; brittle	Normal
Skin color	Dependent rubor; pallor on elevation	Cyanotic if dependent; brown pigmentation
Skin texture	Thin, shiny, dry	Scaling eczema; stasis dermatitis; veins may be visible
Skin temperature	Cool	Warm

the time symptoms occur, the vessel is about 75% narrowed. The femoral-popliteal area is the site most commonly affected in the nondiabetic population. The patient with diabetes tends to develop disease in the arteries below the knee (specifically, the anterior tibial, posterior tibial, and peroneal arteries). In advanced stages, multiple levels of occlusions are seen.

The three most significant risk factors for peripheral arterial disease are cigarette smoking, hyperlipidemia, and hypertension. Others are diabetes mellitus, a positive family history, obesity, and a sedentary lifestyle.

Chronic arterial obstruction leads to progressively inadequate oxygenation of the tissues supplied by the obstructed arteries. The pain attributable to ischemia is produced by end products of anaerobic cellular metabolism, such as lactic acid. This usually occurs in the larger muscle groups of the legs (buttocks, thighs, or calves) during exercise. Once the patient stops exercising, the metabolites are cleared and the pain subsides. As the disease process becomes advanced, pain develops at rest. "Rest pain" most often occurs in the feet or toes and indicates insufficient blood flow to the nerves supplying the distal extremity. The patient may notice rest pain more often at night and achieve partial relief by lowering the limb below heart level (e.g., dangling the leg over the side of the bed).[8]

Clinical Manifestations

The severity of the clinical manifestations depends on the site and extent of the obstruction and the extent and amount of collateral circulation (Table 36-4). The classic symptom of peripheral arterial disease is intermittent claudication, ischemic muscle ache or pain that is precipitated by a predictable amount of exercise, relieved by resting, and reproducible. Disease involving the femoral or popliteal arteries may cause claudication in the calf. Occlusive disease of the aortoiliac arteries may produce claudication in the buttocks and upper part of the thighs. If disease extends into the internal iliac (hypogastric) arteries, impotence may result. Sexual dysfunction occurs in as many as 30% to 50% of patients with aortoiliac occlusion.[12,13]

Pain at rest occurs as the disease becomes more severe. This is an ominous symptom. Without revascularization the limb may progress to ulceration and gangrenous changes may occur. Every attempt is made to save the limb, and surgery is usually indicated unless the patient is at exceedingly high risk or has numerous comorbidities.

Paresthesia, manifested as numbness or tingling occurring in the toes or feet, may result from nerve tissue ischemia. True peripheral neuropathy occurs more commonly in patients with diabetes and in those with progressive long-standing ischemia. The neuropathy produces excruciating shooting or burning pain in the extremity. It does not follow any particular nerve roots but may be present near ulcerated areas. Gradually diminishing perfusion to neurons produces loss of both sensation and deep pain. Therefore injuries to the extremity often go unnoticed.

The physical appearance of the limb as a result of postural changes provides important information about the adequacy of blood flow. Pallor or blanching on elevation indicates significant arterial ischemia. Hyperemia (redness) and a bluish or dusky appearance are observed when the limb is allowed to hang in a dependent position (dependent rubor). The skin becomes shiny and taut and there is a loss of hair on the lower legs. Diminished or absent pedal, popliteal, or femoral pulses may be noted.

Complications

Chronic peripheral arterial disease progresses slowly. Prolonged ischemia leads to atrophy of the skin and underlying structures. Because of the decreased ability to heal, infection and necrosis may result from even minor trauma to the feet, especially in the diabetic patient. Ischemic ulcers caused by arterial insufficiency most commonly occur over bony prominences on the toes and feet. (This differs from ulcers of venous insufficiency, which occur around the malleoli and lower parts of the leg [see Table 36-4]). Ischemic ulcers and gangrene are the most serious complications of chronic arterial disease and may result in lower extremity amputation if blood flow is not restored. If atherosclerosis has been present for an extended period, collateral circulation may prevent gangrene of the extremity.

Diagnostic Studies

Various tests have been developed to assess blood flow and to outline the vascular system (Table 36-5). Doppler ultrasound

COLLABORATIVE CARE

Table 36-5 Chronic Arterial Occlusive Disease

Diagnostic
- History and physical examination, including palpation of peripheral pulses
- Doppler ultrasound studies
- Duplex imaging
- Angiography
- Magnetic resonance angiography

Collaborative Therapy

Ambulatory/Home Care
- Reverse Trendelenburg's position 10 degrees while in bed
- Walking exercises 15-30 min twice daily as tolerated
- Foot care*
- Avoidance of thermal, chemical, and mechanical trauma
- No tobacco

Acute Care
- Percutaneous transluminal angioplasty with or without stent
- Atherectomy
- Arterial bypass
- Patch graft angioplasty, often in conjunction with bypass
- Thrombolytic therapy/anticoagulation
- Endarterectomy (done rarely, with localized stenosis)
- Amputation

*See Table 46-25

consists of a probe transducer containing a crystal that emits sound waves toward moving blood cells. It measures the velocity of blood flow through a vessel and emits an audible signal. Directional flow can be measured antegrade or retrograde. The Doppler is extremely sensitive to movement of blood. When arterial palpation is difficult or impossible because of severe occlusive disease, the Doppler can be useful in determining blood flow. A palpable pulse and a Doppler pulse are not equivalent and should not be used interchangeably. In addition, segmental blood pressures are also obtained (using a Doppler and sphygmomanometer) at the thigh, below the knee, and at ankle level. Pressures in the leg should equal pressures in the arm. As disease develops in the arteries of the legs the blood pressures drop.

Dividing the ankle pressure by the highest brachial pressure yields the ankle-brachial index (ABI). A normal ABI is 1.0. An ABI between 0.8 and 0.95 indicates minimal disease, an index of 0.4 to 0.8 indicates moderate disease, and 0 to 0.4 indicates severe arterial disease. This technique is also used to follow patients postoperatively after revascularization to monitor patency of bypass grafts. This procedure has limited usefulness when arteries are calcified and noncompressive, as occurs in a diabetic patient. In the diabetic patient the ABI is frequently falsely elevated. Plethysmography detects volume changes in limbs and is useful in detecting disease when vessels are calcified.

Duplex imaging, a noninvasive test, uses a Doppler system to systematically map blood flow throughout the entire region of an artery. It provides anatomic and physiologic information about the blood vessels.

Angiography (aortography and femoral arteriography) is used to further delineate the location and extent of the disease process. In addition, it provides information on inflow and outflow vessels to plan for surgery. Angiography is useful when an intervention (i.e., surgery or angioplasty) is indicated. Magnetic resonance angiography has improved significantly and is sometimes used instead of angiography, especially in patients with renal insufficiency or dye allergy.[14]

Collaborative Care

Conservative management goals of chronic peripheral artery disease include protecting the extremity from trauma, slowing the progression of atherosclerosis, decreasing vasospasm, preventing and controlling infection, and improving collateral circulation (see Table 36-5). The patient's risk factors should be assessed, and proper intervention should be begun regarding cessation of smoking, weight reduction (if indicated), and control of lipid disorders. Hypertension also must be properly managed (see Chapter 31).

Slow, progressive physical activity should be encouraged to help develop collateral circulation. For example, the patient should walk for 15 to 30 minutes several times a day, or as tolerated. Exercise should be stopped if pain occurs and resumed after a rest break when the pain subsides.

Careful inspection, cleansing, and lubrication of both feet is advised to prevent cracking of the skin and infection. Although cleansing is important, soaking of the affected foot should be avoided to prevent skin maceration (or breakdown). If ulceration is present, the affected foot should be kept clean and dry. Covering the ulcer with a dry, sterile dressing helps maintain cleanliness and protects the limb. Ulcers with any significant depth may be treated with a variety of wound care products, but without restoration of blood flow healing is unlikely. Footwear should be soft, roomy, and protective. Chemicals, heat, and cold should be avoided.

Interventional radiologic procedures or surgery is indicated when (1) the symptoms of intermittent claudication become incapacitating, (2) the limb is so ischemic that the patient experiences pain at rest, or (3) ulceration or gangrene is severe enough to threaten the viability of the limb. The latter problem will likely progress unless arterial circulation can be restored.[15]

Interventional Radiologic Procedures. *Percutaneous transluminal angioplasty* involves the use of a special catheter with a cylindrical balloon. When inflated, the balloon dilates the vessel by cracking the confining atherosclerotic intimal shell while also stretching the underlying media (Fig. 36-7). This procedure is used in certain patients who have localized, accessible lesions (less than 10 cm in length). Iliac artery lesions have responded most successfully to percutaneous transluminal angioplasty. Smaller vessels below the knee (tibial arteries) have the least favorable patency rates.

Other devices, called *atherectomy catheters,* are also used inside the artery to "shave" or pulverize the plaque lining the arterial wall. Atherectomy is often performed in conjunction with angioplasty. Once the plaque is "debulked," dilation is performed using a balloon catheter.

Intravascular stents help relieve the problems of restenosis and arterial dissection following percutaneous balloon angioplasty.

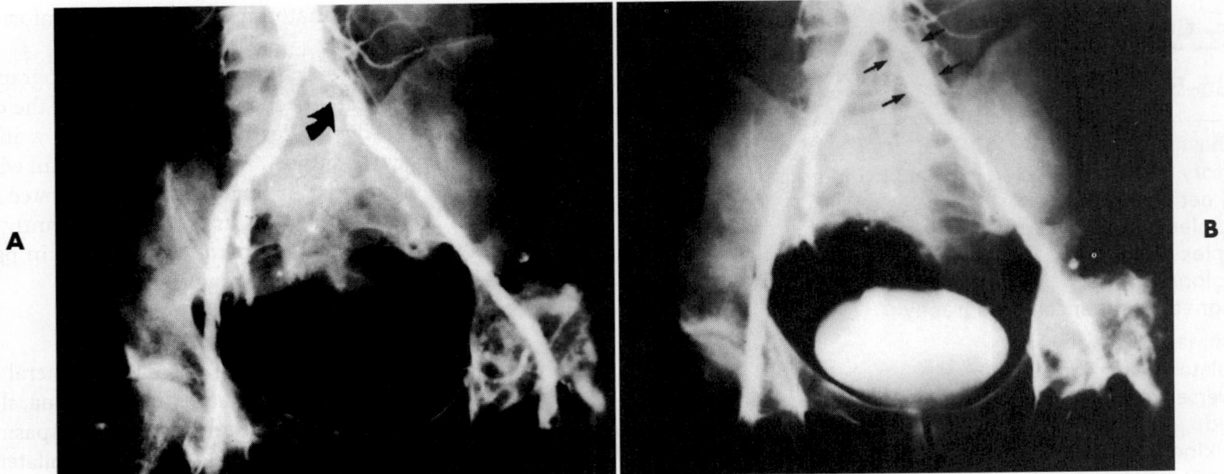

Fig. 36-7 A, Tight stenosis of the left common iliac artery *(arrow)*. B, Dilation of the left common iliac artery lumen following percutaneous transluminal angioplasty *(arrows)*.

Stents are rigid or flexible and are positioned percutaneously within arteries. Stents are most frequently used in the iliac and renal arteries.[16]

Surgical Therapy. Various surgical approaches can be used to improve arterial blood flow beyond a stenotic or occluded artery. The most common is an arterial bypass operation with autogenous vein or synthetic graft material to bypass or carry blood around the lesion (Fig. 36-8).

Other surgical options include endarterectomy (opening the artery and removing the obstructing plaque) and patch graft angioplasty (opening the artery, removing plaque, and sewing a patch to the opening to widen the lumen).[17]

Amputation is the least desired surgical option, but it may be required if gangrene is extensive, infection is present in bone (osteomyelitis), or all major arteries in the limb are occluded, precluding the possibility of bypass surgery. Every effort is made to preserve as much of the limb as possible so that the potential for rehabilitation with an orthotic shoe or prosthesis is optimized (see Chapter 60).

Drug Therapy. Although various drugs are commonly prescribed to treat peripheral arterial occlusive disease, no specific agent is considered to be effective except pentoxifylline (Trental), which increases erythrocyte flexibility and reduces blood viscosity, thus improving the supply of oxygenated blood to ischemic muscle. Although it is not conclusive that antiplatelet aggregating agents such as aspirin, ticlopidine (Ticlid), and clopidogrel (Plavix) improve circulation through diseased arteries or prevent intimal hyperplasia leading to stenosis, they are sometimes used after arterial bypass surgery to promote graft patency. Anticoagulation with warfarin (Coumadin) is sometimes instituted in the patient who has a tendency to occlude grafts secondary to a clotting abnormality.

Cilostazol (Pletal) is a new drug for the treatment of peripheral artery disease. It inhibits platelet aggregation, increases vasodilation, and inhibits smooth muscle cell proliferation. It relieves the symptoms of intermittent claudication.

Nutritional Therapy. The patient with atherosclerosis should be taught and encouraged to do the following:

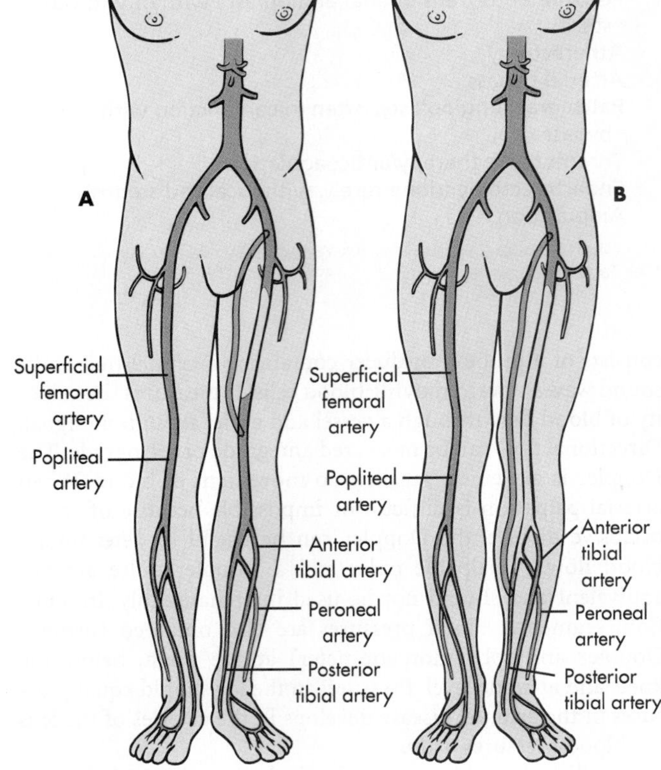

Fig. 36-8 A, Femoral-popliteal bypass graft around an occluded superficial femoral artery. B, Femoral-posterior tibial bypass graft around occluded superficial femoral, popliteal, and proximal tibial arteries.

1. Adjust caloric intake so that optimum weight can be achieved and maintained
2. Decrease dietary cholesterol to less than 200 mg/day
3. Substantially reduce saturated dietary fat (see Table 32-5)
4. Restrict sodium to 2 g per day if edema is present (see Table 33-10)

RESEARCH
IMPLICATIONS FOR NURSING PRACTICE

Exercise Program for Arterial Claudication

Citation Patterson RB and others: Value of a supervised exercise program for the therapy of arterial claudication, *J Vasc Surg* 25:312, 1997.

Purpose To test the effectiveness of a formal supervised exercise program as compared with a home-based exercise program for both walking ability and quality of life in patients with intermittent claudication.

Methods Patients with intermittent claudication were randomized to either a 12-week supervised exercise program (SUPEX) with weekly lectures relating to peripheral vascular disease or to a home exercise group (HOMEX) who attended an identical lecture program and received weekly exercise instruction. The study population included 29 men and 26 women, with a mean age of 69 years. Forty-seven patients completed the 12-week program, and 38 were available for 6-month testing. Claudication pain time (CPT) and maximum walking time (MWT) on a progressive treadmill exercise test were assessed at baseline, program completion, and 6 months. The Medical Outcomes Study Short Form-36 (SF-36) was administered at these intervals to assess effects on quality of life.

Results and Conclusions Each group improved in both CPT and MWT at the completion of the 12-week program, which was sustained at the 6-month follow-up. Although the increase in HOMEX CPT from baseline to 6-month follow-up was less than for the SUPEX group, similar results were obtained for MWT. For both groups, measures of health perception based on the SF-36 demonstrated improvement in the Physical Function Subscale, Bodily Pain Subscale, and Physical Component Score.

Implications for Nursing Practice Supervised exercise programs provide superior increased walking ability in the therapy of intermittent claudication, and both supervised and home-based exercise therapy result in improved SF-36 functional measures. The lack of intergroup differences in these measures may be a result of the high degree of interaction with health care providers in the HOMEX group. Although a supervised program results in optimal walking benefits, a highly structured home-based program provides similar functional improvement and may be a satisfactory alternative for patients.

NURSING MANAGEMENT: CHRONIC ARTERIAL OCCLUSIVE DISEASE

■ Nursing Assessment

Subjective and objective data that should be obtained from a patient with chronic arterial occlusive disease are presented in Table 36-6.

■ Nursing Diagnoses

Nursing diagnoses for the patient with chronic arterial occlusive disease may include, but are not limited to, those presented in NCP 36-2.

■ Planning

The overall goals are that the patient with chronic arterial occlusive disease will have (1) adequate tissue perfusion; (2) relief of pain; (3) increased exercise tolerance; and (4) intact, healthy skin on extremities.

■ Nursing Implementation

Health Promotion. The patient should be assessed for risk factors and should be taught how to control them (see Table 32-4). The nurse's role in the inpatient care facility includes identifying at-risk patients. The nurse should also be involved at the community level, such as in screening clinics for peripheral arterial disease, hypertension, and diabetes. Young people and adults should be educated about the hazards of cigarette smoking. The nurse should also assist in teaching diet modification to reduce the intake of animal fat and refined sugars, proper care of the feet, and the avoidance of injury to the extremities. Patients with positive family histories of cardiac, diabetic, or vascular disease should be encouraged to obtain regular follow-up care.

Acute Intervention. After surgical intervention the patient is placed in a recovery area for close observation. The operative extremity should be checked every 15 minutes initially and then hourly for color, temperature, capillary refill, and the presence of peripheral pulses distal to the operative site. Loss of palpable pulses necessitates immediate intervention. Ankle-brachial index (ABI) measurements may be ordered, and the indices should increase from the patient's preoperative baseline. They should remain constant if the bypass remains patent. All of these findings should be compared with the patient's preoperative baseline and with findings in the opposite limb.[18]

When the patient is transferred from the recovery room, nursing care should focus on continued circulatory assessment and monitoring for the development of potential complications. These include bleeding, hematoma, thrombosis, embolization, and compartment syndrome. Severe ischemic pain, loss of palpable pulse or pulses, pallor, decreasing ABIs, numbness or tingling, or cold temperature may indicate occlusion of the bypass graft and should be reported to the surgeon immediately.

The patient's heels should be kept free of pressure. Knee-flexed positions should be avoided except for exercise. The patient should be turned and positioned frequently with pillows to cushion the incision. On the second or third postoperative day, the patient should be out of bed three to four times daily. Sitting for long periods of time should be discouraged because leg dependency may cause significant edema, resulting in discomfort and stress to suture lines, and increases the risk of deep vein thrombosis. If significant swelling develops, a reclining position is preferred, with the edematous leg elevated above heart level. Occasionally Ace bandages or elastic support stockings are used to help

NURSING ASSESSMENT

Table 36-6 Chronic Arterial Occlusive Disease

Subjective Data	Objective Data
Important Health Information *Past health history:* Hypertension, obesity, diabetes mellitus, hypercholesterolemia, sedentary lifestyle, smoking **Functional Health Patterns** *Health perception–health management:* Family history of vascular disease; smoking *Nutritional-metabolic:* High fat intake *Activity-exercise:* Exercise intolerance *Cognitive-perceptual:* Buttock, thigh, and calf pain that is precipitated by exercise and that subsides with rest (intermittent claudication) or progresses to pain at rest; burning pain in forefeet and toes that increases with activity and decreases with rest; numbness, tingling, sensation of cold in legs or feet; progressive loss of sensation and deep pain in extremities *Sexuality-reproductive:* Impotence	**Integumentary** Loss of hair on legs and feet; thick toenails; pallor with elevation; dependent rubor; thin, cool, shiny skin with muscle atrophy; skin breakdown and ulcerations, especially over bony areas; gangrene **Cardiovascular** Decreased or absent peripheral pulses; bruits may be present at pulse sites **Neurologic** Mobility impairment **Possible Findings** Positive arterial duplex, Doppler pressures, or angiography indicative of occlusive disease

ESR, erythrocyte sedimentation rate.

control edema of the limb. Walking even short distances is desirable. The use of a walker may be helpful initially, especially in the older patient. If no complications are present, discharge from the hospital can be anticipated 3 to 5 days postoperatively.

Ambulatory and Home Care. Atherosclerosis is a systemic disease process and not just localized to the lower extremities. Therefore the overall approach to the control of atherosclerotic occlusive disease involves management of risk factors (see Table 32-4). Tobacco in any form is totally contraindicated, not only because of the vasoconstrictive effects of nicotine, but also because tobacco smoke impairs transport and cellular utilization of oxygen and increases blood viscosity. Continuance of cigarette smoking adversely affects the long-term function of the bypass graft and may result in the development of symptomatic disease in other major arterial beds (e.g., carotid artery disease, coronary artery disease). The health care team must consistently encourage the patient to abstain from smoking. The nurse should tell the patient about various community agencies and support groups, such as behavior modification and antismoking clinics.[15]

If the patient does not undergo surgical repair, a plan of care can be implemented to optimize the patient's arterial circulation. A progressive exercise program often increases the patient's tolerance for exercise and enhances venous return. Collateral vessels—usually small, insignificant branches of major arteries—often enlarge and carry more blood "around" an occlusive lesion as a compensatory mechanism. The demand for blood and oxygen beyond an arterial blockage is believed to enhance collateral vessel development.

Walking is an effective exercise. The patient should be instructed to walk to the point of discomfort, stop and rest, then resume walking until the discomfort recurs. Walking should be done for a prescribed time, usually 30 to 40 minutes a day, in addition to normal activity.

All patients should be taught the importance of meticulous foot care to prevent injury. The patient should learn to inspect the legs and feet daily for skin color changes, mottling, alterations in the texture of the skin and subcutaneous fat, and reduction or absence of hair growth. Any ulceration or inflammation must be reported to the health care provider. Skin temperature should be noted, and capillary refill of the fingers and toes should be tested. In addition, selected patients may be taught to palpate pulses and report any changes to the health care provider. Thick or overgrown toenails and calluses are potentially serious lesions that require regular attention by a skilled health care provider.

Emphasis on foot care is especially important in the diabetic patient with arterial occlusive disease because diabetic neuropathy (i.e., diminished peripheral sensation) increases the susceptibility to traumatic injury and results in delay in seeking treatment (see Table 46-25).

The patient should be instructed to wear clean, light-colored all-cotton or all-wool socks. In addition, comfortable shoes with rounded (not pointed) toes and soft insoles should be worn. Shoes should not be laced tightly, and new shoes should be broken in gradually. Frequent inspection of the feet should be of paramount importance to this patient population so that prompt attention to problems can be facilitated. Patients with poor eyesight, back problems, obesity, or arthritis may need assistance with foot care.[19]

■ Evaluation

Expected outcomes for the patient with chronic arterial occlusive disease are addressed in NCP 36-2. 

36-2 NURSING CARE PLAN PATIENT WITH CHRONIC ARTERIAL OCCLUSIVE DISEASE

Expected Patient Outcomes	Nursing Interventions and *Rationales*
NURSING DIAGNOSIS	**Altered peripheral tissue perfusion** *related to* decreased arterial blood flow *as manifested by* pain in buttocks, thigh, or calf; diminished or absent peripheral pulses; paresthesia in toes or feet; pallor or blanching on elevation of limb; hyperemia when limb is dependent; shiny, taut skin and loss of hair on lower extremities.
▪ Able to identify interventions, activities that promote vasodilation. ▪ Identification of factors that impair peripheral circulation. ▪ Decreased pain.	▪ Assess lower extremities for evidence of altered peripheral tissue perfusion *to provide appropriate interventions.* ▪ Explain the importance of smoking cessation *to increase patient cooperation and reduce vasoconstrictive effects of nicotine.* ▪ Encourage patient to walk to the point of pain *because this exercise promotes the development of collateral circulation.* ▪ Teach patient to stop and rest if pain occurs while walking *to allow increased circulation to deprived areas.* ▪ Teach patient to avoid dependent position of lower extremities *because this position promotes venous stasis.* ▪ Teach patient to avoid tight girdles, garters, or socks *because they impair collateral circulation.*
NURSING DIAGNOSIS	**Impaired skin integrity** *related to* decreased peripheral circulation, altered sensation, and increased susceptibility to infection *as manifested by* ulcerations, nonhealing wounds, or gangrenous areas on lower extremities.
▪ No wounds on lower extremities. ▪ No evidence of infection of wounds on lower extremities.	▪ Teach patient to avoid trauma to lower extremities *because tissue is very fragile and wounds heal poorly due to circulatory insufficiency.* ▪ Teach patient to check temperature of bath water with fingers rather than toes *since sensation may be diminished.* ▪ Teach patient and significant other proper foot care and inspection, including roomy, soft footwear and callus and toenail care by a professional only. ▪ Assess ulcers for signs of infection and treat ulcer with appropriate wound care *to promote wound healing.* ▪ Teach patient to avoid use of chemicals on feet and to keep feet warm.
NURSING DIAGNOSIS	**Pain** *related to* ischemia and exercise *as manifested by* complaints of pain during exercise that is relieved by rest.
▪ Relief of pain.	▪ Assess location, onset, degree, and duration of pain *so appropriate interventions are planned.* ▪ Encourage rest when pain occurs *so that tissue ischemia and pain are relieved or reduced* and explain rationale to patient *to increase cooperation.* ▪ Teach relaxation techniques, *since stress increases vasoconstriction and pain.* ▪ Teach patient to report rest pain *because this is an indication of worsening of the arterial blockages.*
NURSING DIAGNOSIS	**Activity intolerance** *related to* imbalance between oxygen supply and demand *as manifested by* claudication.
▪ Improved ability to ambulate without pain.	▪ Monitor the amount of exercise patient can tolerate before the onset of pain *to provide a baseline for evaluation.* ▪ Assist patient in developing a progressive exercise program *to promote collateral circulation and enhance venous return.* ▪ Explain that patient should walk to point of pain, rest until pain subsides, and resume walking *so endurance can be increased as collateral circulation develops.*

Continued

36-2 NURSING CARE PLAN PATIENT WITH CHRONIC ARTERIAL OCCLUSIVE DISEASE—continued

Expected Patient Outcomes	Nursing Interventions and *Rationales*
NURSING DIAGNOSIS	**Ineffective management of treatment plan** *related to* lack of knowledge of disease and self-care measures *as manifested by* questions about disease process, wound, and treatment.
▪ Able to describe disease and treatment plan. ▪ Able to demonstrate how to care for leg ulcers.	▪ Identify factors that influence learning such as perception of severity, available support systems, cognitive ability, and physical ability *so that teaching plan can be individualized.* ▪ Assess patient's knowledge of disease and its treatment *to determine extent of the problem and plan appropriate interventions.* ▪ Teach patient about the disease, treatment, activity restrictions, and ulcer care *so patient will be less anxious, be more cooperative with treatment plan, and make accurate adjustments in lifestyle.* ▪ Explain the importance of smoking cessation *so patient understands the effects of nicotine.* ▪ Emphasize the importance of meticulous foot care *to reduce the risk of infection and injury to feet.*

THROMBOANGIITIS OBLITERANS

Thromboangiitis obliterans (Buerger's disease) is an inflammatory, thrombotic disorder of the medium-sized arteries and veins of the upper or lower extremities. Occlusion of the vessel occurs with development of collateral circulation around areas of obstruction. The basic cause is unknown. However, there is a direct relationship to cigarette smoking: the disease occurs only in smokers, and when smoking is stopped, the disease improves. Unlike atherosclerosis, lipid accumulation does not occur in the vessel media in thromboangiitis obliterans. The disorder, generally asymmetric, occurs predominantly in men between 25 and 40 years of age who smoke. A familial tendency has also been observed.

The symptom complex of Buerger's disease is often confused with that of atherosclerotic occlusive disease. The patient may have intermittent claudication. The development of rest pain is a premonitory sign of gangrene and may develop in advanced stages of the disease process. Other signs and symptoms may include color and temperature changes in the affected limb or limbs, paresthesia, thrombophlebitis, and cold sensitivity. Painful ulceration and gangrene may necessitate toe amputations.

Treatment includes complete cessation of smoking and avoidance of trauma to the extremity. Patients are often told that they have a choice between their cigarettes and their legs; they cannot have both. Supportive psychotherapy and pharmacologic treatment of underlying anxiety disorders are sometimes helpful in assisting the patient to stop smoking. Although this disorder is difficult to treat, anticoagulants and vasodilator therapy have been used. Amputation, generally below the knee, may be necessary in advanced cases.

RAYNAUD'S PHENOMENON

Raynaud's phenomenon (arteriospastic disease) is an episodic vasospastic disorder of small cutaneous arteries, most frequently involving the fingers and toes. The exact etiology is not known, although there is support for the theory that it occurs secondary to exaggerated reflex sympathetic vasoconstriction.

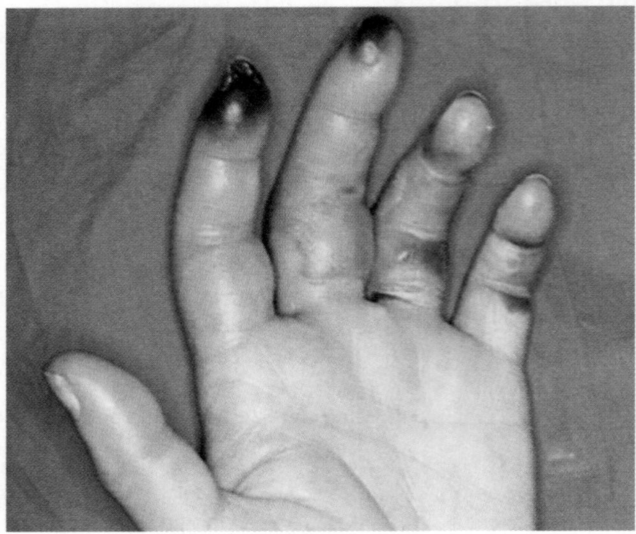

Fig. 36-9 Raynaud's phenomenon.

Raynaud's phenomenon occurs primarily in young women. It is seen frequently in association with collagen diseases such as rheumatoid arthritis, scleroderma, and systemic lupus erythematosus. Other contributing factors include occupationally related trauma and pressure to the fingertips as noted in typists, pianists, and those who use handheld vibrating equipment. Exposure to heavy metals may also be a contributing etiologic factor. The symptoms are usually precipitated by exposure to cold, emotional upsets, caffeine, and tobacco use.

The disorder is characterized by three color changes (white, red, and blue) (Fig. 36-9). Initially the vasoconstrictive effect produces pallor (white), followed by cyanosis (bluish-purple). These changes are subsequently followed by rubor or hyperemia. Because Raynaud's phenomenon is a vasospastic disorder of small blood vessels, the radial and ulnar pulses are never lost. The patient usually describes cold and numbness in the vasocon-

Table 36-7 Clinical Manifestations of Thrombophlebitis

	Superficial	Deep	
		Small Veins	Major Venous Trunks
Usual causes	Varicose veins; direct trauma; IV catheters; thromboangiitis obliterans; caustic IV medications such as chemotherapy, radiopaque contrast material; IV drug use	Postoperatively, before and after childbirth, direct or distant trauma, congestive heart failure, prolonged bed rest, acute febrile disease, sepsis, debilitating disease, malignant disease, blood dyscrasias	Systemic lupus erythematosus, pressure of tumors on veins, estrogen therapy, malignant disease, blood dyscrasias, idiopathic cause
Usual location	Saphenous veins and their tributaries, forearm	Soleal; posterior tibial, other deep calf veins; popliteal; pelvis	Femoral, iliac, inferior or superior vena cava, axillary, subclavian
Clinical findings	Tender, red, inflamed induration along course of subcutaneous vein (visible and palpable)	Possible tenderness to deep pressure, induration of overlying muscle, minimal or no venous distention	Swelling, cyanosis, venous distention, mild to moderate pain, tenderness over involved vein (groin or axilla)
Edema of extremities	Almost never	Occasionally	Frequently
Embolization	Almost never	Always a threat	Always a threat
Chronic venous insufficiency	Almost never	Usually not	Frequently

strictive phase and throbbing, aching pain; tingling; and swelling in the hyperemic phase. This type of episode usually lasts only minutes but in severe cases may persist for several hours. Complications include punctate (small hole) lesions of the fingertips and superficial gangrenous ulcers in advanced stages.

If the symptoms persist for several years in the absence of an associated underlying disorder, the diagnosis of primary Raynaud's disease may be made. It is of diagnostic importance to search for an underlying disease so that appropriate treatment can be instituted. Otherwise, treatment is generally not required because the symptoms are self-limiting. However, treatment of symptoms with certain calcium channel blockers has been encouraging. β-Adrenergic blocking agents have been used with variable success. Sympathectomy is considered only in advanced cases.

Patient education should be directed toward reassurance that no serious underlying disorder is present and that prevention of recurrent episodes is possible. Loose, warm clothing should be worn as protection from the cold, including gloves when the refrigerator-freezer is used or when cold objects are being handled. Temperature extremes should be avoided. Moving to a warmer climate is not necessarily beneficial because symptoms may still occur during cooler weather and in an air-conditioned environment. The patient should stop smoking, avoid caffeine, and develop techniques to cope with anxiety-producing situations. Immersion of the hands in warm water often decreases the spasm.

DISORDERS OF THE VEINS

THROMBOPHLEBITIS

The most common disorder of the veins is thrombophlebitis, the formation of a thrombus (clot) in association with inflammation of the vein. The initiating event is usually thrombus formation. Thrombophlebitis is classified as either *superficial* or *deep* (Table 36-7).

In about 65% of all patients receiving IV therapy, superficial thrombophlebitis develops, and in at least 5% of all surgical patients, deep vein thrombophlebitis (DVT) develops. Superficial thrombophlebitis is often of minor significance and is treated with elevation, antiinflammatory agents, and warm compresses. DVT is of greater significance and can result in embolization of thrombi from deep veins to the lungs. This can be fatal and, at the least, results in prolonged hospitalization.

Etiology

Three important factors (Virchow's triad) in the etiology of thrombophlebitis are (1) venous stasis, (2) damage of the endothelium (inner lining of the vein), and (3) hypercoagulability of the blood. The patient at risk for the development of thrombophlebitis usually has predisposing conditions to these three disorders (Table 36-8).

Venous Stasis. Normal blood flow in the venous system depends on the action of muscles in the extremities and the functional adequacy of venous valves, which allow unidirectional flow. Venous stasis occurs when the valves are dysfunctional or the muscles of the extremities are inactive. Venous stasis occurs more frequently in people who are obese, have CHF, have been on long trips without regular exercise, or are immobile for long periods (e.g., with spinal cord injuries or fractured hips). Also at risk are pregnant women and women in the postpartum period.[20]

The patient with atrial fibrillation is also at high risk because of stagnation of blood and the eddying in blood flow caused by irregular ventricular contractions in response to the fibrillation. Some medications, such as corticosteroids and quinine, predispose a patient to venous stasis and clot formation.

Endothelial Damage. Damage to the endothelial surface of the vein may be caused by trauma or external pressure and occurs any time a venipuncture is performed. Damaged endothelium has decreased fibrinolytic properties, predisposing to the development of thrombus. Increased endothelial

Table 36-8 Risk Factors for Deep Vein Thrombophlebitis and Thromboembolism

Abdominal and pelvic surgery
Advanced age
Antithrombin III deficiency
Atrial fibrillation
Cerebrovascular disease
Cigarette smoking
Congestive heart failure
Drug abuse
Estrogen therapy, including oral contraceptives
Excessive vitamin E intake
History of thrombophlebitis
Hypercoagulable states
Polycythemia vera
Severe anemias
Dehydration or malnutrition
IV therapy
Myocardial infarction
Neoplasms, especially hepatic and pancreatic
Obesity
Postpartum period
Pregnancy
Prolonged immobility
Bed rest
Long trip without adequate exercise
Spinal cord injury
Fractured hip
Sepsis
Suprapubic prostatectomy
Trauma
Venous cannulation or catheterization

damage is sustained when patients on IV therapy are receiving high-dose antibiotics, potassium, chemotherapeutic agents, or hypertonic solutions such as contrast media.

Other factors predisposing to endothelial inflammation and damage include prolonged presence (longer than 48 hours) of an IV catheter in the same site, the use of contaminated IV equipment, a fracture that causes damage to the blood vessels, diabetes mellitus, blood pooling, burns, and any unusual physical exertion that results in muscular strain.

Hypercoagulability of Blood. Hypercoagulability of blood occurs in many hematologic disorders, particularly polycythemia, severe anemias, various malignancies, and antithrombin III deficiency. A patient with systemic infections in which endotoxins are released also has hypercoagulability. Hypercoagulability also seems to be the contributing factor in idiopathic thrombophlebitis.

The patient who takes estrogen-based oral contraceptives is at increased risk for thromboembolic disease. Women who take contraceptives and smoke double their risk because of the constricting effect of nicotine on the blood vessel wall. Smoking may also cause hypercoagulability.[21]

Pathophysiology

Red blood cells (RBCs), WBCs, platelets, and fibrin adhere to form a thrombus. A frequent site of thrombus formation is the valve cusps of veins, where venous stasis allows accumulation of blood products. As the thrombus enlarges, increased amounts of blood cells and fibrin collect behind it, producing a larger clot with a "tail" that eventually occludes the lumen of the vein.

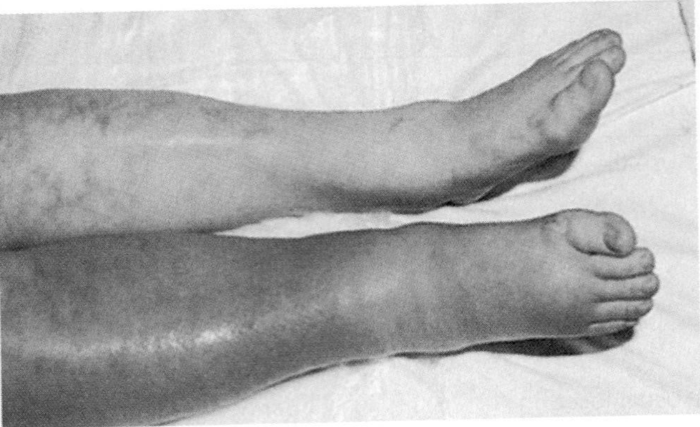

Fig. 36-10 Deep vein thrombophlebitis.

If a thrombus only partially occludes the vein, the thrombus becomes covered by endothelial cells and the thrombotic process stops. If the thrombus does not become detached, it undergoes lysis or becomes firmly organized and adherent within 5 to 7 days. The organized thrombi may detach and result in emboli. Turbulence of blood flow is a major factor contributing to detachment of the thrombus from the vein wall. The thrombus can become an embolus that generally flows through the venous circulation, to the heart, and lodges in the pulmonary circulation.

Clinical Manifestations

Clinical manifestations of thrombophlebitis vary according to the size and location of the thrombus and the adequacy of collateral circulation (see Table 36-7). The patient with superficial thrombophlebitis may have a palpable, firm, subcutaneous cordlike vein. The area surrounding the vein may be tender to the touch, reddened, and warm. A mild systemic temperature elevation and leukocytosis may be present. Edema of the extremity may or may not occur. The most common cause of superficial thrombophlebitis in the upper extremities is IV therapy. The most common cause of superficial thrombophlebitis in the lower extremities is related to varicose veins.

The patient with deep thrombophlebitis may have no symptoms or have unilateral leg edema (Fig. 36-10), pain, warm skin, and a temperature greater than 100.4° F (38° C). If the calf is involved, tenderness may be present on palpation. Homans' sign, pain on dorsiflexion of the foot when the leg is raised, is a classic but unreliable sign because it is not specific for deep vein thrombosis. If the inferior vena cava is involved, the lower extremities may be edematous and cyanotic. If the superior vena cava is involved, the upper extremities, neck, back, and face may be edematous and cyanotic.[22]

Complications

The most serious complications of thrombophlebitis are pulmonary embolism, chronic venous insufficiency, and phlegmasia cerulea dolens. Pulmonary embolism is a life-threatening complication of thrombophlebitis (see the section on pulmonary embolism).

DIAGNOSTIC STUDIES

Table 36-9 Deep Vein Thrombophlebitis and Pulmonary Embolism

Study	Description and Abnormal Findings
Coagulation Studies	
Platelet count, bleeding time, INR, PTT, APTT	Elevation if patient has underlying blood dyscrasia; decrease possible if patient has polycythemia; alteration possible because of medication interaction
Noninvasive Venous Studies	
Venous Doppler evaluation	Determination of venous flow in deep femoral, popliteal, and posterior tibial veins; normal finding of spontaneous flow with variation transmitted by respiration cycle; abnormal finding of absence of flow augmentation with distal compression and proximal release
Duplex scanning	Combination of ultrasound imaging techniques and Doppler capabilities to determine location and extent of thrombus within veins (most widely used test to diagnose deep vein thrombosis)
Plethysmography	Measurement of increase in leg volume induced by obstruction of venous outflow by inflation of thigh cuff (maximum venous capitance), measurement of speed at which volume decreases on thigh cuff release (venous outflow), abnormal finding of slow outflow
Venogram (phlebogram)	X-ray determination of location and extent of clot using contrast media to outline filling defects. Development of collateral circulation defined
Lung Scan (ventilation and perfusion)	Means of determining presence of pulmonary embolism and extent of resulting lung damage, abnormal finding of mismatch between ventilation and perfusion components; frequently inconclusive
Pulmonary Arteriogram	X-ray determination (using contrast media) of location and size of pulmonary embolism

APTT, activated partial thromboplastin time; *INR*, international normalized ratio; *PTT*, partial thromboplastin time.

Chronic venous insufficiency, a common complication resulting from recurrent thrombophlebitis, results in valvular destruction, allowing retrograde flow of blood. Persistent edema, increased pigmentation, secondary varicosities, ulceration, and cyanosis of the limb when it is placed in a dependent position may develop in a person with this complication. Signs and symptoms of chronic venous insufficiency often do not develop until many years following DVT.

Phlegmasia cerulea dolens (swollen, blue, painful leg) may develop in a patient with severe thrombophlebitis of the lower extremities. It causes sudden, massive swelling and intense bluish discoloration of the extremity. Gangrene may occur as a result of arterial occlusion secondary to venous outflow obstruction.

Diagnostic Studies

Various diagnostic studies are used to determine the site or location and extent of the thrombus or emboli (Tables 36-9 and 36-10).

Collaborative Care

The treatment of superficial thrombophlebitis includes elevation of the affected extremity until the tenderness has subsided and the application of warm, moist heat. Heat is used to relieve the pain and treat the inflammation.

If edema still persists when the patient is ambulatory, elastic compression stockings are recommended. Ideally they should be measured to fit the patient once the edema has resolved. The use of elastic compression stockings is recommended for several months (usually at least 3 to 6 months) to support the vein walls and valves and decrease swelling and pain on ambulation.

COLLABORATIVE CARE

Table 36-10 Deep Vein Thrombophlebitis

Diagnostic
- History and physical examination
- Chest x-ray
- Complete blood count with WBC differential
- PT, INR, PTT, APTT, platelet count, bleeding time
- Electrocardiogram
- Venous studies (see Table 36-9)
- Venogram of affected limb (rarely performed)

Collaborative Therapy

Conservative
- Continuous IV heparin
- Bed rest with bathroom privileges
- Elevation of legs above heart level
- Anticoagulant therapy
- Elastic compression stockings
- Measurement and charting of size of both thighs and calves every morning

Surgical
- Intracaval filter insertion
- Venous thrombectomy (rarely done)

PT, prothrombin time.

Drug Therapy. Mild oral analgesics such as aspirin and codeine are used to relieve pain. Nonsteroidal antiinflammatory agents such as ibuprofen (Motrin, Advil) have been used to treat the inflammatory process and accompanying pain. Anticoagulant therapy is usually not indicated for superficial

DRUG THERAPY

Table 36-11 Anticoagulant Therapy

Drug	Route of Administration	Comments
Heparin		
Panheparin	Continuous IV infusion by infusion pump	Initial bolus dose of heparin is required. Protamine sulfate should be available as an antidote. Cannot be mixed with antibiotics or other medications. Frequent clotting studies required.
Lipo-Hepin	Intermittent IV infusion q4hr	Clotting status is monitored by whole blood clotting time (Lee-White clotting time), PTT, activated clotting time, and APTT.
Liquaemin Sodium	Intermittent subcutaneous infusion q6hr	Aspirin should not be administered to a patient taking heparin.
Coumarin Derivatives		
Warfarin (Coumadin, Panwarfin), dicumarol, acenocoumarol (Sintrom)	Oral	Vitamin K injection should be available as an antidote. Plasma levels may be maintained for up to 5 days. Clotting status is monitored by INR. INR (usually 2-3) considered more accurate than PT.

thrombophlebitis but is routinely used for DVT (see Table 36-10). The goals of anticoagulation therapy in the treatment of DVT are to prevent propagation of the clot, development of a new thrombus, and embolization. Anticoagulant therapy does not dissolve the clot. Lysis of the clot begins spontaneously through the body's intrinsic fibrinolytic system (see Chapter 28).

The most commonly used anticoagulants are heparin and coumarin compounds (Table 36-11). Heparin acts directly on the intrinsic and common pathways of blood coagulation. Heparin inhibits thrombin-mediated conversion of fibrinogen to fibrin. It also potentiates the actions of antithrombin III, inhibits the activation of factor IX, and neutralizes activated factor X by activating factor X inhibitor.

In DVT heparin, which is administered by continuous IV infusion after an initial bolus dose, is given for up to 7 days and is followed by oral anticoagulants for 3 to 6 months. Bed rest with elevation of the affected extremity above the level of the heart is indicated until therapeutic levels of anticoagulation are achieved and the edema subsides.

Low-molecular-weight heparin (LMWH) is effective for the prevention of venous thrombosis, as well as prevention of extension or recurrence. Enoxaparin (Lovenox), dalteparin (Fragmin), and ardeparin (Normiflo) are three types of LMWH. LMWH has greater bioavailability, more predictable dose response, and longer half-life than heparin. LMWH has the practical advantage that it does not require anticoagulant monitoring and dose adjustment.[23] LMWH is administered subcutaneously in fixed doses, once or twice daily. Danaparoid (Orgaran), known as a heparinoid, does not contain heparin or heparin fragments. However, like heparain, it has antithrombotic action. It is administered subcutaneously.

Coumarin compounds, of which warfarin (Coumadin) is the most commonly used, exert their action indirectly on the coagulation pathway. Warfarin inhibits the hepatic synthesis of the vitamin K–dependent coagulation factors II, VII, IX, and X by competitively interfering with vitamin K. Vitamin K is normally required for the synthesis of these factors.

Oral anticoagulants are administered concurrently with heparin. Warfarin requires 48 to 72 hours to influence prothrombin time (PT), but may take as long as 3 to 5 days before maximum effect is achieved. Therefore an overlap of heparin and warfarin is required for 3 to 5 days. The clotting status should be monitored by activated partial thromboplastin time (APTT) for heparin therapy and PT or international normalized ratio (INR) for coumarin derivatives. The INR is a standardized system of reporting PT based on a referenced calibration model and calculated by comparing the patient's PT with a control value. Other tests to monitor anticoagulation can be used (Table 36-12).

A careful history of childbearing status and medications should be taken before initiating anticoagulation. Because coumarin compounds are contraindicated in pregnancy, these patients requiring anticoagulation often receive subcutaneous heparin. Antiplatelet agents (e.g., aspirin) are generally contraindicated while on anticoagulation. Other medications that interact with coumarin compounds include ibuprofen (Advil, Motrin), phenytoin (Dilantin), and barbiturates (Table 36-13). Changes in diet can also interact with coumarin compounds. A diet high in vitamin K (e.g., green leafy vegetables) can make it difficult to maintain a patient within a therapeutic range. The patient should be instructed to follow a diet that includes foods containing vitamin K in moderate amounts and to avoid additional vitamin supplements with vitamin K. In addition, the patient should be instructed to avoid excessive amounts of vitamin E.

Surgical Therapy. Although most patients are managed conservatively, a small percentage require surgical intervention (see Table 36-10). The primary indication for surgery is to prevent pulmonary emboli. Surgical procedures include venous thrombectomy (rarely performed) and inferior vena cava interruption (Fig. 36-11). Venous thrombectomy involves the removal of an occluding clot through an incision in the vein. This procedure is done to prevent pulmonary embolism or to decrease the risk of the development of chronic venous insufficiency.

Table 36-12 Tests of Blood Coagulation

Test	Drug Monitored	Normal Value	Therapeutic Value
Lee-White whole blood clotting time	Heparin	9-14 min	20-30 min
INR	Warfarin	0.75-1.25	2-3
APTT	Heparin	24-36 sec	48-60 sec
ACT	Heparin	80-135 sec	3 min

Table 36-13 Drugs Interacting with Oral Anticoagulants

Drugs Potentiating Response	Drugs Diminishing Response
Anabolic steroids (e.g., Dianabol)	Barbiturates (e.g., secobarbital, phenobarbital)
Clofibrate (Atromid-S)	Cholestyramine (Questran)
Dextrothyroxine (Choloxin)	Ethchlorvynol (Placidyl)
Disulfiram (Antabuse)	Glutethimide (Doriden)
Metronidazole (Flagyl)	Griseofulvin (Grifulvin)
Neomycin	Rifampin (Rifadin, Rimactane)
Nonsteroidal anti-inflammatory drugs	
Oxyphenbutazone (Tandearil)	
Phenylbutazone (Butazolidin)	
Phenytoin (Dilantin)	
Phenyramidol (Analexin)	
Salicylates	
Sulfonamides	

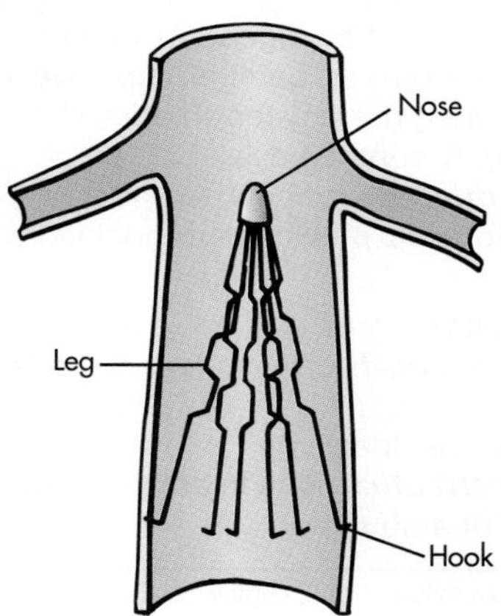

Fig. 36-11 Inferior vena caval interruption technique using Greenfield stainless steel filter to prevent pulmonary embolism.

Vena cava interruption devices, including the Greenfield filter, can be inserted percutaneously through superficial femoral veins. The filter device is opened and the spokes penetrate the vessel walls (Fig. 36-11). These devices result in "sieve-type" obstruction, permitting filtration of clots without interruption of blood flow.

Complications after the insertion of the intravascular filter device are rare. They include air embolism, improper placement, and migration of the filter more distally into the venous system. Venous congestion is common and results from the accumulation of trapped clots at the filter site. Over time these clots may clog the filter and completely occlude the vena cava. Since this process is gradual, collateral vessels usually develop to maintain venous flow. However, these collateral venous pathways may also provide an alternate route for pulmonary emboli.

NURSING MANAGEMENT: THROMBOPHLEBITIS

Nursing Assessment

Subjective and objective data that should be obtained from a patient with thrombophlebitis are presented in Table 36-14.

Nursing Diagnoses

Nursing diagnoses for the patient with thrombophlebitis include, but are not limited to, those presented in NCP 36-3.

Planning

The overall goals are that the patient with thrombophlebitis will have (1) relief of pain, (2) decreased edema, (3) no skin ulceration, and (4) no evidence of pulmonary emboli.

Nursing Implementation

Health Promotion. Thrombus formation can be prevented in many situations. In surgical patients prophylactic measures include early ambulation, leg exercises postoperatively, use of compression stockings, adequate hydration, and low-dose anticoagulant therapy. Heparin (5000 units subcutaneously every 8 to 12 hours) or oral anticoagulants are often recommended for the high risk patient who is predisposed to thrombus formation.[22] LMWH is being used with increasing frequency to prevent thrombus formation in high risk patients.

Mechanical methods of prophylaxis, such as the use of intermittent pneumatic compression stockings or boots, promote venous return and stimulate fibrinolytic activity within the vein. These devices are commonly used on high risk hospitalized patients. These devices are not used on patients with active clotting processes.

Another important preventive measure is to avoid prolonged standing or sitting in a motionless, leg-dependent position. Frequent knee flexion, ankle rotation, and active walking should be done during long periods of sitting or standing, especially on long trips.

The patient should be taught to quit smoking because it increases the viscosity of the blood. The patient should also perform deep-breathing exercises and range-of-motion leg exercises. In addition, the nurse should identify the patient at high risk for deep vein thrombophlebitis and institute appropriate preventive measures.

NURSING ASSESSMENT

Table 36-14 Thrombophlebitis

Subjective Data	Objective Data
Important Health Information *Past health history:* Trauma to vein, varicose veins, childbirth, bacteremia, obesity, prolonged bed rest, irregular heartbeat (e.g., atrial fibrillation), COPD, CHF, malignancies, hematologic disorders, systemic lupus erythematosus, MI, spinal cord injury, prolonged travel *Medications:* Use of estrogens (including oral contraceptives), corticosteroids, quinine, excessive amounts of vitamin E, IV drug therapy (antibiotics, chemotherapy, potassium), IV contrast dyes *Surgery or other treatments:* Any recent surgery, especially orthopedic; previous surgery involving veins, IV therapy **Functional Health Patterns** *Health perception–health management:* IV drug abuse, smoking *Activity-exercise:* Inactivity *Cognitive-perceptual:* Pain in area surrounding vein or on palpation or ambulation	**General** Fever, anxiety, pain **Integumentary** Red, linear streaks at involved vein; increased size of extremity when compared with other side; taut, shiny skin, tenderness on palpation; distention and warmth of superficial veins; edema and cyanosis of extremities, neck, back, and face (superior vena cava involvement) **Cardiovascular** Firm, palpable cord in vein **Possible Findings** Leukocytosis, abnormal coagulation, anemia or elevated hematocrit and RBC count, positive venous duplex or Doppler studies, positive venogram

CHF, congestive heart failure; *COPD,* chronic obstructive pulmonary disease.

Acute Intervention. Nursing care for the patient with thrombophlebitis is directed toward the prevention of emboli formation and the reduction of inflammation (see NCP 36-3). Acute intervention for superficial thrombophlebitis involves the use of warm moist packs or soaks, elevation of the affected extremity, removal of an IV catheter if present, and provision of analgesia to minimize pain and inflammation. Some physicians advocate surgical intervention if the greater saphenous system of the lower extremity is involved. The greater saphenous vein may be ligated to prevent extension of thrombus into the deep venous system.

Acute intervention for DVT involves IV and oral anticoagulation, 3 to 6 days of bed rest with elevation of the affected extremity, and the use of elastic support (elastic bandages or compression stockings) to promote venous return.

While the patient is receiving anticoagulation therapy, the nurse should closely observe for any indication of bleeding, including epistaxis and bleeding gingiva.[24] Urine should be assessed for gross or microscopic hematuria. A smoky appearance to the urine is sometimes noted if blood is present. A specimen should be checked daily for hematuria. Particular attention should be paid to the protection of skin areas that may be traumatized. Surgical incisions should be closely observed for evidence of bleeding. Stools should be tested to determine the presence of occult blood from the gastrointestinal tract. Mental status changes, especially in the older patient, should be assessed as a possible indication of cerebral bleeding.

The nurse should review with the patient any medications currently being taken that may interfere with anticoagulant therapy. The nurse should monitor PTT, INR, hemoglobin, hematocrit, and platelet levels when a patient is receiving anticoagulant drugs. Medication doses are titrated according to the results of clotting studies. The nurse should be cautious about administering either heparin or Coumadin without first checking the results of the clotting studies. The antidote for heparin is protamine sulfate, and the antidote for Coumadin is vitamin K. These drugs must be immediately available if bleeding occurs.

Ambulatory and Home Care. Compression stockings should be properly measured and fitted. They should be worn when the patient becomes ambulatory. These stockings compress superficial veins and prevent venous stasis. The nurse should take care to prevent any pressure under the knee. The patient also should be taught to avoid crossing the legs at the knees. These measures will place pressure on the popliteal space and decrease venous return to the heart.

During all phases of care the nurse should evaluate the patient's psychologic response. Many patients are apprehensive that clots will move to the heart or lungs and cause sudden death. Every patient should be allowed to verbalize concerns, and an attempt should be made to clarify misconceptions. The patient hospitalized for an extended period of time should be provided with diversional activities.

Discharge teaching should stress the hazards of smoking, the importance of compression stockings, the need to avoid constrictive girdles or garters, and the avoidance of contraceptives for the patient with recurrent thrombophlebitis. Exercise programs should be developed with an emphasis on swimming and wading, which are particularly beneficial because of the gentle, even pressure of the water. A balanced program of rest and exercise, along with proper posture and avoiding long periods of sitting, improves arterial filling and venous return. The older patient should be taught safety precautions to prevent injuries, such as falls.

If the patient is continuing on anticoagulant therapy, the patient and family need careful explanations of medication dosage, actions, and side effects, as well as the importance of routine blood tests and the need to report symptoms to the health care provider (Table 36-15). Home monitoring devices are now available for immediate testing of PT.

36-3 NURSING CARE PLAN PATIENT WITH THROMBOPHLEBITIS

Expected Patient Outcomes	Nursing Interventions and *Rationales*
NURSING DIAGNOSIS **Pain** *related to* edema from impaired circulation in extremities *as manifested by* complaints of pain in extremity and presence of edema in extremity.	
▪ Relief of pain.	▪ Keep affected leg elevated above heart level *to promote venous return and decrease swelling.* ▪ Maintain bed rest or activity level in accordance with acuteness of condition *to relieve pain and decrease swelling.* ▪ Apply continuous warm, moist heat (e.g., K-pad at low heat) if ordered *to relieve pain, reduce inflammation, and improve circulation by vasodilation.* ▪ Administer mild analgesics as ordered *to relieve pain.* ▪ Measure thighs and calves daily at a marked site *to provide quantitative measures to assess increase or decrease in edema.* ▪ Instruct patient not to cross legs at knees *to prevent further restriction of circulation to and from legs.*
NURSING DIAGNOSIS **Altered health maintenance** *related to* lack of knowledge about disorder and its treatment *as manifested by* patient asking many questions or no questions about condition.	
▪ Understanding of disease process and treatment, including anticoagulation management, clothing, activity, and diet.	▪ Teach patient signs and symptoms of thrombophlebitis and of abnormal bleeding to report to physician *to enable early diagnosis and treatment.* ▪ Encourage patient to take anticoagulants according to prescribed schedule *to prevent dosing errors resulting in extension of the clot or bleeding.* ▪ Instruct patient on need for routine blood work (INR, platelet count) *to monitor response to treatment and risk of bleeding.* ▪ Assist patient with obtaining Medic Alert identification *to alert others to anticoagulant therapy.* ▪ Teach patient not to wear garters, girdles, or any constrictive clothing *to avoid restriction of blood flow and venous pooling.* ▪ Teach patient to avoid rubbing or massaging extremity *to prevent dislodging a thrombus.* ▪ Teach patient to avoid sitting with legs crossed or in a dependent position, *which increases venous stasis.* ▪ Encourage patient to maintain regular activity on daily basis *to promote blood flow and prevent venous stasis.* ▪ Encourage proper diet to lose weight if indicated *because obesity increases compression of vessels.*
NURSING DIAGNOSIS **Risk for impaired skin integrity** *related to* alteration in peripheral tissue perfusion and possible valvular destruction.	
▪ No evidence of ulcer formation in legs.	▪ Assess patient for altered skin pigmentation in lower extremity, pain, open ulcer, and edema of lower extremity *to identify signs of impaired skin integrity.* ▪ Teach patient to wear elastic compression stockings when ordered by physician except when sleeping *to provide compression of superficial veins and improve venous flow in deep veins.* ▪ Teach patient to change positions when sitting or standing for prolonged periods and to elevate leg when sitting *to reduce venous stasis.* ▪ Lubricate skin regularly *because this minimizes itching that leads to trauma.*

Continued

36-3 NURSING CARE PLAN PATIENT WITH THROMBOPHLEBITIS—continued

Expected Patient Outcomes	Nursing Interventions and *Rationales*

COLLABORATIVE PROBLEMS

Nursing Goals	Nursing Interventions and *Rationales*
POTENTIAL COMPLICATION	Pulmonary embolism *related to* dehydration, immobility, and embolization of thrombus.
▪ Monitor patient for signs of pulmonary embolism. ▪ Report deviations from acceptable parameters. ▪ Carry out appropriate medical and nursing interventions.	▪ Monitor for signs of pulmonary embolism such as sudden onset of dyspnea, tachypnea, tachycardia, hemoptysis; pleuritic chest pain; and apprehension *to identify the problem and ensure immediate treatment.* ▪ Take vital signs as ordered by physician *to provide data on patient's response.* ▪ Administer anticoagulants as ordered *to prevent extension of thrombi.* ▪ Use stool softeners or laxative to reduce straining *because Valsalva's maneuver may cause a venous thrombosis to dislodge.* ▪ Maintain adequate hydration *to prevent increasing coagulability of the blood.* ▪ Maintain bed rest in the acute phase *to minimize risk of embolization of thrombus by promoting venous stasis.* ▪ Use elastic compression stockings when ambulation is started *to provide venous support and prevent venous stasis.*
POTENTIAL COMPLICATION	Anticoagulant therapy adverse effects *related to* use of anticoagulants.
▪ Monitor for signs of hemorrhage. ▪ Report deviations from acceptable parameters. ▪ Carry out medical and nursing interventions.	▪ Assess for signs of hemorrhage such as bright-red bleeding from any body orifice; decreased BP; increased pulse and respiration *to ensure early diagnosis and treatment.* ▪ Monitor hemoglobin or hematocrit levels *to assess possible blood loss.* ▪ Avoid any IM medications *to decrease the possibility of localized hemorrhage.* ▪ Check INR before giving warfarin and PTT before giving heparin *because elevated values can increase risk of hemorrhage.* ▪ Administer anticoagulant therapy only if clotting studies are within prescribed limits *to prevent overdosing and increased risk of hemorrhage.* ▪ Avoid activities such as hard nose blowing and straining at stool *to prevent bleeding.* ▪ Avoid use of aspirin or other over-the-counter drugs *that increase the tendency to bleed.* ▪ Teach dietary restrictions (foods high in vitamin K) *that counteract the effects of warfarin (Coumadin).*

Dietary considerations for the overweight patient are aimed at limiting caloric intake to achieve and then maintain desired weight. Fat intake should be reduced if lipid or triglyceride levels are above normal. Occasionally, sodium limitation is necessary if edema is present. Proper fluid balance is required to prevent additional hypercoagulability of the blood, which may occur in the presence of deficient fluid intake. A well-balanced diet is important because calcium, vitamin E, and vitamin K all play active roles in the clotting mechanism.

▪ Evaluation

Expected outcomes for the patient with thrombophlebitis are addressed in NCP 36-3.

VARICOSE VEINS

Varicose veins, or varicosities, are dilated, tortuous subcutaneous veins most frequently found in the saphenous system. They may be small and innocuous or large and bulging. Primary varicosities are those in which the superficial veins are dilated and the valves may or may not be rendered incompetent. This condition tends to be familial, is characteristically found bilaterally, and is probably caused by congenital weakness of the veins. Secondary varicosities result from previous thrombophlebitis of the deep femoral veins, with subsequent valvular incompetence. Secondary varicose veins may occur in the esophagus (esophageal varices), in the anorectal area (hemorrhoids), and as abnormal arteriovenous connections (fistulas and malformations).

PATIENT & FAMILY TEACHING GUIDE

Table 36-15 Anticoagulant Therapy

1. Reasons for and basic mechanism of action of anticoagulant therapy and how long anticipated therapy will last
2. Need to take medication at same time each day (preferably in afternoon or evening)
3. Close follow-up with blood tests to assess blood clotting and whether change in drug dosages required
4. Side effects and adverse effects of drug therapy requiring medical attention:
   - Any bleeding that does not stop after a reasonable amount of time (usually 10-15 min)
   - Blood in urine or stool, or black, tarry stools
   - Unusual bleeding from gingivae, throat, skin, or nose, or vaginal bleeding
   - Severe headaches or stomach pains
   - Weakness, dizziness, mental status changes
5. Avoidance of any trauma or injury that might cause bleeding (e.g., vigorous brushing of teeth, contact sports)
6. Avoidance of aspirin-containing drugs, nonsteroidal antiinflammatory drugs
7. Limitation of alcohol intake to small to moderate amount
8. Wearing of Medic Alert bracelet or necklace indicating what anticoagulant is being taken
9. Avoidance of marked changes in eating habits, such as food fads and crash diets; no supplemental vitamin K
10. Consultation with physician before beginning or discontinuing any medication
11. Informing all health care providers that patient is on anticoagulant therapy
12. Correct dosing essential—some patients may require supervision (e.g., elderly, demented)

Etiology and Pathophysiology

The etiology of varicose veins is unknown. Superficial veins in the lower extremities become dilated and tortuous, with increased venous pressure. This increased venous pressure may result from a congenital weakness of the vein structure, obesity, pregnancy, venous obstruction resulting from thrombosis or extrinsic pressure by tumors, or occupations that require prolonged standing. As the veins enlarge, the valves are stretched and become incompetent, allowing blood flow to be reversed. As back pressure increases and the calf muscle pump (muscle movement that squeezes venous blood back toward the heart) fails, further venous distention results. The increased venous pressure is transmitted to the capillary bed, and edema develops.

Clinical Manifestations

Discomfort from varicose veins varies dramatically among people and tends to be worsened by superficial thrombophlebitis. In addition, many patients voice concern about cosmetic disfigurement (Fig. 36-12). The most common symptom of varicose veins is an ache or pain after prolonged standing, which is relieved by walking or by elevating the limb. Some patients feel pressure or a cramplike sensation. Swelling may accompany the discomfort. Nocturnal leg cramps, especially in the calf area, may occur.

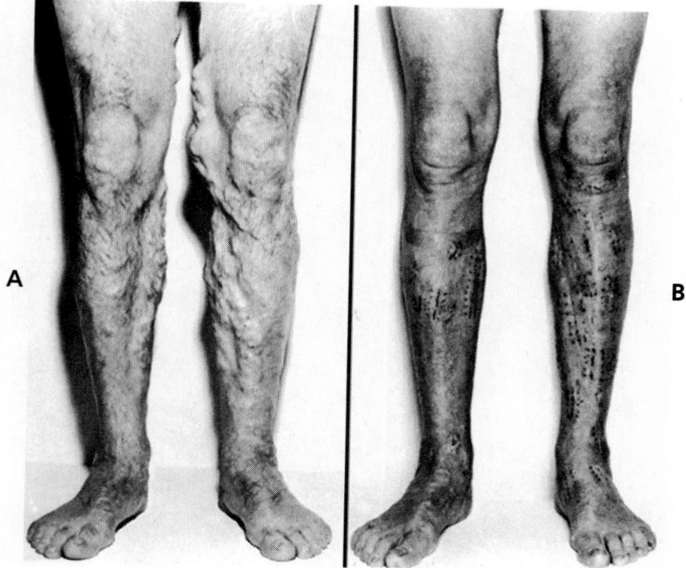

Fig. 36-12 Extensive varicosities (incompetency of the greater saphenous systems). **A,** Appearance preoperatively. **B,** Appearance 2 weeks postoperatively.

Complications

Superficial thrombophlebitis is a serious consequence of varicose veins and may occur either spontaneously or after trauma, surgical procedures, or pregnancy. Rupture of varicose veins (although not common) occurs because of weakening of the vessel wall. Ulceration as a result of skin infections or trauma may also develop.

Areas of chronic venous stasis ulceration (damaged dermis as a result of decreased tissue perfusion) are usually located near the inner aspect of the ankle, above and behind the medial malleolus (see section on venous stasis ulcers).

Diagnostic Studies

A duplex ultrasound can detect obstruction and reflux in the venous system with considerable accuracy. It is the most widely used test to diagnose deep varicose veins.

Collaborative Care

Treatment is usually not indicated if varicose veins are only a cosmetic problem. If incompetency of the venous system develops, collaborative care involves rest with the affected limb elevated, compression stockings, and exercise, such as walking.

Sclerotherapy is a technique used in the treatment of unsightly superficial varicosities (Fig. 36-13).[25] Direct IV injection of a sclerosing agent such as sodium tetradecyl (Sotradecol) induces inflammation and results in eventual thrombosis of the vein. This procedure can be performed safely in an office setting and causes minimal discomfort. After injection the leg is wrapped with an elastic bandage for 24 to 72 hours to maintain pressure over the vein. Local tenderness

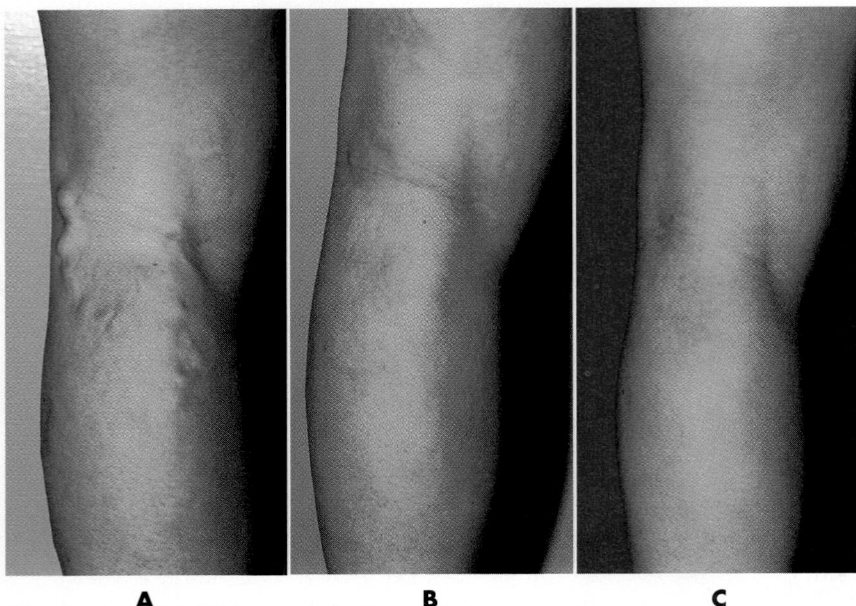

Fig. 36-13 Varicose veins and treatment with sclerotherapy. **A,** Before treatment. **B,** Six weeks after treatment. **C,** Clinical appearance 2½ years after treatment.

subsides within 2 to 3 weeks, and eventually the thrombosed vein disappears. After sclerotherapy the patient should be advised to wear compression stockings to help prevent the development of further varicosities.

Surgical intervention for varicose veins involves ligation of the entire vein (usually saphenous) and dissection and removal of its incompetent tributaries. Surgical intervention is indicated when chronic venous insufficiency cannot be controlled with conservative therapy. Recurrent thrombophlebitis in varicose veins is another indication for surgery.

NURSING MANAGEMENT: VARICOSE VEINS

Prevention is a key factor related to varicose veins. The nurse should instruct the patient to avoid sitting or standing for long periods of time, maintain ideal body weight, take precautions against injury to the extremities, and avoid wearing constrictive clothing.

After vein ligation surgery, the nurse should encourage deep breathing, which helps promote venous return to the right side of the heart. The extremities should be checked regularly for color, movement, sensation, temperature, presence of edema, and pedal pulses. Bruising and discoloration are considered normal.

Postoperatively, the extremities are elevated at a 15-degree angle to prevent the development of venous stasis and edema. Compression stockings are applied and removed every 8 hours for short periods and reapplied.

Long-term management of varicose veins is directed toward improving circulation, relieving discomfort, improving cosmetic appearance, and avoiding complications, such as superficial thrombophlebitis and ulceration. Varicose veins can recur in other veins after vein ligation. The patient should be taught proper care of the lower extremities, including cleanliness and the use of individually fitted compression stockings. The patient should be taught to put on the stockings while still lying down just before rising in the morning. The importance of periodic positioning of the legs above the heart should be stressed. The overweight patient may need assistance with weight reduction. The patient whose occupation requires prolonged periods of standing or sitting should be encouraged to change position as frequently as possible.

VENOUS STASIS ULCERS

Chronic venous insufficiency can lead to venous stasis ulceration, which may occur as a result of previous deep venous thrombosis. The basic dysfunction is incompetent valves of the deep veins. As capillaries rupture, RBCs break down and release hemosiderin, causing a brownish discoloration of the skin due to the deposition of melanin and hemosiderin. The venous stasis ulcers usually develop around the ankles, especially in the area of the medial malleoli (Fig. 36-14). Loss of epidermis occurs, and portions of the dermis may also be involved, depending on the degree of venous stasis.

Clinical Manifestations and Complications

The skin of the lower leg is leathery, with a characteristic brownish or "brawny" appearance. Edema has usually been present for a prolonged period. The ulcer is a concave lesion below the margin of the skin surface. Pain may occur when the limb is in a dependent position or during ambulation. Pain is usually relieved by elevation of the foot.

If the venous ulcer is untreated, the lesion becomes more extensive, eroding wider and deeper and increasing the likelihood of infection. Scar tissue is formed around the rim of the ulcer. Poor hygiene, debilitation, and inadequate nutritional status contribute to the severity of the ulcerative lesion.

Collaborative Care

The patient is instructed to elevate the extremity as much as possible and to maintain extrinsic compression to minimize ve-

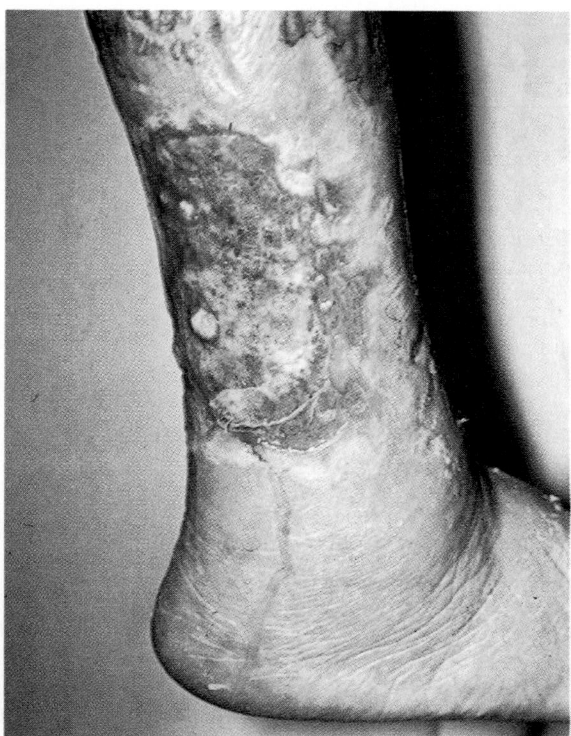

Fig. 36-14 Stasis ulcer.

nous stasis, venous hypertension, and edema. Extrinsic compression methods used include compression stockings, elastic bandages, Circaid dressings (a Velcro wrap), and Unna boot. There are benefits to each type of compression therapy, and the nurse must consider the principles of wound healing, the current status of the wound, and desired goals for healing when choosing an extrinsic compression method for the patient.

Newer therapies, focused on promoting healing in a moist environment, are showing increasing promise. Several adhesive hydrocolloid dressings are currently available and, when used in conjunction with extrinsic compression, have proven to be effective in hastening the healing of venous leg ulcers. (Hydrocolloid dressings are discussed in Chapter 11.)

Routine prophylactic antibiotic therapy is not typically indicated. However, if signs of infection are present (e.g., increased pain, temperature elevation, leukocytosis, purulent drainage from the site), a culture is obtained and appropriate antibiotic therapy is then instituted. Wet to moist dressings are indicated until the infection clears, when hydrocolloid dressings may be used.

If the ulcer fails to respond to conservative therapy, skin grafting may be indicated. The ulcer is debrided and tissue from a donor site is used (see Chapter 23). Any varicosities in the area of the lesion are removed, and veins are ligated as necessary.

NURSING MANAGEMENT: VENOUS STASIS ULCERS

The patient with venous stasis ulcers should elevate the ulcerated leg as much as possible. The nurse should change the dressings as ordered and perform prescribed wound care measures, including observation for signs of infection. A balanced diet is encouraged, with protein and vitamin supplements to promote wound healing.

Long-term management of venous stasis ulcers should focus on educating the patient in self-care measures because the incidence of recurrence is high.[26] Discharge teaching should include avoidance of trauma to the limbs, proper skin care measures, and application of prescribed compression stockings after complete healing has occurred and swelling is minimized. Rest periods with elevation of the extremities should also be encouraged. A balanced nutritional program incorporating protein-vitamin supplementation should be instituted. Caloric limitation for weight reduction and diabetic diet management are taught when indicated. Once scar formation has occurred, the patient should return to a regimen of regular exercise (walking) and periods of leg elevation above the level of the heart.

PULMONARY EMBOLISM

Etiology and Pathophysiology

Pulmonary embolism is the most common pulmonary complication in hospitalized patients. Although the actual incidence of mortality and morbidity from pulmonary embolism is unknown, it is estimated that nearly 50,000 people die of pulmonary embolism each year in the United States and another 650,000 have nonfatal pulmonary embolisms.[27]

Most pulmonary emboli arise from thrombi in the deep veins of the legs. Other sites of origin include the right side of the heart (especially with atrial fibrillation), upper extremities (rare), and the pelvic veins (especially after surgery or childbirth). Lethal pulmonary emboli originate most commonly in the femoral or iliac veins. Emboli are mobile clots that generally do not stop moving until they lodge at a narrowed part of the circulatory system. The lungs are an ideal location for emboli to lodge because of their extensive arterial and capillary network. The lower lobes are most frequently affected because they have a higher blood flow than the other lobes. Occasionally, the presence of deep vein thrombosis is unsuspected until a pulmonary embolism occurs.

Thrombi in the deep veins can dislodge spontaneously. However, a more common mechanism is jarring of the thrombus by mechanical forces, such as sudden standing, and changes in the rate of blood flow, such as those that occur with Valsalva's maneuver.

In addition to dislodged thrombi, less common causes of pulmonary emboli include fat emboli (from fractured long bones), air emboli (from improperly administered IV therapy), amniotic fluid, and tumors. Tumor emboli may originate from primary or metastatic malignancies.

Clinical Manifestations

The severity of clinical manifestations of pulmonary embolism depends on the size of the emboli and the size and number of blood vessels occluded. The most common manifestations of pulmonary embolism are the sudden onset of unexplained dyspnea, tachypnea, or tachycardia. Other manifestations are cough, chest pain, hemoptysis, crackles, fever, accentuation of the pulmonic heart sound, and sudden change in mental status as a result of hypoxemia.

Massive emboli may produce sudden collapse of the patient with shock, pallor, severe dyspnea, and crushing chest pain. However, some patients with massive emboli do not have pain. The pulse is rapid and weak, the BP is low, and an ECG indicates right ventricular strain. When rapid obstruction of 50% or more of the pulmonary vascular bed occurs, acute cor pulmonale may result because the right ventricle can no longer pump blood into the lungs. Death occurs in more than 60% of patients with massive emboli.

Medium-sized emboli often cause pleuritic chest pain accompanied by dyspnea, slight fever, and a productive cough with blood-streaked sputum. A physical examination may indicate tachycardia and a pleural friction rub.

Small emboli frequently are undetected or produce vague, transient symptoms. The exception to this is the patient with underlying cardiopulmonary disease, in whom even small or medium-sized emboli may result in severe cardiopulmonary compromise. However, repeated small emboli gradually cause a reduction in the capillary bed and eventual pulmonary hypertension. An ECG and chest x-ray may indicate right ventricular hypertrophy secondary to pulmonary hypertension.

Complications

Pulmonary Infarction. Pulmonary infarction (death of lung tissue) occurs in less than 10% of patients with emboli. Infarction is more likely when (1) occlusion of a large or medium-sized pulmonary vessel (greater than 2 mm in diameter), (2) insufficient collateral blood flow from the bronchial circulation, or (3) preexisting lung disease is present. Infarction results in alveolar necrosis and hemorrhage. Occasionally the infarcted tissue becomes infected and an abscess may develop. Concomitant pleural effusion is frequently found.

Pulmonary Hypertension. Pulmonary hypertension occurs when more than 50% of the area of the normal pulmonary bed is compromised. Pulmonary hypertension also results from hypoxemia. As a single event an embolus does not cause pulmonary hypertension unless it is massive. However, recurrent small to medium-sized emboli may result in chronic pulmonary hypertension. Pulmonary hypertension eventually results in dilation and hypertrophy of the right ventricle. Depending on the degree of pulmonary hypertension and its rate of development, death may result rapidly or only mild or transient alterations may occur (see Chapter 26).

Diagnostic Studies

An ECG is not a very sensitive or specific diagnostic measure to detect pulmonary embolism. With small to medium-sized pulmonary emboli an ECG may remain normal or show a combination of changes transiently. These include sinus tachycardia and new-onset atrial fibrillation or flutter. Recurrent small pulmonary emboli may eventually produce chronic pulmonary hypertension and ECG changes of right axis deviation with enlargement of the right atrium and right ventricle.

A lung scan is useful in screening for initial (or recurrent) pulmonary embolism, assessing the natural history of the lesion, and evaluating the effectiveness of therapy. The lung scan has two components and is most accurate when both are performed:

COLLABORATIVE CARE

Table 36-16 Acute Pulmonary Embolism

Diagnostic
- History and physical examination
- Venous studies (see Table 36-9)
- Chest x-ray
- Continuous ECG monitoring
- ABGs
- CBC count with WBC differential
- Lung scan (perfusion and ventilation)
- Pulmonary angiography

Collaborative Therapy
- Oxygen by mask or cannula
- Establishment of IV route for drugs and fluids
- Continuous IV heparin
- Bed rest
- Narcotics for pain relief
- Thrombolytic agents in certain patients
- Vena caval filter
- Pulmonary embolectomy in life-threatening situation

1. *Perfusion scanning* involves IV injection of a radioisotope. A scanning device detects the adequacy of the pulmonary circulation.
2. *Ventilation scanning* involves inhalation of a radioactive gas such as xenon. Scanning reflects the distribution of gas through the lung. The ventilation component requires the cooperation of the patient and may be difficult or impossible to perform in the critically ill patient, particularly if the patient is intubated.

Venous studies (see Table 36-9) are helpful in diagnosing deep vein thrombosis as the likely source of a pulmonary embolism.

ABG analysis is important. The arterial oxygen pressure (PaO_2) is below normal because of inadequate oxygenation secondary to an occluded pulmonary vasculature. The arterial carbon dioxide pressure ($PaCO_2$) is usually below normal because of tachypnea and hyperventilation, which occur with pulmonary emboli. The pH remains normal unless respiratory alkalosis develops as a result of prolonged hyperventilation or to compensate for lactic acidosis caused by shock. ABGs may be greatly influenced by the presence of underlying cardiac and pulmonary disease.

Pulmonary angiography is an invasive procedure that involves the insertion of a catheter through the antecubital or femoral vein and advancement to the pulmonary artery. Contrast medium is injected to visualize the pulmonary vascular system.

A chest x-ray is usually not diagnostic unless an infarction has occurred. Even with pulmonary infarction, the chest x-ray is nondiagnostic in many patients. Positive findings are best visualized 12 to 24 hours after embolism because variably shaped (round, linear, or occasionally wedge) areas of consolidation are sometimes found in the periphery or lower lobes. Pleural effusions are often noted.

Collaborative Care

When the diagnosis of thromboembolic disease has been made, treatment should be instituted immediately (Table 36-16). The objectives of treatment are to (1) prevent further growth or multiplication of thrombi in the lower extremities, (2) prevent embolization from the upper or lower extremities to the pulmonary vascular system, and (3) provide cardiopulmonary support if indicated.

Conservative Therapy. Supportive therapy for the patient's cardiopulmonary status varies according to the severity of the pulmonary embolism. The administration of oxygen by mask or cannula may be adequate for some patients. Oxygen is given in a concentration determined by ABG analysis. In some situations, endotracheal intubation and mechanical ventilation may be needed to maintain adequate oxygenation. Respiratory measures such as turning, coughing, and deep breathing are necessary to prevent or treat atelectasis. If shock is present, vasopressor agents may be necessary to support systemic circulation (see Chapter 61). If heart failure is present, digitalis and diuretics are used (see Chapter 33). Pain resulting from pleural irritation or reduced coronary blood flow is treated with narcotics, usually morphine.

Drug Therapy. Properly managed anticoagulant therapy is effective in the treatment of many patients with pulmonary emboli. Heparin and warfarin (Coumadin) are the anticoagulant drugs of choice. Heparin should be started immediately and is continued while oral anticoagulants are initiated. The dosage of heparin is adjusted according to its effect on the PTT, and that of warfarin is regulated by the INR.

Anticoagulant therapy for thromboembolic conditions may not be indicated if the patient has blood dyscrasias, hepatic dysfunction causing alteration in the clotting mechanism, injury to the intestine, overt bleeding, a history of hemorrhagic cerebrovascular accident, or neurologic conditions.

Thrombolytic agents, such as r-tPA, dissolve pulmonary emboli and the source of the thrombus in the pelvis or deep leg veins, thereby decreasing the likelihood of recurrent pulmonary emboli. Patients appear to respond to thrombolysis for up to 14 days after pulmonary emboli have occurred. Contraindications to thrombolysis include intracranial disease, recent surgery, or trauma. (Thrombolytic therapy is discussed in Chapter 32.)

Surgical Therapy. If the degree of pulmonary arterial obstruction is severe (usually greater than 50%) and the patient does not respond to conservative therapy, an immediate embolectomy may be indicated. Pulmonary embolectomy is possible with the use of temporary cardiopulmonary bypass. However, its role is limited because of a high mortality rate. Preoperative pulmonary angiography is necessary to identify and locate the site of the embolus. Fortunately, the need for pulmonary embolectomy is rare.

To prevent further pulmonary embolization, the surgical procedures appropriate for thrombophlebitis may be used (see the section on surgical interventions for thrombophlebitis earlier in this chapter). These include the insertion of intracaval filter devices (see Fig. 36-11).

CRITICAL THINKING EXERCISES

CASE STUDY

Arterial Occlusive Disease

Patient Profile

Mr. J., a 76-year-old man, was admitted to the hospital with rest pain and a nonhealing ulcer of the big toe on the right foot.

Subjective Data

- Has had a myocardial infarction, stroke, and arthritis
- Underwent a left femoral-popliteal bypass 5 years ago
- Has a smoking history of 45 pack-years
- Has been a type 1 diabetic for 30 years
- Complains of intense right foot pain for past 6 weeks
- Sleeps in recliner with right leg in dependent position

Objective Data

Physical Examination

- Has a diminished right femoral pulse with no palpable pulses below that level
- Has a small necrotic ulcer on the tip of the right big toe
- Has thickened toenails and the absence of hair on feet

Critical Thinking Questions

1. What are Mr. J.'s risk factors for peripheral vascular disease?
2. Are Mr. J.'s signs and symptoms evidence of acute or chronic arterial disease? Explain your answer.
3. What is the pathophysiology of rest pain?
4. What treatment modalities are appropriate for the ulcer on the toe?
5. What are the primary nursing responsibilities in caring for Mr. J.?
6. Based on the assessment data presented, write one or more appropriate nursing diagnoses. Are there any collaborative problems?

NURSING RESEARCH ISSUES

1. What changes in quality of life occur following vascular surgery (e.g., bypass surgery, aneurysm repair, or amputation)?
2. What is the effect of structured exercise programs in the rehabilitation of vascular surgery patients?
3. Can complications of peripheral vascular disease be prevented in high risk patients?
4. What are the most effective educational tools to teach emergency department nurses to promptly recognize a patient with a ruptured aortic aneurysm?
5. Can a smoking cessation program delay the need for arterial bypass surgery in patients with peripheral vascular disease?
6. Can a smoking cessation program combined with a structured exercise program delay the need for distal arterial bypass?
7. What measures can be taken to increase the compliance of foot care in patients with peripheral vascular disease?

NURSING MANAGEMENT: PULMONARY EMBOLISM

Nursing Implementation

Health Promotion. Nursing measures aimed at prevention of pulmonary embolism parallel those for prophylaxis of deep vein thrombophlebitis (see earlier in this chapter).

Acute Intervention. The prognosis of a patient with pulmonary emboli is good if therapy is promptly instituted. The patient should be kept on bed rest in a semi-Fowler's position to facilitate breathing. An IV line should be maintained for medications and fluid therapy. The nurse should know the side effects of medications and observe for them. Oxygen therapy should be administered as ordered. Careful monitoring of vital signs, ECG, ABGs, and lung sounds is critical to assess the patient's status.

The patient is usually anxious because of pain, sense of doom, inability to breathe, and fear of death. The nurse should carefully explain the situation and provide emotional support and reassurance to help relieve the patient's anxiety. During the acute phase, someone should be with the patient as much as possible.

Ambulatory and Home Care. The patient affected by thromboembolic processes may require psychologic and emotional support. In addition to the thromboembolic problems, the patient may have an underlying chronic illness requiring long-term treatment. To provide supportive therapy, the nurse must understand and differentiate between the various problems caused by the underlying disease and those related to thromboembolic disease.

Long-term management is similar to that for the patient with thrombophlebitis (see NCP 36-3). Discharge planning is aimed at limiting progression of the condition and preventing complications. The nurse must reinforce the need for the patient to return to the health care facility for regular follow-up examination.

Evaluation

The expected outcomes are that the patient who has a pulmonary embolus will have 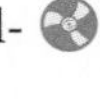

- adequate tissue perfusion and respiratory function
- adequate cardiac output
- increased level of comfort

REVIEW QUESTIONS

The number of the question corresponds to the same-numbered objective at the beginning of the chapter.

1. A patient is being prepared for an abdominal aortic aneurysm repair. The nurse suspects rupture of the aneurysm when
   a. the patient complains of sudden, severe back pain.
   b. the patient becomes dizzy and short of breath.
   c. a bruit and thrill are present at the site of the aneurysm.
   d. the patient develops blue, patchy mottling of the feet and toes.
2. An important nursing measure after an aortic aneurysm repair is to
   a. administer anticoagulant therapy.
   b. apply elastic stockings to both feet.
   c. palpate the peripheral pulses frequently.
   d. position the legs in Trendelenburg's position.
3. Specific symptoms of aortic dissection vary depending on
   a. the medications that are administered.
   b. how elevated the blood pressure becomes.
   c. the aortic branches affected in the descent of the dissection.
   d. the respiratory status of the patient before dissection occurs.
4. A 62-year-old woman weighs 92 kg and has a history of daily alcohol intake, smoking, high blood pressure, high sodium intake, and sedentary lifestyle. The nurse identifies the risk factors most highly related to peripheral atherosclerosis in this patient as
   a. sex and age.
   b. weight and alcohol intake.
   c. cigarette smoking and hypertension.
   d. sedentary lifestyle and high sodium intake.
5. Rest pain is a manifestation of chronic arterial occlusive disease that occurs as a result of
   a. the beginning of gangrene in the toes.
   b. inadequate blood flow to the nerves of the foot.
   c. inadequate blood flow to the muscles during exercise.
   d. inadequate blood flow to the skin after application of heat.
6. A patient with infective endocarditis develops sudden left leg pain with pallor, paresthesia, and a loss of peripheral pulses. The nurse's initial action should be to
   a. notify the physician.
   b. elevate the leg to promote venous return.
   c. wrap the leg in a blanket to provide warmth.
   d. perform passive range of motion to stimulate circulation to the leg.
7. The patient who is most likely to have the highest risk for deep vein thrombophlebitis is a
   a. 25-year-old obese woman who is 3 days postpartum.
   b. 62-year-old man who has a cerebrovascular accident with left-sided hemaparesis.
   c. 40-year-old woman who smokes and uses oral contraceptives.
   d. 72-year-old man who had a suprapubic prostatectomy for cancer of the prostate.
8. The nurse suspects the presence of a deep vein thrombophlebitis based on the findings of
   a. paresthesia and coolness of the leg.
   b. generalized edema of the involved extremity.
   c. pallor and cyanosis of the involved extremity.
   d. pain in the calf that occurs with exercise.
9. Nursing interventions indicated in the plan of care for the patient with acute lower extremity deep vein thrombophlebitis include
   a. administering anticoagulants as ordered.
   b. applying elastic compression stockings.
   c. positioning the leg dependently to promote arterial circulation.
   d. encouraging walking and leg exercises to promote venous return.
10. The nurse instructs the patient discharged on anticoagulant therapy to
    a. limit intake of vitamin C.
    b. report symptoms of nausea to the physician.

c. have blood drawn routinely to check electrolytes.
d. be aware of and report signs or symptoms of bleeding.

11. A patient with a deep vein thrombophlebitis suddenly develops dyspnea, tachypnea, and chest pain. Initially the most appropriate action by the nurse is to
a. auscultate for abnormal lung sounds.
b. administer oxygen and notify the physician.
c. ask the patient to cough and deep breathe to clear the airways.
d. elevate the head of the bed 30 to 45 degrees to facilitate respiration.

12. In planning care and patient teaching for the patient with venous stasis ulcers, the nurse recognizes that the most important intervention in healing and control of this condition is
a. debridement of the ulcers with skin grafting.
b. meticulous cleaning of the ulcers to prevent infection.
c. elevation of the extremities to increase venous return.
d. performance of leg exercises to increase collateral circulation.

References

1. Santilli JD, Santilli SM: Clinical criteria and management strategies for abdominal aortic aneurysms, *Am Fam Physician* 56:1081, 1997.
2. Hollier LH, Wisselink W: Abdominal aortic aneurysm. In Haimovic H, editor: *Vascular surgery,* ed 4, Cambridge, 1996, Blackwell Science.
3. O'Hara PJ: Arterial aneurysms. In Young JR, Olin JW, Bartholomew JR, editors: *Peripheral vascular diseases,* ed 2, St Louis, 1996, Mosby.
4. Anderson LA: An update on the cause of abdominal aortic aneurysms, *J Vasc Nurs* 12:4, 1994.
5. Cohn LH: Aortic dissection: new aspects of diagnosis and treatment, *Hosp Pract* 29:47, 1994.
6. Coselli JS, Biiket S, Crawford ES: Thoracic aortic aneurysm. In Haimovic H, editor: *Vascular surgery,* ed 4, Cambridge, 1996, Blackwell Science.
7. Phillips JK: Abdominal aortic aneurysm, *Nursing* 28:35, 1998.
8. Graham LM, Ford MB: Arterial disease. In Fahey VA, editor: *Vascular nursing,* ed 2, Philadelphia, 1994, Saunders.
9. Inoue K and others: Clinical application of transluminal endovascular graft placement for aortic aneurysms, *Ann Thorac Surg* 63:522, 1997.
10. Lombardo KM: Endovascular grafting of abdominal aortic aneurysms, *J Vasc Nurs* 15:3, 1997.
11. Warbinek E, Wyness MA: Caring for patients with complications after elective abdominal aortic surgery, *J Vasc Nurs* 12:3, 1994.
12. Rice KL, Walsh ME: Peripheral arterial occlusive disease, part I: navigating a bottleneck, *Nursing* 28:33, 1998.
13. Brewster DC: Aortoiliac, aortofemoral, and iliofemoral arteriosclerotic occlusive diseases. In Haimovic H, editor: *Vascular surgery,* ed 4, Cambridge, 1996, Blackwell Science.
14. Foldes MS: Postoperative lower extremity bypass surveillance: beyond ankle arm blood pressure, *J Vasc Nurs* 13:3, 1995.
15. Nunnelee JD: Patient education: hospital to home. In Fahey VA, editor: *Vascular nursing,* ed 2, Philadelphia, 1994, Saunders.
16. Bacharach JM, Sullivan TM: Endovascular treatment of peripheral vascular disease. In Young JR, Olin JW, Bartholomew JR, editors: *Peripheral vascular disease,* ed 2, St Louis, 1996, Mosby.
17. Ferguson JM, Stonebridge PA: Endovascular surgery, *J R Coll Surg Edinb* 41:223, 1996.
18. Capasso VC, Cote K: The management of patients undergoing arterial reconstructive surgery, *Medsurg Nurs* 2:11, 1993.
19. Childs MB: Foot care for the diabetic patient, *J Vasc Nurs* 12:3, 1994.
20. Falter HJ: Deep vein thrombosis in pregnancy and the puerperium, *J Vasc Nurs* 15:2, 1997.
21. Daly E and others: Risk of venous thromboembolism in users of hormone replacement therapy, *Eur Menopause J* 3:260, 1996.
22. Hirsh J: Deep vein thrombosis: recovery or recurrence? *Hosp Pract* 30:71, 1995.
23. Raskob GE: Low molecular weight heparin for the prevention and treatment of venous thromboembolism, *Current Opinion in Pulmonary Medicine* 2:305, 1996.
24. Raimer F, Thomas M: Clot stoppers: using anticoagulants safely and effectively, *Nursing* 25:34, 1995.
25. Green D: Sclerotherapy for the permanent eradication of varicose veins: theoretical and practical considerations, *J Am Acad Dermatol* 38:461, 1998.
26. Cahall E, Spence R: Nursing management of venous ulceration, *J Vasc Nurs* 12:2, 1994.
27. Launius BK, Graham BD: Understanding and preventing deep vein thrombosis and pulmonary embolism, *AACN Clin Issues* 9:91, 1998.

Resources

American Association of Cardiovascular and Pulmonary Rehabilitation
7611 Elmwood, Suite 201
Middleton, WI 53562
609-831-6989
http://www.aacvpr.org/

American Venous Forum
13 Elm Street
Manchester, MA 01944
978-526-8330
http://www.venous-info.com/

Council on Cardiovascular Nursing
American Heart Association
7320 Greenville Avenue
Dallas, TX 75231
214-373-6300
http://www.amhrt.org/Scientific/council/cvn/index.html

Mayo Health Oasis Heart Resource Center
http://www.mayohealth.org/mayo/common/htm/heartpg.htm

National Heart, Lung, and Blood Institute
National Institutes of Health
4733 Bethesda Avenue, Suite 530
Bethesda, MD 20814
301-951-3260
http://www.nhlbi.nih.gov/nhlbi/nhlbi.htm

Society for Vascular Medicine and Biology
13 Elm Street
Manchester, MA 01944-1314
978-526-8330
Fax: 978-526-4018
http://www.svmb.org/

Society for Vascular Nursing
7794 Grow Dr.
Pensacola, FL 32514
850-474-6963

Society for Vascular Surgery
13 Elm Street
Manchester, MA 01944-1314
978-526-8330
Fax: 978-526-4018

Society of Vascular Technology
4601 Presidents Drive, Suite 260
Lanham, MD 20706
301-459-7550

***For additional Internet resources, see the website for this book at* www.mosby.com/MERLIN/medsurg_lewis**

SECTION

8

PROBLEMS OF INGESTION, DIGESTION, ABSORPTION, AND ELIMINATION

SECTION OUTLINE

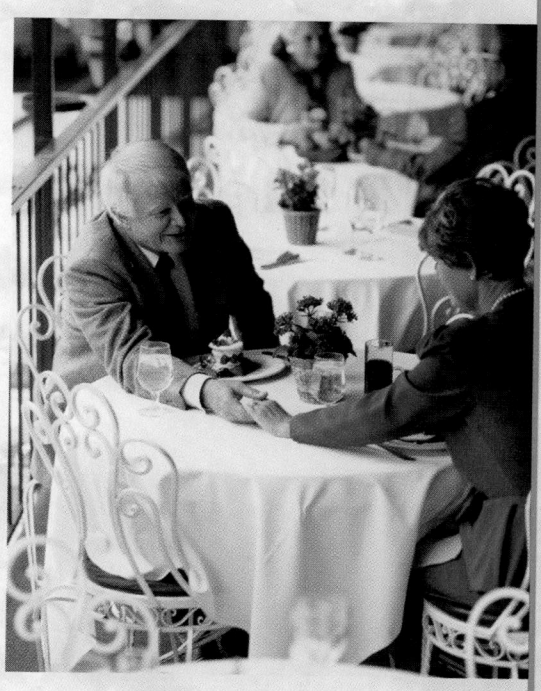

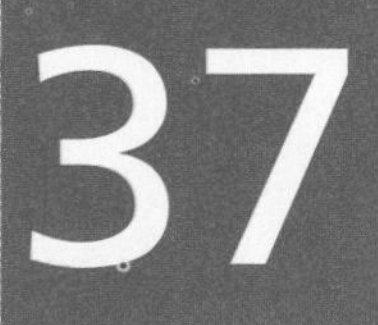

REMEMBER to check out your **companion CD-ROM**

37 NURSING ASSESSMENT Gastrointestinal System

Rachel Elrod

www.mosby.com/MERLIN/medsurg_lewis

LEARNING OBJECTIVES

1. Describe the structures and functions of the organs of the gastrointestinal tract.
2. Describe the structures and functions of the liver, gallbladder, biliary tract, and pancreas.
3. Explain the processes of ingestion, digestion, absorption, and elimination.
4. Explain the processes of biliary metabolism, bile production, and bile excretion.
5. Describe age-related changes in the gastrointestinal system and differences in assessment findings.
6. Identify the significant subjective and objective data related to the gastrointestinal system that should be obtained from a patient.
7. Describe the appropriate techniques used in the physical assessment of the gastrointestinal system.
8. Differentiate normal from common abnormal findings of a physical assessment of the gastrointestinal system.
9. Describe the purpose, significance of results, and nursing responsibilities related to diagnostic studies of the gastrointestinal system.

The main function of the gastrointestinal (GI) system is to supply nutrients to body cells. This is accomplished through the processes of *ingestion* (taking in food), *digestion* (breakdown of food), and *absorption* (transfer of food products into circulation). *Elimination* is the process of excreting the waste products of digestion.

The GI system (also called the *digestive system*) consists of the GI tract and its associated organs and glands. Included in the GI tract are the mouth, esophagus, stomach, small intestine, large intestine, rectum, and anus. The associated organs are the liver, pancreas, and gallbladder (Fig. 37-1).

Psychologic or emotional factors, such as stress and anxiety, influence GI functioning in many people. Stress may be manifested as anorexia, epigastric and abdominal pain, or diarrhea. However, GI problems should never be solely attributed to psychologic factors. Organic and psychologically based problems can exist independently or concurrently. Physical factors, such as dietary intake, ingestion of alcohol and caffeine-containing products, cigarette smoking, and fatigue, may also affect GI function. Some organic diseases of the GI system, such as peptic ulcer disease and ulcerative colitis, may be aggravated by stress. Thus both physical and emotional factors affect GI function.

STRUCTURES AND FUNCTIONS OF THE GASTROINTESTINAL SYSTEM

The GI tract is a tube approximately 30 feet (9 m) long extending from the mouth to the anus. The entire tract is composed of four common layers. From the inside to the outside, these layers are (1) mucosa, (2) submucosa, (3) muscle, and (4) serosa (Fig. 37-2). In the esophagus the outer coat is fibrous tissue rather than serosa. The muscular coat consists of two layers: the circular (inner) and the longitudinal (outer).

The GI tract is innervated by the parasympathetic and the sympathetic branches of the autonomic nervous system. The parasympathetic system is mainly excitatory, and the sympathetic system is mainly inhibitory. For example, peristalsis is increased by parasympathetic stimulation and decreased by sympathetic stimulation. Pain is relayed through sensory fibers of the sympathetic nervous system.

The GI tract also has its own nervous system: the enteric, or intrinsic, nervous system. The enteric nervous system is composed of two nerve layers that lie between the mucosa and the circular muscle layer and the circular and longitudinal muscle layers. These neurons contribute to the coordination of GI motor and secretory activities. The enteric nervous system is also known as the "gut brain." It contains 10^8 neurons (about as many as the spinal cord) and has the ability to control movement and secretion of the GI tract.

The GI tract and accessory organs receive approximately 25% to 30% of the cardiac output. Circulation in the GI system is unique in that venous blood draining the GI tract organs empties into the portal vein, which then perfuses the liver. The upper portion of the GI tract receives its blood supply from the splanchnic artery. The small intestine receives its blood supply from branches of the hepatic and superior mesenteric artery. The large intestine receives its blood supply mainly from the superior and inferior mesenteric arteries. Because such a large percentage of the cardiac output perfuses these organs, the GI tract is a major source from which blood flow can be diverted during exercise or stress.

Reviewed by Linda Monfore Fluke, RN, MN, ARNP, Adult and Geriatric Nurse Practitioner, State of Washington, Seattle, Wash.

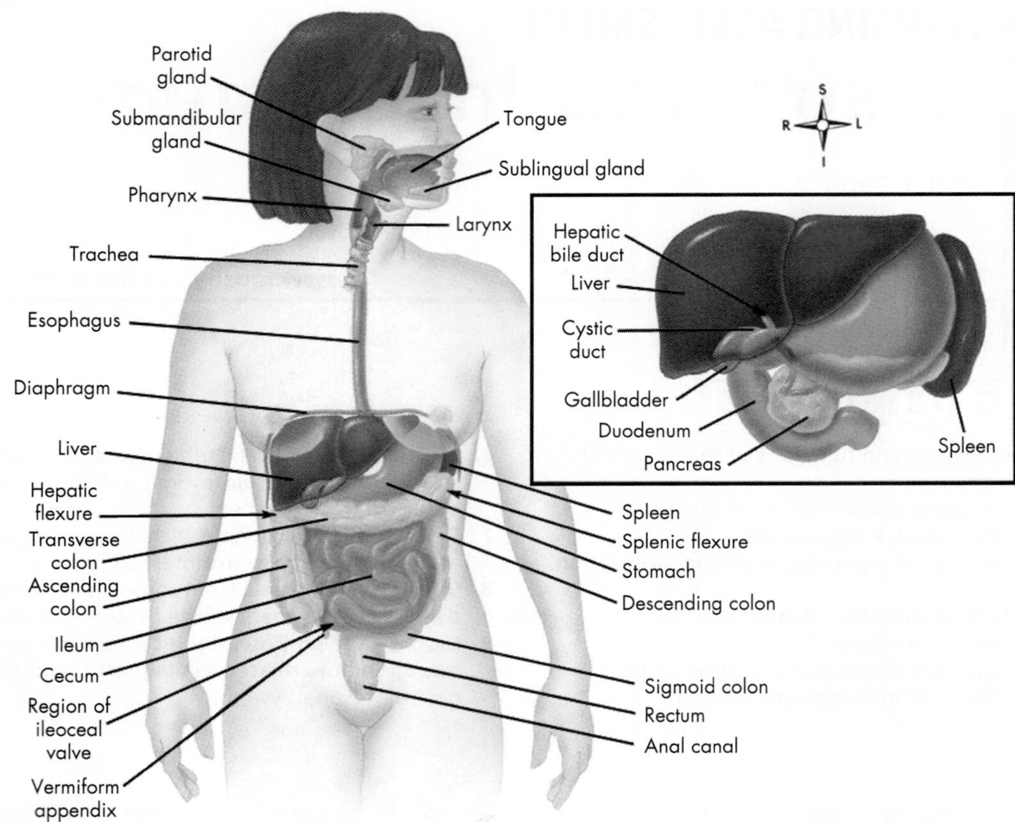

Fig. 37-1 Location of organs of the gastrointestinal system.

The two types of movement of the GI tract are mixing and propulsion. These movements are accomplished by segmentation and peristalsis. The secretions of the GI system consist of enzymes and hormones for digestion, mucus to provide protection and lubrication, and water and electrolytes.

The abdominal organs are almost completely covered by the peritoneum. The two layers of the peritoneum are the parietal, which lines the abdominal cavity wall, and the visceral, which covers the abdominal organs. The peritoneal cavity is the potential space between the parietal and visceral layers. The two folds of the peritoneum are the mesentery and omentum. The mesentery attaches the small intestine and part of the large intestine to the posterior abdominal wall and contains blood and lymph vessels. The lesser omentum goes from the lesser curvature of the stomach and upper duodenum to the liver, and the greater omentum hangs from the stomach over the intestines like an apron. The omentum contains fat and lymph nodes.

The primary functions of the GI system are (1) ingestion and propulsion (movement) of food, (2) digestion, (3) absorption, and (4) elimination. Each part of the GI system performs different activities to accomplish these functions.

Ingestion and Propulsion of Food

Ingestion is the intake of food. A person's appetite or desire to ingest food is a significant factor in how much food is eaten. Multiple factors are involved in the control of appetite. An appetite center is located in the hypothalamus. It is directly or indirectly stimulated by hypoglycemia, an empty stomach, decrease in body temperature, and input from higher brain centers. The sight, smell, and taste of food frequently stimulate appetite. Appetite may be inhibited by stomach distention, illness (especially accompanied by fever), hyperglycemia, nausea and vomiting, and certain drugs (e.g., amphetamines).

Deglutition (swallowing) is the mechanical component of ingestion. The organs involved in the deglutition of food are the mouth, pharynx, and esophagus.

Mouth. The mouth consists of the lips and oral (buccal) cavity. The lips surround the orifice of the mouth and function in speech. The roof of the oral cavity is formed by the hard and soft palate. The oral cavity contains the teeth, used in mastication (chewing), and the tongue. The tongue is a solid muscle mass and assists in mastication by keeping food between the teeth during chewing and moving the food to the back of the throat for swallowing (deglutition). Taste receptors are found on the sides and tip of the tongue. The tongue is also important in speech.

Within the oral cavity are three pairs of salivary glands: the parotid, submaxillary, and sublingual. These glands produce saliva, which consists of water, protein, mucin, inorganic salts, and salivary amylase. Approximately 1 liter of saliva is produced each day.

Pharynx. The pharynx is a musculomembranous tube that may be divided into the nasopharynx, oropharynx, and laryngeal pharynx. The mucous membrane of the pharynx is continuous with the nasal cavity, mouth, auditory tubes, and larynx. The oropharynx secretes mucus, which aids in swal-

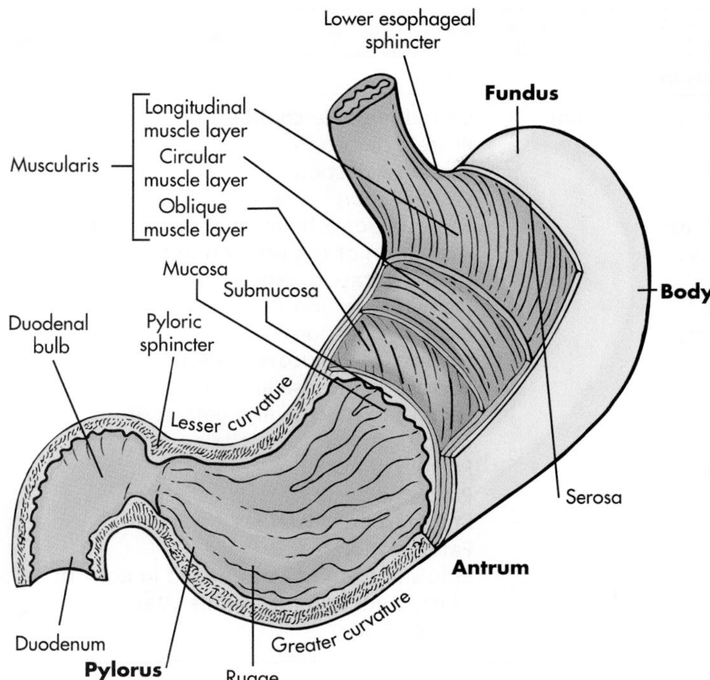

Fig. 37-2 Parts of the stomach.

lowing. The *epiglottis* is a lid of fibrocartilage that closes over the larynx during swallowing. During ingestion the oropharynx provides a route for the food from the mouth to the esophagus. When receptors in the oropharynx are stimulated by food or liquid, the swallowing reflex is initiated.

Esophagus. The esophagus is a hollow, muscular tube that receives food from the pharynx and moves it to the stomach by peristaltic contractions. It is 9.2 to 10.0 inches (23 to 25 cm) long and 0.8 inches (2 cm) in diameter. The esophagus is located in the thoracic cavity and starts behind the trachea at the lower end of the pharynx and extends to the stomach. The upper one third of the esophagus is composed of striated skeletal muscle and the distal two thirds is composed of smooth muscle.

With swallowing, the upper esophageal sphincter (cricopharyngeal muscle) relaxes and a peristaltic wave moves the bolus into the esophagus. The muscular layers contract (peristalsis) and propel the food to the stomach. The lower esophageal sphincter (LES) at the distal end of the esophagus remains contracted except during swallowing, belching, or vomiting. The LES is an important barrier that prevents reflux of acidic gastric contents into the esophagus.

Digestion and Absorption

Mouth. Digestion begins in the mouth. It involves both mechanical (mastication) and chemical digestion. Saliva is the first secretion involved in digestion, and its main function is to lubricate and soften the food mass, thus facilitating swallowing. Saliva contains amylase (ptyalin), which hydrolyzes starches to maltose. However, salivary amylase is not necessary for the digestion of carbohydrates.

Stomach. The functions of the stomach are to store food, mix the food with gastric secretions, and empty contents into the small intestine at a rate at which digestion can occur. The stomach absorbs only small amounts of water, alcohol, electrolytes, and certain drugs.

The stomach lies obliquely in the epigastric, umbilical, and left hypochondriac regions of the abdomen (see Fig. 37-7). The shape and position of the stomach change based on the degree of gastric distention. It always contains gastric fluid and mucus. The three main parts of the stomach are the fundus, body, and antrum (see Fig. 37-2). The pylorus is a small portion of the antrum that lies proximal to the pyloric sphincter. Sphincter muscles (the LES and the pyloric sphincter) guard the entrance to and exit from the stomach. The cardiac orifice is the opening between the esophagus and the stomach.

The serous (outer) layer of the stomach is formed by the peritoneum. The muscular layer consists of the longitudinal (outer) layer, circular (middle) layer, and oblique (inner) layer. The mucosal layer forms folds called *rugae* that contain many small glands. In response to nutrient intake, these glands secrete most of the gastric juice. In the fundus the glands contain chief cells, which secrete pepsinogen, and parietal cells, which secrete hydrochloric acid, water, and intrinsic factor. The secretion of hydrochloric acid makes gastric juice acidic in comparison to other body fluids. This acidic pH aids in the protection against ingested organisms. Intrinsic factor promotes cobalamin absorption in the small intestine. Mucus is secreted by glands in the cardiac and pyloric areas.

Small Intestine. The two primary functions of the small intestine are digestion and absorption. The small intestine is a coiled tube approximately 23 feet (7 m) in length and from 1 to 1.1 inch (2.5 cm to 2.8 cm) in diameter, diminishing in diameter at the lower end. It extends from the pylorus to the ileocecal valve. The small intestine is composed of the duodenum, jejunum, and ileum. The ileocecal valve, which separates the small intestine from the large intestine, prevents reflux of large intestine contents into the small intestine.

Table **37-1** Gastrointestinal Secretions Related to Digestion

Location	Daily Amount (ml)	Secretion/Enzymes	Action
Salivary glands	1000-1500	Salivary amylase (ptyalin)	Initiation of starch digestion
Stomach	2500	Pepsinogen	Protein digestion
		HCl	Protein digestion
		Lipase	Fat digestion
		Intrinsic factor	Essential for cobalamin absorption in ileum
Small intestine	3000	Enterokinase	Activation of trypsinogen to trypsin
		Amylase	Carbohydrate digestion
		Peptidases	Protein digestion
		Aminopeptidase	Protein digestion
		Maltase	Maltose to 2 glucose molecules
		Sucrase	Sucrose to glucose and fructose
		Lactase	Lactose to glucose and galactose
		Lipase	Fat digestion
Pancreas	700	Trypsinogen	Protein digestion
		Chymotrypsin	Protein digestion
		Amylase	Starch to disaccharides
		Lipase	Fat digestion
Liver and gallbladder	1000	Bile	Emulsification of fats and aid in absorption of fatty acids and fat-soluble vitamins (A, D, E, K)

The serous coat of the small intestine is formed by the peritoneum. The mucosa is thick, vascular, and glandular. The circular folds in the mucous and submucous layers provide a greater surface area for digestion and absorption.

The functional units of the small intestine are *villi.* They are present in the entire small intestine. Villi are minute, finger-like projections in the mucous membrane. They contain goblet cells that secrete mucus and epithelial cells that produce the intestinal digestive enzymes. The epithelial cells on the villi also have microvilli, which compose the brush border. Thus the presence of villi and microvilli greatly increases the surface area for absorption.

The digestive enzymes on the brush border of the microvilli chemically break down nutrients so that they can be absorbed. The villi are surrounded by the crypts of Lieberkühn, which contain the base columnar cells that are the stem cells for the other epithelial cell types. Brunner's glands in the submucosa of the duodenum secrete mucus.

Physiology of Digestion. *Digestion* is the physical and chemical breakdown of food into absorbable substances. Digestion in the GI tract is facilitated by the timely movement of food through the various organs and the secretion of specific enzymes. These enzymes break down foodstuffs to appropriate size particles for absorption (Table 37-1).

The process of digestion begins in the mouth, where the food is chewed, mechanically broken down, and mixed with saliva. The saliva lubricates the food. In addition, salivary amylase begins the breakdown of starch. Salivary gland secretion is stimulated by chewing movements and the sight, smell, thought, and taste of food. The food is swallowed and passes into the esophagus where peristaltic waves propel it to the stomach. No digestion or absorption occurs in the esophagus.

In the stomach the digestion of proteins begins with the release of pepsinogen from chief cells. The acidic environment of the stomach results in the conversion of pepsinogen to its active form, pepsin. Pepsin begins the initial breakdown of proteins. In the stomach there is minimal digestion of starches and fats. The food is mixed with gastric secretions, which are under neural and hormonal control (Tables 37-2 and 37-3). The stomach also serves as a reservoir for food, which is slowly expelled into the small intestine. The length of time food remains in the stomach depends on the composition of the food, but average meals remain from 3 to 4 hours.

Digestion is completed in the small intestine, where carbohydrates are hydrolyzed to monosaccharides, fats to glycerol and fatty acids, and proteins to amino acids. The physical presence of chyme (food mixed with gastric secretions), along with its chemical nature in the small intestine, stimulates motility and secretion. Secretions involved in digestion include enzymes from the pancreas, bile from the liver (see Table 37-1), and intestinal secretions from glands in the small intestine. Both secretion and motility are under neural and hormonal control.

When food enters the stomach and small intestine, hormones are released into the bloodstream (see Table 37-3). The hormone secretin stimulates the pancreas to secrete fluid with a high concentration of bicarbonate. This alkaline secretion enters the duodenum and neutralizes acid in the chyme. The duodenal mucosa also secretes mucus to protect against the hydrochloric acid. In response to the presence of chyme, the hormone cholecystokinin (CCK), produced by the duodenal mucosa, enters the bloodstream and stimulates contraction of the gallbladder and relaxation of the sphincter of Oddi. These actions permit bile to flow from the common bile duct into the duodenum. Bile is necessary for the digestion of fats. CCK also stimulates the pancreas to synthesize and secrete enzymes for enzymatic digestion of carbohydrates, fats, and proteins.

Enzymes present on the brush border of the microvilli complete the digestion process. These enzymes hydrolyze disaccharides to monosaccharides and peptides to amino acids for absorption.

Absorption is the transfer of the end products of digestion across the intestinal wall to the circulation. Most absorption oc-

Table 37-2 Phases of Gastric Secretion

Phase	Stimulus to Secretion	Secretion
Cephalic (nervous)	Sight, smell, taste of food (before food enters stomach); initiated in the CNS and mediated by the vagus nerve	Hydrochloric acid, pepsinogen, mucus
Gastric (hormonal and nervous)	Food in antrum of stomach, vagal stimulation	Release of gastrin hormone from antrum into circulation to stimulate gastric secretions and motility
Intestinal (hormonal)	Presence of chyme in small intestine	Acidic chyme (pH <2) release of secretin, gastric inhibitory polypeptide, cholecystokinin into circulation to decrease acid secretion Chyme (pH >3) release of duodenal gastrin to increase acid secretion

CNS, central nervous system.

Table 37-3 Major Hormones Controlling Gastrointestinal Secretion and Motility

Hormone	Source	Activating Stimuli	Function
Gastrin	Gastric and duodenal mucosa	Stomach distention, partially digested proteins in pylorus	Gastric acid secretion, increased motility, maintenance of lower esophageal sphincter tone
Secretin	Duodenal mucosa	Acid entering small intestine	Inhibition of gastric motility and acid secretion, pancreatic bicarbonate secretion
Cholecystokinin	Duodenal mucosa	Fatty acids and amino acids in small intestine	Contraction of gallbladder and relaxation of sphincter of Oddi, allowing increased flow of bile into duodenum; release of pancreatic digestive enzymes
Gastric inhibitory peptide	Duodenal mucosa	Fatty acids and lipids in the small intestine	Inhibition of gastric acid secretion and gastric motility

curs in the small intestine. The surface area of the small intestine is greatly increased by its circular folds, villi, and microvilli. The movement of the villi provides for exposure of the end products of digestion to be in contact with the absorbing membrane. Monosaccharides (from carbohydrates), fatty acids (from fats), amino acids (from proteins), water, electrolytes, and vitamins are absorbed.

Elimination

Large Intestine. The large intestine is a hollow muscular tube approximately 5 to 6 feet (1.5 to 2 m) long and 2 inches (5 cm) in diameter. The four parts of the large intestine are (1) the cecum and appendix, a narrow tube at the end of the cecum; (2) the colon (ascending colon on the right side, transverse colon across the abdomen, descending colon on the left side, and the sigmoid colon); (3) the rectum; and (4) the anus, the terminal portion of the large intestine (Fig. 37-3).

The most important function of the large intestine is the absorption of water and electrolytes. It also forms feces and serves as a reservoir for the fecal mass until defecation occurs. Feces is composed of water (75%), bacteria, unabsorbed minerals, undigested foodstuffs, bile pigments, and desquamated epithelial cells. The large intestine secretes mucus, which acts as a lubricant and protects the mucosa.

Microorganisms in the colon are responsible for the breakdown of proteins not digested or absorbed in the small intestine. These amino acids are deaminated by the bacteria, leaving ammonia, which is carried to the liver and converted to urea. Bacteria in the colon also synthesize vitamin K and some of the B vitamins. Bacteria also play a part in the production of flatus.

The movements of the large intestine are usually slow. When the circular muscles contract, they produce a kneading action termed *haustral churning.* Propulsive (mass movements) peristalsis also occurs. When food enters the stomach and duodenum, the gastrocolic and duodenocolic reflexes are initiated, resulting in peristalsis in the colon. These reflexes are more active after the first daily meal and frequently result in bowel evacuation.

Defecation is a reflex action involving voluntary and involuntary control. Feces in the rectum stimulate sensory nerve endings that produce the desire to defecate. The reflex center for defecation is in the sacral portion of the spinal cord (parasympathetic nerve fibers). These fibers produce contraction of the rectum and relaxation of the internal anal sphincter. Defecation is controlled voluntarily by relaxing the external anal sphincter when the desire to defecate is felt. An acceptable environment for defecation is usually necessary or the urge to defecate will be ignored. If defecation is suppressed over long

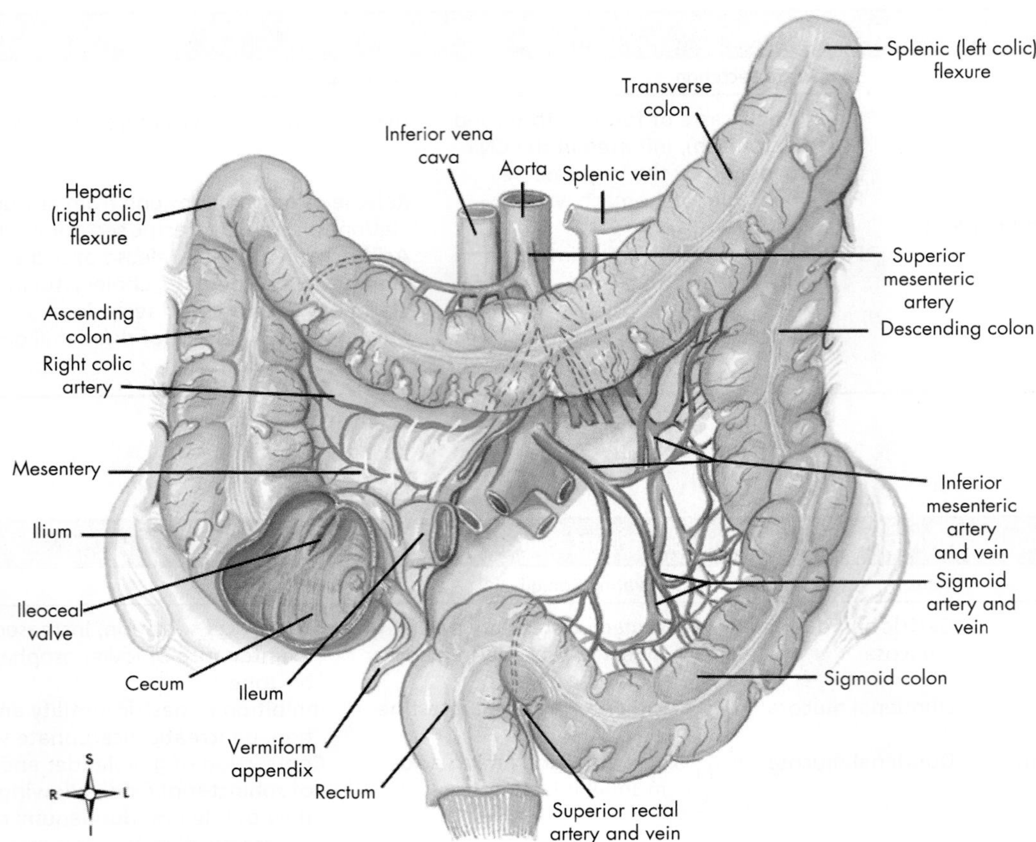

Fig. 37-3 Anatomic locations of the large intestine.

periods of time, problems can occur, such as constipation or stool impaction.

Defecation can be facilitated by Valsalva's maneuver. This maneuver involves contraction of the chest muscles on a closed glottis with simultaneous contraction of the abdominal muscles. These actions result in increased intraabdominal pressure. Valsalva's maneuver is contraindicated in the patient with a head injury, eye surgery, cardiac problems, hemorrhoids, abdominal surgery, or liver cirrhosis with portal hypertension. Constipation is common in the older adult and is due to many factors, including slower peristalsis, inactivity, decreased dietary fiber, decreased fluids, depression, constipating medications, and laxative abuse.[1] (Constipation is discussed in Chapter 40.)

Liver, Biliary Tract, and Pancreas

Liver. The liver is the largest internal organ in the body, weighing approximately 3 lb (1.37 kg) in the adult. It lies in the right hypochondriac and epigastric regions (see Fig. 37-7). Most of the liver is enclosed in peritoneum. It has a fibrous capsule that divides it into the right and left lobes (Fig. 37-4).

The functional units of the liver are lobules (Fig. 37-5). The lobule consists of rows of hepatic cells (hepatocytes) arranged around a central vein. The capillaries (sinusoids) are located between the rows of hepatocytes and are lined with Kupffer cells, which carry out phagocytic activity (removal of bacteria and toxins from the blood). Interlobular bile ducts form from bile capillaries (canaliculi). The hepatic cells secrete bile into the canaliculi.

The nerve supply to the liver is from the left vagus and sympathetic celiac plexus. About one third of the blood supply comes from the hepatic artery (branch of the celiac artery), and two thirds comes from the portal vein.

The portal circulatory system (enterohepatic) brings blood to the liver from the stomach, intestines, spleen, and pancreas. This blood enters the liver through the portal vein. The portal vein carries absorbed products of digestion directly to the liver. In the liver the portal vein branches and comes in contact with each lobule. The blood in the sinusoids is a mixture of arterial and venous blood.

The liver is essential for life. It functions in the manufacture, storage, transformation, and excretion of a number of substances involved in metabolism. The functions of the liver are numerous but can be classified into four main areas, as identified in Table 37-4.

Biliary Tract. The biliary tract consists of the gallbladder and the duct system. The gallbladder is a pear-shaped sac located below the liver. The function of the gallbladder is to concentrate and store bile. It can hold approximately 45 ml of bile.

Bile is produced by the hepatic cells and secreted into the biliary canaliculi of the lobules. Bile then drains into the interlobular bile ducts, which unite into the two main left and right

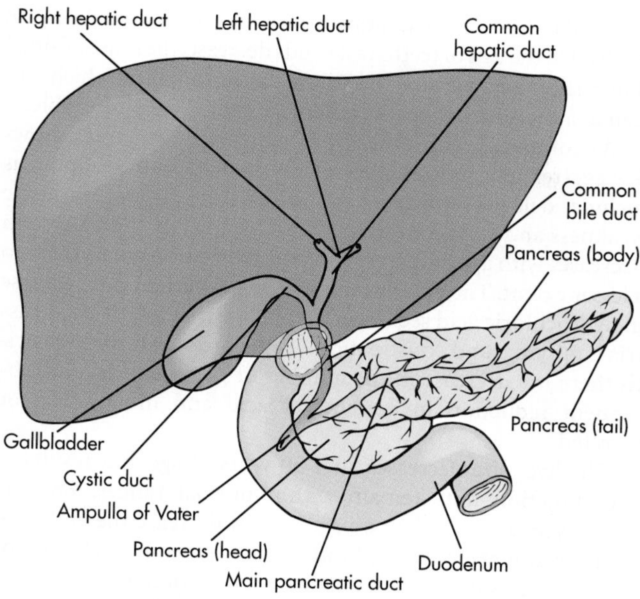

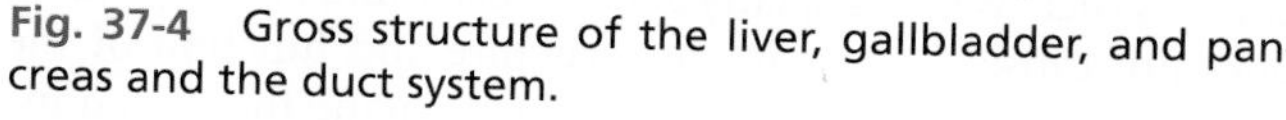
Fig. 37-4 Gross structure of the liver, gallbladder, and pancreas and the duct system.

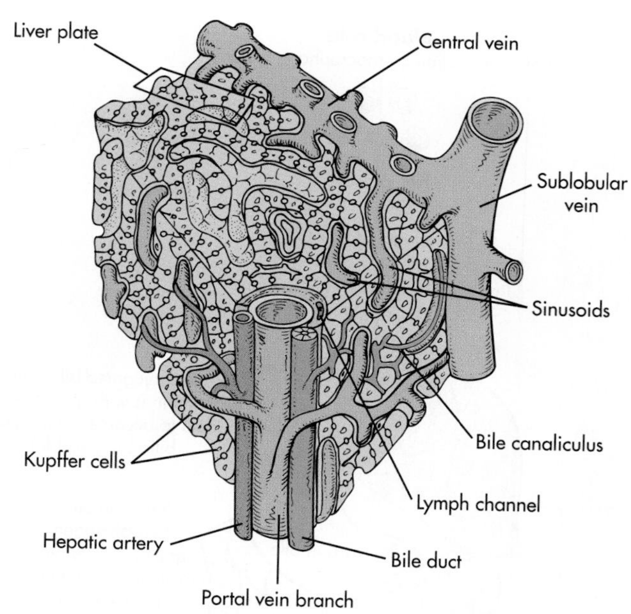

Fig. 37-5 Microscopic structure of liver lobule.

Table 37-4 Major Functions of the Liver

Function	Description
Metabolic functions	
Carbohydrate metabolism	Glycogenesis (conversion of glucose to glycogen), glycogenolysis (process of breaking down glycogen to glucose), gluconeogenesis (formation of glucose from amino acids and fatty acids)
Protein metabolism	Synthesis of nonessential amino acids, synthesis of plasma proteins (except γ-globulin), synthesis of clotting factors, urea formation from NH_3 (NH_3 formed from deamination of amino acids by action of bacteria on proteins in colon)
Fat metabolism	Synthesis of lipoproteins, breakdown of triglycerides into fatty acids and glycerol, formation of ketone bodies, synthesis of fatty acids from amino acids and glucose, synthesis and breakdown of cholesterol
Detoxification	Inactivation of drugs and harmful substances and excretion of their breakdown products
Steroid metabolism	Conjugation and excretion of gonadal and adrenal steroids
Bile synthesis	
Bile production	Formation of bile, containing bile salts, bile pigments (mainly bilirubin), and cholesterol
Bile excretion	Bile excretion by liver about 1 L/day
Storage	Glucose in form of glycogen; vitamins, including fat soluble (A, D, E, K) and water soluble (B_1, B_2, cobalamin, and folic acid); fatty acids; minerals (iron and copper); amino acids in form of albumin and β-globulins
Mononuclear phagocyte system	
Kupffer cells	Breakdown of old RBCs, WBCs, bacteria, and other particles, breakdown of hemoglobin from old RBCs to bilirubin and biliverdin

RBC, red blood cell; *WBC,* white blood cell.

hepatic ducts. The hepatic ducts merge with the cystic duct from the gallbladder to form the common bile duct (see Fig. 37-4). This duct enters the duodenum at the ampulla of Vater. The sphincter of Oddi keeps the ampulla closed except when stimulated by the presence of food in the GI tract.

Bilirubin metabolism. Bilirubin, a pigment derived from the breakdown of hemoglobin, is constantly produced (Fig. 37-6). Because it is insoluble in water, it is bound to albumin for its transport to the liver. This form of bilirubin is referred to as *unconjugated.* In the liver bilirubin is conjugated with glucuronic acid. Conjugated bilirubin is soluble and is excreted in bile. Bile also consists of water, cholesterol, bile salts, electrolytes, and phospholipids. Bile salts are needed for fat emulsification and digestion.

Bile initially enters the duct system in the canaliculi and flows through the interlobular ducts to the hepatic ducts. From the hepatic duct it can move to the cystic duct or down the common bile duct. Most bile is stored and concentrated in the gallbladder. It is then released into the cystic duct and moves down the common bile duct to enter the duodenum at the ampulla of Vater. In

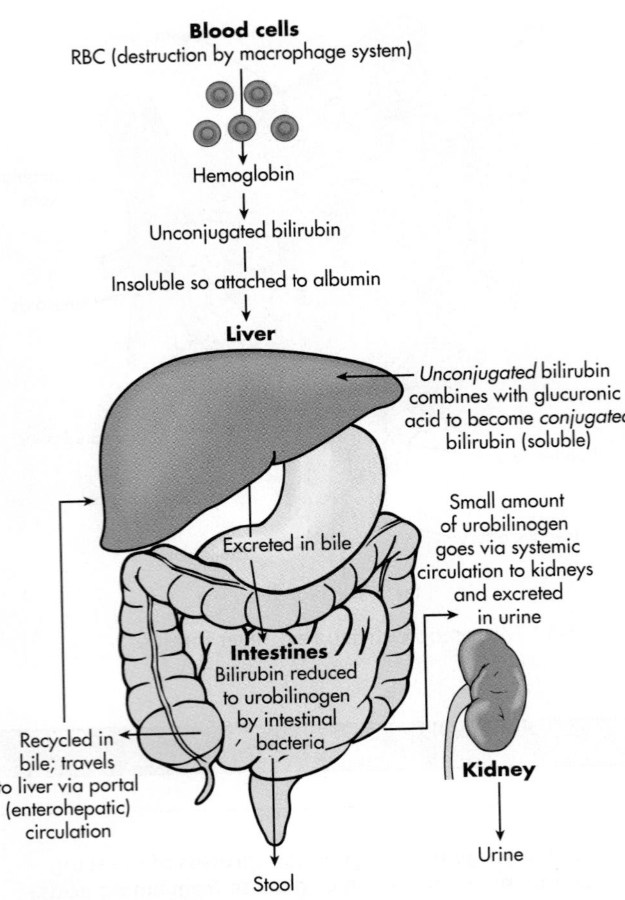
Blood cells
RBC (destruction by macrophage system)
Hemoglobin
Unconjugated bilirubin
Insoluble so attached to albumin
Liver
Unconjugated bilirubin combines with glucuronic acid to become conjugated bilirubin (soluble)
Small amount of urobilinogen goes via systemic circulation to kidneys and excreted in urine
Excreted in bile
Intestines
Bilirubin reduced to urobilinogen by intestinal bacteria
Recycled in bile; travels to liver via portal (enterohepatic) circulation
Kidney
Urine
Stool

Fig. 37-6 Bilirubin metabolism and conjugation.

the intestines, most of the bilirubin is reduced to stercobilinogen and urobilinogen by bacterial action. Stercobilinogen accounts for the brown color of stool. A small amount of conjugated bilirubin is reabsorbed by the blood. Some urobilinogen is reabsorbed by the blood and returned to the liver through the portal circulation (enterohepatic) and excreted in the bile. An insignificant amount of urobilinogen is excreted in the urine.[2]

Pancreas. The pancreas is a long, slender gland lying behind the stomach and in front of the first and second lumbar vertebrae. It consists of the head, body, and tail. The anterior surface is covered by peritoneum. The pancreas contains lobes and lobules. The pancreatic duct extends along the gland and enters the duodenum through the common bile duct (see Fig. 37-4). The pancreas has both exocrine and endocrine functions. It is the exocrine function of the pancreas that contributes to the process of digestion. Exocrine cells in the pancreas secrete pancreatic enzymes (see Table 37-1). The endocrine function occurs in the islets of Langerhans, whose beta cells secrete insulin; alpha cells secrete glucagon; delta cells secrete somatostatin; and F cells secrete pancreatic polypeptide (see Chapter 45).

GERONTOLOGIC CONSIDERATIONS

Effects of Aging on the Gastrointestinal System

The process of aging causes changes in the functional ability of the GI system (Table 37-5). Tooth enamel and dentin wear down and make the teeth susceptible to cavities. Periodontal disease can lead to the loss of teeth. Taste buds decrease, the sense of smell diminishes, and salivary secretions diminish, all of which can lead to a decrease in appetite and make eating less pleasurable.

As compared with other body systems the GI tract shows few age-related changes. Age-related changes in the esophagus include delayed emptying resulting from smooth muscle weakness and an incompetent LES.[1] Motility of the GI system decreases with age, but secretion and absorption are affected to a lesser extent. The elderly patient often experiences a decrease in hydrochloric acid secretion (hypochlorhydria), delayed gastric emptying, and constipation. With chronic atrophic gastritis there is a decrease in the number of parietal cells and subsequent reduction in amount of acid and intrinsic factor secreted.

The liver size decreases after 50 years of age, but results of liver function tests remain within normal ranges. Enzyme changes in the liver that are age related decrease the ability of the liver to metabolize medications and hormones. The size of the pancreas is unaffected by aging but does undergo structural changes such as fibrosis, fatty acid deposits, and atrophy. Aging does not cause changes in the structure and function of the gallbladder and bile ducts. However, with aging there is an increase in the incidence of gallstones.[3]

The economic inability to purchase food supplies may affect nutritional intake, especially in the older adult. Economic constraints may also reduce the number of fresh fruits and vegetables consumed and thus the amount of fiber. A reduction in dietary fiber, along with reduced fluid intake and decreased physical activity, contributes to constipation. Age-related changes in the GI system and differences in assessment findings are presented in Table 37-5.

ASSESSMENT OF THE GASTROINTESTINAL SYSTEM

Subjective Data

Important Health Information

Past health history. Information should be gathered from the patient about the history or existence of the following diseases or problems related to GI functioning: abdominal pain, gastritis, nausea and vomiting, diarrhea and constipation, hepatitis, colitis, peptic ulcer, abdominal distention, jaundice, anemia, hiatal hernia, gallbladder disease, dysphagia, heartburn, dyspepsia, changes in appetite, hematemesis, food intolerance, indigestion, excessive gas, bloating, melena, hemorrhoids, hernia, or rectal bleeding.

The patient should be questioned about weight history. Any unexplained or unplanned weight loss or weight gain within the past 12 months should be explored in detail. A history of chronic dieting and repeated weight loss and gain should be documented.

Medications. The health history should include an assessment of the patient's past and current use of medications. This is an important part of the assessment, particularly in relation to liver problems. It should include over-the-counter and prescription drugs. Many chemicals and drugs are potentially hepatotoxic (Table 37-6). The nurse should ask the patient if laxatives or antacids are taken, including the kind and frequency. Some people take baking soda (sodium bicarbonate) for an

GERONTOLOGIC DIFFERENCES IN ASSESSMENT

Table 37-5 Gastrointestinal System

Changes	Differences in Assessment Findings
Mouth	
Loss of teeth	Presence of dentures, difficulty chewing
Decreased taste buds, decreased sense of smell	Diminished sense of taste (especially salty and sweet)
Decreased volume of saliva	Dry oral mucosa
Atrophy of gingival tissue	Poor-fitting dentures
Esophagus	
Decreased tone and motility	Complaints of pyrosis (heartburn), dysphagia, eructation
Abdominal Wall	
Thinner and less taut	More visible peristalsis, easier palpation of organs
Decrease in number and sensitivity of sensory receptors	Less sensitivity to surface pain
Stomach	
Decreased acid secretion, atrophy of gastric mucosa	Food intolerances, signs of anemia as result of cobalamin malabsorption
Small Intestines	
Decreased secretion of most digestive enzymes, decreased motility	Complaints of indigestion
Liver	
Decreased size and lowered in position	Easier palpation
Large Intestine, Anus, Rectum	
Decreased anal sphincter tone and nerve supply to rectal area	Fecal incontinence
Decreased muscular tone, decreased motility	Flatulence, abdominal distention, relaxed perineal musculature
Increase in transit time	Constipation, fecal impaction

Table 37-6 Hepatotoxic Chemicals and Drugs

Alcohol	Halothane
Arsenic	Isoniazid
Carbon tetrachloride	Propylthiouracil
Chloroform	Sulfonamides
Gold compounds	Thiazide diuretics
Mercury	6-Mercaptopurine
Phosphorus	Methotrexate
Anabolic steroids	Acetaminophen

upset stomach. This can be dangerous because it is a systemic antacid that is readily absorbed and can cause metabolic alkalosis. Sodium bicarbonate is also in many over-the-counter effervescent drugs, such as Alka-Seltzer.

The use of prescription or over-the-counter appetite suppressant medication should be noted. The names of drugs and frequency and duration of use are also important. The patient should also be asked about herbal medicines that may be used to relieve GI symptoms such as nausea and constipation.

Surgery or other treatments. Information should be obtained about hospitalizations for any problems related to the GI system. Data should also be obtained related to any abdominal or rectal surgery, including year, reason for surgery, postoperative course, and possible blood transfusions. Terminology related to surgery of the GI system is presented in Table 37-7.

Functional Health Patterns. Key questions to ask a patient with a GI problem are presented in Table 37-8.

Table 37-7 Surgeries of the Gastrointestinal System

Antrectomy: Removal of antrum portion of stomach
Cecostomy: Opening into cecum
Cholecystectomy: Removal of gallbladder
Cholecystostomy: Opening into gallbladder
Choledochojejunostomy: Opening between common bile duct and jejunum
Choledocholithotomy: Opening into common bile duct for removal of stones
Colostomy: Opening into colon
Esophagoenterostomy: Removal of portion of esophgus with segment of colon attached to remaining portion
Esophagogastrostomy: Removal of esophagus and anastomosis of remaining portion to stomach
Gastrectomy: Removal of stomach
Gastrostomy: Opening into stomach
Glossectomy: Removal of tongue
Hemiglossectomy: Removal of half of tongue
Ileostomy: Opening into ileum
Mandibulectomy: Removal of mandible
Pyloroplasty: Enlargement and repair of pyloric sphincter area
Vagotomy: Resection of branch of vagus nerve

Health perception–health management pattern. The nurse should ask about the patient's health practices related to the GI system, such as maintenance of normal body weight, attention to proper dental care, maintenance of adequate nutrition, and effective elimination habits.

HEALTH HISTORY

Table 37-8 Gastrointestinal System

Health Perception–Health Management Pattern
- Describe any measures used to treat gastrointestinal symptoms such as diarrhea or vomiting.
- Do you smoke?* Do you drink alcohol?*
- Are you exposed to any chemicals on a regular basis?* Have you been exposed in the past?*
- Have you recently traveled outside the United States?*

Nutritional-Metabolic Pattern
- Describe your usual daily food and fluid intake.
- Do you take any supplemental vitamins or minerals?*
- Have you experienced any changes in appetite or food tolerance?*
- Has there been a weight change in the past?*
- Are you allergic to any foods?*

Elimination Pattern
- Describe the frequency and time of day you have bowel movements. What is the consistency of the bowel movement?
- Do you use laxatives or enemas?* If so, how often?
- Have there been any recent changes in your bowel pattern?*
- Describe any skin problems caused by gastrointestinal problems.
- Do you need any assistive equipment, such as ostomy equipment?

Activity-Exercise Pattern
- Do you have limitations in mobility that make it difficult for you to procure and prepare food?*
- Are you able to feed yourself?
- Do you have any gastrointestinal symptoms, such as vomiting or diarrhea, that affect your activity?*
- Do you have any difficulty accessing a toilet when needed?*
- Is a safe and comfortable environment for elimination available?

Sleep-Rest Pattern
- Do you experience any difficulty sleeping because of a gastrointestinal problem?*
- Are you awakened by symptoms such as gas or esophageal burning?*

Cognitive-Perceptual Pattern
- Have you experienced any change in taste or smell that has affected your appetite?*
- Do you have any heat or cold sensitivity that affects eating?*
- Does pain interfere with food preparation, appetite, or chewing?*
- Do pain medications cause constipation or appetite suppression?*

Self-Perception–Self-Concept Pattern
- Describe any changes in your weight that have affected how you feel about yourself.
- Have you had any changes in normal elimination that have affected how you feel about yourself?*
- Have any symptoms of gastrointestinal disease caused physical changes that are a problem for you?*

Role-Relationship Pattern
- Describe the impact of any gastrointestinal problem on your usual roles and relationships.
- Have any changes in elimination affected your relationships?*
- Do you live alone? Describe how your family or others assist you with your gastrointestinal problems.

Sexuality-Reproductive Pattern
- Describe the effect of your gastrointestinal problem on your sexual activity.

Coping–Stress Tolerance Pattern
- Do you experience gastrointestinal symptoms in response to stressful or emotional situations?*
- Describe how you deal with any gastrointestinal symptoms that result.

Value-Belief Pattern
- Describe any culturally specific health beliefs regarding food and food preparation that may influence the treatment of this gastrointestinal problem.

*If yes, describe.

The patient should be asked about exposure to hepatotoxic chemicals such as arsenic, phosphorus, and mercury. The nurse should also ask about foreign travel with possible exposure to hepatitis or parasitic infestation.

The patient should be assessed in relation to certain habits that have a direct effect on GI functioning. The consumption of alcohol in large quantities has detrimental effects on the mucosa of the stomach and also increases the secretion of hydrochloric acid and pepsinogen. Chronic alcohol exposure causes fatty infiltration of the liver. The nurse should obtain a history of cigarette smoking. Nicotine is irritating to the entire GI tract mucosa. Cigarette smoking is related to various GI cancers (especially mouth and esophageal cancers), esophagitis, and ulcers. Smoking will also delay the healing of ulcers.

Nutritional-metabolic pattern. A thorough nutritional assessment is essential. A dietary history should be taken and compared with the food pyramid (Fig. 38-1). The nurse should ask open-ended questions that will allow the patient to express beliefs and feelings about the diet. The nurse may need to ask the patient to do a 24-hour dietary recall to analyze the adequacy of the diet. The nurse should assist the patient in recalling the preceding day's food intake, including early-morning and nighttime intake. The nurse should find out about the intake of snacks, liquids, and vitamin supplements. The nurse must then evaluate the diet in terms of the recommended groups and servings on the food pyramid and try to determine whether the 24-hour recall is typical of the patient's usual eating habits. If weekend eating habits vary greatly, the nurse should obtain a separate weekend diet history and assess the patient's intake for both quality and quantity of food.

The nurse should ask the patient about the use of sugar and salt substitutes, caffeine, and amount of fluid and fiber intake. The patient should be questioned about any changes in appetite, food tolerance, and weight. Anorexia and weight loss may indicate carcinoma. The nurse should ask the patient about allergies to any food and determine what GI symptoms such allergic responses cause.

Elimination pattern. A detailed account of the patient's bowel elimination pattern should be elicited. The frequency, time of day, and usual consistency of stool should be noted. The use of laxatives and enemas, including type, frequency, and results, should be documented. Any recent change in bowel patterns should be investigated.

The amount and type of fluid and fiber intake should be determined because they have an important effect on the frequency and consistency of stools. Inadequate intake of fiber can be associated with constipation. Analysis of fluid intake and output could indicate the presence of a urinary problem and the possibility of fluid retention.

Skin problems can be associated with GI problems. Food allergies can cause lesions, pruritus, and edema. Diarrhea can result in redness, irritation, and pain in the perianal area. External drainage systems such as an ileostomy or ileal conduit can cause local skin irritation. The possible association between a skin problem and a GI problem should be investigated.

Activity-exercise pattern. The patient's ambulatory status should be assessed to determine if the patient is capable of securing and preparing food. If the patient is unable to do these tasks, it should be determined if family or an outside agency is meeting this need. Any limitation in the patient's ability to feed self independently should be noted. Any difficulty accessing a safe environment of elimination should be assessed. Use of and access to elimination supplies should be assessed, such as commode or ostomy supplies. Activity and exercise may affect GI motility. Immobility is a risk factor for constipation.

Sleep-rest pattern. Many food-related events can interrupt and interfere with the quality of sleep. Nausea, vomiting, diarrhea, indigestion, bloating, and hunger can produce sleep problems and should be investigated. The patient should be asked if GI symptoms affect sleep or rest. For example, a patient with a hiatal hernia may be awakened because of burning pain; sleep may be improved by elevating the head of the bed for this patient.

A patient often has a bedtime ritual that involves the use of a particular food or beverage. Warm milk is known to induce sleep through the effect of the serotonin precursor L-tryptophan. Herbal teas and melatonin are often sleep inducing. Individual routines should be noted and complied with whenever possible to avoid sleeplessness. Hunger can prevent sleep and should be relieved by a light, easily digested snack unless contraindicated.

Cognitive-perceptual pattern. Decreases in sensory adequacy can result in problems related to the acquisition, preparation, and ingestion of food. Changes in taste or smell can affect appetite and eating pleasure. Vertigo can make shopping and standing at a stove difficult and dangerous. Heat or cold sensitivity could make certain foods painful to eat. Problems in expressive communication could make it difficult and frustrating for the patient to make personal desires and preferences known. The nurse should assess the patient in this pattern to judge the effect of deficiencies on adequate nutritional intake. If the patient has been diagnosed as having a GI disorder, the nurse should ask questions to determine the patient's understanding of the illness and its treatment.

Pain is another area that requires careful assessment related to its effect on the GI system and nutrition. Relevant behaviors associated with chronic pain include avoidance of activity, fatigue, and disruption of eating patterns. The possible effects of pain medication related to constipation, sedation, and appetite suppression should be assessed.

Self-perception–self-concept pattern. Many GI and nutritional problems can have serious effects on the patient's self-perception. Overweight and underweight persons often have problems related to self-esteem and body image. Repeated attempts to achieve a personally acceptable weight can be discouraging and depressing for the patient. The manner in which a person recounts a weight history can alert the nurse to potential problems in this area.

Another potentially problematic area is the need for external devices to manage elimination, such as a colostomy or an ileostomy. The patient's willingness to engage in self-care and to discuss this situation should provide the nurse with valuable information related to body image and self-esteem.

The altered physical changes often associated with liver disease can be problematic for the patient. Jaundice and ascites cause significant changes in external appearance. The patient's attitude toward these changes should be assessed.

Role-relationship pattern. Problems related to the GI system such as cirrhosis, alcoholism, hepatitis, ostomies, obesity, and carcinoma can have a major impact on the patient's ability to maintain usual roles and relationships. A chronic illness may necessitate leaving a job or reducing the number of hours worked. Changes in body image and self-esteem can affect relationships. The availability of and satisfaction with support should be determined. It is important that the nurse be aware of these possible consequences and assess for their presence.

Sexuality-reproductive pattern. Changes related to sexuality and reproductive status can result from problems of the GI system. For example, obesity, jaundice, anorexia, and ascites could decrease the acceptance of a potential sexual partner. The presence of an ostomy could affect the patient's confidence related to sexual activity. Chronic alcoholism could discourage a meaningful relationship that could develop into a sexual relationship. Sensitive questioning by the nurse could determine the presence of potential problems.

Anorexia can affect the reproductive status of a female patient. Alcoholism can affect the reproductive status of both men and women. A poor nutritional intake before and during pregnancy can result in a low-birth-weight infant. The nurse should determine the patient's desires in the area of reproduction and direct the assessment based on the patient's responses.

Coping–stress tolerance pattern. The nurse should try to determine what is a stressor for the patient and what coping mechanisms the patient uses to function with these stressors. GI symptoms such as epigastric pain, nausea, and diarrhea develop in many people in response to stressful or emotional situations. Some organic GI problems such as peptic ulcers are aggravated by stress.

Value-belief pattern. The patient's spiritual and cultural beliefs regarding food and food preparation should be assessed. Whenever possible, these preferences should be respected by the health care provider. In addition, it should be determined if any value or belief could interfere with planned interventions. For example, if the patient with anemia is a vegetarian, the prescription of a high-meat diet would be met with patient resistance. Likewise, the recovering alcoholic could not take an alcohol-based cough medicine. Thoughtful assessment and consideration of the patient's beliefs and values will usually increase patient compliance and satisfaction.

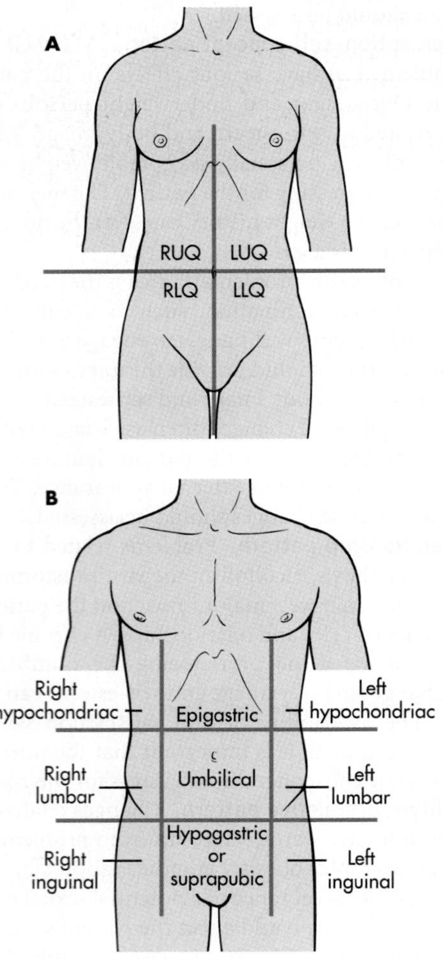

Fig. 37-7 **A,** Abdominal quadrants. **B,** Abdominal regions.

Objective Data

In addition to collecting subjective data related to a diet history and functional health patterns, objective data related to a nutritional assessment should be collected. Anthropometric measurements (height, weight, skinfold thickness) and blood studies such as serum protein, albumin, and hemoglobin are examples of important objective data related to the GI system. A physical examination also adds valuable information.

Physical Examination

Mouth

Inspection. The lips should be inspected for symmetry, color, and size. They should be observed for abnormalities such as pallor or cyanosis, cracking, ulcers, or fissures. The dorsum (top) of the tongue should have a thin white coating; the undersurface should be smooth. The nurse should observe for any lesions. Using a tongue blade, the nurse should inspect the buccal mucosa and note the color, any areas of pigmentation, and any lesions. Dark-skinned individuals normally have patchy areas of pigmentation. In assessing the teeth and gums, the nurse should look for caries; loose teeth; abnormal shape and position of teeth; and swelling, bleeding, discoloration, or inflammation of the gingivae. Any distinctive breath odor should be noted.

The pharynx is inspected by tilting the patient's head back and depressing the tongue with a tongue blade. The tonsils, uvula, soft palate, and anterior and posterior pillars should be observed. The nurse should have the patient say "ah." The uvula and soft palate should rise and remain in the midline.

Palpation. The nurse should palpate any suspicious areas in the mouth. Ulcers, nodules, indurations, and areas of tenderness should be palpated.

The mouth of the older adult requires careful assessment. Particular attention should be given to dentures (e.g., fit, condition), ability to swallow, and lesions. The patient who has dentures must remove the dentures during an oral examination to allow for good visualization and palpation of the area.

Abdomen. Two systems are used to anatomically describe the surface of the abdomen. One system divides the abdomen into four quadrants by a perpendicular line from the sternum to the pubic bone and a horizontal line across the abdomen at the umbilicus (Fig. 37-7, *A*, and Table 37-9). The other system divides the abdomen into nine regions (Fig. 37-7, *B*), but only

Table 37-9 Abdominal Structures in Regions of the Abdomen

Right Upper Quadrant	Left Upper Quadrant	Right Lower Quadrant	Left Lower Quadrant
Liver and gallbladder	Left lobe of liver	Lower pole of right kidney	Lower pole of left kidney
Pylorus	Spleen	Cecum and appendix	Sigmoid flexure
Duodenum	Stomach	Portion of ascending colon	Portion of descending colon
Head of pancreas	Body of pancreas	Bladder (if distended)	Bladder (if distended)
Right adrenal gland	Left adrenal gland	Right ovary and salpinx	Left ovary and salpinx
Portion of right kidney	Portion of left kidney	Uterus (if enlarged)	Uterus (if enlarged)
Hepatic flexure of colon	Splenic flexure of colon	Right spermatic cord	Left spermatic cord
Portion of ascending and transverse colon	Portion of transverse and descending colon	Right ureter	Left ureter

the epigastrium, umbilical, and suprapubic or hypogastric regions are commonly addressed.

For the abdominal examination, good lighting should shine across the abdomen. The patient should be in the supine position and as relaxed as possible. To help relax the abdominal muscles, the patient should slightly flex the knees and the head of the bed should be raised slightly. The patient should have an empty bladder. The examiner should use warm hands when doing the abdominal examination to avoid eliciting muscle guarding. The patient should be asked to breathe slowly through the mouth.

Inspection. The nurse should assess the abdomen for skin changes (color, texture, scars, striae, dilated veins, rashes, and lesions), umbilicus (location and contour), symmetry, contour (flat, rounded [convex], concave, protuberant, distention), observable masses (hernias or other masses), and movement (pulsations and peristalsis). A normal aortic pulsation may be seen in the epigastric area. The nurse should look across the abdomen tangentially (across the abdomen in a line) for peristalsis. Peristalsis is not normally visible in an adult but may be visible in a thin person.

Auscultation. During examination of the abdomen, auscultation is done before percussion and palpation because these latter procedures may alter the bowel sounds. Auscultation of the abdomen includes listening for increased or decreased bowel sounds and vascular sounds. The diaphragm of the stethoscope is used to auscultate bowel sounds because they are relatively high pitched. The bell of the stethoscope is used to detect lower-pitched sounds. Normal bowel sounds occur 5 to 35 times per minute and sound like high-pitched clicks or gurgles.[4] Before auscultation, warming the stethoscope in the hands helps prevent abdominal muscle contraction. The nurse should listen in the epigastrium and in all four quadrants. The nurse should listen for bowel sounds for 2 to 5 minutes. Bowel sounds cannot be described as absent until no sound is heard for 5 minutes (in each quadrant).[5] The frequency and intensity of bowel sounds will vary, depending on the phase of digestion. Normally they will sound relatively high pitched and gurgling. Loud gurgles indicate hyperperistalsis and are termed *borborygmi* (stomach growling). The bowel sounds will be more high pitched (rushes and tinkling) when the intestines are under tension, such as in intestinal obstruction. The nurse should listen for decreased or absent bowel sounds. Terms used to describe bowel sounds include *present, absent, increased, decreased, high pitched, tinkling, gurgling,* and *rushing.* Normally no aortic bruits should be heard. A *bruit,* best heard with the bell of the stethoscope, is a swishing or buzzing sound and indicates turbulent blood flow.

Percussion. The purpose of percussion of the abdomen is to determine the presence of fluid, distention, and masses. Sound waves vary according to the density of underlying tissues; the presence of air produces a higher-pitched, hollow sound termed *tympany*; the presence of fluid or masses produces a short, high-pitched sound with little resonance termed *dullness.* The nurse should lightly percuss all four quadrants of the abdomen and assess the distribution of tympany and dullness. Tympany is the predominant percussion sound of the abdomen.

To percuss the liver, the nurse should start below the umbilicus in the right midclavicular line and percuss lightly upward until dullness is heard, thus determining the lower border of liver dullness. After the lower border of the liver has been determined, the nurse should start at the nipple line in the right midclavicular line and percuss downward between ribs to the area of dullness indicating the upper border of the liver. The height or vertical space between the two areas should be measured to determine the size of the liver. The normal range of liver height in the right midclavicular line is 2.4 to 5 inches (6 to 12 cm).

Palpation. Light palpation is used to detect tenderness or cutaneous hypersensitivity, muscular resistance, masses, and swelling. It also helps in relaxation for deeper palpation. The nurse should keep fingers together and press gently with the pads of the fingertips, depressing the abdominal wall about 0.4 inches (1 cm). Smooth movements should be used and all quadrants palpated (Fig. 37-8, *A*).

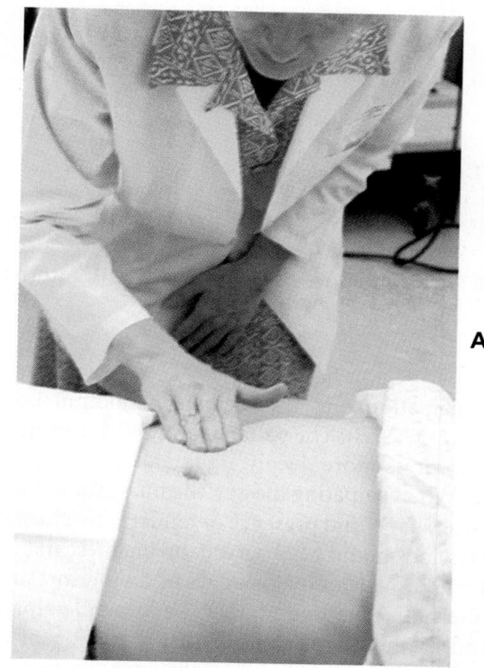

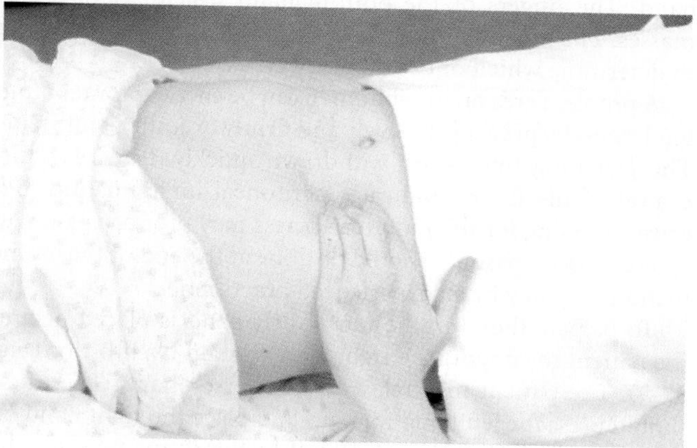

Fig. 37-8 **A,** Technique for light palpation of the abdomen. **B,** Technique for deep palpation.

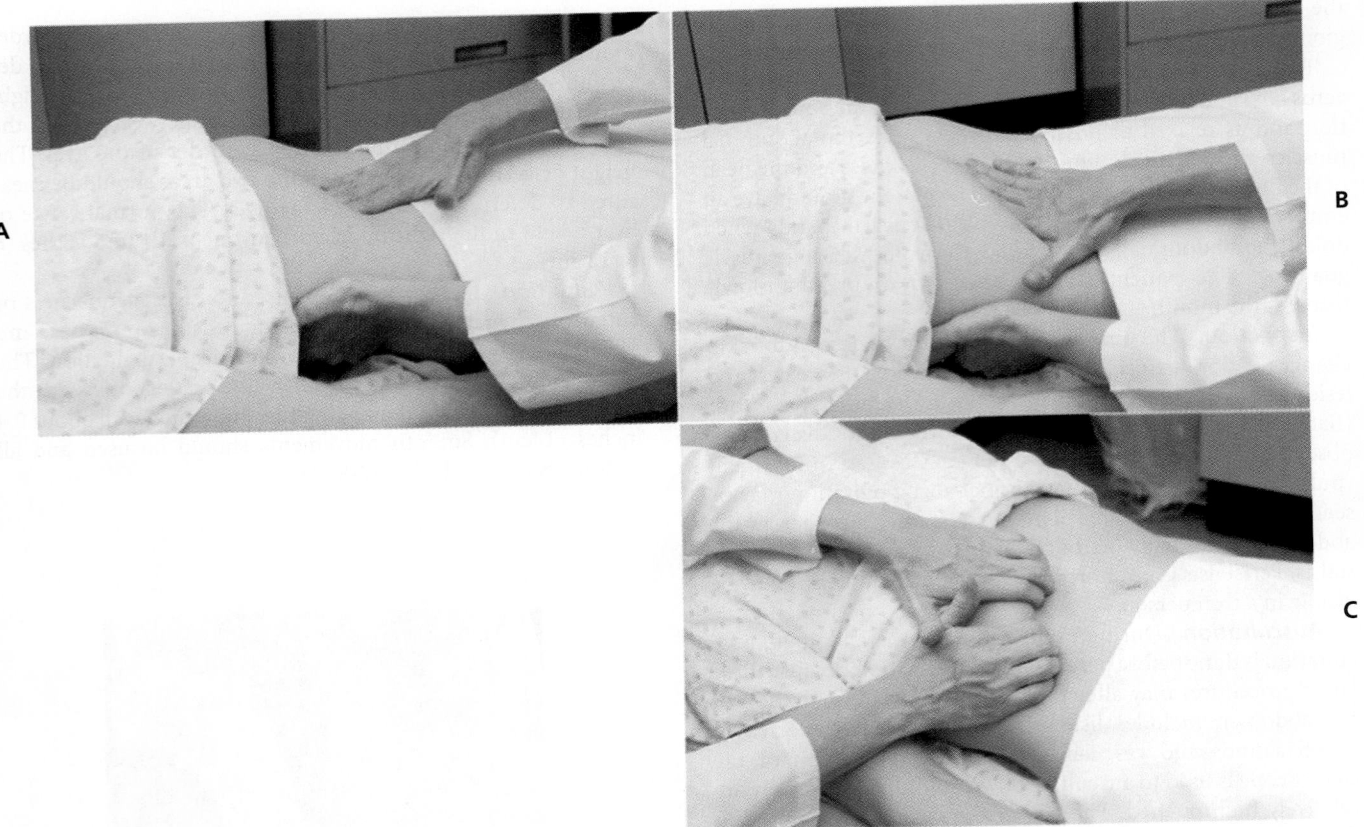

Fig. 37-9 **A,** Technique for liver palpation. **B,** Alternative technique. **C,** Palpating liver with fingers hooked over the costal margin.

Deep palpation is used to delineate abdominal organs and masses (Fig. 37-8, *B*). The palmar surfaces of the fingers should be used to press more deeply. Again, all quadrants should be palpated. When palpating masses, the nurse should note the location, size, shape, and presence of tenderness. The patient's facial expression should be observed during these maneuvers because it will provide nonverbal cues of discomfort or pain.

An alternative method for deep abdominal palpation is the two-hand method. One hand is placed on top of the other. The fingers of the top hand apply pressure to the bottom hand. The fingers of the bottom hand feel for organs and masses. The nurse should practice both methods of palpation to determine which one is most effective.

A problem area on the abdomen can be checked for rebound tenderness by pressing in slowly and firmly over the painful site. The palpating fingers are withdrawn quickly. Pain on withdrawal of the fingers indicates peritoneal inflammation. Because assessing for rebound tenderness may produce pain and severe muscle spasm, it should be done at the end of the examination and only by an experienced practitioner.

To palpate the liver, the nurse's left hand is placed behind the patient to support the right eleventh and twelfth ribs (Fig. 37-9). The patient may relax on the nurse's hand. The nurse should press the left hand forward and place the right hand on the patient's right abdomen lateral to the rectus muscle. The fingertips should be below the lower border of liver dullness and pointed toward the right costal margin. The nurse should gently press in and up. The patient should take a deep breath with the abdomen so that the liver drops and is in a better position to be palpated. The nurse should try to feel the liver edge as it comes down to the fingertips. The liver edge should feel

Table 37-10 Normal Physical Assessment of the Gastrointestinal System

Mouth	Moist and pink lips; pink and moist buccal mucosa and gingivae without plaques or lesions; teeth in good repair; protrusion of tongue in midline without deviation or fasciculations; pink uvula midline; soft palate, tonsils, and posterior pharynx; swallows smoothly without coughing or gagging
Abdomen	Flat without masses or scars, no abdominal tenderness, no bruises, bowel sounds in all quadrants, nonpalpable liver and spleen, liver 10 cm in right midclavicular line, generalized tympany
Rectum/Anus	Absence of lesions, fissures, hemorrhoids; good sphincter tone; rectal walls smooth/soft; no masses; stool soft, brown, and heme-negative

COMMON ASSESSMENT ABNORMALITIES

Table 37-11 Gastrointestinal System

Finding	Description	Possible Etiology and Significance
Mouth		
Ulcer, plaque on lips or in mouth	Sore or lesion	Carcinoma, viral infections
Cheilosis	Softening, fissuring, and cracking of lips at angles of mouth	Riboflavin deficiency
Cheilitis	Inflammation of lips (usually lower) with fissuring, scaling, crusting	Often unknown
Geographic tongue	Scattered red, smooth (loss of papillae) areas on dorsum of tongue	Unknown
Smooth tongue	Red, slick appearance	Cobalamin deficiency
Leukoplakia	Thickened white patches	Premalignant lesion
Pyorrhea	Recessed gums, purulent pockets	Periodontitis
Herpes simplex	Benign vesicular lesion	Herpesvirus
Candidiasis	White, curdlike lesions surrounded by erythematous mucosa	*Candida albicans*
Glossitis	Reddened, ulcerated, swollen tongue	Exposure to streptococci, irritation, injury, vitamin B deficiency, anemia
Acute marginal gingivitis	Friable, edematous, painful, bleeding gingivae	Irritation from ill-fitting dentures, calcium deposits on teeth, food impaction
Esophagus and Stomach		
Dysphagia	Difficulty in swallowing, sensation of food sticking in esophagus	Esophageal problems, cancer of esophagus
Hematemesis	Vomiting of blood	Esophageal varices, bleeding peptic ulcer
Pyrosis	Heartburn, burning in epigastric or substernal area	Hiatal hernia, esophagitis, incompetent lower esophageal sphincter
Dyspepsia	Burning or indigestion	Peptic ulcer, gallbladder disease
Odynophagia	Painful swallowing	Cancer of esophagus, esophagitis
Eructation	Belching	Gallbladder disease
Nausea and vomiting	Feeling of impending vomiting, expulsion of gastric contents through mouth	GI infections, common manifestation of many GI diseases; stress, fear, and pathologic conditions

Continued

firm, sharp, and smooth. The surface and contour and any tenderness should be described.

To palpate the spleen, the nurse moves to the left side of the patient. The nurse places the left hand under the patient and supports and presses the patient's left lower rib cage forward. The right hand is placed below the left costal margin and presses it in toward the spleen. The nurse should ask the patient to breathe deeply. The tip or edge of an enlarged spleen will be felt by the fingertips. The spleen is normally not palpable. If it is palpable, the nurse should not continue because manual compression of an enlarged spleen may cause it to rupture.

The standard approach for examining the abdomen can be used on the older adult. Palpation is important because it may reveal a tumor. The abdomen may be thinner and more lax unless the patient is obese. If the patient has chronic obstructive pulmonary disease, large lungs, or a low diaphragm, the liver may be palpated 0.4 to 0.8 inches (1 to 2 cm) below the right costal margin.

Rectum and anus. The perianal and anal area should be inspected for color, texture, lumps, rashes, scars, erythema, fissures, and external hemorrhoids. Any lumps or unusual areas should be palpated with a gloved hand.

For the digital examination of the rectum the gloved, lubricated index finger is placed against the anus while the patient strains (Valsalva's maneuver). Then, as the sphincter relaxes, the finger is inserted. The finger is pointed toward the umbilicus. The nurse should try to get the patient to relax. The finger is inserted into the rectum as far as possible, and all surfaces are palpated. Nodules, tenderness, or any irregularities should be assessed. A sample of stool can be removed with the gloved finger and should be checked for occult blood.

Recording of the normal physical assessment of the GI system is found in Table 37-10. Gerontologic differences in the GI system and differences in assessment findings are described in Table 37-5. Common assessment abnormalities are presented in Table 37-11.

COMMON ASSESSMENT ABNORMALITIES

Table 37-11 Gastrointestinal System—cont'd

Finding	Description	Possible Etiology and Significance
Abdomen		
Distention	Excessive gas accumulation, enlarged abdomen; generalized tympany	Obstruction, paralytic ileus
Ascites	Accumulated fluid within abdominal cavity; eversion of umbilicus (usually)	Peritoneal inflammation, congestive heart failure, metastatic carcinoma, cirrhosis
Bruit	Humming or swishing sound heard through stethoscope over vessel	Partial arterial obstruction (narrowing of vessel), turbulent flow (aneurysm)
Hyperresonance	Loud, tinkling rushes	Intestinal obstruction
Borborygmi	Waves of loud, gurgling sounds	Hyperactive bowel as result of eating
Absent bowel sounds	No auscultation of bowel sounds	Peritonitis, paralytic ileus, obstruction
Absence of liver dullness	Tympany on percussion	Air from viscus (e.g., perforated ulcer)
Masses	Lump on palpation	Tumors, cysts
Rebound tenderness	Sudden pain when fingers withdrawn quickly	Peritoneal inflammation, appendicitis
Nodular liver	Enlarged, hard liver with irregular edge or surface	Cirrhosis, carcinoma
Hepatomegaly	Enlargement of liver, liver edge >1-2 cm below costal margin	Metastatic carcinoma, hepatitis, venous congestion
Splenomegaly	Enlargement of spleen	Chronic leukemia, hemolytic states, portal hypertension, some infections
Hernia	Bulge or nodule in abdomen, usually appearing on straining	Inguinal (in inguinal canal), femoral (in femoral canal), umbilical (herniation of umbilicus), or incisional (defect in muscles after surgery)
Rectum and Anus		
Hemorrhoids	Thrombosed veins in rectum and anus (internal or external)	Portal hypertension, chronic constipation, prolonged sitting or standing, pregnancy
Mass	Firm, nodular edge	Tumor, carcinoma
Pilonidal cyst	Opening of sinus tract, cyst in midline just above coccyx	Probably congenital
Fissure	Ulceration in anal canal	Straining, irritation
Melena	Abnormal, black, tarry stool containing digested blood	Cancer, bleeding in upper GI tract from ulcers, varices
Tenesmus	Painful and ineffective straining at stool	Ulcerative colitis, diarrhea secondary to GI infection such as food poisoning
Steatorrhea	Fatty, frothy, foul-smelling stool	Chronic pancreatitis, biliary obstruction, malabsorption problems

DIAGNOSTIC STUDIES OF THE GASTROINTESTINAL SYSTEM

Diagnostic studies provide important information to the nurse in monitoring the patient's condition and planning appropriate interventions. These studies are considered to be objective data. Table 37-12 presents diagnostic studies common to the GI system. For most diagnostic studies nurses should make sure a signed consent form for the procedure has been completed and is in the medical record. It is the responsibility of the health care provider doing the procedure to explain the procedure and obtain the written consent. However, nurses play an important role in educating patients regarding the procedures.

Many of the diagnostic procedures of the GI system require measures to cleanse the GI tract, as well as the ingestion or injection of a contrast medium or a radiopaque dye. Often the patient has a series of GI diagnostic tests done. The nurse must monitor the patient closely to ensure adequate hydration and nutrition during the tests. Some diagnostic studies of the GI system are especially difficult and uncomfortable for the older adult. It may be necessary to individualize and make adjustments. It is particularly important to prevent diarrhea from bowel cleansing procedures and dehydration from prolonged fluid restriction.

Many radiologic studies use either barium sulfate or meglumine diatrizoate (Gastrografin) as a contrast medium. Barium sulfate is more effective for visualizing mucosal detail. Gastrografin is water soluble and rapidly absorbed, so it is preferred when a perforation is suspected. Spillage of barium into the peritoneal cavity can result in peritonitis, which is difficult to manage.[6] Under other circumstances in a person at high risk for aspiration, water-soluble media are contraindicated and barium is preferred.

Text continued on p. 1033

DIAGNOSTIC STUDIES

Table 37-12 Gastrointestinal System

Study	Description and Purpose	Nursing Responsibility
Radiologic		
Upper GI or Barium Swallow	X-ray study with fluoroscopy with contrast medium. Study is used to diagnose structural abnormalities of the esophagus, stomach, and duodenal bulb.	Explain procedure to patient and that patient will need to drink contrast medium and assume various positions on x-ray table. Keep patient NPO for 8-12 hr before procedure. Tell patient to avoid smoking after midnight the night before the study. After x-ray test, take measures to prevent contrast medium impaction (fluids, laxatives). Tell patient that stool may be white up to 72 hr after test.
Small Bowel Series	Contrast medium is ingested and flat film taken q20min until medium reaches terminal ileum.	Same as for upper GI.
Lower GI or Barium Enema	Fluoroscopic x-ray examination of colon uses contrast medium, which is administered rectally (enema). Double contrast or air contrast barium enema is test of choice. Air is infused after barium is evacuated.	Before the procedure, administer laxatives and enemas until colon is clear of stool evening before procedure. Administer clear liquid diet evening before procedure. Keep patient NPO for 8 hr before test. Instruct patient about being given barium by enema. Explain that cramping and urge to defecate may occur during procedure and that patient may be placed in various positions on tilt table. After the procedure, give fluids, laxatives, or suppositories to assist in expelling barium. Observe stool for passage of contrast medium.
Oral Cholecystogram (GB Series)	X-ray examination visualizes GB after radiopaque dye such as iopanoic acid (Telepaque) has been ingested orally. Study determines GB's ability to concentrate and store dye and patency of biliary duct system.	Assess patient for sensitivity to iodine. Administer radiopaque dye evening before test. Give 6 tablets (3 g), 1 q5min. Explain that patient may need 2 consecutive days of dye ingestion. Keep patient NPO after ingestion of dye. Observe for side effects of dye such as nausea, vomiting, diarrhea. May give fatty test meal after x-ray test to check for GB emptying. Assess patient's medication for possible contraindications, precautions, or complications with the use of dye.
Cholangiography ▪ IV Cholangiogram	X-rays are used to visualize biliary duct system after IV injection of radiopaque dye.	Keep patient NPO for 8 hr. Assess sensitivity to iodine dye. During injection of dye, assess for urticaria, extreme flushing, respiratory distress. Assess patient's medication for possible contraindications, precautions, or complications with the use of dye.
▪ Percutaneous transhepatic cholangiogram	After local anesthesia, liver is entered with long needle (under fluoroscopy), bile duct is entered, bile withdrawn, and radiopaque dye injected. Fluoroscopy is used to determine filling of hepatic and biliary ducts.	Observe patient for signs of hemorrhage or bile leakage. Assess patient's medication for possible contraindications, precautions, or complications with the use of dye.
▪ Surgical cholangiogram	Study is performed during surgery on biliary structures, such as GB. Contrast medium is injected into common bile duct.	Explain to patient that anesthetic will be used. Assess patient's medication for possible contraindications, precautions, or complications with the use of dye.

Continued

DIAGNOSTIC STUDIES

Table 37-12 Gastrointestinal System—cont'd

Study	Description and Purpose	Nursing Responsibility
Radiologic—continued		
Ultrasound	This noninvasive procedure uses high-frequency sound waves (ultrasound waves), which are passed into body structures and recorded as they are reflected (bounded). A conductive gel (lubricant jelly) is applied to the skin and a transducer is placed on the area.	Be aware that bowel must be cleansed because presence of solid material in GI tract causes changes in reflected sounds and that ultrasound is not transmitted well through gas or air. Schedule test before upper GI or barium enema.
▪ Abdominal ultrasound	Study detects abdominal masses (tumors and cysts) and is also used to assess ascites.	Same as above.
▪ Hepatobiliary ultrasound	Study detects subphrenic abscesses, cysts, tumors, cirrhosis and is used to visualize biliary ducts.	Be aware that bowel must be cleansed. Explain procedure to patient.
▪ GB ultrasound	Study detects gallstones (high degree of accuracy) and can be used for a patient with jaundice or allergic reaction to GB contrast media.	Administer clear liquids for 24 hr before examination. Give laxative evening before and cleansing enema morning of examination. Keep patient NPO 8 hr before procedure.
Nuclear Imaging Scans	Purpose is to show size, shape, and position of organ. Functional disorders and structural defects may be identified. Radionuclide (radioactive isotope) is injected IV and a counter (scanning) device picks up radioactive emission, which is recorded on paper. Only tracer doses of radioactive isotopes are used.	Tell patient that substances contain only traces of radioactivity and pose little to no danger. Schedule no more than one radionuclide test on the same day. Explain to patient need to lie flat during scanning.
▪ Gastric emptying studies	Radionuclide study is used to assess ability of stomach to empty solids or liquids. In solid-emptying study, cooked egg white containing Tc-99m is eaten. In liquid-emptying study, orange juice with Tc-99m is drunk. Sequential images from gamma camera are recorded q2min for up to 60 min. Study is used in patients with emptying disorders from peptic ulcer, ulcer surgery, diabetes, or gastric malignancies.	Same as above.
▪ Liver and spleen scans	Patient is given IV injection of Tc-99m and positioned under camera to record distribution of radioactivity in liver and spleen. In normal person, intensity of liver and spleen images is equal. Test is useful in detecting hepatomegaly, hepatocellular diseases, hepatic malignancies, and splenomegaly.	Same as above.
Computed Tomography (CT)	Noninvasive radiologic examination combines special x-ray machine used for CT (exposures at different depths) with computer. Study detects mainly biliary tract, liver, and pancreatic disorders. Use of contrast medium accentuates density differences and helps detect biliary problems.	Explain procedures to patient. Determine sensitivity to iodine if contrast material used.
Magnetic Resonance Imaging (MRI)	Noninvasive procedure using radiofrequency waves and a magnetic field. Procedure is used to detect hepatic metastases, sources of GI bleeding, and to stage colorectal cancer.	Patient is NPO for 6 hr before procedure. Explain procedure to patient. Contraindicated in patient with metal implants (e.g., pacemaker) or who is pregnant.

Continued

DIAGNOSTIC STUDIES

Table 37-12 Gastrointestinal System—cont'd

Study	Description and Purpose	Nursing Responsibility
Endoscopic		
Upper GI Endoscopy ■ Esophagogastro-duodenoscopy	Technique directly visualizes mucosal lining of esophagus, stomach, and duodenum with flexible, fiberoptic endoscope. Test may use video imaging to visualize stomach motility. Inflammations, ulcerations, tumors, varices, or Mallory-Weiss tear may be detected.	Before the procedure, keep patient NPO for 8 hr. Make sure signed consent is on chart. Give preoperative medication if ordered (diazepam, midazolam, or meperidine). Explain to patient that local anesthetic may be sprayed on throat before insertion of scope, and that patient will be sedated during the procedure. After the procedure, keep patient NPO until gag reflex returns. Gently tickle back of throat to determine reflex. Use warm saline gargles for relief of sore throat. Check temperature q15-30min for 1-2 hr (sudden temperature spike is sign of perforation).
Colonoscopy	Study directly visualizes entire colon up to ileocecal valve with flexible fiberoptic scope. Patient's position is changed frequently during procedure to assist with advancement of scope to cecum. Test is used to diagnose inflammatory bowel disease, detect tumors, and dilate strictures. Procedure allows for removal of colonic polyps without laparotomy.	Before the procedure, keep patient on clear liquids 1-3 days and NPO for 8 hr. Administer laxatives 1-3 days before and enemas night before. Explain to patient same information regarding insertion of scope as for sigmodoscopy. Explain to patient that sedation will be given. Administer alternate preparation of 1 gal of Golytely or Colyte evening before (8 oz glass q10min). On morning of procedure, allow clear liquids. After the procedure, be aware that patient may experience abdominal cramps caused by stimulation of peristalsis because the patient's bowel is constantly inflated with air during procedure. Observe for rectal bleeding and signs of perforation (e.g., malaise, abdominal distention, tenesmus). Check vital signs.
Proctosigmoidoscopy	Study directly visualizes rectum and sigmoid colon with lighted endoscope. It is usually done with rigid metal scope but may be done with flexible fiberscope. Sometimes special table is used to tilt patient into knee-chest position. Test may detect tumors, polyps, inflammatory and infectious diseases, fissures, hemorrhoids.	Administer enemas evening before and morning of procedure. Be aware that patient may have clear liquids day before or that no dietary restrictions may be necessary. Explain to patient knee-chest position (unless patient is older or very ill), need to take deep breaths during insertion of scope, and possible urge to defecate as scope is passed. Encourage patient to relax—let abdomen go limp. Observe for rectal bleeding after polypectomy or biopsy.
Endoscopic Retrograde Cholangiopancreatography (ERCP)	Fiberoptic endoscope is inserted through the oral cavity into descending duodenum, then common bile and pancreatic ducts are cannulated. Contrast medium is injected into ducts and allows for direct visualization of structures. Technique can also be used to retrieve a gallstone from distal CBD, dilate strictures, biopsy tumors, diagnose pseudocysts.	Before the procedure, explain procedure to patient, including patient role. Keep patient NPO 8 hr before procedure. Ensure consent form signed. Administer sedation immediately before and during procedure. Administer antibiotics if ordered. After the procedure, check vital signs. Check for signs of perforation or infection. Be aware that pancreatitis is most common complication. Check for return of gag reflex.

Continued

DIAGNOSTIC STUDIES

Table 37-12 Gastrointestinal System—cont'd

Study	Description and Purpose	Nursing Responsibility
Endoscopic—continued		
Peritoneoscopy (Laparoscopy)	Peritoneal cavity and contents are visualized with laparoscope. Biopsy specimen may also be taken. Double-puncture peritoneoscopy permits better visualization of abdominal cavity, especially liver. Technique can eliminate need for exploratory laparotomy in many patients.	Make sure signed permit is on chart. Keep patient NPO 8 hr before study. Administer preoperative sedative medication. Ensure that bladder and bowel are emptied. Instruct patient that local anesthetic is used before scope insertion. Observe for possible complications of bleeding and bowel perforation after the procedure.
Blood Chemistries		
▪ Serum amylase	Study measures secretion of amylase by pancreas and is important in diagnosing acute pancreatitis. Level of amylase peaks in 24 hr and then drops to normal in 48-72 hr. Depending on method, *normal finding* is 0-130 U/L (0-2.17 μkat/L).	Obtain blood sample in acute attack of pancreatitis. Explain procedure to patient.
▪ Serum lipase	Study measures secretion of lipase by pancreas. Level stays elevated longer than serum amylase. *Normal finding* is 0-160 U/L (0-2.66 μkat/L).	Explain procedure to patient.
Liver Biopsy	Invasive procedure uses needle inserted between sixth and seventh or eighth and ninth intercostal spaces on the right side to obtain specimen of hepatic tissue.	Before the procedure, check patient's coagulation status (PT, clotting or bleeding time). Ensure that patient is typed and crossmatched. Take vital signs as baseline data. Explain holding of breath after expiration when needle is inserted. Ensure that informed consent has been signed. After the procedure, check vital signs to detect internal bleeding q15min × 2, q30min × 4, q1hr × 4. Keep patient lying on right side for minimum of 2 hr to splint puncture site. Keep patient in bed in flat position for 12-14 hr. Assess patient for complications such as bile peritonitis, shock, pneumothorax.
Miscellaneous Tests		
▪ Gastric analysis	Purpose is to analyze gastric contents for acidity and volume. NG tube is inserted and gastric contents are aspirated. Contents are analyzed mainly for hydrochloric acid, but pH, pepsin, and electrolytes may be determined. Histalog and pentagastrin may be used to stimulate hydrochloric acid secretion. Exfoliative cytology may be done to determine whether malignant cells are present. With fasting, *normal acidity* is 2.5 mEq/L (2.5 mmol/L) and *normal volume* is 62 ml/hr; 30 min after Histalog or pentagastrin administration, normal acidity is 1.5 mEq/L (1.5 mmol/L) and normal volume is 110 ml/hr.	Keep patient NPO for 8-12 hr. Explain insertion of NG tube. Withhold drugs affecting gastric secretions 24-48 hr before test. Ensure no smoking morning of test (nicotine increases gastric secretion).
▪ Fecal analysis	Form, consistency, color are noted. Specimen examined for mucus, blood, pus, parasites, and fat content. Tests for occult blood (guaiac test, Hemoccult, Hematest) are done.	Observe patient's stools. Collect stool specimens. Check stools for blood with Hemoccult or Hematest. Keep diet free of red meat for 24-48 hr before guaiac test.

Continued

DIAGNOSTIC STUDIES

Table 37-12 Gastrointestinal System—cont'd

Study	Description and Purpose	Nursing Responsibility
Miscellaneous Tests—continued		
▪ D-Xylose	Absorption test involves xylose, a monosaccharide, given orally in water. All urine is collected for 5 hr and amount of D-Xylose excreted is measured. *Normal finding* is 20% of xylose excreted in 5 hr. Blood levels of xylose may also be obtained 1 hr after ingestion (especially in elderly).	Keep patient NPO for 10-12 hr before test. Ensure that patient empties bladder before xylose given orally.
▪ Duodenal drainage	Duodenal contents are aspirated by double-lumen NG tube—one lumen in stomach, the other in duodenum. Stimulant IV drug is given (usually CCK). Duodenal contents are analyzed for enzymes, blood, bile, malignant cells, cholesterol crystals, and volume.	Explain procedure to patient. Insert NG tube. Keep patient on NPO status.

CBD, common bile duct; *CCK,* cholecystokinin; *GB,* gallbladder; *NG,* nasogastric; *Tc-99m,* technetium-99m.

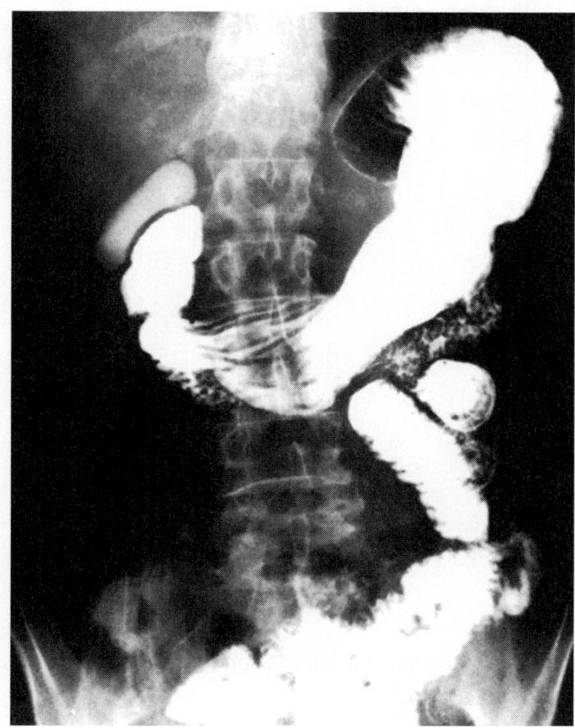

Fig. 37-10 Upper gastrointestinal tract x-ray.

Radiologic Studies

Upper Gastrointestinal Series. The purpose of an upper GI series (barium swallow) is to observe the movement of a contrast medium through the esophagus and into the stomach by means of fluoroscopy and x-ray examination. It is used to identify esophageal and stomach disorders such as esophageal strictures, varices, polyps, tumors, hiatal hernia, and peptic ulcers in the stomach or duodenum (Fig. 37-10).

The procedure consists of the patient swallowing contrast medium and then assuming different positions on the x-ray table. The movement of the contrast medium is observed with fluoroscopy, and several x-rays are taken (see Table 37-12).

Lower Gastrointestinal Series. The purpose of a lower GI series (barium enema) x-ray examination is to observe by means of fluoroscopy the filling of the colon with contrast medium and to observe by x-ray the filled colon. This procedure identifies polyps, tumors, and other lesions in the colon. It consists of administering an enema of contrast medium to the patient. The air-contrast barium enema provides better visualization of an inflammatory bowel disease, polyps, and tumors (Fig. 37-11). It is not tolerated as well in an older or immobile patient.

Oral Cholecystogram. The purpose of an oral cholecystogram (gallbladder series) is to visualize the gallbladder. It is used to determine the gallbladder's ability to concentrate and store dye and to observe the patency of the biliary duct system. It may be used to detect gallstones, obstructions of the biliary tract, and other gallbladder disorders.

The procedure consists of an x-ray examination after the oral ingestion of a radiopaque dye. The radiopaque dye used is an organic-insoluble iodide such as iopanoic acid (Telepaque, Priodax, or Oragrafin) (see Table 37-12).

Endoscopy

Endoscopy refers to the direct visualization of a body structure through a lighted instrument (scope). Most of the GI tract can be visualized by endoscopy, especially with the flexible fiberoptic scopes. The GI structures that can be examined by fiberoptic endoscopy include the esophagus, stomach, duodenum, colon, and, with the aid of fluoroscopy and x-rays, the pancreas and biliary tree. It is now possible to visualize the pancreatic, hepatic, and common bile ducts with sideviewing flexible endoscopes.[5]

The fiberscope is an instrument channel through which biopsy forceps and cytology brushes may be passed. Cameras may be attached and pictures taken. Endoscopy of the GI tract

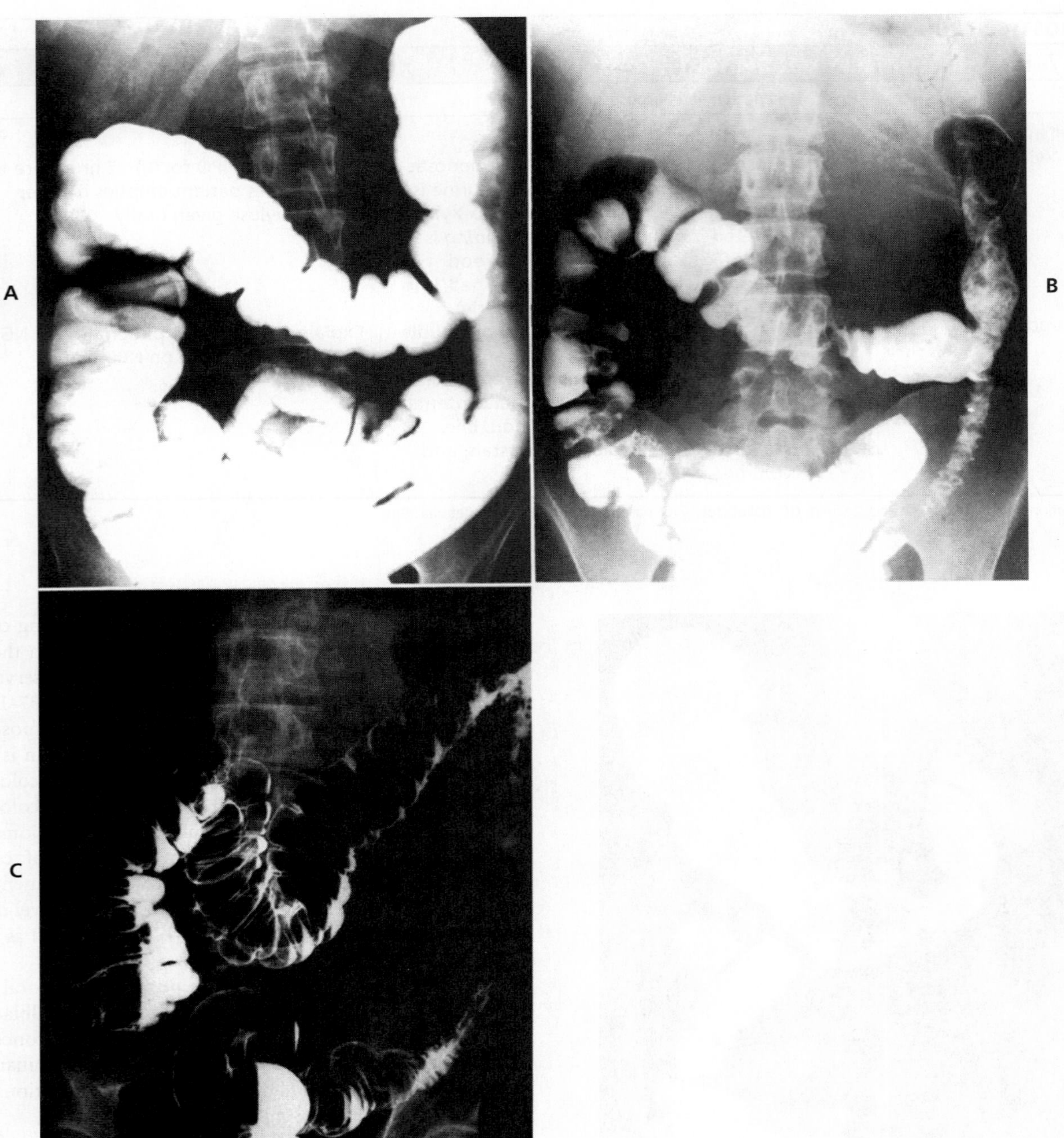

Fig. 37-11 Barium enema x-ray. **A,** Colon filled with barium. **B,** Colon after evacuation of barium. **C,** Air-contrast study of colon.

is frequently done in combination with biopsy and cytologic studies. The major complication of GI endoscopy is perforation through the structure being scoped. This complication is decreased with the use of the flexible fiberoptic scopes. All endoscopic procedures require informed, written consent. Specific endoscopy procedures are discussed in Table 37-12. In addition to diagnostic procedures, many invasive and therapeutic procedures may be done with endoscopes. These include procedures such as polypectomy, sclerosis of varices, laser treatment, cauterization of bleeding sites, papillotomy, common bile duct stone removal, and balloon dilations. A new and valuable diagnostic procedure is video endoscopy. In this procedure an electronic video endoscope converts electronic signals that can be seen on a television screen.

Liver Biopsy

The purpose of a liver biopsy is to obtain hepatic tissue to be used in establishing a diagnosis such as cirrhosis, hepatitis, and neoplasms. It may also be useful for following the progress of liver disease.

Table 37-13 Liver Function Tests

Test	Description and Purpose
Bile Formation and Excretion	
▪ Serum bilirubin	Measurement of ability of liver to conjugate and excrete bilirubin, allowing differentiation between unconjugated (indirect) and conjugated (direct) bilirubin in plasma
Total	Measurement of direct and indirect total bilirubin *Normal finding* of 0.2-1.3 mg/dl (3.4-22.0 μmol/L)
Direct	Measurement of conjugated bilirubin, elevation in obstructive jaundice *Normal finding* of 0.1-0.3 mg/dl (1.7-5.1 μmol/L)
Indirect	Measurement of unconjugated bilirubin, elevation in hepatocellular and hemolytic conditions *Normal finding* of 0.1-1.0 mg/dl (1.7-17 μmol/L)
▪ Urinary bilirubin	Measurement of urinary excretion of conjugated bilirubin *Normal finding* of 0
▪ Urinary urobilinogen	Measurement of urinary excretion of urobilinogen; maximum excretion midafternoon to early evening, collection of total urinary output for 2 hr in afternoon, sent to laboratory in dark container immediately because of oxidation of urobilinogen to urobilin on exposure to air *Normal finding* of 0.5-4 mg/day (0.8-6.8 μmol/day)
▪ Fecal urobilinogen	Measurement of fecal urobilinogen in stool specimen *Normal finding* of 30-220 mg/100 g stool (55-372 μmol/100 g of stool)
Dye Excretion Tests (Detoxification)	
▪ Indocyanine green	Determination of liver's ability to take up and excrete dye given IV, drawing of blood samples every 5 min for 20-30 min *Normal finding* of 500-800 ml/m^2 of body surface/min
Protein Metabolism	
▪ Serum protein levels	Measurement of serum proteins that are manufactured by the liver; measurement of albumin, *normal finding* of 3.5-5.0 g/dl (35-50 g/L); measurement of globulin, *normal finding* of 2.0-3.5 g/dl (20-35 g/L) *Normal total protein* of 6-8 g/dl (60-80 g/L) *Normal A/G ratio* of 1.5:1-2.5:1
▪ α-Fetoprotein	Indication of hepatic cancer *Normal finding* of <25 ng/ml (<25 μg/L)
▪ Blood ammonia levels	Conversion of ammonia to urea normally occurs in the liver, elevation can result in hepatic encephalopathy secondary to liver cirrhosis *Normal finding* of 30-70 μg/dl (17.6-41.1 μmol/L)
Hemostatic Functions	
▪ Prothrombin	Determination of prothrombin activity *Normal finding* of 12-15 sec
▪ Vitamin K production	Determination of response of liver to vitamin K, checking of PT necessary 24 hr after injection of vitamin K

Continued

The two types of liver biopsy are open and closed. The open method involves making an incision and removing a wedge of tissue. It is done in the operating room with the patient under general anesthesia, often concurrently with another surgical procedure. The closed, or needle, biopsy is an invasive procedure in which the site is infiltrated with a local anesthetic and a needle is inserted between the sixth and seventh or eighth and ninth intercostal spaces on the right side. The patient lies supine with the right arm over the head. The patient should be instructed to expire fully and not breathe while the needle is inserted. Nursing assessment before and after a liver biopsy is important (see Table 37-12).

Liver Function Studies

Liver function tests are usually described separately from other GI diagnostic studies. Liver function tests are basically biochemical determinations that reflect hepatic disease. Table 37-13 describes some common liver function tests.

Table 37-13 Liver Function Tests—cont'd

Test	Description and Purpose
Serum Enzyme Tests	
▪ Alkaline phosphatase (ALP)	Originating in bone and liver. Serum levels rise when excretion is impaired as a result of obstruction in the biliary tract. *Normal finding* of 30-120 U/L (0.5-2.0 μkat/L), depending on method and age
▪ Aspartate aminotransferase (AST) or serum glutamic-oxaloacetic transaminase (SGOT)	Elevation in liver damage and inflammation *Normal finding* of 7-40 U/L (0.12-0.67 μkat/L)
▪ Alanine aminotransferase (ALT) or serum glutamic-pyruvic transaminase (SGPT)	Elevation in liver damage and inflammation *Normal finding* of 5-36 U/L (0.08-0.6 μkat/L)
▪ δ-Glutamyl transpeptidase (GGT)	Present in biliary tract (not in skeletal muscle or cardiac), increase in hepatitis and alcoholic liver disease. More sensitive for liver dysfunction than ALP. *Normal finding* of 0-30 U/L (0-.5 μkat/L)
Lipid Metabolism	
▪ Serum cholesterol	Synthesis and excretion by liver, increase in biliary obstruction, decrease in extensive liver disease and malnutrition *Normal finding* of 140-200 mg/dl (3.6-5.2 mmol/L), varying with age

REVIEW QUESTIONS

The number of the question corresponds to the same-numbered objective at the beginning of the chapter.

1. A patient is admitted to the hospital with a diagnosis of diarrhea with dehydration. The nurse recognizes that increased peristalsis resulting in diarrhea can be related to
   a. sympathetic inhibition.
   b. mixing and propulsion.
   c. sympathetic stimulation.
   d. parasympathetic stimulation.
2. A patient has an elevated blood level of indirect bilirubin. One cause of this finding is that
   a. the gallbladder is unable to contract to release stored bile.
   b. bilirubin is not being conjugated and excreted into the bile by the liver.
   c. the Kuppfer cells in the liver are unable to remove bilirubin from the blood.
   d. there is an obstruction in the biliary tract preventing flow of bile into the small intestine.
3. As gastric contents move into the small intestine the bowel is normally protected from the acidity of gastric contents by the
   a. inhibition of secretin release.
   b. release of bicarbonate by the pancreas.
   c. release of pancreatic digestive enzymes.
   d. release of gastrin by the duodenal mucosa.
4. A patient is jaundiced and her stools are clay colored (gray). This is most likely related to
   a. decreased bile flow into the intestine.
   b. increased production of urobilinogen.
   c. increased production of cholecystokinin.
   d. increased bile and bilirubin in the blood.
5. An 80-year-old man states that although he adds a lot of salt to his food it still does not have much taste. The nurse's response is based on the knowledge that the older adult
   a. should not experience changes in taste.
   b. has some loss of taste but no difficulty chewing food.
   c. has a loss of taste buds, especially for sweet and salt.
   d. loses the sense of taste because the ability to smell is decreased.
6. When assessing the health promotion–health maintenance pattern as related to GI function an appropriate question by the nurse is,
   a. "What is your usual bowel elimination pattern?"
   b. "What percentage of your income is spent on food?"
   c. "Have you traveled to a foreign country in the last year?"
   d. "Do you have diarrhea when you are under a lot of stress?"
7. During an examination of the abdomen the nurse should
   a. position the patient in the supine position with the bed flat and knees straight.
   b. listen in the epigastrium and all four quadrants for 2 to 5 minutes for bowel sounds.
   c. use the following order of techniques: inspection, palpation, percussion, auscultation.
   d. describe bowel sounds as absent if no sound is heard in the lower right quadrant after 2 minutes.
8. A normal physical assessment finding of the GI system is
   a. tympany on percussion of the abdomen.
   b. liver edge (1-2 cm below the costal margin).
   c. finding of a firm, nodular edge on the rectal examination.
   d. easy palpation of the spleen edges with moderate pressure.
9. In preparing a patient for a colonoscopy the nurse explains that
   a. a signed permit is not necessary.
   b. sedation may be used during the procedure.
   c. only one cleansing enema is necessary for preparation.
   d. a light meal should be eaten the day before the procedure.

References

1. Eliopoulos C: *Gerontological nursing,* ed 4, Philadelphia, 1997, Lippincott.
2. Porth CM: *Pathophysiology concepts of altered health states,* ed 5, Philadelphia, 1999, Lippincott.
3. Burke MM, Walsh MB: *Gerontologic nursing: wholistic care of the older adult,* ed 2, St Louis, 1997, Mosby.
4. Bates B: *A guide to physical examination and history taking,* ed 7, Philadelphia, 1999, Lippincott.
5. Seidel HM and others: *Mosby's guide to physical examination,* ed 4, St Louis, 1999, Mosby.
6. Karanikas ID and others: Barium peritonitis: a rare complication of upper gastrointestinal contrast investigation, *Postgrad Med J* 73:297, 1997.
7. Thibodeau G, Patton KT: *Anatomy and physiology,* ed 4, St. Louis, 1999, Mosby.
8. Barkausus V and others: *Health and physical assessment,* ed 2, St Louis, 1998, Mosby.
9. Ebersole P, Hess P: *Toward healthy aging,* ed 5, St Louis, 1998, Mosby.
10. McCance KL, Huether SE: *Pathophysiology: the biologic basis for disease in adults and children,* ed 3, St Louis, 1998, Mosby.

Resources

Resources for this chapter are listed after Chapter 38 on p. 1079.

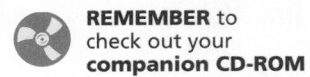

38 NURSING MANAGEMENT Nutritional Problems

Una Elizabeth Westfall

www.mosby.com/MERLIN/medsurg_lewis

LEARNING OBJECTIVES

1. Describe the essential components of a nutritionally sound diet and their importance to good health.
2. Describe possible adverse interactions between drugs and various foods.
3. Describe the common etiologic factors, clinical manifestations, and management of malnutrition.
4. Compare the etiologic factors, clinical manifestations, and collaborative and nursing management of bulimia and anorexia nervosa.
5. Differentiate between central and peripheral total parenteral nutrition administration and tube feedings, including the indications for use, complications, and collaborative and nursing management.
6. Describe the types of gastrostomy tubes and related nursing care.
7. Discuss the multiple etiologies, complications, and collaborative care approaches to the management of obesity.
8. Describe the nursing care related to conservative and surgical management of obesity.

The focus of this chapter is on problems related to nutrition. The primary nutritional problems discussed are malnutrition and obesity.

NUTRITIONAL PROBLEMS

Nutritional problems are present in all age-groups, cultures, ethnic groups, and socioeconomic classes in all parts of the world. Intelligence and wealth do not necessarily preclude the development of poor nutritional habits. The nurse in the roles of caregiver, teacher, and resource person can have a profound influence on the nutritional practices of patients and their families. A strong foundation in the principles of sound nutrition is essential. Together with the physician and the registered dietician, the nurse is in a strategic position to assess the dietary practices of the patient and provide important information, as well as link an individual with nutritional resources within and outside the institutional setting.

The nutritional state of a person or a family may be influenced by many factors. Attitudes toward the importance of food and eating habits are established early. Cultural or religious preferences and requirements are frequently reflected in dietary intake. The financial condition of a family or an individual often determines the type and amount of nutritionally sound food that can be purchased. Findings support that, generally, the lower the socioeconomic status, the poorer the nutritional state.[1] The availability of food sources also contributes to the nutritional state of people. This is usually not a problem in developed countries in which agriculture is well established and productive, but it may be a problem in underdeveloped countries.

NORMAL NUTRITION

Nutrition is the process by which the body uses food for energy, growth, and maintenance and repair of body tissues. Good nutrition in the absence of any underlying disease process results from the ingestion of a balanced diet. The United States Department of Agriculture (USDA) has adopted the food guide pyramid, which consists of food groups that are presented in proportions appropriate for a healthful diet. Figure 38-1 and Table 38-1 show these food groups with the recommended daily requirements and examples of common sources.

The essential components of the basic food groups are carbohydrates, fats, proteins, vitamins, and minerals. Carbohydrates, the body's primary source of energy, yield approximately 4 kilocalories per gram. (Kilocalorie is the correct unit to designate caloric intake and expenditure. However, calorie is more commonly used.) Carbohydrates are either simple or complex. Simple carbohydrates come in two forms: monosaccharides (e.g., glucose and fructose), found in fruits and honey; and disaccharides (e.g., sucrose, maltose, and lactose), found in such substances as table sugar, malted cereal, and milk, respectively. Complex carbohydrates or polysaccharides commonly appear in the diet as starches, such as cereal grains, potatoes, and legumes. Carbohydrates are the chief protein-sparing ingredient in a nutritionally sound diet and compose approximately 47% of the daily caloric needs of the body. The National Research Council recommends that, after infancy, at least half

Reviewed by Kathryn Hennessy, RN, MS, CNSN, Adult Nurse Practitioner, Manager, Clinical and Nursing Services, Nestle Clinical Nutrition, Deerfield, Ill.

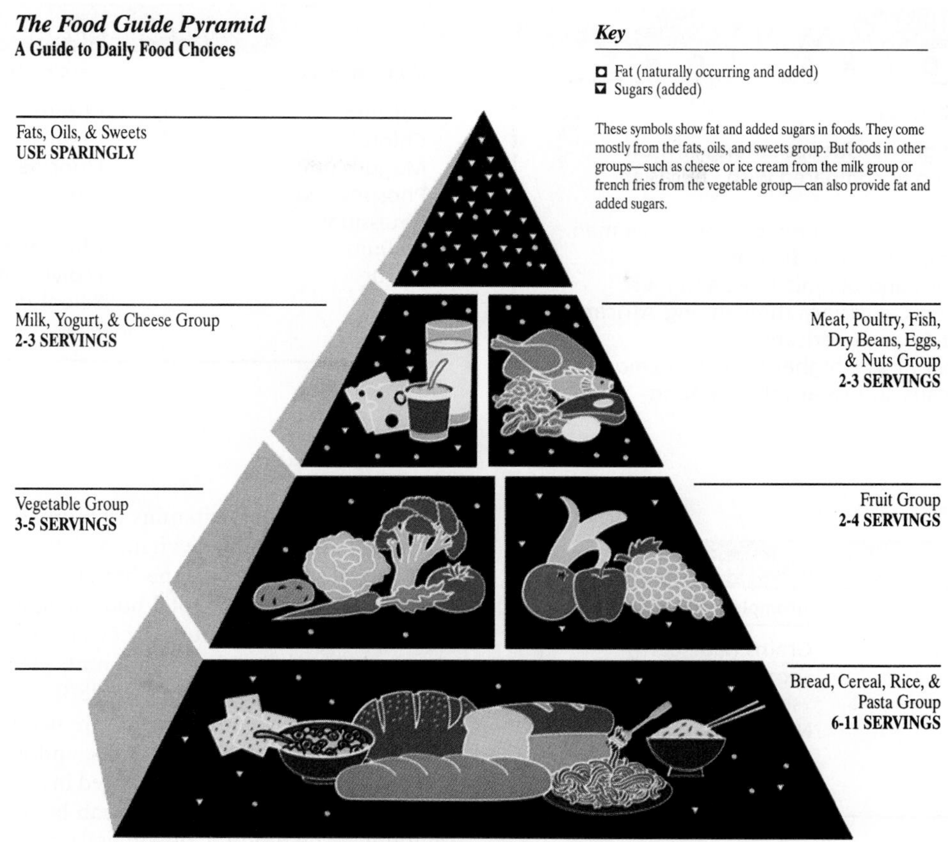

Fig. 38-1 Food guide pyramid: a guide to daily food choices and number of servings.

Table 38-1 Pyramid Food Groups and Recommended Number of Servings

Group	Nutrients Provided	Number of Servings Daily	Serving Size
▪ Bread, cereal, rice, pasta	Thiamine, niacin, iron, protein	6-11	1 slice of bread 1 oz ready-to-eat cereal ½ cup of cooked cereal, rice, or pasta
▪ Vegetable	Vitamins A and C, folic acid	3-5	1 cup of raw leafy vegetables ½ cup of other vegetables, cooked or raw ¾ cup of vegetable juice
▪ Fruit	Vitamins A and C	2-4	1 medium apple, banana, or orange ½ cup of chopped, cooked, or canned fruit ¾ cup of fruit juice
▪ Milk, yogurt, cheese	Calcium, protein, riboflavin, vitamin B_6, and cobalamin	2-3	1 cup of milk or yogurt 1½ oz of natural cheese 2 oz of processed cheese
▪ Meat, poultry, fish, dry beans, eggs, nuts	Protein, niacin, thiamine, iron, zinc, cobalamin, folic acid	2-3	2-3 oz of cooked lean meat, poultry, or fish ½ cup of cooked dry beans, 1 egg, or 2 tbsp of peanut butter (count as 1 oz lean meat)

From Human Nutrition Information Service: *Food guide pyramid,* Hyattsville, Md, 1992, USDA.

of the body's energy needs should come from carbohydrates, especially complex carbohydrates.[2]

Approximately 36% of the daily caloric intake in current American diets is derived from fat.[2] This level is considerably higher than that found in many other societies and is a cause for national concern. The Food and Nutrition Board's Committee on Diet and Health recommends that people reduce their fat intake to 30% of their total daily caloric intake.[3] One gram of fat yields 9 calories. Fats are stored in adipose tissue and in the abdominal cavity. Besides being a major source of energy, fats act as insulation, which reduces loss of body heat in cold environments and provides padding and protection for

CULTURAL & ETHNIC CONSIDERATIONS

Nutritional Problems

- Obesity has a higher incidence among African-American women as compared with Caucasian women.
- Anorexia nervosa is most common among women from middle and upper middle classes.
- Anorexia nervosa and bulimia have a higher incidence among Caucasians than among African-Americans and Asian-Americans.
- Lactase deficiency has a higher incidence among African-Americans and Asians than among Caucasians.

Table 38-2 Good Sources of Protein

Complete Proteins	Incomplete Proteins
Milk and milk products (e.g., cheese)	Grains (e.g., corn)
Eggs	Legumes (e.g., navy beans, soybeans, peas)
Fish	Nuts (e.g., peanuts)
Meats	Seeds (e.g., sesame seeds, sunflower seeds)
Poultry	

vital organs. Fats also act as carriers of essential fatty acids and fat-soluble vitamins. Fats provide a feeling of satiety after eating, partly from the flavor added and partly from their slow rate of digestion, which delays hunger.

Proteins, another essential component of a well-balanced diet, are obtained from both animal and plant sources. Ideally, proteins provide 15% to 20% of daily caloric needs of the body. The recommended daily maintenance protein intake is 0.8 to 1.0 g/kg of body weight. One gram of protein yields 4 calories. Proteins are complex nitrogenous organic compounds, of which amino acids are the fundamental units of structure. The 22 amino acids can be classified as essential and nonessential. The body is capable of synthesizing nonessential amino acids if an adequate supply of nitrogen is available. However, the nine essential amino acids cannot be synthesized, and their availability depends totally on dietary sources. Protein sources containing all the essential amino acids are called complete proteins. Proteins that lack one or more of the essential amino acids are called incomplete proteins. Table 38-2 lists good sources of protein. Proteins are essential for tissue growth, repair, and maintenance; body regulatory functions; and energy production.

Vitamins are organic compounds required in small amounts by the body for normal metabolism. Vitamins function primarily in enzyme reactions that facilitate the metabolism of amino acids, fats, and carbohydrates. The body must rely on a dietary source to meet requirements for some vitamins, such as cobalamin (vitamin B_{12}). Vitamins are divided into two categories: water-soluble vitamins (vitamin C and the B-complex vitamins) and fat-soluble vitamins (vitamins A, D, E, and K).

Table 38-3 Major Minerals and Trace Elements

Major Minerals	Trace Elements
Calcium	Chromium
Chloride	Copper
Magnesium	Fluoride
Phosphorus	Iodine
Potassium	Iron
Sodium	Manganese
Sulfur	Molybdenum
	Selenium
	Zinc

Mineral salts (e.g., magnesium, iron, calcium) make up approximately 4% of the total body weight. When minerals are present in minute amounts, they are referred to as trace elements. Minerals required in amounts greater than 100 mg per day are called major minerals. Table 38-3 lists the major minerals and trace elements. Minerals are necessary for the body to build tissues, regulate body fluids, and assist in various body functions. Some minerals are stored in a manner similar to that of the fat-soluble vitamins and can be toxic if taken in excess amounts. The amount of minerals needed in the daily diet varies greatly from a few micrograms of trace minerals to 1 g or more of the major minerals, such as calcium, phosphorus, and sodium. A well-balanced diet can usually meet the daily requirements of needed minerals. However, deficiency states can occur.

The daily caloric requirements of a person are influenced by body build, age, gender, physical activity, and level of physical and emotional health. Adjustments in caloric intake are necessary, depending on changes in health status and daily activity level. Table 38-4 summarizes the recommended daily caloric and protein intake. Table 38-5 gives an example of caloric and protein needs under normal and stress conditions.

NUTRITIONAL NEEDS

Children and Adolescents

Parents are responsible for setting an example of good nutritional habits for their children. Parental eating habits and attitudes toward food are readily passed on to their children. Parents who have little understanding of what constitutes a well-balanced diet or who cannot or will not learn good nutritional habits influence their children to follow the same poor dietary practices. The nurse is in a good position to help parents understand the changing food requirements of their children from infancy through adolescence.

Infants and children differ from adults in several ways. In the first months of life, the infant's gastrointestinal (GI) tract and kidneys are not functionally mature and therefore are limited in the kinds and quantities of nutrients that should be given. The metabolic rate of infants is higher and they have smaller nutritional reserve as compared with adults.

Table 38-4 **Recommended Daily Protein and Caloric Intake by Median Heights and Weights**

Category	Age (yr)	Weight (lb)	Weight (kg)	Height (in)	Height (cm)	Protein (g)	Average Daily Energy Allowance* (calories)
■ Men	19-24	160	72	70	177	58	2900
	25-50	174	79	70	176	63	2900
	51 and over	170	77	68	173	68	2300
■ Women	19-24	128	58	65	164	46	2200
	25-50	138	63	64	163	50	2200
	51 and over	143	65	63	160	50	1900

Modified from Food and Nutrition Board, National Research Council, National Academy of Sciences: *Recommended dietary allowances,* ed 10, Washington, DC, 1989, National Academy Press.
*For light to moderate activity.

Table 38-5 **Caloric and Protein Needs of a 150 lb (68 kg) Man**

Activity	Calories	Protein (g)
Basal	1400	49
Moderate activity (activities of daily living)	2500	70
Postoperative (no complications)	3150	105
Stress response (e.g., to chemotherapy, radiation therapy)	3500	140
Infection	>4500	>175

Table 38-6 **Low-Cost Protein Supplements**

Brewer's yeast	2⅓ tbs
Cheese	1-in cube
Cottage cheese	¼ cup
Egg	1
Milk (whole, low fat, or skim)	⅞ cup
Peanut butter	2 tbs
Pinto beans	¼ cup
Poultry	1 oz
Soybeans (cooked)	1 cup and 2 tsp
Split peas, lentils (cooked)	½ cup

Adolescence is a particularly vulnerable time for the development of nutritional deficiencies because this is a time of rapid growth and bodily changes. It is a period during which there is extreme concern with body appearance and social acceptability. Teenage girls are often attracted to fad diets as a means of weight control. Unfortunately, fad diets are often nutritionally unsound. Unless good nutritional habits are encouraged and supervised by peers and parents during this developmental period, poor nutritional patterns may become established as a way of life. A state of chronic inadequate nutrition may result.

Socioeconomic Status

Because individuals and families from the lower socioeconomic class spend a greater percentage of their limited income on food, there is a tendency to seek out cheaper foods as the cost of food increases. These foods may not provide adequate or balanced nutrition. In contrast, some lower-income persons may prefer to select foods that are more expensive, but only marginally nutritious, because of their prestige value. The nurse and the registered dietician can assist the poor in making food choices that meet nutritional requirements while staying within their limited resources. Table 38-6 lists low-cost protein supplements.

Older Adults

The unique nutritional requirements of an older adult are often overlooked. It is more common to find an undernourished older person than an obese one. As a person grows older there are decreases in lean body mass (the metabolically active tissue), basal metabolic rate, and physical activity. Combined, these factors decrease the caloric needs for energy. The older person frequently reduces the consumption of needed protein, vitamins, and minerals and may take in "empty calories," such as candy and pastries. The reasons given for such alterations are varied. Table 38-7 outlines factors affecting nutritional intake in older adults.

As a group, older adults may be less well informed about what constitutes a well-balanced diet. The older adult may be induced to purchase more costly "health foods" at specialty stores under mistaken assumptions, such as that these foods offer more nutrients than foods bought at the local market, or that the food supply is nutritionally inadequate.[4]

When these factors are added to already existing medical problems, it is easy to see why poor dietary practices develop. In addition, poor dentition, ill-fitting dentures, anorexia, multiple losses affecting the social setting of meals, low income, and medical conditions involving the GI tract contribute to the type and amount of foods that is eaten. The nurse, working with the registered dietician, must be aware of common medical and psychosocial factors in the older adult and should incorporate interventions for overcoming these problems in the plan of care.

Patients with Physical Illnesses

Regardless of the cause of the illness, the sick person has increased nutritional needs. Pathologic conditions are frequently aggravated by undernutrition, and an existing deficiency state is

Table 38-7 Factors Affecting Nutritional Intake in Older Adults

Age	Feelings of being valued
Anorexia	Food fads
Availability of desired foods	Food intolerance
Availability of transportation to food stores	Gender
Available time for preparation and eating	Health status
Chronic conditions	Importance of food in the past
Decrease in number of taste buds	Income level
Degree of physical activity	Lack of food preparation equipment
Dental problems	Loneliness or loss
Education level and nutritional knowledge	Mental awareness
	Physical disability
	Prescribed diets
	Prescribed or over-the-counter medicines
	Social isolation

likely to become more severe during illness. Malnutrition is not an uncommon consequence of illness, surgery, injury, or hospitalization. Anorexia, nausea, vomiting, diarrhea, abdominal distention, and abdominal cramping may accompany diseases of the GI system. Any combination of these symptoms interferes with normal food consumption and metabolism. Additionally, a patient may restrict the dietary intake to a few foods or fluids that may not be nutritionally sound out of fear of aggravating the already disturbed GI function.

Malabsorption syndrome is defined as the impaired absorption of nutrients from the GI tract. It may result from decreased amounts of necessary enzymes or a reduced bowel surface area and can quickly lead to a deficiency state. Many pharmacologic agents may result in undesirable GI side effects, as well as alter normal digestive and absorptive processes. For example, antibiotics change the normal flora of the intestines, decreasing the body's ability to synthesize biotin.

Fever accompanies many illnesses, injuries, and infections, with a concomitant increase in the body's basal metabolic rate (BMR). Each degree of temperature increase on the Fahrenheit scale raises the BMR by 7%.[2] Without an increase in the amount of calories ingested in the diet, body protein stores will be used to supply calories, and protein depletion can become a problem.

The hospitalized patient, especially the older adult, is at risk of becoming malnourished. Prolonged illness, major surgery, sepsis, draining wounds, burns, hemorrhage, fractures, and immobilization can all contribute to malnutrition. The nurse must assume responsibility, along with the physician and the dietician, for meeting the patient's nutritional needs. The nurse must also be knowledgeable of the requirements of a patient who is not overtly ill but who is undergoing diagnostic studies. This patient may be nutritionally fit on entering the hospital but can develop nutritional problems because of the dietary restrictions imposed by multiple diagnostic studies.

The role of nutrition in the development of diseases has long been studied. Studies of the association of personal dietary habits with the development of selected cancers and cardiovascular diseases have been widely published in recent years. There now appear to be links between some types of cancers and dietary intake; for example, high ingestion of fatty foods is linked with breast and endometrial cancer, and a low fiber intake may be linked with colon cancer (see Chapter 40). Further research in this area is needed for a better understanding of diet and the development of disease, especially cancer.

VITAMIN IMBALANCES

Vitamin deficiencies are rare in most of the developed countries of the world. When vitamin deficiencies are present, several vitamins are usually involved rather than a single vitamin deficiency. The recommended dietary allowance (RDA) for essential vitamins and minerals can be obtained by eating a diet consisting of foods from the basic five food groups. RDAs from the Food and Nutrition Board have a safety margin because the levels exceed minimum daily requirements for most people. When vitamin imbalances do occur, they are usually found among persons with a pattern of alcohol and drug abuse, persons who are chronically ill, and individuals who follow poor dietary practices. Followers of fad diets or poorly planned vegetarian diets are also subject to a potential deficiency state. Clinical manifestations of vitamin imbalances are most commonly exhibited as neurologic manifestations (Table 38-8). In the growing child, the central nervous system (CNS) is primarily involved, while the peripheral nervous system is most affected in the adult.

Vegetarian Diets

The common element among all vegetarians is the exclusion of red meat from the diet. Vegetarianism cannot be considered a nutritional fad because it is found in all age-groups, occupations, and lifestyles. A variety of reasons have been given for following this type of dietary practice, including religious or cultural beliefs that it is a better way of attaining total health, respect for all living beings, ethical-ecologic ideals, and economics.

The two large classes of vegetarians are *vegans,* who are pure or total vegetarians and use only plant food, and *lacto-ovo-vegetarians,* who use plant foods and sometimes dairy products and eggs. There are several other types, including the fruitarians, but they constitute only a small percentage of the total group.

Vegetarian diets can result in a potential vitamin deficiency state. In well-planned vegetarian diets the essential vitamins and minerals are easily obtained. Plant protein, although of a lesser quality than that of animal origin, fulfills most of the protein requirements. Combinations of vegetable protein foods (e.g., cornmeal, kidney beans) can increase the nutritional value. Lacto-ovo-vegetarians obtain additional protein sources from dairy products and eggs. Milk made from soybeans is an excellent protein source, especially for the true vegan. The primary deficiency of a strict vegan is lack of cobalamin (vitamin B_{12}). This vitamin can be obtained only from animal protein, special supplements, or foods that have been fortified with the

Table **38-8** Recommended Dietary Vitamin Allowances and Signs of Imbalance

Vitamin	Recommended Dietary Allowances	Symptoms of Overdose	Manifestations of Deficiencies
Fat Soluble			
■ A	Men: 1000 μg/Retinol equivalents* Women: 800 μg/Retinol equivalents	Hair loss, dry skin; headaches; dry mucous membranes; liver damage; bone and joint pain; blurred vision; nausea and vomiting	Dry, scaly skin; increased susceptibility to infection; night blindness; anorexia; eye irritation; xerosis; keratinization of respiratory and GI mucosa; bladder stones; anemia; retarded growth
■ D	Adults 5-10 μg of cholecalciferol†	Deposits of calcium and phosphorus in soft tissue; kidney and heart damage; bone fragility; constipation; anorexia, nausea, vomiting; headache	Muscular weakness; excessive sweating; diarrhea and other GI disturbances; bone pain; active rickets; healed rickets; osteomalacia
■ E	Men: 10 mg Women: 8 mg	Relatively nontoxic	Neurologic defects; hemolytic anemia (only in newborns)
■ K	Men: 70-80 μg Women: 60-65 μg	Anemia	Defective blood coagulation
Water Soluble			
■ B_1	Men: 1.2-1.5 mg Women: 1.0-1.1 mg	Not stored in body, therefore overdose does not occur	Loss of appetite; fatigue; nervous irritability; constipation; paresthesias; insomnia
■ B_6	Men: 1.7-2.0 mg Women: 1.4-1.6 mg	Not stored in body, therefore overdose does not occur	Seizures; dermatitis; anemia; neuropathy with motor weakness; anorexia
■ Cobalamin (B_{12})	Adults: 2-10 μg	Not stored in body, therefore overdose does not occur	Megaloblastic anemia; inadequate myelin synthesis; anorexia; glossitis; sore mouth and tongue; pallor; neurologic problems such as depression and dizziness; weight loss; nausea; constipation
■ C	Adults: 50-60 mg	Not stored in body, therefore overdose does not occur	Bleeding gums; loose teeth; easy bruising; poor wound healing; scurvy; dry, itchy skin
■ Folic acid	Men: 200 μg Women: 180 μg	Not stored in body, therefore overdose does not occur	Impaired cell division and protein synthesis; megaloblastic anemia; anorexia; fatigue; sore tongue; diarrhea; forgetfulness

Modified from Food and Nutrition Board, National Academy of Sciences, National Research Council: *Recommended dietary allowances,* ed 10, Washington DC, 1989, National Academy Press.
*1 Retinol Equivalent = 10 IU vitamin A activity from β-carotene or 3.33 IU vitamin A activity from retinol.
†1μg of cholecalciferol = 40 IU vitamin D.
GI, gastrointestinal.

vitamin. Vegans not using cobalamin supplements are susceptible to the development of megaloblastic anemia and the neurologic signs of cobalamin deficiency. Strict vegetarians and lacto-ovo-vegetarians are also at risk for iron deficiency. Iron-enriched foods or iron supplements are often prescribed during pregnancy, early childhood, adolescence, and after major blood loss. Table 38-9 lists examples of foods high in iron. Other deficiencies that may be present in a vegan include calcium, zinc, vitamins A and D, and protein.

Megavitamin Therapy

Megavitamin therapy refers to the administration of high doses of one or more vitamins, usually 10 to 20 times the RDA. Unless there are serious vitamin deficiencies, megavitamin therapy has a limited place in maintaining nutrition. The beneficial effects derived from the ingestion of commercially prepared daily vitamins are negligible if a balanced diet is eaten.

The water-soluble vitamins (vitamins C and B complex) are absorbed only as needed by the body, and the excess is excreted rapidly in the urine. Toxicity from overdoses is rare. However, because the excess is excreted through the kidney and urinary tract, detrimental effects may occur. Vitamin C is uricosuric (increases the renal excretion of uric acid) and may cause the formation of urinary tract stones (uric acid stones) in susceptible persons when taken in megadoses. When taken in large doses, vitamins can function as drugs rather than as nutrients and can cause toxic manifestations.

The fat-soluble vitamins (vitamins A, D, E, and K) are readily stored and can accumulate to toxic levels. Because most vitamins can be purchased without a prescription, high doses of

NUTRITIONAL THERAPY

Table 38-9 Foods High in Iron

Food	Selected Serving Size	% of U.S. RDA
Breads, Cereals, and Grain Products		
Farina, regular or quick cooked (enriched)	⅔ cup	25-39
Oatmeal, instant, fortified, prepared (enriched)	⅔ cup	25-39
Ready-to-eat cereals, fortified (enriched)	1 oz	25-39
Meat, Poultry, Fish, and Alternatives		
Beef liver, braised	3 oz	25-39
Pork liver, braised	3 oz	>39
Chicken or turkey liver, braised	½ cup diced	25-39
Clams; steamed, boiled, or canned, drained	3 oz	>39
Oysters; baked, broiled, steamed or canned, undrained	3 oz	25-39
Soybeans, cooked	½ cup	25-39

From Human Nutrition Information Service: *Good sources of nutrients,* Washington, DC, 1990, USDA.
NOTE: Vitamin C improves iron absorption.
RDA, recommended dietary allowance.

vitamins A, D, and E can result in serious health hazards because the excess is not eliminated (see Table 38-8). Toxic levels of the fat-soluble vitamins can be reached within a matter of weeks, especially in infants and children.

DRUG-FOOD INTERACTIONS

When health conditions require drug therapy, drug and food or nutrient interactions may not be explored before starting a prescription. Adverse interactions can include incompatibilities, altered drug effectiveness, and impaired nutritional status. Table 38-10 outlines examples of common drug and food-nutrient interactions. As members of the health team, nurses have a responsibility for monitoring and preventing potential interactions for patients while in the hospital and at home.

EATING DISORDERS

Anorexia Nervosa

Anorexia nervosa, sometimes called anorexia, is a specific psychiatric diagnosis. Anorexia nervosa is characterized by refusal to maintain body weight to greater than 85% of that expected for age and height.[5] This condition results in a severely malnourished state characterized by the vigorous pursuit of thinness and a morbid fear of becoming fat. Restricted intake occurs even in the presence of hunger.

The two subgroups of anorexia nervosa are termed the *bulimic type* and the *restrictive type,* depending on whether there are cycles of binging and purging. This condition is found predominantly in adolescent girls. The disorder was first recorded in England in 1684 and was misnamed anorexia nervosa because it was thought to be secondary to severe sadness and anxiety. The name has persisted to the present day even though current research indicates a different cause. Anorexia nervosa usually begins during adolescence or early adulthood. It is a chronic illness that can place the patient at high risk for serious complications, affecting multiple organ systems. Life-threatening cardiac complications include hypotension, bradycardia, and malignant arrhythmias. It is rare for the illness to occur for the first time in a woman who is more than 25 years old.

Anorexia nervosa is now recognized as occurring more often among persons whose sisters and mothers have the disorder than among the general population. Patients usually come from a middle- or upper-class background.[6] They often are perfectionists and tend to be high achievers. At the same time, they may be dependent and experience insecurity in social situations. In some patients the disorder is associated with stressful life situations with which they are unable to cope. In addition, many patients are somewhat overweight at the onset of their illness.

Common physical signs and symptoms of anorexia nervosa include amenorrhea, bradycardia, orthostatic hypotension, cold intolerance, breast atrophy, lanugo (soft, downlike hair normally associated with a fetus), dry skin, hair loss, severe constipation, and edema with altered fluid balance. Diagnostic studies often show iron deficiency anemia and an elevated blood urea nitrogen that is reflective of marked intravascular volume depletion and prerenal azotemia. Lack of potassium in the diet and loss of potassium in the urine lead to potassium deficiency in blood and tissues, leading to weakness, cardiac arrhythmias, and renal failure. If the eating pattern is permitted to continue for a prolonged time, body wasting and signs of severe malnutrition are evident.

Once anorexia nervosa has developed, the person will go to almost any extreme to hide the eating behavior from parents or peers. Eating habits are severely disturbed. If purging is present, it is often accomplished by self-induced vomiting or the use of cathartics or enemas.

Multidisciplinary treatment must involve a combination of nutrition support and psychiatric care. Hospitalization may be necessary if there are severe physical complications that cannot be managed in an outpatient therapy program. Nutritional replenishment must be closely supervised to ensure consistent and ongoing weight gains. The use of tube or parenteral feedings may be necessary. Improved nutrition, however, is not a cure for anorexia nervosa. The underlying psychiatric problem must be addressed by identification of the disturbed patterns of individual and family interactions, followed by individual and family counseling.

Table 38-10 Common Drug and Food/Nutrient Interactions

Drug Category/Drug	Food/Nutrient	Drug-Food Effects or Cautions
Anticoagulants	Dietary vitamin K (e.g., green leafy vegetables, green tea, dairy products/meats)	Decrease or loss of anticoagulant effect
Antiseizure agents ▪ Phenytoin (Dilantin)	Folic acid	Long-term drug use may increase folic acid requirement
Antidepressants		
▪ Trazodone (Desyrel)	Food	Food slows drug absorption
▪ Tricyclic antidepressants	Riboflavin	Riboflavin requirements may increase with amitriptyline (Elavil) or imipramine (Tofranil)
Antidiabetic agents ▪ Glyburide (Micronase, DiaBeta)	High fat diet	Drug should not be taken with high fat diet
Antithyroid agents ▪ Methimazole (Tapazole)	Food	Foods may inconsistently alter bioavailability of methimzaole
Barbiturates ▪ Phenobarbital ▪ Mephobarbitol (Mebaral)	Folic acid	Drugs may increase folic acid requirements; long-term therapy may require vitamin D supplements for osteomalacia
β-adrenergic blocking agents ▪ Labetalol (Normodyne) ▪ Metaproterenol (Alupent) ▪ Carteolol (Cartrol) ▪ Sotalol (Betapace)	Food	Bioavailability of drug may be enhanced when taken with food
Bronchodilators ▪ Theophylline ▪ Oxtriphylline (Choledyl) ▪ Dyphylline (Lufyllin)	High-carbohydrate, low-protein diets Caffeine-containing foods and fluids	Decrease drug elimination Caffeine may increase CNS stimulant effects of xanthine-derivative bronchodilators
Cholestyramine (Questran)	Fat-soluble vitamins	Drug may interfere with their absorption
Corticosteroids (prolonged therapy)	Salt seasonings	May require sodium limits and/or potassium supplements
Erythropoietin	Folic acid and/or cobalamin	Nutrient deficiencies may reduce/delay drug response
Etidronate (Didronel)	Foods, fluids, or drugs high in calcium	May prevent drug absorption
Furazolidone (Furoxone)	Food and fluids containing tyramine (e.g., aged cheese, smoked or pickled meats or poultry, fermented meat, overripe fruit, beer, wine, liqueurs)	MAO-inhibiting effects may last at least 2 wk after stopping drug. Dietary restrictions need to continue for at least 2 wk after MAO inhibitors discontinued if received large doses or prolonged therapy
Isoniazid (INH)	Cheese (e.g., Swiss or Cheshire) or fish (e.g., tuna, skipjack)	Concurrent ingestion may lead to redness or itching, HR changes, sweating, chills or clammy feeling, headache or light-headedness; thought to be related to altered metabolism of tyramine in foods
Parkinson's drug ▪ Selegiline (Eldepryl)	Food and fluids containing tyramine (e.g., aged cheese, smoked or pickled meats or poultry, fermented meat, overripe fruit, beer, wine, liqueurs)	When used concurrently, may cause sudden and severe hypertensive reactions; dietary restrictions need to continue for at least 2 wk after MAO inhibitors discontinued
Phenothiazines	Riboflavin	Drugs may increase riboflavin requirements
Procarbazine (Matulane)	Food and fluids containing tyramine or other high pressor amines (e.g., aged cheese, smoked or pickled meats or poultry, fermented meat, overripe fruit, beer, wine, liqueurs)	When used concurrently, may cause sudden and severe hypertensive reactions; dietary restrictions need to continue for at least 2 wk after MAO inhibitors discontinued
Ticlopidine (Ticlid)	Food	Drug absorption increased when taken after a meal
Zafirlukast (Accolate)	High-fat and high protein meal	When taken concurrently drug bioavailability reduced by about 40%
Zinc supplements	Foods	Many foods impair zinc absorption

MAO, monoamine oxidase.

Bulimia

Bulimia is a chronic disorder that is often confused with anorexia nervosa. Concern about body image is a key feature in both bulimia and anorexia nervosa; however, the syndrome of bulimia is different from anorexia nervosa. Bulimia is characterized by compulsive binge eating and purging (through self-induced vomiting, laxative abuse, excessive exercise, and diuretics). Food becomes an obsession and an addiction—an escape from the pressures of life. Unlike the person with anorexia, the patient caught up in the syndrome of bulimia usually maintains a normal or near-normal body weight, and the primary symptom is gorging rather than starvation.

Bulimia is increasing in incidence and may be even more prevalent than anorexia nervosa. Female college students seem to be susceptible to this syndrome. The cause remains unclear but is thought to be similar to that of anorexia nervosa. Substance abuse, anxiety, affective disorders, and personality disturbances have been reported among persons with bulimia.

In addition to the psychologic considerations, bulimia may lead to some physical effects in those persons who binge and purge on a daily basis. Characteristic skin lesions on the back of the hand, which are often over the metacarpophalangeal joint and called Russell's sign, can result from repeated trauma to the skin from self-induced vomiting. In addition, dental problems may develop from constant vomiting. Swollen glands or salivary gland hypertrophy, sore throat, facial puffiness, chronic indigestion, irregular menstrual periods, electrolyte imbalances, and dehydration can also occur. Sudden death from cardiac arrest or a fatal arrhythmia is not uncommon. Although rare, esophageal tears and gastric rupture secondary to overdistention can occur. However, most bulimics have few, if any, noticeable signs of the illness.[7]

The patient with bulimia, similar to the one with anorexia nervosa, goes to great lengths to conceal abnormal eating habits. As the behavior persists, many problems associated with the condition become increasingly hard to deal with effectively.

Treatment of bulimia is similar to that described for anorexia nervosa. The multidisciplinary approach consists of strategies that include individual psychotherapy, nutritional counseling (including discussion of the dangers involved in binge eating and purging), cognitive behavior therapy, and drug therapy. Antidepressants (e.g., fluoxetine [Prozac], amitriptyline [Elavil]) are useful for the depression associated with both anorexia nervosa and bulimia. Vitamin, mineral, and iron supplements may be prescribed. However, iron supplementation is not generally required if amenorrhea is present. The return to normal eating habits may take several months to years to accomplish because relapses are frequent. Recovery is difficult; the abnormal eating behavior is hard to change because binge eating and purging provide the person with a feeling of satisfaction and of control over the body. For help and support, several organizations for eating disorders have been formed, including American Anorexia/Bulimia Association; Anorexia Nervosa and Related Eating Disorders, Inc.; National Eating Disorders Organization; National Association of Anorexia Nervosa and Associated Disorders, Inc.; and Overeaters Anonymous. (See Resources at end of chapter.)

MALNUTRITION

Malnutrition may be defined as an excess, a deficit, or an imbalance in the essential components of a balanced diet. Terms such as *undernutrition* and *overnutrition* are also used to describe malnutrition. Undernutrition describes a state of poor nourishment as a result of inadequate diet or diseases that interfere with normal appetite and assimilation of ingested food. Overnutrition refers to the ingestion of more food than is required for body needs, as in obesity.

Malnutrition is most prevalent in developing countries in which adequate food sources do not exist, the inhabitants are not well educated about their nutritional needs, and economic conditions often preclude the purchase of a balanced diet. Undernutrition does exist in scattered parts of the United States, and it is usually found in individuals or groups from the lower socioeconomic class.

Types of Malnutrition

Protein-Calorie Malnutrition. Protein-calorie malnutrition (PCM) is the most common form of undernutrition and can result from either primary or secondary factors. Primary PCM is present when nutritional needs are not met as a result of poor eating habits. Secondary PCM is the result of an alteration or defect in ingestion, digestion, absorption, or metabolism. In this type of malnutrition, tissue needs are not met even though the dietary intake would be satisfactory under normal conditions. Secondary malnutrition may occur as a result of GI obstruction, surgical treatment (e.g., after peptic ulcer surgery), cancer, malabsorption syndromes, medications, and infectious diseases.

PCM may also be due to the ingestion of foods deficient in protein. In addition to decreased quantities of protein, the diet is generally low in necessary vitamins and minerals. PCM is a serious nutritional problem common throughout the world, affecting every socioeconomic group and age-group. In the United States and Canada, where protein intake is high and of good quality, severe malnutrition is less of a problem, but it can occur in high-risk groups.

Marasmus and Kwashiorkor. Malnutrition has long been recognized in infants and children throughout the world by the terms *marasmus* and *kwashiorkor*. Malnutrition in adults may also be classified by this terminology. Marasmus is the result of a concomitant deficiency of both caloric and protein intake leading to generalized loss of body fat and muscle. Kwashiorkor is caused by a deficiency of protein intake that is superimposed on a catabolic stress event, such as a GI obstruction, a surgical procedure, cancer, a malabsorption syndrome, or an infectious disease.

Etiology and Pathophysiology

The following factors increase the potential for the development of malnutrition:

1. Major surgery, radiation therapy, or chemotherapy
2. Severe burns with exudate high in protein
3. Draining wounds, including pressure ulcers
4. Chronic renal or liver diseases
5. Hemorrhage

6. Bone fractures with prolonged immobilization
7. Malabsorption syndrome
8. Presence of infectious diseases such as tuberculosis or acquired immunodeficiency syndrome (AIDS)

The nitrogen loss after severe injury or major surgery may be as much as 20 g per day, excreted as urea, creatinine, and creatine.

Knowledge of the phases of the starvation process is essential to better understand the physiologic changes that occur in PCM. Initially, the body selectively uses carbohydrates (glycogen) rather than fat and protein to maintain metabolic function. These carbohydrate stores, found in the liver and muscles, are minimal and may be totally depleted within 18 hours. During this early phase of starvation, the only use of protein is in its obligatory participation in cellular metabolism. However, once carbohydrate stores are depleted, protein begins to be converted to glucose for energy. Alanine and glutamine are the first amino acids to be used by the liver for the formation of glucose in a process termed *gluconeogenesis.* The resulting available plasma glucose allows the metabolic processes to continue. With these amino acids being used as energy sources, the person is in negative nitrogen balance (greater nitrogen excretion). However, within 5 to 9 days, body fat is fully mobilized to supply much of the needed energy.

In prolonged starvation up to 97% of calories are provided by fat, and protein is conserved. Depletion of fat stores depends on the amount available, but fat stores are generally used up in 4 to 6 weeks. Once fat stores are used, body proteins, including those in internal organs and plasma, can no longer be spared and rapidly decrease because they are the only remaining body source of energy available.

If the malnourished patient has surgery, experiences bodily trauma, or has an infection, the stress response with concomitant increase in energy expenditure is superimposed on the starvation response. These body insults cause an increase in the metabolic rate, with a subsequent increase in energy requirements. Protein stores are no longer spared and are used with increasing frequency for body energy because of the increased metabolic energy needs.

As the protein depletion continues, liver function is impaired, and synthesis of proteins is diminished. The plasma oncotic pressure is decreased because of decreased protein synthesis. A major function of plasma proteins, primarily of albumin, is the maintenance of the osmotic pressure of the blood. Because of this decreased pressure, a shift in body fluids occurs from the vascular space into the interstitial compartment. As protein ingestion decreases and body stores are depleted, albumin eventually leaks into the interstitial space along with the fluid. Edema becomes clinically observable. Often the edema present in the face and legs of the patient masks the muscle wasting that occurs. Ascites (abnormal intraperitoneal accumulation of fluid containing large amounts of protein and electrolytes) is a classic manifestation of kwashiorkor.

As the total blood volume is reduced, the skin appears dry and wrinkled. Along with the shift of fluids to the interstitial space, ions also move. Sodium (a predominant extracellular ion) is found in increased amounts within the cell, and potassium (a predominant intracellular ion) and magnesium are shifted to the extracellular space. The sodium-potassium exchange pump, which is dependent on adenosine triphosphatase (ATPase), has high energy needs, using 20% to 50% of all calories ingested. When the diet is extremely deficient in calories and essential proteins, the pump will fail, leaving sodium inside the cell (along with water), and the cell will expand.

The liver is the body organ that loses the most mass during protein deprivation. It gradually becomes infiltrated with fat secondary to decreased synthesis of lipoproteins. Immediate restoration to the diet of protein and other necessary constituents must be instituted or death will rapidly ensue. The most serious problem associated with PCM in the young is the probability of mental retardation. In severe malnutrition the development of brain cells is greatly slowed down. Brain cells increase most rapidly during fetal life and in the first 5 to 6 months after birth. Once this critical time for brain development has passed, improvement in the nutritional state of the infant will not correct any mental deficiency already incurred.

Clinical Manifestations

The adult who is deprived of adequate protein and calories will have many of the clinical manifestations presented in Table 38-11. The most obvious clinical signs on physical examination are apparent in the skin, eyes, mouth, muscles, and CNS. The speed at which the protein deficiency develops depends on the quantity and quality of the protein intake, caloric value, and the age of the person.

Clinical manifestations of malnutrition are the result of numerous interactions occurring at the cellular level. As protein intake is severely reduced, the muscles, which make up the largest reservoir of protein in the body, become wasted and flabby, leading to weakness, fatigability, and decreased endurance. There is decreased protein available for repair, and as a result, wound healing may be delayed. Malnutrition in the hospitalized patient may result in delayed recovery and prolonged hospitalization. The person is more susceptible to all types of infections. Both humoral and cell-mediated immunity are deficient in PCM. There is a decrease in leukocytes in the peripheral blood. Phagocytosis is altered as a result of the lack of energy (ATP) necessary to drive the process. Most malnourished persons are anemic. Anemia resulting from PCM is usually caused by nutritional deficiencies such as iron and folic acid, the necessary building blocks for red blood cells (RBCs).

Complications

The severity of complications ranges from mild to emaciation and death. Major complications center around delayed wound healing and increased susceptibility to infection from decreased immune function.

Diagnostic Studies

The diagnosis of PCM can be determined by a variety of laboratory studies used in conjunction with physical examination. Serum albumin is useful in the diagnosis of malnutrition. The degree of protein depletion can be identified with the use of the scale in Table 38-12. Serum albumin has a half-life of

Table **38-11** Signs of Protein-Calorie Malnutrition

Body System	Subclinical Signs	Clinical Signs
Integumentary	Slowed tissue turnover rate, surface temperature 1° F-2° F cooler	Brittle nails, decreased tone and elasticity of skin, xeroderma (dry skin), pigment changes (brown-gray), erythematous seborrheic dermatitis, scrotal dermatitis
Visual	Night blindness	Hair: easy loss of hair, color changes, lack of luster Blood vessel growth in cornea, Bitot's spots (gray keratinized epithelium on conjunctiva), dryness of conjunctiva and cornea, pale to red conjunctiva
Gastrointestinal		
Mouth and lips	Reduction in saliva production	Cheilosis (crusting and ulceration at angle of mouth)
Tongue	Mucosa more permeable to bacteria	Raw and beefy red, edematous and smooth, atrophy or hypertrophy of papillae
Teeth	Improper development, delayed eruption	Caries, loose teeth, discolored enamel
Gingivae		Periodontal disease, tendency to bleed easily, receding, pale, and soft
Stomach	Decreased gastric acidity, delayed gastric emptying	Constant hunger, increased incidence of ulcers
Intestines	Decreased motility and absorption, normal flora causing infection from increased permeability of mucosa	Diarrhea and flatulence, protruding abdomen, increased incidence of parasitic diseases
Liver-biliary	Fatty liver, decreased absorption of fat-soluble vitamins	Hepatomegaly
Cardiovascular	Decreased cardiac output, decreased hemoglobin, shift in heart position, increased risk of thrombophlebitis	Decreased blood pressure and pulse, slight cyanosis, anemia, body edema
Endocrine	Decreased insulin production	Thyroid enlargement, polydipsia, polyuria, increased sensitivity to cold
Immunologic	Decreased lymphocyte proliferation, decreased albumin levels, decreased antibody production, decreased total protein, diminished febrile response to infection, delayed immune response	Increased number of infections, decreased response to skin tests
Musculoskeletal	Decreased growth rate, decreased body stature with chronic PCM, decreased muscle mass	Prominence of bony structures such as face, clavicle, scapula, ribs, iliac crests, and spinal vertebrae, due to subcutaneous tissue loss, weak and spindly arms and legs, flat buttocks, weak and flabby muscles, decreased physical activity and ability to work, severe weight loss
Neurologic	Loss of ambition, feeling of being tired	Depression, confusion, decreased reflexes in legs and ankles, decreased position sense, decreased vibratory sense, paresthesias of hands and feet, syncope, motor weakness
Renal	Negative nitrogen balance, decreased BUN and creatinine levels	Nocturia, decreased urinary output
Reproductive	Decreased gonadotropin levels	Amenorrhea, impotence, atrophied breasts
Respiratory	Pulmonary edema, decreased strength of respiratory muscles	Increased susceptibility to respiratory infection, decreased respiratory rate, decreased vital capacity

BUN, blood urea nitrogen; *PCM,* protein-calorie malnutrition.

approximately 20 to 22 days. In the absence of marked fluid loss, such as from hemorrhage or burns, the serum albumin value lags behind actual protein changes by more than 2 weeks and therefore is not a good indicator of acute changes in nutrition status. Prealbumin, which has a half-life of 2 days, is a better indicator of recent or current nutritional status. Serum transferrin level is another indicator of protein status. Transferrin, a protein synthesized by the liver and used to transport iron, decreases during states of protein deficiency. Serum electrolyte levels reflect changes taking place between the intracellular and the extracellular spaces. The serum potassium level is often elevated. The RBC count and the hemoglobin level will indicate the presence and degree of anemia. The total lymphocyte count decreases during malnutrition states. The total lymphocyte count is calculated by multiplying the percent of lymphocytes times total white blood cell (WBC) count.

Liver enzyme levels, a reflection of liver function, may be elevated during malnutrition. Serum levels of both fat-soluble

Table 38-12 Serum Albumin and Prealbumin Levels

Albumin	
Normal value	3.5-5.0 g/dl (35-50 g/L)
Mild depletion	3.0-3.4 g/dl (30-34 g/L)
Moderate depletion	2.5-2.9 g/dl (25-29 g/L)
Severe depletion	<2.5 g/dl (<25 g/L)
Prealbumin	
Normal value	20 mg/dl (200 mg/L)
Mild depletion	10-15 mg/dl (100-150 mg/L)
Moderate depletion	5-10 mg/dl (50-100 mg/L)
Severe depletion	<5 mg/dl (<50 mg/L)

and water-soluble vitamins are usually diminished in malnutrition. The lowered levels of the fat-soluble vitamins correlate with the clinical signs of steatorrhea (fatty stools).

Collaborative Care

The patient with PCM is often below the ideal on weight-for-height scales according to age and gender. Inspection of the unclothed body reveals loss of muscle mass, muscle wasting, and marked reduction in body fat. Diagnosis may be masked, however, when edema is present. The management of early uncomplicated PCM can be achieved without hospitalization by means of a diet high in calories and protein and by close supervision. Table 38-13 gives an example of a high-calorie, high-protein diet.

In severe PCM the patient may be hospitalized for correction of fluid and electrolyte imbalances and for treatment of infections secondary to a compromised immune system. Enteral feeding, both oral and tube feedings, can be used to provide total nutrition or to supplement calories and protein. In cases of severe PCM, total parenteral nutrition (TPN) may be initiated if enteral feedings are not feasible.

NURSING MANAGEMENT: MALNUTRITION

■ Nursing Assessment

Across all settings of care delivery, the nurse must be aware of the nutritional status of the patient. Nursing assessment of the patient with malnutrition is presented in Table 38-14. The recording of the patient's height and weight is an important component of this assessment. The patient's current weight relative to usual body weight and ideal body weight such as the Metropolitan Life Insurance tables (see Table 38-22 later in this chapter) are determined. The percent change in body weight over time provides information on the degree of weight loss. In addition, the nurse should get a record of the complete diet history from the patient or the family. The patient's nutritional state may not be the reason medical assistance was sought. However, it may well be a major factor in the outcome and perhaps may be the underlying reason for the patient's illness. A registered dietician should also be involved in the planning of care. However, the nurse, as the first health care professional dealing with the patient, should take the initiative in determining the seriousness of the nutritional problems.

The nurse should be aware that psychosocial problems have a direct effect on appetite. This is often overlooked as a cause of undernourishment. A diet history of foods eaten over the past week will reveal a great deal about the patient's dietary habits and knowledge of good nutrition. In addition to the height and weight and vital signs, the patient's physical state should be thoroughly assessed and documented. Each body system should be assessed. Table 38-15 summarizes conditions that can predispose persons to malnutrition.

Anthropometric measurements may be ordered. These measurements tend to be most beneficial in evaluating long-term effects of malnutrition or responses to nutritional interventions. Serial measures of skinfold thickness at various sites, an indicator of subcutaneous fat stores, and midarm muscle circumference, an indicator of protein stores, are compared with standards for healthy persons of the same age and gender. Training and practice are required to perform these measurements accurately and reliably. To provide information on the patient's nutritional status in response to treatment, serial measurements are needed. Sites most reflective of body fat are those over the biceps and the triceps, below the scapula, above the iliac crest, and the upper thigh. Both skinfold thickness and midarm muscle circumference measurements are decreased in chronic PCM and acute protein malnutrition. These measurements may also be influenced by shifts in hydration status. The exact relationship of the midarm circumference measure to body composition of functional protein, both muscle and non-muscle, remains to be established.

■ Nursing Diagnoses

Nursing diagnoses for the patient with malnutrition include, but are not limited to, the following:

- Altered nutrition: less than body requirements *related to* decreased access, ingestion, digestion, or absorption of food or to anorexia
- Self-care deficits *related to* decreased strength and endurance, fatigue, and apathy
- Constipation or diarrhea *related to* poor eating patterns, immobility, or medication effects
- Risk for fluid volume deficit *related to* factors affecting access to or absorption of fluids
- Risk for impaired skin integrity *related to* poor nutritional state
- Noncompliance *related to* alteration in perception, lack of motivation, or incompatibility of regimen with lifestyle or resources
- Activity intolerance *related to* weakness, fatigue, and inadequate caloric intake or iron stores

■ Planning

The overall goals are that the patient with malnutrition will (1) achieve weight gain, (2) consume a specified number of calories per day (with a diet individualized for the patient), and (3) have no adverse consequences related to malnutrition.

■ Nursing Implementation

Health Promotion. The nurse is in a good position to teach and reinforce healthy eating habits with individuals and groups of persons throughout their life span. In the 1990s the

NUTRITIONAL THERAPY

Table 38-13 High-Caloric, High-Protein Diet

General Principles

1. A normal diet is supplemented with larger portions to increase the protein and caloric content. It is used for patients with hypermetabolism, burns, excessive stress, and cancer.
2. It is important to eat regularly and not to skip meals or snacks.

Meal	Protein Content (g)	Sample Menu Plan 1	Sample Menu Plan 2	Sample Menu Plan 3
Breakfast				
Fruit	2	Large orange juice	Large apple juice	1/2 grapefruit
Starch, fat		1 toast with butter or jelly	Flour tortilla with butter	Biscuits and gravy
Starch, protein supplement	4	Cream of wheat with 2 tbs skim milk powder	Atole with 2 tbs skim milk powder	Grits with 2 tbs margarine
2 meat		2 poached eggs	2 fried eggs	Omelet with 2 eggs
Milk, protein supplement	14 10	High-protein milk shake (2 tbs skim milk powder added)	High-protein milk shake	High-protein milk shake
Lunch				
4 meat 4 starches Vegetable	28 8 2	Cheeseburger on bun with double meat patty, lettuce, tomato	2 burritos with extra cheese, meat Lettuce and tomato salad with dressing	Split pea soup with ham hocks Grilled cheese sandwich Watermelon wedge
4 fats	10	French fried potatoes	Biscochitos	Sugar cookies
Milk, protein supplement		High-protein milk shake	High-protein milk shake	High-protein milk shake
Dinner				
4 meat 3 starches	28 6	Spaghetti with 4 oz meat sauce, Parmesan cheese	2 tamales with red chili sauce	4 oz fried chicken Sweet potato
Vegetable	2	Green beans with 2 tbs margarine	Spanish rice Peas with 2 tbs butter	Mustard greens with 2 tbs butter
7 fats		Bread with butter Tapioca pudding	Custard	Biscuit Vanilla ice cream
Milk, protein supplement	10	High-protein milk shake	High-protein milk shake	High-protein milk shake
Snack				
Milk Fruit	8	Fruit yogurt	Cottage cheese with fruit	1/2 sandwich with peanut butter Banana
	Total 132			

gap between perceived importance of nutrition and care in selecting foods has widened.[8] To assist in these efforts are the mandatory food labels that are now on all packaged food. These provide more useful and accurate nutritional information than labeling before 1994. The latest *Surgeon General's Report on Nutrition and Health* offers key recommendations for improving nutrition that are useful points for a teaching program.[9] The following recommendations are applicable to most people:

1. Reduce consumption of fat and cholesterol
2. Achieve and maintain a desirable weight
3. Increase energy expenditure through regular and sustained physical activity
4. Increase consumption of whole grain foods and cereal products, vegetables, and fruits
5. Reduce intake of sodium
6. Take alcohol only in moderation, if at all

Acute Intervention. The nurse must assess the patient's nutritional state, as well as focus on the other physical problems of the patient. The incidence of nutritional deficiency, especially PCM, is high in hospitalized patients. A number of nutritional studies have indicated that PCM may develop in as many as 50% of medical and surgical patients.[10] As a direct consequence of these findings, the nurse must become more aware of who is at risk, why, and how to intervene appropriately. In states of increased stress, such as surgery, severe trauma, and sepsis, more calories and protein are required. Wound healing requires increased protein synthesis. In cases of cancer, there may be additional demands made by tumor growth at the same time that appetite is reduced. When fever is present, the metabolic rate is increased and nitrogen loss is accelerated. Despite the return of body temperature to normal, the rate of protein breakdown and resynthesis may be accelerated for several weeks. After major surgery several weeks of

NURSING ASSESSMENT

Table 38-14 Malnutrition

Subjective Data

Important Health Information

Past health history: Severe burns, major trauma, hemorrhage, draining wounds, bone fractures with prolonged immobility, chronic renal or liver disease, cancer, malabsorption syndrome, GI obstruction, infectious diseases (TB, AIDS)

Medications: Corticosteroids, chemotherapeutic agents, diet pills

Surgery or other treatments: Recent surgery, radiation

Functional Health Patterns

Health perception–health management: Alcohol or drug abuse; malaise, apathy

Nutritional-metabolic: Increase or decrease in weight, weight problems; increase or decrease in appetite, typical dietary intake; food preferences and aversions; food allergies or intolerance; ill-fitting or absent dentures; dry mouth, difficulty in chewing or swallowing; bloating or gas; increased sensitivity to cold; delayed wound healing

Elimination: Constipation; diarrhea; nocturia, decreased urinary output

Activity-exercise: Increase or decrease in activity patterns; weakness, fatigue, decreased endurance

Cognitive-perceptual: Pain in mouth; paresthesias; loss of position and vibratory sense

Role-relationship: Change in family (e.g., loss of a spouse); financial resources

Sexual-reproductive: Amenorrhea, impotence, decreased libido

Objective Data

General

Listless; cachectic; underweight for height

Integumentary

Dry, brittle, sparse hair with color changes and lack of luster, alopecia; dry, scaly lips, fever blisters, angular crusts and lesions at corners of mouth (cheilosis); brittle, ridged nails; decreased tone and elasticity of skin; cool, rough, dry, scaly skin with brown-gray pigment changes; reddened, scaly dermatitis, scrotal dermatitis; slight cyanosis; peripheral edema

Eyes

Pale or red conjunctivae, gray keratinized epithelium on conjunctiva (Bitot's spots); dryness and dull appearance of conjunctiva and cornea, soft cornea; blood vessel growth in cornea; redness and fissuring of eyelid corners

Respiratory

Decreased respiratory rate, decreased vital capacity, crackles, weak cough

Cardiovascular

Increase or decrease in heart rate, decreased blood pressure, arrhythmias

Gastrointestinal

Swollen, smooth, raw, beefy red tongue (glossitis), hypertrophic or atrophic papillae; dental caries, absent or loose teeth, discolored tooth enamel; spongy, pale, receded gums with a tendency to bleed easily, periodontal disease; ulcerations, white patches or plaques, redness, swelling of oral mucosa; distended, tympanic abdomen, ascites, hepatomegaly, decreased bowel sounds; steatorrhea

Neurologic

Decreased or loss of reflexes, tremor; inattention, irritability, confusion, syncope

Musculoskeletal

Decreased muscle mass with poor tone, "wasted" appearance; bowlegs, knock-knees, beaded ribs, chest deformity, prominent bony structures

Possible Findings

Decreased hemoglobin and hematocrit; decreased MCV, MCH, or MCHC (iron deficiency); increased MCV or MCHC (folic acid or cobalamin deficiency); altered serum electrolyte levels, especially hyperkalemia; decreased BUN and creatinine; decreased serum albumin, transferrin, and prealbumin; decreased lymphocytes; increased liver enzymes; decreased serum vitamin levels

AIDS, acquired immunodeficiency syndrome; *MCH,* mean corpuscular hemoglobin; *MCHC,* mean corpuscular hemoglobin concentration; *MCV,* mean corpuscular volume; *TB,* tuberculosis.

Table 38-15 Conditions That Increase the Risk for Malnutrition

- Chronic alcoholism
- Drugs with antinutrient or catabolic properties, such as corticosteroids and oral antibiotics
- Gross underweight or overweight with recent weight loss exceeding 5% of usual body weight or 10 lb (4.5 kg) per month for several months
- No oral intake or receiving standard intravenous solutions (5% dextrose) for 10 days or in older adults for 5 days
- Extreme need for nutrients because of hypermetabolism or stresses such as infection, burns, trauma, or fever
- Nutrient losses from malabsorption, dialysis, fistulas, or wounds
- Decreased mobility that limits access to food and its preparation

Table 38-16 Commonly Used Elemental Diets

Product	Protein (g/L)	Carbohydrates (% total kcal)	Lipids (% total kcal)	Protein (% total kcal)	kcal/ml	Osmolarity (mOsm/kg)
Criticare HN	38.0	81.5	4.5	14.0	1.1	650
Reabilan	31.5	52.5	35.0	12.5	1.0	350
Reabilan HN	58.5	47.5	35.0	17.5	1.3	490
Tolerex	21.0	91.0	1.0	8.0	1.0	550
Vital HN	41.7	73.6	9.7	16.7	1.0	500
Vivonex TEN	38.0	82.0	3.0	15.0	1.0	630
Peptamen	40.0	51.0	33.0	16.0	1.0	270
Crucial	93.8	36.0	39.0	25.0	1.5	490

increased protein and calorie intake are needed to promote healing and replenish body stores.

The nurse must have a thorough understanding of nutritional support and the rationale for recording the daily weight, intake, and output. Daily weights can give an ongoing record of body weight gain or loss. However, rapid gains and losses are usually the result of shifts in fluid balance. The body weight, in conjunction with accurate recording of food and fluid intake, provides a clearer picture of the patient's fluid and nutritional state. To obtain an accurate weight, the nurse should weigh the patient at the same time each day, on the same scale, with the same type or amount of clothing, and preferably with the bladder recently emptied.

The protein and calorie intake required in the malnourished patient depends on the cause of the malnutrition, the treatment being employed, and other stressors affecting the patient. If the patient is able to take food by mouth, a daily calorie count and diet diary can be obtained to give an accurate record of food intake.

The nurse and the dietician working with the patient and family can assist in the selection of high-caloric and high-protein foods (unless medically contraindicated). Preparation of foods preferred by the patient enhances the daily intake. Discussion with the patient and family about foods that should be eaten to provide high-protein, high-calorie content is important. The family can be encouraged to bring the patient's favorite foods from home while the patient is still hospitalized.

The undernourished patient usually receives between-meal supplements. These may consist of items prepared in the dietary department or commercially prepared products. Eating these items between meals increases the total daily intake and provides extra calories, proteins, fluids, and nutrients. In addition, multiple small feedings improve the tolerance for food intake by distributing the amount more evenly throughout the day.

Elemental diets are chemically defined, nutritionally sound diets that contain glucose, glucose derivatives, dextrin, amino acids, peptides, essential fatty acids, vitamins, and minerals. They are lactose free and easily absorbed in the small intestine. The nurse should be familiar with the commercial products being used in the particular setting, their ingredients, and whether the products can be used as complete meal replacements or only as dietary supplements. (See Table 38-16 for information about sample elemental formulas.) Disease-specific elemental formulas are also available for special patient groups (e.g., Amin-Aid for patients with renal failure).

Ambulatory and Home Care. With shortened hospital stays, many patients are discharged home on a therapeutic diet. Discharge preparation for both the patient and the family is important. They must be carefully instructed on the cause of the undernourished state and ways to avoid the problem in the future. The patient must be made aware that undernourishment, whatever the cause, can recur and that adhering to a diet high in protein and calories for a few weeks cannot restore a normal nutritional state. Many months are needed to reach this goal. Diet instruction is usually carried out by the dietician, but it is important for the nurse to assess the patient's understanding and reinforce the information whenever possible. The patient's ability to comply with the dietary instructions must be examined in light of past eating habits, religious and ethnic preferences, age, income, other resources, and state of health.

Unless the patient and the family can be convinced of the necessity for dietary change and have the resources to effect change, it is likely that no long-term benefits will be achieved. Ways should be found in which the patient can become involved in the recovery. The need for continuous follow-up care must be strongly emphasized if rehabilitation is to be accomplished and maintained.

The nurse is in an ideal position to determine the need for nutritious meals and snacks after discharge from the hospital. In addition, it is important to consider the availability and acceptability of nutritionally based community resources. Such aspects can be integrated into discharge planning and follow-up home visits by the nurse.

Keeping a diet diary or a calorie count for 3 days at a time is one way to analyze and reinforce healthful eating patterns. These records are also helpful to the health care team in the follow-up care. Self-assessment of progress can be encouraged by having the patient weighed once or twice a week and keeping a weight record.

Evaluation

The expected outcomes are that the patient who is malnourished will

- achieve and maintain body weight
- consume a well-balanced diet
- experience no adverse outcomes related to malnutrition

GERONTOLOGIC CONSIDERATIONS

Malnutrition

The eating patterns established in youth and earlier years usually extend into old age. However, adjustments in the type of food ingested may be made as adaptations to age-related physiologic changes. These changes can result either in obesity or loss of weight depending on individual circumstances.

Some of the physiologic changes associated with aging affect the nutritional status of older adults. The following changes are of particular interest:

1. Changes in the oral cavity (e.g., change in bite surfaces of the teeth, periodontal disease, drying of the mucous membrane of the mouth and tongue, poorly fitting dentures, decreased muscle strength for chewing, decreased number of taste buds, decreased saliva production)
2. Changes in digestion and motility (e.g., decreased absorption of cobalamin, vitamin A, and folic acid and decreased GI motility)
3. Changes in the endocrine system (e.g., decreased tolerance to glucose)
4. Changes in the musculoskeletal system (e.g., decreased bone density, degenerative joint changes)
5. Decrease in vision and hearing (e.g., procurement and preparation of food are more difficult)

Certain illnesses that are more prevalent in the older population are considered to be diet related. These include atherosclerosis, osteoporosis, diabetes mellitus, and diverticulosis. The need to treat these and other common chronic illnesses of the older patient often requires the use of multiple medications. These medications often have an adverse effect on the appetite of older adults, increasing the possibility of inadequate intake caused by anorexia.

To date, with the exception of calories, it has not been determined that older adults have requirements for specific nutrients that are different from those of middle-aged adults. Caloric intake should be decreased with age because there is a progressive loss of lean body mass and a decrease in basal metabolic rate. Therefore fewer calories are needed to meet nutritional needs. Unless caloric intake is decreased by careful attention to food intake, or energy expenditure is increased through greater physical activity and exercise, obesity will result.

Socioeconomic factors are important variables when assessing the nutritional status of an older adult. Because more than one third of older adults have incomes below the poverty level, it would follow that obtaining adequate and nutritious food can be an ongoing problem. In many cases the older person cannot afford to purchase meat, fresh vegetables, and fruits that provide many necessary nutrients.

Lifestyle changes such as relocation to a nursing home or retirement can have a significant impact on the eating habits of the older adult. Other important considerations that should be assessed when evaluating the nutritional status of an older adult include the ethnic background, previous dietary practices, food preferences, knowledge of proper diet, availability and accessibility of food stores, transportation, and health status. Problems related to any or all of these areas can alert the nurse to the possibility of a nutritional problem.

Malnutrition can occur in an older person even though the caloric requirements decrease with age. If malnutrition is present, few malnourished older persons are able to ingest enough food to correct the malnourished state. Special strategies, such as adaptive devices (e.g., large-handled eating utensils), often are helpful in increasing dietary intake. Some older persons may require nutritional support therapies until their strength and general health are improved.

Many community nutritional programs are available to the older person to make mealtime a pleasant, social event. Improving the social setting of a meal often improves the dietary intake. Home-delivered meals and meal sites in a central location are popular meal alternatives for many older adults. The use of food stamps is another alternative that allows low-income households, regardless of age, to buy more food of a greater variety.

TYPES OF SUPPLEMENTAL NUTRITION

ORAL FEEDING

High-calorie supplemental oral feedings may be used in the patient whose nutritional intake is deficient. This may include dietary items such as milk shakes, puddings, eggnogs, or commercially available products (e.g., Ensure, Sustacal, NuBasics).

TUBE FEEDING

Tube feedings may be ordered for the patient who has a functioning GI tract but is unable to take oral nourishment. Indications for tube feeding, besides PCM, may include those persons with anorexia, orofacial fractures, head and neck cancer, neurologic or psychiatric conditions that prevent oral intake, extensive burns, and those who are receiving chemotherapy or radiation therapy. Tube feedings are easily administered, safer, more physiologically efficient, and less expensive than parenteral nutrition. They are used to provide nutrients by way of the GI tract (alone or as a supplement to oral or parenteral nutrition) or as a treatment for malnutrition.

Common delivery options are continuous infusion by pump, intermittent by gravity, intermittent bolus by syringe, and cyclic intermittent by infusion pump.[11] Continuous infusion is most often used with critically ill patients and feedings into the small intestine. Intermittent feeding may be preferred as the patient improves or is receiving such feedings at home.

A nasogastric (NG) tube is most commonly used for short-term feeding problems. If the feedings are necessary for an extended time, other means of feeding may be used, such as an esophagostomy tube, a gastrostomy tube (placed surgically, endoscopically, or percutaneously), or a jejunostomy tube that empties directly into the jejunum. Transpyloric (nasointestinal) tube placement or placement into the jejunum is used when physiologic conditions warrant feeding the patient below the pyloric sphincter. (Figure 38-2 shows the locations of commonly used enteral feeding tubes.)

Nasogastric and Nasointestinal Tubes

Feeding tubes made of polyurethane or silicone materials have added to the comfort level of the patient in tolerating extended periods of feeding. These tubes are long, small in diameter, soft, and flexible, thereby decreasing the risk of mucosal damage from prolonged placement. The older tubes made of rubber or polyvinyl chloride tend to stiffen with time. Polyurethane and

RESEARCH
IMPLICATIONS FOR NURSING PRACTICE

Feeding Tube Location

Citation Metheny NA and others: pH and concentrations of pepsin and trypsin in feeding tube aspirates as predictors of tube placement, *J Parenter Enteral Nutr* 21:279, 1997.

Purpose To determine the extent to which the concentrations of pepsin and trypsin, as well as pH in feeding tube aspirates, predict tube position.

Methods Feeding tube aspirates from 742 feeding tubes (343 nasogastric; 399 nasointestinal) and 146 samples of tracheobronchial and pleural fluids were tested for pH and enzyme concentrations. Tube position was verified by x-ray visualization.

Results and Conclusions As expected, the stomach had a low pH and high pepsin and low trypsin contents. In contrast the intestine had a high pH and low pepsin and high trypsin contents. Respiratory fluids had a high pH and contained little pepsin or trypsin. Using a logistic regression model with pH, trypsin, and pepsin levels, the investigators were able to correctly identify 100% of the respiratory aspirates and 91% of the gastric and intestinal placements.

Implications for Nursing Practice Correct placement of a feeding tube before initiating enteral feeding is extremely important. Although x-ray verification is considered the "gold standard," the development of a bedside monitoring system is both clinically important and cost-effective. Further refinement of bedside tools such as enzyme level determinations may provide a useful and practical clinical tool.

silicone tubes are radiopaque, making their position readily identified by x-ray. Many of these tubes also have weighted tips, allowing for easier passage of the tube through the pylorus into the duodenum. Placement into the intestine decreases the likelihood of regurgitation of contents into the esophagus and subsequent aspiration. With the use of a stylet these tubes can be placed in an uncooperative or comatose patient because the ability to swallow is not essential during insertion.

Although the smaller feeding tubes have many advantages over wider-lumen tubes, such as the Levine tube, there are some disadvantages that the nurse must keep in mind. Because of the small diameter, these tubes are more easily clogged when feedings are thick and are more difficult to use for checking residual volumes. They are particularly prone to obstruction when oral medications have not been thoroughly crushed and dissolved in water before administration. They can become dislodged by vomiting or coughing and can also become knotted or kinked in the GI tract. Failure to flush the tubing after both medication administration and residual volume determinations can result in tube clogging. When the tube becomes clogged, it may necessitate removal and insertion of a new tube, adding to cost and patient discomfort.

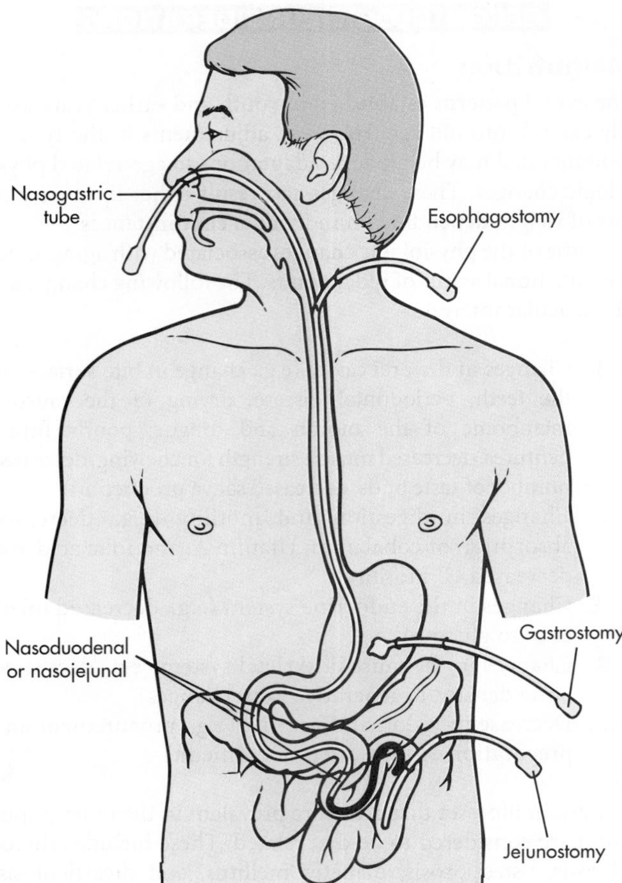

Fig. 38-2 Common enteral feeding tube placement locations.

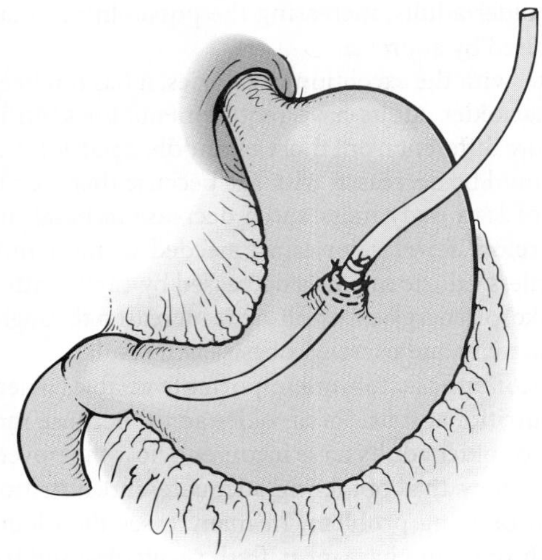

Fig. 38-3 Placement of a gastrostomy tube.

Gastrostomy and Jejunostomy

A permanent gastrostomy, such as a Janeway gastrostomy, may be used for a patient who requires tube feedings over an extended time (Figs. 38-3 and 38-4). A tunnel of gastric tissue is formed and brought out to form a stoma at the skin surface. A small catheter (5F to 10F) is inserted at the skin surface. The

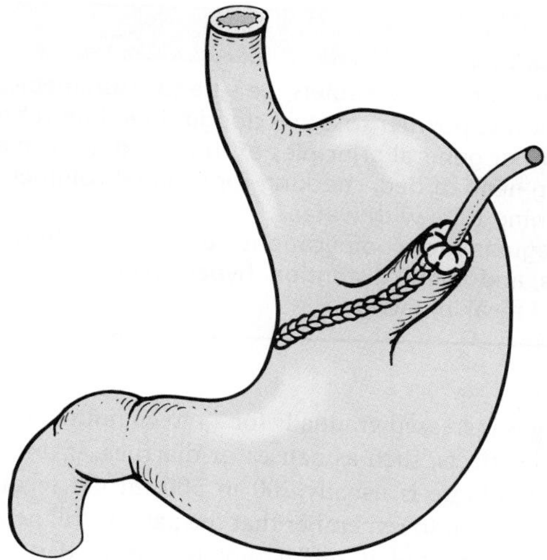

Fig. 38-4 Janeway gastrostomy.

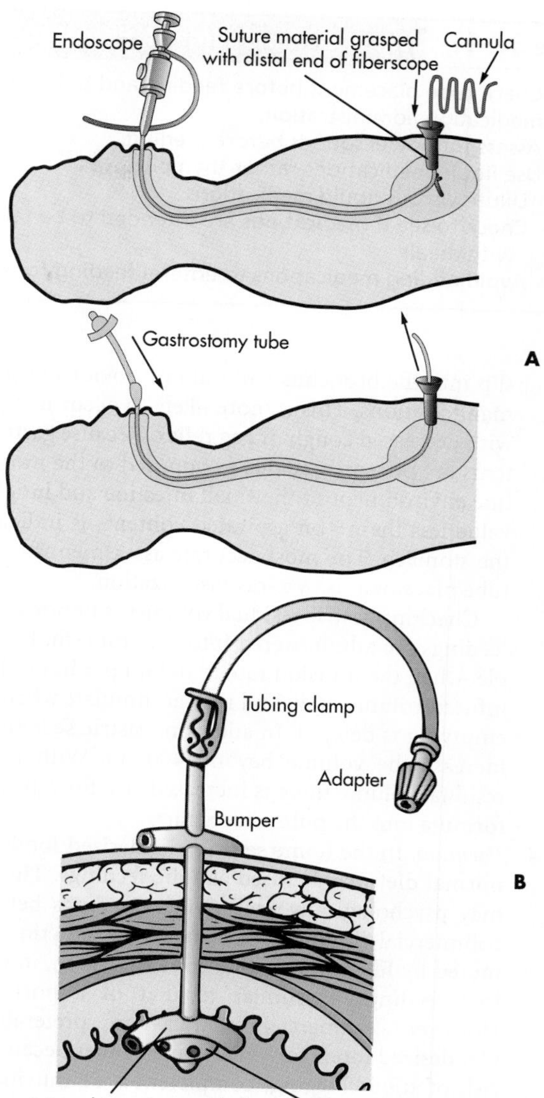

Fig. 38-5 Percutaneous endoscopic gastrostomy. **A,** Gastrostomy tube placement via percutaneous endoscopy. Using endoscopy, a gastrostomy tube is inserted through the esophagus into the stomach and then pulled through a stab wound made in the abdominal wall. **B,** A retention disk and bumper secure the tube.

stoma closes when the catheter is removed. Problems of leakage and skin irritation are decreased or eliminated.[12]

A gastrostomy tube may be placed by means of percutaneous endoscopic gastrostomy (PEG) (Fig. 38-5). The patient must have an intact, unobstructed GI tract, and the esophageal lumen must be wide enough to pass the endoscope. A PEG has several advantages. The procedure itself has fewer risks (no general anesthesia or laparotomy), it can be done at a lower cost, and it requires minimum or no sedation of the patient who is severely compromised. The most common complications of gastrostomy feedings include aspiration, pneumonia, accidental tube removal, wound cellulitis, and clogged tubes.[12]

Feedings can usually be started when bowel sounds are present, usually within 24 hours after catheter placement. Immediately after tube insertion, the tube length from the insertion site to the distal end should be measured and recorded. The tube is then marked at the skin insertion site.[12] At regular intervals the tube insertion length should be rechecked. The catheter is frequently connected to a pump for continuous feeding. Tap water may be infused within 2 hours after placement. For the patient with chronic reflux, a jejunostomy tube with jejunostomy feedings may be necessary to reduce reflux. Some important nursing implications for care and feeding of patients with PEGs are listed in Table 38-17.

Procedures for Tube Feedings

The procedure for the administration of tube feeding through an NG tube is standard. The following principles apply:

1. *Patient position.* The patient should be sitting or lying with the head of the bed elevated 30 to 45 degrees to prevent aspiration. If intermittent delivery, the head should remain elevated for 30 to 60 minutes after feeding.
2. *Patency of tube.* If feedings are intermittent, the tube should be irrigated with water before and after each feeding to ensure that the tube is patent and to prevent blockage of the tube. If the feedings are continuous, they should be administered by using an electric or a battery-operated feeding pump with a built-in alarm that will sound if the tubing becomes occluded. If no pump is available, the feedings require frequent monitoring of the drip rate so that blockage does not occur from the patient lying on the tubing inadvertently or from too slow a drip rate.
3. *Tube position.* Proper placement of the tube in the stomach should be checked before each feeding or every 4 hours with continuous feedings. Methods used to check for tube placement can include aspiration of stomach contents and checking the pH of contents using a pH meter or pH paper. Two advantages of a pH meter over pH paper are that neither the formula nor the added food coloring affect the pH meter results, and the smaller feeding tubes may be passed directly into the bronchus on insertion or may become dislodged and

Table 38-17 Nursing Management: Percutaneous Endoscopic Gastrostomy

- Check tube placement before feeding and before each medication administration.
- Assess for bowel sounds before feeding.
- Use liquid medications rather than pills.
  Dilute viscous liquid medications.
  Check to see if medications are intended to be taken with meals.
  Avoid adding medications to enteral feeding formula.
- If it is necessary to use tablets, be sure to crush medications to a fine powder to avoid clogging feeding tubes.
- Follow other general principles of tube feeding such as elevating head of bed, checking for residual volumes, and flushing tube with water.
- Assess regularly for complications, such as aspiration, diarrhea, abdominal distention, hyperglycemia, constipation, and fecal impaction.

slip into the bronchus without any obvious respiratory manifestations. This is more likely to occur in a patient with decreased cough or gag reflex. Because gastric contents are primarily acidic, as opposed to the more alkaline environment of the small intestine and lungs, a pH value less than 5 on aspirated contents is indicative of the stomach. The most accurate assessment for correct tube placement is by x-ray visualization.

Checking gastric residual volumes is important when feedings are administered into the stomach. For example, when the infusion rate is 100 ml per hour, the total infused volume of 400 ml may accumulate when gastric emptying is delayed. In addition, gastric secretions can increase the volume beyond 400 ml. With increased residual volume there is increased risk for aspiration of formula into the pulmonary tract.

4. *Formula.* In the home setting blenderized foods from a normal diet may be used as tube feedings. The patient may psychologically accept these feedings better than commercial products. Normal bowel function is promoted by fiber and residue content, which, in blenderized feedings, is similar to that of a normal diet. However, commercial formulas are preferable over blenderized foods for small-lumen tubes because of the risk of tube clogging, completeness of nutrition, and decreased risk of formula contamination.

   The feeding should be given at room or body temperature to decrease the likelihood of diarrhea and other GI complaints. The pleasurable aspects of eating, such as smelling, seeing, tasting, and chewing the food, are frequently denied the tube-fed patient. If clinical condition permits, the patient may be allowed to smell, taste, and even chew small amounts of food before the feeding, and then the chewed food must be spit out. The patient may hesitate to do this because it is not esthetic, but it stimulates salivary and gastric secretions and provides the pleasurable sensations associated with oral intake. Before initiating the feeding, the nurse should aspirate gastric contents and measure the amount. If greater than 100 ml and there are clinical signs of intolerance, including report of nausea or increase in abdominal girth, the next feeding is held for 1 hour and then the residual volume is rechecked. The aspirate should be reinstilled.

5. *Administration of feeding.* Feedings are administered either by gravity drip method or by feeding pump. Applying pressure to force the feeding can damage the gastric mucosa. If the feedings have been refrigerated, they should be warmed to room temperature. The feeding is increased gradually for 24 to 48 hours to minimize side effects, such as nausea or diarrhea. If intermittent, the volume is usually 200 to 500 ml per feeding. It is important to remember that the patient still needs water replacement of 30 ml/kg body weight per day.

6. *General nursing considerations.* The patient should be weighed daily or several times a week, and accurate intake and output records should be maintained. These measures provide information on weight gain or loss, as well as tolerance of the feedings. Initially blood glucose checks to assess glucose tolerance are performed at the bedside. An older patient who has glucose intolerance is particularly vulnerable. Feedings that have been opened and not refrigerated or feedings that have been infusing longer than 8 hours should be discarded to minimize bacterial growth and to prevent the administration of contaminated feeding. Feedings should, therefore, be labeled with the date and time they are initially used. If a pump is used, pump tubing should be changed every 24 hours or per manufacturer's guideline. See NCP 38-1 for care of the patient receiving enteral nutrition.

Complications Related to Tubes and Feedings

The types of problems encountered in patients receiving tube feedings and corrective measures are presented in Table 38-18.

When commercial products are used, the concentration, taste, osmolarity, and amounts of protein, sodium, and fat vary according to the manufacturer. Most if not all commercial formulas are lactose free. The concentrations range from 0.5 to 2.0 kcal/ml, with most between 1.0 and 1.5 kcal/ml. A limited number of flavors are available, and the overuse of one or two flavors, even in tube feedings, can lead to dislike and less tolerance with time.

The osmolality of the solution is determined by the number and size of particles in solution. With regard to feeding formulas, the more hydrolyzed the nutrients, the greater the osmolality. Many tube feeding formulas are isotonic, although some are hypertonic. The more calorically dense the formula, the less water it contains. Protein content greater than 16% can lead to dehydration unless the patient is given supplemental fluids or is sufficiently alert to request additional fluids. The nurse must be aware of this potential problem and must provide extra fluids through the feeding tube or, if permitted, by mouth. Tube feedings with high sodium content are contraindicated in the patient with cardiovascular problems, such as congestive heart failure. High fat content is not advocated for a patient suffering from short bowel syndrome or ileocecal resections because of impaired fat absorption.

38-1 NURSING CARE PLAN PATIENT RECEIVING ENTERAL NUTRITION

NURSING DIAGNOSIS **Altered nutrition: less than body requirements** *related to* enteral feeding problems *as manifested by* body weight ≤10% less than ideal, diarrhea, abdominal distention.

Expected Patient Outcomes	Nursing Interventions and *Rationales*
▪ Stable or gain in weight. ▪ No diarrhea or abdominal distention.	▪ Monitor weight and compare with baseline *to make adjustments as needed in calorie intake.* ▪ Progress the patient slowly from clear liquids to blenderized foods that are added to clear liquids *to prevent gastric distention.* ▪ Gradually add high-calorie foods to patient's blenderized foods *to maintain body weight while preventing distention.*

NURSING DIAGNOSIS **Impaired skin integrity** *related to* enzymatic action of gastric juices, which may leak around tube *as manifested by* red, irritated tissue around the tube.

Expected Patient Outcomes	Nursing Interventions and *Rationales*
▪ No skin breakdown around gastrostomy tube. ▪ Daily inspections of skin performed and problems reported.	▪ Assess skin daily for signs of irritation or redness *so that early treatment is provided.* ▪ Wash skin around the tube with soap and water daily; apply a protective skin barrier such as zinc oxide or petrolatum or a Stomahesive wafer *to maintain skin integrity.* ▪ Teach patient and family to assess and provide care *to ensure involvement in self-care and early detection of problems.*

NURSING DIAGNOSIS **Body image disturbance** *related to* presence of feeding tube *as manifested by* refusal to participate in own feeding, verbalization of fear of rejection by family and friends, avoidance of any social activities associated with food and eating.

Expected Patient Outcomes	Nursing Interventions and *Rationales*
▪ Participation in self-care related to feedings. ▪ Verbalization of acceptance of enteral feeding. ▪ Support systems established.	▪ Encourage patient to express feelings about the enteral feedings *to increase the patient's self-awareness.* ▪ Provide information about the tube, feedings, purpose, and patient progress *so that the patient makes decisions based on correct information.* ▪ Acknowledge the patient's fears *to establish a trusting nurse-patient relationship.* ▪ Incorporate the patient in care of operative site; gradually encourage patient to assume full self-care responsibility *to promote positive coping with the change.*

NURSING DIAGNOSIS **Risk for fluid volume deficit** *related to* diarrhea or inadequate fluid intake.

Expected Patient Outcomes	Nursing Interventions and *Rationales*
▪ No signs of fluid volume deficit. ▪ Adequate fluid intake.	▪ Monitor patient for poor skin turgor, decreased blood pressure, tachycardia, decreased urine output, and dry mucous membranes *to identify signs of fluid volume deficit.* ▪ Provide adequate fluid intake, including water, as determined by intake records. ▪ Monitor urine output for osmotic diuresis, *which may occur secondary to high glucose load of feedings or too rapid infusion.* ▪ Identify possible cause of diarrhea *so that appropriate treatment is started.*

NURSING DIAGNOSIS **Ineffective management of therapeutic regimen** *related to* care required for skin around tubing and tube feedings *as manifested by* questioning about self-care.

Expected Patient Outcomes	Nursing Interventions and *Rationales*
▪ Demonstration of skin care and tube feeding before discharge.	▪ Assess the patient's home environment and lifestyle *to make teaching relevant to individual requirements.* ▪ Provide detailed information about how to prepare the formula and manage the tube feeding *to facilitate self-care.* ▪ Use return demonstration technique *to validate patient's and family's learning of the necessary skills.*

NURSING DIAGNOSIS **Risk for aspiration** *related to* enteral tube with tube feedings.

Expected Patient Outcomes	Nursing Interventions and *Rationales*
▪ No aspiration. ▪ Able to describe measures to prevent aspiration.	▪ During feeding have the patient's head elevated at least 30 degrees; remain in this position 30 minutes after feeding *to prevent aspiration.* ▪ Aspirate gastric contents before feeding *to validate gastric emptying.* ▪ Reinstill the residual gastric contents *to prevent excessive fluid and electrolyte losses.*

Table 38-18 Common Problems of Patients Receiving Tube Feedings

Problems and Possible Causes	Corrective Measures
Vomiting or Aspiration	
Improper placement of tube	Replace tube in proper position. Check tube position before beginning feeding and every 4 hr if continuous feedings.
Delayed gastric emptying, increased residual volume	Hold feeding 1 hr; then, if residual volume is less than previous rate, resume feeding.
Potential for aspiration	Keep head of bed elevated to 30° to 45° angle. Have patient lie on right side for ½ hr after feeding. Have patient sit up on side of bed or in chair. Encourage ambulation unless contraindicated.
Contamination of formula	Refrigerate unused formula and record date opened. Discard outdated formula every 24 hr. Discard formula left standing for longer than manufacturer's guidelines: 8-12 hr for ready-to-feed formulas (cans), or 4 hr for reconstituted formula. Use closed system to prevent contamination.
Air in stomach	Clear tubing of air before feeding. Keep tube feeding container filled so air does not enter through feeding set.
Diarrhea	
Feeding too fast, hypertonic formula	Decrease rate of feeding. Change to continuous-drip feedings. Check for drugs that may cause diarrhea (e.g., antibiotics, sorbitol).
Lactose intolerance	Consult physician for change in formula to lactose-free solution.
Contamination of formula or tubing	Change tubing every 24 hr. Hang 8 hr formula at a time. Do not exceed manufacturer's guidelines.
Low-fiber formula	Change to formula with more fiber.
Tube moving distally	Properly secure tube before beginning to feed. Check before each feeding or at least every 24 hr if receiving continuous feedings.
Constipation	
Formula components	Consult physician for change in formula to one with more fiber content. Obtain laxative order.
Poor fluid intake	Increase fluid intake if not contraindicated. Give free water as well as formula. Total fluid 30 ml/kg body weight.
Drugs	Check for drugs that may be constipating.
Impaction	Rectal examination to check and manually remove feces if present.
Dehydration	
Excessive diarrhea, vomiting	Decrease rate or change formula. Check drugs patient is receiving, especially antibiotics. Take care to prevent bacterial contamination of formula and equipment.
Poor fluid intake	Increase intake and check amount and number of feedings. Increase amount of intake if appropriate.
High-protein formula	Change formula
Hyperosmotic diuresis	Frequent blood glucose checks. Change formula.

The registered dietician can be of considerable assistance to the nursing staff. When close consultation with the nursing staff occurs, existing problems with tube feedings can be quickly and efficiently addressed and resolved. Some institutions have nutrition support teams composed of a physician, nurse, dietician, and pharmacist whose function is to oversee the nutrition support of select inpatients and outpatients.

In patients receiving gastrostomy feeding, the nurse is alert to two possible problems: (1) skin irritation and (2) pulling out of the tube. Skin care around the gastrostomy opening is important because the action of the gastric juice is irritating to the skin. The skin around the gastrostomy should be assessed daily for signs of redness and maceration. To keep the skin clean and dry, initially it should be rinsed with sterile water and dried. Once the site has healed, it can be washed with mild soap and water. A protective ointment (zinc oxide, petroleum gauze) or a skin barrier (karaya, Stomahesive) may be used on the skin around the gastrostomy. A small dressing may be placed around the tube until the site is healed. It must be changed promptly if it gets wet. Other types of drain or tube pouches may be used if there is a problem with skin irritation. The patient and family members can be taught how to care for the gastrostomy. Teaching should include skin care, care of the tube, and complete information about feedings.

GERONTOLOGIC CONSIDERATIONS

Enteral Nutrition

Enteral nutrition strategies, including nasogastric, nasointestinal, and gastrostomy feedings, are frequently used in the older patient to improve nutritional status. Because of physiologic changes associated with aging, the older adult is more vulnerable to complications associated with these interventions, especially fluid and electrolyte imbalances. Complications such as diarrhea can leave the patient dehydrated and saline depleted. Decreased thirst perception or impaired cognitive function de-

ETHICAL DILEMMAS

Withholding Treatment

SITUATION

A 26-year-old patient in a permanent vegetative state is diagnosed with her fifteenth bladder infection. Her home care nurse must determine whether or not to seek antibiotics for this infection. The family members have expressed a concern that no *heroic* measures be used to extend the biologic life of their daughter and sister, but they have been unwilling to withdraw the existing treatment, which is enteral nutrition. Should antibiotics be withheld?

DISCUSSION

The questions that arise when discussing heroic measures are of degree and intent. Is the intent not to prolong the patient's life or not to extend any suffering that the patient might experience? Does antibiotic treatment constitute treatment above and beyond the normal care of the patient, or is it simply appropriate treatment of a manageable condition? The family's resistance to the withdrawal of enteral nutrition may stem from discomfort and revulsion about starving the patient to death, or from strong beliefs about the importance of maintaining her biologic existence. The nurse must clarify what the patient's wishes were, if they are known. The family's values and their concerns about the patient, especially about her ability to feel pain or discomfort and about her quality of life, also should be discussed.

ETHICAL AND LEGAL PRINCIPLES

- Medical treatment may be withheld if a competent patient refuses to consent to it, if it is medically futile treatment, or if the burden of its provision outweighs its benefit.
- If withholding treatment or support leads to death, the underlying disease or condition is the cause. Technologic intervention simply prolongs life.
- Patients in a permanent vegetative state cannot be cured of that brain damage. Any treatable comorbidities related to this condition will not lead to a recovery from the permanent vegetative state.

creases the ability of the patient to seek additional fluids. With aging there is decreased ability to handle glucose loads (glucose intolerance). As a result, the older patient may be more susceptible to problems of hyperglycemia in response to the high carbohydrate load of some enteral feeding formulas. If the older adult has compromised cardiovascular function (e.g., congestive heart failure) there will be a decreased ability to handle large volumes of formula, in which case the use of more concentrated formulas may be warranted. The older adult also is at increased risk for aspiration caused by gastroesophageal reflux disease, hiatal hernia, or diminished gag reflex. Physical mobility, fine motor movement, and visual system changes associated with aging may contribute to difficulties in managing enteral nutrition equipment at home. In addition, age-related changes such as a decrease in lean muscle mass influence the reliability of measures used for nutritional assessment.

RESEARCH

IMPLICATIONS FOR NURSING PRACTICE

Fiber and Tube Feeding

Citation Bass DJ, Forman LP, Abrams SE, Hsueh AM: The effect of dietary fiber in tube-fed elderly patients, *J Gerontol Nurs* 22:37, 1996.

Purpose To describe the pattern of stools in patients receiving tube feeding with or without fiber-containing formula.

Methods Retrospective chart review of 50 (29 males and 21 females) tube-fed long-term care patients. The number and consistency of each bowel movement were recorded. Antibiotic use was monitored.

Results and Conclusions Patients on fiber-containing formula had a lower frequency of liquid or loose stools and a higher frequency of formed stools as compared with those on the fiber-free formula. There was no correlation between stool characteristics and antibiotic use.

Implications for Nursing Practice Patients receiving long-term tube feedings may be at risk for constipation as a result of the low fiber content of most formulas. These patients may benefit from the inclusion of fiber in their enteral feeding formula.

TOTAL PARENTERAL NUTRITION

When the GI tract cannot be used for the ingestion, digestion, and absorption of essential nutrients, TPN may be substituted. Parenteral nutrition has become a relatively safe and practical method of delivering total nutritional needs by an IV route.

The goal of using TPN is to meet the patient's nutritional needs and to allow for growth of new body tissue. Regular IV solutions of 5% dextrose (5 g dextrose/100 ml) in water (D_5W) or 5% dextrose in lactated Ringer's solution (D_5LR) contain no protein and have approximately 170 calories per liter. The normal adult requires a minimum of 1200 to 1500 calories per day to carry out normal physiologic functions. Patients who sustain severe injury, surgery, or burns, and those who are malnourished as a result of medical treatment or disease processes, have greatly increased nutritional needs. The volume of regular dextrose solutions needed to meet these high caloric requirements could exceed the capacity of the cardiovascular system. Table 38-19 lists common indications for the use of TPN.

Composition

Commercially prepared TPN base solutions are available for both central and peripheral use (explained on p. 1060). These base solutions contain dextrose and nitrogen in the form of amino acids or protein hydrolysates. The hospital pharmacy adds the prescribed electrolytes (e.g., sodium, potassium, chloride, calcium, magnesium, and phosphate), vitamins, and trace elements (e.g., zinc, copper, chromium, and manganese) to customize the solution for the patient. A three-in-one, or total nutrient, mixture containing an IV fat emulsion, dextrose, and amino acids has become widely available, especially in the

Table 38-19 Common Indications for Total Parenteral Nutrition
Acute or chronic renal failure*
Gastrointestinal tract anomalies and fistula
Burns
Chronic diarrhea and vomiting
Complicated surgery or trauma
Diverticulitis
Failure to thrive
Gastrointestinal obstruction
Granulomatous enterocolitis
Hepatic failure (reversible)*
Hypermetabolic states (sepsis, fractures)
Inflammatory bowel disease (Crohn's disease and ulcerative colitis)
Malabsorption
Malnutrition
Pancreatitis
Severe anorexia nervosa
Severe peptic ulcer disease
Short bowel syndrome

*Total parenteral nutrition should be used with extreme caution in this situation.

home setting. In hospital settings this total nutrient mixture is less likely to be used.

Calories. Calories in TPN are supplied primarily by carbohydrates in the form of dextrose (20% to 50% of total calories). The administration of between 100 and 150 g of dextrose (1 g provides approximately 3.4 calories, as opposed to oral carbohydrates, which provide 4 calories) daily has a protein-sparing effect. Protein should be provided at the rate of 1.0 to 1.5 g/kg per day depending on the patient's needs. Adequate nonprotein calories in the form of glucose and lipids must be provided to allow metabolism of amino acids for wound healing and not as energy. However, overfeeding can lead to multiple organ failure. To minimize these problems, an energy intake of 25 to 30 calories per kilogram per day in a nonobese patient is often recommended. Providing both lipid and amino acid components meets the energy requirement while minimizing problems of overfeeding.

Nitrogen. The normal healthy person of average body size needs approximately 45 to 65 g of protein daily (see Table 38-4). In a nutritionally depleted patient under the stress of illness or surgery, requirements can exceed 150 g per day to ensure a positive nitrogen balance. However, in the most recent guidelines, protein intake levels of 1.5 to 2.0 g per kilogram per day are suggested for most patients with moderate to severe stress.[13]

Electrolytes. The assessment of individual requirements should take place daily at the beginning of therapy and then several times a week as the treatment progresses. The following are ranges for average daily electrolyte requirements for adult patients:

Sodium: 60 to 200 mEq
Potassium: 50 to 160 mEq
Chloride: 100 to 200 mEq
Magnesium: 20 to 30 mEq
Calcium: 5 to 15 mEq
Phosphate: 30 to 100 mEq

The exact amount needed depends on the patient's health problem and on electrolyte levels as determined by blood testing.

Trace Elements. Zinc, copper, manganese, cobalt, selenium, and iodine supplements must be ordered according to the patient's condition and needs. Levels of these elements are monitored in the patient receiving TPN. The physician may order additional amounts of these elements to be added to the solutions according to the patient's requirements.

Vitamins. The daily addition of a multivitamin preparation to 1 L of TPN generally meets the vitamin requirements. If multivitamin infusion is used, the cobalamin (vitamin B_{12}) requirement may be met without the need for supplemental injections. It is necessary for the physician to order vitamin K and folic acid separately. Folic acid 500 μg is given daily. Intramuscular (IM) vitamin K may be ordered depending on the results of the prothrombin time.

Methods of Administration

TPN may be administered by central or peripheral veins. Central parenteral nutrition is given through a catheter whose tip lies in the superior vena cava. The central catheter often originates at the subclavian vein. More recently single- or double-lumen peripherally inserted central catheters (PICCs) are being placed, usually into the basilic or cephalic vein and then advanced into the central circulation. Such catheters are made of soft, flexible material (silicon, polymer) and are 20 to 24 inches long. Ease of placement, cost, and limited complications make this an attractive alternative to a centrally placed line. Central TPN is indicated when long-term nutritional support is necessary, when the patient has high protein and caloric requirements, and when suitable peripheral veins are not available.

Peripheral parenteral nutrition (PPN) is administered through a peripherally inserted catheter or vascular access device (VAD), which uses a large peripheral vein. PPN is used when (1) nutritional support is needed for only a short time (up to 2 weeks), (2) protein and caloric requirements are not excessively high, (3) the risk of a central catheter is too great, or (4) nutritional support is used to supplement inadequate oral intake. Both central and peripheral TPN are used in a patient who is not a candidate for enteral support.

Central and peripheral parenteral nutrition differ in tonicity, which is measured in milliosmoles (mOsm), the concentration of particles in a fluid. Blood is isotonic and measures approximately 280 mOsm per liter. The standard IV solutions of D_5W and normal saline are essentially isotonic. Central TPN solutions are hypertonic, measuring approximately 1600 mOsm per liter. The high glucose content ranges from 20% to 50%. Thus nutrients can be infused using smaller fluid volumes than PPN. Central TPN must be infused in a large central vein so that rapid dilution can occur. The use of a peripheral vein causes irritation and thrombophlebitis. PPN is less hypertonic (using as much as 20% glucose) and can be safely administered through a large peripheral vein, although phlebitis can occur. Another potential complication is fluid overload.

All TPN solutions should be prepared by a pharmacist or a trained technician using strict aseptic techniques under a laminar flow hood. Nothing should be added to parenteral nutrition solutions after they are prepared in the pharmacy. The danger of drug incompatibilities and contamination is high.

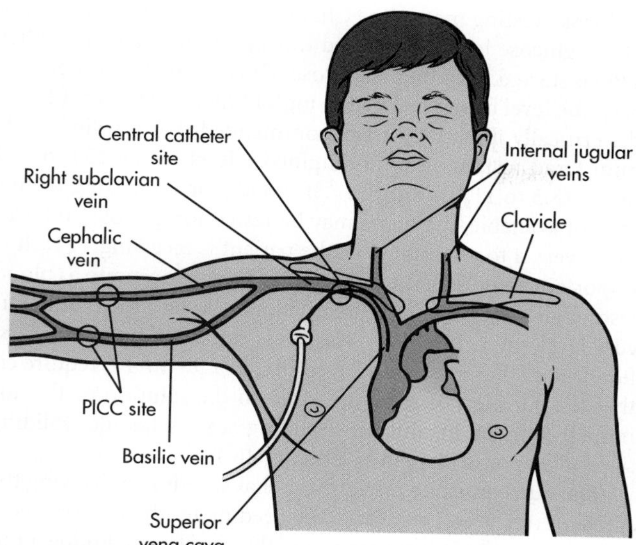

Fig. 38-6 Placement of a catheter for total parenteral nutrition using subclavian vein. Peripherally inserted central catheters (PICC) inserted using the basilic or cephalic veins.

The fewer the personnel involved in the preparation and administration of TPN, the lower the risk of infection for the patient. In most hospitals the physician must order the TPN solution daily. In this way the solution and additives can be adjusted to the patient's current needs. Each bottle of solution indicates the glucose and protein content, all additives, the time mixed, and the date and time of expiration. In general, solutions are good for 24 to 36 hours and must be refrigerated until one-half hour before use.

Catheter Placement

The central placement of the catheter into a large main vein for TPN is performed by the physician or a specially trained advanced practice nurse. The vein most commonly used is the subclavian, although the innominate or the jugular vein may be used. The procedure is the same as for the insertion of a central venous pressure line and should be done under strict aseptic conditions.

A standard isotonic IV solution is infused through the central line until x-ray confirms proper placement of the catheter tip in the superior vena cava and not in the jugular vein or the heart. The catheter insertion site is covered with an iodine ointment, and an occlusive dressing is placed over it. The date is marked on the dressing.

Placement of a PICC catheter is done under sterile conditions, often by a specially trained nurse. A baseline measurement of the upper arm circumference is recommended. A tourniquet is then placed around the upper arm near the axilla to allow examination of the antecubital fossa and selection of a vein. If possible, the patient should be supine with the arm straight and at a 90-degree angle. Preparation of the insertion site should be done according to institutional policy. The sterile catheter will need to be cut to the predetermined length, depending on the vein selected.

Table 38-20 Complications of Total Parenteral Nutrition

- **Infection**
  - Fungus
  - Gram-positive bacteria
  - Gram-negative bacteria
- **Metabolic Problems**
  - Glucose metabolism
    - Hyperglycemia, hypoglycemia, and hyperosmolar nonketotic coma
    - Glycosuria
    - Osmotic diuresis
    - Ketoacidosis
  - Amino acid metabolism
    - Serum amino acid imbalances
    - Elevated serum ammonia
    - Prerenal azotemia
  - Essential fatty acid deficiency
  - Electrolyte and vitamin excesses and deficiencies
  - Trace mineral deficiencies
- **Mechanical Problems**
  - Insertion
    - Air embolus
    - Pneumothorax, hemothorax, and hydrothorax
    - Hemorrhage
  - Dislodgement
  - Thrombosis of great vein
  - Phlebitis

A local anesthetic is usually used at the insertion site. This site should be cleaned, protected, and maintained according to institutional policy. As with the centrally placed line, chest x-ray is needed to verify proper tip placement before administering any TPN solution.

Proper placement of a catheter for central TPN is illustrated in Fig. 38-6. Once established for TPN, a single-lumen central catheter should not be used for the administration of blood or antibiotics, the drawing of blood samples, or the monitoring of central venous pressure.

Administration of Solution

Because TPN solutions are excellent media for microbial growth, it is essential that proper aseptic techniques be followed. The Food and Drug Administration (FDA) recommends that 0.22 μm millipore filters be placed on all parenteral lines. When the filter is used, it should be placed proximal to the catheter hub. Filters are changed every 24 hours, and new IV tubing is changed with each new bottle of TPN. The tubing and the filter should be clearly labeled with the date and the time they are put into use.

Complications

Complications of TPN can be divided into three categories: (1) infectious, (2) metabolic, and (3) mechanical. The major complications of each category are presented in Table 38-20.

NURSING MANAGEMENT: TOTAL PARENTERAL NUTRITION

PPN is a form of IV nutrition that may be given concurrently with oral nourishment. A large peripheral vein can be used because the solution is less hypertonic and therefore less irritating. The peripheral injection site should be observed for signs of phlebitis (redness and swelling). The insertion site dressing is changed at least every 48 hours, depending on established hospital policy and type of peripheral access device. The preparation and administration of PPN follow the same criteria as outlined for central TPN (see NCP 38-2).

Vital signs should be monitored every 2 to 4 hours in the patient receiving TPN. Daily weights give an indication of the patient's hydration status as therapy progresses. Body weight is considered the sum of the changes in protein, fat, and water. On a daily basis, body water fluctuates more than protein or fat. Analysis must be made of whether gains or losses in weight are caused by fluid gained from edema, fluid lost through diuresis, or actual increase or decrease in tissue weight. Blood levels of glucose, electrolytes, protein, a complete blood count, and enzyme studies are followed daily until stable and then weekly as the patient's condition warrants. Assessment of these important values assists the nurse in assessing the patient's tolerance of parenteral nutrition.

Dressings covering the catheter site are changed according to institutional protocol, ranging from every other day to once a week. Frequently, specially trained nurses from the IV team or the nutritional support team are responsible for these dressing changes. Some institutions allow a staff nurse to do the dressing changes after special instruction. The procedure for changing the dressing is similar to that followed after catheter insertion. The institutional routine should be followed with respect to the appropriate use of solutions for the dressing change. The site is carefully observed for signs of inflammation and infection. Phlebitis can readily occur in the vein as a result of the hypertonic infusion, and the area can become infected. The patient receiving central TPN may be immunosuppressed and thus more susceptible to opportunistic infections. In this patient signs of inflammation or infection can be subtle, if present at all. Many patients receiving TPN are receiving chemotherapy, corticosteroids, or antibiotics, which can mask signs of infection.

If sutures are used to anchor the catheter, they may become infected. If an infection is suspected during dressing change, a culture specimen of the site and drainage should be sent for analysis, and the physician should be notified immediately. The use of an occlusive dressing protects the wound from contamination.

Complications frequently associated with catheter placement are hemorrhage, hydrothorax and pneumothorax, hemothorax, air embolus, and venous thrombosis. It is important that the tip of the catheter not lie within the right atrium. The TPN solution is hyperosmolar, and the catheter tip can cause erosions of the atrial tissue with subsequent infection.

Hyperglycemia is a metabolic complication of parenteral nutrition. At the beginning of TPN therapy, the solution is infused at a gradually increasing rate for 24 to 48 hours. This allows the pancreas to adapt to the increased amount of glucose in the circulation by producing more insulin. Blood glucose levels should be checked at the bedside every 4 to 6 hours with a glucose-testing meter (see Chapter 46). Some increase in the blood glucose level is expected during the first few days after TPN is started. A sliding scale dose of insulin may be ordered to keep the level below 180 to 200 mg/dl (9.8 to 10.9 mmol/L). In the critically ill patient it is recommended that insulin be administered to maintain blood glucose level below 150 to 200 mg/dl (8.3 to 11.1 mmol/L).[14] If blood glucose–testing meters are not available, the urine may be tested for glucose and acetone every 4 to 6 hours while the patient is receiving TPN. It is important to note that urine testing is not as accurate as blood testing and thus is not frequently done. As with the blood glucose level, glycosuria of 1+ or 2+ is expected during the first few days of therapy. However, readings of 3+ or 4+ require either the addition of regular insulin to the solution or the administration of insulin on a sliding-scale schedule. (Sliding scale insulin is explained in Chapter 46.)

The nurse must be made aware that speeding or slowing the infusion rate is contraindicated. Speeding up the rate results in a large amount of glucose entering the circulation. Endogenous insulin levels often are not adequate to handle this increase in glucose, and a hyperglycemic state results. The renal tubules are unable to reabsorb the glucose and it spills into the urine. Conversely, slowing the rate may result in a hypoglycemic state because it takes time for the pancreatic islet cells to adjust to a reduced glucose level. Checking the amount infused and the rate every 30 minutes to 1 hour is recommended. An infusion pump should be used during administration of TPN so that the infusion rate can be maintained, and an alarm will sound if the tubing becomes obstructed. Even when using an infusion pump, the nurse should periodically check the volume infused because pump malfunctions can alter the rate.

Before setting up and administering TPN, the nurse must check the label and ingredients in the solution to see that they are what the physician ordered. Solutions must also be examined for signs of contamination, such as a cloudy appearance. If contamination is suspected, the solution should be promptly returned to the pharmacy for replacement. It is the nurse's responsibility to ensure that the TPN solution is discontinued and replaced with a new solution if it is still infusing at the end of 24 hours. At room temperature, the solution is an excellent medium for microorganism growth.

Catheter-related infection and septicemia can occur in patients receiving TPN through both peripherally and centrally placed lines. Local manifestations of infection include erythema, tenderness, and exudate at the catheter insertion site. Systemically the patient may have fever, chills, nausea, vomiting, and malaise. If no other causes can be identified, a catheter-related infection is suspected. Because of the risk of infection, catheters with antibiotic or antiseptic surfaces are frequently used. To diagnose the presence of infection and to determine the causative organism, cultures are performed of the catheter tip if the catheter has been removed or the blood in the catheter if still in place. Blood cultures are drawn simultaneously from the catheter and a peripheral vein. A chest x-ray is taken to detect changes in pulmonary status. The current bottle of TPN solution with tubing and filter should also be cultured and replaced with an entirely new setup. When the catheter tip is the source of infection, antibiotic therapy is generally not necessary because removal of the catheter will eliminate the problem. A

38-2 NURSING CARE PLAN PATIENT RECEIVING TOTAL PARENTERAL NUTRITION

Expected Patient Outcomes	Nursing Interventions and *Rationales*
NURSING DIAGNOSIS	**Risk for infection** *related to* placement of a central venous access catheter, inadequate aseptic practices, and decreased defense mechanisms.
■ No manifestations of infection. ■ Normal body temperature. ■ Negative blood cultures.	■ Assess for altered defense mechanisms caused by inadequate nutrition, compromised health status, open wound for TPN line *to plan for prevention of infection.* ■ Refrigerate solution until 30 minutes before using *to prevent bacterial growth in the solution.* ■ Use protocols for tubing and filter changes; change dressing over catheter site according to institution policy *to minimize the possibility of infection.* ■ Observe for signs of inflammation and infection; monitor vital signs q4hr *to ensure early detection of infection.*
NURSING DIAGNOSIS	**Impaired physical mobility** *related to* muscle or nerve trauma *as manifested by* decreased muscle strength and control, neuromuscular impairment (e.g., brachial plexus injury).
■ Satisfactory movement of upper body. ■ Satisfactory pain control.	■ Observe patient for pain in shoulder and sensory changes *to determine possible nerve damage or faulty catheter placement.* ■ Assist with range of motion within position restrictions *to maintain normal range of motion of shoulder.* ■ Administer pain medication as ordered *to maintain patient's comfort.*
NURSING DIAGNOSIS	**Anxiety** *related to* inability to ingest food and fluids; lack of knowledge regarding catheter, benefits and management of TPN *as manifested by* restlessness and apprehension; frequent questioning regarding care of catheter and TPN line.
■ Statement of rationale for and demonstration of care of TPN line.	■ Instruct patient on rationale and benefits of TPN and care of line *because knowledge and facts may reduce anxiety.* ■ Illustrate catheter position by drawings and pictures *to increase patient understanding.*

COLLABORATIVE PROBLEMS

Nursing Goals	Nursing Interventions and *Rationales*
POTENTIAL COMPLICATION	**Hyperglycemia, hypoglycemia, and electrolyte imbalances** *related to* administration of TPN.
■ Monitor blood glucose and serum electrolytes. ■ Report deviations from acceptable parameters. ■ Carry out medical and nursing interventions.	■ Monitor for signs of hyperglycemia such as thirst, polyuria, confusion, elevated fasting blood glucose, blurred vision, dizziness, nausea and vomiting, dehydration, and deep labored breathing *to plan appropriate treatment.* ■ Monitor for signs of hypoglycemia such as sweating, hunger, weakness, and tremors *to ensure early intervention.* ■ Monitor serum electrolyte levels daily *to identify and treat complications early.* ■ Check for symptoms of hyperkalemia (e.g., muscle weakness, flaccid paralysis, cardiac arrhythmias, abdominal cramps, diarrhea) and hypokalemia (e.g., general weakness, decreased muscle tone, weak or irregular pulse, low blood pressure, shallow respirations, abdominal distention, and ileus). (Other manifestations of electrolyte imbalances are discussed in Chapter 15.) ■ Check blood glucose q4hr. Notify physician of increased levels *so that regular insulin may be added to the solution or administered on a sliding scale basis.* ■ Maintain accurate infusion rate *to control the amount of glucose administered and prevent fluctuations in blood glucose levels.* ■ Check every 30 minutes or use an infusion pump *to ensure accurate administration.* ■ Never increase or decrease flow rate by more than 10% *to prevent fluctuations in blood glucose levels.* ■ Never stop TPN abruptly unless it is replaced by another glucose source *to prevent hypoglycemia.*

Continued

38-2 NURSING CARE PLAN PATIENT RECEIVING TOTAL PARENTERAL NUTRITION—continued

Expected Patient Outcomes	Nursing Interventions and *Rationales*
POTENTIAL COMPLICATION	**Air embolus** *related to* incorrect position of TPN catheter.
▪ Monitor for and report signs of air embolus. ▪ Carry out medical and nursing interventions.	▪ On catheter insertion, place patient in Trendelenburg's position with rolled towel between scapulae *to distend subclavian vein by increasing venous pressure.* ▪ Instruct patient to take a deep breath (Valsalva's maneuver) and hold while needle is inserted into subclavian vein. ▪ Use same position and Valsalva's maneuver when changing tubing *to prevent air from being sucked into vein.* ▪ If air embolism is suspected, place patient in Trendelenburg's position with left side down *to trap "air" in right atria.* ▪ Continue to observe for shock, cough, and shortness of breath. ▪ Notify physician immediately *so definitive diagnosis and treatment can be initiated.* ▪ Monitor for signs of air embolus such as abnormal blood gases, cough, cyanosis, pain, anxiety, fatigue, respiratory rate and depth changes, altered chest excursion, shortness of breath *to ensure early identification and treatment.*

Table 38-21 Common Characteristics of a 20% Intralipid Fat Emulsion in Water*

Soybean triglycerides	20%*
Egg yolk phospholipids	1.20%
Glycerin	2.25%
Electrolytes	1.50 mm phosphorus/100 ml
Total kilocalories	2 cal/ml
Typical pH	8
Osmolarity	260 mOsm/L

*Other stock lipids are 10% and 30%.

new central line may be immediately established or replaced by a peripheral route. It is important that a glucose source be maintained to prevent rebound hypoglycemia.

Weaning. The same precautions should be followed in weaning from TPN as when therapy is being initiated, except in the reverse order. The flow rate must be gradually decreased for 4 to 6 hours, while oral intake is increased. If an emergency situation precludes a slow weaning process, other dextrose-containing fluids should be administered without interruption. When the catheter is removed, the dressing should be changed daily until the wound heals. Oral nourishment should be encouraged, and a careful record of intake should be maintained. Body weight recording and laboratory analysis of serum electrolyte and glucose levels may continue.

Home Parenteral Nutrition. Home parenteral nutrition is an accepted mode of nutritional therapy for the person who does not require hospitalization but who benefits from continued nutritional support. Some patients have been successfully treated at home for many months and even years. It is important to educate the patient or the family about catheter care, aseptic technique in mixing and handling of the IV solutions and tubing, and side effects.

Intravenous Fat Emulsion

The first infusion of fat emulsions occurred during the 1920s in Japan. Further research was delayed until after World War II. The FDA has currently approved the use of 10%, 20%, and 30% intralipid fat emulsion solutions. These lipid emulsions provide approximately 1 calorie per milliliter (10% solution) or 2 calories per milliliter (20% solution). The contents of intralipid fat emulsion are listed in Table 38-21. The use of IV fat emulsions is indicated for the following patients:

1. Those receiving peripheral parenteral nutrition who require an additional source of calories
2. Those receiving long-term (more than 5 days) parenteral nutrition who require a source of essential fatty acids
3. Those receiving central TPN who have high caloric needs

Using daily IV fat emulsions provides another nonprotein energy source. In practice, the conservative approach is IV-administered fat emulsions providing not more than 20% to 30% of the total energy to minimize possible linoleic acid immunosuppressive effects. The maximum fat emulsion amount should not exceed a dose of 2.5 g/kg per day.[15] It is administered slowly over 12 to 24 hours to minimize immune suppression. Nausea, vomiting, and elevated temperature have been reported, especially when lipids are infused quickly.

The administration of fat emulsion is contraindicated in the patient with a disturbance in fat metabolism. It should also be used with caution in the patient who is in danger of fat embolism (e.g., fractured femur) and the patient with an allergy to eggs.

Intralipid solution (10%) is isotonic and in balanced combination with other proteins and carbohydrates contributes to complete peripheral TPN solutions. It can be infused separately. When it is used with TPN, the fat emulsion provides essential fatty acids that are not included in the standard dextrose–amino acid preparations of TPN. Prolonged use of TPN can lead to a fatty acid deficiency, which is manifested by dermatitis and loss of hair. Recent pharmacologic advances now permit the direct mixing of lipid emulsion with dextrose and amino acids in a single bag suitable for infusion in some situations.

Unopened intralipid solutions do not require refrigeration. However, those that have been opened or mixed with other nutrients do require refrigeration and should be refrigerated until 1 hour before administration. Special tubing is provided by the manufacturer, and new tubing is used with each bottle. Nothing is to be added to the solution before administration. Lipid solutions can be filtered but require a 1.2 μm filter. When PPN is being run concurrently, the fat emulsion should be connected below the filter through a Y-injection site as close as possible to the injection site. The preferred delivery method is a continuous low volume, such as 20% lipids delivered at 10 to 30 ml per hour depending on patient needs. Adverse reactions that can occur are allergic manifestations, dyspnea, cyanosis, fever, flushing, phlebitis, chest and back pain, and pain at the IV site. A major benefit derived from IV fat administration is that a large number of calories can be provided in a relatively small amount of fluid. This is especially beneficial when the patient is at risk for fluid overload.

OBESITY

Obesity has reached epidemic proportions in our society.[16] In the United States obesity is the most common nutritional problem. Among adults age 20 years and older, 33% of men and 36% of women are overweight.[17] The prevalence of overweight increases with age, for both men and women, but to a greater degree in women. African-American and Hispanic women have a higher prevalence of being overweight than do Caucasian women.[17]

The calculated body mass index (BMI) is a common clinical index of obesity or altered body fat distribution. A well-accepted scale has been developed to calculate BMI by gender using weight-to-height ratios (Fig. 38-7).[18] Individuals with a BMI of 25 to 29.9 kg/m^2 are classified as being overweight, and those with values of 30 kg/m^2 or more are classified as obese.

The waist-to-hip ratio is another way to define obesity. This ratio is a method of describing the distribution of both subcutaneous and intraabdominal adipose tissue. The waist measurement is divided by the hip measurement to calculate the ratio. A number greater than 1.0 in men and 0.8 in women indicates overweight. This ratio increases with age and excessive weight.[18]

Anthropometric measurements can also be used to define the different levels of overweight. A patient with body weight 10% above the ideal for height and frame is considered overweight. A patient with body weight 20% above the ideal for height and frame is considered obese. Triceps skinfold greater than 15 mm in men and 25 mm in women would classify the person as overweight. When body weight exceeds 100% of the ideal body weight it is classified as morbid obesity.

In obese persons a variety of problems occur at a rate higher than the expected rate. These include hypertension, hyperlipidemia, type 2 diabetes mellitus, degenerative joint disease, gout, insulin resistance with hyperinsulinemia, cardiovascular disease, gallbladder disease, stroke, some kinds of cancer (breast,

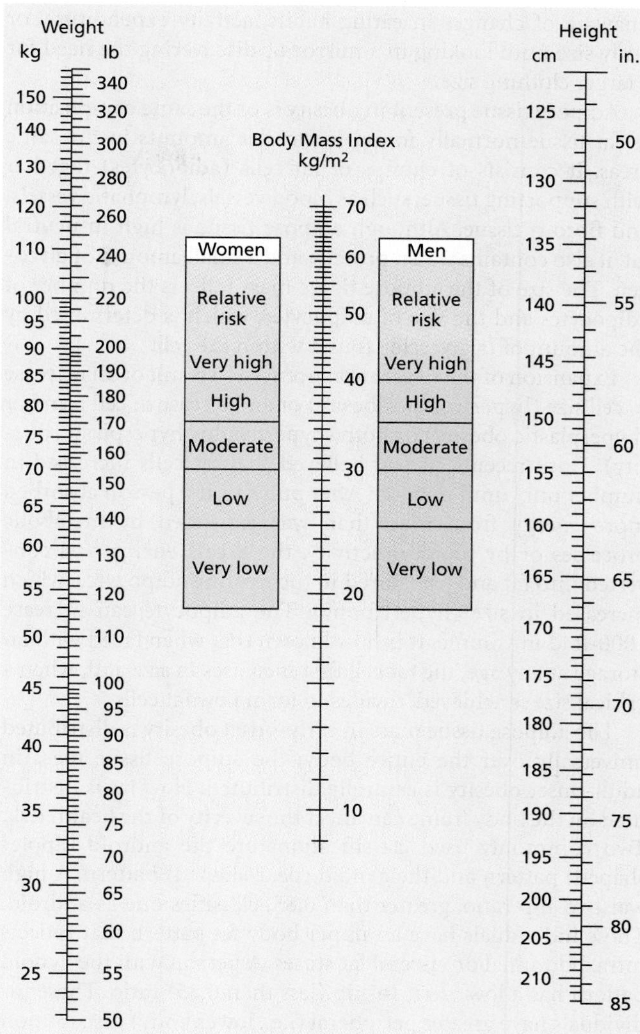

Fig. 38-7 A nomogram for determining body mass index (BMI). To use this nomogram, place a rule or other edge between the column for height and the column for weight connecting an individual's numbers for these two variables. Read the BMI in kg/m^2 where the straight line crosses the middle lines when the height and weight are connected. Overweight: BMI of 25 to 29.9 kg/m^2; obesity: BMI 30 kg/m^2 or more. Heights and weights are without shoes or clothes. Relative risk for health problems associated with obesity are shown.

colon), and menstrual irregularities.[19] These conditions generally improve if weight loss occurs.

Formation of Adipose Tissue

The formation of adipose tissue, unless determined to be secondary to an organic cause, can occur only when a person consumes more food than is required to carry out normal physiologic functions and growth. The excess energy is converted to fat and is stored in adipose tissue in layers beneath the skin surface, the omentum, the mesentery, and in fat pads that normally surround the kidneys and the heart. The process of reaching an obese state is usually insidious. The person may be completely unaware of changes in eating habits, activity expenditure, or body size until looking in a mirror or discovering the need for a larger clothing size.

Adipose tissue present in obesity is of the same composition as fat tissue normally found in smaller amounts in the same areas. It consists of clumps of fat cells (adipocytes) together with supporting tissue, such as blood vessels, lymphatic vessels, and fibrous tissue. Although adipose tissue is high in neutral fat, it also contains water, protein, and a small amount of glycogen. The size of the adipose tissue mass reflects the number of adipocytes and the size of adipocytes, which is determined by the amount of triglyceride found within the cell.

Expansion of the tissue mass occurs as a result of an increase in cell size (hypertrophic obesity) or an increase in cell number (hyperplastic obesity) or both (hypertrophic hyperplastic obesity). Until recently it was believed that fat cells increased in number only until puberty. After puberty, if a person absorbed more energy from food than was expended by metabolic processes or by physical activity, the excess energy was converted into fat and was stored in the existing adipocytes, which increased in size (hypertrophy). The adipocyte can increase 1000-fold in volume. It is now known that when faced with fat storage at any age, the fat cell first increases in size and, when a critical size is achieved, divides to form new fat cells.

The adipose tissue mass in early-onset obesity is distributed universally over the entire body; the adipose tissue mass in adult-onset obesity is centrally distributed. How fat is distributed on the body frame can affect the severity of the health risk. Two commonly used classifications are the android (apple-shaped) pattern and the gynoid (pear-shaped) pattern. A high waist-to-hip ratio, greater than 0.85, classifies one as android. These individuals have an upper body fat pattern that reflects intraabdominal or visceral fat stores. A person with the gynoid pattern has a low waist-to-hip (less than 0.85) ratio. These individuals have greater peripheral (i.e., lower body) distribution of fat, including gluteal and femoral prominence. The android pattern is associated with a higher risk of coronary artery disease, hypertension, and disorders of glucose tolerance and hyperlipidemia.

An understanding of how adipose tissue is formed has considerable impact on methods of weight loss and of reduction of the adipose tissue mass in the adult. Severe dietary restrictions do not decrease the number of fat adipocytes present but do result in a decrease in the size of the cells.

Etiology and Pathophysiology

Many factors have been investigated in an effort to identify the critical elements in the development and maintenance of obesity. Once obesity is present, the number of calories consumed must exceed the energy expended for the condition to continue. However, there is debate about processes leading to obesity.[20] When assessing the obese patient, the nurse should consider several different types of questions, such as the following:

1. What is the psychologic importance of food to the patient?
2. Is the patient's food intake influenced by hunger?
3. Do the taste and appearance of food or other physical factors in the environment stimulate the patient to eat?
4. Is there an emotional problem that stimulates the patient to eat?
5. Are there any stressors influencing the patient's eating patterns?
6. Is there a tendency in the patient's family for members to be overweight?

The nurse must recognize that environmental and genetic factors are important. The children of obese parents tend to be obese. Obesity tends to affect several persons within a family. Evidence of a genetic component is suggested in twin and adoptive children studies.[21] More recently, obesity genes have been identified in rodents. Further research is needed to determine whether similar genes are involved in human obesity.[22,23]

There are a growing number of theories related to etiology of obesity.[24] It is likely that the human obesity genotypes will be complex multigenic systems with networks of gene-gene and gene-environment interactions. The etiology of obesity is complex. The body fat content and, more specifically, an excess of body fat result from an intricate network of additive and interactive causes that may be related to DNA sequence variation but may also be associated with behavior and lifestyle. Obesity is a heterogeneous phenotype, and evidence is growing that each phenotypic entity is modulated by a different set of causal factors. These factors include energy intake, resting metabolic rate, level of habitual physical activity, chemical signals, and nutrient partitioning (tendency to store ingested energy in the form of fat or lean tissue).

Research on the pathophysiology of obesity has focused on multiple factors, including genetics and the role of the hypothalamus and energy balance. The lateral and ventral-medial parts of the hypothalamus control appetite and, as a result, influence eating behavior. It is hypothesized that the hypothalamus has a set point for energy balance, above which energy conservation becomes increasingly less efficient and below which energy conservation becomes increasingly more efficient. This homeostatic mechanism accounts for the fact that most adults keep their weight remarkably constant, despite large swings in energy input and expenditure.

This ability of the body to conserve energy as dieting continues may account for the failure of sustained weight loss to occur even though caloric intake is drastically curtailed. It could also account for why the obese person, no matter what dietary regimen is followed, tends to remain overweight.

A sedentary lifestyle including a nonstrenuous indoor occupation and engagement in few, if any, spirited recreational activities is associated with the development of excess body weight and obesity. Thus an obese person with sedentary habits only adds to an already positive energy balance by not engaging in activities that burn off some excess fatty tissue through energy-consuming exercises.

The emotional component of the tendency to overeat is powerful. People use food for many reasons, including comfort and reward. Some people are triggered by specific foods to continue eating beyond satiety. The social component of eating develops early in life when food is associated with pleasure and fun at such events as birthday parties, Thanksgiving, and religious holidays. All of these factors must be included when considering the etiology of obesity.

Complications

The medical and social problems associated with obesity are numerous. These problems are more common in a patient who exceeds ideal body weight by greater than 20%. The medical problems associated with obesity may be a direct result of too much fat. In addition, medical problems such as hypothyroidism can have an adverse effect on energy balance and result in excess body weight gain. Cardiovascular and respiratory problems are common in the obese person. Many patients experience dyspnea on exertion, orthopnea, paroxysmal nocturnal dyspnea, drowsiness, and somnolence. Obstructive sleep apnea is more prevalent in overweight or obese older men.

In addition, the obese patient is prone to the development of polycythemia secondary to low oxygenation of arterial blood. Polycythemia results in an increased viscosity of the circulating blood and sluggish flow through all vessels and capillaries. As a result, an obese patient may have occluded vessels and clotting abnormalities. Varicose veins, as well as venous leg ulcers, are common partly because of increased back pressure on the venous return from the lower limbs by excess intraabdominal adipose tissue. Heart size increases as body weight increases because the heart must work harder to maintain adequate circulation. Hypertension is the most common cardiovascular problem associated with obesity. The presence of polycythemia creates considerable strain on the heart because of the increased RBC count and plasma volume. Therefore obesity can precipitate hypertrophy of the heart, especially of the left ventricle.

The pickwickian syndrome, which is known as obesity hypoventilation, has long been recognized as a result of morbid obesity. The bellows action of the chest wall is compromised, and there is dysfunction of the central respiratory control center. The movement of the muscles of the chest wall and the diaphragm is reduced because of the weight of the fatty tissue mass. Hypoventilation results in a state of chronic hypercapnia manifested by cyanosis, dyspnea, edema, and somnolence. In addition, most patients have a reduced vital capacity and polycythemia. Blood gas exchange is also directly affected. Although the pickwickian syndrome is rare, caution should always be used when sedatives are used for the morbidly obese person because these drugs can precipitate severe respiratory complications.

Impaired glucose tolerance is common with obesity. The incidence of type 2 diabetes mellitus is high in obese persons. Excessive food intake stimulates hyperinsulinemia. Through a negative-feedback mechanism, excessive insulin levels decrease the number of insulin-receptor sites on the cell membrane. The loss of insulin-receptor sites decreases the amount of glucose that can enter the cells. This promotes high levels of blood glucose. Thus the obese patient is often hyperglycemic and hyperinsulinemic. Weight reduction appears to reverse these effects by increasing insulin receptors and enhancing the movement of glucose into cells.

Gallstone formation in the obese patient is also common. The incidence of gallstones rises as the body weight increases. There is a concomitant rise in the serum cholesterol and triglyceride levels, as well as an increase in body weight. These substances precipitate in the gallbladder, resulting in cholelithiasis and cholecystitis. With weight loss, cholesterol and triglyceride levels often decrease, resulting in decreased risk of gallstone formation. The high levels of cholesterol and triglycerides can also contribute to the development of coronary artery disease (see Chapter 32).

Excessive weight on the weight-bearing joints (hips and knees) and the lower spine can cause pain and discomfort. Although obesity has not been implicated as a cause of degenerative joint disease, it is a predisposing factor. Obesity may contribute to the pathogenesis of osteoarthritis in multiple joints when the disease process has already started.

Other complications associated with obesity are menstrual irregularities, infertility, endometrial cancer, and fatty liver infiltration. Understandably, the life expectancy of an obese person can be shortened as a result of the medical problems.

In addition to the many physical complications associated with obesity, the person may suffer from long-standing emotional and social problems. Society today puts great emphasis on attaining and maintaining a slim and vigorous look. Those who deviate from this prescribed standard often meet with discrimination and disdain. The morbidly obese person may find it difficult to obtain a desired job, social acceptance, or membership in organizations. Choice of clothing is often limited in style, color, size, and quantity. These socioemotional problems may be manifested in poor self-esteem and body image.

Diagnostic Studies

The overwhelming majority of obese persons have primary obesity, that is, excess calorie intake for the body's metabolic demands. Others have secondary obesity, which can result from various congenital anomalies, chromosomal anomalies, metabolic lesions, or CNS lesions and disorders. A first step in the treatment process is to determine whether any such physical conditions are present. A thorough history and physical examination are necessary and will reveal the extent and duration of the obese state.

There is no definite agreement on a technique for determining who is obese. Several methods are currently in use. One widely used method is to compare the patient's weight to a standardized weight-for-height chart and then designate the patient to be overweight by a certain percentage. Table 38-22 provides a standardized weight-for-height chart. Normal weight depends largely on body build. A limitation of this method of assessing obesity can be seen from the following example: A person who inherits a medium frame and develops a bulky muscle mass may be considered 20% overweight according to the standardized chart and yet not be obese.

A more sensitive approach to determine the presence of obesity is the BMI discussed earlier in this chapter. The BMI (see Fig. 38-7) is not dependent on frame size. Because the BMI value rises with age, it has been suggested that age-specific guidelines for older adults be established. A more individualized method of determining the amount of body fat is by measuring skinfold thickness with special calipers at one or more of four body sites: the biceps, the triceps, the subscapular site, or the suprailiac site. Estimates of body fat are then derived as a result of correlations established with body density from anthropometric charts. Although considered a more exact technique, this method also has limitations. The disadvantage of this method of calculating the degree of obesity is that the standards for the skinfold thickness are generally obtained from healthy young men and women, 20 to 30 years of age, and do not consider age-related changes. As a person ages, the percent of total body fat increases, as does the skinfold thickness for the fatty tissue at each site.[25] This measure is not as reliable in an obese individual as in midrange body weights. These measurements should be performed by trained clinicians. The

Table 38-22 Desirable Weights for Men and Women*

Height	Small	Medium	Large
Men			
5′2″	128-134	131-141	138-150
5′3″	130-136	133-143	140-153
5′4″	132-138	135-145	142-156
5′5″	134-140	137-148	144-160
5′6″	136-142	139-151	146-164
5′7″	138-145	142-154	149-168
5′8″	140-148	145-157	152-172
5′9″	142-151	148-160	155-176
5′10″	144-154	151-163	158-180
5′11″	146-157	154-166	161-184
6′	149-160	157-170	164-188
6′1″	152-164	160-174	168-192
6′2″	155-168	164-178	172-197
6′3″	158-172	167-182	176-202
6′4″	162-176	171-187	181-207
Women			
4′10″	102-111	109-121	118-131
4′11″	103-113	111-123	120-134
5′	104-115	113-126	122-137
5′1″	106-118	115-129	125-140
5′2″	108-121	118-132	128-143
5′3″	111-124	121-135	131-147
5′4″	114-127	124-138	134-151
5′5″	117-130	127-141	137-155
5′6″	120-133	130-144	140-159
5′7″	123-136	133-147	143-163
5′8″	126-139	136-150	146-167
5′9″	129-142	139-153	149-170
5′10″	132-145	142-156	152-173
5′11″	135-148	145-159	155-176
6′	138-151	148-162	158-179

*From 1983 Metropolitan Life Insurance Company weight tables by height and size of frame for people aged 25 to 59, in 1-inch shoes and wearing 5 pounds of indoor clothing for men or 3 pounds for women.

hip-to-waist ratio described earlier is another useful assessment technique.

The least reliable technique and yet perhaps the most frequently used is direct observation of the patient. A subjective assessment of total body fat is made. The ideal body is one that has only a thin layer of adipose tissue covering the skeletal frame. When a roll of excess subcutaneous adipose tissue is seen, the patient is often considered obese.

More sophisticated measures of obesity utilize densitometry, dual photon absorption, magnetic resonance imaging, and ultrasonography. However, such measures are generally used only for research purposes.

The physician explores genetic and endocrine factors in the workup. Etiologic factors such as hypothyroidism, hypothalamic tumors, Cushing's syndrome, hypogonadism in men, or polycystic ovarian disease in women are studied. Laboratory tests of liver function, fasting glucose level, triglyceride level, and low- and high-density lipoprotein cholesterol levels assist in evaluating the cause and effects of obesity.

Collaborative Conservative Care

When no organic cause can be found for obesity, it should be considered a chronic, complex illness. Any supervised plan of care should be directed at (1) successful weight loss, requiring a short-term energy deficit, and (2) successful weight control, requiring long-term behavior changes. These are two different processes. A multipronged approach ought to be used with attention to multiple elements in the fat cycle, such as dietary intake, physical activity, behavioral-cognitive modification, and perhaps drug therapy. Focusing on more than one aspect will likely give better balance to weight-loss and weight-control efforts.

Nutritional Therapy. Restricted food intake is a cornerstone for any weight loss or maintenance program. A good weight loss plan should contain foods from the basic food groups. Diets may be classified as low calorie (800 to 1200 calories per day) or very low calorie (less than 800 calories per day). Persons on low and very low calorie diets need frequent professional monitoring because the severe energy restriction places them at risk for multiple nutrient deficiencies. A diet that includes adequate amounts of fruits and vegetables provides enough bulk to prevent constipation and meets daily vitamin A and vitamin C requirements. Lean meat, fish, and eggs provide sufficient protein, as well as the B-complex vitamins. The caloric intake may need to be restricted to 800 to 1200 calories per day, depending on the patient's age, weight, nutritional status, activity level, and length of time estimated for the ideal weight to be achieved. Table 38-23 contains a sample 1200-calorie reducing diet.

The only effective method of treating primary obesity is to restrict dietary intake so that it is below energy requirements. It is rare to find an overweight person who has not at some time attempted to lose weight. Some have met with limited and temporary success, and others have met only with failure. It is likely that the great majority of these persons attempted weight loss by trying out at least one of the many fad diets that offer the enticement to eat and get slim. Fad diets in general claim weight loss quickly, easily, and inexpensively. Although it is true that initially weight is lost, it is not fat but body water that is lost. The normal fat cell is composed of approximately 80% fat, 18% water, and 2% protein. It is also a storage area for small amounts of glycogen. Glycogen is known to bind with water. When reducing diets severely restrict carbohydrates, the body's glycogen stores become depleted within a few days. It is only when the glycogen-water pool is almost depleted of energy that protein and adipose tissue are burned to release energy for bodily functions.

An obese patient must understand that following a well-balanced, low-calorie diet is an essential part of weight loss. Continuing to follow a well-balanced food plan will have a more satisfying and long-lasting result than fad diets.

The degree of success of any reducing diet depends in part on the amount of weight to be lost. A moderately obese person will obviously attain the goal more easily than will a massively obese person. Men are able to lose weight more quickly than women. Women have a higher percentage of metabolically less active body fat, whereas men have a higher percentage of metabolically more active lean body mass. Adult-onset obesity is often more amenable to successful treatment than the obesity of juvenile onset. In juvenile-onset obesity, the eating patterns

NUTRITIONAL THERAPY

Table 38-23 1200-Calorie-Restricted Weight-Reduction Diet*

General Principles

1. Eat regularly. Do not skip meals.
2. Measure foods to determine the correct portion size.
3. Avoid concentrated sweets, such as sugar, candy, honey, pies, cakes, cookies, and regular sodas.
4. Reduce fat intake by baking, broiling, or steaming foods.
5. Maintain a regular exercise program for successful weight loss.

Meal	Exchanges	Meal Plan 1	Meal Plan 2	Meal Plan 3
Breakfast	1 meat 2 bread	1 scrambled egg 1 slice toast ¾ cup dry cereal (unsweetened)	1 hard-boiled egg 1 flour tortilla ½ cup Cream of Wheat	1 oz ham 2 griddle cakes with diet syrup
	1 fruit	½ small banana	⅓ cup orange juice	⅓ cup pineapple juice
	1 fat	1 tsp margarine	1 slice bacon	1 tsp margarine
	1 dairy	1 cup low-fat milk	1 cup low-fat milk	1 cup low-fat milk
	Beverage	Coffee	Coffee	Coffee
Lunch	2 meat	1 slice bologna 1 slice cheese	Cheese enchiladas (made with 2 oz cheese, 2 corn tortillas, chili sauce)	2 oz baked breaded pork chop
	2 bread	2 slices bread		1 corn muffin
	Vegetable	Lettuce, pickles	Tomato wedges	Spinach
	1 fruit	Fresh grapes (12)	2 canned peach halves (packed in water)	Fresh orange
	Beverage	Diet soda	Artificially sweetened lemonade	Unsweetened iced tea
Dinner	2 meat	1 oz roast beef	Chili con carne (made with ½ cup ground beef, ½ cup pinto beans, and chili powder)	2 oz baked chicken
	1 bread	Baked potato (with 1 tsp margarine[†]		Corn on the cob with 1 tsp margarine
	Vegetable	Cooked carrots	Tossed salad and 1 tbs salad dressing[†]	Okra
	1 fruit	¾ cup strawberries	Fresh apple	Fruit cocktail (packed in water)
	1 milk	1 cup low-fat milk	1 cup low-fat milk	1 cup low-fat milk

*For 1000 calories, omit 1 fruit exchange and change low-fat milk to skim milk. For 1500 calories, add 1 meat, 1 fruit, and 2 fat exchanges; change low-fat milk to whole milk. For 1800 calories, add 2 bread, 3 meat, 3 fat, and 1 fruit exchanges; change low-fat milk to whole milk.

†One extra fat exchange allowed for each cup of 2% low-fat milk; 2 extra fat exchanges allowed for each cup of skim milk.

have been present longer, and the number of fat cells is often higher. As a result, more drastic dieting efforts and perseverance are necessary to achieve weight reduction.

Motivation is an essential ingredient for achievement of success. The obese patient must see the need for weight loss and weight control and the advantages that will accrue. The nurse can assist by helping the patient track eating patterns by keeping a diet diary. A frank discussion of eating habits helps the patient realize that often eating is the result of bad habits picked up with time and not of hunger. The bad habits must be changed, or weight loss will be only temporary.

Setting a realistic goal, such as losing 1 to 2 pounds per week, must be mutually agreed on at the outset. Trying to lose too much too fast usually results in a sense of frustration and failure for the patient. The nurse can help the patient understand that losing large amounts of weight in a short period of time causes skin and underlying tissue to lose elasticity and tone and become unsightly folds of flabby tissue. Slower weight loss offers better cosmetic results. Inevitably, the patient reaches plateau periods during which no weight is lost. These plateaus may last from several days to several weeks. It is especially important that the patient realize that these are normal occurrences during weight reduction, so that discouragement, frustration, and giving up of the prescribed dietary plan is prevented. A weekly check of body weight is a good method of monitoring progress. Daily weighing is not recommended because of the frequent fluctuations resulting from retained water (including urine) and elimination of feces. The patient should be instructed to record the weight at the same time each day, wearing the same type of clothing.

There is no firm agreement on the number of meals to be eaten when a person is on a diet. Some nutritionists advocate several small meals per day because the body's metabolic rate is temporarily increased immediately after eating. When several small meals a day are ingested, more calories are used. There seems to be general agreement that consumption of most of the daily caloric intake at a large evening meal results in less weight loss than when the calories are evenly distributed throughout the day.

When a person is first starting on a weight reduction program, food portions should be weighed in order to stay within the dietary guidelines. After a time, weighing may not be necessary because the patient can make more accurate judgments of size and weight. A list of permitted foods serves as a good reference and permits an occasional meal to be eaten at a restaurant. The patient who carefully follows the prescribed diet will not need to take vitamin supplements. Appropriate fluid intake should be encouraged. Alcoholic beverages are usually not permitted on a reducing diet because they increase the caloric intake and are low in nutritional value.

Exercise. Exercise is an essential part of a weight control program. There is no evidence that increased activity promotes an increase in appetite or leads to dietary excess. In fact, exercise frequently has the opposite effect.

The addition of exercise to diet intervention produces more weight loss than does dieting alone. Exercise has a favorable effect on body fat distribution, with a reduction in waist-to-hip ratio with increased exercise.

Exercise is especially important in maintaining weight loss in overweight persons. Overweight men and women who are active and fit have lower rates of morbidity and mortality than overweight persons who are sedentary and unfit. Therefore exercise is of benefit to overweight persons even if it does not make them lean.

Behavior-Cognitive Modification. For successful long-term weight loss management, behavior modification or cognitive therapy should be integrated into the management plan. Useful basic techniques include (1) self-monitoring, (2) stimulus control, and (3) rewards. Self-monitoring can focus on a record that shows what and when foods are eaten, as well as how the person was feeling when the foods were consumed. Stimulus control is aimed at separating events that trigger eating from the act of eating. Rewards may be used as incentive for weight loss. Short- and long-term goals are useful benchmarks for earning rewards. It is important that the reward for a specified weight loss not be associated with food, such as dinner out or a favorite treat. Reward items do not have to have a monetary component. For instance, time for a hot bath or an hour of pleasure reading would be an enjoyable reward for many people. People may participate in group or individual sessions, or both, as they work toward their goals.

Drug Therapy. Medications have been used in the treatment of obesity but only as adjuncts to a good diet and exercise program. Although effective and safe drugs are available for obesity treatment, multiple barriers exist to their proper and effective use. Adverse experiences with "diet drugs" such as amphetamines and fenfluramine have contributed to reluctance by health care providers and many in the public to explore newer pharmacologic agents that could be part of obesity treatment.

Appetite suppressant drugs reduce food intake through noradrenergic (drugs that mimic norepinephrine) or serotonergic mechanisms. Abuse of noradrenergic agents such as amphetamine, methamphetamine, and phenmetrazine has given the entire group of drugs a bad name. These drugs have been replaced by newer drugs, although no perfect drug currently exists. The chemical manipulation of amphetamine has resulted in drugs that have less risk for CNS stimulation and abuse but that have retained the appetite-suppressing effects. Drugs such as benzphetamine (Didrex) and phendimetrazine (Anorex, Obalan) are examples of this type of drug. Adverse effects of these drugs include palpitations, tachycardia, overstimulation, restlessness, dizziness, insomnia, weakness, and fatigue.

In 1998 the FDA approved sibutramine (Meridia) for use in management of obesity, including weight loss and maintenance of weight loss. This agent works by blocking the uptake of norepinephrine, serotonin, and dopamine centrally. These actions ultimately decrease appetite. Its use is recommended in conjunction with reduced calorie intake. Because this drug has been shown to increase blood pressure in some patients, blood pressure must be monitored in patients taking the drug. This drug should not be taken by patients with congestive heart failure, arrhythmias, or coronary artery disease.

In 1997 fenfluramine (Pondimin) and d-fenfluramine (Redux), serotonergic drugs that act as appetite suppressants, were recalled by the FDA after reported cardiac side effects, especially valvular heart disease. They are mentioned to advise patients that their use is dangerous.

Orlistat (Xenical), a new drug that was developed for weight loss and maintenance, works by blocking fat absorption in the intestine. It inhibits the action of pancreatic and gastric lipases. The undigested fat is excreted in the feces.

Because drugs will not cure obesity without substantial changes in food intake and increased physical activity, weight gain will occur when short-term drug therapy is stopped. Supervised long-term drug therapy with safe compounds can contribute to weight management, as well as loss. As with any pharmacologic treatment, there are side effects. Careful evaluation for the presence of other medical conditions can help determine which drugs, if any, would be advisable for a given patient.

The role of the nurse in relation to drug therapy should center around teaching the patient about proper administration and side effects and how the drugs fit into the larger weight loss plan. The modification of dosage without consultation with the physician or the nurse can have detrimental effects. The nurse should reemphasize that the diet and exercise regimens are the cornerstones of permanent weight loss. Medications may be helpful, but they do not help the patient change eating behavior. The purchase of over-the-counter diet aids should be discouraged. Emphasis here should be on the dangers of drug dependence and tolerance.

Even with a comprehensive action plan, there is a high rate of recidivism (weight regain) among all age-groups. For successful management of obesity, it helps if obesity is viewed as a chronic condition that needs day-to-day attention to maintain weight loss.

Collaborative Surgical Care

Many different types of surgical techniques have been described for treating obesity. These techniques can be classified as physical or mechanical (e.g., lipectomy), malabsorptive (e.g., gastric bypass), and regulator (e.g., banding gastroplasty). Though used in the past, jaw wiring and placement of an intragastric balloon are being used less frequently, if at all. Disappointing long-term results, complications from these techniques, and improved effectiveness of other surgical approaches, especially gastric bypasses, have made bypass surgeries the techniques of choice for morbid obesity.

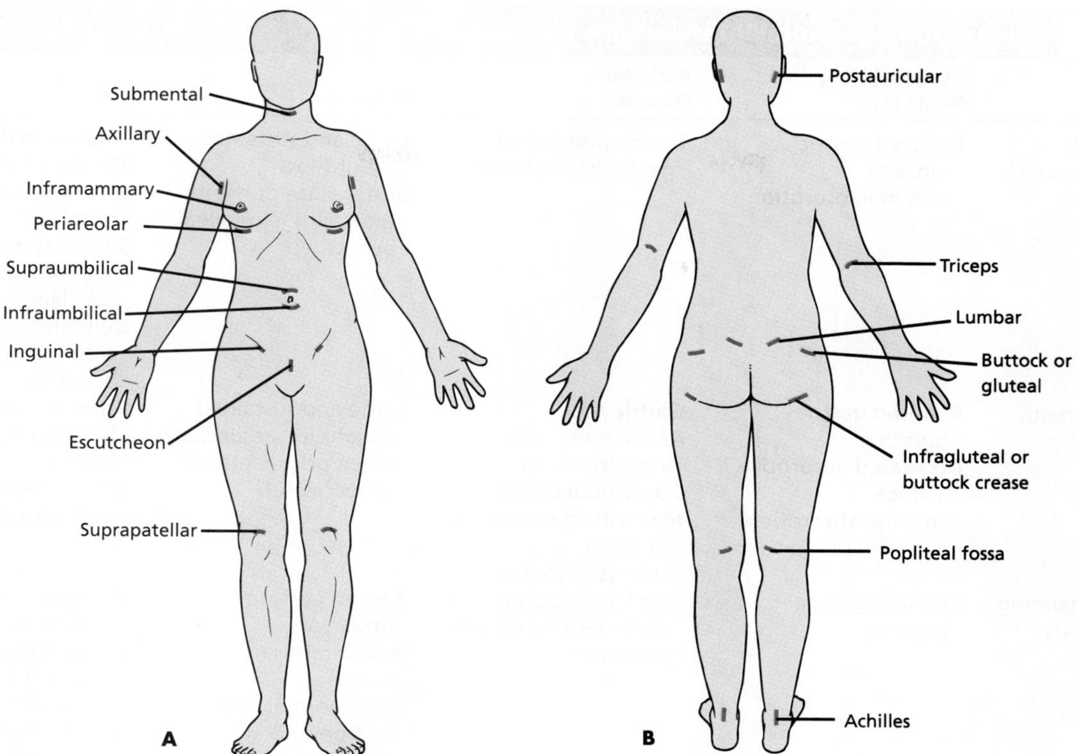

Fig. 38-8 Incision area for suction-assisted lipectomy.

For a patient to be selected for any of the operations for morbid obesity, the following criteria are considered:

1. Gross obesity for 5 years
2. Failure to reduce weight with other forms of therapy
3. Body weight 100% above the ideal for age, gender, and height
4. No serious endocrine problem causing the obesity
5. Absence of other medical conditions (liver disease, alcoholism, cardiovascular or pulmonary disease, inflammatory bowel disease, cancer)
6. Psychiatric and social stability and willingness to cooperate with long-term follow-up
7. Availability of a team of health care providers (nurses, physicians, dieticians) to provide immediate and long-term care
8. Presence of a high-risk condition (degenerative joint disease) that weight loss would ameliorate

Patients older than age 50 are frequently discouraged from seeking surgical treatment because the complications that accompany these procedures are more devastating with age.

Lipectomy. Lipectomy (adipectomy) is performed to remove unsightly flabby folds of adipose tissue. The patient who chooses adipectomies does so for cosmetic reasons. In some patients, up to 15% of the total fat cells are removed from the breasts, abdomen, and lumbar and femoral areas. There is no evidence that a regeneration of adipose tissue occurs at the surgical sites. However, it must be emphasized to the patient that surgical removal does not prevent obesity from recurring, especially if lifetime eating habits remain the same. Although body image and self-esteem may be enhanced by such procedures, these operations are not without complications. The dangerous effects of general anesthesia and the potential for poor wound healing in the obese patient cannot be overemphasized. It is more useful for the majority of patients contemplating adipectomy to be instructed in preventive health measures, such as slow weight reduction to maintain and preserve tissue integrity, the value of exercise, and behavior-modification techniques.

Liposuction. Another surgical procedure is liposuction, or suction-assisted lipectomy. The current use is for cosmetic purposes and not for weight reduction. This surgical intervention helps improve facial appearance or body contours. A candidate for this type of surgery is one who has achieved weight reduction but who has excess fat under the chin, along the jawline, in the nasolabial folds, over the abdomen, or around the waist and upper thighs. The procedure is relatively easy to perform and generally free of major complications; Fig. 38-8 shows incision areas for this procedure. A long, hollow, stainless steel cannula is inserted through a small incision over the fatty tissue to be suctioned. The purpose of this type of surgery is to improve body appearance, thereby enhancing body image and self-concept. It is not usually recommended for the older person because the skin is less elastic and will not accommodate to the new underlying shape.

Gastrointestinal Surgeries. Many different types of GI surgery have been tried for severe obesity and rejected primarily because of complications or because they were not effective. However, three procedures endorsed for clinical use are vertical banded gastroplasty, Roux-en-Y gastric bypass,[26] and

Table 38-24 Comparison of Surgical Interventions for Morbid Obesity

Procedure	Method of Weight Loss	Anatomic Changes	Advantages	Risks
▪ Roux-en-Y gastric bypass*	Reduced gastric capacity Some malabsorption	Gastric pouch and gastrojejunostomy	Large and sustained weight loss Better state of health than with jejunoileal bypass	Staple line dehiscence Marginal ulceration Altered gastric histology Stomal stenosis Iron, calcium, and cobalamin deficiency Dumping syndrome with refined carbohydrates
▪ Biliopancreatic diversion*	Reduced gastric capacity Decreased absorptive surface Some malabsorption	Gastric pouch Anastomosis to Y intestinal loop Duodenum closed Jejunum anastomosed to ileum cholecystectomy	Large and sustained weight loss, especially when prior methods unsuccessful	Same as above, for Roux-en-Y gastric bypass Protein-calorie malnutrition
▪ Vertical banding gastroplasty*	Reduced gastric capacity	Small gastric pouch along lesser stomach curvature	Easy to perform procedure Anastomosis not necessary More normal anatomy and physiology maintained	Disrupted staple line Stomach stenosis Dilated pouch Erosion at band into stomach (rare) Maladaptive eating (calorically dense food intake)

*See Fig. 38-9.

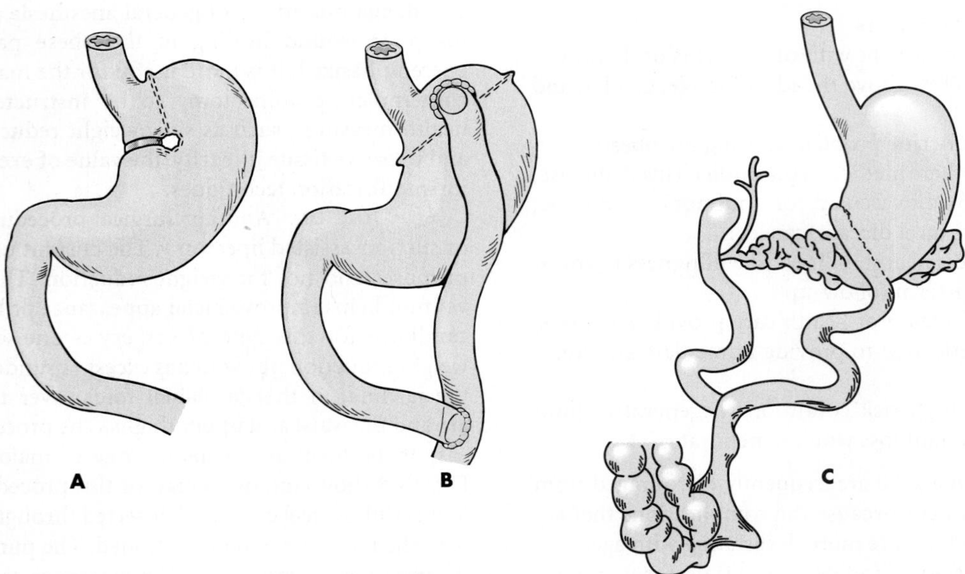

Fig. 38-9 Three gastrointestinal surgical procedures currently being used in the treatment of morbid obesity. **A,** Vertical banded gastroplasty consists of constructing a small pouch with a restricted outlet along the lesser curvature of the stomach. This outlet may be externally reinforced to prevent disruption or dilation. **B,** Roux-en-Y gastric bypass procedure involves constructing a proximal gastric pouch whose outlet is a Y-shaped limb of small bowel. **C,** Biliopancreatic diversion in addition to a proximal gastric pouch involves removal of gallbladder, closure of duodenum, and anastomosis of jejunum to the ileum.

biliopancreatic diversion[27] (Table 38-24 and Fig. 38-9). For these procedures, weight loss results depend more on the patient's motivation and behavior than on metabolic, GI, or technical factors.[27]

Surgical approaches within the GI tract have been directed toward either limiting food intake or producing malabsorption. An early surgery that led to malabsorption was the jejunoileal bypass.[27] This procedure resulted in excellent weight loss. However, because of frequent serious health-related complications, including electrolyte imbalance, osteoporosis, bypass enteritis, and liver failure, this surgery is no longer performed. Many patients had surgical procedures done to reverse the bypass. Nonetheless, a group of patients may still have a jejunoileal bypass in place.

Gastric bypass. The gastric bypass operation now being performed leads to weight loss by reducing food intake. Some malabsorption results. With the Roux-en-Y surgical procedure, the stomach size is decreased with a gastric pouch anastomosis emptying directly into the jejunum. Variations of this procedure include (1) stapling the stomach without transection to create a small, 30 to 45 ml gastric pouch; (2) creating an upper and a lower gastric pouch and totally disconnecting the pouches; and (3) creating an upper gastric pouch and completely removing the lower pouch. In the first two variations, the surgical changes can be reversed. The greatest rate of weight loss is usually achieved during the first year after surgery. Weight tends to stabilize after 18 months.[27] The chief contraindications to this surgical procedure are a history of peptic ulcer disease, coronary artery disease, malignant lesions, drug dependence, alcohol abuse, or psychiatric problems. A complication of this procedure is dumping syndrome, in which gastric contents empty too rapidly into the small intestine, overwhelming its ability to digest nutrients. This operation is more likely to cause iron or calcium deficiency and cobalamin hypovitaminosis, which can require lifelong supplementation.

Biliopancreatic diversion. Biliopancreatic diversion, introduced in 1968 by Scopinaro, is a more severe operation that may be used if other procedures are not successful.[28] In addition to a partial gastric resection, the gallbladder is removed, and bile and pancreatic juices are diverted into the ileum. With this surgery, there is greater potential for metabolic complications and nutritional deficiencies, including protein malnutrition.[28]

Vertical banded gastroplasty. Vertical banded gastroplasty is not used frequently to induce weight loss in the morbidly obese person. This approach leads to physical restriction of food intake. Previously, horizontal banding procedures were also done. However, lack of long-term weight loss coupled with complications such as disrupted staple lines and dilated pouch and stoma led to discontinuing the use of horizontal banding in the treatment of morbid obesity. In vertical banded gastroplasty, the stomach is partitioned into a small (usually about 30 ml) upper portion along the lesser curvature of the stomach. This small pouch drastically limits capacity. Additionally the stoma opening to the rest of the stomach is banded to delay emptying of solid food from the proximal pouch. This procedure has achieved considerable success in management of weight loss. Problems associated with gastric restriction operations include intractable vomiting from too rapid intake of solids,[29] distention of the wall of the proximal pouch, rupture of the staple line, and erosion of the band into the stomach.

Gastroplasty has some advantages over the gastric bypass operation for acceptable candidates. It is technically easier to perform, especially when stapling is used. If reversal of the procedure is required, removal of the staples is easier than the difficult procedure of converting the gastric bypass. In addition, symptoms of the dumping syndrome and malabsorption are eliminated. However, the weight loss record is often disappointing.[30]

NURSING MANAGEMENT: OBESE PATIENT

■ Nursing Assessment

The nurse, working closely with the physician and dietician, plays a major role in the planning and management of the obese patient. To be effective, the nurse must be aware of perceptions of and beliefs about obesity. If a care provider associates this condition with lack of will power and gluttony, the patient can experience shame in a setting that claims to be a caring one. By being sensitive when asking specific and leading questions, the nurse can often obtain information that the patient may withhold out of embarrassment or shyness or because of being a poor historian. Information that can assist the nurse in understanding an obese patient and provide a basis for intervention is presented in Table 38-25. The nurse must provide acceptable reasons for such personally intrusive questions, respond to the patient's concerns about diagnostic tests, and interpret test outcomes. The patient's answers to questions must be treated with respect, understanding, and a nonjudgmental attitude, regardless of negative personal feelings the nurse may have about obesity and working with "fat" people.

Anthropometric measurements are an integral part of the assessment of an obese person. The nurse may perform these measurements and explain their significance to the patient. Measurements used with the obese person include skinfold thickness, height, weight, and BMI. Accumulation of fat cells in the gluteal-femoral area may be metabolically inert, except during the latter part of pregnancy and during lactation. Android obesity, in which fat is distributed over the abdomen and upper body (neck, arms, and shoulders), is associated with a greater cardiovascular risk of hypertension, type 2 diabetes mellitus, dyslipidemia, ischemic heart disease, stroke, and death. The nurse should emphasize the importance of vigorous treatment of this type of obesity. The patient should be informed that gynecoid obesity carries a better prognosis but may be more difficult to reduce.

As part of the initial nursing physical assessment, each body system should be examined with particular attention to the organ system in which the patient has expressed a problem or concern. Providing specific documentation on these areas assists the physician with a more in-depth history and physical examination.

■ Nursing Diagnoses

Nursing diagnoses for the patient with obesity include, but are not limited to, the following:

- Altered nutrition: more than body requirements *related to* excessive intake in relation to metabolic need and decreased activity
- Impaired physical mobility *related to* excessive body weight

NURSING ASSESSMENT

Table 38-25 Obese Patient

Subjective Data

Important Health Information

Past health history: Time of obesity onset; diseases related to metabolism and obesity such as hypertension, cardiovascular problems, stroke, cancer, chronic joint pain, respiratory problems, diabetes mellitus, cholelithiasis

Medications: Thyroid preparations, diet pills

Surgery or other treatments: Weight reduction procedures

Functional Health Patterns

Health perception–health management: Family history of obesity; perception of problem; methods of weight loss attempted

Nutritional-metabolic: Amount and frequency of eating; overeating in response to boredom, stress, specific times or activities

Elimination: Constipation

Activity-exercise: Typical physical activity; drowsiness, somnolence; dyspnea on exertion, orthopnea, paroxysmal noctural dyspnea

Sleep-rest: Sleep apnea

Cognitive-perceptual: Feelings of rejection, isolation, guilt, or shame; meaning or value of food, compliance with prescribed reducing diets, degree of long-term commitment to a weight-loss program

Role-relationship: Change in financial status or family; personal, social, and financial resources to support a reducing diet

Sexuality-Reproductive: Menstrual irregularity, heavy menstrual flow in women, infertility; effect of obesity on sexual activity

Objective Data

General

Body mass index ≥ 30 kg/m^2; waist-to-hip ratio greater than 0.8 (women) or 1.0 (men), body weight 20% above ideal for height and frame, triceps skinfold greater than 25 (women) or 15 (men)

Respiratory

Hypoventilation

Cardiovascular

Hypertension

Musculoskeletal

Decreased joint mobility

Possible Findings

Elevated serum glucose, cholesterol, triglycerides; polycythemia

- Social isolation *related to* alterations in physical appearance and perceived unattractiveness
- Risk for impaired skin integrity *related to* alterations in nutritional state (obesity), immobility, excess moisture, and multiple skinfolds
- Ineffective breathing pattern *related to* decreased lung expansion from obesity
- Noncompliance *related to* alteration in perception or lack of motivation
- Body image disturbance *related to* deviation from usual or expected body size and inability to lose or retain weight loss

Planning

The overall goals are that the obese patient will (1) achieve weight loss to a specified level, (2) maintain weight loss at a specified level, (3) modify eating levels, and (4) participate in a regular physical activity program.

Nursing Implementation

Health Promotion. In collaboration with nutritionists, the nurse is in a prime position to participate in formal and informal health and nutritional teaching activities. This teaching can span the entire life span, including prenatal instruction. Targeting groups in the work setting is one way health promotion activities can be conducted and reinforced. Group competition within the work environment has been reported to offer moderate success for participants. Interrelated key factors are group support coupled with competition.

Acute Intervention

Preoperative care. Special considerations are necessary in the care of the patient who is admitted to the hospital for surgical treatment of obesity, especially the morbidly obese. Most nursing units are not prepared to meet the needs of a patient who is often too large for a typical hospital or recovery room bed or who has arms or legs that even a large-size blood pressure cuff will not fit. To eliminate embarrassment for the patient and frustration for the staff, plans for these special needs should be made before the patient's admission. Oversized blood pressure cuffs should be ready for use when the patient arrives. A private room may be necessary for privacy of the patient and to accommodate the bed and sitting arrangements. A strongly reinforced trapeze bar should be placed over the bed to facilitate movement and positioning. In some cases a specially constructed chair may have to be built and beds joined together to allow the patient to sit and sleep in comfort.

A care-planning conference should be a priority so that even simple nursing care measures do not become impossible tasks. Consideration should be given to questions such as how the patient will be weighed, how the patient will be transported throughout the hospital, and how simple physical assessment strategies may have to be adjusted to accommodate the morbidly obese patient. Anticipation of the need to use the hospital's meat or freight scales saves time and energy later for both the staff and the patient. Another need is a wheelchair with removable arms that is large enough to safely accommodate the patient and that will pass easily through doorways. Strategies for bathing, turning, and ambulating the patient, including the number of extra hands needed to carry out these measures, are invaluable when the actual need arises. Special gowns are also needed for the patient. Routine physical assessment strategies do not work well with a morbidly obese female patient who has numerous layers of skinfolds covering the chest and abdomen in addition to huge, pendulous breasts obscuring the area to be assessed. Without identifying alternatives or unique methods of dealing with this problem, assessment of respiratory status and bowel sounds or even wound inspection could be awkward for the nurse and embarrassing for the patient.

Wound infection is one of the most common complications after surgery. Because of the many layers of flabby skinfolds, especially in the abdominal area, preoperative skin preparation is important. Frequently the patient is instructed to take several showers a day for several days before admission to the hospital. Careful cleansing with soap and warm water of the abdominal area from the breasts to below the waist is emphasized.

The patient must be instructed in the proper coughing technique, deep breathing, and methods of turning and positioning to prevent pulmonary complications after surgery. The use of a spirometer may be introduced before surgery. Because most obese patients breathe shallowly, use of the spirometer helps prevent and alleviate postoperative lung congestion. Practicing these strategies preoperatively can aid in performing them correctly postoperatively.

All patients admitted for major bypass surgery, gastroplasty, or partitioning procedures have an NG tube inserted during surgery and attached to low suction after surgery. Allowing the patient to see a typical tube and explaining why it is necessary is a good method of involving the patient in the plan of care. The patient should know that oral nourishment will be impossible for a few days after the surgery and that IV fluids will be the main source of intake. Parenteral nutrition support may be necessary for some patients.

Early ambulation is mandatory for the obese patient. It is essential that the patient know that it is usually necessary to get out of bed soon after surgery and with increasing frequency thereafter, generally three to four times each day. The dangers of thrombophlebitis and measures to counteract its development are a routine part of preoperative teaching. The patient should know that elastic stockings, elastic compression stockings, or elastic wraps will be applied to the legs and that active and passive range-of-motion exercises will be a frequent part of daily care. Low-dose heparin often will be ordered. (General preoperative nursing care is discussed in Chapter 16.)

Postoperative care. The patient experiences considerable abdominal pain after surgery. Administration of pain medications should be given as frequently as necessary during the immediate postoperative period. If pain medication is not given by patient-controlled analgesia (PCA), the nurse must remember that IM medications must be given with an extra-long needle, such as a spinal needle, so that the medication is administered into the muscle and not into the adipose or subcutaneous tissue, which will delay absorption. Because prevention of pulmonary complications is a major nursing goal, it can be anticipated that the patient will not fully cooperate with respiratory strategies. In addition, the large amount of truncal adipose tissue, especially on the abdomen and chest, compromises respiratory ability. Keeping the head of the bed elevated at a 30-degree angle at all times facilitates ventilatory efforts. Encouraging and assisting the patient to turn, cough, and deep breathe at least every 1 to 2 hours minimizes the risk for atelectasis and pneumonia. Frequent mouth and nose care also helps breathing efforts because the NG tube is inserted through one nostril.

Position changes and range-of-motion exercises are instituted immediately after surgery and carried out every 1 to 2 hours. Ambulatory efforts generally are begun on the evening of surgery. For patient safety, the nurse should enlist the assistance of other staff members during these initial efforts, while encouraging the patient to help.

The abdominal wound requires frequent observation for the amount and type of drainage, condition of the sutures, and signs of infection. The incision must be protected against undue straining that accompanies turning and coughing. Wound dehiscence and wound healing are potential problems for all obese patients. Monitoring the vital signs assists in identifying problems such as infection.

It is important that the NG tube be kept patent and in the correct position. Vomiting is common following gastroplasty, gastric bypass, and gastric partitioning procedures. If patency is blocked or the tube requires repositioning, the physician should be notified at once. The upper gastric pouch is small (usually 15 to 40 ml), and irrigating the tube with too much solution or manipulating tube position can lead to disruption of the anastomosis or staple line. In most cases the NG tube can be removed in approximately 48 hours, or when bowel sounds have resumed.

Skin care should be carried out several times each shift. Perspiration may be excessive at times. The many layers of flabby skin should be kept clean and dry so that this source of irritation is eliminated. The patient who has gastric bypass may experience severe diarrhea early in the postoperative period. This is caused by malabsorption created by surgical shortening of the small intestine. Meticulous care should be taken of the skin around the anal area, and antidiarrheal medications should be administered immediately. For the patient who has an indwelling catheter, perineal care is important so that a urinary tract infection can be avoided.

Clear liquids are given orally when tolerance is established. The amount offered at first is necessarily limited to approximately 1 ounce, which is to be sipped slowly. More solid types of food are given to the patient who has had bypass surgery as progress is made through the postoperative recovery period. The patient who has had gastroplasty surgery is kept on a fluid diet for a longer time. The need for a liquid diet only is based on the rationale that the ingestion of too much fluid or foods can cause disruption of the staple or suture line, leading to leakage and possible peritonitis.

Discharge teaching. The patient who has undergone major surgical treatment for obesity has not, in the past, been successful in following or maintaining a prescribed diet. Now the patient is forced to reduce the oral intake as a result of the anatomic changes brought about by the operation. This patient finds that adherence to a reduced intake is necessary because of the concern for abdominal distention, cramping abdominal pain, increased and foul-smelling flatus, and frequent diarrhea.

Weight loss is considerable during the first 6 to 12 months. More weight is lost by those who have bypass surgery than by those who undergo gastric partitioning procedures. It is during this time that the patient must learn to adjust intake sufficiently to maintain a stable weight. Although behavior modification was not an intended outcome when these surgical procedures were devised, it becomes an unexpected secondary gain. The diet generally prescribed should be high in protein and low in carbohydrates, fat, and roughage and consist of six small feedings daily. Fluids should not be ingested with the meal, and in some cases, fluids should be restricted to less than 1000 ml per day. Fluids and foods high in carbohydrate tend to promote diarrhea and symptoms of the dumping syndrome. Generally calorically dense foods (foods high in fat) should be avoided to permit more nutritionally sound food to be consumed.

Vitamin deficiencies are a long-term concern after bypass surgery because of the induced malabsorption and the body's inability to absorb important vitamins such as vitamins A, C, and D. Parenteral cobalamin supplements are usually prescribed on a permanent basis because absorption of this vitamin takes place in the ileum. Ileal absorption capacity is drastically reduced by the surgical intestinal bypass. The patient should be aware of the signs and symptoms of vitamin deficiencies, as well as of electrolyte imbalances (see Table 38-8). It is often necessary to replace iron, calcium, and potassium to maintain required physiologic levels.

Proper diet and use of antidiarrheal medications must be clearly understood by the patient. Late complications can be anticipated after gastric bypass or gastroplasty, including anemia, vitamin deficiencies, diarrhea, and psychiatric problems. Failure to lose weight or loss of too much weight may be caused by the surgical formation of too large a stomach pouch or of an outlet that is much too small, respectively. Peptic ulcer formation, dumping syndrome, and small bowel obstruction may be seen late in the recovery and rehabilitative stage.

Long-term follow-up care must be stressed, in part because of complications late in the recovery period. The patient must be encouraged to adhere strictly to the prescribed diet and to keep the physician informed of any changes in physical or emotional condition. Some patients have been known to overeat when they return home and to gain rather than lose weight.

Reversal of the surgical procedures may be required for some patients. Reversal of the gastric bypass may be difficult because of the technical nature of the procedure. Reasons for revisional surgery include hepatic failure, weight loss below ideal weight, debilitating weakness, severe psychiatric problems, intractable electrolyte deficiencies, pulmonary tuberculosis, and renal failure.

The nurse must anticipate and recognize several potential psychologic problems after surgery. Some patients express guilt feelings concerning the fact that the only way they could lose weight was by surgical means rather than by the "sheer will power" of reduced dietary intake. The nurse should be ready to provide support so that this patient does not dwell on negative feelings.

Many morbidly obese patients who blamed their feelings of social inferiority or inadequacies on their appearance before bypass surgery may suffer from episodes of depression. By 6 to 8 months after surgery, considerable weight loss has occurred, and they are able to see clearly how much their appearance has changed. Massive weight loss often leaves the patient with large quantities of flabby skin that result in problems of both body image and hygiene. Reconstructive surgery at least 1 full year after the initial surgery may alleviate this unsightly situation. Reduction of the breasts, upper arms, thighs, and excess abdominal skinfolds are possible solutions. Discussion of this possible outcome with the patient before surgery and again during the rehabilitation phase of recovery helps facilitate the patient's adjustment to a new body image and social reintegration.

Ambulatory and Home Care

Physical activity teaching. Once a physical activity program has been outlined for the patient, the nurse can reinforce instruction and help individualize it to the patient's time schedule and physical limitations. The nurse should point out that engaging in weekend exercise only or in spurts of strenuous activity is not advantageous and can actually be dangerous. Joining a health club can be one mechanism of getting exercise. However, sitting in a sauna and trying to spot-reduce a specific part of the body do not constitute an appropriate daily physical activity program. Walking, swimming, and cycling are more sensible forms of exercise and have more long-term benefits. The combination of a good reducing diet and an increased physical activity program can have profound effects on the patient's achievement of weight loss. When large muscles are involved in the exercise program, a primary benefit is cardiovascular conditioning.

Many psychologic benefits can be derived from an increased physical activity program. Reduction in tension and stress, better-quality sleep and rest, decreased desire to eat excessively, increased stamina and energy, improved self-concept and self-confidence, better attitudes toward work and play, and increased optimism about the future can be achieved.

Behavior-modification and cognitive training. The person who is on any type of restrictive dietary program is often encouraged to join a group of other obese persons who are receiving professional counseling to help them modify their eating habits. The assumption behind behavior modification is that obesity is a learned disorder caused by overeating, and that the critical difference between an obese person and a nonobese person are the cues that stimulate eating behavior. Therefore most behavior-modification programs deemphasize the diet and focus on how and when the person eats. Participants often are taught to restrict their eating to designated meals and to increase the amount of physical activity in their lives. Persons who have undergone behavior therapy are more successful in maintaining their losses over an extended time than those who do not participate in such training.

Many self-help groups are available to the person who wants to learn more about successful dieting and who likes the support of others having the same problems and experiences. Take Off Pounds Sensibly (TOPS) is the oldest nonprofit organization of this type. Behavioral modification is an integral part of the program, along with nutrition education. Weight Watchers International, Inc., is probably the most successful commercial weight-reduction enterprise. Weight Watchers offers a food plan that is nutritionally balanced and practical to follow, and it has used behavior-modification techniques since 1974. Other self-help groups and organizations are Overeaters Anonymous; Weight Losers; Trim Clubs, Inc.; and the Diet Workshop, Inc. These groups offer diet education, exercise plans, and behavior modification.

There has been a proliferation of commercial weight-reduction centers across the nation. Many of these programs are staffed by nurses or nutritionists, or both, and require an initial physical examination by a physician before a candidate is accepted for weight reduction. These weight-reduction centers are costly and therefore are cost prohibitive for those with limited financial resources. Many of these programs also offer special prepackaged foods and supplements that must be purchased as part of the weight-reduction plan. Only these prescribed foods and drinks are to be consumed until an agreed-on amount of weight is lost. The patient is encouraged to buy the same type of foods for the maintenance phase of the program, lasting from 6 months to 1 year. Behavior-modification training is incorporated within these programs as well. Research has shown that, regardless of the commercial products used, successful weight loss and control were limited and required individualized programs consisting of restricted caloric intake, behavior modification, and exercise.[29] Although persons who follow this type of program are likely to lose weight, once they leave the program the weight is usually regained because they tend to resume previous eating behaviors and return to the foods previously eaten.

A new concept of influencing health behavior and better employee health has occurred recently. Programs on health teaching and maintenance have been started at places of employment. The rationale for such programs is that better health repays the cost of the programs through improved work performance, decreased absenteeism, and eventually less hospitalization. Weight-reduction and hypertension-reduction programs have been instituted and are popular with employees.

Evaluation

The expected outcomes are that the obese patient will

- experience long-term weight loss
- have improvement in obesity-related comorbidities
- integrate healthy practices into daily routines
- monitor for adverse side effects of surgical therapy

CRITICAL THINKING EXERCISES

CASE STUDY

Obesity

Patient Profile

Mrs. R. is a 60-year old woman who is 5′ 4″ tall and weighs 190 pounds.

Subjective Data

- Reports gradual weight gain during past 40 years
- Spends most of her free time watching television
- Reports health problems related to type 2 diabetes mellitus, shortness of breath, hypertension, and chest pressure
- Had knee replacement surgery at age 56

Objective Data

Physical Examination

- Has obese, nontender, soft abdomen
- BP is 150/90

Laboratory Results

- Fasting blood glucose 250 mg/dl (13.9 mmol/L)
- Total cholesterol 205 mg/dl (5.3 mmol/L)
- Triglyceride 298 mg/dl (3.36 mmol/L)
- HDL cholesterol 31 mg/dl (0.8 mmol/L)

Critical Thinking Questions

1. What are Mrs. R.'s obesity risk factors?
2. What is her estimated BMI (use Fig. 38-7)?
3. What are the primary types of body fat distribution? Which type do you think Mrs. R. has, and why?
4. Of the possible complications of obesity, which ones does Mrs. R. have? What is the pathophysiology of Mrs. R.'s type 2 diabetes mellitus? Of her cardiovascular symptoms? Of her knee replacement surgery?
5. What would you, as the nurse, include in a successful weight loss and weight management program for Mrs. R.?
6. Is Mrs. R. a candidate for surgical intervention for obesity? If so, why? If not, why not?
7. Based on the assessment data presented, write one or more appropriate nursing diagnoses. Are there any collaborative problems?

NURSING RESEARCH ISSUES

1. What impact does rapid gastric emptying of protein have on protein absorption, protein utilization, and subsequent nutritional status?
2. What mechanisms beyond physical activity maintain body weight in obese people when they generally consume fewer carbohydrates than do slender people?
3. How can fat-soluble vitamins be maintained within the RDA when population groups increase their use of fat substitutes in dietary patterns?
4. What happens to serum calcium and bone density in vegetarian patients over time?
5. What is the effect of surgical procedures for obesity on the quality of life or on functional abilities?
6. Does early enteral feeding reduce the risk of sepsis in critically ill patients?
7. Are there valid and reliable bedside methods for determining NG and NI tube placement?
8. What are the ways to reduce the risk of catheter sepsis in a patient receiving TPN?
9. What characteristics (medical condition, antibiotic therapy) are associated with diarrhea in the patient receiving tube feeding?

REVIEW QUESTIONS

The number of the question corresponds to the same-numbered objective at the beginning of the chapter.

1. The nurse identifies a need for dietary teaching for the patient whose daily intake of food groups consists of
   a. 2 to 4 servings of the fruit group.
   b. 2 to 3 servings of the milk, yogurt, and cheese group.
   c. 4 to 5 servings of the bread, cereal, rice, and pasta group.
   d. 2 to 3 servings of the meat, poultry, fish, beans, egg, and nut group.
2. In general, nutrient or food interactions with medications can result in all of the following except
   a. enhancing drug absorption.
   b. retarding drug bioavailability.
   c. increasing a nutrient requirement.
   d. all of the above can happen.
3. During the first 24 hours of starvation the order in which the body obtains substrate for energy is
   a. glycogen, skeletal protein.
   b. visceral protein, fat stores, glycogen.
   c. fat stores, skeletal protein, visceral protein.
   d. liver protein, muscle protein, visceral protein.
4. The nurse recognizes that the major goal of treatment for a patient with anorexia nervosa is being met when the patient
   a. demonstrates a rapid weight gain.
   b. consumes the required daily intake of nutrients.
   c. commits to long-term individual and family counseling.
   d. verbalizes feelings regarding self-image and fears of becoming obese.
5. A nutritionally stressed patient weighing 60 kg is receiving nothing by mouth (NPO) and total parenteral nutrition (TPN). In evaluating the patient's nutritional intake the nurse calculates that the daily TPN solution should provide
   a. 40 g fat.
   b. 80 g protein.
   c. 20 calories per kilogram.
   d. 1000 calories from carbohydrate.
6. One advantage of a percutaneous endoscopic gastrostomy tube placement relative to nasogastric feedings for the patient receiving long-term enteral nutrition is that
   a. it increases patient comfort.
   b. it eliminates the risk of aspiration.
   c. feedings can be initiated before bowel sounds are present.
   d. more calories can be delivered as compared with nasogastric feeding.
7. The obesity aspect that is most often associated with cardiovascular health problems is
   a. primary obesity.
   b. secondary obesity.
   c. gynoid fat distribution.
   d. android fat distribution.
8. A morbidly obese patient has undergone Roux-en-Y gastric bypass surgery. In planning postoperative care the nurse anticipates that the patient
   a. may have severe diarrhea early in the postoperative period.
   b. will not be allowed to ambulate for 5 to 7 days postoperatively.
   c. will require nasogastric suction until healing of the site occurs.
   d. may have only liquids orally, and in very limited amounts, during the postoperative period.

References

1. VanItallie TB: Prevalence of obesity, *Endocrinol Metab Clin North Am* 25:887, 1996.
2. Townsend CD: *Nutrition and diet therapy,* Albany, NY, 1994, Delmar.
3. Food and Nutrition Board, National Research Council, National Academy of Sciences: *Recommended dietary allowances,* ed 10, Washington DC, 1989, National Academy Press.
4. Barrett S: Nutrition quakery, *Sci Med* 4:6, 1997.
5. Garfinkel P, Kennedy S, Kaplan A: Views on classification and diagnosis of eating disorders, *Can J Psychiatry* 40:445, 1995.
6. Gard M, Freeman C: The dismantling of a myth: a review of eating disorders, *Int J Eat Disord* 20:1, 1996.
7. Rock C, Curran-Celentano J: Nutritional management of eating disorders, *Psychiatr Clin North Am* 19:701, 1996.
8. Morreale SJ, Schwartz NE: Helping Americans eat right: developing practical and actionable public nutrition education messages based on the ADA survey of American dietary habits, *J Am Diet Assoc* 95:305,1995.
9. *Surgeon General's report on nutrition and health,* Rocklin, Calif, 1989, Prima Publishing and Communications.
10. McWhirter JP, Pennington CR: Incidence and recognition of malnutrition in hospital patients, *BMJ* 308:945, 1994.
11. Forloines-Lynn S: How to smooth the way for cyclic tube feedings, *Nursing* 50:57, 1996.
12. Caring for a gastrostomy: guidelines and troubleshooting tips, *Nursing* 24:48, 1994.
13. ASPEN Board of Directors: Guidelines for the use of parenteral and enteral nutrition in adult and pediatric patients, *JPEN J Parenter Enteral Nutr* 17:21SA, 1993.
14. Shuster MH: Parenteral nutrition. In Hennessey KA, Orr ME, editors: *Nutrition support nursing core curriculum,* ed 3, Silver Spring, Md, 1996, ASPEN.
15. Bradford S: Method of nutritional support. In Mahan LK, Escott-Stump S, editors: *Krause's food, nutrition, and diet,* ed 9, Philadelphia, 1996, Saunders.
16. Dwyer J: Policy and healthy weight, *Prev Med* 25:30, 1996.
17. Update: prevalence of overweight among children, adolescents, and adults—United States, 1988-1994, *MMWR Morb Mortal Wkly Rep* 46:199, 1997.
18. Bray G: Obesity: part 1—pathogenesis, *West J Med* 149:431, 1988.
19. Dwyer J: Medical evaluation and class of obesity. In Blackburn GL, Kanders BS, editors: *Obesity pathophysiology, psychology and treatment,* New York, 1994, Chapman & Hall.
20. Trayburn P: Socratic debate: obesity is predominantly a problem of food intake—the case against. In Angel A and others, editors: *Progress in obesity research,* London, 1996, John Libbey.
21. Allison DB and others: A genetic analysis of relative weight among 4020 twin pairs with an emphasis on sex effects, *Health Psychol* 13:362, 1994.
22. Roberts S, Greenberg A: The new obesity genes, *Nutr Rev* 54:41, 1996.
23. Weigle DS, Kuijoer J: Obesity genes and the regulation of body fat content, *Bioessays* 18:867, 1996.
24. Angel A and others, editors: *Progress in obesity research,* London, 1996, John Libbey.
25. Heshka S, Buhl K, Heymsfield SB: Obesity: clinical evaluation of body composition and energy expenditure. In Blackburn GL, Kanders BS, editors: *Obesity pathophysiology, psychology, and treatment,* New York, 1994, Chapman & Hall.
26. NIH, NHLBI: *Clinical guidelines on the identification of overweight and obesity in adults: the evidence report,* 1998, NIH, Bethesda, MD.
27. Benotti PN, Forse RA: The role of gastric surgery in the multidisciplinary management of severe obesity, *Am J Surg* 169:361, 1995.
28. Scopinaro N and others: Biolipopancreatic diversion for obesity at 18 years, *Surgery* 119:261, 1996.
29. Kolanowski J: Surgical treatment for morbid obesity, *Br Med Bull* 53:433, 1997.
30. Brolin RE: Update: NIH consensus conference. Gastrointestinal surgery for severe obesity, *Nutrition* 12:403, 1996.

Resources

American Society for Parenteral and Enteral Nutrition
8630 Fenton Street, Suite 412
Silver Spring, MD 20910
301-587-6215
http://www.clinnutr.org/

American Association of Family and Consumer Sciences
1555 King Street
Alexandria, VA 22314
703-706-4600
fax: 703-706-4663
http://www.aafcs.org

American Dietetic Association—Government Affairs
The American Dietetic Association
216 W. Jackson Blvd.
Chicago, IL 60606-6995
312-899-0040
fax: 312-899-1979
http://www.eatright.org

American Society for Clinical Nutrition/American Society for Nutritional Sciences and *The American Journal of Clinical Nutrition*
9650 Rockville Pike
Bethesda, MD 20814-3998
301-530-7110
fax: 301-571-1863
http://www.faseb.org/ascn/

Food and Nutrition Information Center
Agricultural Research Service, USDA
National Agricultural Library, Room 304
10301 Baltimore Avenue
Beltsville, MD 20705-2351
301-504-5719
fax: 301-504-6409
http://www.nal.usda.gov/fnic

FDA Center for Food Safety and Applied Nutrition
200 C Street SW
Washington, DC 20204
http://vm.cfsan.fda.gov/index.html

Nutrition Links—Kansas State University
http://www.oznet.ksu.edu/ext_f&n/nutlink/n2.htm

***For additional Internet resources, see the website for this book at* www.mosby.com/MERLIN/medsurg_lewis**

REMEMBER to check out your **companion CD-ROM**

39 NURSING MANAGEMENT Upper Gastrointestinal Problems

Margaret M. Heitkemper

www.mosby.com/MERLIN/medsurg_lewis

LEARNING OBJECTIVES

1. Describe the etiology, prevention, and treatment of common dental problems.
2. Describe the etiology, clinical manifestations, and treatment of common oral inflammations and infections.
3. Describe the etiology, clinical manifestations, complications, collaborative care, and nursing management of carcinoma of the oral cavity.
4. Describe the nursing management after surgical stabilization of a mandibular fracture.
5. Explain the types, pathophysiology, clinical manifestations, complications, and collaborative care, including surgical therapy, of gastroesophageal reflux disease and hiatal hernia.
6. Describe the nursing management of the patient with gastroesophageal reflux disease and hiatal hernia.
7. Explain the pathophysiology, clinical manifestations, complications, collaborative care, and nursing management of cancer of the esophagus.
8. Describe the clinical manifestations, complications, and management of esophageal diverticula, achalasia, esophageal strictures, and esophagitis.
9. Describe the pathogenesis, complications, collaborative care, and nursing management of nausea and vomiting.
10. Differentiate between acute and chronic gastritis, including the causes, pathophysiology, collaborative care, and nursing management.
11. Explain the common causes, clinical manifestations, collaborative care, and nursing management of upper gastrointestinal bleeding.
12. Compare and contrast gastric and duodenal ulcers, including pathogenesis, clinical manifestations, complications, and collaborative and nursing management.
13. Explain the anatomic and physiologic changes and the common complications that result from surgical procedures for gastric and duodenal ulcers.
14. Describe the clinical manifestations and collaborative, surgical, and nursing management of cancer of the stomach.
15. Identify the common types of food poisoning and the nursing responsibilities related to food poisoning.

Ingestion is the process of taking food and fluids into the body via the gastrointestinal (GI) tract. It begins in the mouth with mastication of food by the teeth. Food then passes down the esophagus and into the stomach. It is important that sufficient nutrients be ingested to meet bodily needs. Oral problems, such as poor dental health, infections and inflammations, and cancer, interfere with ingestion. Esophageal problems may also interfere with swallowing food and fluids and with passage of food to the stomach.

Digestion is the breakdown of foodstuffs to smaller components so that absorption of nutrients can occur. Problems with the stomach and, to a greater extent, the small intestine can profoundly impact the nutritional status of the patient. The older individual is particularly vulnerable to problems related to alterations in both ingestion and digestion.

Reviewed by Diane Britt, RN, MN, CS, CDE, Medical-Surgical Clinical Nurse Specialist, University of Washington Medical Center, Seattle, Wash.

DENTAL PROBLEMS

Dental Caries

Dental caries (decay of teeth) is a general term applied to the decalcification of the mineral components and dissolution of the organic matrix of the teeth. Cavity formation is the clinical evidence of the progression of this process. Although there has been a marked decline in dental caries in recent years, it remains a problem that affects millions of individuals, particularly those from lower socioeconomic groups.[1]

Caries development starts when *plaque* builds up and adheres to the teeth. Plaque is a gelatinous substance consisting of bacteria, saliva, and epithelial cells. The tight adherence of plaque to the teeth provides protection for the bacteria (usually *lactobacilli* and *Streptococcus mutans*). Within 30 minutes after eating, these bacteria produce acids from the breakdown of sugars in food deposits on the teeth. The acids destroy the outer enamel and, later, the underlying dentin of the tooth (Fig. 39-1). The decay proceeds and can progress to the pulp of the tooth.

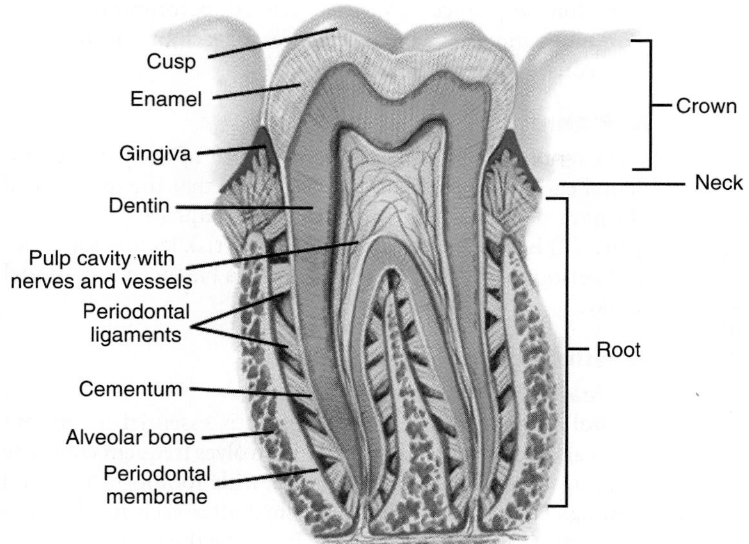

Fig. 39-1 Normal tooth structure.

If the decay is not treated, a *pulpitis* develops and extends to the alveolar bone, forming an abscess. This results in pain, facial edema, and sometimes malaise and fever. During the early stages of pulpitis, pain may be induced by temperature changes, especially cold drinks. In the later stages of pulpitis, heat or reclining may stimulate the onset of severe pain. At this stage, damage to the pulp is irreversible. Treatment consists of tooth removal or root canal therapy (removal of the pulp and filling of the pulp canal with inert material).

Periodontal Disease

The *periodontium* is the tissue surrounding and supporting the teeth. It is composed of the gingivae (gums), cementum, alveolar bone, and the periodontal ligament, which helps to fix the tooth firmly in its bony socket. Periodontal disease is the major cause of tooth loss in adults. The majority of adults have some form of periodontal disease.[1] Periodontal disease begins with gingivitis and eventually involves the periodontal ligament and the alveolar bone. Periodontal disease is the clinical result of a complex interplay between bacterial infection and host response often modified by bacterial factors.[2]

Dental plaque is the most important etiologic factor in periodontal disease. When plaque calcifies, it forms *calculus,* which is a hard, tenacious mass on the crowns of teeth. *Malocclusion* (faulty relationships between the teeth when the jaws are closed), margins of overextended fillings, and impacted food are other etiologic factors that can cause local irritation to the gingivae. Systemic conditions such as poorly controlled diabetes mellitus, thyroid diseases, pregnancy, HIV infection, and vitamin and nutritional deficiencies may modify the person's response to the local etiologic factors and make them more susceptible to periodontal disease. The exact role of systemic conditions is unknown.

Certain drugs cause changes, such as inflammation and hyperplasia of the gingiva, which may be related to periodontal disease. A common drug known to produce these effects is phenytoin (Dilantin). Smoking is a known risk factor for periodontal disease.[2]

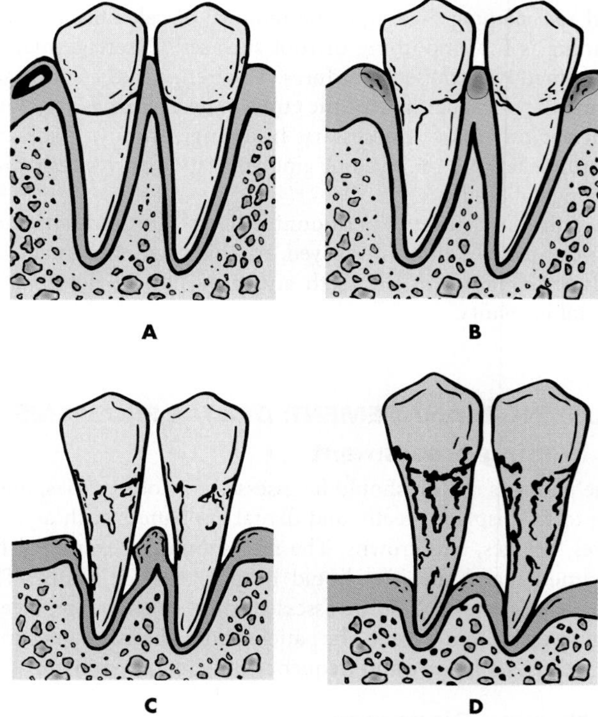

Fig. 39-2 Progression of periodontal disease. **A,** Calculus deposits on teeth at gingival line, causing gingivitis. **B,** Gingivae become swollen and tender with spread of inflammation. **C,** Inflammation spreads and pockets develop between teeth and gingivae, which are receding. **D,** The alveolar bone is destroyed and teeth become loose.

When the gingivae are irritated, they become inflamed (Fig. 39-2). The inflammation causes the gingiva to separate from the surface of the tooth. Pockets created between the teeth and the gingivae can collect pus and bacteria (periodontitis). At this stage, bleeding occurs easily, and pus may ooze from the gingiva. Gradually the bone supporting the teeth is destroyed, and

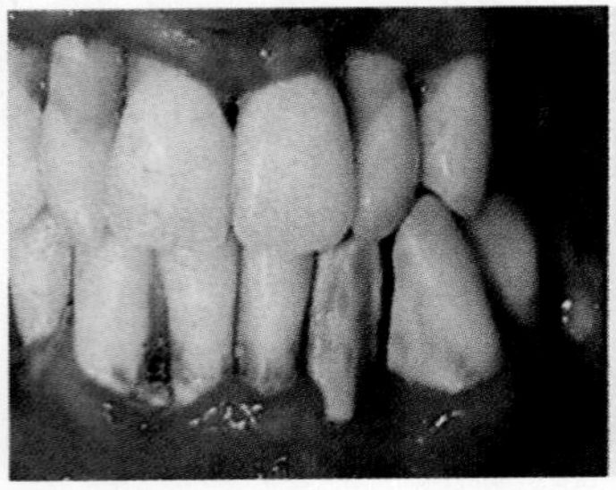
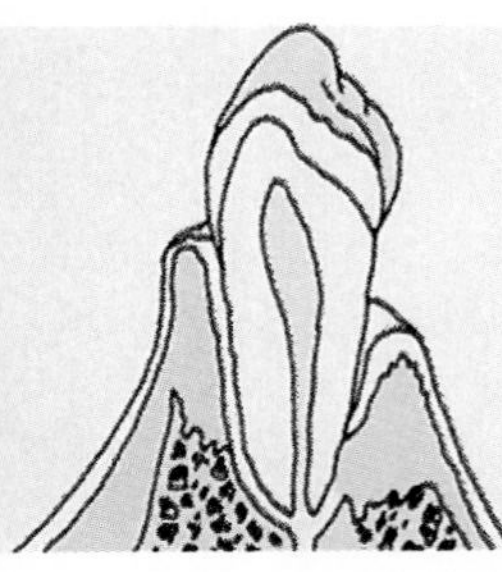

Fig. 39-3 Periodontitis. Signs include edema, periodontal abscess, hemorrhage on slight pressure, tissue recession with retraction of gingival margin, color change from light pink to deep red, loss of tissue in interdental area, horizontal bone loss, and widening of periodontal space.

the teeth become loose. As the periodontal pockets deepen and seal themselves off, periodontal abscesses may occur (Fig. 39-3). At this stage the usual treatment is extraction of the involved tooth or teeth.

Early treatment of periodontal disease consists of *scaling* and *root planing*. Scaling is the removal of calculus, and root planing is the smoothing of root surfaces. Curettage may be combined with these procedures. This removes the soft tissue lining the pocket and helps the gums to heal. *Gingivectomy* and *gingivoplasty* may be necessary. In a gingivectomy, tissue and deep pockets are removed. A gingivoplasty involves reshaping of gingival tissue.

In the later stages of periodontal disease, the bone supporting the teeth is often destroyed. At this stage, treatment involves extraction of the teeth and provision of dentures or dental implants.

NURSING MANAGEMENT: DENTAL PROBLEMS

■ Nursing Assessment

The patient's mouth should be assessed for tooth caries, missing teeth, displaced teeth, and dental appliances such as dentures, bridges, and crowns. The face should be examined for symmetry, and the jaw should be palpated for lumps. The gingivae (gums) should be assessed for redness, pallor, bleeding, recession, and ulcers. The patient should be asked questions regarding dental care and frequency of dental examinations.

■ Nursing Diagnoses

Nursing diagnoses for the patient with dental problems include, but are not limited to, the following:

- Altered oral mucous membrane *related to* caries, ineffective oral hygiene, periodontal disease, or ill-fitting dentures
- Altered nutrition: less than body requirements *related to* inability to ingest adequate nutrients because of ill-fitting dentures, displaced teeth, gingival disease, dental caries, sensitive teeth, edentulous condition, or oral pain
- Body image disturbance *related to* change in appearance of or unattractive teeth, difficulty with eating, or halitosis
- Noncompliance *related to* altered perception, lack of motivation, inadequate finances, or lack of knowledge of consequences of noncompliance

■ Planning

The overall goals of nursing management of the patient with dental caries and periodontal disease are that the patient will (1) have a decrease in caries through improved dental hygiene, (2) be able to identify and reduce risk factors for caries and periodontal diseases, and (3) have a balanced nutritional intake.

■ Nursing Implementation

Health Promotion

Oral hygiene. Proper oral hygiene is essential to prevent caries and periodontal disease. This involves frequent complete cleaning of the teeth and gingivae with toothbrushing and flossing. The teeth should be brushed after each meal with a soft, rounded-bristle toothbrush. Brushing the teeth should remove food debris and plaque and stimulate the gingivae. The teeth should be brushed by first placing the bristles of the toothbrush next to the gum line and then brushing with a motion away from the gum line.

Flossing should be done at least once a day. It is an important measure to remove plaque between teeth, an area that is not easily accessible when brushing. Flossing is done by gently forcing the floss between the teeth and moving the floss up and down the tooth surface a few times until it reaches the gum line.

During illness the patient may not salivate as usual, thereby reducing the natural cleaning process of the teeth and mouth. The nurse may need to assume responsibility for dental care and oral hygiene. Swabbing the patient's mouth and rinsing it with mouthwash are inadequate measures. Mechanical cleansing is essential to remove the plaque. Either a regular or an electric toothbrush should be used on all surfaces to remove plaque and mechanically stimulate the gingivae to increase blood supply. The patient's mouth should be assessed each time oral care is given.

Dental examinations. Regular, periodic dental examinations are important to maintain a healthy mouth and teeth. At the time of a dental examination a thorough cleaning with removal of plaque and calculus is done. Caries and early signs of periodontal disease can be detected and treated. The mouth is examined for any signs of oral cancer. For most adults, an examination every 6 to 12 months is adequate. Some persons may require more frequent visits. Persons at risk for infective endocarditis (e.g., those with prolapsed mitral valve) require prophylactic antibiotics for dental procedures such as teeth cleaning that may provoke bleeding (see Chapter 35).

Nutrition. Caries develop with increasing frequency in persons who ingest diets high in refined carbohydrates. In addition, the cariogenicity (caries promotion) of diet is also related to the frequency of carbohydrate ingestion and eating patterns.[3] A prevention program should, therefore, include reduction in sugar intake. If sugars are eaten, the teeth should be brushed within 30 minutes of eating. Another aspect of diet therapy that seems to reduce plaque formation is increased vi-

CULTURAL & ETHNIC CONSIDERATIONS

Oral, Pharyngeal, and Esophageal Problems

- Periodontal disease is more prevalent among African-Americans than among Caucasians.
- Cancers of the oral cavity and pharynx are the fourth leading cause of death in African-American men 35 to 54 years of age.
- Death rates as a result of oral cancer are decreasing in Caucasians but increasing in non-Caucasians.
- Esophageal cancer has a higher incidence among African-Americans and Asian-Americans than among Caucasians.

tamin C intake. There has been increasing interest in the development of sugar substitutes that are noncariogenic.

Fluoride. Fluoridation makes tooth enamel more resistant to the acids produced from the action of bacteria on sugars in the mouth. In drinking water, one part fluoride per million parts water results in a significant decrease in the decay rate.[1] Many communities consider the fluoridation of drinking water a municipal responsibility and have enacted the necessary legislation. Currently 56% of the U.S. population lives in fluoridated communities.[4] A fluoride solution can be applied topically on the teeth during a dental office visit. In addition, many toothpastes have fluoride added to them, and the American Dental Association recommends them. Fluoride rinses and tablets are also available for at-home use.

Sealants. In addition to fluoride, sealants can be applied to the pits and fissures of teeth in children following the eruption of the teeth or in young adults to reduce caries. Sealant is a coating material that is applied directly to teeth surfaces in the dentist's office. Sealants reduce the attachment of plaque and have been found to be effective in reducing caries.[5]

New techniques. Some chemical methods to inhibit plaque formation and accumulation offer promise. Antimicrobial agents such as chlorhexidine have been used in mouthwashes and varnishes to reduce the *S. mutans* bacterial count in high-risk individuals.[6,7]

Acute Intervention. The nurse may need to refer the patient for intervention and care of an acute dental problem. Local manifestations of dental problems include pain that is intermittent and caused by sensitivity to heat or cold stimulation, dull and continuous pain, facial swelling, halitosis, and bleeding or drainage of pus from the mouth. Systemic manifestations include fever, nausea, vomiting, and malaise.

If pulpitis and abscess develop, immediate dental care is needed to prevent further spread of infection to the bone. An opening may be drilled into the pulp chamber, or the gingivae may be incised to provide drainage for the abscess. Sometimes a root canal procedure or extraction of a tooth is necessary. After treatment of an abscess, the patient can use warm saline rinses. Analgesics may also be required to alleviate the pain.

A damaged or defective tooth or a tooth that has a severe abscess may need to be extracted. After the extraction, the patient should apply cold compresses (e.g., ice bag, cold washcloth) to the side of the face to reduce swelling and relieve discomfort. Some oozing of blood is expected the first 1 to 2 days. If there is loss of large amounts of bright-red blood, direct pressure should be applied to the bleeding site by the patient biting on a gauze pad, and the dentist should be notified. During the first 24 hours the patient should not suck (e.g., smoke or use a straw) because this increases the risk of clot disruption.

Ambulatory and Home Care. Day surgery is used for the extraction of several teeth, such as when impacted molars are excised or when dentures are required. Postoperatively the patient will experience pain and soreness. Ice packs and analgesics are used to relieve the discomfort. Nutrients should be liquid or semisoft for a few days. The dentist or oral surgeon may order mouthwashes for cleansing and relief of soreness.

Dentures. There are approximately 17 million Americans who are edentulous and 10 million of these are more than 65 years of age.[1] The decision to obtain dentures is not easy for most people. They are concerned about changes in cosmetic appearance and the ability to chew food. They must be assured that dentures usually decrease the spread of infection, improve nutritional intake, and improve appearance, especially if they have had multiple dental problems preceding the decision to obtain dentures.

Patience must be stressed in the adjustment phase to dentures. It takes time to get used to a different feel and way of chewing. The gingivae should be checked for proper fit and for any signs of gingival irritation. Dentures should be cleaned at least twice a day with salt and sodium bicarbonate or a dentifrice. When the dentures are removed, the patient should massage the gums for a few minutes. Some patients prefer to wear their dentures at all times, and there are generally no contraindications to this. In fact, facial contour is better maintained by this practice. If dentures are removed at night, they should be covered with water (especially if they are made of vulcanite) and stored in a safe place.

The patient who wears dentures should be encouraged to obtain regular dental care. Dentures will need to be modified because tissue changes occur from aging, weight changes, or disease processes. Poorly fitting dentures can cause pain and oral ulceration leading to poor nutrition.

Dental implants are being used in some patients who require tooth extractions. An implant involves insertion of a titanium post into the bone. The bone fuses with the post and then techniques of restorative dentistry are used to create a crown that is attached to the post. An advantage of dental implants is that the patient experiences less mandibular bone loss compared with dentures.[8]

Evaluation

The expected outcomes for the patient with dental problems are that the patient will

- have a decrease in incidence of active disease
- comply with dental hygiene measures including regular dental examinations
- have balanced nutritional intake

Table 39-1 Infections and Inflammations of the Mouth

Condition	Etiology	Clinical Manifestations	Treatment
▪ Gingivitis	Neglected oral hygiene, malocclusion, missing or irregular teeth, faulty dentistry, eating of soft rather than fibrous foods	Inflamed gingivae and interdental papillae; bleeding during toothbrushing; development of pus, formation of abscess with loosening of teeth (periodontitis)	Prevention through health teaching, dental care, gingival massage, professional cleaning of teeth, fibrous foods, conscientious brushing habits with flossing
▪ Vincent's infection (acute necrotizing ulcerative gingivitis, trench mouth)	Fusiform bacteria; Vincent spirochetes; predisposing factors of stress, excessive fatigue, poor oral hygiene, nutritional deficiencies (B and C vitamins)	Painful, bleeding gingivae; eroding necrotic lesions of interdental papillae; ulcerations that bleed; increased saliva with metallic taste; fetid mouth odor; anorexia, fever, and general malaise	Rest (physical and mental); avoidance of smoking and alcoholic beverages; soft, nutritious diet; correct oral hygiene habits; topical applications of antibiotics; mouth irrigations with hydrogen peroxide and saline solutions
▪ Oral candidiasis (moniliasis or thrush)	*Candida albicans* (a yeastlike fungus), debilitation, prolonged high-dose antibiotic or corticosteroid therapy	Pearly, bluish white "milk-curd" membranous lesions on mucosa of mouth and larynx; sore mouth; yeasty halitosis	Nystatin or amphotericin B as oral suspension or buccal tablets, good oral hygiene
▪ Herpes simplex (cold sore, fever blister)	Herpes simplex virus, type I or II; predisposing factors of upper respiratory infections, excessive exposure to sunlight, food allergies, emotional tension, onset of menstruation	Lip lesions, mouth lesions, vesicle formation (single or clustered), shallow, painful ulcers	Spirits of camphor, corticosteroid cream, mild antiseptic mouthwash, viscous lidocaine; removal or control of predisposing factors, antiviral agents (e.g., acyclovir [Zovirax])
▪ Aphthous stomatitis (canker sore)	Recurrent and chronic form of infection secondary to systemic disease, trauma, stress, or unknown causes	Ulcers of mouth and lips, causing extreme pain; ulcers surrounded by erythematous base	Corticosteroids (topical or systemic), tetracycline oral suspension
▪ Parotitis (inflammation of parotid gland, surgical mumps)	Usually *Staphylococcus* species, *Streptococcus* species occasionally, debilitation and dehydration with poor oral hygiene, NPO status for an extended time	Pain in area of gland and ear, absence of salivation, purulent exudate from duct of gland	Antibiotics, mouthwashes, warm compresses; preventive measures such as chewing gum, sucking on hard candy (lemon drops), adequate fluid intake
▪ Stomatitis (inflammation of mouth)	Trauma; pathogens; irritants (tobacco, alcohol); renal, liver, and hematologic diseases; side effect of many cancer chemotherapy drugs	Excessive salivation, halitosis, sore mouth	Removal or treatment of cause, oral hygiene with soothing solutions, topical medications; soft, bland diet

ORAL INFLAMMATIONS AND INFECTIONS

Oral infections and inflammations may be specific mouth diseases, or they may occur in the presence of some systemic diseases such as leukemia or vitamin deficiency. When oral inflammations and infections are present, they can severely impair the ingestion of food and fluids. Common inflammations and infections of the oral cavity are presented in Table 39-1. The patient who is immunosuppressed (patient with acquired immunodeficiency syndrome or receiving chemotherapy) is most susceptible to oral infections.

CARCINOMA OF THE ORAL CAVITY

Carcinoma of the oral cavity may occur on the lips or anywhere within the mouth (e.g., tongue, floor of the mouth, buccal mucosa, hard palate, soft palate, pharyngeal walls, and tonsils). Oropharyngeal cancer is diagnosed in 30,300 Americans annually, and it is estimated that 8000 persons a year die from the disease.[9] It is more common after 40 years of age, with 60 years being the average age at onset. Carcinoma of the oral cavity occurs in all ethnic groups. It is more common in men (male-to-female ratio of 2:1). Squamous cell carcinoma is the most common oral malignant tumor (more than 90%). The 5-year survival for all stages of cancer of the oral cavity and pharynx combined is 53% and the 10-year rate is 43%.[9]

Most of the malignant lesions occur on the lower lip in men. Other common sites are the lateral border and undersurface of the tongue, the labial commissure, and the buccal mucosa. Carcinoma of the lip has the most favorable prognosis of any of the oral tumors. This is probably because lip lesions are more ap-

Table 39-2 Oral Tumors

Location	Predisposing Factors	Clinical Manifestations	Treatment
▪ Lip	Constant overexposure to sun, ruddy and fair complexion, recurrent herpetic lesions, irritation from pipe stem, syphilis, immunosuppression	Indurated, painless ulcer	Surgical excision, radiation
▪ Tongue	Tobacco, alcohol, chronic irritation, syphilis	Ulcer or area of thickening; soreness or pain; increased salivation, slurred speech, dysphagia, toothache, earache (later signs)	Surgery (hemiglossectomy or glossectomy), radiation
▪ Oral cavity	Poor oral hygiene, tobacco usage (pipe and cigar smoking, snuff, chewing tobacco), chronic alcohol intake, chronic irritation (jagged tooth, ill-fitting prosthesis, chemical or mechanical irritants)	Leukoplakia; erythroplakia; ulcerations; sore spot; rough area; pain, dysphagia, difficulty in chewing and speaking (later signs)	Surgery (mandibulectomy, radical neck dissection, resections of buccal mucosa), internal and external radiation

parent to the patient than other oral lesions and are usually diagnosed earlier.

Etiology and Pathophysiology

Although the cause of carcinoma of the oral cavity is not definitive, there are a number of predisposing factors (Table 39-2). Constant overexposure to ultraviolet radiation from the sun is also a factor in the development of cancer of the lip. Irritation from the pipe stem resting on the lip is a factor in pipe smokers. Factors that influence intraoral cancer include tobacco use (cigar, cigarette, pipe, snuff), excessive alcohol intake, and chronic irritation such as from a jagged tooth or poor dental care. A positive history of tobacco and alcohol use, in the past or currently, is the most significant etiologic factor in oral cancer.[10]

Clinical Manifestations

The common manifestations of carcinoma of the oral cavity are leukoplakia, erythroplakia, ulcerations, a sore spot, and a rough area (felt with the tongue). Later symptoms are pain, dysphagia, and difficulty in chewing and speaking. *Leukoplakia*, called "white patch" or "smoker's patch," is frequently considered a precancerous lesion, although less than 5% of these lesions actually transform into malignant cells. It is a whitish patch on the mucosa of the mouth or tongue. The patch becomes keratinized (hard and leathery) and is sometimes described as hyperkeratosis. Leukoplakia is the result of chronic irritation, especially from smoking. *Erythroplasia* (erythroplakia), which is seen as a red velvety patch on the mouth or tongue, is also considered a precancerous lesion. Areas of erythroplakia have a 90% chance of becoming malignant.

Cancer of the lip usually appears as an indurated, painless ulcer on the lip. The first sign of carcinoma of the tongue is an ulcer or area of thickening. Soreness or pain of the tongue may occur, especially on eating hot or highly seasoned foods. Cancerous lesions are most likely to develop in the proximal half of the tongue. Some patients experience limitation of movement of the tongue. Later symptoms of cancer of the tongue include increased salivation, slurred speech, dysphagia, toothache, and earache. Approximately 30% of patients with oral cancer present with an asymptomatic neck mass.

COLLABORATIVE CARE

Table 39-3 Oral Carcinoma

Diagnostic
- Biopsy
- Oral exfoliative cytology
- CT and MRI scans (for metastases)

Collaborative Therapy*
- Surgical excision of the tumor
- Radical neck dissection
- Radiation (internal or external)
- Combined surgical resection with radiation
- Chemotherapy

*Any of the following approaches may be used, depending on the primary lesion and the extent of metastasis.
CT, computed tomography; *MRI*, magnetic resonance imaging.

Diagnostic Studies

Biopsy of the suspected lesion with cytologic examination is the best definitive diagnostic measure for oral cancer. Oral exfoliative cytology involves scraping of a suspicious lesion and spreading this scraping on a slide. Unlike biopsy, a negative cytologic smear does not reliably rule out the possibility of a malignant condition, but it may be used as a screening test. The toluidine blue test may also be used as a screening test for oral cancer. Toluidine blue is applied topically to stain an area of carcinoma.[11]

Collaborative Care

Collaborative care of oral carcinoma usually consists of surgery, radiation, chemotherapy, or a combination of these (Table 39-3).

Surgical Therapy. Surgery remains the most effective treatment, especially for removing the central core of the tumor. Many of the operations are radical procedures involving extensive resections. Various surgical procedures may be performed, depending on the location and extent of the tumor. Some examples are partial *mandibulectomy* (removal of the mandible), *hemiglossectomy* (removal of half of the tongue), *glossectomy* (removal of the tongue), resections of the buccal mucosa and floor of the mouth, and radical neck dissection. Composite resections, which are combinations of the various surgical procedures, may be performed.

Because cancers of the oral cavity metastasize early to the cervical lymph nodes, a *radical neck dissection* is commonly performed. It includes wide excision of the involved primary lesion with removal of the regional lymph nodes, the deep cervical lymph nodes, and their lymphatic channels. In addition, the following structures may also be removed or transected (depending on the extent of the primary lesion): the sternocleidomastoid muscle and other closely associated muscles, the internal jugular vein, the mandible, the submaxillary gland, part of the thyroid and parathyroid glands, and the spinal accessory nerve. A tracheostomy is commonly performed along with the radical neck dissection. Drainage tubes are inserted into the surgical area and connected to suction to remove fluid and blood.

Chemotherapy and radiation therapy are used together when the lesions are more advanced or involve several structures of the oral cavity. Chemotherapy may also be used when surgery and radiation therapy fail or as the initial therapy for smaller tumors. Chemotherapeutic agents used include 5-fluorouracil (5-FU), cyclophosphamide (Cytoxan), bleomycin (Blenoxane), vinblastine (Velban), hydroxyurea (Hydrea), and cisplatin (Platinol) (see Chapter 14).

Palliative treatment may be the best management when the prognosis is poor, the cancer is inoperable, or the patient decides against surgery. Palliation aims to treat the symptoms and make the patient more comfortable. If it becomes difficult for the patient to swallow, a gastrostomy may be performed to allow for adequate nutritional intake (see Gastrostomy, Chapter 38). Analgesic medication should be given freely to this patient. Frequent suctioning of the oral cavity becomes necessary when swallowing becomes difficult. (Other nursing measures for the terminally ill patient are discussed in Chapter 14.)

Nutritional Therapy. Because of depression, alcoholism, or presurgery radiation treatment, patients may be malnourished even before surgery. After radical neck surgery, the patient may be unable to take in nutrients through the normal route of ingestion because of swelling, the location of sutures, or difficulty with swallowing. Parenteral fluids will be given for the first 24 to 48 hours. After this time, tube feedings are usually given via a nasogastric (NG) or nasointestinal tube that was placed during surgery. Sometimes a temporary feeding gastrostomy may be used. (Nasogastric and gastrostomy feedings are described in Chapter 38.) Cervical esophagostomy and pharyngostomy have also been used. The nurse must observe for tolerance of the feedings and adjust the amount, time, and formula if nausea, vomiting, diarrhea, or distention occurs. The patient is usually instructed about the tube feedings. When the patient can swallow, small amounts of water are given. Close observation for choking is essential. Suctioning may be necessary to prevent aspiration.

NURSING MANAGEMENT: CARCINOMA OF THE ORAL CAVITY

■ Nursing Assessment

Subjective and objective data that should be obtained from a patient with carcinoma of the oral cavity are presented in Table 39-4.

■ Nursing Diagnoses

Nursing diagnoses for the patient with carcinoma of the oral cavity may include, but are not limited to, the following:

- Altered nutrition: less than body requirements *related to* oral pain, difficulty chewing and swallowing, surgical resection, and radiation treatment
- Pain *related to* the tumor and surgical radiation
- Anxiety *related to* diagnosis of cancer, uncertain future, potential for disfiguring surgery, potential for recurrence, and prognosis
- Ineffective individual coping *related to* body image change, smoking, and alcohol cessation
- Altered health maintenance *related to* lack of knowledge of disease process and therapeutic regimen, and unavailability of a support system

■ Planning

The overall goals are that the patient with carcinoma of the oral cavity will (1) have a patent airway, (2) be able to communicate, (3) have adequate nutritional intake to promote wound healing, and (4) have relief of pain and discomfort.

■ Nursing Implementation

Health Promotion. The nurse has a significant role in early detection and treatment of carcinoma of the oral cavity. The nurse should provide the patient with information regarding predisposing factors, such as constant overexposure to the sun, tobacco, and other irritants. Smoking and the long-term use of smokeless tobacco are the major risk factors for oral cancer. A patient identified as a smoker should be informed about smoking cessation programs available in the community. (Smoking cessation is discussed in the section on lung cancer in Chapter 26 and in Table 26-19.)

It is important that adolescents and teenagers be informed about the danger of using "snuff" and chewing tobacco. In addition, oral cancers have an increased chance of recurrence if risk factors are not reduced. The nurse should also teach correct oral hygiene and dental care and encourage the patient to seek preventive dental care. Risk factors must be identified. Because early detection of oral carcinoma is important, the patient should be taught to examine the mouth and to recognize danger signals of oral cancer. If any of these signals are present, the patient should be instructed to visit a doctor. Danger signals are as follows:

- Unexplained pain or soreness in the mouth
- Unusual bleeding from the oral cavity
- Dysphagia
- Swelling or lump in the neck

NURSING ASSESSMENT

Table 39-4 Cancer of the Mouth

Subjective Data

Important Health Information

Past health history: Recurrent herpetic lesions, syphilis, exposure to sunlight

Medications: Immunosuppressants

Surgery or other treatments: Removal of prior tumors or lesions

Functional Health Patterns

Health perception–health management: Use of alcohol and tobacco, pipe smoking; poor oral hygiene

Nutritional-metabolic: Reductions in oral intake, weight loss; difficulty in chewing food; increased salivation; intolerance to certain foods or temperatures of food

Cognitive-perceptual: Mouth or tongue soreness or pain, toothache, earache, neck stiffness, dysphagia, difficulty speaking

Objective Data

Integumentary

Indurated, painless ulcer on lip; painless neck mass

Gastrointestinal

Areas of thickening or roughness, ulcers, leukoplakia, or erythroplakia on the tongue or oral mucosa; limited movement of the tongue; increased salivation, drooling; slurred speech, foul breath odor

Possible Findings

Positive exfoliative smear cytology; positive biopsy

Any individual with an ulcerative lesion that does not heal within 2 to 3 weeks should be referred to a physician, and a biopsy of the lesion should probably be performed. The nurse should inspect the patient's oral cavity to detect suspicious lesions.

Acute Intervention. Preoperative care for the patient who is having a radical neck dissection involves consideration of the patient's physical and psychosocial needs (see the nursing care plan for the patient with a radical neck dissection on p. 604, NCP 25-6). Physical preparation is the same as for any major surgery, with special emphasis on oral hygiene. Thorough assessment of alcohol intake should be done and measures to assess and treat withdrawal, if it occurs, should be implemented early. Explanations and emotional support are of special significance and should include postoperative measures relating to communication and feeding. The surgical procedure should be explained to the patient, and the nurse should make sure that the patient understands the information.

Care of the patient following radical neck dissection is presented in Chapter 25 and NCP 25-6.

■ Evaluation

The expected outcomes are that the patient with oral carcinoma will

- maintain a patent airway
- be able to communicate
- have adequate nutritional intake to promote wound healing
- have relief of pain and discomfort

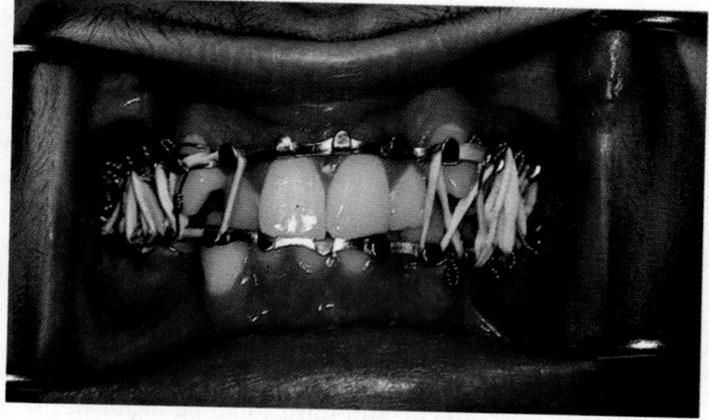

Fig. 39-4 Intermaxillary fixation.

MANDIBULAR FRACTURE

Fracture of the mandible may result from trauma to the face or jaws. Maxillary fractures may also occur, but they are less common than mandibular fractures. The fracture may be simple, with no bone displacement, or it may involve loss of tissue and bone. The fracture may require immediate and sometimes long-term treatment to ensure survival and restore satisfactory appearance and function. Mandibular fracture may also be therapeutically performed to correct an underlying malocclusion problem that cannot be corrected by orthodontic procedures alone. In these conditions, the mandible is split during surgery and moved forward or backward depending on the occlusion problem. For this patient, the procedure is performed on an elective basis.

Surgery consists of immobilization, usually by wiring the jaws (intermaxillary fixation). Internal fixation may be accomplished with screws and plates. In a simple fracture with no loss of teeth, the lower jaw is wired to the upper jaw. First, wires are placed around the teeth; then cross-wires or rubber bands are used to hold the lower jaw tight against the upper jaw (Fig. 39-4). Arch bars may be used and placed on the maxillary and mandibular arches of the teeth. Vertical wires are placed between the arch bars holding the jaws together. When teeth are missing or if there is bone displacement, other forms of fixation such as metal arch bars in the mouth or insertion of a pin in the bone may be used. The immobilization is usually necessary for only 4 to 6 weeks because the fractures heal rapidly.

NURSING MANAGEMENT: MANDIBULAR FRACTURE

■ Preoperative Care

The patient should be told preoperatively about the surgical procedure, including what it involves, how the face will look, and alterations the surgery will cause. The patient must be reassured about the ability to breathe normally, speak, and swallow liquids. Usually hospitalization is brief unless there are other injuries or problems.

■ Postoperative Care

Postoperative care should focus on a patent airway, oral hygiene, communication, and adequate nutrition. Two major potential problems in the immediate postoperative period are airway obstruction and aspiration of vomitus. Because the patient cannot open the jaws, measures to ensure an airway are essential. The nurse must observe for signs of respiratory distress. The patient should be placed on the side with the head slightly elevated immediately after surgery. A wire cutter or scissors (for rubber bands) must be taped to the head of the bed. These may be used to cut the wires or elastic bands in case of an emergency. The wires should be cut only as a last resort. Once the patient is awake the wires should be cut only in case of cardiac or respiratory arrest.

The physician should explain, by using a picture, the appropriate wire or wires to cut, and this should be included in the care plan. In some cases, cutting the wires may cause the entire facial and upper jaw structure to collapse and worsen the problem. A tracheostomy or an endotracheal tray should always be available.

If the patient begins to vomit or choke, the nurse should try to clear the mouth and airway. Suctioning may be necessary and may be done by the nasopharyngeal or oral route, depending on the extent of injury and the type of repair. An NG tube may be used for decompression to remove fluids and gas from the stomach to help prevent aspiration. It also helps prevent vomiting. Antiemetics may also be used. The NG tube can later be used as a feeding tube. The nurse should teach the patient to clear secretions and vomitus.

Oral hygiene is an important part of the nursing care. The mouth should be rinsed frequently, particularly after meals and snacks, to remove food debris. Warm normal saline solution, water, or alkaline mouthwashes may be used. A soft rubber catheter or a Water-Pik is effective for a thorough oral cleansing. The nurse should inspect the mouth several times a day to see that it is clean. A flashlight is necessary, and a tongue depressor is used to retract the cheeks. The lips and corners of the mouth should be kept moist.

Communication may be a problem, particularly in the early postoperative period. An effective way of communication must be established preoperatively (e.g., use of picture board, pad and pencil, small chalkboard). Usually the patient can speak well enough to be understood, especially after the first few postoperative days.

Ingestion of sufficient nutrients poses a challenge because the diet must be liquid. The patient easily tires of sucking through a straw or laboriously using a spoon. The diet must be planned to include adequate calories, protein, and fluids. Liquid protein supplements may be helpful for improving the nutritional status. The nurse works with the dietician and the patient to ensure adequate nutrition. The low-bulk, high-carbohydrate diet and the intake of air through the straw create a problem with flatus and constipation. Ambulation, prune juice, and bulk-forming laxatives may help relieve these problems.

The patient is usually discharged with the wires in place. The nurse should allow the patient to verbalize feelings about the altered appearance. Discharge teaching should include oral care, techniques of handling secretions, diet, and how and when to use wire cutters.

NAUSEA AND VOMITING

Nausea and vomiting are the most common manifestations of GI diseases. Although each symptom can occur independently, they are usually closely related and usually treated as one problem. They are also found in a wide variety of conditions that are unrelated to GI disease. These include pregnancy, infectious diseases, central nervous system (CNS) disorders (e.g., meningitis, CNS lesion), cardiovascular problems (e.g., myocardial infarction, congestive heart failure), side effects of drugs (e.g., digitalis, antibiotics), metabolic disorders (e.g., uremia), and psychologic factors (e.g., stress, fear).

Nausea is a feeling of discomfort in the epigastrium with a conscious desire to vomit. Anorexia usually accompanies nausea and is brought on by unpleasant stimulation involving any of the five senses. Generally, nausea occurs before vomiting and is characterized by contraction of the duodenum and by slowing of gastric motility and emptying. A single episode of nausea accompanied by vomiting in an adult may not be significant. However, if vomiting occurs several times it is important that the cause be identified.

Vomiting is the forceful ejection of partially digested food and secretions from the upper GI tract. It occurs when the gut becomes overly irritated, excited, or distended. It can be a protective mechanism to rid the body of spoiled or irritating foods and liquids. Immediately before the act of vomiting, the person becomes aware of the need to vomit. The autonomic nervous system is activated resulting in both parasympathetic and sympathetic nervous system stimulation. Sympathetic activation produces tachycardia, tachypnea, and diaphoresis. Parasympathetic stimulation causes relaxation of the lower esophageal (cardiac) sphincter, an increase in gastric motility, and a pronounced increase in salivation. These manifestations are experienced immediately before vomiting.

Vomiting is a complex act that requires the coordinated activities of several structures: closure of the glottis, deep inspiration with contraction of the diaphragm in the inspiratory position, closure of the pylorus, relaxation of the stomach and lower esophageal sphincter, and contraction of the abdominal muscles with increasing intraabdominal pressure. These simultaneous activities force the stomach contents up through the esophagus, into the pharynx, and out the mouth.

Etiology and Pathophysiology

There is a vomiting center in the brainstem that coordinates the multiple components involved in vomiting. This center receives input from various stimuli. Neural impulses reach the vomiting center via afferent pathways through branches of the autonomic nervous system. Visceral receptors for these afferent fibers are located in the GI tract, kidneys, heart, and uterus. When stimulated, these receptors relay information to the vomiting center, which then initiates the vomiting reflex (Fig. 39-5).

In addition, the chemoreceptor trigger zone (CTZ) located on the floor of the fourth ventricle in the brain responds to chemical stimuli of drugs and toxins. The CTZ also plays a role in vomiting when it is due to labyrinthine stimulation (e.g., motion sickness). Once stimulated, the CTZ transmits impulses directly to the vomiting center. Emotions, stress, unpleasant sights

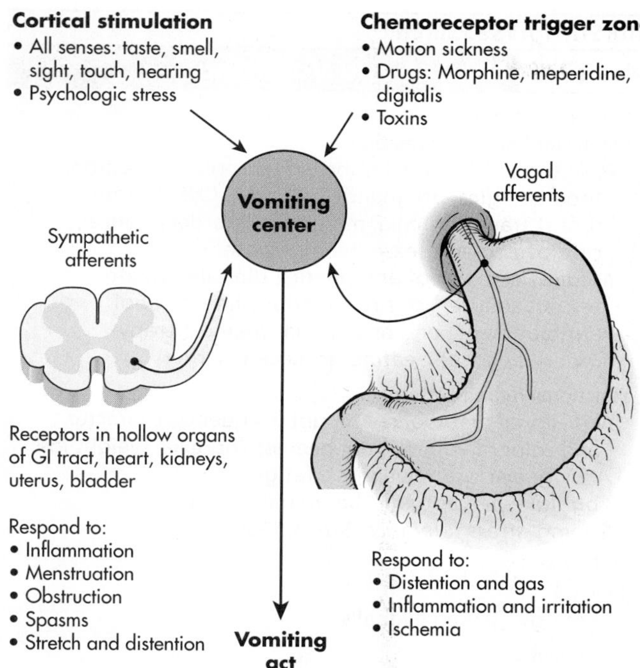

Fig. 39-5 Stimuli involved in the act of vomiting.

and odors, and pain are all capable of triggering vomiting. Nausea and vomiting are frequently associated with uremia, hyperthyroidism, hyperparathyroidism and hypoparathyroidism, diabetic acidosis, Addison's disease, and hypertensive crisis.

When nausea and vomiting are prolonged, dehydration can rapidly occur. In addition to water, essential electrolytes (e.g., potassium) are also lost. As vomiting persists, there may be severe electrolyte imbalances, loss of extracellular fluid (ECF) volume, decreased plasma volume, and eventually circulatory failure. Metabolic alkalosis can result from loss of gastric hydrochloric acid. Metabolic acidosis can occur because of the loss of bicarbonate when contents from the small intestine are vomited. However, metabolic acidosis as a result of severe vomiting is less common than metabolic alkalosis. Weight loss is evident in a short time when vomiting is severe.

The threat of aspiration is a constant concern when vomiting is severe. Aspiration is especially a risk in the older adult and in the patient who is weak and debilitated. The patient who cannot adequately manage self-care should be put in a semi-Fowler's or side-lying position to prevent aspiration.

Collaborative Care

The goals of collaborative care are to determine and treat the underlying cause of the nausea and vomiting and to provide symptomatic relief of nausea and vomiting. Determining the cause is often difficult because nausea and vomiting are manifestations of many conditions of the GI tract and of disorders of other body systems.

A careful history elicits important information regarding times when the vomiting occurs, precipitating factors, and a description of the contents of the vomitus. Differentiation must be made between vomiting, regurgitation, and projectile vomiting. *Regurgitation* is a process in which partially digested food is slowly brought up from the stomach. Retching or vomiting seldom precedes it. *Projectile vomiting* is a very forceful projection of stomach contents without nausea and is characteristic of CNS lesions.

The presence of fecal odor and bile after prolonged vomiting is indicative of intestinal obstruction beyond the pylorus. A functioning ileocecal valve ordinarily prevents the backflow of fecal contents from the colon into the small intestine. The presence of bile may suggest obstruction below the ampulla of Vater or bile reflux gastritis. The presence of partially digested food several hours after a meal is indicative of gastric outlet obstruction or delay in gastric emptying.

The color of the emesis aids in determining the presence and source of bleeding. Vomitus with a "coffee ground" appearance is associated with bleeding in the stomach, where blood changes to dark brown as a result of its interaction with gastric acid. Bright red blood indicates active bleeding suggestive of a tear in the mucosal lining of the lower esophagus or fundus of stomach, bleeding gastric or duodenal ulcer or neoplasm, or bleeding esophageal varices.

The time of day at which the vomiting occurs is often helpful in determining the cause. Early morning vomiting is a frequent occurrence in pregnancy and in uremia associated with renal disease. Emotional stressors with no evident functional disorder may elicit vomiting during or immediately after the ingestion of a meal.

Drug Therapy. The use of drugs in the treatment of nausea and vomiting depends on the cause of the problem. Many different drugs can be used (Table 39-5). Because the cause cannot always be readily determined, medications must be used with caution. The use of antiemetics before the cause of the vomiting is established can lead to masking of the underlying disease process and delay of diagnosis and treatment. Many of the antiemetic drugs act on the CNS at the level of the CTZ. In general, they block the neurochemicals that appear to trigger nausea and vomiting. Drugs that control nausea and vomiting include antimuscarinics (e.g., scopolamine), antihistamines (e.g., diphenhydramine), and phenothiazines (e.g., chlorpromazine, prochlorperazine). Because many of these drugs have anticholinergic actions, they are contraindicated for the patient with glaucoma, prostatic hyperplasia, pyloric or bladder neck obstruction, or biliary obstruction. They share many common side effects, which include dry mouth, hypotension, sedative effects, rashes, and GI disturbances such as constipation. Consultation with a clinical pharmacist may be indicated before administering these medications to the patient with multiple medical problems. Other drugs with antiemetic properties include metoclopramide (Reglan) and ondansetron (Zofran), which act peripherally to block serotonin receptors. These drugs are considered prokinetic agents because they stimulate gastric emptying and are used prophylactically to reduce nausea and vomiting associated with cancer chemotherapy and postanesthesia.

Nutritional Therapy. The patient with severe vomiting requires intravenous (IV) fluid therapy with electrolyte replacement until able to tolerate oral intake. In some cases an

DRUG THERAPY

Table 39-5 Nausea and Vomiting

Classification	Generic Name	Trade Name
▪ Antiemetic and antipsychotic	Chlorpromazine	Thorazine
	Haloperidol	Haldol
	Perphenazine	Trilafon
	Prochlorperazine	Compazine
	Promazine	Sparine
	Trifluoperazine	Stelazine
	Triflupromazine	Vesprin
▪ Antihistamine	Buclizine	Bucladin-S
	Cyclizine	Marezine, meclizine
	Dimenhydrinate	Dramamine
	Diphenhydramine	Benadryl
	Promethazine	Phenergan
▪ Prokinetics	Metoclopramide	Reglan
	Ondansetron	Zofran
	Granisetron	Kytril
	Dolasetron	Anzemet
▪ Antimuscarinic	Scopolamine transdermal	Transderm-Scop
▪ Others	Benzquinamide	Emete-Con
	Diphenidol	Vontrol
	Thiethylperazine	Torecan
	Trimethobenzamide	Tigan

NURSING ASSESSMENT

Table 39-6 Nausea and Vomiting

Subjective Data

Important Health Information

Past health history: GI disorders, chronic indigestion, food allergies, pregnancy, infection, CNS disorders, recent travel, bulimia, metabolic disorders, cancer, cardiovascular disease, renal disease

Medications: Use of antiemetics, digitalis, opiates, ferrous sulfate, aspirin, aminophylline, alcohol, antibiotics; general anesthesia, chemotherapy

Surgery or other treatments: Recent surgery

Functional Health Patterns

Nutritional-metabolic: Amount, frequency, character, and color of vomitus; dry heaves; anorexia; weight loss

Activity-exercise: Weakness, fatigue

Cognitive-perceptual: Abdominal tenderness

Coping–stress tolerance: Stress, fear

Objective Data

General

Lethargy, sunken eyeballs

Integumentary

Pallor, dry mucous membranes, poor skin turgor

Gastrointestinal

Amount, frequency, character (e.g., projectile), content (undigested food, blood, bile, feces), and color of vomitus (red, "coffee ground," green-yellow)

Urinary

Decreased output, concentrated urine

Possible Findings

Altered serum electrolytes (especially hypokalemia), metabolic alkalosis, abnormal upper GI findings or abdominal x-rays

CNS, central nervous system.

NG tube and suction are used to decompress the stomach. Once the symptoms have subsided, oral nourishment beginning with clear liquids is started. Extremely hot or cold liquids are not usually well tolerated. Carbonated beverages at room temperature and with the carbonation gone and warm tea are more easily tolerated. The addition of dry toast or crackers may alleviate the feeling of nausea and help prevent vomiting. Although broth and Gatorade have been used widely for the patient with severe vomiting, these substances are high in sodium and should be administered with caution. Water is the fluid of choice for rehydration by mouth.

As the patient's condition improves, a diet high in carbohydrates and low in fatty foods should be provided. Items such as a baked potato, plain gelatin, cereal with milk and sugar, and hard candy may be added. Foods that are known to be poorly tolerated include coffee, spicy foods, and highly acidic foods. Food should be eaten slowly and in small amounts so that overdistention of the stomach is avoided. When solid foods have been reintroduced, fluids should be taken between meals rather than with meals. It is advised that the patient remain quietly relaxed for approximately 1 hour after meals. A registered dietician may be consulted regarding appropriate foods that have nutritional value and are well tolerated by the patient during the recovery process.

NURSING MANAGEMENT: NAUSEA AND VOMITING

■ Nursing Assessment

Each patient with a history of prolonged and persistent nausea or vomiting requires a thorough nursing assessment before a specific plan of care is developed. Although the conditions associated with nausea and vomiting are numerous, the nurse should have a basic understanding of the more common conditions and should be able to identify the patient who is at high risk. Knowledge of the physiologic mechanisms involved in nausea and vomiting and the demonstration of a genuine regard for the patient are essential. Table 39-6 presents subjective and objective data that should be obtained from a patient with nausea and vomiting, regardless of the underlying cause.

■ Nursing Diagnoses

Nursing diagnoses for the patient with nausea and vomiting may include, but are not limited to, those presented in NCP 39-1. Additional nursing diagnoses may include the following:

- Self-care deficits *related to* fatigue and discomfort of prolonged nausea and vomiting
- Altered oral mucous membrane *related to* persistent vomiting and inadequate oral hygiene

■ Planning

The overall goals are that the patient with nausea and vomiting will (1) experience minimal or no nausea and vomiting, (2) have

39-1 NURSING CARE PLAN PATIENT WITH NAUSEA AND VOMITING

Expected Patient Outcomes	Nursing Interventions and *Rationales*
NURSING DIAGNOSIS **Vomiting** *related to* multiple etiologies *as manifested by* episodes of nausea and vomiting.	
▪ Minimal or no nausea or vomiting. ▪ Verbalization of satisfaction with care.	▪ Assess duration, frequency, and nature of vomitus, and aggravating and alleviating factors *to plan appropriate interventions.* ▪ Offer reassurance and explanations *to increase patient cooperation.* ▪ Remove visual stimuli and source of odors *to avoid precipitating factors of nausea and/or vomiting.* ▪ Provide mouth care; change soiled gown and linens *to ensure patient comfort.* ▪ Use diversional activities (if appropriate) *to decrease awareness of nausea.* ▪ Maintain quiet environment, restrict visitors, and avoid unnecessary procedures or activities *to minimize triggers of vomiting.* ▪ Administer antiemetics as ordered. ▪ Instruct patient to take several deep breaths; prevent sudden changes in position; keep head of bed elevated *to decrease stimulation of the vomiting center.* ▪ Instruct patient to avoid foods and beverages *that stimulate nausea and vomiting.*
NURSING DIAGNOSIS **Fluid volume deficit** *related to* prolonged vomiting and inability to ingest, digest, or absorb food and fluids *as manifested by* decreased urine output and increased urine concentration, increased pulse rate, hypotension (postural), decreased intake, decreased skin turgor, dry skin and mucous membranes.	
▪ No signs of dehydration.	▪ Assess for signs of dehydration *to plan appropriate care.* ▪ Administer and monitor amount and type of IV fluid *to maintain fluid and electrolyte balance.* ▪ Administer antiemetic as prescribed. ▪ Provide small amounts of clear liquids when vomiting stops *to maintain hydration.* ▪ Record amount and frequency of vomitus; maintain accurate intake and output records; weigh daily in acute phase *to accurately monitor fluid balance.* ▪ Monitor laboratory results of serum sodium, potassium, and chloride *as indicators of electrolyte balance.*
NURSING DIAGNOSIS **Anxiety** *related to* lack of knowledge of cause of problem, treatment plan, and follow-up care *as manifested by* verbalization of lack of knowledge, apprehension.	
▪ Decrease in anxiety. ▪ Verbalization of understanding of causative factors and therapeutic interventions.	▪ Explain rationale for plan of care and diagnostic tests *to increase patient's understanding and reduce anxiety.* ▪ Teach about relationship between nausea and vomiting and foods, medications, treatment regimens, and psychosocial factors *to elicit patient's cooperation in avoiding potential causative factors.*
NURSING DIAGNOSIS **Altered nutrition: less than body requirements** *related to* nausea and vomiting *as manifested by* lack of interest in or aversion to food, perceived or actual inability to ingest food, weight loss.	
▪ Gradual return to usual weight and eating habits.	▪ Assess patient's interest in food, ability to ingest food, and weight *to determine if a problem is present.* ▪ Assure patient that appetite will return when nausea and vomiting are controlled. ▪ Maintain IV feedings or total parenteral nutrition until oral intake is possible *to provide necessary fluids, electrolytes, calories, and protein intake.* ▪ Instruct patient to resume eating cautiously with bland, nonirritating foods *to avoid irritating the stomach and initiating recurrence of nausea and vomiting.*

normal electrolyte levels and hydration status, and (3) return to a normal pattern of fluid balance and nutrient intake.

Nursing Implementation

Acute Intervention. The majority of individuals with nausea and vomiting can be managed at home. However, when nausea and vomiting persist regardless of home treatment strategies, hospitalization may be necessary for diagnosis of the underlying problem. Until a diagnosis is confirmed, the patient is kept on NPO status and given IV fluids. An NG tube connected to suction may be necessary for the patient with persistent vomiting as well as for the patient in whom the possible diagnosis may be bowel obstruction or paralytic ileus. Keeping the stomach empty reduces the stimulus to vomit. The NG tube should be stabilized to eliminate its movement in the nose and back of the throat because this can stimulate nausea and vomiting.

With prolonged vomiting, there is a possibility of dehydration and electrolyte imbalances. The nurse plans care that includes accurate recording of intake and output, monitoring vital signs, assessing for signs of dehydration, proper positioning to prevent possible aspiration in the susceptible patient, and observing for changes in the patient's general physical comfort and mentation. The nurse must take responsibility for providing physical and emotional support, maintaining a quiet, odor-free environment, and giving explanations regarding any diagnostic tests or procedures performed.

Those who are already hospitalized for other health problems are also prone to episodes of nausea and vomiting. These individuals include the postoperative patient who is recovering from the effects of a surgical procedure, anesthesia, and pain, and who is experiencing adverse reactions to medications and treatment. Nausea and vomiting are common side effects in the cancer patient receiving chemotherapeutic drugs or radiation therapy. (Nursing care for the patient who is receiving chemotherapy and radiation therapy is found in Chapter 14.)

Ambulatory and Home Care. The patient and family may need instructions on how to deal successfully with the unpleasant sensations of nausea, discussion of methods of preventing nausea and vomiting, and strategies to maintain fluid and nutritional intake during periods of nausea. The occurrence of nausea or vomiting may be minimized if measures are taken to keep the immediate environment quiet, free of noxious odors, and well ventilated. The avoidance of sudden changes of position and unnecessary activity is also helpful. Use of relaxation techniques, frequent rest periods, and diversional tactics help prevent nausea and vomiting or facilitate a more rapid recovery from their effects. Cleansing the face and hands with a cool washcloth and mouth care between episodes increase the person's comfort level. When the symptoms occur, all foods and medications should be stopped until the acute phase is past.

If a medication is suspected as the cause, the physician should be notified immediately so that either the dosage can be altered or a new medication can be prescribed. The patient should be reminded that stopping the drug without consulting the physician may eliminate the immediate cause of the nausea and vomiting but that omission of the prescribed medication may have detrimental effects on health or the disease state.

When food is identified as the precipitating cause of nausea and vomiting, the nurse should help the patient solve the problem. What food was it? When was it eaten? Has this food caused problems in the past? Is anyone else in the family sick?

When the patient believes some foods and fluids can be tolerated, the nurse might suggest that it would be helpful to begin with clear liquids or warm cola beverages, Gatorade, tea or broth, dry crackers or toast, and then plain gelatin. Bland foods, such as pasta, rice, and cooked chicken, are generally well tolerated in small amounts. An antiemetic drug should be taken only if prescribed by the physician. Taking over-the-counter (OTC) drugs for relief of symptoms may make the condition worse.

Evaluation

The expected outcomes are that the patient with nausea and vomiting will

- experience minimal or no nausea and vomiting
- have normal electrolyte levels and hydration status
- return to a normal pattern of fluid balance and nutrient intake

GERONTOLOGIC CONSIDERATIONS

Nausea and Vomiting

The older patient experiencing nausea and vomiting requires careful assessment and monitoring, particularly during periods of fluid loss and subsequent rehydration therapy. The older patient is at increased risk for preexisting conditions, such as cardiac or renal failure, and may experience a sudden compromise in renal or cardiac system functioning during episodes of fluid volume deficit.[12] In addition, the electrolyte imbalances that often accompany dehydration may result in life-threatening consequences for the elderly person who is already experiencing conditions such as congestive heart failure. Finally, the older adult with a decreased level of consciousness may be at high risk for aspiration of vomitus. Close monitoring of the patient's physical status and level of consciousness during episodes of nausea and vomiting must be a primary concern for the nurse.

In addition, the elderly are particularly susceptible to the CNS side effects of antiemetic medications; these medications may produce confusion. Dosages should be reduced and efficacy closely evaluated. Safety precautions should be instituted for frail patients taking these medications.

GASTROESOPHAGEAL REFLUX DISEASE

Etiology and Pathophysiology

Gastroesophageal reflux disease (GERD) is not a disease but a syndrome produced by conditions that result in reflux of gastric secretions into the esophagus. More than 60 million Amer-

Table 39-7 Factors Affecting Lower Esophageal Sphincter Pressure

Increase Pressure	
Bethanechol (Urecholine)	
Cisapride (Propulsid)	
Metoclopramide (Reglan)	
Decrease Pressure	
Fatty foods	Theophylline
Chocolate (theobromine, caffeine)	Diazepam (Valium)
	Morphine sulfate
Peppermint, spearmint	β-Adrenergic blocking drugs
Alcohol	
Nicotine	Calcium channel blockers
Anticholinergics	Nitrates
Progesterone	
Tea, coffee (caffeine)	

icans periodically experience symptoms of gastroesophageal reflux and approximately 17.5 million (or 7%) experience symptoms daily.[13] Predisposing conditions include hiatal hernia, incompetent lower esophageal sphincter (LES), decreased esophageal clearance, and decreased gastric emptying. In GERD there is reflux of gastric contents into the lower portion of the esophagus. The acidity of the gastric secretion results in esophageal irritation and inflammation (esophagitis). In addition, the presence of intestinal secretions such as trypsin and bile salts are also corrosive to the esophageal mucosa. The degree of inflammation is dependent on the amount of acid refluxed as well as on the ability of the esophagus to clear the acid (esophageal clearance).

One of the primary factors in GERD is an incompetent LES. An incompetent LES results in a decrease in pressure in the distal portion of the esophagus. As a result, gastric contents are able to move from an area of higher pressure (stomach) to an area of lower pressure (esophagus) when the patient is in a supine position or there is an increase in intraabdominal pressure. A common cause of GERD is a hiatal hernia, which is discussed in the next section.

Clinical Manifestations

Heartburn (*pyrosis*) from gastroesophageal reflux is the most common clinical manifestation. It is caused by irritation of the esophagus by the gastric secretions. Heartburn is described as a burning, tight sensation that appears intermittently beneath the lower sternum and spreads upward to the throat or jaw. Heartburn occurs following ingestion of substances that decrease the LES pressure (Table 39-7). Heartburn is relieved with milk, alkaline substances, or water. Pulmonary symptoms including wheezing, coughing, and dyspnea are secondary to microaspiration of gastric contents into the pulmonary system. Otolaryngologic symptoms include hoarseness, sore throat, a globus sensation, and choking. Gastric symptoms including early satiety, posteating bloating, nausea, and vomiting are related to gastric stasis, which is common in patients with GERD.[13]

COLLABORATIVE CARE

Table 39-8 Gastroesophageal Reflux Disease and Hiatal Hernia

Diagnostic
- Barium swallow
- Radionuclide tests
- Esophagoscopy with biopsy and cytologic analysis
- Motility (manometry) studies
- pH monitoring (laboratory or 24 hr ambulatory)

Collaborative Therapy

Conservative
- Elevation of head of bed on 4- to 6-inch blocks
- High-protein, low-fat diet with avoidance of foods that decrease LES pressure or irritate acid-sensitive esophagus
- Antacids/Gaviscon
- Cholinergic drugs
- Antisecretory agents
  - Histamine H_2-receptor antagonists (cimetidine, ranitidine)
  - Proton pump inhibitors (omeprazole)
- Prokinetic drug therapy
  - Metoclopramide (Reglan)

Surgical
- Nissen fundoplication
- Hill gastropexy
- Belsey fundoplication
- Antireflux prosthesis

LES, lower esophageal sphincter.

Regurgitation (effortless return of material from stomach into esophagus or mouth) is a fairly common manifestation of an incompetent LES. It is often described as hot, bitter, or sour liquid coming into the throat or mouth. Other symptoms include feelings of a lump in the throat or of food stopping, *dysphagia* (difficulty in swallowing), painful swallowing, and bleeding. An individual with GERD may also experience respiratory complications including bronchospasm, laryngospasm, and cricopharyngeal spasm because of movement of gastric contents into the upper airway.[14]

Complications

Complications of GERD are related to the direct local effects of gastric acid on the esophageal mucosa. As a result of repeated exposure, there may be scar tissue formation and decreased distensibility (esophageal stricture) of the esophagus. This may result in dysphagia. In addition, esophageal metaplasia (Barrett's esophagus, which is a precancerous lesion) may occur. There is also the potential for pulmonary complications (pneumonia) as a result of aspiration of gastric contents into the pulmonary system.

Diagnostic Studies

Diagnostic studies are performed to determine the cause of the GERD (e.g., hiatal hernia) (Table 39-8). Barium swallow is done to determine if there is protrusion of the upper part of the stomach (called the gastric cardia). Radionuclide tests may also

DRUG THERAPY

Table 39-9 Gastroesophageal Reflux Disease (GERD)

Mechanism of Action	Examples
Increase LES Pressure	
Cholinergic	Bethanechol (Urecholine)
Dopamine antagonist	Metoclopramide (Reglan)
Acid Neutralizing	
Antacids	Gelusil, Maalox, Mylanta
Antisecretory	
Histamine H_2-receptor antagonists	Ranitidine (Zantac) Cimetidine (Tagamet) Famotidine (Pepcid) Nizatidine (Axid)
Proton pump inhibitors	Omeprazole (Prilosec) Lansoprazole (Prevacid) Pantoprazole (Pantoloc)
Cytoprotective	
Alginic acid-antacid	Gaviscon
Antacids	Gelusil, Maalox, Mylanta
Acid-protective	Sucralfate (Carafate)

LES, lower esophageal sphincter.

be performed to detect reflux of gastric contents and the rate of esophageal clearance. Esophagoscopy is useful in determining the incompetence of the LES and the extent of inflammation, potential scarring, and strictures. Biopsy and cytologic specimens can be taken to differentiate hiatal hernia from carcinoma of the stomach or esophagus and Barrett's esophagus. Esophageal motility studies are performed to measure pressure in the esophagus as well as the LES. The determination of pH using specially designed probes in the laboratory or using ambulatory monitoring systems may demonstrate the presence of acid in the normally alkaline esophagus.

Collaborative Care

A four-phase management approach is often used. Phase 1 is lifestyle modification (see Tables 39-7 and 39-8); Phase 2 involves drug therapy; Phase 3 is intensified drug therapy; and Phase 4 is antireflux surgery.[14]

Drug Therapy. Pharmacologic management is focused on improving LES function, increasing esophageal clearance, decreasing volume and acidity of reflux, and protecting esophageal mucosa. Antacids are used to relieve heartburn by their neutralizing effect on hydrochloric acid. They should be taken 1 to 3 hours after meals and at bedtime. Alginic acid and an antacid (Gaviscon) are sometimes given together. The alginic acid reacts with sodium bicarbonate and forms a viscous solution that floats to the surface of the gastric contents and coats the esophagus, acting as a mechanical barrier to reflux. However, antacids alone are often not effective in relieving symptoms or healing erosive lesions.[14]

In Phase 2, agents that decrease gastric hydrochloric acid secretion are used in the management of reflux esophagitis. Histamine H_2-receptor blockers (e.g., ranitidine [Zantac] or cimetidine [Tagamet]) have no effect on LES pressure but do decrease gastric acid production. They are particularly helpful for the patient with high acid outputs. Prokinetic drugs, such as cisapride (Propulsid), facilitate gastric emptying and thus reduce the volume of reflux. Prokinetic agents are often administered with antisecretory agents to promote esophageal healing.

If Phase 2 drug therapy is ineffective, patients may begin Phase 3 antisecretory drugs such as omeprazole (Prilosec) and lansoprazole (Prevacid).[15] These agents act by inhibiting the proton pump mechanism responsible for the secretion of H^+ ions, decreasing acid secretion, and facilitating the healing of erosive reflux esophagitis.

Other agents that may be used in both Phase 2 and 3 include sucralfate (Carafate), an antiulcer drug used for its cytoprotective properties, and cholinergic drugs, such as bethanechol (Urecholine), which may be used to increase LES pressure, improve esophageal emptying in the supine position, and increase gastric emptying. A summary of the drug therapy is shown in Table 39-9.

The nurse should observe for and instruct the patient about side effects of the medications being taken. Antacids have minimal side effects. Antacids that contain aluminum tend to cause constipation, whereas those that contain magnesium tend to cause diarrhea. Several of the antacids are combinations of aluminum and magnesium designed to minimize these side effects. If the patient is taking bethanechol, side effects to observe for include urinary urgency, increased salivation, abdominal cramping with diarrhea, nausea, vomiting, and hypotension. Such side effects often limit the effectiveness of cholinergic agents in the treatment of GERD. Side effects of metoclopramide, a prokinetic drug, include restlessness, anxiety, and insomnia. Side effects of metoclopramide (Reglan) a prokinetic agent that increases gastric emptying, include restlessness, anxiety, and insomnia. Side effects of sucralfate include drowsiness, dizziness, nausea, vomiting, constipation, urticaria, and rash.

Nutritional Therapy. A diet high in protein and low in fats is recommended for GERD. Fatty foods stimulate the release of cholecystokinin, which decreases LES pressure. Foods that decrease LES pressure, such as chocolate, peppermint, coffee, and tea (see Table 39-7), should be avoided because they cause reflux. Milk products should be avoided, especially at bedtime, because milk increases gastric acid secretion. Small, frequent meals are advised to prevent overdistention of the stomach. The patient should avoid late meals and nocturnal snacking. Fluids should be taken between rather than with meals to reduce distention. Certain foods (e.g., spicy tomato juice and orange juice) may irritate the acid-sensitive esophagus and thus may have to be avoided. No specific diet is necessary, but foods that cause reflux should be avoided. Weight reduction is recommended if the patient is obese.

NURSING MANAGEMENT: GASTROESOPHAGEAL REFLUX DISEASE

Patients with GERD must avoid factors that cause reflux. A patient teaching guide is provided in Table 39-10. The patient who is a smoker should stop smoking. Smoking causes an almost immediate drop in LES pressure. The patient may need to be referred to other members of the health care team or to community resources for assistance in stopping smoking. Substances

PATIENT & FAMILY TEACHING GUIDE

Table 39-10 Prevention of Gastroesophageal Reflux

The following are teaching guidelines for patient and family:

1. Explain the rationale for a high-protein, low-fat diet.
2. Encourage the patient to eat small, frequent meals to prevent gastric distention.
3. Explain the rationale for avoiding alcohol, smoking (causes an almost immediate, marked decrease in LES pressure), and beverages that contain caffeine.
4. Teach the patient not to lie down for 2 to 3 hours after eating, wear tight clothing around the waist, or bend over (especially after eating).
5. Encourage the patient to sleep with head of bed elevated on 4- to 6-inch blocks (gravity fosters esophageal emptying).
6. Teach regarding medications including rationale for their use and common side effects.
7. Discuss strategies for weight reduction if appropriate.
8. Encourage patient and family to share concerns about lifestyle changes and living with a chronic problem.

that decrease LES pressure and tone should be avoided (see Table 39-7). If stress seems to bring on symptoms, measures to cope with stress should be discussed.

Nursing care for the patient who is having acute symptoms consists mainly of teaching and encouraging the patient to follow the necessary regimen. The nurse should ensure that the head of the bed is elevated to approximately 30 degrees (usually on 4- to 6-inch blocks) and that the patient does not lie down during the first 2 to 3 hours after eating. Teaching the patient to avoid food and activities that cause reflux is important (e.g., late-night eating should be avoided). The patient may be taking medications to relieve heartburn, so the nurse must observe for side effects and evaluate whether the medications are relieving symptoms. The patient should also be taught possible side effects of medications.

Surgical therapy (antireflux surgery) may be necessary if conservative therapy fails, if a hiatal hernia is present, or if complications, such as stenosis, chronic esophagitis, and bleeding exist. The objective of surgery is to restore gastroesophageal integrity. Procedures used for the management of hiatal hernia including surgery are discussed below.

HIATAL HERNIA

Hiatal hernia is herniation of a portion of the stomach into the esophagus through an opening, or hiatus, in the diaphragm. It is also referred to as *diaphragmatic hernia* and *esophageal hernia.*

The incidence of hiatal hernia is difficult to determine. Although it is said to be the most common abnormality found on x-ray examination of the upper GI tract, the hernia is often asymptomatic. Hiatal hernias are common in older adults and occur more frequently in women than in men.

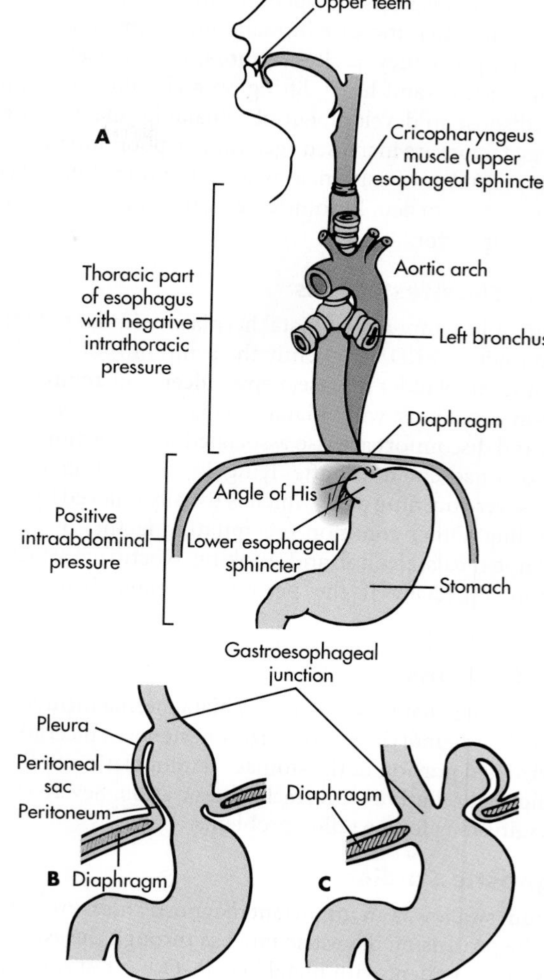

Fig. 39-6 **A,** Normal esophagus. **B,** Sliding hiatal hernia. **C,** Rolling or paraesophageal hernia.

Types

Hiatal hernias are classified into two types (Fig. 39-6):

1. *Sliding:* The junction of the stomach and esophagus is above the hiatus of the diaphragm, and a part of the stomach slides through the hiatal opening in the diaphragm. It "slides" into the thoracic cavity when the patient is supine and usually goes back into the abdominal cavity when the patient is standing upright. This is the most common type.
2. *Paraesophageal or rolling:* The esophagogastric junction remains in the normal position, but the fundus and the greater curvature of the stomach roll up through the diaphragm, forming a pocket alongside the esophagus.

Etiology and Pathophysiology

The actual cause of hiatal hernia is unknown. Many factors contribute to the development of hiatal hernia. Structural changes, such as weakening of the muscles in the diaphragm around the esophagogastric opening, are usually contributing factors. Factors that increase intraabdominal pressure, including obesity, pregnancy, ascites, tumors, tight corsets, intense physical exertion, and heavy lifting on a continual basis, may also predispose to development of a hiatal hernia. Other predisposing factors are increased age, trauma, poor nutrition, and a forced recumbent position, as when a prolonged illness confines the person to bed. In some cases, congenital weakness is a contributing factor.

Clinical Manifestations

The signs and symptoms of hiatal hernia are similar to that described under GERD. Frequently the symptoms of hiatal hernia mimic gallbladder disease, peptic ulcer, and angina. However, some patients with hiatal hernia have no symptoms. Reflux and discomfort are also associated with position, occurring soon or several hours after lying down. Bending over may cause a severe burning pain, which is usually relieved by sitting or standing. Other common precipitating factors of pain include large meals, alcohol, and smoking. Nocturnal attacks are common, especially if the person has eaten before going to sleep.

Complications

Complications that may occur with hiatal hernia include problems such as hemorrhage from erosion, stenosis, ulcerations of the herniated portion of the stomach, strangulation of the hernia, and regurgitation with tracheal aspiration. Severe chronic esophagitis may follow reflux problems.

Diagnostic Studies

A barium swallow is an important diagnostic measure that may show the protrusion of gastric mucosa through the esophageal hiatus in the patient with hiatal hernia. Other tests are similar to those described in Table 39-8.

Collaborative Care

Conservative Therapy. Conservative therapy of hiatal hernia includes administration of antacids and antisecretory agents, elimination of constricting garments, avoidance of lifting and straining, elimination of alcohol and smoking, and elevation of the head of the bed. Elevation of the bed on 4- to 6-inch blocks assists gravity in maintaining the stomach in the abdominal cavity and also helps prevent reflux and tracheal aspiration. If obese, the patient is encouraged to lose weight.

Surgical Therapy. The objective of surgical interventions for hiatal hernia is to reduce reflux by enhancing the integrity of the LES. Surgical procedures are termed *valvuloplasties* or *antireflux* procedures. There are three slightly varied procedures: the Nissen fundoplication, the Hill gastropexy, and the Belsey's fundoplication. These three surgical procedures are all variations of fundoplication, which involves "wrapping" the fundus of the stomach around the lower portion of the esophagus in varying degrees. These procedures reduce the hernia, provide an acceptable LES pressure, and prevent movement of the gastroesophageal junction. The Nissen fundoplication is shown in Fig. 39-7. The Nissen fundoplication procedure is being performed laparoscopically with increasing frequency. The use of laparoscopic techniques has reduced the overall morbidity associated with abdominal surgery.[14] A thoracic or open abdominal approach may also be used.

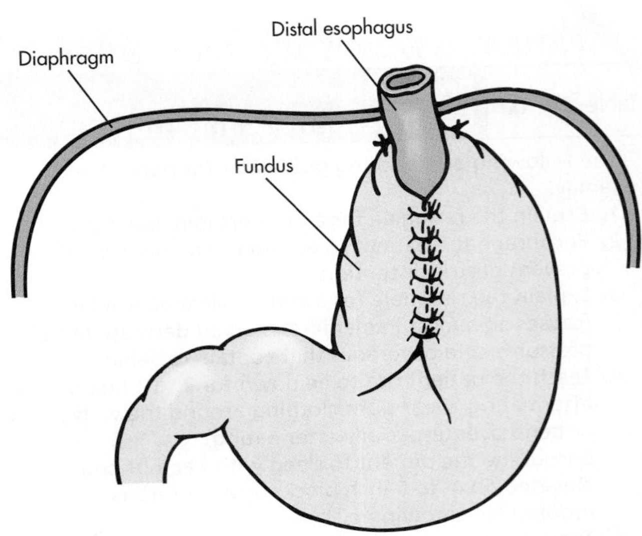

Fig. 39-7 Nissen fundoplication for repair of hiatal hernia. Fundus of stomach is wrapped around distal esophagus and sutured to itself.

Fundoplication prevents reflux in 90% of the patients. The success of fundoplication depends on achieving correct tightness of the fundal wrap. If it is too loose, reflux is not prevented. If it is too tight, dysphagia and the gas-bloat syndrome are problems.

NURSING MANAGEMENT: SURGICAL INTERVENTIONS FOR HIATAL HERNIA

Postoperative care focuses on concerns related to prevention of respiratory complications, maintenance of fluid and electrolyte balance, and prevention of infection. If a thoracic approach is used, a chest tube is inserted. Assessment and management related to closed chest drainage are important (see Chapter 26).

Respiratory complications can occur in a patient treated by an abdominal approach because of the high abdominal incision. Respiratory assessment should include respiratory rate and rhythm, chest reexpansion, pulse rate and rhythm, and signs of pneumothorax (e.g., dyspnea, chest pain, and cyanosis). Deep breathing is essential to fully expand the lungs.

The patient receives IV fluids and electrolytes until the return of peristalsis. Care should be taken to maintain patency of the NG tube (if present) to prevent the need to reinsert the tube. It is dangerous to attempt to replace the tube because of the possibility of perforation of the surgical repair. When peristalsis returns, only fluids are initially given. Solids are added gradually so that the stomach is not overdistended. The nurse must maintain an accurate recording of intake and output and observe for fluid and electrolyte imbalances (see Chapter 15). (Care of the patient undergoing a laparotomy procedure is described in the NCP 40-2 on p. 1147.)

After surgical intervention, there should be no symptoms of gastric reflux. The patient should be instructed to report symptoms such as heartburn and regurgitation. In the early postoperative period there is usually mild dysphagia caused by edema, but it should resolve. The patient should report persistent dysphagia, epigastric fullness, and bloating. Immediately after the surgical procedure, the patient cannot voluntarily vomit or belch, and this may cause the bloating and abdominal discomfort. A normal diet can be resumed within 6 weeks. The patient should avoid foods that are gas forming and should try to prevent gastric distention. Food should be thoroughly chewed.

GERONTOLOGIC CONSIDERATIONS

Gastroesophageal Reflux Disease and Hiatal Hernia

The incidence of hiatal hernia increases with age. It is associated with weakening of the diaphragm, obesity, kyphosis, and use of corsets or other factors that increase intraabdominal pressure. Some older adults with hiatal hernia are asymptomatic. The first indications may include esophageal bleeding secondary to esophagitis or pulmonary complications (e.g., aspiration, pneumonia) related to aspiration of gastric contents. The lower esophageal sphincter may become less competent with aging in some individuals.

The clinical course and management of these problems are similar to that for the younger adult. With the increased use of laparoscopic procedures, surgical risks have been reduced. However, an older adult with cardiovascular and pulmonary problems may not be a good candidate for surgical intervention. In addition, changes in lifestyle, including elimination of dietary factors, such as caffeine-containing beverages and chocolate, and elevating the head of the bed on blocks, may be more difficult.

ESOPHAGEAL CANCER

Carcinoma of the esophagus is unique in its geographic distribution. There are portions of Asia in which the rate of esophageal cancer is extremely high while in Western societies the incidence is relatively low. For example, esophageal cancer is the second most common type of cancer in China.[16] In the United States it is estimated that there will be 12,300 new cases of esophageal cancer (9300 will be men) and that 11,900 Americans will die in 1998 from esophageal cancer.

The incidence of squamous cell esophageal cancer is currently decreasing in the United States, whereas the incidence of adenocarcinoma of the distal esophagus is increasing. However, squamous cell carcinoma remains the most common form of esophageal cancer. The incidence of esophageal cancer increases with age. There is a higher incidence of squamous cell carcinoma in African-Americans and in men. The incidence of esophageal cancer is higher in Alaska Native men and women compared with Caucasians.[17] Because esophageal cancer is rarely diagnosed in early stages, the 5-year prognosis is poor.

A condition called *Barrett's esophagus* is considered a metaplastic change that may progress to adenocarcinoma of the esophagus. This syndrome is characterized by replacement of areas of the normal squamous epithelium of the esophagus with columnar epithelium. It may result from severe reflux esophagitis and is considered an important complication of GERD. Signs and symptoms of Barrett's esophagus can range from none to mild to bleeding and perforation.[14] Because patients with Barrett's esophagus are at risk for adenocarcinoma, they must be monitored on an annual basis by endoscopy and biopsy.

Etiology and Pathophysiology

The cause of cancer of the esophagus is unknown. Possible predisposing factors are cigarette smoking, excessive alcohol intake, chronic trauma, poor oral hygiene, and spicy foods. The two most important risk factors are smoking and excessive alcohol intake. Other risk factors include exposure to asbestos and metal and low intake of fresh fruits and vegetables.[18]

The majority of tumors are located in the middle and lower portions of the esophagus. The malignant tumor usually appears as an ulcerated lesion. It may have advanced to this stage before the appearance of symptoms. The tumor may penetrate the muscular layer and even extend outside the wall of the esophagus. Obstruction of the esophagus occurs in the later stages.

Clinical Manifestations

The onset of symptoms is usually late in relation to the extent of the tumor. Progressive dysphagia is the most common symptom and may be expressed as a substernal feeling as if food is not passing. Initially the dysphagia occurs only with meat, then with soft foods, and eventually with liquids.

Pain develops late and is described as occurring in the substernal, epigastric, or back areas and usually increases with swallowing. The pain may radiate to the neck, jaw, ears, and shoulders. If the tumor is in the upper third of the esophagus, symptoms such as sore throat, choking, and hoarseness may occur. Weight loss is fairly common. When esophageal stenosis is severe, regurgitation of blood-flecked esophageal contents is common.

Complications

Hemorrhage may occur if the cancer erodes through the esophagus and into the aorta. Esophageal perforation with fistula formation into the lung or trachea sometimes develops. The tumor may enlarge enough to cause esophageal obstruction. Esophageal carcinoma has a poor prognosis because of early lymphatic spread and late development of symptoms. The liver and lung are common metastatic sites.

Diagnostic Studies

Barium swallow with fluoroscopy may demonstrate a narrowing of the esophagus at the site of the tumor (Table 39-11). Sometimes a crater is visible. Esophagoscopy with biopsy is necessary to make a definitive diagnosis of carcinoma by identification of malignant cells. Endoscopic ultrasonography is also used to detect tumor invasion into the muscle layer. A bronchoscopic examination may be performed to detect malignant involvement of the trachea. Computerized tomography (CT) scanning and magnetic resonance imaging (MRI) are also used to assess the extent of the disease.

Collaborative Care

The treatment of carcinoma of the esophagus depends on the location of the tumor and whether invasion or metastasis has

COLLABORATIVE CARE

Table 39-11 Esophageal Cancer

Diagnostic
- Barium swallow
- Esophagoscopy with biopsy
- CT and MRI
- Ultrasonography
- Bronchoscopy

Collaborative Therapy
- Surgical resection
  - Esophagectomy
  - Esophagogastrostomy
  - Esophagoenterostomy
- Radiation
- Palliative
  - Dilation
  - Stent or prosthesis
  - Gastrostomy
  - Laser therapy

occurred (see Table 39-11). Surgical removal and radiation are the two methods used. Cancer of the esophagus has a poor prognosis, mainly because in most cases it is not diagnosed until the disease is advanced. Relatively few people are cured. The best results have been obtained with a combination of surgery and radiation. Chemotherapeutic agents, cisplatin (Platinol), and 5-FU in combination with radiation are currently under investigation.[19]

If the tumor is in the cervical section (upper third) of the esophagus, radiation is usually indicated. A tumor in the lower third of the esophagus is usually resected surgically. In addition, radiation may be used either before or after surgery.

The types of surgical procedures that can be performed are (1) removal of part or all of the esophagus (*esophagectomy*) with use of a Dacron graft to replace the resected part, (2) resection of a portion of the esophagus and anastomosis of the remaining portion to the stomach (*esophagogastrostomy*), and (3) resection of a portion of the esophagus and anastomosis of a segment of colon to the remaining portion (*esophagoenterostomy*). The surgical approaches may be thoracic or both abdominal and thoracic.

Surgery may not be performed if the patient is an older adult or in poor physical health. Palliative therapy consists of restoration of the swallowing function and maintenance of nutrition and hydration. Dilation, stent placement, or both can relieve obstruction. Laser therapy or vaporization of the tumor by means of endoscopy may be used in combination with dilation. Obstruction recurs as the tumor grows, but laser therapy can be repeated. Sometimes these procedures are combined with radiation therapy. Other measures for palliation include gastrostomy or esophagostomy tube placements for nutrition support and pain management.

Dilation is done with various types of dilators (e.g., Celestin tube). Dilation often relieves dysphagia and allows for improved nutrition. Placement of a stent or prosthesis may help when dilation is no longer effective. The prostheses are composed of silicone rubber or nylon-reinforced latex tubes with distal and proximal collars. The prosthesis is placed in the esophagus so that food and fluids can pass through the stenotic segment of the esophagus. The prosthesis can be placed endoscopically.

Nutritional Therapy. After esophageal surgery, parenteral fluids are given. When fluids are allowed after bowel sounds have returned, 30 to 60 ml of water are given hourly, with gradual progression to small, frequent bland meals. The patient should be in an upright position to prevent regurgitation of the fluid. The patient is observed for signs of intolerance to the feeding or leakage of the feeding into the mediastinum. Symptoms that indicate leakage are pain, increased temperature, and dyspnea. Symptoms of food intolerance include vomiting and abdominal distention. A gastrostomy may be performed for the purpose of feeding the patient. (Gastrostomy tubes are discussed in Chapter 38.)

NURSING MANAGEMENT: ESOPHAGEAL CANCER

Nursing Assessment

The patient should be assessed for progressive dysphagia and odynophagia (burning, squeezing pain while swallowing). The nurse should question the patient regarding the type of substances ingested that cause dysphagia, such as meat, soft foods, and liquids. The patient should also be assessed for pain (substernal, epigastric, or back areas), choking, hoarseness, cough, anorexia, weight loss, and regurgitation (sometimes bloody). The patient should also be questioned regarding tobacco and alcohol use.

Nursing Diagnoses

Nursing diagnoses for the patient with esophageal cancer include, but are not limited to, the following:

- Altered nutrition: less than body requirements *related to* dysphagia, odynophagia, weakness, and radiation therapy
- Pain *related to* tumor
- Fluid volume deficit *related to* inadequate intake
- Risk for aspiration *related to* impaired esophageal function
- Anxiety *related to* diagnosis of cancer, uncertain future, and poor prognosis
- Anticipatory grieving *related to* diagnosis of life-threatening malignancy
- Altered health maintenance *related to* lack of knowledge of disease process and therapeutic regimen, unavailability of a support system, and chronic debilitating disease

Planning

The overall goals are that the patient with esophageal cancer will (1) have relief of symptoms including pain and dysphagia, (2) achieve optimal nutritional intake, (3) understand the prognosis of the disease, and (4) experience a quality of life appropriate to disease progression.

Nursing Implementation

Health Promotion. Because the cause of esophageal cancer is not definitive, it is difficult to identify preventive measures. Health counseling should focus on elimination of smoking and excessive alcohol intake. Maintenance of good oral hygiene and dietary habits (intake of fresh fruits and vegetables) may also be helpful.

Having the patient obtain treatment of esophageal problems, such as Barrett's esophagus, is helpful because this is considered a premalignant condition. Early diagnosis of esophageal tumors is important but difficult because the onset of symptoms is usually late. The patient should be encouraged to have regular physical examinations and to seek medical attention for any esophageal problems, especially dysphagia. The patient who is at risk of esophageal adenocarcinoma, such as those with Barrett's esophagus, need regular (yearly) endoscopic screening with biopsy and cytologic study.

Acute Intervention

Preoperative care. In addition to general preoperative teaching and preparation, particular attention to the patient's nutritional needs and oral care is important. Many patients are poorly nourished because of the inability to ingest adequate amounts of food and fluids before surgery. A high-calorie, high protein diet is recommended. It may have to be in liquid form. Some patients may need IV fluid replacement or total parenteral nutrition. The patient and or family member is instructed on how to keep an intake and output record and assess for signs of fluid and electrolyte imbalance.

Meticulous oral care is essential. A thorough cleaning of the mouth, including tongue, gingivae, and teeth or dentures, is necessary. It may be necessary to use swabs or a gauze pad and to really scrub the mouth, including the tongue. Milk of magnesia with mineral oil may be used to remove crust formation. A mixture of mouthwash, ice, and water makes a refreshing rinse for the patient.

Teaching should include information about chest tubes (if a thoracic approach is used), IV lines, NG tube, gastrostomy feeding, turning, coughing, and deep breathing. (General preoperative care is presented in Chapter 16.)

Postoperative care. The patient usually has an NG tube in place, and there may be bloody drainage for 8 to 12 hours. The drainage gradually changes to greenish yellow. Assessment of the drainage, maintenance of the tube, and oral and nasal care are nursing responsibilities. The NG tube should not be repositioned or reinserted without consulting with the surgeon.

Because of the location of the incision and the general condition of the patient, special emphasis must be placed on prevention of respiratory complications. Turning and deep breathing should be done every 2 hours. Use of an incentive spirometer helps in preventing respiratory complications.

The patient should be positioned in a semi-Fowler's or Fowler's position to prevent reflux and aspiration of gastric secretions. When the patient can drink fluids or eat, the upright position should be maintained for at least 2 hours after eating to assist the movement of food through the GI tract.

Ambulatory and Home Care. Many patients require long-term follow-up care after surgery for esophageal cancer. The patient may undergo radiation treatment following surgery. The patient needs encouragement and assistance in maintaining adequate nutrition. The patient may need a permanent feeding gastrostomy. The patient usually has fears and anxieties about a diagnosis of cancer. The nurse should know what the doctor has told the patient regarding the prognosis and then provide appropriate counseling. Some communities have resource groups consisting of persons with cancer who can serve as support systems. Groups can usually be contacted through the local chapter of the American Cancer Society.

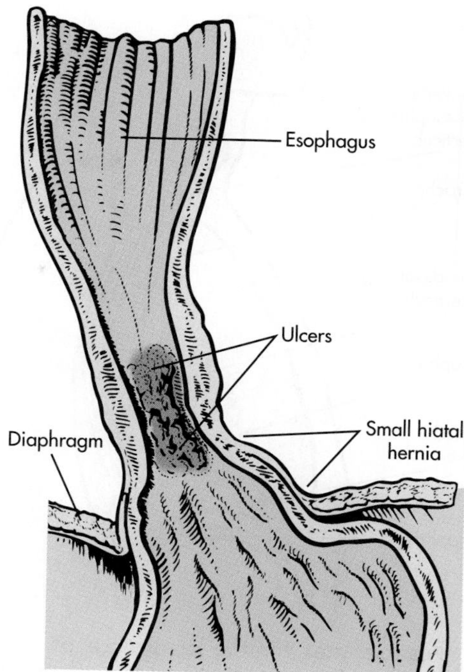

Fig. 39-8 Esophagitis with esophageal ulcerations.

Referral to a home health nurse may be necessary for continued care of the patient (e.g., gastrostomy teaching and follow-up wound care). (Management of the terminally ill cancer patient is discussed in Chapter 14.)

■ Evaluation

The expected outcomes are that the patient with esophageal cancer will

- have relief of symptoms including pain and dysphagia
- achieve optimal nutritional intake
- understand the prognosis of the disease
- experience quality of life appropriate to disease progression

OTHER ESOPHAGEAL DISORDERS

Esophagitis

Esophagitis (inflammation of the esophagus) is a frequent condition and may occur as a result of chemical irritation from lye or dust or physical irritants such as smoking, cold or hot liquids, and excessive alcoholic intake. Trauma to the esophagus may also produce inflammation. *Achalasia* (cardiospasm) and carcinoma may lead to esophagitis. Esophagitis with esophageal ulcerations is shown in Fig. 39-8.

Reflux esophagitis is common. It results from the reflux of gastric contents into the esophagus (see section on Gastroesophageal Reflux Disease). A sliding hiatal hernia is a common cause of reflux esophagitis (see section on Hiatal Hernia),

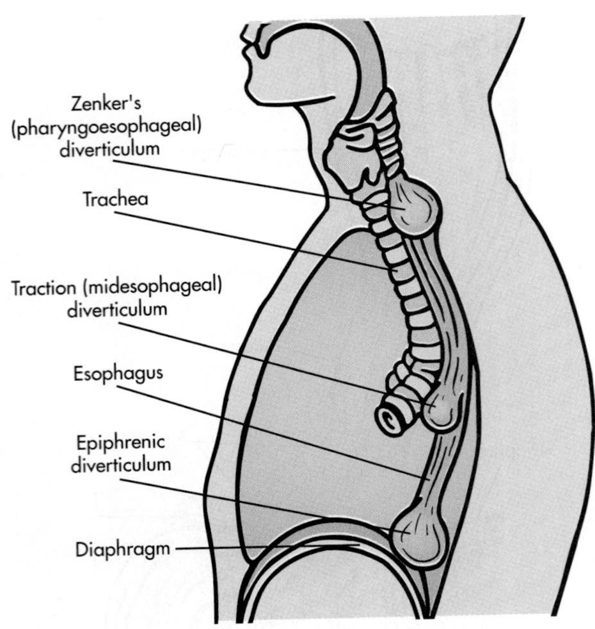

Fig. 39-9 Possible sites for the occurrence of esophageal diverticula. These hollow outpouchings may occur just above the upper esophageal sphincter (Zenker's, the most common type of pulsion diverticulum), near the midpoint of the esophagus (traction), and just above the lower esophageal sphincter (epiphrenic).

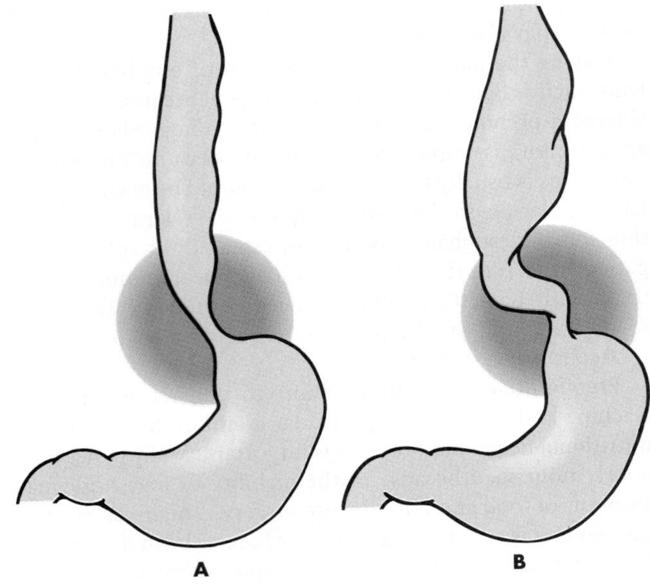

Fig. 39-10 Esophageal achalasia. **A,** Early stage, showing tapering of lower esophagus. **B,** Advanced stage, showing dilated, tortuous esophagus.

although it occurs in many patients without hiatal hernia. Esophagitis results from an incompetent LES.

Treatment of esophagitis depends on the cause. If strong alkalis or acids cause acute esophagitis, prompt, vigorous treatment is necessary. The treatment of chronic esophagitis includes oral antacids, agents that decrease acid secretion (histamine H_2-antagonists, proton pump inhibitors), dietary alterations (Table 39-8), and sleeping with the head of the bed elevated. The goal of treatment is to prevent gastric juices from damaging the esophageal mucosa.

Diverticula

Diverticula are saclike outpouchings of one or more layers of the esophagus. They occur in three main areas: (1) above the upper esophageal sphincter (Zenker's diverticulum), which is the most common location; (2) near the esophageal midpoint (traction); and (3) above the LES (epiphrenic) (Fig. 39-9). The main symptoms are dysphagia and regurgitation, especially with Zenker's diverticulum. Traction diverticula may not cause signs and symptoms. The patient frequently complains of tasting sour food and smelling a foul odor caused by the stagnant food. Complications include malnutrition, aspiration, and perforation.

There is no specific treatment for diverticula. Some patients find they can empty the pocket of food that collects by applying pressure at a point on the neck. The diet may have to be limited to foods that pass more readily (e.g., blenderized foods). Surgical removal of the diverticulum may be necessary if nutrition becomes disrupted. An alternative to surgery is endoscopic division of the septum between the diverticulum and the esophagus.

Esophageal Strictures

The most common causes of esophageal strictures are strong acids or alkalis that have been ingested and reflux or peptic strictures. Trauma such as throat lacerations and gunshot wounds may also lead to strictures as a result of scar formation from healing. The strictures usually develop over a long period of time. Strictures can be dilated endoscopically using bougies (dilating instruments). Another technique is balloon dilation, which is done under endoscopy and does not require fluoroscopy. Surgical excision with anastomosis is sometimes necessary. The patient may have a temporary or permanent gastrostomy.

Achalasia

In achalasia (*cardiospasm*), peristalsis of the lower two-thirds (smooth muscle) of the esophagus is absent. Pressure in the LES is increased, along with incomplete relaxation of the LES. Obstruction of the esophagus at or near the diaphragm occurs. Food and fluid accumulate in the lower esophagus. The result of this condition is dilation of the lower esophagus (Fig. 39-10). The altered peristalsis is a result of impairment of the autonomic nervous system innervating the esophagus. Achalasia affects all ages and both genders. The course of the disease is chronic.

Dysphagia is the most common symptom and occurs more frequently with liquids. Substernal chest pain (similar to the pain of angina) occurs during or immediately after a meal. Halitosis and the inability to eructate are other symptoms. Another common symptom is regurgitation of sour-tasting food and liquids, especially when the patient is in a horizontal position. Weight loss is typical.

Treatment consists of dilation, surgery, and use of drugs. All these therapies are directed at relieving the stasis caused by the increased LES pressure, nonrelaxing LES, and aperistaltic esophagus. The aim of management is to relieve symptoms.

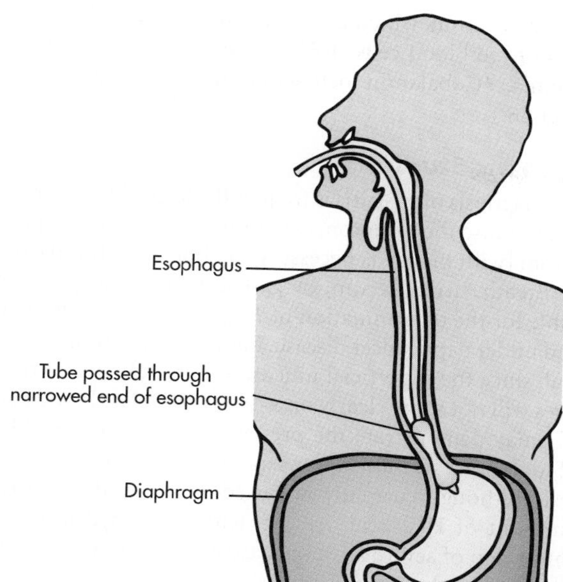

Fig. 39-11 Pneumatic dilation attempts to treat achalasia by maintaining an adequate lumen and decreasing lower esophageal sphincter (LES) tone.

Symptomatic treatment consists of a semisoft bland diet, eating slowly and drinking fluid with meals, and sleeping with the head elevated.

Esophageal dilation (*bougienage*) is an effective treatment measure for many patients. Pneumatic dilation of the LES with a balloon-tipped dilator passed orally is usually used. Commonly used dilators for pneumatic dilation are the Mosher bag, the Tucker mercury dilator, and the Browne-McHardy dilator. They all depend on forcible expansion of a balloon in the LES (Fig. 39-11). The forceful dilation does not restore normal esophageal motility, but it does provide for emptying of the esophagus into the stomach.

Surgical intervention may become necessary. An *esophagomyotomy* may be performed. In this procedure the muscle fibers that enclose the narrowed area of the esophagus are divided. This allows the mucosa to pouch out through the division in the muscle layer to allow food to be swallowed without obstruction.

A similar procedure is Heller's myotomy (cardiomyotomy), which disrupts the LES in a similar manner and reduces LES pressure. An antireflux procedure is frequently done with the myotomy. This procedure can be performed laparoscopically, reducing the potential for postoperative complications.

Classes of drugs used in the treatment of achalasia include anticholinergics, calcium channel blockers (e.g., nifedipine [Procardia]), and long-acting nitrates. Recent studies indicate a role for botulinum toxin injection, which relaxes esophageal muscle, delivered endoscopically in the management of achalasia.[20]

Esophageal Varices

Esophageal varices are dilated, tortuous veins occurring in the lower portion of the esophagus as a result of portal hypertension. Esophageal varices are a common complication of liver cirrhosis and are discussed in Chapter 41.

Table 39-12 Causes of Gastritis

Aspirin	Smoking
Nonsteroidal anti-inflammatory drugs	Physiologic stress
Corticosteroid drugs	Shock
Alcohol	Sepsis
Radiation	Burns
Helicobacter pylori	Psychologic stress
Staphylococcus organisms	Renal failure (uremia)
Salmonella	Spicy, irritating food
Reflux of bile and pancreatic secretions	Trauma
	Nasogastric suction
	Large hiatal hernia
	Endoscopic techniques

GASTRITIS

Types

Gastritis, an inflammation of the gastric mucosa, is one of the most common problems affecting the stomach. Gastritis may be *acute* or *chronic* and may be diffuse or localized. Chronic gastritis can be further classified as type A (fundal) and type B (antral). Presently, the causes of gastritis and its relationship to other gastric disorders, such as gastric cancer, are the focuses of intensive research.

Etiology and Pathophysiology

Gastritis occurs as the result of a breakdown in the normal gastric mucosal barrier. This mucosal barrier normally protects the stomach tissue from autodigestion by acid and the enzyme pepsin. When the barrier is broken, acid can diffuse back into the mucosa. This allows hydrochloric (HCl) acid to enter. The HCl acid stimulates the conversion of pepsinogen to pepsin and stimulates the release of histamine from mast cells. The combined result of these occurrences is tissue edema, disruption of capillary walls with loss of plasma into the gastric lumen, and possible hemorrhage.

Causes of gastritis are listed in Table 39-12. Corticosteroids and nonsteroidal antiinflammatory drugs (NSAIDs) are known to inhibit the synthesis of prostaglandins, which then results in increased HCl acid secretion. Drugs such as aspirin, digitalis, and NSAIDs are directly irritating to the gastric mucosa. The ingestion of even small amounts of aspirin by the susceptible person is known to result in asymptomatic GI bleeding manifested by positive stool tests for occult blood. After an alcoholic drinking binge, acute damage to the gastric mucosa can range from local destruction of superficial epithelial cells to desquamation and destruction of the mucosa, with mucosal congestion, edema, and hemorrhage. Eating large quantities of spicy, irritating foods and metabolic conditions such as uremia can also cause acute gastritis.

Gastritis can occur from reflux of bile salts from the duodenum into the stomach as a result of anatomic changes following surgical procedures such as gastroduodenostomy and gastrojejunostomy. Prolonged vomiting may also cause reflux of bile salts. Intense emotional responses and CNS lesions may also produce inflammation of the mucosal lining as a result of hypersecretion of HCl acid.

Chronic exposure to the factors previously described (e.g., chronic alcohol abuse, excess ingestion of aspirin, reflux of duodenal contents after gastric surgery, uremia) will result in inflammation and eventual loss of viable mucosal tissue. This form of chronic gastritis can result from repeated episodes of acute gastritis.

Chronic gastritis, type A, is likely to be an autoimmune disorder. Approximately 95% of patients with pernicious anemia and 60% of patients with chronic atrophic gastritis have antibodies to parietal cells in their serum. Autoimmune atrophic gastritis affects both the fundus and body of the stomach and is associated with an increased risk of gastric malignancy.

Chronic gastritis, Type B, is related to the presence of *Helicobacter pylori* (*H. pylori*). Type B gastritis primarily involves the antrum of the stomach and is a common problem in adults.[21]

The presence of *H. pylori* also has been correlated with the presence of other gastric disorders, including gastric and duodenal ulcers and gastric cancer. A description of the epidemiolgogy of *H. pylori* and its proposed role in the promotion of gastric disorders is discussed in the sections on peptic ulcers and gastric cancer. This section describes the current understanding of the mechanism by which *H. pylori* functions as a causative agent in chronic gastritis.

It is currently thought that *H. pylori* is acquired in childhood and is able to survive in the hostile environment of the gastric lumen. For reasons not clearly understood, *H. pylori* are capable of promoting the breakdown of the gastric mucosal barrier, given certain "triggers" or conditions. Thus given time, *H. pylori* will eventually have a destructive effect on its host environment. This is congruent with the finding that the incidence of chronic gastritis increases with age. However, studies also have shown that not all persons infected with *H. pylori* go on to develop chronic gastritis. Thus it may be that a combination of factors is at work to "turn on" the virulent process by which *H. pylori* damages the gastric mucosal barrier.

Progressive gastric atrophy from chronic alterations in the protective mucosal barrier causes the chief and parietal cells to eventually die. As the number of the acid-secreting parietal cells decreases with atrophy of the gastric mucosa, *hypochlorhydria* (decreased acid secretion) or *achlorhydria* (lack of acid secretion) occurs.

Clinical Manifestations

The symptoms of acute gastritis include anorexia, nausea and vomiting, epigastric tenderness, and a feeling of fullness. Hemorrhage is commonly associated with alcohol abuse and at times may be the only symptom. Acute gastritis is self-limiting, lasting from a few hours to a few days, with complete healing of the mucosa expected.

The manifestations of chronic gastritis are similar to those described for acute gastritis. Some patients have no symptoms directly associated with the gastric lesion. However, when the acid-secreting cells are lost or do not function as a result of atrophy, the source of intrinsic factor is also lost. Intrinsic factor, which normally combines with cobalamin (vitamin B_{12}), is unavailable, and thus cobalamin cannot be absorbed in the ileum. The intrinsic factor protects cobalamin from digestion by the GI enzymes. Eventually the body's storage of cobalamin in the liver is depleted and a deficiency state exists. Lack of this important vitamin, which is essential for the growth and maturation of red blood cells (RBCs), results in the development of anemia. (Cobalamin deficiency anemia is discussed in Chapter 28.)

Diagnostic Studies

Proper diagnosis of gastritis is frequently delayed or completely missed because the symptoms are nonspecific. Endoscopic examination with biopsy is necessary to obtain a definitive diagnosis. Breath, urine, serum, or gastric tissue biopsy tests are available for the determination of *H. pylori*. These tests are described under peptic ulcer disease. Radiographic studies are not helpful, since the superficial mucosa is generally involved, and changes will not show clearly on x-ray. A complete blood count (CBC) may demonstrate the presence of anemia from blood loss. Stools are tested for the presence of occult blood. A gastric analysis, although currently not used as much, demonstrates the amount of HCl acid present, with achlorhydria being a common sign of severe atrophic gastritis. Serum tests for antibodies to parietal cells and intrinsic factor may be performed. Cytologic examination is needed to rule out gastric carcinoma.

Collaborative Care

Elimination of the cause and preventing or avoiding it in the future are generally all that is needed to treat acute gastritis. The plan of care is supportive and similar to that described for nausea and vomiting. During the acute phase, bed rest, NPO status, and IV fluids may be prescribed. Fluids and electrolytes lost through vomiting and, occasionally, diarrhea are replaced. In severe cases an NG tube may be used, either for lavage of the precipitating agent from the stomach or in conjunction with suction to keep the stomach empty and free of noxious stimuli. Antiemetics are given for nausea and vomiting. Antacids have proved beneficial in the relief of abdominal discomfort by raising intragastric pH to above 6. H_2 antagonists, such as ranitidine (Zantac) or cimetidine (Tagamet), or proton pump inhibitors, such as omeprazole (Prilosec) or lansoprazole (Prevacid), may be prescribed to reduce gastric HCl acid secretion. Once *H. pylori* has been diagnosed, antibiotic therapy is initiated. Clear liquids are resumed when acute symptoms have subsided, with gradual reintroduction of solid, bland foods. Acute gastritis with hemorrhage is treated with blood transfusion and fluid replacement. Surgical intervention with partial gastrectomy, vagotomy, or pyloroplasty may be necessary if treatment fails.

The treatment of chronic gastritis focuses on evaluating and eliminating the specific cause (e.g., cessation of alcoholic intake, abstinence from drugs). Currently, double and triple antibiotic combinations are used to eradicate infection with *H. pylori* (Table 39-13). Triple therapy containing lansoprazole, clarithromycin, and amoxicillin is now available as Prevpac in one convenient package. For the patient with pernicious anemia, regular injections of cobalamin are needed (see Chapter 29). An individualized bland diet and use of antacids are recommended. Smoking is contraindicated in all forms of gastritis. The patient undergoing treatment for gastritis may have to adapt to many lifestyle changes and adopt a strict adherence to a medication regimen. An interdisciplinary team approach in which the physician, nurse, dietician, and pharmacist provide consistent information and support may increase the patient's success in making these alterations.

DRUG THERAPY

Table 39-13 *Helicobacter Pylori* Infection

Treatment	Duration	Eradication Rate
Original Triple Therapy		
Tetracycline		
Metronidazole (Flagyl)	14 days	>90%
Bismuth subsalicylate		
New Triple Therapy		
Amoxicillin		
Clarithromycin (Biaxin)	7 days	>90%
Omeprazole (Prilosec)		
Dual Therapy		
Amoxicillin or clarithromycin (Biaxin)		
Omeprazole (Prilosec)	14 days	60 - 80%

Table 39-14 Types of Upper Gastrointestinal Bleeding

Type	Clinical Manifestations
Obvious bleeding	
▪ Hematemesis	Bloody vomitus appearing as fresh, bright red blood or "coffee ground" appearance (dark, grainy digested blood)
▪ Melena	Black, tarry stools (often foul smelling) caused by digestion of blood in the GI tract. The black appearance is from the presence of iron
Occult bleeding	Small amounts of blood in gastric secretions, vomitus, or stools not apparent by appearance; detectable by guaiac test

NURSING MANAGEMENT: ACUTE GASTRITIS

▪ Nursing Assessment

Dehydration can occur rapidly in severe gastritis that is accompanied by vomiting. Keeping the patient quiet, maintaining NPO status, and monitoring IV fluids are essential. If hemorrhage is considered likely, frequent checking of vital signs and testing the vomitus for blood are indicated. Elimination of the cause of the gastritis results in rapid improvement in the patient's condition. Identification of the causative agent is important to prevent future gastric irritation.

▪ Nursing Diagnoses

The nursing diagnoses for the patient with nausea and vomiting (see NCP 39-1) are also applicable to the patient with gastritis.

▪ Planning

The overall goals are that the patient with gastritis will (1) experience minimal or no symptoms of gastritis, (2) have no recurrent episodes of acute gastritis, and (3) achieve an optimal pattern of gastric function relative to the stage of the disease.

▪ Nursing Implementation

The patient with gastritis should be encouraged to avoid causative factors and to follow the prescribed diet and medication regimen. Because the incidence of gastric cancer is higher in the patient who has a history of chronic gastritis, especially atrophic gastritis, close medical follow-up should be stressed.

Most patients with gastritis receive care in the home, and chronic management may be necessary for extended periods of time. A bland diet consisting of six small feedings a day and the use of an antacid after meals may help provide symptomatic relief. It is essential that the nurse have knowledge of the action and therapeutic effects of antisecretory and H_2 antagonists to teach the patient and to monitor drug effects. The care of the patient with chronic atrophic gastritis and gastric atrophy is also supportive. With advanced gastric atrophy, cobalamin injections may be necessary for the lifetime of the patient. Discussion of the continued need for this essential vitamin must be included in the plan of care.

The patient with severe dehydration and gastric bleeding may require acute intervention. All of the management strategies discussed in the section on gastric bleeding are also applicable to the patient with severe gastritis.

UPPER GASTROINTESTINAL BLEEDING

Etiology and Pathophysiology

Although the most serious loss of blood from the upper GI tract is characterized by a sudden onset, insidious occult bleeding can also be a major problem. The severity of bleeding depends on whether the origin is venous, capillary, or arterial. (Types of upper GI bleeding are presented in Table 39-14.) Bleeding from an arterial source is profuse, and the blood is bright red. The bright red color indicates that the blood has not been in contact with the stomach's acid secretions. In contrast, "coffee ground" vomitus reveals that the blood and other contents have been in the stomach for some time and have been changed by contact with gastric secretions. A massive upper GI hemorrhage is generally defined as a loss of more than 1500 ml of blood or a loss of 25% of intravascular blood volume. Despite improvements in detection and treatment of acute upper GI bleeding, the mortality rate remains around 10%. *Melena* (black, tarry stools) indicates slow bleeding from an upper GI source. The longer the passage of blood through the intestines, the darker the color of the stool as a result of the degradation of hemoglobin and the release of iron.

Discovering the cause of the bleeding is not always an easy task. A variety of areas in the GI tract may be involved, and there may be many different reasons for the blood loss. Table 39-15 lists the common causes of bleeding.

Esophageal Origin. Bleeding from an esophageal source is most likely the result of chronic esophagitis, bleeding from a tear in the mucosa near the esophagogastric junction (Mallory-Weiss tear or syndrome), or esophageal varices. Chronic esophagitis can be caused by the ingestion of chemicals including medications irritating to the mucosa or hot, spicy, irritating foods. Alcohol and cigarettes are known irritants of the esophageal mucosa. An incompetent lower

Table 39-15 Common Causes of Upper Gastrointestinal Bleeding

Drug Induced	Stomach and Duodenum
Salicylates	Peptic ulcer disease
Corticosteroids	Stress ulcer
Nonsteroidal antiinflammatory agents	Hemorrhagic gastritis
	Carcinoma
Esophagus	Polyps
Esophageal varices	**Systemic Diseases**
Esophagitis	Blood dyscrasias
Mallory-Weiss syndrome	Leukemia
	Uremia

esophageal sphincter, which permits reflux of the acidic stomach contents into the esophagus, can lead to chronic irritation and erosion. Severe retching and vomiting can cause a tear in the esophageal mucosa resulting in severe bleeding.

Esophageal varices usually occur secondary to cirrhosis of the liver. Branches of the vena cava and the azygos vein from the systemic circulation converge with the smaller vessels of the lower esophagus. These vessels are inelastic and become engorged and tortuous because of increased pressure exerted on them secondary to portal hypertension. Anything that may increase the pressure (e.g., coughing, sneezing, trauma) or result in mechanical irritation (e.g., vomiting, irritation, erosion) may result in sudden, massive bleeding. (Esophageal varices are discussed in Chapter 41.)

Stomach and Duodenal Origin. Erosion of a blood vessel by a peptic ulcer located in the stomach or duodenum must always be considered as a possible cause of upper GI bleeding. Peptic ulcers account for more than 50% of cases of upper GI bleeding.[22] Ulcers frequently penetrate blood vessels. A gastric ulcer may penetrate the left gastric artery, and a duodenal ulcer may penetrate the superior pancreaticoduodenal artery.

Some medications, either prescribed by the physician or self-administered, have been implicated as a cause of upper GI bleeding. The patient who regularly takes aspirin or aspirin-containing compounds may be at risk for bleeding episodes. Aspirin, NSAIDs (e.g., ibuprofen), and corticosteroids, can cause irritation and disruption of the gastric mucosal barrier.[23] Aspirin-containing products are sold without prescriptions as OTC drugs (see Table 29-15). It is not unusual for a patient to deny the use of aspirin yet be self-medicating with aspirin-containing drugs, such as Alka-Seltzer, Bufferin, and Excedrin. A careful history of all commonly used medications is therefore necessary whenever upper GI bleeding is suspected.

Stress ulcers, which may occur after severe burn, trauma, or major surgery, erode more superficial blood vessels than does a peptic ulcer. They may also cause bleeding from erosion of a larger blood vessel. Gastritis produced by ingestion of drugs or alcohol or the reflux of bile from the small intestine can result in bleeding. Gastric carcinoma can be the cause of a steady blood loss as it grows and ulcerates through the mucosa and blood vessels located in its path. Hematemesis and melena are commonly associated with cancer of the stomach.

Systemic Diseases. Systemic diseases (e.g., leukemia, blood dyscrasias) that interfere with normal blood clotting must be considered whenever upper GI bleeding occurs.

Emergency Assessment and Management

Although approximately 80% of patients who have massive hemorrhage spontaneously stop bleeding, the cause must be identified and treatment initiated immediately. In spite of advances in intensive care, hemodynamic monitoring, and fiberoptic endoscopy, there has been little change in the mortality rate for upper GI bleeding, which has remained approximately 10% for the past 40 years. This is due in part to the greater incidence of upper GI bleeding in older adults, especially women, related to the use of NSAIDs agents.

Although a complete history of events leading to the bleeding episode is important in discovering the cause of the blood loss, it should be deferred until emergency care has been initiated. The immediate physical examination must include a systemic evaluation of the patient's condition with emphasis on blood pressure, rate and character of pulse, peripheral perfusion with capillary refill, and observation for the presence or absence of neck vein distention. Vital signs should be monitored every 15 to 30 minutes. Signs and symptoms of shock must be evaluated, and treatment should be started as soon as possible (see Chapter 61). The patient's respiratory status is carefully assessed, along with a thorough abdominal examination. The presence or absence of bowel sounds should be assessed and noted. A tense, rigid, boardlike abdomen may indicate a perforation and peritonitis.

Once the immediate interventions have begun, the patient or family should answer the following questions. Is there a history of previous bleeding episodes? Has weight loss been a recent problem? Has the patient received blood transfusions in the past, and were there any transfusion reactions? Is there a religious preference that prohibits the use of blood or blood products? Are there any other illnesses that may contribute to bleeding or interfere with treatment (e.g., congestive heart failure, diabetes mellitus)?

Laboratory studies are ordered, including a CBC, blood urea nitrogen (BUN), serum electrolytes, blood glucose, prothrombin time, liver enzymes, arterial blood gases (ABGs), and a type and cross-match for possible blood transfusions. All vomitus and stools should be tested for the presence of gross and occult blood. A urinalysis provides information on the presence of blood in the urine, and the specific gravity gives an immediate indication of the patient's hydration status.

IV lines, preferably two, with a 16- or 18-gauge needle should be established for fluid and blood replacement. The type and amount of fluids infused are dictated by physical and laboratory findings. It is generally best to begin with an isotonic crystalloid solution (e.g., lactated Ringer's solution). Whole blood, packed RBCs, and fresh frozen plasma may be used for replacement of lost volume in massive hemorrhage. Because of the potential for fluid overload and immunologic reactions, packed RBCs are often preferred over whole blood.[24] (The use of blood transfusions and volume expanders is discussed in Chapter 29.) The hemoglobin and hematocrit values are not of immediate assistance in estimating the degree of blood loss, but they provide a baseline for guiding further treatment. The initial hematocrit may be normal and may not reflect the loss until 4 to 6 hours after fluid replacement has taken place, since initially the loss of plasma and RBCs is equal. When upper GI bleeding is less profuse, infusion of isotonic saline solution followed by packed RBCs permits restoration of the hematocrit more quickly and does not create complications related to fluid volume overload. The use of supplemental oxygen delivered by face mask or nasal cannula may help increase blood oxygen saturation.[24]

For most patients who are bleeding profusely, an indwelling urinary catheter is inserted so that urine volume can be accurately assessed hourly. A central venous pressure line may be inserted so that the patient's fluid volume status can be monitored easily. A central venous pressure line is capable of monitoring right-sided heart pressure and function but does not reflect accurate left ventricular function. When a history of valvular heart disease, coronary artery disease, or congestive heart failure is elicited or when pulmonary edema is a factor, a pulmonary artery catheter may be necessary. An NG tube is indicated when the patient is vomiting blood. A large tube passed through the mouth may be more beneficial than a small one passed through the nose. Passage through the mouth is easier, but no tube should ever be advanced against resistance because of the likelihood of damaging the gastric mucosa or causing perforation. Aspiration of stomach contents through a large bore tube such as an Ewald tube facilitates the removal of clots from the stomach and alleviates the patient's need to vomit. In addition, the removal of gastric contents allows the stomach wall to collapse, contributing to hemostasis.

In 80% of cases, bleeding ceases spontaneously without any intervention. However, for many years it has been common practice to lavage the stomach with cool or ice water or saline solution through an NG tube to induce local vasoconstriction of the bleeding vessel. The value of lavage is now in question. Recent studies indicate that ice water lavage has no effect on the rate of bleeding from gastric ulcers and may actually impede the body's normal coagulation mechanism by inhibiting platelet function.[24] The major use for lavage is to ensure that blood will not interfere with emergency endoscopic visualization of the gastric mucosa. If used, the usual procedure for gastric lavage is to instill approximately 50 to100 ml of tap water or saline solution each time, leave it in place for several minutes, and then allow drainage by gravity or low suction. This procedure may be repeated every 30 to 45 minutes.

Diagnostic Studies

Fiberoptic Panendoscopy. In addition to using endoscopic procedures to stop bleeding, these procedures also allow for direct visualization of the bleeding site. Fiberoptic panendoscopy, which should be used before either angiography or barium studies, is quite accurate in identifying the specific source of the bleeding. When a skilled practitioner performs the procedure, bleeding from severe gastritis can be easily distinguished from that of a gastric or duodenal ulcer.

Angiography. Angiography is used in diagnosing upper GI bleeding. It is used most commonly when the bleeding site is not seen by endoscopic procedures.[25] The procedure requires preparation and setup time and may not be appropriate for a high risk, unstable patient. In this procedure a catheter is placed into the left gastric or superior mesenteric artery and advanced until the site of bleeding is discovered. Angiography is an invasive procedure and should be undertaken only if the patient has no allergies to the contrast medium, has adequate hydration and urinary output, and has no cardiovascular contraindications.

Barium Contrast Studies. Barium contrast studies have less immediate value in the identification of major bleeding sites during the acute phase of treatment. These studies are of little value if the bleeding is the result of gastritis or a shallow superficial ulcer. Barium studies can document an actual lesion but cannot verify that it is the bleeding source. If barium is used initially as a diagnostic tool and the bleeding intensifies, the barium will obscure and delay endoscopy and angiography until it has been cleared from the stomach.

Collaborative Care

Endoscopic Therapy. The goal of endoscopic hemostasis is to coagulate or thrombose the bleeding artery and then reduce the necessity of a surgical procedure. This procedure has proved useful in stopping the bleeding of gastritis, Mallory-Weiss syndrome, esophageal and gastric varices, bleeding peptic ulcers, and polyps. Several techniques are used including (1) thermal (heat) probe, (2) electrocoagulation probe, and (3) neodymium: yttrium-aluminum-garnet (Nd-YAG) laser. The heat probe is considered faster, safer, and more effective than the laser. It coagulates tissue by directly applying a heating element to the bleeding site. Endoscopic therapy is more effective than medical management alone in reducing bleeding episodes.[26]

Surgical Therapy. Surgical intervention is indicated when bleeding continues regardless of the therapy provided and when the site of the bleeding has been identified. A high percentage of patients are known to have another massive hemorrhage within 5 years after the first bleeding episode. Some physicians regard surgical therapy as necessary when the patient continues to bleed after rapid transfusion of up to 2000 ml of whole blood or remains in shock after 24 hours. The site of the hemorrhage determines the choice of operation. In addition, the surgeon must consider the age of the patient, since mortality rates increase considerably over the age of 60 years. It is essential that the operation be performed as soon as the need has been established.

Drug Therapy. During the acute phase, drugs are used to decrease bleeding, decrease HCl acid secretion, and neutralize the HCl acid that is present. Table 39-16 reviews their mechanism of action in relation to upper GI bleeding. Histamine H_2-receptor antagonists cimetidine (Tagamet), ranitidine (Zantac), famotidine (Pepcid), and nizatidine (Axid) and the proton pump inhibitors (e.g., omeprazole [Prilosec]) are well established in the treatment of peptic ulcer disease and in the prophylactic treatment of the patient at risk of stress-related upper GI hemorrhage. Although these drugs have no proven ability to control active bleeding, they have become part of standard treatment protocols. H_2-receptor antagonists inhibit the action of histamine at the H_2 receptors of parietal cells and thereby decrease acid secretion. Omeprazole inhibits the pump that is necessary for the secretion of HCl acid. The neutralizing effects of each of these medications are much longer than those of antacid therapy.

Vasopressin (Pitressin), which is posterior pituitary extract, can produce vasoconstriction and has been used to treat upper

DRUG THERAPY

Table 39-16 Gastrointestinal Bleeding

Drug	Source of GI Bleeding	Mechanism of Action
Antacids*	Duodenal ulcer, gastric ulcer, acute gastritis (corrosive, erosive, and hemorrhagic)	Neutralizes acid and maintains gastric pH above 5.5, elevated pH inhibits activation of pepsinogen
Histamine H_2-receptor antagonists Cimetidine (Tagamet), ranitidine (Zantac), famotidine (Pepcid), nizatidine (Axid)	Duodenal ulcer, gastric ulcer, esophagitis, acute gastritis (especially hemorrhagic)	Inhibits action of histamine at H_2-receptors of parietal cells and decreases acid secretion
Proton pump inhibitors Omeprazole (Prilosec), lansoprazole (Prevacid), pantoprazole (Pantoloc)	Same as above	Inhibits the cellular pump that is necessary for secretion of HCl acid
Vasopressin (Pitressin)	Acute gastritis (corrosive, erosive, and hemorrhagic), esophageal varices	Causes vasoconstriction and increases smooth muscle activity of the GI tract, reduces pressure in the portal circulation and arrests bleeding
Somatostatin analogue octreotide (Sandostatin)	Upper GI bleeding, esophageal varices	Decreases splanchnic blood flow, decreases acid secretion via decrease in release of gastrin

*See Table 39-21.

GI bleeding, especially in those patients who do not respond to other therapies and are poor surgical risks. It is administered systemically through a vein or intraarterially at the local site of actual bleeding. However, vasopressin should be used with caution in the patient with a known history of vascular disease. Other side effects of intravenously administered vasopressin include decreased myocardial contractility and decreased coronary blood flow. The patient undergoing vasopressin therapy must be closely monitored for its myocardial, visceral, and peripheral ischemic side effects.[27]

Early administration of the somatostatin analog octreotide (Sandostatin) has been shown to reduce upper GI bleeding related to esophageal varices and nonvariceal upper GI hemorrhage. This drug is given in IV boluses up to 5 to 6 days after the initiation of bleeding. Octreotide reduces splanchnic blood flow as well as inhibits the release of GI hormones such as gastrin, thereby decreasing HCl secretion.[28]

The injection of a vasoconstricting agent into the bleeding site has provided limited improvement in controlling upper GI bleeding. It is a simple procedure that requires little patient preparation. An agent such as epinephrine or norepinephrine (vasoconstrictors) is diluted and injected through the biopsy portal of the endoscope, causing the formation of submucosal deposits around the bleeding site. The resultant vasoconstriction and local inflammation compress the site, and bleeding is controlled.

Antacids have long been known to neutralize HCl acid and are used prophylactically in the management of peptic ulcer disease. Antacids are also beneficial to the healing process as well. Because antacids neutralize HCl acid and increase the pH of gastric contents to above 5, there is inhibition of the conversion of pepsinogen to its active form pepsin. The most frequently used antacid preparations are magnesium hydroxide, magnesium trisilicate, aluminum hydroxide, calcium carbonate, and sodium bicarbonate (see Table 39-21 later in this chapter). Aluminum hydroxide and magnesium trisilicates are the most useful because they are nonabsorbable. Calcium carbonate and sodium bicarbonate are absorbable, and prolonged use can lead to systemic alkalosis.

The neutralizing effects of antacids taken on an empty stomach last only 20 to 30 minutes. When antacids are taken after meals, the effects may last as long as 3 to 4 hours. After the acute phase of bleeding has diminished, antacids are generally administered hourly, either orally or through the NG tube. If the tube is in place, the stomach contents should be aspirated and tested periodically for pH. If pH is less than 5, intermittent suction may be used, or the frequency or dosage of the antacid may be increased.

Sedatives to control agitation and restlessness should be administered cautiously. They make accurate assessment of the patient's condition more difficult. Anticholinergic drugs are contraindicated in acute upper GI bleeding episodes.

NURSING MANAGEMENT: UPPER GASTROINTESTINAL BLEEDING

■ Nursing Assessment

As the nurse begins care of the patient admitted with upper GI bleeding, a thorough and accurate nursing assessment is an essential first step. Subjective and objective data that should be obtained from the patient or significant others are presented in Table 39-17.

The patient experiencing upper GI bleeding may not be able to provide specific information about the cause of the bleeding until the immediate physical needs are met. An immediate nursing assessment should be performed while getting the patient ready for initial treatment. The assessment should include the patient's level of consciousness, vital signs, appearance of neck veins, skin color, and capillary refill. The abdomen should be checked for distention, guarding, and peristalsis. Immediate determination of vital signs indicates whether the patient is in

NURSING ASSESSMENT

Table 39-17 Upper Gastrointestinal Bleeding

Subjective Data

Important Health Information

Past health history: Precipitating events before bleeding episode, previous bleeding episodes and treatment, peptic ulcer disease, esophageal varices, esophagitis, chronic gastritis, stress ulcers

Medications: Use of aspirin, nonsteroidal antiinflammatory drugs, corticosteroids, anticoagulants

Functional Health Patterns

Health perception–health management: Family history of bleeding, smoking, alcohol use

Nutritional-metabolic: Nausea, vomiting, weight loss; thirst

Elimination: Diarrhea; black, tarry stools; decreased urinary output; sweating

Activity-exercise: Weakness, dizziness, fainting

Cognitive-perceptual: Epigastric pain, abdominal cramps

Coping–stress tolerance: Acute or chronic stressors

Objective Data

General

Fever

Integumentary

Clammy, cool, pale skin; pale mucous membranes, nailbeds, and conjunctivae; spider angiomas; jaundice; peripheral edema

Respiratory

Rapid, shallow respirations

Cardiovascular

Tachycardia, weak pulse, orthostatic hypotension, slow capillary refill

Gastrointestinal

Red or coffee-ground vomitus; tense, rigid abdomen, ascites; hypoactive or hyperactive bowel sounds; black, tarry stools

Urinary

Decreased urinary output, concentrated urine

Neurologic

Agitation, restlessness; decreasing level of consciousness

Possible Findings

Decreased hematocrit and hemoglobin; hematuria; guaiac-positive stools, emesis, or gastric aspirate; decreased levels of clotting factors; elevated liver enzymes; abnormal upper GI studies or endoscopy results

shock from blood loss and also provides a baseline blood pressure and pulse by which to monitor the progress of treatment. Signs and symptoms of shock include low blood pressure; rapid, weak pulse; increased thirst; cold, clammy skin; and restlessness. Vital signs should be monitored every 15 to 30 minutes, and the physician should be informed of any significant changes.

When obtaining vital signs, the nurse should consider the patient's age and physical condition. Taking the blood pressure and pulse with the patient lying down and then sitting will indicate postural changes that occur after acute blood loss. The older the patient, the more changes in vital signs should be expected.

Nursing Diagnoses

Nursing diagnoses for the patient with upper GI bleeding include, but are not limited to, the following:

- Fluid volume deficit *related to* acute loss of blood
- Altered peripheral tissue perfusion *related to* loss of circulatory volume
- Altered renal and cerebral tissue perfusion *related to* decreased blood volume
- Anxiety *related to* upper GI bleeding, hospitalization, uncertain outcome, source of bleeding
- Ineffective individual coping *related to* situational crisis and personal vulnerability
- Risk for aspiration *related to* active bleeding and altered level of consciousness
- Potential complication: hypovolemic shock *related to* loss of blood

Planning

The overall goals are that the patient with upper GI bleeding will (1) have no further GI bleeding, (2) have the cause of the bleeding identified and treated, (3) experience a return to a normal hemodynamic state, and (4) experience minimal or no symptoms of pain or anxiety.

Nursing Implementation

Health Promotion. Although not all cases of upper GI bleeding can be anticipated and prevented, the nurse shares responsibility with the physician in trying to identify the patient who is at high risk. The patient with a history of chronic gastritis or peptic ulcer disease should always be considered in the high-risk category because of the increased incidence of bleeding associated with chronic irritation or chronic ulcers. The patient who has had one major bleeding episode is likely to have another within 5 years. This patient must be instructed to avoid irritating foods, prevent or decrease stress-inducing situations at home or at work, and take only prescribed medications. OTC medications can be harmful, since their contents may include drugs that are contraindicated because of their potentially irritating effects on the mucosa. This patient should be instructed in the methods of testing vomitus or stools for the presence of occult blood. Positive results should be promptly reported to the physician or the nurse. Close and frequent follow-up care is very important for all patients with ulcers because recurrence rates are high.

The patient who requires regular administration of ulcerogenic drugs, such as aspirin, corticosteroids, or NSAIDs, should receive instructions regarding the potential adverse effects these agents may have on the GI mucosa. These drugs should be avoided if at all possible. However, if aspirin must be prescribed, enteric-coated tablets can be substituted for regular tablets. Taking the medications with meals or snacks lessens the potential irritating effects. The use of an antacid along with the prescribed medication is usually beneficial.

For the patient at risk for gastric ulcers because of NSAID use, misoprostol (Cytotec) may be prescribed. In addition to inhibiting acid secretion, this prostaglandin analog may have a protective effect on the gastric mucosal barrier. This drug may reduce upper GI bleeding episodes associated with NSAID use. However, the drug has several important side effects including uterine cramping and diarrhea. Because of its effects on the uterus, it is contraindicated in women of childbearing age.[23]

When the nurse is working with the patient who has a history of cirrhosis of the liver with esophageal varices, the instructions must be specific regarding the importance of avoiding known irritants, such as alcohol and hot, spicy, irritating foods. The prompt treatment of an upper respiratory tract infection should be stressed. Severe coughing or sneezing can create increased pressure on the already fragile varices and may result in massive hemorrhage.

The patient who is known to have blood dyscrasias or liver dysfunction or who is taking cancer chemotherapeutic drugs has a potential bleeding problem because of altered hemostasis caused by a decrease in clotting factors and platelets. When these patients also have a history of ulcer disease, gastritis, varices, or drug and alcohol abuse, they should be carefully instructed regarding their disease process and medications, and they should be closely observed for bleeding.

Acute Intervention. The patient should be approached in a calm and assured manner to help decrease the level of anxiety. Caution should be used before administering sedatives for restlessness because it is one of the warning signs of shock and may be masked by the medication.

Once an infusion has been started, the IV line must be maintained for fluid or blood replacement. An accurate intake and output record is essential so that the patient's hydration status can be assessed. Urine output should be measured hourly. A rate of at least 0.5 ml/kg per hour indicates adequate renal perfusion. Lesser amounts may indicate renal ischemia secondary to loss of blood volume. Urine specific gravity should be measured because it gives additional information regarding the patient's hydration status. Consistent readings greater than 1.025 (normal is 1.005 to 1.025) indicate that the urine is extremely concentrated and that there is probably a low blood volume. The physician must be kept informed of these important parameters so that the IV solutions can be increased or decreased accordingly. If the patient has a central venous pressure line or pulmonary artery catheter in place, readings should be recorded every 1 to 2 hours. Hemodynamic monitoring provides an accurate and quick assessment of blood flow and pressure within the cardiovascular system (see Chapter 63).

The older adult or the patient with a history of cardiovascular problems should be observed closely for signs of fluid overload. However, the threat of volume overload and pulmonary edema must be a constant concern in all patients who are receiving large amounts of IV fluids within a short time. Therefore, auscultation of breath sounds and close observation of respiratory effort are important. Electrocardiographic (ECG) monitoring can also be used to evaluate cardiac function.

Foods such as beets or even swallowed mouthwash can give vomitus a bloody appearance. Unless the contents of the vomitus are checked for occult blood, false information may be recorded. Swallowed blood from a nosebleed must also be accurately noted to avoid misdiagnosis of an upper GI bleeding episode. When an NG tube is inserted, the nurse must pay special attention to keeping it in proper position and observing the aspirate for blood.

The majority of upper GI bleeding episodes cease spontaneously, even without intervention. Although the use of cool or iced gastric lavage is used in some institutions, its effectiveness is of questionable value. Therefore the nurse must understand the rationale for this therapy and the results that are anticipated. Either cool or iced tap water or saline solution may be used. Water has the advantage of being able to break up large clots more easily than saline solution, is less expensive, and is always available. A disadvantage of tap water is that it may create more electrolyte imbalance than would an isotonic saline solution.

When lavage is used, approximately 50 to 100 ml of fluid is instilled at a time into the stomach. The lavage fluid may be aspirated from the stomach or drained by gravity. When aspiration is the method used, it is important not to aspirate if resistance is felt. The tip of the NG tube may be up against the gastric mucosal lining. The constant pressure from attempts to aspirate the lavage fluid may cause erosion of the mucosa. When resistance is a factor, the nurse should use gravity as the alternative method of gastric drainage. Close monitoring of vital signs, especially in the patient with a heart problem, is important because arrhythmias may occur. Keeping the patient warm and the head of the bed elevated provide comfort and prevent possible aspiration problems.

The nurse caring for a patient with upper GI bleeding should be well informed as to what constitutes blood in the stools. Black, tarry stools are not usually associated with a brisk hemorrhage but are indicative of the presence of bleeding of prolonged duration. Bright red blood in the stool is usually from a source in the lower bowel. When vomitus contains blood but the stool contains no gross or occult blood, the hemorrhage is considered to have been of short duration. Menses and bleeding hemorrhoids should be ruled out as possible sources of blood in the stools.

Monitoring the patient's laboratory studies enables the nurse to estimate the effectiveness of therapy. The hemoglobin and hematocrit are usually evaluated about every 4 to 6 hours if the patient is actively bleeding. At first the hematocrit may not accurately reflect the amount of blood lost or the amount of blood replaced and will appear falsely high or low. The patient's BUN level is assessed. It is generally elevated with a significant hemorrhage, since blood proteins are subjected to bacterial breakdown in the GI tract. However, renal disease may also result in an elevated BUN level. Many patients receive oxygen by mask or nasally so that the circulating blood is ensured of an adequate oxygen content.

When oral nourishment is begun, the patient is observed for symptoms of nausea and vomiting and a recurrence of bleeding. Feedings initially consist of clear fluids or milk and are given hourly until tolerance is determined. These feedings help neutralize the gastric secretions and assist in the mucosal repair. Gradual introduction of bland foods follows if the patient exhibits no signs of discomfort.

Antacids are sometimes used after upper GI bleeding to reduce the acidity of gastric contents. Anticipating the effects of the prescribed preparations can be helpful in providing better care. The nurse should know that preparations containing calcium or aluminum may result in constipation, whereas those

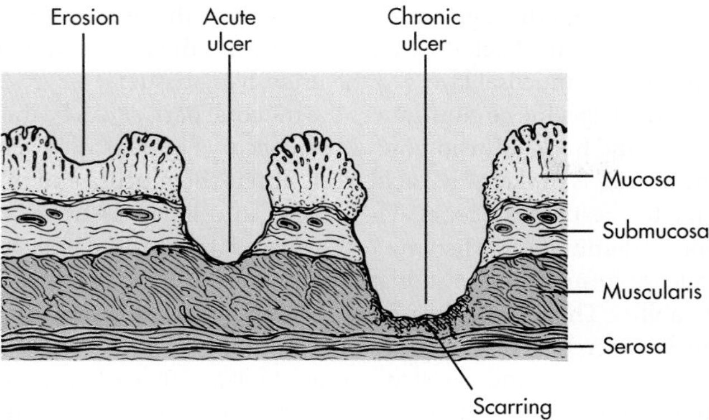

Fig. 39-12 Peptic ulcers, including an erosion, acute ulcer, and chronic ulcer. Both the acute and chronic ulcer may penetrate the entire wall of the stomach.

with magnesium cause diarrhea. Although these preparations are generally nonabsorbable and result in fewer systemic problems, magnesium products must be used cautiously in the patient with renal insufficiency. Administering the antacid preparation accurately and on schedule is important if the stomach pH is to be maintained at a level no lower than 5.

The patient in whom hemorrhage was the result of chronic alcohol abuse requires close observation for the beginning of delirium tremens as withdrawal from alcohol takes place. Symptoms indicating the beginning of delirium tremens are agitation, uncontrolled shaking, sweating, and vivid hallucinations. (Alcohol withdrawal is discussed in Chapter 10.)

Ambulatory and Home Care. The patient and family must be taught how to avoid future bleeding episodes. Ulcer disease, drug or alcohol abuse, and liver and respiratory diseases can all result in upper GI bleeding. The patient and family must be made aware of the consequences of noncompliance with diet and drug therapy. It must be emphasized that no medications (especially aspirin) other than those prescribed by the physician should be taken. Smoking and alcohol should be eliminated because they are sources of irritation and interfere with tissue repair. The need for long-term follow-up care may be necessary because of the possibility of another bleeding episode. The patient and family should be instructed on what to do if an acute hemorrhage occurs in the future.

■ Evaluation

The expected outcomes are that the patient with upper GI bleeding will

- have no further GI bleeding
- have the cause of the bleeding identified and treated
- experience a return to a normal hemodynamic state
- experience minimal or no symptoms of pain or anxiety

PEPTIC ULCERS

Peptic ulcer is an erosion of the GI mucosa resulting from the digestive action of HCl acid and pepsin. Any portion of the GI tract that comes into contact with gastric secretions is susceptible to ulcer development, including the lower esophagus, stomach, duodenum, and margin of gastrojejunal anastomosis after surgical procedures. It is estimated that approximately 10% of men and 4% of women in the United States will have duodenal ulcers during their lifetimes.

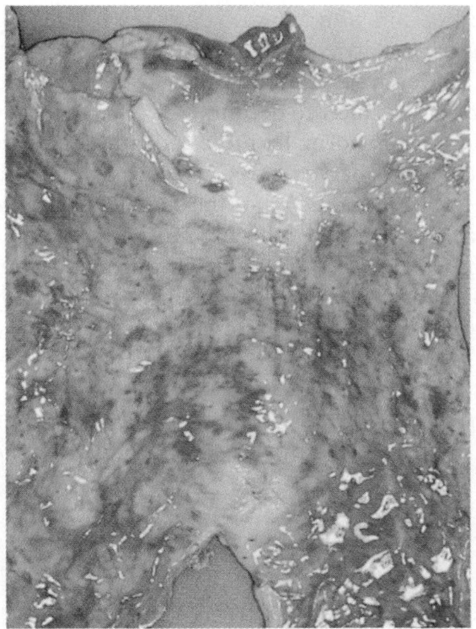

Fig. 39-13 Acute erosive gastritis. Acute erosive gastritis is shown in the opened stomach. The mucosa appears hyperemic, and the foci of superficial ulceration are manifest as scattered, small, red areas termed erosions.

Types

Peptic ulcers can be classified as *acute* or *chronic*, depending on the degree of mucosal involvement (Fig. 39-12), and *gastric* or *duodenal*, according to the location. The acute ulcer (Fig. 39-13) is associated with superficial erosion and minimal inflammation. It is of short duration and resolves quickly when the cause is identified and removed. A chronic ulcer (Fig. 39-14) is one of long duration, eroding through the muscular wall with the formation of fibrous tissue. It is present continuously for many months or intermittently throughout the person's lifetime. A chronic ulcer is at least four times as common as acute erosion. Gastric and duodenal ulcers, although defined as peptic ulcers, are distinctly different in their etiology and incidence (Table 39-18). Generally, the treatment of all types of ulcers is quite similar.

Etiology and Pathophysiology

Pepsinogen, the precursor of pepsin, is activated to pepsin in the presence of HCl acid and a pH of 2 to 3. HCl acid is secreted by the parietal cells at a pH of 0.8. After mixing with the stomach contents, the pH reaches 2 to 3, a highly favorable range of acidity for pepsin activity. When the stomach acid level is neutralized by the presence of food or antacids, the pH is increased to 3.5 or more. At a pH of 3.5 or more, pepsin has little or no proteolytic activity.

Peptic ulcers develop only in the presence of an acid environment. It has been well established that the patient with pernicious anemia and achlorhydria rarely has gastric ulcers. An excess of gastric acid may not be necessary for ulcer development.

The typical person with a gastric ulcer has normal to less than normal gastric acidity compared with the person with a duodenal ulcer. However, some intraluminal acid does seem to be essential for a gastric ulcer to occur.

The stomach is normally protected from autodigestion by the gastric mucosal barrier. The GI tract has a high cell turnover rate, and the surface mucosa of the stomach is renewed about every 3 days. As a result of this high turnover rate, the mucosa can continually repair itself except in extreme instances when the cell breakdown surpasses the cell renewal rate. Normally, water, electrolytes, and water-soluble substances (e.g., glucose) can easily pass through the barrier. However, the mucosal barrier prevents the back diffusion of acid from the gastric lumen through the mucosal layers to the underlying tissue.

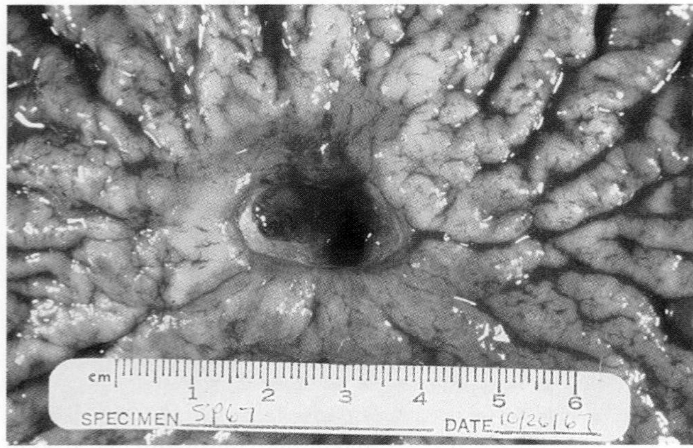

Fig. 39-14 Photograph of a chronic peptic ulcer located in lesser curvature of stomach.

Under specific circumstances the mucosal barrier can be impaired and back-diffusion of acid can occur (Fig. 39-15). When the barrier is broken, HCl acid freely enters the mucosa and injury to the tissues occurs. This results in cellular destruction and inflammation. Histamine is released from the damaged mucosa, resulting in vasodilation and increased capillary permeability. The released histamine is then capable of stimulating further secretion of acid and pepsin.

As described under gastritis, a variety of agents are known to destroy the mucosal barrier. By generating ammonia in the mucous layer, *H. pylori* may create a condition of chronic inflammation, rendering the mucosa especially vulnerable to other noxious substances.[10] Ulcerogenic drugs, such as aspirin and aspirin-like agents, inhibit synthesis of mucus and prostaglandins and cause abnormal permeability. Corticosteroids have the ability to decrease the rate of mucous cell renewal and thereby decrease its protective effects. Lipid-soluble cytotoxic drugs can pass through the barrier and destroy it.

When the mucosal barrier is disrupted, there is a compensatory increase in blood flow. This phenomenon can occur in several ways. Prostaglandin-like substances and histamine act as vasodilators, thus increasing capillary blood flow. As blood flow increases within the affected mucosa, hydrogen ions are rapidly removed from the area, buffers are delivered to help neutralize the hydrogen ions present, nutrients necessary for cell function arrive, and the rate of mucosal cell replication increases. When blood flow is not sufficient to carry out these events, tissue in-

Table 39-18 Comparison of Gastric and Duodenal Ulcers

	Gastric Ulcers	Duodenal Ulcers
Lesion	Superficial; smooth margins; round, oval, or cone-shaped	Penetrating (associated with deformity of duodenal bulb from healing of recurrent ulcers)
Location of lesion	Predominantly antrum, also in body and fundus of stomach	First 1-2 cm of duodenum
Gastric secretion	Normal to decreased	Increased
Incidence	▪ Greater in women ▪ Peak age fifth to sixth decade ▪ More common in persons of lower socioeconomic status and in unskilled laborers ▪ Increased with smoking, drug, and alcohol use ▪ Increased with incompetent pyloric sphincter ▪ Increased with stress ulcers after severe burns, head trauma, and major surgery	▪ Greater in men, but increasing in women especially postmenopausal ▪ Peak age 35-45 yr ▪ Associated with psychologic stress ▪ Increased with smoking, drug, and alcohol use ▪ Associated with other diseases (e.g., chronic obstructive pulmonary disease, pancreatic disease, hyperparathyroidism, Zollinger-Ellison syndrome, chronic renal failure)
Clinical manifestations	▪ Burning or gaseous pressure in high left epigastrium and back and upper abdomen ▪ Pain 1-2 hr after meals; if penetrating ulcer, aggravation of discomfort with food ▪ Occasional nausea and vomiting, weight loss	▪ Burning, cramping, pressurelike pain across midepigastrium and upper abdomen; back pain with posterior ulcers ▪ Pain 2-4 hr after meals and midmorning, midafternoon, middle of night, periodic and episodic ▪ Pain relief with antacids and food; occasional nausea and vomiting
Recurrence rate	High	High
Complications	Hemorrhage, perforation, outlet obstruction, intractability	Hemorrhage, perforation, obstruction

jury results. When the increase is sufficient to dilute, buffer, and remove the excess hydrogen ions, tissue damage may be minimal or may result in no injury at all. Figure 39-16 shows a representation of the interrelationship between the mucosal blood flow and disruption of the gastric mucosal barrier.

Although gastric ulcers are characterized by a normal to low secretion of gastric acid, the back-diffusion of acid is greater with chronic gastric ulcers than with duodenal ulcers or in the normal person. Therefore the critical pathologic process in gastric ulcer formation may not be the amount of acid that is secreted but the amount that is able to penetrate the mucosal barrier.

The gastric mucosa is also protected from the damage of ulceration by two other mechanisms. First, mucus is secreted by superficial mucous cells and forms a layer that can entrap or slow the diffusion of hydrogen ions across the mucosal barrier. Second, bicarbonate is secreted by the gastric and duodenal mucosa, and this helps neutralize HCl acid in the lumen of the GI tract.

Increased vagal nerve stimulation from a variety of causes (e.g., emotions) causes hypersecretion of HCl acid. Increased concentrations of HCl acid can alter the mucosal barrier. Duodenal ulcers are associated with high acid content. The fact that the person with duodenal ulcers is more vulnerable to the effects of emotional stressors may be one reason acid levels are above normal. It has been suggested that the continual response of the parietal cells to maximal stimulation results in hyperplasia of the cell mass. There is also an increase in gastrin levels in most persons with duodenal ulcers.

Gastric Ulcers. Although gastric ulcers can occur in any portion of the stomach, they are most commonly found on the lesser curvature in close proximity to the antral junction. Before 1900, gastric ulcers were more common than duodenal ulcers, and they were found predominantly in young women. Since the turn of the century, the incidence of gastric ulcers has decreased, and they are now surpassed in incidence by duodenal ulcers by a ratio of 4:1. Gastric ulcers remain more prevalent in women and in older adults.

The mortality rate from gastric ulcers is greater than that from duodenal ulcers because the peak incidence of gastric ulcers occurs in persons over 50 years of age. Contrary to common belief, gastric ulcers are not more prevalent among those in executive or managerial positions. Persons from the lower socioeconomic class and manual or unskilled workers are more prone to gastric ulcers.

The understanding of the factors that contribute to ulcer formation is developing rapidly at the present time. As described previously in the section concerning gastritis (p. 1102), the discovery of the bacterium *H. pylori* provides a new understanding of ulcer formation. *H. pylori* are thought to be a dominant factor in the promotion of peptic ulcer formation. Although many questions remain to be answered regarding *H. pylori,* it survives in the human upper GI tract for long periods of time as a result of its ability to move in mucus and attach to mucosal cells. In addition, it secretes a substance called urease, which buffers the area around the bacterium and protects it from destruction in an acidic environment. Infection with *H. pylori* is highest in underdeveloped countries and in persons of low socioeconomic status. Although the routes of transmission are largely unknown, it is thought that infection occurs during childhood via transmission from family members to the child, possibly through an oral-oral route. In the United States and Canada, persons born before 1940 have a significantly higher risk of carrying *H. pylori* than persons in younger age groups.[29] This enhanced prevalence in older persons has been attributed to the presence of crowded living conditions and poor sanitation practices, which were more common in the earlier part of the 1900s.

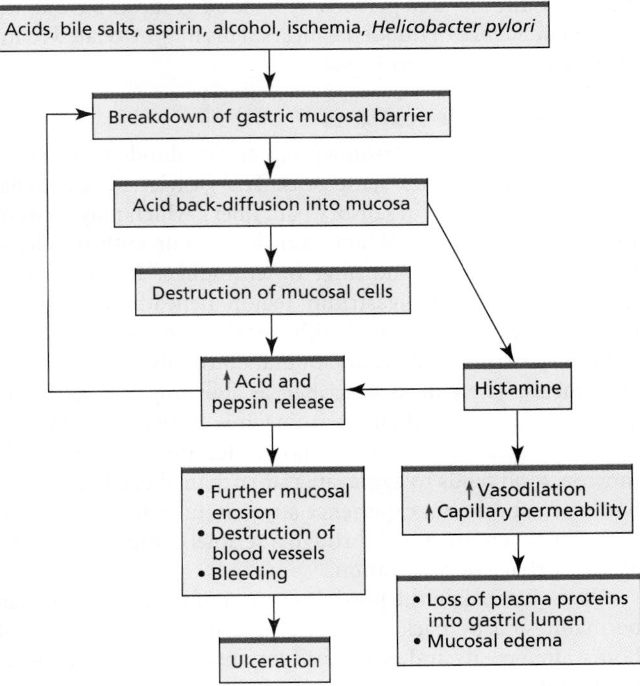

Fig. 39-15 Disruption of gastric mucosa and pathophysiologic consequences of back diffusion of acids.

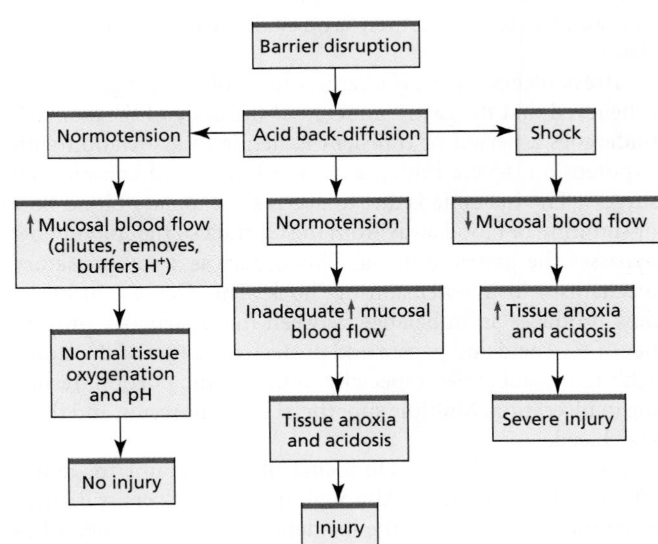

Fig. 39-16 The relationship between mucosal blood flow and disruption of the gastric mucosal barrier.

Research into a genetic cause for ulcers has shown that some members of the same family are more prone to develop gastric or duodenal ulcers. Evidence is not complete, however, and the ulcer development could just as well be due to the sharing of the same environment. For example, the transmission of *H. pylori* may be increased by crowded living conditions. Gastric ulcer personality has not been demonstrated, yet ulcer-prone persons do appear to react to stress with more frustration, fear, anxiety, and guilt than do those who are less predisposed to ulcer formation. It is thought that destruction of the gastric mucosa by noxious agents such as drugs or smoking may be enhanced by the presence of *H. pylori,* which further promotes gastric mucosal destruction as described in the previous section on gastritis.

It is rare for gastric ulcers to become malignant, but transformation may occur in about 1% of all cases. When there is any doubt, a biopsy of the gastric mucosa should be performed during endoscopy to differentiate between a benign ulcer and a malignant neoplasm.

Gastric ulcers have also been attributed to various factors that can lead to acute episodes or to chronic involvement. Drugs and physiologically stressful situations can precipitate acute gastric lesions.

Medication-induced ulcers. Medications can cause acute gastric ulcers and in some cases can lead to the development of chronic ulcers. The drugs most often implicated include aspirin, corticosteroids, NSAIDs (e.g., ibuprofen), and reserpine. It is estimated that 2% to 4% of patients taking NSAIDs for 1 year experience serious GI complications including gastric ulcer, upper GI hemorrhage, or perforation.[22] Other known causative factors of gastric ulcer formation are chronic alcohol abuse, gastritis, and bile reflux gastritis from an incompetent pyloric sphincter. Caffeine is known to stimulate gastric acid secretion. Cigarette smoking is positively linked with gastric ulcer. One proposed theory is that smoking causes a reduction of pancreatic bicarbonate secretion, thus creating a decreased pH in the duodenum. In addition, nicotine seems to enhance reflux of duodenal contents into the antrum of the stomach. The ingestion of hot, rough, or spicy foods has been suggested as a causative factor, but there is no evidence to substantiate this claim.

Stress ulcers. A *stress ulcer* is a form of erosive gastritis. It is believed that the gastric mucosa of the body of the stomach undergoes a period of transient ischemia in association with hypotension, severe injury, extensive burns, and complicated surgery. The ischemia is due to decreased capillary blood flow or shunting of blood away from the GI tract so that blood flow bypasses the gastric mucosa. This occurs as a compensatory mechanism in hypotension or shock. The decrease in blood flow produces an imbalance between the destructive properties of HCl acid and pepsin and protective factors of the stomach's mucosal barrier, especially in the fundic portion, resulting in ulceration. Multiple superficial erosions result, and these may bleed.

Duodenal Ulcers. Duodenal ulcers account for about 80% of all peptic ulcers. Although duodenal ulcers still affect more men than women, the incidence of duodenal ulcers has followed a downward trend in men and a steady increase in women. The explanation for this change has not been clearly identified. However, it is possible that the overuse of aspirin and NSAIDs and increased consumption of alcohol by women may partially account for this increased incidence. Duodenal ulcers may occur at any age, but the incidence is especially high between the ages of 35 and 45 years.

Whereas many factors are thought to contribute to the formation of duodenal ulcers, *H. pylori* has been identified as playing a key role. The prevalence of *H. pylori* infection in duodenal ulcer patients has consistently been found to be between 95% and 100%. However, a clear-cut direct causal relationship between *H. pylori* and duodenal ulcer formation has not yet been proven. Although duodenal ulcers often occur in persons susceptible to psychologic pressures and anxieties, this theory of causation requires more study. It is known that a duodenal ulcer can develop in anyone, regardless of occupation or socioeconomic group. The development of duodenal ulcers is associated with a high HCl acid secretion. Several diseases have been identified with a high risk of duodenal ulcer development, including chronic obstructive pulmonary disease, cirrhosis of the liver, chronic pancreatitis, hyperparathyroidism, chronic renal failure, and the Zollinger-Ellison syndrome. A high HCl acid concentration is believed to be the factor common to all these conditions. It is possible that the treatment of these conditions may also have detrimental effects on the gastric mucosa. Alcohol ingestion and heavy smoking habits are also associated with duodenal ulcer formation, since both are known irritants to the GI mucosa.

Pregnancy appears to protect women from developing ulcers. Estrogen and progesterone have demonstrated positive effects on ulcer healing. Progesterone has also been noted to lower acid secretion to a small degree. There is evidence that women past menopause, who no longer have this endocrine protection, develop ulcers at the same rate as men.

As with gastric ulcers, some persons in certain families are more prone to duodenal ulcer formation. Supporting a genetic etiology is the fact that persons with blood group O have an increased incidence of duodenal ulcers. This may be related to increased susceptibility to *H. pylori.*

Clinical Manifestations

It is common for the person with gastric or duodenal ulcers to have no pain or other symptoms. The gastric and duodenal mucosas are not rich in sensory pain fibers, which may account for this phenomenon. When pain does occur with duodenal ulcer, it is described as "burning" or "cramplike." It is most often located in the midepigastrium region beneath the xiphoid process. The pain associated with gastric ulcers is located high in the epigastrium and occurs spontaneously about 1 to 2 hours after meals. The pain is described as "burning" or "gaseous." The pain can occur when the stomach is empty or when food has been ingested. If the ulcer has eroded through the gastric mucosa, food tends to aggravate rather than alleviate the pain. Some persons do not experience any pain until the presence of the ulcer is demonstrated through a serious complication such as hemorrhage or perforation.

Ulcers located on the posterior aspect of the duodenum can be manifested by back pain. The pain usually occurs 2 to 4 hours after meals and is relieved by antacids and sometimes foods that neutralize and dilute the HCl acid. A characteristic of duodenal ulcer is its tendency to occur continuously for a few weeks or months and then disappear for a time, only to recur

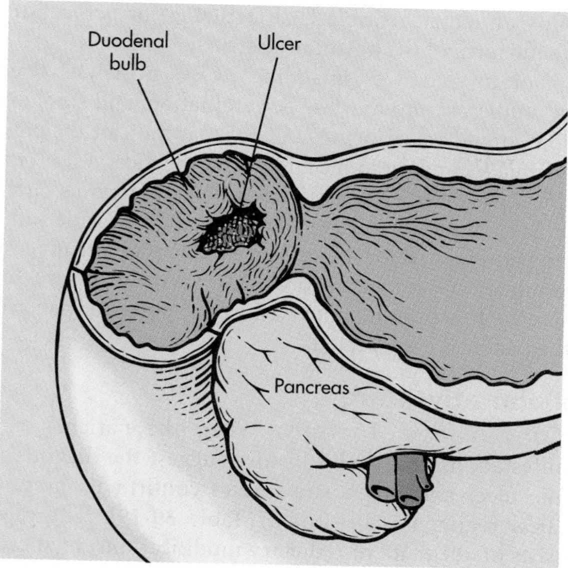

Fig. 39-17 Duodenal ulcer of the posterior wall penetrating into the head of the pancreas, resulting in walled-off perforation.

some months later. Some patients claim their symptoms worsen in the spring and fall of the year, thus strengthening the concept of a seasonal trend in occurrence. This course of events usually lasts throughout the entire life span of the ulcer.

Complications

The three major complications of chronic peptic ulcer disease are hemorrhage, perforation, and gastric outlet obstruction. All are considered emergency situations and are initially treated conservatively. However, surgery may become necessary at any time during the course of the therapy.

Hemorrhage. Hemorrhage is the most common complication of peptic ulcer disease. It develops from erosion of the granulation tissue found at the base of the ulcer during healing or from erosion of the ulcer through a major blood vessel. Duodenal ulcers account for a greater percentage of upper GI bleeding episodes than gastric ulcers.

Perforation. Perforation is considered the most lethal complication of peptic ulcer. Perforation is commonly seen in large penetrating duodenal ulcers that have not healed and are located on the posterior mucosal wall (Fig. 39-17). Perforated gastric ulcers are most frequently located on the lesser curvature of the stomach. Even though duodenal ulcers are more prevalent and perforate more frequently, mortality rates associated with perforation of gastric ulcers are higher. The older age of the patient with gastric ulcers, who often has other concurrent medical problems, is thought to be the crucial factor.

Perforation of a peptic ulcer occurs when the ulcer penetrates the serosal surface, with spillage of either gastric or duodenal contents into the peritoneal cavity. The size of the perforation is directly proportional to the length of time the patient has had the ulcer. The larger the perforation, the longer the history of the ulcer. Small perforations seal themselves and result in a cessation of symptoms; larger perforations require immediate surgical closure. Spontaneous sealing occurs as a result of large amounts of fibrin being produced in response to the perforation. This leads to fibrinous fusion of the duodenum or gastric curvature to adjacent tissue, mainly the liver.

The clinical manifestations of perforation are characterized by their sudden and dramatic onset. The patient experiences sudden, severe upper abdominal pain that quickly spreads throughout the abdomen. The visceral and parietal layers of the peritoneum have an abundance of pain receptors, and this contributes to the abrupt, intense pain experienced. There may be shoulder pain if the spillage causes irritation to the phrenic nerve. The abdominal muscles contract, appearing rigid and boardlike as they attempt to protect the abdomen from further injury. The patient's respirations become shallow and rapid. Bowel sounds are usually absent. Nausea and vomiting may occur but are generally absent. Many patients report a history of ulcer disease or recent symptoms of indigestion.

The contents entering the peritoneal cavity from the stomach or duodenum contain a variety of ingredients that include air, saliva, food particles, HCl acid, pepsin, bacteria, bile, and pancreatic fluid and enzymes. A bacterial peritonitis may occur within 6 to 12 hours, followed by paralytic ileus. The intensity of the peritonitis is proportional to the amount and duration of the spillage through the perforation. It is difficult to determine from the sudden onset of symptoms whether gastric or duodenal ulcer is the cause, since the clinical characteristics of intestinal perforation are the same (see Chapter 40).

Gastric Outlet Obstruction. Ulcers located in the antrum and the prepyloric and pyloric areas of the stomach and the duodenum are predisposed to obstruction. In the early phase of obstruction (often referred to as the *compensated phase*), gastric emptying is normal to near normal. This phase may be associated with large peristaltic waves. Over time, excessive peristalsis creates hypertrophy of the stomach wall. After long-standing obstruction the stomach enters the *decompensated phase,* which results in dilation and atony. The obstruction is not totally due to fibrous scar tissue because active ulcer formation is associated with edema, inflammation, and pylorospasm, all of which contribute to the narrowing of the pylorus.

The patient with gastric outlet obstruction generally has a long history of ulcer pain. Ulcerlike pain of short duration or complete absence of pain is more indicative of a malignant obstruction. The pain progresses to a more generalized upper abdominal discomfort that becomes worse toward the end of the day as the stomach fills and dilates. Relief may be obtained by belching or by self-induced vomiting. Vomiting is common and often projectile. The vomitus contains food particles that were ingested many hours or even a day or two before the vomiting episode. There is often an offensive odor if the contents have been dormant in the stomach for a time. The patient who vomits frequently will be anorectic, with evident weight loss, and will complain of thirst and an unpleasant taste in the mouth. Constipation is a common complaint that usually results from dehydration and lack of roughage in the diet.

The patient with gastric outlet obstruction may show a swelling in the upper abdomen indicating dilation of the stomach. Loud peristalsis can be heard, and visible peristaltic waves are often observed passing across the abdomen from left to right. If the stomach is grossly dilated, it is possible to palpate it as well.

An upper GI examination with barium as contrast medium is helpful in making a diagnosis, and it demonstrates the presence of an active ulcer crater or scarring from previously healed ulcers. Barium normally should pass from the stomach within 2 hours, but with gastric outlet obstruction, 50% of the barium remains on follow-up films up to 6 hours later.

Diagnostic Studies

The diagnostic measures used to determine the presence and location of a peptic ulcer are similar to those with acute upper GI bleeding. *Fiberoptic endoscopy* is the procedure most often used. It is more reliable than barium contrast studies because of the maneuverability of fiberoptic scopes for viewing the entire gastric and duodenal mucosa. This procedure can also be used to determine the degree of ulcer healing after treatment. During endoscopy, specimens can be obtained for identification of *H. pylori*. When gastric malignancy is a possibility, the endoscope also can be used in obtaining tissue specimens for biopsy.

There are currently four diagnostic tests available to confirm *H. pylori* infection: serologic (blood) test, ^{13}C-urea breath test, histology of mucosa, and the Campylobacter-like organism test.[28] The blood test measures anti–*H. pylori* IgG, IgA, and IgM and is useful in patients who have not been treated with antibiotics. However, because of the length of time that IgG levels remain elevated in the blood after the infection, the serologic tests will not distinguish active from recently treated disease. The breath test determines the presence of active infection. The invasive tests (Campylobacter-like organism, culture, and histology) require endoscopy. The Campylobacter-like organism test is a rapid test that can determine the presence of active infection. The mucosa histology examination remains the most sensitive test.

Barium contrast studies, although widely used, are not accurate in identifying shallow, superficial ulcers because of failure of the barium to properly fill the ulcer crater. X-ray studies are also ineffective in differentiating a peptic ulcer from a malignant tumor. In addition, x-rays do not as readily demonstrate the degree of healing that can be visually determined with the endoscope. Barium studies are of benefit in the diagnosis of pyloric obstruction caused by recurrent ulcers.

Gastric analysis has questionable value in the diagnosis of peptic ulcer disease because in many patients gastric secretions are normal in amount and composition. However, it can provide important data in (1) identifying a possible gastrinoma (Zollinger-Ellison syndrome), (2) determining the degree of gastric hyperacidity, and (3) evaluating the results of therapy such as vagotomy and antisecretory drug therapy. Several methods may be used to determine the amount of gastric secretions. An NG tube can be placed into the antrum with the use of fluoroscopy, and the secretions can be collected overnight for a 12-hour period. The HCl acid concentration is calculated and compared with equivalents already established for persons who do not have ulcers, those with gastric and duodenal ulcers, and those with Zollinger-Ellison syndrome. This method is not extremely accurate because the NG tube may become plugged or aspiration methods may be inconsistent. Augmented histamine or pentagastrin stimulation may be more accurate in estimating the degree of acid secretion. In these tests the stomach's ability to secrete HCl acid is studied after stimulation with either betazole HCl (Histalog) or pentagastrin (a synthetic form of the hormone gastrin).

Laboratory analyses, including a CBC, urinalysis, liver enzyme studies, serum amylase determination, and stool examination, should be performed. A CBC may indicate the presence of anemia secondary to bleeding from the ulcer. Liver enzyme studies help determine any liver problems, such as cirrhosis, that may complicate the treatment of the ulcer. Urine and stool are routinely tested for the presence of blood. A serum amylase determination is frequently ordered to provide information on pancreatic function in patients in whom posterior penetration of the pancreas is suspected.

Collaborative Care

Conservative Therapy. When the patient's clinical manifestations and health history suggest the diagnosis of a peptic ulcer and diagnostic studies confirm its presence, a medical regimen is instituted (Table 39-19). The regimen consists of adequate rest, dietary modifications, medications, elimination of smoking, and long-term follow-up care. The aim of the treatment program is to decrease the degree of gastric acidity, enhance mucosal defense mechanisms, and minimize the harmful effects on the mucosa. Patients are often treated in ambulatory care clinics.

Adequate rest, both physical and emotional, is important in the treatment process. A quiet, calm environment at home or on the job is not easy to achieve and may require some modifications in the patient's daily routine. The benefits derived from the elimination of stressors help decrease the stimulus for overproduction of HCl acid. Moderation in daily activity is essential.

Dietary modifications may be necessary so that foods and beverages irritating to the patient can be avoided or eliminated. A bland diet consisting of six small meals a day may be recommended to the patient during the symptomatic phase. However, there is considerable controversy over the actual therapeutic benefits derived from a bland diet, since the rationale is not supported by scientific evidence. Each patient should be instructed to eat and drink foods and fluids that do not cause any distressing or harmful side effects. Alcohol and caffeine-containing products should be eliminated because of their irritating effects.

Smoking has an irritating effect on the mucosa, increases gastric motility, and delays mucosal healing. It should be eliminated completely or severely reduced. The combination of adequate rest and abstinence from smoking accelerates ulcer healing.

Medications are a vital part of therapy. The patient must be well informed about each drug prescribed, why it is ordered, and the expected benefits. Strict adherence to the prescribed regimen of drugs is mandatory. Drug therapy that includes the use of antacids, histamine H_2-receptor antagonists, antisecretory agents, antibiotics, and anticholinergics is presented in Tables 39-19, 39-20, 39-21, and 39-22. Aspirin and NSAIDs should be discontinued. When these medications must be continued, enteric-coated or highly buffered preparations are more suitable.

Antibiotics to eradicate *H. pylori* infection are prescribed. When *H. pylori* is present, ulcer recurrence rates with H_2-receptor antagonists alone can be as high as 75% to 90% while

COLLABORATIVE CARE

Table 39-19 Peptic Ulcer Disease

Diagnostic
- Complete blood count
- Urinalysis
- Liver enzymes
- Serum electrolytes
- Fiberoptic endoscopy with biopsy
- Upper GI barium-contrast study
- Gastric analysis
- Exfoliative cytology
- *H. pylori* testing of breath, urine, blood, stool

Collaborative Therapy

Conservative Therapy
- Adequate rest
- Bland diet (six small meals a day)
- Cessation of smoking
- Medications
  - Antacids (Table 39-21)
  - H_2-receptor blocking agents (Table 39-20)
  - Anticholinergics (Table 39-20)
  - Cytoprotective drugs (Table 39-20)
  - Proton pump inhibitors (Table 39-20)
  - Misoprostol (Cytotec)
  - Antibiotics for *H. pylori* (Table 39-13)
- Stress reduction

Acute Exacerbation Without Complications
- NPO
- NG suction
- Bed rest to moderate light activity
- Cessation of smoking
- IV fluid replacement
- Medications
  - Antacids
  - H_2-receptor antagonist
  - Proton pump inhibitor (omeprazole)
  - Anticholinergics
  - Sedatives

Acute Exacerbation with Complications (Hemorrhage, Perforation, Obstruction)
- NPO
- NG suction
- Bed rest
- IV fluid replacement (lactated Ringer's solution)
- Blood transfusions
- Stomach lavage (possible)

Surgical Therapy
- Perforation—simple closure with omentum graft
- Gastric outlet obstruction—pyloroplasty and vagotomy
- Ulcer cure
  - Billroth I and II
  - Vagotomy and pyloroplasty

NG, nasogastric; *NPO*, nothing by mouth.

DRUG THERAPY

Table 39-20 Peptic Ulcer Disease

Antisecretory
- H_2-receptor antagonists
  - Cimetidine (Tagamet)
  - Ranitidine (Zantac)
  - Famotidine (Pepcid)
  - Nizatidine (Axid)
- Proton pump inhibitors
  - Omeprazole (Prilosec)
  - Lansoprazole (Prevacid)
  - Pantoprazole (Pantoloc)
- Anticholinergics

Antisecretory and Cytoprotective
- Misoprostol (Cytotec)

Cytoprotective
- Sucralfate (Carafate)
- Bismuth subsalicylate (Pepto-Bismol)

Neutralizing
- Antacids*

Antibiotics for *H. pylori*†
- Amoxicillin
- Metronidazole
- Tetracycline

Others
- Tricyclic antidepressants
  - Imipramine (Tofranil)
  - Doxepin (Sinequan)

*See Table 39-21.
†See Table 39-13.

with antibiotic treatment the recurrence rate may be as low as 2%. Antibiotic therapy for *H. pylori* is shown in Table 39-13.[30]

The healing of a peptic ulcer requires many weeks of therapy. Pain disappears after 3 to 6 days, but ulcer healing is much slower. Complete healing may take 3 to 9 weeks, depending on ulcer size and treatment regimen employed. Healing of the ulcer should be assessed by means of x-rays or endoscopic examination. Barium-contrast films can be used to provide a rough estimate of the degree of gastric ulcer healing. However, it should be noted that endoscopic examination is the only accurate method to monitor for duodenal ulcer healing.

Because recurrence of peptic ulcer is frequent, interruption or discontinuation of therapy can have detrimental results. The patient must be encouraged to comply with therapy and continue with follow-up care for at least 1 year. If changes in lifestyle were part of the prescribed therapy, they should be maintained. Antacids, H_2-receptor antagonists, and proton pump inhibitors may be stopped after the ulcer has healed or may be prescribed in the form of low-dose maintenance therapy. No other medications, unless prescribed by the physician, should be taken because they may have an ulcerogenic effect. Finally, the patient and family should be told what to do in the event pain and discomfort recur or blood is noted in the vomitus or stools.

Acute Exacerbation. The patient with an acute exacerbation of peptic ulcer can usually be treated with the same regimen used for conservative management. However, the situation is considered more serious because of the possible complications of perforation, hemorrhage, and obstruction.

An acute exacerbation is frequently accompanied by bleeding, increased pain and discomfort, and nausea and vomiting. If the patient experiences recurrent vomiting or pyloric outlet obstruction, an NG tube is placed into the stomach with intermittent suction for about 24 to 48 hours.

DRUG THERAPY

Table 39-21 Antacid Preparations

Ingredient	Trade Name
Single Substance	
Aluminum carbonate	Basaljel
Aluminum hydroxide gel tablets	Amphojel, Alu-Cap
Aluminum phosphate	Phosphaljel
Calcium carbonate	Alka-2, Tums
Dihydroxyaluminum aminoacetate	Robalate
Dihydroxyaluminum sodium carbonate	Rolaids
Magaldrate	Riopan
Magnesium hydroxide	Mag-Ox
Sodium bicarbonate	Alka-Seltzer
Mixtures of Aluminum Hydroxide and Magnesium Salts	
	Aludrox
	A-M-T
	Cremalin
	Delcid
	Gaviscon
	Gelusil and Gelusil M
	Maalox
	Mylanta
	WinGel
Mixtures of Calcium Carbonate and Aluminum and Magnesium Hydroxides	
	Camalox
	Ducon
Mixtures of Calcium Carbonate, Magnesium Carbonate, and Magnesium Oxide	
	Alkets

DRUG THERAPY

Table 39-22 Side Effects of Antacid Therapy

Antacid	Reactions
Aluminum hydroxide gels	Constipation, phosphorus depletion with chronic use
Calcium carbonate	Constipation or diarrhea, hypercalcemia, milk-alkali syndrome, renal calculi
Magnesium preparations	Diarrhea, hypermagnesemia
Sodium preparations	Milk-alkali syndrome if used with large amounts of calcium; used with caution in patients on sodium restrictions

If there is a history of an incompetent pyloric sphincter allowing reflux of duodenal contents into the stomach, an NG tube will remove intestinal contents from the stomach. The maintenance of an empty stomach decreases the stimulus for pancreatic enzyme secretion as well. This period of stomach rest eliminates any causative factors that may have precipitated the acute exacerbation and permits the resolution of edema and inflammation of the mucosa. Fluids and electrolytes are replaced by IV infusion until the patient is able to tolerate oral feedings without distress.

Blood or blood products may be administered, depending on the amount of blood loss. Careful monitoring of the vital signs, intake and output, laboratory studies, and signs of impending shock are important during this acute episode.

Endoscopic evaluation is performed to reveal the degree of inflammation or bleeding, as well as the ulcer location. It is important to ascertain the presence of a prepyloric or pyloric ulcer that can cause gastric outlet obstruction. When endoscopic examination reveals no major problems and the patient's physical condition stabilizes, the plan of care for the patient should follow the same regimen of diet, activity, and medications used in conservative therapy. A 5-year follow-up program is recommended after acute exacerbation. An increase in the healing rate is achieved after conservative treatment, but the treatment plan cannot prevent the scar formation that can result in gastric outlet obstruction. Approximately 42% to 88% of ulcers recur.

Perforation. The immediate focus of management of a patient with a perforation is to stop the spillage of gastric or duodenal contents into the peritoneal cavity and restore blood volume. An NG tube is inserted into the stomach to provide continuous aspiration and gastric decompression to halt spillage through the perforation. Although duodenal aspiration is not achieved as promptly, placement of the tube as near to the perforation site as possible facilitates decompression.

Circulating blood volume must be replaced with lactated Ringer's and albumin solutions. These solutions substitute for the fluids lost from the vascular and interstitial space as the peritonitis develops. Blood replacement in the form of packed RBCs may be necessary. Unless contraindicated, a central venous pressure line and an indwelling urinary catheter should be inserted and monitored hourly. The patient with a history of cardiac disease requires ECG monitoring or placement of a pulmonary artery catheter for more accurate assessment of left ventricular function. Broad-spectrum antibiotic therapy should be started immediately to treat bacterial peritonitis. Administration of pain medications provides comfort.

The operative procedure involving the least risk to the patient is simple oversewing of the perforation and reinforcement of the area with a graft of omentum. The excess gastric contents are suctioned from the peritoneal cavity during the surgical procedure. Before surgical closure some surgeons irrigate with warm lactated Ringer's solution or instill an antibiotic solution into the abdominal cavity to help counteract the peritonitis.

There is controversy regarding the need for more definitive surgical treatment of a perforated ulcer than can be achieved with simple closure. Other types of surgical procedures depend on the location of the peptic ulcer and the surgeon's preference. If cure of the ulcer is the ultimate goal, the surgical procedures may include gastric resection or vagotomy and pyloroplasty.

Gastric Outlet Obstruction. The aim of therapy for gastric outlet obstruction is to decompress the stomach, correct any existing fluid and electrolyte imbalances, and improve the patient's general state of health. An NG tube is inserted into the stomach and attached to continuous suction to remove excess fluids and undigested food particles. With continuous decompression for several days the stomach has the opportunity to regain its normal muscle tone, the ulcer can begin healing, and the inflammation and edema will subside.

The tube is clamped after several days of suction, and gastric residue is measured periodically. The frequency and amount of time the tube remains clamped are proportional to the amount of aspirate obtained and the comfort level of the patient. A method commonly followed is to clamp the tube overnight for approximately 8 to 12 hours and to measure the gastric residue in the morning. When the aspirate falls below 200 ml, it is considered to be within a normal range and the patient can begin oral intake of clear liquids. Initially, oral fluids are begun at 30 ml per hour and then gradually increased in amount. The patient must be watched carefully for signs of distress or vomiting. As the amount of gastric residue decreases, solid foods are added and the tube is removed.

IV fluids and electrolytes are administered according to the degree of dehydration, vomiting, and electrolyte imbalance indicated by laboratory studies. Pain relief results from the decompression measures, and analgesics are usually not necessary. Antacid and antisecretory drug therapy (i.e., histamine H_2-receptor antagonists, proton pump inhibitors) is an integral part of treatment if the obstruction has been determined on endoscopic examination to be the result of an active ulcer. Pyloric obstruction may be removed nonsurgically by balloon dilations performed through the endoscope. Surgical intervention may be necessary to remove scar tissue.

Drug Therapy

Drug therapy for peptic ulcer disease is outlined in Table 39-20.

Antacids. Antacids are one of the initial drugs of choice in the treatment of peptic ulcers.[14] They decrease gastric acidity and the acid content of chyme reaching the duodenum. By raising the pH level to above 3.5, antacids effectively block the conversion of pepsinogen to its active form pepsin. In addition to their neutralizing effects, some antacids, such as aluminum hydroxide, can bind to bile salts, thus decreasing the salts' detrimental effects on the gastric mucosa.

Antacids consist of systemic and nonsystemic types. Systemic antacids, such as sodium bicarbonate, are extremely soluble and are absorbed into the circulation. Their long-term use can lead to systemic alkalosis; therefore they are rarely used in ulcer treatment. The nonsystemic antacids are insoluble and poorly absorbed. The common commercial nonsystemic antacids consist of magnesium hydroxide or aluminum hydroxide as single preparations or in various combinations (see Table 39-21).

The antacid preparation may be in liquid or tablet form. A large number of tablets may be required to equal the same dose of a liquid preparation. Since the tablets are chewable, some of the medication is left coating the teeth and gingivae instead of the stomach.

It has long been recognized that antacids ingested on an empty stomach are quickly evacuated and only partially used. Because the duration of action is only about 30 minutes, best results are obtained when they are prescribed 1 and 3 hours after meals and at bedtime. More frequent administration has resulted in poor tolerance and reduced long-term compliance. Acid secretion is also known to occur with higher doses and frequency by maintaining a high antral pH, which in turn stimulates release of gastrin.

The type and dosage of antacid prescribed depends on the adverse effects some of these preparations have on the health status or on other medications the patient may be taking (see Table 39-22). Preparations high in sodium, such as Titralac, Di-Gel, and Amphojel, should be used with caution in older adults and in the patient with cirrhosis of the liver, hypertension, congestive heart failure, and renal disease. Magnesium preparations should not be prescribed for the patient in renal failure because of the risk of magnesium toxicity. The most frequent side effect experienced with magnesium antacids is diarrhea. Aluminum hydroxide causes constipation. An antacid combination of aluminum and magnesium salts seems to lessen the side effects of both. Side effects of antacids are shown in Table 39-22.

Antacids have the capacity to interact unfavorably with some medications. They can enhance the absorption of drugs such as dicumarol and amphetamines. The action of digitalis preparations can be potentiated when taken in combination with calcium or magnesium antacids. In some instances, antacids may decrease the absorption rates of prescribed drugs, such as tetracycline. Therefore it is important to inform the physician of any drugs that are being taken before antacid therapy is begun.

The physician must often adjust the dosage of antacid so that the amount prescribed has the capacity of neutralizing the acid present. It is generally recommended that each dose of an antacid be capable of neutralizing 100 mEq of HCl acid. Any alteration in dosage should be carefully communicated to the patient and family, along with the rationale for the change so that compliance is more likely. The adjustment of antacids by the patient must be avoided. Taking too much or too little of an antacid can compromise its effectiveness and may lead to unpleasant side effects or an increase in ulcer discomfort.

For active gastric and duodenal ulcers, the prescribed treatment period varies from 4 to 8 weeks or until healing is demonstrated through endoscopic or barium-contrast studies. Many physicians recommend daily maintenance doses of an antacid to minimize ulcer recurrence.

Compliance with long-term antacid therapy seems to diminish with time. The patient fails to take the correct dose or stops taking the drug altogether. Many persons stop therapy because they find it inconvenient to keep the necessary daily supply at work, when traveling, or at home. For some patients it is embarrassing to be seen taking medications generally known to be prescribed for people with ulcers.

Histamine H_2-receptor Antagonists. The use of the histamine H_2-receptor antagonists cimetidine (Tagamet), ranitidine (Zantac), famotidine (Pepcid), and nizatidine (Axid) is now a standard component of most ulcer treatment regimens. Histamine is believed to be the final intracellular activator of HCl acid secretion. These drugs block the action of histamine on the H_2 receptors and thus reduce HCl acid secretion and accelerate ulcer healing. Antihistamine drugs used to treat allergies are H_1-receptor antagonists and thus have no effect on gastric acid secretion.

Histamine H_2-blocker drugs may be administered orally or IV. Their therapeutic effects are considerably longer than are those of antacids, some lasting for up to 12 hours. However, the onset of action (i.e., symptom relief) is longer than antacids. In addition, the drugs have demonstrated capabilities in the healing of gastric and duodenal ulcers. When the oldest of the H_2 blockers, cimetidine and ranitidine, are compared, the latter clearly has several advantages: (1) it is 5 to 12 times more potent and therefore has a longer duration of action; (2) optimal dosage can be achieved on a bid (twice a day) schedule versus qid (four times a day) schedule for cimetidine; (3) it inhibits nocturnal acid secretion for a longer time period; and (4) it has fewer side effects (headache, dizziness, malaise, neutropenia, thrombocytopenia, and elevated liver enzyme levels) than cimetidine (granulocytopenia, gynecomastia, diarrhea, fatigue, dizziness, rash, and mental confusion in the older adult).

Famotidine (Pepcid) and nizatidine (Axid) are the most recently available of these drugs. They are considered more potent at reduced dosage levels. Side effects appear to be minimal. Muscle cramps, headache, and constipation have been associated with the use of famotidine. Somnolence, sweating, and urticaria have occurred with nizatidine. Both drugs can be administered with antacids. Several of these preparations (e.g., Pepcid-AC, Tagamet) are now available as OTC drugs.

Proton Pump Inhibitors. Proton pump inhibitors, such as omeprazole (Prilosec), lansoprazole (Prevacid), and pantoprazole (Pantoloc), block the ATPase enzyme that is important for the secretion of gastric acid. These agents tend to be more effective than H_2-receptor antagonists are in reducing gastric acid secretion and promoting ulcer healing. Proton pump inhibitors are also used in combination with antibiotics to treat ulcers caused by *H. pylori.*

Antibiotic Therapy. Once the presence of *H. pylori* has been determined, antibiotic treatment is instituted. It has been recommended that only those patients with verified *H. pylori* be treated with antibiotics to reduce the potential for drug resistance. As shown in Table 39-13 triple and double drug therapies are used because no single agent has been found effective in eliminating *H. pylori.*

Anticholinergic Drugs. Anticholinergic drugs are only occasionally ordered in the treatment of peptic ulcer disease. These drugs decrease cholinergic stimulation of HCl acid. There is divided opinion concerning their efficacy in preventing recurrences and their therapeutic effectiveness in alleviating symptoms and preventing complications. Because of their tendency to decrease gastric motility, they should be avoided in gastric ulcers in which stasis of secretions increases the patient's pain and discomfort. Anticholinergics are associated with a high number of side effects, such as dry mouth and skin, flushing, thirst, tachycardia, dilated pupils, blurred vision, and urine retention. Anticholinergics must be prescribed with caution in the patient with narrow-angle glaucoma, prostatic hyperplasia, and gastric outlet obstruction. The use of anticholinergics has decreased as a result of histamine H_2-receptor antagonists and proton pump inhibitors.

Other Drug Therapy. Several other medications are used in the management of ulcers. Sucralfate (Carafate) is used for the short-term treatment of ulcers. It has proven to be cytoprotective of the esophagus, stomach, and duodenum. Its ability to accelerate ulcer healing is thought to be a result of the formation of an ulcer-adherent complex covering the ulcer and thereby protecting it from erosion caused by pepsin, acid, and bile salts. Sucralfate does not have acid-neutralizing capabilities. Its action is most effective at a low pH, and it should be given at least 30 minutes before or after an antacid. Adverse side effects are minimal. However, it does bind with cimetidine, digoxin, warfarin (Coumadin), phenytoin (Dilantin), and tetracycline, causing reduced bioavailability of these drugs.

Colloidal bismuth or bismuth subsalicylate (Pepto-Bismol) has demonstrated the ability to facilitate healing of peptic ulcer. It is thought to be partially effective against *H. pylori* infection. This drug is nonabsorbable and causes black stools.

Misoprostol (Cytotec) is a synthetic prostaglandin analog. It has protective and some antisecretory effects on gastric mucosa. Misoprostol is the only drug approved in the United States for the prevention of gastric ulcers induced by NSAIDs and aspirin. A major advantage of misoprostol is that it does not interfere with the therapeutic effects of aspirin and NSAIDs. It is believed that persons who require chronic NSAID therapy, such as those with osteoarthritis, benefit from the use of misoprostol because it reduces the risk of gastric ulcers and their complications.

Tricyclic antidepressants (e.g., imipramine, doxepin) have duodenal ulcer healing rates close to those obtained with cimetidine. The mode of action is not fully understood but appears similar to that of anticholinergic agents.

Nutritional Therapy Related to Conservative Therapy

Food acts as a buffer for gastric secretions. The buffering action of food lasts about 60 minutes and is then followed by an increase in the concentration of acid in the secretions. There are no specific diets or foods that are totally effective in treating peptic ulcer disease. The patient is encouraged to eat as normally as possible. If certain foods result in pain or discomfort, they should be avoided. The critical aspect is individualization of the dietary plan. Dietary orders may also vary according to the preference of the physician. Small, frequent meals (six per day) may be recommended. The rationale for ingesting six meals a day instead of three large ones is that the stomach should never be totally empty. In this way, gastric acid is neutralized.

Dietary instructions should include a sample diet with a list of foods that usually cause distress and should therefore be eliminated from the diet. Foods known to irritate the gastric mucosa include hot, spicy foods and pepper, alcohol, carbonated beverages, tea, coffee, and broth (meat extract). These foods also have limited buffering ability in addition to stimulating gastric acid secretion. Foods high in roughage, such as raw fruit, salads, and vegetables, may irritate an inflamed mucosa. If these foods are well chewed, this seems to be less of a problem.

Protein is considered the best neutralizing food, but it also stimulates gastric secretions. Carbohydrates and fats are the least stimulating to HCl acid secretion, but they do not neutralize well. The patient must determine a suitable combination of these essential nutrients without causing undue distress.

Historically, milk was an essential part of ulcer therapy until it was learned that milk proteins and calcium stimulate gastric acid production. For this reason, milk as part of diet therapy for ulcers was out of favor for a time. However, milk is again used as part of the diet plan because it can neutralize gastric acidity and contains prostaglandins and growth factors, both of which are known to protect the GI mucosa from injury.

NURSING MANAGEMENT: PEPTIC ULCER

■ Nursing Assessment

Subjective and objective data that should be obtained from a patient with peptic ulcer disease are presented in Table 39-23.

■ Nursing Diagnoses

Nursing diagnoses related to peptic ulcer may include, but are not limited to, those presented in NCP 39-2.

■ Planning

Overall goals are that the patient with peptic ulcer disease will (1) experience a reduction or absence of discomfort related to peptic ulcer disease, (2) exhibit no signs of GI complications related to the ulcerative process, (3) have complete healing of the peptic ulcer, (4) make appropriate lifestyle changes to prevent recurrence, and (5) comply with the prescribed therapeutic regimen.

■ Nursing Implementation

Health Promotion. Nurses are involved in identifying patients at risk for ulcer development. Early detection and treatment of ulcers are important aspects of reducing morbidity associated with ulcers. Patients who are taking ulcerogenic medications such as aspirin and NSAIDs are at risk for ulcer development. Patients are encouraged to take these medications with food or milk. Patients are also taught to report symptoms related to gastric irritation including epigastric pain to their care provider.

Acute Intervention. During the acute exacerbation of an ulcer, the patient generally complains of increased pain and nausea and vomiting, and some may have evidence of bleeding. Initially many patients attempt to cope with the symptoms at home before seeking medical assistance.

Very often during this acute phase all that is necessary for the patient's immediate recovery is to maintain NPO status for a few days, have an NG tube inserted and connected to intermittent suction, and replace fluids intravenously. The rationale for this therapy must be conveyed to the anxious patient and family. They must understand that the advantages far outweigh any temporary discomfort imposed by the presence of the tube. Regular mouth care alleviates the dry mouth. Cleansing and lubrication of the nares facilitates breathing and decreases soreness. Gastric contents should be analyzed for pH, blood, bile, or other irritating substances. When the stomach is kept empty of gastric secretions, the ulcer pain diminishes and ulcer healing begins. Usually this form of intervention is effective.

Because the patient is on NPO status, IV fluids are ordered. The type and amount administered are directly related to the fluid lost, the manifestations exhibited by the patient, and the results of the hemoglobin, hematocrit, and electrolyte determinations. The nurse should be aware of any other current health problem that could be adversely affected by the type of fluid used or the rate of the infusion. Repeated monitoring of these parameters provides information on the hydration status and the effectiveness of treatment. Vital signs are initially taken at least hourly so that shock can be detected and treated.

Physical and emotional rest are conducive to ulcer healing. The patient's immediate environment should be quiet and restful, and visitors should be restricted. The use of a mild sedative or tranquilizer has beneficial effects when the patient is anxious and apprehensive. The nurse must use good judgment before sedating a person who is becoming increasingly restless. There is danger that the medication will mask the signs of shock secondary to upper GI bleeding.

If the patient's condition improves without progression of symptoms (e.g., increased pain, vomiting, and hemorrhage), the regimen outlined for conservative therapy is followed. All too frequently an acute exacerbation is accompanied by one or more complications, especially hemorrhage and perforation and, to a lesser extent, obstruction.

Hemorrhage. Changes in the vital signs and an increase in the amount and redness of the aspirate often signal massive upper GI bleeding. When there is an increased amount of blood in the gastric contents, the patient's pain is often decreased because the blood helps to neutralize the acidic gastric contents. It is important to maintain the patency of the NG tube so that blood clots do not obstruct the tube. If the tube becomes blocked, the patient can develop abdominal distention.

NURSING ASSESSMENT

Table 39-23 Peptic Ulcer

Subjective Data

Important Health Information

Past health history: Chronic renal failure, pancreatic disease, chronic obstructive pulmonary disease, serious illness or trauma, hyperparathyroidism, cirrhosis of the liver, Zollinger-Ellison syndrome

Medications: Use of aspirin, corticosteroids, nonsteroidal antiinflammatory drugs, reserpine

Surgery or other treatments: Complicated or prolonged surgery

Functional Health Patterns

Health perception–health management: Chronic alcohol abuse, smoking, caffeine use; family history of peptic ulcer disease

Nutritional-metabolic: Weight loss, anorexia; nausea and vomiting, hematemesis; dyspepsia, heartburn, belching

Elimination: Black, tarry stools

Cognitive–perceptual: **Duodenal ulcers**—Burning, midepigastric or back pain occurring 2 to 4 hours after meals and relieved by food; nocturnal pain common; **Gastric ulcers**—High epigastric pain occurring 1 to 2 hours after meals; pain may be precipitated or aggravated by food

Coping-stress tolerance: Acute or chronic stress

Objective Data

General

Anxiety, irritability

Gastrointestinal

Epigastric tenderness

Possible Findings

Anemia; guaiac-positive stools; gastric analysis indicating high gastric acid secretion; positive *H. pylori* culture from gastric tissue, abnormal upper gastrointestinal endoscopic and barium studies

39-2 NURSING CARE PLAN PATIENT WITH PEPTIC ULCER

Expected Patient Outcomes	Nursing Interventions and *Rationales*
CONSERVATIVE MANAGEMENT	
NURSING DIAGNOSIS	**Pain** *related to* increased gastric secretions, decreased mucosal protection, and ingestion of gastric irritants *as manifested by* burning cramplike pain in epigastrium and abdomen; pain onset 1 to 2 hr after meals with gastric ulcer; pain onset 2 to 4 hr after meals (midmorning, midafternoon) and middle of night with duodenal ulcer.
▪ Verbalization of satisfaction with pain control.	▪ Determine pain characteristics from verbal description and physical assessment data *so appropriate interventions can be planned.* ▪ Administer antacids, H_2 antagonists, proton pump inhibitors, anticholinergics, and protective agents as ordered *to reduce pain.* ▪ Teach patient to avoid smoking and ingesting spicy, hot or cold foods, coffee, tea and cola drinks, and alcoholic beverages *to prevent increasing acid production.* ▪ Teach patient stress reduction *as relaxation results in decreased acid production and reduction in pain.*
NURSING DIAGNOSIS	**Ineffective management of therapeutic regimen** *related to* lack of knowledge of long-term management of peptic ulcer disease, not following treatment plan, and unwillingness to modify lifestyle *as manifested by* frequent questions about home care, incorrect responses to questions about peptic ulcer disease, noncompliance with medical regimen.
▪ Verbalization of plan to modify lifestyle and incorporate therapeutic regimen into lifestyle.	▪ Explain ulcer disease process at patient's level *to foster understanding.* ▪ Help patient identify stressors and initiate modifications in daily routine *as stress causes hypersecretion of HCl acid and pepsin, which can alter the mucosal barrier.* ▪ Discuss diet plan and assist with implementation at home and in work setting. ▪ Explain rationale for the elimination of alcohol, spicy foods, coffee, tea, and colas from diet; explain the harmful effects of smoking *as these agents increase acid production and directly irritate gastric mucosa.* ▪ Provide information on medication actions and side effects *to ensure safe self-administration.* ▪ Inform patient what to do if symptoms related to ulcers reoccur *to ensure early initiation of treatment.*
EXACERBATION MANAGEMENT	
NURSING DIAGNOSIS	**Pain** *related to* acute exacerbation of disease process and inadequate comfort measures *as manifested by* verbalization of increase in pain, nonverbal indicators of pain (e.g., moaning, crying, doubling up).
▪ Expression of satisfaction with pain management.	▪ Encourage bed rest or light activity *to conserve energy and promote comfort.* ▪ Provide quiet, relaxed environment and limit visitors *to decrease stress and other factors that increase acid secretion.* ▪ Administer medications as ordered *to relieve pain.*
NURSING DIAGNOSIS	**Vomiting** *related to* acute exacerbation of disease process and inadequate comfort measures *as manifested by* increase in nausea and/or vomiting.
▪ Decrease in or absence of nausea and vomiting.	▪ Maintain NPO status *to prevent irritation of GI mucosa.* ▪ Maintain NG tube to suction *to keep stomach empty and remove any stimulus for HCl acid and pepsin secretion.* ▪ Check vomitus or aspirate for occult blood *to assess for hemorrhage.*

Continued

39-2 NURSING CARE PLAN PATIENT WITH PEPTIC ULCER—continued

Expected Patient Outcomes	Nursing Interventions and *Rationales*

COLLABORATIVE PROBLEMS

POTENTIAL COMPLICATION **Hemorrhage** *related to* eroded mucosal tissue.

Nursing Goals	Nursing Interventions and *Rationales*
▪ Monitor for signs of hemorrhage. ▪ Carry out medical and nursing interventions if hemorrhage occurs.	▪ Assess for evidence of hematemesis, bright red or melena stool, abdominal pain or discomfort, symptoms of shock (e.g., decreased blood pressure; cool, clammy skin; cyanosis; dyspnea; tachycardia; decreased urine output); *to plan appropriate interventions.* ▪ If ulcer is actively bleeding, observe NG tube aspirate or emesis for amount and color *to assess degree of bleeding.* ▪ Take vital signs every 15 to 30 min *to determine patient's hemodynamic status and as indicators of shock.* ▪ Maintain IV infusion line *to provide ready access for blood and fluid replacement.* ▪ If RBC transfusion is given, observe for transfusion reaction *so appropriate actions can be taken immediately.* ▪ Monitor hematocrit and hemoglobin *as indicators of severity of hemorrhage and need for fluid and blood replacement.* ▪ Record intake and output *to monitor fluid balance.* ▪ Reassure patient and family *to decrease their anxiety.* ▪ Remain calm and confident in plan of care *to foster calm and confidence in patient and family.*

POTENTIAL COMPLICATION **Perforation of GI mucosa** *related to* impaired mucosal tissue integrity.

Nursing Goals	Nursing Interventions and *Rationales*
▪ Monitor for signs of perforation. ▪ Report deviations from expected parameters. ▪ Carry out appropriate medical and nursing interventions.	▪ Observe for manifestations of perforation (e.g., sudden, severe abdominal pain; rigid, boardlike abdomen; pain to shoulders; increasing distention; decreasing bowel sounds) *to ensure early recognition and intervention.* ▪ Monitor vital signs every 15 to 30 min *as indicators of shock.* ▪ Maintain NG tube to suction *to provide continuous aspiration and gastric decompression to prevent further leakage of gastric fluid through the perforation.* ▪ Administer pain medication *to promote comfort and reduce anxiety.* ▪ Prepare patient for emergency diagnostic tests and possible surgical intervention *to foster timely intervention.*

The nurse must monitor the results of the hemoglobin and hematocrit determinations. Awareness of the significance of these laboratory results and ability to correlate the data to the patient's signs and symptoms can be lifesaving.

Perforation. When there is sudden, severe abdominal pain unrelated in intensity and location to the pain that brought the patient to the hospital, the nurse must recognize the possibility of ulcer perforation. When any person with an ulcer, particularly a chronic duodenal ulcer, demonstrates these manifestations, perforation should be suspected and the physician notified immediately.

Perforation is indicated by a rigid, boardlike abdomen; severe generalized abdominal and shoulder pain; drawing up of the knees; and shallow, grunting respirations. The bowel sounds that may have been previously normal or hyperactive may diminish and become absent.

Vital signs are important parameters and should be promptly recorded and taken every 15 to 30 minutes. The nurse should temporarily stop all oral or NG medications and feedings until the physician can be notified and a definitive diagnosis made. If perforation does exist, anything taken internally can add to the spillage into the peritoneal cavity and increase discomfort. If IV fluids are being administered at the time of the perforation, the rate should be maintained or increased to replace the depleted plasma volume.

The symptoms experienced by the patient are very frightening. The reaction of the nursing staff must be one of calm reassurance in spite of the seriousness of the situation. Simple explanations of the need for chest and abdominal x-rays help diminish the patient's anxiety and give some insight into the diagnostic plan. Indicating why frequent samples of blood are necessary lessens confusion and resistance.

When perforation is confirmed, the nurse should ensure that any known allergies the patient has have been recorded on the chart. This is important because antibiotic therapy is usually started, and careful observation for allergic reactions must

PATIENT & FAMILY TEACHING GUIDE

Table 39-24 Peptic Ulcer Disease

The following are teaching guidelines for patient and family:

1. Explain dietary modifications, including avoidance of foods that cause epigastric distress. This may include black pepper, spicy foods, and acidic foods. Small frequent meals may be better tolerated than large meals.
2. Explain the rationale for avoiding cigarettes. In addition to promoting ulcer development, smoking will delay ulcer healing.
3. Encourage the need to reduce or eliminate alcohol ingestion.
4. Explain the rationale for avoiding OTC medications unless approved by the patient's care provider. Many preparations contain ingredients, such as aspirin, that should not be taken unless approved by the physician. Check with the care provider regarding the use of nonsteroidal antiinflammatory drugs.
5. Explain the rationale for not interchanging brands of antacids and H_2-antagonists that can be purchased without a prescription without checking with the physician or nurse. This can lead to harmful side effects.
6. Teach the need to take all medications as prescribed. This includes both antisecretory and antibiotic medications. Failure to take medications as prescribed can result in relapse.
7. Explain the importance of reporting any of the following:
   - increased nausea and/or vomiting
   - increase in epigastric pain
   - bloody emesis or tarry stools
8. Explain the relationship between symptoms and stress. Stress-reducing activities or relaxation strategies are encouraged.
9. Encourage patient and family to share concerns about lifestyle changes and living with a chronic illness.

OTC, over-the-counter.

be made. When the perforation fails to seal spontaneously, surgical closure is necessary and is performed as soon as possible. There is often little time to prepare the patient and family thoroughly for the surgical intervention, yet some instructions can be carried out while the immediate therapy is begun. If major reconstructive surgery is anticipated, the patient and family may question the need when the problem is only a small hole. To answer this type of question, the nurse must first have an understanding of the usual operative procedures being used and, in addition, must know that unless the surgery can cure the ulcer that caused the perforation, the patient may need more surgery in the future. (Nursing management of peritonitis is discussed in Chapter 40.)

Gastric outlet obstruction. Gastric outlet obstruction is a complication of peptic ulcer disease that can occur at any time. Obstruction is a possible complication, particularly in the patient whose ulcer is located close to the pylorus. Because the onset of symptoms is usually gradual, the condition is not generally as serious an emergency as hemorrhage or perforation. Relief of symptoms may be achieved by constant NG aspiration of stomach contents. This allows edema and inflammation to subside and then permits normal flow of gastric contents through the pylorus.

Obstruction can also occur during the treatment of an acute episode of peptic ulcer exacerbation. If these symptoms are experienced while the patient is still on NPO status, the patency of the NG tube should be suspected. Regular irrigation of the tube with a saline solution facilitates proper functioning. It may be helpful to reposition the patient from side to side so that the tube tip is not constantly lying against the mucosal surface.

When oral feedings have been resumed and symptoms of obstruction are observed, the physician should be promptly informed. Generally, all that is necessary to treat the problem is to resume gastric aspiration so that the edema and inflammation resulting from the acute episode have time to resolve. IV fluids with electrolyte replacement keep the patient hydrated during this period. The NG tube can be clamped and gastric fluids can be aspirated to check for retention. It is important to maintain accurate intake and output records, especially of the gastric aspirate. The patient should be kept aware of why these symptoms are being experienced. In some instances in which treatment is not successful, surgery may be performed after the acute phase has passed.

Ambulatory and Home Care. The patient in whom peptic ulcer disease has been diagnosed has specific needs that must be met to prevent and avoid recurrence or complications. General instructions should cover aspects of the disease process itself, medications, possible changes in lifestyle (including diet), and regular follow-up care. Table 39-24 provides a patient teaching guide for the patient with peptic ulcer disease.

Knowing the cause of the ulcer and understanding the disease process may motivate the patient to become more involved in care and increase compliance with therapy. The patient must understand the dietary modifications and why they are important for recovery and health maintenance. The nurse and the dietician should elicit a dietary history from the patient and plan for ways that dietary modifications can be easily incorporated into the patient's home and work setting. The patient who is following a diet prescribed for another illness needs to know how to balance the two so that neither condition is harmed by dietary interventions.

The patient does not always provide the physician with accurate information regarding habitual use of alcohol or cigarettes. The nurse may be looked on as less threatening and more understanding of these habits than the physician may be. The nurse should provide useful information about the detrimental effects of alcohol and cigarettes on ulcer disease and ulcer healing.

The nurse should instruct the patient about prescribed medications, including their actions, side effects, and inherent dangers if omitted for any reason. The patient should know why OTC medications (e.g., aspirin) should not be taken unless approved by the physician. Because antacids and some H_2-receptor antagonists may be bought without a prescription, the patient must be informed that interchanging brands without checking with the physician or nurse can lead to harmful side effects.

Efforts should be made to obtain more information about the patient's psychosocial status. Knowledge of lifestyle, occupation, and coping behaviors can be helpful to the plan of care. The patient may be reluctant to talk about personal subjects, the stress experienced at home or on the job, the usual methods of coping, or dependence on drugs or alcohol. Unfortunately, the patient does not often see the relationship between lifestyle or occupation and ulcer disease. It is important to listen for subtle clues from the patient's statements and to observe for behaviors that broaden this database.

When the occupation, related work habits, home, or environment have been implicated as factors in peptic ulcer development, the patient must be made aware of these stressors, how to avoid them in the future, or how to cope with them successfully if they cannot be altered. Vocational or psychologic counseling may be necessary so that fatigue and repeated emotional upsets can be avoided when possible.

The need for long-term follow-up care must be stressed. Because successful treatment is frequently followed by a recurrence of the ulcer disease, the patient should be encouraged to seek immediate intervention if symptoms of the disease recur. The patient who has recurrence of ulcer disease following initial healing must learn to live with a disease that is chronic. The patient may be angry and frustrated, especially if the prescribed mode of therapy has been faithfully followed yet has failed to prevent the recurrence or extension of the disease process.

Unfortunately, many patients do not comply with the plan of care originally designed, and they experience repeated exacerbations. Patients quickly learn that they often experience no discomfort when they omit prescribed medications or indulge in occasional dietary indiscretions. Consequently they make no or little alteration in lifestyle. After an acute exacerbation the patient is often more amenable to following the plan of care and open to suggestions for changes in lifestyle. Changes are difficult for most people and may be met with resistance. If the patient has been instructed to stop smoking or to avoid the use of alcohol, this request may be met with resistance. The patient may fare better from a reduction in his or her use of these substances rather than from total elimination. Although alcohol and smoking are known to interfere with ulcer healing, they frequently serve as coping mechanisms. From the patient's point of view, the distress caused by their total elimination may outweigh the benefits to be gained from abstention. The goal, however, should always be total cessation. A patient with chronic ulcers must be aware of the complications that may result from the disease, the clinical manifestations indicating their presence, and what to do until the physician can be seen.

■ Evaluation

Expected outcomes for the patient with a peptic ulcer are addressed in NCP 39-2 on p. 1120.

Surgical Therapy for Peptic Ulcers

Approximately 20% of patients with ulcers need surgical intervention. Because there is a high recurrence rate for both duodenal and gastric ulcers and complications increase with the duration of the ulcer, many physicians believe that surgery is necessary after therapy has been tried and proved unsuccessful. The following criteria are used as general indications for surgical intervention:

1. Intractability: failure of the ulcer to heal or recurrence of the ulcer after therapy
2. History of hemorrhage or increased risk of bleeding during treatment
3. Prepyloric or pyloric ulcers (both have high recurrence rates)
4. Concurrent condition, such as severe burns, trauma, or sepsis
5. Multiple ulcer sites
6. Drug-induced ulcers, especially when withdrawal from the drug may put the person at risk
7. Possible existence of a malignant ulcer
8. Obstruction

A variety of surgical procedures are used to treat ulcer disease. They usually involve a partial gastrectomy, vagotomy, or pyloroplasty. Partial gastrectomy with removal of the distal two thirds of the stomach and anastomosis of the gastric stump to the duodenum is called a *gastroduodenostomy* or *Billroth I operation* (Fig. 39-18). Partial gastrectomy with removal of the distal two thirds of the stomach and anastomosis of the gastric stump to the jejunum is called a *gastrojejunostomy* or *Billroth II operation.* In both procedures the antrum and the pylorus are removed. Because the duodenum is bypassed, the Billroth II operation is the preferred surgical procedure to prevent recurrence of duodenal ulcers.

Vagotomy is the severing of the vagus nerve, either totally (truncal) or selectively at some point in its innervation to the stomach. In a truncal vagotomy the nerve is severed bilaterally in both the anterior and the posterior trunk. Selective vagotomy consists of cutting the nerve at a particular branch of the vagus nerve, resulting in denervation of only a portion of the stomach, such as the antrum or the parietal cell mass.

Pyloroplasty consists of surgical enlargement of the pyloric sphincter to facilitate the easy passage of contents from the stomach. It is most commonly done after vagotomy or to enlarge an opening that has been constricted from scar tissue. A vagotomy causes decreased gastric motility. A pyloroplasty accompanying vagotomy increases gastric emptying.

The combination of a Billroth I or II procedure with vagotomy has the advantage of eliminating the ulcer and the stimulus for acid secretion. Surgical removal of the antrum results in removal of the source of gastrin secretion. (Gastrin normally stimulates parietal and chief cells.) Vagotomy eliminates the stimulus of HCl acid and gastrin hormone secretion caused by vagal stimulation.

Postoperative Complications. The most common postoperative complications from peptic ulcer surgery are (1) dumping syndrome, (2) postprandial hypoglycemia, and (3) bile reflux gastritis.

Dumping syndrome. Dumping syndrome is the direct result of surgical removal of a large portion of the stomach and the pyloric sphincter. These changes drastically reduce the reservoir capacity of the stomach. Although dumping syndrome is more commonly experienced after a Billroth II procedure, it can occur after any gastric reconstruction and vagotomy.

Dumping syndrome is associated with meals having a hyperosmolar composition. Normally, gastric chyme enters the small intestine in small amounts, and shifts in fluid from the extracellular space are minimal. After surgery, however, the stomach no longer has control over the amount of gastric chyme entering the small intestine. Consequently a large bolus

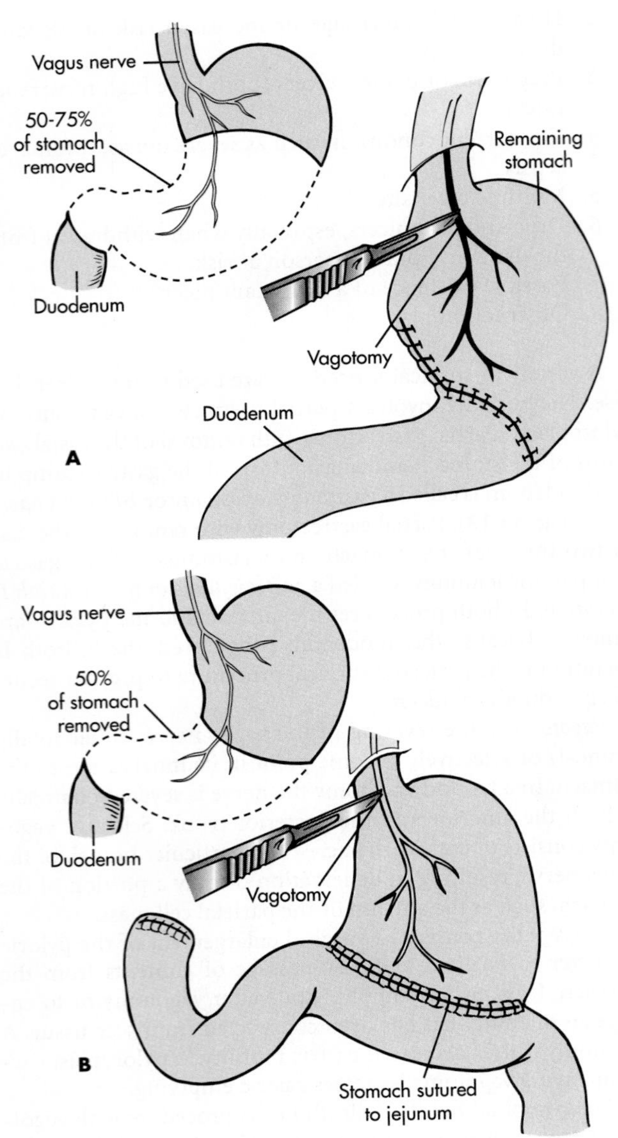

Fig. 39-18 **A,** Billroth I procedure (subtotal gastric resection with gastroduodenostomy anastomosis). **B,** Billroth II procedure (subtotal gastric resection with gastrojejunostomy anastomosis).

of hypertonic fluid enters the intestine and results in fluid being drawn into the bowel lumen. This creates a decrease in plasma volume. A secondary consequence of this fluid shift is distention of the bowel lumen, which stimulates intestinal motility and the urge to defecate.

Approximately one third to one half of patients experience dumping syndrome after peptic ulcer surgery. The onset of symptoms occurs at the end of a meal or within 15 to 30 minutes after eating. The patient usually describes feelings of generalized weakness, sweating, palpitations, and dizziness. These symptoms are attributed to the sudden decrease in plasma volume. The patient complains of abdominal cramps, borborygmi, and the urge to defecate. These manifestations usually last for no longer than an hour after meals.

Postprandial hypoglycemia. Postprandial hypoglycemia is considered a variant of the dumping syndrome, since it is the result of uncontrolled gastric emptying of a bolus of fluid high in carbohydrate into the small intestine. The bolus of concentrated carbohydrate results in hyperglycemia and the release of excessive amounts of insulin into the circulation. A secondary hypoglycemia then occurs, with symptoms appearing about 2 hours after meals. The symptoms experienced are the ones observed in any hypoglycemic reaction and include sweating, weakness, mental confusion, palpitations, tachycardia, and anxiety.

The immediate ingestion of sugared fluids or candy relieves the hypoglycemic symptoms. The treatment of this type of hypoglycemia is similar to that of the dumping syndrome. To avoid similar occurrences the patient should be instructed to limit the amount of sugar consumed with each meal and to eat small, frequent meals with moderate amounts of protein and fat.

Bile reflux gastritis. Gastric surgery that involves the pylorus, either reconstruction or removal, can result in reflux alkaline gastritis. Prolonged contact of bile, especially bile salts, causes damage to the gastric mucosa. Chronic gastritis of this form may result in the back-diffusion of hydrogen ions through the gastric mucosa. Paradoxically, peptic ulcer may recur after surgical treatment that was intended as a cure.

The symptoms associated with reflux alkaline gastritis are continuous epigastric distress that increases after meals. Vomiting relieves the distress but only temporarily. The administration of cholestyramine (Questran), either before or with meals, has met with considerable success. Cholestyramine binds with the bile salts that are the source of irritation in this condition. Aluminum hydroxide antacids have also been used in the treatment of this condition.

Nutritional Therapy Related to Surgical Therapy. Discharge planning and instruction should be started as soon as the immediate postoperative period is successfully passed. Dietary instructions may be given by the dietician and reinforced by the nursing staff. Because the stomach's reservoir has been greatly diminished after gastric resection, the meal size must be reduced accordingly. The patient must be advised to eliminate drinking fluids with meals as had been done in the past. Dry foods with a low-carbohydrate content and moderate protein and fat content are better tolerated initially. These dietary changes, with the incorporation of a short rest period after each meal, reduce the likelihood of dumping syndrome. Reassurance that following these dietary measures will result in cessation of these symptoms within a few months is essential to long-term compliance.

Postprandial hypoglycemic reaction can be avoided if these dietary instructions are followed with special emphasis on eating foods low in sugar content. Although only a small percentage of patients experience bile reflux gastritis, the patient must be cautioned to notify the physician of any continuous epigastric distress after meals that is similar to that felt before surgery.

With regard to dumping syndrome, the symptoms are self-limiting and frequently disappear within several months to a year after surgery. Interventions prescribed for the patient are diet instruction, rest, and reassurance. The diet should consist of small dry feedings daily that are low in carbohydrate, restricted in refined sugars, and contain moderate amounts of protein and fat. Sample menu plans are presented in

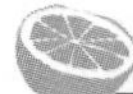

NUTRITIONAL THERAPY

Table 39-25 Postgastrectomy Dumping Syndrome

Purpose

To slow the rapid passage of food into the intestine; to control symptoms of the dumping syndrome (dizziness, sense of fullness, diarrhea, tachycardia), which sometimes occur following a partial or total gastrectomy

Diet Principles

1. Meals are divided into six small feedings to avoid overloading intestines at mealtimes.
2. Fluids should not be taken with meals but at least 30 to 45 minutes before or after meals; this helps prevent distention or a feeling of fullness.
3. Concentrated sweets (e.g., honey, sugar, jelly, jam, candies, sweet pastries, sweetened fruit) are avoided because they sometimes cause dizziness, diarrhea, and a sense of fullness.
4. Protein and fats are increased to promote rebuilding of body tissues and to meet energy needs. Meat, cheese, eggs, and milk products are specific foods to increase in the diet.
5. Amount of time these restrictions should be followed varies. The health care provider decides the proper amount of time to remain on this prescribed diet according to the patient's clinical condition and progress.

Exchanges	Sample Menu 1	Sample Menu 2	Sample Menu 3
Breakfast			
1 meat 1 starch Fat	1 poached egg 1 slice toast 2 sausage Margarine	1 fried egg 1 corn tortilla 2 slices bacon Margarine	1 oz ham 2 biscuits with 2 tsp gravy
10 AM snack			
1 starch ½ cup milk 1 fruit	¾ cup dry cereal ½ cup milk ½ fresh banana Sugar substitute	½ cup atole ½ cup milk 2 unsweetened canned peach halves Sugar substitute	½ cup grits with 2 tbs margarine added ⅛ cantaloupe ½ cup buttermilk
Lunch			
2 meat 2 starch 1 vegetable 1 fruit Fat	Grilled cheese sandwich with 2 oz cheese, lettuce 2 unsweetened pear halves	1 burrito with 1 oz meat, 1 oz cheese, ½ cup pinto beans, 1 flour tortilla ½ diet gelatin dessert with fruit cocktail added	2 oz fried fish ½ cup buttered rice ½ cup mustard greens 1 fresh apple 1 slice bread
2 PM snack			
1 meat or substitute 1 starch	½ cup plain yogurt 2 graham crackers	½ cup cottage cheese 5 soda crackers	2 tsp peanut butter 1 slice bread
Dinner			
2 meat 1 starch Vegetable 1 fruit Fat	2 oz tomato meatloaf ½ cup mashed potatoes with gravy ½ cup buttered green beans ½ cup unsweetened apple sauce	2 tamales ½ cup buttered corn 1 fresh orange	2 oz fried pork chop ½ cup black-eyed peas ½ cup buttered carrots 1 fresh plum
8 PM snack			
1 meat 1 starch Vegetable Fat	½ sandwich with 1 slice bread, 1 oz roast beef, lettuce, mayonnaise	1 corn tortilla with 1 oz melted cheese and green chili	½ sandwich with 1 slice bread, 1 slice salami, lettuce, mayonnaise

Table 39-25. Fluids should be taken between meals but not with the meal and the patient should plan rest periods of at least 30 minutes after each meal. The recumbent position is the most beneficial if the patient can arrange for it. Reassuring the patient that the unpleasant symptoms are usually of short duration is helpful in gaining cooperation. A small percentage of patients experience long-term problems and may require further reconstructive surgery.

NURSING MANAGEMENT: SURGICAL THERAPY FOR PEPTIC ULCERS

■ Preoperative Care

When surgery is planned with the goal of curing the ulcer disease, the surgeon should provide necessary information about the procedure and the expected outcome so that the patient can make an informed decision. The nurse can help the patient and family by clarifying and interpreting their questions. A discussion of the surgical procedure accompanied by a diagram or picture showing the anatomical changes that will result should be incorporated into the preoperative teaching plan. Instructions should be clear on what to expect after surgery, including comfort measures, pain relief, coughing and breathing exercises, use of an NG tube, and IV fluid administration (see Chapter 16).

Postoperative Care

Care of the patient after major abdominal surgery is similar to the postoperative care after abdominal laparotomy (see Chapter 40). An NG tube is used to decompress the remaining portion of the stomach to decrease pressure on the suture line and to allow for resolution of edema and inflammation resulting from surgical trauma.

The gastric aspirate must be carefully observed for color, amount, and odor during the immediate postoperative period. The color of the aspirate is expected to be bright red at first, with a gradual darkening within the first 24 hours after surgery. Normally the color changes to yellow-green within 36 to 48 hours. If the tube becomes clogged during this period, the physician may order periodic gentle irrigations with normal saline solution. It is essential that the NG suction is working and that the tube remains patent so that accumulated gastric secretions do not put a strain on the anastomosis. This can lead to distention of the remaining portion of the stomach and result in (1) rupture of the sutures, (2) leakage of gastric contents into the peritoneal cavity, (3) hemorrhage, and (4) possible abscess formation. If the tube must be replaced or repositioned, the physician must be called to perform this task because of the danger of perforating the gastric mucosa or disrupting the suture line.

The nurse should observe the patient for signs of decreased peristalsis and lower abdominal discomfort that may indicate impending intestinal obstruction. Accurate intake and output records must be kept. Vital signs are monitored and recorded every 4 hours.

The patient should be kept comfortable and free of pain by the administration of the prescribed medications and by frequent changes in position. The incision is relatively high in the epigastrium and may interfere with deep-breathing and coughing measures. Splinting the area with a pillow while gently and persistently encouraging the patient to put forth the best efforts possible helps prevent pulmonary complications. Splinting also protects the abdominal suture line from rupturing during coughing. The dressing must be observed for signs of bleeding or odor and drainage indicative of an infection. Ambulation is encouraged and is increased daily.

While the NG tube is connected to suction, IV therapy is maintained. Potassium and vitamin supplements are added to the infusion until oral feedings are resumed. Before the NG tube is removed, the patient is started on oral feedings of clear liquids to determine the tolerance level. The stomach is aspirated within 1 or 2 hours to assess the amount remaining and its color and consistency. When fluids are well tolerated, the tube is removed and fluids are increased in frequency with a slow progression to regular foods. The regimen of six small meals a day is begun.

Pernicious anemia is a long-term complication that may occur after partial gastrectomy. However, it is seen more often when the entire stomach is surgically removed. Pernicious anemia is caused by the loss of intrinsic factor, which is produced by the parietal cells. Depending on the amount of parietal cell mass removed in surgery, the patient may eventually require regular injections of cobalamin. (Cobalamin deficiency and pernicious anemia are discussed in Chapter 29.)

Because the patient is generally returning to the same home and work environment, there is always the danger of ulcer redevelopment, especially at the site of the anastomosis. Adequate rest, nutrition, and avoidance of known stressors are keys to complete recovery. Avoiding the use of medications not prescribed by the physician should be reemphasized, along with restrictions on smoking and alcohol use. If the patient is willing to make these kinds of adjustment in lifestyle, a successful rehabilitation is more likely.

GERONTOLOGIC CONSIDERATIONS

Peptic Ulcer Disease

The incidence of gastric ulcers in patients over 60 years of age is increasing. This is related to the increased use of NSAIDs. In the elderly patient pain may not be the first symptom associated with an ulcer. For some patients the first indication may be frank gastric bleeding (e.g., hematemesis, melena) or a subtle decrease in hematocrit. The morbidity and mortality rates associated with gastric ulcers in the elderly patient are higher than younger adults because of concomitant health problems (e.g., cardiovascular, pulmonary) and a decreased ability to withstand hypovolemia. The treatment and management of gastric ulcers in the older adult are similar to that in younger adults. An emphasis is placed on prevention of gastritis and gastric ulcers. This includes teaching the patient to take NSAIDs and other gastric-irritating medications with food, milk, or antacids. If necessary, the patient may be treated with antisecretory agents (i.e., proton pump inhibitors or H_2-receptor antagonists). The patient should be instructed to avoid irritating substances, such as alcohol and smoking, and to report abdominal pain or discomfort to his or her health care provider.

CANCER OF THE STOMACH

Although the rate of stomach cancer has been steadily declining in the United States since the 1930s, it is the seventh leading cause of cancer mortality in the United States, accounting for more than 13,700 deaths and 22,600 new cases annually.[9] Worldwide gastric adenocarcinoma is the second most common malignant growth. Costa Rica and Japan have the highest incidence rates in the world. Cancer of the stomach is more prevalent in men of the lower socioeconomic class, primarily those living in urban areas. Stomach cancer is typically at an advanced stage when diagnosed and is not usually amenable to surgical resection. Only 10% to 20% of patients develop disease confined to the stomach. Survival of patients with nonlocalized gastric cancer is less than 10% 5 years after diagnosis.

Etiology and Pathophysiology

Many factors have been implicated in the development of gastric cancer, yet no single causative agent has been identified. It is believed that a diet of smoked, highly salted, or spiced foods may have a carcinogenic effect. A genetic etiology has been postulated because of the greater than normal occurrence of stomach cancer in immediate family members. Persons with blood group A have a greater incidence of gastric cancer than the general population. At the present time there is no universally accepted genetic connection.

Gastric carcinogenesis probably begins with a nonspecific mucosal injury as a result of aging, autoimmunity, or repeated exposure to irritants such as bile, antiinflammatory agents, or alcohol. Nutritional or other undetermined genetic deficiencies may impede mucosal repair, resulting in chronic gastritis and subsequent proliferation of *H. pylori.* It is possible that *H. pylori* and resulting metabolic changes can induce a sequence of transitions from dysplasia to carcinoma *in situ.*

Other predisposing factors associated with a high incidence of gastric cancer are atrophic gastritis, pernicious anemia, benign gastric polyps, and achlorhydria. The relationship between chronic peptic ulcers of the stomach and the development of gastric cancer is still controversial. Malignant transformation of a benign chronic ulcer does occur but accounts for less than 5% of all gastric cancers. It is known that the person with achlorhydria or pernicious anemia is more likely to develop gastric cancer than is the person with normal gastric acid production.

Malignant tumors of the stomach may be present for a long time and may have spread to adjacent organs before any distressing symptoms occur. The tumor may grow to large dimensions without obstructing the lumen of the stomach simply because the lumen itself is so large. The mean interval from onset of symptoms to consultation with a physician may be as long as 6 months. This long delay is largely attributed to the vague, intermittent abdominal distress experienced by the patient. Unfortunately, most healthy persons at one time or another experience this type of early symptom as a result of dietary indiscretions, nervous tension, and anxiety.

Gastric cancer can occur in any portion of the stomach. In the past, cancers of the pyloric antral region were most common. Recently there has been an increase in the incidence of proximal gastric cancer. Tumors located at the cardia and fundus are associated with a poor prognosis. These tumors typically infiltrate rapidly to the surrounding tissue, the regional lymph nodes, and the liver. The patient with tumor growth along the lesser curvature has a better survival rate. Adenocarcinomas account for more than 95% of the cancers, and sarcomas (comprising lymphomas and leiomyomas) make up the rest.

The tumor growth is insidious and follows a pattern of continuous infiltration. Cancer of the stomach may spread by direct extension along the mucosal surface and infiltrate through the gastric wall. The rich lymphatic plexuses in the stomach wall facilitate distant metastasis. Seeding of tumor cells into the peritoneal cavity may occur late in the course of the disease. Evidence of spread to the peritoneal cavity is manifested by ascites and by spread to the ovaries.

Clinical Manifestations

The clinical manifestations exhibited by persons with gastric cancer can be categorized by signs and symptoms of anemia, peptic ulcer disease, or indigestion. Anemia is a common occurrence with stomach cancer. It is caused by chronic blood loss as the lesion erodes through the mucosa or as a direct result of pernicious anemia, which develops when intrinsic factor is lost. The person appears pale and weak and complains of fatigue, weakness, dizziness, and, in extreme cases, shortness of breath. The stool may be positive for occult blood.

The symptoms of gastric malignancy are sometimes identical to those of peptic ulcer disease. The pain and discomfort may be alleviated by belching and by the use of antacids, antisecretory agents and diet modifications.

Manifestations related to indigestion include vague epigastric fullness with feelings of early satiety after meals. Weight loss, dysphagia, and constipation frequently accompany epigastric distress. When nausea, vomiting, and hematemesis occur, they may indicate obstruction at the gastric outlet or may be a warning of impending hemorrhage.

The early detection of gastric cancer is difficult because of the vagueness of the symptoms. On physical examination the patient may be pale and lethargic if anemia is present. When the appetite has been poor and weight loss has been considerable, the patient may appear cachectic. A mass can often be detected beneath the abdominal wall and is seen to move with each inspiration. On palpation the mass may be felt in the epigastrium. Masses that are predominantly in the antrum of the stomach are generally found to the left of the midline. Masses located to the right of midline usually tend to be metastases to the liver or indicate involvement of the perigastric lymph nodes. Supraclavicular lymph nodes that are hard and enlarged and located on the left side are suggestive of metastasis via the thoracic duct from the stomach lesion. The presence of ascites is a poor prognostic sign.

Diagnostic Studies

The diagnostic studies for gastric malignancy include laboratory analysis of blood, stool, and gastric secretions (Table 39-26). Blood chemistry studies assist in the determination of anemia and its severity. Liver enzymes and serum amylase may indicate liver and pancreatic involvement or other abnormalities related to their dysfunction. Stool examination provides evidence of occult or gross bleeding. A gastric analysis indicates the level of HCl acid present in the stomach after fasting. Washings obtained during the gastric analysis can be used for the exfoliative cytologic examination. The test demonstrates the histologic changes indicative of malignancy. However, this test should never be used as the sole diagnostic criterion because false readings are sometimes obtained.

The carcinoembryonic antigen (CEA) test is used as an adjunctive diagnostic tool for cancer of the GI tract. CEA is a glycoprotein that is found in significant amounts in embryonic life, especially in the large intestine. It is also found in some adult patients with GI carcinomas. Elevated levels of CEA may indicate malignancy, yet CEA may be elevated in persons who smoke and also in those with benign lesions. Therefore, whereas the CEA test may be of some use in the preoperative workup of a patient with suspected cancer of the stomach, it

COLLABORATIVE CARE

Table 39-26 Gastric Cancer

Diagnostic
- History and physical examination
- Complete blood count
- Urinalysis
- Stool examination
- Liver enzymes
- Serum amylase
- Upper gastrointestinal barium study
- Carcinoembryonic antigen
- Exfoliative cytology
- Fiberoptic endoscopy and biopsy
- Gastric analysis

Collaborative Therapy
- Surgery
  - Subtotal gastrectomy—Billroth I or II procedure
  - Total gastrectomy with esophagojejunostomy
- Adjuvant therapy
  - Radiation therapy
  - Chemotherapy
  - Combination radiation therapy and chemotherapy

should never be used as the only diagnostic tool. (CEA is also discussed in Chapters 14 and 40.) Another more promising tumor marker for gastric cancer is carbohydrate antigen 19-9 (CA 19-9), which correlates with advanced stages and poorer prognosis.[31]

Upper GI barium studies may demonstrate defects in tone, secretion, motility, and spasm of the stomach. On x-ray examination the malignant ulcer crater is more irregular around the edges and more elevated than the craters found with benign peptic ulcers. Barium studies do not always detect small lesions of the cardia and fundus.

Endoscopic examination of the stomach remains the best diagnostic tool. Lesions that go undetected on x-ray can be more easily viewed and biopsied when the fiberoptic scope is used. The stomach can be distended with air during the procedure so that the mucosal folds can be stretched. Fixation of the mucosa is indicative of malignancy.

Collaborative Care

When the diagnosis of gastric malignancy has been confirmed, the treatment of choice is surgical removal of the tumor. The preoperative management of the patient with gastric cancer focuses on the correction of nutritional deficits, treatment of anemia, and replacement of blood volume.

Transfusions of packed RBCs correct the anemia. If a gastric lesion has been located at or near the pylorus and is causing gastric outlet obstruction, gastric decompression may be necessary before surgery. When the tumor has extended into the transverse colon and partial colon resection is also required, special preparation of the bowel is necessary. This preparation may include a low-residue diet, enemas to cleanse the bowel, and the use of antibiotics to reduce the intestinal bacteria. Correction of malnutrition is important if surgery is planned. Malnutrition is associated with increased postoperative complications and mortality rates.

RESEARCH

IMPLICATIONS FOR NURSING PRACTICE

Patients with Colorectal and Gastric Cancer

Citation Forsberg C, Bjovell H, Cedermark B: Well-being and its relation to coping ability in patients with colorectal and gastric cancer before and after surgery, *Scand J Caring Sci* 10:35-44, 1996.

Purpose To describe and compare the perceived well-being and general health, symptoms, and coping ability of a group of patients with colorectal and gastric cancer before and after surgery. In addition, to describe the patients' perceptions of their postoperative recovery and to determine the relationship between sense of coherence and well-being.

Methods The sample included 79 patients diagnosed with either colorectal or gastric cancer. The Health Index, symptom checklist, and Sense of Coherence Scale were used to measure responses before surgery and 6 weeks after surgery.

Results and Conclusions Compared with presurgery, patients experienced a decrease in pain and improvement in bowel function postoperatively. However, patients had greater problems related to energy level, sleep, and mobility postoperatively. Patients living with relatives rated their well-being as better than those who lived alone did. A stronger sense of coherence was related to sense of well-being.

Implications for Nursing Practice Patients undergoing surgery for GI malignancies have a number of postoperative care needs. Instruments used in this study may be helpful when used in the preoperative period to plan nursing care and in particular patient teaching during the postoperative period.

Surgical Therapy. The surgical intervention used in the treatment of stomach cancer may be the same surgical procedures used for peptic ulcer disease. The location and extent of the lesion, the patient's physical condition, and preference of the surgeon determine the specific surgery employed. When metastasis is widespread at the time of diagnosis, surgical intervention may be only palliative.

The surgical aim is to remove as much of the stomach as necessary to remove the tumor and a margin of normal tissue. When the lesion is located in the cardia or high in the fundus, a total gastrectomy with esophagojejunostomy is performed. This procedure involves anastomosis of the lower end of the esophagus to the jejunum (Fig. 39-19). Lesions located in the antrum or the pyloric region are generally treated by either a Billroth I or Billroth II procedure. When metastasis has occurred to adjacent organs, such as the spleen, ovaries, or bowel, the surgical procedures must be modified and extended as necessary.

The chance of a complete cure by surgical means is decreased considerably when the lymph nodes are involved. Sur-

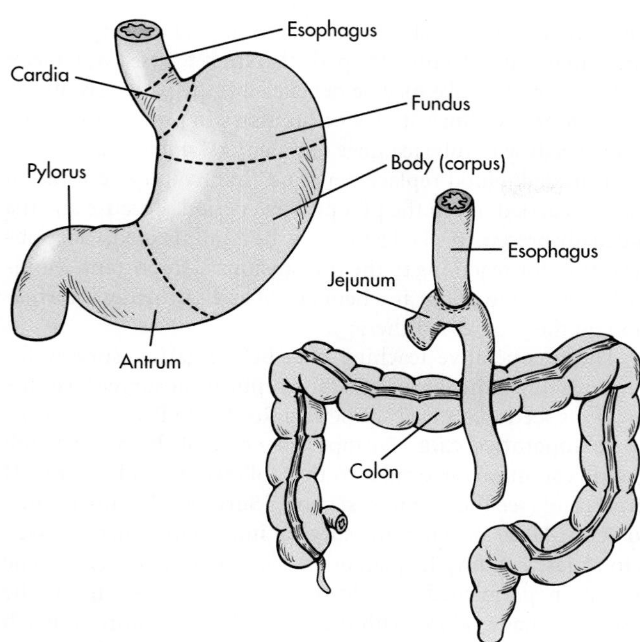

Fig. 39-19 A total gastrectomy for gastric cancer (total gastrectomy with esophagojejunostomy).

vival rates are considerably shortened when organs adjacent to the stomach show evidence of invasion at the time of surgery.

Adjuvant Therapy. Surgery is the only definitive means of achieving a cure. However, when the patient cannot physically withstand a surgical procedure or when surgical cure is not feasible, radiation or chemotherapy alone or in combination may be used. Neither radiation therapy nor chemotherapeutic agents have been very successful when used as the primary mode of treatment. Because the radiosensitivity of gastric cancers is low, radiation therapy has proved to be of little value.

When radiation is used as a palliative measure, the tumor mass can be decreased, with temporary relief of the cardia or pyloric obstruction. The combination of chemotherapy and radiation is now being used for patients who are not candidates for surgical excision. Combination chemotherapy only causes a temporary relief of symptoms, and long-term survival rates have not shown significant improvement.

Until recently, single-agent chemotherapy for gastric cancer has proved of little value. Agents that have been identified as having some effect on gastric cancer are 5-FU, BCNU, methyl CCNU, doxorubicin (Adriamycin), and triazinate (TZT). A better response rate in patients with advanced gastric cancer is now found when chemotherapeutic agents are used in combination, such as FAT (5-FU, doxorubicin, and triazinate). The hope for better outcomes with the use of chemotherapy depends on finding new ways of administering old drugs, finding new drugs, and determining new drug combinations. The hope for the ultimate cure of patients with gastric cancer now seems to lie in the combined efforts of surgery, radiation, and chemotherapy. The role of biologic therapy is still under investigation for use in gastric cancer. (These therapies are discussed in Chapter 14.)

NURSING MANAGEMENT: GASTRIC CANCER

■ Nursing Assessment

The assessment of a person with possible gastric cancer is similar to that for one with peptic ulcer disease (see Table 39-23). Important data to be obtained from the patient and the family should include a nutritional assessment, a psychosocial history, the patient's perceptions of the health problem and need for hospitalization, and the physical examination of the patient.

The nutritional assessment must elicit information regarding appetite, changes in eating patterns over the previous 6 months, and the role of highly seasoned or salty foods as a regular part of the diet. It is necessary to determine the patient's normal weight and any changes that may have occurred in the past few months. Unexplained weight loss is common in many types of cancer before diagnosis. A history of vague symptoms of dyspepsia, early satiety, feeling full after consuming even a small amount of food, or reporting symptoms of gas pain should help the nurse differentiate these typical gastric cancer symptoms from those of peptic ulcer. As with peptic ulcer patients, the nurse should determine whether pain is present, where and when it occurs, and how it is relieved. When the pain has been controlled with ingestion of foods, fluids, or antacids for a period of time but now continues or worsens regardless of interventions, gastric cancer may be the underlying cause.

Psychosocial and demographic data include age, present or previous occupation, and financial status. Gastric cancer can occur at any age, but the risk is more prevalent in men in the fifth to the sixth decade of life. A family history of cancer, especially gastric cancer, puts a person at greater than normal risk.

It is important to determine the patient's personal perception of the health problem and method of coping with hospitalization, diagnostic tests, and procedures. The possibility of a diagnosis of cancer and a treatment regimen that may include surgery, chemotherapy, or radiation treatment forecasts a prolonged stressful period and a possibly fatal outcome. Therefore it is important for the nurse to support the patient and family if tests result in an unfavorable diagnosis and complex treatment interventions are planned. If surgery is probable, the nurse should assess what the patient expects from surgery (cure or palliation) and how that patient has responded to any previous surgical procedures.

A complete physical examination reveals the patient's current functional abilities, the presence of other health problems, and an estimate on how well the patient may respond to therapy. Cachexia may be evident if the nutritional state has been compromised for an extended time. A malnourished patient does not respond well to chemotherapy or radiation therapy and is a poor surgical risk.

■ Nursing Diagnoses

Nursing diagnoses for the patient with gastric cancer include, but are not limited to, the following:

- Altered nutrition: less than body requirements *related to* inability to ingest, digest, or absorb nutrients
- Activity intolerance *related to* generalized weakness, abdominal discomfort, and nutritional deficits

- Anxiety *related to* lack of knowledge of diagnostic tests, unknown diagnostic outcome, disease process, and therapeutic regimen
- Pain *related to* underlying disease process and side effects of surgery, chemotherapy, or radiation therapy
- Anticipatory grieving *related to* perceived unfavorable diagnosis and impending death

Planning

The overall goals are that the patient with gastric cancer will (1) experience minimal discomfort, (2) achieve optimal nutritional status, and (3) maintain a degree of spiritual and psychologic well-being appropriate to the disease stage.

Nursing Implementation

Health Promotion. The nursing role in the early detection of cancer of the stomach is focused primarily on identification of the patient at risk because of specific disorders such as pernicious anemia and achlorhydria. The nurse should be aware of symptoms associated with gastric cancer, method of spread, and the significant findings on physical examination. The nurse should understand that the cure rate is often quite dismal because symptoms arise late in the course of the disease process, are vague, and often mimic other conditions, such as peptic ulcers.

The nurse must be alert to problems suggesting gastric cancer, such as poor appetite, weight loss, fatigue, and persistent gastric distress. If any of these manifestations are present, medical attention should be obtained and the necessary diagnostic tests performed.

In addition, any patient with a positive family history of gastric cancer should be encouraged to undergo diagnostic evaluation if manifestations of anemia, peptic ulcer, or vague epigastric distress are present. It is important that the nurse recognize the possible existence of stomach cancer in a patient who is treated for peptic ulcer and who fails to gain relief after 3 weeks of diet and prescribed medications. The ulcer, if it is benign, should show signs of healing on x-ray examination.

Acute Intervention

Preoperative care. When the diagnostic tests confirm the presence of a malignancy, the patient and the family generally react with shock, disbelief, and depression, regardless of how thoroughly they may have been prepared for this possible outcome. Throughout this period the nurse must give emotional and physical support, provide information, clarify test results, and maintain a positive attitude with respect to the patient's immediate recovery and long-term survival.

On admission to the hospital, the patient may be in poor physical condition. Surgery may have to be delayed while the patient becomes more physically able to withstand the strain of major surgery. A positive nutritional state enhances wound healing as well as the ability to withstand infection and other possible postoperative complications. Often the patient is better able to tolerate several small meals a day rather than three regular meals. The diet may be supplemented by a variety of commercial liquid supplements (see Chapter 38) and vitamins. The nurse is challenged to find innovative ways of persuading the patient to eat when lack of appetite and state of mind make eating difficult and unrewarding. Getting the patient's family to assist with meals and encourage intake may be beneficial. If the patient is unable to ingest oral feedings, it may be necessary to provide for nutritional needs with tube feedings or parenteral nutrition.

If needed, blood replacement and fluid volume restoration may be carried out in the preoperative period. Because anemia is usually present, packed RBCs may be administered. Close observation for reactions to the transfusions is important. Monitoring the hemoglobin and hematocrit levels provides information on the progress of therapy.

The preoperative teaching plan before gastric surgery for cancer is much the same as that for peptic ulcer surgery (see the previous section, "Surgical Therapy Related to Peptic Ulcer").

Postoperative care. Postoperative care of the patient with gastric carcinoma is similar to that following a Billroth I or II procedure (see the previous section, "Surgical Therapy Related to Peptic Ulcer"). When the surgical intervention has involved a total gastrectomy, the plan of care is somewhat different. The operation performed usually requires some resecting of the lower esophagus along with the removal of the entire stomach and anastomosis of the esophagus to the jejunum. The chest cavity must be entered, and drainage is accomplished by the insertion of chest tubes. (Chest surgery and drainage tubes are discussed in Chapter 26.) After total gastrectomy, the NG tube does not drain a large quantity of secretions because removal of the stomach has eliminated the reservoir capacity. The NG tube is removed after several days, when peristalsis has resumed. Small amounts of clear fluid may then be started. The patient requires close observation for signs of leakage of the fluids at the anastomosis as evidenced by an elevation in the temperature and increasing dyspnea. When fluids are well tolerated without distress, the amount may be increased along with the addition of some solid foods.

As a consequence of a total gastrectomy, a patient experiences the symptoms of the dumping syndrome. Unfortunately, weight loss is very common, and poor nutritional intake often contributes. Postoperative wound healing may be impaired because of inadequate dietary intake. This necessitates the IV or oral replacement of vitamins C, D, K, and the B complex vitamins and IM or intranasal administration of cobalamin. Because these vitamins are absorbed primarily in the upper part of the small intestine, they must be replaced, since the duodenum has been bypassed in the surgical procedure.

A patient who has a Billroth I or II operative procedure should receive the same postoperative care as one who has had peptic ulcer surgery. This patient is also subject to the same type of postoperative complications as dumping syndrome and postprandial hypoglycemia.

The patient with advanced malignant disease can be offered only palliative treatment. The chemotherapy agent found most useful for controlling symptoms of gastric cancer is 5-FU. When this medication or any of the combination drugs is prescribed, the nurse must have current information regarding the action and side effects of the drugs. The patient should be made aware of the potential benefits and hazards that can result from the chemotherapy. (The care of the patient receiving chemotherapy is discussed in detail in Chapter 14.)

Radiation therapy can be used as an adjuvant to surgery or for palliation. A patient is generally quite fearful of radiation and may develop many misconceptions regarding its value and dangers. To reassure the patient and ensure completion of the designated number of treatments, the nurse must provide detailed instruction. Because most therapy is completed on an outpatient basis, the nurse should assess the patient's knowledge of radiation, care of the skin, the need for good nutrition and fluid intake during therapy, and the appropriate use of antiemetic drugs. (Specific care of the patient receiving radiation therapy is discussed in Chapter 14.)

Ambulatory and Home Care. Before the patient is discharged, the need for teaching should be reviewed. Most dietary measures useful after peptic ulcer surgery are applicable after surgery for gastric carcinoma. Plans should be made for the relief of pain, including comfort measures and the judicious use of analgesics. Wound care, if needed, must be taught to the primary caregiver in the home situation. Dressings, special equipment, or special services may be required for the patient's continued care at home. A list of community agencies that are available for assistance can be provided before the patient goes home. The services of the American Cancer Society are especially helpful.

When treatment in the form of chemotherapy or radiation therapy is to be continued after discharge, a referral to the home health nurse may be beneficial. The home health nurse can assist with recovery, determine the degree of patient compliance, and be a sympathetic health care provider with whom the patient can consult.

Long-term follow-up must be stressed. The patient must be encouraged to comply with the prescribed dietary and medication regimens, keep appointments for chemotherapy administration or radiation treatments, and keep the physician informed of changes in physical condition. (Long-term management of the cancer patient is discussed in Chapter 14.)

■ Evaluation

Expected outcomes are that the patient with gastric cancer will

- experience minimal discomfort
- achieve optimal nutritional status
- maintain a degree of spiritual and psychologic well-being appropriate to the disease stage

FOOD POISONING

Food poisoning is a nonspecific term that describes acute GI symptoms such as nausea, vomiting, diarrhea, and colicky abdominal pain caused by the intake of contaminated food. Food most commonly causes illness if it is contaminated with microorganisms or their products. The GI tract is frequently the portal of entry for the microorganisms. The epidemiology of food-borne illness is changing. There are new organisms and many have spread worldwide. The two main types of food poisoning are (1) acute gastroenteritis from bacteria and (2) neurologic symptoms from botulism. The most common bacterial food poisonings are presented in Table 39-27.

Poisonous chemicals, such as mercury, arsenic, zinc, and potassium chlorate may contaminate foods. Poisoning can also occur from ingestion of poisonous plants (e.g., certain mushroom species).

Prevention of occurrence is the focus of interventions. Teaching should include correct food preparation and cleanliness, adequate cooking, and refrigeration. If the patient is hospitalized, care focuses on correction of fluid and electrolyte imbalance from diarrhea and vomiting. With botulism, additional assessment and care relative to neurologic symptoms are indicated (see Chapter 57).

Escherichia Coli Food Poisoning

Of recent importance is the increase in number of cases of hemorrhagic colitis caused by the presence of the bacterial strain *Escherichia coli* 0157:H7. Widespread outbreaks in the United States and Japan have increased the public's awareness of this organism. *E. coli* 0157:H7 is found primarily in undercooked meats, such as roast beef, ham, and turkey. However, other sources include cheese sandwiches, apple cider, and unpasteurized milk. *E. coli* can also be transmitted from person to person, particularly in settings such as nursing homes and day care centers. Recent studies suggest that *E. coli* 0157:H7 may be responsible for 0.6% to 2.4% of all nonbloody diarrhea and 15% to 36% of all cases of bloody diarrhea.[32]

The clinical manifestations of *E. coli* 0157:H7 vary from mild diarrhea to bloody diarrhea and systemic complications including hemolytic uremia and thrombocytopenic purpura and even death. The diarrhea may start out as watery but may progress to bloody. Treatment involves use of antibiotics and supportive care to maintain intravascular volume.

Table 39-27 Bacterial Food Poisoning

Type	Causative Agent	Sources	Onset of Symptoms (hr)	Symptoms	Treatment	Prevention
Staphylococcal	Toxin from *Staphylococcus aureus*	Meat, bakery products, cream fillings, salad dressings, milk; skin and respiratory tract of food handlers	30 min-7 hr	Vomiting, nausea, abdominal cramping, diarrhea	Symptomatic, fluid and electrolyte replacement, antiemetics	Immediate refrigeration of foods, monitoring of food handlers
Clostridial	*Clostridium perfringens*	Meat or poultry dishes cooked at lower temperature (stew or pot pie), rewarmed meat dishes, gravies, improperly canned vegetables	8-24 hr	Diarrhea, nausea, abdominal cramps, vomiting (rare); midepigastrium pain	Symptomatic, fluid replacement	Correct preparation of meat dishes, serving of food immediately after cooking or rapid cooling of food
Salmonella	*Salmonella typhimurium* (grows in gut)	Improperly cooked poultry, pork, beef, lamb, and eggs	8 hr-several days	Nausea and vomiting, diarrhea, abdominal cramps, fever and chills	Symptomatic, fluid and electrolyte replacement	Correct preparation of food
Botulism	Toxin from *Clostridium botulinum,* ingested toxin absorbed from gut and blocks acetylcholine at neuromuscular junction	Improperly canned or preserved food, home-preserved vegetables (most common), preserved fruits and fish, canned commercial products	12-36 hr	GI symptoms of nausea, vomiting, abdominal pain, constipation, distention Central nervous system symptoms of headache, dizziness, muscular incoordination, weakness, inability to talk or swallow, diplopia, breathing difficulties, paralysis, delirium, coma	Maintenance of ventilation, polyvalent antitoxin, guanidine hydrochloric acid (enhances acetylcholine release)	Correct processing of canned foods, boiling of suspected canned foods for 15 min before serving
Escherichia coli	*E. coli* serotype 0157:H7	Contaminated beef, pork, milk, cheese, fish	Varies by strain: 8 hr-1 wk	Bloody stools, hemolytic uremic syndrome, abdominal cramping, profuse diarrhea	Symptomatic, fluid and electrolyte replacement	Correct preparation of food

CRITICAL THINKING EXERCISES

CASE STUDY

Hiatal Hernia

Patient Profile

Mary, 63 years old, has had a sliding hiatal hernia for 10 years. Mary is admitted to the hospital for a hiatal hernia repair.

Subjective Data

- Reports increasing heartburn, especially at night
- Is currently on a bland diet and taking antacids
- Complains of substernal pain and heartburn
- Reports some problems with regurgitation

Objective Data

Physical Examination

- 5 feet 2 inches tall and weighs 195 pounds

Diagnostic Study

- Barium swallow and an esophagoscopy revealed a large sliding hiatal hernia.

Collaborative Care

- Mary had a Nissen fundoplication through a laparoscopic approach.

Critical Thinking Questions

1. Explain the pathophysiology of a hiatal hernia. What is the difference between a sliding and a paraesophageal hiatal hernia?
2. What are the characteristic symptoms of a hiatal hernia? Which of these did Mary have?
3. Describe a Nissen fundoplication procedure. What is the objective of this surgical procedure?
4. What are potential postoperative complications, and what nursing measures prevent them?
5. What should be included in a teaching plan for Mary?
6. Based on the assessment data presented, write one or more nursing diagnoses. Are there any collaborative problems?

NURSING RESEARCH ISSUES

1. What are the most effective methods to get an individual to comply with dental and oral hygiene care?
2. What are the most effective topical methods to relieve pain related to stomatitis secondary to infection?
3. Are dietary interventions successful in improving symptoms in the patient with gastroesophageal reflux disease?
4. What are optimal strategies to promote multiple lifestyle changes in a patient with peptic ulcer disease?
5. What are environmental manipulations that could be used to promote decreased nausea in patients receiving chemotherapy?
6. What sensory stimuli in the environment, including sight, smell, and sound, could promote optimal nutrient intake in the chemotherapy patient who is experiencing nausea?
7. What is the most effective way to obtain a nutritional assessment from a patient with gastric carcinoma?

REVIEW QUESTIONS

The number of the question corresponds to the same-numbered objective at the beginning of the chapter.

1. The most appropriate nursing intervention to provide oral care for a patient unable to do this for himself or herself involves
   a. brushing and flossing the patient's teeth.
   b. applying a fluoride solution to the surface of the teeth.
   c. using oral antimicrobial agents to reduce local bacterial counts.
   d. swabbing the patient's mouth with soft foam applicators soaked with mouthwash.
2. The nurse explains to the patient with Vincent's infection that treatment will include
   a. smallpox vaccinations.
   b. viscous lidocaine rinses.
   c. amphotericin B suspension.
   d. topical application of antibiotics.
3. A patient with oral cancer returns from the postanesthesia care unit awake and alert following a partial mandibulectomy and radical neck resection. An appropriate nursing intervention to facilitate the patient's respiratory function at this time is to
   a. elevate the head of the bed.
   b. assess chest expansion and symmetry.
   c. perform oral hygiene with half-strength hydrogen peroxide.
   d. position the patient supine with the head turned to one side.
4. A patient with wired intermaxillary fixation to stabilize a fractured mandible vomits following removal of the NG tube on the second postoperative day. The nurse should
   a. cut the wires to allow the patient to open the mouth.
   b. teach the patient to clear the vomitus from the mouth.
   c. turn the patient's head to the side and suction the vomitus.
   d. notify the physician and prepare the patient for a tracheostomy.
5. The nurse explains to the patient with gastroesophageal reflux disease that this disorder
   a. will require surgical wrapping or repair of the pyloric sphincter to control the symptoms.
   b. results in acid erosion and ulceration of the esophagus caused by the frequent vomiting.
   c. is the protrusion of a portion of the stomach into the esophagus through an opening in the diaphragm.
   d. often involves relaxation of the lower esophageal sphincter allowing stomach contents to back up into the esophagus.

6. To help the patient with a hiatal hernia control the symptoms of this disorder the nurse teaches the patient to
   a. drink a glass of milk at bedtime to coat the esophagus.
   b. lie down after eating to promote relaxation of the GI tract.
   c. avoid tight clothing and bending to decrease intraabdominal pressure.
   d. drink several glasses of liquids with meals to promote stomach emptying.
7. A patient who has undergone an esophagectomy for esophageal cancer develops increasing pain, fever, and dyspnea when a full liquid diet is started postoperatively. The nurse recognizes that these symptoms are most indicative of
   a. an intolerance to the feedings.
   b. extension of the tumor into the aorta.
   c. leakage of fluid or foods into the mediastinum.
   d. esophageal perforation with fistula formation into the lung.
8. During assessment of the patient with esophageal achalasia the nurse would expect the patient to report
   a. a history of alcohol use.
   b. a sore throat and hoarseness.
   c. dysphagia, especially with liquids.
   d. relief of pyrosis with the use of antacids.
9. Mrs. J. calls to tell you that her elderly mother, who is 85 years of age, has been nauseated all day and has vomited twice. Before you hang up and telephone the physician to communicate your assessment data, you instruct Mrs. Jones to
   a. administer antispasmodic medications and observe skin turgor.
   b. give her mother sips of water and elevate the head of her bed to prevent aspiration.
   c. offer her mother a high-protein liquid supplement to drink to maintain her nutritional needs.
   d. offer her mother large quantities of Gatorade to drink, since elderly people are at risk for sodium depletion.
10. The pernicious anemia that may accompany gastritis is due to which of the following?
    a. Chronic autoimmune destruction of cobalamin stores in the body
    b. Progressive gastric atrophy from chronic breakage in the mucosal barrier and blood loss
    c. A lack of intrinsic factor normally produced by acid-secreting cells of the gastric mucosa
    d. Hyperchlorhydria resulting from an increase in acid-secreting parietal cells and degradation of RBCs
11. Your teaching plan for the patient being discharged following an acute episode of GI bleeding will include information concerning the importance of
    a. taking only medications prescribed by the physician.
    b. avoiding taking aspirin with acidic beverages such as orange juice.
    c. taking all medications 1 hour before mealtime to prevent further bleeding.
    d. reading all OTC medication labels to avoid medications containing stearic acid and calcium.
12. You are teaching your patient and her family about possible causative factors for peptic ulcers. You explain that ulcer formation is
    a. caused by a stressful lifestyle and other acid-producing factors such as *C. pylori.*
    b. inherited within families and reinforced by bacterial spread of *Staphylococcus aureus* in childhood.
    c. promoted by factors that tend to cause oversecretion of acid, such as excess dietary fats, smoking, and *B. pylori.*
    d. promoted by a combination of possible factors that may result in erosion of the gastric mucosa, including certain medications, and alcohol.
13. The dumping syndrome is associated with large
    a. hyperosmolar volumes emptying rapidly into the intestine.
    b. isotonic volumes stimulating increased GI motility.
    c. hypertonic volumes promoting third-spacing in the intestinal cavity.
    d. hyposmolar volumes drawing fluid out of the plasma space and into the bowel.
14. An optimal teaching plan for an outpatient with gastric carcinoma receiving radiation therapy should include information about
    a. cancer support groups, alopecia, and stomatitis.
    b. avitaminosis, ostomy care, and community resources.
    c. prosthetic devices, skin conductance, and grief counseling.
    d. wound and skin care, nutrition, medications, and community resources.
15. Several patients are seen at an urgent care center with symptoms of nausea, vomiting, and diarrhea that began while attending a large family reunion potluck dinner. The nurse questions the patients specifically about foods they ingested containing
    a. beef.
    b. meat and milk.
    c. poultry and eggs.
    d. home-preserved vegetables.

References

1. Brown LJ, Brunelle JA, Kingman A: Periodontal status in the United States, 1988-1991: prevalence, extent, and demographic variation, *J Dent Res,* 75:672, 1996.
2. Position paper: Epidemiology of periodontal diseases, American Academy of Periodontology, *J Periodontol* 67:935, 1996.
3. Kandelman D: Sugar, alternative sweeteners and meal frequency in relation to caries prevention: new perspectives, *Brit J Nutr* 77 (suppl 1):S121, 1997.
4. Horowitz HS: The effectiveness of community water fluoridation in the United States, *J Public Health Dent* 56:253, 1996.
5. Brown LJ, Selwitz RH: The impact of recent changes in the epidemiology of dental caries on guidelines for the use of dental sealants, *J Public Health Dent* 55:274, 1995.
6. Twetman S, Peterson LG: Effect of different chlorhexidine varnish regimens on mutans streptococci levels in interdental plaque and saliva, *Caries Res* 31:189, 1997.
7. Anderson GB and others: Clinical effects of chlorhexidine mouthwashes on patients undergoing orthodontic treatment, *Am J Orthod Dentofacial Orthop* 111:606, 1997.
8. Cosci F, Cosci B: A 7-year retrospective study of 423 immediate implants, *Compend Contin Educ Dent* 18:940, 1997.
9. Cancer Facts and Figures-1998, American Cancer Society.
10. NIH Consensus Conference. *Helicobacter pylori* in peptic ulcer disease, *JAMA* 272:65, 1994.
11. Epstein JB and others: The utility of toluidine blue application as a diagnostic aid in patients previously treated for upper oropharyngeal carcinoma, *Oral Surgery, Oral Medicine, Oral Pathology, Oral Radiology and Endodontics* 83:537, 1997.
12. Hampton JK, Craven R, Heitkemper MM: *The biology of human aging,* ed 2, Dubuque, Iowa, 1996, Brown Publishers.
13. Greenberger NJ: *Helicobacter pylori* and peptic ulcer disease: current status, *Hosp Pract* 30:11, 1995.
14. Horwitz BJ, Fisher RS: Intervening in GERD: the phases of management, *Hosp Pract* 30:43, 1995.

15. Johnson DA: Medical therapy of GERD: current state of the art, *Hosp Pract,* 31:135, 1996.
16. Dawsey SM, Shen Q, Neiberg RK: Studies of esophageal balloon cytology in Linxian, China, *Cancer Epidemiology, Biomarkers and Prevention* 6:121, 1997.
17. Miller BA and others: Human papillomavirus type 16 DNA in esophageal cancer from Alaska Natives, *Int J Cancer* 71:218, 1997.
18. Kang SK and others: Gastrointestinal cancer mortality of workers in occupations with high asbestos exposures, *Am J Industrial Med* 31:713, 1997.
19. Ilson DH, Kelsen CP: Management of esophageal cancer, *Oncology* 10:1385, 1996.
20. Birgisson S, Richter JE: Achalasia: what's new in diagnosis and treatment? *Dig Dis* 15 (suppl 1): 1, 1997.
21. McQuaid KR: Dyspepsia and nonulcer dyspepsia. In *Current diagnosis and treatment in gastroenterology,* Stamford, Conn, 1996, Appleton & Lange.
22. Peura DA and others: The American College of Gastroenterology Bleeding Registry: Preliminary findings. 92:924, 1997.
23. Wolfe MM: NSAIDs and the gastrointestinal mucosa, *Hosp Pract* 32:37, 1997.
24. Lichtenstein DR, Berman MD, Wolfe MM: Approach to the patient with acute upper gastrointestinal hemorrhage. In Taylor MB: *Gastrointestinal emergencies,* ed 2, Baltimore, 1997, Williams & Wilkins.
25. Porter DH, Ducksoo K: Angiographic intervention in upper gastrointestinal bleeding. In Taylor MB: *Gastrointestinal emergencies,* ed 2, Baltimore, 1997, Williams & Wilkins.
26. Savides TJ, Jensen DM: Severe gastrointestinal hemorrhage. In Ayres SM and others: *Textbook of critical care,* ed 3, Philadelphia, 1995, WB Saunders.
27. Bracy W, Peterson WL: Medical therapy of nonvariceal upper gastrointestinal hemorrhage. In Taylor MB: *Gastrointestinal emergencies,* ed 2, Baltimore, 1997, Williams & Wilkins.
28. Imperiale TF, Birgisson S: Somatostatin or octreotide compared with H_2 antagonists and placebo in the management of acute nonvariceal upper gastrointestinal hemorrhage: a meta-analysis, *Ann Intern Med* 127:1062, 1998.
29. Cave DR, Hoffman JS: Management of *Helicobacter pylori* infection in ulcer disease, *Hosp Pract* 31:63, 1996.
30. Greenberger NR: *Helicobacter pylori* and peptic ulcer disease: current status, *Hosp Pract* 30:11, 1995.
31. Grem J: The prognostic importance of tumor markers in adenocarcinomas of the gastrointestinal tract, *Curr Opin Oncol* 9:380, 1997.
32. Greenwald DA, Brandt LJ: Recognizing *E. coli* 0157:H7 infection, *Hosp Pract* 32:123, 1997.

Resources

American College of Gastroenterology
4900 B South 31st Street
Arlington, VA 22206
703-820-7400
fax: 703-931-4520
http://www.acg.gi.org/

American Gastroenterological Association
7910 Woodmont Ave., 7th Floor
Bethesda, MD 20814
301-654-2055
fax: 301-652-3890
http://www.gastro.org/

American Society for Gastrointestinal Endoscopy
13 Elm Street
Manchester, MA 01944-1314
978-526-8330
fax: 978-526-4018
http://www.asge.org/

Digestive Disease National Coalition
711 2nd Street, NE, Suite 200
Washington, DC 20002
202-544-7497
fax: 202-546-7105

National Digestive Diseases Information Clearinghouse
2 Information Way
Bethesda, MD 20892-3570
301-654-3810
fax: 301-907-8906
http://www.niddk.nih.gov/health/digest/nddic.htm

National Institute of Diabetes & Digestive & Kidney Diseases (NIDDK)
Building 31, Room 9A-52
Bethesda, MD 20892
301-496-5877
http://www.niddk.nih.gov/index.htm

Society of Gastroenterology Nurses & Associates, Inc.
401 North Michigan Avenue
Chicago, IL 60611-4267
800-245-7462
In Illinois: 312-321-5165
fax: 312-321-51941070
http://www.sgna.org

For additional Internet resources, see the website for this book at **www.mosby.com/MERLIN/medsurg_lewis**

REMEMBER to check out your companion CD-ROM

40 NURSING MANAGEMENT Lower Gastrointestinal Problems

Donna Zimmaro Bliss & Linda Sawchuk

www.mosby.com/MERLIN/medsurg_lewis

LEARNING OBJECTIVES

1. Explain the common etiologies, collaborative care, and nursing management of diarrhea, fecal incontinence, and constipation.
2. Formulate a teaching plan for the patient with constipation.
3. Describe common causes of acute abdominal pain and nursing care of the patient following an exploratory laparotomy.
4. Describe the nursing management of a patient with acute appendicitis.
5. Describe the collaborative care and nursing management of peritonitis.
6. Describe the common etiologies, clinical manifestations, and nursing management of gastroenteritis.
7. Compare and contrast ulcerative colitis and Crohn's disease, including pathophysiology, clinical manifestations, complications, collaborative care, and nursing management.
8. Differentiate among mechanical, neurogenic, and vascular bowel obstructions, including causes and collaborative care and nursing management.
9. Describe the clinical manifestations and surgical and nursing management of cancer of the colon and rectum.
10. Explain the anatomic and physiologic changes that result from a sigmoid colostomy, a transverse colostomy, and an ileostomy.
11. Describe the preoperative and postoperative nursing management of a patient having bowel surgery.
12. Compare and contrast a colostomy and an ileostomy in relation to nursing care and patient teaching.
13. Differentiate between diverticulosis and diverticulitis, including clinical manifestations, collaborative care, and nursing management.
14. Compare and contrast the types of hernias, including etiology and surgical and nursing management.
15. Describe the types of malabsorption syndrome and appropriate management of sprue syndrome, lactase deficiency, and short bowel syndrome.
16. Describe the types, clinical manifestations, collaborative care, and nursing management of anorectal conditions.

DIARRHEA, FECAL INCONTINENCE, AND CONSTIPATION

Diarrhea is not a disease but a symptom. The term *diarrhea* may mean different things to different patients. It is commonly used to denote an increase in stool frequency or volume and an increase in the looseness of stool.

DIARRHEA

Etiology

Causes of diarrhea can be divided into the general classifications of decreased fluid absorption, increased fluid secretion, motility disturbances, or a combination of these (Table 40-1). Causes of acute infectious diarrhea are listed in Table 40-2.

Clinical Manifestations and Complications

Diarrhea may be acute or chronic. *Acute* diarrhea most commonly results from infection. Bacterial or viral infection of the intestine may result in explosive watery diarrhea, *tenesmus* (spasmodic contraction of anal sphincter with pain and persistent desire to defecate), and abdominal cramping pain. Perianal skin irritation may also develop. Systemic manifestations include fever, nausea, vomiting, and malaise. Leukocytes, blood, and mucus may be present in the stool, depending on the causative agent (see Table 40-2). Acute diarrhea is often self-limiting in the adult. Symptoms continue until the irritant or causative agent is excreted. The mucous membrane lining of the gastrointestinal (GI) tract is composed of epithelial cells, which regenerate following the inflammatory response.

Diarrhea is considered *chronic* when it persists for at least 2 weeks or when it subsides and returns more than 2 to 4 weeks after the initial episode. Severe diarrhea may be debilitating and life threatening. A patient may have severe dehydration (water and sodium loss) and electrolyte disturbances. Malabsorption and malnutrition are also sequelae of chronic diarrhea. Throughout the world diarrhea is one of the major causes of death, especially in infants.

Reviewed by Priscilla Ann Taylor, RN, MN, CGRN, Clinical Nurse Specialist in Gastroenterology, Tacoma, Wash.

Table **40-1** Causes of Diarrhea

Decreased Fluid Absorption
- Oral intake of poorly absorbable solutes (e.g., laxatives)
- Maldigestion and malabsorption
  - Mucosal damage: tropical sprue, Crohn's disease, radiation injury, ulcerative colitis, ischemic bowel disease
  - Pancreatic insufficiency
  - Intestinal enzyme deficiencies (e.g., lactase)
  - Bile salt deficiency
  - Decreased surface area (e.g., intestinal resection)

Increased Fluid Secretion
- Infectious: bacterial endotoxins (e.g., *Cholera, Escherichia coli, Shigella, Salmonella, Staphylococcus, Clostridium difficile,* viral agents [rotavirus], and parasitic agents *[Giardia lamblia]*)
- Drugs: laxatives, antibiotics, suspensions or elixirs containing sorbitol (e.g., acetaminophen)
- Hormonal: vasoactive intestinal polypeptide secretion from adenoma of the pancreas; gastrin secretion caused by Zollinger-Ellison's syndrome; calcitonin secretion from carcinoma of the thyroid
- Tumor: villous adenoma

Motility Disturbances
- Irritable bowel syndrome
- Diabetic enteropathy
- Visceral scleroderma
- Carcinoid syndrome
- Vagotomy

Diagnostic Studies

Accurate diagnosis and management require a thorough history, physical examination, and, when indicated, laboratory tests. A history of travel, medication use, diet, previous surgery, interpersonal contacts, and family history should be obtained. Blood tests may identify anemia, elevated white blood cell (WBC) count, iron and folate deficiencies, elevated liver enzyme levels, and electrolyte disturbances. Stools may be examined for the presence of blood, mucus, WBCs, and parasites. Stool cultures help in identifying infectious organisms.

In a patient with chronic diarrhea, measurement of stool electrolytes, pH, and osmolality may help determine whether the diarrhea is related to decreased fluid absorption or increased fluid secretion (secretory diarrhea). Measurement of stool fat and undigested muscle fibers may indicate fat and protein malabsorption conditions, including pancreatic insufficiency. Elevated serum levels of GI peptides such as vasoactive intestinal polypeptide (VIP) and gastrin may be present in some patients with secretory diarrhea. Endoscopy may be used to examine the mucosa and to obtain specimens for examination. Upper and lower barium studies may be helpful in detecting mucosal disease.

Collaborative Care

The treatment of diarrhea is based on the cause and is aimed at replacement of fluid and electrolytes and decreasing the number, volume, and frequency of stools. Oral solutions containing glucose and electrolytes (e.g., Gatorade, Pedialyte) may be sufficient to replace losses from mild diarrhea. In situations

Table **40-2** Causes of Acute Infectious Diarrhea

	Onset	Duration	Symptoms and Signs
Viral			
Rotavirus, Norwalk	18-24 hr	24-48 hr	Explosive, watery diarrhea; nausea; vomiting; abdominal cramps
Bacterial			
Escherichia coli	4-24 hr	3-4 days	Four or five loose stools per day, nausea, malaise, low-grade fever
Enterohemorrhagic *E. coli* (0157:H7)	4-24 hr	4-9 days	Bloody diarrhea, severe cramping, fever
Shigella	24 hr	7 days	Watery stools containing blood and mucus, tenesmus, urgency, severe cramping, fever
Salmonellae	6-48 hr	2-5 days	Watery diarrhea, nausea, vomiting, abdominal cramps, fever
Campylobacter species	24 hr	<7 days	Profuse, watery diarrhea; malaise, nausea, abdominal cramps, low-grade fever
Clostridium perfringens	8-12 hr	24 hr	Watery diarrhea, abdominal cramps, vomiting
Clostridium difficile	4-9 days after start of antibiotics	24 hr	Associated with antibiotic treatment; symptoms range from mild, watery diarrhea to severe abdominal pain, fever, leukocytosis, leukocytes in stool
Parasitic			
Giardia lamblia	1-3 wk	Few days to 3 months	Sudden onset; malodorous, explosive, watery diarrhea; flatulence, epigastric pain and cramping, nausea
Entamoeba histolytica	4 days	Weeks to months	Frequent soft stools with blood and mucus (in severe cases, watery stools), flatulence, distention, abdominal cramps, fever, leukocytes in stool
Cryptosporidium	2-10 days	1-6 months	Watery diarrhea, nausea, vomiting, abdominal cramps, weight loss in AIDS

AIDS, acquired immunodeficiency syndrome.

DRUG THERAPY

Table 40-3 Antidiarrheal Drugs

Type	Mechanism of Action	Examples
Demulcent	Soothes, coats, and protects mucous membranes	Bismuth subsalicylate* (Pepto-Bismol); calcium polycarbophil (Mitrolan-OTC); activated charcoal; kaolin†, pectin, hyoscyamine sulfate, and hyoscine hydrobromide (Donnagel)*†; Donnagel and opium (Donnagel-PG)*†
Anticholinergic	Inhibits GI motility	Donnagel*†, Donnagel-PG*†, diphenoxylate with atropine sulfate (Lomotil, Colonaid), loperamide (Imodium)†‡
Antisecretory	Decreases intestinal secretion	Octreotide (Sandostatin), a synthetic analog of somatostatin
Narcotic	Decreases CNS stimulation of GI tract motility and secretion	Camphorated tincture of opium (paregoric); Donnagel-PG†; paregoric, pectin, and kaolin (Parepectolin)†; tincture of opium, homatropine methylbromide, and pectin (Dia-Quel liquid OTC)§

*Also inhibits bacterial activity.
†Also absorbent, which contributes to the adhesiveness of the stool.
‡Has cholinergic and noncholinergic actions.
§Also an anticholinergic.
CNS, central nervous system; *GI,* gastrointestinal.

NURSING ASSESSMENT

Table 40-4 Diarrhea

Subjective Data

Important Health Information

Past health history: Recent travel, infections, stress; diverticulitis or malabsorption; metabolic disorders; inflammatory bowel disease; irritable bowel syndrome

Medications: Use of laxatives, magnesium-containing antacids, sorbitol-containing suspensions or elixirs, antibiotics, methyldopa, digitalis, colchicine; OTC antidiarrheal medications

Surgery or other treatments: Stomach or bowel surgery, radiation

Functional Health Patterns

Health perception–health management: Chronic laxative abuse, malaise

Nutritional-metabolic: Ingestion of coarse and spicy foods, food intolerances; anorexia, nausea, vomiting; weight loss; thirst

Elimination: Increased stool frequency, volume, and looseness; change in color and character of stools; abdominal bloating; decreased urinary output

Cognitive-perceptual: Abdominal tenderness, abdominal pain and cramping; tenesmus

Objective Data

General

Lethargy, sunken eyeballs, fever, malnutrition

Integumentary

Pallor, dry mucous membranes, poor skin turgor, perianal irritation

Gastrointestinal

Frequent soft to liquid stools that may alternate with constipation; altered stool color; abdominal distention, hyperactive bowel sounds; presence of pus, blood, mucus, or fat in stools; fecal impaction

Urinary Tract

Decreased output, concentrated urine

Possible Findings

Abnormal serum electrolyte levels; anemia; leukocytosis; eosinophila, hypoalbuminemia; positive stool cultures; presence of ova, parasites, leukocytes, blood, or fat in stools; abnormal sigmoidoscopic or colonoscopic findings; abnormal lower GI series

OTC, over-the-counter.

of severe diarrhea, parenteral administration of fluids, electrolytes, vitamins, and, potentially, nutrition is warranted.

Once the cause of the diarrhea has been determined, antidiarrheal agents may be given to coat and protect mucous membranes, absorb irritating substances, inhibit GI motility, decrease intestinal secretions, and decrease central nervous system (CNS) stimulation of the GI tract (Table 40-3). Antiperistaltic agents are not given to a patient who has infectious diarrheal syndromes because of the potential of prolonging exposure to the infectious agent. Antidiarrheal medications should not be given for a prolonged time.

Antibiotics are reserved for treating specific bacterial organisms. Antibiotics can cause diarrhea by altering the normal bowel flora. Patients receiving antibiotics (e.g., clindamycin [Cleocin]), are susceptible to *Clostridium difficile* infection. Health care workers who do not adhere to infection control precautions can transmit *C. difficile* from patient to patient. Some strains of *C. difficile* release a toxin that causes mucosal damage resulting in cramps, pain, and diarrhea that may be bloody. *C. difficile* infection can lead to mucosal damage, pseudomembranous enterocolitis, and intestinal perforation.[1] Vancomycin (Vancocin) or metronidazole (Flagyl) is used to treat *C. difficile.*

NURSING MANAGEMENT: ACUTE INFECTIOUS DIARRHEA

■ Nursing Assessment

Nursing assessment should begin with a thorough history and physical examination (Table 40-4). The patient should be asked to describe the stool pattern and associated symptoms. Questions should focus on the duration, frequency, character,

40-1 NURSING CARE PLAN PATIENT WITH ACUTE INFECTIOUS DIARRHEA

Expected Patient Outcomes	Nursing Interventions and *Rationales*
NURSING DIAGNOSIS	**Diarrhea** *related to* acute infectious process *as manifested by* frequent loose, watery stools.
▪ Normal bowel elimination. ▪ Afebrile.	▪ Monitor frequency, amount, color, consistency of stools *to determine severity of diarrhea and need for intervention.* ▪ Record intake and output *to monitor fluid balance.* ▪ Follow hospital procedure for infection control precautions; use strict medical asepsis when handling bedpan, linens, or patient *to prevent spread of infection.* ▪ Monitor vital signs q4hr *as changes can indicate development of hypovolemia.* ▪ Administer antiinfective and antidiarrheal medications as ordered *to treat bacterial infection and relieve diarrhea.*
NURSING DIAGNOSIS	**Fluid volume deficit** *related to* excessive fluid loss and decreased fluid intake secondary to diarrhea *as manifested by* dry skin and mucous membranes, poor skin turgor, hypotension, tachycardia, decreased urine output, electrolyte imbalance.
▪ Normal vital signs. ▪ Normal skin turgor. ▪ Moist mucous membranes. ▪ Urine output >0.5 ml/kg/hr. ▪ Normal serum electrolytes.	▪ Assess for skin turgor changes, sunken eyes, rapid pulse, and anorexia *as indicators of fluid volume deficit.* ▪ Monitor intake and output *to determine fluid balance.* ▪ Monitor serum sodium and potassium levels *so abnormalities can be reported to physician.* ▪ Monitor vital signs q4hr. ▪ Weigh patient daily *to monitor fluid loss.* ▪ Administer IV fluids as ordered and increase intake of fluids as tolerated to at least 3000 ml/day *to replace fluids and electrolytes lost in stools.* ▪ Assess mouth for dryness and note patient's complaints of thirst *as dry mucous membranes and thirst are indicators of dehydration.* ▪ If patient is not vomiting, administer fluids, such as Gatorade or Pedialyte *to replace electrolytes lost in stools.* ▪ Medicate with antidiarrheals as ordered *to decrease diarrhea.*
NURSING DIAGNOSIS	**Impaired skin integrity** *related to* perianal contact with diarrheal stools and inadequate perianal hygiene *as manifested by* redness, irritation, swelling, possible ulceration of skin, pain during elimination.
▪ No evidence of skin breakdown in perianal area.	▪ Assess skin of perianal area *to plan appropriate interventions.* ▪ Cleanse area with warm water after each bowel movement, rinse well and dry with a soft towel *to prevent skin excoriation and promote patient comfort.* ▪ Apply ointment (e.g., A and D, zinc oxide) *to protect skin and promote healing.* ▪ Use an anesthetic ointment or spray foam *to decrease local discomfort.*
NURSING DIAGNOSIS	**Risk for infection transmission** *related to* lack of knowledge about prevention of reinfection or transmission of infectious disease.
▪ No recurrence of symptoms. ▪ Knowledgeable about disease process and preventive measures.	▪ Teach patient to be alert for recurrence of diarrhea, fever, and other presenting symptoms; evidence of same symptoms in family members *as signs of possible infection transmission.* ▪ Assist patient in identifying factors that precipitated diarrhea *to avoid causing reinfection of self or transmission to others.* ▪ Stress importance of good hand-washing techniques *to prevent spread of diarrhea to others.* ▪ Explain importance of seeking medical care when diarrhea and other symptoms begin *so early treatment can be initiated.*

and consistency of stool. A medication history should include use of antibiotics, laxatives, and other drugs known to cause diarrhea. Recent travel, stress, and health and family history should be discussed. Dietary history should include questions about eating habits, appetite, and food intolerances, especially milk and dairy products, and food preparation practices.

Physical examination begins with obtaining vital signs, height, and weight. The patient's skin should be inspected for decreased turgor, dryness, and areas of breakdown. The abdomen should be inspected for distention, auscultated for bowel sounds, and palpated for tenderness.

Nursing Diagnoses

Nursing diagnoses for the patient with acute infectious diarrhea may include, but are not limited to, those presented in NCP 40-1 on p. 1139.

Planning

The overall goals are that the patient with diarrhea will (1) not transmit the microorganism causing the infectious diarrhea, (2) cease having diarrhea and resume normal bowel patterns, (3) have normal fluid and electrolyte and acid-base balance, (4) have normal nutritional intake, and (5) have no perianal skin breakdown.

Nursing Implementation

Adherence to infection control precautions for infectious diseases (see Table 11-19) is important because some cases of acute diarrhea are infectious. All cases of acute diarrhea should be considered infectious until the cause is determined. The use of precautions is effective in reducing the spread of infectious diarrhea.

Hand washing is the most important measure in prevention of the transfer of microorganisms. Hands should be washed before and after contact with each patient and when body fluids of any kind are handled. The patient should be taught the principles of hygiene, infectious control precautions, and the potential dangers of an illness that is infectious to themselves and others. Proper handling, cooking, and storage of food should be discussed with the patient suspected of having infectious diarrhea.

FECAL INCONTINENCE

Etiology and Pathophysiology

Fecal incontinence, or the involuntary passage of stool, may be due to multiple causes (Table 40-5). Knowledge of the mechanisms involved in fecal continence is helpful in understanding fecal incontinence. Normally, fecal contents pass from the sigmoid colon into the rectum, causing rectal distention. Sensory (stretch) receptors in the muscles surrounding the rectum provide the sensation of rectal filling. This causes a reflex relaxation of the internal anal sphincter and contraction of the external anal sphincter. Sensory receptors in the epithelium of the anal canal can usually distinguish among solid, liquid, and gas. The combination of contraction of the abdominal muscles, relaxation of the pelvic muscles, squatting (which straightens the anorectal angle), and voluntary relaxation of the external anal sphincter allows for elimination of feces.

Table 40-5 Causes of Fecal Incontinence

Traumatic	Inflammatory
Obstetric	Infection
Postsurgical	Trauma
Hemorrhoidectomy	Radiation
Anterior resection	**Other**
Fistulectomy	Pelvic floor relaxation
Anorectal surgery	Perineal descent
Spinal cord injuries	Loss of elasticity of rectum
Neurologic	Decreased sphincter tone (age-related)
Stroke	Rectal prolapse
Tumor	Fecal impaction
Degenerative diseases	Diarrhea
Iatrogenic drug intoxication	Medications
Multiple sclerosis	
Diabetes mellitus	
Dementia	

Diagnostic Studies and Collaborative Care

The diagnosis and effective management of fecal incontinence require a thorough health history and physical examination with appropriate diagnostic studies. In all cases a rectal examination should be performed, followed by examination with a flexible sigmoidoscope. Fecal impaction, internal prolapse, increased perineal descent, and rectocele may be identified by rectal examination. If the impaction is higher in the colon, an abdominal x-ray may be helpful. Flexible sigmoidoscopy may identify inflammation, tumors, fissures, and other sigmoid-rectum pathology. Other studies may include barium enema, colonoscopy, and anorectal manometry.

Treatment of incontinence depends on the underlying cause. If fecal incontinence is related to noninfectious diarrhea, antidiarrheal agents may be prescribed. For example, loperamide (Imodium) may be useful in reducing diarrhea and increasing sphincter tone.

Fecal incontinence caused by fecal impaction can be a common problem in the older adult. Fecal impaction usually resolves after manual disimpaction and cleansing enemas. To prevent recurrence, a high-fiber diet (see Table 40-9 later in this chapter), along with increased fluid intake, should be given unless contraindicated. Dietary fiber supplements (e.g., psyllium in Metamucil) can improve continence by increasing stool bulk and promoting sensation of rectal filling.

Biofeedback therapy is aimed at improving awareness of rectal sensation and coordination of the internal and external anal sphincters and increasing the strength of contraction of the external sphincter.[2] Biofeedback training requires adequate mental status and motivation to learn. Components of biofeedback include education, reinforcement, and concentration. It is a safe, painless, and inexpensive treatment for fecal incontinence. (Biofeedback is discussed further in Chapter 8.)

Surgery (e.g., sphincter repair procedures) should be considered only when conservative treatment fails, in cases of full-thickness prolapse, and when the sphincter needs repair.

NURSING MANAGEMENT: FECAL INCONTINENCE

■ Nursing Assessment

Fecal incontinence is not only an embarrassment to the patient but also a potential hazard to normal skin integrity. It is necessary to make an assessment of the patient's general condition to identify the best alternative for managing the patient with fecal incontinence. The nurse should identify normal bowel habits and current symptoms, including frequency and nature of the stools.

A neurologic assessment that includes evaluation of mental status can be helpful in identifying the most effective treatment for the patient. Assessment should also include history of multiple or traumatic childbirths, previous anorectal surgery, and injury.

■ Nursing Diagnoses

Nursing diagnoses for the patient with fecal incontinence include, but are not limited to, the following:

- Impaired skin integrity *related to* incontinence of stool and irritation of perianal area
- Social isolation *related to* embarrassment and odor
- Self-esteem disturbance *related to* inability to control bowel functions
- Self-care deficits *related to* inability to manage bowel evacuation independently

■ Planning

The overall goals are that the patient with fecal incontinence will (1) have normal bowel control, (2) maintain perianal skin integrity, and (3) not suffer any self-esteem problems related to problems with bowel control.

■ Nursing Implementation

Prevention and treatment of fecal incontinence may be managed by implementing a bowel-training program. The patient should be put on a bedpan, assisted to a bedside commode, or walked to the bathroom at a regular time daily to assist with reestablishment of bowel regularity. A good time to establish this pattern is within 30 minutes after breakfast. Most individuals experience an urge to defecate following the first meal of the day because of the gastrocolic reflex. If the usual bowel habits differ from this pattern, efforts should be made to adhere to the patient's individual timing.

If these techniques are ineffective in reestablishing bowel regularity, a bisacodyl (Dulcolax) or glycerin suppository or "mini-enema" may be given 15 to 30 minutes before the usual evacuation time. A mini-enema is a small (4 ml) gelatin capsule with an enema tip for instilling its contents (e.g., Therevac Plus contains docusate, soft-soap, and xylocaine).[3] These preparations stimulate the anorectal reflex and often can be discontinued when a regular pattern is reestablished.

Maintenance of skin integrity is of utmost importance, especially in the bedridden and older adult patient. Nursing management may necessitate drainage tubes or catheters, use of incontinence briefs, and meticulous skin care. Tubes and catheters are usually not recommended because their use for an extended period may decrease responsiveness of the rectal sphincter and cause ulceration of the rectal mucosa. Use of incontinence briefs may be helpful in maintaining skin integrity if changed frequently, but this can be demeaning and humiliating to the patient. Meticulous cleaning after each stool is required. Washing, rinsing, thorough drying, and application of a protective barrier are essential to the maintenance of skin integrity. Because the patient may have several stools each day, maintaining skin integrity is a time-consuming task for the nurse and the family.

Perianal pouching is an alternative in the management of fecal incontinence. Pouching provides skin protection and fecal containment as well as comfort and dignity. Because odor is often a problem, deodorant sprays and room deodorizers may be used. For the patient who is ambulatory, a chair (regular or special commode wheelchair) may be used. Regardless of the patient's mobility, the nurse must make sure the skin is clean, odorless, and intact.

CONSTIPATION

Constipation may be defined as a decrease in frequency of bowel movements from what is "normal" for the individual, hard, difficult-to-pass stools, a decrease in stool volume, and retention of feces in the rectum. Normal bowel elimination may vary from three times a day to once every 3 days.[4] Because of this variability, it is important to determine the severity of constipation on the basis of the patient's normal pattern of elimination. It is important to remember that changes in bowel habits may also indicate bowel obstruction produced by a tumor. Millions of people suffer from constipation.

Etiology

Frequently constipation may be due to insufficient dietary fiber, inadequate fluid intake, medication use, and lack of exercise. If proper preventive measures are subsequently taken, constipation should not recur. Constipation may also be due to sociocultural beliefs, environmental constraints, ignoring the urge to defecate, chronic laxative abuse, and multiple organic causes (Table 40-6). Changes in diet, in mealtime, or in daily routines are a few environmental factors that may cause constipation. Depression and stress can also result in constipation. For many patients with constipation, however, it is not possible to identify the underlying cause.[4]

Some patients believe that they are constipated if they do not have a daily bowel movement. This can result in chronic laxative use and subsequent *cathartic colon syndrome.* In this condition, the colon becomes dilated and atonic.

Ignoring the urge to defecate for a period of time causes the muscles and mucosa in the rectal area to become insensitive to the presence of feces. In addition, the prolonged retention of feces in the rectum results in drying of stool because of the absorption of water. The harder and drier the feces, the more difficult it is to expel.

Clinical Manifestations and Complications

The clinical presentation of constipation may vary from a chronic discomfort to an acute event mimicking an "acute abdomen." Other clinical manifestations are presented in Table 40-7.

Table 40-6 **Causes of Constipation**

Colonic Disorders	Systemic Disorders
Luminal or extra-luminal obstructing lesions	**Metabolic/Endocrine**
Inflammatory strictures	Diabetes mellitus
Volvulus	Hypothyroidism
Intussusception	Pregnancy
Irritable bowel syndrome	Hypercalcemia/hyper-parathyroidism
Diverticular disease	Pheochromocytoma
Rectocele	**Collagen Vascular Disease**
Drug Induced	Scleroderma
Antacids (calcium and aluminum)	Amyloidosis
Antidepressants	**Neurogenic Disorders**
Anticholinergics	Hirschsprung's megacolon
Antipsychotics	Neurofibromatosis
Antihypertensives	Autonomic neuropathy (pseudoobstruction)
Barium sulfate	Multiple sclerosis
Iron supplements	Parkinson's disease
Bismuth	Spinal cord lesions or injury
Calcium supplements	Cerebrovascular accident
Laxative abuse	

Hemorrhoids are the most common complication of chronic constipation. They result from venous engorgement caused by repeated *Valsalva's maneuvers* (straining) and venous compression from hard impacted stool.

Valsalva's maneuver, which occurs during straining to pass a hardened stool, may cause serious problems in patients with congestive heart failure, cerebral edema, hypertension, and coronary artery disease. During straining, the patient takes a deep inspiration, the breath is held, and the glottis closes and traps the air. The abdominal muscles contract and try to push against the colon. Increases in intraabdominal pressure and intrathoracic pressure occur, reducing venous return to the heart. The heart slows temporarily (bradycardia), the cardiac output is decreased, and there is a transient drop in arterial pressure. When the patient relaxes, there is decreased thoracic pressure and a sudden flow of blood into the heart, causing distention and an increase in heart rate. Immediately the arterial pressure rises momentarily. These changes may be fatal for the patient who cannot compensate for sudden overload of blood flow returning to the heart.

Diverticulosis is another potential complication of chronic constipation. This is a relatively common complication in an older adult. Diverticuli or outpouchings of the colon wall are thought to be due to the increased intraluminal pressure

DRUG THERAPY

Table 40-8 **Cathartic Agents**

Category	Mechanisms of Action	Example	Onset of Action	Comments
▪ Bulk forming	Absorbs water; increases bulk, thereby stimulating peristalsis	Metamucil, Perdiem, Konsyl, Hydrocil, Citrucil, Fibercon	Usually within 24 hr	Contraindicated in patients with abdominal pain, nausea, and vomiting and in patients suspected of having appendicitis, biliary tract obstruction, or acute hepatitis; needs to be taken with fluids
▪ Stimulants	Increase peristalsis by irritating colon wall and stimulating enteric nerves	Antraquinone drugs: Cascara sagrada, senna Phenolphthalein drugs Ex-Lax, Correctol, Feen-a-Mint, Bisacodyl, Dulcolax	Usually within 12 hr	Cause melanosis coli (brown or black pigmentation of colon); are most widely abused laxatives; should not be used in patients with impaction or obstipation
▪ Stool softeners and lubricants	Lubricate intestinal tract and soften feces, making hard stools easier to pass; do not affect peristalsis	Mineral oil, dioctyl sodium, sulfosuccinate, Colace, Peri-Colace, Doxidan	Softeners up to 72 hr, lubricants up to 8 hr	Can block absorption of fat-soluble vitamins such as vitamin K, which may increase risk of bleeding in patients on anticoagulants
▪ Saline and osmotic solutions	Cause retention of fluid in intestinal lumen caused by osmotic effect	Magnesium salts: Magnesium citrate, Milk of Magnesia Sodium phosphates: Fleets enema, Phospho-soda Lactulose Polyethylene glycolsaline solutions Go-Lytely, Colyte	15 min to 3 hr	Magnesium-containing products may cause hypermagnesemia in patients with renal insufficiency

Table 40-7 Clinical Manifestations of Constipation

Hard, dry stool	Increased flatulence
Abdominal distention	Nausea
Abdominal pain	Anorexia
Decreased frequency of bowel movements	Headache
Straining	Palpable mass
Rectal pressure	Stool with blood
Tenesmus	Dizziness
	Urinary retention

needed to expel hard stool. Diverticulosis and diverticulitis are described later in this chapter.

In the presence of *obstipation,* or fecal impaction secondary to constipation, colonic perforation may occur. Perforation, which is life threatening, causes abdominal pain, nausea, vomiting, fever, and an elevated WBC count. An abdominal x-ray shows the presence of free air, which is diagnostic of perforation. Rectal mucosal ulcers may also occur as a result of stool stasis or straining. These complications are most common in older patients.

Diagnostic Studies and Collaborative Care

A thorough history and physical examination should be performed so that the underlying cause of constipation can be identified and treatment started. Abdominal x-rays, barium enema, colonoscopy, sigmoidoscopy, and anorectal manometry may be helpful in the diagnosis. Most cases of constipation can be managed with diet therapy including fiber and fluids and an exercise program. Laxatives (Table 40-8) should always be used cautiously because with chronic overuse they may become a cause of constipation. Enemas are fast acting and are beneficial in the immediate treatment of constipation but should be limited in their use for long-term treatment of constipation. Soapsuds enemas should be avoided because they may lead to inflammation of colon mucosa. Oil-retention enemas may be used to soften fecal impactions. Biofeedback therapy may benefit patients who are constipated as a result of *anismus* (uncoordinated contraction of the anal sphincter during straining).[5]

For the patient in whom perceived constipation is related to rigid beliefs regarding bowel function, the nurse should initiate a discussion about these beliefs with the patient. Appropriate information on normal bowel function is given and discussed along with the adverse consequences of excessive use of laxatives and enemas.

A patient with severe constipation related to motility or mechanical disorders may require more intensive treatment. Studies such as anorectal manometry, GI tract transit studies, and sigmoidoscopic rectal biopsies should be performed before treatment. In a patient with unrelenting constipation, a subtotal colectomy with ileorectal anastomosis is the procedure of choice.[4]

Nutritional Therapy. Diet is an important factor in the prevention of constipation. Many patients experience an improvement in their symptoms when they simply increase their intake of dietary fiber and fluids. Dietary fiber is found in two forms: insoluble and soluble in water. Both are contained in most foods, but some foods are higher in soluble fiber (Table 40-9).

NUTRITIONAL THERAPY

Table 40-9 High Fiber Foods*

	Fiber Per Serving (g)	Size of Serving	Calories Per Serving
Vegetables			
Asparagus	3.5	½ cup	18
Beans			
Navy	8.4	½ cup	80
Kidney	9.7	½ cup	94
Lima	8.3	½ cup	63
Pinto	8.9	½ cup	78
String	2.1	½ cup	18
Broccoli	3.5	½ cup	18
Carrots, raw	1.8	½ cup	15
Corn	2.6	½ medium ear	72
Peas, canned	6.7	½ cup	63
Potatoes			
Baked	1.9	½ medium	72
Sweet	2.1	½ medium	79
Squash			
Acorn	7.0	1 cup	82
Tomato, raw	1.5	1 small	18
Fruits			
Apple	2.0	½ large	42
Banana	1.5	½ medium	48
Blackberries	6.7	¾ cup	40
Orange	1.6	1 small	35
Peach	2.3	1 medium	38
Pear	2.0	½ medium	44
Raspberries	9.2	1 cup	42
Strawberries	3.1	1 cup	45
Grain Products			
Bread			
Rye	0.8	1 slice	62
White	0.7	1 slice	64
Whole wheat	1.3	1 slice	59
Cereal			
All Bran (100%)	8.4	⅓ cup	70
Corn Flakes	2.6	¾ cup	70
Shredded Wheat	2.8	1 biscuit	70
Crackers			
Graham	1.4	2 squares	53
Popcorn	3.0	3 cups	62
Rice			
Brown	1.6	⅓ cup	72
White	0.5	⅓ cup	76

*Recommended for patients with diverticulosis, irritable bowel syndrome, constipation, hemorrhoids, colon cancer, atherosclerosis, hyperlipidemia, and diabetes mellitus.

Insoluble fiber remains essentially unchanged by the time it reaches the colon, and it is found in higher concentrations in whole wheat and bran. *Soluble fibers* form gel-like substances that add viscosity to the digested contents, causing decreased gastric emptying and increased transit in the small intestine. When these fibers are fermented, they increase stool bulk,

NURSING ASSESSMENT

Table 40-10 Constipation

Subjective Data	Objective Data
Important Health Information *Past health history:* Colorectal disease, neurologic dysfunction, bowel obstruction, environmental changes, cancer *Medications:* Use of aluminum antacids, anticholinergics, antidepressants, antihistamines, antipsychotics, diuretics, narcotics, iron, laxatives, enemas **Functional Health Patterns** *Health perception–health management:* Chronic laxative or enema abuse; rigid beliefs regarding bowel function; malaise *Nutritional-metabolic:* Changes in diet or mealtime; inadequate fiber and fluid intake; anorexia, nausea *Elimination:* Change in usual elimination patterns; hard, difficult to pass stool, decrease in frequency and amount of stools; flatus, abdominal distention; tenesmus, rectal pressure; fecal incontinence (if impacted) *Activity-exercise:* Change in daily activity routines; immobility; sedentary lifestyle *Cognitive-perceptual:* Dizziness, headache, anorectal pain; abdominal pain on defecation *Coping–stress tolerance:* Acute or chronic stress	**General** Lethargy **Integumentary** Anorectal fissures, hemorrhoids, abscesses **Gastrointestinal** Abdominal distention; hypoactive or absent bowel sounds; palpable abdominal mass; fecal impaction, small, hard, dry stool, stool with blood **Possible Findings** Guaiac-positive stools, abdominal x-ray demonstrating stool in lower colon

promoting defecation and sequestering fluid, which softens stools. Soluble fiber is found in oat bran, fruits, vegetables, and psyllium. Patients should be told that initially fiber will increase gas production but that this effect decreases with time.

The diet should also include a fluid intake of at least 3000 ml per day, unless contraindicated by cardiac or renal disease. Increasing fiber intake without increasing fluids may predispose the patient to impaction or obstruction. The nurse should encourage the selection of foods that the patient likes, is able to prepare, and can afford. The patient's understanding of the diet and the importance of dietary fiber is important to ensure compliance.

NURSING MANAGEMENT: CONSTIPATION

■ Nursing Assessment

Subjective and objective data that should be obtained from a patient with constipation are presented in Table 40-10.

■ Nursing Diagnoses

Nursing diagnosis for the patient with constipation includes, but is not limited to, the following:

- Constipation *related to* inadequate intake of dietary fiber and fluid and decreased physical activity

■ Planning

The overall goals are that the patient with constipation will (1) increase dietary intake of fiber and fluids; (2) have the passage of soft, formed stools; and (3) not have any complications, such as bleeding hemorrhoids.

■ Nursing Implementation

Nursing management should be based on the patient's symptoms (see Table 40-7) and the assessment of the patient (see Table 40-10). An important role of the nurse is teaching the patient the importance of dietary measures to prevent constipation. A patient teaching guide for constipation is presented in Table 40-11. Emphasis should be placed on maintenance of a high-fiber diet, increasing fluid intake, and a regular exercise program. The patient should be taught to establish a regular time to defecate and not to suppress the urge to defecate. In many persons the urge to defecate occurs after breakfast because of the stimulation of the gastrocolic reflex. The patient should be discouraged from using laxatives and enemas to achieve fecal elimination.

Proper position is important when defecating. For a patient in bed, the bedpan should be placed and the head of the bed should be elevated as high as the patient can tolerate. For the person who can sit on a toilet, a footstool may be placed in front of the toilet. Placing the feet on the footstool promotes flexion of the thighs, which assists in defecation.

The patient with poor muscle tone should be encouraged to exercise the abdominal muscles and can be taught to contract the abdominal muscles several times a day. Sit-ups and straight leg raises can also be used to improve abdominal muscle tone.

Some patients may have to be encouraged to increase their social activities, as well as their physical activity. This is especially true for older adults who may become depressed and socially isolated because of multiple factors. Inactivity can lead to constipation. This patient should be encouraged and assisted in establishing social contacts and activities outside the home.

PATIENT TEACHING GUIDE

Table 40-11 Constipation

The following are teaching guidelines for the patient:

1. **Eat dietary fiber**
   Eat 20 to 30 g of fiber per day. Gradually increase amount of fiber eaten over 1 to 2 weeks. Fiber softens hard stools and adds bulk to stool, promoting evacuation.
   - Foods high in fiber: raw vegetables and fruits, beans, breakfast cereals (All Bran, oatmeal)
   - Fiber supplements: Metamucil, Citrucel, and FiberCon
2. **Drink fluids**
   Drink 3 quarts per day. Drink water or fruit juices; avoid caffeinated coffee, tea, and cola. Fluid softens hard stools; caffeine stimulates fluid loss through urination.
3. **Exercise regularly**
   Walk, swim, or bike at least three times per week. Contract and relax abdominal muscles when standing or by doing sit-ups to strengthen muscles and prevent straining. Exercise stimulates bowel motility and moves stool through the intestine.
4. **Establish a regular time to defecate**
5. **Do not delay defecation**
   Respond to the urge to have a bowel movement as soon as possible. Delaying defecation results in hard stools and a decreased "urge" to defecate. Water is absorbed from stool by the intestine over time. The intestine becomes less sensitive to the presence of stool in the rectum.
6. **Record your bowel elimination pattern**
   Develop a habit of recording when you have a bowel movement on your calendar. Regular monitoring of bowel movement will assist in early problem identification.
7. **Avoid laxatives and enemas**
   Do not overuse laxatives and enemas as they can actually cause constipation. The normal motility of the bowel is interrupted and bowel movements slow or stop.

ABDOMINAL PAIN

ACUTE ABDOMINAL PAIN

Etiology

The patient with an *acute abdomen* has an acute onset of abdominal pain requiring prompt decision making. Causes of an acute abdomen are varied (Table 40-12). Many disorders must be ruled out before a diagnosis is confirmed.

Table 40-12 Causes of Acute Abdomen

Abdominal penetrating trauma	Peptic ulcer
Acute ischemic bowel	Perforated gastrointestinal malignancy
Appendicitis	Peritonitis
Bowel obstruction with perforation or necrosis	Ruptured abdominal aneurysm
Cholecystitis	Ruptured ectopic pregnancy
Crohn's disease	Ruptured ovarian cyst
Diverticulitis with peritonitis	Ulcerative colitis
Foreign body perforation	Uterine rupture
Gastritis	Volvulus
Gastroenteritis	
Mesenteric adenitis	
Pancreatitis	
Pelvic inflammatory disease	

Clinical Manifestations

Pain is the most common presenting symptom. The patient may also complain of abdominal tenderness, vomiting, diarrhea, constipation, flatulence, fatigue, fever, and an increase in abdominal girth.

Diagnostic Studies and Collaborative Care

Diagnosis begins with a complete history and physical examination. Physical examination should include a rectal and pelvic examination. A complete blood count (CBC), urinalysis, abdominal x-ray, and an electrocardiogram (ECG) are done initially. Pregnancy tests should be performed in women of childbearing age who have acute abdominal pain. The findings of these studies may provide some information as to the cause of the acute abdomen.

Emergency management of the patient with an acute abdomen is presented in Table 40-13. The goal of management is to identify and treat the cause. The physician attempts to make a differential diagnosis when the patient is seen with an acute abdomen because many causes of abdominal pain do not require surgery (see Table 40-12). It was previously thought that pain medication should be withheld because analgesics might obscure progression of clinical manifestations and impede diagnosis. Appropriate pain management that does not result in altered consciousness (e.g., ketorolac [Toradol]) can decrease diffuse pain and abdominal rigidity and help localize the pain. This can lead to earlier diagnosis and treatment.[6]

In addition to being a therapeutic measure, surgery can also be diagnostic. Operative exploration is usually done after a careful examination of the patient and is justified when "look and see" is better than "wait and see." The surgical procedure is an *exploratory laparotomy,* in which an opening is made through the abdominal wall into the peritoneal cavity to determine the cause of an acute abdomen. If the cause of the acute abdomen can be surgically removed (e.g., inflamed appendix) or surgically repaired (e.g., ruptured abdominal aneurysm), surgery is considered definitive therapy.

EMERGENCY MANAGEMENT

Table 40-13 Acute Abdomen

Etiology	Assessment Findings	Interventions
Inflammation Appendicitis Cholecystitis Pancreatitis Ulcerative colitis/Crohn's disease Gastritis Pyelonephritis **Vascular Problems** Ruptured aortic aneurysm Mesenteric vascular occlusion **Gynecologic Problems** Ruptured ectopic pregnancy Ruptured ovarian cyst Pelvic inflammatory disease **Infectious Disease** *Giardia* *Salmonella* **Other** Obstruction or perforation of abdominal organ Gastrointestinal bleeding	**Abdominal/Gastrointestinal Findings** ▪ Diffuse, localized, dull, burning, or sharp abdominal pain or tenderness ▪ Rebound tenderness ▪ Abdominal distention ▪ Abdominal rigidity ▪ Nausea, vomiting ▪ Diarrhea ▪ Hematemesis ▪ Melena **Hypovolemic Shock** ▪ Decreased blood pressure ▪ Decreased pulse pressure ▪ Tachycardia ▪ Cool, clammy skin ▪ Decreased level of consciousness	**Initial** ▪ Ensure patent airway. ▪ Administer oxygen via nasal cannula or nonrebreather mask. ▪ Establish IV access with large bore catheter and infuse warm normal saline or lactated Ringer's solution. Insert additional large bore catheter if shock present. ▪ Obtain blood for CBC, electrolytes. ▪ Anticipate order for amylase, pregnancy tests, clotting studies, and type and crossmatch as appropriate. ▪ Insert indwelling urinary catheter. ▪ Obtain urinalysis. ▪ Insert NG tube as needed. **Ongoing Monitoring** ▪ Monitor vital signs, level of consciousness, oxygen saturation, and intake and output. ▪ Assess quality and amount of pain. ▪ Assess amount and character of emesis. ▪ Anticipate surgical intervention. ▪ Keep NPO.

NG, nasogastric.

NURSING MANAGEMENT: ACUTE ABDOMEN

■ Nursing Assessment

Vital signs should be taken immediately. Blood pressure and pulse rate should be obtained to determine hypovolemic changes. An elevated temperature may indicate an inflammatory or infectious process. The abdomen should be inspected for distention, masses, abnormal pulsation, rashes, scars, and pigmentation changes. Bowel sounds should be auscultated. Bowel sounds that are diminished or absent in a quadrant may indicate a complete bowel obstruction, acute peritonitis, or paralytic ileus. Palpation should be gentle.

A thorough assessment of the patient's symptoms should be made to determine the onset, location, intensity, duration, frequency, and character of pain. The nurse should determine whether the pain has spread or moved to new locations (quadrants), as well as what makes the pain worse or better. It should also be determined whether the pain is associated with other symptoms, such as nausea, vomiting, changes in bowel and bladder habits, or vaginal discharge in women. Assessment of vomiting should include the amount, color, consistency, and odor of the vomitus. Bowel patterns and habits should also be carefully assessed.

■ Nursing Diagnoses

Nursing diagnoses for the patient with acute abdomen peritonitis include, but are not limited to, the following:

- Pain *related to* inflammation of the peritoneum and abdominal distention
- Risk for fluid volume deficit *related to* collection of fluid in peritoneal cavity secondary to inflammation or infection
- Altered nutrition: less than body requirements *related to* anorexia, nausea, and vomiting
- Anxiety *related to* uncertainty of cause or outcome of condition and pain

■ Planning

The overall goals are that the patient with acute abdomen will have (1) resolution of inflammation, (2) relief of abdominal pain, (3) freedom from complications (especially hypovolemic shock), and (4) normal nutritional status.

■ Nursing Implementation

Nursing interventions are based on the diagnosis and medical or surgical management of the patient. General care for the patient involves management of fluid and electrolyte imbalances, pain, and anxiety.

Preoperative Care. Emergency preparation of the patient with an acute abdomen is usually limited to a CBC, typing and crossmatching of blood, and clotting studies. Catheterization, preparation of the abdominal skin, and the passage of a nasogastric (NG) tube may be done in the emergency department or operating room. (General care of the preoperative patient is discussed in Chapter 16.)

40-2 NURSING CARE PLAN PATIENT FOLLOWING LAPAROTOMY

Expected Patient Outcomes	Nursing Interventions and *Rationales*
NURSING DIAGNOSIS	**Pain** *related to* surgical incision and inadequate pain control measures *as manifested by* complaints of pain, body posturing, unwillingness to move in bed or to ambulate.
▪ Satisfactory level of pain control.	▪ Assess for pain and give pain medication every 3 to 4 hr as ordered for first 72 hr *to treat pain appropriately.* ▪ Splint incision with pillows during coughing, deep breathing, and moving *to relieve pain while performing these activities.* ▪ Position patient comfortably *to relieve pain.*
NURSING DIAGNOSIS	**Nausea and vomiting** *related to* decreased GI motility, GI distention, and narcotics *as manifested by* nausea, vomiting, lack of or diminished bowel sounds, abdominal distention.
▪ Relief of nausea and vomiting.	▪ Administer antiemetic medications (as ordered) *to relieve nausea and vomiting.* ▪ Assess response to pain medications *to determine if this is a possible cause of nausea and vomiting.* ▪ Maintain patency of NG tube (if present) *to prevent accumulation of gastric juices and subsequent vomiting.* ▪ Assess for bowel sounds and abdominal distention *to determine return of peristalsis.* ▪ Keep patient on NPO status until bowel sounds return *to prevent vomiting.* ▪ Limit unpleasant sights, smells, and stimuli *to prevent initiating episodes of nausea and vomiting.*
NURSING DIAGNOSIS	**Constipation** *related to* immobility, pain, medication, and decreased GI motility *as manifested by* decreased or absent bowel sounds, abdominal pain, abdominal distention, inability to pass flatus or stool.
▪ Normal bowel sounds within 72 hr after surgery. ▪ Soft, formed bowel movement within 4 days.	▪ Assess abdomen for distention and bowel sounds every shift *to determine need for intervention.* ▪ Administer cathartic as ordered if patient has not had bowel movement in 4 days *to soften fecal mass or promote elimination.* ▪ Encourage frequent position changes and ambulation as tolerated *to increase peristalsis.* ▪ Encourage increased fluid intake as tolerated *to soften fecal material.*

*General nursing care for the postoperative patient is presented in NCP 18-1 in Chapter 18 on p. 401.

Postoperative Care. Postoperative care depends on the type of surgical procedure performed. The increased use of laparoscopic procedures has reduced the risk of postoperative complications related to wound care and altered GI motility. These procedures generally result in shorter hospital stays.

A general nursing care plan for the postoperative patient is presented in Chapter 18. Nursing care for the patient following a laparotomy is presented in NCP 40-2.

An NG tube may or may not be present in the patient returning from surgery. If present, the NG tube is connected to suction as ordered. The purpose of the NG tube is to empty the stomach of secretions and gas to prevent gastric dilation. GI peristaltic activity is often impaired because of the manipulative procedures of the surgery and anesthesia. Low intermittent suctioning is ordered to prevent trauma to the gastric mucosa.

Drainage from the NG tube may be dark brown to dark red for the first 12 hours. Later it should be light yellowish brown, or it may have a greenish tinge because of the presence of bile. If a dark red color continues or if bright red blood is observed, the physician should be notified at once of the possibility of hemorrhage. "Coffee ground" granules in the drainage are due to the presence of small amounts of blood that have been chemically acted on by gastric secretions.

The NG tube is checked frequently for patency. The tube may become obstructed with mucus, sediment, or old blood. An order is usually written to irrigate the tube with 20 to 30 ml of normal saline solution if needed. Repositioning the tube may facilitate drainage.

An accurate record of intake and output, including emesis and gastric drainage, is essential. The nurse should assess serum electrolyte values and acid-base balance because prolonged gastric suctioning results in loss of sodium, chloride, potassium, water, and hydrochloric acid.

The NG tube is removed when intestinal peristalsis returns, usually 24 to 72 hours after surgery. Motility of the stomach normally returns within 24 to 48 hours. Motility of the small intestine usually resumes within 24 hours, whereas return of large intestine motility may take as long as 3 to 5 days. Peristaltic activity is assessed by auscultation for bowel sounds.

Mouth care and nasal care are essential. The patient tends to breathe through the mouth while the NG tube is in place. In addition, increased nasal secretions and crusting result from mechanical stimulation of the NG tube.

Parenteral fluids are administered to provide the patient with fluids and electrolytes until bowel sounds return. Occasionally, ice chips may be ordered because they aid in the flow of saliva and prevent dry mouth. When bowel sounds return, fluids and food are increased gradually. The diet may be supplemented with multivitamins and iron.

Nausea and vomiting are not uncommon after abdominal surgery. These problems are often self-limiting. Observation is important in determining the cause. Antiemetics such as promethazine (Phenergan), hydroxyzine (Vistaril), prochlorperazine (Compazine), or trimethobenzamide (Tigan) may be ordered.

Abdominal distention and gas pains are also common after surgery; these are due to swallowed air and impaired peristalsis resulting from immobility, manipulation of abdominal contents during surgery, and side effects of anesthesia. The pain can be so uncomfortable that medications to stimulate peristalsis, such as bethanechol (Urecholine) or neostigmine methylsulfate (Prostigmin), may be given. A rectal tube or moist heat on the abdomen may be effective in relieving distention. The physician should be informed of abdominal distention and rigidity. Gradually, as intestinal activity increases, distention and gas pains decrease.

Emotional support from the nursing staff is important. Honest, clear, concise explanations of all procedures in language the patient and the family can understand may assist in allaying anxiety.

Ambulatory and Home Care. Preparation for discharge begins when the patient returns from the operating room. Instructions to the patient and the family should include any modifications in activity, care of the incision, diet, and drug therapy. Small, frequent meals high in calories should be taken initially, with a gradual increase in intake of food as tolerated.

Normal activities should be resumed gradually, with planned rest periods. The patient should be aware of possible complications after surgery and should notify the physician immediately if vomiting, pain, weight loss, incisional drainage, or changes in bowel functions occur.

■ Evaluation

The expected outcomes are that the patient with acute abdomen will have

- resolution of inflammation
- relief of abdominal pain
- freedom from complications (especially hypovolemic shock)
- normal nutritional status

CHRONIC ABDOMINAL PAIN

Chronic abdominal pain may originate from abdominal structures or may be referred from a site with the same or a similar nerve supply. Some common causes are irritable bowel syndrome (IBS), peptic ulcer disease, diverticulitis, chronic pancreatitis, hepatitis, cholecystitis, pelvic inflammatory disease, and vascular insufficiency. Psychogenic pain should also be considered.

Diagnosis of chronic abdominal pain presents a challenge. Assessment should begin with a thorough history and identification of the specific pain pattern. Character and severity of pain, location, duration, and onset should be determined. The assessment should also include the relationship of pain to meals, defecation, activity, and factors that increase or decrease the pain. Chronic abdominal pain is often described as dull, aching, or diffuse.

Endoscopy, computed tomography (CT) scans, magnetic resonance imaging (MRI), laparoscopy, and radiographic barium studies have decreased the need for exploratory laparotomy. Treatment for chronic abdominal pain is comprehensive and directed toward palliation of symptoms using analgesics and antiemetics as well as psychologic or behavioral therapies (e.g., relaxation).[7]

ABDOMINAL TRAUMA

Etiology

Injuries to the abdominal area most often occur as a result of *blunt trauma* (e.g., motor vehicle accident) or *penetration injuries,* primarily gunshot wounds or stab wounds to the abdomen. Blunt trauma is most common. Regardless of whether it is a blunt or penetration injury, the result is often the same damage to or alteration of the internal organs.

Common injuries of the abdomen include lacerated liver, ruptured spleen, pancreatic trauma, mesenteric artery tears, diaphragmatic rupture, urinary bladder rupture, great vessel tears, renal injury, and stomach or intestinal rupture. These injuries may result in massive blood loss and hypovolemic shock. Surgery must be performed as early as possible to repair the damaged organs and to stop the bleeding. Common sequelae of intraabdominal trauma are peritonitis and massive infection, particularly when the bowel is perforated.

Clinical Manifestations

Clinical manifestations of abdominal trauma are (1) guarding and splinting of the abdominal wall; (2) a hard, distended abdomen (indicating intraabdominal bleeding); (3) decreased or absent bowel sounds; (4) contusions, abrasions, or bruising over the abdomen; (5) abdominal pain; (6) pain over the scapula caused by irritation of the phrenic nerve by free blood in the abdomen; (7) hematemesis or hematuria; and (8) signs of hypovolemic shock (Table 40-14). An ecchymotic discoloration around the umbilicus (Cullen's sign) can indicate intraabdominal or retroperitoneal hemorrhage.

Intraabdominal injuries are often associated with low rib fractures, fractured femur, fractured pelvis, and thoracic injury. If any of these injuries are present, the patient should be observed for abdominal trauma.

EMERGENCY MANAGEMENT

Table 40-14 Abdominal Trauma

Etiology	Assessment Findings	Interventions
Blunt Falls Motor vehicle collisions Pedestrian event Assault with blunt object Crush injuries Explosions **Penetrating** Knife Gunshot wounds Other missiles	**Hypovolemic Shock** ▪ Decreased level of consciousness ▪ Tachypnea ▪ Tachycardia ▪ Decreased blood pressure ▪ Decreased pulse pressure **Surface Findings** ▪ Abrasions or ecchymoses on abdominal wall, flank, or peritoneum. ▪ Open wounds—lacerations, eviscerations, puncture wounds, gunshot wounds ▪ Impaled object ▪ Healed incisions or old scars **Abdominal/Gastrointestinal Findings** ▪ Nausea and vomiting ▪ Bloody urine ▪ Abdominal distention ▪ Abdominal rigidity ▪ Abdominal pain with palpation ▪ Rebound tenderness ▪ Pain radiation to shoulder and back	**Initial** ▪ Ensure patent airway. ▪ Administer oxygen via nonrebreather mask. ▪ Control external bleeding with direct pressure or sterile pressure dressing. ▪ Establish IV access with two large bore catheters and infuse warm normal saline or lactated Ringer's solution. ▪ Obtain blood for type and crossmatch and CBC. ▪ Remove clothing. ▪ Stabilize impaled objects with bulky dressing—*do not remove.* ▪ Cover protruding organs or tissue with sterile, saline dressing. ▪ Insert indwelling urinary catheter if there is no blood at the meatus, pelvic fracture, or boggy prostate. ▪ Obtain urine for urinalysis. ▪ Insert NG tube if no evidence of facial trauma. ▪ Anticipate diagnostic peritoneal lavage. **Ongoing Monitoring** ▪ Monitor vital signs, level of consciousness, oxygen saturation, and urine output. ▪ Maintain patient warmth using blankets, warm IV fluids, or warm humidified oxygen.

Diagnostic Studies

Specific diagnostic procedures include CBC, urinalysis, x-ray of the abdomen, CT scan, and peritoneal lavage. In peritoneal lavage the abdomen below the umbilicus is locally anesthetized, and a large angiocatheter or peritoneal dialysis catheter is inserted into the abdomen. A syringe is attached to the catheter, and an attempt is made to gently aspirate any blood. If less than 10 ml of blood is aspirated, a liter of saline solution is then infused into the abdomen and drained. The fluid is observed for gross abnormalities, especially blood, and is sent to the laboratory for microscopic evaluation. Positive findings may include (1) RBC count greater than 100,000/µl, (2) WBC count greater than 500/µl, (3) high amylase level, and (4) presence of bacteria, bile, or fecal material. If the results are positive, immediate surgery is indicated. If the results are negative, continued observation of the patient is warranted. An impaled object should never be removed until skilled care is available. Removal may cause further injury and bleeding.

NURSING AND COLLABORATIVE MANAGEMENT: ABDOMINAL TRAUMA

Emergency management of abdominal trauma focuses on establishing a patent airway and adequate breathing, fluid replacement, and prevention of hypovolemic shock (see Table 40-14). IV lines are inserted, and volume expanders or blood is given if the patient is hypotensive. An NG tube is inserted to decompress the stomach and prevent the aspiration of vomitus.

Regardless of the mechanism of injury, physical evidence of abdominal trauma in a patient who is hemodynamically unstable mandates immediate laparotomy. In other cases the indications for laparotomy must be correlated with the mechanism of injury. For example, if an individual has a gunshot wound or impaled object, surgery is usually indicated. If surgery is performed, the postoperative nursing care is for the patient after laparotomy (see NCP 40-2).

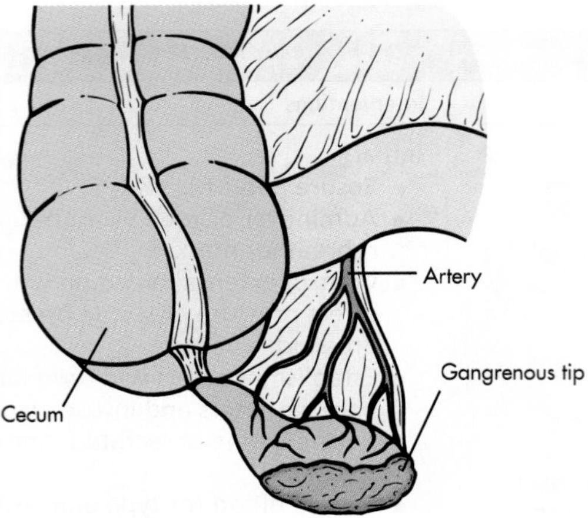

Fig. 40-1 In appendicitis the blood supply of the appendix is impaired by inflammation and bacterial infection in the wall of the appendix, which may result in gangrene.

INFLAMMATION

APPENDICITIS

Appendicitis is an inflammation of the appendix, a narrow blind tube that extends from the inferior part of the cecum. It occurs in 6% of the general population. Peak incidence is between the ages of 11 and 30 years, and the condition occurs equally in both sexes.[8]

Etiology

The most common causes of appendicitis are obstruction of the lumen by a *fecalith* (accumulated feces) (Fig. 40-1), foreign bodies, tumor of the cecum or appendix, or intramural thickening caused by lymphoid hyperplasia. After age 30 years, the number of appendicular lymph follicles declines until they are nearly absent at age 60 years.[8] Obstruction results in distention, venous engorgement, and the accumulation of mucus and bacteria, which can lead to gangrene and perforation.

Clinical Manifestations

Appendicitis typically begins with periumbilical pain, followed by anorexia, nausea, and vomiting. The pain is persistent and continuous, eventually shifting to the right lower quadrant and localizing at McBurney's point (located halfway between the umbilicus and the right iliac crest). Further assessment of the patient reveals localized tenderness, rebound tenderness, and muscle guarding. The patient usually prefers to lie still, often with the right leg flexed. Low-grade fever may or may not be present, and coughing aggravates pain. Rovsing's sign may be elicited by palpation of the left lower quadrant, causing pain to be felt in the right lower quadrant. Complications of acute appendicitis are perforation, peritonitis, and abscesses.

Diagnostic Studies and Collaborative Care

Examination of the patient includes a complete history and physical examination (particularly palpation of the abdomen) and a differential WBC count. A urinalysis may be done to rule out genitourinary (GU) conditions that mimic the manifestations of appendicitis.

The treatment of appendicitis is immediate surgical removal (*appendectomy*) if the inflammation is localized. If the appendix has ruptured and there is evidence of peritonitis or an abscess, conservative treatment, consisting of antibiotic therapy and parenteral fluids, may be used to prevent sepsis and dehydration for 6 to 8 hours before an appendectomy is performed.

Table 40-15 Causes of Peritonitis

Primary	Secondary
Blood-borne organisms Genital tract organisms Cirrhosis with ascites	Appendicitis with rupture Blunt or penetrating trauma to abdominal organs Diverticulitis with rupture Ischemic bowel disorders Obstruction in the gastrointestinal tract Pancreatitis Perforated peptic ulcer Peritoneal dialysis Postoperative (breakage of anastomosis)

NURSING MANAGEMENT: APPENDICITIS

The patient with abdominal pain is encouraged to see a physician and to avoid self-treatment, particularly the use of laxatives and enemas. The increased peristalsis from these procedures may cause perforation of the appendix. Until the patient is seen by a physician, nothing should be taken by mouth (NPO) to ensure that the stomach is empty in the event surgery is needed. An ice bag may be applied to the right lower quadrant to decrease the flow of blood to the area and impede the inflammatory process. Heat is never used because it may cause the appendix to rupture. Surgery is usually performed as soon as a diagnosis is made.

Postoperative nursing management is similar to postoperative care of the patient after laparotomy (see NCP 40-2). In addition, the patient should be observed for evidence of peritonitis. Ambulation begins the day of surgery or the first postoperative day. The diet is advanced as tolerated. The patient is usually discharged on the first or second postoperative day, and normal activities are resumed 2 to 3 weeks after surgery.

PERITONITIS

Peritonitis results from a localized or generalized inflammatory process of the peritoneum.

Etiology and Pathophysiology

Causes of peritonitis are listed in Table 40-15. Peritonitis may appear in acute and chronic forms, and trauma or rupture of an organ containing chemical irritants or bacteria (which are released into the peritoneal cavity) may cause it. Examples of a chemical peritonitis include gastric ulcer perforation and ruptured ectopic pregnancy. A chemical peritonitis is commonly followed by bacterial invasion. Bacterial peritonitis can be caused by a traumatic injury (e.g., gunshot wound, ruptured appendix), or it can be secondary to other diseases or conditions (e.g., pancreatitis, peritoneal dialysis).

COLLABORATIVE CARE

Table 40-16 Peritonitis

Diagnostic
- CBC
- Serum electrolytes
- Abdominal x-ray
- Abdominal paracentesis and culture of fluid
- CT scan or ultrasound
- Peritoneoscopy

Collaborative Therapy

Preoperative or Nonoperative
- NPO status
- Fluid replacement
- Antibiotic therapy
- NG suction
- Analgesics
- Preparation for surgery to include the above and total parenteral nutrition

Postoperative
- NPO status
- NG tube to low-intermittent suction
- Semi-Fowler's position
- IV fluids with electrolyte replacement
- Total parenteral nutrition as needed
- Antibiotic therapy
- Blood transfusions as needed
- Sedatives and narcotics

CBC, complete blood count; *CT,* computed tomography; *IV,* intravenous; *NPO,* nothing by mouth.

The response of the peritoneum to the leakage of GI contents is localization of the offending agent by attempting to "wall it off" by exuding fibrin-containing fluids and swelling. Adhesions may form. These adhesions may shrink and disappear when the infection is eliminated. Normally, peritoneal injuries heal without formation of adhesions unless other factors, such as infection, ischemia, or foreign substances, are present.

Clinical Manifestations

Abdominal pain is the most common symptom of peritonitis.[9] A universal sign of peritonitis is tenderness over the involved area. Rebound tenderness, muscular rigidity, and spasm are other major signs of irritation of the peritoneum. Abdominal distention or ascites, fever, tachycardia, tachypnea, nausea, vomiting, and altered bowel habits may also be present. These manifestations vary, depending on severity and acuteness of the underlying cause. Complications of peritonitis include hypovolemic shock, septicemia, intraabdominal abscess formation, paralytic ileus, and organ failure.

Diagnostic Studies

A CBC is done to determine leukocytosis and hemoconcentration (Table 40-16). Peritoneal aspiration may be performed and the fluid analyzed for blood, bile, pus, bacteria, fungus, and amylase content. An x-ray of the abdomen may show dilated loops of bowel consistent with paralytic ileus, free air if perforation has occurred, or air and fluid levels if an obstruction is present. Ultrasound and CT scans may be useful in identifying the presence of ascites and abscesses. Peritoneoscopy may be helpful in the patient without ascites. Direct examination of the peritoneum can be obtained, along with biopsy specimens for diagnosis.

Collaborative Care

The goals of management of peritonitis are to identify and eliminate the cause, combat infection, and prevent complications. Patients with milder cases of peritonitis or those who are poor surgical risks may be managed nonsurgically. Treatment consists of antibiotics, NG suction, analgesics, and IV fluid administration. Patients who require surgery need preoperative preparation as previously described. Those patients may be placed on total parenteral nutrition (TPN) because of increased nutritional requirements.

NURSING MANAGEMENT: PERITONITIS

Nursing Assessment

Assessment of the patient's pain, including the location, is important and may help in determining the cause of peritonitis. The patient should be assessed for the presence and quality of bowel sounds, increasing abdominal distention, abdominal guarding, nausea, fever, and manifestations of hypovolemic shock.

Nursing Diagnoses

Nursing diagnoses for the patient with peritonitis include, but are not limited to, the following:

- Pain *related to* inflammation of the peritoneum and abdominal distention
- Risk for fluid volume deficit *related to* collection of fluid in peritoneal cavity secondary to trauma, infection, or ischemia
- Altered nutrition: less than body requirements *related to* anorexia, nausea, and vomiting
- Anxiety *related to* uncertainty of cause or outcome of condition and pain
- Potential complication: hypovolemic shock *related to* loss of circulatory volume

Planning

The overall goals are that the patient with peritonitis will have (1) resolution of inflammation, (2) relief of abdominal pain, (3) freedom from complications (especially hypovolemic shock), and (4) normal nutritional status.

Nursing Implementation

The patient with peritonitis is extremely ill and needs skilled supportive care. The patient is monitored for pain and response to analgesic therapy. The patient may be positioned with knees flexed to increase comfort. The nurse should provide rest and a quiet environment. Sedatives may be given to allay anxiety.

Accurate monitoring of fluid intake and output and electrolyte status is necessary to determine replacement therapy. Vital signs are monitored frequently. Antiemetics may be administered to decrease nausea and vomiting and further fluid losses. The patient is on NPO status and may have an NG tube in place to decrease gastric distention.

If the patient has an open surgical procedure, drains are inserted to remove purulent drainage and excessive fluid. Postoperative care of the patient is similar to the care of the patient with an exploratory laparotomy (see NCP 40-2).

GASTROENTERITIS

Gastroenteritis is an inflammation of the mucosa of the stomach and small intestine. Clinical manifestations include nausea, vomiting, diarrhea, abdominal cramping, and distention. Fever, leukocytosis, and blood or mucus in the stool may be present. Causative agents are varied (see Table 40-2). Most cases are self-limiting and do not require hospitalization. However, older adults and chronically ill patients may be unable to consume sufficient fluids orally to compensate for fluid loss. Until vomiting has ceased, the patient should be on NPO status. If dehydration has occurred, IV replacement of fluids may be necessary. As soon as tolerated, fluids containing glucose and electrolytes (e.g., Pedialyte) should be given. If the causative agent is identified, appropriate antibiotic, antimicrobial, or antiinfective medication is given.

CULTURAL & ETHNIC CONSIDERATIONS

Colon Disorders

- Inflammatory bowel disease (IBD) is more common among Caucasians than African-Americans and Asian-Americans.
- IBD is more common among Jewish people and those of middle European origin.
- Colorectal cancer is higher in the United States and Canada than in Japan, Finland, or Africa.
- Incidence of colorectal cancer is declining in the United States except for African-American men.

NURSING MANAGEMENT: GASTROENTERITIS

Accurate monitoring of intake and output is important for successful replacement of lost fluid. Strict medical asepsis and infection control precautions should be instituted when indicated. The patient should be instructed in the importance of proper food handling and preparation of food to prevent infections such as salmonellosis and trichinosis (see Chapter 39).

Symptomatic nursing care is given for nausea, vomiting, and diarrhea. The importance of rest and increased fluid intake should be stressed. The nurse should assess complaints of pain, vomiting, and diarrhea because gastroenteritis is often confused with appendicitis. To allay the patient's apprehension, the nurse should explain that gastroenteritis usually runs an acute course with no sequelae.

IRRITABLE BOWEL SYNDROME

Irritable bowel syndrome (IBS) is a symptom complex characterized by intermittent and recurrent abdominal pain associated with an alteration in bowel function (diarrhea or constipation). Other symptoms commonly found include abdominal distention, excessive flatulence, urge to defecate, and sensation of incomplete evacuation. IBS is a common problem affecting approximately 10% to 17% of the population in the United States.[10] In western societies, approximately two times as many women as men seek health care services for IBS. Stress, psychologic factors, and specific food intolerances have been identified as major factors that precipitate IBS symptoms.

The key to accurate diagnosis is a thorough health history and physical examination. Emphasis should be on symptoms, past health history (including psychosocial aspects including physical or sexual abuse), family history, and drug and dietary history. Diagnostic tests should be selectively used to rule out more serious life-threatening disorders with symptoms similar to those of IBS, such as colon cancer, peptic ulcer disease, and malabsorption disorders.

The health care provider should establish a trusting relationship with the patient at the onset of treatment. The patient needs reassurance that the symptoms are functional. The patient should be encouraged to verbalize concerns and anxiety. A diet containing at least 20 g per day of dietary fiber should be initiated (see Table 40-9). This may also include the addition of psyllium-containing products (e.g., Metamucil).

The patient whose primary symptoms are abdominal distention and increased flatulence should be advised to eliminate common gas-producing foods such as broccoli and cabbage from the diet and to substitute yogurt for milk products if there is lactose intolerance. Anticholinergic agents, such as dicyclomine (Bentyl), may be helpful if taken before meals to alleviate the pain associated with ingestion of food. For the patient with a high level of anxiety, a mild sedative or tranquilizer may be ordered but should be prescribed for only a short time. Additional therapies include relaxation and stress management techniques, although no single therapy has been found to be effective for all patients with IBS.

INFLAMMATORY BOWEL DISEASE

Crohn's disease and *ulcerative colitis* are immunologically related disorders that are referred to as *inflammatory bowel disease* (IBD). These disorders are characterized by chronic, recurrent inflammation of the intestinal tract. For both conditions, the clinical manifestations are varied, with long periods of remission interspersed with episodes of acute inflammation. Both diseases can be debilitating.

Although there has been extensive research on the etiology of IBD, the cause of both ulcerative colitis and Crohn's disease remains unknown. Possible causes include (1) an infectious agent (e.g., virus, bacteria) because IBD produces mucosal changes in the colon similar to those of infectious diarrhea, although no consistent pathogen has been identified; (2) an autoimmune reaction from the presence of other immune-related disorders, such as systemic lupus erythematosus, ankylosing spondylitis, and erythema nodosum in patients with IBD; (3) food allergies (although this has not been substantiated); and (4) heredity. (Both Crohn's disease and ulcerative colitis occur more commonly in related families.[11]) In one study, 84% of identical twins of patients who had Crohn's disease also had the disorder.[12] For years IBD (especially ulcerative colitis) was thought to be due to psychosomatic factors, such as severe emotional stress. It is now believed that these emotional changes result from and are not the cause of the disease.

ULCERATIVE COLITIS

Ulcerative colitis is characterized by inflammation and ulceration of the colon and rectum. It may occur at any age but peaks

Table 40-17 Comparison of Ulcerative Colitis and Crohn's Disease

Characteristic	Ulcerative colitis	Crohn's disease
Clinical		
Age at onset	Young to middle age	Young
Diarrhea	Common	Common
Abdominal crampy pain	Possible	Common
Fever (intermittent)	During acute attacks	Common
Weight loss	Common	Severe
Rectal bleeding	Common	Infrequent
Tenesmus	Severe	Rare
Malabsorption and nutritional deficiencies	Minimal incidence	Common
Pathologic		
Location	Starts distally and spreads in a continuous pattern up the colon	Occurs anywhere along GI tract in characteristic skip lesions; most frequent site is terminal ileum
Distribution	Continuous	Segmental
Depth of involvement	Mucosa and submucosa	Entire thickness of bowel wall (transmural)
Granulomas	Absent	Common
Cobblestoning of mucosa	Rare	Common
Pseudopolyps	Common	Rare
Small-bowel involvement	Minimal	Common
Complications		
Fistulas	Rare	Common
Strictures	Rare	Common
Anal abscesses	Rare	Common
Perforation	Common	Common
Toxic megacolon	Common	Rare
Carcinoma	Increased incidence after 10 yr of disease	Slightly greater than general population
Recurrence after surgery	Cure with colectomy	70% or more recurrence after segmental resections of small or large intestine

between the ages of 15 and 25 years. There is a second, smaller peak onset between 50 and 80 years of age. Ulcerative colitis affects both sexes but has a higher incidence in women. It is more common in Jewish and upper-middle-class urban populations.

Etiology and Pathophysiology

The inflammation of ulcerative colitis is diffuse and involves the mucosa and submucosa, with alternate periods of exacerbations and remissions (Table 40-17). The disease usually begins in the rectum and sigmoid colon and spreads up the colon in a continuous pattern.

The mucosa of the colon is hyperemic and edematous in the affected area (Fig. 40-2). Multiple abscesses develop in the crypts of Lieberkühn (intestinal glands). As the disease advances, the abscesses break through the crypts into the submucosa, leaving ulcerations. These ulcerations also destroy the mucosal epithelium, causing bleeding and diarrhea. Losses of fluid and electrolytes occur because of the decreased mucosal surface area for absorption. Breakdown of cells results in protein loss through the stool. Areas of inflamed mucosa form *pseudopolyps,* tonguelike projections into the bowel lumen. Granulation tissue develops, and the mucosa musculature becomes thickened, shortening the colon.

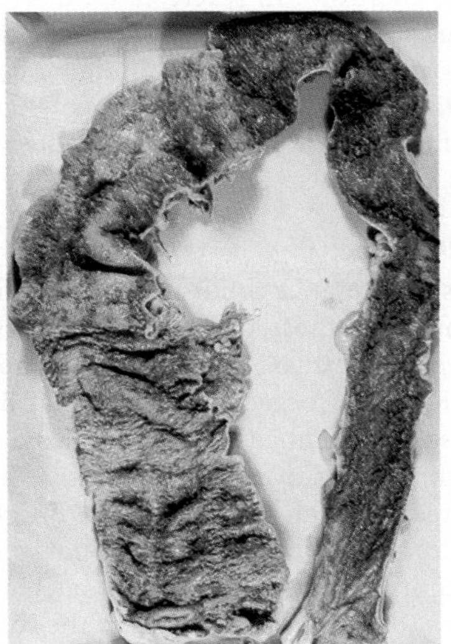

Fig. 40-2 Acute ulcerative colitis. Colitis with extensive mucosal ulceration involving the entire colon.

Clinical Manifestations

Ulcerative colitis may appear as an acute fulminating crisis or, more commonly, as a chronic disorder with mild to severe acute exacerbations that occur at unpredictable intervals over many years. The major symptoms of ulcerative colitis are bloody diarrhea and abdominal pain. Pain may vary from the mild lower-abdominal cramping associated with diarrhea to the severe, constant abdominal pain associated with acute perforations. With mild disease, diarrhea may consist of one or two semiformed stools containing small amounts of blood per day.

Table 40-18 Extraintestinal Complications of Ulcerative Colitis

Colitis Related
- Joints
  - Peripheral arthritis (colitic)
  - Ankylosing spondylitis
  - Sacroiliitis
  - Finger clubbing
- Skin
  - Erythema nodosum
  - Pyoderma gangrenosum
- Mouth
  - Aphthous ulcers
- Eye
  - Conjunctivitis
  - Uveitis
  - Episcleritis

Related to Small Bowel Pathology
- Malabsorption
- Gallstones
- Kidney stones

Nonspecific
- Liver disease—primary sclerosing cholangitis
- Osteoporosis
- Amyloidosis
- Peptic ulcer disease

COLLABORATIVE CARE

Table 40-19 Ulcerative Colitis

Diagnostic
- Fiberoptic colonoscopy
- Sigmoidoscopy
- Barium enema
- CBC
- Stool for blood, culture and sensitivity

Collaborative Therapy

Mild and Moderate Disease
- Low-roughage diet and no milk or milk products
- Antimicrobial therapy*
- Corticosteroids
- Anticholinergic therapy*
- Antidiarrheal agents*

Severe (Fulminant) Disease
- IV fluids with electrolytes
- Blood transfusions
- NPO status
- NG tube to low suction
- Antimicrobial therapy*
- Corticosteroids
- Parenteral nutritional therapy
- Surgery if no improvement (colon resection with ileostomy)

*See Table 40-20.

The patient may have no other systemic manifestations. In moderate ulcerative colitis there is increased stool output (4 to 5 stools per day), increased bleeding, and systemic symptoms (fever, malaise, anorexia). In severe cases, diarrhea is bloody, contains mucus, and occurs 10 to 20 times a day. In addition, fever, weight loss greater than 10% of total body weight, anemia, tachycardia, and dehydration are present. Acute fulminant colitis is present in only 6% to 10% of patients with severe ulcerative colitis.[11]

Complications

Complications of ulcerative colitis may be classified into those that are *intestinal* and those that are *extraintestinal.* Intestinal complications of ulcerative colitis include hemorrhage, strictures, perforation, toxic megacolon, and colonic dilation. Hemorrhage is a result of inflamed, ulcerated mucosa and is usually controlled with conservative therapy. Massive hemorrhage is unusual and requires emergency surgery. Strictures are less common in ulcerative colitis than in Crohn's disease and are seen most often in patients with severe, long-standing disease. *Toxic megacolon* (dilation and paralysis of the colon) occurs in approximately 5% of patients with ulcerative colitis.[13] Colonic dilation, most often in the transverse colon, occurs as a result of severe acute inflammation of the entire colon wall. Perforation is most often associated with toxic megacolon but may occur alone. Most cases of perforation occur in the left side of the colon.

A patient who has had ulcerative colitis for more than 10 years is at greater risk of colon cancer. The risk of cancer depends on age at onset, duration, and extent of disease. The patient should be periodically screened with surveillance colonoscopy. During this procedure, biopsy specimens should be taken every 10 cm throughout the entire colon.

Extraintestinal complications may be directly related to the colitis and small intestine pathology (malabsorption), or they may be nonspecific complications mediated by a disturbance in the immune system (Table 40-18). Colitis-related complications are associated with active inflammation and often respond to treatment of the underlying bowel disease. These manifestations can involve the joints, skin, mouth, and eyes as well as disturbances of the hematologic system including anemia, leukocytosis, and thrombocytosis.[14] Skin lesions such as erythema nodosum and pyoderma gangrenosum are among the most frequently seen extraintestinal manifestations. Uveitis is the most common eye problem.

Diagnostic Studies

Several studies are appropriate for diagnosis of ulcerative colitis (Table 40-19). Blood studies should include a CBC, serum electrolyte levels, and serum protein levels. A CBC typically shows iron deficiency anemia from blood loss. An elevated WBC count may indicate toxic megacolon or perforation. Decreases in serum electrolytes, such as sodium, potassium, chloride, bicarbonate, and magnesium, are due to fluid and electrolyte losses from diarrhea and vomiting. Hypoalbuminemia is present with severe disease and is due to protein loss from the bowel. The stool should be examined for blood, pus, and mucus. Stool cultures should be obtained to rule out infectious causes of inflammation.

Examinations with a flexible sigmoidoscope and a colonoscope allow direct examination of the mucosa of the large

DRUG THERAPY

Table 40-20 Ulcerative Colitis

Category	Action	Examples
▪ Antimicrobial	Prevention or treatment of secondary infection	Cephalothin sodium (Keflin) Sulfasalazine (Azulfidine)* Mesalamine (Rowasa)* Olsalazine (Dipentum)
▪ Corticosteroids	Antiinflammatory	Corticosteroids (cortisone, prednisone)
▪ Anticholinergic	Decrease in GI motility and secretions and relief of smooth muscle spasms[†]	Methantheline bromide (Banthine) Propantheline (Pro-Banthine) Oxyphencyclimine (Daricon)
▪ Sedatives	Quieting of CNS without inducing sleep or analgesia	Diazepam (Valium) Flurazepam (Dalmane)
▪ Antidiarrheal	Decrease in GI motility[†]	Diphenoxylate (Lomotil)
▪ Immunosuppressives	Suppression of immune response	Azathioprine (Imuran), cyclosporine
▪ Hematinics and vitamins	Correction of iron deficiency anemia and promotion of healing	Iron dextran injection (Imferon) Cobalamin, zinc

*Mechanism of action unknown, likely to be antiinflammatory as well as antimicrobial.
[†]Used with caution during severe disease because of potential to produce toxic megacolon.
CNS, central nervous system; *GI,* gastrointestinal.

intestine. Using a sigmoidoscope the physician can view the rectum, the sigmoid colon, and the descending colon. The colonoscope allows for examination of the entire large intestine. The extent of inflammation, ulcerations, pseudopolyps, strictures, and lesions may be identified. Biopsy specimens should be taken for definitive diagnosis.

A double-contrast barium enema may show areas of granular inflammation with ulcerations. The colon may appear narrow and shortened, and pseudopolyps may be present. A double-contrast study (in which air is introduced into the bowel after the expulsion of barium) is effective in detecting mucosal abnormalities in ulcerative colitis.

Collaborative Care

The goals of treatment are to (1) rest the bowel, (2) control the inflammation, (3) combat infection, (4) correct malnutrition, (5) alleviate stress, and (6) provide symptomatic relief using drug therapy (see Table 40-20). The mainstays of drug therapy are sulfasalazine (Azulfidine) and corticosteroids. Hospitalization is indicated if the patient fails to respond to corticosteroid therapy or if complications are suspected.

Drug Therapy. Drug therapy is an extremely important aspect of treatment (see Table 40-20).[15] Sulfasalazine, a combination of sulfapyridine and 5-aminosalicylic acid (5-ASA), is the principal drug used. It is effective in the maintenance of clinical remission and in the treatment of mild to moderately severe attacks. After remission is obtained, therapy is continued with a gradual reduction over several months. The maintenance dose is usually continued for at least 1 year.

During active disease 5-ASA (the active form of sulfasalazine) and 4-ASA, given as retention enemas, are effective in the treatment of left-sided ulcerative colitis and proctitis. Topical salicylate therapy is the treatment of choice in patients with localized disease. 5-ASA (mesalamine [Rowasa]) can also be administered orally. The acrylic-coated tablets provide delivery of the drug more distally in the intestine.

Corticosteroids are of proven benefit in the management of active ulcerative colitis. Oral prednisone or prednisolone is effective in treatment of mild to moderate disease without systemic manifestations. If remission is not achieved, the patient requires hospitalization and IV corticosteroid therapy. The patient is placed on a regimen of bowel rest. Fluids and electrolytes are administered intravenously. Hydrocortisone enemas and foams are effective in the treatment of colitis limited to the rectosigmoid area. Rectal foams are usually administered in 5 ml volumes and are generally preferred over enemas because of the ease of administration. However, enemas are the preferred choice if the disease spreads beyond the sigmoid colon. Retention enemas have been shown to deliver medication into the descending colon and beyond in patients with active disease. Although corticosteroids are reported to bring remission in 60% to 89% of cases, they do not necessarily prolong remission.[15] The patient on corticosteroids is to be monitored for signs of Cushing's syndrome, hypertension, hirsutism, and mood swings. In some cases, psychosis may develop.[16]

Immunosuppressive drugs (e.g., 6-mercaptopurine [6-MP]) have been used in severe cases of ulcerative colitis when a patient has failed to respond to any of the usual medications and before surgery is considered. Side effects of 6-MP, including bone marrow suppression and increased risk of infection, necessitate that it be used cautiously in these patients. Patients receiving this medication need to maintain an adequate fluid intake of 1800 to 2400 ml to reduce the risk of nephrotoxicity.[15] The drug should be taken with food and milk to reduce gastric irritation. Cyclosporine (discussed in Chapter 44) and methotrexate have been evaluated for their effectiveness in the treatment of severe ulcerative colitis that is unresponsive to corticosteroid treatment. New therapies such as monoclonal antibodies against tumor necrosis factor [TNF] or the antiinflammatory cytokine interleukin-10 [IL-10] that are used to modify the inflammatory response in IBD are under investigation.[17]

Epidemiologic studies showing a low incidence of ulcerative colitis among smokers has led to investigation of nicotine transdermal patches or gum to induce remission.[18] For distal ulcerative colitis, rectal enemas containing short chain fatty acids

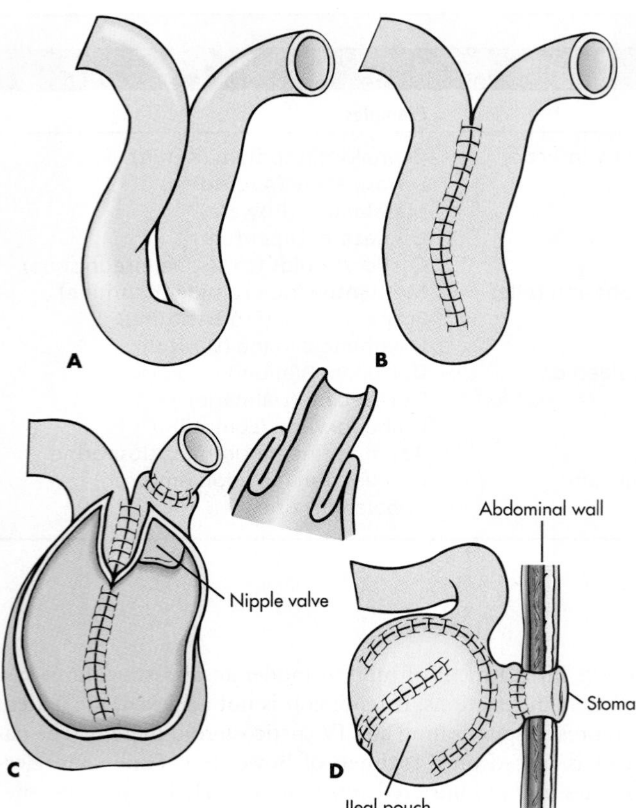

Fig. 40-3 Surgical formation of continent ileostomy (Kock pouch). **A,** Loop of terminal ileum. **B,** Both limbs sutured together and incised in a *U shape*. **C,** Pouch created with nipple valve. **D,** Pouch sutured to abdominal wall.

have been evaluated for their antiinflammatory effects. Short chain fatty acids are important fuels supporting colonic cell function and are naturally produced from fiber fermentation.[19]

Surgical Therapy. Approximately 85% of patients with ulcerative colitis go into remission with conservative therapy and nursing care, but 15% to 20% require surgery. Surgery is indicated if (1) the patient fails to respond to treatment; (2) exacerbations are frequent and debilitating; (3) massive bleeding, perforation, strictures, or obstruction occur; (4) changes that suggest dysplasia are occurring; or (5) carcinoma develops.

Surgical procedures used to treat chronic ulcerative colitis include (1) total proctocolectomy with permanent ileostomy, (2) total proctocolectomy with continent ileostomy (Kock pouch), and (3) total colectomy with rectal mucosal stripping and ileoanal reservoir.

Total proctocolectomy with permanent ileostomy. Total proctocolectomy with an ileostomy, is a one-stage operation involving the removal of the colon, rectum, and anus with closure of the anus. The end of the terminal ileum is brought out through the abdominal wall and forms a stoma, or ostomy. The stoma is usually placed in the right lower quadrant below the belt line.

Total proctocolectomy with continent ileostomy. Kock pouch is a continent ileostomy, which is a variation from the traditional ileostomy (Fig. 40-3). This method eliminates the need for the patient to wear an external pouch over the stoma. The stoma is usually covered with a cap or dressing in case of mucus leakage. This procedure is considered curative for ulcerative colitis but has a higher complication rate than the traditional ileostomy.

In this procedure an internal pouch in the distal segment of the ileum is made surgically, the intestine is split, a fold is made, and a one-way nipple valve is created and sutured into place on the abdomen. The pouch acts as a reservoir and is drained at regular intervals on insertion of a catheter. During surgery, a catheter is inserted into the pouch to allow suture lines to heal and to allow fixation of scar tissue around the valve to prevent slippage. Postoperative irrigations are performed every 2 to 4 hours to rinse mucus from the pouch. The catheter may stay in place for up to 3 to 4 weeks. Once the catheter is removed, insertion of a catheter to remove contents begins every 2 hours and is gradually decreased until it is needed only three to six times a day. The patient eventually determines the frequency by the changes in sensation of pressure in the pouch. A continuous leakage of fluid is prevented by the one-way valve created at the internal end of the ileum from the stoma to the ileal pouch. Pressure created when the pouch fills with feces forces the valve to close. The majority of complications that arise are a result of valve failure, which has been reported to be as high as 40%.

The primary late complications of the procedure include pouchitis, fistula development, and nipple valve extrusion. These complications affect function by increasing intubation frequency and compromising pouch continence. Manifestations of pouchitis are fever, malaise, and watery diarrhea. The lining appears red and inflamed, and biopsy shows nonspecific inflammation. Patients usually respond to treatment with metronidazole (Flagyl).

Total colectomy and ileal reservoir. A more widely performed procedure involves total colectomy and ileoanal anastomosis with the formation of an ileal reservoir (Fig. 40-4). The ileoanal surgical procedure is usually a combination of two procedures performed approximately 8 to 12 weeks apart. The initial procedure includes colectomy, rectal mucosectomy, ileal reservoir construction, ileoanal anastomosis, and temporary ileostomy. The second surgery involves closure of the ileostomy, which functionalizes the reservoir. Adaptation of the reservoir occurs over the next 3 to 6 months, which usually results in the ability to control and have decreased numbers of bowel movements over a 24-hour period.

Patient selection criteria include absence of colon cancer, small intestine free of disease (e.g., Crohn's), competent anorectal sphincter, and physical status adequate to permit lengthy surgery. In addition, the patient needs to be motivated and capable of understanding self-care instructions.

Postoperative Care. Postoperative care following surgical procedures to treat ulcerative colitis includes routine observations for patients who have had abdominal surgery. Stoma viability, mucocutaneous juncture, and peristomal skin integrity must be monitored. Because a more proximal portion of the bowel is used to create the ileostomy, output initially may be as high as 1500 to 2000 ml per 24 hours. The patient must be observed for signs of hemorrhage, abdominal abscess, small bowel obstruction, dehydration, and other related complications. If an NG tube is used, it will be removed

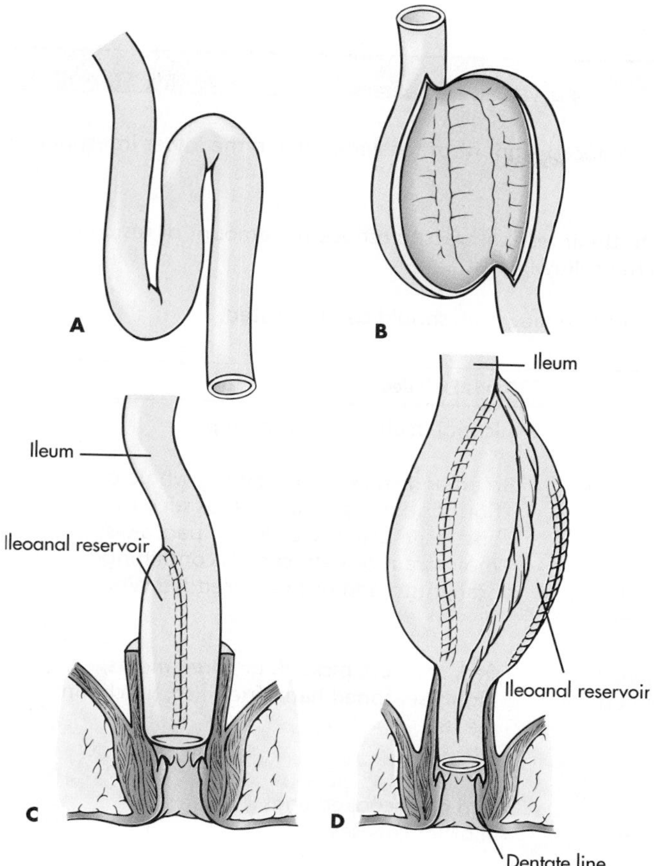

Fig. 40-4 Ileoanal reservoir. **A,** Formation of a reservoir. **B,** Posterior suture lines completed. **C,** J-shaped configuration for ileoanal reservoir. **D,** S-shaped configuration for ileoanal reservoir.

when bowel function returns and oral intake is instituted. Drainage of serosanguineous fluid from the abdominal drain site may vary from 100 to 150 ml per 24 hours. The drain is usually removed within 4 days of surgery. The urinary catheter is removed 2 to 5 days after surgery. Systemic antibiotics are discontinued within 24 hours of the operation and corticosteroids, if used, are tapered.

Transient incontinence of mucus is a result of intraoperative manipulation of the anal canal. The patient should be reassured before the operation regarding this potential transient problem. Kegel exercises are recommended later on (several weeks postoperatively) to strengthen the pelvic floor and sphincter muscles. They are not recommended in the immediate postoperative period. Perianal skin care must be implemented to protect the epidermis from mucous drainage and maceration. The patient should be instructed to gently rinse the skin with water and dry thoroughly. A moisture barrier ointment may be used, and a perineal pad may be required.

The most frequent type of ileostomy that is constructed is a loop. This frequently presents a pouching challenge because it retracts or drains inferiorly, resulting in effluent contact with the skin and predisposing to a denuded epidermis. An enterostomal therapy nurse is an appropriate referral for these challenging problems. Self-care instructions should be reviewed and written information provided before discharge. Stoma care is presented later in this chapter (see p. 1174).

Nutritional Therapy. An important component in the treatment of ulcerative colitis is diet. The dietician is an important member of the team and should be consulted regarding dietary recommendations. The goals of diet management are to provide adequate nutrition without exacerbating symptoms, to correct and prevent malnutrition, to replace fluid and electrolyte losses, and to prevent weight loss. The diet for each patient must be individualized.

Traditionally during the acute phase the patient may be on NPO status. When food is permitted, a high-calorie, high-protein, low-residue diet with vitamin and iron supplements is frequently prescribed. (A low-residue diet is presented in Table 40-21.) Special dietary restrictions are not usually necessary. Some physicians allow the patient to eat anything that does not cause symptoms. Cold foods, high-residue foods (whole-wheat bread, cereal with bran, nuts, raw fruit), and smoking increase GI motility and should be avoided.

Often enteral supplements and parenteral nutrition are necessary. Patients with systemic manifestations, significant fluid and electrolyte losses, or malabsorption may need parenteral nutrition or enteral feedings, such as elemental diets. Elemental diets are high in calories and nutrients, lactose-free, and absorbed in the proximal small intestine, which allows the more distal bowel to rest. (Elemental diets are discussed in Chapter 38.)

Parenteral nutrition allows for a positive nitrogen balance while resting the bowel. Vitamins, minerals, electrolytes, and other important nutrients can be administered to promote healing and correct nutritional deficiencies.

Iron dextran (Imferon) intramuscularly (IM) by Z-track or IV may be necessary if anemia is severe. In patients receiving long-term sulfasalazine therapy, folic acid deficiency may develop and supplementation may be necessary. Patients with small bowel disease, ileal resection, or malabsorption, which affects the absorption of cobalamin (vitamin B_{12}), may need monthly injections of cobalamin. Potassium supplements may be necessary if corticosteroid therapy is used because hypokalemia can lead to toxic megacolon. Zinc deficiency can result from severe or chronic diarrhea and supplementation may be necessary.

NURSING MANAGEMENT: ULCERATIVE COLITIS

■ Nursing Assessment

Subjective and objective data that should be obtained from a person with ulcerative colitis are presented in Table 40-22.

■ Nursing Diagnoses

Nursing diagnoses for the patient with ulcerative colitis include, but are not limited to, those presented in NCP 40-3.

■ Planning

The overall goals are that the patient with ulcerative colitis will (1) experience a decrease in number and severity of acute exacerbations, (2) maintain normal fluid and electrolyte balance, (3) be free from pain or discomfort, (4) comply with medical regimens, and (5) maintain nutritional balance.

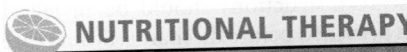

Table 40-21 Low-Residue Diet

Purpose

Low-residue diet provides foods low in fiber, which will result in a reduced amount of fecal material in the lower intestinal tract.

General Principles

1. This diet eliminates foods that are indigestible or stimulating to the intestinal tract to reduce the amount of residue in the colon. Foods should be included or excluded according to the following list.
2. Hot and cold foods should be eaten slowly.
3. Milk products are limited to 2 cups daily. For a more restricted-residue diet, milk should be eliminated.

Food	Foods Included	Foods Excluded
Beverages	Carbonated drinks, coffee, tea, cocoa, strained fruit juices	Alcohol, fruit juices with pulp
Bread	White bread, rolls, rusk, melba toast, crackers	Bread and crackers containing whole grain flour or bran; any hot breads such as biscuits, muffins, waffles, or pancakes
Cereals	Cooked, refined, or strained cereals: Cream of Wheat, Cream of Rice, farina, grits, dry cereals without bran, noodles, spaghetti, and macaroni	Whole grain cereals; cereals containing bran, nuts, and raisins; Shredded Wheat
Meat	Lean, tender ground beef, lamb, pork, veal or fish, broiled, stewed, or baked; canned tuna or salmon; shellfish; crisp bacon, chicken or turkey without skin, liver; creamy peanut butter	Fried, smoked, pickled, or cured meats, highly seasoned ham, fried fish, luncheon meats
Egg	All but fried	Fried or uncooked eggs
Cheese	Milk, cheese (American, cheddar), cottage cheese	All other cheeses
Milk	Limit to 1-2 cups (if tolerated), including that used in cooking; plain yogurt	Fruit yogurt
Fats	Butter, margarine, cream, oil, crisp bacon, mayonnaise, plain gravy	Any other; rich or spiced gravies
Soup	Cream and vegetable soups made from foods allowed and with milk allowed, bouillon, broth; strained vegetable juices	Cream and vegetable soups from foods not allowed (peas and dried beans)
Vegetables	Tender carrots, beets, or asparagus; strained vegetables; potatoes without skins; vegetable juices	Raw vegetables, all vegetables not strained, dried beans, peas, and legumes
Fruits	Strained fruit juices, ripe bananas, applesauce, pears, peaches, peeled apricots, Napoleon cherries, baked apple (no skin)	Raw fruits, fruits with skins, seeds
Desserts	Plain desserts (custards and puddings, plain ice cream from milk allowance), sherbet, plain gelatin desserts, angel food cake, sponge cake, plain butter cake, plain cookies	Nuts, coconut, raisins, rich desserts (pies, rich cakes, cobblers)
Condiments	Allspice, cinnamon, mace, paprika, salt, ground thyme, sugar, vinegar, lemon juice	All others

Sample Menu Plan

Breakfast	Lunch	Dinner
½ cup applesauce ½ cup Cream of Wheat Scrambled egg White toast Butter or jelly 1 cup milk Coffee	Roast beef sandwich on 2 slices white bread (no lettuce or tomato) 1 tbs mayonnaise 2 sugar cookies Canned peach halves Coffee	Baked chicken Mashed potato Cooked carrots White bread Butter Angel food cake 1 cup milk Coffee

NURSING ASSESSMENT

Table 40-22 Ulcerative Colitis

Subjective Data	Objective Data
Important Health Information	**General**
Past health history: Infection, autoimmune disorders	Intermittent fever; emaciated appearance
Medications: Use of antidiarrheal medications	**Integumentary**
Functional Health Patterns	Pale skin with poor turgor, dry mucous membranes; rash, nodules, or blisters; anorectal excoriation
Health perception–health management: Family history of ulcerative colitis; fatigue, malaise	**Gastrointestinal**
Nutritional-metabolic: Nausea, vomiting; anorexia; weight loss	Abdominal distention, hyperactive bowel sounds
Elimination: Frequent bloody stools containing mucus and pus	**Cardiovascular**
Cognitive-perceptual: Lower abdominal pain (worse before defecation), cramping, tenesmus	Tachycardia, hypotension
	Possible Findings
	Anemia; leukocytosis; electrolyte imbalance; hypoalbuminemia; vitamin and trace metal deficiencies; guaiac-positive stool; abnormal proctosigmoidoscopic, colonoscopic, and barium enema findings

■ Nursing Implementation

During the acute phase, attention is focused on hemodynamic stability, pain control, fluid and electrolyte balance, and nutritional support. Accurate intake and output records must be maintained. The number and appearance of stools are monitored. Nursing care of the patient with ulcerative colitis is directed toward an intensive therapeutic and supportive program (see NCP 40-3). Emotional support is important because the patient with ulcerative colitis may feel insecure, dependent, and sensitive. It is important that the nurse establishes a good working relationship and encourages the patient to talk about self and daily activities. Honesty, patience, and understanding are crucial in the relationship with the patient. An explanation of all procedures and treatment is necessary and may allay some apprehension.

Appropriate diversional activity should be used to move the patient's attention away from the intestinal tract. Psychotherapy may be indicated if the patient is experiencing emotional problems, but the nurse must recognize that the patient's behavior may result from factors other than emotional ones. Any person who has 10 to 20 bowel movements a day and has rectal discomfort may be anxious, frustrated, discouraged, and depressed. Along with other team members, the nurse can assist the patient to accept the chronic condition and have an optimistic view with the possibility of cure after surgery. The nurse may find that inadequate coping mechanisms in the patient with ulcerative colitis are due to early onset of the disease (often at 10 to 15 years of age), which may have interfered with usual growth, development, and maturation.

Bed rest may be ordered if the patient has a severe exacerbation. Nursing interventions to prevent complications of immobility should be instituted. A sedative or tranquilizer may be prescribed to ensure rest. In addition to teaching related to treatment, medications, diet, diagnostic tests, and the disease and its management, discussion of everyday topics should also be a part of diversional therapy.

Rest is important in the management of ulcerative colitis. Patients may lose much sleep because of frequent episodes of diarrhea and abdominal pain. Nutritional deficiencies and anemia leave the patient feeling weak and listless. Activities should be scheduled around rest periods. The nurse should also set limits and follow through because the patient can be demanding. The patient needs to know and understand that the nurse wants to help and does not consider the care repugnant.

Until diarrhea is controlled, the patient must be kept clean, dry, and free of odor. A bedpan and wipes should be kept within reach of the patient. The bedpan should be emptied as soon as possible. A deodorizer should be placed in the room. Antidiarrheal agents should be administered as ordered. If the patient has continuous diarrhea, the enterostomal therapy nurse may give helpful suggestions. Meticulous perianal skin care using plain water (no harsh soap) is necessary to treat and prevent skin breakdown. Dibucaine (Nupercaine), witch hazel, or other soothing compresses or prescribed ointment and sitz baths may reduce irritation and relieve discomfort of the anus.

■ Evaluation

The expected outcomes for the patient with ulcerative colitis are presented in NCP 40-3.

CROHN'S DISEASE

Crohn's disease is a chronic, nonspecific inflammatory bowel disorder of unknown origin that can affect any part of the GI tract. It was once thought to be a disease specific to the small intestine and was called *regional enteritis.*

Crohn's disease may occur at any age but occurs most often between the ages of 15 and 30 years. When it occurs in older adults, the morbidity and mortality rates are higher because of other chronic problems that may be present. Both sexes are affected, with a slightly higher incidence in women. Similar to ulcerative colitis, it occurs more often in Jewish and upper-middle-class urban populations. The incidence of Crohn's disease is slightly lower than that of ulcerative colitis.

40-3 NURSING CARE PLAN PATIENT WITH ULCERATIVE COLITIS

Expected Patient Outcomes	Nursing Interventions and *Rationales*
NURSING DIAGNOSIS	**Diarrhea** *related to* irritated bowel and intestinal hyperactivity *as manifested by* frequent diarrheal stools (>10 per day).
▪ Fewer, firmer stools.	▪ Monitor frequency and character of stools *to evaluate effectiveness of antidiarrheal agents and dietary restrictions.* ▪ Maintain food and fluid restrictions *to rest bowel during exacerbations.* ▪ Teach patient to avoid caffeine and foods or fluids that are *irritating to bowel or cause increased motility.* ▪ Rarely administer antidiarrheal medications *as they may precipitate colonic dilation.*
NURSING DIAGNOSIS	**Anxiety** *related to* possible social embarrassment, unfamiliar environment, diagnostic tests, and treatment *as manifested by* expression of concerns about effect of disease on social relationships, questions about disease and treatment.
▪ Less anxious feelings.	▪ Monitor signs of anxiety *to plan appropriate interventions.* ▪ Encourage open discussion of feelings about diagnosis *to demonstrate acceptance and concern for patient and allow verbalization of concerns.* ▪ Explain disease treatments, diagnostic tests, and medications *as understanding may reduce anxiety.* ▪ Provide privacy *to reduce embarrassment and anxiety associated with frequent bowel movements.*
NURSING DIAGNOSIS	**Altered nutrition: less than body requirements** *related to* decreased intake, increased nutrient loss through diarrhea and decreased absorption *as manifested by* anorexia, weight loss, weakness, lethargy, anemia.
▪ Maintenance of body weight within normal range. ▪ Adequate nutritional intake. ▪ Increased strength and activity tolerance.	▪ Assess and document signs of malnutrition (e.g., hair loss, dry skin, bleeding, fatigue) *to direct plan for treating the problem.* ▪ Record daily weights *to evaluate nutritional status and response to treatment.* ▪ Perform ongoing calorie counts *to determine adequacy of caloric intake.* ▪ Administer IV fluids and TPN as ordered *to provide nutrients for healing* and *promote fluid balance while resting the bowel.* ▪ Administer and instruct patient on high-calorie, nonspicy, caffeine-free, low-residue diet with small, frequent feedings *to reduce the amount of fecal material in the lower intestinal tract.* ▪ Administer nutritional supplements (as ordered) *to provide additional calories, protein, and fluid.* ▪ Teach patient to take small bites, eat slowly, and chew well *to facilitate digestion by slowing GI activity and breaking food down first in the mouth.*
NURSING DIAGNOSIS	**Impaired skin integrity** *related to* diarrhea and altered nutritional status *as manifested by* erythema of perianal area, discomfort around perianal area during and after evacuation, poor nutritional intake.
▪ No evidence of skin breakdown.	▪ Assess skin for signs of breakdown *to ensure early intervention.* ▪ Cleanse perianal area after each bowel movement with mild soap and warm water and dry thoroughly *to remove bacteria, provide comfort, and stimulate circulation to treat and prevent skin breakdown.* ▪ Provide sitz baths for comfort and hygiene and apply protective ointment. ▪ Encourage increased intake of proteins *to promote healing.* ▪ Instruct patient and family on proper skin care techniques *to enable them to participate fully in treatment plan.*

Continued

40-3 NURSING CARE PLAN PATIENT WITH ULCERATIVE COLITIS—continued

Expected Patient Outcomes	Nursing Interventions and *Rationales*
NURSING DIAGNOSIS	**Ineffective individual coping** *related to* chronic disease, lifestyle changes, stress, and pain *as manifested by* inability to express feelings and concerns; display of dependent, attention-getting behavior.
▪ Development of healthy coping behaviors.	▪ Identify ineffective behaviors and institute plan *to assist patient in learning more effective behaviors.* ▪ Include other staff members and family in setting limits *to provide a consistent approach.* ▪ Encourage patient's expression of feelings *to provide support as patient explores areas of concern and add to patient's feelings of self-worth.* ▪ Offer reassurance and psychologic support *to demonstrate caring and concern.* ▪ Know limitations and refer to counseling when appropriate *as more intensive treatment may be required to deal with specific stress or problem areas.*
NURSING DIAGNOSIS	**Ineffective management of therapeutic regimen** *related to* lack of knowledge of course of disease, appropriate lifestyle adjustments, and nutritional and drug interventions *as manifested by* questioning about disease and treatment, poor decisions about activities of daily living.
▪ Able to repeat correct information about disease and treatment.	▪ Provide information about the disease *to ensure patient has adequate knowledge about the disease and treatment.* ▪ Refer to dietician if complex dietary changes are necessary *to provide patient with expert counseling.* ▪ Teach about the relationship of stress to the disease *as stress may stimulate hyperreactivity of the colon in susceptible persons.* ▪ Teach stress-reduction techniques *to assist patient in developing positive ways to reduce stress.* ▪ Recommend regular appointments for colon cancer screening *as there is an increased risk of colon cancer.*

COLLABORATIVE PROBLEMS

POTENTIAL COMPLICATION	**Hypovolemia and electrolyte imbalances** *related to* fluid and electrolyte losses from diarrhea.
Nursing Goals	**Nursing Interventions and *Rationales***
▪ Monitor for signs of hypovolemia and electrolyte imbalances. ▪ Report deviations from acceptable parameters. ▪ Carry out medical and nursing interventions.	▪ Monitor for tachycardia, hypotension, weakness, dizziness, poor skin turgor, pallor, sunken eyes, rectal bleeding, abnormal serum electrolytes, urine output <0.5 ml/kg/hr *to identify hypovolemia and electrolyte imbalances and guide treatment.* ▪ Maintain accurate intake and output records; include stool volumes *to enable appropriate fluid replacement.* ▪ Administer IV fluids as ordered *to restore fluid volume.* ▪ Encourage oral intake (at least 3000 ml/day) when tolerated *to maintain fluid balance.*

TPN, total parenteral nutrition.

Etiology and Pathophysiology

Crohn's disease is characterized by inflammation of segments of the GI tract. It can affect any part of the GI tract but is most often seen in the terminal ileum, jejunum, and colon. Involvement of the esophagus, stomach, and duodenum is rare. The inflammation involves all layers of the bowel wall (i.e., transmural). Areas of involvement are usually discontinuous, with segments of normal bowel occurring between diseased portions (Table 40-17). Typically, ulcerations are deep and longitudinal and penetrate between islands of inflamed edematous mucosa, causing the classic cobblestone appearance (Fig. 40-5). Thickening of the bowel wall occurs, as well as narrowing of the lumen with stricture development. Abscesses or fistula tracts that communicate with other loops of bowel, skin, bladder, rectum, or vagina may develop. Histologically, granulomas are present in 50% of patients and may be located in any layer of the bowel wall.

Clinical Manifestations

The manifestations depend largely on the anatomical site of involvement, extent of the disease process, and presence or absence of complications. The onset of Crohn's disease is usually insidious, with nonspecific complaints such as diarrhea, fatigue, abdominal pain, weight loss, and fever. Early diagnosis

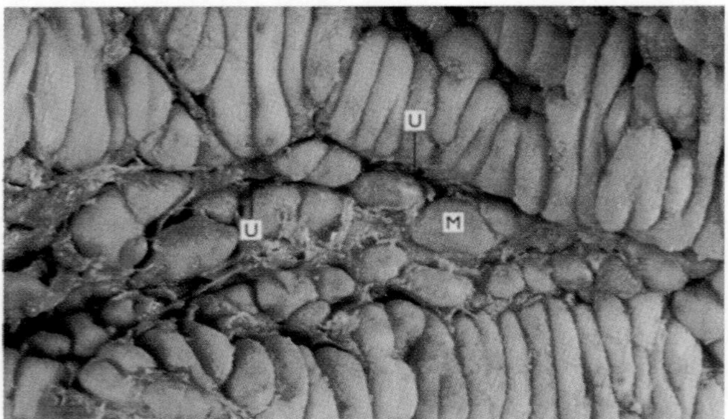

Fig. 40-5 Crohn's disease. The mucosa in Crohn's disease demonstrates a cobblestone pattern as a result of fissured ulcers (U) with intervening areas of edematous mucosa (M).

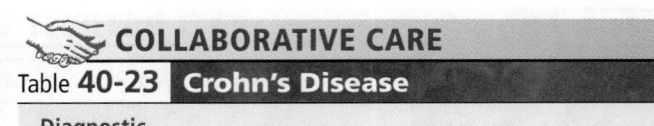

Table 40-23 Crohn's Disease

Diagnostic
- Complete blood cell count
- Serum chemistries
- Stool for occult blood
- Barium enema of small and large intestine
- Proctosigmoidoscopic examination
- Sigmoidoscopy and colonoscopy with biopsy

Collaborative Therapy
- High-calorie, high-vitamin, high-protein, low-residue, milk-free diet
- Antimicrobial agents*
- Corticosteroid drugs
- Supplementary parenteral nutrition
- Elemental diet
- Physical and emotional rest
- Surgery†

*See Table 40-20.
†See Table 40-24.

may be more difficult than for ulcerative colitis. The principal symptoms of Crohn's disease are diarrhea and abdominal pain. Diarrhea is usually nonbloody and is a result of the inflammatory process or malabsorption. Pain may be severe and intermittent or constant, depending on the cause. Other manifestations include abdominal cramping and tenderness, abdominal distention, fever, and fatigue. Extraintestinal manifestations, such as arthritis and finger clubbing, may precede the onset of bowel disease. As the disease progresses, there is weight loss, malnutrition, dehydration, electrolyte imbalances, anemia, increased peristalsis, and pain around the umbilicus and right lower quadrant.

Crohn's disease is a chronic disorder with unpredictable periods of recurrence and remission. Attacks are intermittent, usually recurring over a period of several weeks to months, with diarrhea and abdominal pain subsiding spontaneously.

Complications

Complications, both gastrointestinal and extragastrointestinal, are common in Crohn's disease. Scar tissue from the inflammation narrows the lumen of the intestine and may cause strictures and obstruction, a frequent complication. *Fistulas* are a cardinal feature and may develop between segments of bowel. Cutaneous fistulas, common in the perianal area, and rectovaginal fistulas also occur. Fistulas communicating with the urinary tract may cause urinary tract infections. Inflammation of the intestines may involve all layers, predisposing the patient to perforation and the formation of intraabdominal abscesses and peritonitis.

Impaired absorption causing various nutritional abnormalities may occur as a result of damage to areas of the intestinal mucosa. Fat malabsorption causes a deficiency in the fat-soluble vitamins (A, D, E, and K). The patient may have an intolerance to gluten (a protein found in barley, rye, and wheat).

Systemic complications are similar to those of ulcerative colitis and include arthritis, liver disease, cholelithiasis (especially with ileal involvement), ankylosing spondylitis, pyoderma gangrenosum, erythema nodosum, and uveitis. Renal disorders are common, especially nephrolithiasis (kidney stones) secondary to increased oxalate absorption.

Diagnostic Studies

Diagnosis of Crohn's disease can be made by means of a thorough history and physical examination to establish clinical signs and symptoms, barium studies, and endoscopy with biopsy (Table 40-23). Laboratory studies may determine electrolyte disturbances and the presence of anemia. Barium studies are useful in determining location and extent of the disease and may reveal classic findings, such as stricturing of the ileum (string sign), cobblestoning of the mucosa, fistulas, and areas of abnormal and normal mucosa. Endoscopic studies, such as colonoscopy and sigmoidoscopy, are useful in detecting such early mucosal changes as patchy inflammation, small ulcerations, and skip areas that may not be seen radiographically. Biopsies may be performed to determine the presence of granulomas. A small-bowel barium enema is preferred over an upper GI x-ray series with small bowel follow-through for defining mucosal abnormalities.

Collaborative Care

The goal of collaborative care is to control the inflammatory process, relieve symptoms, correct metabolic and nutritional problems, and promote healing. Drug therapy and nutritional support are the mainstays of treatment.

Drug Therapy. Sulfasalazine is effective when the disease involves the large intestine but is much less effective when only the small intestine is involved. Corticosteroid therapy is effective in reducing inflammation and suppressing disease. The dosage and the route of administration depend on the severity of the illness and the area involved. Once clinical symptoms subside, the dosage should be tapered. Immunosuppressive agents (6-MP, azathioprine) may be tried if repeated trials with corticosteroids fail. Patients require close monitoring because of the serious side effects of these drugs.

Table 40-24 Indications for Surgical Management of Crohn's Disease

Drainage of abdominal abscess	Intestinal obstruction
Failure to respond to conservative therapy	Massive hemorrhage
Fistulas	Perforation
Growth retardation	Secondary hydronephrosis
Inability to decrease corticosteroids	Severe anorectal disease
	Suspicion of carcinoma

Metronidazole (Flagyl) is useful in treating Crohn's disease of the perianal area. Marked exacerbations have been reported when the drug is stopped. Fish oil preparations have been evaluated for their ability to prevent recurrence of inflammation in Crohn's patients in remission; however, their palatability has been low.[20]

Balloon dilation of strictures may be effective in relieving symptoms in some patients. This is usually performed through a colonoscope or under fluoroscopic guidance. Strictures most often dilated are those in the colon or small bowel.

Nutritional Therapy. Elemental diets and parenteral nutrition may be used in the patient with Crohn's disease (see Chapter 38). Parenteral nutrition may be given to patients with severe disease, small-bowel fistulas, or short bowel syndrome (described later in this chapter). It is given before and after surgery to promote wound healing, reduce complications, and hasten recovery. The elemental diet provides a high-calorie, high-nitrogen, fat-free, no-residue substrate that is absorbed in the proximal small bowel. This diet can be given to most patients with Crohn's disease, even during acute exacerbations.

The diet should otherwise be low in residue, roughage, and fat but high in calories and protein. It may be difficult to maintain adequate absorption during periods of disease exacerbation and even during periods of remission. Milk and milk products may need to be excluded from the diet. Lactose, the primary disaccharide found in milk, may not be adequately absorbed because of the inability of the damaged mucosa of the intestine to produce adequate amounts of lactase. High-fat diets are poorly tolerated because of the loss of absorbing mucosa and altered bile salt metabolism and absorption.

Vitamin deficiencies may develop as a result of malabsorption. Cobalamin (vitamin B_{12}) injections every month may be needed because of the inability of the terminal ileum (if affected) to absorb this vitamin.

Surgical Therapy. Surgery is used in patients with severe symptoms that are unresponsive to therapy and in those with life-threatening complications. The majority of patients with Crohn's disease eventually require surgery at least once in the course of their disease. Indications for surgery are outlined in Table 40-24. Unlike ulcerative colitis, which can be cured by total proctocolectomy, Crohn's disease is not cured by surgery. The recurrence rate after surgery is high. The surgical procedure depends on the affected area and the condition of the patient. Conservative intestinal resection with anastomosis of healthy bowel is the procedure of choice.

NURSING MANAGEMENT: CROHN'S DISEASE

Care of the patient is similar to that of the patient with ulcerative colitis (see NCP 40-3 and p. 1160). As the patient's condition improves, the nurse should allow for more self-care, provide frequent rest periods, and advise the patient of the importance of rest and avoidance or control of emotional stress. Initially this may be difficult for the patient when told the nature of the disease and the limitations of the treatment. Patients who have perianal fistulas or abscesses may need special skin care. Postoperative care should be the same as for exploratory laparotomy.

In the majority of patients with Crohn's disease the course is chronic and intermittent, regardless of the site of involvement. The patient and significant others may need help in setting realistic short-term and long-term goals. Teaching is important and should include (1) the importance of rest and diet management, (2) perianal care, (3) action and side effects of medications, (4) symptoms of recurrence of disease, (5) when to seek medical care, and (6) use of diversional activities to reduce stress.

GERONTOLOGIC CONSIDERATIONS

Inflammatory Bowel Disease

Although inflammatory bowel diseases (i.e., ulcerative colitis and Crohn's disease) are considered diseases of young adults, a second peak in the distribution of these inflammatory conditions occurs around the age of 70 years. The pathogenesis, natural history, and clinical course of ulcerative colitis and Crohn's disease in older adults are similar to those observed in younger patients. However, the distribution of the inflammation appears to be somewhat different. In the older patient with ulcerative colitis the distal colon (proctitis) is usually involved. In the older patient with Crohn's disease the colon rather than the small intestine tends to be involved. There tends to be less recurrence of Crohn's disease in older patients treated with surgical resection. The degree of inflammation associated with both conditions tends to be less in the older adult than in the younger patient.

Collaborative care of the older patient with one of these conditions is similar to the younger patient. However, because of increased risk of cardiovascular and pulmonary complications, older adults tend to have increased morbidity associated with surgical procedures.

In addition to Crohn's disease and ulcerative colitis, older adults are also vulnerable to inflammation of the colon (colitis) from medication use and systemic vascular disease. Drugs such as nonsteroidal antiinflammatory drugs (NSAIDs), digitalis, vasopressin, estrogen, and allopurinol (Zyloprim) have been associated with colitis development in the elderly patient. Colitis may also be secondary to ischemic bowel disease related to atherosclerosis and congestive heart failure.

Inflammation of the colon as a result of IBD or colitis results in diarrhea, which may be bloody. The loss of fluid and electrolytes and possibly blood may leave the older adult more vulnerable to problems related to volume depletion and dehydration. This may be particularly problematic in the patient with diminished renal and cardiovascular function. Thus

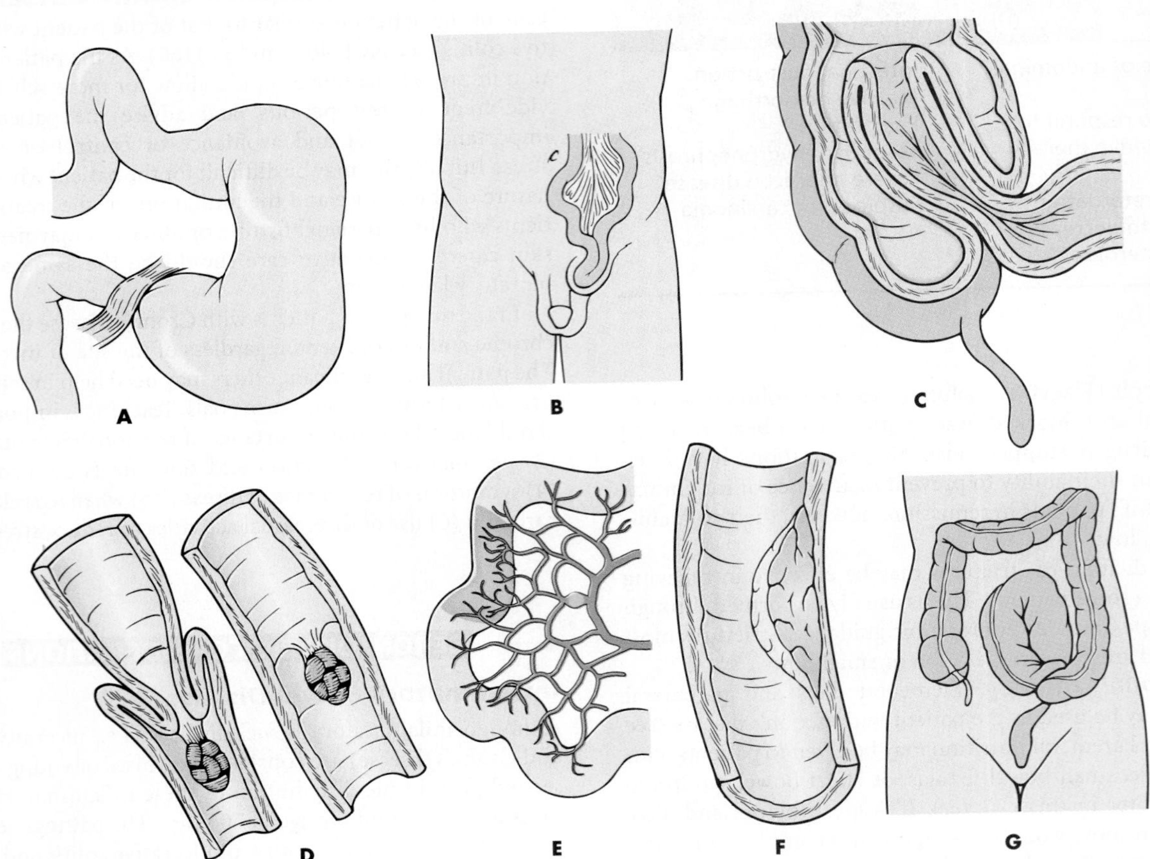

Fig. 40-6 Bowel obstructions. **A,** Adhesions. **B,** Strangulated inguinal hernia. **C,** Ileocecal intussusception. **D,** Intussusception from polyps. **E,** Mesenteric occlusion. **F,** Neoplasm. **G,** Volvulus of the sigmoid colon.

nursing management is focused on careful assessment of fluid and electrolyte status and evaluation of the replacement therapies.

INTESTINAL OBSTRUCTION

Intestinal obstruction occurs when intestinal contents cannot pass through the GI tract, and it requires prompt treatment. The obstruction may be partial or complete. The causes of intestinal obstruction can be classified as *mechanical* or *nonmechanical.*

Types of Intestinal Obstruction

Mechanical. Mechanical obstruction may be caused by an occlusion of the lumen of the intestinal tract. Most intestinal obstructions occur in the small intestine, most often in the ileum. Mechanical obstruction accounts for 90% of all intestinal obstructions (Fig. 40-6).[21] Adhesions account for 50%, hernias for 15%, and neoplasms for 15% of obstructions of the small intestine. Adhesions can develop after abdominal surgery. Obstruction can occur within days of surgery or years later. Carcinoma is the most common cause of large bowel obstruction, followed by volvulus and diverticular disease.

Nonmechanical. A nonmechanical obstruction may result from a neuromuscular or vascular disorder. *Paralytic (adynamic) ileus* is the most common form of nonmechanical obstruction. It occurs to some degree after any abdominal surgery. Other causes of paralytic ileus include inflammatory responses (e.g., acute pancreatitis, acute appendicitis), electrolyte abnormalities, and thoracic or lumbar spinal fractures.

Pseudoobstruction is an apparent mechanical obstruction of the intestine without demonstration of obstruction by radiographic methods. Collagen vascular diseases and neurologic and endocrine disorders may cause pseudoobstruction, but mostly it is found to be idiopathic.

Vascular obstructions are rare and are due to an interference with the blood supply to a portion of the intestines. The most common causes are emboli and atherosclerosis of the mesenteric arteries. The celiac, inferior, and superior mesenteric arteries supply blood to the bowel. Emboli may originate from thrombi in patients with chronic atrial fibrillation, diseased heart valves, and prosthetic valves. Venous thrombosis may be seen in low-blood-flow states, such as heart failure and shock.

Etiology and Pathophysiology

Normally 6 to 8 L of fluid enters the small bowel daily. Most of the fluid is absorbed before it reaches the colon. Approximately 75% of intestinal gas is swallowed air. Bacterial metabolism produces methane and hydrogen gases. Fluid, gas, and intestinal contents accumulate proximal to the intestinal obstruction. This causes distention, and the distal bowel may collapse. The distention reduces the absorption of fluids and

Table 40-25 Clinical Manifestations of Small and Large Intestinal Obstructions

Clinical Manifestation	Small Intestine	Large Intestine
Onset	Rapid	Gradual
Vomiting	Frequent and copious	Rare
Pain	Colicky, cramplike, intermittent	Low-grade, crampy abdominal pain
Bowel movement	Feces for a short time	Absolute constipation
Abdominal distention	Minimally increased	Greatly increased

stimulates intestinal secretions. As the fluid increases, so does the pressure in the lumen of the bowel. The increased pressure leads to an increase in capillary permeability and extravasation of fluids and electrolytes into the peritoneal cavity. Edema, congestion, and necrosis from impaired blood supply and possible rupture of the bowel may occur. The retention of fluid in the intestine and peritoneal cavity can lead to a severe reduction in circulating blood volume and result in hypotension and hypovolemic shock.

The electrolyte-rich fluids, which are normally absorbed in the bowel, are retained in the bowel and subsequently lost into the peritoneal cavity. The location of the obstruction determines the extent of fluid, electrolyte, and acid-base imbalances. If the obstruction is high, as in the pylorus, metabolic alkalosis may result from the loss of hydrochloric acid from the stomach through vomiting or NG intubation.

When the obstruction is located in the small bowel, dehydration occurs rapidly. Dehydration and electrolyte imbalances do not occur early in large bowel obstruction. If the obstruction is below the proximal colon, most GI fluids have been absorbed before reaching the point of the obstruction. Solid fecal material accumulates until symptoms of discomfort appear. Reverse peristalsis may cause vomiting of fecal material very late in the bowel obstruction.

Simple obstructions of the intestine involve blockage of the lumen in one spot. A closed-loop obstruction occurs when the lumen is blocked in two different spots (e.g., volvulus). This results in an isolated segment of bowel and obstruction proximal to that segment. Strangulation and gangrene are likely to develop if treatment is not immediate. A strangulated obstruction occurs when the circulation to the obstructed intestine is impaired. This is the most dangerous form of obstruction because it may lead to necrosis of the intestine (incarcerated). Volvulus, hernias, or adhesions are the most common causes.

Clinical Manifestations

The clinical manifestations of intestinal obstruction vary, depending on the location of the obstruction, and include nausea, vomiting, abdominal pain, distention, inability to pass flatus, and obstipation (Table 40-25). Obstruction located high in the small intestine produces rapid-onset, sometimes projectile vomiting with bile-containing vomitus. Vomiting from more distal obstructions of the small intestine is more gradual in onset. The vomitus may be orange-brown and foul smelling because of bacterial overgrowth. Vomiting may be entirely absent in large bowel obstruction if the ileocecal valve is competent; otherwise, the patient may eventually vomit feculent material.

Vomiting usually relieves abdominal pain in high intestinal obstructions. Persistent, colicky abdominal pain is seen with lower intestinal obstruction. A characteristic sign of mechanical obstruction is pain that comes and goes in waves. This is due to intestinal peristalsis trying to move bowel contents past the obstructed area. In contrast, paralytic ileus produces a more constant generalized discomfort. Strangulation causes severe, constant pain that is rapid in onset. Abdominal distention is a common manifestation of intestinal obstructions. It is usually absent or minimally noticeable in high obstructions of the small intestine and greatly increased in lower intestinal obstructions. Abdominal tenderness and rigidity are usually absent unless strangulation or peritonitis has occurred.

Auscultation of bowel sounds reveals high-pitched sounds above the area of obstruction. The patient often notes audible borborygmi. The patient's temperature rarely rises above 100° F (37.8° C) unless strangulation or peritonitis has occurred.

Diagnostic Studies

A thorough history and physical examination should be performed. Abdominal x-rays are the most useful diagnostic aids. Upright and lateral abdominal x-rays show the presence of gas and fluid in the intestines. The presence of intraperitoneal air indicates perforation. Barium enemas are helpful in locating large intestinal obstructions. However, barium is not used if perforation is suspected. If the location is unknown, a lower GI tract study is done before an upper GI series. Sigmoidoscopy or colonoscopy may provide direct visualization of an obstruction in the colon.

Laboratory tests are important and provide essential information. A CBC and serum electrolyte, amylase, and blood urea nitrogen (BUN) determinations should be performed. An elevated WBC count may indicate strangulation or perforation; elevated hematocrit values may reflect hemoconcentration. Decreased hemoglobin and hematocrit values may indicate bleeding from a neoplasm or strangulation with necrosis. Serum electrolytes should be monitored frequently. They provide essential information on the patient's fluid and electrolyte balance. Serum sodium, potassium, and chloride concentrations are decreased in small bowel obstruction. The BUN value may be increased because of dehydration. The stool should be checked for occult blood.

Collaborative Care

Treatment is directed toward decompression of the intestine by removal of gas and fluid, correction and maintenance of fluid and electrolyte balance, and relief or removal of the obstruction. NG or intestinal tubes (Fig. 40-7) may be used to decompress the bowel. NG tubes should be inserted before surgery to empty the stomach and relieve distention. They are also used instead of nasointestinal tubes to treat partial or complete small-bowel obstruction. Intestinal tubes, such as the Cantor or Miller-Abbott tubes, are passed into the small intestine. They are 10 feet (300 cm) long and mercury weighted.

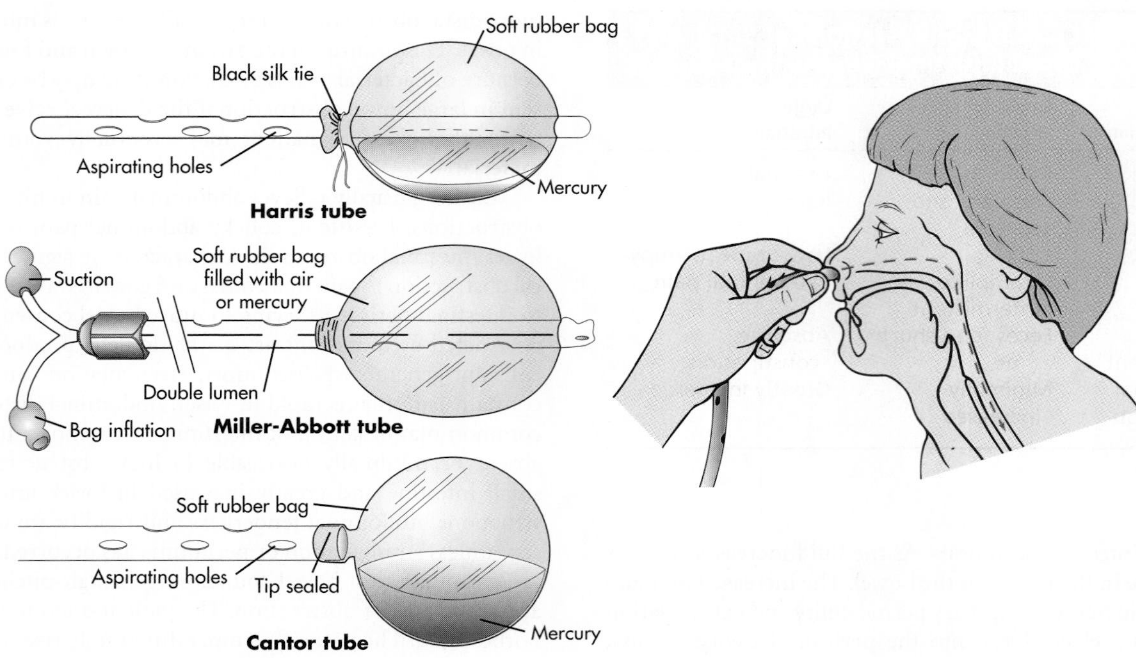

Fig. 40-7 Intestinal tubes used for decompression.

Insertion of an intestinal tube is controversial. Use of a long intestinal tube is difficult and time consuming. Some clinicians believe there is inadequate gastric decompression once the tube is in the small intestine. NG or intestinal tubes are effective in the treatment of patients with neurogenic obstruction who do not require surgery.

Sigmoidoscopy may successfully reduce a sigmoid volvulus. Colon-decompression catheters may be passed through partially obstructed areas via a colonoscope to decompress the bowel before surgery.

IV infusions that contain normal saline solution and potassium should be given to maintain fluid and electrolyte balance. Total parenteral nutrition may be necessary in some cases to correct nutritional deficiencies, improve the patient's nutritional status before surgery, and promote postoperative healing.

Most mechanical obstructions are treated surgically. They may involve simply resecting the obstructed segment of bowel and anastomosing the remaining healthy bowel. Partial or total colectomy, colostomy, or ileostomy may be required when extensive obstruction or necrosis is present. Occasionally obstructions can be removed nonsurgically. A colonoscope can be used to remove polyps, dilate strictures, and remove and necrose tumors with a laser.

NURSING MANAGEMENT: INTESTINAL OBSTRUCTION

■ Nursing Assessment

Intestinal obstruction is a potentially life-threatening condition. Signs and symptoms are varied. Nursing assessment must begin with a detailed patient history and physical examination. The type and location of obstruction usually cause characteristic symptoms. The nurse should determine the location, duration, intensity, and frequency of abdominal pain and whether abdominal tenderness or rigidity is present. Onset, frequency, color, odor, and amount of vomitus should be recorded. Bowel function, including passage of flatus, should be determined. The nurse should auscultate for bowel sounds and document character and location; inspect the abdomen for scars, palpable masses, and distention; and observe for muscle guarding and tenderness.

■ Nursing Diagnoses

Nursing diagnoses for the patient with intestinal obstructions include, but are not limited to, the following:

- Pain *related to* abdominal distention and increased peristalsis
- Fluid volume deficit *related to* decrease in intestinal fluid absorption and loss of fluids secondary to vomiting
- Altered nutrition: less than body requirements *related to* intestinal obstruction and vomiting

■ Planning

The overall goals are that the patient with an intestinal obstruction will have (1) relief of the obstruction and return to normal bowel function, (2) minimal to no discomfort, and (3) normal fluid and electrolyte status.

■ Nursing Implementation

The patient should be monitored closely for signs of dehydration and electrolyte imbalance. A strict intake and output record should be maintained. All vomitus and tube drainage should be included. IV fluids should be administered as ordered. Serum electrolyte levels should be monitored closely. A patient with a high obstruction is more likely to have metabolic alkalosis; a patient with a low obstruction is at greater risk of

Table 40-26 Types of Polyps of the Large Intestine

Neoplastic	Nonneoplastic
Epithelial polyps (adenomatous)	Epithelial polyps (hyperplastic)
Tubular adenoma	Hereditary polyposis syndromes (hamartomatous polyposis syndrome)
Tubular villous adenoma	Familial juvenile polyposis
Villous adenoma	Peutz-Jeghers syndrome
Hereditary polyposis syndromes (adenomatous polyposis syndrome)	Inflammatory polyps
Familial adenomatous polyposis	Pseudopolyps
Gardner syndrome	Benign lymphoid polyp
	Submucosal polyps
	Lipomas
	Leiomyomas
	Fibromas

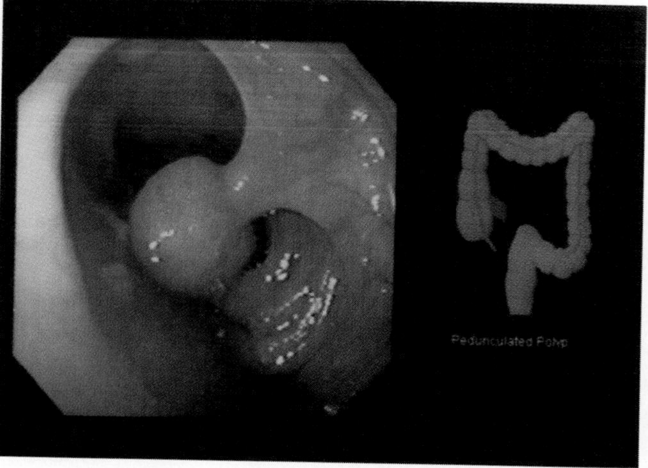

Fig. 40-8 Endoscopic image of pedunculated polyp in descending colon.

metabolic acidosis. The patient is often restless and constantly changes position to relieve the pain. Analgesics may be withheld until the obstruction is diagnosed because they may mask other signs and symptoms and decrease intestinal motility. The nurse should provide comfort measures, promote a restful environment, and keep distractions and visitors to a minimum. Nursing care of the patient after surgery for an intestinal obstruction is similar to care of the patient after a laparotomy (see NCP 40-2).

Care of Nasogastric and Intestinal Tubes. Although the physician usually inserts intestinal tubes, the nurse assists with the procedure. Insertion is easier if the patient relaxes, takes deep breaths, and swallows when instructed. If insertion of the tube to the small intestine is desired, the patient may be instructed or positioned to lie on the right side to facilitate tube passage through the pylorus. In some situations a prokinetic drug such as metoclopramide (Reglan) may be used to facilitate tube movement.

Once the tube is in place, mouth care is extremely important. Vomiting leaves a terrible taste in the patient's mouth, and fecal odor may be present. When an NG tube is in place, the patient breathes through the mouth, drying the mouth and lips. The nurse should encourage and assist the patient to brush the teeth frequently. Mouthwash and water for the patient to use in rinsing the mouth and petroleum jelly or water-soluble lubricant for the lips should be provided at the bedside.

The patient's nose should be checked for signs of irritation from the NG tube. This area should be cleaned and dried daily with application of a water-soluble lubricant and retaping of the tube. NG and intestinal tubes should be checked every 4 hours for patency. The patient may be placed on a schedule to clamp the tube for 1 hour out of every 3 hours or for 3 out of every 4 hours before removal of the tube.

POLYPS OF THE LARGE INTESTINE

Colonic polyps arise from the mucosal surface of the colon and project into the lumen. They may be *sessile* (flat, broad-based, and attached directly to the intestinal wall) or *pedunculated* (attached to the intestinal wall by a thin stalk). Polyps tend to be sessile when small and become pedunculated as they enlarge, especially if they are in the left or descending colon (Fig. 40-8).[22] They may be found anywhere in the large intestine but are most commonly found in the rectosigmoid area. Although most polyps are asymptomatic, rectal bleeding or occult blood in the stool are the most common symptoms.

TYPES OF POLYPS

The most common types of polyp are *hyperplastic* and *adenomatous.* Hyperplastic polyps originate from the epithelium and are nonneoplastic growths. They rarely grow larger than 5 mm in size and never cause clinical symptoms. Other benign (nonneoplastic) polyps include inflammatory polyps, lipomas, and juvenile polyps (Table 40-26).

Adenomatous polyps are characterized by neoplastic changes in the epithelium. They are closely linked to colorectal adenocarcinoma. Structurally, there are three types, with tubular adenomas being the most prevalent. The risk of cancer in the polyp increases with polyp size and villous structure. Villous adenomas have a higher risk of turning cancerous than tubular adenomas.[22]

Although there are several polyposis syndromes, they are relatively rare. Of these, *familial adenomatous polyposis* (FAP) is the most common. This disorder is characterized by multiple polyps that at times number in the thousands and that are located in the large intestine and sometimes in other areas of the GI tract. Patients with a history of FAP have lifetime risk of developing colorectal cancer that approaches 100%. They also develop cancer at an earlier age (i.e., 40 years of age) than patients with non-FAP colon cancer. For children of patients with FAP, screening must be initiated at puberty and then conducted annually. There is a 50% risk for these children to develop FAP. When there is indication of disease, total colectomy with ileostomy is the treatment of choice.[22]

Diagnostic Studies and Collaborative Care

Barium enema, sigmoidoscopy, and colonoscopy are used to make diagnosis of polyps. All polyps are considered abnormal

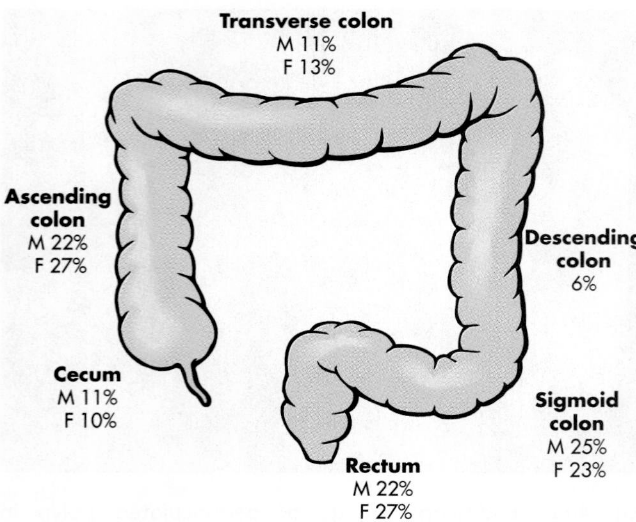

Fig. 40-9 Incidence of cancer. Approximately one half of all colon cancers occur in the rectosigmoid area. Percentages are listed for men and women.

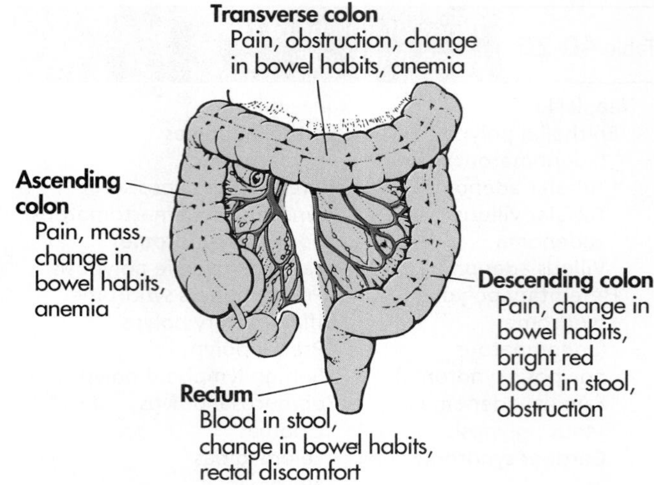

Fig. 40-10 Signs and symptoms of colorectal cancer by location of primary lesion.

Table 40-27 Risk Factors for Colorectal Cancer

Age
Familial polyposis
Colorectal polyps
Chronic IBD
Family history of colorectal cancer or adenomas
Previous history of colorectal cancer
History of genital or breast cancer (women)
High-fat and/or low-fiber diet

IBD, inflammatory bowel disease.

and should be removed. In patients whose polyps are identified through barium enema, removal (polypectomy) should be done through a colonoscope or a sigmoidoscope. If the polyp is not removable, a biopsy specimen should be taken for tissue examination. Surgery is not indicated unless carcinoma is present or in certain cases of polyposis syndromes. The patient should be observed for rectal bleeding, fever, severe abdominal pain, and abdominal distention, which may indicate hemorrhage or perforation.

CANCER OF THE COLON AND RECTUM

Colorectal cancer is the second most common cause of cancer death in the United States.[23] Death rates from colorectal cancer in the United States and Canada are approximately 16.5 per 100,000 males and 11 per 100,000 females, accounting for approximately 56,500 deaths.[24] In 1998, there were approximately 131,600 new cases of colorectal cancer in the United States.[24] Cancer of the colon and rectum may occur at any age but is most prevalent over the age of 50 years. The 5-year survival rate for early, localized colorectal cancers is 91% and 63% for cancer spread to adjacent organs and lymph nodes.[24]

The incidence of cancer at specific sites in the colon varies (Fig. 40-9). In both sexes, the incidence of right colon cancers has increased and cancers in the rectum have decreased. The highest percentages of colorectal cancers in the United States are currently located in the cecum, ascending colon, and sigmoid colon. Approximately 20% of colorectal cancers are within reach of the examining finger, and 50% are within reach of the sigmoidoscope.

Etiology and Pathophysiology

The causes of colorectal cancer remain unclear. Groups at high risk of colorectal cancer have been identified (Table 40-27). Age is a risk factor in both men and women. The risk for development in the general population increases slightly after the age of 40 years and then rises rapidly in the following decades. Diet is the most important environmental factor associated with colorectal cancer. The high-calorie, high-fat Western diet has been closely associated with development of colon cancer.

Adenocarcinoma is the most common type of colon cancer. Most colorectal cancers appear to arise from adenomatous polyps. All tumors tend to spread through the walls of the intestine and into the lymphatic system. Tumors commonly spread to the liver because the venous blood flow from the colorectal tumor is through the portal vein.

Clinical Manifestations

Clinical manifestations of colon cancer are usually nonspecific or do not appear until the disease is advanced. Cancer on the right side of the colon gives rise to clinical manifestations that are different from those on the left side of the colon.[25] Rectal bleeding, the most common symptom of colorectal cancer, is most often seen with left-sided lesions. Other commonly seen manifestations of left-sided lesions include alternating constipation and diarrhea, change in stool caliber (narrow, ribbon-like), and sensation of incomplete evacuation. Obstruction symptoms appear earlier with left-sided lesions because of the smaller lumen size (Fig. 40-10).

Cancers of the right side of the colon are usually asymptomatic. Vague abdominal discomfort or crampy, colicky abdominal pain may be present. Iron deficiency anemia and occult bleeding dictate further investigation. Weakness and fatigue result from anemia.

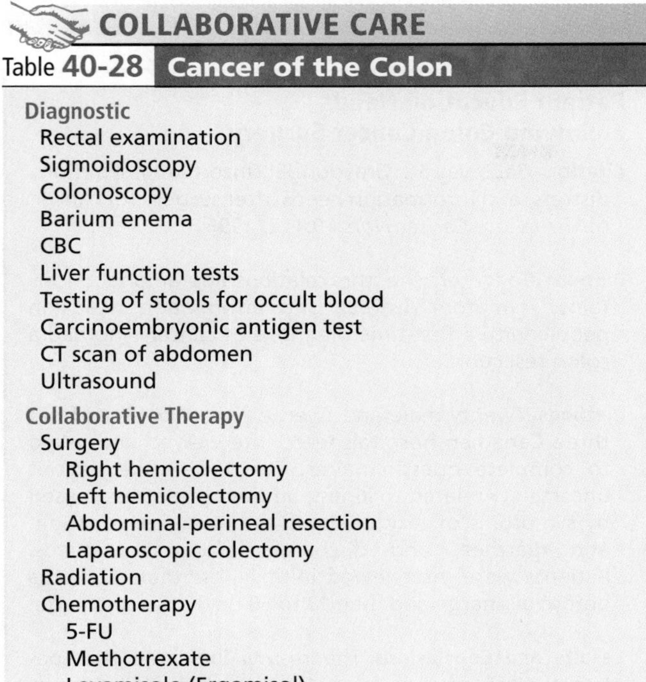

COLLABORATIVE CARE

Table 40-28 Cancer of the Colon

Diagnostic
- Rectal examination
- Sigmoidoscopy
- Colonoscopy
- Barium enema
- CBC
- Liver function tests
- Testing of stools for occult blood
- Carcinoembryonic antigen test
- CT scan of abdomen
- Ultrasound

Collaborative Therapy
- Surgery
  - Right hemicolectomy
  - Left hemicolectomy
  - Abdominal-perineal resection
  - Laparoscopic colectomy
- Radiation
- Chemotherapy
  - 5-FU
  - Methotrexate
  - Levamisole (Ergamisol)
  - Irinotecan (Camptosar)

Diagnostic Studies

A thorough history with close attention to family history should be obtained, and a physical examination should be performed initially (Table 40-28). The digital rectal examination is the most important aspect of the physical examination because many rectal cancers are within reach of the finger. In the asymptomatic person who is 50 years or older with no risk factors (other than age), fecal occult blood testing once a year and flexible sigmoidoscopy every 5 years beginning at age 50 years are important aspects of the examination.[26] If colorectal cancer is suspected, examinations with the flexible sigmoidoscope and an air-contrast barium enema (in combination) are often performed. Colonoscopy is the procedure of choice if a questionable lesion is seen on barium enema or sigmoidoscopy. Other procedures include endorectal ultrasonography and a CT scan of the abdomen and pelvis to localize the lesion or determine its size. Synchronous lesions may be present at other sites in the colon, and tissue diagnosis may be made by brushing or biopsy during the procedure.

Laboratory studies should include a CBC to check for anemia, clotting studies, and liver function tests. A CT scan of the abdomen may be helpful in detecting liver metastases, retroperitoneal and pelvic disease, and depth of penetration of tumor into the bowel wall. A CT scan should be done before surgery. Liver function tests are performed to determine liver metastases.

A carcinoembryonic antigen (CEA) test is often performed, although it is not specific for colon cancer. A normal level of CEA does not exclude the possibility of a malignant condition. This test is used most effectively in following the progress of a patient after surgery. Return to normal of a previously elevated CEA indicates successful removal of the tumor. In contrast, persistent postoperative elevated or increasing CEA levels suggest residual tumor or tumor spread.

Table 40-29 Dukes' Staging System for Colorectal Carcinoma

Classification	Description
A	Negative nodes, limitation of lesion to mucosa
B_1	Negative nodes, extension of lesion through mucosa but still within bowel wall
B_2	Negative nodes, extension through entire bowel wall
C_1	Positive nodes, limitation of lesion to bowel wall
C_2	Positive nodes, extension of lesion through entire bowel wall
D	Presence of distant, unresectable metastases

Collaborative Care

Prognosis and treatment correlate with pathologic staging of the disease. Several methods of staging are currently being used. The most widely known is Dukes' classification (Table 40-29). Surgical removal of the primary lesion is the treatment for Dukes' stages A, B, and C. Prognosis for Dukes' stage A is 90% to 100% 5-year survival compared with less than 15% with Dukes' stage D.

The most recent classification of colorectal cancer is the TNM system (Table 40-30), which is based on pathologic assessment and includes data from the history and physical examination and presurgical endoscopic and laboratory evaluations. Cancer of the colon can also be divided into stages, with stage 0 representing cancer in situ, stage I corresponding to Dukes' A and B_1, stage II corresponding to B_2, stage III corresponding to C_1 and C_2, and stage IV corresponding to Dukes' D.

Several noninvasive procedures may be performed through a colonoscope to effectively treat certain types of colorectal cancer. Endoscopic polypectomy is a highly effective and safe procedure. Adequate treatment is thought to be obtained if the resected margin of the polyp is free of cancer, the cancer is well differentiated, and there is no apparent lymphatic or blood vessel involvement. Laser therapy may be used to ablate nonresectable tumors. This is usually used only as palliative therapy in patients with obstructive symptoms.

Surgical Therapy. Surgery is the only curative treatment of colorectal cancer. The location and extent of the cancer determine the type of surgery performed. Success of surgery depends on resection of the tumor with an adequate margin of healthy bowel and resection of the regional lymph nodes.

Right hemicolectomy is performed when the cancer is located in the cecum, ascending colon, hepatic flexure, or transverse colon to the right of the middle colic artery. A portion of the terminal ileum, the ileocecal valve, and the appendix are removed, and an ileotransverse anastomosis is performed. A *left hemicolectomy* involves resection of the left transverse colon, the splenic flexure, the descending colon, the sigmoid colon, and the upper portion of the rectum.

Table 40-30 Tumor-Node-Metastasis (TNM) Classification of Colon and Rectal Cancer

T	**Primary Tumor**
TX	Primary tumor cannot be assessed
TO	No evidence of primary tumor
Tis	Carcinoma in situ
T1	Tumor invades submucosa
T2	Tumor invades muscularis propria
T3	Tumor invades through the muscularis propria into the subserosa, or into nonperitonealized pericolic or perirectal tissues
T4	Tumor perforates the visceral peritoneum, or directly invades other organs or structures
N	**Regional Lymph Node Involvement**
NX	Regional lymph node cannot be assessed
NO	No regional lymph node metastasis
N1	Metastasis in 1 to 3 pericolic or perirectal lymph nodes
N2	Metastasis in 4 or more pericolic or perirectal lymph nodes
N3	Metastasis in any lymph node along the course of a named vascular trunk
M	**Distant Metastasis**
MX	Presence of distant metastasis cannot be assessed
MO	No distant metastasis
MI	Distant metastasis

RESEARCH
IMPLICATIONS FOR NURSING PRACTICE

Patient Education Needs Following Colon Cancer Surgery

Citation Galloway SC, Graydon JE: Uncertainty, symptom distress, and information needs after surgery for cancer of the colon, *Cancer Nurs* 19:112, 1996.

Purpose To determine the relationships among uncertainty, symptom distress, and information needs in people with a first-time diagnosis of cancer who had a colon resection.

Methods Twenty male and twenty female patients from three Canadian hospitals were interviewed and asked to complete questionnaires. The tools asked about uncertainty related to illness; amount of distress caused by symptoms of fatigue, pain, anorexia, constipation, and diarrhea; and discharge information needs. Patients were interviewed initially less than 72 hours before discharge and then 13 to 60 days after discharge.

Results and Conclusions The results indicated that patients after surgery for colon cancer had moderate levels of uncertainty and low levels of symptom distress. The most distressing symptom was fatigue followed by pain. As uncertainty increased, patients had a greater need for discharge information. Patients perceived information related to treatment, actions to take if a complication occurred, guidelines about diet and activity, and management of symptoms as important.

Implications for Nursing Practice Information about the impact of cancer on physical functioning appears to take priority over information about community resources and how to handle feelings about cancer in the early postoperative period. Discharge teaching should include explanations of follow-up treatments, possible complications, and how to manage symptoms such as pain and fatigue. Discharge teaching should be individualized, since many patients can predict their needs for information at the time of discharge.

Clear margins are most difficult to obtain with rectal carcinoma. Location of the rectal lesion determines the surgical procedure to be performed. There must be enough rectum left to ensure a secure anastomosis, or an abdominal-perineal resection is indicated. *Abdominal-perineal resection* is most often performed when the cancer is located within 5 cm of the anus.

In the abdominal-perineal resection, an abdominal incision is made and the proximal sigmoid is brought through the abdominal wall in a permanent colostomy. The distal sigmoid, rectum, and anus are removed through a perineal incision. The perineal wound may be closed around a drain or left open with packing to allow healing by granulation. Complications that can occur are delayed wound healing, hemorrhage, persistent perineal sinus tracts, infections, and urinary tract and sexual dysfunctions.

Low anterior resection may be indicated for tumors of the rectosigmoid and the mid-to-upper rectum. The use of EEA (end-to-end anastomosis) staplers has allowed lower and more secure anastomoses. The stapler is passed through the anus, where the colon is stapled to the rectum. This technique has made it possible to resect lesions as low as 5 cm from the anus.

Sphincter-sparing procedures are being performed on the patient who is a poor operative risk and for the patient with early disease. The number of these procedures may increase with continued early detection and surveillance. In these procedures a local resection is performed and the anal sphincters are left intact.

Laparoscopic colectomy is being evaluated for its effectiveness in eliminating cancer and improving survival. Potential benefits are reduced pain, shortened hospital stay, and improved cosmetic appearance.[27]

Radiation Therapy and Chemotherapy. Radiation may be used preoperatively or as a palliative measure for patients with advanced lesions. As a palliative measure, its primary objective is to reduce tumor size and provide symptomatic relief. (For discussion on radiation therapy, see Chapter 14.) Chemotherapy is recommended when a patient has positive lymph nodes at the time of surgery or has metastatic disease. No drug is available that can cure malignant colon or rectal tumors. The most commonly used drugs are 5-fluorouracil (5-FU) and methotrexate. Levamisole (Ergamisol), BCNU, and MeCCNU are sometimes used in combination with 5-FU. Irinotecan (Camptosar) is used for the treatment of metastatic colorectal cancer. New agents being examined for adjuvant therapy of colorectal cancer include leucovorin, monoclonal antibody to epithelial antigen 17-1A, and tegafur-4M uracil (UFT).[28]

NURSING ASSESSMENT

Table 40-31 Colorectal Cancer

Subjective Data	Objective Data
Important Health Information *Past health history:* Previous breast or gynecologic cancer; familial polyposis; villous adenoma; adenomatous polyps; inflammatory bowel disease *Medications:* Use of any medications affecting bowel function (e.g., cathartics, antidiarrheal medication) **Functional Health Patterns** *Health perception–health management:* Family history of cancer, especially colon or breast; weakness, fatigue *Nutritional-metabolic:* High-calorie, high-fat, low-fiber diet; anorexia, weight loss; nausea and vomiting *Elimination:* Change in bowel habits; alternating diarrhea and constipation, defecation urgency; rectal bleeding; mucoid stools; black, tarry stools; increased flatus, decrease in stool caliber; feelings of incomplete evacuation *Cognitive-perceptual:* Abdominal and low back pain, tenesmus	**General** Pallor, cachexia, lymphadenopathy (later signs) **Gastrointestinal** Palpable abdominal mass, distention, ascites and hepatomegaly (liver metastasis) **Possible Findings** Anemia; guaiac-positive stools, palpable mass on digital rectal examination; positive proctosigmoidoscopy, colonoscopy, barium enema, or CT scan; positive biopsy

NURSING MANAGEMENT: COLON AND RECTAL CANCER

■ Nursing Assessment

Subjective and objective data that should be obtained from a patient with cancer of the colon or rectum are presented in Table 40-31.

■ Nursing Diagnoses

Nursing diagnoses for the patient with cancer of the colon or rectum include, but are not limited to, the following:

- Diarrhea or constipation *related to* altered bowel elimination patterns
- Pain *related to* difficulty in passing stools because of partial or complete obstruction from tumor
- Fear *related to* diagnosis of colon cancer, surgical or therapeutic interventions, and possible terminal illness
- Ineffective individual coping *related to* diagnosis of cancer and side effects of treatment

■ Planning

The overall goals are that the patient with cancer of the colon or rectum will have (1) no metastasis or recurrence of the cancer, (2) normal bowel elimination patterns, (3) quality of life appropriate to disease progression, (4) relief of pain, and (5) feelings of comfort and well-being.

■ Nursing Implementation

Health Promotion. The current recommendations from the American Cancer Society for colorectal cancer screening in patients who are not at high risk include annual digital rectal examination beginning at the age of 40 years. Starting at the age of 50 years, fecal testing for occult blood should be done every year, and flexible sigmoidoscopy should be performed every 5 years. Positive findings should be followed with colonoscopy or air-contrast barium enema.[26]

Screening for high-risk patients usually begins with colonoscopy and continues at more frequent intervals that vary according to risk factors.[29] Participation in early cancer screening is effective in decreasing mortality, but barriers exist including lack of information and fear of diagnosis.[30]

Recent epidemiology studies reported that use of nonsteroidal antiinflammatory drugs (e.g., sulindac [Clinoril])[31] or long-term use of aspirin (four to six tablets per day)[32] may reduce the risk of colorectal cancer.

Acute Intervention

Preoperative care. Acute nursing care for the patient with a colon resection is similar to care of the patient having a laparotomy (see NCP 40-2). In addition to general preoperative teaching and ostomy care instructions, the patient undergoing abdominal-perineal resection should be informed of the extent of the surgical procedure and the amount of care necessary to facilitate complete wound healing. The patient should be taught side-to-side positioning and made to understand that short walks are better than sitting. The nurse should teach and assist the patient in proper positioning for taking a sitz bath. The patient may not know that the sitz bath and positioning are sources of comfort. The patient may experience phantom rectal sensation because the sympathetic nerves responsible for rectal control are not severed during the surgery. The nurse must be astute in distinguishing phantom sensations from perineal abscess pain.

A well-developed, consistent nursing care plan should be coordinated early. The implementation of this plan will facilitate the healing process and hasten the patient's rehabilitation.

Postoperative care. After an abdominal-perineal resection, there are two wounds and a stoma is surgically constructed in the left lower quadrant. There is an abdominal incision through which the colon is resected and an incision is made in the perineum. The management of a perineal incision differs depending on the type of wound. Three techniques are used: (1) packing of the entire open wound; (2) partial closure with Penrose drains for open drainage; and (3) primary closure of the perineal wound with closed-suction drainage of the pelvic cavity. The type of management of the perineal wound is individualized. The open and packed method is used in patients with extensive surgery or uncontrollable bleeding in the pelvic wound. When infection or contamination is minimal, a partial closure with drains is used. Wound sites connected to low intermittent suction or a Jackson Pratt or Hemovac suction placed in the perineal wound is commonly used to provide drainage of the operative site during the early postoperative period. This usually remains until drainage is less than 50 ml per 24 hours, which occurs after approximately 3 to 5 days.

A patient who has open and packed wounds requires meticulous postoperative care. During the immediate postoperative period the perineal dressing is reinforced and changed frequently because drainage can be profuse for several hours after surgery. All drainage is carefully assessed for amount, color, and consistency. The drainage is usually serosanguineous.

The packing is usually left in place for 2 to 3 days. Packing the pelvic cavity for prolonged periods may result in sepsis and rigidity of the cavity wall and thus impede the healing process. The nurse should examine the wound regularly and record bleeding, excessive drainage, and unusual odor. The perineal wound is usually irrigated with a normal saline solution when the dressings are changed. Dressings are changed several times a day, and aseptic technique is always used.

If the wound is partially closed and drains are in place, the nurse assesses the incision for suture integrity and signs and symptoms of wound inflammation and infection. The drainage is examined for amount, color, and characteristics. When the primary closure technique is used, the catheters are left in place for approximately 3 to 5 days, and during this time the drainage is examined and observations recorded. The area around the catheter is observed for signs of inflammation and kept clean and dry. The nurse should observe for signs of edema, erythema, drainage around the suture line, fever, and elevated WBC count. If the perineal wound was not closed, warm sitz baths at 100.4° to 106° F (38° to 41° C) for 10 to 20 minutes three to four times a day assist in tissue debridement, provide comfort, and increase circulation to the area. Moist heat causes vasodilation, which allows more oxygen to flow to the affected area. Sitz baths of more than 20 minutes may result in too much vasodilation, causing congestion and discomfort.

The patient may complain of pain and itching in and around the wound. There is no physiologic explanation of sensations that are felt, but a careful examination should be made to rule out delayed wound healing. Antipruritic agents and sitz baths are usually ordered. Use of a pressure-reducing chair cushion provides comfort when sitting. Sitting on a toilet for prolonged periods is discouraged until the perineal wound is well healed.

Sexual dysfunction is a possible complication of an abdominal-perineal resection and should be included in the plan of care. Although the effect of the procedure depends on the technique used, the surgeon should discuss the subject intelligently and tactfully, with follow-up as necessary by other members of the health care team. The nurse should understand that erection, ejaculation, and orgasm involve different nerve pathways and that a dysfunction of one does not mean total sexual dysfunction. The enterostomal therapy nurse is an important member of the team and can often provide correct and factual information concerning sexual dysfunction resulting from an abdominal-perineal resection.

Ambulatory and Home Care. Psychologic support for the patient and family is important. The recovery period is long, and the possibility of recurrence of cancer is always present. The overall 5-year survival rate for all patients undergoing resection for colon cancer is less than 50%. This presents a problem for the patient and health care providers because of the often painful, debilitating, and demoralizing manifestations produced by the recurrent disease and the lack of any effective palliative therapy. Chemotherapy may be used as an adjuvant measure for the patient with evidence of local or distant metastasis. (The special needs of the cancer patient are discussed in Chapter 14.)

The perineal wound may not be completely healed before discharge. After discharge the physician, the home health nurse, and the enterostomal therapist in an outpatient clinic usually see the patient. The wound is usually irrigated and debrided. The skin around the wound should be assessed for loose hair. Shaving may be necessary to prevent the development of a chronic draining sinus. The nurse should report the drainage because it may also indicate the presence of a foreign body, fistula, osteomyelitis, or rectal tissue not removed during surgery. The patient and significant others are taught management of the wound and the procedure to take a sitz bath at home. The patient and the family should be aware of all community services available for assistance.

Evaluation

The expected outcomes for the patient with cancer of the colon or rectum are that the patient will have

- no alterations in bowel elimination patterns
- relief of pain
- balanced nutritional intake
- quality of life appropriate to disease progression
- feelings of comfort and well-being

OSTOMY SURGERY

TYPES

An *ostomy* is a surgical procedure in which an opening is made to allow the passage of intestinal contents from the bowel to an incision or *stoma.* The stoma, which is the opening on the surface of the abdomen is created when the intestine is brought through the abdominal wall and sutured to the skin. It may be permanent or temporary. Fecal matter is diverted through the stoma to the outside of the abdominal wall.

An *ileostomy* is an opening from the ileum through the abdominal wall and is also referred to as a *conventional* or *Brooke* ileostomy (Fig. 40-11). It is most commonly used in surgical treatment of ulcerative colitis, Crohn's disease, and familial polyposis.

A *cecostomy* is an opening between the cecum and the abdominal wall. Both cecostomies and ascending colostomies are uncommon. They are usually temporary and most often are used for fecal diversion before surgery or for palliation.

A *colostomy* is an opening between the colon and the abdominal wall. The proximal end of the colon is sutured to the skin. Locations for colostomies are shown in Fig. 40-11. A

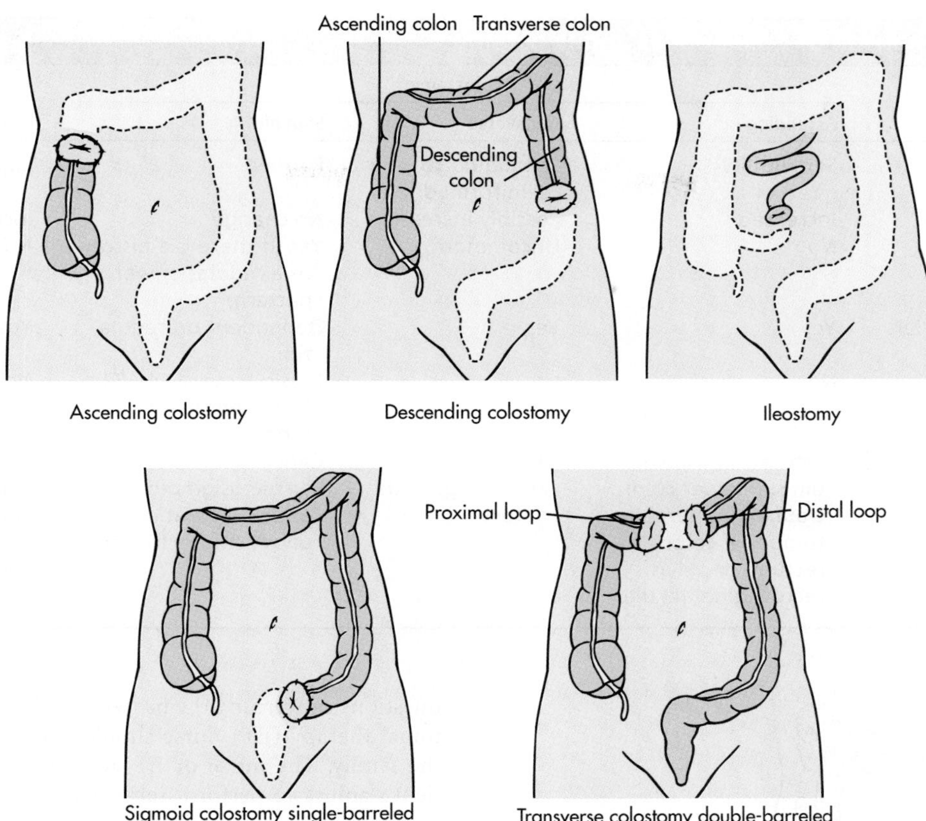

Fig. 40-11 Types of ostomies.

temporary colostomy is usually performed to protect an end-to-end anastomosis after a bowel resection or is an emergency measure following bowel obstruction (e.g., malignant tumor), abdominal trauma (e.g., gunshot wound), or a perforated diverticulum. Temporary colostomies are usually located in the transverse colon. *Loop colostomy* (Fig. 40-12) and *double-barrel colostomy* (see Fig. 40-11) are most commonly performed as temporary colostomies, but they may be permanent. A comparison of colostomies and ileostomy is shown in Table 40-32.

Surgical Therapy

End stoma. An end stoma is surgically constructed by dividing the bowel and bringing out the proximal end as a single stoma. The distal portion of the GI tract is surgically removed, or the distal segment is oversewn and left in the abdominal cavity with its mesentery intact. An end colostomy or ileostomy is then constructed. When the distal bowel is oversewn rather than removed, the procedure is known as a *Hartmann's pouch* (Fig. 40-13). If the distal bowel is removed, the stoma is permanent; if the distal bowel remains intact and oversewn, the potential exists for the bowel to be reanastomosed and the stoma to be closed (referred to as a *takedown*).

Loop stoma. A loop stoma is constructed by bringing a loop of bowel to the abdominal surface and then opening the anterior wall of the bowel to provide fecal diversion. This results in one stoma with a proximal and distal opening and an intact posterior wall that separates the two openings. The loop of bowel is frequently held in place with a plastic rod for 7 to 10 days after surgery to prevent it from slipping back into the abdominal cavity (see Fig. 40-12). A loop stoma is usually temporary.

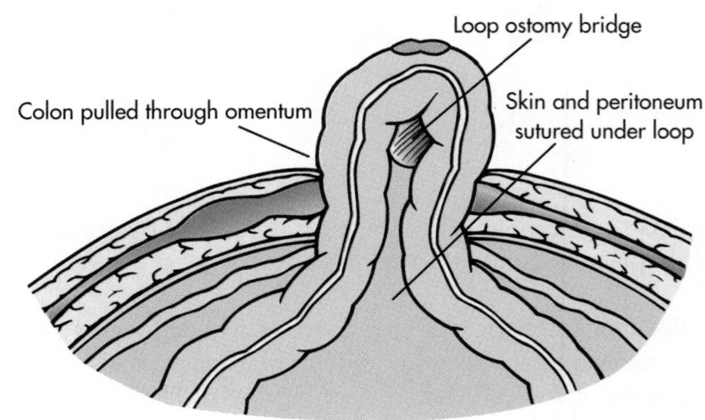

Fig. 40-12 Loop colostomy.

Double-barrel stoma. When the bowel is divided, both the proximal and distal ends are brought through the abdominal wall as two separate stomas (see Fig. 40-11). The proximal one is the functioning stoma; the distal, nonfunctioning stoma is referred to as the *mucus fistula.* The double-barrel stoma is usually temporary.

Kock pouch. As described previously in this chapter the *Kock pouch* is a continent ileostomy, which is a variation from the traditional ileostomy (see Fig. 40-3). This method eliminates the need for the patient to wear an external pouch over the stoma. The stoma is usually covered with a cap or dressing in case of mucus leakage. Additional information is provided on p. 1156.

Table **40-32** Comparison of Colostomies and Ileostomy

	Colostomy			
	Ascending	Transverse	Sigmoid	Ileostomy
Stool consistency	Semiliquid	Semiliquid to semiformed	Formed	Liquid to semiliquid
Fluid requirement	Increased	Possibly increased	No change	Increased
Bowel regulation	No	Uncommon	Yes (if there is a history of a regular bowel pattern)	No
Pouch and skin barriers	Yes	Yes	Dependent on regulation	Yes
Irrigation	No	No	Possible every 24-48 hr (if patient meets criteria)	No
Indications for surgery	Perforating diverticulitis in lower colon; trauma; inoperable tumors of colon, rectum, or pelvis; rectovaginal fistula	Same as for ascending; birth defect	Cancer of the rectum or rectosigmoidal area; perforating diverticulum; trauma	Ulcerative colitis, Crohn's disease, diseased or injured colon, birth defect, familial polyposis, trauma, cancer

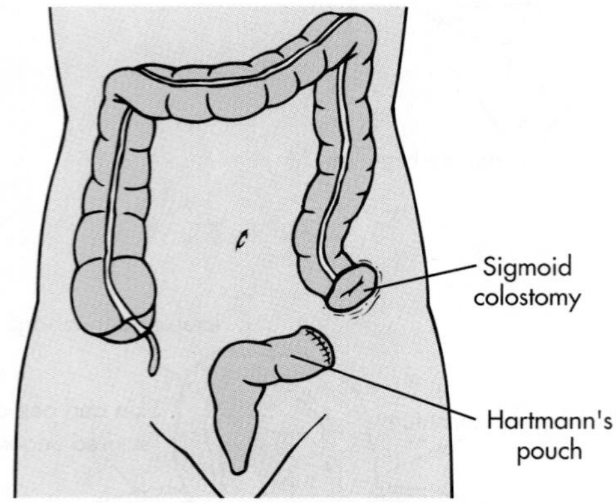

Fig. 40-13 Sigmoid colostomy. Distal bowel is oversewn and left in place to create Hartmann's pouch.

Ileoanal reservoir. Another more widely performed procedure involves total colectomy and ileoanal anastomosis with the formation of an ileal reservoir (see Fig. 40-4). The ileoanal surgical procedure is usually a combination of two procedures performed approximately 8 to 12 weeks apart. The initial procedure includes colectomy, rectal mucosectomy, ileal reservoir construction, ileoanal anastomosis, and temporary ileostomy. The second surgery involves closure of the ileostomy, which functionalizes the reservoir. Adaptation of the reservoir occurs over the next 3 to 6 months, which usually results in the ability to control and have decreased numbers of bowel movements over a 24-hour period. Additional information is provided on p. 1156.

NURSING MANAGEMENT: OSTOMY SURGERY

■ Preoperative Care

It is important to review the information the patient has received from the physician. Psychologic preparation is very important. The family and the patient usually have many questions concerning the procedures. If available, an enterostomal therapy (ET) nurse should visit with the patient and the family. The nurse or ET nurse must determine the patient's ability to perform self-care, identify support systems, and determine potential adverse factors that could be modified to facilitate learning during rehabilitation. Preoperative assessment must be comprehensive and include physical, psychologic, social, cultural, and educational components. Assessment is ongoing, including both the patient and family. The ET nurse marks the stoma site before surgery. An improperly placed stoma complicates rehabilitation by increasing time and expense of pouch change routine. It can also contribute to skin irritation and poor adaptation. The patient and the family should understand the extent of surgery and the type of stoma and its care.

If the patient desires a referral and the physician agrees, a trained ostomy visitor from the United Ostomy Association can provide meaningful psychologic support. The patient has the opportunity to see a person who has adjusted well and who has experienced some of the same feelings and concerns. The family will also benefit from the visit.

Bowel preparation before surgery decreases the chance of a postoperative infection by cleansing the bowel of feces and bacteria. Orally administered osmotic lavages (e.g., Go-Lytely) have shortened the classic 72-hour preparation with clear liquids, cathartics, and enemas. IV and oral antibiotics are given. Nonabsorbable neomycin and erythromycin are given orally to decrease the number of intracolonic bacteria.

■ Colostomy Care

Postoperative nursing care should focus on assessing the stoma, protecting the skin, selecting the pouch, and assisting the patient to adapt psychologically to a changed body. Nursing care for the patient with a colostomy is presented in NCP 40-4.

40-4 NURSING CARE PLAN PATIENT WITH A COLOSTOMY/ILEOSTOMY

Expected Patient Outcomes	Nursing Interventions and *Rationales*
NURSING DIAGNOSIS	**Risk for impaired skin integrity** *related to* irritation from fecal drainage, irritation of pouch, and lack of knowledge of skin care.
▪ Normal skin integrity. ▪ Intact pouch seal.	▪ Have enterostomal therapy nurse see patient before surgery *to mark stoma site in area free of creases and folds for better seal of appliance.* ▪ After surgery assess peristomal skin for erythema with burning and itching, poorly fitting appliance with leakage, lack of adequate skin care, and failure to use skin barrier *to initiate treatment if indicated.* ▪ During pouch change assess skin for signs of breakdown *to initiate treatment if indicated.* ▪ Clean area with mild soap and water and dry thoroughly *to prevent irritation from intestinal contents or pouch adhesive.* ▪ Apply skin barrier *to protect skin and prevent direct contact with intestinal contents.* ▪ Teach patient proper skin and pouch care *to ensure proper technique for long-term care.* ▪ Plan for outpatient or home visit *for continued teaching and monitoring.* ▪ Empty pouch when it is one-third full *to prevent seal from leaking.*
NURSING DIAGNOSIS	**Body-image disturbance** *related to* presence of stoma and malodor *as manifested by* verbalization of embarrassment or shame due to malodor or presence of stoma.
▪ Adjustment to altered body image. ▪ Satisfactory plan for control of odor.	▪ Assess patient's attitude toward stoma *to determine if problem is present* and, if indicated, *plan appropriate intervention.* ▪ Instruct patient on measures for odor control, use of odor-proof pouch, pouch deodorants, and use of room deodorants when pouch is emptied *to minimize embarrassing odors from drainage.* ▪ Teach patient to use loose clothing *to conceal pouch.* ▪ Discuss normal emotional response to stoma and encourage patient to express feelings *to assist patient in adjusting to change in body.* ▪ Encourage family members to participate in care *to foster patient's support system.* ▪ Provide patient with information on local United Ostomy Association *to offer patient and family an opportunity for education and support.* ▪ Prepare patient to do own stoma and pouch care *to increase independence and enhance self-esteem.*
NURSING DIAGNOSIS	**Altered nutrition: less than body requirements** *related to* lack of knowledge of appropriate foods and decreased appetite *as manifested by* weight loss, vitamin and mineral deficiencies, inability to tolerate certain foods.
▪ Dietary intake to maintain weight at optimum level.	▪ Assess nutritional intake *to determine need for intervention.* ▪ Gradually introduce foods one at a time *to identify individual foods that may be problematic* and begin with low-residue diet, *which is usually well-tolerated.* ▪ Teach patient to chew food slowly and thoroughly *to facilitate digestion and prevent gas.* ▪ Give list of foods to avoid *so patient has a ready source of referral.* ▪ Arrange visit with dietician if indicated.
NURSING DIAGNOSIS	**Altered sexuality patterns** *related to* perceived loss of sexual appeal and possibility of accidental seepage of fecal material during sexual activity *as manifested by* verbalization of concern about intimate relations with spouse or significant other.
▪ Confidence in ability to resume previous sexual activity.	▪ Assess patient's attitude about impact of ostomy on sexual functioning *to determine if a problem exists and if there is a need to plan interventions.* ▪ Encourage discussion of meaning of sexuality to patient and significant other *to allow patient opportunity to discuss sensitive topic in a nonthreatening situation.*

Continued

40-4 NURSING CARE PLAN PATIENT WITH A COLOSTOMY/ILEOSTOMY —continued

Expected Patient Outcomes	Nursing Interventions and *Rationales*
NURSING DIAGNOSIS **Altered sexuality patterns** *—continued*	
	■ Discuss ways to avoid seepage and conceal stoma and/or pouch during intimate relations *to decrease fear of embarrassment or withdrawal from intimate situations because of anxiety over "accidents."* ■ If appropriate, arrange visit with person of same sex and condition *to discuss sexual concerns and share potential solutions, to provide an opportunity to ask questions, and get practical, realistic answers from a supportive, understanding other.*
NURSING DIAGNOSIS **Risk for fluid volume deficit** *related to* excess fluid loss from ileostomy or diarrhea with a colostomy and inadequate oral intake.	
■ Normal serum electrolytes. ■ Normal vital signs. ■ Good skin turgor. ■ Urine output >0.5 ml/kg/hr.	■ Assess for signs of weakness, poor skin turgor, sunken eyes, hypotension, tachycardia, hypokalemia, hyponatremia, oliguria *to determine presence of fluid volume deficit and, if present, plan appropriate interventions.* ■ Record intake and output and include ileostomy drainage *to have an accurate record of fluid balance.* ■ Ensure fluid intake of at least 3000 ml/day in the initial postoperative period *to prevent dehydration.* ■ Instruct patient to maintain high fluid intake and to increase it during hot weather, when patient is perspiring excessively, and during episodes of diarrhea *to ensure adequate fluid intake in various situations.* ■ Monitor serum electrolytes *as inadequate fluid volume will be reflected in changed electrolyte values.* ■ Instruct patient on signs and symptoms of sodium, potassium, and fluid deficits *to ensure early reporting and correction of underlying electrolyte problem.*

The stoma should be pink. A dusky-blue stoma indicates ischemia, and a brown-black stoma indicates necrosis. The nurse should assess and document stoma color every 8 hours. There is mild to moderate swelling of the stoma the first 2 to 3 weeks after surgery (Table 40-33). A skin barrier should be applied to protect the peristomal suture line and skin surrounding the stoma. Solid skin barriers include Stomahesive (Convatec), Coloplast, and Hollister skin barriers. The skin should be washed with warm water and dried thoroughly before the barrier is applied.

With an open-ended, transparent, plastic, odor-proof pouch it is easy to protect the skin and to observe and collect the drainage. The pouch must fit snugly to prevent leakage around the stoma. The size of the stoma is determined with a stoma-measuring card. Although the pouch is applied after surgery, the colostomy functions when peristalsis has been adequately restored. When a temporary colostomy is performed and the stoma is opened in the operating room with no bowel preparation being done previously the stoma functions immediately.

The volume, color, and consistency of the drainage are recorded. Each time the pouch is changed, the condition of the skin is observed for irritation. A pouch should *never* be placed directly on irritated skin without the use of a skin barrier.

A colostomy in the ascending and transverse colon has semiliquid stools. The patient needs to be instructed to use a drainable pouch. A colostomy in the sigmoid or descending colon has semiformed or formed stools and can sometimes be regulated by the irrigation method. The patient may or may not wear a drainage pouch. A nondrainable pouch should have a gas filter.

For most patients with colostomies, there are few, if any, dietary restrictions. A well-balanced diet and adequate fluid in-

Table 40-33 Characteristics of Stoma

Characteristic	Description or Cause
Color*	
Rose to brick red	Viable stoma mucosa
Pale	May indicate anemia
Blanching, dark red to purple	Indicates inadequate blood supply to the stoma or bowel from adhesions, low flow state, or excessive tension on the bowel at the time of construction
Edema†	
Mild to moderate edema	Normal in the initial postoperative period Trauma to the stoma Any medical condition that results in edema
Moderate to severe edema	Obstruction of the stoma Allergic reaction to food Gastroenteritis
Bleeding	
Small amount	Oozing from the stoma mucosa when touched is normal because of its high vascularity
Moderate to large amount‡	Moderate to large amount‡ of bleeding from the stoma mucosa could indicate coagulation factor deficiency; stomal varices secondary to portal hypertension Moderate to large amount from intestinal stoma opening could indicate lower gastrointestinal bleeding

*Sustained color changes must be reported to surgeon.
†Closely observe and report to the surgeon and adjust the stoma opening size in the pouch.
‡Report moderate to large amounts of bleeding to surgeon.

NUTRITIONAL THERAPY

Table 40-34 Effects of Food on Stoma Output

Odor Producing*	Diarrhea Causing*
Eggs	Alcohol
Garlic	Beer
Onions	Cabbage family
Fish	Spinach
Asparagus	Green beans
Cabbage	Coffee
Broccoli	Spicy foods
Alcohol	Fruits (raw)
Gas Forming*	**Potential Obstruction in Ileostomy****
Beans	Nuts
Cabbage family	Raisins
Onions	Popcorn
Beer	Seeds
Carbonated beverages	Vegetables (raw)
Cheeses, strong	Celery
Sprouts	Corn

*The effect of food on stoma output is individual. Patients are not discouraged from eating the above listed foods and beverages.
**Patients are encouraged to chew high roughage food well, drink increased fluids, and initially limit the amount.

take is important. The patient's medical and surgical history must be considered when individualizing dietary instructions. Table 40-34 lists foods and their effects on stoma output.

Colostomy Irrigations

Colostomy irrigations are intended to regulate bowel function, treat constipation, or prepare the bowel for surgery. When irrigating to achieve a regular bowel pattern, the irrigations stimulate the bowel to function at a specific time every day or every other day. If control is achieved, there should be little or no spillage between irrigations. The patient who establishes regularity may need to wear only a pad or cover over the stoma. The patient who cannot or chooses not to establish regularity by irrigations must wear a pouch at all times. The procedure for colostomy irrigation is presented in Table 40-35.

All equipment should be assembled before the irrigation. A commercially obtained irrigation set usually has all the equipment needed. The nurse should encourage the patient to watch the procedure and should explain each step to the patient. The cone tip on the tubing controls the depth of insertion and prevents the water from coming out from the stoma and not going into the colon. If resistance is met, force should not be used because perforation of the intestine can result. However, this is unlikely when using a stoma cone. A hard plastic catheter is not recommended because of the risk of intestinal perforation. The procedure should not be rushed; the patient should feel relaxed. The patient or family member must be instructed in the procedure and must be able to demonstrate the ability to irrigate before being independent. This can be done in the outpatient setting.

The patient should be able to perform skin care, control odor, care for the stoma, and identify signs and symptoms of complications. The patient should know the importance of fluids and food in the diet, have names and addresses of the United Ostomy Association, and know when to seek medical care. Home care and outpatient follow-up by an ET nurse is highly recommended. Patients should be discharged with written pouch change instructions, teaching literature relevant to the type of stoma they have, a list of equipment they use, a list of equipment retailers (including names and phone numbers), outpatient follow-up appointments with the surgeon and ET nurse, and the phone numbers of the surgeon and nurse. The patient and family teaching guidelines are included in Table 40-36.

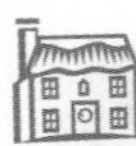

PATIENT & FAMILY HOME CARE GUIDE

Table 40-35 Colostomy Irrigation

Equipment

Lubricant
Irrigation set (1000-2000 ml container, tubing with irrigating cone, clamp)
Irrigating sleeve with adhesive or belt
Toilet tissue to clean around the stoma
Disposal sack for soiled dressing

Procedure

1. Place 500-1000 ml of lukewarm water (not to exceed 105° F) [40.5° C] in container. The volume is titrated for the individual; use enough irrigant to distend the bowel but not enough to cause cramping pain. Most adults use 500-1000 ml of water.
2. Ensure comfortable position. Patient may sit in chair in front of toilet or on the toilet if the perineal wound is healed.
3. Clear tubing of all air by flushing it with fluid.
4. Hang container on hook or IV pole (18-24 in) above stoma (about shoulder height).
5. Apply irrigating sleeve and place bottom end in toilet bowl.
6. Lubricate cone and insert cone tip gently into the stoma and hold tip securely in place.
7. Allow irrigation solution to flow in steadily for 5-10 min.
8. If cramping occurs, stop the flow of solution for a few seconds, leaving the cone in place.
9. Clamp the tubing and remove irrigating cone when the desired amount of irrigant has been delivered or when the patient senses colonic distention.
10. Allow 30-45 minutes for the solution and feces to be expelled. Initial evacuation is usually complete in 10-15 min. Close off the irrigating sleeve at the bottom to allow ambulation.
11. Clean, rinse, and dry peristomal skin well.
12. Replace the colostomy drainage pouch or desired stoma covering.
13. Wash and rinse all equipment and hang to dry.

PATIENT & FAMILY TEACHING GUIDE

Table 40-36 Ostomy Self-Care

The following are guidelines to include for patient and family teaching:

1. Explain the following principles of ostomy and pouch care:
   - Apply and change pouch to collect intestinal drainage.
   - Empty pouch before it is full to prevent leakage.
   - Cleanse skin and use skin barriers and deodorizers to prevent skin breakdown and malodor.
   - Irrigate colostomy to regulate bowel elimination (optional).
   - Explain how to contact enterostomal therapist with questions.
   - Explain how to obtain additional supplies.
2. Instruct the following dietary and fluid intake guidelines:
   - Identify a well-balanced diet and dietary supplements to prevent nutrition deficiencies.
   - Identify foods to avoid to reduce diarrhea, gas, malodor, or obstruction.
   - Drink at least 3000 ml/day of fluid to prevent dehydration (unless contraindicated).
   - Increase fluid intake during hot weather, excessive perspiration, and diarrhea to replace losses and prevent dehydration.
   - Explain how to contact registered dietitian with questions.
3. Describe potential resources to assist with emotional and psychologic adjustment:
   - Identify persons available to provide emotional support.
   - Identify community resources for psychologic counseling.
   - Contact United Ostomy Association for information or peer support.
   - Inform that treatment for potential depression is available if needed.
4. Explain the importance of follow-up care:
   Report signs and symptoms of:
   - Fluid and electrolyte deficits
   - Fever
   - Diarrhea
   - Skin irritation
   - Other stoma problems including inversion, eversion, discoloration, abscess, or infection

■ Ileostomy Care

Care of the ileostomy is presented in NCP 40-4. An ileostomy stoma protrusion of at least 1 to 1.5 cm makes care easier. When the stoma is flat, seepage occurs resulting in altered skin integrity. Drainage is constant and extremely irritating to the skin. Regularity cannot be established. A pouch must be worn at all times. An open-ended, drainable pouch is worn by the patient so that drainage can be emptied when one-third full. The drainable pouch is usually worn for 4 to 7 days before being changed as long as leakage does not occur around the stoma. If pouch leakage occurs, the pouch should be promptly removed and the skin should be cleansed and a new pouch placed. A solid skin barrier should always be used. A transparent pouch should be used in the initial postoperative period to facilitate assessment of stoma viability.

Immediately after surgery, intake and output must be accurately monitored. The patient should be observed for signs and symptoms of fluid and electrolyte imbalance, particularly potassium, sodium, and fluid deficits. In the first 24 to 48 hours after surgery the amount of drainage from the stoma may be negligible. A person with an ileostomy has lost the absorptive functions provided by the colon, as well as the delay feature provided by the ileocecal valve. Once peristalsis returns, the patient may experience a period of high-volume output of 1000 to 1800 ml per day. Later on, the average amount can be 800 ml daily because the proximal small bowel adapts. If the small bowel has been shortened as a result of surgical resections in Crohn's or other disease, the drainage from the ileostomy may be greater. The patient must understand the importance of fluid and electrolyte balance.

The patient should be instructed to drink at least 2 to 3 L of fluid daily; more may be necessary when diarrhea occurs and in the summer, when perspiration is increased. Diarrhea from an ileostomy produces acidosis from the loss of bicarbonate. The physician may instruct the patient to take an electrolyte solution at home (e.g., 1 teaspoon of salt and 1 teaspoon of baking soda in 1 quart of water). Fluids rich in electrolytes should be encouraged.

Usually a low-roughage diet is ordered initially. Fiber-containing foods are reintroduced gradually. Later there are no dietary restrictions except for foods that are troublesome (e.g., high-roughage popcorn). The goal for the patient is a return to a normal, presurgical diet.

The stoma often bleeds easily when it is touched because it has a high vascular supply. The patient should be told that minimal oozing of blood is normal. If the terminal ileum has been removed, the patient may need cobalamin injections or use intranasal cobalamin.

Adaptation to an Ostomy

Adaptation to the ostomy is a gradual process. The patient experiences a grief reaction to the loss of a body part and an alteration in body image. Each person uses different coping mechanisms. The adjustment period for the person depends on the individual. Psychologic support during the grieving process is needed. There are concerns about body image, sexual activity, family responsibilities, and changes in lifestyle. The patient may become resentful and have fears of odor or soiling. Supportive measures by nurses include helping the patient acquire knowledge, providing or recommending support services, and identifying coping mechanisms that are effective. The nurse provides support by responding to the physiologic needs of stoma care and the psychosocial needs of self-esteem.

The patient should not be forced to learn to care for the stoma. The nurse should watch for clues that the patient is ready. Teaching at the appropriate time is an important part of the care and can contribute to a smooth adjustment process.

Activities of daily living are resumed within 6 to 8 weeks. Heavy lifting should be avoided. The patient's physical condition determines when sports may be resumed. Bathing and swimming are not prohibited. Water does not harm the stoma.

A clinical pathway for home care of the patient with an ostomy is provided on p. 1180.

Sexual Dysfunction After Ostomy Surgery

Discussion of sexuality and sexual function must be incorporated in the plan of care. The nurse can help the patient understand that sexual function or sexual activity may be affected, but sexuality does not have to be altered.

Pelvic surgery can disrupt nerve and vascular supply to the genitals. Radiation, chemotherapy, and medications can also alter sexual function. Hormones and overall physical health of the patient influence desire. Certain pain medications and antiemetics can lower the sex drive. Generalized fatigue caused by illness can also influence desire. By communicating this information to patients, they can plan sexual activity around a medication schedule and energy levels. Any pelvic surgery that removes the rectum has the potential of damaging the parasympathetic nerve plexus. Erection in men depends on the parasympathetic nerves that control blood flow and vascular supply to the pelvis and the pudendal nerves that transmit sensory responses from the genital area. Nerve-sparing surgical techniques are used when possible to preserve sexual function. Radiation therapy to the pelvis can reduce blood vascularity to the pelvis by causing scarring in the small blood vessels. A woman's sexual functioning after healing includes expansion and lubrication of the vagina. Pelvic surgery usually does not affect a woman's arousal unless part or the entire vagina is removed. Radiation therapy can affect the small blood vessels, which reduces available blood supply and can affect vaginal expansion and lubrication.

Muscular contraction and genital pleasure that occur during orgasm are not disrupted by pelvic surgery. If the sympathetic nerves in the presacral area are damaged, the male mechanism of emission can be disrupted. This can occur in an abdominal-perineal resection. Orgasms can occur in both men and women with stoma surgery, although other aspects of the response cycle may be affected.

The psychologic impact of the stoma and how it affects the patient's body image and self-esteem must be discussed. Emotional factors can contribute to sexual problems. A life-threatening illness can override concerns about sexual function. The nurse can assist a patient to identify ways of coping with depression and anxiety resulting from illness, surgery, or postoperative problems.

The social impact of the stoma is interrelated with the psychologic, physical, and sexual aspects. Concerns of people with stomas include the ability to resume sexual activity, altering clothing styles, the effect on daily activities, sleeping while wearing a pouch, passing gas, the presence of odor, cleanliness, and deciding when or if to tell others about the stoma. The fear of rejection from a partner or the fear that others will not find them desirable as a sexual partner can be a concern. The nurse should encourage open communication about feelings and should realize that the patient needs time to adjust to the pouch and to body changes before feeling secure in his or her sexual functioning.

Although pregnancy is possible, the physician may recommend a limited number of pregnancies on the basis of the patient's physical condition. The person with an ostomy who becomes pregnant should have regular medical care.

CLINICAL PATHWAY Home Care of Ostomy (attention to colostomy)

ICD-9 Code(s) V55.3

Patient Name ________ Pt. ID No. ________ SOC Date ________ Discharge Date ________

Date Noted	Expected Outcomes	Achieved Y	Achieved N	Achieved Date	Variance Codes	Date Noted	Nursing/Functional Diagnoses	Date Closed
	1. Wound site stabilized with no signs of infection (per agency clinical parameters) by visit no. ____ .						Body image disturbance Outcome(s) no. ____ :	
	2. Patient/caregiver/family demonstrates compliance with ostomy therapeutic care plan, as evidenced by clinical assessment of patient, by visit no. ____ .						Knowledge deficit: self-management, observation skills. Outcome(s) no. ____ :	
	3. Patient demonstrates skills needed to cope with lifestyle adjustment by visit no. ____ .						Skin integrity, impaired Outcome(s) no. ____ :	
	4. Other:						Social interaction, impaired Outcome(s) no. ____ :	
	5. Other:						Other: Outcome(s) no. ____ :	
	6. Other:						Other: Outcome(s) no. ____ :	

Assessments/Instructions/Interventions	VS No. _	VS No. _	VS No. _	VS No. _	VS No. _	VS No. _	VS No. _	VS No. _	VS No. _	VS No. _
Explain patient rights and responsibilities.										
Assess for home safety management.										
Assess ostomy/wound.										
Assess gastrointestinal status.										
Assess vital signs.										
Assess skin integrity.										
Assess hydration and nutrition status.										
Assess coping skills of patient and caregiver.										
Assess patient/caregiver's willingness and ability to provide home therapeutic regimen.										
Assess patient/caregiver's strengths/weaknesses related to therapeutic regimen.										
Assess patient/caregiver's need for personal care assistance.										
Refer to: Enterostomal nurse for ostomy and wound care.										
Refer to: Dietitian for nutritional assessment (especially if receiving tube feedings).										
Refer to: Social worker for linkage to appropriate community resources.										
Instruct patient/caregiver on home safety.										
Instruct patient/caregiver on use of ostomy supplies and lifestyle adjustment.										

Medical Supplies/Home Medical Equipment Needs

1. Ostomy supplies
2. Wound care supplies
3. Other ________

Variance codes
1. Patient related
2. Situation related
3. Systems related

Team member signature ________ Initials ____
Team member signature ________ Initials ____
Team member signature ________ Initials ____

Case manager name ________

____
Patient signature (involved in care planning)

From Marrelli TM, Hilliard LS: *Home care and clinical paths: effective care across the continuum,* St Louis, 1996, Mosby.

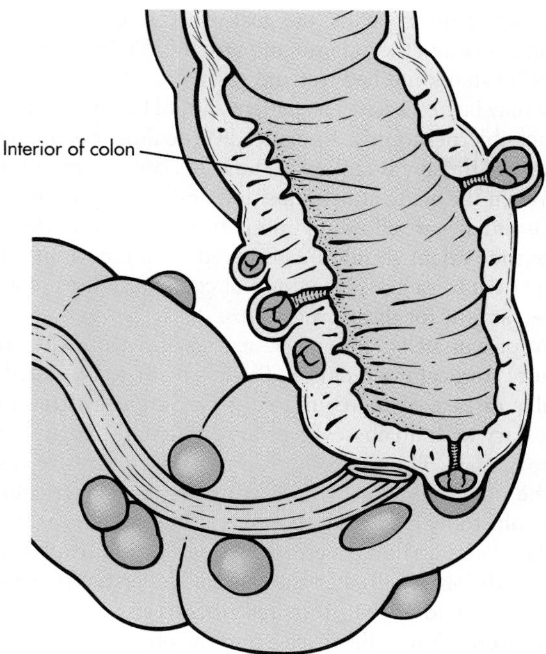

Fig. 40-14 Diverticula are outpouchings of the colon. When they become inflamed, the condition is diverticulitis. The inflammatory process can spread to the surrounding area in the intestine.

DIVERTICULOSIS AND DIVERTICULITIS

A *diverticulum* is a saccular dilation or outpouching of the mucosa through the circular smooth muscle of the intestinal wall. Clinically, diverticular disease occurs in two forms: diverticulosis and diverticulitis. Multiple noninflamed diverticula are present with diverticulosis. The patient is most often free of symptoms but may have some abdominal discomfort. In diverticulitis, inflammation of the diverticula occurs (Fig. 40-14). Diverticula may occur at any point within the GI tract but are most commonly found in the sigmoid colon.

Etiology and Pathophysiology

Diverticular disease is a common GI disorder that affects 5% of the population by the age of 40 years, and 50% are affected by the age of 80 years.[33] It affects men and women equally, but men seem to have a higher complication rate. Although it affects almost 30 million Americans, most are asymptomatic.

There is no known cause of diverticular disease, but deficiency in dietary fiber has been associated with it. The disease is more prevalent in Western populations that consume diets low in fiber and high in refined carbohydrates, and it is virtually unknown in areas of the world, such as rural Africa, where high-fiber diets are consumed.

When diverticula form, the smooth muscle of the colon wall becomes thickened (Fig. 40-15). Lack of dietary fiber slows transit time and more water is absorbed from the stool, making it more difficult to pass through the lumen. Decreased bulk of the stool, combined with a more narrowed lumen in the sigmoid colon, causes high intraluminal pressures. These factors are believed to contribute to the formation of diverticula.

The cause of diverticulitis is related to the retention of stool and bacteria in the diverticulum, forming a hardened mass called a *fecalith*. This causes inflammation and usually small perforations. Inflammation of the diverticulum spreads to the surrounding area in the intestines (Fig. 40-16), causing the tissue to become edematous. Abscesses may form, or complete perforation with peritonitis may occur.

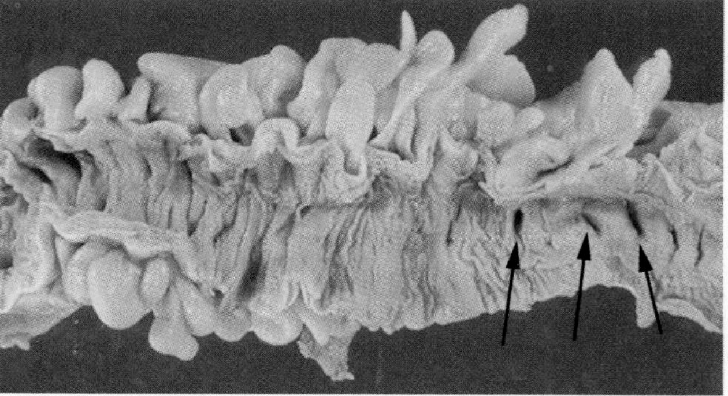

Fig. 40-15 In diverticular disease, the outpouches (arrows) of mucosa appear as slitlike openings from the mucosal surface of the open bowel.

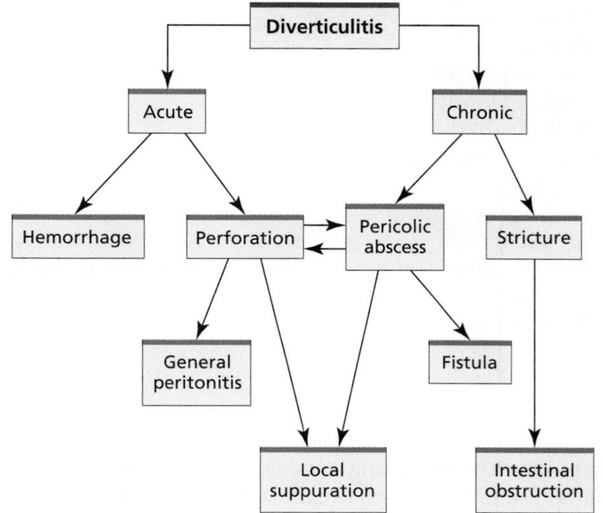

Fig. 40-16 Complications of diverticulitis.

Clinical Manifestations

The majority of patients with diverticulosis have no symptoms. Those with symptoms typically have crampy abdominal pain located in the left lower quadrant that is usually relieved by passage of flatus or bowel movement. Alternating constipation and diarrhea may be present.

Approximately 15% of patients with diverticulosis progress to acute diverticulitis. In patients with diverticulitis, abdominal pain is localized over the involved area of the colon. A tender, left lower quadrant mass may be felt on palpation of the abdomen. Fever, chills, nausea, anorexia, and leukocytosis may be present. Elderly patients with diverticulitis are frequently afebrile, with a normal WBC, and little, if any, abdominal tenderness.

Complications of diverticulitis include perforation with peritonitis, abscess and fistula formation, bowel obstruction, ureteral obstruction, and bleeding. Bleeding is a common

COLLABORATIVE CARE

Table 40-37 Diverticulosis and Diverticulitis

Diagnostic
- Stool for occult blood
- Barium enema
- Sigmoidoscopy
- Colonoscopy
- CBC
- Urinalysis
- Blood culture

Collaborative Therapy

Ambulatory and Home Care
- High-residue diet
- Dietary fiber supplements
- Stool softeners
- Anticholinergics
- Mineral oil
- Bed rest
- Clear liquid diet
- Oral antibiotics
- Bulk laxatives

Acute Care: Diverticulitis
- Antibiotics
- NPO status
- IV fluids
- Possible colon resection for obstruction or hemorrhage
- Bed rest
- NG suction

complication of diverticulitis and is manifested by *hematochezia* (maroon stools). Bleeding usually stops spontaneously.

Diagnostic Studies

A barium enema is typically used to diagnose diverticular disease. A CBC, urinalysis, and fecal occult blood test should be performed (Table 40-37). A colonoscopy should be performed on patients with symptoms to rule out possible hidden polyps or lesions. A patient with acute diverticulitis should not have a barium enema or colonoscopy because of the possibility of perforation and peritonitis.

NURSING AND COLLABORATIVE MANAGEMENT: DIVERTICULOSIS AND DIVERTICULITIS

Uncomplicated diverticular disease is treated with a high-fiber diet (see Table 40-9) and bulk laxatives, such as psyllium hydrophilic mucilloid (Metamucil). Anticholinergic drugs such as dicyclomine (Bentyl) and Donnatal may be used to relieve discomfort from spasm of the bowel (see Table 40-37).

Fluids should be increased because fibers retain water, thus decreasing the amount absorbed by the body. If the patient is obese, a reduction in weight is needed. Increased intraabdominal pressure should be avoided because it may precipitate an attack. Factors that increase intraabdominal pressure are straining at stool, vomiting, bending, lifting, and tight, restrictive clothing.

In acute diverticulitis, the goal of treatment is to allow the colon to rest and the inflammation to subside. The patient is kept on NPO status and bed rest and given parenteral fluids. An NG tube may be necessary. The patient should be observed for signs of possible peritonitis. In acute diverticulitis, broad-spectrum antibiotic therapy is required. The WBC count is monitored.

When the acute attack subsides, oral fluids progressing to a semisolid diet are allowed. Ambulation is also permitted. At this stage the patient should be observed for a recurrent attack. If the patient has a bowel resection or colostomy, the nursing care is the same as for these procedures.

Approximately 30% of patients with acute diverticulitis require surgical intervention. Patients with complicated diverticular disease often require surgery. Surgical intervention is necessary to drain abscesses or to resect an obstructing inflammatory mass. The usual surgical procedures involve resection of the involved colon with a temporary diverting colostomy. The colostomy is reanastomosed after the colon is healed.

The patient should be provided with a full explanation of the condition. The better the patient understands the disease process and adheres to the prescribed regimen, the less likely the exacerbation of the disease and the onset of complications.

HERNIAS

A hernia is a protrusion of a viscus through an abnormal opening or a weakened area in the wall of the cavity in which it is normally contained. A hernia may occur in any part of the body, but it usually occurs within the abdominal cavity. If the hernia can be placed back into the abdominal cavity, it is known as *reducible.* The hernia can be reduced by manipulation, or it can occur without manipulation when the person lies down. If the hernia cannot be placed back into the abdominal cavity, it is known as *irreducible,* or *incarcerated.* In this situation the intestinal flow may be obstructed. When the hernia is irreducible and the intestinal flow and blood supply are obstructed, the hernia is *strangulated.* The result is an acute intestinal obstruction.

Types

The *inguinal* hernia is the most common type of hernia and occurs at the point of weakness in the abdominal wall where the spermatic cord in men and the round ligament in women emerge (Fig. 40-17). When the protrusion escapes through the inguinal ring and follows the spermatic cord or the round ligament, it is termed an *indirect* hernia. When it escapes through the posterior inguinal wall, it is a *direct* hernia. An inguinal hernia is more frequent in men.

A *femoral* hernia occurs when there is a protrusion through the femoral ring into the femoral canal. It occurs below the inguinal (Poupart's) ligament as a bulge. It becomes strangulated easily and occurs more frequently in women. The *umbilical* hernia occurs when the rectus muscle is weak or the umbilical opening fails to close after birth. This type is found most commonly in children.

Ventral, or *incisional,* hernia is due to weakness of the abdominal wall at the site of a previous incision. It is found most commonly in patients who are obese, who have had multiple surgical procedures in the same area, and who have had inadequate wound healing because of poor nutrition or infection.

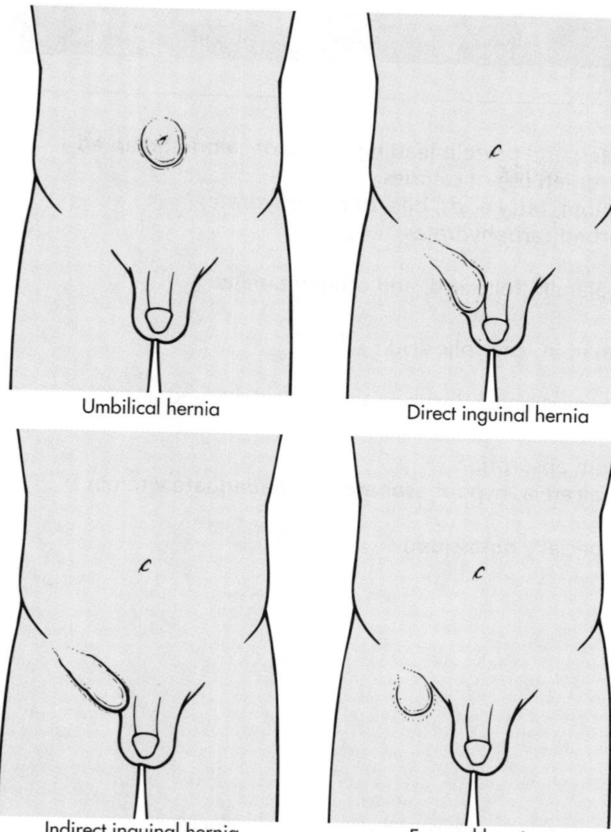

Fig. 40-17 Types of hernias.

Clinical Manifestations

A hernia commonly occurs over the involved area when the patient stands or strains. There may be some discomfort as a result of tension. Severe pain is caused if the hernia becomes strangulated. In this situation the clinical manifestations of a bowel obstruction, such as vomiting, crampy abdominal pain, and distention, are found.

NURSING MANAGEMENT: HERNIAS

Diagnosis is based on history and physical examination findings. Surgery is the treatment of choice for hernias to prevent the possible complication of strangulation. An umbilical hernia is not usually repaired surgically because it may reduce itself if left alone until the child gets older. The surgical repair of a hernia is known as a *herniorrhaphy.* The reinforcement of the weakened area with wire, fascia, or mesh is known as a *hernioplasty.* When there is strangulation, necrosis and gangrene may develop if immediate care is not given. A bowel resection of the involved area or a temporary colostomy may be needed to treat a strangulated hernia.

Some patients with hernias wear a *truss,* a pad placed over the hernia and held in place with a belt. The truss is worn to keep the hernia from protruding. If a patient wears a truss, the nurse should check for skin irritation caused by the continual rubbing of the truss.

Table 40-38 Common Causes of Malabsorption

Biochemical or Enzyme Deficiencies
Lactase deficiency
Biliary tract obstruction
Pancreatic insufficiency
Cystic fibrosis
Chronic pancreatitis
Zollinger-Ellison syndrome
Bacterial Proliferation
Tropical sprue
Parasitic infection
Small Intestinal Mucosal Disruption
Celiac disease
Whipple's disease
Crohn's disease
Disturbed Lymphatic and Vascular Circulation
Lymphoma
Ischemia
Lymphangiectasia
Heart failure
Surface Area Loss
Billroth II gastrectomy
Short bowel syndrome
Distal ileal resection, disease, or bypass

After a hernia repair, the patient may have difficulty voiding. Therefore the nurse should observe for a distended bladder. An accurate intake and output record is important. Scrotal edema is a painful complication after an inguinal hernia repair. A scrotal support with application of an ice bag may help relieve pain and edema. Coughing is not encouraged, but deep breathing and turning should be done. If the patient needs to cough or sneeze, the incision should be splinted during coughing, and sneezing should be done with the mouth open.

After discharge the patient may be restricted from heavy lifting for 6 to 8 weeks. Some surgeons do not put any limitations on physical activities.

MALABSORPTION SYNDROME

Malabsorption results from impaired absorption of fats, carbohydrates, proteins, minerals, and vitamins. The stomach, small intestine, liver, and pancreas regulate normal digestion and absorption. Digestive enzymes ordinarily break down nutrients so that absorption can take place through the intestinal mucosa and nutrients can get into the bloodstream. If there is an interruption in this process at any point, malabsorption may occur. Several problems can cause malabsorption (Table 40-38). They can be classified into malabsorptions caused by (1) biochemical or enzyme deficiencies, (2) bacterial proliferation, (3) disruption of small intestine mucosa, (4) disturbed lymphatic and vascular circulation, or (5) surface area loss. Lactose intolerance is the most common malabsorption disorder, followed by inflammatory bowel disease, nontropical (celiac) and tropical sprue, and cystic fibrosis.

Table 40-39 Clinical Manifestations of Malabsorption

Manifestations	Pathophysiology
Gastrointestinal	
Weight loss	Malabsorption of fat, carbohydrates, and protein leading to loss of calories; marked reduction in caloric intake or increased use of calories
Diarrhea	Impaired absorption of water, sodium, fatty acids, bile, or carbohydrates
Flatulence	Bacterial fermentation of unabsorbed carbohydrates
Steatorrhea	Undigested and unabsorbed fat
Glossitis, cheilosis, stomatitis	Deficiency of iron, riboflavin, cobalamin, folic acid, and other vitamins
Hematologic	
Anemia	Impaired absorption of iron, cobalamin, and folic acid
Hemorrhagic tendency	Vitamin C deficiency Vitamin K deficiency inhibiting production of clotting factors II, VII, IX, and X
Musculoskeletal	
Bone pain	Osteoporosis from impaired calcium absorption Osteomalacia secondary to hypocalcemia, hypophosphatemia, inadequate vitamin D
Tetany	Hypocalcemia, hypomagnesemia
Weakness, muscle cramps	Anemia, electrolyte depletion (especially potassium)
Muscle wasting	Protein malabsorption
Neurologic	
Altered mental status	Dehydration
Paresthesias	Cobalamin deficiency
Peripheral neuropathy	Cobalamin deficiency Thiamine deficiency
Night blindness	Vitamin A deficiency
Integumentary	
Bruising	Vitamin K deficiency
Dermatitis	Fatty acid deficiency, zinc deficiency, niacin and other vitamin deficiencies
Brittle nails	Iron deficiency
Hair thinning and loss	Protein deficiency
Cardiovascular	
Hypotension	Dehydration
Tachycardia	Hypovolemia, anemia
Peripheral edema	Protein malabsorption, protein loss in diarrhea

The most common clinical manifestation of malabsorption is *steatorrhea* (fatty stools). Bulky, foul-smelling stools that float in water and are difficult to flush are characteristic of steatorrhea (Table 40-39). However, steatorrhea does not occur with lactose intolerance.

Screening tests available for malabsorption include qualitative examination of stool for fat (Sudan stain), a 72-hour stool collection for quantitative measurement of fecal fat, and the d-xylose absorption-excretion test, which is a good screening test for carbohydrate absorption (see Table 37-11). Other diagnostic studies include three different kinds of breath tests: (1) the bile acid breath test, which is used to evaluate bile salt malabsorption or malabsorption from bacterial overgrowth; (2) the triolein breath test, which measures carbon dioxide excretion after ingestion of a radioactive triglyceride; and (3) the excretion of breath hydrogen after ingestion of lactose, which is a sensitive, specific, and noninvasive test for detection of lactase deficiency. The rationale for the hydrogen breath test is that bacterial metabolism is the only source of hydrogen production in humans, and most of this occurs in the colon.

A pancreatic secretion test using secretion may be performed to rule out pancreatic insufficiency. Endoscopy may be used to obtain a small bowel biopsy specimen for diagnosis. Radiographic studies of the esophagus, stomach, and small intestine may be indicated. A small bowel barium enema is frequently performed to identify abnormal mucosal patterns.

Laboratory studies that are frequently ordered include a CBC, determination of prothrombin time, serum vitamin A and carotene levels, serum electrolytes, cholesterol, and calcium.

SPRUE

Two closely related malabsorption conditions are *nontropical sprue* and *tropical sprue.* Tropical and nontropical sprue are found in adults. Nontropical sprue is most commonly referred to as *celiac sprue* (especially in children) but is also called *adult celiac disease* and *gluten-induced enteropathy.*

Etiology and Pathophysiology

In celiac disease there is marked atrophy and flattening of the villi. As a result, absorption within the small intestine is reduced. The proposed reason for the injury to the villi is a hypersensitivity response initiated by gluten and gliadin (a breakdown product of gluten). Gluten is a protein found in wheat, rye, barley, and oats. The hypersensitivity leads to an inflammatory response of the mucosa.

Tropical sprue is a chronic disorder acquired in endemic tropical areas. The exact cause is unknown, but the disorder has been linked to an infectious agent. Folate deficiency is also believed to play a role in the development of this disease. Clinically, it resembles nontropical sprue.

Clinical Manifestations

A patient may become symptomatic at any age with celiac sprue, but the incidence peaks in childhood when gluten is first introduced and then during the fourth and fifth decades.[34] Symptoms include steatorrhea (bulky, foul-smelling, yellow-gray, greasy stools with puttylike consistency), diarrhea, weight loss, abdominal distention, and excessive flatulence. There may also be signs of multiple vitamin deficiencies (e.g., glossitis, cheilosis).

Diagnostic Studies and Collaborative Care

Diagnosis of sprue may be made by stool content analyses or intestinal biopsy. Barium enema may demonstrate abnormalities, including obliteration of intestinal folds. Treatment of sprue syndrome is based on the underlying cause. In nontropical sprue, a gluten-free diet usually leads to clinical recovery. Wheat, barley, oats, and rye products should be avoided. Soybean flours may be used. Foods must be scrutinized for the gluten content. Additives such as hydrolyzed vegetable proteins are often derived from cereal grains, including wheat. For those patients who are unresponsive to dietary exclusion therapy (gluten-free diet), corticosteroids may be used to treat nontropical sprue. The basis for this treatment is that the inflammatory response is mediated by an immunologic response.

Tropical sprue is treated with broad-spectrum antibiotics (e.g., tetracycline) in conjunction with folic acid therapy. The patient who responds to this therapy and achieves a remission is usually maintained on folic acid.

LACTASE DEFICIENCY

Lactase deficiency is a condition in which the lactase enzyme is deficient or absent. Lactase is the enzyme that breaks down lactose into two simple sugars—glucose and galactose. Although primary lactase deficiency seems to be hereditary, milk intolerance may not become clinically evident until late adolescence or early adulthood. About 5% of the adult population have primary lactase deficiency. The highest incidence is found in African-Americans, Native-Americans, Mexican-Americans, and persons of Jewish descent. Acquired lactase deficiency is often seen in other GI diseases in which the mucosa has been damaged, including ulcerative colitis, Crohn's disease, gastroenteritis, and sprue syndrome.

Clinical Manifestations

The symptoms of lactose intolerance include bloating, flatulence, crampy abdominal pain, and diarrhea. They may occur within one half hour to several hours after drinking a glass of milk or ingesting a milk product. The diarrhea of lactose intolerance results from fluid secretion into the small intestines, responding to the osmotic action of undigested lactose.

NURSING AND COLLABORATIVE MANAGEMENT: LACTASE DEFICIENCY

Many lactose-intolerant persons are aware of their milk intolerance and avoid milk. A lactose intolerance test can be performed to rule out milk allergies. The patient is given 50 g of lactose orally. Blood samples are drawn before the consumption of lactose and at 15-, 30-, 60-, and 90-minute intervals. Failure of the blood glucose level to increase more than 20 mg/dl is suggestive of lactase deficiency. Results of the hydrogen breath test after ingestion of lactose are abnormal.

Treatment consists of eliminating lactose from the diet by avoiding milk and milk products. A lactose-free diet is given initially and is gradually advanced to a low-lactose diet as tolerated by the patient. The objective of care is to teach the importance of adherence to the diet. Many lactose-intolerant persons may not exhibit symptoms if lactose is taken in small amounts. In some persons, lactose may be tolerated better if taken with meals.

The patient needs to be aware that milk, ice cream, cottage cheese, and cheese have a high lactose content. If the milk has been fermented (e.g., cultured buttermilk, yogurt, sour cream), the patient with low lactase levels may tolerate it better.

Lactase enzyme (Lactaid) is available commercially as an over-the-counter (OTC) product. It is mixed with milk and breaks down the lactose before the milk is ingested.

SHORT BOWEL SYNDROME

Short bowel syndrome (SBS) results from extensive resection of the small intestine. Rapid intestinal transit, impaired digestive and absorption processes, and fluid and electrolyte losses characterize the syndrome. In adults, resection of the small intestine may be necessary for bowel infarction because of vascular thrombosis or insufficiency, abdominal trauma, cancer, radiation enteritis, or Crohn's disease.

The amount and portions of small bowel resected are associated with the number and severity of symptoms. Resections of up to 50% of the small intestine cause little disturbance of bowel function, especially if the terminal ileum and ileocecal valve remain intact. After large resections, the remaining intestine undergoes adaptive changes that are more pronounced in the ileum. The villi and crypts increase in size, and absorptive capacity of the remaining intestine increases. Intestinal adaptation is enhanced by the presence of food, fiber, bile, and pancreatic secretions in the lumen and continues for up to 2 years. Resection of the ileum, ileocecal valve, or colon results in a rapid intestinal transit, decreasing absorption time. Ileal resection causes malabsorption of cobalamin, bile salts, and fat, resulting in steatorrhea.

Clinical Manifestations

The predominant manifestations of SBS are diarrhea or steatorrhea.[35] There may be signs of malnutrition and multiple vitamin and mineral deficiencies (e.g., weight loss, cobalamin, and zinc deficiency, hypocalcemia). The patient may develop lactase deficiency and bacterial overgrowth. Oxalate kidney stones may form from increased colonic absorption of oxalate.

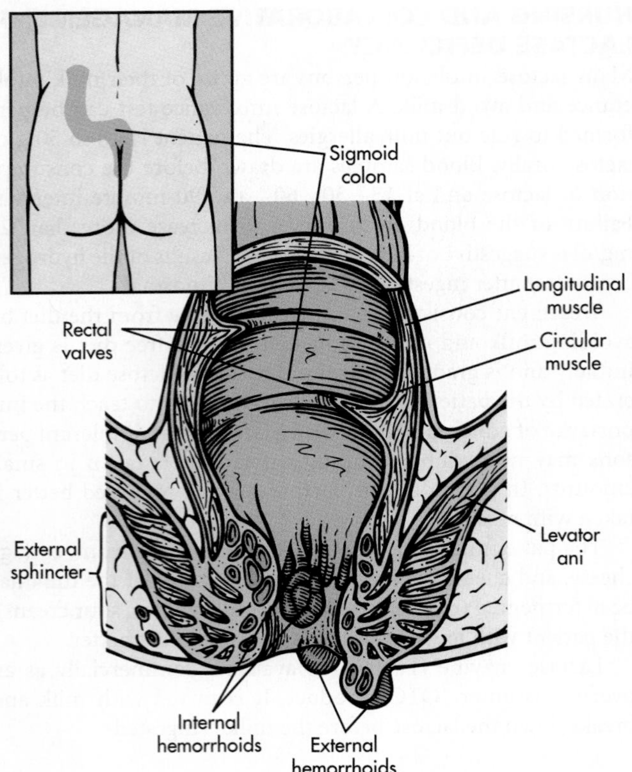

Fig. 40-18 Anatomic structures of the rectum and anus with external and internal hemorrhoids.

Collaborative Care

The overall goals are that the patient with SBS will have fluid and electrolyte balance, normal nutritional status, and control of diarrhea. In the period immediately following massive bowel resection, patients receive total parenteral nutrition to replace fluid, electrolyte, and nutrient losses and to rest the bowel. Hypersecretion of gastric acid, whose cause is unknown, is reduced by H_2-receptor antagonists (e.g., cimetidine [Tagamet]).

A diet high in carbohydrate and low in fat is recommended. A high-carbohydrate, low-fat diet supplemented with soluble fiber, pectin, the amino acid glutamine, and parenteral growth hormone improved nutrient absorption, decreased stool output, and enabled patients to wean off parenteral nutrition.[35] The patient with SBS is encouraged to eat at least six meals per day to increase the time of contact between food and the intestine. Oral intake can be supplemented with elemental nutrient formulas and tube feeding during the night. For patients with severe malabsorption, total parenteral nutrition may be reinstituted. Intestinal transplantation is an experimental procedure primarily used for patients with severe SBS complicated by liver failure.[36]

Narcotic antidiarrheal drugs are the most effective in decreasing intestinal motility (see Table 40-3). For patients with limited ileal resections (<100 cm), cholestyramine (Questran) reduces diarrhea resulting from unabsorbed bile acids and increasing their excretion in feces. Bile acids stimulate intestinal fluid secretion and reduce colonic fluid absorption.

ANORECTAL PROBLEMS

HEMORRHOIDS

Hemorrhoids are dilated hemorrhoidal veins. They may be *internal* (occurring above the internal sphincter) or *external* (occurring outside the external sphincter) (Fig. 40-18). Symptoms of hemorrhoids, including bleeding, pruritus, prolapse, and pain, are common in all age groups. In affected persons, hemorrhoids appear periodically, depending on amount of anorectal pressure.

Etiology and Pathophysiology

Hemorrhoids develop when the flow of blood through the veins of the hemorrhoidal plexus is impaired. Internal hemorrhoids may become constricted and painful. They are the most common cause of bleeding with defecation. The amount of blood lost at one time may be small but may lead to iron deficiency anemia over time. External hemorrhoids are reddish blue and seldom bleed or cause pain unless a vein ruptures. If the blood clots in external hemorrhoids, they become inflamed, painful, and are said to be *thrombosed.*

Hemorrhoids may be caused by many factors, including pregnancy, prolonged constipation, straining in an effort to defecate, heavy lifting, prolonged standing and sitting, and portal hypertension (as found in cirrhosis).

Collaborative Care

Hemorrhoids are diagnosed by inspection, digital examination, proctoscopy, or examination with the flexible sigmoidoscope. Therapy should be directed toward the causes and the patient's symptoms. A high-fiber diet and increased fluid intake prevents constipation and reduces straining, which allows engorgement of the veins to subside. Ointments such as Nupercaine; creams, suppositories, and impregnated pads that contain antiinflammatory agents (e.g., hydrocortisone); or astringents and anesthetics (e.g., witch hazel, pramoxine, and benzocaine) may be used to shrink the mucous membranes and relieve discomfort. Stool softeners may be ordered to keep the stools soft, and sitz baths may be ordered to relieve pain.

Application of ice packs for a few hours, followed by warm packs, may be used for thrombosed hemorrhoids. Another conservative treatment involves use of a sclerosing solution, such as 5% phenol in oil, or a combined solution of quinine and urea may be injected into the submucous tissue surrounding the hemorrhoids, causing a fibrosing and shrinking of the supporting tissues.

Internal hemorrhoids may be ligated with a rubber band. The constrictive effect impairs circulation, and the tissue becomes necrotic, separates, and sloughs off. There is some local discomfort with this procedure, but no anesthetic is required. Aspirin or propoxyphene (Darvon) is usually given for discomfort. Anal dilation and lateral sphincterotomy may be performed to reduce vascular engorgement by reducing sphincter pressure. Other methods, such as infrared photocoagulation, bipolar diathermy, and cryotherapy, are used to treat the mucosa.

A *hemorrhoidectomy* is the surgical excision of hemorrhoids. Surgery is indicated when there is prolapse, excessive pain or bleeding, or large hemorrhoids. In general, hemorrhoidectomy is reserved for patients with severe symptoms related to multiple thrombosed hemorrhoids or marked protrusion. Surgical removal may be done by cautery, clamp, or excision. One surgical approach is to leave the area open so that healing takes place by secondary intention. In another approach the hemorrhoids are removed, the tissue is sutured, and healing takes place by primary-intention wound healing.

NURSING MANAGEMENT: HEMORRHOIDS

Conservative nursing management for the patient with hemorrhoids includes teaching measures to prevent constipation, avoidance of prolonged standing or sitting, proper use of OTC medications available for hemorrhoidal symptoms, and the need to seek medical care for severe symptoms of hemorrhoids (e.g., excessive pain and bleeding, prolapsed hemorrhoids) when necessary.

Pain is a common problem after a hemorrhoidectomy. The nurse must be aware that although the procedure is minor the pain is severe, and narcotics are usually given initially.

Sitz baths are started 1 to 2 days after surgery. A warm sitz bath provides comfort and keeps the anal area clean. A sponge ring in the sitz bath helps relieve pressure on the area. Initially the patient should not be left alone because of the possibility of weakness or fainting.

Packing may be inserted into the rectum to absorb drainage. A T-binder may hold the dressing in place. If packing is inserted, it usually is removed the first or second postoperative day. The nurse should assess for rectal bleeding. The patient may be embarrassed when the dressing is changed, and privacy should be provided. The patient usually dreads the first bowel movement and often resists the urge to defecate. Pain medication may be given before the bowel movement to reduce discomfort.

A stool softener such as docusate (Colace) is usually ordered the first few postoperative days. If the patient does not have a bowel movement within 2 to 3 days, an oil retention enema is given.

Discharge teaching includes the importance of the diet, care of the anal area, symptoms of complications (especially bleeding), and avoidance of constipation and straining. Sitz baths are recommended for 1 to 2 weeks. The physician may order a stool softener to be taken for a time. Hemorrhoids may recur. Occasionally anal strictures develop and dilation is necessary. Regular checkups are important in the prevention of any further problems.

ANAL FISSURE

An *anal fissure* (*fissura in ano*) is a skin ulcer or a crack in the lining of the anal wall that is caused by trauma or local infection. It is frequently associated with constipation and subsequent stretching of the anus from hard feces. The most common clinical manifestations are painful spasms of the anal sphincter and severe, burning pain during defecation. Some bleeding may occur, and constipation results because of fear of pain associated with bowel movements.

Conservative treatment consists of bowel regulation with mineral oil and stool softeners. Sitz baths and anal anesthetic suppositories (Anusol) are also ordered. Surgical treatment usually consists of excision of the fissure. Postoperative nursing care is the same as the care for the patient who has had a hemorrhoidectomy.

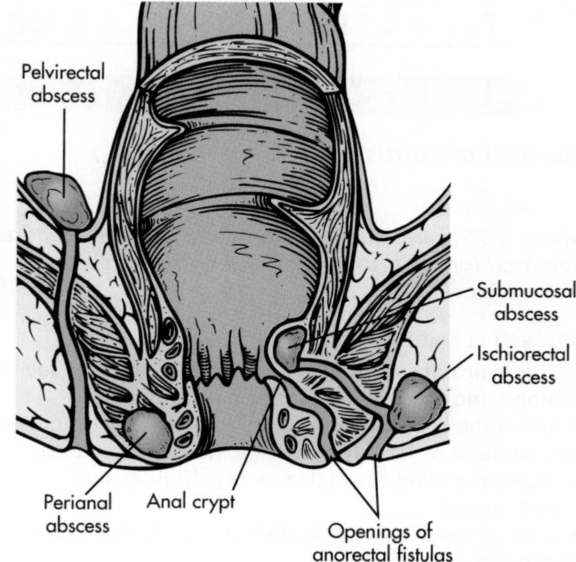

Fig. 40-19 Common sites of anorectal abscesses and fistula formation.

ANORECTAL ABSCESS

Anorectal abscesses are defined as undrained collections of perianal pus (Fig. 40-19). They are due to perirectal infections in patients who have compromised local circulation or active inflammatory disease. The most common causative organisms are *Escherichia coli*, staphylococci, and streptococci. Clinical manifestations include local pain and swelling, foul-smelling drainage, tenderness, and elevated temperature. Sepsis can occur as a complication.

Surgical therapy consists of drainage of abscesses. If packing is used, it should be impregnated with petroleum jelly and the area should be allowed to heal by granulation. The packing is changed every day, and moist, hot compresses are applied to the area. Care must be taken to avoid soiling the dressing during urination or defecation. A low-residue diet is given. The patient may leave the hospital with the area open. Discharge teaching should include wound care, the importance of sitz baths, thorough cleaning after bowel movements, and follow-up visits to the physician.

ANORECTAL FISTULA

An anal fistula is an abnormal tunnel leading out from the anus or rectum. It may extend to the outside of the skin, vagina, or buttocks. Anorectal fistulas are a complication of Crohn's disease. This condition often precedes an anorectal abscess.

Feces may enter the fistula and cause an infection. There may be persistent, bloodstained, purulent discharge or stool leakage from the fistula. The patient may have to wear a pad to prevent staining of clothes.

CRITICAL THINKING EXERCISES

CASE STUDY

Ulcerative Colitis

Patient Profile

Marie, a 37-year-old mother to two school-aged children, is admitted for the fifth time in 11 months with acute ulcerative colitis.

Subjective Data

- Complains of severe diarrhea (10 to 15 stools a day with blood and mucous) and intestinal cramping.
- States she has lost 8 lb (3.6 kg) in the past 11 months.
- Complains of fatigue, anorexia, nausea, vomiting.
- States she takes sulfasalazine (Azulfidine) and prednisone.
- Has not taken any medication in past 72 hours because of nausea and vomiting.
- Tearfully states she is "tired of this disease interfering with her life."

Objective Data

Physical Examination

- Temperature of 100.4°F (38°C)
- Heart rate of 110 beats per minute; BP of 115/70 mm Hg
- Weight 109 lb (50 kg)
- Palpation over the colon reveals abdominal tenderness.

Laboratory Tests

Hct 26%
Hb 9 g/dl (90 g/L)
Serum albumin 2.3 g/dl (23 g/L)

Critical Thinking Questions

1. How do the pathophysiologic changes of ulcerative colitis differ from those of Crohn's disease?
2. Explain the reason for Marie's anemia and low serum albumin.
3. What is the significance of Marie's tachycardia?
4. What nursing interventions are indicated for Marie at this stage of her illness?
5. Explain the actions of sulfasalazine and prednisone in treating ulcerative colitis.
6. What are complications of ulcerative colitis and the role of the nurse in preventing their occurrence?
7. Based on the assessment data, write one or more nursing diagnoses. Are there any collaborative problems?

NURSING RESEARCH ISSUES

1. What are the primary problems related to sexuality and sexual function in patients with an ostomy?
2. Are the psychologic responses and coping strategies of younger patients "receiving" an ostomy different from those of older patients?
3. What can a nurse do to help improve the self-image of patients with ostomies?
4. Do psychosocial factors have a significant role in the exacerbation of IBD?
5. Do nonpharmacologic, complementary therapies alleviate the symptoms of a patient with IBS?
6. Which sources of dietary fiber are most effective in treating fecal incontinence and IBS?
7. Which strategies can increase screening behaviors for colorectal cancer, especially among minority groups?
8. How can a nurse facilitate self-care among older adults with chronic IBD?

Surgical therapy involves a fistulotomy or a fistulectomy. In a fistulotomy the fistula is opened and healthy tissue is allowed to granulate. A fistulectomy is an excision of the entire fistulous tract. Gauze packing is inserted and the wound is allowed to heal by granulation. Care is the same as after a hemorrhoidectomy.

PILONIDAL SINUS

A *pilonidal sinus* is a small tract under the skin between the buttocks in the sacrococcygeal area. It is thought to be of congenital origin. It may have several openings and is lined with epithelium and hair, thus the name pilonidal ("a nest of hair").

The skin is moist, and movement of the buttocks causes the short, wiry hair to penetrate the skin. The irritated skin becomes infected and forms a pilonidal cyst or abscess. There are no symptoms unless there is an infection. If it becomes infected, the patient complains of pain and swelling at the base of the spine.

The formed abscess requires incision and drainage. The wound may be closed or left open to heal by secondary intention. The wound is packed and sitz baths are ordered.

Nursing care includes hot, moist heat applications when an abscess is present. The patient is usually more comfortable lying on the abdomen or side. The patient should be instructed to avoid contaminating the dressing when urinating or defecating and to avoid straining whenever possible.

REVIEW QUESTIONS

The number of the question corresponds to the same-numbered objective at the beginning of the chapter.

1. Common treatment measures for the patient with constipation include
   a. enemas and high fluid intake.
   b. anticholinergic drugs and low fiber diet.
   c. antiemetics and high fluid intake.
   d. stool softeners and high fiber diet.
2. In teaching the patient with chronic constipation, the nurse instructs the patient to
   a. drink at least 3 quarts of liquids daily.
   b. avoid intake of insoluble fiber to prevent gas production.
   c. use laxatives until the bowel establishes a regular emptying pattern.
   d. schedule enemas three to four times a week to completely empty the large bowel.

3. During the first 12 hours following an exploratory laparotomy for an acute abdomen the nurse anticipates that drainage from the NG tube will be
   a. yellowish in color.
   b. clear gastric secretion.
   c. dark brown to dark red.
   d. bright red with blood clots.
4. The nurse notifies the physician, suspecting a possible ruptured appendix when the patient has
   a. a low-grade fever with a leukocytosis.
   b. a distended, rigid abdomen and muscle spasms.
   c. right lower quadrant pain on palpation of the left lower quadrant.
   d. localized abdominal pain halfway between the umbilicus and the right iliac crest.
5. A patient is admitted to the emergency department with right lower abdominal pain of 6 hours duration. During the examination of the patient to establish a diagnosis the nurse would expect medical orders to include
   a. application of a heating pad to relax the abdominal muscles.
   b. obtaining a urine specimen to rule out genitourinary conditions.
   c. encouraging oral fluids to prevent dehydration and hypovolemia.
   d. administration of cleansing enemas in preparation for colonoscopy.
6. On assessment of the patient with gastroenteritis the nurse would expect to find
   a. fever, diarrhea, and leukopenia.
   b. anorexia, pain, and constipation.
   c. vomiting, fever, and constipation.
   d. abdominal cramps, nausea, and vomiting.
7. In planning care for the patient with ulcerative colitis the nurse recognizes that a major difference between ulcerative colitis and Crohn's disease is that ulcerative colitis
   a. causes more nutritional deficiencies than does Crohn's disease.
   b. causes more abdominal pain and cramping than does Crohn's disease.
   c. is curable with a colectomy while Crohn's disease often recurs after surgery.
   d. is more highly associated with a familial relationship than is Crohn's disease.
8. The nurse performs a detailed assessment of the abdomen of a patient with a possible bowel obstruction knowing that a manifestation of an obstruction high in the small intestine is
   a. orange-brown, feculent vomitus.
   b. widespread abdominal distention.
   c. persistent, colicky abdominal pain.
   d. projectile vomiting that relieves abdominal pain.
9. A patient with cancer of the rectum is scheduled for an abdominal-perineal resection. Preoperatively the nurse teaches the patient that postoperative measures will include
   a. positioning from side-to-side to prevent perineal pressure.
   b. care of an abdominal ileostomy site that drains fecal material.
   c. administration of medicated enemas to prevent anal infections.
   d. maintenance of portable suctions draining the abdominal incision.
10. The nurse explains to the patient undergoing ostomy surgery that the procedure that maintains the most normal functioning of the bowel is
    a. a sigmoid colostomy.
    b. a transverse colostomy.
    c. a descending colostomy.
    d. an ascending colostomy.
11. The use of nonabsorbable antibiotics as preparation for bowel surgery is done primarily to
    a. reduce the bacterial flora in the colon.
    b. prevent additional formation of ammonia.
    c. prevent postoperative formation of intestinal gas.
    d. stimulate bowel bacteria to increase production of Vitamin K.
12. The patient with an ileostomy is more likely than a patient with transverse colostomy to require
    a. ostomy irrigations.
    b. solid skin barriers.
    c. drainable pouches.
    d. increased fluid intake.
13. In contrast to diverticulitis, the patient with diverticulosis
    a. has rectal bleeding.
    b. often has no symptoms.
    c. has localized crampy pain.
    d. frequently develops peritonitis.
14. A nursing intervention that is most appropriate to decrease postoperative edema and pain following an inguinal herniorrhaphy is
    a. applying a truss to the hernia site.
    b. allowing the patient to stand to void.
    c. elevation of the scrotum with a support or small pillow.
    d. supporting the incision during routine coughing and deep breathing.
15. The nurse determines that the goals of dietary teaching have been met when the patient with nontropical sprue selects from the menu
    a. cornmeal mush and sausage.
    b. yogurt, fresh fruit, and rye toast.
    c. oatmeal, skim milk, and orange juice.
    d. pancakes with syrup and scrambled eggs.
16. A patient undergoes a hemorrhoidectomy in a day surgery unit. To promote bowel movements the first several days postoperatively the nurse teaches the patient to
    a. take a sitz bath in the morning before defecating.
    b. administer an oil-retention enema to empty the bowel.
    c. use prescribed pain medication before the bowel movement.
    d. avoid straining and increasing abdominal pressure during defecation.

References

1. Kelly CP, LaMont JT: *Clostridium difficile* infection, *Ann Rev Med* 49:375, 1998.
2. Bentsen D, Braun JW: Controlling fecal incontinence with sensory retraining managed by advanced practice nurses, *Clin Nurs Specialist* 10:171, 1996.
3. Doughty D: A physiologic approach to bowel training, *J WOCN* 23:46, 1996.
4. Norton C: The causes and nursing management of constipation, *Br J Nurs* 5:1252, 1996.
5. Storrie JB: Biofeedback: a first line treatment for idiopathic constipation, *Br J Nurs* 6:152, 1997.
6. Town J: Bringing acute abdomen into focus, *Nursing* 27:52, 1997.
7. Drossman DA: Diagnosing and treating patients with refractory functional gastrointestinal disorders, *Ann Intern Med* 123:688, 1995.
8. Sabiston DC: Appendicitis. In Sabiston DC, editor: *Textbook of surgery: the biological basis of modern surgical practice,* ed 15, Philadelphia, 1997, WB Saunders.
9. Hau T: Biology and treatment of peritonitis: the historic development of current concepts, *J Am Coll Surg* 186:475, 1998.

10. Drossman DA and others: US householder survey of functional gastrointestinal disorders: prevalence, sociodemography, and health impact, *Dig Dis Sci* 38:1569, 1993.
11. Moses PL and others: Inflammatory bowel disease: 1. Origins, presentation, and course, *Postgrad Med* 103:77, 1998.
12. Tayoda H and others: Distinct associations of HLA class II genes with inflammatory bowel disease, *Gastroenterology* 104:741, 1993.
13. Jewell DP: Ulcerative colitis. In Feldman M and others, editors: *Sleisenger and Fardtran's gastrointestinal and liver disease,* ed 6, Philadelphia, 1998, WB Saunders.
14. Zlatanic J and others: Inflammatory bowel disease and immune thrombocytopenic purpura: is there a correlation? *Am J Gastroenterol* 92:2285, 1997.
15. Hanauer SB: Drug therapy: inflammatory bowel disease, *N Engl J Med* 334:841, 1996.
16. Rogler G, Andus T: Cytokines in inflammatory bowel disease, *World J Surg,* 22:382, 1998.
17. Sachar DB: Maintenance strategies in Crohn's disease, *Hosp Prac* 31:99, 1996.
18. Birtwistle J, Hall K: Does nicotine have beneficial effects in the treatment of certain diseases? *Br J Nurs* 5:1195, 1996.
19. Cummings JH: Short-chain fatty acid enemas in the treatment of distal ulcerative colitis, *Europ J Gastroenterol Hepatol* 9:149, 1997.
20. Belluzzi A and others: Effect of an enteric-coated fish-oil preparation on relapses in Crohn's disease, *N Engl J Med* 334:1557, 1996.
21. McCloy C and others: The etiology of intestinal obstruction in patients without prior laparotomy or hernia, *Am Surg* 64:19, 1998.
22. Markowitz A, Winawer SJ: Management of colorectal polyps, *CA-A Cancer Journal for Clinicians* 47:93, 1997.
23. American Cancer Society: Cancer facts and figures—1998, Atlanta, 1998, American Cancer Society.
24. Parker SL and others: Cancer statistics 1997, *CA-A Cancer Journal for Clinicians* 47:5, 1997.
25. Meissner JE: Caring for patients with colorectal cancer, *Nursing* 26:60, 1996.
26. Bond JH: Screening for colorectal cancer, *Hosp Prac* 32:59, 1997.
27. Hammerhofer-Jereb A: Laparoscopic bowel resection? *RN* 59:22, 1996.
28. Diaz-Canton E, Pazdur R: Adjuvant medical therapy for colorectal cancer, *Surg Clin North Am* 77:211, 1997.
29. Byers T and others. American Cancer Society guidelines for screening and surveillance for early detection of colorectal polyps and cancer: update 1997, *CA-A Cancer Journal for Clinicians* 47:154, 1997.
30. Powe BD: Fatalism among elderly African-Americans. Effects on colorectal cancer screening, *Cancer* 18:385, 1995.
31. Vainio H, Morgan G, Kleihues P: An international evaluation of the cancer-preventive potential of nonsteroidal antiinflammatory drugs, *Cancer Epidemiol Biomarkers Prev* 6:749, 1997.
32. Sandler RS and others: Aspirin and nonsteroidal antiinflammatory agents and risk for colorectal adenomas, *Gastroenterology* 114:441, 1998.
33. Roberts P and others: Practice parameters for sigmoid diverticulitis-supporting documentation, *Dis Colon Rectum* 38:126, 1995.
34. Murphy D: Celiac sprue, *Gastroenterology Nursing* 18:133, 1995.
35. Thompson JS: Management of the short bowel syndrome, *Postsurgical Syndromes* 23:403, 1994.
36. Byrne TA and others: Growth hormone, glutamine and a modified diet enhance nutrient absorption in patients with severe short bowel syndrome, *JPEN* 19:296, 1995.

Resources

American Cancer Society
1599 Clifton Rd NE
Atlanta, GA 30329
404-320-3333
http://www.acs.org

American Gastroenterological Association
7910 Woodmont Ave, 7th Floor,
Bethesda, MD 20814
301-654-2055
fax: 301-652-3890
http://www.gastro.org/

American Society for Gastrointestinal Endoscopy
13 Elm Street
Manchester, MA 01944-1314
978-526-8330
fax: 978-526-4018
http://www.asge.org/

Crohn's & Colitis Foundation of America (CCFA)
386 Park Avenue South, 17th Floor
New York, NY 10016-8804
212-685-3440
800-932-2423
fax: 212-779-4098
http://www.ccfa.org

Crohn's & Colitis Foundation of Canada (CCFC)
21 St. Clair Avenue East, Suite 301
Toronto, Ontario M4T 1L9 CANADA
416-920-5035
800-387-1479
fax: 416-929-0364
http://www.ccfc.org

United Ostomy Association (UOA)
19772 MacArthur Blvd, Suite 200
Irvine, CA 92612-2405
800-826-0826
http://www.uoa.org/

Wound, Ostomy & Continence Nurses Society
2755 Bristol Street, Suite 110
Costa Mesa, CA 92626
714-476-0268
fax: 714-545-3643

***For additional Internet resources, see the website for this book at* www.mosby.com/MERLIN/medsurg_lewis/**

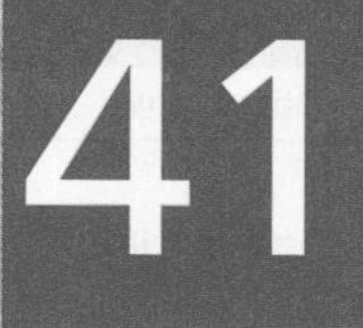

REMEMBER to check out your **companion CD-ROM**

41 NURSING MANAGEMENT Liver, Biliary Tract, and Pancreas Problems

Rachel Elrod

www.mosby.com/MERLIN/medsurg_lewis

LEARNING OBJECTIVES

1. Define jaundice and describe signs and symptoms that may occur with the different types of jaundice.
2. Differentiate among the types of viral hepatitis, including etiology, pathophysiology, clinical manifestations, complications, and collaborative care.
3. Describe the nursing management of the patient with viral hepatitis.
4. Explain the etiology, pathophysiology, clinical manifestations, complications, and collaborative care of the patient with cirrhosis of the liver.
5. Describe the nursing management of the patient with cirrhosis.
6. Describe the clinical manifestations and management of carcinoma of the liver.
7. Describe the pathophysiology, clinical manifestations, complications, and collaborative care of acute and chronic pancreatitis.
8. Describe the nursing management of the patient with pancreatitis.
9. Explain the clinical manifestations and collaborative care of the patient with carcinoma of the pancreas.
10. Explain the pathophysiology, clinical manifestations, complications, and collaborative care including surgical therapy of gallbladder disorders.
11. Describe the nursing management of the patient undergoing conservative or surgical treatment of cholecystitis and cholelithiasis.

JAUNDICE

Jaundice, a yellowish discoloration of body tissues, results from an alteration in normal bilirubin metabolism or flow of bile into the hepatic or biliary duct systems. It is a symptom rather than a disease. Jaundice results when the concentration of bilirubin in the blood becomes abnormally increased. The bilirubin level has to be approximately three times normal levels (2 to 3 mg/dl [34 to 51 mol/L]) for jaundice to occur. Jaundice can usually first be detected in the sclera and skin (Fig. 41-1).

Most of the body's bilirubin is formed from the breakdown of hemoglobin (from erythrocytes) by macrophages (see Fig. 37-6). This unconjugated (indirect) bilirubin is released into the circulation bound to albumin and is not water soluble. Because unconjugated bilirubin is not water soluble and cannot be filtered in the kidneys, it is not excreted in the urine. In the liver the unconjugated bilirubin is conjugated with glucuronic acid to form conjugated (direct) bilirubin, which is water soluble. Conjugated bilirubin is secreted into bile, which flows through the hepatic and biliary duct system into the small intestine. In the large intestine, bilirubin is converted to stercobilinogen and urobilinogen by bacterial action. Stercobilinogen gives the characteristic brown color to feces. Some urobilinogen is reabsorbed into the portal circulation and returned to the liver. Normally a very small amount of urobilinogen is excreted in urine.

The three types of jaundice are classified as hemolytic, hepatocellular, and obstructive. Diagnostic findings associated with these types of jaundice are shown in Table 41-1.

Hemolytic Jaundice

Hemolytic (prehepatic) jaundice is due to an increased breakdown of red blood cells (RBCs), which produces an increased amount of unconjugated bilirubin in the blood (see Table 41-1). The liver is unable to handle this increased load. Causes of hemolytic jaundice include blood transfusion reactions, sickle cell crisis, and hemolytic anemia.

Hepatocellular Jaundice

Hepatocellular (hepatic) jaundice results from the liver's altered ability to take up bilirubin from the blood or to conjugate or excrete it. Both unconjugated and conjugated bilirubin serum levels increase (see Table 41-1). Because conjugated bilirubin is water soluble, it is excreted in the urine. The most common causes of hepatocellular jaundice are hepatitis, cirrhosis, and hepatic carcinoma.

Obstructive Jaundice

Obstructive (posthepatic) jaundice is due to impeded or obstructed flow of bile through the liver or biliary duct system.

Reviewed by Deborah L. Martin, RN, MN, Chief Executive Officer, Infection Control and Prevention Analysis, Inc., Austin, Tex.

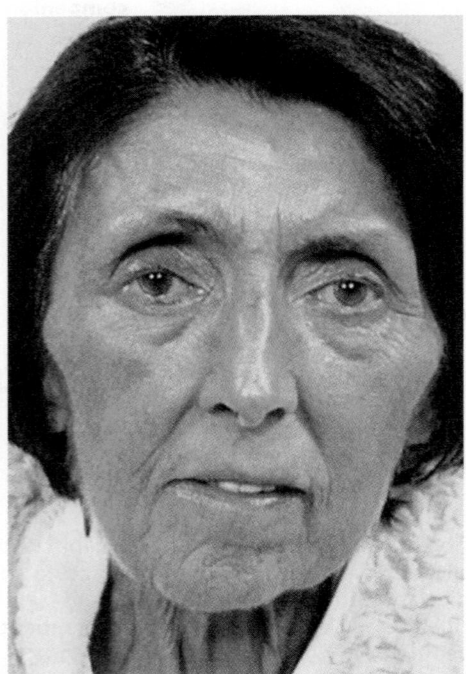

Fig. 41-1 Severe jaundice.

The obstruction may be intrahepatic or extrahepatic. Intrahepatic obstructions are due to swelling or fibrosis of the liver's canaliculi and bile ducts. This can be caused by damage from liver tumors, hepatitis, or cirrhosis. Causes of extrahepatic obstruction include common bile duct obstruction from a stone, sclerosing cholangitis, and carcinoma of the head of the pancreas. Laboratory findings show an elevation of both unconjugated and conjugated bilirubin and urine bilirubin (see Table 41-1). Because bilirubin does not enter the intestines, there is decreased to no fecal or urinary urobilinogen. With complete obstruction, the stools are clay colored.

VIRAL HEPATITIS

Hepatitis is an inflammation of the liver. Acute viral hepatitis is the most common cause of hepatitis. The types of infectious viral hepatitis are A, B, C (formerly called post-transfusion non-A, non-B), D, E, and G. Noninfectious hepatitis may also be caused by drugs and other chemicals (see Table 37-6). Rarely, hepatitis is caused by bacteria, such as streptococci, salmonellae, and *Escherichia coli.*

Viral hepatitis is a major public health concern in the United States. Approximately 152,000 cases of hepatitis A occur annually in the United States and 10 million worldwide. It is nearly universal during childhood in developing countries. There is an estimated 140,000 cases of hepatitis B annually in the United States. In the 1990s the incidence of hepatitis B decreased overall, partly because of the hepatitis B vaccine. However, since 1993 there has been an increase in the incidence of hepatitis B in homosexual men, injecting drug users, and sexually active heterosexuals.

Approximately 35,000 Americans contract hepatitis C annually.[1] Each year 8000 to 12,000 persons chronically infected

Table 41-1 Diagnostic Findings in Jaundice

	Hemolytic	Hepatocellular	Obstructive
Serum bilirubin			
Unconjugated (indirect)	↑	↑	Somewhat ↑
Conjugated (direct)	Normal	↑	Moderately ↑
Urine bilirubin	Negative	↑	↑
Urobilinogen			
Stool	↑	Normal to ↓	Negative
Urine	↑	Normal to ↑	Negative

CULTURAL & ETHNIC CONSIDERATIONS

Disorders of the Liver, Pancreas, and Gallbladder

- Mortality from cirrhosis occurs more frequently among African-Americans than in other ethnic groups.
- Primary hepatic cancer has a higher incidence among African-Americans, Asian-Americans, and Eskimos than Caucasians.
- Pancreatic cancer occurs more frequently among African-Americans and Asian-Americans than Caucasians.
- Caucasians and Native-Americans have a higher incidence of gallbladder disease than African-Americans or Asian-Americans.

with hepatitis C die of a liver-related complication of their infection.[2,3] Chronic hepatitis C infection is now the most common liver disease in the United States.[3] Fortunately, there has been a decline in the incidence of hepatitis C in recent years, which is due in part to screening of the blood supply for anti-HCV (antibody to hepatitis C virus) and safer needle-using practices by injecting drug users.

Etiology

Viral hepatitis can be caused by one of five major viruses: A, B, C, D, and E. Hepatitis G has recently been described. Approximately 90% of post-transfusion and community-acquired hepatitis cases are due to viruses A to E.[1] Other viruses known to damage the liver include cytomegalovirus, Epstein-Barr virus, herpes virus, coxsackievirus, and rubella virus.

The only definitive way to distinguish the various forms of viral hepatitis is by the presence of the antigens and antigenic subtypes and the subsequent development of antibodies to them. Outbreaks of hepatitis are consistently caused by hepatitis A virus. Approximately 50% of viral hepatitis cases in adults in the United States are hepatitis B, 20% are hepatitis C, and 30% are hepatitis A.[4] Infection with each virus provides immunity to that virus (homologous immunity). However, the patient can still develop another type of viral hepatitis. Characteristics of hepatitis viruses are summarized in Table 41-2.

Hepatitis A Virus. The hepatitis A virus (HAV) is an RNA virus that is transmitted through the fecal-oral route. It

Table 41-2 Characteristics of Hepatitis Viruses

	Incubation Period	Mode of Transmission	Sources of Infection and Spread of Disease	Infectivity
Hepatitis A virus (HAV)	15-50 days (average 28)	Fecal-oral (fecal contamination and oral ingestion)	Crowded conditions; poor personal hygiene; poor sanitation; contaminated food, milk, water, and shellfish; persons with subclinical infections; infected food handlers; sexual contact	Most infectious during 2 weeks before onset of symptoms; infectious until 1-2 weeks after symptoms start
Hepatitis B virus (HBV)	45-180 days (average 56-96)	Percutaneous (parenteral)/permucosal exposure to blood or blood products Sexual contact Perinatal transmission Human bile	Contaminated needles, syringes, and blood products; sexual activity with infected partners; asymptomatic carriers Tattoo/body piercing, bites	Before and after symptoms appear; infectious for 4-6 months; in carriers continues for patient's lifetime
Hepatitis C virus (HCV)	14-180 days (average 56)	Percutaneous (parenteral)/permucosal exposure to blood or blood products High-risk sexual contact Perinatal contact	Blood and blood products, needles and syringes, sexual activity with infected partners	1-2 weeks before symptoms; continues during clinical course; indefinitely with carriers
Hepatitis D virus (HDV)	2-26 weeks HBV must precede HDV; chronic carriers of HBV are always at risk	Can cause infection only together with HBV; routes of transmission same as for HBV	Same as HBV	Blood is infectious at all stages of HDV infection
Hepatitis E virus (HEV)	15-64 days (average 26-42 days in different epidemics)	Fecal-oral Outbreaks associated with contaminated water supply in developing countries	Contaminated water; poor sanitation; found in Asia, Africa, and Mexico; not common in the United States and Canada	Not known; may be similar to HAV

frequently occurs in small outbreaks caused by fecal contamination of food or drinking water. It is found in feces 2 or more weeks before the onset of symptoms and up to 1 week after the onset of jaundice (Fig. 41-2). It is present in the blood only briefly. Anti-HAV (antibody to hepatitis A virus) IgM appears in the serum as the stool becomes negative for the virus. Detection of IgM anti-HAV indicates acute hepatitis, and IgG anti-HAV is an indicator of past infection. The presence of IgG antibody provides lifelong immunity.

The mode of transmission of HAV is predominantly fecal-oral (mainly by ingestion of food or liquid infected with the virus) and rarely parenteral. Poor hygiene, crowded situations, and poor sanitary conditions are all factors related to hepatitis A. Transmission occurs between family members, institutionalized individuals, and from common-source outbreaks. The disease occurs more frequently in underdeveloped countries. The eating of raw shellfish from contaminated waters can also be a source of infection. Food-borne hepatitis A outbreaks are usually due to contamination of food during preparation by an infected food handler.

There is no chronic carrier state for HAV. The virus is present in feces during the incubation period, so it can be carried by persons who have undetectable, subclinical infections. The greatest risk of transmission occurs before clinical symptoms are apparent. It can also be transmitted by patients with anicteric (nonjaundice) hepatitis A.

Hepatitis B Virus. Hepatitis B virus (HBV) is a DNA virus that is transmitted by percutaneous (IV drug use, accidental needle-stick punctures) or permucosal exposure to infectious blood, blood products, or other body fluids (semen, vaginal secretions, saliva). Perinatal transmission is also possible. In persons who have HBV, hepatitis B surface antigen (HBsAg) has been detected in almost every body fluid, including vaginal secretions, menstrual fluids, semen, saliva,

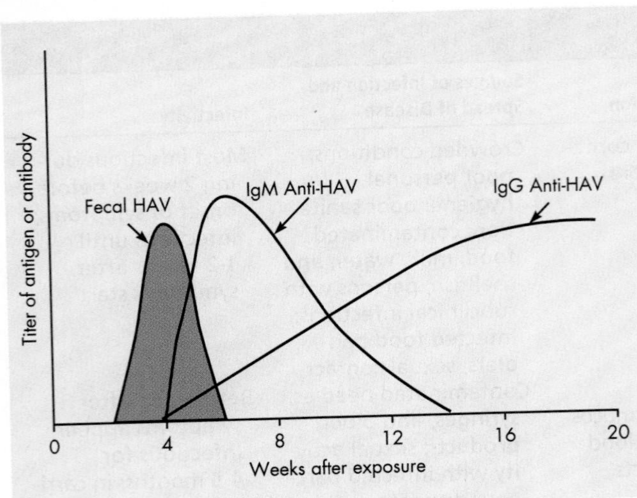

Fig. 41-2 Clinical and serologic events of a typical patient infected with hepatitis A virus (HAV). Elevated alanine aminotransferase (ALT) levels are present by 4 weeks and jaundice appears by about 5 weeks after exposure to the virus.

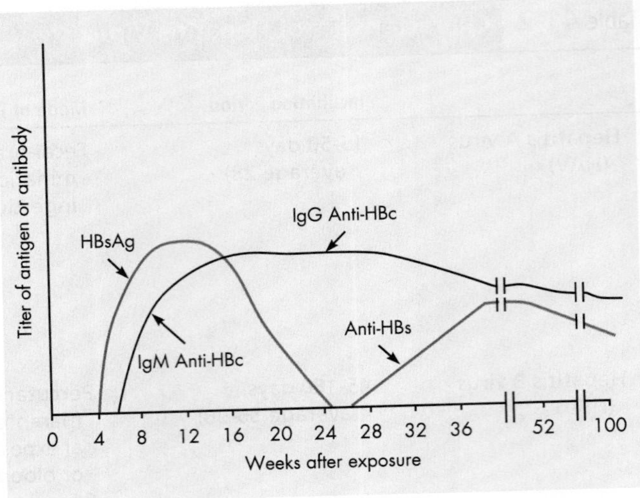

Fig. 41-3 Clinical and serologic events of a typical patient infected with acute hepatitis B virus (HBV). Elevated alanine aminotransferase (ALT) levels are present by about 8 weeks and jaundice appears by about 10 weeks after exposure to the virus. *HBc,* hepatitis B core antigen; *HBsAg,* hepatitis B surface antigen.

respiratory secretions, tears, gastric juice, synovial fluid, and cerebrospinal fluid. Infected semen and saliva contain much lower concentrations of HBV than blood, but the virus can be transmitted via these secretions. If GI bleeding occurs, feces can be contaminated with the virus from the blood. There is no evidence that urine, feces, breast milk, tears, and sweat are infective. Sometimes HBV is transmitted by unidentified means. In 20% to 30% of patients with acute hepatitis B there are no readily identifiable risk factors.[5]

Hepatitis B is a sexually transmitted disease. Approximately 30% of HBV cases are related to heterosexual activity, either with multiple sexual partners or unprotected sex with an infected person.[6] Male homosexuals (especially those practicing anal intercourse) are at risk for HBV infection. Although there is a much lower risk of transmission, kissing and sharing of food items may spread the virus via saliva. The hepatitis B virus can live on a dry surface for at least 7 days. HBV is considered to be 100 times more infectious than human immunodeficiency virus (HIV).[6]

HBV is a complex structure with three distinct antigens: the surface antigen (HBsAg), the core antigen (HBcAg), and the e antigen (HBeAg). The persistence of HBsAg in the serum for 6 to 12 months or longer indicates a carrier state of hepatitis B. Each antigen has a corresponding antibody that may be elicited during an attack of acute viral hepatitis B. These antibodies can be detected in the serum of persons with prior exposure to the antigenic virus (Fig. 41-3). The presence of anti-HBsAg indicates immunity to hepatitis B.

From 2% to 10% of adults who become infected with HBV become chronic HBV carriers and may transmit the virus.[6] The HBsAg level remains elevated in carriers (HBsAg-positive on at least two occasions at least 6 months apart). With carrier status, liver enzyme values may be normal. The carriers of hepatitis B may have low-grade disease, a normal liver, or severe chronic active liver disease. α-Interferon is now being used to try to eliminate the chronic HBV carrier state. A positive test for anti-HBsAg in adults indicates that they have had hepatitis B or the vaccine.

Hepatitis C Virus. Hepatitis C virus (HCV) is an RNA virus that is primarily transmitted percutaneously. Thus the major risk factor for infection is direct percutaneous exposure, such as injecting drugs, transfusion of blood products, hemodialysis, tattooing, high-risk sexual behavior, organ transplants, and exposure to blood and blood products by health care workers. Less frequent routes of transmission are sexual and perinatal. However, 40% to 50% of patients with HCV have no known source of infection.[7]

Hepatitis D Virus. Hepatitis D virus (HDV), also called delta virus, is a defective RNA virus that cannot survive on its own. The importance of HDV relates to its clinical virulence. It can transform asymptomatic or mild chronic hepatitis B infection to severe, progressive chronic active hepatitis and cirrhosis and can accelerate the course of chronic active hepatitis B. Delta virus is also a contributing factor in a substantial number of cases of fulminant hepatitis B. Delta hepatitis can occur as a primary infection along with HBV (coinfection) or in a carrier of hepatitis B (superinfection). HDV is transmitted percutaneously.

Hepatitis E Virus. Hepatitis E virus (HEV) is an RNA virus that is transmitted by the fecal-oral route. The most common mode of transmission is drinking contaminated water. Hepatitis E is also called enteric non-A, non-B hepatitis. Hepatitis E occurs primarily in developing countries. There have been reported epidemics in India, Asia, Mexico, and Africa. Only a few cases have been reported in the United States. Occurrence in the United States is almost always in persons who have recently traveled to HEV-endemic areas.[8] Although not yet commercially available, there is an assay test to determine the antibody to HEV.

Hepatitis G Virus. Recently hepatitis G virus (HGV), an RNA virus, has been discovered. HGV has been found in some

Table 41-3 Clinical Manifestations of the Phases of Hepatitis

Preicteric	Icteric	Posticteric
Anorexia Nausea, vomiting Right upper quadrant discomfort Constipation or diarrhea Decreased sense of taste and smell Malaise Headache Fever Arthralgias Urticaria Hepatomegaly Splenomegaly Weight loss	Jaundice Pruritus Dark urine Bilirubinuria Light stools Fatigue Continued hepatomegaly with tenderness Weight loss	Malaise Easy fatigability Hepatomegaly

blood donors and can be transmitted by transfusion.[9,10] It frequently coexists with other hepatitis viruses, such as HCV. However, most HGV infections are not associated with chronic hepatitis.[9] Thus at this time HGV association with liver disease is uncertain.

Pathophysiology

Liver. The pathophysiologic changes in the various types of viral hepatitis are similar. Hepatitis involves widespread inflammation of liver tissue. Liver cell damage consists of hepatic cell degeneration and necrosis. There is proliferation and enlargement of the Kupffer cells. Inflammation of the periportal areas may interrupt bile flow. Cholestasis may occur. The liver cells regenerate in an orderly manner, and if no complications occur, they should resume their normal appearance and function during convalescence.

Systemic Effects. The antigen-antibody complexes between the virus and its corresponding antibody form a circulating immune complex in the early phases of hepatitis. The presence of circulating immune complexes activates the complement system (see Chapter 12). The clinical manifestations of this activation are rash, angioedema, arthritis, fever, and malaise. Glomerulonephritis and vasculitis have also been found secondary to immune complex disease.

Clinical Manifestations

A large number of patients, especially the younger ones, have no symptoms. The clinical manifestations of viral hepatitis may be classified into three phases: (1) preicteric or prodromal phase, (2) icteric phase, and (3) posticteric or convalescent phase (Table 41-3).

Preicteric Phase. The preicteric phase precedes jaundice and lasts from 1 to 21 days. This is the period of maximal infectivity for hepatitis A. Hepatitis B patients who are HBcAg positive can be infective for years. Gastrointestinal (GI) symptoms include anorexia, nausea, abdominal (right upper quadrant) discomfort, and sometimes vomiting, constipation, or diarrhea. The anorexia is frequently severe and is thought to be caused by a toxin produced by the diseased liver. The patient may find food repugnant and, if a smoker, may have a distaste for cigarettes. There is also a decreased sense of smell. Weight loss occurs during the preicteric phase. Other symptoms during this phase are malaise, headache, low-grade fever, arthralgias, and skin rashes. Physical examination reveals hepatomegaly, lymphadenopathy, and sometimes splenomegaly.

Icteric Phase. The icteric phase lasts 2 to 4 weeks and is characterized by jaundice. Jaundice results when bilirubin diffuses into the tissues. The urine may darken because of excess bilirubin being excreted by the kidneys. If conjugated bilirubin cannot flow out of the liver because of obstruction or inflammation of the bile ducts, the stools will be light or clay colored. Pruritus sometimes accompanies the jaundice, especially if cholestasis is present. The pruritus occurs as a result of the accumulation of bile salts beneath the skin.

When jaundice occurs, the fever usually subsides. The GI symptoms usually remain, and some fatigue may continue. The liver is usually enlarged and tender.

Posticteric Phase. The convalescent stage of the posticteric phase begins as jaundice is disappearing and lasts weeks to months, with an average of 2 to 4 months. During this period the patient's major complaint is malaise and easy fatigability. Hepatomegaly remains for several weeks, but splenomegaly subsides during this period. Relapses may occur, and the disappearance of jaundice does not mean the patient has totally recovered.

General Considerations

Not all patients with viral hepatitis have jaundice. This is termed *anicteric hepatitis* and occurs more frequently in children. A high percentage of persons with HAV are anicteric and do not have symptoms.

There is some slight variation in manifestations between the types of hepatitis. In hepatitis A the onset is more acute and the symptoms are usually mild, flulike manifestations. In hepatitis B the onset is more insidious and the symptoms are usually more severe. There may be fewer GI symptoms. In hepatitis C, although the majority of cases are asymptomatic or mild, HCV has a high rate of persistence and can induce chronic liver disease.

Complications

Most patients with acute HAV and HBV hepatitis recover completely with no complications. The overall mortality rate for hepatitis is less than 1%. The mortality rate is higher in older adults and those with underlying debilitating diseases. Complications that can occur include chronic persistent hepatitis, chronic active hepatitis, fulminant viral hepatitis, and cirrhosis of the liver.

Chronic Persistent Hepatitis. The most common complication of viral hepatitis is chronic persistent hepatitis in which there is a delayed convalescent period. It is usually benign and is characterized by fatigue and hepatomegaly. However, no treatment is required. Liver function tests may remain abnormal for several years.

Table 41-4 Tests for Viral Hepatitis

Virus	Tests	Significance
A	Anti-HAV IgM	Acute infection
	Anti-HAV IgG	Previous infection and long-term immunity
B	HBsAg (hepatitis B surface antigen)	Current infection (but not necessarily acute)* Positive in chronic carriers
	Anti-HBs (antibody to surface antigen)	Indicates previous infection with hepatitis B or immunization Marker for response to vaccine
	HBeAg (hepatitis B e antigen)	Indicates high infectivity; present in acute, active infection
	Anti-HBe (antibody to e antigen)	Indicates previous infection
	HBcAg	Ongoing infection with hepatitis B
	Anti-HBc IgM	Acute infection*
	Anti-HBc IgG (antibody to HB core antigen)	Indicates previous infection or ongoing infection with hepatitis B Does not appear after vaccination
	HBV-DNA	Indicates active ongoing viral replication Best indicator of viral replication
C	Anti-HCV (antibody to hepatitis C)	Marker for acute or chronic infection with HCV Coexisting infection with HBV
	HCV RNA	Indicates active ongoing viral replication
D	Anti-HDV	Present in past or current infection with hepatitis D

*If positive HBsAg and anti-HBc IgM, it indicates the presence of acute infection.
DNA, deoxyribonucleic acid.

Chronic Active Hepatitis. Chronic active hepatitis is characterized by the persistence of signs and symptoms of hepatitis and abnormal liver function tests for more than 6 months. Chronic active hepatitis is seen in hepatitis B and C but not in hepatitis A or E. It is seen in patients with hepatitis D only if they also have hepatitis B. A high percentage of persons with HCV infection (at least 85%) become chronically infected.[11] HBsAg persists longer than 6 months in approximately 10% of patients with hepatitis B. It is distinguished from chronic persistent hepatitis by liver biopsy. The ongoing process of liver necrosis may progress to cirrhosis.

The HBsAg-positive patient whose serum remains positive for HBeAg is more likely to have chronic active hepatitis. In addition, alteration in the patient's cellular immune response may be important in the development of the chronic HBsAg carrier state and consequent progression from acute hepatitis B to chronic active hepatitis. This finding may explain why the patient with chronic renal failure who is undergoing dialysis when hepatitis B develops is more at risk for chronic active hepatitis. (Persons with chronic renal failure are known to have a depressed cellular immune response.)

There is a greater risk for HCV infection to become chronic as compared with HBV. Approximately 85% of patients who have acute HCV will go on to develop chronic infection.[3]

Fulminant Hepatitis. Fulminant viral hepatitis is a clinical syndrome that results in severe impairment or necrosis of liver cells and potential liver failure. Fulminant viral hepatitis develops in a small percentage of patients. The disorder may occur as a complication of hepatitis B, particularly hepatitis B accompanied by infection with delta virus (HDV). Fulminant hepatitis occurs much less frequently with hepatitis C. Toxic reactions to drugs and congenital metabolic disorders may also cause fulminant hepatitis and fulminant liver failure. Hepatocellular failure with death usually occurs.

Diagnostic Studies

Tests for the different types of viral hepatitis are presented in Table 41-4. In viral hepatitis many of the liver function tests show significant abnormalities. The common abnormalities are identified in Table 41-5.

Antibodies to HCV are not protective and are often an indication of active disease. For the patient who has a positive anti-HCV test by enzyme immunoassay (EIA) or if HCV is suspected and there is a false HCV antibody test (only 90% of patients with hepatitis C are positive for anti-HCV), the hepatitis C virus recombinant immunoblot assay (HCV-RIBA) is used to make the diagnosis. There are tests to detect HCV RNA (the virus); however, because of their expense and the possibility of false-negative results, they are not used as the primary tests to confirm or rule out a diagnosis.[12]

Physical assessment reveals hepatic tenderness, hepatomegaly, and splenomegaly. The liver is palpable. A liver biopsy is not indicated unless the diagnosis is in doubt or a more severe form of hepatitis is suspected.

Collaborative Care

There is no specific treatment or therapy for viral hepatitis. Most patients can be managed at home. Emphasis is on measures to rest the body and assist the liver in regenerating (Table 41-6). Adequate nutrients and rest seem to be most beneficial for healing and liver cell (hepatocyte) regeneration. Dietary emphasis is on a well-balanced diet that the patient can tolerate.

Rest reduces the metabolic demands on the liver and promotes cell regeneration. Bed rest may be indicated while the patient is symptomatic. The degree of rest ordered depends on the severity of symptoms, but usually alternating periods of activity and rest are adequate.

Drug Therapy. There are no specific drug therapies for the treatment of acute viral hepatitis. Corticosteroid therapy

Table 41-5 Diagnostic Findings in Hepatitis

Test	Abnormal Finding	Etiology
Transaminases (aminotransferases)		
Aspartate aminotransferase (AST) or serum glutamic-oxaloacetic transaminase (SGOT)	Elevation in preicteric phase; decrease as jaundice disappears	Liver cell injury
Alanine aminotransferase (ALT) or serum glutamic-pyruvic transaminase (SGPT)	Elevation in preicteric phase; decrease as jaundice disappears	Liver cell injury
γ-Glutamyl transpeptidase (GGT)	Elevation	Liver cell injury
Alkaline phosphatase	Some elevation	Impaired excretory function of the liver
Serum proteins		
γ-Globulin	Normal or increased	Impaired clearance of the liver
Albumin	Normal or decreased	Liver damage
Serum bilirubin (total)	Elevation to about 8-15 mg/dl (137-257 μmol/L)	Hepatocellular damage
Urinary bilirubin	Elevation	Conjugated hyperbilirubinemia
Urinary urobilinogen	Elevation 2-5 days before jaundice	Diminished reabsorption of urobilinogen
Prothrombin time	Prolonged	Decreased absorption of vitamin K in intestine with decreased production of prothrombin by liver

COLLABORATIVE CARE

Table 41-6 Viral Hepatitis

Diagnostic
- Liver function studies
- Hepatitis serology
  - HBsAg (HBeAg in some cases)
  - Anti-HBs
  - Anti-HBc—IgM and IgG
  - Anti-HAV—IgM and IgG
  - Anti-HCV

Collaborative Therapy
- High-calorie, high-protein, high-carbohydrate, low-fat diet
- Vitamin supplements
- Rest—degree of strictness varying
- Avoid alcohol intake and drugs detoxified by the liver
- α-Interferon

is controversial. Supportive drug therapy may include antiemetics, such as dimenhydrinate (Dramamine) or trimethobenzamide (Tigan). Phenothiazines should not be used because of their possible cholestatic and hepatotoxic effects. If the patient requires a sedative or hypnotic drug, diphenhydramine (Benadryl) or chloral hydrate may be used.

α-Interferon. α-Interferon (antiviral or immune-modulating drug) has been approved to treat hepatitis B and C. It is primarily used in the treatment of chronic hepatitis. The efficacy of α-interferon is greater in the treatment of HBV than in HCV infections. α-Interferon is considered effective if the patient with HBV becomes negative for HBsAg. Ribavirin (Virazole), given in combination with α-interferon, has a synergistic effect.

Treatment protocols for hepatitis B and C using α-interferon are variable. In approximately 30% to 40% of patients with HBV treated with α-interferon 5 million units per day for 16 weeks, there will be loss of HBeAg and undetectable HBV DNA levels. In patients with chronic HCV a typical treatment protocol might include 3 million units three times weekly for 6 months. Approximately 40% to 50% of these patients will initially respond with a decrease in HCV DNA. However, 50% of these patients will relapse in 6 months, indicating that interferon therapy is effective in less than 25% of patients with chronic HCV.[13] Combination therapy using ribavirin with α-interferon is used in some medical centers to reduce the rate of relapse following α-interferon therapy for hepatitis C. Although not as high as with hepatitis C, relapse is also a problem in patients with chronic hepatitis B receiving α-interferon.

α-Interferon treatment is associated with a number of side effects (Table 41-7). These side effects are dose related and tend to decrease in severity with continued treatment. Newer antiviral drugs such as lamivudine (3TC) and famciclovir may be used to inhibit HBV replication.[14]

Hepatitis A vaccine and immune globulin. Immune globulin is used in the prevention and modification of viral hepatitis. Immune globulin (IG) is effective for hepatitis A if given up to 2 weeks after exposure. It provides temporary passive immunity. IG is recommended in cases of exposure to hepatitis A from close (household, day care center) contact in persons who are not positive for anti-HAV and for travelers to countries with high endemic levels of hepatitis A.

DRUG THERAPY

Table 41-7 Side Effects of α-Interferon

- Flulike symptoms
  - Myalgia
  - Arthralgia
  - Headache
  - Nausea
  - Fatigue
- Other effects
  - Decline in platelet and neutrophil counts
  - Weight loss
  - Hair loss
  - Thyroid disease
- Less common effects
  - Diarrhea
  - Seizures
  - Severe depression
  - Vasculitis
  - Retinopathy
  - Peripheral neuropathy

Both IG and hepatitis A vaccine are used for prevention of hepatitis A. The vaccine is used for preexposure prophylaxis, and IG can be used either before or after exposure. Because patients with hepatitis A are most infectious just before the onset of symptoms, those exposed through household contact or food-borne outbreaks should be given IG within 1 to 2 weeks of exposure. If the exposed person has anti-HAV antibodies, the IG is not necessary. When given within 2 weeks of exposure, IG can prevent infection in most people. Although IG may not prevent infection in all persons, it may modify the illness to a subclinical infection. IG provides 6 to 8 weeks of passive protection. It may also be used as a prophylactic measure for travelers to countries that have a high incidence of hepatitis A.

There are currently three hepatitis A vaccines, Havrix, Vaqta, and Avaxim. This active immunization can be a means to control the disease from a public health perspective. Primary immunization consists of a single dose administered intramuscularly in the deltoid. A booster is recommended any time between 6 and 12 months after the initiation of the primary dose to ensure adequate antibody titers and long-term protection. However, a primary immunization provides immunity within 30 days after a single dose. The vaccine may be administered concomitantly with IG, although the ultimate antibody titer obtained is likely to be lower than if the vaccine is given alone.

The side effects of the vaccine are mild and are usually limited to soreness and redness at the injection site. It is recommended that until routine vaccination of children is feasible, the following persons who are at risk for infection be vaccinated for hepatitis A: persons traveling to countries where hepatitis A is endemic; sexually active homosexual and bisexual men; injecting drug users; patients with chronic liver disease; and persons at risk for occupational infection, suchas those who work with hepatitis A in research laboratory settings.[15]

Hepatitis B vaccine and immune globulin. The first line of defense against hepatitis B is the hepatitis B vaccine. Immunization with hepatitis B vaccine is the most effective method of preventing HBV infection. Recommendations of the Centers for Disease Control and Prevention (CDC) Immunization Practices Advisory Committee include making hepatitis B vaccine a part of routine vaccination schedules for all newborns and adolescents.

In addition to immunizing newborns and adolescents, it is important to vaccinate adolescents and adults in the major risk groups. It may be helpful to screen for the antibody before vaccination because past infection is high in sexually active homosexual men and injecting drug users. It is hoped that universal vaccination will lead to eventual prevention and control of hepatitis B.

Hepatitis B vaccine is produced through recombinant DNA technology (see Fig. 12-12). The vaccines are Recombivax HB and Engerix-B. The vaccine is given in a series of three intramuscular (in the deltoid) injections. The second dose is administered within 1 month of the first one, and the third one within 6 months of the first. The cost is about $150 for the series. The vaccine is greater than 95% effective.[1] Successful vaccination should result in anti-HBsAg titers of 10 mIU/ml or greater. Only minor adverse reactions have been reported with vaccination, including transient fever and soreness at the injection site. The vaccine is not contraindicated in pregnancy.

It has not been definitely determined what level of antibody is required to provide protection. Therefore it remains to be determined how frequently boosters (additional doses) are necessary. For postexposure prophylaxis, the vaccine and hepatitis B immune globulin (HBIG) are used. HBIG contains antibodies to HBV and confers temporary passive immunity. HBIG is given to persons who have been exposed to HBV (needle stick, sexual exposure, infants born to mothers who are positive for HBsAg) and who have not been vaccinated. It should be given after exposure, preferably within 24 hours. The vaccine series should also be started.

For acute one-time exposure to the virus in individuals who have been vaccinated against HBV, HBIG plus the vaccine can be administered. HBIG is prepared from plasma of donors with a high titer of anti-HBsAg and is expensive. HBIG provides temporary passive immunity and is recommended for postexposure prophylaxis in cases of needle stick, mucous membrane contact, or sexual exposure.

Hepatitis C vaccine and immune globulin. Currently there are no products to prevent hepatitis C; however, several vaccines are in development. The CDC does not recommend immune globulin or antiviral agents such as α-interferon for postexposure prophylaxis (e.g., needle-stick exposure from an infected patient) for HCV infection.[16] Immune globulin is of no proven benefit for hepatitis C postexposure prevention.[17] Instead the exposed person should have baseline and 6-month follow-up testing for antibodies to HCV.

Nutritional Therapy. An important measure in assisting hepatocytes to regenerate is adequate nutrition. No special diet is required in the treatment of viral hepatitis. However, a diet high in carbohydrates and proteins with low fat content is usually recommended. Adequate calories are important because the patient usually loses weight. If fat content is poorly tolerated because of decreased bile production, it should be reduced. Basically the specific foods in the diet are dictated by the patient. Vitamin supplements, particularly B-complex vitamins and vitamin K, are frequently used. If anorexia, nausea, and vomiting are severe, intravenous (IV) solutions of glucose or supplemental tube feedings may be used. Fluid and electrolyte balance must be maintained.

NURSING ASSESSMENT

Table 41-8 Hepatitis

Subjective Data

Important Health Information

Past health history: Hemophilia; exposure to infected persons; ingestion of contaminated food or water; sexual promiscuity; exposure to benzene, carbon tetrachloride, or other hepatotoxic agents; crowded, hepatotoxic, unsanitary living conditions; exposure to contaminated needles; recent travel; organ transplant recipient; exposure to new drug regimens

Medications: Use and misuse of acetaminophen, phenytoin, halothane, methyldopa

Functional Health Patterns

Health perception–health management: IV drug and alcohol abuse; malaise, distaste for cigarettes (in smokers)

Nutritional-metabolic: Weight loss, anorexia, nausea, vomiting; feeling of fullness in right upper quadrant

Elimination: Dark urine; light-colored stools, constipation or diarrhea; skin rashes, hives

Activity-exercise: Fatigue, arthralgias, myalgias

Cognitive-perceptual: Right upper quadrant pain and liver tenderness, headache; pruritis

Role-relationship: Exposure as health care worker, chronic care institution resident

Objective Data

General

Low-grade fever, lethargy, lymphadenopathy

Integumentary

Rash, angioedema, jaundice, icteric sclera, injection sites

Gastrointestinal

Hepatomegaly, splenomegaly

Possible Findings

Abnormal liver enzyme studies; elevated serum bilirubin, hypoalbuminemia, anemia, bilirubin in urine and increased urobilinogen, prolonged prothrombin time, serologic tests positive for hepatitis, including anti-HAV IgM, HBsAg, HBeAg, anti-HBc IgM, anti-HCV, anti-HDV, abnormal liver scan, positive liver biopsy

NURSING MANAGEMENT: HEPATITIS

Nursing Assessment

Subjective and objective data that should be obtained from a person with hepatitis are presented in Table 41-8.

Nursing Diagnoses

Nursing diagnoses for the patient with hepatitis may include, but are not limited to, those presented in NCP 41-1.

Planning

The overall goals are that the patient with viral hepatitis will (1) have relief of discomfort, (2) be able to resume normal activities, and (3) return to normal liver function without complications.

Nursing Implementation

Health Promotion. Viral hepatitis is a community health problem. The nurse must assume a significant role in the control and prevention of this disease. It is helpful to first understand the epidemiology of the different types of viral hepatitis before considering appropriate control measures.

Hepatitis A. Outbreaks of viral hepatitis are usually due to HAV. Preventive measures include personal and environmental hygiene and health education to promote good sanitation (see Table 41-9). Hand washing is essential and is probably the most important precaution. Health teaching should include careful hand washing after bowel movements and before eating. When hepatitis A occurs in a food handler, IG should be administered to all other food handlers at the establishment. Patrons may also need to be given IG.

Isolation is not required for hepatitis A. For a patient with hepatitis A, infection control precautions should be used (see Table 11-19). A private room is indicated if the patient is incontinent of stool or has poor personal hygiene. Hand washing is essential.

Hepatitis B. Control and prevention of hepatitis B focuses on identification of possible exposure via percutaneous and sexual transmission (Table 41-9). The nurse must be aware of the individuals at high risk of contracting hepatitis B and teach methods to reduce risks. These include patients receiving frequent transfusions or hemodialysis, workers in hemodialysis units and blood chemistry laboratories, IV drug users, persons with multiple sexual partners, prison inmates, and household members and sexual partners of HBV carriers.

Good hygienic practices, including hand washing and the use of gloves when expecting contact with blood, are important. A condom is advised for sexual intercourse, and the partner should be vaccinated. Razors, toothbrushes, and other personal items should not be shared. Close contacts of the patient with hepatitis B who are HBsAg negative and antibody negative should be vaccinated.

According to CDC guidelines, infection control precautions should be followed for the patient with hepatitis B. This includes the use of disposable needles and syringes, which should be disposed of in puncture-resistant disposal units without recapping, bending, or breaking. (See Table 11-19 for various types of infection control precautions.) Preventive and control measures for hepatitis A and B are summarized in Table 41-9.

Hepatitis C. The primary measures to prevent hepatitis C are screening of blood, organ, and tissue donors; use of infection control precautions; and modification of high-risk behavior (see Table 41-9).

Acute Intervention

Jaundice. The nurse should assess for the degree of jaundice. In light-skinned persons the jaundice is usually observed first in the sclera of the eyes and later in the skin. In dark-skinned persons, jaundice is observed in the hard palate of the mouth and inner canthus of the eyes. Ictotest reagent tablets may be used to detect urinary bilirubin. The urine may be cola colored or mahogany because of the presence of bilirubin. Comfort measures to relieve pruritus (if present), headache, and arthralgias are helpful (see NCP 41-1).

Ensuring that the patient receives adequate nutrients is not always easy. The anorexia and extreme distaste for food cause nutritional problems. Dietary assessment must be considered. The nurse should try to determine whether there is something that appeals to the patient in spite of the anorexia. Small,

41-1 NURSING CARE PLAN PATIENT WITH VIRAL HEPATITIS

Expected Patient Outcomes	Nursing Interventions and *Rationales*
NURSING DIAGNOSIS	**Altered nutrition: less than body requirements** *related to* anorexia, nausea, and altered metabolism of nutrients by liver *as manifested by* inadequate food intake; aversion to eating; actual or potential metabolic needs in excess of intake.
▪ Adequate nutritional intake. ▪ Maintenance of normal body weight.	▪ Assess patient's appetite and adequacy of intake *so appropriate interventions can be planned.* ▪ Offer frequent small feedings, provide oral care before meals *to enhance patient's dietary intake.* ▪ Allow patient to choose food items; serve high-carbohydrate and high-protein foods at time of day patient feels most like eating *to increase likelihood of adequate intake.* ▪ Provide attractively served meals in pleasant surroundings *to stimulate patient's appetite.* ▪ Take weight daily on same scale, at same time, with same clothing *to monitor weight loss secondary to poor appetite.*
NURSING DIAGNOSIS	**Activity intolerance** *related to* fatigue and weakness *as manifested by* verbal report of fatigue or weakness, altered response to activity (as measured by BP, pulse, respiratory rate).
▪ Increased tolerance for activity.	▪ Provide rest periods. ▪ Increase patient's activity gradually as allowed and tolerated *so previous activity pattern can be resumed.* ▪ Conserve patient's strength by careful monitoring activity *to prevent increasing weakness and fatigue.* ▪ Teach patient to monitor and control activities that provoke fatigue *so patient can be an active participant in plan.*
NURSING DIAGNOSIS	**Body image disturbance** *related to* stigma of having a communicable disease, change in appearance (jaundice), and possible alterations in lifestyle and roles (alcohol consumption, drug use, restriction of sexual activity) *as manifested by* negative verbal or nonverbal response to actual or perceived changes.
▪ Positive adaptation to changes in appearance. ▪ Verbalization of understanding of body changes.	▪ Assist patient in expressing feelings and assess patient's feelings about disease process and appearance *to plan appropriate interventions.* ▪ Clarify misconceptions regarding limitations *to avoid unnecessary restrictions on patient's activities.* ▪ Encourage participation in self-care *to foster independence and self-esteem.* ▪ Instruct patient in ways to prevent spread of hepatitis *to reduce fear and guilt associated with potential for infecting others.* ▪ Encourage patient to ask questions *because accurate information fosters good decision making.*
NURSING DIAGNOSIS	**Ineffective management of therapeutic regimen** *related to* lack of knowledge of follow-up care *as manifested by* frequent questions about transmission of disease, activities allowed, and general follow-up care.
▪ Verbalization of understanding of follow-up care. ▪ Plan for follow-up visit with health care provider.	▪ Teach patient basic facts about illness, modes of transmission, diet, activities allowed, avoidance of alcohol, and need for follow-up care *so appropriate follow-up care will be planned and carried out.* ▪ Teach patient to watch for and report signs of complications such as bleeding gums or bloody stools, worsening of symptoms *to enable prompt intervention.* Emphasize the importance of adequate rest *to enable liver to repair itself and to prevent relapse.*
NURSING DIAGNOSIS	**Risk for infection transmission** *related to* lack of knowledge about source of and prevention of infection.
▪ Able to explain methods of disease transmission and methods of preventing transmission to others.	▪ Teach about the causative agent *because teaching varies depending on the specific cause.* ▪ Teach use of infection control precautions *to reduce risk of cross-contamination.* ▪ Explain the mode of infection transmission *to enable patient to prevent spread of hepatitis.* ▪ Depending on type of hepatitis, for example, encourage possible hepatitis A contact to have immune globulin *to prevent infection from hepatitis A virus.*

Table 41-9 Preventive Measures for Viral Hepatitis

Hepatitis A	Hepatitis B and C
General Measures Hand washing Proper personal hygiene Environmental sanitation Control and screening (signs, symptoms) of food handlers Serologic screening while carrying virus Active immunization: HAV vaccine to anyone over age 2 **Use of Immune Globulin** Early administration (1-2 wk after exposure) to those exposed Use of prophylaxis for travelers to areas where hepatitis A is common	**Percutaneous Transmission** Screening of donated blood B—HBsAg C—anti-HCV Use of disposable needles and syringes **Sexual Transmission** Acute exposure: HBIG administration to sexual partner of HBsAg-positive person Administer hepatitis B vaccine series to uninfected sexual partners Use condoms for sexual intercourse **General Measures** Hand washing Avoid sharing toothbrushes and razors HBIG administration for one-time exposure (needle stick, contact of mucous membranes with infectious material) Active immunization: HBV vaccine

Table 41-10 Measures to Prevent Transmission of Hepatitis Viruses from Patients to Health Care Personnel*

Hepatitis A	Hepatitis B	Hepatitis C
Always maintain good personal hygiene. Wash hands after contact with a patient or removal of gloves. Use infection control precautions.[†]	Use infection control precautions.[†] Wash hands. Reduce contact with blood or blood-containing secretions. Handle the blood of patients as potentially infective. Dispose of needles properly. Administer HBV vaccine to all health care personnel. Use needleless IV access devices when available.	Use infection control precautions.[†] Wash hands. Reduce contact with blood or blood-contaminated secretions. Handle the blood of patients as potentially infective. Dispose of needles properly. Use needleless IV access devices when available.

*A suggested guideline for general practice to prevent the nurse from contracting viral hepatitis from diagnosed and undiagnosed patients and carriers is for the nurse to wear disposable gloves, goggles, gowns (sometimes) when fecal or blood contamination is likely in handling (1) soiled bedpans, urinals, and catheters and (2) patient's bed linens soiled by body excreta or secretions.
[†]See Table 11-19.

frequent meals may be preferable to three large ones and may also help prevent nausea. Frequently, a patient with hepatitis finds that anorexia is not as severe in the morning, so it is easier to eat a good breakfast than a large dinner. Measures to stimulate the appetite, such as mouth care, antiemetics, and attractively served meals in pleasant surroundings, should be included in the nursing care plan. Other measures that may be tried to counteract the anorexia are carbonated beverages and avoidance of very hot or very cold foods. Adequate fluid intake is important (2500 to 3000 ml per day).

Rest. Rest is essential and is an important factor in promoting liver cell regeneration. The nurse must assess the patient's response to the rest and activity plan and modify it accordingly. The care plan should include appropriate time schedules for rest and activity, with scheduled rest periods uninterrupted by visitors or nursing staff. If the patient is on strict bed rest, measures to prevent respiratory and circulatory complications should be initiated. Assessment of the liver function tests and symptoms should continue as a guide to activity.

Psychologic and emotional rest are as essential as physical rest. Strict bed rest may produce anxiety and extreme restlessness in some patients and may be more damaging than reasonable ambulation. Diversional activities, such as reading and hobbies (e.g., knitting, stamp collecting), may help the patient. The patient should be assisted to understand the temporary nature of symptoms during the period of communicability.

Ambulatory and Home Care. Most patients with viral hepatitis will be cared for at home, so the nurse must assess the patient's knowledge of nutrition and provide the necessary dietary teaching. Rest and adequate nutrition are especially important until studies show that liver function has returned to normal. The patient must be cautioned about overexertion and the need to follow the physician's advice about when it is safe to return to work. The nurse must also teach the patient and family about preventive measures and how to prevent transmission to other family members. The patient should know what symptoms need to be reported to the physician.

The patient should be assessed for any manifestations indicative of complications. Bleeding tendencies with increasing prothrombin time values, symptoms of encephalopathy, or abnormal liver function tests indicate problems, and the patient should be assessed and treated promptly.

The patient should be instructed to have regular follow-up for at least 1 year after the diagnosis of hepatitis. Because relapses are fairly common with hepatitis B and C, the patient should be instructed about symptoms of recurrence. Alcohol should be avoided for 1 year because it is detoxified in the liver and may interfere with recovery.

A patient who remains positive for HBsAg is a carrier and should never be a blood donor. The patient with hepatitis B should also be instructed to use condoms when engaging in sexual intercourse until tests for HBsAg are negative.

The patient who is receiving α-interferon for the treatment of hepatitis B or C requires education regarding the medication. α-Interferon is administered intramuscularly or subcutaneously, and thus the patient or family member needs to be taught how to administer the drug. There are numerous side effects with the therapy, including flulike symptoms (fever, malaise, fatigue, chills). The physician may recommend that acetaminophen be administered 30 to 60 minutes before injection to reduce these symptoms. Other significant side effects include thrombocytopenia, neutropenia, psychologic disturbances (mood swings, depression) and limited alopecia (see Table 41-7). (Additional information on α-interferon is presented in Chapters 10 and 12.)

■ Evaluation

Expected outcomes for the patient with hepatitis are addressed in NCP 41-1.

Control of Hepatitis in Health Care Personnel

Hepatitis A. Hepatitis A is rarely transmitted from patients to health care personnel. When this does occur, it is associated with patients with undiagnosed hepatitis A who are treated for other problems. Usually these patients are incontinent of feces. The use of infection control precautions should prevent transmission of HAV to health care personnel.

Hepatitis B. Health care workers may be exposed to HBV from needle sticks or blood contamination to mucous membranes or nonintact skin. If a health care worker is exposed to HBV through a needle stick and does not receive the vaccine, there is a 6% to 30% chance of infection with hepatitis B.[1] Vaccination is the most effective method to prevent hepatitis B in health care workers. Employers are required by the Occupational Safety and Health Administration (OSHA) to provide free HBV immunization to employees at risk for infection.

The principal mode of transmission of HBV for health care personnel is parenteral. Examples of parenteral transmission include accidental needle sticks and, rarely, transfusion of contaminated blood or blood products. Because all blood and blood products are tested for HBV and anti-HCV, there is diminishing risk of this latter mode of transmission. Other forms of transmission include contamination of fresh cutaneous scratches or abrasions, burns, and contamination of mucosal surfaces with infective blood, blood products, saliva, or semen.

Hepatitis C. Transmission is usually due to percutaneous needle exposure or other blood exposure and undetected parenteral transmission. Measures to prevent transmission of the viruses from patients to health care personnel are presented in Table 41-10. Very rarely do health care workers infect patient contacts.

TOXIC AND DRUG-INDUCED HEPATITIS

Liver injury and death may occur after the inhalation, parenteral injection, or ingestion of certain chemical substances (see Table 37-6). The two major types of chemical hepatotoxicity are toxic and drug-induced hepatitis. Agents producing toxic hepatitis are generally systemic poisons (e.g., carbon tetrachloride, gold compounds) or are converted in the liver to toxic metabolites (e.g., acetaminophen). Liver necrosis generally occurs within 2 to 3 days of acute exposure to a toxic substance.

Idiosyncratic drug reactions produce drug-induced hepatitis. Such agents as halothane, isoniazid (INH), chlorothiazides (e.g., Diuril), methotrexate, and methyldopa (Aldomet) may produce idiosyncratic reactions because of patient susceptibility (metabolic reactivity) to these agents or immunologically mediated hypersensitivity responses. Liver injury may occur at any time during or shortly after exposure. Some responses occur 2 to 5 weeks after exposure.

Older patients are particularly vulnerable to drug-induced hepatitis. This is due to several factors, including increased use of prescription and over-the-counter drugs, which can lead to drug interactions and potential drug toxicity. Age-related decreases in liver function caused by decreased liver blood flow and enzyme activity result in decreased drug metabolism. In addition, with aging there is a decreased ability of the liver to recover from drug-induced injury.

Toxic and drug-induced hepatitis are similar to viral hepatitis in the pathophysiologic changes in the liver and the clinical manifestations. The usual presenting clinical findings are anorexia, nausea, vomiting, hepatomegaly, splenomegaly, and abnormal liver function studies. Treatment is largely supportive as in acute viral hepatitis. Recovery may be rapid if the hepatotoxin is identified and removed. Liver transplantation may be necessary.

IDIOPATHIC HEPATITIS

Chronic active hepatitis may also occur in a number of patients who have no known risk factors for the development of viral hepatitis. The cause of this form of hepatitis is idiopathic. However, because many of these patients often have a number of systemic problems, including glomerulonephritis and arthritis, the disease is thought to be autoimmune. The presenting signs and symptoms are variable and similar to viral hepatitis. Laboratory tests (elevation of liver enzymes) reveal liver inflammation without evidence of viral antigens. The majority (70% to 80%) of patients who are diagnosed with autoimmune hepatitis are women. The course of the disease is also variable, with the majority of the patients exhibiting chronic active hepatitis.

Unlike viral hepatitis, autoimmune hepatitis (in which there is evidence of necrosis and cirrhosis) is treated with cortico-

A

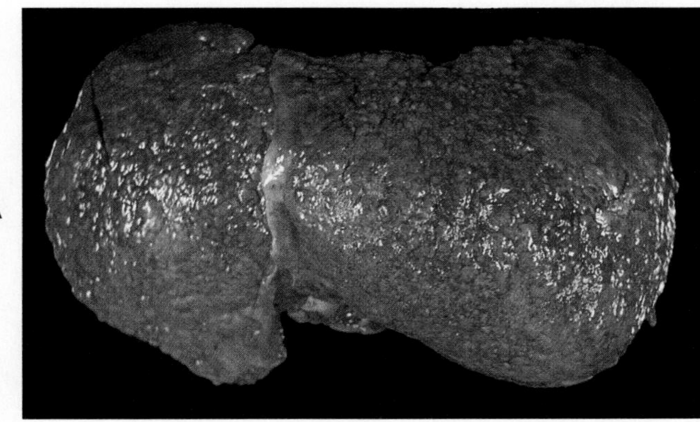

B

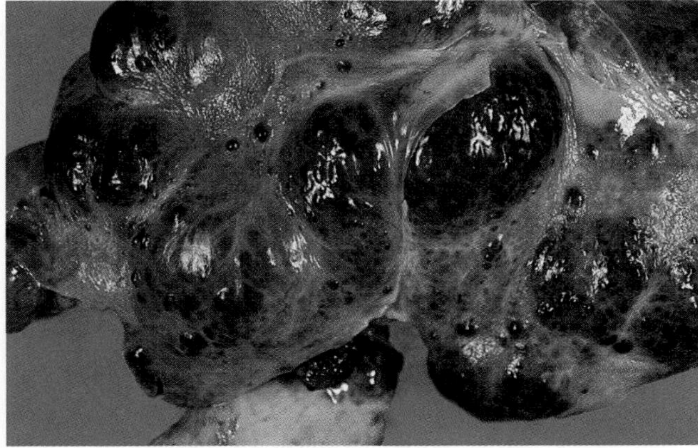

Fig. 41-4 Cirrhosis. **A,** Micronodular cirrhosis. **B,** Macronodular cirrhosis.

steroids or other immunosuppressive agents. Daily treatment with methylprednisolone is the first line of therapy for nonviral chronic active hepatitis. Azathioprine (Imuran) may also be used to treat the disease.

CIRRHOSIS OF THE LIVER

Cirrhosis is a chronic progressive disease of the liver characterized by extensive degeneration and destruction of the liver parenchymal cells (Fig. 41-4). The liver cells attempt to regenerate, but the regenerative process is disorganized, resulting in abnormal blood vessel and bile duct relationships from the fibrosis. The overgrowth of new and fibrous connective tissue distorts the liver's normal lobular structure, resulting in lobules of irregular size and shape with impeded vascular flow. Cirrhosis may have an insidious, prolonged course.

Cirrhosis is ranked as the ninth leading cause of death in the United States and the fourth leading cause of death in persons between 35 and 54 years of age. The highest incidence occurs between the ages of 40 and 60, and it is twice as common in men as in women. Excessive alcohol ingestion is the single most common cause of cirrhosis.

Etiology and Pathophysiology

The four types of cirrhosis, in order of incidence, are as follows:

1. *Alcoholic* (previously called *Laënnec's*), also called portal or nutritional cirrhosis, is usually associated with alcohol abuse. The first change in the liver from excessive alcohol intake is an accumulation of fat in the liver cells. Uncomplicated fatty changes in the liver are potentially reversible if the person stops drinking alcohol. If the alcohol abuse continues, widespread scar formation occurs throughout the liver.
2. *Postnecrotic cirrhosis* is a complication of viral, toxic, or idiopathic (autoimmune) hepatitis. Broad bands of scar tissue form within the liver.
3. *Biliary cirrhosis* is associated with chronic biliary obstruction and infection. There is diffuse fibrosis of the liver with jaundice as the main feature.
4. *Cardiac cirrhosis* results from long-standing, severe right-sided heart failure in patients with cor pulmonale, constrictive pericarditis, and tricuspid insufficiency.

In cirrhosis, cell necrosis occurs, and the destroyed liver cells are replaced by scar tissue. The normal lobular architecture becomes nodular. Eventually irregular, disorganized regeneration; poor cellular nutrition; and hypoxia caused by inadequate blood flow and scar tissue result in decreased functioning of the liver.

The specific cause of cirrhosis may not be determined in all patients. It is known that cirrhosis occurs with greatest frequency among alcoholics. There continues to be some controversy as to whether the cause is the alcohol or the malnutrition that frequently coexists with chronic ingestion of alcohol. A common problem in alcoholics is protein malnutrition. There have been cases of nutritional cirrhosis resulting from extreme dieting or malnutrition. It is believed that the combined impact of malnutrition and alcohol is especially damaging to hepatocytes. Alcohol alone has a direct hepatotoxic effect. It is known to produce necrosis of cells and fatty infiltration with formation of fibrous septa. Some persons seem to have a predisposition to cirrhosis, regardless of their dietary or alcohol intake.

Clinical Manifestations

Early Manifestations. The onset of cirrhosis is usually insidious. Occasionally there is an abrupt onset of symptoms. GI disturbances are common early symptoms and include anorexia, dyspepsia, flatulence, nausea and vomiting, and change in bowel habits (diarrhea or constipation). These symptoms occur as a result of the liver's altered metabolism of carbohydrates, fats, and proteins. The patient may complain of abdominal pain described as a dull, heavy feeling in the right upper quadrant or epigastrium. The pain may be due to swelling and stretching of the liver capsule, spasm of the biliary ducts, and intermittent vascular spasm. Other early manifestations are fever, lassitude, slight weight loss, and enlargement of the liver and spleen. The liver is palpable in many patients with cirrhosis.

Later Manifestations. Later symptoms may be severe and result from liver failure and portal hypertension. Jaundice, peripheral edema, and ascites develop gradually. Other late symptoms include skin lesions, hematologic disorders, endocrine disturbances, and peripheral neuropathies (Fig. 41-5). In the advanced stages the liver becomes small and nodular.

Jaundice. Jaundice results from the functional derangement of liver cells and compression of bile ducts by connective tissue overgrowth. Jaundice occurs as a result of the decreased

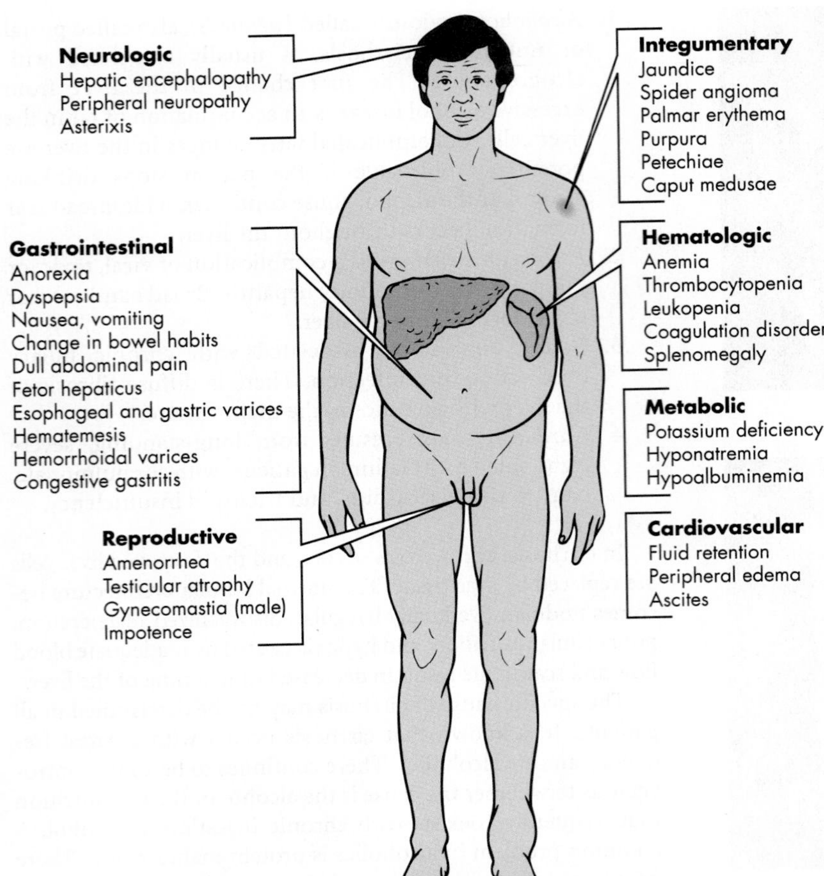

Fig. 41-5 Systemic clinical manifestations of liver cirrhosis.

ability to conjugate and excrete bilirubin (hepatocellular jaundice). The jaundice may be minimal or severe, depending on the degree of liver damage. If obstruction of the biliary tract occurs, obstructive jaundice may also occur and is usually accompanied by pruritus. The pruritus is due to an accumulation of bile salts underneath the skin.

Skin lesions. Various skin manifestations are commonly seen in cirrhosis. *Spider angiomas* (*telangiectasia* or *spider nevi*) are small, dilated blood vessels with a bright-red center point and spider-like branches. They occur on the nose, cheeks, upper trunk, neck, and shoulders. *Palmar erythema* (a red area that blanches with pressure) is located on the palms of the hands. Both of these lesions are attributed to an increase in circulating estrogen as a result of the damaged liver's inability to metabolize steroids.

Hematologic problems. Hematologic problems include thrombocytopenia, leukopenia, anemia, and coagulation disorders. Thrombocytopenia, leukopenia, and anemia are probably caused by the splenomegaly. Splenomegaly results from backup of blood from the portal vein into the spleen. Overactivity of the enlarged spleen results in increased removal of blood cells from circulation. The anemia is also due to inadequate red blood cell production and survival. Other factors involved in the anemia relate to poor diet, poor absorption of folic acid, and bleeding from varices.

The coagulation problems result from the liver's inability to produce prothrombin and other factors essential for blood clotting. Coagulation problems are manifested by hemorrhagic phenomena or bleeding tendencies, such as epistaxis, purpura, petechiae, easy bruising, gingival bleeding, and heavy menstrual bleeding.

Endocrine disturbances. Several signs and symptoms relating to the metabolism and inactivation of adrenocortical hormones, estrogen, and testosterone occur in cirrhosis. Normally the liver metabolizes these hormones. When the damaged liver is unable to do this, various manifestations occur. In men, gynecomastia, loss of axillary and pubic hair, testicular atrophy, and impotence with loss of libido may occur as a result of estrogen accumulation. In younger women amenorrhea may occur, and in older females there may be vaginal bleeding. The liver fails to metabolize aldosterone adequately, and this results in hyperaldosteronism with subsequent sodium and water retention and potassium loss.

Peripheral neuropathy. Peripheral neuropathy is a common finding in alcoholic cirrhosis. It is probably due to a dietary deficiency of thiamine, folic acid, and cobalamin (vitamin B_{12}). The neuropathy usually results in mixed nervous system symptoms, but sensory symptoms may predominate. Clinical manifestations of cirrhosis of the liver are numerous and may eventually involve the total body (see Fig. 41-5).

Complications

Major complications of cirrhosis are portal hypertension with resultant esophageal varices, peripheral edema and ascites, hepatic encephalopathy (coma), and hepatorenal syndrome.

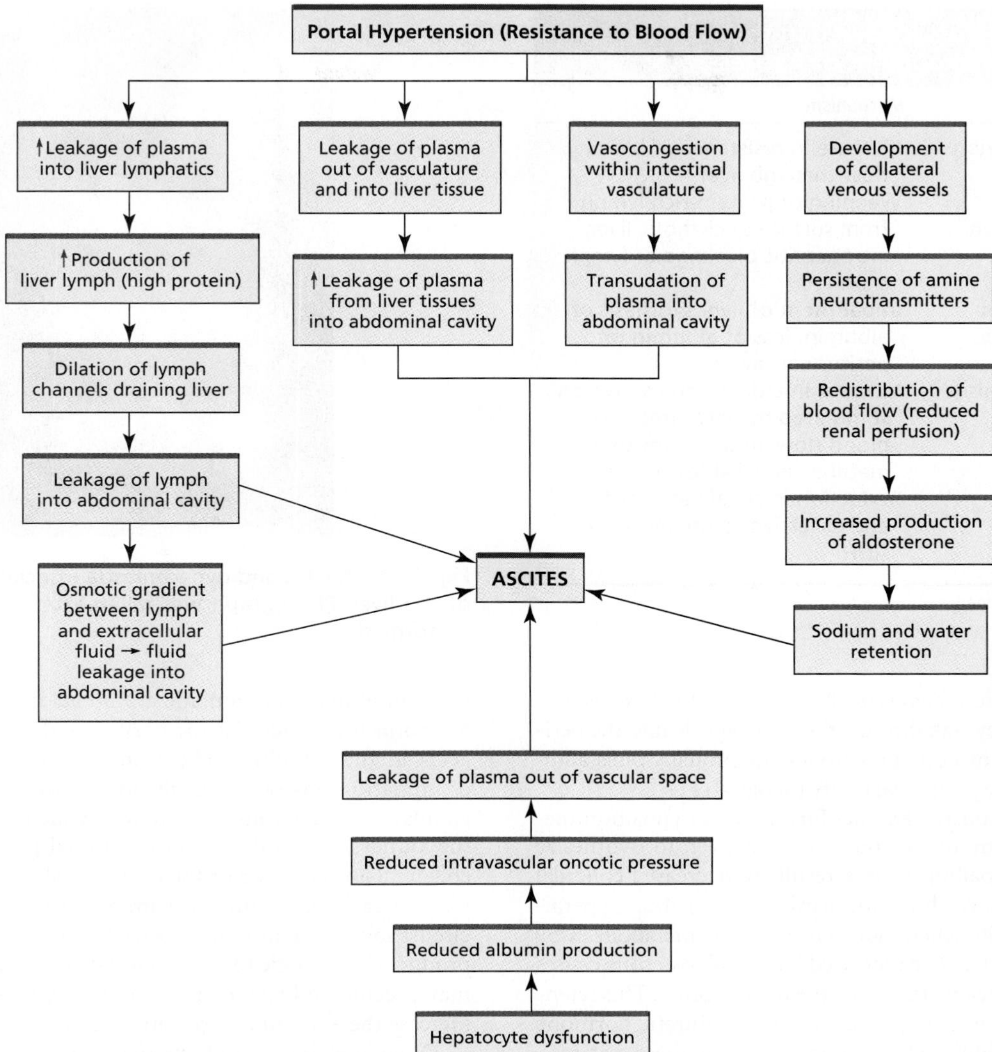

Fig. 41-6 Mechanisms for development of ascites.

Portal Hypertension and Esophageal Varices. Because of the structural changes in the liver from the cirrhotic process, there is compression and destruction of the portal and hepatic veins and sinusoids. These changes result in obstruction to the normal flow of blood through the portal system, resulting in portal hypertension. Many pathophysiologic changes result from portal hypertension. Collateral circulation develops in an attempt to reduce this high portal pressure and also to reduce the increased plasma volume and lymphatic flow. The common areas where the collateral channels form are in the lower esophagus (the anastomosis of the left gastric vein and the azygos veins), the anterior abdominal wall, the parietal peritoneum, and the rectum. Varicosities may develop in areas where the collateral and systemic circulations communicate, resulting in esophageal and gastric varices, caput medusae (ring of varices around the umbilicus), and hemorrhoids.

Esophageal varices are a common complication, occurring in two thirds to three fourths of patients with cirrhosis. These collateral vessels contain little elastic tissue and are quite fragile. They tolerate the high pressure poorly, and the result is distended, tortuous veins that bleed easily. Large varices are more likely to bleed.

Bleeding esophageal varices are the most life-threatening complication of cirrhosis. The mortality rate for hemorrhage of esophageal varices is 30% to 60%.[18] The varices rupture and bleed in response to ulceration and irritation. Factors producing ulceration and irritation include alcohol ingestion; swallowing of poorly masticated food; ingestion of coarse food; acid regurgitation from the stomach; and increased intraabdominal pressure caused by nausea, vomiting, straining at stool, coughing, sneezing, or lifting heavy objects. The patient may have melena or hematemesis. There may be slow oozing or massive hemorrhage. Massive hemorrhage is a medical emergency.

Peripheral Edema and Ascites. Peripheral edema sometimes precedes ascites, but in some patients its development coincides with or occurs after ascites. Edema results from decreased colloidal osmotic pressure from impaired liver synthesis of albumin and increased portocaval pressure from portal hypertension. Peripheral edema occurs as ankle and presacral edema.

Ascites is the accumulation of serous fluid in the peritoneal or abdominal cavity. It is a common manifestation of cirrhosis. When the blood pressure is elevated in the liver, as occurs in portal cirrhosis, proteins move from the blood vessels via the larger pores of the sinusoids (capillaries) into the lymph space (Fig. 41-6).

Table 41-11 Factors Involved in the Development of Ascites

Factor	Mechanism
Portal hypertension	Increase in resistance of blood flow through liver
Increased flow of hepatic lymph	Weeping of protein-rich lymph from surface of cirrhotic liver, intrahepatic blockage of lymph channels
Decreased serum colloidal oncotic pressure	Impairment of liver synthesis of albumin, loss of albumin into peritoneal cavity
Hyperaldosteronism	Increase in aldosterone secretion stimulated by decreased renal blood flow, impairment of liver metabolism of aldosterone
Impaired water excretion	Reduction in renal vascular flow and excessive serum levels of ADH

ADH, antidiuretic hormone.

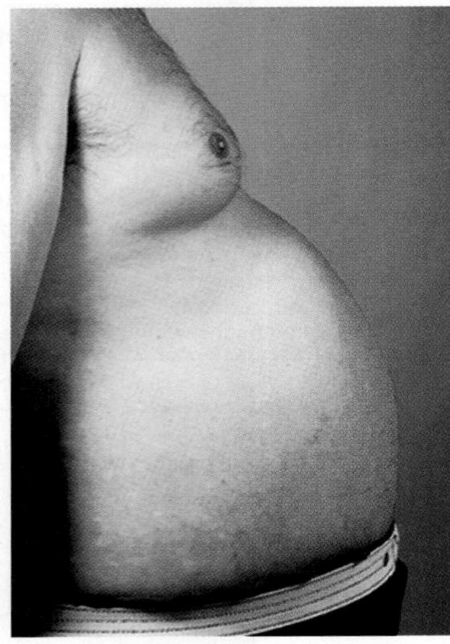

Fig. 41-7 Ascites and gynecomastia associated with cirrhosis of the liver. Photograph was taken after a paracentesis was performed.

When the lymphatic system is unable to carry off the excess proteins and water, they leak through the liver capsule into the peritoneal cavity. The osmotic pressure of the proteins pulls additional fluid into the peritoneal cavity (Table 41-11).

A second mechanism of ascites formation is hypoalbuminemia resulting from the inability of the liver to synthesize albumin. The hypoalbuminemia results in decreased colloidal osmotic pressure. A third mechanism of ascites, hyperaldosteronism, results when aldosterone is not metabolized by damaged hepatocytes. The increased level of aldosterone causes increased sodium reabsorption by the renal tubules. This retention of sodium, as well as an increase in antidiuretic hormone (ADH), causes additional water retention in these patients. Because of edema formation there is decreased intravascular volume and subsequently decreased renal blood flow and glomerular filtration.

Ascites is manifested by abdominal distention with weight gain (Fig. 41-7). If the ascites is severe, the umbilicus may be everted. Abdominal striae with distended abdominal wall veins may be present. The patient has signs of dehydration (e.g., dry tongue and skin, sunken eyeballs, muscle weakness). There is also a decrease in urinary output. Hypokalemia is common and is due to an excessive loss of potassium because of the effects of aldosterone. Low potassium levels can also result from diuretic therapy used to treat the ascites.

Hepatic Encephalopathy. Hepatic encephalopathy, or coma, is a frequent terminal complication in liver disease. *Encephalopathy* is a more descriptive term than *coma*. Hepatic encephalopathy can occur in any condition in which liver damage causes ammonia to enter the systemic circulation without liver detoxification. There is a high mortality rate associated with hepatic encephalopathy.

The pathogenesis of hepatic encephalopathy is incompletely understood at this time. A number of etiologic factors may be involved. It is basically a disorder of protein metabolism and excretion. The main pathogenic agents appear to be nitrogenous ammonia and aromatic amino acids. A major source of ammonia is the bacterial and enzymatic deamination of amino acids in the intestines. The ammonia that results from this deamination process normally goes to the liver via the portal circulation and is converted to urea, which is then excreted by the kidneys. When the blood is shunted past the liver via the collateral anastomoses or the liver is unable to convert ammonia to urea, large quantities of ammonia remain in the systemic circulation. The ammonia crosses the blood-brain barrier and produces neurologic toxic manifestations. A number of factors may precipitate hepatic encephalopathy, mostly because they increase the amount of circulating ammonia (Table 41-12).

Other metabolic products that may contribute to hepatic encephalopathy are mercaptans (such as methionine) and short-chain fatty acids. Another theory is that the liver may produce substances necessary for normal brain functioning. When the diseased liver can no longer produce these substances, encephalopathy may result.

Clinical manifestations of encephalopathy are changes in neurologic and mental responsiveness, ranging from lethargy to deep coma. Changes may occur suddenly because of an increase in ammonia in response to bleeding varices or gradually as blood ammonia levels slowly increase. In the early stages, manifestations include euphoria, depression, apathy, irritability, memory loss, confusion, yawning, drowsiness, insomnia, agitation, slow and slurred speech, emotional lability, impaired judgment, hiccups, slow and deep respirations, hyperactive reflexes, and a positive Babinski's reflex.

Clinical manifestations of impending coma include disorientation as to time, place, or person. A characteristic symptom is *asterixis,* or flapping tremors (liver flap). This may take several forms, the most common involving the arms and hands. When asked to hold the arms and hands stretched out, the patient is unable to hold this position and there will be a series of rapid flexion and extension movements of the hands. Other signs of asterixis are rhythmic movements of the legs with dorsiflexion

Table 41-12 Factors Precipitating Hepatic Encephalopathy

Factor	Mechanism
GI hemorrhage	Increase in ammonia in GI tract
Constipation	Increase in ammonia from bacterial action on feces
Hypokalemia	Potassium ions are needed by brain to metabolize ammonia
Hypovolemia	Increase in blood ammonia by causing hepatic hypoxia; impairment of cerebral, hepatic, and renal function because of decreased blood flow
Infection	Increase in catabolism, increase in cerebral sensitivity to toxins
Cerebral depressants (e.g., narcotics)	No detoxification by liver, causing increase in cerebral depression
Metabolic alkalosis	Facilitation of transport of ammonia across blood-brain barrier, increase in renal production of ammonia
Paracentesis	Loss of sodium and potassium ions, decrease in blood volume
Dehydration	Potentiation of ammonia toxicity
Increased metabolism	Increase in workload of liver
Diuretics	Increase in renal formation of ammonia, possibly resulting in azotemia, which increases endogenous ammonia production; hypokalemia also possible
Uremia (renal failure)	Retention of nitrogenous metabolites

of the foot and rhythmic movements in the face with strong closure of the eyelids. Impairments in writing involve difficulty in moving the pen or pencil from left to right and apraxia (the inability to construct simple figures). Other signs include hyperventilation, hypothermia, and grimacing and grasping reflexes.

Fetor hepaticus occurs in some patients with encephalopathy. It is a musty, sweet odor of the patient's breath. This odor is from the accumulation of digestive by-products that the liver is unable to degrade.

Hepatorenal Syndrome. Hepatorenal syndrome is a serious complication of cirrhosis. It is characterized by functional renal failure with advancing azotemia, oliguria, and intractable ascites. There is no structural abnormality of the kidneys. The exact cause of the decreased renal function is unknown but is thought to be related to a redistribution of blood flow from the kidneys to peripheral and splanchnic circulations or hypovolemia secondary to ascites. In the patient with cirrhosis the syndrome frequently follows diuretic therapy, GI hemorrhage, or paracentesis. Hepatic encephalopathy is also associated with the deterioration in renal function. Treatment measures include salt-poor albumin, salt and water restrictions, and diuretic therapy. However, treatment is usually unsuccessful.

Table 41-13 Bilirubin Metabolism Abnormalities in Cirrhosis*

Type	Finding
Serum bilirubin	
Unconjugated	↑↓
Conjugated	↑↓
Urine bilirubin	↑↓
Urobilinogen	
Stool	Normal, ↓↑
Urine	Normal, ↑↓

*These are bilirubin metabolism abnormalities occurring with hepatocellular jaundice, the most frequent type of jaundice with cirrhosis.

Diagnostic Studies

A liver profile in cirrhosis demonstrates abnormalities in most of the liver function studies (see Table 37-13). Enzyme levels, including alkaline phosphatase, aspartate aminotransferase (AST) (serum glutamic-oxaloacetic transaminase [SGOT]), alanine aminotransferase (ALT) (serum glutamate pyruvate transaminase [SGPT]), and γ-glutamyltransferase (GGT), are elevated because of the release of these enzymes from damaged liver cells. Protein metabolism tests show decreased total protein, decreased albumin, and increased globulin levels. The liver does not synthesize γ-globulins but does synthesize albumin. γ-Globulins (antibodies) are produced by B lymphocytes in the lymphatic system and spleen. The globulin level often increases in cirrhosis and indicates increased synthesis or decreased removal. Fat metabolism abnormalities are reflected by decreased cholesterol levels. The prothrombin time is prolonged, and bilirubin metabolism is altered (Table 41-13). Liver biopsy may be performed to identify liver cell changes and alterations in the lobular structure. Differential analysis of ascitic fluid may be helpful in establishing a diagnosis.

Collaborative Care

Rest. Although there is no specific therapy for cirrhosis, certain measures can be taken to promote liver cell regeneration and prevent or treat complications (Table 41-14). Rest is significant in reducing metabolic demands of the liver and allowing for recovery of liver cells. At various times during the progress of cirrhosis the rest may have to take the form of complete bed rest.

Ascites. Management of ascites is focused on sodium restriction, diuretics, and fluid removal. A low-sodium diet is prescribed (250 to 500 mg per day). The patient is usually not on restricted fluids unless severe ascites develops. There should be accurate assessment and control of fluid and electrolyte balance. Bed rest initially produces diuresis, which increases fluid excretion. Salt-poor albumin may be used to help maintain intravascular volume and adequate urinary output by increasing plasma colloid osmotic pressure.

Diuretic therapy is an important part of management. Frequently a combination of drugs that work at multiple sites in the nephron is more effective. Spironolactone (Aldactone) is an effective diuretic, even in patients with severe sodium retention. Spironolactone is an antagonist of aldosterone and is

COLLABORATIVE CARE

Table 41-14 Cirrhosis of the Liver

Diagnostic
- Liver function studies
- Liver biopsy (percutaneous needle)
- Esophagogastroduodenoscopy
- Angiography (percutaneous transhepatic portography)
- Liver scan
- Serum electrolytes
- Prothrombin time
- Serum albumin
- CBC
- Stool for occult blood
- Upper GI barium swallow

Collaborative Therapy

Conservative Therapy
- Administration of B-complex vitamins
- Rest
- Avoidance of alcohol and aspirin

Ascites
- Administration of 3000-calorie, high-carbohydrate, protein (depends on stage), low-fat diet, low sodium for ascites
- Diuretics
  - Spironolactone (Aldactone)
  - Amiloride (Midamor)
  - Triamterene (Dyrenium)
  - Furosemide (Lasix)
- Paracentesis (if indicated)
- Peritoneovenous shunt (if indicated)

Esophageal Varices
- β-adrenergic blockers
- Vasopressin (Pitressin)
- Endoscopic sclerotherapy or ligation
- Balloon tamponade
- Somatostatin
- Surgical shunting procedure
- Transjugular intrahepatic portosystemic shunt

Hepatic Encephalopathy
- Sterilization of GI tract with antibiotics
- Lactulose (Cephulac)
- Levodopa

CBC, complete blood count.

potassium sparing. Other potassium-sparing diuretics are amiloride (Midamor) and triamterene (Dyrenium). A high-potency loop diuretic, such as furosemide (Lasix), is frequently used in combination with a potassium-sparing drug. Chlorothiazide (Diuril) or hydrochlorothiazide may also be used, but the thiazide diuretics are not as potent as the loop diuretics.

A paracentesis (needle puncture of the abdominal cavity) may be performed to remove ascitic fluid. However, it is reserved for the patient with impaired respiration or abdominal pain caused by severe ascites. It is only a temporary measure because the fluid tends to reaccumulate.

Peritoneovenous shunt. A surgical procedure, peritoneovenous shunt, provides for the continuous reinfusion of ascitic

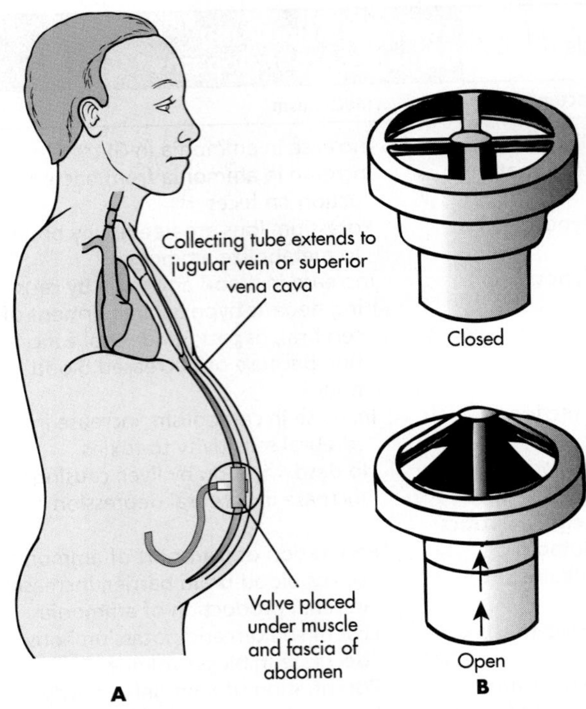

Fig. 41-8 LaVeen continuous peritoneovenous shunt. **A,** Collecting tube. **B,** Valve in closed and open positions.

fluid into the venous system. One type, the LaVeen peritoneovenous shunt, consists of a tube and a one-way valve. The tube runs from the abdominal cavity through the peritoneum, under the subcutaneous tissue, and into the jugular vein or superior vena cava (Fig. 41-8). The valve opens when the pressure in the peritoneal cavity is 3 to 5 cm H_2O higher than that in the superior vena cava. This allows the ascitic fluid to flow into the venous system. The patient's inspiration increases the intraperitoneal pressure, causing the valve to open. Another shunt, the Denver shunt, has a subcutaneous pump that irrigates the tubing when manually compressed. This shunting of the ascitic fluid causes an improvement in hemodynamic factors and increases sodium and fluid excretion. Urine output is also increased.

Esophageal Varices. The main therapeutic goal related to esophageal varices is avoidance of bleeding and hemorrhage. The patient who has esophageal varices should avoid ingesting alcohol, aspirin, and irritating foods. Upper respiratory infections should be treated promptly, and coughing should be controlled.

Management related to bleeding esophageal varices includes emergency, therapeutic, and prophylactic interventions. Management measures used are vasopressin (VP) and nitroglycerin (NTG), β-adrenergic blockers, balloon tamponade, sclerotherapy, ligation of varices, and shunt therapy.

When esophageal variceal bleeding occurs, the first step is to stabilize the patient and manage the airway. IV therapy is initiated and may include administration of blood products. The next step is to make a definitive diagnosis. This is important because patients with cirrhosis can also bleed from erosive

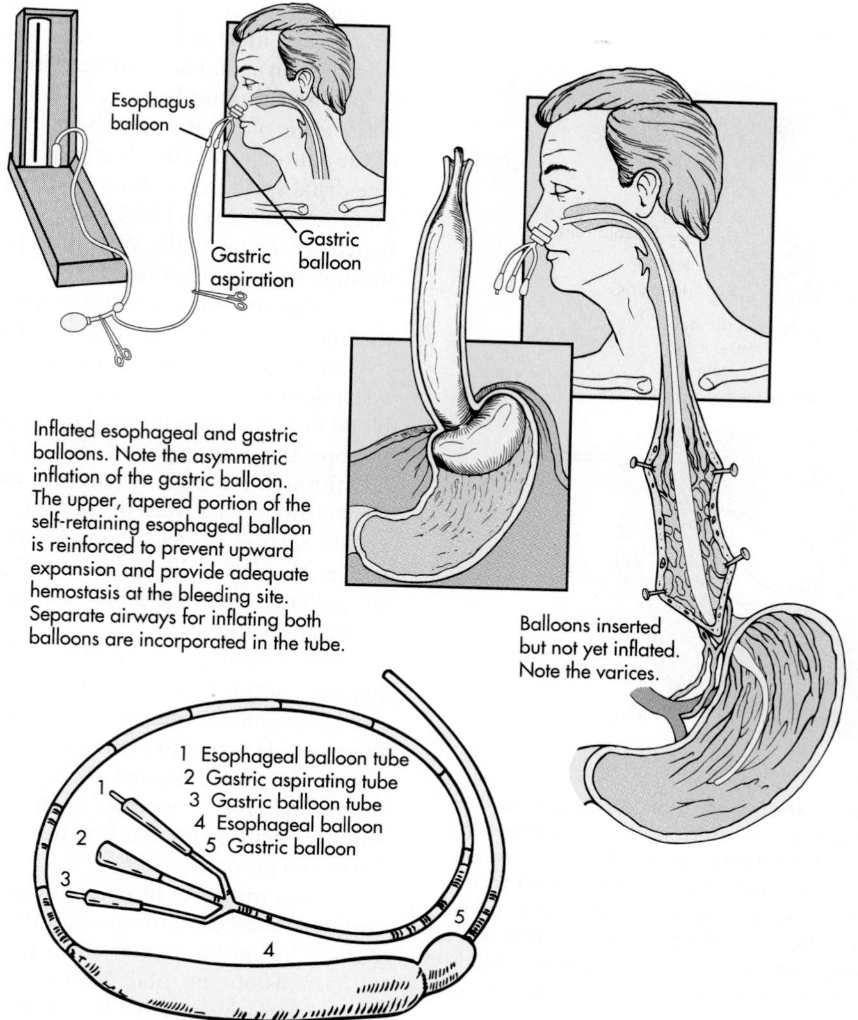
Esophagus balloon
Gastric aspiration
Gastric balloon
Inflated esophageal and gastric balloons. Note the asymmetric inflation of the gastric balloon. The upper, tapered portion of the self-retaining esophageal balloon is reinforced to prevent upward expansion and provide adequate hemostasis at the bleeding site. Separate airways for inflating both balloons are incorporated in the tube.
Balloons inserted but not yet inflated. Note the varices.
1 Esophageal balloon tube
2 Gastric aspirating tube
3 Gastric balloon tube
4 Esophageal balloon
5 Gastric balloon
1
2
3
4
5

Fig. 41-9 Esophageal tamponade accomplished with Sengstaken-Blakemore tube.

gastritis, peptic ulcers, and Mallory-Weiss tears. The diagnosis is made by endoscopic examination as soon as possible. Lavage with a wide-bore nasogastric (NG) tube (e.g., Ewald) may be done to remove blood and clots to prepare the patient for endoscopy.

The main goal of drug therapy is to stop bleeding so treatment measures can be done. The initial measures to stop the bleeding include IV administration of VP. VP produces vasoconstriction of the splanchnic arterial bed, decreased portal blood flow, and decreased portal hypertension. It has many side effects, including decreased coronary blood flow and heart rate and increased blood pressure. Current drug therapy in some institutions is a combination of VP and NTG. The NTG reduces the detrimental effects of the VP while enhancing its beneficial effect.

Endoscopic sclerotherapy is a treatment method for both acute and chronic bleeding varices in many institutions. The sclerosing agent, introduced via endoscopy, thromboses and obliterates the distended veins.

Another procedure for managing acute variceal bleeding is endoscopic ligation or banding of the varices. A small rubber band (elastic O-ring) is slipped around the base of the varix. Endoscopic variceal ligation can be done using clips instead of the O-rings (endoscopic clipping). Endoscopic ligation is as effective as endoscopic sclerotherapy with fewer complications. A combination of endoscopic sclerotherapy and ligation may be used and seems to be more effective than either treatment alone.[19]

Balloon tamponade may be used if sclerotherapy or ligation is unsuccessful. Balloon tamponade controls the hemorrhage by mechanical compression of the varices. The Minnesota or Sengstaken-Blakemore tube is used for this purpose (Fig. 41-9). These tubes have two balloons: gastric and esophageal. The Sengstaken-Blakemore has three lumens: one for the gastric balloon, one for the esophageal balloon, and one for gastric aspiration. The Minnesota tube has an esophageal aspiration port. When inflated, the gastric and esophageal balloons put mechanical compression on the varices. The gastric balloon anchors the tube in position and also applies pressure to any bleeding gastric varices.

Supportive measures during an acute variceal bleed include administration of fresh frozen plasma and packed RBCs, vitamin K (Aquamephyton), and histamine (H_2)

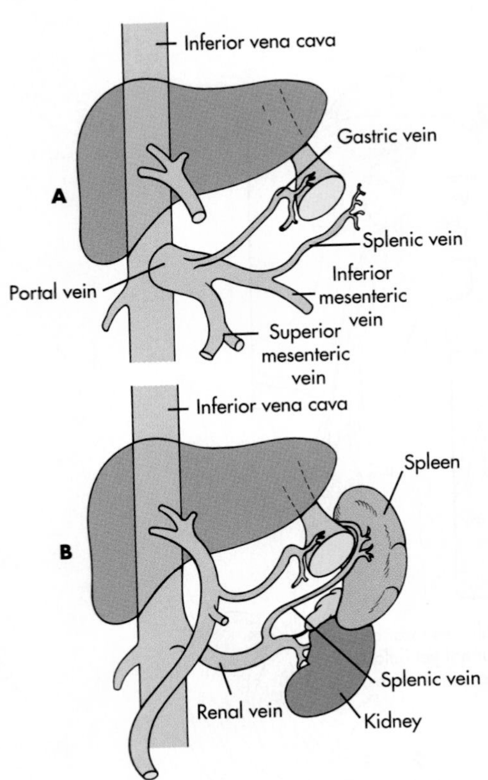

Fig. 41-10 Portosystemic shunts. **A,** Portacaval shunt. The portal vein is anastomosed to the inferior vena cava, diverting blood from the portal vein to the systemic circulation. **B,** Distal splenorenal shunt. The splenic vein is anastomosed to the renal vein. The portal venous flow remains intact while esophageal varices are selectively decompressed. (The short gastric veins are decompressed.) The spleen conducts blood from the high pressure of the esophageal and gastric varices to the low-pressure renal vein.

blockers such as cimetidine (Tagamet). Neomycin administration may be started to prevent hepatic encephalopathy from breakdown of blood and the release of ammonia in the intestine.

Long-term management. Long-term management of patients who have had an episode of bleeding includes β-adrenergic blockers, repeated sclerotherapy, endoscopic ligation, and portosystemic shunts. There is a high incidence of recurrent bleeding with a high mortality risk with each bleeding episode, so continued therapy is necessary. Repeated endoscopic sclerotherapy and ligation is commonly used.

Propranolol (Inderal), a β-adrenergic blocker, can be given orally to prevent recurrent GI bleeding. It reduces portal venous pressure. This effect is due to reduced cardiac output and possibly constriction of splanchnic vessels. However, because it reduces hepatic blood flow, it can enhance the possibility of hepatic encephalopathy.

Various surgical shunting procedures may be used to decrease portal hypertension by diverting some of the portal blood flow while at the same time allowing adequate liver perfusion. Currently, the shunts most commonly used are the portacaval shunt and the distal splenorenal shunt (Fig. 41-10). Shunts are indicated more after a second major bleeding episode than an initial bleeding episode. Although a prophylactic portacaval shunt lessens bleeding, it does not prolong life. Patients die of hepatic encephalopathy caused by the diversion of the ammonia past the liver and into the systemic circulation. The distal splenorenal shunt (Warren shunt) leaves portal venous flow intact (see Fig. 41-10), so it has a lower incidence of hepatic encephalopathy. With time, however, the flow of blood through the liver decreases.

Another procedure for the treatment of esophageal varices is the transjugular intrahepatic portosystemic shunt (TIPS). TIPS is a nonsurgical procedure in which a tract (shunt) between the systemic and portal venous systems is created to redirect portal blood flow. A stent is inserted to support the tract. Under fluoroscopy, the stent is passed via the right internal jugular vein and through the right atrium into the inferior vena cava. The stent is inserted between the hepatic and portal veins. This procedure reduces portal venous pressure and decompresses the varices, thus controlling bleeding. This procedure is used more for patients requiring short-term control while waiting for a liver transplant.

Hepatic Encephalopathy. The goal of management of hepatic encephalopathy is the reduction of ammonia formation. This consists mainly of protein restriction and reduction of ammonia formation in the intestines. The degree of protein restriction is determined by the severity of mental change. The protein restriction may range from 0 to 40 g per day. With improvement of mental function, dietary protein content is increased gradually over days.

Several measures to reduce ammonia formation in the intestines are used. Sterilization of the intestines with antibiotics such as neomycin sulfate, which are poorly absorbed from the GI tract, is one method. Neomycin is given orally or rectally. This reduces the bacterial flora of the colon. Bacterial action on protein in the feces results in ammonia production. Cathartics and enemas are also used to decrease bacterial action. Constipation should be prevented.

Lactulose (Cephulac) may also be used to treat hepatic encephalopathy. This is a synthetic keto-analog of lactose. In the colon, it is split into lactic acid and acetic acid, which decreases the pH from 7.0 to 5.0. The acidic environment discourages bacterial growth. The lactulose traps the ammonia in the gut, and the laxative effect of the drug expels the ammonia from the colon. It is usually given orally but may be given as a retention enema or via NG tube. Because neomycin may cause renal toxicity and hearing impairments, lactulose is frequently the preferred drug.

Levodopa has been used in the treatment of hepatic encephalopathy. It is a precursor of dopamine and norepinephrine. Use of levodopa is based on the theory that there is a deficiency of dopamine and norepinephrine in encephalopathy because they are replaced by false transmitters (amines from breakdown of dietary proteins). Normally these false transmitters are destroyed by liver enzymes, but when the liver is diseased, this no longer happens. The use of levodopa prolongs the lives of patients with coma resistant to other measures.

Control of hepatic encephalopathy also involves treatment of precipitating causes (see Table 41-12). This involves control-

DRUG THERAPY

Table 41-15 Cirrhosis

Medication	Mechanism of Action
Vasopressin (Pitressin)	Hemostasis and control of bleeding in esophageal varices, constriction of splanchnic arterial bed
Propranolol (Inderal)	Reduction of portal venous pressure, prevention of gastrointestinal bleeding
Neomycin sulfate	Decrease in bacterial flora, decreasing formation of ammonia
Lactulose (Cephulac)	Acidification of feces in bowel and trapping of ammonia, causing its elimination in feces
Levodopa	Conversion to dopamine, which has been displaced with amines from protein breakdown, to increase vascular resistance
Cimetidine (Tagamet)	Decrease in gastric acidity
Diuretics	
Spironolactone (Aldactone)	Blocking of action of aldosterone, potassium sparing
Amiloride (Midamor)	Inhibits reabsorption of sodium and secretion of potassium
Chlorothiazide (Diuril)	Thiazide that acts on proximal tubule to decrease reabsorption of sodium and water
Furosemide (Lasix)	Rapid action on distal tubule and loop of Henle to prevent reabsorption of sodium and water
Triamterene (Dyrenium)	Inhibits reabsorption of sodium and secretion of potassium
Magnesium sulfate	Magnesium replacement; hypomagnesemia occurs with liver dysfunction
Vitamin K (Synkavite)	Correction of clotting abnormalities

ling GI hemorrhage and removing the blood from the GI tract to decrease the protein in the intestine. Electrolyte and acid-base imbalances and infections should also be treated.

Liver transplantation should be considered in patients with recurring hepatic encephalopathy and end-stage liver disease. The use of liver transplantation depends on a number of factors, including the cause of the cirrhosis and other systemic medical problems.

Drug Therapy. There is no specific drug therapy for cirrhosis. However, a number of medications are used to treat symptoms and complications of advanced liver disease (Table 41-15). Some drug therapies are being used in the treatment of cirrhosis to try to prevent or reverse the fibrosis that occurs in the liver. The use of Colbenemid (combination of colchicine and probenecid) has shown an improvement in survival in cirrhotic patients. Propylthiouracil (PTU) has been used to reduce hepatic hypermetabolism, which occurs in alcoholic liver disease. More studies are needed before PTU can be recommended for routine use in these patients.[20]

Nutritional Therapy. The diet for the patient with cirrhosis without complications is high in calories (3000 kcal per day) with high carbohydrate content and moderate to low fat levels. The amount of protein varies depending on the degree of liver damage and the danger of encephalopathy. When the patient is symptomatic (e.g., ascites, edema, mental changes), a low-protein diet is indicated. When there is reduced risk of encephalopathy, 1.5 g of protein per kilogram of body weight may be ordered to maintain plasma osmotic balance and promote liver cell regeneration. Vitamin supplements are usually given. Foods high in protein include meat, fish, poultry, eggs, and dairy products. High-protein nourishment in the form of eggnogs, milkshakes, or protein supplements may be used, particularly for the patient who is malnourished.

The patient with hepatic encephalopathy is on a very-low-protein to no-protein diet (Table 41-16). Foods allowed include toast, cereal, rice, tea, fruit juices, and hard candies. Sufficient carbohydrate intake must be provided to maintain an intake of 1500 to 2000 calories to prevent hypoglycemia and catabolism. Glucose polymer (Polycose) is protein free and can be used as a source of calories. It can be given orally or via NG tube. A patient with alcoholic cirrhosis frequently has protein-calorie malnutrition. For the patient with protein malnutrition, enteral formulas such as Travasorb Hepatic or Hepatic-Aid may be used. These supplements contain protein from branched-chain amino acids that are metabolized by the muscles. They provide protein but put less burden on the liver. IV or tube feedings may be required.

The patient with ascites and edema is on a low-sodium diet. The degree of sodium restriction varies depending on the patient's condition. The patient needs instruction regarding the degree of restriction. Table salt is the most common source of sodium. Sodium is also present in baking soda and baking powder. Foods that are high in sodium content include canned soups and vegetables, salted snacks such as potato chips, nuts, smoked meats and fish, crackers, breads, olives, pickles, ketchup, and beer.

Sodium is also present in many over-the-counter medications (e.g., antacids). However, most antacids are now lower in sodium than previously. Carbonated beverages tend to be high in sodium, and low-sodium and sodium-free carbonated drinks are available. The patient should be advised to read labels. Foods high in protein usually have large amounts of sodium. Alternative protein supplements that are low in sodium may have to be used. The patient and the family need assistance to make the diet more palatable by the use of seasonings such as garlic, parsley, onion, lemon juice, and spices.

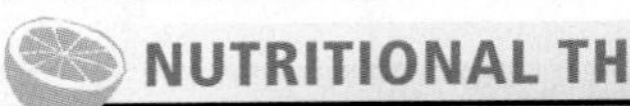

NUTRITIONAL THERAPY

Table 41-16 Low-Protein Diet for Hepatic Failure*

General Principles

Limit protein to 20 g per day at onset of severe hepatic failure.
Protein must be from protein sources with high biologic value.
Diet must be high in calories.
Fat is limited only to prevent early satiety.
Protein is increased in diet by 10 g increments as tolerated without causing signs and symptoms of hepatic encephalopathy.
Sodium is also usually restricted as well as fluid when edema and ascites are present.

Meal	Menu Plan 1	Menu Plan 2	Menu Plan 3
Breakfast			
1 fruit, calorie supplement 1 low-protein bread 1 egg (protein) Fat, calorie supplement ¼ cup milk (2 g protein)	½ cup grape juice with 2 tbs Polycose powder† French toast made with low-protein bread, 1 egg, 3 tsp salt-free butter and syrup ¼ cup milk	¼ cup cranberry juice with 2 tbs Polycose powder Low-protein toast with 3 tsp salt-free butter and 2 tsp jelly 1-egg omelet with 3 tsp salt-free butter ¼ cup milk	¼ cup prune juice with 2 tbs Polycose powder Low-protein toast with 3 tsp salt-free butter 1 egg fried in 3 tsp salt-free butter ¼ cup milk
Snack			
Calorie supplement	Jelly beans	Hard candy	Sugar mints
Lunch			
2 starch (4 g protein) 1 vegetable (2 g protein) 1 fruit, calorie supplement Fat, calorie supplement	¼ cup half and half ½ cup Cream of Wheat with 3 tsp salt-free butter Applesauce with whipped topping or Lipomul‡ Small tossed salad with 3 tbs oil and vinegar§ Peas with 3 tsp salt-free butter	¼ cup half and half ½ cup cornmeal (atole) with 3 tsp salt-free butter Small guacamole salad Gelatin with whipped topping or Lipomul Corn with 3 tsp salt-free butter	¼ cup half and half ½ cup grits with 3 tsp salt-free butter Cucumbers in sour cream Peaches with whipped topping or Lipomul Sweet potatoes with brown sugar and 3 tsp salt-free butter
Snack			
Calorie supplement	Low-protein cookies	Low-protein bread cubes with whipped cream and strawberries	Popsicles made with Polycose
Dinner			
1 starch (2 g protein) 1 vegetable (2 g protein) 1 low-protein bread ¼ cup milk (2 g protein) Fat, calorie supplement	½ baked potato 3 tsp salt-free butter Low-protein bread ¼ cup sour cream ½ cup green beans with 3 tsp salt-free butter and 2 tsp jelly ¼ cup milk	½ cup fried potatoes with 1 tsp melted salt-free butter ½ cup zucchini with 3 tsp salt-free butter Low-protein toast with 3 tsp salt-free butter and 2 tsp marmalade ¼ cup milk	½ cup mashed potatoes ½ cup fried okra Low-protein toast with 3 tsp salt-free butter and 2 tsp jam ¼ cup milk

*The diet plan contains approximately 20 g protein.
†Polycose is a brand-name product made by Ross Laboratories.
‡Lipomul is a fat emulsion made by Upjohn.
§Crisp food should be avoided because of the possibility of esophageal varices.

NURSING MANAGEMENT: CIRRHOSIS

■ Nursing Assessment

Subjective and objective data that should be obtained from an individual with cirrhosis are presented in Table 41-17.

■ Nursing Diagnoses

Nursing diagnoses for the patient with cirrhosis include, but are not limited to, those presented in NCP 41-2.

■ Planning

The overall goals are that the patient with cirrhosis will (1) have relief of discomfort; (2) have minimal to no complications (ascites, esophageal varices, hepatic encephalopathy); and (3) return to as normal a lifestyle as possible.

■ Nursing Implementation

Health Promotion. The common etiologies of cirrhosis are alcohol, malnutrition, hepatitis, biliary obstruction, and

NURSING ASSESSMENT

Table 41-17 **Cirrhosis**

Subjective Data	Objective Data
Important Health Information *Past health history:* Previous viral, toxic or idiopathic hepatitis; chronic biliary obstruction and infection; severe right-sided heart failure *Medications:* Adverse reaction to any medication; use of anticoagulants, aspirin, acetaminophen **Functional Health Patterns** *Health perception–health management:* Chronic alcoholism; weakness, fatigue *Nutritional-metabolic:* Anorexia, weight loss, dyspepsia, nausea and vomiting; gingival bleeding *Elimination:* Dark urine, decreased urinary output; light-colored or black stools, flatulence, change in bowel habits; dry, yellow skin, bruising *Cognitive-perceptual:* Dull, right upper quadrant or epigastric pain; numbness, tingling of extremities; pruritis *Sexuality-reproductive:* Impotence, amenorrhea	**General** Fever, cachexia, wasting of extremities **Integumentary** Icteric sclera, jaundice, petechiae, ecchymoses, spider angiomas, palmar erythema, alopecia, loss of axillary and pubic hair; peripheral edema **Respiratory** Shallow, rapid respirations; epistaxis **Gastrointestinal** Abdominal distention, ascites, distended abdominal wall veins, palpable liver and spleen, foul breath; hematemesis; black, tarry stools; hemorrhoids **Neurologic** Altered mentation, asterixis **Reproductive** Gynecomastia and testicular atrophy (men), impotence (men), loss of libido (men and women), amenorrhea or heavy menstrual bleeding (women) **Possible Findings** Anemia, thrombocytopenia; leukopenia; decreased serum albumin, potassium; abnormal liver function studies; elevated coagulation studies, ammonia, and bilirubin levels; abnormal abdominal ultrasound and liver scan; positive liver biopsy

right-sided heart failure. Prevention and early treatment of cirrhosis must focus on the primary etiology. Alcoholism must be treated (see Chapter 10). Patients should be urged to avoid alcohol ingestion, and their efforts should be supported. Adequate nutrition, especially for the alcoholic and other individuals at risk for cirrhosis, is essential to promote liver regeneration. Hepatitis must be identified and treated early so that it does not progress to chronic hepatitis. Biliary disease must be treated so that the stones do not cause obstruction and infection. The underlying cause (e.g., chronic lung disease) of right-sided heart failure must be treated so that the heart failure does not lead to cirrhosis.

Acute Intervention. The focus of nursing care for the patient with cirrhosis is on conserving the patient's strength (see NCP 41-2). Rest enables the liver to restore itself. Complete bed rest may not always be necessary. When the patient requires complete bed rest, measures to prevent pneumonia, thromboembolic problems, and pressure ulcers should be taken. The activity and rest schedule may be modified according to signs of clinical improvement (e.g., decreasing jaundice, improvement in liver function studies). Major concerns of the nurse in determining appropriate nursing care measures to meet the need for rest involve regulation of the physical, emotional, and social climate.

Anorexia, nausea and vomiting, pressure from ascites, and poor eating habits all create problems in maintenance of an adequate intake of nutrients. The nursing measures relating to nutrition for patients with hepatitis also apply here. Oral hygiene before meals may improve the patient's taste sensation. Between-meal nourishments should be available so that they can be provided at times when the patient can best tolerate them. Food preferences should be provided whenever possible. Explanations to the patient and the family of the reason for any dietary restrictions should be provided.

Nursing assessment and care should include the patient's physiologic response to cirrhosis. Is jaundice present? Where is it observed—sclera, skin, hard palate? What is the progression of jaundice? If the jaundice is accompanied by pruritus, measures to relieve itching should be carried out. Cholestyramine (Questran) may be ordered to help relieve the pruritus. The color of the urine and stools should be noted. With jaundice the urine is often cola colored or mahogany and the stool gray or tan.

Edema and ascites are frequent manifestations of cirrhosis and require nursing assessments and interventions. Accurate calculation and recordings of intake and output, daily weights, and measurements of extremities and abdominal girth help in the ongoing assessment of the location and extent of the edema. If the patient can assume a kneeling position when abdominal girth measurement is taken, the abdominal fluid will go to the most dependent part of the abdomen. This gives the best measurement of abdominal girth. For many patients, girth must be measured in the standing or lying position. Where the measurements are taken should be recorded and should be a part of the nursing care plan.

When a paracentesis is done, the nurse must have the patient void immediately before the procedure to prevent puncture of the bladder. The patient should sit on the side of the bed or be placed in high Fowler's position. Following the procedure the

41-2 NURSING CARE PLAN PATIENT WITH CIRRHOSIS

Expected Patient Outcomes	Nursing Interventions and *Rationales*
NURSING DIAGNOSIS	**Altered nutrition: less than body requirements** *related to* anorexia, impaired utilization and storage of nutrients, nausea, and vomiting *as manifested by* lack of interest in food, aversion to eating, reported inadequate food intake.
▪ Adequate intake of nutrients. ▪ Maintenance of normal body weight.	▪ Monitor weight *to evaluate nitrogen balance.* ▪ Provide oral care before meals *to remove foul tastes and improve taste of food.* ▪ Administer antiemetics as ordered *to relieve nausea and vomiting.* ▪ Provide small, frequent meals with nourishments *to prevent feeling of fullness and maintain nutritional status.* ▪ Determine food preferences and allow these whenever possible *to increase nutritional appeal for patient, since a low- or no-protein diet is not very palatable.*
NURSING DIAGNOSIS	**Impaired skin integrity** *related to* edema, ascites, and pruritus *as manifested by* complaints of itching; areas of excoriation from scratching; taut, shiny skin over edematous areas; areas of skin breakdown.
▪ Maintenance of skin integrity. ▪ Relief of pruritus.	▪ Restrict sodium intake and fluids as ordered *to reduce fluid retention.* ▪ Administer prescribed diuretics *to prevent fluid retention and promote diuresis.* ▪ Monitor intake and output *to assess fluid balance and renal function.* ▪ Assess location and extent of edema by weighing patient at the same time each day, taking daily measurements of extremities and of abdominal girth (same location each time) *to determine patient's response to treatment.* ▪ Provide meticulous skin care *because edematous tissues are easily traumatized and subject to breakdown.* ▪ Reposition patient at least q2hr *to relieve pressure over bony prominences.* ▪ Elevate edematous areas *to promote venous drainage.* ▪ Have patient use special mattress, such as alternating-air pressure mattress or egg crate mattress, *to reduce the risk of skin breakdown from prolonged pressure.* ▪ Clip patient's nails short and keep clean *to prevent excoriation from pruritus secondary to deposit of bile salts on skin.* ▪ Administer antipruritic medication as ordered *to relieve itching.* ▪ Provide diversions and distractions *to assist patient in coping with the discomfort of itching and edema.*
NURSING DIAGNOSIS	**Ineffective breathing pattern** *related to* pressure on diaphragm and reduced lung volume secondary to ascites *as manifested by* dyspnea, cyanosis, cough, changes in pulse or respiratory rate, depth, or pattern.
▪ Able to breathe with minimal difficulty. ▪ Effective breathing pattern. ▪ Absence of cyanosis and other signs and symptoms of hypoxia.	▪ Place patient in semi-Fowler's or Fowler's position; support the arms and chest with pillows *to facilitate breathing by relieving pressure on diaphragm.* ▪ Auscultate chest for crackles *to identify fluid in lungs.* ▪ Assess respiratory rate and rhythm *to identify increasing dyspnea.*
NURSING DIAGNOSIS	**Risk for injury** *related to* diminished sensory perception secondary to peripheral neuropathy.
▪ No injury due to decreased sensory perception.	▪ Assess for numbness and tingling of lower extremities, decreased sensation in lower extremities *to determine risk of injury.* ▪ Prevent excess stimulation or trauma to extremities *because patient may not be able to detect harmful stimuli.* ▪ Do not use restrictive bed linens *because they reduce circulation and place pressure on edematous tissue.* ▪ Instruct patient to avoid tight clothing *because it impedes circulation.* ▪ Use care with heat and cold applications *because patient's ability to perceive temperature is impaired.* ▪ Assist with ambulation *to assess patient's ability to safely ambulate and to prevent injury.*

Continued

41-2 NURSING CARE PLAN PATIENT WITH CIRRHOSIS—continued

Expected Patient Outcomes	Nursing Interventions and *Rationales*
NURSING DIAGNOSIS	**Activity intolerance** *related to* fatigue, anemia, ascites, dyspnea, treatment schedule, and cardiac deconditioning *as manifested by* fatigue or weakness, abnormal heart rate or blood pressure, altered response to activity and weakness.
▪ Increased tolerance for activity.	▪ Assess patient's ability to perform activities *to plan appropriate interventions.* ▪ Conserve patient's strength *to minimize cardiac and respiratory work.* ▪ Provide activity and rest as required *to reduce metabolic demands on the liver, reduce hepatic blood flow, and allow for recovery of liver cells.* ▪ Monitor hemoglobin and hematocrit levels *to detect GI hemorrhage.* ▪ Assist with ADLs as needed *to ensure patient's needs are met.*
NURSING DIAGNOSIS	**Risk for infection** *related to* leukopenia and increased susceptibility to environmental pathogens.
▪ No signs or symptoms of infections.	▪ Use appropriate infection control measures. ▪ Assess patient for evidence of risk factors, including leukopenia, and altered circulation *to ensure early identification of infection.* ▪ Monitor patient's temperature every 2 to 4 hr *because fever is an indicator of infection.* ▪ Observe for any local and systemic manifestations of infection *to enable early diagnosis and treatment.* ▪ Protect patient from others with infections *to reduce the risk of infection secondary to decreased resistance.* ▪ Monitor white blood cell count *to assess patient's response to treatment.*
NURSING DIAGNOSIS	**Ineffective airway clearance** *related to* inability to remove and swallow secretions and bleeding from esophageal varices *as manifested by* ineffective cough; inability to remove airway secretions; abnormal breath sounds; abnormal respiratory rate, rhythm, depth.
▪ Patent airway. ▪ Normal breath sounds.	▪ Suction patient (oral and pharyngeal areas) frequently *to reduce risk of aspiration because patient is unable to swallow with Sengstaken-Blakemore (S-B) tube in place.* ▪ Place in semi-Fowler's position *to facilitate drainage from mouth and ease breathing by reducing intraabdominal pressure.* ▪ Have scissors near bed to cut S-B tube (if necessary) *to prevent a displaced esophageal balloon from obstructing the airway.* ▪ Encourage patient to expectorate, *since the patient is unable to swallow saliva because the inflated esophageal balloon occludes the esophagus.* ▪ Offer frequent oral and nasal care *to provide relief from taste of blood and irritation from mouth bleeding.*

COLLABORATIVE PROBLEMS

Nursing Goals	Nursing Interventions and *Rationales*
POTENTIAL COMPLICATION	**Hepatic encephalopathy** *related to* increased formation of ammonia and aromatic amino acids.
▪ Monitor for signs of hepatic encephalopathy. ▪ Report deviation from acceptable parameters. ▪ Carry out appropriate medical and nursing interventions.	▪ Monitor for encephalopathy by assessing patient's general behavior, orientation to time and place, speech, blood pH, and ammonia levels *because liver is unable to convert accumulating ammonia to urea for renal excretion.* ▪ Encourage fluids (if not restricted) and give laxatives and enemas as ordered *to decrease production of ammonia.* ▪ Provide low-protein or no-protein diet as ordered *because ammonia (a breakdown product of protein) is responsible for mental changes.* ▪ Limit physical activity *because exercise produces ammonia as a by-product of metabolism.*

Continued

41-2 NURSING CARE PLAN PATIENT WITH CIRRHOSIS—continued

Expected Patient Outcomes	Nursing Interventions and *Rationales*
POTENTIAL COMPLICATION	**Hemorrhage** *related to* bleeding tendency secondary to liver's inability to make clotting factors.
▪ Monitor for signs of hemorrhage. ▪ Initiate appropriate medical and nursing interventions.	▪ Monitor for hemorrhage by assessing for epistaxis, purpura, petechiae, easy bruising, gingival bleeding, heavy menstrual bleeding, hematuria, melena *because liver disease results in impaired synthesis of clotting factors.* ▪ Provide gentle nursing care *to minimize the risk of tissue trauma.* ▪ Observe for bleeding from body orifices, urine, and stool *to detect bleeding early and allow prompt intervention.* ▪ Use smallest-gauge needle possible when giving injection and apply gentle but prolonged pressure after injection *to minimize risk of bleeding into tissue.* ▪ Advise use of soft-bristle toothbrush *to reduce trauma to mouth because mucous membranes have increased risk of injury.* ▪ Teach patient to avoid straining at stool, vigorous blowing of nose, and coughing *to reduce risk of hemorrhage from these areas.* ▪ Observe for bruising on the forearms, axillae, and skin. ▪ Monitor laboratory results (hematocrit, hemoglobin, and prothrombin time) *as indicators of anemia, active bleeding, or impending complications.*

nurse should monitor for hypovolemia and electrolyte imbalances and check the dressing for bleeding and leakage.

Dyspnea is a frequent problem for the patient with ascites. A semi-Fowler's or Fowler's position allows for maximal respiratory efficiency. Pillows can be used to support the arms and chest and may increase the patient's comfort and ability to breathe.

Meticulous skin care is essential because the edematous tissues are subject to breakdown. An alternating–air pressure mattress or other special mattress should be used. A turning schedule (minimum of every 2 hours) must be adhered to rigidly. The abdomen may be supported with pillows. If the abdomen is taut, cleansing must be done very gently. This patient tends to move very little because of the abdominal discomfort and dyspnea. Therefore range-of-motion exercises are helpful, and measures such as coughing and deep breathing to prevent respiratory problems should be implemented. The lower extremities may be elevated. If scrotal edema is present, a scrotal support provides some comfort.

When the patient is taking diuretics, the serum levels of sodium, potassium, chloride, and bicarbonate should be monitored. The patient should be observed for signs of fluid and electrolyte imbalance, especially hypokalemia. Hypokalemia may be manifested by cardiac arrhythmias, hypotension, tachycardia, and generalized muscle weakness. Water excess is manifested by muscle cramping, weakness, lethargy, and confusion.

Observations and nursing care in relation to hematologic disorders (bleeding tendencies, anemia, increased susceptibility to infection) are the same as for the patient with advanced liver disease (see NCP 41-2).

The nurse must assess the patient's response to altered body image resulting from jaundice, spider angiomas, palmar erythema, ascites, and gynecomastia. The patient may experience a great deal of anxiety regarding these changes. The nurse should explain these phenomena and should be a supportive listener. Nursing care with concern and warmth regardless of physical changes helps the patient maintain self-esteem.

Bleeding esophageal varices. If the patient has esophageal varices in addition to cirrhosis, the nurse must be observant of any signs of bleeding from the varices, such as hematemesis and melena. If hematemesis occurs, the nurse should assess the patient for hemorrhage, call the physician, and be ready to assist with whatever treatment is used to control the bleeding. The patient will be admitted to the intensive care unit (ICU). The patient's airway must be maintained.

When balloon tamponade is used, the initial nursing task related to insertion of the tube is to explain the use of the tube and how it will be inserted. The balloons should be checked for patency. Sometimes the stomach is lavaged with saline solution before insertion of the tube. It is usually the physician's responsibility to insert the tube. It may be inserted via the nose or the mouth (see Fig. 41-9). The placement of the tube is ascertained by x-ray. Then the gastric balloon is inflated with approximately 250 ml of air and the tube is retracted until resistance (gastroesophageal junction) is felt. The tube is secured by placement of a piece of sponge or foam rubber at the nostrils (nasal cuff). This protects the mucosal surfaces from irritation and injury. For continued bleeding the esophageal balloon is then inflated. A sphygmomanometer is used to measure and maintain the desired pressure at 20 to 40 mm Hg. The position of the balloons is verified by x-ray. Sometimes it is helpful to have the patient wear a football helmet with the tube secured to the mouth guard. This stabilizes the tube and applies traction. Traction may also be applied (0.75 to 1.25 pounds [0.3 to 0.6 kg]) to hold the tube securely in place and prevent downward movement. Traction causes ulceration of the nasal mucosa and can be used only for short intervals (2 to 3 hours) at a time.

ETHICAL DILEMMAS

Rationing

SITUATION

A 43-year-old patient with cirrhosis of the liver is frequently admitted to the hospital. She has been told that her continued drinking will inevitably lead to her death. Now she has been admitted for GI bleeding and needs blood transfusions. She has a rare blood type and it is frequently difficult to get compatible blood. Should the nurse call an ethics consultation?

DISCUSSION

A noncompliant patient whose behavior has led to a worsening of the disease process raises difficult ethical problems regarding rationing care. Rationing treatment of a manageable presenting problem probably would not be discussed for a cancer or a trauma patient. However, since alcoholism is understood as a disease with a behavioral component, this patient could be seen to be both noncompliant and unworthy of additional treatment. If the GI problem can be treated and transfusions are integral to that treatment, will that change the overall condition of the patient in regard to her cirrhosis? Will it extend her life or improve the quality of her life? If her underlying disease and quality of life cannot be treated or improved, this treatment could be seen as medically futile and therefore not required. Rationing decisions should be made based on triage, when necessary, rather than assessments of compliance or moral weakness. If the blood supply is very low and desperately needed by a patient whose disease or condition *can* be effectively treated by transfusions, rationing treatment to the patient with cirrhosis might be appropriate. However, if the blood supply is sufficient and no other patients are in competition for it, this is not a rationing decision. Regardless of the availability of resources, this continues to be a medical futility issue, and that may eventually be the basis for decisions about which treatments can be withheld for the greater benefit of all patients.

ETHICAL AND LEGAL DECISIONS

- Rationing is the distribution of scarce resources to an individual patient or a class of patients and the denial of those resources to others. It is based on a limited amount of technology, specific resources (e.g., blood, organs, ICU beds), or financing allocated at the societal level.
- Triage is the priority of care given to patients in an emergency or disaster situation based on the utility of providing the greatest good for the greatest number of patients.
- Prior noncompliant behavior should not be grounds for denying care of the present, acute problem. If the noncompliance is expected to continue and will affect the goals of this medical treatment, it can be grounds for decisions about whether or how to treat the presenting problem.

Sometimes saline lavage is used to remove blood from the stomach. (Nursing care of upper GI bleeding is discussed in Chapter 39.) This helps prevent the blood from degrading to ammonia, leading to encephalopathy. The nurse must ensure that the right amount of pressure is maintained for the correct time. Constant tension and an upward pull on the stomach initiate contraction of the stomach, which may lead to retching and increased portal pressures. The esophageal balloon should be deflated every 8 to 12 hours to avoid necrosis. Each lumen must be labeled to avoid confusion. The NG lumen may be connected to suction to remove blood and keep the stomach empty to reduce the risk of aspiration. The most common complication of balloon tamponade therapy is aspiration pneumonia.

Nursing care includes monitoring for complications of rupture or erosion of the esophagus, regurgitation and aspiration of gastric contents, and occlusion of the airway by the balloon. If the gastric balloon breaks or is deflated, the esophageal balloon will slip upward, obstructing the airway and causing asphyxiation. If this happens, the nurse must cut the tube or deflate the esophageal balloon. Scissors should be kept at the bedside. Regurgitation can be minimized by oral and pharyngeal suctioning and by keeping the patient in a semi-Fowler's position.

The patient is unable to swallow saliva because of the inflated esophageal balloon occluding the esophagus. With the Minnesota tube, which has an esophageal aspiration lumen, this problem can be alleviated. The nurse should encourage the patient to expectorate and should provide an emesis basin and tissues. Frequent oral and nasal care provides relief from the taste of blood and irritation from mouth breathing.

The patient is extremely ill at this stage. The crisis of the bleeding and the ordeal of the tube create a great deal of psychologic trauma. Emotional support and gentle caring must be provided.

Hepatic encephalopathy. The focus of nursing care of the patient with hepatic encephalopathy is on sustaining life and assisting with measures to reduce the formation of ammonia. The nurse should assess (1) the patient's level of responsiveness (e.g., reflexes, pupillary reactions, orientation); (2) sensory and motor abnormalities (e.g., hyperreflexia, asterixis, motor coordination); (3) fluid and electrolyte imbalances; (4) acid-base imbalances; and (5) the effect of treatment measures.

The neurologic status, including an exact description of the patient's behavior, should be assessed and recorded at least every 2 hours. Care of the patient with neurologic problems should be based on the severity of the encephalopathy.

Nursing measures to prevent constipation should be instituted to decrease ammonia production. Drugs, laxatives, and enemas should be given as ordered. Encouragement of fluids may also help if not contraindicated. The patient should not strain at stool because this may cause bleeding of hemorrhoidal varices. Any GI bleeding may worsen the coma. The patient who is taking lactulose should be assessed for diarrhea. Some physicians have diarrhea as a goal when treating with lactulose. The drug's laxative action expels the ammonia from the colon. Because lactulose can cause severe purging, the nurse should observe the patient for excessive fluid and electrolyte loss.

Factors that are known to precipitate coma should be controlled as much as possible (see Table 41-12). Because exercise

PATIENT & FAMILY TEACHING GUIDE

Table 41-18 Cirrhosis

1. Explain to the patient and family the importance of continuous health care so they understand that cirrhosis is a chronic illness.
2. Teach the patient and family symptoms of complications and when to seek medical attention to enable prompt treatment of complications.
3. Teach proper diet because a low-protein, high-carbohydrate diet is usually indicated and can be difficult to follow.
4. Teach the patient to avoid potentially hepatotoxic over-the-counter drugs since the diseased liver is unable to metabolize these medications.
5. Encourage abstinence from alcohol because continued use of alcohol will increase the risk of liver complications.
6. Instruct the patient to avoid aspirin and control cough to prevent hemorrhage when esophageal or gastric varices are present.
7. Teach the patient to avoid spicy and rough foods and activities that increase portal pressure, such as straining at stool, coughing, sneezing, and retching and vomiting because hemorrhage is a danger due to inability of the liver to produce clotting factors.

produces ammonia as a by-product of metabolism, the physical activity of the patient must be limited. Hypokalemia should be controlled.

The patient is on either a very low-protein or a no-protein diet, neither of which is very palatable. Vegetable protein is better tolerated than meat protein. Foods and fluids high in carbohydrate should be given because the liver is not synthesizing and storing glucose. The patient may require tube feedings if an adequate diet cannot be ingested.

Ambulatory and Home Care. The patient with cirrhosis may be faced with a prolonged course and the possibility of serious, life-threatening problems and complications. The nurse should be a resource person in helping the patient achieve the highest level of wellness. The patient and the family need to understand the importance of continuous health care and medical supervision. They should be taught symptoms of complications and when to seek medical attention. Patients with cirrhosis should refrain from eating raw shellfish and avoid activities that place them at risk for contracting viral hepatitis.

Measures to achieve and maintain a remission should be encouraged. These include proper diet, rest, avoidance of potentially hepatotoxic over-the-counter drugs such as acetaminophen, and abstinence from alcohol. Abstinence from alcohol is important and results in improvement in most patients. The nurse must realize the difficulty this poses for some patients. The nurse's own attitude regarding the patient whose cirrhosis is attributed to alcohol abuse should be explored. Care should be given without rejection and moralizing. The alcoholic patient should be treated with a caring attitude.

Cirrhosis is a chronic disease. The patient is affected not only physically but also psychologically, socially, and economically. Major adjustments may be required to make lifestyle changes, especially if alcohol abuse is the primary etiologic factor. The nurse should provide information regarding community support programs, such as Alcoholics Anonymous, for help with alcohol abuse.

Adequate explanations, along with written instructions, related to fluid or dietary restrictions should be given to the patient and the family (Table 41-18). Other health teaching should include instruction about adequate rest periods, how to detect early signs of complications, skin care, drug therapy precautions, observation for bleeding, and protection from infection. Counseling information regarding sexual problems may be needed. Referral to a community or home health nurse may be helpful to ensure adequate patient compliance with prescribed therapy. The emphasis of home care for the patient with cirrhosis should be on helping the patient maintain the highest level of wellness possible and initiate and maintain necessary lifestyle changes.

Evaluation

Expected outcomes for the patient with cirrhosis are addressed in NCP 41-2.

FULMINANT HEPATIC FAILURE

Fulminant hepatic failure is a clinical syndrome characterized by severe impairment of liver function associated with hepatic encephalopathy. In fulminant hepatic failure the encephalopathy occurs within 8 weeks of the first symptoms. The most common cause is viral hepatitis, in particular HBV, but it may also occur with HAV and less frequently with HCV.

Medications are the second most common cause of fulminant hepatic failure. Acetaminophen (Tylenol) in combination with alcohol is a common offending agent. Persons who abuse alcohol are particularly susceptible to detrimental effects of acetaminophen on the liver. Other drugs include INH, halothane, sulfa-containing drugs, and nonsteroidal antiinflammatory drugs.

The patient has jaundice and signs of encephalopathy. Laboratory tests reveal elevated liver function tests and increased bilirubin. Depending on the degree of liver failure, treatment may involve liver transplantation.

CARCINOMA OF THE LIVER

Primary carcinoma (originating in the liver) is rare. Metastatic carcinoma of the liver is more common. Hepatocellular carcinoma is the most common malignant tumor of the liver. The remaining primary tumors are cholangiomas or bile duct carcinomas. A high percentage of patients with primary cell carcinoma have cirrhosis of the liver. Some cases of hepatocellular carcinoma are associated with chronic hepatitis B or C.[21] Men have a higher incidence of primary liver cancer than women.

The liver is a common site of metastatic growth because of its high rate of blood flow and extensive capillary network. Cancer cells in other parts of the body are commonly carried to the liver via the portal circulation.

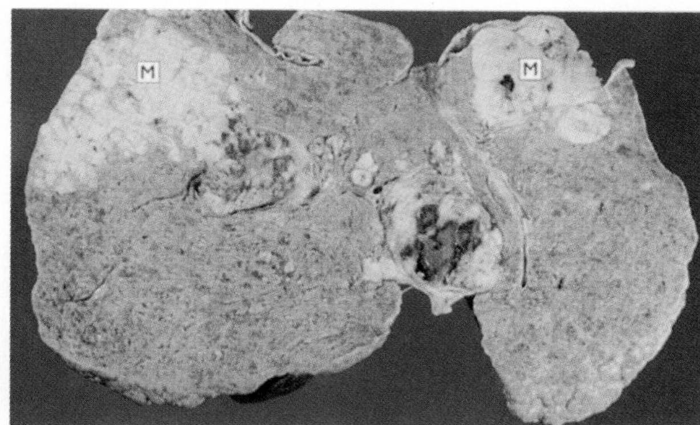

Fig. 41-11 Hepatocellular carcinoma. Macroscopically hepatocellular carcinoma may be single or multifocal. They usually develop in a liver already affected by cirrhosis. Tumor appears as an abnormal mass *(M)* within the liver.

The malignant cells cause the liver to be enlarged and misshapen. Hemorrhage and necrosis in the liver are common (Fig. 41-11). Lesions may be singular or numerous and nodular or diffusely spread over the entire liver. Some tumors infiltrate into other organs such as the gallbladder or into the peritoneum or diaphragm. Primary liver tumors commonly metastasize to the lung.

Clinical Manifestations

It is difficult to diagnose carcinoma of the liver. It is particularly difficult to differentiate it from cirrhosis in its early stages because many of the clinical manifestations (e.g., hepatomegaly, weight loss, peripheral edema, ascites, portal hypertension) are similar. Other common manifestations include dull abdominal pain in the epigastric or right upper quadrant region, jaundice, anorexia, nausea and vomiting, and extreme weakness. Patients frequently have pulmonary emboli. Tests used to assist in the diagnosis are a liver scan, hepatic arteriography, endoscopic retrograde cholangiopancreatography (ERCP), and a liver biopsy. The test for α-fetoprotein (AFP) may be positive in hepatocellular carcinoma. AFP helps distinguish primary cancer from metastatic cancer.

NURSING AND COLLABORATIVE MANAGEMENT: CANCER OF THE LIVER

Treatment of cancer of the liver is largely palliative. Surgical excision (lobectomy) is sometimes performed if the tumor is localized to one portion of the liver. Only 30% to 40% of patients have surgically resectable disease. Usually surgery is not feasible because the cancer is too far advanced when it is detected. Surgical excision offers the only chance for cure of liver cancer. Management is similar to that for cirrhosis. Chemotherapy may be used, but there is usually a poor response. Portal vein or hepatic artery perfusion with 5-fluorouracil (5-FU) may be attempted.

Nursing intervention for the patient with liver carcinoma focuses on keeping the patient as comfortable as possible. Because this patient manifests the same problems as any patient with advanced liver disease, the nursing interventions discussed for cirrhosis of the liver apply. (See Chapter 14 for care of the patient with cancer.)

The prognosis for cancer of the liver is poor. The cancer grows rapidly, and death may occur within 4 to 7 months as a result of hepatic encephalopathy or massive blood loss from GI bleeding.

RESEARCH
IMPLICATIONS FOR NURSING PRACTICE

Sexual Functioning After Transplant Surgery

Citation Hart LK and others: Survey of sexual concerns among organ transplant recipients, *J Transpl Coord* 7:82, 1997.

Purpose To identify the frequency of sexual dysfunction, degree of satisfaction, overall satisfaction, and life quality in desire for and receipt of instruction regarding sexual dysfunction in organ transplant recipients.

Methods A survey was mailed to 768 adult liver, kidney, and pancreas/kidney recipients (39% responded) to determine satisfaction, quality of life, and sexual functioning among transplant recipients.

Results and Conclusions Of those who responded there were no differences among the transplant groups with respect to satisfaction, quality of life, or sexual functioning. The degree of relationship satisfaction was related to frequency of intercourse, sexual desire, orgasm, and acceptance of partners' advances. Sixty-seven percent of the patients received no instruction related to sexuality or fertility.

Implications for Nursing Practice The results of this survey indicate that many transplant recipients receive little or no information related to sexuality and fertility. This is an important area for nursing intervention. In addition, efforts should be made to validate and support sexual identity in this patient population.

LIVER TRANSPLANTATION

The first human liver transplant was performed in 1963 at the University of Colorado by Thomas Starzl. In the last decade, liver transplantation has become a practical therapeutic option for many adults and children with irreversible liver disease. It improves the quality of life for end-stage liver patients and is an accepted treatment modality for these patients. Indications for liver transplantation include congenital biliary abnormalities, inborn errors of metabolism, hepatic malignancy (confined to the liver), sclerosing cholangitis, and chronic end-stage liver disease.[23] Cirrhosis of the liver, primarily as a result of hepatitis viruses, is a major indication for transplantation in adults. Liver transplants are not recommended for the patient with widespread malignant disease.

The major postoperative complications are rejection and infection. Rejection is not as major a problem as in kidney transplants. The liver seems to be less susceptible to severe

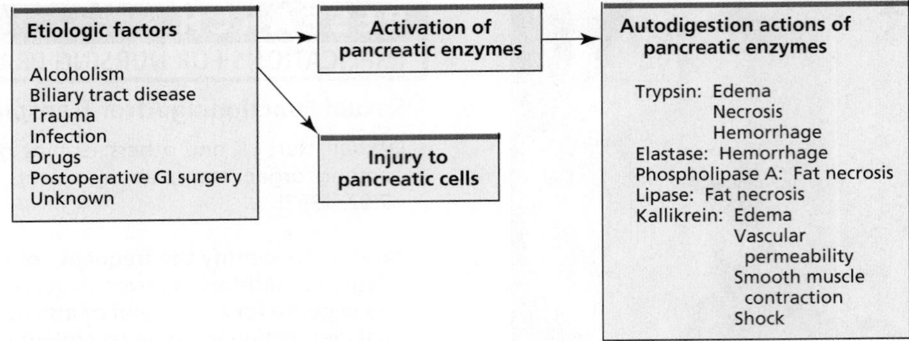

Fig. 41-12 Pathogenic process of acute pancreatitis.

rejection than the kidney. Cyclosporine is an effective immunosuppressant drug. The use of cyclosporine has been a major factor in the success rates of liver transplantation. The mechanism of action and side effects of cyclosporine are discussed in Chapter 44 and Table 44-12. It does not cause bone marrow suppression and does not impede wound healing. Other immunosuppressants used include azathioprine (Imuran), corticosteroids, and the monoclonal antibody OKT3 (see Table 44-12). Other factors in the improved success rate are advances in surgical techniques, better selection of potential recipients, and improved management of the underlying liver disease before surgery.

Patients who have liver disease secondary to viral hepatitis often experience reinfection of the graft with hepatitis C or B following transplantation. Despite this, the 5-year survival rate of patients with hepatitis C undergoing transplantation is 78%.[22]

The patient who has had a liver transplant requires competent and highly skilled nursing care, either in an ICU or in some other specialized unit. Postoperative nursing care includes assessing neurologic status; monitoring for signs of hemorrhage; preventing pulmonary complications; monitoring drainage, electrolytes, and urinary output; and monitoring for signs and symptoms of infection and rejection. Common respiratory problems are pneumonia, atelectasis, and pleural effusions. The nurse should have the patient use measures such as coughing, deep breathing, incentive spirometry, and repositioning to prevent these complications. Drainage from the Jackson-Pratt drain, NG tube, and T-tube should be measured and the color and consistency of drainage noted. A critical aspect of nursing care following liver transplantation is monitoring for infection. The first 2 months after the surgery are critical. Infection can be viral, fungal, or bacterial. Fever may be the only sign of infection. Emotional support and teaching the patient and family are essential.

ACUTE PANCREATITIS

Acute pancreatitis is an acute inflammatory process of the pancreas. The degree of inflammation varies from mild edema to severe hemorrhagic necrosis.

Acute pancreatitis is most common in middle-aged men and women, but it affects more men than women. The severity of the disease varies according to the extent of pancreatic destruction. Some patients recover completely, others have recurring attacks, and chronic pancreatitis develops in others. Acute pancreatitis can be life threatening.

Etiology and Pathophysiology

Many factors can cause injury to the pancreas. The primary etiologic factors are biliary tract disease and alcoholism. In the United States the most common cause is alcoholism, followed by gallbladder disease. Other, less common, causes of acute pancreatitis include trauma (postsurgical, abdominal); viral infections (mumps, coxsackievirus B); penetrating duodenal ulcer; cysts; abscesses; cystic fibrosis; Kaposi's sarcoma; certain drugs (corticosteroids, thiazide diuretics, oral contraceptives, sulfonamides, nonsteroidal antiinflammatory drugs); and metabolic disorders (hyperparathyroidism, hyperlipidemia, renal failure). Pancreatitis may occur after surgical procedures on the pancreas, stomach, duodenum, or biliary tract. Pancreatitis can also occur after ERCP. In some cases the cause is not known (idiopathic).

The most common pathogenic mechanism is believed to be autodigestion of the pancreas (Fig. 41-12). The etiologic factors cause injury to pancreatic cells or activation of the pancreatic enzymes in the pancreas rather than in the intestine. It is not clear how the activation of pancreatic enzymes occurs. One possible cause is believed to be the reflux of bile acids into the pancreatic ducts through an open or distended sphincter of Oddi. This reflux may occur because of gallstones impacted at the ampulla of Vater, atony and edema of the sphincter, or obstruction of pancreatic ducts and pancreatic ischemia.

Trypsinogen is an inactive proteolytic enzyme produced by the pancreas. Normally it is released into the small intestine via the pancreatic duct. In the intestine it is activated to trypsin by enterokinase. Normally, trypsin inhibitors in the pancreas and plasma bind and inactivate any trypsin that is inadvertently produced. In pancreatitis, activated trypsin is present in the pancreas. This enzyme can digest the pancreas and can activate other proteolytic enzymes such as elastase and phospholipase.

Elastase and phospholipase A play a major role in autodigestion of the pancreas. Elastase is activated by trypsin and causes hemorrhage by producing dissolution of the elastic fibers of blood vessels. Phospholipase A is probably activated by trypsin and bile acids and causes fat necrosis.

It is not entirely clear how alcohol causes acute pancreatitis. One theory is that it stimulates secretion and excess production of hydrochloric acid. A decrease in the gastric pH results in the release of the hormone secretin from the intestinal mucosa.

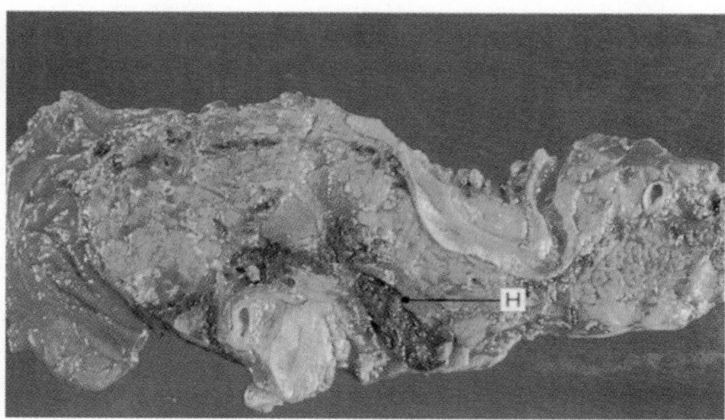

Fig. 41-13 In acute pancreatitis the pancreas appears edematous and is commonly hemorrhagic (H).

This hormone then stimulates pancreatic secretions. Alcohol may also cause regurgitation of duodenal contents into the pancreatic duct, resulting in inflammation.

The pathophysiologic involvement of acute pancreatitis ranges from edematous pancreatitis (which is mild and self-limiting) to necrotizing pancreatitis (in which the degree of necrosis correlates with the severity of manifestations) (Fig. 41-13).

Clinical Manifestations

Abdominal pain is the predominant symptom of acute pancreatitis. The pain is usually located in the left upper quadrant but may be in the mid-epigastrium. It commonly radiates to the back because of the retroperitoneal location of the pancreas. The pain has a sudden onset and is described as severe, deep, piercing, and continuous or steady. It is aggravated by eating and frequently has its onset when the patient is recumbent; it is not relieved by vomiting. The pain may be accompanied by flushing, cyanosis, and dyspnea. The patient may assume various positions involving flexion of the spine in an attempt to relieve the severe pain. The pain is due to distention of the pancreas, peritoneal irritation, and obstruction of the biliary tract.

Other manifestations of acute pancreatitis include nausea and vomiting, low-grade fever, leukocytosis, hypotension, tachycardia, and jaundice. Abdominal tenderness with muscle guarding is common. Bowel sounds may be decreased or absent. Ileus may occur and causes marked abdominal distention. The lungs are frequently involved, with crackles present. Intravascular damage from circulating trypsin may cause areas of cyanosis or greenish to yellow-brown discoloration of the abdominal wall. Other areas of ecchymoses are the flanks (Grey Turner's spots or sign, a bluish flank discoloration) and the periumbilical area (Cullen's sign, a bluish periumbilical discoloration). These result from seepage of blood-stained exudate from the pancreas and may occur in severe cases.

Shock may occur because of hemorrhage into the pancreas or toxemia from the activated pancreatic enzymes. The increased formation of kinin peptides (activated by trypsin), such as kallikrein and bradykinin, causes vasodilation, increased capillary permeability, and altered vasomotor tone. Hypovolemia also occurs as a result of exudation of blood and plasma proteins into the retroperitoneal space (massive fluid shifts).

Complications

Two significant local complications of acute pancreatitis are pseudocyst and abscess. A pancreatic pseudocyst is a cavity continuous with or surrounding the outside of the pancreas. The pseudocyst is filled with necrotic products and liquid secretions, such as plasma, pancreatic enzymes, and inflammatory exudates. As pancreatic enzymes escape from the pseudocyst, the serosal surfaces next to the pancreas become inflamed, with subsequent formation of granulation tissue leading to encapsulation of the exudate. Symptoms of pseudocyst are abdominal pain, palpable epigastric mass, nausea, vomiting, and anorexia. The serum amylase level frequently remains elevated. These cysts usually resolve spontaneously within a few weeks but may perforate, causing peritonitis, or rupture into the stomach or duodenum. Treatment consists of an internal drainage procedure with a Roux-en-Y anastomosis between the pancreatic duct and the jejunum.

A pancreatic abscess is a large fluid-containing cavity within the pancreas. It results from extensive necrosis in the pancreas. It may become infected or perforate into adjacent organs. Manifestations of an abscess include upper abdominal pain, abdominal mass, high fever, and leukocytosis. Pancreatic abscesses require prompt surgical drainage to prevent sepsis.

The main systemic complications of acute pancreatitis are pulmonary complications (pleural effusion, atelectasis, and pneumonia) and tetany caused by hypocalcemia. The pulmonary complications are probably caused by the passage of the exudate containing pancreatic enzymes from the peritoneal cavity through transdiaphragmatic lymph channels. When hypocalcemia occurs, it is a sign of severe disease. It is due in part to the combining of calcium and fatty acids during fat necrosis. The exact mechanisms of how or why hypocalcemia occurs are not well understood.

Diagnostic Studies

The primary diagnostic tests for acute pancreatitis are serum amylase (pancreatic isoamylase) and lipase and urinary amylase levels (Table 41-19). The serum amylase level is the criterion most commonly used. It may elevate to levels greater than 200 U/L (3.34 μkat/L). The serum amylase is usually elevated early and remains elevated for 24 to 72 hours.

The serum lipase is also elevated in acute pancreatitis and is a helpful complementary test because other disorders (e.g., mumps, cerebral trauma, renal transplantation) may also cause an increase in serum amylase.

There is an increase in urinary amylase, which may persist several days beyond the elevation of serum amylase. Urinary amylase may be increased to more than 3600 U per day. Normally a timed collection (e.g., a 2-hour collection) is a more dependable measure than a randomly collected urinary specimen.

The renal amylase-creatinine clearance test estimates the amount of blood cleared of amylase by the kidney per minute. The finding that the renal clearance of amylase is higher than the creatinine clearance in acute pancreatitis has led to the suggestion that the amylase-creatinine clearance ratio is a more specific test than urinary amylase levels alone.

Other laboratory abnormalities include hyperglycemia, hyperlipidemia, and hypocalcemia (see Table 41-19). There is a high incidence of hyperlipidemia with recurrent pancreatitis.

DIAGNOSTIC STUDIES

Table 41-19 Acute Pancreatitis

Laboratory Test	Abnormal Finding	Etiology
Primary Tests		
Serum amylase	Increased (>200 U/L [3.34 μkat/L])	Pancreatic cell injury
Serum lipase	Elevated	Pancreatic cell injury
Urinary amylase	Elevated	Pancreatic cell injury
Secondary Tests		
Blood glucose	Hyperglycemia	Impairment of carbohydrate metabolism due to β-cell damage and release of glucagon
Serum calcium	Hypocalcemia	Saponification of calcium by fatty acids in areas of fat necrosis
Serum triglycerides	Hyperlipidemia	Release of free fatty acids by lipase

ERCP is the definitive diagnostic test for gallstones, pancreatic cysts, and abscesses. A combination of laboratory studies and ERCP is usually used to help make the diagnosis. Abdominal x-ray and ultrasound scan of the pancreas may also be performed.

Collaborative Care

Objectives of collaborative care for acute pancreatitis include (1) relief of pain; (2) prevention or alleviation of shock; (3) reduction of pancreatic secretions; (4) control of fluid and electrolyte imbalance; (5) prevention or treatment of infections; and (6) removal of the precipitating cause, if possible (Table 41-20).

Conservative Therapy. A primary consideration in the treatment of acute pancreatitis is the relief and control of pain. Meperidine (Demerol) is preferred because it causes less spasm of the smooth muscles of the ducts than morphine. It may be combined with an antispasmodic. However, atropine-like drugs should be avoided when paralytic ileus is present because they may contribute to the problem. Other medications that relax smooth muscles (spasmolytics), such as nitroglycerin or papaverine, may be used.

If shock is present, blood volume replacements are used. Plasma or plasma volume expanders such as dextran or albumin may be given. Fluid and electrolyte imbalances are corrected with lactated Ringer's solution or other electrolyte solutions. Central venous pressure readings may be used to assist in determination of fluid-replacement requirements.

It is important to reduce or suppress pancreatic enzymes to decrease stimulation of the pancreas and allow it to rest. This is accomplished in several ways. First, the patient is allowed to take nothing by mouth (NPO). Second, NG suction may be used to reduce vomiting and gastric distention and to prevent gastric acidic contents from entering the duodenum. These measures suppress pancreatic secretion. Certain drugs may also be used for this purpose (Table 41-21).

COLLABORATIVE CARE

Table 41-20 Acute Pancreatitis

Diagnostic
- Serum amylase
- Serum lipase
- 2-hour urinary amylase and renal amylase clearance
- Blood glucose
- Serum calcium
- Triglycerides
- Flat plate of the abdomen
- Pancreatic ultrasound scan
- CT scan of the pancreas
- ERCP

Collaborative Therapy
- Meperidine
- NPO with NG tube to suction
- Cimetidine (Tagamet) or ranitidine (Zantac) IV
- Albumin (if shock present)
- IV calcium gluconate (10%) (if tetany present)
- Lactated Ringer's solution

CT, computed tomography; *ERCP,* endoscopic retrograde cholangiopancreatography; *NPO,* nothing by mouth.

The inflamed and necrotic pancreatic tissue is a good medium for bacterial growth. Therefore it is important to prevent infections. There is some controversy about the prophylactic use of antibiotics. It is important to monitor the patient closely so that antibiotic therapy can be instituted early if infection occurs.

Peritoneal lavage or dialysis has been used to remove the kinin and phospholipase A–containing exudate from the peritoneal cavity. This has proved beneficial in some cases of severe acute pancreatitis. It prevents early death but has little effect on overall mortality rate. Endoscopic papillotomy may be used to remove an impacted gallstone from the common bile duct when the pancreatitis is due to the stone.

Surgical Therapy. Surgical intervention may be indicated when the diagnosis is uncertain and in patients who do not respond to conservative therapy. Surgery is necessary for an abscess, acute pseudocyst, and severe peritonitis. Percutaneous drainage of a pseudocyst can be performed, and a drainage tube is left in place. Surgical treatment of associated biliary tract disease may be necessary.

Drug Therapy. Several different drugs may be used in the treatment of both acute and chronic pancreatitis (see Table 41-21). A number of drugs are used in an effort to suppress pancreatic secretion, but these drugs have not proved effective in the management of pancreatitis.

Nutritional Therapy. Initially the patient with acute pancreatitis is on NPO status to reduce pancreatic secretion. When food is allowed, small, frequent feedings are given. The

DRUG THERAPY

Table 41-21 Acute and Chronic Pancreatitis

Drug	Mechanisms of Action
Acute Pancreatitis	
Meperidine (Demerol)	Relief of pain
Nitroglycerin or papaverine	Relaxation of smooth muscles and relief of pain
Antispasmodics (e.g., dicyclomine [Bentyl], propantheline bromide [Pro-Banthine])	Decrease of vagal stimulation, motility, pancreatic outflow (inhibition of volume and concentration of bicarbonate and enzymatic secretion); contraindicated in paralytic ileus
Carbonic anhydrase inhibitor (acetazolamide [Diamox])	Reduction in volume and bicarbonate concentration of pancreatic secretion
Antacids	Neutralization of gastric secretions; decrease in hydrochloric acid stimulation of secretin, which stimulates production and secretion of pancreatic secretions
Histamine H_2-receptor antagonists (cimetidine [Tagamet], ranitidine [Zantac])	Decrease in hydrochloric acid by inhibiting histamine (hydrochloric acid stimulates pancreatic activity)
Calcium gluconate	Treatment of hypocalcemia to prevent or treat tetany
Corticosteroids	Use only for seriously ill patients with hypotension or shock
Aprotinin (Trasylol)	Antitryptic and antikallikreinic actions
Glucagon	Reduction in pancreatic inflammation and decrease in serum amylase, suppression of pancreatic secretions
Somatostatin	Inhibition of pancreatic secretions
Chronic Pancreatitis	
Pancreatin (Viokase), pancrelipase (Cotazym)	Replacement therapy for pancreatic enzymes
Insulin	Treatment for diabetes mellitus if it occurs or for hyperglycemia

diet is usually high in carbohydrate content because that is the least stimulating to the exocrine portion of the pancreas. The diet combines high carbohydrate intake with low fat and high protein intake. It is bland, with no stimulants (e.g., caffeine) or alcohol. Supplemental fat-soluble vitamins may be given. The patient may require supplemental commercial liquid preparations. If severe nutritional deficiencies exist, total parenteral nutrition (TPN) may be used (see Chapter 38).

NURSING MANAGEMENT: ACUTE PANCREATITIS

■ Nursing Assessment

Subjective and objective data that should be obtained from a person with acute pancreatitis are presented in Table 41-22.

■ Nursing Diagnoses

Nursing diagnoses for the patient with acute pancreatitis may include, but are not limited to, those presented in NCP 41-3.

■ Planning

The overall goals are that the patient with acute pancreatitis will have (1) relief of pain, (2) return of fluid and electrolyte balance, (3) minimal to no complications, and (4) no recurrent attacks.

■ Nursing Implementation

Health Promotion. The major factors involved in health promotion are assessment of the patient for predisposing and etiologic factors of pancreatitis and encouragement of early treatment of these factors to prevent occurrence of acute pancreatitis. The nurse should encourage the early diagnosis and treatment of biliary tract disease, such as cholelithiasis. The patient should be encouraged to eliminate alcohol intake, especially if there have been any previous episodes of pancreatitis. Attacks of pancreatitis become milder or disappear with the discontinuance of alcohol use.

Acute Intervention. During the acute phase, it is important to monitor vital signs. Hemodynamic stability may be compromised by hypotension, fever, and tachypnea, which may result in fluid volume deficit. IV fluids are ordered and the response to therapy is monitored. A vital part of the nursing care plan for this patient is observation for electrolyte imbalances. Frequent vomiting, along with gastric suction, may result in decreased chloride, sodium, and potassium levels.

Respiratory failure may develop in the patient with severe acute pancreatitis. It is important that respiratory function be assessed (e.g., lung sounds). If acute respiratory distress syndrome develops, the patient may require intubation and mechanical ventilatory support.

Because hypocalcemia can also occur, the nurse must observe for symptoms of tetany, such as jerking, irritability, and muscular twitching. Numbness or tingling around the lips and in the fingers is an early indicator of hypocalcemia. The patient should be assessed for a positive Chvostek's or Trousseau's sign (see Chapter 15). Calcium gluconate as ordered should be given to treat symptomatic hypocalcemia. In addition, hypomagnesemia may develop, necessitating the observation of serum magnesium levels.

Because abdominal pain is a prominent symptom of pancreatitis, a major focus of nursing care is the relief of pain (see NCP 41-3). Giving the prescribed medications before the

NURSING ASSESSMENT

Table 41-22 Acute Pancreatitis

Subjective Data	Objective Data
Important Health Information *Past health history:* Biliary tract disease, abdominal trauma, duodenal ulcers, infection, metabolic disorders *Medications:* Use of thiazides, estrogens, corticosteroids, azathioprine, sulfonamides, nonsteroidal antiinflammatory agents *Surgery and other treatments:* Surgical procedures on the pancreas, stomach, duodenum, or biliary tract; endoscopic retrograde cholangiopancreatography **Functional Health Patterns** *Health perception–health management:* Alcohol abuse; weakness *Nutritional-metabolic:* Nausea and vomiting; anorexia *Activity-exercise:* Dyspnea *Cognitive-perceptual:* Severe midepigastric or left upper quadrant pain that may radiate to the back, aggravated by food and alcohol intake and unrelieved by vomiting	**General** Restlessness, anxiety, low-grade fever **Integumentary** Flushing, diaphoresis, discoloration of abdomen and flanks, cyanosis, jaundice; decreased skin turgor, dry mucous membranes **Respiratory** Tachypnea, basilar crackles **Cardiovascular** Tachycardia, hypotension **Gastrointestinal** Abdominal distention, tenderness, and muscle guarding; diminished bowel sounds **Possible Findings** Elevated serum amylase and lipase, leukocytosis, hyperglycemia, elevated urine amylase, hyperlipidemia, hypocalcemia, abnormal ultrasound and CT scans of pancreas

pain becomes too severe makes the medication more effective. Meperidine (Demerol) or pentazocine (Talwin) may be used for pain relief because morphine may cause spasm of the sphincter of Oddi. The nurse should ascertain how long the pain medication provides relief. Measures such as comfortable positioning, frequent changes in position, and relief of nausea and vomiting assist in reducing the restlessness that usually accompanies the pain. Some patients experience lessened pain by assuming positions that flex the trunk and draw the knees up to the abdomen. A side-lying position with the head elevated 45 degrees decreases tension on the abdomen and may help ease the pain. It is important to control the pain and restlessness because they increase body metabolism and subsequent stimulation of pancreatic secretions.

Nursing measures for the patient who is on NPO status or has an NG tube should be employed. Frequent oral and nasal care to relieve the dryness of the mouth and nose is comforting to the patient. Oral care is essential to prevent parotitis. If the patient is taking anticholinergics to decrease GI secretions, there will be additional dryness of the mouth caused by the side effects of the drug. If the patient is taking antacids to suppress secretions, they should be sipped slowly or inserted in the NG tube. The nurse must regularly assess the functioning of the suction.

The patient with acute pancreatitis is susceptible to infections. The nurse should observe for fever and other manifestations of infection. Respiratory infections are common because the retroperitoneal fluid raises the diaphragm, which causes the patient to take shallow, guarded abdominal breaths. Measures to prevent respiratory infections include turning, coughing, deep breathing, and assuming a semi-Fowler's position.

Other important assessments are observation for signs of paralytic ileus, renal failure, and mental changes. Determination of the blood glucose level should be done to assess damage to the β-cells of the islets of Langerhans in the pancreas.

After pancreatic surgery the patient may require special wound care for an anastomotic leak or a fistula. Measures to prevent skin irritation should be used. These include skin barriers such as Stomahesive, karaya paste, or Colley-Seel; pouching; and drains. In addition to protecting the skin, pouching also provides a more accurate determination of fluid and electrolyte losses and increases patient comfort. Sterile pouching systems are available. The nurse may want to consult with a clinical specialist or an enterostomal therapist, if available.

Ambulatory and Home Care. After acute pancreatitis most patients will need home care follow-up. The patient may have lost physical reserve and muscle strength. Physical therapy may be needed. Continued care to prevent infection and detect any complications is important. Because frequent doses of narcotics may be required for this patient during the acute stage, follow-up for assessment of possible narcotic addiction may be indicated. This is a more likely problem with chronic pancreatitis than in the patient with acute pancreatitis. Counseling regarding abstinence from alcohol is important to prevent the patient from experiencing future attacks of acute pancreatitis and development of chronic pancreatitis. Beverages with caffeine should not be consumed. Because smoking and stressful situations can overstimulate the pancreas, they should be avoided.

Dietary teaching should include restriction of fats because they stimulate the secretion of cholecystokinin, which then stimulates the pancreas. Carbohydrates are less stimulating to the pancreas, so they should be encouraged. The patient should be instructed to avoid crash dieting and bingeing because these can precipitate attacks.

Early detection makes it possible to correct neurologic changes by treating the cause before overt psychotic behavior is manifested. Possible causes of neurologic changes include sepsis, anorexia, toxicity from cellular breakdown products, and withdrawal from alcohol.

41-3 NURSING CARE PLAN PATIENT WITH ACUTE PANCREATITIS

Expected Patient Outcomes	Nursing Interventions and *Rationales*
NURSING DIAGNOSIS	**Pain** *related to* inflammation of pancreas, peritoneal irritation, and ineffective pain and comfort measures *as manifested by* communication of pain descriptors, guarding behavior, behaviors indicative of pain (e.g., moaning), diaphoresis, changes in blood pressure, pulse, and respiratory rate.
▪ Minimal to no pain.	▪ Assess degree and nature of pain *to plan appropriate interventions.* ▪ Give ordered analgesic and antispasmodic medications before pain becomes severe *to ensure more effective relief of pain.* ▪ Ascertain how long the medication provides relief *to adjust pain medication administration in order to provide ongoing relief of pain.* ▪ Provide comfort measures, such as positioning patient comfortably with frequent changes in position, and diversional activities *to assist in reducing the restlessness that usually accompanies the pain and to demonstrate caring behaviors by the nurse.*
NURSING DIAGNOSIS	**Fluid volume deficit** *related to* nausea, vomiting, nasogastric suction, and restricted oral intake *as manifested by* thirst, increased fluid output, altered intake, dry skin and mucous membranes, decreased skin turgor, decreased oral intake.
▪ Adequate intake of fluids and electrolytes as evidenced by normal skin turgor. ▪ Moist mucous membranes. ▪ Stable weight. ▪ Normal serum electrolyte levels.	▪ Give antiemetics as ordered *to reduce fluid loss by preventing vomiting.* ▪ Measure and describe emesis *as indicators of replacement needs and effectiveness of treatment.* ▪ Observe for manifestations of metabolic alkalosis such as confusion, irritability, tachycardia, nausea, vomiting, muscle cramps, and tetany due to loss of chloride, sodium, and potassium with severe vomiting *so appropriate replacements can be started promptly.*
NURSING DIAGNOSIS	**Altered nutrition: less than body requirements** *related to* anorexia, dietary restrictions, nausea, loss of nutrients from vomiting, and impaired digestion *as manifested by* weight loss, weakness, fatigue, weight below normal for height and age.
▪ Weight appropriate for height. ▪ No further weight loss.	▪ Monitor weight and laboratory values *as indicators of patient's response to treatment.* ▪ Observe stools for steatorrhea, *which may develop from incomplete digestion of fats.* ▪ Administer total parenteral nutrition if ordered *to provide carbohydrates and amino acids to prevent negative nitrogen balance.* ▪ Implement measures to reduce pain and nausea *to increase patient's desire to eat.* ▪ Provide oral care before and after meals *to decrease foul taste and odor that inhibit appetite.* ▪ If oral intake is allowed, provide small portions of high-carbohydrate, low-protein, low-fat foods.
NURSING DIAGNOSIS	**Ineffective management of therapeutic regimen** *related to* lack of knowledge of preventive measures, diet restrictions, restriction of alcohol intake, and follow-up care *as manifested by* verbalization of the problem, request for information, inaccurate follow-through on instructions.
▪ Verbalization of understanding of condition or disease process and treatment. ▪ Initiation of lifestyle changes. ▪ Participation in treatment regimen.	▪ Teach patient to (1) abstain from alcohol *to prevent the patient from experiencing future attacks of acute pancreatitis and development of chronic pancreatitis;* (2) restrict fats and avoid rich, rough, and stimulating foods *to decrease stimulation of the pancreas and allow it to rest;* (3) use more carbohydrates in diet *because these are less stimulating to pancreas;* and (4) correctly measure blood glucose levels and observe for steatorrhea *because high blood glucose and fatty stools indicate destruction of pancreatic tissue.* ▪ Assess patient's understanding of prescribed regimen; provide details on follow-up care *to increase likelihood of successful convalescence and to minimize the possibility of recurrence.* ▪ Suggest follow-up if alcohol use is problematic *because continued use of alcohol will result in additional attacks of acute pancreatitis and eventual chronic pancreatitis.*

Continued

41-3 NURSING CARE PLAN PATIENT WITH ACUTE PANCREATITIS—continued

Expected Patient Outcomes	Nursing Interventions and *Rationales*

COLLABORATIVE PROBLEMS

Nursing Goals	Nursing Interventions and *Rationales*
POTENTIAL COMPLICATION	**Fluid and electrolyte imbalance** *related to* loss of fluids into peritoneal cavity.
▪ Monitor for signs of hypokalemia, hyponatremia, hypocalcemia, and hypochloremia. ▪ Report deviations from acceptable parameters. ▪ Carry out medical and nursing interventions.	▪ Observe for signs of fluid and electrolyte imbalance such as confusion, anorexia, diarrhea, seizures, muscle weakness, paralytic ileus, arrhythmias, metabolic alkalosis, muscle cramps, mental changes, tetany; monitor serum laboratory reports *to aid in early detection and prompt intervention.* ▪ Give calcium gluconate as ordered *to treat symptomatic hypocalcemia.*
POTENTIAL COMPLICATION	**Hemorrhagic shock** *related to* destruction of blood vessel walls by proteolytic enzymes.
▪ Monitor for signs of hemorrhagic shock. ▪ Report deviations from acceptable parameters. ▪ Carry out appropriate medical and nursing interventions.	▪ Assess for continuing or increasing signs of shock such as pallor; cool, clammy skin; hypotension; tachycardia; increased respirations *to ensure prompt detection and intervention.* ▪ Monitor vital signs every 1-2 hr *to evaluate patient's response to treatment.* ▪ Assess hourly for decreased urinary output *as an indicator of circulating blood volume and renal perfusion.*

The patient and the family should be given instructions regarding the recognition and reporting of symptoms of infection, diabetes mellitus, or steatorrhea (foul-smelling, frothy stools). These changes indicate possible destruction of pancreatic tissue. The nurse should make sure the patient fully understands the prescribed regimen. Each aspect must be explained. The importance of taking the required medications and following the recommended diet should be stressed.

■ Evaluation

Expected outcomes for the patient with acute pancreatitis are presented in NCP 41-3.

CHRONIC PANCREATITIS

Etiology and Pathophysiology

Chronic pancreatitis is progressive destruction of the pancreas with fibrotic replacement of pancreatic tissue. Strictures and calcifications may also occur in the pancreas. There are several types of chronic pancreatitis, but they all have a common underlying pathophysiologic disorder. The two major types are chronic obstructive pancreatitis and chronic calcifying pancreatitis. Chronic pancreatitis may follow acute pancreatitis, but it may also occur in the absence of any history of an acute condition.

Chronic obstructive pancreatitis is associated with biliary disease. The most common cause is inflammation of the sphincter of Oddi associated with cholelithiasis. Cancer of the ampulla of Vater, duodenum, or pancreas can also cause this type of chronic pancreatitis.

In chronic calcifying pancreatitis there is inflammation and sclerosis, mainly in the head of the pancreas and around the pancreatic duct. This type of chronic pancreatitis is the most common form. It is also called alcohol-induced pancreatitis. Increases in heavy social drinking have produced a higher incidence in countries in which the disease was previously considered rare. In the United States chronic pancreatitis is found almost exclusively in alcoholics. As with cirrhosis there seems to be a metabolic abnormality that predisposes a person who drinks to the direct toxic effect of the alcohol on the pancreas.

In chronic calcifying pancreatitis the ducts are obstructed with protein precipitates. These precipitates block the pancreatic duct and eventually calcify. This is followed by fibrosis and glandular atrophy. Pseudocysts and abscesses commonly develop.

Clinical Manifestations

As with acute pancreatitis, a major manifestation of chronic pancreatitis is abdominal pain. The patient may have episodes of acute pain, but it usually is chronic (recurrent attacks at intervals of months or years). The attacks may become more and more frequent until they are almost constant, or they may diminish as the pancreatic fibrosis develops. The pain is located in the same areas as in acute pancreatitis but is usually described as a heavy, gnawing feeling or sometimes as burning and cramplike. The pain is not relieved with food or antacids.

Other clinical manifestations include symptoms of pancreatic insufficiency, including malabsorption with weight loss, constipation, mild jaundice with dark urine, steatorrhea, and diabetes mellitus. The steatorrhea may become severe, with voluminous, foul, fatty stools. Urine and stool may be frothy. Some abdominal tenderness may be present.

Diagnostic Studies

Laboratory findings in chronic pancreatitis include increased serum amylase (200 to 600 U/L [3.34 to 10.0 μkat/L]), increased serum bilirubin, and increased alkaline phosphatase levels. There is usually mild leukocytosis and an elevated sedimentation rate.

The secretin stimulation test is probably the most useful test in diagnosing chronic pancreatitis. Secretin is given IV, and gastric-duodenal secretions are collected with a double-lumen tube for separate gastric and duodenal aspiration. In chronic pancreatitis there is reduced volume of secretions and reduced bicarbonate concentration (less than 90 mEq/L). Normally, secretin stimulates the production of pancreatic fluid high in bicarbonate content.

Other abnormal diagnostic findings are hyperglycemia and fatty stools (steatorrhea) found in fecal fat determination. Neutral fat indicates maldigestion. Arteriography and x-rays may demonstrate fibrosis and calcification.

ERCP involves cannulation and visualization of the pancreatic and common bile ducts through a fiberoptic endoscope that is inserted into the esophagus and then into the duodenum. The common bile duct and the pancreatic duct are then cannulated. Contrast dye can be injected into the ducts for visualization. Changes in the pancreatic ductal system, such as gross dilation and microcysts, can be visualized through the use of ERCP.

Collaborative Care

When the patient with chronic pancreatitis is experiencing an acute attack, the therapy is identical to that for acute pancreatitis. At other times the focus is on prevention of further attacks, relief of pain, and control of pancreatic exocrine and endocrine insufficiency. It sometimes takes large, frequent doses of analgesics to relieve the pain.

Diet, pancreatic enzyme replacement, and control of the diabetes are measures used to control the pancreatic insufficiency. The diet is a bland, low-fat, high-carbohydrate, and high-protein diet. The patient does not tolerate fatty, rich, and stimulating foods, and these should be avoided to decrease pancreatic secretions and demands on the pancreas. Alcohol must be totally eliminated.

Antacids and anticholinergic drugs may be given to decrease hydrochloric acid, which stimulates pancreatic activity. Cimetidine (Tagamet) and ranitidine (Zantac), which block histamine receptors and thus decrease hydrochloric acid secretion, may be used for the same purpose. Pancreatic enzymes such as pancreatin (Viokase) and pancrelipase (Cotazym) contain amylase, lipase, and trypsin and are used to replace the deficient pancreatic enzymes. They are usually enteric coated to prevent their breakdown or inactivation by gastric acid. Bile salts are sometimes given to facilitate the absorption of the fat-soluble vitamins (A, D, E, and K) and prevent further fat loss. If diabetes develops, it is controlled with insulin or oral drugs.

Treatment of chronic pancreatitis sometimes requires surgery. When biliary disease is present or if obstruction or pseudocyst develops, surgery may be indicated. Operations performed are procedures to divert bile flow or relieve ductal obstruction. A choledochojejunostomy diverts bile around the ampulla of Vater, where there may be spasm or hypertrophy of the sphincter. In this procedure the common bile duct is anastomosed into the jejunum. If the pancreatic sphincter is fibrotic, a sphincterotomy enlarges it. Pancreatic drainage procedures relieve ductal obstruction. One type is the Roux-en-Y pancreatojejunostomy, in which the pancreatic duct is opened and an anastomosis is made with the jejunum.

NURSING MANAGEMENT: CHRONIC PANCREATITIS

Except during an acute episode, the focus of nursing management is on chronic care and health promotion. The patient should be instructed to take measures to prevent further attacks. Dietary control, along with consistency of other treatment measures, such as taking pancreatic enzymes, is essential. The pancreatic extracts are usually given with meals or can be given with a snack. The nurse should observe the patient's stools for steatorrhea to help determine the effectiveness of the enzymes. The patient and the family need instructions regarding observation of stools.

If diabetes has developed, the patient will need instruction regarding testing of blood glucose levels and medications (see Chapter 46). The patient who is taking liquid antacids should be instructed to sip the medication slowly, and the nurse should make certain it is taken as ordered to help control gastric acidity. Antacids should be taken after meals. Both the antacid and the pancreatic enzymes may be left at the bedside to prepare the patient for self-management at home.

Alcohol must be avoided, and the patient may need assistance with this problem. If the patient has developed a dependence on alcohol or narcotics, referral to other agencies or resources may be necessary (see Chapter 10).

CARCINOMA OF THE PANCREAS

In the United States more than 29,000 people are diagnosed with cancer of the pancreas each year.[23] It is the fifth leading cause of death from cancer. It is more common in men and more common in African-Americans than Caucasians. The risk increases with age, with the peak incidence occurring between 65 and 80 years of age.[24]

Most of the tumors are adenocarcinomas originating from the epithelium of the ductal system. More than half the tumors occur in the head of the pancreas. As the tumor grows, the common bile duct becomes obstructed and obstructive jaundice develops. Tumors starting in the body or tail often remain silent until their growth is advanced. The majority of cancers have metastasized at the time of diagnosis. The signs and symptoms of pancreatic cancer are often similar to chronic pancreatitis. The prognosis of a patient with cancer of the pancreas is poor. Most patients die within 5 to 12 months of the initial diagnosis, and the 5-year survival rate is only about 10%.[25] The prognosis is related to the location of the tumor.

Etiology and Pathophysiology

The cause of cancer of the pancreas remains unknown. There may be some relationship between cancer, diabetes mellitus, and chronic pancreatitis. However, it is not clear whether the cancer follows these diseases or whether these diseases occur as a result of pancreatic cancer. It is known that pancreatic cancer can be induced with chemicals such as nitrosoureas. Major risk factors seem to be cigarette smoking, high-fat diet, diabetes, and exposure to chemicals such as benzidine and coke. The most firmly established risk factor is cigarette smoking. Pancreatic cancer develops twice as frequently in persons with a history of heavy cigarette use (more than two packs a day) than in nonsmokers. The carcinogens from the tobacco probably reach the pancreatic ducts by bile reflux or via the bloodstream. Another risk factor is the Western diet, particularly the high fat content. High consumption of meat has also been implicated. Methods of processing foodstuffs may also be involved as a possible risk factor for cancer of the pancreas.

Clinical Manifestations

Common manifestations of pancreatic cancer include abdominal pain (dull, aching), anorexia, rapid and progressive weight loss, nausea, and jaundice. Pain is common and is related to the location of malignancy. Extreme, unrelenting pain is related to extension of the cancer into the retroperitoneal tissues and nerve plexuses. The pain is frequently located in the upper abdomen or left hypochondrium and frequently radiates to the back. It is commonly related to eating, and it also occurs at night. Weight loss is due to poor digestion and absorption caused by lack of digestive juices from the pancreas.

Diagnostic Studies

Better diagnostic measures are needed for detection of pancreatic cancer because most of the current methods detect only advanced stages. Cytologic examination of the pancreatic juice may reveal malignant cells. The secretin test frequently indicates a decreased volume of pancreatic juice with normal bicarbonate and enzyme production. Carcinoembryonic antigen (CEA) is elevated in a high percentage of patients with advanced disease, but it is also increased with other types of cancers and even some benign conditions. The CEA plasma level is therefore probably more useful in assessing the patient's response to treatment than in diagnosis. CA19-9 is a more specific tumor marker because it is associated with pancreatic cancer in particular.

Ultrasonography detects abnormalities of the pancreas but cannot distinguish cancer from other pancreatic disorders such as pancreatitis. Since this is a noninvasive procedure, it may be used in some situations. Computed tomography scans are effective in identifying a solid tumor mass and changes such as lymph node spread. Pancreatic arteriography demonstrates occlusion of the celiac axis and the superior mesenteric artery.

With ERCP it is possible to get excellent x-ray visualization of the pancreatic ducts. In pancreatic cancer, findings include obstruction or narrowing of a major duct and, frequently, saccular dilations of smaller peripheral ducts. Material for cytology and biopsy may show malignant cells. ERCP is usually considered to be the best diagnostic test.

Collaborative Care

Surgery provides the most effective treatment of cancer of the pancreas. The classic surgery is a radical pancreaticoduodenectomy, or Whipple's procedure (Fig. 41-14). This entails resection of the proximal pancreas (proximal pancreatectomy), the adjoining duodenum (duodenectomy), the distal portion of the stomach (partial gastrectomy), and the distal segment of the common bile duct. An anastomosis of the pancreatic duct, common bile duct, and stomach to the jejunum is done. A total pancreatectomy is performed in some institutions for cancers of the head of the pancreas. Sometimes a simple bypass procedure, such as a cholecystojejunostomy to relieve biliary obstruction, may be used as a palliative measure. Some surgeons suggest a more radical resection, such as a total pancreaticoduodenectomy with splenectomy. Biliary stents (e.g., Cotton-Leung stent) can be used as a palliative measure when tumors compress the bile duct.

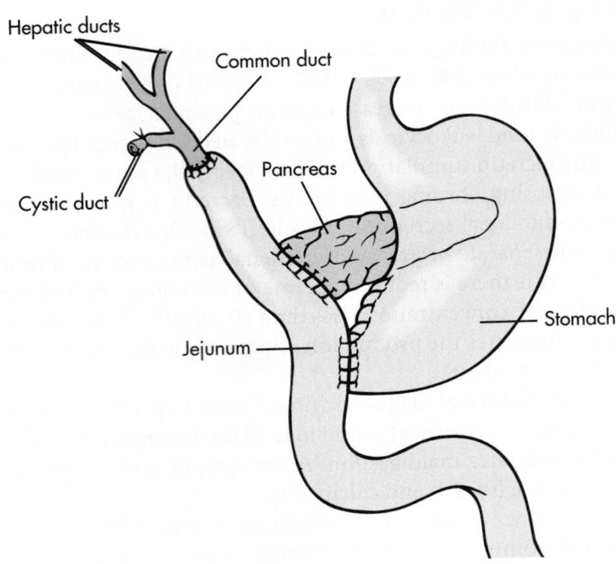

Fig. 41-14 Whipple procedure or radical pancreaticoduodenectomy. This surgical procedure involves resection of the proximal pancreas, adjoining duodenum, distal portion of the stomach, and distal portion of the common bile duct. An anastomosis of the pancreatic duct, common bile duct, and stomach to the jejunum is done.

Radiation therapy alters survival rates little but is effective for pain relief. External radiation is usually used, but implantation of internal radiation seeds into the tumor has also been used. Chemotherapy has limited success. Combinations of drugs such as 5-FU and carmustine (BCNU) produce a better response than single chemotherapeutic agents. Gemcitabine (Gemzar) is used in advanced pancreatic cancer. Biologic therapy is sometimes attempted (see Chapter 14). Adjuvant therapy, which uses surgical resection, radiation, and chemotherapy, is believed by some to be the most effective way to manage the almost always fatal cancer of the pancreas.

NURSING MANAGEMENT: CARCINOMA OF THE PANCREAS

Because the patient with carcinoma of the pancreas has many of the same problems as the patient with pancreatitis, nursing care includes the same measures (see NCP 41-3). The nurse should provide symptomatic and supportive nursing care. Medications and comfort measures to relieve pain should be provided before the patient reaches the peak of pain. Psycho-

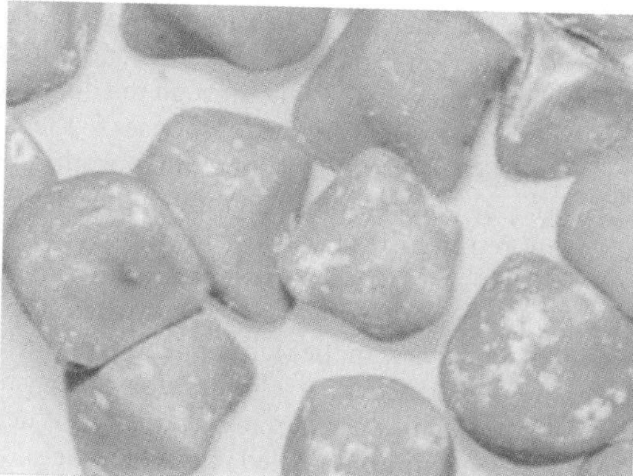

Fig. 41-15 Gallstones.

logic support is essential, especially during times of anxiety or depression, which seem to occur frequently in these patients.

Adequate nutrition is an important part of the nursing care plan. Frequent and supplemental feedings may be necessary. Measures to stimulate the appetite as much as possible and to overcome anorexia, nausea, and vomiting should be included in the nursing care. Because bleeding can result from impaired vitamin K production, the nurse should assess for bleeding from body orifices and mucous membranes. If the patient is undergoing radiation therapy, the nurse must observe for adverse reactions, such as anorexia, nausea, vomiting, and skin irritation.

The prognosis for a patient with pancreatic cancer is not good. A significant component of the nursing care is helping the patient and the family or significant others through the grieving process.

DISORDERS OF THE BILIARY TRACT

The most common disorder of the biliary system is cholelithiasis (stones in the gallbladder) (Figs. 41-15 and 41-16). Cholecystitis (inflammation of the gallbladder) is usually associated with cholelithiasis. The stones may be lodged in the neck of the gallbladder or in the cystic duct. Cholecystitis may be acute or chronic. These conditions usually occur together.

Gallbladder disease is a common health problem in the United States. It is estimated that 8% to 10% of the adults in the United States have cholelithiasis. The actual number is not known because many persons are asymptomatic with stones. Cholecystectomy (removal of the gallbladder) ranks among the most common surgical procedures performed in the United States. The incidence of cholelithiasis is higher in women, multiparous women, and persons over 40 years of age. Postmenopausal women on estrogen therapy are at somewhat greater risk of having gallbladder disease than are women who are taking birth control pills. Oral contraceptives alter the character of bile, resulting in increased cholesterol saturation. Other factors that seem to increase the occurrence of gallbladder disease are a sedentary lifestyle, a familial tendency, and obesity. Obesity causes increased secretion of cholesterol in bile. Gallbladder disease is more common in Caucasians than in Asians and African-Americans. There is an especially high incidence in

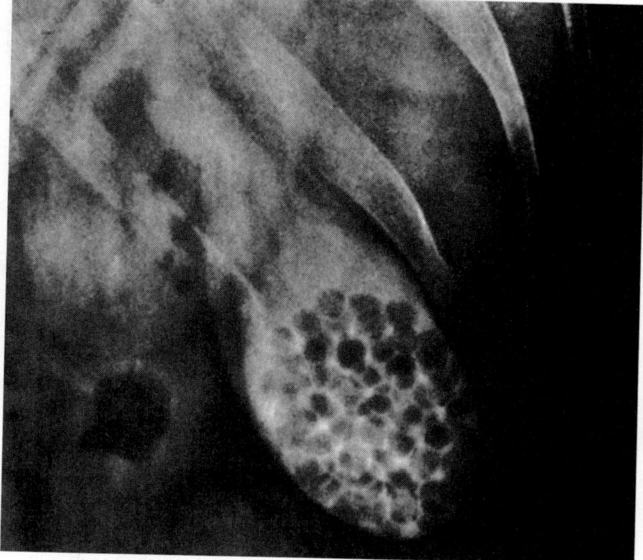

Fig. 41-16 X-ray of a gallbladder with gallstones.

the Native-American population, particularly in the Navajo and Pima tribes.

Etiology and Pathophysiology

Cholecystitis. Cholecystitis is most commonly associated with stones. When it occurs in the absence of stones, it is thought to be caused by bacteria reaching the gallbladder via the vascular or lymphatic route or chemical irritants in the bile. *Escherichia coli* is the most common bacterium involved. Streptococci and salmonellae are also common causative bacteria. Other etiologic factors include adhesions, neoplasms, extensive fasting, frequent weight fluctuations, anesthesia, and narcotics.

Inflammation is the major pathophysiologic condition and may be confined to the mucous lining or involve the entire wall of the gallbladder. During an acute attack of cholecystitis the gallbladder is edematous and hyperemic. It may be distended with bile or pus. The cystic duct is also involved and may become occluded. The wall of the gallbladder becomes scarred after an acute attack. Decreased functioning occurs if large amounts of tissue are fibrosed.

Cholelithiasis. The actual cause of gallstones is unknown. Basically, cholelithiasis develops when the balance that keeps cholesterol, bile salts, and calcium in solution is altered so that precipitation of these substances occurs. Conditions that upset this balance include infection and disturbances in the metabolism of cholesterol.

It is known that in patients with cholelithiasis the bile secreted by the liver is supersaturated with cholesterol (lithogenic bile). The bile in the gallbladder also becomes supersaturated with cholesterol. Whenever bile is supersaturated with cholesterol, precipitation of cholesterol will occur.

A high percentage of gallstones are precipitates of cholesterol. Other components of bile that precipitate into stones are bile salts, bilirubin, calcium, and protein. The stones sometimes have a mixed consistency. Mixed cholesterol stones, which are predominantly cholesterol, are the most common gallstones.

Table **41-23** Clinical Manifestations Caused by Obstructed Bile Flow

Clinical Manifestation	Etiology
Obstructive jaundice	No bile flow into duodenum
Dark amber urine, which foams when shaken	Soluble bilirubin in urine
No urobilinogen in urine	No bilirubin reaching small intestine to be converted to urobilinogen
Clay-colored stools	Same as above
Pruritus	Deposition of bile salts in skin tissues
Intolerance for fatty foods (nausea, sensation of fullness, anorexia)	No bile in small intestine for fat digestion
Bleeding tendencies	Lack of or decreased absorption of vitamin K, resulting in decreased production of prothrombin
Steatorrhea	No bile salts in duodenum, preventing fat emulsion and digestion

The changes in the composition of bile are probably significant in the formation of gallstones. Stasis of bile leads to progression of the supersaturation and changes in the chemical composition of the bile. Immobility, pregnancy, and inflammatory or obstructive lesions of the biliary system decrease bile flow. Hormonal factors during pregnancy may cause delayed emptying of the gallbladder.

The stones may remain in the gallbladder or migrate to the cystic duct or to the common bile duct. They cause pain as they pass through the ducts and may lodge in the ducts and produce an obstruction. Small stones are more likely to move into a duct and cause obstruction. Table 41-23 depicts the changes and manifestations that occur when the stones obstruct the common bile duct. If the blockage occurs in the cystic duct, the bile can continue to flow into the duodenum directly from the liver. When the bile in the gallbladder cannot escape, however, this stasis of bile may lead to cholecystitis.

Clinical Manifestations

Manifestations of cholecystitis vary from indigestion to moderate to severe pain, fever, and jaundice. Initial symptoms of acute cholecystitis include indigestion and pain and tenderness in the right upper quadrant, which may be referred to the right shoulder and scapula. The pain may be acute and be accompanied by nausea and vomiting, restlessness, and diaphoresis. Manifestations of inflammation, such as leukocytosis and fever, occur. Physical findings include right upper quadrant tenderness and abdominal rigidity. Symptoms of chronic cholecystitis include a history of fat intolerance, dyspepsia, heartburn, and flatulence.

Cholelithiasis may produce severe symptoms or none at all. Many patients have "silent cholelithiasis." The severity of symptoms depends on whether the stones are stationary or mobile and whether obstruction is present. When a stone is lodged in the ducts or when stones are moving through the ducts, spasms may result. The spasms are the tissues' responses to the stone in an attempt to move it forward. This sometimes produces severe pain, which is termed *biliary colic* even though the pain is rarely colicky; it is more often steady. The pain can be excruciating and accompanied by tachycardia, diaphoresis, and prostration. The severe pain may last up to an hour, and when it subsides there is residual tenderness in the right upper quadrant. The attacks of pain frequently occur 3 to 6 hours after a heavy meal or when the patient assumes a recumbent position. When total obstruction occurs, symptoms related to bile blockage are manifested (see Table 41-23).

Complications

Complications of cholecystitis include subphrenic abscess, pancreatitis, cholangitis (inflammation of biliary ducts), biliary cirrhosis, fistulas, and rupture of the gallbladder, which can produce bile peritonitis.

Many of the same complications can occur from cholelithiasis, including cholangitis, biliary cirrhosis, carcinoma, and peritonitis. Choledocholithiasis (stone in the common bile duct) may occur, producing symptoms of obstruction.

Diagnostic Studies

Ultrasonography is probably the best means of diagnosing gallstones (see Table 37-12). It is 90% to 95% accurate in detecting stones. It is especially useful for patients with jaundice (because it does not depend on liver function) and for patients who are allergic to contrast medium.

An oral cholecystogram allows for the detection of stones when they are radiopaque. An IV cholangiogram outlines both the gallbladder and the ducts, so gallstones that have moved into the ductal system can be detected. Percutaneous transhepatic cholangiography may be used to diagnose obstructive jaundice and to locate stones within the bile ducts. Bile taken during ERCP is sent for culture to identify any possible infecting organism.

Laboratory tests may demonstrate abnormalities in some of the liver function tests and an increased WBC count as a result of inflammation. Both the direct and indirect bilirubin levels are elevated, as is the urinary bilirubin level if there is an obstructive process present. If the common bile duct is obstructed, no bilirubin will reach the small intestine to be converted to urobilinogen. Serum enzymes, such as alkaline phosphatase and AST (SGOT), may be elevated. The serum amylase is increased if there is pancreatic involvement.

Collaborative Care

Conservative Therapy

Cholecystitis. During an acute episode of cholecystitis the focus of treatment is on control of pain, control of possible infection with antibiotics, and maintenance of fluid and electrolyte balance (Table 41-24). Treatment is mainly supportive and symptomatic. If nausea and vomiting are severe, gastric decompression may be used to prevent further gallbladder stimulation. Anticholinergics to decrease secretions (which prevents

COLLABORATIVE CARE

Table 41-24 Cholelithiasis

Diagnostic
- Ultrasound
- Cholecystogram or IV cholangiogram
- Liver function studies
- WBC count
- Serum bilirubin

Collaborative Therapy

Conservative Therapy
- IV fluid
- NPO with NG tube, later progressing to low-fat diet
- Antiemetics
- Analgesics (e.g., meperidine)
- Fat-soluble vitamins (A, D, E, and K)
- Anticholinergics (antispasmodics)
- Hydrocholetic drugs
  - Dehydrocholic acid (Decholin)
  - Florantyrone (Zanchol)
- Antibiotics
- ERCP with sphincterotomy (papillotomy)
- Cholesterol solvents
- Extracorporeal shock-wave lithotripsy

Dissolution Therapy
- Ursodeoxycholic acid (UDCA)
- Ursodiol (Actigall)
- Chenodeoxycholic acid (CDCA)

Surgical Therapy
- Laparoscopic cholecystectomy
- Incisional cholecystectomy
- See Table 41-25

biliary contraction) and counteract smooth muscle spasms may be administered. Analgesics are given to decrease the pain.

Cholelithiasis. There are currently several options for management of cholelithiasis. These include cholesterol solvents such as methyl tertiary terbutyl ether (MTBE), oral drugs that dissolve stones, endoscopic sphincterotomy, extracorporeal shock-wave lithotripsy (ESWL), and surgery. Supportive treatment, similar to that given for cholecystitis, may also be necessary. If the stones cause an obstruction, additional treatment consists of replacement of fat-soluble vitamins, administration of bile salts to facilitate digestion and vitamin absorption, and a low-fat diet.

A direct-contact dissolving agent such as MTBE can be instilled into the gallbladder via a percutaneous catheter. MTBE dissolves cholesterol stones within hours. The gallstones may recur. Oral bile acids are also used to dissolve stones.

Endoscopic sphincterotomy (papillotomy) is especially effective in removing common bile duct stones (Fig. 41-17). The endoscope is passed to the duodenum. With an electrodiathermy knife attached to the endoscope, the sphincter of Oddi is widened by incision of the sphincter muscle (sphincterotomy). A basket is used to retrieve the stone. The stone may be removed in the basket, but more commonly it is left in the duodenum and will be passed naturally in the stool.

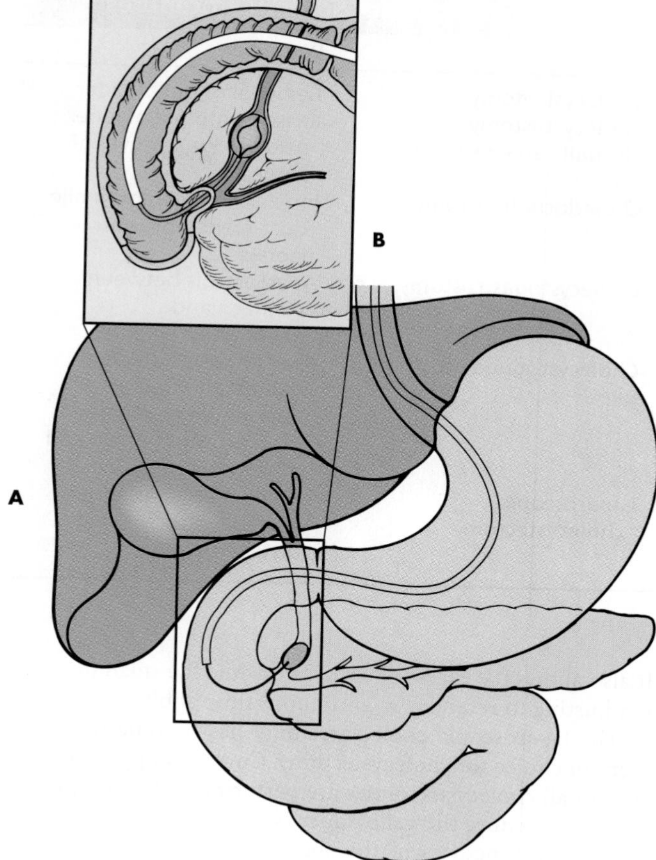

Fig. 41-17 **A,** During endoscopic sphincterotomy, a flexible endoscope is advanced through the mouth and stomach until its tip sits in the duodenum opposite the common bile duct. **B,** After widening the duct mouth by incising the sphincter muscle, the physician advances a basket attachment into the duct and snags the stone.

In ESWL a biliary lithotriptor uses high-energy shock waves to disintegrate gallstones. The patient must have a functioning gallbladder. An ultrasound scan is first done to locate the stones and to determine where to direct the shock waves. The shock waves are directed through the abdomen as a water-filled cushion is pressed against the area. It usually takes 1 to 2 hours to disintegrate the stones. After they are broken up, the fragments pass through the common bile duct and into the small intestine. There has been mixed success with ESWL.

Surgical Therapy. Surgical intervention for cholelithiasis is frequently indicated and may consist of any one of several procedures (Table 41-25). The procedure of choice for most patients is still a cholecystectomy. This is a safe procedure with minimal morbidity, and it requires only a brief hospitalization. One procedure is removal of the gallbladder through a right subcostal incision. A T-tube is inserted into the common bile duct during surgery when a common bile duct exploration is part of the surgical procedure (Fig. 41-18). This ensures patency of the duct until the edema produced by the trauma of exploring and probing the duct has subsided.

Table 41-25 Gallbladder Surgery Procedures

Name	Description
Cholecystectomy	Removal of gallbladder
Cholecystostomy (usually an emergency)	Incision into gallbladder (usually for removal of stones)
Choledocholithotomy	Incision into common bile duct for removal of stones
Cholecystogastrostomy	Anastomosis between stomach and gallbladder
Cholecystoduodenostomy	Anastomosis between gallbladder and duodenum to relieve obstruction at distal end of common bile duct
Laparoscopic cholecystectomy	Removal of gallbladder via laparoscopy using a dissecting laser

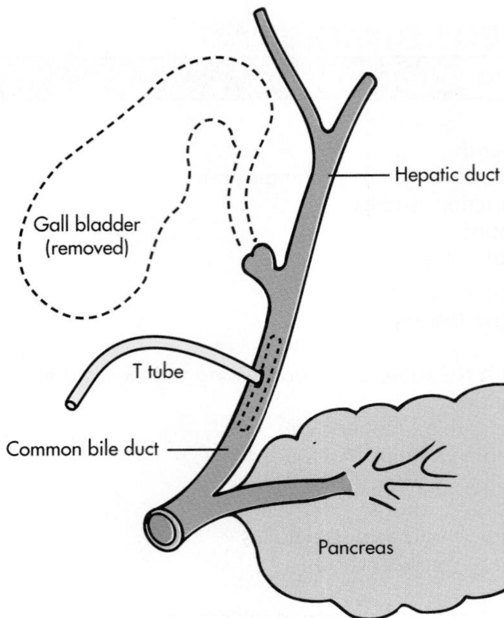

Fig. 41-18 Placement of T tube. Dotted lines indicate parts removed.

It also allows the excess bile to drain while the small intestine is adjusting to receiving a continuous flow of bile.

The laparoscopic cholecystectomy has become the treatment of choice for cholecystectomy. Currently approximately 90% of all cholecystectomies are performed laparoscopically. In this procedure the gallbladder is removed through one of four small punctures in the abdomen. A 1 cm puncture is made slightly above the umbilicus, and the surgeon inflates the abdominal cavity with 3 to 4 L of carbon dioxide to improve visibility. A laparoscope, which has a camera attached, is then inserted into the abdomen. Two additional punctures are made just below the ribs, one on the right anterior axillary line and the other on the right midclavicular line. These punctures are used for insertion of grasping forceps. A dissection laser is inserted into the fourth puncture, which is made just right of the midsection. (The incision sites may vary.) Using closed-circuit monitors to view the abdominal cavity, the surgeon retracts and dissects the gallbladder and removes it with grasping forceps.

This procedure is relatively minor with few complications. Most patients experience minimal postoperative pain and are discharged the day of surgery or the day after. In most cases they are able to resume normal activities and return to work after 2 or 3 days.

Advantages to the laparoscopic cholecystectomy include decreased postoperative pain, shorter hospital stay, and earlier return to work and full activity. The main complication is injury to the common bile duct. There are few contraindications to laparoscopic cholecystectomy. The primary ones are peritonitis, cholangitis, gangrene or perforation of the gallbladder, portal hypertension, and serious bleeding disorders.

Transhepatic Biliary Catheter. The transhepatic biliary catheter can be used preoperatively in biliary obstruction and in hepatic dysfunction secondary to obstructive jaundice. It can also be inserted when inoperable liver, pancreatic, or bile duct carcinoma obstructs bile flow. The catheter is inserted under fluoroscopy and involves percutaneous insertion across the liver parenchyma into the common bile duct and duodenum. It decompresses obstructed extrahepatic bile ducts so that bile can flow freely. After insertion, the catheter is connected to a drainage bag. The skin around the catheter insertion site has to be cleansed daily with an antiseptic. It is important to observe for bile leakage at the insertion site. Depending on the reason the catheter was inserted, the patient may be discharged with it in place.

Drug Therapy. The most common drugs used in the treatment of gallbladder disease are analgesics, anticholinergics (antispasmodics), fat-soluble vitamins, and bile salts. Meperidine (Demerol) is used if a narcotic analgesic is required. This causes less spasm in the ducts than opiates such as morphine sulfate. Anticholinergics such as atropine and other antispasmodics may be used to relax the smooth muscle and decrease ductal tone.

If the patient has chronic gallbladder disease or any biliary tract obstruction, fat-soluble vitamins (A, D, E, and K) will probably be given. Bile salts may be administered to facilitate digestion and vitamin absorption.

Hydrocholeretic drugs, which stimulate the production of bile with a low specific gravity, may be administered following gallbladder surgery when a T-tube is in place or with conservative therapy as long as there is no obstruction. These drugs stimulate the production of bile of a low specific gravity. Examples are bile salts such as dehydrocholic acid (Decholin) and florantyrone (Zanchol).

For treatment of pruritus, cholestyramine (Questran) may provide relief. This is a resin that binds bile salts in the intestine, increasing their excretion in the feces. Cholestyramine is administered in powder form and should be mixed with milk or

NURSING ASSESSMENT

Table 41-26 Cholecystitis or Cholelithiasis

Subjective Data	Objective Data
Important Health Information *Past health history:* Obesity, multiparity, infection, cancer, extensive fasting, pregnancy *Medications:* Use of estrogen or oral contraceptives *Surgery and other treatments:* Previous abdominal surgery **Functional Health Patterns** *Health perception–health management:* Positive family history; sedentary lifestyle *Nutritional-metabolic:* Weight loss, anorexia; indigestion, fat intolerance, nausea and vomiting, dyspepsia; chills *Elimination:* Clay-colored stools, steatorrhea, flatulence; dark urine *Cognitive-perceptual:* Moderate to severe pain in right upper quadrant that may radiate to the back or scapula; pruritus	**General** Fever, restlessness **Integumentary** Jaundice, icteric sclera; diaphoresis **Respiratory** Tachypnea, splinting during respirations **Cardiovascular** Tachycardia **Gastrointestinal** Palpable gallbladder, abdominal guarding and distention **Possible Findings** Elevated serum liver enzymes and bilirubin, absence of urobilinogen in urine, increased urinary bilirubin; leukocytosis, abnormal gallbladder ultrasound, positive oral cholecystogram or IV cholangiogram

juice. Side effects include nausea, vomiting, diarrhea or constipation, and skin reactions.

Medical dissolution therapy is recommended for patients with small radiolucent stones who are mildly symptomatic and are poor surgical risks. Ursodeoxycholic acid (UDCA), ursodiol (Actigall), and chenodeoxycholic acid (CDCA, chenodiol, Chenix) may be used to dissolve the stones. The main side effects of CDCA are cramps and diarrhea, but these are usually not severe. A more serious side effect is hepatotoxicity. UDCA has fewer side effects than CDCA. Dissolution therapy may take anywhere from 6 months to 2 years for dissolution of the stones, and low-dose therapy is recommended to prevent recurrence. Results are often better in nonobese patients. These drugs may be used after ESWL to prevent formation of other stones. The drugs to dissolve the gallstones are not used as much currently because of high use of laparoscopic cholecystectomy.

Nutritional Therapy. The major dietary modification for a patient with cholelithiasis and cholecystitis is a low-fat diet (see Table 32-5). If obesity is a problem, a reduced-calorie diet is indicated. The low-fat diet decreases stimulation of the gallbladder. Foods that are avoided include dairy products such as whole milk, cream, butter, whole milk cheese, and ice cream; fried foods; rich pastries; gravies; and nuts. Many patients have fewer problems if they eat smaller, more frequent meals.

After a laparoscopic cholecystectomy the patient is instructed to have liquids for the rest of the day and eat light meals for a few days. If an incisional cholecystectomy is done, the patient will progress from liquids to a bland diet once bowel sounds have returned. The amount of fat in the postoperative diet depends on the patient's tolerance of fat. A low-fat diet may be helpful if the flow of bile is reduced (usually only in the early postoperative period) or if the patient is overweight. Sometimes the patient is instructed to restrict fats for 4 to 6 weeks. Otherwise no special dietary instructions are needed other than to eat nutritious meals and avoid excessive fat intake.

NURSING MANAGEMENT: GALLBLADDER DISEASE

Nursing Assessment

Subjective and objective data that should be obtained from a person with gallbladder disease are presented in Table 41-26.

Nursing Diagnoses

Nursing diagnoses for the patient with gallbladder disease treated surgically include, but are not limited to, the following:

- Pain *related to* surgical procedure
- Ineffective management of therapeutic regimen *related to* lack of knowledge of diet and postoperative management

Planning

The overall goals are that the patient with gallbladder disease will have (1) relief of pain and discomfort, (2) no complications postoperatively, and (3) no recurrent attacks of cholecystitis or cholelithiasis.

Nursing Implementation

Health Promotion. The nurse should assume responsibility for recognition of predisposing factors of gallbladder disease in general health screening. Ethnic groups in which the disease is more common, such as Native-Americans, should be taught initial manifestations and instructed to seek medical care if these manifestations occur. The patient with chronic cholecystitis does not have acute symptoms and may not seek help until jaundice and biliary obstruction occur. Earlier detection in these patients is beneficial so that they can be treated with a low-fat diet and monitored more closely.

Acute Intervention. Nursing objectives for the patient undergoing conservative therapy include relieving pain, relieving nausea and vomiting, providing comfort and emotional support, maintaining fluid and electrolyte balance and nutrition, making accurate assessments for effectiveness of treatment, and observing for complications.

The patient with cholecystitis or cholelithiasis is frequently experiencing severe pain. The medications ordered to relieve the pain should be given as required by the patient and before the pain becomes more severe. The nurse should assess what medications relieve the pain and how much medication is required. Observations for side effects of the medications must be part of the continued assessment. Nursing comfort measures, such as a clean bed, comfortable positioning, and oral care, are appropriate.

Some patients have more severe nausea and vomiting than others. For these patients it may be necessary to use gastric decompression. The elimination of intake of food and fluids also prevents further stimulation of the gallbladder. Oral hygiene, care of nares, accurate intake and output measurements, and maintenance of suction should be a part of the nursing care plan for this patient. For patients with less severe nausea and vomiting, antiemetics are usually adequate. When the patient is vomiting, comfort measures such as frequent mouth rinses should be provided. Any vomitus should be immediately removed from the patient's view.

If pruritus occurs with jaundice, measures to relieve itching are necessary. Such measures include baking soda or Alpha Keri baths; lotions, such as those containing calamine; antihistamines; soft, old linen; and control of the temperature (not too hot and not too cold). The patient's nails should be kept short and clean. Patients should be taught to rub with their knuckles rather than scratch with their nails when they cannot resist scratching.

A significant portion of the nursing care plan for this patient centers on accurate assessment of progression of the symptoms and development of complications. The nurse must be knowledgeable of and observe for signs of obstruction of the ducts by stones. These include jaundice; clay-colored stools; dark, foamy urine; steatorrhea; fever; and increased WBC count.

When symptoms of obstruction are present (see Table 41-23), the nurse must be aware of the possibility of bleeding as a result of decreased prothrombin production. Common sites to observe for bleeding are the mucous membranes of the mouth, nose, gingivae, and injection sites. If injections are given, a small-gauge needle should be used and gentle pressure applied after the injection. The nurse should know what the patient's prothrombin time is and use this as a guide in the assessment process.

Assessment for infections includes monitoring of vital signs. A temperature elevation with chills and jaundice may indicate choledocholithiasis.

Nursing care of the patient after endoscopic papillotomy includes assessment to detect complications such as pancreatitis, perforation, infection, and bleeding. The patient's vital signs should be monitored. Abdominal pain and fever may indicate pancreatitis. The patient should be on bed rest for several hours and should have nothing by mouth until the gag reflex returns.

Postoperative care. Postoperative nursing care following a laparoscopic cholecystectomy includes monitoring for complications such as bleeding, making the patient comfortable, and preparing the patient for discharge. A common postoperative problem is referred pain to the shoulder because of the CO_2 that was not released or absorbed by the body. The CO_2 can irritate the phrenic nerve and the diaphragm, causing some difficulty breathing. Placing the patient in Sim's position (left side with right knee flexed) helps move the gas pocket away from the diaphragm. Deep breathing should be encouraged, along with movement and ambulation. There is usually minimal pain that can be relieved by narcotic analgesics such as oxycodone and acetaminophen with codeine. The patient is allowed clear liquids and can walk to the bathroom to void. Many patients go home the same day, but some will stay overnight.

Postoperative nursing care for incisional surgery (cholecystectomy) focuses on adequate ventilation and prevention of respiratory complications. Other nursing care is the same as general postoperative nursing care (see Chapter 18).

If the patient has a T-tube, part of the nursing care plan is related to maintaining bile drainage and observation of the T-tube functioning and drainage. The T-tube is connected to a closed gravity drainage system. If the Penrose or Jackson-Pratt drain or the T-tube is draining large amounts, it is helpful to use a sterile pouching system to protect the skin.

Ambulatory and Home Care. When the patient has conservative therapy, long-term nursing management depends on symptoms and on whether surgical intervention is being planned. Dietary teaching is usually necessary. The diet is usually low in fat, and sometimes a weight-reduction diet is also recommended. The patient may need to take fat-soluble vitamin supplements. The nurse should provide instructions regarding observations the patient should make indicating obstruction (stool and urine changes, jaundice, and pruritus). Continued health care is important, and its significance should be explained and stressed.

The patient who undergoes a laparoscopic cholecystectomy is discharged soon after the surgery, so home care is important. Teaching is essential (Table 41-27).

PATIENT & FAMILY TEACHING GUIDE

Table 41-27 Postoperative Laparoscopic Cholecystectomy

1. Instruct patient to remove the bandages on the puncture site the day after surgery and bathe or shower.
2. Explain the need to report the following signs and symptoms:
   - Redness, swelling, bile-colored drainage or pus from any incision
   - Severe abdominal pain, nausea, vomiting, fever, chills
3. Explain that normal activities can be resumed gradually.
4. Instruct that returning to work can occur within 1 week of surgery.
5. Instruct to resume usual diet; may need to be a low-fat diet for several weeks following surgery.

CRITICAL THINKING EXERCISES

CASE STUDY

Cirrhosis of the Liver

Patient Profile

Mr. R. is a 55-year-old man admitted with a diagnosis of cirrhosis of the liver.

Subjective Data

- Has had cirrhosis for 12 years
- Acknowledges that he had been drinking heavily for 20 years but has been sober for the past 2 years
- Complains of anorexia, nausea, and abdominal discomfort

Objective Data

Physical Examination

- Thin and malnourished
- Has moderate ascites
- Has jaundice of sclera and skin
- Has 4+ pitting edema of the lower extremities
- Liver and spleen are palpable

Laboratory Values

- Total bilirubin 15 mg/dl (257 μmol/L)
- Serum ammonia 220 μg/dl (122 μmol/L)
- AST 190 U/L (3.2 μkat/L)
- ALT 210 U/L (3.5 μkat/L)

Critical Thinking Questions

1. What are possible causes of cirrhosis? What type of cirrhosis does Mr. R. probably have?
2. Describe the pathophysiologic changes that occur in the liver as cirrhosis develops.
3. List Mr. R.'s clinical manifestations of liver failure. For each manifestation, explain the pathophysiologic bases.
4. Explain the significance of the results of his laboratory values.
5. If Mr. R. begins to manifest signs and symptoms of hepatic encephalopathy, what would you monitor? What measures should be instituted to control or decrease the ammonia level?
6. Mr. R. was being closely observed for the possibility of gastrointestinal bleeding. Why is this considered a possible complication?
7. In the early stages of cirrhosis, what can be done to control the disease?
8. Based on the assessment data presented, write one or more nursing diagnoses. Are there any collaborative problems?

NURSING RESEARCH ISSUES

1. What is the most effective way to assess jaundice in a dark-skinned person?
2. What are the most significant psychosocial problems experienced by a patient with viral hepatitis?
3. What are the best ways to treat pruritus associated with jaundice in patients with hepatitis?
4. What is the quality of life for a patient after a liver transplant?
5. Can nutritional support improve outcomes in patients with alcohol-related cirrhosis?
6. What support resources are needed by the family of a patient with pancreatic cancer?

After an open-incision cholecystectomy, the patient may be discharged as soon as 3 to 5 days. The patient should be instructed to avoid heavy lifting for 4 to 6 weeks. Usual sexual activities, including intercourse, can be resumed as soon as the patient feels ready unless given other instructions by the physician.

Sometimes the patient is required to remain on a low-fat diet for 4 to 6 weeks. If so, a dietary teaching plan is necessary. A weight-reduction program may be helpful if the patient is overweight. Most patients tolerate a regular diet with no difficulties but should avoid excessive fats.

■ Evaluation

The overall expected outcomes are that the patient with gallbladder disease will

- appear comfortable and verbalize pain relief
- verbalize knowledge of activity level and dietary restrictions

CANCER OF THE GALLBLADDER

Primary cancer of the gallbladder is uncommon. The majority of gallbladder carcinomas are adenocarcinomas. There seems to be a definite relationship between cancer of the gallbladder and chronic cholecystitis and cholelithiasis.

The early symptoms of carcinoma of the gallbladder are insidious and are similar to those of chronic cholecystitis and cholelithiasis, which makes diagnosis difficult. Later symptoms are usually those of biliary obstruction. Cancer of the gallbladder has a poor prognosis.

Treatment is mainly symptomatic and supportive. Sometimes the tumor is resected. Chemotherapy and radiotherapy are seldom used because they are neither curative nor palliative.

Nursing management involves supportive care with special attention to nutrition, hydration, skin care, and pain relief. Many of the nursing care measures used for patients with cholecystitis and cholelithiasis are frequently applied, as well as nursing care measures for the patient with cancer (see Chapter 14).

REVIEW QUESTIONS

The number of the question corresponds to the same-numbered objective at the beginning of the chapter.

1. During assessment of a patient with obstructive jaundice the nurse would expect to find
   a. serum bilirubin of 1 mg/dl.
   b. pyrexia and severe pruritus.
   c. elevated urinary urobilinogen.
   d. dark urine and clay-colored stools.
2. A patient with hepatitis A is in the prodromal (preicteric) phase. The nurse plans care for the patient based on the knowledge that
   a. pruritus is a common problem with the jaundice of this phase.
   b. the patient is most likely to transmit the disease during this phase.
   c. gastrointestinal symptoms are not as severe in hepatitis A as they are in hepatitis B.
   d. extrahepatic manifestations of glomerulonephritis and polyarteritis are common in this phase.
3. A patient with hepatitis B is being discharged in 2 days. The nurse includes in his discharge teaching plan instructions to
   a. avoid alcohol for 3 weeks.
   b. use a condom during sexual intercourse.
   c. have family members get an injection of immunoglobulin.
   d. follow a low-protein, moderate-carbohydrate, moderate-fat diet.
4. The patient with advanced cirrhosis asks the nurse why his abdomen is so swollen. The nurse's response to the patient is based on the knowledge that
   a. a lack of clotting factors promotes the collection of blood in the abdominal cavity.
   b. portal hypertension and hypoalbuminemia cause a fluid shift into the peritoneal space.
   c. decreased peristalsis in the GI tract contributes to gas formation and distention of the bowel.
   d. bile salts in the blood irritate the peritoneal membranes, causing edema and pocketing of fluid.
5. When caring for a patient with hepatic encephalopathy the nurse may give enemas, provide a low-protein diet, and limit physical activity. These measures are done to
   a. promote fluid loss.
   b. eliminate potassium ions.
   c. decrease portal pressure.
   d. decrease the production of ammonia.
6. In planning care for a patient with metastatic cancer of the liver the nurse includes interventions that
   a. focus primarily on symptomatic and comfort measures.
   b. reassure the patient that chemotherapy offers a good prognosis for recovery.
   c. promote the patient's confidence that surgical excision of the tumor will be successful.
   d. provide information necessary for the patient to make decisions regarding liver transplantation.
7. The nurse explains to the patient with acute pancreatitis that the most common pathogenic mechanism of the disorder is
   a. cellular disorganization.
   b. overproduction of enzymes.
   c. lack of secretion of enzymes.
   d. autodigestion of the pancreas.
8. Nursing management of the patient with acute pancreatitis includes
   a. checking for signs of hypercalcemia.
   b. observing stools for signs of steatorrhea.
   c. providing a diet low in carbohydrates with moderate fat.
   d. monitoring for infection, particularly respiratory infection.
9. A patient with pancreatic cancer is admitted to the hospital for evaluation for treatment. The patient asks the nurse to explain the Whipple procedure the surgeon has described. The nurse's explanation includes the information that a Whipple procedure involves
   a. creating a bypass around the obstruction caused by the tumor by joining the gallbladder to the jejunum.
   b. resection of the entire pancreas and the distal portion of the stomach, with anastomosis of the common bile duct and stomach into the duodenum.
   c. removal of part of the pancreas, part of the stomach, the duodenum, and the gallbladder, with joining of the pancreatic duct, common bile duct, and stomach into the jejunum.
   d. radical removal of the pancreas, duodenum, and spleen, attaching the stomach to the jejunum, which requires oral supplementation of pancreatic digestive enzymes and insulin replacement therapy.
10. The nursing management of the patient with cholecystitis associated with cholelithiasis is based on the knowledge that
    a. the disorder can be successfully treated with oral bile salts that dissolve gallstones.
    b. morphine is the drug of choice to relieve the pain of bile duct spasms during an acute attack.
    c. a heavy meal with a high fat content may precipitate the signs and symptoms of the disease.
    d. a low-cholesterol diet is indicated to reduce the availability of cholesterol for gallstone formation.
11. Teaching in relation to home management following a laparoscopic cholecystectomy should include
    a. keeping the bandages on the puncture sites for 48 hours.
    b. reporting any bile-colored drainage or pus from any incision.
    c. using over-the-counter antiemetics if nausea and vomiting occur.
    d. emptying and measuring the contents of the bile bag from the T-tube every day.

References

1. *Hepatitis statistics,* 1997, Hepatitis Foundation International. http://www.hepsi.org/stats.htm
2. Idilman R and others: Interferon treatment of cirrhotic patients with chronic hepatitis C, *J Viral Hepatitis* 4:81, 1997.
3. Koff RS: Chronic hepatitis C: early intervention, *Hosp Pract* 33:101, 1998.
4. Seeff LB: Acute viral hepatitis. In Kaplowtiz N, editor: *Liver and biliary diseases,* ed 2, Baltimore, 1996, Williams & Wilkins.
5. Lee WK: Hepatitis B virus infection, *N Engl J Med* 337:1733, 1997.
6. Bryan JP and others: Hepatitis B vaccine booster dose: low-dose recombinant hepatitis B vaccines as a booster dose, *Am J Infect Control* 25:215, 1997.
7. Sharara AI, Hunt CM, Hamilton JD: Hepatitis C, *Ann Intern Med* 125:658, 1996.
8. Hepatitis Branch, Centers for Disease Control and Prevention: Epidemiology and prevention of viral hepatitis A to E: an overview. http://www.cdc.gov/httoc.htm

9. Alter HJ and others: The incidence of transfusion-associated hepatitis G virus infection and its relation to liver disease, *N Engl J Med* 336:747, 1997.
10. Tacke M and others: Detection of antibodies to a putative hepatitis G virus envelope protein, *Lancet* 349:318, 1997.
11. Centers for Disease Control and Prevention: Notice to readers. Recommendations for follow-up of health-care workers after occupational exposure to hepatitis C virus, *MMWR* 46:26, 1997.
12. The hepatitis place. http://www.hepplace.com/tests/html
13. Woo MH, Burnakis TG: Interferon alpha in the treatment of chronic viral hepatitis B and C, *Ann Pharmacol* 31:330, 1997.
14. Perrillo RP: Mechanisms of anti-viral therapy for HBV: interferons; nucleoside analogues; immunomodulators. Internet: http://www.hepnet.com/boca/perrillo.html.
15. Centers for Disease Control and Prevention: Prevention of hepatitis A through active or passive immunization, *MMWR* 45(no. RR-15):1, 1996.
16. Centers for Disease Control and Prevention: Notice to readers. Interferon may be used in the treatment of chronic hepatitis C, *MMWR* 46:26, 1997.
17. Freitag-Koontz MJ: Prevention of hepatitis B and C transmission during pregnancy and the first year of life, *J Perinat Neonat Nurs* 10:40, 1996.
18. O'Hanlon-Nichols T: Clinical snapshot: portal hypertension, *AJN* 95:38, 1995.
19. Koutsomanis D: Endoscopic clipping for bleeding varices, *Gastrointest Endosc* 40:126, 1994.
20. Sogni P and others: Acute effects of propylthiouracil on hemodynamics and oxygen content in patients with alcoholic cirrhosis, *J Hepatol* 26:628, 1997.
21. Holland JF and others, editors: *Cancer medicine,* vol II, ed 4, Baltimore, 1997, Williams & Wilkins.
22. Feray SD, Bismuth H: HCV infection and liver transplantation, *Acta Gastroenterol Belg* 60:214, 1997.
23. *Cancer facts and figures—1998,* American Cancer Society, Atlanta, Ga.
24. Holland JF and others, editors: *Cancer medicine,* vol II, ed 4, Baltimore, 1997, Williams & Wilkins.
25. DeVita VT and others: *Cancer principles and practice of oncology,* ed 5, Philadelphia, 1997, Lippincott-Raven.

Resources

American Association for the Study of Liver Diseases (AASLD)
c/o American Gastroenterological Association
7910 Woodmont Ave, 7th Floor
Bethesda, MD 20814
301-654-2055
Fax: 301-652-3890

American Liver Foundation
1425 Pompton Avenue
Cedar Grove, NJ 07009
800-GO-LIVER (465-4837)
http://sadieo.ucsf.edu/alf/alffinal/homepagealf.html

United Ostomy Association
19772 MacArthur Boulevard, Suite 200
Irvine, CA 92612-2405
800-826-0826
http://www.uoa.org/

***For additional Internet resources, see the website for this book at* www.mosby.com/MERLIN/medsurg_lewis**

SECTION

9

PROBLEMS OF URINARY FUNCTION

SECTION OUTLINE

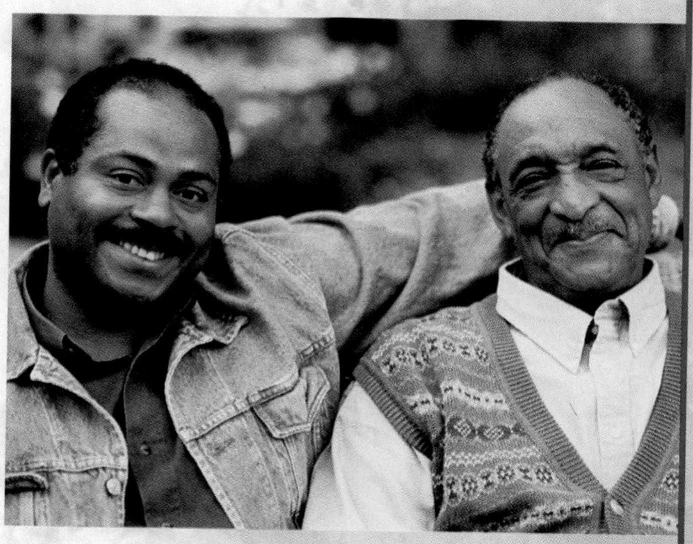

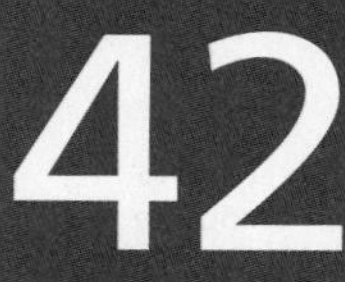

REMEMBER to check out your **companion CD-ROM**

42 NURSING ASSESSMENT Urinary System

Patricia Bates

www.mosby.com/MERLIN/medsurg_lewis

LEARNING OBJECTIVES

1. Describe the anatomic location and functions of the kidneys, ureters, bladder, and urethra.
2. Explain the physiologic events involved in the formation and passage of urine from glomerular filtration to voiding.
3. Identify the significant subjective and objective data related to the urinary system that should be obtained from a patient.
4. Describe age-related changes in the urinary system and differences in assessment findings.
5. Describe the appropriate techniques used in the physical assessment of the urinary system.
6. Differentiate normal from common abnormal findings of a physical assessment of the urinary system.
7. Describe the purpose, significance of results, and nursing responsibilities related to diagnostic studies of the urinary system.
8. Describe the normal physical and chemical characteristics of urine.

"Bones can break, muscles can atrophy, glands can loaf, even the brain can go to sleep without immediate danger to survival. But should the kidneys fail . . . neither bone, muscle, gland, nor brain could carry on."[1] This statement underlines the importance of kidneys to our lives. Adequate functioning of the kidneys is essential to the maintenance of a healthy body. If there is complete kidney failure and treatment is not given, death is inevitable.

The kidneys are the principal organs of the urinary system. Besides the two kidneys, there are two ureters, a urinary bladder, and a urethra in the urinary system (Fig. 42-1). The other organs can be thought of as storage and drainage channels for the urine after it is formed by the kidneys.

The primary function of the kidneys is to regulate the volume and composition of extracellular fluid (ECF). The excretory function of kidneys is secondary to this regulatory function. Other major functions of the kidneys include renin secretion and blood pressure control, erythropoietin production, vitamin D activation, and acid-base balance regulation.

STRUCTURES AND FUNCTIONS OF THE URINARY SYSTEM

Kidneys

Macrostructure. The kidneys are bean-shaped organs that are retroperitoneal (behind the peritoneum) on either side of the vertebral column at about the level of the twelfth thoracic (T12) vertebra to the third lumbar (L3) vertebra. Each kidney weighs 4 to 6 ounces (120 to 170 g) and is about 5 inches (12 cm) long. The right kidney, with the liver above it, is lower than the left. The right kidney is at the level of the twelfth rib. An adrenal gland lies on top of each kidney.

Each kidney is surrounded by a considerable amount of fat and connective tissue that serves to support and maintain its position. The surface of the kidney is covered by a thin, smooth layer of fibrous membrane called the *capsule.* The *hilus* on the medial side of the kidney serves as the entry site for the renal artery and nerves, as well as the exit site for the vein and ureter.

On a longitudinal section of the kidney (Fig. 42-2), the internal structures can be visualized. The outer layer is termed the *cortex,* and the inner layer is called the *medulla.* The medulla consists of a number of *pyramids.* The apices of these pyramids are called *papillae,* through which urine passes to enter the *calyces.* The minor calyces widen and merge to form major calyces, which form a funnel-shaped sac called the *renal pelvis.* The minor and major calyces and the renal pelvis are holding areas for urine before it exits the kidney via the ureter. The capacity of the renal pelvis is about 3 to 5 ml. The lumen of the renal pelvis decreases to form the ureter.

Microstructure. The functional unit of the kidney is termed the *nephron.* Each kidney has more than 1 million nephrons. A nephron is composed of a glomerulus, Bowman's capsule, and tubular system. The tubular system consists of the proximal convoluted tubule, the loop of Henle, and the distal convoluted tubule (Fig. 42-3). Several nephrons converge into a collecting duct, which eventually merges into a pyramid and empties via the papilla into a minor calyx.

The glomeruli, Bowman's capsule, proximal tubule, and distal tubule are located in the cortex of the kidney. The loop of Henle and the collecting ducts are located in the medulla.

Reviewed by Diane M. Fesler, RN, MSN, PhD Candidate, Assistant Professor, Northern Illinois University, Dekalb, Ill.

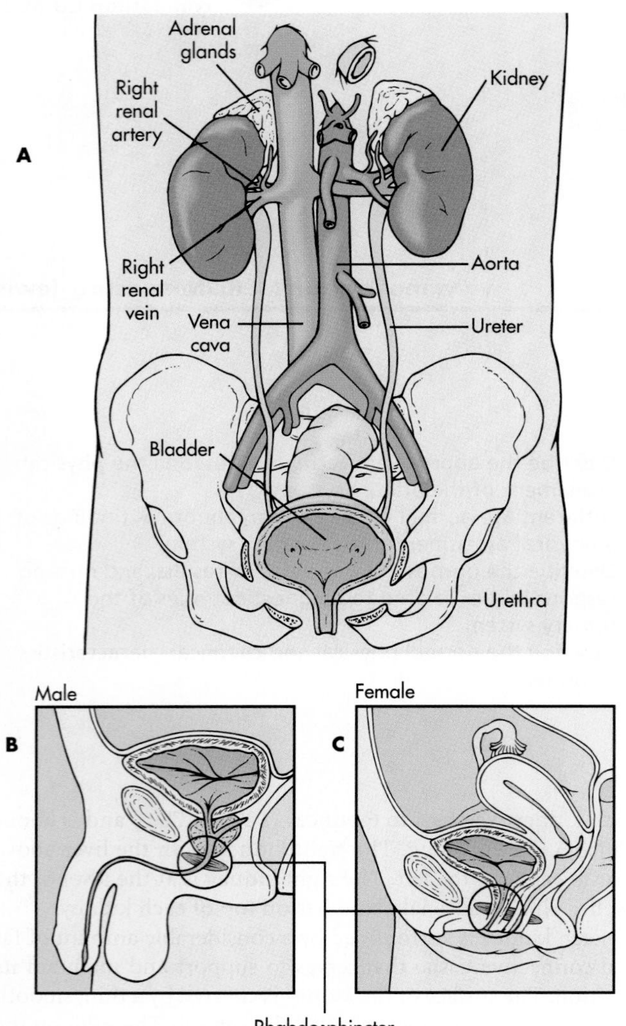

Fig. 42-1 Organs of the urinary system. **A,** Upper urinary tract in relation to other anatomic structures. **B,** Male urethra in relation to other pelvic structures. **C,** Female urethra.

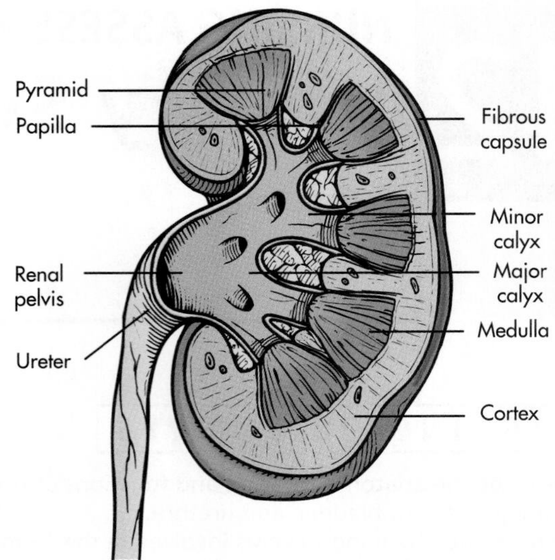

Fig. 42-2 Longitudinal section of the kidney.

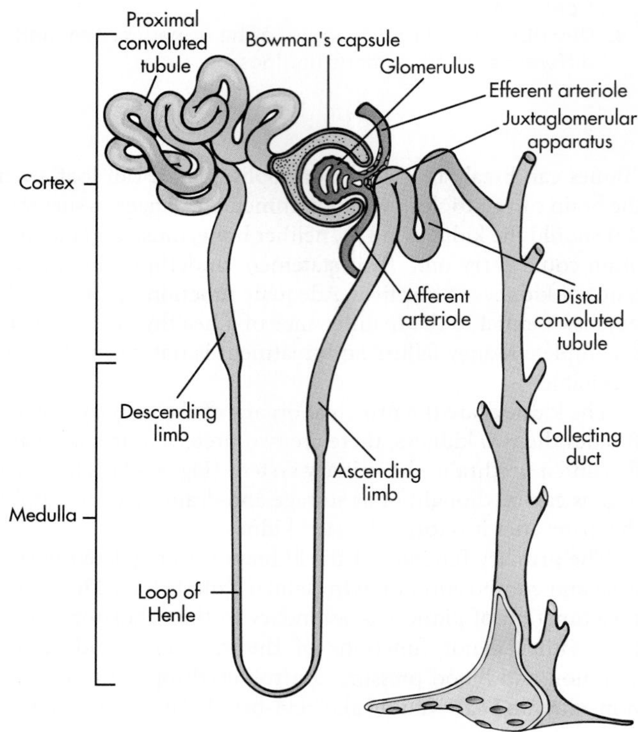

Fig. 42-3 Nephron of the kidney.

Blood Supply. A blood supply of about 1200 ml/min, which is 20% to 25% of the cardiac output, flows to the two kidneys. Blood reaches the kidneys via the renal artery, which arises from the aorta and enters the kidney through the hilus. The renal artery divides into secondary branches and then into still smaller branches, each of which eventually forms an *afferent arteriole* (Fig. 42-4). The afferent arteriole divides into a capillary network termed the *glomerulus,* which is a tuft of up to 50 capillaries. The capillaries of the glomerulus eventually unite in the *efferent arteriole.* This arteriole splits to form a capillary network called the *peritubular capillaries,* which, as the name suggests, surround the tubular system. All peritubular capillaries eventually drain into the venous system. The renal vein empties into the inferior vena cava.

Physiology of Urine Formation

Normal Glomerular Function. Urine formation starts at the glomerulus where blood is filtered. The glomerulus, which is a semipermeable membrane, allows for filtration (see Fig. 42-3). The hydrostatic pressure of the blood within the glomerular capillaries causes a portion of blood to be filtered across the semipermeable membrane into Bowman's capsule, where the filtered portion of the blood called the *glomerular filtrate* begins to pass down to the tubule. Filtration is more rapid in the glomerulus than in ordinary tissue capillaries because of the porosity of the glomerular membrane. The ultrafiltrate is similar in composition to blood except that it lacks blood cells, platelets, and large plasma proteins. Under normal conditions the capillary pores are too small to allow the

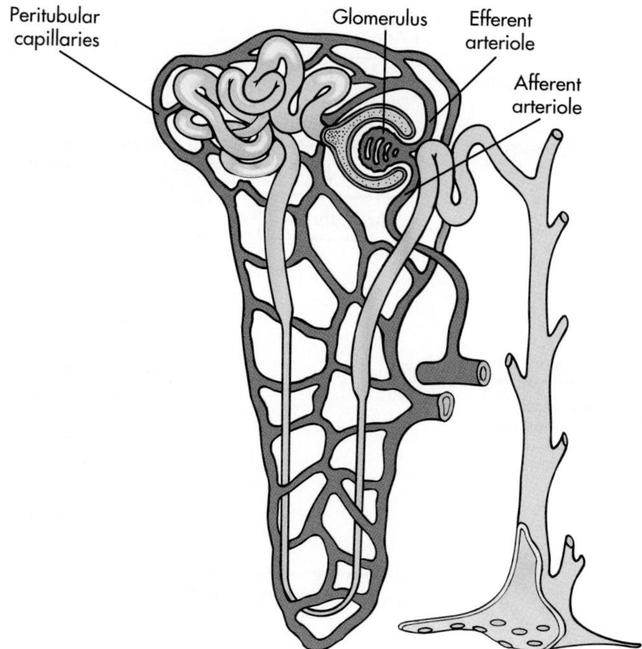

Fig. 42-4 Blood supply of the nephron.

Table 42-1 Functions of the Segments of the Nephron

Component	Function
▪ Glomerulus	Selective filtration
▪ Proximal tubule	Reabsorption of 80% of electrolytes and water, reabsorption of all glucose and amino acids, reabsorption of HCO_3^-, secretion of H^+ and creatinine
▪ Loop of Henle	Reabsorption of Na^+ and Cl^- in ascending limb, reabsorption of water in descending loop, concentration of filtrate
▪ Distal tubule	Secretion of K^+, H^+, ammonia; reabsorption of water (regulated by ADH); reabsorption of HCO_3^-; regulation of Ca^{2+} and PO_4^{2-} by parathyroid hormone, regulation of Na^+ and K^+ by aldosterone
▪ Collecting duct	Reabsorption of water (ADH required)

ADH, antidiuretic hormone; *Ca^{2+}*, calcium ions; *Cl^-*, chloride ions; *H^+*, hydrogen ions; *HCO_3^-*, bicarbonate ions; *K^+*, potassium ions; *Na^+*, sodium ions; *PO_4^{2-}*, phosphate ions.

loss of these large blood components. Capillary permeability is increased in many renal diseases, permitting plasma proteins to pass into the urine.

The amount of blood filtered by the glomeruli in a given time is termed the *glomerular filtration rate* (GFR). The normal GFR is about 125 ml per minute. However, on the average only 1 ml per minute is excreted as urine because most glomerular filtrate is reabsorbed by the peritubular capillary network before it reaches the end of the collecting duct.

Tubular Function. Because the glomerular membrane is a selective filtration membrane that filters primarily by size, provision is made for the reabsorption of essential materials and the excretion of nonessential ones (Table 42-1). The tubules and collecting ducts carry out these functions by means of reabsorption and secretion (Fig. 42-5). *Reabsorption* is the passage of a substance from the lumen of the tubules through the tubule cells and into the capillaries. This process involves both active and passive transport. *Tubular secretion* is the passage of a substance from the capillaries through the tubular cells into the lumen of the tubule. Reabsorption and secretion occur along the entire length of the tubule, causing numerous changes in the composition of the glomerular filtrate as it moves through the tubules.

In the proximal convoluted tubule, about 80% of the electrolytes are reabsorbed. Normally, all the glucose, amino acids, and protein are reabsorbed. For the most part reabsorption occurs by active transport. Hydrogen ions (H^+) and creatinine are secreted into the filtrate.[2]

The loop of Henle is important in conserving water and thus concentrating the filtrate. In the loop of Henle, reabsorption continues. The descending loop is permeable to water and moderately permeable to sodium, urea, and other solutes. In the ascending limb, chloride ions (Cl^-) are actively reabsorbed, followed passively by sodium ions (Na^+). About 25% of the filtered sodium is reabsorbed here.

Two important functions of the distal convoluted tubules are final regulation of water balance and acid-base balance. Antidiuretic hormone (ADH), released by the posterior pituitary gland, is required for water reabsorption. The stimuli for ADH release is increased serum osmolality and decreased blood volume. ADH makes the distal convoluted tubules and the collecting ducts permeable to water, allowing it to be reabsorbed into the peritubular capillaries and to be eventually returned to circulation. In the absence of ADH the tubules are practically impermeable to water, and any water in the tubules leaves the body as urine.

In the presence of aldosterone (released from the adrenal cortex) acting on the distal tubule, reabsorption of Na^+ and water occurs. In exchange for Na^+, potassium ions (K^+) are excreted. The secretion of aldosterone is influenced by both circulating blood volume and plasma concentrations of Na^+ and K^+.

Acid-base regulation involves reabsorbing and conserving most of the bicarbonate (HCO_3^-) and secreting excess H^+. The distal tubule functions in different ways to maintain the pH of ECF within a range of 7.35 to 7.45 (see Chapter 15).

Atrial natriuretic factor (ANF) is a hormone secreted from cells in the right atrium when right atrial blood pressure increases. ANF inhibits the secretion and effect of ADH and results in a large volume of dilute urine (see Chapter 45).

Parathyroid hormone (parathormone) is released from the parathyroid gland in response to low serum calcium levels. It causes increased tubular reabsorption of calcium ions (Ca^{2+}) and decreased tubular reabsorption of phosphate ions (PO_4^{-2}). Therefore serum Ca^{2+} levels are increased.

The basic function of nephrons is to clean or clear blood plasma of unnecessary substances. After the glomerulus has

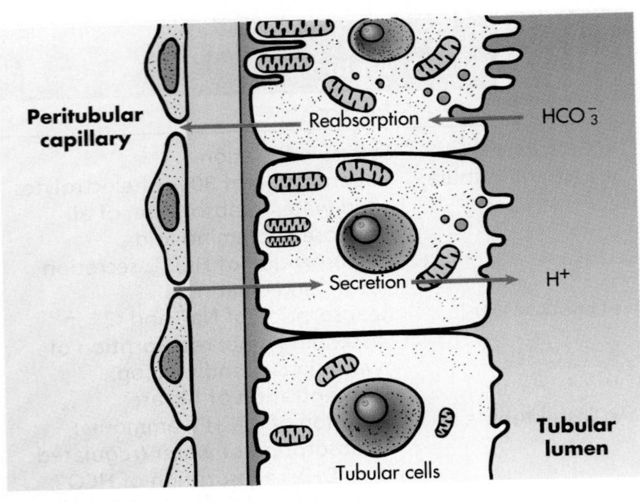

Fig. 42-5 Reabsorption and secretion in the tubules.

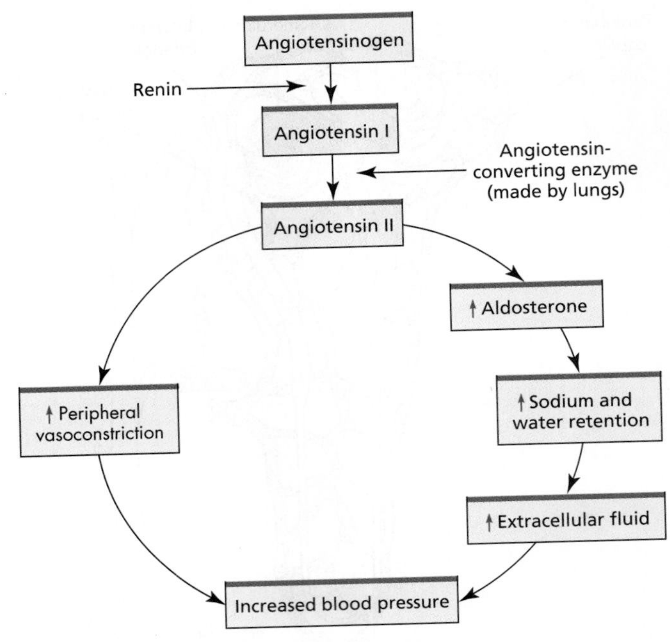

Fig. 42-6 Renin-angiotensin mechanism.

filtered the blood, the tubules separate the unwanted from the wanted portions of tubular fluid. The necessary portions are returned to the blood, and the unnecessary portions pass into urine.

Other Renal Functions

In addition to their function in regulating the volume and composition of ECF, the kidneys also have other vital functions, including the production of erythropoietin, production and secretion of renin, and activation of vitamin D.

Erythropoietin is produced and released in response to decreased oxygen tension in the renal blood supply, which is usually caused by a loss of red blood cells (RBCs). Erythropoietin stimulates the production of RBCs in the bone marrow. A deficiency of erythropoietin leads to anemia in renal failure.

Vitamin D is a hormone that can be obtained in the diet or synthesized by the action of ultraviolet radiation on cholesterol in the skin. These forms of vitamin D are inactive and require two more steps to become metabolically active. The first step in activation occurs in the liver. The second step occurs in the kidneys. Active vitamin D is essential for the absorption of calcium from the gastrointestinal (GI) tract. The patient with renal failure has a deficiency of the active metabolite of vitamin D and manifests problems of altered calcium and phosphate balance (see Chapter 44).

Renin is important in the regulation of blood pressure (Fig. 42-6). It is released from the granular cells of the afferent arteriole. These cells, together with the macula densa cells of the distal convoluted tubule and the mesangial cells, form the juxtaglomerular apparatus. Renin is released in response to decreased arterial blood pressure, renal ischemia, ECF depletion, increased norepinephrine, and increased urinary Na^+ concentration. Renin catalyzes the splitting of the plasma protein angiotensinogen into angiotensin I, which is subsequently converted to angiotensin II by a converting enzyme made in the lungs. Angiotensin II stimulates the release of aldosterone from the adrenal cortex, which causes Na^+ and water retention, leading to an increased ECF volume. Angiotensin II also causes increased peripheral vasoconstriction. The increase in ECF and vasoconstriction causes an elevation in blood pressure, which should inhibit renin release. Excessive renin production caused by impaired renal perfusion may be a contributing factor in the etiology of hypertension (see Chapters 31 and 44).

Prostaglandins. Prostaglandins (PGs) are synthesized by most body tissues from the precursor, arachidonic acid, in response to appropriate stimuli. PGs, which are involved in the regulation of cell function and host defenses, exert their influence primarily on cells or tissues that are close to the site where they are synthesized. (See Chapter 11 and Fig. 11-7 for a more detailed discussion of PGs.)

In the kidney, PG synthesis (primarily PGE_2 and PGI_2) occurs primarily in the medulla. These PGs have a vasodilating action in addition to increasing renal blood flow and promoting Na^+ excretion. They counteract the vasoconstrictor effect of substances such as angiotensin and norepinephrine. Renal PGs may have a systemic effect in lowering blood pressure by decreasing systemic vascular resistance.[3]

The significance of these PGs is related to the role of the kidneys in causing hypertension. In renal failure with a loss of functioning tissue, these renal vasodilator factors are also lost. This may be one factor that contributes to the common finding of hypertension in renal failure (see Chapter 44).

Ureters

The ureters are tubes approximately 10 to 12 inches (25 to 35 cm) long and 0.08 to 0.3 inch (0.2 to 0.8 cm) in diameter that carry urine from the renal pelvis to the bladder. The narrow area where the ureter joins the renal pelvis is termed the *ureteropelvic junction* (UPJ). After coursing down along the psoas muscle, the ureter crosses over the pelvic brim and iliac artery and inserts into the base of the bladder at the *ureterovesical junction* (UVJ). The ureteral lumen is narrowest at these junctions; consequently, they are often the sites of urinary stone (calculi) obstruction. Since the lumen of the ureter is narrow, it can be easily occluded internally (e.g., calculi) or externally (e.g., tumors, adhesions, inflammation).

Sympathetic and parasympathetic nerves, along with the vascular supply, surround the mucosal lining of the ureter. Circular and longitudinal smooth muscle fibers are arranged in a meshlike outer layer and contract to promote the peristaltic one-way flow of urine. These muscle contractions can be affected by distention and neurologic, endocrine, and pharmacologic factors. Stimulation of these nerves during passage of a stone or clot may cause acute, severe pain termed *renal colic.*

Because the renal pelvis holds only 3 to 5 ml of urine, kidney damage can result from a backflow of more than that amount of urine. The UVJ relies on the ureter's angle of bladder penetration and muscle fiber attachments with the bladder to prevent the backflow of urine (reflux) and ascending infection. The distal ureter entering the bladder has more longitudinal muscle fibers than the upper ureter. This segment enters the bladder laterally at its base, courses along obliquely through the bladder wall for about 1.5 cm, and intermingles with muscle fibers of the bladder base. Circular and longitudinal bladder muscle fibers adjacent to the imbedded ureter help secure it. When bladder pressure rises (e.g., during voiding or coughing), muscle fibers that the ureter shares with the bladder base contract first to help promote ureteral lumen closure. The bladder then contracts against its base to further close the UVJ and prevent urine from moving back through the junction.

Bladder

The urinary bladder is a distendible organ positioned behind the symphysis pubis and anterior to the vagina and rectum. Its primary functions are to serve as a reservoir for urine and to help the body eliminate waste products. Normal adult urine output is approximately 1500 ml per day, which varies with food and fluid intake. The volume of urine produced at night is less than half of that formed during the day because of hormonal influences (e.g., ADH). This diurnal pattern of urination is normal. Most persons urinate five to six times during the day and occasionally at night.

The triangular area formed by the two ureteral openings and the bladder neck at the base of the bladder is termed the *trigone.* It is affixed to the pelvis by many ligaments, and it does not change its shape during bladder filling or emptying. The bladder muscle, termed the *detrusor,* is composed of layers of intertwined smooth muscle fibers and is capable of considerable distention during bladder filling and contraction during emptying. It is affixed to the abdominal wall by an umbilical ligament. Consequently, as the bladder fills, it rises toward the umbilicus. The dome, anterior, and lateral aspects of the bladder expand and contract. When the bladder is empty, it appears as multiple folds within the pelvis.

On the average, 200 to 250 ml of urine in the bladder causes moderate distention and the urge to urinate. When the quantity of urine reaches about 400 to 600 ml, the person feels uncomfortable. Bladder capacity varies with the individual, usually ranging from 600 to 1000 ml. Evacuation of urine is termed *urination, micturition,* or *voiding.*

The bladder has the same mucosal lining as that of the renal pelvis, ureter, and bladder neck. It is called *transitional cell epithelium* or *urothelium* and is unique to the urinary tract. Transitional cell epithelium is resistant to absorption of urine. Therefore urinary wastes produced by the kidneys do not leak out of the urinary system after they leave the kidneys. Microscopically, transitional cell epithelium is several cells deep. These cells stretch out in the bladder to only a few cells deep as it accommodates filling. As the bladder empties, the epithelium resumes its multicellular layer formation.

Because the lining is the same, transitional cell tumors that occur in one section of the urinary tract can easily metastasize to other urinary tract areas. Malignant cells may move down from upper urinary tract tumors and imbed in the bladder, or large bladder tumors can invade the ureter. Tumor recurrence within the bladder is common. Intact urothelium also has phagocytic properties, although the exact mechanism is unknown.

Interstitial cystitis, a syndrome unique to the bladder, causes chronic inflammation of the bladder lining and wall. Histologic changes may be evident in the bladder epithelium. (Interstitial cystitis is discussed in Chapter 43.)

Urethra

The urethra is a small muscular tube that leads from the bladder neck to the external meatus. Its primary function is to serve as a conduit for urine to the bladder and then to the outside of the body.

The urothelium and submucosal layers are the same as that of the bladder. Smooth muscle fibers extend from the bladder neck down into the urethra and are further supported by circular smooth muscle fibers around the urethra. Special C-shaped striated muscle fibers (the rhabdosphincter, or external sphincter) surround a portion of the urethra and voluntarily contract and prevent leaking when bladder pressure increases.

The female urethra is 1 to 2 inches (3 to 5 cm) long and lies behind the symphysis pubis but anterior to the vagina. The rhabdosphincter encircles the middle third of the urethra. The short urethra is a contributing factor to the increased incidence of urinary tract infections in women.

The male urethra, which is about 8 to 10 inches (20 to 25 cm) long, originates at the bladder neck and extends the length of the penis. It is often separated into three parts. The prostatic urethra extends from the bladder neck through the prostate to the urogenital diaphragm. The membranous urethra passes through the urogenital diaphragm. The rhabdosphincter encircles this portion. Because of the concentrated muscular support, this short portion is not as expandable; consequently, stricture formation in this area after instrumentation is common. The penile urethra continues through the corpora spongiosum, a cavernous penile body, from the urogenital diaphragm to a distal dilated area, the fossa navicularis, before terminating at the meatus.

Urethrovesical Unit Function

Together, the bladder, bladder neck, urethra, and pelvic floor muscles form what is called the *urethrovesical unit.* Normal voluntary control of this unit is defined as continence. Various areas of the brain send stimulating and inhibiting impulses to the thoracolumbar (T11–L2) and sacral (S2–S4) areas of the spinal cord to control voiding. Distention of the bladder stimulates stretch receptors within the bladder wall. Impulses are transmitted to the sacral spinal cord and then to the brain, causing a desire to urinate. If the time to void is not appropriate, inhibitor impulses in the brain are stimulated and transmitted back to the thoracolumbar and sacral nerves innervating the bladder. In a coordinated fashion, the detrusor accommodates to the pressure (does not contract) while the sphincter and pelvic floor muscles tighten to resist bladder

GERONTOLOGIC DIFFERENCES IN ASSESSMENT

Table 42-2 Urinary System

Changes	Differences in Assessment Findings
Kidney	
Decrease in amount of renal tissue	Less palpable
Decrease in number of nephrons and renal vascular bed; thickened basement membrane of Bowman's capsule and glomeruli	Decrease in creatinine clearance, increase in BUN level
Decrease in function of loop of Henle and tubules	Alterations in drug excretion; nocturia; loss of normal diurnal excretory pattern because of decreased ability to concentrate urine; less concentrated urine
Ureter, Bladder, and Urethra	
Decrease in elasticity and muscle tone	Palpable bladder after urination because of retention
Weakening of urinary sphincter	Stress incontinence (especially during Valsalva maneuver), dribbling of urine after urination
Decrease in bladder capacity and sensory receptors	Frequency, urgency, nocturia, overflow incontinence
Estrogen deficiency leading to thin, dry vaginal tissue	Stress or urge incontinence, dysuria, positive urine culture
Uninhibited bladder contractions	Urge incontinence
Prostatic enlargement	Hesitancy, frequency, urgency, nocturia, straining to urinate, retention, dribbling

BUN, blood urea nitrogen.

pressure. If voiding is appropriate, cerebral inhibition is voluntarily suppressed, and impulses are transmitted via the spinal cord for the bladder neck, sphincter, and pelvic floor muscles to relax and for the bladder to contract. The sphincter closes and the detrusor muscle relaxes when the bladder is empty.

Any disease or trauma that affects function of the brain, spinal cord, or nerves that directly innervate the bladder, bladder neck, external sphincter, or pelvic floor can affect bladder function. These conditions include diabetes mellitus, paraplegia, and quadriplegia. Medications affecting nerve transmission also can affect bladder function.

GERONTOLOGIC CONSIDERATIONS

Effects of Aging on the Urinary System

Anatomic changes in the aging kidney include a 20% to 30% decrease in size and weight between the ages of 30 and 90 years. This loss in renal mass is predominantly in the cortex. The aging nephron fails as a unit because glomerular and tubular function appear to decrease at the same rate. By the seventh decade of life, 30% to 50% of glomeruli have lost their function because of sclerosis or other abnormalities. Despite losing this original kidney volume, older individuals maintain body fluid homeostasis unless they encounter diseases or other physiologic stressors.[4]

Blood flow to and within the kidneys also decreases. There is no evidence that atherosclerotic vascular disease is primarily responsible for the age-related changes in the kidneys.

Physiologic changes in the aging kidney include decreased renal blood flow; decreased GFR; and decreased ability to conserve Na^+, dilute or concentrate urine, and excrete an acid load. Under normal conditions, the aging kidney is able to maintain homeostasis, but after abrupt changes in blood volume, acid load, or other insults, the kidneys may not be able to function effectively because much of its renal reserve has been lost.

Physiologic changes also occur in the aging bladder and urethra.[5,6] Estrogen receptors exist in the female urethra, bladder, vagina, and pelvic floor. As estrogen levels decrease with age, tissues become less elastic, thin, and less vascular.[7] Periurethral striated muscle fibers and muscles supporting the bladder relax. Consequently, older women are more prone to urethral irritation, urethral and bladder infections, and urinary incontinence.

Men's prostates enlarge as they age, and since the prostate surrounds the proximal urethra, increasing prostate size may affect urinary patterns in men, causing hesitancy, retention, slow stream, and bladder infections.

Constipation, a complaint often expressed by the elderly, can also affect urination. Partial urethral obstruction may occur because of the rectum's close proximity to the urethra.

Age-related changes in the urinary system and differences in assessment findings are presented in Table 42-2.

ASSESSMENT OF THE URINARY SYSTEM

Subjective Data

Important Health Information

Past health history. The patient should be questioned about the presence or history of diseases that are known to be related to renal or other urologic problems. Some of these diseases are hypertension, diabetes mellitus, gout and other metabolic problems, connective tissue disorders (e.g., systemic lupus erythematosus, scleroderma), skin or upper respiratory infections of streptococcal origin, tuberculosis, viral hepatitis, congenital disorders, neurologic conditions (e.g., stroke, back injury), or trauma. Specific urinary problems such as cancer, infections, benign prostatic hyperplasia, and calculi should be noted.

Medications. An assessment of the patient's current and past use of medications is important. This should include over-the-counter drugs, as well as prescription medications and

Table 42-3 **Nephrotoxic Agents**

Antibiotics	Other Agents
Amikacin	Captopril
Amphotericin B	Cimetidine
Bacitracin	Cisplatin
Cephalosporins	Cocaine
Colistin	Contrast medium
Gentamicin	Cyclosporine
Kanamycin	Ethylene glycol
Neomycin	Gold
Polymyxin B	Heavy metals
Streptomycin	Heroin
Sulfonamides	Lithium
Tobramycin	Methotrexate
Vancomycin	Nitrosoureas (e.g., carmustine)
	Nonsteroidal antiinflammatory agents (e.g., ibuprofen, indomethacin)
	Phenacetin
	Quinine
	Rifampin
	Salicylate (large quantities)

herbs. Drugs affect the urinary tract in several ways. Many drugs are known to be nephrotoxic (Table 42-3). Certain drugs may alter the quantity and character of urine output (e.g., diuretics). Numerous drugs such as phenazopyridine (Pyridium) and nitrofurantoin (Macrodantin) change its color. Anticoagulants may cause hematuria. Many antidepressants, calcium channel blockers, antihistamines, and medications used for neurologic and musculoskeletal disorders affect the ability of the bladder or sphincter to contract or relax normally.

Surgery or other treatments. The patient should also be questioned about any previous hospitalizations related to renal or urologic diseases and all urinary problems during past pregnancies. The duration, severity, and patient's perception of any problem and its treatment should be elicited. Past surgeries, particularly pelvic surgeries, or urinary tract instrumentation should be documented. Information should be obtained from the patient about any radiation or chemotherapy treatment for cancer.

Functional Health Patterns. Key questions to ask a patient with problems related to the urinary system are listed in Table 42-4.

HEALTH HISTORY

Table 42-4 **Urinary System**

Health Perception–Health Management Pattern
- How is your energy level compared with a year ago?
- Do you notice any visual changes?*
- Have you ever smoked? If yes, how much?

Nutritional-Metabolic Pattern
- How is your appetite?
- Has your weight changed over the past year?*
- Do you take vitamin or mineral supplements?*
- How much and what kinds of fluids do you drink daily?
- How much dairy products or meat do you eat?
- Do you drink coffee? Colas?
- Do you eat chocolate?
- Do you spice your food heavily?*

Elimination Pattern
- How often do you urinate during the day and night?
- Is the color normal for you?
- Do you ever notice blood in your urine?* If so, at what point in the urination does it occur?
- Do you find it difficult to postpone urination when you feel the urge to urinate?*
- Do you ever leak urine? If so, when does it occur?
- Do you ever have pain when you urinate?*
- Have you ever experienced urinary incontinence? If so, please describe specifically.
- Do you use special devices or supplies for urine elimination or control?*
- Do your bowels move regularly?

Activity-Exercise Pattern
- Have you noticed any changes in your ability to do your usual daily activities?*
- Do certain activities aggravate your urinary problem?*
- Has your urinary problem caused you to alter or stop any activity or exercise?*
- Do you require assistance in moving or getting to the bathroom?*

Cognitive-Perceptual Pattern
- Describe any pain you have in relation to urination.

Self-Perception–Self-Concept Pattern
- How does your urinary problem make you feel about yourself?
- Do you perceive your body differently since you have developed a urinary problem?

Role-Relationship Pattern
- Does your urinary problem interfere with your relationships with family or friends?*
- Has your urinary problem caused a change in your job status or affected your ability to carry out job-related responsibilities?*

Sexuality-Reproductive Pattern
- Has your urinary problem caused any change in your sexual pleasure or performance?*
- Do you have hygiene problems related to sexual activities that cause you concern?*

Coping–Stress Tolerance Pattern
- Do you feel able to manage the problems associated with your urinary problem? If not, explain.
- What strategies are you using to cope with your urinary problem?

Values-Beliefs Pattern
- Has your present illness affected your belief system?*
- Are your treatment decisions related to your urinary problem in conflict with your value system?*

*If yes, describe.

Table 42-5 Clinical Manifestations of Disorders of the Urinary System

General Manifestations	
Fatigue	Itching
Headaches	Excess thirst
Blurred vision	Chills
Elevated blood pressure	Change in body weight
Anorexia	Change in mentation
Nausea and vomiting	
Related to Urinary System	
Pain	**Changes in Urine Output**
Dysuria	Polyuria
Flank or costovertebral angle	Oliguria
	Anuria
Groin	**Changes in Urine Consistency**
Suprapubic	
Changes in Patterns of Urination	Hematuria
	Pyuria
Frequency	Concentrated
Nocturia	Dilute
Dysuria	Color (red, brown, yellowish green)
Hesitancy of stream	
Change in stream	**Edema**
Urgency	Facial (periorbital)
Retention	Ankle
Incontinence	Ascites
Stress incontinence	Anasarca
Enuresis	Sacral
Dribbling	

Health perception–health management pattern. The nurse may want to ask about the patient's general health. Sometimes responses such as "feeling tired all of the time," changes in weight or appetite, excess thirst, fluid retention, and complaints of headache, pruritus, or blurred vision may be related to abnormal kidney function.

An occupational history should be taken. Exposure to certain chemicals can affect the kidneys and urinary tract system. Phenol and ethylene glycol are examples of nephrotoxic chemicals. Aromatic amines and certain organic chemicals may increase the risk of bladder cancers. Textile workers, painters, hairdressers, and industrial workers have a high incidence of bladder tumors.[8]

A smoking history should be obtained. Cigarette smoking is a major factor in the risk for bladder cancer. Tumors occur four times more frequently in cigarette smokers than in nonsmokers.[8]

Places where a patient has lived may be important information to obtain. It has been shown that persons living in certain parts of the United States (Great Lakes, Southwest, Southeast) have a higher than normal incidence of urinary calculi. This may be caused by the higher mineral content of the soil and water. A person living in Middle Eastern countries or Africa can acquire certain parasites that can cause cystitis or bladder cancer.

The presence of certain renal or urologic problems in a family history increases the likelihood of similar problems occurring in the patient. The nurse should ask about family members who have had any of the diseases referred to in the past health history, as well as polycystic renal disease, congenital urinary tract abnormalities, and Alport's syndrome (hereditary nephritis).

Nutritional-metabolic pattern. The usual quantity and types of fluid a patient drinks are important information related to urinary tract disease. Dehydration may contribute to urinary infections, calculi formation, and renal failure. Large intake of particular foods, such as dairy products or foods high in proteins, may also lead to calculi formation. Coffee, alcohol, carbonated beverages, or spicy foods often aggravate urinary inflammatory diseases. An unexplained weight gain may be the result of fluid retention secondary to a renal problem. Anorexia and nausea and vomiting can dramatically affect fluid status and require careful assessment. Information on vitamin and mineral supplements and herbal therapies should be obtained. The patient may not think of these supplements and therapies when listing over-the-counter drugs; supplements are often considered part of nutritional intake.

Elimination pattern. The patient should be questioned about urinary patterns such as frequency or urgency and the amount of urine output. Table 42-5 lists some of the common clinical manifestations of urinary tract disorders. Changes in the color and appearance of urine are often significant and should be evaluated. If blood is visible in the urine, it should be determined if it occurs at the beginning, throughout, or at the end of urination.

Bowel function should also be investigated. Problems with fecal incontinence may signal neurologic causes for bladder problems because of shared nerve pathways. Constipation and fecal impaction can partially obstruct the urethra, causing inadequate bladder emptying and overflow incontinence.

The nurse should find out the patient's method of handling a urinary problem. A patient may already be using a catheter or collection device. Sometimes a patient has to assume a particular position to urinate or perform such maneuvers as pressing on the abdomen (Valsalva's maneuver), straining, or stretching the rectum to empty the bladder.

Activity-exercise pattern. The patient's level of activity should be assessed. A sedentary person is more likely than an active one to have stasis of urine, which can predispose to infection and calculi. Demineralization of bones in a person with limited physical activity causes increased urine calcium precipitation.

An active person may find that increasing activity aggravates the urinary problem. The patient who has had prostate surgery or who has weakened pelvic floor muscles may leak urine when attempting particular activities such as running. Some men may develop chronic inflammatory prostatitis or epididymitis after heavy lifting or long-distance driving.

Sleep-rest pattern. Lower urinary tract disorders, such as infections, neurologic conditions, or bladder outlet obstructions, often necessitate a person getting up as much as every hour at night. This situation can lead to sleep deprivation. Sleep problems associated with a urinary disorder should be documented. The older adult may awaken many times during the night to urinate and may need to be assured that this may be normal. However, a complete assessment should be made to rule out any problem.

Cognitive-perceptual pattern. Level of mobility, visual acuity, and dexterity are important factors to determine for a patient with urologic problems when managing his or her own care at home, particularly when bladder retention or inconti-

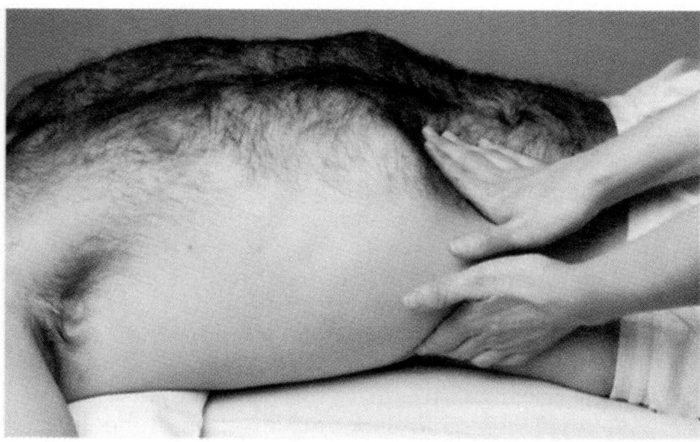

Fig. 42-7 Palpating the right kidney.

nence is a problem. It should be determined if the patient is alert, is able to understand instructions, and can recall the instructions when necessary.

If urinary incontinence is present, a thorough history of the problem should be elicited to assist in determining the type of incontinence. It is important to document what the patient has tried in order to manage the problem. Incontinence is a distressing problem and calls for great sensitivity on the part of the nurse if accurate information is to be obtained.

Pain is a frequent symptom of urinary tract disease. Types of pain associated with renal and urologic problems include dysuria, groin pain, costovertebral pain, and suprapubic pain. If present, the location, character, and duration should be assessed. The absence of pain when other urinary symptoms exist is also significant. Many urinary tract tumors are painless in the early stages.

Self-perception–self-concept pattern. Problems associated with the urinary system, such as incontinence, urinary diversion procedures, and chronic fatigue, can result in loss of self-esteem and a negative body image. Sensitive questioning may elicit cues to problems in this area.

Role-relationship pattern. Urinary problems can affect many aspects of a person's life, including the ability to work and relationships with others. These factors will have important implications on future treatment and management. The nurse must be aware of cues from the patient.

Urinary system problems may be serious enough to cause problems in job- and social-related situations. Chronic dialysis therapy often makes regular employment or full-time homemaking difficult. Also, the concurrent poor health and negative body image can seriously alter existing roles. The nurse should assess this area to plan appropriate interventions.

Sexuality-reproductive pattern. The patient should be questioned about the effect of a renal or urologic problem on her or his sexual patterns and satisfaction. Problems related to personal hygiene and fatigue can seriously affect a sexual relationship. Counseling of both the patient and partner may be indicated.

Objective Data

Physical Examination

Inspection. The nurse should assess for changes in the following:

Skin: pallor, yellow-gray cast, excoriations, changes in turgor, bruises, texture (e.g., rough, dry skin)
Mouth: stomatitis, ammonia breath odor
Face, abdomen, and extremities: generalized edema, peripheral edema, bladder distention, masses, enlarged kidneys
Weight gain: secondary to edema
General state of health: fatigue, lethargy, and diminished alertness

Palpation. The kidneys are posterior organs protected by the abdominal organs, the ribs, and the heavy back muscles. A landmark useful in locating the kidneys is the costovertebral angle (CVA) formed by the rib cage and the vertebral column. The normal-sized left kidney is rarely palpable because the spleen lies directly on top of it. Occasionally the lower pole of the right kidney is palpable.

To palpate the right kidney, the examiner's left hand is placed behind and supports the patient's right side between the rib cage and the iliac crest (Fig. 42-7). The right flank is elevated with the left hand, and the right hand is used to palpate deeply for the right kidney. The lower pole of the right kidney may be felt as a smooth, rounded mass that descends on inspiration. If the kidney is palpable, its size, contour, and tenderness should be noted. Kidney enlargement is suggestive of neoplasm or other serious renal pathology.

The urinary bladder is normally not palpable unless it is distended with urine. If the bladder is full, it may be felt as a smooth, round, firm organ and is sensitive to palpation.

Percussion. Tenderness in the flank area may be detected by fist percussion. This technique is performed by striking the fist (kidney punch) of one hand against the dorsal surface of the other hand, which is placed flat along the posterior CVA margin. Normally a firm blow in the flank area should not elicit pain. If CVA tenderness and pain are present, it may indicate a kidney infection or polycystic kidney disease.

Normally a bladder is not percussible until it contains 150 ml of urine. If the bladder is full, dullness is heard above the symphysis pubis. A distended bladder may be percussed as high as the umbilicus.

Auscultation. The diaphragm of the stethoscope may be used to auscultate over both CVAs and in the upper abdominal quadrants. With this technique, the abdominal aorta and renal arteries are auscultated for a bruit (an abnormal murmur), which indicates impaired blood flow to the kidneys.

Table 42-6 shows how to record the normal physical assessment findings of the urinary system. Table 42-7 presents common assessment abnormalities of the urinary system. Normally, assessment findings may vary in the older adult. Table 42-2 shows the age-related changes in the urinary system and differences in assessment findings.

Table 42-6 Normal Physical Assessment of the Urinary System
No costovertebral angle tenderness
Nonpalpable kidney and bladder
No palpable masses

COMMON ASSESSMENT ABNORMALITIES

Table 42-7 Urinary System

Finding	Description	Possible Etiology and Significance
▪ Dysuria	Painful or difficult urination	Sign of urinary tract infection and wide variety of pathologic conditions
▪ Frequency	Increased incidence of urinating	Acutely inflamed bladder, retention with overflow, excess fluid intake
▪ Enuresis	Involuntary nocturnal urinating	Symptomatic of lower urinary tract disorder
▪ Hesitancy	Delay or difficulty in initiating urination	Partial urethral obstruction
▪ Urgency	Strong desire to urinate	Inflammatory lesions in bladder or urethra, acute bacterial infections
▪ Hematuria	Blood in the urine	Cancer of genitourinary tract, blood dyscrasias, renal disease, urinary tract infection, stones in kidney or ureter, medications (anticoagulants)
▪ Burning on urination	Stinging pain in urethral area	Urethral irritation, urinary tract infection
▪ Pneumaturia	Passage of urine containing gas	Fistula connections between bowel and bladder, gas-forming urinary tract infections
▪ Retention	Inability to urinate, even though bladder contains excessive amount of urine	Finding after pelvic surgery, childbirth, catheter removal; urethral stricture or obstruction; neurogenic bladder; postanesthesia
▪ Pain	Presence over suprapubic area (related to bladder), urethral pain (irritation of bladder neck), flank (CVA) pain	Infection, urinary retention, foreign body in urinary tract, urethritis, pyelonephritis, renal colic or stones
▪ Incontinence	Inability to voluntarily control discharge of urine	Neurogenic bladder, bladder infection, injury to external sphincter
▪ Stress incontinence	Involuntary urination with increased pressure (sneezing or coughing)	Weakness of sphincter control
▪ Nocturia	Frequency of urination at night	Renal disease with impaired concentrating ability, bladder obstruction, congestive heart failure, diabetes mellitus, finding after renal transplant
▪ Polyuria	Large volume of urine in a given time	Diabetes mellitus, diabetes insipidus, chronic renal failure, diuretics, excess fluid intake
▪ Anuria	Technically no urination (24 hr urine output <100 ml)	Acute renal failure, end-stage renal disease, bilateral ureteral obstruction
▪ Oliguria	Diminished amount of urine in a given time (24 hr urine output of 100-400 ml)	Severe dehydration, shock, transfusion reaction, kidney disease, end-stage renal disease

CVA, costovertebral angle.

DIAGNOSTIC STUDIES OF THE URINARY SYSTEM

Table 42-8 contains diagnostic studies common to the urinary system. Diagnostic studies are important in locating and understanding problems of the urinary system. The accuracy of the results is influenced by (1) adherence to the proper procedures related to the study and (2) cooperation of the patient in restricting fluids, collecting urine specimens, lying quietly on the examination table, or following other instructions.

Many radiologic studies require the use of a bowel preparation the evening before the study to clear the lower GI tract of feces and flatus. Because the kidneys lie in a retroperitoneal location, the contents of the colon may obstruct visualization of the urinary tract. If a bowel preparation is not properly done, the study may be unsuccessful and have to be rescheduled. Commonly used bowel preparations include enemas, castor oil, magnesium citrate, and bisacodyl (Dulcolax) tablets or suppositories. Sometimes a further bowel preparation is required the morning of the study. Some bowel preparations, such as magnesium citrate and Fleet Enema, are contraindicated in the patient with renal failure. Magnesium cannot be excreted by patients with renal failure (see Chapter 44).

When a patient has repeated diagnostic studies on consecutive days, it is important to prevent dehydration. It is not uncommon to have a patient take nothing by mouth (NPO) after midnight, spend all morning in the x-ray department, return too late for lunch or too tired to eat, sleep all afternoon, and be on NPO status after midnight again because of studies the next day. Severe dehydration, especially in a diabetic, debilitated, or older patient, may lead to acute renal failure. The nurse is responsible for ensuring that a patient undergoing diagnostic studies is properly hydrated and given adequate nourishment between studies. The nurse should also check with the physician regarding the insulin dose for the diabetic patient who is NPO.

Another important nursing responsibility related to diagnostic studies is providing the patient with an adequate explanation of the procedure. The period during a diagnostic workup is typically a time of anxiety for most patients. The fear inherent in not knowing what is wrong is often worse than the diagnosis itself. Additional anxiety is caused by the unknown

DIAGNOSTIC STUDIES

Table 42-8 Urinary System

Study	Description and Purpose	Nursing Responsibility
Urine Studies		
▪ Urinalysis	Study is a general examination of urine to establish baseline information or provide data to establish a tentative diagnosis and determine whether further studies are to be ordered. (See Table 42-9)	Try to obtain first urinated morning specimen. Ensure that specimen is examined within 1 hr of urinating. Wash perineal area if soiled with menses or fecal material.
▪ Creatinine clearance	Creatinine is a waste product of protein breakdown (primarily body muscle mass). Clearance of creatinine by the kidney approximates the GFR. *Normal finding* is 85-135 ml/min.	Collect 24 hr urine specimen. Discard first urination when test is started. Save urine from all subsequent urinations for 24 hr. Instruct patient to urinate at end of 24 hr, and add specimen to collection. Ensure that serum creatinine is determined during 24 hr period.
▪ Urine culture ("clean catch," "midstream")	Study is done to confirm suspected urinary tract infection and identify causative organisms. *Normally,* bladder is sterile, but urethra contains bacteria and a few WBCs. If properly collected, stored, and handled: <10,000 organisms/ml usually indicates no infection; 10,000-100,000/ml is usually not diagnostic, and test may have to be repeated; >100,000/ml indicates infection.	Use sterile container for collection of urine. Touch only outside of container. For women, separate labia with one hand and clean meatus with other hand, using at least three sponges (saturated with cleansing solution) in a front-to-back motion. For men, retract foreskin (if present) and cleanse glans with at least three cleansing sponges. After cleaning, instruct patient to start urinating and then continue voiding in sterile container. (The initial voided urine flushes out most contaminants in the urethra and perineal area.) Inform physician of need for catheterization if patient is unable to cooperate with this procedure.
▪ Concentration test	Study evaluates renal concentration ability. Concentration is measured by specific gravity readings. *Normal finding* is 1.020-1.035.	Instruct patient to fast after given time in evening (in usual procedure). Collect three urine specimens at hourly intervals in morning.
▪ Residual urine	Study determines amount of urine left in bladder after urinating. Finding may be abnormal in problems with bladder innervation, sphincter impairment, BPH, or urethral strictures. *Normal finding* is ≤50 ml urine (increases with age).	If residual urine test is ordered, catheterize patient immediately after urinating or use bladder ultrasound equipment. If a large amount of residual urine is obtained, physician may want catheter left in bladder.
▪ Protein determination—Dipstick (Albustix, Combistix)	Test detects protein (primarily albumin) in urine. *Normal finding* is 0-trace.	Dip end of stick in urine, and read result by comparison with color chart on label as directed. Grading is from 0 to 4+. Interpret with caution. A positive result may not indicate significant proteinuria; some medications may give false-positive readings.
Quantitative test for protein	A 12- or 24-hr collection gives a more accurate indication of the amount of protein in urine. Persistent proteinuria usually indicates glomerular renal disease. *Normal finding* is <150 mg/24 hr (<0.15 g/24 hr), consisting mainly of albumin.	Perform 12 or 24 hr urine collection.
▪ Urine cytology	Study is used to identify changes in cellular structure indicative of malignancy, especially bladder cancer.	Obtain urine and send immediately to lab. The first morning specimen should *not* be used.
Blood Chemistries		
▪ BUN	Study is most commonly used to identify presence of renal problems. Concentration of urea in blood is regulated by rate at which kidney excretes urea. *Normal finding* is 10-30 mg/dl (1.8-7.1 mmol/L).	Be aware that when interpreting BUN, nonrenal factors may cause increase (e.g., rapid cell destruction from infections, fever, GI bleeding, trauma, athletic activity with excessive muscle breakdown, corticosteroid therapy).

Continued

DIAGNOSTIC STUDIES

Table 42-8 Urinary System—cont'd

Study	Description and Purpose	Nursing Responsibility
Blood Chemistries—cont'd		
▪ Creatinine	Study is more reliable than BUN as a determinant of renal function. Creatinine is end-product of muscle and protein metabolism and is liberated at a constant rate. *Normal finding* is 0.5-1.5 mg/dl (44-133 μmol/L). Results are higher in men.	Explain test, and watch for postpuncture bleeding.
▪ BUN/creatinine ratio	*Normal finding* is 10:1.	
▪ Uric acid	Study is used as a screening test primarily for disorders of purine metabolism but can indicate kidney disease as well. Values depend on renal function and rate of purine metabolism and dietary intake of food rich in purines. *Normal finding* is 2.5-5.5 mg/dl (149-327 μmol/L) for women and 4.5-6.5 mg/dl (268-387 μmol/L) for men.	Explain test, and watch for postpuncture bleeding.
▪ Sodium	Sodium is main extracellular electrolyte determining blood volume. Usually, values stay within normal range until late stages of renal failure. *Normal finding* is 135-145 mEq/L (135-145 mmol/L).	Explain test, and watch for postpuncture bleeding.
▪ Potassium	Kidneys are responsible for excreting majority of body's potassium. In renal disease, K^+ determinations are critical because K^+ is one of the first electrolytes to become abnormal. Elevated K^+ levels of >6 mEq/L can lead to muscle weakness and cardiac arrhythmias. *Normal finding* is 3.5-5.5 mEq/L (3.5-5.5 mmol/L).	Explain test, and watch for postpuncture bleeding.
▪ Calcium	Calcium is main mineral in bone and aids in muscular contraction, neurotransmission, and clotting. In renal disease, decreased absorption of Ca^{2+} leads to renal osteodystrophy. *Normal finding* is 9-11 mg/dl (4.5-5.5 mEq/L, 2.25-2.74 mmol/L).	Explain test, and watch for postpuncture bleeding.
▪ Phosphorus	Phosphorus balance is inversely related to Ca^{2+} balance. In renal disease, phosphorus levels are elevated because the kidney is the primary excretory organ. Soft tissue calcification may occur if both Ca^{2+} and phosphorus are elevated. *Normal finding* is 2.8-4.5 mg/dl (0.9-1.45 mmol/L).	Explain test, and watch for postpuncture bleeding.
▪ Bicarbonate	Most patients in renal failure have metabolic acidosis and low serum HCO_3^- levels. *Normal finding* is 20-30 mEq/L (20-30 mmol/L).	Explain test, and watch for postpuncture bleeding.
Radiologic Procedures		
▪ Kidneys, ureters, bladder (KUB)	Study involves flat-plate x-ray examination of abdomen and pelvis and delineates size, shape, and position of kidneys.	Perform bowel preparation (if ordered).
▪ IVP or excretory urogram	X-ray examination visualizes urinary tract after IV injection of contrast material.	Evening before procedure, give cathartic or enema to empty colon of feces and gas. Keep patient on NPO status 8 hr before procedure. Before procedure, assess patient for iodine sensitivity to avoid anaphylactic reaction. Inform patient that procedure involves lying on table and having serial x-rays taken. After procedure, force fluids (if permitted) to flush out contrast material.

Continued

DIAGNOSTIC STUDIES

Table 42-8 Urinary System—cont'd

Study	Description and Purpose	Nursing Responsibility
Radiologic Procedures—cont'd		
▪ Nephrotomogram	X-ray is taken with rotating tubes. Test delineates segments of the kidney at different levels. Multiple exposures are taken to visualize specific sections of the kidney after IV injection of contrast material.	Explain procedure, and prepare patient as for IVP.
▪ Retrograde pyelogram	X-ray of urinary tract is taken after injection of contrast material into kidneys. Cystoscope is inserted, and ureteral catheters are inserted through it into renal pelvis. Contrast material is injected through catheters.	Prepare patient as for IVP. Inform patient that pain may be experienced from distention of pelvis and discomfort from cystoscope. Inform patient that general anesthesia may be given for procedure.
▪ Cystogram	Contrast material is instilled into bladder via cystoscope or catheter. Purpose is to visualize bladder and evaluate vesicoureteral reflux.	Explain procedure to patient. If done via cystoscope, follow nursing care related to cystoscopy.
▪ Renal arteriogram (angiogram)	Study is performed by injecting contrast material into renal artery via catheter inserted into femoral artery. Purpose is to visualize renal blood vessels.	Prepare patient evening before procedure by giving cathartic or enema. Before injection of contrast material, test for iodine sensitivity. After procedure, check insertion site for bleeding, and take peripheral pulses in involved leg every 30-60 min to detect occluded blood flow.
▪ Ultrasound	Small external ultrasound probe is placed on patient's skin. Conductive gel is applied to the skin. Noninvasive procedure involves passing sound waves into body structures and recording images as they are reflected back. Computer interprets tissue density based on sound waves and displays it in picture form. Study is most valuable in detection of renal or perirenal masses, differential diagnosis of renal cysts, solid masses, and identification of obstructions. It can be used safely in patients with renal failure.	Explain procedure to patient.
▪ CT scan	Study provides excellent visualization of kidneys. Kidney size can be evaluated; tumors, abscesses, suprarenal masses (e.g., adrenal tumors, pheochromocytomas), and obstructions can be detected. Advantage of CT over ultrasound is its ability to distinguish subtle differences in density. Use of IV-administered contrast material during CT accentuates density of renal tissue and helps differentiate masses.	Explain procedure to patient.
▪ MRI	Computer-generated films rely on radio waves and alteration in magnetic field. Useful for visualization of kidneys. Not proven useful for detecting urinary calculi or calcified tumors.	Explain procedure to patient. Have patient remove all metal objects. Patients with a history of claustrophobia may need to be sedated.
Renal Radionuclide Imaging		
▪ Renal scan	Radioactive isotopes are injected IV. Radiation detector probes are placed over kidney, and scintillation counter monitors radioactive material in kidney. Purpose is to show blood flow, glomerular filtration, tubular function, and excretion. Radioisotope distribution in kidney is scanned and mapped. Test is useful in showing location, size, and shape of kidney and, in general, assessing blood perfusion and its ability to secrete urine. Abscesses, cysts, and tumors may appear as cold spots because of presence of nonfunctioning tissue.	Requires no dietary or activity restriction. Inform patient that no pain or discomfort should be felt during test.

Continued

DIAGNOSTIC STUDIES

Table 42-8 Urinary System—cont'd

Study	Description and Purpose	Nursing Responsibility
Endoscopy		
▪ Cystoscopy	Study involves use of tubular lighted scope to inspect bladder. Lithotomy position is used. It may be done using local or general anesthesia.	Before procedure, force fluids or give IV fluids if general anesthesia is to be used. Ensure consent form is signed. Explain procedure to patient. Give preoperative medication. After procedure, explain that burning on urination, pink-tinged urine, and urinary frequency are expected effects after cystoscopy. Do not let patient walk alone immediately after procedure because orthostatic hypotension may occur. Offer warm sitz baths, heat, mild analgesics to relieve discomfort.
Urodynamics		
▪ Cystometrogram	Study involves insertion of catheter and instillation of water or saline solution into bladder. Measurements of pressure exerted against bladder wall are recorded. Purpose is to evaluate bladder tone, sensations of filling, and bladder (detrusor) stability.	Explain procedure to patient. Observe patient for manifestations of urinary infection after procedure.
Invasive Procedure		
▪ Renal biopsy	Technique is usually done as a skin (percutaneous) biopsy through needle insertion into lower lobe of kidney. Purpose is to obtain renal tissue for examination to determine type of renal disease or to follow progress of renal disease.	Before procedure, ascertain coagulation status through patient history, medication history, CBC, hematocrit, prothrombin time, and bleeding and clotting time. Type and crossmatch patient for blood. Ensure consent form is signed. Be aware that IVP or ultrasound study is done before biopsy. After procedure, apply pressure dressing to biopsy site, and check frequently for bleeding. Keep patient on bed rest up to 24 hr. Take vital signs frequently. Observe urine for gross bleeding. Determine microscopic bleeding by use of dipstick. Assess patient for flank pain. Monitor hematocrit levels.

†See Chapter 44.
BPH, benign prostatic hyperplasia; *CBC,* complete blood count; *CT,* computed tomography; *GFR,* glomerular filtration rate; *IVP,* intravenous pyelogram; *KUB,* kidneys, ureters, bladder; *MRI,* magnetic resonance imaging; *NPO,* nothing by mouth; *WBC,* white blood cell.

nature of the procedure. The patient needs to know what the procedure involves and its basic purpose, where it will be done, how long it will take, and whether it will hurt. These things should be explained at a level appropriate to the patient's understanding. The patient should also be instructed on personal responsibility during a particular study (e.g., to lie flat on the table or to keep the legs straight).

Diagnostic studies of the urinary system often cause embarrassment and emotional stress. Examination of the urinary system may be perceived as an intrusion on a personal body area. The nurse should alleviate anxiety by providing privacy and protecting the patient's modesty.

Urine Studies

Urinalysis. In evaluating disorders of the urinary tract, one of the first studies done is a urinalysis (Tables 42-8 and 42-9). This test may provide information about possible abnormalities, indicate what further studies need to be done, and supply information on the progression of a diagnosed disorder.

For a routine urinalysis, a specimen may be collected at any time of the day. However, it is best to obtain the first specimen urinated in the morning. This concentrated specimen is more likely to contain abnormal constituents if they are present in the urine. The specimen should be examined within 1 hour of urinating. If it is not, bacteria multiply rapidly, RBCs hemolyze, casts disintegrate, and the urine becomes alkaline as a result of urea-splitting bacteria. If it is not possible to send the specimen to the laboratory immediately, it should be refrigerated. However, to obtain the best results, the nurse should coordinate specimen collection with routine laboratory hours.

Multiple reagent strips (also called urine dipsticks) are commonly used by laboratories and in outpatient settings to provide chemical analysis of urine along with a microscopic interpretation. The results of a urinalysis usually include a description of the appearance, specific gravity (mass and density), pH, glucose, ketones, and protein in the urine and a microscopic examination of urine sediment for white blood cells (WBCs), RBCs, crystals, and casts (see Table 42-9).

Table **42-9** Urinalysis Findings

Test	Normal	Abnormal Finding and Significance
Color	Amber yellow	▪ Dark, smoky color suggests hematuria. Yellow brown to olive green indicates excessive bilirubin. Orange red or orange brown caused by phenazopyridine (Pyridium) or urobilin in excess. Cloudiness of freshly voided urine indicates infection. Colorless urine indicates excessive fluid intake, renal disease, or diabetes insipidus.
Smell	Aromatic	▪ On standing, urine becomes more ammonia-like in smell. In urinary tract infections, urine smells unpleasant.
Protein	0-150 mg/24 hr 0-18 mg/dl	▪ Persistent proteinuria is characteristic of acute and chronic renal disease, especially involving glomeruli. In absence of disease, positive reading may be caused by high-protein diet, strenuous exercise, dehydration, fever, or emotional stress. Vaginal secretions may contaminate urine specimen and give positive reading.
Glucose	None	▪ Glycosuria indicates diabetes mellitus or low renal threshold for glucose reabsorption (if blood glucose level is normal). Small amounts may be found after glucose loading (e.g., glucose tolerance test).
Ketones	None	▪ Altered carbohydrate and fat metabolism indicates diabetes mellitus and starvation. Findings can also be seen in dehydration, vomiting, and severe diarrhea.
Bilirubin	None	▪ Presence of bilirubinuria is as significant as jaundice in detection of liver disorders. Bilirubin may appear in urine before jaundice becomes visible or may be present in persons with hepatic disorders who do not have recognizable jaundice.*
Nitrite	None	▪ Gram-negative bacteria commonly cause urinary infection and have an enzyme that produces nitrite in the urine. When nitrite is positive and WBCs are present, the probability of urinary infection is high. A negative nitrite, however, does not rule out infection because gram-positive organisms and yeast do not contain the converting enzyme.
Specific gravity	1.003-1.030	▪ Specific gravity of morning urine specimen reflects maximum concentrating ability of kidney and is 1.025-1.030. Low specific gravity indicates dilute urine and possibly excessive diuresis. High specific gravity indicates dehydration. If it becomes fixed at about 1.010, this indicates renal inability to concentrate urine, suggesting that kidney is progressing to end-stage renal disease.
Osmolality	300-1300 mOsm/kg (300-1300 mmol/kg)	▪ Measurement is a more accurate method than specific gravity for determining diluting and concentrating ability of kidneys. Deviations from normal indicate tubular dysfunction. Findings indicate if kidney has lost ability to concentrate or dilute urine. (Not part of routine urinalysis.)
pH	4.0-8.0 (average, 6.0)	▪ If >8.0, finding may be the result of standing of urine or urinary tract infections because bacteria decompose urea to form ammonia. If <4.0, may indicate respiratory or metabolic acidosis.
RBC	0-4/hpf	▪ Bleeding in urinary tract is caused by calculi, cystitis, neoplasm, glomerulonephritis, tuberculosis, kidney biopsy, or trauma.
WBC	0-5/hpf	▪ Increased number of WBCs in urine (pyuria) indicates urinary tract infection or inflammation.
Casts	None-occasional hyaline	▪ Casts are molds of the renal tubules and may contain protein, WBCs, RBCs, or bacteria. Noncellular casts are hyaline in appearance, and a few may be found in normal urine. Casts indicate renal dysfunction or urinary tract infections.
Culture for organisms	No organisms in bladder, $<10^4$ organisms/ml result of normal urethral flora	▪ Bacteria counts $>10^5$/ml indicate urinary tract infection. Organisms most commonly found in urinary tract infections are *Escherichia coli,* enterococci, *Klebsiella, Proteus,* and streptococci.

*See Chapter 41 for further discussion.
hpf, high-powered field.

Composite Urine Collections. Composite urine specimens are collected over a period that may range from 2 to 24 hours. The purpose of a composite specimen is to examine or measure specific components, such as electrolytes, sugar, protein, 17-ketosteroids, catecholamines, creatinine, and minerals. These specimens may have to be refrigerated, or preservatives may have to be added to the container used for collecting urine.

For collection of a composite urine specimen, the patient is instructed to urinate and discard this first urine specimen. This time is noted as the start of the test. All urine from subsequent urinations is saved in a container for the designated period. Finally, at the end of the period, the patient is asked to urinate and this urine is added to the container. Incomplete collections do not provide valid results. Reminding the patient to save all urine during the study period is critical.

Creatinine Clearance. One of the most common composite indicators used to analyze urinary system disorders is creatinine clearance. Creatinine is a waste product produced by muscle breakdown. Urinary excretion of creatinine is a measure of the amount of active muscle tissue in the body, not of body weight. Therefore people with larger muscle mass have higher values. Because almost all creatinine in the blood is normally excreted by the kidneys, creatinine clearance is the most accurate indicator of renal function. The result of a creatinine clearance closely approximates that of the GFR. A blood specimen for serum creatinine determination should be obtained during the period of urine collection. Creatinine clearance is calculated as follows:

$$\text{Creatinine clearance (ml/min)} = \frac{\text{Urine creatinine (mg/ml)} \times \text{Urine volume (ml/min)}}{\text{Serum creatinine (mg/ml)}}$$

Creatinine levels remain remarkably constant for each person because they are not significantly affected by protein ingestion, muscular exercise, water intake, or rate of urine production. Normal creatinine clearance values range from 85 to 135 ml per minute. After age 40, the creatinine clearance rate decreases at a rate of about 1 ml per minute per year.

Urine Cytology. Urine can be checked for abnormal cellular structures that occur with bladder cancer. Specimens may be obtained by voiding, catheterization, or bladder irrigation (bladder washing). The first morning's voided specimen should not be used because epithelial cells may change in appearance in urine held in the bladder overnight. As with urinalysis, the specimen should be fresh or brought to the lab within the hour. An alcohol-based fixative is then added to preserve the cellular structure. Urine cytology is currently being used for detection of and following the prognosis of bladder cancer.[9,10]

Radiologic Studies

Kidney, Ureter, and Bladder Film. The kidney, ureter, and bladder (KUB) film is an abdominal view taken without using a contrast medium to show the renal outline, psoas shadow, and the bladder, if full. Radiopaque stones and foreign bodies can be seen on this x-ray. The form, size, and position of the kidneys can also be seen. Abscesses, tumors, and cysts may distort anatomic relationships on the KUB. Sometimes tomograms (sectional views that focus on a single plane of the kidney) are ordered at the same time as the KUB x-ray.

Intravenous Pyelogram. The purpose of an intravenous pyelogram (IVP), or excretory urogram, is to visualize the urinary tract. The presence, position, size, and shape of the kidneys, ureters, and bladder can be evaluated. Cysts, tumors, lesions, and obstructions cause a distortion in the normal appearance of these structures. The IVP also gives clues to renal function since sequential films are taken, but other tests (discussed later) are more accurate for this purpose.

The procedure consists of injecting an IV dose of contrast material, which circulates in the blood and is excreted by the kidneys into the urine. During injection, the patient may experience warmth, a flushed face, and a salty taste. After injection, films are taken sequentially. (A rapid-sequence IVP has x-ray films taken every minute for the first 5 minutes.) The sequencing of films is planned so that contrast excretion can be followed from the cortex of the kidney to the bladder. A film taken at 45 minutes allows visualization of the bladder. The presence of bladder atony or outlet obstruction also can be detected by a film taken after urination, which shows the residual volume of urine in the bladder.

Preparation of the patient the evening before the test includes giving a cathartic or an enema to eliminate feces and air from the colon. The patient with neurologic bowel dysfunction may require more vigorous routines. Fluids are withheld for 8 hours before testing to produce slight dehydration so that the contrast material will concentrate and therefore improve visualization. The patient with significantly decreased renal function should not have an IVP because the contrast material will not be properly excreted by the kidneys. Contrast medium can also be nephrotoxic and can worsen renal function. An IVP should be avoided on a pregnant patient, particularly in the first trimester, because of radiation exposure and harm to the fetus.

The patient should be assessed for any possible allergic reactions to the contrast material. The contrast medium is typically an iodine derivative of shellfish. A person with iodine sensitivity may have an anaphylactic reaction after contrast material is injected. If known to have an allergy to iodine or seafood, the patient should not have an IVP, or it can be done using prophylactic diphenhydramine (Benadryl) and corticosteroids.

During contrast material injection, the patient should be observed for signs of respiratory distress, urticaria, decrease in blood pressure, and other signs of anaphylaxis. Emergency drugs such as diphenhydramine (Benadryl), corticosteroids, and epinephrine (Adrenalin) and cardiopulmonary resuscitation equipment should be available. A patient may experience transient hypersensitivity reactions (e.g., nausea, itching), but these are not considered serious reactions contraindicating future IVPs.

After the procedure, the nurse should encourage the patient to force fluids to dilute and flush out the contrast material. Dilution of the contrast medium makes it less nephrotoxic. The patient should be monitored for delayed reactions such as itching, nausea, respiratory problems, and decreased urine output.

Retrograde Pyelogram. A retrograde pyelogram evaluates the same structures as an IVP. This is an x-ray visualization of the kidneys, ureter, and bladder after direct injection of a contrast material into the kidney via a ureteral catheter introduced through a cystoscope. It may be done if an IVP does not visualize the urinary tract or if the patient is allergic to the contrast material or has decreased renal function. The dangers associated with a retrograde pyelogram are similar to those related to cystoscopy, including the risk of infection and the use of anesthesia.

Antegrade Pyelogram. Sometimes an antegrade pyelogram is done to evaluate the upper urinary tract when there is allergy to contrast material or decreased renal function and when abnormalities prevent passage of a ureteral catheter. Contrast may be injected percutaneously into the renal pelvis or via a nephrostomy tube that is already in place (also called a nephrostogram) when determining tube function or ureteral integrity after trauma or surgery. Complications of an antegrade pyelogram include hematuria, infection, and hematoma.

Renal Ultrasound. A renal ultrasound uses high-frequency waves to image the kidneys, ureter, and bladder. Because radiation exposure is avoided, a number of images can be obtained, and repeat studies over a brief period of time can be done. Images can be obtained from both the prone and supine positions. A bowel preparation is not required for a renal ultrasound.

Computed Tomography Scan. Computed tomography (CT) of the abdomen and pelvis may be done to detect tumors and possible metastases. The CT scan can differentiate these from cysts or abscesses. Contrast material may be used to help visualize urinary structures more clearly in the computer-generated images produced by the machine. The patient is instructed to lie very still during the procedure while the machine takes precise transaxial images. Sedation may be required if the patient is unable to cooperate.

Magnetic Resonance Imaging. Specific structures such as the kidney or prostate can be visualized by disturbing the electromagnetic fields generated by different body tissues and converting this to computer-generated images. This is done using radiofrequency waves. Magnetic resonance imaging (MRI) helps evaluate genitourinary tumors and abdominal or pelvic masses. The patient must lie still in an enclosed cylinder while these images are being produced. Some patients cannot tolerate being in the small MRI chamber, and sedation may be required. All metal objects must be removed because they interfere with the radiofrequency. The MRI is contraindicated in a patient with a pacemaker or with certain kinds of internal metallic vascular surgical clips.

Cystogram. The purpose of a cystogram is to outline and visualize the bladder and evaluate the UVJ for reflux. In addition to suspected vesicoureteral reflux, indications for a cystogram include a neurogenic bladder and recurrent urinary tract infections. A cystogram can also delineate abnormalities of the bladder, such as diverticuli, calculi, and tumors. The procedure involves instillation of a contrast material into the bladder, which may be done via a cystoscope or catheter.

A voiding cystourethrogram is a voiding study of the bladder opening and urethra. The bladder is filled with contrast material. During urination, films are taken to visualize the bladder and urethra. After urination, another film is taken to assess for residual urine. A voiding cystourethrogram can detect abnormalities of the lower urinary tract, urethral stenosis, bladder neck obstruction, and prostatic enlargement.

Urethrogram. A urethrogram is similar to a cystogram. Contrast material is injected retrograde into the urethra to identify strictures, diverticula, or other urethral pathology. When urethral trauma is suspected, a urethrogram is done before catheterization.

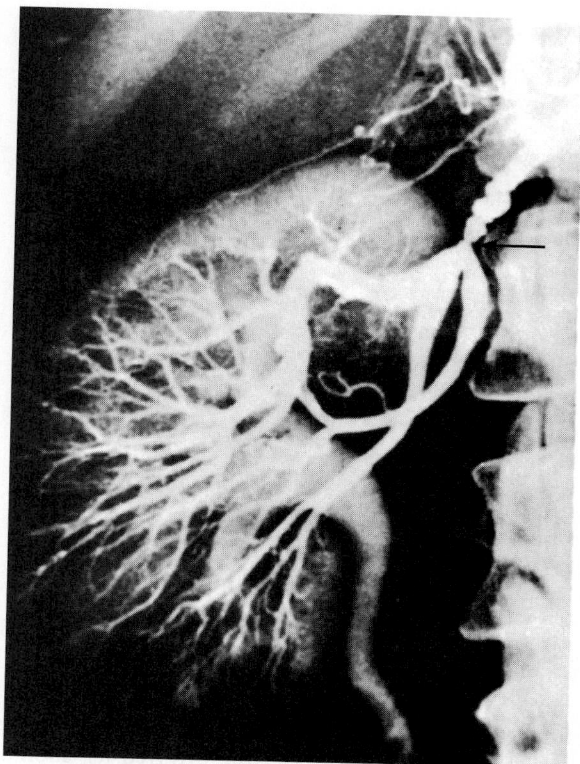

Fig. 42-8 Renal arteriogram showing stenosis of the right renal artery.

Loopogram. A loopogram is used to detect obstructions, anastomotic leaks, stones, reflux, and other uropathology when a patient has a urinary pouch or ileal conduit. Since urinary diversions are created with bowel, there is risk of contrast absorption. The patient should be closely monitored for contrast reactions.

Renal Arteriogram. The purpose of a renal arteriogram (angiogram) is to visualize the renal blood vessels. The findings of an arteriogram can assist in diagnosing renal artery stenosis (Fig. 42-8), additional or missing renal blood vessels, and renovascular hypertension and can assist in differentiating between a renal cyst and a renal tumor. Renal arteriograms are also included in the workup of a potential renal transplant donor.

The evening before the procedure, the patient is given a cathartic to eliminate fecal material from the colon. The morning of the procedure, a preoperative medication is given to relax and sedate the patient.

Most arteriograms are done in the x-ray department by a specially trained physician. The patient is given a local anesthetic at the site of catheter insertion. A catheter is usually inserted into the femoral artery and passed up the aorta to the level of the renal arteries (Fig. 42-9). Contrast material is then injected to outline the renal blood supply, and x-rays are taken. The patient may experience a transient warm feeling along the course of the blood vessel when the contrast material is injected. As with all contrast studies, possible iodine and shellfish allergies should be determined before the study.

After the catheter is removed, a pressure dressing is placed over the femoral injection site. It is important to observe the

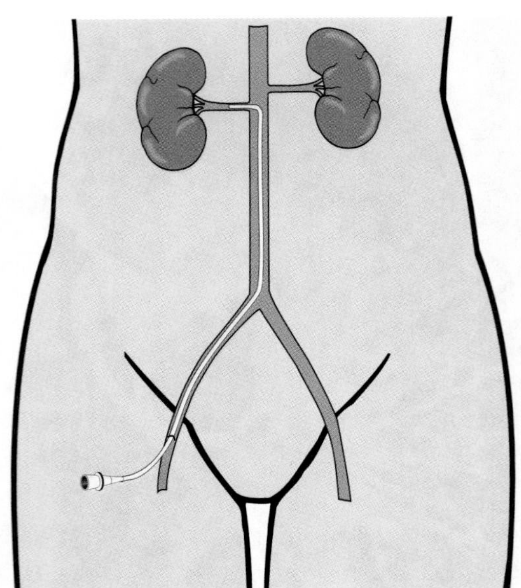

Fig. 42-9 Catheter insertion for a renal arteriogram.

site for bleeding. Bed rest is usually prescribed with the affected leg straight. Peripheral pulses in the involved leg should be taken at least every 30 to 60 minutes to detect occlusion of blood flow caused by a thrombus. Complications that may result from a renal arteriogram include thrombus, embolus, local inflammation, and hematoma. The patient with baseline renal insufficiency may experience a decrease in renal function secondary to the nephrotoxic contrast material.

Digital Subtraction Angiography. Because of potential complications, the renal arteriogram is sometimes replaced by digital subtraction angiography (DSA) in many hospitals that have the facilities to perform this procedure. Using computer technology, this procedure permits visualization of the arteries after an IV injection of contrast material. A primary advantage of DSA is that it requires small peripheral venous injections of contrast medium compared with the relatively large doses that must be injected via arterial cannulation for a renal arteriogram. (See Table 30-7 for a further description of DSA.)

Renal Radionuclide Imaging. Renal scans involving the use of radionuclides are useful in evaluating the anatomic structures, perfusion, and function of the kidneys. Different institutions use different imaging techniques. In general, the following radionuclides are used for these purposes:

Anatomic structures: technetium 99m (^{99m}Tc)–labeled compounds such as dimercaptosuccinic acid (DMSA) or glucoheptonate

Perfusion and function: iodine 131 (^{131}I)–labeled orthoiodohippurate (Hippuran) and ^{99m}Tc-labeled diethylenetriamine pentaacetic acid (DTPA)

Infection or abscesses: gallium 67 citrate

For this procedure a radioactive isotope is injected intravenously. Radiation detector probes are placed over the kidneys, and a scintillation counter monitors the appearance and disappearance of the radioactive material in the kidney.

The results reveal the difference between the two kidneys with respect to blood flow, tubular function, and excretion. A normal scan shows symmetric functioning of both kidneys. Normally the distribution of activity is recorded throughout the kidneys. A lesion (e.g., a tumor) is indicated by the absence of radioactivity in the involved area and the appearance of the resultant defect on the scan. In renovascular disease, an area with decreased blood flow can be readily visualized. This study is particularly useful in detecting renal vascular disease, acute renal failure, and upper urinary tract obstruction, as well as useful in monitoring the function of a transplanted kidney.

Usually there are no dietary or activity restrictions related to preparation of the patient. During the test the patient should feel no pain or discomfort. No special precautions are needed in the use of radioactive material since only tracer doses are used.

Renal Biopsy. The purpose of a renal biopsy is to determine the nature and extent of renal disease. This information can be used in establishing a diagnosis and following the progress of a disease, as well as determining the treatment. Biopsy material can be obtained through an open biopsy or a closed percutaneous needle biopsy. An open biopsy is rarely performed because it requires a surgical procedure with anesthesia. A percutaneous needle biopsy is more common. It is usually done in the x-ray department or in the patient's room, although it may be done in the operating room.

Absolute contraindications to a percutaneous renal biopsy are bleeding disorders, the presence of a single kidney, and uncontrolled hypertension. Relative contraindications include suspected renal infection, hydronephrosis, and possible vascular lesions.

Because hemorrhage is one danger of biopsy, the patient's coagulation status should be assessed before the procedure. This includes a health history, complete blood count, hematocrit, prothrombin time, and bleeding or clotting time determinations. The patient may also be typed and crossmatched for blood. The patient who is to be biopsied should not be taking aspirin or warfarin (Coumadin) before the procedure.

An IVP or ultrasound examination is done to determine the position and location of the kidneys as a guide to needle insertion. Preparation also includes explaining the procedure to the patient and discussing all concerns. A signed consent form is required before a biopsy is performed.

The procedure consists of having the patient lie prone with a pillow or sandbag to elevate the abdomen and kidneys. Using the IVP or ultrasound findings as a guide, the position of the kidney is marked on the body. Local anesthesia is used, and a biopsy needle is inserted into the kidney just below the twelfth rib. The patient is instructed to hold his or her breath while the biopsy specimen is being taken.

After the procedure, a pressure dressing is applied, and the patient is kept prone for 30 to 60 minutes. Usually bed rest is prescribed for 24 hours. Vital signs should be taken every 5 to 10 minutes during the first hour and then with decreasing frequency, if no problems are noted. The biopsy site should be inspected frequently for bleeding. Serial urine specimens should be assessed for gross and microscopic hematuria. A dipstick can be used to test for bleeding, even when hematuria is not obvious. The physician may order all urine sent for laboratory analysis to detect possible hematuria. The patient should also

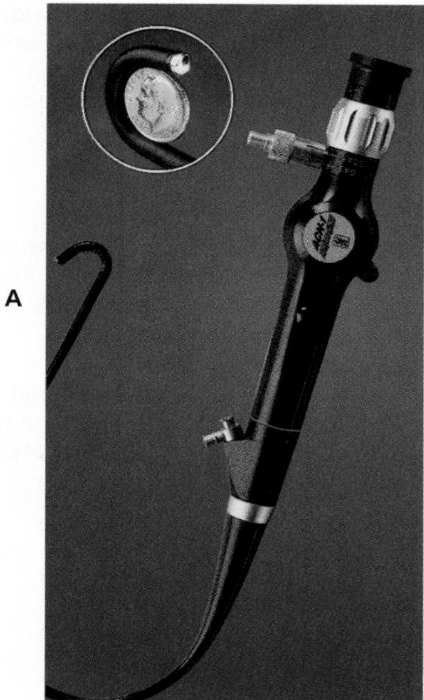

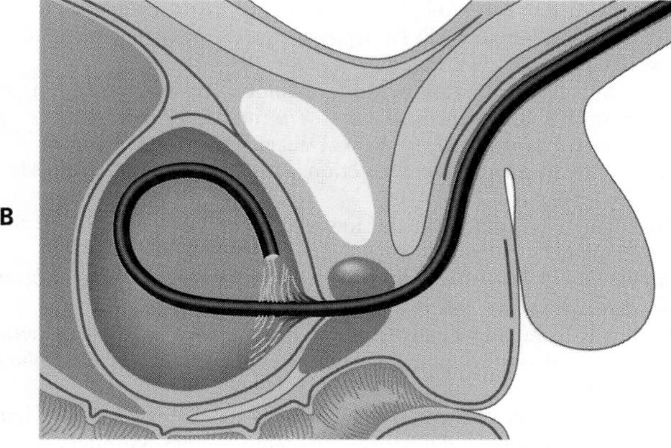

Fig. 42-10 Cystoscopic examination of the bladder in a man. **A,** Flexible Cysto Nephroscope. **B,** Scope inserted into bladder.

be assessed for flank pain, hypotension, decreasing hematocrit, and temperature elevation. The patient should be observed for chills, urinary frequency, and dysuria.

Complications of a renal biopsy include renal hemorrhage, hematoma, and infection. Even if no complications occur, the patient should be instructed to avoid lifting heavy objects for 5 to 7 days. The patient should be instructed not to take any anticoagulant medication until permission is given by the physician who performed the biopsy.

Endoscopy

Cystoscopy. The main purpose of cystoscopy is to inspect the interior of the bladder with a tubular lighted scope called a *cystoscope* (Fig. 42-10). Cystoscopes can be used to insert ureteral catheters, remove calculi, obtain biopsy specimens of bladder lesions, and treat bleeding lesions. In most cases, bladder disorders can be determined by cystoscopic examination. Although rigid instruments still are used, newer flexible cystoscopes (and ureteroscopes) make visualization easier for the urologist and the procedure more comfortable for the patient.

Cystoscopy is usually done in a cystoscopy room in the x-ray department, in urology clinics, or in the operating room. A signed consent form may be required. The cystoscopic examination may be performed with local or general anesthesia, depending on the needs and condition of the patient. The patient may be put in a lithotomy position. Most of the pain associated with cystoscopy results from spasms and contractions of bladder and sphincter. Relaxation and deep breathing by the patient alleviate some of the bladder and sphincter spasms. A local anesthetic is instilled into the urethra before scope insertion. During the examination, saline solution is inserted slowly to distend the bladder. This allows better visualization but causes an urge to urinate.

After the procedure the patient can expect to have some burning on urination, blood-tinged urine, and urinary frequency from the irritation of scope insertion and manipulation. The nurse should observe for bright-red bleeding, which is not normal. The patient should not be allowed to walk without assistance immediately after the procedure because postural hypotension may result from blood flow back to the legs after the patient has been in a lithotomy position. After the procedure the nurse is responsible for keeping the patient well hydrated, administering mild analgesics, providing sitz baths, and applying heat to decrease the patient's discomfort. Complications that may result from cystoscopy include urinary retention, urinary tract hemorrhage, bladder infection, and perforation of the bladder.

Urodynamics

Urodynamics can involve many tests that are used to evaluate voiding problems. The extent of testing depends on the patient's problems and access to urodynamic laboratories. Complex urodynamics are done in special clinics. Two common urodynamic tests done in hospitals or clinics are the urinary flow rate and cystometrogram.

Urinary Flow Rate. The urinary flow rate study measures urine volume in a single voiding expelled in a period of time and is expressed as milliliters per second. As the patient voids, the stream pattern is depicted graphically on a printout.

The patient is asked to start the test with a full bladder, urinate into a special container, and try to empty completely. This test is used to (1) assess the degree of outflow obstruction caused by such conditions as benign prostatic hyperplasia or stricture, (2) assess bladder or sphincter dysfunction effects on voiding such as occurs with neuropathology, and (3) evaluate the effects of treatment for lower urinary tract problems. A residual urine volume may be obtained after a urinary flow rate using ultrasound or catheterization.

A normal maximum flow rate for men is about 20 to 25 ml/sec and about 25 to 30 ml/sec for women. However, the volume voided and the patient's age can affect the flow rate, so normal variations are common. Graphic displays can illustrate straining and intermittent flow patterns or other abnormal voiding disorders.[11]

Cystometrogram. The purpose of a cystometrogram is to evaluate bladder tone and neurologic bladder dysfunction. It is usually ordered if a patient has incontinence or neurogenic dysfunction of the bladder.

The procedure consists of insertion of a retention catheter while the patient is in a supine position. A liter bottle of saline solution or water and a cystometer are connected to the catheter and taped to an IV pole for measurement. Fluid is instilled at a constant rate, and the pressure exerted against the bladder wall is measured. The patient is asked to indicate when the urge to void is first experienced (usually after 100 to 200 ml has been instilled). Fluids are instilled until urgency occurs (350 to 450 ml) or until it is determined that this sensation is absent. After the catheter is withdrawn the patient is asked to empty the bladder, and the amount of residual urine is determined. During the study a cholinergic drug such as bethanechol (Urecholine) may be given to determine whether it will enhance the tone of a flaccid bladder. However, an anticholinergic drug may be given to promote relaxation of a hyperactive bladder. Water or carbon dioxide gas may be used for this examination. Complete urodynamic studies are often done simultaneously using specialized equipment and catheters.

REVIEW QUESTIONS

The number of the question corresponds to the same-numbered objective at the beginning of the chapter.

1. A renal stone in the pelvis of the kidney will alter the function of the kidney by interfering with
   a. the structural support of the kidney.
   b. regulation of the concentration of urine.
   c. the entry and exit of blood vessels at the kidney.
   d. collection and drainage of urine from the kidney.
2. A patient with renal disease has oliguria and a creatinine clearance of 40 ml/min. The nurse recognizes that these findings most directly reflect abnormal function of
   a. tubular secretion.
   b. glomerular filtration.
   c. capillary permeability.
   d. concentration of filtrate.
3. The nurse identifies a risk for urinary calculi in a patient who relates a past health history that includes
   a. measles.
   b. gastric ulcer.
   c. diabetes mellitus.
   d. hyperparathyroidism.
4. Normal changes associated with aging of the urinary system that the nurse expects to find include
   a. decreased levels of BUN.
   b. postvoiding urine residual.
   c. increased bladder capacity.
   d. more easily palpable kidneys.
5. During physical assessment of the urinary system the nurse
   a. percusses the flank area with a firm blow.
   b. palpates an empty bladder as a small nodule.
   c. positions the patient prone to palpate the kidneys.
   d. uses auscultation to determine the level of urine in the bladder.
6. Normal findings expected by the nurse on physical assessment of the urinary system include
   a. nonpalpable left kidney.
   b. auscultation of renal artery bruit.
   c. CVA tenderness elicited by a kidney punch.
   d. palpable bladder to the level of the pubic symphysis.
7. An important nursing responsibility after an intravenous pyelogram is to
   a. assess the patient for flank pain.
   b. encourage extra oral fluid intake.
   c. observe urine for remaining contrast material.
   d. encourage ambulation 2 to 3 hours after the study.
8. On reading the urinalysis results of a dehydrated patient the nurse would expect to find
   a. a pH of 8.4.
   b. RBC of 4/hpf.
   c. color: yellow, cloudy.
   d. specific gravity of 1.035.

References

1. Smith HW: *Fish to philosopher,* Boston, 1953, Little, Brown.
2. McCance KL, Huether SE: *Pathophysiology: the biologic basis for disease in adults and children,* ed 3, St Louis, 1998, Mosby.
3. Smith MC, Dunn MJ: Role of kidney in blood pressure regulation. In Jacobson HR and others, editors: *The principles and practice of nephrology,* Philadelphia, 1993, BC Decker.
4. Beck LH: Changes in renal function with aging, *Clin Geriatr Med* 14:199, 1998.
5. Ouslander JG: Aging and the lower urinary tract, *Am J Med Sci* 314:214, 1997.
6. Samsioe G: Urogenital aging—a hidden problem, *Am J Obstet Gynecol* 178:S245, 1998.
7. Bernier F, Jenkins P: The role of vaginal estrogen in the treatment of urogenital dysfunction in postmenopausal women, *Urol Nurs* 17:92, 1997.
8. Reilly NJ: Cancer of the bladder. In Karlowicz KA, editor: *Urologic nursing—principles and practice,* Philadelphia, 1995, Saunders.
9. Goldstein ML, Whitman T, Renshaw AA: Significance of cell groups in voided urine, *Acta Cytol* 42:290, 1998.
10. Wiener HG and others: Can urine bound diagnostic tests replace cystoscopy in the management of bladder cancer? *J Urol* 159:1876, 1998.
11. Karlowicz KA, Meredith CE: Adult voiding dysfunction. In Karlowicz KA, editor: *Urologic nursing—principles and practice,* Philadelphia, 1995, Saunders.

Resources

Resources for this chapter are listed after Chapter 43 on p. 1298.

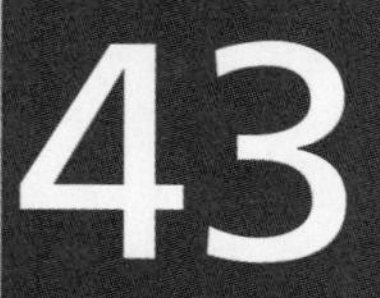

REMEMBER to check out your **companion CD-ROM**

43 NURSING MANAGEMENT Renal and Urologic Problems

Patricia Bates

www.mosby.com/MERLIN/medsurg_lewis

LEARNING OBJECTIVES

1. Describe the pathophysiology, clinical manifestations, collaborative care, and drug therapy of cystitis, urethritis, and pyelonephritis.
2. Explain the nursing management of urinary tract infections.
3. Describe the immunologic mechanisms involved in glomerulonephritis.
4. Explain the clinical manifestations and nursing and collaborative management of acute poststreptococcal glomerulonephritis, Goodpasture's syndrome, and chronic glomerulonephritis.
5. Describe the common causes, clinical manifestations, collaborative care, and nursing management of nephrotic syndrome.
6. Compare and contrast the etiology, clinical manifestations, collaborative care, and nursing management of various types of urinary calculi.
7. Explain the common causes and management of renal trauma, renal vascular problems, and hereditary renal problems.
8. Describe the mechanisms of renal involvement in metabolic and connective tissue disorders.
9. Describe the clinical manifestations and collaborative care of renal and bladder cancer.
10. Describe the common causes and management of bladder dysfunctions.
11. Differentiate among ureteral, suprapubic, nephrostomy, and urethral catheters with regard to indications for use and nursing responsibilities.
12. Explain the nursing management of the patient undergoing nephrectomy or urinary diversion surgery.

Renal and urologic disorders encompass a wide spectrum of clinical problems. The diverse causes of these disorders may involve infectious, immunologic, obstructive, metabolic, collagen-vascular, traumatic, congenital, neoplastic, and neurologic mechanisms. This chapter discusses specific disorders of the kidneys, ureters, bladder, and urethra. Acute and chronic renal failure are discussed in Chapter 44. Female reproductive problems are discussed in Chapter 51. Male genitourinary problems are discussed in Chapter 52.

INFECTIOUS AND INFLAMMATORY DISORDERS OF THE URINARY SYSTEM

Urinary tract infections (UTIs) are the second most common bacterial disease. More than 1 million people are hospitalized annually because of UTIs. Nosocomial urinary infections are responsible for 40% of all hospital-acquired infections, and the majority of these are related to catheterization.[1] More than 15% of patients who develop gram-negative bacteremia die, and one third of these are caused by bacterial infections originating in the urinary tract. UTIs are the most common source of bacteremia in older adults.[2]

Reviewed by Mikel Gray, RN, PhD, CUNP, CCCN, FAAN, Associate Professor, Department of Urology and School of Nursing, University of Virginia Medical Center, Charlottesville, Va.

Infections of the urinary tract may appear as a variety of disorders. The common factor is a microbial invasion of the tissues of the urinary tract, most often by *Escherichia coli* (Table 43-1). Bacterial counts of 10^5 organisms or more generally indicate a UTI. However, bacterial counts as low as 10^2 to 10^3 in a person with symptoms are indicative of UTI. Viral, fungal, and parasitic infections are not as common but are seen most frequently in the patient who is immunosuppressed, has diabetes mellitus, or has taken multiple courses of antibiotics.

Classification

Infections may be broadly classified as upper and lower UTIs (Fig. 43-1) based on the patient's symptoms. Terminology may specifically delineate the site of inflammation or infection. Examples of terms are *pyelonephritis* (involvement of kidney and kidney pelvis) and *cystitis* (involvement of bladder). However, it may be difficult to determine the specific location of a UTI. A patient may have a simultaneous infection in both the upper and lower urinary tract, an infection of adjacent organs causing urinary infection–like symptoms, or no symptoms at all.

Determining whether a UTI is complicated or uncomplicated is a significant factor in determining the treatment plan. Uncomplicated infections are those that occur in an otherwise normal urinary tract. First-time infections in young women are usually uncomplicated. Complicated infections include the coexisting presence of obstruction, stones, or catheters; when

Table 43-1 Common Microorganisms Causing Urinary Tract Infections

*Escherichia coli**	*Proteus*
Enterococci	*Pseudomonas*
Klebsiella	*Staphylococci*
Enterobacter	*Candida*
Serratia	

*Causes about 80% of cases in persons who do not have urinary tract structural abnormalities or calculi.

diabetes or neurologic diseases exist; or when an infection is a recurrent one. The individual with a complicated infection is at risk for renal damage.

Only about one fourth of individuals who develop an acute infection go on to develop a recurrent UTI.[3] Recurrent UTIs can be classified as *relapses* (recurrence with the same strain of bacteria from within the urinary tract that occurs within 1 to 2 weeks of stopping antibiotic therapy) or *reinfections* (recurrence with a new organism following successful treatment).

Relapse can be further defined as states of unresolved bacteriuria or true bacterial persistence. Unresolved bacteriuria occurs when bacteria are resistant to the antibiotic used to treat an infection or when the infection is undertreated. Some bacteria, although initially sensitive to a drug, can mutate during therapy. Insufficient antibiotic concentrations in the urinary system may be attributed to renal insufficiency or an inability of the antibiotic to infiltrate the tissues (such as the prostate or urethra). Often the patient feels better and stops medication before an adequate course is completed. Bacterial persistence occurs when the infection is successfully treated but a persistent source of infection remains. This may result from infected stones, chronic pyelonephritis, obstructive uropathies, or foreign bodies. Urine cultures may be negative immediately following antibiotic therapy but will show growth again when cultured about 1 week after treatment.

Etiology

Defense Mechanisms. The urinary tract above the urethra is normally sterile. Several physiologic and mechanical defense mechanisms assist in maintaining sterility and preventing UTIs. These defenses include normal voiding with complete emptying of the bladder, normal antibacterial ability of the bladder mucosa and urine, ureterovesical junction competence, and peristaltic activity that propels urine toward the bladder. An alteration in any of these defense mechanisms increases the risk of contracting a UTI. Table 43-2 lists predisposing factors to urinary tract infections.

Source of Urinary Tract Infections. The organisms that usually cause UTIs are introduced via the ascending route from the urethra. Less common routes are via the bloodstream or lymphatic system. Most infections are due to gram-negative aerobic bacilli normally found in the gastrointestinal (GI) tract, although gram-positive organisms such as streptococci, enterococci, and *Staphylococcus saprophyticus* also can cause urinary infections. A common factor contributing to ascending infection is urologic instrumentation (e.g., catheterization, cystoscopic examinations). Instrumentation allows bacteria that are normally present at the opening of the urethra to enter the urethra or bladder. Sexual intercourse promotes milking of bacteria from the vagina and perineum

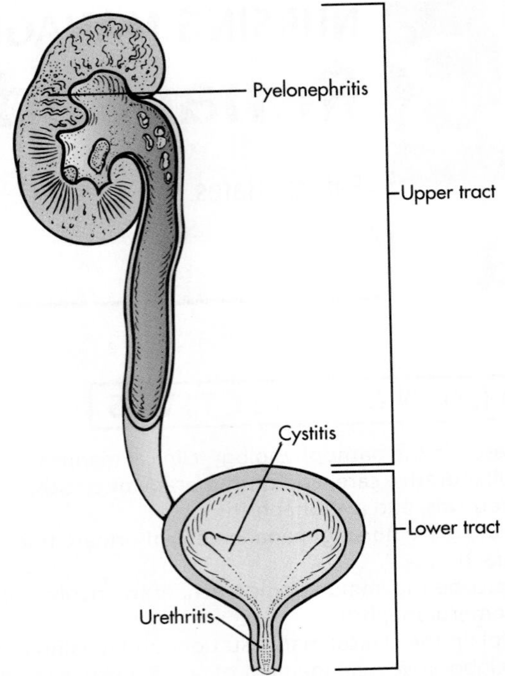

Fig. 43-1 Sites of infectious processes in the urinary tract.

Table 43-2 Predisposing Factors to Urinary Tract Infections

1. Renal scarring from previous UTI
2. Diminished ureteral peristalsis (e.g., pregnancy)
3. Compression of growing uterus against ureters (e.g., tumor, fibroids)
4. Urinary retention for any reason
5. Presence of a foreign body (e.g., urinary catheter)
6. Vesicoureteral reflux of urine in a retrograde direction from bladder toward the kidney
7. Humoral or cellular immunodeficiency in an otherwise normal urinary tract
8. Shorter urethra in females
9. Presence of urinary calculi
10. Neurogenic bladder
11. Congenital defects
12. Diabetes mellitus

and may cause minor urethral trauma that predisposes women to UTIs.

Rarely do UTIs result from a hematogenous route, where blood-borne bacteria secondarily invade the kidneys, ureters, or bladder from elsewhere in the body. For a kidney infection to occur from hematogenous transmission, there must be prior injury to the urinary tract, such as obstruction of the ureter, damage caused by stones, or renal scars.

An important source of UTIs is hospital-acquired, or nosocomial, infection. The cause of nosocomial infection is often *E. coli* and, less frequently, *Pseudomonas* organisms. Urologic instrumentation, particularly with an indwelling urinary catheter, is the most common predisposing factor.

The occurrence of UTIs is often related to the presence of abnormalities of the urinary tract, such as strictures and

CULTURAL & ETHNIC CONSIDERATIONS

Urologic Disorders

- Urinary tract calculi are more common among Caucasians than African-Americans.
- Jewish men have a high incidence of uric acid stones.
- Bladder cancer has a higher incidence among Caucasian men than African-American men. In all ethnic groups it affects men about three times more often than women.

obstructions. An untreated UTI can lead to chronic pyelonephritis and a progressive decrease in renal function. If no abnormality exists, uncomplicated pyelonephritis rarely leads to progressive renal damage and renal failure.

CYSTITIS

Etiology and Pathophysiology

Although the majority of patients with cystitis are women, other groups with a high incidence are older men and young children (especially girls). These age and sex variations in the frequency of cystitis are related to anatomic differences or pathologic changes in the groups at risk. The adult female urethra is short, and its proximity to the rectum and vagina predisposes women to the risk of bladder contamination. Bacterial contamination of the bladder can be the result of poor personal hygiene practices and sexual intercourse.

In children and older men, UTIs are often associated with other preexisting problems. In children, vesicoureteral reflux is usually the preexisting abnormality. In men, the longer urethra (of which the proximal two thirds is normally sterile) and the antibacterial property of prostatic secretions provide protection from bacterial infections unless there are predisposing causes, such as benign prostatic hyperplasia.

Not all bacterial invasions of the bladder result in lower UTI or cause spread to the upper urinary tract (pyelonephritis). Once cystitis has occurred, it may remain localized in the urinary bladder for years without ascension to the kidneys or may be completely resolved after initial treatment. Although the bacterial infection may be self-limiting, the urinary tract should be evaluated if there is recurrence, even in the patient who has no symptoms. The risk of recurrent symptomatic infection is increased when there are urinary tract abnormalities.

Asymptomatic bacteriuria can occur and is not synonymous with UTI. It indicates that bacteria are present in the urine. Tissue invasion must occur for an infection to exist. Pyuria (the presence of white blood cells [WBCs] in the urine) usually signals this occurrence and is the characteristic laboratory finding in symptomatic UTI. Asymptomatic bacteriuria is more likely to occur in women over 65 years of age.[1] Asymptomatic bacteriuria may be important in a patient of any age if that person is at risk for complicated urinary infection and resultant renal damage.

Clinical Manifestations

The manifestations of cystitis are frequency and urgency of urination, suprapubic pain, dysuria, foul-smelling urine, and pyuria. Hematuria may or may not occur in symptomatic UTI.

COLLABORATIVE CARE

Table 43-3 Cystitis

Diagnostic
- Urinalysis
- Urine for Gram's stain
- Urine for culture and sensitivity (if indicated)
- Evaluation of urinary tract (e.g., IVP, cystoscopy) (if indicated)

Collaborative Therapy

Uncomplicated
- Single-dose regimen
  - Trimethoprim-sulfamethoxazole (Bactrim, Septra)
- 1- to 3-day regimen
  - Nitrofurantoin (Macrodantin, Furadantin)
  - Cephalexin (Keflex)
  - Ciprofloxacin (Cipro)
  - Norfloxacin (Chibroxin, Noroxin)
  - Ofloxacin (Floxin)
- Encouragement of high fluid intake

Recurring
- Continuous prophylaxis
  - Trimethoprim-sulfamethoxazole (Bactrim, Septra)
  - Nitrofurantoin (Macrodantin, Furadantin)
  - Cephalexin (Keflex)
- Repeat of urine culture

IVP, intravenous pyelogram.

The presence of fever, nausea and vomiting, and flank tenderness usually indicates pyelonephritis. About one half of all persons with significant bacteriuria have no symptoms or may report nonspecific signs such as increased fatigue, anorexia, or changes in cognitive ability. The incidence of asymptomatic bacteriuria increases greatly with age.[4]

Diagnostic Studies

Examining the urine for the presence of WBCs by means of either a microscope or a urine dipstick is important in evaluating a person who complains of dysuria. The definitive diagnosis of cystitis is made on examination of a urine Gram's stain or by urine culture. Urine is usually cultured if the UTI is complicated or is unresponsive to therapy or if the diagnosis is questionable.[5] The best method for obtaining the urine culture is the midstream technique called *clean-catch urine.* (See Table 42-8 for an explanation of this technique.) If a satisfactory specimen cannot be obtained with this method, catheterization may be used.

The nurse should be aware that noninfectious agents also cause irritative bladder symptoms similar to UTI. The patient with a bladder tumor or the individual receiving intravesical chemotherapy or pelvic radiation often experiences urinary frequency, urgency, and dysuria. Nonbacterial inflammatory lesions such as interstitial cystitis also cause these symptoms.

Collaborative Care and Drug Therapy

Once cystitis has been diagnosed, appropriate antimicrobial therapy is initiated. The collaborative care and drug therapy of cystitis are summarized in Table 43-3. Uncomplicated cystitis

NURSING ASSESSMENT

Table 43-4 Urinary Tract Infection

Subjective Data

Important Health Information

Past health history: Previous urinary tract infections; urinary calculi, stasis, reflux, strictures, or retention; neurogenic bladder; pregnancy; prostatic hyperplasia; sexually transmitted disease; bladder cancer

Medications: Use of antibiotics, anticholinergics, antispasmodics

Surgery or other treatments: Recent urologic instrumentation (catheterization, cystoscopy, surgery)

Functional Health Patterns

Health perception–health management: Urinary hygiene practices; lassitude, malaise

Nutritional-metabolic: Nausea, vomiting, and anorexia; chills

Elimination: Urinary frequency, urgency, hesitancy; nocturia

Cognitive-perceptual: Suprapubic or low back pain, costovertebral tenderness; bladder spasms, dysuria, burning on urination

Objective Data

General

Fever

Urinary

Hematuria; cloudy, foul-smelling urine; tender, enlarged kidney

Possible Findings

Leukocytosis; urinalysis positive for bacteria, pyuria, RBCs, and WBCs; positive urine culture; IVP, CT scan, ultrasound, voiding cystourethrogram and cystoscopy demonstrating abnormalities of urinary tract

CT, computed tomography; *RBCs,* red blood cells; *UTI,* urinary tract infection; *WBCs,* white blood cells.

can be treated with short-term antibiotics, which consists of single-dose therapy or 1 to 3 days of therapy.[6]

Sulfamethoxazole combined with trimethoprim (Bactrim, Septra) has proved to be effective in treating UTIs. When these drugs are combined, resistance seems to develop less rapidly. Systemic antibiotics such as cephalexin (Keflex), nitrofurantoin (Macrodantin, Furadantin), and fluoroquinolones (ciprofloxacin [Cipro], norfloxacin [Chibroxin, Noroxin], enoxacin [Penetrex], levofloxacin [Levaquin], ofloxacin [Floxin]) can also be used.

High single-dose therapy has been effective when the infection is localized to the bladder and the organism is sensitive to antibiotics. Single-dose therapy results in lowered cost, increased compliance, and decreased potential for resistant organisms. Fosfomycin (Monurol) is a single-dose medication indicated exclusively for treatment of UTI. It has antibacterial activity for up to 3 to 5 days. However, if there is involvement of the kidney or if the patient is an older adult or has diabetes, single-dose therapy is not appropriate.

Phenazopyridine (Pyridium) may be used in cystitis to provide an analgesic effect on the urinary mucosa. This drug should relieve the burning sensation. The azo dye in the drug stains the urine reddish orange. It is important to tell the patient about the color change so that she or he does not think it is related to the infection. Phenazopyridine stain is also fairly permanent on underclothing.

Other drugs that may be used are methenamine mandelate (Mandelamine), methenamine hippurate (Hiprex), hyoscyamine sulfate (Cystospaz), and flavoxate (Urispas). Methenamine achieves its desired effect by decomposing to formaldehyde and ammonia. The urinary pH should be less than 6 for methenamine to be effective, so urinary pH should be tested to ensure the activity of the drug. Hyoscyamine and flavoxate help decrease bladder muscle irritability and spasm.

Many clinicians are now treating uncomplicated lower UTI with a 1 to 3 day course of antibiotics. As with single-dose therapy, the candidate for 1 to 3 day therapy must be chosen to exclude the patient with UTI associated with fever or flank or back pain.

Patients with chronic UTIs require longer periods of treatment, sometimes several months. Initial treatment dosages are usually followed by smaller dosages of the same drug or a different drug to prevent reinfection or relapse (suppression therapy).

Antibiotic therapy is not usually recommended for asymptomatic bacteriuria unless symptoms develop or there is evidence of obstructive uropathy in the symptom-free patient. The risk of developing bacterial resistance and the inability to treat the patient when symptoms do occur is great. In general, asymptomatic bacteriuria in the older adult should not be treated. Prophylactic antibiotics may be ordered when a patient with asymptomatic bacteriuria undergoes surgery or genitourinary instrumentation.

Prophylactic antibiotic therapy is given to prevent recurrence after treatment of UTI. Women who have had more than three episodes of cystitis per year are considered candidates for prophylaxis. The three most common antibiotics used for prophylaxis are trimethoprim-sulfamethoxazole, nitrofurantoin, and cephalexin. In postmenopausal women, estrogen replacement therapy, particularly vaginally applied creams or estrogen rings, may also reduce the rate of recurrent UTI.[7]

NURSING MANAGEMENT: CYSTITIS

■ Nursing Assessment

Subjective and objective data that should be obtained from a patient with cystitis are presented in Table 43-4.

■ Nursing Diagnoses

Nursing diagnoses for the patient with cystitis may include, but are not limited to, those presented in NCP 43-1.

43-1 NURSING CARE PLAN PATIENT WITH A URINARY TRACT INFECTION

Expected Patient Outcomes	Nursing Interventions and *Rationales*
NURSING DIAGNOSIS	**Hyperthermia** *related to* infection *as manifested by* elevation in temperature, tachycardia, tachypnea, chills, malaise.
▪ Normal body temperature. ▪ No chills.	▪ Assess vital signs q2-4hr *to plan appropriate intervention.* ▪ Administer antipyretics and antibiotics as ordered *to control fever and infection and promote comfort.* ▪ Ensure adequate hydration via oral or IV route *because fever increases fluid loss through insensible perspiration.* ▪ Monitor intake and output *to ensure adequate hydration and monitor renal function.* ▪ Cover patient lightly and keep patient dry *to prevent chilling and promote comfort.* ▪ Provide cooling sponge baths or compresses *to assist in temperature reduction by evaporation of moisture on skin.*
NURSING DIAGNOSIS	**Pain** *related to* inflammation of mucosal tissue of urinary tract *as manifested by* pain on urination, flank pain, suprapubic pain, lower back pain, bladder spasms.
▪ Satisfaction with pain control. ▪ No pain.	▪ Assess pain for location and severity *to plan appropriate interventions.* ▪ Position patient *for comfort.* ▪ Administer analgesics, antispasmodics, and phenazopyridine (Pyridium) as ordered *to promote comfort,* and note their effectiveness. ▪ Alert patient that phenazopyridine will color urine orange *to prevent concern over unusual appearance of urine.* ▪ Apply heating pad to painful area *because heat relieves pain associated with UTI.*
NURSING DIAGNOSIS	**Altered urinary elimination** *related to* UTI *as manifested by* urgency, frequency, nocturia, incontinence, or hematuria; verbalization of concern over altered elimination pattern.
▪ Normal urination pattern.	▪ Assess for changes in usual voiding pattern *to determine presence of UTI.* ▪ Instruct patient regarding reason for symptoms *to promote understanding and cooperation.* ▪ Encourage high fluid intake or administer IV fluids as ordered *to maintain a dilute, nonirritating urine and decrease bacterial concentration.* ▪ Obtain urine for culture and sensitivity *to determine cause of UTI or monitor effectiveness of treatment.* ▪ Administer antimicrobial medication as ordered *to eliminate symptoms by inhibiting bacterial growth.* ▪ Instruct patient about good perineal care and cleansing after each bowel movement *to prevent reintroducing infection.* ▪ Observe urine for color, odor, amount, and frequency *to evaluate effectiveness of treatment plan.*
NURSING DIAGNOSIS	**Risk for reinfection** *related to* lack of knowledge regarding measures to prevent recurrence (see Table 43-5).

Planning

The overall goals are that the patient with cystitis will have (1) relief from dysuria, (2) no upper urinary tract complications, and (3) no recurrent episodes of UTI.

Nursing Implementation

Health Promotion. Health promotion measures include recognizing the groups with a higher than normal incidence of UTIs. Especially for these individuals, health promotion activities can help decrease the frequency of infections and promote early detection of infection. These activities include teaching preventive measures, such as emptying the bladder regularly and completely, evacuating the bowel regularly, wiping the perineal area from front to back after urination and defecation, and drinking an adequate amount of liquid each day. The standard adult requirement for daily liquid intake is approximately 15 ml per pound of body weight.[8] For example, a 135-pound person would require a minimum 2025 ml or more than eight 8-ounce glasses of liquids each day. Fluids such as coffee or colas containing caffeine, alcohol, and citrus juices may irritate the bladder and should be limited. In addition, it is important to teach the patient to seek early treatment once symptoms are identified.

The nurse can play a major role in the prevention of nosocomial infections. Debilitated persons, older adults, patients with severe underlying disease (cancer, cirrhosis, diabetes), and patients treated with immunosuppressive drugs, long-term corticosteroid therapy, or radiation are at high risk for UTIs. The patient undergoing instrumentation of the urinary tract is also at risk for developing nosocomial infections, and aseptic technique should always be followed for these procedures. Washing hands before and after contact with each patient and wearing gloves for care involving the urinary system are especially important. In general, catheterization of the bladder should be avoided if possible.

For the patient at risk for a nosocomial UTI, it is important to provide good perineal hygiene, especially after a bedpan is used. Incontinence should be avoided by answering the call light quickly or offering the bedpan or urinal at frequent intervals to the bedridden patient. If a catheter has been inserted, special catheter care measures must be employed as explained in the section on urethral catheterization (see p. 1289).

Acute Intervention. Acute intervention for a patient with cystitis includes an adequate fluid intake if this is not contraindicated. This means drinking more than the standard daily requirement. It is sometimes difficult to get the patient to maintain an adequate fluid intake because the person may think it will increase a feeling of urgency. Explain to the patient that fluids will increase frequency at first but will also dilute the urine, making the bladder less irritable. Fluids will help flush out bacteria before they have a chance to colonize in the bladder. Caffeine, alcohol, citrus juices, chocolate, and highly spiced foods or beverages should be avoided because they are potential bladder irritants. A heating pad or sitz bath may also help reduce discomfort. Treatment of cystitis does not usually require hospitalization.

The patient should be instructed about the prescribed drug therapy. Common side effects of the drugs should be explained, and the patient should be told to notify the health care provider if they occur. It is important for the patient to take the full course of antibiotics. Often patients stop antibiotic therapy once symptoms disappear. This practice can lead to inadequate treatment and recurrence of infection or to bacterial resistance to antibiotics. Sometimes a second medication or a reduced dose of medication is ordered after the initial course to suppress bacterial growth in certain patients susceptible to recurrent UTI.

The urine should be examined for gross or microscopic hematuria, presence of WBCs, malodor, and sediment. The patient should be instructed to watch for any changes in the color or consistency of the urine and a decrease in or cessation of symptoms as a sign of the effectiveness of therapy.

Ambulatory and Home Care. Home care for the patient with a UTI should emphasize the patient's compliance with the medication regimen. It is the nurse's responsibility to educate the patient about the need for ongoing care (Table 43-5). This includes taking antimicrobial medication as ordered, maintaining more than an adequate daily fluid intake, emptying the bladder when the urge to urinate occurs or at least every 2 to 4 hours, urinating after intercourse, and discontinuing use of a diaphragm (if used).

PATIENT TEACHING GUIDE

Table 43-5 Urinary Tract Infection

The following are important to teach to the patient with a UTI to prevent recurrence:

1. Explain importance of taking all antibiotics as prescribed. Symptoms will improve after 1-2 days of therapy, but organisms may still be present.
2. Instruct the patient on appropriate hygiene, including
   - careful cleansing of perineal region
   - wiping from front to back after urinating
   - cleansing with soap and water after each bowel movement
3. Explain the importance of emptying the bladder before and after intercourse.
4. Instruct the patient to urinate when the urge occurs or at least every 2-4 hr during the day.
5. Instruct the patient about the need to maintain high fluid intake (seven to eight 8-ounce glasses of water per day).
6. Instruct the patient to avoid harsh soaps, bubble baths, powders, and sprays in the perineal area.
7. Instruct the patient to avoid tight-fitting pants and clothing on lower part of body.
8. Have the patient report symptoms or signs of recurrent urinary tract infection (e.g., cloudy urine, pain on urination, urgency, frequency).

The patient must understand the need for follow-up care with urine culture to determine that the infection has been adequately treated. Relapse with bacteria of the same species usually occurs within 1 to 2 weeks after completion of therapy. If the patient has been compliant, relapse suggests possible renal involvement or other uropathology in the infectious process. For the individual who has more than three episodes of cystitis in 1 year, the use of prophylactic antibiotic therapy may be ordered.

Evaluation

The expected outcomes for the patient with a urinary tract infection are presented in NCP 43-1.

ACUTE PYELONEPHRITIS

Etiology and Pathophysiology

Pyelonephritis is an acute or chronic inflammatory process of the renal pelvis and parenchyma of the kidney. Generally the inflammatory process is caused by bacterial invasion. Most infections are caused by the normal inhabitants of the intestinal tract (e.g., *E. coli, Proteus, Klebsiella, Enterobacter*).

Pyelonephritis usually ascends from the lower urinary tract. A preexisting factor is often present. In children it is usually associated with vesicoureteral reflux or other urinary tract abnormalities. In adults common preexisting factors are bladder tumors, prostatic hyperplasia, strictures, urinary stones, and pregnancy. Repeated attacks of acute pyelonephritis, especially in the presence of these abnormalities, can result in chronic pyelonephritis. The infection commonly starts in the renal medulla and spreads to the adjacent cortex. The infected portion of the kidney heals, resulting in fibrosis and scarring.

Clinical Manifestations

The clinical manifestations of acute pyelonephritis vary from mild lassitude to the sudden onset of chills, fever, vomiting, malaise, flank pain, dysuria, and frequent urination. Symptoms of cystitis may or may not be present. Costovertebral tenderness will be present on the affected side. The clinical manifestations usually subside within a few days, even without specific therapy. However, bacteriuria or pyuria may persist.

The results of a CBC show leukocytosis and a shift to the left with an increase in banded neutrophils. Urinalysis shows pyuria, bacteriuria, and varying degrees of hematuria. White cell casts may be found in the urine.

Bacteremia (presence of bacteria in blood) can occur secondary to a UTI ascending to the kidney and can result in sepsis. Some patients develop septic shock as a result of endotoxins produced by gram-negative bacteria that are released in the blood. (Septic shock is discussed in Chapter 61.) If bacteremia is a possibility, close observation and vital sign monitoring are essential. Prompt recognition and treatment of septic shock may prevent irreversible damage.

Collaborative Care and Drug Therapy

The diagnostic tests and collaborative therapy of acute pyelonephritis are summarized in Table 43-6. Severe infections or complicating factors require hospital admission. Urine cultures should always be obtained when pyelonephritis is suspected. In patients with more severe illness who are hospitalized, blood cultures should also be obtained. Intravenous pyelograms (IVPs) or excretory urograms are usually not obtained in the early stages of pyelonephritis to prevent the possible spread of infection.

An essential principle of management is to consider factors that may be contributing to the infection, such as an obstruction or a urinary tract anomaly. In addition to an IVP, other diagnostic procedures such as a cystourethrogram and cystoscopy may be used to evaluate any uropathies. It is essential to obtain follow-up urine cultures to determine the effectiveness of therapy.

The patient with mild symptoms may be treated as an outpatient with antibiotics for 14 to 21 days (see Table 43-6). IV antibiotics are often given initially in the hospital to achieve quick, high serum and urinary drug levels. If this treatment appears to be successful, the patient may be discharged on oral antibiotics for 14 to 21 days. Symptoms and signs typically improve or resolve within 48 to 72 hours after starting therapy.

Relapses may be treated with a 6-week course of antibiotics. Reinfections may be treated as individual episodes of disease or managed with long-term antibiotic therapy. Antibiotic prophylaxis may also be used for recurrent infections. The effectiveness of therapy is evaluated in accordance with the presence or absence of bacterial growth on urine culture.

COLLABORATIVE CARE

Table 43-6 Acute Pyelonephritis

Diagnostic
- Urinalysis
- Urine for culture and sensitivity, Gram's stain
- IVP, ultrasound, or CT scan
- WBC count
- Blood culture (if bacteremia suspected)
- Palpation for flank pain

Collaborative Therapy

Mild Symptoms
- Outpatient management or short hospitalization for IV antibiotics
- Administration of oral antibiotics for 14-21 days
  - Trimethoprim-sulfamethoxazole (Bactrim, Septra)
  - Cephalexin (Keflex)
  - Ciprofloxacin (Cipro)
  - Nitrofurantoin (Furadantin, Macrodantin)
  - Norfloxacin (Chibroxin, Noroxin)
  - Ofloxacin (Floxin)
- High fluid intake
- Follow-up urine cultures

Severe Symptoms
- Hospitalization
- Parenteral antibiotics
  - Ampicillin and aminoglycoside (e.g., gentamicin)
  - Ciprofloxacin (Cipro)
  - Ofloxacin (Floxin)
  - Trimethoprim-sulfamethoxazole (Bactrim, Septra)
- High fluid intake
- Follow-up urine cultures

NURSING MANAGEMENT: PYELONEPHRITIS

■ Nursing Assessment

Subjective and objective data that should be obtained from a patient with a UTI are presented in Table 43-4.

■ Nursing Diagnoses

Nursing diagnoses for the patient with a UTI include, but are not limited to, those presented in NCP 43-1.

■ Planning

The overall goals are that the patient with pyelonephritis will have (1) relief of pain, (2) normal body temperature, (3) no complications, and (4) no recurrence of symptoms.

■ Nursing Implementation

Health Promotion. Health promotion and maintenance measures are similar to those for cystitis (see Health Promotion under Cystitis, p. 1265). In addition, it is important that the patient receive early treatment for cystitis to prevent ascending infections. Because the patient with structural abnormalities of the urinary tract is at high risk for infection, the need for regular medical care should be stressed.

Acute Intervention and Home Care. Nursing interventions vary depending on the severity of symptoms. These interventions include teaching the patient about the disease process with emphasis on (1) the need to continue medications as prescribed, (2) the need for a follow-up urine culture to ensure proper management, and (3) identification of recurrence of infection or relapse (see Table 43-5 and NCP 43-1). In addition to antibiotic therapy, the patient should be encouraged to drink at least eight glasses of fluid every day. Increased fluid intake should be continued, even after the infection has been treated. Rest is often indicated to increase patient comfort. The patient with frequent relapses or reinfections may be treated with long-term, low-dose antibiotics. Understanding the rationale for therapy is important to enhance patient compliance.

■ Evaluation

The expected outcomes for the patient with a UTI are presented in NCP 43-1.

CHRONIC PYELONEPHRITIS

Chronic pyelonephritis (also called chronic interstitial nephritis) is not the result of an isolated episode of acute pyelonephritis unless there are predisposing factors such as obstruction, neurogenic bladder, or vesicoureteral reflux. Chronic pyelonephritis is usually the end result of long-standing UTIs with relapses and reinfections.

The pathologic changes indicate that there have been repeated episodes of chronic inflammation and scarring. Grossly, both kidneys are irregularly and asymmetrically scarred. The renal pelvis and calyces are deformed, blunted, and dilated.

Clinical features of chronic pyelonephritis include a history of recurrent acute infections leading to progressive destruction of functioning nephrons resulting in chronic renal insufficiency. During active infection, urine cultures are positive and leukocyte casts are found on urinalysis. End-stage chronic pyelonephritis is not easily distinguished from other causes of chronic renal failure. IVP, renal biopsy, renal ultrasound, or computed tomography (CT) scan may be useful in delineating the severity of renal involvement after the infection has been resolved.

The level of renal function can vary in chronic pyelonephritis. The patient may have improvement in function after an acute exacerbation. Chronic pyelonephritis may progress to chronic renal failure. (Nursing and collaborative management of the patient with chronic renal failure is discussed in Chapter 44.)

URETHRITIS

Urethritis (inflammation of the urethra) is often difficult to diagnose, but the clinical manifestations are the same as those for cystitis. The female urethra may be extremely tender, or there may be a discharge, especially in men. Inflammatory changes may make recovery of bacteria difficult because they become entrapped in urethral tissue and do not appear in the urine. Urethritis may coexist with cystitis. Cultures on split urine collections (taken at beginning of urine flow and then midstream) or any urethral discharge may confirm a diagnosis of urethral infection. Causes of urethritis include a bacterial or viral infection, *Trichomonas* and monilial infection (especially in women), *Chlamydia,* and gonorrhea (especially in men). (Gonococcal urethritis is discussed in Chapter 50.)

Detection of chlamydial organisms requires tissue culture or immunologic testing for chlamydial antigen in urethral or cervical specimens. Chlamydial infection is less likely to cause hematuria and suprapubic pain than bacterial infection.

Treatment is based on identifying and treating the cause and providing symptomatic relief. Sulfamethoxazole with trimethoprim or nitrofurantoin are examples of medications used for bacterial infections. Metronidazole (Flagyl) and clotrimazole (Mycelex) may be used for treating *Trichomonas.* Medications such as nystatin (Mycostatin) or fluconazole (Diflucan) may be prescribed for monilial infections. In chlamydial infections, doxycycline may be used. Women with negative urine cultures and no pyuria do not usually respond to antibiotics. Hot sitz baths without perfumed bath oil or bath salts may relieve the symptoms. The patient should be instructed to avoid the use of vaginal deodorant sprays, to properly cleanse the perineal area after bowel movements and urination, and to avoid intercourse until symptoms subside.

URETHRAL SYNDROME

Symptoms of dysuria, urgency, and frequency unaccompanied by significant bacteriuria (i.e., less than 10^2 to 10^3 per ml of urine) have been termed *acute urethral syndrome.* Clinically these patients cannot be readily distinguished from those with cystitis. When present, bacteria are usually *E. coli,* enterococci, or staphylococci. If few or no bacteria are detected, *Chlamydia trachomatis* or *Neisseria gonorrhoeae* (both sexually transmitted pathogens) may be the cause.

Vaginitis must be ruled out. If vaginitis is the cause, the symptoms may have a more gradual onset, and pruritis or vaginal discharge may be present.

Treatment depends on the causative agent. If bacteria are involved, the treatment is similar to that for cystitis. This patient responds well to single-dose therapy. Simultaneous treatment of the individual's sexual partner may be recommended. Heat or sitz baths may help alleviate symptoms. Acute symptoms of urethral syndrome tend to recur. The patient needs a great deal of reassurance.

INTERSTITIAL CYSTITIS

Interstitial cystitis is a chronic, painful inflammatory disease of the bladder that most commonly occurs in women. The etiology is unknown. Once thought to be psychologic in etiology, interstitial cystitis is now considered a physiologic syndrome with multifactorial etiologies.[9] The disease is characterized by severe bladder and pelvic pain, urinary frequency, and urgency. The inflammation can lead to scarring and stiffening of the bladder, decreased bladder capacity, bleeding, and ulcers of the bladder lining. Pyuria is usually not present. Hematuria is sometimes present. (The presence of hematuria more commonly suggests a lower urinary tract infection or tumor.) Urine cultures are negative.

The diagnosis is made following cystoscopy with the characteristic findings of reduced bladder capacity and the presence of superficial, often stellate, ulcers. In the earlier stages of the disease, only multiple petechiae-like hemorrhages may be found and the bladder capacity may be normal. A bladder biopsy may be done to rule out carcinoma in situ.

Specific treatments do not help all patients, but they are based on theories of physiologic causes and directed toward symptom relief. Hydraulic distention of the bladder under anesthesia, intravesical instillation of dimethyl sulfoxide (DMSO) and other medications, electrostimulation, and oral medications such as tricyclic antidepressants (which have anticholinergic, antihistamine effects on the bladder), antispasmodics, bladder anesthetics, and nonsteroidal anti-inflammatory drugs are often used as initial treatments. Pentosan polysulfate (Elmiron) is a newer oral medication that acts as a bladder protectant and brings symptom relief to many patients. This drug has a mild anticoagulant effect, and any bleeding (e.g., epistaxis, gum hemorrhage) should be noted. Dietary and activity changes, biofeedback, application of heat, diversional activities, and involvement in interstitial cystitis support groups are also helpful approaches for decreasing symptoms and managing the disease.

Cystectomy with urinary diversion is an approach occasionally used when other measures fail to control severe pain and when the patient is willing to risk the consequences and potential complications of this surgery. Even after surgery, some individuals continue to have pain.[10] No matter what treatment course is chosen, nurses caring for patients with interstitial cystitis must offer a great deal of support, empathy, and education about managing symptoms.

RENAL TUBERCULOSIS

Renal tuberculosis (TB) is rarely a primary lesion. It is usually secondary to TB of the lung. In a small percentage of patients with pulmonary TB, the tubercle bacilli reach the kidneys via the bloodstream. Onset occurs 5 to 8 years after the primary infection. The patient is often asymptomatic when the kidney is initially infiltrated with bacilli. Sometimes the patient complains of fatigue and develops a low-grade fever. As the lesions ulcerate, infection descends to the bladder, and the patient experiences frequent urination, burning on voiding, and epididymitis (in men). Symptoms of cystitis are the first sign in the majority of patients with renal TB. Renal lesions may calcify as they heal. Infrequently, renal colic, lumbar and iliac pain, and hematuria may be present. A diagnosis is based on localization of tubercle bacilli in the urine and on IVP findings.

Long-term complications of renal TB depend on the duration of the disease before treatment. Scarring of the renal parenchyma and the development of ureteral strictures occur. The earlier treatment is initiated, the less likely renal failure will develop. Reduced bladder volume may be irreversible in advanced disease. The patient may require long-term urologic follow-up. (Nursing and collaborative management for the patient with TB is discussed in Chapter 26.)

IMMUNOLOGIC DISORDERS OF THE KIDNEY

GLOMERULONEPHRITIS

Immunologic processes involving the urinary tract predominantly affect the renal glomerulus. The disease process results in glomerulonephritis (inflammation of the glomeruli), which affects both kidneys equally. Although the glomerulus is the primary site of inflammation, tubular, interstitial, and vascular changes also occur. Glomerulonephritis is divided into a number of classifications, which may describe (1) the extent of damage (diffuse or focal), (2) the initial cause of the disorder (systemic lupus erythematosus, scleroderma, streptococcal infection), or (3) the extent of changes (minimal or widespread).

Etiology and Pathophysiology

Two types of antibody-induced injury can initiate glomerular damage. In the first type, the antibodies have specificity for antigens within the glomerular basement membrane (GBM). These are termed *anti-GBM antibodies.* Immunoglobulins and complement are deposited along the basement membrane. The mechanism that causes a person to develop antibodies against its GBM is not known. Production of autoantibodies (antibodies to one's own tissue) may be stimulated by a structural alteration in the GBM or by a reaction of the basement membrane with an exogenous agent (e.g., hydrocarbon, viruses).

In the second type of immune process, the antibodies react with circulating nonglomerular antigens and are randomly deposited as immune complexes along the GBM. On electron microscopy of renal tissue sections, the deposits appear "lumpy-bumpy." In this immune complex process, the antigens do not come from the glomeruli but from either endogenous circulating native deoxyribonucleic acid (DNA) or exogenous sources (e.g., bacteria, viruses, chemicals, drugs). Bacterial products appear to be important in poststreptococcal glomerulonephritis. Viral agents have been recognized in certain cases of glomerulonephritis that develop after hepatitis A, B, or C and rubella (measles).

All forms of immune complex disease are characterized by an accumulation of antigen, antibody, and complement in the glomeruli, which can result in tissue injury. The immune complexes activate complement (see Chapter 12). Complement activation results in the release of chemotactic factors that attract polymorphonuclear leukocytes and causes the release of histamine and other vasoactive amines. The intrinsic clotting pathway may also be activated. The end result of these processes is glomerular injury as a result of inflammation.

Clinical Manifestations

There are many clinical manifestations of glomerulonephritis. They may include varying degrees of hematuria (ranging from microscopic to gross) and urinary excretion of various formed elements, including red blood cells (RBCs), WBCs, and some granular casts. Proteinuria and elevated blood urea nitrogen (BUN) and serum creatinine levels are other manifestations. In most cases, recovery from the acute illness is complete. However, if progressive involvement occurs, the result is destruction of renal tissue and marked renal insufficiency.

The patient's history provides important information related to glomerulonephritis. It is necessary to assess exposure to drugs, immunizations, microbial infections, and viral infections such as hepatitis. It is also important to evaluate the patient for more generalized conditions involving immune disorders, such as systemic lupus erythematosus and systemic progressive sclerosis (scleroderma).

ACUTE POSTSTREPTOCOCCAL GLOMERULONEPHRITIS

Acute poststreptococcal glomerulonephritis (APSGN) is most common in children and young adults, but all age-groups can be affected. APSGN develops 5 to 21 days after an infection of

COLLABORATIVE CARE

Table 43-7 Acute Glomerulonephritis

Diagnostic
- History and physical examination
- Urinalysis
- CBC
- BUN, serum creatinine and albumin
- Complement levels and ASO titer
- Renal biopsy (if indicated)

Collaborative Therapy
- Rest
- Sodium and fluid restriction
- Diuretics
- Antihypertensive therapy
- Adjustment of dietary protein intake to level of proteinuria and uremia

ASO, antistreptolysin; *BUN,* blood urea nitrogen; *CBC,* complete blood count.

the pharynx or skin (e.g., streptococcal sore throat, impetigo) by certain nephrotoxic strains of group A β-hemolytic streptococci. The person produces antibodies to the streptococcal antigen. Although the specific mechanism is not known with certainty, the antigen-antibody complexes are deposited in the glomeruli and activate complement. Complement activation causes an inflammatory reaction to the injury. The response to the injury is also a decrease in the filtration of metabolic waste products from the blood and an increase in the permeability of the glomerulus to larger protein molecules.

Clinical Manifestations and Complications

The clinical manifestations of APSGN appear as a variety of signs and symptoms, which may include generalized body edema, hypertension, oliguria, hematuria with a smoky or rusty appearance, and proteinuria. Fluid retention occurs as a result of decreased glomerular filtration. The edema appears initially in low-pressure tissues, such as around the eyes (periorbital edema), but later progresses to involve the total body as ascites or peripheral edema in the legs. Smoky urine is indicative of bleeding in the upper urinary tract. The degree of proteinuria varies with the severity of the glomerulonephropathy. Hypertension primarily results from increased extracellular fluid volume.

The patient with APSGN may have abdominal or flank pain. At times the patient has no symptoms, with the problem found on routine urinalysis.

More than 95% of patients with APSGN recover completely or improve rapidly with conservative management. The prognosis for adults is less favorable than for children. Chronic glomerulonephritis develops in 5% to 15% of the affected persons, and irreversible renal failure occurs in less than 1% of patients.

Diagnostic Studies

The diagnosis of APSGN is based on a complete history and physical examination and laboratory studies (Table 43-7) to determine the presence or history of a group A β-hemolytic streptococcus in a throat or skin lesion. An immune response to the streptococcus is often demonstrated by assessment of antistreptolysin O (ASO) titers. The finding of decreased complement components (especially C3 and CH50) is indicative of an immune-mediated response. A renal biopsy may be performed to confirm the presence of the disease.

Dipstick and urine sediment microscopy will reveal the presence of erythrocytes in significant numbers. Erythrocyte casts are highly suggestive of acute glomerulonephritis. Proteinuria may range from mild to severe. Screening blood tests include BUN and serum creatinine to assess the extent of renal impairment.

NURSING AND COLLABORATIVE MANAGEMENT: ACUTE POSTSTREPTOCOCCAL GLOMERULONEPHRITIS

The management of APSGN focuses on symptomatic relief (see Table 43-7). Rest is recommended until the signs of glomerular inflammation (proteinuria, hematuria) and hypertension subside. Edema is treated by restricting sodium and fluid intake and by administrating diuretics. Severe hypertension is treated with antihypertensive drugs. Dietary protein intake may be restricted if there is evidence of an increase in nitrogenous wastes (e.g., elevated BUN value). The restriction varies with the degree of proteinuria. (Low-protein, low-sodium, fluid-restricted diets are discussed in Chapter 44.)

Antibiotics should be given only if the streptococcal infection is still present. Corticosteroids and cytotoxic drugs have not been shown to be of value.

One of the most important ways to prevent the development of APSGN is to encourage early diagnosis and treatment of sore throats and skin lesions. If streptococci are found in the culture, treatment with appropriate antibiotic therapy (usually penicillin) is essential. The patient must be encouraged to take the full course of antibiotics to ensure that the bacteria have been eradicated. Good personal hygiene is an important factor in preventing the spread of cutaneous streptococcal infections.

GOODPASTURE'S SYNDROME

Goodpasture's syndrome, an example of cytotoxic (type II) autoimmune disease, is characterized by the presence of circulating antibodies against GBM and alveolar basement membrane.[11] Although the primary target organ is the kidney, the lungs are also involved. The pathologic nature of the syndrome results when binding of the antibody causes an inflammatory reaction mediated by complement fixation and activation (see Chapter 12). The causative factors for development of autoantibody production are unknown, although type A influenza viruses, hydrocarbons, penicillamine, and unknown genetic factors may be involved.

Goodpasture's syndrome is a rare disease that is seen mostly in young male smokers. The clinical manifestations include hemoptysis, pulmonary insufficiency, crackles, rhonchi, renal involvement with hematuria and renal failure, weakness, pallor, and anemia. Pulmonary hemorrhage usually occurs and may precede glomerular abnormalities by weeks or months. Abnormal diagnostic findings include low hematocrit and hemoglobin levels, elevated BUN and serum creatinine levels, hematuria, and proteinuria. Circulating serum anti-GBM antibodies parallel the activity of the renal disease and are diagnostic of this syndrome.

NURSING AND COLLABORATIVE MANAGEMENT: GOODPASTURE'S SYNDROME

Until recently, the prognosis for the patient with Goodpasture's syndrome was poor. Management consists of corticosteroids, immunosuppressive drugs (e.g., cyclophosphamide [Cytoxan], azathioprine [Imuran]), plasmapheresis (see Chapter 12), and dialysis. Plasmapheresis removes the circulating anti-GBM antibody, and immunosuppressive therapy inhibits further antibody production. Renal transplantation can be attempted once the circulating anti-GBM antibody titer decreases. Although recurrences may develop, the disease is not a contraindication to transplantation. In selected patients with severe pulmonary hemorrhage, bilateral nephrectomy has been helpful. The exact mechanism for improvement has not been determined.

Nursing management appropriate for a critically ill patient who is experiencing symptoms of acute renal failure and respiratory distress is instituted. Death is often secondary to hemorrhage in the lungs and respiratory failure. (Nursing interventions for a patient in acute renal failure are discussed in Chapter 44, and nursing interventions for a patient with respiratory failure are discussed in Chapter 62.) Because this syndrome is rare and primarily affects previously healthy young men, support and understanding of the patient and family are of major importance. The patient and family need instructions concerning current therapy, medications, and complications of the disease process.

RAPIDLY PROGRESSIVE GLOMERULONEPHRITIS

Rapidly progressive glomerulonephritis (RPGN) is glomerular disease associated with rapid, progressive loss of renal function over days to weeks. Renal failure may occur within weeks to months in contrast to chronic glomerulonephritis, which develops insidiously and progresses over many years. The manifestations of RPGN are hypertension, edema, proteinuria, hematuria, and RBC casts.

RPGN can occur in a variety of situations: (1) as a complication of inflammatory or infectious disease (e.g., APSGN), (2) as a complication of a multisystemic disease (e.g., systemic lupus erythematosus, Goodpasture's syndrome), (3) as an idiopathic disease, or (4) in association with the use of certain drugs (e.g., penicillamine).

Treatment is directed toward correction of fluid overload, hypertension, uremia, and inflammatory injury to the kidney. Treatment includes corticosteroids, cytotoxic agents, and plasmapheresis. Dialysis therapy and transplantation are used to maintain the patient with RPGN. Following renal transplantation, RPGN may recur.

CHRONIC GLOMERULONEPHRITIS

Chronic glomerulonephritis is a syndrome that reflects the end stage of glomerular inflammatory disease. Most types of glomerulonephritis and nephrotic syndrome can eventually lead to chronic glomerulonephritis.

Table 43-8 Causes of Nephrotic Syndrome

Primary Glomerular Disease
Membranous proliferative glomerulonephritis
Primary nephrotic syndrome
Focal glomerulonephritis
Inherited nephrotic disease
Extrarenal Causes
Multisystem Disease
Systemic lupus erythematosus
Diabetes mellitus
Amyloidosis
Infections
Bacterial (streptococcal, syphilis)
Viral (hepatitis, human immunodeficiency virus infection)
Protozoal (malaria)
Neoplasms
Hodgkin's disease
Solid tumors of lungs, colon, stomach, breast
Leukemias
Allergens (e.g., Bee Sting, Pollen)
Drugs
Penicillamine
Nonsteroidal antiinflammatory drugs
Captopril (Capoten)
Heroin

The syndrome is characterized by proteinuria, hematuria, and the slow development of uremic syndrome (see Chapter 44) as a result of decreasing renal function. Chronic glomerulonephritis does not usually follow an acute course. It progresses insidiously toward renal failure over a few to as many as 30 years.

Chronic glomerulonephritis is often found coincidentally when an abnormality on a urinalysis or elevated blood pressure is detected. It is common to find that the patient has no recollection or history of acute nephritis or any renal problems. A renal biopsy may be performed to determine the exact cause and nature of the glomerulonephritis. However, many institutions now prefer to use ultrasound and CT scanning as diagnostic measures.

Treatment is supportive and symptomatic. Hypertension and urinary tract infections should be treated vigorously. Protein and phosphate restrictions may slow the rate of progression of renal failure. (Management of chronic renal failure is discussed in Chapter 44.)

NEPHROTIC SYNDROME

Etiology and Clinical Manifestations

The term *nephrotic syndrome* describes a clinical course that can be associated with a number of disease conditions. Some of the more common causes of nephrotic syndrome are listed in Table 43-8. In adults about one third of patients with nephrotic syndrome will have a systemic disease such as diabetes or systemic lupus erythematosus. The remainder will be categorized as having idiopathic nephrotic syndrome.[12]

The characteristic manifestations include peripheral edema, massive proteinuria, hyperlipidemia, and hypoalbuminemia.

Characteristic blood chemistries include decreased serum albumin, decreased total serum protein, and elevated serum cholesterol. The increased glomerular membrane permeability found in nephrotic syndrome is responsible for the massive excretion of protein in the urine. This results in decreased serum protein and subsequent edema formation. Ascites and anasarca develop if there is severe hypoalbuminemia.

The diminished plasma oncotic pressure from the decreased serum proteins stimulates hepatic lipoprotein synthesis, which results in hyperlipidemia. Initially, cholesterol and low-density lipoproteins are elevated. Later the triglyceride level is also increased. Fat bodies (fatty casts) commonly appear in the urine.

Immune responses, both humoral and cellular, are altered in nephrotic syndrome. As a result, infection is an important cause of morbidity and mortality. Calcium and skeletal abnormalities may occur, including hypocalcemia, blunted calcemic response to parathyroid hormone, hyperparathyroidism, and osteomalacia.

With nephrotic proteinuria, loss of clotting factors can result in a relative hypercoagulable state. Hypercoagulability with thromboembolism is potentially the most serious complication of nephrotic syndrome. The renal vein is the site most commonly involved for thrombus formation. Pulmonary emboli occur in about 40% of nephrotic patients with thrombosis.

Collaborative Care

Treatment of nephrotic syndrome is symptomatic. The goals are to relieve edema and cure or control the primary disease. Management of the edema includes the cautious use of angiotensin-converting enzyme (ACE) inhibitors, nonsteroidal antiinflammatory drugs, and a low-sodium (2 to 3 g per day), low- to moderate-protein diet (0.5 to 0.6 kg per day). Dietary salt restrictions are a key to managing edema. In some individuals thiazide or loop diuretics may be needed. If urine protein loss exceeds 10 g/24 hr, additional dietary protein may be needed.

The treatment of hyperlipidemia is frequently unsuccessful. However, treatment with lipid-lowering agents, such as colestipol (Colestid), probucol (Lorelco), and lovastatin (Mevacor), may result in moderate decreases in serum cholesterol levels. If thrombosis is detected, anticoagulant therapy may be necessary for up to 6 months.

Corticosteroids and cyclophosphamide (Cytoxan) may be used for the treatment of severe cases of nephrotic syndrome. Prednisone has been effective to varying degrees in persons with lipoid nephrosis, membranous glomerulonephritis, proliferative glomerulonephritis, and lupus nephritis. Management of diabetes and treatment of edema are the only measures used for nephrotic syndrome related to diabetes.

NURSING MANAGEMENT: NEPHROTIC SYNDROME

A major nursing intervention for a patient with nephrotic syndrome is related to edema. It is important to assess the edema by weighing the patient daily, accurately recording intake and output, and measuring abdominal girth or extremity size. Comparing this information daily provides the nurse with a tool for assessing the effectiveness of treatment. The edematous skin needs careful cleaning. Trauma should be avoided, and the effectiveness of diuretic therapy must be monitored.

The patient has the potential to become malnourished from the excessive loss of protein in the urine. Maintaining a low- to moderate-protein diet that is also low in sodium is not always easy. The patient is usually anorexic. Serving small, frequent meals in a pleasant setting may encourage better dietary intake.

Because the patient is susceptible to infection, measures should be taken to avoid exposure to persons with known infections. The person with nephrotic syndrome is often ashamed of an edematous appearance and needs support in dealing with an altered body image.

RENAL DISEASE AND ACQUIRED IMMUNODEFICIENCY SYNDROME

The patient with human immunodeficiency virus (HIV) infection can have a variety of renal manifestations, ranging from mild fluid and electrolyte abnormalities to progressive renal impairment resulting in end-stage renal disease.[13] The incidence of renal disease associated with HIV infection is about 10% and is highest among IV drug users.

HIV-associated renal syndromes include the following:

1. *Proteinuria and nephrotic syndrome,* which occurs in about 10% of patients with HIV infection. It may be the initial sign of HIV infection in some persons.
2. *HIV-associated nephropathy* (HIVAN), which is characterized by proteinuria, progressive azotemia, absence of hypertension, large kidney size on renal imaging studies, and unusually rapid progression to end-stage renal disease.
3. *Acute renal failure,* which is most commonly seen in the patient with acquired immunodeficiency syndrome (AIDS) who is critically ill with HIV-related infection or malignancy. Both oliguric and nonoliguric forms of renal failure can occur. The natural cause of acute renal failure secondary to AIDS is similar to acute renal failure associated with other acute illnesses (see Chapter 44). Survival and recovery usually depend on the treatment of the primary cause of renal failure and support of renal function by dialysis. (HIV infection is discussed in Chapter 13.)

OBSTRUCTIVE UROPATHIES

Obstruction of the urinary system may occur at any point from the kidney to the urethral meatus (Fig. 43-2). It may be congenital or acquired. Obstruction may be due to intrinsic causes such as anomalies, diverticuli, tumors, or benign growth within the urinary tract; extrinsic causes such as tumors, adhesions, retroperitoneal fibrosis, or prolapsed adjacent organs; or functional causes as a result of neurologic or psychogenic factors. Some common intrinsic obstructions are narrowing of the ureteropelvic junction, bladder neck contracture, benign prostatic hyperplasia, urethral stricture, and meatal stenosis. Common extrinsic causes include pelvic and abdominal tumors or a prolapsed uterus. Examples of functional causes are vesicosphincter dyssynergia after spinal cord injury and neurogenic bladder secondary to diabetes.

Damaging effects from urinary tract obstruction affect the system above the level of the obstruction. The severity of these

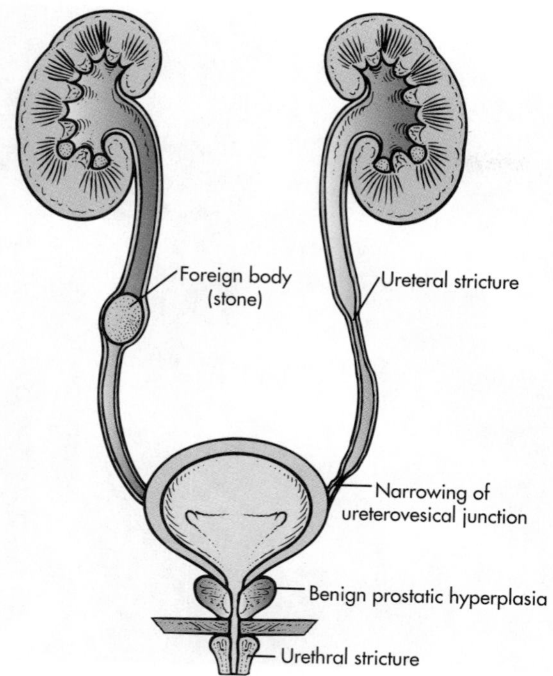

Fig. 43-2 Common causes of urinary tract obstruction.

effects depends on the location, duration of obstruction, amount of pressure or dilation, presence of urinary stasis, and whether infection is present. Infection increases the risk of irreversible consequences.

Although obstruction distal to the prostate in men or the bladder neck in women causes mucosal scarring and a slower stream, it rarely results in major obstructive uropathy because the urethral wall pressure is less than that of the bladder neck and bladder. Urethral obstruction may contribute to outlet resistance and cause lower or upper urinary tract damage when other obstructive or dysfunctional factors are also present. For example, there is an increased risk of compromised renal function in the patient with a spinal cord injury with vesicosphincter dyssynergia.

When obstruction occurs at the level of the bladder neck or prostate, significant bladder changes can occur. Detrusor muscle fibers hypertrophy (increase in size) in order to contract harder to push urine out a narrower pathway. Over a long period of time, the detrusor loses its ability to compensate for this resistance. Muscle bundles separate and become less compliant. This separation is termed *trabeculation.* Trabeculaton is caused by the deposition of collagen in the bladder wall that separates the smooth muscle fascicles. Trabeculation may hasten the decompensation of the detrusor. The areas between these muscle bundles are called *cellules.* Because these areas have no muscle support, the bladder mucosa can herniate between detrusor muscle bundles, forming sacs that drain poorly, called *diverticuli.* Residual urine can be very high in a noncompensating bladder.

Pressure increases during bladder filling or storage and can be transmitted to the ureter when bladder outlet obstruction is present. This pressure overcomes the normal peristaltic pressure and leads to reflux (a backflow of urine); ureteral dilation, kinking, and tortuosity; hydroureter (dilation of the renal pelvis); and hydronephrosis (dilation of the calyces) and consequent chronic pyelonephritis and renal atrophy (Fig. 43-3). If only one kidney is obstructed, the other kidney may try to compensate by hypertrophy, but the ureter will not be dilated on this contralateral side.

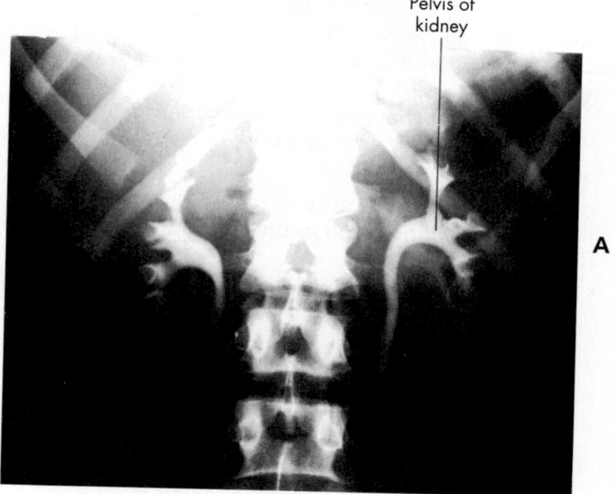

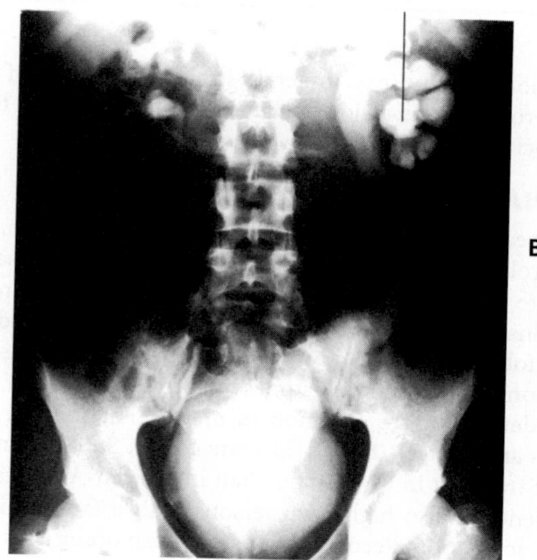

Fig. 43-3 **A,** Normal intravenous pyelogram (IVP). **B,** IVP showing hydronephrosis and hydroureter.

Partial obstruction may occur in the ureter or at the ureterovesical junction (UVJ). If the pressure remains low or moderate, the kidney may continue to dilate with no noticeable loss of function. There is an increased risk of pyelonephritis because of urinary stasis and reflux. If only one kidney is involved and the other kidney is functioning, the patient may be free of symptoms. If both kidneys or only one functioning kidney is involved (e.g., if the patient has only one kidney), alterations in renal function (e.g., increased BUN or serum creatinine levels) are found. If the obstruction progresses, oliguria or anuria develops. Often episodes of oliguria are followed by polyuria if the obstruction is a stone that becomes dislodged. Treatment requires locating and relieving the blockage. This can include

Table 43-9 Risk Factors for the Development of Urinary Tract Calculi

Metabolic
Abnormalities that result in increased urine levels of calcium, oxaluric acid, uric acid, or citric acid
Climate
Warm climates that cause increased fluid loss, low urine volume, and increased solute concentration in urine
Diet
Large intake of dietary proteins that increases uric acid excretion
Excessive amounts of tea or fruit juices that elevate urinary oxalate level
Large intake of calcium and oxalate
Low fluid intake that increases urinary concentration
Genetic Factors
Family history of stone formation, cystinuria, gout, or renal acidosis
Lifestyle
Sedentary occupation, immobility

insertion of a tube (e.g., ureteral), surgical correction of the disease process, or diversion of the urinary stream above the level of blockage.

URINARY TRACT CALCULI

Each year an estimated 500,000 people in the United States have nephrolithiasis (kidney stone disease).[14] Many of these people require hospitalization. In the United States the incidence of urinary stone disease is highest in the Southeast and Southwest, followed by the Midwest. Except for struvite (magnesium-ammonium-phosphate) stones associated with UTI, stone disorders are more common in men.[15] The majority of patients are between 20 and 55 years of age. Stone formation is more frequent in Caucasians than in African-Americans. The incidence is also higher in persons with a family history of stone formation. Recurrence of stones can occur in up to 50% of patients.[14] There is seasonal variation, with stone formation occurring more often in the summer months, thus supporting the role of dehydration in this process. Stone formation in the kidney also seems to increase in incidence as countries become more industrialized, whereas the incidence of bladder stones decreases.

Etiology and Pathophysiology

Many factors are involved in the incidence and type of stone formation, including metabolic, dietary, genetic, climatic, lifestyle, and occupational influences (Table 43-9). Many theories have been proposed to explain the formation of stones in the urinary tract. No single theory can account for stone formation in all cases. Crystals, when in a supersaturated concentration, can precipitate and unite to form a stone. Keeping urine dilute and free-flowing reduces the risk of recurrent stone formation in many individuals. It is known that a mucoprotein (the matrix for the stone) is formed in the kidneys that form stones. Urinary pH, solute load, and inhibitors in the urine affect the formation of stones. The higher the pH, the less soluble are calcium and phosphate. The lower the pH, the less soluble are uric acid and cystine.

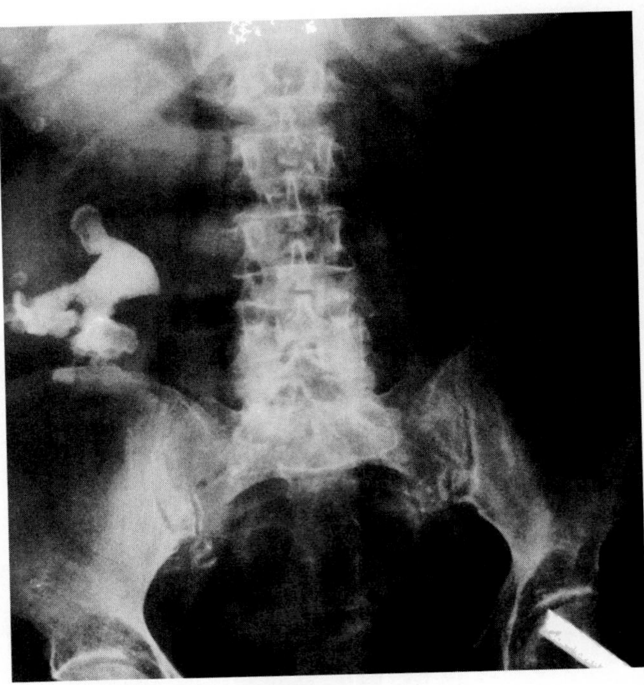

Fig. 43-4 X-ray of a staghorn calculus.

Other important factors in the development of stones include obstruction with urinary stasis and urinary infection with urea-splitting bacteria (e.g., *Proteus, Klebsiella, Pseudomonas,* and some species of staphylococci). These bacteria cause the urine to become alkaline and contribute to the formation of calcium-magnesium-ammonium phosphate stones (struvite or triple phosphate stones).[15] Infected stones, when they are entrapped in the kidney, may assume a staghorn configuration as they enlarge (Fig. 43-4). Infected stones are frequent in the patient with an external urinary diversion, long-term indwelling catheter, neurogenic bladder, or urinary retention. Genetic factors may also contribute to urine stone formation. Cystinuria is an autosomal recessive disorder. In this disorder there is greatly increased excretion of cystine.

Types

The term *calculus* refers to the stone and *lithiasis* refers to stone formation. There are five major categories of stones: (1) calcium phosphate, (2) calcium oxalate, (3) uric acid, (4) cystine, and (5) struvite (magnesium-ammonium phosphate) (Table 43-10). Stone composition may be mixed, although calcium stones are the most common. Calculi can be found in various locations in the urinary tract (Fig. 43-5).

Clinical Manifestations

Urinary stones cause clinical manifestations when they cause obstruction to urinary flow. Common sites of complete obstruction are at the ureteropelvic junction (UPJ), in the ureter at the point it crosses the iliac vessels, and at the ureterovesical junction (UVJ). Symptoms include abdominal or flank pain (usually severe), hematuria, and renal colic. The pain may be associated with nausea and vomiting. The type of pain is determined by the location of the stone (see Fig. 43-5). If the stone is nonobstructing, pain may be absent. If it produces obstruction in a calyx or at the UPJ, the patient may experience

Table 43-10 Types of Urinary Tract Calculi

Urinary Stone	Incidence (%)	Characteristics	Predisposing Factors	Therapeutic Measures
Calcium oxalate*	35-40	Small, often possible to get trapped in ureter; more frequent in men than in women	Idiopathic hypercalcuria, hyperoxaluria, independent of urinary pH, family history	Increase hydration. Reduce dietary oxalate.‡ Give thiazide diuretics. Give cellulose phosphate to chelate calcium and prevent GI absorption. Give potassium citrate to maintain alkaline urine. Give cholestyramine to bind oxalate. Give calcium lactate to precipitate oxalate in GI tract.
Calcium phosphate	8-10	Mixed stones (typically), with struvite or oxalate stones	Alkaline urine, primary hyperparathyroidism	Treat underlying causes and other stones.
Struvite ($MgNH_4PO_4$)	10-15	Three to four times as common in women than men, always in association with urinary tract infections, large staghorn type (usually)†	Urinary tract infections (usually *Proteus* organisms)	Administer antimicrobial agents, acetohydroxamic acid. Use surgical intervention to remove stone. Take measures to acidify urine.
Uric acid	5-8	Predominant in men, high incidence in Jewish men	Gout, acid urine, inherited condition	Reduce urinary concentration of uric acid. Alkalinize urine with potassium citrate. Administer allopurinol. Reduce dietary purines.‡
Cystine	1-2	Genetic autosomal recessive defect, defective absorption of cystine in GI tract and kidney, excess concentrations causing stone formation	Acid urine	Increase hydration. Give α-penicillamine and tiopronin to prevent cystine crystallization. Give potassium citrate to maintain alkaline urine.

*Calcium stones can exist as calcium oxalate, calcium phosphate, or a mixture of both. Calcium stones account for the majority of all stones.
†See Fig. 43-4.
‡See Table 43-11.

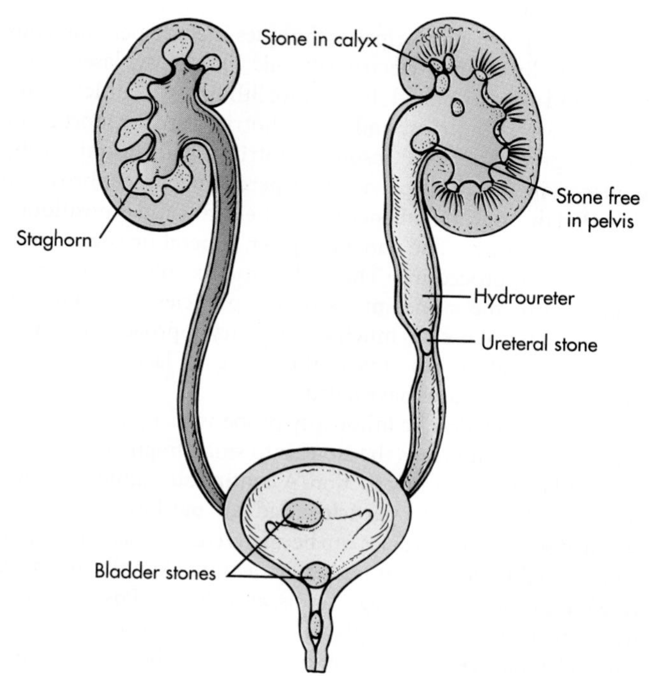

Fig. 43-5 Location of calculi in the urinary tract.

dull costovertebral flank pain or even colic. Pain resulting from the passage of a calculus down the ureter is intense and colicky. The patient may be in mild shock with cool, moist skin. As a stone nears the UVJ, pain will be felt in the lateral flank and sometimes down into the testicles, labia, or groin. Other clinical manifestations include the presence of urinary infection accompanied by fever, vomiting, nausea, and chills.

Diagnostic Studies

Diagnostic studies useful in the evaluation and management of renal lithiasis include urinalysis, urine culture, IVP, retrograde pyelogram, ultrasound, and cystoscopy. A plain film of the abdomen and renal ultrasound will usually diagnose most stones. An IVP or retrograde pyelogram can further localize the degree and site of obstruction and confirm the presence of nonradiopaque stones (uric acid, cystine). CT scans may be used to differentiate a nonopaque stone from a tumor.

Measurement of the urine and serum levels of various substances involved in stone formation (e.g., calcium, phosphate, oxalate, uric acid) is often done after a stone is discovered to determine possible metabolic causes and preventive management strategies. BUN and serum creatinine are determined to assess renal function. A careful history, including previous stone formation, prescribed and over-the-counter medications and dietary supplements, and familial stone formation, is useful.

Measurement of urine pH is useful in the diagnosis of struvite stones and renal tubular acidosis (tendency to alkaline pH) and uric acid stones (tendency to acidic pH). Retrieval and analysis of the stones are important in the diagnosis of the underlying problem contributing to stone formation. Chemical and crystallographic analyses are done.

Collaborative Care

Evaluation and management of a patient with renal lithiasis consist of two concurrent approaches. The first approach is directed toward management of the acute attack. This involves treating the symptoms of pain, infection, or obstruction as indicated for the individual patient. At frequent intervals, narcotics are typically required for relief of renal colic pain. Many stones pass spontaneously. However, stones larger than 4 mm are unlikely to pass through the ureter.

The second approach is directed toward evaluation of the etiology of the stone formation and the prevention of further development of stones. Information to be obtained from the patient includes family history of stone formation, geographic residence, nutritional assessment including the intake of vitamins A and D, activity pattern (active or sedentary), history of periods of prolonged illness with immobilization or dehydration, and any history of disease or surgery involving the GI or genitourinary (GU) tract.

Proper therapy for active stone formers requires a concerted management approach, with primary emphasis on teaching and on developing a therapeutic regimen with which the patient can reasonably comply (see Table 43-10). Adequate hydration, dietary sodium restrictions, dietary changes (Table 43-11), and the use of medications minimize urinary stone formation. Various medications are prescribed, depending on the specific problem underlying stone formation (see Table 43-10). These medications prevent stone formation in various ways, including altering urine pH, preventing excessive urinary excretion of a substance, or correcting a primary disease (e.g. hyperparathyroidism).

Treatment of struvite stones requires control of infection. This may be difficult if the stone remains in place. In addition to antibiotics, acetohydroxamic acid may be used in the treatment of kidney infections that result in the continual formation of struvite stones. Acetohydroxamic acid, an inhibitor of the chemical action caused by the persistent bacteria, can be used effectively to retard struvite stone formation. If the infection cannot be controlled, the stone may have to be removed surgically.

Indications for endourologic, lithotripsy, or open surgical stone removal include the following:

1. Stones too large for spontaneous passage
2. Stones associated with bacteriuria or symptomatic infection
3. Stones causing impaired renal function
4. Stones causing persistent pain, nausea, or ileus
5. Inability of patient to be treated medically
6. Patient with one kidney

Endourologic Procedures. If the stone is located in the bladder, a cystoscopy is done to remove small stones. For large stones a cystolitholapaxy is done. In this procedure large stones can be broken up with an instrument called a lithotrite (stone crusher). The bladder is then irrigated and the crushed stones washed out. A cystoscopic lithotripsy uses an ultrasonic lithotrite to pulverize stones. Complications associated with these cystoscopic procedures include hemorrhage, retained stone fragments, and infection.

Flexible ureteroscopes, inserted via a cystoscope, can be used to remove stones from the renal pelvis and upper urinary tract. Ultrasonic, laser, or electrohydraulic lithotripsy can be used in conjunction with the ureteroscope to pulverize and break the stone into fragments.[16]

In percutaneous nephrolithotomy (PNL) a nephroscope is inserted through a sinus tract from the skin into the kidney pelvis.[17] Stones can be fragmented using ultrasound, electrohydraulic, or laser lithotripsy. The stone fragments are removed and the pelvis irrigated. A percutaneous nephrostomy tube is usually left in place to ensure that the ureter is not obstructed. Complications include bleeding, injury to adjacent structures, and infection.

Lithotripsy. Lithotripsy techniques include percutaneous ultrasonic lithotripsy, electrohydraulic lithotripsy, laser lithotripsy, and extracorporeal shock-wave lithotripsy. Extracorporeal shock-wave lithotripsy and laser lithotripsy are the most common. In percutaneous ultrasonic lithotripsy an ultrasonic probe is placed in the renal pelvis via a percutaneous nephroscope (inserted through a small incision in the flank) and is positioned against the stone. (The patient is given general or spinal anesthesia for this procedure.) The probe produces ultrasonic waves, which break the stone into sandlike particles. Percutaneous lithotripsy is not used as much as a primary approach to renal or upper ureteral stones unless the stone is large and other lithotripsy procedures have failed.

The electrohydraulic lithotripsy probe is also placed directly on a stone, but it breaks the stone into small fragments that are removed by forceps or by suction. A continuous saline irrigation flushes out the stone particles, and all outflow drainage is strained so that the particles can be analyzed. The calculi can also be removed by forceps or basket extraction. Complications are rare but include hemorrhage, sepsis, and abscess. Postoperatively, the patient usually complains of moderate to severe colicky pain. The first few voidings are bright red; as the bleeding subsides, the urine becomes dark red or turns a smoky color. Antibiotics are usually given for 2 weeks to reduce the risk of infection.

NUTRITIONAL THERAPY

Table 43-11 Urinary Tract Calculi

The following is a list of foods high in purine, calcium, or oxalate content

Purine

High: Sardines, herring, mussels, liver, kidney, goose, venison, meat soups, sweetbreads

Moderate: Chicken, salmon, crab, veal, mutton, bacon, pork, beef, ham

Calcium

Milk, cheese, ice cream, yogurt, sauces containing milk; all beans (except green beans), lentils; fish with fine bones (e.g., sardines, kippers, herring, salmon); dried fruits, nuts; chocolate, cocoa, Ovaltine

Oxalate

Spinach, rhubarb, asparagus, cabbage, tomatoes, beets, nuts, celery, parsley, runner beans; chocolate, cocoa, instant coffee, Ovaltine, tea; Worcestershire sauce

Laser lithotripsy probes are used to fragment lower ureteral and large bladder stones. The medium used, a coumarin-based pulsed dye, works on a wavelength that fragments stones but does not injure the surrounding tissue.

In extracorporeal shock-wave lithotripsy, a noninvasive procedure, the patient is anesthetized (spinal or general) and placed in a water bath. Anesthesia is necessary to keep the patient very still during the procedure. Some of the newer-generation lithotripters do not require submersion and use other means of initiating shock waves. The lithotripters are categorized as electrohydraulic, electromagnetic, and piezoelectric. The second-generation lithotripters use less power to fragment stones. Lower power reduces a patient's pain, but usually some sedation or analgesia is necessary.

Fluoroscopy or ultrasound is used to focus the lithotripter on the affected kidney, and a high-voltage spark generator produces high-energy acoustic shock waves that shatter the stone without damaging the surrounding tissues. The stone is broken into fine sand, which is excreted into the patient's urine within a few days after the procedure.

Hematuria is common after lithotripsy procedures. A self-retaining ureteral stent is often placed after the procedure to promote passage of this sand and to prevent obstruction caused by *Steinstrasse* (a buildup of sand in the ureter). The stent is removed 1 to 2 weeks after lithotripsy. A primary advantage of these techniques compared with open surgery is the decrease in the length of hospitalization and the patient's earlier return to normal activities. Retreatment may be necessary, especially if a stone is large and in the mid or distal ureter.

Surgical Therapy. There are a small group of select patients who need open surgical procedures, such as the very obese patient or the individual with complex abnormalities in the calyces or at the UPJ. The type of open surgery needed depends on the location of the stone. A nephrolithotomy is an incision into the kidney to remove a stone. A pyelolithotomy is an incision into the renal pelvis to remove a stone. If the stone is located in the ureter, a ureterolithotomy is performed. A cystotomy may be indicated for bladder calculi. For open surgery on the kidney or ureter, a flank incision directly below the diaphragm and across the side is usually the preferred surgical approach. Complications related to hemorrhage are the most common following these surgical procedures.

Nutritional Therapy. A high fluid intake (at least 3000 ml per day) is recommended after an episode of urolithiasis to produce a urine output of at least 2 L per day. High urine output prevents supersaturation of minerals (i.e., dilutes the concentration) and flushes them out before the minerals have a chance to precipitate. Increasing the fluid intake is especially important for the patient who is active in sports, lives in a dry climate, performs physical exercise, has a family history of stone formation, or works in an occupation that requires outdoor work or a great deal of physical activity that can lead to dehydration.

Dietary intervention may be important in the management of urolithiasis. In the past, calcium restriction was routinely implemented for the patient with kidney stones. Recent research suggests that a high dietary calcium intake, which was previously thought to contribute to kidney stones, may actually lower the risk by reducing the urinary excretion of oxalate, a common factor in many stones. Initial nutritional management should include limiting oxalate-rich foods and thereby reducing oxalate excretion. Foods high in calcium, oxalate, and purines are presented in Table 43-11.

NURSING MANAGEMENT: RENAL CALCULI

■ Nursing Assessment

Subjective and objective data that should be obtained from a patient with urinary tract lithiasis are presented in Table 43-12.

■ Nursing Diagnoses

Nursing diagnoses for the patient with urinary tract lithiasis include, but are not limited to, those presented in NCP 43-2.

NURSING ASSESSMENT

Table 43-12 Urinary Tract Calculi

Subjective Data

Important Health Information

Past health history: Recent or chronic UTI; bed rest; immobilization; previous urinary tract stones, obstruction, or kidney disease with urinary stasis; gout; prostatic hyperplasia; hyperparathyroidism

Medications: Prior use of medication for prevention of stones or treatment of UTI; allopurinol, analgesics

Surgery or other treatments: External urinary diversion, long-term indwelling urinary catheter

Functional Health Patterns

Health perception–health management: Family history of renal calculi; sedentary lifestyle

Nutritional-metabolic: Nausea, vomiting: dietary intake of purines, calcium, oxalates, phosphates; low fluid intake; chills

Elimination: Decreased urinary output, urinary urgency, frequency, feeling of bladder fullness

Cognitive-perceptual: Acute, severe, colicky pain in flank, back, abdomen, groin, or genitalia; burning on urination, dysuria, anxiety

Objective Data

General

Guarding, fever

Integumentary

Warm, flushed skin or pallor with cool, moist skin (mild shock)

Gastrointestinal

Abdominal distention, absence of bowel sounds

Urinary

Oliguria, hematuria, tenderness on palpation of renal areas, passage of stone or stones

Possible Findings

Elevated BUN and serum creatinine levels; RBCs, WBCs, pyuria, crystals, casts, minerals, bacteria on urinalysis; elevated creatinine, uric acid, calcium, phosphorus, oxalate, or cystine values on 24 hr urine sample; calculi or anatomic changes on IVP or KUB x-ray; direct visualization of obstruction on cystoureteroscopy

BUN, blood urea nitrogen; *KUB,* kidneys, ureters, bladder; *UTI,* urinary tract infection.

43-2 NURSING CARE PLAN PATIENT WITH ACUTE RENAL LITHIASIS

Expected Patient Outcomes	Nursing Interventions and *Rationales*
NURSING DIAGNOSIS **Pain** *related to* irritation of stone and inadequate pain control or comfort measures *as manifested by* complaints of pain, facial grimacing, restlessness.	
▪ Minimal or no pain. ▪ Decrease in pain and satisfaction with pain control.	▪ Assess for pain location and severity *to plan appropriate interventions.* ▪ Encourage high fluid intake unless contraindicated *to promote passage of stone, dilute the urine, and reduce risk of additional stone formation.* ▪ Administer pain medication as ordered *to promote comfort.* ▪ Apply moist heat to flank area as needed *because heat reduces inflammation and reflex muscle spasm and promotes comfort.*
NURSING DIAGNOSIS **Anxiety** *related to* uncertain outcome and lack of knowledge regarding possible surgery *as manifested by* expressions of concern about future treatments.	
▪ Relief of anxiety. ▪ Expression of confidence in treatment plan.	▪ Assess cause and level of anxiety *to plan appropriate interventions.* ▪ Explain surgical or nonsurgical procedure (include insertion of ureteral catheters) *because accurate information often decreases anxiety and fosters control.* ▪ Encourage patient to express feelings of anxiety, fear of surgery *to validate feelings and provide support.*
NURSING DIAGNOSIS **Ineffective management of therapeutic regimen** *related to* lack of knowledge about prevention of recurrence, diet, fluid requirements, and symptoms of recurrence *as manifested by* questions that indicate inadequate knowledge of disorder.	
▪ Verbalization of correct self-care measures. ▪ Able to list symptoms of recurrence.	▪ Instruct patient during initial hospital stay regarding increasing fluids unless contraindicated and diet restrictions and rationale *to prepare for home self-care.* ▪ Inform patient about rationale, dose, frequency, and side effects of medication *to foster adherence to medication regimen.* ▪ Tell patient to strain all urine through a urine strainer or piece of gauze (if necessary) *to determine if stones are passed,* and to bring stone to physician for analysis. ▪ Educate patient about symptoms of recurrence (e.g., hematuria, flank pain) *to ensure early reporting and initiation of treatment.*
NURSING DIAGNOSIS **Altered urinary elimination** *related to* trauma or blockage of ureters or urethra *as manifested by* decrease in urinary output, bloody urine.	
▪ Free flow of urine. ▪ Minimal to no hematuria.	▪ Monitor urine amount and character *to ensure patency in urinary system and that hematuria is not excessive.* ▪ Encourage increased fluid intake *because increased hydration flushes bacteria and blood and may facilitate passage of stone fragments.*
NURSING DIAGNOSIS **Risk for infection** *related to* introduction of bacteria following manipulations of the urinary tract.	
▪ No urinary tract infections.	▪ Assess for elevation in temperature; chills; cloudy, foul-smelling urine *as indicators of potential infection.* ▪ Monitor vital signs and observe for fever *because abnormalities may indicate infection.* ▪ Report any fever or chills to physician *so prompt treatment can be initiated.* ▪ Administer antipyretics and antibiotics as ordered *to reduce fever and treat infection.* ▪ Encourage high fluid intake unless contraindicated *because stones form more rapidly in concentrated urine and increased fluids help the stone fragments pass down urinary tract.*

Continued

43-2 NURSING CARE PLAN PATIENT WITH ACUTE RENAL LITHIASIS—continued

Expected Patient Outcomes	Nursing Interventions and *Rationales*
COLLABORATIVE PROBLEMS	
Nursing Goals	**Nursing Interventions and *Rationales***
POTENTIAL COMPLICATION	**Urinary obstruction** *related to* presence of stone in path of urine flow.
▪ Monitor for signs of urinary obstruction and report occurrence. ▪ Carry out medical and nursing interventions.	▪ Assess patient for signs of urinary obstruction such as complaints of persistent pain, urgency along with inability to void and bladder distention *to ensure early identification of the problem.* ▪ Monitor urine output and fluid intake *because decreased output relative to intake can suggest urinary obstruction.* ▪ Notify physician of oliguria *so treatment can be started promptly.* ▪ Strain all urine *to determine if stones are passed.* ▪ Save stones *so they can be sent for analysis to determine chemical composition.*

Planning

The overall goals are that the patient with urinary tract calculi will have (1) relief of pain, (2) no urinary tract obstruction, and (3) an understanding of measures to prevent further recurrence of stones.

Nursing Implementation

Preventive measures relate to the person who is on bed rest or is relatively immobile for a prolonged time. It is important to maintain a high fluid intake and to prevent urinary stasis by turning the patient every 2 hours and helping the patient to sit or stand if possible. In the acute phase it is important to retrieve the stone if passed. All urine voided by the patient should be strained through gauze or a special urine strainer in an effort to detect the stone. Increased intake of fluids and ambulation help the stone pass down the urinary tract. The patient should not walk if pain is present during an attack of renal colic. Narcotics will be required for renal colic because the pain is excruciating. Pain management and patient comfort are primary nursing responsibilities (see NCP 43-2).

Stone formation can be prevented, and the recurrence rate can be greatly reduced. After the acute phase, it is important for the nurse to teach the patient ways to prevent recurrence. Dietary restriction of oxalate is important for the patient who has calcium oxalate stones. Diets that restrict purines may be helpful to the patient at risk for developing uric acid stones. Follow-up care includes monitoring the patient's compliance with fluid, dietary, and medication recommendations. Periodic urine cultures may be indicated. Testing the pH of the urine is important, especially to assess the effectiveness of acidifying or alkalinizing agents. It is important to emphasize the need to avoid inadvertent dehydration from excessive exercise and to increase fluid needs during illness and hot weather.

Evaluation

The expected outcomes for the patient with urinary calculi are presented in NCP 43-2.

STRICTURES

A *stricture* is a narrowing of the lumen and is sometimes congenital but is usually acquired. Strictures may occur in the bladder neck, urethra, or ureters. Strictures of the bladder neck may be congenital or may result from chronic prostatitis in men or cystitis in women. Causes of urethral strictures include trauma from accidents (e.g., those resulting in fractured pelvis), gonorrheal infections, and urethral instrumentation. The membranous urethra is a common site of stricture caused by instrumentation because of its location (the urethral curve just below the prostatic urethra) and because the surrounding rhabdosphincter muscles prevent easy distention. Meatal stenosis, a narrowing of the urethral opening, is also common. Ureteral strictures may be caused by severe or chronic infection, radiation therapy, and retroperitoneal abscess formation from inflammatory bowel disease and perforation.

Strictures can sometimes be avoided by the proper management of inflammatory processes or traumatic injuries. Treatment of existing strictures includes dilation, use of a catheter for temporary or permanent drainage for ureteral or urethral strictures, and surgery. Some patients are taught to dilate the urethra themselves between office visits to keep strictured areas open. Nursing interventions include informing the patient about the procedure; preparing the patient for the procedure; and assessing the patient's need for management, education, and follow-up care.

RENAL TRAUMA

A continual increase in the incidence of traumatic renal injuries is related to an increase in the mechanization and speed of transportation and to the increase in violent crimes and injuries. The majority of incidents occur in men younger than 30 years of age. Blunt trauma is the most frequent cause. Injury to the kidney should be considered in multiple or sports injuries, traffic accidents, and falls. It is especially likely when the patient injures the abdomen, flank, or back. Penetrating injuries may result from violent encounters (e.g., gunshot or stabbing incidents) or from surgical errors.

Clinical findings include a history of trauma to the area of the kidneys. Gross or microscopic hematuria may be present. Diagnostic studies include urinalysis, IVP with cystography, ultrasound, CT, or MRI evaluation. Renal arteriography may also be used. Both the injured kidney and the noninvolved kidney should be evaluated to provide information for further management.

The severity of renal trauma depends on the extent of the injury. Treatments range from bed rest, fluids, and analgesia to surgical exploration and repair or nephrectomy.

Nursing interventions vary with the type and extent of associated injuries. Specific interventions related to renal trauma include ensuring increased fluid intake, providing comfort measures, monitoring intake and output, observing for hematuria, determining the presence of myoglobinuria, assessing the cardiovascular status, and monitoring potentially nephrotoxic antibiotics.

RENAL VASCULAR PROBLEMS

Vascular problems involving the kidney include (1) nephrosclerosis, (2) renal artery stenosis, and (3) renal vein thrombosis.

NEPHROSCLEROSIS

Nephrosclerosis consists of sclerosis of the small arteries and arterioles of the kidney. There is decreased blood flow, which results in patchy necrosis of the renal parenchyma. Ischemic necrosis and destruction of glomeruli with subsequent fibrosis also occur.

Benign nephrosclerosis usually occurs in adults 30 to 50 years of age. It is caused by vascular changes resulting from hypertension and from the arteriosclerotic process. Arteriosclerotic vascular changes account for most of the loss of renal function associated with aging. There is a direct relation between the degree of nephrosclerosis and the severity of hypertension. The patient with benign nephrosclerosis may have normal renal function in the early stages. The only detectable abnormality may be hypertension.

Accelerated nephrosclerosis, or malignant nephrosclerosis, is associated with malignant hypertension, a complication of hypertension characterized by a sharp increase in blood pressure with a diastolic pressure greater than 130 mm Hg. The patient is usually a young adult, with a male-to-female predominance of 2:1. Renal insufficiency progresses rapidly.

Treatment of benign nephrosclerosis is the same as that of essential hypertension (see Chapter 31). Malignant nephrosclerosis is treated with aggressive antihypertensive therapy (see Chapter 31). The availability and use of antihypertensives have improved the prognosis for the patient with benign nephrosclerosis. Renal dysfunction and renal failure (in some persons) constitute two of the major complications of hypertension. The prognosis for the patient with malignant hypertension is poor, with the major cause of death related to renal failure.

RENAL ARTERY STENOSIS

Renal artery stenosis is a partial occlusion of one or both renal arteries and their major branches. It can be due to atherosclerotic narrowing or fibromuscular hyperplasia. Renal artery stenosis accounts for 1% to 2% of all cases of hypertension.

Renal artery stenosis is considered a major cause of hypertension when it develops abruptly, especially in the patient under 30 or over 50 years of age and in the patient with no familial history of hypertension. This contrasts with the age distribution for essential hypertension, which is 30 to 50 years of age. A renal arteriogram is the best diagnostic tool for identifying renal artery stenosis.

The goals of therapy are control of blood pressure and restoration of perfusion to the kidney. Surgical revascularization of the kidney is indicated when blood flow is decreased enough to cause renal ischemia or when evidence indicates that renovascular hypertension is present and surgical intervention may result in the patient becoming normotensive. The surgical procedure usually involves anastomoses between the kidney and another major artery, usually the splenic artery or aorta. Percutaneous transluminal angioplasty may be used as an alternative to surgery, especially in older patients who are poor surgical risks. In selected cases of unilateral renal involvement with high renin production, unilateral nephrectomy may be indicated.

RENAL VEIN THROMBOSIS

Renal vein thrombosis may occur unilaterally or bilaterally. Trauma, extrinsic compression (e.g., tumor, aortic aneurysm), renal cell carcinoma, pregnancy, contraceptive use, and nephrotic syndrome are associated with renal vein thrombosis.

The patient has symptoms of flank pain, hematuria, or fever or has nephrotic syndrome. Anticoagulation is important in treatment because there is a high incidence of pulmonary emboli. Corticosteroids may be used in the patient with nephrosis. Surgical thrombectomy may be performed instead of or along with anticoagulation.

HEREDITARY RENAL DISEASES

Hereditary renal diseases involve developmental abnormalities of the renal parenchyma. These abnormalities are either isolated or part of more complex malformation syndromes. The majority of inherited structural abnormalities are cystic. However, cysts may also develop as a result of obstructive uropathies, metabolic derangements, or neurologic diseases. Cysts may be evaluated to rule out any tumor content.

POLYCYSTIC RENAL DISEASE

Polycystic renal disease is one of the most common genetic diseases in humans and affects 600,000 people in the United States.[18] There are two forms of hereditary polycystic renal disease. It may be manifested in childhood or adulthood. The childhood form of polycystic disease is a rare autosomal recessive disorder that is often rapidly progressive.

The adult form of polycystic disease is an autosomal dominant disorder. It is latent for many years and is usually manifested between 30 and 40 years of age. It involves both kidneys and occurs in both men and women. The cortex and the medulla are filled with thin-walled cysts that are several millimeters to several centimeters in diameter (Fig. 43-6). The cysts enlarge and destroy surrounding tissue by compression. They are filled with fluid and may contain blood or pus.

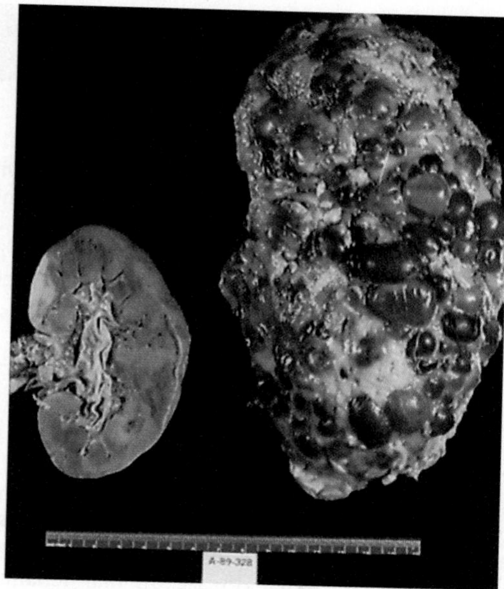

Fig. 43-6 Comparison of polycystic kidney with normal kidney.

Clinical Manifestations

In the patient with polycystic disease, symptoms appear when the cysts begin to enlarge. A common early symptom of adult cystic disease is abdominal or flank pain, which is either steady and dull or abrupt in onset, as well as episodic and colicky. This pain is often caused by bleeding into the cysts. On physical examination, palpable bilateral enlarged kidneys are often found. Other clinical manifestations include hematuria (from rupture of cysts), UTI, and hypertension. Diagnosis is based on clinical manifestations, family history, IVP, ultrasound, or CT scan. Usually the disease progresses to chronic renal failure, although some individuals have relatively mild disease and die from unrelated problems. Loss of kidney function to the point of end-stage renal disease occurs by age 60 in 50% of patients.[18]

Collaborative Care

There is no specific treatment for polycystic kidney disease. A major aim of treatment is to prevent infections of the urinary tract or to treat them with appropriate antibiotics if they occur. Nephrectomy may be necessary if pain, bleeding, or infection becomes a chronic, serious problem.

When the patient begins to experience progressive renal failure, the interventions are determined by the remaining renal function. Nursing measures are those used for management of end-stage renal disease (see Chapter 44). They include diet modification, fluid restriction, medications (e.g., antihypertensives), assisting the patient to accept the chronic disease process, and assisting the patient and family to deal with financial concerns and other issues related to the hereditary nature of the disease.

The patient who has adult polycystic disease often has children by the time the disease is diagnosed. Each child of a parent with polycystic kidney disease has a 50% chance of having the disease. The patient will need appropriate counseling regarding plans for having more children. In addition, genetic counseling resources should be provided for the children.

MEDULLARY CYSTIC DISEASE

Medullary cystic disease is a hereditary disorder that occurs in two forms. The recessive form is associated with renal failure before age 20; the dominant form is associated with renal failure after age 20. Most cysts are located in the medulla. The kidneys are asymmetric in shape and are significantly scarred. There are defects in the concentration ability of the kidneys. Polyuria, progressive renal failure, severe anemia, metabolic acidosis, and poor sodium conservation are common. Hypertension can be a terminal event. Genetic counseling may be helpful in family planning. Treatment measures are those related to end-stage renal disease (see Chapter 44).

ALPORT'S SYNDROME

Alport's syndrome is also known as chronic hereditary nephritis. Two forms of the disease exist: (1) classic Alport's syndrome, which is inherited as a sex-linked disorder with hematuria, sensorineural deafness, and deformities of the anterior surface of the lens; and (2) nonclassical Alport's syndrome, which is inherited as an autosomal trait that causes hematuria but not deafness or lens deformities. Men are affected earlier and more severely than women. The disease is frequently diagnosed in the first decade of life. The basic defect is altered synthesis of the glomerular basement membrane (GBM). The patient most commonly has hematuria and progressive uremia. Treatment is supportive. Corticosteroids and cytotoxic drugs are not effective. The disease does not recur after kidney transplantation.

RENAL INVOLVEMENT IN METABOLIC AND CONNECTIVE TISSUE DISEASES

Various metabolic and connective tissue disease processes may have an effect on renal function. The pathophysiologic effects on the renal parenchyma are not always specific to each process. The clinical course of renal involvement is that of chronic progressive nephropathy, which can result in uremia and death. Management includes treatment of the primary disorder along with symptomatic relief of renal involvement. If renal involvement progresses to chronic renal failure, management includes dialysis or transplantation (see Chapter 44). Nursing interventions include teaching the patient about the primary disease process, the renal involvement, and the resulting need to comply with dietary and fluid restrictions and medication.

Diabetic nephropathy is the major cause of end-stage renal failure in the United States. Diabetes mellitus may affect the kidneys in several ways. Microangiopathic changes in diabetes consist of diffuse glomerulosclerosis, involving thickening of the GBM and nodular glomerulosclerosis (Kimmelstiel-Wilson syndrome), which is characterized by nodular lesions. Nodular glomerulosclerosis is reasonably specific for type 1 diabetes mellitus. The diabetic patient prone to glomerulonephropathy (e.g., the presence of trace proteinuria or retinopathy) requires careful monitoring of glucose levels and insulin requirements.

Diabetic nephropathy can result in chronic renal failure. The patient with diabetes is especially susceptible to UTIs. Primary nursing interventions include teaching the patient about the increased risk of UTIs, the appropriate preventive measures, and when to seek additional medical care. (Diabetes mellitus is discussed in Chapter 46.)

Gout is a syndrome of acute attacks of arthritis caused by hyperuricemia (see Chapter 60). Monosodium urate crystals deposited in joints are responsible for the syndrome. Renal disease may develop as a result of damage caused by deposition of uric acid crystals in the renal interstitium and tubules.

Amyloidosis is a group of disorders manifested by impaired organ function from the infiltration of tissues with a hyaline substance (amyloid). The hyaline consists largely of protein. Kidney involvement is common in amyloidosis. Proteinuria is often the first clinical manifestation.

Systemic lupus erythematosus (SLE) is a connective tissue disorder characterized by the involvement of several tissues and organs, particularly the joints, skin, and kidneys (SLE is discussed in Chapter 60). Clinical manifestations of lupus nephritis are similar to those of other forms of glomerulonephritis. Most frequently found are microscopic hematuria and significant proteinuria. Renal failure frequently occurs in systemic lupus erythematosus and has a poor prognosis. The long-term course of the disorder is extremely variable. Corticosteroids are effective for the patient with severe renal disease. Recently, plasmapheresis therapy has been used.

Scleroderma (progressive systemic sclerosis) is a disease of unknown etiology characterized by widespread alterations of connective tissue and by vascular lesions in many organs (see Chapter 60). In the kidney, vascular lesions are associated with fibrosis. An immune complex mechanism has been postulated as a possible etiologic factor. The severity of renal involvement varies. The patient who develops severe renal lesions has a poor prognosis. Once uremia develops, about 70% die within 3 years.

NEOPLASTIC DISORDERS OF THE URINARY TRACT

RENAL TUMORS

Tumors of the kidney are responsible for approximately 12,000 deaths per year, and 30,000 new cases are diagnosed each year.[19] Renal tumors arise from the cortex or pelvis (and calyces). Tumors arising from both areas may be benign or malignant. However, malignant tumors are more frequent. Renal cell carcinoma (adenocarcinoma) is the most common type. Adenocarcinoma is twice as frequent in men as in women and is typically discovered when the person is 50 to 70 years old. Cigarette smoking is the most significant risk factor for the development of renal cell carcinoma. Other risk factors are the use of phenacetin-containing analgesics and exposure to asbestos, cadmium, and gasoline.

There are no characteristic early symptoms. Generalized symptoms of weight loss, weakness, and anemia are the earliest manifestations. The classic manifestations of gross hematuria, flank pain, and a palpable mass are those of advanced disease.[20] The most common sites of metastases include the lungs, liver, and long bones. Local extension of renal cancer into the renal vein and vena cava is common. Renal cystic disease and renal-associated carcinomas may develop in the patient with end-stage renal disease on maintenance renal dialysis (see Chapter 44).

Several studies are used to diagnose adenocarcinoma of the kidney. IVP with nephrotomography is the primary examination by which most masses are detected and evaluated. Ultrasounds have improved the ability to differentiate between a tumor and a cyst. Angiography, percutaneous needle aspiration, CT, and magnetic resonance imaging (MRI) are also used in the diagnosis of renal tumors. Small renal tumors are found earlier because of the increased use of CT scans and MRI. Radionuclide isotope scanning is used to detect metastases.

Robson's system of staging renal carcinoma is presented in Table 43-13. Tumor, node, metastases (TNM) classification is also used for renal cancer staging. The treatment of choice is a radical nephrectomy. Radical nephrectomy is the removal of the kidney, adrenal gland, surrounding fascia, part of the ureter, and draining lymph nodes. Radiation therapy is used palliatively in inoperable cases and when there are metastases to bone or lungs. No effective chemotherapy is available for metastatic renal cell carcinoma. Biologic therapy, including α-interferon and interleukin-2 (IL-2), are most promising in the treatment of metastatic disease.[21] Side effects of IL-2 include capillary leakage syndrome, fever, chills, fatigue, and hypotension.

Table 43-13 Robson's System of Staging Renal Carcinoma

Stage	Description
I	Limitation to renal capsule
II	Spreading to perirenal fat, but confined within fascia; includes metastasis to adrenal gland
III	Regional lymph node involvement, tumor thrombus in renal vein or vena cava, involvement of lymph nodes and renal vein or vena cava
IV	Presence of distant metastases

WILMS' TUMOR

Wilms' tumor is a common renal tumor of infants and children. Of these tumors, 40% are hereditary, with an autosomal dominant mode of transmission. The most common clinical manifestation is abdominal swelling or distention. This distention is often noticed by the parents or is found on a routine examination. Other symptoms include pain, fever, hematuria, and hypertension. Diagnostic studies for Wilms' tumor include ultrasound and renal arteriography.

These tumors respond well to multimodality therapy. Therapeutic treatment includes surgical removal of the involved kidney and radiation therapy. Radiation therapy is used postoperatively and for inoperable tumors, bilateral tumors, and

Table 43-14 Tumor–Node–Metastasis (TNM) Staging System for Bladder Cancer

Primary Tumor (T)

- TX: Primary tumor cannot be assessed
- T0: No evidence of primary tumor
- Ta: Noninvasive papillary carcinoma
- Tis: Carcinoma in situ ("flat tumor")
- T1: Tumor invades subepithelial connective tissue
- T2: Tumor invades superficial muscle (inner half)
- T3: Tumor invades deep muscle or perivesical fat
- T3a: Tumor invades deep muscle (outer half)
- T3b: Tumor invades perivesical fat
- T4: Tumor invades any of the following: prostate, uterus, vagina, pelvic wall, or abdominal wall
- T4a: Tumor invades the prostate, uterus, or vagina
- T4b: Tumor invades the pelvic wall or abdominal wall

Nodal Involvement (N)

Regional lymph nodes are those within the true pelvis; all others are distant nodes.

- NX: Regional lymph nodes cannot be assessed
- N0: No regional lymph node metastasis
- N1: Metastasis in a single lymph node, 2.0 cm or less in greatest dimension
- N2: Metastasis in a single lymph node, more than 2.0 cm but not more than 5.0 cm in greatest dimension; or multiple lymph nodes, none more than 5.0 cm in greatest dimension
- N3: Metastasis in a lymph node more than 5.0 cm in greatest dimension

Distant Metastasis (M)

- MX: Presence of distant metastasis cannot be assessed
- M0: No distant metastasis
- M1: Distant metastasis

American Joint Committee on Cancer Stage Groupings of Bladder Cancer

Stage 0a
- Ta, N0, M0

Stage 0is
- Tis, N0, M0

Stage I
- T1, N0, M0

Stage II
- T2, N0, M0
- T3a, N0, M0

Stage III
- T3b, N0, M0
- T4a, N0, M0

Stage IV
- T4b, N0, M0
- Any T, N1, M0
- Any T, N2, M0
- Any T, N3, M0
- Any T, any N, M1

metastases. Chemotherapy with actinomycin D and vincristine (Oncovin) is also frequently used.

BLADDER CANCER

In 1998 there were an estimated 54,400 new cases of bladder cancer and 12,500 deaths related to bladder cancer. Bladder cancer accounts for nearly 1 in every 20 cancers diagnosed in the United States.[19] The most frequent malignant tumor of the urinary tract is transitional cell carcinoma of the bladder. Most bladder tumors are papillomatous growths within the bladder. Cancer of the bladder is most common between the ages of 60 and 70 years and is at least three times as common in men as in women. Risk factors for bladder cancer include cigarette smoking, exposure to dyes used in the rubber and cable industries, and chronic abuse of phenacetin-containing analgesics. Women treated with radiation for cervical cancer and patients receiving cyclophosphamide (Cytoxan) also have increased risk, but the reason is unknown.[22]

Individuals with chronic, recurrent stones (often bladder) and chronic lower urinary infections have an increased risk of squamous cell cancer of the bladder. Patients who have indwelling catheters for long periods of time can develop these chronic conditions.

Clinical Manifestations and Diagnostic Studies

Gross, painless hematuria (chronic or intermittent) is the most common clinical finding and the first in 85% to 90% of patients. Bladder irritability with dysuria, frequency, and urgency may also occur. When cancer is suspected, urine specimens for cytology can be obtained to determine the presence of neoplastic or atypical cells. Exfoliated cells from the epithelial surface of the bladder can readily be detected in voided specimens. Other recent urine tests assess for specific factors associated with bladder cancer, such as bladder tumor antigens. Bladder cancers can be detected using IVP, ultrasound, CT, or MRI. However, the presence of cancer is confirmed by cytoscopy and biopsy.

The clinical staging of carcinoma of the bladder is determined by the depth of invasion of the bladder wall and surrounding tissue (Table 43-14). The Jewett-Strong-Marshall classification system broadly classifies bladder cancer as superficial (CIS, O, A), invasive (B1, B2, C), or metastatic (D1–D4) disease. Pathologic grading systems are also used to classify the malignant potential of tumor cells, indicating a scale from well-differentiated to anaplastic categories. Low-stage, low-grade bladder cancers are the most responsive to treatment and are more easily cured.

NURSING AND COLLABORATIVE MANAGEMENT: BLADDER CANCER

Collaborative care of bladder cancer is outlined in Table 43-15.

■ Surgical Therapy

Surgical therapies include a variety of procedures. Transurethral resection (TUR) with fulguration (electrocautery) is used for

COLLABORATIVE CARE

Table 43-15 Bladder Cancer

Diagnostic
- Urinalysis
- Intravenous pyelogram
- Cystoscopy with biopsy
- Cytology studies
- Ultrasound
- CT scan

Collaborative Therapy
- Surgical treatment
  - Transurethral resection with fulguration
  - Laser photocoagulation
  - Open loop resection or fulguration
  - Segmental cystectomy
  - Radical cystectomy
- Radiation
- Intravesical immunotherapy
  - Bacille Calmette-Guérin (BCG)
- Intravesical chemotherapy
  - Thiotepa
  - Mitomycin (Mutamycin)
  - Doxorubicin (Adriamycin)
- Systemic chemotherapy

the diagnosis and treatment of superficial lesions with a low recurrence rate. This procedure is also used to control bleeding in the patient who is a poor operative risk or who has advanced tumors. With this technique the tumor mass is excised by means of a blade inserted through the cystoscope. The remaining portions of the tumor are cauterized.

A second technique, laser photocoagulation, is also used to treat superficial bladder cancers. This procedure can be repeated a number of times for recurrence. The advantages of laser include bloodless destruction of the lesion, minimal risk of perforation, and lack of need for a urinary catheter. Because laser destroys tumor tissue, pathologic evaluation cannot be done after this procedure.

A third technique used is open loop resection (snaring of polyp types of lesion) with fulguration. It is used for the control of bleeding, for large superficial tumors, and for multiple lesions. Treatment of large lesions entails a segmental resection of the bladder (segmental cystectomy).

Postoperative management of the patient who has had any of these surgical procedures includes instructions to drink large amounts of fluid each day, measurement of intake and output, avoidance of alcoholic beverages, use of analgesics and stool softeners (if necessary), and sitz baths to promote muscle relaxation and reduce urinary retention. The nurse should also help the patient and family cope with fears about cancer, surgery, and sexuality and should emphasize the importance of regular follow-up care. Frequent routine cystoscopies are required.

When the tumor is invasive or involves the trigone (the area where the ureters insert into the bladder) and the patient otherwise has a good life expectancy and has demonstrated no metastases beyond the pelvic area, a radical cystectomy with urinary diversion is the treatment of choice (see the following section on urinary diversion). A radical cystectomy involves the removal of bladder, prostate, seminal vesicles (in men) and uterus, cervix, urethra, and usually ovaries (in women).

Radiation Therapy and Chemotherapy

Radiation therapy is used with cystectomy or as the primary therapy when the cancer is inoperable or when surgery is refused. Increasingly radiation therapy is being combined with systemic chemotherapy. Sometimes combination systemic chemotherapy is used for bladder cancer, usually preoperatively or before radiation therapy, or is used to treat distant metastases.[23] Chemotherapy drugs used in treating invasive bladder cancer include cisplatin (Platinol), vinblastine (Velban), doxorubicin (Adriamycin), and methotrexate.

Intravesical therapy

Chemotherapy with local instillation of chemotherapeutic or immune-stimulating agents can be delivered directly into the bladder by a urethral catheter. Protocols vary, but intravesical therapy is usually initiated at weekly intervals for 6 to 12 weeks. They are instilled directly into the patient's bladder and retained for about 2 hours. The patient's position may be changed every 15 minutes for maximum contact in all areas of the bladder, especially if the tumor occurred on the bladder dome. The use of maintenance therapy after the initial induction regimen may be beneficial.

Bacille Calmette-Guérin (BCG), a weakened strain of *Mycobacterium bovis,* is the treatment of choice. It differs from other agents in that BCG stimulates the immune system rather than acting directly on cancer cells in the bladder. Thiotepa is an alkylating agent that is pharmacologically related to nitrogen mustard. Thiotepa may be used if BCG fails and a patient's bladder cancer returns.

Most patients have irritative voiding symptoms and hemorrhagic cystitis following intravesical therapy. Thiotepa can significantly reduce WBC and platelet counts in some individuals. BCG may cause flulike symptoms, hematuria, or systemic infection. Systemic side effects usually associated with chemotherapy, such as nausea, vomiting, and hair loss, are not experienced with intravesical chemotherapy.

Nursing responsibilities include encouraging the patient to increase the daily fluid intake and to quit smoking, assessing the patient for secondary urinary tract infection, and stressing the need for routine urologic follow-up. The patient may have fears or concerns about sexual activity or bladder function that will need to be addressed.

URINARY INCONTINENCE AND RETENTION

An estimated 13 million people (of which 11 million are women) in the United States suffer from urinary incontinence, or the unintentional loss of urine that is sufficient to be a problem.[24] Although about half of older people have episodes of incontinence, bladder problems are not a natural consequence of aging, and they are not exclusively a problem of older adults.[25]

Incontinence exacts physical (infection, pressure sores, perineal rashes), psychosocial (embarrassment, isolation, depression), and economic costs. However minor the problem, incontinence can cause severe psychologic distress. Incontinence is not an inevitable consequence of aging; in most cases among older adults, it can be significantly improved or corrected. *Retention* is the inability to urinate in spite of the presence of urine in the bladder. Both incontinence and retention may occur in the same person.

NORMAL BLADDER FUNCTION

Storage of urine in the bladder is mediated by relaxation of the detrusor muscle (which provides the propulsive force for emptying the bladder) and closure of the sphincters. The detrusor muscle is controlled by the parasympathetic nervous system through the pelvic nerves from sacral spinal cord segments S2, S3, or S4. These spinal segments are modulated by the pons (brainstem) and cortical centers in the brain. The smooth muscle of the trigonal portion of the bladder between the ureteral orifices and the posterior area of the bladder outlet is innervated by the sympathetic nervous system, in which α-receptors predominate. This layer of muscle acts as an involuntary internal sphincter. The external urethral sphincter and perineal muscles are under voluntary control.

The sensation of bladder fullness is transmitted via sensory nerves to the sacral cord. If not suppressed by cortical control, the sacral cord discharges motor impulses by reflex that cause powerful sustained detrusor contraction. Urination can be prevented by means of cortical suppression of the reflex arc or voluntary contraction of the external sphincter and perineal muscles. Urination occurs when detrusor contraction is coordinated with sphincter relaxation.

CAUSES OF URINARY INCONTINENCE AND RETENTION

Anything that interferes with bladder or urethral sphincter control can result in urinary incontinence. Causes may be transient (e.g., caused by confusion or depression, infection, medications, restricted mobility, or stool impaction). Congenital disorders that produce incontinence include exstrophy of the bladder, epispadias, spina bifida with myelomeningocele, and ectopic ureteral orifice. Acquired disorders are described in Table 43-16. Patients may have more than one type of incontinence.

Neurogenic Bladder

Neurogenic bladder is a general term referring to any bladder dysfunction resulting from a central nervous system (CNS) neurologic disorder. There are numerous causes of this condition, including such problems as CNS tumors, cerebrovascular accidents, multiple sclerosis, diabetic neuropathy, and spinal cord injury. A person with a neurogenic bladder may have problems with urgency, frequency, incontinence, inability to urinate, and obstruction-like symptoms. Long-term problems include formation of calculi, urinary tract infection, and progressive deterioration in renal function.

A simple way to classify neurogenic dysfunction is to identify whether there is a failure to store, failure to empty, or both problems and whether the dysfunction is of the bladder or urethra. Either or both problems lead to urinary tract damage if not treated. The type of dysfunction usually depends on where the problem affects the brain or spinal cord (e.g., cerebral centers, suprasacral spinal cord, sacral cord area). Lesions in the brain or upper spinal cord usually cause hyperreflexic symptoms, whereas lesions in the sacral cord cause arreflexia. Detrusor sphincter dyssynergia (the bladder and sphincter contract at the same time) is often associated with lesions in the suprasacral spinal cord. (A more detailed description of neurogenic bladder is found in Chapter 57.)

Urinary Retention

Retention can be found in association with incontinence but can also be independent of incontinence. Drugs that may cause retention include (1) antihypertensives (methyldopa [Aldomet], hydralazine [Apresoline]), (2) antiparkinsonian drugs (levodopa), (3) antihistamines, (4) anticholinergics (e.g., atropine, belladonna), (5) antispasmodics, (6) sedatives, and (7) anesthesia (especially spinal anesthesia).

Postoperative urinary retention is not uncommon and is related to preoperative medication (atropine and sedatives are frequently used), anesthesia, supine position after surgery, and low fluid intake. Postoperative retention may also be related to the effects of surgical manipulation of the bladder nerves.

Another cause of retention is urethral obstruction, which may be caused by congenital urethral stenosis, prostate cancer, benign prostatic hyperplasia, fecal impaction, or tumors (involving bladder outlet or large, displaced uterine myomas). Psychologic problems may also contribute to urinary retention. Psychogenic urinary retention is found more commonly in women than in men.

Diagnostic Studies

A complete history and physical examination (with particular attention to the GU system) are essential to obtain information on the patient's past and current urination patterns, current physical health, and underlying reasons for incontinence or retention. A drug history, including both prescription and over-the-counter drugs, should be obtained. It is advisable to ask the patient to keep a bladder diary that logs the times and precipitating factors for incontinence.

Diagnostic tests of urologic dysfunction are important in the evaluation of the function and structure of the urinary tract, especially the bladder. A urinalysis is essential. These tests may include IVP, cystoscopy (including urethroscopy), urodynamic studies (to assess sphincter, perineal, and muscle activity), and catheterization or ultrasound for residual urine.

Collaborative Care

An estimated 80% of incontinence can be improved.[25] Treatment should correct the factors responsible for incontinence or retention, if possible (see Table 43-16). Treatment includes

Table 43-16 Acquired Disorders Causing Urinary Incontinence

Type	Description	Causes	Treatment
■ Stress incontinence*	Sudden increase in intraabdominal pressure causes involuntary passage of urine. It can occur during coughing, heavy lifting, straining, or laughing.	Condition is found most commonly in women with relaxed pelvic musculature (frequently from obstetric complications or multiple pregnancies). Structures of the female urethra atrophy when estrogen de creases. Condition is found in men after prostate surgery for benign prostatic hyperplasia or prostatic carcinoma.	Perineal muscle exercises (e.g., Kegel exercises), weight loss if patient is obese, insertion of vaginal pessary, estrogen vaginal creams, condom catheters or penile clamp, surgery Urethral inserts, patches, or bladder neck support devices to correct underlying problem
■ Urge incontinence*	Condition occurs randomly when involuntary urination is preceded by warning of few seconds to few minutes. Leakage is periodic but frequent. Nocturnal frequency and incontinence are common. Condition may appear with varying severity during psychologic stress.	Condition is caused by uncontrolled contraction or overactivity of detrusor muscle. Bladder escapes central inhibition and contracts reflexively. Conditions include central nervous system disorders (e.g., cerebrovascular disease, Alzheimer's disease, brain tumor, Parkinson's disease), bladder disorders (e.g., carcinoma in situ, radiation effects, interstitial cystitis), interference with spinal inhibitory pathways (e.g., malignant growth in spinal cord, spondylosis), and bladder outlet obstruction, as well as conditions of unknown etiology.	Treatment of underlying cause, instruction to have patient urinate more frequently or on time schedule, anticholinergic drugs (e.g., propantheline), imipramine at bedtime, calcium channel blockers, condom catheters, vaginal estrogen creams
■ Overflow (paradoxic) incontinence	Condition occurs when the pressure of urine in overfull bladder overcomes sphincter control. Leakage of small amounts of urine is frequent throughout the day and night. Urination may also occur frequently in small amounts. Bladder remains distended and is usually palpable.	Disorder is caused by outlet obstruction (prostatic hyperplasia, bladder neck obstruction, urethral stricture) or by underactive detrusor muscle caused by myogenic or neurogenic factors (e.g., herniated disk, diabetic neuropathy). It may also occur after anesthesia and surgery (especially procedures such as hemorrhoidectomy, herniorrhaphy, cystoscopy). Neurogenic bladder (flaccid type) is another cause.	Urinary catheterization to decompress bladder, implementation of Credé's or Valsalva's maneuver, α-adrenergic blocker (e.g., prazosin) to decrease outlet resistance, bethanechol to enhance bladder contractions, intermittent catheterization, surgery to correct underlying problem
■ Reflex incontinence	Condition occurs when no warning or stress precedes periodic involuntary urination. Urination is frequent, is moderate in volume, and occurs equally during the day and night.	Spinal cord lesion above S2 interferes with central nervous system inhibition. Disorder results in detrusor hyperreflexia and interferes with pathways coordinating detrusor contraction and sphincter relaxation.	Treatment of underlying cause, bladder decompression to prevent ureteral reflux and hydronephrosis, intermittent self-catheterization, α-adrenergic blocker (e.g., prazosin) to relax internal sphincter, diazepam or baclofen to relax external sphincter, prophylactic antibiotics, surgical sphincterotomy
■ Incontinence after trauma or surgery	Vesicovaginal or urethrovaginal fistula may occur in women. Alteration in continence control in men involves proximal urethral sphincter (bladder neck and prostatic urethra) and distal urethral sphincter (external striated muscle).	Fistulas may occur during pregnancy, after delivery of baby, as a result of hysterectomy or invasive cancer of cervix, or after radiation therapy. Incontinence is found as postoperative complication after transurethral, perineal, or retropubic prostatectomy.	Surgery to correct fistula, urinary diversion surgery to bypass urethra and bladder, external condom catheter, penile clamp, placement of artificial implantable sphincter
■ Functional incontinence	Loss of urine due to problems of patient mobility or environmental factors	Elderly often have problems that affect balance and mobility	Modifications of environment or care plan that facilitate regular, easy access to toilet and promote patient safety (e.g., better lighting, ambulatory assistance equipment, clothing alterations, timed voiding, different toileting equipment)

*Patients can have combination of stress and urge incontinence that is referred to as mixed incontinence.

DRUG THERAPY

Table 43-17 Urinary Incontinence*

Muscarinic receptor antagonists and anticholinergics
Oxybutynin (Ditropan)
Tolterodine (Detrol)
Propantheline (Pro-Banthine)
α-Adrenergic blockers
Prazosin (Minipress)
Phenoxybenzamine (Dibenzyline)
α-Adrenergic agonists
Phenylpropanolamine
Tricyclic antidepressants
Imipramine (Tofranil)
Desipramine (Norpramin)
Nortriptyline (Aventyl)
Calcium channel blockers
Nifedipine (Adalat)
Diltiazem (Cardizem)
Verapamil (Calan, Isoptin)
Hormone replacement therapy

*The type of drug therapy depends on the type of incontinence.

behavioral techniques, electrostimulation, surgery, and medications.

Behavioral therapies help people regain control of their bladder. Bladder training teaches people to resist the urge to void and gradually expand the intervals between voiding. (Bladder training programs are described in Chapter 57.)

Pelvic floor electrical stimulation uses mild electrical pulses to stimulate muscle contractions. Electrical stimulation should be performed in conjunction with Kegel exercises (explained in next column).

Surgical approaches vary, depending on the underlying problem. For example, a transurethral resection of the prostate is used to treat benign prostatic hyperplasia. Urethral strictures are dilated. Several surgical procedures help correct anatomic malposition of the bladder neck and urethra that causes female stress incontinence. The Marshall-Marchetti procedure involves suspending the urethra and bladder neck by suturing the anterior vaginal wall on each side to the periosteum of the pubic bones and lower rectum through an abdominal incision. The Pereyra procedure and subsequent modifications involve suspending the tissues adjacent to the bladder neck to the abdominal fascia, mainly through a transvaginal approach.

Injection of urethral bulking agents, such as Teflon or collagen, and implantation of a prosthetic urethral sphincter are also done for stress incontinence in selected cases. There is risk of Teflon particles migrating to lungs; consequently, alternatives are more favorable. Augmentation enterocystoplasty (enlarging the bladder with a segment of bowel or stomach) may be attempted for severe urge incontinence when the disorder does not respond to other treatment measures and when kidney function may be compromised as a result of reflux.

Drug Therapy (Table 43-17)

Muscarinic receptor antagonists. This group of drugs is used to treat hyperreflexic bladders by suppressing the unwanted contractions that occur when the bladder has only a small volume of urine. Oxybutynin (Ditropan), which has both anticholinergic and direct smooth-muscle relaxing properties, has been the gold standard of drug therapy for many years.[24] Oxybutynin is a nonselective muscarinic receptor antagonist that tends to produce significant anticholinergic effects such as drying of the mouth and eyes. Tolterodine (Detrol), a selective antimuscarinic agent, has recently been approved for use for treatment of overactive bladder. Propantheline (Pro-Banthine), an anticholinergic, inhibits the action of acetylcholine.

Other drug therapy. α-Adrenergic blockers such as prazosin (Minipress) and phenoxybenzamine (Dibenzyline) can be used to relax spastic bladder necks and prostatic smooth muscle. α-Adrenergic agonists, such as phenylpropanolamine, also increase urethral resistance. Imipramine and calcium channel blockers (see Table 43-17) reduce detrusor contractions and improve continence. Vaginal or oral estrogen replacement is often prescribed for postmenopausal women to restore urethral suppleness.

NURSING MANAGEMENT: URINARY INCONTINENCE

The nurse must recognize both the physical and the emotional problems that accompany incontinence. The patient's dignity, privacy, and feelings of self-worth must be maintained or enhanced. Most persons suffering from incontinence can be helped with proper diagnosis and modern therapeutic approaches.

A patient with stress incontinence can be taught to do pelvic floor (perineal) muscle exercises (Kegel exercises). The patient should contract the pelvic muscles, as though trying to stop the flow of urine, while relaxing the abdomen, thighs, and buttocks. Each contraction is held for a few seconds and followed by relaxation for the same period of time. Contraction and relaxation times are gradually increased. These exercises should be repeated in sets of 10 or more contractions and done four to five times each day over several weeks. Consistency and persistence are necessary for success, and exercise regimens have to be individualized. Vaginal weights (cones) or biofeedback may help patients gain awareness and control of their pelvic muscles. Vaginal weight training involves holding small weights within the vagina by tightening the vaginal muscles. These exercises should be performed for 15 minutes, twice daily, for 4 to 6 weeks.

The nurse has a major responsibility to help the patient with incontinence problems in a variety of settings. In the hospital, nursing measures aimed at maintaining urinary continence include identifying transient causes and assessing the patient for signs of bladder infection, fecal impaction, or bladder distention. The nurse should offer the urinal or bedpan or help the patient to the bathroom every 2 hours or at scheduled times.

Assuming the usual position for urination (standing for the man and sitting and leaning forward for the woman) or using relaxation techniques often help a patient urinate successfully, particularly in unfamiliar settings. Applying pressure over the bladder area (Credé's maneuver) may be helpful when bladder outlet obstruction is not a problem. The nurse should be sure the patient has privacy and is not rushed when trying to urinate. Techniques to stimulate urination include running water in the sink, placing hands in water, and pouring warm water over the perineum. Fluid intake patterns can be monitored and fluids encouraged.

The patient should be taught that incontinence is not a normal part of aging and that it can be eliminated or controlled in most cases. Local medical supply resources and suggestions for improving urinary control, including having the problem further evaluated, are helpful in discharge planning. The patient may feel more comfortable talking about incontinence when given this kind of permission to talk about a problem that is embarrassing to most people.

Fluid restriction, incontinence pads, and keeping a urinal in place at all times are only temporary measures to reduce the occurrence or effects of incontinence. Long-term use of these measures discourages continence and can lead to dehydration and skin problems.

If bladder retraining cannot be achieved, external appliances or intermittent self-catheterization may be indicated. Several external appliances that prevent soiling, decrease odor, and improve body image are available for men. External appliances for women are not useful in most situations. However, newly developed inserts, patches, pessaries, and bladder neck support devices are useful for some women with stress urinary incontinence.[26,27] Intermittent self-catheterization using a clean technique can be taught to selected patients. Keeping the skin clean and dry is essential to prevent skin irritation and breakdown. (Intermittent-catheterization is discussed on p. 1290)

INSTRUMENTATION

A catheter is a tubular instrument made of rubber, plastic, metal, or other material used to drain or inject gases or fluids through a body passage. The process of inserting the catheter into a body cavity or passage is termed *catheterization.* Indwelling catheters often have self-retaining balloons to keep the catheter in place. Nursing responsibility includes understanding the reason for catheterization, the scientific principles involved, aseptic technique, and the appropriate care of the patient after catheterization.

Table 43-18 Indications for Urinary Catheterization

1. Relief of urinary retention caused by lower urinary tract obstruction, paralysis, or inability to void
2. Bladder decompression preoperatively and operatively for lower abdominal or pelvic surgery
3. Facilitation of surgical repair of urethra and surrounding structures
4. Splinting of ureters or urethra to facilitate healing after surgery or other trauma in area
5. Instillation of medications into bladder
6. Accurate measurement of urinary output in critically ill patient
7. Measurement of residual urine after urination
8. Study of anatomic structures of urinary system
9. Urodynamic testing
10. Collection of sterile urine sample in selected situations

The reasons for urinary catheterization are listed in Table 43-18. Two reasons that are *not* indications for catheterization are (1) routine acquisition of a sterile specimen for laboratory analysis and (2) convenience of the nursing staff or the patient's family. The risks of nosocomial infection are too high to allow catheterization of a patient for the convenience of hospital personnel or family members. Catheterization for sterile urine specimens may occasionally be indicated when patients have complicated urinary infection histories. These specimens have to be as free of contaminants as possible. A catheter should be the final means of providing the patient with a dry environment for prevention of skin breakdown and protection of dressings or skin lesions.

Urinary catheterization is commonly used in the management of the hospitalized patient. However, it is not without serious risks. The urinary tract is the most common site of nosocomial infections. Urinary catheterization is a major cause of UTIs. Scrupulous aseptic technique is mandatory when a urinary catheter is inserted. After insertion, maintenance and protection of the closed drainage system are major nursing responsibilities. Irrigation of the catheter should *not* be routinely performed.

While the patient has a catheter in place, nursing actions should include maintaining patency of the catheter, managing fluid intake, providing for the comfort and safety of the patient, and preventing infection. Attention should be given to the psychologic implications of urinary drainage. Concerns of the patient can include embarrassment related to exposure of the body, an altered body image, and fear concerning the care of the catheter that results in increased dependency.

Catheters vary in construction materials, tip shape (Fig. 43-7), and size of the lumen. Catheters are sized according to

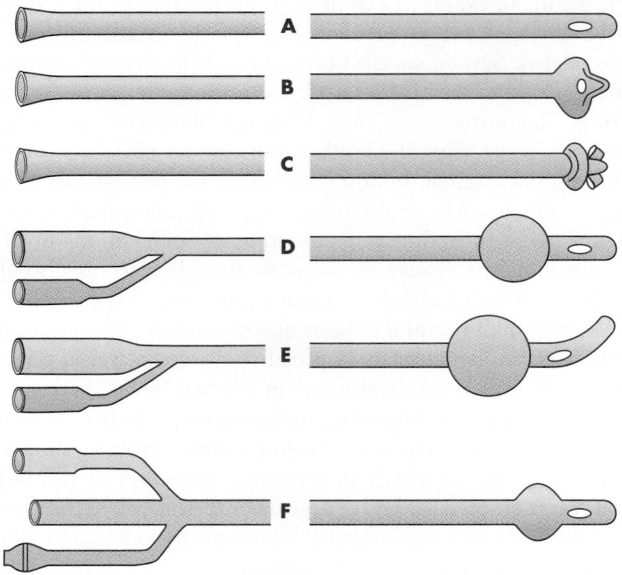

Fig. 43-7 Different types of commonly used catheters. **A,** Simple urethral catheter. **B,** Mushroom or dePezzar (can be used for suprapubic catheterization). **C,** Winged-tip or Malecot. **D,** Indwelling with inflated balloon. **E,** Indwelling with Coudé tip or Tiemann. **F,** Three-way indwelling (the third lumen is used for irrigation of the bladder).

the French scale. Each French unit equals 0.33 mm of diameter. The diameter measured is the internal diameter of the catheter. The size used varies with the size of the individual and the purpose for catheterization. In women, urethral catheter sizes 14F to 16F are the most common; in men, sizes 16F to 18F are used. Problems resulting from too small a catheter include possible obstruction of the urinary flow by blood clots, mineral sediment, or mucous plugs and difficulty in passing the catheter if resistance is met in the urethra. The primary problem resulting from too large a catheter is tissue erosion secondary to excessive pressure on the meatus or urethra. Four routes are used for urinary tract catheterization: urethral, ureteral, suprapubic, and via a nephrostomy tube.

URETHRAL CATHETERIZATION

The most common route of catheterization is insertion of the catheter through the external meatus into the urethra, past the internal sphincter, and into the bladder. Principles that should be considered in the management of the patient with a urethral catheter include the following:

1. The indwelling urinary catheter should be used *only* when absolutely necessary and never solely for the convenience of the caregivers. Its use should be discontinued as early as possible.
2. The catheterized patient, particularly the person who is ambulatory, should receive appropriate instruction regarding catheter care.
3. A sterile, closed drainage system should always be used in short-term catheterization. The distal urinary catheter and the proximal drainage tube should not be disconnected except for necessary catheter irrigation. Unobstructed downhill flow must be maintained. The collecting bag should be emptied regularly and kept below the level of the bladder. A poorly functioning catheter should be replaced. The leg bag should not be used for the short-term patient in the hospital setting because the risk of bacterial infection is great when the catheter is disconnected and the drainage bags are exchanged.
4. Perineal care (one to two times per day and when necessary) should include cleaning of the meatus-catheter junction with soap and water. Following this, an antimicrobial ointment may be applied. Lotion or powder should not be used near the catheter. The catheter should be properly secured to the leg to prevent movement and urethral traction.
5. Sterile technique must be used whenever the collecting system is opened. Catheter irrigation is performed only when obstruction or blood clots are suspected or, in the case of long-term catheterization, to reduce sediment buildup. If frequent irrigations are necessary in short-term catheterization for catheter patency, a triple-lumen catheter may be preferable, permitting continuous irrigations within a closed system. Small volumes of urine for culture can be aspirated from the distal catheter by means of a sterile syringe and a 21-gauge needle after the drainage tubing is clamped. The puncture site must first be prepared with a tincture of iodine or alcohol solution. Many drainage systems are now equipped with a sampling port. Silicone or plastic catheters do not self-seal. Urine for chemical analysis (e.g., electrolytes) can be obtained from the drainage bag.
6. When the patient is catheterized for less than 2 weeks, routine catheter change is not necessary. For long-term use of an indwelling catheter, replacement is necessary when concretions can be palpated in the catheter or when the catheter malfunctions. With long-term use of a catheter, the leg bag may be used. If the collection bag is reused, it should be washed in soap and water and rinsed thoroughly. When not reused immediately, it should be filled with ½ cup of vinegar and drained. The vinegar is effective against *Pseudomonas* and other organisms and eliminates odors.

URETERAL CATHETERS

The ureteral catheter is placed through the ureters into the renal pelvis. The catheter is inserted either (1) by being threaded up the urethra and bladder to the ureters under cystoscopic observation or (2) by surgical insertion through the abdominal wall into the ureters. The ureteral catheter is used after surgery to splint the ureters and to prevent them from being obstructed by edema. The urine volume from the ureteral catheter should be recorded separately from other urinary catheters. The patient is usually kept on bed rest while a ureteral catheter is in place until specific orders indicate that ambulation is permissible. The self-retaining ureteral catheter is often inserted after a lithotripsy procedure or when ureteral obstruction from adjacent tumors or fibrosis threatens renal function. The double-J ureteral catheter is often used and allows the patient to ambulate. One end coils up in the kidney pelvis, while the other coils in the bladder.

The placement of the ureteral catheter should be checked frequently, and tension on the catheter should be avoided. The catheter drains urine from the renal pelvis, which has a capacity of 3 to 5 ml. If the volume of urine in the renal pelvis increases, tissue damage to the pelvis will result from pressure. Therefore the ureteral catheter should not be clamped. If the physician orders irrigation of the ureteral catheter, strict aseptic technique is required. If output is decreased, the physician should be notified immediately. Drainage should be checked often (at least every 1 to 2 hours). It is normal for some urine to drain around the ureteral catheter into the bladder. Accurate recording of urine output from both the ureters and the urethral catheter is essential. Sometimes a ureteral catheter may be used as a stent and is not expected to drain. It is important to check with the physician as to the type of catheter and what to expect.

SUPRAPUBIC CATHETERS

Suprapubic catheterization is the simplest and oldest method of urinary diversion. The two methods of insertion of a suprapubic catheter into the bladder are (1) through a small incision in the abdominal wall and (2) by the use of a trocar. A suprapubic catheter is placed while the patient is under general anesthesia for another surgical procedure or at the bedside with a local anesthetic. The catheter may be sutured into place, but a Foley catheter is usually used. The nursing responsibility includes taping the catheter to prevent dislodgment. The care of the tube and catheter is similar to that of the urethral catheter. A pectin-base skin barrier (e.g., Stomahesive) is effective around the insertion site in protecting the skin from breakdown.

The suprapubic catheter is used in temporary situations such as bladder, vesical neck, prostate, and urethral surgery. Suprapubic catheterization may be used instead of urethral catheterization, especially in the young or infant boy and when a urethral catheter cannot be inserted. The suprapubic catheter is also used long-term in selected patients (e.g., male quadriplegic patient who tends to form penoscrotal fistulas).

A suprapubic catheter is prone to poor drainage because of mechanical obstruction of the catheter tip by the bladder wall, sediment, and clots. Nursing interventions to ensure patency of the tube include (1) preventing tube kinking by coiling the excess tubing and maintaining gravity drainage, (2) having the patient turn from side to side, and (3) milking the tube. If these measures are not effective, the catheter is irrigated with sterile technique after a physician's order has been obtained.

If the patient experiences bladder spasms that are difficult to control, urinary leakage may result. Oxybutynin (Ditropan) or other oral antispasmodics or belladonna and opium (B & O) suppositories may be prescribed to decrease bladder spasms.

NEPHROSTOMY TUBES

The nephrostomy tube (catheter) is inserted on a temporary basis to preserve renal function when a complete obstruction of the ureter is present. It is inserted directly into the pelvis of the kidney and attached to connecting tubing for closed drainage. The principle is the same as with the ureteral catheter; that is, the catheter should never be kinked, laid or leaned on, or clamped. If the patient complains of excessive pain in the area or if there is excessive drainage around the tube, the catheter should be checked for patency. If irrigation is ordered, strict aseptic technique is required. No more than 5 ml of sterile saline solution is gently instilled at one time to prevent overdistention of the kidney pelvis and renal damage. Infection and secondary stone formation are complications associated with the insertion of a nephrostomy tube.

INTERMITTENT CATHETERIZATION

An alternative approach to a long-term indwelling catheter is intermittent catheterization.[28] It is being used with increasing frequency in conditions characterized by neurogenic bladder (e.g., spinal cord injuries, chronic neurologic diseases) or bladder outlet obstruction in men. This type of catheterization may also be used in the oliguric and anuric phases of acute renal failure to reduce the possibility of infection from an indwelling catheter. Intermittent catheterization is also used postoperatively, often after a surgical procedure for female incontinence or radioactive seed implantation into the prostate for cancer. The main goal of intermittent catheterization is to prevent urinary retention, stasis, and compromised blood supply to the bladder caused by prolonged pressure.

The technique consists of inserting a urethral catheter into the bladder every 3 to 5 hours. Some patients do intermittent catheterization only once or twice a day to measure residual urine and to ensure an empty bladder. Patients should be instructed to wash and rinse the catheter and their hands with soap and water before and after catheterization. Lubricant is necessary for men and may make catheterization more comfortable for women. The catheter may be inserted by the patient or the care provider. The bladder is emptied and the catheter is removed. The catheter can be dried and placed in a carrying pouch, purse, or folded in a paper towel until it is next needed. The same catheter can be used for weeks at a time. In general, patients should change the catheter every 2 to 4 weeks.

In the hospital, sterile technique is used. For home care, a clean technique that includes good hand washing with soap and water is used. There has been no significant increase in infection with the use of an appropriate clean technique as compared with sterile technique.[28] The patient is taught to observe for signs of UTI so that treatment can be instituted early. If indicated, some patients are placed on a regimen of prophylactic antibiotics.

SURGERY OF THE URINARY TRACT

RENAL AND URETERAL SURGERY

The most common indications for nephrectomy are a renal tumor, polycystic kidneys that are bleeding or severely infected, massive traumatic injury to the kidney, and the elective removal of a kidney from a donor. Surgery involving the ureters and kidneys is most commonly performed to remove calculi that become obstructive, correct congenital anomalies, and divert urine when necessary.

Preoperative Management

The basic needs of the patient undergoing renal and ureteral surgery are similar to those of any patient who experiences surgery (see Chapters 16 through 18). In addition, it is especially important preoperatively to ensure adequate fluid intake and a normal electrolyte balance. The patient should be told that there will probably be a flank incision on the affected side and that surgery will require a hyperextended, side-lying position. This position frequently causes the patient to experience muscle aches after surgery. If a nephrectomy is planned, the patient must be assured that one working kidney is sufficient to maintain normal renal function.

Postoperative Management

Specific postoperative needs of a patient are related to urine output, respiratory status, and abdominal distention.

Urine Output. In the immediate postoperative period, urine output should be determined at least every 1 to 2 hours. Drainage from various catheters should be recorded separately. The catheter or tube should not be clamped or irrigated without a specific order. The total urine output should be at least 30 to 50 ml per hour. It is also important to assess for urine drainage on the dressing and to estimate the amount. Daily weighing of the patient is important. The same scale should be used, properly balanced, and the patient should wear similar clothing and dressings each time.

It is important to observe and monitor the color and consistency of urine. Urine with increased amounts of mucus, blood, or sediment may occlude the drainage tubing or catheter.

Respiratory Status. Renal surgery is frequently performed through a flank incision just below the diaphragm and frequently involves removal of the twelfth rib. Postoperatively, it is important to ensure adequate ventilation. The patient is often reluctant to turn, cough, and deep breathe

Table 43-19 Types of Urinary Diversion Surgery Requiring Collection Devices

Type	Description	Advantages	Disadvantages	Special Considerations
▪ Ileal conduit	Ureters are implanted into part of ileum or colon that has been resected from intestinal tract. Abdominal stoma is created.	Relatively good urine flow with few physiologic alterations	External appliance necessary to continually collect urine	Surgical procedure is more complex. Postoperative complications may be increased. Reabsorption of urea by ileum occurs. Meticulous attention is necessary to care for stoma and collecting device.
▪ Cutaneous ureterostomy	Ureters are excised from bladder and brought through abdominal wall, and stoma is created. Ureteral stomas may be created from both ureters, or ureters may be brought together and one stoma created.	No need for major surgery as required with ileal conduit	External appliance necessary because of continuous urine drainage; possibility of stricture or stenosis of small stoma	Periodic catheterizations may be required to dilate stomas to maintain patency.
▪ Nephrostomy	Catheter is inserted into pelvis of kidney. Procedure may be done to one or both kidneys and may be temporary or permanent. It is most frequently done in advanced disease as palliative procedure.	No need for major surgery	High risk of renal infection; predisposition to calculus formation from catheter	Nephrostomy tube may have to be changed every month. Catheter must never be clamped.

because of the incisional pain. Adequate pain medication should be given to ensure the patient's comfort and ability to perform coughing and deep-breathing exercises. Frequently, additional respiratory devices such as an incentive spirometer are used every 2 hours while the patient is awake. In addition, early and frequent ambulation assists in maintaining adequate respiratory function.

Abdominal Distention. Abdominal distention is present to some degree in most patients who have had surgery on their kidneys or ureters. It is most commonly due to paralytic ileus caused by manipulation and compression of the bowel during surgery. Oral intake is restricted until bowel sounds are present (usually 24 to 48 hours after surgery). IV fluids are given until the patient can take oral fluids. Progression to a regular diet follows.

Laparoscopic Nephrectomy

Laparoscopic nephrectomy can be performed in selected situations to remove a diseased kidney. Laparoscopic nephrectomy can also be used to obtain a kidney from a living related donor to be transplanted into a person with end-stage renal disease. In contrast to the open incision of about 7 in (18 cm) required in a conventional nephrectomy, a laparoscopic nephrectomy is performed using five puncture sites of less than 0.5 inches (12 mm). One incision is to view the kidney and the other is to dissect it. The laparoscope contains a miniature camera so the surgeons can watch what they are doing on a video monitor. Once dissected, the kidney is maneuvered into a nylon impermeable sack, and its contents can then be safely removed from the patient. As compared with a conventional nephrectomy, the laparoscopic approach is less painful and requires no sutures or staples, a shorter hospital stay, and a much faster recovery.

URINARY DIVERSION

Urinary diversion may be performed with and without cystectomy. Urinary diversion procedures are performed to treat cancer of the bladder, neurogenic bladder, congenital anomalies, strictures, trauma to the bladder, and chronic infections with deterioration of renal function. Numerous urinary diversion techniques and bladder substitutes are possible, including an incontinent urinary diversion, continent urinary diversion catheterized by patient, or an orthotopic bladder so the patient voids urethrally.[29] Types of these surgical procedures are presented in Table 43-19 and Fig. 43-8.

Incontinent Urinary Diversion

Incontinent urinary diversion is diversion to the skin, requiring an appliance. The simplest form is the cutaneous ureterostomy, but scarring and strictures led to the use of ileal or colonic conduits. The most commonly performed incontinent urinary diversion procedure is the ileal conduit (ileal loop). In this procedure a 6- to 8-inch (15 to 20 cm) segment of the ileum is converted into a conduit for urinary drainage. The colon (colon conduit) can be used instead of the ileum. The ureters are anastomosed into one end of the conduit, and the other end of the bowel is brought out through the abdominal

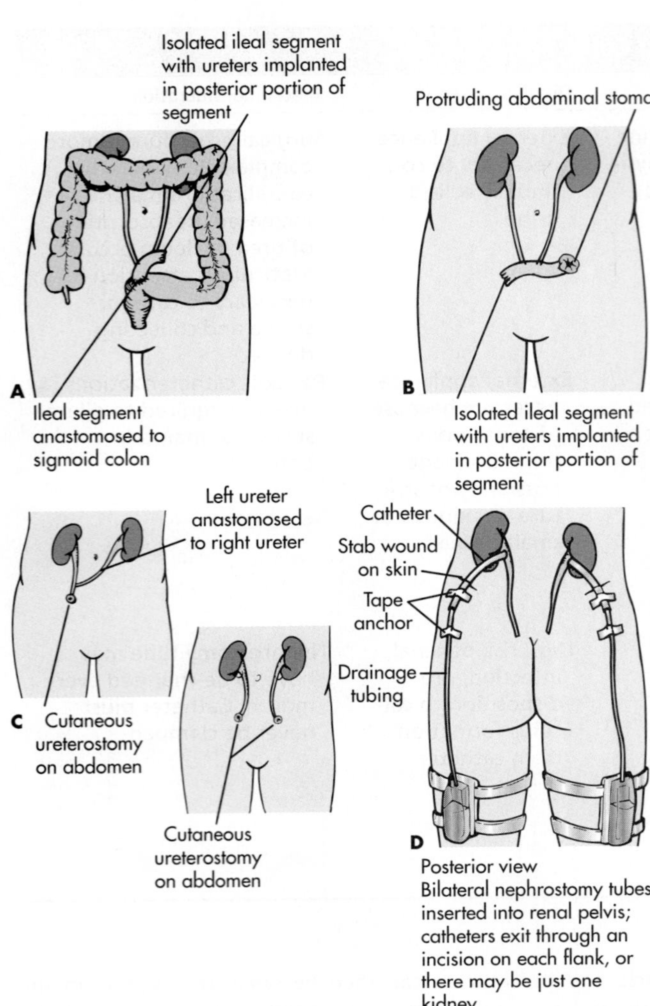

Fig. 43-8 Methods of urinary diversion. **A,** Ureteroileosigmoidostomy. **B,** Ileal loop (or ileal conduit). **C,** Ureterostomy (transcutaneous ureterostomy and bilateral cutaneous ureterostomies). **D,** Nephrostomy.

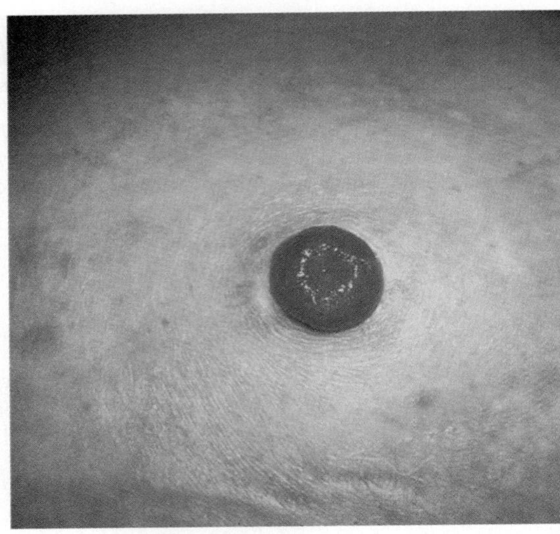

Fig. 43-9 Ideal urinary stoma. It is symmetric, has no skin breakdown, and protrudes about 1.5 cm; the mucosa is a healthy red and the configuration is flat when the patient is upright and supine.

wall to form a stoma (Fig. 43-9). Although the segment of bowel remains supported by the mesentery, it is completely isolated from the intestinal tract. The bowel is anastomosed and continues to function normally. Because there is no valve and no voluntary control over the stoma, drops of urine flow from the stoma every few seconds, requiring the use of a permanent external collecting device. The visible stoma and the need for external collection devices are obvious disadvantages of this procedure. The lifelong care and dealing with the stoma and collection devices may be psychologically difficult. These problems have stimulated the increasing use of continent diversions and orthotopic bladder substitutes.

Continent Urinary Diversions

A *continent urinary diversion* is an intraabdominal urinary reservoir that is catheterizable or with an outlet controlled by the anal sphincter. Continent diversions are internal pouches created similarly to the ileal conduit. Reservoirs have been constructed from the ileum, ileocecal segment, or colon. Large segments of bowel are altered to prevent peristaltic action. A continence mechanism is formed between this large, low-pressure reservoir and the stoma by intussuscepting a portion of bowel. In this way, a patient does not leak involuntarily. The patient with a continent reservoir needs to self-catheterize every 4 to 6 hours but does not need to wear external attachments. Examples of continent diversions are the Kock (Fig. 43-10), Mainz, Indiana, and Florida pouches. A main difference between the various diversions is the segment of bowel used. For example, the Indiana pouch uses the right colon as

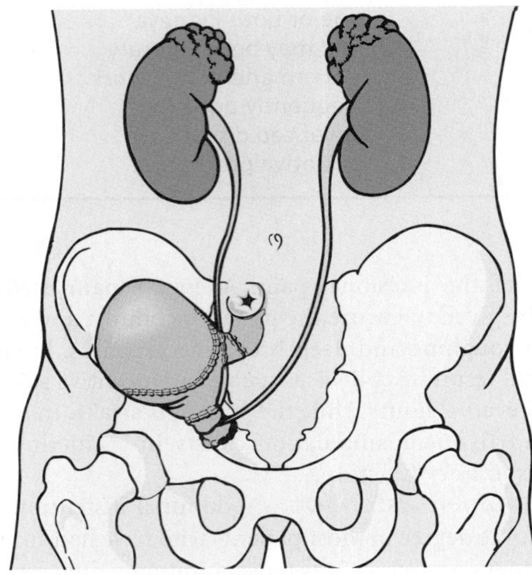

Fig. 43-10 Creation of a Kock pouch with implantation of ureters into one intussuscepted portion of the pouch and creation of a stoma with the other intussuscepted portion.

RESEARCH
IMPLICATIONS FOR NURSING PRACTICE

Quality of Life with Continent Urinary Diversion

Citation Sullivan LD and others: An evaluation of quality of life in patients with continent urinary diversions after cystectomy, *Br J Urol* 81:699, 1998.

Purpose To determine the long-term results and assess the quality of life in patients with continent urinary diversions after cystectomy.

Methods Eighty-six patients who received a continent urinary diversion were evaluated. The evaluation comprised a review of their hospital charts and clinic visits at 3 months and then yearly. Quality of life issues were assessed using a questionnaire pertaining to the patient's urinary symptoms, activity level, and overall well-being while living with a continent urinary diversion.

Results and Conclusions There was an acceptable rate of complications, with stone formation and urinary tract infection as the most common. Continence was rated as good in most patients, with no patient reporting complete incontinence. Undesirable urinary symptoms occurred less often than 20% of the time in most patients. Although there was a significant effect on sex life, the overall quality of life appeared to be very good, as 70% of the patients had no limitations to their activities.

Implications for Nursing Practice Bladder removal and urinary diversion result in significant physiologic and psychoemotional issues. Continent urinary diversions provide both a functional and a psychologic advantage to patients who have undergone a cystectomy. Patient counseling, education, and follow-up care and support can contribute to facilitating a positive outcome for patients.

a reservoir and has become a popular form of continent urinary diversion.

Orthotopic Bladder Substitution

Orthotopic bladder substitutes can be derived from various segments of the intestines. An isolated segment of the distal ileum is often preferred. Various procedures include the hemi-Kock pouch, Studer pouch, and the ileal W-neobladder. In these procedures the bowel is surgically reshaped to become a neobladder. The ureters and urethra are sutured into the neobladder. Orthotopic bladder substitution has been more commonly done in men because in women the urethra is usually removed when the bladder is resected.[30] The advantage of orthotopic bladder substitution is that it allows for natural micturition. Incontinence is a possible problem with this technique, and intermittent catheterization may need to be used.

NURSING MANAGEMENT: URINARY DIVERSION

■ Preoperative Management

The patient awaiting cystectomy and urinary diversion must be given a great deal of information. The nurse must assess ability and readiness to learn before initiating a teaching program. If the patient is not ready to learn, the teaching plan should be adjusted. The patient's anxiety and fear may be decreased by the information. However, the anxiety and fear may also interfere with learning. The patient's family should be involved in the teaching process. A discussion of the social aspects of living with a stoma (including clothing, changes in body image and sexuality, exercise, and odor) provides the patient with facts that may allay some fears. The patient who will have a continent diversion must be taught to catheterize and irrigate the pouch and be able to adhere to a strict catheterization schedule. The patient with an orthotopic neobladder may have problems with incontinence. Concerns about the effect on sexual activities should be discussed. The enterostomal therapy nurse should be involved in the preoperative phase of the patient's care. A visit from an ostomate or enterostomal therapy nurse can be helpful. Additional interventions are presented in NCP 43-3.

■ Postoperative Management

Nursing interventions during the postoperative period (see NCP 43-1 for care after an ileal conduit) should be planned to prevent surgical complications such as postoperative atelectasis and shock (see Chapter 18). After pelvic surgery, there is an increased incidence of thrombophlebitis. With removal of part of the bowel, there is an increased incidence of paralytic ileus and small bowel obstruction, the patient is NPO, and a nasogastric tube is necessary for 3 to 5 days.

Specific attention should be given to preventing injury to the stoma and maintaining urine output. Mucus is present in the urine because it is secreted by the intestines as a result of the irritating effect of the urine. The patient should be told that this is a normal occurrence. A high fluid intake is encouraged to "flush" the ileal conduit or continent diversion.

When an ileal conduit is created, the skin around the stoma requires meticulous care. Alkaline encrustations with dermatitis may occur when alkaline urine comes in contact with exposed skin (Fig. 43-11). Other common peristomal skin problems include yeast infections, product allergies, and shearing effect excoriations. Changing appliances (pouches) is discussed in Table 43-20. A properly fitting appliance is essential to prevent skin problems. The appliance should be about 0.1 inch (0.2 cm) larger than the stoma. It is normal for the stoma to shrink within the first few weeks after surgery. The urine is kept acidic to prevent alkaline encrustations.

Acceptance of the surgery and of alterations in body image is needed to ensure the patient's best adjustment. Concerns of the patient include fear that the stoma will be offensive to others and will interfere with sexual, personal, professional, and recreational activities. The patient should know that few activities, if any, will be restricted as a result of the urinary diversion.

43-3 NURSING CARE PLAN PATIENT WITH AN ILEAL CONDUIT

Expected Patient Outcomes	Nursing Interventions and *Rationales*
NURSING DIAGNOSIS	**Anxiety** *related to* effects of ileal conduit on lifestyle and relationships; lack of knowledge regarding surgical procedure, appliance (pouch), and its use *as manifested by* frequent questions about surgical procedure; drawn facies; pallor, restlessness, inability to sleep.
▪ Knowledgeable about preoperative, operative, and postoperative procedures, including both stoma and appliance.	▪ Instruct patient in preoperative, operative, and postoperative procedures including diet, medications, nasogastric tubes, IVs, NPO status, pain management, turning, deep breathing, and leg exercises *to reduce anxiety and facilitate patient's progress through postoperative recovery.* ▪ Demonstrate how to apply appliance and use equipment *because knowledge before surgery reduces patient's postoperative concerns.* ▪ Answer questions honestly and provide emotional support *to reduce fear of the unknown and convey a caring attitude.* ▪ Arrange for visit with person with an ileal conduit or with enterostomal therapist *to provide patient with significant information related to ostomy care.*
NURSING DIAGNOSIS	**Risk for UTI** *related to* surgical procedure, ureteral obstruction, chronic use of external appliance, and incorrect or inadequate stoma care.
▪ No urinary tract infection.	▪ Assess patient for elevation in body temperature, pain in back or abdomen, bloody or cloudy urine, decrease in urinary output *to ensure early detection of UTI.* ▪ Empty appliance q2-3hr or when one-third full of urine *to reduce risk of urinary reflux.* ▪ Use bedside drainage bag at night *to prevent reflux of urine into conduit.* ▪ Instruct patient about symptoms to be reported *as indicators of possible infection.* ▪ Encourage high fluid intake *to maintain adequate urine flow.*
NURSING DIAGNOSIS	**Body image disturbance** *related to* effects of change in body function on lifestyle or relationships *as manifested by* negative feelings about self, refusal to look at or touch stoma or participate in self-care, expression of concern about effect on family and lifestyle.
▪ Acceptance of changes in body image and function.	▪ Encourage patient to share feelings *to provide opportunity to assist with issues and misconceptions and plan appropriate interventions.* ▪ Demonstrate willingness to listen and answer questions *to convey interest in the patient's concerns and to provide needed information.* ▪ Provide information about surgery and expected effects *to reduce anxiety associated with the unknown and altered body function.* ▪ Determine the need for additional support (e.g., psychiatric support, visit by an ostomate) *because these persons may provide new information and suggestions for ways to modify lifestyle.* ▪ Encourage gradual involvement in self-care *because independence in self-care helps improve self-esteem.*
NURSING DIAGNOSIS	**Ineffective management of therapeutic regimen** *related to* lack of knowledge regarding stoma and appliance care *as manifested by* expression of concern about how to manage ileal conduit, frequent questions or inaccurate responses regarding stoma care.
▪ Able to change stoma bag and cleanse stoma. ▪ Able to maintain permanent appliance.	▪ Demonstrate proper method of changing stoma bag and have patient give return demonstration *to teach correct care and evaluate learning.* ▪ Teach measures such as high fluid intake, regular activity, and urine acidification *to prevent urinary calculi and infection.* ▪ Teach practices such as proper stoma and pouch care; empty or change pouch when one-third to one-half full; avoid odor-producing foods such as onions, fish, eggs, cheese; drink cranberry juice or use a liquid appliance deodorant *to enable satisfactory self-care.*

Continued

43-3 NURSING CARE PLAN PATIENT WITH AN ILEAL CONDUIT—continued

Expected Patient Outcomes	Nursing Interventions and *Rationales*
NURSING DIAGNOSIS	**Risk for impaired skin integrity** *related to* ill-fitting appliance, inadequate hygiene, and lack of knowledge regarding stoma care.
▪ Intact, viable stoma. ▪ Clean and intact skin surrounding stoma.	▪ Assess for improperly fitted appliance, reddened and irritated skin around stoma *to ensure prompt identification of the problem.* ▪ Check appliance position *to prevent leakage of caustic drainage onto skin.* ▪ Observe stoma for any bleeding or eroded areas *for early identification and treatment of complications.* ▪ Cleanse stoma as ordered *to reduce encrustations and bacterial contact with the stoma and surrounding skin.* ▪ Allow no tight clothing or binders over stoma *to enable unobstructed circulation of blood and flow of urine.*
NURSING DIAGNOSIS	**Risk for altered sexuality patterns** *related to* perceived or actual effects of surgery on sexual activity.
▪ Satisfaction with sexual practices.	▪ Assess patient's concerns related to sexuality such as future sexual functioning and lack of understanding by significant other *to determine presence or extent of problem.* ▪ Provide accurate information related to sexual activity *so patient will know the effect of this surgery on sexual activities/practices.* ▪ Inform female patient about water-based vaginal lubricant for intercourse *to reduce dyspareunia related to inadequate vaginal lubrication;* teach Kegel exercises *to promote control of the pubococcygeal muscles around the vagina to ease dyspareunia.*

COLLABORATIVE PROBLEMS

Nursing Goals	Nursing Interventions and *Rationales*
POTENTIAL COMPLICATION	**Thrombophlebitis** *related to* surgery involving pelvic manipulation.
▪ Monitor for signs of thrombophlebitis. ▪ Report deviations from acceptable parameters. ▪ Initiate appropriate medical and nursing interventions.	▪ Assess for signs of thrombophlebitis such as swelling, warmth, and pain in legs *to ensure early identification and treatment.* ▪ Teach patient method to do range-of-motion exercises for legs while in bed and instruct patient to keep legs uncrossed *to improve circulation in legs and reduce venous stasis.* ▪ Turn patient q2hr while in bed *to improve circulation to all body systems.* ▪ Increase activity level gradually and have patient ambulate as soon as possible *to improve circulation, especially in lower extremities.* ▪ Provide elastic compression stockings for legs as ordered *to provide support around veins and improve venous return of blood.* ▪ Administer anticoagulants if ordered *to reduce risk of thrombophlebitis by increasing clotting time.*
POTENTIAL COMPLICATION	**Paralytic ileus** *related to* surgical manipulation of bowel.
▪ Monitor for signs of paralytic ileus. ▪ Report deviations from acceptable parameters. ▪ Initiate appropriate medical and nursing interventions.	▪ Assess patient for signs of paralytic ileus such as absence of bowel sounds, abdominal distention, cramping pain, nausea and vomiting *to enable early identification and treatment.* ▪ Maintain patency of nasogastric tube *to prevent accumulation and ensure removal of gastric secretions.* ▪ Encourage early ambulation *to promote peristalsis.* ▪ Administer IV fluids as ordered *to maintain fluid and electrolyte balance.* ▪ Monitor fluid and electrolyte levels *to identify imbalance and enable prompt treatment.* ▪ Assess for presence of bowel sounds, flatus, and bowel movements *as indicators of peristalsis.*

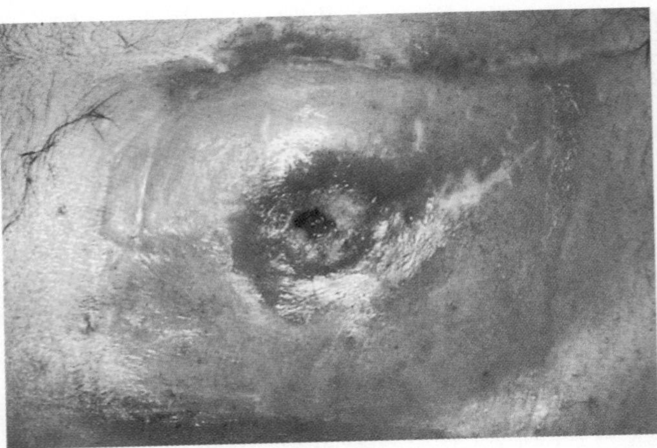

Fig. 43-11 Ammonia salt encrustation secondary to alkaline urine.

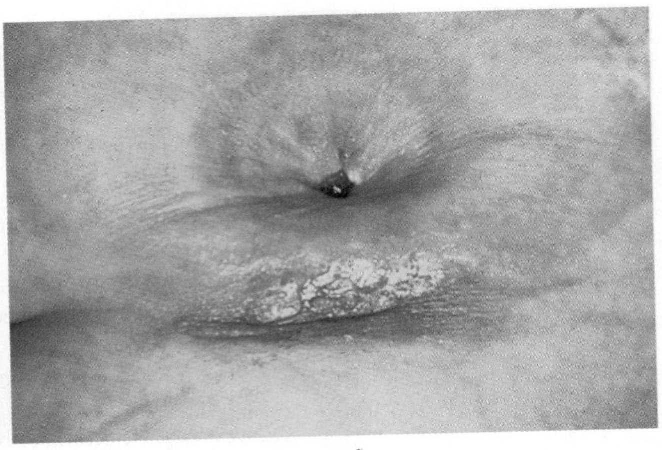

Fig. 43-12 Retracted urinary stoma with pressure sore from faceplate above stoma.

PATIENT & FAMILY TEACHING GUIDE

Table 43-20 Changing Ileal Conduit Appliances

Temporary Appliance

1. Cut hole in pouch to fit over stoma (pouch 3.2 mm [⅛ in] larger than stoma).
2. Remove old pouch.
3. Clean area gently and remove old adhesive.
4. Wash area with warm water.
5. Place wick (rolled-up 4 × 4 in pad) over stoma to keep area dry during rest of procedure.
6. Dry skin around stoma.
7. Apply tincture of benzoin or other skin protectant around stoma to area where pouch will be placed.
8. Apply pouch by first smoothing its edges toward side and lower portion of body.
9. Remove wick and complete application of bag.
10. If patient is usually in bed, apply bag so that it lies toward side of body.
11. If patient is ambulatory, apply bag so that it lies vertically.
12. Connect drainage tubing to pouch.
13. Keep drainage pouch on same side of bed as stoma.

Permanent Appliance*

1. Keep appliance in place for 2-14 days.
2. Change appliance when fluid intake has been restricted for several hours.
3. Have patient sit or stand in front of mirror.
4. Moisten edge of faceplate with adhesive solvent and gently remove.
5. Clean skin with adhesive solvent.
6. Wash skin with warm water. (Patient may shower.)
7. Dry skin and inspect.
8. Place wick (rolled up 4 × 4 in pad) over stoma to keep skin free of urine.
9. Apply skin cement to faceplate and skin.
10. Place appliance over stoma.
11. Wash removed appliance with soap and lukewarm water; soak in distilled vinegar; rinse with lukewarm water and air dry.

*Many disposable appliances with self-adhesive backing are used as permanent appliances.

Discharge planning after an ileal conduit includes teaching the patient symptoms of obstruction or infection and care of the ostomy. The patient with an ileal conduit is fitted for a permanent appliance 7 to 10 days after surgery and may need to be refitted at a later time, depending on the degree of stoma shrinkage. Appliances are made of a variety of products, including natural and synthetic rubbers, plastics, and metals. Most appliances have a faceplate that adheres to the skin, a collecting pouch, and an opening to drain the pouch. The faceplate may be secured to the skin with glues, adhesives, or adhering synthetic wafers. Some appliances do not require adhesives, but their design relies on pressure to keep the pouch in place. If improperly fitted or applied, the faceplate may cause skin problems (Fig. 43-12). The patient needs information on where to purchase supplies, emergency telephone numbers, location of ostomy clubs, and follow-up visits with an enterostomal therapist. Physician follow-up is imperative to monitor and correct homeostatic abnormalities and to prevent complications and renal function deterioration.

CRITICAL THINKING EXERCISES

CASE STUDY

Urinary Tract Infection

Patient Profile

Sue, a 28-year-old woman, was seen in the nurse practitioner's office for a history of painful, frequent urination.

Subjective Data

- Has had a history of painful, frequent urination with passage of small volumes of urine for 3 days
- Has had intermittent fever, chills, and back pain during these 3 days
- Was frightened when she saw blood in her urine
- Is anxious because her father died of kidney cancer

Objective Data

Physical Examination

- Complains of bilateral flank pain and abdominal tenderness to palpation
- Temperature is 100.4° F (38° C)

Diagnostic Study

- Urinalysis : pyuria and hematuria

Critical Thinking Questions

1. What are the most common organisms that cause UTIs?
2. What factors predispose a patient to a UTI?
3. What is the difference between upper and lower UTIs?
4. What nursing interventions will help Sue cope with her symptoms?
5. What can the nurse do to help Sue prevent another UTI?
6. Based on the data presented, write one or more appropriate nursing diagnoses. Are there any collaborative problems?

NURSING RESEARCH ISSUES

1. In the patient with UTI, what are the most effective methods to ensure compliance with therapy and follow-up care?
2. What therapeutic measures are most effective in treating stress incontinence?
3. What are the differences in quality of life of the patient with an ileal conduit as compared with the patient with a continent urinary diversion?
4. What are the most effective ways to manage pain following lithotripsy?
5. Does biofeedback improve the effectiveness of pelvic muscle exercises?

REVIEW QUESTIONS

The number of the question corresponds to the same-numbered objective at the beginning of the chapter.

1. In teaching a patient with pyelonephritis about the disorder, the nurse informs the patient that the organisms that cause pyelonephritis most commonly reach the kidneys through
   a. the bloodstream.
   b. the lymphatic system.
   c. a descending infection.
   d. an ascending infection.
2. The nurse teaches the female patient who has frequent urinary tract infections that she should
   a. urinate after sexual intercourse.
   b. take tub baths with bubble bath.
   c. take prophylactic sulfonamides for the rest of her life.
   d. restrict fluid intake to prevent the need for frequent voiding.
3. The immunologic mechanisms involved in glomerulonephritis include
   a. tubular blocking by precipitates of bacteria and antibody reactions.
   b. deposition of immune complexes and complement along the GBM.
   c. thickening of the GBM from autoimmune microangiopathic changes.
   d. destruction of glomeruli by proteolytic enzymes contained in the GBM.
4. One of the most important roles of the nurse in relation to acute poststreptococcal glomerulonephritis is to
   a. promote early diagnosis and treatment of sore throats and skin lesions.
   b. encourage patients to request antibiotic therapy for all upper respiratory infections.
   c. teach patients with APSGN that long-term prophylactic antibiotic therapy is necessary to prevent recurrence.
   d. monitor patients for respiratory symptoms that indicate that the disease is affecting the alveolar basement membrane.
5. The edema that occurs in nephrotic syndrome is due to
   a. decreased aldosterone secretion from adrenal insufficiency.
   b. increased hydrostatic pressure caused by sodium retention.
   c. increased fluid retention caused by decreased glomerular filtration.
   d. decreased colloidal osmotic pressure caused by loss of serum albumin.
6. A patient is admitted to the hospital with severe renal colic caused by renal lithiasis. The nurse's first priority in management of the patient is to
   a. administer narcotics as prescribed.
   b. obtain supplies for straining all urine.
   c. encourage fluid intake of 3 to 4 liters per day.
   d. keep the patient NPO in preparation for surgery.
7. The nurse recommends genetic counseling for the children of a patient with
   a. nephrotic syndrome.
   b. chronic pyelonephritis.
   c. malignant nephrosclerosis.
   d. adult-onset polycystic renal disease.
8. The nurse encourages strict diabetic control in the patient prone to diabetic nephropathy knowing that the renal tissue changes that may occur in this condition include
   a. uric acid calculi and nephrolithiasis.
   b. renal sugar-crystal calculi and cysts.
   c. lipid deposits in the glomeruli and nephrons.
   d. thickening of the GBM and glomerulosclerosis.

9. The nurse identifies a risk factor for kidney and bladder cancer in a patient who relates a history of
   a. aspirin use.
   b. tobacco use.
   c. chronic alcohol abuse.
   d. use of artificial sweeteners.
10. In planning nursing interventions to increase bladder control in the patient with urinary incontinence the nurse includes
   a. restricting fluid intake after dinner in the evening.
   b. using incontinence pads to prevent patient embarrassment.
   c. clamping and releasing a catheter to increase bladder tone.
   d. teaching the patient biofeedback mechanisms to suppress the urge to void.
11. A patient with a ureterolithotomy returns from surgery with a nephrostomy tube in place. Postoperative nursing care of the patient includes
   a. encouraging the patient to drink fruit juices and milk.
   b. forcing fluids of at least 2 to 3 L per day after nausea has subsided.
   c. notifying the physician if nephrostomy tube drainage is more than 30 ml/hr.
   d. irrigating the nephrostomy tube with 10 ml of normal saline solution as needed.
12. A patient has had a cystectomy and ileal conduit diversion performed. Four days postoperatively, mucous shreds are seen in the drainage bag. The nurse should
   a. notify the physician.
   b. notify the charge nurse.
   c. irrigate the drainage tube.
   d. chart it as a normal observation.

References

1. Marchiondo K: A new look at urinary tract infection, *AJN* 98:34, 1998.
2. Barnett BJ, Stephens DS: Urinary tract infection: an overview, *Am J Med Sci* 314:245, 1997.
3. Schaeffer AJ: Infections of the urinary tract. In Walsh PC and others, editors: *Campbell's urology,* ed 7, Philadelphia, 1998, Saunders.
4. Nicolle LE: Asymptomatic bacteriuria in the elderly, *Infect Dis Clin North Am* 11:647, 1997.
5. Hooton TM, Stamm WE: Diagnosis and treatment of uncomplicated urinary tract infection, *Infect Dis Clin North Am* 11:551, 1997.
6. Karlowicz KA: Pharmacologic therapy for acute cystitis in adults: a review of treatment options, *Urol Nurs* 17:106, 1997.
7. Stapleton A, Stamm WE: Prevention of urinary tract infection, *Infect Dis Clin North Am* 11:719, 1997.
8. Pearson BD: Liquidate a myth: reducing liquid intake is not advisable for elderly with urine control problems, *Urol Nurs* 13:86, 1993.
9. Kaufman MW and others: Caring for the patient with interstitial cystitis, *Medsurg Nurs* 6:203, 1997.
10. Irwin P, Galloway N: Surgical management of interstitial cystitis, *Urol Clin North Am* 21:145, 1994.
11. Wiseman KC: New insights on Goodpasture's syndrome, *ANNA J* 20:17, 1993.
12. Orth SR, Ritz E: The nephrotic syndrome, *N Engl J Med* 338:1202, 1998.
13. Humphreys MH: Human immunodeficiency virus–associated glomerulosclerosis, *Kidney Int* 48:311, 1995.
14. Kupin WL: A practical approach to nephrolithiasis, *Hosp Pract* 30:57, 1995.
15. Sosa RE, Martin TV: Critical challenges of renal calculi in women, *Medscape Women's Health* 1:8, 1996.
16. Wolf JS, Clayman RV: Percutaneous nephrostolithotomy. What is its role in 1997? *Urol Clin North Am* 24:43, 1997.
17. Nakada SY: The surgical management of renal stones: selecting what is best, *Infect Urol* 10:42, 1997.
18. Miller-Hjelle MA and others: Polycystic kidney disease: an unrecognized emerging infectious disease? *Emerg Infect Dis* 3:113, 1997.
19. American Cancer Society: *Cancer facts and figures,* Atlanta, 1998.
20. Lerner L, Heaney J: Incidentally detected renal tumors, *Hosp Pract* 32:53, 1997.
21. Bukowski RM, Novick AC: Clinical practice guidelines: renal cell carcinoma, *Cleve Clin J Med* 64(suppl 1):S1, 1997.
22. Cohen SM: Urinary bladder carcinogenesis, *Toxicol Pathol* 26:121, 1998.
23. McCaffrey JA, Bajorin DF, Scher HI, Bosl GJ: Combined-modality therapy for bladder cancer, *Oncology* 11(suppl 9):18, 1997.
24. Fourcroy JL: Urogynecology update: incontinence, *Hosp Pract* 33:63, 1998.
25. Urinary Incontinence Guideline Panel: *Urinary incontinence in adults: clinical practice guideline,* AHCPR pub no 92-0038, Rockville, Md, 1996, Agency for Health Care Policy and Research, Public Health Service, US Department of Health and Human Services.
26. Bernier F, Harris L: Treating stress incontinence with the bladder neck support device, *Urol Nurs* 15:5, 1995.
27. Gallo ML and others: Quality of life improvement and the reliance urinary control insert, *Urol Nurs* 17:146, 1997.
28. Hollander JB, Biokno AC: Clean intermittent catheterization: an update, *Infect Urol* 9:118, 1996.
29. Turner WH, Studer UE: Cystectomy and urinary diversion, *Semin Surg Oncol* 13:350, 1997.
30. Montie JE, Park JM: Orthotopic diversion in women, *Semin Urol Oncol* 15:184, 1997.

Resources

American Urological Association
1120 North Charles Street
Baltimore, MD 21201
410-727-1100
Fax: 410-223-4370
http://www.auanet.org/

Bladder Health Council
American Foundation for Urologic Disease
300 West Pratt Street, Suite 401
Baltimore, MD 21201
410-727-2908
800-242-2383

National Association for Continence (NAFC)
PO Box 8310
Spartanburg, SC 29305
864-579-7900
800-BLADDER (252-3337)
http://www.medhelp.org/agsg/agsg1172.htm

Simon Foundation for Continence
PO Box 835
Wilmette, IL 60091
800-23-SIMON (237-4666)
708-864-3913
http://www.simonfoundation.org/html/

Society of Urological Nurses and Associates
East Holly Avenue, Box 56
Pitman, NJ 08071-0056
East Holly Avenue
888-827-7862
Fax: 609-589-7463

United Ostomy Association
19772 MacArthur Boulevard, Suite 200
Irvine, CA 92612-2405
800-826-0826
http://www.uoa.org/

Also see Resources for Chapter 44 on p. 1341.

For additional Internet resources, see the website for this book at **www.mosby.com/MERLIN/medsurg_lewis**

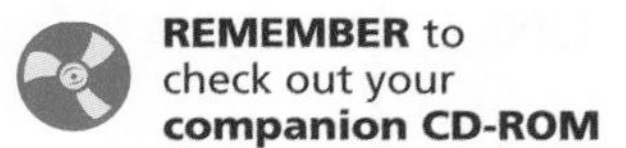

REMEMBER to check out your **companion CD-ROM**

44 NURSING MANAGEMENT Acute and Chronic Renal Failure

Gillian Brunier & Marilyn Bartucci

www.mosby.com/MERLIN/medsurg_lewis

LEARNING OBJECTIVES

1. Differentiate between acute and chronic renal failure.
2. Differentiate among the causes of prerenal, intrarenal, and postrenal acute renal failure.
3. Describe the clinical course of reversible acute renal failure.
4. Explain the collaborative care and nursing management of a patient in the oliguric and diuretic phases of acute renal failure.
5. Describe the systemic effects of chronic renal failure.
6. Explain the conservative collaborative care and the related nursing management of the patient with chronic renal failure.
7. Differentiate between peritoneal dialysis and hemodialysis in terms of purpose, indications for use, advantages and disadvantages, and nursing responsibilities.
8. Compare common vascular access sites used for hemodialysis.
9. Compare dialysis and renal transplantation as methods of treatment for end-stage renal disease.
10. Describe the nursing management of patients in the preoperative, intraoperative, and postoperative stages of kidney transplantation.
11. Explain the long-term problems of the patient with a kidney transplant.

Renal failure is severe impairment or total lack of kidney function. In renal failure there is an inability to excrete metabolic waste products and water, as well as functional disturbances of all body systems. Renal failure is classified as acute or chronic. Acute renal failure most commonly has a rapid onset. Although acute renal failure is potentially reversible, the mortality rate remains distressingly high in spite of advances in treatment.

Chronic renal failure usually develops insidiously over time and necessitates the initiation of dialysis or transplantation for long-term survival. The focus in chronic renal failure has changed from treating a terminally ill patient to dealing with a person who has a manageable chronic disease that requires long-term care. In dialysis, the change in focus is a result of technical advances. In renal transplant, the change in focus is a result of improved surgical techniques and immunosuppressive therapy.

ACUTE RENAL FAILURE

Acute renal failure is a clinical syndrome characterized by a rapid decline in renal function with progressive azotemia (an accumulation of nitrogenous waste products such as blood urea nitrogen [BUN]) and increasing levels of serum creatinine. *Uremia* is the condition in which azotemia progresses to a symptomatic state. Acute renal failure is usually associated with a decrease in urinary output to less than 400 ml per day, although it is possible to have normal or increased urinary output. There is no correlation between the amount of urine produced and the severity of the renal failure.

Acute renal failure usually develops over hours or days with progressive elevations of BUN, creatinine, and potassium with or without oliguria. Most commonly, acute renal failure follows severe, prolonged hypotension or hypovolemia or contact with a nephrotoxic agent.

Etiology and Pathophysiology

The etiologies of acute renal failure are multiple and complex. They are categorized according to similar pathogenesis into prerenal, intrarenal (or renal parenchymal), and postrenal causes (Table 44-1).

Prerenal causes consist of factors outside the kidneys that reduce renal blood flow and lead to decreased glomerular perfusion and filtration. Hypovolemia can lead to decreased renal perfusion, as can cardiac failure, which decreases the effective circulating volume of the blood. Drugs that may start or complicate prerenal azotemia include nonsteroidal antiinflammatory drugs (NSAIDs), which block synthesis of vasodilating prostaglandins, and angiotensin-converting enzyme (ACE) inhibitors, which block synthesis of angiotensin II. Prerenal disease can lead to intrarenal disease (tubular necrosis) if renal ischemia is prolonged. Prerenal causes are the most common cause of acute renal failure, accounting for approximately 70% of all cases.[1]

Reviewed by Mary Jo Holechek, MS, CRNP, CS, CNN, Transplant Nurse Coordinator, Johns Hopkins Hospital, Baltimore, Md.

Table 44-1 Common Causes of Acute Renal Failure

Prerenal	Intrarenal	Postrenal
▪ Hypovolemia Hemorrhage Burns Dehydration Prolonged diarrhea or vomiting ▪ Decreased cardiac output Myocardial infarction Cardiac arrhythmias Congestive heart failure Cardiogenic shock Pericardial tamponade Surgery (e.g., open heart) ▪ Decreased peripheral vascular resistance Septic shock Anaphylaxis Neurologic injury ▪ Renal vascular obstruction Thrombosis of renal arteries Bilateral renal vein thrombosis Embolism	▪ Nephrotoxic injury Drugs (aminoglycosides [gentamicin, tobramycin, amikacin], amphotericin B, cisplatin) Radiographic contrast agents Hemolytic blood transfusion reaction (hemoglobin blocks tubules) Severe crushing injury (myoglobin released from muscles blocks tubules) Chemicals (ethylene glycol, mercuric chloride, carbon tetrachloride, lead, arsenic) ▪ Acute glomerulonephritis ▪ Acute pyelonephritis ▪ Toxemia of pregnancy ▪ Malignant hypertension ▪ Systemic lupus erythematosus ▪ Interstitial nephritis Allergic (antibiotics [sulfonamides, rifampin], nonsteroidal antiinflammatory drugs, ACE inhibitors) Infection (bacterial [e.g., acute pyelonephritis], viral [e.g., CMV], fungal [e.g., candidiasis])	▪ Calculi formation ▪ Benign prostatic hyperplasia ▪ Prostate cancer ▪ Bladder cancer ▪ Trauma (to back, pelvis, or perineum) ▪ Strictures ▪ Spinal cord disease

ACE, angiotensin-converting enzyme; *CMV*, cytomegalovirus.

Intrarenal causes include conditions that cause direct damage to the renal tissue (parenchyma) resulting in malfunctioning of nephrons. Intrarenal causes account for approximately 25% of all cases of acute renal failure.[1] Primary renal diseases such as acute glomerulonephritis and acute pyelonephritis may lead to acute renal failure. More commonly, acute tubular necrosis (ATN) is the predisposing insult. ATN may be caused by ischemia, nephrotoxins (e.g., antibiotics), hemoglobin released from hemolyzed red blood cells (RBCs), or myoglobin released from necrotic muscle cells. Nephrotoxic chemicals and drugs can cause obstruction of intrarenal structures by crystallization or actual damage to the epithelial cells of the tubules. The most common drugs that cause nephrotoxic injury are aminoglycoside antibiotics and radiocontrast agents. Hemoglobin and myoglobin block the tubules and cause renal vasoconstriction.

Postrenal causes involve mechanical obstruction of urinary outflow. As the flow of urine is blocked, urine backs up into the renal pelvis, ultimately resulting in renal failure. The most common causes are benign prostatic hyperplasia, calculi, trauma, prostate cancer, and tumors. Postrenal causes of acute renal failure account for less than 5% of cases, with a higher incidence among the elderly.[1] These causes are almost always treatable if identified before permanent kidney damage occurs.

The two major mechanisms that lead to acute renal failure are renal ischemia and nephrotoxic injury (Fig. 44-1). Acute renal failure that results from these two causes is usually referred to as ATN. Severe renal ischemia causes a disruption in the basement membrane and patchy destruction of the tubular epithelium. Nephrotoxic agents cause necrosis of tubular epithelial cells, which slough off and plug the tubules. Nephrotoxic injury usually leaves the basement membrane intact. ATN is potentially reversible if the basement membrane is not destroyed and if the necrotic tubular epithelium regenerates.

Possible pathologic processes involved in acute renal failure include the following:

1. *Renal vasoconstriction.* Hypovolemia and decreased renal blood flow stimulate renin release, which activates the angiotensin-aldosterone system (see Fig. 42-6) and results in constriction of the peripheral arteries and the renal afferent arterioles. With decreased renal blood flow, there is decreased glomerular capillary pressure and glomerular filtration rate (GFR), as well as tubular dysfunction and, ultimately, oliguria.
2. *Cellular edema.* Ischemia causes anoxia, which leads to endothelial cell edema. Cellular edema raises tissue pressures above capillary flow pressure; consequently, blood flow through the arterioles may still be altered after treatment of the underlying condition. Inadequate renal blood flow further depresses the GFR.
3. *Decreased glomerular capillary permeability.* Ischemia alters glomerular epithelial cells and thus decreases glomerular capillary permeability. This in turn reduces the GFR, which significantly reduces blood flow and leads to tubular dysfunction.
4. *Intratubular obstruction.* When tubules are damaged, interstitial edema occurs, and necrotic epithelial cells accumulate in the tubules. This accumulated debris also lowers the GFR by obstructing the tubules and increasing intratubular pressure.

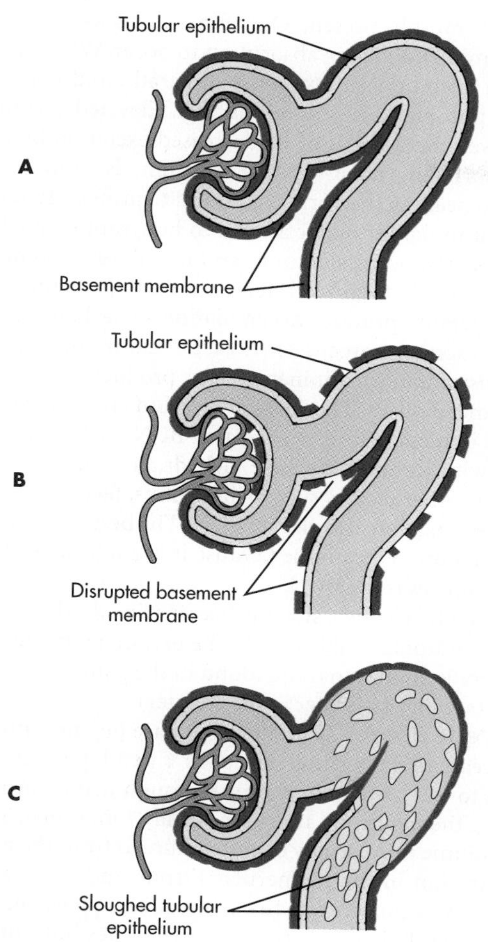

Fig. 44-1 Nephron destruction in acute renal failure. **A,** Normal nephron. **B,** Damage from renal ischemia results in disrupted basement membrane. **C,** Nephrotoxic agents can cause tubular injury.

5. *Leakage of glomerular filtrate.* Glomerular filtrate leaks back into plasma through holes in the damaged tubular membranes, which decreases intratubular fluid flow.

Clinical Course

Clinically acute renal failure may progress through the phases of oliguria, diuresis, and recovery. In some situations the patient does not recover from acute renal failure, and chronic renal failure results.

Oliguric Phase. The most common initial manifestation of acute renal failure is oliguria caused by a reduction in the GFR. The oliguria usually occurs within 1 to 7 days of the causative event. If the cause is ischemia, oliguria may occur within 24 hours, but when nephrotoxic drugs are involved, the onset may be delayed for as long as a week. Initially, the presence of anuria (≤400 ml urine output per 24 hours) is rare unless the precipitating cause is a urinary obstructive disorder. (Acute nonoliguric renal failure may also occur. In this situation, the onset may be less obvious with hypervolemia or an elevated BUN as the first presenting abnormality.) The duration of the oliguric phase may range from a few days to several weeks. Some cases have lasted for several months. The average duration is about 10 to 14 days, but it rarely exceeds 4 weeks. The longer the oliguric phase lasts, the poorer the prognosis for recovery of renal function.

It is important to distinguish prerenal oliguria from oliguria of acute intrarenal failure. In prerenal oliguria there is no damage to the renal tissue. The oliguria is caused by a decrease in circulating blood volume (e.g., as a result of shock, burns, severe dehydration, decreased cardiac output) and is usually reversible. (Many causes of intrarenal failure are also potentially reversible.) With a decrease in circulating blood volume, autoregulatory mechanisms such as increases in angiotensin II, norepinephrine, and antidiuretic hormone (ADH) attempt to preserve blood flow to essential organs. Vasoconstriction occurs with sodium and water retention. Therefore prerenal oliguria is characterized by urine with a high specific gravity and a low sodium concentration.

In contrast, oliguria of intrarenal failure is characterized by urine with a normal specific gravity and a high sodium concentration, indicating that the injured tubules cannot respond to autoregulatory mechanisms. In addition, oliguria of intrarenal failure caused by ATN due to ischemia or toxins is characterized by the presence of granular or epithelial cell casts in the urine. The casts are formed from mucoprotein impressions of the necrotic renal tubular epithelial cells, which detach or slough into the tubules.

The manifestations of the oliguric phase are changes in urinary output, fluid and electrolyte abnormalities, and uremia. The nurse must be alert for the signs and symptoms of these changes.

Urinary changes. Urinary output decreases to less than 400 ml per 24 hours. The urine may be bloody but is usually not. A urinalysis may show casts, RBCs, white blood cells (WBCs), a specific gravity fixed at around 1.010, and urine osmolality at about 300 mOsm/kg (300 mmol/kg). This is the same specific gravity and osmolality as for plasma, reflecting tubular damage with a loss of concentrating ability by the kidney. Proteinuria may be present if the renal failure is related to glomerular membrane dysfunction.

Fluid volume excess. When urinary output decreases, fluid retention occurs. The severity of the symptoms depend on the extent of the fluid overload. The neck veins may become distended, the pulse may become more bounding, and peripheral and central edema and hypertension may develop. Fluid overload can eventually lead to congestive heart failure, pulmonary edema, and pericardial and pleural effusions.

Metabolic acidosis. In renal failure the kidneys cannot synthesize ammonia, which is needed for H^+ excretion, or excrete acid metabolites. The serum bicarbonate level decreases because bicarbonate is used up in buffering hydrogen ions. In addition, defective reabsorption and regeneration of bicarbonate occur. The patient may develop Kussmaul's respirations (rapid, deep respirations) to increase the excretion of carbon dioxide.

Sodium balance. Damaged tubules cannot conserve sodium. Consequently, the urinary excretion of sodium may increase, resulting in normal or below normal levels of serum sodium. Elevated sodium levels may be masked by hypervolemia (dilutional hyponatremia). However, excessive intake of sodium should be avoided because it can lead to volume expansion, hypertension, and congestive heart failure.

Potassium excess. The serum potassium levels increase, since the normal ability of the kidneys to excrete 80% to 90% of

Table 44-2 **Clinical Manifestations of Acute Renal Failure**

Body System	Clinical Manifestations
Urinary	↓ Urinary output Proteinuria Casts ↓ Specific gravity ↓ Osmolality ↑ Urinary sodium
Cardiovascular	Volume overload Congestive heart failure Hypotension (early) Hypertension (after development of fluid overload) Pericarditis Pericardial effusion Arrhythmias
Respiratory	Pulmonary edema Kussmaul's respirations Pleural effusions
Gastrointestinal	Nausea and vomiting Anorexia Stomatitis Bleeding Diarrhea Constipation
Hematologic	Anemia (development within 48 hr) Leukocytosis Defect in platelet functioning
Neurologic	Lethargy Convulsions Asterixis Memory impairment
Others	↑ Susceptibility to infection ↑ BUN ↑ Creatinine ↑ Potassium ↓ pH ↓ Bicarbonate ↓ Calcium ↑ Phosphate

BUN, blood urea nitrogen.

the body's potassium is impaired. If the acute renal failure was caused by massive tissue trauma, the damaged cells release additional potassium to the extracellular fluid. Thus the patient with tissue injury may have an even higher serum potassium level. In addition, acidosis enhances the movement of potassium from intracellular to extracellular fluid.

When potassium levels exceed 6 mEq/L (6 mmol/L), treatment must be initiated immediately to prevent cardiac arrhythmias. Before clinical signs of hyperkalemia are apparent, the electrocardiogram (ECG) will show tall, peaked T waves, widening of the QRS complex, and ST depression. Progressive changes in the ECG, which are related to increasing potassium levels, are depicted in Fig. 15-13. The cardiac muscle is very intolerant of acute increases in potassium.

Calcium deficit and phosphate excess. A low serum calcium level results from decreased gastrointestinal (GI) absorption of calcium. To absorb calcium from the GI tract, activated vitamin D must be present. Only functioning kidneys can activate vitamin D, allowing absorption to occur. When calcium is removed from bones in response to parathyroid hormone secretion, phosphate is released as well. Elevated serum phosphate levels are a result of its decreased excretion by the kidneys. Normally most plasma calcium is found ionized (physiologically active form) or bound to protein. In renal failure it is unusual for hypocalcemia to be symptomatic because acidosis keeps more calcium in an ionized form. Sometimes a low serum level of ionized calcium can lead to tetany.

Nitrogenous product accumulation. The kidneys are the primary excretory organs for urea, an end product of protein metabolism, and creatinine, an end product of endogenous muscle metabolism. The BUN and serum creatinine levels are elevated in renal failure. An elevated BUN level must be interpreted with caution because dehydration and catabolism, caused by other factors such as infections, fever, severe injury, or GI bleeding, can also elevate BUN. The best serum indicator of renal failure is creatinine because it is not usually altered by other factors as is the BUN.

Eventually all body systems become involved in the acute uremic syndrome (Table 44-2). The extrarenal manifestations are generally similar to those found in the patient with chronic uremia (see Fig. 44-3 later in the chapter).

Diuretic Phase. The diuretic phase begins with a gradual increase in daily urine output of 1 to 3 L per day but may reach 3 to 5 L per day or more. Although urine output is increasing, the nephrons are still not fully functional. The high urine volume is caused by osmotic diuresis from the high urea concentration in the glomerular filtrate and the inability of the tubules to concentrate the urine. In this phase the kidneys have recovered their ability to excrete wastes but not to concentrate the urine. In this phase hypovolemia and hypotension can occur from massive fluid losses.

At this stage the uremia may still be severe, as reflected by low creatinine clearances and elevated serum creatinine and BUN levels. Because of the large losses of fluid and electrolytes, the patient must be monitored for hyponatremia, hypokalemia, and dehydration. The diuretic phase may last 1 to 3 weeks. Near the end of this phase the patient's acid-base, electrolyte, and waste product parameters begin to normalize.

Recovery Phase. The recovery phase begins when the GFR increases so that BUN and serum creatinine levels start to stabilize and then decrease. Although the major improvements occur in the first 1 to 2 weeks of this phase, renal function can continue to improve for up to 12 months after acute renal failure.

The outcome of acute renal failure is influenced by the patient's overall health, the severity of renal failure, and the number and type of complications. The mortality rate from acute renal failure varies from 30% to 60%, depending on the cause. Patients with ATN and oliguria have a 50% risk of mortality, especially when there is an underlying disease.[1] Many deaths are related to the underlying disease. However, the most common cause of death is infection. Infection occurs in 30% to 70% of individuals who develop acute renal failure. The incidence of infection is highest in the individual in whom surgery or traumatic injury contributed to renal failure.

Some individuals do not recover and progress to chronic renal failure. The older adult patient is less likely to recover normal renal function than the younger patient. Among the individuals who recover, the vast majority achieve clinically normal renal function with no complications (e.g., hypertension).

Diagnostic Studies

The most important tool for distinguishing prerenal, intrarenal, and postrenal causes is the history, including a thorough review of recent clinical events and drug therapy. Prerenal causes should be suspected when there is a history of heart disease or extracellular fluid volume loss or depletion. Intrarenal causes may be suspected if the patient has been taking potentially nephrotoxic medication or has a history of systemic disorders such as systemic lupus erythematosus. Postrenal causes are suggested by a history of changes in urinary stream, hematuria or pyuria, or cancer of the bladder or prostate.

Urinalysis is an important diagnostic test. Urine sediment containing abundant cells, casts, or proteins suggests intrarenal disorders. ATN is associated with abundant urinary casts. Normal urine sediment is possible in both prerenal and postrenal causes. Hematuria, pyuria, and crystals may be associated with postrenal causes.

If the cause of acute renal failure is difficult to determine from the history and physical examination, further testing may be necessary, such as a renal ultrasound, renal scan, retrograde pyelogram, computed tomography (CT) scan, or magnetic resonance imaging (MRI).

Collaborative Care

Because acute renal failure is potentially reversible, the primary goal of treatment is to maintain the patient in as normal a state as possible while the kidneys are repairing themselves (Table 44-3). The precipitating cause is determined and corrected if possible. Management is focused on controlling the patient's symptoms and preventing complications.

The first step is to determine if there is adequate intravascular volume and cardiac output to ensure adequate perfusion of the kidneys. Diuretic therapy is often administered along with volume expanders to prevent volume overload. Diuretic therapy includes loop diuretics (furosemide [Lasix], ethacrynic acid [Edecrin], bumetanide [Bumex]) or an osmotic diuretic (mannitol). If acute renal failure is already established, forcing fluids and diuresis is not effective and may in fact be harmful. Conservative therapy may be all that is necessary until renal function resumes. However, the general trend is to initiate early and frequent dialysis to minimize symptoms and prevent complications.

Fluid intake must be closely monitored during the oliguric phase. The common rule for calculating fluid replacement is to consider all losses for the previous 24 hours (e.g., urine, diarrhea, vomitus, blood) plus 500 to 600 ml for insensible losses (e.g., respirations, diaphoresis). For example, if a patient excreted 300 ml of urine on Tuesday with no other losses, fluid replacement on Wednesday would be 800 to 900 ml.

Hyperkalemia is one of the most dangerous complications in acute renal failure because it can cause life-threatening cardiac arrhythmias. The various therapies used to decrease potassium levels are listed in Table 44-4. Sodium polystyrene sulfonate (Kayexalate) should never be given to a patient with paralytic ileus.

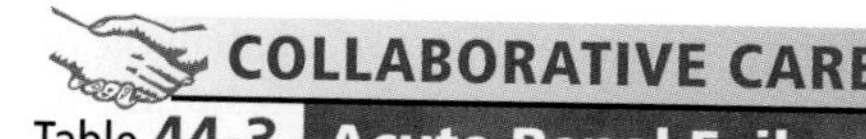

Table 44-3 Acute Renal Failure

Diagnostic
- History and physical examination
- Identification of precipitating cause
- Serum creatinine and BUN levels
- Serum electrolytes
- Urinalysis
- Renal ultrasound
- Retrograde pyelogram (as indicated)
- Renal scan (as indicated)
- CT scan or MRI (as indicated)

Collaborative Therapy
- Treatment of precipitating cause
- Fluid restriction (500-600 ml plus previous 24 hr fluid loss)
- Nutritional therapy
  - Adequate protein provision (1.0-1.5 g/kg/day)
  - Potassium restriction
  - Phosphate restriction
  - Sodium restriction
- Measures to lower potassium (if elevated)*
- Calcium supplements or phosphate-binding agents
- Total parenteral nutrition (if indicated)†
- Enteral nutrition (if indicated)†
- Initiation of dialysis (if necessary)
- Continuous renal replacement therapy (if necessary)

*See Table 44-4.
†Renal formulations of these two forms of nutrition are available.

Table 44-4 Therapies to Lower Serum Potassium Levels

1. **Regular Insulin Administration IV**
   Potassium moves into cells when insulin is given. Glucose is given concurrently to prevent hypoglycemia. When effects of insulin diminish, potassium shifts back out of cells.
2. **Sodium Bicarbonate**
   Therapy can correct acidosis and causes shift of potassium into cells.
3. **Calcium Gluconate IV**
   Therapy is given IV and generally used in advanced cardiac toxicity. Calcium raises the threshold for excitation resulting in arrhythmias.
4. **Dialysis**
   Hemodialysis can bring potassium levels to normal within 30 min to 2 hr. Peritoneal dialysis takes longer.
5. **Sodium Polystyrene Sulfonate (Kayexalate)**
   Cation-exchange resin is administered by mouth or retention enema. When resin is in the bowel, potassium is exchanged for sodium. Therapy removes 1 mEq of potassium per gram of drug. It is mixed in water with sorbitol to produce osmotic diarrhea, allowing for evacuation of potassium-rich stool from body.
6. **Dietary Restrictions**
   Daily potassium intake is limited to 40-50 mEq.

IV, intravenous.

The most common indications for the use of dialysis in acute renal failure include (1) volume overload resulting in congestive heart failure and pulmonary edema; (2) potassium level greater than 6 mEq/L (6 mmol/L) with ECG changes; (3) metabolic acidosis (serum bicarbonate level less than 15 mEq/L [15 mmol/L]); (4) BUN level greater than 120 mg/dl (43 mmol/L); (5) significant change in mental status; and (6) pericarditis, pericardial effusion, or cardiac tamponade. Laboratory values are only rough parameters, and clinical assessment is the most important guide in determining the need for dialysis.

If dialysis is required, there are two options available—hemodialysis (HD) and peritoneal dialysis (PD). HD has the advantage of efficiency and shorter duration compared with PD. However, it is technically more complicated because specialized equipment and vascular access is required and may require anticoagulation therapy to prevent blood clotting in the dialysis blood circuit. Rapid biochemical changes on HD may induce side effects such as hypotension. In most situations, HD is preferred to PD for treatment of acute renal failure because it is efficient and metabolic problems can be corrected safely and quickly. PD is simpler than HD but carries the risk of peritonitis, is less efficient in the catabolic patient, and takes longer. PD may be preferred for the individual with intracranial bleeding or cardiovascular instability. HD is preferred for the hypercatabolic patient and for the individual who has had abdominal or thoracic trauma or surgery. (HD and PD are discussed later in this chapter.)

Continuous renal replacement therapy (CRRT) may also be used in the treatment of acute renal failure.[2] (CRRT is discussed later in this chapter.) In the hemodynamically unstable patient, CRRT provides gradual removal of excess fluid and solutes. It is technically similar to HD and requires extracorporeal blood circulation via cannulation of an artery and vein or two veins. Blood removed from the artery or vein passes through a hemofilter where solutes and water are removed, and then the blood is returned to the patient. CRRT is used continuously and requires at least 12 to 24 hours to accomplish what can be done with 3 to 4 hours of HD. Larger amounts of fluid may be removed than with intermittent HD. It is the preferred treatment in the hemodynamically unstable patient with mild to moderate acute renal failure or fluid overload.

Nutritional Therapy. In the past, the regimen of fluid restriction and nutritional therapy was designed so that body weight would decrease by 0.25 to 0.5 kg per day from the loss of body tissue catabolized on the low-protein diet. Today, these severe restrictions are usually not necessary except during the interval between the diagnosis of oliguria and the establishment of dialysis and a nutritional regimen. However, a stable weight or a weight gain during this interval usually indicates hypervolemia.

If the patient does not receive adequate nutrition, catabolism of body protein will occur.[3] This process causes increased urea, phosphate, and potassium levels. The major goal of nutritional therapy is to decrease catabolism of the body's protein. Adequate energy must be provided from carbohydrate and fat sources to prevent ketosis from fat breakdown and gluconeogenesis from protein breakdown.[4] Nonprotein calories (35 to 55 kcal/kg body weight) should be provided daily. Protein intake is generally 1.0 to 1.5 g/kg. Essential amino acid supplements (e.g., Amin-Aid) may be given for amino acid and caloric supplementation, either orally or through tube feedings.

Potassium and sodium are regulated in accordance with plasma levels. Sodium is restricted as needed to prevent edema, hypertension, and congestive heart failure. Dietary fat intake is increased so that the patient receives at least 30% to 40% of total calories from fat. Intralipid (fat emulsions) infusions can also be given as a nutritional supplement, and it provides a good source of nonprotein calories (see Chapter 38). If a patient cannot obtain an adequate oral intake, enteral nutrition is the preferred route for nutritional support (see Chapter 38). When the GI tract is not functional, total parenteral nutrition (TPN) is necessary for the provision of adequate nutrition. TPN is most commonly used in the patient who has had extensive surgical procedures or multiple trauma. The patient treated with TPN may need daily HD or CRRT to remove the excess fluid. However, concentrated TPN formulas are available to minimize fluid volume.[4]

NURSING MANAGEMENT: ACUTE RENAL FAILURE

■ Nursing Assessment

An assessment of the patient in acute renal failure includes the specific areas presented in Table 44-2. It is important to monitor the blood pressure, pulse, respiratory rate and pattern, and temperature. The patient's general appearance should be assessed, including skin color, peripheral edema, neck vein distention, and bruises.

If HD is used for treating acute renal failure, the vascular access site should be observed for signs of inflammation. The patient's mental status and level of consciousness should also be determined. The oral mucosa should be examined for dryness and presence of inflammation. The lungs should be auscultated for the presence of crackles and rhonchi. Heart sounds should be monitored for the presence of S_3 sounds and murmurs. If a pulmonary artery catheter is inserted, the pulmonary artery pressures should be obtained. ECG readings should be obtained to assess for the presence of arrhythmias. Any urine output should be assessed, including volume, color, specific gravity, and the presence of blood, glucose, sediment, or protein.

■ Nursing Diagnoses

Nursing diagnoses for the patient with acute renal failure include, but are not limited to, the following:

- Fluid volume excess *related to* renal failure and fluid retention
- Risk for infection *related to* invasive lines, uremic toxins, and altered immune responses secondary to renal failure
- Altered nutrition: less than body requirements *related to* altered metabolic state and dietary restrictions
- Sensory-perceptual alterations *related to* uremic toxins and fluid and electrolyte and acid-base imbalances
- Altered thought processes *related to* effects of uremic toxins on central nervous system (CNS)
- Impaired skin integrity *related to* sites for vascular access or peritoneal dialysis and renal failure
- Fatigue *related to* anemia and uremic toxins
- Anxiety *related to* disease process, therapeutic interventions, and uncertainty of prognosis

- Potential complication: hyperkalemia *related to* decreased renal excretion of potassium
- Potential complication: arrhythmias *related to* electrolyte imbalances

Planning

The overall goals are that the patient with acute renal failure will (1) completely recover with no residual loss of kidney function, (2) be maintained in normal fluid and electrolyte balance, (3) have decreased anxiety, and (4) comply with and understand the need for careful follow-up care.

Nursing Implementation

Health Promotion. Prevention of acute renal failure is essential because of the high mortality rate and is primarily directed toward identifying and monitoring high risk populations, controlling industrial chemicals and nephrotoxic drugs, and preventing prolonged episodes of hypotension and hypovolemia. In the hospital the patient at greatest risk for developing acute renal failure is the person who has experienced massive trauma, major surgical procedures, extensive burns, cardiac failure, sepsis, or obstetric complications or the individual who has a baseline renal insufficiency as a result of chronic diseases such as hypertension, diabetes mellitus, or systemic lupus erythematosus. This patient must be monitored carefully for intake and output, fluid and electrolyte balance, and possible blood transfusion reactions. Extrarenal losses of fluid from vomitus, diarrhea, hemorrhage, and increased insensible losses must be assessed and recorded. Prompt replacement of lost extracellular fluids will help prevent ischemic tubular damage associated with trauma, burns, and extensive surgery. Intake and output records and the patient's weight provide valuable indicators of fluid volume status. Aggressive diuretic therapy for the patient with fluid overload as a result of any cause can lead to inadequate renal vascular perfusion.

Streptococcal infections must be identified and treated with antibiotics. Compliance with the antibiotic regimen is critical to eliminate the source of infection. Complications of streptococcal infections include acute poststreptococcal glomerulonephritis and rheumatic heart disease.

The older adult patient and the individual with diabetes who is undergoing multiple diagnostic studies, especially those requiring IV dye injection, need special attention to prevent the patient from sustaining a nephrotoxic injury secondary to the dye. Adequate hydration is critical. The individual with urinary tract infections needs prompt treatment and careful follow-up care. Other persons who are considered at risk are those taking chemotherapeutic drugs that cause hyperuricemia.

Industrial and agricultural chemicals and products (organic solvents, insecticides, cleaning agents) must be monitored regularly regarding their safety for both the employee and the general population. The individual who is taking drugs that are potentially nephrotoxic (see Table 42-3) must have renal function monitored with serum creatinine and BUN determinations. Nephrotoxic medications should be used sparingly in the high risk patient. When they must be used, nephrotoxic medications should be given in the smallest effective doses for the shortest possible periods. The patient should be cautioned about the abuse of over-the-counter analgesics (especially NSAIDs), since some of these may precipitate renal failure in the patient with borderline renal insufficiency.

Acute Intervention. The patient with acute renal failure is critically ill and suffers not only from the effects of a renal disease but often from those effects of the nonrenal disease or condition (e.g., trauma, cardiac disease) that contributed to the renal failure. The nursing staff may become overly concerned with the patient's urinary output and forget to focus on the patient as a total person with many physical and emotional needs. Usually the changes caused by renal failure come on suddenly. Both the patient and the family need assistance in understanding that the functioning of the whole body can be disrupted by renal failure. However, these changes are potentially reversible.

The nursing role in managing fluid and electrolyte balance is important during the oliguric and diuretic phases. Observing and recording the accurate intake and output of fluids cannot be overemphasized. Daily weights measured with the same scale at the same time each day are essential in evaluating and detecting excessive gains or losses of body fluid (1 kg is equivalent to 1000 ml of fluid). The nurse must be knowledgeable about the common signs and symptoms that result from hypervolemia (in the oliguric phase) or hypovolemia (in the diuretic phase), hypernatremia or hyponatremia, hyperkalemia or hypokalemia, and other electrolyte imbalances that may occur in acute renal failure (see Chapter 15). Hyperkalemia is a leading biochemical cause of death in the oliguric phase of acute renal failure. Most typically, hyperkalemia is manifested by impairment of neuromuscular function and arrhythmias. Muscle weakness, abdominal cramps, flaccid paralysis, and absence of deep tendon reflexes are signs of neuromuscular impairment. Cardiac conduction abnormalities to watch for include a prolonged PR interval, prolonged QRS interval, peaked T wave, and depressed ST segment.

Because infection is the leading cause of death in acute renal failure, meticulous aseptic technique is critical. The patient should be protected from other individuals with infectious diseases. The nurse should be alert for local manifestations of infection (e.g., swelling, redness, pain) and systemic manifestations (e.g., anorexia, malaise, leukocytosis) because an elevated temperature may not be present in the patient with renal failure. (Patients with renal failure are usually hypothermic relative to healthy individuals.) If antibiotics are used to treat an infection, the type and dosage must be carefully considered because the kidneys are the route of excretion for many antibiotics.

Respiratory complications, especially pneumonitis, can be prevented. Humidified oxygen, intermittent positive-pressure breathing, turning, deep breathing, and ambulation are measures the nurse can use to help the patient maintain adequate respiratory ventilation.

Skin care and measures to prevent pressure ulcers should be performed, since the patient usually develops edema, as well as decreased muscle tone. Mouth care is important to prevent stomatitis, which develops when ammonia (produced by bacterial breakdown of urea) in saliva irritates the mucous membranes.

Ambulatory and Home Care. Recovery from acute renal failure is highly variable and depends on the underlying illness, the general condition and age of the patient, the length of the oliguric phase, and the management of the patient. The rest of the body, as well as the kidneys, has experienced a major insult. Good nutrition, rest, and limited activity are necessary to restore patients to their previous level of functioning. The diet should be high in calories, and protein and potassium intake should be regulated in accordance with renal function. Follow-up care and regular evaluation of renal function are necessary. The patient should be taught the signs and symptoms of recurrent renal disease, especially manifestations of fluid and electrolyte imbalances. Measures to prevent the recurrence of acute renal failure must be emphasized.

The long-term convalescence of 3 to 12 months may cause social and financial hardships for the family, and appropriate counseling and referrals should be done. Occasionally, renal function deteriorates, and manifestations of chronic renal failure develop. If the kidneys do not recover, the patient progresses to chronic renal failure.

■ Evaluation

The expected outcomes are that the patient with acute renal failure will

- regain and maintain normal fluid and electrolyte balance
- comply with treatment regimen
- experience no infectious complications
- have complete recovery

GERONTOLOGIC CONSIDERATIONS

Acute Renal Failure

The older adult is more susceptible than the younger adult to acute renal failure. Although decreased renal reserve function in advancing age is the primary risk factor, age itself and impaired function of other organ systems are independent risk factors. The aging kidney is less able to compensate for changes in fluid volume, solute load, and cardiac output. Common causes of acute renal failure in the older adult include dehydration, hypotension, diuretic therapy, aminoglycoside therapy, obstructive disorders (e.g., prostatic hyperplasia), surgery, infection, and radiocontrast agents. The prognosis after acute renal failure is generally worse in the older adult than in the younger person. The mortality rate after acute renal failure is 5% to 25% higher in the older adult than in the younger person, and death is usually caused by infection, GI hemorrhage, or myocardial infarction.[4]

CHRONIC RENAL FAILURE

Chronic renal failure involves progressive, irreversible destruction of the nephrons in both kidneys. The disease process progresses until most nephrons are destroyed and replaced by nonfunctional scar tissue. Although there are many different causes of chronic renal failure (Fig. 44-2), the end result is a systemic disease involving every body organ. (The specific disease processes are discussed in Chapter 43.)

The kidneys have remarkable functional reserve. Up to 80% of the GFR (reflected in creatinine clearance measurements) may be lost with few overt changes in the functioning of the body. A person is born with 2 million nephrons and can survive (albeit with difficulty) with as few as 20,000. In the vast majority of cases the individual passes through the early stages of chronic renal failure without recognizing the disease state because the remaining nephrons hypertrophy to compensate. The prognosis and course of chronic renal failure are highly variable. Some individuals live normal, active lives with compensated renal failure, whereas others may rapidly progress to end-stage renal failure. When the creatinine clearance falls below 10 ml per minute (from the norm of 85 to 135 ml per minute for the average adult), some form of dialysis or transplantation is required for survival.

Although there are no distinct stages in chronic renal failure, the disease progression may be divided into three stages:

1. *Diminished renal reserve.* This stage is characterized by normal BUN and serum creatinine levels and an absence of symptoms.
2. *Renal insufficiency.* This stage occurs when the GFR is about 25% of normal. BUN and serum creatinine levels are increased. Easy fatigue and weakness are common symptoms. As the renal failure progresses, headaches, nausea, and pruritus may occur. Nocturia and polyuria occur as a result of the kidneys' loss of ability to concentrate urine.
3. *End-stage renal disease (ESRD) or uremia.* The last stage occurs when the GFR is less than 5% to 10% of normal or when creatinine clearances are less than 5 to 10 ml/min. It is at this stage that most patients have great difficulty carrying out basic activities of daily living (ADLs) because of the cumulative effect and extent of the symptoms.

Significance

In the United States over 290,000 individuals with ESRD are being treated with dialysis or have kidney transplants. This number could double in the next 7 years if current trends continue. Each year over 30,000 people die from various diseases of the kidneys.[5] During the 1970s, dramatic changes in the focus of treatment of chronic renal disease occurred. In July 1973 the federal government enacted a law that provided financial assistance through Medicare for all eligible persons who had ESRD and required treatment. (Medicare pays 80% of the cost of health care for ESRD patients.)

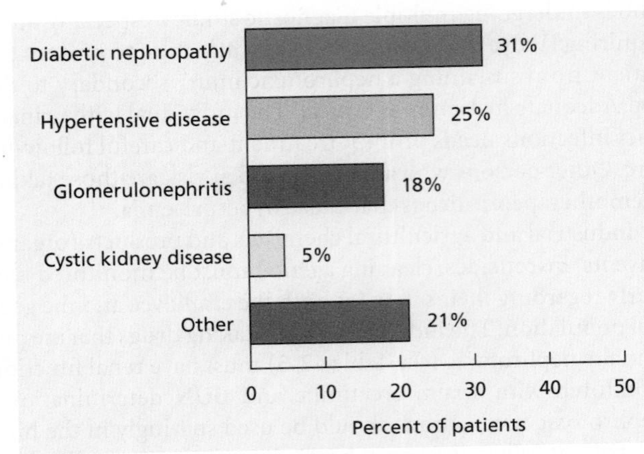

Fig. 44-2 Primary renal disease leading to end-stage renal failure.

Since 1973 many deaths have been prevented through the use of maintenance dialysis and renal transplantation. The majority of patients are treated with dialysis because (1) there is a lack of donated organs, (2) many patients do not want transplants, or (3) patients are medically unsuitable for the transplantation procedure. With the advancement of medical science each year, an increasing percentage of older individuals and patients with systemic disease (diabetics and patients with stable cancer) are being maintained on dialysis.

Every patient with ESRD, regardless of age, should be offered dialysis unless it is medically contraindicated or the patient refuses treatment. The Medicare program covers the cost of dialysis for most patients. For those not covered by Medicare, a variety of state and private programs are available. The incidence of patients being treated for ESRD is rising by an average of 9% per year. Older patients remain the fastest growing group entering the Medicare Renal Disease Program, with 34% of patients now over age 65.[5]

The increasing number of older adults with ESRD has changed the data related to the most common causes of chronic renal failure. Before the mid 1970s, glomerulonephritis and interstitial nephritis were the most common causes. Currently, diabetes and hypertension are the leading causes of chronic renal failure in the United States (see Fig. 44-2). In Canada the leading causes of ESRD are diabetes and glomerulonephritis.

Clinical Manifestations

As renal function progressively deteriorates, every body system becomes involved. The clinical manifestations are a result of retained substances, including urea, creatinine, phenols, hormones, electrolytes, water, and many other substances. Uremia is a syndrome that incorporates all the disturbances seen in the various systems throughout the body in chronic renal failure (Fig. 44-3). It is important to recognize that the manifestations of uremia vary among patients, according to the etiology of the renal failure, comorbid conditions, age, and degree of compliance with the prescribed medical regimen.

Urinary System. In the stage of renal insufficiency, the most noticeable sign is polyuria that is caused by the inability of the kidneys to concentrate urine. The patient will notice this most frequently at night when she or he must arise several times to urinate (nocturia). Because of the decrease in renal concentrating ability, the specific gravity of urine gradually becomes fixed at around 1.010 (the osmolar concentration of plasma). As renal failure progresses, oliguria develops, and later, anuria may develop. If the patient is still producing urine, common findings are proteinuria with casts, pyuria, and hematuria.

Metabolic Disturbances

Waste product accumulation. As the GFR decreases, the BUN and serum creatinine levels increase. The BUN influenced

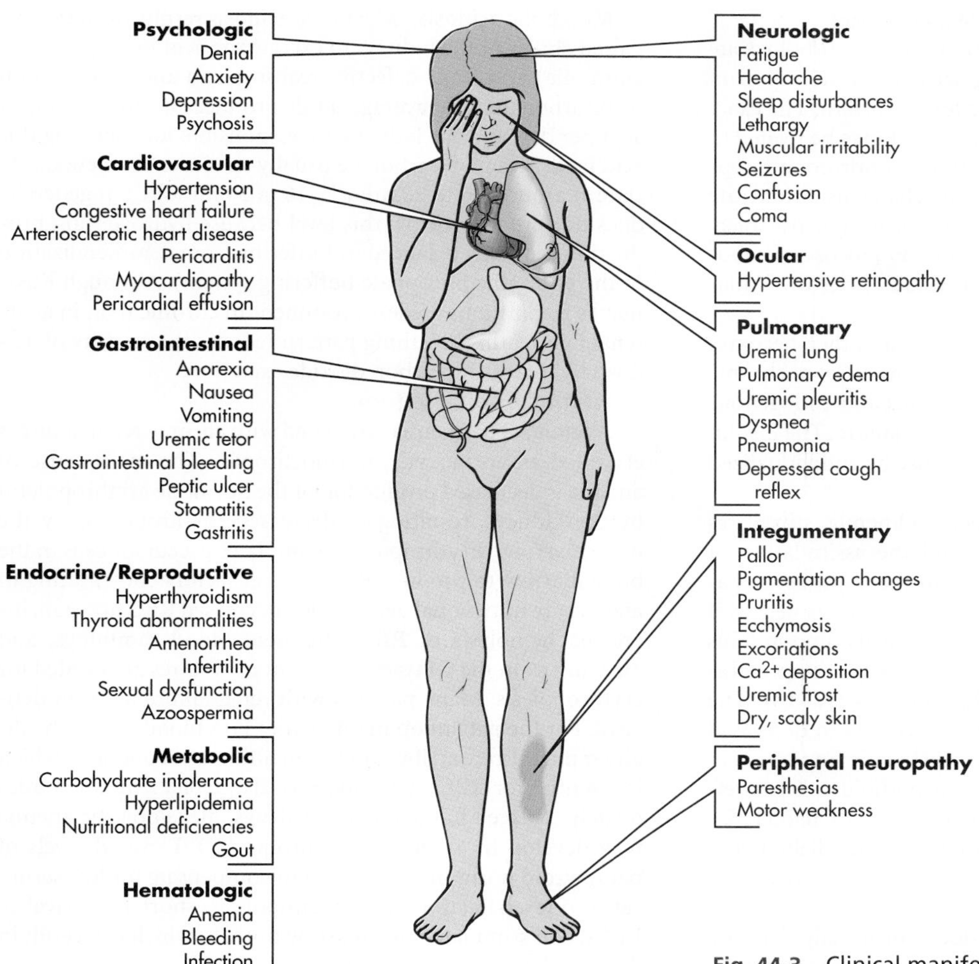

Fig. 44-3 Clinical manifestations of chronic uremia.

CULTURAL & ETHNIC CONSIDERATIONS

End-stage Renal Disease

- End-stage renal disease (ESRD) is more common among African-Americans and Native Americans than Caucasians. A history of hypertension and diabetes is also more common in these high risk groups.
- Risk of ESRD from hypertension is significantly increased in African-Americans.
- Risk of ESRD from diabetes is significantly increased in Native Americans.
- African-Americans live longer and have better outcomes on chronic dialysis than Caucasians.

not only by renal failure but by protein intake, fever, and catabolic rate. For this reason serum creatinine and creatinine clearance determinations are considered more accurate indicators of renal function than BUN. As the BUN increases, nausea, vomiting, lethargy, fatigue, impaired thought processes, and headaches become common complaints.

The serum creatinine level in an older adult patient with ESRD is lower than the level expected in a younger person with the same degree of renal dysfunction. Decreased muscle mass and decreased muscle activity account for this finding because creatinine is an end product of muscle metabolism.

Altered carbohydrate metabolism. Defective carbohydrate metabolism is caused by impaired glucose use resulting from cellular insensitivity to the normal action of insulin. The exact nature of this insulin resistance is unclear but may be related to circulating insulin antagonists, alterations in hormone receptors, or abnormalities of transport mechanisms. Moderate hyperglycemia, hyperinsulinemia, and abnormal glucose tolerance tests are common findings. Insulin and glucose metabolism may improve (but not to normal values) after the initiation of dialysis.

The individual who has diabetes mellitus and then becomes uremic may require less insulin than before the onset of chronic renal failure. This is because both exogenous and endogenous insulin remain in circulation longer in renal failure. The insulin doses of insulin-dependent diabetics must be individualized and monitored carefully.

Elevated triglycerides. The hyperinsulinemia stimulates hepatic production of triglycerides, and the assimilation of triglycerides by peripheral tissues is diminished. Almost all patients with uremia develop hyperlipidemia, which is usually a type IV profile with elevated very-low-density lipoproteins (VLDLs), normal or decreased low-density lipoproteins (LDLs), and lowered high-density lipoproteins (HDLs). The reason for the altered lipid metabolism is related to decreased levels of the enzyme lipoprotein lipase, which is important in the breakdown of lipoproteins. Type IV hyperlipidemia is a definite risk factor for accelerated atherosclerosis (see Chapter 32). This dysfunction compounds the problem in the diabetic patient with renal disease who already has increased atherosclerotic changes.

The serum level of triglycerides does not usually decrease after dialysis is started. In the patient who is on chronic peritoneal dialysis, the level frequently becomes higher as a result of the increased amounts of glucose absorbed from the peritoneal dialysate fluid.

Electrolyte and Acid-Base Imbalances

Potassium. Hyperkalemia is the most serious electrolyte problem associated with renal failure. Fatal arrhythmias can occur when the serum potassium level reaches 7 to 8 mEq/L (7 to 8 mmol/L). Hyperkalemia results from the failure of the excretory ability of the kidneys, the breakdown of cellular protein with the subsequent release of potassium, and acidosis, which contributes to the shift of potassium from intracellular to extracellular spaces. Potassium can come from the diet, dietary supplements, medications, and intravenous infusions.

Calcium and phosphate. Calcium and phosphate alterations are discussed in the section on acute renal failure (p. 1302) and in the section on the musculoskeletal system (p. 1309).

Magnesium. Magnesium is primarily excreted by the kidneys. Hypermagnesemia is generally not a problem unless the patient is taking magnesium (e.g., milk of magnesia, magnesium citrate, antacids containing magnesium).

Sodium. Sodium levels can range from low to normal. Hypernatremia is unusual because whenever sodium is retained, so is water, resulting in a dilutional hyponatremia. Sodium retention can contribute to edema, hypertension, and congestive heart failure. Sodium intake must be individually determined but is generally restricted in all patients.

Metabolic acidosis. Metabolic acidosis results from the impaired ability of the kidneys to excrete the acid load (primarily ammonia) and from defective reabsorption and regeneration of bicarbonate. The average adult produces 80 to 90 mEq of acid per day, and the kidneys are responsible for excreting this acid load. Plasma bicarbonate usually stabilizes at a new steady state at around 16 to 20 mEq/L (16 to 20 mmol/L). It generally does not progress below this level because hydrogen ion production is usually balanced by buffering from demineralization of the bone (the phosphate buffering system). Although Kussmaul's respirations are less prominent in chronic than in acute renal failure, this breathing pattern reduces the severity of acidosis by increasing carbon dioxide excretion.

Hematologic System

Anemia. The anemia associated with chronic renal failure is classified as normocytic, normochromic. The main cause of anemia is decreased production of the hormone erythropoietin by the kidneys, resulting in decreased erythropoiesis by the bone marrow.[6] Erythropoietin stimulates precursor cells in the bone marrow to produce RBCs. Other factors contributing to anemia are nutritional deficiencies, decreased RBC life span, increased hemolysis of RBCs, frequent blood samplings, and bleeding from the GI tract. Sufficient iron stores are needed for erythropoiesis. Many patients with renal failure are iron deficient. For the patient on maintenance HD, blood loss in the dialyzer may also contribute to the anemic state. Folic acid, which is essential for RBC maturation, is dialyzable. If it is not adequately replaced in the diet or by drugs, megaloblastic anemia may develop in a patient on chronic HD. Elevated levels of parathyroid hormone (produced to compensate for low serum calcium levels) can inhibit erythropoiesis, shorten survival of RBCs, and stimulate bone marrow fibrosis, which can result in decreased numbers of hematopoietic cells.

Bleeding tendencies. The most common cause of bleeding in uremia is a qualitative defect in platelet function. This dysfunction is caused by impaired platelet aggregation and impaired release of platelet factor 3. The altered platelet function, hemorrhagic tendencies, and GI bleeding are usually reversible by HD or PD. In addition, there are alterations in the coagulation system with increased concentrations of both factor VIII and fibrinogen found in the serum of these patients.

Infection. Infectious complications are caused by changes in leukocyte function and altered immune response and function. A diminished inflammatory response occurs as a result of an altered chemotactic response by both neutrophils and monocytes. This impairment significantly decreases the accumulation of WBCs at the site of injury or infection. Both cellular and humoral immune responses are also suppressed. Characteristic clinical findings include lymphopenia, lymphoid atrophy (especially of the thymus), decreased antibody production, and suppression of the delayed hypersensitivity response. Other factors contributing to the increased risk of infection include protein malnutrition, hyperglycemia, and external trauma (e.g., catheters, needle insertions into vascular access sites).

Increased incidence of cancer. There is a significant increase in the incidence of neoplasms in the patient with renal failure who has not had transplants as compared with the general population. Lung, breast, uterus, colon, prostate, and skin malignancies are most commonly found.

Cardiovascular System. The most common cardiovascular abnormality is hypertension, which is usually caused by sodium retention and increased extracellular fluid volume. In some individuals, increased renin production contributes to the problem (see Fig. 42-6). Hypertension accelerates atherosclerotic vascular disease, produces intrarenal arterial spasm, and eventually leads to left ventricular hypertrophy and congestive heart failure.[7] Hypertension also causes retinopathy and encephalopathy.

Congestive heart failure from left ventricular hypertrophy can lead to pulmonary edema. Peripheral edema is also commonly present. Cardiac arrhythmias may result from hyperkalemia, hypocalcemia, and decreased coronary artery perfusion.

Uremic pericarditis develops and occasionally progresses to pericardial effusion and cardiac tamponade. Pericarditis is manifested by a friction rub, chest pain, and low-grade fever.

The vascular changes from long-standing hypertension and the accelerated atherosclerosis from elevated triglyceride levels are responsible for many of the cardiovascular complications (e.g., myocardial infarction, cerebrovascular accident), which are the leading causes of death for patients on chronic dialysis. Diabetes mellitus is also a major risk factor for the development of vascular problems.

Respiratory System. Respiratory changes include Kussmaul's respirations, dyspnea from congestive heart failure, pulmonary edema, uremic pleuritis (pleurisy), pleural effusion, and a predisposition to respiratory infections, which may be related to decreased pulmonary macrophage activity. The sputum is thick and tenacious. The cough reflex is depressed. "Uremic lung," or uremic pneumonitis, is typically found in chronic renal failure and shows up as an interstitial edema on chest x-ray. This condition usually responds to vigorous fluid removal during dialysis treatments.

Gastrointestinal System. Every part of the GI system is affected as a result of inflammation of the mucosa caused by excessive urea. Mucosal ulcerations, found throughout the GI tract, are caused by the increased ammonia produced by bacterial breakdown of urea. Stomatitis with exudates and ulcerations, a metallic taste in the mouth, and uremic fetor (a urinous odor of the breath) are commonly found. Anorexia, nausea, and vomiting caused by irritation of the GI tract by waste products contribute to weight loss. Diarrhea may occur because of hyperkalemia and altered calcium metabolism. Constipation or diarrhea may be a complication of taking iron salts, which are taken as part of anemia therapy, or a complication of taking calcium-containing phosphate binders, which are taken to facilitate phosphate excretion.

Neurologic System. Neurologic changes are expected as renal failure progresses. The exact cause of these changes is unknown, but they may be partially attributed to increased nitrogenous waste products, electrolyte imbalances, and axonal atrophy and demyelination of nerve fibers.[8] High levels of uremic toxins have been implicated in axonal damage.

In renal failure a general depression of the CNS results in lethargy, apathy, decreased ability to concentrate, fatigue, and altered mental ability. Seizures and coma may result from a rapidly increasing BUN and hypertensive encephalopathy.

Dialysis encephalopathy (dialysis dementia), a progressive neurologic impairment, is characterized by speech disturbances, dementia, lack of muscle coordination, and myoclonic seizures. A frequent cause of this problem is aluminum toxicity, which may result from ingestion of aluminum-containing antacids and a decreased ability of the kidneys to excrete aluminum. Phosphate-binding antacids (e.g., calcium acetate, calcium carbonate) that are not aluminum based are usually administered.

Peripheral neuropathy is initially manifested by a slowing of nerve conduction to the extremities. The patient complains of a restless leg syndrome and may describe it as "bugs crawling inside the leg." Paresthesias, especially of both feet and legs, may be described by the patient as a burning sensation. Eventually, motor involvement may lead to bilateral footdrop, muscular weakness and atrophy, and loss of deep tendon reflexes. Muscle twitching, jerking, asterixis (hand-flapping tremor), and nocturnal leg cramps also occur.

The treatment for neurologic problems is dialysis and, ultimately, transplantation. Altered mental status is often the signal that dialysis must be initiated. Dialysis should improve the general CNS symptoms and may halt the progression of neuropathies, but not necessarily. Motor neuropathy may not be reversible. The problem of uremic neuropathy is compounded in the diabetic patient who has diabetic neuropathy as well.

Musculoskeletal System. Renal osteodystrophy is a syndrome of skeletal changes found in chronic renal failure.[9] This syndrome is a result of alterations in calcium and phosphate metabolism (Fig. 44-4). Normally the calcium/phosphate ratio maintains the electrolytes in a soluble state. As the GFR decreases, phosphate cannot be excreted by the kidneys, thus increasing the serum phosphate.

Normally the kidneys metabolize vitamin D (formed in the skin or ingested) to its active form. The active form of vitamin D is needed for calcium absorption from the GI tract. In renal failure the kidneys fail to activate vitamin D, and calcium

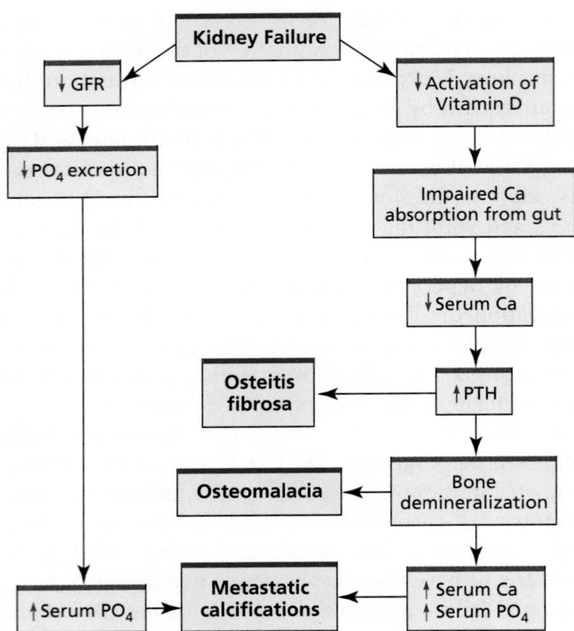

Fig. 44-4 Mechanisms of renal osteodystrophy.

absorption is impaired, thus lowering serum calcium. Low serum calcium stimulates the release of parathyroid hormone (PTH), which causes resorption of calcium and phosphate from the bone. This release increases serum calcium, as well as serum phosphate. When the phosphate level is high, it complexes with calcium, leading to the formation of metastatic calcifications that are deposited throughout the body.

The changes resulting from increased phosphate retention, bone resorption of calcium, inadequate calcium absorption, and elevated PTH levels lead to the following conditions:

1. *Osteomalacia.* This condition results from lack of mineralization of newly formed bone. It can be a result of hypocalcemia. It can also be caused by aluminum accumulation, since the primary route for aluminum excretion is through the kidneys. The primary source of aluminum is aluminum-based phosphate binders. Over the past decade, there has been a decreased use of aluminum-based phosphate binders and a concomitant decrease in the incidence of osteomalacia.
2. *Osteitis fibrosa.* This condition results from calcium resorption from the bone and replacement with fibrous tissue. Osteitis fibrosa is primarily a result of markedly elevated levels of PTH that cause bone resorption.[9]
3. *Metastatic calcification (soft-tissue calcification).* This condition results from calcium-phosphate deposits in soft tissues of the body. Common sites are the blood vessels, joints, lungs, muscles, myocardium, and eyes. "Uremic red eye" is caused by the irritation of the deposits in the eye. Metastatic calcifications in the arteries of the fingers and toes may cause gangrene. Intracardiac calcifications can disrupt the conduction system and cause cardiac arrest.

Integumentary System. The most noticeable change in the integumentary system is a yellowish discoloration of the skin. This change is a result of the absorption and retention of urinary chromogens that normally give the characteristic color to urine. The skin also appears pale as a result of anemia and is dry and scaly because of a decrease in oil and sweat gland activity. Decreased perspiration results from a decrease in the size of the sweat glands.

Pruritus most commonly results from a combination of the dry skin, calcium-phosphate deposition in the skin, and sensory neuropathy. The itching may be so intense that it can lead to bleeding or infection secondary to scratching. Uremic frost is a condition in which urea crystallizes on the skin and is usually seen only when BUN levels are extremely high. This is almost never seen unless the patient refuses dialysis or is withdrawn from dialysis.

The hair is dry and brittle and may fall out. The nails are thin, brittle, and ridged. Petechiae and ecchymoses may be present and are caused by clotting abnormalities.

Reproductive System. Both sexes characteristically experience infertility and a decreased libido. Women usually have decreased levels of estrogen, progesterone, and luteinizing hormone, causing anovulation and menstrual changes (usually amenorrhea). Menses and ovulation may return after dialysis is started. Men experience loss of testicular consistency, decreased testosterone levels, and low sperm counts. Sexual dysfunction in both sexes may also be caused by anemia, which causes fatigue and decreased libido. In addition, peripheral neuropathy can cause impotence in men and anorgasmy in women. Additional factors that may cause changes in sexual function are psychologic problems (e.g., anxiety, depression), physical stress, and side effects of medication.

Sexual function may improve with maintenance dialysis and may return to normal with successful transplantation. In rare cases pregnant dialysis patients have been able to carry a fetus to term, but there is significant risk to the mother and infant. Pregnancy in transplant patients is more common, but in this situation there is also a risk to both the mother and fetus.

Endocrine System. Many patients with chronic renal failure exhibit some clinical manifestations of hypothyroidism. Tests of thyroid function may yield low to low-normal levels for serum triiodothyronine (T_3) and thyroxine (T_4) levels. Neither the clinical significance nor the exact reason for these findings is known.

Psychologic Changes. Personality and behavior changes, emotional lability, withdrawal, and depression are commonly observed. Fatigue and lethargy contribute to the patient's feeling of sickness. The changes in body image caused by edema, integumentary disturbances, and access devices (e.g., fistulas, catheters) lead to further anxiety and depression. Decreased ability to concentrate and lessened mental activity can make the patient appear dull and disinterested in the environment. The patient is faced with significant changes in lifestyle, occupation, family responsibilities, and financial status. The patient's future depends on medications, dietary restrictions, dialysis, and possibly transplantation of another person's kidney. The patient will grieve the loss of renal function. This can be a prolonged process for some individuals.

Collaborative Conservative Care

When a patient is diagnosed as having chronic renal insufficiency, conservative therapy is attempted before maintenance

COLLABORATIVE CARE

Table 44-5 Chronic Renal Failure

Diagnostic
- Identification of reversible renal disease
  - Renal ultrasound
  - Renal scan (if indicated)
  - CT scan (if indicated)
- Hematocrit and hemoglobin level
- BUN, serum creatinine, and creatinine clearance levels
- Serum electrolytes
- Urinalysis and urine culture

Collaborative Therapy
- Correction of extracellular fluid volume overload or deficit
- Nutritional therapy*
- Erythropoietin therapy
- Calcium supplementation, phosphate binders, or both
- Antihypertensive therapy
- Measures to lower potassium†
- Adjustment of drug dosages to degree of renal function

*See Tables 44-6, 44-7, and 44-8.
†See Table 44-4.
BUN, blood urea nitrogen.

dialysis begins (Table 44-5). Every effort is made to detect and treat potentially reversible causes of renal failure (e.g., cardiac failure, dehydration, pyelonephritis, nephrotoxins, urinary tract obstruction, renal artery stenosis). Conservative therapy is directed toward preserving existing renal function, treating the symptoms, preventing complications, and providing for the patient's comfort.[10] Conservative therapy primarily consists of drug and nutritional therapy and supportive care. Patients with chronic renal insufficiency should be cautioned to avoid NSAIDs, since NSAIDs may block synthesis of prostaglandins in the kidney that promote vasodilation and thus may induce renal hypoperfusion.

Drug Therapy

Hyperkalemia. Acute hyperkalemia is usually treated with intravenous (IV) glucose and insulin or IV 10% calcium gluconate (see Table 44-4). Dietary restriction of foods high in potassium is needed. (Foods high in protein content are usually high in potassium.) Sodium polystyrene sulfonate (Kayexalate), a cation-exchange resin, is commonly used to lower potassium levels. The exchange resin, administered orally or rectally, exchanges 1 mEq of sodium for 1 mEq of potassium. The potassium is bound to the resin, which is excreted in the stool. To ensure excretion of potassium, a bulk laxative (usually sorbitol) is mixed with Kayexalate. The patient should be told to expect some diarrhea. Kayexalate should never be given to a patient with hypoactive bowels because fluid shifts could lead to bowel necrosis. As Kayexalate exchanges sodium for potassium the patient should be observed for sodium and water retention.

Hypertension. The progression of chronic renal failure can be delayed by controlling hypertension.[10] Treatment of hypertension initially consists of sodium and fluid restriction and the administration of antihypertensives. The antihypertensive drugs most commonly used are calcium channel blockers (e.g., nifedipine [Procardia], nicardipine [Cardene]) and ACE inhibitors (e.g., captopril [Capoten], enalapril [Vasotec]) (see Chapter 31). Calcium channel blockers have renoprotective properties. In addition to their antihypertensive action, ACE inhibitors decrease proteinuria and delay the progression of renal failure. ACE inhibitors should be used cautiously when ESRD occurs because they can further decrease GFR and increase serum potassium levels. The blood pressure should be measured in supine, sitting, and standing positions to effectively monitor the antihypertensive drugs. Treatment that is too vigorous can cause a hypotensive reaction in a patient who has compensated for long-standing hypertension. A significant decrease in blood pressure can lead to further renal problems because kidneys may be dependent on high blood pressure to be perfused via atherosclerotic blood vessels. Blood pressure control is essential to slow atherosclerotic changes that could further impair renal function.

Renal osteodystrophy. Phosphate intake is generally restricted to less than 1000 mg/day. Calcium-based phosphate binders such as calcium carbonate (e.g., Tums) and calcium acetate (e.g., PhosLo) are used frequently to bind the phosphate, which is then excreted in the stool. Giving a calcium-based binder when the phosphate levels are still high (6 mg/dl [1.98 mmol/L]) may cause the formation of calcium-phosphate deposits.

Because of dementia and bone disease (osteomalacia) associated with excessive absorption of aluminum, aluminum hydroxide gels or antacids (e.g., Alu-Cap, Amphojel, Basaljel, and Alternagel) are used less frequently to bind the phosphate. Magnesium-containing antacids (Maalox, Mylanta) should not be given because magnesium is dependent on the kidneys for excretion. Phosphate binders should be administered with each meal to be effective because most phosphate is absorbed within 1 hour after eating. Hypercalcemia may occur with calcium binders. Constipation is a frequent side effect of phosphate binders and may necessitate the use of stool softeners.

Hypocalcemia is often a problem because of the inability of the GI tract to absorb calcium in the absence of vitamin D. If hypocalcemia occurs in the setting of controlled serum phosphate levels and supplemental calcium, the active form of vitamin D should be given. It is commercially available in oral preparations such as calcitriol (Rocaltrol) and in IV form as calcitriol (Calcijex). Paricalcitol (Zemplar), a synthetically manufactured vitamin D analog, is also used to prevent and treat secondary hyperparathyroidism associated with renal failure. It is important to lower the phosphate level before administering calcium or vitamin D because these drugs may contribute to soft-tissue calcification if both calcium and phosphate levels are elevated.

If renal osteodystrophy remains severe, a subtotal parathyroidectomy may be performed to decrease the synthesis and secretion of PTH. In some situations a total parathyroidectomy is performed and some parathyroid tissue is transplanted into the forearm. The transplanted cells produce PTH as needed. If production of PTH becomes excessive, some of the cells can be removed using local anesthesia.

The most common methods for evaluating the status of the bone disease are skeletal x-ray, bone scans, bone biopsy, and bone densitometry. PTH and alkaline phosphatase levels should also be measured. The enzyme alkaline phosphatase is elevated when there is demineralization of the bone.

NUTRITIONAL THERAPY

Table 44-6 Daily Requirements for the Patient with Chronic Renal Failure

	Conservative Management	Hemodialysis	Peritoneal Dialysis
Fluid allowance	Urine output plus 500-600 ml	Urine output plus 1000 ml	Frequently no restriction
Protein*	0.6-0.8 g/kg body weight	1.0-1.5 g/kg IBW	1.2-2.0 g/kg IBW
Calories	35-40 kcal/kg EDW	35-40 kcal/kg EDW†	35-40 kcal/kg IBW†
Fat	Determined by caloric requirement	Determined by caloric requirement	Determined by caloric requirement
Carbohydrate	Unlimited intake of sugars and starches; bread and cereal products limited because of protein limit	Same as for conservative management	Dependent on individual patient needs
Iron	No supplementation	900 mg supplement	500-900 mg supplement
Potassium	2-3 g	2-3 g	3-4 g, no restrictions
Sodium	1-3 g	2 g	2-4 g
Phosphorus	700-1200 mg	700-1200 mg	700-1200 mg
Calcium	1000-2000 mg	1000-1500 mg	1000-1500 mg
Folic acid	1.0 mg supplement	1.0 mg supplement	1.0 mg supplement

*At least 70% of protein intake should be of high biologic value (e.g., coming from eggs, milk, and meat).
†Includes dialysate calories.
EDW, estimated dry weight; *IBW,* ideal body weight.

Anemia. The most important cause of renal anemia is a decreased production of erythropoietin. With the use of recombinant deoxyribonucleic acid (DNA) technology (see Chapter 12), human erythropoietin can now be made in large amounts and is available for the treatment of anemia.[6] It can be administered IV at the end of HD or subcutaneously for the PD patient. Erythropoietin has been effective in treating anemia. Clinically, a significant increase in hematocrit is usually not seen for 2 to 3 weeks. The patient who is receiving erythropoietin has an improved cardiac performance and exercise tolerance and an enhanced quality of life.

A common adverse effect of exogenous erythropoietin is the development or aggravation of hypertension. The underlying mechanism is related to the hemodynamic changes (e.g., increased whole blood viscosity) that occur as the patient's anemia is corrected. Another side effect of erythropoietin therapy is the development of functional iron deficiency as a result of the increased demand for iron to support erythropoiesis. Most patients receive oral iron supplements; however, the GI side effects of iron supplements may lead to patients not taking the medication. Parenteral iron is used if iron deficiencies persist in spite of oral iron intake. Orally administered iron should not be taken at the same time as phosphate binders because the aluminum and calcium bind the iron. Supplemental folic acid (1 mg or more daily) is usually given because it is needed for RBC formation and is usually deficient in these patients.

Blood transfusions should be avoided in treating anemia unless the patient experiences an acute blood loss or has symptomatic anemia (i.e., dyspnea, excess fatigue, tachycardia, palpitations, chest pain). Undesirable effects of transfusions are the suppression of erythropoiesis as a result of a decrease in the hypoxic stimulus, the possible transmission of hepatitis or human immunodeficiency virus (HIV), and the possibility of iron overload because each unit of blood contains about 250 mg of iron.

Complications of drug therapy. Most drugs are excreted partially or totally by the kidneys. Drug dosages must be adapted to the degree of renal failure. Drug toxicity is a serious problem in the patient with uremia. Delayed and decreased elimination leads to an accumulation of drugs in the body. Increased sensitivity to the drug may result as drug levels increase in the blood and tissues. Drugs of particular concern include digitalis preparations, antibiotics, and pain medication.

Digitalis preparations are excreted largely by the kidneys. Loading doses may not have to be changed, but maintenance dosages may have to be adjusted. Dialysis does not affect body levels of digoxin, but it does affect potassium levels, which can potentiate the action of digitalis.

Aminoglycosides (gentamicin, kanamycin, tobramycin [Nebcin]), penicillin in high doses, and tetracyclines are potentially nephrotoxic. The frequency of doses or the dose of many antibiotics, such as vancomycin (Vancocin) and gentamicin, must be decreased because they are dependent on the kidney for excretion. These drugs can accumulate to toxic levels if appropriate precautions are not taken.

Meperidine should never be administered to a patient with chronic renal failure because the liver metabolizes it to normeperidine, which is dependent on the kidneys for excretion. If normeperidine accumulates, seizures can result. Other pain medications are appropriate, but they may need to be given less frequently and in smaller doses.

Nutritional Therapy

Protein restriction. Before the use of maintenance dialysis, Giovannetti and Giordano designed a 20 g, high-quality protein diet to prevent the accumulation of nitrogenous waste products. This diet provided the essential amino acids from eggs and milk. No meat was allowed. In addition to eggs and milk, low-protein vegetables, noodles, butter balls, and high-carbohydrate foods were included. Patient acceptance of this dietary regimen was poor, and patients were malnourished and vitamin deficient.

The current diet is designed to be as normal as possible to maintain good nutrition (Table 44-6). For the patient who is not undergoing dialysis, one guide is to restrict protein intake

NUTRITIONAL THERAPY

Table 44-7 Chronic Renal Failure*

General Principles

1. Protein, sodium, potassium, phosphorus, and fluids are controlled to meet each patient's needs.
2. Protein sources should be of high biologic value.
3. High-sodium and high-potassium foods should be avoided.
4. Sufficient calories and nutrients are provided to meet daily requirements.

Meal	Exchanges	Sample Menu 1	Sample Menu 2	Sample Menu 3
Breakfast	1 fruit	60 ml grape juice	60 ml apple juice	Applesauce
	1 bread	Toast or corn flakes	Tortilla	Grits
	1 meat	Scrambled egg	Fried egg	Poached egg
	3 fats	2 tsp margarine or butter	2 tsp butter	2 tsp butter
		30 ml cream	30 ml cream	30 ml cream
		Jelly	Jam	Jam
	Beverage	250 ml decaf coffee	250 ml decaf coffee	250 ml decaf coffee
	Dairy	120 ml milk	120 ml milk	120 ml milk
Lunch	1 meat	Salt-free tuna (¼ cup)	2 enchiladas (using ¼ cup ground beef, 2 corn tortillas, and shredded lettuce)	Fried chicken leg
	2 breads	2 slices bread		Cornbread ½ cup rice
	Vegetable	Lettuce and cucumber	Chili sauce	Zucchini
	Fruit	Canned plums	Canned pears	Canned peaches
	2 fats	2 tbs salt-free mayonnaise	2 tbs oil for cooking	1 tsp butter 1 tbs oil for cooking
		Hard candy	Jelly beans	Hard candy
	Beverage	250 ml carbonated beverage	250 ml carbonated beverage	250 ml carbonated beverage
Dinner	1 meat	1 oz fried fresh fish	1 oz chicken	1 oz pork
	1 bread	½ cup mashed potatoes (using presoaked potatoes)	1 salt-free corn or flour tortilla to make chicken taco	Salt-free corn on the cob
	Vegetable	Salt-free green peas	Tossed salad	Salt-free green beans
	Fruit	Fruit cocktail	Canned pineapple	Grapes
	3 fats	30 ml cream	30 ml cream	2 tsp butter
		1 tbs fat for cooking	2 tbs salt-free dressing	
		1 tsp butter		
	Beverage	250 ml fruit punch	250 ml fruit punch	250 ml fruit punch
		250 ml decaf coffee	250 ml decaf coffee	250 ml decaf coffee
Snack		120 ml gelatin dessert with whipped topping	180 ml Popsicle	Butter balls
		140 ml carbonated beverage†	80 ml carbonated beverage	320 ml carbonated beverage

*Each diet plan contains 40 g protein, 40 mEq potassium, 2 g sodium, and 1500 ml fluid. To increase the protein to 60 g, the dietician can add 3 oz meat; 1 egg and 2 oz meat; 120 ml milk, 1 egg, and 1½ oz meat; or 120 ml milk and 2½ oz meat. With the increase in protein, the potassium level also increases to 60 mEq.

†Coke is an acceptable beverage.

to 0.6 to 0.8 g/kg of ideal body weight (IBW) per day when the creatinine clearance is less than 25 ml per minute.[10] Some treatment centers use a routine 40 g protein diet (Table 44-7). Because this diet is deficient in vitamins, multivitamins are prescribed.

Protein restriction may reduce the decline of renal function in the patient with chronic renal insufficiency. A low-protein (0.6 to 0.8 g/kg body weight per day), low-phosphorus diet supplemented with amino acids and their ketoanalogues can slow the progression of renal failure.[11] Keto acids of essential amino acids are a dietary supplement. The rationale for using this treatment is that in the body, nonessential amino acids transfer amine groups to the essential keto acids synthesizing essential amino acids. Thus the nitrogen present in nonessential amino acids is used, and the total nitrogen intake is kept to an absolute minimum. Keto acid supplements are available in liquid preparations. Modest protein restriction (0.6 to 0.8 g/kg per day) appears to be a relatively safe therapeutic option for patients with moderate renal insufficiency. For patients with more severe renal insufficiency, low-protein diets should be used with caution, since these patients are at risk for developing malnutrition.

Once the patient is started on dialysis, protein intake can be increased to 1.0 to 1.5 g/kg of IBW per day. Dietary protein guidelines for the patient on PD differ from those for the patient on HD. Because excessive amounts of protein are lost in the dialysate during peritoneal dialysis, the protein intake must be high enough to compensate for the losses so that the nitrogen balance is maintained. The recommended protein intake is 1.2 to 2.0 g/kg of IBW per day, depending on the individual needs of the patient. For all patients with renal failure, at least 70% of protein intake should come from eggs, milk, poultry, and meat; these foods are considered to have high biologic value because they contain all of the essential amino acids.

Sufficient calories from carbohydrates and fat are needed to minimize catabolism of body protein and to maintain body weight. Therefore 100 g of carbohydrates and an appropriate amount of fat are prescribed to maintain an intake of 2000 to 2500 calories per day (35 kcal/kg body weight per day). See Table 44-6 for specific guidelines.

Lowering the protein intake decreases the metabolic end products of urea, potassium, phosphate, and hydrogen. As the BUN level decreases, the symptoms of nausea, vomiting, fatigue, and headache become less troublesome. However, dietary protein restriction should not be prescribed for chronic renal failure patients who are malnourished, and the ongoing assessments of a skilled dietician are necessary. A patient experiences increased anorexia from the progression of chronic renal failure and may spontaneously decrease protein intake to a low level in spite of nutritional counseling. Dialysis for this type of patient may need to be started early to prevent severe malnutrition and increased risk of morbidity and mortality.

Commercially prepared products that are high in calories and low in protein, sodium, and potassium are available. Liquid and powder preparations include Nepro, Microlipid, SumaCal, Suplena, and Polycose. Products containing only the essential amino acids (Amin-Aid) can also be used as dietary supplements.

Water restriction. Water intake depends on the daily urine output. Generally, 500 to 600 ml (from insensible loss) plus an amount equal to the urine output is allowed for a patient with chronic renal failure who is not on dialysis. This amount of fluid is in addition to the fluid found in food. Foods that are liquid at room temperature (e.g., Jell-O and ice cream) should be counted as fluid intake. The fluid allotment should be spaced throughout the day so that the patient does not become uncomfortable from thirst. During chronic HD, fluid intake is adjusted so that ideally the patient gains no more than 1.0 to 1.5 kg between dialyses.

NUTRITIONAL THERAPY

Table 44-8 High-Potassium Foods

100-250 mg K^+	250-350 mg K^+	>350 mg K^+
Fruits		
1 medium tangerine	½ cup prune juice	1/10 honey dew melon
½ cup fresh pineapple	3 apricots	1 medium banana
1 medium orange	1 fresh peach	10 dried prunes
1 dried fig	½ fresh papaya	10 dates
½ grapefruit	¼ cantaloupe	½ cup raisins
1 fresh pear		½ avocado
½ cup grapefruit juice		1 nectarine
½ cup orange juice		
½ cup pineapple juice		
½ cup apricot nectar		
Cooked Vegetables		
½ cup broccoli	½ cup tomato juice	½ cup parsnips
½ cup rutabagas	½ cup vegetable juice	Artichokes
½ cup pared and boiled potatoes	½ cup rhubarb	1 baked potato
½ cup yams	½ cup pumpkin	
2½-in diameter tomato	½ cup winter squash	
½ cup brussels sprouts		
½ cup pinto beans		
Miscellaneous		
2 tbs wheat germ	1 oz chocolate	1 cup milk
2 slices whole grain bread		1 tbs dark molasses
2 ounces meat		
2 tbs cocoa		
1 cup bran cereal		
20 pecans		
10 peanuts		
10 walnuts		
1 tbs light molasses		

Sodium and potassium restriction. The amount of sodium and potassium restriction depends on the ability of the kidneys to excrete these electrolytes. Sodium-restricted diets may vary from 1000 to 4000 mg (1 mEq = 23 mg of sodium), depending on the degree of edema and hypertension. (The average daily intake of sodium is 3 g to 7 g.) Sodium and salt should not be equated because the sodium content in 1 g of sodium chloride is equivalent to 400 mg of sodium. The patient should be instructed to avoid foods known to be high in sodium such as cured meats, pickled foods, canned soups and stews, frankfurters, cold cuts, soy sauce, and salad dressings (see Table 33-11). Most salt substitutes should not be used because they contain potassium chloride.

Controlled dietary restrictions of potassium range from 1500 to 4000 mg (1 mEq = 39 mg of potassium). Some PD patients do not need potassium restrictions. For every 20 g increase in dietary protein, the potassium intake is increased by 500 mg. This makes it virtually impossible to restrict potassium to 40 mEq (1.6 g) in an 80 g protein diet because most foods that are high in protein are also high in potassium. Foods with high potassium levels that should be avoided are dried fruits, legumes, oranges, bananas, melons, deep green and deep yellow vegetables, beans, and peas (Table 44-8).

NURSING MANAGEMENT: CONSERVATIVE THERAPY OF CHRONIC RENAL FAILURE

Nursing Assessment

The nurse should obtain a complete history of any existing renal disease or family history of renal disease because many renal disorders have a hereditary basis. Information on long-term health problems such as hypertension, diabetes, recurrent urinary tract infections, and systemic lupus erythematosus must be obtained. Because many medications are potentially nephrotoxic, both current and past use of prescription and over-the-counter medications must be determined.

The nurse should assess the patient's dietary habits and discuss any problems. Accurate height and weight assessment and information about recent weight gain or loss must be obtained.

Clinical manifestations of chronic renal failure are related to alterations in multiple body systems (see Fig. 44-3). The nurse must be aware of the wide diversity of problems in the patient. Fatigue, lethargy, and pruritus are often the early symptoms of chronic renal failure; hypertension and changes in urine characteristics are often the first signs.

Family and other support systems should be assessed. The chronicity of renal disease and the long-term nature of treatment modalities affect every area of a person's life, including family relationships, social and work activities, and self-image. The choice of treatment modality may be related to support systems available to the patient.

■ Nursing Diagnoses

Nursing diagnoses for chronic renal failure may include, but are not limited to, those presented in NCP 44-1.

■ Planning

The overall goals are that a patient with chronic renal failure will (1) demonstrate knowledge and ability to comply with the therapeutic regimen, (2) participate in decision making for the plan of care and future treatment modality, (3) demonstrate effective coping strategies, and (4) continue with activities of daily living within physiologic limitations.

■ Nursing Implementation

Health Promotion. Individuals must be instructed on the importance of maintaining an adequate fluid intake each day (at least 2 L). They should be advised that any changes in urine appearance (color, odor), frequency, or volume must be reported to the health care provider.

If a patient has a history of renal disease, hypertension, or diabetes mellitus or a family history of renal disease, regular checkups including serum creatinine, BUN, and urinalysis are essential. If a patient must be prescribed a potentially nephrotoxic drug, it is important to monitor renal function with serum creatinine and BUN determinations.

Acute Intervention. The specific nursing management related to various problems is included in NCP 44-1. In addition, it is important to educate the patient and family because diet, medications, and follow-up medical care are the responsibilities of the patient (Table 44-9). The patient should obtain a daily weight, learn to take daily blood pressures, and be able to identify signs and symptoms of edema, hyperkalemia, and other electrolyte imbalances. The patient and family must understand the importance of strict dietary adherence. The dietician and the nurse should meet with the patient and family on a continuing basis to assist in diet planning. A diet history and consideration of cultural variations make diet planning and adherence more easily achieved goals.

The patient needs a complete understanding of the drugs, the dosages, and the common side effects. It may be helpful to make a list of the medications and the times of administration that can be posted in the home in a convenient location. The patient must be instructed to avoid certain over-the-counter drugs such as laxatives and antacids that contain magnesium.

It is important that the patient be motivated to assume the primary role in the management of the disease. The period of conservative management provides a good opportunity to evaluate each patient's ability to manage the disease. This is a critical factor in considering each patient as a candidate for home dialysis or transplantation.

Ambulatory and Home Care. The length of time a patient can be maintained on conservative therapy is highly variable and depends on the progression of renal failure. When conservative therapy is no longer effective, hemodialysis, peritoneal dialysis, and transplantation are the available treatment options.

While the patient is being maintained on conservative therapy, the decision regarding future therapies, if any, should be made. This should be done before complications such as mental status changes, bleeding, progressive neuropathies, and persistent congestive heart failure occur.

The patient and family need a clear explanation of what is involved in dialysis and transplantation. If alternative treatments

44-1 NURSING CARE PLAN PATIENT WITH CHRONIC RENAL FAILURE

Expected Patient Outcomes	Nursing Interventions and *Rationales*
NURSING DIAGNOSIS	**Fluid volume excess** *related to* inability of kidneys to excrete fluid, inadequate dialysis, and excessive fluid intake *as manifested by* edema, hypertension, bounding pulse, weight gain, shortness of breath, pulmonary edema.
▪ No edema. ▪ No evidence of dyspnea. ▪ Dry weight remaining within 2 lb (1 kg) of patient's dry weight. ▪ Blood pressure within limits for patient.	▪ Monitor for increase in blood pressure, periorbital sacral and peripheral edema, dyspnea, and pericardial friction rub, *which are indicators of fluid excess.* ▪ Auscultate lungs for crackles *to identify fluid in the lungs.* ▪ Teach patient how to maintain a low-sodium diet *to help control edema and hypertension.* ▪ Teach patient fluid control measures and importance of daily weights *to help monitor and control fluid overload and related hypertension.* ▪ Teach patient on hemodialysis or peritoneal dialysis what the individual goal weight or dry weight is and how this may change *to help maintain better fluid balance.* ▪ Provide skin care with special emphasis on edematous areas *because these areas are prone to breakdown.*
NURSING DIAGNOSIS	**Impaired skin integrity** *related to* decrease in oil and sweat gland activity, deposition of calcium-phosphate precipitates, capillary fragility, excess fluid, and neuropathy *as manifested by* itching, bruising, dry skin, edema, excoriation.
▪ No itching or skin dryness. ▪ Intact, clean skin.	▪ Assess skin for changes in color, texture, turgor, and vascularity *to provide direction for appropriate interventions.* ▪ Inspect patient for bruises, purpura, and signs of infection *to detect early signs of problems.* ▪ Provide skin care with tepid water, xipamide (Aquaphor), or bath oils *to relieve itching and moisturize dry, cracked skin.* ▪ Apply ointments or creams (lanolin, Aquaphor) following bath or shower *to relieve itching and promote comfort.* ▪ Administer antihistamines and antipruritics as prescribed *to relieve itching.* ▪ Trim patient's nails short and keep them clean *to reduce tissue damage from scratching and prevent infection.* ▪ Monitor serum calcium and phosphate levels *since elevated blood levels may lead to calcium-phosphate precipitation in the skin.*
NURSING DIAGNOSIS	**Risk for injury: fracture** *related to* alterations in the absorption of calcium and excretion of phosphate, altered vitamin D metabolism.
▪ Slowing of bone disease. ▪ Serum calcium levels >8 mg/dl (2.0 mmol/L) and phosphate levels <5.5 mg/dl (1.8 mmol/L). ▪ No bone fractures.	▪ Assess for hypocalcemia, elevated serum phosphate levels, muscle pain, and limited mobility of joints *to detect potential risks for injury.* ▪ Observe for manifestations of bone pain *as a possible indicator of bone injury.* ▪ Provide range-of-motion exercises and encourage ambulation *to foster osteoblast activity and decrease bone resorption.* ▪ Provide safe environment *to reduce the risk of injury.* ▪ Administer calcium supplements, vitamin D, and phosphate binders as ordered *to prevent or treat the bone demineralization.* ▪ Give calcium supplements or phosphate binders with meals *to increase their effectiveness by binding dietary phosphorus to form insoluble calcium phosphate or aluminum phosphate, which is excreted in feces.* ▪ Instruct patient in the importance of taking these drugs with meals *to facilitate compliance with therapeutic regimen.* ▪ Ensure that patient understands and follows dietary restrictions of phosphate. ▪ Observe for hypocalcemia when using calcium supplements. ▪ Explain to patient the potential for fracture *to reduce the risk of unsafe practices that might result in a traumatic or pathologic fracture.*

Continued

44-1 NURSING CARE PLAN PATIENT WITH CHRONIC RENAL FAILURE—continued

Expected Patient Outcomes	Nursing Interventions and *Rationales*
NURSING DIAGNOSIS	**Activity intolerance** *related to* anemia secondary to uremia and blood loss during dialysis *as manifested by* fatigability, shortness of breath, pallor, dyspnea, tachycardia.
▪ Hematocrit in acceptable range. ▪ Able to perform activities of daily living without undue fatigue.	▪ Monitor hematocrit and hemoglobin levels *as an indicator of the patient's oxygen-carrying capacity.* ▪ Administer iron between meals and erythropoietin as ordered *to maintain normal erythropoiesis and stimulate production of RBCs.* ▪ Do not administer folic acid before or during hemodialysis *because folic acid is dialyzable and would be lost in the dialysate.* ▪ Provide adequate periods of rest *to enable patient to recuperate from past activities and participate in future activity.* ▪ Teach patient to plan activities *to avoid fatigue.* ▪ Minimize blood loss during dialysis and watch for any bleeding sites *because bleeding reduces RBCs and can result in decreased O_2 at cellular level.* ▪ Assess patient's response to activity *to make appropriate adjustments in plan of care.*
NURSING DIAGNOSIS	**Altered nutrition: less than body requirements** *related to* restricted level of nutrients (especially protein), nausea, vomiting, anorexia, stomatitis, and altered metabolism of nutrients *as manifested by* loss of appetite, loss of weight, alterations in electrolyte balance.
▪ Maintenance of ideal body weight. ▪ Albumin and total protein within acceptable limits.	▪ Monitor weight, BUN, serum creatinine, albumin, total protein, and serum electrolytes *as indicators of effectiveness of dialysis, nutritional status, and response to treatment.* ▪ Provide frequent mouth care *to prevent stomatitis, remove foul tastes, and increase patient's comfort.* ▪ Provide small, frequent meals *because smaller, more frequent feedings reduce nausea and vomiting.* ▪ Allow patient freedom in choosing food and fluid intake within limitations *to increase the patient's sense of control.* ▪ Provide at least 2000-2500 kcal/day with a high-carbohydrate intake *to minimize catabolism of body protein and maintain body weight.* ▪ Restrict protein and phosphate to prescribed amount *to decrease the metabolic end products of urea, potassium, phosphate, and hydrogen.* ▪ Provide hard candy, gum, and lollipops *to improve taste and increase carbohydrate intake if patient is not a diabetic.*
NURSING DIAGNOSIS	**Constipation** *related to* decreased mobility, antacid intake, fluid restrictions, dietary modification, or electrolyte imbalances *as manifested by* lack of usual bowel elimination.
▪ Usual bowel elimination pattern.	▪ Administer stool softeners as prescribed *to prevent constipation by maintaining soft stools.* ▪ Teach patient to avoid over-the-counter laxatives that contain magnesium *since hypermagnesemia could develop.* ▪ Encourage ambulation to patient's ability *to increase bowel peristalsis.*
NURSING DIAGNOSIS	**Diarrhea** *related to* GI inflammation secondary to urea or as side effect of sorbitol-Kayexalate treatment *as manifested by* frequent, loose-to-watery stools.
▪ Usual bowel elimination pattern.	▪ Record and measure stool *to monitor fluid and electrolyte losses.* ▪ Monitor serum electrolytes (especially potassium, calcium, and bicarbonate levels) when patient has persistent diarrhea *because altered levels can result in significant problems.* ▪ Encourage oral intake of fluids containing electrolytes *to replace losses.* ▪ Clean perianal area gently and apply lotions *to maintain perianal skin integrity.* ▪ Increase oral fluid intake to prescribed maximum and return to normal diet as tolerated *to promote return to normal bowel functioning.*

Continued

44-1 NURSING CARE PLAN PATIENT WITH CHRONIC RENAL FAILURE —continued

Expected Patient Outcomes	Nursing Interventions and *Rationales*
NURSING DIAGNOSIS	**Anticipatory grieving** *related to* loss of kidney function *as manifested by* expression of feelings of sadness, anger, inadequacy, hopelessness.
▪ Acceptance of chronic disease.	▪ Listen to concerns of patient *to convey a caring attitude and foster the nurse-patient relationship and to determine how patient is handling the situation.* ▪ Allow patient time to mourn loss of body function *so patient can deal with feelings and identify ways of coping with losses more effectively.* ▪ Include family members in discussions of patient's concerns *to enable them to assist the patient and foster their support and understanding.*
NURSING DIAGNOSIS	**Self-esteem disturbance** *related to* enforced lifestyle changes, dependency on dialysis, chronic fatigue, body image changes, occupational problems, and role maintenance *as manifested by* expression of feelings of inadequacy and unworthiness, concerns about family finances and functioning.
▪ Positive feelings about self. ▪ Participation in treatment regimen. ▪ Adaptation of lifestyle to changing health status.	▪ Provide opportunity for patient to discuss concerns *to determine how patient is dealing with the changes in her or his life.* ▪ Refer patient to social worker and for counseling if indicated *to provide additional assistance for management of chronic illness.* ▪ Assure patient of self-worth *to raise self-esteem by reinforcing positive attributes.* ▪ Encourage patient and significant others to share feelings *because verbalization helps clarify feelings and may provide insight into solutions.* ▪ Arrange for patient to talk with other patients in similar circumstances *to provide support and understanding.*
NURSING DIAGNOSIS	**Sensory-perceptual alterations** *related to* CNS changes induced by uremic toxins *as manifested by* confusion, slowing of thought processes, decreased attention and memory span, disorientation, changes in sensorium (e.g., somnolence, stupor), changes in mood (e.g., irritability, depression), changes in behavior (e.g., withdrawal).
▪ Mental alertness and appropriate interaction with environment.	▪ Provide explanation to patient and family of effects of uremia on nervous system *to reduce anxiety over changes in mentation.* ▪ Assess patient's level of consciousness and mental status at regular intervals *because minor confusion and irritability can progress and indicate a worsening of condition.* ▪ Discuss significant material for brief rather than long time periods *to reduce confusion and increase possibility that information will be understood and retained.* ▪ Provide calm, nonstimulating environment *to prevent increasing patient's confusion and agitation.*
NURSING DIAGNOSIS	**Risk for sexual dysfunction** *related to* effects of uremia on reproductive and endocrine systems and the psychosocial impact of renal failure and its treatment.
▪ Satisfaction with sexual relationship by patient and significant other.	▪ Assess female patients for amenorrhea and decreased libido; assess male patients for impotence, atrophy of testicles, and gynecomastia *to determine presence and extent of risk factors for sexual dysfunction and plan appropriate interventions.* ▪ Discuss meaning of sexuality with patient and significant other *to determine significance of problem.* ▪ Encourage patient and partner to discuss feelings openly and to use other means of sexual expression besides intercourse; explore new patterns of sexual activity if previous patterns lead to anxiety *to ensure continued expression of sexual feelings.*

Continued

44-1 NURSING CARE PLAN PATIENT WITH CHRONIC RENAL FAILURE —continued

Expected Patient Outcomes	Nursing Interventions and *Rationales*

NURSING DIAGNOSIS **Risk for infection** *related to* suppressed immune system, access sites, and malnutrition secondary to dialysis and uremia.

Expected Patient Outcomes	Nursing Interventions and *Rationales*
▪ No infections. ▪ WBC count within normal range.	▪ Assess for chills, fever, tachycardia; redness, swelling, or drainage in area of break in skin *to detect signs of possible infection.* ▪ Provide frequent oral and personal hygiene *to reduce risk of self-contamination.* ▪ Instruct patient to avoid exposure to people with infections *because the patient has an altered immune response and therefore has an increased risk of infection.* ▪ Watch for local and systemic manifestations of infection *to promote early identification and treatment.* ▪ Maintain aseptic technique when performing dialysis *to prevent the introduction of organisms.* ▪ Avoid invasive procedures such as catheterization *to avoid introduction of organisms.*

COLLABORATIVE PROBLEMS

POTENTIAL COMPLICATION **Hypertension** *related to* sodium and water retention and alterations of renin-angiotensin system.

Nursing Goals	Nursing Interventions and *Rationales*
▪ Monitor for hypertension. ▪ Report deviations from acceptable parameters. ▪ Carry out appropriate medical and nursing interventions.	▪ Assess patient for elevated blood pressure, headache, dizziness, shortness of breath, chest pain, edema *to identify the presence and effects of hypertension.* ▪ Take vital signs q4hr *to provide a database for ongoing analysis of patient's response to treatment.* ▪ Administer antihypertensive medications as ordered. ▪ Observe for orthostatic hypotension and other side effects of medication *because overtreatment may cause problems.* ▪ Instruct patient to change positions slowly *to minimize dizziness caused by orthostatic hypotension.* ▪ Explain the actions and side effects of drugs and risks of uncontrolled hypertension (e.g., stroke) *to foster adherence to medication regimen.*

POTENTIAL COMPLICATION **Hyperkalemia** *related to* decreased renal function, increased tissue catabolism, and shift of potassium into extracellular fluid *related to* metabolic acidosis.

Nursing Goals	Nursing Interventions and *Rationales*
▪ Monitor for signs of hyperkalemia. ▪ Report deviations from acceptable parameters. ▪ Carry out appropriate medical and nursing interventions.	▪ Assess for signs of hyperkalemia such as serum potassium >5.5 mEq/L (5.5 mmol/L), muscle weakness, arrhythmias, paresthesias, intestinal colic and diarrhea, peaked T waves on ECG *to ensure early identification and treatment.* ▪ Discuss importance of following prescribed diet and avoiding foods high in potassium *to prevent complications of hyperkalemia.* ▪ Monitor serum potassium and notify physician of elevated levels and ECG results *because elevated potassium can cause life-threatening cardiac arrhythmias.* ▪ Be prepared to administer treatment for hyperkalemia *because this is a medical emergency requiring prompt treatment.*

POTENTIAL COMPLICATION **Peripheral neuropathy** *related to* effects of uremia on peripheral nerves.

Nursing Goals	Nursing Interventions and *Rationales*
▪ Monitor for peripheral neuropathies. ▪ Report deviations from acceptable parameters. ▪ Carry out appropriate medical and nursing interventions.	▪ Assess patient for decreased sensation, numbness, burning of feet, muscle cramps, restlessness of legs, loss of muscle strength, footdrop *to identify presence of peripheral neuropathy.* ▪ Explain to patient reason for neuropathy *to increase understanding and decrease anxiety.* ▪ Prevent trauma and excess stimulation to extremities *because areas with diminished sensation are extremely prone to injury.* ▪ Instruct patient to avoid tight clothing and restricting bed linens *to prevent inadvertent injury since the affected areas have decreased sensation.* ▪ Teach patient to examine areas of decreased sensation *to observe for injury.* ▪ In collaboration with physical therapy department, develop exercise regimen *to maintain prescribed level of activity.* ▪ Assess adequacy of dialysis therapy *because dialysis may reduce the symptoms and halt the progress of neuropathies.*

PATIENT & FAMILY TEACHING GUIDE

Table 44-9 Chronic Renal Failure

1. Explain dietary (protein, sodium, potassium, phosphate) and fluid restrictions.
2. Encourage discussion of difficulties in modifying diet and fluid intake.
3. Explain signs and symptoms of electrolyte imbalance, especially high potassium.
4. Teach alternative ways of reducing thirst, such as sucking on ice cubes, lemon, or hard candy.
5. Explain the rationale for prescribed medications and common side effects. Examples:
   - Calcium supplements or phosphate binders should be taken with meals.
   - Iron supplements should be taken between meals.
6. Explain the importance of reporting any of the following:
   - Weight gain greater than 2 lb (1 kg)
   - Increasing blood pressure
   - Shortness of breath
   - Edema
   - Increasing fatigue or weakness
   - Confusion or lethargy
7. Encourage patient and family to share concerns about lifestyle changes, living with a chronic illness, decisions about type of dialysis or transplantation.

are presented early in the course of therapy, the patient will have an opportunity to carefully consider choices. The patient will feel more control over her or his life and health care when educated about treatment and treatment options and when active in the decision-making process. The patient should be informed that if dialysis is chosen, the option of transplantation still remains. It should be emphasized that if a transplanted organ fails, the patient can return to dialysis. Some individuals with chronic renal failure have received more than one kidney transplant.

■ Evaluation

The expected outcomes for the patient with chronic renal failure are presented in NCP 44-1.

DIALYSIS

Dialysis is the movement of fluid and molecules across a semipermeable membrane from one compartment to another. Clinically, dialysis is a technique in which substances move from the blood through a semipermeable membrane and into a dialysis solution (dialysate). Dialysis is used to correct fluid and electrolyte imbalances and to remove waste products in renal failure. Dialysis can also be used to treat drug overdoses. The two methods of dialysis are peritoneal dialysis (PD) and hemodialysis (HD) (Table 44-10). In PD the peritoneal membrane is used as the semipermeable membrane. In HD an artificial membrane (usually made of cellulose-based or synthetic materials) is used as the semipermeable membrane that is in contact with the patient's blood.

Dialysis is begun when the patient's uremic state can no longer be adequately managed conservatively. A general guideline is to start dialysis when the GFR (or creatinine clearance) is less than 5 to 10 ml per minute. However, this criterion varies widely in different clinical situations, and the physician determines when to start dialysis based on the patient's clinical status. Certain uremic complications, including encephalopathy, neuropathies, uncontrollable hyperkalemia, pericarditis, and accelerated hypertension, indicate a need for immediate dialysis.

GENERAL PRINCIPLES

Solutes and water move across the membrane from the blood to the dialysate or from the dialysate to the blood in accordance with concentration gradients. The principles of diffusion, osmosis, and ultrafiltration are involved in dialysis (Fig. 44-5). *Diffusion* is the movement of solutes from an area of greater concentration to an area of lesser concentration. In renal failure, urea, creatinine, uric acid, and electrolytes (potassium, phosphate) move from the blood to the dialysate with the net effect of lowering their concentration in the blood. RBCs, WBCs, and large plasma proteins are too large to diffuse through the pores of the membrane.

Osmosis is the movement of fluid from an area of lesser to an area of greater concentration of solutes. Glucose is added to the dialysate bath and creates an osmotic gradient across the membrane to remove excess fluid from the blood.

Ultrafiltration (water and fluid removal) results when a pressure gradient across the dialyzer membrane is created by an increased pressure in the blood compartment (positive pressure) or a decreased pressure in the dialysate compartment (negative pressure). Extracellular fluid moves into the dialysate because of the pressure gradient. In peritoneal dialysis, excess fluid is removed by increasing the osmolality of the dialysate with the addition of glucose. In HD, excess fluid is removed by creating a pressure differential between the blood and the dialysate solution with a combination of positive pressure in the blood compartment or a negative pressure in the dialysate compartment.

PERITONEAL DIALYSIS

Although PD was first used in 1923, it did not come into widespread use for chronic treatment until the 1970s with the development of soft, pliable peritoneal solution bags and the introduction of the concept of continuous PD. In the United States, approximately 15% of patients receiving dialysis treatments are on peritoneal dialysis.[5] In Canada, approximately 36% of patients are on PD because of the decreased availability of HD. In recent years the use of PD to treat chronic renal failure has increased considerably. The large surface area of the peritoneum makes it a good semipermeable membrane for performing clinical dialysis.

Table 44-10 Comparison of Peritoneal Dialysis and Hemodialysis

Peritoneal Dialysis		Hemodialysis	
Advantages	**Disadvantages**	**Advantages**	**Disadvantages**
Immediate initiation in almost any hospital Less complicated than hemodialysis Portable system with CAPD Fewer dietary restrictions Relatively short training time Usable in the patient with vascular access problems Less cardiovascular stress Home dialysis possible Preferable for the diabetic patient	Bacterial or chemical peritonitis Protein loss into dialysate Exit-site and tunnel infections Self-image problems with catheter placement Hyperglycemia Aggravated hyperlipidemia Surgery for catheter placement Contraindication in the patient with multiple abdominal surgery or trauma Specially trained personnel needed	Rapid fluid removal Rapid removal of urea and creatinine Effective potassium removal Less protein loss Lowering of serum triglycerides Home dialysis possible Temporary access can be placed at bedside	Vascular access problems Dietary and fluid restrictions Heparinization may be necessary Extensive equipment necessary Hypotension during dialysis Added blood loss that contributes to anemia Specially trained personnel necessary

CAPD, continuous ambulatory peritoneal dialysis.

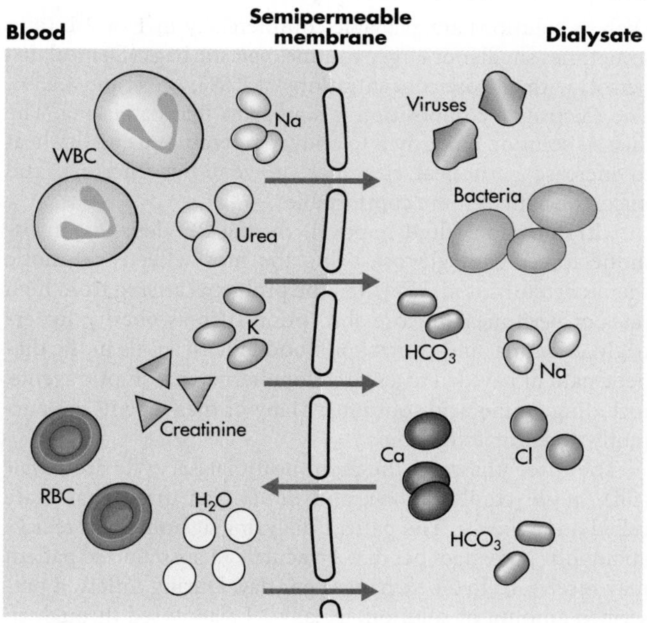

Fig. 44-5 Osmosis and diffusion across a semipermeable membrane.

Catheter Placement

Peritoneal access is obtained by inserting a catheter through the anterior abdominal wall (Fig. 44-6). The prototype of the catheter that is used was developed by Tenckhoff in 1968 and is made of silicone rubber tubing (see Fig. 44-6). The current version of this catheter is about 25 cm long and has one or two Dacron cuffs at the subcutaneous and peritoneal ends of the catheter that anchor it securely and prevent the migration of microorganisms down the shaft from the skin. Within a few weeks, fibrous tissue grows into the Dacron cuff, anchors the catheter in place, and prevents bacterial penetration into the peritoneal cavity. The tip of the catheter rests in the peritoneal cavity and has many perforations spaced throughout the distal end of the tubing to allow fluid to flow in and out of the catheter. Other types of catheters for chronic PD are variations of the Tenckhoff catheter, including the Toronto-Western, Purdue-Column Disc, and Gore-Tex catheters (Fig. 44-7).

The technique for catheter placement varies. Although it is possible to place a permanent catheter in the peritoneal cavity with a trocar, it is usually done via surgery so that its placement can be directly visualized, thus minimizing potential complications. Preparation of the patient for catheter insertion includes emptying the bladder and bowel, weighing the patient, and obtaining a signed consent form. In the nonsurgical approach, an area approximately 2 cm below the umbilicus is anesthetized with a local anesthetic, and the abdomen is distended with dialysis solution. A trocar, with the catheter threaded through or over it, is inserted into the peritoneal cavity. When the patient feels pressure in the rectal area and has the urge to defecate, the trocar is withdrawn, and the catheter is in place.

In the surgical approach a midline umbilical incision is made, and a small puncture is made to one side and below this incision. The distal end of the catheter is placed in the peritoneum and it is tunneled under the skin to the puncture site. After the catheter is inserted, the skin is cleaned with an antiseptic solution, and a sterile dressing is applied. Complications of catheter insertion include perforation of the bladder, the bowel, or a blood vessel and the introduction of bacteria.

The catheter is connected to a sterile tubing system and anchored to the abdomen with tape. The catheter is irrigated immediately with heparinized dialysate (usually 500 ml) to clear blood and fibrin from it. The irrigations may continue for 12 to 24 hours using small volumes of dialysate. This procedure helps prevent the catheter from clogging, resulting in poor drainage

RESEARCH
IMPLICATIONS FOR NURSING PRACTICE

Self-care Knowledge Among Elderly Dialysis Patients

Citation Badzek L, Hines SC, Moss AH: Inadequate self-care knowledge among elderly hemodialysis patients: assessing its prevalence and potential causes, *ANNA J* 25:293, 1998.

Purpose To determine how well informed elderly hemodialysis (HD) patients are about information needed for self-care and to identify factors contributing to their inadequate knowledge.

Methods The sample included 142 patients over the age of 65 in 17 outpatient hemodialysis units in three Eastern states. Interviews were conducted to test factual knowledge of dialysis and to assess how well informed the subjects thought they were about self-care related issues. Interviewers also asked demographic questions and administered the Mini-Mental State Exam (MMSE) to assess cognitive capacity.

Results and Conclusions Seventy-five percent of patients believed they were well informed; however, only 14% answered all three questions correctly. The average number correct on a three-question, self-care knowledge measure was only 1.67. Knowledge was lowest for older, poorly-educated patients with diminished cognitive capacity who had recently begun dialysis (mean correct score 1.1). The majority of these elderly HD patients lacked information needed for self-care.

Implications for Nursing Practice Nurses should not unquestionably accept patient's claims that they are well informed. Older patients especially may require extra teaching efforts, closer monitoring, and more family involvement in care and decision making. The Mini-Mental State Exam may be a valuable way to help identify patients with cognitive impairments. Educational programs may need to be adjusted to accomodate cognitive impairment.

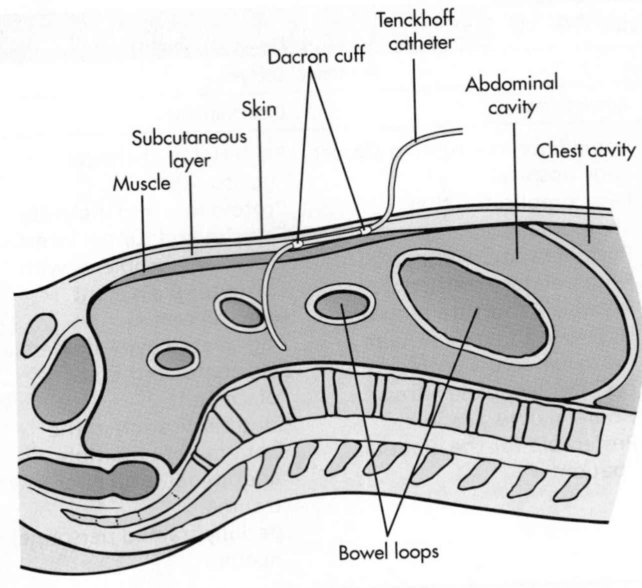

Fig. 44-6 Tenckhoff catheter used in peritoneal dialysis.

and inflow. More frequently today, this procedure is carried out as day surgery and the patient is discharged home with a sterile dressing covering the PD catheter. The patient then needs explicit instructions on keeping the dressing dry and an appointment to visit the dialysis clinic in a few days.

Before the start of PD, it is preferable to allow a waiting period of 7 to 14 days for proper sealing of the catheter and for tissue ingrowth into the cuffs. However, some centers start dialysis 5 to 7 days after catheter insertion. About 2 to 4 weeks after catheter implantation, the exit site should be clean, dry, and free of redness and tenderness (Fig. 44-8). Once the catheter incision site is healed, the patient may shower and then pat the catheter and exit site dry. Daily catheter care includes the application of an antiseptic solution and a clean dressing, as well as examination of the catheter site for signs of infection.

Dialysis Solutions and Cycle

Dialysis solutions are available commercially in 1 or 2 L (and sometimes smaller or larger volumes) plastic bags (Dianeal, Inpersol) with glucose concentrations of 1.5%, 2.5%, and 4.25%. The electrolyte composition is similar to that of plasma. The dialysis solution is warmed to body temperature using dry heat to increase peritoneal clearance, prevent hypothermia, and make the patient more comfortable.

Ultrafiltration (fluid removal) during PD depends on osmotic forces with glucose being the most effective osmotic agent currently used. However, the problems arising from high rates of peritoneal glucose absorption such as obesity, hypertriglyceridemia, and control of blood glucose levels in the diabetic patient have led to a search for alternative osmotic agents, including amino acid solutions. Many of these agents are currently under investigation.

The three phases of the peritoneal dialysis cycle are *inflow* (fill), *dwell* (equilibration), and *drain.* The three phases are called an *exchange.* The patient dialyzing at home will receive about four exchanges per day. An acutely ill hospitalized patient may receive 12 to 24 exchanges per day. During inflow, a prescribed amount of solution, usually 2 L, is infused through an established catheter over about 10 minutes. The flow rate may be decreased if the patient becomes uncomfortable. After the solution has been infused, the inflow clamp is closed before air enters the tubing.

The next part of the cycle is the dwell phase, or equilibration, during which diffusion and osmosis occur between the patient's blood and the peritoneal cavity. The duration of the dwell time can last 20 to 30 minutes to 8 or more hours, depending on the method of PD. Drain time takes 15 to 30 minutes and may be facilitated by gently massaging the abdomen or changing the patient's position. The cycle starts again with the infusion of another 2 L of solution. For manual PD, a period of about 30 to 50 minutes is required to complete an exchange.

A

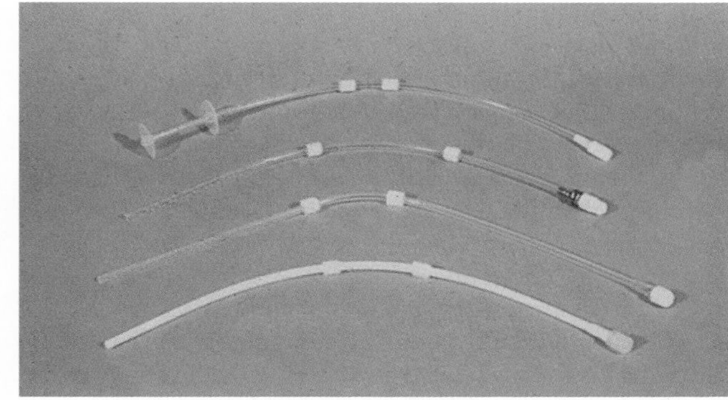

B

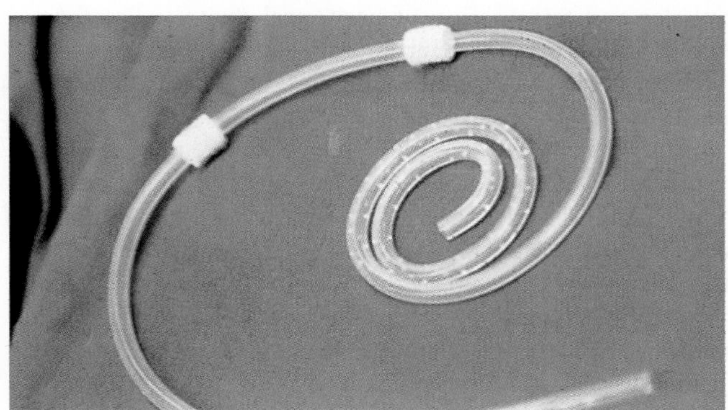

C

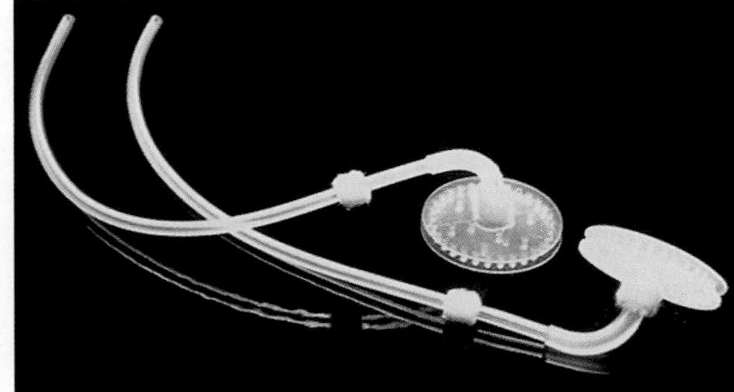

Fig. 44-7 **A,** Peritoneal catheters used for peritoneal dialysis. **B,** Bent neck curl catheters. **C,** Disk catheters.

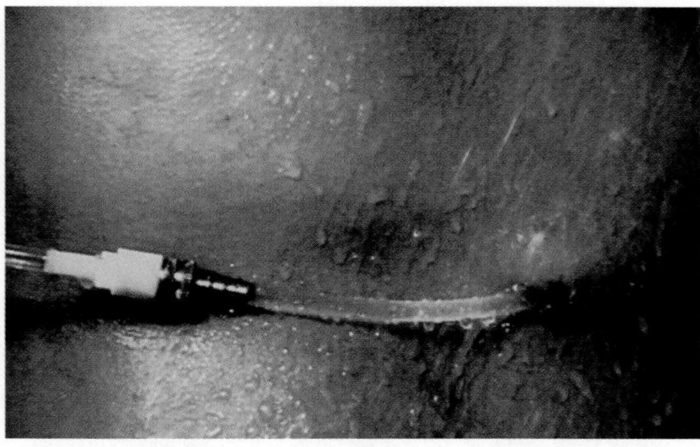

Fig. 44-8 Placement of peritoneal catheter.

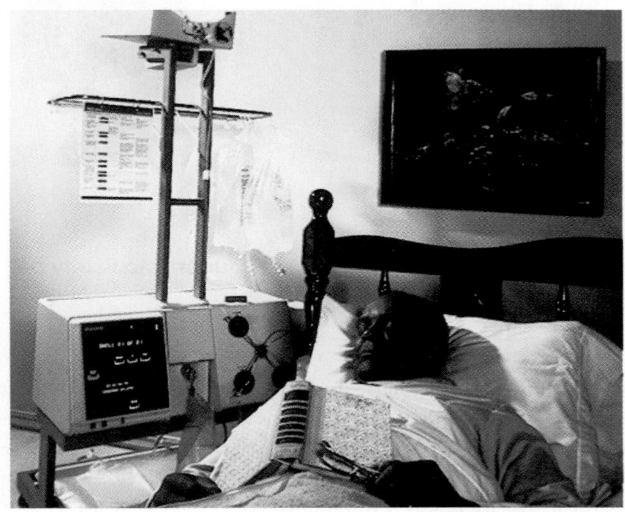

Fig. 44-9 Automated peritoneal dialysis cycler that can be used while the patient is sleeping or for hospitalized patients who require frequent exchanges.

Peritoneal Dialysis Systems

Two types of PD currently being used are automated peritoneal dialysis (APD) and continuous ambulatory peritoneal dialysis (CAPD).

Automated Peritoneal Dialysis. An automated device called a *cycler* is used to deliver the dialysate for APD (Fig. 44-9). The automated cycler times and controls the fill, dwell, and drain phases. The machine cycles four to eight exchanges per night with 1 to 2 hours per exchange. Alarms and monitors are built into the system to make it safe for the patient to dialyze while sleeping. It may be easier to teach the patient and family to use the PD machine at home compared with the HD equipment. APD includes the following variations: continuous cyclic peritoneal dialysis (CCPD), intermittent peritoneal dialysis (IPD), and nightly peritoneal dialysis (NPD). In CCPD the dialysis solution can be left in the peritoneal cavity during the day between nightly cycling, or the peritoneal cavity can be left "dry" during the day. With IPD and NPD, cycling is performed five to seven nights per week, and the abdomen is left empty between dialysis.

Continuous Ambulatory Peritoneal Dialysis. CAPD is carried out manually by exchanging 1.5 to 3 L (usually 2 L) of peritoneal dialysate usually four times daily with dwell times of 4 to 10 hours. One schedule, for example, starts the exchanges at 7 AM, 12 noon, 5 PM, and 10 PM. In this procedure the person instills 2 L of dialysate from a collapsible plastic bag into the peritoneal cavity through a disposable plastic tube.

Technical advances in CAPD systems, including Y sets and twin bag systems, allow the bag and line to be disconnected after the instillation of the fluid and decrease the risk of peritonitis. After the equilibration period the line is reconnected to

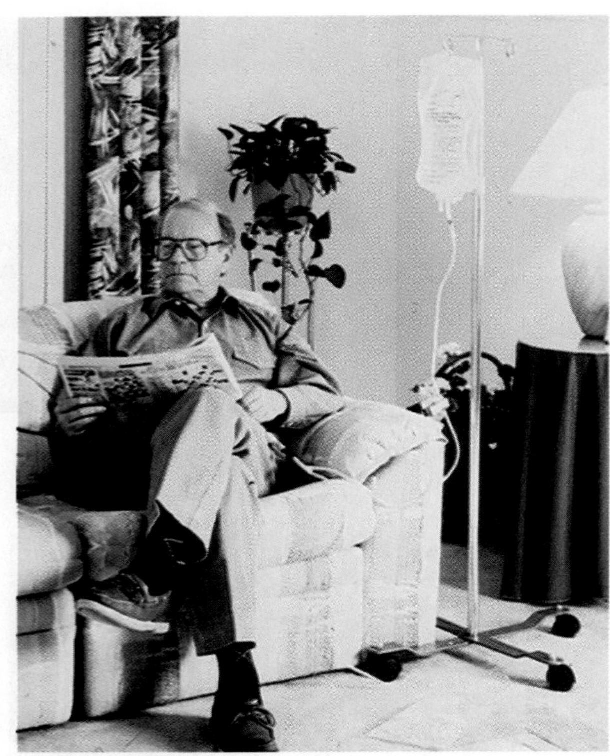

Fig. 44-10 Infusion period for a continuous ambulatory peritoneal dialysis patient.

the catheter, and the dialysate (effluent) is drained from the peritoneal cavity, and a new 2 L bag of dialysate solution is infused (Fig. 44-10). It is critical in PD to maintain aseptic technique to avoid peritonitis. Several tubing connections and devices are commercially available to help maintain an aseptic system.

Contraindications for PD include the following:

1. History of multiple abdominal surgical procedures or severe abdominal pathology (e.g., severe pancreatitis, diverticulitis)
2. Recurrent abdominal wall or inguinal hernias
3. Excessive obesity with large abdominal wall and fat deposits
4. Preexisting vertebral disease (e.g., chronic back problems)
5. Severe obstructive pulmonary disease

Complications of Peritoneal Dialysis

Exit Site Infection. Infection of the peritoneal catheter exit site is most commonly caused by *Staphylococcus aureus* or *S. epidermidis* (from skin flora). Superficial exit-site infections caused by these organisms are generally resolved with antibiotic therapy. Clinical manifestations of an exit site infection include redness at site, tenderness, and drainage. If not treated immediately, subcutaneous tunnel infections usually result in abscess formation and may cause peritonitis and necessitate catheter removal.

Peritonitis. Peritonitis results from contamination of the dialysate or tubing or from progression of exit site or tunnel infections. Less commonly peritonitis results from bacteria in the intestine crossing over into the peritoneal cavity. Peritonitis is usually caused by *S. aureus* or *S. epidermidis.*[12] The primary clinical manifestation of peritonitis is a cloudy peritoneal effluent that has a WBC count of over 100 cells per microliter (particularly neutrophils). GI manifestations may also be present, including diffuse abdominal pain, diarrhea, vomiting, abdominal distention, and hyperactive bowel sounds. Fever may or may not be present. Cultures, Gram's stain, and a cell count and a differential of peritoneal effluent are used to confirm the diagnosis of peritonitis. Antibiotics are given by mouth, IV, or, most commonly, intraperitoneally. The patient is usually treated on an outpatient basis. Repeated infections may necessitate the removal of the peritoneal catheter and termination of peritoneal dialysis. The formation of adhesions in the peritoneum can result from repeated infections and can interfere with the peritoneal membrane's ability as a dialyzing surface.

Abdominal Pain. Although not severe, pain is a common complication caused by the low pH of the dialysate solution, peritonitis, intraperitoneal irritation (which usually subsides in 1 to 2 weeks), and placement of the catheter. Pain can also occur when the tip of the catheter touches the bladder, bowel, or peritoneum. A change in the position of the catheter should correct this problem. Accidental infusion of air or infusing the dialysate too rapidly may cause referred pain in the shoulder. If the infusion rate is decreased, the pain usually subsides.

Outflow Problems. When outflow is less than 80% of inflow immediately after catheter placement, it may be caused by a kink in the tunnel segment of the catheter, omentum wrapped around the catheter, or migration of the catheter out of the pelvic region. Persistent outflow problems may require radiologic or surgical manipulation of the catheter. Outflow problems after the catheter has settled into place are often a result of a full colon; bowel evacuation frequently relieves the problem.

Hernias. Because of increased intraabdominal pressures secondary to the dialysate infusion, hernias can develop in predisposed individuals such as multiparous women and older men. However, in most situations after hernia repair, peritoneal dialysis can be restarted after several days using small dialysate volumes and keeping the patient supine.

Lower Back Problems. Increased intraabdominal pressure can cause or aggravate lower back pain. The lumbosacral curvature is increased by intraperitoneal infusion of dialysate. Orthopedic binders and a regular exercise program for the back muscles have been beneficial for some patients.

Bleeding. Effluent drained after the first few exchanges may be pink or slightly bloody because of the trauma of catheter insertion. Bloody effluent over several days or the new appearance of blood in the effluent can indicate active intraperitoneal bleeding. If this occurs, the blood pressure and hematocrit should be checked. Blood may also be present in the effluent of women who are menstruating or ovulating, but this requires no intervention.

Pulmonary Complications. Atelectasis, pneumonia, and bronchitis may occur from repeated upward displacement of the diaphragm, resulting in decreased lung expansion. The longer the dwell time, the greater the likelihood of pulmonary complications. Frequent repositioning and deep-breathing exercises can help alleviate pulmonary complications. When lying in bed, elevation of the head of the bed may prevent these problems.

Protein Loss. The peritoneal membrane is permeable to plasma proteins, amino acids, and polypeptides. Therefore these substances are lost in the dialysate fluid. The amount of loss may be as much as 9 to 12 g per day. This protein loss may be increased up to 40 g per day during episodes of peritonitis as the membrane becomes more permeable. The patient can maintain a positive nitrogen balance with satisfactory protein intake.

Carbohydrate and Lipid Abnormalities. Dialysate glucose is absorbed via the peritoneum and may amount to as much as 100 to 150 g per day. Continuous absorption of glucose results in increased insulin secretion and increased plasma insulin levels. The hyperinsulinemia stimulates hepatic production of triglycerides (see p. 1308).

Encapsulating Sclerosing Peritonitis and Loss of Ultrafiltration. *Encapsulating sclerosing peritonitis* is a term applied to the development of a thick fibrous membrane that surrounds and compresses the bowel. Intestinal obstruction and strangulation are common complications. This condition generally necessitates changing the patient to HD because of the loss of ultrafiltration. It can also occur as a result of unknown reasons or accidental infusion of disinfecting agents. Loss of ultrafiltration is associated with rapid glucose absorption.

Effectiveness of and Adaptation to Chronic Peritoneal Dialysis

The use and popularity of chronic PD is increasing. The technique is associated with a short training program, independence, and ease of traveling. Clinically, the patient on PD does at least as well as the patient on HD and sometimes better. There are fewer dietary restrictions, and greater mobility is possible than with conventional HD. The major disadvantage is the possibility of developing peritonitis. As further improvements in techniques are made (e.g., improved connecting and sterilizing devices, in-line filters, improved catheters), the incidence of peritonitis should decrease.

PD is especially indicated for the individual who has vascular access problems and responds poorly to the hemodynamic stresses of HD (e.g., the older adult patient with diabetes and cardiovascular disease). The diabetic patient with ESRD does better on PD than on HD. The advantages of PD for the diabetic patient include better blood pressure control, stable cardiovascular status without rapid fluid shifts, better control of blood glucose by intraperitoneal insulin (which can often eliminate the need for subcutaneous insulin), and avoidance of the risk of retinal hemorrhage from heparin use during HD.

HEMODIALYSIS

In 1943 Willem Kolff in the Netherlands performed the first successful dialysis on a human being with the use of a rotating-drum dialyzer. He initiated dialysis treatment in the United States in the 1950s.

Vascular Access Sites

Vascular access is one of the major problems with HD. To carry out HD, a high blood flow is required. Before 1960, HD required the insertion of needles into arteries and veins for each dialysis. Chronic dialysis was not possible with this technique.

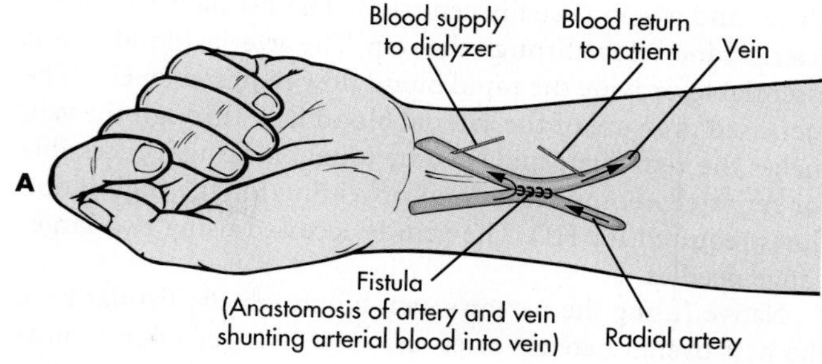

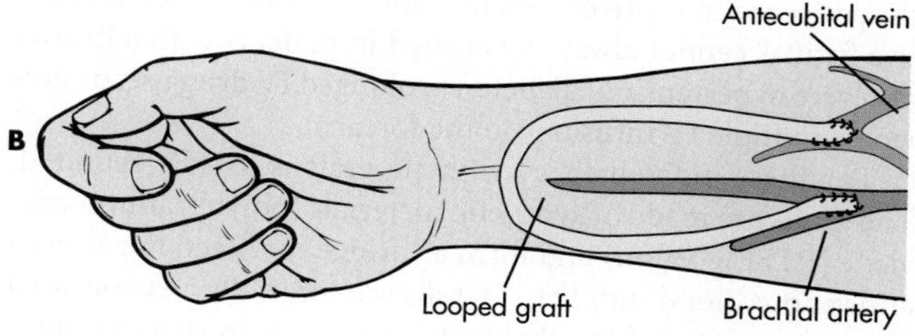

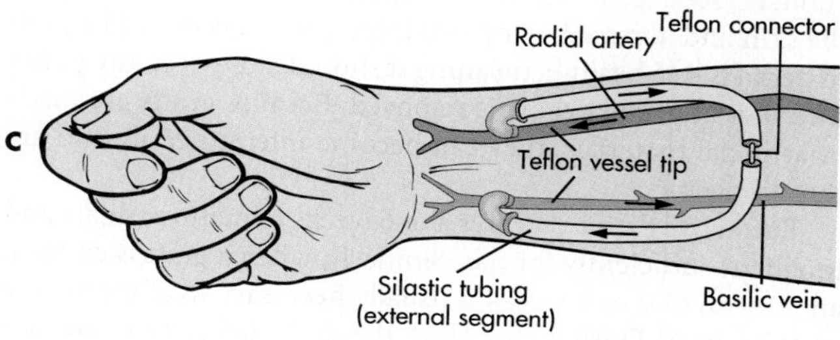

Fig. 44-11 Methods of vascular access for hemodialysis. **A,** Internal arteriovenous fistula. **B,** Looped graft in forearm. **C,** External cannula or shunt.

Shunts. In 1960 Scribner developed a Teflon silicone rubber cannula that could be inserted into the radial artery and into an adjacent forearm vein (Fig. 44-11, *C*). The cannula is implanted subcutaneously in both the artery and vein and is connected to a silicone rubber tubing that exits from the skin. The two ends are connected by a U-shaped shunt that has a connector at its midpoint. The U portion of the shunt is external. This connection can be opened after clamping on both sides to attach the patient to the dialysis machine. The external access cannula is commonly referred to as an *external shunt* and can be used immediately. The external shunt is associated with many complications, including infection and bleeding. Because of these complications and the availability of other access alternatives, it is very rarely used for chronic dialysis. Although not commonly used, it can be used as a temporary access for continuous renal replacement therapy (see p. 1329).

Internal Arteriovenous Fistulas and Grafts. In 1966 the use of the subcutaneous internal arteriovenous native fistula (see Fig. 44-11, *A*) was introduced by Cimino and Brescia. An arteriovenous (AV) fistula is created most commonly in the forearm by a side-to-side, end-to-side, or end-to-end anastomosis between an artery (usually radial or ulnar) and a vein (usually cephalic). The fistula provides for arterial blood flow through the vein. The arterial blood flow is essential to provide the rapid blood flow required by HD. The increased pressure of the arterial blood flow through the vein makes the vein dilate and become tough, making it accessible for repeated venipuncture and providing for the high blood flows required for HD. The vein is accessed using two large-gauge needles.

Native (using the person's own blood vessels) fistulas have the best overall patency rates and least number of complications of all vascular accesses; however, they are suitable only for the patient with relatively healthy blood vessels.[13] Therefore native fistulas cannot always be created in patients with a history of severe hypertension, diabetes, prolonged IV drug use, or previous multiple IV infusions in the forearm.

For these individuals a synthetic graft is usually required. The grafts are made of synthetic materials (polytetrafluoroethylene [PTFE], Teflon) and form a "bridge" between the arterial and venous blood supplies.[13] Grafts are surgically anastomosed between an artery (usually brachial) and a vein (usually antecubital) (see Fig. 44-11, *B*). The graft, like the fistula, is under the skin and accessed using two large-gauge needles. The graft material is self-healing, meaning it should close over any puncture sites after the needle is removed. Because grafts are made of artificial materials, they can become infected easily and are thrombogenic.

The native fistula requires 4 to 6 weeks to mature (dilate and toughen) sufficiently for use. Similarly, when a graft is created, an interval of 2 to 4 weeks is usually necessary to allow for the graft to heal. During this time the endothelial cells are deposited on the inside of the graft, and these cells help seal the needle puncture site after the dialysis needle is removed. Some dialysis centers use the graft earlier.

Two 14- to 16-gauge needles are inserted into the fistula or graft (local anesthesia may be used) to obtain vascular access. One needle is placed to pull blood from the circulation to the HD machine, and the other needle is used to return the dialyzed blood to the patient. The needles are attached via tubing to dialysis lines. Normally, a thrill can be felt by palpating the area of anastomosis, and a bruit can be heard with a stethoscope. The bruit and thrill are created by arterial blood rushing into the vein. Blood pressures, IV insertion, and venipuncture should not be performed on the affected extremity. This prevents infection and potential sources of clotting of the vascular access. Vascular access can be difficult to obtain in patients with ESRD. Protection of the vascular access site is of paramount importance.

The subcutaneous AV fistula is much less likely to clot and become infected than a graft. Native fistulas seem to get better as the years go by. Thrombosis in grafts is common. Grafts can lead to the development of distal ischemia (steal syndrome) because arterial blood is being shunted. This is usually seen soon after surgery and may require surgical correction. Another complication is the development of an aneurysm at the fistula site. When a graft becomes infected, it is a serious problem that is frequently associated with bacteremia and may require the removal of the graft.

Temporary Vascular Access. In some situations when temporary vascular access is required quickly, percutaneous cannulation of the subclavian, internal jugular, or femoral vein is used. A flexible Teflon, silicone rubber, or polyurethane catheter is inserted into one of these large veins and provides easy immediate access to circulation without the need for the patient to have surgery or to sacrifice a peripheral artery or vein. The catheters usually have a double lumen with an internal septum separating the two segments (Fig. 44-12). One lumen is used for blood removal and the other for blood return. The procedure for percutaneous cannulation is similar to the method of insertion of a pulmonary artery catheter (see Chapter 63).

Percutaneous cannulas in the subclavian or jugular veins can be left in place for 1 to 3 weeks. Femoral-vein cannulas can remain in place for up to 1 week.

Technical complications of subclavian vein catheterization include brachial plexus problems, hemothorax, and pneumothorax. A moderate risk of infection also exists. While the catheter is in place, the patient is usually comfortable and can be ambulatory. No medications should be administered or blood withdrawn from this catheter by nondialysis staff. Trained dialysis staff may inject heparin into the lumen of the catheter at the end of dialysis and remove the heparin before starting dialysis. Subclavian vein thrombosis and stenosis is a complication of subclavian cannulation.

Although jugular vein cannulation is associated with a low incidence of thrombosis, short-term jugular vein access with stiff catheters is often unacceptable to the patient since the catheter is in the patient's neck and can cause discomfort and restrict movement.

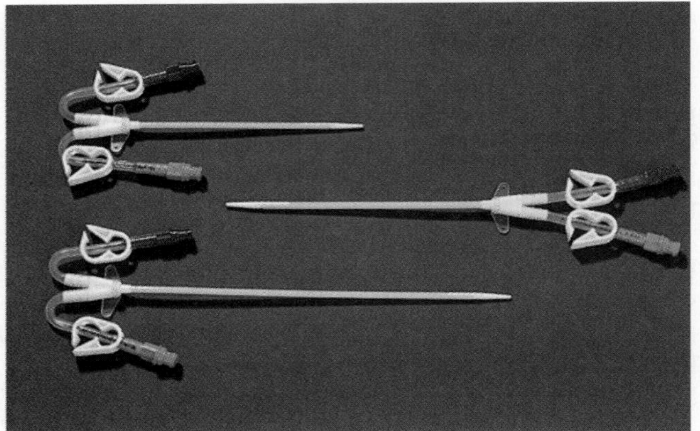

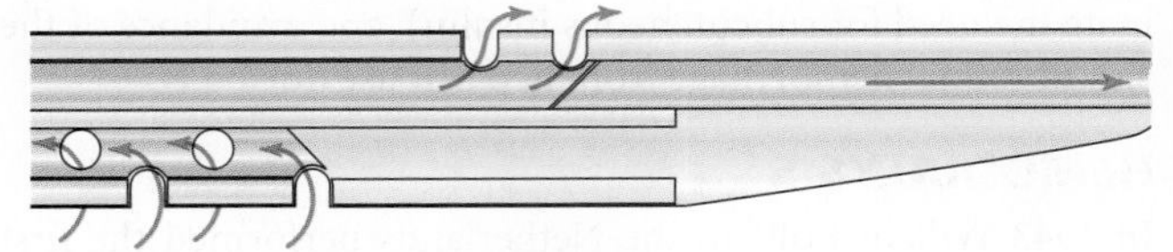

Fig. 44-12 Temporary double-lumen, single-needle vascular access catheter for acute hemodialysis. **A,** The soft, flexible dual-lumen polyurethane tube is attached to a Y hub. **B,** Blood is withdrawn continuously through the outer lumen upstream and returned through the inner lumen downstream, thus reducing recirculation.

Disadvantages of femoral-vessel cannulization include the following: (1) the catheter can remain in place only a short time, (2) the location encourages catheter kinking, and (3) the groin is not a clean site. Complications of femoral catheterization consist of femoral vein thrombosis with pulmonary emboli (especially if the treatment is prolonged), infections, immobility, and inadvertent blood vessel punctures with hematoma formation.

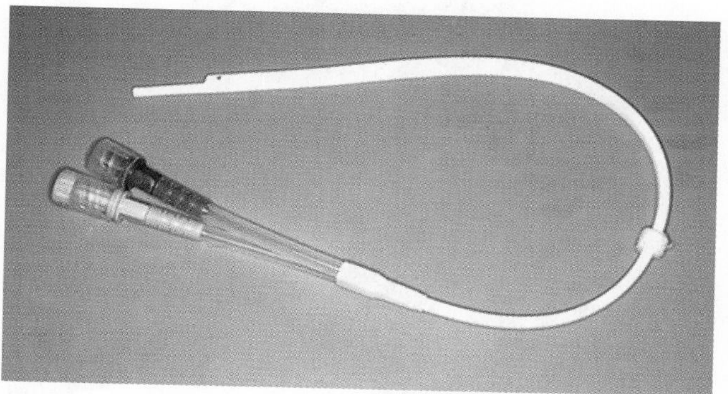

Fig. 44-13 Silastic permanent catheter used for permanent or temporary access.

A permanent, soft, flexible Silastic double-lumen catheter is being used more commonly (Fig. 44-13). It exits on the upper chest wall and is tunneled subcutaneously to the internal or external jugular vein. It has two Dacron cuffs, which reside subcutaneously to prevent infection and anchor the catheter, thus eliminating the need for sutures. The catheter must be placed radiologically. It is used as a temporary access while awaiting fistula placement and development or long-term access when other forms of vascular access have failed.

When dialysis is indicated, a permanent access is created, and a temporary access is used until the permanent access is ready to use. A subcutaneous AV fistula is created or a graft inserted, and the patient is hemodialyzed via a subclavian or jugular catheter until the AV fistula or graft is ready. Preferably the AV fistula or graft will be surgically created while the patient is being maintained on conservative therapy, well in advance of ESRD.

Dialyzers

The coil dialyzer was the first type of dialyzer used in which blood flowed through a series of cellophane tubes. Historically, this was later replaced by a flat plate dialyzer (Kiil) in which blood flowed between sheets of membrane outside of which the dialysate passed. Today the dialyzer is a long plastic cartridge that contains thousands of parallel hollow tubes or fibers (Fig. 44-14).

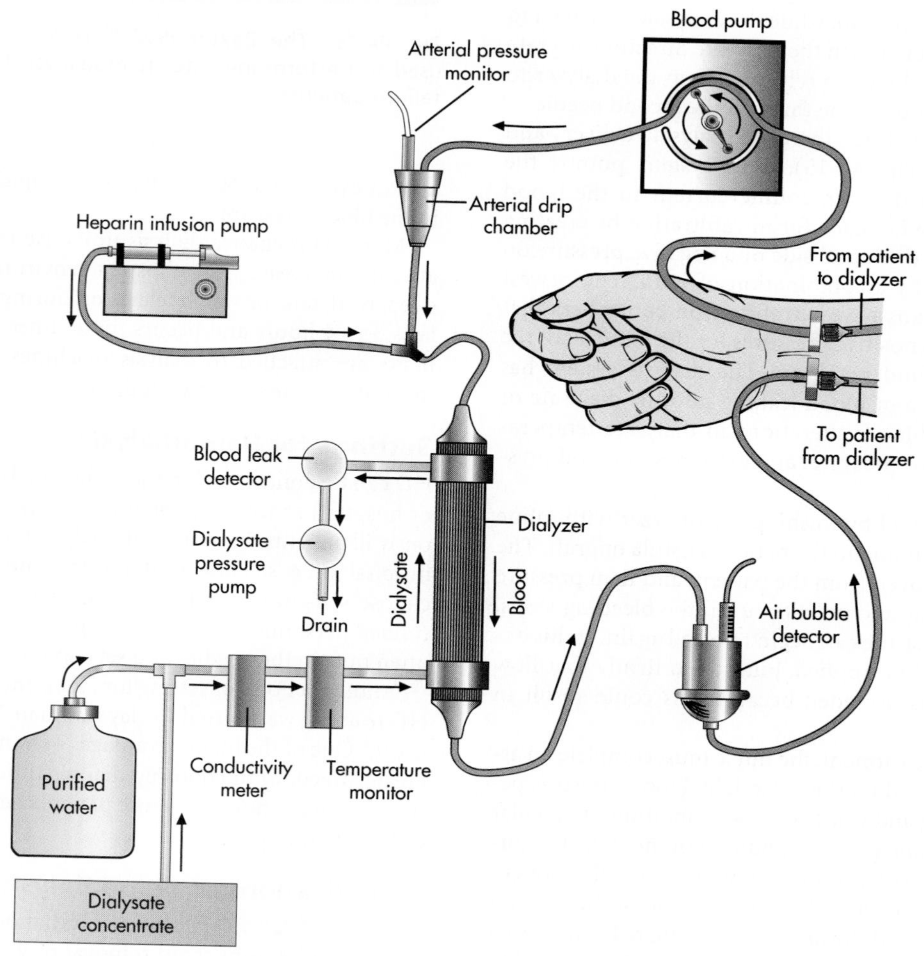

Fig. 44-14 Components of a hemodialysis system.

The fibers are the semipermeable membrane made of cellulose-based or other synthetic materials. The blood is pumped into the top of the cartridge and is dispersed to all of the fibers. Dialysis fluid (dialysate) is pumped into the cartridge and bathes the outside of the fibers with dialysis fluid. Ultrafiltration, diffusion, and osmosis occur across the pores of this semipermeable membrane. When the dialyzed blood reaches the end of the thousands of semipermeable fibers, it converges into a single tubing that returns it to the patient. Various dialyzers differ in regard to surface area, membrane composition and thickness, clearance of waste products, and removal of fluid.

Procedure

To initiate chronic dialysis, two needles are placed in the fistula or graft. The needle closest to the fistula is used to obtain "arterial" blood from the patient and send it to the dialyzer with the assistance of a blood pump. The dialyzer and blood lines are usually primed with up to 1000 ml of saline solution so no air is in the system. On initiation of hemodialysis, the saline solution is discarded as blood fills the dialyzer circuit. Heparin is added to the blood as it flows into the dialyzer because any time blood contacts a foreign substance it has a tendency to clot. Once the blood enters the extracorporeal circuit, it is propelled through the top of the dialyzer by a blood pump at a flow rate of 200 to 500 ml/min, while the dialysate (warmed to body temperature) circulates in the opposite direction at a rate of 300 to 900 ml/min. Blood is returned from the dialyzer to the patient via the "venous" line through the second needle.

In addition to the dialyzer, there is a dialysate delivery and monitoring system (Fig. 44-15). This system pumps the dialysate through the dialyzer, countercurrent to the blood flow. Adjustments can be made for ultrafiltration by creating a positive pressure in the blood side or a negative pressure on the dialysate side or by a combination of both. The newest dialysis delivery systems have ultrafiltration controllers that equalize negative and positive pressures for the removal of the precise amount of fluid per hour. The dialysis system has alarm systems to warn of blood leaking into the dialysate or air leaking into the blood; alterations in dialysate temperature, concentration, or pressure; and extremes in blood pressure readings.

Dialysis is terminated by flushing the dialyzer with saline solution to return all blood to the patient's fistula or graft. The needles are then removed from the patient, and firm pressure is applied to the venipuncture sites until the bleeding stops. On occasion the access site can begin to bleed again. If this occurs, pressure should be applied, but not so firmly that flow through the access is occluded because this could result in clotting.

Before beginning treatment, the nurse must complete an assessment that includes fluid status (weight, blood pressure, peripheral edema, lung and heart sounds), condition of vascular access, temperature, and general condition of the skin. The difference between the last postdialysis weight and the present predialysis weight determines the ultrafiltration or the amount of weight to be removed. Ideally, no more than 1.0 to 1.5 kg should be gained between treatments to avoid causing hypotension associated with the removal of larger volumes of fluid. While the patient is on dialysis, vital signs should be taken at least every 30 to 60 minutes, since rapid changes may occur in the blood pressure.

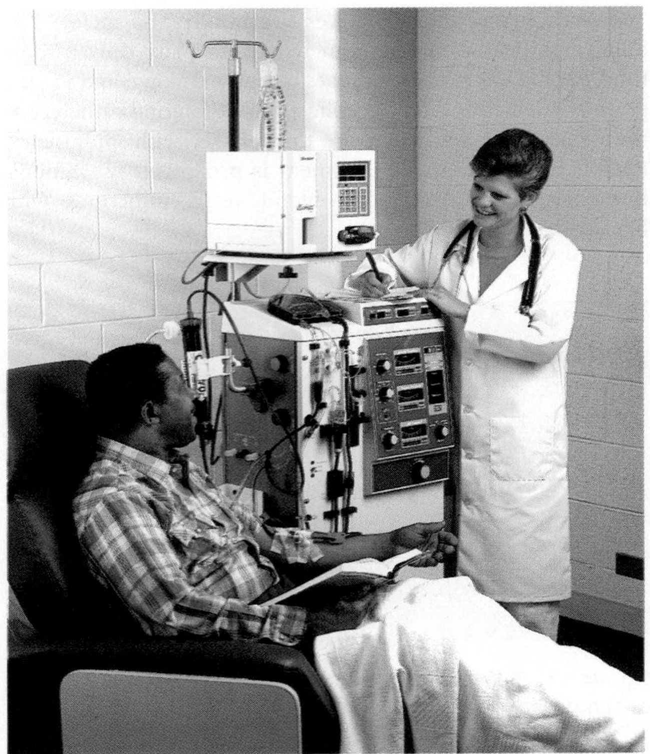

Fig. 44-15 The Baxter ISSO™ Hemodialysis Instrument is used to perform in-center hemodialysis treatments on renal failure patients.

Most maintenance dialysis units use reclining chairs in an attempt to create a nonhospital environment. Most people sleep, read, talk, or watch television during dialysis. HD usually lasts 3 to 4 hours and occurs three times per week. While patients are attached to dialysis machines, they can engage in meaningful interaction with the staff.

Settings for Hemodialysis

HD can be done in an inpatient (hospital) or outpatient (clinic or hospital) setting. Inpatient dialysis is used for treating seriously ill patients. In outpatient dialysis the patient comes to the hospital or a satellite unit for treatment. The patient may choose self-care in either setting with backup support from trained personnel if needed. The patient who chooses self-care often puts in the needles and sets up the machine.

Another choice of setting for HD is the home. In 1963 home HD training was started. Today less than 2% of patients on HD use it.[5] One of the main advantages of home HD is that it allows greater freedom in choosing dialysis times. Today home PD is the treatment choice for more patients because it is less technically demanding.

Complications of Hemodialysis

Hypotension. Hypotension that occurs during HD primarily results from rapid removal of vascular volume (hypovolemia), decreased cardiac output, and decreased systemic vascular resistance. The drop in blood pressure during dialysis may precipitate light-headedness, nausea, vomiting, seizures, vision changes, and coronary ischemia. The usual treatment for hypotension includes decreasing the volume of fluid being removed and infusion of 0.9% saline solution (100 to 300 ml). If a patient experiences recurrent hypotensive episodes, a reassessment may have to be done of dry weight and blood pressure medications. Blood pressure medications should be held before dialysis if there is hypotension during dialysis.

Muscle Cramps. Muscle cramps are a common problem in the patient on dialysis and are associated with significant discomfort and pain. They result from too rapid removal of sodium and water or from neuromuscular hypersensitivity. Treatment includes reducing the ultrafiltration rate and administering a hypertonic solution or normal saline bolus.

Loss of Blood. Blood loss may result from residual blood not being rinsed from the dialyzer, from accidental separation of blood tubing or dialysis membrane rupture, or from bleeding after the removal of needles at the end of dialysis. In a patient who has received too much heparin or has clotting problems, there can be significant postdialysis bleeding. It is essential to rinse back all blood, to closely monitor heparinization to avoid excess anticoagulation, and to hold pressure on access sites until the risk of bleeding has passed.

Hepatitis. The cause of hepatitis in the patient on dialysis is related to blood transfusions, IV drug abuse, or the lack of adherence to precautions used to prevent the spread of infection. Although the patient is frequently free of symptoms if he or she develops hepatitis B as a result of the immunocompromised state, the patient can become a carrier of hepatitis B. The incidence of hepatitis B has decreased with frequent testing for hepatitis B surface antigen (HBsAg) in patients, isolation of dialysis patients who are positive for hepatitis B, the use of disposable equipment, and the use of infection control precautions. All patients and personnel in dialysis units should receive hepatitis B vaccine.

Currently hepatitis C is responsible for the majority of cases of hepatitis in dialysis patients. (Hepatitis is discussed in more detail in Chapter 41.) Currently the Centers for Disease Control and Prevention (CDC) does not recommend isolation of the HD patient positive for hepatitis C antibody. Infection control precautions are mandated in the care of the patient with hepatitis C to protect the patient and staff. (Infection control precautions are discussed in Chapter 11.) There is currently no vaccine for hepatitis C.

Sepsis. Sepsis is most often related to infections of vascular access sites. Bacteria can also be introduced during the dialysis treatment as a result of poor technique or interruption of blood tubings or dialyzer membranes. Bacterial endocarditis can occur because of the frequent and prolonged access to the vascular system. Aseptic technique is essential to prevent this problem. Nurses must monitor patients for signs and symptoms of sepsis HD such as fever accompanied by decreasing blood pressure.

Disequilibrium Syndrome. Disequilibrium syndrome develops as a result of rapid changes in the composition of the extracellular fluid. Urea, sodium, and other solutes are removed more rapidly from the blood than from the cerebrospinal fluid and the brain. This creates a high osmotic gradient in the brain resulting in the shift of fluid into the brain, causing cerebral edema. Manifestations include nausea, vomiting, confusion, restlessness, headaches, twitching and jerking, and seizures. In addition, the rapid changes in osmolality may cause muscle cramps and contribute to hypotension. Treatment consists of slowing or stopping dialysis and infusing hypertonic saline solution, albumin, or mannitol to draw fluid from the brain cells back into circulation. It is more commonly observed in the initial treatment of the patient when the BUN level is high. First dialyses are purposely short and inefficient to limit total solute removal.

Effectiveness of and Adaptation to Hemodialysis

HD is still an imperfect technique in treating ESRD. It cannot fully replace the metabolic and hormonal functions of the kidneys. HD can relieve most of the symptoms of chronic renal failure and, if started early, can prevent certain complications. However, it does not alter the accelerated atherosclerosis.

The yearly death rate of patients on maintenance dialysis has increased from about 10% to almost 20%.[5] The major reason for this is the increased proportion of older adult patients who are now receiving dialysis as maintenance therapy. The majority of deaths are caused by cardiovascular-related disease (cerebrovascular accident or myocardial infarction). Infectious complications are the second leading cause of death. Many of the complications associated with chronic renal failure continue after the transplantation period and can affect the success of a kidney transplant.

Individual adaptation to maintenance HD varies considerably. Initially many patients feel positive about the machine because it makes them feel better. Some people come to hospitals or satellite units for dialysis because they know that if they are not treated, they will become sicker and die. Dependence on a machine is a reality. Many patients have dreams about being tied to the machine. Depression and suicidal tendencies may be manifested in noncompliance with diet or drug therapy or in a large weight gain. A primary nursing goal is to help the patient regain or maintain positive self-esteem and continue to be productive in society.

CONTINUOUS RENAL REPLACEMENT THERAPY

CRRT is an alternative or adjunctive method for treating acute renal failure.[14] CRRT provides a means by which solutes and fluids can be removed slowly and continuously in the hemodynamically unstable patient. CRRT is especially useful in the individual with fluid overload regardless of the cause of the overload (e.g., acute renal failure with or without hemodynamic instability, pulmonary edema).[15] If a patient with acute renal failure has life-threatening manifestations of uremia (e.g., hyperkalemia, pericarditis), HD is indicated for therapy rather than any of the continuous renal replacement therapies. However, CRRT can be used in conjunction with HD for continuous fluid removal.

There are several technical variations of CRRT. Both fluid and solute removal can be achieved with continuous therapies. There are two types of CRRT differentiated by whether arterial or venous access is required (Table 44-11). The continuous arteriovenous therapies (CAVTs) require arterial access because arterial pressure is needed to pump blood through the circuit. Vascular access is achieved by means of an

Table 44-11 Types of Continuous Renal Replacement Therapies

Term	Description
SCUF	Slow continuous ultrafiltration
CAVH	Continuous arteriovenous hemofiltration
CVVH	Continuous venovenous hemofiltration
CAVHD	Continuous arteriovenous hemodialysis
CVVHD	Continuous venovenous hemodialysis
CAVHDF	Continuous arteriovenous hemodiafiltration
CVVHDF	Continuous venovenous hemodiafiltration

AV Scribner external shunt (rarely used) or cannulation of the femoral artery and vein or a subclavian vein. The CAVTs include slow continous ultrafiltration (SCUF), continuous arteriovenous hemofiltration (CAVH), and continuous arteriovenous hemodialysis (CAVHD). Continuous venovenous therapies (CVVT) achieve the same goals as CAVT but use venous access necessitating the use of a blood pump to propel the blood through the circuit. In many clinical situations CVVT is preferred because it is difficult to obtain and maintain arterial access for long periods of time.

In CRRT a highly permeable hollow fiber hemofilter removes plasma water and nonprotein solutes, which are collectively termed *ultrafiltrate*. When the hydrostatic pressure exceeds the oncotic pressure, water and nonprotein solutes pass out of the filter into the extracapillary space and drain through the ultrafiltrate port into a collection device (Fig. 44-16). The remaining fluid continues through the filter and returns to the patient through the venous access site. While the ultrafiltrate pours out of the hemofilter, fluid and electrolyte replacements can be infused into the venous port. This fluid is designed to replace volume and solutes such as sodium, chloride, bicarbonate, and glucose and is free of unwanted solutes such as creatinine, urea, potassium, and phosphates. The infusion rate of replacement fluids is determined in accordance with the ultrafiltration rate to control weight reduction and fluid and electrolyte elimination. Replacement fluid may also be infused into the arterial port. This method of fluid replacement allows for greater clearance of urea and can decrease filter clotting. Like HD, CRRT provides for the removal of fluid, electrolytes, and solutes. However, several of its features differ from HD, including the following:

1. It is continuous rather than intermittent.
2. Solute removal occurs by means of convection rather than by osmosis and diffusion (no dialysate required).
3. It has fewer or no effects on cardiovascular stability (e.g., hypotension).
4. It does not require the specialized skills of an HD nurse.
5. It does not require complicated HD equipment.

CRRT can be continued as long as 30 to 40 days, but the hemofilter is changed about every 24 to 48 hours because of loss of filtration efficiency or clotting. The ultrafiltrate should be clear yellow, and specimens may be obtained for evaluation of serum chemistries. If the ultrafiltrate becomes bloody or blood tinged, a possible rupture in the filter membrane should be suspected, and treatment should be suspended immediately to prevent blood loss and infection.[16]

During CRRT the nurse must monitor fluid and electrolyte balance. Hourly intake and output measurements and daily weights must be recorded. Vital signs and hemodynamic status should be monitored hourly. Although reductions in central venous pressure and pulmonary artery pressure are expected, there should be little change in mean arterial pressure or cardiac output. Assessment and care of the vascular access sites are important.

An alternative to CAVH is CAVHD. During CAVHD a bag of PD solution is connected to the end of the hemofilter opposite the ultrafiltration port and infused, creating a diffusion gradient. The advantage of CAVHD is that urea and creatinine clearances are greater than during CAVH. The increased rate of solute removal can reduce the incidence of uremia, acidosis, and electrolyte imbalances. High ultrafiltration rates can be achieved by changing the glucose concentration of the dialysis solution to create a greater osmotic gradient.

KIDNEY TRANSPLANTATION

Major advances have been made in the art and science of organ transplantation since the first kidney transplant was performed in 1954 in Boston between identical twins. The advances made in organ procurement and preservation, surgical techniques, tissue typing and matching, understanding the immune system, immunosuppressant therapy, and preventing and treating rejection have dramatically increased the demand for organs for transplantation.

The supply and demand discrepancy is most severe in kidney transplantation because almost 210,000 patients are on dialysis. Kidney transplantation is extremely successful, with 1-year graft survival rates at almost 90% for cadaver-donated kidneys and 90% to 95% for recipients of live donor kidneys. At the end of 1997 nearly 35,000 patients were awaiting cadaveric kidney transplants, but less than 8600 cadaveric kidney transplants were performed during the same year.[17] Transplantation from a cadaver donor usually requires a prolonged waiting period, averaging close to 2 years. In 1997 there were approximately 3100 living related and 650 living unrelated (spousal and biologically unrelated) kidney transplants.[5]

The advantages of kidney transplantation as compared with dialysis include the reversal of many of the pathophysiologic changes associated with renal failure as normal kidney function is restored. It also eliminates the dependence on dialysis and the accompanying dietary restrictions, provides the opportunity to return to normal life activities (including work), and is less expensive than dialysis after the first year.

RECIPIENT SELECTION

Appropriate recipient selection is important for a successful outcome. Candidacy is determined by a variety of medical and psychosocial factors that vary among transplant centers. A careful evaluation is completed in an attempt to identify and minimize potential complications after transplantation. Certain patients, particularly those with cardiovascular disease and those with diabetes mellitus, are considered high risk. However, with a careful evaluation and monitoring, these high-risk patients can achieve the same success rates as other patients.[18] Some patients who are approaching ESRD may undergo transplant

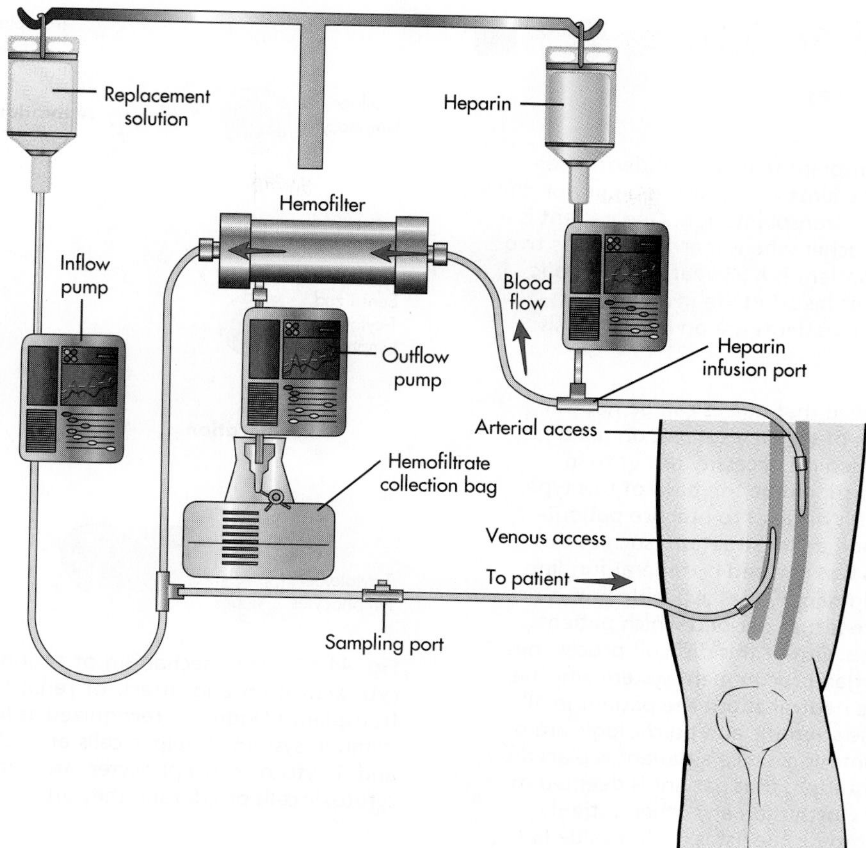

Fig. 44-16 Continuous arteriovenous hemofiltration.

surgery before they require dialysis. This approach is most advantageous for patients with diabetes, who have a much higher mortality rate on dialysis than nondiabetics.

Contraindications to transplantation include disseminated malignancies, refractory cardiac failure, chronic respiratory failure, extensive vascular disease, chronic infection (including HIV), and unresolved psychosocial disorders (e.g., noncompliance with medical regimens, alcoholism, drug addiction). Having hepatitis B or C is not an absolute contraindication to transplantation.

Surgical procedures may be required before transplantation based on the results of the recipient evaluation. For example, a bilateral nephrectomy may be considered in a patient with (1) intractable hypertension secondary to renin activity in the person's own kidneys, (2) any problem causing repeated urinary tract or kidney infections, and (3) polycystic kidney disease with grossly enlarged kidneys or repeated infection or bleeding in the cysts. However, pretransplant nephrectomies are rarely performed. Some patients may undergo coronary artery bypass graft surgery for advanced coronary artery disease in preparation for kidney transplantation.

Histocompatibility Studies

ABO blood group antigens must be compatible (see Table 28-8). Histocompatibility testing is performed to determine the degree of genetic similarity between the donor and recipient. Human leukocyte antigens (HLAs), which identify the individual's genetic makeup, are determined to assess histocompatibility (see Chapter 12). All recipients and donors express HLA antigens on all nucleated cells. The recognition of non-self HLA antigens by the recipient's immune system initiates the attack against the transplanted organ (Fig. 44-17).

The HLA antigens are located on chromosome 6. Major HLA loci that have been identified in this region include A, B, C, D, and D-related (DR) (see Fig. 12-10). Each locus may have multiple alleles (antigens). Each person has two antigens at each locus, one inherited from each parent. Because the genes that code for HLA are closely linked, they are inherited as a group or haplotype. One haplotype is inherited from each parent (see Fig. 12-10).

The purpose of histocompatibility testing is to identify the two antigens at each locus for both donors and potential recipients. A serologic test is used to type for the antigens at all five loci (A, B, C, D, and DR) with lymphocytes taken from peripheral blood. Currently only the A, B, and DR antigens are thought to be clinically significant for renal transplantation. Because there are two antigens at each of the loci, a total of six antigens are identified. The total time required for HLA typing is about 4 to 6 hours.

In cadaveric transplantation an attempt is made to match as many antigens as possible between the HLA-A, HLA-B, and HLA-DR loci. Antigen matches of five and six antigens and certain four-antigen matches have been found to have better outcomes. A good match is less important if a donor is available because limited "cold times" (i.e., the time from when the kidney is removed from the donor and revascularized in the recipient) allow for better outcomes.

ETHICAL DILEMMAS

Allocation of Resources

SITUATION

The nurse on the transplant team is considering her feelings about two patients who want to be put on the waiting list for kidney transplantation. One patient is a 40-year-old school teacher who is married and has two children. The other patient is a 58-year-old alcoholic who has spent most of his adult life in and out of prison. Currently both patients are on hemodialysis.

DISCUSSION

It is tempting to believe that nurses can be neutral, basing our allocation of scarce resources on need rather than worth. Medical necessity rather than societal contribution should be the basis of this type of decision. However, it is difficult to practice patient-neutral care in life and death situations such as this. Before renal dialysis was covered by federal funding and before the equipment was as available as it is now, there were committees that decided which patients would receive dialysis. Out of this difficult process has grown a national organ procurement system which is, in itself, set up to be neutral about the patient in all respects except those scientific and psychologic areas relevant to transplantation. Once a patient is placed on the list for transplantation, that patient is deemed of no greater or lesser worth than any other patient. However, being placed on the list is itself a value laden process, not just a neutral medical assessment. In kidney transplantation, there is no option but to transplant the organ into the best matched patient, regardless of the person's position on the list or the health professional's opinion of the patient's worth.

ETHICAL AND LEGAL ISSUES

- Blaming the patient for his disease and his lifestyle choices does not contribute to the appropriate professional detachment owed to all patients. Unless past medical history or current compliance will affect treatment decisions, they are best left out of consideration for allocation of scarce resources.
- Organ transplantation systems are based on medical necessity, prognosis, and need. If two patients of equal medical standing are on the list for organ transplantation, the first one on the list has priority unless the patient's tissue type does not appropriately match that of the donor kidney.
- Any attempt to bring moral judgments about the worth of patients into the selection process for allocation of scarce resources raises the questions of criteria and authority.
- Since organ donation is voluntary and altruistic in the United States, any concerns that the system of procurement and transplantation is not fair may negatively affect the pool of available organs.

Another test done is termed a *crossmatch.* This is done at the time a living donor is being evaluated and just before surgery for live and cadaver donors. A crossmatch uses serum from the recipient mixed with donor lymphocytes to test for any preformed cytotoxic (anti-HLA) antibodies to the potential donor kidney. A positive crossmatch indicates that the recipient has cytotoxic antibodies to the donor and is an absolute contraindication to transplantation. The potential recipient may have been exposed to antigens similar to those of the donor by means of previous blood transfusions, pregnancy, or a previous kidney transplant. If transplanted, the kidney would undergo hyperacute rejection. This procedure takes about 3 to 5 hours. A negative crossmatch indicates that no preformed antibodies are present and it is safe to proceed with transplantation.

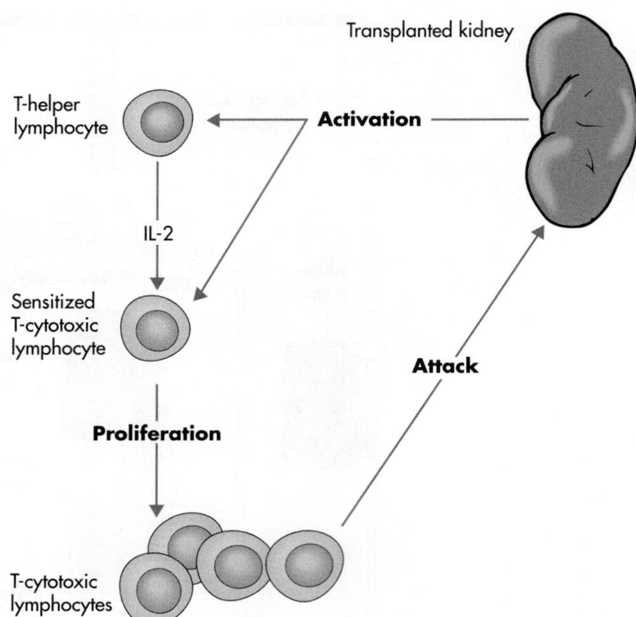

Fig. 44-17 The mechanism of action of T-cytotoxic lymphocyte activation and attack of renal transplanted tissue. The transplanted kidney is recognized as foreign and activates the immune system. T-helper cells are activated to produce IL-2, and T-cytotoxic lymphocytes are sensitized. After these T-cytotoxic cells proliferate, they attack the transplanted kidney.

Crossmatching is also performed to detect preformed cytotoxic antibodies in the recipient serum to HLA antigens on lymphocytes from random donors. In this situation, rather than using specific donor lymphocytes, the recipient serum is mixed with a randomly selected panel of donor lymphocytes to determine reactivity. This is called the panel of reactive antibodies (PRA) and indicates the recipient's sensitivity to various HLA antigens. The results are calculated in percentages. A high PRA indicates that the person has a large number of cytotoxic antibodies, which means that there is a poor chance of finding a crossmatch-negative donor. In patients awaiting transplantation a PRA panel is usually done on a monthly basis.

All patients wishing to be transplanted must have these tests done. If a patient is awaiting a cadaveric kidney, the information related to HLA will be entered into the national transplant database.

Donor Sources

Kidneys for transplantation may be obtained from blood type–compatible cadavers, blood relatives, or emotionally related individuals, such as spouses, adoptive parents or children, and, less commonly, friends. In 1997 about 25% of the total number of kidney transplants performed involved living related donors, and about 5% were from living unrelated donors.[5]

Live Donors. Advantages of a live donor include the following:

1. Patient and graft survival rates are improved, even with unrelated donors who may have no HLA antigens in common with the recipient.
2. The kidney is immediately available (no 2- to 3-year wait).
3. It is elective surgery with the recipient in the best possible medical condition.
4. The kidney usually functions immediately because there is minimal cold time.

Live donors must undergo extensive evaluation to be certain that they are in good general health and have no history of diseases that would place them at risk for developing kidney or other significant diseases later on, such as diabetes, hypertension, or cystic kidney disease. In addition to a compatible blood type, the recipient must have a negative crossmatch with the donor indicating there are no preformed antibodies to the donor's HLA.

Crossmatches for live donors are done at the time of evaluation and 1 day before the transplant. The second crossmatch ensures that no new antibodies have developed in the interval. Once donor and recipient compatibility are confirmed, the donor is scheduled to see the nephrologist for a complete history and physical examination and laboratory studies. Laboratory studies include a 24-hour urine study for creatinine clearance and total protein, complete blood count (CBC), and chemistry and electrolyte profile. Blood tests to rule out the presence of infectious diseases that could be transmitted from the donor to the recipient are also obtained. These include hepatitis B and C, HIV, and cytomegalovirus (CMV). An ECG and chest x-ray are also done. The next phase of the evaluation involves a renal ultrasound and a renal arteriogram to ensure that the blood vessels supplying each kidney are normal. An arteriogram is done to determine which kidney will be removed for transplantation and to ensure that there are no anatomic abnormalities that would preclude transplantation.

The donor must also be evaluated by a transplant psychologist or social worker who will determine if the individual is emotionally stable and can deal with the issues related to organ donation. All donors must be informed regarding the risks and benefits of donation, the potential short- and long-term complications, what the evaluation entails, and what can be expected during the hospitalization and recovery phases. Although the cost of the evaluation and surgery are covered by the recipient's insurance, there is no compensation available for lost wages during the posthospitalization recovery period, which can be as long as 6 weeks for jobs requiring heavy manual labor. Most transplant centers have an interdisciplinary team comprising transplant surgeons, nephrologists, nurse coordinators, psychologists, and social workers who participate in the donor evaluation and selection process.

Cadaver Donors. Cadaver kidney donors are previously healthy individuals who have suffered an irreversible brain injury. The most common causes of injury are cerebral trauma from motor vehicle accidents or gunshot wounds, intracerebral or subarachnoid hemorrhage, and anoxic brain damage resulting from a cardiac arrest. The brain-dead donor must have effective cardiovascular function and must be supported on a ventilator to preserve organ viability. The age range of most suitable kidney donors is 2 to 70 years of age. The age of the donor is generally less important than the quality of kidney function. The donor must be free of IV drug abuse, malignancies, sepsis, chronic diseases that result in renal damage (e.g., diabetes mellitus, hypertension, systemic lupus erythematosus), and communicable diseases, including HIV, hepatitis, syphilis, and tuberculosis. Permission from the donor's legal next-of-kin is required after brain death is determined even if the donor carried a signed donor card.

The kidneys are removed attached to the aorta and vena cava and flushed with a sterile, cold preservation solution and either preserved in the iced solution or on a pulsatile perfusion machine that continuously pumps the preservation solution through the kidneys. Kidneys can be preserved for up to 72 hours, but most transplant surgeons prefer to transplant kidneys before the cold time reaches 24 hours. Experience has shown that longer cold time increases the likelihood that the kidney will not function immediately, and the transplant recipient will require dialysis until the acute tubular necrosis (ATN) caused by the prolonged cold time resolves.

Kidneys are distributed by the United Network for Organ Sharing (UNOS) using an objective computerized point system. All kidney transplant candidates' ABO and HLA typing are entered into the national computer at the time they are listed. When a donor becomes available, the donor's HLA, ABO, and other key information are compared through the computer with the ABO and HLA typing of all patients awaiting transplantation in the local area where the donor is hospitalized. ABO compatibility between donor and recipient is mandatory. A national search is also conducted. If a six HLA-antigen match is identified nationally, one of the donor kidneys must be sent to that recipient's transplant center. If there is no six HLA-antigen match, the potential recipient with the best HLA match in the local area receives the most points. Additional points are given for waiting time compared with other recipients in the same locale. Potential recipients who have a high PRA ($> 80\%$) also receive extra points because the presence of these antibodies severely limits the number of kidneys for which they would be eligible. Once the patient with the most points is identified, she or he is called in for the transplant. The transplant is not done until the final crossmatch comes back negative.

SURGICAL PROCEDURE

Live Donor

The donor nephrectomy is usually performed by a urologist or transplant surgeon at the same time that the recipient is being surgically prepared for the kidney transplant in an adjoining operating room. After routine operative preparation and induction of general anesthesia for a conventional nephrectomy, the donor is placed in a lateral decubitus position on the operating table so the flank is presented laterally. An incision is made at the level of the eleventh rib. The rib is often removed to provide adequate visualization of the kidney. The kidney is carefully dissected free with its renal artery and vein. The ureter is also dissected with great care to preserve the periureteral vascular supply. The renal artery and vein are clamped and divided. The kidney is removed; flushed with a chilled, sterile electrolyte solution; and prepared for transplant into the recip-

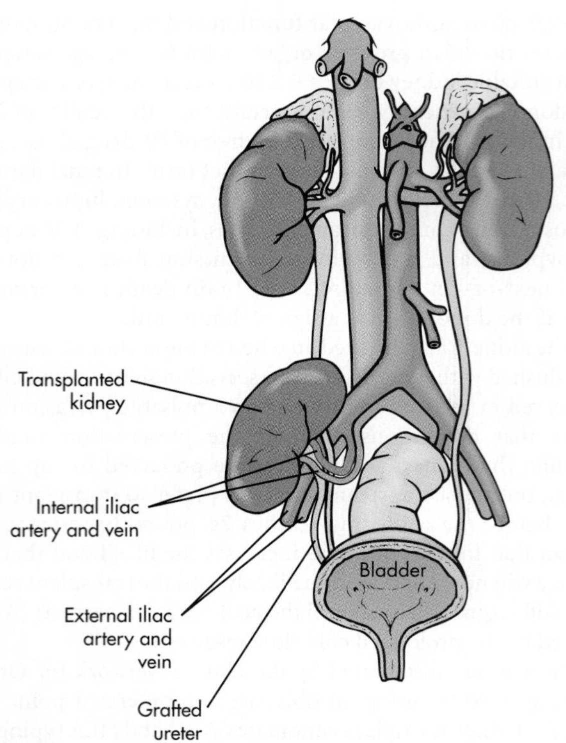

Fig. 44-18 Surgical placement of transplanted kidney.

ient. The whole procedure takes about 2 hours. Immediately after removal the organ is carried to the recipient's operating room for placement. This very limited cold time is a key reason for the success of living donor transplants.

Laparoscopic donor nephrectomy is an alternative to a conventional nephrectomy. (Laparoscopic nephrectomy is discussed in Chapter 43.) The laparoscopic approach significantly decreases the hospital stay, pain, debilitation, and length of time off work. For this reason it has increased the number of people willing to donate a kidney.

Kidney Transplant

The transplanted kidney is placed extraperitoneally in the iliac fossa. Intraperitoneal placement may be indicated in certain circumstances, such as in a small person for whom the transplanted kidney is too large to fit in the extraperitoneal space or in individuals who have received previous transplants or have inadequate extraperitoneal vascular access.[19]

Before any incisions are made, a urinary catheter is placed into the bladder. An antibiotic solution is instilled to distend the bladder and decrease the risk of infection. An incision is made extending from the iliac crest to the symphysis pubis. The peritoneum is left intact and retracted upward while the common iliac, external iliac, and hypogastric arteries and common and external iliac veins are dissected free.

Efficient revascularization is critical to prevent ischemic injury to the kidney. In the live donor kidney transplant, an end-to-side anastomosis between the donor renal artery and the recipient hypogastric artery or internal iliac artery is made. In the cadaver transplant, the donor renal artery is anastomosed to the side of the recipient hypogastric artery or internal iliac artery (Fig. 44-18).

The kidney is positioned in the iliac fossa, and the iliac vein is clamped until the donor renal vein is anastomosed to the recipient iliac vein. When the clamp is released and blood flow to the kidney is reestablished, the kidney becomes firm and pink. Urine may begin to flow from the ureter immediately. Mannitol or furosemide (Lasix) may be administered intravenously to promote diuresis.

The donor ureter in most cases is tunneled through the bladder submucosa before entering the bladder cavity and sutured in place. This is termed *ureteroneocystostomy.* This allows the bladder to clamp down on the ureter as it contracts for micturition, thereby preventing reflux of urine up the ureter into the transplanted kidney. On closing, a drain is inserted adjacent to the incision to facilitate removal of excess blood and serum from the operative site. The transplant surgery takes approximately 3 to 4 hours.

NURSING MANAGEMENT: KIDNEY TRANSPLANT RECIPIENT

Nursing care of the kidney transplant recipient is challenging, complex, and rewarding. The successful recovery and rehabilitation of the recipient is made possible with careful nursing assessment, diagnosis, intervention, and evaluation of all body systems. With a hospital length of stay averaging 7 days, time and attention must be paid to discharge planning and teaching needs early in the hospital course.

■ Preoperative Care

Nursing care of the patient in the preoperative phase includes emotional and physical preparation for surgery. Since the patient and family may have been waiting 2 to 3 years for the kidney transplant, a review of the operative procedure and what can be expected in the immediate postoperative recovery period is necessary. It is important to stress that there is a 20% chance the kidney will not function immediately and dialysis may be required for the first few weeks. In addition, the need for immunosuppressive medications and the importance of preventing infection after surgery must be stressed.

To ensure the patient is in optimal physical condition for surgery, an ECG, chest x-ray, and laboratory studies are ordered. Dialysis may be required before surgery to achieve optimal fluid, electrolyte, and acid-base balance, as well as remove excess nitrogenous wastes. A patient on peritoneal dialysis must empty the peritoneal cavity of all dialysate solution before going to surgery. Because dialysis may be required after transplant, the patency of the vascular access must be maintained. Before surgery, the extremity containing the vascular access should be lightly wrapped with Kerlix and labeled "dialysis access." This identification will remind all health care professionals to avoid using the affected extremity for blood pressure measurement, blood drawing, or IV infusions.

■ Postoperative Care

Live Donor. The usual postoperative care is similar to that after a conventional or laparoscopic nephrectomy (see Chapter 43). Often the donor is the forgotten person because most of the attention is focused on the kidney recipient. The pain of a conventional nephrectomy is greater than that of the iliac fossa incision used for the recipient. Most donors are ready to be discharged from the hospital in 3 to 5 days and can usually return to work in 4 to 6 weeks. Patients with laparoscopic nephrectomy have much less pain than with conventional nephrectomy, are able to be discharged from the hospital in 2 to 3 days, and return to work in 2 to 3 weeks. Renal function studies and a complete blood count are performed before discharge. The donor is seen by the surgeon within 2 weeks after discharge.

The majority of kidney donors feel good about donation because of the improved health of their close family member or friend. If the kidney does not function immediately or is rejected, the donor may feel disappointed, angry, or guilty. The donor is a healthy individual who donated a kidney and took a leave from work and family to do so. Nurses caring for live donors need to acknowledge the precious gift they have given.

Recipient. The first priority of care during this period is maintenance of fluid and electrolyte balance. In many centers, kidney transplant recipients spend the first 24 hours in the intensive care unit because of the close monitoring required. Renal function with rapid diuresis may begin soon after the blood supply to the transplanted kidney is reestablished. This diuresis is due to (1) the new kidney's ability to filter blood urea nitrogen, which acts as an osmotic diuretic; (2) the abundance of fluids administered intravenously during the operation; and (3) the renal tubular dysfunction, which inhibits the kidney from concentrating urine normally. Urine output during this phase may be as high as 1 L per hour, slowing down as the BUN and serum creatinine levels return toward normal. For every ml of urine output, IV fluid is administered hourly for the first 12 to 24 hours. Central venous pressure readings are essential for monitoring postoperative fluid status. Dehydration must be avoided to prevent subsequent renal hypoperfusion and renal tubular damage. Electrolyte monitoring to assess for hypokalemia often associated with rapid diuresis and for hyponatremia resulting from the inability of the kidney tubules to concentrate urine is critical. Treatment with potassium supplements or 0.9% normal saline solution infusion may be indicated. Intravenous sodium bicarbonate may also be required.

As mentioned earlier, 20% of patients receiving cadaver kidneys preserved for longer than 24 hours experience delayed graft function. The ischemic damage from prolonged preservation results in ATN. The period of ATN can last anywhere from several days to weeks, with gradually improving kidney function. Most of these patients will be discharged from the hospital on dialysis. This is extremely discouraging for the patient, who needs reassurance that renal function usually improves. Dialysis will be discontinued when urine output increases and serum creatinine and urea nitrogen begin to normalize. Some patients have high-output ATN; that is, they are able to excrete the fluid but unable to excrete metabolic wastes and control electrolytes. Other patients have oliguric or anuric ATN. These patients are at risk for fluid overload in the immediate postoperative period.

A sudden decrease in urine output in the early postoperative period warrants concern. It may be caused by dehydration, rejection, a technical complication, or an obstruction that impedes urine flow. A common cause of early obstruction is a blood clot in the urinary catheter. Because the catheter remains in the bladder for 3 to 5 days to allow the bladder anastomosis to heal, patency must be maintained. If blood clots are suspected, careful sterile catheter irrigation can dislodge the occluding clots. This should not be attempted without an order from the physician.

Most patients undergo ultrasonography within 24 hours of transplantation to assess vascular supply and to look for any fluid collections such as hematoma, lymphocele, or urine leak. Hydronephrosis, with or without a dilated ureter, may indicate obstruction. A radionucleotide renal scan is performed to assess blood supply to the kidney, as well as the kidney's ability to concentrate and then excrete the radioisotope iodohippurate sodium iodine 131 (Hippuran^{131}). Hippuran^{131} is injected through a peripheral vein and timed scanning is performed over the kidney, ureter, and bladder. Abnormal results can include minimal isotope filtering into the kidney, indicating an inadequate blood supply; isotope slowly filtering through the kidney into the ureter, demonstrating ATN; isotope being filtered only to a certain point in the urinary tract, suggesting obstruction; or isotope filtering outside the urinary tract, demonstrating urine leakage or extravasation.

Once the patient has sufficiently recovered from the operative procedure, nursing care involves ongoing assessment, diagnosis, intervention, and evaluation of the patient's response to the transplant. These include the prevention and treatment of rejection, infection, complications of surgery, and complications of immunosuppression. Patient education to ensure a smooth transition from hospital to home is an integral part of the nursing care.

IMMUNOSUPPRESSIVE THERAPY

The goal of immunosuppression is to adequately suppress the immune response to prevent rejection of the transplanted kidney while maintaining sufficient immunity to prevent overwhelming infection. Many of the medications used to achieve immunosuppression have adverse effects. By using a combination of medications that work in different phases of the immune response, lower doses of each drug produce effective immunosuppression while minimizing side effects.[20] Immunosuppressive protocols are highly variable among transplant centers, with different combinations of medications used. Most kidney transplant patients are initially on triple therapy consisting of combination of drugs that suppress the immune system in different ways. Doses of maintenance drugs may be decreased over time, and some patients can be weaned off corticosteroids (prednisone) after 1 to 2 years.

The major groups of immunosuppressive agents are (1) cyclosporine (Sandimmune, Neoral), tacrolimus (Prograf/FK506), or sirolimus (Rapamune); (2) mycophenolate mofetil (CellCept), azathioprine (Imuran), or cylophosphamide (Cytoxan); and (3) corticosteroids. Antithymocyte globulin (ATG), antilymphocyte globulin (ALG), and muromonab-CD3 are IV medications used for short periods to prevent or reverse acute rejection. The drugs, route of administration, mechanism of action, and adverse side effects are presented in Table 44-12.

Cyclosporine and Similar Drugs

Cyclosporine (Sandimmune), first used in Europe in 1978, is now being used in most kidney transplant centers in the United

DRUG THERAPY

Table 44-12 **Immunosuppressive Therapy for Renal Transplant Recipients**

Agent	Route of Administration	Mechanism of Action	Adverse Side Effects
Azathioprine (Imuran)	IV, PO	Antimetabolite that suppresses proliferation of rapidly dividing cells, including sensitized T and B lymphocytes	Bone marrow suppression (leukopenia, anemia, thrombocytopenia), drug-induced hepatitis, oral lesions, increased susceptibility to infection, alopecia, malignancies, pancreatitis
Corticosteroids Prednisone, Deltasone Methylprednisolone (Solu-Medrol)	 PO IV	Suppresses inflammatory response; prevents proliferation of T-cytotoxic lymphocytes; inhibits cytokine production	Cushingoid syndrome (peptic ulcer, hypertension, GI bleeding, aseptic necrosis, sodium and water retention, acne, muscle weakness, fat dystrophy, capillary fragility, delayed healing, hyperglycemia, mood alterations); bacterial, fungal, and viral infections
Cyclophosphamide (Cytoxan)	PO	Alkylating agent that interferes with DNA, RNA, and protein synthesis	Alopecia, leukopenia, hemorrhagic cystitis
ATG, ALG	IV	Polyclonal antibody directed against lymphocytes, reduces circulating lymphocytes, decreases lymphocyte proliferation	Serum sickness (fever, chills, malaise, joint and muscle pain), leukopenia, anaphylactic shock, rash, local phlebitis, thrombocytopenia, infection, lymphoma
Cyclosporine (Sandimmune)	PO, IV	Prevents production and release of interleukin 2 (IL-2) and gamma interferon; inhibits maturation of T-cytotoxic lymphocyte precursors	Hepatotoxicity, nephrotoxicity, lymphomas, infections, hirsutism, hypertension, tremors, gingival hyperplasia, hypermagnesemia, seizures
Cyclosporine (Neoral)	PO	Microemulsion available in capsules or oral solution with more consistent absorption than Sandimmune	Same as above
Tacrolimus (Prograf, FK506)	PO	Prevents production and release of IL-2 and gamma interferon; inhibits maturation of T-cytotoxic lymphocyte precursors	Hepatotoxicity, nephrotoxicity, neurotoxicity, hyperglycemia, gastrointestinal toxicity, alopecia, seizures, hypertension, lymphoma
Mycophenolate mofetil (CellCept)	PO	Antimetabolite that inhibits purine synthesis; suppresses proliferation of T and B cells	Gastrointestinal toxicity (diarrhea, nausea, vomiting), leukopenia, thrombocytopenia
Sirolimus (Rapamune)	PO	Suppresses lymphocyte proliferation; inhibits B cells from synthesizing antibodies	Gastrointestinal toxicity (diarrhea, nausea, vomiting)
Muromonab-CD3 (Orthoclone OKT3)	IV	Monoclonal antibody that binds to CD3 receptors on lymphocytes and lyses cells	Fever, tachycardia, infections, headache, vomiting, chills, joint and muscle pain, diarrhea, hypertension, hypotension, bronchospasm, infection, aseptic meningitis, malignancies
Daclizumab (Zenapax)	IV	Monoclonal antibody (hybrid of human and mouse) that acts as an IL-2 receptor antagonist by inhibiting the binding of IL-2; inhibits T cell activation and proliferation	Gastrointestinal toxicity (nausea, diarrhea, constipation, abdominal pain)
Basiliximab (Simulect)	IV	Same as above	Same as above

ALG, antilymphocytic globulin; *ATG*, antihymocytic globulin; *DNA*, deoxyribonucleic acid; *HLA*, human leukocyte antigen; *PO*, oral; *RNA*, ribonucleic acid.

States. The mechanism of action of this fungus extract is to prevent the production and release of interleukin-2 (IL-2) from T-helper lymphocytes (see Fig. 44-17). Since the proliferation and maturation of T-cytotoxic lymphocytes is mediated by IL-2, cyclosporine alters the cell-mediated immune attack against the transplanted kidney. This drug does not cause bone marrow depression or alter the normal inflammatory response. Cyclosporine is used in conjunction with corticosteroids or with a combination of corticosteroids and mycophenolate mofetil. Many of the side effects of cyclosporine are dose related. Cyclosporine is nephrotoxic, and absorption is incomplete and inconsistent from dose to dose. For this reason, drug levels are followed closely to prevent toxicity. Neoral, a microemulsion of cyclosporine, is replacing Sandimmune because of better and more consistent absorption.[24] Neoral and Sandimmune are not biocompatible and should never be given in exchange for the other.

Like cyclosporine, tacrolimus (Prograf, FK506) inhibits cytokine production (including IL-2), inhibits expression of IL-2 receptors, and blocks cell division. It is 100 times more potent than cyclosporine. It is never used in combination with cyclosporine because of the nephrotoxicity of both drugs. Tacrolimus does not cause hirsutism or gingival hyperplasia and is often selected over cyclosporine for women and adolescents because of these body image effects.

Sirolimus (Rapamune, rapamycin) is a new immunosuppressive agent with structural similarities to tacrolimus. Sirolimus suppresses lymphocyte proliferation and inhibits B cells from synthesizing antibodies. In relatively low doses it has a synergistic effect with cyclosporine, corticosteroids, or both.

Mycophenolate Mofetil

Mycophenolate mofetil (CellCept) is a lymphocyte-specific inhibitor of purine synthesis with antiproliferative effects on both T and B lymphocytes.[22] This drug appears to be most effective when used in combination with the immunosuppressant agents cyclosporine, tacrolimus, or sirolimus. Its effects are additive because it acts later in the lymphocyte activation pathway by an entirely different mechanism. Mycophenolate mofetil is being used in place of azathioprine (Imuran) at many transplant centers in the immunosuppressive regimen because of its greater lymphocyte-specific effects.

Antithymocyte Globulin and Antilymphocyte Globulin

ALG and ATG are also used as immunosuppressive therapy in many transplant centers. These agents are prepared by immunizing horses, rabbits, or goats with human lymphoblasts (for ALG) or thymocytes (for ATG). The antibody made against human lymphocytes is then purified and administered intravenously. The actual mechanism of action of ATG and ALG is not known. These polyclonal antibody preparations, which are directed against lymphocytes, induce lymphopenia and decrease the proliferative response of T lymphocytes, possibly as a result of the generation of T-suppressor lymphocytes. ATG and ALG are used for induction to prevent rejection immediately after transplantation or less commonly to treat an acute rejection episode.

Allergic reactions to the foreign proteins, manifested by fever, arthralgias, and tachycardia, are common but usually not severe enough to preclude use. These reactions can be attenuated by administering the preparation slowly, over 4 to 6 hours, and premedicating patients with acetaminophen (Tylenol), diphendydramine HCl (Benadryl), or methylprednisolone (Solu-Medrol). Patients may develop antibodies against the antisera, limiting the drugs' effectiveness during subsequent courses of treatment. The main toxicities of these antisera are lymphopenia and thrombocytopenia caused by antibody contaminants that are not completely removed during preparation of the antisera.

Monoclonal Antibodies

Monoclonal antibodies are used for preventing and treating acute rejection episodes. (Monoclonal antibodies are discussed in Chapter 12.) Muromonab-CD3 was the first of these monoclonal antibodies to be used in clinical transplantation. It is a mouse monoclonal antibody that reacts with the CD3 antigen found on the surface of human thymocytes and mature T cells. Therefore muromonab-CD3 is an anti–antigen-receptor antibody that interferes with the function of the T lymphocyte, the pivotal cell in the response to graft rejection. This agent reverses 95% of acute rejection episodes. Muromonab-CD3 is administered via IV push daily for 10 to 14 days.

Unfortunately all T cells are affected rather than just the subset active in graft rejection. Within minutes after the initial infusion of muromonab-CD3, circulating T cells become essentially undetectable.

A flulike syndrome occurs that lasts through the first few days of treatment. Side effects include fever, rigors, headache, myalgias, and various gastrointestinal disturbances. To reduce the expected side effects of CD3, patients should receive acetaminophen, diphenhydramine, and corticosteroids at the time of IV infusion. Newer-generation monoclonal antibodies include daclizumab (Zenapax) and basiliximab (Simulect). These monoclonal antibodies are a hybrid of mouse and human antibodies and have fewer side effects than muromonab-CD3.

COMPLICATIONS OF TRANSPLANTATION

Rejection

Rejection is one of the major problems following kidney transplantation. Rejection can be hyperacute, acute, or chronic.

Hyperacute Rejection. Hyperacute (antibody-mediated) rejection occurs minutes to hours after transplantation. Preformed cytotoxic antibodies from pregnancy, blood transfusions, or previous transplants bind to donor antigens in the kidney. Renal vessels thrombose and the kidney dies. There is no treatment and the transplanted kidney is removed. Hyperacute rejection can usually be prevented by avoiding the transplantation of a kidney with HLA antigens to which the recipient has been sensitized. However, on occasion the final crossmatch does not detect these preformed antibodies.

Acute Rejection. Acute rejection most commonly occurs 4 days to 4 months after transplantation. This type of rejection is mediated by the recipient's T-cytotoxic cells, which attack the foreign kidney. It is not uncommon to have at least one rejection episode, especially with cadaver kidneys. These episodes are usually reversible with additional immunosuppressive therapy, which consists of increased doses of corticosteroids, muromonab-CD3, ALG, or ATG. Signs of rejection include increasing serum creatinine, elevated BUN, fever, weight gain, decreased urine output, increasing blood pressure, and tenderness over the transplanted kidney. It is sometimes difficult to distinguish between acute rejection and nephrotoxicity from cyclosporine or tacrolimus.

Chronic Rejection. Chronic rejection is a process that occurs over months or years and is irreversible. The kidney is infiltrated with large numbers of T and B cells characteristic of an ongoing, low-grade immunologically mediated injury. Chronic rejection is associated with a gradual occlusion of the renal blood vessels. Signs include proteinuria, hypertension, and increasing serum creatinine levels. There is no definitive therapy for this type of rejection. Switching immunosuppressive therapy has brought some improvement for some patients. Treatment is mainly supportive. This type of rejection is difficult to manage and is not associated with the optimistic prognosis of acute rejection. Patients with chronic rejection should be put on the transplant list in the hope that they can be retransplanted before dialysis is required.

Infection

Infection remains a major cause of morbidity and mortality after transplantation.[23] The transplant recipient is at risk for infection because of alteration of the body's normal defense mechanisms by surgery, immunosuppressive medications, and the effects of ESRD. Any underlying systemic illness such as diabetes mellitus, systemic lupus erythematosus, malnutrition, and older age further compounds the effects on the immune response. The signs and symptoms of infection can be subtle. Nurses caring for transplant recipients must be astute in their observation and assessment because prompt diagnosis and treatment of infectious disease can improve patient outcomes.

The most common infections observed in the first month after transplantation are similar to those acquired by any postoperative patient, such as pneumonia, wound infections, IV line and drain infections, and urinary tract infections.[24] In addition, fungal and viral infections are prevalent secondary to the patient's immunosuppressed state. Fungal infections from *Candida, Cryptococcus, Pneumocystis carinii,* and other fungi are difficult to treat.

Viral infections, especially the herpesvirus group—CMV, Epstein-Barr virus (EBV), herpes simplex virus (HSV), and varicella-zoster virus (VZV)—may be primary or reactivated.[25] Primary infections occur as new infections after transplantation from an exogenous source such as the donated organ or blood transfusion. Reactivation occurs when a virus exists in a patient and becomes reactivated after transplantation because of immunosuppression.

Because of the donor shortage and high frequency of CMV in donors, it is not practical to match CMV status between the donor and recipient. If a CMV-negative recipient receives a CMV-positive organ, he or she is given CMV immune globulin that contains CMV antibodies. This therapy will prevent the disease from occurring or at least decrease the severity of the disease. If primary CMV is diagnosed or there is symptomatic reactivation of CMV, ganciclovir (Cytovene) will be given along with immune globulin.

Hypertension

Hypertension is a well-known complication of kidney failure that unfortunately is rarely cured by kidney transplant. In fact, hypertension occurs in approximately 70% of kidney transplant recipients. In kidney transplant recipients, hypertension has been attributed to acute or chronic rejection episodes, the effects of antirejection drugs (corticosteroids, cyclosporine, and tacrolimus), the presence of diseased native kidneys, and weight gain following the transplant. Less common factors include blockage of the artery perfusing the transplanted kidney (renal artery stenosis) and recurrence of the original kidney disease in the transplanted kidney.

Malignancies

The incidence of malignancies (approximately 5% of patients) in kidney transplant recipients is 100 times greater than that in the general population. In general, the primary reason for this increased incidence is related to an altered immune system secondary to immunosuppressive therapy. The malignancies include cancer of the skin and lips, lymphomas, and cervical cancer.

Recurrence of Renal Disease

Recurrence of the same type of renal disease that destroyed the original kidney takes place in some kidney transplant recipients. It is most common with certain types of glomerulonephritis and can result in the loss of a functioning kidney transplant. Patients must be advised before transplant if they have a disease known to recur.

Vascular Disease

Patients who receive transplants have an increased incidence of atherosclerotic vascular disease. Coronary artery disease is a leading cause of death after renal transplantation. Atherosclerotic vascular disease is a problem because of an inability to alter the process that started with renal failure, and because hypertension and hyperlipidemia are present and enhanced by immunosuppression with corticosteroids, cyclosporine, and tacrolimus.

ETHICAL DILEMMAS

Withdrawing Treatment

SITUATION

A 70-year-old patient with diabetes mellitus and chronic renal failure who has been on dialysis for 10 years tells the nurse he wants to discontinue his dialysis. His quality of life has diminished during the past 2 years since his wife died. He is not a prospective transplant patient. How should the nurse respond to the patient's request?

DISCUSSION

The first concern about a patient's wish to discontinue life support treatment should be his or her mental state. Is the patient clinically depressed, mentally affected by the progress of the disease or condition, or affected by the medication or treatment? If a psychiatric consultation finds that the patient is not impaired, then a competent adult patient has expressed a legally valid treatment directive. The nurse should explain the consequences of withdrawing treatment to the patient and the family, and offer a referral to hospice care. The physician should be contacted to confer with the patient and his family, and should offer palliative support.

ETHICAL AND LEGAL ISSUES

- There is no ethical responsibility to continue or finish a treatment once it has begun, especially if the patient no longer consents to it or it is no longer having the intended outcome.
- Dialysis therapy may treat renal failure, but it cannot cure it. The goal of technologic intervention is to relieve the patient's pain and suffering. But once the patient perceives that the burden of the treatment itself outweighs the benefits, a competent adult patient may decide to request the withdrawal of treatment.
- Competent adults have the legal right to have any form of treatment withheld or withdrawn, including life-sustaining treatment.

Aseptic Bone Necrosis

Aseptic necrosis of the hips, knees, and other joints can occur in kidney transplant recipients. This problem is primarily the result of chronic corticosteroid therapy and may be potentiated by altered calcium metabolism. The incidence of aseptic necrosis has decreased in the last 10 years because of lower corticosteroid doses with the discovery of cyclosporine and tacrolimus. Some patients have been successfully withdrawn from corticosteroids 1 to 2 years after transplantation and eliminated the risk of this complication.[26]

GERONTOLOGIC CONSIDERATIONS

Chronic Renal Failure

The incidence of ESRD in the United States and Canada is increasing most rapidly in older patients. Currently the average age of patients on dialysis is 60.2 years. In 1986 the average age of patients on dialysis was 56.[5] The most common diseases leading to renal failure in the older adult are hypertension and diabetes.

The health problems of the older ESRD patient differ significantly from the younger patient. For example, the incidence of other chronic illnesses increases with advancing age. Physiologic changes of clinical importance in the older ESRD patient include diminished cardiopulmonary function, bone loss, immunodeficiency, altered protein synthesis, and altered drug metabolism. Malnutrition is common in the older ESRD patient for a variety of reasons, including lack of mobility, lack of understanding of basic nutritional requirements, social isolation, physical disability, impaired cognitive function, and malabsorption problems.[27]

The older patient and the family need to consider what is the best form of dialysis. Home peritoneal dialysis allows the patient to be more mobile and to enjoy an increased sense of control over the illness. Peritoneal dialysis is not as hemodynamically stressful as HD. On the other hand, PD requires self-care or assistance from a family member. The older adult may not want to burden the family to get involved in the medical care. Establishing vascular access for HD may be difficult in an older patient.

Withdrawal from dialysis accounts for 9% of deaths in ESRD patients in the United States and Canada. For patients over 70 years old, voluntary withdrawal is the most common cause of death in U.S. dialysis patients.[5] If a patient decides to withdraw from dialysis, it is crucial to support the patient, family, and dialysis staff. In the early years of the ESRD program, the older adult was not placed on dialysis. The availability of chronic PD changed this situation. The increasing number of elderly, debilitated ESRD patients on dialysis has raised a number of ethical concerns about the appropriateness of using scarce technical resources in a population with limited life expectancy.

On the other hand, substantial evidence exists showing success of dialysis (especially PD) in the elderly. Quality of life has also been reported to be good to excellent in many older ESRD patients. There appears to be no justification for excluding the older adult from dialysis programs. Rationing dialysis on the basis of age alone is not supported based on currently available outcome and quality of life data.

CRITICAL THINKING EXERCISES

CASE STUDY

Chronic Renal Failure

Patient Profile

Sue, a 46-year-old school teacher, has been treated for type 1 diabetes mellitus since the age of 15. She has been followed by her nephrologist for the past several years for manifestations of increasing chronic renal failure. Eight weeks ago she had an AV fistula created in day surgery in preparation of needing hemodialysis. Over the past week she has experienced anorexia, nausea, vomiting, and headaches.

Subjective Data

- Complains of swelling in her feet and hands
- Has gained 10 pounds (4.5 kg) in the past 2 weeks
- Complains of dyspnea and weakness when walking

Objective Data

Laboratory Data

- Creatinine clearance 8.2 ml/min
- Serum creatinine 12.8 mg/dl (1132 μmol/L)
- BUN 125 mg/dl (45 mmol/L)
- Potassium 6 mEq/L (6 mmol/L)
- Hematocrit 20%

Chest X-ray

- Pulmonary edema and cardiomegaly

Critical Thinking Questions

1. Explain the basic pathologic changes that resulted in the development of diabetic nephropathy.
2. What are the indications for dialysis in this patient?
3. Identify the abnormal diagnostic study results and why each would occur.
4. Explain why Sue developed each of her clinical manifestations.
5. What are important nursing interventions for Sue and her family?
6. Based on the assessment data provided, write one or more nursing diagnoses. Are there any collaborative problems?

NURSING RESEARCH ISSUES

1. What is the psychosocial impact of home peritoneal dialysis on the spouse and family?
2. What nursing strategies promote compliance in the dialysis patient?
3. Are the stressors for older (>65 years) dialysis patients different from those of younger patients?
4. What is the impact of kidney transplantation on rehabilitation and functional capacity?
5. What is the quality of life for a living-related donor following surgery?
6. What are the needs of the family when a patient chooses to withdraw from dialysis treatment?

REVIEW QUESTIONS

The number of the question corresponds to the same-numbered objective at the beginning of the chapter.

1. A patient is admitted to the hospital in chronic renal failure. The nurse understands that this condition is characterized by
   a. a rapid decrease in urinary output with azotemia.
   b. progressive irreversible destruction of the kidneys.
   c. an increasing creatinine clearance with a decrease in urinary output.
   d. prostration, somnolence, and confusion with coma and imminent death.
2. Prerenal causes of acute renal failure include
   a. hypovolemia and cardiogenic shock.
   b. prostate cancer and calculi formation.
   c. acute glomerulonephritis and neoplasms.
   d. septic shock and nephrotoxic injury from drugs.
3. During the oliguric phase of acute renal failure the nurse monitors the patient for
   a. hypernatremia and CNS depression.
   b. Kussmaul's respirations and hypotension.
   c. pulmonary edema and electrical changes in cardiac activity.
   d. urine with high specific gravity and low sodium concentration.
4. If a patient is in the diuretic phase of acute renal failure, the nurse must monitor for which serum electrolyte imbalances?
   a. Hyperkalemia and hyponatremia
   b. Hyperkalemia and hypernatremia
   c. Hypokalemia and hyponatremia
   d. Hypokalemia and hypernatremia
5. A systemic effect of chronic renal failure that is usually reversed by the initiation of dialysis is
   a. anemia.
   b. hyperlipidemia.
   c. psychologic changes.
   d. nausea and vomiting.
6. Measures indicated in the conservative therapy of chronic renal failure include
   a. decreased fluid intake, carbohydrate intake, and protein intake.
   b. increased fluid intake, decreased carbohydrate intake and protein intake.
   c. decreased fluid intake and protein intake, increased carbohydrate intake.
   d. decreased fluid intake and carbohydrate intake, increased protein intake.
7. One of the major disadvantages of peritoneal dialysis is that
   a. hypotension is a constant problem because of continuous fluid removal.
   b. blood loss can be extensive because of the use of heparin to keep the catheter patent.
   c. solutes are removed more rapidly from the blood than from the CNS, causing disequilibrium syndrome.
   d. high glucose concentrations of the dialysate necessary for ultrafiltration cause carbohydrate and lipid abnormalities.
8. To assess the patency of a newly placed arteriovenous graft for dialysis the nurse should
   a. irrigate the graft daily with low-dose heparin.
   b. monitor for any increase in blood pressure in the affected arm.
   c. listen with a stethoscope over the graft for the presence of a bruit.
   d. frequently monitor the pulses and neurovascular status distal to the graft.
9. A patient in end-stage renal disease on hemodialysis is considering asking a relative to donate a kidney for transplant. In assisting the patient to make a decision about his treatment, the nurse informs the patient that
   a. successful transplantation usually provides better quality of life than that offered by dialysis.
   b. if rejection of the transplanted kidney occurs, no further treatment for the renal failure is available.
   c. the immunosuppressive therapy that is required following transplantation causes fatal malignancies in many patients.
   d. hemodialysis replaces the normal functions of the kidneys and patients do not have to live with the continual fear of rejection.
10. Following a kidney transplant the nurse teaches the patient that signs of rejection include
    a. fever, weight loss, increased urinary output, increased blood pressure.
    b. fever, weight gain, increased urinary output, increased blood pressure.
    c. fever, weight loss, increased urinary output, decreased blood pressure.
    d. fever, weight gain, decreased urinary output, increased blood pressure.
11. Most of the long-term problems that occur in the patient with a kidney transplant are a result of
    a. chronic rejection.
    b. immunosuppressive therapy.
    c. recurrence of the original renal disease.
    d. failure of the patient to follow the prescribed regimen.

References

1. Biology of acute renal failure: therapeutic implications, *Kidney Int* 52:1102, 1997.
2. Stark J: Dialysis choices: turning the tide in acute renal failure, *Nursing* 27:41, 1997.
3. Franz M, Horl WH: Protein catabolism in acute renal failure, *Miner Electrolyte Metab* 23:189, 1997.
4. Ikizler TA, Himmelfarb J: Nutrition in acute renal failure patients, *Advances in Renal Replacement Therapy* 4:54, 1997.
5. *United States Renal Data System,* Washington, DC, 1998, Department of Health and Human Services.
6. Henry DH, Spivak JL: Clinical use of erythropoietin, *Curr Opin Hematol* 2:118, 1995.
7. Calkins ME: Pathophysiology of congestive heart failure in ESRD, *ANNA J* 23:457, 1996.
8. Pirzada NA, Morgenlander JC: Peripheral neuropathy in patients with chronic renal failure. A treatable source of discomfort and disability, *Postgrad Med* 102:249, 1997.
9. Headley CM: Osteitis fibrosa: treatment trends, *ANNA J* 25:21, 1998.
10. Kobrin S, Aradhye S: Preventing progression and complications of renal disease, *Hosp Med* 33:11, 1997.
11. Levey AS and others: Effects of dietary protein restriction on the progression of advanced renal disease in the modification of diet in renal disease study, *Am J Kidney Dis* 27:652, 1996.
12. Brunier G: Peritonitis in patients on peritoneal dialysis: a review of pathophysiology and treatment, *ANNA J* 22:575, 1995.
13. Berkoben M, Schwab SJ: Maintenance of permanent hemodialysis vascular access patency, *ANNA J* 22:17, 1995.
14. Gretz N, Quintel M, Kranzlin B: Extracorporeal therapies in acute renal failure: different therapeutic options, *Kidney Int* 64(suppl):S57, 1998.

15. Giuliano KK, Pysznik EE: Renal replacement therapy in critical care: implementation of a unit-based continuous venovenous hemodialysis program, *Crit Care Nurse* 18:40, 1998.
16. Joy MS and others: A primer on continuous renal replacement therapy for critically ill patients, *Ann Pharmacother* 32:362, 1998.
17. United Network for Organ Sharing (UNOS) Scientific Registry, 1998.
18. Cecka M: Clinical outcome of renal transplantation. Factors influencing patient and graft survival, *Surg Clin North Am* 78:133, 1998.
19. Odland MD: Surgical technique/post-transplant surgical complications, *Surg Clin North Am* 78:55, Richmond, VA, 1998.
20. First MR: Clinical application of immunosuppressive agents in renal transplantation, *Surg Clin North Am* 78:61, 1998.
21. Corbett J, Ross K: Neoral: the new cyclosporine, *ANNA J* 25:71, 1998.
22. Hoffmann RL, Reeder SJ: Mycophenolate mofetil (CellCept): the newest immunosuppressant, *Crit Care Nurse* 18:50, 1998.
23. Sia IG, Paya CV: Infectious complications following renal transplantation, *Surg Clin North Am* 78:95, 1998.
24. Schlatter S, McNatt GE: Risk of community infections in transplant patients: a literature review, *ANNA J* 22:590, 1995.
25. Lott S: Cytomegalovirus prophylaxis in kidney transplant recipients, *ANNA J* 22:599, 1995.
26. Is corticosteroid withdrawal after kidney transplantation a good idea? *Drugs and Therapy Perspectives* 11:13, 1998.
27. Winchester JF, Rakowski TA: End-stage renal disease and its management in older adults, *Clin Geriatr Med* 14:255, 1998.

Resources

American Council on Transplantation
700 N. Fairfax Street, Suite 505
Alexandria, VA 22314

American Kidney Fund
7315 Wisconsin Avenue
Bethesda, MD 20814-3266
800-638-8299
http://www.arbon.com/kidney/info.htm

American Nephrology Nurses' Association
ANNA National Office
East Holly Avenue, Box 56
Pitman, NJ 08071-0056
800-203-5561
Fax: 609-589-7463
http://www.inurse.com/~anna/

American Society for Artificial Internal Organs
P.O. Box C
Boca Raton, FL 33429-0468
561-391-8589
Fax: 561-368-9153
http://www.asaio.com

American Society of Transplant Physicians
6900 Grove Road
Thorofare, NJ 08086-9447
609-848-6205
Fax: 609-848-4016
http://www.astp.org/

American Society of Transplant Surgeons
P.O. Box 510
Thorofare, NJ 08086-0510
609-384-8256
Fax: 609-251-0278
http://www.asts.org

International Society for Peritoneal Dialysis
c/o Georgetown University Hospital
3800 Reservoir Road NW, PHC-6003
Washington, DC 20007
202-784-3662
Fax: 202-687-2808
http://www.ispd.org

International Society of Nephrology
http://www.med.ualberta.ca/isn/

National Association for Patients on Hemodialysis and Transplantation (NAPHT)
211 East 43rd Street, Suite 301
New York, NY 10017
212-867-4486

National Kidney Foundation
30 East 33rd St.
New York, NY 10016
212-889-2210
800-622-9010
http://www.kidney.org/

National Kidney and Urologic Diseases Information Clearinghouse (NKUDIC)
9000 Rockville Pike
Bethesda, MD 20892
301-468-6345
http://www.niddk.nih.gov/health/kidney/nkudic.htm

Nephroworld
http://www.nephroworld.com

Renalnet
http://www.renalnet.org/renalnet/renalnet.cfm

***For additional Internet resources, see the website for this book at* www.mosby.com/MERLIN/medsurg_lewis**

SECTION

10

PROBLEMS RELATED TO REGULATORY MECHANISMS

SECTION OUTLINE

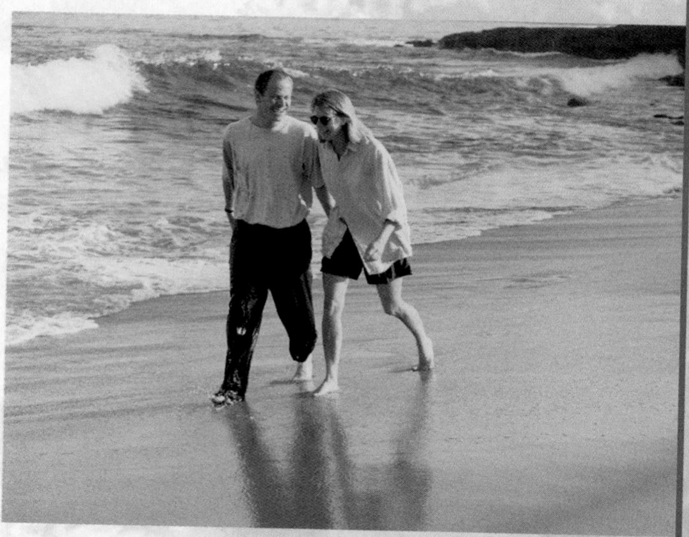

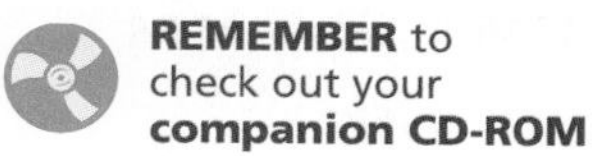

45 NURSING ASSESSMENT Endocrine System

Linda B. Haas

www.mosby.com/MERLIN/medsurg_lewis

LEARNING OBJECTIVES

1. Identify the common characteristics and functions of hormones.
2. Identify the locations of the endocrine glands.
3. Describe the functions of hormones secreted by the pituitary, thyroid, parathyroid, and adrenal glands and the pancreas.
4. Describe the locations and roles of hormone receptors.
5. Identify the significant subjective and objective assessment data related to the endocrine system that should be obtained from a patient.
6. Describe the appropriate technique used in the physical assessment of the thyroid gland.
7. Describe age-related changes in the endocrine system and differences in assessment findings.
8. Differentiate normal from common abnormal findings in the assessment of the endocrine system.
9. Describe the purpose, significance of results, and nursing responsibilities related to diagnostic studies of the endocrine system.

The endocrine system is an integrated chemical communication and coordination system that enables reproduction, growth and development, and regulation of energy. With the nervous and immune systems, the endocrine system maintains the internal homeostasis of the body and coordinates responses to external and internal environmental changes. The endocrine system is composed of glands or glandular tissues that synthesize, store, and secrete chemical messengers (hormones) that travel through the blood to specific target cells throughout the body. The specificity of this system is determined by the affinity of receptors on the target organs and tissues for a particular hormone, the "lock-and-key" mechanism (Fig. 45-1).

The endocrine glands include the hypothalamus, pituitary, thyroid, parathyroids, adrenals, pancreas, ovaries, testes, pineal, and thymus[1] (Fig. 45-2). The pineal gland, which secretes melatonin (a hormone that is secreted in response to light/dark cycles) is not discussed, because the significance of this gland in humans is not well understood.[2,3] The thymus gland, which secretes hormones (e.g., thymosin), is important in the function of the immune system and is discussed in Chapter 12. In addition to the glands mentioned above, other organs of the body secrete hormones. For example, the kidneys secrete erythropoietin, the heart secretes atrial natriuretic factor, and the gastrointestinal tract secretes numerous peptide hormones (e.g., gastrin). These hormones are discussed in the respective assessment chapters.

Reviewed by Susan Harrington, RN, MN, ARNP, Family Nurse Practitioner, University of Washington, Seattle, Wash.

STRUCTURES AND FUNCTIONS OF THE ENDOCRINE SYSTEM

Glands

Endocrine organs (glands and cells) are ductless but highly vascularized. They synthesize hormones and secrete them into blood, where they eventually affect specific target tissues. For instance, the thyroid (gland) synthesizes thyroxine (the hormone), which influences all body tissues (target tissue).

Hormones

Characteristics. A *hormone* is a chemical substance synthesized and secreted by a specific organ or tissue. Hormones are carried by the blood to other sites in the body where their actions are exerted. Most hormones have common characteristics, including (1) secretion in minute but effective amounts at variable but predictable rates, (2) circulation through the blood, and (3) binding to specific cellular receptors either in the cell membrane or within the cell.

Many hormones (e.g., somatostatin, vasoactive intestinal peptide) are synthesized and secreted by several tissues and stimulate different physiologic responses depending on the source and target tissue. For example, somatostatin is found in several areas of the brain, including the part of the hypothalamus that controls the anterior pituitary. In this instance, somatostatin inhibits growth hormone and thyroid-stimulating hormone (TSH) release. Somatostatin is also synthesized and secreted by the delta cells of the pancreas where it inhibits insulin and glucagon release.

Structure. Structurally the major hormones are amines, peptides (proteins), and steroids. Amine hormones are derived from the amino acid tyrosine. For example, catecholamines released from the adrenal medulla are derived

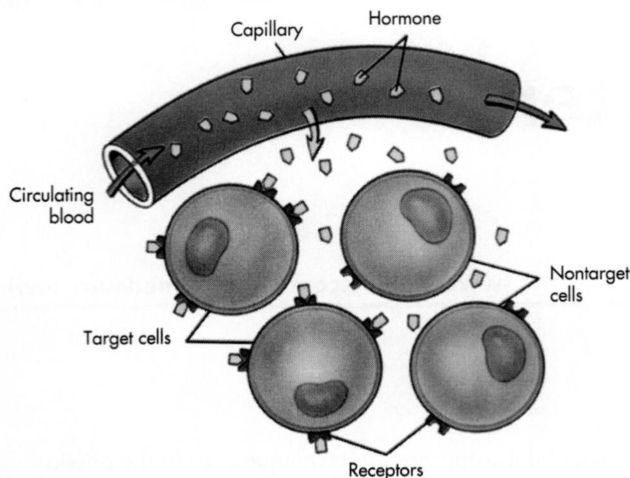

Fig. 45-1 The target cell concept. A hormone acts only on cells that have receptors specific to that hormone, because the shape of the receptor determines which hormone can react with it. This is an example of the lock-and-key model of biochemical reactions.

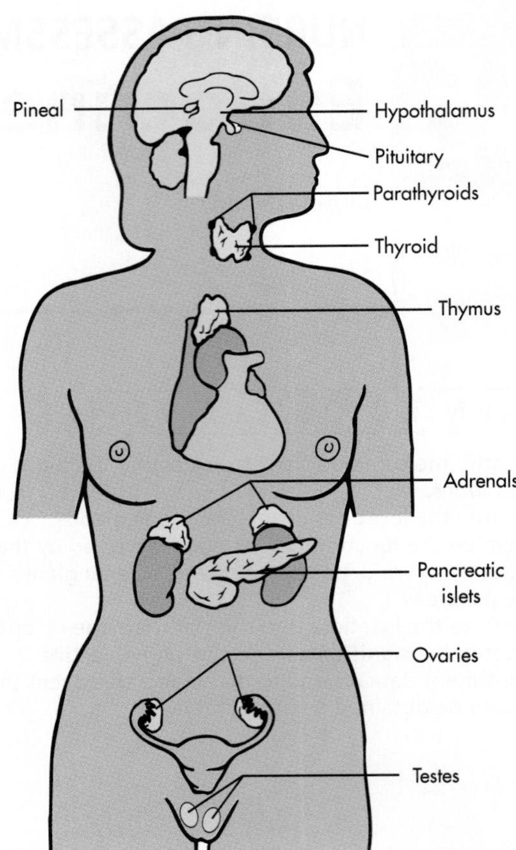

Fig. 45-2 Location of the major endocrine glands. The parathyroid glands actually lie on the posterior surface of the thyroid.

from the amino acid tyrosine. Catecholamines produce their effects by binding to receptors located on cell membranes. Thyroid hormones are also derived from the amino acid tyrosine. However, thyroid hormones bind to receptors in the cell nucleus.

Peptide hormones, which are strings of amino acids in various configurations, are unable to penetrate cell membranes because of their large size and lipid insolubility. Therefore they bind to cell membrane receptors. Some protein hormones are initially synthesized as part of larger structures (prohormones) and are not active until they have been cleaved from the prohormone. For example, proinsulin has little biologic activity, and insulin cannot exert its action until it is cleaved from proinsulin.

Steroid hormones, which have 17 carbon atoms arranged in three or four rings, are secreted by the adrenal cortices and gonads. Steroid hormones are synthesized from cholesterol, are lipid soluble, and are able to diffuse into cells and bind with cytoplasmic receptors. This hormone-receptor complex translocates to the cell nucleus to produce changes.

Transport. Steroid and thyroid hormones are not water soluble. Therefore the majority of these hormones are bound to plasma proteins for transport in the blood. When the hormones are bound to transport proteins, they can travel in the blood and not be degraded by the liver. The hormone/transport complex also acts as a reservoir. Although hormones are inactive when bound to plasma proteins, they can be released when appropriate and immediately exert their action at the target tissue. Peptide hormones and catecholamines are water soluble. Thus they do not need to be bound to proteins and circulate freely in the blood.

Functions. Hormones modulate or control a number of physiologic activities. Important hormonal functions are related to reproduction, responses to stress and injury, electrolyte balance, energy metabolism, growth, maturation, and aging. For examples, the thyroid hormone triiodothyronine regulates cellular metabolic rates, and insulin activates intracellular glucose transport proteins, which in turn enable glucose to enter cells. Table 45-1 summarizes the major hormones, glands or tissues from which they are synthesized, target organs or tissues, and functions.

Mechanism of Action. Hormones can produce their effects in several different ways, including the activation of second messengers such as cyclic adenosine monophosphate (cAMP), the synthesis of protein via increases in messenger ribonucleic acid (mRNA) levels, and directly within the cell. Hormones initiate these effects via the binding with a receptor.

Hormone Receptors

Specificity. The specificity of hormone–target cell interaction is determined by receptors. *Receptors,* or *hormone-binding sites,* are glycoprotein macromolecules of the target cell that interact with a hormone in the first step of the hormone's action. The receptor allows the hormone to recognize the cell. Steroid hormone receptors are in the cytoplasm of the target cell, thyroid and some steroid hormone receptors are in the nucleus, and receptors for other hormones are in the cell membrane.[1]

Intracellular hormone-receptor complexes, such as those seen in steroid hormone action, translocate to the cell nucleus where they bind to specific sites on DNA to stimulate or inhibit the synthesis of mRNA. When new mRNA is synthesized, it migrates to the cytoplasm, where it stimulates the synthesis of new protein. These new proteins produce specific effects in the target cell (Fig. 45-3).[4] This process requires minutes to days. In

Table 45-1 Major Endocrine Glands and Hormones

Hormones	Target Tissue	Functions
Anterior Pituitary (adenohypophysis)		
Growth hormone (GH) or somatotropin	All body cells	Promotes protein anabolism (growth, tissue repair) and lipid mobilization and catabolism
Thyroid-stimulating hormone (TSH) or thyrotropin	Thyroid gland	Stimulates synthesis and release of thyroid hormones, growth and function of thyroid
Adrenocorticotropic hormone (ACTH) or corticotropin	Adrenal cortex	Fosters growth of adrenal cortex; stimulates secretion of glucocorticoids
Gonadotropic hormones ▪ Follicle-stimulating hormone (FSH) ▪ Luteinizing hormone (LH)	Reproductive organs	Stimulates sex hormone secretion, reproductive organ growth, reproductive processes
Melanocyte-stimulating hormone (MSH)	Melanocytes in skin	Increases melanin production in melanocytes to make skin darker in color
Prolactin	Ovary and mammary glands in females	Stimulates milk production in lactating women; increases response of follicles to LH and FSH; has unclear function in men
Posterior Pituitary (neurohypophysis)		
Oxytocin	Uterus; mammary glands	Stimulates milk secretion, uterine motility
Antidiuretic hormone (ADH) or vasopressin	Renal tubules, vascular smooth muscle	Promotes reabsorption of water
Thyroid		
Thyroxine (T_4)	All body tissues	Precursor to T_3
Triiodothyronine (T_3)	All body tissues	Regulates metabolic rate of all cells and processes of cell growth and tissue differentiation
Calcitonin (CT)	Bone tissue	Regulates calcium and phosphorus blood levels, lowering of blood Ca^{2+} levels
Parathyroids		
Parathyroid hormone (PTH) or parathormone	Bone, intestine, kidneys	Regulates calcium and phosphorus blood levels (bone demineralization and increased intestinal absorption)
Adrenal Medulla		
Epinephrine (adrenalin)	Sympathetic effectors	Enhances and prolongs effects of sympathetic nervous system
Norepinephrine	Sympathetic effectors	Response to stress; enhances and prolongs effects of sympathetic nervous system
Adrenal Cortex		
Corticosteroids (e.g., cortisol, hydrocortisone)	All body tissues	Promotes metabolism, response to stress
Androgens (e.g., testosterone and androsterone) and estrogen	Sex organs	Promotes masculinization in men, growth and sexual activity in women
Mineralocorticoids (e.g., aldosterone)	Kidney	Regulates sodium and potassium balance and thus water balance
Pancreas		
Islets of Langerhans		
Insulin (from beta cells)	General	Promotes movement of glucose out of blood and into cells
Glucagon (from alpha cells)	General	Promotes movement of glucose from storage and into blood
Somatostatin	Pancreas	Inhibits insulin and glucagon secretion
Gonads		
Women: Ovaries		
Estrogen	Reproductive system, breasts	Stimulates development of secondary sex characteristics, preparation of uterus for fertilization and fetal development; stimulates bone growth
Progesterone	Reproductive system	Maintains lining of uterus necessary for successful pregnancy
Men: Testes		
Testosterone	Reproductive system	Stimulates development of secondary sex characteristics, spermatogenesis

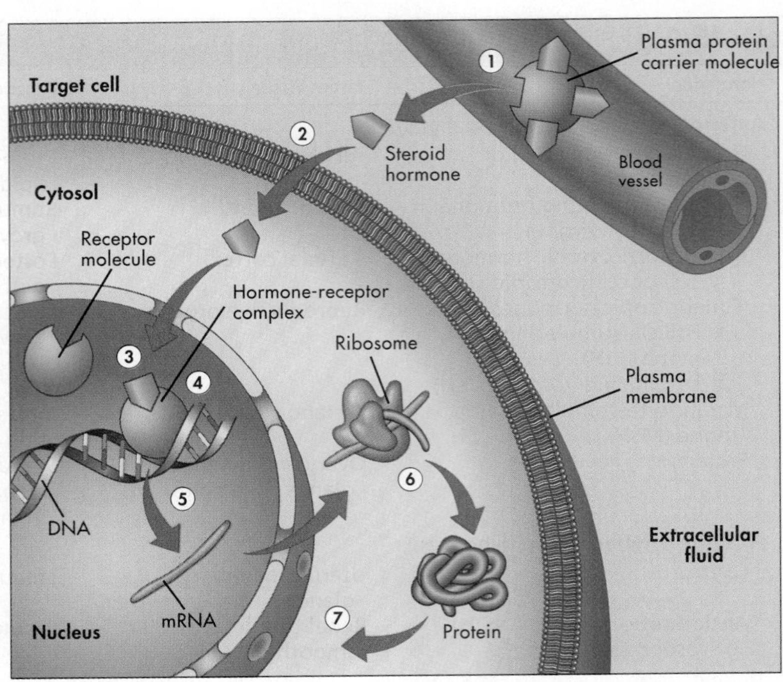

Fig. 45-3 Steroid hormone mechanism. According to the mobile-receptor hypothesis, lipid-soluble hormone molecules detach from a carrier protein *(1)* and pass through the plasma membrane *(2)*. The hormone molecules then pass into the nucleus where they bind with a mobile receptor to form a hormone-receptor complex *(3)*. This complex then binds to a specific site on a DNA molecule *(4)*, triggering transcription of the genetic information encoded there *(5)*. The resulting mRNA molecule moves to the cytosol, where it associates with a ribosome, initiating synthesis of a new protein *(6)*. This new protein—usually an enzyme or channel protein—produces specific effects in the target cell *(7)*.

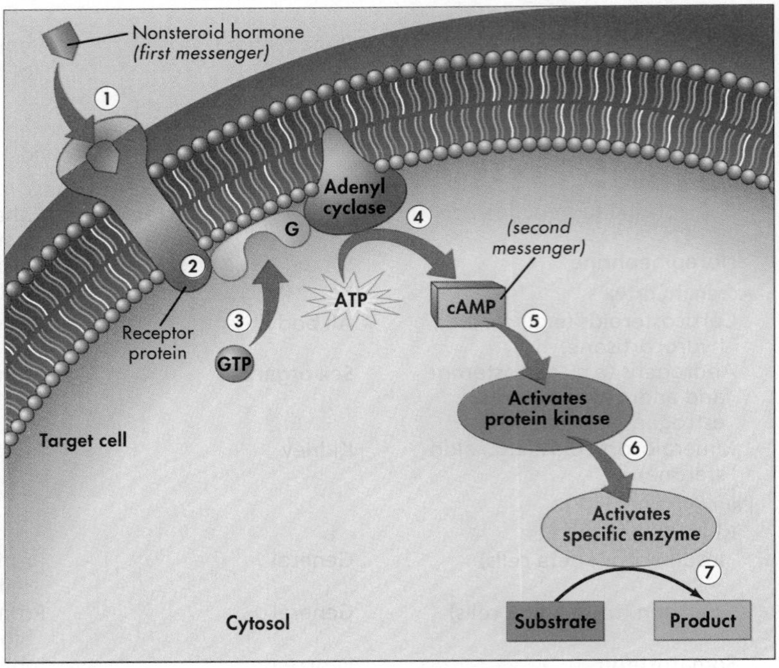

Fig. 45-4 Example of a second-messenger mechanism. A nonsteroid hormone (first messenger) binds to a fixed receptor in the plasma membrane of the target cell *(1)*. The hormone-receptor complex activates the G protein *(2)*. The activated G protein reacts with guanosine triphosphate (GTP), which in turn activates the membrane-bound enzyme adenyl cyclase *(3)*. Adenyl cyclase removes phosphates from ATP, converting it to cAMP (second messenger) *(4)*. cAMP activates protein kinases *(5)*. Protein kinases activate specific intracellular enzymes *(6)*. These activated enzymes then influence specific cellular reactions, thus producing the target cell's response to the hormone *(7)*.

contrast, thyroid hormones bind to receptors in the cell nucleus.[5] Thyroid hormone promotes synthesis of structural and functional cellular components.

Peptide (protein) and amine hormone receptors are located in the cell membrane. The hormone-receptor complex is then linked to effector molecules via coupling by G proteins.[6] The effector molecules can stimulate or inhibit secondary messengers within the cell, which in turn alter the cell's metabolism or gene expression. These intracellular effector molecules activate secondary messengers such as cAMP and nitric oxide (NO). cAMP exerts its action by activating kinases to regulate intracellular activity (Fig. 45-4). NO activates cyclic guanosine monophosphate (cGMP) and is a major regulator of peripheral blood flow. NO is also an important messenger in the brain.

Regulation of Hormonal Secretion. The regulation of endocrine activity is controlled by specific mechanisms of varying levels of complexity. These mechanisms stimulate or inhibit hormone synthesis and secretion. One such mechanism, simple feedback, which may be negative or positive, is based on the blood level of a particular substance. This substance may be a hormone or other chemical compound regulated by, or responsive to, a hormone.

Negative feedback. In negative feedback, high levels of the substance inhibit hormone synthesis and secretion, and low

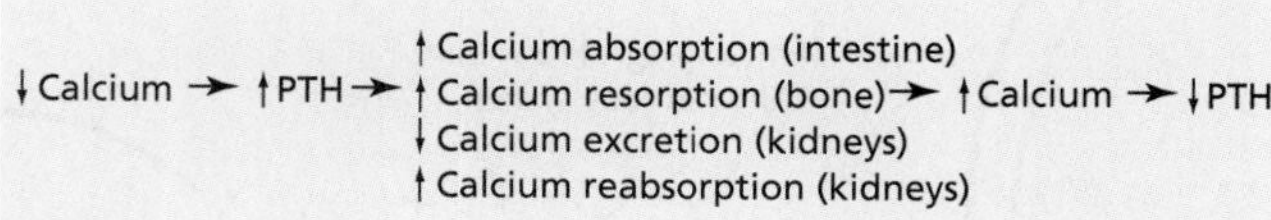

Fig. 45-5 Simple negative feedback: calcium and parathyroid hormone (PTH).

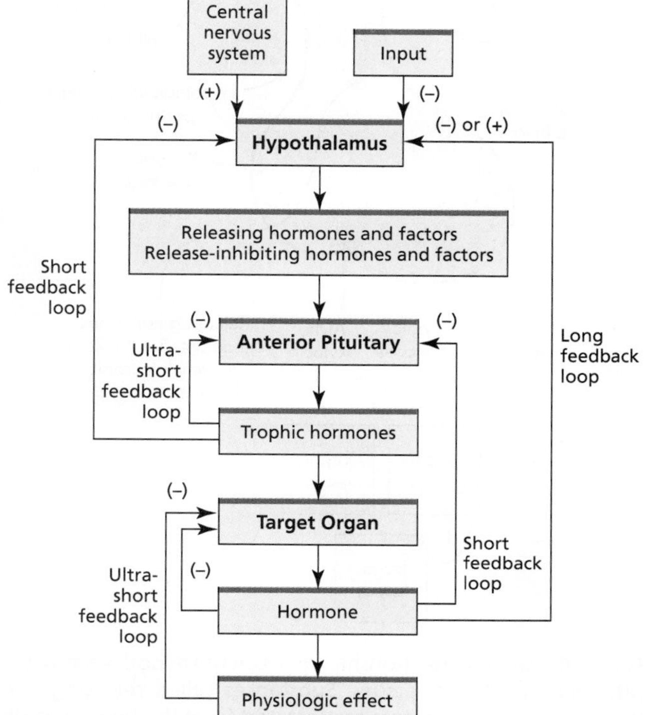

Fig. 45-6 General model for control and negative feedback to hypothalamus-pituitary target organ systems. Negative feedback regulation is possible at three levels: target organ (ultrashort feedback), anterior pituitary (short feedback), and hypothalamus (long feedback).

levels stimulate hormone synthesis and secretion. Negative feedback is similar to the functioning of a thermostat in which cold air in a room activates the thermostat to release heat, and hot air turns off the thermostat to prevent more warm air from entering the room. A physiologic example of this is the relationship between calcium and parathyroid hormone (PTH). Low blood calcium levels stimulate the parathyroid glands to release PTH, which acts on bone, the intestine, and the kidneys to increase blood calcium levels. The increased blood calcium levels then inhibit further PTH release (Fig. 45-5).

Positive feedback. In positive feedback, high levels of a substance stimulate hormone synthesis and secretion, and low levels inhibit hormone synthesis and secretion. An example of positive feedback is the stimulatory effect of increased luteinizing hormone (LH) levels on ovarian estradiol secretion during the menstrual cycle.

Complex feedback system. Another level of complexity exists in feedback systems. An example of this is regulation of thyroid hormones (Fig. 45-6). The synthesis and release of TSH or thyrotropin from the anterior pituitary is stimulated by thyrotropin-releasing hormone (TRH), which is secreted by the hypothalamus. The thyroid hormones, T_3 and T_4, have an inhibitory effect on the secretion of both TRH from the hypothalamus and TSH from the anterior pituitary.

Another example of a complex feedback system is insulin regulation (Table 45-2). High levels of circulating glucose, amino acids, and fats (as seen after a meal) stimulate insulin secretion. In addition, gastrointestinal or enteric hormones such as gastrin and gastric inhibitory polypeptide enhance insulin release after a meal, as does vagal stimulation. After a high-protein meal, the secretion of both glucagon and insulin increases. Glucagon increases gluconeogenesis and insulin has an anabolic effect on protein synthesis. Insulin secretion is inhibited by low circulating levels of glucose and amino acids, high circulating levels of steroids and catecholamines (as seen in stress), hypokalemia, and other pancreatic hormones such as glucagon and somatostatin.

Table 45-2 Factors Influencing Insulin Secretion

Stimulate Secretion	Inhibit Secretion
↑ Glucose levels	↓ Glucose levels
↑ Amino acid levels	↓ Amino acid levels
↑ Gastrointestinal hormone levels	↓ Potassium levels
↑ Vagal stimulation	↑ Steroid hormone levels
↑ Fats	↑ Catecholamine levels
	↑ Somatostatin levels
	↑ Glucagon levels (usually)
	↑ Insulin levels

Nervous system control. In addition to chemical regulation, some endocrine glands are directly affected by the activity of the nervous system. Pain, emotion, sexual excitement, and stress can stimulate the nervous system to modulate hormone secretion. Neural involvement is initiated by the central nervous system (CNS) and implemented by the autonomic nervous system (ANS). For example, stress is sensed by the CNS and the ANS secretes catecholamines to inhibit insulin secretion so that the liver can produce glucose to enable the individual to physiologically deal with stress.

Rhythms. Another regulatory mechanism affecting many hormonal secretions involves the rhythms of secretions. These rhythms originate in brain structures. A common physiologic rhythm is the diurnal (circadian) rhythm, in which a hormone level fluctuates predictably during a 24-hour period. These rhythms may be related to sleep-wake or dark-light cycles. For example, cortisol rises early in the day, declines toward evening, and rises again toward the end of sleep to peak by morning (Fig. 45-7). Growth hormone (GH) and prolactin secretion peak during sleep. TSH secretion is also maximal during sleep and ebbs 3 hours after a person awakens in the morning. The menstrual cycle is an example of a body rhythm that is longer than 24 hours (infradian). These rhythms must be considered when interpreting hormone levels on laboratory results. (See diagnostic studies section in this chapter and Chapter 48.)

Neuroendocrine System

The ANS and endocrine system are interrelated and interdependent, and together integrate stimuli to allow a coordinated response to internal or external environmental changes. The ANS controls endocrine gland blood flow and hormone

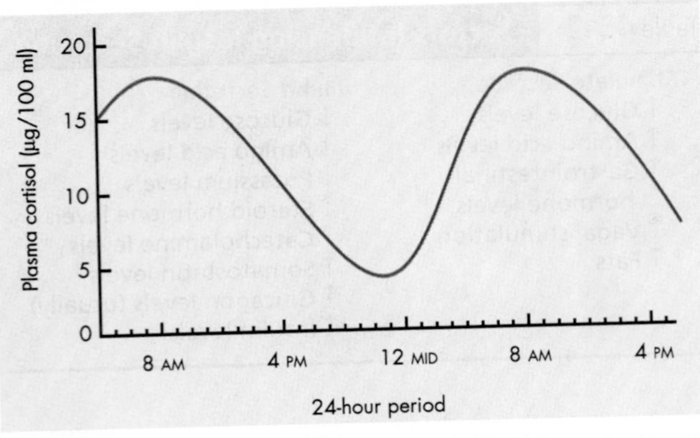

Fig. 45-7 Circadian rhythm of cortisol secretion.

Table 45-3 Hormones of the Hypothalamus

Releasing Hormones
Corticotropin-releasing hormone (CRH)
Thyrotropin-releasing hormone (TRH)
Growth hormone–releasing factor or somatotropin-releasing hormone
Gonadotropin-releasing hormone
Prolactin-releasing hormone
Inhibiting Hormones
Somatostatin (inhibits growth hormone release)
Prolactin-inhibiting hormone

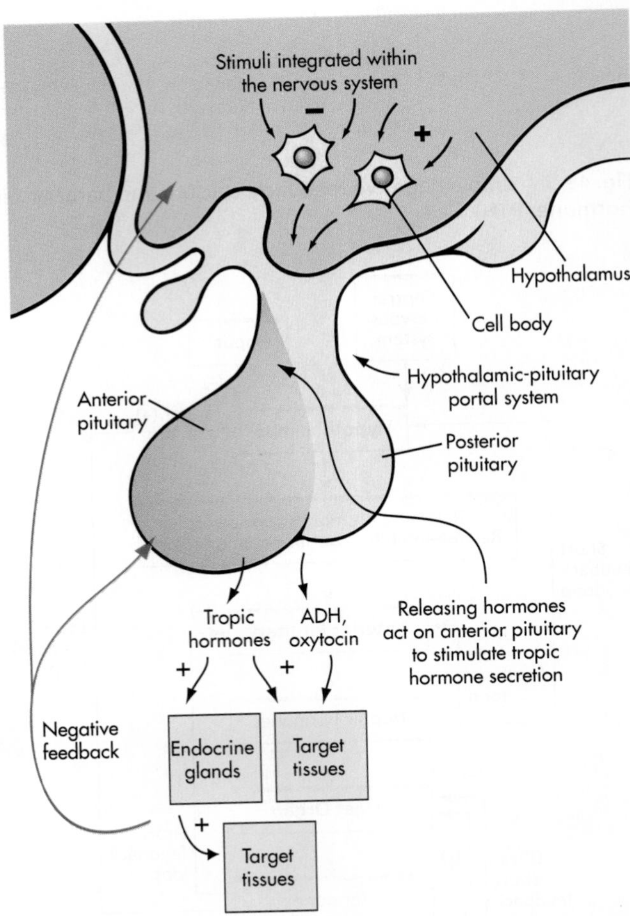

Fig. 45-8 General relationship between the hypothalamus, the pituitary, and target tissues. Substances called releasing hormones or releasing factors are secreted from the hypothalamic neurons as a result of certain stimuli. They pass through the hypothalamic-pituitary portal system to the anterior pituitary. The releasing hormones either stimulate or inhibit the secretion of anterior pituitary hormones. Secreted hormones from cells within the anterior pituitary pass through the blood and influence the activity of their target tissues. In response to stimulation of hypothalamic neurosecretory cells, action potentials pass along the axons of the neurosecretory cells to the posterior pituitary. The action potentials cause the release of neurohormones from the posterior pituitary and pass through the blood to target tissues. *ADH,* antidiuretic hormone.

secretion, and hormones have a regulatory effect on nervous tissue. For example, testosterone and estrogen affect the hypothalamic neuronal synthesis and release of gonadotropin-releasing hormone (GnRH), which in turn affects the release of follicle-stimulating hormone (FSH) and LH. Hormones can also influence behavior.[7] For example, excess growth hormone, cortisol, and PTH can cause mood swings. Depression has been associated with adrenal insufficiency.

Substances can be hormones in one instance and neurotransmitters or modulators in another. For example, catecholamines are hormones when they are secreted by the adrenal medulla and neurotransmitters when they are secreted by nerve cells in the brain and peripheral sympathetic nervous system. The differentiating factor is the mode of transport. When epinephrine travels through the blood, it is a hormone and affects a number of organs and tissues. When it travels across synaptic junctions, it acts as a neurotransmitter producing a specific effect on the effector tissue.

Hypothalamus. The hypothalamus is the most central part of the diencephalon area of the brain. The hypothalamus and the pituitary gland integrate communication between the nervous and endocrine systems.[8] CNS input is mediated by hypothalamic hormones and neurotransmitters (norepinephrine, dopamine, serotonin, and acetylcholine), which helps regulate pituitary hormone secretion. Hypothalamic hormones can stimulate or inhibit the synthesis and release of anterior pituitary hormones (Table 45-3). Two major hormones synthesized in the hypothalamus are antidiuretic hormone (ADH, vasopressin) and oxytocin.

The hypothalamus and pituitary gland communicate via veins called the median eminence portal system (Fig. 45-8). ADH and oxytocin are secreted into the portal vessels and travel to the posterior pituitary, where they are stored until needed. A major function of the hypothalamus is the secretion of releasing and inhibiting hormones that travel through this portal system to the anterior pituitary. There they interact with specific receptors and rapidly stimulate or inhibit the synthesis and release of anterior pituitary hormones (see Table 45-3).

The hypothalamus also contains neurons, which receive data from the brainstem and limbic system. These neurons also influence the limbic system, the brainstem, and spinal cord. This creates a circuit to facilitate the coordination of the endocrine system, ANS, and expression of complex behavioral responses, such as anger and feelings of fear and pleasure, to ensure homeostasis. The hypothalamus may also have a role in libido.[8]

Pituitary Gland

The pituitary gland (hypophysis) weighs approximately 0.6 g and is located in the sella turcica at the base of the brain above the sphenoid bone. It is connected to the hypothalamus by the infundibular (hypophyseal) stalk. The pituitary consists of two parts, the anterior (adenohypophysis) and the posterior (neurohypophysis) lobes, which are derived from different embryonic tissue.

Anterior Pituitary. The anterior lobe accounts for 80% of the gland by weight. Anterior pituitary function is regulated by the integrated effects of hypothalamic releasing and inhibiting hormones and feedback effects from circulating hormones. Hormones secreted by the anterior pituitary include GH, TSH, adrenocorticotropic hormone (ACTH), prolactin, gonadotropic hormones (e.g., FSH, LH), and β-lipotropin (see Table 45-1).

Posterior Pituitary. The posterior pituitary is an extension of the hypothalamus. The cell bodies of neurons that carry posterior pituitary hormones are in the hypothalamus, and the axons terminate in the posterior pituitary or neurohypophysis. The posterior pituitary lies behind the anterior pituitary and consists of unmyelinated nerve fibers and the terminals of axons. The hormones of the posterior pituitary, ADH or vasopressin and oxytocin, are produced in the hypothalamus as prohormones, travel down the nerve fibers, and are stored in the posterior pituitary near capillaries. The hormones are released into the general circulation after appropriate stimulation.

Antidiuretic hormone. The major physiologic role of ADH is regulation of fluid volume by stimulating reabsorption of water in the renal tubules. ADH, also called vasopressin, can be a potent vasoconstrictor. The most important stimulus to ADH secretion is increased osmotic pressure of body fluid as reflected by increased plasma osmolality (a measure of solute concentration of circulating blood). Plasma osmolality is increased by decreased extracellular fluid or increased sodium concentration. The increased plasma osmolality activates osmoreceptors, which are extremely sensitive, specialized neurons near the supraorbital nucleus of the hypothalamus. These activated osmoreceptors then stimulate ADH release. Therefore when body fluids become highly concentrated, osmoreceptors stimulate ADH release. In the absence of ADH, dilute urine is excreted.

Nonosmotic stimuli to ADH secretion include decreased blood volume, orthostatic changes in blood pressure, hypotension, pain, nausea, vomiting, hypoglycemia, and many pharmacologic agents (e.g., epinephrine, general anesthesia, lithium, narcotics, nicotine, tricyclic antidepressants). ADH release is inhibited by an increase in fluid volume, hypothermia, β-adrenergic agonists, and alcohol.[9]

Oxytocin. Oxytocin stimulates ejection of milk into mammary ducts and contraction of uterine smooth muscle. Oxytocin secretion is increased by stimulation of touch receptors in the nipples of lactating women. Oxytocin secretion is inhibited by endorphins and alcohol.[9]

Thyroid Gland

The thyroid gland is located in the anterior portion of the neck in front of the trachea. It consists of two encapsulated lateral lobes connected by a narrow isthmus (Fig. 45-9). The thyroid is a highly vascular organ and is regulated by TSH from the anterior pituitary.

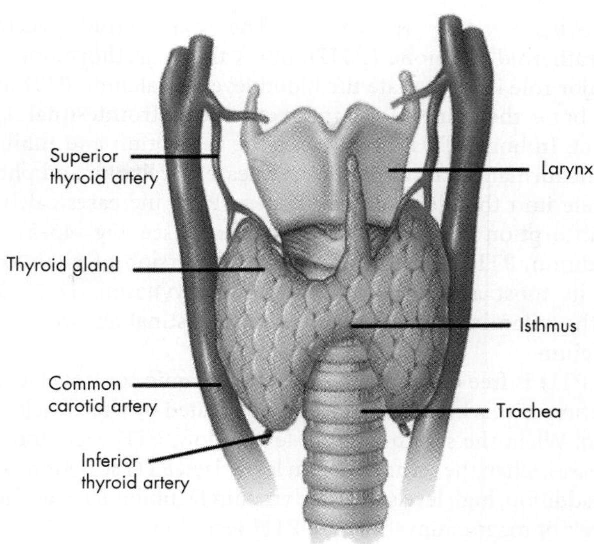

Fig. 45-9 Frontal view of thyroid gland.

Thyroxine (T_4) and Triiodothyronine (T_3). The major function of the thyroid gland is the production, storage, and release of the thyroid hormones, T_4 (thyroxine) and T_3 (triiodothyronine). T_4 is the precursor for T_3, which is the more active hormone. About 10% of circulating T_3 is secreted directly by the thyroid gland, and the remainder is obtained by peripheral conversion of T_4. Iodine is necessary for the synthesis of thyroid hormones. T_4 and T_3 affect metabolic rate, caloric requirements, oxygen consumption, carbohydrate and lipid metabolism, growth and development, brain functions, and nervous system activity. More than 99% of thyroid hormones are bound to plasma proteins, especially thyroxine-binding globulin synthesized by the liver. Only the unbound "free" hormones are biologically active.

Thyroid hormone production and release is stimulated by TSH from the anterior pituitary gland. Low circulating levels of thyroid hormone stimulate the release of TRH by the hypothalamus and TSH by the anterior pituitary. High circulating thyroid hormone levels have an inhibitory effect on the secretion of both TRH from the hypothalamus and TSH from the adenohypophysis.

Calcitonin. Calcitonin is a hormone produced by C cells (parafollicular cells) of the thyroid gland in response to high circulating calcium levels. Secretion is inhibited by somatostatin. In pharmacologic doses, calcitonin inhibits calcium resorption from bone, increases calcium storage in bone, and increases renal excretion of calcium and phosphorus, thereby lowering serum calcium levels.[10]

Parathyroid Glands

The parathyroid glands are small, oval structures arranged in pairs behind each thyroid lobe. Occasionally they are found in the chest. There are usually four glands. The major cell type of the glands is epithelial, and the gland is richly supplied with blood by fenestrated capillaries from the inferior and superior thyroid arteries.

Parathyroid Hormone. The parathyroids secrete parathyroid hormone (PTH), also called parathormone. Its major role is to regulate the blood level of calcium. PTH acts on bone, the kidneys, and indirectly the gastrointestinal (GI) tract. In bone, PTH stimulates bone resorption and inhibits bone formation, resulting in the release of calcium and phosphate into the blood. In the kidney, PTH increases calcium reabsorption and phosphate excretion (see Fig. 45-5). In addition, PTH stimulates the renal conversion of vitamin D to its most active form (1,25-dihydroxyvitamin D_3). This active vitamin D then enhances the intestinal absorption of calcium.

PTH is free of pituitary and hypothalamic control. The secretion of this hormone is directly regulated by a feedback system. When the serum calcium level is low, PTH secretion increases; when the serum calcium level rises, PTH secretion falls. In addition, high levels of active vitamin D inhibit PTH and low levels of magnesium stimulate PTH secretion.

Adrenal Glands

The adrenal glands are small, paired, highly vascularized glands located near the upper poles of each kidney and lateral to the lower thoracic and upper lumbar vertebrae. Each gland weighs about 4 g and consists of two parts, the inner medulla and the outer cortex. Each has distinct functions.

Adrenal Medulla. The adrenal medulla constitutes 10% to 20% of the gland and consists of sympathetic postganglionic neurons. The medulla secretes the catecholamines epinephrine (the major hormone [75%]), norepinephrine (25%), and dopamine. Catecholamines, usually considered neurotransmitters, are hormones when secreted by the adrenal medulla, because they are released into the circulation and transported to their target organs. Catecholamines exert their effects after binding to adrenergic receptors on cells, and they have widespread effects on all body systems.

Adrenal Cortex. The adrenal cortex, the outer part of the adrenal gland, constitutes 80% to 90% of the gland. It secretes more than 50 steroid hormones, which are classified as glucocorticoids, mineralocorticoids, and androgens. Cholesterol is a precursor for steroid hormone synthesis. Glucocorticoids (e.g., cortisol) are named for their effects on glucose metabolism. Mineralocorticoids are essential for the maintenance of fluid and electrolyte balance. Adrenal androgens and estrogens (sex steroids) are produced and secreted in small but significant amounts.

Cortisol, the most abundant and potent glucocorticoid, is necessary to maintain life. Approximately 75% to 80% of circulating cortisol is bound to transcortin (corticosteroid-binding globulin) and about 15% to albumin. The free cortisol (5% to 10% of total) binds with receptors in the cytoplasm and nucleus of a target cell.[11] The hormone-receptor complex exerts cortisol's effects within the nucleus of the target tissue. Cortisol is secreted in a diurnal pattern (see Fig. 45-7). Major functions of cortisol are to facilitate hepatic gluconeogenesis by facilitating conversion of protein to glucose and inhibiting protein synthesis and to decrease peripheral glucose use in the fasting state. In addition, cortisol contributes to lipid and nucleic acid metabolism and physiologic responses to many hormones. Cortisol is also critical in the body's response to stress. Glucocorticoids stimulate lipolysis in adipose tissue, thereby mobilizing glycerol and free fatty acids.[12]

Other effects of glucocorticoids include their antiinflammatory action and supportive actions in stressful situations. Cortisol decreases the inflammatory response by stabilizing the membranes of cellular lysosomes and preventing increased capillary permeability. The lysosomal stabilization reduces the release of proteolytic enzymes and thereby their destructive effects on surrounding tissue. Cortisol can also inhibit production of prostaglandins, thromboxanes, and leukotrienes and alter the cell-mediated immune response. Cortisol helps maintain vascular integrity and responsiveness and fluid volume, and it has mineralocorticoid effects because it can bind to mineralocorticoid receptors. A marked increase in the rate of cortisol secretion by the adrenal cortex can aid the body in coping more effectively with stressful situations (see Chapter 7).

The major control of cortisol is by means of a negative feedback mechanism that involves the secretion of corticotropin-releasing hormone (CRH) from the hypothalamus. CRH stimulates the secretion of ACTH by the anterior pituitary. Cortisol levels are also increased by surgical stress, burns, infection, fever, psychoses, acute anxiety, and hypoglycemia.

Aldosterone, a potent mineralocorticoid, maintains extracellular fluid volume. It acts at the renal tubule to promote renal reabsorption of sodium and excretion of potassium and hydrogen ions. Aldosterone synthesis and secretion are stimulated by angiotensin II (see Fig. 42-6), hyponatremia, and hyperkalemia and inhibited by atrial natriuretic factor and hypokalemia.

Adrenal androgens are the third class of steroids synthesized and secreted by the adrenal cortex. The normal adrenal cortex secretes small amounts of androgens. Adrenal androgens stimulate pubic and axillary hair growth and sex drive in females. In the female, androgens are converted to estrogen in the peripheral tissues. In postmenopausal women the adrenal cortex is the major source of endogenous estrogen (see Chapters 48 and 49). Adrenal androgen effects in men are negligible in comparison with testosterone secreted by the testes.

Pancreas

The pancreas is a long, tapered, lobular, soft gland that weighs between 60 and 90 g. It lies behind the stomach and anterior to the first and second lumbar vertebrae. The pancreas performs exocrine and endocrine functions (see Chapter 37). The islets of Langerhans are the areas of endocrine activity; they release their secretions into the portal circulation. However, the secretions are also paracrine. (Paracrine secretions diffuse to neighboring cells to exert their action, rather than traveling to their target tissues through the blood like endocrine secretions.) The islets account for less than 2% of the gland and consist of alpha, beta, and delta cells. Glucagon is synthesized by the alpha cells, insulin by the beta cells, and gastrin and somatostatin by the delta cells.

Glucagon. Glucagon is synthesized and released from pancreatic alpha cells in response to low levels of blood glucose, protein ingestion, and exercise. Glucagon stimulates hepatic glycogenolysis and gluconeogenesis and ketogenesis. Usually, glucagon and insulin function in a reciprocal manner to maintain normal blood glucose levels (euglycemia). The exception is after ingestion of a high-protein carbohydrate-free diet, in which case both hormones are secreted. In this instance, glucagon counteracts the inhibitory effect of insulin on gluconeogenesis, and euglycemia is maintained.[13]

Insulin. Insulin is the principal regulator of the metabolism and storage of ingested carbohydrates, fats, and proteins.[14] Insulin facilitates glucose transport across cell membranes in most tissues. However, the brain, nerves, the lens of the eye, hepatocytes, erythrocytes, and cells in the intestinal mucosa and kidney tubules are not dependent on insulin for glucose uptake. An increased blood glucose level is the major stimulus for insulin synthesis and secretion. Other stimuli to insulin secretion are increased amino acid levels; specific GI hormones, which enhance the response to glucose; and vagal stimulation. Insulin secretion is usually inhibited by low blood glucose levels, glucagon, somatostatin, hypokalemia, and catecholamines (see Table 45-2).

A major effect of insulin on glucose metabolism occurs in the liver, where the hormone enhances glucose incorporation into glycogen and triglyceride by altering enzymatic activity and inhibiting gluconeogenesis. Another major effect occurs in peripheral tissues where insulin facilitates glucose transport into cells, transport of amino acids across muscle membranes and their synthesis into protein, and transport of triglyceride into adipose tissue. Thus insulin is a storage, or anabolic, hormone.

The endocrine system is concerned with the regulation of body processes and the maintenance of internal homeostasis despite vastly changing substrates, as is seen in glucose homeostasis after food ingestion. After a meal, insulin is responsible for the storage of nutrients (anabolism). In the fasting state (during which ingested glucose is not readily available), hormones such as catecholamines, cortisol, epinephrine, and glucagon break down stored complex fuels (catabolism) to provide simple glucose as fuel for energy.

Heart

Atrial Natriuretic Factor. Naturietic hormones are a family of peptides; the most abundant is atrial natriuretic factor (ANF). ANF is produced by right atrial myocytes; it helps maintain fluid homeostasis. Its release is stimulated by an increase in the stretch of the atrial wall caused by an abnormally high blood volume or blood pressure. These receptors in the atrial myocytes are also stimulated by high serum sodium levels. ANF acts on the kidneys to inhibit the reabsorption of sodium ions. When sodium is lost, water follows, resulting in a decrease in blood volume and a decrease in blood pressure. ANF also inhibits renin, ADH, and the action of angiotensin II on the adrenal glands, thereby suppressing aldosterone secretion. ANF also causes vasodilation.[15]

GERONTOLOGIC CONSIDERATIONS

Effects of Aging on the Endocrine System

Normal aging has many effects on the endocrine system (Table 45-4). General changes include increased connective tissue in the glands, decreased blood supply, and decreased metabolism resulting in an increased half-life. This can be manifested by events such as changes in a hormone's basal level, response to stimuli, transport of the hormone, target organ responsiveness, and catabolism. Often one change such as decreased response to stimuli is offset by another such as decreased metabolic clearance rate so that the net effect is normal hormone levels. Because radioimmunoassays of hormone levels have become widely available, problems previously attributed to age-related endocrine changes have been found to be the effects of specific illnesses, health problems, or nutritional deficits affecting the endocrine system.

Assessment of the effects of aging on the endocrine system is difficult because the subtle changes of aging often mimic symptoms of endocrine disorders. However, there are endocrine changes with clinical significance. Aging is associated with altered hypothalamic neurotransmitters, and the hypothalamus is less sensitive to feedback inhibition. In addition, increased PTH secretion is often seen and may be related to the bone changes seen in older adults. In addition to endocrine changes related to aging, the nurse must be aware that endocrine problems may occur differently in an older adult than in a younger person.[16] Altered PTH secretion usually manifests as hyperparathyroidism. Because of altered PTH secretion the older adult often has altered mental status, fatigue, and generalized weakness rather than the kidney stones and peptic ulcers seen in a younger person.

Some symptoms of hypothyroidism in the older adult are similar to those in a younger person but are more likely to be overlooked because the symptoms, such as fatigue, mental impairment, sluggishness, and constipation, are often attributed solely to aging.[17] The older person with hypothyroidism has symptoms unique to the age set, including more disturbances of the CNS, such as syncope, convulsions, dementia, and coma. There is often pitting edema and deafness. The older patient with hyperthyroidism frequently has manifestations related only to the cardiovascular system, such as palpitations, angina, atrial fibrillation, and breathlessness. The older adult may also have depression, anorexia, and constipation (apathetic hyperthyroidism). Thus signs and symptoms often attributed to "old age" may actually indicate an endocrine problem.

ASSESSMENT OF THE ENDOCRINE SYSTEM

Hormones affect every body tissue and system, causing great diversity in the signs and symptoms of endocrine dysfunction.[7] Therefore assessment of the endocrine system is often difficult and requires keen clinical skills to detect manifestations of disorders (Table 45-5). Endocrine dysfunction may result from deficient or excessive hormone secretion, transport abnormalities, an inability of the target tissue to respond to a hormone, or inappropriate stimulation of the target-tissue receptor. If the patient has a specific problem, an appropriate health history should be taken and the system involved should be assessed. For instance, a chief complaint of tachycardia indicates the need for a cardiovascular assessment and for information related to stress, diet, exercise, and sleep. The nurse must also remember the possibility of endocrine dysfunction and assess for hyperthyroidism.

Endocrine disorders may have nonspecific or specific manifestations. For example, weight loss may be a sign of panhypopituitarism, hyperthyroidism, occasionally hypothyroidism, Addison's disease, pheochromocytoma, relative or absolute insulin deficiency, or hyperparathyroidism. Alternatively, it may

GERONTOLOGIC DIFFERENCES IN ASSESSMENT

Table 45-4 Effects of Aging on the Endocrine System

Hormone	Basal Level	Secretion	MCR	Target Organ Response	Clinical Significance
Posterior Pituitary					
ADH	↑	↑	—	↓ (renal)	Sodium imbalance, syndrome of inappropriate ADH, hyponatremia
Anterior Pituitary					
GH	↓	↓	—	—	Unknown significance
TSH	—	—	—	—	
ACTH	—	—	—	—	
Prolactin	—	—	?	?	
LH and FSH	↑	↑	?	↓	
Thyroid					
T_4	—	↓	↓	↓	Atypical presentation of hyperthyroidism
T_3	—	—	↓	↓	Increased hypothyroidism
Parathyroids					
PTH	↑	↑	?	↓ (renal)	Hypercalcemia, hypercalciuria, increased bone resorption
Adrenal Cortex					
Cortisol	—	↓	↓	↓	
Androgens	↓	↓	?	?	
Aldosterone	↓	↓	↓	?	Decreased response to sodium restriction and upright posture
Adrenal Medulla					
Epinephrine	—		—	↓	Decreased response to β-blockers (e.g., less of a decrease in heart rate and cardiac output)
Norepinephrine	↑	↑	↑	↓	Increased sympathetic nervous system activity, possible increase in hypertension
Pancreas					
Insulin	↑	↓	—	↓	Impaired glucose tolerance
Gonads					
Estrogen	↓	↓	—	?	Increased hot flashes, decreased vaginal secretions, increased risk for atherosclerosis, osteoporosis
Testosterone	↓	↓	?	?	Decreased ejaculatory force
Kidneys					
Renin	↓	↓	?	?	Decreased response to sodium restriction, upright posture
Vitamin D	↓	N/A	?	↓	Decreased intestinal absorption of calcium

↑, increased; ↓, decreased; —, no change; ?, no data or conflicting data.
ACTH, adrenocorticotropic hormone; *ADH*, antidiuretic hormone; *FSH*, follicle-stimulating hormone; *GH*, growth hormone, *LH*, luteinizing hormone; *MCR*, metabolic clearance rate; *N/A*, not applicable; *TSH*, thyroid stimulating hormone.

be due to malignancy, GI or emotional problems, or a well-planned weight reduction program. A careful health history will yield data to help sort out possible causes. Some signs of endocrine dysfunction are specific, such as the classic "polys" (polyuria, polydipsia, and polyphagia) in diabetes mellitus and exophthalmos in hyperthyroidism. Specific signs make the assessment easier; nonspecific signs and symptoms such as tachycardia and fatigue are more problematic. The lack of clear-cut manifestations of endocrine problems requires a conscientious and detailed health history.

Certain guidelines should be used in the assessment of endocrine dysfunction. Nonspecific changes should alert the clinician to the possibility of an endocrine disorder. The most common nonspecific symptoms are fatigue and depression, often accompanied by other manifestations. The latter includes changes in energy level, alertness, sleep patterns, mood, affect, weight, skin, hair, personal appearance, and sexual function (Table 45-6).

Subjective Data

Important Health Information

Past health history. During an assessment, the patient should be questioned about the general state of health and if there have been any changes. In addition, the patient or significant other should be specifically questioned about previous or concurrent endocrine abnormalities. The presence of delay or acceleration in growth and development and abnormal secondary sex characteristics (e.g., facial hair in a woman or decreased need for shaving in a man) should also be documented.

Medications. The patient should be questioned as to whether any hormone replacements are being taken, and the reasons for these hormones. This is particularly important if

HEALTH HISTORY

Table 45-5 Endocrine System

Health Perception–Health Management
- What is your usual day like?
- Have you noticed any changes in your ability to perform your usual activities compared with last year, 5 years ago?*

Nutritional-Metabolic
- What is your weight and height?
- How much do you want to weigh?
- Have there been any changes in your appetite or weight?*
- Have you noticed any changes in the distribution of the hair anywhere on your body?*
- Have you noticed any changes in the color of your skin, particularly on your face, neck, hands, or body creases?*
- Has the texture of your skin changed? For example, does it seem thicker and drier than it used to?*
- Have you noticed any difficulty swallowing, or are your shirts more difficult to button?*
- Do you feel more nervous than you used to? Do you notice your heart pounding, or that you sweat when you do not think you should be sweating?
- Do you have difficulty holding things because of shakiness of your hands?*
- Do you feel that most rooms are too hot or too cold? Do you frequently have to put on a sweater, or feel as though you need to open windows when others in the room seem comfortable?*

Elimination
- Do you have to get up at night to urinate? If so, how many times? Do you keep water by your bed at night?
- Have you ever had a kidney stone?*
- Describe your usual bowel pattern. Have you noted any bowel changes?*
- Do you use anything, such as laxatives, to help you move your bowels?*

Activity-Exercise
- What is your usual activity pattern during a typical day?
- Do you have a planned exercise program? If yes, what is it and have you had to make any changes in this routine lately? If so, why and what kinds of changes?
- Do you experience fatigue with or without activity?*

Sleep-Rest
- How many hours do you sleep at night? Do you feel rested on awakening?
- Are you ever awakened by sweating during the night?*
- Do you have nightmares?*
- Does anyone in your family complain about your snoring?*

Cognitive-Perceptual
- How is your memory? Have you noticed any changes?
- How long can you concentrate on any one thing? Has this changed lately?
- Have you experienced any blurring or double visions?*
- When was your last eye examination?

Self-Perception–Self-Concept
- Have you noticed any changes in your physical appearance or size?*
- Are you concerned about your weight?*
- Do you feel you are able to do what you think you should be capable of doing? If not, why not?
- Does your health problem affect how you feel about yourself?*

Role-Relationship
- Are you married? Do you have any children? Do you think you are able to take care of your family, home? If no, why not?
- Have there been any changes in your ability to function at work, at school?*

Sexuality-Reproductive

Women
- When did you start to menstruate? Was this earlier or later than other women in your family? Do you have scant, heavy, or irregular menstrual flows?
- How many children have you had? How much did they weigh at birth? Were you told you had diabetes during any pregnancy?*
- Were you able to nurse your children if you wanted to?
- Are you attempting to get pregnant but cannot?*

Men
- Have you noticed any changes in your ability to have an erection?*
- Are you trying to have children but cannot?*

Coping–Stress Tolerance
- Where do you work? What kind of work do you do? Are you able to do what is expected of you and what you expect of yourself?
- What kind of stressors do you have at work (school)?
- If retired, what do you do with your time? What did you do before you retired?
- If unemployed, are you looking for work?
- Is your income adequate for your needs?
- How do you deal with stress or problems?
- What is your support system? Whom do you turn to when you have a problem?

Value-Belief
- Do you think medicine should still be taken even though you feel OK?
- Does your health plan cause any conflict in your value-belief system?*

*If yes, describe.

Table 45-6 Nonspecific Manifestations of Hormone Dysfunction

Manifestations	Panhypopituitary Hormone	ADH		Thyroid Hormone		Cortisol		Mineralocorticoids		Insulin		PTH	
	Hypo	*Hyper*	*Hypo*	*Hyper*	*Hypo*	*Hyper*	*Hypo*	*Hyper*	*Hypo*	*Hyper*	*Hypo*	*Hyper*	*Hypo*
Nutrition and elimination													
Weight	↓	↑	↓	↓	↑	↑	↓	↑		↓	↓	↓	
Appetite	↓			↑	↓	↑	↓			↑	↓	↓	
Growth abnormality (children)	+				+	+	+				+		+
Abdominal pain				+	+		+				+	+	
Stool output	↓			↑	↓							↓	
Urine output		↓	↑					↑			↑	↑	
Cardiovascular system													
Blood pressure		↑	↓			↑		↑		↑			
Pulse				↑	↓		↑			↑			
Anemia	+			+	+		+					+	
Neurologic system													
Temperature				↑	↓		↑			↓	↑		
Sleep disturbances	+		+	+		+	+			+		+	
Seizures	+	+			+		+			+			+
Mood													
Depression or apathy	+	+	+		+	+	+			+		+	+
Skin													
Body hair	↓			↓	↓	↑							↓
Pigmentation	↓			↓		↑	↓						↓
Reproductive or sexual system													
Male dysfunction	+			+	+	+	+	+		+		+	
Female dysfunction	+			+	+	+	+			+			

↑, increased; +, present; ↓, decreased.

the patient is taking large doses of glucocorticoids because abrupt discontinuance of these medications may cause an Addisonian crisis. In addition, regular long-term glucocorticoid therapy can result in potentially serious side effects and complications (see Table 47-19).

Insulin replacement should be identified in terms of type, amount, and timing of replacement. In addition, some medications may adversely affect endocrine function. Corticosteroids may cause glucose intolerance in the susceptible patient by increasing glycogenolysis and insulin resistance. There is a greater glucose-lowering effect of sulfonylureas and insulin when taken with large doses (>4 g per day) of aspirin. Dicumarol can cause adrenal hemorrhage and resultant adrenal insufficiency. Lithium carbonate has many adverse effects on the endocrine system, including diffuse nontoxic goiter, hypercalcemia, hyperparathyroidism, transient hyperglycemia, and impotence or sexual dysfunction. Many medications affect blood glucose levels (see Table 47-10).

Surgery or other treatments. The nurse should inquire about previous hospitalizations, surgeries, chemotherapies, and radiation treatments (especially of the neck). A history of a severe blow to the head could indicate pituitary or hypothalamic trauma.

Functional Health Patterns

Health perception–health management pattern. The nurse should ask about energy levels, particularly as compared with the patient's past energy level. Fatigue and hyperactivity are two common problems associated with endocrine problems. Inquiry should also be made about the patient's general health care and health care behaviors. Such an inquiry might result in the identification of vague, nonspecific symptoms that could suggest an endocrine problem.

Heredity and general health can play a major role in the occurrence of endocrine problems. The patient should be questioned about the following conditions in family members: diabetes mellitus or insipidus; hyperthyroidism or hypothyroidism, goiter; hypertension or hypotension; obesity; infertility; growth problems; pheochromocytoma (neoplastic tumor of the adrenal medulla or sympathetic ganglia); autoimmune diseases (e.g., Addison's disease); and adrenal hyperplasia. Further information may be elicited by asking additional questions such as the following: Are there any other members of your family who have, or have had, a similar problem? This frequently uncovers evidence of a familial tendency that cannot be found in any other way.

Nutritional-metabolic pattern. Because a major function of the endocrine system is regulating metabolism and maintenance of homeostasis, the patient with endocrine dysfunction will often experience alterations in nutritional-metabolic patterns. Changes in appetite and weight can indicate endocrine dysfunction. Weight loss with increased appetite may indicate hyperthyroidism or diabetes mellitus, particularly type 1. Weight loss with decreased appetite may indicate hypopituitarism, hypocortisolism, or gastroparesis from diabetes mellitus. Weight gain may indicate hypothyroidism and, if the weight gain is concentrated in the truncal area, hypercortisolism. In addition, weight gain in a genetically susceptible patient may increase the risk for type 2 diabetes mellitus.

Assessment of the endocrine system includes growth and development patterns, weight distribution and changes, and comparisons of these factors with normal findings. Height should be measured in all patients. The charts used should be race specific because significant racial differences exist in normal children. For example, Caucasian children usually are smaller than African-American children but larger than Asian children. Familial patterns should always be assessed. A helpful guide in growth assessment is that approximate normal growth rates are 3 inches (7.5 cm) per year from ages 1 to 7 and 2 inches (5 cm) per year from ages 8 to 15. Heights more than 3 standard deviations below the mean should be investigated.[18] Approximate average heights for children and young teenagers can be estimated on the basis of age using the following formula:

$$\text{Height (inches)} = 2.5 \times \text{Age (years)} + 30$$

In adults, weight changes may indicate endocrine dysfunction. Body mass index (BMI) is a common way to assess obesity (see Table 38-7). This estimation takes height into account. It is derived by dividing the weight (in kilograms) by the height (in meters squared): BMI = Weight (kg)/Height (m^2). A BMI of 25 is the upper limit of normal; 25 to 29.9 indicates that a patient is overweight; and 30 or above indicates obesity. A weight increase of more than 1 kg per day usually indicates fluid retention.

Changes in hair distribution and skin and hair color and texture can all indicate endocrine dysfunction. Hair loss can indicate hypopituitarism, hypothyroidism, hypoparathyroidism, or increased testosterone and other androgens. Increased body hair may indicate hypercortisolism. Decreased skin pigmentation can occur in hypopituitarism, hypothyroidism, and hypoparathyroidism, whereas increased skin pigmentation, particularly in sun-exposed areas, can indicate hypocortisolism. A patient with hypothyroidism or excess growth hormone may complain of coarse, leathery skin. A patient with hyperthyroidism may comment about fine, silky hair. A history of hypertension may indicate excess ADH, aldosterone, or cortisol.

Difficulty swallowing or a change in neck size may indicate thyroid hyperplasia or inflammation. Questions related to increased sympathetic nervous system activity (e.g., nervousness, palpitations, sweating, tremors) may assist the nurse in identifying a thyroid disorder or pheochromocytoma. Heat or cold intolerance may indicate hyperthyroidism or hypothyroidism, respectively. The patient should be questioned about dietary intake. This record should be examined for the presence of foods that contain thyroid-inhibiting substances (goitrogens) (see Table 47-7).

Elimination pattern. Because maintenance of fluid balance is a major role of the endocrine system, questions related to elimination patterns may uncover endocrine dysfunction. For instance, increased thirst and urination can indicate diabetes mellitus or insipidus. A history of nephrolithiasis (kidney stones) may indicate excess PTH. The patient should be asked about the frequency and consistency of bowel movements. Hyperdefecation may indicate hyperthyroidism. Large-volume, watery stools or fecal incontinence may indicate autonomic gastroenteropathy of diabetes mellitus. Constipation is also seen in the gastroenteropathy of diabetes mellitus, as well as in hypothyroidism, hypoparathyroidism, and hypopituitarism.

Activity-exercise pattern. The major effect of endocrine dysfunction on activity-exercise pattern will be an inability to maintain previous activity levels. Although a patient with hyperthyroidism may seem to have excess energy, fatigue is common. A patient with an endocrine dysfunction will almost always manifest apathy and frequently depression. This indicates the need for the nurse to specifically question the patient or significant other to describe current activity in relation to previous activity patterns. In addition, in diabetes mellitus, the patient's activity-exercise patterns will help determine diabetes management, including insulin therapy.

Sleep-rest pattern. It is important that the nurse obtain a detailed sleep history. Sleep disturbances are frequently seen in endocrine dysfunction. The patient with diabetes mellitus or insipidus will complain of nocturia, which can severely disrupt normal sleep patterns. The patient with tightly controlled type 1 diabetes mellitus who complains of sweating or nightmares may be experiencing hypoglycemia. The hyperthyroid patient may complain of inability to sleep, as may one with hypercortisolism. The patient with hypothyroidism, hypocortisolism, or hypopituitarism may tell the nurse of sleeping all the time, yet still being fatigued. The significant other of a patient with excess growth hormone may tell the nurse of an inability to sleep because of the patient's snoring.

Cognitive-perceptual pattern. The nurse can question both the patient and significant other to determine if any cognitive changes are present. Memory deficits, inability to concentrate, and decreased energy levels are common in endocrine disorders. As mentioned, depression and apathy are frequent in endocrine disorders. Visual changes can also occur. A patient with hyperglycemia may complain of blurred vision. Diplopia may indicate pressure from a pituitary tumor. Exophthalmos secondary to hyperthyroidism can cause corneal drying and other visual disturbances.

Self-perception–self-concept pattern. Endocrine disorders may affect the patient's self-perception because of associated physical changes. Changes in weight, size, and level of fatigue should be determined. Weight changes often occur, and both increases and decreases can affect self-perception. Increases in the size of the head, hands, or feet in the adult (e.g., change in ring, glove, or shoe size) may indicate excess growth hormone. In addition, the fatigue so often experienced by a patient with an endocrine disorder often affects feelings about self.

The chronicity of many endocrine disorders and need for continued therapy can affect the patient's self-perception. The patient can be asked to describe the effects of the present illness on self-perception.

Role-relationship pattern. The nurse should ask whether there have been any changes in the patient's ability to maintain roles at home, at work, or in the community. Often the patient with an endocrine disorder will be unable to sustain life's roles. However, in most cases the patient can be advised that, with adequate management, previous roles can be resumed. This can be very reassuring for the patient and family.

Sexuality-reproductive pattern. Problems with menstruation and pregnancy in a woman may indicate an endocrine disorder. Consequently, a detailed history of menstruation and pregnancy should be obtained. Menstrual irregularities are seen in disorders of the ovaries, pituitary, thyroid, and adrenal glands. A female patient with a history of large babies may have had undiagnosed gestational diabetes, which may put her at a higher risk to develop type 2 diabetes mellitus. A history of inability to lactate may indicate a pituitary disorder.

Male sexual dysfunction is also frequently seen in endocrine disorders. It usually takes the form of impotence, although retrograde ejaculation can occur in diabetes mellitus. Infertility in either sex warrants a full reproductive and endocrine workup.

Coping–stress tolerance pattern. Stressors of all kinds affect the endocrine system. Areas that can cause a great deal of stress should be investigated. The patient should be asked about place of employment, kind of work, ability to meet job requirements, and the amount of stress involved. The nurse should ask whether the job provides an adequate income to identify financial stressors. Usual coping patterns are also discussed. The nurse then determines whether previous coping patterns are still successful. It is often useful to ask family members or a significant other about the patient's coping strategies and reaction to stress.

Value-belief pattern. When dealing with a patient with a chronic condition, identification of the patient's value-belief patterns can assist the health care team to identify appropriate regimens. This is particularly important in a condition such as diabetes mellitus, which may require major lifestyle changes for successful management. Other endocrine disorders, such as hypothyroidism or hypocortisolism, can be easily managed with oral medication taken faithfully. Identification of a patient's ability to make lifestyle changes or take daily medication (and increase this medication as indicated) is an important nursing function.

Objective Data

Physical Examination

Mental-emotional status. Throughout the examination the patient's orientation, alertness, memory, affect, personality, anxiety, and speech pattern should be objectively assessed. Endocrine disorders commonly cause changes in mental status and level of consciousness.

General appearance

Inspection. The nurse should observe the patient's general appearance, including physical growth and development, level of consciousness and orientation, and appearance and appropriateness of dress for ambient temperature. Endocrine dysfunction can subtly or markedly affect the size, shape, color, and maturation of the body. Assessment should include the following:

1. *Body size:* height and weight compared with a table of standards or estimation of normality; size of head and extremities, proportionality and posture; facial features
2. *Integumentary system:* skin color, pigmentation, texture, coarseness, leathery texture, excessive thinness, size of sweat glands, diaphoresis, acne, striae, ecchymosis, vitiligo (patchy loss of pigmentation)
3. *Hair:* texture, distribution, brittleness, alopecia (patchy baldness)
4. *Face:* color; erythema, especially on cheeks (plethora); pained, anxious expression
5. *Eyes:* eyebrows, hair distribution; visual acuity, lens opacity; shape, position, movement of eyelids; lid lag; visual fields; extraocular movements; edema
6. *Nose:* mucosa, noisy breathing
7. *Mouth:* buccal mucosa, condition of teeth, malocclusion and mottling, tongue size and fasciculations (local-

ized, uncoordinated, uncontrollable twitching of a single muscle group), size and shape of jaw
8. *Voice:* huskiness or hoarseness, volume, pitch, slurring
9. *Neck:* symmetry, alignment; forceful carotid pulsations; unusual bulging of the thyroid lobes behind the sternocleidomastoid muscles; trachea in midline; dullness, thickening, flabbiness of vocal chords; polyps; gray-brown hyperpigmentation on posterior neck and axillae (acanthosis nigricans); when inspecting the thyroid gland, observation should be made first in the normal position, preferably with side lighting, then in slight extension, and then as the patient swallows some water
10. *Extremities:* size, shape, symmetry, proportionality (distance from symphysis pubis to foot: approximately half of total height), edema
    a. *Hands:* tremors (a piece of paper is placed on outstretched fingers, palm down, to assess fine tremors); muscle strength, grip, thenar (ball of the thumb) wasting, Dupuytren's contracture, clubbing, muscle wasting
    b. *Legs:* muscle weakness (assessed by having the seated patient extend one leg to a horizontal position; ability to hold this position for 2 minutes usually indicates normal muscle strength), bowing, color and amount of hair, size of feet, corns, calluses, pedal pulses
    c. *Toes:* maceration, fissures, deformities, toenails with fungal infection
11. *Reflexes:* particularly deep tendon reflexes, relaxation time
12. *Pulses:* rate and force
13. *Thorax:* gynecomastia in men
14. *Abdomen:* increased pigmentation of scars, purplish striae, pain on light palpation
15. *Genitalia:* decreased hair distribution (diamond pattern in women may indicate virilizing adrenal tumor), size of testes, clitoral enlargement

Palpation. The thyroid is the only palpable endocrine gland. Thyroid palpation requires considerable practice, as well as validation by an experienced examiner. Palpation can cause the release of thyroid hormone into the circulation, increasing the patient's symptoms and potentially causing a thyroid storm. (Hyperthyroidism is discussed in Chapter 47.) In the patient with a visibly enlarged thyroid, palpation of the thyroid should be deferred if a more experienced clinician will be examining the patient.

To palpate the thyroid, the nurse identifies other midline neck structures (see Fig. 45-9). The thyroid can be palpated anteriorly and posteriorly. Water should always be available for the patient to swallow as part of this examination.

For anterior palpation the nurse stands in front of the patient, with the patient's neck flexed. The nurse places the thumb horizontally with the upper edge along the lower border of the cricoid cartilage. The thumb is then moved over the isthmus as the patient swallows water. The fingers are then placed laterally to the anterior border of the sternocleidomastoid muscle, and each lateral lobe is palpated before and while the patient swallows water.

For posterior palpation the examiner stands behind the patient. With the thumbs of both hands resting on the nape of the patient's neck, the nurse uses the index and middle fingers of both hands to feel for the thyroid isthmus and for the anterior

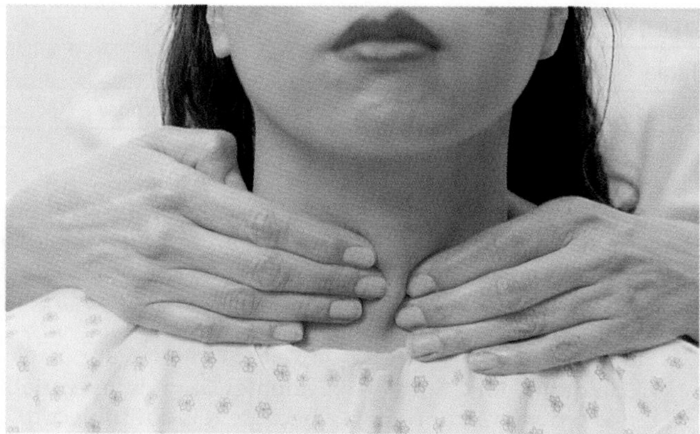

Fig. 45-10 Posterior palpation of the thyroid gland.

surfaces of the lateral lobes. To facilitate the examination of each lobe and to relax the neck muscles, the nurse asks the patient to flex the neck slightly forward and to the right. The thyroid cartilage is displaced to the right by the left hand and fingers. The nurse palpates with the right hand after placing the thumb deep and behind the sternocleidomastoid muscle with the index and middle fingers in front of it; the area is palpated with the right hand (Fig. 45-10). While this is done, the patient is asked to swallow water. This procedure is then repeated on the left side. The thyroid is palpated for its size, shape, symmetry, tenderness, and for any nodules. In the average person the thyroid is often not palpable. If palpable, it usually feels smooth with a firm consistency and is not tender with gentle pressure. Nodules, enlargement, asymmetry, or hardness is abnormal, and the patient should be referred for further evaluation.

Other assessment skills. Percussion and auscultation are not normally part of an endocrine assessment. When an enlarged thyroid has been noted, however, the lateral lobes should be auscultated with the stethoscope bell to determine the presence of a bruit.

Assessment of vital signs should include the following:

1. Temperature: Hyperthermia or hypothermia
2. Pulse: Rate and rhythm
3. Respirations: Change in rate or rhythm
4. Blood pressure: Widening of the pulse pressure, hypotension, hypertension, or orthostatic hypotension (see Chapter 31)
5. Heart sounds: Systolic murmur at apex or pulmonic area (possible indication of increased blood flow as a result of hyperthyroidism)

DIAGNOSTIC STUDIES OF THE ENDOCRINE SYSTEM

Diagnostic studies common to the endocrine system are presented in Table 45-7. Accurately performed laboratory tests aid and confirm diagnoses of problems of the endocrine system.[19]

Hormone Assays

These tests can measure absolute hormone levels and estimate the production, transport, and catabolism of hormones.

Text continues on p. 1365

DIAGNOSTIC STUDIES

Table 45-7 Endocrine System

Study	Description and Purpose	Nursing Responsibility
Pituitary Studies		
Serum Studies		
▪ Growth hormone (GH) (somatotropin)	Evaluates GH hypersecretion. After an overnight fast, GH should be <5 ng/ml (5.0) in men and <10 ng/ml (10.0) in women. Values >50 ng/ml (50.0) suggest acromegaly.	Inform patient that blood sample will be drawn. Make sure that patient takes nothing by mouth after midnight and does not smoke. Send samples to laboratory immediately. Observe venipuncture site for bleeding or hematoma formation.
▪ Somatomedin C (insulin-like growth factor I [IGF-I], growth factor I)	Evaluates GH; it is less variable than GH because it is not subject to circadian rhythm and fluctuations. *Normal values* are 135-250 ng/ml; low levels indicate GH deficiency, and high levels indicate GH excess. Values increase during puberty and pregnancy.	Observe venipuncture site for bleeding or hematoma formation.
▪ GH release after exercise	Evaluates GH reserve in suspected hypopituitarism. Exercise stimulates GH secretion. Patient exercises vigorously for ½ hour before blood sample drawn. GH values should rise above 20 ng/ml after exercise.	Have patient fast for 12 hours. Explain procedure. Monitor pulse rate before and after exercise. May be contraindicated in patient with coronary artery insufficiency or exercise-induced asthma. Send sample to laboratory immediately.
▪ Insulin-induced hypoglycemia	Used in examination of patients with suspected hypopituitarism. IV injection of regular insulin is given, based on body weight (usually 0.1 U/kg). Basal samples of GH, cortisol, and glucose are drawn. Blood samples are drawn at 30, 45, 60, and 90 minutes after injection. If test is terminated because of hypoglycemia (glucose level less than 40 mg/dl [40 ng/L]), samples are drawn for GH and cortisol levels 30 minutes after IV dextrose. GH level should rise twofold to threefold over baseline levels. Response is subnormal or absent in GH deficiency.	Ensure that patient fasted overnight (water is allowed) and that bed rest was prescribed. Have 5% cortisone, 20 ml of 50% dextrose, and IV solution of 5% glucose at bedside for use if severe hypoglycemia occurs and test will continue. Weigh patient. Continually assess patient's mental status because seizures, cardiac arrhythmias, and coma can result from hypoglycemia (test is contraindicated in patients with seizure disorders, cardiac disease, hypocortisolism, and hypothyroidism.) Assess capillary glucose levels immediately with BGM. Note on laboratory slips times that blood is drawn. Provide 25 g glucose and breakfast after last sample.
▪ Prolactin level	Evaluates prolactin levels. Decreased levels in postpartum women attempting to nurse may be associated with Sheehan's syndrome. *Normal values* <20 ng/ml (<20 µg/L) (nonlactating); levels greater than 200 ng/ml (200 µg/L) indicate pituitary tumors.	Have patient fast. Inform patient that blood sample will be drawn. Draw blood within 3-4 hours after patient awakens. Observe venipuncture site for bleeding or hematoma formation.
▪ Gonadotropin levels Follicle-stimulating hormone (FSH) Luteinizing hormone (LH)	Useful in distinguishing primary gonadal problems from pituitary insufficiency. Normal levels vary according to age and sex. In women, there are marked differences during menstrual cycle and in postmenopausal period. Levels are low in pituitary insufficiency and high in primary gonadal failure. In women, values for FSH are basal rate—2-15 mIU/ml (2-15 IU/L); ovulatory surge—8-40 mIU/ml (8-40 IU/L); and postmenopausal level—greater than 50 mIU/ml (40 IU/L). In women, values for LH are basal rate—2-20 mIU/ml (2-20 IU/L); ovulatory surge—30-140 mIU/ml (30-140 IU/L); and postmenopausal level—greater than 50 mIU/ml (50 IU/L). In men, values for FSH are 2-15 mIU/ml (2-15 IU/L) and LH 3-25 mIU/ml (3-25 IU/L).	Ensure that patient has fasted. Inform patient that three blood samples may be drawn 30 minutes apart for FSH. For women, note on laboratory slip time of menstrual cycle or whether she is postmenopausal.

Continued

DIAGNOSTIC STUDIES

Table 45-7 Endocrine System—cont'd

Study	Description and Purpose	Nursing Responsibility
Serum Studies—cont'd		
■ Water deprivation test	Used to differentiate causes of polyuria, including pituitary diabetes insipidus (DI), nephrogenic DI, syndrome of inappropriate ADH, and psychogenic polydipsia. ADH or vasopressin diluted in saline solution are administered intravenously over a 2-hour period. With normal patients and with patients with psychogenic DI, urine osmolality is >600 mOsm/kg and plasma osmolality <300 mOsm/kg after ADH administration. With pituitary DI, plasma osmolality is >300 mOsm/kg; with dilute urine, it is <270 mOsm/kg. With nephrogenic DI, there is little or no response to ADH.	Have patient discontinue tea, coffee, alcohol, and smoking after midnight. Obtain baseline weight and urine and plasma osmolality. Ensure that fluid is withheld. Weigh patient and take three postural BP measurements (lying and standing BP measurements separated by 2 minutes) hourly. Assess urine hourly for volume and specific gravity. Send hourly samples for urine osmolality. Draw sample for plasma osmolality when (1) urine samples are collected and (2) orthostatic hypotension and postural tachycardia appear. Assess weight at 4, 6, 7, and 8 hours. Patients must be very closely supervised during this test.
Radiologic Studies		
■ Skull x-ray, CT scan, MRI	Useful in evaluating sella turcica for volume, enlargement, or erosion when disease of hypothalamic-pituitary axis is suspected. Compare with normal measurement of sella turcica in relation to patient's height.	Inform patient of the need to lie as still as possible during test; explain that tests are painless and noninvasive. Explain procedure.
Thyroid Studies		
Serum Studies		
■ T_4	Measures total serum level of T_4. Useful in evaluating thyroid function and monitoring thyroid therapy. *Normal values* are 5-12 μg/dl (51-142 nmol/L).	Inform patient that fasting is not necessary. Inform patient that blood samples will be drawn. Observe venipuncture site for bleeding or hematoma formation.
■ T_3	Measures serum levels of T_3. It is helpful in diagnosing hyperthyroidism if T_4 levels are normal. *Normal values* are 65-195 ng/dl (1.0-3.0 nmol/L).	Same as above.
■ T_3 resin uptake (T_3RU)	This study indirectly measures binding capacity of thyroid-binding globulin. *Normal values* are 25-35% (0.25-0.35).	Same as above.
■ Free T_4	Measures active component of total T_4. *Normal values* are 1.0-3.5 ng/dl (12.9-45.0 pmol/L).	Same as above.
■ Free T_3	Measures active component of total T_3. *Normal values* are 0.26-0.65 ng/dl.	Same as above.
■ Thyroid ^{131}I uptake (radioactive iodine uptake)	Provides direct measure of thyroid activity. Useful for evaluation of functional activity of solitary thyroid nodules. Small tracer dose of ^{131}I is given orally or intravenously. Serum uptake measurements are drawn at 2 to 4 and at 24 hours. *Normal serum values* for 2-4 hours are 3-10%; for 24 hours, they are 5-30%. Values are affected by drugs, seafood, certain radiographic contrast media, and antiseptics containing iodine.	Instruct patient to discontinue thyroid medication and to start T_3 (Cytomel) 2-3 times/day for 4 weeks. Tell patient to report for further testing in 10-14 days. Collect 24-hour urine specimen.
■ Thyroid-stimulating hormone (TSH)	This test measures level of TSH, which is markedly elevated in primary hypothyroidism. *Normal values* are 0.3-5.4 μU/ml (0.3-5.4 mU/L).	Inform patient that fasting is not necessary. Inform patient that blood sample will be drawn. Observe venipuncture site for bleeding or hematoma formation.
■ Calcitonin	High calcitonin level with normal serum calcium level is associated with medullary thyroid carcinoma. *Normal values* are ≤155 pg/ml (155 ng/L) for men and 105 pg/ml (105 ng/L) for women.	Ensure that patient has fasted. Inform patient that blood sample will be drawn. Observe venipuncture site for bleeding or hematoma formation.

Continued

DIAGNOSTIC STUDIES

Table 45-7 Endocrine System—cont'd

Study	Description and Purpose	Nursing Responsibility
Thyroid Studies—cont'd		
Radiologic Studies		
▪ Thyroid scan	Used to evaluate nodules of the thyroid. Tracer dose of technetium is given intravenously. Scanner passes over thyroid and makes graphic record of radiation emitted. Normal thyroid scan reveals homogeneous pattern with symmetric lobes.	Determine whether other tests requiring iodine preparation (IV pyelogram, saturated solution of potassium iodine, or barium enema) have been done within 30 days (can invalidate test). Explain procedure to patient.
Parathyroid Studies		
Serum Studies		
▪ Parathyroid hormone (PTH)	Measures PTH level in serum. Normal range depends on assay used (check with laboratory). This study must be interpreted in terms of concomitantly drawn serum calcium level.	Fasting specimen preferred. Inform patient that blood sample will be drawn. Sample must be kept on ice. Observe venipuncture site for bleeding or hematoma formation.
▪ Total serum calcium	Measures total serum calcium to help detect bone and parathyroid disorders. Hypercalcemia can indicate primary hyperparathyroidism, and hypocalcemia can indicate hypoparathyroidism. *Normal values* are 9.0-11.0 mg/dl or 4.5-5.5 mEq/L (2.25-2.74 mmol/L).	Fasting specimen preferred. Inform patient that blood sample will be drawn. Observe venipuncture site for bleeding or hematoma formation. Ensure that prolonged tourniquet application does not cause falsely elevated values. Adjust total calcium for albumin levels. Using following formula: Total serum calcium (mg/dl) − Albumin (g/dl) + 4.0 = Adjusted total serum calcium.
▪ Phosphorus	Measures inorganic phosphorus. Hyperphosphatemia indicates primary hypoparathyroidism or secondary causes (e.g., renal failure); hypophosphatemia indicates hyperparathyroidism. Phosphorus and calcium levels are inversely related. *Normal values* are 2.8-4.5 mg/dl (0.90-1.45 mmol/L).	Need for fasting varies with lab. Determine fasting requirement. Inform patient that blood sample will be drawn. Observe venipuncture site for bleeding or hematoma formation.
▪ 1,25-Dihydroxyvitamin D_3	This test is used to evaluate calcium and phosphorus levels and bone disease. *Normal values* are 15-60 pg/ml.	Inform patient that blood sample will be drawn. Observe venipuncture site for bleeding or hematoma formation.
Radiologic Studies		
▪ Skeletal x-ray, CT scans	Used to determine bone disease and osteoporosis. Fractures or deformities can be caused by the demineralization produced by excessive PTH.	Monitor patient's exposure to x-rays. Inform patient that tests are painless and noninvasive and that no special preparation is required for x-ray studies. For CT scan, give patient radiolabeled agent 4 hours before scan.
Adrenal Studies		
Serum Studies		
▪ Cortisol	Measures amount of cortisol in serum and evaluates status of adrenocortical function. *Normal values* are 5-25 μg/dl (0.14-0.69 μmol/L) at 8 AM, <10 μg/dl (<0.28 μmol/L) at 8 PM.	Inform patient that blood sample will be taken. Observe venipuncture site for bleeding and hematoma formation. Ensure collection of properly timed blood sample. Draw specimen early in morning when cortisol levels are highest. Mark time on laboratory slip. Minimize stress to avoid raising level.
▪ Aldosterone	Normal values are 5-20 ng/dl (140-556 pmol/L) (upright posture) and 8.5 ng/dl (237 pmol/L) supine position.	Increases with low-salt diet (less than 2 g/day), stress, an upright posture, and diuretics; decreases with a high-salt diet, ACE inhibitors such as captopril, and lying in supine position. Determine which maneuvers will be done and advise patient.

Continued

DIAGNOSTIC STUDIES

Table 45-7 Endocrine System—cont'd

Study	Description and Purpose	Nursing Responsibility
Adrenal Studies—cont'd		
Serum Studies—cont'd		
▪ ACTH stimulation	Used to evaluate adrenal function. After baseline samples are drawn, 250 μg synthetic ACTH is given as IV or IM bolus; samples are drawn 30 and 50 minutes after bolus. Baseline ACTH sample is often drawn in case results are abnormal. Plasma cortisol at 60 minutes should be (1) greater than baseline and (2) greater than 20 μg/dl.	Inject ACTH with a plastic syringe and collect samples for ACTH in plastic, heparinized tubes. Administer test with continuous-infusion method. Monitor site and rate of IV infusion. Ensure sample collection at appropriate times.
▪ Dexamethasone suppression (overnight)	Assesses adrenal function and is especially helpful if hyperactivity is suspected. Useful in evaluation of Cushing's syndrome. Dexamethasone (Decadron) 2 mg is given at 11 PM to suppress secretion of corticotropin-releasing hormone. Plasma cortisol sample is drawn at 8 AM. Cortisol level less than 5 μg/dl (138 nmol/L) indicates normal adrenal response (50% decrease in cortisol production).	Ensure that patient has fasted. Inform patient that blood sample will be taken. Observe venipuncture site for bleeding and hematoma formation. Do not test acutely ill patients; those under stress are not tested. ACTH may override suppression. Screen patient for drugs such as estrogen and glucocorticoids, which may give false-positive results. Ensure accurate timing of medication and sample collection.
▪ Metyrapone suppression	Used to evaluate feedback response of hypothalamus and pituitary and adrenal glands and to differentiate causes of endogenous glucocorticoid overproduction. Metyrapone (30 mg/kg) is given at midnight. Sample is drawn at 8 AM for plasma 11-deoxycortisol (Compound S), cortisol, and ACTH. Normal response is 11-deoxycortisol: 7-232 μg/dl (202-6696 nmol/L) and ACTH >250 pg/ml (55.1 pmol/L). To validate blockage by metyrapone, cortisol must be (1) less than 8 μg/dl (220 nmol/L) and (2) less than 45% of Compound S level.	Weigh patient. Administer metyrapone with milk and snack at midnight. (Note that metyrapone can cause gastrointestinal distress and confusion.) Draw ACTH into heparinized plastic tube with plastic syringe. Ensure that patient has not ingested estrogens, phenytoin, and phenobarbital because these substances invalidate test.
Urine Studies		
▪ 17-Ketosteroids	Measures androgen metabolites in urine and evaluates adrenal cortical and gonadal function. *Normal values* are 10-22 mg/day (35-76 μmol/day) for men and 6-16 mg/day (21-55 μmol/day) for women.	Instruct patient regarding 24-hour urine collection. Tell patient that specimen must be kept refrigerated or iced during collection. Determine whether preservative is required for method used.
▪ Aldosterone	Measures urinary aldosterone level to evaluate adrenal function. Useful in determining therapy for hypertension. *Normal values* are 2-26 μg/24 hours (5.5-72 nmol/day).	Ensure that patient is on unrestricted diet with normal salt intake and no medication for 3 weeks before collection. Instruct patient regarding 24-hour urine collection.
▪ Free cortisol	Preferred test to evaluate hypercortisolism. Can also be used to screen for endogenous glucocorticoids. *Normal values* are less than 100 mg/24 hours.	Instruct patient regarding 24-hour urine collection and avoidance of stressful situations and excessive physical exercise. Tell patient that some drugs (e.g., reserpine, diuretics, phenothiazines, and amphetamines) may elevate levels. Ensure that patient is on low-sodium diet.
▪ Vanillylmandelic acid	Measures urinary excretion of catecholamine metabolite and is helpful in diagnosing pheochromocytoma. *Normal values* are less than 8 mg/14 hours (40 μmol/day); pheochromocytoma is indicated with values of 10-250 mg/24 hours (51-126 μmol/day).	Keep 24-hour urine collection at pH of less than 3.0 with hydrochloric acid as preservative. Know that newer methods are not affected by dietary intake. Consult with laboratory or physician about patient discontinuing any drugs 3 days before urine collection.

Continued

DIAGNOSTIC STUDIES

Table 45-7 Endocrine System—cont'd

Study	Description and Purpose	Nursing Responsibility
Pancreatic Studies		
Serum Studies		
▪ Fasting blood sugar (FBS) levels	Measures circulating glucose level. *Normal serum values* for adults are 70-110 mg/dl (3.9-6.7 mmol/L); for pregnant women they are 60-90 mg/dl (3.3-5 mmol/L).	Ensure that patient has fasted at least 4 hours. Inform patient that blood sample will be drawn. Observe venipuncture site for bleeding or hematoma formation.
▪ Oral glucose tolerance	**A.** This 2-hour test is used to diagnose diabetes mellitus if FBS is equivocal. Patient drinks 75 g of glucose; samples for glucose are drawn immediately and at 30, 60, and 120 minutes. *Normal values* are <200 mg/dl (11.1 mmol/L) at 30, 60, and 90 minutes and <140 mg/dl (7.8 mmol/L) at 120 minutes.	Ensure that tests are not done on patients who are malnourished, confined to bed for over 3 days, or severely stressed. Instruct patient to refrain from smoking and caffeine and to fast for 12 hours before test. Ensure that patient's diet 3 days before test included 150-300 g of carbohydrate with intake of at least 1500 calories per day. Screen for estrogens, phenytoin, and corticosteroids, and check for hypokalemia, which may impair glucose tolerance.
	B. This 5-hour test is used to evaluate hypoglycemia. Patient drinks 100 g of glucose; samples of glucose are drawn immediately and at 30, 60, 90, 120, 180, 240, and 300 minutes. Baseline cortisol level test is done if patient becomes symptomatic. Patients with reactive hypoglycemia have adrenergic symptoms and glucose less than 60 mg/dl (3.3 mmol/L) between 30 minutes and 5 hr after glucose ingestion.	Simultaneously monitor glucoses with capillary BGM.
▪ Capillary glucose monitoring	Used to give immediate glucose values with glucose oxidase or electrochemical methods. Capillary values (whole blood) are usually 10-15% less than serum values.	Obtain large drop of blood from clean finger, touch strip to drop of blood (not finger), time accurately, and compare colors in good lighting, if using visual method. Use digital readout if available. Use automatic finger-puncture device if available. Be sure to change section of device that touches patients' fingers between patients.
▪ Glycosylated hemoglobin	Measures degree of glucose control during previous 3 months (life span of hemoglobin molecule). *Normal values* are 4-6% (values vary widely, check with laboratory.)	Inform patient that fasting is not necessary and that blood sample will be drawn. Observe venipuncture site for bleeding or hematoma formation.
Urine Studies		
▪ Glucose (Clinistix, Labstix, Multistix, Clinitest)	Estimates amount of glucose in urine by using reducing substance. Results have wide range from negative (no glucose) to 2% (large amount of glucose).	Use freshly voided urine specimen collected at appropriate time. Know that many different drugs alter glucose readings and that errors are great if directions for timing are not followed exactly. Follow package directions.
▪ Ketone (Acetest, Ketostix, Labstix, Multistix)	Measures amount of acetone excreted in urine as result of incomplete fat metabolism. Positive result can indicate lack of insulin and diabetic acidosis.	Use freshly voided urine specimen. Test is often done with glucose test. Directions must be followed exactly. Certain drugs can produce false-positive and false-negative results.
▪ Glucose and acetone (Ketodiastix)	Measures glucose and acetone levels.	Know that large amounts of urinary acetone may depress glucose measurement.

ACE, angiotensin-converting enzyme; *BGM*, blood glucose monitoring.

Hormones with fairly constant basal levels (e.g., T_4) require only a single measurement. Hormones with pulsatile secretion (e.g., LH) may require multiple samples with a measurement taken from pooled aliquots. Notation of sample time on the laboratory slip and sample is important for hormones with circadian or sleep-related secretion (e.g., cortisol, GH).

On occasion, multiple blood sampling is indicated, such as in suppression tests (e.g., dexamethasone suppression) and stimulation tests (e.g., glucose tolerance). To decrease patient discomfort and minimize the effects of stress hormones, the nurse initiates an intravenous infusion of normal saline solution with a stopcock between the extension and the infusion tubing. After insertion of the infusion, 15 to 30 minutes should be allowed for stress hormones to normalize. Baseline samples are then drawn, the appropriate medication is given through the stopcock, and samples are withdrawn through the stopcock at the appropriate times. A heparin lock may be used in place of the saline infusion. It is necessary to draw and discard 1.5 to 3 ml of blood from the patient before drawing the sample for measurement. This prevents saline or heparin dilution.

In general, tests of endocrine function require patient fasting and the elimination of as many environmental stimuli as possible. This necessitates inactivity throughout the test; such inactivity can be achieved with bed rest with the head of the bed elevated or through the use of a recliner chair. The patient should refrain from smoking or taking food or fluids by mouth. A thorough explanation of the test and the reasons for reducing environmental stimuli reassures patients and helps them cooperate. The patient should be monitored frequently during the test and not just when samples are being taken.

During endocrine testing there are instances in which simultaneous blood and urine samples or special preservatives are needed for samples. The nurse ensures thorough patient instruction, as well as correct and complete sample collection. When a patient is having multiple endocrine testing, such as with suspected pituitary disease, a fluid volume deficit may occur. Nursing interventions in this instance include recording the amount of blood and urine taken per test, assessing for dehydration, and promptly notifying the physician if blood loss through sample collection is excessive or the patient becomes dehydrated. Using the saline infusion method helps offset fluid volume deficit.

Types of Laboratory Tests. Several types of laboratory tests are used to determine endocrine status, including immunoassay, immunometric, receptor, chromatographic, and in vitro bioassays.[20] The immunoassay, a displacement assay, uses antibodies specific for a hormone or parts of a hormone and can measure very small amounts of circulating hormones. It is used for peptide, steroid, and thyroid hormones. Immunometric assays can measure minute hormone levels and are used for TSH measurements. Radioreceptor assays measure the ability of a hormone to bind to its receptor. Receptor measurements are useful in states of hormone resistance such as those seen with insulin, PTH, and vitamin D. Chromatographic assay allows measurement of several hormones in the same sample. In vitro bioassays can provide information about the transport, clearance rate, and enzymatic transformation of a substance before it binds to its receptor.

Specific diagnostic studies related to the endocrine system are summarized in Table 45-7. Because of the interrelatedness of the endocrine system, nursing interventions are focused on reducing the stress and anxiety often associated with diagnostic testing. Unless nursing measures related to patient instruction and expectations are initiated, the effect of stress hormones can produce inaccurate and misleading results.

Normal values and collection procedures vary among laboratories. It is therefore important to check with the laboratory doing the testing to determine the correct collection and transport procedures and normal values.

REVIEW QUESTIONS

The number of the question corresponds to the same-numbered objective at the beginning of the chapter.

1. A characteristic common to all hormones is that they
   a. circulate in the blood bound to plasma proteins.
   b. influence cellular activity of specific target tissues.
   c. accelerate the metabolic processes of all body cells.
   d. enter cells to alter the cell's metabolism or gene expression.
2. A patient is receiving radiation therapy for cancer of the kidney. The nurse monitors the patient for signs and symptoms of damage to the
   a. pancreas.
   b. thyroid gland.
   c. adrenal glands.
   d. posterior pituitary gland.
3. A patient has a serum sodium level of 152 mEq/L (152 mmol/L). The normal hormonal response to this situation is
   a. release of ADH.
   b. release of renin.
   c. secretion of aldosterone.
   d. secretion of corticotropin-releasing hormone.
4. All cells in the body are believed to have intracellular receptors for
   a. insulin.
   b. cortisone.
   c. growth hormone.
   d. thyroid hormones.
5. When obtaining subjective data from a patient during assessment of the endocrine system, the nurse asks specifically about
   a. energy level.
   b. intake of vitamin C.
   c. employment history.
   d. frequency of sexual intercourse.
6. An appropriate technique to use during physical assessment of the thyroid gland is
   a. asking the patient to hyperextend the neck during palpation.
   b. percussing the neck for dullness to define the size of the thyroid.
   c. having the patient swallow water during inspection and palpation of the gland.
   d. using deep palpation to determine the extent of a visibly enlarged thyroid gland.
7. The older adult with hypothyroidism is more likely than a younger person to have disturbances of
   a. bone metabolism.
   b. cardiovascular function.
   c. gastrointestinal function.
   d. central nervous system function.

8. An abnormal finding by the nurse during an endocrine assessment would include
   a. joint pain.
   b. blood pressure of 100/70.
   c. decreased skin pigmentation.
   d. soft, formed stool every other day.
9. A patient has a serum cortisol level of 3 μg/dl at 8 AM. If this finding reflects a primary dysfunction of the adrenal glands, the nurse would expect further diagnostic testing to reveal
   a. increased serum ACTH.
   b. decreased urinary aldosterone.
   c. increased urine 17-ketosteroids.
   d. serum cortisol level less than 5 μg with dexamethasone suppression.

References

1. Baxter JD, Frohman L, Felig P: Introduction to the endocrine system. In Felig P, Baxter JD, Frohman L, editors: *Endocrinology and metabolism,* ed 3, New York, 1995, McGraw-Hill.
2. Hagan RM, Oakley NR: Melatonin comes of age? *Trends Pharmacol Sci* 16:50, 1995.
3. Reppert SM, Weaver RR: Melatonin madness, *Cell* 83:1059, 1995.
4. Gill GN: Biosynthesis, secretion, and metabolism of hormones. In Felig P, Baxter JD, Frohman LC, editors: *Endocrinology and metabolism,* ed 3, New York, 1995, McGraw-Hill.
5. Oppenheimer JH, Schwartz HL, Strait KA: The molecular basis of thyroid hormone action. In Braverman LE, Utiger RD, editors: *Werner and Ingbar's the thyroid, a fundamental and clinical text,* ed 7, Philadelphia, 1996, Lippincott.
6. Catt KJ: Molecular mechanisms of hormone action: control of target cell function by peptide and catecholamine hormones. In Felig P, Baxter JD, Frohman LA, editors: *Endocrinology and metabolism,* ed 3, New York, 1995, McGraw-Hill.
7. Loriaux TC: Endocrine assessment: red flags for those on the front lines, *Nurs Clin North Am* 31:695, 1996.
8. Cooper PF, Martin JB: Physiology and pathophysiology of the endocrine brain and hypothalamus. In Becker KL, editor: *Principles and practices of endocrinology and metabolism,* ed 2, Philadelphia, 1995, Lippincott.
9. Robertson GL: Posterior pituitary. In Felig P, Baxter JD, Frohman LA, editors: *Endocrinology and metabolism,* ed 3, New York, 1995, McGraw-Hill.
10. Baran DT: The skeletal system in thyrotoxicosis. In Braverman LE, Utiger RD, editors: *Werner and Ingbar's the thyroid: a fundamental and clinical text,* ed 7, Philadelphia, 1996, Lippincott.
11. Carlstedt-Duke J and others: Molecular mechanisms of hormone action: regulation of target cell function by the steroid hormone receptor supergene family. In Felig P, Baxter JD, Frohman LA, editors: *Endocrinology and metabolism,* ed 3, New York, 1995, McGraw-Hill.
12. Miller WL, Tyrell JB: The adrenal cortex. In Felig P, Baxter JD, Frohman LA, editors: *Endocrinology and metabolism,* ed 3, New York, 1995, McGraw-Hill.
13. Felig P, Bergman M: The endocrine pancreas: diabetes mellitus. In Felig P, Baxter JD, Frohman LC, editors: *Endocrinology and metabolism,* ed 3, New York, 1995, McGraw-Hill.
14. Scheen AJ, Lefebvre PJ: Insulin action in man, *Diabetes Metab* 22:105, 1996.
15. Seely EW, Williams GH: The endocrine heart. In Becker KL, editor: *Principles and practice of endocrinology and metabolism,* ed 2, Philadelphia, 1995, Lippincott.
16. Winger JM, Hornick T: Age-associated changes in the endocrine system, *Nurs Clin North Am* 31:827, 1996.
17. Grunewald DA, Matsumoto AM: Aging and endocrinology. In Becker KL, editor: *Principles and practice of endocrinology and metabolism,* ed 2, Philadelphia, 1995, Lippincott.
18. Aceto TJ and others: Short stature and slow growth in the infant and child. In Becker KL, editor: *Principles and practice of endocrinology and metabolism,* ed 2, Philadelphia, 1995, Lippincott.
19. Rusterholtz A: Interpretation of diagnostic laboratory tests in selected endocrine disorders, *Nurs Clin North Am* 31:715, 1996.
20. Pekary AE, Hershman JM: Hormone assays. In Felig P, Baxter JD, Frohman LC, editors: *Endocrinology and metabolism,* ed 3, New York, 1995, McGraw-Hill.

Resources

Resources for this chapter are listed after Chapter 47 on p. 1448.

REMEMBER to check out your companion CD-ROM

46 NURSING MANAGEMENT Patient with Diabetes Mellitus

Virginia Valentine

www.mosby.com/MERLIN/medsurg_lewis

LEARNING OBJECTIVES

1. Describe the pathophysiology and clinical manifestations of diabetes mellitus.
2. Describe the differences between type 1 and type 2 diabetes mellitus.
3. Identify the pathophysiology and manifestations of the acute and chronic complications of diabetes mellitus.
4. Describe the components of the collaborative care for diabetes mellitus.
5. Describe the role of nutrition in the management of diabetes.
6. Describe the nursing management of a patient with newly diagnosed diabetes mellitus.
7. Describe the nursing responsibilities in the ambulatory and home management of the patient with diabetes.

DIABETES MELLITUS

Diabetes mellitus is a serious health problem throughout the world. An estimated 15.7 million people have diabetes mellitus in the United States alone. It is estimated that, counting both diagnosed and undiagnosed diabetes, as many as 5.9% of the United States population has diabetes mellitus.[1] Diabetes mellitus contributed to more than 162,000 deaths in 1996. Diabetes is the seventh leading cause of death listed on U.S. death certificates, but diabetes is believed to be underreported on death certificates, both as a condition and as cause of death.[1] Diabetes is the leading cause of new cases of blindness. African-Americans are 1.7 times more likely than Caucasians to have diabetes.[1] It increases the risk of coronary artery disease twofold or more. More than 60% to 65% of people with diabetes mellitus have hypertension.[1] The staggering cost from both direct and indirect medical expenditures attributable to diabetes in 1997 was estimated at $98 billion. Hospitalization costs accounted for the greatest proportion of direct medical costs (62%).[2] These dollar amounts do not reflect the impact that the diagnosis of diabetes has on the lives of patients and their families.

Etiology and Pathophysiology

Diabetes mellitus is not a single disease. Rather, it is a group of genetically and clinically heterogeneous disorders characterized by abnormalities in glucose homeostasis resulting in hyperglycemia. The hyperglycemia of diabetes is caused by a decrease in the secretion or activity of insulin. These insulin alterations result in disordered metabolism of carbohydrate, fat, and protein. In time, structural abnormalities in a variety of organs and organ systems, especially the heart, kidneys, and eyes, develop. The complications arise primarily from microangiopathy, macroangiopathy, and neuropathy. Chronic hyperglycemia is generally recognized as contributing to the development of these complications. In addition, diabetes mellitus is associated with complications in pregnancy.

Diabetes mellitus is a heterogeneous syndrome for which several theories of etiology have been proposed. Current theories link the causes of diabetes, singly or in combination, to genetic, autoimmune, viral, and environmental factors such as obesity and stress. There are primarily two types of diabetes mellitus: type 1, in which insulin production by the β-cells is reduced or completely absent and for which the management requires insulin replacement; and type 2, which is the more prevalent type of diabetes mellitus (approximately 90% of patients). Table 46-1 depicts the distinguishing characteristics of type 1 and type 2 diabetes mellitus.

Normal Insulin Metabolism. Insulin is a hormone produced by the β-cells in the islets of Langerhans of the pancreas. Under normal conditions, insulin is continuously released into the bloodstream in small pulsatile increments (a basal rate), with increased release (bolus) when food is ingested (Fig. 46-1). The activity of released insulin lowers blood glucose and facilitates a stable, normal glucose range of approximately 70 to 110 mg/dl (3.9 to 6.0 mmol/L). The average amount of insulin secreted daily by an adult is approximately 40 to 50 U or 0.6 U/kg of body weight. Other hormones (glucagon, epinephrine, growth hormone, cortisol, and somatostatin) work to counter the effects of insulin and are often referred to as counterregulatory hormones because they stimulate glycogen release and breakdown or antagonize the effect of insulin and thereby increase blood glucose levels. Insulin and these counterregulatory substances provide a sustained but regulated release of glucose for energy during

Reviewed by Carol Blainey, RN, MN, Associate Professor, Biobehavioral Nursing and Health Systems, University of Washington School of Nursing, Seattle, Wash.

Table 46-1 Characteristics of Type 1 and Type 2 Diabetes Mellitus

Factor	Type 1 Diabetes Mellitus	Type 2 Diabetes Mellitus
▪ Age at onset	Usually in young person but possible at any age	Usually age 35 yr or older but possible at any age
▪ Type of onset	Signs and symptoms abrupt, but disease process may be present for several years	Insidious
▪ Genetic susceptibility	HLA-DR3, HLA-DR4, and others	Frequent genetic tendency, no relation to HLA
▪ Environmental factors	Virus, toxins	Obesity, lack of exercise
▪ Islet cell antibodies	Often present at onset	Absent
▪ Endogenous insulin	Minimal or absent	Possibly excessive; adequate but delayed secretion or reduced but not absent secretion
▪ Nutritional status	Thin, catabolic state	Obese or possibly normal
▪ Symptoms	Thirst, polyuria, polyphagia, fatigue	Frequently none or mild
▪ Ketosis	Prone at onset or during insulin deficiency	Resistant except during infection or stress
▪ Dietary management	Essential	Essential, possibly sufficient for glycemic control
▪ Insulin	Required for all	Required for 30-40%
▪ Oral agents	Not beneficial	Usually beneficial
▪ Vascular and neurologic complications	In majority of patients after ≥5 yr	Frequent

HLA, human leukocyte antigen.

CULTURAL & ETHNIC CONSIDERATIONS

Diabetes Mellitus

- The highest incidence of diabetes is among Native-Americans.
- There is a higher incidence of diabetes among African-Americans and Hispanics than Caucasians.
- Complications of diabetes are more common in Native-Americans and African-Americans than Caucasians.
- Type 2 diabetes tends to affect a younger-age population in non-Caucasians than Caucasians.

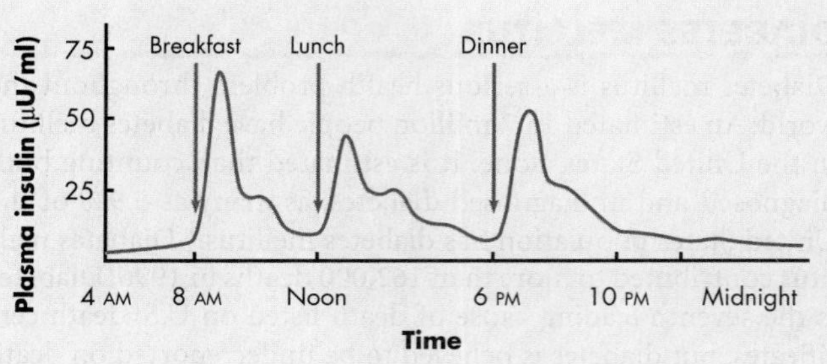

Fig. 46-1 Normal endogenous insulin secretion. In the first hour or two after meals, insulin concentrations rise rapidly in blood and peak at about 1 hour. After meals, insulin concentrations promptly decline toward preprandial values as carbohydrate absorption from the gastrointestinal tract declines. After carbohydrate absorption from the gastrointestinal tract is complete and during the night, insulin concentrations are low and fairly constant, with a slight increase at dawn.

food intake and periods of fasting and usually maintain blood glucose levels within the normal range. Abnormal production of any or all of these hormones may be present in diabetes.

Once insulin is released into the bloodstream from the β-cells as proinsulin, it is routed through the liver. Within the liver, approximately 50% to 70% of received insulin is extracted from the blood. Insulin is formed from proinsulin after cleavage of the C-peptide chain.[3] The presence of C peptide in serum and urine is a useful indicator of β-cell function. The remaining insulin (now active A- and B-peptide chains) functions to promote glucose transport from the bloodstream across the cell membrane to the cytoplasm of the cell. The rise in plasma insulin after a meal stimulates storage of glucose as glycogen in liver and muscle, enhances fat deposition in adipose tissue, inhibits protein degradation, and accelerates the processes of amino acid transport into cells and protein synthesis. The fall in insulin level during normal overnight fasting facilitates the release of stored glucose from the liver, protein from muscle, and fat from adipose tissue.[4] For this reason insulin is known as the storage hormone.

Skeletal muscle and adipose tissue have specific receptors for insulin and are considered to be insulin-dependent tissues. Other tissues (e.g., brain, liver, and blood cells) do not directly depend on insulin for glucose transport but require an adequate glucose supply.

Classification of Diabetes Mellitus

The diagnostic label of diabetes mellitus carries many psychologic and socioeconomic ramifications and therapeutic requirements. Therefore accurate classification of the degree of glucose intolerance and the type of diabetes is important. In 1997 an expert committee supported by the American Diabetes Association (ADA), the National Institute of Diabetes and Digestive and Kidney Diseases at the National Institutes of Health, and the Division of Diabetes Translation at the Centers

Table 46-2 Types of Diabetes Mellitus and Other Categories of Glucose Intolerance

Types	Characteristics
▪ Type 1	May be of any age, is usually thin, and usually has abrupt onset of signs and symptoms with insulinopenia before age 30. Patient often has strongly positive urine ketone tests in conjunction with hyperglycemia and depends on insulin therapy to prevent ketoacidosis and to sustain life.
▪ Type 2	Is usually older than 30 yr at diagnosis, often obese, and has relatively few classic symptoms. Patient is not prone to ketoacidosis except during periods of stress. Although not dependent on exogenous insulin for survival, patient may require it for adequate control of hyperglycemia. Primarily insulin resistant.
▪ Impaired glucose tolerance	Has plasma glucose levels that are higher than normal but not diagnostic for diabetes mellitus. In response to glucose challenge, 2 hr plasma glucose ≥140 mg/dl (7.8 mmol/L) and <200 mg/dl (11.1 mmol/L).
▪ Impaired fasting glucose	Fasting plasma glucose ≥110 mg/dl (6.1 mmol/L) and <126 mg/dl (7.0 mmol/L).
▪ Gestational diabetes mellitus	Has onset or discovery of glucose intolerance during pregnancy.

for Disease Control and Prevention revised the classification system and diagnostic criteria for diabetes, marking the first changes since 1979.[5] The classification system is based not on the treatment of the disease but on the presence and degree of hyperglycemia and the presenting history and symptoms (Table 46-2). The classification scheme also includes the person who has had or who is having glucose intolerance without overt signs of diabetes mellitus. Recognition of this difference allows a person at risk for diabetes to be followed up without being misclassified or mismanaged.

According to the new criteria, the diagnosis of diabetes mellitus is made when the fasting plasma glucose level equals or exceeds 126 mg/dl (7.0 mmol/L), when a random plasma glucose measurement equals or exceeds 200 mg/dl (11.1 mmol/L), or when plasma glucose 2 hours after a glucose challenge is equal or greater than 200 mg/dl (11.1 mmol/L). When the fasting blood glucose level is greater than 110 mg/dl (6.1 mmol/L) but less than 126 mg/dl (7.0 mmol/L), the individual is considered to have impaired fasting glucose. *Impaired glucose tolerance* is classified as a 2 hour plasma glucose level higher than normal but lower than that considered diagnostic for diabetes mellitus (≥140 mg/dl [7.8 mmol/L] and less than 200 mg/dl [11.1 mmol/L]).

As shown in Fig. 46-2 there are altered mechanisms in type 1 and type 2 diabetes in different tissue sites. The development of hyperglycemia arises from different causes. Type 1 diabetes results from progressive destruction of β-cell function as a result of an autoimmune process in a susceptible individual. Islet cell antibodies and insulin autoantibodies cause a reduction in β-cells of 80% to 90% of normal before hyperglycemia and symptoms occur. Type 2 diabetes is a combination of genetically determined defects in skeletal muscle, fat, and liver receptors for insulin and β-cell secretory exhaustion. Excessive hepatic glucose production eventually adds to the fasting and postprandial hyperglycemia.[4] Because of these possibilities for malfunctioning, diabetes mellitus must be considered a heterogeneous disease that cannot be managed by only one treatment regimen.

Type 1 Diabetes Mellitus. Type 1 diabetes is characterized by autoimmune β-cell destruction, which is attributed to a genetic predisposition coupled with one or more viral agents and possibly chemical agents. It is not known conclusively that these are the only factors involved.

The complexity may be better appreciated in relationship to information about human leukocyte antigens (HLAs), which are proteins on the cell surface controlled by genes on chromosome 6. (See Chapter 12 for a discussion of HLAs and disease associations.) Five groups of these antigens have been recognized (A, B, C, D, and DR), and these groups can appear in many variations. Results of family studies confirm that susceptibility to type 1 diabetes is strongly linked to the HLA-DR3 and DR4 loci.[6,7] The individual at highest risk for type 1 diabetes has one or more of the following HLA types: B8, DR3, B15, DR4.[6,7] Theoretically, when an individual with these genetic characteristics is exposed to viral infections, the β-cells are destroyed directly, or an autoimmune process is triggered, which in turn destroys the β-cells. A combination of both processes may occur. Current research continues to seek genetic markers to identify a person at risk for type 1 diabetes who is free of symptoms and to study immunologic parameters that may be manipulated to prevent or cure type 1 diabetes.

Genetic counseling for parents is based on statistical risk. If one child has type 1 diabetes, other siblings have a 5% to 10% chance of type 1 diabetes developing (up to 45% if the sibling is an identical twin). The offspring of a father with type 1 diabetes has a risk of 4% to 6%, double that of offspring of type 1 diabetic mothers (2% to 3%).[7]

The onset and progression of hyperglycemic symptoms are usually more rapid and acute in type 1 diabetes as compared with type 2, and successful treatment depends on insulin replacement. If the disease process is allowed to progress without treatment, diabetic ketoacidosis with nausea and vomiting, electrolyte imbalance, weight loss, and muscle wasting may develop. Without treatment (i.e., insulin) ketoacidosis can progress to coma and death.

Once treatment is initiated, the patient with type 1 diabetes may go into a remission (often called the "honeymoon" period). During this time, the patient needs very little insulin to control blood glucose. The honeymoon period occurs because, even as insulin islet cell antibodies destroy β-cells, β-cells continue to produce insulin. Eventually, blood glucose levels climb, more insulin is needed, and the honeymoon period ends. The honeymoon period may last up to a year, depending on the patient.

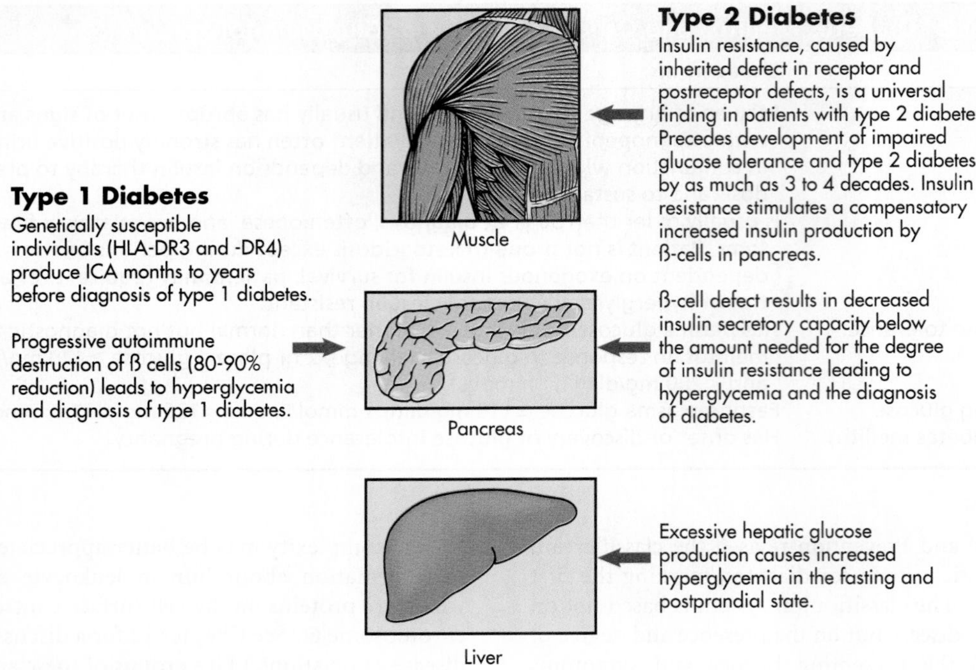

Type 2 Diabetes
Insulin resistance, caused by inherited defect in receptor and postreceptor defects, is a universal finding in patients with type 2 diabetes. Precedes development of impaired glucose tolerance and type 2 diabetes by as much as 3 to 4 decades. Insulin resistance stimulates a compensatory increased insulin production by β-cells in pancreas.
Type 1 Diabetes
Genetically susceptible individuals (HLA-DR3 and -DR4) produce ICA months to years before diagnosis of type 1 diabetes.
Muscle
Progressive autoimmune destruction of β cells (80-90% reduction) leads to hyperglycemia and diagnosis of type 1 diabetes.
β-cell defect results in decreased insulin secretory capacity below the amount needed for the degree of insulin resistance leading to hyperglycemia and the diagnosis of diabetes.
Pancreas
Excessive hepatic glucose production causes increased hyperglycemia in the fasting and postprandial state.
Liver

Fig. 46-2 Altered mechanisms in type 1 and type 2 diabetes. *ICA,* islet cell antibodies.

Type 2 Diabetes Mellitus. Approximately 90% of people with diabetes mellitus have type 2. Type 2 diabetes has a strong genetic influence (almost 100% concordance in monozygotic twins), but no correlation with HLA type has been found.

Genetic counseling for the type 2 group is based on a known higher familial risk. The siblings of a person with type 2 diabetes have a 7% to 14% risk for type 2 diabetes developing. The offspring of parents who both have type 2 diabetes have a 15% to 45% chance of the disease developing. Children and young adults with type 2 diabetes have a 50% chance of transmitting the disease to their children.[7]

Prevalence of diabetes increases with age, with about half of cases in people older than age 55. It was formerly called non–insulin-dependent diabetes mellitus or maturity-onset diabetes. These names are no longer used because they do not accurately characterize the treatment or the pathophysiology. Prevalence of type 2 varies by race and is highest among Native-Americans such as the Pima tribe (one out of two adults has type 2 diabetes mellitus). Hispanic populations are two times as likely to develop diabetes as non-Hispanic whites. Overall, the prevalence of diagnosed and undiagnosed diabetes in adults is about 30% higher in African-Americans than in Caucasians.[1] Obesity appears to play a major role in type 2 diabetes.

In addition to older age at onset, type 2 diabetes mellitus is distinguished by an endogenous insulin supply sufficient to inhibit the development of diabetic ketoacidosis (DKA), which occurs when endogenous insulin is markedly reduced or absent. The pathophysiologic factors that have been identified in type 2 diabetes include (1) decreased tissue (e.g., fat, muscle) responsiveness to insulin as a result of receptor or postreceptor defects; (2) overproduction of insulin early in the disease, but eventual decreased secretion of insulin from β-cell exhaustion; and (3) abnormal hepatic glucose regulation. These factors result in what is often referred to as peripheral insulin resistance. This resistance stimulates increased insulin production as a compensatory response, which may also predispose the patient to weight gain. A reduced-calorie diet for the obese patient with type 2 diabetes tends to reverse this phenomenon.[4] The patient with type 2 diabetes may benefit from oral antidiabetic agents, which have been found to be physiologically effective in several ways, including increasing insulin production, improving cell receptor binding, and regulating hepatic glucose production.

In type 2 diabetes mellitus the onset of hyperglycemic symptoms may occur over a long period. The person may "adjust" to the persistent feelings of fatigue, thirst, polyuria, and blurred vision without realizing that the diabetic disease process is producing the symptoms.[8] If the patient with type 2 diabetes has marked hyperglycemia (e.g., 500 to 1000 mg/dl; 27.6 to 55.1 mmol/L), a sufficient endogenous insulin supply may prevent DKA from occurring, but fluid and electrolyte loss may become severe and lead to hyperosmolar coma. (See Fig. 46-13 for the sequence of events associated with hyperosmolar hyperglycemia.) During precipitating and acute situations (such as acute illness), the patient with type 2 diabetes may briefly require insulin administration. It is also possible for the type 2 patient to have DKA if a precipitating stress event is severe and strains the available endogenous insulin supply. The fact that some persons with type 2 diabetes may require insulin during times of stress or for treatment of hyperosmolar nonketotic hyperglycemia does not mean that these persons are "insulin dependent" or will require long-term insulin treatment.[9]

Clinical Manifestations

Normally, insulin and its counterregulatory hormones maintain blood glucose within a range of 70 to 110 mg/dl (3.9 to 6.0 mmol/L). Elevated blood glucose levels produce symptoms related to the degree of actual or relative insulin deficiency. When an absolute insulin deficiency or decreased insulin activ-

COLLABORATIVE CARE

Table 46-3 Diabetes Mellitus

Diagnostic

- Complete history and physical examination
- Blood tests, including fasting blood glucose, postprandial blood glucose, glycosylated hemoglobin, cholesterol and triglyceride levels, blood urea nitrogen and serum creatinine, electrolytes
- Urine for complete urinalysis, microalbuminuria, culture and sensitivity, glucose and acetone
- Funduscopic examination—dilated eye examination
- Neurologic examination
- Blood pressure
- Monitoring of weight
- Doppler scan

Collaborative Therapy

- Calculated food plan
- Exercise plan
- Insulin or oral hypoglycemia agent (if indicated)
- Dental examination
- Podiatric examination
- Specific teaching and follow-up programs

ity occurs, glucose is not used properly. Glucose remains in the bloodstream and produces an osmotic effect on intracellular and interstitial fluid. This shift in fluid balance results in clinical symptoms of frequent urination (polyuria) and thirst (polydipsia). Without sufficient insulin the patient may experience hunger (polyphagia) as the body turns to other energy sources besides glucose: first fat and then protein. Varying degrees of polyuria, polydipsia, and polyphagia are the hallmark symptoms of diabetes mellitus. Acute and chronic complications from hyperglycemia are closely associated with the type of diabetes mellitus and the circumstances in which it occurs.

Diagnostic Studies

The classification of diabetes depends on appropriate and accurate diagnostic studies (Table 46-3). Urine tests are not sufficient for diagnosing diabetes mellitus because variables such as age, medications, and a normally low renal threshold for glucose may show glycosuria without the presence of diabetes or glucose intolerance.

When overt symptoms of hyperglycemia (polyuria, polydipsia, and polyphagia), together with fasting blood glucose levels of 126 mg/dl (7.0 mmol/L) or greater are present, further glucose tolerance tests are usually not warranted. However, when oral glucose tolerance tests are used, the accuracy of test results depends on adequate patient preparation and attention to the many factors that may influence the outcome of such tests. For example, factors that can cause falsely elevated values include recent severe restrictions of dietary carbohydrate, acute illness, medications such as contraceptives and glucocorticoids, and restricted activity such as bed rest. A patient with impaired gastrointestinal (GI) absorption may also have false-negative test results.

Because diabetes is a multisystem, multiproblem disease, all laboratory studies must be correlated with clinical findings. The most common finding in overt diabetes mellitus is an elevated blood glucose level (≥126 mg/dl [7.0 mmol/L]). Glucose values differ depending on the source of the sample and the site from which the blood is taken, the timing in relation to meals, and the time of day. Arterial blood values tend to be higher than venous blood samplings. Postprandial (after meals) and late afternoon values also tend to be higher.

In the presence of abnormal insulin use, fat metabolism is altered. This results in elevations of lipid, cholesterol, and triglyceride levels that are associated with the vascular disorders of diabetes.

The results of urine tests for glucose and acetone depend on age, severity of diabetes, and renal function. Blood glucose is a better measurement of glycemic status because glycosuria may not be evident when hyperglycemia is present. The presence of ketonuria and elevated serum ketones accompanied by marked hyperglycemia is the heralding sign of DKA. When a person without diabetes fasts, ketonuria also develops as a result of fat breakdown but without accompanying hyperglycemia.

Glycosylated hemoglobin is a measurement that is useful in determining glycemic levels over time. The hemoglobin of red blood cells (RBCs) attracts a certain amount of glucose (approximately 4% to 6% in the nondiabetic person). When blood glucose is elevated over time, or when the person has frequent wide fluctuations in glycemic levels, the amount of glucose attached to the hemoglobin molecule increases. The glucose remains attached to the RBC for the life of the cell (120 days). Therefore a glycosylated hemoglobin test indicates the overall glucose control for the past 120 days. Laboratory methods may differ in this assay because some methods measure the entire glycosylated hemoglobin molecule, whereas other methods measure only a specific glycosylated hemoglobin, hemoglobin A1, or hemoglobin A1c. The ideal goal range for glycosylated hemoglobin is a value that is less than 1% to 2% above the laboratory normal. Diseases affecting RBCs (e.g., sickle cell anemia) also affect the glycosylated hemoglobin results and should be taken into consideration in the interpretation of this test result. The glycosylated albumin (fructosamine), a glycosylated serum protein test, reflects blood glucose control over the preceding 7 to 10 days. The reliability and clinical applicability of these tests is under evaluation.[10]

Proteinuria is a sign of early nephropathy. Analysis for microalbuminuria may show early nephropathy long before routine urinalysis displays proteinuria.[11] Microalbuminuria tests are now the recommended method for early detection of nephropathy. The presence of protein in the urine as detected by microalbuminuria urinalysis should be followed with a 24-hour urine collection for determination of creatinine clearance and serum creatinine. It is important to monitor renal function because the patient with diabetes in the later stages of renal disease may require a reduction in insulin dose as a result of both a decrease in caloric intake and an alteration in insulin function and metabolism in chronic renal failure[11] (see Chapter 44).

The Doppler instrument is used to diagnose the presence or degree of peripheral vascular disease. It is a device similar to an electronic stethoscope that amplifies sound. The procedure is noninvasive and can measure blood pressure in the lower extremities and blood flow velocity. It can indicate areas of stenosis or occlusion and is useful as an indicator of the need for additional vascular tests.

Collaborative Care

Management of diabetes mellitus is primarily aimed at achieving a balance of diet, activity, and medications together with

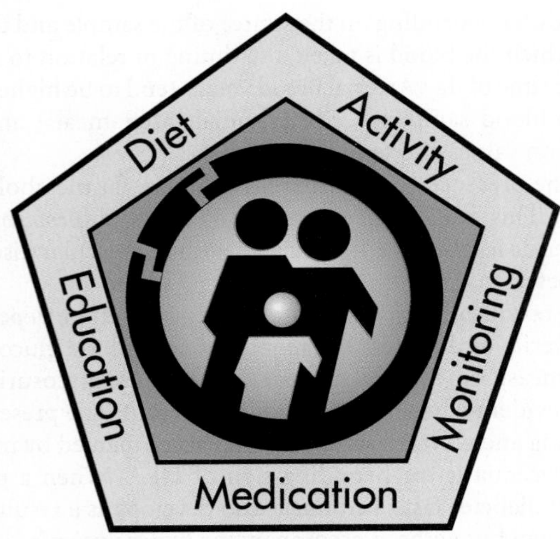

Fig. 46-3 The five aspects of diabetes management make up the complete program for good control.

appropriate monitoring and patient and family education (Table 46-3 and Fig. 46-3). These components are equally necessary for effective control of diabetes.

Nutritional Therapy. Nutritional therapy is the cornerstone of care for the person with diabetes. Achieving nutritional goals requires a coordinated team effort that includes the person with diabetes. Today there is no one "diabetic" or "ADA" diet. In an institutional setting, the prescribed diet is often labeled "ADA," indicating that the meal plan follows the American Diabetes Association's current nutritional recommendations.

The recommended diet can only be defined as a dietary prescription based on nutritional assessment and goals. Because of the complexity of nutritional issues, it is recommended that a registered dietician, with expertise in diabetes management, be a member of the treatment team. Effective self-management training requires an individualized approach that is appropriate for the personal lifestyle and diabetes management goals of the patient. Monitoring of glucose and glycosylated hemoglobin, lipids, and renal status is essential to evaluate nutrition-related outcomes. Nutritional assessment is used to determine what the individual with diabetes is able and willing to do. Sensitivity to cultural, ethnic, and financial considerations is important when developing individual meal planning approaches.

Goals of nutritional therapy. The overall goal is to assist people with diabetes in making changes in nutrition and exercise habits leading to improved metabolic control. Additional specific goals include the following:

1. Maintenance of as near-normal blood glucose levels as possible by balancing food intake with insulin (either endogenous or exogenous) or oral glucose-lowering medications and activity levels.
2. Achievement of optimal serum lipid levels.
3. Provision of adequate calories for maintaining or attaining reasonable weights for adults, normal growth and development rates in children and adolescents, increased metabolic needs during pregnancy and lactation, or recovery from catabolic illnesses. *Reasonable weight* is defined as the weight an individual and health care provider acknowledge as achievable and maintainable, both short-term and long-term. This may not be the same as the usually defined desirable or ideal body weight.
4. Prevention and treatment of acute complications, such as hypoglycemia, and long-term complications, such as renal disease, neuropathy, hypertension, and cardiovascular disease.
5. Improvement of overall health through optimal nutrition. The food guide pyramid summarize and illustrate nutritional guidelines and nutrient needs for all healthy Americans and can be used by the patient with diabetes (see Chapter 38).

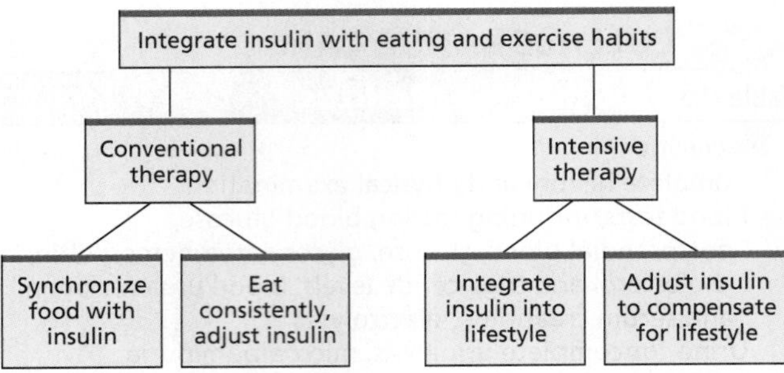

Fig. 46-4 Nutritional therapy for type 1 diabetes.

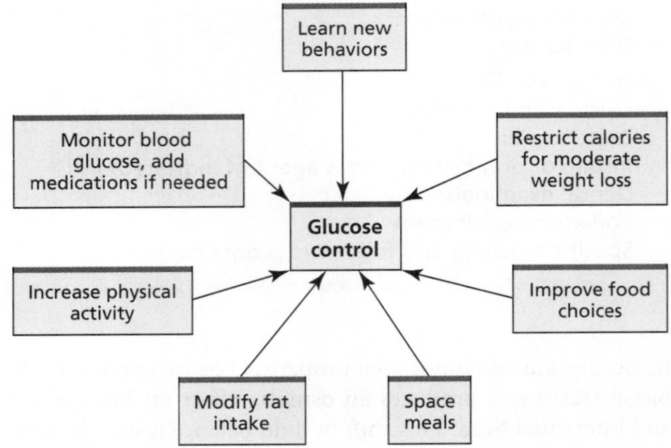

Fig. 46-5 Nutritional therapy for type 2 diabetes.

Type 1 diabetes. Meal planning should be based on the individual's usual food intake with insulin therapy integrated into the usual eating and exercise patterns. It is recommended that the individual using insulin therapy eat meals at consistent times synchronized with the action time of the insulin preparation used. Additionally, the individual must monitor blood glucose levels and adjust insulin doses for the amount of food eaten. Intensified insulin therapy, such as multiple daily injections or use of an insulin pump, allows considerable flexibility in food selection and can be adjusted for deviations from usual eating and exercise habits (Fig. 46-4).

Type 2 diabetes. The emphasis for nutritional therapy in type 2 diabetes should be placed on achieving glucose, lipid, and blood pressure goals. Weight loss and hypocaloric diets usually improve short-term glycemic levels and have the potential to increase long-term metabolic control. However, traditional dietary strategies and even very-low-calorie diets have usually

NUTRITIONAL THERAPY

Table 46-4 Diabetes Mellitus

Factor	Type 1 Diabetes Mellitus	Type 2 Diabetes Mellitus
▪ Total calories	Increase in caloric intake possibly necessary to achieve desirable body weight and restore body tissues	Reduction in caloric intake desirable for the obese patient
▪ Effect of diet	Diet and insulin necessary for glucose control	Diet alone possibly sufficient for glucose control
▪ Distribution of calories	Equal distribution of carbohydrates through meals or adjustment of carbohydrates for insulin activity	Equal distribution not essential; low-fat desirable; consistency of carbohydrate intake at meals desirable
▪ Consistency in daily intake	Necessary for glucose control	Desirable for weight reduction
▪ Uniform timing of meals	Crucial for NPH/Lente insulin programs; flexibility with multidose rapid-acting insulin	Desirable but not essential
▪ Intermeal and bedtime snacks	Frequently necessary	Not recommended
▪ Nutritional supplement for exercise programs	Carbohydrates 20 g/hr for moderate physical activities	Necessary if patient controlled on sulfonylurea or insulin

not been effective in achieving long-term weight loss, and the focus is more rationally placed on glucose and lipid goals.

Although weight loss is desirable, and some individuals are able to lose weight and maintain weight loss, several strategies can be implemented to improve metabolic control. No one proven strategy or method can be uniformly recommended. A nutritionally adequate meal plan with a reduction of total fat, especially saturated fats, can be employed. Spacing meals is another strategy that can be adopted to spread nutrient intake throughout the day. A weight loss of 11 to 22 lb (5 to 10 kg) has been shown to improve diabetes control, even if desirable body weight is not achieved. Weight loss is best attempted by a moderate decrease in calories and an increase in caloric expenditure. Regular exercise and learning new behaviors and attitudes can help facilitate long-term lifestyle changes. Monitoring of blood glucose levels, glycosylated hemoglobin, lipids, and blood pressure is essential (Fig. 46-5). Table 46-4 describes dietary strategies for type 1 and type 2 diabetes. General guidelines for patient teaching are shown in Table 46-5.

Food composition. Distribution of nutrients is based on guidelines for all adults. There are limited data on which to establish firm nutritional recommendations for protein. Dietary protein derived from both animal and vegetable sources should make up about 10% to 20% of calories. The remaining 80% to 90% of calories should be distributed between dietary fat and carbohydrates. Less than 10% of these calories should be from saturated fats. The distribution of calories from fat and carbohydrates can vary and can be individualized based on the nutritional assessment and treatment goals. Consideration of the individual's usual eating habits, lifestyle, body weight, and quality of life is essential for successful meal planning.

Another topic to consider is the glycemic index, which refers to the ranking of foods by comparing the glycemic effect on blood glucose in reference to white bread. This type of information is useful in considering ways to select and prepare foods for more predictable glycemic control. It has been concluded that starches and sucrose do not act differently in the context of a mixed meal when it comes to glycemic effect. It is important for patients to understand the principles underlying the glycemic index, or how foods of different composition affect blood glucose. Mixed meal, method of food preparation, and fiber content also play an important role.[12]

Scientific research has not supported the belief that simple sugars should be avoided and replaced with complex carbohydrates. Fruits and milks have been shown to have a lower glycemic response than most starches, and sucrose produces a glycemic response similar to that of bread, rice, and potatoes. Even though various starches do have different glycemic responses, from a clinical perspective, priority should be given to the total amount of carbohydrate consumed rather than the source of carbohydrate. The American Diabetes Association advises that the use of sucrose as a part of the meal plan does not impair blood glucose control in individuals with type 1 or type 2 diabetes. Sucrose and sucrose-containing foods must be substituted for other carbohydrates and not simply added to the meal plan. In making such substitutions, the nutrient content of concentrated sweets and sucrose-containing foods, as well as the presence of other nutrients frequently ingested with sucrose such as fat, must be considered.[12]

Diet teaching. Most often the dietician initially teaches the principles of the dietary prescription. However, the nurse should be knowledgeable about diabetes dietary principles to answer questions and to help the patient make appropriate selections and decisions. The nurse should include the family of the patient when teaching the diet plan. Particular attention and teaching efforts are effectively directed to the person who will be cooking. It is important, however, that the responsibility for maintaining a diabetic diet not fall to someone other than the patient with diabetes. Reliance on another person to make health decisions fosters dependence and should be avoided except in special situations.

Areas of concern

Alcohol. Alcohol is high in calories, has no nutritive value, and promotes hypertriglyceridemia. In addition, it has detrimental effects on the liver (see Chapter 41). The

PATIENT TEACHING GUIDE

Table 46-5 Diet Guidelines

Principles that both the nurse and dietician should teach and reinforce include the following:

1. **Eat according to the prescribed meal plan.** A dietary prescription is individualized to reflect the dietary needs related to a specific patient's body weight, occupation, age, activities, and type of diabetes. Individual responses to a dietary prescription should be monitored, and appropriate adjustments should be made when necessary.
2. **Never skip meals.** This is particularly important for the patient taking insulin or oral agents (OAs). The body requires food at regularly spaced intervals throughout the day. Insulin and OAs are prescribed to fit this schedule. Omission or delay of meals can result in hypoglycemia.
3. **Learn to recognize appropriate food portions.** Practice can result in accurate portion allotments.

inhibitory effect of alcohol on gluconeogenesis can cause severe hypoglycemia in patients on glucose-lowering agents. A patient can reduce this risk by eating carbohydrates when drinking alcohol. Alcohol may produce a disulfiram (Antabuse) effect (nausea and vomiting, flushing, respiratory distress, chest pain) proportional to the amount ingested with certain oral agents.

However, if the patient chooses, a drink can be included in the meal plan. One drink has approximately 135 calories. The patient with diabetes should drink alcohol with food, use sugar-free mixes, and drink dry, light wines.

Dietetic foods. The word *dietetic* is confusing because it does not always refer to a lack of calories. The caloric value of dietetic foods should be considered if weight loss is a dietary goal. Dietetic foods are expensive and, although convenient, are not necessary. The patient can be taught to make intelligent decisions regarding the use of nondietetic foods by reading labels. The increasing availability of foods prepared with artificial sweeteners allows greater freedom in the diet. Recipes that use artificial sweeteners are also available.

Drug Therapy: Insulin. The two types of glucose-lowering agents (GLAs) used in the treatment of diabetes are insulin and oral antidiabetes agents (OAs).

Indications for use. Exogenous insulin is needed when a patient has inadequate insulin to meet specific metabolic needs, and the combination of nutritional therapy, exercise, and OAs cannot maintain a satisfactory blood glucose level. Exogenous insulin is required for the management of type 1 diabetes. Exogenous insulin may be prescribed for the patient with type 2 diabetes during periods of severe stress, such as illness or surgery, or when attempts at glycemic control by means of diet, exercise, or OAs fail.

Types of insulin. Exogenous insulin has commonly been obtained from the pancreases of pigs and cows. These two forms of insulin are similar to human insulin protein chains, with pork insulin being more similar to human insulin. However, these sources have become expensive to obtain. Also, although the purification process for extracting the insulin islets has improved to where only minuscule amounts of foreign protein are present, these substances can initiate insulin allergies. Insulins marked "purified" have had nearly all extraneous pancreatic proteins removed.

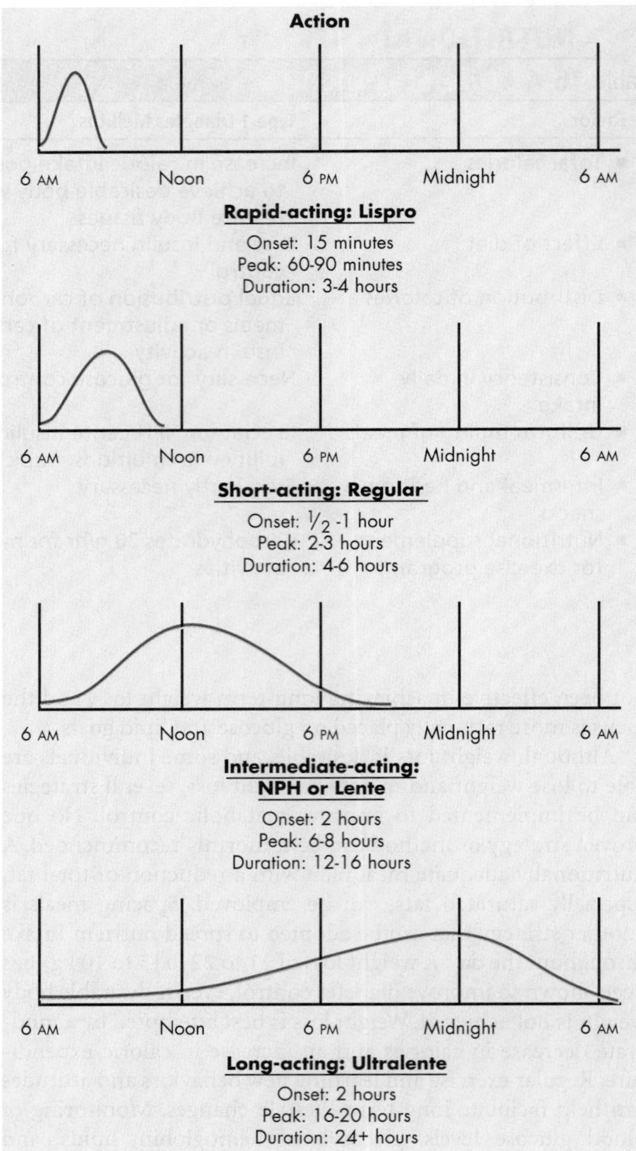

Fig. 46-6 Commercially available insulin preparations showing onset, peak, and duration.

Today, biosynthetic insulin is used almost exclusively. Human insulin is produced by genetically altering common bacteria or yeast using recombinant deoxyribonucleic acid (DNA) technology (see Fig. 12-12). This insulin exhibits chemical and biologic properties identical to human insulin produced by human β-cells. The advantage of these new insulins is a reduced allergic response and a more predictable insulin activity. The purified and human insulins are the preferred type of drug.

In addition to origin and purity, insulins differ in regard to onset, peak action, and duration (Fig. 46-6). The specific properties of each type of insulin are matched with the patient's diet and activity. Not all patients respond to insulin exactly as shown in Table 46-6. The action times are listed as approximate guidelines. Human insulin may have slightly less activity time.

Table 46-6 Insulin Regimens

Regimen	Type of Insulin Used	Time Administered and Expected Time-Action Curve*	Advantages	Disadvantages
Single dose	Intermediate insulin (I)	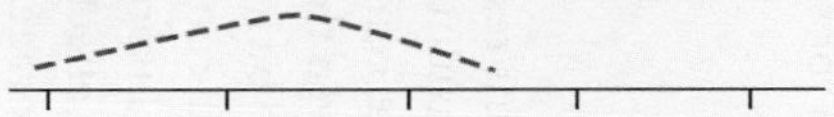 7 AM (I); Noon; 6 PM; Midnight; 7 AM	One injection should cover noon and PM meal. Hypoglycemia during sleep is not a problem.	No fasting, breakfast, or nighttime coverage of hyperglycemia is available.
Split-mixed dose (70/30 premix)	Intermediate and regular or Humalog insulin (I + R or I + H)	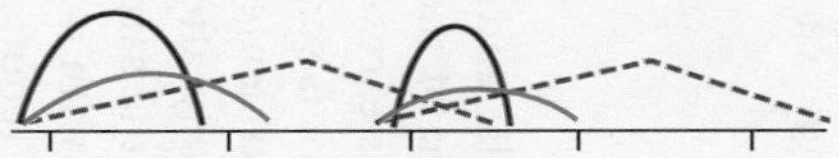 7 AM (I + R) (I + H); Noon; 6 PM (I + R) (I + H); Midnight; 7 AM	Two injections provide coverage for 24 hr.	Two injections are required. Patient must adhere to a set meal pattern.
Split-mixed dose	Intermediate and regular or Humalog insulin (I + R or I + H)	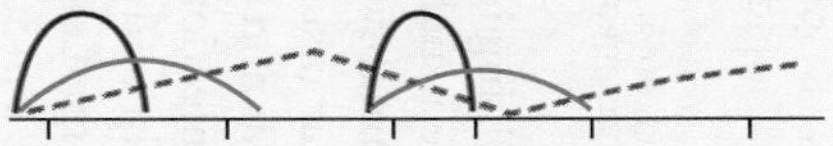 7 AM (I + R) (I + H); Noon; 7 PM (R) (H); 9 PM (I); Midnight; 7 AM	Three injections provide coverage for 24 hr, particularly during early AM hours. Potential is reduced for 2-3 AM hypoglycemia.	Three injections are required.
Multiple dose	Intermediate and regular or Humalog insulin (I + R or I + H)	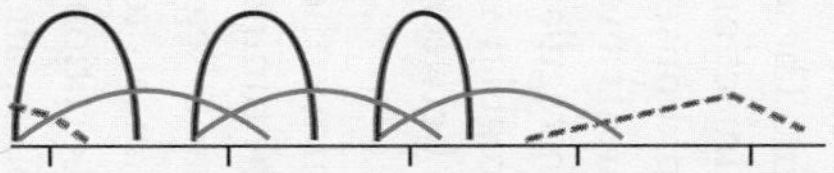 7 AM (R) (H); Noon (R) (H); 7 PM (R) (H); 9 PM (I); 7 AM	More flexibility is allowed at mealtimes and for amount of food intake.	Four injections are required. Premeal blood glucose checks, establishing and following individualized algorithm are necessary. Patients with type 1 will require basal insulin (I or LA) during the day.
Multiple dose† (split dose long-acting insulin [Ultra Lente])	Regular or Humalog and long acting insulin (R + LA or H + LA)	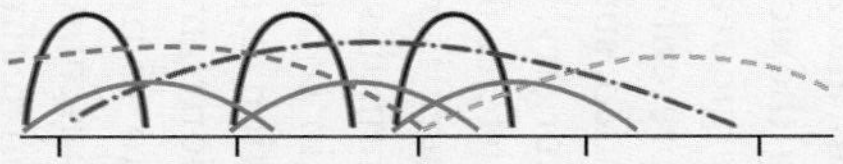 7 AM (H + LA) (R + LA); Noon (H) (R); 7 PM (H + LA) (R + LA); Midnight; 7 AM	Insulin delivery pattern more closely simulates normal endogenous insulin pattern. Some flexibility is allowed in food intake pattern. Regimen gives a basal insulin coverage and regular or Humalog insulin covers meal blood glucose excursions.	Required three or four injections and blood glucose check premeal and on retiring. Establishing and following individualized algorithm are necessary.

*H = lispro (Humalog) or rapid-acting insulin (R) = ———
I = intermediate insulin = - - - -
LA = long-acting insulin = — · — ·
R = regular insulin = ———
†Insulin delivery through a pump is similar to this regimen.

By adding zinc, acetate buffers, and protamine to insulin in various ways, the onset of activity, peak, and duration times can be manipulated.[13] A new class of insulins, synthetic analogs, were introduced in 1996 with the advent of lispro insulin (Humalog). Lispro is a synthetic product made by exchanging the amino acids proline and lysine at positions 28 and 29 on the beta chain of the insulin molecule.[14] This change in structure results in a change in time of action. Regular human insulin self-associates into hexameric structures that require 30 minutes to 1 hour to break apart in subcutaneous deposits. This is the cause of the 30- to 60-minute delay in onset of action for regular insulin. Lispro's structure permits rapid dissociation and therefore an onset of action of approximately 15 minutes. This rapid-acting insulin has a peak of 30 to 90 minutes and duration of 4 hours or less. This time action profile makes lispro a preferred meal coverage insulin. Lispro can be used wherever regular insulin is used, but because of its limited duration of action, a basal background insulin must be used in conjunction with the meal coverage when lispro is used for patients with type 1 diabetes.[14] Different combinations of insulins can be used to tailor treatment to the patient's specific pattern of blood glucose levels. Formulas are classified as rapid acting (e.g., lispro insulin [Humalog]), short acting (e.g., regular insulin [Humulin]), intermediate acting (e.g., NPH insulin [Humulin L]), and long acting (Ultralente insulin [Humulin U]). In the future the same technology used to make lispro insulin will be used to create new insulins with different times of action.

All insulin preparations start with regular insulin as a base; zinc is added to make Lente insulin, and zinc and protamine are added to make NPH to prolong the action of insulin. These binding agents can cause an allergic reaction at the injection site. Lispro or regular insulin is prescribed when a rapid onset of glucose-lowering action is needed, such as before meals and during periods of acute illness, surgery, or stress. Both regular and lispro insulin can be administered IV; however, regular is used in emergencies because there is no difference between lispro and regular in half-life (9 minutes).

Insulins are commonly used in combination to mimic the normal endogenous insulin secretion (see Fig. 46-1). The timing of insulin administration in relation to meals is important. Regular insulin should be taken 30 to 45 minutes before meals to ensure the onset of action in conjunction with meal absorption. Examples of insulin combination regimens, onset, peak, and descriptions of the advantages and disadvantages of each regimen are presented in Table 46-6. Ideally, regimens should be mutually selected by the patient and the health care provider. The criteria for selection are based on the type of diabetes and the required, desired, and feasible levels of glycemic control.

Because a single injection of a modified insulin rarely provides adequate glycemic control for most insulin-dependent patients, lispro or regular insulin is mixed with the modified insulin in the same syringe to avoid unnecessary injections. On the basis of current insulin formulations and use, the effect of NPH and lispro or regular insulin mixed in any proportion is the same as if the two were injected separately. The commercially available 70/30 or 50/50 mixtures of NPH and regular insulin appear to have the same activity as their component insulins given at separate injection sites. Stable mixtures with lispro and intermediate-acting insulin will probably be on the market in the near future.

PATIENT TEACHING GUIDE

Table 46-7 Insulin Therapy

1. Wash hands thoroughly.
2. Roll intermediate or long-acting insulin bottle between palms of hands to mix insulin. *Note:* Always inspect insulin bottle before using it for first time. Make sure that it is of proper type and concentration, expiration date has not passed, and top of bottle is in perfect condition.
3. Prepare insulin injection in same manner as for any injection.
4. Select proper injection site and inject following procedure for any SC injection.* In sites where SC tissue is adequate, inject commercial insulin needles at 90-degree angle. For sites with minimal SC tissue, pinch up skin and insert needle at 45-degree angle.
5. If blood appears in syringe after needle is inserted, select new site for injection. Aspiration is not necessary.
6. After injecting insulin, apply some pressure with dry cotton ball (or 2 × 2) at site when withdrawing needle.
7. Hold ball in place for a few seconds but do not massage.
8. Destroy and dispose of single-use syringe safely. *Note:* When instructing patient to self-inject insulin, use the following guidelines (if appropriate):
   - Aspiration does not need to be done before injection.
   - Disposable syringes can be reused for several injections.

*See Fig. 46-8.
SC, subcutaneous.

Mixing human regular and lente insulins results in blunting of the usual peak action of the regular insulin, but not lispro, presumably because the excess zinc in the Lente insulin binds regular insulin. A patient is sometimes given the option to mix regular and Lente or Ultralente and should be instructed to give the injection immediately after mixing if combining a Lente insulin and regular in the same syringe. Lispro can be mixed with the Lente insulins with no change in effect.

As a protein, insulin requires special storage considerations. Heat and freezing alter the insulin molecule. Insulin in use may be left at room temperature for up to 4 weeks unless the room temperature is higher than 70° F (21° C) or below freezing. Extra insulin may be stored in the refrigerator. The same principles apply for a patient with diabetes who is traveling. Insulin can be stored in a thermos or cooler to keep it cool (not frozen) if the patient is traveling in hot climates.

Administration of insulin

Injection. Because insulin is inactivated by gastric juices, it must be administered by injection. Daily administration of insulin is most commonly done by means of subcutaneous (SC) injection, although intramuscular (IM) or IV administration of regular insulin can be done when immediate onset of action is desired. The half-life of regular insulin in the circulation is 9 minutes, necessitating a continuous IV infusion for administration rather than a bolus IV injection. The steps in administering an SC insulin injection are outlined in Table 46-7. The tech-

1. Wash hands.
2. Gently rotate NPH insulin bottle.
3. Wipe off tops of insulin vials with alcohol sponge.
4. Draw back amount of air into the syringe that equals total dose.
5. Inject air equal to NPH dose into NPH vial. Remove syringe from vial.
6. Inject air equal to regular dose into regular vial.

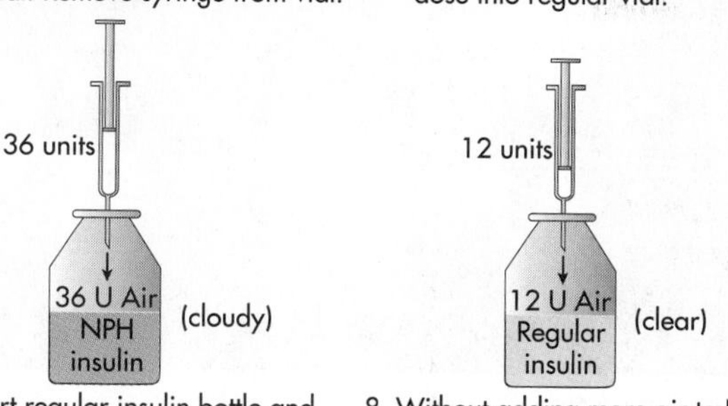

7. Invert regular insulin bottle and withdraw regular insulin dose.
8. Without adding more air to NPH vial, carefully withdraw NPH dose.

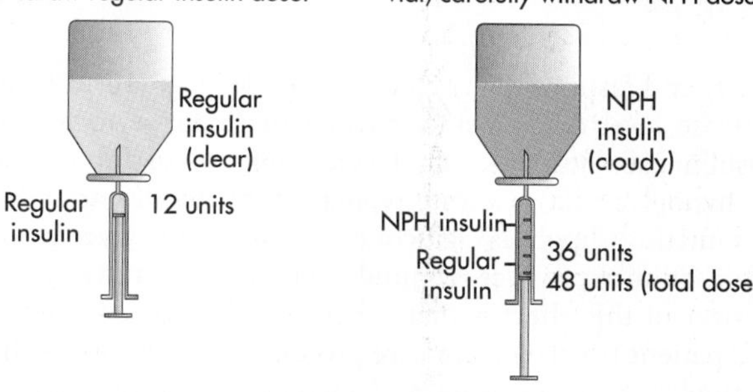

Fig. 46-7 Mixing insulins. This step-order process avoids the problem of contaminating regular insulin with intermediate-acting insulin.

nique should be taught to new insulin users and reviewed periodically with long-term users. It should never be assumed that because insulin is being used, the patient knows and practices the correct insulin injection technique. Inaccurate preparation is often caused by poor eyesight. Air bubbles in the syringe may not be seen, or the scale on the syringe may be read improperly. Administration systems, such as the insulin "pen," or "prefilled syringe," are available for patient convenience and are sometimes useful for visually or manually impaired persons.

The patient receiving mixed insulins (e.g., regular and an intermediate-acting insulin) must learn the proper technique for combining both in the same syringe if commercially prepared premixed insulins are not used (Fig. 46-7). Insulins should not be mixed if they differ in purity or species of origin.

Recommended sites for insulin injection are noted in Fig. 46-8. The speed with which peak serum concentrations are reached varies with the anatomic site for injection. The fastest absorption is from the abdomen, then the arm, thigh, and buttock. Because of the variability in absorption and the decreased frequency of lipoatrophy in a patient treated with human or purified pork insulins, rotation of injection sites is no longer the recommended injection technique when these types of insulin are used. The patient should rotate the injection sites within a particular area, such as the abdomen, for a period, and then, if rotation to the thigh is desired, the patient can adjust the regimen to the new peak and action times for the new site.

The patient should also be cautioned about injecting into a site that is to be exercised. For example, the patient should not

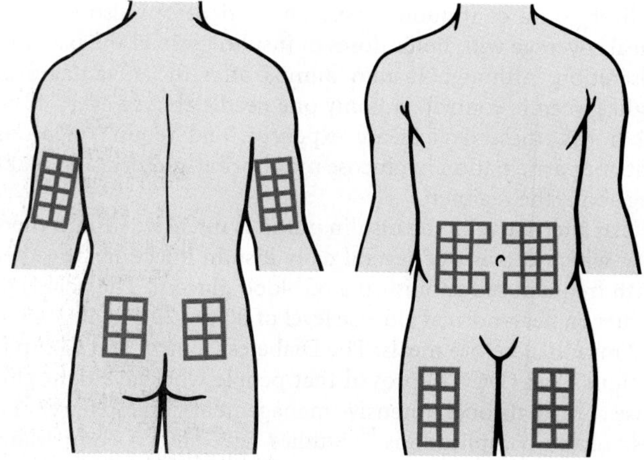

Fig. 46-8 Injection sites for insulin.

inject insulin into the thigh and then go jogging. Exercise of the area containing the injection site together with the increased body heat generated by the exercise may increase the rate of absorption and speed the onset of insulin action.

Insulin administration also requires the appropriate syringe. Most commercial insulin is available as U100, indicating that each milliliter contains 100 U of insulin. U100 insulin must be used with an U100-marked syringe. For a user taking smaller doses of insulin, insulin syringes with larger black lines are marked for 25, 30, or 50 U and are available for use with U100 insulin. One important distinction regarding the different-size syringes is that the 100 U syringe is marked in 2 U increments, whereas the 50 U and 30 U syringes are marked in 1 U increments. To avoid serious dosing errors, the patient must use the correct syringe and not switch back and forth between different-size syringes. Before the development of U100 insulin, insulin was available in concentrations of U40 and U80. U500 insulin is available for patients requiring very large doses of insulin.

Some patients may prefer to use their syringe more than once. Insulin preparations have bacteriostatic additives that inhibit growth of bacteria commonly found on the skin. Many studies have shown that it is both safe and practical for the syringe to be reused if the patient desires. The syringe should be discarded when the needle becomes dull, has been bent, or has come in contact with any surface other than the skin. If reuse is planned, the needle must be recapped after each use.[15]

Another change in the insulin injection routine relates to the use of the alcohol swab on the skin before injection. When instructing a patient on the technique of insulin injection, the use of the alcohol wipe is optional. Routine hygiene such as washing with soap and rinsing with water is adequate.[16]

Alternative delivery methods. Continuous SC insulin infusion is currently being accomplished through insulin pumps. The pump devices are able to deliver insulin continuously in titrated amounts through tubing attached to a small pump device on one end and to a needle on the other end, which is placed subcutaneously in the skin. The pump delivers a preprogrammed dose of insulin that is designed to match the patient's basal profile to achieve a nearly normal insulin delivery on a continuous basis. The patient can also regulate meal coverage with bolus doses of insulin given at the patient's discretion. Although insulin pumps offer the advantages of tight glycemic control and only one needle change every 48 to 72 hours, these devices are expensive and require vigorous patient participation in glucose monitoring and decision making about the regimen.

An alternative to the insulin pump is intensive insulin therapy, which consists of several daily insulin injections together with frequent self-monitoring of blood glucose. The goal is to achieve a near-normal glucose level of 80 to 120 mg/dl (4.45 to 6.7 mmol/L) before meals. The Diabetes Control and Complications Trial (DCCT) proved that people who have tight glucose control through intensive management develop fewer and less severe complications.[17] Studies have shown comparable control outcomes in patients receiving intensive therapy and patients with an insulin pump. Because the required patient participation is similar, intensive therapy may be instituted before the initiation of pump use.[17] Because of the specialized nature of these insulin delivery systems and devices, expert guidance from a physician and a nurse educator is essential.

Intensive insulin therapy is not for everyone. Children are already at increased risk for low blood glucose (hypoglycemia), which can impair normal brain development. This risk is increased with intensive insulin therapy. In the elderly, intensive insulin therapy increases the risk of hypoglycemia, which could result in heart attacks or strokes during periods of low blood glucose in older adults with atherosclerosis.[18]

Another insulin administration technique under investigation is aerosol inhalation. In a small study, aerosol insulin, inhaled in 5 to 10 times the amount of insulin found in normal injections, effectively controlled blood glucose levels.[19] No adverse respiratory tract or hypoglycemic symptoms were reported. If further studies of aerosol insulin prove the effectiveness of this method, persons with diabetes may have a more convenient method to control their blood glucose levels.

Problems with insulin therapy. Hypoglycemia, allergic reactions, lipodystrophy, and the Somogyi effect are the problems associated with insulin therapy. Hypoglycemia is discussed in detail later in this chapter.

Allergic reactions. There are three types of allergic reactions to insulin. Local reactions may occur as itching, erythema, and burning around the injection site. Local reactions may be self-limiting within 1 to 3 months or may improve with a low dose of antihistamine.

A "true" insulin allergy is a systemic response with urticaria and possibly anaphylactic shock generally resulting from the use of animal insulins. Fortunately, this type of allergy is rare, particularly since human insulin has become available.

Lipodystrophy. Lipodystrophies (hypertrophy or atrophy of SC tissue; lipoatrophy) may occur if the same injection sites are used frequently (Fig. 46-9). Hypertrophy, a thickening of the SC tissue, eventually regresses if the patient does not use the site for at least 6 months. The use of hypertrophied sites may result in erratic insulin absorption. Lipoatrophies have been most commonly associated with beef or beef and pork insulin and rarely with human insulin. Site rotation on a daily or weekly basis is not necessary with human insulin.

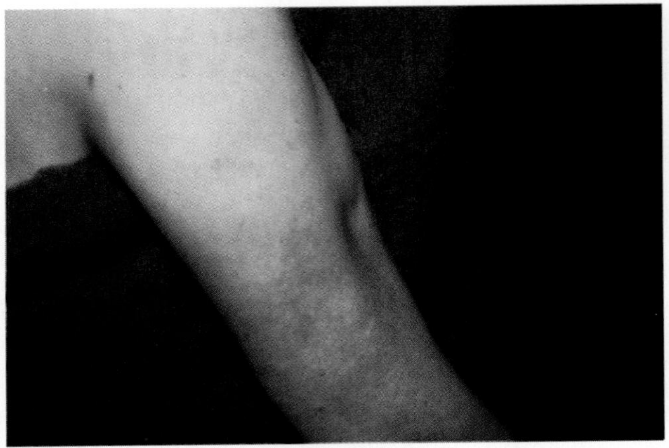

Fig. 46-9 Lipodystrophy of the arm.

Somogyi effect and dawn phenomenon. The Somogyi effect is characterized by wide differences in early morning (low) and fasting (high) glucose levels (Fig. 46-10). The blood glucose level drops below normal in response to too much insulin usually in the night (see Table 46-20 for the causes of hypoglycemia). Counterregulatory hormones are released, stimulating lipolysis, gluconeogenesis, and glycogenolysis, which in turn produce rebound hyperglycemia and ketosis. The danger of this effect is that, when blood glucose is measured, the patient (or the health care professional) may assess the situation as hyperglycemia and increase the insulin dose. The Somogyi effect is associated with the occurrence of undetected hypoglycemia during sleep, although it can happen at any time. The patient may report headaches on awakening and may recall night sweats or nightmares. When the Somogyi effect occurs at night, the patient's blood glucose is elevated on awakening in the morning.

With the dawn phenomenon, hyperglycemia is also present on awakening in the morning and ketonuria may be present. The cause is theorized to be a dawn release of endogenous growth hormone or cortisol, diurnal variation of insulin clearance, and insulin sensitivity. Both growth hormone and cortisol are counterregulatory hormones to insulin and raise the blood glucose level. The dawn phenomenon affects the majority of diabetics and tends to be most severe when growth hormone is at its peak in adolescence and young adulthood.

Careful assessment is required to document each phenomenon because the treatment for each differs. The treatment for the Somogyi effect is less insulin. The treatment for the dawn phenomenon is an adjustment in the timing of insulin administration or an increase in insulin. The assessment must include insulin dose, injection sites, and variability in the time of meals or insulin administration. In addition, the patient is asked to measure and document bedtime, between 2 and 4 AM, and morning fasting blood glucose levels on several occasions. If the predawn levels are below 60 mg/dl (3.3 mmol/L) and signs and symptoms of hypoglycemia are present, the insulin dosage should be reduced. If the 2 to 4 AM blood glucose is high, the insulin dosage should be increased.[20] In addition, the patient should be counseled on appropriate bedtime snacks.

Drug Therapy: Oral Agents. Currently, four classes of medications are available to improve diabetes control for patients with type 2 diabetes. Oral agents are listed in Table 46-8.

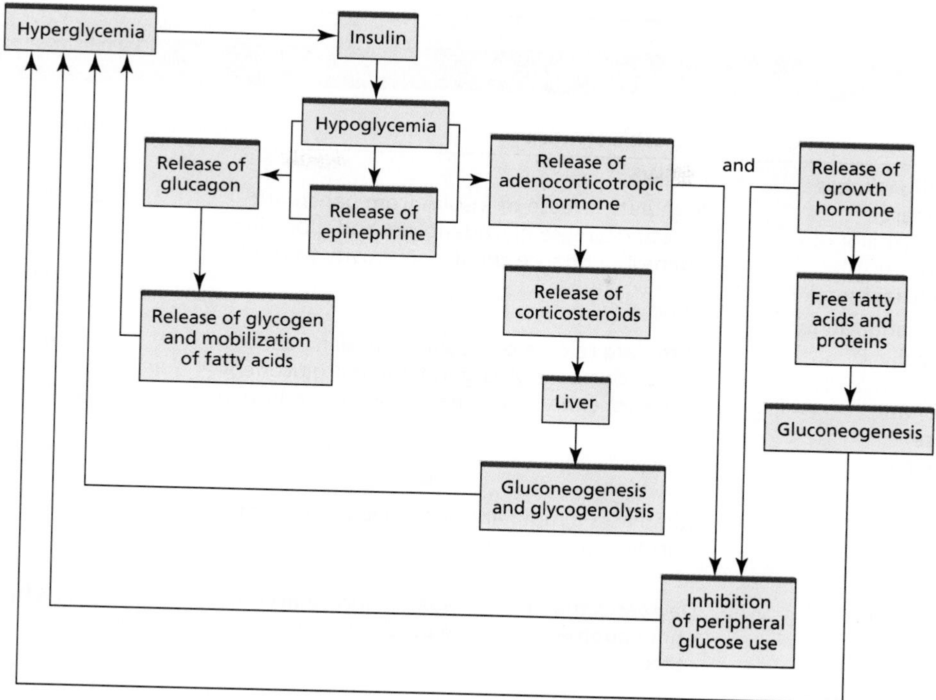

Fig. 46-10 The Somogyi effect.

Sulfonylureas. Sulfonylureas were found to have blood glucose–lowering effects during research on their antibiotic properties in the 1940s. They are called first generation or second generation depending on when they were introduced into clinical use in the United States. The first generation of these drugs used in the treatment of diabetes mellitus included tolbutamide (Orinase), acetohexamide (Dymelor), tolazamide (Tolinase), and chlorpropamide (Diabinese). A second generation of sulfonylureas, approved for use in the United States more recently, includes glipizide (Glucotrol and Glucotrol XL), glyburide (Micronase, DiaBeta, Glynase), and glimepiride (Amaryl).

Second-generation drugs have fewer adverse effects, are about 100 times more potent by weight, and have more predictable action times and half-lives.[21] Their drug interaction potential is lower because they bind to circulating proteins differently. The main disadvantage of second-generation drugs is their increased expense.

Meglitinides. Repaglinide (Prandin), classified as a meglitinide, stimulates the pancreas to secrete insulin, which is an action similar to that of the sulfonylureas. However, it has a more rapid onset and shorter duration of action. It is most effectively used before meals.

Biguanides. Metformin (Glucophage) is a biguanide glucose-lowering agent. Worldwide, metformin is widely used as a monotherapy and in combination with a sulfonylurea. Unlike sulfonylureas, metformin is not bound to plasma proteins, is not metabolized, and is eliminated rapidly by the kidney. The glucose-lowering effect occurs without stimulation of insulin secretion and results mainly by decreasing the rate of hepatic glucose production (gluconeogenesis). The presence of insulin is required for metformin to be effective. Metformin may also act by augmenting glucose uptake by muscle tissues. Because metformin does not cause clinical hypoglycemia, it is actually an antihyperglycemic drug. It does not cause weight gain and helps combat hypertriglyceridemia.[20] Side effects include GI problems such as nausea, diarrhea, and flatulence. Lactic acidosis is also a potential side effect for which the patient and nurse should monitor. Metformin is contraindicated in patients with renal insufficiency (serum creatinine >1.5 mg/dl for men and >1.4 mg/dl for women), congestive heart failure, or alcohol abuse.[22]

Alpha glucosidase inhibitors. Carbohydrate absorption inhibitors is another class of oral antidiabetes agents that work in the small intestine. Alpha glucosidase inhibitors, such as acarbose (Precose) and miglitol (Glyset), slow the breakdown of disaccharides and polysaccharides and other complex sugars into monosaccharides on the brush border of the small intestine. The enzymatic generation and subsequent absorption of glucose is delayed, and the postprandial blood glucose, which is usually high after a meal high in carboyhydrates, is improved. The most common side effects of these medications include flatulence and mild abdominal pain. Many of the symptoms are dose related and transient, occurring with the highest frequency during the first few weeks of therapy. Titration of acarbose up from 25 mg with the first bite of a meal to 50 to 100 mg with each meal will help minimize the GI side effects. Dosages at different meals can be determined and adjusted by postprandial monitoring of blood glucose, usually 1 to 2 hours after meals. This drug can be used as a monotherapy or in combination with other oral agents or insulin.

Thiazolidinediones. Thiazolidinediones are a new class of agents that improve peripheral insulin resistance in skeletal muscle without stimulating insulin secretion. These agents work

DRUG THERAPY

Table 46-8 Oral Agents for Diabetes Mellitus*

Type	Mechanism of Action	Duration of Action
First-Generation Sulfonylureas		
Tolbutamide (Orinase)	Stimulate release of insulin from pancreatic islets; decrease glycogenolysis and gluconeogenesis; enhance cellular sensitivity to insulin	6-12 hr
Acetohexamide (Dymelor)		12-24 hr
Tolazamide (Tolinase)		12-24 hr
Chlorpropamide (Diabinese)		36-60 hr
Second-Generation Sulfonylureas		
Glipizide (Glucotrol, Glucotrol XL)	Stimulate release of insulin from pancreatic islets; decrease glycogenolysis and gluconeogenesis; enhance cellular sensitivity to insulin	10-24 hr
Glyburide (Micronase, DiaBeta, Glynase)		24 hr
Glimepiride (Amaryl)		24 hr
Meglitinides		
Repaglinide (Prandin)	Stimulates a rapid and short-lived release of insulin from the pancreas	2-3 hr
Biguanide		
Metformin (Glucophage)	Decreases the rate of hepatic glucose production; augments glucose uptake by muscle tissues	12-24 hr
Alpha-Glucosidase Inhibitors		
Acarbose (Precose) Miglitol (Glyset)	Works on the brush border of the small intestine to slow the breakdown of disaccharides and polysaccharides into monosaccharides; delays subsequent absorption of glucose	Affects postprandial absorption of carbohydrates
Thiazolidinediones		
Rosiglitazone (Avandia) Pioglitazone (Actos)	Decreases peripheral insulin resistance in skeletal muscle without stimulating insulin secretion	>24 hr

*Side effects can be minimized if OA choice is matched appropriately to patient's needs. OAs are not appropriate for ketosis-prone patients and pregnant patients and should be used cautiously if at all in patients with renal or hepatic dysfunction.

using a novel action that stimulates glucose transport in muscle and, to a lesser degree, hepatic tissues. Fasting and glucose-stimulated insulin levels are reduced while glucose disposal is increased in obese, insulin-resistant patients. Thus these agents reduce insulin resistance and improve glycemia both as monotherapy and in combination with sulphonylureas or metformin. Troglitzone (Rezulin), the first thiazolidinedione, was approved in 1997. However, because of reported cases of hepatic failure, this agent was removed from the market in 1999. Newer thiazolidinediones include rosiglitazone (Avandia) and pioglitazone (Actos). There are still potential liver problems with these agents. Liver function tests are required at baseline, then every 2 months for the first year and periodically thereafter.

Indication for use. OAs are not oral insulin or a substitute for insulin. The patient must have some functioning endogenous insulin for OAs to be effective. They may be used in combinations of oral agents or with insulin to achieve goal-range control. Guidelines for assessing patients receiving OAs are shown in Table 46-9.

In the patient with newly diagnosed diabetes, therapy with OAs may not be started until the patient has been given an opportunity to try dietary control. Even if OA therapy is initially successful, the patient may eventually fail to maintain control and insulin therapy may have to be initiated.

The hypoglycemic action of OAs can be enhanced and prolonged by means of the concurrent administration of drugs such as anticoagulants, salicylates, alcohol, and propranolol. Drugs that can oppose OA action include thyroid preparations, corticosteroids, and thiazide diuretics.

Other Drugs Affecting Blood Glucose Levels. The patient with diabetes may be concurrently taking other medications. Both the patient and the health care provider must be aware of drug interactions that can potentiate hypoglycemic and hyperglycemic effects. For example, beta-adrenergic drugs block the hepatic glycogenolytic response that occurs in response to hypoglycemia. Thiazide diuretics can also potentiate hyperglycemia by inducing potassium loss. A list of medications that may influence glycemic control is pre-

Table 46-9 Assessing the Patient Treated with Glucose-Lowering Agents

For patient with newly diagnosed diabetes or for reevaluation of GLA regimen	
Cognitive	Is patient or responsible other able to understand why insulin or OAs are being used as part of diabetes management? Is patient or responsible other able to understand concepts of asepsis, combining insulins, insulin-OA actions, and side effects? Is patient able to remember to take >1 dose/day? Does patient take medications at right times in relation to meals?
Psychomotor	Is patient or responsible other physically able to prepare and administer accurate doses of GLA?
Affective	What emotions and attitudes are patient and responsible others displaying in regard to diagnosis of diabetes and insulin or OA treatment?
For follow-up of GLA-treated patient	
Effectiveness of therapy	Is patient having symptoms of hyperglycemia? Does blood glucose and urine record show good or poor control? Is glycosylated hemoglobin consistent with glucose records?
Side effects of GLA therapy	Is atrophy or hypertrophy present at injection sites? Has patient had hypoglycemic episodes? If so, how often? What time of day? Are there complaints of nightmares, night sweats, or early morning headaches? Has patient had skin rash or GI upset since taking OA?
Self-management behaviors	If patient is having hypoglycemic episodes, how are those episodes managed? How much insulin or OA is patient taking and at what times of day? Is patient adjusting insulin or OA dose? Under what circumstances and by how much? Has exercise pattern changed? Is patient adhering to number of prescribed calories? Are meals taken at times corresponding to peak insulin action?

GLA, glucose lowering agent.

DRUG THERAPY

Table 46-10 Blood Glucose Level Effects

Glucose-Lowering Effect

Acetaminophen	Clofibrate	Potassium salts
Alcohol	Dicumarol	Probenecid
Allopurinol (Zyloprim)	Fenfluramine	Salicyclates in large doses
α-Glucosidase inhibitors	Histamine antagonists	Sulfonylureas
Anabolic steroids	Insulin	Thiazolidinediones (rosiglitazone)
β-Adrenergic blockers	Monoamine oxidase inhibitors	Tricyclic antidepressants
Biguanides	Phenylbutazone	Urinary acidifiers
Chloramphenicol		

Glucose-Raising Effect

Acetazolamide (Diamox)	Ethacrynic acid (Edecrin)	Marijuana
Asparaginase (Elspar)	Morphine	Nicotine
Caffeine in large doses	Epinephrine	Nifedipine (Procardia)
Arginine HCl	Furosemide (Lasix)	Phenobarbital
Barbiturates	Glucagon	Phenothiazines
β-Adrenergic blockers	Glucose	Phenytoin (Dilantin)
Birth control pills	Glycerin	Rifampin
Cholestyramine (Questran)	Glycerol	Thiazide diuretics
Corticosteroids	Levodopa	Urinary alkalizing agents
Calcitonin	Lithium	

sented in Table 46-10. Medications may have to be changed or dosages adjusted if the patient is also taking GLAs.

Exercise

Regular, consistent exercise is considered an essential part of diabetic management. Exercise contributes to weight loss, reduces triglycerides and cholesterol, increases muscle tone, and improves circulation. In type 1 diabetes, exercise may increase insulin sensitivity, thereby allowing a lowering of the insulin dose. In type 2 diabetes, exercise contributes to weight loss and improves insulin binding on cell receptors. However, the patient should be aware that exercise is perceived by the body as a stress, and that counterregulatory hormones are increased to ensure that adequate glucose is readily available.

PATIENT TEACHING GUIDE

Table 46-11 **Exercise**

1. Exercise does not have to be vigorous to be effective. The blood glucose–reducing effects of exercise can be attained with mild exercise such as brisk walking. The exercises selected should be enjoyable to foster regularity.
2. Exercise is best done after meals, when the blood glucose level is rising.
3. Exercise plans should be individualized for each patient and monitored by the health care provider.
4. It is important to self-monitor blood glucose levels before, during, and after exercise to determine the effect exercise has on blood glucose level at particular times of the day.
5. Be alert to the possibility of delayed exercise-induced hypoglycemia, which may occur several hours after the completion of exercise.
6. Taking a GLA does not mean that planned or spontaneous exercise cannot occur. It is important to compensate for extensive planned and spontaneous activity by monitoring blood glucose level to make adjustments in the insulin dose (if taken) and food intake.

Table 46-12 **Activities That Affect Caloric Expenditure**

Light Activity (100-200 cal/hr)	Moderate Activity (200-350 cal/hr)	Vigorous Activity (400-900 cal/hr)
Driving a car	Active housework	Aerobic exercise
Fishing	Bicycling	Bicycling
Light housework	Bowling	Hard labor
Secretarial work	Brisk walking	Ice skating
Teaching	Dancing	Outdoor sports
Walking casually	Gardening	Running
	Golf	Soccer
	Roller skating	Tennis
		Wood chopping

As a result, hyperglycemia may occur in situations of poorly controlled diabetes or in insulin-dependent patients who exercise at a time of day when insufficient insulin is available. Additional information about exercise and diabetes that is important for both the patient and the health care provider is provided in Table 46-11.

Hypoglycemia is likely to occur if the insulin-dependent patient exercises at a time when the GLA action is peaking or if exercise is strenuous and prolonged and carbohydrate is not replaced. This can also occur if a normally sedentary patient with diabetes has an unusually active day. Exercise can be scheduled about 1 hour after a meal, or a 10 to 15 g carbohydrate snack can be eaten before exercising to avoid hypoglycemia. For every 45 minutes to 1 hour of strenuous exercise such as tennis, the patient should repeat the 10 to 15 g carbohydrate snack. (See Table 46-12 for guidelines on calories burned per hour for different activities.)

Hyperglycemia may occur if exercise is scheduled at a time when insulin action is waning. When the insulin dose is insufficient to cover the amount of exercise, the increase in blood glucose created by the counterregulatory hormones may not be curtailed. Again, the patient can guard against this situation by scheduling exercise when sufficient insulin is available. Some patients may have to inject a small bolus of regular insulin if the blood glucose level is elevated before exercising to prevent progressive hyperglycemia.[24]

Monitoring Blood Glucose

Glucose levels must be determined daily to monitor the interactions and effect of diet, exercise, and medication on an individual diabetic regimen. Detection of extreme or episodic hyperglycemia is necessary to avoid DKA and hyperglycemic hyperosmolar nonketosis (HHNK). Traditionally, monitoring has been accomplished by checking for the presence and degree of glycosuria. This technique provides only gross, semiquantitative information. Many factors affect urine test results, such as age, medications, disease, and the individual renal threshold. Urine testing also cannot measure the presence or degree of hypoglycemia. Urine testing for ketonuria, however, is a valuable aid in determining the advent of DKA and is recommended for every patient with type 1 diabetes when the patient is experiencing hyperglycemia or acute illness. Second-voided specimens, which were previously recommended for the patient using urine testing, have been shown to constitute an unnecessary step.

Self-Monitoring. Self-monitoring of blood glucose using capillary blood glucose monitoring (CBGM) technology is a more reliable technique for measuring blood glucose. Commercially available glucose-testing products, including disposable lancets and lancet holders, are widely available. A small drop of capillary blood (usually from a finger stick) is dropped onto a reagent strip. After a specified time, the strip is read either visually or by a machine. The machines are either reflectance meters or sensors. Reflectance meters work by measuring the amount of light reflected onto a strip that has reacted with a color change in response to the reaction of glucose with the reagent strip. Sensors use the measurement of conductivity of electricity as it is affected by the glucose in the blood. The technology of CBGM is a rapidly changing field with newer and more convenient systems being introduced every year. Blood glucose monitoring technology uses a noninvasive spectroscopy, or the use of laser light on a skin surface. Implantable sensors for continuous glucose monitoring are also being considered in research trials.[25] A diabetes educator should be consulted to learn the latest in monitoring technology.

Many meters are computerized and are becoming increasingly sophisticated. Some models are capable of storing results of previous blood glucose tests. These tests can be retrieved to provide a more complete picture of blood glucose fluctuations over time and to guide adjustment to the regimen.

The blood glucose level reported by a laboratory is often higher than the patient's home glucose monitor or the hospital's portable meter. This is because a finger stick is based on a capillary whole blood sample rather than a plasma sample, so it may be approximately 10% to 15% lower. Plasma or serum gives a higher glucose reading.[3] To further complicate this

PATIENT TEACHING GUIDE

Table 46-13 Capillary Blood Glucose Monitoring

1. Hands are washed in warm water. Cleaning the site with alcohol is not necessary and may even interfere with test results.
2. If it is difficult to obtain an adequate drop of blood for testing, the patient should warm the hands in warm water or let the arms hang dependently for a few minutes before the finger puncture is made.
3. The puncture is made on the side of the finger pad rather than near the center. Fewer nerve endings are along the side of the finger pad.
4. The puncture should be only deep enough to obtain a sufficiently large drop of blood. Unnecessarily deep punctures may cause pain and bruising.

process, some monitors are calibrated to give whole blood results while other meters are calibrated to give values equivalent to plasma concentrations. This must be determined by reading the literature accompanying the particular monitor and strips being used by the patient. Finally, home monitoring equipment must be cleaned and calibrated regularly to maintain its accuracy.

The technique for using a blood glucose–monitoring product accompanies each product. Because errors in monitoring technique can cause errors in clinical management strategies that may be based on erroneous CBGM information, patient training should be emphasized not only at the initial session but at follow-up visits with any member of the health care team. Patient technique should be reassessed at 30 to 180 days after initial training and yearly thereafter.[26] The major source of variability in results obtained with CBGM devices is attributable to the user.[27] Table 46-13 lists the steps that the patient performing CBGM should be taught.

The advantages of CBGM are that it ensures immediate information about blood glucose levels and produces accurate records with daily glucose fluctuations and trends.[28] CBGM is the preferred glucose-monitoring method for the patient with type 1 diabetes. The type 2 diabetic patient may also benefit from CBGM by seeing the correlation between dietary choices and blood glucose levels. As weight is lost and blood glucose levels are lowered, the obese type 2 patient may also gain reinforcement from CBGM.

The frequency of monitoring depends on the glycemic goals the patient and health care provider set and the intensity of the treatment regimen. The patient receiving two or more injections per day may want to test before meals every day. If the glycemic control is relatively stable, the patient may elect to test two or more times a day on certain days of the week. Testing is most often done before meals but can be done any time the patient needs to know the way a factor, such as exercise or stress, is affecting the blood glucose level. The frequency of recording CBGM results to guide therapy decisions should be mutually determined by the health care provider and the patient.

Ideally, a patient should be motivated to learn not only CBGM technique but also how to interpret the results. Most patients find that CBGM brings about physiologic and emotional benefits, as well as a willingness to be an active partner in the treatment. Achieving the desired level of patient participation also requires time and effort from the health care professional. The nurse involved in this aspect of management should anticipate a close working relationship with the patient for a period of 3 to 6 months as the patient learns refinements of the technique and appropriate decision making regarding changes in diet, medication, and exercise. A patient who is visually impaired, color blind, or limited in manual dexterity needs careful evaluation of the glucose-monitoring method most appropriate for that patient's needs. Glucose monitors are now commercially available for the visually impaired.

NURSING MANAGEMENT: DIABETES MELLITUS

■ Nursing Assessment

Initial subjective and objective data that should be obtained from a person with diabetes mellitus are presented in Table 46-14. After the initial assessment, periodic patient assessments should be done on a schedule as outlined in Table 46-15.

■ Nursing Diagnoses

Nursing diagnoses for the patient with diabetes mellitus may include, but are not limited to, those found in NCP 46-1.

■ Planning

The overall goals are that the patient with diabetes mellitus will (1) be an active participant in the management of the diabetes regimen; (2) experience minimal or no episodes of DKA, HHNK, or hypoglycemia; (3) prevent or delay the occurrence of chronic complications of diabetes; and (4) adjust lifestyle to accommodate diabetes regimen with a minimum of stress.

■ Nursing Implementation

Health Promotion. The role of the nurse in health promotion and maintenance relates to the identification, monitoring, and education of the patient at risk for the development of diabetes mellitus. The American Diabetes Association now recommends routine screening for diabetes for all adults over age 45, and if normal, it should be repeated at 3-year intervals. This screening should include a fasting plasma glucose, although a screening may be done by capillary glucose in some instances. Testing should be considered at a younger age or be carried out more frequently in individuals who meet the criteria listed in Table 46-16.[5]

A person with impaired glucose tolerance with plasma levels of glucose that are higher than normal is also at increased risk for diabetes. In addition, the presence of pancreatic or endocrine disease or the use of certain medications such as corticosteroids also alerts the nurse to evaluate this person for diabetes.

Acute Intervention. The nurse is involved with the care of a patient with diabetes in many acute situations, such as DKA, hypoglycemia, and HHNK. Nursing management for hypoglycemia, DKA, and HHNK are discussed starting on p. 1396. Other areas of acute intervention relate to management during stress, such as during acute illness and surgery.

Stress of acute illness and surgery. Both emotional and physical stress can increase the blood glucose level and result in hyperglycemia. However, it is impossible to avoid stress totally

NURSING ASSESSMENT

Table 46-14 Diabetes Mellitus

Subjective Data	Objective Data
Important Health Information *Past health history:* Mumps, rubella, coxsackievirus or other viral infections; recent trauma, infection, or stress; pregnancy, gave birth to infant >9 lb; chronic pancreatitis; Cushing's syndrome, acromegaly *Family history:* History of type 1 or type 2 diabetes mellitus *Medications:* Use of and compliance with insulin or OAs; use of glucocorticoids, diuretics, phenytoin (Dilantin) *Surgery and other treatments:* Any recent surgery **Functional Health Patterns** *Health perception–health management:* Positive family history; malaise *Nutritional-metabolic:* Obesity; weight loss (type 1), weight gain (type 2): thirst, hunger; nausea and vomiting; poor healing especially involving the feet, compliance with diet in patients with previously diagnosed diabetes *Elimination:* Constipation or diarrhea; frequent urination, nocturia, incontinence; skin infections *Activity-exercise:* Muscle weakness, fatigue *Cognitive-perceptual:* Abdominal pain, headache; blurred vision; numbness or tingling of extremities; pruritus *Sexuality-reproductive:* Impotence; frequent vaginal infections; decreased libido *Coping–stress tolerance:* Depression, irritability, apathy *Value-belief:* Commitment to lifestyle changes involving diet, medication, and activity patterns	**Eyes** Soft, sunken eyeballs; vitreal hemorrhages, cataracts **Integumentary** Dry, warm, inelastic skin; pigmented lesions (on legs); ulcers (especially on feet), loss of hair on toes **Respiratory** Rapid, deep respirations (Kussmaul respirations) **Cardiovascular** Hypotension; weak, rapid pulse **Gastrointestinal** Dry mouth, vomiting, fruity breath **Neurologic** Altered reflexes, restlessness, confusion, stupor, coma **Musculoskeletal** Muscle wasting **Possible Findings** Serum electrolyte abnormalities; fasting blood glucose level ≥126 mg/dl (7.0 mmol/L); glucose tolerance test ≥200 mg/dl (11.1 mmol/L); leukocytosis; elevated blood urea nitrogen, creatinine, triglycerides, cholesterol, LDL, VLDL; glycosylated hemoglobin ≥6%; glycosuria; ketonuria; albuminuria; acidosis

LDL, low density lipoproteins; *VLDL*, very low density lipoproteins.

in life situations such as deaths in the family, job interviews, and final examinations. These situations may require extra insulin to avoid hyperglycemia.

Common stress-evoking situations include acute illness and the controlled stress of surgery. The patient with diabetes who has a minor illness such as a cold or the flu should continue drug therapy and food intake. A carbohydrate liquid substitution such as regular soft drinks, gelatin dessert, or beverages such as Gatorade may be necessary. The patient should understand that food intake is important during this time because the body requires extra energy to deal with the stress of the illness. Extra insulin may be necessary to meet this demand without DKA concurrently developing.

Blood glucose monitoring should be done every 1 to 2 hours by either the patient or a person who can assume responsibility for care during the illness. Urine output and the presence and degree of ketonuria should be monitored, particularly when fever is present. Fluid intake should be increased to prevent dehydration, with a minimum of 4 oz per hour for an adult.

The patient should be instructed to contact the health care provider when a blood glucose level more than 250 mg/dl (13.9 mmol/L), fever, ketonuria, and nausea and vomiting occur. The health care provider should supervise the necessary adjustments in the treatment regimen during times of stress. Eventually, the well-informed patient will be able to make most adjustments independently on the basis of past successful experiences.

Surgery is controlled stress, and adjustments in the diabetes regimen can be planned to ensure glycemic control. The patient is given IV fluids and insulin immediately before, during, and after surgery when there is no oral intake. The type 2 diabetic patient receiving OAs usually has the OAs discontinued 48 hours before surgery and is treated with insulin during the surgical period. The patient should understand that this is a temporary measure and is not to be interpreted as a worsening of diabetes.

The nurse caring for an unconscious surgical patient receiving insulin must be alert for hypoglycemic signs such as sweating, tachycardia, and tremors. The nurse should be aware that blood glucose monitoring must also be done frequently.

Ambulatory and Home Care. The nurse may be involved in any or all aspects of management, but the focus of nursing care has two aims: to care for the patient during acute episodes and to assist the patient in learning to live with diabetes every day. Both aims require the nurse to be thoroughly familiar with diabetes and its management and to educate the patient with diabetes about all aspects of the disease.

Patients are often treated in outpatient diabetes clinics. Frequently these clinics are staffed by diabetes nurse specialists. These specialists have preparation beyond the baccalaureate degree in diabetes and work collaboratively with physicians to manage patients with diabetes. The diabetes nurse specialist is also often available to the nursing staff for consultation in the acute care setting.

Table 46-15 Standards of Medical Care for a Patient with Diabetes Mellitus

Item	Initial Visit	Every 3 Mo	Every 12 Mo
Assessment of Glycemic Control			
Symptoms of hypoglycemia	X	X	
Symptoms of hyperglycemia	X	X	
Record of blood tests	X	X	
Glycosylated hemoglobin	X	X	
Assessment for Complications			
Postural blood pressure and pulse (BP goal <130/85)	X	X	
Weight	X	X	
Funduscopic—dilated eye examination	X	X	
Ophthalmologist or optometrist			X
Cardiac examination	X		X
Neurologic examination			
Sensory: monofilament foot examination	X		X
Motor: ankle reflexes, muscle bulk and tone	X		X
Pelvic examination as indicated for vaginal discharge		As needed	
Extremities			
Feet: calluses, toenails, ulcers	X	X	
Peripheral pulses			
Dorsalis pedis	X		X
Posterior tibial	X		X
Popliteal	X		X
Femoral	X		X
Assessment of Educational Needs			
Diet	X	X	
Medication management	X	X	
Monitoring skills	X	X	
Diagnostic Studies			
Blood glucose level	X	X	
Blood urea nitrogen and creatinine level	X		X
Urinalysis for microalbuminuria	X		X
Electrocardiogram	X*		X
Lipid profile	X		X
Fasting triglyceride level	X		X

*If appropriate to age and history.

The nurse may request consultation with a diabetes educator who is certified by the National Certification Board for Diabetes Educators. Certified diabetes educators (CDEs) have met stringent preparation and experience criteria and have demonstrated expertise in the field of diabetes education. Nurses, dieticians, pharmacists, physicians, and other health care professionals who make up the diabetes management team are eligible to apply for the CDE credential. The certified diabetes educator is designated with the initials CDE after the name.

The effect of the diagnosis of diabetes cannot be overestimated. An assessment of the patient's perception of what it means to have diabetes must be carefully assessed before patient education is designed and implemented. The nurse should foster a positive attitude about the prescribed regimen and assist the patient in developing an individualized management plan. Learning goals should be mutually determined by the patient and the nurse on the basis of individual needs and therapeutic requirements. The nurse should assess the patient's feelings and facilitate acceptance of diabetes mellitus and its treatment over time.

A clinical pathway for home care of the patient with diabetes mellitus is provided on p. 1389.

Insulin therapy. Nursing responsibilities for the patient receiving insulin include proper administration, assessment of the patient's use of and response to insulin therapy, and education of the patient regarding administration, adjustment to, and side effects of insulin (see Table 46-6). Table 46-9 lists guidelines for the nurse assessing a patient using glucose-lowering agents, including insulin and OAs.

The patient with newly diagnosed diabetes should be assessed for the ability to understand the purpose of insulin therapy; the interaction of insulin, diet, and activity; and the ways side effects may be manifested. The patient or significant other also has to be able to prepare and inject the insulin. If the patient or family lacks the psychomotor skills to prepare insulin, the nurse may have to find additional resources to assist the patient.

Some patients find it difficult to inject themselves. This may be due to fear of the needle or anger and lack of acceptance of the disease. The nurse should determine the emotions and attitude of the patient and family regarding insulin therapy.

46-1 NURSING CARE PLAN PATIENT WITH DIABETES MELLITUS*

Expected Patient Outcomes | **Nursing Interventions and *Rationales***

Ambulatory and Home Care

NURSING DIAGNOSIS **Ineffective management of therapeutic regimen** *related to* inadequate knowledge of adequate exercise program, diet and weight control, administration and potential side effects of glucose-lowering agents (GLAs), glucose monitoring, and care during acute minor illness *as manifested by* frequent questioning regarding diabetic management, inaccurate responses to questions about diabetic management.

Expected Patient Outcomes

- Participation in exercise program.
- Appropriate dietary preparation and intake.
- Safe, effective administration of GLA.
- Demonstration of proper blood glucose testing and recording of measurements.
- Plan of action for self in event of illness and symptoms lasting >24 hr.

Nursing Interventions and *Rationales*

- Plan individualized exercise program with patient *because exercise is an integral part of diabetic management.*
- Review steps to prevent hyperglycemia and hypoglycemia *because activity changes can cause changes in insulin needs.*
- Review diet and problem areas with patient *to provide appropriate teaching.*
- Counsel on weight loss if appropriate *because excess weight complicates diabetic management.*
- Refer to dietician *because dietary management of diabetes can be complex and requires ongoing monitoring.*
- Review GLA administration; have patient give return demonstration of insulin injection *to ensure proper technique.*
- Assess injection sites *to determine need for changing sites or initiating treatment to problematic areas.*
- Review symptoms and treatment of hypoglycemia *so early treatment can be initiated.*
- Demonstrate glucose testing; have patient give return demonstration *to ensure proper technique.*
- Review glucose records with patient and explain how to identify trends *to improve glucose control.*
- Remind patient to call physician if blood glucose is >250 mg/dl (13.9 mmol/L) and ketonuria is present *so appropriate adjustments can be made to prevent development of diabetic ketoacidosis (DKA).*
- Review effect of stress on glycemic control *so patient is aware that stress can increase glucose level.*
- Review sick-day care *so patient can make appropriate adjustments in diabetic management.*
- Assist patient in devising a sick-day plan, including foods to have on hand and family member or friend who can be with patient during illness episode, *to be ready to properly manage diabetes when illness occurs.*
- Review symptoms needing attention of physician, including blood glucose level >250 mg/dl (13.9 mmol/L), ketonuria, fever, nausea, and vomiting *so patient can contact physician when necessary to prevent occurrence of DKA and hyperglycemic hyperosmolar nonketosis (HHNK).*

NURSING DIAGNOSIS **Risk for infection** *related to* depressed immune system, inadequate circulation, and environmental pathogens.

Expected Patient Outcomes

- Verbalization of steps to prevent infection (skin care, foot care, regular dental care).
- Recognition of signs of infection and need for intervention.

Nursing Interventions and *Rationales*

- Assess for signs of infection such as fever, redness, swelling, or pus at trauma or pressure site; fever *to ensure early recognition and treatment.*
- Assess oral cavity, skin, pulses, particularly lower extremities and pedal pulses, *to detect areas of infection or poor circulation.*
- Review skin and foot care; have patient give return demonstration of foot care *to ensure patient understanding.*
- Review signs of infection, including redness, swelling, pus, and when to contact health care provider *to ensure patient recognizes infection and notifies health care provider if indicated so treatment can be initiated.*

Continued

46-1 NURSING CARE PLAN PATIENT WITH DIABETES MELLITUS*—continued

Expected Patient Outcomes	Nursing Interventions and *Rationales*
NURSING DIAGNOSIS	**Self-esteem disturbance** *related to* lifestyle changes imposed by diabetes and its treatment and frustration at progression of disease *as manifested by* negative feelings about self, resistance to incorporating treatment regimen into lifestyle.
▪ Verbalization of positive attitude about self and ability to manage disease. ▪ Plan for continued contact with health care provider for health monitoring.	▪ Encourage patient to discuss diagnosis and its implications *so appropriate counseling and interventions can be planned.* ▪ Suggest individualized diabetes education and support group *to increase patient's knowledge base and meet other people with diabetes.* ▪ Suggest creative approaches to problems with patient *because patient may be overwhelmed initially by complexity of disease management.* ▪ Assure patient of continued value and self-worth *to minimize impact of diabetes on patient's self-esteem.*

COLLABORATIVE PROBLEMS

Nursing Goals	Nursing Interventions and *Rationales*
	Acute Management
POTENTIAL COMPLICATION	**DKA and HHNK** *related to* inadequate insulin and excess blood glucose secondary to increased caloric intake, physical or emotional stress, or undiagnosed diabetes.
▪ Monitor for signs of DKA and HHNK. ▪ Report deviations from acceptable parameters. ▪ Carry out appropriate medical and nursing interventions.	▪ Assess for signs of DKA such as increase in urination; vomiting; somnolence; dehydration; dry, loose skin; hypotension with weak, rapid pulse; coma; hyperglycemia >250 mg/dl (13.9 mmol/L); presence of urine ketones; pH <7.3 *to ensure early recognition and intervention.* ▪ Assess for signs of HHNK such as hyperglycemia >500 mg/dl (27.8 mmol/L), serum osmolality >300 mOsm/kg (300 mmol/kg), absence of ketonuria *to detect signs of HHNK.* ▪ Administer insulin per physician order *to stabilize blood glucose level.* ▪ Administer fluid and electrolyte replacement as ordered *to correct dehydration.* ▪ Monitor input and output and vital signs *to detect signs and symptoms of inadequate tissue perfusion.* ▪ Assess for precipitating factors *to prevent recurrence and identify teaching needs.*
POTENTIAL COMPLICATION	**Hypoglycemia** *related to* low blood glucose secondary to too much insulin.
▪ Monitor for signs of hypoglycemia. ▪ Report deviations from acceptable parameters. ▪ Carry out appropriate medical and nursing interventions.	▪ Assess for signs of hypoglycemia such as cold sweats; weakness; trembling; nervousness; irritability; pallor; increase in heart rate; confusion; fatigue; abnormal behavior *to ensure prompt identification and treatment.* ▪ Check blood glucose if time permits (e.g., when symptoms are mild) *to provide an indicator for treatment.* ▪ Provide quick-acting carbohydrate source such as 6-8 oz orange juice, 1 cup milk, or 6-8 oz soft drink *to quickly reverse hypoglycemia;* give orally only if patient is alert enough to swallow *to prevent aspiration.* ▪ Repeat oral dose in 10-15 min if no improvement. If no improvement or patient is comatose, administer 1 mg glucagon subcutaneously or 30-50 ml of 50% IV dextrose per physician order *to stimulate hepatic response to convert glycogen to glucose.* ▪ When patient improves and is alert, provide long-acting carbohydrate or next scheduled meal *to keep blood glucose level within acceptable range.* ▪ Assess for precipitating factors such as history of too much insulin, too little food, unusual amounts of exercise, or delayed eating *to prevent recurrence and identify precipitating factors.*

*This care plan is intended to be used for persons with newly diagnosed diabetes.

Table 46-16 Criteria for Testing in Asymptomatic, Undiagnosed Individuals

Type 1 diabetes: Testing presumably healthy individuals for the presence of any immune markers, outside of a clinical trials setting, is not recommended.

Type 2 diabetes: In asymptomatic, undiagnosed individuals, testing for diabetes should be considered in all individuals at age 45 years and above; if normal, it should be repeated at 3-year intervals.

Testing* should be considered at a younger age, or be carried out more frequently, in individuals who

- are obese (≥120% desirable body weight or a body mass index ≥27 kg/m^2)
- have a first-degree relative with diabetes
- are members of a high risk ethnic population (African-American, Hispanic, Native-American, Asian)
- delivered a baby weighing >9 lb or were diagnosed with gestational diabetes mellitus
- are hypertensive (≥140/90 mm Hg)
- have an HDL cholesterol level ≤35 mg/dl (9.1 mmol/L) or a triglyceride level ≥250 mg/dl (2.82 mmol/L)
- on previous testing had impaired glucose tolerance or impaired fasting glucose

Adapted from American Diabetes Association Clinical Practice Recommendations.
*The fasting plasma glucose is the preferred diagnostic test because of its ease of administration, convenience, acceptability to patients, and lower cost.

Name Phone
Address
Physician Phone
Address

INSULIN	DOSAGE	TIME	ORAL MEDICATION	DOSAGE	TIME
Regular			Orinase		
PZI			Diabinese		
Globin			Dymelor		
NPH			Tolinase		
Lente			DBI		
Semilente			DBI TD		
Ultralente					

Date

I am a DIABETIC

If unconscious or behaving abnormally, I may be having a reaction associated with diabetes or its treatment.

If I can swallow give me sugar, candy, or a sweet drink. If I do not recover promptly, call a physician or send me to the hospital.

If I am unconscious or cannot swallow, do not attempt to give me anything by mouth, but call a physician or send me to the hospital immediately.

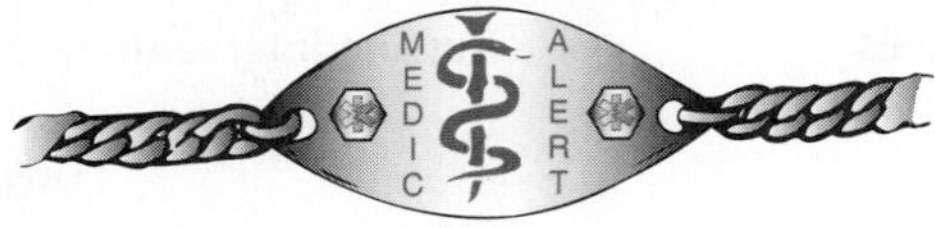

Fig. 46-11 Medical alerts. A patient with diabetes should carry a card and wear a bracelet or necklace that indicates diabetes. If the patient with diabetes is unconscious, these measures will ensure prompt and appropriate attention.

Follow-up assessment of the patient who has been using insulin therapy also includes an inspection of injection sites for allergic reactions, a review of insulin preparation and injection technique, a history pertaining to the occurrence of hypoglycemic episodes, and the patient's method for handling hypoglycemic episodes. A review of the patient's record of urine and blood glucose tests is also important in assessing overall glycemic control.

Oral agents. Nursing responsibilities for the patient taking OAs are similar to those for the patient taking insulin. Proper administration, assessment of the patient's use of and response to the OA, and education of the patient and the family about OAs are all part of the nurse's function. Table 46-9 lists guidelines for the nurse assessing a patient starting therapy with OAs and the follow-up assessment. The assessment done by the nurse can be invaluable in determining the most appropriate oral agent for a patient. The assessment includes the patient's mental status, eating habits, home environment, attitude toward diabetes, and use of oral agents. For example, if the patient is older, lives alone, or has difficulty remembering to follow a medication and diet schedule, a shorter-acting OA may be preferable. Some patients may assume that their diabetes is not a serious condition if they are taking only a pill for glycemic control. The patient needs to understand the importance of diet and not skipping meals. The patient should not take extra pills if overeating has occurred. The patient also needs to know that if on sulfonylureas, hypoglycemic reactions may be severe and prolonged and that health care provider supervision may be necessary, particularly for the older patient.

The patient should also be instructed to contact a physician if periods of illness or extreme stress occur. During such a period, insulin therapy may be required to prevent or treat hyperglycemic symptoms and HHNK.

Personal hygiene. The potential chronic complications of infections, neuropathy, and microangiopathy require the patient with diabetes to participate in effective hygiene practices related to skin and dental care. Because of susceptibility to periodontal disease and pyorrhea, daily brushing and flossing should be encouraged. When dental work must be done, the dentist should be informed that the patient has diabetes.

Daily baths should be part of routine care, with particular emphasis given to foot care. (See Table 46-25 for patient teaching guide.) If cuts, scrapes, or burns occur, they should be treated promptly. The area should be washed, and a nonabrasive or nonirritating antiseptic ointment must be applied. The area should be covered with a dry, sterile pad. If the injury does not begin to heal within 24 hours or if signs of infection develop, the health care provider should be notified immediately.

Medical identification and travel. The patient should be instructed to carry medical identification at all times indicating diabetes. An identification card (Fig. 46-11) can supply valuable information, such as the name of the health care provider and the type and dose of insulin or OA. A Medic Alert bracelet or necklace should be worn by every person with diabetes. Police, paramedics, and many private citizens are aware of the need to look for this identification when working with sick or unconscious persons.

Travel for a patient with diabetes requires planning in advance. The patient should have all supplies in carry-on luggage and keep them at hand at all times. This includes insulin, syringes, quick-acting carbohydrate, and glucagon. Extra insulin should be available in case a bottle breaks or gets lost. If

CLINICAL PATHWAY Home Care of Diabetes Mellitus

ICD-9 Code(s) 250.9, 250.91, 250.11, 250.70

Patient Name ____________ **Pt. ID No.** ________ **SOC Date** ________ **Discharge Date** ________

Date Noted	Expected Outcomes	Achieved			Variance Codes	Date Noted	Nursing Diagnoses	Date Closed
		Y	N	Date				
	1. Stable endocrine status by visit no. ___ as noted by blood glucose in range of ___ to ___.						Cardiac output, decreased Outcome(s) no. ____ :	
	2. Patient/caregiver demonstrates compliance with treatment regimen to include dietary and exercise requirements, as well as general health issues by visit no.___						Coping, ineffective family/patient Outcome(s) no. ____ :	
	3. Patient/caregiver demonstrates understanding and compliance with blood glucose testing, insulin administration, and medication regimens as evidenced by return demonstration by visit no. ___						Denial, ineffective Outcome(s) no. ____ :	
							Knowledge deficit: medication and therapeutic regimen Outcome(s) no. ____ :	
	4. Patient/caregiver demonstrates understanding of home safety, general emergency measures related to disease condition, infection control, and proper disposal of contaminated wastes by visit no. ___.						Management of therapeutic regimen, ineffective Outcome(s) no. ____ :	
							Nutrition, altered: risk for more than body requirements Outcome(s) no. ____ :	
	5. Other:						Tissue perfusion, altered: peripheral, renal Outcome(s) no. ____ :	
	6. Other:						Noncompliance (specify) Outcome(s) no. ____ :	
	7. Other:						Other: Outcome(s) no. ____ :	

Adapted from Marrelli TM, Hilliard LS: *Home care and clinical paths: effective care across the continuum,* St Louis, 1996, Mosby.

Continued

the patient is planning a trip out of the country, it is wise to have a letter from the physician explaining that the patient has diabetes and requires all the materials, particularly syringes, for ongoing health care.

Some travel involves time changes such as traveling coast to coast or across the international date line. The patient should contact the health care provider to plan an appropriate insulin schedule. Many patients find it easier and more predictable to take only regular insulin every 4 to 6 hours to cover insulin needs while on long airplane trips instead of trying to anticipate the peak of intermediate insulin and the availability of meals. During travel, most patients find it helpful to keep watches set to the time of the city of origin until they reach their destination. The key to travel when taking insulin is to know the type of insulin being taken, its onset of action, and the anticipated peak time. Meals or carry-along food can then be planned around this schedule.

Patient Teaching. The major educational objective is to match the level of self-management to the ability of the individual patient. Ideally, the patient should be taught about the disease and encouraged to achieve self-management with guidance only from the health care provider. The more in control the patient with diabetes can feel, the more likely the patient is to accept and adhere to the management program. The basis of self-management is a sound educational program related to diabetes. A knowledgeable patient

CLINICAL PATHWAY Home Care of Diabetes Mellitus—continued

Assessments/Instructions/Interventions	VS No. _	VS No. _	VS No. _	VS No. _	VS No. _	VS No. _	VS No. _	VS No. _	VS No. _	VS No. _
Explain patient rights and responsibilities.										
Assess for home safety management.										
Assess vital signs.										
Assess endocrine status.										
Assess hydration and nutrition status.										
Assess weight.										
Assess coping skills of patient/family/caregiver.										
Assess patient/caregiver's strengths/weaknesses related to therapeutic regimen.										
Assess patient/caregiver's willingness and ability to provide home therapeutic regimen.										
Assess patient/caregiver's understanding of disease process and compliance with therapeutic regimen.										
Refer to dietician for nutritional needs.										
Instruct on home safety.										
Instruct on medication regimen and compliance issues.										
Instruct patient/caregiver on signs of hypoglycemia and hyperglycemia and emergency measures related to those conditions.										
Instruct patient/caregiver on blood glucose testing.										
Instruct patient/caregiver on self/caregiver administration of insulin.										
Instruct patient/caregiver on home maintenance program (including exercise and correct nutritional intake). ______ on visit no. ____.										
Venipuncture for ordered laboratory tests.										
Other:										

Medical Supplies/Home Medical Equipment Needs

1. Blood glucose meter
2. Insulin syringes/insulin
3. Other ______

Variance codes

1. Patient related
2. Situation related
3. Systems related

Team member signature ______ Initials ____
Team member signature ______ Initials ____
Team member signature ______ Initials ____

Case manager name______

______
Patient signature
(involved in care planning)

should be able to make minor adjustments in insulin dosage and diet prescription to compensate for special circumstances, such as illness or increased exercise.

Not all patients with diabetes are capable of self-management. If the patient is not able to manage the disease, a family member may be able to assume this role. If the patient or the family cannot make decisions related to diabetes management, the nurse may identify appropriate resources outside the family. These resources can assist the patient and the family in outlining a feasible treatment program that meets their capabilities. Patient and health care provider resources are listed at the end of this chapter.

The American Diabetes Association offers pamphlets, booklets, and a bimonthly magazine called Diabetes Forecast for patients of all ages. Affiliates of the American Diabetes Association are located in all states, and most can be reached by dialing 800-DIABETES. The American Diabetes Association also publishes materials and sponsors conferences for health care professionals concerned with diabetes education, research, and management of patients. It gives recognition to education programs that meet the national standards of diabetes education and can provide a list of these programs. Drug companies manufacturing diabetes-related products also have free educational material for patients and health care providers.

Treatment programs take time to learn. The theory and textbook information are only the beginning. The information must then be incorporated into the patient's lifestyle. The health care provider who educates the patient and family understands that the education process initially takes weeks to months and provides periodic reassessment after the basics have been learned and integrated.

Another useful strategy is to divide the teaching content into the level that must be learned right away and the level

Table 46-17 Levels of Diabetes Education

Level 1

Educational Guidelines for Initial Management of Diabetes

Provide content required at time of diagnosis and represent basic or survival needs. Level is based on limitations of patient and family to accept and assimilate all there is to know about diabetes at time of diagnosis and limitations of some settings to provide additional education.

Example

Capillary blood glucose monitoring and insulin administration and hypoglycemia prevention and management.

Level 2

Educational Guidelines for Home Management of Diabetes

Place emphasis on increasing knowledge and flexibility as some experience is gained in living with diabetes. This is perceived as essential for every patient but must be tailored to individual needs and capacity. This type of educational experience is preferably offered in a nonhospital environment as close to home as possible.

Example

Goals for control, diabetes diet management, and sick-day guidelines.

Level 3

Education Guidelines for Improvement of Lifestyle

Present form of advanced learning viewed as enriching patient's life with flexibility, insight, and self-determination. Most patients are forced to discover this information by trial and error through experience. Although no educational program can or should entirely replace personal experience, the process need not be experienced by each person.

Example

Exercise, adjusting insulin and lifestyle, stress management.

RESEARCH

IMPLICATIONS FOR NURSING PRACTICE

Diabetes Self-Care

Citation Coates VE, Boore JR: The influence of psychological factors on the self-management of insulin-dependent diabetes mellitus, *J Adv Nurs* 17:528, 1998.

Purpose To determine the influence that perceived health beliefs, perceived control of diabetes, and knowledge have on the practice and outcomes of diabetes self-management.

Methods A mailed survey was completed by 263 patients (ages 18 to 35) with type 1 diabetes mellitus who were treated in a diabetes clinic. The questionnaires included items related to health beliefs, perceived control, and knowledge of diabetes. Glycosylated hemoglobin levels and clinic attendance as obtained from the medical records were used as indicators of self-care practice.

Results and Conclusions Most patients shared the belief that the consequences of diabetes were serious, and most had a sense of internal control and a high level of knowledge about diabetes. However, neither perceptions of control nor health belief had a demonstrable effect on either of the outcome measures (glycosylated hemoglobin or clinic attendance). Only 22% attended the clinic on all six appointment days.

Implications for Nursing Practice Although assessment of knowledge and beliefs is useful to planning care, it may not be predictive of how well patients followed through with prescribed therapy. Additional markers of patient compliance or outcomes are also needed. These results support the notion that care for diabetic patients must be tailored to meet their individual needs.

that can be scheduled for another time. Levels of diabetes education include survival, home management, and improvement of lifestyle. These levels are outlined in Table 46-17. The levels provide the diabetes educator with some structure for patient education and relieve the expectation that the patient will have to be taught everything in a short time.

In 1984 the National Diabetes Advisory Board established a set of standards to be used for ensuring the quality of diabetes patient education programs. The American Diabetes Association then developed a set of review criteria that specify the conditions under which each standard is to be met for a diabetes education program to be "recognized." It is believed that meeting the national standards and obtaining recognition will result in improvement in the overall quality of diabetes patient education programs.[29]

After the initial diagnosis of diabetes has been made, the lifelong process of patient education begins. The nurse's understanding of diabetes mellitus is central to a successful teaching program. An assessment of the patient's knowledge of diabetes and lifestyle preferences is useful in planning the teaching program. Table 46-18 is an example of a diabetes patient education record that can provide the nurse with a framework related to the patient's learning needs. Based on the information obtained from the record, an educational plan can be developed to meet the patient's individual needs. Table 46-19 is a summary of educational needs that can be used to track the progress of the patient's educational program. The nurse should assess the patient's knowledge base frequently so that gaps in knowledge or incorrect or inaccurate ideas can be quickly corrected. The record can be reviewed with the patient to outline and contract for additional educational information. The record can also provide an efficient way for other health care providers to be aware of what the patient knows or needs to learn.

Follow-up Nursing Management. Although the educational emphasis is on self-care, the patient should be encouraged to also be a partner in care with the health care provider. In addition to carrying out the daily management routines, maintaining a schedule of regular follow-up to assess the progress of the disease and additional education are necessary. Table 46-15 outlines a suggested follow-up schedule to aid in the long-term care of a patient with diabetes and to meet American Diabetes Association Standards of Care.

Table 46-18 Diabetes Patient Education Record

1. Demographic information Date: ______
Name: ______ Age: ______
Race: ______ Sex (circle): M F Participant status (circle): Inpatient Outpatient
Level of education: ______ Occupation: ______
Physician's name: ______ Marital status (circle): Single Married Widowed Divorced

2. General medical condition
Height: ______ Weight: ______ %Ideal weight: ______ Blood pressure: ______
Hb_{A1c}: ______ Total cholesterol level: ______ HDL: ______ Triglyceride level: ______
Allergies: ______
Other medications: ______
Other medical problems: ______
Present health status: ______

3. Diabetes history
Types of diabetes: ______ Duration of diabetes: ______
Treatment plan (check): ______ Insulin ______ OAs ______ Diet alone
Monitoring system: Type: ______ Test times: ______ Product: ______ Usual AM glucose level: ______
Attach monitoring log, if appropriate.
Name and type of insulin or OA: Dose Times taken
______ ______ ______
______ ______ ______
Describe any side effects of OAs/insulin: ______
Complications (check):
______ Retinopathy ______ Neuropathy ______ Renal ______ Foot ______ Macrovascular ______ Other (specify) ______
Describe: ______
Incidences of DKA, hypoglycemia, hyperglycemia (date, etc.): ______

4. Dietary habits
If prescribed, daily caloric intake: ______ Food or foods to avoid: ______
Indicate times of Breakfast ______ Lunch ______ Dinner ______
Attach dietary recall data or nutrition workup, if appropriate.

5. Physical activity habits
Does patient have regular exercise program (20 min, 3 days/wk)? Yes ______ No ______
If yes, indicate:

Type	Duration	Intensity (Circle)
______	______	Light Medium Heavy
______	______	Light Medium Heavy
______	______	Light Medium Heavy

6. Diabetes education history
Prior diabetes education? Patient/NP ______ Yes ______ No Significant other ______ Yes ______ No
Prior education: ______
Special educational needs: ______
Will significant other participate in program? Yes ______ No ______ Relationship: ______

7. Source of referral (check one)
______ Physician/NP ______ Self-referred ______ Facility staff ______ Community agency ______ Other (specify): ______

8. Social history
Cigarettes/day: ______ Alcoholic drinks/wk: ______
No. in household: ______ Relationship: ______
Types of health/medical insurance: ______

Modified from *Meeting the standards: a manual for completing the ADA application for recognition*, ed 5, American Diabetes Association, 1998.

COMPLICATIONS OF DIABETES

With the discovery and initial administration of insulin, it was believed that a cure for diabetes had been found. However, 70 years of insulin therapy has proved that insulin is not the total answer in the treatment of diabetes. Hyperglycemia-related problems do not cause death as often as they did before insulin was discovered. Other chronic complications of long-term disease are responsible for more than 75% of all diabetic deaths.

The acute problems of diabetes are associated with severe, untreated hyperglycemia (e.g., DKA, HHNK) or the hypoglycemic side effects of treatment with GLAs. Chronic problems are primarily those of end organ disease from microangiopathy, macroangiopathy, and neuropathy. Hyperglycemia plays a significant role in these complications as shown by the DCCT. Hyperglycemia may damage cells and tissue in at least two ways:

1. Metabolic dysfunction in the breakdown of glucose may lead to accumulation of damaging by-products (e.g., sorbitol).
2. Glucose becomes abnormally bound to protein structures of the body and produces deleterious effects in nerves and blood vessels over time.

In June 1993 the National Institute of Diabetes and Digestive and Kidney Diseases announced the results of a landmark medical study that began in 1983. Called the Diabetes Control

Table 46-19 Summary of Educational Needs Assessment and Progress Form

Content Area	Preprogram*		Taught†	Postprogram‡	
Patient			Date/initial/method		
1. Understands general facts of diabetes	Y	N		Y	N
2. Is well adjusted psychologically in relation to diabetes	Y	N		Y	N
3. Adequately or appropriately involves family in diabetes care	Y	N		Y	N
4. Understands and practices effective nutritional management	Y	N		Y	N
5. Understands benefits of and engages in appropriate exercise	Y	N		Y	N
6. Monitors blood or urine glucose levels appropriately	Y	N		Y	N
7. Properly uses insulin or OAs	Y	N		Y	N
8. Knows relationship among nutrition, exercise, and medication	Y	N		Y	N
9. Recognizes and responds appropriately to symptoms of hypoglycemia and hyperglycemia	Y	N		Y	N
10. Understands effects of illness on diabetes management and responds appropriately	Y	N		Y	N
11. Practices proper hygiene (skin care, foot care, dental care) to prevent complications of diabetes	Y	N		Y	N
12. Cooperates in therapeutic management and rehabilitation of diabetes complications	Y	N		Y	N
13. Understands benefits and responsibilities of self-management in diabetes	Y	N		Y	N
14. Effectively uses available health care systems	Y	N		Y	N
15. Makes appropriate use of community resources	Y	N		Y	N

Modified from *Meeting the standards: a manual for completing the ADA application for recognition*, ed 5, American Diabetes Association, 1998.
*Preprogram: Did patient know content before education?
†Taught: Was content taught? Put date, initials (instructor's name must accompany initials at least once); method of instruction (L, lecture; D, demonstration; R, return demonstration; V, video; X, other); and format (1/1, one to one; CL, classroom; G, group; SI, self-instruction module).
‡Postprogram: Did patient know content after education?

and Complications Trial (DCCT), it compared different forms of diabetes treatment in preventing or slowing the complications of diabetes. The trial included more than 1400 people with insulin-dependent diabetes at 29 medical centers in the United States and Canada, half with no retinopathy at baseline (the primary prevention cohort) and the other half with mild retinopathy (the secondary intervention cohort). Patients were randomly assigned to one of two groups: intensive or standard treatment. The intensive treatment group took three or more insulin injections a day or used an insulin pump. The patients in the standard treatment group took one to two injections a day and tested their blood glucose once or twice a day. The intensive group was distinguished from the standard treatment group in terms of glycosylated hemoglobin levels and capillary blood glucose values throughout the study (average glycosylated hemoglobin in the intensive treatment group was about 7.2% and the standard treatment group was about 9% on a normal range of 4.0% to 6.05%).

The results found that in the primary prevention cohort, intensive therapy reduced the adjusted mean risk for the development of retinopathy by 76%, as compared with conventional therapy. In the secondary intervention cohort, intensive therapy slowed the progression of retinopathy by 54%. In the two cohorts combined, intensive therapy reduced the occurrence of microalbuminuria by 39% and of albuminuria (urinary albumin excretion of 300 μg per 24 hours) by 54%, and that of clinical neuropathy by 60%. The chief adverse event associated with intensive therapy was a twofold to threefold increase in severe hypoglycemia.[30]

The American Diabetes Association issued a position statement regarding the DCCT:

> A primary treatment goal should be blood glucose control at least equal to that achieved in the intensively treated cohort. This goal may not apply to all patients with diabetes and must be based on clinical judgment. Of importance, intensively treated patients had a threefold greater risk of hypoglycemia than did patients in the control group. Because serious hypoglycemia is dangerous, "tight" control goals may have to be sacrificed in people in whom frequent or severe hypoglycemia cannot be avoided by treatment modification.[31]

ACUTE METABOLIC COMPLICATIONS

The acute problems of DKA and HHNK coma arise from events associated with hyperglycemia and insufficient insulin. A problem that may arise from too much insulin or an excessive dose of an OA is hypoglycemia (also referred to as insulin reaction or low blood glucose), which occurs when the level of available blood glucose falls. It is important for the health care provider to be able to distinguish between hyperglycemia and hypoglycemia because hypoglycemia can constitute a serious threat and requires immediate attention. Table 46-20 compares the manifestations, causes, management, and prevention of hyperglycemia and hypoglycemia.

Diabetic Ketoacidosis

DKA, also referred to as diabetic acidosis and diabetic coma, may develop quickly or over several days or weeks. It can be caused by too little insulin accompanied by increased caloric intake, physical or emotional stress, or undiagnosed diabetes. DKA is most likely to occur in type 1 diabetes but may be seen in type 2 in conditions of severe illness or stress when extra demand for insulin cannot be met by the pancreas.

Table 46-20 Comparison of Hyperglycemia and Hypoglycemia

Hyperglycemia	Hypoglycemia
Manifestations*	
Elevated blood glucose[†] Increase in urination Increase in appetite followed by lack of appetite Weakness, fatigue Blurred vision Headache Glycosuria Nausea and vomiting Abdominal cramps Progression to DKA or HHNK	Blood glucose <50 mg/dl (2.8 mmol/L) Cold, clammy skin Numbness of fingers, toes, mouth Rapid heartbeat Emotional changes Headache Nervousness, tremors Faintness, dizziness Unsteady gait, slurred speech Hunger Changes in vision Seizures, coma
Causes	
Too much food Too little or no diabetes medication Inactivity Emotional, physical stress Poor absorption of insulin	Alcohol intake with food Too little food—delayed, omitted, inadequate intake Too much diabetic medication Too much exercise without compensation Diabetes medication or food taken at wrong time Loss of weight with change in medication Use of β-blockers interfering with recognition of symptoms

Hyperglycemia	Hypoglycemia
Treatment	
Physician's attention Continuance of diabetes medication as ordered Frequent checking of blood and urine specimens and recording of results Hourly drinking of fluids	Immediate ingestion of 5-20 g of simple carbohydrates Ingestion of another 5-20 g of simple carbohydrates in 15 min if no relief obtained Contacting of physician if no relief obtained Discussion with physician about medication dosage
Preventive Measures	
Taking of prescribed dose of medication at proper time Accurate administration of insulin/OA Maintenance of diet Maintenance of good personal hygiene Adherence to sick-day rules when ill Checking of blood for glucose as ordered Contacting of physician regarding ketonuria Wearing of diabetic identification	Taking of prescribed dose of medication at proper time Accurate administration of insulin/OA Ingestion of all ordered diet foods at proper time Provision of compensation for exercise Ability to recognize and know symptoms and treat them immediately Carrying of simple carbohydrates Education of friends, family, fellow employees about symptoms and treatment Checking blood glucose as ordered

*There is usually a gradual onset of symptoms in hyperglycemia and a rapid onset in hypoglycemia.
[†]Specific clinical manifestations related to elevated levels of blood glucose vary according to the patient.

When the insulin supply is insufficient, glucose cannot be properly used for cellular energy. In response to cellular starvation, the body releases and breaks down stored fats and protein to provide the needed energy. Free fatty acids from stored triglycerides are released and metabolized in the liver in such large quantities that ketones are formed (ketonemia). Excess ketones alter the pH balance, and acidosis develops. More water is lost as ketones are excreted (ketonuria) in an attempt to balance the pH (Fig. 46-12).

Gluconeogenesis from protein is the last resource used by the body as a compensatory response to provide a cellular energy source. The result is an increase in blood glucose and nitrogen. However, because of the prevailing insulin deficiency, this glucose resource cannot be used and the blood glucose level rises further, adding to the osmotic diuresis. Dehydration and loss of electrolytes, particularly potassium, ensue. The patient's skin becomes dry and loose, and the eyeballs become soft and sunken. Hypotension with a weak, rapid pulse may develop.

Vomiting caused by the acidosis results in more fluid and electrolyte losses. The continual bicarbonate loss adds to the acidosis. Finally, Kussmaul's respirations (rapid, deep breathing associated with dyspnea) begin to remove carbonic acid through the exhalation of carbon dioxide. Acetone is noted on the breath as a sweet, fruity odor.

Renal failure may eventually occur from hypovolemic shock. This failure causes the retention of ketones and glucose, and the acidosis progresses. The patient becomes comatose as a result of the neurologic stressors of dehydration, electrolyte imbalance, and acidosis. If the condition is not treated, death is inevitable.

Collaborative Care

Before the advent of self-monitoring of blood glucose, patients with DKA required hospitalization for treatment. Today, hospitalization may not be required. In instances where fluid and electrolyte imbalance is not severe and self-monitoring of blood glucose can be done by the patient or someone in the household, less severe forms of DKA may be managed on an outpatient basis. However, other factors, such as the presence of fever, nausea and vomiting, or diarrhea; altered mental status; nature of the cause of the ketoacidosis; and availability of frequent communication with the physician (every few hours), must also be considered in this decision.

Regardless of the setting in which it occurs, DKA is a serious condition that proceeds rapidly and must be treated promptly. (See Table 46-21 for the emergency management of a patient with DKA.) Treatment is aimed at immediate administration of insulin, replacement of fluid to correct hypovolemia, and replacement of electrolytes to correct imbalances.

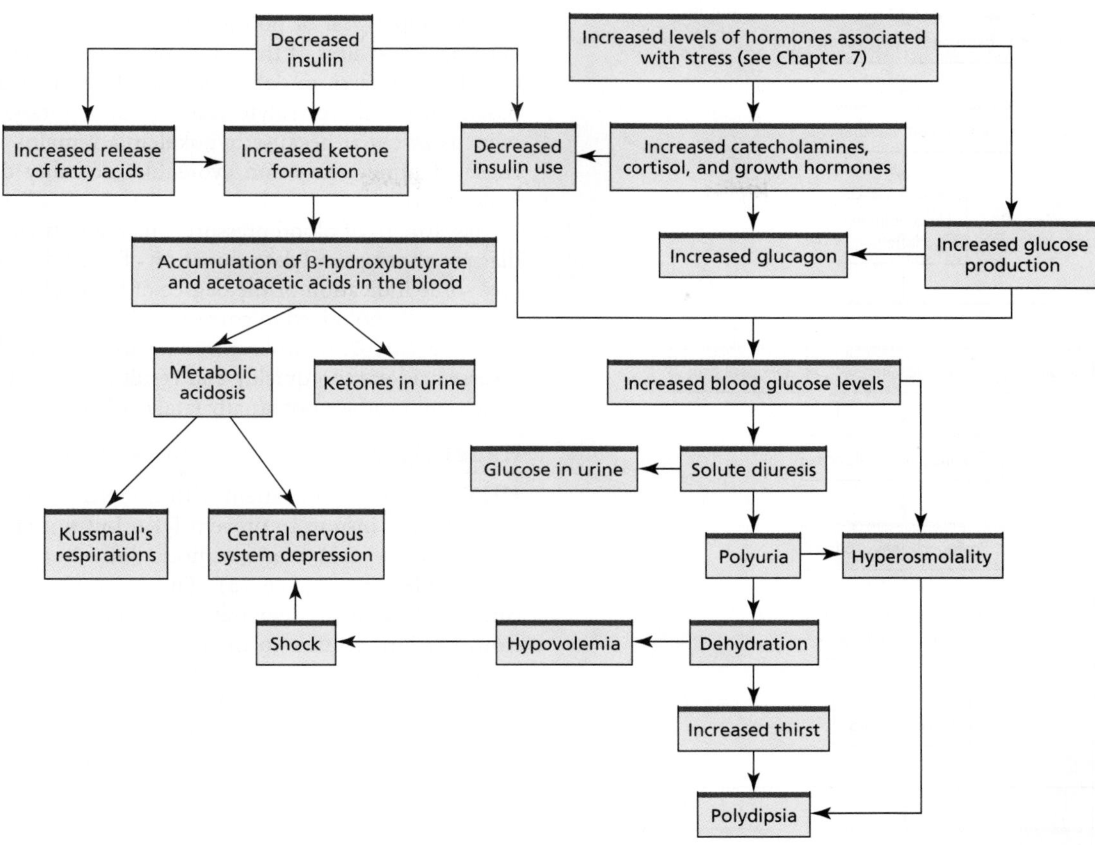

Fig. 46-12 Diabetic ketoacidosis.

EMERGENCY MANAGEMENT

Table 46-21 Diabetic Ketoacidosis

Etiology	Assessment Findings	Interventions
Undiagnosed diabetes mellitus Inadequate treatment of existing diabetes mellitus Insulin not taken as prescribed Infection Change in diet, insulin, or exercise regimen	▪ Dry mouth ▪ Thirst ▪ Abdominal pain ▪ Nausea and vomiting ▪ Gradually increasing restlessness, confusion, lethargy ▪ Flushed, dry skin ▪ Eyes appear sunken ▪ Breath odor of ketones ▪ Rapid, weak pulse ▪ Labored breathing (Kussmaul's respirations) ▪ Fever ▪ Urinary frequency ▪ Serum glucose >300 mg/dl (16.7 mmol/L) ▪ Glucosuria and ketonuria	**Initial** ▪ Ensure patient airway. ▪ Administer oxygen via nasal cannula or non-rebreather mask. ▪ Establish IV access with large-bore catheter. ▪ Begin fluid resuscitation with normal saline solution 1 L/hr until BP stabilized and urine output 60 ml/hr. ▪ Begin continuous IV insulin (0.1 U/kg/hr). ▪ Identify history of diabetes, time of last food, and time/amount of last insulin injection. **Ongoing Monitoring** ▪ Monitor vital signs, level of consciousness, cardiac rhythm, oxygen saturation, and urine output. ▪ Assess breath sounds for fluid overload. ▪ Monitor serum glucose and serum potassium. ▪ Anticipate possible administration of sodium bicarbonate with severe acidosis (pH <7.0).

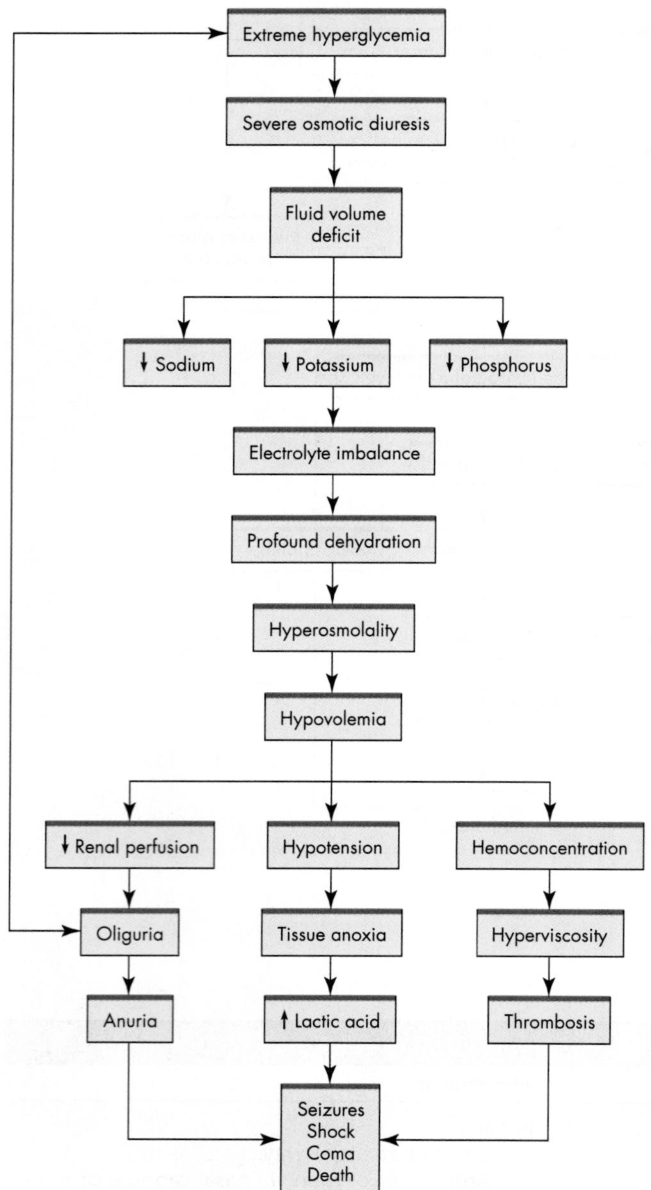

Fig. 46-13 Pathophysiology of hyperglycemic hyperosmolar nonketosis (HHNK).

The preferred treatment for DKA is the low-dose insulin IV infusion method. In this method 5 to 10 U of insulin per hour in normal saline solution is administered until ketoacidosis is reversed.[32] This insulin therapy is continued until a blood glucose level of 250 mg/dl (13.9 mmol/L) is reached. When the blood glucose level reaches 250 mg/dl (13.9 mmol/L), a solution containing 5% to 10% glucose (e.g., 5% dextrose in saline solution) is given to prevent hypoglycemia along with IV or SC insulin as needed to maintain blood glucose control.

Fluid and electrolyte therapy is aimed at replacing extracellular and intracellular water and deficits of sodium, chloride, bicarbonate, potassium, phosphate, magnesium, and nitrogen. The principal goal of potassium therapy is to prevent hypokalemia. Regardless of the initial plasma potassium value, the total body potassium deficit is large. Treatment decisions are based on serial electrolyte results. Early potassium replacement is essential because hypokalemia remains a significant cause of unnecessary and avoidable mortality during treatment of DKA.

Assessment of blood pressure, pulse, and tissue turgor; cardiac monitoring; and determination of central venous pressure give some indication of the degree of hypovolemia. Bicarbonate is usually not given to correct acidosis unless the condition is severe (pH 7.0). Indiscriminate use of bicarbonate may reverse acidosis too quickly and result in severe hypokalemia, which can produce potentially fatal cardiac arrhythmias.

Hyperglycemic Hyperosmolar Nonketosis

HHNK occurs in the patient with diabetes who is able to produce enough insulin to prevent DKA but not enough to prevent severe hyperglycemia, osmotic diuresis, and extracellular fluid depletion (Fig. 46-13). The increasing hyperglycemia causes intracellular dehydration because of a shift of fluid from the intracellular to the extracellular space. This causes neurologic abnormalities such as somnolence, coma, seizures, hemiparesis, and aphasia. HHNK often occurs in the older adult patient with type 2 diabetes. There is usually a history of inadequate fluid intake, increasing mental depression, and polyuria.

Collaborative Care

HHNK constitutes a medical emergency. This acute complication has a mortality rate greater than 50%.[33] The immediate therapy to reverse this hyperosmolar state consists of the rapid administration of IV solutions. From 6 to 20 L of fluid may have to be given during the first 24 to 48 hours. Depending on the degree of dehydration, either 0.9% or 0.45% sodium chloride is used. Regular insulin is given IV to aid in reducing the hyperglycemia. When blood glucose levels fall to 250 mg/dl (13.9 mmol/L), IV fluids containing glucose should be administered. Electrolytes are monitored and replaced as needed. Vital signs, intake and output, tissue turgor, and cardiac monitoring are assessed to monitor fluid and electrolyte replacement.

The management for both DKA and HHNK is similar except that HHNK requires greater fluid replacement (Table 46-22). Once the patient is stabilized, attempts to detect and correct the underlying precipitating cause should be initiated. 

NURSING MANAGEMENT: DIABETIC KETOACIDOSIS AND HYPERGLYCEMIC HYPEROSMOLAR NONKETOSIS

When hospitalized, the patient is closely monitored with appropriate blood and urine tests. The nurse is responsible for monitoring blood glucose and urine for output and ketones, as well as using laboratory data to direct care.

Areas that need monitoring are administration of IV fluids to correct dehydration, administration of insulin therapy to reduce blood glucose and serum acetone, administration of

COLLABORATIVE CARE

Table 46-22 **Diabetic Ketoacidosis and Hyperglycemic Hyperosmolar Nonketosis**

Diagnostic
- Blood work, including immediate blood glucose, complete blood count, ketones, pH, electrolytes, blood urea nitrogen, arterial blood gases
- Urinalysis, including specific gravity, pH, sugar, acetone

Collaborative Therapy
- Administration of rapid-acting insulin IV
- Administration of IV fluids
- Electrolyte replacement
- Assessment of mental status
- Recording of intake and output
- Central venous pressure monitoring (if indicated)
- Assessment of blood glucose level
- Assessment of blood and urine for ketones
- Electrocardiogram monitoring

electrolytes to correct electrolyte imbalance, assessment of renal status, assessment of the cardiopulmonary status related to hydration and electrolyte levels, and monitoring of the level of consciousness.

The nurse must also monitor the signs of potassium imbalance resulting from hypoinsulinemia and osmotic diuresis (see Chapter 15). When treatment for hyperglycemia is begun with insulin, potassium loss may initially be increased. As insulin is replaced, potassium moves back into the cell. This movement of potassium into and out of extracellular fluid influences cardiac functioning. For this reason, cardiac monitoring is a useful aid in detecting hyperkalemia and hypokalemia because characteristic changes indicating potassium excess or deficit are observable on electrocardiographic readings. Vital signs should be assessed often to determine the presence of fever, hypovolemic shock, tachycardia, and Kussmaul's breathing.

HYPOGLYCEMIA

Hypoglycemia, or low blood glucose, occurs when proportionately too much insulin is in the blood for the available glucose. This causes the blood glucose level to drop to less than 50 mg/dl (2.8 mmol/L). This type of hypoglycemia is different from the condition commonly termed *reactive hypoglycemia* (see p. 1402).

Hypoglycemic symptoms may also occur when a very high blood glucose level falls too rapidly (e.g., a blood glucose level of 300 mg/dl [16.7 mmol/L] falling quickly to 180 mg/dl [10 mmol/L]). Although the blood glucose level is above normal by definition and measurement, the sudden metabolic shift can evoke hypoglycemic symptoms. This type of situation can be induced by too vigorous management of hyperglycemia with insulin.

The balance between blood glucose and insulin can be disrupted by the administration of too much insulin, the ingestion of too little food, unusual amounts of exercise, and delayed eating. Insulin reactions can occur at any time, but most reactions occur when the GLA is at its peak of action or when the patient's daily routine is disrupted without adequate adjustments in diet, medications, and activity. Although hypoglycemia is more common with insulin therapy, it can occur with OAs and may be severe and persist for an extended time as a result of the longer half-lives of active metabolites of some OAs.

A decrease in available blood glucose can result in sympathetic nervous system activation with the release of epinephrine. This results in manifestations of cold sweats, weakness, trembling, nervousness, irritability, pallor, and increased heart rate. The clinical manifestations of hypoglycemia vary with each patient. The brain depends on a constant supply of glucose because it is unable to store glucose or glycogen. If that supply is inadequate, the patient will experience confusion, fatigue, and abnormal behavior that can resemble alcohol intoxication.

In recent years the physiology of glucose recovery has been shown to depend on glucagon and epinephrine. In type 1 diabetes, secretion and use of one or both of these substances may be impaired. As a result, some type 1 patients do not have the early warning symptoms produced by epinephrine. Rather, they have neuroglycopenia, that is, the more advanced symptoms of cerebral glucose deficit. The symptoms of this condition are irritability, irrational behavior, dizziness, tremors, and loss of consciousness. This may result from the development of autonomic neuropathy or from treatment with beta-adrenergic blocking agents. These patients must be managed with intensive education and instruction in the prevention of hypoglycemia.

NURSING AND COLLABORATIVE MANAGEMENT: HYPOGLYCEMIA

The preferred treatment of hypoglycemia is prevention. However, if hypoglycemia occurs, the patient should be able to reverse the situation before medical assistance is required. The patient's ability to do this depends on the state of alertness and ability to swallow and the availability of a quick-acting carbohydrate source.

At the first sign of hypoglycemia the patient should ingest 5 to 20 g of a simple (fast-acting) carbohydrate, such as 120 to 180 ml of orange juice, 180 to 240 ml of regular soft drink, two packets of sugar, or five or six hard candies. Overtreatment with large quantities of quick-acting carbohydrates such as a whole candy bar should be avoided.

If the symptoms are still present after 10 to 15 minutes, ingestion of 5 to 20 g of carbohydrate should be repeated.[34] Once the symptoms have improved, the patient should eat a longer-lasting carbohydrate such as bread or milk to prevent symptoms from recurring. Commercial products such as gels or tablets containing specific amounts of quick-acting carbohydrate are convenient for carrying in a purse or pocket to be used in such situations. High-fat foods and high-protein foods should not be used initially to correct hypoglycemia. These

COLLABORATIVE CARE

Table 46-23 Hypoglycemia

Diagnostic
Stat blood glucose
History (if possible)
Collaborative Therapy
Determination of cause of hypoglycemia (after correction of condition)
Conscious Patient
Administration of 5-20 g of quick-acting CHO (e.g., 6-8 oz of regular soda, 1 tbs syrup or honey, 4 tsp jelly, 4-6 oz orange juice, 8 oz milk, 2½ tsp sugar, commercial dextrose products [per label instructions])
Repetition of treatment in 15 min (if no improvement)
Administration of additional food of longer-acting CHO (e.g., slice of bread, crackers) after subsiding of symptoms
Immediate notification of health care provider or emergency service (if patient outside hospital) if symptoms not subsiding after 2 to 3 administrations of quick-acting CHO
Worsening Symptoms or Unconscious Patient
SC or IM injection of 1 mg glucagon
Administration of 50 ml 50% IV glucose

CHO, carbohydrate.

food sources are metabolized too slowly to be effective as immediate treatment.

If there is little discernible improvement in the patient's condition after two to three doses of 5 to 20 g of simple carbohydrate within 30 minutes or if the patient is not alert enough to swallow, 1 mg of glucagon may be administered with the same technique used for an insulin injection, although an IM injection in a site such as the deltoid will result in a quicker response. Glucagon stimulates a strong hepatic response to convert glycogen to glucose and therefore make glucose rapidly available. Once the patient is receiving medical care, a concentrated glucose solution may also be administered slowly IV until the patient regains consciousness. Blood glucose level must be carefully monitored during the treatment. (See Table 46-23 for a summary of collaborative care of hypoglycemia.)

With effective treatment, hypoglycemia can be quickly reversed. Once the acute hypoglycemia has been reversed, the nurse should explore with the patient the reasons why the situation developed. This assessment may indicate the need for additional education of the patient and the family to avoid future episodes of hypoglycemia. The danger of hypoglycemic reactions must be stressed because memory and learning impairment can result from repeated episodes of severe hypoglycemia.

DKA, HHNK, and hypoglycemia constitute potentially life-threatening situations and may be frightening to the patient and the family. The nurse should attempt to keep the family members informed about the patient's progress to relieve their anxiety. The nurse's calm, competent manner in caring for the patient can provide assurance to the acutely ill patient and the family.

Table 46-24 Mechanisms of Macrovascular Disease in Diabetes

Cellular Mechanisms
Arterial endothelial cell injury (sorbitol accumulation, hypoxia, hypertension, immune complexes)
Foam cell activation (smooth muscle cell migration, monocyte/macrophage activation)
Hemostatic Mechanisms
Platelet dysfunction (aggregation, thromboxane production, growth factor release)
Clotting factor abnormalities (raised fibrinogen, factor VII, factor VIII, reduced fibrinolysis)
Cell-cell forces (RBC rigidity)
Lipoprotein Abnormalities
Hypertriglyceridemia (increased VLDL, remnant particles, reduced lipoprotein lipase activity, reduced HDL in type 2 diabetes mellitus)
Hypercholesterolemia (increased LDL in type 2 diabetes mellitus)
Apolipoprotein abnormalities (e.g., glycosylation)
Other Mechanisms
Chronic renal disease secondary to diabetes (raised VLDL, LDL; lowered HDL; hypertension)
Increased arterial wall proteoglycans (trapping of lipoproteins, local cell activation)
Abnormalities of collagen, fibronectin (synthesis, glycosylation)
Insulin-induced lipogenesis, esterification
Intramural coronary vascular (macro and micro) disease

HDL, high density lipoproteins; *LDL,* low density lipoproteins; *VLDL,* very low density lipoproteins.

CHRONIC COMPLICATIONS

Angiopathy

Angiopathy, or blood vessel disease, is estimated to account for the majority of deaths among patients with diabetes. Many factors, including genetics, diet, and lipid metabolism, are being investigated for their role in the development of angiopathy. These chronic blood vessel dysfunctions are divided into two categories: macroangiopathy and microangiopathy.

Macroangiopathy. Macroangiopathy, or disease of large and medium-sized blood vessels, is essentially atherosclerosis and arteriosclerotic vascular disease characterized by a higher frequency and earlier onset than in the nondiabetic population. The degree of vascular damage appears to be related to the duration of the diabetes and not to its severity. Although atherosclerotic plaque formation is believed to have a genetic origin, its development seems to be promoted by the altered lipid metabolism common to diabetes (Table 46-24). Tight glucose control may help delay the atherosclerotic process.[30]

The complications resulting from macroangiopathy are cerebrovascular, cardiovascular, and peripheral vascular disease. Although genetic makeup cannot be altered, a patient with diabetes can diminish other risk factors associated with macroangiopathy, such as obesity, smoking, hypertension, high fat intake, and low activity level.

In addition to the association of type 1 and type 2 diabetes with ischemic heart disease, some have suggested that insulin resistance may be implicated in the pathogenesis of essential

PATIENT TEACHING GUIDE

Table **46-25** **Foot Care**

1. Wash feet daily with a mild soap and *warm* water. Test water temperature with hands first.
2. Pat feet dry gently, especially between toes.
3. Examine feet daily for cuts, blisters, swelling, and red, tender areas. Do not depend on feeling sores. If eyesight is poor, have others inspect feet.
4. Use lanolin on feet to prevent skin from drying and cracking. Do not apply between toes.
5. Use mild foot powder on sweaty feet. Powder feet only, not shoes.
6. Do not use commercial remedies to remove calluses or corns.
7. Cleanse cuts with *warm* water and mild soap, covering with clean dressing. Do not use iodine, rubbing alcohol, or strong adhesives.
8. Report skin infections or nonhealing sores to health care provider immediately.
9. Cut toenails even with rounded contour of toes. Do not cut down corners. Soak nails before cutting.
10. Separate overlapping toes with cotton or lamb's wool.
11. Break in new shoes slowly. Avoid open-toe, open-heel, and high-heel shoes. Leather shoes are preferred to plastic ones. Wear slippers with soles. Do not go barefoot. Shake out shoes before use.
12. Wear clean, absorbent (cotton or wool) socks or stockings that have not been mended. Colored socks must be colorfast.
13. Do not wear clothing that leaves impressions, hindering circulation.
14. Do not use hot water bottles or heating pads to warm feet. Wear socks for warmth.
15. Guard against frostbite.
16. Exercise feet daily either by walking or by flexing and extending feet in suspended position. Avoid prolonged sitting, standing, and crossing of legs.

hypertension and dyslipidemia. The term *syndrome X* is applied to the clinical association of insulin resistance, hypertension, and increased very-low-density lipoprotein (VLDL) and decreased high-density lipoprotein (HDL) cholesterol concentrations. The role of insulin resistance in the pathogenesis of cardiovascular disease is not well understood; in the United States, insulin resistance probably combines with dyslipidemia in contributing to greater risk of cardiovascular disease in patients with diabetes mellitus.[35]

Microangiopathy. Microangiopathy, or disease of the small blood vessels, is different from macroangiopathy in that it is specific to diabetes. Microangiopathy is the result of thickening of the basement membranes in the capillaries and arterioles, a highly characteristic concomitant of long-term diabetes mellitus. Although microangiopathy can be found throughout the body, the areas most noticeably affected are the eyes (retinopathy), the kidneys (nephropathy), and the skin (dermopathy). Thickening of the basement membrane has been found in some persons with diabetes before or at the time of diagnosis or before the onset of symptoms of diabetes

Table **46-26** **Types of Diabetic Retinopathy**

Type	Pathologic Alteration
Background	Microvasculature of retina of eye is damaged. Capillaries become damaged, resulting in development of microaneurysms (seen as tiny red dots on retina).
Preproliferative	Possible progression from background retinopathy represents further destruction of retinal capil- l-aries and development of capillary dropout.
Proliferative	Abnormal blood vessels (neovascularization) grow on surface of retina. Vessels can grow into chamber of vitreous surface and can hemorrhage, filling vitreous chamber with blood.

Modified from Peragallo V: *A core curriculum for diabetes education,* Chicago, 1993, American Association of Diabetes Educators.

mellitus. However, clinical manifestations usually do not appear until 15 to 20 years after the onset of diabetes.[36] However, Native-Americans with diabetes mellitus have an earlier onset of microangiopathy relative to other groups.

Peripheral Vascular Disease

Peripheral vascular disease (PVD) is a combination of microangiopathy and macroangiopathy, as well as clotting abnormalities. The legs and feet are most often affected in diabetes mellitus, and associated problems account for 20% of hospitalizations of patients with diabetes. The sequelae of PVD can lead to infection, gangrene, and amputation. Signs of PVD include intermittent claudication, pain at rest, cold feet, loss of hair, delayed capillary filling, and dependent rubor. The disease is diagnosed by history, Doppler findings, and angiography. Management centers on control or reduction of risk factors, particularly smoking, high cholesterol intake, and hypertension. Antibiotics are necessary when infection is present. If the infection cannot be reversed with antibiotic therapy, amputation may be necessary. Proper care of the feet is crucial for the patient with PVD; guidelines for patient teaching regarding foot care are listed in Table 46-25. Approximately 6% of the U.S. diabetic population (14 million) experience lower-extremity amputation because of diabetic foot ulcers.[37]

Diabetic Retinopathy

The term *retinopathy* literally means disease of the retina; however, diabetic retinopathy refers to the microangiopathic process seen in a patient with diabetes. After 10 years with diabetes mellitus, 50% of patients demonstrate diabetic retinopathy; after 15 years, approximately 80% of patients have some retinal disease.

The primary problems in diabetic retinopathy are microvascular damage and occlusion of retinal capillaries. Retinopathy can be classified as background retinopathy, preproliferative retinopathy, and proliferative retinopathy. The types are outlined in Table 46-26. In background retinopathy, the most common form, partial occlusion of the small blood vessels in the retina causes the development of microaneurysms in the capillary walls. These microaneurysms are so weak that capillary fluid leaks out, causing retinal edema and eventually hard exudates or intraretinal hemorrhages. Vision may be affected if the macula is involved. Preproliferative retinopathy is distinct from background retinopathy and indicates further destruction of retinal capillaries.

Proliferative retinopathy, the most severe form, involves the retina and the vitreous. When retinal capillaries become occluded, new blood vessels are formed (neovascularization) to supply the retina with blood. These new vessels hemorrhage easily and may produce vitreous contraction. The vessels are torn and bleed into the vitreous cavity, preventing light from reaching the retina. The patient sees black or red spots or lines. If these new blood vessels pull the retina while the vitreous contracts, causing a tear, partial or complete retinal detachment will occur. If the macula is involved, vision is lost. Without treatment, more than half of patients with proliferative diabetic retinopathy will be blind.[38]

The earliest and most treatable stages of diabetic retinopathy often produce no visual symptoms. Because of this, the patient with diabetes must have regular examinations by an ophthalmologist for early detection and appropriate treatment. Careful ophthalmoscopic and slit lamp microscopic retinal examinations are the most important diagnostic tools to identify diabetic fundus changes. Fluorescein angiography demonstrates dye leakage from abnormal retinal and subretinal vessels and identifies retinal areas amenable to focal laser treatment. If the vitreous humor is opaque in advanced disease, ultrasonography may be useful to identify retinal detachments.

The two most common forms of treatment of diabetic retinopathy are early photocoagulation of the retina and vitrectomy. Photocoagulation by laser converts light energy into heat and coagulates the tissue in the area where the light is directed. It is particularly useful with neovascularization because the laser obliterates new vessels, stopping the hemorrhage. Panretinal photocoagulation (PRP) is a scatter technique in which thousands of laser burns are placed in the retinal periphery. PRP is generally recommended when there is moderate to severe neovascularization. PRP destroys the hypoxic retina, reducing its oxygen requirement and reducing the stimulus for new blood vessel growth.

Topical anesthetic is generally adequate for laser treatment. Pain is usually transient but occasionally requires retrobulbar anesthesia. The patient may experience some loss of peripheral or central vision, and the dark adaptation may be affected.

Photocoagulation is not possible when there is significant vitreous or retinal hemorrhage. In these cases, vitrectomy is useful. *Vitrectomy* is the aspiration of blood, membrane, and fibers from the inside of the eye through a small incision just behind the cornea. Vitrectomy is indicated when there is vitreal hemorrhage that does not clear or when the hemorrhage is obscuring the retina in the patient who needs photocoagulation. This type of surgery is also helpful in patients with traction retinal detachments. Vitrectomy is an intraocular procedure, and possible complications include the risk of further vitreous hemorrhage, cataract formation, glaucoma, and infection. Despite the risks, vitrectomy has been an important development in treating the ocular complications of diabetes mellitus.

Persons with diabetes are also prone to other visual problems. Glaucoma occurs as a result of the occlusion of the outflow channels secondary to neovascularization. This type of glaucoma is difficult to treat and often results in blindness. Cataracts occur with increasing frequency in the patient with diabetes. Although the process is similar to that of senile cataracts, it occurs at an earlier age in the patient with diabetes. Diabetic retinopathy may occur concurrently with nephropathy and parallel its progression. Although the vast majority of diabetic patients have some degree of retinopathy, nephropathy develops in only 35% to 45% of patients with type 1 diabetes.[36]

Nephropathy

Diabetic nephropathy is now the leading cause of end-stage renal disease (ESRD) in the United States.[38] Mild proteinuria develops in 70% of persons with diabetes mellitus and may progress to more serious involvement and ESRD. This occurs as a result of microvascular abnormalities associated with diabetes mellitus, but these processes are not clearly understood.

Microangiopathy in the kidneys causes diffuse and nodular glomerulosclerosis. Diffuse glomerulosclerosis affects the basement membranes of all glomerular capillaries, usually in both kidneys. The basement membranes become thickened and leaky. Sclerosis of glomerular vascular tufts leads to progressive renal failure. In nodular glomerulosclerosis (Kimmelstiel-Wilson lesions), nodules develop in the glomeruli. In advanced cases most glomeruli are involved. In more than 70% of patients, the course of diabetic nephropathy is complicated by the presence of hypertension. The monitoring and treatment of hypertension are important parts of diabetes management and are believed to be significant factors in controlling the progression of nephropathy. (See Chapter 31 for a discussion of hypertension and Chapter 44 for a discussion of acute and chronic renal failure.) The majority of type 1 diabetes patients with diabetic nephropathy die of cardiovascular disease. The risk of cardiovascular disease is 30 to 40 times higher in patients with nephropathy than in those diabetics who did not develop renal diseases.[38]

ESRD requires treatment by either dialysis or kidney transplantation. A patient in the later stages of nephropathy may require an adjustment in insulin and OAs because of a loss of the insulin-degradative function of the kidneys and an abnormal peripheral insulin response.

Neuropathy

Neuropathy is probably one of the most common complications of diabetes in adults. However, its cause is unclear. Mononeuropathic conditions (i.e., single nerve branch involvement) are theorized to develop from microangiopathy, whereas the more diffuse neuropathic conditions are attributed to metabolic defects and the accumulation of by-products in the nerve tissue. The result is reduced nerve conduction and demyelinization. Neuropathy can precede, accompany, or follow the diagnosis of diabetes.

The two major categories of diabetic neuropathy are neuropathic conditions of the peripheral nervous system, includ-

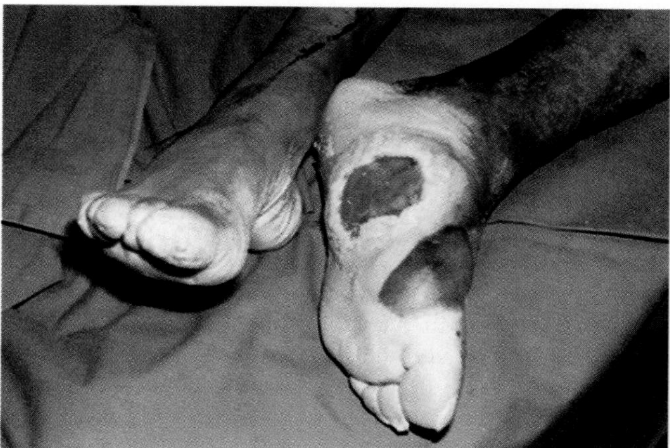

Fig. 46-14 Neuropathy: neurotrophic ulceration.

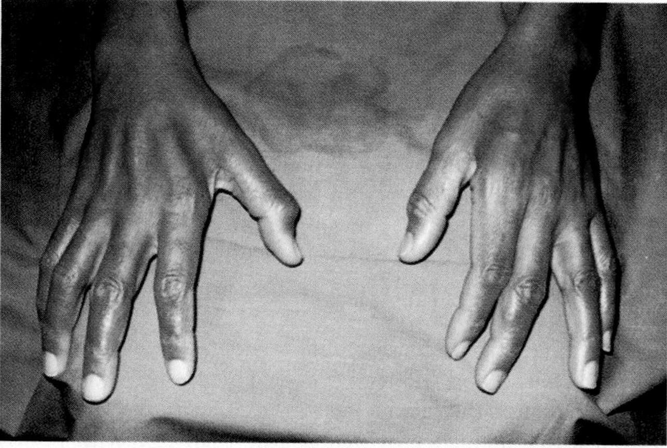

Fig. 46-15 Diabetic neuropathy: muscle atrophy.

ing symmetric peripheral polyneuropathy, mononeuropathic disorders, and diabetic amyotrophy; and autonomic neuropathic conditions, including cardiovascular abnormalities, GI abnormalities, urinary bladder abnormalities, and sexual dysfunction. Symmetric peripheral polyneuropathy affects all the extremities but most often affects the legs. Symmetric peripheral polyneuropathy is usually bilateral and symmetric and is thought to be due to both metabolic and vascular mechanisms. The patient has pain and paresthesias. The pain, described as burning, cramping, crushing, or tearing, is usually worse at night and may occur only at that time. It may be relieved by walking.

The paresthesias are associated with tingling, burning, and itching sensations. Complete or partial loss of sensitivity to touch and temperature is common. Foot injury and ulcerations can occur without the patient ever having pain (Fig. 46-14). The patient may report a feeling of walking on pillows or numb feet. At times the skin becomes so sensitive (hyperesthesia) that even light pressure from bed sheets cannot be tolerated. Neuropathy in the hands causes atrophy of the small muscles, limiting fine movement (Fig. 46-15).

Mononeuropathic conditions tend to occur unilaterally and are characterized by a sudden onset of pain with weakness or paralysis. Although the extremities are most often affected, cranial nerves III, IV, and VI may be involved.

No direct treatment for neuropathy is known. Treatment is aimed at relief of symptoms, particularly pain. Medications commonly used include tricyclic antidepressants (e.g., amitriptyline [Elavil]) and topical creams (e.g., capsaicin [Zostrix]). Better glucose control may also aid in the reduction of symptoms. As nerve conduction improves, the pain may initially increase before relief is noted.

Neuropathy affecting the autonomic nervous system may produce nocturnal diarrhea, postural hypotension, impotence, and neurogenic bladder. Nocturnal diarrhea is not associated with abdominal cramping. It affects few persons with diabetes and does not disturb diabetic control. *Gastroparesis diabeticorum* is delayed gastric emptying that can produce anorexia, nausea, vomiting, and persistent feelings of fullness. Gastroparesis can trigger hypoglycemia by delaying food absorption. Metoclopramide (Reglan), a dopamine receptor antagonist and serotonin antagonist, stimulates esophageal and gastric emptying and has been used in the treatment of gastroparesis. Other drugs that are sometimes useful to increase intestinal motility are domperidone (Motilium) and cisapride (Propulsid).

The cardiovascular abnormalities associated with autonomic neuropathy are postural hypotension, resting tachycardia, and painless myocardial infarction. A patient with postural hypotension should be instructed to change from a lying or sitting position slowly.

Reports of the prevalence of erectile dysfunction (ED) among men with diabetes vary from 30% to 60%. ED associated with diabetes mellitus is believed to result from damage to the sacral parasympathetic nerves. Determining whether ED is of organic or psychologic origin is an important part of the assessment. Organic ED usually develops insidiously, whereas psychologic ED is often acute in onset. Measuring nocturnal penile tumescence (extent and duration of penile erection) during rapid eye movement phases of sleep is one assessment method to establish the presence of organic disease. Nonsurgical devices and surgical prosthetic implantations have been developed that make vaginal penetration possible. Decreased libido is a problem with some women with diabetes. Monilial and nonspecific vaginitis are also common. Organic ED or sexual dysfunctioning in either the male or the female patient requires sensitive therapeutic counseling for both the patient and the patient's partner. (See Chapter 52 for a further discussion of erectile dysfunction.)

A neurogenic bladder develops as sensation in the inner bladder wall decreases, causing urinary retention. A patient with retention has infrequent voiding, difficulty in voiding, and a weak stream of urine. Emptying the bladder every 3 hours in a sitting position helps prevent stasis and subsequent infection. Tightening the abdominal muscles during voiding and using the Credé maneuver (mild massage downward over the lower abdomen and bladder) may also help with complete bladder emptying. Cholinergic drugs such as bethanechol (Urecholine) may be used. The patient may also have to learn self-catheterization (see Chapter 43).

Neuropathic arthropathy, or Charcot's joints, results in ankle and foot changes that ultimately lead to joint dysfunction and footdrop. These changes occur gradually and promote an abnormal distribution of weight over the foot. New pressure points emerge, and neuropathic ulcers often develop. The ulcers resemble a "BB-shot" or "punched-out" wound and are initially painless when peripheral polyneuropathy is present. Infection is a danger and may penetrate to underlying bone tissue, necessitating the long-term use of antibiotics and weeks of avoidance of weight bearing on the affected limb. The ideal treatment is prevention. Table 46-25 outlines rules for foot care that can reduce the patient's risk for infection and possible amputation.

The treatment of neuropathic disorders involves effective diabetic control and supportive care. There is no known cure. The patient under relatively good glycemic control appears to have a lower incidence of neuropathy than one with poorly controlled disease. However, neuropathy can occur despite good control.

Skin Changes

Skin disorders such as diabetic dermopathy and *necrobiosis lipoidica diabeticorum* are attributed to microangiopathy. Shin spots are brown spots located on the anterior surfaces of the lower extremities. They are harmless and painless and initially measure less than 1 cm in diameter. Necrobiosis lipoidica diabeticorum, which is believed to be the result of trauma, consists of lesions similar to those of diabetic dermopathy but is more likely to be associated with ulcerations and necrosis. The lesions are reddish yellow and atrophic. Skin grafts are sometimes required because of the slow healing of the lesions. Necrobiosis lipoidica diabeticorum is present most often in women with type 1 diabetes and may precede the onset of overt diabetes.

Infection

A patient with diabetes is more susceptible to infections than other patients. The mechanisms for this phenomenon include a defect in the mobilization of inflammatory cells and an impairment of white blood cells in the process of phagocytosis. Recurring or persistent infections such as *Candida albicans,* as well as boils and furuncles in the undiagnosed patient, often lead the health care provider to suspect diabetes. Loss of sensation (neuropathy) may delay the detection of an infection.

Persistent glycosuria may encourage bladder infections, especially in a neurogenic bladder. Decreased circulation as a result of angiopathy can prevent or delay the healing process. Protein waste during hyperglycemia and DKA is also responsible for poor healing. Antibiotic therapy has prevented infection from being a major cause of death in diabetic patients. The treatment of infections must be prompt and vigorous.

GERONTOLOGIC CONSIDERATIONS

Diabetes Mellitus

The prevalence of diabetes is about 18% in persons between age 65 and 74. The increased blood glucose levels and decreased glucose tolerance make diabetes more difficult to diagnose in the older adult. Aging is also associated with an increase in the prevalence of other factors that tend to impair carbohydrate metabolism and are more likely to be treated with medications that impair insulin action (e.g., corticosteroids, antihypertensives, phenothiazines). The clinical manifestations of renal, retinal, and neurologic complications of diabetes generally take 10 to 20 years to develop. Attempts to normalize glucose are associated with an increased frequency of hypoglycemia. Therefore in the older patient there is less reason for treatment of hyperglycemia based on the prevention of these specific diabetic complications. Whereas it is generally agreed that treatment is usually indicated for this patient, the goals for control probably do not need to be as near normoglycemia as in the younger population. Because of the physiologic changes that occur with aging, the therapeutic outcome for the older adult with diabetes who receives OAs may be altered. The second-generation OAs such as glyburide and glipizide have increased potency but appear to have fewer side effects and fewer drug interaction problems when compared with the first-generation agents. Insulin therapy may be instituted if OAs fail. However, for accurate insulin administration, it is important to recognize the limitations among some individuals related to manual dexterity and visual acuity.

The patient education issues for the older patient that should be addressed are self-care in terms of vision, mobility, mental status, functional ability, and finances; the effect of multiple medications; eating habits; undetected hypoglycemia; and quality of life issues.

Patient teaching should be based on the individual's needs, using a slower pace with simple printed or audio materials. It is important to include family or a support person in the teaching.

REACTIVE HYPOGLYCEMIA

Many people claim to have reactive hypoglycemia. However, reactive hypoglycemia occurs infrequently in persons other than those with diabetes treated with insulin or sulfonylureas. Reactive hypoglycemia results from an uncompensated reduction in blood glucose level. The symptoms are similar to those of the hypoglycemia of diabetes: sudden onset of hunger, diaphoresis, tremulousness, weakness, nervousness (adrenergic) and headache, confusion, slurred speech, behavioral aberrations, focal neurologic signs, and coma (neuroglycopenic). These symptoms mimic the effects of anxiety and stress and are often misinterpreted.

Idiopathic hypoglycemia (i.e., hypoglycemia of no known cause) is particularly difficult to document. Various physiologic disturbances have been suggested, but subtle abnormalities of insulin response to food (particularly excessive or delayed secretion) seem the most likely possibilities. A definite diagnosis can be made only if the plasma glucose concentration is less than 50 mg/dl (2.8 mmol/L) accompanied by symptoms of hypoglycemia and relieved by eating. The usual treatment is a diet balanced in protein and carbohydrate with frequent small meals.

If a patient claims to have reactive hypoglycemia, it should be determined whether this has been medically diagnosed or self-diagnosed. Because of the similarity to symptoms of anxiety reaction, careful assessment of the symptoms and the treatment is important.

CRITICAL THINKING EXERCISES

CASE STUDY

Diabetic Ketoacidosis

Patient Profile

John, a 34-year-old man, was admitted to the emergency department after he was found comatose in his apartment by his wife.

Subjective Data (provided by wife)

- Was diagnosed with diabetes mellitus 12 months ago
- Was taking 48 U of insulin daily: 12 U of regular insulin plus 20 U of NPH before breakfast, 8 U of regular insulin before dinner, and 8 U of NPH at bedtime
- Has history of flu for 1 week with vomiting and anorexia
- Stopped taking insulin 2 days ago when he was unable to eat

Objective Data

Physical Examination

- Breathing is deep and rapid
- Acetone smell on breath
- Skin flushed and dry

Diagnostic Studies

- Blood glucose level of 730 mg/dl (40.5 mmol/L)
- Urine acetone of 3+ with Acetest tablets
- Blood pH of 7.26

Critical Thinking Questions

1. Briefly explain the pathophysiology of the development of diabetic ketoacidosis (DKA) in this patient.
2. What clinical manifestations of DKA does this patient exhibit?
3. What factors precipitated this patient's DKA?
4. What distinguishes this case history from one of hyperglycemic hyperosmolar nonketosis or hypoglycemia?
5. What educational needs must be met before the patient's discharge?
6. What role does John's wife play in the management of his diabetes?
7. Based on the assessment data presented, write one or more appropriate nursing diagnoses. Are there any collaborative problems?

NURSING RESEARCH ISSUES

1. What degree of pain does the patient associate with capillary blood glucose monitoring?
2. How often does the patient make phone contact with a diabetes patient educator when this service is available free as compared with when there is a charge?
3. Is the patient willing to maintain tight glycemic control in the present to prevent chronic complications from diabetes in the future?
4. Does the frequency of review of major diabetes education issues affect the frequency of occurrence of acute complications of diabetes?

REVIEW QUESTIONS

The number of the question corresponds to the same-numbered objective at the beginning of the chapter.

1. The polydipsia and polyuria related to diabetes are caused primarily by
   a. the release of ketones from cells during fat metabolism.
   b. fluid shifts resulting from the osmotic effect of hyperglycemia.
   c. damage to the kidneys from exposure to high levels of glucose.
   d. changes in RBCs resulting from attachment of excessive glucose to hemoglobin.
2. In planning care for a patient with type 2 diabetes admitted to the hospital with pneumonia, the nurse recognizes that the patient
   a. must receive insulin therapy to prevent the development of ketoacidosis.
   b. has islet cell antibodies that have destroyed the ability of the pancreas to produce insulin.
   c. has minimal or absent endogenous insulin secretion and requires daily insulin injections.
   d. may have sufficient endogenous insulin to prevent ketosis but is at risk for development of hyperosmolar coma.
3. A diabetic patient has a serum glucose level of 824 mg/dl (45.7 mmol/L) and is somnolent and unresponsive. Following assessment of the patient the nurse suspects diabetic ketoacidosis rather than hyperglycemic hyperosmolar nonketosis based on the finding of
   a. polyuria.
   b. severe dehydration.
   c. rapid, deep respirations.
   d. decreased serum potassium.
4. A diabetic patient takes a combination of regular and NPH insulin twice a day for glucose control. The nurse teaches the patient to be alert for hypoglycemia
   a. immediately after breakfast and dinner.
   b. immediately after lunch and dinner.
   c. in the late afternoon and at bedtime.
   d. immediately after dinner and at bedtime.
5. The nurse assists the patient with dietary management of diabetes with the knowledge that a diabetic diet is designed
   a. to be used only for type 1 diabetes.
   b. for use during periods of high stress.
   c. to normalize blood glucose by elimination of sugar.
   d. to help normalize blood glucose through a balanced diet.
6. In teaching a newly diagnosed type 1 diabetic "survival skills," the nurse includes information about
   a. weight-loss measures.
   b. elimination of sugar from diet.
   c. need to reduce physical activity.
   d. capillary blood glucose monitoring.

7. An appropriate instruction for the patient with diabetes related to care of the feet is
   a. use heat to increase blood supply.
   b. avoid softening lotions and creams.
   c. inspect all surfaces of the feet daily.
   d. use iodine to disinfect cuts and abrasions.

References

1. Centers for Disease Control and Prevention: *National diabetes fact sheet—1998,* Atlanta, Ga, 1998.
2. Report from the American Diabetes Association: Economic consequences of diabetes mellitus in the US in 1997, *Diabetes Care* 21:246, 1998.
3. Davidson MB: *Diabetes mellitus: diagnosis and treatment,* ed 4, Philadelphia, 1998, Saunders.
4. DeFronzo R: Pathogenesis of type 2 diabetes: metabolic and molecular implications for identifying diabetes genes, *Diabetes Rev* 5:177, 1997.
5. Report of the expert committee on the diagnosis and classification of diabetes mellitus, *Diabetes Care* 21(suppl 1):55, 1998.
6. Peakman M and others: Persistant activation on $CD8^+$ T-cells characterizes prediabetic twins, *Diabetes Care* 19:1177, 1996.
7. Dorman JS and others: *Risk factors for insulin dependent diabetes, diabetes in America,* NIH pub no 95-1468, 1995, National Diabetes Data Group, Bethesda, MD.
8. Leahy JL: Impaired beta-cell function with chronic hyperglycemia "overworked beta-cell" hypothesis, *Diabetes Rev* 4:298, 1996.
9. Kelley DB, editor: *American Diabetes Association complete guide to diabetes,* Alexandria, 1997, American Diabetes Association.
10. Goldstein DE: How much do you know about glycated hemoglobin testing? *Clinical Diabetes* 13:60, 1995.
11. Mahnensmith RL: Diabetic nephropathy: a comprehensive approach, *Hosp Pract* 28:129, 1993.
12. American Diabetes Association position statement: nutritional recommendations and principles for people with diabetes mellitus, *Diabetes Care* 21(suppl 1):32, 1998.
13. Kestel F: Are you up to date on diabetes medications? *AJN* 94:48, 1994.
14. Herter CD: Insulin lispro: the next step, *Clinical Diabetes* 15:51, 1997.
15. Position statement on insulin administration by the American Diabetes Association, *Diabetes Care* 21(suppl 1):72, 1998.
16. McCarthy JA, Covarrubias B, Sink P: Is the traditional alcohol wipe necessary before an insulin injection? Dogma disputed, *Diabetes Care* 16:402, 1993.
17. Farkas-Hirsch R, editor: *Intensive diabetes management,* Alexandria, 1995, American Diabetes Association.
18. American Diabetes Association position statement: implications of the Diabetes Control and Complication Trial, *Diabetes Care* 21(suppl 1):88, 1998.
19. Valensi P and others: Effect of insulin concentration on bioavailability during nasal spray administration, *Pathol Biol* 44:235, 1996.
20. Ahern JA: Steps to reduce the risks of severe hypoglycemia, *Diabetes Spectrum* 10:39, 1997.
21. Edelman SV: Prescribing oral antidiabetic agents: general considerations, *Clinical Diabetes* 16:37, 1998.
22. Bihm B, Wilson BA: Metformin (Glucophage): new treatment for NIDDM, *Medsurg Nurs* 4:236, 1995.
23. Bressler R, Johnson DG: Pharmacologic regulation of blood glucose levels in non–insulin dependent diabetes mellitus, *Arch Intern Med* 157:836, 1997.
24. Jakicic JM, Leermakers EA: Commit to get fit: exercise for life, *Diabetes Spectrum* 9:202, 1996.
25. Shichiri M and others: Enhanced, simplified glucose sensors: long-term clinical application of wearable artificial endocrine pancreas, *Artif Organs* 22:32, 1998.
26. The National Steering Committee for Quality Assurance in Capillary Blood Glucose Monitoring: Proposed strategies for reducing user error in capillary blood glucose monitoring, *Diabetes Care* 16:493, 1993.
27. American Diabetes Association technical review: tests of glycemia in diabetes, *Diabetes Care* 18:1896, 1995.
28. Position statement of the American Diabetes Association: tests of glycemia in diabetes, *Diabetes Care* 21(suppl 1):69, 1998.
29. American Diabetes Association national standards for diabetes self-management education programs and American Diabetes Association review criteria, *Diabetes Care* 21(suppl 1):95, 1998.
30. The Diabetes Control and Complications Trial Research Group: The effect of intensive treatment of diabetes on the development and progression of long-term complications in insulin-dependent diabetes mellitus, *N Engl J Med* 329:977, 1993.
31. American Diabetes Association position statement: implications of the Diabetes Control and Complications Trial, *Diabetes Care* 21(suppl 1):88, 1998.
32. Genuth S: Diabetic ketoacidosis and hyperosmolar hyperglycemic nonketotic syndrome in adults. In Lebovitz HE, editor: *Therapy for diabetes mellitus and related disorders,* ed 2, Alexandria, 1994, American Diabetes Association.
33. Foster DW: Diabetes mellitus. In Isselbacher KJ and others, editors: *Harrison's principles of internal medicine,* ed 14, New York, 1998, McGraw-Hill.
34. Reising DL: Acute hypoglycemia, *Nursing* 25:41, 1995.
35. American Diabetes Association Consensus Development Conference on Insulin Resistance, *Diabetes Care* 21:310, 1998.
36. Nathan DM: Long-term complications of diabetes mellitus, *N Engl J Med* 328:1676, 1993.
37. Kaufman MW, Bowsher JE: Preventing diabetic foot ulcers, *Medsurg Nurs* 3:204, 1994.
38. Seaquist ER: Microvascular complications of diabetes. Strategies for managing retinopathy, nephropathy, and neuropathy, *Postgrad Med* 103:61, 1998.

Resources

Academy for the Advancement of Diabetes Research and Treatment
http://drinet.med.miami.edu

American Association of Clinical Endocrinologists
1000 Riverside Ave., Suite 205
Jacksonville, FL 32204
http://www.aace.com

American Association of Diabetes Educators (AADE)
100 W Monroe, 4th floor
Chicago, IL 60603
312-424-2426
800-338-3633
http://www.diabetesnet.com/aade.html

American Diabetes Association—National Service Center
1660 Duke Street
Alexandria, VA 22314
800-232-3472
http://www.diabetes.org/default.htm

Canadian Diabetes Association
15 Toronto Street, Suite #800
Toronto, Ontario M5C 2E3
CANADA
416-363-3373
800-226-8464
http://www.diabetes.ca

Diabetes Mall on the Net
http://www.diabetesnet.com/

Diabetes Resources on the Internet
http://vigora.com/resources/

Endocrine Society
4350 East West Highway
Bethesda, MD 20814-4410
301-941-0252
Fax: 301-941-0259
http://www.endo-society.org/

Joslin Diabetes Center DNA Core Facility
Room 616
One Joslin Place
Boston, MA 02215
617-735-1932
Fax: 617-735-1915
http://dnacore.joslab.harvard.edu/core/home.html

Juvenile Diabetes Foundation International—The Diabetes Research Foundation
120 Wall Street
New York, NY 10005-4001
800-JDF-CURE
212-785-9500
Fax: 212-785-9595
http://www.jdfcure.org

National Diabetes Information Clearinghouse
1 Information Way
Bethesda, MD 20892-3570
301-654-3327
Fax: 301-907-8906
http://www.niddk.nih.gov/health/diabetes/ndic.htm

National Institute of Diabetes, and Digestive and Kidney Diseases
Building 31, Room 9A-52
Bethesda, MD 20892
301-496-5877
http://www.niddk.nih.gov

Pituitary Tumor Network Association
P.O. Box 1958
Thousand Oaks, CA 91358
805-499-2262
Fax: 805-499-1523
http://www.pituitary.com

Thyroid Foundation of Canada
96 Mack Street
Kingston, Ontario K7L 1N9
CANADA
613-544-8364
800-267-8822
Fax: 613-544-9731
http://home.ican.net/~thyroid/Canada.html

For additional Internet resources, see the website for this book at **www.mosby.com/MERLIN/medsurg_lewis**

REMEMBER to check out your **companion CD-ROM**

47 NURSING MANAGEMENT Endocrine Problems

Linda B. Haas

www.mosby.com/MERLIN/medsurg_lewis

LEARNING OBJECTIVES

1. Describe the pathophysiology, clinical manifestations, collaborative care, and nursing management of the patient with an imbalance of hormones produced by the anterior pituitary gland.
2. Describe the pathophysiology, clinical manifestations, collaborative care, and nursing management of the patient with an imbalance of hormones produced by the posterior pituitary gland.
3. Describe the pathophysiology, clinical manifestations, collaborative care, and nursing management of the patient with thyroid enlargement or dysfunction.
4. Describe the pathophysiology, clinical manifestations, collaborative care, and nursing management of the patient with an imbalance of the hormone produced by the parathyroid glands.
5. Describe the pathophysiology, clinical manifestations, collaborative care, and nursing management of the patient with an imbalance of hormones produced by the adrenal cortices.
6. Describe the pathophysiology, clinical manifestations, collaborative care, and nursing management of the patient with an excess of hormones produced by the adrenal medullae.
7. Name the endocrine disorders characterized by excesses and deficits in fluid volume, and describe the appropriate nursing interventions.
8. Describe the systemic effects of replacement and pharmacologic use of corticosteroid therapy.
9. List the nursing assessments, interventions, rationales, and expected outcomes related to patient education for chronic management of endocrine problems.

DISORDERS OF THE ANTERIOR PITUITARY GLAND

GROWTH HORMONE EXCESS

Etiology and Pathophysiology

Growth hormone (GH), an anabolic hormone, promotes protein synthesis and mobilizes glucose and free fatty acids. Overproduction of GH, which is usually caused by a benign pituitary adenoma (tumor), causes gigantism or acromegaly characterized by soft tissue and boney overgrowth.

Gigantism results when the onset occurs before closure of the epiphyses, while the long bones are still capable of longitudinal growth. The onset usually occurs in early childhood but may occur at puberty. The excessive growth is usually proportional. These children may grow as tall as 8 feet (240 cm) and weigh more than 300 lb (136 kg).[1]

Acromegaly, with a prevalence of approximately 60 cases per million and an incidence of 1000 cases per million per year in the United States, is rare, but it is more common than gigantism.[1]

Reviewed by Susan Harrington, RN, MN, ARNP, Family Nurse Practitioner, University of Washington, Seattle, Wash.

Clinical Manifestations

Symptoms of acromegaly begin insidiously in the third and fourth decades of life, and both genders are affected equally. When the problem develops after epiphyseal closure, bones increase in thickness and width. Physical features include enlargement of the hands, feet, and paranasal and frontal sinuses and deformities of the spine and mandible (Fig. 47-1). In addition, enlargement of soft tissue (e.g., tongue, skin, abdominal organs) causes manifestations such as speech difficulties and hoarseness, coarsening of facial features, abdominal distention, and sleep apnea. The sleep apnea may be related to upper airway narrowing or may be central in origin.[2] Persons with acromegaly may have hypertension, cardiomegaly, left ventricular hypertrophy, diaphoresis, oily skin, peripheral neuropathy, proximal muscle weakness, and joint pain. Women exhibit menstrual disturbances.[1]

The enlarged pituitary gland can exert pressure on surrounding structures, leading to visual disturbances and headaches. Because GH mobilizes stored fat for energy, it increases free fatty acids levels in the blood and predisposes the patient to atherosclerosis. The hormone also antagonizes the action of insulin and can cause hyperglycemia. Prolonged secretion of GH is diabetogenic (see Chapter 46).

Diagnostic Studies

In addition to the history and physical examination, diagnosis of GH excess requires evaluation of plasma GH and somatomedin

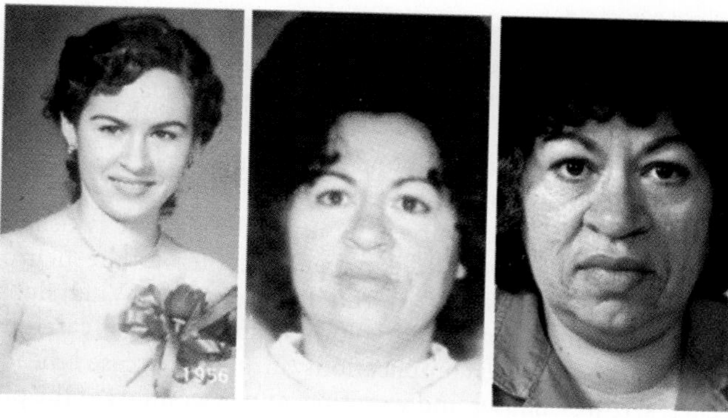

Fig. 47-1 Progressive development of facial features of acromegaly.

C (insulin-like growth factor 1 [IGF-1]) levels, IGF binding protein 3 (IGFBP-3) levels, and GH response to an oral glucose challenge.[2] Magnetic resonance imaging (MRI), used for further evaluation and tumor localization, is a sensitive method for identification, localization, and determination of extension of the tumor into surrounding tissue.[3] High-resolution computed tomography (CT) scanning with contrast media may also be used to localize the tumor. The patient with macroadenoma (10 mm) will require a complete ophthalmologic examination, including visual fields, because of potential pressure of the tumor on the optic chiasm or nerve.

Collaborative Care

The therapeutic goal in gigantism and acromegaly is to return GH levels to normal. This is accomplished by surgery, radiation, drug therapy, or a combination of these three. The prognosis depends on age at onset, age when treatment is initiated, and tumor size. Usually bone growth can be arrested, and soft tissue hypertrophy can be reversed. However, sleep apnea and diabetic and cardiac complications may persist in spite of treatment.

Surgical Therapy. Surgery is the usual treatment and offers the best hope for a cure, especially for microadenomas (<10 mm). Surgery is most commonly accomplished with the transsphenoidal approach, in which an incision is made in the inner aspect of the upper lip and gingiva. The sella turcica is entered through the floor of the nose and sphenoid sinuses (Fig. 47-2). The goal of transsphenoidal microsurgery is to remove only the GH-secreting adenoma. However, the pituitary gland may be destroyed or removed in some instances. Removal of the entire gland results in permanent deficiencies of hormones of the anterior pituitary. Rather than replacing the tropic hormones, which requires parenteral administration, the essential hormones produced by target organs (glucocorticoids, thyroid hormone, and certain sex hormones) can be given orally. Testosterone can be administered to men via a transdermal patch or self-administered intramuscularly (IM) every 2 weeks. Hormone replacement must be continued throughout life.

Radiation Therapy. External radiation normalizes GH levels in 30% to 70% of patients treated in this manner, although it may be months to years before GH levels normalize.[4] If a tumor is large or has a great deal of supersellar extension, surgery may be followed by radiation. Depending on the amount of radiation and the patient's susceptibility, the patient may experience local skin changes, alopecia, or oral complications. Hypopituitarism is a common sequela that often requires hormone replacement therapy.

Stereotactic radiosurgery (gamma surgery) may be applied to small, surgically inaccessible pituitary tumors. This procedure consists of radiation delivered to a single site from multiple angles and can be used to occlude blood vessels feeding the tumor, thereby starving it. The radiation source is arranged on a helmet device on the patient's head and focused on the tumor.[5]

Drug therapy may include the use of bromocriptine (Parlodel), a dopamine agonist, or octreotide (Sandostatin), a somatostatin analog that reduces GH levels to within the normal range in many patients. The GH-lowering effects of these drugs are seldom complete or permanent, and they are often used as adjuncts to other therapies or to reduce tumor size before surgery.[6]

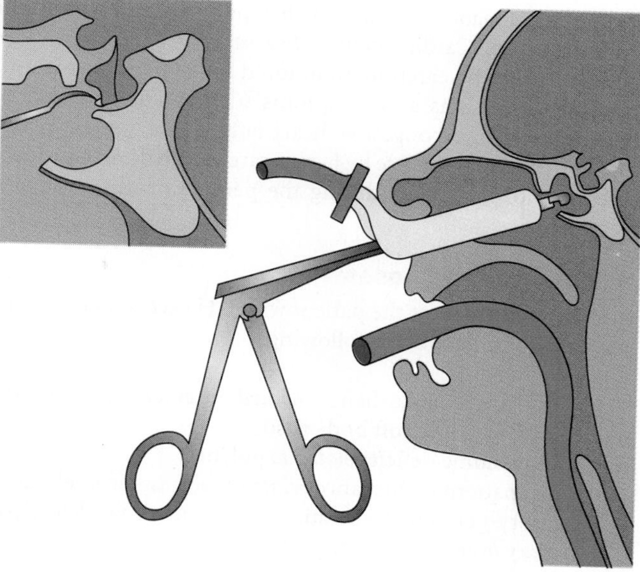

Fig. 47-2 Surgery on the pituitary gland is most commonly performed with the transsphenoidal approach. An incision is made in the inner aspect of the upper lip and gingiva. The sella turcica is entered through the floor of the nose and sphenoid sinuses.

NURSING MANAGEMENT: GROWTH HORMONE EXCESS

■ Nursing Assessment

The nurse assesses for signs and symptoms of abnormal tissue growth and evaluates the physical size of each patient. Assessment of children includes evaluation of growth and development with the use of growth charts (see Chapter 45). Accelerated growth, especially if greater than 5 to 6 inches (12 to 15 cm) per year and if inconsistent with familial patterns, constitutes cause for medical referral. The adult should be questioned about increases in hat, ring, glove, and shoe sizes. The patient can be questioned about changes in appearance noted in serial photographs.

When first seen, the patient usually has experienced undesirable changes in appearance and may have substantial alterations in self-image. The individual also commonly exhibits symptoms of diabetes mellitus such as polydipsia, polyuria, and blurred vision. Cardiovascular disease may be present. The patient should be carefully monitored for hyperglycemia and cardiovascular signs and symptoms such as angina pectoris, hypertension, and congestive heart failure. The patient needs unconditional acceptance by health care workers and considerable emotional support during the periods of diagnosis and treatment.

Nursing Diagnoses

Nursing diagnoses for the patient with GH excess may include, but are not limited to, the following:

- Body image disturbance *related to* enlargement of the hands, feet, jaw, soft body tissue
- Fluid volume deficit *related to* polyuria
- Sleep pattern disturbance *related to* soft tissue swelling
- Sensory-perceptual alteration *related to* visual defect *secondary to* enlarged pituitary gland

Planning

The overall goals are that the patient with GH excess will (1) accept and cope effectively with altered body image, (2) maintain adequate fluid volume, (3) experience restful sleep patterns, (4) develop no complications, and (5) state and accept the need for long-term follow-up.

Nursing Implementation

Health Promotion. At this time there are no known preventive measures for GH excess. Efforts are directed at early detection of the GH excess and treatment of the underlying cause.

Acute Intervention

Surgical care. The individual treated surgically needs skilled neurosurgical nursing care and must be prepared before surgery for postoperative care. Nursing interventions include preoperative installation of bacitracin nose drops,[5] discussion of mouth breathing, mouth care, ambulation, pain control, activity, and hormone replacement. The patient should be instructed to avoid vigorous coughing, sneezing, and straining at stool (Valsalva's maneuver) to prevent cerebrospinal fluid leakage from the point at which the sella turcica was entered.[5]

After surgery in which a transsphenoidal approach has been used, the head of the patient's bed should be elevated at a 30-degree angle at all times. This elevation avoids pressure on the sella turcica and decreases headaches, a frequent postoperative problem. Mild analgesia is given for headaches. The nurse should perform mouth care every 4 hours to keep the surgical area clean and free of debris and to promote patient comfort. Tooth brushing should be avoided for at least 10 days to prevent disrupting the suture line and to avoid discomfort.

Any clear nasal drainage should be sent to the laboratory to be tested for glucose. A level greater than 30 mg/dl (1.67 mmol/L) indicates cerebrospinal fluid leakage from an open connection to the brain, which places the patient at an increased risk for meningitis. Complaints of persistent and severe generalized or supraorbital headache may indicate cerebrospinal fluid leakage into the sinuses. A cerebrospinal fluid leak usually resolves within 72 hours when treated with head elevation and bed rest. If the leak persists, daily spinal taps may be done to reduce pressure to below normal levels and allow the fossa to heal. Intravenous (IV) antibiotics are usually administered when there is a cerebrospinal fluid leak to prevent meningitis. If the leak does not respond to treatment in 48 to 72 hours, surgical intervention may be required.

If stereotactic radiosurgery is used, the patient is usually moved from the specialized radiation center to the neurosurgical nursing unit for overnight observation. Vital signs, neurologic status, and fluid volume status must be carefully monitored. Possible complications include increased headaches, seizures, nausea and vomiting, and discomfort at the pin sites. All staff members should know how to remove a stereotactic frame in case of an emergency. The patient with a history of seizures is at increased risk for seizures for 24 hours after the procedure. The anterior and posterior pin sites should be cleaned with hydrogen peroxide and covered with clean dressings. Family members can be instructed in pin-site care if the patient is discharged the day after the procedure.[7]

A common postoperative occurrence is transient diabetes insipidus (DI).[5] The signs of DI are discussed in more detail later in this chapter. To assess for DI, serum sodium and fluid balance must be closely monitored. The DI may occur because of the loss of antidiuretic hormone (ADH), which is stored in the posterior lobe of the pituitary gland or cerebral edema related to manipulation of the pituitary stalk during surgery. If DI develops and ingestion of free water and nonsalty fluids does not allow the patient to keep up with urinary water losses, IV fluids are indicated. Vasopressin (Pitressin) is given IM, subcutaneously (SC), or intranasally as needed if the urine output exceeds 800 to 900 ml over 2 hours or if the urine specific gravity is less than 1.005. When vasopressin is used in a patient with known cardiovascular disease, the patient should be closely monitored because this drug may lead to vasoconstriction and angina.

Ambulatory and Home Care. If a hypophysectomy (removal of pituitary gland) is performed or the pituitary is damaged, hormone replacement will be necessary.[4] Permanent ADH, cortisol, and thyroid hormone replacement will be needed. Because these medications must be taken for life, careful patient education is necessary when replacement of these hormones is necessary.

Hypopituitarism causes infertility because of deficient sex hormones secondary to loss of gonadotropins. In addition, gamete (ova and sperm) production ceases because of a lack of stimulation from the gonadotropins, follicle-stimulating hormone (FSH), and luteinizing hormone (LH). However, if an individual with deficient FSH and LH wishes to have children, these hormones can be replaced with intermittent SC injections with possible restoration of fertility.

Because surgery may result in pituitary destruction with permanent hormone deficiencies and possible altered fertility, the patient needs assistance in working through the grieving process associated with these losses. It is important that the patient be aware of the disease progression if surgery is not done so that an informed decision can be made. The need for continued drug therapy reduces the patient's perception of independence and requires considerable emotional adjustment. The nurse must consider the emotional impact of a hypophysectomy when counseling the patient and planning the educational program related to hormone replacement. Referral to the Acromegaly Network Association (619-431-2625) may be helpful.

■ Evaluation

The expected outcomes are that the patient

- is adequately prepared for all collaborative care therapies
- experiences a complication-free postoperative course
- maintains adequate fluid and electrolyte balance
- is able to cope with altered body image
- knows how and when to take hormone replacement (if indicated)
- states the importance of long-term follow-up and has a follow-up medical appointment

EXCESSES OF OTHER TROPIC HORMONES

Excesses of other tropic hormones and overproduction of a single anterior pituitary hormone usually produce syndromes related to hormone excess from the target organ. If adrenocorticotropic hormone (ACTH) is involved, Cushing's disease (hypercortisolism) results; if thyroid-stimulating hormone (TSH) levels are excessive, hyperthyroidism develops.

In some instances, excess secretion of a pituitary hormone may be appropriate, such as when there are alterations in the negative feedback system. (See Chapter 45 for a discussion of negative feedback.) In the adult, hypersecretion of FSH and LH occurs in primary gonadal failure. The resultant low levels of sex hormones cause oversecretion of gonadotropins by the pituitary gland and are not indicative of intracranial disease. Thus excess FSH and LH may indicate a pathologic gonadal process such as orchitis (testicular inflammation resulting in decreased testosterone), or the excess may be a normal consequence of aging such as menopause. Sex hormone replacement therapy normalizes gonadotropin activity but does have side effects (see Chapters 48 and 51).

Sometimes symptoms of excess gonadotropins signify pituitary disease and require prompt referral for a definitive diagnosis. This is true of inappropriate lactation in either gender and precocious puberty in children.

Prolactin-secreting adenomas (prolactinomas) are the most frequently occurring pituitary tumor. The affected patient may experience headaches and visual problems. The visual problems are secondary to pressure on the optic chiasm. Women may have galactorrhea, menstrual abnormalities, or infertility. In men, impotence and decreased libido and sperm density may result. Treatment is achieved with surgery, radiation, or drug therapy using bromocriptine (Parlodel) or cabergoline (Doxtinex).[8]

HYPOFUNCTION OF THE PITUITARY GLAND

Hypopituitarism is a rare disorder that involves a decrease in one or more of the anterior pituitary hormones.

Etiology and Pathophysiology

Primary hypofunction may be a result of developmental or autoimmune disorders, infections, tumors, vascular diseases, or destruction of the gland. The most common cause of pituitary hypofunction is a tumor, but destruction of the pituitary can also result from trauma, radiation, and surgical procedures. Cranial radiation used in the treatment of other conditions may cause hypothalamic dysfunction, which often results in pituitary dysfunction. Failure to secrete GH and gonadotropins is the most common abnormality, followed by deficiencies of TSH, ACTH, and prolactin.[9] The manifestations of hypopituitarism depend on the specific pituitary hormones that are lacking. Infertility may be caused by primary gonadal failure or may be the first indication of pituitary hypofunction. In the latter case the gonads lack tropic hormone stimulation.

Clinical Manifestations

Clinical findings associated with pituitary hypofunction vary with the degree and speed of onset of pituitary dysfunction and are related to hyposecretion of the target glands. The symptoms are often nonspecific and commonly include weakness, fatigue, headache, sexual dysfunction, fasting hypoglycemia, dry and sallow skin, diminished tolerance for stress, and poor resistance to infection. In the adult, premature, fine wrinkling around the eyes and mouth is common. Psychiatric symptoms include apathy, mental slowness, and delusions. Orthostatic hypotension may also occur. If a pituitary tumor exerts pressure on the optic chiasm, there may be asymmetric visual field changes. If the tumor is large, blindness in one or both eyes may occur.

Hyposecretion of GH during childhood results in growth retardation. Growth may be normal for the first 1 or 2 years but then slows progressively. Intelligence is usually normal. Adults with GH deficiency have an increased cardiovascular mortality rate. In addition, they have decreased muscle strength, defective renal function and thermoregulation, altered thyroid metabolism, and reduced basal metabolic rate. These adults are also easily fatigued and have truncal obesity and altered body image.[10,11]

Anorexia and bulimia (see Chapter 38) are associated with decreased pituitary hormone secretion. These conditions usually affect young women with distorted body images. The patient decreases caloric intake and may increase exercise levels to the point where body weight and body fat percentage fall below a critical level for normal hypothalamic-pituitary-gonadotropin function, leading to amenorrhea. Decreased circulating thyroid hormone with inadequate TSH response and glucocorticoid and androgen abnormalities can also occur.

In women, hypofunction can follow a postpartum hemorrhage. This is called *postpartum pituitary necrosis,* or *Sheehan's syndrome.* Sheehan's syndrome should be suspected when failure to lactate and amenorrhea occur in a patient with a history of postpartum hemorrhage. The vascularity of the pituitary gland increases during pregnancy, making it vulnerable to hemorrhage. If hemorrhagic shock occurs during childbirth, the pituitary gland can become hypoxic, causing a slow degeneration and necrosis of the gland.[12] Panhypopituitarism may develop over a span of 10 to 15 years. The patient does not lactate secondary to postpartum hemorrhage after childbirth and is subsequently infertile because of prolactin, FSH, and LH deficiencies. Later, hypothyroidism develops and is followed by corticosteroid deficiency. Mental disorders are common, and because lethargy and apathy are characteristic of thyroid and corticosteroid hormone deficiencies, affected women rarely seek treatment. Many women with Sheehan's syndrome are diagnosed only after an acute Addisonian crisis (discussed later in this chapter). Some are never diagnosed or treated and succumb to this life-threatening condition.

When pituitary hypofunction affects FSH and LH, sexual development is impaired and features remain childlike. FSH and LH deficiencies in the adult woman are first manifested as menstrual irregularities, diminished libido, and changes in secondary sex characteristics (e.g., decreased breast size). If the cause is Sheehan's syndrome, lactation fails and infertility occurs. Men with FSH and LH deficiencies experience testicular atrophy, diminished spermatogenesis, loss of libido, impotence, and decreased facial hair and muscle mass.

If hypopituitarism is not detected and treated, the patient eventually develops deficiencies of thyroid hormone and the adrenal corticosteroids. The latter deficiency causes a tendency toward shock and may result in an episode of acute adrenal insufficiency (refractory and life-threatening shock from sodium and water depletion).

Collaborative Care

For GH deficiency, replacement therapy with recombinant GH is available. Prepubertal children, whose bones are undergoing more rapid growth spurts, respond better than postpubertal children do. GH therapy is costly, but it is recommended for children with growth retardation caused by GH deficiency and children with chronic renal failure before renal transplantation, and it may be useful in Turner's syndrome.[13] Adults with GH deficiency respond well to GH replacement and experience increased energy and lean body mass and improved body image.[10,11] The major side effect of GH replacement is fluid retention.

Treatment of hypopituitarism consists of surgery or radiation for tumor removal, permanent target gland hormone replacement, and a nutritious dietary plan. Replacement therapy is carried out with corticosteroids, thyroid hormone, and sex hormones. Gonadotropins can sometimes restore fertility.

NURSING MANAGEMENT: HYPOFUNCTION OF THE PITUITARY GLAND

A primary nursing role in anterior pituitary insufficiency is assessment and recognition of subtle signs and symptoms. The patient with hypopituitarism may first exhibit symptoms in stressful situations such as trauma or surgery. In addition, hypopituitarism may be detected in the patient with symptoms of failure to grow, infertility, or amenorrhea. Failure to grow may indicate pituitary dwarfism, and infertility and amenorrhea can be signs of Sheehan's syndrome or a pituitary adenoma.

Children affected by pituitary dwarfism exhibit slow but proportional growth. Except for their small size, they may appear completely normal. When the age of puberty is reached, however, sexual maturation may not occur. If it does occur, the epiphyses will close, ending the possibility of further longitudinal bone growth despite hormone replacement. For this reason and because normal stature and psychosocial development are more likely to be achieved with early initiation of treatment, these children must be identified and treated early. (See a pediatric text for a complete discussion of pituitary dwarfism.)

The nurse should be alert for the possibility of Sheehan's syndrome and refer any woman with the following characteristics for diagnosis and treatment:

1. History of hemorrhage or other hypoxic episode during the birth of youngest child
2. Failure to lactate after birth—this is usually the preeminent clue
3. Scanty, irregular, or absent menses
4. Decrease in secondary sex characteristics (or complaints of being "less womanly" than before)
5. Signs and symptoms of hypothyroidism
6. Signs and symptoms of glucocorticoid insufficiency without the "bronzing" of the skin associated with the condition

Although Sheehan's syndrome has been considered a relatively rare condition, there is evidence that it has been seriously underdiagnosed. The disease is devastating to affected women but is largely reversible with hormone replacement.[12] If the disease is not detected and treated early, the woman is likely to need considerable help in rebuilding her life. Marital, vocational, or psychologic counseling may be needed, and appropriate referrals should be made. The nature of the physiologic problem should be explained to significant others, and their help should be enlisted in the rehabilitative process.

DISORDERS OF THE POSTERIOR PITUITARY GLAND

The hormones secreted by the posterior pituitary are antidiuretic (ADH), also called arginine vasopressin (AVP), and oxytocin. These hormones are formed in the hypothalamus and stored in the posterior pituitary. ADH contributes to fluid balance by controlling renal reabsorption of free water (Fig. 47-3). It also has potent vasoconstrictive properties. Oxytocin controls lactation and uterine contractions. Oxytocin excess is not recognized as a clinical problem. This hormone is administered pharmacologically in the management of labor.

SYNDROME OF INAPPROPRIATE ANTIDIURETIC HORMONE

Etiology and Pathophysiology

Syndrome of inappropriate antidiuretic hormone (SIADH), also called Schwartz-Bartter syndrome, occurs when ADH is released in amounts far in excess of those indicated by the plasma osmotic pressure (Fig. 47-4). This syndrome is associated with diseases that affect osmoreceptors in the hypothalamus and is more common in the elderly.[14] SIADH is characterized by fluid retention, serum hypoosmolality, dilutional hyponatremia, hypochloremia, concentrated urine in the presence of normal or increased intravascular volume, and normal renal function.

SIADH has various causes (Table 47-1). Although ectopic ADH production by carcinomas is not a primary pituitary disorder, it has similar clinical manifestations and nursing management. The most common ADH-secreting tumor is bronchogenic carcinoma. Other pulmonary conditions, such as pneumonia, tuberculosis, lung abscess, and positive-pressure

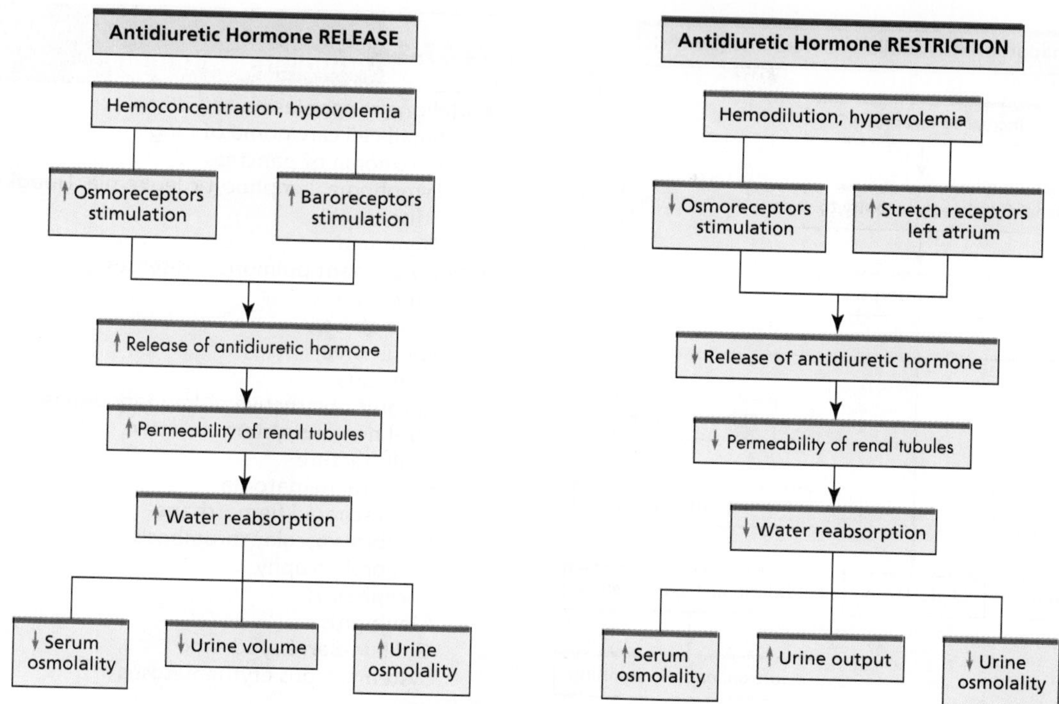

Fig. 47-3 Physiology of the release and restriction of antidiuretic hormone.

breathing, have been associated with SIADH. The syndrome is also associated with such diverse conditions as trauma (all types but most frequently head trauma), meningitis, subarachnoid hemorrhage, acquired immunodeficiency syndrome (AIDS), peripheral neuropathy, delirium tremens, Addison's disease, psychoses, vomiting, stress, and many medications.[15]

SIADH tends to be self-limiting when caused by head trauma or drugs but chronic in nature when associated with tumors or metabolic diseases. Treatment of the underlying cause or discontinuing the causal medication is indicated to improve the clinical course.

Clinical Manifestations

The excess ADH increases renal tubular permeability and reabsorption of water into the circulation. Consequently, extracellular fluid (ECF) volume expands, plasma osmolality declines, the glomerular filtration rate rises, and sodium levels decline (dilutional hyponatremia). This hyponatremia causes muscle cramps and weakness. The patient with SIADH will experience low urinary output and increased body weight without edema. As plasma osmolality and serum sodium levels continue to decline, cerebral edema may occur, leading to lethargy, anorexia, confusion, headache, seizures, and coma.

Diagnostic Studies

The diagnosis of SIADH is made by simultaneous measurements of urine and serum osmolality. The dilutional hyponatremia is indicated by serum sodium less than 134 mEq/L, serum osmolality less than 280 mOsm/kg (280 mmol/kg), and urine specific gravity greater than 1.005.[16] A serum osmolality much lower than the urine osmolality indicates the inappropriate excretion of concentrated urine in the presence of very dilute serum. Associated manifestations correlate with the serum sodium level. Initially, thirst, dyspnea on exertion, fatigue, and dulled sensorium may be evident. As the serum sodium level falls (usually below 120 mEq/L [120 mmol/L]), symptoms become more severe and include vomiting, abdominal cramps, muscle twitching, and seizures.[15] Other laboratory findings are a decreased blood urea nitrogen (BUN), creatinine clearance, hemoglobin, and hematocrit.[16]

Collaborative Care

The treatment goal is to restore normal fluid volume and osmolality. If symptoms are mild and serum sodium is greater than 125 mEq/L (125 mmol/L), the only treatment may be restriction of fluids to 800 to 1000 ml per day. This restriction should result in gradual, daily reductions in weight, a progressive rise in serum sodium concentration and osmolality, and symptomatic improvement. If fluid restriction alone does not improve the symptoms, 3% to 5% (hypertonic) saline solution may be administered IV. A diuretic such as furosemide (Lasix) may be used to promote diuresis if the serum sodium is less than 105 mEq/L (105 mmol/L) or cardiac symptoms or seizures develop. Because furosemide increases potassium excretion, potassium supplements may be needed.

In chronic SIADH, water restriction of 800 to 1000 ml/day is recommended. Regardless of the etiology, demeclocycline (Declomycin), a tetracycline that causes nephrogenic diabetes insipidus, is useful. This drug blocks the action of ADH at the level of the distal and collecting tubules, regardless of the ADH source.

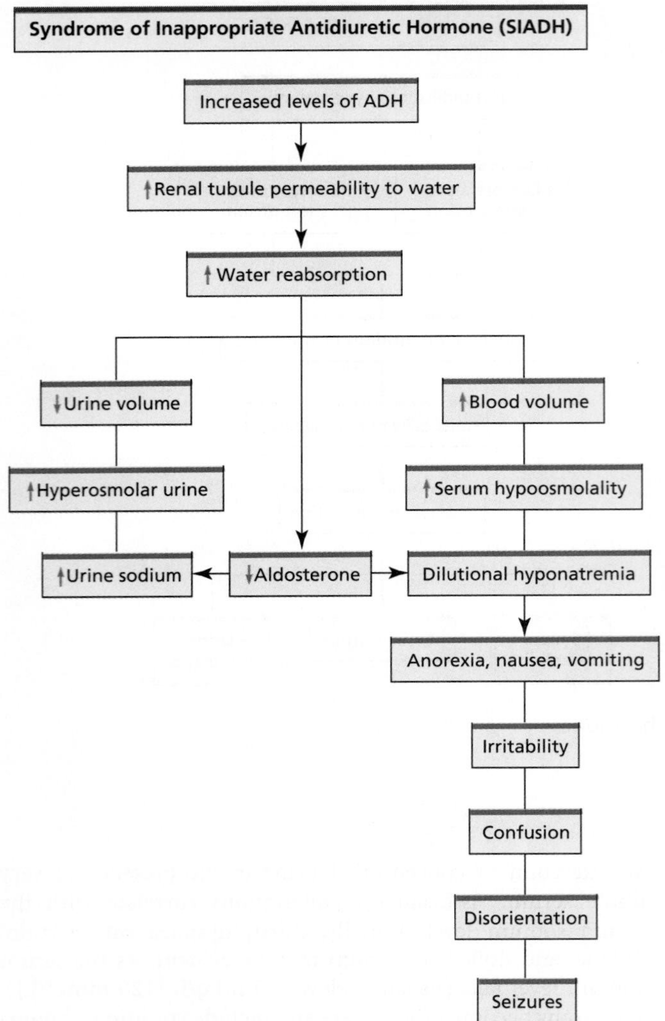

Fig. 47-4 Pathophysiology of syndrome of inappropriate antidiuretic hormone (SIADH).

Table 47-1 Causes of Syndrome of Inappropriate Antidiuretic Hormone

- Malignant neoplasms
  - Small-cell carcinoma of lung
  - Carcinoma of pancreas
  - Lymphoma, lymphocytic leukemia, Hodgkin's disease
  - Thymoma
- Nonmalignant pulmonary diseases
  - Tuberculosis
  - Lung abscess
  - Pneumonia
  - Empyema
  - Chronic obstructive pulmonary disease
- Central nervous system disorders
  - Skull fracture
  - Subdural hematoma
  - Subarachnoid hemorrhage
  - Cerebral vascular thrombosis
  - Cerebral atrophy
  - Encephalitis
  - Meningitis
  - Guillain-Barré syndrome
  - Systemic lupus erythematosus
- Drugs
  - Chlorpropramide
  - Vincristine
  - Vinblastine
  - Cyclophosphamide
  - Carbamazepine
  - Oxytocin
  - General anesthesia
  - Narcotics
  - Tricyclic antidepressants
- Miscellaneous causes
  - Hypothyroidism
  - Positive pressure mechanical ventilation

From Moses A, Streeten D: Disorders of the neurohypophysis. In Isselbacher K and others, editors: *Harrison's principles of internal medicine,* ed 14, New York, 1998, McGraw-Hill.

NURSING MANAGEMENT: SYNDROME OF INAPPROPRIATE ANTIDIURETIC HORMONE

Nursing Assessment

Careful nursing assessment of the patient who has had surgery or is susceptible to the syndrome (Table 47-2) can help in the early detection of SIADH. The nurse should be alert for low urinary output with a high specific gravity, a sudden weight gain, or a serum sodium decline.

Nursing Diagnoses

Nursing diagnoses for the patient with SIADH may include, but are not limited to, the following:

- Altered urinary elimination *related to* excess ADH levels
- Fluid volume excess *related to* excess ADH

Planning

The overall goals are that the patient with SIADH will (1) maintain fluid and electrolyte balance and (2) adhere to fluid restriction and drug therapy.

Nursing Implementation

Health Promotion. At this time there are no known preventive measures for SIADH. Health promotion is focused on early identification of those at risk and appropriate interventions. Patients at risk include those who have had intracranial trauma or surgery and those who have tumors or infections (e.g., meningitis).

Acute Intervention. If a patient has SIADH, nursing measures include the assessments and interventions presented in Table 47-2.

Ambulatory and Home Care. When SIADH is chronic, the patient must learn to self manage treatment regimens. Fluids are restricted to 800 to 1000 ml per day. Sucking on hard candy or ice chips can help decrease thirst. If drinking liquids is an aspect of socialization, the patient should be assisted in planning fluid intake so liquid allowances are saved for social occasions. The patient may be treated with a diuretic to remove excess fluid volume. The diet should be supplemented with sodium and potassium, especially if diuretics are

Table 47-2 Syndrome of Inappropriate Antidiuretic Hormone

Assessment*
- Accurate hourly intake (oral and parenteral) and output
- Hourly measurement of urine specific gravity
- Daily weights
- Level of consciousness
- Observation for signs of hyponatremia every 2 hr (decreased neurologic function, seizures, nausea and vomiting, muscle cramping)
- Monitoring of heart and lung sounds and blood pressure

Interventions
- Restriction of total fluid intake to no more than 1000 ml/day (including that taken with medications); restriction of oral intake to 700 ml < urine output until normalization of serum sodium (if appropriate)
- Positioning head of bed flat or with no more than 10° of elevation to enhance venous return to heart and increase left atrial filling pressure, reducing antidiuretic hormone release
- Positioning side rails up because of potential alterations in mental status
- Turning of patient every 2 hr, proper positioning, range-of-motion exercise, massage (if patient bedridden)
- Use of seizure precautions such as padded side rails and dim lighting
- Assistance with ambulation
- Provision of frequent oral hygiene

*Use a flow sheet for assessment documentation.

prescribed. Solutions of these electrolytes must be well diluted to prevent gastrointestinal (GI) irritation or damage. They are best taken at mealtime to allow mixing with and dilution by food. The patient should be taught the symptoms of fluid and electrolyte imbalances, especially those involving sodium and potassium, so that responses to treatment can be monitored (see Chapter 15). If a patient is to be treated with demeclocycline (Declomysin) the need for close follow-up care should be stressed because of the nephrotoxic side effects and the potential for fungal infections associated with this drug.

■ Evaluation

The expected outcomes are that the patient with SIADH

- has an adequate fluid and electrolyte balance
- understands the need for, and has a plan for, adhering to the meal plan and drug regimen

DIABETES INSIPIDUS

Etiology and Pathophysiology

Central DI occurs when any organic lesion of the hypothalamus, infundibular stem, or posterior pituitary interferes with ADH synthesis, transport, or release. Brain tumors, pituitary or other cranial surgery, closed head trauma, granulomatous disease, central nervous system (CNS) infections, and vascular disorders may cause DI. Central DI may also be caused by osmoreceptor destruction or have no apparent cause (idiopathic).[17]

Clinical Manifestations

DI is characterized by increased thirst (polydipsia) and increased urination (polyuria) (Fig. 47-5). The primary characteristic of DI is the excretion of large quantities of urine (5 to 20 L per day) with a very low specific gravity (less than 1.003) and urine osmolality of <100 mOsm/kg (<100 mmol/kg). Serum osmolality is usually greater than 295 mOsm/kg (295 mmol/kg). In the milder form, urinary output may be lower (2 to 4 L per day). Most patients compensate for fluid loss by drinking large amounts of water so that serum osmolality is normal or only moderately elevated. The patient with central DI particularly favors cold or iced drinks. The patient is usually fatigued from nocturia and may experience generalized weakness.

Central DI usually occurs suddenly. After intracranial surgery, central DI usually has a triphasic pattern: the acute phase, with abrupt onset of polyuria; an interphase, where urine volume apparently normalizes; and a third phase, where central DI is permanent. The third phase is usually apparent within 10 to 14 days postoperatively. Neurogenic DI that results from head trauma is usually self-limiting and improves with treatment of the underlying problem. DI following cranial surgery is more likely to be permanent.

If oral fluid intake cannot keep up with urinary losses, severe fluid volume deficit results. This deficit is manifested by weight loss, poor tissue turgor, hypotension, tachycardia, constipation, and shock. In addition, the patient shows CNS manifestations, ranging from irritability and mental dullness to coma. These symptoms are related to rising serum osmolality and hypernatremia. Because of the polyuria, severe dehydration and hypovolemic shock may occur.

Diagnostic Studies

Because DI may be pituitary (central, neurogenic), renal (nephrogenic), or psychologic (psychogenic) in origin, identification of the cause of the DI is the initial step. A complete history and physical is done. An attempt is made to rule out psychogenic DI related to emotional disturbances. Psychogenic DI is associated with overhydration and hypervolemia rather than with dehydration and hypovolemia seen in other forms of DI. A water deprivation test is usually done to confirm the diagnosis of central DI (see Table 45-7).

Collaborative Care

The therapeutic goal is maintenance of fluid and electrolyte balance. This goal may be accomplished by IV administration of fluid (saline and glucose) and by hormone replacement, with ADH (vasopressin) administered either SC, IM, or IV. In acute DI, fluids should be administered at a rate that decreases the serum sodium by about 1 mEq/L every 2 hours.[16] Clofibrate (Atromid), carbamazepine (Tegretol), and thiazide diuretics may also be prescribed for symptomatic DI. For long-term therapy, desmopressin acetate (DDAVP), an analog of ADH that is administered as a nasal preparation and does not have the vasoconstrictive effect, is the preferred therapy.

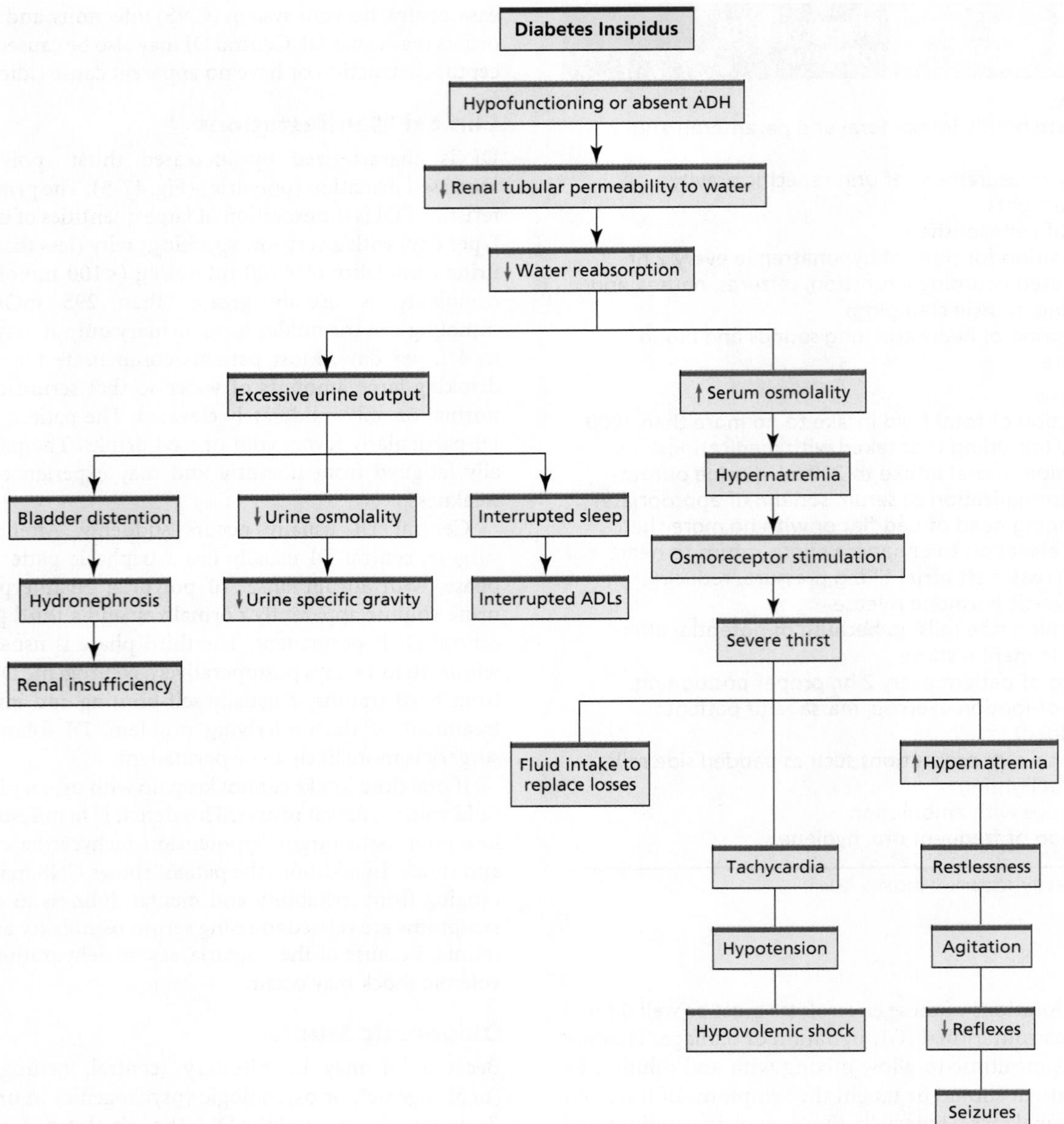

Fig. 47-5 Pathophysiology of diabetes insipidus (DI). *ADH,* antidiuretic hormone; *ADLs,* activities of daily living.

NURSING MANAGEMENT: DIABETES INSIPIDUS

Nursing Assessment

Nursing care of the patient with DI is based on the clinical symptoms. Fluid volume deficit manifested by hypotension, tachycardia, and rapid, shallow respirations can be detected early by frequent assessment. Polyuria and nocturia can cause disturbances in rest and sleep patterns.

Nursing Diagnoses

The nursing diagnoses for the patient with DI may include, but are not limited, to the following:

- Altered urinary elimination *related to* inadequate secretion of, or renal sensitivity to, ADH
- Sleep pattern disturbance *related to* nocturia

Planning

The overall goals are that the patient with DI will (1) maintain fluid and electrolyte balance, (2) have normal sleep patterns, and (3) comply with drug therapy.

Nursing Implementation

Health Promotion. At this time there are no known preventive measures for DI. Health promotion is focused on early identification of those at risk and appropriate interventions. Patients at risk include those who have had intracranial trauma or surgery, brain tumors, infections, and vascular diseases.

Acute Intervention. Fluids must be replaced orally or intravenously, depending on the patient's condition and ability to drink copious amounts of fluids. Adequate fluids should be kept at the bedside. If IV glucose is used, urine should be assessed for glucose. If positive, the physician should be notified, because glucosuria causes an osmotic diuresis, which increases the fluid volume deficit. Accurate records of intake and output, urine specific gravity, and daily weights are mandatory in the assessment of fluid volume status. The patient is often listless, tired, and discouraged. Support and reassurance that the sleep disturbances are temporary may be helpful. Perineal care should be done at least twice daily for the bedridden female patient to cleanse urine from the perineum.

If a water deprivation test is done, the patient's baseline weight, heart rate, urine and plasma osmolalities, urine specific gravity, and blood pressure are obtained. All fluids are withheld for 8 to 16 hours. The patient may be anxious and should be reassured that the test will be stopped if fluid volume deficit becomes severe. The patient should be observed throughout the test because of the craving to drink. During the test, the patient's blood pressure, weight, and urine osmolality are assessed hourly. The test continues until urine osmolalities stabilize (hourly increase less than 30 mOsm/kg [30 mmol/kg] in 2 consecutive hours) or body weight declines by 5%, or orthostatic hypotension develops.[18] Aqueous vasopressin is then given IV, and urine osmolality is measured 1 hour later. In central DI, the rise in urinary osmolality after vasopressin exceeds 9%.[17]

When the patient affected by DI is hospitalized, often for emergency treatment of hypertonic encephalopathy, the therapeutic goal is to restore fluid balance. Desmopressin acetate is administered as a nasal or subcutaneous preparation. Overmedication can precipitate volume excess. The patient should be assessed for weight gain, headache, restlessness, and chest pain. The adequacy of treatment is assessed by monitoring fluid intake and output and by urine specific gravity. Increased urine volume with lower specific gravity is related to an inadequate pharmacologic effect, and the physician should be notified immediately.

Ambulatory and Home Care. The patient who requires long-term ADH replacement needs instruction in self-management. Desmopressin acetate is usually taken intranasally twice daily. Nasal irritation, headache, and nausea may indicate overdosage, whereas failure to improve may indicate underdosage. The patient should be instructed to report any of these symptoms. The need for close follow-up should be stressed.

DISORDERS OF THE THYROID GLAND

Thyroid hormones, thyroxine (T_4) and triiodothyronine (T_3), which is the more active form, regulate energy metabolism and growth and development. Thyroid disorders are manifested as hyperfunction (thyrotoxicosis), hypofunction, inflammation, or enlargement (goiter). A goiter may interfere with surrounding structures and can be associated with increased, normal, or decreased hormone production.

HYPERTHYROIDISM

Hyperthyroidism is defined as sustained increased synthesis and release of thyroid hormones by the thyroid gland. *Thyrotoxicosis* is hypermetabolism that results from excess circulating levels of T_4, T_3, or both. Hyperthyroidism and thyrotoxicosis usually occur together as in Graves' disease. However, in some forms of thyroiditis, thyrotoxicosis may occur without hyperthyroidism.[19]

Hyperthyroidism is second only to diabetes mellitus among noniatrogenic-occurring endocrine diseases. The incidence of hyperthyroidism is 4 to 10 times greater in women, and the highest frequency is in the 30- to 50-year-old age-group. Iodine deficiency is believed to predispose the patient to thyrotoxicosis and other thyroid diseases with a greater incidence in iodine-poor geographic locations. The most common form of thyrotoxicosis is Graves' disease, followed by multinodular goiter, thyroiditis, and exogenous thyroid administration.[20]

Etiology and Pathophysiology

Graves' Disease. *Graves' disease* (diffuse toxic goiter) is a multisystem autoimmune disease of unknown etiology marked by diffuse thyroid enlargement, increased production of thyroid hormone, and usually ophthalmopathy. The patient who is genetically susceptible becomes sensitized to and develops antibodies against various antigens within the thyroid gland and often to other tissues as well. The hyperthyroidism and diffuse thyroid hyperplasia are caused by antibodies that attack thyroid tissue and thus stimulate hyperplasia. These antibodies are found in the serum of the individual with Graves' disease and are known collectively as thyroid-stimulating antibodies (TSAbs). TSAbs stimulate the TSH receptor on the thyroid and by acting like TSH, inappropriately activate the production of thyroid hormones.

Graves' disease occurs more frequently in women in their fourth to sixth decades. A concordance rate of 50% in identical twins indicates genetic and environmental components in the expression of the disease. The disease is characterized by remissions and exacerbations, with or without treatment. It may progress to destruction of thyroid tissue, causing hypothyroidism. Precipitating factors such as insufficient iodine supply, infections, and stressful life events may interact with genetic factors that control immunology and metabolic abnormalities to cause Graves' disease.[20]

Nodular Goiters. Nodular goiters are characterized by small, discrete, autonomously functioning (not TSH dependent) nodules that secrete thyroid hormone. If associated with signs of hyperthyroidism, a nodule is termed *toxic.* There may be multiple nodules (multinodular goiter) or a single nodule (uninodular goiter, thyroid adenoma).

The frequency of toxic multinodular goiter is highest in women in the sixth and seventh decades of life, and it is more common in iodine-deficient areas. There is usually a history of preexisting simple goiter for years before the onset of demonstrable thyrotoxicosis. The manifestations are slower to develop and usually less severe than in Graves' disease. Multinodular goiter is usually not associated with exophthalmos (eyeball protrusion from the orbit). These nodules may be benign or malignant. Uninodular goiter is characterized by a single nodule. These single adenomas are usually larger than 3 cm in diameter, and although encapsulated and benign, they are considered true tumors.[21]

Clinical Manifestations

The clinical manifestations of hyperthyroidism are related to the effects of excess thyroid hormones in two ways. The first is

Table 47-3 Clinical Manifestations: Thyroid Hormone Dysfunction

Hypofunction	Hyperfunction
Cardiovascular System	
Increased capillary fragility Decreased pulse rate Varied changes in blood pressure Cardiac hypertrophy, weak contractility Distant heart sounds Anemia Tendency to develop congestive heart failure, angina, myocardial infarction	Systolic hypertension Increased rate and force of cardiac contractions Bounding, rapid pulse Increased cardiac output Cardiac hypertrophy Systolic murmurs Arrhythmias Palpitations Atrial fibrillation (more common in the older adult) Angina
Respiratory System	
Dyspnea Decreased breathing capacity	Increased respiratory rate Dyspnea on mild exertion
Gastrointestinal System	
Decreased appetite Nausea and vomiting Weight gain Constipation Distended abdomen Enlarged, scaly tongue	Increased appetite, thirst Weight loss Increased peristalsis Diarrhea, frequent defecation Increased bowel sounds Splenomegaly Hepatomegaly
Integumentary System	
Dry, thick, inelastic, cold skin Thick, brittle nails Dry, sparse, coarse hair Poor turgor of mucosa Generalized interstitial edema Puffy face Decreased sweating Pallor	Warm, smooth, moist skin Thin, brittle nails detached from nail bed (onydrolysis) Hair loss (may be patchy) Acropachy (clubbing) Palmar erythema Fine silky hair Premature graying (in men) Diaphoresis Vitiligo
Musculoskeletal System	
Fatigue Weakness Muscular aches and pains Slow movements Arthralgia	Fatigue Muscle weakness (especially proximal) Proximal muscle wasting Pretibial myxedema Dependent edema Osteoporosis
Nervous System	
Apathy Lethargy Forgetfulness Slowed mental processes Hoarseness Slow, slurred speech Prolonged relaxation of deep tendon muscles Stupor, coma Paresthesias Anxiety, depression Polyneuropathy	Difficulty in focusing eyes Nervousness Fine tremor (of fingers and tongue) Insomnia Lability of mood, delirium Restlessness Personality changes of irritability, agitation Exhaustion Hyperreflexia of tendon reflexes Depression, fatigue, apathy (in the older adult) Lack of ability to concentrate Stupor, coma
Reproductive System	
Prolonged menstrual periods or amenorrhea Decreased libido Infertility	Menstrual irregularities Amenorrhea Decreased libido Impotence in men Gynecomastia Decreased fertility
Other	
Increased susceptibility to infection Increased sensitivity to narcotics, barbiturates, anesthesia Intolerance to cold Decreased hearing Sleepiness Goiter	Intolerance to heat Increased sensitivity to stimulant drugs Elevated basal temperature Lid lag, stare Eyelid retraction Exophthalmos Goiter Rapid speech

their direct effect of increasing metabolism. The second is an increased tissue sensitivity to stimulation by the sympathetic division of the autonomic nervous system. Thyroid hormones increase the number of β-adrenergic receptors, thereby increasing sensitivity to the activity of catecholamines (epinephrine and norepinephrine), although the absolute levels of these hormones are not elevated.[20] (The manifestations of thyroid hyperfunction are summarized in Table 47-3.) A patient with advanced disease may exhibit many of the symptoms, whereas a patient in the early stages of hyperthyroidism may exhibit only weight loss and increased nervousness. In the elderly patient with this disorder the only symptoms may be those related to cardiovascular function (apathetic hyperthyroidism).[22] Table 47-4 compares features of hyperthyroidism in young and older adult patients.

Ophthalmopathy. Ophthalmopathy may be infiltrative or noninfiltrative.[20] In infiltrative ophthalmopathy, the eyeballs protrude from the orbits (exophthalmos, proptosis). This exophthalmos is due to impaired venous drainage from the orbit, which causes increased fat deposits and fluid (edema) in the retroorbital tissues (Fig. 47-6). Because of increased pressure, the eyeballs are forced outward and protrude. This sign, which is seen in 20% to 40% of patients with Graves' disease, is autoimmune in nature. It is usually bilateral

Table 47-4 Comparison of Hyperthyroidism in Younger and Older Patients

	Young Adult	Older Adult
▪ Common causes	Graves' disease in >90% of cases	Graves' disease or toxic nodular goiter
▪ Syndrome	Nervousness, irritability, weight loss, palpitations, heat intolerance, and warm, fine skin	Cardiac (angina, arrhythmia, congestive heart failure) Weight loss Myopathy
▪ Goiter	In >90% of cases	In about 50% of cases
▪ Eye signs	Endocrine exophthalmos reflects autoimmune pathogenesis of Graves' disease	Eye signs less frequent
▪ Cardiac features	Tachycardia without heart disease	Underlying cardiac disease common
▪ Thyroxine (T_4)	Elevated in >90% of cases	Elevated somewhat less often
▪ Triiodothyronine (T_3)	Elevated	Elevated
▪ Thyroid-stimulating hormone	Low	Low

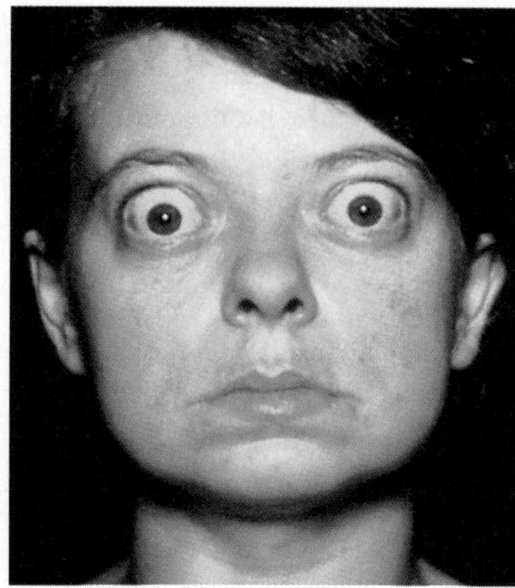

Fig. 47-6 Exophthalmos secondary to Graves' disease.

but can be unilateral or asymmetric. In noninfiltrative ophthalmopathy, the upper lids are usually retracted and elevated, with the sclera above the iris visible. When the eyelids do not close completely, the exposed corneal surfaces become dry and irritated. Serious consequences, such as corneal ulcers and eventual loss of vision, can occur.

Complications

Thyrotoxic crisis (thyroid storm) is an acute but rare condition in which all hyperthyroid manifestations are heightened. It is potentially fatal, but death is rare when treatment is vigorous and initiated early. The cause is presumed to be stressors such as infection, trauma, or surgery in a patient with preexisting hyperthyroidism, either diagnosed or undiagnosed. The physiologic factor or factors that initiate thyrotoxic crisis are unknown.

Manifestations include severe tachycardia, heart failure, shock, hyperthermia (up to 105.3° F [40.7° C]), restlessness, agitation, abdominal pain, nausea, vomiting, diarrhea, delirium, and coma. Measures must be taken to prevent death. Treatment is aimed at reducing circulating thyroid hormone levels and the clinical manifestations of this disorder by appropriate drug therapy. Therapy is directed at fever reduction, fluid replacement, and elimination or management of the initiating stressor(s).[23]

Diagnostic Studies

Serum T_4 and T_3 can be measured with radioimmunoassay techniques (see Table 45-7) and will be elevated. TSH levels, the most sensitive marker, are low in hyperthyroidism. T_3 resin uptake (T_3RU) is also elevated. T_3RU varies inversely with the amount of thyroid hormone that is protein bound and therefore inactive; that is, a high T_3RU indicates that more hormone than normal is biologically active. Free T_4 and T_3 are usually elevated in thyrotoxicosis. The electrocardiogram (ECG) may show tachycardia, atrial fibrillation, and alterations in P and T waves.

In the nonpregnant, nonlactating patient, a 6- or 24-hour radioactive iodine uptake (RAIU) may be done. This test is contraindicated for pregnant or lactating women because radioactive iodine can cross the placenta and destroy the fetal thyroid or enter breast milk and destroy the infant's thyroid. This test can differentiate Graves' disease from other forms of thyroiditis. The patient with Graves' disease will show a diffuse, homogeneous uptake of 35% to 95%, whereas the patient with thyroiditis will show an uptake of less than 2%. The person with nodular goiter will show an uptake in the high normal range.[24,25]

Collaborative Care

The therapeutic goals are to block the adverse effects of thyroid hormones and stop their oversecretion. The diagnostic studies and collaborative care measures are summarized in Table 47-5. Therapy involves drug therapy with antithyroid medications and β-adrenergic receptor blockers, thyroid ablation with radioactive iodine, and subtotal thyroidectomy after adequate preparation. The choice of treatment is influenced by the patient's age, severity of the disorder, complicating features

COLLABORATIVE CARE

Table 47-5 Hyperthyroidism

Diagnostic Studies
History and physical examination
Ophthalmologic examination
ECG
Laboratory tests
Serum T_3RU, T_4, free T_3, TSH levels
TRH stimulation test
Nuclear medicine—thyroid scan
Collaborative Therapy
Graves' Disease
Antithyroid drugs
Propylthiouracil
Methimazole (Tapazole)
β-Adrenergic blockers such as propranolol (Inderal)
Ablation of thyroid tissue
Radioactive iodine (^{131}I)
Subtotal thyroidectomy
High-caloric diet
Multinodular Goiter
Antithyroid drugs
Propylthiouracil
Methimazole (Tapazole)
Ablation of thyroid tissue by radioactive iodine

ECG, electrocardiogram; *TRH*, thyrotropin-releasing hormone; *T_3RU*, T_3 resin uptake; *TSH*, thyroid-stimulating hormone.

(including pregnancy), and patient's preferences. If surgery is to be performed, the patient is usually given antithyroid drugs to produce a euthyroid state and possibly iodine and β-adrenergic blockers to relieve symptoms preoperatively.

Surgical Therapy. Preoperatively, any other associated disorders, such as cardiac disease or diabetes mellitus, must be controlled before surgery. For thyroidectomy to be effective, approximately 90% of thyroid tissue must be removed. If too much tissue is taken, the gland will not regenerate after surgery and hypothyroidism will develop. Occasionally the recurrent laryngeal nerve or parathyroid glands may be damaged during surgery.

Drug Therapy

Thioamides. The most commonly used antithyroid drugs are classified as thioamides. Propylthiouracil (PTU) and methimazole (Tapazole) are clinically the most commonly used drugs. These drugs inhibit the synthesis of thyroid hormones. PTU also blocks peripheral conversion of T_4 to T_3. Although there is considerable individual variation, improvement usually begins 1 to 2 weeks after the initiation of therapy, and good results are seen within 4 to 8 weeks. Therapy is usually continued for 6 months to 2 years to allow for spontaneous remission. The major disadvantages of antithyroid drugs are patient noncompliance and a high rate of recurrence of hyperthyroidism when the drugs are discontinued. In addition, agranulocytosis may occur in rare situations. Indications for use of antithyroid drugs include Graves' disease in the young patient, hyperthyroidism during pregnancy, and the need to make a patient euthyroid before surgery or radiation.

Iodine. Iodine (e.g., Lugol's solution, potassium iodide) in large doses inhibits synthesis of active thyroid hormones T_3 and T_4 and blocks the release of these hormones into circulation. Its maximal effect is usually seen within 1 to 2 weeks. After that time, a reduction in the therapeutic effect may be seen, and long-term iodine therapy is not effective in controlling hyperthyroidism. Usually one drop of a saturated solution of potassium iodide is administered three times daily before surgery. Iodine decreases the size and vascularity of the thyroid, making resection safer and easier. Administration of PTU, with iodine therapy added 10 days before surgery, is a common method for surgical preparation of a patient with hyperthyroidism.

β-Adrenergic blockers. Propranolol (Inderal) is the most frequently used β-adrenergic blocker. It relieves the symptoms of thyrotoxicosis that result from increased β-adrenergic receptors caused by excess thyroid hormones. These symptoms include heat intolerance, palpitations, nervousness, tremor, and muscle weakness. Propranolol is used with other antithyroid treatment and rapidly relieves the symptoms that cause such discomfort to the patient with hyperthyroidism. Propranolol is not used in the patient with asthma or heart disease. Atenolol (Tenormin) may be used instead.

Radioactive iodine. Radioactive iodine (radioiodine) limits thyroid hormone secretion by damaging or destroying thyroid tissue. Between 8 and 12 mCi (296 and 444 MBq) is administered orally. This treatment is effective but often results in hypothyroidism.[25] Radioactive iodine has a delayed response, and maximum effects may not be seen for 2 to 3 months. However, it is effective and inexpensive and can be administered on an outpatient basis. The patient is treated with PTU or propranolol before and during the first 3 months after the initiation of radioactive iodine therapy and for relief of hypermetabolic symptoms until the effects of irradiation become apparent. Thyroid ablation with ^{131}I is not indicated in pregnant women because radioactive iodine crosses the placenta and destroys the fetal thyroid.

Nutritional Therapy. The potential for nutritional deficits is high when an increased metabolic rate is present. A high-caloric diet (4000 to 5000 kcal/day) may be ordered to satisfy hunger and prevent tissue breakdown. This is accomplished with six full meals a day and snacks high in protein, carbohydrates, minerals, and vitamins, particularly vitamin A, thiamin, vitamin B_6, and ascorbic acid. The protein allowance should be 1 to 2 g/kg of ideal body weight. Increased carbohydrates should compensate for disturbed metabolism, provide energy, and spare protein. A registered dietician should be consulted for guidance in meeting the nutritional needs of a patient with hyperthyroidism.

Highly seasoned and high-fiber foods should be avoided because they stimulate the already hyperactive gastrointestinal tract. Substitutes should be provided for caffeine-containing liquids such as coffee, tea, and cola because the stimulating effects of these fluids increase the restlessness and sleep disturbances. Milk is an excellent food source that provides calcium and protein.

NURSING ASSESSMENT

Table 47-6 Hyperthyroidism

Subjective Data	Objective Data
Important Health Information *Past health history:* Preexisting goiter; recent infection or trauma, immigration from iodine-deficient area, autoimmune disease *Medications:* Use of thyroid hormones **Functional Health Patterns** *Health perception–health management:* Positive family history of thyroid or autoimmune disorders *Nutritional-metabolic:* Insufficient iodine intake; weight loss; increased appetite, thirst; nausea *Elimination:* Diarrhea; polyuria; sweating *Activity-exercise:* Dyspnea on exertion; palpitations; muscle weakness, fatigue *Sleep-rest:* Insomnia *Cognitive-perceptual:* Chest pain; nervousness; heat intolerance, pruritis *Sexuality-reproductive:* Decreased libido; impotence; gynecomastia (in men); amenorrhea (in women) *Coping–stress tolerance:* Emotional lability, irritability, restlessness, personality changes, delirium	**General** Agitation, rapid speech and body movements; hyperthermia, enlarged or nodular thyroid gland **Eyes** Exophthalmos, eyelid retraction; infrequent blinking **Integumentary** Warm, diaphoretic, velvety skin; thin, loose nails; fine, silky hair and hair loss; palmar erythema; clubbing; white pigmentation of skin (vitiligo), diffuse edema of legs and feet **Respiratory** Tachypnea **Cardiovascular** Tachycardia, bounding pulse, systolic murmurs, arrhythmias, hypertension **Gastrointestinal** Increased bowel sounds; hepatosplenomegaly **Neurologic** Hyperreflexia, diplopia, fine tremors of hands, tongue, eyelids; stupor, coma **Musculoskeletal** Muscle wasting **Reproductive** Menstrual irregularities, infertility; decreased libido; impotence, gynecomastia in men **Possible Findings** Elevated serum T_3, T_4, and T_3 resin uptake; decreased serum TSH; chest x-ray showing cardiac hypertrophy

NURSING MANAGEMENT: HYPERTHYROIDISM

Nursing Assessment

Subjective and objective data that should be obtained from an individual with hyperthyroidism are presented in Table 47-6.

Nursing Diagnoses

Nursing diagnoses for the patient with hyperthyroidism may include, but are not limited to, those presented in NCP 47-1.

Planning

The overall goals are that the patient with hyperthyroidism will (1) experience relief of symptoms, (2) have no serious complications related to the disease or treatment, and (3) cooperate with the therapeutic plan.

Nursing Implementation

Health Promotion. There are currently no preventive measures for hyperthyroidism. Health promotion is focused on preventing relapse in patients who have been treated for hyperthyroidism. Thyrotoxicosis may recur after a period of time, requiring further treatment. Factors that may precipitate relapse include exposure to dietary sources of iodine. Iodine is widespread and can be found in red food dye, preservatives such as iodates in flour, some public drinking systems, health food products such as kelp tablets, and milk from cows treated with iodine or iodophors used to clean milk vats.[26]

Acute Intervention. A restful, calm, quiet room should be provided because increased metabolism causes sleep disturbances. Provision of adequate rest may be a challenge because of the patient's irritability and restlessness. Interventions may include (1) placing the patient in a cool room, away from very ill patients and noisy, high-traffic areas; (2) using light bed coverings and changing the linen frequently if the patient is diaphoretic; (3) encouraging and assisting with exercise involving large muscle groups (tremors can interfere with small-muscle coordination) to allow the release of nervous tension and restlessness; (4) restricting visitors who upset the patient; and (5) establishing a supportive, trusting relationship to help the patient cope with aggravating events and lessen anxiety.

If exophthalmos is present there is a potential for corneal injury related to irritation and dryness. The patient may also have orbital pain. Nursing interventions to relieve eye discomfort and prevent corneal ulceration include applying artificial tears to soothe and moisten conjunctival membranes. Salt restriction may help reduce periorbital edema. Elevation of the patient's head promotes fluid drainage from the periorbital

47-1 NURSING CARE PLAN PATIENT WITH HYPERTHYROIDISM

Expected Patient Outcomes	Nursing Interventions and *Rationales*
NURSING DIAGNOSIS	**Activity intolerance** *related to* fatigue, exhaustion, and heat intolerance secondary to hypermetabolism *as manifested by* complaints of weakness, inability to perform usual activities, short attention span, memory lapses, dyspnea, tachycardia, irritability.
▪ Decreased perception of weakness and fatigue.	▪ Assess for signs of activity intolerance *because hyperthyroidism results in protein catabolism, overactivity, and increased metabolism leading to exhaustion.* ▪ Monitor vital signs q4hr and before and after activities *because tachycardia and BP elevations can indicate excessive activity.* ▪ Assist patient with self-care as needed *to make certain patient's daily needs are met.* ▪ Limit ambulation to short walks *to avoid fatiguing patient.* ▪ Schedule activities of daily living and treatments *to promote adequate rest periods.*
NURSING DIAGNOSIS	**Risk for injury: corneal ulceration** *related to* decreased blinking or inability to close eyelids secondary to exophthalmos.
▪ No evidence of corneal damage.	▪ Assess patient for complaints of eye pain, feeling of grittiness or "sand" in eyes, proptosis, inability to close eyelids completely, lid lag, lid retraction, visible sclera above iris, and "stare" *to determine if risk factors are present and initiate appropriate interventions.* ▪ Restrict patient's salt intake *to reduce periorbital edema.* ▪ Raise head of bed at night *to promote fluid drainage.* ▪ Teach patient to exercise extraocular muscles daily *to maintain flexibility.* ▪ Cover patient's eyes with mask or tape shut if eyes will not close if exophthalmos is severe *to prevent corneal drying and, at night, to promote sleep.* ▪ Apply methylcellulose eyedrops (artificial tears) *to soothe and moisten conjunctival membranes.*
NURSING DIAGNOSIS	**Risk for injury** *related to* fine muscle tremors, fatigue, inattentiveness, incoordination.
▪ No accidental injury.	▪ Assess for complaints of inability to perform tasks requiring small muscles; restlessness, fatigue; fine muscle tremors; uncoordinated movements; pretibial myxedema *to determine risk for injury and plan appropriate interventions.* ▪ Assist patient as necessary with tasks requiring fine motor skill; reduce environmental hazards *to reduce exposure to high-risk activities.* ▪ Assist patient with ambulation *to prevent injury from falling or bumping into items.* ▪ Teach patient safety practices *to reduce possibility of injury and increase patient's sense of control.* ▪ Avoid use of caffeine *because it stimulates catecholamines, which can increase fine muscle tremors.*
NURSING DIAGNOSIS	**Altered nutrition: less than body requirements** *related to* hypermetabolism and inadequate diet *as manifested by* complaints of weight loss; body weight 20% less than ideal.
▪ Maintenance of weight (or gain weight). ▪ Alleviation (or prevention) of nutritional deficiency.	▪ Assess patient's eating habits and weight pattern *to determine extent of the problem and plan appropriate interventions.* ▪ Teach and provide high-calorie, high-vitamin, high-mineral diet that includes between meal and bedtime snacks *because hyperthyroidism increases metabolic rate with resulting need to prevent muscle breakdown and weight loss.* ▪ Weigh patient daily *to evaluate effectiveness of nutritional plan.* ▪ Monitor BUN and albumin levels *to evaluate protein levels to determine extent of protein malnutrition.*

Continued

area; the patient should sit upright as much as possible. Dark glasses reduce glare and prevent irritation from smoke, air currents, dust, and dirt. If the eyelids cannot be closed, they should be lightly taped shut for sleep. To maintain flexibility, the patient should be taught to exercise the intraocular muscles several times a day, by turning the eyes in the complete range of motion. Good grooming can be helpful in reducing the loss of self-esteem that can result from an altered body image. If the exophthalmos is severe, treatment may involve suturing the eyelids together, administering corticosteroids,

47-1 NURSING CARE PLAN PATIENT WITH HYPERTHYROIDISM—continued

Expected Patient Outcomes	Nursing Interventions and *Rationales*
NURSING DIAGNOSIS	**Anxiety** *related to* lack of knowledge about management and course of disease, hypermetabolism, and presence of hypertension *as manifested by* inability to verbalize information regarding medication, verbalization of inability to cope with stress.
▪ Verbalization of knowledge of management and course of disease. ▪ Verbalization of decrease in anxiety.	▪ Teach patient about disease management, including medication regimen, potential for hypertension, chronic nature of disease, and dietary implications, *because knowledge decreases anxiety and increases a sense of control.* ▪ Assist patient to develop strategies for behavior change *to incorporate medication regimen into lifestyle.* ▪ Promote rest and relaxation *because anxiety often causes difficulty with rest and sleep.* ▪ Teach patient strategies for coping with stress *to prevent increasing anxiety.* ▪ Administer medications as ordered *because decrease in disease activity will decrease anxiety.*
NURSING DIAGNOSIS	**Hyperthermia** *related to* impaired temperature adaptation, hypermetabolism; and altered perception of ambient temperature *as manifested by* verbalization of feelings of excess warmth; elevated temperature; diaphoresis.
▪ Decrease in perspiration. ▪ Increase in comfort.	▪ Assess for elevated temperature, diaphoresis, and heat intolerance *to determine extent of problem and plan interventions.* ▪ Maintain cool environmental temperature; provide light, loose clothing; bathe patient and change linen frequently *to promote patient comfort.* ▪ Encourage fluids to 3 L/day *to replace fluid loss.*

COLLABORATIVE PROBLEMS

Nursing Goals	Nursing Interventions and *Rationales*
POTENTIAL COMPLICATION	**Congestive heart failure** *related to* cardiac hypertrophy, hypertension, arrhythmias.
▪ Monitor for signs of congestive heart failure. ▪ Report deviations from acceptable parameters. ▪ Carry out appropriate medical and nursing interventions.	▪ Assess for complaints of dyspnea, fatigue, chest pain; edema; cardiac enlargement; atrial fibrillation; diaphoresis *to determine presence of congestive heart failure.* ▪ Reduce environmental stressors; promote rest and relaxation *to reduce cardiac workload.* ▪ Assess tolerance to activity *so appropriate assistance can be provided.* ▪ Discourage physical activity that is not well tolerated *to prevent stressing heart beyond its limit to respond.* ▪ Administer cardiotonics (e.g., digoxin [Lanoxin]) as ordered *to stabilize cardiac status.* ▪ Monitor vital signs and cardiac status frequently *to evaluate effectiveness of plan.*

radiation of retroorbital tissues, orbital decompression, or corrective lid or muscle surgery.

Thyroid surgery. When subtotal thyroidectomy is the treatment of choice, the patient must be adequately prepared to avoid postoperative complications. The signs and symptoms of thyrotoxicosis must be alleviated as much as possible, and cardiac problems must be controlled before surgery. If iodine is used to relieve hyperthyroid symptoms, it should be mixed with water or juice, sipped through a straw, and administered after meals. The patient must be assessed for signs of iodine toxicity such as swelling of buccal mucosa and other mucous membranes, excessive salivation, nausea and vomiting, and skin reactions. If toxicity occurs, iodine administration should be discontinued and the physician notified.

Preoperative teaching should include comfort and safety measures in which the patient can participate. Coughing, deep breathing, and leg exercises should be practiced and their importance explained. The patient should be taught how to support the head manually while turning in bed, because this maneuver minimizes stress on the suture line after surgery. Range-of-motion exercises of the neck should be practiced. The nurse should explain routine postoperative care such as IV infusions. The patient should be told that talking is likely to be difficult for a short time after surgery.

The hospital room must be prepared before the patient's return from surgery. Oxygen, suction equipment, and a tracheostomy tray should be readily available. A tracheostomy tray is required in case airway obstruction occurs. Although this rarely happens, it is an emergency situation. Recurrent laryngeal nerve damage leads to vocal cord paralysis. If there is paralysis of both cords, spastic airway obstruction will occur, requiring an immediate tracheostomy.

Respiration may also become difficult because of excess swelling of the neck tissues, hemorrhage, hematoma formation,

RESEARCH
IMPLICATIONS FOR NURSING PRACTICE

Patients with Thyroid Cancer

Citation Dow KH, Ferrell BR, Anello C: Balancing demands of cancer surveillance among survivors of thyroid cancer, *Cancer Practice* 5:289, 1997.

Purpose To explore and describe the demands of long-term cancer surveillance among survivors of thyroid cancer and how these perceived demands influenced their quality of life.

Methods The sample included 34 patients with a history of thyroid cancer on thyroid hormone replacement therapy. The mean age of the patients was 40 years. Patients participated in the study at the time they were undergoing thyroid hormone withdrawal for the purpose of body scanning for detection of cancer recurrence or metastatic disease. In addition to completing a demographic data collection tool, the participants were asked three open-ended questions about their quality of life during the thyroid hormone withdrawal period.

Results and Conclusions The patients experienced profound changes in quality of life during the withdrawal phase. Patients reported changes in physical, psychologic, and social well-being related to the thyroid hormone withdrawal (hypothyroidism). Regardless of the prognosis, patients expressed concerns about the possibility of disease recurrence.

Implications for Nursing Practice Symptoms related to thyroid hormone withdrawal (which is necessary for diagnostic testing) can produce profound and debilitating symptoms in hypothyroid patients. Because thyroid cancer tends to affect young to middle-aged adults, the withdrawal of thyroid hormone can greatly affect work and life schedules. These withdrawal effects occur at the same time the patient is coping with the stress of additional testing.

and laryngeal stridor. Laryngeal stridor (harsh, vibratory sound) may occur during respiration as a result of tetany, which occurs if the parathyroid glands are removed or damaged during surgery. To treat tetany, calcium salts such as calcium gluconate and calcium chloride should be readily available for IV administration.

After a thyroidectomy the nurse should do the following:

- Assess the patient every 2 hours for 24 hours for signs of hemorrhage or tracheal compression such as irregular breathing, neck swelling, frequent swallowing, sensations of fullness at the incision site, choking, and blood on the anterior or posterior dressings.
- Place the patient in a semi-Fowler's position and support the head with pillows, avoiding flexion of the neck and any tension on the suture lines.
- Monitor vital signs. Complete the initial assessment by checking for signs of tetany secondary to hypoparathyroidism (e.g., tingling in toes, fingers, or around the mouth; muscular twitching; apprehension) and by evaluating difficulty in speaking and hoarseness. Trousseau's sign and Chvostek's sign should be monitored for 72 hours (see Fig. 15-14). Some hoarseness is to be expected for 3 to 4 days after surgery because of edema.
- Control postoperative pain by giving medication.[27]

The neck incision should be supported and range-of-motion exercises should be carried out three or four times daily to promote comfort and the return of full range of motion. The patient should be taught to avoid movements that cause flexion, extension, rotation, and lateral bending of the neck. The appearance of the incision may be distressing. The patient can be reassured that the scar will fade in color and eventually look like a normal neck wrinkle. A scarf, jewelry, high collar, or other covering can effectively camouflage a fresh scar.

If postoperative recovery is uneventful, the patient is ambulated the first day, takes fluid as soon as tolerated, and eats a soft diet by the second day after surgery. Recommended foods should be kept readily available.

Ambulatory and Home Care. Nursing interventions with the patient's significant others include assisting them to perform the nursing interventions. In addition, the nurse should instruct them about the nature of the patient's illness to enable them to understand the physical and emotional manifestations that the patient experiences. Exploring or suggesting ways they can help reduce stressful situations and providing a nonjudgmental atmosphere for them to express difficulties in accepting and dealing with the patient's demands and behavior can be helpful.

Follow-up care is important for the patient who has undergone thyroid surgery. Hormone balance should be monitored periodically to ensure that normal function has returned. Most patients experience a period of relative hypothyroidism soon after surgery because of the substantial reduction in the size of the thyroid. However, the remaining tissue usually hypertrophies, recovering the capacity to produce the hormone needed by the body; but this takes time. The administration of thyroid hormone is avoided because exogenous hormone inhibits pituitary production of TSH and delays or prevents the restoration of normal gland function and thyroid tissue regeneration.

The patient can do a great deal to prevent complications and promote a return to normal function during the hypothyroid period after surgery. Caloric intake must be reduced substantially below the amount that was required before surgery to prevent weight gain. The surgeon may suggest avoiding foods that contain thyroid-inhibiting substances (goitrogens) (Table 47-7). Adequate iodine is necessary to promote thyroid function, but excesses inhibit the thyroid. Seafood once or twice a week or normal use of iodized salt should provide sufficient intake. Regular exercise helps stimulate the thyroid and should be encouraged. Exposure to alternating extremes of temperature, such as hot and cold showers, also promotes thyroid hyperplasia but is not acceptable to many individuals because of cold intolerance. High environmental temperature should be avoided because it inhibits thyroid regeneration.

Regular follow-up care is necessary. The patient should be seen biweekly for a month and then at least semiannually to assess for the development of hypothyroidism. If a complete

Table 47-7 Common Exogenous Goitrogens

Foods
Potent goitrogens
Turnips
Rutabagas
Soybeans (especially when fed to infants in formula)
Skins of peanuts
Milk from kale-fed cattle
Less potent goitrogens
Seafood
Green leafy vegetables
Peanuts
Peaches
Peas
Strawberries
Carrots
Cabbage
Mustard seed
Radishes
Drugs
Thyroid inhibitors
Propylthiouracil
Methimazole
Carbimazole
Iodine in large doses
Others
Sulfonamides
Salicylates
p-Aminosalicylic acid
Phenylbutazone
Lithium
Amiodarone

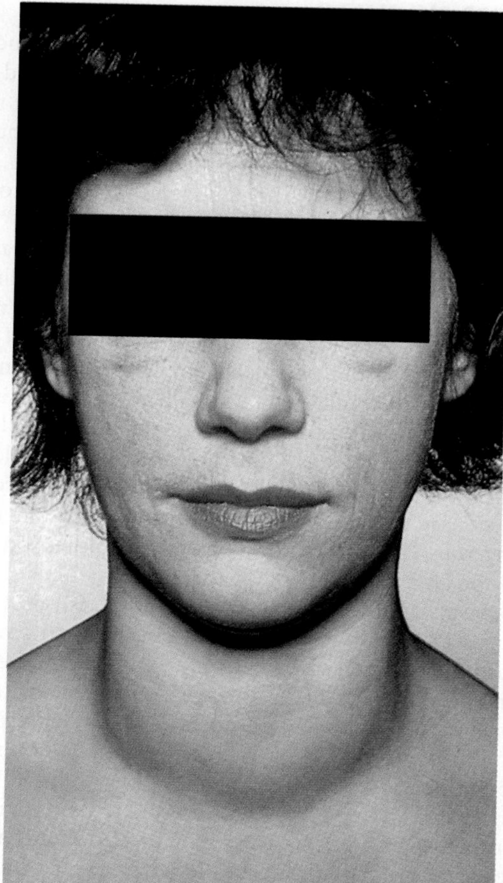

Fig. 47-7 Simple goiter.

thyroidectomy has been performed, the patient needs instruction in lifelong pharmacologic thyroid replacement. Failure of thyroid function is considered by some authorities to be the normal end stage of Graves' disease. The patient should be taught the signs and symptoms of progressive thyroid failure and instructed to seek medical care if these develop. Hypothyroidism is relatively easy to control with oral administration of thyroid preparations.

Radioactive iodine therapy. Radioactive iodine therapy (ablation) is usually administered on an outpatient basis and is the therapy of choice for the adult beyond childbearing years. Because the usual therapeutic dose of radioactive iodine is only 7 to 10 mCi, no radiation safety precautions are necessary. The patient should be instructed that radiation thyroiditis and parotiditis are possible and may cause dryness and irritation of the mouth and throat. Relief may be obtained with frequent sips of water, ice chips, or the use of a salt and soda gargle three to four times per day. This gargle is made by dissolving 1 teaspoon of salt and 1 teaspoon of baking soda in 2 cups of warm water. The discomfort should subside in 3 to 4 days. If dryness and irritation persist, the patient should contact a clinician. Because of the high frequency of hypothyroidism after radioactive iodine therapy, the patient and significant others should be taught the symptoms of hypothyroidism and instructed to seek medical help if these symptoms occur.

■ Evaluation

The expected outcomes are that the patient with hyperthyroidism

- experiences relief of symptoms
- has no serious complications related to the disease or treatment
- cooperates with the therapeutic plan

THYROID ENLARGEMENT

Enlargement of the thyroid gland is called *goiter* (Fig. 47-7). Goiter may result from hypertrophy caused by excess TSH stimulation, which in turn can be caused by inadequate circulating thyroid hormones. Goiter may also be caused by growth-stimulating immunoglobulins and other growth factors. Goitrogens (see Table 47-7), which inhibit synthesis of thyroid hormone, can cause goiter but usually only in the individual who lives in an iodine-deficient area (endemic goiter).

TSH and T_4 are measured to determine whether a goiter is associated with hyperthyroidism, hypothyroidism, or normal thyroid function. Thyroid antibodies are measured to assess for thyroiditis. Treatment with thyroid hormone may prevent further thyroid enlargement. Surgery to remove large goiters may be necessary.

THYROID NODULES

A thyroid nodule, a palpable deformity of the thyroid gland, may be benign or malignant. Malignant tumors of the thyroid gland are rare. Both single and multinodular thyroids carry a risk of cancer. The major sign of thyroid cancer is the appearance of a hard, painless nodule in an enlarged thyroid.

A thyroid scan shows whether nodules on the thyroid are "hot" or "cold." When a person is given tracer doses of ^{131}I, thyroid tumors on the thyroid may or may not take up the radioactive iodine. Tumors that take up the radioactive iodine are termed *hot nodules* and are nearly always benign. If the nodule does not take up the radioactive iodine, it is termed a *cold nodule* and has a higher risk of being malignant. High-resolution ultrasonography and MRI may also be used to aid in diagnosis. Needle biopsy (fine-needle aspiration) of the nodule is usually done to identify malignant tissue.[28] Measurement of serum calcitonin is also helpful in diagnosis, since increased levels are associated with medullary thyroid carcinoma. Benign nodules are usually not dangerous, but they can cause tracheal compression if they become too large.

Neoplasms are treated by surgical removal. Surgical procedures may range from unilateral total lobectomy with removal of the isthmus to total thyroidectomy with bilateral neck dissection. Many thyroid cancers are TSH dependent, and thyroid hormone in hyperphysiologic doses is often prescribed to inhibit pituitary secretion of TSH. External radiation may be used to prolong survival.

Nursing care for the patient with thyroid tumors is similar to care for the patient who has undergone thyroidectomy and also includes general nursing measures for the patient with cancer (see Chapter 14).

THYROIDITIS

Thyroiditis is an inflammatory process in the thyroid and can have several causes. Subacute granulomatous thyroiditis (de Quervain's thyroiditis), which causes thyrotoxicosis, is thought to be caused by a viral infection. Acute thyroiditis is due to bacterial or fungal infection. Subacute and acute forms of thyroiditis have abrupt onsets and the thyroid is painful. Chronic autoimmune thyroiditis (Hashimoto's thyroiditis), leading to hypothyroidism, is insidious in onset. Hashimoto's thyroiditis is a chronic autoimmune disease in which thyroid tissue is replaced by lymphocytes and fibrous tissue. It is the most common cause of goiterous hypothyroidism in the United States. Silent thyroiditis, a form of lymphocytic thyroiditis, has a variable onset. This condition may occur in the postpartal period. It is believed to be an autoimmune disease and may be early Hashimoto's thyroiditis.

T_4 and T_3 are initially elevated in subacute, acute, and silent thyroiditis but may become depressed with time. TSH levels are low and then elevated. Thyroid hormone levels are usually low in chronic Hashimoto's thyroiditis, and TSH is high. Suppression of RAIU is seen in subacute and silent thyroiditis. Antithyroid antibodies are present in Hashimoto's thyroiditis.

NURSING AND COLLABORATIVE MANAGEMENT: THYROIDITIS

Recovery from thyroiditis may be complete in weeks or months without treatment. If the condition is bacterial in origin, treatment may include specific antibiotics or surgical drainage. In subacute and acute forms, salicylates and nonsteroidal anti-inflammatory drugs (NSAIDs) are used. If there is no response to these drugs in 48 hours, corticosteroids are given. Propranolol or atenolol may be used for the cardiovascular symptoms of a hyperthyroid condition. Thyroid hormone is used if the patient is hypothyroid.

Nursing care of the patient with thyroiditis includes education regarding normal thyroid function and what is happening in the patient's specific instance. Other nursing interventions depend in part on the therapeutic management. Nursing interventions include reassurance, support, and assistance during the recovery period. The patient should be instructed to remain under close health supervision so that progress can be monitored and to report any change in symptoms to the health care provider.

The patient with thyroiditis of autoimmune origin may be susceptible to other autoimmune diseases such as Addison's disease, pernicious anemia, or premature gonadal failure or Graves' disease. The patient should be taught the signs and symptoms of these disorders, particularly Addison's disease. Because stress may aggravate these autoimmune diseases, stress management is an important part of patient education (see Chapter 7). The patient should also be given a list of common goitrogens (see Table 47-7) and encouraged to avoid them as much as possible.

A patient receiving thyroid hormone replacement or corticosteroids must be taught the expected side effects of these drugs and measures to manage them. The patient should also be instructed in unexpected side effects and told when and to whom these should be reported. Toxic symptoms should be clearly defined, and the patient should be instructed to report them. Table 47-3 lists signs of hyperthyroidism that are the same as toxic symptoms of thyroid hormone replacement. Patient handouts written in understandable language should accompany verbal instruction. The handouts should be reviewed with the patient to assess understanding, and information should be clarified when necessary. The patient treated surgically needs care similar to that given to the person undergoing thyroidectomy.

HYPOTHYROIDISM

Etiology and Pathophysiology

Hypothyroidism usually results from insufficient circulating thyroid hormone as a result of a variety of abnormalities. Hypothyroidism can be primary, related to destruction of thyroid tissue or defective hormone synthesis, or secondary, related to pituitary disease with decreased TSH secretion or to hypothalamic problems with decreased TRH secretion. It may also be transient, related to a thyroiditis or discontinuance of thyroid hormone therapy.[29] All hypothyroid states have certain features in common, regardless of the cause. Some differences depend on the patient's age at onset of the deficiency.

Hypothyroidism may occur in infancy (cretinism), childhood, or adulthood. Cretinism is caused by thyroid hormone deficiencies during fetal or early neonatal life. It can be caused by maternal iodine deprivation or congenital thyroid abnormalities. Cretinism occurs in 1 of 3700 births in the United States and is more frequent in females.[30] Juvenile hypothyroidism has causes similar to those seen in the adult and requires prompt diagnosis and treatment to prevent developmental retardation.

ETHICAL DILEMMAS

Alternative Healers

SITUATION

Although thyroid replacement therapy is the planned treatment, the patient's cultural healer tells her not to take the medication and that she should begin an herbal regimen instead. Should the nurse intervene?

DISCUSSION

Knowledge of a patient's cultural background and setting is important to a successful treatment plan. If the nurse can learn about the healing practices and come to know the healers in the community, a partnership can develop between traditional and allopathic (Western) medicine. Education can be conducted in both directions, and the cultural healer's methods can be used in conjunction with the prescribed treatment. However, if the nurse reacts negatively and denigrates or condemns traditional healing, the patient may be forced to choose between what is culturally appropriate, acceptable, and known, and that which is required by the Western medical establishment. Hostility between Western medical professionals and traditional healing does not benefit the patient and may, in fact, dissuade the community from seeking medical attention. It is always in the patient's best interests for providers to be knowledgeable of the cultures of the people they serve and to develop relationships with traditional healers.

ETHICAL AND LEGAL PRINCIPLES

- Patient autonomy (the right of a patient to decide for himself or herself) should be upheld.
- Planning appropriate and effective health care should take into consideration a patient's religious and cultural values and beliefs.
- In some situations, Western (allopathic) medicine can no longer provide definitive care (e.g., terminally ill cancer patient), and alternative medicine may provide the patient with hope and support.

In areas where iodine intake is adequate, such as the United States, the most common cause of primary hypothyroidism in the adult is atrophy of the thyroid gland. This atrophy is the end result of both Hashimoto's thyroiditis and Graves' disease. These autoimmune diseases destroy the thyroid gland. Thyroid deficiency also occurs when pituitary TSH production is inadequate. Iatrogenic causes of hypothyroidism include surgical removal of the thyroid, destruction of the thyroid gland by radiation, and surgical removal of the pituitary gland. Occasionally, hypothyroidism develops as a result of the ingestion of excessive amounts of goitrogens (see Table 47-7). The person with underlying autoimmune disease is particularly susceptible to goitrogens.

Although the typical patient with hypothyroidism is a woman over age 50, the disease can occur at any age and in either sex. An increased incidence has been correlated with the previous therapeutic use of radioactive iodine. Hypothyroidism is more common in iodine-deficient areas of the world, such as Zaire and Nepal, and iodine deficiency is the most common cause of hypothyroidism worldwide.[30]

Clinical Manifestations

The major manifestations of cretinism are defective physical development and mental retardation. Although affected infants usually appear normal at birth, cretinism should be suspected when there is a long gestational period and a large infant who fails to thrive. Affected infants may exhibit a large posterior fontanel, squinting, excessive sleeping, thickened skin and lips, enlarged tongue, abdominal distention with vomiting, a hoarse cry, dull facial expression, feeding and respiratory difficulty, peripheral cyanosis, supraclavicular and periorbital edema, umbilical hernia, and hypothermia.

Hypothyroidism in childhood is usually due to autoimmune thyroiditis. Intellectual development is normal, but the child may seem mentally sluggish. Physical and sexual development are altered. Although there is generalized muscle hypertrophy, the face remains childlike, and eruption of permanent teeth, linear growth, and sexual maturation are delayed. In addition, there is a high frequency of other autoimmune diseases.[30,33]

Hypothyroidism in the adult is characterized by an insidious and nonspecific slowing of body processes. The adult with hypothyroidism often is fatigued and lethargic and may experience personality changes. The mental changes seen in hypothyroidism include impaired memory, slowed speech, decreased initiative, and somnolence. In addition, cold intolerance, hair loss, dry and coarse skin, brittle nails, hoarseness, muscle weakness and swelling, overall weakness, constipation, weight gain, and menorrhagia are common.

Unless hypothyroidism occurs after thyroidectomy or thyroid ablation, or during treatment with antithyroid drugs, the onset of symptoms may occur over months to years. The symptoms are so insidious that medical attention is seldom sought. The patient's family and friends are often unaware of the changes. The severity of the symptoms depends on the degree of thyroid hormone deficiency and results from the long-term physiologic effects of thyroid hormone deficiency. They may involve any body system but are more pronounced in cardiovascular, GI, reproductive, and hematopoietic systems.

Hypothyroid heart disease includes cardiomyopathy, pericardial effusion, and coronary atherosclerosis. Bradycardia and weakened cardiac contractility lead to decreased cardiac output. Pericardial effusion, however, seldom results in hemodynamic compromise. Increased serum cholesterol and triglyceride levels and the accumulation of mucopolysaccharides in the intima of small blood vessels can result in coronary atherosclerosis. This accumulation is seldom symptomatic (i.e., characterized by angina) because of the decreased myocardial oxygen consumption that has been observed in hypothyroidism.

The brain is affected by diminished cerebral blood flow related to decreased cardiac output. This is manifested by mental sluggishness, inattentiveness, memory loss, lethargy, and changes in affect. Although some individuals with hypothyroidism exhibit a jocular air regarding their condition, others appear depressed. They express distress and describe an impaired self-image in regard to their disabilities and altered appearance. Although the patient with hypothyroidism sleeps long hours, stage 3 and stage 4 sleep are reduced.

GI motility is decreased in hypothyroidism, and achlorhydria (absence of hydrochloric acid) is common. Constipation, which is a common complaint, may progress to obstipation and, rarely, to intestinal obstruction. The underlying metabolic disease makes the individual a high-risk candidate for intestinal surgery.

Women with hypothyroidism frequently complain of menorrhagia. Some affected individuals have been treated for menorrhagia for years and may have undergone hysterectomy before the hypothyroidism was diagnosed. In addition, anovulatory cycles with subsequent infertility may occur.

Anemia is a common feature of hypothyroidism. Erythropoietin levels may be low or normal. Oxygen demand is decreased in the periphery, and there is hypocellular bone marrow. The result is a low hematocrit. Other hematopoietic problems are cobalamin, iron, and folate deficiencies and a predisposition to bruising.

The term *myxedema* is often used synonymously with hypothyroidism but actually connotes severe, long-standing hypothyroidism. Myxedema is the accumulation of hydrophilic mucopolysaccharides in the dermis and other tissues. This mucinous edema causes the characteristic facies of hypothyroidism and puffiness, periorbital edema, and masklike affect.

Complications

The mental sluggishness, drowsiness, and lethargy of hypothyroidism may progress gradually or suddenly to a notable impairment of consciousness or coma. This situation, termed *myxedema coma,* constitutes a medical emergency. Myxedema coma can be precipitated by infection, drugs (especially narcotics, tranquilizers, and barbiturates), exposure to cold, and trauma. It is characterized by subnormal temperature, hypotension, and hypoventilation. For the patient to live, vital functions must be supported, and IV thyroid hormone must be administered.

Diagnostic Studies

T_4, T_3, and T_3RU levels are usually low in hypothyroidism. These values, correlated with symptoms gathered from the history and physical examination, confirm the diagnosis. Serum TSH levels help determine the cause of hypothyroidism. Serum TSH is high when the defect is in the thyroid and low when it is in the pituitary or hypothalamus. An increase in TSH after TRH injection suggests hypothalamic dysfunction, whereas no change suggests anterior pituitary dysfunction (Table 47-8). In the well elderly, T_3, T_4, and TSH levels are unchanged.

Clinical diagnosis of hypothyroidism in the elderly adult can be difficult. The typical manifestations of hypothyroidism, which are often considered normal changes of aging, include fatigue; cold, dry skin; hoarseness; hair loss; constipation; and cold intolerance.

DIAGNOSTIC STUDIES

Table 47-8 Hypothyroidism

Study	Finding
Serum T_3RU	Low
Serum T_3	Low
Serum T_4	Low
Serum cholesterol	Increased
ECG	Bradycardia, low voltage
Serum TSH	High (if thyroid diseased), low (if pituitary diseased)
TRH stimulation test	Increase in TSH if hypothalamus diseased, no change in TSH if pituitary diseased

Collaborative Care

The therapeutic objective in hypothyroidism is restoration of a euthyroid state as safely and rapidly as possible with hormone replacement therapy. In the adult a low-calorie diet is indicated to promote weight loss.

Synthetic oral thyroxine (Synthroid, Levothroid, Noroxine) is the drug of choice to treat hypothyroidism. In the young, otherwise healthy patient, the maintenance replacement dose can be started at once.[25] In the older adult patient and the person with compromised cardiac status, a small initial dose is recommended because the usual dose may increase myocardial oxygen consumption.[34] The resultant oxygen demand may cause angina and cardiac arrhythmias. Any chest pain experienced by a patient starting thyroid replacement should be reported immediately, and ECG and serum cardiac enzyme tests must be performed. The dose is increased at 1- to 4-week intervals. It is important that the patient take replacement medication regularly. Lifelong thyroid replacement therapy is usually required for both adults and children.

NURSING MANAGEMENT: HYPOTHYROIDISM

■ Nursing Assessment

Assessment of the patient who is suspected of having hypothyroidism should include questions about weight gain, mental changes, fatigue, slowed and slurred speech, cold intolerance, skin changes such as increased dryness or thickening, constipation, and dyspnea. In addition, the nurse should assess for recent introduction of iodine-containing medications or ingestion of large amounts of goitrogens.[31,35] The patient should be assessed for bradycardia; distended abdomen; dry, thick, cold skin; thick, brittle nails; paresthesias; and muscular aches and pains.

■ Nursing Diagnoses

Nursing diagnoses for the patient with hypothyroidism may include, but are not limited to, those presented in NCP 47-2.

■ Planning

The overall goals are that the patient with hypothyroidism will (1) experience relief of symptoms, (2) maintain a euthyroid state, (3) maintain a positive self-image, and (4) comply with lifelong thyroid replacement therapy.

■ Nursing Implementation

Health Promotion. The nurse plays an important role in the detection of hypothyroidism. Careful assessment may reveal the early and subtle changes that indicate dysfunction, particularly when caring for the patient with a condition, such as family history, that may predispose him or her to endocrine dysfunction. Promotion and maintenance of thyroid function requires an adequate dietary intake of iodine for hormone production. The importance of adequate nutrition is illustrated by

47-2 NURSING CARE PLAN PATIENT WITH HYPOTHYROIDISM

Expected Patient Outcomes	Nursing Interventions and *Rationales*
NURSING DIAGNOSIS	**Hypothermia** *related to* cold intolerance *as manifested by* complaints of feeling cold, shivering.
▪ Satisfaction with temperature of environment. ▪ Personal comfort.	▪ Provide extra clothing, blankets, warm environment *to increase patient's comfort.* ▪ Explain to patient and significant others that decreased heat production causes discomfort *to increase understanding of and empathy for patient's condition.*
NURSING DIAGNOSIS	**Altered nutrition: more than body requirements** *related to* hypometabolism *as manifested by* weight gain greater than 10% more than ideal body weight.
▪ Maintenance of weight in usual range.	▪ Provide low-calorie, high-protein diet; include foods high in cobalamin, folic acid, iron, and vitamin C *to reduce tendency for weight gain while preventing muscle wasting and anemia.* ▪ Explain the need for fewer calories *so patient will be more agreeable to dietary restrictions.* ▪ Assist patient to develop method of monitoring weight and caloric intake *so excess weight gain can be avoided.* ▪ Encourage small, frequent meals *because early satiety and decreased gastrointestinal motility can cause gas and discomfort.*
NURSING DIAGNOSIS	**Constipation** *related to* gastrointestinal hypomotility *as manifested by* irregular, hard stools.
▪ Daily soft formed stool.	▪ Assess bowel pattern and characteristics *to plan appropriate interventions.* ▪ Provide 2-3 L of fluids per day *to maintain soft stool.* ▪ Encourage activity *to stimulate peristalsis.* ▪ Administer laxatives or stool softeners if necessary *to stimulate GI motility.* ▪ Offer foods high in bulk and roughage *to increase fecal mass.*
NURSING DIAGNOSIS	**Activity intolerance** *related to* decreased metabolic rate and mucin deposits in joints and interstitial spaces *as manifested by* generalized weakness and muscle and joint stiffness.
▪ Able to participate in self-care activities with minimal discomfort and fatigue.	▪ Assess ability to participate in self-care activities *to determine extent of problem and plan appropriate interventions.* ▪ Monitor vital signs and comfort level *to determine effect of activities and plan activity increases.* ▪ Administer thyroid hormone as ordered *to correct hypometabolic state.* ▪ Plan frequent rest periods *to improve patient's tolerance and comfort level.* ▪ Apply splints and hot packs if appropriate *to relieve joint stiffness and pain by immobilization.* ▪ Pace activities to match patient's abilities *to allow maximum participation.*
NURSING DIAGNOSIS	**Altered thought processes** *related to* diminished cerebral blood flow secondary to decreased cardiac output *as manifested by* forgetfulness, memory loss, and personality changes.
▪ Maintenance of orientation to reality at highest level possible.	▪ Assess thinking processes such as memory; attention span; orientation to time, person, and place *to enable appropriate planning.* ▪ Repeat information to patient *because this person requires more time to comprehend.* ▪ Explain cause of symptoms to patient and family *to reduce anxiety and frustration.* ▪ Provide clock and calendar *to maintain orientation to time and day.* ▪ Provide written handouts with all instructions *to help patient remember and thereby enhance adherence to regimen.*

the thyroid enlargement and marginal hypothyroidism that can develop in the individual with iodine deficiencies (endemic goiter). Thyroid hormone production also requires an adequate intake of protein.

Acute Intervention. If the patient has myxedema coma, mechanical respiratory support will be necessary, as well as cardiac monitoring. The nurse will be administering all medications IV since the paralytic ileus associated with myxedema coma causes unreliable absorption of oral medications. If the patient is hyponatremic, hypertonic saline may be administered until the serum sodium reaches 130 mEq/L (130 mmol/L). The nurse should monitor core temperature because the patient with myxedema coma is often extremely hypothermic.[36]

For assessment of the patient's progress, vital signs, body weight, fluid intake and output, and visible edema should be monitored. Cardiac assessment is especially important because the cardiovascular response to the hormone determines the medication regimen. Energy level and mental alertness should be noted. These should increase within 2 to 14 days and continue to rise steadily to normal levels.

Ambulatory and Home Care. Repeated patient education is imperative (Table 47-9). Initially the hypothyroid patient needs more time than usual to comprehend all of the necessary information. It is important to provide written instructions, repeat the information often, and assess the patient's comprehension level regularly. The need for lifelong drug therapy must be stressed. The signs and symptoms of hypothyroidism or hyperthyroidism that indicate hormone imbalance should be included in the teaching plan. It is sometimes difficult for the patient to recognize signs of overdosage or underdosage; therefore a family member or friend should be included in the instruction process. Forgetfulness is an early indication of thyroid deficiency.

The patient must be taught to contact a clinician immediately if signs of overdose such as orthopnea, dyspnea, rapid pulse, palpitations, nervousness, or insomnia appear. The patient with diabetes mellitus should test his or her capillary blood glucose at least daily because return to the euthyroid state frequently increases insulin requirements. In addition, thyroid preparations potentiate the effects of other common drug groups, such as anticoagulants, antidepressants, and digitalis compounds. Thus the patient should be taught the toxic signs and symptoms of these medications and should remain under close medical observation until stable.

With treatment, striking transformations occur in both appearance and mental function. Most adults return to a normal state. Cardiovascular conditions and (occasionally) psychosis may persist despite corrections of the hormonal imbalance. Relapses occur if treatment is interrupted.

■ Evaluation

The expected outcomes are that the patient with hypothyroidism will

- have relief from symptoms
- maintain a euthyroid state as evidenced by normal thyroid hormone and TSH levels
- state the need for and a plan to adhere to lifelong therapy

PATIENT TEACHING GUIDE

Table 47-9 Hypothyroidism

1. Provide a comfortable, warm environment because of intolerance to cold.
2. Take measures to prevent skin breakdown. Use soap sparingly, and apply an emollient or lotion. An alternating-pressure mattress may be helpful.
3. Avoid using sedatives. If they must be used, use the lowest possible dose, and family members should closely monitor mental status, level of consciousness, and respirations.
4. Prevent constipation by a gradual increase in exercise, increased fiber in diet, stool softeners as advised, and maintenance of a regular bowel elimination time (usually in the morning). Avoid enemas because they produce vagal stimulation, which can be hazardous if cardiac disease is present.
5. Understand the nature of the thyroid hormone deficiency and the self-care practices necessary to prevent complications.

DISORDERS OF THE PARATHYROID GLANDS

HYPERPARATHYROIDISM

Etiology and Pathophysiology

Hyperparathyroidism is a condition involving increased secretion of parathyroid hormone (PTH). PTH helps regulate calcium and phosphate levels by stimulating bone resorption, renal tubular reabsorption of calcium, and activation of vitamin D. Until recently, this dysfunction was considered rare. However, with the increased use of routine evaluation of serum calcium levels the prevalence in the general population is estimated to be 0.04%, and the annual incidence in persons over 40 years of age ranges between 0.1% and 0.5%.[37,38]

Hyperparathyroidism is classified as primary, secondary, or tertiary. Primary hyperparathyroidism is due to an increased secretion of PTH leading to disorders of calcium, phosphate, and bone metabolism. The excessive concentration of circulating PTH usually leads to hypercalcemia and hypophosphatemia. The most common cause is a benign neoplasm or a single adenoma (80% of cases) in the parathyroid gland. Secondary hyperparathyroidism appears to be a compensatory response to states that induce or cause hypocalcemia, the main stimulus of PTH secretion. Disease conditions associated with secondary hyperparathyroidism include vitamin D deficiencies, malabsorption, chronic renal failure, and hyperphosphatemia. Tertiary hyperparathyroidism occurs when there is hyperplasia of the parathyroid glands and a loss of negative feedback from circulating calcium levels. Thus there is autonomous secretion of PTH, even with normal calcium levels. It is observed in the patient who has had a kidney transplant after a long period of dialysis treatment for chronic renal failure (see Chapter 44).

Primary hyperparathyroidism is more common in women and usually occurs between 30 and 70 years of age. The peak incidence is in the fifth and sixth decades of life. Previous head and neck radiation may predispose a patient to the

Table 47-10 Clinical Manifestations: Parathyroid Dysfunction

System	Hypofunction	Hyperfunction
Cardiovascular	Decreased contractility of heart muscle Decreased cardiac output Prolongation of QT and ST intervals on ECG Arrhythmias	Arrhythmias Shortened QT interval on ECG Hypertension
Gastrointestinal	Abdominal cramps Urinary and fecal incontinence (in older adult)	Vague abdominal pain Anorexia Nausea and vomiting Constipation Pancreatitis Peptic ulcer disease Cholelithiasis Weight loss
Integumentary	Dry, scaly skin Hair loss on scalp and body Brittle nails, transverse ridging Changes in developing teeth, lack of tooth enamel	Skin necrosis Moist skin
Musculoskeletal	Fatigue Weakness Painful muscle cramps Skeletal x-ray changes, osteosclerosis Soft-tissue calcification Difficulty in walking	Skeletal pain Backache Weakness, fatigue Pain on weight bearing Osteoporosis Pathologic fractures of long bones Compression fractures of spine Decreased muscle tone
Neurologic	Personality changes Psychiatric manifestations of depression, anxiety Irritability Memory impairment Headache Seizures Positive Chvostek's sign or Trousseau's phenomenon Tremor Paresthesias of perioral area, hands, feet Hyperactive deep-tendon reflexes Disorientation, confusion (in older adult)	Personality disturbances Emotional irritability Memory impairment Psychosis Delirium, confusion, coma Incoordination Hyperactive deep-tendon reflexes Abnormalities of gait Psychomotor retardation Headache
Renal	Urinary frequency	Hypercalciuria Kidney stones (nephrolithiasis) Urinary tract infections Polyuria
Other	Eye changes, including lenticular opacities, cataracts, papilledema	Corneal calcification on slit-lamp examination

development of parathyroid adenoma in a small group of patients.[38] Increased PTH has a multisystem effect (Table 47-10). In the bones, subperiosteal bone resorption, decreased bone density, cyst formation, and general weakness can occur as a result of the effect of PTH on osteoclastic (bone resorbers) and osteoblastic (bone formers) activity.

In the kidneys the excess calcium cannot be reabsorbed, leading to increased levels of calcium in the urine (hypercalciuria). This urinary calcium, along with a large amount of urinary phosphate, can lead to calculi formation. In addition, in the kidneys, PTH stimulates the synthesis of a biologically active form of vitamin D, a potent stimulator of calcium transport in the intestine. In this way, PTH indirectly increases GI absorption of calcium, contributing further to the high serum calcium levels.

Clinical Manifestations and Complications

Hyperparathyroidism has varying symptoms (see Table 47-10). The major symptoms include weakness, loss of appetite, constipation, increased need for sleep, emotional disorders, and shortened attention span. Major signs include loss of calcium from bones (osteoporosis), broken bones, and kidney stones (nephrolithiasis). Neuromuscular abnormalities are characterized by muscle weakness, particularly in the proximal muscles of the lower extremities. Asymptomatic cases are being identified with increasing frequency with routine calcium screening.

Serious complications of hyperparathyroidism are renal failure, pancreatitis, collapse of vertebral bodies, cardiac changes, and long bone and rib fractures.

Diagnostic Studies

PTH, as measured by radioimmunoassay, will be elevated. Serum calcium levels usually exceed 10 mg/dl (2.50 mmol/L). Because of its inverse relation with calcium, the serum phosphorus level is usually below 3 mg/dl (0.1 mmol/L). Elevations in other laboratory tests include urine calcium, serum chloride, uric acid, creatinine, amylase (if pancreatitis is present), and alkaline phosphatase (if bone disease has begun). If bone changes are present, radiologic studies may reveal subperiosteal resorption. Imaging such as MRI, CT scanning, and ultrasound may be used for localization of the adenoma.[39]

Collaborative Care

The treatment objectives are to relieve symptoms and prevent complications caused by excess PTH. The choice of therapy depends on the urgency of the clinical situation, the degree of hypercalcemia, the underlying disorder, the status of renal and hepatic function, the clinical presentation of the patient, and the particular advantages and disadvantages of the different therapeutic modalities.

If the symptoms are mild or if the patient is elderly or at increased surgical risk from other health problems, a conservative management approach is used. This includes an annual examination with tests for serum PTH, calcium, phosphorus, and alkaline phosphatase levels and renal function, x-rays to assess for metabolic bone disease, and measurement of urinary calcium excretion. Continued ambulation and the avoidance of immobility are critical aspects of management.

Parathyroid tumors should be removed surgically. The parathyroid glands occasionally lie in ectopic sites such as the mediastinum. This situation requires a highly skilled surgeon to open the chest and explore the area behind the sternum. Generally, a single gland is removed if an adenoma is the cause of the hyperparathyroidism. When cancer is the cause, all the parathyroid glands are removed. With a total parathyroidectomy, the patient will need to take calcium supplements for life.

Specific management measures include maintenance of a high fluid intake and a moderate calcium intake. The diet should contain 8 to 10 g of sodium per day to replace losses from increased urine output. Phosphorus is usually supplemented, unless contraindicated by an increased risk for urinary calculi formation.

Drug Therapy. Plicamycin (Mithracin), an antihypercalcemic agent, lowers serum calcium within 48 hours. However, because of toxic side effects, its use is limited to the patient with metastatic parathyroid carcinoma and severe bone disease. Biphosphonates such as pamidronate (Aredia) may be used. They inhibit osteoclastic bone resorption and rapidly normalize serum calcium levels. Estrogen or progestin therapy can reduce serum and urinary calcium levels in the postmenopausal woman and may retard demineralization of the skeleton.[39] Oral phosphate may be used to inhibit the calcium-absorbing effects of vitamin D in the intestine. Phosphates should be used only if a patient has normal renal function and low serum phosphate levels. Diuretics may be given to increase the urinary excretion of calcium.

In severe hyperparathyroidism, normal saline is given IV to correct fluid volume deficit and promote calcium excretion. Furosemide (Lasix) is given orally or IV to promote sodium loss and decrease renal tubular reabsorption of calcium. Plicamycin (Mithracin) may be administered IV to inhibit osteoclastic bone resorption.[40]

NURSING MANAGEMENT: HYPERPARATHYROIDISM

■ Nursing Assessment

Subjective and objective data that should be obtained from an individual with hyperparathyroidism are presented in Table 47-11.

■ Nursing Diagnoses

Nursing diagnoses for the patient with hyperparathyroidism may include, but are not limited to, those presented in NCP 47-3.

■ Planning

The overall goals are that the patient with hyperparathyroidism will (1) maintain satisfactory activity level, (2) keep a consistently high fluid intake, (3) not experience any serious complications related to the disease or its treatment, (4) maintain a positive self-image, and (5) accept and comply with the long-term nature of the problem.

■ Nursing Implementation

If surgery is performed, close monitoring of the patient's vital signs is required. Other aspects of care are similar to that after thyroidectomy. The major postoperative complications are tetany and fluid and electrolyte disturbances. Tetany is usually apparent early in the postoperative period but may develop over several days. Mild tetany, characterized by unpleasant tingling of the hands and around the mouth, may be present but should abate without problems. If tetany becomes more severe (e.g., muscular spasms or laryngospasms develop), IV calcium may be given. Strict monitoring of intake and output is necessary to evaluate fluid status. Calcium, potassium, phosphate, and magnesium levels are assessed frequently, as well as Chvostek's and Trousseau's signs (see Fig. 15-14). Mobility is encouraged to promote bone calcification.

If surgery is not performed, treatment to relieve symptoms and prevent complications is carried out. The nurse can assist the patient with hyperparathyroidism to adapt the meal plan to her or his lifestyle. A referral to a dietician may be useful. Since immobility can aggravate the bone loss, the nurse can assist the patient to implement an exercise prescription and identify resources, such as shopping malls and YMCAs or YWCAs, as places to exercise safely. The patient should be encouraged to keep the annual appointments, and the tests being performed should be explained. The patient should also be instructed in the symptoms of hypocalcemia and hypercalcemia and to report these should they occur. Hypocalcemia and hypercalcemia are discussed in Chapter 15.

■ Evaluation

Expected outcomes for the patient with hyperparathyroidism are addressed in NCP 47-3.

NURSING ASSESSMENT

Table 47-11 Hyperparathyroidism

Subjective Data	Objective Data
Important Health Information *Past health history:* Vitamin D deficiency; malabsorption, malnutrition; chronic renal failure *Medications:* Compliance with renal failure medication (e.g., phosphate binders, calcium supplements) *Surgery or other treatments:* Previous head or neck radiation **Functional Health Patterns** *Health perception–health management:* Malaise *Nutritional-metabolic:* Anorexia, nausea, vomiting, weight loss *Elimination:* Polyuria, dysuria, constipation *Activity-exercise:* Weakness, fatigue *Sleep:* Increase in sleeping *Cognitive-perceptual:* Irritability, depression; generalized skeletal pain with pain on weight bearing, headache, abdominal and back pain, arthralgias; renal colic *Coping–stress tolerance:* Irritability, memory impairment, personality changes	**General** Apathy **Integumentary** Moist skin, skin necrosis **Cardiovascular** Hypertension, arrhythmias (especially bradycardias) **Neurologic** Drowsiness, slow mentation, confusion, delirium, poor coordination, hyperactive deep tendon reflexes **Musculoskeletal** Fractures, decreased muscle tone, abnormal gait **Possible Findings** Elevated serum calcium (>10 mg/dl), parathyroid hormone, chloride, alkaline phosphatase, uric acid, creatinine; decreased serum phosphate (<3 mg/dl); hypercalciuria; guaiac-positive stool and emesis (peptic ulcer); subperiosteal bone resorption and demineralization on x-ray examination; enlarged parathyroids on ultrasonography

HYPOPARATHYROIDISM

Etiology and Pathophysiology

Hypoparathyroidism, or inadequate circulating PTH, is uncommon. It is characterized by hypocalcemia resulting from a lack of PTH to maintain serum calcium levels. PTH resistance at the cellular level may also occur (pseudohypoparathyroidism). This is caused by a genetic defect resulting in hypocalcemia in spite of normal or high PTH levels and is often associated with hypothyroidism and hypogonadism.

The most common cause of hypoparathyroidism is iatrogenic, that is, accidental removal of the parathyroids or damage to the vascular supply of the glands during neck surgery (e.g., thyroidectomy, radical neck surgery). Idiopathic hypoparathyroidism resulting from the absence, fatty replacement, or atrophy of the glands is a rare disease that usually occurs early in life and may be associated with other endocrine disorders. Affected patients may have antiparathyroid antibodies. Hypomagnesemia is increasingly being recognized as a cause of hypoparathyroidism. Hypomagnesemia, as seen in alcoholism or malabsorption, impairs PTH secretion and its action on bone and kidneys.[37]

Clinical Manifestations

The clinical features of acute hypoparathyroidism are due to a low serum calcium level (see Table 47-10). Sudden decreases in calcium concentration give rise to a syndrome called *tetany.* This state is characterized by tingling of the lips, fingertips, and occasionally feet and increased muscle tension leading to paresthesias and stiffness. Painful tonic spasms of smooth and skeletal muscles (particularly of the extremities and face), dysphagia, a constricted feeling in the throat, and laryngospasms are also present. Chvostek's sign (facial muscle spasm when the face is tapped below the temple) and Trousseau's sign (carpopedal spasm when arterial circulation is interrupted by applying a blood pressure cuff for 3 minutes; see Fig. 15-14) are usually positive. Respiratory function may be severely compromised by accessory muscle spasm and laryngeal spasm–induced airway obstruction. Patients are usually anxious and apprehensive. Abnormal laboratory findings include decreased serum calcium and PTH levels and increased serum phosphate levels. Other causes of chronic hypocalcemia include chronic renal failure, vitamin D deficiency, and hypomagnesemia.

Collaborative Care

The main objectives of treatment are to treat tetany when present and prevent long-term complications by maintaining normal serum calcium levels (eucalcemia).

Tetany is treated with IV infusion or slow push of calcium salts. Long-term therapy consists of the administration of vitamin D and possibly supplemental calcium and oral phosphate binders.[41]

Emergency treatment of tetany requires the administration of IV calcium. Generally, in adults, 10 to 20 ml of a 10% solution of calcium gluconate is infused over 10 minutes. Calcium salts can cause hypotension and cardiac arrest; thus a slow IV push is required.[41] In addition, these salts can cause venous irritation and inflammation if leakage occurs into extravascular tissues. For long-term management, oral calcium supplements may be prescribed. Calcium carbonate, an antacid, is readily available but may alter acid-base balance. It also stimulates secretion of hydrochloric acid, which could be a problem for the patient with an ulcer. Calcium gluconate, which is available in tablet form, should be chewed into fine particles before swallowing. Acid aids in the gastrointestinal absorption of calcium

47-3 NURSING CARE PLAN PATIENT WITH HYPERPARATHYROIDISM

Expected Patient Outcomes	Nursing Interventions and *Rationales*
NURSING DIAGNOSIS **Activity intolerance** *related to* muscle weakness and fatigue *as manifested by* complaints of weakness and fatigue, pain on weight bearing.	
■ Decreased fatigue and weakness. ■ Activities of daily living needs met by self or others.	■ Assist with ambulation and limit ambulation to short walks *to demonstrate a caring attitude and prevent fatigue.* ■ Assist patient with self-care as needed *to ensure activities of daily living needs are met and to conserve energy.* ■ Plan activities of daily living and treatment *to allow for adequate rest periods.* ■ Provide patient with walker or cane as necessary *as aids to safe ambulation and to keep patient ambulatory.*
NURSING DIAGNOSIS **Altered urinary elimination** *related to* renal involvement secondary to hypercalcemia *as manifested by* hypercalciuria, renal stones.	
■ No renal stones. ■ Prompt detection and early treatment of renal stones.	■ Instruct patient about symptoms of renal stones such as flank pain and hematuria *to ensure early reporting of symptoms.* ■ Strain urine *to detect stones.* ■ Keep fluids within easy reach and offer frequently; encourage fluid intake to point of moderate overhydration (4000 ml or more fluid output per day) *to keep fluid level high so kidneys are flushed and stone formation is less likely.*
NURSING DIAGNOSIS **Altered nutrition: less than body requirements** *related to* anorexia and nausea *as manifested by* loss of weight and complaints of loss of appetite and nausea.	
■ Maintenance of adequate food and fluid intake. ■ Maintenance of stable weight.	■ Administer mouth care frequently with use of flavored mouthwash or toothpaste *to keep mouth fresh.* ■ Eliminate noxious odors from environment *to prevent this potential cause of a decreased appetite.* ■ Reduce milk products *to reduce nausea.* ■ Teach calorie counting *so that caloric intake is sufficient to maintain weight.* ■ Serve small amounts of food frequently *to prevent bloating and a premature sense of fullness.*
NURSING DIAGNOSIS **Constipation** *related to* dehydration and inactivity *as manifested by* complaints of rectal fullness and pressure, pain on defecation, hard stools, <3 stools per week.	
■ Regular evacuation (preferably daily) of soft or formed stools. ■ Prompt detection of constipation or impaction.	■ Encourage fluid intake to 3000 ml per day *to increase fluid content of fecal mass.* ■ Administer prune juice daily *because it contains dihydroxyphenyl isatin, which acts as a laxative.* ■ Maintain diet high in bulk *to increase fecal mass.* ■ Request order for stool softener from physician. ■ Encourage frequent, short walks *to promote increased peristalsis and movement of fecal mass.* ■ Promote maintenance of regular habit of defecation consistent with preadmission pattern *to foster bowel regularity.*
NURSING DIAGNOSIS **Risk for injury: fractures and joint contractures** *related to* decreased bone density, weakness, improper body alignment, and immobility.	
■ No occurrence of deformity or accidental injury.	■ Monitor for complaints of bone and joint pain, weakness, backache, impaired mobility, unsteady gait *to detect potential for injury.* ■ Assist patient with ambulation, reduce safety hazards in environment, and maintain bed in low position *to reduce potential for injury.* ■ Alert other hospital departments about handling and positioning patient during tests *to avoid accidental injury caused by lack of knowledge of patient's musculoskeletal fragility.*

Continued

47-3 NURSING CARE PLAN PATIENT WITH HYPERPARATHYROIDISM —continued

Expected Patient Outcomes	Nursing Interventions and *Rationales*
NURSING DIAGNOSIS	**Body image disturbance** *related to* weight loss, weakness, fatigue, and mental status changes *as manifested by* verbalization of negative feelings about self; expression of feelings of hopelessness; hostile, angry behavior; self-isolation.
▪ Statements and actions indicative of improved self-image. ▪ More positive mental outlook.	▪ Encourage patient to ventilate feelings about physical and emotional changes *because venting of feelings helps clarify issues.* ▪ Compliment patient when appropriate *to promote a positive body image.* ▪ Reassure patient that fatigability and depression will improve when hormone imbalance is corrected *to foster hope and a positive attitude.* ▪ Encourage short walks to social areas *to prevent isolation.* ▪ Ascertain which activities the patient has enjoyed in past; encourage continued involvement in those activities that are appropriate to setting and patient's condition.
NURSING DIAGNOSIS	**Altered thought processes** *related to* slowed mentation, depression, and drowsiness *as manifested by* disorientation, inappropriate behavior or response, difficulty in concentrating.
▪ Maintenance of reality-based orientation. ▪ Appropriate actions and reactions.	▪ Assess sensory-perceptual status *to plan appropriate interventions.* ▪ Orient patient as indicated *to assist with reality orientation.* ▪ Provide calm, restful environment *to minimize confusion and foster rest.* ▪ Explain actions in simple language *to avoid increasing patient's confusion.* ▪ Monitor and record level of consciousness and orientation every shift *to evaluate effectiveness of plan and alter as appropriate.*

COLLABORATIVE PROBLEMS

Nursing Goals	Nursing Interventions and *Rationales*
POTENTIAL COMPLICATION	**Tetany** *related to* hypocalcemia secondary to low serum calcium following parathyroidectomy.
▪ Monitor for signs of tetany, including neuromuscular irritability, Chvostek's sign, and Trousseau's sign. ▪ Report deviations from acceptable parameters. ▪ Carry out appropriate nursing and medical interventions.	▪ Assess the patient for circumoral and hand paresthesias that do not subside *as a precursor to tetany.* ▪ Be prepared to administer calcium gluconate intravenously if ordered *to treat hypocalcemia.*

gluconate, so it should be taken at the end of a meal. Oral calcium supplements are given four times a day.

Specific hormone replacement of PTH is not used to treat hypoparathyroidism because of expense and the need for parenteral administration. Vitamin D is used in chronic and resistant hypocalcemia to enhance intestinal calcium absorption and bone resorption. The preferred preparations are dihydrotachysterol (Hytakerol) and calcitriol (1,25-dihydroxycholecalciferol [Rocaltrol]). These drugs are more potent, raise calcium levels rapidly, and are quickly metabolized. Rapid metabolism is desired because vitamin D is a fat-soluble vitamin and toxicity can cause irreversible renal impairment. Oral vitamin D (ergocalciferol) may also be prescribed.

NURSING MANAGEMENT: HYPOPARATHYROIDISM

■ Nursing Assessment

Nursing care of a patient with hypoparathyroidism requires close assessment for signs of tetany. The patient should be observed closely for carpopedal spasm (Trousseau's phenomenon) while blood pressures are being taken because this is an early sign of tetany. Periodic assessment for Chvostek's sign is advisable. Tingling in the fingertips and around the mouth, irritability, anxiety, apprehension, muscular hypertonicity, and cramps may precede acute tetany. It is important to note any allergy to iodine because it may be used in associated diagnostic testing, such as an intravenous pyelogram (IVP).

Nursing Diagnoses

Nursing diagnoses for the patient with hypoparathyroidism may include, but are not limited to, the following:

- Impaired skin integrity *related to* dry, scaly skin
- Activity intolerance *related to* fatigue, weakness, and painful muscle cramps
- Altered thought processes *related to* personality and psychiatric changes and memory impairment
- Ineffective management of therapeutic regimen *related to* lack of knowledge regarding signs and symptoms of calcium deficiency, calcium-rich foods and supplements, and chronic nature of the problem
- Potential complication: arrhythmia
- Potential complication: tetany

Planning

The overall goals are that the patient with hypoparathyroidism will (1) develop no complications such as tetany or arrhythmias, (2) recognize signs and symptoms of hypoparathyroidism and hyperparathyroidism, and (3) comply with periodic assessment of calcium level.

Nursing Implementation

Health Promotion. Health promotion is directed at identifying patients at risk. This includes patients who have undergone thyroid removal (thyroidectomy).

Acute Intervention. If tetany or generalized muscle cramps develop, rebreathing may partially alleviate the symptoms. The patient who can cooperate should be instructed to breathe in and out of a paper bag or breathing mask. This reduces carbon dioxide excretion from the lungs, increases carbonic acid levels in the blood, and lowers body pH. Because an acidic environment enhances both solubility and the degree of ionization of calcium, the proportion of total body calcium available in physiologically active form (i.e., ionized calcium) is increased, temporarily relieving the functional hypocalcemia.

IV calcium salts should be available at the bedside for treatment of acute tetany. Calcium salts must be infused slowly because high blood levels can cause serious cardiac arrhythmias or cardiac arrest. The patient who has been digitalized is particularly vulnerable. Because calcium-induced ventricular standstill occurs in systole, this type of arrest is less likely than other types to respond to resuscitation. ECG monitoring is indicated. Side rails should be padded as a seizure precaution. The patient should be kept in a nonstimulating environment, assisted with hygienic needs, and given support and encouragement until free of symptoms.

Ambulatory and Home Care. The patient with hypoparathyroidism needs instruction in the management of long-term nutrition and drug therapy. A high-calcium meal plan includes foods such as dark green vegetables, soy beans, and tofu. The patient should be told that foods containing oxalic acid (e.g., spinach and rhubarb), phytic acid (e.g., bran and whole grains), and phosphorus reduce calcium absorption. Calcium supplements of at least 1 g per day for the patient under 40 years of age and 2 g per day for the patient more than 40 years of age are usually prescribed. These supplements are best administered 2 to 3 hours after meals. Although calcium carbonate often leads to constipation and flatulence, bran and whole grain foods should not be used for treatment. Alternative nursing interventions include providing stool softeners, adequate fluids, and fresh fruits.

The patient should be instructed with written handouts about the signs and symptoms of hypocalcemia and hypercalcemia and to report these to a clinician as soon as possible if they occur. If manifestations of hypocalcemia occur, calcium supplementation should be increased. The need for lifelong treatment and health supervision should be stressed. The patient's calcium levels should be monitored three to four times a year. Treatment modification is often necessary because hypercalcemia can develop without apparent cause. Thorough patient instruction and frequent serum calcium assessment should allow a normal life expectancy. The patient needs support and encouragement to continue with the regimen. The patient may dislike taking so many pills.

Evaluation

The expected outcomes are that the patient with hypoparathyroidism

- experiences no complications of the disease
- states the signs and symptoms of hypoparathyroidism
- has a follow-up appointment and states the importance of periodic assessment of calcium levels

DISORDERS OF THE ADRENAL CORTEX

There are three main classifications of adrenal steroid hormones. Glucocorticoids regulate metabolism, increase blood glucose levels, and are critical in the physiologic stress response. In humans the primary glucocorticoid is cortisol. Mineralocorticoids regulate sodium and potassium balance. The primary mineralocorticoid is aldosterone. Androgens contribute to growth and development in both genders and to sexual activity in adult women. The term *corticosteroid* refers to any one of these three types of hormones produced by the adrenal cortex.

CUSHING'S SYNDROME

Etiology and Pathophysiology

Cushing's syndrome is a spectrum of clinical abnormalities caused by excess corticosteroids, particularly glucocorticoids. Several conditions can cause Cushing's syndrome (Table 47-12). The most common cause is iatrogenic administration of exogenous cortisol. Approximately 85% of endogenous Cushing's syndrome is due to an ACTH-secreting pituitary tumor (Cushing's disease). Other causes include adrenal tumors and ectopic ACTH production by tumors outside the hypothalamic-pituitary-adrenal axis (usually of the lung or pancreas). Cushing's disease and primary adrenal tumors are more common in women 20 to 40 years of age (Fig. 47-8), whereas ectopic ACTH production is more common in men.[42]

Clinical Manifestations

The clinical manifestations of Cushing's syndrome can be seen in most body systems and are related to excess levels of corti-

Table 47-12 Causes of Cushing's Syndrome

Prolonged administration of high doses of corticosteroids
ACTH-secreting pituitary tumor (Cushing's disease)
Cortisol-secreting neoplasm within the adrenal cortex that can be either carcinoma or adenoma
Excess secretion of ACTH from carcinoma of lung or other malignant growth outside pituitary or adrenals

ACTH, adrenocorticotropic hormone.

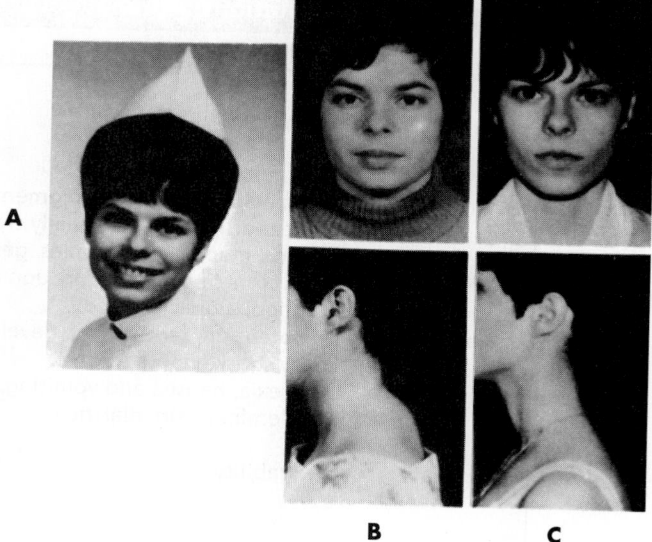

Fig. 47-8 A woman with Cushing's syndrome resulting from right adrenal cortical adenoma. **A,** Patient at age 18, 2 years before surgery. **B,** Patient at age 20, 1 month before surgery. **C,** Patient at age 21, 1 year after surgery. (From Williams GH, Dluhy RG: Diseases of the adrenal cortex. In Isselbacher K and others, eds: *Harrison's principles of internal medicine,* ed 14, New York, 1998, McGraw-Hill.)

costeroids (Table 47-13). Although manifestations of glucocorticoid excess usually predominate, symptoms of mineralocorticoid and androgen excess may also be seen.

Glucocorticoid excess causes pronounced changes in personal appearance (Fig. 47-9). These signs and symptoms logically flow from the known actions of glucocorticoids. Weight gain, the most common feature, results from the accumulation of adipose tissue in the trunk, face, and cervical area. Transient weight gain from sodium and water retention may be present because of the mineralocorticoid effects of cortisol. Glucose intolerance occurs because of cortisol-induced insulin resistance and increased gluconeogenesis by the liver.

Protein wasting is caused by the catabolic effects of cortisol on peripheral tissue. Muscle wasting leads to muscle weakness, especially in the extremities. Loss of protein matrix in bone leads to osteoporosis with subsequent pathologic fractures, vertebral compression fractures, and bone and back pain. Loss of collagen makes the skin weaker and thinner; therefore it bruises easier. Catabolic processes predominate, and wound healing is delayed. Mood disturbances (irritability, anxiety, euphoria), insomnia, irrationality, and occasionally psychosis may occur. The skin and mucous membranes may take on a bronze or brownish color because of the melanotropic activity of ACTH.

Mineralocorticoid excess may cause hypertension, whereas adrenal androgen excess may cause pronounced acne, virilization in women, and feminization in men. Menstrual disorders and hirsutism in women and gynecomastia and impotence in men are seen more commonly in adrenal carcinomas.

The clinical presentation, as revealed by the history and physical examination, is the first indication of Cushing's syndrome. Of particular importance are (1) centripedal (truncal) obesity or generalized obesity; (2) "moon facies" (fullness of the face) with facial plethora; (3) purplish-red striae, which are usually depressed below the skin surface, on the abdomen, breast, or buttocks; (4) hirsutism; (5) menstrual disorders; (6) hypertension; and (7) unexplained hypokalemia.

Diagnostic Studies

Abnormal findings include granulocytosis, lymphocytopenia, eosinopenia, hyperglycemia, glycosuria, hypercalciuria, and osteoporosis (as observed on x-rays). Hypokalemia and alkalosis are seen in ectopic ACTH syndrome and adrenal carcinoma. Plasma ACTH may be low, normal, or elevated depending on the underlying problem. High or normal levels indicate ACTH-dependent Cushing's syndrome, whereas low or undetectable levels indicate an adrenal or exogenous etiology. When Cushing's syndrome is suspected, a 24-hour urine collection for free cortisol and a low-dose dexamethasone suppression test (see Chapter 45) are done. If these results are borderline, a high-dose dexamethasone suppression test is done.[43] False-positive results can occur in depressed patients, those under acute stress, and those who are active alcoholics. Plasma cortisol (the primary glucocorticoid) levels may be elevated, with loss of diurnal variation. CT scanning and MRI may be used for tumor localization.

Collaborative Care

The treatment of choice for Cushing's disease is transsphenoidal surgical removal of the pituitary adenoma (hypophysectomy) (see earlier in this chapter). Adrenalectomy is indicated for adrenal tumors or hyperplasia. Currently transperitoneal or retroperitoneal laparoscopic surgery is performed to remove adrenal tumors less than 5 cm in size. Occasionally, bilateral adrenalectomy is necessary (Table 47-14). Patients with ectopic ACTH-secreting tumors are managed with treatment of the neoplasm.

If surgery is anticipated, the patient should be brought to optimal physical condition. Hypertension and hyperglycemia must be controlled, and hypokalemia is corrected with diet and potassium supplements. A high-protein meal plan helps correct the protein depletion. Vitamin A supplementation may be given to counteract the problem of delayed wound healing.[43]

Drug Therapy. In inoperable cases or in cases in which residual disease remains, treatment with mitotane (Lysodren) may be used. This drug suppresses cortisol production, alters peripheral metabolism of cortisol, and decreases plasma and urine corticosteroid levels. The action of this drug results in a "medical adrenalectomy." Metyrapone, ketoconazole (Nizoral),

Table 47-13 Clinical Manifestations: Adrenal Cortical Hormone Dysfunction

System	Hypofunction	Hyperfunction
Glucocorticoids		
General appearance	Weight loss	Truncal (centripedal) obesity, thin extremities, rounding of face (moon face), fat deposits on back of neck and on shoulders ("buffalo hump")
Integumentary	Bronzed or smoky hyperpigmentation of face, neck, hands (especially creases), buccal membranes, nipples, genitalia, and scars (if pituitary function normal); vitiligo, alopecia	Thin, fragile skin; purplish-red striae; petechial hemorrhages; bruises; florid cheeks (plethora); acne; poor wound healing
Cardiovascular	Hypotension, tendency to develop refractory shock, vasodilation	Hypervolemia, hypertension, edema of lower extremities
Gastrointestinal	Anorexia, nausea and vomiting, cramping abdominal pain, diarrhea	Increase in secretion of pepsin and hydrochloric acid, anorexia
Urinary		Glycosuria, hypercalciuria, kidney stones
Musculoskeletal	Fatigability	Muscle wasting in extremities, proximal muscle weakness, fatigue, osteoporosis, awkward gait, back and joint pain, weakness, growth retardation (in children)
Immune	Propensity toward autoimmune diseases	Inhibition of immune response, suppression of allergic response, inhibition of inflammation
Hematologic	Anemia, lymphocytosis	Leukocytosis, lymphopenia, polycythemia, increased coagulability
Fluids and electrolytes	Hyponatremia, hypovolemia, dehydration, hyperkalemia	Sodium and water retention, edema, hypokalemia
Metabolic	Hypoglycemia, insulin sensitivity, fever	Hyperglycemia, negative nitrogen balance, dyslipidemia
Emotional	Neurasthenia, depression, exhaustion or irritability, confusion, delusions	Psychic stimulation, euphoria, irritability, hypomania to depression, emotional lability
Mineralocorticoids		
Fluid and electrolytes	Sodium loss, decreased volume of extracellular fluid, hyperkalemia, salt craving	Marked sodium and water retention, tendency toward edema, marked hypokalemia
Cardiovascular	Hypovolemia, tendency toward shock, decreased cardiac output, decreased heart size	Hypertension, hypervolemia
Androgens		
Integumentary	Decreased axillary and pubic hair (in women)	Hirsutism, acne
Reproductive	No effect in men, decreased libido in women	Menstrual irregularities and enlargement of clitoris (in females); gynecomastia and testicular atrophy (in males)
Musculoskeletal	Decrease in muscle size and tone	Increase in muscle development

and aminoglutethimide (Cytadren) may be used to inhibit cortisol synthesis. The relatively common side effects of these agents include anorexia, nausea and vomiting, GI bleeding, depression, vertigo, skin rashes, and diplopia. The GI side effects may be minimized by administering mitotane (Lysodren) with meals and with a bedtime snack. Ketoconazole, which inhibits synthesis of gonadal and adrenal corticosteroids, may also be used. The side effects from this medication are fewer than those of other adrenal suppressants.

If Cushing's syndrome has developed during the course of prolonged administration of glucocorticoids (e.g., cortisol), one or more of the following alternatives may be tried: (1) gradual discontinuance of glucocorticoid therapy, (2) reduction of the glucocorticoid dose, and (3) conversion to an alternate-day regimen. Gradual tapering of the glucocorticoids is necessary to avoid potentially life-threatening adrenal insufficiency. An alternate-day regimen is one in which twice the daily dosage of a shorter-acting glucocorticoid is given every other morning to minimize hypothalamic-pituitary-adrenal suppression, growth suppression, and altered appearance. This regimen is not used when the corticosteroids (i.e., cortisol and aldosterone mimicking drugs) are given as physiologic replacements.

NURSING MANAGEMENT: CUSHING'S SYNDROME

■ Nursing Assessment

Subjective and objective data that should be obtained from a patient with Cushing's syndrome are presented in Table 47-15.

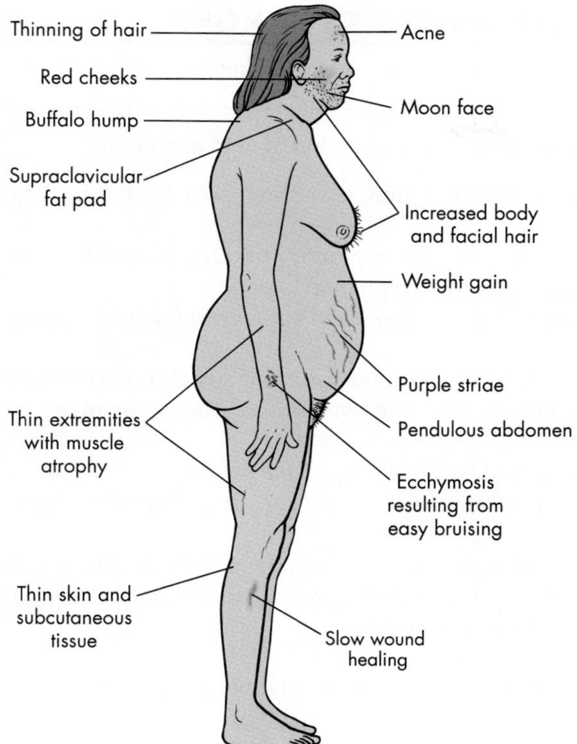

Fig. 47-9 Common characteristics of Cushing's syndrome.

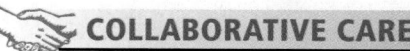

COLLABORATIVE CARE

Table 47-14 Cushing's Syndrome

Diagnostic

- History and physical examination
- Mental status examination
- Plasma cortisol levels for diurnal variations
- Plasma ACTH level
- Complete blood count
- Blood chemistries for sodium, potassium, glucose
- Dexamethasone suppression test
- 24-hour urine for free cortisol
- Examination of visual fields
- CT scan, MRI

Collaborative Therapy

- Adrenal cortical adenoma, carcinoma, or hyperplasia
  - Surgical adrenalectomy
    - Laparoscopic adrenalectomy
  - Medical adrenalectomy
- Pituitary corticotropin (ACTH) hypersecretion
  - Transsphenoidal resection of microadenoma
  - Radiation
  - Treatment with hypothalamic serotonin antagonist (cyproheptadine)
- Surgical removal of nonendocrine ACTH-producing tumors, adrenalectomy (if pituitary tumor inoperable)
- Discontinuance of or alteration in administration of exogenous corticosteroids

NURSING ASSESSMENT

Table 47-15 Cushing's Syndrome

Subjective Data

Important Health Information

Past health history: Pituitary tumor (Cushing's disease); adrenal, pancreatic, or pulmonary neoplasms; GI bleeding; frequent infections

Medications: Use of corticosteroids

Functional Health Patterns

Health perception–health management: Malaise

Nutritional-metabolic: Weight gain, anorexia

Elimination: Polyuria; prolonged wound healing, easy bruising

Activity-exercise: Weakness, fatigue

Sleep: Insomnia, poor sleep quality

Cognitive-perceptual: Headache; back, joint, bone, and rib pain; poor concentration and memory

Self-perception–self-concept: Negative feelings regarding changes in personal appearance

Sexuality-reproductive: Amenorrhea, impotence, decreased libido

Coping–stress tolerance: Anxiety, mood disturbances, emotional lability, psychosis

Objective Data

General

Truncal obesity, supraclavicular fat pads, buffalo hump, moon facies

Integumentary

Plethora; hirsutism of body and face, thinning of head hair; thin, friable skin; acne; petechiae; purpura; hyperpigmentation; purplish-red striae on breasts, buttocks, and abdomen; edema of lower extremities

Cardiovascular

Hypertension

Musculoskeletal

Muscle wasting, thin extremities, awkward gait

Reproductive

Gynecomastia, testicular atrophy (in men), enlarged clitoris (in women)

Possible Findings

Hypokalemia, hyperglycemia, dyslipidemia; polycythemia, granulocytosis, lymphocytopenia, eosinopenia; elevated plasma cortisol; high, low, or normal ACTH levels; abnormal dexamethasone suppression test; elevated urine free cortisol, 17-ketosteroids; glycosuria, hypercalciuria; osteoporosis on x-ray

47-4 NURSING CARE PLAN PATIENT WITH CUSHING'S SYNDROME

Expected Patient Outcomes	Nursing Interventions and *Rationales*
NURSING DIAGNOSIS	**Risk for infection** *related to* lowered resistance to stress and suppression of immune system.
▪ No infection. ▪ Early detection and treatment of any infectious process.	▪ Assess for inadequate protein stores, proteinuria, muscle wasting, poor wound healing *as indicators of risk for infection.* ▪ Assess potential infection sites such as urinary and respiratory tracts, skin, and IV lines *so infection can be detected early and treatment initiated promptly.* ▪ Note pain, loss of function, and purulent drainage *because other signs and symptoms of infection may be minimal or absent.* ▪ Provide private room, if possible; maintain meticulous asepsis and prevent contact with contagious individuals *to reduce the risk of cross-contamination because patient has an increased susceptibility to infection.* ▪ Instruct patient in self-care practices *to avoid infection (e.g., hand washing).* ▪ Refer patient to dietician for high-protein diet instruction *to help correct the protein depletion caused by excess glucocorticoids.* ▪ Instruct patient and family to be alert for slight changes in signs and symptoms of infection *since the usual immune and inflammatory responses are suppressed* and to report these to clinician immediately *so treatment can be initiated promptly.*
NURSING DIAGNOSIS	**Risk for injury: fracture** *related to* decreased muscle strength, fatigue, osteoporosis, and increased protein catabolism.
▪ No accidental injury.	▪ Assess for complaints of weakness, fatigue, back and rib pain; difficulty in ambulating, impairment in mobility; impairment in judgment; drowsiness; hypocalcemia *to detect injury risk factors.* ▪ Provide cane or walker as necessary *to provide patient with stabilizing device.* ▪ Keep side rails up if patient's judgment is impaired *to reduce possibility of falls.* ▪ Instruct patient in high-calcium diet *to replace lost calcium and prevent increasing the severity of osteoporosis.* ▪ Reinforce dietary instructions. Instruct patient and family in provisions of a safe environment (e.g., nonskid surfaces in wet areas, use of railings, good lighting).
NURSING DIAGNOSIS	**Altered nutrition: more than body requirements** *related to* increased appetite, high caloric content of foods, and inactivity *as manifested by* statement of increased appetite; weight greater than 10% optimum for height.
▪ Maintenance of body weight if appropriate or no more than 1-2 lb loss per week.	▪ Obtain dietary consult for instruction in low-caloric, high-nutrition diet (including protein and calcium) *because excess glucocorticoids produce weight gain and calcium and protein loss.* ▪ Assist with appropriate menu choices *to reinforce dietary instructions.* ▪ Provide low-calorie, high-vitamin snacks.
NURSING DIAGNOSIS	**Self-esteem disturbance** *related to* altered body image, emotional lability, and diminished physical capabilities *as manifested by* verbalization of negative feelings regarding personal appearance and inability to perform usual activities.
▪ Verbalization of acceptance of appearance by patient and family. ▪ Self-care methods to improve appearance.	▪ Explain to patient and family that physical and emotional changes are related to hormone imbalance and that most will disappear when hormone imbalance is corrected *to increase their understanding and assist with coping.* ▪ Accept and respect patient as a person *to maintain patient's self-worth.* ▪ Encourage good grooming and use of attractive attire *to improve patient's appearance and self-esteem.* ▪ Compliment patient when appropriate *to boost morale by providing positive feedback.*

Continued

47-4 NURSING CARE PLAN PATIENT WITH CUSHING'S SYNDROME—continued

Expected Patient Outcomes	Nursing Interventions and *Rationales*
NURSING DIAGNOSIS	**Impaired skin integrity** *related to* excess corticosteroids, immobility, and altered skin fragility *as manifested by* edema; thin, fragile skin; impaired healing.
▪ Intact skin.	▪ Assess skin *for early detection of trauma.* ▪ Protect patient from bumping and bruising *to prevent injury to easily traumatized tissue.* ▪ Change patient's position frequently *to minimize pressure over bony prominences and improve circulation in edematous tissue.* ▪ Provide good skin care, particularly to edematous areas and areas over bony prominences *because these areas have decreased circulation.*

■ Nursing Diagnoses

Nursing diagnoses for the patient with Cushing's syndrome may include, but are not limited to, those presented in the NCP 47-4.

■ Planning

The overall goals are that the patient with Cushing's syndrome will (1) experience relief of symptoms, (2) experience no serious complications, (3) maintain a positive self-image, and (4) actively participate in the therapeutic plan.

■ Nursing Implementation

Health Promotion. Health promotion is focused on identifying patients at risk for Cushing's syndrome. Patients receiving long-term, exogenous cortisol for a variety of diseases are at risk. Careful patient teaching related to the medication usage and monitoring of side effects are important preventive measures.

Acute Intervention. The patient with Cushing's syndrome is seriously ill. Because the therapeutic interventions have many side effects, the focus of daily assessment is on signs and symptoms of hormone and drug toxicity and complicating conditions such as cardiovascular disease, diabetes mellitus, infection, nephrolithiasis, and pathologic fractures. Daily nursing assessment includes the following:

1. Vital signs every 4 hours, particularly blood pressure
2. Daily weights (gain possibly indicates volume excess)
3. Signs and symptoms of infection, especially pain, loss of function, and purulent drainage, because other signs and symptoms of inflammation such as fever and redness may be minimal or absent
4. Location, time, and duration of abdominal pain
5. Signs and symptoms of abnormal thromboembolic phenomena, such as sudden chest pain, dyspnea, or tachypnea
6. Capillary blood glucose monitoring
7. Bone pain or limitations of range of motion, especially in the lower back
8. Changes in mental status, particularly depression

The patient needs a great deal of emotional support. Changes in appearance such as centripedal obesity, multiple bruises, hirsutism in women, and gynecomastia in men can be distressing. The patient may feel unattractive, repulsive, or unwanted. A survey of patients with Cushing's syndrome showed that 71% reported that their lives had been very adversely affected by this condition.[44] The nurse can help by remaining sensitive to patients' feelings and offering respect and unconditional acceptance.[45] The patient can be reassured that the physical changes and much of the emotional lability are related to side effects of drug therapy and will resolve when hormone levels return to normal.

If treatment involves surgical removal of a pituitary adenoma, an adrenal tumor, or one or both adrenal glands, nursing care will have an additional focus on preoperative and postoperative care. Before surgery the patient should be brought to optimal physical condition. Hypertension and hyperglycemia must be controlled, and hypokalemia is corrected with diet and potassium supplements. A high-protein meal plan helps correct the protein depletion. Surgery on glandular structures poses risks beyond those of other types of operations. Because glands are highly vascular, the risk of hemorrhage is increased. Manipulation of glandular tissue during surgery may release large amounts of hormone into the circulation, producing marked fluctuations in the metabolic processes affected by these hormones.

Preoperative teaching for an adrenalectomy should include information that intermittent pneumatic leg compression may be used to prevent venous thrombosis.[43] In addition, teaching should include that IV infusion and nasogastric suctioning are likely after surgery. Information and instruction about exercises, coughing, and deep breathing are particularly important because patients are prone to thrombosis and infection. If an open surgical approach is used, an upper abdominal incision will be made, increasing the difficulty of coughing and deep breathing. Except for the patient with adrenal cancer or a tumor larger than 5 cm, a laparoscopic adrenalectomy may be performed. This procedure is done via a transperitoneal or retroperitoneal approach. Because this procedure is associated with a faster and less complicated recovery, its use is increasing.[46]

Postoperatively, blood pressure, fluid balance, and electrolyte levels tend to be unstable because of hormone fluctuations. High doses of glucocorticoids (e.g., cortisone) are administered IV during surgery and for several days afterward to ensure adequate responses to the stress of the procedure. If large amounts of endogenous hormone have been released into the systemic circulation during surgery, the patient is likely to develop hypertension, increasing the risk of hemorrhage. High levels of glucocorticoids also increase susceptibility to infection and delay healing.

Any rapid or significant changes in blood pressure, respirations, or heart rate should be reported. Fluid intake and output should be monitored carefully and assessed for potential imbalance. The critical period for circulatory instability ranges from 24 to 48 hours after surgery. IV glucocorticoids are given, and the dose and rate of flow are adjusted to the patient's clinical manifestations and fluid and electrolyte balance. Oral doses are given as tolerated. The IV line may be kept in place after IV glucocorticoids are withdrawn to keep a line open for quick administration of glucocorticoids or vasopressors. Morning urine levels of cortisol (obtained at the same time each morning) are measured to evaluate the effectiveness of the surgery.

If glucocorticoid dosage is tapered too rapidly after surgery, acute adrenal insufficiency may develop. Vomiting after the nasogastric tube is removed, increased weakness, dehydration, and hypotension may indicate hypocortisolism. In addition, the patient may complain of painful joints, pruritus, or peeling skin and may experience severe emotional disturbances. These signs and symptoms should be reported so that drug doses can be adjusted. The nurse must constantly be alert for signs of glucocorticoid imbalance. After surgery the patient is usually maintained on bed rest until the blood pressure stabilizes. The nurse must be alert for subtle signs of postoperative infections because the usual immune and inflammatory responses are suppressed. Meticulous care must be used when changing the dressing and during any other procedures that necessitate access to body cavities, circulation, or areas under the skin so that infection is prevented.

Ambulatory and Home Care. The discharge instructions are based on the patient's lack of endogenous corticosteroids and resulting inability to react to stressors physiologically. Patients should wear Medic Alert bracelets at all times and carry medical identification and instructions in a wallet or purse. Exposure to extremes of temperature, infections, and emotional disturbances should be avoided as much as possible. Stress may produce or precipitate acute adrenal insufficiency because the remaining adrenal tissue cannot meet an increased hormonal demand. Many patients can be taught to adjust their corticosteroid replacement therapy in accordance with their stress levels. The nurse should consult with each patient's physician to determine the parameters for dosage changes if this plan is feasible. If the patient cannot adjust his or her own medication or if weakness, fainting, fever, or nausea and vomiting occur, the patient should contact the clinician for a possible adjustment in corticosteroid dosage. Lifetime replacement therapy is required by many patients, but it may take several months to adjust the hormone dose satisfactorily, and patients should be prepared for this.

■ Evaluation

Expected outcomes for the patient with Cushing's syndrome are addressed in NCP 47-4.

ADRENOCORTICAL INSUFFICIENCY/ADDISON'S DISEASE

Etiology and Pathophysiology

Adrenocortical insufficiency (hypofunction of the adrenal cortex) may be primary (Addison's disease) or secondary, from a lack of pituitary ACTH. In Addison's disease, all three classes of adrenal corticosteroids (glucocorticoids, mineralocorticoids, and androgens) are reduced. In secondary adrenocortical insufficiency, corticosteroids and androgens are deficient but mineralocorticoids rarely are. ACTH deficiency may be caused by pituitary disease or suppression of the hypothalamic-pituitary axis as a result of the administration of exogenous glucocorticoids.[47]

In the United States, the most common cause of primary Addison's disease (which is a rare condition) is autoimmune. Adrenal tissue is destroyed by antibodies against the patient's own adrenal cortex. Often, other endocrine conditions are present and Addison's disease is considered a component of polyendocrine deficiency syndrome. Tuberculosis can cause Addison's disease, but this is now rare in areas in which tuberculosis is controlled. Less common causes include infarction, fungal infections (e.g., histoplasmosis), AIDS, and metastatic cancer. Iatrogenic Addison's disease may be due to adrenal hemorrhage, often related to anticoagulant therapy, antineoplastic chemotherapy, ketoconazole (Nizoral) therapy for AIDS, or bilateral adrenalectomy.

Clinical Manifestations

Progressive weakness, fatigue, weight loss, and anorexia are primary features. Skin hyperpigmentation, a striking feature, is seen primarily in sun-exposed areas of the body, at pressure points, over joints, and in creases, especially palmar creases. It is most likely due to increased secretion of melanocyte stimulating hormone and ACTH. These tropic hormones are increased because of low glucocorticoid levels. Other frequent manifestations are hypotension, hyponatremia, hyperkalemia, nausea and vomiting, and diarrhea. The most dangerous feature of Addison's disease is hypotension, which may cause shock, especially during stress. Circulatory collapse from this cause is unresponsive to the usual treatment (vasopressors and fluid replacement) and requires glucocorticoid administration to reverse the hypotension.

Patients with secondary adrenocortical hypofunction may have many signs and symptoms in common with patients with Addison's disease but are characteristically not hyperpigmented because ACTH and related peptide levels are low. When severe dehydration, hyponatremia, and hyperkalemia are present, a diagnosis of primary adrenocortical insufficiency is favored because of the severe mineralocorticoid insufficiency associated with this disorder.

Complications

Patients with adrenocortical insufficiency are at risk for acute adrenal insufficiency (Addisonian crisis), which is a life-threatening emergency caused by insufficient adrenocortical hormones or a sudden sharp decrease in these hormones. It may occur during stress (e.g., from infection, surgery, trauma, hemorrhage, or psychologic distress); following sudden withdrawal of corticosteroid hormone replacement therapy (which

COLLABORATIVE CARE

Table 47-16 Addison's Disease

Diagnostic
History and physical examination
Plasma cortisol levels
Serum electrolytes
ACTH-stimulation test
Tuberculin test
CT scan, MRI
Collaborative Therapy
Daily glucocorticoid replacement (two thirds on awakening in morning, one third in late afternoon)*
Daily mineralocorticoid in morning*
Salt additives for excess heat or humidity

*For conditions of normal daily stress in individuals with usual daytime activity.

PATIENT TEACHING GUIDE

Table 47-17 Addison's Disease

1. Names and dosages of drugs
2. Actions of drugs
3. Symptoms of overdosage and underdosage
4. Conditions requiring increased medication (e.g., trauma, infection, surgery, emotional crisis)
5. Course of action to take relative to changes in medication
   - Increase in dose of corticosteroid
   - Administration of large dose of corticosteroid IM—including demonstration and return demonstration
   - Consultation with clinician
6. Prevention of infection and need for prompt and vigorous treatment of existing infections
7. Need for lifelong replacement therapy
8. Need for lifelong medical supervision
9. Need for medical identification device

is often done by a patient who lacks knowledge of the importance of replacement therapy); after adrenal surgery; or following sudden pituitary gland destruction (pituitary apoplexy).

Severe manifestations of glucocorticoid and mineralocorticoid deficiencies are exhibited, including hypotension (particularly postural), tachycardia, dehydration, hyponatremia, hyperkalemia, hypoglycemia, fever, weakness, and confusion. GI manifestations include nausea, vomiting, diarrhea, and vague abdominal pain.

Diagnostic Studies

In addition to clinical features, a diagnosis of Addison's disease can be made when cortisol levels are subnormal or fail to rise over basal levels with an ACTH stimulation test. Other abnormal laboratory findings include hyperkalemia, hypochloremia, hyponatremia, hypoglycemia, anemia, and increased blood urea nitrogen levels. Urine levels of free cortisol are low. A failure of cortisol levels to rise in response to ACTH stimulation indicates primary adrenal disease. A positive response to ACTH stimulation indicates a functioning adrenal gland and points to probable pituitary disease (see Chapter 45). An ECG may show low voltage and a vertical QRS axis. In addition, peaked T waves caused by hypokalemia may be evident.[42] CT scans and MRI are used to localize tumors or identify adrenal calcifications or enlargement (Table 47-16).

Collaborative Care

Treatment of adrenocortical insufficiency is focused on management of the underlying cause when possible. The mainstay of treatment for adrenocortical insufficiency is replacement therapy with glucocorticoids and mineralocorticoids. Hydrocortisone, the most commonly used form of replacement therapy, also has mineralocorticoid properties (Table 47-17). Management of Addisonian crisis requires immediate glucocorticoid replacement therapy. Treatment must be vigorous and directed toward shock management. IV hydrocortisone 100 mg every 6 hours, sodium, fluids, and dextrose (for hypoglycemia) are necessary for 24 hours or until blood pressure returns to normal.[48]

NURSING MANAGEMENT: ADDISON'S DISEASE

Nursing Assessment

Nursing assessment related to the patient with Addison's disease includes assessment of subjective data such as weight loss, hyperpigmentation, loss of body hair, anorexia, salt craving, nausea and vomiting, cramping abdominal pain, and diarrhea. Patients may also complain of exhaustion, profound weakness, inability to perform usual activities, muscle aches, light-headedness, lack of interest in usual activities and relationships, confusion, inability to tolerate any stress, decreased libido, and amenorrhea.

Objective data noted during the physical examination include emaciation, pale skin (but bronzed in sun-exposed areas, scars, buccal mucosa, and genitalia), and sparse body hair (particularly axillary and genital). Irritability, confusion, disorientation, or depression may also be noted. Skin tenting (delayed return of skin to flat position after pinching) may be observed with poor skin turgor. Hypotension (particularly postural), decreased cardiac output and heart size, muscle wasting, and weakness may also be present. Laboratory values may indicate hyponatremia, hyperkalemia, hypoglycemia, low serum cortisol, increased serum ACTH, decreased 24-hour urine free cortisol, and lack of response to an ACTH stimulation test (see Table 45-7).

Nursing Diagnoses

Nursing diagnoses for the patient with Addison's disease may include, but are not limited to, the following:

- Activity intolerance *related to* weakness and hypotension
- Self-care deficits *related to* weakness, lack of interest, and depression
- Altered nutrition: less than body requirements *related to* weakness, anorexia, and nausea and vomiting
- Self-esteem disturbance *related to* inability to perform usual activities, loss of hair, skin hyperpigmentation, and diagnosis of chronic illness

- Altered health maintenance *related to* lack of knowledge of management of lifelong hormone replacement therapy
- Decreased cardiac output *related to* hypotension and volume depletion
- Altered sexuality patterns *related to* weakness, malaise, depression, and changing self-concept
- Potential complication: hypotension

Planning

The overall goals are that the patient with Addison's disease will (1) manage self-care activities, (2) experience relief of symptoms, (3) learn to adjust medication dosage to life situations, (4) avoid acute adrenocortical insufficiency, and (5) actively participate in long-term therapeutic plan.

Nursing Implementation

Acute Intervention. When the patient with Addison's disease is hospitalized, whether for diagnosis, an acute crisis, or some other health problem, frequent nursing assessment is necessary. Vital signs and signs of fluid volume deficit and electrolyte imbalance should be assessed every 30 minutes to 4 hours for the first 24 hours depending on the patient's instability. In addition, the following nursing assessments and orders should be included: daily weights, diligent corticosteroid administration, protection against exposure to infection (reverse isolation), and complete assistance with daily hygiene. The patient should be protected from noise, light, and environmental temperature extremes. The patient cannot cope with these stresses because she or he cannot produce corticosteroids, in particular glucocorticoids.

If the hospitalization was due to adrenal crises, the patient usually responds by the second day and can start oral corticosteroid replacement. Because discharge frequently occurs before the usual maintenance dose of corticosteroids is reached, the patient should be instructed on the importance of keeping scheduled follow-up appointments.

Ambulatory and Home Care. The nurse has an important role in the long-term management of Addison's disease. Because of the serious nature of the disease and the need for lifelong replacement therapy, a well-organized and carefully presented teaching plan is vital to the health of the patient. Table 47-18 outlines the major areas that must be included in the teaching plan.

Glucocorticoids are usually given in divided doses, two thirds in the morning and one third in the afternoon. Mineralocorticoids are given once daily, usually in the morning. This dosage schedule reflects normal circadian rhythm in endogenous hormone secretion and decreases the side effects associated with steroid replacement therapy. A hormone-deficit patient receiving glucocorticoid replacement is less apt to exhibit harmful symptoms from the medication than a patient receiving pharmacologic doses of these drugs. Because the aim of replacement therapy is to return to normal hormone levels, nursing care is designed to help the patient maintain hormone balance and manage the medication regimen. Glucocorticoids are stimulating to the CNS and thus may cause insomnia if taken late in the evening.

Because the patient with Addison's disease is unable to tolerate physical or emotional stress, without additional exogenous corticosteroids, long-term care revolves around recognizing the need for extra medication and techniques for stress management. The need for glucocorticoid hormone is proportional to stress levels. A patient who cannot produce endogenous hormone must adjust the dose of exogenous hormone to the stress level. Examples of situations requiring glucocorticoid adjustment are fever, influenza, extraction of teeth, and rigorous physical activity, such as playing tennis on a hot day or running a marathon. Doses are usually doubled when minor stress occurs (e.g., a respiratory infection or dental work) and tripled when major stress occurs. When in doubt, it is better to err on the side of overreplacement. If vomiting or diarrhea occurs, as

DRUG THERAPY

Table 47-18 Use of Corticosteroids

Hormone Replacement

Adrenal insufficiency
Congenital adrenal hyperplasia

Therapeutic Effect

- Allergic reactions
  - Anaphylaxis
  - Bee stings
  - Contact dermatitis
  - Drug reactions
  - Serum sickness
  - Urticaria
- Collagen diseases
  - Giant cell arteritis
  - Mixed connective tissue disorders
  - Polymyositis
  - Polyarteritis nodosa
  - Systemic lupus erythematosus
- Eye disease
  - Inflammation
- Gastrointestinal diseases
  - Inflammatory bowel disease
  - Nontropical sprue
- Hypercalcemia
  - Thyroid storm
- Endocrine diseases
  - Hypercalcemia
  - Hashimoto's thyroiditis
  - Thyroid storm
- Immunosuppression (after organ transplantation)
- Liver diseases
  - Alcoholic hepatitis
  - Autoimmune hepatitis
- Nephrotic syndrome
- Neurologic disease
  - Prevention of cerebral edema and increased intracranial pressure
  - Malignancies, leukemia, lymphoma
  - Head trauma
- Pulmonary diseases
  - Aspiration pneumonia
  - Asthma
  - Chronic obstructive pulmonary disease
- Rheumatoid arthritis
- Skin diseases

may happen with influenza, the clinician must be notified immediately because electrolyte replacement may be necessary. In addition, these symptoms may be early indicators of crisis. Overall, however, patients who take their medications consistently can anticipate a normal life expectancy.

Patients must be taught the signs and symptoms of glucocorticoid deficiency and excess and to report to their clinicians so that dosages can be adjusted to each patient's need. It is critical that the patient wear an identification bracelet and carry a wallet card stating that the patient has Addison's disease so that appropriate therapy can be initiated in case of an unexpected trauma, accident, or crisis. The patient should be instructed in and given handouts related to other medications that cause a need to increase glucocorticoid dosage (e.g., phenytoin [Dilantin], barbiturates, rifampin [Rifadin], and antacids).[43] Estrogen inhibits steroid metabolism. Patients using mineralocorticoid therapy should be instructed how to take their blood pressure and given parameters to report to their clinicians, because untoward changes may indicate a need for dosage adjustment.

The patient should carry an emergency kit at all times. The kit should consist of 100 mg of IM hydrocortisone, syringes, and instructions for use. The patient and significant others should be instructed in how to give an IM injection in case the replacement therapy cannot be taken orally. The patient should verbalize instructions, practice IM injections with saline, and have written instructions as to when to alter the dose.[49]

■ Evaluation

The expected outcomes are that the patient with adrenal insufficiency

- is able to manage self-care activities
- experiences relief of symptoms
- states and demonstrates how to adjust medication doses for potential stressors
- states how to avoid acute adrenal insufficiency
- states the importance of lifelong follow-up medical care and has an appointment for follow-up

DRUG THERAPY

Table 47-19 Side Effects of Corticosteroids

- Susceptibility to infection is increased. Infection develops more rapidly and spreads more widely in the cushingoid individual.
- Blood pressure is increased because of excess blood volume and potentiation of vasoconstrictor effects. Hypertension in turn predisposes patient to cardiac failure.
- Glucose intolerance affects more than 90% of individuals with cushingoid patterns.
- Protein depletion decreases bone formation, density, and strength and predisposes patient to pathologic fractures, especially compression fractures of the vertebrae (osteoporosis).
- Hypocalcemia related to anti–vitamin D effect may occur.
- Decreased mucus production predisposes patient to stomach and duodenal ulceration (peptic ulcer).
- Patients undergoing surgery are at increased risk for dehiscence and evisceration. Healing is delayed.
- Hypokalemia may develop, and potassium supplements may be indicated.
- Skeletal muscle atrophy occurs, and muscle weakness predisposes patient to accidental injury.
- Suppression of pituitary ACTH synthesis occurs. Glucocorticoid deficiency is likely if hormones are withdrawn abruptly.
- Mood and behavior changes (feelings of invulnerability and depression) may be observed.
- Fat from extremities is redistributed to trunk and face.

CORTICOSTEROID THERAPY

Cortisol and related glucocorticoids are used to relieve the signs and symptoms associated with many diseases (see Table 47-18). The long-term administration of glucocorticoids in therapeutic doses often leads to serious complications and side effects (Table 47-19). Therefore glucocorticoid therapy is not recommended for minor chronic conditions. Rather, therapy should be reserved for diseases in which there is a risk of death or permanent loss of function and conditions in which short-term therapy is likely to produce remission or recovery. The potential benefits of treatment must always be weighed against the risks.

Effects of Corticosteroid Therapy

The therapeutic actions of glucocorticoids include the following:

1. *Antiinflammatory action.* Glucocorticoids decrease the number of circulating lymphocytes, monocytes and macrophages, and eosinophils. They enhance the release of polymorphonuclear leukocytes from bone marrow, inhibit the accumulation of leukocytes at the site of inflammation, and inhibit the release of substances involved in the inflammatory response (e.g., kinins, prostaglandins, and histamine) from the leukocytes. Therefore manifestations of inflammation, including redness, tenderness, heat, swelling, and local edema, are suppressed.
2. *Immunosuppression.* Glucocorticoids cause atrophy of lymphoid tissue, suppress cell-mediated immune responses, and decrease production of antibodies.
3. *Maintenance of normal blood pressure.* Glucocorticoids potentiate the vasoconstrictor effect of norepinephrine and act on the renal tubules to increase sodium reabsorption and enhance potassium and hydrogen excretion. Retention of sodium (and subsequently water) increases blood volume and helps maintain blood pressure. Mineralocorticoids have a direct effect on sodium reabsorption in the distal tubule of the kidney and as a result increase sodium and water retention.
4. *Carbohydrate and protein metabolic effects.* Glucocorticoids antagonize the effects of insulin and can induce glucose intolerance by increasing hepatic glycogenolysis and insulin resistance. They also stimulate the breakdown of protein for gluconeogenesis, which can lead to skeletal muscle wasting. Although glucocorticoids mobilize free fatty acids and redistribute fat in cushingoid patterns, the mechanism for this process is unknown. Glucocorticoids also decrease the conversion of T_4 to T_3.[50]

Complications of Corticosteroid Therapy

Beneficial and harmful effects of the corticosteroids relate to their physiologic actions. A beneficial effect in one situation may be a harmful one in another. For example, the vasopressive effect of the hormone is critical in enabling the organism to function in stressful situations but can produce hypertension when the substance is used for drug therapy. Inhibition of cell division is therapeutic and sometimes curative in the treatment of malignancies, but it slows healing after trauma or surgery. Suppression of inflammation and the immune response may help save the life of the victim of anaphylaxis and the transplant recipient, but it causes reactivation of latent tuberculosis and greatly reduces resistance to other infections. In addition, glucocorticoids inhibit the antibody response to vaccines. Specific side effects related to corticosteroid therapy are listed in Table 47-19.

NURSING AND COLLABORATIVE MANAGEMENT: CORTICOSTEROID THERAPY

Many patients receive corticosteroid therapy, in particular glucocorticoid therapy, for nonendocrine reasons (see Table 47-18), and thorough instruction is necessary to ensure patient cooperation. Corticosteroids are taken once daily or once every other day. They should be taken early in the morning with food to decrease gastric irritation. Because exogenous corticosteroid administration may suppress endogenous ACTH and therefore endogenous cortisol (suppression is time and dose dependent), the danger of abrupt cessation of corticosteroid therapy must be emphasized to patients and significant others.

Because patients often receive corticosteroid treatment for prolonged periods of time (more than 3 months), glucocorticoid-induced osteoporosis is an important concern. Therapies to reduce the resorption of bone may include increased calcium intake, vitamin D supplementation, biphosphonates, and institution of a low-impact exercise program. Further instruction and interventions to minimize the side effects and complications of corticosteroid therapy are shown in Table 47-20.

PATIENT TEACHING GUIDE

Table 47-20 Corticosteroid Therapy

1. Provide a diet plan high in protein, calcium (at least 1500 mg per day), and potassium but low in fat and concentrated simple carbohydrates such as sugar, honey, syrups, and candy.
2. Identify measures to ensure adequate rest and sleep, such as daily naps and avoidance of caffeine late in the day.
3. Develop and maintain an exercise program to help maintain bone integrity.
4. Instruct on how to recognize edema and ways to restrict sodium intake to less than 2000 mg per day if edema occurs.
5. Monitor glucose levels, symptoms and signs of hyperglycemia (e.g., polydipsia, polyuria, blurred vision), and glycosuria (glucose in the urine). Need to report hyperglycemic symptoms or capillary glucose levels greater than 180 mg/dl (10 mmol/L) or urine positive for glucose.
6. Notify a clinician if experiencing postprandial heartburn or epigastric pain that is not relieved by antacids.
7. See an eye specialist yearly to assess for possible cataracts.
8. Get up slowly from bed or a chair, and use good lighting to avoid accidental injury.
9. Maintain good hygiene practices. Avoid contact with persons with colds or other contagious illnesses to avoid infection.

PRIMARY HYPERALDOSTERONISM

Etiology and Pathophysiology

Primary hyperaldosteronism (aldosteronism, Conn's syndrome) is characterized by excessive aldosterone secretion caused by an adenoma of the adrenal zona glomerulosa or bilateral adrenal hyperplasia. This disorder is seen in approximately 2.0% of patients with hypertension.[51] It is more common in women, and the usual age of diagnosis is between 20 and 40 years.[47] The main effects of aldosterone are sodium retention and potassium and hydrogen ion excretion. Thus the hallmark of this disease is hypertension with hypokalemic alkalosis.

Clinical Manifestations

The sodium retention leads to hypernatremia, hypertension, and headache. Edema does not usually occur because the rate of sodium excretion is reset, which prevents more severe sodium retention. However, there is an increased loss of potassium. The potassium wasting leads to hypokalemia, which causes generalized muscle weakness, tiredness, cardiac arrhythmias, glucose intolerance, and metabolic alkalosis that may lead to tetany.[51]

Diagnostic Studies

The diagnosis of hyperaldosteronism should be suspected in all patients with hypokalemia and hypertension who are not being treated with diuretics. Diagnostic tests show increased plasma aldosterone and serum sodium levels and decreased serum potassium levels. An IV saline infusion test is often performed. In this test, 2 L of normal saline is infused over 4 hours, with plasma aldosterone levels measured at the beginning and end of the infusion. If aldosterone fails to suppress (i.e., is <10 ng/dl [277 pmol/L]), the patient probably has hyperaldosteronism. Adenomas are localized by means of a CT scan. If a tumor is not found, plasma 18-hydroxycorticosterone is measured after overnight bed rest. A level greater than 50 ng/dl (1387 pmol/L) indicates an adenoma.

NURSING AND COLLABORATIVE MANAGEMENT: PRIMARY HYPERALDOSTERONISM

The treatment for adenoma is unilateral adrenalectomy. Before surgery, patients should be treated with a low-sodium diet, potassium-sparing diuretics, and antihypertensive agents to control serum potassium levels and blood pressure. Spironolactone (Aldactone) binds to the mineralocorticoid receptor in the terminal distal tubules and collecting ducts of the kidney and increases excretion of sodium and water and retention of potassium.[52] Oral potassium supplements and sodium restrictions are also necessary. Potassium supplementation and a potassium-sparing diuretic should not be started simultaneously because of the danger of hyperkalemia. Patients with bilateral hyperplasia are treated with spironolactone (Aldactone); amiloride (Midamor), another potassium-sparing diuretic; or aminoglutethimide (Cytadren), which blocks aldosterone synthesis. Calcium channel blockers may also be used.[51]

Nursing care includes careful assessment for signs of hypokalemia, tetany (Chvostek's sign, Trousseau's sign), fluid and electrolyte balance, and cardiovascular status. Blood pressure should be monitored frequently before and after surgery because unilateral adrenalectomy is successful in controlling hypertension in only 50% of patients with adenoma.

Patients receiving maintenance therapy with spironolactone (Aldactone) or amiloride need instruction about the possible side effects of gynecomastia, impotence, and menstrual disorders, as well as knowledge about the signs and symptoms of hypokalemia and hyperkalemia. Patients should be taught how to monitor their own blood pressure and the need for frequent monitoring. The need for continued health supervision should be stressed.

SECONDARY HYPERALDOSTERONISM

Secondary hyperaldosteronism occurs in response to an extra-adrenal stimulus (often angiotensin), renal artery stenosis, or juxtaglomerular cell tumors. If treatment of the primary disorder is not possible, angiotensin-converting enzyme inhibitors are useful in inhibiting the powerful mineralocorticoid.

CONGENITAL ADRENAL HYPERPLASIA SYNDROMES

The adrenal glands normally produce small amounts of androgens. Overproduction of these hormones can be caused by adrenogenital syndromes. Causes of these syndromes are congenital enzymatic deficiencies leading to hypocortisolism. The hypocortisolism causes increased ACTH secretion, which overstimulates the adrenals and causes hypertrophy and excess androgen production. The onset of symptoms may occur from birth to early adult life and depends on the enzymes affected. In some deficiencies, males show precocious sexual development, whereas in others, sexual development may fail to occur. Females can show signs of masculinization and menstrual irregularities.

DISORDERS OF THE ADRENAL MEDULLA

PHEOCHROMOCYTOMA

Etiology and Pathophysiology

Disorders of the adrenal medulla are uncommon. Defects in norepinephrine release in autonomic nervous system failure may be associated with orthostatic hypotension, and defective adrenal epinephrine secretion and pancreatic glucagon secretion may affect the recovery from hypoglycemia in persons with diabetes mellitus.[53] However, the most common of these rare disorders of the adrenal medulla is pheochromocytoma, a neoplasm that produces excessive catecholamines. Most of these tumors (95%) are benign and encapsulated. Pheochromocytoma can occur at any age and in either gender, but it is found most commonly in patients between 30 and 50 years of age.[54]

Clinical Manifestations

The most striking clinical features of pheochromocytoma are severe, episodic hypertension accompanied by the classic triad of severe, pounding headache, tachycardia, and profuse sweating. Attacks of episodic hypertension are due to sympathetic nervous system stimulation usually from norepinephrine and are often accompanied by anxiety and palpitations. Attacks may be provoked by many medications, including antihypertensives, opiates, radiographic contrast media, and tricyclic antidepressants.[54] The duration of the attacks may vary from a few minutes to several hours. Untreated, pheochromocytoma may lead to diabetes mellitus, cadiomyopathy, and manifestations of uncontrolled hypertension and death.

Diagnostic Studies

Measurement of urinary metanephrines (catecholamine metabolites) is the simplest and most reliable test. Values are elevated in at least 90% of persons with pheochromocytoma. Vanillylmandelic acid (VMA) may also be measured in a 24-hour urine sample. However, this test has more false-negative results than urine metanephrines.[53] Plasma catecholamines are also elevated. It is preferable to measure catecholamines during an attack. CT scans and MRI are used for tumor localization.

Collaborative Care

Treatment consists of surgical removal of the tumor. Surgery may be done via laparoscopic adrenalectomy or by open abdominal incision. Regardless of the approach, this is one of the few conditions in which dangerously high blood pressure may be corrected surgically. Before surgery the patient is hospitalized for treatment to correct hypovolemia and cardiovascular complications to decrease the risk of surgery. Complete removal of the tumor cures the hypertension in the majority of individuals. In the others, hypertension persists or returns but is usually well controlled by standard therapy.

Preoperatively, sympathetic blocking agents (e.g., phenoxybenzamine [Dibenzyline], prazosin [Minipress], terazosin [Hytrin], or doxazosin [Cardura]) are administered to reduce the blood pressure and alleviate other symptoms of catecholamine excess. Because this management may result in orthostatic hypotension, the patient must be advised to make postural changes cautiously. Calcium channel blockers may be used to treat the hypertension and avoid the orthostatic hypotension in patients with cardiovascular disease. If surgery is not an option, metyrosine (Demser) is used to diminish catecholamine production by the tumor and simplify chronic management.

NURSING MANAGEMENT: PHEOCHROMOCYTOMA

■ Nursing Assessment

Case finding is an important nursing function. Any patient with hypertension accompanied by symptoms of sympathoadrenal discharge should be referred to a physician for definitive diagnosis. An important part of the nursing assessment is observation of the patient for the classic triad of symptoms of pheochromocytoma; severe, pounding headache; tachycardia; and profuse sweating. Blood pressure should be monitored immediately if the patient is experiencing an attack. The nurse should be prepared to check blood pressure when any of the drugs that might precipitate an attack are given.

■ Nursing Diagnoses

Nursing diagnosis for the patient with pheochromocytoma may include, but are not limited to, the following:

- Decreased cardiac output *related to* variations in blood pressure
- Sleep pattern disturbance *related to* interrupted sleep
- Body image disturbance *related to* anxiety caused by catecholamine surges.

■ Planning

The goals are that the patient with pheochromocytoma will (1) experience relief of symptoms, (2) experience no serious complications, and (3) maintain a positive self-image.

■ Nursing Implementation

The nurse should attempt to make the patient with pheochromocytoma as comfortable as possible. All diagnostic samples should be collected appropriately. Capillary blood glucose levels should be monitored to assess for diabetes mellitus. Patients should be monitored closely if any medications are used that may precipitate an attack. Patients need rest, nourishing food, and emotional support during this period. Preoperative and postoperative care is similar to that for any patient undergoing adrenalectomy except that blood pressure fluctuations from catecholamine imbalances tend to be severe and must be carefully monitored. In addition, blood may be transfused preoperatively to reduce postoperative hypotension.[55]

Since the hypertension may persist, even when the tumor is removed, the nurse should stress the importance of follow-up care and routine blood pressure monitoring. If metyrosine is being used, the patient should be instructed to rise slowly and hold onto a secure object, because this medication can cause orthostatic hypotension.

■ Evaluation

The expected outcomes are that the patient with pheochromocytoma

- experiences relief of symptoms
- does not experience any complications
- maintains a positive self-image

CRITICAL THINKING EXERCISES

CASE STUDY

Graves' Disease

Patient Profile

Sally C., a 43-year-old woman, was admitted to the hospital with a high fever. Following an endocrine workup, she was diagnosed as having Graves' disease.

Subjective Data

- Reports recent job loss because of inability to cope with job stress
- Reports symptoms that include fatigue, unintentional weight loss, insomnia, palpitations, and heat intolerance

Objective Data

Physical Examination

- Has a fever of 105° F (40.6° C)
- Has blood pressure of 150/78, pulse of 118, and respiratory rate of 24
- Has hot, moist skin
- Has fine tremors of the hands
- Has 4+ deep tendon reflexes and muscle strength of 1 to 2

Collaborative Care

- Subtotal thyroidectomy planned for 2 months later
- Started on propylthiouracil and propranolol

Critical Thinking Questions

1. What is the etiology of the patient's symptoms?
2. What diagnostic studies were probably ordered? What would the results have been to establish the diagnosis of Graves' disease?
3. Why was surgery delayed?
4. What was the purpose of the pharmacologic intervention?
5. What are the patient's immediate learning needs and her learning needs preoperatively and postoperatively?
6. What are the nursing interventions for successful long-term management of this patient after the subtotal thyroidectomy?
7. Based on the assessment data presented, write one or more appropriate nursing diagnoses pertinent to this patient while hospitalized. Are there any collaborative problems?

NURSING RESEARCH ISSUES

1. Is sucking on hard candy or ice chips more effective in decreasing the subjective sensation of thirst in patients with SIADH?
2. Do patients with hyperthyroidism sleep better in a private hospital room than in a hospital room shared with another patient?
3. What is the difference in the mental status of hypothyroid patients before and after thyroid replacement therapy?
4. What are the presenting symptoms of infection in patients with Cushing's syndrome?
5. Is a nurse-directed dosage adjustment more effective in preventing symptoms in the patient lacking endogenous cortisol who is exposed to stress than a patient-directed dosage adjustment?
6. Does regular exercise prevent bone loss in patients receiving glucocorticoid therapy?

REVIEW QUESTIONS

The number of the question corresponds to the same-numbered objective at the beginning of the chapter.

1. Following a hypophysectomy for treatment of acromegaly a patient develops hypopituitarism. The nurse teaches the patient that
   a. hormone replacement with ACTH, TSH, FSH, and LH will be necessary.
   b. permanent ADH replacement will be needed if the postoperative diabetes insipidus does not reverse.
   c. frequent monitoring of blood and urine glucose is needed to identify the development of diabetes mellitus.
   d. the elimination of the source of excess growth hormone will reverse the physiologic effects of acromegaly.
2. A patient with a head injury develops SIADH. Symptoms the nurse would expect to find include
   a. edema.
   b. weight gain.
   c. serum sodium of 140 mEq/L (140 mmol/L).
   d. urine specific gravity of 1.004.
3. The physician prescribes levothyroxin for a patient with myxedema. Following teaching regarding this therapy the nurse determines that further instruction is needed when the patient says,
   a. "I can expect to return to normal function with the use of this drug."
   b. "I can expect the medication dose to be increased every several weeks."
   c. "I will only need to take this medication until my symptoms are improved."
   d. "I will report any chest pain or difficulty breathing to the doctor right away."
4. Following thyroid surgery the nurse suspects damage or removal of the parathyroid glands when the patient develops
   a. laryngeal stridor.
   b. muscle weakness.
   c. hoarseness and difficulty swallowing.
   d. hyperthermia and severe tachycardia.
5. An important nursing intervention when caring for a patient with Cushing's syndrome is to
   a. restrict protein intake.
   b. observe for signs of hypotension.
   c. administer corticosteroids in equal doses.
   d. protect the patient from exposure to infection.
6. After an adrenalectomy for pheochromocytoma, the patient is most likely to experience
   a. hypokalemia.
   b. hyperglycemia.
   c. marked sodium and water retention.
   d. marked fluctuations in blood pressure.
7. Before surgery a patient with hyperaldosteronism is being treated with spironolactone (Aldactone). The nurse evaluates a successful response to this therapy when the
   a. blood pressure increases.
   b. urine output decreases.
   c. urine sodium decreases.
   d. serum potassium increases.
8. To control the side effects of pharmacologic corticosteroid therapy the nurse teaches the patient to
   a. increase calcium intake to 1500 mg per day.
   b. perform glucose monitoring for hypoglycemia.
   c. carry an emergency kit of hydrocortisone in case of severe stress.
   d. avoid abrupt position changes because of orthostatic hypotension.
9. The nurse teaches the patient that the best time to take cortisone for replacement purposes is
   a. once a day at bedtime.
   b. every other day on awakening.
   c. on arising and in the late afternoon.
   d. at consistent intervals every 6 to 8 hours.

References

1. Melmed S: Acromegaly. In Melmed S, editor: *The pituitary,* Cambridge, Mass, 1995, Blackwell Science.
2. Melmed S and others: Recent advances in pathogenesis, diagnosis, and management of acromegaly, *J Clin Endocrinol Metab* 80:3395, 1995.
3. Mohammed-Zadeh L: MR imaging of macroadenomas, *Radiol Technol* 67:29, 1995.
4. O'Halloran DJ, Shalet SM: Radiotherapy for pituitary adenomas: an endocrinologist's perspective, *Clin Oncol* 8:79, 1996.
5. Counsell C: Management of the patient with a pituitary tumor resection, *DCCN* 15:75, 1996.
6. Sherman RG, Lasseter DH: Pharmacologic management of patients with the diseases of the endocrine system, *Dent Clin North Am* 40:727, 1996.
7. Krause EA: Radiosurgery: a nursing perspective, *J Neurosci Nurs* 23:24, 1991.
8. Vance ML: New directions in the treatment of hyperprolactinemia, *Endocrinologist* 7:153, 1997.
9. Dexter RN: Hypopituitarism. In Becker KL, editor: *Principles and practice of endocrinology and metabolism,* ed 6, Philadelphia, 1995, Lippincott.
10. Jorgenson JOL and others: Adult growth hormone deficiency, *Horm Res* 42:235, 1994.
11. Wallymahmed M: Growth hormone deficiency in adults, *Nurs Times* 9:50, 1997.
12. Carlson HE: The pituitary gland in pregnancy and the puerperium. In Melmed S, editor: *The pituitary,* Cambridge, Mass, 1995, Blackwell Science.
13. Furlanetto RW and others: Guidelines for the use of growth hormone in children with short stature. A report by the Drug and Therapeutics Committee of the Lawson Wilkins Pediatric Endocrine Society, *J Pediatr* 127:857, 1995.
14. Winger JM, Hornick T: Age-associated changes in the endocrine system, *Nurs Clin North Am* 31:827, 1996.
15. Miller M: Inappropriate antidiuretic hormone secretion. In Bardin CW, editor: *Current therapy in endocrinology and metabolism,* ed 6, St Louis, 1997, Mosby.
16. Parobek V, Alaimo I: Fluid and electrolyte management in the neurologically-impaired patient, *J Neurosci Nurs* 28:322, 1996.
17. Robertson GL: Posterior pituitary. In Felig P, Baxter JD, Frohman LA, editors: *Endocrinology and metabolism,* ed 3, New York, 1995, McGraw-Hill.
18. Chernecky CC, Berger BJ: *Laboratory tests and diagnostic procedures,* Philadelphia, 1997, Saunders.
19. Braverman LE, Utiger RD: Introduction to thyrotoxicosis. In Braverman LE, Utiger RD, editors: *Werner and Ingbar's the thyroid: a fundamental and clinical text,* ed 7, Philadelphia,1996, Lippincott-Raven.
20. Utiger RD: The thyroid: physiology, thyrotoxicosis, hypothyroidism, and the painful thyroid. In Felig P, Baxter JD, Frohman LA, editors: *Endocrinology and metabolism,* ed 3, New York, 1995, McGraw-Hill.
21. Hay ID, Morris JC: Toxic adenoma and toxic multinodular goiter. In Braverman LE, Utiger RD, editors: *Werner and Ingbar's the thyroid: a fundamental and clinical text,* ed 7, Philadelphia, 1996, Lippincott-Raven.
22. Mariotti S and others: The aging thyroid, *Endocr Rev* 16:686, 1995.
23. Dillman WH: Thyroid storm. In Bardin CW, editor: *Current therapy in endocrinology and metabolism,* ed 7, St Louis, 1997, Mosby.
24. Ladenson PW: Diagnosis of thyrotoxicosis. In Braverman LE, Utiger RD, editors: *Werner and Ingbar's the thyroid: a fundamental and clinical text,* ed 7, Philadelphia, 1996, Lippincott-Raven.
25. Streff MM, Pachucki-Hyde LC: Management of the patient with thyroid disease, *Nurs Clin North Am* 31:779, 1996.
26. Wartofsky L: Treatment options for hyperthyroidism, *Hosp Pract* 31: 69, 1996.

27. McKennis A, Waddington C: Nursing interventions for potential complications after thyroidectomy, *ORL Head Neck Nurs* 15:27, 1997.
28. Gharib H: Management of thyroid nodules: another look, *Thyroid Today* 20: 1, 1997.
29. Bravermann LE, Utiger RD: Introduction to hypothyroidism. In Braverman LE, Utiger RD, editors: *Werner and Ingbar's the thyroid: a fundamental and clinical text,* ed 7, Philadelphia, 1996, Lippincott-Raven.
30. Moltz KC, Postellon DC: Congenital hypothyroidism and mental development, *Compr Ther* 20:342, 1994.
31. Braverman LE, Roti E: Effects of iodine on thyroid function, *Acta Med Austriaca* 23:4, 1996.
32. Aceto TJ and others: Short stature and slow growth in the infant and child. In Becker KL, editor: *Principles and practice of endocrinology and metabolism,* ed 2, Philadelphia, 1995, Lippincott.
33. MacGillivray MH: Disorders of growth and development. In Felig P, Baxter JD, Frohman LC, editors: *Endocrinology and metabolism,* ed 3, New York, 1996, McGraw-Hill.
34. Finucane P, Anderson C: Thyroid disease in older patients. Diagnosis and treatment, *Drugs Aging* 6:268, 1996.
35. Wartofsky L: The scope and impact of thyroid disease, *Clin Chem* 42:121, 1996.
36. Pittman CS, Zayed AA: Myxedema coma. In Bardin CW, editor: *Current therapy in endocrinology and metabolism,* ed 6, St Louis, 1997, Mosby.
37. Strewler GJ, Rosenblatt M: Mineral metabolism. In Felig P, Baxter JD, Frohman LC, editors: *Endocrinology and metabolism,* ed 3, New York, 1995, McGraw-Hill.
38. Silverberg SJ, Fitzpatrick LA, Bilezikian JP: Primary hyperthyroidism. In Becker KL, editor: *Principles and practice of endocrinology and metabolism,* ed 2, Philadelphia, 1995, Lippincott.
39. Horowitz M and others: Primary hyperparathyroidism, *Clin Geriatr Med* 10:757, 1994.
40. Attie JN: Primary hyperparathyroidism. In Bardin CW, editor: *Current therapy in endocrinology and metabolism,* ed 6, St Louis, 1997, Mosby.
41. Zeiger MA: Hypoparathyroidism, pseudohypoparathyroidism, and pseudopseudohypoparathyroidism. In Clark OH, Duh QY, editors: *Textbook of endocrine surgery,* Philadelphia, 1997, Saunders.
42. Miller WL, Tyrell JB: The adrenal cortex. In Felig P, Baxter JD, Frohman LA, editors: *Endocrinology and metabolism,* New York, 1995, McGraw-Hill.
43. Prinz RA, Falimirski ME: Operative approaches to the adrenal gland. In Clark OH, Duh QY, editors: *Textbook of endocrine surgery,* Philadelphia, 1997, Saunders.
44. Gotch P: Cushing's syndrome from the patient's perspective, *Endocrinol Metab Clin North Am* 23:607, 1994.
45. Davis-Martin S: Disorders of the adrenal glands, *J Am Acad Nurse Pract* 8:323, 1996.
46. Gagner M: Laparoscopic adrenalectomy. In Clark OH, Duh QY, editors: *Textbook of endocrine surgery,* Philadelphia, 1997, Saunders.
47. Gumowski J, Loughran M: Diseases of the adrenal gland, *Nurs Clin North Am* 31:747, 1996.
48. Malcoff CD, Carey RM: Adrenal insufficiency. In Bardin CW, editor: *Current therapy in endocrinology and metabolism,* St Louis, 1997, Mosby.
49. Braatvedt GD, Newrick PG, Corrall RJM: Patient's self administration of hydrocortisone, *BMJ* 301:1312, 1990.
50. Magiakou MA, Chrousos GP: Corticosteroid therapy, nonendocrine disease, and corticosteroid withdrawal. In Bardin CW, editor: *Current therapy in endocrinology and metabolism,* ed 6, St Louis, 1997, Mosby.
51. Gill JR: Hyperaldosteronism. In Becker KL, editor: *Principles and practice of endocrinology and metabolism,* ed 2, Philadelphia, 1995, Lippincott.
52. Obara T, Ito Y, Fujimoto Y: Hyperaldosteronism. In Clark OH, Duh QY, editors: *Textbook of endocrine surgery,* Philadelphia, 1997, Saunders.
53. Cryer PE: Disease of the sympathochromaffin system. In Felig P, Baxter JD, Frohman LC, editors: *Endocrinology and metabolism,* ed 3, New York, 1995, McGraw-Hill.
54. Keiser HR: Pheochromocytoma and other diseases of the sympathetic nervous system. In Becker KL, editor: *Principles and practice of endocrinology and metabolism,* ed 2, Philadelphia, 1995, Lippincott.
55. Bravo EL: Pheochromocytoma. In Bardin CW, editor: *Current therapy in endocrinology and metabolism,* ed 6, St Louis, 1997, Mosby.

Resources

Addison's Disease, National Institute of Diabetes and Digestive and Kidney Diseases
2 Information Way
Bethesda, MD 20892-3570
http://www.niddk.nih.gov

American Association of Clinical Endocrinologists
1000 Riverside Avenue, Suite 205
Jacksonville, FL 32204
http://www.aace.com

American Society for Bone and Mineral Research
1200—19th Street NW, Suite 300
Washington, DC 20036-2401
202-857-1161
Fax: 202-223-4579
http://www.asbmr.org/

American Thyroid Association
Montefiore Medical Center
111 East 210th Street
Bronx, NY 10467
Fax: 718-882-6085
http://www.thyroid.org

Endocrine Nurses Society
2258 SE Darline Avenue
Gresham, OR 97080
503-215-1082
http://www.endo-nurses.org/

Endocrine Society
4350 East West Highway
Bethesda, MD 20814-4410
301-941-0252
Fax: 301-941-0259
http://www.endo-society.org/

Pituitary Tumor Network Association
http://www.pituitary.com/

Thyroid Foundation of Canada
96 Mack Street, Kingston, Ontario K7L 1N9
613-544-8364
800-267-8822
Fax: 613-544-9731
http://home.ican.net/~thyroid/Canada.html

For additional Internet resources, see the website for this book at **www.mosby.com/MERLIN/medsurg_lewis**

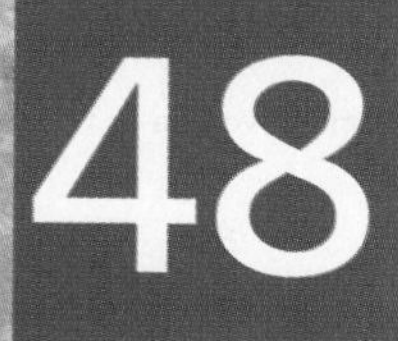

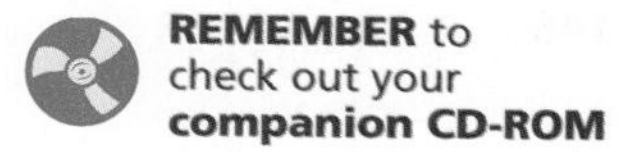

48 NURSING ASSESSMENT Reproductive System

Nancy MacMullen & Laura Dulski

www.mosby.com/MERLIN/medsurg_lewis

LEARNING OBJECTIVES

1. Describe the structures and functions of the male and female reproductive systems.
2. Explain the functions of the major hormones essential for the structure and function of the reproductive systems.
3. Describe the physiologic and psychologic changes of a man and of a woman during the stages of sexual response.
4. Describe age-related changes in the reproductive systems and differences in assessment findings.
5. Identify significant subjective and objective data related to the reproductive systems and information about sexual function that should be obtained from a patient.
6. Describe noninvasive techniques used in the physical assessment of the reproductive systems.
7. Differentiate normal from abnormal findings obtained from a physical assessment of the reproductive systems.
8. Describe the purpose, significance of results, and nursing responsibilities related to diagnostic studies of the reproductive systems.

STRUCTURES AND FUNCTIONS OF THE MALE AND FEMALE REPRODUCTIVE SYSTEMS

The reproductive system is interrelated with other systems, including the neurologic, endocrine, and urinary systems, and also with general physiologic function. For example, estrogen (produced primarily in a woman's ovaries) influences bone density and testosterone (produced primarily in a man's testes) influences muscle mass. The reproductive system is responsible for the perpetuation of the species through fertilization, implantation, maintenance of pregnancy, and birth of a baby. The reproductive system is also directly related to sexual function and is therefore intricately interwoven into the complex, sensitive, and frequently stress-laden area of psychosocial mores and cultural values regarding sex.

Male Reproductive System

The male reproductive system consists of the external structures—the penis and the scrotum—and the internal structures, including the prostate gland, the seminal vesicles, and several ducts (Fig. 48-1). The scrotum lies within the scrotal sac, which is a thin, loose outer layer of skin over a more muscular internal layer. The scrotum consists of two halves divided by a septum; each half contains a testis, an epididymis, and a spermatic cord. The testis is an ovoid, smooth, firm organ measuring 3.5 to 5.5 cm deep and 2 to 3 cm wide.[1] Within the testes are the seminiferous tubules, where spermatozoa (immature sperm) are formed at a rate of 10 to 30 billion per month. The tubules lead into a system of small ducts that conduct sperm to the epididymis.

The epididymis is a soft, cordlike structure that measures almost 212 inches (530 cm) in length if stretched out. It lies in the anterior plane and along the posterolateral surface of each testis. This organ may be considered to be a large duct. It stores the sperm as they mature and until they are released by ejaculation or until they disintegrate and are reabsorbed by the body. The ductus deferens (vas deferens) begins in the epididymis within the scrotal sac, goes up, goes through the scrotum and continues proximally through the inguinal ring, and then posteriorly above the bladder and down again behind the bladder, where it is joined by ducts from the seminal vesicles. It then continues down through the prostate gland, connecting with the urethra (Fig. 48-2). The duct system emerging from each testis conveys sperm into the urethra.

The spermatic cord is composed of the ductus deferens and the arteries, veins, and lymph vessels supplying the testes and the epididymis. All of these structures are enclosed by the cremaster muscle and by layers of fascia. The spermatic cord extends from the scrotum up to the external inguinal ring. The cord ends there, and its components, primarily the ductus deferens, continue along a backward course toward the scrotum.

The prostate gland, the seminal vesicles, and Cowper's (bulbourethral) glands are the accessory glands of the male reproductive system. These glands produce and secrete seminal fluid, which surrounds the sperm and forms the ejaculate. The prostate gland lies underneath the bladder. Its posterior surface approximates the rectal wall. The normal prostate measures 2 cm wide and 3 cm long and is divided into the right and left lateral lobes and an anteroposterior median lobe. As the ejaculate passes through the urethra, it receives an alkaline secretion

Reviewed by Linda Monfore Fluke, RN, MN, ARNP, Adult and Geriatric Nurse Practitioner, State of Washington, Seattle, Wash.

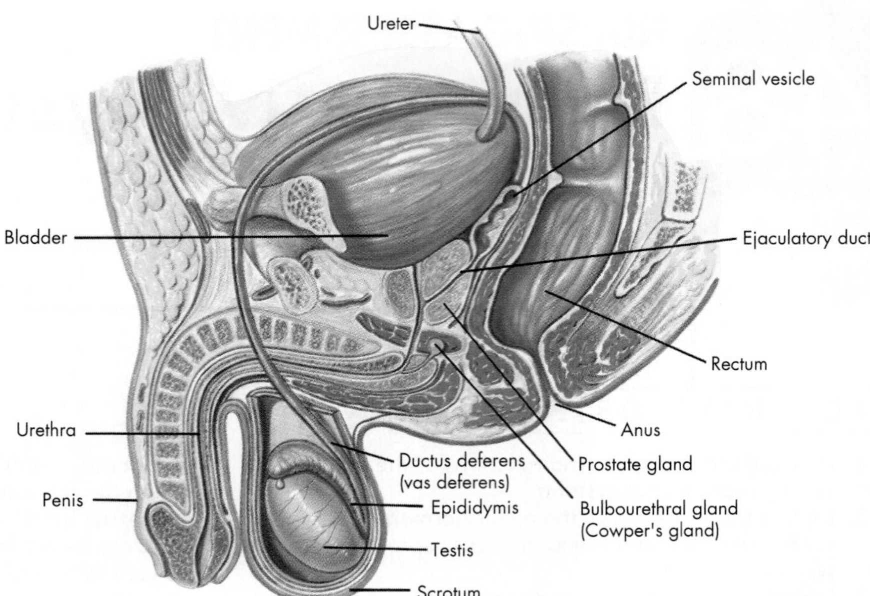

Fig. 48-1 External and internal male sex organs.

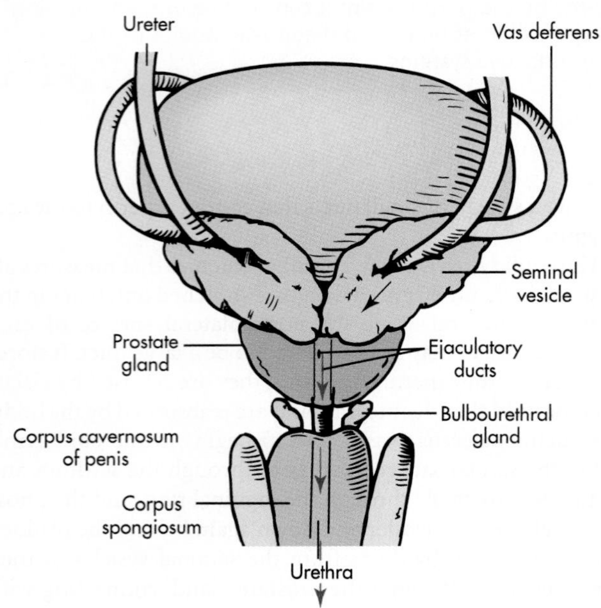

Fig. 48-2 Formation of the ejaculatory ducts by union of the seminal vesicles with the ductus deferens just before entrance into the prostate gland. The ejaculatory ducts open into the prostatic portion of the urethra.

from the prostate gland. The seminal vesicles lie just behind the bladder and between the rectum and the bladder. The ducts of the seminal vesicles fuse with the ductus deferens to form the ejaculatory ducts that enter the prostate gland. Cowper's glands lie on each side of the urethra and slightly posterior to it, just below the prostate. The ducts of these glands enter directly into the urethra. The secretion from the prostate makes up most of the fluid in the ejaculate. By comparison, the seminal vesicles and Cowper's glands contribute a minimum amount of fluid to the ejaculate. These various secretions serve as a medium for the transport of sperm and create an alkaline, nutritious environment that promotes sperm motility and survival.

The urethra extends from the bladder, through the prostate, and ends in a slitlike opening (the meatus) on the ventral side of the glans, the end of the penis. The glans is covered by a fold of skin, the prepuce (or foreskin), which forms at the junction of the glans and the shaft of the penis. In circumcised men the prepuce has been removed. The broadened segment of the glans at the junction is the corona. The shaft of the penis consists of erectile tissue composed of the corpus cavernosum and corpus spongiosum, the fibrous sheath that encases the erectile tissue, and the urethra. The skin covering the penis is thin, loose, and essentially hairless.

Female Reproductive System

The female reproductive system consists of the breasts, the uterus, the ovaries, the fallopian tubes, the vagina, and the external genitalia (the vulva), as well as ligaments and pelvic bones.

Breasts. The breasts are a secondary sex characteristic that develops during puberty in response to estrogen and progesterone. Cyclic hormonal changes lead to regular changes in breast tissue to prepare it for lactation when fertilization and pregnancy occur. The breasts are also considered a major organ of sexual stimulation and response among some cultures.

The breasts extend from the second to the sixth ribs, with the tail reaching the axilla (Fig. 48-3). The fully mature breast is dome shaped and contains a pigmented center termed the *areola.* The areolar region contains Montgomery's tubercles, which are similar to sebaceous glands and assist in moistening the nipple. During lactation, the alveoli or acini secrete milk. The milk then flows into a ductal system and is transported to the lactiferous sinuses. The nipple contains 15 to 20 tiny openings through which the milk flows during breastfeeding. The breast's rich lymphatic network drains primarily into the axillary, the infraclavicular, and the supraclavicular channels. This system is often responsible for the metastasis of a malignant tumor from the breast to other parts of the body (Fig. 48-4). The fibrous and fatty tissue that supports and separates the channels of the mammary duct system is primarily responsible for the varying sizes and shapes of the breasts in different individuals.

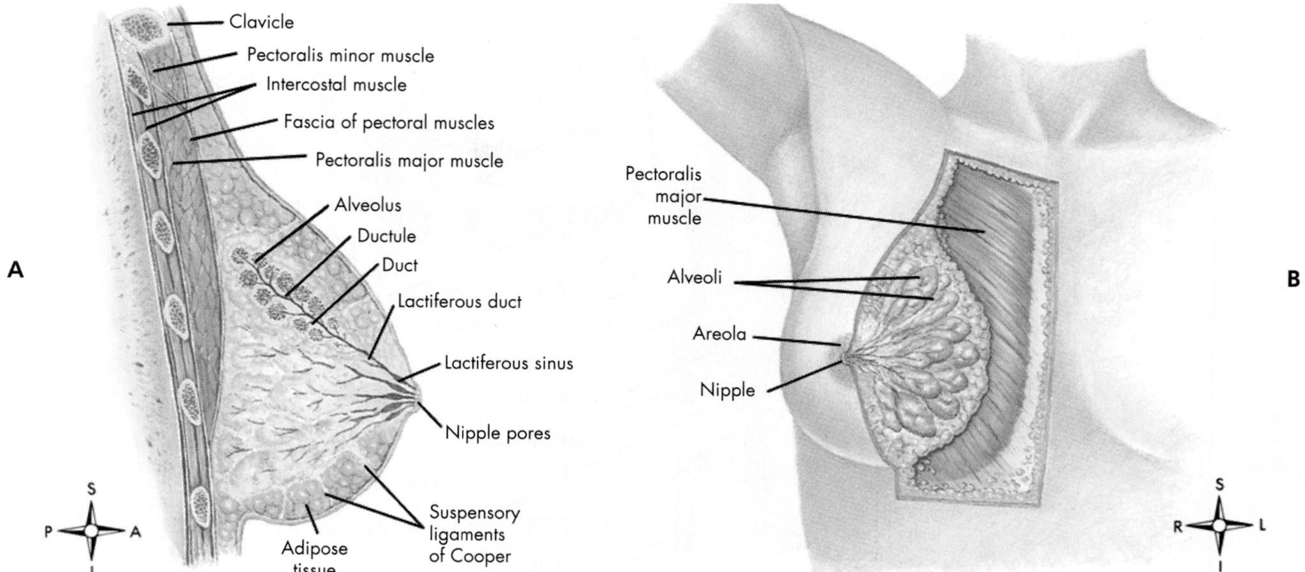

Fig. 48-3 The female breast. **A,** Sagittal section of a lactating breast. Notice how the glandular structures are anchored to the overlying skin and to the pectoral muscles by suspensory ligaments of Cooper. Each lobule of glandular tissue is drained by a lactiferous duct that eventually opens through the nipple. **B,** Anterior view of a lactating breast. In nonlactating breasts the glandular tissue is much less prominent, with adipose tissue comprising most of each breast.

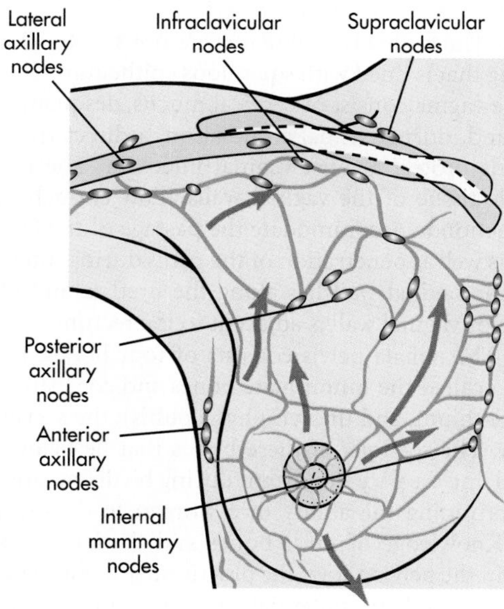

Fig. 48-4 Lymphatic drainage of the breast. *Arrows* indicate direction of drainage.

Pelvic Organs

Ovaries. The ovaries are usually located on either side of the uterus, just behind and below the fallopian (uterine) tubes (Fig. 48-5). The ovaries are firm and solid, averaging 1.5 cm wide, 3 cm long, and 2 cm deep. Their functions include ovulation, as well as secretion of the two major reproductive hormones, estrogen and progesterone. The outer zone of the ovary contains follicles with germ cells, or oocytes. Each follicle contains a primordial (immature) oocyte surrounded by granulosa and theca cells. These two layers protect and nourish the oocyte until the follicle reaches maturity and ovulation occurs. However, not all follicles reach maturity. In a process termed *atresia,* most of the primordial follicles become smaller and are reabsorbed by the body; thus the number of follicles declines from 2 to 4 million at birth to approximately 300,000 to 400,000 at menarche. This number continues to decrease throughout a woman's reproductive years.[2] The vast majority of oocytes are destroyed by atresia. Fewer than 500 are actually released by ovulation during the reproductive years of the normal healthy woman.

Fallopian tubes. Normally, each month during a woman's reproductive years, one ovarian follicle reaches maturity, and the ovum is ovulated, or expelled, from the ovary through the stimulus of the gonadotropic hormones, follicle-stimulating hormone (FSH) and luteinizing hormone (LH). The ovum then travels up a fallopian tube where fertilization by a sperm may occur, assuming that sperm are present. An ovum can be fertilized up to 72 hours after its release. Sperm are viable for 24 to 48 hours.[3]

The distal ends of the fallopian tubes consist of fingerlike projections called *fimbriae* that "massage" the ovaries at ovulation to help extract the mature ovum. The tubes, which average 4.8 inches (12 cm) in length, extend from the fimbriae to the superior lateral borders of the uterus. Fertilization usually takes place within the outer one third of the tubes.

Uterus. The uterus is a pear-shaped, hollow, muscular organ (see Fig. 48-5). It is located between the bladder and the rectum. In the mature nulliparous (never pregnant) female the uterus is approximately 6 cm long and 4 cm wide. The uterine walls consist of an outer serosal layer, the perimetrium, a middle muscular layer, the myometrium, and an inner mucosal layer, the endometrium.

The uterus consists of the fundus, the body (or the corpus), and the cervix. The body makes up about 80% of the uterus and connects with the cervix at the isthmus, or the neck. The cervix

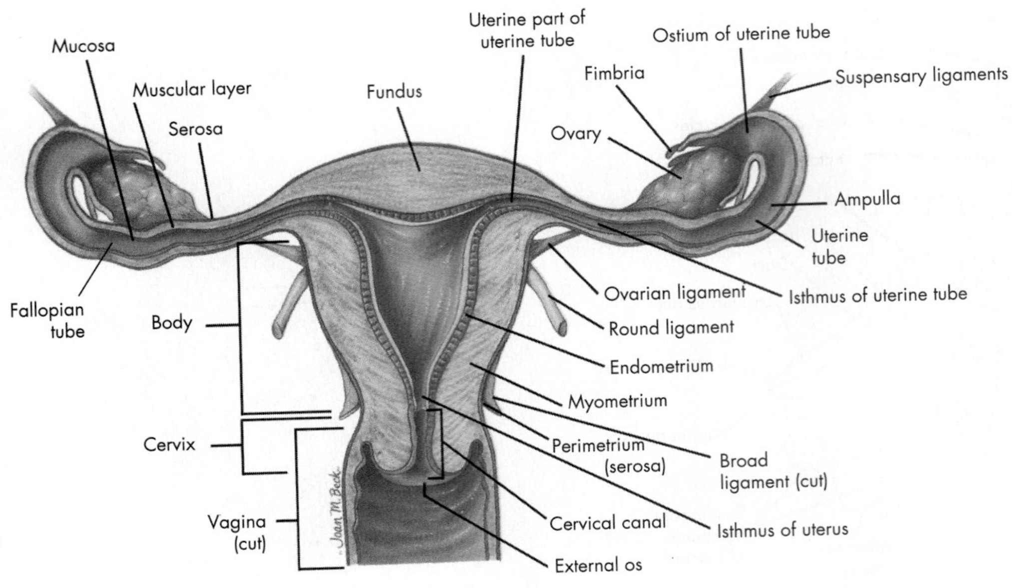

Fig. 48-5 Anatomy of the female reproductive tract.

is the lower portion that invaginates (projects) into the anterior wall of the vaginal canal. It makes up about 15% to 20% of the uterus in the nulliparous female. The cervix consists of the ectocervix, the outer portion that protrudes into the vagina, and the endocervix, the canal in the opening of the cervix. The ectocervix is covered with squamous epithelial cells, which give it a smooth, pinkish appearance. The endocervix contains a lining of columnar epithelial cells, which give it a rough, reddened appearance. The junction at which the two types of epithelial cells meet is termed the *squamocolumnar junction* and contains the optimal types of cells needed for an accurate Papanicolaou (Pap) smear to screen for malignancies. The presence of endocervical cells in the sample taken for a Pap smear ensures that the squamocolumnar junction, or the transformation zone, has been sampled. Cells taken from the vagina provide a less accurate diagnosis and therefore are not included in the routine Pap smear.[2] The cervical canal is 2 to 4 cm long and is relatively tightly closed. The cervix, however, allows sperm to enter the uterus and also allows menses to be expelled. The columnar epithelium, under hormonal influence, provides enough elasticity at labor for the cervix to stretch so that a fetus can pass. The entrance of sperm into the uterus is facilitated by mucus produced by the cervix under the influence of estrogen. Under normal conditions, the cervical mucus becomes watery and more abundant at ovulation. This mucus can stretch several inches (spinnbarkeit) and allows for the easy entrance of sperm into the uterus. The postovulatory cervical mucus, under the influence of progesterone, is thick and inhibits sperm passage. Knowledge of these physiologic changes is used in natural approaches to family planning.

The anterior and posterior peritoneal covering of the uterus is called the *broad ligament*. It separates the uterus from the bladder and the rectum but does not provide support for the uterus or the adnexa (ovaries and tubes). The cardinal ligaments, which extend from the isthmus of the uterus to the pelvic wall, also offer only minimal support. The round ligament, which extends anteriorly to the labia majora, provides some support but is easily weakened by pregnancy. The firmest support for the uterus is provided by the uterine sacral ligaments, which pull the uterus back and away from the vaginal orifice.

Vagina. The vagina is a tubular structure 3 to 4 inches (8 to 10 cm) long that is lined with squamous epithelium. The secretions of the vagina consist of cervical mucus, desquamated epithelium, and, during sexual stimulation, a direct transudate. These fluids protect against vaginal infection. The muscular and erectile tissue of the vaginal walls allow enough dilation and contraction to accommodate the passage of the fetus during labor, as well as penetration of the penis during intercourse. The anterior vaginal wall lies along the urethra and bladder. The posterior vaginal wall is adjacent to the rectum.

Pelvis. The female pelvis consists of four bones: two hipbones (also called the innominate bones and consisting of the ilium, the ischium, and the symphysis pubis), the sacrum, and the coccyx. The sections of these bones that lie below the iliopectineal line are very important during birth and are often a factor determining the ability of a woman to deliver a child vaginally. Knowledge of these bones and the landmarks that they form in the pelvis allows the practitioner to estimate pelvic measurements and the potential for a woman's pelvis to accommodate the birth of a full-term fetus. Specialty references discuss the specific techniques of clinical pelvimetry.

The pelvis is also divided into the true pelvis and the false pelvis. The true pelvis encompasses the brim, the cavity, and the outlet and is the bony passageway through which the fetus passes during birth. The false pelvis consists of the superior portion of the iliac bones, above the brim or the iliopectineal line.[2]

External Genitalia. The external portion of the female reproductive system (Fig. 48-6), commonly called the *vulva*, consists of the mons pubis, the labia majora, the labia minora, the clitoris, the urethral meatus, the ducts of Skene's glands, the vaginal orifice, and the Bartholin's glands.

The mons pubis is a fatty layer lying over the pubic bone. It contains coarse hair that lies in an upside-down triangular pat-

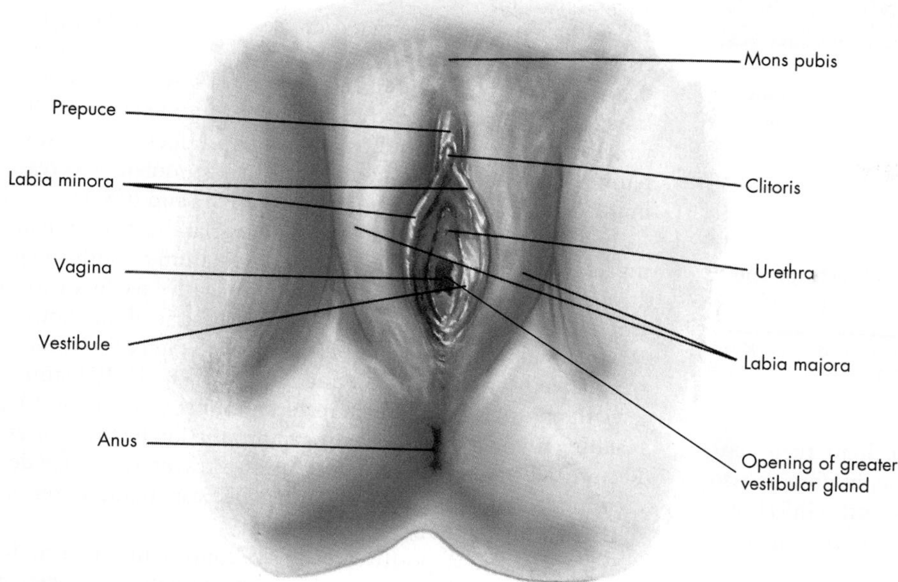

Fig. 48-6 External female genitalia.

tern. (The male hair pattern is diamond shaped.) The labia majora are folds of adipose tissue that form the outer borders of the vulva. These hair-covered folds contain sweat glands and sebaceous glands. The hairless labia minora form the borders of the vaginal orifice and extend anteriorly to enclose the clitoris. The vestibule is a boat-shaped fossa between the labia minora, extending from the clitoris at the anterior end to the vaginal opening at the posterior end. The perineum is the area between the vagina and the anus.

In a virgin the vaginal orifice usually but not always contains a thin membrane called the *hymen,* which varies the size of the vaginal orifice in individuals from that of a pinhole to an opening large enough to allow two fingers to enter. Frequently, the hymen is torn during first sexual intercourse, and only tags remain. In many societies, the bleeding that occurs with this tearing has been used to validate virginity. However, not all hymens are torn by the first intercourse. Some are already well stretched or are torn because of childhood activity, tampon usage, or accidents.

The clitoris is homologous (similar) to the male penis; it is the erectile tissue that becomes engorged during sexual excitation. It lies anterior to the urethral meatus and the vaginal orifice and is usually covered by the prepuce or hood. Clitoral stimulation is an important part of sexual activity for many women.

Skene's glands and ducts lie alongside the urethral meatus and have no known function. They are homologous to the male prostate. Bartholin's glands, which are at the posterior and lateral aspects of the vaginal orifice, secrete a thin, mucoid material believed to contribute slightly to lubrication during sexual intercourse. These glands are not usually palpable unless sebaceous-like cysts form or an infection, especially a sexually transmitted disease, arises.

Neuroendocrine Regulation

The hypothalamus and pituitary gland (see Chapter 45) and the gonads (organs of reproduction) secrete numerous hormones (Fig. 48-7). These hormones regulate the processes of ovulation, spermatogenesis (formation of sperm), and fertilization, as well as the formation and function of the secondary sex characteristics. The cyclic changes in the amounts of these hormones secreted by the anterior pituitary gland cause cyclic changes in the ovaries. The hypothalamus secretes gonadotropin-releasing hormones (GnRHs), which stimulate the pituitary gland to secrete its hormones, including FSH and LH. LH in males is sometimes called interstitial cell–stimulating hormone (ICSH). The gonadal hormones are estrogen, progesterone, and testosterone.

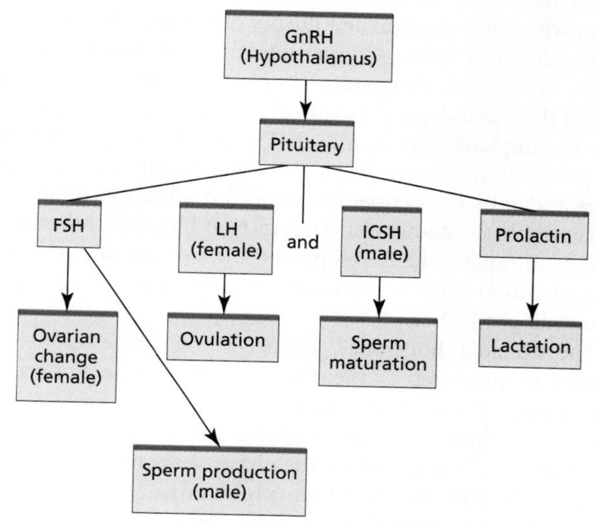

Fig. 48-7 The hypothalamic-pituitary-gonadal axis. Only the major pituitary hormone actions are depicted. *FSH,* follicle-stimulating hormone; *GnRH,* gonadotropin-releasing hormone; *ICSH,* interstitial cell–stimulating hormone; *LH,* luteinizing hormone.

In women, FSH production by the pituitary stimulates the growth and maturity of the ovarian follicles to cause ovulation.

Table 48-1 Gonadal Feedback Mechanisms

Negative Feedback			
↓ Estrogen	→ ↑ GnRH (hypothalamus)	→ ↑ FSH (pituitary)	→ ↑ Estrogen (ovaries)
Positive Feedback			
↑ Estrogen	→ ↑ GnRH (hypothalamus)	→ ↑ LH (pituitary)	
Testes (Negative Feedback)			
↓ Testosterone	→↑ GnRH (hypothalamus)	→↑ FSH and ICSH (pituitary)	→↑ Testosterone (testes)

FSH, follicle-stimulating hormone; *GnRH,* gonadotropin-releasing hormone; *ICSH,* interstitial cell–stimulating hormone; *LH,* luteinizing hormone.

The mature follicle produces estrogen, which in turn suppresses the release of FSH. Another hormone, inhibin, is also secreted by the ovarian follicle and inhibits both GnRH and FSH secretion. In men, FSH stimulates the seminiferous tubules to produce sperm.

LH contributes to the ovulatory process because it causes follicles to complete maturation and undergo ovulation. It also causes the development of a ruptured follicle, or the area on the ovum where the ovum exited during ovulation. The ruptured follicle develops into a corpus luteum, from which progesterone is secreted. Progesterone maintains the rich vascular state of the uterus (secretory phase) in preparation for fertilization and implantation. In men, LH or ICSH is responsible for the production of testosterone by the interstitial cells of the testes and thus is essential for the full maturation of sperm. Prolactin has no known function in men but, with other hormones, stimulates the development and growth of the mammary glands in women. During lactation, it initiates and maintains milk production.

The gonadal hormones, estrogen and progesterone, in women are produced by the ovaries. Small amounts of an estrogen precursor are also produced in the adrenal cortices. Estrogen is essential to the development and maintenance of the secondary sex characteristics, the phase of the menstrual cycle immediately after menstruation (proliferative phase), and the uterine changes essential to pregnancy. Estrogen has also been found in the urine of men, although its role and importance are not well understood. In men, this hormone is produced predominantly in the adrenal cortex.

Progesterone plays a major role in the menstrual cycle but most specifically in the secretory phase. Like estrogen, progesterone is involved in the bodily changes associated with pregnancy. Adequate progesterone is necessary to maintain an implanted egg.

The major gonadal hormone of men, testosterone, is produced by the testes. Testosterone is responsible for the development and maintenance of secondary sex characteristics, as well as for adequate spermatogenesis. Androgens are produced in females by the adrenal glands and ovaries, though in small amounts.

The circulating levels of gonadal hormones are controlled primarily by a negative feedback process. Receptors within the hypothalamus and pituitary are sensitive to the circulating blood levels of the hormones (Table 48-1). Increased levels of hormones stimulate a hypothalamic response to decrease the high circulating levels. Likewise, low circulating levels provoke a hypothalamic response that increases the low circulating levels. For example, if the circulating level of testosterone is low, the hypothalamus is stimulated to secrete GnRH. This stimulates the pituitary to secrete greater amounts of FSH and ICSH, which in turn causes an increase in the production of testosterone. The high levels of testosterone then stimulate a decrease in the production of GnRH and thus of FSH and ICSH.

In women, however, there is a slight variation. The circulating levels are controlled through a combination of both a negative and a positive feedback system. A negative feedback control mechanism exists, similar to that described previously. When circulating estrogen levels are low, the hypothalamus is stimulated to increase its production of GnRH. GnRH stimulates the pituitary to secrete greater amounts of FSH and LH, resulting in higher levels of estrogen production by the ovaries. Reciprocally higher levels of circulating estrogen result in a decreasing secretion of GnRH and thus a decrease in the secretion of FSH by the pituitary.

There is also a positive feedback control mechanism in women. Thus, with increasing levels of circulating estrogen, a greater level of GnRH is produced, resulting in an increased level of LH from the pituitary. Likewise, lowered levels of estrogen result in a lowered level of LH.

Menarche

Menarche is the first episode of menstrual bleeding, indicating a female has reached puberty. This usually occurs around 13 years of age, although there is individual variation according to race, nutrition, health, and heredity.

As puberty approaches, there are changes associated with the elevated rate of estrogen and progesterone secretion by the ovaries. These changes include the development of breast buds, the development of pubic hair, and later the development of axillary hair. During this time, there is a decrease in the sensitivity of the hypothalamic-pituitary axis that allows for increased secretion of FSH and LH and a resultant increase in estrogen. It is during this time that the adult pattern of gonadotropin secretion occurs, resulting in the menstrual cycle. Menstrual cycles are often irregular during the first few years of menarche because of anovulation.

Menstrual Cycle

The major functions of the ovaries are ovulation and the secretion of hormones. These functions are accomplished during the normal menstrual cycle, a monthly process mediated by the hormonal activity of the hypothalamus, the pituitary gland, and the ovaries. Menstruation occurs during each month in which an egg is not fertilized (Fig. 48-8). The endometrial cycle is divided into three phases labeled in relation to uterine and ovarian changes: (1) the proliferative or follicular phase, (2) the secretory or luteal phase, and (3) the menstrual or ischemic phase. The length of the menstrual cycle ranges from 20 to 40 days, the average being 28 days.

The menstrual cycle begins on the first day of menstruation, which usually lasts 3 to 5 days. During this time, estrogen and progesterone levels are low, but FSH levels begin to increase. During the follicular phase, a single follicle matures fully under the stimulation of FSH. (The mechanism that ensures that usually only one follicle reaches maturity is not known.) The ma-

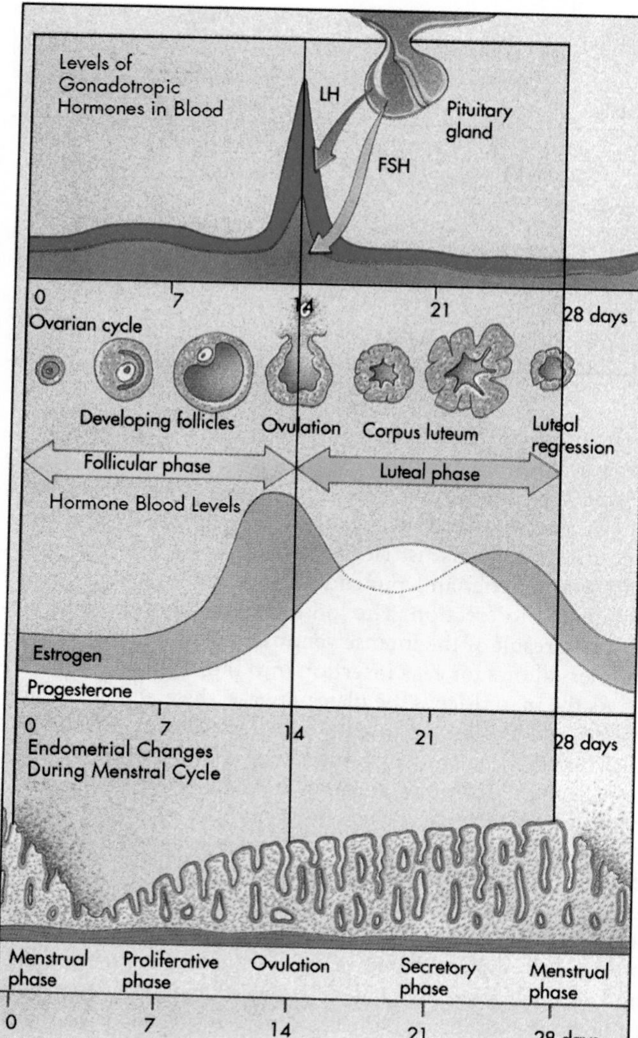

Fig. 48-8 Events of the menstrual cycle. The various lines depict the changes in blood hormone levels, the development of the follicles, and the changes in the endometrium during the cycle. *FSH,* follicle-stimulating hormone; *LH,* luteinizing hormone.

ture follicle stimulates estrogen production, causing a negative feedback with resulting decreased FSH secretion.

Although the initial stage of follicular maturation is stimulated by FSH, complete maturation and ovulation occur only with the presence of LH. When estrogen levels peak on about the twelfth day of the cycle, there is a surge of LH, which triggers ovulation a day or two later. After ovulation (maturation and release of an ovum), LH promotes the development of the corpus luteum.

The fully developed corpus luteum continues to secrete estrogen and initiates progesterone secretion. If fertilization occurs, high levels of estrogen and progesterone continue to be secreted as a result of the continued activity of the corpus luteum from stimulation by human chorionic gonadotropin (hCG). If fertilization does not take place, menstruation occurs because of a decrease in estrogen production and progesterone withdrawal.

Table 48-2 Common Manifestations During the Climacteric

Premenopausal	Postmenopausal
Irregular menses	Atrophic vaginitis
Vasomotor instability (hot flashes)	Occasional vasomotor symptoms
Nervousness	Atrophy of genitourinary tissue with decreased support
Perimenopausal	Osteoporosis
Cessation of menses	
Frequent vasomotor symptoms	
Atrophy of genitourinary tissue (e.g., vaginal epithelium)	
Stress and urge incontinence	

During the follicular phase, the endometrial lining of the uterus also undergoes change. As larger amounts of estrogen are produced, the endometrial lining undergoes proliferative changes, and there is an increase in cellular growth, including an increase in the length of blood vessels and glandular tissue.

With ovulation and the resulting increased levels of progesterone, the luteal, or secretory, phase begins. In this phase, the blood vessels begin to coil, increasing the surface area of the vascular supply. The glandular tissues mature and secrete a glycogen-rich substance, and the glandular ducts dilate. If the corpus luteum regresses (when fertilization does not occur) and estrogen and progesterone levels fall, the endometrial lining can no longer be supported. As a result, the blood vessels contract, and tissue begins to slough (fall away). This sloughing results in the menses and the start of the menstrual phase.

Menopause

Menopause is the cessation of the menses for the remainder of a woman's lifetime. It is usually considered complete after 1 year of amenorrhea (absence of menstruation). The average age at which menopause occurs is 52 years, but this can vary.[4] The climacteric, also commonly known as the perimenopause, is the period during which symptoms of approaching menopause begin, menopause actually occurs, and equilibrium after menopause is established (Table 48-2). Ovulation decreases over a period of years. In a way, the factors that result in menopause are established during fetal life. Approximately 2 to 4 million oocytes are present by the 20th week of gestation, after which time the number begins to decline. The average woman ovulates 400 to 500 times during a lifetime. Most follicles undergo atresia and are then called atretic follicles.[2] In 40 to 50 years after birth the full store of oocytes is greatly depleted. Because the number of oocytes decreases during the climacteric, the amount of estrogen produced also begins to decrease.

The decreasing level of estrogen causes a gradual increase in FSH and LH as a result of the negative feedback process. By the time menopause occurs, there is a tenfold to twentyfold increase in FSH. These elevated FSH levels may take several years to return to premenopausal levels. The reduced estrogen level also causes a decrease in the frequency of ovulation and results in atrophy of the secondary sex characteristics.

The reason for "hot flashes" or vasomotor instability is not clearly understood. It has been theorized that temperature regulators in the brain are in proximity to the area where GnRH is released. However, lowered estrogen levels are correlated with dilation of cutaneous blood vessels, resulting in "hot flashes" and increased sweating. The more sudden the withdrawal of estrogen (e.g., surgical removal of the ovaries), the more likely the symptoms will be severe if no replacement is provided. These symptoms subside over time, with or without hormone replacement therapy. Autonomic nervous system instability may also be related to emotional irritability during the climacteric, but this "symptom" has been greatly exaggerated in literature and myth. Atrophy of the vaginal epithelium often causes vaginal dryness that is responsible for mild to moderate dyspareunia (painful intercourse). This can lead to unnecessary and premature cessation of sexual activity. Dryness is a problem that can be easily corrected with water-soluble lubricants or, if needed, with hormonal creams or systemic hormone replacement therapy. In general, the extent and severity of the symptoms of the climacteric vary and are not easily predicted, even with a detailed history of family patterns.

Osteoporosis, a condition in which the bone mass is decreased because of increased bone resorption, is prevalent in menopausal women. This condition puts women at a much greater risk for sustaining fractures of the spine, vertebrae, wrists, and hips. Such fractures can be life threatening in older women. Although the exact mechanism is not known, cessation of estrogen production is associated with accelerated bone loss. Hormone replacement therapy in the postmenopausal period can help protect women from osteoporosis and cardiovascular disease. Combined estrogen and progesterone therapy reduces the risk of endometrial cancer associated with the use of estrogen alone. Research on hormonal replacement therapy and breast cancer is underway; past study results have been equivocal.[5]

The changes of menopause and particularly the risk of osteoporosis create a dilemma in the care of menopausal women. The use of estrogen replacement therapy often reduces the risk of such symptoms but can create other potentially serious side effects. Adequate calcium intake and exercise both before and after menopause are also important factors in the prevention of osteoporosis (see Chapter 59).

Phases of the Sexual Response

It is helpful to look at the structural homologues in the male and female reproductive systems to understand the sexual response (Table 48-3). Masters and Johnson described the sexual response in terms of the excitement, plateau, orgasmic, and resolution phases.[6] These phases are discussed for the male and the female as the sexual response.

Orgasm does not occur in every sexual encounter. In addition, orgasm does not depend on anatomic features such as the size of the penis or of the vaginal canal. The sexual response is a complex interplay of psychologic and physiologic phenomena and is therefore influenced by daily stress, as well as by illness and crisis.

Male Sexual Response. The penis and the urethra are essential to the transport of sperm into the vagina and the cervix during intercourse. This transport is facilitated by penile erection in response to sexual stimulation during the excitement phase. Erection results from the filling of the large venous sinuses within the erectile tissue of the penis. In the flaccid state the sinuses hold only a small amount of blood, but during the erection stage they are congested with blood. Because the penis is richly endowed with sympathetic, parasympathetic, and pudendal nerve endings, it is readily stimulated to erection. The loose skin of the penis becomes taut as a result of the intense venous congestion. This erectile tautness allows for easy insertion into the vagina.

Table 48-3 Structural Homologues of the Male and Female Reproductive Systems

Male	Female
Penis	Clitoris
Scrotal ridge	Labia minora
Scrotum	Labia majora
Testes	Ovaries
Cowper's glands	Bartholin's glands
Prostate gland	Skene's ducts
Prostatic utricle (blind pouch of urethra)	Vagina

As the man reaches the plateau phase, the erection is maintained, and a small increase in diameter occurs as a result of a slight increase in vasocongestion. There is also an increase in testicle size. Sometimes a change in color occurs in the glans penis, which becomes more reddish-purple.

The subsequent contraction of the penile and urethral musculature during the orgasmic phase propels the sperm outward through the meatus. In this process, termed *ejaculation,* sperm are released into the ductus deferens during contractions. They advance through the urethra, where fluids from the prostate and seminal vesicles are added to the ejaculate. The sperm continue their path through the urethra, receiving a small amount of fluid from the Cowper's glands, and are finally ejaculated through the urinary meatus. Orgasm is characterized by the rapid release of the vasocongestion and myotonia that have developed. The rapid release of muscular tension (through rhythmic contractions) occurs primarily in the penis, the prostate gland, and the seminal vesicles.

After ejaculation, a man enters the resolution phase. During this phase the penis undergoes involution, gradually returning to its unstimulated, flaccid state.

Female Sexual Response. The changes that occur in a woman during sexual excitation are similar to those in a man. In response to stimulation the clitoris swells (becomes congested, as does the penis in a man), and vaginal lubrication increases from secretions from the cervix and Bartholin's glands and sweating of the vaginal walls. This initial response is the excitation phase.

As excitation is maintained in the plateau phase, the vagina expands and the uterus is elevated (in the man, correspondingly, there is an increase in testicular size). In the orgasmic phase, contractions occur in the uterus from the fundus to the lower uterine segment. There is a slight relaxation of the cervical os, which helps the entrance of the sperm, and rhythmic contractions of the vagina. Muscular tension is rapidly released through rhythmic contractions in the clitoris, the vagina, and the uterus. This phase is followed by a resolution phase in which these organs return to their preexcitation state. However,

GERONTOLOGIC DIFFERENCES IN ASSESSMENT

Table 48-4 Reproductive System

Changes	Differences in Assessment Findings
Male	
Penis	
Decreased subcutaneous fat, decreased skin turgor	Easily retractable foreskin (if uncircumcised), decrease in size, fewer sustained erections
Testes	
Decreased testosterone production	Decrease in size, change in position (lower), increase in firmness
Prostate	
Benign hyperplasia	Enlargement
Breasts	
Enlargement	Gynecomastia (abnormal enlargement)
Female	
Breasts	
Decreased subcutaneous fat, increased fibrous tissue, decreased skin turgor	Less resilient, looser, more pendulous tissue, decreased size, duct around nipple may feel like stringy strand
Vulva	
Decreased skin turgor	Atrophy, decreased amount of pubic hair, decreased size of clitoris, decreased size of labia
Vagina	
Atrophy of tissue, decreased muscle tone	Pale mucosa, dryness of mucosa, less intense sexual response, relaxation of outlets, mucosa thins, vagina narrower and shorter
Urethra	
Decreased muscle tone	Cystocele (protrusion of bladder through vaginal wall)
Uterus	
Decreased thickness of myometrium	Decrease in size, uterine prolapse
Ovaries	
Decreased ovarian function	Nonpalpable ovaries, decreased size

women do not have to go through the resolution (refractory) recovery state before they can be orgasmic again. They can be multiorgasmic without resolution between orgasms.

GERONTOLOGIC CONSIDERATIONS

Effects of Aging on the Reproductive Systems and the Sexual Response

With advancing age, changes occur in the male and female reproductive systems. In women, many of these changes are related to the altered estrogen production that is associated with menopause. Age-related changes in the reproductive systems and differences in assessment findings are presented in Table 48-4.

Gradual changes resulting from advancing age occur in the sexual responses of men and women (Table 48-5). These changes occur at different rates and to varying degrees. The cumulative effects of these changes, as well as the negative social attitude toward sexuality in older adults, can affect the sexual practices of people in this age-group. Nurses have an important role in providing accurate and unbiased information about sexuality and age. Nurses should emphasize the normalcy of sexual activity in older adults. Counseling may be necessary to help older patients accommodate to these normal physiologic changes.[7]

GERONTOLOGIC DIFFERENCES IN ASSESSMENT

Table 48-5 Sexual Function

Sexual Function
Male
Increased stimulation necessary for erection
Decreased need to ejaculate
Decreased ability to attain erection
Possible decreased response to sexual stimuli
Female
Decreased vaginal lubrication
Possible decreased response to sexual stimuli

ASSESSMENT OF THE MALE AND FEMALE REPRODUCTIVE SYSTEMS

Subjective Data

Important Health Information. Problems in other systems are often interrelated with problems and stresses within the reproductive system. The nurse must elicit general information, as well as information specifically relating to the reproductive system. Reproduction and sexual issues are often considered extremely personal and private. The nurse must develop trust to elicit such information. A professional demeanor is important when taking a reproductive or sexual history.

Past health history. Every woman who enters the health care system should have a complete obstetric and gynecologic history taken (Table 48-6). The gynecologic history provides information related to such problems as pelvic pain, exposure to sexually transmitted diseases, vaginal infections, and the presence of symptoms such as vaginal discharge and dyspareunia that need treatment. An obstetric history provides important information related to family planning and fertility counseling most relevant to the individual.

In addition, the nurse should obtain data related to in utero exposure to diethylstilbestrol (DES). DES was frequently administered to women to prevent spontaneous abortions during the 1940s and 1950s, with a national decline in use during the 1960s. It is associated with cervical adenosis and cervical and vaginal adenocarcinoma in women who were exposed to it in utero. Male offspring of mothers given DES experience congenital anomalies such as structural defects of the genitourinary tract and decreased sperm levels, as well as an increase in the incidence of penile cancer.

Table 48-6 Gynecologic and Obstetric History Format

General Gynecologic Information

External genitalia

______ Pain
______ Rashes
______ Lesions
______ Other
______ Vaginal discharge
Amount ______
Color ______
Consistency ______
Odor ______
Past history of vaginal infection ______Yes ______No
If yes, type ______
______ Pain during intercourse
______ Bleeding after intercourse

Sexually transmitted diseases (STDs)

______ Chlamydia ______ Syphilis
______ Genital herpes ______ Yeast infection *(Candida albicans)*
______ Gonorrhea
______ HIV
______ Other (specify) ______

Gynecologic history

Last Pap Smear ______ Abnormal ______ (Yes or No)
______ Uterine fibroids Treatment if any ______
______ Endometriosis Treatment if any ______
______ Ovarian cyst ______
Did your mother take hormones when she was pregnant with you? (Yes, No, or Not Sure)
Any difficulties in getting pregnant? (Yes, No, or Has not attempted)
Gynecologic surgery (e.g., D&C, cryosurgery)
Type ______
Reason ______
Year ______

Obstetric Information

______ Number of pregnancies
______ Number of full-term births
______ Number of preterm births
______ Number of live births
______ Number of spontaneous abortions (miscarriages)
______ Number of therapeutic abortions
______ Number of ectopic (tubal) pregnancies
______ Number of cesarean sections
Problems during pregnancy, if any ______

Menstrual Information

Age at onset ______
Last menstrual period ______
Cycle (frequency) ______ Irregular periods ______ Length ______
Duration of each menses ______
Number of pads or tampons used on heaviest days ______
Clots ______ Spotting (other than during menses) ______
Dysmenorrhea (describe) ______
Treatment ______
Change in flow or amount (yes or no)
Explain ______
Menopause ______ Menopausal symptoms ______
Hormonal replacement ______ (yes or no)
What ______ Dose ______
If menopausal, have you noticed any vaginal bleeding? ______
Birth control method (if applicable) ______
Length ______ Previous methods ______

Breast Information

______ Monthly breast self-exam (yes or no)
Breast lumps (location) ______
Treatment, if any
______ Mammogram (date) ______
______ Breast pain
Onset ______
Severity ______
Previous occurrence ______
______ Breast discharge
Onset ______
Amount ______
Color ______
Odor and consistency ______
Breastfeeding ______ (yes or no)
Where are you in your menstrual cycle (in case any breast abnormality is found)? ______

D&C, dilation and curettage.

Common pediatric illnesses that affect reproductive function are mumps and rubella. The occurrence of mumps in young men has been associated with an increase in sterility because of bilateral testicular atrophy secondary to orchitis. In the health history, the nurse should elicit whether male patients have had mumps, been immunized, or had any indications of sterility.

Rubella is of primary concern to women of childbearing age. If rubella occurs during the first 3 months of pregnancy, the possibility of congenital anomalies is increased. For this reason, nurses should encourage immunization for all women of childbearing age who have not been immunized for rubella or have not already had the disease. However, women should not be immunized if they are already pregnant. Women are also advised not to conceive for at least 3 months after immunization.

The presence of a chronic disease such as diabetes mellitus that can affect the functioning of the reproductive system must be determined. Men who have diabetes mellitus frequently experience impotency problems because of associated neuropathies. Impotence and retrograde ejaculation are additional manifestations of diabetes mellitus in men. In women with uncontrolled diabetes mellitus, pregnancy and the use of oral contraceptives may constitute significant risks to health. Likewise, in women, a history of cardiovascular disease, including hypertension, thrombophlebitis, and angina, causes a higher incidence of morbidity and mortality with pregnancy or oral con-

Table 48-7 Surgeries of the Reproductive System

Surgery	Definition
Men	
Herniorrhaphy	Repair of hernia
Orchiectomy	Removal of a testis
Prostatectomy	Removal of prostate gland
Repair of testicular torsion	Correction of axial rotation of spermatic cord, which cuts off blood supply to the testicle, epididymis, and other structures
Varicocelectomy	Repair of varicose vein of scrotum
Vasectomy	Removal of part of vas deferens, can be an elective procedure for sterilization or contraception
Women	
Cryosurgery	Use of subfreezing temperature to destroy tissue, especially in treatment of abnormal cells
Dilation and curettage	Dilation of uterus and scraping of endometrium, performed to diagnose disease of uterus, correct heavy or prolonged vaginal bleeding, or empty uterus of products of conception; also used in the treatment of infertility to correlate state of endometrium and time of cycle
Hysterectomy	Removal of uterus
Oophorectomy	Removal of one or both ovaries
Repair of cystocele	Correction of protrusion of urinary bladder through vaginal wall
Repair of rectocele	Correction of protrusion of rectum and posterior vaginal wall into vagina
Salpingectomy	Removal of one or both fallopian tubes
Tubal sterilization	Ligation of fallopian tubes

traceptive use. Anemia is also relevant to women's reproductive health. Anemia can result from or be aggravated by menstrual flow. Fear of painful intercourse can occur in women because of the physiologic changes of vaginal atrophy and decreased vaginal lubrication.

A history of a stroke (cerebrovascular accident [CVA]) should be determined. In men, strokes may cause physiologic or psychologic impotence. Men who have suffered heart attacks frequently experience impotence. This impotence is often caused by the fear of precipitating another heart attack as a result of the increased heart rate associated with sexual activity. This same concern is shared by the woman both as a partner and as the person recovering from a heart attack. The interviewer must be sensitive to this concern. Questions asked about the original cardiac event may elicit fear and thus indicate a need for counseling and support regarding safe sexual practices related to cardiac health.

Questions relating to endocrine disorders, particularly hypothyroidism and hyperthyroidism, must also be asked because these disorders directly interfere with women's menstrual cycles and with sexual performance in men. Finally, men and women should be assessed for kidney and urinary tract disorders because sexual functioning and reproductive capacity can be affected by genitourinary problems. When taking a sexual or reproductive history, it is helpful to begin with the least sensitive information (e.g., menstrual history) before asking questions regarding more sensitive issues such as sexual practices or sexually transmitted diseases.

Medications. A pharmacologic profile of prescribed and over-the-counter drugs is necessary for all patients. Particularly relevant in assessment of the reproductive system is the use of diuretics (sometimes prescribed for premenstrual edema), psychotropic agents (which may interfere with sexual performance), and antihypertensives (some of which have been implicated in impotence). Thus patients who use drugs such as methyldopa (Aldomet), clonidine (Catapres), guanethidine (Ismelin), and hydralazine (Apresoline) must be closely assessed for these problems. All drugs taken by female patients should be evaluated for possible teratogenic effects in women of childbearing age.

In women, the use of oral contraceptives or other hormones should be noted. The use of estrogen replacement therapy is relevant for women because of its effect on the prevention of osteoporosis and coronary artery disease. Recent data suggest that estrogen may also have beneficial effects on memory and cognitive function in older women.[8] In women with a uterus, the concurrent use of a progestational agent should be documented. The use of estrogen alone has been shown to increase the incidence of endometrial cancer. The nurse must also note the use of drugs such as alcohol, marijuana, barbiturates, amphetamines, and phencyclidine hydrochloride (PCP), or "angel dust," which can have serious behavioral or physiologic effects on the functioning of the reproductive system.

Oral contraceptive use can aggravate the symptoms of certain neurologic dysfunctions, such as seizures or migraine headaches. However, the use of lower doses in current contraceptives makes these side effects less problematic. A history of cholecystitis and hepatitis is important information because these conditions may be contraindications for oral contraceptives; cholecystitis is often aggravated by oral contraceptives, and chronic active inflammation of the liver generally precludes the use of estrogen products because they are metabolized by the liver. Other contraindications to oral contraceptive use may be chronic obstructive pulmonary disease because progesterone thickens respiratory secretions.

Surgery or other treatments. Any hospitalizations or surgeries should be noted in the health history. In particular, certain types of surgeries should be noted (Table 48-7). Therapeutic or spontaneous pregnancy interruptions are also documented at this time.

HEALTH HISTORY

Table 48-8 Reproductive System

Health Perception–Health Management
- Have you had or been immunized for rubella?
- Are you currently attempting to become pregnant?
- Explain how you examine your breasts (testes).
- When was your last mammogram? Pap smear? Rectal exam? What were the results?
- Do you have any chronic illnesses such as diabetes?
- Do you have any vaginal or urethral discharge?
- What is "safe sex"?
- Do you protect yourself from unwanted pregnancy, HIV, and sexually transmitted diseases? How?

Nutritional-Metabolic
- Have you ever been told you were anemic?
- Do you think you get enough calcium in your diet? What calcium-rich foods do you eat regularly? Do you take a calcium supplement?
- What is your average daily caloric intake? (For pregnant, lactating, obese, or underweight patients)
- How do you feel about your weight? Would you like to be thinner/heavier? Are you on a diet currently?

Elimination
- Do you have any problems with urination? Bowel movements?
- Have you ever had a bladder infection? If so, when? How often does this problem occur? Does anything make it better?
- Do you use laxatives? How often? Have you ever made yourself vomit after eating?

Activity-Exercise
- Tell me what activities you typically do each day.
- Can you dress yourself? Feed yourself? Walk without help?

Cognitive-Perceptual
- Do you have any problems with your balance?
- Are you having any pain in your private parts?
- Do you have pain during sexual activity or intercourse?
- Are you forgetful at times?

Self-Perception–Self-Concept
- Has the problem in your reproductive system affected how you feel about yourself as a woman/man?
- Tell me how your problem has affected your sex life.

Role-Relationship
- What effect has your reproductive problem/pregnancy had on your work, family, or social life?
- Are you experiencing any role-associated problems in your family?*

Sexuality-Reproductive
- Are you satisfied with your present means of sexual expression? If no, explain.
- Have you had any recent changes in your sexual practices?
- Does your problem of your reproductive system affect your ability to have a satisfactory sex life?

Coping–Stress Tolerance
- What is stressful in your life right now?
- How do you handle your health problem(s)?
- Whom do you go to for support? Does this help?

Value-Belief
- What do you believe about your health problem(s)?
- Does your medical treatment contradict your personal beliefs?
- Do you use home remedies? What are they?
- Have you been seen by a homeopath, naturopath, or chiropractor?

Note: Some questions apply only to a woman or a man.
*If yes, describe.
HIV, human immunodeficiency virus

Functional Health Patterns. The key questions to ask a patient with a reproductive problem are presented in Table 48-8.

Health perception–health management pattern. The patient's sexual and contraceptive practices are important aspects of health management (Table 48-9). The patient's knowledge of safe sexual practices should be determined. Exposure to environmental toxins and sexually transmitted diseases can adversely affect fertility and reproductive health. Monthly breast self-examination (BSE), mammography according to age-specific guidelines, and routine Pap smears are integral to a woman's health. Testicular self-examination (TSE) should be practiced by all men, starting in adolescence. Prostate examination should be done annually by a health care professional for all men over age 40.

Initial questions asked of the female patient usually refer to the breast. The nurse asks the patient whether she performs a monthly BSE (see Chapter 49). If a lump is present, its onset, size, and consistency should be noted. The nurse also asks whether there has been an increase or a decrease in the size and shape of the lump since its onset or discovery. The patient is also questioned about breast pain or tenderness. She should describe the degree and severity of pain; breast pain or tenderness is not usually present with a malignant mass, particularly in the early stages.

The nurse should also inquire about a history of breast cancer in a woman's mother, maternal aunt, or sister because such a history increases the patient's risk of developing breast cancer. A family history of cancer, particularly cancer of the reproduc-

Table 48-9 Sexual History Format

How long have you been sexually active?
How frequently do you have penile-vaginal intercourse?
How frequently do you masturbate?
How many sexual partners do you have?
What is your sexual preference?
How frequently do you have oral sex?
How frequently do you have rectal intercourse?
Have you ever had an STD? If yes, what?
Are you using a contraceptive method? If yes, what kind? How often? Is it satisfactory?
Do you consider your sex life satisfactory?
How often have you experienced impotence or difficulty with vaginal lubrication or pain with intercourse?
Has your sex life changed? If yes, how?
Would you like to see your sex life change? If yes, how?
How would your partner rate your sex life?

STD, sexually transmitted disease.

tive organs, is important information related to health counseling. Determination of a familial tendency for diabetes mellitus, hypothyroidism, hyperthyroidism, hypertension, stroke, angina, myocardial infarction, endocrine disorders, or anemia is also important.

The nurse must determine if the patient is allergic to sulfonamides, penicillin, rubber, or latex. Sulfonamides and penicillin are used frequently in the treatment of reproductive and genitourinary problems such as vaginitis and gonorrhea. Rubber or latex are commonly used in diaphragms and condoms. An allergy to these substances precludes their use as contraceptive methods.

Assessment of the reproductive system is incomplete without a knowledge of the patient's lifestyle choices. The nurse should know whether a woman uses cigarettes, alcohol, caffeine, or other drugs because these substances can be detrimental to both mother and fetus. Cigarette smoking may delay conception. Maternal smoking during pregnancy may result in an infant of low birth weight and increases the risk of spontaneous abortion, fetal death, neonatal death, and sudden infant death syndrome (SIDS). Cigarette smoking can increase the risk of morbidity in women using contraceptives and is associated with early menopause. These substances may also adversely affect the sperm count in men and cause impotence or decreased libido.

Nutritional-metabolic pattern. Anemia is a common problem in women in their reproductive years, particularly during pregnancy and the postpartum period. The adequacy of the diet should be evaluated with this problem in mind. Women should be encouraged to gain adequate but not excessive weight during pregnancy. The nurse should determine whether specific dietary recommendations from the health care provider are being followed throughout pregnancy.

A thorough nutritional and psychologic history should be taken to assess for the presence of an eating disorder. Anorexia can cause amenorrhea and the subsequent problems, such as osteoporosis, that are related to estrogen cessation. The nurse has the opportunity to help prevent the debilitating condition of osteoporosis. From early adolescence, women can be counseled regarding adequate calcium intake and the role of calcium in the prevention of osteoporosis. The patient's daily calcium intake should be estimated to determine whether there is a need for supplementation. Folic acid intake for women in their reproductive years should be evaluated because a deficiency can result in spina bifida and other neural tube defects in the fetus.[9,10]

Elimination pattern. Many gynecologic problems can result in genitourinary problems. Stress and urge incontinence are common in older women because of relaxation of the pelvic musculature caused by multiple births or advancing age. Vaginal infections predispose patients to chronic or recurrent urinary tract infections. The proximity of the reproductive organs and the genitourinary tract make metastasis of malignant tumors to this site a possibility to be considered. Benign prostatic hyperplasia is a common problem of aging in men. It can impede normal urination, causing retention and difficulty in initiating the stream.

Activity-exercise pattern. Weight-bearing exercise decreases the risk of osteoporosis in women. The amount, type, and intensity of exercise should be documented. Lack of stress on bones, secondary to lack of exercise, is an important factor in the development of osteoporosis. Anemia, secondary to menorrhagia, can result in fatigue and activity intolerance and can interfere with satisfactory performance of the activities of daily living. Exercise should be encouraged during pregnancy, following guidelines regarding the type of exercise, the intensity, and the frequency of workouts.

Sleep-rest pattern. Sleep disturbances occur during pregnancy because of nocturia and the woman's inability to find a comfortable sleeping position. Sleep patterns may be affected during the postpartum period and also while raising young children. The hot flashes and sweating often present during the perimenopause can cause serious sleep interruption when the woman is awakened in a drenching sweat. The need to change her nightgown and bedding further disrupts her sleep. Insomnia is also a common complaint of perimenopausal women. Daytime fatigue often results from such nighttime awakenings.

Cognitive-perceptual pattern. Changes in balance and sensory perception accompany normal pregnancy. Aches and pains during gestation are caused by stretching of muscles and ligaments to accommodate the growing fetus. Pelvic pain is associated with various gynecologic disorders such as pelvic inflammatory disease, ovarian cysts, and endometriosis.

Reproduction and sexual issues are often considered highly personal and private and are not easily discussed by many patients. The nurse must strive to develop trust and must maintain a professional demeanor when eliciting a reproductive history.

Dyspareunia (painful intercourse) can be particularly problematic for a woman. The pain associated with intercourse can make her reluctant to participate in sexual activity and strain her relationship with her sexual partner. The woman should be referred to her health care provider if dyspareunia is present.

Self-perception–self-concept pattern. For both men and women, there may be body image changes associated with developmental changes. Menarche and puberty herald the appearance of secondary sexual characteristics, which may result in either pride or embarrassment. Adolescent problems related to body image include acne, myopia, obesity, anorexia nervosa, bulimia, and scoliosis.

Pregnancy may affect a woman's body image in a negative way as her size increases and her functional abilities decrease. Changes in body shape become more threatening to the woman as the pregnancy progresses.

The reproductive changes of aging such as pendulous breasts and vaginal dryness in women and decreased size of the penis in men may lead to emotional distress. The subtle changes associated with sexuality and advancing age may challenge the self-concept of many persons.

Role-relationship pattern. The addition of a new baby into the family may change family dynamics. Indeed, one maternal task is to integrate the new member of the household into the family.

The changes occurring during adolescence and the need to challenge parental authority may lead to stress among family members. Conflicts that arise during the adolescent's quest for identity can add further tension. Risk-taking behaviors, such as smoking and substance abuse on the part of the adolescent, are often symptomatic of the problem.

As the years go by, role relationship patterns change as children begin their careers and move away from home. This again rearranges the family configuration.

The nurse seeks information about the type of family to which the patient belongs. Questions regarding recent changes or family conflicts should be asked. It is important to ascertain the patient's role in the family as a starting point in determining family dynamics.

A thorough health history also includes information about the patient's occupation and potential hazards associated with it. For example, exposure to toxic chemicals can affect sexual functioning and reproductive capacity.

Sexuality-reproductive pattern. The extent and depth of the interview about a patient's sexuality depend primarily on the expertise of the interviewer and on the needs and the willingness of the patient. Before taking a sexual history, interviewers should assess their comfort with their own sexuality, because any discomfort in questioning becomes obvious to the patient. Interviews must be carried out in an environment that provides reassurance, confidentiality, and a nonjudgmental attitude. It is best to begin with the least sensitive areas and then move to more sensitive areas. For this reason, sexual histories are frequently initiated during the review of the genitourinary and gynecologic systems. Early questioning can relate to menstruation, the onset of puberty, and the presence or absence of symptoms of genitourinary problems. These questions thus serve as an introduction for both the care provider and the patient before they move into more sensitive areas. Questions about sexuality should always be asked in a straightforward and nonjudgmental manner. Table 48-9 outlines questions appropriate for an initial assessment or annual examination. Both men and women should be asked about their general satisfaction with sexuality. Indications of sexual dysfunction may require referral or consultation with a sex counselor. A thorough genitourinary history must also be collected for the assessment of the reproductive system to be complete.

Problems of the reproductive system can cause physiologic or psychologic problems that can lead to painful intercourse, impotence, sexual dysfunction, or infertility. Both the cause and the effect of such problems should be determined.

The patient should be questioned about sexual beliefs and practices and whether orgasm is achieved. The patient's satisfaction with the opportunities for sexual gratification is important information that should be elicited. Any unexplained change in sexual practices or performance should be explored. This is an appropriate time to discuss methods of birth control and safe sex.

Menstrual history data are used in the detection of pregnancy, infertility, and numerous other gynecologic concerns. Changes in the usual menstrual pattern must be explicitly described to determine whether the change is transient and unimportant or connected with a more serious gynecologic problem. Metrorrhagia (spotting or bleeding between menstruations), menorrhagia (excessive menstrual bleeding), amenorrhea (lack of menstruation), and postcoital bleeding are examples of such problems. Changes in menstrual patterns associated with the use of contraceptive pills, intrauterine devices (IUDs), subdermal estrogen-only implant (Norplant), or medroxyprogesterone (Depo-Provera) injections must be identified. Contraceptive pills usually decrease the amount and duration of flow, whereas IUDs may cause an increase in the amount and duration. IUDs also frequently increase the severity of dysmenorrhea.

Patterns of sexual relationships also provide important information. A history of multiple sex partners increases the risk of contracting a sexually transmitted disease. For a woman, this can increase the risk of pelvic inflammatory disease, which can compromise her ability to become pregnant.

Coping–stress tolerance pattern. The stress related to situational or maturational crises such as pregnancy, menopause, or the climacteric may cause an increased dependence on support systems. It is essential for the nurse to ascertain who the support people are in the patient's life. The diagnosis of a sexually transmitted disease can cause stress to the patient and the partner. Means to manage such stress should be explored.

Value-belief pattern. Sexual and reproductive functioning is closely related to cultural, religious, moral, and ethical values. The nurse should be aware of his or her own beliefs in these areas and should recognize and sensitively react to the patient's personal beliefs associated with reproductive issues.

Objective Data

Physical Examination. The examination of the external genitalia uses inspection and palpation.

Male genitalia. An examination may be performed with the patient lying or standing. The standing position is generally preferred. The examiner should be seated in front of the standing patient. Gloves should be used during examination of the male genitalia.

Pubes. The nurse observes the diamond-shaped pattern of hair distribution. The absence of hair is not normal. The skin is also evaluated.

Penis. The nurse notes the size and skin texture of the penis and any lesions, scars, or swelling. The location of the urethral meatus, as well as the presence or absence of a foreskin, should be noted. If present, the foreskin should be retracted to note cleanliness and replaced over the glans after observation. The glans are compressed to note any discharge and its amount, color, and odor if present. The nurse also palpates the penile shaft for tenderness or masses and observes the ventral and dorsal aspects.

Scrotum and testes. The nurse performs a complete skin examination by lifting each testis to inspect all sides of the scrotal sac. Palpation of the scrotum is done to note changes in consistency or the presence of masses. It is important to note if the testes are descended. The left testis usually hangs lower than the right. Undescended testis is a major risk factor for testicular cancer, as well as a potential cause of male infertility. The patient should also be taught TSE (see Chapter 52).

Inguinal region and spermatic cord. The examiner inspects the inguinal regions for rashes, lesions, or lymphadenopathy, which may suggest pelvic organ infection. The nurse has the patient cough or bear down and notes any conspicuous bulging in the inguinal canals. The nurse also palpates the area for any bulging as the patient again coughs or bears down. The nurse palpates the inguinal and femoral pulses and the local lymph nodes.

The spermatic cord is located posteriorly in the scrotal sac. The nurse follows the cord on each side. The inguinal region is gently palpated using the forefinger or small finger and by pushing up through the loose scrotal skin to the abdominal wall along the inguinal region. The internal inguinal ring meets and impedes the finger. At this point, the patient again bears down and coughs. The nurse determines whether the strain produces a bulging of the intestines through the ring, indicating the presence of a hernia, a condition that requires follow-up.

Anus and prostate. The anal sphincter and perineal regions are inspected for lesions, masses, and hemorrhoids. A digital examination is required for all patients who have symptoms of prostate trouble, such as difficulty in initiating the flow and the urge to void frequently; this examination should be performed annually for all men over 40 years of age.

Female breasts and external genitalia. Physical examination of women often begins with inspection and palpation of the breasts and then proceeds to the abdomen. Examination of the abdomen provides an opportunity to detect pain or any masses that may involve the genitourinary system.

Breasts. Breasts are examined first by visual inspection. The nurse, with the patient seated, observes the breasts for symmetry, size, shape, skin color and texture, vascular patterns, and the presence of unusual lesions. The patient is asked to put her arms at her sides, arms overhead, lean forward, and press hands on hips. The nurse observes for any abnormalities during these maneuvers. The axillae and the clavicular areas are then palpated for enlarged lymph nodes.

After the patient assumes a supine position, a pillow is placed under the back on the side to be examined. The patient is asked to put the arm above and behind the head. These maneuvers flatten breast tissue and make palpation easier. The breast is then palpated in a systematic fashion using a vertical line, a clockwise, or a spoke approach. The nurse should use the distal finger pads for palpation. The tail of Spence should be included in the examination because this area and the upper outer quadrant are the areas where most breast malignancies develop.

Finally, the nurse should palpate the area around the areolae for masses. The nipple should be compressed to determine the presence of discharge or any masses. The color, consistency, and odor of any discharge should be documented.

External genitalia. The nurse uses gloves for examination of the external genitalia. The mons pubis, the labia majora, the labia minora, the perineum, and the anal region are inspected for characteristics of skin, hair distribution, and contour. Lesions, swelling, and discharge are noted.

The nurse separates the labia to fully inspect the clitoris, the urethral meatus, the vaginal orifice, the hymen, the perineum, and the anal region. Any inflammation or cysts on Bartholin's glands or Skene's glands are noted.

Internal pelvic examination. During the speculum examination, the nurse observes the walls of the vagina and the cervix for inflammation, discharge, polyps, and suspicious growths. During this examination, it is possible to take a Pap smear and collect secretions for culture and study under the microscope (i.e., wet smears).

After the speculum examination, a bimanual examination is performed to allow assessment of the size, shape, and consistency of the uterus, ovaries, and tubes. The tubes are not normally palpable. Details of the pelvic and bimanual examinations are described in physical assessment textbooks. Because these skills are not usually within the scope of the nurse generalist, they are not described here.

Table 48-10 illustrates a recording format for the physical assessment findings of the male and female reproductive

Table 48-10 Recording the Normal Physical Assessment of the Reproductive System

Male	Female
Penis and Scrotum	**Breasts**
Diamond-shaped hair distribution	Symmetric or slightly asymmetric
Testes	Nipples everted
Descended bilaterally	No nipple discharge
3 cm wide, 4.5 cm long	No dimpling or retraction
Smooth, firm	No masses, lesions, or tenderness
Skin	No axillary nodes
No lesions, redness, swelling, masses, or inflammation	Appropriate for age and parity
Circumcised penis	**Vulva**
Meatus patent, no discharge	Triangular hair distribution
No masses, slight tenderness	No lesions, redness, swelling, masses, or inflammation
No inguinal hernias	Patent vaginal orifice, no discharge
Epididymis	Nonpalpable Skene's ducts and Bartholin's glands, no tenderness
Nontender	Intact clitoris and urethral meatus
No masses	
Rectum	
No hemorrhoids	

COMMON ASSESSMENT ABNORMALITIES

Table 48-11 Breast

Finding	Description	Possible Etiology and Significance
▪ Nipple inversion or retraction	Recent onset, erythematous, pain, unilateral	Abscess, inflammation, cancer
	Recent onset (usually within past year), unilateral presentation, lack of tenderness	Neoplasm
▪ Nipple secretions		
Galactorrhea (female)	Milky, no relationship to lactation, unilateral or bilateral or intermittent or consistent presentation	Drug therapy, particularly phenothiazines, tricyclic antidepressants, methyldopa; hypofunction or hyperfunction of thyroid or adrenal glands; tumors of hypothalamus or pituitary gland; excessive estrogen; prolonged suckling or breast foreplay
Galactorrhea (male)	Milky, bilateral presentation	Chorioepithelioma of testes
Purulent	Gray-green or yellow color; frequent unilateral presentation; association with pain, erythema, induration, nipple inversion	Puerperal (after birth) mastitis (inflammatory condition of breast) or abscess
	Same as above but usually without nipple inversion	Infected sebaceous cyst
Serous discharge	Clear appearance, unilateral or bilateral or intermittent or consistent presentation	Intraductal papilloma
Dark green or multicolored discharge	Thick, sticky, and frequently bilateral	Mammary duct ectasia (dilation of mammary ducts)
Serosanguineous or bloody drainage	Unilateral presentation	Papillomatosis (widespread development of nipplelike growths), intraductal papilloma, carcinoma (male and female)
▪ Scaling or irritation of nipple	Unilateral or bilateral presentation, crusting, possible ulceration	Paget's disease, eczema, infection
▪ Nodules, lumps, or masses	Multiple, bilateral, well-delineated, soft or firm, mobile cysts; pain; premenstrual occurrence	Fibrocystic changes
	Rubbery consistency, fluid-filled interior, pain	Mammary duct ectasia
	Soft, mobile, well-delineated cyst, absence of pain	Lipoma, fibroadenoma
	Erythema, tenderness, induration	Infected sebaceous cysts, abscesses
	Usually singular, hard irregularly shaped, poorly delineated, nonmobile	Neoplasm

systems. Tables 48-11 through 48-13 summarize common assessment abnormalities of the breasts, the female reproductive system, and the male reproductive system, respectively.

DIAGNOSTIC STUDIES OF THE REPRODUCTIVE SYSTEM

Many diagnostic tests that are performed to assess problems occurring in other body systems also provide valuable data on the condition of the reproductive system. Table 48-14 summarizes the most commonly used diagnostic studies in the assessment of the reproductive system and the nurse's responsibility regarding these diagnostic tests.[11,12]

To understand many of the diagnostic studies of the reproductive system, it is important to understand the concepts of sensitivity and specificity. *Sensitivity* addresses the issue of how well a test identifies people with a particular disease. The goal of sensitivity testing is to avoid the occurrence of false-negative results, that is, to avoid saying that someone does not have a particular health problem when, in fact, the disease is present. It is considered a screening test. *Specificity* testing answers the question of how well a test eliminates those individuals without the disease. The goal of sensitivity testing is to avoid false-positive results. It is the nurse's responsibility to ensure that the patient understands the purpose of any test being performed.

Urine Studies

Pregnancy Testing. Occurrence of pregnancy is generally validated by measuring the output of human chorionic gonadotropin (hCG) in the urine by means of an immunologic test. A solution containing monoclonal antibodies specific for

COMMON ASSESSMENT ABNORMALITIES

Table 48-12 Female Reproductive System

Finding	Description	Possible Etiology and Significance
▪ Vulvar discharge	Plaquelike consistency, frequent itching and inflammation, lack of odor	Candidiasis (*Candida* or yeast infection), vaginitis
	Grayish color, copious flow, frothy appearance, vulvar irritation	Bacterial vaginosis infection
	Purulent odor, grayish-green or yellow color	*Trichomonas vaginalis*
	Bloody color	*Chlamydia trachomatis* or *Neisseria gonorrhoeae* infection, menstruation, trauma, cancer
▪ Vulvar erythema	Bright or beefy red color, itching	*Candida albicans,* allergy, chemical vaginitis
	Reddened base, painful vesicles or ulcerations	Genital herpes
	Macules or papules, itching	Chancroid (STD), contact dermatitis, scabies, pediculosis
▪ Vulvar growths	Soft, fleshy growth; nontender	Condyloma acuminatum
	Flat and warty appearance, nontender	Condyloma latum
	Same as either of above, possible pain	Neoplasm
	Reddened base, vesicles, and small erosions; pain	Lymphogranuloma venereum, genital herpes, chancroid
	Indurated, firm ulcers; lack of pain	Chancre (syphilis), granuloma inguinale
▪ Abdominal pain or tenderness	Intermittent or consistent tenderness in right or left lower quadrant	Salpingitis (infection of fallopian tube), ectopic pregnancy, ruptured ovarian cyst, PID, tubal or ovarian abscess
	Periumbilical location, consistent occurrence	Cystitis, endometritis (inflammation of endometrium), ectopic pregnancy

PID, pelvic inflammatory disease.

hCG is mixed with a small amount of urine. The presence of hCG causes a change in color of the tested urine. To reduce cross-reactivity with LH and other pituitary hormones, the beta subunit of hCG is measured.

Home pregnancy test kits use the same assay principle described in the preceding paragraph. Positive results are based on the presence of hCG in urine. Some tests can detect pregnancy as early as the first day after the expected period. These tests are 97% accurate, but a negative test should be repeated in 2 weeks to achieve the greatest accuracy.[13] Serum pregnancy tests have also been developed, and they are almost 100% accurate.

Hormone Studies. Although estrogen studies are performed on urine, the results are frequently inaccurate because of variable estrogen levels during the normal cycle and the difficulty in estimating the day of the cycle in women with irregular menses. Adrenal androgens are precursors of estrogens and can be measured in the urine of both men and women. FSH can be measured in a 24-hour urine specimen. Increased and decreased FSH levels can indicate gonad failure resulting from pituitary dysfunction.

Blood Studies

Recently, serum pregnancy tests using radioimmunoassays have been developed. One test, a radioimmunoassay for the beta subunit of hCG, is so sensitive that a pregnancy can be detected before a woman misses her menstrual period.

The prolactin assay is used primarily in the workup of a patient with amenorrhea. High levels of prolactin are normally associated with low levels of estrogen, such as those that occur during lactation. However, the same finding can occur with pituitary adenomas, especially with otherwise unexplained galactorrhea.

Serum progesterone and estradiol are sometimes tested in ovarian function assessment, particularly for amenorrhea. In addition, hormonal blood studies are essential components of a thorough fertility workup.

Biologic tumor markers are often secreted by germinal cell cancers of the testis. The two most common markers are alphafetoprotein (AFP) and hCG. Measurement of these markers is useful in monitoring therapy (marker levels rise as disease progresses and fall with disease regression) because marker levels may rise months before new disease or metastasis is evident.

Syphilis Studies

The types of tests performed to diagnose syphilis can be classified as nontreponemal or treponemal. Nontreponemal tests such as the Venereal Disease Research Laboratory (VDRL) test and the rapid plasma reagin (RPR) test are inexpensive and reliable but have high levels of false-positive results (i.e., good sensitivity but poor specificity). These tests detect the presence of antibodies in the serum of infected patients. Nonspecific antibodies can be produced during many pathologic processes, especially some types of autoimmune diseases, and can yield false-positive test results.

Treponemal tests such as the fluorescent treponemal antibody absorption (FTAAbs) test are highly reliable and should be used after a positive nontreponemal test, even if it is weakly positive or questionable. This test measures specific antibodies to *Treponema pallidum.* The FTAAbs test does not assess the

COMMON ASSESSMENT ABNORMALITIES

Table 48-13 Male Reproductive System

Finding	Description	Possible Etiology and Significance
▪ Penile growths or masses	Indurated, smooth, disklike appearance; absence of pain; singular presentation	Chancre
	Papular to irregularly shaped ulceration with pus, lack of induration	Chancroid
	Ulceration with induration and nodularity	Cancer
	Flat, wartlike nodule	Condyloma latum
	Elevated, fleshy, moist, elongated projections with single or multiple projections	Condyloma acuminatum
	Localized swelling with retracted, tight foreskin	Paraphimosis (inability to replace foreskin to its normal position after retraction), trauma
▪ Vesicles, erosions, or ulcers	Painful, erythematous base; vesicular or small erosions	Genital herpes, balanitis (inflammation of glans penis), chancroid
	Painless, singular, small erosion with eventual lymphadenopathy	Lymphogranuloma venereum, cancer
▪ Scrotal masses	Localized swelling with tenderness, unilateral or bilateral presentation	Epididymitis (inflammation of epididymis), testicular torsion, orchitis (mumps)
	Swelling, tenderness	Incarcerated hernia
	Unilateral or bilateral presentation; swelling without pain; translucent, cordlike or wormlike appearance	Hydrocele (accumulation of fluid in outer covering of testes), spermatocele (firm, sperm-containing cyst of epididymis), varicocele (dilation of veins that drain testes), hematocele (accumulation of blood within scrotum)
	Firm, nodular testes or epididymis; frequent unilateral presentation	Tuberculosis, cancer
▪ Penile discharge	Clear to purulent color, minimal to copious flow	Urethritis or gonorrhea, *Chlamydia trachomatis* infection, trauma
▪ Penile or scrotal erythema	Macules and papules	Scabies, pediculosis
▪ Inguinal masses	Bulging, unilateral presentation during straining	Inguinal hernia
	Shotty, 1-3 cm nodules	Lymphadenopathy

adequacy of treatment of syphilis; the test remains reactive even after treatment. Antibody titers obtained with a VDRL test are used to measure the adequacy of therapy.

The most specific and direct examination for syphilis is dark-field microscopy of a specimen obtained from a potential syphilitic lesion (chancre). Unfortunately, the chancre is frequently gone by the time other symptoms occur, so the test cannot be performed. Other miscellaneous tests of secretions involve wet mounts, cultures, and stains to detect specific reproductive problems (see Table 48-14).

Cytologic Studies

The Pap smear is a screening test to detect abnormal cells obtained from the cervix, vagina, or nipple. It is performed by obtaining cells from the cervical canal, preferably the endocervix, as well as from the vagina, and placing these cells in a fixative for examination by a cytologist for cellular abnormalities. Pap smears are more accurate if performed at midcycle or during the secretory phase of the menstrual cycle because there is a greater likelihood that abnormal cells will be detected during these times. A Pap smear should be performed annually or more frequently in women with a history of dysplasia or exposure to DES. Pap smears are necessary in women who have had a hysterectomy because abnormal vaginal cells can sometimes be detected.

Although a Pap smear is highly accurate in detecting cervical cancer, a negative Pap test does not rule out endometrial cancer. Specific tests are available to obtain a smear directly from the endometrium. Uterine aspiration and cannulation into the uterine cavity make it possible to obtain endometrial tissue. Cytologic studies are also performed on any nipple discharge.

Radiologic Studies

Mammography has become one of the most frequently used diagnostic tools in reproductive system assessment (see Chapter 49). Unfortunately, its frequent use has been highly criticized because of the potential risks of radiation. However, increased awareness of the risks from radiographic studies has resulted in valuable improvements in the technique of mammography, particularly in lowering the exposure per examination. The American Cancer Society recommends that a screening mammogram be performed every 1 to 2 years for women between the ages of 40 and 49 and yearly after age 50.[14]

DIAGNOSTIC STUDIES

Table 48-14 Male and Female Reproductive Systems

Study	Description and Purpose	Nursing Responsibility
Urine Studies		
▪ Pregnancy testing	hCG is detected in urine to ascertain whether a woman is pregnant. Hydatidiform mole and chorioepithelioma (in men and women) may also be detected.	Obtain thorough menstrual history from patient, including birth control methods. Determine presence or absence of presumptive signs of pregnancy (e.g., breast changes or increased whitish vaginal discharge).
▪ Hormone testing		
Testosterone levels	Tumors and developmental anomalies of the testes can be detected.	Instruct patient to collect 24-hr urine specimen. Keep it refrigerated.
Follicle-stimulating hormone (FSH) assay	Test indicates gonadal failure because of pituitary dysfunction. Female: Follicular phrase: 2-5 IU/24 hr Midcycle: 8-40 IU/24 hr Luteal phase: 2-10 IU/24 hr Menopause: 35-100 IU/24 hr Male: 2-15 IU/24 hr	Instruct patient to collect 24-hr urine specimen. Indicate phase of menstrual cycle, if menopausal, and if on oral contraceptives or hormones.
Blood Studies		
▪ Prolactin assay	This test detects pituitary dysfunction that can cause amenorrhea.	Observe venipuncture site for bleeding or hematoma formation.
▪ Serum hCG assay	hCG is detected in serum to ascertain whether a woman is pregnant (see entry on pregnancy testing).	Instruct patient to have blood drawn in laboratory. Elicit where she is in her menstrual cycle, whether she has missed menses, and if so, how late she is.
▪ Serum androstenedione and testosterone levels	These tests ascertain whether elevated androgens are due to adrenal or ovarian dysfunction. Serum testosterone is also drawn to assess cause of amenorrhea.	Collect health history to eliminate potential sources of interference with accuracy of results (e.g., use of steroids or barbiturates or presence of hypothyroidism or hyperthyroidism).
▪ Serum progesterone	This test is frequently used to detect functioning corpus luteum cyst.	Observe venipuncture site for bleeding or hematoma formation. Include last menstrual period and trimester of pregnancy since progesterone levels vary with gestation.
▪ Serum estradiol	This test measures ovarian function. It is particularly useful in assessing estrogen-secreting tumors and states of precocious female puberty. Normal values depend on laboratory that performs test and should be obtained from that laboratory. May be used to confirm perimenopausal time. Increased serum estradiol levels in men may be indicative of testicular tumors.	Observe venipuncture site for bleeding or hematoma formation.
▪ Serum FSH	This test indicates gonadal failure due to pituitary dysfunction; used to validate menopause. Female: Follicular phase: 4-30 mIU/ml Midcycle: 10-90 mIU/ml Luteal phase: 4-30 mIU/ml Menopause: 40-250 mIU/ml Male: 4-25 mIU/ml	No food or fluid restrictions required. State phase of menstrual cycle, if menopausal, or if on oral contraceptive or hormones

Continued

DIAGNOSTIC STUDIES

Table 48-14 Male and Female Reproductive Systems—cont'd

Study	Description and Purpose	Nursing Responsibility
Syphilis Studies		
▪ Nontreponemal serologic tests: Wassermann (complement fixation) Venereal Disease Research Laboratory (VDRL) (flocculation) Rapid plasma reagin (RPR) (agglutination)	These tests are nonspecific antibody tests used to screen for syphilis. Positive readings can be made within 1-2 wk after appearance of primary lesion (chancre) or 4-15 wk after initial infection.	Tell the patient that fasting is unnecessary. Inform patient that blood sample will be drawn. Observe venipuncture site for bleeding or hematoma formation. Obtain data to determine presence or absence of problems such as hepatitis, pregnancy, and autoimmune diseases that may interfere with the accuracy of results.
▪ Treponemal test Fluorescent treponemal antibody absorption (FTAAbs)	This test detects syphilis antibodies. It also detects early syphilis with great accuracy. It is usually performed if results of nontreponemal testing are questionable.	Tell the patient that fasting is unnecessary. Inform patient that blood sample will be drawn. Observe venipuncture site for bleeding or hematoma formation.
Miscellaneous Studies		
▪ Dark-field microscopy	Direct examination of specimen obtained from potential syphilitic lesion (chancre) is performed to detect treponema.	Avoid direct skin contact with open lesion.
▪ Wet mounts	Direct microscopic examination of specimen of vaginal discharge is performed immediately after collection. This determines presence or absence and number of *Trichomonas* organisms, bacteria, white and red blood cells, and candidal buds or hyphae. Other clues or causes of inflammation or infection may be determined.	Explain procedure and purpose to patient. Instruct patient not to douche before examination. Prepare for collection of specimens (glass slide, 10-20% potassium hydroxide [KOH] solution, sodium chloride [NaCl] solution, and cotton-tipped applicators).
▪ Cultures	Culture of specimens of vaginal, urethral, or cervical discharge are taken and used to assess presence of gonorrhea or chlamydia. Rectal and throat cultures may also be taken, depending on data obtained from sexual history.	Obtain specific contact and sexual history inclusive of oral and rectal intercourse. Instruct against douching before examination. Obtain urethral specimen from men before they void. Instruct women who are sexually active with multiple partners to have at least a yearly culture for gonorrhea and chlamydia. Instruct sexually active men to have any discharge evaluated immediately to rule out gonorrhea strains that do not cause classic symptoms of dysuria.
▪ Gram's stain	This presumptive test is used for rapid detection of gonorrhea. Presence of gram-negative intracellular diplococci generally warrants initiation of treatment. Not highly accurate for women.	Same as above.
Cytologic Studies		
▪ Pap smear	Microscopic study of exfoliated cells via special staining and fixation technique detects abnormal cells. Cells most commonly studied are those obtained directly from endocervix, cervix, vaginal pool, and endometrial lining of uterine cavity.	Instruct women who are sexually active and who are over age 18 to have Pap smears according to American Cancer Society guidelines. Arrange for smear at midcycle time. Instruct patients not to douche for at least 24 hr before examination. Collect careful menstrual and gynecologic history.
▪ Nipple discharge test	Cytologic study of nipple discharge is performed.	Indicate whether hormonal preparations or other drugs are being taken, breastfeeding, or history of amenorrhea. Instruct patient during demonstration of breast self-examination or examination of breasts that nipple discharge should always be evaluated.

Continued

DIAGNOSTIC STUDIES

Table 48-14 Male and Female Reproductive Systems—cont'd

Study	Description and Purpose	Nursing Responsibility
Radiologic Studies		
▪ Soft tissue mammography	Low-dose x-ray image of breast tissue on photographic film is used to assess breast masses, recent breast enlargement, and nipple discharge to detect malignancy. It is usually an outpatient procedure.	Instruct patient about risks (radiation) and advantages of the examination. Instruct regarding American Cancer Society recommendations.
▪ Contrast mammography	This test is used to evaluate abnormal nipple discharge. It is particularly effective in detecting nonpalpable intraductal papillomas. Test consists of injection of radiopaque dye in breast duct.	Determine actual or possible allergy to contrast medium.
▪ Ultrasound	This test measures and records high-frequency sound waves as they pass through tissues of variable density. It is very useful in detecting masses greater than 3 cm, such as ectopic pregnancies, IUDs, ovarian cysts, and hydatidiform moles.	Instruct patient that a full bladder may be required depending on the reason for the study.
Invasive Procedures		
▪ Breast biopsy	Histologic examination of excised breast tissue is performed, either by needle-aspiration or excisional biopsy.	Before surgery, instruct patient about operative procedures and sedation. After surgery, perform wound care and instruct patient about breast self-examination.
▪ Hysterosalpingogram	This test involves instillation of radioscopic dye through cervix into uterine cavity and subsequently through and out fallopian tubes. Spot x-ray images are taken to detect abnormalities of uterus and its adnexa (ovaries and tubes) as dye progresses through them. Test may be most useful in diagnostic assessment of fertility (e.g., to detect adhesions near ovary, an abnormal uterine shape, or blockage of tubal pathways).	Inform patient about procedure and that it may be fairly uncomfortable, especially shoulder pain. Determine possibility of dye allergy.
▪ Colposcopy	Direct visualization of cervix with binocular microscope that allows magnification and study of cellular dysplasia and vascular and tissue abnormalities of cervix. This test is used as a follow-up study for abnormal Pap smears and for examination of women exposed to DES in utero. Biopsy of cervix may be taken during colposcopic examination. This test is valuable in decreasing number of false-negative cervical biopsies.	Instruct patient about this outpatient procedure. Inform patient that this examination is similar to speculum examination. Explain purpose of procedure and prepare patient for it.
▪ Conization	Cone-shaped sample of squamocolumnar tissue of cervix is removed for direct study.	Explain purpose and method of procedure and that it requires use of surgical facilities and anesthesia. Instruct patient to rest for at least 3 days after procedure. Also discuss necessity for 3-wk follow-up check.
▪ Loop electrosurgical excision of transformation zone (LEETZ)	Excision of cervical tissue via an electrosurgical instrument.	Explain purpose and method of procedure and that it may be done in the physician's office for further diagnostic testing.
▪ Loop electrosurgical excision procedure (LEEP)	Same as above.	Same as above.

Continued

DIAGNOSTIC STUDIES

Table 48-14 Male and Female Reproductive Systems—cont'd

Study	Description and Purpose	Nursing Responsibility
Operative Procedures—cont'd		
■ Culdotomy, culdoscopy, and culdocentesis	Culdotomy is an incision made through posterior fornix of cul-de-sac and allows visualization of peritoneal cavity (i.e., uterus, tubes, and ovaries). Culdoscope can then be used to study these structures closely. This technique is valuable in fertility evaluations. Withdrawal of fluid (culdocentesis) allows examination of fluid characteristics.	Explain purpose and method of procedure. Prepare patient for vaginal operation with preoperative instruction and sedation. Perform assessment of bleeding and discomfort after surgery.
■ Laparoscopy (peritoneoscopy)	This method of entry into the abdomen allows visualization of pelvic structures via fiberoptic scopes inserted through small abdominal incisions. Instillation of carbon dioxide into cavity improves visualization. This technique is used in diagnostic assessment of uterus, tubes, and ovaries. Can be used in conjunction with tubal sterilization.	Explain purpose and method of procedure. Before surgery, instruct patient about procedure, prepare abdomen, and reassure patient about sedation. Tell patient to rest for 1-3 days after surgery. Inform patient of probability of shoulder pain because of air in the abdomen.
■ Dilation and curettage	The operative procedure dilates cervix and allows curetting of endometrial lining. This test is used in assessment of abnormal bleeding patterns and cytologic evaluation of lining.	Before surgery, instruct patient about procedure and sedation. Tell patient that overnight hospitalization is occasionally required. Perform postoperative assessment of degree of bleeding (frequent pad check during first 24 hr).
Fertility Studies		
■ Semen analysis	Semen is assessed for volume (2-5 ml), viscosity, sperm count (>20 million/ml), sperm motility (60% motile), and percent of abnormal sperm (60% with normal structure).	Instruct patient to bring in fresh specimen within 2 hr after ejaculation.
■ Basal body temperature assessment	This measurement indicates indirectly whether ovulation has occurred. (Temperature rises at ovulation and remains elevated during secretory phase of normal menstrual cycle.)	Instruct woman to take her temperature using special basal temperature thermometer (calibrated in tenths of degrees) every morning before getting out of bed. Tell woman to record temperature on graph.
■ Huhner test or Sims-Huhner	Mucus sample of cervix is examined within 2-8 hr after intercourse. Total number of sperm is assessed in relation to number of live sperm. This test is performed to determine whether cervical mucus is "hostile" to passage of sperm from vagina into uterus.	Instruct couples to have intercourse at estimated time of ovulation and be present for test within 2-8 hr after intercourse.
■ Endometrial biopsy	In this outpatient procedure, small curette is used to obtain piece of endometrial lining to assess endometrial changes common to progesterone secretion after ovulation.	Tell patient that test must be performed postovulation. Explain that procedure should cause only short period of uterine cramping.
■ Hysterosalpingogram	Same as operative procedures.	Same as operative procedures.
■ Serum progesterone	Same as blood studies.	Same as blood studies.

DES, diethylstilbestrol; *hCG*, human chorionic gonadotropin; *IUDs*, intrauterine device

REVIEW QUESTIONS

The number of the question corresponds to the same-numbered objective at the beginning of the chapter.

1. A normal reproductive function that may be altered in a patient who undergoes a prostatectomy is
   a. sperm production.
   b. production of testosterone.
   c. production of seminal fluid.
   d. release of sperm from the epididymis.
2. Estrogen production by the mature ovarian follicle causes
   a. decreased secretion of FSH and LH.
   b. increased production of GnRH and FSH.
   c. release of GnRH and increased secretion of LH.
   d. decreased release of FSH and decreased progesterone production.
3. Female orgasm is the result of
   a. clitoral swelling and increased vaginal lubrication.
   b. vaginal enlargement and secretion with penile insertion.

c. clitoral swelling, vaginal lubrication, and uterine elevation.
d. rapid release of vasocongestion and myotonia in the reproductive structures.

4. An age-related finding noted by the nurse during assessment of the older woman's reproductive system would include
   a. gynecomastia.
   b. presence of a cystocele.
   c. soft, nontender, fleshy vulvar lesions.
   d. soft, mobile, well-delineated cysts in the breast.
5. Significant data collection regarding past health history during assessment of male and female reproductive systems should include
   a. extent of sexual activity.
   b. general satisfaction with sexuality.
   c. self-image and relationships with others.
   d. in utero exposure to diethylstilbestrol (DES).
6. After age 40 every man should have an annual examination involving palpation of the
   a. testes.
   b. prostate.
   c. spermatic cord.
   d. inguinal canals.
7. An abnormal finding noted during physical assessment of the male reproductive system is
   a. slight clear urethral discharge.
   b. the glans covered with prepuce.
   c. rubbery feeling of the testes on palpation.
   d. urethral meatus on the ventral side of the glans.
8. The American Cancer Society's criteria for mammography include
   a. a baseline mammogram for all women at age 50.
   b. a yearly mammogram for women over age 50.
   c. mammography only when a discernible mass is found.
   d. a mammogram every 1 to 2 years for women over age 40 only if they are at high risk for breast cancer.

References

1. Bates B, Bickley LS, Hoekelman RA: *A guide to physical examination and history taking,* ed 6, Philadelphia, 1995, Lippincott.
2. Seeley R, Stephens T, Tate P: *Anatomy and physiology,* ed 3, St Louis, 1995, McGraw-Hill.
3. Scanlon VC, Saunders T: *Understanding human structure and function,* Philadelphia, 1997, Davis.
4. Benson R, Pernoll M: *Handbook of obstetrics and gynecology,* ed 9, New York, 1994, McGraw-Hill.
5. Allen KM, Phillips JM: *Women's health across the lifespan: a comprehensive perspective,* Philadelphia, 1997, Lippincott.
6. Masters WH, Johnson E: *Human sexual response,* Boston, 1966, Little, Brown.
7. Bolten A and others: Love and sex after 60: how physical changes affect intimate expression, *Geriatrics* 49:21, 1994.
8. Henderson VW: Estrogen, cognition, and a woman's risk of Alzheimer's disease, *Am J Med* 103:11S, 1997.
9. Butterworth CE, Bendich A: Folic acid and the prevention of birth defects, *Annu Rev Nutr* 16:73, 1996.
10. Jorde LB, Carey JC, White RL: *Medical genetics,* ed 2, St Louis, 1998, Mosby.
11. Tilkian SM, Conover MB, Tilkian AG: *Clinical and nursing implications of laboratory tests,* St Louis, 1996, Mosby.
12. Corbett JV: *Laboratory tests and diagnostic procedures with nursing diagnoses,* East Norwalk, Conn, 1996, Appleton & Lange.
13. Munroe W: Home diagnostic kits, *Am Pharm* 34:50, 1994.
14. Youngkin EQ, Davis MS: *Women's health: a primary care clinical guide,* East Norwalk, Conn, 1994, Appleton & Lange.

Resources

Resources for this chapter are listed after Chapter 51 on p. 1552.

REMEMBER to check out your companion CD-ROM

49 NURSING MANAGEMENT Breast Disorders

Shannon Ruff Dirksen & Sharon Mantik Lewis

www.mosby.com/MERLIN/medsurg_lewis

LEARNING OBJECTIVES

1. Assess breast tissue by inspection and palpation using appropriate examination techniques.
2. Teach breast health awareness and breast self-examination, including rationale, technique, and reasons for referral.
3. Describe the types, causes, clinical manifestations, and appropriate nursing and collaborative management of common benign breast disorders.
4. Identify the known risk factors for breast cancer.
5. Describe the pathophysiology, clinical manifestations, and collaborative care of breast cancer.
6. Identify the types of, indications for, and complications of surgical interventions for breast cancer.
7. Explain the physical and psychologic preoperative and postoperative aspects of nursing management for the patient undergoing a mastectomy.
8. Describe the indications for reconstructive breast surgery; types, potential risks, and complications of reconstructive breast surgery; and nursing management after reconstructive breast surgery.

Breast disorders are a significant health concern to women. In a woman's lifetime, there is a one in eight chance that she will be diagnosed with breast cancer. An estimated 178,700 new cases of breast cancer were diagnosed in women in the United States in 1998.[1] About 1000 new cases were diagnosed in men. Whether benign or malignant, intense feelings of shock, fear, and denial often accompany the initial discovery of a lump or change in the breast. These feelings are associated both with the fear of survival and with the possible loss of a breast. Throughout history, the female breast has been regarded as a symbol of beauty, sexuality, and motherhood. The potential loss of a breast, or part of a breast, may be devastating for many women because of the significant psychologic, social, sexual, and body image implications associated with it.

HEALTH PROMOTION

Early Detection

Health promotion practices apply to all women, regardless of their age or menstrual status. It is critical that breast disorders be detected early, diagnosed accurately, and treated promptly. A variety of factors influence the potential for cure, the length of a disease-free period, and the overall length of survival after a diagnosis of breast cancer. Research indicates that 97% of patients diagnosed with localized breast cancer with little or no axillary node involvement will be alive in 5 years. Conversely, only 21% of patients diagnosed with advanced-stage breast cancer with metastases to distant sites will survive 5 years.[2] The essential factors in the early detection of breast cancer and other breast-related problems are the regular performance of routine mammography, regular clinical breast examination (CBE), and breast self-examination (BSE). The frequency of these examinations is determined by the woman's age, the presence of significant risk factors, and her past medical history (Table 49-1). Current guidelines established in the United States by the American Cancer Society and the National Cancer Institute regarding breast surveillance practices include the following:

1. Annual screening mammography for asymptomatic women beginning at age 40 every 1 to 2 years and an annual mammogram for women 50 years of age or older[3]
2. Physical examination of the breasts by a trained health professional (CBE) every 3 years between ages 20 and 40 and every year thereafter
3. Monthly BSE over age 18

The benefits of early detection of breast cancer are well established. The use of a screening mammography has significantly improved early and accurate detection of breast malignancies. Mammography can identify breast abnormalities that may be cancer before physical symptoms appear.[2] Women at high risk for disease, such as those with a family history of breast cancer, should consult their physician about having mammograms earlier and more frequently. Women who have regular mammograms starting when they are 40 to 49 years old have 17% fewer breast cancer deaths.[3] Despite the promise of reduced mortality rates, only 31% of all women follow mammography guidelines.

Reviewed by Rebecca Crane, RN, PhD, AOCN, Oncology Clinical Nurse Specialist, John Wayne Cancer Institute, Saint John's Health Center, Santa Monica, Calif; and Marci Lovett, RN, MN, FNP, CS, Project Manager, Iris Cantor Center for Breast Imaging, UCLA Medical Center, Los Angeles, Calif.

Table 49-1 Risk Factors for Breast Cancer

Increased Risk	Comments
Female	Women account for 99% of breast cancer cases.
Age 50 or over	Nearly two thirds of breast cancers are found in postmenopausal women.
Family history	Breast cancer in a maternal first-degree relative, particularly when premenopausal or bilateral, increases risk; 85-90% of women with breast cancer have no family history. Gene mutations (BRCA-1 or 2) play a role in 5-10% of breast cancer cases.
Personal history of breast cancer, colon cancer, endometrial cancer	Personal history significantly increases risk of breast cancer, risk of cancer in other breast, and recurrence.
Onset of menarche at age 12 yr or younger; onset of menopause at age 55 years or older	Active menstruation for 40 yr or more results in twice the breast cancer risk.
First full-term pregnancy after age 30; nulliparity	Prolonged exposure to unopposed estrogen increases risk for breast cancer.
Benign breast disease with atypical epithelial hyperplasia	Atypical changes in breast biopsy increase the risk of breast cancer fivefold.
Obesity	Fat cells store estrogen.
Exposure to ionizing radiation	Radiation damages DNA.

Improved imaging techniques have reduced the radiation exposure that accompanies mammography to insignificant levels. Therefore the benefits of mammography outweigh the risks from radiation exposure. Ultrasound (echogram, sonogram) is another diagnostic procedure that can be used to differentiate a benign cyst (fluid filled) from a malignant mass (solid). An ultrasound will not detect microcalcifications, which are often the only indicators of very small tumors. Thermography is not currently recommended as a screening method for a breast mass because the results are inconclusive. (See Table 48-14 for a more detailed discussion of diagnostic studies of the breast.)

Education and encouraging women to perform BSE are recommended to decrease mortality rates from breast cancer. In recent years there has been some controversy regarding the value of BSE and its role in reducing mortality rates from breast cancer in women.[4] Until the issue is resolved, BSE should be used as a supplement rather than a substitute for screening by mammography and CBE.

Although the reasons that women report for failing to practice regular BSE have changed somewhat over the years, many women still do not regularly examine their breasts. Some reasons cited by women for not practicing BSE are embarrassment, lack of confidence in ability to do BSE, inadequate knowledge of the procedure, and not remembering to do BSE. Factors that increase BSE compliance include a reminder system, confidence in BSE skill, encouragement from health care providers and significant others, and BSE instruction that involves the woman's active participation.[5,6]

The nurse who is teaching BSE must emphasize that early detection and treatment enhance survival rates. Efforts must be directed toward teaching women the importance of BSE, how to perform it, and what to do if a problem is detected. BSE teaching techniques should include allowing time for the woman to ask questions about the procedure and to perform a return demonstration. The technique for BSE has been established by the American Cancer Society and the National Cancer Institute (Fig. 49-1). BSE should be done monthly at a regular time when the breasts are not tender. In premenopausal women, the best time is 7 days after the start of menstruation. At this time, hormonal stimulation of the breasts is at its lowest point. In most women, nodularity and tenderness will be minimal. For women on oral contraceptives (about 20% to 25% of women ages 15 to 45) the first day of a new package may be a helpful reminder. Postmenopausal women and women who have had hysterectomies should set a regular date for monthly BSE. The monthly date of a birthday or the first day of the month are common choices for many women.

BSE should be done in good light and should include inspection before a mirror and careful, systematic palpation. The entire breast, axilla, and clavicle should be examined. The woman should be taught the BSE procedure by a health care provider using the woman's own hand on her breast. A gentle circular motion over wet, soapy skin is particularly useful if she is in the shower. The woman should be told what to look for, such as a lump, nipple discharge, nipple retraction, redness, pain or tenderness, dimpling of the skin, or edema. Some teaching techniques involve using silicone breast models that simulate normal and abnormal breast tissue to help women learn to identify problems. The woman should be shown the normal variations in her own breasts so that she will be able to detect changes. Finally, she should be reminded that most breast problems are not related to malignancy.

Follow-up Care

If a problem is suspected, the woman should see her primary care provider or contact a comprehensive breast center as soon as possible so that additional diagnostic studies can be promptly initiated. If the problem is not serious, the woman's anxiety can be quickly relieved. If a serious problem is suspected or diagnosed, definitive treatment should not be delayed. Even when the woman faithfully practices BSE, she should have an annual breast examination by a qualified health care provider and a mammogram if age appropriate. The care and attention to detail shown by the clinician in performing BSE reinforces the practice of BSE by the patient.

ASSESSMENT OF BREAST DISORDERS

The most frequently encountered breast disorders in women are fibrocystic changes, carcinoma, fibroadenoma, intraductal papilloma, and ductal ectasia including dilated ducts

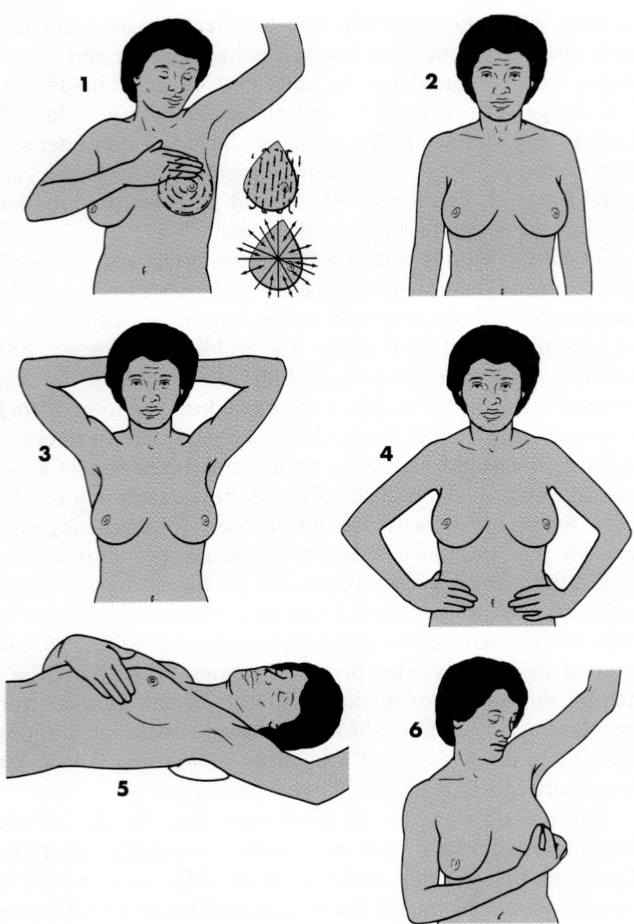

Fig. 49-1 Breast self-examination and patient instruction. *(1)* While in the shower or bath, when the skin is slippery with soap and water, examine your breasts. Use the pads of your second, third, and fourth fingers to firmly press every part of the breast. (While examining your left breast, use your right hand, and use your left hand to examine your right breast.) Check for any lump, hard knot, or thickening of the tissue. *(2)* Look at your breasts in a mirror. Stand with your arms at your side. *(3)* Raise your arms overhead and check for any changes in the shape of your breasts, dimpling of the skin, or any changes in the nipple. *(4)* Next, place your hands on your hips and press down firmly, tightening the pectoral muscles. Observe for asymmetry or changes, keeping in mind that your breasts probably do not exactly match. *(5)* Feel your breasts while lying down. When examining your right breast, place a folded towel under your right shoulder and put your right hand behind your head. Using the pads of the fingers on your left hand, examine the entire breast using small circular motions in a spiral or in an up-and-down motion so that the entire breast area is examined. Repeat the procedure using your right hand to examine your left breast. Repeat pattern of palpation under the arm. *(6)* Finally, gently squeeze the nipple of each breast between your thumb and index finger to check for any discharge.

(Table 49-2). In men, gynecomastia is overwhelmingly the most frequently observed breast disorder.

Many factors must be considered when the nurse is assessing a breast problem. Gender and age are important variables. Only 1% of breast carcinomas occur in males. Benign lesions occur more frequently in premenopausal women. Breast cancer is predominantly found in postmenopausal women, and the incidence increases with age. Family history is also a significant risk factor. Although it is not as common, premenopausal breast cancer tends to be more aggressive.

The history of the breast disorder assists in establishing the diagnosis. The presence of nipple discharge, pain, rate of growth of the lump, and correlation with the menstrual cycle should all be investigated (see Table 49-2).

The size and location of the lump or lumps should be carefully documented, and the physical characteristics of the lesion, such as consistency, mobility, and shape, should be assessed. If nipple discharge is present, the color and consistency should be noted, as well as whether it occurs from single or multiple ducts or from one or both breasts.

Diagnostic Studies

Several techniques can be used to screen for breast disease or provide a diagnosis of a suspicious physical finding. Mammography is a method used to visualize the internal structure of the breast using low-dose x-rays (Fig. 49-2). This simple, safe procedure can detect tumors and cysts that cannot be felt by palpation. The minimum size detectable by physical examination is 1 cm. It may take 10 years or longer to grow a tumor this size. Mammography can detect masses of 0.5 cm.

Calcifications are the most easily recognized mammogram abnormality. These deposits of calcium crystals form in the breast for many reasons, such as inflammation, trauma, and aging. Although most calcifications are benign, they also may be associated with preinvasive cancer.[7]

A comparison of current and prior mammograms may show early cancer tissue changes. Because some tumors metastasize late in the preclinical course, early detection by mammography allows for early treatment and the prevention of metastasis of these smaller lesions. In younger women mammography is less sensitive because of the greater density of breast tissue, resulting in more false-negative results.[8] From 10% to 15% of breast cancers cannot be seen on mammography and are detected only by palpation. Suspicious masses should be biopsied even if mammogram findings are unremarkable.

Definitive diagnosis of a mass can be made only by means of histologic examination of biopsied tissue. Biopsy techniques include fine-needle aspiration (FNA) biopsy, stereotactic core biopsy, or open surgical biopsy.

FNA biopsy is performed by inserting a needle into the lesion and aspirating tissue into a syringe. Three or four passes are usually made. FNA and cytologic evaluation may be helpful in making a diagnosis and planning treatment. It should be done only if an experienced cytologist is available and all suspicious lesions read as negative are followed with a more definitive biopsy procedure. If the aspirated specimen is positive for malignancy, the patient can be given this information at the same visit and begin learning about the treatment options.

Stereotactic core biopsy is a reliable diagnostic technique for obtaining a biopsy. In this procedure mammography is used to locate the lesion. The skin is anesthetized, and a small skin incision is made to allow the entrance of a biopsy gun device. The gun is fired and removes a core sample of the lesion. This is repeated several times, and the core samples are sent for pathologic analysis. This technique has several advantages over an

Table 49-2 Differential Diagnosis of Selected Breast Masses

Condition	Risk Factors	Clinical Picture
■ Breast cancer	Genetic predisposition Radiation Advanced age or over age 50 Menarche/menopausal ages Proliferative breast disease (atypia) Alcohol intake	Breast mass (movable or fixed) Abnormal breast findings may also accompany mass, such as increase in breast size, dimpling, nipple inversion, or bloody discharge
■ Puerperal mastitis	Lactating woman Occurs spontaneously in approximately 2% of all postpartum lactating mothers (both primipara and multipara), usually 2-4 weeks after birth	Warm to touch Indurated Usually unilateral Most common etiology is *Staphylococcus aureus*
■ Nonpuerperal mastitis	Rare condition Usually women in late adolescence or midyears	Palpable mass Usually an obscure organism Should rule out syphilis or tuberculosis
■ Ductal ectasia (plasma cell mastitis or comedomastitis)	Perimenopausal woman—most common in women in their 50s Previous lactation Inverted nipples	Fixation of nipple Usually accompanied by nipple discharge of thick gray material Often associated with breast pain
■ Physiologic nodularity (fibrocystic breast changes)	Most common between ages 35 and 50	Not usually discrete masses, nodularity instead; usually accompanied by cyclic pain and tenderness; mass(es) usually cyclic in occurrence
■ Cysts	Most common between ages 30 and 50	Palpable mass; may have multiple microcysts
■ Fibroadenoma	Peak age range between ages 21 and 25 Most occur before age 30 Most common among African-American women	Often bilateral Most common size at diagnosis is 2-3 cm Rapid growth
■ Fat necrosis	50% report previous history of trauma to breast	Accounts for 2-3% of all breast masses Usually a hard, tender, mobile, indurated mass with irregular borders
■ Intraductal papilloma (benign lesion of lactiferous duct)	Peak age at 40	Usually associated with serous, serosanguineous, or bloody nipple discharge on affected side

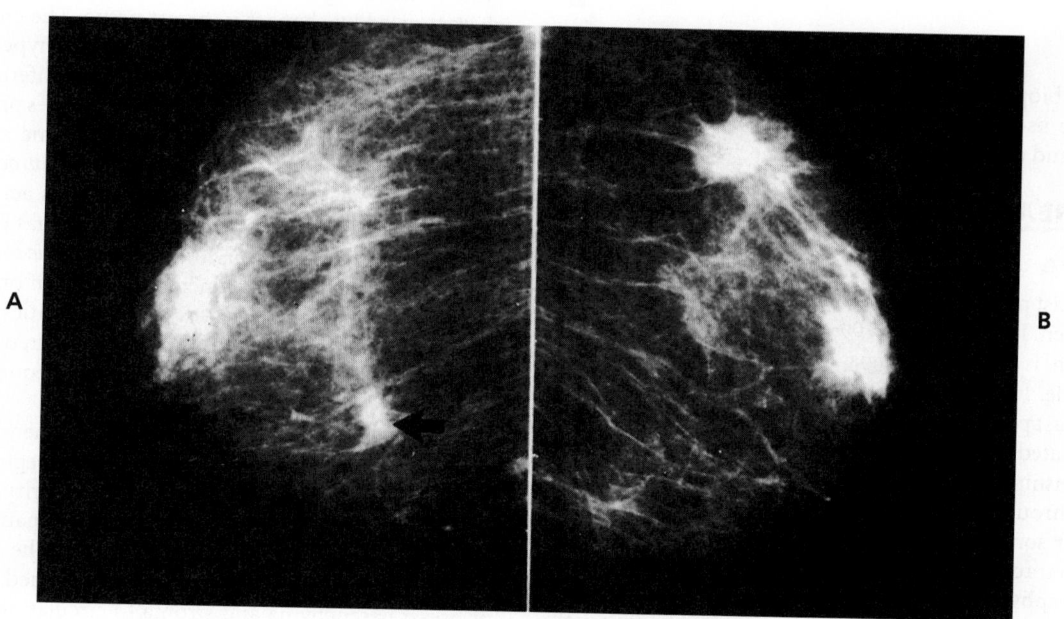

Fig. 49-2 Mammogram showing bilateral invasive ductal carcinoma. **A,** The larger left mass was palpable. **B,** The smaller right mass was clinically occult.

RESEARCH
IMPLICATIONS FOR NURSING PRACTICE

Experience of Women Attending Breast Cancer Screening

Citation Bakker D and others: The experience and satisfaction of women attending breast cancer screening, *Oncol Nurs Forum* 25:115, 1998.

Purpose To determine women's satisfaction and experience with breast cancer screening and associated factors.

Methods Asymptomatic women ($n = 315$), age 50 years or older, with no previous history of breast malignancy participated in the study. Data were collected from the entire sample immediately after screening using a self-report questionnaire and from a subgroup of 256 women by telephone interview 3 weeks after screening.

Results and Conclusions Women reported a high level of satisfaction with their screening experience, including respect for privacy, encouragement to ask questions, and provision of information. Two areas of concern that participants identified were mammogram discomfort and fear about radiation risks. Since the degree of satisfaction that participants in health services report has been shown to influence attendance patterns, assessing breast screening programs from the perspective of attendees is necessary.

Implications for Nursing Practice As health educators, nurses play an important role in providing breast cancer screening information to women. As well as being knowledgeable about screening guidelines and the benefits of screening, nurses also must recognize women's concerns about radiation risks and pain or discomfort with the procedure and be prepared to provide teaching and support for these women.

open surgical biopsy, including decreased length of time for procedure, the use of local anesthesia, outpatient procedure, reduced cost, and decreased recovery time.[9]

BENIGN BREAST PROBLEMS

MASTALGIA

Mastalgia (breast pain) is the most common breast-related complaint in women. It affects up to 70% of all women.[10] The most common form is cyclic mastalgia, which coincides with the menstrual cycle. It is described as diffuse breast tenderness or heaviness. Breast pain may last 2 to 3 days or most of the month. The pain is related to hormonal sensitivity. Noncyclic mastalgia has no relationship to the menstrual cycle. It may be constant or intermittent throughout the month. Symptoms include a burning, aching, or soreness in the breast. The etiology of the pain may be due to trauma, fat necrosis, or duct ectasia.

Mammography is frequently done to exclude cancer and provide information on the etiology of mastalgia. Some relief may occur with caffeine and dietary fat reduction and the continual wearing of a support bra. Hormonal therapy may be recommended, including oral contraceptives, gamma-linolenic acid (evening primrose oil), tamoxifen (Nolvadex), and danazol (Danocrine).[11]

BREAST INFECTIONS

Mastitis

Mastitis is an inflammatory condition that occurs most frequently in lactating women. Lactational mastitis manifests as a localized area that is erythematous, painful, and tender to palpation. Fever is usually present. The infection develops when organisms, usually staphylococci, gain access to the breast through a cracked nipple. In its early stages, mastitis can be cured with antibiotics. Breastfeeding should continue unless an abscess is forming or a purulent drainage is noted. The mother may wish to use a nipple shield or to hand-express milk from the involved breast until the pain subsides. The woman should see her health care provider promptly to begin a course of antibiotic therapy. Any breast that remains red, tender and not responsive to antibiotics needs follow-up care for inflammatory breast cancer.

Lactational Breast Abscess

If lactational mastitis persists after several days of antibiotic therapy, a lactational breast abscess may have developed. In this condition the skin may become red and edematous over the involved breast, often with a corresponding palpable mass, and the patient may have an elevated temperature. Antibiotics alone constitute insufficient treatment for a breast abscess. Surgical incision and drainage is necessary. The drainage is cultured, sensitivities are obtained, and therapy with an appropriate antibiotic is begun. Often the woman will find it necessary to express and discard milk from the affected breast until the abscess is resolved.

FIBROCYSTIC CHANGES

Fibrocystic changes in the breast constitute a benign condition characterized by changes in breast tissue. The changes include the development of excess fibrous tissue, hyperplasia of the epithelial lining of the mammary ducts, proliferation of mammary ducts, and cyst formation. These changes produce pain by nerve irritation from connective tissue edema and by fibrosis from nerve pinching. The use of the term *fibrocystic disease* is incorrect because the cluster of problems is actually an exaggerated response to hormonal influence. It has been suggested that the term *fibrocystic condition* or *fibrocystic complex* be used. Fibrocystic changes do not increase the risk of breast cancer for the majority of patients. Masses or nodularities can appear in both breasts and are often found in the upper, outer quadrants and usually occur bilaterally. It is the most frequently occurring breast disorder.

Fibrocystic changes occur most frequently in women between 35 and 50 years of age but often begin in women as young as 20 years of age. Pain and nodularity often increase over time but tend to subside after menopause unless high doses of estrogen replacement are used. The cause of these fibrocystic changes is thought to be heightened responsiveness of breast parenchyma and stroma to circulating estrogens and progesterones. Predominantly affected are women with premenstrual abnormalities, nulliparous women, women with a history of spontaneous abortion, nonusers of oral contraceptives, and women with early menarche and late menopause. Fibrocystic changes often exacerbate in the premenstrual phase and subside after menstruation.

Manifestations of fibrocystic breast changes include one or more palpable lumps that are usually round, well delineated, and freely movable within the breast. Some lumps are fibrous and do not contain cysts. There may be accompanying discomfort ranging from tenderness to pain. The lump is usually observed to increase in size and perhaps in tenderness before menstruation. Cysts may enlarge or shrink rapidly. Nipple discharge associated with fibrocystic breasts is often milky, watery-milky, yellow, or green.

Mammography may be helpful in distinguishing fibrocystic changes from breast cancer. However, in some women the breast tissue is so dense that it is difficult to obtain a worthwhile mammogram study. In these situations, ultrasound may be more useful in differentiating a cystic mass from a solid mass.

NURSING AND COLLABORATIVE MANAGEMENT: FIBROCYSTIC CHANGES

With the initial discovery of a discrete mass in the breast by a woman or her health care provider, aspiration or surgical biopsy may be indicated. A wait of 7 to 10 days may be planned if the nodularity is recurrent to note changes as the menstrual cycle changes. With large or frequent cysts, surgical removal may be favored over repeated aspiration. An excisional biopsy should be done if no fluid is found on aspiration, if the fluid that is found is hemorrhagic, or if a residual mass remains. This surgery is performed in an office or day surgery unit with the patient under local anesthesia.

Biopsies in women with fibrocystic disease may be indicated for women with an increased risk for breast cancer (see Table 49-1). Hyperplastic changes approximating the histologic appearance of carcinoma in situ (atypical hyperplasia) and a family history of breast cancer increase the probability of developing breast cancer.

The woman with cystic changes should be encouraged to return regularly for follow-up examinations throughout life. She should also be taught BSE to self-monitor the problem. Severe fibrocystic changes may make palpation of the breast more difficult. Any new lumps or changes in the breasts should be evaluated, and changes in symptoms should be reported and investigated.

Many types of treatment have been suggested for a fibrocystic condition. These include the use of a good support bra, dietary therapy (low-salt diet, restriction of methylxanthines such as coffee and chocolate), vitamin E therapy, analgesics, danazol (Danocrine), diuretics, hormone therapy, antiestrogen therapy, and surgical therapy (subcutaneous mastectomy).[12] Although many of these treatments have not been scientifically proven to be beneficial, many women report less discomfort with these measures. Danazol has been used for patients with severe pain. It decreases follicle-stimulating hormone (FSH) and luteinizing hormone (LH), resulting in reduced estrogen production and subsequent decreased pain and nodularity. The androgenic side effects of danazol (acne, edema, hirsutism) often make this therapy intolerable for many women.

Because stress can be a contributing factor in breast discomfort, efforts should be directed toward the reduction of stress. Many of these approaches are considered experimental. The large number of possible interventions indicates the uncertainty surrounding the causes and treatment of fibrocystic conditions.

The role of the nurse in the care of the patient with fibrocystic breast changes is primarily one of teaching. A woman with fibrocystic breasts should be told that she may expect recurrence of the cysts in one or both breasts until menopause and that cysts may enlarge or become painful just before menstruation. Additionally, she should be reassured that cysts do not "turn into" cancer. Any new lump that does not respond in a cyclic manner over 1 to 2 weeks should be examined promptly. The woman should be carefully instructed in BSE, using her own breasts. Teaching breast models can also be helpful.

FIBROADENOMA

Fibroadenoma is a common cause of discrete benign breast lumps in young women. It generally occurs in women between 15 and 25 years of age and is the most frequent cause of breast tumors in women under 25 years of age. Fibroadenomas tend to develop more frequently and at a younger age in African-American women.[13] The possible cause of fibroadenoma may be increased estrogen sensitivity in a localized area of the breast. Fibroadenomas are usually small, painless, round, well delineated, and very mobile. They may be soft but are usually solid, firm, and rubbery in consistency. There is no accompanying retraction or nipple discharge. The lump is often painless. The fibroadenoma may appear as a single unilateral mass, although multiple bilateral fibroadenomas have been reported. Growth is slow and often ceases when size reaches 2 to 3 cm. Size is not affected by menstruation. However, pregnancy can stimulate dramatic growth. Fibroadenomas are rarely associated with cancer.

NURSING AND COLLABORATIVE MANAGEMENT: FIBROADENOMA

Fibroadenomas are easily detected by physical examination and are often visible on mammography. Definitive diagnosis, however, requires biopsy and tissue examination by a pathologist. Treatment is by excision, which is not urgent in women under 25 years of age. In women over 35 years of age all new lesions should be examined using an excisional biopsy. Fibroadenomas are not reduced by radiation and are not affected by hormone therapy. The nurse frequently has the opportunity to counsel a young woman with fibroadenomas. During this contact the benign nature of the lesion should be stressed and follow-up examinations and BSE should be encouraged.

NIPPLE DISCHARGE

Nipple discharge may occur spontaneously or as a result of nipple manipulation. A milky secretion is due to inappropriate lactation (galactorrhea) as a result of such problems as drug therapy, endocrine problems, and neural disorders. It may also be idiopathic.

Secretions can also be serous, grossly bloody, or brown to green. These may be caused by either benign or malignant disease. A slide can be made of the secretion to detect specific disease. Diseases associated with nipple discharge include malignancies, cystic disease, intraductal papilloma, and ductal ectasia. Treatment depends on identification of the cause. In most cases, nipple discharge is not related to malignancy. If galactorrhea is accompanied by amenorrhea, various gynecologic endocrinopathies should be explored.

Intraductal Papilloma

Intraductal papillomas are benign, wartlike growths found in the mammary ducts, usually near the nipple. Typically, there is an associated bloody nipple discharge, a mass, or both. Intraductal papillomas usually affect women 40 to 60 years of age. A single duct or several ducts may be involved. Treatment includes excision of the papilloma and the involved duct or duct system.

Ductal Ectasia

Ductal ectasia is a benign breast disease of perimenopausal and postmenopausal women involving the ducts in the subareolar area. It usually involves several bilateral ducts. Nipple discharge is the primary symptom. This discharge is multicolored and sticky. Ductal ectasia is initially painless but may progress to burning, itching, and pain around the nipple, as well as swelling in the areolar area. Inflammatory signs are often present, the nipple may retract, and the discharge may become bloody in more advanced disease. Ductal ectasia is not associated with malignancy. If an abscess develops, warm compresses and antibiotics are usually effective treatments. Therapy consists of close follow-up examinations or surgical excision of the involved ducts.

GYNECOMASTIA IN MEN

Gynecomastia, a transient enlargement of one or both breasts, is the most common breast problem in men. The condition is usually temporary and benign. Gynecomastia in itself is not an established risk factor for breast cancer. The most common cause of gynecomastia is a disturbance of the normal ratio of active androgen to estrogen in plasma or within the breast itself. Other causes include tumor of the testes or pituitary, medication with estrogen or steroidal compounds, or failure of the liver to inactivate circulating estrogen, as in liver failure (e.g., cirrhosis).[14]

Gynecomastia may also be a symptom of other problems. It is seen accompanying developmental abnormalities of the male reproductive organs. It may also accompany organic diseases, including testicular tumors, cancer of the adrenal cortex, pituitary adenomas, hyperthyroidism, and liver disease. Gynecomastia may occur as a side effect of drug therapy, particularly with administration of estrogens and androgens, digitalis, isoniazid (INH), ranitidine (Zantac), and spironolactone (Aldactone). Use of heroin and marijuana can also cause gynecomastia.

Pubertal Gynecomastia

Pubertal gynecomastia caused by increased estrogen production is seen most often in boys between the ages of 13 and 17. It is usually limited, although occasionally the localized hyperplasia may measure 2 to 3 cm in size. Pubertal gynecomastia is almost always self-limiting, and disappears within 4 to 6 months of onset. Parents and the affected boy should be reassured that in almost all cases this is a normal physiologic phenomenon that will disappear spontaneously and will require no treatment. Rarely, unilateral gynecomastia in the young male may be marked and fail to regress. This is the only indication for surgical intervention.

Senescent Gynecomastia

Senescent gynecomastia occurs in 40% of older men. A probable cause is the elevation in plasma estrogen in older adult men as the result of an increase in the peripheral conversion of androgens to estrogens with age. Although initially unilateral, the tender, firm, centrally located enlargement may become bilateral. When gynecomastia is characterized by a discrete, circumscribed mass, it must be diagnosed to differentiate it from the rarer breast cancer in males. Senescent hyperplasia requires no treatment and generally regresses within 6 to 12 months.

GERONTOLOGIC CONSIDERATIONS

Age-Related Breast Changes

Loss of subcutaneous fat and structural support and atrophy of mammary glands often result in pendulous breasts in the postmenopausal woman. The nurse should encourage older women to wear a well-fitting bra. Adequate support can improve physical appearance and reduce pain in the back, shoulders, and neck. It can also prevent intertrigo (dermatitis caused by friction between opposing surfaces of skin). Surgical lifting of sagging breasts is possible and may be desirable when reconstruction after a mastectomy is performed.

The decrease in glandular tissue in older women makes a breast mass easier to palpate. This decreased density is probably age related and occurs even with women on hormone replacement therapy. Rib margins may be palpable in the older adult woman and can be confused with a mass. As a woman becomes more familiar with her own breasts and is reassured about her findings, the anxiety about this finding should decrease. The nurse should encourage the older woman to continue BSE and to have annual mammograms and clinical examinations because the incidence of breast cancer increases with age.

BREAST CANCER

Breast cancer is the most common malignancy in American women. It is second only to lung cancer as the leading cause of death from cancer in women. The number of deaths of women from breast cancer appears to be leveling off.[1] Each year in the United States, approximately 184,000 cases of breast cancer occur in women and about 46,000 women die of the disease. At the present time the American Cancer Society predicts that one of every eight American women will develop breast cancer during her lifetime.[2]

Although the vast majority of breast problems occur in women, men can also have breast cancer. Therefore it is critical that men know the importance of reporting any change in their breasts. One out of every 100 cases of breast cancer occurs in men. Predisposing risk factors include states of hyperestrogenism, a family history of breast cancer, and radiation exposure. A thorough examination of the male breast should be a routine part of a physical examination.

Etiology and Risk Factors

Although the etiology is not completely understood, a number of factors are thought to relate to the cause of breast cancer.

CULTURAL & ETHNIC CONSIDERATIONS

Breast Cancer

- African-American women have lower survival rates from breast cancer than Caucasian women, even when diagnosed at an early stage.
- African-American women are diagnosed at a later stage of breast cancer than Caucasian women, but this fact alone does not account for the higher mortality rate.
- Caucasian women have a higher incidence of breast cancer than non-Caucasians.

Table 49-3 Types of Breast Cancer

Type	Frequency of Occurrence
Infiltrating ductal carcinoma	
(not otherwise specified)	80%
Medullary	5-8%
Colloid (mucinous)	2-4%
Tubular	1-2%
Papillary	1-2%
Infiltrating lobular carcinoma	10-15%
Noninvasive	4-6%
Ductal carcinoma in situ	2-3%
Lobular carcinoma in situ	2-3%

Heredity or genetically related susceptibility is considered to play a role. Hormonal regulation of the breast is related to the development of breast cancer, but the mechanisms are poorly understood. Sex hormones may act as tumor promoters if initiating agents have induced malignant changes. Additional factors under study include physical inactivity, dietary fat intake, obesity, and alcohol intake.[2] Environmental factors such as chemical and pesticide exposure and radiation may also play a role.

Some factors that place a woman at higher risk for breast cancer have been identified (see Table 49-1). Women are at far greater risk than men because 99% of breast cancers occur in women. Increasing age also increases the risk of developing breast cancer. The incidence of breast cancer in women under 25 years of age is very low and increases gradually until age 60. After age 60 the incidence increases dramatically.[9] Positive family history is an important risk factor, especially if the involved member with breast cancer was premenopausal, had bilateral disease, and is a first-degree relative (i.e., mother, sister, daughter). Having any first-degree relative with breast cancer increases a woman's risk of breast cancer 1.5 to 3 times, depending on age.[11] Controversy exists as to whether hormone replacement therapy (HRT), primarily estrogen, in postmenopausal women increases breast cancer risk. Some studies suggest that risk increases only with prolonged HRT use.[15] Other studies suggest that adding progesterone to the estrogen decreases risk.[16] The Nurses' Health Study has linked long-term oral contraceptive use to an increased risk of breast cancer.[17] Given that estrogen protects against heart disease and hip fractures, each woman and her health care provider must weigh the risk of these problems against the risk of developing breast cancer.

Risk factors appear to be cumulative. Therefore the presence of other risk factors may greatly increase the overall risk, especially for those with a positive family history. Identification of risk factors indicates an increased need for careful clinical surveillance of the patient and participation in cancer screening measures. However, about 60% of women who develop breast cancer have none of the identifiable risk factors.[18]

As many as 5% to 10% of all breast cancer patients may have inherited a specific genetic abnormality contributing to the development of their breast cancer.[19] The first genetic alteration to be identified was in the tumor suppressor gene, p53. The BRCA-1 gene, located on chromosome 17, is a tumor suppressor gene which inhibits tumor development when functioning normally. Women who have BRCA-1 mutations have an 85% to 90% lifetime chance of developing breast cancer. The BRCA-2 gene, located on chromosome 11, is another tumor suppressor gene.[20] Mutations in the two known BRCA genes may cause 90% of all inherited breast cancers. As many as 1 in 200 to 400 women in the United States may be carriers. Women with a strong family history of breast cancer may wish to consider testing in a program that includes pre- and post-test counseling. Routine screening for genetic abnormalities in women without evidence of a strong family history of breast cancer is not warranted. Genetic screening is expensive and often not covered by insurance.

Pathophysiology

Various types of breast cancer have been identified based on their histologic characteristics and growth pattern of the tumor (Table 49-3). The main components of the breast are lobules (milk-producing glands) and ducts (milk passages that connect the lobules and the nipple). In general breast cancer arises from the epithelial lining of the ducts (ductal carcinoma) or from the epithelium of the lobules (lobular carcinoma). Breast cancers may be invasive or in situ. Most breast cancers arise from the ducts and are invasive. Subtypes of invasive ductal cancer with unusual growth patterns include medullary, colloid, tubular, and papillary. Lobular carcinomas may be either infiltrating or in situ.

The natural history of breast cancer varies considerably from patient to patient. Cancer growth can range from slow to rapid. Factors that affect cancer prognosis are size, axillary node involvement (the more nodes involved, the worse the prognosis), tumor differentiation, DNA content (characteristics of malignant cells), and estrogen and progesterone receptor status. The histologic type of breast cancer seems to have little prognostic significance once the tumors are truly invasive.

Noninvasive Breast Cancer. The increased use of screening mammography has led to more women being diagnosed with noninvasive breast cancer. These intraductal cancers include ductal carcinoma in situ (DCIS) and lobular carcinoma in situ (LCIS). While DCIS behaves as an early malignancy, LCIS would be better called lobular neoplasia. DCIS tends to be unilateral and most likely would progress to invasive cancer if left untreated. LCIS appears to be more of a risk factor for breast cancer, and women with this condition have a higher risk of developing an invasive breast cancer in the same or opposite breast.

Although the management of these two disorders is controversial, patients with DCIS and LCIS have historically been treated with mastectomy. Once diagnosed, all treatment options should be discussed with the patient, including prophylactic bilateral mastectomy with breast reconstruction, breast-conserving treatment (lumpectomy), and radiation therapy.

Paget's Disease. Paget's disease is a breast malignancy characterized by a persistent lesion of the nipple and areola with or without a palpable mass. Itching, burning, bloody nipple discharge with superficial erosion, and ulceration may be present. Diagnosis of Paget's disease is confirmed by pathologic examination of the erosion. Nipple changes are often diagnosed as an infection or dermatitis, which can lead to treatment delays. (This is different from Paget's disease of the bone that is discussed in Chapter 59.) The treatment of Paget's disease is a simple or modified radical mastectomy. Prognosis is good when the cancer remains in the nipple only. The nursing care for the patient with Paget's disease is the same as the care for a patient with any breast carcinoma.

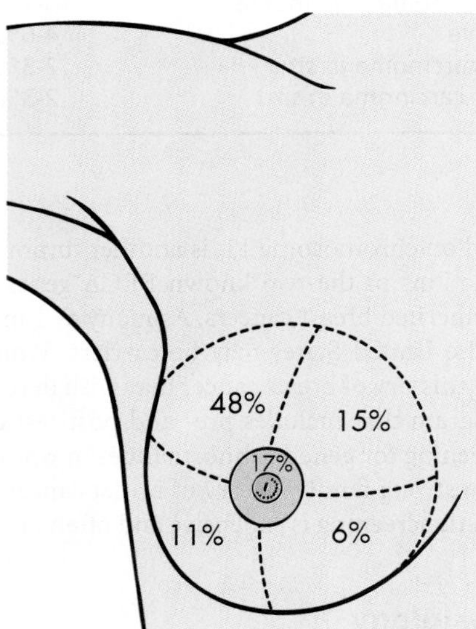

Fig. 49-3 Distribution of carcinomas in different areas of the breast.

Inflammatory Breast Cancer. Inflammatory breast cancer, the most malignant form of all breast cancers, is rare. It is an aggressive and fast-growing cancer. The skin of the breast looks red, feels warm, and has a thickened appearance that is often described as resembling an orange peel. Sometimes the breast develops ridges and small bumps that look like hives. The inflammatory changes, often mistaken for an infection, are caused by cancer cells blocking lymph channels. Metastases occurs early and widely. Radiation, chemotherapy, and hormone therapy are more likely to be used for treatment than surgery.

Clinical Manifestations

Breast cancer is detected as a single lump or mammographic abnormality in the breast. It occurs most often in the upper, outer quadrant of the breast because most of the glandular tissue is there (Fig. 49-3). The rate at which the lesion grows varies considerably. Slow-growing lesions are often associated with a lower mortality rate. If palpable, breast cancer is characteristically hard, irregularly shaped, poorly delineated, nonmobile, and nontender.

Table 49-4 Common Sites of Breast Cancer Recurrence and Metastasis

Site	Clinical Presentation
Local Recurrence	
Skin	Firm, discrete nodules; occasionally pruritic, usually painless
Regional Recurrence	
Lymph nodes	Enlarged nodes in axilla or supraclavicular area, usually nontender, superior vena caval obstruction from enlarged supraclavicular nodes (oncologic emergency), pain in shoulder and arm of affected side
Distant Metastases	
Skeletal metastasis	Localized pain of gradually increasing intensity, percussion tenderness at involved sites, pathologic fracture caused by involvement of bone cortex, hypercalcemia from skeletal metastasis or endocrine therapy
Spinal cord metastasis	Progressive back pain, localized and radicular; muscular weakness, usually in lower extremities; paresthesias in one or more extremities; bowel or bladder sphincter dysfunction; paralysis from epidural spinal cord compression
Brain metastasis	Headache, unilateral sensory loss, focal muscular weakness, hemiparesis, incoordination (ataxia), visual defects, speech disorder (dysphasia), impaired cognition, behavioral or mental changes, loss of sphincter control, papilledema, persistent nausea and vomiting, seizure activity, progressive decrease in level of consciousness
Pulmonary metastasis (including lung nodules and pleural effusions)	Dependent on sites and extent of pulmonary metastases; chest pain, dyspnea on exertion, shortness of breath, tachypnea, nonproductive cough (not present in all patients); adventitious breath sounds, dullness to percussion, restricted chest-wall expansion on affected side with pleural effusion
Liver metastasis	Abdominal distention; right lower quadrant abdominal pain sometimes with radiation to scapular area; nausea and vomiting, anorexia, weight loss; weakness and fatigue; hepatomegaly, ascites, jaundice; peripheral edema; elevated liver enzymes
Bone marrow metastasis	Anemia; infection; increased bleeding, bruising, petechiae; weakness and fatigue; mild confusion, light-headedness; dyspnea

A small percentage of breast cancers cause nipple discharge. The discharge is usually unilateral and may be clear or bloody. Nipple retraction may occur. Plugging of the dermal lymphatics can cause skin thickening and exaggeration of the usual skin markings, giving the skin the appearance of an orange peel (peau d'orange). In large cancers, infiltration, induration, and dimpling (pulling in) of the overlying skin may occur.

Complications

The main complication of breast cancer is recurrence (Table 49-4). Recurrence may be local or regional (skin or soft tissue near the mastectomy site, axillary or internal mammary lymph nodes) or distant (most commonly bone, lung, brain, and liver). However, metastatic disease can be found in any distant site.

About 50% to 75% of patients with node-positive disease have recurrences, compared with about 25% to 33% of those with negative nodes. Seventy percent of all recurrences occur during the 3 to 4 years following diagnosis.

Widely disseminated or metastatic disease involves the growth of colonies of cancerous breast cells in parts of the body distant from the breast. Metastases primarily occur through the lymphatic chains, principally those of the axilla (see Fig. 48-4). However, the cancer can spread to other parts of the body without invading the axillary nodes even when the primary breast tumor is small. Even in node-negative breast cancer, there is a possibility of distant metastasis. Prognosis is directly related to the number of nodes involved and other factors discussed in the section on diagnostic studies.

Chemotherapy is the usual treatment for recurrent disease. Hormonal therapy or radiation therapy may be used alone or in combination with chemotherapy when recurrent disease occurs.

Diagnostic Studies

In addition to tissue studies used to diagnose breast cancer, other tests done on breast tissue are useful in predicting the risk of recurrence or metastatic breast disease. These tests include axillary lymph node status, tumor size and histologic characteristics, estrogen and progesterone receptor status, DNA content analysis (ploidy status), and cell proliferative indices (Table 49-5).

Axillary lymph node involvement is one of the most important prognostic factors in early-stage breast cancer.[21] The presence of metastasis in axillary nodes can be determined by pathologic examination of as few as 6 to 10 nodes. The more nodes involved, the greater the risk of relapse. Nodal status is often grouped into three subsets: negative nodes (30% to 35% recurrence at 10 years), one to three positive nodes (55% to 65% recurrence at 10 years), and four or more positive nodes (80% to 90% recurrence at 10 years).

New studies are addressing better methods to identify key lymph nodes for removal. A new technique called *lymphatic mapping* and *sentinel lymph node biopsy* helps the surgeon identify the lymph node(s) that drain first from the tumor site (sentinel node).[22] A radioisotope with blue dye is injected into the tumor site, and with the aid of a gamma probe, it is determined in which node(s) the radioisotope is located. A local incision is made and the surgeon dissects the blue-stained sentinel node, which is then subsequently analyzed by pathologic studies.

Tumor size is a valuable prognostic variable: the larger the tumor, the greater the risk of relapse. The wide variety of histologic types of breast cancer explains the heterogeneity of the disease. In general, the more well differentiated the tumor, the less aggressive it is. Poorly differentiated tumors appear morphologically disorganized and aggressive.

Another diagnostic test useful both for treatment decisions and prediction of prognosis is estrogen and progesterone receptor status. Receptor-positive tumors commonly (1) show histologic evidence of being well differentiated, (2) frequently have a diploid DNA content and low proliferative indices, (3) have a low propensity for visceral recurrence, and (4) are frequently hormone dependent and responsive to hormonal therapy. Receptor-negative tumors (1) are frequently poorly differentiated histologically, (2) have a high incidence of aneuploidy (abnormally high or low DNA content) and higher proliferative indices, (3) frequently recur at visceral sites, and (4) are usually unresponsive to hormonal therapy.

Flow cytometry can be used to measure DNA content (ploidy status) and cell proliferation. The technique uses a flow cytometer to measure certain characteristics of malignant cells that are difficult to measure by microscopy. This test quantifies

COLLABORATIVE CARE

Table 49-5 Breast Cancer

Diagnostic
- History including risk factors
- Physical examination of breast and lymphatics
- Mammography
- Ultrasound
- Biopsy
- Estrogen-progesterone receptor assays
- Other molecular studies (DNA ploidy, S phase, p53, HER-2/neu)

Staging Workup
- Complete blood count, platelet count
- Calcium and phosphate levels
- Liver function tests
- Sentinel lymph node biopsy
- Chest x-ray
- Bone scan
- CT scan of chest, abdomen, pelvis
- MRI (if indicated)

Collaborative Therapy
- Surgery
  - Breast-conserving (lumpectomy) with or without axillary node sampling or dissection
  - Modified radical mastectomy (may include reconstruction)
- Radiation therapy
  - Primary radiotherapy
  - Adjuvant radiotherapy
  - Palliative radiotherapy
- Chemotherapy
  - Adjuvant chemotherapy
  - Chemotherapy of recurrent disease
- Hormonal therapy
  - Hormones (e.g., tamoxifen [Nolvadex])
- Surgical hormonal therapy

CT, computed tomography; *DNA*, deoxyribonucleic acid; *MRI*, magnetic resonance imaging.

cellular DNA content and determines if a tumor is diploid (DNA content equal to that in normal cells) or aneuploid (abnormally high or low DNA content). Ploidy correlates with tumor aggressiveness. Diploid tumors have been shown to have a significantly lower risk of relapse than aneuploid tumors.

Cell-proliferative indices indirectly measure the rate of tumor cell proliferation. The percent of tumor cells in the S phase of the cell cycle (see Fig. 14-1) is another important prognostic indicator. Patients with cells that have high S-phase fractions have a higher risk for recurrence and earlier cancer death.

Another prognostic indicator is the genetic marker HER-2/neu (also called c-erb-B2 or neu). Amplification and overexpression of this gene have been associated with a poor prognosis in breast cancer, advanced-stage ovarian cancer, and endometrial cancer.[23] People with this gene have tumors that are routinely resistant to some forms of chemotherapy and more responsive to others.

Collaborative Care

Historically, radical ablative surgery was the standard of care. Presently there is a wide range of treatment options available to both the patient and the care providers attempting to make critical decisions about what treatment to select (see Table 49-5). Many prognostic factors are considered when treatment decisions are made about a specific breast cancer. These factors include lymph node status, tumor size, histologic classification, and the identification of special histologic subtypes. All of these factors enter into the staging of breast cancer. The most widely accepted staging method is the American Joint Committee on Cancer's (AJCC's) TNM system (Table 49-6).[24] This system uses tumor size (T), nodal involvement (N), and presence of metastasis (M) to determine the stage of disease. The stages range from I to IV, with stage I being very small tumors (less than 2 cm) with no lymph node involvement and no metastasis. Classification within these stages depends on the size of the tumor and the number of lymph nodes involved. Stage IV indicates the presence of metastatic spread, regardless of tumor size or lymph node involvement. The therapeutic regimen is often dictated by the clinical stage classification of the cancer. (Side effects and appropriate nursing management of general treatment modalities for cancer are discussed in Chapter 14.)

In spite of the advent of new prognostic indicators such as flow-cytometric determination of DNA content and analysis of cell-cycle phases, the single most powerful prognostic factor related to local recurrence or metastasis after primary therapy is still the presence or absence of malignant cells in axillary lymph nodes.

Surgical Therapy. Breast conservation surgery with radiation therapy and modified radical mastectomy with or without reconstruction are currently the most common options for resectable breast cancer.[25] Most women diagnosed with early-stage breast cancer (tumors smaller than 4 to 5 cm) are candidates for either treatment choice. Ten-year overall survival with lumpectomy and radiation is about the same as that with modified radical mastectomy.[21]

Axillary node dissection. Axillary lymph node dissection is often performed regardless of the treatment option selected. Examination of nodes provides the most powerful prognostic data currently available. Knowing the status of the lymph nodes helps determine further treatment (chemotherapy, hormone therapy, or both). For all cases of invasive breast cancer, a typical lymph node dissection has always involved the removal of 10 to 15 lymph nodes. However, this technique may not be necessary or appropriate for some women with very small invasive breast cancers or with noninvasive (in situ) cancers.

Sentinel lymph node biopsy shows promise for reducing unnecessary lymph node dissection. If the sentinel node does not show any signs of cancer, no further lymph nodes are removed. Because this technique is still under study, ongoing research will reveal which patients are most appropriate for lymph node preservation.

Lymphedema (accumulation of lymph in soft tissue) can occur as a result of the excision or radiation of lymph nodes.[26] When the axillary nodes cannot return lymph fluid to the central circulation, the fluid accumulates in the arm, causing obstructive pressure on the veins and venous return. The patient may experience heaviness, pain, impaired motor function in the arm, and numbness and paresthesia of the fingers as a result of lymphedema. Cellulitis and progressive fibrosis can result from lymphedema.

Although lymphedema is not always preventable, it can be controlled somewhat after surgery or radiation. Frequent and sustained elevation of the arm, exercises, regular use of a custom-fitted pressure sleeve, and treatment with an inflatable sleeve (pneumomassage) are all helpful in preventing or reducing lymphedema.[18]

Table 49-6 TNM Classification of Breast Cancer

Primary Tumor (T)			
T0	No evidence of primary tumor		
Tis	Carcinoma in situ		
T1	Tumor ≤2 cm		
T2	Tumor >2 cm but ≤5 cm		
T3	Tumor >5 cm		
T4	Extension to chest wall, inflammation		
Regional Lymph Nodes (N)			
N0	No tumor in regional lymph nodes		
N1	Metastasis to movable ipsilateral nodes		
N2	Metastasis to matted or fixed ipsilateral nodes		
N3	Metastasis to ipsilateral internal mammary nodes		
Distant Metastasis (M)			
M0	No distant metastasis		
M1	Distant metastasis (includes spread to ipsilateral supraclavicular nodes)		
Stage Grouping			
Stage 0	TIS	N0	M0
Stage I	T1	N0	M0
Stage IIA	T0	N1	M0
	T1	N1	M0
	T2	N0	M0
Stage IIB	T2	N1	M0
	T3	N0	M0
Stage IIIA	T0	N2	M0
	T1	N2	M0
	T2	N2	M0
	T3	N1, N2	M0
Stage IIIB	T4	Any N	M0
	Any T	N3	M0
Stage IV	Any T	Any N	M1

Breast conservation surgery. Breast conservation surgery (lumpectomy) involves the removal of the entire tumor along with a margin of normal tissue. Following surgery, radiation therapy is delivered to the entire breast, ending with a boost to the tumor bed. This treatment method is an option when the tumor is less than 4 cm and can be totally removed. If there is evidence of systemic disease, chemotherapy may be given before radiation therapy. Contraindications to breast conservation surgery include breast size too small to yield an acceptable cosmetic result, tumor exceeding 4 cm, masses and calcifications that are multifocal (within the same breast quadrant), masses that are multicentric (in more than one quadrant), or diffuse calcifications in more than one quadrant.

One of the main advantages of breast conservation surgery and radiation is that it preserves the breast, including the nipple. The goal of the combined surgery and radiation is to maximize the benefits of both cancer treatment and cosmetic outcome while minimizing risks. Disadvantages of this surgery include the increased cost of the surgery plus radiation over surgery alone and the possible side effects of radiation. Table 49-7 describes treatment options, side effects, complications, and patient issues related to the most common surgical procedures currently used to treat breast cancer.

Modified radical mastectomy. The modified radical mastectomy includes removal of the breast and axillary lymph nodes, but it preserves the pectoralis major muscle. This surgery would be selected over breast conservation therapy if the tumor is too large to excise with good margins and attain a reasonable cosmetic result. Some patients may select this surgical procedure over lumpectomy when presented with the choice of either procedure.

When a modified radical mastectomy is performed, the patient has the option of breast reconstruction. If the patient chooses to have reconstructive surgery, it can be performed immediately following the mastectomy or it can be delayed until postoperative recovery is complete (about 6 months).

Follow-up care. After surgery, the woman must be followed up for the rest of her life at regular intervals. Most women have professional examinations every 3 months for 2 years, every 6 months for the next 3 years, and then annually thereafter. In addition, the woman must continue to practice a monthly BSE on both breasts or the remaining breast and the mastectomy site. The most common sites of recurrence of breast cancer are at the surgical site and in the opposite breast. The woman should also have yearly mammography of the remaining breast or breast tissue.

Adjuvant Therapy. The decision to recommend adjuvant (additional) therapy after surgery depends on the number of involved nodes, menstrual status, age, cell type, size and extent of the cancer, presence or absence of estrogen receptors, and other preexisting health problems that can complicate treatment. Adjuvant therapies include radiation therapy and systemic therapies such as chemotherapy, hormonal manipulation, and biologic therapy. Adjuvant therapy for men with breast cancer is the same as adjuvant therapy for women.[27]

Radiation therapy. The three situations in which radiation therapy may be used for breast cancer are (1) as the primary treatment to destroy the tumor or as a companion to surgery to prevent local recurrence, (2) to shrink a large tumor to operable size, and (3) as the palliative treatment for pain caused by local recurrence and metastases. Lumpectomy is almost always followed by radiation.

Primary radiation therapy. When radiation therapy is the primary treatment, it is usually performed after local excision of the breast mass. The breast (and the regional lymph nodes in some cases) are radiated daily over the course of approximately 5 to 6 weeks. An external beam of radiation is used to deliver an approximate total dose of 4500 to 5000 cGy (4500 to 5000 rads; 1 rad = 1 cGy). A "boost" treatment to the full breast may also be given, either before or after therapy has been completed. The boost is a dose of radiation delivered to the area in which the original tumor was located. It can be given by external beam and usually adds 10 treatments to the total number given. Esophagitis, tracheitis, fatigue, skin changes, and breast edema may be temporary side effects of external beam radiation therapy. Radiation of the axilla is also effective in decreasing the incidence of axillary recurrence. Chemotherapy may be used systemically to enhance the local effects of radiation. (Nursing management of the patient receiving radiation therapy is discussed in Chapter 14.)

Radiation therapy as adjunct to surgery. Although an uncommon treatment mode, preoperative radiation therapy can be used to reduce the size of a large tumor mass to operable proportions by destroying the cancer cells. Additionally, because the malignant cells are partially or completely destroyed, the rate of local recurrence decreases. The disadvantages of potential delayed wound healing and increased lymphedema do not seem to outweigh the advantages of preoperative radiation in cases in which the cancer is locally advanced.

The decision to use radiation therapy after mastectomy is based on the probability of the presence of local residual cancer cells. Radiating the area will not prevent the appearance of distant metastasis at a later date. The site of radiation therapy (lymph nodes, chest wall, or both) depends on the degree of possible spread of the cancer.

Palliative radiation therapy. In addition to reducing the primary tumor mass with a resultant decrease in pain, radiation therapy is also used to stabilize symptomatic metastatic lesions in such sites as bone, soft-tissue organs, the brain, and the chest. Radiation therapy relieves pain and is often successful in controlling recurrent or metastatic disease for long periods.

Systemic therapy. The goal of systemic therapy is to destroy or control tumor cells that have spread to distant sites. The vast majority of women with breast cancer have no evidence of metastatic disease at the time of diagnosis. However, micrometastases have probably occurred even in stage I disease and especially in stage II disease, making breast cancer a systemic disease at the time of diagnosis. Because of the high risk for recurrent disease, nearly all women with evidence of node involvement, particularly those who are hormone-receptor negative, will have some type of systemic therapy. Certain women, particularly those who are premenopausal, are known to be at higher risk for recurrent or metastatic disease. These women are often recommended for systemic therapy even when no evidence of node involvement is found. Weighing the different risk factors to determine the need for adjuvant therapy in a node-negative patient is a complex process.[27]

Systemic therapy as an adjuvant to primary local treatment, in the absence of demonstrable metastases, significantly decreases

Table 49-7 Breast Cancer: Treatment Options, Side Effects, Complications, and Patient Issues

Procedure	Description	Hospitalization	Side Effects	Potential Complications: Short Term	Potential Complications: Long Term	Patient Issues
Modified radical mastectomy	Removal of breast, preservation of pectoralis muscle, axillary node dissection	Hospital stay is 1-2 days	Chest wall tightness Phantom breast sensations Arm swelling Sensory changes	Skin flap necrosis Seroma Hematoma Infection	Muscle atrophy Muscle weakness Lymphedema	Loss of breast Incision Body image Need for prosthesis Impaired arm mobility
Breast conservation surgery (lumpectomy) with radiation therapy	Wide excision of tumor, axillary node dissection, radiation therapy	Hospital stay is 1-2 days Radiation 5-6 weeks	Breast soreness Breast edema Skin reactions Arm swelling Sensory changes in breast and arm Fatigue	Moist desquamation* Hematoma Seroma Infection	Fibrosis Rib fractures* Lymphedema Myositis Pneumonitis*	Prolonged treatment* Impaired arm mobility Change in texture and sensitivity of breast
Tissue expansion and breast implants	Expander used to slowly stretch tissue; saline gradually injected into reservoir over weeks to months Insertion of implant under musculofascial layer of chest wall	Outpatient or overnight hospital stay	Discomfort	Skin flap necrosis Wound separation Seroma Hematoma Infection	Capsular contractions	Body image Prolonged physician visits (expander implants)
Musculocutaneous flap procedures	A musculocutaneous flap (muscle, skin, blood supply) is transposed from latissimus dorsi or transverse rectus abdominis to chest wall	Hospital stay is 3-5 days	Pain related to two surgical sites and extensive surgery	Delayed wound healing Cellulitis Skin flap necrosis Abdominal hernia		Prolonged postoperative recovery New breast tissue Similar to normal breast

Sources: Bostwick J, Carlson GW: Reconstruction of the breast, *Surg Oncol Clin North Am* 6:71, 1997; and Knobf MT: Treatment options for early stage breast cancer, *Medsurg Nurs* 3:249, 1994.
*Specific to radiation therapy.

cancer recurrence rates and increases survival. Current types of systemic therapy available for breast cancer treatment include chemotherapy, hormonal manipulation, and biologic therapy.

Chemotherapy. Chemotherapy refers to the use of cytotoxic drugs to destroy cancer cells. The greatest benefits from chemotherapy have been achieved among premenopausal women with node findings that are positive for malignancy. Some studies indicate improved outcomes for postmenopausal women as well.

In some instances chemotherapy is being used preoperatively. Preoperative chemotherapy may be more convenient than postoperative administration and can decrease the size of the primary tumor, possibly permitting less extensive surgery. Also, it has been shown that preoperative chemotherapy suppresses tumor growth and prolongs survival.

Breast cancer is one of the solid tumors that is most responsive to chemotherapy. The use of combinations of drugs is clearly superior to the use of a single drug. The benefit of combination treatment results from the use of drugs that have different actions on cell growth and division. Two common combination-therapy protocols are cyclophosphamide (Cytoxan), methotrexate, 5-fluorouracil (5-FU), vincristine (Oncovin), and prednisone (CMFVP); and cyclophosphamide, doxorubicin (Adriamycin), and 5-FU (CAF). Paclitaxel (Taxol) and docetaxel (Taxotere) show promise for treating metastatic breast cancer.[28] Capecitabine (Xeloda), used to treat metastatic breast cancer, is administered orally and causes minimal hair loss and limited bone marrow depression. Vinorelbine (Navelbine), a relatively new chemotherapeutic drug for treating metastatic breast cancer, is well tolerated with fewer and milder side effects than other chemotherapy drugs.

Because healthy cells are also affected by chemotherapy, a variety of side effects accompany this treatment modality. The incidence and severity of predictable and commonly observed side effects will be influenced by the specific drug combination, drug schedule, and dose intensity of the drug or drugs. Usually body organs with rapidly growing cells are the most strongly affected. The most common side effects involve the gastrointestinal (GI) tract, bone marrow, and hair follicles, resulting in nausea, anorexia, weight loss, bone marrow suppression and subsequent fatigue, and alopecia (hair loss). When prednisone is added to the chemotherapy regimen, the side effects related to myelosuppression and GI toxicity are reduced.

Herceptin is an antibody to HER-2/neu, an antigen that often appears on the surface of breast cancer cells. After the antibody attaches to the antigen, it is taken into the cells and eventually kills them. It can be used in combination with standard therapy to treat patients with metastatic breast cancer.

Hormonal therapy. Estrogen can promote growth of breast cancer cells if the cells are estrogen-receptor positive. If the source of estrogen is removed, tumor regression may occur. The source of estrogen (especially estradiol) can be greatly reduced by surgical ablation (e.g., oophorectomy, adrenalectomy, hypophysectomy) or with additive hormonal therapy.[18] Hormonal therapy is widely used to treat recurrent or metastatic cancer but may occasionally be used as an adjuvant to primary treatment.

Two advances have increased the use of hormone therapy. First, hormone receptor assays, which are reliable tests, have been developed to identify women who are likely to respond to hormone therapy. Both estrogen and progesterone receptor status of the tumor can be determined. The importance of these assays is their ability to predict whether hormone manipulation is a treatment option for women with breast cancer, either at the time of initial therapy or if the cancer recurs. Second, drugs have been developed that can inactivate the hormone-secreting glands as effectively as surgery or radiation, without the side effects of these therapies or the need to supplement other hormones no longer secreted by the ablated gland.

Not all breast malignancies are estrogen dependent. Although normal breast tissue contains receptor sites for hormones, malignant cell transformation alters these receptor sites in some cells. If a malignant cell retains hormone receptor sites, it continues to depend on estrogen for cell division. The receptor sites that are altered as a result of malignant transformation are no longer controlled by hormones. Premenopausal and perimenopausal women are more likely to have tumors that are not hormone dependent, whereas women who are postmenopausal are more likely to have hormone-dependent tumors. Chances of tumor regression observed with hormone manipulation are minimal in women whose tumors are lacking estrogen and progesterone receptors. Receptor status probably has no relation to response to chemotherapy. Receptor status may change following hormonal therapy, radiotherapy, or chemotherapy.

Tamoxifen citrate (Nolvadex) is the usual first choice of treatment in postmenopausal, estrogen receptor–positive women with or without nodal involvement. Tamoxifen, an antiestrogen drug, blocks the estrogen receptor sites of malignant cells and thus inhibits the growth-stimulating effects of estrogen. It is commonly used to prevent or treat recurrent breast cancer. Side effects of tamoxifen are minimal but include hot flashes, nausea, vomiting, dry skin, vaginal bleeding, menstrual irregularities, and other effects commonly associated with decreased estrogen.

Women with breast cancer have an increased risk of a second primary breast tumor. Tamoxifen reduces not only the risk of recurrent breast cancer but also that of new primary tumors. Although originally prescribed for 1 to 2 years, it is often used now for longer periods of time.[27] The risk for endometrial cancer increases following tamoxifen therapy for invasive breast cancer. However, it is generally agreed that the net benefit greatly outweighs the risk. Endometrial cancers occurring after tamoxifen therapy do not appear to be of a different type than endometrial cancers in non–tamoxifen-treated patients.

Initial results from clinical trials have shown that tamoxifen may significantly prevent breast cancer in high risk individuals.[29] Women who took tamoxifen in these trials had a rate of breast cancer half as high as women taking a placebo. Side effects from tamoxifen in postmenopausal women include blood clots and increased risk for endometrial cancer. Current trials are examining the effect of taking tamoxifen for 2 years versus 3 to 5 years to prevent cancer relapse. Raloxifene (Evista), a drug used to prevent bone loss, may also reduce the risk of breast cancer without stimulating endometrial growth. Raloxifene acts as an estrogen antagonist at hormone-sensitive breast cancer tissue. (Raloxifene is discussed in the section on osteoporosis in Chapter 59.)

Toremifene citrate (Fareston), an antiestrogen agent similar to tamoxifen, is indicated as first-line treatment for

NURSING ASSESSMENT

Table 49-8 Breast Cancer

Subjective Data

Important Health Information

Past health history: Benign breast disease with atypical changes; previous unilateral breast cancer; menstrual history (early menarche with late menopause); pregnancy history (nulliparity or first full-term pregnancy after age 30); previous endometrial, ovarian, or colon cancer; hyperestrogenism and testicular atrophy (in men)

Medications: Use of estrogens, especially as post-menopausal hormone replacement therapy and in oral contraceptives

Surgery and other treatments: Exposure to excessive radiation

Functional Health Patterns

Health perception–health management: Positive family history (especially mother or sister); alcohol use; mammography history; palpable change found on BSE

Nutritional-metabolic: Obesity; anorexia (possible indicator of metastasis)

Cognitive-perceptual: Headache, back, arm, or bone pain (possible indicators of metastasis)

Sexuality-reproductive: Unilateral nipple discharge (clear, milky, or bloody); change in breast contour, size, or symmetry

Coping–stress tolerance: Chronic psychologic stress

Self-perception–self-concept: Anxiety regarding threat to self-esteem

Objective Data

General

Axillary and supraclavicular lymphadenopathy

Integumentary

Firm, discrete nodules at mastectomy site (possible indicator of local recurrence); peripheral edema (possible indicator of metastasis)

Respiratory

Pleural effusions (possible indicator of metastasis)

Gastrointestinal

Hepatomegaly, jaundice; ascites (possible indicators of liver metastasis)

Reproductive

Hard, irregular, nonmobile breast lump most often in upper, outer sector, possibly fixated to fascia or chest wall; nipple inversion or retraction, erosion; edema ("orange peel"), erythema, induration, infiltration, or dimpling (in later stages)

Possible Findings

Finding of mass or change in tissue on breast examination; positive results of mammography or ultrasonography; positive results of FNA or surgical biopsy or similar results with a needle biopsy

FNA, fine needle aspiration.

metastatic breast cancer in postmenopausal women with estrogen receptor–positive or estrogen receptor–unknown tumors. Aromatase inhibitor drugs, which block the synthesis of estrogen from precursor molecules, are used in the treatment of advanced breast cancer in postmenopausal women with disease progression. These drugs include aminoglutethimide (Cytadren), anastrozole (Arimidex), and letrozole (Femara).

Additional drugs that may be used to suppress hormone-dependent breast tumors include megestrol (Megace), diethylstilbestrol (DES), and fluoxymesterone (Halotestin). Less common hormone-deprivation strategies include bilateral oophorectomy, adrenalectomy, and hypophysectomy.

Biologic Therapy. The use of biologic therapy represents an attempt to stimulate the body's natural defenses to recognize and attack cancer cells. (The use of these therapies is discussed in Chapter 14.)

Bone Marrow and Stem Cell Transplantation. Autologous bone marrow or stem cell transplantation combined with high-dose chemotherapy has been used to treat patients with advanced metastatic breast cancer. In this technique patients donate their own bone marrow or peripheral blood from which stem cells are harvested. Then they receive high doses of chemotherapy, which causes bone marrow suppression. The patient subsequently undergoes autologous bone marrow or stem cell transplantation. (Bone marrow and stem cell transplantation are discussed in Chapter 14.)

NURSING MANAGEMENT: BREAST CANCER

■ Nursing Assessment

Subjective and objective data that should be obtained from an individual suspected of having or diagnosed as having breast cancer are presented in Table 49-8.

■ Nursing Diagnoses

Nursing diagnoses related to the care of a patient diagnosed with breast cancer vary. Following diagnosis and before a treatment plan has been selected, the following diagnoses would apply:

- Decisional conflict *related to* lack of knowledge about treatment options and their effects
- Fear *related to* diagnosis of breast cancer
- Body image disturbance *related to* anticipated physical and emotional effects of treatment modalities

If a mastectomy is planned, the nursing diagnoses may include, but are not limited to, those presented in NCP 49-1. Nursing diagnoses for the patient receiving radiation therapy or chemotherapy are presented in NCP 14-1.

■ Planning

The overall goals are that the patient with breast cancer will (1) actively participate in the decision-making process related to treatment options, (2) fully comply with the therapeutic plan, (3) manage the side effects of adjuvant therapy, and (4) be

49-1 NURSING CARE PLAN PATIENT AFTER A MODIFIED RADICAL MASTECTOMY*

Expected Patient Outcomes	Nursing Interventions and *Rationales*
NURSING DIAGNOSIS Pain *related to* surgical incision and manipulation of tissue *as manifested by* verbalization regarding presence and degree of pain at operative area.*	
▪ Absence of or tolerable level of pain. ▪ Satisfaction with pain control.	▪ Administer analgesics as prescribed *to relieve pain.* ▪ Position arm *to prevent tension on suture line and provide support.* ▪ Encourage use of noninvasive pain management strategies such as distraction, guided imagery, and relaxation *to complement analgesics and decrease need for analgesia.*
NURSING DIAGNOSIS Fear *related to* diagnosis of cancer *as manifested by* questioning, insomnia, reduced attention span, crying.*	
▪ Verbalization of fear. ▪ Support of significant others. ▪ Confidence in ability to cope.	▪ Encourage woman to talk about feelings and diagnosis of cancer *to promote successful resolution of fear and establish effective coping mechanisms.* ▪ Provide accurate information *to promote understanding, clarify information, and reduce anxiety.* ▪ Provide opportunity for significant others to discuss situation and learn about support groups *because their fear about the diagnosis and outcome can decrease their effectiveness as a support system.*
NURSING DIAGNOSIS **Body image disturbance** *related to* loss of body part *as manifested by* verbalization of concern about appearance and feelings of loss of femininity, refusal to view incision, fear of intimacy.	
▪ Verbalization of feelings about surgery and change in body image. ▪ Indication of beginning of resolution of negative feelings toward self. ▪ Acceptance of altered body image.	▪ Assess degree of self-esteem disturbance *so appropriate interventions can be initiated.* ▪ Arrange for Reach for Recovery visitor or similar community resource *to serve as a role model and provide hope for recovery and a normal future.* ▪ Provide information regarding prosthesis fitting and breast reconstruction (if patient is interested) *so patient can make informed decisions regarding options.* ▪ Assist patient to verbalize feelings and encourage open communication with significant others *to promote grief work and maintain support from family/friends.* ▪ Share information regarding community resources (e.g., support groups, information services) *to enable patient to find a place to exchange concerns and feelings about the experience.*
NURSING DIAGNOSIS **Ineffective management of therapeutic regimen** *related to* lack of knowledge regarding BSE and signs and symptoms to report to health care provider *as manifested by* lack of knowledge of or confidence in performing BSE; lack of information about plans for follow-up care, signs and symptoms of recurrent or metastatic disease.*	
▪ Practice of monthly BSE. ▪ Early recognition of recurrent or metastatic disease.	▪ Teach or evaluate BSE performance *to ensure that patient is performing correctly.* ▪ Reinforce importance of annual mammogram *because it is a recommended screening technique for identification of local recurrence after mastectomy and for assessing other breast.* ▪ Provide information about signs and symptoms to report to health care provider (e.g., new and persistent problems such as skin changes at surgical site, new changes in breast or chest wall).
NURSING DIAGNOSIS **Impaired physical mobility** *related to* pain *as manifested by* limitation in movement or upper extremity on surgical side.	
▪ Return to usual arm and shoulder function.	▪ Assess degree of mobility impairment *to provide baseline data and to plan appropriate interventions.* ▪ Treat pain *to promote participation in exercise plan.* ▪ Flex and extend fingers in postoperative period *to maintain range of motion and promote arm circulation.* ▪ Carry out postmastectomy exercises *to prevent contractures and muscle shortening, maintain muscle tone, and improve lymph and blood circulation.* ▪ Assist woman to resume activities of daily living as tolerated or as directed by physician *to reduce dependent behaviors, raise self-esteem, and maintain mobility of affected arm.* ▪ Emphasize bilateral activity of upper extremities *to prevent guarding of operative side and loss of function.*

Continued

49-1 NURSING CARE PLAN PATIENT AFTER A MODIFIED RADICAL MASTECTOMY*—continued

Expected Patient Outcomes	Nursing Interventions and *Rationales*

COLLABORATIVE PROBLEMS

Nursing Goals	Nursing Interventions and *Rationales*
POTENTIAL COMPLICATION	**Lymphedema** *related to* impaired lymphatic drainage and lack of knowledge of preventive measures.
■ Monitor for signs of lymphedema. ■ Report deviations from acceptable parameters. ■ Carry out appropriate medical and nursing interventions.	■ Assess woman for signs of lymphedema such as edema in hand or arm on operative side, heaviness, or localized pain *to enable early diagnosis and intervention to prevent and treat the complication.* ■ Instruct patient about self-care strategies and precautions to reduce risk of lymphedema *so patient will be an active, informed participant in self-care.* ■ Do not perform venipunctures or take BP measurements on affected arm *to reduce risk of constriction, infection, and lymphedema in affected arm.* ■ Avoid dependent arm position *to allow proper wound healing and decrease stress to incision site.* ■ Elevate arm and hand on pillow *to use gravity to assist with drainage of fluid.* ■ Perform hand and wrist movements, elbow flexion, and extension hourly or as indicated *to maintain circulation and range of motion of affected arm.* ■ Encourage participation in activities of daily living and self-care as much as possible *to promote patient's independence and maintain use of affected arm.* ■ Use elastic sleeve if ordered *to apply mechanical pressure to reduce fluid collection in affected arm and promote venous return.*

*Nursing diagnoses with an asterisk also apply to the patient following breast conservation therapy.

satisfied with the support provided by significant others and health care providers.

Nursing Implementation

Acute Intervention. The time between the diagnosis of breast cancer and the selection of a treatment plan is a difficult period for the woman and her family. Although the primary care provider has discussed treatment options, the woman often relies on the nurse to clarify and expand on these options. During this time, the woman may be very self-focused, verbalizing her conflict and indecision frequently. Appropriate nursing interventions during this period include exploring the woman's usual decision-making patterns, helping the woman accurately evaluate the advantages and disadvantages of the options, providing information relevant to the decision, and supporting the patient once the decision is made.

During this period the woman may exhibit signs of distress or tension, such as tachycardia, increased muscle tension, and restlessness, whenever she focuses on the decision to be made. The nurse should assess the woman's body language, motor activity, and affect during periods of high stress and indecision so appropriate interventions can be carried out.

Regardless of the surgery planned, the patient must be provided with sufficient information to ensure informed consent. Some patients need extensive, detailed information. For others, this only increases anxiety. Sensitivity to individual needs is essential. Preoperative diagnostic studies must be completed. Teaching in the preoperative phase includes instruction in turning, coughing and deep breathing, a review of postoperative exercises, and an explanation of the recovery period from the time of surgery until discharge.

The woman who has breast conservation surgery usually has an uneventful postoperative course with only a moderate amount of pain. If an axillary lymph node dissection has occurred or if a woman has had a modified radical mastectomy, specific interventions will be needed.

Restoring arm function on the affected side after mastectomy and axillary lymph node dissection is one of the most important goals of nursing activities. The woman should be placed in a semi-Fowler's position with the arm on the affected side elevated on a pillow. Flexing and extending the fingers should begin in the recovery room with progressive increases in activity encouraged. (Information pertaining to arm exercises and care also apply to women who have had an axillary node dissection after lumpectomy or total mastectomy.) Postoperative mastectomy exercises are instituted gradually at the surgeon's direction (Fig. 49-4). These exercises are designed to prevent contractures and muscle shortening, maintain muscle tone, and improve lymph and blood circulation. The difficulty and pain encountered by the woman in performing the previously simple tasks included in the exercise program may cause

ETHICAL DILEMMAS

Passive Euthanasia and Suffering

SITUATION

A terminally ill 50-year-old woman with metastatic breast cancer resistant to chemotherapy and radiation has developed severe bone pain that is not being managed adequately by her present dose of IV morphine. This is exhibited by moaning at rest and verbalizing severe pain from any movement to reposition her. Even though she appears to sleep at intervals, she requests pain medicine frequently, and her family is demanding additional pain medicine for her. At the team conference the nurses have discussed concerns that additional pain medicine could hasten her death.

DISCUSSION

A medical intervention for the purpose of causing death in order to reduce a patient's suffering is *active euthanasia* and is not legal in the United States. The *intent* in active euthanasia is that the patient die. In *passive euthanasia*, the intent is to reduce pain and suffering and to allow the disease to take its course; the *consequence* may be a hastened death. Although most cancer pain can be managed by health care professionals trained in pain management, a specific patient's suffering may not be helped significantly. Relieving this patient's pain may cause her death to come earlier, but alleviation of pain and suffering is the goal.

ETHICAL AND LEGAL PRINCIPLES

- Euthanasia (good death) can be classified as active or passive. Active euthanasia involves the intentional act to cause the death of another. Passive euthanasia results from the omission of treatment that would sustain life or from the provision of pain medication at a dose that could hasten death. The difference is ambiguous and is often thought to be irrelevant.
- In the theory of double effect it is permissible to provide high levels of medication to provide pain relief even if the secondary effect of that medication is to hasten death.
- The principles of beneficence and nonmaleficence may be considered to conflict in this case. Providing pain relief is beneficent, but hastening a death by an increased dosage could be viewed as harmful. Refusing to give adequate pain relief is harmful to the patient, but not hastening the patient's death is beneficent.

frustration and depression. The goal of all exercise is a return to full range of motion gradually within 4 to 6 weeks.

Postoperative discomfort can be minimized by administering analgesics about 30 minutes before initiating exercises. When showering is appropriate, the flow of warm water over the involved shoulder often has a soothing effect and reduces joint stiffness. Whenever possible, the same nurse should work with the woman so that progress can be monitored and problems can be identified.

Measures to prevent or reduce lymphedema must be used by the nurse and taught to the woman. The affected arm should never be dependent, even while the person is sleeping. Blood pressure readings, venipunctures, and injections should not be done on the affected arm. Elastic bandages should not be used in the early postoperative period because they inhibit collateral lymph drainage. The woman must be instructed to protect the arm on the operative side from even minor trauma such as a pinprick or sunburn. If trauma to the arm occurs, the area should be washed thoroughly with soap and water. A topical antibiotic ointment and a bandage or other sterile dressing should be applied. The surgeon must be advised of the trauma, and the site of injury must be observed closely for evidence of inflammation. The patient must know and understand that she is at risk of developing lymphedema for the rest of her life.[26]

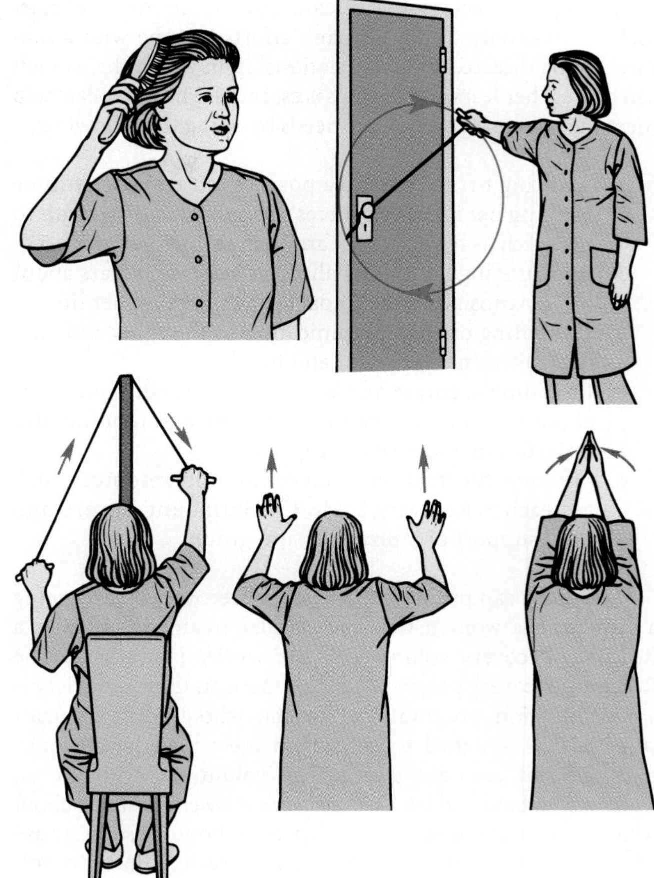

Fig. 49-4 Postoperative mastectomy exercises.

When lymphedema is acute, an intermittent pneumatic compression sleeve may be prescribed. This device applies mechanical massage to the arm. Manual massage is also effective in mobilizing subcutaneous accumulations of fluid. Elevation of the arm so that it is level with the heart, diuretics, and isometric exercises may be recommended to reduce the fluid volume in the arm. The patient may need to wear a fitted elastic pressure-gradient sleeve during waking hours to maintain maximum volume reduction.

Psychologic care. Throughout interactions with a woman with breast cancer, the nurse must keep in mind the extensive psychologic impact of the disease. All aspects of care must include sensitivity to the woman's efforts to cope with a life-threatening disease. An open relationship in which the woman can express her fears and feelings is essential. The nurse can help meet the woman's psychologic needs by doing the following:

1. Assisting her to develop a positive but realistic attitude
2. Helping her identify sources of support and strength to her, such as her partner, family, and spiritual practices
3. Encouraging her to verbalize her anger and fears about her diagnosis and the impact it will have on her life
4. Promoting open communication of thoughts and feelings between the patient and her family
5. Providing accurate and complete answers to questions about her disease, treatment options, and reproductive or lactation issues (if appropriate)
6. Offering information about community resources, such as Reach to Recovery, Y-Me, CanSurmount, Encore, and local support organizations and groups

The nurse can promote the woman's recovery by arranging a visit from a woman who had similar treatment, such as a Reach to Recovery volunteer, if the service is available. The Reach to Recovery program of the American Cancer Society is a rehabilitation program for women who have had breast surgery. It is designed to help them meet their psychologic, physical, and cosmetic needs. The volunteers, who are all women who have had breast cancer, can answer questions about what to expect at home, how to tell people about the surgery, and what prosthetic devices are available. If a Reach to Recovery volunteer is not available, it is the nurse's responsibility to be knowledgeable about the needs of the woman after breast surgery. The American Cancer Society and the National Cancer Institute can provide excellent materials to assist the nurse in meeting the special needs of women with breast cancer.

The professional staff must never underestimate the tremendous psychologic impact that a diagnosis of cancer and subsequent breast surgery can have on a woman. Emotional complications are common. The nurse's accepting, concerned attitude can do a great deal to relieve the feelings of anger and depression experienced by many patients.

Ambulatory and Home Care. The nurse should explain the follow-up routine to the patient and emphasize the importance of beginning and continuing BSE and annual mammography. Immediately after surgery, symptoms that should be reported to the clinician include fever, inflammation at surgical site, erythema, and unusual swelling. Other changes to report are new back pain, weakness, constipation, shortness of breath, and confusion. If adjuvant therapy is to be used, the woman should have specific instructions about appointment times and treatment locations and management of side effects.

For women who have had a mastectomy, the nurse should stress the importance of wearing a well-fitting prosthesis. A variety of products are available to meet the specific needs of the individual woman. A well-trained salesperson can help the woman select a suitable prosthesis. There are both physical and psychologic advantages to the use of a prosthesis; the return of a normal external appearance is especially important to most women.

The implications of the loss of a breast on the sexual identity and relationships of the woman vary. A preoperative sexual assessment provides helpful baseline data that the nurse can use to plan postoperative interventions. Often the husband, sexual partner, or family members may need assistance in dealing with their emotional reactions to the diagnosis and surgery for them to act as effective means of support for the patient.[30] There are no physical reasons for a mastectomy to prevent sexual satisfaction. The woman taking tamoxifen may have a decreased sexual drive or vaginal dryness. She may need to use lubrication to prevent discomfort during intercourse. If difficulty in adjustment or other problems develop, counseling may be necessary to deal with the emotional component of a mastectomy and the diagnosis of cancer.

Depression may occur with the continued stress and uncertainty of a cancer diagnosis. A woman's self-esteem and identity may also be threatened. Special nursing interventions are necessary in terms of both psychologic support and self-care teaching, if a recurrence of cancer is found. The support of family and friends and participation in a cancer support group are important aspects of care that are helpful in improving quality of life and have been found to have a clinically significant impact on survival.[31]

■ Evaluation

The expected outcomes for the patient after a modified radical mastectomy are presented in NCP 49-1.

MAMMOPLASTY

Mammoplasty is the surgical change in the size or shape of the breast. It may be done electively for cosmetic purposes to either enlarge or reduce the size of the breasts. It may also be done to reconstruct the breast after a mastectomy.

Health care providers should remain nonjudgmental toward women who desire mammoplasty. The desire to alter the appearance of the breasts has special significance for each woman as she attempts to alter or re-create her body image. It is important for the nurse to be aware of the cultural value placed on the breast by the woman. It is important that the woman have a realistic idea about what mammoplasty can accomplish and about possible complications, such as hematoma formation, hemorrhage, and infection. If an implant is involved, capsular contracture and loss of the implant are possible.

Breast Augmentation

In augmentation mammoplasty (the procedure to enlarge the breasts), an implant is placed in a surgically created pocket between the capsule of the breast and the pectoral fascia. Most implants are silicone envelopes filled with a fluid such as dextran, saline, or silicone. Because of their resemblance to the human breast, implants filled with silicone were the most widely used. In 1992 the Food and Drug Administration suspended the routine use of silicone implants in response to potential hazards related to silicone leakage. Allegations of associated immune-related diseases caused or exacerbated by the presence of silicone gel implants have caused considerable controversy and litigation. Their use is approved only when medically prescribed in clinical trials.

In the United States saline-filled implants are usually used. Saline-filled implants are silicone shells filled with normal saline. Soybean implants are an alternative form of implant. This implant has an outer shell of silicone and is filled with highly refined soybean oil. A major advantage of soybean implants is that it is easier for x-rays to penetrate the implant, so better visualization of breast tissue is possible with mammography.

Breast Reduction

For some women, large breasts can be a source of pain and embarrassment. They can interfere with normal daily activities such as walking, typing, and driving a car. Overly large breasts can interfere with self-esteem and self-image and can lead to back, shoulder, and neck problems. They may make stylish dressing more difficult. Reduction in the size of the breasts can have positive effects on both the psychologic and the physical health of the patient. Reduction mammoplasty is performed by resecting wedges of tissue from the upper and lower quadrants of the breast. The excess skin is removed, and the areola and nipple are relocated on the breast. Lactation can usually be accomplished if massive amounts of tissue are not removed and the nipples are left connected during surgery.

NURSING MANAGEMENT: BREAST AUGMENTATION AND REDUCTION

Breast augmentation and breast reduction may be done in the outpatient surgical area, or it may involve overnight hospitalization. General anesthesia is used. Drains are generally placed in the surgical site to prevent hematoma formation and then removed 2 to 3 days after surgery or when drainage is under 20 ml per day. The drainage must be examined for color and odor to detect postoperative infection or hemorrhage. The woman's temperature should also be monitored. Dressings should be changed as necessary and prescribed using sterile technique. After surgery the woman should be assured that the appearance of the breast will improve when healing is completed. Depending on physician instructions, the patient may be instructed to wear a bra that provides good support continuously for 2 to 3 days after breast reduction or augmentation. Depending on the extent of the operation, most women can resume normal activities within 2 to 3 weeks. Strenuous exercise may not be appropriate until several weeks later.

Breast Reconstruction

Breast reconstruction can be done at the time of mastectomy or any time after mastectomy. Recent advances in techniques have made breast reconstruction a satisfactory alternative for many women. The possibility of breast reconstruction may encourage women to seek professional help if a breast lump is detected. Women are demanding more information about and participation in treatment decisions, and breast reconstruction is becoming more common and accepted.

Indications. The main indication for breast reconstruction is to improve the woman's self-image and regain a sense of normality.[32] Present techniques cannot restore lactation, nipple sensation, or erectility. Therefore the erotic functions of the breast are not present. Although the breast will not fully resemble its premastectomy appearance, the reconstructed appearance usually represents an improvement over the mastectomy scar (Fig. 49-5). The contour of the breast is restored without the use of an external prosthesis.

Timing of Reconstruction. Reconstructive surgery may be done simultaneously with a mastectomy or some time afterward to achieve symmetry and to restore or preserve body image. The timing of reconstruction surgery should be individualized, based on the psychologic needs of the patient. The timing of reconstruction ranges from during the initial mastectomy surgery to many years after surgery. Immediate breast reconstruction after mastectomy is being performed with increasing frequency.[33] The advantages to immediate

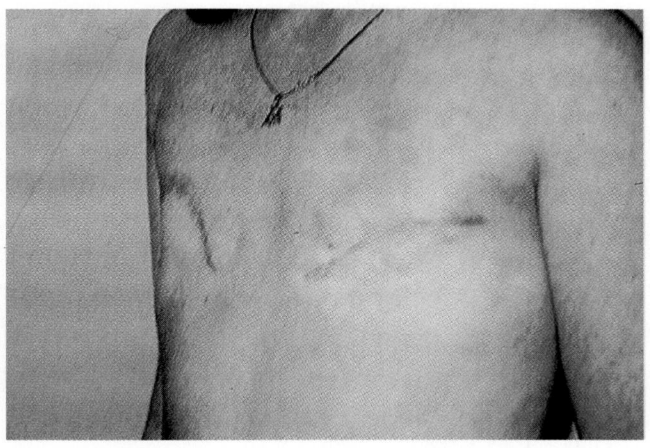

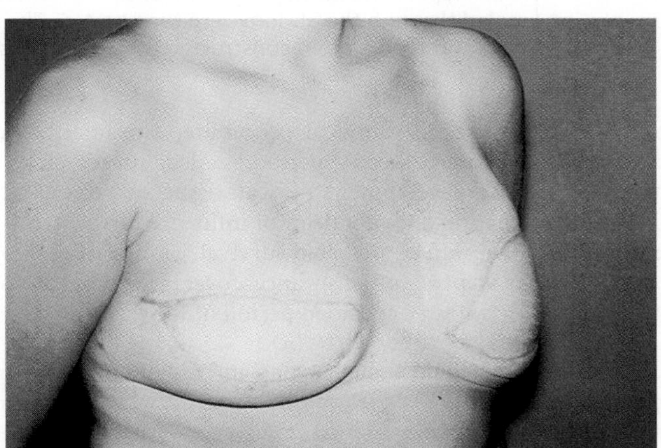

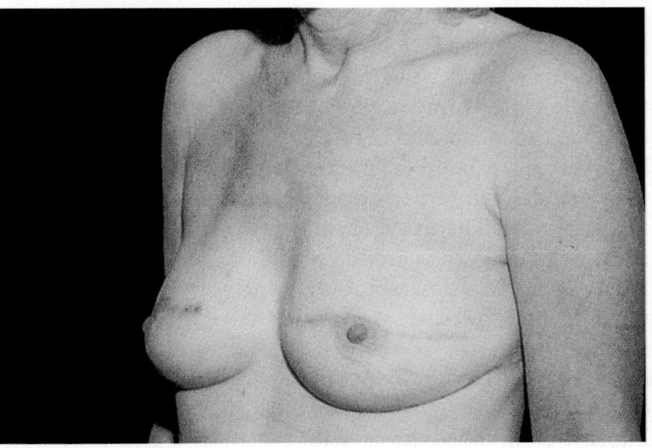

Fig. 49-5 **A,** Appearance of chest following bilateral mastectomy. Postoperative breast reconstruction before, **B,** and after, **C,** nipple-areolar reconstruction.

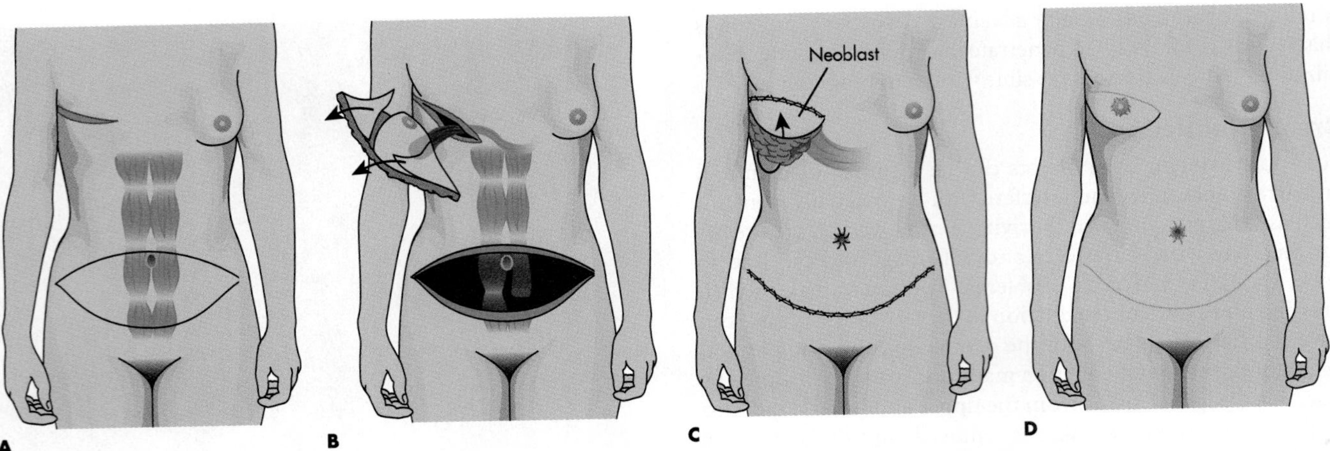

Fig. 49-6 TRAM flap. **A,** TRAM flap is planned. **B,** The abdominal tissue, while attached to the rectus muscle, nerve, and blood supply, is tunneled through the abdomen to the chest. **C,** The flap is trimmed to shape the breast. The lower abdominal incision is closed. **D,** Nipple and areola are reconstructed after the breast is healed.

reconstruction are one surgical procedure, one anesthesia induction, and one recovery period.[33] Also, surgery takes place before the development of scar tissue or adhesions. Early reconstruction does not delay or influence further treatment or adversely affect predicted survival. Timing of reconstruction may depend on insurance coverage. Some plans reimburse only within a specified period of time.

Techniques of Reconstruction

Breast implants and tissue expansion. Breast implants are placed in a pocket under the pectoralis muscle, which protects the implant and provides soft tissue coverage over the implant. Implants can be placed either at the time of mastectomy or later. Because many mastectomy patients have insufficient tissue, simple placement of an implant may lead to small breast reconstruction that is tight or firm.

A tissue expander can be used to stretch the skin and muscle at the mastectomy site before inserting implants. The use of tissue expanders and breast implants is the most common breast reconstruction technique currently used. Placement of the expander can be performed at the time of mastectomy or at a later date. The tissue expander, which is fully deflated at the time of surgery, is gradually filled by weekly injections of sterile water or saline solution, which stretch the skin and muscle. Once the tissue is adequately stretched and the anticipated breast size is reached, the expander is surgically removed and a permanent implant is inserted. Some expanders are designed to remain in place and become the implant, eliminating the need for a second surgical procedure. Tissue expansion does not work well in individuals with extensive scarred tissue from surgery or radiation therapy.

The body's natural response to the presence of a foreign substance is the formation of a fibrous capsule around the implant. If excessive capsular formation occurs as a result of infection, hematoma, trauma, or reaction to a foreign body, a contracture can develop, resulting in a deformed breast. Surgeons differ in their approaches to the prevention of contracture formation, although gentle manual massage around the implant is routine. Prevention of the problems that cause excessive capsule formation is critical. Other postoperative complications include skin ulceration, hypertrophic scar formation, intercostal neuralgia, and wound infection.

Musculocutaneous flap techniques. If insufficient muscle is left after mastectomy or if the chest wall has been radiated, the person's own musculocutaneous flaps may be used to repair the soft-tissue defects. Current restrictions on the use of silicone implants have resulted in an increased use of autologous tissue reconstruction.[33] Flaps are most often taken from the back (latissimus dorsi muscle) or the abdomen (transverse rectus abdominis muscle). In the latissimus dorsi musculocutaneous flap a block of skin and muscle from the patient's back is used to replace tissue removed during mastectomy. A small implant may be needed beneath the flap to gain reasonable breast shape and size. A disadvantage of this technique is an additional scar on the back.

The transverse rectus abdominis musculocutaneous (TRAM) flap is the most frequently used flap operation.[33] The rectus abdominis muscles are paired flat muscles running from the rib cage down to the pubic bone. Arteries running inside the muscle provide branches at many levels, and these branches supply the fat and skin across a large expanse of the abdomen. With this technique the surgeon elevates a large block of tissue from the lower abdominal area, but leaves it attached to the rectus muscle (Fig. 49-6). This tissue is then tunneled under the skin up to the area where the breast will be reconstructed. Then it is molded and fashioned to form a breast. The abdominal incision is closed, giving the patient a result that is similar to having an abdominoplasty. This surgical procedure can last 2 to 4 hours, with recovery taking 4 to 6 weeks. Complications include bleeding, hernia, and infection. An implant may be used in addition to the flap if the flap does not provide the desired cosmetic result alone.

Nipple-areolar reconstruction. The majority of patients who have breast reconstruction also have nipple-areolar reconstruction. Nipple reconstruction gives the reconstructed breast a much more natural appearance. Nipple-areolar reconstruction is usually done a few months after breast reconstruction. Tissue to construct a nipple may be taken from the opposite breast or from a small flap of tissue on the reconstructed breast mound. The areola may be grafted from the labia, skin in area of the groin, or lower abdominal skin, or it may be tattooed with a permanent pigmented dye. In some patients a small implant may be placed under the completed nipple areolar reconstruction to add additional projection.

CRITICAL THINKING EXERCISES

CASE STUDY

Breast Cancer

Patient Profile

Karen G., a 46-year-old woman, discovered a large lump in the upper outer quadrant of her left breast while showering.

Subjective Data

- Has family history of breast cancer—mother diagnosed at age 48
- Had onset of menarche at age 11
- Has two daughters, first birth at age 33
- Has no previous history of breast cancer
- States she is afraid she has cancer

Objective Data

- Palpable 1.5 cm mass in upper outer quadrant of left breast
- Left breast mass confirmed by mammogram
- Otherwise normal physical examination
- Fine-needle aspiration biopsy of mass indicates diagnosis of cancer

Collaborative Care

- Scheduled for lumpectomy and axillary lymph node dissection

Critical Thinking Questions

1. What characteristics of malignancy could be determined by palpation of Karen's breast mass?
2. What information would the nurse provide to Karen about her planned therapy?
3. What information about breast cancer risks is important to provide to Karen and her daughters? What early detection measures are important for them to know?
4. What are the possible complications the patient may face after a lumpectomy?
5. What are common postoperative exercises that Karen will need to practice?
6. What community resources are available to help Karen and her family adjust to the change in her body and to cope with the diagnosis of cancer? How can the nurse access these resources?
7. Based on the assessment data presented, write one or more appropriate nursing diagnoses. Are there any collaborative problems?

NURSING RESEARCH ISSUES

1. What are the major concerns of women who are diagnosed with breast cancer?
2. Does attendance at a cancer support group decrease anxiety in women who elect to have breast conservation surgery and radiation?
3. What are the informational and support needs of family members of the woman with cancer?
4. Do elderly women experience more or less sensory changes after breast surgery than young women?
5. Does perceived susceptibility to breast cancer increase a woman's motivation to participate in breast cancer screening?
6. What effect does dietary intake of caffeine have on a woman's perception of the severity of fibrocystic changes in the breast?
7. What influence does immediate versus delayed reconstruction have on the psychosocial adjustment of a woman after a mastectomy?
8. What is the influence of individualized teaching by a health professional on the frequency of breast self-examination practice in women?

REVIEW QUESTIONS

The number of the question corresponds to the same-numbered objective at the beginning of the chapter.

1. The nurse teaches a patient that BSE involves both the palpation of the breast tissue and
   a. hard squeezing of the breast tissue.
   b. palpation of cervical lymph nodes.
   c. a mammogram to evaluate breast tissue.
   d. inspection of the breasts for any changes.
2. An occupational health nurse is planning a program on BSE for women in the company. To best promote learning and compliance of the participants the nurse includes
   a. a movie that demonstrates the procedure of BSE.
   b. distribution of detailed written instructions for use at home.
   c. explanations emphasizing the value of early detection of breast cancer.
   d. an opportunity to practice BSE on themselves with individual guidance from the nurse.
3. In teaching a patient with painful fibrocystic breast changes about the condition, the nurse explains that
   a. all discrete breast lumps must be biopsied to rule out malignant changes.
   b. the lumps will become progressively larger and more painful, eventually necessitating surgical removal.
   c. the symptoms will probably subside following menopause unless hormone replacement is used.
   d. restrictions of coffee and chocolate and supplements of vitamin E are effective treatments for most postmenopausal patients.
4. While discussing risk factors for breast cancer with a group of women, the nurse stresses that the greatest risk factor for breast cancer is
   a. being a female over the age of 50.
   b. experiencing menstruation for 40 years or more.
   c. using estrogen replacement therapy during menopause.
   d. having a paternal grandmother with postmenopausal breast cancer.
5. A patient has an excisional biopsy of a breast nodule that is positive for cancer. The nurse explains that of the other tests done to determine the risk for cancer recurrence or spread, the result that supports the most favorable prognosis is
   a. cells with low S-phase fractions.
   b. absence of an HER-2/neu genetic marker.
   c. absence of axillary lymph node involvement.
   d. estrogen and progesterone receptor–positive tumors.

6. A patient diagnosed with breast cancer has been offered the treatment choice of breast conservation surgery with radiation or a modified radical mastectomy. When questioned by the patient about these options, the nurse informs the patient that the lumpectomy with radiation
   a. preserves the normal appearance and sensitivity of the breast.
   b. provides a shorter treatment period with fewer long-term complications.
   c. has about the same 10-year survival rate as the modified radical mastectomy.
   d. reduces the fear and anxiety that accompany the diagnosis and treatment of cancer.
7. Postoperatively the nurse teaches the patient with a modified radical mastectomy to prevent lymphedema by
   a. using a sling to keep the arm flexed at the side.
   b. exposing the arm to sunlight to increase circulation.
   c. wrapping the arm with elastic bandages during the night.
   d. avoiding unnecessary trauma (e.g., venipuncture, BP) to the arm on the operative side.
8. To prevent capsular formation following breast reconstruction with implants, the nurse teaches the patient to
   a. bind the breasts tightly with elastic bandages.
   b. gently massage the area around the implant.
   c. avoid strenuous exercise until implant healing has occurred.
   d. exercise the arm on the affected side to promote drainage.

References

1. Landis SH and others: Cancer statistics 1998, *CA Cancer J Clin* 48:1, 1998.
2. American Cancer Society: *Cancer facts and figures 1998: selected cancers,* Atlanta, 1998, American Cancer Society.
3. National Institutes of Health Consensus Development Panel: National Institutes of Health Consensus Development Conference Statement: breast cancer screening for women ages 40–49, *J Natl Cancer Inst* 89:1, 1998.
4. National Cancer Institute: PDQ: detection and prevention, *http://www.icic.nci.nih.gov/clinpdg/screening/breastcancer-physician.html#1.*
5. Champion V, Menon U: Predicting mammography and breast self-examination in African-American women, *Cancer Nurs* 20:315, 1997.
6. Womeodu RJ, Bailey JE: Barriers to cancer screening, *Med Clin North Am* 80:115, 1996.
7. Harvard Women's Health Watch: *Benign breast conditions 5:4,* Boston, 1998, Harvard Women's Health.
8. Weber E: Questions and answers about breast cancer diagnosis, *AJN* 97:34, 1997.
9. Witmer DR, Dickson-Witmer D, Teixido R: Initial 100 consecutive stereotactic core breast biopsies in a private breast center setting, *Del Med J* 69:297, 1997.
10. Adner D, Shriver C: Cyclical mastalgia: prevalence and impact in an outpatient breast clinic sample, *Am Coll Surg* 185:466, 1997.
11. Perna W: Mastalgia: diagnosis and treatment, *J Am Acad Nurse Pract* 8:579, 1996.
12. Cady B and others: Evaluation of common breast problems: guidance for primary care providers, *CA Cancer J Clin* 48:49, 1998.
13. Robinson K, McCance K: Alterations of the reproductive systems. In McCance K, Huether S, editors: *Pathophysiology—biologic basis for disease in adults and children,* ed 3, St Louis, 1998, Mosby.
14. Thompson J, Wilson S: *Health assessment for nursing practice,* St Louis, 1996, Mosby.
15. Colditz G: The benefits of hormone replacement therapy do not outweigh the increased risk of breast cancer, *J NIH Research* 8:41, 1996.
16. Stanford J: The benefits of hormone replacement therapy outweigh the breast cancer risks for some women, *J NIH Research* 8:40, 1996.
17. Nurses Health Study: Risks and benefits of oral contraceptives and postmenopausal hormones, *Nurses' Health Study Newsletter* 5:6, 1998.
18. Dow K: Breast cancer. In Varrichio C and others, editors: *A cancer source book for nurses,* ed 7, Atlanta, 1997, American Cancer Society.
19. Lessick M, Wickham R, Rehwaldt M: Breast and ovarian cancer: genetic update and implications for nursing, *Medsurg Nurs* 6:341, 1997.
20. Calzone K: Issues in breast cancer susceptibility testing, *Innovations in Breast Cancer Care* 2:66, 1997.
21. Moore M, Kinne D: The surgical management of primary invasive breast cancer, *CA Cancer J Clin* 45:279, 1995.
22. Harvard Women's Health Watch: Sentinel node biopsy, 5:7 Boston, 1998, Harvard Women's Health.
23. Cirisano F, Karlan B: The role of HER-2/neu oncogene in gynecologic cancers, *J Soc Gynecol Investig* 3:99, 1996.
24. American Joint Committee on Cancer: *Manual for staging of cancer,* ed 4, Philadelphia, 1992, Lippincott.
25. Gross R: Current issues in the surgical treatment of early stage breast cancer, *Clin J Oncol* 2:55, 1998.
26. Price J, Purtell J: Prevention and treatment of lymphedema after breast cancer, *AJN* 97:34, 1997.
27. Hortobaggi G, Buxdar A: Current status of adjuvant systemic therapy for breast cancer: progress and controversy, *CA Cancer J Clin* 45:199, 1995.
28. Marty M and others: Prospects with docetaxel in the treatment of patients with breast cancer, *Eur J Cancer* 33(suppl 7):526, 1997.
29. Early Breast Cancer Trialists: Tamoxifen for early breast cancer: an overview of the randomized trials, *Lancet* 351:9114, 1998.
30. Pelushi J: The lived experience of surviving breast cancer, *Oncol Nurs Forum* 24:1343, 1997.
31. Ferrell B and others: Quality of life in breast cancer survivors: implications for developing support services, *Oncol Nurs Forum* 25:887, 1998.
32. Neil K, Armstrong N, Burnett C: Choosing reconstruction after mastectomy: a qualitative analysis, *Oncol Nurs Forum* 25:743, 1998.
33. Bostwick J, Carlson GW: Reconstruction of the breast, *Surg Oncol Clin North Am* 6:71, 1997.

Resources

American Cancer Society—Reach to Recovery
1599 Clifton Road NE
Atlanta, GA 30329
404-320-3333
http://www.cancer.org

Breast Cancer Information Center
http://breast-cancer.sciweb.com/index.html

Breast Cancer Information Clearinghouse (BCIC)
http://nysernet.org/bcic/

National Alliance of Breast Cancer Organizations
9 East 37th Street, 10th Floor
New York, NY 10016
212-719-0154
800-719-9154
Fax: 212-689-1213
http://www.nabco.org

National Breast Cancer Coalition
1707 L Street, NW, Suite 1060
Washington, DC 20036
202-296-7477
Fax: 202-265-6854
http://www.natlbcc.org/

National Lymphedema Network
2211 Post Street, Suite 404
San Francisco, CA 94115-3427
415-921-1306
800-541-3259
Fax: 415-921-4284
http://www.wenet.net/~lymphnet/

OncoLink (cancer information site)
http://www.oncolink.upenn.edu

***For additional Internet resources, see the website for this book at* www.mosby.com/MERLIN/medsurg_lewis**

REMEMBER to check out your **companion CD-ROM**

50 NURSING MANAGEMENT Sexually Transmitted Diseases

Janis Luft

www.mosby.com/MERLIN/medsurg_lewis

LEARNING OBJECTIVES

1. Identify the factors contributing to the high incidence of sexually transmitted diseases.
2. Explain the etiology, clinical manifestations, complications, and diagnostic abnormalities of gonorrhea, syphilis, genital herpes, chlamydial infections, and condylomata acuminata.
3. Compare primary genital herpes with recurrent genital herpes.
4. Explain the collaborative care and drug therapy of gonorrhea, syphilis, genital herpes, chlamydial infections, and condylomata acuminata.
5. Identify nursing assessment and nursing diagnoses for patients who have a sexually transmitted disease.
6. Describe the nursing role in the prevention and control of sexually transmitted diseases.
7. Describe the nursing management of patients with sexually transmitted diseases.

SEXUALLY TRANSMITTED DISEASES

Sexually transmitted diseases (STDs) are infectious diseases usually associated with intimate sexual contact. Historically they have been referred to as venereal diseases. Many diseases can be sexually transmitted (Table 50-1). Some STDs, such as chancroid and granuloma inguinale, are more common in tropical and semitropical areas. However, with the mobility of modern society, their occurrence in other areas of the world is increasing. Diseases that are associated with sexual transmission can also be contracted by other routes such as through blood, blood products, and accidental inoculation. Common STDs are discussed in this chapter. Human immunodeficiency virus (HIV) infection and related problems are discussed in Chapter 13. Hepatitis B and hepatitis C infection and related problems are discussed in Chapter 41.

Significance

In the United States all cases of gonorrhea and syphilis must be reported to the state or local health officer. In spite of this requirement, there are many unreported and undiagnosed cases. Often, various STDs coexist; for instance, if a person has gonorrhea, chlamydial infection may also be present. In 1994 and again in 1996, reported cases of chlamydia exceeded those of gonorrhea in the United States. The incidence of gonorrhea steadily increased after 1966 but began to decline in 1975. This trend continued throughout the past two decades, possibly influenced by more focused control activities, changes in surveillance and reporting procedures, and changes in host factors. There were 325,883 cases of gonorrhea reported in the United States in 1996. This was a 17% decrease from 1995.[1]

Resistant strains of gonorrhea accounted for almost 30% of all cases.[1] In 1996 29% of isolates collected by the Gonococcal Isolate Surveillance Project (GISP) were resistant to penicillin, tetracycline, or both. Between 1991 and 1996, the percentage of GISP isolates that were penicillinase-producing *Neisseria gonorrhoeae* (PPNG) declined from 13.1% to 5.8%.[1] In contrast, isolates with chromosomally mediated resistance to penicillin increased from 6.4% in 1991 to 9.1% in 1996. The prevalence of chromosomally mediated tetracycline resistance, 14.3% in 1996, has been relatively stable since 1992. The proportion of GISP isolates demonstrating decreased susceptibility to ciprofloxacin (Cipro), one of the currently recommended treatments for gonorrhea, has decreased from a high of 1.3% in 1994 to 0.5% in 1996.[1] Teenagers and young adults account for 25% to 40% of all gonorrhea cases reported. Most states have enacted laws that permit examination and treatment of minors without parental consent.

The incidence of primary and secondary syphilis has changed since 1941 (Fig. 50-1), mainly because of the availability of penicillin. In 1996 11,387 cases of primary and secondary syphilis were reported to the Centers for Disease Control and Prevention (CDC), the lowest rate of infection since 1960.[1] The reasons for this decline are unclear, but the recognition of the epidemic rise of syphilis and a renewed priority in screening, treating, and educating high risk populations by health care providers may have been factors. Still this disease remains an important health problem. Syphilis is an ulcerative disease, and as such facilitates transmission of HIV infection during sexual

Reviewed by Stephine Heitkemper, RN, ARNP, Nurse Practitioner, Women's Health Care Specialist, Washington State Health Department, Olympia, Wash.

Table 50-1 Microorganisms Responsible for Diseases Transmitted by Sexual Activity

Organism	Disease
Chlamydia trachomatis	Nongonococcal urethritis (NGU); cervicitis; lymphogranuloma venereum
Cytomegalovirus (CMV)	Multiple diseases
Hepatitis B virus	Hepatitis B
Herpes simplex virus (HSV)	Genital herpes
Human immuno-deficiency virus (HIV)	HIV infection, acquired immuno-deficiency syndrome (AIDS)
Human papillomavirus	Genital and anal warts
Molluscum contagiosum virus	Molluscum contagiosum
Neisseria gonorrhoeae	Gonorrhea
Treponema pallidum	Syphilis

contact. If untreated in early pregnancy, syphilis can lead to fetal infection or perinatal death.

Because genital herpes and condylomata acuminata (genital warts) are not reportable diseases in most states, their true incidence is difficult to determine. It is estimated that more than 45 million people in the United States are infected with genital herpes. Since the early 1970s, the prevalence of herpes simplex virus type 2 (HSV-2) has risen by 30%.[2]

Infections caused by bacterium *Chlamydia trachomatis* are the most prevalent bacterial STDs in the United States today. In 1996 490,000 cases of chlamydia were reported to the CDC.[1] Chlamydial infections are a major contributor to pelvic inflammatory disease (PID), ectopic pregnancy, and infertility among women and nongonococcal urethritis in men, and perinatal transmission of the organism can cause neonatal conjunctivitis and pneumonia.[3] Genital warts, the primary clinical manifestation of human papillomavirus (HPV), have become increasingly common with an estimated annual incidence of 500,000 to 1 million cases.

Factors Affecting Incidence of Sexually Transmitted Diseases

There are contributing factors to the increased incidence of STDs. Earlier reproductive maturity and increased longevity have resulted in a longer sexual life span. The increase in the total population has resulted in an increase in the number of susceptible hosts. Other factors include greater sexual freedom, changing roles of women, changes in the institutions of marriage and the family, decreased social control by religious institutions, and an increased emphasis on sexuality on the part of the media. In many studies, the incidence of drug abuse is closely correlated with increasing numbers of cases of STDs.[4] In addition, increased leisure time, inexpensive travel, and

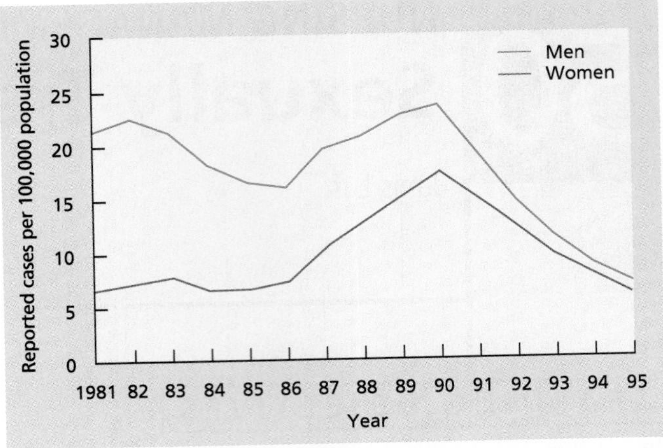

Fig. 50-1 Syphilis. Reported by sex: United States, 1981 to 1995.

urbanization have brought together people of varying cultural backgrounds and value systems.

Changes in the methods of contraception are also reflected in the incidence of STDs. The condom is considered to be the only contraceptive device that is prophylactic in regard to STDs. Although condom use is increasing in selected populations, it is not used frequently in the general population.[5,6] Commonly used oral contraceptives cause the secretions of the cervix and the vagina to become more alkaline. This change produces a more favorable environment for the growth of organisms that cause STDs at these sites. Women who take oral contraceptives have a lower risk of PID as a result of the ability of the cervical mucus to act as a barrier against bacteria. However, the proliferation of chlamydia, the leading cause of nongonococcal PID, may be enhanced by oral contraceptive use. Whether or not intrauterine device (IUD) users are at increased risk of PID is controversial,[7,8] but it is clear that IUDs confer no protection against STDs. Long-acting contraceptives such as levonorgestrel (Norplant) and medroxyprogesterone (Depo-Provera) have been shown to lower concurrent use of condoms, even among women with risk factors for STDs.[4] Both Norplant and Depo-Provera confer no protection against STDs. Lack of awareness of this fact may be a factor leading to STDs in persons using these products.

GONORRHEA

Etiology and Pathophysiology

Gonorrhea is caused by *Neisseria gonorrhoeae*, a gram-negative diplococcus. Mucosa with columnar epithelium is susceptible to gonococcal infection. This tissue is present in the genitalia (the urethra in men, the cervix in women), the rectum, and the oropharynx. The disease is spread by direct physical contact with an infected host, usually during sexual activity. Neonates can develop a gonococcal infection after passage through an infected birth canal. The delicate gonococcus is easily killed by drying, heating, or washing with an antiseptic solution. Consequently, indirect transmission by instruments or linens is rare. The incubation period is 3 to 4 days. The disease confers no immunity to subsequent reinfection. Gonococcal infection elicits an inflammatory response, which, if left untreated, leads to the formation of fibrous tissue and adhesions. This fibrous scarring is subsequently responsible for many complications such as strictures and tubal abnormalities, which can lead to tubal pregnancy, chronic pelvic pain, and infertility.

Clinical Manifestations

Men. The initial site of infection in heterosexual men is usually the urethra. Symptoms of urethritis consist of dysuria and profuse, purulent urethral discharge developing 2 to 5 days after infection. Men generally seek medical assistance early in the disease because their symptoms are usually obvious and distressing. It is very unusual for men with gonorrhea to be asymptomatic.

Women. Most women who contract gonorrhea are asymptomatic or have minor symptoms that are often overlooked, making it possible for them to remain a source of infection. A few women may complain of vaginal discharge, dysuria, or frequency of urination. Changes in menstruation may be a symptom, but these changes are often disregarded by the woman. After the incubation period, redness and swelling occur at the site of contact, which is usually the cervix or urethra. A purulent exudate often develops with a potential for abscess formation. The disease may remain local or can spread by direct tissue extension to the uterus, fallopian tubes, and ovaries. Although the vulva and vagina are uncommon sites for a gonorrheal infection, they may become involved when little or no estrogen is present, as is the case in prepubertal girls and postmenopausal women. Because the vagina acts as a natural reservoir for infectious secretions, transmission is often more efficient from men to women than it is from women to men.

General. Anorectal gonorrhea may be present, particularly in homosexual men, and is usually caused by anal intercourse. Gonococcal proctitis in women probably results from rectal coitus, as well as contamination from infected vaginal secretions. Most patients with rectal infections have no significant symptoms. A small percentage of individuals develop gonococcal pharyngitis resulting from orogenital sexual contact. When the gonococcus can be demonstrated by culture, individuals of either gender are infectious to their sexual partners.

Complications

Because men often seek treatment early in the course of the disease, they are less likely to develop complications. The complications that do occur in men are prostatitis, urethral strictures, and sterility from orchitis or epididymitis. Because women who are free of symptoms seldom seek treatment, complications are more common and usually constitute the reason for seeking medical attention. PID, Bartholin abscess, ectopic pregnancy, and infertility are the main complications of gonorrhea in women. A small percentage of infected persons, mainly women, may develop a disseminated gonococcal infection (DGI). In disseminated infection the appearance of skin lesions, fever, arthralgia, or arthritis usually causes the patient to seek medical help.

Eye Infections in Newborns. Almost all states have a health department regulation or law requiring the instillation of a prophylactic drug such as erythromycin (0.5%) or silver nitrate into the eyes of all newborns.[9] The incidence of gonorrheal eye infections in newborns (ophthalmia neonatorum) is therefore relatively rare today. Untreated infected infants develop permanent blindness.

Diagnostic Studies

The most reliable way to confirm gonococcal infection is to isolate the organism in culture. The immediate identification of *N. gonorrhoeae* is usually made with a Gram's stain of smears made from the exudate. The slides should be interpreted by an experienced technician so that a correct diagnosis is made initially, since some patients fail to return for follow-up care. Cultures of the discharge or secretion can provide a definitive diagnosis after incubation for 24 to 48 hours. For culture, a specific medium (Thayer-Martin), which encourages the growth of the gonococcus, is used. If laboratory facilities are not readily accessible, special holding media are available.

Newer nonculture techniques, including DNA probe techniques and polymerase chain reaction (PCR), do not involve bacterial culture and are useful in situations where culture facilities are unavailable. The new tests are rapidly approaching the specificity and sensitivity of culture methods. The use of DNA amplification techniques (PCR) holds promise for noninvasive testing of genital secretions or urine in the near future. These techniques offer a quicker approach to detecting infection with high rates of sensitivity and specificity.[10,11]

For men, a presumptive diagnosis of gonorrhea is made if there is a history of sexual contact with an infected individual followed within a few days by a urethral discharge. Typical clinical manifestations, combined with a positive finding in a gram-stained smear of the purulent discharge from the penis, gives an almost certain diagnosis. Culture of the discharge is indicated for men whose smears are negative in the presence of strong clinical evidence.

Making a diagnosis of gonorrhea in women on the basis of symptoms is difficult because most women are symptom free or have complaints that may be confused with other conditions. Smears and purulent discharge do not establish a diagnosis of gonorrhea because the female genitourinary tract normally harbors a large number of organisms that resemble *N. gonorrhoeae.* A culture must be performed to confirm the diagnosis. Although the cervix is the most common site of sampling, specimens may also be taken from the urethra, anus, or oropharynx to confirm the diagnosis. The CDC recommends that all women treated for gonorrhea have a rectal culture done.

Collaborative Care

Drug Therapy. A history of sexual contact with a partner known to have gonorrhea is considered good evidence for the presence of gonorrhea. Because of a short incubation period and high infectivity, treatment is instituted without awaiting culture results, even in the absence of any signs or symptoms. The treatment of gonorrhea in the early stage is curative. Traditionally, the drug of choice for gonorrheal therapy had been penicillin, but changes have been made because of resistant strains of *N. gonorrhoeae* and the presence of coexisting chlamydial infection (Table 50-2).

Recently, a rapid increase in the number of cases of gonorrhea caused by resistant strains of *N. gonorrhoeae* has been identified

(Fig. 50-2). Antibiotic resistance can occur as a result of the bacteria producing penicillinase (these strains first appeared in 1976), as well as chromosomally mediated resistance to penicillin (strains displaying this mechanism first appeared in 1983). The recent increase in the rate of chromosomally mediated penicillin-resistant strains of *N. gonorrhoeae* is a worrisome trend. Resistance to ciprofloxacin (Cipro) was first reported in certain strains in 1991, and although still somewhat rare is a cause for concern.

There is no clinical distinction between infections caused by drug-resistant or drug-sensitive strains of *N. gonorrhoeae.* It was therefore anticipated that there would be increased numbers of disease-related complications (e.g., PID, DGI), extended periods of infectiveness resulting in increased numbers of sex partners becoming infected, and increased cost of treatment. As a result, ceftriaxone (Rocephin), a penicillinase-resistant cephalosporin, became part of the treatment plan. Cefixine (Suprax) given orally one time is also effective. The high frequency (up to 45%) of coexisting chlamydial and gonococcal infections has led to the addition of doxycycline (Vibramycin) to the treatment regimen. The expense of diagnosing chlamydial infection and the sequelae of chlamydial infection make this strategy cost-effective. Patients with coexisting syphilis are likely to be cured by the same drugs.

All sexual contacts of patients with gonorrhea must be treated to prevent reinfection after resumption of sexual relations. The "ping-pong" effect of reexposure, treatment, and reinfection can cease only when infected partners are treated simultaneously. Additionally, the patient should be counseled to abstain from sexual intercourse and alcohol during treatment. Sexual intercourse allows the infection to spread and can retard complete healing as a result of vascular congestion. Alcohol has an irritant effect on the healing urethral walls. Men should be cautioned against squeezing the penis to look for further discharge. Follow-up examination and reculture should be done at least once after treatment, usually in 4 to 7 days. Relapse, reinfection, and complications should be treated appropriately.

COLLABORATIVE CARE

Table 50-2 Gonorrhea

Diagnostic
- History and physical examination
- Gram-stained smears of urethral or endocervical exudate
- Cultures for *N. gonorrhea*
- Testing for other STDs (syphilis, HIV, chlamydia)

Collaborative Therapy
- Uncomplicated gonorrhea: cefixine (Suprax) 400 mg orally in a single dose or ceftriaxone (Rocephin) 125 mg IM in a single dose or ciprofloxacin (Cipro) 500 mg orally in a single dose PLUS azithromycin (Zithromax) 1 gm orally in a single dose or doxycycline (Vibramycin) 100 mg orally twice a day for 7 days
- Follow-up cultures after completion of treatment (usually 7 days)
- Case finding
- Treatment of contacts
- Instruction on abstinence from sexual intercourse and alcohol
- Reexamination if symptoms persist or recur after completion of treatment
- Repeat of serologic test for syphilis at 1 month

Modified from Centers for Disease Control: STD treatment guidelines, *MMWR* 47(RR-1):1, 1998.
IM, intramuscular.

SYPHILIS

Etiology and Pathophysiology

The causative organism of syphilis is *Treponema pallidum,* a spirochete. It is extremely fragile and easily destroyed by drying, heating, or washing. The organism is thought to enter the body through very small breaks in the skin or mucous membranes. Its entry is facilitated by the minor abrasions that often occur during intercourse. Not all people who are exposed to syphilis acquire the disease; about one third become infected after intercourse with an infected person. In addition to sexual contact, syphilis may be spread through contact with infectious lesions and sharing of needles among drug addicts. Congenital syphilis is transmitted from an infected mother to the fetus in utero. The incubation period for syphilis ranges from 10 to 90 days but is usually considered to be 3 weeks.

Data from the CDC show the number of reported syphilis cases in 1996 to be the lowest since 1959.[1] However, the disease remains a significant problem among African-Americans (Fig. 50-3). More so than for gonorrhea, persons with untreated syphilis tend to be young persons of a low educational and socioeconomic level, a group that also has high rates of prostitution and drug abuse. This group of people has been extremely hard to reach for education and case finding.

Syphilis is a disease of the blood vessels. The tissue reaction to the presence of *T. pallidum* multiplying in the lymphatics and the perivascular spaces is characterized by dilation and

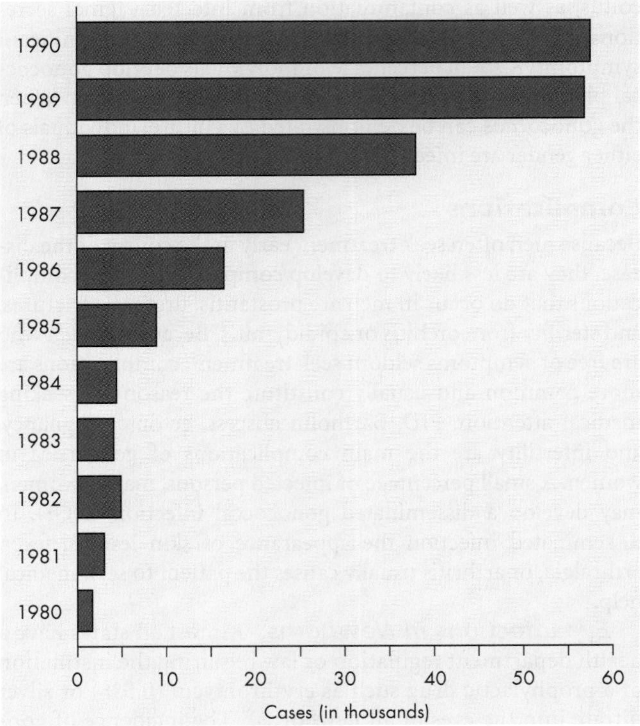

Fig. 50-2 Antibiotic-resistant gonorrhea. Reported cases: United States, 1980 to 1990.

swelling of the capillaries and proliferation of the endothelium and a perivascular infiltration of lymphocytes, giant cells, and fibroblasts, with the formation of new blood vessels. Scar tissue formation is the method of healing in syphilis. The severity and extent of the damage vary.

There is an association between syphilis and HIV infection. Persons at high risk for acquiring syphilis are also at an increased risk for acquiring HIV. Often, both infections are present in the same person. The presence of syphilitic lesions on the genitals enhances HIV transmission. HIV-infected patients with syphilis appear to be at greatest risk for clinically significant central nervous system (CNS) involvement and may require more intensive treatment with penicillin than do other patients with syphilis. Therefore the evaluation of all patients with syphilis should also include testing for HIV antibodies with the patient's consent.

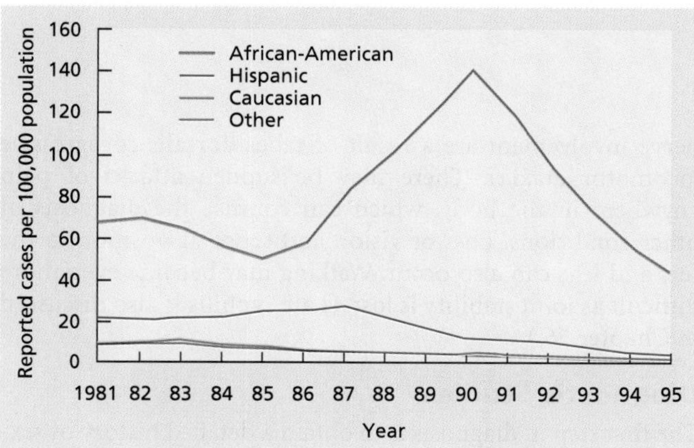

Fig. 50-3 Rate of primary and secondary syphilis in men and women in the United States, by ethnic origin, 1981 to 1995.

Clinical Manifestations

Syphilis has a variety of signs and symptoms that can mimic a number of less serious diseases. Consequently, compared with other venereal diseases, it is more difficult to recognize syphilis. If it is not treated, specific clinical stages are characteristic of the progression of the disease (Table 50-3). Chancres, which are painless indurated lesions found on the penis, vulva, and lips and in the mouth, vagina, and rectum, are seen in the primary stage at the site of bacterial invasion (Fig. 50-4). There, *T. pallidum* multiples in the epithelium, producing a granulomatous tissue reaction (chancre). Some of these microorganisms drain with the lymph into adjacent lymph nodes.

Secondary syphilis is systemic. During this stage bloodborne bacteria spread to all major organ systems. Manifestations characteristic of the secondary stage include cutaneous eruptions, alopecia (hair loss), and generalized adenopathy. The cutaneous eruptions include a bilateral, symmetric rash usually involving the palms and soles; mucous patches in the mouth, tongue, or cervix; and condylomata (moist papules) in the anal and genital area (Fig. 50-5). Latent syphilis follows the secondary stage and is a period during which the immune system is able to suppress the infection. There are no signs or symptoms of syphilis during this time. The diagnosis is established by the finding of a positive specific treponemal antibody test for syphilis together with a normal cerebrospinal fluid (CSF) examination and the absence of clinical manifestations of syphilis on physical examination and chest radiograms. About 70% of untreated patients with latent syphilis never develop clinically evident late syphilis, but the occurrence of a spontaneous cure is in doubt.[12]

Late syphilis (also called tertiary syphilis) is the most severe stage of the disease. Because antibiotics can cure syphilis, manifestations of late syphilis are rare. However, when it does occur, it is responsible for significant morbidity and mortality. The

Table 50-3 Stages of Syphilis

Clinical Stage	Characteristic Findings	Communicability	Duration of Stage
Primary	Chancre	Exudate from chancre highly infectious; blood is infectious	3-8 wk
Secondary	Cutaneous eruptions, alopecia, systemic symptoms (malaise, arthralgia, headache, occasionally liver and kidney dysfunction), regional adenopathy 6-12 wk after chancre	Exudate from skin and mucous membrane lesions highly infectious	1-2 yr
Latent	Absence of signs or symptoms	Noninfectious after 4 yr, possible placental transmission	Throughout life or progression to late stage
Late*	Appearance 3-20 yr after initial infection	Noninfectious	Chronic (without treatment), possibly fatal
Benign	Gummas (chronic, destructive lesions affecting any organ of body, especially skin, bone, liver, mucous membranes)	Spinal fluid possibly containing organism	
Cardiovascular	Aortic valve insufficiency or saccular aneurysm of thoracic aorta, aortitis		
Neurosyphilis	General paresis (personality changes from minor to psychotic, tremors, physical and mental deterioration)		
	Tabes dorsalis (ataxia, areflexia, paresthesias, lightning pains, damaged joints [Charcot's joints])		

*Several forms such as cardiovascular and neurosyphilis occur together in approximately 25% of untreated cases.

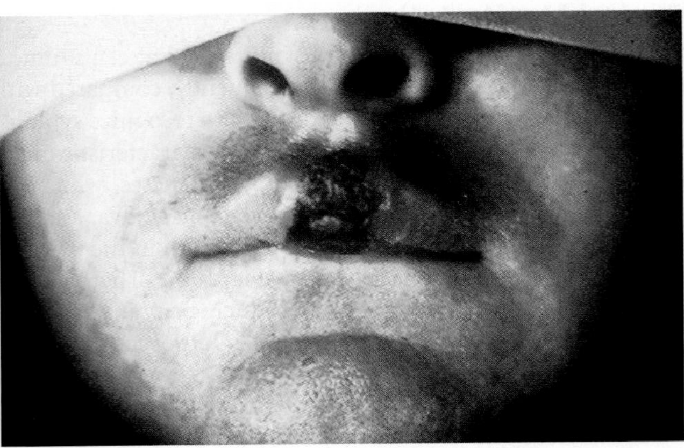

Fig. 50-4 Primary syphilis chancre on upper lip.

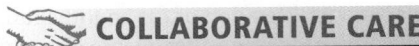

COLLABORATIVE CARE

Table 50-4 Primary Syphilis

Diagnostic
- History and physical examination
- Dark-field microscopy
- Nontreponemal or treponemal serologic testing
- Testing for other STDs (HIV, gonorrhea, chlamydia)

Collaborative Therapy
- Appropriate drug therapy (See Table 50-5)
- Confidential counseling and testing for HIV infection
- Case finding
- Surveillance
  - Repeat of quantitative nontreponemal tests at 3, 6, and 12 mo
  - Examination of cerebrospinal fluid at 1 year if treatment involves alternative antibiotics

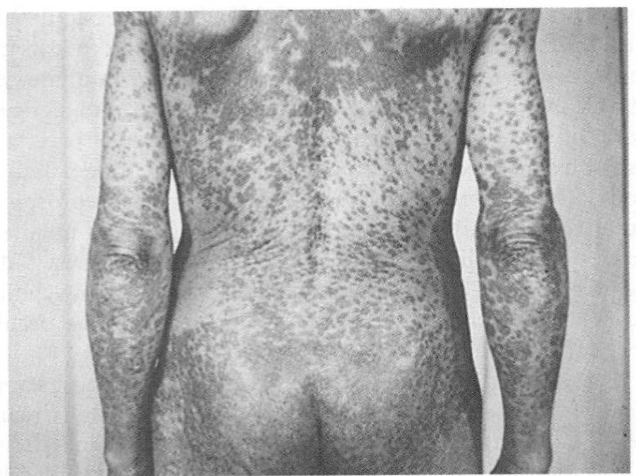

Fig. 50-5 Generalized posterior cutaneous eruptions in secondary syphilis. Distribution of lesions is bilateral and symmetric.

pathogenesis of the manifestations of this stage is unclear. Gummas (destructive skin, bone, and soft-tissue lesions associated with late syphilis) are probably caused by a severe hypersensitivity reaction to the microorganism. Within the cardiovascular system late syphilis may cause aneurysms, heart valve insufficiency, and heart failure. Within the CNS the presence of *T. pallidum* in CSF may cause manifestations of neurosyphilis (see Table 50-3).

Complications

Complications of the disease occur chiefly in late syphilis. The gummas of benign late syphilis may produce irreparable damage to bone, liver, or skin but seldom result in death. In cardiovascular syphilis, the resulting aneurysm may press on the structures such as intercostal nerves, causing pain. The possibility of rupture exists as the aneurysm increases in size. Scarring of the aortic valve results in aortic valve insufficiency and eventually heart failure.

Neurosyphilis (general paresis) is responsible for degeneration of the brain with mental deterioration. Evidence of other neurologic deficits may be present. Problems related to sensory nerve involvement are a result of tabes dorsalis (progressive locomotor ataxia). There may be sudden attacks of pain anywhere in the body, which can confuse the diagnosis of other conditions. Loss of vision and sense of position in the feet and legs can also occur. Walking may become even more difficult as joint stability is lost. (Late syphilis is also discussed in Chapter 56.)

Diagnostic Studies

The first step in diagnosis is to obtain a detailed history of sexual behavior. A physical examination should be done to identify any suspicious lesions, as well as to note other significant signs and symptoms.

The presence of spirochetes on dark-field microscopy of tissue scrapings from primary or secondary lesions can confirm a clinical diagnosis of syphilis. However, syphilis is more commonly diagnosed by a serologic test. Tests for syphilis may be classified as those performed for screening and those performed for confirmation of a positive screening test. Nonspecific antitreponemal antibodies can be detected by tests such as the Venereal Disease Research Laboratory (VDRL) test and the rapid plasma reagin (RPR) test. These nontreponemal tests are suitable for screening purposes and usually become positive 10 to 14 days after the appearance of a chancre. The fluorescent treponemal antibody absorption (FTAAbs) test and the microhemagglutination (MHA) test detect specific antitreponemal antibodies and are suitable for confirming the diagnosis.

False-negative and false-positive test results do occur with the nontreponemal tests (VDRL, RPR). A false-negative result may be obtained during primary syphilis if the test is done before the individual has had time to produce antibody. A false-positive finding may occur with other diseases or conditions such as hepatitis, infectious mononucleosis, after smallpox vaccination, collagen diseases (systemic lupus erythematosus), narcotic addiction, pregnancy, or aging. Positive nontreponemal test results should be confirmed by more specific treponemal tests to rule out other causes. In the CSF, changes such as increased white blood cell count, increased total protein, and a positive treponemal antibody test are diagnostic of asymptomatic neurosyphilis.

DRUG THERAPY

Table 50-5 Syphilis

Stage	Benzathine Penicillin G (IM)	Aqueous Crystalline Penicillin (IV)	Other Antibiotics*
Early syphilis (primary, secondary, and early latent)	At single visit		Doxycycline, tetracycline, erythromycin
Syphilis lasting >1 year	Three weekly injections		
Symptomatic neurosyphilis		Daily for 14 days followed by penicillin G benzathine weekly for 3 doses	Doxycycline, tetracycline, erythromycin

Modified from Centers for Disease Control: *STD treatment guidelines of USPHS,* Atlanta, 1998, Centers for Disease Control and Prevention.
*Given when penicillin is contraindicated.

If a patient is treated with antibiotics early in the course of the disease on the basis of the history and the symptoms, the serologic testing may not indicate the presence of syphilis. Once a person has positive serologic findings for syphilis, indicating the presence of antibodies, these findings may remain positive for an indefinite period in spite of successful treatment.

Collaborative Care

Drug Therapy. Management of syphilis is aimed at eradication of all syphilitic organisms (Table 50-4). However, treatment cannot reverse damage that is already present in the late stage of the disease. Parenteral penicillin remains the treatment of choice for all stages of syphilis. To date, there is no evidence to suggest a decrease in the effectiveness of penicillin against *T. pallidum.* Table 50-5 describes therapy for the various stages of syphilis and is in accordance with U.S. Public Health Service recommendations. All stages of syphilis should be treated.

Appropriate antibiotic treatment of maternal syphilis before the eighteenth week of pregnancy prevents infection of the fetus. Appropriate treatment after 18 weeks of pregnancy cures both mother and fetus because the antibiotics can cross the placental barrier. Treatment administered in the second half of pregnancy may pose a risk of premature labor. Some authorities recommend hospitalization and fetal monitoring of women at 20 weeks of gestation or greater.[13] All patients with neurosyphilis must be carefully monitored, with periodic serologic testing, clinical evaluation at 6-month intervals, and repeat CSF examinations for at least 3 years. Specific management is based on the presenting symptoms.

GENITAL HERPES

Etiology and Pathophysiology

There are two different strains of herpes simplex virus (HSV) that cause infection—type 1 and type 2. In general, HSV type 1 (HSV-1) causes infection above the waist, involving the gingivae, the dermis, the upper respiratory tract, and the CNS. HSV type 2 (HSV-2) most frequently infects the genital tract and the perineum (i.e., locations below the waist). However, either strain can cause disease on the mouth or the genitals. HSV-1 can be transmitted from mouth to genitals, and HSV-2 can be transmitted from genitals to mouth through oral-genital contact.

In the course of the primary infection, HSV is established in the sensory nerve ganglion innervating the primary site. The virus remains dormant within sensory and autonomic nerve ganglia and can cause recurrence of the disease. Upon activation, the virus travels down the nerve axon to the skin or to the mucous membrane. Additional sexual contact is therefore not necessary for a recurrence of HSV infection. The recurrent infection produces a syndrome similar to but less intense than the primary infection.

Because HSV is readily inactivated at room temperature and by drying, airborne and fomitic spread have not been documented as significant means of transmission. The virus enters through the mucous membrane or through breaks in the skin during contact with an infected person. When a person is infected with HSV, the virus usually persists within the individual for life. Approximately 500,000 people a year contract genital herpes. The incubation period ranges from 1 to 45 days with an average of 6 days. Viral shedding even in the absence of an identifiable lesion is a well-established phenomenon. It is estimated that up to 80% of those infected with HSV are asymptomatic or unaware of their infection.[14]

Clinical Manifestations

A patient with primary HSV-2 infections may initially complain of burning or tingling at the site of inoculation. Vesicular lesions, which may occur on the penis, scrotum, vulva, perineum, perianal region, vagina, or cervix, contain large quantities of infectious viral particles (Fig. 50-6). The lesions rupture and form shallow, moist ulcerations. Finally, crusting and epithelialization of the erosions occur. Primary infections tend to be associated with local inflammation and pain, accompanied by systemic manifestations of fever, headache, malaise, myalgia, and regional lymphadenopathy.

Urination may be painful from urine touching active lesions. Retention may occur as a result of HSV urethritis or cystitis. A purulent vaginal discharge may develop with HSV cervicitis. The duration of symptoms is longer and the frequency of complications is greater in women. Many HSV-2 infections, both primary and secondary, are asymptomatic; the exact percentage is unknown. Transmission of genital herpes therefore can occur by sexual contact with an excretor of virus who is free of symptoms. Primary lesions are generally present for 17 to 20 days, but new lesions sometimes continue to develop for 6 weeks.

After the first infection, HSV-2 establishes latency in the sacral ganglia and may be reactivated periodically. Recurrent attacks occur in about 50% to 80% of individuals during the

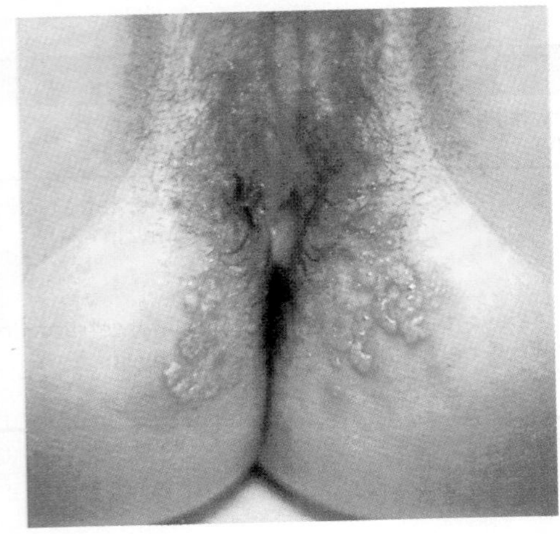
A

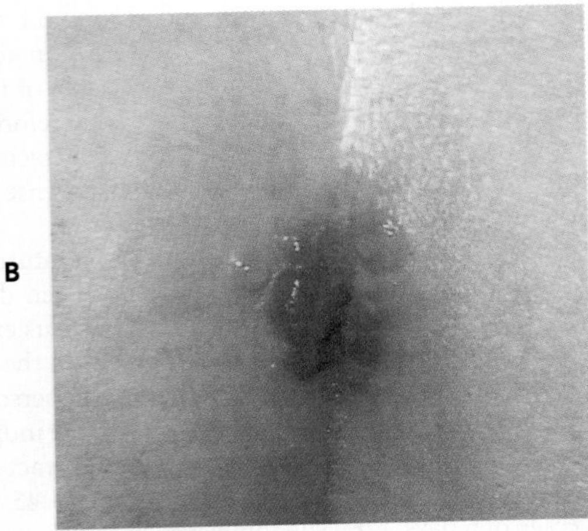
B

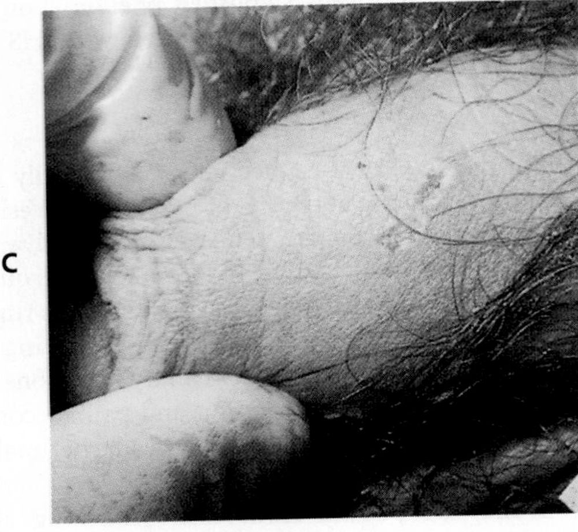
C

Fig. 50-6 Unruptured vesicles of herpes simplex virus type 2. **A,** Vulvar and **B,** perianal area. **C,** Penile herpes simplex, ulcerative stage.

year following the primary episode. Stress, sexual activity, sunburn, and fever tend to trigger recurrence. Many patients can predict a recurrence by noticing early symptoms of tingling, burning, and itching at the site where lesions eventually arise. The symptoms of recurrent episodes are less severe, and the unilateral lesions heal within 8 to 12 days. With time the recurrent lesions generally occur less frequently.

Although viral transmission is easier when overt genital lesions are present, there does not appear to be any predictability as to when viral transmission is possible once the primary HSV-2 infection has occurred. It has been shown that women with recurrent symptomatic genital herpes shed the virus up to 1% of the time even when no visible lesions are present. The person with HSV is capable of transmitting the virus at any time, even when he or she is asymptomatic. Suppressive therapy with antiviral agents can reduce but not eradicate asymptomatic shedding. Barrier forms of contraception, especially condoms, used during asymptomatic periods decrease transmission of the disease. When lesions are present, the patient should avoid sexual activity altogether because even barrier protection is not satisfactory in eliminating disease transmission.

Complications

Although most infections are of a relatively benign nature, complications of genital herpes may involve the CNS, causing aseptic meningitis and lower motor neuron damage.[15] Neuron damage may result in atonic bladder, impotence, and constipation. The most common complication is autoinoculation of the virus to extragenital sites such as fingers (whitlow), lips, and breasts.

Herpes Simplex Virus Infection in Pregnancy. Studies indicate no difference in the length or severity of symptoms in pregnant or nonpregnant women.[16] Some studies have suggested that HSV increases the incidence of spontaneous abortion. However, a recent large prospective study of high risk pregnant women showed that while 2% or more of susceptible women become infected during pregnancy, acquisition of new disease before labor does not seem to adversely affect pregnancy outcome. New infections near the time of labor increase the risk of neonatal herpes and perinatal morbidity.[17] Although women with recurrent HSV infections are not at higher risk for transmitting the virus to their infants, an active genital lesion at the time of delivery is usually an indication for cesarean section delivery, since most infections to neonates occur during passage through an infected birth canal.

Diagnostic Studies

Diagnosis of genital herpes is usually based on the patient's symptoms and history. The diagnosis can be confirmed through isolation of the virus from active lesions by means of tissue culture. Tzanck- or Pap-stained smears from lesions may show the cellular characteristics of viral infection, including multinucleated giant cells and intranuclear inclusions. Rapid testing using anti-HSV antibodies in direct immunofluorescence tests or in an enzyme-linked immunosorbent assay (ELISA), and DNA hybridization is now available with sensitivity ranging from 75% to 90%. Herpes antibody tests are unreliable for distinguishing between HSV-1 and HSV-2 antibodies. Highly accurate serologic methods have been developed, based on identification of specific antibody to the glycoprotein G component of the outer membrane of the virus. The Western blot technique is becoming more available but remains very expensive. Thus these tests have limited availability.

Collaborative Care

Drug Therapy. The skin lesions of genital herpes heal spontaneously unless secondary infection occurs. Symptomatic

COLLABORATIVE CARE

Table 50-6 Genital Herpes

Diagnostic

History and physical examination
Viral isolation by tissue culture
Cytologic examination of vesicular exudate for multinucleated giant cells

Collaborative Therapy

Primary Infection

Acyclovir (Zovirax) 400 mg orally three times a day for 7-10 days OR acyclovir 200 mg orally five times a day for 7-10 days OR famciclovir (Famvir) 250 mg orally three times a day for 7-10 days OR valcyclovir (Valtrex) 1 gm orally twice a day for 7-10 days.

Recurrent Infection

Acyclovir 400 mg orally three times a day for 5 days OR acyclovir 200 mg orally five times a day for 5 days OR famciclovir 125 mg orally twice a day for 5 days OR valcyclovir 500 mg orally twice a day for 5 days
Attempt to identify trigger mechanisms
Yearly Pap smear
Abstinence from sexual contact while lesions are present; however, may shed virus without lesions
Provision of symptomatic interventions
Confidential counseling and testing for HIV

Daily Suppressive Therapy for Frequent Recurrence

Acyclovir 400 mg orally twice a day OR famciclovir 250 mg orally twice a day OR valcyclovir 250 mg twice a day

Severe Infection

Acyclovir (Zovirax) 5-10 mg/kg IV for 5-7 days

Modified from Centers for Disease Control: STD treatment guidelines, *MMWR* 47(RR-1): 1, 1998.
*When treatment is started during the prodrome or within 1 day after onset of lesions, many patients who have recurrent disease benefit from episodic therapy.

Table 50-7 Comparison of Gonorrhea and Chlamydia

Site of Infection	*N. gonorrhoeae*	*C. trachomatis*
Men		
Urethra	Urethritis	Nongonococcal urethritis; post-gonococcal urethritis
Epididymis	Epididymitis	Epididymitis
Rectum	Proctitis	Proctitis
Conjunctiva	Conjunctivitis	Conjunctivitis
Systemic	Disseminated gonococcal infection	Reiter syndrome
Women		
Urethra	Acute urethral syndrome	Acute urethral syndrome
Bartholin's gland	Bartholinitis	Bartholinitis
Cervix	Cervicitis	Cervicitis; atypical cervical cells
Fallopian tube	Salpingitis	Salpingitis
Conjunctiva	Conjunctivitis	Conjunctivitis
Liver capsule	Perihepatitis	Perihepatitis
Systemic	Disseminated gonococcal infection	Arthritis-dermatitis syndrome

From McCance KL, Huether SE: *Pathophysiology: the biologic basis for disease in adults and children,* ed 3, St Louis, 1998, Mosby.

treatment such as good genital hygiene and the wearing of loose-fitting cotton undergarments should be encouraged (Table 50-6). The lesions should be kept clean and dry. To ensure complete drying of the perineal area, women may use a hair dryer set on a cool setting. Frequent sitz baths may soothe the area and reduce inflammation. Techniques to reduce pain on urination include pouring a pitcher of water onto the perineal area while voiding to dilute the urine and voiding in a warm tub of water. Pain may require a local anesthetic such as lidocaine (Xylocaine) or systemic analgesics such as codeine and aspirin. Patients are advised to abstain from sexual contact while lesions are present. However, sexual transmission of HSV has been documented even in the absence of clinical lesions, and the use of condoms should be encouraged.

Three antiviral agents are available for the treatment of HSV: acyclovir (Zovirax), valacyclovir (Valtrex), and famciclovir (Famvir). These purine analogues inhibit herpetic viral replication and are prescribed for primary and recurrent infections. Acyclovir, valacyclovir, and famciclovir are also used to suppress frequent recurrences (more than six episodes per year). Although not a cure, these drugs shorten the duration of viral shedding and the healing time of genital lesions and suppress 75% of recurrences with daily use. Continued use of oral acyclovir for up to 5 years is safe and effective, but it should be interrupted after 1 year to assess the patient's rate of recurrent episodes. Adverse reactions are mild and include headache, occasional nausea and vomiting, and diarrhea. The safety of these drugs for treatment of pregnant women has not been established. Acyclovir ointment appears to be of no clinical benefit in the treatment of recurrent lesions, either in speed of healing or in resolution of pain, and is not commonly recommended. IV acyclovir is reserved for severe or life-threatening infections in which hospitalization is required for treatment of disseminated infections, CNS (meningitis), or pneumonitis. With high-dose IV use nephrotoxicity has been observed.

CHLAMYDIAL INFECTIONS

Urogenital Infections

Chlamydia trachomatis, a gram-negative bacterium, is recognized as a genital pathogen that is responsible for an increasing variety of clinical illnesses. Numerous different serotypes, or strains, of *C. trachomatis* cause urogenital infection (e.g., nongonococcal urethritis [NGU] in men and cervicitis in women), ocular trachoma, and lymphogranuloma venereum. Between 1987 and 1996 reported rates of genital chlamydia soared from 47.8 cases per 100,000 to 194.5 cases per 100,000.[1]

Chlamydia trachomatis is now a reportable disease in all states except Alaska and the District of Columbia. It is the most prevalent bacterial STD in the United States.[1] Symptoms, however, may be absent or minor in most infected women and in many men.

Because chlamydial infections are closely associated with gonococcal infections, clinical differentiation may be difficult (Table 50-7). Both infections are therefore usually treated

Table 50-8 Risk Factors for Chlamydial Infection

Risk Factors
Age <25 years
Multiple sex partners
Sex partners who have had multiple partners
History of STDs
Use of nonbarrier contraception
Bleeding inducible by swabbing of cervical mucosa

concurrently even without diagnostic evidence. The incubation period of 1 to 3 weeks for chlamydial infection is longer than that for gonorrhea, and the symptoms are often milder. The high incidence of recurrence may be because of failure to treat the sexual partners of infected persons. Table 50-8 lists the risk factors for chlamydial infection. Because of the high prevalence of asymptomatic infections, screening of high risk populations is needed to identify those infected.

Clinical Manifestations and Complications

As with gonorrhea, chlamydial infections result in a superficial mucosal infection that can become more invasive. Infections and associated signs and symptoms in men include urethritis (dysuria, urethral discharge), epididymitis (unilateral scrotal pain, swelling, tenderness, fever), and proctitis (rectal discharge and pain during defecation). Infections and associated signs and symptoms in women include cervicitis (mucopurulent discharge and hypertrophic ectopy [area that is edematous and bleeds easily]), urethritis (dysuria, frequent urination, and pyuria), bartholinitis (purulent exudate), pelvic inflammatory disease (abdominal pain, nausea, vomiting, fever, malaise, abnormal vaginal bleeding, and menstrual abnormalities), and perihepatitis (fever, nausea, vomiting, and right upper quadrant pain).[18] A large number of women with chlamydial cervicitis have been found to have a male partner with NGU.

Complications often develop from poorly managed, inaccurately diagnosed, or undiagnosed chlamydial infections. Infection in men may result in epididymitis, with possible infertility and Reiter's disease (a systemic condition characterized by urethritis, conjunctivitis, arthritis, and mucocutaneous lesions). Complications from chlamydial infections in men are rare; in women, infection with *C. trachomatis* is a major cause of PID and ectopic pregnancy. For this reason, in 1993 the CDC issued a recommendation that all females younger than 20 years of age be routinely screened for chlamydia at their annual gynecologic examination. They further advised annual screening of all sexually active women older than 20 years of age with one or more risk factors for disease (e.g., new sexual partner in the past 3 months, multiple sexual partners, lack of barrier contraception.) Chlamydial infection can also be transmitted from a mother to the newborn, causing neonatal inclusion conjunctivitis or pneumonia.

Diagnostic Studies and Collaborative Care

Chlamydial infections in men can be diagnosed by excluding gonorrhea. If no gram-negative intracellular diplococci are found on the gram-stained smear of male urethral discharge or the sediment of first-catch urine specimen, a culture is done. If both are negative and signs of inflammation are present (e.g., polymorphonuclear leukocytes [PMNs] on the gram-stained smear), a diagnosis of NGU *Chlamydia* infection can be made. The availability of nonculture tests has made the screening of both men and women more effective. Direct fluorescent antibody (DFA) tests, enzyme immunoassay (EIA), and DNA hybridization tests (using specific DNA probes) do not require special handling of specimens, are less expensive, and are easier to perform than are cell cultures. New techniques using nucleic acid amplification including PCR and ligase chain reaction promise to surpass culture as the gold standard of chlamydial testing. Tests being developed are highly sensitive and specific and may not require pelvic examination for obtaining appropriate sample material.[10,19]

Drug Therapy. Chlamydial infections respond to treatment with doxycycline (Vibramycin), azithromycin (Zithromax), or ofloxacin (Floxin). For doxycycline, the dosage is 100 mg two times a day. The dosage of ofloxacin is 300 mg twice a day. Both drugs are taken for 7 days. Azithromycin (1 g in a single dose) offers the advantage of ease of administration, but the safety and efficacy in patients under 15 years of age has not been established. Both of these medications are contraindicated in pregnancy. Erythromycin or amoxicillin is the drug of choice for use in pregnant patients. Follow-up care should include advising the patient to return if symptoms persist or recur, treatment of sex partners, and encouraging the use of condoms during all sexual contacts.

Lymphogranuloma Venereum

Lymphogranuloma venereum (LGV) is a chronic sexually transmitted disease caused by specific strains of *C. trachomatis.* LGV is rare in the United States. LGV is endemic in other areas of the world, including Africa, India, Southeast Asia, South America, and the Caribbean.

The strain of *C. trachomatis* that causes LGV probably enters the skin and mucous membranes through tiny abrasions. LGV begins as a skin lesion and spreads via the regional lymphatics. It may also spread systemically through the bloodstream and enter the CNS. Penile, vulvar, and anal infection can lead to inguinal and femoral lymphadenopathy. Marked inflammation occurs, resulting in necrosis, buboes (greatly enlarged, inflamed lymph nodes), abscesses of inguinal lymph nodes, and infection of surrounding tissue. Healing occurs by fibrosis after several weeks or months and results in scarring, which damages the lymph nodes and disrupts nodal function.

Constitutional symptoms that occur during the stage of regional lymphadenopathy include fever, chills, headache, meningismus (meningitis-like symptoms), anorexia, myalgia, and arthralgia. Complications of untreated anorectal infection include perirectal abscess; fistula in ano; and rectovaginal, rectovesical, and ischiorectal fistulas. LGV is treated with a 2-week course of tetracycline. Sex partners should also be treated.

CONDYLOMATA ACUMINATA

Condylomata acuminata (genital warts) is caused by human papilloma virus (HPV) and is a highly contagious STD seen frequently in young, sexually active adults. It is often found in conjunction with other STDs. Accurate incidence data are not available because it is not a reportable condition. The genitalia and anorectal region, as well as the urethra, bladder, and oral mucosa, may be affected. The incubation period of the virus is generally 1 to 6 months, but may be longer. Prevention is hampered by a high proportion of asymptomatic infections and lack of curative treatment.

Minor trauma during intercourse can cause abrasions that allow HPV to enter the body. The epithelial cells infected with HPV undergo transformation, proliferate, and form a warty growth. Immunosuppressed persons, pregnant women, and diabetics are the individuals most susceptible to HPV.

Clinical Manifestations and Complications

Condylomata acuminata lesions are discrete single or multiple papillary growths that are white to gray. The warts may grow and coalesce to form large, cauliflower-like masses. In men, the warts may occur on the penis and scrotum, around the anus, or in the urethra. In women, the warts may be located on the vulva, the vagina, and the cervix and in the perianal area (Fig. 50-7).

During pregnancy, genital warts tend to grow rapidly. An infected mother may transmit the condition to her newborn. Cesarean delivery is not routinely indicated unless the birth canal becomes blocked by massive warts. Bleeding on defecation may occur with anal warts.

Subclinical Human Papillomavirus Infections. Research has linked HPV infection with cervical and vulvar cancer in women and with anorectal and squamous cell carcinoma of the penis in men. To date more than 60 types of HPV have been identified, at least 15 of which invade the genital tract. Some of these types appear to be harmless and self-limiting (e.g., types 6 and 11 commonly found in genital warts), while others seem to have oncogenic (cancer-causing) potential (e.g., types 16, 18, and 31).[20] Up to two thirds of the early lesions caused by these viruses are undetectable by visual examination. Flat subclinical lesions are commonly found on the cervix, introitus, and perianal and intraanal mucosa of women and on the penis, perianal, and anal mucosa of men[21,22] and are strongly associated with the development of dysplasia and neoplasia at these sites.

Diagnostic Studies and Collaborative Care

Diagnosis of condylomata can be made on the basis of the gross appearance of the lesions. However, the warts may be confused with condylomata lata of secondary syphilis, carcinoma, or benign neoplasms. Serologic and cytologic testing should be done to rule out these conditions. If dysplasia is confirmed by the Pap smear, a colposcopic examination and directed biopsies should be performed. Virapap, a test that uses DNA hybridization techniques, can be used to determine some molecular types of HPV present in a lesion. Currently, HPV cannot be confirmed by culture.

The primary goal when treating visible genital warts is the removal of symptomatic warts. The removal may or may not decrease infectivity. Genital warts are difficult to treat and often require multiple office visits with a variety of treatment modalities. One common treatment is the use of 80% to 90% trichloroacetic acid (TCA) applied directly to the wart surface. Petroleum jelly is applied to the surrounding normal skin to minimize irritation before a small amount of TCA is applied to the wart with a cotton swab. A sharp stinging pain is often felt with initial acid contact, but this quickly subsides. TCA is not washed off after treatment. It can be used in pregnant women.

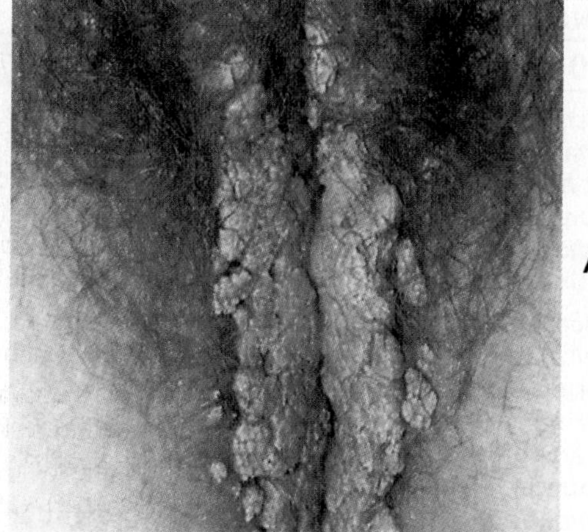

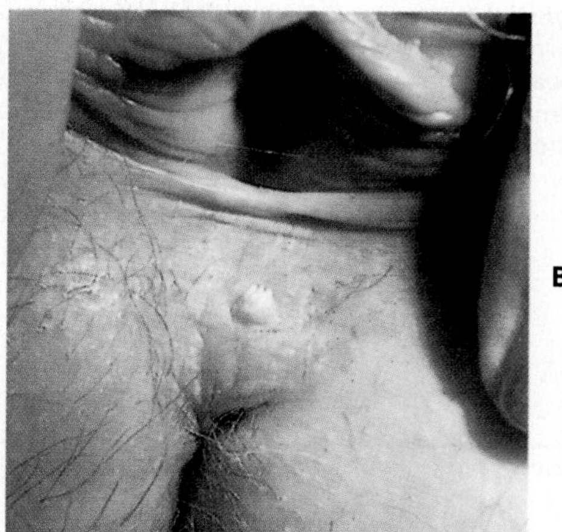

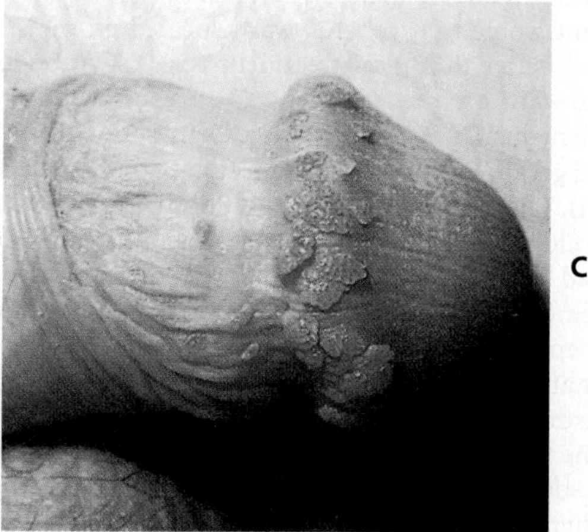

Fig. 50-7 Condyloma. **A,** Severe vulvular condyloma; **B,** perineal wart; **C,** multiple genital warts (condylomata acuminata) of the glans penis.

Podophyllin (10% to 25%), a cytotoxic agent, is recommended therapy for small external genital warts. When podophyllin is used, it is applied carefully to each wart, with normal tissue being avoided, and is then thoroughly washed off in 1 to 4 hours. This substance encourages the sloughing off of skin containing viral particles. Podophyllin has local (e.g., pain, burning) and systemic (e.g., nausea, dizziness, leukopenia,

NURSING ASSESSMENT

Table 50-9 Sexually Transmitted Disease

Subjective Data	Objective Data
Important Health Information *Past health history:* Contact with individuals with STDs, multiple sexual partners, pregnancy *Medications:* Use of oral contraceptives; allergy to any antibiotics, especially penicillin **Functional Health Patterns** *Health perception–health management:* Shared needles during IV drug use; malaise *Nutritional-metabolic:* Nausea, vomiting, anorexia; pharyngitis, oral lesions, itching at infected site; chills; alopecia *Elimination:* Dysuria, urinary frequency, retention; urethral discharge; tenesmus, proctitis *Cognitive-perceptual:* Arthralgia; headache; painful, burning lesions *Sexuality-reproductive:* Dyspareunia; vaginal discharge, menstrual abnormalities; presence of genital or perianal lesions	**General** Fever, lymphadenopathy (generalized or inguinal) **Integumentary** *Syphilis:* Primary: painless, indurated genital, oral, or perianal lesions; secondary: bilateral, symmetric rash on palms, soles, or entire body, mucous patches on mouth or tongue, alopecia *Genital herpes:* Painful genital or anal vesicular lesions *Condylomata:* Single or multiple gray or white genital or anal warts (possibly becoming massive) **Gastrointestinal** Purulent rectal discharge (indicator of gonorrhea), rectal lesions, proctitis **Urinary** Urethral discharge, erythema **Reproductive** Cervical discharge, lesions, inflamed Bartholin's glands **Possible Findings** *Gonorrhea:* Positive Gram's stain, smears, and cultures for *N. gonorrhoeae* *Syphilis:* Positive findings on VDRL and RPR, spirochetes on dark-field microscopy *Genital herpes:* Positive tissue culture for HSV-2, anti–HSV-2 antibody assay *Chlamydia:* Positive culture for *Chlamydia* organism

HSV-2, herpes simplex virus type 2; *RPR,* rapid plasma reagin; *STD,* sexually transmitted disease; *VDRL,* venereal disease research laboratory.

respiratory distress) toxic symptoms. It is contraindicated in pregnant women. In general, warts located on moist surfaces respond better to topical treatment (e.g., TCA, podophyllin) than do warts on drier surfaces.

Patient-managed treatment is also an option. Podofilox liquid and gel are available by prescription (Condylox and Condylox Gel). The patient applies the solution or gel for 3 successive days followed by 4 days of no treatment. Treatment can be repeated up to 4 weeks or until resolution of the lesions. Imiquimod cream (Aldara) is an immune response modifier that is applied every other day for up to 16 weeks or until the lesions are resolved. None of these treatments is recommended for use during pregnancy or lactation.

If the warts do not regress with any of these therapies, treatments such as cryotherapy with liquid nitrogen, electrocautery, laser therapy, 5-fluorouracil (5% cream), and surgical excision may be indicated. Because treatment does not destroy the virus, merely the infected tissue, recurrences and reinfection are possible, and careful long-term follow-up is advised.

NURSING MANAGEMENT: SEXUALLY TRANSMITTED DISEASES

■ Nursing Assessment

Subjective and objective data that should be obtained from a person with a sexually transmitted disease are presented in Table 50-9.

■ Nursing Diagnoses

Nursing diagnoses for the patient with a sexually transmitted disease include, but are not limited to, the following:

- Risk for infection *related to* lack of knowledge about mode of transmission, inadequate personal and genital hygiene, and failure to practice precautionary measures
- Anxiety *related to* impact of condition on relationships, disease outcome, and lack of knowledge of disease
- Altered health maintenance *related to* lack of knowledge about disease process, appropriate follow-up measures, and possibility of reinfection

■ Planning

The overall goals are that the patient with a sexually transmitted disease will (1) demonstrate understanding of the mode of transmission of STDs and the the risk posed by STDs, (2) complete treatment and return for appropriate follow-up, (3) notify or assist in notification of contacts about their need for testing and treatment, (4) abstain from intercourse until infection is resolved, and (5) demonstrate knowledge of safer sex practices.

■ Nursing Implementation

Health Promotion. Many approaches to curtailing the spread of STDs have been advocated and have met with varying degrees of success. Nurses should be prepared to discuss

PATIENT TEACHING GUIDE

Table 50-10 Sexually Transmitted Disease

1. Instruct patient in hygienic measures, such as washing and urinating after intercourse to destroy many causative organisms.
2. Explain the importance of taking all antibiotics as prescribed. Symptoms will improve after 1-2 days of therapy, but organisms may still be present.
3. Teach patient about the need for treatment of sexual partners with antibiotics to prevent transmission of disease.
4. Instruct patient to abstain from sexual intercourse during treatment and to use condoms when sexual activity is resumed to prevent spread of infection and prevent reinfection.
5. Explain the importance of follow-up examination and reculture at least once after treatment if appropriate to confirm complete cure and prevent relapse.
6. Allow patient and partner to verbalize concerns to clarify areas that need explanation.
7. Instruct patient about symptoms of complications and need to report problems to ensure proper follow-up and early treatment of reinfection.
8. Explain precautions to take, such as being monogamous; asking potential partners about sexual history; avoiding sex with partners who use IV drugs or who have visible oral, inguinal, genital, perineal, or anal lesions; using condoms; voiding and washing genitalia after coitus to reduce the occurrence of reinfection.
9. Inform patient regarding state of infectivity to prevent a false sense of security, which might result in careless sexual practices and poor personal hygiene.

practices with all patients, not only those who are perceived to be at risk. These "safe" sex practices include abstinence, monogamy with an uninfected partner, avoidance of certain high risk sexual practices, and use of condoms and other barriers to limit contact with potentially infectious body fluids or lesions. Sexual abstinence is a certain method of avoiding all STD's, but few adults consider this a feasible alternative to sexual expression. Limiting sexual intimacies outside of a well-established monogamous relationship can reduce the risk of contracting a STD. A patient teaching guide related to the patient with an STD is presented in Table 50-10.

All sexually active women should be screened for cervical cancer. Women with a history of STDs are at greater risk for cervical cancer than those women without this history. Pap smears are discussed in Chapter 51.

Measures to prevent infection. An inspection of the sexual partner's genitals before coitus is recommended. The presence of discharge, sores, blisters, or rash should be viewed with concern. A patient who is aware of specific signs and symptoms of infection can intelligently make the decision to continue the sexual interaction with modifications or elect not to have sexual relations. The patient should remember that, when engaging in sex, there is exposure to the infections of everyone with whom the partner has ever had sex. Men should be told that some protection is provided if they void immediately following intercourse and wash their genitalia and the adjacent areas with soap and water. Women may also benefit from postcoital voiding and washing. However, it should not be assumed that this provides adequate protection against STDs after exposure to infection. Although spermicidal jellies and creams have a mild detergent effect that may reduce the risk of contracting STDs, this has not been proven. These same barriers can serve as supplementary lubrication, thereby decreasing irritation and friction and chances for development of a minor laceration that could serve as an entry point for the organism.

Proper use of a latex condom provides a highly effective mechanical barrier to infection. The condom should be undamaged and correctly in place throughout all phases of sexual activity. The use of a spermicide such as nonoxynol-9 (which inactivates most STD organisms) in the vagina and concurrent use of a condom may further reduce the risk of disease.[22] Some studies have shown that condoms are less likely to be used by couples using a nonbarrier method of birth control (such as oral contraceptives, contraceptive injections or implants, IUD, or sterilization.)[4,6] The patient should be strongly cautioned that although these methods are highly effective in preventing pregnancy, they do not protect against STDs. Another deterrent to condom usage is alcohol and drug use. In one survey by the CDC, one fourth of high school students questioned reported that they had used drugs or alcohol with previous sexual intercourse.[4] Use of barrier contraceptives requires planning and motivation, both of which are impaired with alcohol or drug ingestion. The patient should be given specific verbal and written instructions on the proper use of condoms (see Chapter 13). The objections to condom usage, such as interference with spontaneity and the presence of a barrier, should be discussed by the partners. Information about the mechanics of sexual arousal and incorporating a condom into lovemaking can help in overcoming patient or partner resistance to its use. The Reality female condom is a lubricated polyurethane sheath with a ring at each end designed for vaginal wear (see Chapter 13). Laboratory studies indicate that it is an effective barrier to microorganisms, including viruses, but clinical trials are currently lacking for STDs.[23]

Sexual contact with persons known or suspected to have HIV infection should be avoided (see Chapter 13). Among couples with one infected partner, consistent and scrupulous condom use can reduce transmission to the uninfected partner. A sexually active homosexual man can reduce risk by minimizing the number of sexual contacts. Unprotected anal intercourse and other high-risk behaviors should be eliminated, and condoms should be used if sexual contact continues. Interpersonal skills necessary for this interview include respect, compassion, and a nonjudgmental attitude. Counseling should be tailored to the individual patient.

The nurse can initiate an interview to establish the patient's risk for contracting an STD. Questions to ask include number of partners, type of birth control used, use of condoms, use of IV drugs, and sexual preference. Patient education can be planned based on the response to these questions.

Screening programs. Screening programs that are used to detect infected patients can also help prevent certain STDs. For

ETHICAL DILEMMAS

Confidentiality

SITUATION

A nurse in a clinic gives the positive results of a test for *Chlamydia* to a patient and advises her to tell her sexual partners that she has this disease. The patient refuses to tell her boyfriend because he will know that she has had sex with another partner. Should the nurse contact the boyfriend?

DISCUSSION

A patient has the right to confidential diagnosis and treatment. However, if the boyfriend is not treated and continues to have sex with this (treated) patient, she will be reinfected. If he has additional partners, he could transmit the disease to them which, if left untreated, could lead to irreversible damage to the reproductive tract. While this disease could potentially endanger others, it is not life threatening. Education, not violation of confidentiality or coercion, is the key issue. The patient should be educated about reinfection and the long-term effects on others that this disease may have. The nurse should discuss the potential for reinfection if the boyfriend is not treated and encourage the patient to inform her partners of her diagnosis.

ETHICAL AND LEGAL PRINCIPLES

- Providers of health care have a legal obligation to maintain their patients' confidentiality unless required by law to report those who pose a risk to the health or life of innocent parties.
- Health care professionals have an ethical obligation to do no harm.
- Health care professionals have a primary responsibility to their patients. If trust cannot be maintained between health care professionals and their patients, patients may choose not to seek medical attention.

many years, there have been various screening programs to find cases of syphilis. With the decline of infection rates across the United States, many states have eliminated laws requiring premarital testing for syphilis. Many institutions offer voluntary prenatal HIV testing and counseling for pregnant women.

Screening programs have been developed and implemented for detection of gonorrhea and chlamydia. These programs are targeted to women because women are more likely to have asymptomatic gonorrhea and thereby serve as sources of infection. Routine gonorrheal and chlamydial testing during pelvic examinations and prenatal visits are being performed as a major part of these programs. Their effectiveness is well documented.[24] Mass application of screening programs for genital chlamydial infections, genital herpes, and HPV infections (warts) may also be possible with the advent of rapid, cost-effective tests.

Case finding. Interviewing and case finding are other processes used to control venereal disease. These activities are directed toward locating and examining all contacts of each known patient with an STD as soon after sexual exposure as possible, so that effective treatment can be initiated. Trained interviewers may often find cases even if they are supplied with only limited information. The caseworkers, who are often nurses, are aware of the social implications of these diseases and the need for discretion. Sexual contacts are often not informed about the origin of the information naming them as a contact so that greater cooperation and privacy is ensured.

Educational and research programs. Nurses can actively encourage their communities to provide better education about STDs for their citizens. Teenagers, who are known to have a high incidence of infection, should be a prime target for such educational programs. Hot-line services, school nurses, nurse practitioners, nurse midwives, and outreach programs sponsored by the CDC in the United States and Canada's Health Protection Branch are effective. The National Gay Task Force and the Herpes Resource Center were established to provide education and support where needed. Knowledge and understanding of the disease can decrease the STD epidemic. Currently, efforts are being made to develop immunizing agents for syphilis, gonorrhea, genital herpes, HPV, and HIV. The development of effective vaccines is viewed by many clinicians as a prerequisite for eradication of sexually transmitted diseases.

Acute Intervention

Psychologic support. The diagnosis of an STD may be met with a variety of emotions, such as shame, guilt, anger, and a desire for vengeance. The nurse should provide counseling and try to help the patient verbalize feelings. Couples in marital or committed relationships are confronted with an added problem when an STD is diagnosed. The implication of sexual activity by one of the partners with a person outside the relationship must be faced. Other concerns relative to their relationship are present, and the acute problem may serve as an incentive for further problem solving. Support and counseling for the couple are needed. A referral for professional counseling to explore the ramifications of an STD in their relationship may be indicated.

A patient who has contracted genital herpes is faced with the fact that repeated infections can occur and that no cure is available. This can be frustrating and disruptive to the patient's physical, emotional, social, and sexual lives. Helping the patient identify and avoid any factors that may precipitate the condition is indicated. Informing the patient that the incidence and severity of recurrences will decrease over time may provide some support.

HPV infections involve a prolonged course of treatment. The patient can become frustrated and distressed because of frequent office visits, associated costs, potential for unpleasant side effects as a result of treatment, and effects of the infection on future health and sexual relationships. Tremendous support and a willingness to listen to the patient's concerns are needed.

Compliance and follow-up. A nurse working in public health facilities, clinics, or other outpatient settings may care for a patient with an STD more often than a nurse in a hospital. This nurse is in a position to explain and interpret treatment measures such as the purpose and possible side effects of prescribed drugs and the need for follow-up care.

Frequently, single-dose treatment for gonorrhea, chlamydial infection, and syphilis helps prevent the problems associated with noncompliance with drug therapy. The patient requiring multiple-dose therapy should be given special instructions in completing the prescribed regimen and should be informed about problems resulting from noncompliance. All patients should return to the treatment center for a repeat culture from the infected sites or for serologic testing at designated times to determine the effectiveness of the treatment. Informing the patient that cures are not always obtained on the first treatment can reinforce the need for a follow-up visit. The patient should also be advised to inform sexual partners of the need for testing and treatment, regardless of whether they are free of symptoms or experiencing symptoms.

Hygiene measures. The patient with an STD should have certain hygiene measures emphasized. An important measure is frequent hand washing and bathing; this results in the destruction of many of the causative organisms of STDs. Bathing and cleaning of the involved areas can provide local comfort and prevent secondary infection. Douching may spread the infection or undermine local immune responses and is therefore contraindicated. The synthetic materials used in most undergarments frequently increase or exacerbate local irritations by trapping moisture. Cotton undergarments provide better absorption and are cooler and more comfortable for the patient with an STD.

Sexual activity. Sexual abstinence is indicated during the communicable phase of the disease. If sexual activity occurs before treatment of the patient has been completed, the use of condoms may prevent the spread of infection and reinfection. Condom usage after treatment should be encouraged to prevent future exposure to infection. The patient can also choose to relate to a partner in an intimate way that avoids both coitus and oral-genital contact. It is important to note that even single-dose treatments can take up to 1 week to be effective and thus the patient is infective during this period.

Ambulatory and Home Care. Because many STDs are cured with a single dose or short course of antibiotic therapy, many persons are casual about the outcome of these diseases. The consequences of this attitude can include delays in treatment, noncompliance with instructions, and subsequent development of complications. The complications are serious and costly; they can result in disfigurement and destruction of important tissues and organs.

Surgery and prolonged therapy are indicated for many patients with disease-related complications. Major surgical procedures such as resection of an aneurysm or aortic valve replacement may be necessary to treat cardiovascular problems caused by syphilis. Pelvic surgery and procedures to correct fertility problems secondary to an STD may include lysis of adhesions, dilation of strictures, reconstructive tuboplasty, and in vitro fertilization.

■ Evaluation

Expected outcomes for the patient with an STD are that the patient

- describes modes of transmission
- uses appropriate hygienic measures
- experiences no reinfection
- demonstrates compliance with follow-up protocol

CRITICAL THINKING EXERCISES

CASE STUDY

Chlamydia

Patient Profile

Sara M. is a 17-year-old female who visits the outpatient Teen Clinic seeking birth control pills.

Subjective Data

- Had first-time intercourse with boyfriend 2 weeks ago
- Did not use condom or spermicide
- Has not asked boyfriend about his sexual practices
- Denies any symptoms

Objective Data

- Has hypertrophic ectopy noted during Pap test
- Tests positive for chlamydia
- Crying and very upset when informed of positive test result

Collaborative Care

- Doxycycline 100 mg bid for 7 days

Critical Thinking Questions

1. What were Sara's risk factors for acquiring chlamydial infection?
2. What complications could have occurred if Sara's infection had not been detected?
3. What impact is her diagnosis likely to have on Sara's self-image? On her relationship with her boyfriend?
4. What instructions should Sara receive to ensure successful treatment? To prevent reinfection? To prevent further transmission of the infection?
5. What does she need to know about other STDs? What other testing would you recommend?
6. Based on the assessment data presented, write one or more nursing diagnoses. Are there any collaborative problems?

NURSING RESEARCH ISSUES

1. What are the best strategies for encouraging safer sex practices and condom use among high risk populations?
2. What is the level of teens' knowledge of risk, transmission, and impact of STDs? How can teaching about STDs best be adapted to their developmental level?
3. Does education about safer sex practices increase preventive behaviors?

REVIEW QUESTIONS

The number of the question corresponds to the same-numbered objective at the beginning of the chapter.

1. The individual with the lowest risk for sexually transmitted pelvic inflammatory disease is a woman who
   a. uses oral contraceptives.
   b. uses an intrauterine device for contraception.
   c. uses barrier methods of contraception.
   d. uses a Norplant implant or injectible Depo-Provera for contraception.
2. While obtaining subjective assessment data from a woman reported as a sexual contact of a man with chlamydia, the nurse understands that symptoms of chlamydial infections in women
   a. are frequently absent.
   b. mimic those of genital herpes.
   c. include a macular palmar rash in later stages.
   d. may involve chancres hidden inside the vagina.
3. A primary HSV infection differs from recurrent episodes in that
   a. it is of shorter duration than recurrent episodes.
   b. only primary infections are sexually transmissible.
   c. systemic manifestations such as fever and myalgia are more common.
   d. transmission of the virus to a fetus is less likely during primary infection.
4. The nurse explains to a patient with gonorrhea that treatment will include both ceftriaxone and a tetracycline agent because
   a. most patients do not respond to ceftriaxone alone.
   b. coverage with more than one antibiotic prevents reinfection.
   c. no single agent successfully eradicates all strains of gonorrhea.
   d. the high rate of coexisting chlamydia and gonorrhea indicates dual coverage.
5. The patient with an STD who is most likely to have a nursing diagnosis of body image disturbance that hinders future sexual relationships is the patient with
   a. gonorrhea.
   b. primary syphilis.
   c. chlamydial infection.
   d. condylomata acuminata.
6. Teaching by the nurse to prevent infection and transmission of STDs includes explanations of
   a. the appropriate use of birth control pills.
   b. sexual positions used to avoid infection.
   c. sexual practices that are considered high risk.
   d. the necessity of annual Pap smears for patients with HPV.
7. An appropriate nursing intervention to provide emotional support to a patient with an STD is to
   a. use concerned listening when the patient expresses negative feelings.
   b. offer many alternatives that the patient can use to change sexual relationships.
   c. reassure the patient that the disease is curable with appropriate treatment.
   d. help the patient who is an innocent sexual partner forgive the infecting partner.

References

1. US Department of Health and Human Services, Division of STD Prevention: *Sexually transmitted disease surveillance, 1996:* Atlanta, 1997, Centers for Disease Control.
2. Fleming DT and others: Herpes simplex virus type 2 in the United States, 1976 to 1994, *N Engl J Med* 337:16, 1997.
3. Centers for Disease Control: *Chlamydia trachomatis* genital infections—United States, 1995, *MMWR* 46:9, 1997.
4. Centers for Disease Control: Youth risk behaviour surveillance—United States, 1995, *MMWR* 44:SS-4, 1996.
5. Centers for Disease Control: Update: barrier protection against HIV infection and other sexually transmitted diseases, *MMWR* 42:30, 1993.

*6. Rannie K, Craig DM: Adolescent females' attitudes, subjective norms, perceived behavioral control, and intention to use latex condoms, *Public Health Nursing* 14:1, 1997.

7. Sarma SP, Garafalo K, Graves WL: Use of intrauterine device by inner city women, *Arch Fam Med* 7:130, 1998.
8. Pasquale S: Clinical experience with today's IUDs, *Obstet Gynecol Surv* 51(12 suppl):S25, 1996.
9. Finelli L and others: Early syphilis: relationship to sex, drugs, and changes in high-risk behavior from 1987–1990, *Sex Transm Dis* 20:2, 1993.
10. Wagar EA: Direct hybridization and amplification application for the diagnosis of infectious diseases, *J Clin Lab Anal* 10:6, 1996.
11. Young H and others: Non-cultural detection of rectal and pharyngeal gonorrhoeae by the Gen-Probe PACE 2 assay, *Genitourin Med* 73:1, 1997.
12. Lukehart SA, Holmes KK: Syphilis. In Fauci AS and others, editors: *Harrison's principles of internal medicine,* ed 14, New York, 1998, McGraw-Hill.
13. Brunham RC and others: Sexually transmitted diseases in pregnancy. In Holmes KK, editor: *Sexually transmitted diseases,* ed 2, New York, 1990, McGraw-Hill.

*14. Andrist LC: Genital herpes: overcoming barriers to diagnosis and treatment, *AJN* 97:10, 1997.

15. Catotti DN and others: Herpes revisited, *Sex Transm Dis* 20:2, 1993.
16. Corey L: Genital herpes. In Holmes KK, editor: *Sexually transmitted diseases,* ed 2, New York, 1990, McGraw-Hill.
17. Brown ZA and others: The acquisition of herpes simplex virus during pregnancy, *N Engl J Med* 337:8, 1997.

*18. Erickson MF: Chlamydial infections: combating the silent threat, *AJN* 94:16B, 1994.

19. LeBar WD: Keeping up with new technology: new approaches to diagnosis of *Chlamydia* infection, *Clin Chem* 42:5, 1996.

*20. Carson S.: Human papillomatous virus infection update: impact on women's health, *Nurs Pract* 22:4, 1997.

21. Beutner KR: Human papilloma virus infection of the vulva, *Semin Dermatol* 15:1, 1996.
22. Mayman R and others: Penile condyloma: a gynecological epidemic disease. A review of the current approach and management aspects, *Obstet Gynecol Surv* 49:11, 1994.
23. US Department of Health and Human Services, Public Health Service: *1998 sexually transmitted diseases treatment guidelines,* Atlanta, 1998, Centers for Disease Control.
24. US Department of Health and Human Services, Public Health Service: *Recommendations for the prevention and management of* Chlamydia trachomatis *infections, 1998,* Atlanta, 1998, Centers for Disease Control.

*Nursing research-based articles.

Resources

American Venereal Disease Association
Box 385
University of Virginia Hospital
Charlottesville, VA 22908

National Herpes Hotline
Herpes Resource Center
13827 Research Triangle Park
Raleigh, NC 27709
800-230-6039
http://www.ashastd.org/herpes/hrc.html

Sex Information and Education Council of the United States
130 West 42nd Street, Suite 350
New York, NY 10036-7802
212-819-9770
Fax: 212-819-9776
http://www.siecus.org

For additional Internet resources, see the website for this book at **www.mosby.com/MERLIN/medsurg_lewis**

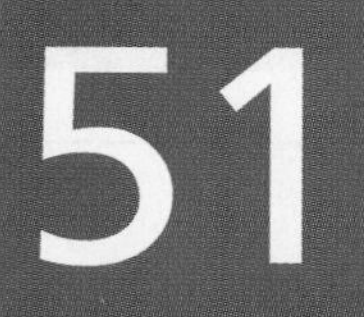

REMEMBER to check out your companion CD-ROM

51 NURSING MANAGEMENT Female Reproductive Problems

Susan Flagler & Kathryn Patterson

www.mosby.com/MERLIN/medsurg_lewis

LEARNING OBJECTIVES

1. Describe the advantages and disadvantages of common contraceptive methods.
2. Identify causative factors and the strategies to diagnose and treat infertility.
3. Discuss the nursing management of women who miscarry or terminate a pregnancy.
4. Describe the etiology, clinical manifestations, and collaborative and nursing management of menstrual problems and irregular vaginal bleeding.
5. Identify the risk factors for and symptoms of ectopic pregnancy.
6. Discuss the changes that accompany perimenopause and postmenopause and their collaborative and nursing management.
7. Identify the clinical manifestations of rape and the appropriate collaborative and nursing management.
8. Differentiate among the common problems that affect the vulva, vagina, and cervix and the related collaborative care and nursing management.
9. Describe the assessment and collaborative care and nursing management of women with pelvic inflammatory disease.
10. Describe the clinical manifestations, complications, collaborative care, and nursing management of endometriosis.
11. Describe the manifestations and collaborative care of benign tumors of the female reproductive system.
12. Identify the clinical manifestations, diagnostic studies, collaborative care, and surgical interventions of malignancies of the uterus, ovaries, and vulva.
13. Describe the preoperative and postoperative nursing management for the patient requiring major surgery of the female reproductive system.
14. Identify the nursing responsibilities in caring for women receiving radiation therapy for cancers of the reproductive system.
15. Describe common problems with cystoceles, rectoceles, and fistulas and the related collaborative care.

CONTRACEPTIVE METHODS

Although contraceptive methods are not reproductive problems, they have an important influence on the health of women in their reproductive years. Pregnancy and childbirth carry a higher risk, although extremely small, of death to a woman than either the use of oral contraceptives or the early termination of pregnancy.[1] Nearly half of the pregnancies occurring in the United States are unintended ones, even with the availability of safe and effective birth control methods. An unintended pregnancy is more likely than an intended pregnancy to compromise a woman's health and socioeconomic status.[2] Most unintended pregnancies occur when a method of birth control is not used or not used correctly. By providing accurate contraceptive information, nurses in all settings can positively influence women's health. Women's knowledge and ability to use contraceptive methods correctly can result in planned pregnancies at desired intervals.

Several contraceptives have health benefits beyond preventing pregnancy. These are referred to as the noncontraceptive benefits. Barrier methods such as condoms and diaphragms reduce the spread of sexually transmitted diseases (STDs). Decreased vaginal and cervical infections reduce the risk of developing more serious conditions such as pelvic inflammatory disease or cervical cancer. Oral contraceptives can improve women's health by decreasing their risk for endometrial and ovarian cancer. In women over 35 years of age, oral contraceptives can have a positive effect on bone calcium content.[3] In addition, women on oral contraceptives report fewer problems with dysmenorrhea (painful uterine cramping) and have lighter menstrual flow resulting in decreased potential for anemia.[4]

Selection of Contraceptive Method

An ideal contraceptive is one that is safe, simple to use, inexpensive, reversible, and does not interfere with sexual activity. No current single method meets all of these criteria. Thus the selection of a method involves the careful consideration of the risks and benefits of the various methods. Each woman's active involvement in selecting the method is essential.[1] Most women use several methods over time. Temporary methods are used to delay or space childbearing. Permanent methods such as voluntary surgical contraception or sterilization (i.e., tubal ligation) are used by women who have completed their childbearing or do not wish to have any children.

Reviewed by Katherine A. Howe, RN, MSN, MEd, Women's Health Nurse Practitioner, Center for Women's Health, The Toledo Hospital, Toledo, Ohio.

Table 51-1 Methods of Birth Control

Description	Side Effects and Complications	Patient Education
Temporary		
Combined Estrogen-Progesterone		
Combination pill contains both estrogen and progesterone (standard and low-dose) taken usually on fifth through twenty-fifth day of each cycle. Prevents ovulation, causes changes in endometrium, alterations in cervical mucus, and tubal transport. Simple and unobtrusive in use, 99% effective. Failure from irregular or incorrect use.	Side effects of nausea, spotting and breakthrough bleeding, postpill amenorrhea, breast tenderness, headache, irritability, nervousness, depression, and decreased libido; complications are benign liver tumors, gallstones, myocardial infarction, thromboembolism, stroke (smokers over age 35 yr at higher risk); contraindications are history of cardiovascular disease, breast or pelvic cancer, and caution with diabetes mellitus, sickle cell disease. Provides no protection against HIV transmission.	Instruct patient in correct use of pills. Tell patient to take pill same time each day; if forgotten one day, take two next day. Review side effects, contraindications. Explain that patient should report cramps or swelling of legs, chest pain. Discuss need for periodic (every 12 mo) checkup that involves weight, BP, Pap smear, hematocrit. Review danger signs of drug. Take drug history, asking about use of phenytoin (Dilantin), phenobarbital, antibiotic (e.g., ampicillin, rifampin [Rifamale]), which decrease contraceptive action. Inform patient that method is usually not recommended for persons over age 35 yr who smoke. Discourage smoking.
Morning-after pill (Ovral) ethinyl estradiol 50 µg and norgestrel 0.5 mg. Another use of combined hormonal contraception. 98.4% effective. Creates hostile uterine lining and alters tubal transport.	Nausea for 1 or 2 days. Would not prevent an ectopic pregnancy.	Take two Ovral within 72 hr of coitus. Repeat if vomiting occurs. Take second dose 12 hr later. Menses should begin within 2-3 wk. Start an ongoing method of contraception immediately after menses.
Progestin Only		
Progestin-only pills (Minipills) are taken daily, with no pill-free days. Preferred for women who are breast feeding. Does not suppress lactation. Inhibits ovulation. Thickens cervical mucus. Alters uterine lining. Lower cardiovascular risk than combined pills.	Menstrual changes; breakthrough bleeding, prolonged cycles or amenorrhea. Increase in functional cysts of the ovary. Increase in ectopic pregnancy.	Use alternate contraception when starting progestin-only pills or if pill is missed. Take pill at same time every day. Keep record of menses and get pregnancy test if 2 wk late.
Depo-Provera (DMPA) is a progestin-only drug given by injection every 3 mo. A private, convenient, and highly effective method.	May cause amenorrhea, headaches, bloating, and weight gain. Return of fertility may be delayed for several months. May cause bone mineral loss.	Return every 3 mo for injection. Discontinue method for several months before planning to conceive.
Norplant is a progestin-only subdermal implant. Six silicone capsules provide protection for 5 yr. Continuous, long-term contraception. Failure rate is extremely low. Does not suppress lactation.	Surgical removal of capsules after 5 yr. Menstrual irregularities, especially during the first year. Later may cause amenorrhea. May cause abdominal pain, headaches, weight gain, acne, and bone mineral loss.	Is effective after 24 hr. Keep arm dry for 48 hr after insertion. Report arm pain. Implants are soft and flexible and cannot break. Expect some irregular bleeding. Report any other changes. Remove implants in 5 yr. Continue to protect against STDs.
Barrier Method		
Cervical cap		
Rubber thimble-shaped shield covering cervix held in place only by suction. Spermicide in inner surface provides mechanical barrier to sperm. Fitting by trained professional. Effectiveness similar to diaphragm; failure from dislodgement and improper fit.	Allergy to latex, rubber, or spermicide, possible cervical irritation or erosion from suction.	Provide sufficient time for practice with insertion and removal (more time than for diaphragm). Give instruction for cleaning, storing, and inspecting for damage. Inform patient that it can be used with abnormalities of vaginal canal but not with cervical inconsistencies, genital infections or cervical malignancy.

Continued

Table 51-1 Methods of Birth Control—cont'd

Description	Side Effects and Complications	Patient Education
Barrier Method—cont'd		
Condom		
Male: thin rubber, latex, or animal membrane sheath fitting over erect penis and providing mechanical barrier to sperm. Simple method to use, no prescription necessary. 85% effective; failure from tearing or slipping during coitus. Used with spermicide. Affords some protection against STDs and HIV transmission.	Possible allergy to latex, rubber, possible decrease in sensation and interference with foreplay.	Advise patient to roll sheath along entire penis, leaving slack at end to receive semen. Inform patient that sharp object (e.g., fingernails) may tear condom. Tell patient to hold sheath in place when penis is withdrawn to prevent emptying of sperm in or near vagina.
Female: double ring system fitted into vagina up to 8 hr before intercourse. No prescription necessary; 88% effective. Affords protection against HIV, cytomegalovirus, and hepatitis B.	No significant side effects; generally acceptable to couple.	Discuss insertion, lubrication, method of removal. More expensive than male condom.
Diaphragm		
Dome-shaped latex cup with flexible metal ring (varies in size) covering cervix. Inner surface coated with spermicide before insertion. Provides mechanical barrier to sperm. Prescription method; fitting by professional; recurrent motivation to use necessary. 87% effective; failure from improper fitting or placement of device.	Allergy to latex, spermicide.	Demonstrate how to hold, insert, and remove device, using model. Allow for insertion and removal practice sessions. Advise patient that insertion may be any time up to 6 hr before coitus, but removal should be 6-8 hr after coitus. Tell patient that bowel and bladder should be emptied before insertion. Give instructions for cleansing and storing, checking for holes or deterioration. Advise patient that diaphragm must be refitted following pregnancy, weight loss, or weight gain. Advise patient that it is not suitable if severe pelvic relaxation is present.
Foam, creams, jellies and suppositories		
Available without prescription. Contain nonoxynol 9 or octoxynol 9; viricidal and bactericidal activity.	Allergy to spermicide. Alteration of normal vaginal flora.	Discuss how to use. Advise patient to void after coitus. Most effective when used in combination with other barrier methods.
Other Methods		
IUD		
Insertion into uterus of flexible objects made of plastic containing fine copper wire or progesterone with string that protrudes into vagina. The method of action is not fully clear. After insertion, no additional equipment necessary; 97-99% effective; failure mainly from undetected expulsion. Most common type used today is Copper T380, effective for 10 years.	Increased menstrual flow and cramping, especially during early months of use; possible complications of ectopic pregnancy, pelvic infection. Undetected expulsion of IUD resulting in pregnancy.	Discuss techniques and experience of insertion and removal. Inform women that the IUD is not advised if future pregnancies are wanted, and about any risk for STDs. Instruct patient to check for string in vagina after each period; report to provider if unable to locate. Discuss need for annual pelvic examination and Pap smear.

Continued

Selecting the method most suitable for her current circumstances should be accomplished when the woman has a full understanding of the benefits, risks, and drawbacks involved with each of the available methods. Benefits might include effectiveness in preventing pregnancy and infection. Drawbacks might include side effects, cost, or messiness of the method. Primary care providers are responsible for ensuring that medical contraindications do not exist for any prescribed contraceptive methods. Table 51-1 presents a description of common contraceptive methods, their side effects, and related patient education. Figure 51-1 shows various temporary contraceptive methods.

Table 51-1 Methods of Birth Control—cont'd

Description	Side Effects and Complications	Patient Education
Other Methods—cont'd		
Natural family planning		
Periodic abstinence during fertile portion of menstrual cycle. Requires strong motivation, self-control; complies with all religious doctrines; 60-65% effective; failure from difficulty in determining precise day of ovulation, irregularity of menses.	Inaccurate or incomplete knowledge of menstrual cycle.	Discuss methods to establish baseline menstrual patterns and identify ovulation. Give instructions in use of calendar, cervical mucus, or basal body temperature method to determine ovulation and fertile period.
Permanent		
Tubal		
Variety of abdominal and vaginal surgical procedures (laparotomy, laparoscopy, culdoscopy) that permanently prevent sperm and ovum from meeting. Crushing, ligating, clipping, or plugging of fallopian tubes (potentially reversible procedure); 99.96% effective; failure due to recanalization of fallopian tubes, erroneous ligation.	Bowel injury, hemorrhage, or infection.	Determine whether temporary contraceptives were used and reason for patient's dissatisfaction. Counsel regarding effects of procedure on physiology and sexual performance. Assist in obtaining written informed consent for procedure. Inform patient that procedure requires short-term hospitalization or can be done on outpatient basis.
Vasectomy		
Bilateral surgical ligation or occlusion of the vas deferens, nearly 100% effective.	Hematoma, swelling, psychologic adjustment.	Inform patient that procedure is usually done as outpatient procedure and takes 15-30 min. Tell patient that alternative form of contraception is needed until no sperm is seen on examination. Explain that procedure does not affect masculinity.

BP, blood pressure; *DES,* diethylstilbestrol; *HIV,* human immunodeficiency virus; *IUD,* intrauterine device; *STD,* sexually transmitted disease.

Hormonal Contraceptive Methods

Oral Contraceptives. Oral contraceptives containing a combination of estrogen and progesterone are the most widely used reversible method of contraception in the United States and Canada. So called "low-dose" pills containing 35 μg or less of estrogen, and new synthetic progesterones provide the same high level of effectiveness as earlier pills while producing fewer side effects. Primary care providers may prescribe progestin-only or minipills for women with cardiovascular problems or who have other contraindications for taking estrogen. Progestin-only pills must be taken at the same time daily and continuously without a break. This differs from combination estrogen-progesterone pills that are taken every day for 3 weeks followed by 1 week of placebo pills. During this week withdrawal bleeding occurs.

Injectable and Subdermal Methods. Progestin-only injectable methods such as medroxyprogesterone acetate (Depo-Provera) and subdermal implants such as levonorgestrel (Norplant) have effectiveness rates greater than the combined oral contraceptives. Depo-Provera injections are prescribed to be given every 3 months in a deep muscle such as the gluteus maximus. Crystals form from the injected solution and create the "deposit" that releases small amounts of progesterone over time. The site should not be massaged after the injection as this could interfere with the crystal formation. Norplant prevents pregnancy for 5 years, but it must be both placed and removed surgically. Progestin-only methods are associated with irregular vaginal bleeding, which is the major reason women discontinue these methods. In addition, progestin-only methods are associated with weight gain, amenorrhea, headaches, and bone mineral loss.[5] Fully informed consent is important for all contraceptives. Failure to fully inform women about what to expect has greater consequences with longer-acting methods. No counterinjection can be given to neutralize Depo-Provera, and surgical removal is necessary to stop the effects of Norplant.

Intrauterine Devices

Intrauterine devices (IUDs) are effective contraceptives that provide long-term pregnancy prevention without unwanted metabolic effects. The mechanism by which IUDs prevent conception is not completely understood. IUDs are thought to prevent fertilization by immobilizing sperm and preventing them from migrating from the vagina to the fallopian tubes and by speeding the transit of the ovum through the fallopian tube. The most often used IUD, the Copper-T 380, is approved for 10 years and has a typical failure rate of less than 1% in the first year of use.[1]

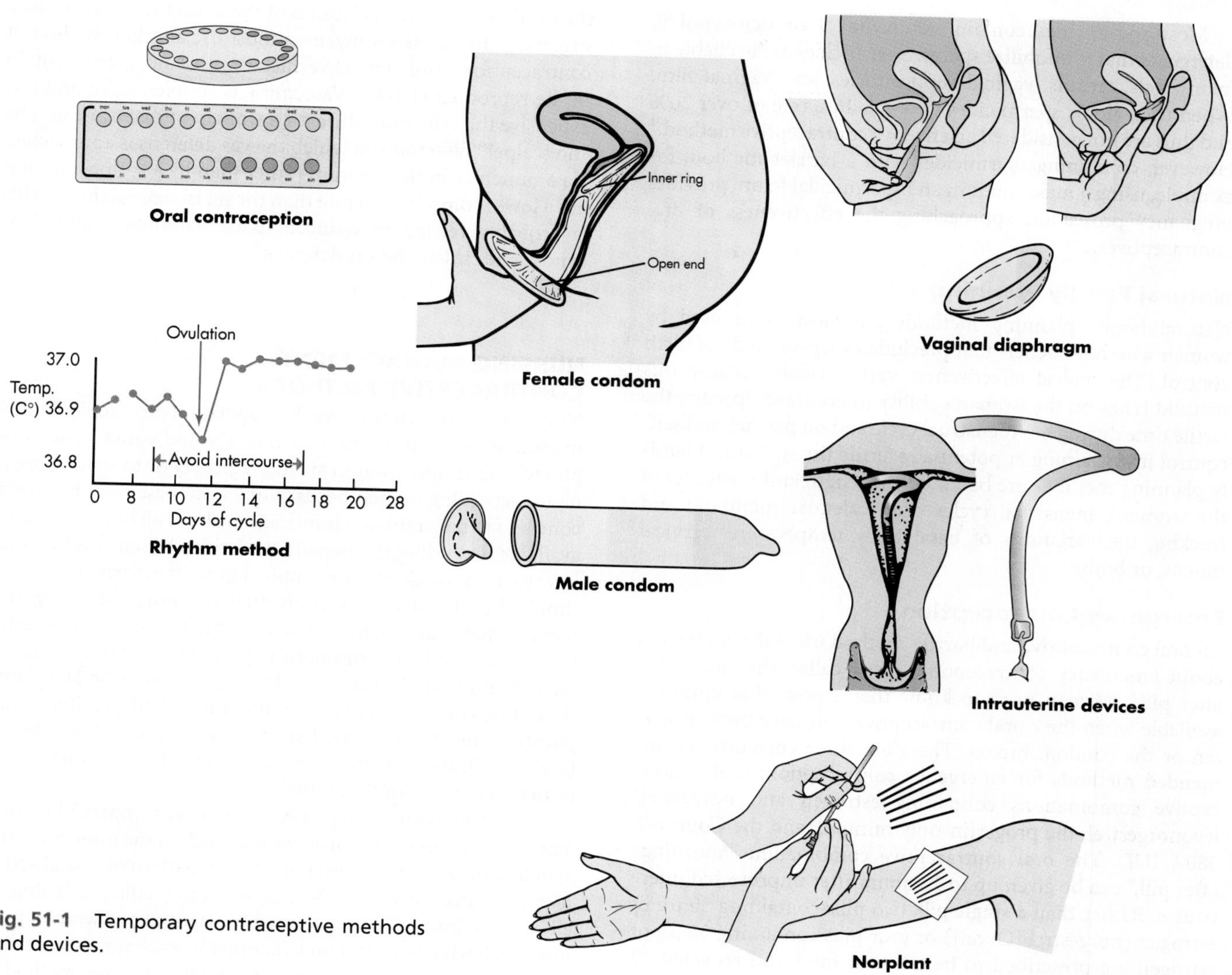

Fig. 51-1 Temporary contraceptive methods and devices.

Two potential problems for IUD users are pelvic infection and ectopic pregnancy. In the past, certain models of IUDs were implicated in causing pelvic infections and subsequent infertility. Now it is clear that the risk of pelvic infection is increased only during the first 3 weeks following IUD insertion. Prophylactic antibiotics may be prescribed at the time of IUD insertion.[4] To reduce the risk of postinsertion infection, women desiring an IUD must be carefully screened and treated for genital tract infections before insertion. Three weeks after insertion, women with IUDs have the same relative risk of pelvic inflammatory disease as other women. The few women who become pregnant with their IUDs in place (typically 2 or less out of 100) have a 25% to 50% chance of losing the pregnancy by spontaneous abortion and approximately 5% chance of having an ectopic pregnancy. Since an ectopic pregnancy can be life threatening, women with IUDs must understand the importance of contacting a primary care provider if their menstrual periods are late or if they experience irregular spotting or bleeding.

Since the IUD offers no protection against STDs, women in long-term, mutually monogamous relationships are the best candidates. Many primary care providers discourage IUDs for women who consider having children in the future. Other providers view the IUD as an option for women who have not completed their childbearing, as long as the risks have been fully discussed. The IUD is not a good choice for women who are at risk for STDs or who have an impaired response to infection (e.g., individuals with diabetes mellitus or who are taking corticosteroids or HIV patients) because of their greater risk for developing a pelvic infection.

Barrier Methods and Spermicides

With typical use, barrier methods are less effective in preventing pregnancy than are hormonal methods. However, condoms are highly effective in preventing the transmission of HIV and other STDs. Hormonal methods provide little or no protection against infection. Male condoms are readily available, inexpensive, and should be used, even during pregnancy, whenever the possibility of an STD exists. Female condoms are more expensive than male condoms but provide another option for women wanting protection from pregnancy and STDs.

Most spermicides contain nonoxynol 9 or octoxynol 9, detergents that immobilize sperm. Spermicides are available in foams, gels, creams, vaginal suppositories, and vaginal film. When used alone, spermicides have a failure rate of over 20% and thus are not considered an effective contraceptive method.[1] However, combining spermicides with a barrier method, for example, using a male condom and spermicidal foam, provides pregnancy protection approaching the effectiveness of oral contraceptives.

Natural Family Planning

Natural family planning methods are most often used by women who have beliefs that preclude other methods of birth control. The typical effectiveness varies widely because this method relies on the woman's ability to accurately predict the fertile time during her menstrual cycle and on partner and self-control in abstaining at potentially fertile times. Natural family planning methods are based on the length and regularity of the woman's menstrual cycles (the "calendar method") and tracking the variations of basal body temperature, cervical mucus, or both.

Emergency Contraception

All oral contraceptive and barrier method users should be told about emergency contraception, often called the "morning-after pill." Women need to know that a postcoital option is available when their oral contraceptive pills have been forgotten or the condom breaks. There are three currently recommended methods for emergency contraception: oral contraceptive combinations containing estrogen and norgestrel/levonorgestrel, the progestin-only minipill, and the Copper-T 380A IUD. The oral contraceptive combination, "morning-after pill," can be given up to 72 hours after unprotected intercourse. Rather than a single pill, two pills containing 50 μg of estrogen (norgestrel [Ovral]) or four pills containing 30 μg of estrogen are prescribed to be taken at once and repeated 12 hours later.[6] The major side effects are nausea and vomiting. This contraceptive combination prevents pregnancy by blocking ovulation.

Recently the progestin minipill has been shown to be more effective than combination contraceptives and produces fewer side effects.[6] Due to the small amount of progestin in each minipill, 20 pills are needed for each dose. Again, therapy must be started within 72 hours of unprotected sex.

Insertion of a copper IUD within 5 to 7 days after unprotected intercourse is also a highly effective postcoital method. It is not clear how the device works but is thought to interfere with sperm transport or implantation.[6] Better utilization of emergency contraceptive methods could significantly reduce unintended pregnancies and, hence, the termination of pregnancies.

Permanent Methods of Contraception

Increasing numbers of men and women are choosing voluntary surgical contraception or sterilization to provide themselves with permanent contraception. Close to 100% effective, the first year failure rate for bilateral tubal ligation is 0.4% and for males with vasectomies only 0.15%.[1] Women who were unknowingly pregnant at the time of surgery and surgical error account for the majority of failures. For males having vasectomies, the failure rate is due to spontaneous recanalization of the vas deferens or the occlusion of the wrong structure during surgery.[1] After a vasectomy, men must use another method of contraception until clinical verification that no sperm remain in the reproductive tract. Vasectomy is simpler, safer, and less expensive than the procedure for a woman's tubal ligation. The "no scalpel" vasectomy in which the vas deferens is approached via a puncture in the scrotum rather than by a scalpel incision has a lower complication rate than the incisional method.[7] This is probably related to reduced tissue handling required to expose and isolate the vas deferens.[8]

NURSING MANAGEMENT: CONTRACEPTIVE METHODS

Nurses in many settings have the opportunity to provide information about contraceptive methods to individuals and couples who currently want to avoid pregnancy or to space a pregnancy according to their needs. Nurses can best assist by giving concise, factual, unbiased information about all of the methods available, including the benefits and risks. When feasible, this information should also be supplied in written form. Emphasis should be placed on the individual or couple selecting the method that is most compatible with current personal circumstances. Individuals considering permanent sterilization or long-term methods, for example, Depo-Provera or Norplant, should be counseled regarding discomfort and possible complications of surgery, as well as the consequences of the choice (e.g., sterilization is not reversible; Depo-Provera may delay return to fertility for 9 months).

Contraceptive needs typically change over a woman's lifetime. The woman's personal considerations such as the importance of avoiding pregnancy at a given time, cost, pattern of sexual activity, risk of exposure to STDs, and access to medical care should all be taken into account. Factors important to one woman may not match what is important to another woman nor match what the nurse thinks is most important. However, the best method is the one the woman will use consistently and safely. Women selecting a hormonal method, diaphragm, IUD, or surgical sterilization should see their primary care providers. Nurses should know the available resources for contraceptive referral within their communities. These resources may include Planned Parenthood, health departments, and community clinics.

Nurses should teach women how to use the method selected. If the method is tied to the act of intercourse (e.g., spermicides, condoms, diaphragms), women must know how and when it should be placed or inserted and how and when it should be removed. Women selecting oral contraceptives should know what to do if a pill is missed and when using a back-up method is indicated. Women taking oral contraceptives should be advised to keep an additional method on hand, such as foam and condoms, so it is readily available when needed. Both barrier and oral contraceptives method users should be told about the availability of emergency contraception.

Nurses can assist women to use their methods safely by giving accurate information. Foremost is educating women about the specific danger signs. This should be done both verbally and in writing. While serious complications are rare, women should know the possible danger signs and what should be done when a danger sign is recognized. For example, women selecting "the pill" may be taught the danger signs using the acronym *ACHES*. ACHES stands for the following signs: *A*, abdominal pain; *C*, chest pain, cough, shortness of breath; *H*, headache, dizziness, weakness, or numbness; *E*, eye problems, speech problems; and *S*, severe leg pain. If any of these danger signs are present, the woman should contact her primary care provider promptly.

Nurses should also educate women that discomforts, such as nausea or breast tenderness, when first starting oral contraceptives are not danger signs. Teaching women what can be done to minimize discomfort is important so they feel better and are less likely to discontinue the method. Also any misconceptions a woman may have about the method should be corrected. For example, some women have the misconception that after several years on oral contraceptives the pills should be discontinued to give the body a break from taking hormones. This is not true. On the contrary, continuing oral contraceptives increases the noncontraceptive benefits, such as reducing the risks for endometrial and ovarian cancer, with no detrimental effects on future fertility.

The woman's safety may also depend on protection from STDs. Women using nonbarrier methods who may be at risk for STDs should be encouraged to use condoms before any penetration with every act of intercourse. Many women are not aware that genital herpes and human papillomavirus (HPV) can be transmitted when their partners are unaware of being infected or have no evidence of disease.

INFERTILITY

Infertility is the inability to achieve a pregnancy after at least 1 year of regular intercourse without contraception.[9] Approximately 15% of couples in North America are involuntarily infertile. Evaluation and therapeutic measures can be invasive, expensive, and take a year or more, with only 50% eventually conceiving.[10] Understandably, infertility can constitute a physical and emotional life crisis.

Etiology

Infertility may be caused by either female factors or male factors. Conditions that cause male infertility are discussed in Chapter 52. In up to 20% of the couples evaluated, the cause of infertility may remain unexplained.[9] The most frequent female causes of infertility include ovulation factors such as anovulation or inadequate corpus luteum, tubal obstruction or dysfunction such as endometriosis or damage from pelvic infection, and uterine or cervical factors such as leiomyoma or structural anomalies.[9] Risk factors for infertility include increasing age, tobacco and illicit drug use, extremes of exercise activity, severe dietary restrictions, and specific occupational and environmental exposures.[9] The infertility risk for women aged 35 to 44 years is double the risk for women 30 to 34 years old.[11] One third of women older than 35 years who desire pregnancy experience infertility.

Diagnostic Studies

Evaluation of infertility is generally conducted over a series of visits (Table 51-2). A detailed history and general physical examination of the woman and her partner provide the basis for selecting diagnostic studies. The possibility of medical or gynecologic diseases is explored before tests are performed to evaluate whether the cause is female infertility. These tests include ovulatory studies, tubal patency studies, and postcoital studies.[11]

Table 51-2 Evaluation of the Infertile Couple

Initial Visit

Clinical
- History/physical for both partners
- Extensive review of menstrual pattern

Laboratory
- Testing to assess specific medical findings
- Assess for sexually transmitted diseases
- Papanicolaou smear
- Semen analysis

Education
- Health maintenance (breast and scrotal self-examinations)
- Discussion of possible future testing options and cost

Ovulation Monitoring
- Instruction for at-home ovulation testing using basal body temperature, cervical mucus evaluation, and urinary LH test kit

Second Visit (scheduled in midcycle, periovulatory phase)

Clinical
- Postcoital test

Laboratory
- Schedule for midluteal progesterone/prolactin level
- Sperm penetration assay

Education
- Review ovulation monitoring data and techniques
- Review laboratory findings from last visit

Third Visit (at postovulatory part of cycle)

Clinical
- Endometrial biopsy

Laboratory
- Draw blood for midluteal progesterone/prolactin levels

Education
- Discuss need to assess tubal/uterine integrity (hysterosalpingogram vs. laparoscopy)

Fourth Visit (conclusion of initial work-up)

Education
- Outline biochemical/physiologic bases of couple's infertility
- Outline management plans with time and cost for each
- Discuss referral for possible assisted reproductive technologies (ART)

Modified from Stenchever MA: *Office gynecology,* ed 2, St Louis, 1997, Mosby.
LH, luteinizing hormone.

Ovulatory Studies. A basal body temperature record is kept to determine whether there is regular ovulation (Fig. 51-2). The woman is instructed to take and graph her temperature on awakening before any activity. The same site (e.g., oral) for taking the temperature should be used each time. Any cause for variation, such as sleeplessness or illness, should be noted. As ovulation approaches, the production of estrogen increases and may cause a drop in temperature. When ovulation occurs, progesterone is produced, causing a rise in temperature. The temperature graph thus helps to detect ovulation and suggest the timing of intercourse if pregnancy is

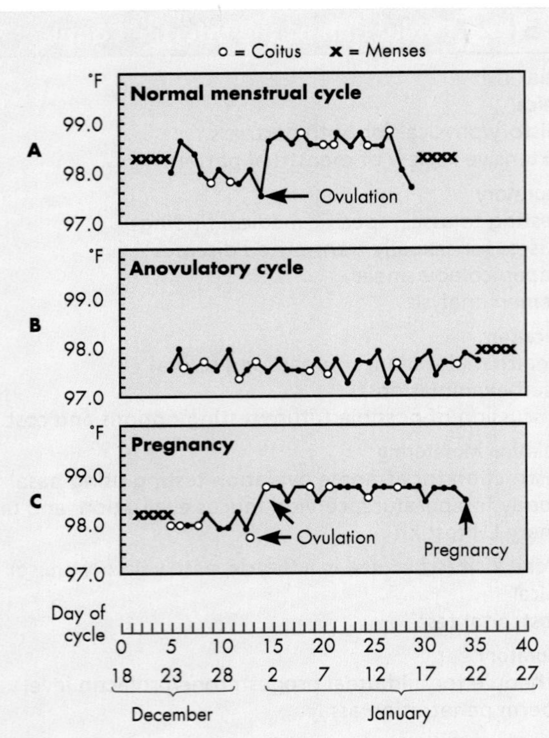

Fig. 51-2 Basal body temperature chart. **A,** Typical biphasic temperature curve indicative of ovulation and normal progesterone effect. **B,** Irregular monophasic curve characteristic of anovulatory cycles. **C,** Ovulatory curve with sustained temperature elevation following conception and the first missed period.

desired. Rigid adherence to a schedule can produce psychologic stress sufficient to inhibit sexual relations.

Simple rapid ovulation prediction kits are now available for use by women at home. These kits are generally used daily to measure luteinizing hormone (LH) levels in urine samples. Ovulation occurs about 28 to 36 hours after the first rise of LH, so intercourse can be timed accordingly. Other tests for ovulation include cervical and vaginal smears, endometrial biopsy, and plasma progesterone levels.

Tubal Patency Studies. Tubal factors (occlusion or deformity) are assessed most commonly by means of hysterosalpingogram. This procedure consists of the radiographic visualization of the uterus and tubes by injecting a radiopaque dye through the cervix. Tubal patency, shape, position, and any distortions of the endometrial cavity can be determined. Laparoscopy may be used when hysterosalpingogram is contraindicated or a pelvic cause appears likely.

Postcoital Studies. Examination of the cervical mucus can reveal whether it undergoes favorable changes at ovulation, enabling penetration, survival, and normal motility of the sperm. A postcoital examination can determine whether the cervical environment is favorable for the sperm. The couple is asked to have intercourse about the time ovulation is expected and 2 to 12 hours before the office visit. Douching or bathing should be avoided before the test. The cervical and vaginal secretions are aspirated and examined for the number and motility of sperm present.

NURSING AND COLLABORATIVE MANAGEMENT: INFERTILITY

The management of infertility problems depends on the cause. If infertility is secondary to an alteration in ovarian function, supplemental hormone therapy to restore and maintain ovulation may be attempted. Drugs used to induce ovulation include clomiphene citrate (Clomid), human menopausal gonadotropin (Pergonal), and bromocriptine (Parlodel). When a tubal blockage exists, the woman should be referred to a specialist to discuss whether surgical correction or in vitro fertilization is more appropriate.[9] Chronic cervicitis and inadequate estrogenic stimulation are cervical factors causing infertility. Antibiotic therapy is indicated for cervicitis. Inadequate estrogenic stimulation is treated by the administration of estrogens.

When a couple has not succeeded in conceiving while under infertility management, an option is intrauterine insemination with the husband's or donor's sperm. If this technique does not succeed, in vitro fertilization (IVF) may be used. IVF is the removal of mature oocytes from the woman's ovarian follicle via laparoscopy, followed by fertilization of the ova with the partner's sperm in a Petri dish. When fertilization and cleavage have occurred, the resulting embryos are transferred into the woman's uterus. The procedure requires 2 to 3 days to complete and is used in cases of fallopian tube obstruction, oligospermia, and unexplained infertility. IVF is costly and emotionally stressful, but it has become a recognized and accepted method of therapy for infertile couples.

Assisted reproductive technologies (ART) continue to develop rapidly since the first IVF baby was born in 1978. ARTs include IVF, gamete intrafallopian transfer (GIFT), zygote intrafallopian transfer (ZIFT), donor gametes, and embryo cryopreservation. With the increasing sophistication of embryo cryopreservation, assisted hatching, and intracytoplasmic sperm injection, couples will have an increased potential for pregnancy. The use of ART poses many ethical, legal, and social concerns.

Nurses can assist women experiencing infertility by providing information about the reproductive process and infertility evaluation and addressing the psychologic and social distress that can accompany infertility. Removing or reducing psychologic stress can improve the emotional climate, making it more conducive to achieving a pregnancy.

The nurse has a major responsibility for teaching and providing emotional support throughout the infertility testing and treatment period. Feelings of anger, frustration, grief, and helplessness may heighten as more and more diagnostic tests are performed. Infertility can generate great tension in a marriage as the couple exhausts their financial and emotional resources. Few insurance carriers cover the high cost of infertility testing or the therapeutic measures associated with infertility. Recognizing and taking steps to deal with the psychologic factors that surface can assist the couple to better cope with the situation. Couples should be encouraged to participate in a support group for infertile couples as well as individual therapy.

ABORTION

An *abortion* is the loss or termination of a pregnancy before 20 weeks or a fetal weight of less than 500 g. Abortions are classified as spontaneous (occurring naturally) or induced (occur-

Table 51-3 Induced Abortion

Method	Length of Pregnancy	Procedure	Advantages	Disadvantages
Early Abortion				
▪ Menstrual extraction	Usually up to 2 wk after first missed period	Catheter is inserted through cervix into uterus, and suction is applied. Endometrium and contents of uterus are aspirated.	Low cost, simple, done at outpatient facility without anesthesia or cervical dilatation, minimally traumatic	Continuation of pregnancy possible, potential for uterine injury and bleeding
▪ Suction curettage	Up to 14 wk	Cervix is usually dilated, uterine aspirator is introduced, and suction is applied, removing endometrial tissue and implanted pregnancy.	Outpatient procedure, most often involving local anesthesia, 1- to 2-day recovery period	Infection, uterine perforation possible
▪ Dilation and evacuation (D & E)	10-16 wk (approximate)	Cervix is dilated, and products of conception are removed by vacuum cannula and the use of other instruments as needed.	Safe and effective procedure for more advanced pregnancy, outpatient procedure with general anesthesia, 2-day recovery period	More psychologic trauma, more expensive, greater risk with general anesthesia and more invasive procedure
Late Abortion				
▪ Instillation of drugs				
Hypertonic saline solution	After 16 wk	About 200 ml of amniotic fluid is withdrawn, and a similar amount of 20% normal saline solution is injected. Uterus is apparently irritated and begins to contract within 12-36 hr. Contractions may be assisted with IV oxytocin.	Inexpensive, readily available, feticidal	Hypernatremia, infection, hemorrhage, disseminated intravascular coagulation, more emotional trauma because of time required
Prostaglandins	After 16 wk	Amniocentesis is done, and 8 ml of prostaglandin is inserted into amniotic sac, resulting in stimulation of smooth muscle of uterus. Expulsion of uterine contents occurs within 24 hr.	Fast induction, no need for surgery	Nausea and vomiting, abdominal cramps, cervical laceration, possible delivery of live fetus, high cost
▪ Hysterotomy	16-20 wk	Miniature cesarean section is performed. Incision is made into uterus and contents are removed.	Concurrent sterilization procedure possible	More difficult and expensive in time and money, surgical incision with possible complications

ring as a result of mechanical or medicinal interruption). Miscarriage is the common term indicating the unintended loss of a pregnancy. Habitual abortion is defined by a history of three or more previous abortions.

Spontaneous Abortion

Approximately 70% of all conceptions never achieve fetal viability with nearly 50% being lost before the first missed menses.[9] Spontaneous abortion is the loss of pregnancy before 20 weeks of gestation that had been clinically recognized by ultrasound or a reliable pregnancy test. Fetal chromosomal anomalies account for 60% of miscarriages before 8 weeks of gestation. Other causes of spontaneous abortions include endocrine abnormalities, maternal infection, acquired anatomic abnormalities (such as uterine fibroids or endometriosis), immunologic factors, and environmental factors.[9]

Uterine cramping in the presence of vaginal bleeding is an indication of a spontaneous abortion. Cramping is usually absent in vaginal bleeding caused by other conditions, such as polyps. Serial serum beta-human chorionic gonadotropin hormone (β-hCG) and vaginal ultrasound examination of the pelvis are the most reliable indicators of an early abortion. The gestational sac can be visualized using ultrasound as early as 6 weeks of gestation.

Treatment for a possible spontaneous abortion is limited. Although bed rest and abstention from sexual activity are often recommended, there is no evidence that these measures or any active medical management improves the outcome. The woman is advised to report any bleeding to her primary care provider. An estimated 80% of patients proceed to abortion regardless of management. If the products of conception do not pass on their own or bleeding becomes excessive, a dilation and curettage (D&C) is generally performed. A D&C procedure involves dilating the uterine cervix and scraping the endometrium of the uterus to empty the uterus of the products of conception.

NURSING MANAGEMENT: SPONTANEOUS ABORTION

Women who are threatening to abort (bleeding and cramping) may be admitted to the hospital. Nurses must attend to both the physical and emotional needs of patients. Vital signs and estimated blood loss are monitored. Any tissue or clots that might contain tissue are saved to be examined for traces of the fetus and placenta. Women may be very distressed and experience both physical and emotional pain. Nurses should use comfort measures to provide the needed physical and mental rest. Arranging for someone significant to the patient to stay with the patient provides important emotional support. The nurse should offer other resources for support of the grieving process that may result from this loss.

Induced Abortion

Pregnancy termination or an abortion that is induced for medical and personal reasons is one of the most commonly performed surgical procedures. In Europe, pharmacologic methods (e.g., RU-486) of abortion induction are available and soon will be approved in the United States. A woman's right to seek safe pregnancy termination and in what circumstances that termination may occur continue to be matters of debate and controversy. Early pregnancy termination involves fewer health risks to a woman than carrying a pregnancy to term.[1]

Techniques. The decision about which technique to use to terminate a pregnancy depends on the length of the pregnancy and the woman's condition. Early abortion methods include menstrual extraction, suction curettage, and dilation and evacuation (D&E). Table 51-3 lists current surgical techniques for abortion.

Suction curettage may be performed up to 14 weeks of gestation and accounts for more than 90% of abortion procedures.[11] Late or second-trimester abortions are most often used to terminate pregnancies when a fetal anomaly has been detected. Late termination procedures involve intrauterine instillation of prostaglandins or hypertonic saline that precipitate uterine contractions and the eventual expulsion of the fetus.

ETHICAL DILEMMAS

Abortion

SITUATION

A recently married, 39-year-old woman is informed that the results of her amniocentesis indicate her fetus has major chromosomal abnormalities and is expected to have severe physical as well as mental disabilities. The patient has no children, but her husband has three children from a previous marriage. She asks the nurse what should she do. How would the nurse respond?

DISCUSSION

The patient has three choices: (1) continue the pregnancy and raise the child, (2) terminate the pregnancy, or (3) continue the pregnancy and relinquish the child for adoption. Although these are all legal and morally acceptable decisions, each is extremely difficult. The patient and her family need support, information, and as much time as is practical to make their decision. Appropriate pregnancy counseling would involve clarification about the nature of this pregnancy (e.g., was it a desired pregnancy), the patient's concerns and desires about having a child with her husband, how she feels about both abortion and the prospects of raising a child with severe disabilities, and education about future pregnancy risk both to a fetus and to the patient. The nurse might suggest counseling for the patient and her husband and a conference with the physician to answer questions about the diagnosis, the prognosis, and their alternatives. It also might be helpful to refer them to agencies that deal with children with disabilities for additional information.

ETHICAL AND LEGAL PRINCIPLES

- Abortion was legalized in the United States in 1973 in the *Roe v. Wade* case heard by the Supreme Court. Abortion in the first trimester is a private matter between a woman and her physician. In the second trimester the state may regulate abortion services for safety concerns. Third trimester abortions may be performed in cases in which the life or health of the woman is endangered by the pregnancy.
- Patient autonomy requires that a woman decide for herself whether or not to continue a pregnancy. She may consult with her family and/or physician before this decision is made.
- Coercion occurs when a health care provider influences a patient to act in a way that the health care provider would choose and not in a manner consistent with the patient's values.

NURSING MANAGEMENT: INDUCED ABORTIONS

Pregnancy terminations are usually sought because women have decided that an abortion is better than any other option. Women seeking abortions experience less distress afterwards if the decision has been freely made after the consideration of the options of keeping the pregnancy and the child as well as keeping the pregnancy and relinquishing the child. Once the decision has been made, the woman and her significant others need support and acceptance. The patient should be prepared in advance for what to expect both emotionally and physically. Grief and sadness are normal postabortion feelings and should not be misconstrued as otherwise. As with any surgical procedure, the patient needs to understand the instructions to be carried out

PATIENT TEACHING GUIDE

Table 51-4 Characteristics of the Menstrual Cycle

Characteristic	Patient Education
Menarche	
Occurs between ages of 9 and 16 yr; average age at onset is 12 or 13 yr	See physician regarding possible endocrine or developmental abnormality when delayed.
Interval	
Usually is 21-35 days, but regular cycles as short as 17 or as long as 45 days are considered normal if pattern is consistent for individual	Keep written record to identify own pattern of menstrual cycle. Expect some irregularity in premenopausal period. Be aware that drugs (phenothiazines, narcotics, contraceptives) and stressful life events can result in missed periods.
Duration	
Menstrual flow generally lasts 2-8 days	Realize that pattern is fairly constant but that wide variations do exist.
Amount	
Menstrual flow varies from 20-80 ml per menses; average is 30 ml; amount varies among women and in the same woman at different times; it is usually heaviest first 2 days	Count pads or tampons used per day. The average tampon or pad completely saturated absorbs 20-30 ml. Very heavy flow is indicated by complete soaking of 2 pads in 1-2 hr. Know that flow increases and then gradually decreases in premenopausal period. IUD or drugs such as anticoagulants and thiazides can produce heavy menses.
Composition	
Menstrual discharge is mixture of endometrium, blood, mucus, and vaginal cells; it is dark red and less viscous than blood and usually does not clot	Realize that clots indicate heavy flow or vaginal pooling.

before and after the procedure. The nurse's compassionate care can be a positive factor in the patient's experience.

Follow-up care includes instructions on signs and symptoms of possible complications, including an increase in vaginal bleeding, severe abdominal cramping, and signs associated with infection, such as fever and foul drainage. The importance of avoiding intercourse, tampons, and douching until reexamination should be stressed. The patient needs to return for reexamination in 2 weeks. Contraception can be started the day of the procedure or during the patient's return visit in accordance with her needs and desires.

PROBLEMS RELATED TO MENSTRUATION

To better understand problems of menstruation, key aspects of normal menstrual cycles must be understood. Menstrual cycles are influenced by hormones from the hypothalamus (gonadotropin-releasing hormone) and anterior pituitary (follicle-stimulating hormone and luteinizing hormone).[12] These hormones influence the development of a dominant follicle and egg within one ovary and the resulting production of estrogen during the follicular phase of the cycle. The estrogen from the ovary causes the growth of the endometrial lining of the uterus. Following ovulation, the corpus luteum (site of ovulation) produces progesterone that further develops and stabilizes the endometrial lining, building a suitable lining to receive a fertilized egg. The progesterone dominant part of the menstrual cycle is called the luteal phase because of the essential part the corpus luteum plays. When a fertilized egg does not implant in the endometrial lining, the corpus luteum is not maintained and production of progesterone falls. In response to decreasing levels of progesterone, the endometrial lining is shed. This shedding is referred to as *menstruation* or the woman's menses or her period. The first day of menses is considered the start or day 1 of the menstrual cycle.

Menses may be irregular during the first few years after menarche and the years preceding menopause. Once established, a woman's menstrual cycles usually have a predictable pattern. However, considerable normal variation exists among women in cycle length as well as in the duration, amount, and character of the menstrual flow (Table 51-4). Women's awareness of normal menstrual variation may reduce unfounded concerns.

PREMENSTRUAL SYNDROME

Premenstrual syndrome (PMS) constitutes a group of somatic, behavioral, cognitive, and mood symptoms distressing enough to impair interpersonal relationships or interfere with usual activities. Because there are many symptoms associated with PMS it is difficult to concisely define it. However, PMS symptoms always occur cyclically during the luteal phase before the onset of menstruation and are not present at other times of the month.[13]

Etiology and Pathophysiology

The etiology and pathophysiology of PMS are not well understood. PMS is thought to have a biologic trigger with compounding psychosocial factors. Women with PMS may have a genetically determined sensitivity to one or more of the neurotransmitter systems, such as serotonin. This sensitivity results in heightened responses to the normal cyclic fluctuations of ovarian hormones.[11] Other proposed causes of PMS include estrogen and progesterone imbalances and nutritional deficiencies of pyridoxine (vitamin B_6) or magnesium.[13]

Clinical Manifestations

PMS is extremely variable in its clinical manifestations. Variation is common between women and, for an individual

RESEARCH
IMPLICATIONS FOR NURSING PRACTICE

Relationship Between Stress, Hormones, and Premenstrual Symptoms

Citation Woods NF and others: Luteal phase ovarian steroids, stress arousal, premenses perceived stress, and premenstrual symptoms, *Res Nurs Health* 21:1269, 1998.

Purpose To examine the relationships among perceived stress, ovarian hormones (estradiol and pregnanediol), stress arousal indicators (urine levels of catecholamines and cortisol), and premenstrual symptoms, including sense of turmoil (e.g., anxiety, irritability, and depression) and fluid retention.

Methods Women (n=74) with low symptom severity, premenstrual syndrome (PMS), or premenstrual magnification of symptoms (PMM) kept a daily diary of symptoms and stress ratings as well as daily urine samples for one menstrual cycle. Multiple regression analyses were performed to test models of premenstrual symptoms in the different groups.

Results and Conclusions In the women with low symptoms and PMS, the premenses global stress rating was the single significant factor accounting for turmoil symptoms. Cortisol levels were also a significant factor in predicting symptoms in women with PMS. Epinephrine and norepinephrine were both associated with symptoms but in opposite directions. Epinephrine was positively related to turmoil ratings while norepinephrine was inversely related.

Implications for Nursing Practice The results support the importance of perceived stress, stress arousal hormones, and ovarian hormone patterns in accounting for two of the more distressing symptoms associated with PMS, which are fluid retention and turmoil. Strategies to reduce stress arousal, including relaxation, biofeedback, and guided imagery techniques, may be useful techniques for further study in this population. Such results also point to the physiologic basis for symptom experiences of PMS.

woman, from one cycle to another. Commonly occurring physical symptoms include breast discomfort, peripheral edema, abdominal bloating, episodes of binge eating, and headache. Abdominal bloating and breast swelling are apparently caused by local fluid shifts because total body weight does not generally change. Symptoms of autonomic nervous system arousal such as heart palpitations and dizziness have been reported by women with PMS. Anxiety, depression, irritability, and mood swings are some of the emotional symptoms women may experience.

Diagnostic Studies and Collaborative Care

PMS can be diagnosed only when other possible causes for the symptoms have been eliminated. A focused health history and physical examination are done to identify any underlying conditions, such as thyroid dysfunction, uterine fibroids, or depression, that may account for the symptoms. While laboratory work such as thyroid function tests can help determine whether the symptoms are attributed to another condition, no definitive diagnostic test is available for PMS.

When PMS is a possible diagnosis, women are given a symptom diary to record their symptoms prospectively for two or three menstrual cycles. Diagnosis is based on an evaluation of the woman's symptoms. Evaluation of at least two cycle records must show no or low symptoms in the follicular phase (first part of menstrual cycle) and presence of symptoms or magnified symptoms in the luteal phase for a diagnosis of PMS.[14]

Nonpharmacologic and pharmacologic strategies that aid in relieving some PMS symptoms are shown in Fig. 51-3. No simple treatment is available. The goal of treatment is to reduce the severity of symptoms and enhance the woman's sense of control and quality of life. The nonpharmacologic approaches include diet changes, exercise, stress management, education, and counseling.[14] To decrease autonomic nervous system arousal women should avoid caffeine, reduce refined carbohydrates, exercise on a regular basis, and practice relaxation techniques. Increasing calcium intake may also help to reduce symptoms associated with PMS. Techniques for stress reduction include yoga, meditation, imaging, and biofeedback training. Eating complex carbohydrates high in fiber, foods rich in vitamin B_6, and sources of tryptophan (dairy and poultry) are thought to promote serotonin production. Vitamin B_6 may be found in foods such as pork, milk, egg yolk, and legumes.

Exercise results in a release of endorphins, leading to mood elevation. Aerobic exercise can also have a relaxing effect. The patient's lifestyle and interests should be considered when an exercise program is being planned. Because fatigue tends to exaggerate the symptoms of PMS, adequate rest in the premenstrual period is a priority.

The patient should be informed about PMS and the current theories on its etiology and treatment. Explanations help the woman with PMS understand the complexity of PMS and ways she can regain a better sense of control. The patient needs to be assured that her symptoms are real, PMS exists, and she is not "crazy." Acknowledgment of her PMS can be therapeutic.[13] Educating the woman's partner about the nature of PMS assists the partner to better understand PMS and to provide support to the woman in making lifestyle changes to reduce her PMS.

Drug Therapy. Pharmacologic treatment strategies should be considered when symptoms persist. Presently, no single drug is being prescribed for the treatment of PMS symptoms. One therapy may be tried for a time and if no improvement is observed, another approach is tried. Some treatments are symptom specific. For fluid retention, diuretics such as spironolactone (Aldactone) are used. For reducing cramps, backache, and headache, prostaglandin inhibitors such as ibuprofen (Motrin, Advil) are used. To improve negative mood, vitamin B_6 supplementation (50 mg daily) may by used. For anxiety, buspirone (BuSpar) taken during the luteal phase or on an as needed basis has helped some women.

Other pharmacologic treatments are directed at PMS in general. Selective serotonin reuptake inhibitors (SSRIs) (sertra-

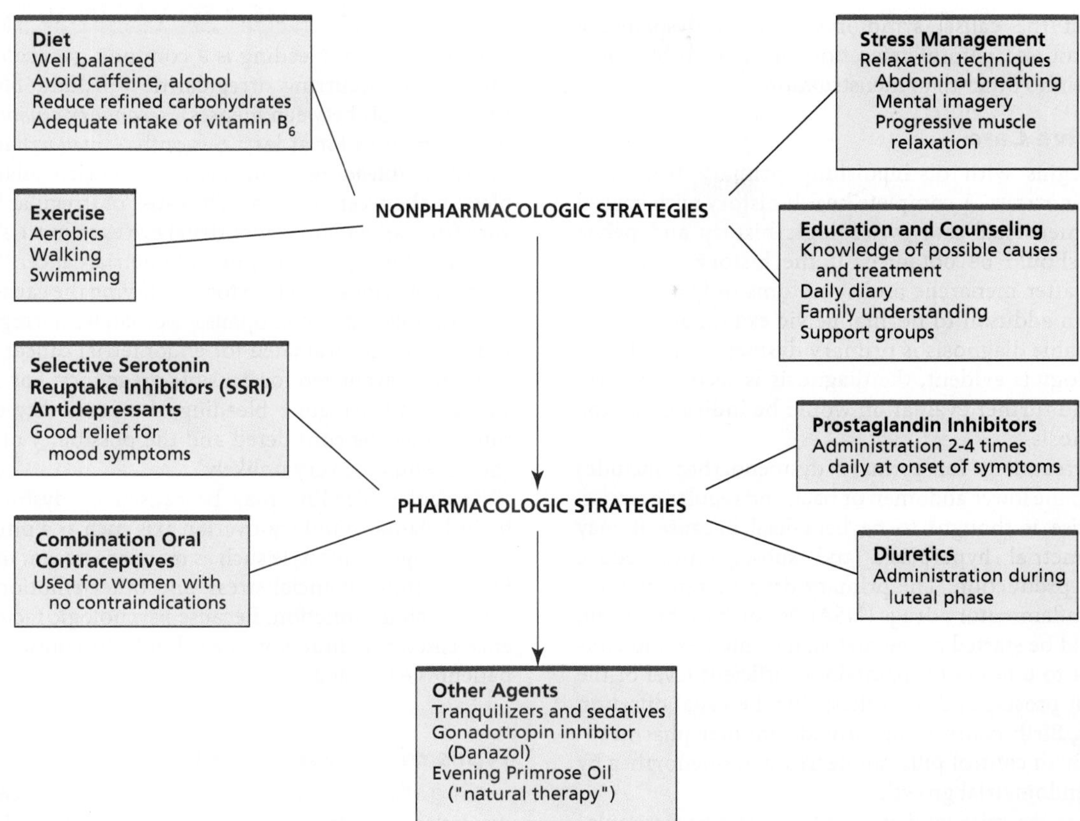

Fig. 51-3 Treatment strategies for premenstrual syndrome.

line [Zoloft]), a type of antidepressant, have provided significant relief to about 60% of women with severe PMS.[14] General treatments include combined oral contraceptives, tranquilizers such as alprazolam (Xanax), and gonadotropin inhibitors such as danazol (Danocrine). Although progesterone was previously used, it is not currently used. Evening Primrose Oil, a natural therapy, may help some women.

DYSMENORRHEA

Dysmenorrhea is defined as abdominal cramping pain or discomfort associated with menstrual flow. The degree of pain and discomfort varies with the individual. The two types of dysmenorrhea are primary (when no pathology exists) and secondary (when a pelvic disease or condition is the underlying cause). Dysmenorrhea is one of the most common gynecologic problems, affecting approximately 50% of all women.[11]

Etiology and Pathophysiology

Primary dysmenorrhea is not a disease. It is caused by either an excess of prostaglandin F_2 alpha (PGF_2 alpha) and/or an increased sensitivity to it. The sequential stimulation of the endometrium by estrogen followed by progesterone results in a dramatic increase in prostaglandin production by the endometrium. With the onset of menses, degeneration of the endometrium releases prostaglandins. Locally, prostaglandins increase myometrial contractions and constriction of small endometrial blood vessels with consequent tissue ischemia and increased sensitization of the pain receptors resulting in menstrual pain. Prostaglandins absorbed into the circulatory system may be responsible for symptoms of headache, diarrhea, and vomiting, which are other manifestations of dysmenorrhea. Primary dysmenorrhea begins in the few years after menarche, typically with the onset of regular ovulatory cycles.

Secondary dysmenorrhea is usually acquired after adolescence, occurring most commonly in the 30s and 40s. Common pelvic conditions that cause secondary dysmenorrhea include endometriosis, chronic pelvic inflammatory disease, uterine leiomyomas, and adenomyosis. Because secondary dysmenorrhea is caused by multiple conditions, symptoms vary. However, a symptom shared in common is increasingly painful menses.[13]

Clinical Manifestations

Primary dysmenorrhea starts 12 to 24 hours before the onset of menses. The pain is most severe the first day of menses and rarely lasts more than 2 days.[11] Characteristic manifestations include lower abdominal pain that is colicky in nature, frequently radiating to the lower back and upper thighs. The abdominal pain is often accompanied by nausea, diarrhea or loose stools, fatigue, headache, and lightheadedness.

Secondary dysmenorrhea usually occurs after the woman has experienced problem-free periods for some time. The pain, which may be unilateral, is generally more constant in nature and usually continues longer than in primary dysmenorrhea.

Depending on the cause, symptoms such as dyspareunia (painful intercourse), painful defecation, or irregular bleeding, may occur at times other than menstruation.[13]

Collaborative Care

Evaluation begins with distinguishing primary from secondary dysmenorrhea. A complete health history with special attention to menstrual and gynecologic history and pelvic examination should be obtained. If the history reveals an onset shortly after menarche and symptoms only associated with menses in addition to normal pelvic examination findings, the probable diagnosis is primary dysmenorrhea. If any cause or etiology is evident, the diagnosis is secondary dysmenorrhea and further evaluation would be indicated by the possible diagnosis.

Nondrug treatment for primary dysmenorrhea includes heat applied to the lower abdomen or back and regular exercise. Regular exercise is thought to be beneficial because it may reduce endometrial hyperplasia and subsequently reduce prostaglandin production. The primary drug therapy is nonsteroidal antiinflammatory drugs (NSAIDs) such as ibuprofen. NSAIDs should be started at the first sign of menses and continued every 4 to 8 hours to maintain a sufficient level of the drug to inhibit prostaglandin synthesis for the usual duration of discomfort. Birth control pills provide another pharmacologic choice. Birth control pills can decrease dysmenorrhea by reducing the endometrial growth.

Acupuncture, exercise, and transcutaneous nerve stimulation provide varying degrees of relief. (See Chapter 8 for discussion of alternative therapies.) These methods may be used for women who obtain inadequate relief from medications or who prefer not to take medications. Patients who are unresponsive to these treatments should be evaluated for chronic pelvic pain.

Treatment of secondary dysmenorrhea depends on the cause. Some but not all individuals with secondary dysmenorrhea will be helped by the approaches used for primary dysmenorrhea. Additional drug or surgical intervention would relate to the underlying causes of dysmenorrhea.

NURSING MANAGEMENT: DYSMENORRHEA

Women often ask nurses what can be done for minor discomforts associated with menstrual cycles. They should be advised that during acute pain, relief may be obtained by lying down for short periods, drinking hot beverages, applying heat to the abdomen or back, and taking an antiinflammatory drug for mild analgesia. The nurse can also suggest noninvasive pain-relieving practices such as distraction and guided imagery.

Other health care measures can reduce the discomfort of dysmenorrhea. These include regular exercise, maintenance of proper nutritional habits, avoidance of constipation, maintenance of good body mechanics, and avoidance of stress and fatigue, particularly during the time preceding menstrual periods. Staying active and interested in activities may also help. Women should be taught why dysmenorrhea occurs as well as how to treat it. Education and supportive therapy can provide women with a foundation for coping with this common occurrence and increase feelings of control and self-reliance.

PROBLEMS RELATED TO VAGINAL BLEEDING

Irregular vaginal bleeding is a common gynecologic concern. Frequently occurring irregularities include *oligomenorrhea* (long intervals between menses), *secondary amenorrhea* (cessation of menses for at least 6 months), *menorrhagia* (excessive menstrual bleeding), and *metrorrhagia* (irregular bleeding or bleeding between menses). The cause of irregular bleeding may vary from anovulatory menstrual cycles to more serious causes such as ectopic pregnancy or endometrial cancer. The age of the woman provides direction for identifying the cause of bleeding. For example, a postmenopausal woman with irregular bleeding must always be evaluated for endometrial cancer but does not need to be evaluated for possible pregnancy. For a 20-year-old woman with irregular bleeding, the possibility of pregnancy must always be considered and the possibility of endometrial cancer would be very unlikely.

Irregular bleeding may be caused by dysfunction of the hypothalamic-pituitary-ovarian axis such as a pituitary adenoma. Changes in lifestyle such as marriage, recent moves, a death in the family, financial stress, and other emotional crises can cause such dysfunction. Because psychologic factors can influence endocrine function, they should be considered when the patient is evaluated.

Types of Irregular Bleeding

Oligomenorrhea and Secondary Amenorrhea. Anovulation is the most common cause for missing menses once pregnancy has been ruled out. Additional causes of amenorrhea are listed in Table 51-5. *Secondary amenorrhea* is cessation of menses after menses have occurred. *Primary amenorrhea* is not having menarche by age 16 years or by age 14 years if secondary sex characteristics are present.[13]

For several years following menarche and then before menopause, ovulation is often erratic. Thus oligomenorrhea resulting from anovulation is common for women at the beginning and end of menstruation. In anovulatory cycles, the corpus luteum that produces progesterone does not form. This may result in a situation referred to as unopposed estrogen. When estrogen is unopposed by progesterone, it can cause excessive build-up of the endometrium. Persistent overgrowth of the endometrium increases a woman's risk for endometrial cancer. To reduce this risk, progesterone or birth control pills are prescribed to ensure that the patient's endometrial lining is shed at least four to six times per year.

Menorrhagia. The excessive bleeding of menorrhagia may be increased duration (more than 7 days), increased amount (more than 80 ml), or both. Approximately 80% of menorrhagia is anovulatory uterine bleeding. Here, an unopposed estrogen state continues to build-up the endometrium until it becomes unstable, resulting in menorrhagia. For young women with excessive bleeding, clotting disorders should be considered. Uterine fibroids (leiomyomas) are a common cause of menorrhagia for women in their 30s and 40s.

Metrorrhagia. *Metrorrhagia,* also referred to as spotting or breakthrough bleeding, is bleeding between menstrual periods. For all reproductive age women, pregnancy complications such as spontaneous abortion or ectopic pregnancy must be considered as a possible cause. Other causes include

Table 51-5 Causes of Amenorrhea

Hypothalamic-Pituitary Axis
Reversible CNS-mediated insults (e.g., emotional stress, anorexia nervosa or severe dieting, strenuous exercise, postpill syndrome, chronic or acute illness)
Prolactinoma and other causes of hyperprolactinemia (e.g., drugs)
Craniopharyngioma and other brainstem or parasellar tumors
Congenital conditions (e.g., isolated gonadotropin deficiency)*
Trauma (e.g., head injury with hypothalamic contusion)
Infiltrative processes (e.g., sarcoidosis)
Vascular disease (e.g., hypothalamic vasculitis)
Pituitary tumors
Sheehan's syndrome
Ovaries
Autoimmune disease (often involving thyroid, adrenal, and islet cells)
Premature menopause (idiopathic) or resistant-ovary syndrome
Polycystic ovary disease
Tumors
Congenital or genetic conditions (e.g., Turner's syndrome)*
Infection (e.g., mumps oophoritis)
Toxins (especially alkylating chemotherapeutic agents)
Radiation
Trauma, torsion (rare)
Uterovaginal Outflow Tract
Asherman's syndrome (postcurettage loss of endometrium)
Müllerian dysgenesis*
Hormonal Synthesis and Action
Male pseudohermaphroditism (e.g., testicular feminization)*
17-Hydroxylase deficiency*

*Usually presents as primary amenorrhea.
CNS, central nervous system.

cervical or endometrial polyps, infection, and carcinoma. Spotting is common during the first four cycles of birth control pills. If spotting continues past the woman's fourth cycle of pills, a different pill formulation can be prescribed when other causes of metrorrhagia have been ruled out. Spotting with long-acting progestin therapy is also common. For postmenopausal women, endometrial cancer must be considered whenever spotting is experienced. In postmenopausal women, exogenous estrogen administration during hormone replacement therapy is a common cause of metrorrhagia. *Menometrorrhagia* is excessive bleeding that occurs at irregular intervals. It may be caused by endometrial cancer or uterine fibroids.

Diagnostic Studies and Collaborative Care

Because irregular vaginal bleeding has multiple causes, diagnostic and collaborative care vary as well. A health history and physical examination directed at the most likely causes of vaginal bleeding for the woman's age-group is the first step. These findings provide the basis for selecting the necessary laboratory tests and diagnostic procedures. Treatment depends on the nature of the problem (menorrhagia or amenorrhea), degree of threat to the patient's health, and whether children are desired in the future.

Birth control pills may be prescribed for a woman with amenorrhea to ensure regular shedding of endometrium if she also wants contraception. If she does not need birth control, progesterone may be prescribed to ensure a shedding of the endometrial lining four to six times per year. On the other hand, if she wants to become pregnant, a fertility drug may be prescribed.

The treatment goal for women with menorrhagia is to minimize further blood loss. If menorrhagia is the result of anovulatory cycles, the endometrium needs to be stabilized by a combination of oral estrogen and progesterone. This can usually be accomplished on an outpatient basis. With severe bleeding, hospitalization is indicated. All patients with menorrhagia should to be evaluated for anemia and treated as indicated.

Surgical Therapy. Surgery may be indicated depending on the underlying cause of the irregular vaginal bleeding. Dilation and curettage (D&C) was once a common therapy for excessive bleeding or for spotting in perimenopausal women. Now D&C is used only in extreme cases of bleeding or for older women when endometrial biopsy and ultrasonography have not provided the necessary diagnostic information.[11] Endometrial ablation done by laser or electrosurgical technique has been successful with 85% of patients with uncontrolled menorrhagia. If menorrhagia is caused by uterine fibroids, a hysterectomy may be performed or a *myomectomy,* removal of fibroids without removal of the uterus, may be performed if the patient wants to preserve her uterus.

NURSING MANAGEMENT: IRREGULAR VAGINAL BLEEDING

For some women, infrequent or no menses might seem a desirable state. Educating women about characteristics of the menstrual cycle assists them to identify normal variations. Table 51-4 includes characteristics of the menstrual cycle and related patient education. This knowledge can help dispel apprehension and misconceptions. If the patient's menstrual cycle pattern does not fall within the range of normal, the nurse should urge her to visit her primary care provider. Myths concerning activities allowed during menstruation are common. The nurse should be prepared to clarify the facts. The patient should be assured that bathing and hair washing are safe. A daily warm tub bath may actually relieve some of the associated pelvic discomfort. Women can swim, exercise, have intercourse, and basically continue their usual daily activities.

Frequent changing of tampons or pads meets comfort and hygiene needs during menstruation. The selection of internal or external sanitary protection is a matter of personal preference. Tampons are convenient and make menstrual hygiene easier, whereas pads may provide better protection. Using a

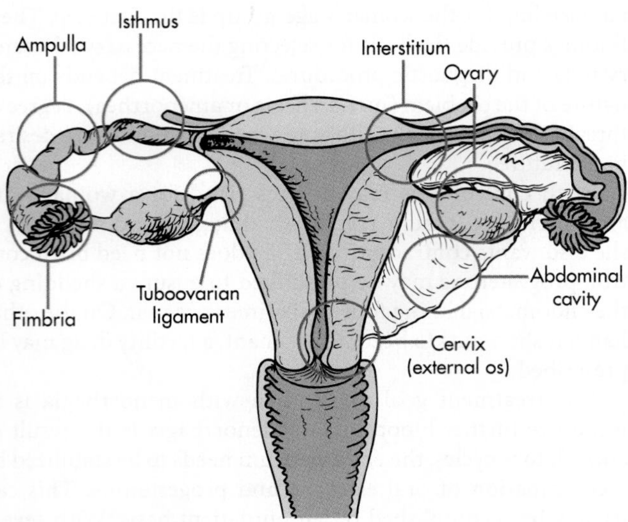

Fig. 51-4 Sites of implantation of ectopic pregnancies. Order of frequency of occurrence is ampulla, isthmus, interstitium, fimbria, tuboovarian ligament, ovary, abdominal cavity, and cervix (external os).

combination of tampons and pads and avoiding superabsorbent tampons may decrease the risk of *toxic shock syndrome* (TSS).[13] TSS is an acute condition caused by the toxin of *Staphylococcus aureus.* TSS causes high fever, vomiting, diarrhea, weakness, myalgia, and a sunburnlike rash.

Whenever excessive, the amount of the patient's vaginal bleeding should be assessed as accurately as possible. The number and size of pads or tampons used and the degree of saturation should be reported and recorded. The patient's fatigue level, along with variations in blood pressure and pulse, should be monitored because anemia and hypovolemia may be present. If a surgical procedure is indicated, the nurse should provide appropriate preoperative and postoperative care.

ECTOPIC PREGNANCY

An *ectopic pregnancy* is the implantation of the fertilized ovum anywhere outside the uterine cavity. Between 97% and 98% of ectopic pregnancies occur in the fallopian tube. The remaining 2% to 3% may be ovarian, abdominal, or cervical (Fig. 51-4). Ectopic pregnancy is a life-threatening condition. Earlier identification has contributed to a decrease in mortality. However, in the United States 40 to 50 deaths per year occur as a result of ectopic pregnancy, and ectopic pregnancy is the leading cause of maternal mortality among African-American women.[15] Any blockage of the tube or reduction of tubal peristalsis that impedes or delays the zygote passing to the uterine cavity can result in tubal implantation. Risk factors for ectopic pregnancy include a history of pelvic inflammatory disease, prior ectopic pregnancy, current progestin-releasing IUD, progestin-only birth control failure, and prior pelvic or tubal surgery.[15] Additional risk factors for ectopic pregnancy include procedures used in infertility treatment including in vitro fertilization procedures, embryo transfer, and ovulation induction. After implantation, the growth of the gestational sac expands the tubal wall until eventually the tube ruptures, causing acute peritoneal symptoms. Less acute symptoms usually begin by 6 to 8 weeks after the last normal menstrual period and weeks before rupture would occur.

Clinical Manifestations

The classic symptoms of ectopic pregnancy are abdominal or pelvic pain, missed menses, and irregular vaginal bleeding.[15] Pain is almost always present and caused by distention of the fallopian tube. It may start unilaterally and then spread to become bilateral. The character of the pain varies among women and can be colicky or vague. If tubal rupture occurs, the pain is intense and may be referred to the right shoulder because of irritation of the diaphragm by blood released into the abdominal cavity. With rupture, the risk of hemorrhage and hypovolemic shock is present. Suspected rupture is treated as an emergency.

More than 75% of women with an ectopic pregnancy realize they have missed their last menstrual period. Vaginal bleeding is most often spotting, but may be heavier and can be confused with menses. Irregular bleeding occurs in 75% of the women with ectopic pregnancy.

Diagnostic Studies

Because of the life-threatening nature of ectopic pregnancy, it should be considered whenever pregnancy is even remotely possible. Ectopic pregnancy can be a diagnostic challenge as a result of its similarity to other pelvic and abdominal disorders, such as salpingitis, spontaneous abortion, ruptured ovarian cyst, appendicitis, and peritonitis. A sensitive serum pregnancy test should be performed. If the test is negative, an ectopic pregnancy is highly unlikely. If ectopic pregnancy cannot be excluded by the pregnancy test, further evaluation is warranted. If the patient is in a stable condition, a combination of serial beta-human chorionic gonadotropin (β-hCG) and vaginal ultrasonography is used. In a normal pregnancy, β-hCG is expected to double about every 48 hours. If the β-hCG level fails to double, the patient may have an ectopic pregnancy. Ultrasound can be used to confirm the presence of an intrauterine pregnancy once the β-hCG level has reached 2000 mIU/ml.

Absence of a normal intrauterine pregnancy means that the diagnosis is very likely spontaneous abortion or ectopic pregnancy. With a spontaneous abortion, serial β-hCG levels decrease over time. Women with bleeding in pregnancy should have their Rh status determined with appropriate follow-up if Rh negative. A complete blood count is obtained when there is any concern regarding the amount of blood loss or if surgery is contemplated. A gradually decreasing hematocrit may indicate internal bleeding.

Collaborative Care

Surgery remains the primary approach for treating ectopic pregnancies and should be performed immediately. However, medical management with methotrexate is being used with increasing success with patients who are hemodynamically stable and have an adnexal mass less than 3 cm in size. The most conservative surgical approach is used to limit damage to the reproductive system as much as possible. Therefore removal of the pregnancy from the tube is preferred to removing the tube. Laparoscopy is preferable to laparotomy, since it decreases blood loss and the hospital stay.[15] If the patient is unstable, as may happen with tubal rupture, conservative surgical approaches may not be possible. Further, the patient may need a blood transfusion and supplemental IV fluid therapy to relieve shock and restore a satisfactory blood volume for safe anesthesia and surgery. The use of microsurgery techniques has resulted in fewer repeated ectopic pregnancies and a higher rate of future successful pregnancies.

NURSING MANAGEMENT: ECTOPIC PREGNANCY

Nursing care depends on the condition of the patient. Before the diagnosis has been confirmed the nurse should be alert to signs of increasing pain and vaginal bleeding, which may indicate that rupture of the tube has occurred. Vital signs are monitored closely, along with observation for signs of shock. Explanations and preparation for diagnostic procedures are given when appropriate. Preparation of the patient for abdominal surgery may follow rapidly. The patient's emotional status should be assessed. Reassurance and support for the surgery should be given to both the patient and her family. Postoperatively, the patient may express a fear of future ectopic pregnancies and have many questions about the impact of this experience on her future fertility.

PERIMENOPAUSE AND POSTMENOPAUSE

The *perimenopause* is a normal life transition that begins with the first signs of change in menstrual cycles and ends 6 to 12 months after menopause. *Menopause* is the single day that marks the last naturally occurring menstrual period. The date of the last menses is determined in retrospect, when a woman has not had a period for 12 months. The average age when natural menopause occurs is 50 years. However, wide variation exists, and menopause during a woman's fourth decade would not be considered premature.[13] *Artificial menopause* results from surgical removal of both ovaries or may occur as a side effect of radiation, chemotherapy, and certain drugs, particularly drugs that inhibit gonadotropin-releasing hormone (e.g., leuprolide [Lupron]). *Postmenopause* refers to any time after menopause.

Changes in the ovary start the cascade of events that finally result in menopause. The regression of the follicles within each ovary begins with puberty and accelerates after age 35 years. With age, fewer and fewer follicles remain that are responsive to follicle-stimulating hormone (FSH). FSH normally stimulates the dominant follicle to secrete estrogen. When the follicles can no longer respond to FSH, ovarian production of estrogen and progesterone decline. However, perimenopausal women can get pregnant until menopause has occurred.

Table 51-6 Signs and Symptoms of Estrogen Deficiency

Vasomotor
Hot flashes
Genitourinary
Atrophic vaginitis
Dyspareunia secondary to poor lubrication
Incontinence
Psychologic
Emotional lability
Change in sleep pattern
Decreased REM sleep
Skeletal
Increased fracture rate, particularly of vertebral bodies but also of humerus, distal radius, and upper femur
Cardiovascular
Decreased high-density lipoproteins (HDL)
Increased low-density lipoproteins (LDL)
Dermatologic
Diminished collagen content of skin
Breast tissue changes

REM, rapid eye movement.

Clinical Manifestations

The perimenopause is a time of erratic hormonal fluctuation. Thus irregular vaginal bleeding is common. With decreasing estrogen, hot flashes and other symptoms begin. The signs and symptoms of diminished estrogen are listed in Table 51-6. Postmenopause is associated with changes in bone density, lipid levels, and skin as discussed in Chapter 48. The loss of estrogen plays a significant role in the cause of age-related alterations. Changes most critical to a woman's well-being are the increased risks for coronary artery disease and osteoporosis secondary to bone density loss. Other changes include a redistribution of fat, a tendency to gain weight more easily, muscle and joint pain, loss of skin elasticity, changes in hair amount and distribution, and atrophy of external genitalia and breast tissue.

Hallmarks of the perimenopause are hot flashes and irregular menses. *Vasomotor* instability (hot flash) is described as a sensation of warmth in the upper part of the chest, neck, and face followed by profuse perspiration and sometimes chilling. These sensations last from several seconds to 5 minutes and occur most often at night, thereby disturbing sleep. Hot flashes can be triggered by situations that affect body temperature, such as eating a hot meal, hot weather, drinking an alcoholic beverage, stress, or warm clothing.

Atrophic vaginal changes secondary to decreased estrogen include thinning of the vaginal mucosa and disappearance of rugae. Vaginal secretions also decrease and become more alkaline. Because of these changes, the vagina is easily traumatized and susceptible to infection. Dyspareunia may also occur.

Atrophic changes in the lower urinary tract also occur with a decrease in estrogen. Bladder capacity decreases and the bladder and urethral tissue lose tone. These changes can cause symptoms that mimic a bladder infection (dysuria, urgency, frequency) when no infection is present.

Whether decreasing estrogen is responsible for the psychologic changes associated with perimenopause is not clear.[16] The attributed depression, irritability, and cognitive problems could result from life stressors or sleep deprivation from hot flashes. Studies conducted in both Canada and the United States have not found a statistically significant relationship between perimenopause and depression.[16] Other studies have found that women who are most likely to be depressed believe depression is related to menopause, are concerned about menopause and aging, or have a previous history of depression or unemployment.

Collaborative Care

Educating women about perimenopausal changes is essential. Women need to be told what to expect and options for symptom management. The advantages and risks of hormone therapy should be discussed thoroughly. This discussion needs to include the individual woman's risks and benefits based on her family and personal medical history. As long as no absolute contraindications exist for hormone therapy, it should be the woman's choice whether or not she takes hormone replacement therapy.

The diagnosis of perimenopause should be made only after careful consideration of other possible causes for the woman's symptoms. Depression, thyroid dysfunction, anemia, or anxiety reactions could be responsible for the same symptoms. Because of the erratic hormonal fluctuations before menopause, routine testing of the serum FSH level is not indicated. After age 50 years, postmenopause can be diagnosed by an FSH of 30 mIU/ml or greater if the woman is not on any hormonal medication.[13]

Nonhormonal Therapy. The frequency and severity of hot flashes can be reduced by avoiding things that increase heat production and by promoting heat loss. Keeping a cool environment as well as reducing caffeine and alcohol intake reduce heat production. Behavioral changes, such as slowing down and reducing tension with relaxation techniques, also help. To promote heat loss at night when hot flashes can disrupt sleep, increase air circulation in the room and avoid bedding that traps the heat such as heavy quilts. Loose fitting clothes do not retain body heat as well as clothes with tight necks and wrists. Cool cloths applied to flushed areas also aid heat loss. Daily Vitamin E in doses up to 600 IU is reported to reduce hot flashes.[17]

Skin and urogenital changes may be self managed by nonhormonal approaches. Dry skin can be improved by reducing the use of soap and the number of showers or baths and using body lotions. Stress incontinence can be decreased with the practice of Kegel exercises. Dyspareunia related to vaginal dryness can be managed with a water-soluble lubricant.

Symptoms of anxiety or depression can be reduced by improving nutrition, exercise, and sleep. For better sleep, alcohol and sleep-interfering drugs should be avoided and techniques employed to reduce hot flashes. Employing techniques to decrease stress also decreases depression and anxiety.

Hormonal Therapy. Significant beneficial effects are associated with postmenopausal hormonal therapy. Initially, the regimen involved estrogen alone, so it was called estrogen replacement therapy (ERT). Concern about the increased risk of endometrial cancer with unopposed estrogen led to development of replacement therapy with estrogen and progesterone. This regimen is referred to as hormone replacement therapy (HRT). Some HRT regimens include low-dose testosterone to increase libido.[18] Women using ERT or HRT have a decrease in heart disease, which is a reason to use HRT even when the woman does not have vasomotor instability. HRT also helps to retard bone loss and prevent osteoporosis. HRT also minimizes atrophic changes to the genitourinary tissues.[11] There is some evidence to suggest that estrogen replacement in women may reduce the risk of Alzheimer's disease.[19]

Whether women on ERT or HRT have an increased risk for breast cancer is still controversial.[11] Known or suspected breast cancer is a contraindication to estrogen use.[13] Long-term use of ERT increases the risk for endometrial cancer, but this increased risk is eliminated with 12 or more days of progesterone per month. The risk for endometrial cancer is present only in those women who still have a uterus. Some women have an increase in their hyperlipidemia with progesterone. However, this is not a contraindication to HRT. The lowest dose of progesterone should be used and serum lipid levels monitored. Women have increased cardiovascular benefit from estrogen replacement, and the addition of progesterone does not decrease the cardioprotective effects of estrogen.

In addition to known or suspected breast cancer, other absolute contraindications for HRT include abnormal vaginal bleeding, pregnancy, active thrombophlebitis or thromboembolic disorder, and current liver dysfunction.[13] Whether a personal history of breast cancer and/or a family history of breast cancer are contraindications for HRT remains controversial. HRT is not contraindicated for women who smoke cigarettes or who have diabetes mellitus.

HRT may be started before menopause to control hot flashes and changes related to decreased estrogen. In the absence of menopausal symptoms, HRT is initiated as soon as possible after menopause to achieve the maximum health benefits. Many different regimens of HRT are available, including continuous combined estrogen and progesterone therapy to various sequential and cyclic patterns. The choice of HRT regimen should be tailored to the individual woman. Factors for consideration include her concern about cancer, previously used regimens and side effects, tolerance of hormonal side effects, and presence of perimenopausal symptoms.

The side effects of estrogen include nausea, fluid retention, headache, and breast enlargement. Side effects of progesterone include increased appetite, weight gain, irritability, depression, spotting, and breast tenderness. To minimize these unwanted side effects, the lowest possible but still beneficial dose of each should be used.

Protective effects from estrogen are achieved by 0.625 mg of conjugated estrogen (Premarin) daily. For symptom relief, a higher dose may be needed. To receive a protective benefit of progesterone, 5 to 10 mg of medroxyprogesterone (Provera) is indicated for 12 days of each month on a cyclic regimen or 2.5 mg if a continuous regimen. If the estrogen needs to be increased for symptom relief, the progesterone should also be increased. Other forms of progesterone include norethindrone (Aygestin) and micronized progesterone (Prometrium).[13] Estrogen comes in a variety of forms: oral tablets, vaginal creams, dermal patches, rings placed around the cervix, and subcutaneous pellets. Vaginal creams are especially useful for urogenital symptoms. Transdermal (skin patches) estrogen has the advantage of bypassing the liver but the disadvantage of causing skin irritation.

A new class of drugs called SERMS (selective estrogen receptor modulators) are now available. These drugs have some of the positive benefits of estrogen, such as preventing bone loss, without the negative effects such as endometrial hyperplasia. Raloxifene (Evista) is a nonsteroidal drug that competes with estrogen for estrogen receptor sites and decreases bone loss and serum cholesterol but has minimal effects on breast and uterine tissue. These drugs are also discussed with respect to their potential role in the management of osteoporosis in Chapter 59.

Nutritional Therapy. Good nutrition can decrease the risk of cardiovascular disease and osteoporosis in addition to assisting with vasomotor symptoms. A daily intake of about 30 kcal/kg body weight with maintenance of sound nutrition is recommended. A decrease in metabolic rate and careless eating habits rather than menopause itself can be the cause for weight gain and related fatigue. An adequate intake of calcium and vitamin D can help maintain healthy bones and thereby counteract the effect of decreased estrogen that makes bones become lighter and more fragile. Postmenopausal women should have a daily calcium intake of 1200 to 1500 mg. Calcium supplements are best absorbed when taken with meals. Either dietary calcium or calcium supplements may be used.

The diet should be high in complex carbohydrates and Vitamin B complex, especially B_6. Phytoestrogens from plant sources have been shown to be beneficial in some women.[20] Examples of foods containing phytoestrogens include soy, tofu, chickpeas, and sunflower seeds.

NURSING MANAGEMENT: PERIMENOPAUSE

Nurses can play a key role in helping women to understand perimenopausal changes and their options to minimize unwanted symptoms and decrease their risk for cardiovascular disease and osteoporosis. Nurses can foster a positive image of perimenopause as a time of vitality and attractiveness. Perimenopause can provide women with an incentive to enhance self-care.

Nurses should provide health education teaching and reassurance to perimenopausal women distraught by their symptoms. The woman should be taught that the symptoms are normal and only temporary. Nondrug approaches to managing symptoms should be taught. Any misconceptions about menopause and HRT should be clarified by the nurse to reduce unnecessary anxiety. The decision to use HRT is personal. The nurse should support a woman's decision not to take HRT by discussing alternative ways (e.g., diet and exercise) to manage symptoms related to decreasing estrogen.

A regular program of exercise and physical activity can improve circulation, maintain good muscle tone, and delay some aspects of aging for postmenopausal women. Exercising for 20 to 60 minutes at least three times a week stimulates osteoblastic activity, thereby stimulating calcium deposition into bone and delaying osteoporosis.

Sexual function can continue with little change in the vast majority of postmenopausal women. Cessation of menstruation and ability to bear children should not be equated with cessation of sexual capability. Femininity and libido do not disappear with menopause. Atrophic changes in vaginal epithelium associated with decreased estrogen may lead to dyspareunia (painful coitus). A water-soluble lubricant (e.g., Replens, Astroglide) is often effective in managing this problem. An active sex life helps increase lubrication and maintain the pliability of vaginal tissues. The patient should be given an opportunity to candidly discuss concerns related to sexual functioning.

The nurse should be alert to the risks, benefits, and possible side effects of the drugs that the patient is taking and should be able to explain them for the patient. Hormonal therapy may be continued indefinitely as part of a plan to prevent the development or worsening of osteoporosis.

RAPE

Rape is defined as any nonconsensual sexual act. Violence against women is a significant health and societal problem. Within the United States, one out of every eight adult women has been forcibly raped sometime in her life.[16] Because over 80% of adult women are raped by an acquaintance or intimate partner, rape is one of the most underreported crimes. Also, women may not report rape because they fear that they would not be able to withstand the stresses of prosecution or that they would be met with disbelief and humiliation from the police, the medical staff, or their peers.

Changes in residency and place of employment may occur as a consequence of the experience because of fear or inability to maintain previous relationships. Rape trauma dramatically disrupts the homemaking and parenting roles normally performed by the adult woman. The survivor's partner and family have a tremendous potential for both negative and positive influence. They can revictimize her and increase her burden in resolving the rape, or they can provide her with support and find support themselves in resolving a shared crisis.

Clinical Manifestations

Physical. Of the rape survivors who seek help immediately after the assault, between one half and two thirds will not have any evidence of physical trauma.[16] Evidence of trauma may be limited because women do not resist for fear of physical danger and injury. When present, physical injuries may include bruising and lacerations to the perineum, hymen, vulva, vagina, cervix, and anus. In general, the more serious injuries involve nongenital areas, such as the face, neck, and extremities, and often occur after the rape. Fractures, subdural hematomas, cerebral concussions, and intraabdominal injuries have resulted in the need for hospitalization. Sexual assault also places women at risk for STDs and pregnancy.

Psychologic. Immediately after the assault, women are often in a state of crisis. They may show shock, numbness, denial, or withdrawal. Some women may seem unnaturally calm; others may be crying or expressing anger.[16] Then feelings of humiliation, degradation, embarrassment, anger, self-blame, and fear of another assault are commonly expressed. These symptoms usually decrease after 2 weeks, and survivors may appear to have adjusted. Yet any time from 2 to 3 weeks

EMERGENCY MANAGEMENT

Table 51-7 Sexual Assault

Etiology	Assessment Findings	Interventions
Sexual molestation Sodomy Assault involving genitalia (male or female) without consent	▪ Emotional or physical manifestations of shock ▪ Hysteria ▪ Crying ▪ Anger ▪ Silence ▪ Decreased level of consciousness ▪ Hyperventilation ▪ Oral, vaginal, and rectal injuries ▪ Extragenital injuries ▪ Pain in genital area or extragenital area	**Initial** ▪ Treat shock and other urgent medical problems, (e.g., head injury, hemorrhage, wounds, fractures). ▪ Assess emotional state. ▪ Contact support person (i.e., social worker, rape advocate, sexual assault nurse examiner). ▪ Do *not* clean the patient until all evidence is collected. Make sure the patient does not wash, douche, urinate, brush teeth, or gargle. ▪ Place sheet on floor. Then have patient stand on sheet to remove clothing. Place sheet with clothing in paper bag. ▪ Obtain forensic evidence per local protocol (i.e., body hair, nail scrapings, tissue, dried semen, vaginal washing, blood samples). ▪ Maintain chain of evidence for all legal specimens. Clearly label evidence and keep in locked cabinet until given to law enforcement agency. ▪ Obtain baseline HIV, syphilis, and other STD screening. ▪ Determine method of contraception, date of last menstrual period, and date of last tetanus immunization. ▪ Consider tetanus prophylactis if lacerations contain soil/dirt. ▪ Vaccinate against Hepatitis B. **Ongoing Monitoring** ▪ Monitor vital signs and emotional status. ▪ Provide clothing as needed. ▪ Counsel patient regarding confidential HIV and STD testing.

to months after the assault, symptoms may return and become more severe. About 50% of women are clinically depressed. Many women experience psychologic effects for 2 years. Suicidal ideation may occur during this time.

Some rape survivors have long-term psychologic problems. The rape trauma syndrome is a classification of posttraumatic stress disorder. Flashbacks, intrusive recall, sleep disturbances, and numbing of feelings are common initial symptoms. Women feel embarrassment, self-blame, and powerlessness. Later symptoms include mood swings, irritability, and anger. Feelings of despair, shame, and hopelessness are often the cause of the anger.[16] These feelings may be internalized and expressed as depression.

Collaborative Care

In the acute care of a rape survivor, ensuring the woman's emotional and physical safety has the highest priority. Other care includes prevention of STDs and pregnancy, collecting evidence for possible prosecution, and arranging both initial and long-term follow-up.[11] The patient's immediate and long-term need for emotional support is given special consideration. Table 51-7 outlines the emergency management of the patient who has been sexually assaulted. Most emergency departments (ED) have identified personnel who have received special training in order to work with women who have been raped. Special procedures are followed in taking the history and conducting the examination in order to preserve all evidence in case of future prosecution.

When the survivor of a rape is admitted to the ED or clinic, a specific chain of events occurs (Table 51-8). A signed informed consent is obtained from the woman before any data are collected. All materials gathered are well documented, labeled, and given to the appropriate person, such as the pathologist or a police officer. The materials are handled by as few people as possible, and signatures of all responsible for keeping and handling the data are obtained. Many items can be used as evidence if the victim chooses to file a complaint. Consequently, the integrity of the material must be maintained. The nurse's involvement in the medicolegal process depends on the policies of the individual institution and state law.

A gynecologic and sexual history and an account of the assault (who, what, when, and where), as well as a general physical and pelvic examination, add further information about the rape incident. Laboratory tests are done primarily to determine the presence of sperm in the vagina and to identify any existing STDs or pregnancy. The woman's physical injuries are attended to and prophylaxis for STDs, tetanus, hepatitis B, and pregnancy are administered.

Table 51-8 Checklist for Evaluation for Alleged Rape

1. **Medicolegal**
   Valid written consent for examination, photographs, laboratory tests, release of information, and laboratory samples
   Appropriate "chain of evidence" documentation
2. **History**
   History of assault (who, what, when, where)
   Penetration, ejaculation, extragenital acts
   Activities since assault (e.g., changed clothes, bathed, douched)
   Inquire about safety
   Menstrual and contraceptive history
   Medical history
   Emotional status
   Current symptoms
3. **General Physical Examination**
   Vital signs and general appearance
   Extragenital trauma—mouth, breasts, neck
   Cuts, bruises, scratches (photograph taken)
4. **Pelvic Examination**
   Vulvar trauma, erythema; hymen, anal, and rectal status
   Matted hairs or free hairs
   Vaginal examination with unlubricated speculum for discharge, blood, lacerations
   Uterine size
   Adnexa, especially hematomas
5. **Laboratory Samples**
   Vaginal vault content sampling
   Vaginal smears—microscope evaluation for trichomonads and semen
   Oral or rectal swabs and smears, if indicated
   Blood samples—VDRL serology, pregnancy test; serologic testing for HIV and hepatitis B infection
   Freeze serum sample for later testing
   Cultures—cervix and other areas (if indicated) for gonorrhea and chlamydia
   Fingernail scrapings
   Pubic hair scrapings
   Clipping of matted pubic hairs
6. **Treatment**
   Care of injuries and emotional trauma
   Antibiotic prophylaxis for venereal disease, if appropriate; ceftriaxone 250 mg IM followed by doxycycline 100 mg PO bid for 7 days
   Protection against pregnancy if any risk with Ovral 2 tabs PO within 72 hr of rape and 2 tabs PO 12 hr later
   Protection of legal rights
   Recommendation of continued follow-up and services of rape crisis center
   Repetition of gonorrhea and chlamydial culture 14-21 days later; consider herpes culture
   Repetition of serologic testing for HIV and hepatitis B 8-12 wk later
   Pregnancy test if appropriate

VDRL, Venereal Disease Research Laboratory.

The health care provider cannot legally state that rape occurred. However, the provider can swear that the findings show that sexual intercourse took place and describe any injury that was inflicted. These findings, along with others such as the police report and examination of the rape scene, can form the foundation for the rapist's conviction.

Follow-up physical and psychologic care is essential. Women should return weekly for the first month following the rape. This includes the time period when women's psychologic reactions may be the most severe.[16] Providers should have the telephone numbers and names of contact persons for local resources for rape survivors, including rape crisis centers, legal and law enforcement authorities, and human services. Follow-up for physical concerns should include a pregnancy test in 2 to 3 weeks. Testing for HIV, syphilis, and hepatitis B may be done at 6 weeks. The HIV test and any other indicated tests should be repeated 3 to 6 months after the rape.

NURSING MANAGEMENT: RAPE

Nurses can assist all women in becoming aware of rape prevention tactics (Table 51-9). They should also be encouraged to learn some basic techniques of self-defense. Local high schools and the YWCA usually have self-defense classes in which formal

PATIENT TEACHING GUIDE

Table 51-9 Rape Prevention

1. See that there are lights at all entrances to your home.
2. Keep your doors locked and do not open them to a stranger; ask for identification if a service person comes to the door.
3. Do not advertise that you live alone; list only your initials with your last name in the telephone directory or on the mailbox; never reveal to a caller that you are home alone.
4. Avoid walking alone in deserted areas; walk to the parking lot with a friend; be sure you see each other leave.
5. Have your keys ready as you approach your car or home.
6. Keep all doors locked and windows up when driving.
7. Never get on an elevator with a suspicious person; pretend you have forgotten something and get off.
8. Say what you mean in social situations; be sure your voice and body language reflect your response.
9. Carry a loud whistle and use it when you think you are in danger.
10. Yell "fire" if you are attacked and run toward a lighted area.

instruction is given. Practicing the various techniques with a friend builds a woman's confidence in her ability to fight back. Learning self-defense can make the woman less vulnerable and more self-reliant.

When a rape survivor is brought to the clinic or emergency room, she should be given the highest priority for care and treatment. A quiet, private area should be used for the initial assessment and the examinations that follow. The patient should not be left alone. Whenever possible, the same nurse should remain with her throughout her stay and provide needed emotional support. The patient's actions and words as she describes the rape incident may be inconsistent, confused, and inappropriate. The nurse should maintain a nonjudgmental attitude.

The patient usually has many feelings and thoughts about the rape and generally wants to talk about them to an interested listener. Talking may help the patient feel better and gain understanding of her reactions to the incident. When the nurse listens carefully, the patient feels that she is not alone and is better able to gain control over the situation.

The nurse should assess the patient's stress level before preparing her for the various procedures that follow. The patient's coping mechanisms are supported when she knows what to expect and what is expected of her, as well as why the particular procedure must be done. Because the pelvic examination may trigger a flashback of the rape, the nurse should answer all related questions before the examination and be a supportive presence during the examination.

Following the examinations, the patient's physical comfort needs should be considered. She may need safety pins or needle and thread for her torn clothing or a cool drink to relieve her thirst. Most women who have been raped feel dirty and would appreciate a place to wash as well as use of mouthwash, especially if oral sex was involved.

The nurse can also further emphasize and elaborate on any prescribed treatment. The patient's understanding of the possible side effects of the medications given should be assessed. The patient is urged to see her own primary care provider if care was given elsewhere. The importance of follow-up should be emphasized. Many rape survivors are unaware of the availability of financial compensation (a law in most states) and appreciate information about the application process. This compensation is to assist them in paying for emergency services and for emotional injuries that may temporarily interfere with their ability to work.

When the patient is discharged, the nurse should make certain the patient has transportation home. If friends or family members are not available, the hospital or clinic should make arrangements with an appropriate community resource. The patient should not be sent home alone.

Many communities today have rape crisis centers. These public service organizations have trained professional and nonprofessional volunteers who provide an emotional support system for rape survivors on request. Their programs provide advocacy to ensure dignified treatment throughout the medical and police procedures, short-term counseling for the woman and her family, and court assistance and public education on rape-related issues. The nurse should be able to give the patient the names and local telephone numbers of such organizations.

CONDITIONS OF THE VULVA, VAGINA, AND CERVIX

Etiology and Pathophysiology

Infection and inflammation of the vagina, cervix, and vulva tend to occur when the natural defenses of the acidic vaginal secretions (maintained by sufficient estrogen levels) and the presence of *Lactobacillus* are disrupted. The woman's resistance may also be decreased as a result of aging, poor nutrition, and the use of drugs that alter the mucosa. Organisms gain entrance to the areas through contaminated hands, clothing, and douche nozzles and during intercourse, surgery, and childbirth. Table 51-10 relates the specific etiologic factors, clinical manifestations and diagnostic methods, and collaborative care of common inflammations and infections.

Most lower genital tract infections are related to sexual intercourse. Intercourse can transmit organisms, injure tissues, and alter the acid-base balance of the vagina. All of these increase risk for inflammations or infections such as bacterial vaginosis or chlamydial cervicitis. Vulvar infections caused by viruses such as herpes and genital warts can be sexually transmitted when no lesions are apparent. Drugs such as oral contraceptives, antibiotics, and corticosteroids may produce changes in the vagina and trigger an overgrowth of the organisms present. For example, *Candida albicans* may be present in small numbers in the vagina. An overgrowth of this organism causes yeast vaginitis.

Clinical Manifestations

Abnormal vaginal discharge and vulvar lesions are the two main classifications of clinical manifestations. Cervicitis and vaginal problems may be accompanied by an abnormal vaginal discharge. In addition to a thick, white, curdy discharge, women with monilial vaginitis often experience intense itching and dysuria, which is the result of urine coming into contact with fissures and irritated areas on the vulva. The hallmark of bacterial vaginosis is the fishy odor of the discharge. Women with cervicitis may notice spotting after intercourse.

Common vulvar lesions include herpes infection and genital warts. Initial or primary herpes infections may be extremely painful and tender, or they may go unnoticed. Herpes begins as a small vesicle followed by superficial red ulcers. Most herpes lesions are painful. Dysuria is common when urine touches the lesion. Genital warts, caused by the human papillomavirus (HPV), vary in appearance. Irregularly shaped "cauliflower" type lesions are common. Genital warts are painless unless traumatized. (See Chapter 50 for discussion of STDs.)

Older women may develop vulvar dystrophies including lichen sclerosis and squamous cell hyperplasia.[11] These conditions are associated with intense itching. The lesions are white initially although scratching in response to itching produces changes in the appearance.

Collaborative Care

Genital problems are evaluated by performing a history and physical examination and obtaining the appropriate laboratory and diagnostic studies. Since many problems may be related to sexual activity, a sexual history is essential. The nature of the problem directs specific aspects of the evaluation. A herpes culture should be taken of any ulcerative lesions. A blood test for syphilis may be done when ulcerative lesions are present. Gen-

Table 51-10 Infections of the Lower Genital Tract

Infection/Etiology	Clinical Manifestations and Diagnostic Methods	Drug Management
▪ Monilial vaginitis *Candida albicans* (fungus)	Commonly found in mouth, gastrointestinal tract, and vagina; pruritus, thick white curd-like discharge; KOH microscopic examination—pseudohyphae; pH 4.0-4.7.	Antifungal agents (e.g., Monistat, Gyne-Lotrimin, Mycelex [available over the counter]) available in cream or suppository.
▪ Trichomoniasis *Trichomonas vaginalis* (protozoa)	Sexually transmitted; pruritus, frothy greenish or gray discharge; hemorrhagic spots on cervix or vaginal walls; saline microscopic examination—swimming trichomonads; pH 5.0-7.0.	Metronidazole (Flagyl) orally in single dose for patient and partner.
▪ Bacterial vaginosis *Gardnerella vaginalis* *Corynebacterium vaginale*	Watery discharge with fishy odor; may or may not have other symptoms; saline microscopic examination—epithelial cells; pH 5.0-5.5.	Sexually transmitted; metronidazole (Flagyl) 500 mg orally or clindamycin (Cleocin) 300 mg orally bid for 7 days; examine and treat partner.
▪ Cervicitis *Chlamydia trachomatis* *Neisseria gonorrhoeae* *Staphylococcus aureus*	Sexually transmitted; mucopurulent discharge with postcoital spotting from cervical inflammation; culture for chlamydia and gonorrhea.	Azithromycin (Zithromax) PO single dose or Doxycycline PO bid for 7 days and Ciprofloxacin (Cipro) PO single dose or Cefriaxone (Rocephin) IM in single dose. Treat partners with same drugs.
▪ Severe recurrent vaginitis *Candida albicans* (most often)	May be indication of HIV infection; all women who are unresponsive to first-line treatment should be counseled and offered HIV testing.	Drug appropriate to opportunistic organism.

ital warts are usually identified by their clinical appearance. Vulva dystrophies may be examined using a colposcope and biopsies taken for diagnosis.

Problems involving vaginal discharge are evaluated by microscopy and cultures. The most common vaginal conditions (bacterial vaginosis, monilial vaginitis, and trichomoniasis) are diagnosed by a procedure called a wet mount. The findings characteristic of each condition are shown in Table 51-10. To assess for cervicitis, endocervical cultures are obtained for chlamydia and gonorrhea. If purulent discharge is observed coming from the cervix, a sample of endocervical cells may be taken to conduct a Gram stain. The gram-stained slide is examined on high power to identify white blood cells and any intracellular gram-negative diplococci (indicative of gonorrhea). STDs are discussed in Chapter 50.

Drug therapy is based on the diagnosis and is shown in Table 51-10.[21] Antibiotics taken as directed will cure bacterial infections. Antifungal preparations, usually creams, are indicated for monilial vaginitis. Women with vaginal conditions or cervical infection should abstain from intercourse for at least 1 week. Douching should be avoided. Douching disrupts the normal protective mechanisms within the vagina and may increase the number of pathogens and move them higher into the genital tract. Sexual partners must be evaluated and treated if the patient is diagnosed with trichomoniasis or cervicitis.

Viral infections such as herpes and genital warts cannot be cured. Systemic antiviral drugs may reduce the duration and severity of recurrent herpes outbreaks. Nondrug measures such as wearing loose fitting clothes and sitz baths may decrease discomfort. Many women with visible genital warts want them removed for cosmetic reasons. Application of liquid nitrogen is a common treatment. Women with genital warts or those who have partners with genital warts are advised to get annual Pap tests. The reason for this is that certain subtypes of the wart virus appear to cause cervical cancer.

Pharmacologic treatment of vulvar dystrophies is symptomatic because no cures are available. Treatment involves controlling the itching and hence the scratching. Interrupting the "itch-scratch cycle" prevents further secondary damage to the skin. Women should be monitored annually for squamous cell cancer, since it also presents as a vulvar lesion.

NURSING MANAGEMENT: CONDITIONS OF THE VULVA, VAGINA, AND CERVIX

Nurses have the opportunity to educate women about common genital conditions and about how they can reduce their risks. Understanding the symptoms that may indicate a problem helps women seek care in a timely manner. Matters involving genitals or sexual intercourse are frequently difficult for people to discuss. The nurse's nonjudgmental attitude in providing information allows women to feel more comfortable and ask the questions that may be especially worrisome.

When a woman is diagnosed with cervicitis or a vaginal or vulvar condition, nurses should ensure that the patient fully understands the directions for treatment. Taking the full course of medication is especially important to decrease the chance of relapse. Because genitals are such a private area, use of graphs and models is especially helpful for patient teaching. When a woman is using a vaginal medication such as an antifungal

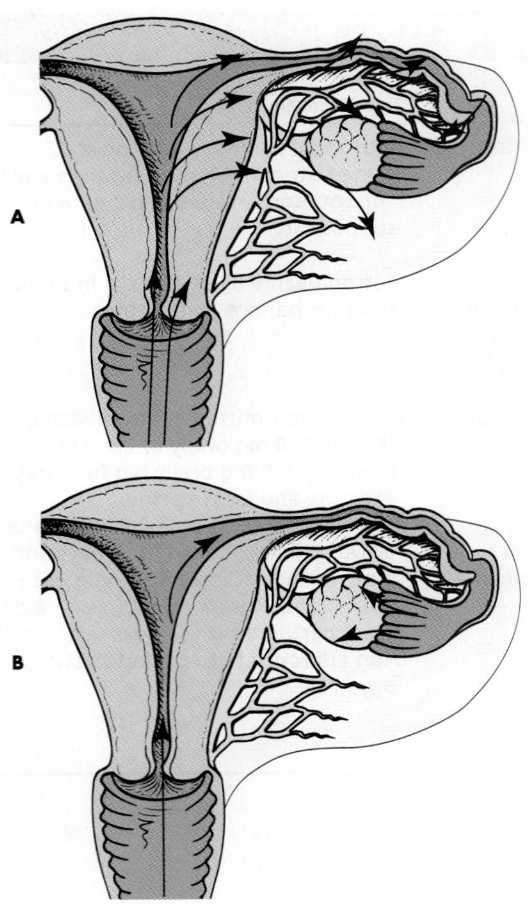

Fig. 51-5 Common routes of the spread of pelvic inflammatory disease. **A,** Direct spread of bacterial infection other than *Neisseria gonorrhoeae*. **B,** Direct spread of *Neisseria gonorrhoeae*.

cream for the first time, showing her the applicator and how to fill it is important. The woman should be taught where and how the applicator should be inserted using visual aids or models. Vaginal creams should be inserted before going to bed so that the medication remains in the vagina for a long period of time. Women using vaginal creams or suppositories may wish to use panty liners during the day, when the residual medication may drain out.

PELVIC INFLAMMATORY DISEASE

Pelvic inflammatory disease (PID) is an infectious condition of the pelvic cavity that may involve infection of the fallopian tubes (salpingitis), ovaries (oophoritis), and pelvic peritoneum (peritonitis). A tuboovarian abscess may also form. PID is referred to as "silent" when women do not perceive any symptoms. Other women with PID are in acute distress.

Etiology and Pathophysiology

PID is often the result of untreated cervicitis. The organism infecting the cervix ascends higher into the uterus, fallopian tubes, ovaries, and peritoneal cavity (Fig. 51-5). *Chlamydia trachomatis* or *Neisseria gonorrhoeae* are the most common causative organisms of PID. These organisms, as well as mycoplasma, streptococci, and anaerobes, may gain entrance during sexual intercourse or after pregnancy termination, pelvic surgery, or childbirth. It is important to remember that not all PID is the result of STDs.

Women at increased risk for chlamydial infections (i.e., those women younger than 24 years of age and having multiple sex partners or a new sex partner) should be routinely tested for chlamydia. Chlamydial infections can be asymptomatic and so unknowingly transmitted during intercourse. Even silent PID can cause damage that cannot be reversed. PID remains a major cause of female infertility.

Clinical Manifestations

Women with PID usually go to a care provider because they are experiencing lower abdominal pain. The pain typically starts gradually and is constant. The intensity may vary from mild to severe, and movements such as walking can increase the pain. Pain increases during intercourse. Spotting after intercourse and abnormal vaginal discharge are common. Fever and chills may also be present. Women with less acute symptoms notice increased cramping pain with menses, irregular bleeding, and some pain with intercourse. Women who have mild symptoms may go untreated either because they did not seek care or the health care provider misdiagnosed the complaints.

PID is a clinical diagnosis based on the patient's signs and symptoms. The diagnosis of PID is based on data obtained during the bimanual portion of the pelvic examination.[21] Women with PID have lower abdominal tenderness, bilateral adnexal tenderness, and tenderness when the cervix is moved. Additional criteria useful for diagnosis include fever and abnormal vaginal or cervical discharge. Cultures for gonorrhea and chlamydia should be obtained from the endocervix. A pregnancy test should always be done. Drug therapy should begin when the minimal criteria are met and should not await culture results.

When the patient's pain or obesity compromise the pelvic examination and a tuboovarian abscess may be present, a vaginal ultrasound is indicated. Although the patient will already have met the minimal criteria for diagnosing and treating PID, if a tuboovarian abscess is present, hospitalization is necessary.

Complications

Immediate complications of PID include septic shock and *Fitz-Hugh-Curtis syndrome,* which occurs when PID spreads to the liver and causes acute perihepatitis. The patient will have symptoms of right upper quadrant pain, but liver function tests will be normal. Pelvic and tuboovarian abscesses may "leak" or rupture, resulting in pelvic or generalized peritonitis. As the general circulation is flooded with bacterial endotoxins from the infected areas, septic shock may result. Also, embolic episodes may occur as the result of thrombophlebitis of the pelvic veins.

Long-term complications include ectopic pregnancy, infertility, and chronic pelvic pain. PID can cause adhesions and strictures to develop in the fallopian tubes. Ectopic pregnancy may result when a tube is partially obstructed because the sperm can pass through the stricture but the fertilized ovum cannot reach the uterus. After one episode of PID, the risk of having an ectopic pregnancy increases tenfold. Further damage can result in closure of the fallopian tubes and cause infertility.

NURSING ASSESSMENT

Table 51-11 Pelvic Inflammatory Disease

Subjective Data	Objective Data
Important Health Information *Past health history:* Use of IUD; previous PID, gonorrhea, or chlamydia; multiple sexual partners; exposure to partner with urethritis; infertility *Medications:* Use of and allergy to any antibiotics *Surgery or other treatments:* Recent abortion or pelvic surgery **Functional Health Patterns** *Health perception-health management:* Malaise *Nutritional-metabolic:* Nausea, vomiting; chills *Elimination:* Urinary frequency, urgency *Cognitive-perceptual:* Lower abdominal and pelvic pain; low back pain; pain on fundal palpation and cervical motion; onset of pain just after a menstrual cycle; dysmenorrhea, dyspareunia, dysuria, vulvar pruritus *Sexuality-reproductive:* Abnormal vaginal bleeding and menstrual irregularity; vaginal discharge	**General** Fever **Reproductive** Mucopurulent cervicitis, vulval maceration, vaginal discharge (heavy and purulent to thin and mucoid), tenderness on motion of cervix and uterus; presence of inflammatory masses on palpation **Possible Findings** Leukocytosis: elevated erythrocyte sedimentation rate; positive culture of secretions or endocervical fluid; pelvic inflammation and positive endometrial biopsy on laparoscopic examination; abscess or inflammation on ultrasonography

PID, pelvic inflammatory disease.

Collaborative Care

PID is usually treated on an outpatient basis. The patient is given a combination of antibiotics such as cefoxitin (Mefoxin) and doxycycline (Vibramycin) to provide broad coverage against the causative organisms. The patient must have no intercourse for 3 weeks. Her partners must be examined and treated. An important part of care is physical rest and oral fluids. The patient's return to the clinic for reevaluation in 48 to 72 hours, even if symptoms are improving, is an essential part of outpatient care.

Some cases of PID require hospitalization. If outpatient treatment is not successful or if the patient is acutely ill or in severe pain, admission to the hospital is indicated. Maximum doses of parenteral antibiotics can be given in the hospital. Some providers believe the addition of corticosteroids to the antibiotic regimen reduces the inflammation, allowing for faster recovery and improvement in subsequent fertility. Application of heat to the lower abdomen or sitz baths may be used to improve circulation and decrease pain. Bed rest in the semi-Fowler's position promotes drainage of the pelvic cavity by gravity and may prevent the development of abscesses high in the abdomen. Analgesics to relieve pain and IV fluids to prevent dehydration are also prescribed.

An indication for surgery is the presence of abscesses that fail to resolve with IV antibiotics. The abscess may be drained by laparoscopy or laparotomy. At one time, a hysterectomy was the standard approach for tuboovarian abscess. Now this is only done in extreme cases. When surgery is necessary, the capacity for childbearing is preserved whenever possible.

NURSING MANAGEMENT: PELVIC INFLAMMATORY DISEASE

Subjective and objective data that should be obtained from the woman with PID are presented in Table 51-11.

Prevention, early recognition, and prompt treatment of vaginal and cervical infections can help prevent PID and its serious complications. Nurses can provide accurate information about factors, such as multiple sexual partners and intercourse without a condom, that place women at increased risk for PID. Nurses should urge women to seek medical attention for any unusual vaginal discharge or possible infection of their reproductive organs. Women should be helped to understand that all discharge is not indicative of infection, but early diagnosis and treatment of an infection, if present, can prevent serious complications. Women should be informed of the methods to decrease the risk of getting STDs and to recognize the signs of infection in their partners.

The patient may have guilt feelings about having PID, especially if it was associated with an STD. She may also be concerned about the complications associated with PID, such as adhesions and strictures of the fallopian tubes, infertility, and the increased incidence of ectopic pregnancy. Discussion with the patient regarding her feelings and concerns can assist her to cope more effectively with them. Nursing diagnoses related to PID may include, but are not limited to, those presented in NCP 51-1.

For patients requiring hospitalization, nurses have an important role in implementing drug therapy, monitoring the patient's health status, and providing symptom relief and patient education. Vital signs and the character, amount, color, and odor of the vaginal discharge should be recorded. Explanations about the need for limited activity, being in a semi-Fowler's position, and increased fluid intake should increase patient cooperation. Assessing the degree of abdominal pain provides information about the effectiveness of drug therapy.

The nurse can use interventions such as applying heat to the lower abdomen, giving sitz baths, and giving analgesics to reduce pain. Usually the pain is dull and constant in character. The location and intensity of the pain may vary. With effective antibiotics the pain should gradually subside. Subsequent use of barrier methods (e.g., condoms and diaphragm) of birth control with spermicide and avoidance of intercourse during menses may reduce the risk of reinfection.[4]

51-1 NURSING CARE PLAN PATIENT WITH PELVIC INFLAMMATORY DISEASE

Expected Patient Outcomes	Nursing Interventions and *Rationales*
NURSING DIAGNOSIS	**Pain** *related to* infectious process *as manifested by* crampy, continuous, bilateral lower abdominal pain, guarding behavior, altered muscle tone.
▪ Satisfactory level of pain control.	▪ Assess degree of pain *to plan appropriate interventions.* ▪ Provide comfort measures (e.g., backrub, nonstimulating environment, heat to lower abdomen) *to increase patient comfort.* ▪ Administer analgesics (e.g., ibuprofen [Motrin]) as ordered *to relieve the pain.* ▪ Instruct patient to restrict movement *to avoid increasing pain.*
NURSING DIAGNOSIS	**Risk for infection transmission** *related to* vaginal discharge and lack of knowledge of proper hygiene and appropriate sexual practices.
▪ Knowledge and use of principles of medical asepsis. ▪ Avoidance of practices that could lead to transmission of disease.	▪ Assess for purulent vaginal discharge, inadequate hand washing, improper disposal of perineal pads, unsafe sexual practices *as possible sources of transmission of infection.* ▪ Use and teach strict medical asepsis when in contact with discharge (e.g., proper hand washing, careful handling and disposal of perineal pads); explain need for precautions related to vaginal discharge and encourage patient's participation in them; advise patient against sexual contact while infected *to prevent transmission of infection.*
NURSING DIAGNOSIS	**Anxiety** *related to* imposed activity restrictions, perceived loss of control, and lack of knowledge of outcome on reproductive status and course of disease *as manifested by* restlessness, frequent questioning about restricted activity and outcome, irritability, crying spells.
▪ Understanding of possible outcomes of disease process on reproductive status.	▪ Assess degree of anxiety and areas of questioning and concern *to plan appropriate interventions.* ▪ Maintain bed rest in semi-Fowler's position *to promote drainage of pelvic cavity by gravity and possibly prevent development of an abscess.* ▪ Explain need for limited activity *to improve patient's understanding and increase cooperation.* ▪ Discuss possible outcomes of disease process *to assist patient in considering a realistic outcome.* ▪ Provide counsel for patient and significant others *to demonstrate caring and understanding.* ▪ Clarify course of disease *so patient can prepare herself and be an informed partner in the plan of care.*

ENDOMETRIOSIS

Endometriosis is the presence of normal endometrial tissue in sites outside the endometrial cavity. The most frequent sites are in or near the ovaries, the uterosacral ligaments, and the uterovesical peritoneum (Fig. 51-6). However, endometrial tissues can be in many other locations such as the stomach, lungs, intestines, and spleen. The tissue responds to the hormones of the ovarian cycle and undergoes a mini–menstrual cycle similar to the uterine endometrium. About 7% to 10% of all women have endometriosis, so it is a common problem for women during their reproductive years.

Endometriosis occurs among all ethnic groups from early adolescence to the perimenopause. However, most typically, the patient with endometriosis is in her late 20s or early 30s, Caucasian, and has never had a full-term pregnancy. While not a life-threatening condition, endometriosis is responsible for considerable pain and loss of work time. Endometriosis is found in 30% to 60% of women who seek evaluation for infertility.[11]

Etiology and Pathophysiology

The etiology of endometriosis is not well understood and many theories about the cause of endometriosis have been proposed. A widely held view is that retrograde menstrual flow passes through the fallopian tubes carrying viable endometrial tissues into the pelvis. Here the tissue attaches to various sites shown in Fig. 51-6. Another theory suggests that undifferentiated celomic cells (embryonic peritoneal cavity cells) remain dormant on the peritoneal surface until the ovaries produce sufficient hormones to stimulate their growth and cyclic changes.[11]

Clinical Manifestations

A wide range of symptoms and severity exist, and the magnitude of a woman's symptoms do not match the clinical extent of her endometriosis. The most common symptoms are secondary dysmenorrhea (50%), infertility (25% to 50%), pelvic pain and dyspareunia (20%), and irregular bleeding (12% to 14%).[11] Less common symptoms include backache, painful bowel movements, and dysuria. These symptoms may or may not correspond to the woman's menstrual cycles. With menopause, estrogen is no longer produced in the ovaries, which may lead to the disappearance of the symptoms.

When the ectopic endometrial implants "menstruate," the blood collects in cystlike nodules that have a characteristic bluish black look. Nodules in the ovaries are sometimes called

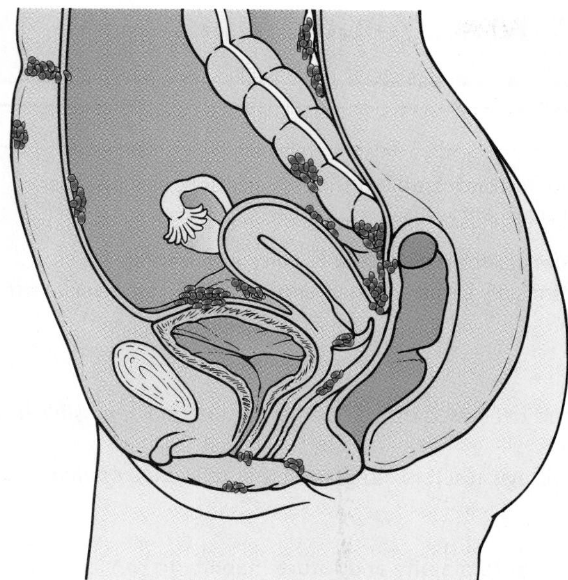

Fig. 51-6 Common sites of endometriosis.

chocolate cysts because of the thick, chocolate-colored material they contain. When a cyst ruptures, the pain may be acute and the resulting irritation promotes the formation of adhesions, which fix the affected area to another pelvic structure. The adhesions may become severe enough to cause a bowel obstruction or painful micturition. Adhesions involving the uterus, tubes, or ovaries may result in infertility.

Collaborative Care

Endometriosis may be suspected from a woman's history of the characteristic symptoms and the health care provider's palpation of firm nodular lumps in the adnexa on bimanual examination. However, laparoscopy is necessary for a definitive diagnosis. The treatment of endometriosis is influenced by the patient's age, desire to get pregnant, symptom severity, and the extent and location of the disease. When symptoms are not disruptive, a watch and wait approach is used. When endometriosis is identified as a possible cause of infertility, therapy will proceed more rapidly.

Surgical Therapy. The only cure for endometriosis is surgical removal of all the implants. Surgical therapy may be conservative or definitive. Conservative surgery is done to confirm the diagnosis or to remove implants. It involves removal or destruction of endometrial implants and lysing or excision of adhesions by means of laparoscopic laser surgery and laparotomy. Gonadotropin-releasing hormone agonist therapy (e.g., leuprolide acetate) can be administered for 4 to 6 months to reduce the size of the lesions before surgery. By reducing the extent of the surgery, this preoperative drug treatment helps reduce the development of adhesions that may further threaten fertility.

For women wishing to get pregnant, conservative surgical therapy is used to remove implants that may block the fallopian tube. Also, adhesions are removed from the tubes, ovaries, and pelvic structures. Efforts are made to conserve all tissues necessary to maintain fertility.

Definitive surgery involves removal of the uterus, tubes, ovaries, and as many endometrial implants as possible. The individual woman should be actively involved in making the decision about preserving part or all of her ovaries, if surgically possible. Her feelings about maintaining her cyclical ovarian function must be explored. The health care provider should assess the woman's risk for ovarian cancer and provide this information for her consideration.

Drug Therapy. Drug therapy is used to reduce symptoms. Drugs are selected to inhibit estrogen production by the ovary so that the endometrial tissue shrinks. The various drugs used imitate a state of pregnancy or menopause, since both natural conditions relieve symptoms. Continuous use (for 9 months) of combined progestin and estrogen causes regression of endometrial tissue. Ovulation is suppressed and pseudopregnancy (hyperhormonal amenorrhea) is produced. Another approach to hormonal treatment is danazol (Danocrine), a synthetic androgen that inhibits the anterior pituitary. When given in dosages of up to 800 mg/day for 6 to 9 months, the drug produces a pseudomenopause (ovarian suppression), with consequent atrophy of ectopic endometrial tissue. Subjective relief of symptoms is noted within 6 weeks of danazol use. Side effects include weight gain, acne, hot flashes, and hirsutism. These side effects and the expense of this drug restrict its use.

The newest and most expensive drug therapy is injectable gonadotropin-releasing hormone analog (leuprolide [Lupron]). It causes a hypoestrogenic state resulting in amenorrhea. The side effects reported by patients are usually the same as menopause (hot flashes, vaginal dryness, and emotional lability). Loss of bone density has also been reported in women who remain on the therapy longer than 6 months. Endometriosis is controlled but not cured by hormonal therapy. Persistent lesions give rise to subsequent recurrences once the menstrual cycle is reestablished.

NURSING MANAGEMENT: ENDOMETRIOSIS

Nurses should educate women about endometriosis with special attention to the common symptoms. Dysmenorrhea after years of relatively pain-free menses and the inability to achieve pregnancy may serve as clues to the presence of endometriosis. When women understand the symptoms that might suggest endometriosis, they are more likely to see their primary care providers sooner when symptoms develop.

Education of the patient and reassurance that a life-threatening situation does not exist may permit her to accept a conservative and progressive treatment. When the symptoms are less severe, teaching about nondrug comfort measures may be very helpful. Nurses often assist patients to fully understand the drugs that have been ordered to treat their condition. The action of the prescribed drug should be explained, as well as the possible side effects. Psychologic support may be needed for the women experiencing severe disabling pain, sexual difficulties secondary to dyspareunia, and infertility.

If conservative surgery is the treatment selected, the nursing care is similar to the general preoperative and postoperative care of a patient undergoing laparotomy. If definitive surgery is planned, the nursing care is similar to the patient undergoing an abdominal hysterectomy (see NCP 51-2 on p. 1538). The nurse must know the extent of the procedure so that appropriate postoperative teaching can be done.

51-2 NURSING CARE PLAN PATIENT WITH A TOTAL ABDOMINAL HYSTERECTOMY

Expected Patient Outcomes	Nursing Interventions and *Rationales*
NURSING DIAGNOSIS **Urinary retention** *related to* loss of bladder tone, uncomfortable urinating position, and pain *as manifested by* distention of bladder, voiding of small amounts.	
■ Able to urinate in sufficient quantities without difficulty.	■ Measure intake and output *to determine if satisfactory fluid balance is maintained.* ■ Encourage fluids orally within limitations of diet *to ensure adequate quantity of urine to stimulate urge to urinate.* ■ Percuss bladder *to detect distention.* ■ Catheterize as ordered. ■ Report any complaints of backache and decreased output *as these are signs of a possible ligation of a ureter.* ■ Provide routine catheter care if indwelling catheter is in place *to ensure catheter patency and free flow of urine.*
NURSING DIAGNOSIS **Body-image disturbance** *related to* perceived loss of femininity and future inability to conceive *as manifested by* crying, weeping, depression; verbalization of perceived loss of femininity and/or ability to conceive.	
■ Accurate statements of effects of hysterectomy. ■ Verbalization of confidence in ability to adjust to postsurgical state.	■ Assess depth of impact of surgery on body image *to determine need and plan for intervention.* ■ Provide factual information regarding anticipated bodily changes *so patient will have accurate information.* ■ Provide information on hormone replacement *so patient is informed about possible treatment of surgical menopause.* ■ Encourage discussion with patient, significant others, and health professionals *to minimize emotional impact of hysterectomy through open discussion.*
NURSING DIAGNOSIS **Altered sexuality patterns** *related to* perceived lack of desirability and lack of knowledge regarding resumption of sexual activity *as manifested by* frequent questioning about future sexual response, lack of desire to resume presurgical sexual practices.	
■ Optimism that satisfactory sexual practices can be resumed when indicated by surgeon.	■ Facilitate discussion of sexuality with significant other *to clarify areas of misunderstanding and foster mutual approach to any problems.* ■ Reassure patient that energy and desire will return after a period of convalescence *to prevent discouragement and depression.* ■ Explain psychologic and physiologic implications of hysterectomy related to a woman's sexuality *to provide accurate facts and decrease fear of consequences of hysterectomy.*
NURSING DIAGNOSIS **Altered health maintenance** *related to* lack of knowledge regarding activity restrictions and hormone replacement therapy (HRT) *as manifested by* questioning about postdischarge plans.	
■ Ability to make appropriate decisions related to occupational and leisure activity and HRT.	■ Encourage expression of concerns *to clarify areas of concern.* ■ Assess knowledge level. ■ Provide information regarding HRT *so patient has accurate knowledge base to make decisions.* ■ Provide timetable for gradual resumption of presurgery activity *so patient does not resume activities too soon or delay resumption of activities unnecessarily.*
NURSING DIAGNOSIS **Pain** *related to* incision and manipulation of internal organs *as manifested by* statements about pain, guarding of incision, reluctance to ambulate, facial grimacing.	
■ Verbalization of satisfactory level of pain control.	■ Assess degree of pain *to plan appropriate interventions.* ■ Provide comfort measures (e.g., backrub, heat to lower abdomen) *to increase patient comfort.* ■ Administer analgesics as ordered *to relieve the pain.* ■ Instruct patient on methods for moving and coughing while supporting abdominal incision.

Continued

51-2 NURSING CARE PLAN PATIENT WITH A TOTAL ABDOMINAL HYSTERECTOMY—continued

Expected Patient Outcomes	Nursing Interventions and *Rationales*
COLLABORATIVE PROBLEMS	
Nursing Goals	**Nursing Interventions and *Rationales***
POTENTIAL COMPLICATION	**Paralytic ileus** *related to* surgical manipulation of bowel and immobility.
▪ Monitor for signs of paralytic ileus and report if present. ▪ Carry out appropriate medical and nursing interventions.	▪ Assess for distended abdomen, complaints of gas pains, decreased bowel sounds *to detect presence of paralytic ileus.* ▪ Encourage ambulation q4hr *to promote bowel peristalsis.* ▪ Insert rectal tube as ordered *to expel flatus and promote patient comfort.* ▪ Withhold food and fluids if paralytic ileus is present *to prevent nausea and vomiting.*
POTENTIAL COMPLICATION	**Thromboembolic phenomenon** *related to* immobility and irritation of vessels of pelvis and upper thigh.
▪ Monitor for signs of thromboembolism and report if present. ▪ Carry out appropriate medical and nursing interventions.	▪ Assess lower extremities for warmth, color, blanching, pain, and sensation q8hr *to detect impaired circulation.* ▪ Assess for signs of pulmonary embolism such as chest pain, tachycardia, and dyspnea. ▪ Report and record signs and symptoms of thrombophlebitis *so early treatment can be initiated.* ▪ Encourage foot-leg exercises while in bed; ambulate q4hr and avoid prolonged sitting *to promote good circulation and prevent stasis.* ▪ Reapply elastic compression gradient stockings every shift *to apply even pressure to veins to prevent venous stasis.*

BENIGN TUMORS OF THE FEMALE REPRODUCTIVE SYSTEM

LEIOMYOMAS

Etiology

Leiomyomas (fibroids, myomas, fibromyomas, fibromas) are the most common benign tumors of the female genital tract (Fig. 51-7). By 30 years of age, 10% of Caucasian women and 30% of African-American women have uterine leiomyomas. The cause of leiomyomas is unknown. They appear to depend on ovarian hormones because they grow slowly during the reproductive years and undergo atrophy after menopause. Leiomyomas consist of smooth muscle cells.

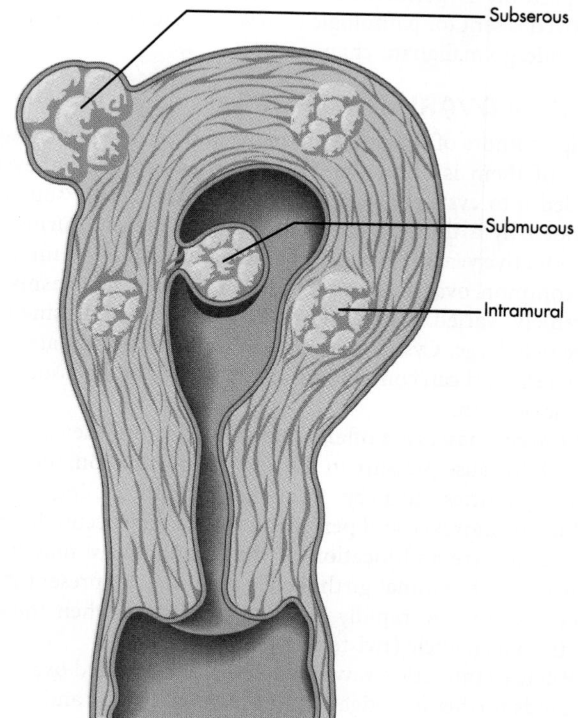

Fig. 51-7 Leiomyomas. Uterine section showing whorl-like appearance and locations of leiomyomas, which are also called uterine fibroids.

Clinical Manifestations

The majority of women with fibroids do not have any symptoms. Of the women with leiomyomas who develop symptoms, the most common is menorrhagia. Although rarely experienced with leiomyomas, pain is associated with infection or twisting of the pedicle from which the tumor is growing. Dysmenorrhea and dyspareunia may occasionally occur. Pressure on surrounding organs may result in rectal, bladder, and lower abdominal discomfort. Large tumors may cause a general enlargement of the lower abdomen. These tumors are sometimes associated with miscarriage and infertility.

Collaborative Care

Clinical diagnosis is based on the characteristic pelvic findings of an enlarged uterus distorted by nodular masses. Treatment depends on the symptoms, the age of the patient, her desire to bear children, and the location and size of the tumor or tumors. If the symptoms are minor, the provider may elect to follow the patient closely for a time. If the woman is experiencing menorrhagia, the use of aspirin is discouraged because of its effect on platelets.

Persistent heavy menstrual bleeding causing anemia and large or rapidly growing fibroids are indications for surgery. The fibroids are removed by hysterectomy or myomectomy. A myomectomy is performed for women who wish to have children. In this case, only the fibroids are removed in order to preserve the uterus. Small fibroids may be removed using a hysteroscope and laser resection instruments.[4] In cases of large leiomyomas, a gonadotropin-releasing hormone agonist (e.g., leuprolide) may be used preoperatively to shrink the size of the leiomyomas. However, the risks and benefits of this drug should be fully discussed, including the potential for irreversible loss of bone mass.

CERVICAL POLYPS

Cervical polyps are benign pedunculated lesions that generally arise from the endocervical mucosa and are seen protruding through the cervical os during a speculum examination. Polyps are a characteristic bright cherry red and are soft and fragile in consistency. They are generally small, measuring less than 3 cm in length, and may be single or multiple. Their origin is unknown. Symptoms are usually not present, but metrorrhagia and bleeding after straining and coitus can occur. Polyps are prone to infection. When the polyp is small, it can be excised in an outpatient procedure. If the point of attachment of the polyp cannot be identified and is not accessible to cautery, a polypectomy is performed in an operating room. All tissue removed is sent for pathologic review because polyps occasionally undergo malignant changes.

BENIGN OVARIAN TUMORS

Benign tumors of the ovary are many and varied. The cause of most of them is unknown. For purposes of clarity, they are divided into cysts and neoplasms. Cysts are usually soft, surrounded by a thin capsule, and are seen mainly during the reproductive years (Fig. 51-8). Follicle and corpus luteum cysts are common ovarian cysts. Epithelial ovarian neoplasms are extremely varied. They may be cystic or solid, small or extremely large. Cystic teratomas or dermoids originate from germ cells and can contain bits of any type of body tissue, such as hair or teeth.

Ovarian masses are often asymptomatic until they are large enough to cause pressure in the pelvis. Constipation, menstrual irregularities, urinary frequency, a full feeling in the abdomen, anorexia, and peripheral edema may occur, depending on the size and location of the tumor. There may be an increase in abdominal girth. Pelvic pain may be present if the tumor is growing rapidly. Severe pain results when the cyst twists on its pedicle (twisted ovarian cyst).

Pelvic examination reveals a mass or an enlarged ovary that demands further investigation. If the mass is cystic and smaller than 8 cm, the patient is asked to return for reexamination in 4 to 6 weeks. If the mass is cystic and greater than 8 cm or is solid, laparoscopic surgery or laparotomy is performed. Immediate surgery is necessary if the ovarian mass causes the ovary to rotate, cutting off circulation. Surgical techniques are used to save as much of the ovary as possible.

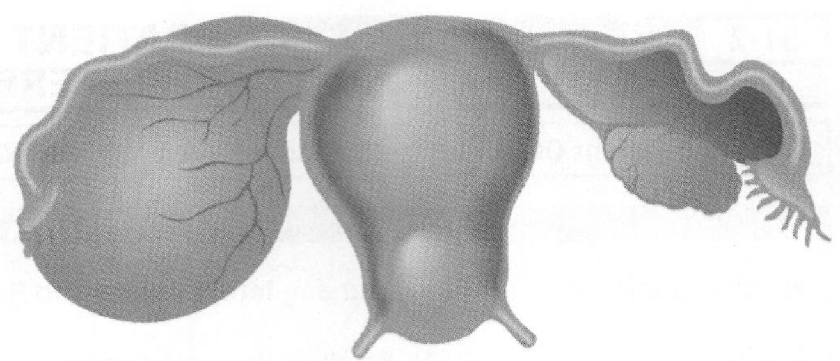

Fig. 51-8 Ovarian cysts can occur on both ovaries and have different sizes.

MALIGNANT TUMORS OF THE FEMALE REPRODUCTIVE SYSTEM

CERVICAL CANCER

In 1998, there were approximately 13,700 cases of invasive cervical cancer diagnosed and approximately 4900 women in the United States died from cervical cancer. The mortality rate was twice as high for African-American women as compared with Caucasian women. The incidence is also higher among Hispanic women than Caucasian women. An increased risk of cervical cancer is associated with low economic status, early sexual activity (before 17 years of age), multiple sexual partners, infection with HPV, and smoking.[9]

The number of deaths from cervical cancer has fallen steadily over the past 40 years. This is attributable to better and earlier diagnosis with the widespread use of the Pap test. In addition to cancer, the Pap test detects precancerous changes called cervical intraepithelial neoplasia (CIN) or dysplasia. By treating dysplasia, progression to cervical cancer can be prevented. The American Cancer Society recommends annual Pap tests beginning with the onset of sexual activity. Following three negative Pap tests, less frequent tests may be recommended by the health care provider.

Etiology and Pathophysiology

The progression from normal cervical cells to dysplasia and on to cervical cancer appears to be related to repeated injuries to the cervix.[22] The progression occurs slowly over years rather than months. There is a relationship between certain subtypes of HPV and cervical cancer.[9] However, a cofactor such as smoking is thought to be needed in addition to the specific subtype of HPV. Women who smoke have a 50% higher risk for developing cervical cancer than nonsmokers. This risk is greatest in those with longer duration of smoking, increased number of cigarettes smoked, and use of unfiltered cigarettes.[11]

Clinical Manifestations

Precancerous changes are asymptomatic, highlighting the importance of routine screening. CIN occurs mainly in young women. The peak incidence of CIN is in women in their early

Table **51-12** Classification of Cytologic Findings of Pap Tests

Papanicolaou Class	Dysplasia	CIN	Bethesda System
Class I Normal smear	Negative	Negative	Within normal limits
Class II Atypical cells, no dysplasia	Reactive atypia Koilocytosis or HPV Mild dysplasia	Koilocytosis or HPV CIN 1	Regeneration, repair Inflammation Low-grade squamous intraepithelial lesion
Class III Abnormal cells consistent with dysplasia	Moderate dysplasia	CIN 2	
Class IV Abnormal cells consistent with CIS	Severe dysplasia, CIS	CIN 2 CIN 3	High-grade squamous intraepithelial lesion
Class V Abnormal cells consistent with invasive or squamous cell origin	Squamous cell carcinoma	Squamous cell carcinoma	Squamous cell carcinoma

CIN, cervical intraepithelial neoplasia; *CIS,* carcinoma in situ; *HPV,* human papillomavirus.

CULTURAL & ETHNIC CONSIDERATIONS

Cancer of the Female Reproductive System

- Japanese women have a low incidence of ovarian cancer. However, second and third generation Japanese women in the United States have much higher rates, similar to Caucasian women born in the United States. Dietary practices may explain this difference.
- Five-year survival rate for endometrial cancer (all stages combined) is 80% for Caucasian women and 55% for African-American women.
- Cervical cancer has a higher incidence among Hispanic, African-American, and Native-American women than Caucasians.
- Mortality rates from cervical cancer are more than twice as high among African-American women as among Caucasian women.

30s. The average age for women with invasive cervical cancer is 50 years. Early cervical cancer is generally asymptomatic, but leukorrhea and intermenstrual bleeding eventually occur. The discharge is usually thin and watery but becomes dark and foul smelling as the disease advances, suggesting the presence of an infection. The vaginal bleeding is initially only spotting, but as the tumor enlarges, it becomes heavier and more frequent. Pain is a late symptom and is followed by weight loss, anemia, and cachexia.

Diagnostic Studies

A Pap test, the Schiller iodine test, colposcopy, and a biopsy may be used to diagnose cervical cancer. (These diagnostic tests are described in Chapter 48.) Various classification systems are used to interpret the cytologic findings. Examples are given in Table 51-12. The current trend is to use the Bethesda system because it improves accuracy and quality of diagnosis by standardizing diagnostic reports. Pap tests are less than 100% accurate. There are problems with both false-positive and false-negative reports. New techniques for cervical cancer screening are being explored.

Collaborative Care

The finding of an abnormal Pap smear indicates the need for follow-up. The type of follow-up depends on the Pap findings. Women with minor changes (Class II) may be followed with a repeated Pap test in 3 to 4 months. Up to 80% may revert to normal spontaneously. Women with more prominent changes (Class III or greater) receive additional procedures, such as colposcopy and biopsy, before a definitive diagnosis can be made. Colposcopy involves examination of the cervix with a binocular microscope with low levels of magnification (10× to 40×). The procedure helps in the identification of possible epithelial abnormalities and suggests areas for biopsy. Biopsies are sent to pathology for evaluation. Colposcopy and biopsy have improved diagnosis and allowed more focused treatments to be selected.

The type and extent of the biopsy vary with the abnormality seen. A punch biopsy may be done on an outpatient basis with special punch biopsy forceps. The excision of a cone-shaped section of the cervix may be used for both diagnosis and treatment. Conization is accomplished using one of several techniques. The choice of procedure is determined by the provider's experience and the availability of equipment. Cryotherapy (freezing) and laser cone vaporization destroy the tissue. Laser cone excision and loop electrosurgery excision procedure (LEEP) remove the identified tissue and allow for histologic examination to ensure that all microinvasive tissue has been removed. These procedures can be performed in the office with some mild analgesics or relaxants. Complications of these procedures include excessive bleeding and possible cervical stenosis with healing.

Table 51-13 International Classification of Clinical Stages of Carcinoma of the Cervix

Stage	Extent	Treatment
Stage 0	In situ, intraepithelial	Cervical conization, total hysterectomy, cryosurgery, laser surgery
Stage I	Strict confinement to cervix (no consideration of extension to corpus)	
Stage IA	Microinvasive (early stromal invasion)	Radiation or surgery
Stage IB	All other cases of stage I	Radiation, Wertheim's hysterectomy
Stage II	Extension beyond cervix but not to pelvic wall, involvement of vagina, but not as far as lower third	
Stage IIA	No obvious parametrial involvement	Radiation, Wertheim's hysterectomy
Stage IIB	Obvious parametrial involvement	Radiation; if this fails, pelvic exenteration may be required
Stage III	Extension to pelvic wall, no cancer-free space between tumor and pelvic wall on rectal examination, involvement of lower third of vagina, hydronephrosis or nonfunctioning kidney	Radiation
Stage IIIA	No extension to pelvic wall	
Stage IIIB	Extension to pelvic wall or hydronephrosis or nonfunctioning kidney	
Stage IV	Extension beyond true pelvis or clinical involvement of the mucosa of bladder or rectum, no stage IV classification with bullous edema alone	Radiation, surgery (e.g., exenteration)
Stage IVA	Spread to adjacent organs	
Stage IVB	Spread to distant organs	

Treatment of cancer of the cervix is guided by the stage of the tumor (Table 51-13) and the patient's age and general state of health. There are four procedures in which fertility can be preserved. Conization may be the only type of therapy needed for CIN if analysis of removed tissue demonstrates that a wide area of normal tissue surrounds the excised tissue. Laser treatments using a directed infrared beam is effective in the destruction of dysplasic tissue. Cautery and cryosurgery may also be used.

Invasive cancer of the cervix is treated with surgery, radiation, or a combination of the two are used to remove or destroy the involved areas and lymphatic drainage. Surgical procedures commonly carried out include hysterectomy, Wertheim or radical hysterectomy (involving adjacent structures), and rarely pelvic exenteration. Radiation may be external (e.g., cobalt) or internal (e.g., cesium or radium). Standard radiation treatment is 4 to 6 weeks of external radiation followed with one or two treatments with internal implants.[22] (Radiation therapy is discussed in Chapter 14.)

ENDOMETRIAL CANCER

Cancer of the endometrium is the most common gynecologic malignancy, accounting for nearly 50% of female genital tract neoplasms. In 1998 there were approximately 36,100 cases of endometrial cancer and 6300 deaths. Endometrial cancer has a relatively low mortality, with a survival rate of 94% if the cancer has not spread at the time of diagnosis.[22] About 25% of endometrial cancer is diagnosed before menopause. The average age at the time of diagnosis is 61 years.

Etiology and Pathophysiology

The major risk factor for endometrial cancer is estrogen, in particular unopposed estrogen. Additional risk factors include increasing age, nulliparity, obesity, hypertension, and diabetes mellitus. Obesity is a risk factor because adipose (fat) cells store estrogen, which increases endogenous estrogen and increases its availability. Pregnancy and birth control pills are protective factors.

Cancer arises from the lining of the endometrium. Most tumors are pure adenocarcinomas. The precursor may be a hyperplasic state that progresses to invasive carcinoma. Hyperplasia occurs when estrogen is not counteracted by progesterone. Direct extension develops into the cervix and through the uterine serosa. As invasion of the myometrium occurs, regional lymph nodes, including the paravaginal and paraaortic, become involved. Hematogenous metastases develop concurrently. The usual sites of metastases are lung, bone, liver, and eventually the brain. Malignant cells can be found in the peritoneal cavity, presumably by tubal transport, and their presence is included in staging. Prognostic factors include histologic differentiation, uterine size at time of diagnosis, myometrial invasion, peritoneal cytology, lymph node and adnexal metastases, and tumor size. Endometrial cancer grows slowly, metastasizes late, and is amenable to therapy if diagnosed early.

Clinical Manifestations

The first sign of endometrial cancer is abnormal uterine bleeding, usually in postmenopausal women. Because perimenopausal women have sporadic periods for a time, it is important that this sign not be ignored or automatically blamed on menopause. Pain occurs late in the disease process, and other symptoms that may arise are related to metastasis to other organs.

Collaborative Care

Endometrial biopsy has replaced a D&C as a diagnostic procedure for endometrial cancer. Endometrial biopsy, often an office procedure, involves obtaining endometrial tissue from the uterus. Any occurrence of spotting or unexpected bleeding in a postmenopausal woman mandates obtaining a tissue sample to exclude endometrial cancer. The American Cancer Society recommends an endometrial biopsy be performed at menopause and then periodically in women who are at risk. The Pap test is not a reliable diagnostic tool for endometrial cancer, but it can rule out cervical cancer.

Treatment of endometrial cancer is a total hysterectomy and bilateral salpingo-oophorectomy with selective node biopsies. Surgery may be followed by radiation, either to the pelvis or abdomen externally or intravaginally, to decrease local recurrence.[22] Treatment of advanced or recurrent disease is difficult. Hormonal therapy (e.g., progesterone) is the treatment of choice when the progesterone receptor status is positive and the tumor is well differentiated. Chemotherapy is considered when progesterone therapy is unsuccessful. The most common agents used are doxorubicin (Adriamycin) and cisplatin (Platinol).[22]

OVARIAN CANCER

Because most women with ovarian cancer have advanced disease at diagnosis, it causes more deaths than any other cancer of the female reproductive system. Ovarian cancer is responsible for 32% of all cancers of the female reproductive system, but carries a mortality rate over 50%.[11] It occurs most frequently in women between 55 and 65 years of age.[11] The median age of women with ovarian cancer is 60 years. Caucasian women of North American or European descent are also at greater risk for ovarian cancer as compared with African-American women.

Etiology and Pathophysiology

Risk factors include family history of ovarian cancer, increasing age, and high-fat diet. However, many women diagnosed with ovarian cancer have none of these risks. Women who have mutations of the BRCA-1 gene have increased susceptibility (60% higher risk) for ovarian cancer.[23] The BRCA genes are tumor suppressor genes. They inhibit tumor growth when functioning normally. When they mutate, they lose their tumor suppressor ability, and hence there is increased risk for women to develop cancer (ovarian and breast). Breast feeding, multiple pregnancies, oral contraceptive use (greater than 5 years), and early age at first birth seem to reduce the risk of ovarian cancer. It is thought that these factors have a protective effect because they reduce the number of ovulatory cycles the woman experiences.

Between 80% and 85% of ovarian cancers are epithelial carcinomas, that is, they arise from malignant transformation of the surface epithelial cells. Germ cell tumors account for another 10%. Histologic grading is an important prognostic determinant. Generally, tumors are divided into well differentiated (grade I), moderately well differentiated (grade II), and poorly differentiated (grade III). Grade III lesions carry a worse prognosis than the other grades.

Ovarian cancer has two patterns of metastasis: lymphatic and direct. Primary lymphatic drainage of the ovary is through the retroperitoneal nodes surrounding the renal hilum. Secondary drainage is through the iliac lymphatics. Tertiary drainage is through the inguinal lymphatics. Ovarian cancer also metastasizes directly to the abdominal cavity, the diaphragm, and the omentum.

Clinical Manifestations

In its early stages, ovarian cancer is usually asymptomatic. As the malignancy grows, a variety of symptoms, such as an increase in abdominal girth, bowel and bladder dysfunction, pain, menstrual irregularities, and ascites, can occur. An ovarian malignancy should be considered when abnormal uterine bleeding occurs.

Diagnostic Studies

Unlike the Pap test used to screen for cervical cancer, no screening test exists for ovarian cancer. For women at risk for ovarian cancer, a combination of serum CA-125 and ultrasound is recommended in addition to a yearly pelvic examination. CA-125 is positive in 80% of women with epithelial ovarian cancer and is used to monitor the course of disease.[22] However, values of CA-125 may be elevated with other nonovarian malignancies or with benign conditions such as fibroids or endometriosis.

Collaborative Care

Since early ovarian cancer is usually asymptomatic, yearly bimanual pelvic examinations should be performed to identify the presence of an ovarian mass. Postmenopausal women should not have palpable ovaries, so a mass of any size should be suspected as possible ovarian cancer. When a suspicious mass in the ovarian area is palpated, laparoscopy is performed to establish the diagnosis. Women identified as high risk based on family and health history may require additional surveillance and counseling regarding options such as prophylactic oophorectomy and birth control pills. It is important to note that while oophorectomy significantly reduces the risk of ovarian cancer it does not completely eliminate the possibility of disease.

If the mass is malignant, staging is critical for guiding treatment decisions. Because of the numerous metastatic pathways for ovarian cancer, accurate staging usually involves multiple biopsies. Stage I describes disease limited to the ovaries; stage II, disease limited to the true pelvis; stage III, disease limited to the abdominal cavity; and stage IV, distant metastatic disease.

The usual treatment for stage I malignancies is a total abdominal hysterectomy and bilateral salpingo-oophorectomy with removal of as much of the tumor as possible (i.e., tumor debulking). The remaining tissues in the abdomen and pelvis are carefully scrutinized. Ascitic fluid is submitted for cytologic study, and appropriate biopsies are performed to determine the stage of the disease.

The addition of chemotherapy or the instillation of intraperitoneal radioisotopes is usually suggested for stage I disease. The patient with stage II disease may receive external abdominal and pelvic radiation, intraperitoneal radiation, or systemic combined chemotherapy after tumor-reducing surgery. After completion of systemic chemotherapy, in the patient who is clinically free of symptoms, a "second-look" surgical procedure is often performed to determine whether there is any evidence of disease. This option does not necessarily improve the outcome. If no disease is found, the patient is monitored for recurrent disease.

Chemotherapy (e.g., cisplatin [Platinol] or carboplatin [Paraplatin]) is used for the treatment of stage III and stage IV diseases. Altretamine (Hexalen) is used for palliative treatment of persistent, recurrent ovarian cancer. Paclitaxel (Taxol) and topotecan (Hycamtin) are used to treat metastatic ovarian cancer. Surgical debulking is often done in conjunction with chemotherapy for advanced disease. Intraperitoneal chemotherapy, although associated with substantial side effects, is coming into wider use for the patient who has minimum residual disease after surgery. Unfortunately, the malignancy may have metastasized to the peritoneum, omentum, or bowel surface before discovery of the tumors. In these situations the prognosis is poor. Recurrent pleural effusion causing shortness of breath and discomfort may require frequent paracenteses, but the fluid accumulates again. Radiation and chemotherapy may be used to shrink the size of the tumor, relieving pressure and pain.

VAGINAL CANCER

Primary vaginal cancers are rare, representing less than 2% of genital cancers. The peak incidence is between 50 and 70 years of age. Vaginal tumors are usually secondary sites or metastases of other cancers such as cervical or endometrial cancer. The most common type of vaginal cancer is squamous cell carcinoma. Intrauterine exposure to diethylstilbestrol (DES) places a woman at risk for clear cell adenocarcinoma of the vagina. Treatment of vaginal cancer depends on the type of cells involved and the stage of the disease, the size of the tumor, and the location of the tumor. Squamous cell carcinomas can be treated with both surgery and radiation.

VULVAR CANCER

Cancer of the vulva is relatively rare, accounting for about 5% of cancers of the female reproductive system.[9] Similar to cervical cancer, preinvasive lesions referred to as vulvar intraepithelial neoplasia (VIN) precede invasive vulvar cancer. The invasive form occurs mainly in women over 60 years of age with the highest incidence being in the 70s.[22] Patients with vulvar neoplasia may have symptoms of vulvar itching or burning, pain, bleeding, or discharge. Women who are immunosuppressed, have diabetes mellitus, hypertension, and chronic vulvar dystrophies are at a higher risk for developing vulvar cancer.[9] Several subtypes of HPV have been identified in some but not all vulvar cancers.[4]

Diagnosis of vulvar cancer is based on the pathology report on the biopsy of the suspicious lesion. VIN is managed by eradicating the lesion medically with 5-fluorouracil (5-FU) or surgical excision. Larger lesions may require more extensive surgery and skin graft. The traditional treatment for vulvar cancer has been radical vulvectomy. However, the procedure results in extensive morbidity related to scarring and wound breakdown. For this reason, more conservative surgical techniques such as radical hemivulvectomy are being used. Cure rates are comparable between the radical vulvectomy and hemivulvectomy. Morbidity and loss of function has been significantly decreased with the hemivulvectomy.

SURGICAL PROCEDURES FOR FEMALE REPRODUCTIVE SYSTEM

A variety of surgical procedures (Table 51-14) are performed when benign or malignant tumors of the genital tract are found. A hysterectomy may be done either vaginally or abdominally. A vaginal route is often used when vaginal repair is to be done in addition to removal of the uterus. The abdominal route is used when large tumors are present and the pelvic cavity is to be explored or when the tubes and ovaries are to be removed at the same time (Fig. 51-9). The abdominal route can present more postoperative problems because it involves an incision and the opening of the abdominal cavity. In both vaginal and abdominal hysterectomies the ligaments that support the uterus are attached to the vaginal cuff so that normal depth of the vagina is maintained. Laparoscopy assisted vaginal hysterectomy is becoming more common as a means of decreasing morbidity associated with abdominal hysterectomy.[24,25]

Table 51-14 Surgical Procedures on the Female Reproductive Tract

Type of Surgery	Description
Subtotal hysterectomy	Removal of uterus without cervix (rarely done today)
Total hysterectomy	Removal of uterus and cervix
Panhysterectomy (TAH-BSO)	Removal of uterus, cervix, fallopian tubes, and ovaries
Simple vulvectomy	Excision of vulva and wide margin of skin
Radical vulvectomy	Excision of tissue from anus to few cm above symphysis pubis (skin, labia majora and minora, and clitoris) with superficial and deep lymph node dissection
Vaginectomy	Removal of vagina
Radical hysterectomy (Wertheim)	Panhysterectomy, partial vaginectomy, and dissection of lymph nodes in pelvis
Pelvic exenteration	Radical hysterectomy, total vaginectomy, removal of bladder with diversion of urinary system and resection of bowel with colostomy
Anterior pelvic exenteration	Above operation without bowel resection
Posterior pelvic exenteration	Above operation without bladder removal

TAH-BSO, total abdominal hysterectomy and bilateral salpingo-oophorectomy.

RADIATION THERAPY FOR CANCERS OF THE FEMALE REPRODUCTIVE SYSTEM

Radiation is used to cure, control, or palliatively treat cancers of the female reproductive system either alone or in combination with other treatments. The goal of radiation therapy is to deliver a specific amount of high-energy (or ionizing) radiation to the cancer with minimal damage to the normal surrounding tissue.[22] Radiation therapy may be external or internal.

External Radiation Therapy

With external radiation therapy, a source outside of the body delivers electromagnetic radiation in the form of waves.[22] The waves are produced by highly specialized machines or from rays emitted from a radioactive source. Higher energy machines, such as the betatron, penetrate deeper with a more sharply

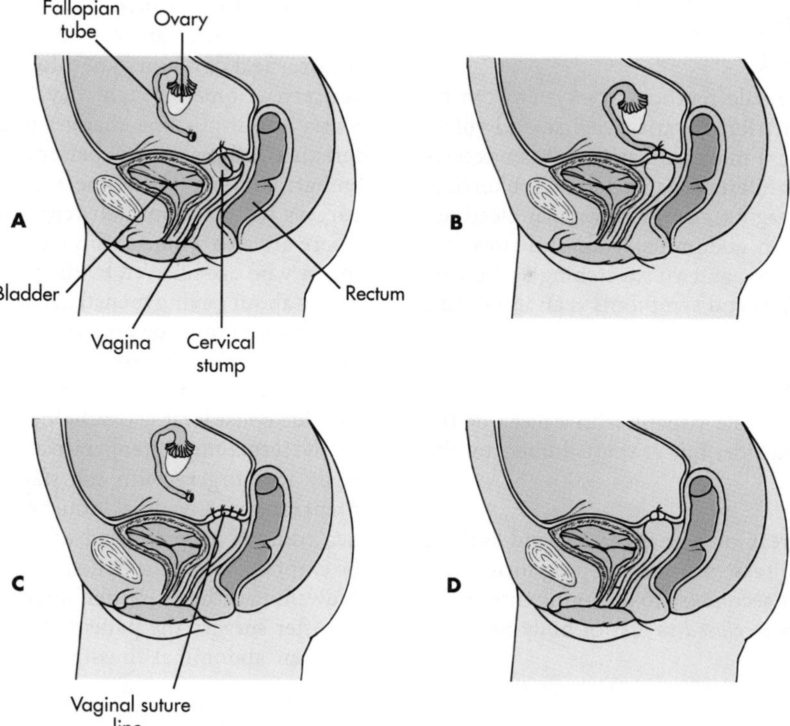

Fig. 51-9 **A,** Cross section of subtotal hysterectomy. Note that cervical stump, fallopian tubes, and ovaries remain. **B,** Cross section of total hysterectomy. Note that fallopian tubes and ovaries remain. **C,** Cross section of vaginal hysterectomy. Note that fallopian tubes and ovaries remain. **D,** Total hysterectomy, salpingectomy, and oophorectomy. Note that uterus, fallopian tubes, and ovaries are completely removed.

defined beam. This reduces the side effects that patients experience. The radiation treatment plan is based on a thorough evaluation of the patient. The plan includes the total amount of radiation to control the tumor, the daily dose, schedule, and arrangement of the radiation beams.[22] (External radiation therapy is discussed in Chapter 14.)

Internal Radiation Therapy

Use of internal radiation therapy allows the radiation to be placed near or into the tumor. This method can deliver a high dose of radiation directly to the tumor. The dose decreases sharply the farther away from the source, causing less damage to the surrounding normal tissue. A variety of forms are used to deliver internal radiation including wires, capsules, needles, tubes, and grains or seeds. Internal radiation is used in the management of cervical and endometrial cancer because of the accessibility of these body parts and the favorable results obtained. Radium and cesium are two commonly used isotopes. In preparation of the patient for the treatment, a cleansing enema is given to prevent straining at stool, which could cause displacement of the isotope. An indwelling catheter is inserted to prevent a distended bladder from coming into contact with the radioactive source.

A variety of applicators have been developed for intrauterine treatment. Applicators are inserted into the endometrial cavity and vagina of an anesthetized patient in the operating room. When the applicator contains the radioactive material, this is known as preloading.[22] In afterloading, the applicator is implanted in the operating room but is not loaded with the radioactive material until its correct placement is verified and the patient has been returned to her room. Radiation exposure to the patient is precisely controlled. The radiation exposure to the physician and other personnel involved in the implantation is reduced when the afterload technique is used. The applicator is secured with vaginal packing and is left in place for 24 to 72 hours. The radiation oncologist determines the exact amount of radioactive substance to be used and the length of time it will be left in place so that destruction of cancer cells can occur with minimal damage to normal cells.

During the treatment the patient is placed in a lead-lined private room and is on absolute bed rest. She may be turned from side to side. The presence of an intrauterine applicator produces uterine contractions that may require analgesics. The destruction of cells results in a foul-smelling vaginal discharge, and a deodorizer is helpful. Nausea, vomiting, diarrhea, and malaise may develop as a systemic reaction to the radiation.

At the end of the prescribed period of radiation, the radioactive material and the catheter are removed. The patient is allowed off bed rest and is discharged from the hospital when stable. Late complications that may arise after radiation of the uterus include fistulas (vesicovaginal, ureterovaginal), cystitis, phlebitis, hemorrhage, and fibrosis. If fibrosis occurs, the vaginal wall becomes smaller in diameter and shorter. Dilation of the vagina through intercourse or the use of a sequentially sized dilators may be indicated. The patient is urged to report any unusual symptoms or complaints to her physician. (Internal radiation and related nursing care are discussed in Chapter 14.)

NURSING MANAGEMENT: CANCERS OF THE FEMALE REPRODUCTIVE SYSTEM

■ Nursing Assessment

Malignant tumors of the female reproductive system can be found in the cervix, endometrium, ovaries, vagina, and vulva. The patient with any of these malignant tumors may experience a variety of clinical manifestations, including leukorrhea (white discharge from the vagina), irregular vaginal bleeding, vaginal discharge, increase in abdominal pain and pressure, bowel and bladder dysfunction, and vulvar itching and burning. Assessment for these signs and symptoms is an important nursing responsibility.

■ Nursing Diagnoses

Nursing diagnoses for the female patient with cancer of the reproductive system may include, but are not limited to, the following:

- Anxiety *related to* threat of a malignancy and lack of knowledge about the disease process and prognosis
- Pain *related to* pressure secondary to enlarging tumor
- Body image disturbance *related to* loss of body part and loss of good health
- Altered sexuality patterns *related to* physiologic alterations and fatigue
- Ineffective breathing pattern *related to* presence of ascites and effusions
- Anticipatory grieving *related to* poor prognosis of advanced disease

■ Planning

The overall goals are that the patient with a malignant tumor will (1) actively participate in treatment decisions, (2) achieve satisfactory pain and symptom management, (3) recognize and report problems promptly, (4) maintain preferred lifestyle as long as possible, and (5) continue to practice cancer detection strategies.

■ Nursing Implementation

Health Promotion. Through their contact with women in a variety of settings, nurses can teach women the importance of routine screening for cancers of the reproductive system. Cancer can be prevented from ever occurring when screening can reveal precancerous conditions of the vulva, cervix, or endometrium. Also, routine screening increases the chance that a cancer will be identified in its early stage. When cancer is identified earlier, treatment can be more conservative and the woman's prognosis is better. A yearly pelvic examination and Pap test allows the health care provider to detect lesions on the vulva or any uterine or ovarian irregularities and screen for cervical cancer. Nurses can assist women to view routine cancer screening as an important self-care activity.

Educating women about risk factors for cancers of the reproductive system is also very important. Limiting sexual activity during adolescence, using condoms, having fewer sexual partners, and not smoking reduce the risk of cervical cancer.[22] A high-fat diet increases risk for ovarian cancer. Therefore, when high risk behaviors are identified, nurses should assist women with behavior change.

Acute Intervention with Surgery. All patients experience a degree of anxiety when surgery is contemplated, but the prospect of major gynecologic surgery may heighten these concerns. Some women may fear a loss of femininity and worry about possible changes in their secondary sex characteristics. Others may experience feelings of guilt, anger, or embarrassment. Still others may focus on the effect the surgery will have on their reproductive and sexual functions. There are also women who view the whole process as annoying or who are relieved by the thought of no longer having to worry about having menstrual periods or becoming pregnant. Each patient must be understood in light of her fears and concerns and must be approached and evaluated individually. The nurse who exhibits interest and a willingness to listen can provide considerable psychologic support.

Hysterectomy. Preoperatively, the patient is prepared physically for surgery with the standard perineal or abdominal preparation. A vaginal douche and enemas may be given, according to the preference of the surgeon. The bladder should be emptied before the patient is sent to the operating room. An indwelling catheter is often inserted preoperatively.

After surgery the patient who has had a hysterectomy will have an abdominal dressing (abdominal hysterectomy) or a sterile perineal pad (vaginal hysterectomy). (See NCP 51-2 for care of the patient after a total abdominal hysterectomy.) The dressing should be observed frequently for any sign of bleeding during the first 8 hours after surgery. A moderate amount of serosanguineous drainage on the perineal pad is expected following a vaginal hysterectomy.

The patient may experience urinary retention postoperatively because of temporary bladder atony resulting from edema or nerve trauma. This problem is more acute when a radical hysterectomy has been performed. At times an indwelling catheter is used for 1 to 2 days postoperatively to maintain constant drainage of the bladder and prevent strain on the suture line. If an indwelling catheter is not used, catheterization may be necessary if the patient has not urinated for 8 hours postoperatively. If residual urine is suspected after the removal of an indwelling catheter, catheterization is done to prevent bladder infection caused by pooling of urine. Accidental ligation of a ureter is a serious surgical complication. Any complaint of backache or decreased urine output should be reported to the surgeon.

Abdominal distention may develop from the sudden release of pressure on the intestines when a large tumor is removed or from paralytic ileus secondary to anesthesia and pressure on the bowel. Food and fluids may be restricted if the patient is nauseated. A rectal tube may be prescribed to relieve abdominal flatus, and ambulation is encouraged. A Fleet enema or suppository is frequently given on the third postoperative day.

Special care must be taken to prevent the development of thrombophlebitis of the veins in the pelvis or legs. Frequent changes of position and the avoidance of high Fowler's position and pressure under the knees minimize stasis and pooling of blood. Special attention must be given to patients with varicosities. Leg exercises to promote circulation and the use of elastic gradient compression stockings or elastic bandages can be helpful.

The loss of the uterus may bring about grief responses similar to any great personal loss. The ability to bear children is central to society's image of being a female. Although not experienced by all women, grief over this loss is normal. Eliciting the woman's feelings and concerns about her surgery, will provide the needed information to give understanding care. When surgery removes the ovaries as well, women experience surgical menopause. Estrogen is no longer available from the ovaries, so symptoms of estrogen deficiency will arise. To counter this, hormone therapy may be initiated in the early postoperative period.

Discharge teaching should prepare the patient for what to expect following surgery (e.g., she will not menstruate). Teaching should include specific activity restrictions. Intercourse should be avoided until the wound is healed (about 4 to 6 weeks). However, intercourse is not contraindicated once healing is complete. Sutures at the top of the vagina can tear and produce considerable bleeding if genital sex is engaged in too early or too vigorously. Secondary sex characteristics are not affected unless the ovaries have been removed. If a vaginal hysterectomy is performed, the woman needs to know that there may be a temporary loss of vaginal sensation. She should be reassured that sensation will return in several months.

Physical restrictions are limited for a short time. Heavy lifting should be avoided for 2 months. Activities that may increase pelvic congestion, such as dancing and walking swiftly, should be avoided for several months, whereas activities such as swimming may be both physically and mentally helpful. Wearing a girdle is allowed and may provide comfort. Once the patient has been assured that healing is complete, all previous activity can be resumed.

Salpingectomy and oophorectomy. Postoperative care of the woman who has undergone removal of a fallopian tube (*salpingectomy*) or an ovary (*oophorectomy*) is similar to that for any patient having abdominal surgery. One exception is that if a large ovarian cyst is removed, there may be abdominal distention caused by the sudden release of pressure on the intestines. An abdominal binder may provide relief until the distention subsides.

When both ovaries are removed (bilateral oophorectomy), surgical menopause results. The symptoms are similar to those of regular menopause but may be more severe because of the sudden withdrawal of hormones. Attempts may be made to leave at least a portion of an ovary. Replacement therapy with estrogen is given to most patients to avoid symptoms of menopause and to prevent bone loss and the development of osteoporosis.

Vulvectomy. Although cancer of the vulva is relatively uncommon, it is important that the nurse recognize the extent of the vulvectomy and the significant effect it is likely to have on the patient's life. An honest, open attitude with the patient and her partner preoperatively can be most helpful in the postoperative period.

After a vulvectomy, the patient returns to the unit with a wound in the perineal area extending to the groin. The wounds may be covered or left exposed and frequently have drains attached to portable suction (e.g., Hemovac). A heavy pressure dressing is often in place for the first 24 to 48 hours. The wounds are cleaned with normal saline solution or an antiseptic twice daily. Solutions can be applied with an aseptic bulb syringe or a WaterPik machine. A heat lamp or a hair dryer is then used to dry the area. Wound care must be meticulous to prevent infection, which results in delayed healing.

Special attention to bowel and bladder care is needed. A low-residue diet and fecal softeners prevent straining at stool and wound contamination. An indwelling catheter is used to provide urinary drainage. Great care is taken not to dislodge the catheter because the extensive edema in the area would make its reinsertion difficult. Heavy, taut sutures are often used to close the wounds, resulting in severe discomfort for the patient. In other instances the wound may be allowed to heal by granulation. Analgesics may be required frequently to control pain. Careful positioning of the patient through the use of strategically placed pillows provides comfort. Ambulation is usually begun on the second postoperative day, but this varies with the preference of the surgeon. Anticoagulant therapy to prevent vascular complications is common.

Because the surgery causes mutilation of the perineal area and the healing process is slow, the patient is likely to become discouraged. Opportunities for the patient to express her feelings and concerns about the operation should be provided. The patient needs specific instructions in self-care before she is discharged. She should be told to report any unusual odor, fresh bleeding, breakdown of incision, or perineal pain. Home care nursing can benefit the patient during her adjustment period. Sexual function is often retained. Whether clitoral sensation is retained may be critical to some women, particularly if it was a primary source of orgasmic satisfaction. A discussion of alternative methods of achieving sexual satisfaction may also be indicated.

Pelvic exenteration. When other forms of therapy are ineffective in checking the spread of cancer and no metastases have been found outside of the pelvis, pelvic exenteration may be performed. Although different types are done, this radical surgery usually involves removal of the uterus, ovaries, fallopian tubes, vagina, bladder, urethra, and pelvic lymph nodes (Fig. 51-10). In some situations, the descending colon, rectum, and anal canal may also be removed. Candidates for this procedure are selected on the basis of their likelihood of surviving the surgery and their ability to adjust to and accept the resulting limitations.

The postoperative care involves that of a patient who has had a radical hysterectomy, an abdominal perineal resection, an ileostomy or colostomy, a cystectomy, and urinary diversion surgery. The physical, emotional, and social adjustments to life on the part of the woman and her family are great. There are urinary or fecal diversions in the abdominal wall, a reconstructed vagina, and the onset of menopausal symptoms.

The patient's rehabilitative process should keep pace with her acceptance of the situation. Much understanding and support is needed from the nursing staff during a long hospital stay. The patient should be gently encouraged to regain her independence. She needs to verbalize her feelings about her altered body structure to an interested and concerned listener. Inclusion of the family in the plan of care is important.

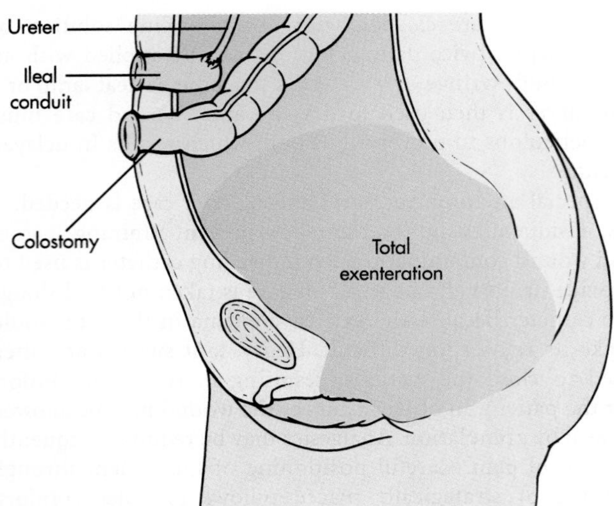

Fig. 51-10 Total exenteration is removal of all pelvic organs with creation of an ileal conduit and colostomy.

The patient needs to return to her physician at specified intervals. Early recurrence of the cancer may then be identified and treated. At this time the patient's physical and emotional adjustment to the changes in body image produced by the surgery and her ability to carry out any treatment measures can also be assessed. Additional teaching and counseling can then be provided.

Acute Intervention with Radiation Therapy. Nursing management of a patient receiving internal radiation therapy requires special considerations. The nurse should not stay in the immediate area any longer than is necessary to give proper care and attention. No individual nurse should attend the patient for more than 30 minutes per day. The nurse should stay at the foot of the bed or at the entrance to the room to minimize radiation exposure. Visitors should be told to stay 6 feet away from the bed and limit visits to less than 3 hours a day. Efficient organization of nursing care is essential so the nurse does not stay in the immediate area of the patient any longer than is necessary. The reasons for these precautions should be explained fully to the patient and her visitors. (A more detailed discussion of nursing care of the patient with an internal implant is given in Chapter 14.)

When the patient is to receive external radiation, she should be told to urinate immediately before the treatment to minimize radiation exposure to the bladder. She should be advised about the radiation side effects, including enteritis and cystitis, that may occur. These are natural reactions to radiotherapy and do not indicate an overdose. The patient should be fully informed of the possible side effects and measures to use to reduce their impact.

■ Evaluation

The expected outcomes are that the patient with a malignant tumor of the reproductive system will

- actively participate in treatment decisions
- achieve satisfactory pain and symptom management
- recognize and report problems promptly
- maintain preferred lifestyle as long as possible
- continue to practice cancer detection strategies

PROBLEMS WITH PELVIC SUPPORT

The most common occurring problems with pelvic support are uterine prolapse, cystocele, and rectocele. Vaginal birth increases the risk for these problems, but women without any children can also have them. Obesity, chronic coughing, and straining during bowel movements can increase the likelihood of these problems. The decreased estrogen that normally accompanies the perimenopause also reduces some connective tissue support.

Uterine Prolapse

Uterine prolapse is the downward displacement of the uterus into the vaginal canal (Fig. 51-11). Prolapse is rated by degrees. In first-degree prolapse, the cervix rests in the lower part of the vagina. Second-degree prolapse means the cervix is at the vaginal opening. A third-degree prolapse means the uterus protrudes through the introitus. Symptoms vary with the degree of prolapse. The patient may describe a feeling of "something coming down." She may have dyspareunia, a dragging or heavy feeling in the pelvis, backache, and bowel or bladder problems if cystocele or rectocele are also present. Stress incontinence is a common and troubling problem. When third-degree uterine prolapse occurs, the protruding cervix and vaginal walls are subjected to constant irritation, and tissue changes may occur.

Therapy depends on the degree of prolapse and how much the woman's daily activities have been affected. Pelvic muscle strengthening exercises (Kegel exercises) may be effective for some women. If not, a pessary may be used. A *pessary* is a devise that is placed in the vagina to help to support the uterus. A wide variety of shapes exist including rings, arches, and balls. Most are made of plastic or wire coated with plastic. When a woman first receives a pessary, she also needs instructions for its cleaning and follow-up. Pessaries that are left in place for long periods are associated with erosion, fistulas, and an increased incidence of vaginal carcinoma. If more conservative measures are not successful, surgery is indicated. Surgery generally involves a vaginal hysterectomy with anterior and posterior repair of the vagina and underlying fascia.

Cystocele and Rectocele

Cystocele occurs when support between the vagina and bladder is weakened (Fig. 51-12). Similarly, a *rectocele* results from weakening between the vagina and rectum. These problems are common and asymptomatic in many women. With large cystoceles, complete emptying of the bladder can be difficult, predisposing women to bladder infections. A woman with a large rectocele may not be able to completely empty her rectum when defecating unless she helps to push the stool out by putting her fingers in her vagina.

As with uterine prolapse, Kegel exercises may be used to strengthen the weakened perineal muscles if the cystocele or rectocele is not too problematic. A pessary may be helpful for cystoceles. Surgery designed to tighten the vaginal wall is generally the method of treatment. A cystocele is corrected with a

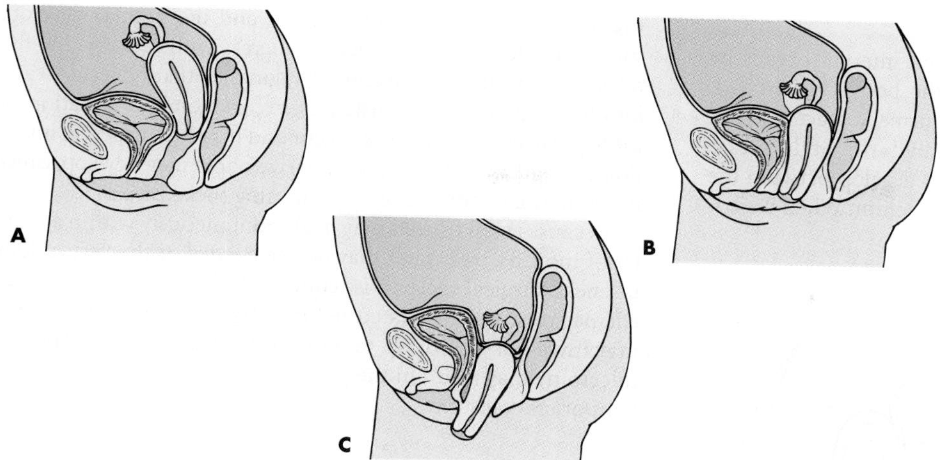

Fig. 51-11 Uterine prolapse. **A,** First-degree prolapse. **B,** Second-degree prolapse. **C,** Third-degree prolapse.

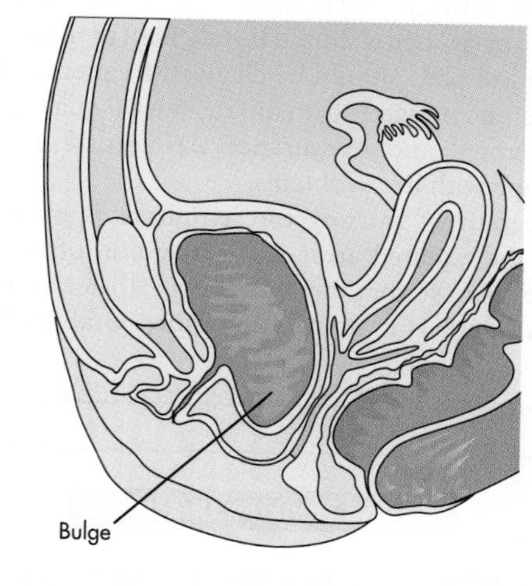

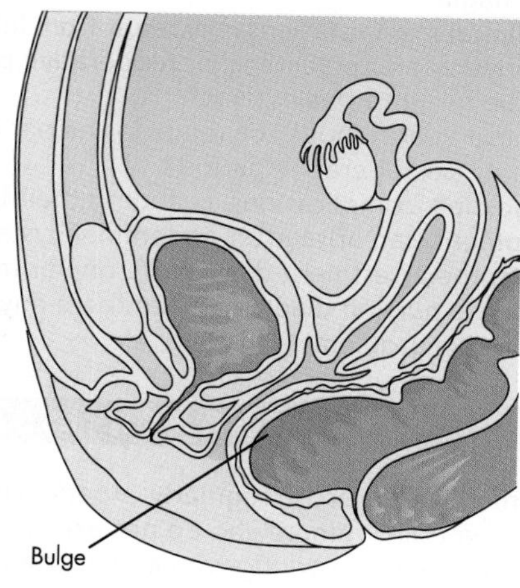

Fig. 51-12 **A,** Cystocele. **B,** Rectocele.

procedure called an anterior colporrhaphy, whereas a posterior colporrhaphy is done for a rectocele. If further surgery is needed to relieve stress incontinence, procedures to support the urethra and restore the proper angle between the urethra and the posterior bladder wall are used.

NURSING MANAGEMENT: PROBLEMS WITH PELVIC SUPPORT

Nurses can assist women to avoid or decrease problems with pelvic support by teaching them how to do Kegel exercises to strengthen their pelvic floor muscles. Women of all ages can benefit from these exercises. However, Kegel exercises are especially important following childbirth or whenever women begin to have incontinence. To instruct a patient in this exercise, she should be told to pull in or contract her muscles as if she were trying to stop the flow of urine. She should hold the contraction for several seconds and then relax. Sets of 5 to 10 contractions each should be done several times daily.

If vaginal surgery is necessary, the preoperative preparation usually includes a cleansing douche the morning of surgery. A cathartic and a cleansing enema are usually given when a rectocele repair is scheduled. A perineal shave is done.

In the postoperative period, the goals of care are to prevent wound infection and pressure on the vaginal suture line. This necessitates perineal care at least twice a day and after each urination or defecation. An ice pack applied locally may relieve the initial perineal discomfort and swelling. A disposable glove filled with ice and covered with a cloth works well in these instances. Later, sitz baths may be used. A heat lamp may be used to help dry the area and enhance the healing process.

After an anterior colporrhaphy, an indwelling catheter is usually left in the bladder for 4 days to allow the local edema to subside. The catheter keeps the bladder empty, thereby preventing strain on the sutures. Catheter care with an antiseptic is generally done twice daily. After posterior colporrhaphy, straining at stool is avoided by means of a low-residue diet and the prevention of constipation. A stool softener is usually given each night.

Discharge instructions should be reviewed before the patient leaves the hospital. They include the use of douches or mild laxatives as needed; restriction of heavy lifting and prolonged standing, walking, or sitting; and avoidance of intercourse until the physician gives permission. There may be a loss of vaginal sensation, which can last for several months. The patient needs to be reassured that this situation is temporary.

FISTULAS

A *fistula* is an abnormal opening between internal organs or between an organ and the exterior of the body (Fig. 51-13). Gynecologic procedures cause 75% of urinary tract fistulas. Other causes include injury during childbirth and disease processes such as carcinoma. Fistulas may develop between the vagina and the bladder, urethra, ureter, or rectum. When vesicovaginal fistulas (between the bladder and the vagina) develop, some urine leaks into the vagina, whereas with rectovaginal fistulas (between the rectum and the vagina), flatus and feces escape into the vagina. In both instances, excoriation and irritation of the vaginal and vulvar tissues occur and may lead to severe infections. In addition to wetness, offensive odors may develop, causing embarrassment and severely limiting socialization.

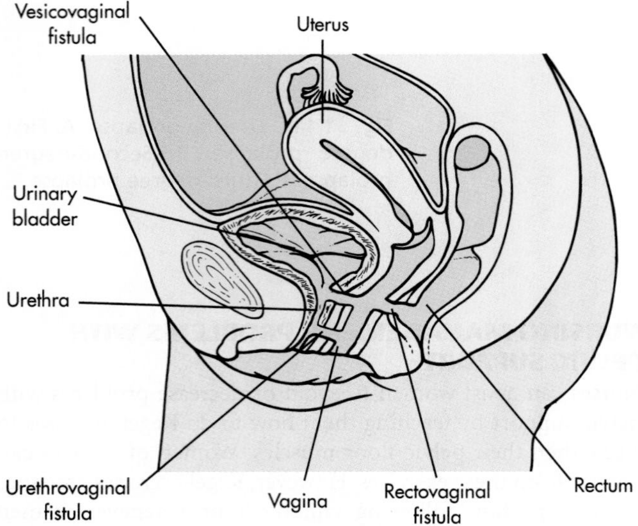

Fig. 51-13 Common fistulas involving the vagina.

Because small fistulas may heal spontaneously within a matter of months, treatment may not be needed. If the fistula does not heal, surgical excision is required. Inflammation and tissue edema must be eliminated before surgery is attempted. This may involve a wait of up to 6 months for the surgery. The fistulectomy may result in the patient's having an ileal conduit or temporary colostomy.

NURSING MANAGEMENT: FISTULAS

Perineal hygiene is of great importance, both preoperatively and postoperatively. The perineum should be cleansed every 4 hours. Warm sitz baths should be taken three times daily if possible. Perineal pads should be changed frequently. The patient should be encouraged to maintain an adequate fluid intake. Encouragement and reassurance are needed in helping the patient cope with her problems.

Postoperatively, nursing care emphasis is on avoidance of stress on the repaired areas and prevention of infection. Care should be taken so that the indwelling catheter, usually in place for 7 to 10 days, is draining at all times. Oral fluids should be

CRITICAL THINKING EXERCISES

CASE STUDY

Total Abdominal Hysterectomy

Patient Profile

Marion P., a 40-year-old woman with two children, consulted her health care provider about experiencing menorrhagia and occasionally metrorrhagia for the past 5 months. She was diagnosed with leiomyomas, and a total abdominal hysterectomy was recommended.

Subjective Data

- Was initially reluctant about surgery
- States family is complete
- Concerned that she may actually have uterine cancer

Objective Data

Physical Examination

- Has several large, firm masses thought to be leiomyomas in body of uterus
- Had otherwise normal physical examination

Postoperative Status

- Returned to room with indwelling urinary catheter in place
- Legs wrapped in full-length elastic compression gradient stockings

Critical Thinking Questions

1. What are the common causes of menorrhagia and metrorrhagia?
2. What clinical manifestations may result from leiomyomas?
3. What physical and psychologic preoperative preparation should be given to this patient?
4. What observation should be made in the patient's immediate postoperative period?
5. What possible complications, including their basis for development, can arise after abdominal hysterectomy?
6. Based on the assessment data, write one or more appropriate nursing diagnoses. Are there any collaborative problems?

NURSING RESEARCH ISSUES

1. Do women who exercise regularly experience less dysmenorrhea than women who do not exercise regularly?
2. Do working or nonworking women experience more episodes of vasomotor instability during the perimenopausal period?
3. Are women who use a female condom satisfied with this form of birth control?
4. Does the emotional response of the nurse caring for a rape victim help or hinder effective intervention?
5. What parameters can a nurse use in deciding how much information to provide to a woman who is to have a pelvic exenteration?

urged to provide for internal catheter irrigation. Minimal pressure and strict asepsis are used if catheter irrigation becomes necessary. The first stool after bowel surgery may be purposely delayed to prevent contamination of the wound. Later, stool softeners or mild laxatives may be given. See Chapter 43 for care of a patient with an ileal conduit and Chapter 40 for care of a patient with a colostomy. Surgical repair of fistulas is not always effective, even in the best conditions. Therefore supportive nursing care for the patient and her significant others is especially important.

REVIEW QUESTIONS

The number of the question corresponds to the same-numbered objective at the beginning of the chapter.

1. In assisting a sexually active woman to choose a birth control method, the nurse advises the patient that taking oral contraceptives may cause
   a. later infertility.
   b. infection of the uterus.
   c. toxic shock syndrome.
   d. thromboembolic disorders.
2. In telling a patient with infertility what she and her partner can expect, the nurse explains that
   a. the cause should be diagnosed by the second visit.
   b. an hysterosalpingogram is a common diagnostic study.
   c. if postcoital studies are normal, infection tests will be done.
   d. the reason will remain unexplained for 50% of couples.
3. A patient with a spontaneous abortion is more likely than the patient with an induced abortion to have
   a. a D&C performed.
   b. feelings of loss and grief.
   c. emotional support from family and friends.
   d. physical complications such as infection.
4. An appropriate question to ask the patient with painful menstruation to differentiate primary dysmenorrhea from secondary dysmenorrhea is
   a. "Does your pain become worse with activity or overexertion?"
   b. "Have you had a recent personal crisis or change in your lifestyle?"
   c. "Is your pain relieved by nonsteroidal antiinflammatory medications?"
   d. "When in your menstrual history did the pain with your period begin?"
5. In caring for a patient after an ectopic pregnancy was surgically removed, the nurse advises the patient that
   a. most ectopic pregnancies attach to the ovary.
   b. she will not be able to get pregnant in the future.
   c. bed rest must be maintained for 24 hours to assist healing.
   d. having one ectopic pregnancy increases her risk for another.
6. To prevent or decrease age-related pathology that occurs after menopause in a patient who chooses not to take hormone therapy, the nurse teaches the patient that the most important self-care measure is
   a. maintaining usual sexual activity.
   b. increasing the intake of dietary calcium.
   c. performing regular aerobic, weight-bearing exercise.
   d. taking vitamin E and vitamin B-complex supplements.
7. The first nursing intervention for the patient who has been raped is to
   a. treat urgent medical problems.
   b. contact a support person for the patient.
   c. provide supplies for the patient to cleanse self.
   d. document bruises and lacerations of the perineum and cervix.
8. The patient's history indicating thick, white, curdlike vaginal discharge and vulvar pruritus is most consistent with
   a. bacterial vaginosis.
   b. chlamydial cervicitis.
   c. monilial vaginitis.
   d. trichomoniasis.
9. The nurse caring for a patient with pelvic inflammatory disease places her in semi-Fowler's position. The rationale for this measure is to
   a. relieve pain.
   b. prevent the complication of sterility.
   c. improve circulation and promote healing.
   d. promote drainage to prevent abscesses.
10. In planning care for the patient receiving medical management of endometriosis, the nurse includes teaching regarding the side effects of
    a. estrogen supplementation.
    b. large doses of vitamins A and E.
    c. hormonal suppression of ovulation.
    d. long-term use of NSAIDs.
11. A 31-year-old woman who wishes to have children is diagnosed with leiomyoma. The nurse plans care for the patient based on the knowledge that
    a. a hysterectomy will be necessary to treat the tumor.
    b. a myomectomy may be performed to maintain fertility.
    c. hormonal therapy to shrink the tumor and increase fertility can be used.
    d. aspirin and other NSAIDs used to control pain may cause fetal defects.
12. A 52-year-old woman who has not had a menstrual period for 18 months tells the nurse she has recently had some spotting. The nurse advises the patient that
    a. she should keep a menstrual calendar for the next 6 months.
    b. this problem should be further investigated by an endometrial biopsy.
    c. this is a common, but not serious, problem that can occur after menopause.
    d. warm douching is recommended to promote healing of fragile vaginal tissue.
13. The nurse plans early and frequent ambulation for the patient who has undergone an abdominal hysterectomy in order to
    a. prevent urinary retention.
    b. promote pelvic circulation.
    c. relieve abdominal distention.
    d. maintain a sense of normalcy.
14. Nursing responsibilities related to the patient receiving internal radiation for uterine cancer include
    a. maintaining absolute bed rest.
    b. allowing the patient bathroom privileges only.
    c. limiting an individual nurse's contact with the patient to 1 hour per day.
    d. allowing visitors to stay as long as desired if they stay 6 feet (2 meters) from the bed.
15. When instructing a woman how to do Kegel exercises, the nurse should advise her
    a. to tighten abdominal muscles and hold her breath.
    b. to tilt the pelvis forward keeping her back as straight as possible.
    c. to bear down like having a bowel movement and hold her breath.
    d. to tighten her perineal muscles as if trying to stop the flow of urine.

References

1. Hatcher RA and others: *Contraceptive technology,* ed 16, New York, 1994, Irvington.
2. Grimes DA: *Contraception Report* 9:4, 1998.
3. DeCherney A: Bone sparing properties of oral contraceptives, *Am J Obstet Gynecol* 174:15, 1996.
4. MacKay H, Trent MD: Gynecology. In Lawrence M: *Current medical diagnosis and treatment,* ed 37, Stamford, Conn, 1998, Appleton & Lange.
5. Kaunitz AM: Long-acting injectable contraception with depot medroxyprogesterone acetate, *Am J Obstet Gynecol* 170:1543, 1994.
6. Stewart F: Promoting emergency contraception, *Hosp Pract* 33:61, 1998.
7. Davis LE, Stockton MD: Office procedures: No scalpel vasectomy, *Prim Care* 24:433, 1997.
8. Holt BA, Higgins AF: Minimally invasive vasectomy, *Br J Urol* 77:585, 1996.
9. Carlson KJ, Eisenstat SA, editors: *Primary care of women,* St Louis, 1995, Mosby.
10. Schroeder CJ, Krysa LW: The comfort and discomfort of infertility, *JOGNN* 25:167, 1996.
11. Johnson CA and others: *Women's health care handbook,* Philadelphia, 1996, Hanley & Belfus/Mosby.
12. Speroff L, Glass RH, Kase NG: *Clinical gynecologic endocrinology and infertility,* ed 5, Baltimore, 1994, Williams & Wilkins.
13. Youngkin EQ, Davis MS: *Women's health,* ed 2, Stamford, Conn, 1998, Appleton & Lange.
14. Freeman EW and others: PMS: new treatments that really work, *Contemp OB/GYN* 41:25, 1996.
15. Leppart PC, Howard FM: *Primary care of women,* Philadelphia, 1997, Lippincott-Raven.
16. Rosenfeld JA: *Women's health in primary care,* Baltimore, 1997, Williams & Wilkins.
17. LeBoeuf, FJ, Carter SG: Discomforts of the perimenopause, *JOGNN* 25:173, 1996.
18. Gelfand MM: Women and androgen—HRT, *Women's Health Digest* 3:236, 1997.
19. Paganini-Hill A, Henderson VW: Estrogen replacement therapy and risk of Alzheimer's disease, *Arch Intern Med* 156:221, 1996.
20. Taylor M: Alternatives to conventional hormone replacement therapy, *Complement Ther* 23:514, 1997.
21. Center for Disease Control and Prevention: 1998 Guidelines for treatment of sexually transmitted diseases, *MMWR* 47, 1998.
22. Moore GJ: *Women and cancer,* Boston, 1997, Jones & Bartlett.
23. Schwartz PE: Prophylactic oophorectomy for the prevention of epithelial ovarian cancer revisited, *Eur Menopause J* 4:105, 1997.
24. Reisner JG, Miollis M: Laparoscopically assisted vaginal hysterectomy in a community hospital, *J Reprod Med* 42:542, 1997.
25. Riza ED: Laparoscopically assisted vaginal hysterectomy: report of 190 cases, *J Laparoendosc Adv Surg Techniques* 7:13, 1997.

Resources

Association of Women's Health, Obstetric, & Neonatal Nurses (AWHONN)
2000 L Street, Suite 740
Washington, D.C. 20036
800-673-8499 (U.S.)
800-245-0231 (Canada)
Fax: 202-737-0575
http://www.awhonn.org/

National Center for Education in Maternal and Child Health
2000 15th Street, North, Suite 701
Arlington, VA 22201-2617
703-524-7802
Fax: 703-524-9335
http://www.ncemch.georgetown.edu/

For additional Internet resources, see the website for this book at www.mosby.com/MERLIN/medsurg_lewis

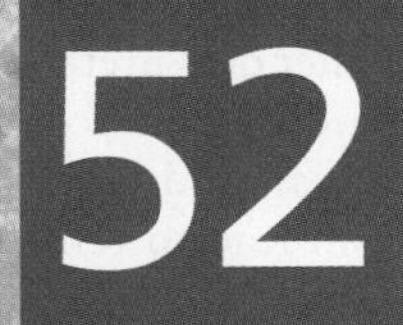

REMEMBER to check out your **companion CD-ROM**

52 NURSING MANAGEMENT Male Genitourinary Problems

Cindy Meredith

www.mosby.com/MERLIN/medsurg_lewis

LEARNING OBJECTIVES

1. Describe the pathophysiology, clinical features, diagnostic studies, and collaborative care of benign prostatic hyperplasia.
2. Describe the nursing management of benign prostatic hyperplasia.
3. Describe the pathophysiology, clinical features, diagnostic studies, and collaborative care of cancer of the prostate.
4. Describe the nursing management of prostate cancer.
5. Describe the pathophysiology, clinical features, diagnostic studies, and collaborative and nursing management of problems of the penis, problems of the scrotum, and prostatitis.
6. Explain the nursing management of problems related to male sexual functioning.
7. Identify the psychologic and emotional implications of problems related to the male genitourinary organs.

Problems of the male genitourinary system can involve a variety of structures (Fig. 52-1) and create anxiety for both the patient and nurse providing care. Anxiety and fear may also cause the patient to delay seeking help for a problem or practicing health-promoting behaviors. Our society often does not encourage men to admit to or seek help for problems related to their sex organs. The nurse should be particularly sensitive to the possible embarrassment associated with a male genitourinary problem.

PROBLEMS OF THE PROSTATE GLAND

BENIGN PROSTATIC HYPERPLASIA

The most common problem of the adult male genitourinary system is *benign prostatic hyperplasia* (BPH), a term referring to an increase in the number of epithelial and especially stromal tissue within the prostate gland. The problem occurs in about 50% of men over 50 years of age and 75% of men over 70 years of age. BPH is most likely to develop in the innermost part of the prostate,[1] and cancer is most likely to develop in the outer part of the prostate gland (Fig. 52-2).[2] Prostatic hyperplasia does not predispose to the development of cancer of the prostate.

Etiology and Pathophysiology

BPH begins with enlargement of the glandular tissue. Although the cause is not completely understood, it is thought that the primary cause is an increased number of cells resulting from endocrine changes associated with the aging process. Excessive accumulation of dihydroxytestosterone (the principal intraprostatic androgen), stimulation of estrogen, and local growth hormone action are proposed causes.

Clinical Manifestations

The patient seeks assistance for relief of the symptoms related to urinary obstruction. Symptoms are usually gradual in onset and may not be noticed until prostatic enlargement has been present for some time. There is no direct relationship between the degree of obstruction and the size of the prostate. Mild hyperplasia can cause severe obstruction, whereas severe hyperplasia can result in few bladder symptoms. It is often the location of the enlargement rather than the size that causes the symptoms. Treatment is generally based on the degree to which the symptoms bother the patient rather than on the size of the prostate alone.

Early symptoms are usually minimal because the bladder can compensate for a small amount of resistance to urine flow.[3] With increasing blockage, obstructive symptoms of BPH develop. Symptoms include a decrease in the caliber and force of the urinary stream, hesitancy in initiating voiding, dribbling at the end of urination, and a feeling of incomplete bladder emptying because of urinary retention. Irritative symptoms include nocturia and urgency, which can develop from inflammatory, infectious, or neoplastic causes.

Self-assessment such as the one developed by the American Urological Association (AUA) (Table 52-1) and quality-of-life questionnaires have been developed to facilitate assessment of the symptom burden. Such tools are also used to facilitate decisions regarding treatment options.

Reviewed by Donna Berry, PhD, RN, AOCN, Research Assistant Professor, University of Washington, School of Nursing, Seattle, Wash.

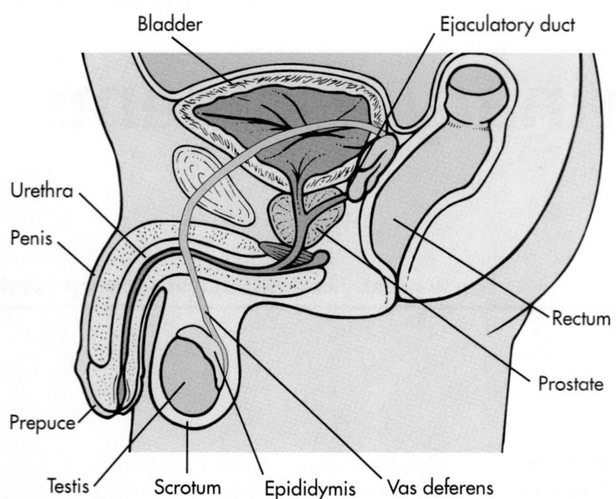

Fig. 52-1 Areas of the male reproductive system in which problems are likely to develop.

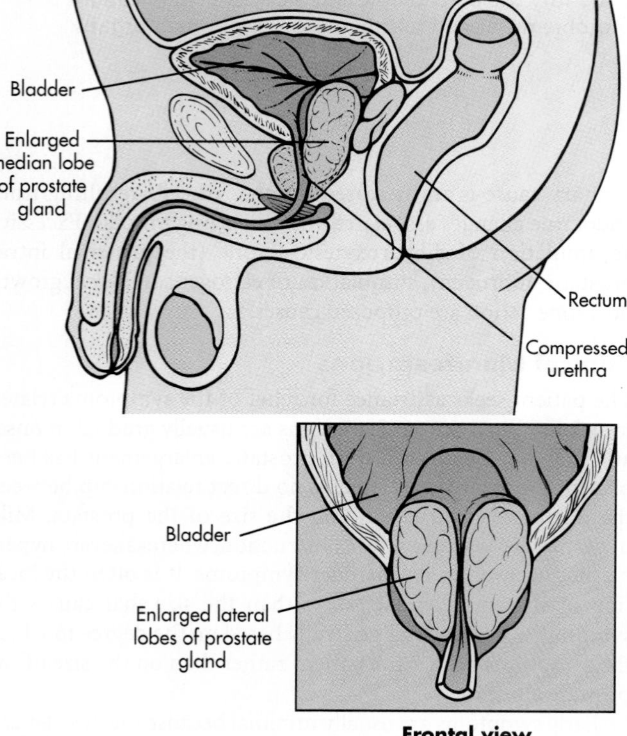

Fig. 52-2 Benign prostatic hyperplasia.

Complications

The patient with BPH is at increased risk for urinary tract infection. The bladder does not empty completely because of partial or complete obstruction of the proximal urethra. The residual urine provides a favorable environment for bacterial growth. Calculi may develop because of the alkalinization of the residual urine. Breakage of tiny overstretched blood vessels in the bladder may produce hematuria. Increased pressure in the bladder can cause wall thickening and the formation of diverticula.

More serious complications resulting from urinary retention are bladder dysfunction, abnormally distended ureters (hydroureters), destruction of the kidney's parenchyma from the back pressure of the urine (hydronephrosis), and infection (pyelonephritis). These complications can lead to renal failure.

Diagnostic Studies

The primary diagnostic test for BPH is a digital rectal examination (DRE) to palpate for enlargement and assess whether the gland is hard, nodular, or "boggy." In the early stages of BPH, the specific gravity of the urine may be unchanged or elevated because the patient may restrict fluid intake to decrease the need to void. If hydronephrosis with renal impairment has occurred, the specific gravity will be about 1.010, which is the specific gravity of plasma. The presence of bacteria, white blood cells, or microscopic hematuria found on urinalysis may indicate the presence of infection or inflammation. If BPH has been a long-standing problem, the blood urea nitrogen (BUN) and serum creatinine levels may be elevated because of renal involvement. The prostate-specific antigen (PSA) blood level is examined as a potential indicator of prostatic cancer.

Secondary diagnostic screening may include a transrectal ultrasound (TRUS) scan of the prostate, urodynamic flow studies, and cystoscopy. A TRUS scan is useful in locating specific areas of enlargement or tumors. A biopsy can be taken during the ultrasound procedure. Locating and possible staging of cancer growths provide important information in deciding whether surgery or another treatment option should be the first approach to care.

Urine flow studies are helpful in determining the extent of obstruction. Measuring the urinary flow rate helps gauge the extent of blockage and aid in determining the type of treatment needed. Cystourethroscopy may be done to evaluate bladder neck obstruction in patients scheduled for surgery. Diagnostic studies are outlined in Table 52-2.

Collaborative Care

The goal of collaborative management is to restore bladder drainage, relieve the patient's symptoms, and prevent or treat the complications of BPH.

Conservative Therapy

The primary treatment for BPH is now referred to as "watchful waiting." When there are no symptoms or only mild ones, a conservative, noninvasive wait-and-see approach is taken. If the patient begins to have signs or symptoms that indicate an increase in uretheral obstruction, further treatment is indicated. The numerous treatment options for BPH can be categorized as pharmacologic, nonsurgical invasive, and surgical invasive options.[4,5]

Drug Therapy. Hormone manipulation can be used to cause regression of hyperplastic tissue through suppression of androgens. Finasteride (Proscar) blocks the enzyme 5-α-reductase, which is necessary for the conversion of testosterone to dihydroxytestosterone, the principal intraprostatic androgen. Studies have shown a decrease in prostate size and an increase in urine flow. This medication must be taken on a continuous

Table 52-1 **American Urological Association Symptom Index to Determine Severity of Prostatic Problems**

Questions to Be Answered	American Urological Association (AUA) Symptom Score* (Circle 1 number on each line)					
	Not At All	Less Than 1 Time in 5	Less Than Half the Time	About Half the Time	More Than Half the Time	Almost Always
Over the past month,						
1. How often have you had a sensation of not emptying your bladder completely after you finished urinating?	0	1	2	3	4	5
2. How often have you had to urinate again, less than 2 hr after you finished urinating?	0	1	2	3	4	5
3. How often have you found you stopped and started again several times when you urinated?	0	1	2	3	4	5
4. How often have you found it difficult to postpone urination?	0	1	2	3	4	5
5. How often have you had a weak urinary stream?	0	1	2	3	4	5
6. How often have you had to push or strain to begin urination?	0	1	2	3	4	5
7. How many times did you most typically get up to urinate from the time you went to bed at night until the time you got up in the morning?	0 (None)	1 (1 Time)	2 (2 times)	3 (3 times)	4 (4 times)	5 (5 times or more)
Sum of circled numbers (AUA Symptom Score):*						

From Barry B and others: The American Urological Association symptom index for benign prostatic hyperplasia, *J Urol* 148:1547, 1992. Used with permission.
*Score is interpreted as: 0-7, mild; 8-19, moderate; and 20-35, severe.

COLLABORATIVE CARE

Table 52-2 **Benign Prostatic Hyperplasia**

Diagnostic

Primary Screening
- History including symptoms of voiding problems
- Physical examination including digital rectal exam (DRE)
- Urinalysis with culture
- Serum creatinine and BUN
- Prostate-specific antigen (PSA)

Secondary Screening
- Urodynamic flow studies
- Transrectal ultrasound
- Cystoscopy (for surgical candidates)

Collaborative Therapy
- "Watchful waiting" and patient education
- Catheterization (intermittent or indwelling)
- High fluid intake
- Antibiotics
- Finasteride (Proscar) therapy
- Alpha-adrenergic receptor blockers
  - Prazosin (Minipress)
  - Terazosin (Hytrin)
  - Tamsulosin (Flomax)
- Coils and stents
- Balloon dilation
- Thermoregulatory procedures (TUMA)
- Laser ablation
- Transurethral incision of the prostate (TUIP)
- Transurethral resection of the prostate (TURP)
- Open prostatectomy (>60 g)
  - Suprapubic
  - Retropubic
  - Perineal

BUN, blood urea nitrogen.

basis to achieve therapeutic results. The major side effects are erectile dysfunction, which develops in about 10% of patients, and decreased libido.[6]

α-Adrenergic receptor blockade is another drug treatment option in the treatment of BPH. This type of drug causes smooth muscle relaxation in the prostate and the bladder neck. This relaxation ultimately facilitates urinary flow through the prostatic urethra. Several alpha-adrenergic blockers, such as prazosin (Minipress), doxazosin (Cardura), terazosin (Hytrin), and tamsulosin (Flomax), are currently being used. Alpha-adrenergic blockers do not decrease the prostate hyperplasia. Side effects, including postural hypotension, dizziness, and fatigue, can be a problem, especially if the patient is also taking cardiac or antihypertensive medication.

Herbal medicines extracted from plants (phytotherapy) have been used in the management of BPH. In particular, phytotherapy involving plant extracts, such as saw palmetto have been used. Although some data suggest improvement of urinary symptoms based on patient self-report, additional studies are needed.[10]

Nonsurgical Invasive Care

Intermittent catheterization or an indwelling catheter can temporarily be used to reduce symptoms and bypass the obstruction. Long-term catheter use should be avoided because of the increased risk of infection. If BPH becomes symptomatic, other nonsurgical invasive options may be tried before surgery. These outpatient options include stents or coils, prostatic balloon dilation, heat, and experimental approaches such as transuretheral needle ablation (TUNA)[7] or percutaneous radical cryosurgical ablation (PRCSA).

One nonsurgical therapeutic option is the placement of stents (stainless steel) or coils (titanium) in the prostatic urethra. These devices hold back the walls of the prostate to allow for the unobstructed flow of urine. In the majority of cases the stents become covered by epithelium, reducing the risk of

Table 52-3 Treatment Options for Benign Prostatic Hyperplasia

Treatment Options	Advantages	Disadvantages
Nonsurgical Invasive		
▪ Stents and coils	Local anesthesia Minimal hemorrhage Short operative time Usually an outpatient procedure	Short-term incontinence
▪ Balloon dilation	Topical or local anesthesia Simple, short procedure Less expensive Outpatient procedure No impotence or retrograde ejaculation	Later treatment may be necessary Long-term effectiveness not known Tissue sample unavailable for histologic examination
▪ Heat (transurethral microwave antenna [TUMA])	Short procedure No retrograde ejaculation Decrease nocturia	Cell death in normal as well as benign and malignant tissue Potential for urinary retention
Surgical		
▪ Laser ablation (transurethral ultrasound-guided laser-induced prostatectomy [TULIP]; visual laser ablation of the prostate [VLAP])	Short procedure Little bleeding No fluid absorption Decreased incidence of retrograde ejaculation	Postoperative urinary retention Tissue sample unavailable for histologic examination
▪ Transurethral resection of the prostate (TURP)	No external incision Erectile dysfunction and long-term incontinence unlikely	Not all prostatic tissue removed Regular follow-up less likely
▪ Transurethral incision of the prostate (TUIP)	Maintenance of antegrade ejaculation Short operating time Minimal complications	Temporary solution Effective on small glands (< 30 g) Cancer can be missed Possible rectal injury
▪ Suprapubic prostate resection	Better exploration and visualization Choice for larger prostate	Increased risk of urinary tract infection, spasms, incontinence, hemorrhage Recovery longer than TURP Difficult in obese patient
▪ Retropubic prostate resection	Removal of large mass high in pelvic area Direct visualization of prostate possible Bladder not incised Voiding problems are rare	Difficult in obese patient High risk for hemorrhage Slight risk of erectile dysfunction
▪ Perineal prostate resection	Able to remove large mass low in pelvic area and lymph nodes Direct visualization of prostate and surrounding tissue	High risk of erectile dysfunction Possible urinary incontinence Higher risk of infection

encrustation and infection. The procedure is used most often for men who have medical contraindications to surgery because only local anesthesia is required for this procedure. The advantages and disadvantages of the various treatment options are compared in Table 52-3.

Another nonsurgical approach is prostatic balloon dilation, which uses a balloon device to dilate the urethra by stretching, fracturing, or compressing the gland to enlarge the passage and allow for free flow of urine. After dilation the balloon is removed, and the urethra is assessed for an increase in diameter. If the procedure is successful, an indwelling catheter is left in place for the first 24 hours to monitor urinary output and the extent of hematuria. The dilation procedure may be repeated if the first attempt is unsuccessful. The procedure is not a permanent solution to the problem of an enlarged prostate but does offer a nonsurgical, cost-saving option to appropriate patients, particularly those who are surgical risks. The balloon technique is contraindicated in patients with atonic bladder because dilation alone will not allow proper emptying of the bladder.

Microwave therapy involves the use of heat to reduce the prostatic tissue.[8,9] There are two basic types of microwave treatment. Hyperthermia involves either a transurethral or transrectal (rarely used today) heated probe. The transurethral probe raises the temperature in the prostate gland to between 107.6° and 111° F (42° and 44° C). The heat causes an inflammatory reaction but is not hot enough to result in tissue necrosis. After a series (between 3 and 20) of 1-hour treatments the obstruction is generally relieved.

In transurethral microwave thermal therapy (sometimes referred to as transurethral microwave antenna [TUMA] therapy, a one-time treatment), a microwave uretheral probe or catheter heats the prostatic tissue above 113° F (45° C) to produce tissue necrosis. A rectal temperature probe is often used during the procedure to be sure that the rectal temperature is kept below 110° F (43.5° C) to prevent rectal tissue damage. The patient is generally sent home with an indwelling catheter for 2 to 7 days to maintain urinary flow and to facilitate the passing of small clots or necrotic tissue. Prescriptions for an antibiotic, pain medication, and bladder antispasmodic medications are generally sent home with the patient. The procedure is not appropriate for men with rectal problems. Anticoagulant therapy should be stopped 10 days before treatment. Mild side effects include occasional problems of bladder spasm, hematuria, dysuria, and retention.

Surgical Therapy

Surgery is indicated when there is a decrease in urine flow sufficient to cause discomfort, persistent residual urine, acute urinary retention because of obstruction with no reversible precipitating cause, or hydronephrosis. Treatment of symptomatic BPH primarily involves resection of the prostate. The selection of a surgical approach to remove the tissue depends on the size and position of the prostatic enlargement (Fig. 52-3). No correlation has been found between symptoms and the size of the prostate.

It is the location of the enlargement rather than the amount that produces symptoms. The nurse can help the patient ask appropriate questions regarding the impact of a particular type of surgery.

Laser Ablation. A transurethral, ultrasound-guided, laser-induced prostatectomy (TULIP) is a specially designed laser used to decrease the obstructive tissue. A second approach is visual laser ablation of the prostate (VLAP), which uses a

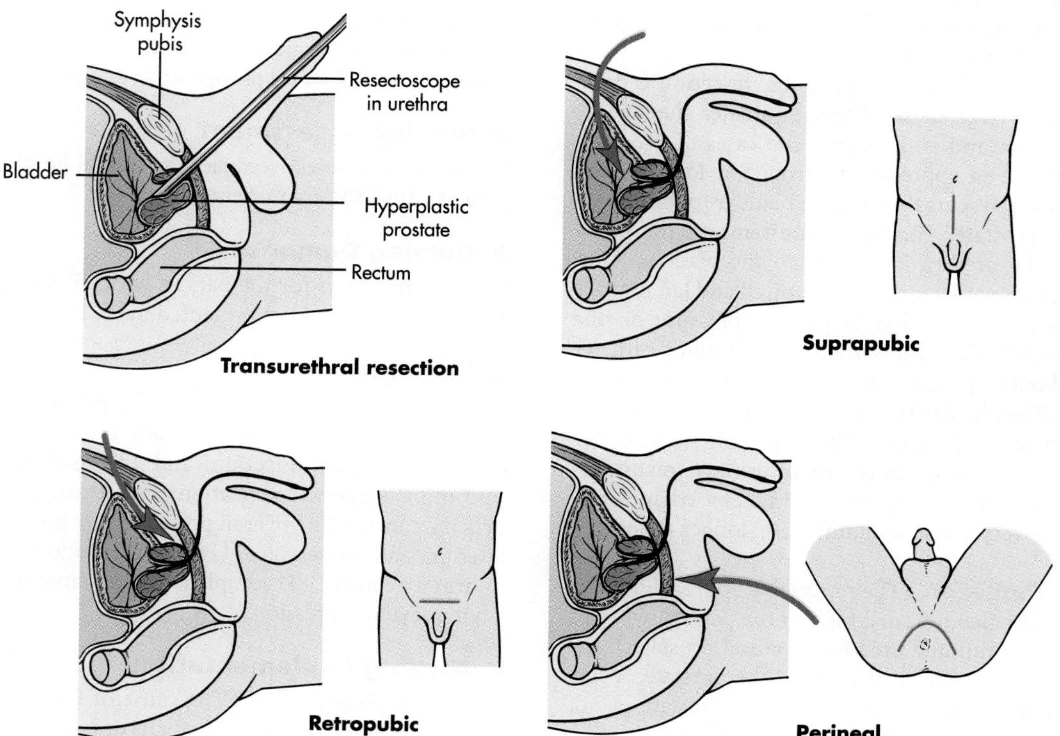

Fig. 52-3 Four types of prostatectomy.

standard cystoscope and allows direct visualization. Both approaches use the neodymium:yttrium-aluminum-garnet (Nd:YAG) laser, which produces coagulation necrosis and ultimately shrinkage of the prostate gland.

Transurethral Resection of the Prostate. Transurethral resection of the prostate (TURP) is the most common route for partial removal of the prostate. No external surgical incision is made because a resectoscope is passed through the urethra to excise and cauterize prostatic tissue. A large (no. 18 to no. 22) three-way indwelling catheter with a 30 ml balloon containing 30 to 60 ml of sterile water is usually inserted into the bladder after the procedure to provide hemostasis and facilitate urinary drainage. The bladder is irrigated, either continuously or intermittently, for approximately the first 24 hours to prevent obstruction from mucus threads and blood clots.

A TURP is often the surgery of choice for the debilitated patient or for the patient with moderate prostatic enlargement. The advantages of a TURP are that it does not involve an external incision and is less likely to result in erectile dysfunction or long-term urinary incontinence. A disadvantage is that it does not completely remove all prostatic tissue, leaving the potential for recurrence of hyperplasia, possible prostatic cancer, and sometimes the false impression that there is no need for yearly DREs.

Transurethral Incision of the Prostate. A transurethral incision of the prostate (TUIP) can be performed in high risk patients, those with mild obstruction, or younger patients. Transurethral slits or incisions are made into the prostatic tissue to relieve bladder neck obstruction. This method is usually used to treat intravesical obstruction related to BPH. The incision can be made unilaterally or bilaterally with a variety of instruments (including laser) at different locations around the bladder neck. The patient is discharged with an indwelling catheter for the first 24 hours to monitor urinary output and hematuria.

Suprapubic Resection. A suprapubic resection is done when an extremely large mass of tissue (greater than 60 g) obstructs the urethra and is done in some cases of prostatic cancer. The prostate is approached through a low midline abdominal incision that cuts through the bladder to the anterior aspect of the prostate. This technique removes the gland completely, and the urethra is sutured to the bladder. After surgery, a suprapubic catheter is often required and left in place through the abdominal incision to prevent pressure on the suture line and to aid in bladder healing. An indwelling catheter with a 30 ml balloon is placed in the bladder via the urethra to avoid strictures. The bladder is irrigated continuously through the urethral catheter for 24 hours. This approach allows better exploration, but it has an increased risk of urinary tract infections, incontinence, bladder spasms, and hemorrhage. The postoperative recovery phase is significantly longer than after a TURP.

Retropubic Resection. The retropubic approach is used to remove a massive gland located high in the pelvic area. This approach is more commonly used for a radical prostatectomy with lymph node dissection for cancer of the prostate. A low midline abdominal incision is made into the prostate gland. After surgery, the patient has a large indwelling catheter with a 30 ml balloon placed in the bladder via the urethra. A surgical drain may be left at the site of the abdominal incision to aid in the removal of drainage from the area. Although the bladder is not incised in this approach, direct visualization of the prostate is possible. The risk of hemorrhage remains high. Both suprapubic and retropubic resections are difficult in the obese patient.

Perineal Resection. The perineal approach is used on rare occasions to remove a large mass located low in the pelvic area or for cancer of the prostate. The incision is made between the scrotum and the anus. Because of the possibility of inadvertently entering the rectum, the bowel is prepared with enemas, antibiotics, and a low-residue diet. After surgery, an indwelling catheter with a 30 ml balloon is left in the urethra. A surgical drain may be placed in the incision site to promote drainage of the area. Careful dressing changes and perineal care after each bowel movement are important for comfort and to prevent incisional infection. Although all open procedures carry some risk of erectile dysfunction, the perineal approach has the highest incidence. Urinary incontinence may also be a problem. This approach also has an increased risk of incisional infection because of the closeness of the anus.

Complications of Prostatic Surgery. The major postoperative complications of these types of surgery are hemorrhage, infection, bladder spasm, urinary incontinence, and erectile problems. The Campbell-Walsh procedure, a nerve-sparing surgical technique, greatly reduces the incidence of erectile dysfunction. Patients should be encouraged to talk with their physician or qualified nurse about postoperative management of urinary incontinence or erectile dysfunction.[13]

NURSING MANAGEMENT: BENIGN PROSTATIC HYPERPLASIA

Because the nurse is most directly involved with care of prostate patients having surgical interventions, the focus of nursing management will be on preoperative and postoperative care.[11]

■ Nursing Assessment

Subjective and objective data that should be obtained from a patient with BPH are presented in Table 52-4.

■ Nursing Diagnoses

Nursing diagnoses for the patient with BPH may include, but are not limited to, those presented in NCP 52-1.

■ Planning

The overall preoperative goals for the patient having prostatic surgery are (1) restoration of urinary drainage, (2) treatment of any urinary tract infection, and (3) understanding of the upcoming surgery, implications for sexual functioning, and urinary control. The overall postoperative goals for the patient after prostate surgery are (1) no complications, (2) restoration of urinary control, (3) complete bladder emptying, and (4) satisfying sexual expression.

■ Nursing Implementation

Health Promotion. The cause of BPH is largely attributed to the aging process. The focus of health promotion is on early detection and treatment. The American Cancer Society,

NURSING ASSESSMENT

Table 52-4 Benign Prostatic Hyperplasia

Subjective Data	Objective Data
Important Health Information *Medications:* Estrogen or testosterone supplementation *Surgery or other treatments:* Previous treatment for BPH **Functional Health Patterns** *Health perception–health management:* Knowledge of the condition *Nutritional-metabolic:* Voluntary fluid restriction *Elimination:* Urinary urgency, diminution in caliber and force of urinary stream; hesitancy in initiating voiding; postvoiding dribbling; urinary retention; incontinence *Sleep:* Nocturia *Cognitive-perceptual:* Dysuria, sensation of incomplete voiding; bladder discomfort *Sexuality-reproductive:* Anxiety about sexual dysfunction	**General** Older adult male **Urinary** Distended bladder on palpation; smooth, firm, elastic enlargement of prostate on rectal examination **Possible Findings** Enlarged prostate on ultrasonography; vesicle neck obstruction on cystourethroscopy; residual urine with postvoiding catheterization; presence of white blood cells, bacteria, or microscopic hematuria with infection; elevated BUN and serum creatinine levels with renal involvement

along with the AUA, recommends a yearly medical history and DRE for men over 40 years of age in an effort to provide early detection of prostate problems. After 50 years of age, and when symptoms of prostatic hyperplasia become evident, further diagnostic screening may be necessary (see Table 52-2).

Some men find that the ingestion of alcohol and caffeine tends to increase prostatic symptoms because the diuretic effect of these substances increases bladder distention. Compounds found in common cough and cold remedies such as pseudoephedrine (in Sudafed) and phenylephrine (in Allerest and Coricidin preparations) often worsen the symptoms of BPH. These drugs are alpha-adrenergic agonists that cause smooth muscle contraction. If this happens, the patient should avoid these drugs.

The patient with obstructive symptoms should be advised to urinate every 2 to 3 hours and when first feeling the urge so urinary stasis and acute urinary retention are minimized. Fluid intake should be maintained at a normal level to avoid dehydration or fluid overload. The patient may believe that if he restricts his fluid intake, symptoms will be less severe, but this only increases the chances of an infection. However, if the patient increases his intake too rapidly, bladder distention can develop because of the prostatic obstruction.

Acute Intervention

Preoperative care. Urinary drainage must be restored before surgery. Prostatic obstruction may have resulted in retention or inability to void. A urethral catheter such as a Coudé (curved-tip) catheter may be needed to restore drainage. If a sizable obstruction of the urethra exists, a filiform catheter with sufficient rigidity to pass the obstruction may be inserted by a urologist. Aseptic technique is important at all times to avoid introducing bacteria into the bladder.

Antibiotics are usually administered before any invasive surgical procedure. Any infection of the urinary tract must be treated before surgery. Restoring urine drainage and encouraging a high fluid intake (2 to 3 L/day, unless contraindicated) are also helpful in managing the infection.

The patient is often concerned about the impact of the impending surgery on his sexual functioning. Data gathered from the health history relating to sexual activities will identify possible problem areas. The nurse should provide an opportunity for the patient and partner to express their concerns. The patient needs to know how the surgery may affect sexual functioning. All types of prostatic surgery generally result in some degree of retrograde ejaculation. The patient should be informed that the ejaculate may be decreased in amount or totally absent. This may decrease orgasmic sensations felt during ejaculation. Retrograde ejaculation is not harmful because the semen is simply eliminated during the next urination.

Postoperative care. The main complications of prostatectomy are hemorrhage, bladder spasms, urinary incontinence, and infection. The plan of care should be adjusted to the type of surgery, the reasons for surgery, and the patient's response to surgery.

After prostatectomy the bladder may be continuously irrigated with sterile normal saline solution or another prescribed solution to remove clotted blood from the bladder and ensure drainage of urine. Some form of irrigation (continuous or intermittent) may be used for 24 hours or until no clots are noted draining from the bladder.

Blood clots are normal after a prostatectomy for the first 24 to 36 hours. However, large amounts of bright red blood in the urine can indicate hemorrhage. Postoperative hemorrhage may occur from displacement of the catheter, dislodging a large clot, or increases in abdominal pressure. Release or displacement of the catheter dislodges the balloon that provides counterpressure on the operative site. Traction on the catheter may be applied to provide counterpressure (tamponade) on the bleeding site in the prostate, decreasing bleeding. Such traction can result in local necrosis if pressure is applied for too long. Pressure should therefore be relieved on a scheduled basis by qualified personnel. Activities that increase abdominal pressure, such as sitting or walking for prolonged periods and straining to have a bowel movement (Valsalva's maneuver), should be avoided in the postoperative recovery period.

Bladder spasms are a distressing complication for the patient after transurethral and suprapubic prostatectomy. They occur as a result of irritation of the bladder mucosa from the

52-1 NURSING CARE PLAN PATIENT UNDERGOING TRANSURETHRAL RESECTION

Expected Patient Outcomes	Nursing Interventions and *Rationales*
Preoperative	
NURSING DIAGNOSIS	**Pain** *related to* bladder distention secondary to enlarged prostate *as manifested by* complaints of discomfort caused by inability to void, palpable bladder, no urine output, diaphoresis, restlessness.
▪ No complaints of pain.	▪ Assist with insertion of indwelling catheter (usually done by urologist) *to reduce pain by providing urinary drainage.* ▪ Monitor intake and output *to evaluate adequacy.* ▪ Percuss bladder for distention *to validate adequate emptying of the bladder.* ▪ Assess comfort status *to continue or revise plan as necessary.* ▪ Maintain patency of catheter *to ensure continuous flow of urine from the bladder.*
NURSING DIAGNOSIS	**Risk for infection** *related to* indwelling catheter, environmental pathogens, and urinary stasis.
▪ No evidence of urinary tract infection.	▪ Assess for elevated temperature and cloudy, foul-smelling urine *to identify symptoms of infection and initiate appropriate interventions.* ▪ Do urinalysis for culture *to determine presence and cause of infection.* ▪ Give patient 8 oz of water or other noncitrus, noncaffeine fluids every waking hour *to prevent urinary stasis and dilute the urine.* ▪ Observe strict aseptic technique for catheter care *to minimize the risk of introducing an infectious organism.*
NURSING DIAGNOSIS	**Fear** *related to* actual or potential sexual dysfunction, possible diagnosis of cancer, and lack of knowledge regarding surgical procedure and postoperative care *as manifested by* verbalization of fear about impact of surgery on sexuality; questioning or inaccurate comments about surgical course.
▪ Decreased fear about effect of surgery on sexuality and surgical course as shown by accurate knowledge base. ▪ Correct responses to questions. ▪ Calm demeanor.	▪ Perform preoperative teaching *to provide information regarding the preoperative and postoperative routines.* ▪ Assess patient's concerns related to sexual functioning and correct misconceptions and inaccuracies *to plan appropriate interventions that address unique concerns.* ▪ Provide opportunity for private conversation for patient to ask personal questions *because a private setting facilitates open discussion.* ▪ Inform patient about retrograde ejaculation *because this often occurs in prostatic surgery and is not harmful because the fluid is eliminated during the next urination.*
Postoperative	
NURSING DIAGNOSIS	**Pain** *related to* irrigations and clots, presence of catheter, and surgical procedure *as manifested by* expression of pain; nonverbal signs of pain such as moaning, crying, legs drawn to abdomen.
▪ Decreased or no pain.	▪ Maintain patency of catheter *because clots cause obstruction of urine flow resulting in bladder spasms.* ▪ Irrigate catheter if occluded with clots (according to aseptic technique and institution protocols) *so urine can flow freely.* ▪ Instruct patient to try not to urinate around catheter *because this increases the occurrence of spasm.* ▪ Give belladonna and opium suppository as needed; instruct patient in relaxation techniques such as deep breathing exercises and distraction therapy or visual imagery *to relieve pain and decrease spasm.*

Continued

52-1 NURSING CARE PLAN PATIENT UNDERGOING TRANSURETHRAL RESECTION—continued

Expected Patient Outcomes	Nursing Interventions and *Rationales*
NURSING DIAGNOSIS	**Ineffective management of therapeutic regimen** *related to* lack of knowledge regarding need for follow-up care and activity restriction postoperatively *as manifested by* questioning or inaccurate comments about postoperative activity.
▪ No postoperative bleeding because of performing activities that increase intraabdominal pressure.	▪ Teach patient that some prostatic tissue is present that could become malignant *so patient understands need for annual prostatic examination.* ▪ Instruct patient to avoid heavy lifting (>10 lb [4.5 kg]), straining during defecation, prolonged periods of travel, stair climbing, driving, and sexual activity until surgeon approves such activity *to prevent increases in intraabdominal pressure and the possibility of bleeding.* ▪ Teach patient to increase fiber in diet, use of stool softeners, and to avoid straining during bowel movements *to prevent constipation and prevent increased intraabdominal pressure.*
NURSING DIAGNOSIS	**Urge incontinence** *related to* poor sphincter control *as manifested by* urinary urgency.
▪ Absence of or satisfactory control of dribbling.	▪ Teach patient Kegel exercises *to strengthen sphincter tone.* ▪ Advise patient about devices to control dribbling and absorbent materials *so patient is aware of various devices and can make an informed decision among alternatives.*
NURSING DIAGNOSIS	**Risk for infection** *related to* indwelling catheter, bladder irrigations, environmental pathogens, inadequate oral intake, and poor catheter care.
▪ No evidence of infection.	▪ Assess for fever, diaphoresis, self-restriction of fluid intake, cloudy urine *to determine if risk factors or signs and symptoms of infection are present.* ▪ Monitor temperature q4hr first 48 hr postoperatively *because fever is a good indicator of infection.* ▪ Give patient 8 oz of water hourly while awake *to maintain good urine flow and dilute the urine.* ▪ Observe strict aseptic technique for catheter care and bladder irrigations *to prevent introducing infectious organisms.*

COLLABORATIVE PROBLEMS

Nursing Goals	Nursing Interventions and *Rationales*
POTENTIAL COMPLICATION	**Hemorrhage** *related to* surgical procedure
▪ Monitor for and report signs of hemorrhage. ▪ Carry out appropriate medical and nursing interventions.	▪ Observe urinary drainage and report bright red bleeding in larger than expected quantities immediately *because this could indicate hemorrhage and the need for immediate intervention.* ▪ Monitor blood pressure, pulse, and respirations and report abnormalities *because increasing pulse and respirations and decreasing BP can indicate hemorrhage.* ▪ Maintain catheter drainage *to prevent obstruction and allow monitoring of bleeding and urine flow.* ▪ Do not perform rectal treatments such as enemas or rectal temperatures (except belladonna and opium suppositories for bladder spasms) *because bleeding could be initiated.* ▪ Teach patient not to strain during bowel movement; limit ambulation and chair sitting to 15 min tid *to decrease pressure on operative area.*

insertion of the resectoscope, the presence of a catheter, or clots leading to obstruction of the catheter. The patient should be instructed not to urinate around the catheter because this increases the likelihood of spasm. If bladder spasms develop, the catheter should be checked for clots. If present, the clots should be removed by irrigation so urine can flow freely. Belladonna and opium suppositories, or other antispasmodics (e.g., oxybutynin [Ditropan]) along with relaxation techniques, are used to relieve the pain and decrease spasm. The catheter is often removed 2 to 4 days after surgery. The patient should urinate within 6 hours after catheter removal. If he cannot, a catheter is reinserted for a day or two. If the problem continues, the nurse may need to instruct the patient in clean intermittent self-catheterization (see Chapter 43).

Sphincter tone may be poor immediately after catheter removal, resulting in urinary incontinence or dribbling. This is a common but distressing situation for the patient. Sphincter tone can be strengthened by having the patient practice Kegel exercises (pelvic floor muscle technique) 10 to 20 times per hour while awake. The patient should be encouraged to practice starting and stopping the stream several times during urination. This facilitates learning the pelvic floor exercises. It usually takes several weeks to achieve urinary continence. In some instances, control of urine may never be fully regained. Continence can improve for up to 12 months. If continence has not been achieved by that time, the patient may be referred to a continence clinic. A variety of methods, including biofeedback, have been used to achieve positive results. The patient can also be instructed to use a penile clamp, condom catheter, or incontinence pads or briefs to avoid embarrassment from dribbling. In severe cases, an occlusive cuff that serves as an artificial sphincter can be surgically implanted to restore continence. The nurse should assist the patient in finding ways to manage the problem that will allow him to continue socializing and interacting with others.

The patient should be observed for signs of postoperative infection. If an external wound is present, the area should be observed for redness, heat, swelling, and purulent drainage. Special care must be taken if a perineal incision is present because of the proximity of the anus. Rectal procedures, such as taking rectal temperatures and administering enemas, should be avoided. The insertion of well-lubricated belladonna and opium suppositories is acceptable.

Careful aseptic technique should be used when irrigating the bladder because bacteria can easily be introduced into the urinary tract. Proper care of the catheter is important. To prevent urethral irritation and minimize the risk of bladder infection, the catheter must be secured to the leg or abdomen with tape or catheter strap. The catheter should be connected to a closed-drainage system and should not be disconnected unless it is being removed, changed, or irrigated. The secretions that accumulate around the meatus can be cleansed daily with soap and water.

Dietary intervention and stool softeners are important in the postoperative period to prevent the patient from straining while having bowel movements. Straining increases the intraabdominal pressure, which can lead to bleeding at the operative site. A diet high in fiber facilitates the passage of stool.

Ambulatory and Home Care. Discharge planning and home care issues are important aspects of care after prostatectomy. Instructions include (1) caring for an indwelling catheter, if one is in place; (2) managing of urinary incontinence; (3) maintaining oral fluids between 2000 and 3000 ml per day; (4) observing for signs and symptoms of urinary tract and wound infection; (5) preventing constipation; (6) avoiding heavy lifting (more than 10 pounds [4.5 kg]); and (7) refraining from driving or intercourse for 6 weeks after surgery or as directed by the surgeon.

After prostatic surgery the patient may be concerned about erectile dysfunction. Physiologic erectile dysfunction may occur when nerves are cut or damaged during surgery. The patient often experiences anxiety over the loss of his sex role, his self-esteem, and the quality of sexual interaction with his sexual partner. Sexual counseling and treatment options may be necessary if erectile dysfunction becomes a chronic or permanent problem. Patients may also require counseling regarding treatment options, which include drug therapy, vacuum or constriction devices, implants, and surgery.

Many men experience retrograde ejaculation after prostatectomy because of trauma to the internal sphincter. Semen is discharged into the bladder at orgasm and may produce cloudy urine when the patient urinates after orgasm. The nurse should discuss these changes with the patient and his partner and allow them to ask questions and express their concerns.

The bladder may take up to 2 months to return to its normal capacity. The patient should be instructed to drink at least 1 to 2 L of fluid per day and to urinate every 2 to 3 hours to flush the urinary tract. Bladder irritants such as caffeine products, citrus juices, and alcohol should be avoided or limited to small amounts. Because the patient may be experiencing incontinence or dribbling, he may incorrectly believe that decreasing fluid intake will relieve this problem. Urethral strictures may result from instrumentation or catheterization. Treatment ranges from teaching the patient intermittent clean catheterization to urethral dilation.

The patient must be advised that he should continue to have a yearly DRE if he has had any procedure other than complete removal of the prostate. Hyperplasia or cancer can occur in the remaining prostatic tissue.

CULTURAL & ETHNIC CONSIDERATIONS

Cancer of the Male Genitourinary System

- Prostate cancer occurs twice as frequently among African-American men as among Caucasian men.
- African-American men tend to be diagnosed with prostate cancer at an earlier age, have more advanced disease at the time of diagnosis, and have a higher mortality rate than do Caucasian men.
- Hispanic and Asian-American men have a lower incidence of prostate cancer and lower mortality rate as compared with Caucasian men.
- Testicular cancer occurs most frequently among Caucasians and is rare in African-Americans.

Evaluation

Expected outcomes for the patient with BPH are addressed in NCP 52-1. 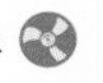

CANCER OF THE PROSTATE

Cancer of the prostate is the most common cancer in men. It is the second leading cause of cancer death in men, after lung cancer. Because of new screening procedures (e.g., prostate-specific antigen), subclinical prostate cancer is being diagnosed with increasing frequency. In 1998 an estimated 184,500 men in the

United States were diagnosed with prostate cancer. Continued increases in prostatic cancer are projected, primarily because of an aging population.

Etiology and Pathophysiology

Prostate cancer is an androgen-dependent adenocarcinoma. Factors such as sexual activity, socioeconomic class, and alcohol use have not been shown to be significant risk factors. In addition, patients with BPH are at no greater risk for prostate cancer. Researchers are now investigating high fat diets and environmental factors for possible links to prostate cancer. A family history of prostate cancer is a major risk factor. Approximately 9% of prostate cancers may be familial.[12]

A higher incidence exists in men 60 years of age or older, in African-American men, and in married men.[13] African-Americans have the highest incidence of prostate cancer, and tend to have more aggressive tumors at diagnosis and higher mortality rates.[14]

The tumor is slow growing and usually begins in the posterior or lateral portions of the prostate. It can spread by three routes: direct extension, via the lymphatics, and via the bloodstream. Direct extension is by continuity to the seminal vesicles, urethral mucosa, bladder wall, and external sphincter. The cancer later spreads through the perineural lymphatic system to the regional lymph nodes. The veins from the prostate seem to be the mode of spread to the pelvic bones, head of the femur, lower lumbar spine, liver, and lungs.

Clinical Manifestations and Complications

Prostate cancer is asymptomatic in the early stages. Eventually the patient may have symptoms similar to those of BPH, including dysuria, hesitancy, dribbling, frequency, urgency, hematuria, nocturia, and retention. The prostate feels hard, enlarged, and fixed on rectal examination. The enlargement is usually unilateral. Pain in the lumbosacral area, which radiates down to the hips or legs, when coupled with urinary symptoms may indicate metastasis.

Early recognition and treatment is required to control growth, prevent metastasis, and preserve quality of life. The tumor can spread to pelvic lymph nodes, bones, bladder, lungs, and liver. Once the tumor has spread to distant sites, the major problem becomes the management of pain. As the cancer spreads to the bones, pain can become severe, especially in the back and the legs because of compression of the spinal cord and osteoblastic lesions.

Diagnostic Studies

Improved diagnostic techniques have greatly enhanced the physician's ability to detect cancer of the prostate at an earlier stage. Primary screening for prostate cancer consists of palpation of the gland during DRE, a blood test for PSA (a glycoprotein that is detected only in the epithelial cells of the prostate), and TRUS. The American Cancer Society and the AUA recommend yearly DREs for all men over age 40. Current evidence strongly suggests that the combination of DRE and serum PSA level measurement increases the chances of early detection of prostate cancer. Ultrasonography of the prostate allows the physician to visualize the outer lobes of the prostate and pinpoint potential cancer sites. When a suspicious area is located, a special biopsy needle can be inserted and the specimen examined.

Elevated levels of PSA (normal level, 0 to 4 ng/ml [0 to 4 μg/L]) and the prostatic isoenzyme of acid phosphatase (prostatic acid phosphatase [PAP]) are both suggestive of cancer of the prostate. Elevated PSA levels indicate prostatic pathology, although not necessarily cancer of the prostate. Mild elevations in PSA may occur in BPH, acute or chronic prostatitis, urinary retention, or infarction of the prostate. In addition, cystoscopy, indwelling urethral catheters, and prostate biopsies may produce an elevation. An elevated PSA alerts the physician to the possibility of cancer of the prostate. In prostate cancer, serum PSA levels are a useful marker of tumor volume. For example, the higher the serum value the greater the tumor mass. Finasteride (Proscar), which is taken to reduce prostatic hyperplasia in men with BPH, may reduce the levels of PSA by almost 50%.[12] This should be considered when evaluating PSA blood levels.

PSA is also useful in following patients after treatment for localized disease. When treatment has been successful in removing all prostatic tissue, the PSA should fall to undetectable levels.

Elevated PAP is specifically indicative of cancer of the prostate. In advanced prostate cancer, serum alkaline phosphatase is increased as a result of bone metastasis. Investigation is now under way to locate a serum marker for prostate cancer similar to CA-125 in ovarian cancer.

When an elevated PSA level or a positive finding on digital rectal examination is noted, the prostate gland is biopsied. This is done through a transrectal needle biopsy. Six systematic samples of prostate tissue are taken for histologic examination. Other tests used to determine the location and extent of the spread of the cancer may include transrectal ultrasound, computed tomography (CT), and magnetic resonance imaging (MRI).

Collaborative Care

The collaborative care of cancer of the prostate depends on the stage of the cancer. Prostatic cancer is staged on the basis of tumor volume and spread (Table 52-5). The TNM staging system is also used to stage prostate cancer (see Chapter 14). Surgery is the most accurate method of staging the extent of the tumor growth and lymph node involvement. At all stages, there is more than one possible treatment option. The decision of which treatment course to pursue is made jointly by the patient and the physician based on a careful analysis of the facts and the patient's unique situation.[15] Table 52-6 summarizes the various treatment options available.

Surgical Therapy. Surgery is often the first line of treatment, particularly in the earlier stages of the disease. In stage A or B a TURP or total prostatectomy may be the treatment depending on the location and symptoms. Patients who are asymptomatic may be observed carefully, with annual DRE and PSA testing. For patients in good health with stage C tumor, surgery is usually a radical prostatectomy involving resection of the prostate gland, seminal vesicles, and part of the ampulla of the vas deferens.[16] Surgery is usually not considered an option for stage D cancer except to relieve obstruction because metastasis has already occurred.

A nerve-sparing surgical technique is sometimes used to decrease the incidence of erectile dysfunction following a radiacal prostatectomy.[17,18] This surgery is useful only for patients

Table 52-5 Whitmore-Jewett Staging Classification of Prostate Cancer

Stage A: Clinically Unrecognized	
A1	<5% of prostatic tissue neoplastic
A2	>5% of prostatic tissue neoplastic, all high-grade tumors
Stage B: Clinically Intracapsular	
B1	Nodule <2 cm and surrounded by palpably normal tissue
B2	Nodule >2 cm or multiple nodules
Stage C: Clinically Extracapsular, Localized to Periprostatic Area	
C1	Minimal extracapsular extension
C2	Large tumors involving seminal vesicles, adjacent structures, or both
Stage D: Metastatic Disease	
D1	Pelvic lymph node metastases or ureteral obstruction causing hydronephrosis
D2	Distant metastases to bone, viscera, or other soft-tissue structures

who are younger and have negative lymph nodes, no elevation of serum alkaline phosphatase levels, and no clinical evidence of extracapsular extension. Patients with extensive disease or older men may not benefit from the nerve-sparing operation. However, a patient with a localized nodule or with small-volume disease may benefit. Up to 70% of patients undergoing a nerve-sparing operation will retain erectile function postoperatively.

Radiation Therapy. External beam radiation therapy is commonly used in the management of prostate cancer, especially in men over age 70. As compared with surgery, there is a reduced risk of erectile dysfunction. Long-term outcomes of radiation therapy compared with prostatectomy show few differences. Potential side effects of radiation include diarrhea, cystitis, and erectile dysfunction. Sexual potency may not be affected when lower-dose, well-controlled radiation therapy is used.[19-21] Radiation therapy may also be combined with the antiandrogen agents such as goserelin (Zoladex).[22]

Interstitial radioactive seed implants (brachytherapy) have been used for the past 25 years to treat prostate cancer. Radioactive implants are placed in the prostate tissue through a transrectal approach. This therapy may be used in conjunction with external beam radiation therapy. Brachytherapy is discussed in Chapter 14.

Drug Therapy. A unique feature of prostate cancer is that cell growth initially depends on the presence of androgens. Hormone therapy is focused on reducing the levels of circulating androgens and is used in the management of extraprostatic (metastatic) disease. Hormone or antiandrogen therapy is rarely used alone in the treatment of prostate cancer.[12]

Current antiandrogen therapy involves agents such as leuprolide (Lupron) and goserelin (Zoladex) that are agonists of luteinizing hormone–releasing hormone (LHRH), a hypothalamic hormone that controls the release of luteinizing hormone (LH) and follicle-stimulating hormone (FSH) from the anterior pituitary. By binding the LHRH receptor sites there is a reduction in release of FSH and LH and as a result a decrease in testosterone levels. Antiandrogen medications are given by

COLLABORATIVE CARE

Table 52-6 Prostate Cancer

Diagnostic
- Digital rectal examination (DRE)
- Prostate specific antigen (PSA)
- Prostatic acid phosphatase (PAP) in advanced stages
- Transrectal ultrasound (TRUS)
- Biopsy, needle aspiration, open biopsy
- Bone scan
- Grading and staging

Collaborative Therapy

Stage A
- Continue medical follow-up, observation, TURP or total prostatectomy
- Radiation therapy

Stage B
- TURP
- Total prostatectomy with or without lymphadenectomy
- Radiation therapy

Stage C
- Hormone manipulation (e.g., luteinizing hormone–releasing hormone analogues) or orchiectomy
- Radical resection of prostate
- Radiation therapy

Stage D
- Hormone therapy
- Radiation to metastatic bone areas
- Chemotherapy

TURP, transurethral resection of prostate.

monthly subcutaneous or intramuscular injections, require monitoring, and must be taken indefinitely. More recent developments include a suspension preparation that can be administered every 3 months.[12] Side effects include hot flashes, loss of libido, and erectile dysfunction.

Another classification of antiandrogens primarily used in combination with LHRH agonists are drugs that compete with circulating androgens at the receptor sites. Flutamide (Eulexin), nilutamide (Nilandron), and bicalutamide (Casodex) are nonsteroidal androgen receptor blockers. They can be used in combination with goserelin or leuprolide. The combination has been found to be safe and well tolerated as a potency-sparing, androgen-ablative therapy. These agents may also be used in combination with finesteride (Proscar) to reduce androgenic effects.[23,24] Adverse effects of antiandrogen drugs are similar to LHRH agonists and include loss of libido, erectile dysfunction, and hot flashes. The loss of libido and erections are not as great when antiandrogens are used alone as when combined with LHRH agonists. However, breast pain and gynecomastia may occur in men treated with antiandrogens.

Surgical removal of the prostate followed by orchiectomy (removal of the testes) removes the source of 90% of circulating androgens. Orchiectomy often provides rapid relief of bone pain. Orchiectomy alone may induce sufficient shrinkage of the prostate to relieve urinary obstruction in later stages of disease when surgery is not an option. While an orchiectomy can cause emotional distress, the physiologic side effects are less than when chemical androgen suppression is used. Men are often

NURSING ASSESSMENT

Table 52-7 Cancer of the Prostate

Subjective Data

Important Health Information

Medications: Testosterone supplements; use of any medications affecting urinary tract such as morphine, anticholinergics, monoamine oxidase inhibitors, and tricyclic antidepressants

Functional Health Patterns

Health perception–health management: Positive family history; increasing fatigue and malaise

Nutritional-metabolic: High-fat diet; anorexia, weight loss (possible indicators of metastasis)

Elimination: Hesitancy or straining to start stream, urinary urgency, frequency, retention with dribbling, weak stream, hematuria

Sleep: Nocturia

Cognitive-perceptual: Dysuria; low back pain radiating to legs or pelvis, bone pain (possible indicators of metastasis)

Self-preception–self-concept: Anxiety regarding self-concept

Objective Data

General

Older adult male; pelvic lymphadenopathy (late sign)

Urinary

Distended bladder on palpation; unilaterally hard, enlarged, fixed prostate on rectal examination

Musculoskeletal

Pathologic fractures (metastasis)

Possible Findings

Elevated serum PSA; elevated serum acid phosphatase PAP (metastasis); nodular and irregular prostate on ultrasonography, positive biopsy results; anemia

PSA, prostate specific antigen.

able to continue having erections and orgasmic sensations, even though ejaculation is absent.

Estrogen (e.g., diethylstilbestrol) treatment may be substituted for orchiectomy. It causes regression of the size of the prostate and of metastatic bone lesions. The minimum dose that is capable of suppressing plasma testosterone to castration levels is used. Estrogen therapy often results in gynecomastia, mood swings, decreased libido, hot flashes, and total loss of erectile functioning. Estrogen treatment is declining in popularity because of more serious side effects such as heart attack, stroke, and pulmonary embolism.

Chemotherapy is occasionally used in late-stage disease with some success. It does appear to reduce pain associated with prostate cancer. However, it has not been shown to improve survival or quality of life.

Other Therapies. Prostatic cryosurgery is an experimental but promising approach to treating cancer of the prostate. The treatment takes about 2 hours under general or spinal anesthesia and does not involve a major abdominal incision. Liquid nitrogen is circulated in probes inserted into the prostate gland through tiny punctures in the perineum. Possible complications of prostatic cryosurgery include the development of a urethrorectal fistula (an opening between the urethra and the rectum) or a urethrocutaneous fistula (an opening between the urethra and the skin), tissue sloughing, erectile dysfunction, urinary incontinence, and hemorrhage.

NURSING MANAGEMENT: PROSTATIC CANCER

Nursing Assessment

Subjective and objective data that should be obtained from an individual with cancer of the prostate are presented in Table 52-7.

Nursing Diagnoses

Nursing diagnoses for the patient with cancer of the prostate depend on the stage of the cancer. General nursing diagnoses, which may or may not apply to every patient with cancer of the prostate, may include, but are not limited to, the following:

- Decisional conflict *related to* numerous alternative treatment options
- Pain *related to* surgery, prostatic enlargement, bone metastasis, and bladder spasms
- Urinary retention *related to* obstruction of urethra or bladder neck by the prostate, blood clots, and loss of bladder tone
- Altered urinary elimination *related to* bladder neck sphincter damage
- Constipation or diarrhea *related to* treatment interventions
- Sexual dysfunction *related to* effects of treatment
- Anxiety *related to* uncertain outcome of disease process on life and lifestyle and effect of treatment on sexual functioning

Planning

The overall goals are that the patient with cancer of the prostate will (1) be an active participant in the treatment plan, (2) have satisfactory pain control, (3) follow the therapeutic plan, (4) accept the effect of the therapeutic plan on sexual function, and (5) find a satisfactory way to manage the impact on bladder or bowel function.

Nursing Implementation

Health Promotion. One of the most important roles for nurses in relation to prostate cancer is to encourage patients to have an annual prostate examination to facilitate early detection of this malignant tumor. Because of their

RESEARCH
IMPLICATIONS FOR NURSING PRACTICE

Uncertainty and Prostate Cancer

Citation Germino BB and others: Uncertainty in prostate cancer: ethnic and family patterns, *Cancer Pract* 6:107, 1998.

Purpose To examine the relationship of sense of uncertainty with family coping, psychologic adjustment to illness, and spiritual factors. In addition, to determine whether these relationships were similar for white and African-American patient and family caregivers.

Method A sample of 403 white and African-American men and their family caregivers were interviewed either 1 week after postsurgical catheter removal or at the beginning of primary radiation treatment. All men were diagnosed with stage B prostate cancer. Tools included measures of uncertainty, adult role behavior, problem solving, social support, importance of God in one's life, family coping, psychologic adjustment to illness, and perceptions of health and illness.

Results and Conclusions In African-American and white family care providers, the more uncertainty experienced, the less positive they felt about treatment and the patient recovering from the illness. For white patients and family members higher levels of uncertainty were related to lower scores on adult role behavior (e.g., shopping), less active problem solving, and less perceived social support. Higher levels of uncertainty were related to poorer social environment for African-American patients and white family members.

Implications for Nursing Practice Uncertainty accompanying the diagnosis and treatment (surgery versus radiation) of prostate cancer is a common experience for both the patient and the family caregivers. This study demonstrates that there are differences between African-Americans and whites in the relationship of uncertainty to a number of coping variables. The results have implications for the assessment and management of psychosocial responses to cancer and cancer treatments. The nurse should consider the sociocultural perspective of the individual patient and his family members when planning care.

increased risk of prostate cancer, African-American men in particular should be encouraged to participate in prostate screening programs or to consult a clinician on an annual basis. All men should have an annual DRE beginning at 40 years of age.

Acute Intervention. Preoperative and postoperative phases of therapy are the same as for BPH. Nursing interventions for the patient who undergoes radiation therapy and chemotherapy are discussed in Chapter 14. An additional consideration is the psychologic response of the patient to a diagnosis of cancer. The nurse should provide sensitive, caring support for the patient and his family to help them cope with the diagnosis of cancer.[25,26] Prostate support groups are available for men and their families to encourage them to be active, informed participants in their own care.

Ambulatory and Home Care. If the patient is discharged with an indwelling catheter in place, the nurse must teach appropriate catheter care. The patient should be instructed to clean the urethral meatus with soap and water once a day; maintain a high fluid intake; keep the collecting bag lower than the bladder at all times; keep the catheter securely anchored to the inner thigh or abdomen; and report any signs of bladder infection, such as bladder spasms, fever, or hematuria. If urinary incontinence is a problem, patients should be encouraged to practice pelvic floor muscle exercises (Kegel exercises) at every urination and throughout the day. Continuous practice during the 4- to 6-week healing process improves the success rate. Products used for incontinence specifically designed for men are available through home care product catalogs and many retail stores.

Cancer of the prostate has a high cure rate if detected and treated early. However, prognosis for stage D prostate cancer is very unfavorable. Pain control is the primary nursing intervention for the terminally ill patient. Hospice care is often appropriate and most beneficial to the patient and family. (Hospice care is discussed in Chapter 2.)

Evaluation

The expected outcomes are that the patient with prostate cancer will

- be an active participant in the treatment plan
- have satisfactory pain control
- follow the therapeutic plan
- accept the effect of the treatment on sexual function
- find a satisfactory way to manage the impact on bladder or bowel function

PROSTATITIS

Etiology and Pathophysiology

A number of inflammatory conditions can affect the prostate gland after a male reaches puberty. The four most common forms of prostatitis are acute bacterial prostatitis, chronic bacterial prostatitis, nonbacterial prostatitis, and prostatodynia. Bacterial prostatitis generally results from organisms reaching the prostate gland by one of the following routes: ascending from the urethra, descending from the bladder, and invasion via the bloodstream or the lymphatic channels.

Bacterial prostatitis is frequently associated with urethritis or an infection of the lower urinary tract. It can also be associated with an indwelling urethral catheter, urethral instrumentation, or trauma. Common causative organisms are *Escherichia coli, Pseudomonas, Enterobacter, Proteus, Chlamydia trachomatis, Neisseria gonorrhoeae,* and group D streptococci. Chronic bacterial prostatitis should be considered in men with a history of recurrent bacteriuria.

Nonbacterial prostatitis may occur after a viral illness, or it may be associated with other sexually transmitted diseases (STDs), particularly in a younger adult. The etiology is not known, and a culture reveals no causative organisms. Prostatodynia has the same symptoms as prostatitis (irritation and pelvic pain on urination) but no evidence of inflammation. The condition is generally limited to younger men.

Clinical Manifestations and Complications

Acute bacterial prostatitis results in manifestations of fever; chills; dysuria; urethral discharge; increased urinary frequency and urgency; low back, rectal, pelvic, and perineal pain; and acute cystitis with cloudy, smelly urine. The prostate is extremely swollen, tender, firm, and warm to touch. The complications of prostatitis are epididymitis and cystitis. Sexual functioning may be affected as manifested by post-ejaculation pain, libido problems, and erectile dysfunction. Prostatic abscess is a rare complication.

The symptoms of chronic prostatitis may be absent or are generally milder than those of acute prostatitis.[27] These include backache, perineal pain, ejaculatory pain, mild dysuria, and increased frequency of urination.[28] Factors that may contribute to chronic prostatitis include urethral obstruction, persistent infections above the urethra, and prostatic pathologic conditions such as congestion, hyperplasia, and prostatic calculi. Chronic prostatitis can predispose the patient to recurrent urinary tract infections. The prostate feels irregularly enlarged, firm, and slightly tender on palpation.

Diagnostic Studies

A prostatitis symptom severity index and symptom frequency assessment questionnaire has been developed as a primary screening tool.[29] Complaints of lower abdominal, testicular, penile, and ejaculatory pain are found more often in prostatitis when compared with BPH. If a patient with prostatitis has a fever, the white blood cell (WBC) count may be elevated. An increased PSA level can be found in acute prostatitis, a moderate increase in chronic prostatitis, and a minimal increase in nonbacterial prostatitis.[30] The urine is often cloudy with a foul odor and may test positive for bacteria. The patient may be instructed to void into two or three separate containers for a split-specimen urinalysis. The first container shows many more WBCs and bacteria than subsequent containers. On palpation, the prostate gland may be normal or may appear enlarged and tender, and in long-standing cases, may reveal the presence of calculi. Cystoscopy, catheterizations, and prostatic massage are avoided during the acute phase to minimize the risk of introducing the organisms into the bladder and to avoid further pain. Prostatic massage may be used in chronic prostatitis to express secretions for culture and sensitivity. A transrectal ultrasound (TRUS) scan may be done before the massage to prevent unnecessary prolonged treatment.

NURSING AND COLLABORATIVE MANAGEMENT: PROSTATITIS

Collaborative care of acute bacterial prostatitis usually consists of administering an antibiotic for 3 to 6 weeks that concentrates in the prostatic tissue. Most antibiotics cannot penetrate the prostate because the low pH of the gland precludes solubility of the drugs. The specific antibiotics for acute bacterial prostatitis are ciprofloxacin (Cipro) and trimethoprim-sulfamethoxazole (Bactrim). Antispasmodics, analgesics, and stool softeners are often prescribed to provide relief from painful symptoms. Other interventions include increasing fluid intake, use of warm sitz baths, antiinflammatory agents, and rest.

Collaborative care of chronic prostatitis may consist of long-term (12 to 16 weeks) administration of antibiotics, antiinflammatory agents, frequent prostatic massage and ejaculations, sitz baths, and stool softeners. Antibiotics include ciprofloxacin, trimethoprim-sulfamethoxazole, carbenicillin, tetracycline, doxycycline, and erythromycin. If the infection is sexually transmitted, both the patient and partner need to be treated.

Nonbacterial prostatitis and prostatodynia are difficult to treat because no bacteria are found in the urine or prostatic fluid. Treatment generally consists of antiinflammatory agents, hot sitz baths, and sexual activities that result in ejaculation. TUMA therapy may be a treatment option when traditional therapy is unsuccessful.[31]

The patient with acute bacterial prostatitis experiences prostate pain when standing, when urinating, and during ejaculation. Nursing interventions are aimed at relief of pain and fever, bed rest, and the maintenance of adequate hydration. The patient with chronic prostatitis should be instructed regarding the long-term nature of the problem. Because the prostate can serve as a source of bacteria, fluid intake should be kept at a high level. Antibiotics may have to be taken for a number of months. Activities that drain the prostate, such as intercourse (use a condom to protect the partner from infection), masturbation, and prostatic massage, are often helpful in the long-term management of this problem. Chronic prostatitis may eventually lead to erectile dysfunction, for which the patient may need to seek treatment.

PROBLEMS OF THE PENIS

Health problems of the penis are rare if sexually transmitted infectious diseases are excluded (see Chapter 50). Problems of the penis may be classified as congenital, problems of the prepuce, problems with the erectile mechanism, and cancer.

CONGENITAL PROBLEMS

Hypospadias is a urologic abnormality in which the urethral meatus is located on the ventral surface of the penis anywhere from the corona to the perineum. Hormonal influences in utero, environmental factors, and genetic factors are possible causes. Surgical repair of hypospadias may be necessary if it is associated with chordee, or if it prevents intercourse or normal urination. Surgery may also be done for cosmetic reasons or emotional well-being.

Epispadias, an opening of the urethra on the dorsal surface of the penis, is a complex birth defect that is usually associated with other genitourinary tract defects. Corrective surgery to place the urethra in a normal position in the penis is usually done in early childhood.

PROBLEMS OF THE PREPUCE

Problems of the prepuce in the United States are rare because circumcision has been a routine procedure for most male infants for many years. The trend is now shifting away from routine circumcision to one of preference, which may result in an increased incidence of problems.

Circumcision, the surgical removal of the foreskin of the penis, may be done for religious, cultural, or hygienic reasons.

Parents are encouraged to make the final decision after consideration of all the advantages and disadvantages.

Phimosis is caused by edema or inflammation of the foreskin of an uncircumcised male. This results in the foreskin constricting around the head of the penis, making retraction difficult. It is generally caused by poor hygiene techniques that allow bacterial and yeast organisms to become trapped under the foreskin.

Paraphimosis is edema of the retracted uncircumcised foreskin, preventing normal return over the glans. This can occur when the foreskin is pulled back during bathing, use of urinary catheters, or intercourse and is not placed back in the forward position. Antibiotics, warm soaks, and sometimes circumcision or dorsal slit of the prepuce may be required. Careful cleaning followed by replacement of the foreskin generally prevents these problems.

PROBLEMS OF THE ERECTILE MECHANISM

Priapism is a painful erection lasting longer than 6 hours. Causes of priapism include thrombosis of the corpora cavernosal veins, leukemia, sickle cell anemia, diabetes mellitus, degenerative lesions of the spine, neoplasms of the brain or spinal cord, prolonged foreplay, injection of vasoactive medications into the corpus cavernosa, and cocaine use. Treatment may include sedatives, injection of smooth muscle relaxants directly into the penis, aspiration and irrigation of the corpora cavernosa with a large-bore needle, or the surgical creation of a shunt to drain the corpora. Prolonged priapism constitutes a medical emergency. Complications may include penile tissue necrosis caused by lack of blood flow or hydronephrosis from bladder distention. After an episode of priapism, the patient may be unable to achieve a normal erection.

Peyronie's disease, sometimes referred to as curved or crooked penis, is caused by plaque formation in one of the corpora cavernosa of the penis. The palpable, nontender, hard plaque formation is usually found on the posterior surface. It may result from trauma to the penile shaft or may occur spontaneously. The plaque prevents adequate blood flow into the spongy tissue, which results in a curvature during erection. The condition is not dangerous but can result in painful erections, erectile dysfunction, or embarrassment. If conservative measures do not correct the problem, surgery may be necessary.

CANCER OF PENIS

Cancer of the penis is rare apart from cancers associated with the STD human papillomavirus (HPV) and in men who were not circumcised as infants. The tumor may appear as a superficial ulceration or a pimple-like nodule. The nontender warty lesion may be mistaken for a venereal wart. The majority of malignancies (95%) are well-differentiated squamous cell carcinomas. Treatment in the early stages is laser removal of the growth. A radical resection of the penis may be done if the cancer has spread. Surgery, radiation, or chemotherapy may be tried depending on the extent of the disease, lymph node involvement, or metastasis.

PROBLEMS OF THE SCROTUM AND ITS CONTENTS

EXTERNAL PROBLEMS

The skin of the scrotum is susceptible to a number of common skin diseases. The most common conditions of the scrotal skin are fungal infections, dermatitis (neurodermatitis, contact dermatitis, and seborrheic dermatitis), and parasitic infections (scabies and lice). These conditions involve discomfort for the patient but are associated with few, if any, severe complications (see Chapter 22).

CONGENITAL PROBLEMS

Cryptorchidism (undescended testes) is failure of the testes to descend into the scrotal sack before birth. It is the most common congenital testicular condition. It may occur bilaterally or unilaterally and may be the cause of infertility if corrective surgery is not done by 2 years of age. The incidence of testicular cancer is also higher if the condition is not corrected before puberty. Surgery is performed to locate and suture the testis or testes to the scrotum.

Absence of the vas deferens is a rare condition associated most often with cystic fibrosis. With the advent of advanced techniques to treat infertility, this defect can be circumvented by aspirating the sperm directly from the testis.

"DES sons" are the male children of women who took diethylstilbestrol (DES) during pregnancy. Until recently it was thought that only females were affected in utero if their mothers took DES during pregnancy. The impact on males is now seen in the form of undescended or underdeveloped testes, a micropenis or small penis, varicocele, or epididymal cysts. These males also have an increased rate of infertility.[32]

ACQUIRED PROBLEMS

Problems that develop within the scrotum usually are first noticed as a mass or as scrotal edema. Some problems produce pain, whereas others do not. Acquired conditions affecting scrotal contents in the adult include epididymitis, hydrocele, spermatocele, varicocele, orchitis, torsion, and testicular cancer (Fig. 52-4).

Epididymitis

Epididymitis is an inflammatory process of the epididymis, usually secondary to an infectious process (sexually or nonsexually transmitted), trauma, or urinary reflux down the vas deferens. When the problem is associated with prostatitis it is usually painful. Swelling may progress to the point that the epididymis and testis are indistinguishable. In younger men, less than 35 years of age, the most common cause is through sexual transmission of either gonorrhea or chlamydia. The use of antibiotics is important for both partners if the transmission is through sexual contact. Patients should be encouraged to refrain from sexual intercourse during the acute phase. If they do engage in intercourse, a condom should be used. Conservative treatment consists of bed rest with elevation of the scrotum, use of ice packs, and analgesics. Ambulation places the scrotum in a dependent position and increases pain. Most tenderness subsides within 1 week, although swelling may last for weeks or months.

Hydrocele

A *hydrocele* is a nontender, fluid-filled mass that results from interference with lymphatic drainage of the scrotum and swelling of the tunica vaginalis that surrounds the testis. Diagnosis is fairly simple because the mass can be seen by shining a

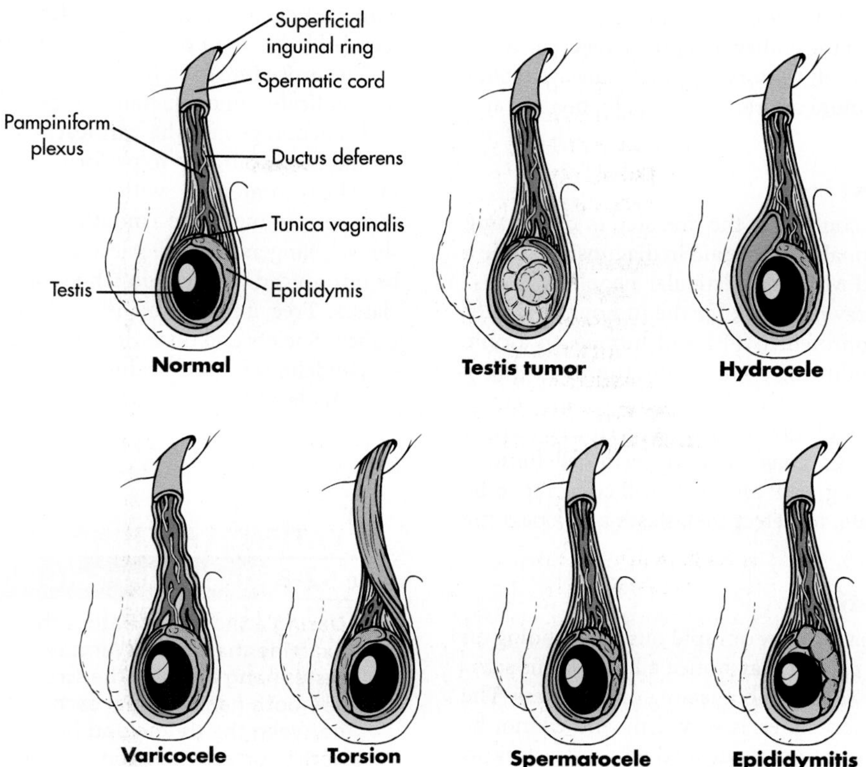

Fig. 52-4 Scrotal masses.

flashlight through the scrotum (transillumination). No treatment is indicated unless the swelling becomes very large and uncomfortable, in which case aspiration or surgical drainage of the mass is performed.

Spermatocele

A *spermatocele* is a firm, sperm-containing, painless cyst of the epididymis that may be visible with transillumination. The cause is unknown, and surgical removal is the treatment. It is important for the patient to see his doctor if he feels any lumps. He would be unable to distinguish this cyst from cancer when performing self-examination.

Varicocele

A *varicocele* is a dilation of the veins that drain the testes. The scrotum feels wormlike when palpated. The cause of the problem is unknown. The varicocele is usually located on the left side of the scrotum as a consequence of retrograde blood flow from the left renal vein. Surgery is indicated if the patient is infertile, since persistent varicoceles are associated with 40% to 50% of the causes of infertility. Repair of the varicocele may be through injection of a sclerosing agent or by surgical ligation of the spermatic vein.

Orchitis

In *orchitis* the testis is acutely inflamed, painful, tender, and swollen. It generally occurs after an episode of bacterial or viral infections such as mumps, pneumonia, tuberculosis, or syphilis. It can also be a side effect of epididymitis, prostatectomy, trauma, infectious mononucleosis, influenza, catheterization, or complicated urinary tract infection. Mumps orchitis is a condition contributing to infertility and could easily be decreased by childhood vaccination against mumps. Treatment involves the use of antibiotics (if the organism is known), pain medications, or bed rest with the scrotum elevated on an ice pack.

Torsion

Testicular torsion involves a twisting of the spermatic cord that supplies blood to the testes and epididymis. It is most commonly seen in young males under the age of 20. Torsion constitutes a surgical emergency. The patient experiences severe scrotal pain, tenderness, swelling, nausea, and vomiting. Urinary complaints, fever, and WBCs or bacteria in the urine are absent. The pain does not usually subside with rest or elevation of the scrotum. Unless it resolves spontaneously, surgery to untwist the cord and restore the blood supply must be performed quickly. The torsion causes ischemia to the testis, leading to necrosis and the possible need for removal.

Testicular Cancer

Etiology and Pathophysiology

Testicular tumors occur primarily in men between 20 and 40 years of age. Testicular tumors are more common in males who have had undescended testes (cryptorchidism) or a family history of testicular cancer or anomalies. Other predisposing factors include a history of mumps, orchitis, inguinal hernia in childhood, maternal exposure to DES, and testicular cancer in the contralateral testis.

Testicular tumors may develop from the cellular components of the testis or from the embryonal precursors (germ cell tumors). Testicular germ cell tumors are almost always malignant. Non–germ cell tumors are rare, are usually benign, and can occur at any age.

Diagnostic Studies

Palpation of the scrotal contents is the first step in diagnosing testicular cancer. Additional tests that aid in diagnosis include a testicular sonogram and MRI. If a testicular neoplasm is suspected, blood may be drawn to look for the tumor markers of glycoproteins alpha-fetoprotein (AFP) and human chorionic gonadotropin (hCG). Following orchiectomy, tumor staging is done on the testicle tissue and lymph node biopsy specimens. Testicular cancer is histologically classified as germ cell tumors (seminomas and nonseminomas) or non–germ cell tumors. After diagnosis and staging, AFP and hCG will continue to be monitored, if appropriate, to detect metastases and assess the response to therapy.

Clinical Manifestations

Germ cell tumors may have a slow or rapid onset depending on the type of tumor. The patient may notice a lump in his scrotum, as well as scrotal swelling and a feeling of heaviness. The scrotal mass usually is nontender, is very firm, and cannot be transilluminated. Manifestations associated with metastasis to other systems include back pain, cough, dyspnea, hemoptysis, dysphagia (difficulty swallowing), alterations in vision or mental status, papilledema, and seizures.

NURSING AND COLLABORATIVE MANAGEMENT: TESTICULAR CANCER

As with many forms of cancer, the survival of the patient is closely associated with early recognition of the tumor. The scrotum is easily examined, and beginning tumors are usually palpable. Every male between puberty and 40 years of age should be taught and encouraged to perform a monthly testicular self-examination for the purpose of detecting testicular tumors or other scrotal abnormalities such as varicoceles. The nurse should teach the patient how to do a self-examination with particular emphasis on males with a history of an undescended testis or a previous testicular tumor.

The procedure for self-examination is not difficult. The male may indicate some reluctance to examine his own genitals, but with encouragement he can learn this simple procedure. He should be encouraged to perform self-examinations frequently until he is comfortable with the procedure. The scrotum should then be examined once a month. Videotapes and illustrations on shower hangers are available as teaching aids and ideally should be introduced during high school or college physical education classes. Free information is available through the American Cancer Society and on various Internet medical websites.

Guidelines for self-examination of the scrotum are presented in Table 52-8 and Fig. 52-5. The nurse should make this pro-

PATIENT TEACHING GUIDE

Table 52-8 Testicular Self-Examination

1. During a shower or bath is the easiest time to examine the testes. Warm temperatures make the testes hang lower in the scrotum (See Fig. 52-5).
2. Use both hands to feel each testis. Roll the testis between the thumb and first three fingers until the entire surface has been covered. Palpate each one separately.
3. Identify the structures. The testis should feel round and smooth, like a hard-boiled egg. Differentiate the testis from the epididymis. The epididymis is not as smooth as the egg-shaped testis. One testis may be larger than the other. Size is not as important as texture. Check for lumps, irregularities, pain in the testes, or a dragging sensation. Locate the spermatic cord, which is usually firm and smooth and goes up toward the groin.
4. Choose a consistent day of the month, such as a birth date, that is easy to remember to examine the testes. The examination can be performed more frequently if desired.
5. Notify the doctor at once if any abnormalities are found.

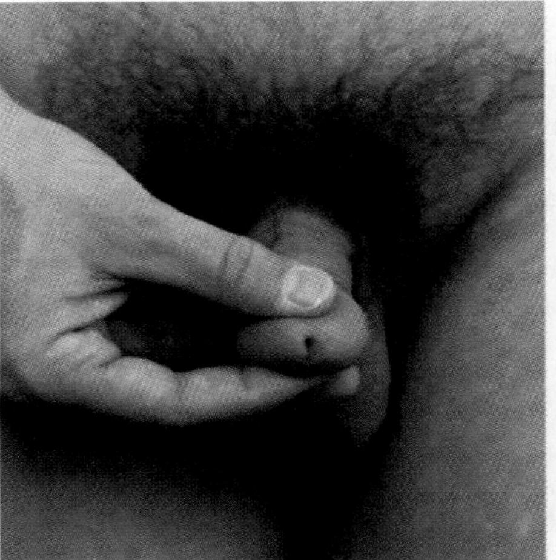

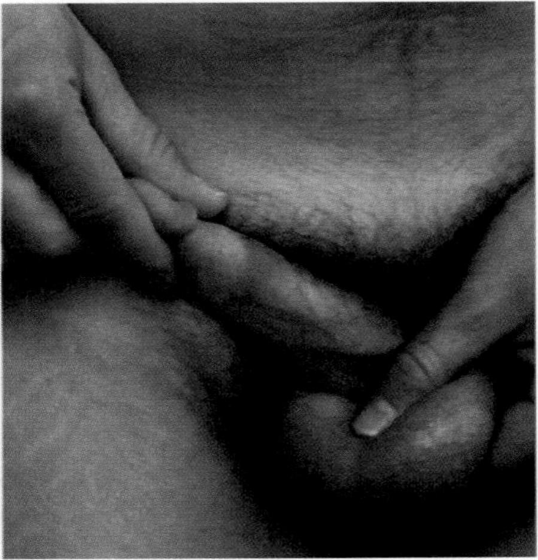

Fig. 52-5 Testicular self-examination.

cedure as simple and uncomplicated for the man as possible. The man should choose a technique that is comfortable and consistent for him. It may be his first step toward a lifetime of healthy living practices.

Collaborative management of testicular cancer generally involves a radical orchiectomy (surgical removal of the affected testis, spermatic cord, and regional lymph nodes). Radiation of the remaining lymph nodes may be used if the tumor is radiosensitive. Single or multiple chemotherapeutic agent regimens, including bleomycin (Blenoxane), vincristine (Oncovin), cisplatin (Platinol), vinblastine (Velban), and etoposide (VePesid), are also used before or after surgery, depending on the histologic conditions and disease stage.[33,34]

The prognosis for patients with testicular cancer has improved, and 75% of the patients obtain complete remission if the disease is detected in the early stages. All patients with testicular cancer, regardless of pathology or stage, require meticulous follow-up and regular physical examinations, chest radiography, CT scan, and assessment of hCG and AFP (if appropriate). The goal is to detect relapse when the tumor burden is minimal. Some studies have indicated a higher risk of second cancers in these men.[35] Secondary malignancies that occur as a result of chemotherapy and radiation are described in Chapter 14. The man with testicular cancer should have the opportunity to discuss fertility and sperm banking before any treatment. The nurse should be sensitive to any psychosocial problems this type of cancer can have on a man's feelings of maleness or self-worth.[36] Treatment has the potential to interfere with both erections and fertility.

SEXUAL FUNCTIONING

VASECTOMY

Vasectomy is the bilateral surgical ligation or resection of the vas deferens performed for the purpose of sterilization (Fig. 52-6). The procedure requires only 15 to 30 minutes and is usually performed with the patient under local anesthesia on an outpatient basis. Vasectomy is considered a permanent form of sterilization, although some successful reversals (vasovasotomy) have been reported.

After vasectomy, the patient should not notice any difference in the look or feel of the ejaculate, because its major component is seminal and prostatic fluid. The patient will need to use an alternative form of contraception until semen examination reveals no sperm. This usually requires at least 10 ejaculations or 6 weeks to evacuate sperm distal to the surgical site. Sperm cells continue to be produced by the testes but are absorbed by the body rather than being passed through the vas deferens. Occasionally postoperative hematoma and swelling of the scrotum occur.

Vasectomy does not affect the production of hormones, ability to ejaculate, or physiologic mechanisms related to erection or orgasm. Psychologic adjustment may be a problem after surgery. It may be very difficult for the patient to separate vasectomy from castration at a subconscious level. Some men may develop erectile dysfunction or may feel the need to become much more sexually active than they were in the past to prove their masculinity. Careful discussion of the procedure and its outcome before the surgery can be helpful in detecting patients who may have problems with psychologic adjustment. Surgery should be delayed for these patients.

ERECTILE DYSFUNCTION

Over 20 million men in the United States experience erectile dysfunction.[37] The problem is increasing in all segments of the sexually active male population and impacts both the man and his partner. In younger men the increase is attributed to an increase in substance abuse, such as recreational drugs and alcohol. Middle-aged men are affected by modern medical technology, such as major organ transplants, bypass surgeries, and chemotherapeutic agents. The older population (men over 70 years of age) are living longer, fuller lives and expect to remain sexually active, regardless of any existing medical conditions. Stress factors associated with modern lifestyles are affecting men of all ages and contribute greatly to the overall causes of erectile failure.

Etiology and Pathophysiology

Erectile dysfunction is the inability to attain or maintain an erect penis that allows satisfactory sexual performance. This problem occurs at some time or other for almost all sexually active males. The problem can occur at any age, although it most often begins among males between 55 and 65 years of age. Erection is a parasympathetic reflex initiated mainly by certain tactile, visual, and mental stimuli. It consists of dilation of the arteries and arterioles of the penis, which in turn fills and distends spaces in its erectile tissue and compresses veins. When this occurs, more blood enters the penis through the dilated arteries than leaves it through the constricted veins. The penis then becomes larger and rigid, or, in other words, erection occurs. Problems occur when these spaces (corporeal bodies) fail to fill when desired or when they empty before orgasm.

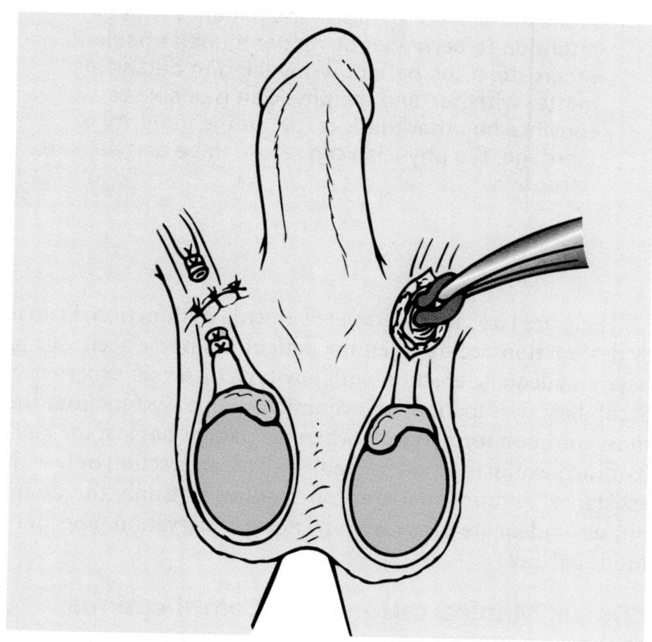

Fig. 52-6 Vasectomy procedure. The vas deferens is ligated or resected for the purpose of sterilization.

ETHICAL DILEMMAS

Sterilization

SITUATION

A 43-year-old male patient is requesting a vasectomy and informs the nurse that he does not wish to discuss this with his wife. The physician's policy is to have the spouse or partner sign a form acknowledging the patient's desire to be sterilized. This patient explains that while his wife wants to have more children, the one they already have is all he wants.

DISCUSSION

Physician practice rather than state law dictates the need for disclosure of the intent to sterilize a patient to that patient's spouse or significant other. Had the patient not informed the physician that he was married, there would be no issue. As it is, he can seek another physician to perform this procedure who has no such reservations, or he may choose to lie about his marital status. Women in most states are not required to prove that their husbands or significant others are aware of their intention to terminate a pregnancy, but the (intended) finality of a vasectomy is considered to be a different case. Professional ethics require that the nurse explain to the patient that he cannot have a vasectomy with this physician without obtaining the needed consultation with his wife. The patient would then be free to determine how to handle this problem.

ETHICAL AND LEGAL PRINCIPLES

- Patient autonomy would require that matters relating to reproduction be left to the privacy and discretion of the individual.
- Competent adults may legally choose to be sterilized for convenience or for medical reasons.
- Nonmaleficence and truth telling, however, would address the need to inform the patient's wife of his intention to permanently render himself unable to procreate. If the patient is unwilling to discuss the matter with her, and the physician is unable to convince him that this is crucial to the integrity of his marriage, the physician can refuse to be party to this deception.

There are two classifications of erectile dysfunction. Primary dysfunction occurs when the patient has never been able to have an adequate erection with any type of sexual experience. Secondary dysfunction, or acquired organic dysfunction, the most common form, occurs when the patient has lost the ability to achieve an erection or is able to have an erection only with assistance. A functional erection requires not only the desire but also adequate blood supply, nerve innervation, and hormone balance.

Clinical Manifestations and Complications

The causative factors for the disorder may be physiologic, psychologic, or both (Table 52-9). The major complication of this problem is that the man's inability to perform sexually can cause great distress in his interpersonal relationships and may interfere with his concept of himself as a man. Our society promotes images of a man being strong, capable, and sexually responsive. Table 52-10 lists normal age-related changes in sexual performance. Explanation of these age-related changes may be necessary to reassure an anxious older man regarding normal changes in his sexual abilities.

Diagnostic Studies

Rapid advances have been made in the diagnosis and treatment of erectile dysfunction. With the advent of modern technology, 80% to 90% of the causes are being attributed to physiologic reasons and can be determined by diagnostic studies. Diagnostic testing is now divided into primary and secondary levels based on findings during the initial assessment (Table 52-11). For primary testing, a complete medical history and physical examination is performed. In addition, self-administered, assessment- and treatment-related questionnaires have been developed and may prove useful as primary screening tools. For example, the International Index of Erectile Function (IIEF)[38] identifies a man's response to five key areas of male sexual function. These areas include erectile function, orgasmic function, sexual desire, intercourse satisfaction, and overall satisfaction. Intracavernosal vasoactive testing is done to help distinguish psychogenic from neurogenic or vascular causes of erectile dysfunction. In this test vasoactive agents such as papaverine, phentolamine (Regitine), or prostaglandin (PGE_1), are given to directly relax the smooth muscle of the corporal erectile tissue, causing an erection within 5 to 10 minutes. Failure of an erection to occur indicates a potential vascular etiology.

Secondary testing may include vascular flow studies (duplex Doppler, cavernosogram). Nocturnal penile tumescence may also be performed to distinguish a psychogenic from neurogenic or vascular cause. This test is based on the theory that normal erections occur during the rapid eye movement phase of sleep. The test involves recording of both sleep and penile changes.

Neurogenic factors can be evaluated using somatosensory evoked potential studies. In this test, electrical activity within the bulbocavernosa muscle is measured in response to stimulation of the penile skin. The presence of electrical activity following tactile stimulation suggests an intact sacral arc.

Collaborative Care

The treatment for erectile dysfunction is based on the cause.[37,39] Treatment of psychogenic erectile dysfunction should be carried out by a qualified therapist. The approach may be behavioral or psychologic, and in some patients it may also involve medical intervention to temporarily restore self-confidence. The goal of all erectile dysfunction therapy is to have the man and his partner develop a satisfactory sexual relationship, including good communication skills.

When the problem is physical, interventions are directed at correcting or eliminating the cause or restoring function by medical means. The results of these interventions are usually most satisfactory when both partners are involved in the deci-

Table 52-9 Risk Factors for Erectile Dysfunction

Anatomic
- Congenital deformities of the penis (e.g., hypospadias)
- Peyronie's disease

Cardiorespiratory
- Angina pectoris
- Atherosclerosis
- Emphysema
- Hypertension
- Myocardial infarction
- Post cardiac surgery

Drug Induced
- 5-alpha-reductase inhibitors (finasteride [Proscar])
- Alcohol
- Antiandrogens
- Antilipidemic agents
- Antihypertensives
- Caffeine
- Diuretics (chlorothiazide [Diuril]; spironolactone [Aldactone])
- Drugs for Parkinson's disease (carbidopa-levodopa [Sinemet])
- Estrogens
- Major tranquilizers (diazepam [Valium]; alprazolam [Xanax])
- Marijuana, cocaine, LSD
- Narcotics
- Nicotine neuroleptics (phenothiazine [Thorazine])
- Tricyclic antidepressants (amitriptyline [Elavil])

Endocrine
- Addison's disease
- Diabetes mellitus
- High levels of prolactin
- Obesity
- Pituitary tumor
- Testosterone deficiency
- Thyrotoxicosis

Genitourinary
- Cystectomy
- Hydrocele
- Perineal or suprapubic prostatectomy
- Phimosis
- Post kidney transplant
- Postpriapism
- Prostatitis
- Renal failure
- Varicocele

Neurologic and nerve conduction
- Central nervous system disorders
- Cerbrovascular accident
- Electroshock therapy
- Multiple sclerosis
- Parkinson's disease
- Peripheral neuropathic conditions
- Spina bifida
- Sympathectomy
- Trauma to the spinal cord
- Tumors or transection of spinal cord

Psychogenic
- Depression
- Excessive stress in family, work, or interpersonal relationships
- Fatigue
- Fear of failure to perform

Vascular
- Aortic aneurysm
- Aortofemoral bypass
- Atherosclerosis of pelvic blood vessels

GERONTOLOGIC DIFFERENCES IN ASSESSMENT

Table 52-10 Sexual Performance

1. Time lag between perceiving sexual opportunity and full erection
2. Diminished size and rigidity of the penis at full erection
3. Increased time interval to ejaculation
4. Changed nature of ejaculation with less spurting and lessened intensity of feeling
5. Shortened period between ejaculation and flaccidity
6. Increase in time to next reaction to sexual stimulation

*For almost all men by the age of 45 to 50 years.

sion-making process and have realistic expectations of the treatment. Many treatment options are available to the man experiencing vascular or neurogenic erectile dysfunction. Clinical practice guidelines on erectile dysfunction were developed by the American Urological Association.[40] Treatment recommendations include vasoactive drug therapy, vacuum constrictive devices, and penile prosthesis. Other invasive and experimental techniques are limited to research centers.

Nonsurgical Management

Drug therapy. Whenever possible, collaboration should occur between the primary physician providing the medical care and the urologist treating the erectile dysfunction. Elimination of or substitution for a medication that causes erectile dysfunction is sometimes all that is necessary to alleviate the problem (see Table 52-9).

When there is an established diagnosis of testicular failure (hypogonadism), androgen replacement therapy may sometimes be effective in improving erectile function. It should be given as an intramuscular injection of testosterone enanthate (Delatestryl) or testosterone cypionate (Virilon). Oral androgens that are currently available are not as effective. The effectiveness of testosterone supplementation for older men experiencing a normal, gradual decline is doubtful. Careful evaluation of the man's serum testosterone level and prostate

DIAGNOSTIC STUDIES

Table 52-11 Erectile Dysfunction

Primary
- Medical history and physical examination
- Detailed sexual history, including practices and techniques
- Psychosocial evaluation
- Testosterone levels
- Prostate-specific antigen
- Intracavernosal vasoactive testing

Secondary
- Hormone profile (e.g., prolactin, FSH, LH)
- Vascular flow studies (e.g., duplex Doppler, cavernosogram)
- Neurologic evaluation
- Sacral evoked potential test
- Nocturnal penile tumescence
- Tests to exclude unrecognized systemic disease: CBC, urinalysis, creatinine, lipid profile, FBS, thyroid function studies

FBS, fasting blood sugar; *FSH,* follicle stimulating hormone; *LH,* luteinizing hormone.

condition must precede introduction of this therapy. Administration of testosterone to a man with normal levels of hormone production may actually suppress the body's natural ability to produce testosterone. Testosterone is contraindicated in men with cancer of the prostate because of its ability to cause proliferation of the prostate cancer cells. For men with hyperprolactinemia, bromocriptine (Parlodel) therapy is often effective in normalizing the prolactin level and improving sexual functioning.

A major breakthrough in the treatment of erectile dysfunction has been in the area of penile vasoactive drug therapy. The medication enhances blood flow into the penile arteries. Until recently the only method available for administration was in the form of penile injections. These medications are now available in pill, gel, patch, pellet, and injection form. Current vasoactive medications include papaverine (topical gel or injection),[41,42] alprostadil (topical, transurethral pellet [e.g., MUSE], or injection),[43-47] phentolamine (Regitine) in combination with other vasoactive medications (injection), vasoactive intestinal peptide (injection), and sildenafil (Viagra, pill).[48]

The vasoactive medication dose is regulated on an individual basis to prevent side effects. Side effects may include penile pain, priapism, corporal fibrosis, fibrotic nodules, and hypotension. It is important to instruct patients carefully on the specific administration techniques and precautions for any of the vasoactive medications.

Home injection therapy instruction is given to those men who are suitable candidates for the therapy. The injection is nearly painless and generally begins to work in 20 to 30 minutes. Success rates have been high when there is adequate patient teaching and follow-up.[49-51] This treatment is not suitable for men with severe vascular problems, intolerance for transient hypotension, severe psychiatric disease, poor manual dexterity, or poor vision or those receiving anticoagulant therapy. The man may discontinue treatment if he perceives a lack of spontaneity, has a needle phobia, or wants a more permanent treatment option.

The latest advances in treatment of erectile dysfunction are the oral vasoactive medications. The most widely prescribed medication is sildenafil (Viagra), a pill that increases smooth muscle relaxation in the penis by blocking specific enzymes.[52] Viagra is generally taken 30 to 60 minutes before engaging in sexual activity. The usual dose is 50 to 100 mg orally and has a success rate of approximately 70% to 80% for psychogenic causes, 50% to 60% in diabetes mellitus, and 40% to 50% in radical prostatectomy patients. It should be avoided in men using nitrates (antianginal agents) such as Isordil, nitroglycerin, Nitro-Bid, and Transderm Nitro and used cautiously in men with retinitis pigmentosa. Other oral medications under investigation include apomorphine (a parkinsonian drug), which affects brain chemistry, and Vasomax, an oral version of an injectable vasodilator.[52]

Aids or devices. Suction devices applied to the flaccid penis produce an erection by pulling blood up into the corporeal bodies. A penile ring or other device is placed around the base of the penis, causing vasoconstriction and preventing detumescence (subsidence of swelling). Special care must be taken in using these devices to prevent tissue damage. Suction devices are sometimes used in conjunction with intracorporeal injection therapy and in those patients with moderate to severe venous leaks of the penile veins.[53]

Alternative methods. Some patients do not require penetration for satisfactory sexual expression, and a vibrator or dildo (rubber penis) could be used by the partner. Patients experiencing temporary loss of erection or who are awaiting surgical interventions can use a variety of methods to achieve sexual satisfaction. Sexual counselors or therapists acting as consultants can provide support and suggest alternative forms of sexual expression.

Surgical Therapy

Penile implants. Penile implants have provided surgical management of erectile dysfunction for more than 25 years. The paired devices can be semirigid, malleable, or inflatable (Fig. 52-7).[54,55] They are implanted into the corporeal bodies to provide an erection firm enough for penetration. All implants provide a usable erection and should be chosen carefully based on the man's mental and physical capabilities, surgical risk factors, personal lifestyle, insurance, and financial resources. The main problems associated with penile prostheses are mechanical failure, infection, and erosions.

For essentially healthy men the surgical procedure may be performed on an outpatient basis, with patients being monitored by home care nurses. Complete recovery time varies from 4 to 6 weeks. Patients considered to be at high risk for complications include those with uncontrolled diabetes mellitus and those with severe circulatory problems.

Patients should be advised that none of the options will restore ejaculation or tactile sensations if they were absent before treatment. Sexual counseling is often recommended before and after treatment. The ability to please both partners enhances satisfaction levels.

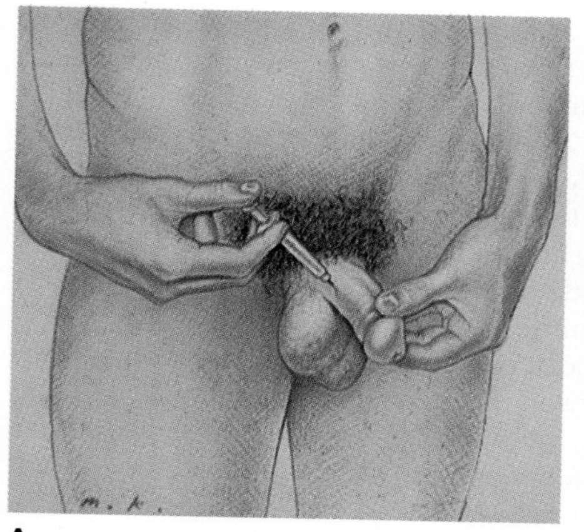
A

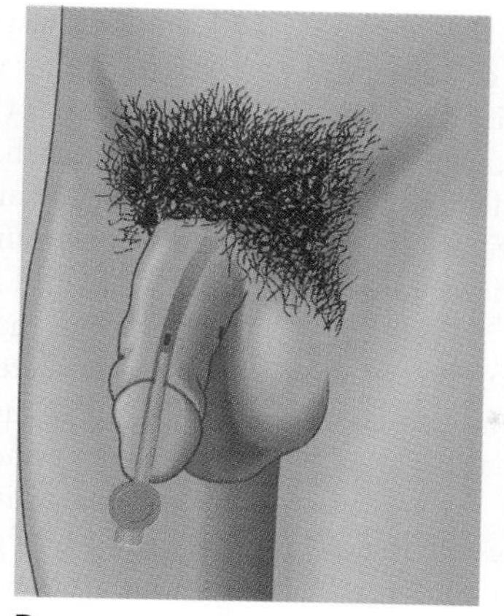
B

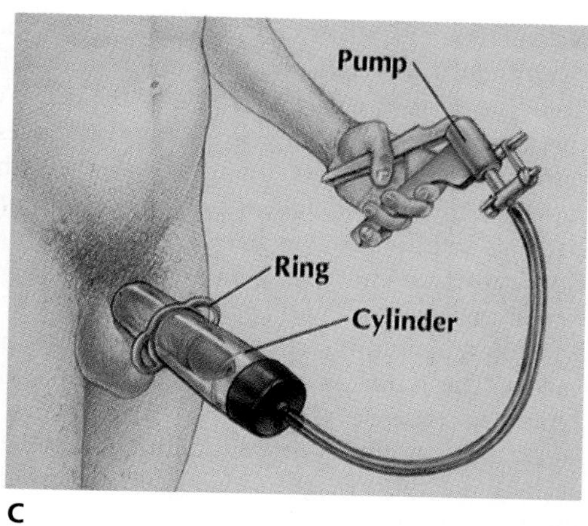

C

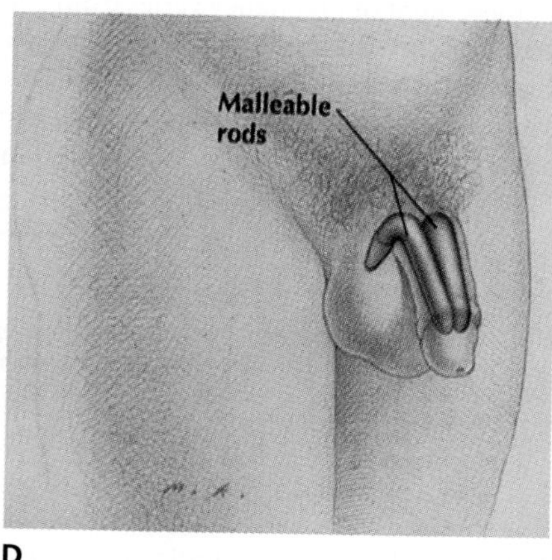

D

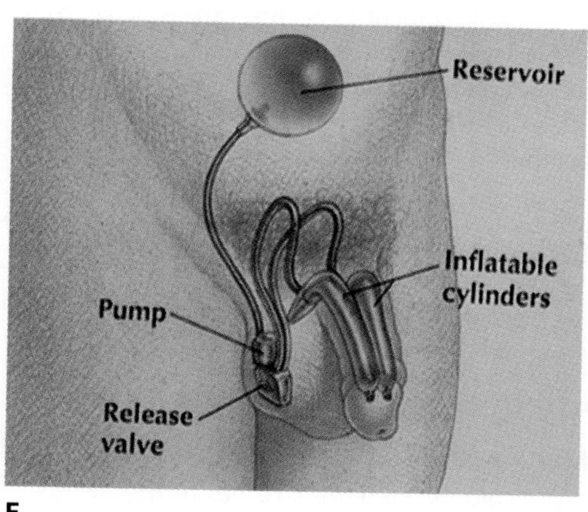

E

Fig. 52-7 **A,** Self-injection therapy involves injecting a medication directly into the penis. This increases blood flow and causes an erection. **B,** Intraurethral pellets are used to deliver drug therapy. **C,** With the vacuum device in place, blood can be drawn into the penis by means of a hand pump. This creates an erection. For intercourse, the ring is slipped to the base of the penis and the cylinder removed. **D,** A malleable implant is always erect but can be bent close to the body for concealment. **E,** Inflatable implants consist of cylinders in the penis, a small pump in the scrotum, and a reservoir in the lower abdomen. When activated, the pump fills the cylinders with fluid from the reservoir. A small release valve permits the fluid to drain back into the reservoir after intercourse.

NURSING MANAGEMENT: ERECTILE DYSFUNCTION

The man experiencing erectile dysfunction requires a great deal of emotional support for both himself and his partner. Men often do not feel comfortable discussing their problems with others because of society's expectations of a man's sexual abilities. The man may experience and demonstrate isolation from support systems, and he may also lose self-esteem, which can eventually lead to loss of role functions.[56]

The patient needs reassurance that confidentiality will be maintained. In conjunction with medical treatment, it often becomes necessary to provide counseling and therapy for the couple to establish realistic expectations and develop meaningful communication patterns. The majority of men wait an average of 2 years before seeking medical assistance. They are often highly motivated and expect immediate solutions to their problems. The health care team should provide a support system and accurate information as soon as possible.[56]

Nurses are in a unique position of conducting routine health assessments on men seeking any form of medical treatment. It provides an opportunity to ask not only general health questions but also those seldom-asked sexual function ones as well. Given the opportunity, most men do not hesitate to answer these questions when they know that someone cares and can provide them with answers.

INFERTILITY

In about one third of childless marriages in which children are desired, the primary cause of infertility is due to male factors.[56] Infertility can be caused by disorders of the hypothalamic-pituitary system, disorders of the testes, and abnormalities of the ejaculatory system.

The physical causes are generally divided into three categories: pre-testicular, testicular, and post-testicular. The pre-testicular or endocrine causes occur only in about 3% of the cases and can generally be treated with medication or surgery. Testicular problems make up 50% of the cases. Varicoceles are the major cause with 60% involving the left testis, 39% both testes, and only 1% involving the right testis. Other factors that influence the testes include infection (e.g., mumps virus, STDs, bacterial infections), congenital anomalies, medications, radiation, substance abuse, and environmental hazards.[57] Post-testicular causes account for approximately 5% to 7% of the cases, with obstruction, infection, or vasectomy being the primary causes. The remaining 40% are classified as idiopathic or of unknown causes.

A careful health history includes occupation; lifestyle issues such as hot tubs, weight training, or wearing tight undergarments; sexual practices; frequency of intercourse; and emotional factors such as stress levels and the desire for children. The use of drugs, such as chemotherapeutic agents, anabolic steroids (testosterone), sulfasalazine (Azulfidine), cimetidine (Tagamet), and recreational drugs, should be documented. A physical examination can disclose a varicocele, Peyronie's disease, or other physical abnormalities.

The first test in an infertility study is a semen analysis. The test determines the sperm concentration (count greater than 20 million/ml), forward progressive motility (at least 60% with a grade greater than 2), and morphology (at least 60% have normal oval head and long tail). Additional tests that may be helpful in determining the etiology include plasma testosterone and serum LH and FSH measurements. A test for sperm penetration abilities may also be done. The specific cause of infertility is often not determined.

The nurse should be concerned and tactful in dealing with the male patient undergoing infertility studies. For many men, fertility and masculinity are equated. The nurse must be sensitive to the problem of gender identity in the infertile man.[56] Treatment options for the man include medications,[58] conservative lifestyle changes (e.g., avoidance of scrotal heat, substance abuse, high stress), in vitro fertilization techniques, and corrective surgery. Achievement of pregnancy varies from 8% to 60% and ranges in cost from several hundred to several thousand dollars. Infertility can seriously strain a marriage, and the couple may require counseling and discussion of alternatives if conception is not achieved. (Female infertility is discussed in Chapter 51.)

CRITICAL THINKING EXERCISES

CASE STUDY

Benign Prostatic Hyperplasia

Patient Profile

Mr. R.K., a 71-year-old married man, comes to the emergency department because of an inability to void for the past 12 hours.

Subjective Data

- Complains of severe bladder pain and pressure
- Is very restless and agitated
- Relates history of three cans of beer at party the previous evening; has not voided since then

Objective Data

Physical Examination

- Has prostate enlargement on rectal examination
- Has hematuria and WBCs in urine
- Has palpable bladder above umbilicus

Laboratory Studies

- PSA: 8 ng/ml (normal: 0 to 4 ng/ml)

Collaborative Care

- Indwelling catheter inserted by a urology resident
- Mr. R.K. admitted to the hospital

Critical Thinking Questions

1. What risk factors for acute urinary retention and BPH are present in Mr. R.K.?
2. Explain the etiology of the objective symptoms Mr. R.K. exhibited.
3. Discuss the pharmacologic options available to Mr. R.K.
4. Discuss the invasive options available to Mr. R.K.
5. Mr. R.K. asks you about the effect of the various treatment options on his ability to have sex. How would you respond?
6. Write one or more appropriate nursing diagnoses based on the assessment data presented. Are there any collaborative problems?
7. On further assessment, you note that Mr. R.K. has a nursing diagnosis of decisional conflict. How would you help him resolve this conflict related to treatment options?

NURSING RESEARCH ISSUES

1. Is a man more likely to report problems related to prostatic enlargement directly to the health care provider or via a printed questionnaire?
2. What percentage of patients with prostatic enlargement have a concurrent urinary tract infection?
3. What is the best strategy to get men over 40 years of age to have an annual digital rectal examination?
4. What relaxation techniques are most effective in relieving bladder spasms after a transurethral or suprapubic prostatectomy?
5. How receptive are men with an erectile dysfunction to the idea of a prosthetic device to accomplish an erection?
6. What is the compliance rate for testicular self-examination at 3, 6, and 12 months following a training program for high school boys?
7. Does awareness of behaviors that can cause acute urinary retention in men with BPH alter the practice of these behaviors?

REVIEW QUESTIONS

The number of the question corresponds to the same-numbered objective at the beginning of the chapter.

1. A patient with BPH experiences hesitancy in initiating voiding and a feeling of incomplete bladder emptying. In assessing for complications related to these symptoms the nurse asks specifically about the presence of
   a. constipation.
   b. dysuria and urgency.
   c. gross blood in the urine.
   d. decreased force of the urinary stream.
2. Postoperatively a patient who has had a transurethral prostatectomy has continuous bladder irrigation with a three-way Foley with a 30 ml balloon and traction applied. The patient complains that he feels the urge to void even with the catheter in place. The nurse should
   a. hand irrigate the catheter to ensure that it is patent.
   b. deflate the catheter balloon to 10 ml to decrease bulk in the bladder.
   c. encourage the patient to try to have a bowel movement to relieve colon pressure.
   d. explain that this feeling is normal and that he should not try to urinate around the catheter.
3. In teaching health promotion related to early detection of prostate cancer the nurse advises that beginning at middle age men should have an annual
   a. urinalysis.
   b. rectal examination.
   c. prostatic ultrasound.
   d. prostatic acid phosphatase (PAP).
4. A patient scheduled for a suprapubic prostatectomy for prostate cancer expresses the fear that he will be impotent. In responding to the patient the nurse explains that
   a. sterility, but not impotence, is common with a suprapubic prostatectomy.
   b. the most common complication of this surgery is postoperative urinary retention.
   c. a penile implant may be an alternative to consider after he has recovered from his surgery.
   d. pain control will be a more important factor than sexual function in the long-term consideration of his condition.
5. The nurse advises the patient with chronic prostatitis that long-term management includes
   a. a permanent indwelling catheter.
   b. regular injection of sclerosing agents.
   c. sexual activities that result in ejaculation.
   d. aspiration or surgical drainage of abscesses.
6. Discharge teaching for the patient who has had a vasectomy includes explaining that
   a. the procedure blocks the production of sperm.
   b. an alternative form of contraception will be necessary for 6 to 8 weeks.
   c. the ejaculate will be about half the volume it was before the procedure.
   d. erectile dysfunction is temporary and will return with continued sexual activity.
7. A nursing measure that can decrease the patient's discomfort over care involving his reproductive organs includes
   a. relating his sexual concerns to his sexual partner.
   b. arranging to have only male nurses care for the patient.
   c. maintaining a nonjudgmental attitude toward his sexual practices.
   d. using only technical terminology when discussing reproductive function.

References

1. McConnell JD and others: *Benign prostatic hyperplasia: diagnosis and treatment. Clinical practice guideline no. 8,* AHCPR publ no 940582, Rockville, Md, 1994, Agency for Health Care Policy and Research, Public Health Service, US Department of Health and Human Services.
2. Prostate Health Council: *Enlarged prostate: BPH and male urinary problems,* Baltimore, 1998, American Foundation for Urologic Disease.
3. Reilly NJ: Benign prostatic hyperplasia. In Meredith CE, Karlowicz KA, editors: *Urologic nursing: a study guide,* New Jersey, 1995, Soc of Urol Nurs Assoc.
4. Barry MJ and others: A nationwide survey of practicing urologists: current management of benign prostatic hyperplasia and clinically localized prostate cancer, *Urology* 158:488, 1997.
5. Oesterling JE: Benign prostatic hyperplasia: medical and minimally invasive treatment options, *N Engl JMed* 332:99, 1995.
6. Albertsen PC: Prostate disease in older men: benign hyperplasia, *Hosp Pract* 32:61, 1997.
7. Campo B and others: Transurethral needle ablation (TUNA) of the prostate: a clinical and urodynamic evaluation, *Urology* 49:847, 1997.
*8. Bartkui TP, Goldfarb B, Trachtenberg J: Understanding microwave therapy as a treatment option for benign prostatic hyperplasia, *Urol Nurs* 17:53, 1997.
9. Ramsey EW, Miller PD, Parsons K: A novel transurethral microwave thermal ablation system to treat benign prostatic hyperplasia: results of a prospective multicenter clinical trial, *J Urol* 158:112, 1997.
10. Anderson RJ: Primary care management of benign prostatic hyperplasia, *Hosp Pract* 33:11, 1998.
11. Angelucci PA: Caring for patients with benign prostatic hyperplasia, *Nursing* 27:54, 1997.
12. Albertsen PC: Prostate disease in older men: cancer, *Hosp Pract* 32:159, 1997.
13. LaFollette SS, Reilly NJ: Cancer of the prostate. In Meredith CE, Karlowicz KA, editors: *Urologic nursing: a study guide,* New Jersey, 1995, Soc of Urol Nurs Assoc.
14. Powell IJ and others: Outcome of African American men screened for prostate cancer: the Detroit Education and Early Detection study, *J Urol* 158:146, 1997.
15. Choday GW and others: Results of conservative management of clinically localized prostate cancer, *N Engl J Med* 330:242, 1994.
16. Zincke H and others: Radical prostatectomy for clinically localized prostate cancer: long-term results of 1,143 patients from a single institution, *J Clin Oncol* 12:2254, 1994.
17. Catalona WJ, Basler JW: Return of erections and urinary continence following nerve sparing radical retropubic prostatectomy, *J Urol* 150:905, 1993.
18. Jonler M and others: Sequelae of radical prostatectomy, *Br J Urol* 74:352, 1994.
19. Lim AJ and others: Quality of life: radical prostatectomy versus radiation therapy for prostate cancer, *J Urol* 154:1420, 1995.
20. Litwin MS and others: Quality of life outcomes in men treated for localized prostate cancer, *JAMA* 273:129, 1995.
21. Helgason AR and others: Factors associated with waning sexual function among elderly men and prostate cancer patients, *J Urol* 158:155, 1997.
22. Bolla M and others: Improved survival in patients with locally advanced prostate cancer treated with radiotherapy and goserelin, *N Engl J Med* 337:295, 1997.
23. Brufsky A and others: Finasteride and flutamide as potency-sparing androgen-ablative therapy for advanced adenocarcinoma of the prostate, *Urology* 49:913, 1997.
24. Kirschenbaum A: Management of hormonal treatment effects, *Cancer* 75:1983, 1995.
*25. Jakobsson L, Hallberg IR, Loven L: Met and unmet nursing care needs in men with prostate cancer: an explorative study, *Eur J Cancer Care* 6:117, 1997.
*26. Davison BJ, Degner LF: Empowerment of men newly diagnosed with prostate cancer, *Cancer Nurs* 20:187, 1997.
27. Thin RN: Diagnosis of chronic prostatitis: overview and update, *Int J STD AIDS* 8:475, 1997.
28. Krieger JN and others: Chronic pelvic pains represent the most prominent urogenital symptoms of "chronic prostatitis," *Urology* 48:715, 1996.

29. Donovan DA, Nicholas PK: Prostatitis: diagnosis and treatment in primary care, *Nurse Pract* 22:144, 1997.
30. Pansadoro V and others: Prostate-specific antigen and prostatitis in men under fifty, *Eur Urol* 30:24, 1996.
31. Nickel JC, Sorensen R: Transurethral microwave thermotherapy for nonbacterial prostatitis: a randomized double-blind sham controlled study using new prostatitis specific assessment questionnaires, *J Urol* 155:1950, 1996.
32. McLachlan JA and others: Are estrogens carcinogenic during development of the testes? *AOMIS* 106:240, 1998.
33. Pont J and others: Chemotherapy should follow orchiectomy in high-risk patients, *J Clin Oncol* 14:441, 1996.
34. Leibovitch I and others: Delayed orchiectomy after chemotherapy for metastatic nonseminomatous germ cell tumors, *J Urol* 155:952, 1996.
35. Travis LB and others: Risk of second malignant neoplasms among long-term survivors of testicular cancer, *J Natl Cancer Inst* 89:1439, 1997.
36. Arai Y and others: Psychosocial aspects in long-term survivors of testicular cancer, *J Urol* 155:574, 1996.
37. Kim ED, Lipshultz LI: Advances in the treatment of organic erectile dysfunction, *Hosp Pract* 32:101, 1997.
38. Rosen RC and others: The international index of erectile function (IIEF): a multidimensional scale for assessment of erectile dysfunction, *Urology* 49:822, 1997.
39. Greiner KA, Weigel JW: Erectile dysfunction, *Am Fam Physician* 54:1675, 1996.
40. Montague DK and others: Clinical guidelines panel on erectile dysfunction: summary report on the treatment of organic erectile dysfunction. The American Urological Association, *J Urol* 156:2007, 1996.
41. Bechara A and others: Comparative study of papaverine plus phentolamine versus prostaglandin-E1 in erectile dysfunction, *J Urol* 157:2132, 1997.
42. Kim ED, el-Rashidy R, McVary KT: Papaverine topical gel for treatment of erectile dysfunction, *J Urol* 153:361, 1995.
*43. Kupecz D: Alprostadil for the treatment of erectile dysfunction, *Nurs Pract* 21:143, 1996.
44. Linet OI, Ogrine FG: Efficacy and safety of intracavernosal alprostadil in men with erectile dysfunction. The Alprostadil Study Group, *N Engl J Med* 334:873, 1996.
45. Kim ED, McVary KT: Topical prostaglandin-E1 for the treatment of erectile dysfunction, *J Urol* 153:182, 1995.
46. Padma-Nathan H and others: Treatment of men with erectile dysfunction with transurethral alprostadil, *N Engl J Med* 336:1, 1997.
47. Hellstrom WJ and others: A double-blind, placebo-controlled evaluation of the erectile response to transurethral alprostadil, *Urology* 48:851, 1996.

*Nursing research-based article.

48. McMahon CG: A pilot study of the role of intracavernous injection of vasoactive intestinal peptide (VIP) and phentolamine mesylate in the treatment of erectile dysfunction, *Int J Impot Res* 8:233, 1996.
49. Truss MC and others: Intracavernous pharmacotherapy, *World J Urol* 15:71, 1997.
50. Sundaram CP and others: Long-term follow-up of patients receiving injection therapy for erectile dysfunction, *Urology* 49:932, 1997.
51. Riley AJ, Athanasiadis L: Impotence and its non-surgical management, *Br J Clin Pract* 51:99, 1997.
52. Boolel M and others: Sildenafil, a novel effective oral therapy for male erectile dysfunction, *Br J Urol* 78:257, 1996.
53. Soderdahl DW, Thrasher JB, Hansberry KL: Intracavernosal drug-induced erection therapy versus external vacuum devices in the treatment of erectile dysfunction, *Br J Urol* 79:952, 1997.
54. Shafik A: Hollow and fenestrated penile prosthesis: a new implant for treatment of impotence, *Arch Androl* 38:93, 1997.
55. Goldstein I and others: Safety and efficacy of mentor alpha-1 inflatable penile prosthesis implantation for impotence treatment, *J Urol* 157:833, 1997.
56. Meredith CE: Erectile dysfunction. In Karlowicz KA, editor: *Urologic nursing: principles and practice*, Philadelphia, 1995, Saunders.
57. Bigelow PL and others: Association of semen quality and occupational factors: comparison of case-control analysis and analysis of continuous variables, *Fertil Steril* 69:11, 1998.
58. Gregoriou O and others: Treatment of idiopathic oligozoospermia with an alpha-blocker: a placebo controlled, double-blind trial, *Int J Fertil Womens Med* 42:301, 1997.

Resources

National Prostate Cancer Coalition
1156 15th Street NW, Suite 905
Washington, DC 20005
202-463-9455
Fax: 202-463-9456
http://www.4npcc.org/

Prostate Cancer Home Page
c/o UMHS
1500 E. Medical Center Dr.
Ann Arbor, MI 48109
734-936-4000
http://www.cancer.med.umich.edu/prostcan/prostcan.html

For additional Internet resources, see the website for this book at www.mosby.com/MERLIN/medsurg_lewis

SECTION

11

PROBLEMS RELATED TO MOVEMENT AND COORDINATION

SECTION OUTLINE

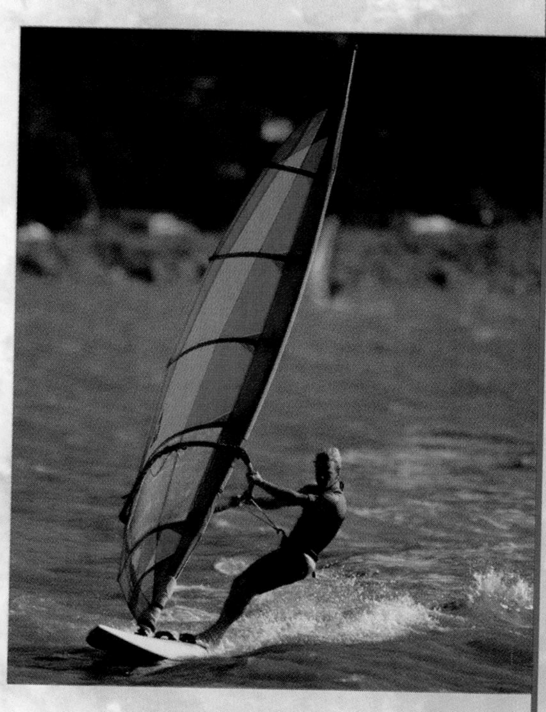

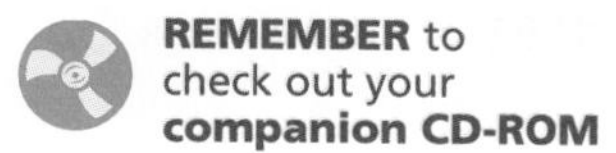

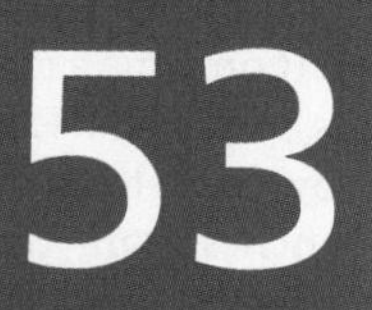

53 NURSING ASSESSMENT Neurologic System

Judith M. Ozuna

www.mosby.com/MERLIN/medsurg_lewis

LEARNING OBJECTIVES

1. Describe the functions of neurons and neuroglia.
2. Explain the electrochemical aspects of nerve impulse transmission.
3. Explain the anatomic location and functions of the cerebrum, brainstem, cerebellum, spinal cord, peripheral nerves, and cerebrospinal fluid.
4. Identify the major arteries supplying the brain.
5. Describe the functions of the 12 cranial nerves.
6. Compare the functions of the two divisions of the autonomic nervous system.
7. Describe age-related changes in the neurologic system and differences in assessment findings.
8. Identify the significant subjective and objective data related to the nervous system that should be obtained from a patient.
9. Describe the techniques used in the physical assessment of the nervous system.
10. Differentiate normal from common abnormal findings of a physical assessment of the nervous system.
11. Describe the purpose, significance of results, and nursing responsibilities related to diagnostic studies of the nervous system.

STRUCTURES AND FUNCTIONS OF THE NERVOUS SYSTEM

The human nervous system is a highly specialized system responsible for the control and integration of the body's many activities. The nervous system can be divided into the central nervous system (CNS) and the peripheral nervous system (PNS). The CNS consists of the brain and spinal cord. The PNS consists of the cranial and spinal nerves and the peripheral components of the autonomic nervous system (ANS). Before considering higher-order structures and their functions, cellular elements and nerve impulse transmission are discussed.

Cells of the Nervous System

The nervous system is made up of two types of cells: neurons and neuroglia. Although neuroglial cells are more numerous, they are mainly supportive to the neuron, the primary functional unit of the nervous system. Neurons are generally nonmitotic; that is, they do not replicate and cannot replace themselves if they are irreversibly damaged. Neuroglia, however, are mitotic and can replicate themselves.

Neurons. The neurons of the nervous system come in many different shapes and sizes, but they all share common characteristics: (1) excitability, or the ability to generate a nerve impulse; (2) conductivity, or the ability to transmit the impulse to other portions of the cell; and (3) the ability to influence other neurons, muscle cells, and glandular cells by transmitting nerve impulses to them.

A typical neuron consists of a cell body, an axon, and several dendrites (Fig. 53-1). The cell body containing the nucleus and cytoplasm is the metabolic center of the neuron. Dendrites are short processes extending from the cell body. They receive nerve impulses from the axons of other neurons and conduct impulses toward the cell body. The nerve axon projects varying distances from the cell body, ranging from several micrometers to more than a meter. Its function is to carry nerve impulses to other neurons or to end organs. The end organs are smooth and striated muscles and glands. Axons may be myelinated or unmyelinated. Many axons present in the CNS and the PNS are covered by a segmentally interrupted myelin sheath composed of a white, lipid substance that acts as an insulator for the conduction of impulses. Generally, the smaller fibers are unmyelinated.

Neuroglia. Neuroglia, or glial cells, provide support, nourishment, and protection to neurons. They constitute almost half the brain and spinal cord mass and are 5 to 10 times more numerous than neurons. Different types of glial cells, including oligodendroglia, astrocytes, ependymal cells, and microglia, have specific functions. Oligodendroglia produce the myelin sheath of nerve fibers in the CNS (Schwann cells myelinate the nerve fibers in the periphery) and are primarily found in the white matter of the CNS. Astrocytes are found primarily in gray matter; however, their physiologic importance is not well understood. They are thought to provide structural support to neurons and their delicate processes, form the blood-brain barrier with the endothelium of the blood vessels, and play an indirect role in synaptic transmission (conduction of impulses between neurons). When the

Reviewed by Mary Baird, RN, MN, ARNP, Nurse Practitioner, Neuromuscular Associates, Olympia, Wash; Lecturer, School of Nursing, University of Washington, Seattle, Wash.

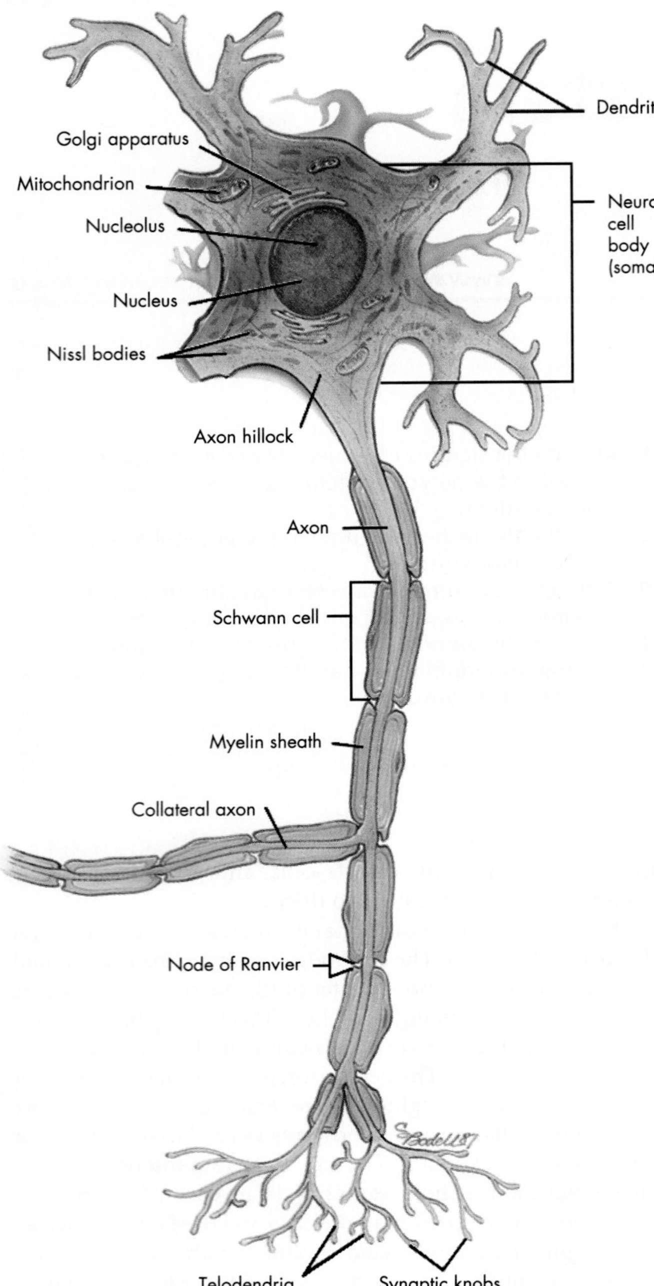

Fig. 53-1 Structural features of neurons: dendrites, cell body, and axons.

brain is injured, astrocytes act as phagocytes for neuronal debris. They help restore the neurochemical milieu and provide support for repair. Proliferation of astrocytes contributes to the formation of scar tissue (gliosis) in the CNS. Ependymal cells line the brain ventricles and aid in the secretion of cerebrospinal fluid. Microglia, a type of macrophage, are relatively rare in normal CNS tissue. They migrate to areas of CNS damage, act as phagocytes, and are important in host defense.

Most primary CNS tumors involve neuroglia. Primary malignancies involving neurons are rare because these cells are usually not mitotic.

Nerve Regeneration

Once a neuron dies, it is generally not replaced. If only the axon of the nerve cell is damaged, the cell attempts to repair itself. When damaged, all nerve cells attempt to grow back to their original destinations by sprouting many branches from the damaged ends of their axons. Unfortunately, axons in the CNS are less successful than peripheral axons in regenerating. This difference may be because of dense scar tissue that develops in the CNS and forms a barrier. Regenerating nerve fibers grow 4 mm per day.

In the PNS (outside the brain and the spinal cord), injured nerve fibers can successfully regenerate by growing within the protective myelin sheath of the supporting Schwann cells if the cell body is intact. The final result of nerve regeneration depends on the number of axon sprouts that join with the appropriate Schwann cell columns and reinnervate appropriate end organs.

Nerve Impulse

The purpose of a neuron is to initiate, receive, and process messages about events both within and outside the body. The initiation of a neuronal message (nerve impulse) involves the generation of an action potential. Once an action potential is initiated, a series of action potentials travels along the axon. When the impulse reaches the end of the nerve fiber, it is transmitted across the junction between nerve cells (synapse) by a chemical interaction involving neurotransmitters. This chemical interaction generates another set of action potentials in the next neuron. These events are repeated until the nerve impulse reaches its destination.

Action Potential. When nerve cells are in a resting (nonactive) state, the inside of the cell carries a negative electric charge relative to the outside of the cell. Sodium ions (Na^+) are in high concentration outside the cell, and potassium ions (K^+) are in high concentration inside the cell. The difference in electric charge across the cell membrane is termed the *resting membrane potential* (Fig. 53-2). An action potential occurs when a stimulus is of sufficient magnitude to alter the membrane potential.

During the action potential, the cell membrane becomes more permeable to Na^+, allowing the Na^+ to move readily into the cell. The resulting change in the voltage across the cell membrane is called *depolarization.* The inside of the cell temporarily becomes positive relative to the outside. After rapid depolarization, *repolarization* (the inside of the cell becoming negative relative to the outside) is facilitated by a slower increase in K^+ permeability, which in turn is caused by the depolarization associated with entry of Na^+ into the cell. The whole process of depolarization and repolarization of the nerve cell membrane takes only 1 to 2 milliseconds. With repeated action potentials the cells accumulate Na^+. An active metabolic process within the cell is required to move Na^+ out of and K^+ back into the cell. This metabolic process is accomplished by the Na^+-K^+ pump, which requires energy from the breakdown of adenosine triphosphate (ATP).

The action potential has an all-or-none quality; that is, once the cell depolarizes enough to cause an action potential, the size of the action potential is independent of the strength of the stimulus. When an action potential is initiated at one point

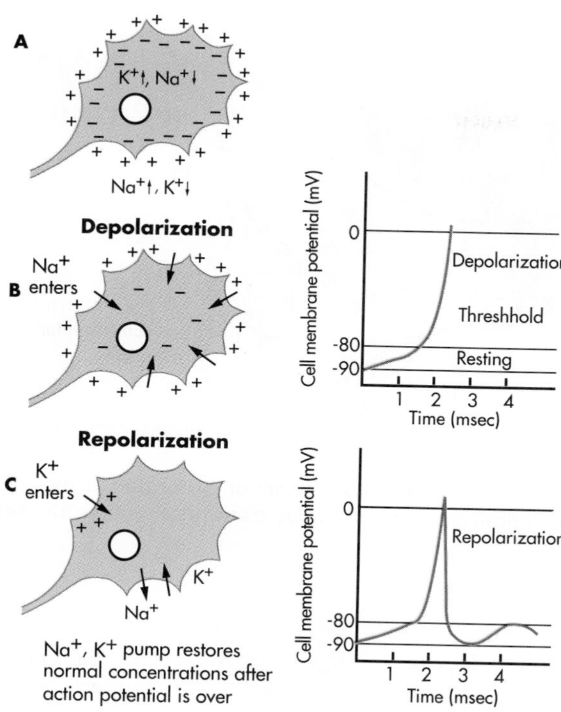

Fig. 53-2 **A,** Resting membrane potential. **B,** Depolarization. **C,** Repolarization.

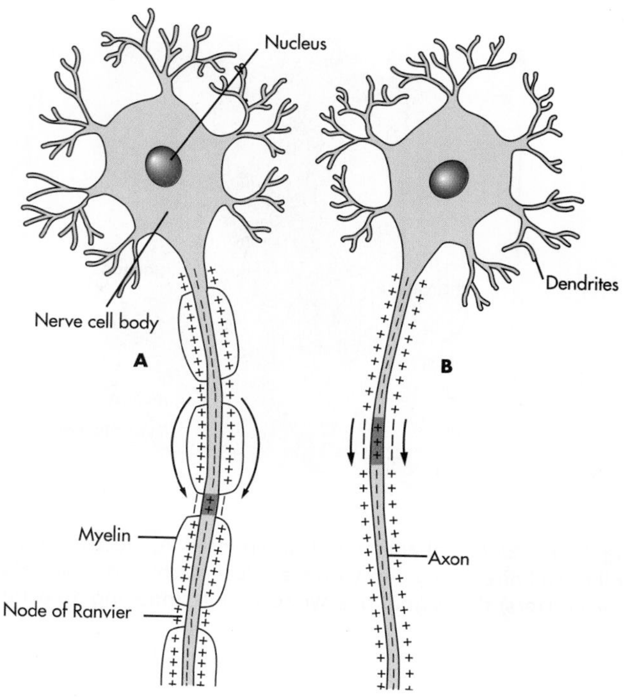

Fig. 53-3 **A,** Saltatory conduction in a myelinated nerve. **B,** Depolarization in an unmyelinated fiber.

of a neuron, it is transmitted along the axon without losing its intensity.

Because of its insulating capacity, myelination of nerve axons facilitates the conduction of an action potential. Many peripheral nerve axons have gaps, termed *nodes of Ranvier,* at regular intervals in the myelin sheath surrounding them. An action potential traveling down one of these axons hops from node to node without traversing the insulated membrane segment between nodes, making the action potential travel much faster than it would otherwise. This is called *saltatory (hopping) conduction.* In an unmyelinated fiber the wave of depolarization traverses the entire length of the axon, each portion of the membrane becoming depolarized in turn. Figure 53-3 compares nerve impulse transmission of myelinated and unmyelinated fibers.

Synapse. A synapse is the structural and functional junction between two neurons. It is the point at which the nerve impulse is transmitted from one neuron to another or from neuron to end or effector organ. The essential structures of synaptic transmission are a presynaptic terminal, a synaptic cleft, and a receptor site on the postsynaptic cell (Fig. 53-4). When a nerve impulse reaches the end of the axon (presynaptic terminal), it causes release of a chemical substance (neurotransmitter) from tiny vesicles within the axon terminal. This release depends on influx of calcium (Ca^+), initiated by depolarization of the nerve terminal. The neurotransmitter then crosses the microscopic space (synaptic cleft) between the two neurons and attaches to receptor sites of the receiving (postsynaptic) neuron. This causes a change in the permeability of the postsynaptic cell membrane to specific ions such as Na^+ and K^+ and a change in the electric potential of the membrane.

Neurotransmitters. Neurotransmitters are chemical agents involved in the transmission of an impulse across the synaptic cleft. Some neurotransmitters are excitatory: they cause an increase in Na^+ permeability at the postsynaptic cell membrane, increasing the likelihood that an action potential will be generated. This type of synaptic input results in an excitatory postsynaptic potential. Other neurotransmitters are inhibitory: they cause an increase in permeability of K^+ and chloride (Cl^-) ions, decreasing the likelihood that an action potential will be generated. This type of synaptic input results in an inhibitory postsynaptic potential.

Each of the hundreds to thousands of synaptic connections of a single neuron has an influence on that neuron. The net effect of the input is sometimes excitatory and sometimes inhibitory. In general, the net effect is dependent on the number of presynaptic neurons that are releasing neurotransmitters on the postsynaptic cell. A presynaptic cell that releases an excitatory neurotransmitter does not always cause the postsynaptic cell to depolarize enough to generate an action potential. However, when many presynaptic cells release excitatory neurotransmitters on a single neuron, the sum of their input is enough to generate an action potential. The presynaptic input can be summed by the number of presynaptic cells firing (spatial summation) or by the frequency of firing of a single presynaptic cell (temporal summation). Summation usually occurs by both events.

The effect of an excitatory or inhibitory neurotransmitter depends on which ion channels in the postsynaptic membrane are influenced by that neurotransmitter. In mammals, the neurotransmitters that are known to generally have an excitatory influence are acetylcholine, norepinephrine, serotonin, dopamine, glutamate, and histamine. The neurotransmitters that generally have an inhibitory influence are gamma-aminobutyric acid (GABA) and glycine.

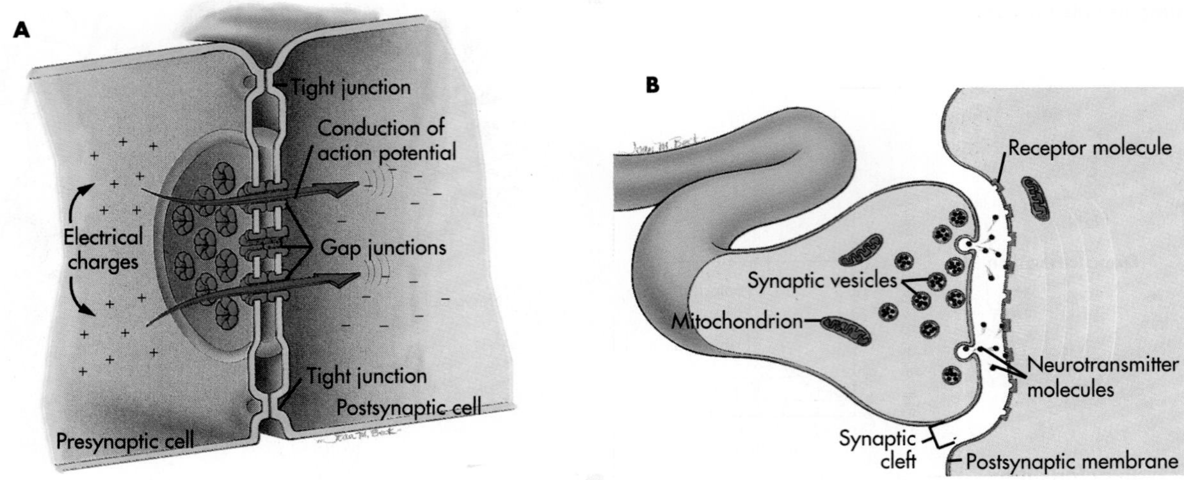

Fig. 53-4 Electrical and chemical synapses. **A,** Electrical synapses involve gap junctions that allow action potentials to move from cell to cell directly by allowing electrical current to flow between cells. **B,** Chemical synapses involve transmitter chemicals (neurotransmitters) that signal postsynaptic cells, inducing an action potential.

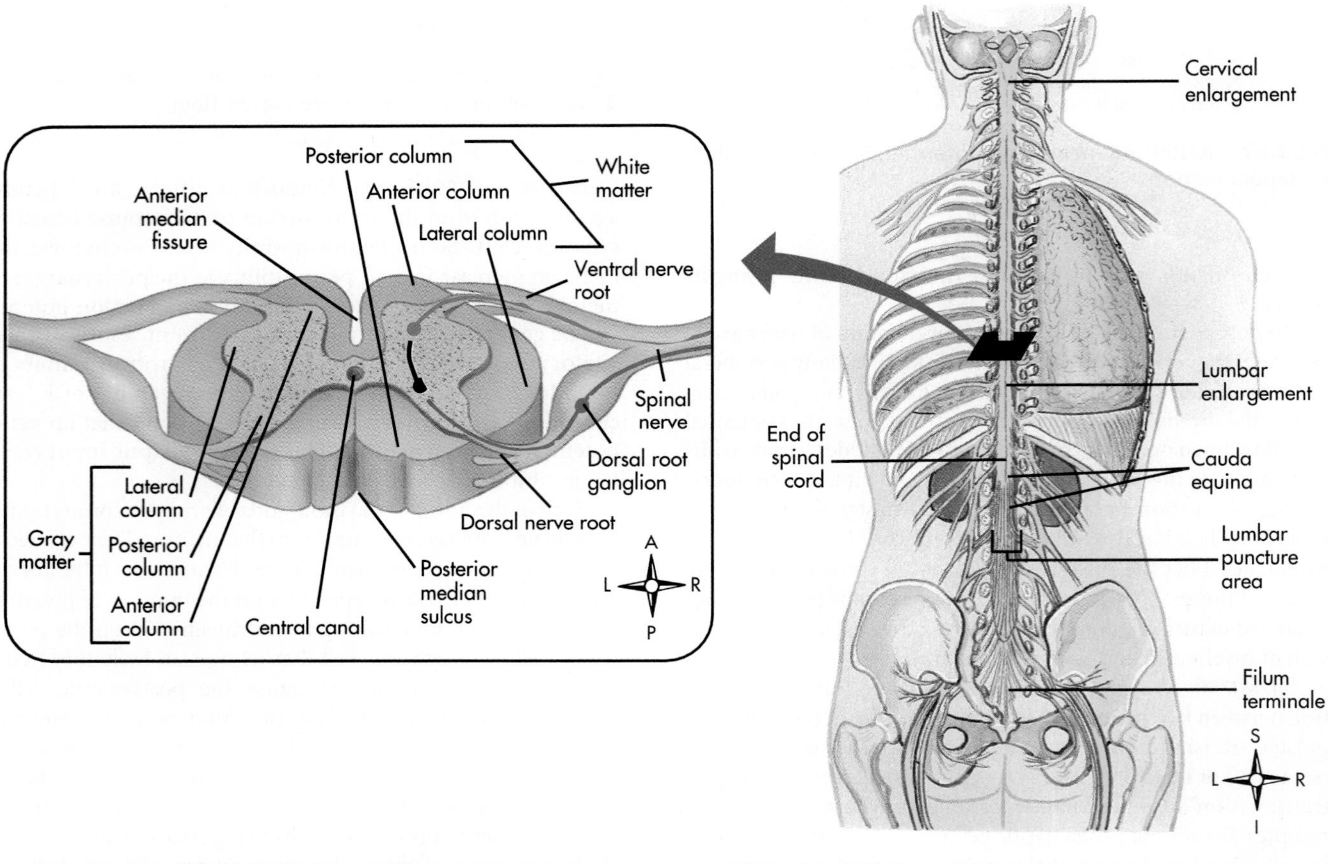

Fig. 53-5 Spinal cord. The inset illustrates a transverse section of the spinal cord shown in the broader view.

Neurotransmitters continue to combine with the receptor sites at the postsynaptic membrane until they are inactivated by enzymes, are taken up by the presynaptic endings, or diffuse away from the synaptic region. In addition, neurotransmitters can be affected by drugs and toxins, which can modify their function or block their attachment to receptor sites on the postsynaptic membrane. Enkephalins and endorphins are also considered neurotransmitters. These substances have opiate-like properties. They are found in multiple areas of the CNS and PNS and act to inhibit pain perception (see Chapter 9).

Central Nervous System

Major structural components of the CNS are the spinal cord and brain. The brain consists of the cerebral hemispheres, the cerebellum, and the brainstem.

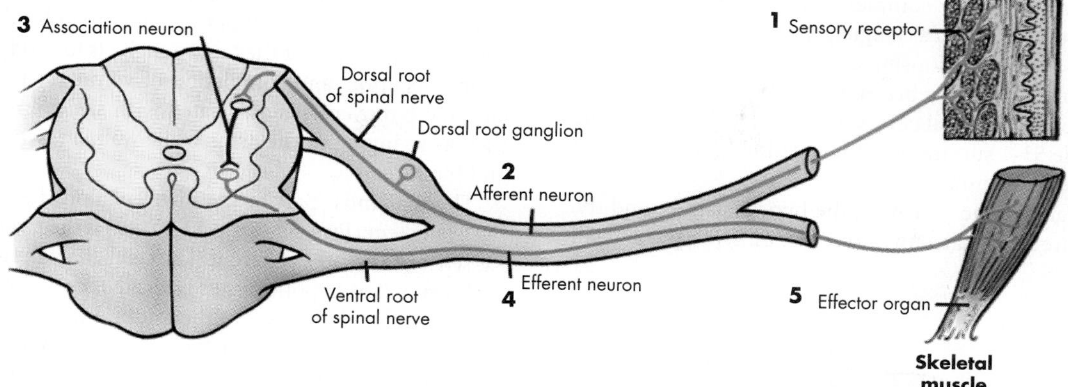

Fig. 53-6 Basic diagram of a reflex arc, including the (1) sensory receptor, (2) afferent neuron, (3) association neuron, (4) efferent neuron, and (5) effector organ.

Spinal Cord. The spinal cord is continuous with the brainstem and exits from the cranial cavity through the foramen magnum. A cross section of the spinal cord reveals gray matter that is centrally located in an H shape and is surrounded by white matter (Fig. 53-5). The gray matter contains the cell bodies of voluntary motor neurons and preganglionic autonomic motor neurons, as well as cell bodies of association neurons (interneurons). The white matter contains the axons of the ascending sensory and the descending (suprasegmental) motor fibers. The myelin surrounding these fibers gives them their white appearance. Specific ascending and descending pathways in the white matter can be identified. The spinal pathways or tracts are named for the point of origin and the point of destination (e.g., spinocerebellar tract [ascending], corticospinal tract [descending]). The major spinal pathways are presented in Fig. 53-5.

Ascending tracts. In general, the ascending tracts carry specific sensory information to higher levels of the CNS. This information comes from special sensory endings (receptors) in the skin, muscles and joints, viscera, and blood vessels, and enters the spinal cord by way of the dorsal roots of the spinal nerves. The fasciculus gracilis and the fasciculus cuneatus (commonly called the dorsal or posterior columns) carry information and transmit impulses concerned with touch, deep pressure, vibration, position sense, and kinesthesia (appreciation of movement, weight, and body parts). The spinocerebellar tracts carry subconscious information about muscle tension and body position to the cerebellum for coordination of movement. This information is not consciously perceived. The spinothalamic tracts carry pain and temperature sensations. Therefore the ascending tracts are organized by sensory modality, as well as by anatomy.

Although the functions of these pathways are generally accepted, other ascending tracts may also carry sensory modalities. The symptoms of various neurologic diseases suggest that additional pathways for touch, position sense, and vibration exist.

Descending tracts. Descending tracts carry impulses that are responsible for muscle movement. Among the most important descending tracts are the corticobulbar and corticospinal tracts, collectively termed the *pyramidal tract.* These tracts carry volitional (voluntary) impulses from the cortex to the cranial and peripheral nerves, respectively. Another group of descending motor tracts carries impulses from the extrapyramidal system, which includes all motor systems (except the pyramidal system) concerned with voluntary movement. It includes descending pathways originating in the brainstem, the basal ganglia, and the cerebellum. The motor output exits the spinal cord by way of the ventral roots of the spinal nerves.

Lower and upper motor neurons. Lower motor neurons (LMNs) are the final common pathway through which descending motor tracts influence skeletal muscle, the effector organ for movement. The cell bodies of LMNs, which send axons to innervate the skeletal muscles of the arms, trunk, and legs, are located in the anterior horn of the corresponding segments of the spinal cord (e.g., cervical segments contain LMNs for the arms). LMNs for skeletal muscles of the eyes, face, mouth, and throat are located in the corresponding segments of the brainstem. These cell bodies and their axons make up the somatic motor components of the cranial nerves. LMN lesions generally cause weakness or paralysis, denervation atrophy, hyporeflexia or areflexia, and decreased muscle tone (flaccidity).

Upper motor neurons (UMNs) originate in the cerebral cortex and project downward. The corticobulbar tract ends in the brainstem, and the corticospinal tract descends into the spinal cord. These neurons influence skeletal muscle movement. UMN lesions generally cause weakness or paralysis, disuse atrophy, hyperreflexia, and increased muscle tone (spasticity).

Reflex arc. A *reflex* is defined as an involuntary response to a stimulus. The components of a monosynaptic reflex arc (the simplest kind of reflex arc) are a receptor organ, an afferent neuron, an effector neuron, and an effector organ (e.g., skeletal muscle). The afferent neuron synapses with the efferent neuron in the gray matter of the spinal cord. A reflex arc is shown in Fig. 53-6. More complex reflex arcs have other neurons (interneurons) in addition to the afferent neuron influencing the effector neuron. In the spinal cord, reflex arcs play an important role in maintaining muscle tone, which is essential for body posture.

Brain. The brain can be divided into three major components: the cerebrum, the brainstem, and the cerebellum.

Cerebrum. The cerebrum is composed of the right and left hemispheres. Both hemispheres can be further divided into four major lobes: frontal, temporal, parietal, and occipital (Fig. 53-7). These divisions are useful to delineate portions of the neocortex (gray matter), which makes up the outer layer of the cerebral hemispheres. Neurons in specific parts of the neocortex are essential for various highly complex and sophisticated aspects of mental functioning, such as language, memory, and appreciation of visual-spatial relationships.

The functions of the cerebrum are multiple and complex. Specific areas of the cerebral cortex are associated with specific functions. Table 53-1 summarizes the location and function of the parts of the cerebrum.

The basal ganglia, the thalamus, the hypothalamus, and the limbic system are also located in the cerebrum. The basal ganglia are a group of paired structures located centrally in the cerebrum and midbrain; most of them are on both sides of the thalamus. The function of the basal ganglia is to modulate the initiation, execution, and completion of voluntary movements and automatic movements associated with skeletal muscle activity, such as swinging of the arms while walking, swallowing saliva, and blinking.

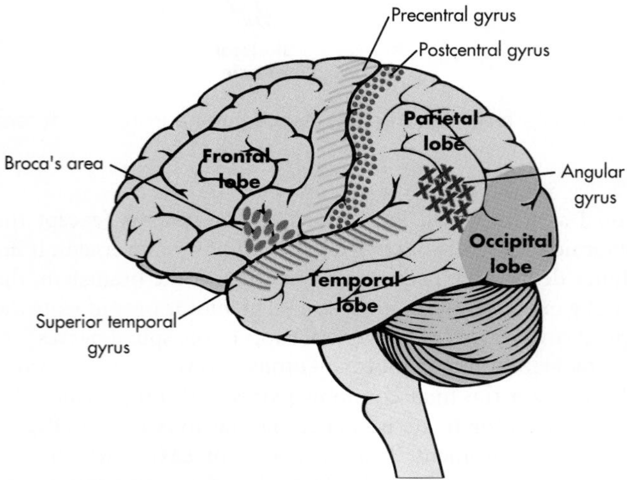

Fig. 53-7 Left hemisphere of cerebrum, lateral surface, showing major lobes and areas of the brain.

The thalamus (part of the diencephalon) lies directly above the brainstem (Figs. 53-8 and 53-9) and is the major relay center for sensory and other afferent (i.e., cerebellar) inputs to the cerebral cortex. The hypothalamus is located just inferior to the thalamus and slightly in front of the midbrain. It regulates the autonomic nervous system and the endocrine system. The limbic system is, phylogenetically, an old part of the human cerebrum. It is located near the inner surfaces of the cerebral hemispheres (Fig. 53-10) and is concerned with emotion, aggression, feeding behavior, and sexual response.

Brainstem. The brainstem includes the midbrain, pons, and medulla (see Figs. 53-8 and 53-9). Ascending and descending fibers pass through the brainstem going to and from the cerebrum and cerebellum. The cell bodies, or nuclei, of cranial nerves III through XII are in the brainstem. Also located in the brainstem is the reticular formation, a diffusely arranged group of neurons and their axons that extends from the medulla to the thalamus and hypothalamus. The functions of the reticular formation include relaying sensory information, influencing excitatory and inhibitory control of spinal motor neurons, and controlling vasomotor and respiratory activity. The reticular activating system is part of a reticular formation and is the regulatory system for arousal, a component of consciousness.

Table 53-1 Location and Function of the Parts of the Cerebrum

Part	Location	Function
Cortical areas		
Motor		
Primary	Precentral gyrus	Controls initiation of movement on opposite side of body
Supplemental	Anterior to precentral gyrus	Facilitates proximal muscle activity, including activity for stance and gait, and spontaneous movement and coordination
Sensory		
Somatic	Postcentral gyrus	Registers body sensations (e.g., temperature, touch, pressure, pain) from opposite side of body
Visual	Occipital lobe	Registers visual images
Auditory	Superior temporal gyrus	Registers auditory inputs
Association areas	Parietal lobe	Integrates somatic and special sensory inputs
	Posterior temporal lobe	Integrates visual and auditory inputs for language comprehension
	Anterior temporal lobe	Integrates past experiences
	Anterior frontal lobe	Controls higher-order processes (e.g., judgment, insight, reasoning, problem solving, planning)
Language		
Comprehension	Angular gyrus	Integrates auditory language (understanding of spoken words)
Expression	Broca's area	Regulates verbal expression
Basal ganglia	Near lateral ventricles of both cerebral hemispheres	Controls and facilitates learned and automatic movements
Thalamus	Below basal ganglia	Relays sensory and motor inputs to cortex and other parts of cerebrum
Hypothalamus	Below thalamus	Regulates endocrine and autonomic functions (e.g., feeding, sleeping, emotional and sexual responses)
Limbic system	Lateral to hypothalamus	Influences affective (emotional) behavior and basic drives such as feeding and sexual behavior

The vital centers concerned with respiratory, vasomotor, and cardiac function are located in the medulla. The brainstem also contains the centers for sneezing, coughing, hiccupping, vomiting, sucking, and swallowing.

Cerebellum. The cerebellum is located in the posterior part of the cranial fossa, along with the brainstem, under the occipital lobe of the cerebrum. The function of the cerebellum is to coordinate voluntary movement and to maintain trunk stability and equilibrium. It influences motor activity through its axonal connections to the motor cortex, brainstem nuclei, and their descending pathways. To perform these functions, the cerebellum receives information from the cerebral cortex, muscles, joints, and inner ear.

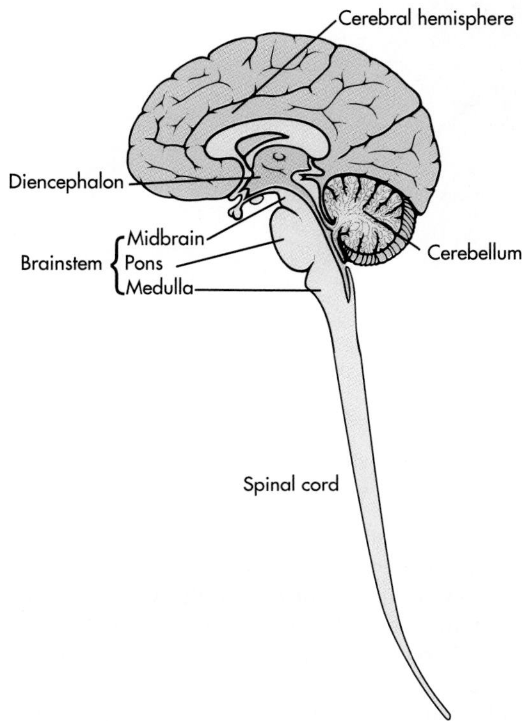

Fig. 53-8 Major divisions of the CNS.

Ventricles and cerebrospinal fluid. Several supporting structures located within the CNS are important in regulating neuronal function and physical support of the brain. The ventricles are four fluid-filled cavities within the brain that connect with one another and with the spinal canal. The lower portion of the fourth ventricle becomes the spinal canal in the lower part of the brainstem. The spinal canal is located in the center and extends the full length of the spinal cord. Figure 53-11 shows the ventricles and the flow of cerebrospinal fluid in the CNS.

The ventricles and spinal canal are filled with an average of 135 ml of cerebrospinal fluid (CSF). CSF circulates within the subarachnoid space that surrounds the brain, brainstem, and spinal cord. This fluid provides cushioning for the brain and spinal cord, allows fluid shifts from the cranial cavity to the spinal cavity, and carries nutrients. The formation of CSF in the choroid plexus in the ventricles involves both passive diffusion and active transport of substances. CSF resembles an ultrafiltrate of blood. Although CSF is continually being formed, many physiologic factors influence its rate of absorption and formation.

The CSF circulates throughout the ventricles and seeps into the subarachnoid space surrounding the brain and spinal cord. It is absorbed primarily through the arachnoid villi (tiny projections into the subarachnoid space) and into the intradural venous sinuses and eventually into the venous system. The analysis of CSF composition provides useful diagnostic information relating to certain nervous system diseases. CSF pressure is sometimes measured in patients with actual or suspected intracranial diseases. Increases in intracranial pressure, indicated by increased CSF pressure, can lead to herniation of the brain and compression of vital brainstem structures. The signs marking this event are part of the herniation syndrome (see Chapter 54).

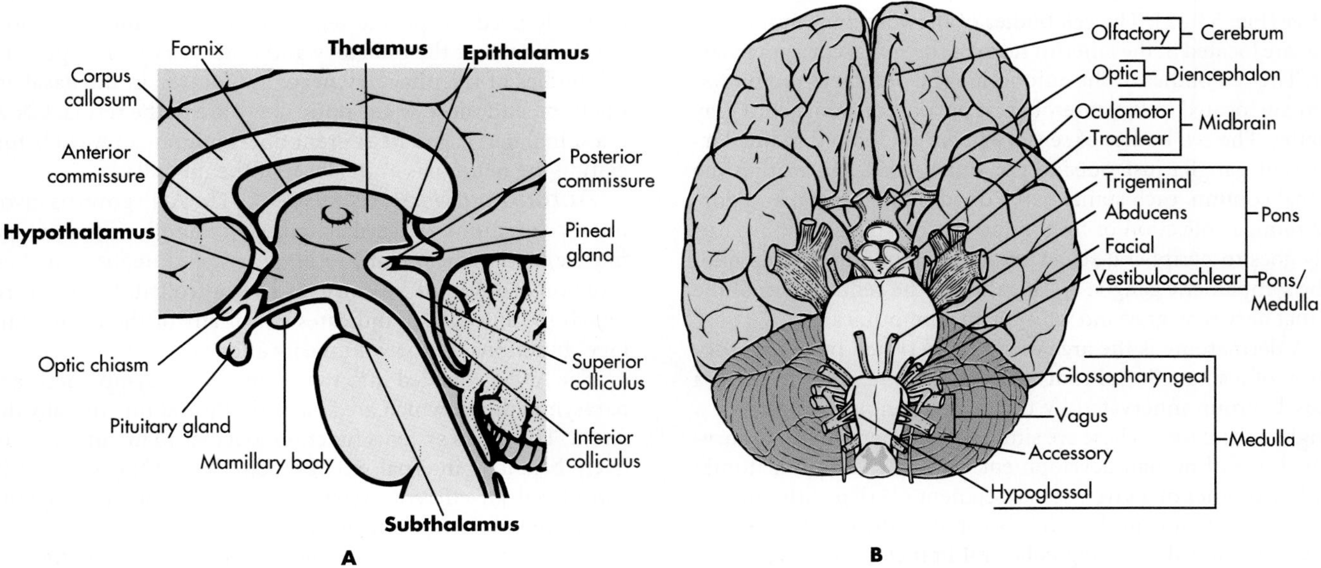

Fig. 53-9 **A,** The diencephalon (thalamus and hypothalamus) and **B,** cranial nerves.

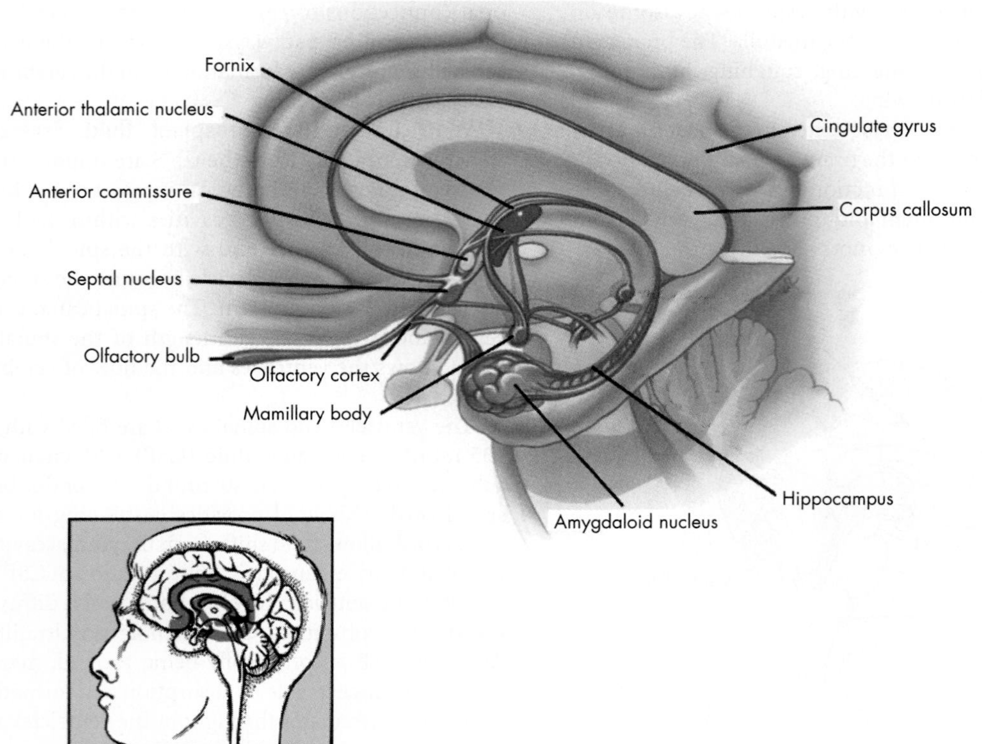

Fig. 53-10 Structures of the limbic system.

Peripheral Nervous System

The PNS includes all the neuronal structures that lie outside the CNS. It consists of the spinal and cranial nerves, their associated ganglia (groupings of cell bodies), and portions of the ANS.

Spinal Nerves. The spinal cord can be seen as a series of spinal segments, one on top of another. In addition to the cell bodies, each segment contains a pair of dorsal (afferent) sensory nerve fibers or roots and ventral (efferent) motor fibers or roots, which innervate a specific region of the neck, trunk, or limbs. This combined motor-sensory nerve is called a *spinal nerve* (Fig. 53-12). The cell bodies of the voluntary motor system are located in the anterior horn of the spinal cord gray matter. The cell bodies of the autonomic (involuntary) motor system are located in the anterolateral portion of spinal cord gray matter. The cell bodies of sensory fibers are located in the dorsal root ganglia just outside the spinal cord. On exiting the spinal column, each spinal nerve divides into ventral and dorsal rami, a collection of motor and sensory fibers that eventually goes to peripheral structures (e.g., skin, muscles, viscera). The sympathetic ganglia are attached to the ventral rami of the spinal nerves by gray and white rami communicans.

A dermatome is the area of skin innervated by the sensory fibers of a single dorsal root of a spinal nerve. A myotome is a muscle group innervated by the primary motor neurons of a single ventral root. These are simple components in the embryonic stage of human development. However, the dermatomes and myotomes of a given spinal segment overlap with those of adjacent segments in the adult because of the development of ascending and descending collateral branches of nerve fibers. The dermatomes give a general picture of somatic sensory innervation by spinal segments.

Cranial Nerves. The cranial nerves (CNs) are the 12 paired nerves composed of cell bodies with fibers that exit from the cranial cavity. Unlike the spinal nerves, which always have both afferent sensory and efferent motor fibers, some CNs have only afferent and some only efferent fibers; others have both. Table 53-2 summarizes the motor and sensory components of the CNs. Figure 53-9 shows the position of the CNs in relation to the brain and spinal cord. Just as the cell bodies of the spinal nerves are located in specific segments of the spinal cord, so are the cell bodies (nuclei) of the cranial nerves located in specific segments of the brain. Exceptions are the nuclei of the olfactory and optic nerves. The primary cell bodies of the olfactory nerve are located in the nasal epithelium, and those of the optic nerve are in the retina. CN XI is a spinal nerve, and its efferent fibers migrate upward before exiting the neuroaxis at the level of the medulla.

Autonomic Nervous System. The ANS governs involuntary functions of cardiac muscle, smooth (involuntary) muscle, and glands. Until recently it was thought that these functions could not be consciously controlled. However, research in biofeedback indicates that many of these "involuntary" functions can be voluntarily affected.[1]

The ANS is divided into two components, sympathetic and parasympathetic, which are anatomically and functionally different. These two systems function together to maintain a relatively balanced internal environment. The ANS is primarily considered an efferent system and consists of preganglionic nerves and postganglionic nerves.

The preganglionic cell bodies of the sympathetic nervous system (SNS) are located in spinal segments T1 through L2. The sympathetic ganglia, which contain the cell bodies of the

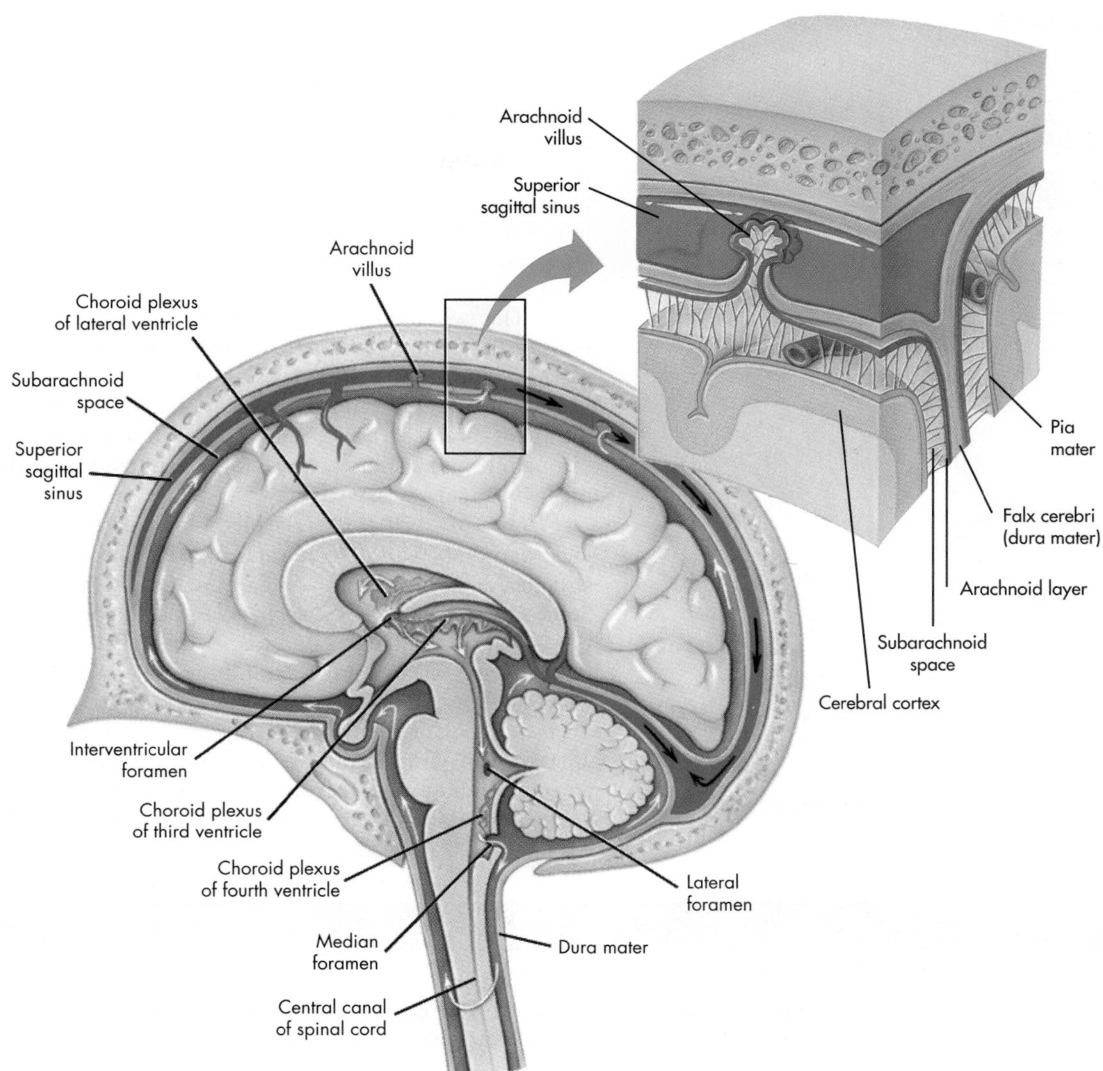

Fig. 53-11 Flow of cerebrospinal fluid. The fluid produced by filtration of blood by the choroid plexus of each ventricle flows inferiorly through the lateral ventricles, interventricular foramen, third ventricle, cerebral aqueduct, fourth ventricle, and subarachnoid space and to the blood.

postganglionic neurons, lie close to the spinal column, along the vertebral bodies in the rami communicans. These ganglia and the connecting nerves are called the *paravertebral chain.* The major neurotransmitter released by the postganglionic fibers of the SNS is norepinephrine, and the neurotransmitter released by the preganglionic fibers is acetylcholine.

In contrast, the preganglionic cell bodies of the parasympathetic nervous system (PSNS) are located in the brainstem and in the sacral spinal segments (S2 through S4). The parasympathetic ganglia are located in or near the structures that they innervate. Acetylcholine is the neurotransmitter released at both preganglionic and postganglionic nerve endings.

The ANS provides dual and often reciprocal innervation to many structures. For example, the SNS increases the rate and force of the heart contraction, and the PSNS decreases the rate and force. The SNS dilates bronchi and bronchioles of the lungs, and the PSNS constricts them. Some structures are innervated by only one system (e.g., the hair follicles and the sweat glands, which are innervated only by the SNS). Table 53-3 compares the SNS and PSNS.

The result of SNS stimulation is activation of mechanisms required for the "fight or flight" response that occurs throughout the body. In contrast, the PSNS is geared to act in localized and discrete regions. It serves to conserve and restore the energy stores of the body.

Cerebral Circulation

The blood supply of the brain arises from the internal carotid arteries (anterior circulation) and the vertebral arteries (posterior circulation), which are shown in Fig. 53-13. Knowledge of the distribution of the major arteries of the brain and the area supplied is essential for understanding and evaluating the signs and symptoms of cerebrovascular disease and trauma.

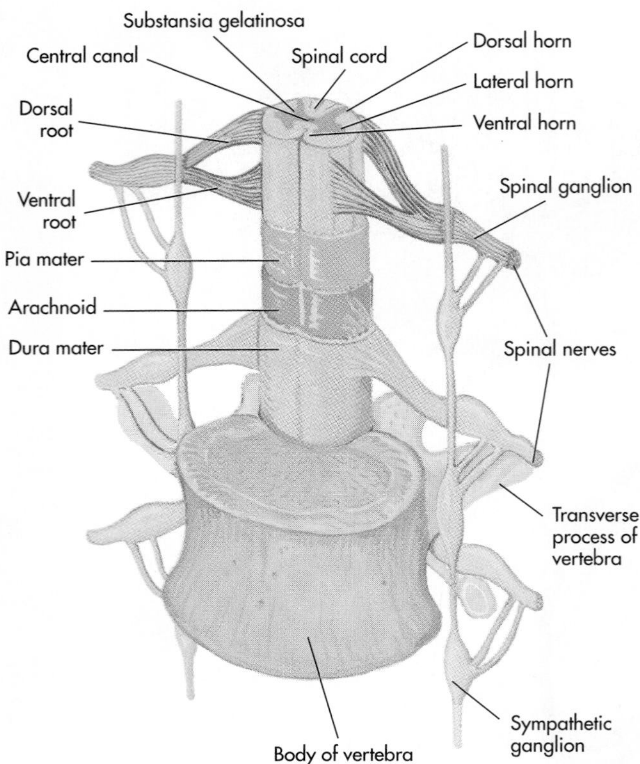

Fig. 53-12 Cross section of spinal cord showing attachments of spinal nerves and coverings of the spinal cord.

Each internal carotid artery supplies the ipsilateral hemisphere, whereas the basilar artery, formed by the junction of the two vertebral arteries, supplies structures within the posterior fossa (cerebellum and brainstem). The circle of Willis arises from the basilar artery and the two internal carotid arteries (Fig. 53-14). This vascular circle may act as a safety valve when differential pressures are present in these arteries. It also may function as an anastomotic pathway when occlusion of a major artery on one side of the brain occurs. In general, the two anterior cerebral arteries supply the medial portion of the frontal lobes. The two middle cerebral arteries supply the outer portions of the frontal, parietal, and superior temporal lobes. The two posterior cerebral arteries supply the medial portions of the occipital and inferior temporal lobes. Figure 53-13 shows the major cerebral arteries. Venous blood drains from the brain through the dural sinuses, which form channels that drain into the two jugular veins.

Blood-Brain Barrier. The blood-brain barrier is a physiologic barrier between blood capillaries and brain tissue. The structure of brain capillaries differs from that of other capillaries. Some substances that normally pass readily into most tissues are prevented from entering brain tissue. This barrier protects the brain from certain potentially harmful agents, while allowing nutrients and gases to enter. Because the blood-brain barrier affects the penetration of pharmaceutical agents, only certain drugs can enter the CNS from the bloodstream. Lipid-soluble compounds enter the brain easily, whereas water-soluble and ionized drugs enter the brain and spinal cord slowly. Damage to the blood-

Table 53-2 Cranial Nerves

Nerve	Connection with Brain	Function
I. Olfactory nerves and tract	Anterior ventral cerebrum	Sensory: from olfactory epithelium of superior nasal cavity
II. Optic nerve	Lateral geniculate body of the thalamus	Sensory: from retina of eyes
III. Oculomotor nerve	Midbrain	Motor: to four eye movement muscles and levator palpebrae Parasympathetic: smooth muscle in eyeball
IV. Trochlear nerve	Midbrain	Motor: to one eye movement muscle, the superior oblique
V. Trigeminal nerve		
Ophthalmic branch	Pons	Sensory: from forehead, eye, superior nasal cavity
Maxillary branch	Pons	Sensory: from inferior nasal cavity, face, upper teeth, mucosa of superior mouth
Mandibular branch	Pons	Sensory: from surfaces of jaw, lower teeth, mucosa of lower mouth, and anterior tongue Motor: to muscles of mastication
VI. Abducens nerve	Pons	Motor: to one eye movement muscle, the lateral rectus
VII. Facial nerve	Junction of pons and medulla	Motor: to facial muscles of expression and cheek muscle, the buccinator Sensory: taste from anterior two thirds of tongue
VIII. Vestibulocochlear nerve Vestibular branch	Junction of pons and medulla	Sensory: from equilibrium sensory organ, the vestibular apparatus
Cochlear branch	Junction of pons and medulla	Sensory: from auditory sensory organ, the cochlea
IX. Glossopharyngeal nerve	Medulla	Sensory: from pharynx and posterior tongue, including taste Motor: superior pharyngeal muscles
X. Vagus nerve	Medulla	Sensory: much of viscera of thorax and abdomen Motor: larynx and middle and inferior pharyngeal muscles Parasympathetic: heart, lungs, most of digestive system
XI. Accessory nerve	Medulla and superior spinal segments	Motor: to several neck muscles, sternocleidomastoid and trapezius
XII. Hypoglossal nerve	Medulla	Motor: to intrinsic and extrinsic muscles of tongue

Table 53-3 Effect of Sympathetic and Parasympathetic Nervous Systems

Visceral Effector	Effect of Sympathetic Nervous System*	Effect of Parasympathetic Nervous System†
Heart	Increase in rate and strength of heartbeat (β-receptors)	Decrease in rate and strength of heartbeat
Smooth muscle of blood vessels		
Skin blood vessels	Constriction (α-receptors)	No effect
Skeletal muscle blood vessels	Dilation (β-receptors)	No effect
Coronary blood vessels	Dilation (β-receptors), constriction (α-receptors)	Dilation
Abdominal blood vessels	Constriction (α-receptors)	No effect
Blood vessels of external genitals	Ejaculation (contraction of smooth muscle in male ducts [e.g., epididymis, ductus deferens])	Dilation of blood vessels causing erection in male
Smooth muscle of hollow organs and sphincters		
Bronchi	Dilation (β-receptors)	Constriction
Digestive tract, except sphincters	Decrease in peristalsis (β-receptors)	Increase in peristalsis
Sphincters of digestive tract	Contraction (α-receptors)	Relaxation
Urinary bladder	Relaxation (β-receptors)	Contraction
Urinary sphincters	Contraction (α-receptors)	Relaxation
Eye		
Iris	Contraction of radial muscle, dilation of pupil	Contraction of circular muscle, constriction of pupil
Ciliary	Relaxation, accommodation for far vision	Contraction, accommodation for near vision
Hairs (pilomotor muscles)	Contraction producing goose pimples or piloerection (α-receptors)	No effect
Glands		
Sweat	Increase in sweat (neurotransmitter, acetylcholine)	No effect
Digestive (e.g., salivary, gastric)	Decrease in secretion of saliva; not known for others	Increase in secretion of saliva and gastric HCl acid
Pancreas, including islets	Decrease in secretion	Increase in secretion of pancreatic juice and insulin
Liver	Increase in glycogenolysis (β-receptors), increase in blood glucose level	No effect
Adrenal medulla‡	Increase in epinephrine secretion	No effect

Modified from Thibodeau GA, Patton KT: *Anatomy and physiology,* ed 4, St Louis, 1999, Mosby.
*Neurotransmitter is norepinephrine unless otherwise stated.
†Neurotransmitter is acetylcholine unless otherwise stated.
‡Sympathetic preganglionic axons terminate in contact with secreting cells of the adrenal medulla. Thus the adrenal medulla functions as a "giant sympathetic postganglionic neuron."

brain barrier results in the penetration of drugs and other substances into brain tissue.

Protective Structures

Meninges. The meninges are three layers of protective membranes that surround the brain and spinal cord. The thick dura mater forms the outermost layer, with the arachnoid layer and pia mater being the next two layers. The falx cerebri is a fold of the dura that separates the two cerebral hemispheres and prevents expansion of brain tissue in situations such as the presence of a rapidly growing tumor or acute hemorrhage. The expanding brain must squeeze under this structure, causing displacement toward the side opposite the lesion. The tentorium cerebelli is a fold of dura that separates the cerebral hemispheres from the posterior fossa (which contains the brainstem and cerebellum). Expansion of mass lesions in the cerebrum forces the brain to herniate through the opening created by the brainstem. This is termed *tentorial herniation.*

The arachnoid layer is a delicate, impermeable membrane that lies between the thick dura mater and the pia mater and directly covers the brain and spinal cord. The subarachnoid space lies between the arachnoid layer and the pia mater. This space is filled with CSF. Structures passing to and from the brain and the skull or its foramina (holes through which blood vessels and nerves enter and exit the intracranial compartment) must pass through the subarachnoid space. Therefore all cerebral arteries and veins lie in this space, as do the cranial nerves. A larger subarachnoid space is present in the region of the third and fourth lumbar vertebrae, which is the area penetrated to obtain CSF during a lumbar puncture. (The spinal cord itself ends between the first and second lumbar vertebrae.)

Skull. The bony skull protects the brain from external trauma. It is composed of 8 cranial bones and 14 facial bones. The structure of the skull cavity explains the physiology of head injuries (see Chapter 54). Although the top and sides of the inside of the skull are relatively smooth, the bottom surface is uneven. It has many ridges, prominences, and foramina. The largest hole is the foramen magnum, through which the brainstem extends to the spinal cord. This foramen offers

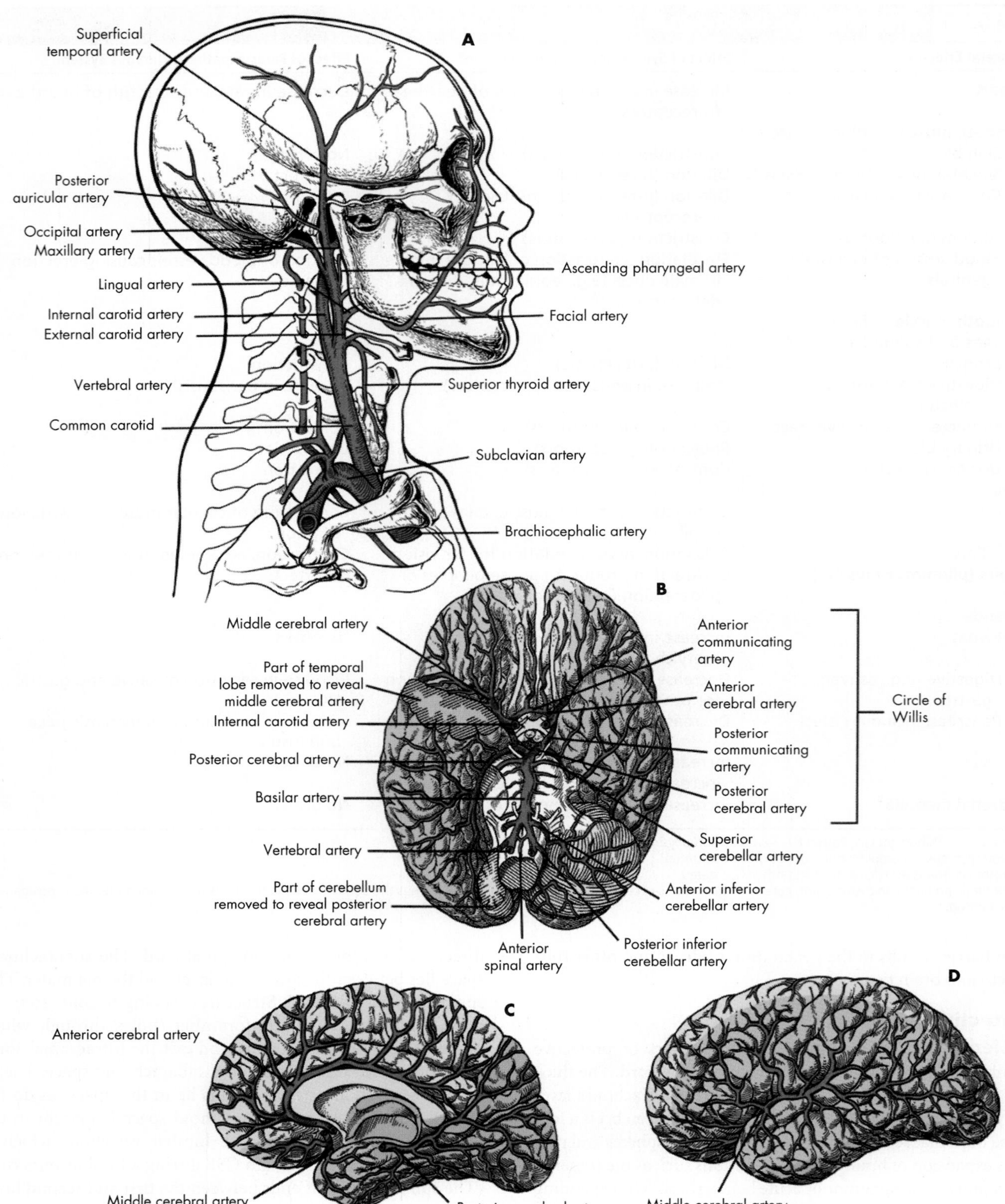

Fig. 53-13 Arteries of the head and neck. **A,** The brachiocephalic artery, the right common carotid artery, the right subclavian artery, and their branches. The major arteries to the head are the common carotid and vertebral arteries. **B,** Inferior view of the brain showing the vertebral, basilar, and internal carotid arteries and their branches. **C,** Medial view of the brain showing middle, anterior, and posterior cerebral arteries. **D,** Lateral view of the brain showing the distribution of the middle cerebral artery. **B** to **D,** Colors indicate brain regions supplied by various arteries—*yellow*, anterior cerebral; *orange*, middle cerebral; *purple*, posterior cerebral.

the only major space for the expansion of brain contents when increased intracranial pressure occurs.

Vertebral Column. The vertebral column protects the spinal cord, supports the head, and provides for flexibility. The vertebral column is made up of 33 individual vertebrae: 7 cervical, 12 thoracic, 5 lumbar, 5 sacral (fused into one), and 4 coccygeal (fused into one). Each vertebra has a central opening through which the spinal cord passes. The vertebrae are held together by a series of ligaments. Intervertebral disks occupy the spaces between vertebrae. Figure 53-15 shows the vertebral column in relation to the trunk.

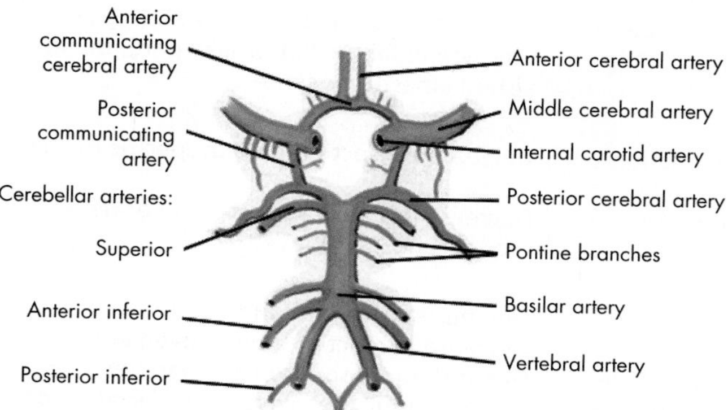

Fig. 53-14 Arteries at the base of the brain. The arteries that compose the circle of Willis are the two anterior cerebral arteries joined to each other by the anterior communicating cerebral artery and to the posterior cerebral arteries by the posterior communicating arteries.

GERONTOLOGIC CONSIDERATIONS

Effects of Aging on the Nervous System

Several parts of the nervous system are affected by aging. In the CNS loss of neurons occurs in certain areas of the brainstem, cerebellum, and cerebral cortex. This is a gradual process that begins in early adulthood. With loss of neurons there is widening or enlargement of the ventricles. Brain weight also decreases as a result of neuron loss. Cerebral blood flow and CSF production decline.[2]

In the PNS there are changes in the anterior horn cells and peripheral nerves, as well as the target organ, muscle. Degenerative changes in myelin cause a decrease in nerve conduction. Coordinated neuromuscular activity such as the maintenance of blood pressure in response to changing from a lying to a standing position is altered with aging. As a result older adults are more vulnerable to problems with orthostatic hypotension. Similarly, coordination of neuromuscular activity to maintain body temperature is also less efficient with aging. Older adults are less able to adapt to extremes in environmental temperature and are more vulnerable to both hypothermia and hyperthermia. Additional relevant changes associated with aging include decreases in memory, vision, hearing, taste, smell, vibration and position sense, muscle strength, and reaction time.

Changes in assessment findings result from age-related alterations in the various components of the nervous system. Age-related changes in the nervous system and differences in assessment findings are presented in Table 53-4.

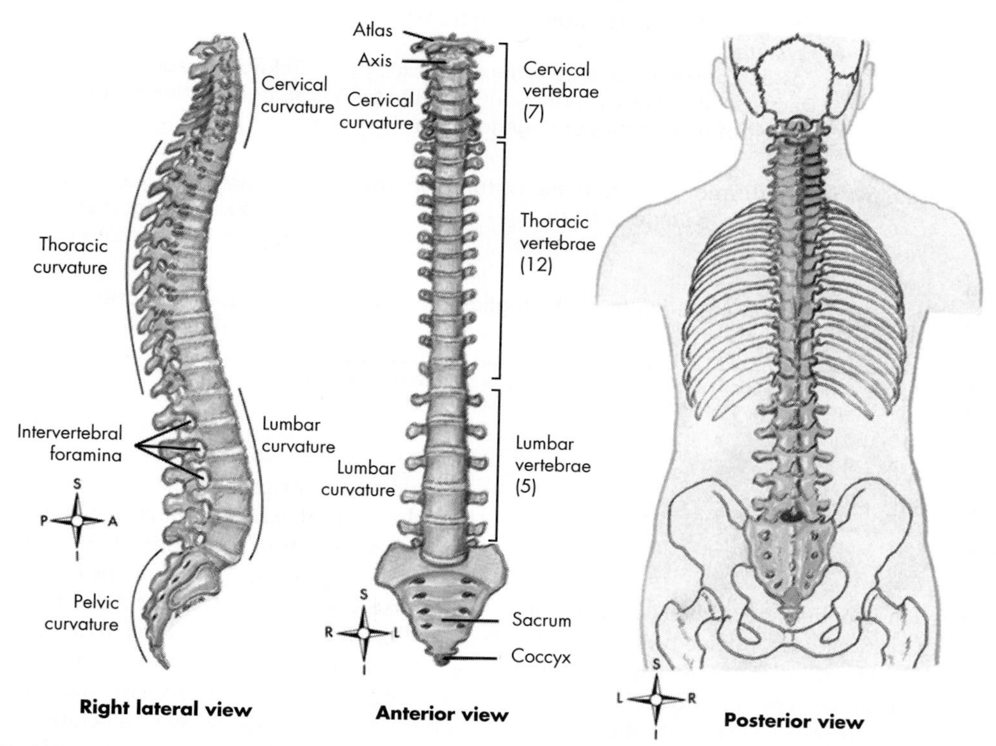

Fig. 53-15 The vertebral column (three views).

GERONTOLOGIC DIFFERENCES IN ASSESSMENT

Table 53-4 Nervous System

Component	Changes	Differences in Assessment Findings
Central Nervous System		
Brain	Reduction in cerebral blood flow and metabolism	Alterations in selected mental functioning
	Decrease in efficiency of temperature-regulating mechanism	Decrease in body temperature, impairment of ability to adapt to environmental temperature
	Decrease in neurotransmitter content, disruption in integration as result of loss of neurons	Repetitive movements, tremors
	Decrease in oxygen supply, changes in basal ganglia caused by vascular changes	Changes in gait and ambulation (e.g., extrapyramidal, Parkinson-like gait); diminished kinesthetic sense
Peripheral Nervous System		
Cranial and spinal nerves	Loss of myelin and decrease in conduction time in some nerves	Decrease in reaction time in specific nerves
	Cellular degeneration, death of neurons	Decrease in speed and intensity of neuronal reflexes
Functional Divisions		
Motor	Decrease in muscle bulk	Diminished strength and agility
	Decrease in electrical activity	Decrease in reactions and movement time
Sensory*	Decrease in sensory receptors caused by degenerative changes and involution of fine corpuscles of nerve endings	Diminished sense of touch; inability to localize stimuli; decrease in appreciation of touch, temperature, and peripheral vibrations
	Decrease in electrical activity	Slowing of or alteration in sensory reception
	Atrophy of taste buds	Signs of malnutrition, weight loss
	Degeneration and loss of fibers in olfactory bulb	Diminished sense of smell
	Degenerative changes in nerve cells in vestibular system of inner ear, cerebellum, and proprioceptive pathways in nervous system	Poor ability to maintain balance, widened gait
Reflexes	Possible decrease in deep tendon reflexes	Below-average reflex score
	Decrease in sensory conduction velocity as result of myelin sheath degeneration	Sluggish reflexes, slowing of reaction time
Reticular Formation		
Reticular activating system	Modification of hypothalamic function, reduction in stage IV sleep	Increase in frequency of spontaneous awakening together with tiredness, interrupted sleep, insomnia
Autonomic Nervous System		
SNS and PSNS	Morphologic features of ganglia, slowing of ANS responses	Orthostatic hypotension, systolic hypertension

*Specific changes related to the eye are in Table 19-1 and specific changes related to the ear are in Table 19-7.
ANS, autonomic nervous system; *PSNS,* parasympathetic nervous system; *SNS,* sympathetic nervous system.

ASSESSMENT OF THE NERVOUS SYSTEM

Subjective Data

Important Health Information

Past health history. Three points should be considered in taking the history of a patient with neurologic problems. The first is to avoid suggesting symptoms to the patient. Caution must be used not to suggest certain symptoms to the patient or ask leading questions such as "Is your headache throbbing?" or "Are you weak on the right side?" It is better to ask open-ended questions such as "What is your headache like?" or "Is there anything about your right side that bothers you?" A second point is that the mode of onset and the course of the illness are especially important aspects of the history. Often the nature of a neurologic disease process can be described by these facts alone, and the nurse should elicit all pertinent data in the history of the present illness, especially data related to the characteristics and progression of the symptoms. The third point is that because many neurologic diseases affect a patient's mental functioning, mental status must be accurately assessed before assuming that the history is factual. If the patient is not considered a reliable historian, the health history should be obtained from a person who has firsthand knowledge of the patient's problems and complaints. In many instances a health history cannot be obtained, and the clinician must proceed with only objective data.

The health history helps guide the approach for the neurologic examination; that is, it can direct the clinician toward the parts of the nervous system that need to be closely assessed. If the patient's primary complaint is dizziness, the examination may be focused on visual, vestibular, and cerebellar functions rather than on somatic motor and sensory functions.

Many complaints, including behavioral changes, alteration in level of consciousness, developmental problems, paroxysmal disorders, infectious processes, pain, motor or sensory aberrations, and trauma, should alert the clinician to the need for a detailed neurologic examination. In addition to being a primary complaint, neurologic problems often result from other problems, such as alcoholism or metastatic lesions.

When eliciting data about the health history, the nurse should ask the patient specific questions about diabetes mellitus, pernicious anemia, cancer, infections, thyroid disease, substance abuse, and hypertension because these conditions can affect the nervous system. Any hospitalizations, injuries, or surgeries related to the nervous system should be noted.

Medications. Particular attention should be given to eliciting a careful medication history, especially the use of sedatives, narcotics, tranquilizers, and mood-elevating drugs. If the patient experiences dizziness as a side effect of a medication, it should be noted. If the drug cannot be changed, the patient will need to be instructed in strategies to cope with dizziness and prevent falls.

Commonly, patients with chronic neurologic conditions will take medications to either treat the disease or manage symptoms. For example, many patients with neurologic problems will be taking antiseizure medications such as phenytoin (Dilantin), carbamazepine (Tegretol), and phenobarbital. The nurse should inquire about the occurrence of common side effects such as diplopia, drowsiness, ataxia, and mental slowing.

If the patient experiences headaches, the medications taken most commonly for the problem should be investigated. Many headache medications have potentially dangerous side effects such as gastric bleeding and coagulation abnormalities. The occurrence of these side effects should be noted.

Surgery or other treatments. The nurse should inquire about any surgery involving any part of the nervous system such as the head, spine, or sensory organs. If a patient had surgery, the date, cause, procedure, recovery, and current status should be investigated.

The perinatal history may reveal exposure to toxic agents such as viruses, alcohol, tobacco, drugs, and radiation, which are known to adversely influence the development of the nervous system. The history may reveal a difficult labor and delivery, which can cause brain damage as a result of hypoxia, forceps delivery, or Rh incompatibility. If the patient is elderly, this line of questioning may be unnecessary.

Growth and developmental history can be important in ascertaining whether nervous system dysfunction was present at an early age. The nurse should specifically inquire about major developmental tasks such as walking and talking. Success at school or identified problems in an educational setting are other important developmental data to gather. Often this information is not available when the older patient is interviewed. If the patient cannot provide a detailed developmental history, the nurse should proceed with the history gathering and avoid distressing the patient by further probing.

Functional Health Patterns. Key questions to ask a patient with a neurologic problem are presented in Table 53-5.

Health perception–health management pattern. The nurse should ask about the patient's health practices related to the nervous system, such as avoidance of substance abuse and smoking, maintenance of adequate nutrition, safe participation in physical and recreational activities, use of seat belts and helmets, and control of hypertension. The nurse should ask about previous hospitalizations for neurologic problems. A careful family history may determine whether the neurologic problem has a hereditary or congenital background. Specifically, the patient should be questioned about a family history of such disorders as epilepsy, amyotrophic lateral sclerosis, multiple sclerosis, Huntington's disease, muscular dystrophy, mental retardation, dementia, stroke, and cancer.

If the patient has an existing neurologic problem, the nurse should ask about how it affects daily living and the ability to carry out self-care. After a careful review of information, the nurse should ask someone who knows the patient well whether any mental or physical changes have been noticed in the patient. The patient with a neurologic problem may not be aware of it or may be unable to provide enough specific data to aid in the diagnosis.

Nutritional-metabolic pattern. Neurologic problems can result in problems of inadequate nutrition. Problems related to chewing, swallowing, facial nerve paralysis, and muscle coordination could make it difficult for the patient to ingest adequate nutrients. Also, certain vitamins such as thiamine (B_1), niacin, and pyridoxine (B_6) are essential for the maintenance and health of the CNS. Deficiencies in one or more of these vitamins could result in such nonspecific complaints as depression, apathy, neuritis, weakness, mental confusion, and irritability.

Elimination pattern. Bowel and bladder problems are often associated with neurologic problems, such as stroke, head injury, spinal cord injury, multiple sclerosis, and dementia. It is important to determine if the bowel or bladder problem was present before or after the neurologic event in order to plan appropriate interventions. Incontinence of urine and feces and urinary retention are the most common elimination problems associated with a neurologic problem. Careful documentation of the details of the problem, such as number of episodes, accompanying sensations or lack of sensations, and measures to control the problem, is important.

Activity-exercise pattern. Many neurologic disorders can cause problems in the patient's mobility, strength, and coordination. These problems can result in changes in the patient's usual activity and exercise patterns. Falls can also result from such problems. Many aspects of daily living such as getting out of a bed or chair, ambulating, preparing meals, and performing personal hygiene can be affected and should be assessed. The ability to perform fine motor tasks may be affected, which increases the possibility of personal injury.

Sleep-rest pattern. Sleep can be disrupted by many neurologically related factors. Discomfort from pain and inability to move and change to a position of comfort because of muscle weakness and paralysis could interfere with sound sleep. Hallucinations resulting from dementia or medications can also

HEALTH HISTORY

Table 53-5 Nervous System

Health Perception–Health Management Pattern
- What are your usual daily activities?
- Do you use any recreational drugs?*
- What safety practices do you perform in a car? On a motorcycle? On a bicycle?
- Do you have hypertension? If so, is it controlled?
- Have you ever been hospitalized for a neurologic problem?*
- How does it affect your daily living?

Nutritional-Metabolic Pattern
- Give a 24 hr dietary recall.
- Do you have any problems getting adequate nutrition because of chewing or swallowing difficulties, facial nerve paralysis, or poor muscle coordination?*
- Are you able to feed yourself?

Elimination Pattern
- Do you have incontinence of bowel or bladder? If yes, explain in detail the onset and pattern of the problem.
- What measures have you used to control the incontinence?
- Do you ever experience problems with hesitancy, urgency, retention?*
- Do you postpone defecation?*
- Does a neurologic problem make it difficult to reach a toilet when needed?
- Do you take any medication to manage neurologic problems? If so, what?

Activity-Exercise Pattern
- Describe any problems you experience with usual activities and exercise as a result of a neurologic problem.
- Do you have weakness or lack of coordination due to a neurologic problem?*
- Does a neurologic problem keep you from performing your personal hygiene needs independently?*

Sleep-Rest Pattern
- Describe any problems you have with sleep.
- If you have trouble falling asleep, what do you do about it? (Ask specifically about use of sleep-inducing medications.)

Cognitive-Perceptual Pattern
- Have you noticed any changes in your memory?*
- Do you experience vertigo, heat or cold sensitivity, numbness, or tingling?*
- Describe any pain you have experienced during the past 6 mo.
- Do you have any difficulty with verbal or written communication?*

Self-Perception–Self-Concept Pattern
- What effect has your neurologic problem had on how you feel about yourself? Your abilities? Your body?
- Describe your general emotional pattern.

Role-Relationship Pattern
- Have you experienced changes in roles such as spouse, parent, breadwinner because of neurologic disease?*
- How do you feel about these changes?

Sexuality-Reproductive Pattern
- Are you satisfied with sexual functioning? Describe any problems you experience related to your sexuality and sexual functioning.
- Are problems related to sexual functioning causing tension in an important relationship?*
- Do you feel the need for professional counseling related to your sexual functioning?*
- Do you use alternative methods of achieving sexual satisfaction?

Coping–Stress Tolerance Pattern
- Describe your usual coping pattern.
- Do you think your present coping pattern is adequate to meet the stressors of your neurologic problem?*
- Is your support system adequate to meet your needs? If not, what needs are unmet?

Value-Belief Pattern
- Describe any culturally specific beliefs and attitudes that may influence the treatment of this neurologic problem.

*If yes, describe.

interrupt sleep. The nurse should carefully document the sleep problem and the patient's methods of dealing with the problem.

Cognitive-perceptual pattern. Because the nervous system controls cognition and sensory integration, many neurologic disorders affect these functions. The nurse should assess memory, language, calculation ability, problem-solving ability, insight, and judgment. Often a structured mental status questionnaire will be used to evaluate these functions and provide baseline data.

Information about sensory changes related to hearing, sight, and touch should be sought. In addition, the patient should be questioned about problems with vertigo and sensitivity to heat and cold.

Ability to both use and understand language is a cognitive function that the nurse should also assess. Appropriateness of responses is a useful indicator of cognitive and perceptual ability.

Pain is a common event associated with many health problems. It is often the reason a patient seeks health care. A careful assessment of the patient's pain should be carried out (see Chapter 9).

Neurologic problems and their treatment can be complex and confusing. The patient's understanding and ability to carry out necessary treatments should be determined. Cognitive changes associated with the problem can also interfere with understanding and compliance.

Self-perception–self-concept pattern. Neurologic disease can drastically alter control over one's life and create dependency on others for daily needs. Also, the patient's physical appearance and emotional control can be affected. The nurse should ask about the patient's evaluation of self-worth, perception of abilities, body image, and general emotional pattern.

Role-relationship pattern. The patient should be asked if changes in roles, such as spouse, parent, or breadwinner, resulting from a neurologic problem have occurred. Physical impairments such as weakness and paralysis can alter or limit participation in usual roles and activities. Cognitive changes, however, can permanently change a person's ability to maintain previous roles. These changes can dramatically affect both the patient and significant others. Spousal relationships often change to dependent relationships.

Sexuality-reproductive pattern. The ability to participate in sexual activity should be assessed because many nervous system disorders can affect sexual response. Cerebral lesions may inhibit the desire phase or the reflex responses of the excitement phase. Brainstem and spinal cord lesions may partially or completely interrupt the connections between the brain and effector systems necessary for intercourse.

Neuropathies and spinal cord lesions that affect sensation, especially in the erotic zones, may decrease desire. Autonomic neuropathies and lesions of the sacral cord and cauda equina may prevent reflex activities of the sexual response. The nurse should determine if the patient and the spouse or significant other are satisfied with their sexual activity. The use or need for alternative methods of achieving sexual satisfaction should be explored. Despite neurologic-related changes in sexual functioning, many persons can achieve satisfying expression of intimacy and affection.

Coping–stress tolerance pattern. The physical sequelae of a neurologic problem can seriously strain a patient's coping patterns. Often the problem is chronic and may require that the patient learn new coping skills. The nurse should assess the patient's usual coping pattern to determine if coping skills are adequate to meet the stress of a problem.

When the problem is a decrease in cognitive functioning, both the patient and the caregiver can be seriously stressed. The nurse should assess for the potential for suicide, abuse, and burnout of the involved parties. The presence of an adequate support system in this type of situation should be assessed.

Value-belief pattern. Many neurologic problems have serious, long-term, life-changing effects. These effects can strain the patient's belief system and should be assessed. The nurse should also determine if any religious or cultural beliefs could interfere with the planned treatment regimen.

Objective Data

Physical Examination. The standard neurologic examination was developed by physicians and clinicians to help determine the presence, location, and nature of disease of the nervous system. The examination assesses six categories of functions: mental status, function of cranial nerves, motor function, cerebellar function, sensory function, and reflex function. The choice of particular parts of the examination depends on the purpose for which it is done. If a comprehensive baseline assessment of neurologic functioning is desired, all components of the examination are done. However, if a specific problem is to be evaluated, only certain components may be assessed. For example, if a patient's primary complaint is lack of feeling in the feet, the examination may be focused only on movement and sensation of the lower limbs. Similarly, if a patient comes into the emergency department after a head injury and is unconscious, a limited examination is conducted because the patient is not able to respond to verbal instructions.

A different approach to the neurologic examination has been proposed for nursing purposes. The primary purposes of the nursing neurologic examination are to determine the effects of neurologic dysfunction on daily living in relation to the patient's and the family's ability to cope with the neurologic deficits. Although the method of gathering data may be the same, the interpretation of the data is different from the medical model. The standard medical model of the neurologic examination can also be used for nursing purposes. Nurses and physicians share the responsibility for assessing life-threatening neurologic dysfunction.

Mental status. Assessment of mental status (cerebral functioning) gives an indication of how the patient is functioning as a whole and how the patient is adapting to the environment. It involves determination of complex and high-level cerebral functions that are governed by many areas of the cerebral cortex. Much of the area covered in this part of the examination is assessed during the history and therefore does not need to be evaluated further. For example, language and memory can be assessed when the patient is asked for details of the illness and significant past events. The patient's cultural and educational background should be taken into account when evaluating mental status.

The components of the mental status examination are as follows:

1. *General appearance and behavior.* This component includes motor activity, body posture, dress and hygiene, facial expression, and speech.
2. *State of consciousness.* The patient must be conscious before other functions can be determined. The nurse should note orientation to time, place, person, and situation, as well as memory, general knowledge, insight, judgment, problem solving, and calculation. Common questions are "Who were the last three presidents?" "What does 'a stitch in time saves nine' mean?" "Subtract 7 from 100, and keep subtracting 7." The nurse should consider whether the patient's plans and goals match the physical and mental capabilities.
3. *Mood and affect.* The nurse should note agitation, anger, depression, or euphoria and the appropriateness of these states. Questions should be directed to bring out the feelings of the patient.
4. *Thought content.* The nurse should note illusions, hallucinations, delusions, or paranoia.
5. *Intellectual capacity.* The nurse should note retardation, dementia, and intelligence.

Cranial nerves. Testing of each CN is an essential component of the neurologic examination (see Table 53-2).

Olfactory nerve. After determining that both nostrils are patent, the olfactory nerve (CN I) is tested by asking the patient to close one nostril, close both eyes, and sniff from a bottle containing coffee, spice, soap, or some other readily recognized odor. The same is done for the other nostril. Generally, olfaction is not tested unless the patient has some disturbance with smell. Chronic rhinitis, sinusitis, and heavy smoking can often decrease the sense of smell. Disturbance in ability to smell may be associated with a tumor involving the olfactory bulb, or it may be the result of a basilar skull fracture that has damaged the olfactory fibers as they pass through the delicate cribriform plate of the skull.

Optic nerve. Visual fields and visual acuity are assessed to test the function of the optic nerve (CN II). Visual fields are assessed by confrontation. The examiner, positioned directly opposite the patient, asks the patient to close one eye, look directly at the bridge of the examiner's nose, and indicate when an object (finger, pencil tip, head of pin) presented from the periphery of each of the four visual field quadrants is seen (Fig. 53-16). The same test is repeated for the other eye. The examiner is used as a control because both examiner and patient are sharing the same visual field. It is important to remember that the nasal side of the visual field is narrower because of the nasal

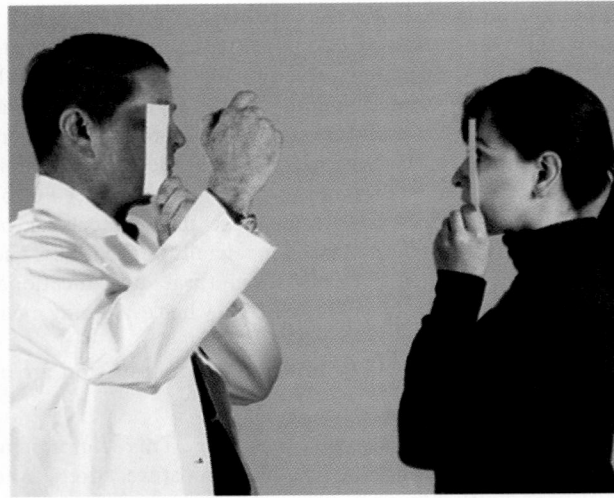

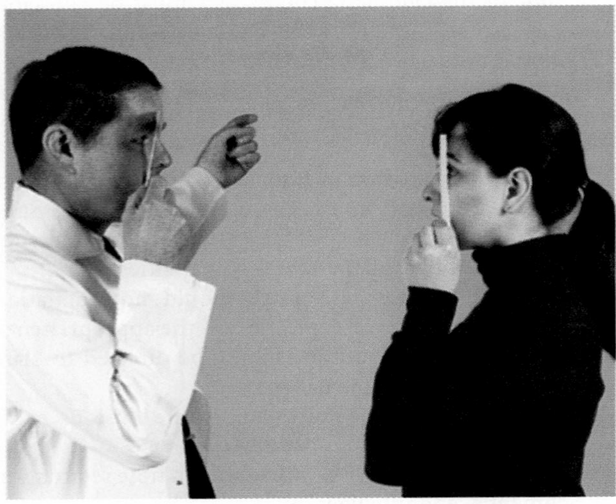

Fig. 53-16 Assessment of visual fields by gross confrontation.

bridge. Visual field defects may arise from lesions of the optic nerve, optic chiasm, or tracts that extend through the temporal, parietal, or occipital lobes. Visual field changes resulting from brain lesions are usually either a hemianopsia (one half of the visual field is affected), a quadrantanopsia (one fourth of the visual field is affected), or monocular.

Visual acuity is tested by asking the patient to read a Snellen chart from 20 feet away. The number on the lowest line that the patient can read with 50% accuracy is recorded. The patient who wears glasses should wear them during testing, unless they are used only for reading. The eyes should be tested individually and together. If a Snellen chart is not available, the patient should be asked to read newsprint for a gross assessment of acuity. The distance from the patient to the newsprint required for accurate reading should be recorded. Acuity may not be testable by these means if the patient does not read English or is aphasic.

Funduscopy reveals the physical condition of the optic disc (head of the optic nerve), as well as the retina and blood vessels. This procedure is routinely performed when the optic nerve is tested. Optic nerve atrophy and papilledema can be detected by this method.

Oculomotor, trochlear, and abducens nerves. Because the oculomotor (CN III), trochlear (CN IV), and abducens (CN VI) nerves all help move the eye, they are tested together. The patient is asked to follow the examiner's finger as it moves horizontally and vertically (making a cross) and diagonally (making an X). If there is weakness or paralysis of one of the eye muscles, the eyes do not move together, and the patient has a disconjugate gaze. The presence and direction of nystagmus (fine, rapid jerking movements of the eyes) is observed at this time, even though it is most often indicative of vestibulocerebellar problems.

Other functions of the oculomotor nerve are tested by checking for pupillary constriction and for convergence (eyes turning inward) and accommodation (pupils constricting with near vision). To test pupillary constriction, the examiner shines a light into the pupil of one eye and looks for ipsilateral constriction of the same pupil and contralateral (consensual) constriction of the opposite eye. The size and shape of the pupils are also noted. The optic nerve must be intact for this reflex to occur. Testing for pupillary constriction is an important component of the neurologic assessment of patients at risk for herniation syndrome (see Chapters 54 and 55). Because the oculomotor nerve exits at the top of the brainstem at the tentorial notch, it can be easily compressed by expanding mass lesions in the cerebral hemispheres. The result is a pupil that does not constrict to light; it may become dilated because the sympathetic input to the pupil acts unopposed. Convergence and accommodation are tested by having the patient focus on the examiner's finger as it moves toward the patient's nose. Another function of the oculomotor nerve is to keep the eyelid open. Damage to the nerve can cause ptosis (drooping eyelid), pupillary abnormalities, and eye muscle weakness.

Trigeminal nerve. The sensory component of the trigeminal nerve (CN V) is tested by having the patient identify light touch (cotton) and pinprick in each of the three divisions (ophthalmic, maxillary, and mandibular) of the nerve on both sides of the face. The patient's eyes should be closed during this part of the examination. The motor component is tested by asking the patient to clench the teeth and palpating the masseter muscles just above the mandibular angle. The corneal reflex test evaluates CN V and CN VII simultaneously. It involves applying a cotton wisp strand to the cornea. The sensory component of this reflex (corneal sensation) is innervated by the ophthalmic division of CN V. The motor component (eye blink) is innervated by the facial nerve (CN VII). This reflex is not normally tested in patients who are awake and alert because other tests evaluate these two nerves. However, for patients with a decreased level of consciousness, the corneal reflex test provides an opportunity to evaluate the integrity of the brainstem at the level of the pons because the fibers of CN V and CN VII have connections in this area.

Facial nerve. The facial nerve (CN VII) innervates the muscles of facial expression. Its function is tested by asking the patient to raise the eyebrows, close the eyes tightly, purse the lips, draw back the corners of the mouth in an exaggerated smile, and frown. The examiner should note any asymmetry in the facial movements because they can indicate damage to the facial nerve. Although taste discrimination of salt and sugar in the anterior two thirds of the tongue is a function of this nerve, it is not routinely tested unless a peripheral nerve lesion is suspected.

Acoustic nerve. The cochlear portion of the acoustic (vestibulocochlear) nerve (CN VIII) is tested by having the patient close the eyes and indicate when a ticking watch or the rustling of the examiner's fingertips is heard as the stimulus is brought closer to the ear. Each ear is tested individually, and the distance from the patient's ear to the sound source when first heard is recorded. This test identifies only gross deficits in hearing. For more precise assessment of hearing, an audiometer is used (see Chapter 19). The vestibular portion of this nerve is not routinely tested unless the patient complains of dizziness, vertigo, or unsteadiness or has auditory dysfunction. If this is the case, caloric testing, which is beyond the scope of routine testing, may be done.

Glossopharyngeal and vagus nerves. The glossopharyngeal and vagus nerves are tested together because both innervate the pharynx. The glossopharyngeal nerve (CN IX) is primarily sensory. In the gag reflex (bilateral contraction of the palatal muscles initiated by stroking or touching either side of the posterior pharynx or soft palate with a tongue blade), the sensory component is mediated by CN IX and the major motor component by the vagus nerve (CN X). It is important to assess the gag reflex in patients who have a decreased level of consciousness, a brainstem lesion, or a disease involving the throat musculature. If the reflex is weak or absent, the patient is in danger of aspirating food or secretions. The strength and efficiency of swallowing is important to test in these patients for the same reason. Another test for the awake, cooperative patient is to have the patient phonate by saying "ah" and to note the bilateral symmetry of elevation of the soft palate. Any asymmetry can indicate weakness or paralysis. Swallowing is also assessed by lightly holding the examiner's hands on either side of the patient's throat and asking the patient to swallow. Any asymmetry is noted.

Spinal accessory nerve. The spinal accessory nerve (CN XI) is tested by asking the patient to shrug the shoulders against resistance and to turn the head to either side against resistance. There should be smooth contraction of the sternomastoid and trapezius muscles. Symmetry, atrophy, or fasciculation of the muscle should also be noted.

Hypoglossal nerve. The hypoglossal nerve (CN XII) is tested by asking the patient to protrude the tongue. It should protrude in the midline. The patient should also be able to push the tongue to either side against the resistance of a tongue blade. Again, any asymmetry, atrophy, or fasciculation should be noted.

Motor system. The motor system examination includes assessment of bulk, tone, and power of the major muscle groups of the body, as well as assessment of balance and coordination. The examiner tests strength by asking the patient to push and pull against the resistance of the examiner's arm as it opposes flexion and extension of the patient's muscle. The patient should be asked to offer resistance at the shoulder, elbow, wrist, hips, knees, and ankles. The patient's grip strength can also be tested. Mild weakness of the upper extremities may be tested by having the patient extend both arms forward at shoulder height with palms up while the eyes are closed. Mild weakness of the arm is demonstrated by downward drifting of the arm or pronation of the palm (pronator drift). Any weakness or asymmetry of strength between the same muscle groups of the right and left side should be noted.

Tone is tested by passively moving the limbs through their range of motion; there should be a slight resistance to these movements. Abnormal tone is described as hypotonia (flaccidity) or hypertonia (spasticity). Involuntary movements (e.g., tics, tremor, myoclonus, athetosis, chorea, dystonia) should be noted.

Cerebellar function is tested by assessing balance and coordination. A good screening test for both balance and muscle strength is to observe the patient's stature (posture while standing) and gait. The examiner should note the pace and rhythm of the gait and observe the arm swing. (The arms should move symmetrically and in the opposite direction of the leg on the same side.) The patient's ability to ambulate is a key factor in determining the amount of nursing care that is needed and the risk of injury from falling. A patient with cerebellar disease may have an ataxic or staggering gait, in which the feet are placed wide apart and the steps are unsteady.

Coordination can be easily tested in several ways. The finger-to-nose test involves having the patient alternately touch the nose with the index finger, then touch the examiner's finger. The examiner repositions the finger while the patient is touching the nose so that the patient must adjust to a new distance each time the examiner's finger is touched. These movements should be performed smoothly and accurately. Other tests include asking the patient to pronate and supinate both hands rapidly and to do a shallow knee bend, first on one leg, and then on the other. Dysarthria or slurred speech should be noted because it is a sign of uncoordination of the speech muscles.

The heel-to-shin test involves having the patient place one heel on the opposite shin below the knee and moving the heel down the shin to the ankle. This is repeated for the other leg. These movements should flow smoothly without jerking or hesitation.

Sensory system. Several modalities are tested in the somatic sensory examination. Each modality is carried by a specific ascending pathway in the spinal cord before it reaches the sensory cortex.

There are some general guidelines for performing the sensory examination. The patient should always have the eyes closed to avoid visual clues. The examiner should avoid giving verbal cues such as "Is this sharp?" The sensory stimulus should be applied in such a way that the patient does not expect it; that is, the examiner should avoid rhythmic application of the stimulus. In the routine neurologic examination, sensory testing of the four extremities is sufficient. However, if a disturbance in sensory function of the skin is identified, the boundaries of that dysfunction should be carefully delineated.

Light touch. Light touch is usually tested first. The examiner gently strokes a cotton wisp over each of the four extremities and asks the patient to indicate when the stimulus is felt by saying "touch." (The sensory examination of the trigeminal nerve may be delayed until this time because the same material for testing sensation is used.)

Pain and temperature. Pain is tested by touching the skin with the sharp end of a pin. This stimulus is irregularly alternated with a simple touch stimulus with the dull end of the pin to determine whether the patient can distinguish the two stimuli. Extinction or inhibition is assessed by simultaneously stimulating opposite sides of the body symmetrically with either a pain or a touch stimulus. Normally, the simultaneous stimuli are perceived (sensed); perception of only one may indicate a parietal lobe lesion.

The sensation of temperature is tested by applying tubes of warm and cold water to the skin and asking the patient to identify the stimuli with the eyes closed. If pain sensation is intact, assessment of temperature sensation may be omitted because both sensations are carried by the same ascending pathways.

Vibration sense. Vibration sense is assessed by applying a vibrating C128 tuning fork to the fingernails and the bony

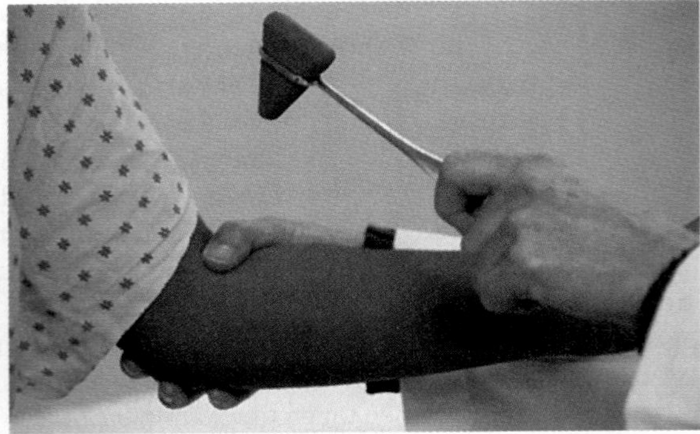

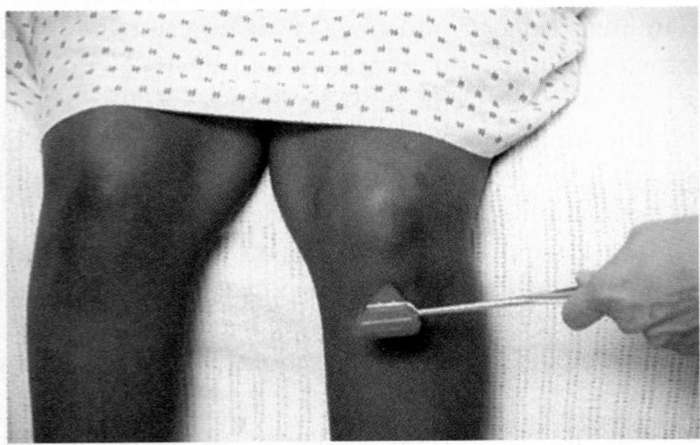

Fig. 53-17 The examiner strikes a swift blow over a stretched tendon to elicit a stretch reflex.

prominences of the hands, legs, and feet with the patient's eyes closed. The examiner asks the patient if the vibration or "buzz" is felt. The examiner then asks the patient to indicate when the vibration ceases. The examiner stops the vibration with the hand as desired.

Position sense. Position sense is assessed by placing the thumb and forefinger on either side of the patient's forefinger or great toe and gently moving the finger up or down. The patient is asked to indicate the direction in which the digit is moved.

Another test of position sense of the lower extremities is the Romberg test. The patient is asked to stand with the feet together and then close his or her eyes. If the patient is able to maintain balance with the eyes open, but sways or falls with the eyes closed (i.e., a positive Romberg test), this may indicate disease in the posterior columns of the spinal cord. It is important that the nurse be aware of patient safety during this test.

Cortical sensory functions. Several tests evaluate cortical integration of sensory perceptions (which occurs in the parietal lobes). Two-point discrimination is assessed by placing the two points of a calibrated compass on the tips of the fingers and toes. The minimum recognizable separation is 4 to 5 mm in the fingertips and a greater degree of separation elsewhere. This test is important in diseases of the sensory cortex and in peripheral nerve disease.

Graphesthesia is tested by having the patient identify numbers traced on the palm of the hands. Stereognosis is tested by having the patient identify the size and shape of easily recognized objects (e.g., coins, keys, a safety pin) placed in the hands. Sensory extinction or inattention is evaluated by touching both sides of the body simultaneously. An abnormal response occurs when the patient perceives the stimulus only on one side. The other stimulus is "extinguished."

Table 53-6 Recording the Normal Neurologic Examination*

Mental Status
Alert and oriented, orderly thought processes, appropriate mood and affect
Cranial Nerves†
Smell intact to soap and coffee; visual fields full to confrontation; visual acuity 20/20 in both eyes; intact extraocular movements; no nystagmus; pupils equal, round, reactive to light and accommodation; intact facial sensation to touch and pinprick; facial movements full; intact gag and swallow reflexes; symmetric elevation of soft palate; full strength with head turning and shrugging of shoulders against resistance; midline protrusion of tongue
Motor System
Normal gait and station; normal tandem walk; negative Romberg test; normal and symmetric muscle bulk, tone, strength; smooth performance of finger-nose, heel-shin movements
Sensory System
Intact sensation to light touch, position sense, vibration, pinprick, heat and cold, two-point discrimination; intact stereognosis and graphesthesia
Reflexes‡
Biceps, triceps, brachioradialis, patellar, and Achilles tendon reflexes 2+ bilaterally; downgoing toes with plantar stimulation

*If some portion of the neurologic examination was not done, this should be indicated (e.g., "Smell not tested").
†May also be recorded as "CN I to XII intact."
‡May also be recorded as drawing of stick figure indicating reflex strength at appropriate sites.

Reflexes. Tendons attached to skeletal muscles have receptors that are sensitive to stretch. A reflex contraction of the skeletal muscle occurs when the tendon is stretched. A simple muscle stretch reflex is initiated by briskly tapping the tendon of a stretched muscle, usually with a reflex hammer (Fig. 53-17). The response (muscle contraction of the corresponding muscle) is measured as follows: 0 = absent, 1 = weak response, 2 = normal response, 3 = exaggerated response, 4 = hyperreflexia with clonus. *Clonus,* an abnormal response, is a continued rhythmic contraction of the muscle after the stimulus has been applied.

In general, the biceps, triceps, brachioradialis, and patellar and Achilles tendon reflexes are tested. The examiner elicits the biceps reflex by placing the thumb over the biceps tendon in the antecubital space and striking the thumb with a hammer. The patient should have the arms partially flexed at the elbow with the palms up. The normal response is flexion of the arm at the elbow or contraction of the biceps muscle that can be felt by the examiner's thumb.

The triceps reflex is elicited by striking the triceps tendon above the elbow while the patient's arm is flexed. The normal response is extension of the arm or visible contraction of the triceps.

The brachioradialis reflex is elicited by striking the radius 3 to 5 cm above the wrist while the patient's arm is relaxed. The normal response is flexion and supination at the elbow or visible contraction of the brachioradialis muscle.

The patellar reflex is elicited by striking the patellar tendon just below the patella. The patient can be sitting or lying as long

COMMON ASSESSMENT ABNORMALITIES

Table 53-7 **Nervous System**

Finding	Description	Possible Etiology and Significance
Altered consciousness	Inability to speak, obey commands, open eyes appropriately with verbal or painful stimulus	Intracranial lesions, metabolic disorder, psychiatric disorders
Anisocoria	Inequality of pupil size	Lesion, injury, or intracranial pressure in area of midbrain
Agnosia	Inability to determine meaning or significance of sensory stimulus	Cerebral cortex lesion
Apraxia	Inability to perform learned movements, defect in motor planning	Cerebral cortex lesion
Aphasia	Loss of language faculty (language comprehension, language expression, or both)	Cerebral cortex lesion
Analgesia	Loss of pain sensation	Lesion in spinothalamic tract or thalamus, lack of or damage to sensory nerve endings
Anesthesia	Absence of sensation	Lesions in spinal cord, thalamus, sensory cortex, or peripheral sensory nerve
Hyperesthesia	Increase in sensation	
Hypoesthesia	Decrease in sensation	
Anosognosia	Inability to recognize bodily defect or disease	Lesions in right parietal cortex, common in right-brain stroke
Astereognosis	Inability to recognize form of object by touch	Lesions in parietal cortex
Ataxia	Lack of coordination of movement	Lesions of sensory or motor pathways, cerebellum; antiseizure drugs, sedative, hypnotic drug toxicity (including alcohol)
Muscle atrophy (disuse or denervation atrophy)	Wasting away or diminution in size of muscle	Suprasegmental (upper motor neuron) lesions, segmental (lower motor neuron) lesions
Bladder dysfunction		
Atonic (autonomous)	Absence of muscle tone and contractility, enlargement of capacity, no sensation of discomfort, overflow with large residual, inability to voluntarily empty or empty by reflex	Early stage of spinal cord injury
Hypotonic	More ability than atonic bladder but less than normal	Interruption of afferent pathways from bladder
Hypertonic	Increase in muscle tone, diminished capacity, reflex emptying, dribbling, incontinence	Lesions in pyramidal tracts (efferent pathways)
Diplopia	Double vision	Lesions affecting nerves of extraocular muscles, cerebellar toxicity
Dysarthria	Lack of coordination in articulating speech	Lesions in cerebellum or pathway of cranial nerves (including brainstem); antiseizure drug, sedative, or hypnotic drug toxicity (including alcohol)
Dyskinesia	Impairment of power of voluntary movement, resulting in fragmentary or incomplete movements	Disorders of basal ganglia, idiosyncratic reaction to psychotropic drugs
Dysphagia	Difficulty in swallowing	Lesions involving motor pathways of CN IX, X (including lower brainstem)
Extensor plantar response (Babinski's sign)	Upgoing toes with plantar stimulation	Suprasegmental or upper motor neuron lesion

Continued

as the leg being tested hangs freely. The normal response is extension of the leg with contraction of the quadriceps.

The Achilles tendon reflex is elicited by striking the Achilles tendon while the patient's leg is flexed at the knee and the foot is dorsiflexed at the ankle. The normal response is plantar flexion at the ankle.

Table 53-6 is an example of how to record a normal neurologic assessment. Common abnormal assessment findings of the neurologic system are presented in Table 53-7.

Nursing Approach. The premise of the nursing approach is that the primary purpose of nursing is to help patients cope effectively with deficits in self-care and in activities of daily living.

COMMON ASSESSMENT ABNORMALITIES

Table 53-7 Nervous System—cont'd

Finding	Description	Possible Etiology and Significance
Homonymous hemianopsia	Loss of vision in one side of visual field	Injury or lesions in area of optic tract or its radiations to occipital cortex
Hemiplegia	Paralysis on one side	Stroke and other lesions involving motor cortex
Nystagmus	Jerking or bobbing of eyes as they track moving object	Lesions in cerebellum, brainstem, vestibular system; antiseizure, sedative, hypnotic toxicity (including alcohol)
Ophthalmoplegia	Paralysis of eye muscles	Lesions in brainstem or CN III, IV, VI
Opisthotonus	Extreme arching of back with retraction of head	Meningitis, tonic phase of grand mal seizure
Papilledema	"Choked disc," swelling of optic nerve head	Increase in intracranial pressure
Paraplegia	Paralysis of lower extremities	Spinal cord transection or mass lesion (thoracolumbar region)
Quadriplegia	Paralysis of all extremities	Spinal cord transection or mass lesion (cervical region) or brainstem

Consequently, the neurologic examination should be viewed in terms of functional disabilities rather than dysfunction of component parts of the nervous system. The effects of the disabilities on the patient's potential for self-care, movement, and desired activities of daily living should be the focus. This includes understanding, communicating, remembering, seeing, speaking, feeling, moving, walking, and using integrated regulatory functions, such as elimination and temperature regulation. In addition, based on knowledge of the location of the problematic area and the functions it controls, the nurse should ask specific questions and perform certain examinations to determine what other effects the condition may have on daily functioning.

All functions of the nervous system can be categorized in six areas: consciousness, mentation, movement, sensation, integrated regulation, and coping with disability. Table 53-8 lists the functions involved in each of these categories and thus forms the basis of a nursing neurologic assessment.

Table 53-8 Functional Categories in Nursing Neurologic Assessment

Consciousness	
Arousal	Self-awareness
Mentation	
Thinking	Language
Remembering	Problem solving
Perceiving	
Movement	
Expressing (facial)	Transferring
Speaking	Eating (chewing, swallowing)
Walking	Blinking (combined movement and sensation)
Sensation	
Seeing	Feeling (e.g., touch, temperature, pain, pressure, position, form, shape)
Smelling	
Hearing	
Integrated Regulatory Function	
Eating (ingesting, digesting)	Circulation
	Temperature control
Eliminating	Sexual response
Breathing	Emotion
Coping with Disability	
Self-care competence	Coping (e.g., adapting, supporting, growing)
Role competence	

DIAGNOSTIC STUDIES OF THE NERVOUS SYSTEM

Diagnostic studies provide important information to the nurse in monitoring the patient's condition and planning appropriate interventions. These studies are considered to be objective data. Diagnostic studies common to the nervous system are presented in Table 53-9.

Cerebrospinal Fluid Analysis

CSF analysis provides information about a variety of CNS diseases. Normal CSF fluid is clear, colorless, and free of red blood cells (RBCs) and contains little protein. Normal CSF values are listed in Table 53-10.

Lumbar Puncture. Lumbar puncture is the most common method of obtaining CSF for analysis. It is contraindicated in the presence of increased intracranial pressure or infection at the site of puncture.

Nurses often assist in this procedure because it is usually performed in the patient's room. Before the procedure, the nurse should have the patient empty the bladder. The patient should lie in the lateral recumbent position, with the back as near as possible to the edge of the bed. The nurse should assist the patient to draw up the knees to the abdomen and flex the head to the chest. This helps separate the vertebrae so that the needle can be inserted more easily.

Using strict sterile technique, the physician inserts a long needle below the third lumbar vertebra. This may cause some local discomfort. There is no danger of injuring the spinal cord, since the cord terminates between the first and second lumbar vertebrae. However, the patient may have some pain radiating

DIAGNOSTIC STUDIES

Table 53-9 Nervous System

Study	Description and Purpose	Nursing Responsibility
Cerebrospinal Fluid Analysis		
▪ Lumbar puncture	CSF is aspirated by needle insertion in L3-4 or L4-5 interspace to assess many CNS diseases. (See Table 53-10.)	Assist patient to assume and maintain lateral recumbent position with knees flexed. Ensure maintenance of strict aseptic technique. Ensure labeling of CSF specimens in proper sequence. Keep patient flat for at least a few hours depending on physician preference. Encourage fluids. Monitor neurologic and VS. Administer analgesia as needed.
Radiologic		
▪ Skull and spine x-rays	Simple x-ray of skull and spinal column is done to detect fractures, bone erosion, calcifications, abnormal vascularity.	Explain that procedure is noninvasive. Explain positions to be assumed.
▪ Cerebral angiography	Serial x-ray visualization of intracranial and extracranial blood vessels is performed to detect vascular lesions and tumors of brain. Radiopaque contrast medium is used.	Withhold preceding meal. Explain that patient will have hot flush of head and neck when dye is injected. Administer premedication. Explain need to be absolutely still during procedure. Monitor neurologic and VS every 15-30 min first 2 hr, every hr next 6 hr, then every 2 hr for 24 hr. Maintain pressure dressing and ice to injection site. Maintain bed rest until patient is alert and VS are stable. Report any signs of change in neurologic status.
▪ Computed tomography (CT) scan	Computer-assisted x-ray of several levels or thin cross sections of body parts are done to detect problems such as hemorrhage, tumor, cyst, edema, infarction, brain atrophy, hydrocephalus.	Explain that procedure is noninvasive (if no dye used). Observe for allergic reaction and note puncture site (if dye used). Explain appearance of scanner. Instruct patient on need to remain absolutely still during procedure.
▪ Myelography	X-ray of spinal cord and vertebral column after injection of dye into subarachnoid space is used to detect spinal lesions (e.g., ruptured disk, tumor).	Administer preprocedure sedation as ordered. Instruct patient to empty bladder. Inform patient that test is performed with patient on tilting table that is moved during test. Encourage fluids. Monitor neurologic and VS.
▪ Magnetic resonance imaging (MRI)	Internal body parts are visualized by means of magnetic energy. No invasive procedures are required unless contrast material is used.	Screen patient for metal parts and pacemaker in body. Instruct patient on need to lie very still for up to 1 hr. Sedation may be necessary if patient is claustrophobic.
▪ Positron emission tomography (PET)	Measures metabolic activity of brain regions to assess cell death or damage. Uses radioactive compounds.	Explain procedure to patient. Explain that two IV lines will be inserted. Instruct patient not to take sedatives or tranquilizers. Empty bladder before procedure. May be asked to perform different activities during test.
Electrographic		
▪ Electroencephalography (EEG)	Electrical activity of brain is recorded by scalp electrodes to evaluate cerebral disease, CNS effects of systemic diseases, brain death.	Inform patient that procedure is painless and without danger of electric shock. Withhold stimulants. Inform that patient may be asked to perform various activities such as hyperventilation during test. Determine whether any medications (e.g., tranquilizers, antiseizure drugs) should be withheld. Resume medications after test. Assist patient to wash electrode paste out of hair.

Continued

DIAGNOSTIC STUDIES

Table 53-9 Nervous System—cont'd

Study	Description and Purpose	Nursing Responsibility
Electrographic—cont'd		
▪ Electromyography/ Nerve conduction	Electrical activity associated with nerve and skeletal muscle is recorded by insertion of needle electrodes to detect muscle and peripheral nerve disease.	Inform patient of slight discomfort associated with insertion of needles.
▪ Evoked potentials	Electrical activity associated with nerve conduction along sensory pathways is recorded by electrodes placed on skin and scalp. Stimulus generates the impulse. Procedure is used to diagnose disease, locate nerve damage, and monitor function intraoperatively.	Explain procedure to patient.
▪ Visual evoked potentials	Electrical activity in visual pathway is recorded with rapidly reversing checkerboard pattern on television screen. One eye is tested at a time.	Explain procedure to patient.
▪ Brainstem auditory evoked potentials	Electrical activity in auditory pathway is recorded with earphones that produce clicking sounds. One ear is tested at a time.	Explain procedure to patient.
▪ Somatosensory evoked potentials	Electrical activity in certain nerve pathways is recorded with mild electrical pulse (several per second).	Inform patient that stimulus may cause mild discomfort or muscle twitch.
Ultrasound		
▪ Carotid duplex studies	Sound waves determine blood flow velocity, which indicates presence of occlusive vascular disease.	Explain procedure to patient.
▪ Transcranial Doppler	Same technology as carotid duplex, but evaluates intracranial vessels.	Explain procedure to patient.

VS, vital signs.

Table 53-10 Normal Cerebrospinal Fluid Values

Parameter	Normal Value
Specific gravity	1.007
pH	7.35
Appearance	Clear, colorless
RBCs	None
WBCs	0-8/μl (0-0.008/L)
Protein	
Lumbar	15-45 mg/dl (0.15-0.45 g/L)
Cisternal	15-25 mg/dl (0.15-0.25 g/L)
Ventricular	5-15 mg/dl (0.05-0.15 g/L)
Glucose	45-75 mg/dl (2.5-4.2 mmol/L)
Microorganisms	None
Opening pressure with lumbar puncture	60-150 mm H_2O

down the leg or muscle twitching if the spinal root is irritated by the needle. The nurse can assure the patient that this is temporary, and that the patient is not in danger of being paralyzed.

A manometer is attached to the needle, and CSF pressure is determined *after* the patient is asked to relax and extend the legs. If this is not done, the pressure appears abnormally high. CSF is withdrawn in a series of tubes and sent for analysis. Some examiners believe that the patient should be kept lying flat for at least a few hours after the procedure to avoid a spinal headache, which is presumably caused by loss of the cushioning effect of CSF as a result of leakage of CSF at the puncture site. The prone position may be effective in preventing CSF leakage. Other clinicians do not believe that the lying position is necessary because headache seems to develop in some patients despite precautions. Meningeal irritation (nuchal rigidity) or signs and symptoms of local trauma (e.g., hematoma, pain) may develop in some patients.

Radiologic Studies

Cerebral Angiography. Cerebral angiography is indicated when vascular lesions or tumors are suspected. A catheter is inserted into the femoral (sometimes brachial) artery. It is then passed up the artery to the aortic arch and into the base of a carotid or a vertebral artery for injection of radiopaque dye. A series of x-rays is taken in a timed sequence so that pictures of the arteries, smaller vessels, and veins can be obtained (Fig. 53-18). This study can help localize and determine the presence of abscesses, aneurysms, hematomas,

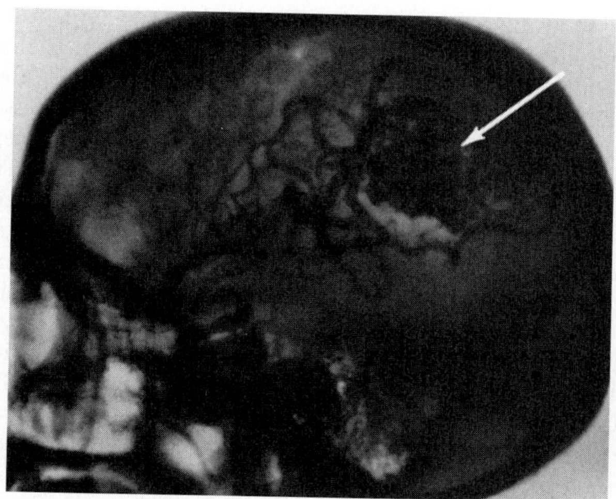

Fig. 53-18 Cerebral angiogram illustrating an arteriovenous malformation *(arrow).*

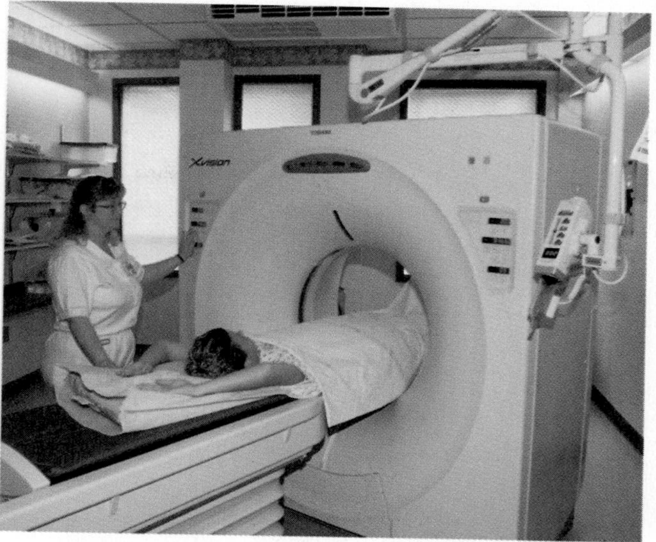

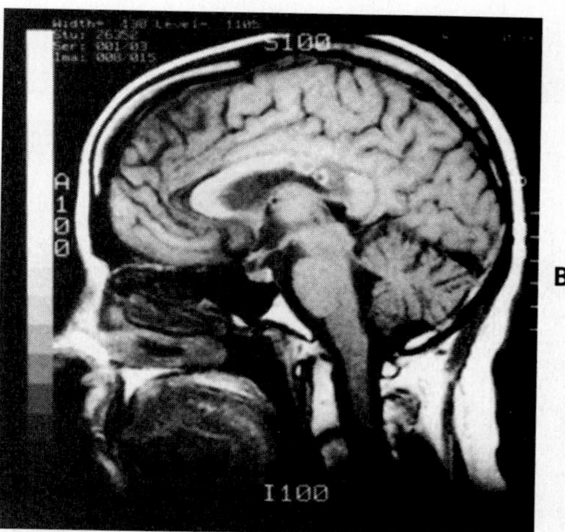

Fig. 53-19 **A,** Clinical setting for magnetic resonance imaging (MRI). **B,** Midline sagittal view of the brain using MRI.

arteriovenous malformations, arterial spasm, and certain tumors.

Because this is an invasive procedure, adverse reactions may occur. The patient may have an allergic (anaphylactic) reaction to the contrast medium. This reaction usually occurs immediately after injection of the contrast medium and may require emergency resuscitation measures in the procedure room. The most common precaution for nurses to take in caring for the patient after the return to the room is observation for bleeding at the catheter puncture site (usually the groin). A pressure dressing and ice are usually placed on the site to promote hemostasis and prevent swelling.

Computed Tomography. Computed tomography (CT) scan is a noninvasive procedure, although intravenous injection of contrast medium may be used to enhance visualization of the blood vessels and identify disruptions in the blood-brain barrier. CT scans can be done on an outpatient basis. A number of x-rays scanning different levels of the brain are compiled with computer assistance and presented in a series of black-and-white pictures. These pictures, which illustrate "slices" of the brain, can show hemorrhages, tumors, cysts, edema, infarction, brain atrophy, and hydrocephalus. CT scans do not illustrate structures in the posterior fossa and the base of the brain as clearly as does magnetic resonance imaging.

Magnetic Resonance Imaging. Magnetic resonance imaging (MRI) became available in the mid-1980s. Rather than using x-rays, this method involves two kinds of magnetism. The patient is placed within a giant magnetic field that aligns the protons of the hydrogen ions in the cells of the body (Fig. 53-19). Bursts of radio-frequency magnetism are introduced to flip the protons out of alignment. When the radio-frequency magnetism is turned off, the protons realign. The resulting magnetic field change is picked up by the machine and is processed by a computer. A vivid black-and-white picture of slices of the brain is then produced.

MRI is useful in evaluating brain and spinal cord edema, hemorrhage, infarction, blood vessels, neoplasms, and bone lesions. Intravenous injection of gadolinium is used to enhance the images obtained with MRI.[3] Because MRI yields greater contrast in the images of soft-tissue structures than does the CT scan, it is the diagnostic test of choice for many neurologic diseases.

Positron Emission Tomography. Positron emission tomography (PET) is used to determine regional metabolism in the brain. PET provides a noninvasive means of determining biochemical processes that occur in the brain. There is increased clinical use of PET scan to monitor select patients following cerebrovascular accident, Alzheimer's disease, epilepsy, and Parkinson' disease.

Myelography. Myelography is used to visualize the spinal column and the subarachnoid space when a spinal lesion is suspected. The most common lesion for which this test is used is a herniated or protruding intervertebral disk. Other lesions include spinal tumors, adhesions, syringomyelia, bony deformations, and arteriovenous malformations. The test involves x-rays of the spinal column after injection of the contrast medium into the subarachnoid space via a catheter. Water-soluble iodine dyes such as iopamidol (Isovue) are used most often because they are absorbed into the bloodstream and excreted by the kidneys.

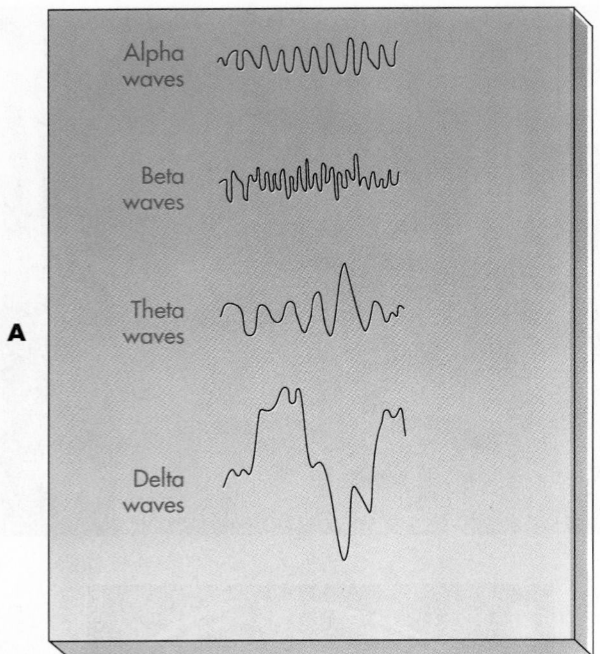

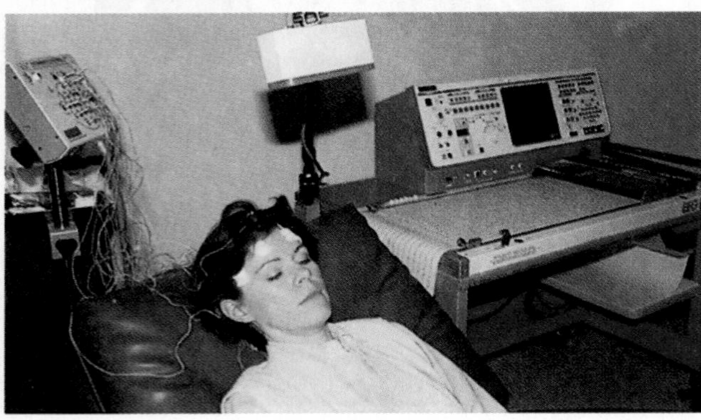

Fig. 53-20 The electroencephalogram (EEG). **A,** Examples of alpha, beta, theta, and delta waves seen on an EEG. **B,** Photograph showing a person undergoing an EEG test. Notice the scalp electrodes that detect voltage fluctuations within the cranium.

Preparation for this procedure is the same as for lumbar puncture. Before the dye is injected, patients must be asked whether they have any allergies, specifically whether they have had any anaphylactic or hypotensive episodes from other dyes. After myelography the patient should be flat for a few hours.

Headache is the most common complaint after myelography. It may be accompanied by nausea and occasionally by vomiting. The nurse should observe the patient for any changes in neurologic status and provide a quiet, comfortable environment after the procedure.

Electrographic Studies

Electroencephalography. The technique of electroencephalography (EEG) involves the recording of the electrical activity of the surface cortical neurons of the brain by 8 to 16 electrodes placed on specific areas of the scalp. This test is done to evaluate not only cerebral disease but also the CNS effects of many metabolic and systemic diseases and to determine brain death. Among the cerebral diseases assessed by EEG are epilepsy, mass lesions (e.g., tumor, abscess, hematoma), cerebrovascular lesions, and brain injury (Fig. 53-20). The procedure is noninvasive. Patients sometimes have the misconception that the recording electrodes will give them an electric shock. They should be assured that this is not true and that the procedure is similar to electrocardiography.

Electromyography and Nerve Conduction Studies. Electromyography (EMG) is the recording of electrical activity associated with innervation of skeletal muscle. The recording is displayed on a cathode-ray oscilloscope and may be played on a loudspeaker for simultaneous analysis. Needle electrodes are inserted into the muscle to record specific motor units because recording from the skin is not sufficient. Normal muscle at rest shows no electrical activity. Typical electrical activity occurs when the muscle contracts. This activity may be altered in diseases of muscle itself (e.g., myopathic conditions) or in disorders of muscle innervation (e.g., segmental or lower motor neuron lesions, peripheral neuropathic conditions). Fibrillations are spontaneous, independent contractions of individual muscle fibers that can be detected only by EMG. They appear on EMG 1 to 3 weeks after a muscle has lost its nerve supply.

Nerve conduction studies involve application of a brief electrical stimulus to a distal portion of a sensory or mixed nerve and recording the resulting wave of depolarization at some point proximal to the stimulation. For example, a stimulus can be applied to the forefinger and a recording electrode placed over the median nerve at the wrist. The time between the onset of the stimulus and the initial wave of depolarization at the recording electrode is measured. This is termed *nerve conduction velocity.* Damaged nerves have slower conduction velocities.

Evoked Potentials. Evoked potentials are recordings of electrical activity associated with nerve conduction along sensory pathways. The activity is generated by a specific sensory stimulus related to the type of study (e.g., checkerboard patterns for visual evoked potentials, clicking sounds for auditory evoked potentials, and mild electrical pulses for somatosensory evoked potentials). Electrodes placed on specific areas of the skin and scalp record the electrical activity, which is stored and averaged by a computerized instrument. A wave pattern appears on a screen and is printed on paper. Peaks in the wave pattern correspond to conduction of the stimulus through certain points along the sensory pathway (e.g., peripheral nerve, brainstem, cortical areas). Increases in the normal time from stimulus onset to a given peak (latency) indicate slowed nerve conduction or nerve damage. Indications for these tests include evaluation of the optic nerve in conditions such as multiple sclerosis (optic neuritis) and the vestibulocochlear nerve in acoustic neuroma.

Combined Doppler and Ultrasound (Duplex) Studies

Carotid Duplex. A carotid duplex study uses combined ultrasound and pulsed Doppler technology. A technician places a probe on the skin over the carotid artery and slowly moves the probe along the course of the common carotid to the bifurcation of the external and internal carotid arteries. The ultrasound signal emitted from the probe reflects off the moving blood cells within the vessel. The frequency of the reflected signal corresponds to the blood velocity. This response is amplified and is registered on a graphic record and also as sound. The graphic record registers blood velocity. Increased blood flow velocity can indicate stenosis of a vessel. Carotid duplex scanning is a noninvasive study that evaluates carotid occlusive disease.

Transcranial Doppler Sonography. Transcranial Doppler (TCD) sonography uses the same technology as carotid duplex studies, except that it records blood flow velocities of the intracranial blood vessels. The probe is placed on the skin at various "windows" in the skull (areas in the skull that have only a thin bony covering) in order to register velocities of the middle cerebral artery, anterior cerebral artery, posterior cerebral artery, terminal carotid artery, and occasionally the anterior and posterior communicating arteries. The temporal, orbital, and suboccipital sites are used. The ultrasound signal received is recorded graphically as a wave form. Peak blood flow velocities and systolic-diastolic ratios can be calculated from this information. TCD sonography is a noninvasive technique that is useful in assessing vasospasm associated with subarachnoid hemorrhage, altered intracranial blood flow dynamics associated with occlusive vascular disease, cerebral autoregulation, presence of emboli, and brain death.

REVIEW QUESTIONS

The number of the question corresponds to the same-numbered objective at the beginning of the chapter.

1. In a patient with a disease that affects the myelin sheath of nerves, such as multiple sclerosis, the glial cells that are affected are the
   a. microglia.
   b. astrocytes.
   c. oligodendroglia.
   d. ependymal cells.
2. A state of hypoxia alters the repeated action potentials necessary for transmission of nerve impulses because energy is required for
   a. repolarization of the cell membrane.
   b. creation of cell membrane permeability.
   c. movement of sodium into the nerve cell.
   d. maintenance of the resting membrane potential.
3. Drugs or diseases that impair the function of the extrapyramidal system may cause loss of
   a. sensations of pain and temperature.
   b. regulation of the autonomic nervous system.
   c. integration of somatic and special sensory inputs.
   d. automatic movements associated with skeletal muscle activity.
4. An obstruction of the anterior cerebral arteries will affect functions of
   a. visual imaging.
   b. balance and coordination.
   c. judgment, insight, and reasoning.
   d. visual and auditory integration for language comprehension.
5. Paralysis of lateral gaze indicates a lesion of cranial nerve
   a. II.
   b. III.
   c. IV.
   d. VI.
6. A result of stimulation of the parasympathetic nervous system is
   a. relaxation of the bladder.
   b. dilation of skin blood vessels.
   c. increased secretion of insulin.
   d. increased blood glucose levels.
7. Assessment of muscle strength of older adults cannot be compared with that of younger adults because
   a. stroke is more common in older adults.
   b. nutritional status is better in young adults.
   c. most young people exercise more than older people.
   d. aging leads to a decrease in muscle bulk and strength.
8. Data regarding mobility, strength, coordination, and activity tolerance are important for the nurse to obtain because
   a. many neurologic diseases affect one or more of these areas.
   b. patients are less able to identify other neurologic impairments.
   c. these are the first functions to be affected by neurologic disease.
   d. aspects of movement are the most important functions of the nervous system.
9. During neurologic testing the patient is able to perceive pain elicited by pinprick. Based on this finding the nurse may omit testing for
   a. position sense.
   b. patellar reflexes.
   c. temperature perception.
   d. heel-to-shin movements.
10. A patient's eyes jerk as they follow the nurse's moving finger. The nurse records this finding as
    a. nystagmus.
    b. normal tracking.
    c. ophthalmoplegia.
    d. ophthalmic dyskinesia.
11. Nursing responsibilities for lumbar puncture include
    a. ensuring the patient has a full bladder.
    b. placing the patient in the lateral recumbent position.
    c. straightening the patient's legs just before the puncture.
    d. having the patient cough when the needle has been inserted.

References

1. Bradley WG and others, editors: *Neurology in clinical practice,* ed 2, Boston, 1996, Butterworth-Heineman.
2. Haerer AF: *DeJong's the neurologic examination,* ed 5, Philadelphia, 1992, Lippincott.
3. Haines DE, editor: *Fundamental neuroscience,* New York, 1997, Churchill Livingstone.
4. Hickey JV: *The clinical practice of neurological and neurosurgical nursing,* ed 4, Philadelphia, 1997, Lippincott.
5. Mitchell PH and others: *Neurologic assessment for nursing practice,* Reston, Va, 1984, Reston.

***For additional Internet resources, see the website for this book at* www.mosby.com/MERLIN/medsurg_lewis**

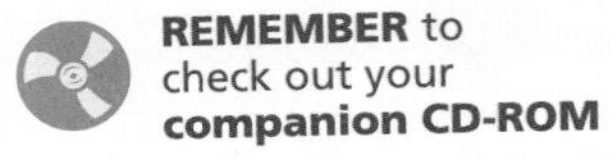

54 NURSING MANAGEMENT Intracranial Problems

Mary E. Kerr

www.mosby.com/MERLIN/medsurg_lewis

LEARNING OBJECTIVES

1. Define unconsciousness.
2. Explain the mechanisms of unconsciousness.
3. Describe the nursing management of the unconscious patient.
4. Define intracranial pressure, including normal values.
5. Identify the physiologic mechanisms of accommodation that maintain normal intracranial pressure.
6. Identify the common etiologies, clinical manifestations, and collaborative care of increased intracranial pressure.
7. Describe the nursing management of the patient with increased intracranial pressure.
8. Differentiate types of head injury by mechanism of injury, clinical manifestations, and treatments.
9. Describe the collaborative care and nursing management of head injury.
10. Compare the types, clinical manifestations, and collaborative care of intracranial tumors.
11. Identify the nursing diagnoses and nursing management of the patient with an intracranial tumor.
12. Describe the nursing management of the patient undergoing cranial surgery.
13. Compare the primary causes, collaborative care, and prognosis of common cerebral inflammatory problems.
14. Explain the general nursing management of the patient with a cerebral inflammatory problem.

UNCONSCIOUSNESS

Unconsciousness is an abnormal state in which the patient is unaware of self or environment.[1] Unconsciousness can range from a brief episode, such as fainting, to the prolonged unconsciousness of coma from which the person cannot be roused, even with vigorous external stimuli. Between these two extremes are degrees of unconsciousness varying in length and severity. Unconsciousness itself is not a diagnosis or a disease but rather a manifestation of a large number of pathophysiologic processes, including trauma, metabolic disturbances, mass lesions, and infections. Collaborative care is aimed at determining and correcting the cause of the unconsciousness, maintaining the bodily functions of the patient, supporting the vital functions, and protecting the patient from injury and the hazards of immobility.

Etiology

Consciousness involves two aspects: arousal and content. The arousal component of consciousness refers to a state of wakefulness dependent on the activity of the reticular activating system (RAS), a network of nerve fibers and cell bodies that is located in the reticular formation in the central part of the brainstem and has neural connections to many parts of the nervous system. An intact RAS can maintain a state of wakefulness, even in the absence of a functioning cortex. The content component of consciousness refers to the ability to reason, think, and feel and to react to stimuli with purpose and awareness. These activities are mediated by the cerebral hemispheres, commonly called the higher centers. Intellect and emotional functions are also controlled by these centers.

Interruption of impulses from the RAS or alteration of the functioning of the cerebral hemispheres can cause unconsciousness. Any condition that markedly alters the function of the hemispheres or that depresses or destroys the upper brainstem results in an impaired consciousness. Many specific etiologic events can result in unconsciousness. Causes can be grouped according to pathophysiologic mechanisms, such as supratentorial mass lesions, subtentorial mass lesions, destructive lesions, or metabolic and diffuse cerebral disorders (Table 54-1). Psychiatric disorders such as depression, catatonia, and schizophrenia can result in failure to respond to the environment.

Supratentorial mass lesions generally interfere with consciousness by compressing and shifting the cerebral contents and causing pressure on the upper brainstem containing the RAS. These lesions, occurring above the tentorium, may include those resulting from trauma (e.g., lacerations or contusions, subdural or epidural hematomas), subarachnoid hemorrhage, intracerebral hemorrhage or infarction, tumors, and abscesses. The most serious consequence of a supratentorial mass lesion is herniation of the cerebral hemisphere through the tentorial notch, causing compression of the brainstem. Another form of herniation can occur if the brain shifts laterally, forcing the cingulate gyrus under the falx and compressing the

Reviewed by Mary Lou Muwaswes, RN, MS, Clinical Nurse Specialist, San Francisco, Calif.

Table 54-1 Causes of Unconsciousness

Supratentorial Mass Lesions	Metabolic and Diffuse Cerebral Disorders
Epidural hematoma	Hypoxia or anoxia
Subdural hematoma	Postictal states and concussion
Intracerebral hematoma	Infection (meningitis, encephalitis)
Cerebral infarction	Subarachnoid hemorrhage
Brain tumor	Exogenous toxins
Brain abscess	Drug overdose
Subtentorial Lesions	Alcohol intoxication
Brainstem infarction	Lead poisoning
Brainstem tumor	Endogenous toxins and deficiencies
Brainstem hemorrhage	Hypoglycemia
Cerebellar hemorrhage	Uremia
Cerebellar abscess	Hepatic encephalopathy
	Thiamine deficiency

blood vessels and brain tissue of the opposite hemisphere. The end result of herniation is ischemia and irreversible infarction (see Fig. 54-5 later in this chapter).

Subtentorial masses or destructive lesions that occur below the tentorium interfere with consciousness by compressing or destroying the RAS above the midpons. Pontine or cerebellar hemorrhage, infarction, tumor, or abscess can affect the subtentorial area of the brain through direct brain compression, upward herniation through the tentorial notch, or downward herniation into the foramen magnum.

Metabolic and diffuse cerebral disorders of either intracranial or extracranial origin can cause alterations in the conscious state. These disorders can disturb cerebral metabolism and thus alter the regulation of cellular nutrition, electrolyte balance, oxygen and carbon dioxide regulation, and enzymatic functions. Specific metabolic problems that can cause unconsciousness include uremia, diabetes mellitus, hypoglycemia, alcohol intoxication, drug (e.g., barbiturate) overdose, and lead poisoning.

Regardless of the cause of the unconscious state, two pathophysiologic processes that affect cerebral metabolism generally occur: cerebral ischemia-anoxia and cerebral edema. The pathophysiologic problem common to all metabolic brain diseases is decreased oxygen uptake. Cerebral ischemia-anoxia, both focal and global, is managed by instituting measures to ensure adequate systemic circulation. Cerebral edema and the resulting increased intracranial pressure may be treated by hyperosmotic drugs and corticosteroids.

Psychiatric or psychogenic disorders can cause unconsciousness. Although the neurologic system is intact, the patient does not react to the environment. A psychiatric referral is appropriate when the possibility of organic disease has been ruled out.

Unconscious State

The patient's state of consciousness is defined by both the behavior and the pattern of brain activity recorded by an electroencephalogram (EEG). In the deepest state of unconsciousness, the patient does not respond to painful stimuli. Corneal and pupillary reflexes are absent. The patient cannot swallow or cough and is incontinent of urine and feces. The EEG pattern demonstrates decreased or absent neuronal activity. This patient is in a coma.

Behavior. The nurse may find it helpful to conceptualize states of consciousness as a continuum. This continuum of electrical activity in the brain ranges from the hyperexcitable state of seizure to the hypoexcitable state of coma. The normal level of alertness is between these two states, with abnormalities ranging from slight disorientation to coma. A variety of terms have been used to describe points on the continuum, but they tend to be confusing. For example, the term *lethargy* has a variety of meanings. Rather than relying on these terms, the nurse must learn appropriate assessment techniques and describe the level of consciousness by noting the specific behaviors observed. When a deviation from the normal state of consciousness occurs, a more structured method of observation should be initiated. This type of systematic approach to nursing assessment is illustrated in Fig. 54-1 and consists of assessing the level of consciousness by the Glasgow Coma Scale (GCS) and by body functions.

Glasgow Coma Scale. Because of the confusion and ambiguity that surround terms describing altered states of consciousness, the GCS was developed in 1974. The three areas assessed in this method correspond to the definition of *coma* as the inability of a patient to speak, obey commands, or open the eyes when a verbal or painful stimulus is applied.[2] Specific assessments evaluate the patient's response to varying degrees of stimuli. Three indicators of response are evaluated: (1) opening of the eyes, (2) the best verbal response, and (3) the best motor response (Table 54-2). Specific behaviors that are seen as responses to the testing stimulus in each of these three areas are given a numeric value and can be plotted on a graph. The clinician's responsibility is to elicit the best response on each of the scales: the higher the scores, the higher the level of brain functioning. The graph visually plots a place on the consciousness continuum to determine whether the patient is stable, improving, or deteriorating. The subscale scores are particularly important if a patient is untestable in one area. For example, severe periorbital edema may make eye opening impossible. The total GCS score is a sum of the numeric values assigned to each of the three areas evaluated. The highest GCS score is 15 for a fully alert person, and the lowest possible score is 3. A GCS score of 8 or less is generally indicative of coma.

The GCS offers several advantages in the assessment of the unconscious patient. It is specific and structured, allowing different clinicians to arrive at the same conclusion regarding the patient's status. It saves time for the assessor because the ratings are done with numbers rather than with lengthy descriptions. The GCS is also specific enough to discriminate between different or changing states.

The GCS is used to assess the arousal aspect of consciousness. Other components of the neurologic assessment include pupillary checks, extremity strength testing, and, if appropriate, corneal reflex testing.

Monitoring of Body Functions. In addition to assessing the neurologic state of the unconscious patient, various body functions, such as respiration and elimination, also must

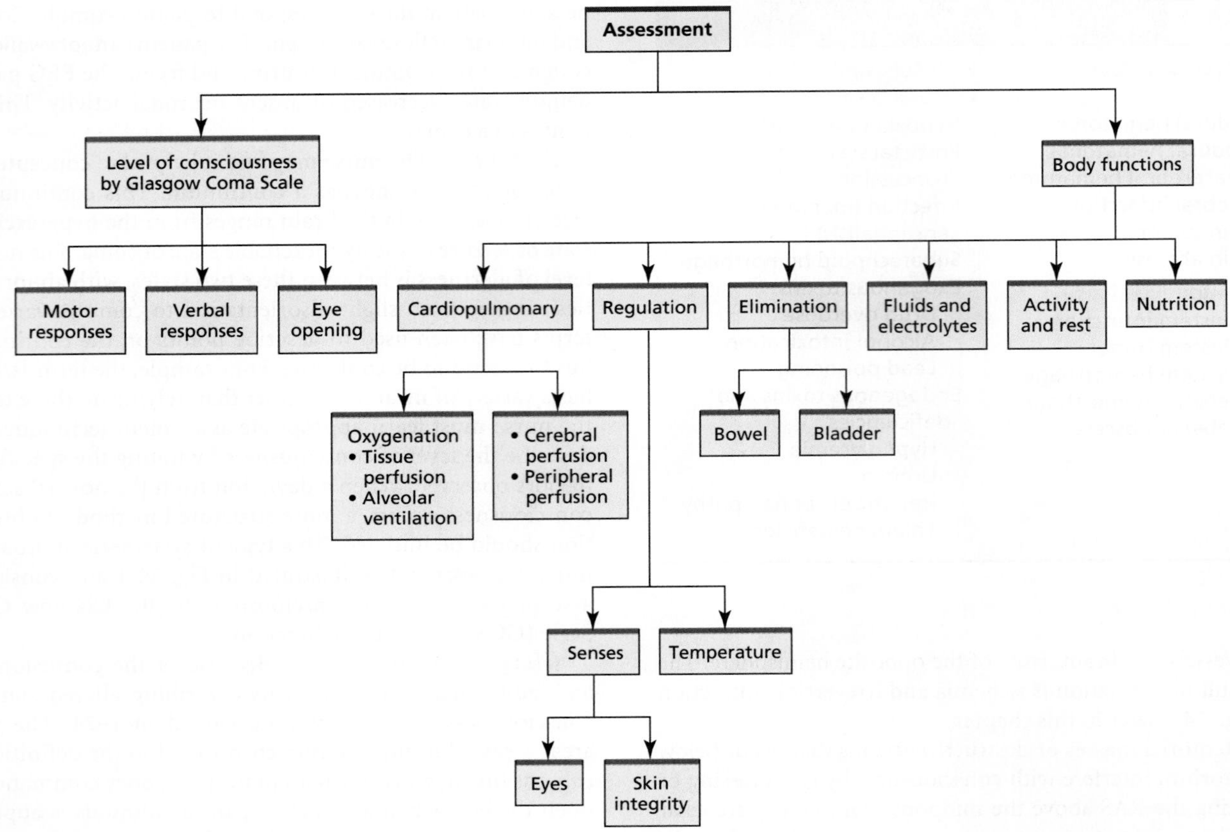

Fig. 54-1 A systematic approach to nursing assessment of the unconscious patient.

Table 54-2 Glasgow Coma Scale

Category of Response	Appropriate Stimulus	Response	Score
■ Eyes open	Approach to bedside	Spontaneous response	4
	Verbal command	Opening of eyes to name or command	3
	Pain	Lack of opening of eyes to previous stimuli but opening to pain	2
		Lack of opening of eyes to any stimulus	1
		Untestable	U
■ Best verbal response	Verbal questioning with maximum arousal	Appropriate orientation, conversant, correct identification of self, place, year, and month	5
		Confusion, conversant, but disorientation in one or more spheres	4
		Inappropriate or disorganized use of words (e.g., cursing), lack of sustained conversation	3
		Incomprehensible words, sounds (e.g., moaning)	2
		Lack of sound, even with painful stimuli	1
		Untestable	U
■ Best motor response	Verbal command (e.g., "raise your arm, hold up two fingers")	Obedience of command	6
		Localization of pain, lack of obedience but presence of attempts to remove offending stimulus	5
	Pain (pressure on proximal nail bed)	Flexion withdrawal,* flexion of arm in response to pain without abnormal flexion posture	4
		Abnormal flexion, flexing of arm at elbow and pronation, making a fist	3
		Abnormal extension, extension of arm at elbow usually with adduction and internal rotation of arm at shoulder	2
		Lack of response	1
		Untestable	U

*Added to the original scale by many centers.

be monitored (see Fig. 54-1). Adequate circulation and respiration are the most vital and should always be the first body functions evaluated.

INTRACRANIAL PRESSURE

Understanding the mechanisms associated with intracranial pressure (ICP) is important in caring for patients with many different neurologic problems. The skull is like a closed box with three essential volume components: brain tissue, blood, and cerebrospinal fluid (CSF) (Fig. 54-2). The total volume in the skull is 1900 ml. The intracellular and extracellular fluids of brain tissue make up approximately 78% of this volume. Blood in the arterial, venous, and capillary network makes up 12% of the volume, and the remaining 10% is the volume of the CSF. Under normal conditions, in which intracranial volume remains relatively constant, the balance between these components maintains the ICP. The modified Monro-Kellie doctrine explains the relatively constant volume of these three components within the rigid skull structure. If the volume added to the cranial vault equals the volume displaced from it, the total intracranial volume will not change.[3] This hypothesis is not applicable in situations in which the skull is not rigid (e.g., in neonates and in adults with unfused skull fractures).

Other factors that influence ICP under normal circumstances are changes in (1) arterial pressure, (2) venous pressure, (3) intraabdominal and intrathoracic pressure, (4) posture, (5) temperature (especially hypothermia), and (6) blood gases, particularly CO_2 levels. The degree to which these factors increase or decrease the ICP depends on the ability of the brain to accommodate to the changes.

Regulation and Maintenance of Intracranial Pressure

Normal Intracranial Pressure. Normal ICP is the pressure exerted by the total volume from the three components within the skull: brain tissue, blood, and CSF. ICP can be measured in the ventricles, subarachnoid space, subdural space, epidural space, or brain parenchymal tissue using a water manometer or a pressure transducer. With the patient in the lateral recumbent position, the pressure is generally recorded at 60 to 150 mm H_2O with the use of the water manometer. When the patient is lying with a 30-degree elevation of the head and the pressure is measured intracranially, it is 0 to 15 mm Hg with the use of the pressure transducer. A sustained pressure above the upper limit is considered abnormal.

Normal Compensatory Adaptations. In applying the modified Monro-Kellie doctrine, the body can compensate for changes in the volume of components of the skull to maintain a normal ICP. The body does this by making small changes in any of the three components. Initial compensatory mechanisms include increased CSF absorption, displacement of CSF into the spinal subarachnoid space, and collapse of the cerebral veins and dural sinuses. Other mechanisms that assist in compensation are (1) dispensability of the dura, (2) increased venous outflow, (3) decreased CSF production, (4) changes in intracranial blood volume through constriction and dilation, and (5) slight compression of brain tissue.[3]

Initially, an increase in volume produces no increase in ICP as a result of the compensatory mechanisms. However, these compensatory adaptations to changes in volume are limited, and as the volume increase continues, the ICP rises and decompensation occurs resulting in compression and ischemia.[3]

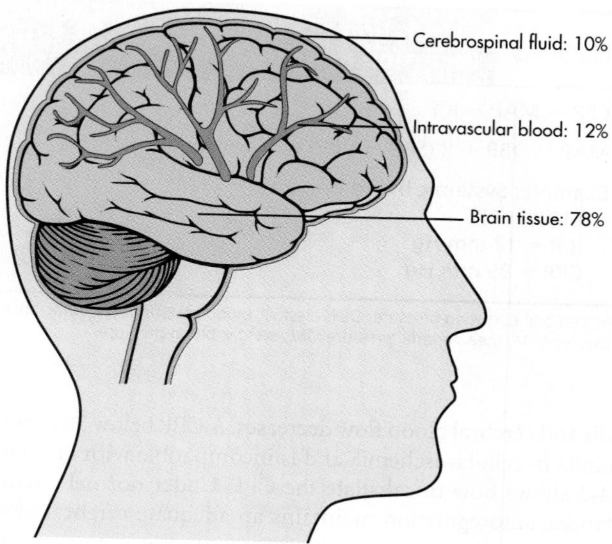

Fig. 54-2 Components of the brain.

Cerebral Blood Flow

Cerebral blood flow (CBF) is the amount of blood in milliliters passing through 100 g of brain tissue in 1 minute. The global cerebral blood flow is approximately 50 ml per minute per 100 g of brain tissue. There is a difference in flow between the white and gray matter of the brain. The white matter has a slower blood flow, approximately 25 ml per minute per 100 g, and the gray matter has a faster blood flow, approximately 75 ml per minute per 100 g. The maintenance of blood flow to the brain is critical because the brain requires a constant supply of oxygen and glucose. The brain uses 20% of the body's oxygen and 25% of its glucose.

Autoregulation of Cerebral Blood Flow. The brain has the ability to regulate its own blood flow in response to its metabolic needs in spite of wide fluctuations in systemic arterial pressure. *Autoregulation* is defined as the automatic alteration in the diameter of the cerebral blood vessels to maintain a constant blood flow to the brain during changes in systemic arterial pressure. The purpose of autoregulation is to ensure a consistent cerebral blood flow to provide for metabolic needs and to maintain cerebral perfusion pressure within normal limits. The lower limit of systemic arterial pressure at which autoregulation is effective in a normotensive person is a mean arterial pressure (MAP) of 50 mm Hg. Below this, cerebral blood flow decreases and symptoms of cerebral ischemia, such as syncope and blurred vision, occur. The upper limit of systemic arterial pressure at which autoregulation is effective is 150 mm Hg. When this pressure is exceeded, the vessels are maximally constricted. Thus further vasoconstrictor response is lost and the blood-brain barrier is disrupted; the result is an increase in ICP.

The cerebral perfusion pressure (CPP) is the pressure needed to ensure blood flow to the brain. CPP is equal to the MAP minus the ICP (CPP = MAP − ICP). This formula is clinically useful, although it does not consider the effect of systemic vascular resistance. As the CPP decreases, autoregulation

Table 54-3 Calculation of Cerebral Perfusion Pressure

CPP = MAP − ICP

MAP = DBP + ⅓ (SBP − DBP) or $\frac{SBP + 2(DBP)}{3}$

Example: Systemic blood pressure = 122/84
MAP = 97
ICP = 12 mm Hg
CPP = 85 mm Hg

CPP, cerebral perfusion pressure; *DBP*, diastolic blood pressure; *ICP*, intracranial pressure; *MAP*, mean arterial pressure; *SBP*, systolic blood pressure.

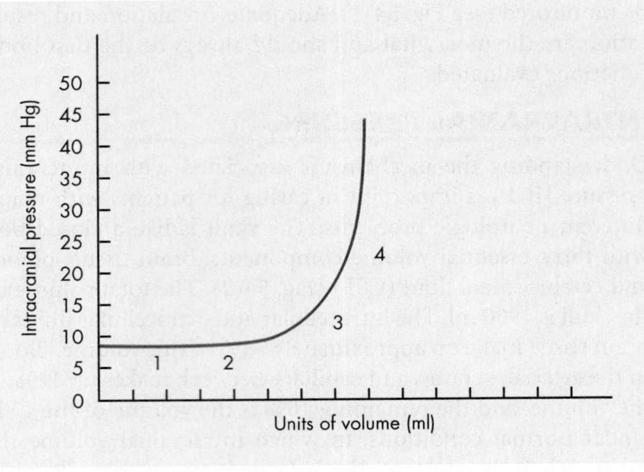

Fig. 54-3 Intracranial volume-pressure curve. (See text for descriptions of 1, 2, 3, and 4.)

fails and cerebral blood flow decreases. A CPP below 30 mm Hg results in cellular ischemia and is incompatible with life. Table 54-3 shows how to calculate the CPP. Under normal circumstances, autoregulation maintains an adequate cerebral blood flow and perfusion pressure by three physiologic mechanisms: changes in ICP, cerebral vasodilation, and metabolic factors.

Pressure Changes. The relationship of pressure to volume is depicted in the pressure-volume curve. The curve is affected by the brain's elastance and compliance. *Elastance* is the brain's ability to accommodate changes in volume. It represents the stiffness of the brain. With high elastance, large increases in pressure occur with small increases in volume.

Elastance = Pressure/Volume

Compliance is the inverse of elastance and is the expandability of the brain. It is represented as the volume increase for each unit increase in pressure. Low compliance is the same as high elastance. With low compliance, high changes in pressure result from small changes in volume.

Compliance = Volume/Pressure

The concept of the pressure-volume curve can be used to represent the stages of increased ICP (intracranial hypertension) (Fig. 54-3). At stage 1 on the curve, there is high compliance and low elastance. The brain is in total compensation, with accommodation and autoregulation intact. An increase in volume does not increase the ICP. At stage 2, the compliance is lower and elastance is increasing. An increase in volume places the patient at risk of increased ICP. At stage 3, there is high elastance and low compliance. Any small addition of volume causes a great increase in pressure. There is a loss of autoregulation, and there may be symptoms indicating increased ICP, such as systolic hypertension with an increasing pulse pressure, bradycardia, and slowing of respiratory rate (Cushing's triad). With the loss of autoregulation and the rise in the systolic blood pressure as a result of the Cushing response, decompensation occurs. The ICP passively mimics the blood pressure. Finally, when the patient is in stage 4, the ICP rises to terminal levels with little increase in volume. Herniation occurs as the brain tissue shifts from the compartment of greater pressure to a compartment of lesser pressure.

Factors Affecting Cerebral Blood Flow. Oxygen tension, carbon dioxide tension, and hydrogen ion concentration affect cerebral vessel tone. Cerebral arteries dilate when the cerebral oxygen tension falls below 50 mm Hg. This dilation decreases cerebral vascular resistance and increases cerebral blood flow in an effort to raise oxygen tension. If oxygen tension is not raised, anaerobic metabolism begins, resulting in an accumulation of lactic acid. In an acid environment, an increase in vasodilation and a further increase in blood flow occur. An increase in the partial pressure of arterial carbon dioxide ($PaCO_2$) is the most potent vasodilator. An increase in $PaCO_2$ relaxes the smooth muscles. This decreases cerebrovascular resistance and increases cerebral blood flow. A severely low arterial oxygen pressure (PaO_2) and a high hydrogen ion concentration (acidosis) are also potent cerebral vasodilators.[3]

Extreme cardiovascular changes such as asystole and pathophysiologic states such as diabetic coma can alter or abolish autoregulation globally. Trauma and tumors can alter autoregulation focally. When autoregulation is lost, cerebral blood flow is no longer maintained at a constant level but is directly influenced by changes in systemic blood pressure, hypoxia, or the effects of catecholamines. Increasing ICP can progress to loss of consciousness, changes in neurologic function, brain herniation, and death.

INCREASED INTRACRANIAL PRESSURE

Increased ICP is a life-threatening situation that results from an increase in any or all of the three components (brain tissue, blood, and CSF) of the skull. Cerebral edema is an important factor contributing to increased ICP.

Cerebral Edema

A variety of conditions are associated with cerebral edema (Table 54-4). Regardless of the cause, cerebral edema results in an increase in tissue volume that carries the potential for increased ICP. The extent and severity of the original insult are factors that determine the degree of cerebral edema.

Three types of cerebral edema have been distinguished: vasogenic edema, cytotoxic edema, and interstitial edema.[4] More than one type may result from a single insult in the same patient.[5]

Vasogenic Cerebral Edema. Vasogenic cerebral edema, the most common type of edema, occurs mainly in the white

Table 54-4 Conditions Associated with Cerebral Edema

Mass lesions	**Vascular insult**
Neoplasm (primary and metastatic)	Infarct (thrombolic and embolic)
Abscess	Venous sinus thrombosis
Hemorrhage (intracerebral and extracerebral)	Anoxic and ischemic episodes
Head injuries	**Toxic or metabolic encephalopathic conditions**
Hemorrhage	Lead or arsenic intoxication
Contusion	Renal failure
Posttraumatic brain swelling	Liver failure
Brain surgery	Reye's syndrome
Infections	

matter and is attributed to changes in the endothelial lining of cerebral capillaries. These changes allow leakage of macromolecules from the capillaries into the surrounding extracellular space, resulting in an osmotic gradient that favors the flow of water from the intravascular to the extravascular space. A variety of insults, such as brain tumors, abscesses, and ingested toxins, may cause an increase in the permeability of the blood-brain barrier and produce an increase in the extracellular fluid volume. The speed and extent of the spread of the edema fluid are influenced by the systemic blood pressure, the site of the brain injury, and the extent of the blood-brain barrier defect. This edema may produce a continuum of symptoms ranging from focal neurologic deficits to disturbances in consciousness, including coma.

Cytotoxic Cerebral Edema. Cytotoxic cerebral edema results from local disruption of the functional or morphologic integrity of cell membranes and occurs most often in the gray matter. Cytotoxic cerebral edema develops from destructive lesions or trauma to brain tissue resulting in cerebral hypoxia or anoxia, sodium depletion, and syndrome of inappropriate antidiuretic hormone (SIADH). Cerebral edema results as fluid and protein shift from the extracellular space directly into the cells, with subsequent swelling and loss of cellular function.

Interstitial Cerebral Edema. Interstitial cerebral edema is the result of periventricular diffusion of ventricular CSF in a patient with uncontrolled hydrocephalus. It can also be caused by enlargement of the extracellular space as a result of systemic water excess (hyponatremia). Fluid moves into the cells to equilibrate with the hypo-osmotic interstitial fluid. Regardless of the cause of cerebral edema, manifestations of increased ICP result, unless compensation is adequate.

Mechanisms of Increased Intracranial Pressure

Sustained elevations of ICP, above the threshold of 20 mm Hg, are associated with a poor prognosis.[6] Increased ICP can be caused by several clinical problems, including a mass lesion, such as a hematoma, contusion, abscess, or rapidly growing tumor; cerebral edema associated with brain tumors, hydrocephalus, head injury, or brain inflammation; or metabolic insult. These cerebral insults may result in hypercapnia, cerebral

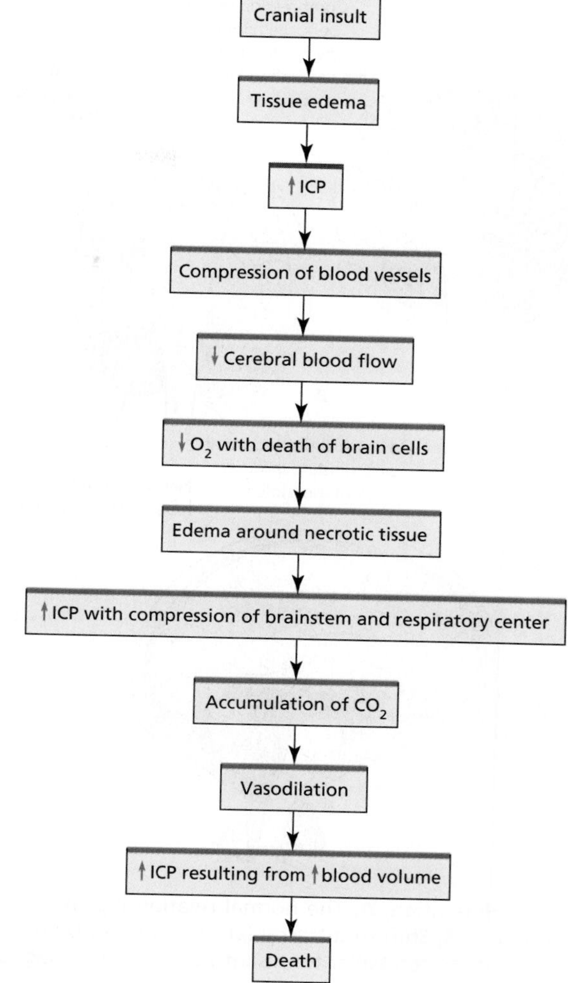

Fig. 54-4 Progression of increased intracranial pressure.

acidosis, impaired autoregulation, and systemic hypertension, which promote the formation and spread of cerebral edema. This edema distorts brain tissue, further increasing the ICP, which leads to even more tissue hypoxia and acidosis. Figure 54-4 illustrates the progression of increased ICP.

Unless there is a reduction in the ICP, the end result is brainstem compression. As the intracranial mass continues to increase, herniation of the brain from one compartment to another can occur.

Complications of Increased Intracranial Pressure

The major complications of uncontrolled increased ICP are inadequate cerebral perfusion and cerebral herniation (Fig. 54-5). The three major patterns of supratentorial brain shift are cingulate (lateral, beneath the falx) herniation, central or transtentorial (downward) herniation, and uncal (lateral and downward) herniation. These patterns are distinguished by the direction of the shift and by the cerebral structures involved. Regardless of the specific intracranial shift, displacement and herniation cause a potentially reversible pathophysiologic process to become irreversible. Ischemia and edema are further

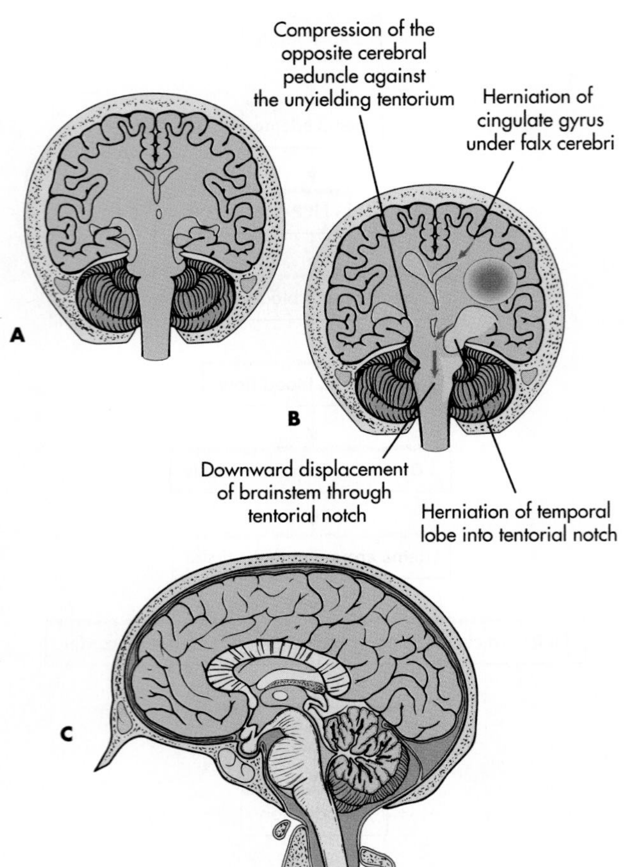

Fig. 54-5 Herniation. **A,** The normal relationship of intracranial structures. **B,** Shift of intracranial structures. **C,** Downward herniation of the cerebellar tonsils into the foramen magnum.

increased, compounding the preexisting problem. Compression of the brainstem and cranial nerves may be fatal. Figure 54-6 illustrates symptoms of supratentorial increased ICP from the early phase through herniation of the brain.

Subtentorial and infratentorial herniations force the cerebellum and brainstem downward through the foramen magnum. If compression of the brainstem is unrelieved, respiratory arrest may occur.

Clinical Manifestations

The clinical manifestations of increased ICP can take many forms, depending on the cause, location, and rate at which the pressure increase occurs. The earlier the condition is recognized and treated, the better the prognosis. The clinical manifestations of increased ICP associated with supratentorial lesions include the following:

1. *Change in level of consciousness.* The level of consciousness (LOC) is a sensitive and important indicator of the patient's neurologic status. The change in consciousness may be dramatic, as in coma, or subtle, such as a flattening of affect, change in orientation, or decrease in level of attention. Changes in LOC are a result of impaired cerebral blood flow, which affects the cells of the cerebral cortex and the RAS.
2. *Changes in vital signs.* Although the complex of increasing systolic pressure (widening pulse pressure), bradycardia with a full and bounding pulse, and irregular respiratory pattern (Cushing's triad) may be present, these symptoms often do not appear until ICP has been increased for some time or markedly increased suddenly (e.g., head trauma). Changes in vital signs are caused by increasing pressure on the thalamus, hypothalamus, pons, and medulla. A change in body temperature may also be noted.
3. *Ocular signs.* Compression of the oculomotor nerve (CN III) results in dilation of the pupil ipsilateral to the mass or lesion, sluggish or no response to light, inability to move the eye upward, and ptosis of the eyelid. These signs can be the result of a shifting of the brain from the midline, a process that compresses the trunk of CN III, paralyzing the pupil sphincter. A fixed, unilaterally dilated pupil is a neurologic emergency that indicates transtentorial herniation of the brain. Other cranial nerves may also be affected, such as the optic (CN II), trochlear (CN IV), and abducens (CN VI) nerves. Signs of dysfunction of these cranial nerves include blurred vision, diplopia, and changes in extraocular eye movements. Central herniation may initially manifest as sluggish but equal pupils. Uncal herniation may cause dilated unilateral pupil. Papilledema, a choked optic disc seen on retinal examination, is also seen and is a nonspecific sign that is associated with long-standing increased ICP.
4. *Decrease in motor function.* As the ICP continues to rise, the patient manifests changes in motor ability. A contralateral hemiparesis or hemiplegia may be seen, depending on the location of the source of the increased ICP. If painful stimuli to elicit a motor response are used, the patient may exhibit a localization to the stimuli or a withdrawal from it. Decorticate (flexor) and decerebrate (extensor) posturing may also be elicited by noxious stimuli (Fig. 54-7). A decorticate posture consists of internal rotation and adduction of the arms with flexion of the elbows, wrists, and fingers as a result of interruption of voluntary motor tracts. Extension of the legs may also be seen. A decerebrate posture may indicate more serious damage and results from disruption of motor fibers in the midbrain and brainstem. In this position, the arms are stiffly extended, adducted, and hyperpronated. There is also hyperextension of the legs with plantar flexion of the feet.
5. *Headache.* Although the brain itself is insensitive to pain, compression of other intracranial structures such as the walls of arteries and veins and the cranial nerves can produce headache. The headache is often continuous but worse in the morning. Straining or movement may accentuate the pain.
6. *Vomiting.* Vomiting, usually not preceded by nausea, is often a nonspecific sign of increased ICP. This is called *unexpected vomiting* and is related to pressure changes in the cranium. Projectile vomiting may also be seen and is related to increased ICP.

It is often difficult to identify increased ICP as the cause of coma. Loss of consciousness also confuses the interpretation of

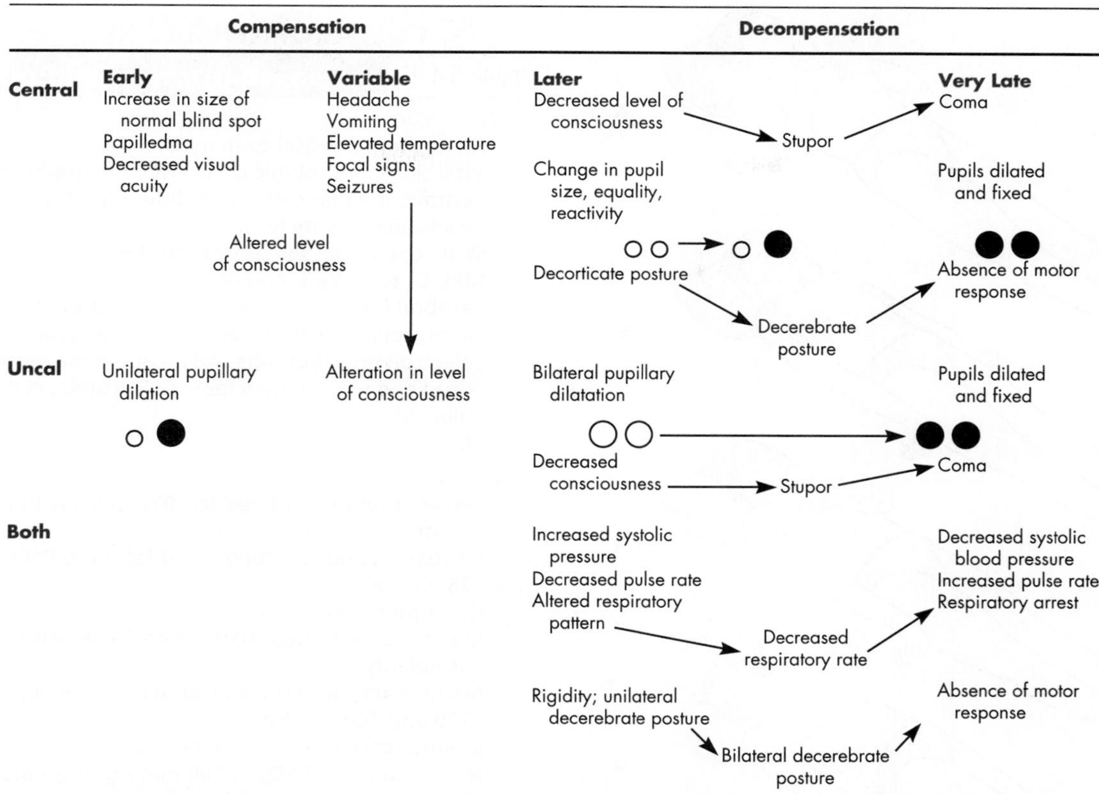

Fig. 54-6 Signs and symptoms of supratentorial increased intracranial pressure.

clinical signs, making it difficult to follow the progression of the increasing ICP.

Diagnostic Studies

Diagnostic studies are aimed at identifying the presence and the underlying cause of increased ICP (Table 54-5). Magnetic resonance imaging (MRI) and computed tomography (CT) have revolutionized the diagnosis of increased ICP. These tests are used to differentiate the many conditions that can cause increased ICP and to evaluate therapeutic options. Other tests that may be used include cerebral angiography, EEG, cerebral blood flow, transcranial Doppler studies, near-infrared spectroscopy for regional cerebral oxygenation, and evoked potential studies. Positron emission tomography (PET) may prove to be even more helpful in diagnosing the cause of increased ICP. In general, a lumbar puncture is not performed when increased ICP is suspected because of the possibility of cerebral herniation from the sudden release of the pressure in the skull from the area above the lumbar puncture.

Collaborative Care

The goals of collaborative care (see Table 54-5) are to identify and treat the underlying cause of increased ICP and to support brain function. A careful history is an important diagnostic aid that can direct the search for the underlying cause.

The emergency management of the patient with actual or potential increased ICP is important to prevent secondary injury to the brain (Table 54-6). Once the patient has been transported to a hospital, aggressive collaborative care is needed.

While the cause of increased ICP is being sought, the condition itself must be treated aggressively to interrupt the cycle. Ensuring adequate oxygenation to support brain function is the first step in the management of increased ICP. An endotracheal tube or tracheostomy may be necessary to maintain adequate ventilation. Arterial blood gas (ABG) analysis guides the oxygen therapy. The goal is to maintain the PaO_2 at 100 mm Hg or greater. It may be necessary to maintain the patient on a mechanical ventilator to ensure adequate oxygenation.

If the condition is caused by a mass lesion, such as a tumor or hematoma, surgical removal of the mass is the best management (see Intracranial Tumors later in this chapter). Nonsurgical intervention for the reduction of tissue volume related to cerebral tissue swelling and cerebral edema includes the use of diuretics and corticosteroids and fluid restriction.

Drug Therapy. Drug therapy plays an important part in the management of increased ICP. Osmotic and loop diuretics are used to reduce the volume of brain water. Corticosteroids are thought to control the vasogenic edema surrounding tumors and abscesses but appear to have limited value in the management of head-injured patients.[7]

Osmotic diuretics. Osmotically active agents have been used for more than 50 years to treat cerebral tissue swelling. The principle governing the use of hypertonic solutions is the removal of fluid from the cerebral tissues in response to a vascular osmotic gradient established between the brain and the intravascular compartment. To be effective, the agent must remain in the

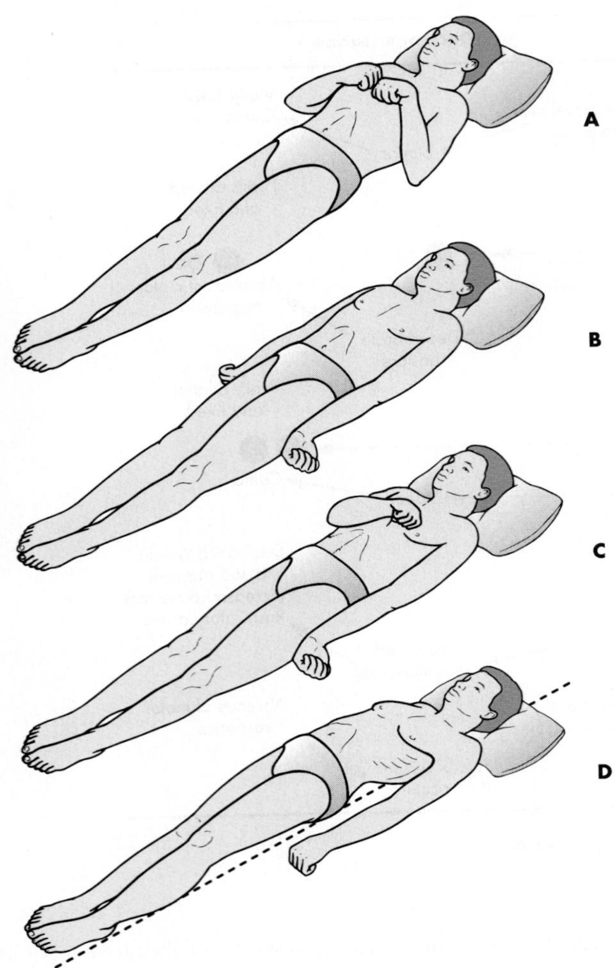

Fig. 54-7 Decorticate and decerebrate posturing. **A,** Decorticate response. Flexion of arms, wrists, and fingers with adduction in upper extremities. Extension, internal rotation, and plantar flexion in lower extremities. **B,** Decerebrate response. All four extremities in rigid extension, with hyperpronation of forearms and plantar extension of feet. **C,** Decorticate response on right side of body and decerebrate response on left side of body. **D,** Opisthotonic posturing.

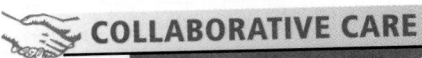

COLLABORATIVE CARE

Table 54-5 Increased Intracranial Pressure

Diagnostic
- History and physical examination
- Vital signs, neurologic checks, ICP measurements (via intraventricular catheter, subdural bolt, or epidural transducer) every hour
- Skull, chest, and spinal x-ray studies
- MRI, CT scan, EEG, angiography
- Cerebral blood flow and velocity studies, PET
- Laboratory studies, including CBC, coagulation profile, electrolytes, creatinine, ABGs, ammonia level, general drug and toxicology screen, CSF protein, cells, and glucose
- ECG

Collaborative Therapy
- Elevation of head of bed to 30 degrees with head in a neutral position
- Intubation and controlled ventilation to $PaCO_2$ of 30 to 35 mm Hg
- Good pulmonary toilet
- Maintenance of fluid balance and assessment of osmolality
- Maintenance of systolic arterial pressure between 100 and 160 mm Hg
- Maintenance of CPP > 70 mm Hg
- Maintenance of PaO_2 at 100 mm Hg or greater
- Maintenance of normothermia
- Adequate sedation
- Drug therapy
  - Osmotic diuretics (mannitol)
  - Loop diuretics (furosemide [Lasix], ethacrynic acid [Edecrin])
  - Corticosteroids (methylprednisone, dexamethasone [Decadron])
  - GI ulcer prophylactics (H_2-receptor antagonist, e.g., cimetidine [Tagamet])
- ICP monitoring

ABGs, arterial blood gases; *CBC,* complete blood count; *CPP,* cerebral perfusion pressure; *CSF,* cerebrospinal fluid; *CT,* computerized tomography; *ECG,* electrocardiogram; *EEG,* electroencephalogram; *ICP,* intracranial pressure; *MRI,* magnetic resonance imaging; *$PaCO_2$,* partial pressure of arterial carbon dioxide; *PaO_2,* partial pressure of arterial oxygen; *PET,* positron emission tomography.

intravascular compartment. In cases of brain injury and damage to the blood-brain barrier, the osmotic withdrawal is from normal tissue, where the vessels and blood-brain barrier are intact, rather than from edematous tissue. The beneficial effects must therefore be attributed to a decrease in the bulk of the normal tissue. However, if a major disruption of the blood-brain barrier occurs, this form of therapy may be more harmful than beneficial, because the hypertonic solution can pass into the edematous tissue and lead to a rebound phenomenon.

Agents such as mannitol (Osmitrol), glycerol, and urea are available for use in osmotherapy. Mannitol (25%) is the most widely used agent and is given intravenously in doses ranging from 0.25 to 1 g/kg. For optimal effect, rapid administration with attention to preventing fluid overload is recommended. Mannitol acts to decrease the ICP in two ways: plasma expansion and osmotic effect. There is an immediate plasma-expanding effect whereby there is a reduction in the hematocrit and blood viscosity that increases cerebral blood flow and cerebral oxygen delivery. The osmotic effect is delayed 15 to 30 minutes until gradients across cerebral vessels and tissues are reestablished. Thus the ICP is altered by a decrease in the total brain water content. Fluid and electrolyte status must be monitored when these drugs are used. Mannitol may be contraindicated if renal disease is present and if serum osmolality is elevated.[8]

Loop diuretics. Loop diuretics such as furosemide (Lasix), bumetanide (Bumex), and ethacrynic acid (Edecrin) may also be used in the management of increased ICP. These diuretics inhibit sodium and chloride reabsorption in the ascending limb of the loop of Henle and thus reduce blood volume and ultimately tissue volume. In addition these agents cause a reduction in the rate of CSF production, which also contributes to the reduction in ICP.[9]

Corticosteroid therapy. Corticosteroid therapy has been used extensively in the treatment of cerebral edema. The mode

EMERGENCY MANAGEMENT

Table 54-6 **Unconscious Patient**

Etiology	Assessment Findings	Interventions
Trauma Head and neck trauma **Infection** Meningitis Encephalitis **Poison** Drug overdose Toxic exposure Carbon monoxide **Metabolic** Diabetic coma Insulin shock Liver failure Uremia Cardiac arrest Cerebrovascular accident	▪ Unresponsive to voice and pain ▪ Dilated or pinpoint pupils, may be unreactive ▪ Involuntary movements ▪ Flaccidity or rigidity of muscles ▪ Depressed or hyperactive reflexes ▪ Decerebrate or decorticate posturing ▪ Diaphoresis ▪ Hyperthermia ▪ Flushed, dry skin ▪ Glasgow Coma Score <12 ▪ Abnormal vital signs ▪ Arrhythmias ▪ Odor of alcohol, acetone on breath ▪ Track marks ▪ Signs of trauma ▪ Petechiae or rash	**Initial** ▪ Ensure patent airway. ▪ Administer oxygen via nasal cannula or non-rebreather mask. ▪ Establish IV access with one large-bore catheter and normal saline. ▪ Administer IV naloxone if narcotic overdose suspected. ▪ Administer thiamine to malnourished or known alcoholic patient to prevent Wernicke's encephalopathy. ▪ Administer one vial 50% dextrose if blood glucose <60 mg/dl (3.3 mmol/L). ▪ Prepare for IV insulin administration if glucose >400 mg/dl (22.2 mmol/L). ▪ Elevate head of bed or position on side to prevent aspiration (unless trauma involved). **Ongoing Monitoring** ▪ Monitor vital signs, level of consciousness, oxygen saturation, cardiac rhythm, Glasgow Coma Score, pupil size and reactivity, respiratory status. ▪ Anticipate need for intubation if gag reflex is absent. ▪ Anticipate gastric lavage if drug overdose is suspected.

of action of corticosteroids is not completely known. It is theorized that they act by their stabilizing effect on the cell membrane and by inhibiting the synthesis of arachidonic acid from cell membranes, thus preventing the formation of proinflammatory mediators.[9] Corticosteroids are also thought to improve neuronal function by improving cerebral blood flow and restoring autoregulation.

Dexamethasone (Decadron), a semisynthetic corticosteroid, is the most commonly used steroid. Corticosteroids are most beneficial in patients who have cerebral edema from vasogenic causes such as brain tumors with peritumoral edema. However, evidence for the efficacy of corticosteroid therapy in trauma or hemorrhage is limited. Clinical trials involving corticosteroid therapy in severe head injury were conducted in the 1980s. Overall these studies demonstrated that corticosteroid therapy did not improve outcomes. However, there were subpopulations that did improve, and these findings warrant further investigation.[10,11]

Complications associated with the use of corticosteroids include hyperglycemia, increased incidence of infections, and gastrointestinal (GI) bleeding. Patients receiving corticosteroids should concurrently be given antacids or histamine H_2 receptor blockers such as cimetidine (Tagamet) or famotidine (Pepcid) to prevent GI bleeding. Fluid intake should be monitored because of the potential for hyponatremia. Since hyperglycemia has also been associated with corticosteroid use, glucose levels of the blood and urine should be monitored regularly.

Other drug therapies. Drug therapy for reducing cerebral metabolism may be an effective strategy to control ICP. The reduction in the metabolic rate decreases the cerebral blood flow and therefore the ICP. High-dose barbiturates (e.g., pentobarbital and thiopental) are used in patients with increased ICP refractory to treatment. Barbiturates produce a decrease in cerebral metabolism and a subsequent decrease in increased ICP. A secondary effect is a reduction in cerebral edema and production of a more uniform blood supply to the brain.[12] Capabilities to monitor the patient's ICP, blood flow, and metabolism should be available when this treatment is used. Other agents may also be used in the management of ICP. These include the antiseizure agent phenytoin (Dilantin) because seizures can further increase ICP.

Hyperventilation Therapy. In the past, aggressive hyperventilation ($PaCO_2$ <25 mm Hg) has been a mainstay treatment of elevated ICP. The lowering of the $PaCO_2$ leads to constriction of the cerebral blood vessels, reducing cerebral blood flow and thereby decreasing the ICP. More recent evidence suggests that aggressive hyperventilation increases the risk of focal cerebral ischemia and may adversely affect outcomes.[13] Prolonged aggressive hyperventilation therapy should be avoided in the absence of increased intracranial pressure, particularly during the first 24 hours following a head injury or when cerebral blood flow (CBF) is low. Brief periods of hyperventilation therapy may be useful for refractory intracranial hypertension.[13]

Nutritional Therapy. All patients must have their nutritional needs met, regardless of their state of consciousness or health. Early enteral feeding following brain injury improves outcomes.[14] The patient with increased ICP is in a hypermetabolic and hypercatabolic state and in need of glucose to provide the necessary fuel for the metabolism of the injured brain. If the patient cannot maintain an adequate oral intake, other means of meeting the nutritional requirements, such as enteral feedings or total parenteral nutrition, should be initiated. Nutritional replacements should begin within 3 days after injury in order to reach full nutritional replacement within 7 days after injury.[14] (Nutritional therapy is discussed in Chapter 38.) Because certain types of feedings are low in sodium, added salt may be necessary. In addition to added minerals, free water may also be needed to meet the fluid needs of the patient. Because malnutrition promotes continued cerebral edema, maintenance of optimal nutrition is imperative.

It is controversial as to whether patients should be maintained in a state of moderate dehydration. On one hand, moderate dehydration is thought to be effective in reducing cerebral edema; in this case fluids are restricted to 65% to 75% of normal requirements. However, the concern is that hypovolemia may result in a decrease in cardiac output and blood pressure, which may have an impact on cerebral perfusion and the amount of oxygen delivered to the brain. There is additional concern that dehydrated patients do not respond well to vasoactive drugs. Because of this the current therapy is directed at keeping patients normovolemic. The use of fluid restriction to reduce tissue volume should be evaluated on the basis of clinical factors such as urine output, insensible fluid loss, serum and urine osmolality, and the condition of the patient.

A lowering of serum osmolarity and an increase in cerebral edema occur if 5% dextrose in water is used for the administration of piggyback medications. If an intravenous (IV) drug routine is used, 0.45% or 0.9% sodium chloride is the preferred solution.

NURSING MANAGEMENT: INCREASED INTRACRANIAL PRESSURE

Regardless of the cause of unconsciousness, the unconscious patient is managed with the assumption that the ICP is increased or has the potential to increase. The primary goals of nursing management are to (1) prevent secondary cerebral damage, (2) maintain function, and (3) prevent complications secondary to immobility and decreased LOC.

■ Nursing Assessment

Subjective data about the unconscious patient can be obtained from family members or other persons who are familiar with the patient. Events preceding the unconscious state should be investigated. Figure 54-1 presents a systematic approach to the assessment of the unconscious patient. This information, together with data for the Glasgow Coma Scale (see Table 54-2), provides the base of knowledge on which a nursing care plan can be formulated.

Ongoing assessment and recording of the ICP is important for evaluating trends and responses to nursing care. Figure 54-8 illustrates a typical neurologic clinical flow sheet used to display a patient's neurologic status over time.

The general plan of the neurologic assessment is to evaluate the patient's mental status, cranial nerve functioning, motor functioning, sensory status, cerebellar functioning, and reflexes. This schema helps the nurse organize the assessment to gather the data needed (see Chapter 53 for a discussion of the neurologic assessment). If the patient is critically ill, an abbreviated neurologic assessment using the GCS, pupillary checks, and certain cranial nerve evaluations is made by the nurse on an ongoing basis.

The pupils are compared to one another for size, movement, and response (Fig. 54-9). If the oculomotor nerve is compressed by supratentorial pressure, the pupil on the affected side (ipsilateral) becomes larger until it fully dilates. If ICP continues to increase, both pupils dilate.

Pupillary reaction is tested with a flashlight. The normal reaction is brisk constriction when the light is shone directly into the eye. A consensual response (a slight constriction in the opposite pupil) should also be noted at the same time. A sluggish reaction can indicate early pressure on CN III. A fixed pupil shows no response to light stimulus, which usually indicates increased ICP.

Evaluation of other cranial nerves can be included in the neurologic check. Eye movements controlled by cranial nerves III, IV, and VI can be examined in the patient who is awake and can be used to assess the function of the brainstem. In the unconscious patient, extraocular eye movements are not specifically tested. Testing the corneal reflex gives information on the functioning of cranial nerves V and VII. If this reflex is absent, routine eye care should be initiated to prevent corneal abrasion (see Chapters 19 and 20).

Eye movements of the uncooperative or unconscious patient can be elicited by reflex with the use of head movements (oculocephalic) and caloric stimulation (oculovestibular) (see Chapters 19 and 20). To test the oculocephalic reflex (doll's head or doll's eyes phenomenon), the nurse rotates the patient's head briskly while holding the eyelids open. A positive response is movement of the eyes across the midline in the direction opposite that of the rotation. Next, the nurse quickly flexes and then extends the neck. Eye movement should be opposite to the direction of head movement—up when the neck is flexed and down when it is extended. Abnormal responses can aid in locating the intracranial lesion. This test should not be attempted if a cervical spine problem is suspected. (The oculovestibular reflex is discussed in Chapter 19.)

Motor strength is tested by asking the patient who is awake to squeeze the nurse's hands to compare strength in the hands. The palmar drift test is an excellent measure of strength in the upper extremities. The patient raises the arms in front of the body with the palmar surface facing upward. If there is any weakness in the upper extremity, the palmar surface turns downward and the arm drifts downward. Asking the patient to raise the foot from the bed or to bend the knees up in bed is a good assessment of lower extremity strength. All four extremities should be tested for strength and evaluated for any asymmetry in strength or movement.

The motor strength of the unconscious or uncooperative patient can be assessed by observation of spontaneous movement. If no spontaneous movement is possible, a pain stimulus should be applied to the patient, and the response should be noted. Resistance to movement during passive range-of-motion exercises is another measure of strength.

The vital signs, including blood pressure, pulse, respiratory rate, and temperature, should also be systematically

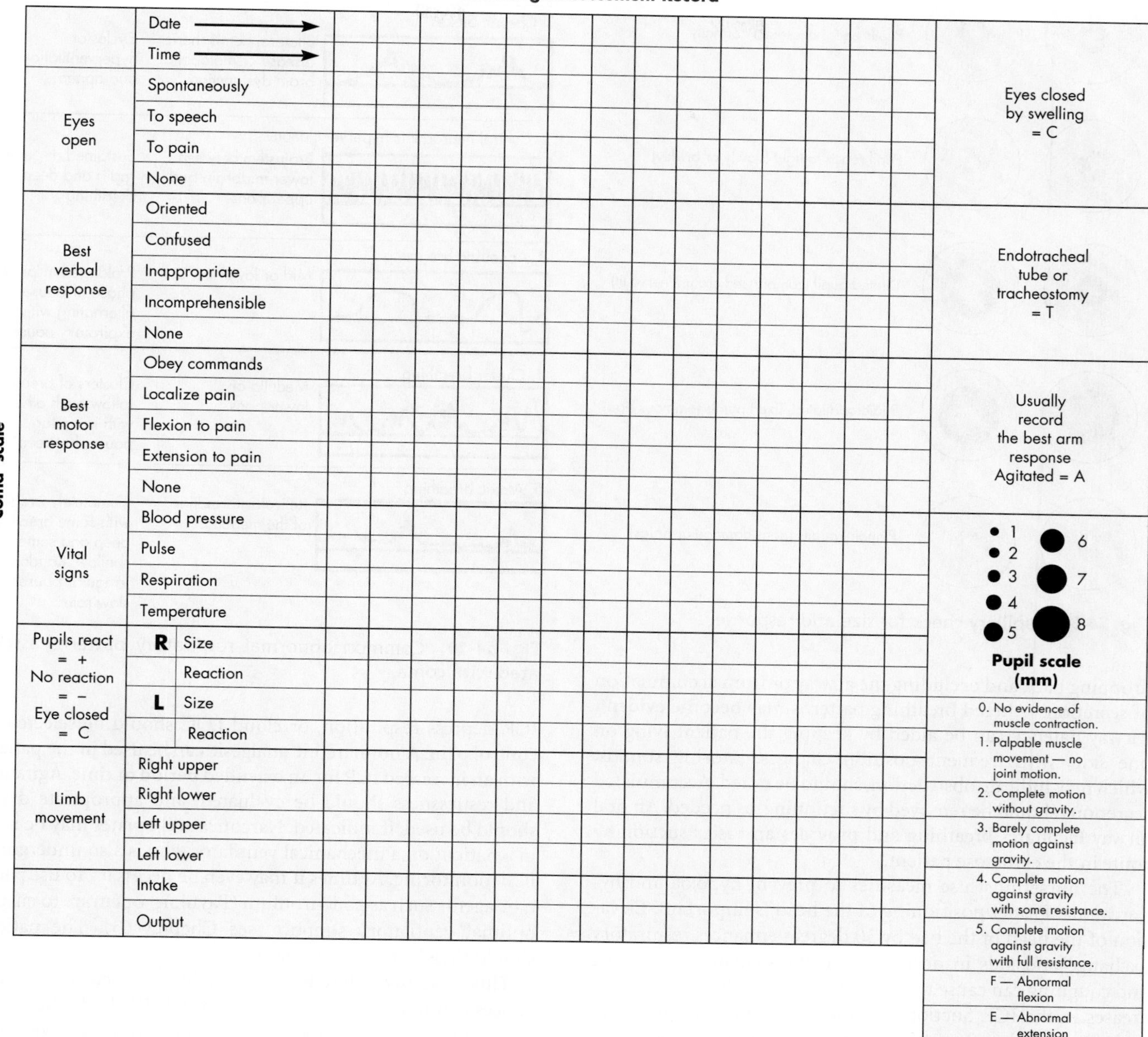

Neurologic Assessment Record

	Date →	
	Time →	
Eyes open	Spontaneously	Eyes closed by swelling = C
	To speech	
	To pain	
	None	
Best verbal response	Oriented	Endotracheal tube or tracheostomy = T
	Confused	
	Inappropriate	
	Incomprehensible	
	None	
Best motor response	Obey commands	Usually record the best arm response Agitated = A
	Localize pain	
	Flexion to pain	
	Extension to pain	
	None	
Vital signs	Blood pressure	• 1 • 2 • 3 • 4 • 5 ● 6 ● 7 ● 8
	Pulse	
	Respiration	
	Temperature	Pupil scale (mm)
Pupils react = + No reaction = − Eye closed = C	R Size	0. No evidence of muscle contraction.
	R Reaction	1. Palpable muscle movement — no joint motion.
	L Size	2. Complete motion without gravity.
	L Reaction	3. Barely complete motion against gravity.
Limb movement	Right upper	4. Complete motion against gravity with some resistance.
	Right lower	5. Complete motion against gravity with full resistance.
	Left upper	F — Abnormal flexion
	Left lower	E — Abnormal extension
	Intake	
	Output	

Coma scale

Fig. 54-8 Neurologic clinical flow sheet.

recorded. The nurse must be aware of Cushing's triad, since this indicates severe increased ICP. Besides recording respiratory rate, the nurse should also note the respiratory pattern (Fig. 54-10).

Nursing Diagnoses

The nursing diagnoses are supported by the data obtained on assessment and include those associated with increased ICP and unconsciousness. Patients with one or both of these serious problems require the highest level of nursing care because they are usually totally dependent on the nurse. Nursing diagnoses related to the unconscious patient are presented in NCP 54-1.

Planning

The overall goals are that the patient with increased ICP and unconsciousness will (1) have decreased ICP to within normal limits, (2) maintain a patent airway, and (3) demonstrate normal fluid and electrolyte balance.

Nursing Implementation

Acute Intervention

Maintenance of respiratory function. Maintenance of a patent airway is critical in the patient with increased ICP and is a primary nursing responsibility. As the LOC decreases, the patient is at increased risk of airway obstruction from the tongue

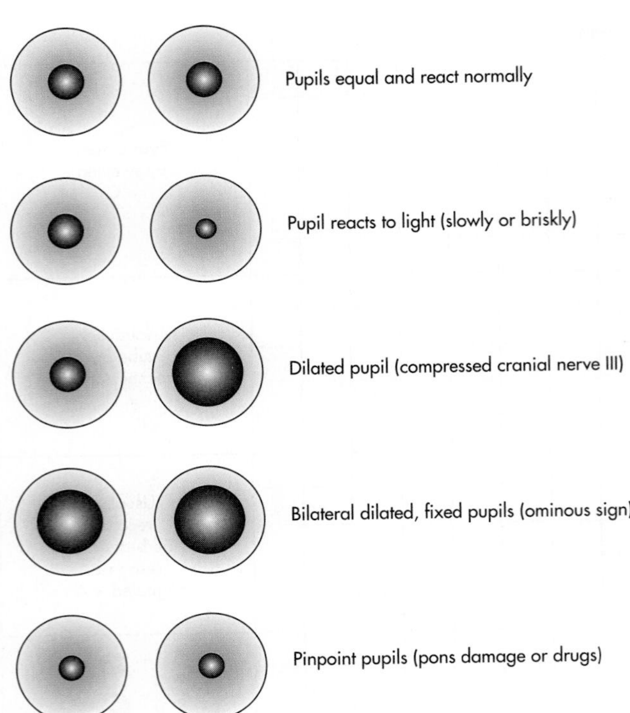

Fig. 54-9 Pupillary check for size and response.

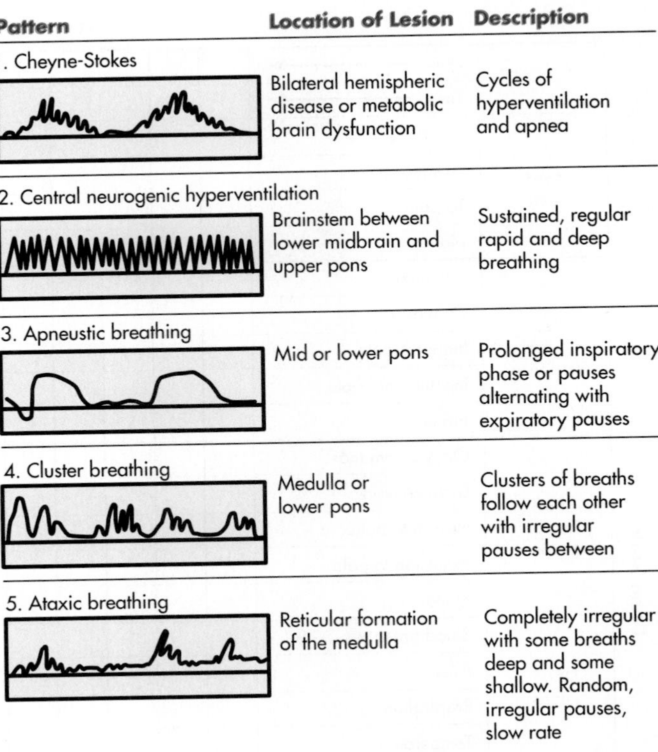

Fig. 54-10 Common abnormal respiratory patterns associated with coma.

dropping back and occluding the airway or from accumulation of secretions. Altered breathing patterns may become evident. Airway patency can be aided by keeping the patient lying on one side, with frequent position changes. Snoring sounds, which may indicate obstruction, should be noted. Accumulated secretions should be removed by suctioning, as needed. An oral airway facilitates breathing and provides an easier suctioning route in the comatose patient.

The nurse must use measures to prevent hypoxia and hypercapnia. Proper positioning of the head is important. Elevation of the head of the bed by 30 degrees enhances respiratory exchange and aids in decreasing cerebral edema. Suctioning and coughing can cause transient decreases in the PaO_2 and increases in the ICP. Suctioning should be kept to a minimum and should be less than 10 seconds in duration, with administration of 100% oxygen before and after to prevent decreases in the PaO_2.[15] To avoid cumulative increases in the ICP with suctioning, suctioning should be limited to two passes per suction procedure. Patients with elevated ICP are at risk for lower CPP during suctioning.[16]

Abdominal distention can interfere with respiratory function and should be prevented. Insertion of a nasogastric tube to aspirate the stomach contents can prevent distention, vomiting, and possible aspiration.

ABGs should be measured and evaluated regularly (see Chapter 24). The appropriate ventilatory support can be ordered on the basis of the PaO_2 and $PaCO_2$ values. The nurse should be aware if moderate hyperventilation ($PaCO_2$ of 30 to 35 mm Hg) is desired.

Unless the patient is on ventilatory support, the use of narcotic sedatives and opiates should be evaluated on an individual basis. Besides depressing respirations, these agents can also cloud the patient's LOC. A narcotic that does not increase the ICP, depress respiration, or cloud LOC should be selected to control pain. A nonnarcotic analgesic can be used in the patient with an increased ICP for an extended period of time. Agitation and restlessness should be evaluated, and appropriate drugs should be used, if indicated. Narcotics and opiates may be used in a patient on a mechanical ventilator who is also undergoing ICP monitoring. At times it may even be necessary to use paralytic agents such as pancuronium (Pavulon) or curare to ensure optimal ventilatory support (see Chapter 63). The patient should then be fully monitored.

Fluid and electrolyte balance. Fluid and electrolyte disturbances can have an adverse effect on ICP. IV fluids should be closely monitored with the use of a limited-volume device or a volume-control apparatus for accuracy. Intake and output, with insensible losses and daily weights taken into account, are important parameters in the assessment of fluid balance.

Electrolyte determinations should be made daily, and any abnormal values should be discussed with the physician. It is especially important to monitor serum glucose, sodium, potassium, and osmolality. Urinary output is monitored to detect problems related to diabetes insipidus (e.g., increased urinary output related to a decrease in antidiuretic hormone secretion) and SIADH, which results in decreased urinary output. Besides urinary output, the serum sodium and osmolality are also used to diagnose diabetes insipidus and SIADH. Diabetes insipidus may result in severe dehydration unless treated. The usual treatment is fluid replacement, vasopressin (Pitressin), or desmopressin acetate (DDAVP) (see Chapter 47). SIADH results in a dilutional hyponatremia that may produce cerebral edema, changes in LOC, seizures, and coma. (Treatment of SIADH is described in Chapter 47.)

54-1 NURSING CARE PLAN UNCONSCIOUS PATIENT

Expected Patient Outcomes	Nursing Interventions and *Rationales*
NURSING DIAGNOSIS	**Ineffective airway clearance** *related to* unconsciousness and inability to mobilize secretions *as manifested by* ineffective cough, inability to clear secretions, crackles on auscultation, thick secretions.
▪ Demonstration of increased air exchange as measured by ABGs within normal limits. ▪ Normal breath sounds in all lobes of the lungs.	▪ Maintain patient's side-lying position, keeping head of bed elevated *to prevent aspiration and tongue from blocking airway and to assist in decreasing cerebral edema.* ▪ Suction as needed *to remove accumulated secretions, reduce risk of aspiration, and ensure patent airway.* ▪ Perform chest physical therapy at least q4hr *to improve ventilation and prevent pulmonary complications.* ▪ Monitor patient for signs of decreased oxygenation, including changes in LOC, decreased PaO_2 or SaO_2, and increased respiratory rate and cyanosis *because low PaO_2 and a high hydrogen ion concentration (acidosis) are potent cerebral vasodilators that increase cerebral flow and may increase ICP.*
NURSING DIAGNOSIS	**Altered tissue perfusion: cerebral** *related to* cerebral tissue swelling *as manifested by* mental state, intracranial pressure > 20 mm Hg, CPP < 60 mm Hg, decreased cerebral blood flow or oximetry.
▪ No further deterioration in LOC. ▪ ICP < 20 mm Hg, CPP > 60 mm Hg. ▪ Stable vital signs.	▪ Monitor patient's neurologic status at least every hour initially; assess level of consciousness and document *to evaluate patient's response to treatment and modify if necessary.* ▪ Monitor ICP and calculate CPP *to evaluate adequacy of cerebral blood perfusion, detect patient's response to treatment, and provide information necessary for clinical decisions.* ▪ Limit care activities that increase ICP (e.g., suctioning, hip flexion) *to prevent increases in ICP.* ▪ Provide comfort measures *because pain or agitation increases ICP.* ▪ Elevate head of bed 30 to 45 degrees *to facilitate reduction of cerebral edema.* ▪ Maintain the $PaCO_2$ at 30 to 35 mm Hg when ICP > 20 mm Hg *because CO_2 is a potent cerebral vasodilator and hyperventilation reduces $PaCO_2$.* ▪ Monitor level of cerebral oximetry and read cerebral blood flow reports *to ensure that global and regional cerebral oxygenation are maintained.* ▪ Monitor reactions to all medications (especially diuretics and sedatives) *to evaluate for signs (change in LOC) of reduced cerebral edema.* ▪ Calibrate and maintain intracranial monitoring device *to provide an accurate indicator of ICP.*
NURSING DIAGNOSIS	**Altered nutrition: less than body requirements** *related to* hypermetabolism and inability to ingest food and fluids *as manifested by* inability to feed self, hyperthermia (>101° F [38.3° C]), metabolic needs in excess of intake, weight loss.
▪ Adequate caloric intake to maintain weight. ▪ Maintenance of weight within 5 lb (2.3 kg) of admission weight.	▪ Assess fluid status and document intake and output hourly initially *to evaluate adequacy of renal perfusion and indicators of fluid balance.* ▪ Assess skin turgor *as an indicator of fluid balance.* ▪ Monitor electrolytes *to identify electrolyte imbalances and initiate treatment.* ▪ Weigh patient daily *as an indicator of fluid balance and nutritional status.* ▪ Maintain oral fluid restrictions as ordered *because pharyngeal reflex may be absent and patient may be unable to swallow.* ▪ Evaluate swallowing abilities *to reduce risk of aspiration when oral intake is resumed.* ▪ Advance patient to high-protein, high-caloric feedings (enteral or oral) as indicated *to provide nutrients needed to prevent wasting and negative nitrogen balance.* ▪ Auscultate bowel sounds before feeding *to ensure presence of peristalsis.* ▪ Elevate head of bed during and after feedings *to reduce risk of regurgitation and aspiration.* ▪ Provide adequate free water if not contraindicated *to maintain a high fluid intake.*

Continued

54-1 NURSING CARE PLAN UNCONSCIOUS PATIENT—continued

Expected Patient Outcomes	Nursing Interventions and *Rationales*
NURSING DIAGNOSIS **Risk for impaired skin integrity** *related to* nutritional deficit, self-care deficit, and immobility.	
■ Absence of skin breakdown. ■ Intact skin.	■ Assess skin frequently, especially over bony prominences and around genitalia and buttocks, *to identify potential or actual skin problems and initiate a plan of care.* ■ Turn patient at least q2hr as indicated *because prolonged pressure decreases capillary circulation and leads to tissue hypoxia and necrosis.* ■ Provide fluids *to prevent dehydration.* ■ Use low-air-loss beds as indicated *to reduce pressure to bony prominences by distributing body weight evenly.* ■ Cleanse all abrasions and lacerations; massage skin as indicated *to reduce risk of infection and stimulate circulation.*
NURSING DIAGNOSIS **Risk of infection** *related to* immobility, invasive monitoring devices and lines, and compromised immune system.	
■ No wound infections. ■ Normal temperature, white blood cell count, and chest x-ray.	■ Assess for hyperthermia (temperature > 101° F [38.4° C]), exudate around catheter insertion sites (IV, indwelling, intracranial), lethargy, abnormal chest x-ray and breath sounds, foul-smelling urine *to determine if risk factors for infection are present.* ■ Observe strict sterile technique when assisting with insertion and maintenance of ICP-monitoring devices and all invasive lines; maintain integrity of all closed systems *to prevent introduction of bacteria.*

Monitoring of intracranial pressure. In 1960 Lundberg refined a technique for the continuous monitoring of ICP by insertion of a catheter into the ventricles.[17] Over the last 35 years, the technology for monitoring ICP has improved greatly and is now regularly used in patients with suspected increased ICP who may benefit from treatment and in whom the underlying process is thought to be self-limiting. Patients with irreversible pathologic processes or advanced neurologic decline caused by primary or metastatic lesions may not be monitored. The measurement of ICP is valuable in detecting the early rise of ICP and the patient's response to treatment and in providing information necessary for clinical decisions.

There are four basic systems used to monitor ICP: a ventricular pressure monitoring system, a subarachnoid pressure monitoring system, an epidural pressure monitoring system, and an intraparenchymal pressure monitoring system. These methods are discussed in detail in Chapter 63.

Prevention of infection. Prevention of infection by use of strict aseptic technique during dressing changes or sampling of CSF is imperative. Maintenance of the intactness of the system is critical to ensure that the ICP readings are accurate, since treatment is initiated on basis of the level of the pressures.

Body position. The patient with increased ICP should be maintained in the head-up position. The nurse must take care to prevent extreme neck flexion, which can cause venous obstruction and contribute to increased ICP. The body position should be adjusted to decrease the ICP maximally and to improve the CPP. Traditional practice has been to elevate the head of the bed to at least 30 degrees, unless a concurrent cervical neck injury has been identified. Research now suggests there is an inconsistent response of the ICP and the CPP to head elevation.[18,19] Elevation of the head of the bed reduces sagittal sinus pressure, promotes venous drainage from the head via the valveless jugular system, and decreases the vascular congestion that can produce cerebral edema. However, raising the head of the bed may decrease the CPP. There is no evidence, however, that head-of-bed elevation decreases cerebral tissue oxygenation. Careful evaluation of the effects of elevation of the head of the bed on both the ICP and the CPP is required. The bed should be positioned so that it lowers the ICP while maintaining the CPP and other indices of cerebral oxygenation.

Care should be taken to turn the patient with slow, gentle movements because rapid changes in position may increase the ICP. Continuous rotation bed therapy allows for frequent position changes and does not increase ICP.[20] Caution should be used to prevent discomfort in turning and positioning the patient because pain or agitation also increases pressure. Increased intrathoracic pressure also contributes to increased ICP by impeding the venous return; thus coughing, straining, and Valsalva's maneuver should be avoided. Extreme hip flexion should be avoided in order to decrease the risk of raising the intraabdominal pressure, which can restrict movement of the diaphragm and cause respiratory distress. The patient should be turned at least every 2 hours.

Decorticate or decerebrate posturing is a reflex response in some patients with increased ICP. Turning, skin care, and even passive range of motion can elicit the posturing reflexes. Attempts should be made to provide needed physical care activities to minimize complications of immobility, such as atelectasis and contractures. In cases of severe posturing reflexes, these

Table 54-7 Etiologic Factors for Increased Intracranial Pressure

- Hypercapnia ($PaCO_2$ >45 mm Hg)
- Hypoxemia (PaO_2 <60 mm Hg)
- Cerebral vasodilating agents (e.g., halothane, antihistamines)
- Valsalva's maneuver
- Body positions (e.g., prone position, flexion of neck, extreme hip flexion)
- Isometric muscle contractions
- Coughing or sneezing
- Rapid-eye-movement sleep
- Emotional upset
- Noxious stimuli
- Arousal from sleep
- Clustering of activities

activities may have to be done less frequently because posturing can cause increases in ICP.

Protection from injury and environmental management. The patient with increased ICP and a decreased LOC needs protection from self-injury. Confusion, agitation, and the possibility of seizures can put the patient at risk of injury. Restraints should be used judiciously in the agitated patient. If restraints are absolutely necessary to keep the patient from removing tubes or falling out of bed, they should be secure enough to be effective, and the skin area under the restraints should be observed regularly for irritation. Agitation may increase with the use of restraints, which indicates the need for other measures to protect the patient from injury. Light sedation with agents such as haloperidol (Haldol) or lorazepam (Ativan) may be needed. Having a family member stay with the patient may have a calming effect. For the patient with seizures or the patient at risk of seizure activity, seizure precautions should be instituted. They include padded side rails, an airway at the bedside, accurate and timely administration of antiseizure medications, and close observation.

The patient can benefit from a quiet, nonstimulating environment. The nurse should always use a calm, reassuring approach. Touching and talking to the patient, even one who is in a coma, is always an appropriate care approach. The nurse must create a balance between sensory deprivation and sensory overload for the patient with increased ICP.

Contributory factors to increased intracranial pressure. There is a relationship between nursing care activities and increases in ICP. Table 54-7 lists some of the factors that have been identified as contributors to increased ICP. Nurses should be alert to these factors and should attempt to minimize them. Nursing management of the patient with increased ICP is one of the most important aspects of the care provided these patients.

Psychologic considerations. Besides the carefully planned physical care provided patients with increased ICP, the nurse must also be aware of the psychologic well-being of the patients and their families. Anxiety over the diagnosis and the prognosis for the patient with neurologic problems can be distressing to the patient, the family, and the nursing staff. The nurse's competent and assured manner in performing the care needed

RESEARCH
IMPLICATIONS FOR NURSING PRACTICE

Impact of Critical Injury on the Family

Citation Leske JS, Jiricka MK: Impact of family demands and family strengths and capabilities on family well-being and adaptation after critical injury, *Am J Crit Care* 7:383, 1998.

Purpose To examine family demands, including prior stressors and severity of patient's injuries, and family strengths and capabilities, including hardiness, coping, problem solving, and on outcomes of family well-being and adaptation after critical illness.

Methods Family members of 21 intensive care unit (ICU) patients were interviewed using standardized questionnaires related to family demands, family strengths and capabilities, family resources, coping, problem-solving communication, and family adaptation outcomes. Patients were admitted to the ICU as a result of injuries from gunshot wounds or motor vehicle accident. The majority of the 21 patients were male (71%), and the majority of the 51 family members interviewed were female (73%).

Results and Conclusions There was no significant relationship between severity of the patient's injury and the family outcomes of well-being and adaptation. Increases in prior stressors, strains, and transitions were negatively related to family outcomes. In addition, family hardiness, resources, coping, and problem-solving communication were positively related to family adaptation scores.

Implications for Nursing Practice Nurses play an important role in helping families adjust to sudden, critical illness. In this role, the nurse must be aware of the negative impact of the patient's condition on the family so that planning for assistance of the family can be initiated. Vulnerable families should be identified early. Increased communication between the family members and health care providers may enhance understanding and decrease family tensions.

by the patient is reassuring to everyone involved. Short, simple explanations are appropriate and allow the patient and the family to acquire the amount of information they desire. There is a need for support, information, and education of both patients and families that begins with the traumatic event and continues for years after the event. The nurse should assess the family members' desire and need to assist in providing care for the patient and allow for their participation as appropriate.

Evaluation

The expected outcomes are that the unconscious patient will

- have ICP within normal limits
- maintain a patent airway
- exhibit no manifestations of infection
- demonstrate normal fluid and electrolyte and nutrition balance
- have no evidence of skin breakdown

Table 54-8 Types of Skull Fractures

Description	Cause
Linear	
Break in continuity of bone without alteration of relationship of parts	Low-velocity injuries
Depressed	
Inward indentation of skull	Powerful blow
Simple	
Linear or depressed skull fracture without fragmentation or communicating lacerations	Low to moderate impact
Comminuted	
Multiple linear fractures with fragmentation of bone into many pieces	Direct, high-momentum impact
Compound	
Depressed skull fracture and scalp laceration with communicating pathway to intracranial cavity	Severe head injury

Table 54-9 Clinical Manifestations of Skull Fractures by Location

Location	Syndrome or Sequelae
Frontal fracture	Exposure of brain to contaminants through frontal air sinus; possible association with air in forehead tissue, CSF rhinorrhea, or pneumocranium
Orbital fracture	Periorbital ecchymosis (raccoon eyes)
Temporal fracture	Boggy temporal muscle because of extravasation of blood, benign oval-shaped bruise behind ear in mastoid region (Battle's sign), CSF otorrhea
Parietal fracture	Deafness, CSF or brain otorrhea, bulging of tympanic membrane caused by blood or CSF, facial paralysis, loss of taste, Battle's sign
Posterior fossa fracture	Occipital bruising resulting in cortical blindness, visual field defects; rare appearance of ataxia or other cerebellar signs
Basilar skull fracture	CSF or brain otorrhea, bulging of tympanic membrane caused by blood or CSF, Battle's sign, tinnitus or hearing difficulty, facial paralysis, conjugate deviation of gaze, vertigo

CSF, cerebrospinal fluid.

HEAD TRAUMA

Head injury includes any trauma to the scalp, skull, or brain. The term *head trauma* is used primarily to signify craniocerebral trauma, which includes an alteration in consciousness, no matter how brief.

Head trauma has a high potential for poor outcome.[21] Deaths from head injury trauma occur at three time points after injury: immediately after the injury, within 2 hours after injury, and approximately 3 weeks after injury.[22] The majority of deaths after a head injury occur immediately after the injury, either from the direct head trauma or from massive hemorrhage and shock. Deaths occurring within a few hours of the trauma are caused by progressive worsening of the head injury or from internal bleeding. An immediate note of changes in neurologic status and surgical intervention are critical in the prevention of deaths at this point. Deaths occurring 3 weeks or more after injury result from multisystem failure. Expert nursing care in the weeks following the injury are crucial in decreasing mortality. Factors that predict a poor outcome include the presence of an intracranial hematoma, increasing age of the patient, abnormal motor responses, impaired or absent eye movements or pupil light reflexes, early sustained hypotension, hypoxemia or hypercapnia, and ICP levels higher than 20 mm Hg.[22]

Statistics regarding the occurrence of head injuries are incomplete because many victims die at the scene of the accident or because the condition is considered minor and health care is not sought. An estimated 3 million persons suffer head injuries each year in the United States.[23] The mortality rate related to head injury is 19.3 per 100,000 persons in the United States and represents a 21% decline in fatalities related to head injury since 1976.[24] In the past, motor vehicle accidents and falls were the most common causes of head injury in both Canada and the United States. More recently, in the United States, deaths from motor vehicle accidents and falls have decreased while firearm-related head injury death rates have increased.[24] Other causes include assaults, sports-related injuries, and recreational accidents.

Types of Head Injuries

Scalp Lacerations. Scalp lacerations are the most minor of the head traumas. Because the scalp contains many blood vessels with poor constrictive abilities, most scalp lacerations are associated with profuse bleeding. The major complication associated with scalp laceration is infection.

Skull Fractures. Skull fractures frequently occur with head trauma. There are several ways to describe skull fractures: (1) linear or depressed; (2) simple, comminuted, or compound; and (3) closed or open (Table 54-8). Fractures may be closed or open, depending on the presence of a scalp laceration or extension of the fracture into the air sinuses or dura. The type and severity of a skull fracture depend on the velocity, the momentum, the direction of injuring agent, and the site of impact. Specific manifestations of a skull fracture are generally associated with the location of the injury (Table 54-9).

The location of the fracture alters the presentation of the clinical signs and symptoms. For example, a specialized type of linear fracture is seen when the fracture occurs at the base of the skull, a basilar skull fracture. This fracture generally crosses a sinus and tears the dura (e.g., the frontal or the temporal) and is associated with leakage of CSF. Rhinorrhea (CSF leakage from the nose) or otorrhea (CSF leakage from the ear) generally confirms that the fracture has traversed the dura (Fig. 54-11). Two methods of testing can be used to determine whether the fluid leaking from the nose or ear is CSF. The first method

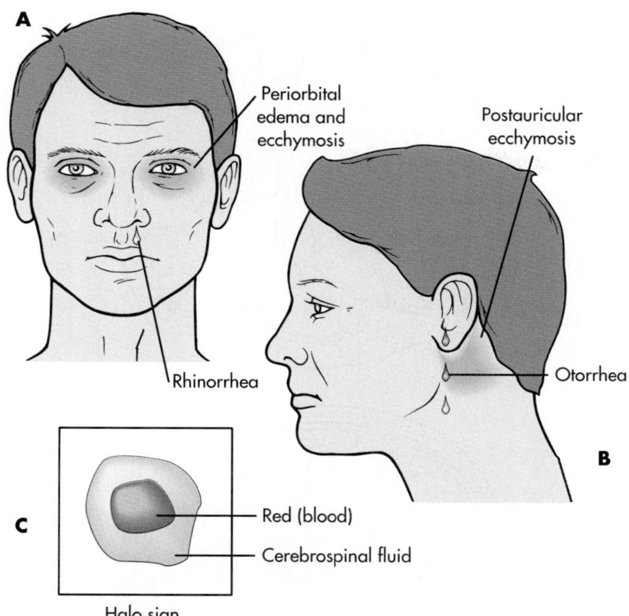

Fig. 54-11 **A,** Raccoon eyes and rhinorrhea. **B,** Battle's sign (postauricular ecchymosis) with otorrhea. **C,** Halo or ring sign (see text).

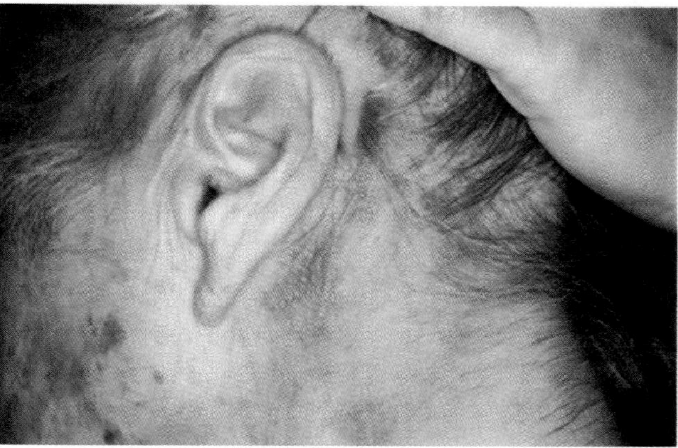

Fig. 54-12 Battle's sign.

is to test the leaking fluid with a Dextrostix or Tes-tape strip to determine whether glucose is present. CSF gives a positive reading for glucose. If blood is present in the fluid, however, testing for the presence of glucose is unreliable because blood contains glucose. In this event, the nurse should look for the "halo" or "ring" sign (Fig. 54-11, *C*). To perform this test, the nurse allows the leaking fluid to drip onto a white pad (4 × 4) or towel and observes the drainage. Within a few minutes the blood coalesces into the center, and a yellowish ring encircles the blood if CSF is present. The color, appearance, and amount of leaking fluid must be noted because both tests can give false-positive results.

The major potential complications of skull fractures are intracranial infections and hematoma, as well as meningeal and brain tissue damage. A frontal or orbital fracture may have CSF leakage along with periorbital ecchymosis (raccoon eyes). A basal skull fracture may result in ecchymosis of the mastoid process of the temporal bone (Battle's sign) (Fig. 54-11, *B*, and Fig. 54-12), conjunctival hemorrhage, or periorbital edema.

Minor Head Trauma. Brain injuries are categorized as being minor or major. Concussion (a sudden transient mechanical head injury with disruption of neural activity and a change in the LOC) is considered a minor head injury. The patient may not lose total consciousness with this injury.

Signs of concussion include a brief disruption in LOC, amnesia regarding the event (retrograde amnesia), and headache. The manifestations are generally of short duration. If the patient has not lost consciousness, or if the loss of consciousness lasts less than 5 minutes, the patient is usually discharged from the care facility with instructions to notify the physician if symptoms persist or if behavior changes are noted.

The postconcussion syndrome is seen anywhere from 2 weeks to 2 months after the concussion. Symptoms include persistent headache, lethargy, personality and behavior changes, shortened attention span, decreased short-term memory, and changes in intellectual ability. This syndrome can significantly affect the patient's abilities to perform the activities of daily living.

Although concussion is generally considered benign and usually resolves spontaneously, the symptoms may be the beginning of a more serious, progressive problem. At the time of discharge it is important to give the patient and the family instructions for observation and accurate reporting of symptoms or changes in neurologic status.

Major Head Trauma. Major head trauma includes contusions and lacerations. Both injuries represent severe trauma to the brain. Contusions and lacerations are generally associated with closed injuries.

A *contusion* is the bruising of the brain tissue within a focal area that maintains the integrity of the pia mater and arachnoid layers. A contusion develops areas of necrosis, infarction, hemorrhage, and edema. A contusion frequently occurs at the site of a fracture. With contusion, the phenomenon of coup-contrecoup injury is often noted. Damage from coup-contrecoup injury occurs because of mass movement of the brain inside the skull. Contusions or lacerations occur both at the site of the direct impact of the brain on the skull and at a secondary area of damage on the opposite side away from injury, leading to multiple contused areas. Bleeding around the contusion site is generally minimal, and the blood is reabsorbed slowly. Neurologic assessment demonstrates focal findings and a generalized disturbance in the LOC. Seizures are a common complication of brain contusion.

Lacerations involve actual tearing of the brain tissue and occur frequently in association with depressed and compound fractures and penetrating injuries. Tissue damage is severe, and surgical repair of the laceration is impossible because of the texture of the brain tissue. If bleeding is deep into the brain parenchyma, focal and generalized signs are noted.

When major head trauma occurs, many delayed responses are seen, including hemorrhage, hematoma formation, seizures, and cerebral edema. Intracerebral hemorrhage is generally associated with cerebral laceration. This hemorrhage manifests as a space-occupying lesion accompanied by unconsciousness, hemiplegia on the contralateral side, and a dilated pupil on the ipsilateral side. As the hematoma expands, symptoms of increased ICP become more severe. Prognosis is generally poor for the patient with a large intracerebral hemorrhage.

Subarachnoid hemorrhage and intraventricular hemorrhage can also occur secondary to head trauma.

Diffuse Axonal Injury. *Diffuse axonal injury* (DAI) is widespread axonal damage occurring after a mild, moderate, or severe traumatic brain injury. The damage occurs primarily around axons in subcortical white matter of the cerebral hemispheres, basal ganglia, thalamus, and brainstem.[25] Initially, DAI was believed to occur from the tensile forces of trauma that sheared axons resulting in axonal disconnection. There is increasing evidence that axonal damage is not preceded by an immediate tearing of the axon from the traumatic impact but rather the trauma changes the function of the axon, resulting in axon swelling (axonal ballooning) and disconnection. This process takes approximately 12 to 24 hours to develop and may persist longer.

An MRI scan is more sensitive in detecting small DAI lesions than the CT scan because of the lack of gross pathologic changes in brain tissue. The clinical signs and symptoms, including a decreased LOC, increased ICP, decerebration or decortication, and global cerebral edema, are important indicators.

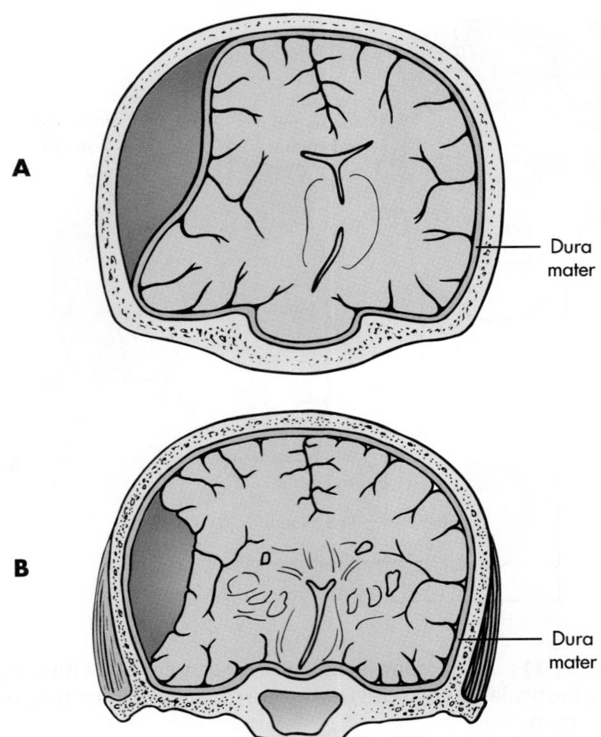

Fig. 54-13 **A,** Epidural hematoma in the temporal fossa, usually a result of laceration of the middle meningeal artery. **B,** Subdural hematoma, usually a result of laceration of the subdural veins.

Complications

Epidural Hematoma. An epidural hematoma results from bleeding between the dura and the inner surface of the skull. An epidural hematoma is a neurologic emergency and is usually associated with a linear fracture crossing a major artery in the dura, causing a tear. It can have a venous or an arterial origin. Venous epidural hematomas are associated with a tear of the dural venous sinus and develop slowly. With arterial hematomas, the middle meningeal artery lying under the temporal bone is frequently torn. Hemorrhage occurs into the epidural space, which lies between the dura and the inner surface of the skull (Fig. 54-13, *A*). Because this is an arterial hemorrhage, the hematoma develops rapidly and under high pressure. Symptoms typically include unconsciousness at the scene, with a brief lucid interval followed by a decrease in LOC. Other symptoms may be a headache, nausea and vomiting, or focal findings. Rapid surgical intervention to prevent cerebral herniation dramatically improves outcomes.[26] Patients over 65 years of age with increased ICP have a higher mortality rate than younger patients.[27]

Subdural Hematoma. A subdural hematoma occurs from bleeding between the dura mater and the arachnoid layer of the meningeal covering of the brain. A subdural hematoma usually results from injury to the brain substance and its parenchymal vessels (Fig. 54-13, *B*). The veins that drain from the surface of the brain into the sagittal sinus are the source of most subdural hematomas. Because a subdural hematoma is usually venous in origin, the hematoma is much slower to develop into a mass large enough to produce symptoms. However, a subdural hematoma may be caused by an arterial hemorrhage, in which case it develops more rapidly. Subdural hematomas may be acute, subacute, or chronic (Table 54-10).

After the initial bleeding of the veins, a subdural hematoma may appear to enlarge over time as the breakdown products of the blood draw fluid into the subdural space to reach isotonicity. An acute subdural hematoma manifests signs within 48 hours of the injury. The signs and symptoms are similar to those associated with brain tissue compression in increased ICP and include decreasing LOC and headache. The patient appears drowsy and confused. The ipsilateral pupil dilates and becomes fixed. A subacute subdural hematoma usually occurs within 2 to 14 days of the injury. Failure to regain consciousness may point to this possibility.

A chronic subdural hematoma develops over weeks or months after a seemingly minor head injury. The peak incidence of chronic subdural hematoma is in the sixth and seventh decades of life when a potentially larger subdural space is available as a result of brain atrophy. With atrophy, the brain remains attached to the supportive structures, but tension is increased, and it is subject to tearing. The larger size of the subdural space also accounts for the presenting complaint to be the focal symptoms, rather than the signs of increased ICP. Chronic alcoholics are also prone to cerebral atrophy and subsequent development of subdural hematoma.

Delay in diagnosis in the older adult can be attributed to the fact that the symptoms mimic other health problems in persons of this age-group, such as vascular disease and senile dementia. Somnolence, confusion, lethargy, and memory loss are associated with health problems other than subdural hematoma. The patient has a history of head trauma in only 60% to 70% of cases.

Intracerebral Hematoma. Intracerebral hematoma occurs from bleeding within the parenchyma and occurs in approximately 16% of head injuries. They usually occur within the frontal and temporal lobes possibly from the rupture of intracerebral vessels at the time of injury. A "burst" lobe is an intracerebral or intracerebellar hematoma that is an extension of a subarachnoid hemorrhage. This type of intra-

Table 54-10 Acute, Subacute, and Chronic Subdural Hematomas

Occurrence after Injury	Progression of Symptoms	Treatment	Type of Trauma
Acute 24-48 hr	Immediate deterioration	Craniotomy, evacuation and decompression	Severe
Subacute 48 hr-2 wk	Initial unconsciousness, gradual improvement, deterioration over hours, dilation of pupils, ptosis	Evacuation and decompression	Severe
Chronic Weeks, months (>20 days)	Nonspecific, nonlocalizing progression; progressive alteration in LOC	Evacuation and decompression, membranectomy	Trivial, nonexistent, or forgotten (recollection of incident by only 60-70% of patients)

✚EMERGENCY MANAGEMENT

Table 54-11 Head Injury

Etiology	Assessment Findings	Interventions
Blunt Motor vehicle collision Pedestrian event Fall Assault Sports injury **Penetrating** Gunshot wound Arrow	**Surface Findings** ▪ Scalp lacerations ▪ Fracture or depressions in skull ▪ Bruises or contusions on face, Battle's sign (bruising behind ears) ▪ Raccoon eyes (dependent bruising around eyes) **Respiratory** ▪ Central neurogenic hyperventilation ▪ Cheyne-Stokes respirations ▪ Decreased oxygen saturation ▪ Pulmonary edema **Central Nervous System** ▪ Unequal or dilated pupils ▪ Asymmetric facial movements ▪ Garbled speech, abusive speech ▪ Confusion ▪ Decreased level of consciousness ▪ Combativeness ▪ Involuntary movements ▪ Seizures ▪ Bowel and bladder incontinence ▪ Flaccidity ▪ Depressed or hyperactive reflexes ▪ Decerebrate or decorticate posturing ▪ Glasgow Coma Scale <12 ▪ CSF leaking from ears or nose	**Initial** ▪ Ensure patent airway. ▪ Stabilize cervical spine. ▪ Administer O_2 via nasal cannula or non-rebreather mask. ▪ Establish IV access with two large-bore catheters to infuse normal saline or lactated Ringer's solution. ▪ Control external bleeding with sterile pressure dressing. ▪ Assess for rhinorrhea, otorrhea, scalp wounds. ▪ Remove patient's clothing. **Ongoing Monitoring** ▪ Maintain patient warmth using blankets, warm intravenous fluids, overhead warming lights, warm humidified oxygen. ▪ Monitor vital signs, level of consciousness, O_2 saturation, cardiac rhythm, Glasgow Coma Score, pupil size and reactivity. ▪ Anticipate need for intubation if gag reflex is absent. ▪ Assume neck injury with head injury. ▪ Administer fluids cautiously to prevent fluid overload and increasing ICP.

cerebral hematoma is thought to result from hemorrhage of supracortical vessels.

Diagnostic Studies and Collaborative Care

Skull x-rays are routinely ordered on any patient with a craniocerebral trauma. This is done to rule out a skull fracture. Skull x-rays are also useful in identifying orbital fractures and other facial fractures. CT scan and MRI are considered the best diagnostic tests to determine craniocerebral trauma. CT scan and MRI allow for rapid diagnosis and intervention. PET and evoked potential studies may also be used in the diagnosis and differentiation of head injuries. Transcranial Doppler studies allow for the measurement of cerebral blood flow velocity. In general, the diagnostic studies are similar to those used for a patient with increased ICP (see Table 54-5).

Emergency management of the patient with a head injury is presented in Table 54-11. In addition to measures to prevent secondary injury by treating cerebral edema and managing increased ICP, the principal treatment of head injuries is timely diagnosis and surgery if necessary. For the patient with concussion and contusion, observation and management of increased ICP are the primary management strategies.

The treatment of skull fractures is usually conservative. For depressed fractures and fractures with loose fragments, a craniotomy is necessary to elevate the depressed bone and remove the free fragments. If large amounts of bone are destroyed, the bone may be removed (craniectomy) and a cranioplasty will be needed at a later time (see Cranial Surgery later in this chapter).

In cases of acute subdural and epidural hematomas the blood must be removed. A craniotomy is generally performed to visualize the bleeding vessels so that the bleeding can be controlled. Burr-hole openings may be used in an extreme emergency for a more rapid decompression, followed by a craniotomy to stop all bleeding. A drain is generally placed postoperatively for several days to prevent any reaccumulation of blood.

NURSING MANAGEMENT: HEAD TRAUMA

■ Nursing Assessment

The patient with a head injury is always considered to have the potential for development of increased ICP. Increased ICP is associated with higher mortality rates and poorer functional outcomes.[28] The data collected generally include information gathered for the unconscious patient (see Fig. 54-1). The most important aspects of the objective data are noting the GCS score (see Table 54-2), monitoring the neurologic status (see Fig. 54-8), and determining whether a CSF leak has occurred.

■ Nursing Diagnoses

Nursing diagnoses for the patient who has sustained a head injury may include, but are not limited to, the following:

- Altered tissue perfusion: cerebral *related to* interruption of cerebral blood flow associated with cerebral hemorrhage, hematoma, and edema
- Hyperthermia *related to* increased metabolism, infection, and loss of cerebral integrative function secondary to possible hypothalamic injury
- Sensory/perceptual alterations *related to* cerebral injury and intensive care unit environment
- Pain *related to* headache, nausea, and vomiting
- Impaired physical mobility *related to* decreased LOC and treatment-imposed bed rest
- Risk for eye injury *related to* loss of protective reflexes
- Risk for infection *related to* environmental contamination secondary to open wound
- Anxiety *related to* abrupt change in health status, hospital environment, and lack of knowledge of seriousness of health problem
- Self-esteem disturbance *related to* altered appearance of head and face and dependence on others

■ Planning

The overall goals are that the patient with an acute head injury will (1) maintain adequate cerebral perfusion; (2) remain normothermic; (3) be free from pain, discomfort, and infection; and (4) attain maximal cognitive, motor, and sensory function.

■ Nursing Implementation

Health Promotion. One of the best ways to prevent head injuries is to prevent car and motorcycle accidents. The nurse can be active in campaigns that promote driving safety and can speak to driver education classes regarding the dangers of unsafe driving and of driving after drinking alcohol. The use of seat belts in cars and the use of helmets for riding on motorcycles are the most effective measures for increasing survival after accidents. Increasingly, individual states are passing legislation requiring the use of automobile safety devices for both children and adults. The wearing of protective helmets by lumberjacks, construction workers, miners, horseback riders, bicycle riders, and sky divers is also recommended. The nurse should be familiar with data on outcomes with and without safety devices in working with groups who oppose safety legislation as an infringement of personal freedom. Parents of young children should be educated in the proper use of car seats and restraints for their children. The nurse should also teach children about safety precautions for bicycle riding, skateboarding, and contact sports. Where appropriate parents and children should also be taught about the importance of handgun safety.

Acute Intervention. Action taken at the scene of the accident can have an important impact on the outcome of the head injury. Emergency management of head injury is discussed in Table 54-11. The general goal of nursing management of the head-injured patient is to maintain cerebral perfusion and prevention of secondary cerebral ischemia. Nursing care may initially consist of surveillance or monitoring for changes in neurologic status. This action is critically important because the patient's condition may deteriorate rapidly, necessitating emergency surgery. Appropriate preoperative and postoperative nursing interventions are initiated if surgery is anticipated.

The nurse should explain the need for frequent neurologic assessments to both the patient and the family. Behavioral manifestations associated with head injury can result in a frightened, disoriented patient who is combative and resists help. The nurse's approach should be calm and gentle. Restraints should be avoided if possible because they often produce agitation, which further increases ICP. A family member may be available to stay with the patient and thus prevent increasing anxiety and fear. Other teaching points are presented in Table 54-12.

The nurse should perform neurologic assessments at intervals, based on the patient's condition. The GCS is useful in assessing the level of arousal (see Table 54-2). Indications of a deteriorating neurologic state, such as a decreasing LOC or a lessening of motor strength, should be reported to the physician, and the patient's condition should be closely monitored.

The major focus of nursing care for the brain-injured patient relates to the unconscious state and increased ICP (see Nursing Management: Increased Intracranial Pressure earlier in this chapter). However, there may be specific problems that require nursing intervention.

Eye problems may include loss of the corneal reflex, periorbital ecchymosis and edema, and diplopia. Loss of the corneal reflex may necessitate administering lubricating eyedrops, taping the eyes shut, or suturing the eyelids to prevent abrasion. Periorbital ecchymosis and edema disappear spontaneously, but cold and, later, warm compresses provide comfort and hasten the process. Diplopia can be relieved by use of an eye patch.

Hyperthermia may occur from infection or injury to the hypothalamus. Increased metabolism secondary to hyperthermia increases metabolic waste, which in turn produces further cerebral vasodilation.

PATIENT & FAMILY HOME CARE

Table 54-12 Head Injury

Teaching guidelines for the patient and family during the initial 2-3 days following a head injury include the following:

1. Notify your health care provider immediately if experiencing signs and symptoms that may indicate complications:
   - Increased drowsiness (e.g., difficulty arousing, confusion)
   - Nausea and vomiting
   - Worsening headache or stiff neck
   - Seizures
   - Vision difficulties (e.g., blurring)
   - Behavior change (e.g., irritability, anger)
   - Motor problems (e.g., clumsiness, difficulty walking, slurred speech, weakness in arms or legs)
   - Sensory disturbances (e.g., numbness)
   - Decreased heart rate
2. Emphasize the importance of having someone stay with the patient.
3. Abstain from alcohol.
4. Check with your health care provider before taking medications that may increase drowsiness, including muscle relaxants, tranquilizers, and narcotic pain medications.
5. Avoid driving, using heavy machinery, contact sports, and warm baths.

If CSF rhinorrhea or otorrhea occurs, the nurse should inform the physician immediately. The patient should lie flat in bed unless this is contraindicated because of increased ICP. The head of the bed may be raised to decrease the CSF pressure so that a tear can seal. A loose collection pad may be placed under the nose or over the ear. No dressing should be placed into the nasal or ear cavities. The patient should be cautioned not to sneeze or blow the nose. Nasogastric tubes should not be used, and nasotracheal suctioning should not be performed on these patients.

Nursing measures specific to the care of the immobilized patient, such as those related to bladder and bowel function, skin care, and infection, are also indicated. Nausea and vomiting may be a problem and can be alleviated by antiemetic medication. Headache can usually be controlled with aspirin or small doses of codeine.

If the patient's condition deteriorates, intracranial surgery may be necessary (see Cranial Surgery later in this chapter). A burr-hole opening or craniotomy may be indicated, depending on the underlying injury that is causing the symptoms.

The patient is often unconscious before surgery, making it necessary for a family member to sign the consent form for surgery. This is a difficult and frightening time for the patient's family and requires sensitive nursing management. The suddenness of the situation makes it especially difficult for the family to cope.

The emergency nature of the surgery may prevent the usual careful preoperative preparation. The nurse should consult with the neurosurgeon to determine specific preoperative nursing measures.

Ambulatory and Home Care. Once the condition has stabilized, the patient is usually transferred for postacute rehabilitation management to prepare the patient for reentry into the community. As with any craniocerebral problem, there may be chronic problems related to motor and sensory deficits, communication, memory, and intellectual functioning. Many of the principles of nursing management of the patient with a stroke are appropriate (see Chapter 55). Conditions that may require nursing and collaborative management include poor nutritional status, bowel and bladder management, spasticity, dysphagia, neurogenic heterotopic ossification (overgrowth of bone), deep vein thrombosis, and communicating hydrocephalus. With time and patience, many of the chronic problems subside or disappear. The patient's outward appearance is not a good indicator of how well the patient will function in the home or work environment.

Seizure disorders are seen in approximately 5% of patients with a nonpenetrating head injury. The most vulnerable period of time for seizures to develop is during the first week after the head injury. In 25% of patients who develop a seizure disorder, the onset is at 4 or more years after the initial injury. Antiseizure agents are not used prophylactically but are generally instituted after a witnessed seizure or if an EEG demonstrates subclinical seizure activity. However, some clinicians recommend that antiseizure drugs be used during the first week and then be discontinued if no seizure activity is observed. Phenytoin (Dilantin) is the antiseizure drug of choice in posttraumatic seizure activity.

The mental and emotional sequelae of brain trauma are often the most incapacitating problems. It is estimated that more than 60% of patients with head injuries who have been comatose for more than 6 hours undergo some personality change. They may suffer loss of concentration and memory and defective memory processing. Personal drive may decrease; apathy and apparent laziness may increase. Euphoria and mood swings, along with a seeming lack of awareness of the seriousness of the injury, mark the affect of patients. The patient's behavior may indicate a loss of social restraint, judgment, tact, and emotional control.

Progressive recovery may continue for 6 months or more before a plateau is reached and a prognosis for recovery can be made. Specific nursing management in the posttraumatic phase depends on specific residual deficits.

In all cases the family must be given special consideration. They need to understand what is happening, and they must be taught appropriate interaction patterns. The nurse must give guidance and referrals for financial aid, child care, and other personal needs and must assist the family in involving the patient in family activities whenever possible. Assisting the patient and family in developing and maintaining hope and keeping communication open are strategies perceived as supportive by families.[29]

The family often has unrealistic expectations of the patient as the coma begins to recede. The family expects full return to pretrauma status. In reality, the patient experiences a reduced awareness and ability to interpret environmental stimuli. The nurse must prepare the family for the emergence of the patient from coma and must explain that the process of awakening often takes several weeks.

When the time for discharge planning arrives, the family and the patient may benefit from very specific posthospital instructions to avoid family-patient friction. Special "no" policies that may be appropriately suggested by the neurosurgeon, neuropsychologist, and nurse include *no* drinking of alcoholic beverages, *no* driving, *no* use of firearms, *no* work with hazardous implements and machinery, and *no* unsupervised smoking.[12] Family members, particularly spouses, go through role transition as the role changes from one of spouse to that of caregiver.[12]

Evaluation

The expected outcomes are that the head-injured patient will

- maintain normal cerebral perfusion pressure
- achieve maximal cognitive, motor, and sensory function
- experience no infection, hyperthermia, or pain

INTRACRANIAL TUMORS

Tumors within the cranial cavity cause approximately 2% of all deaths. It is estimated that in 1998 there were 17,400 primary brain cancers diagnosed in the United States.[30] The brain is also a frequent site for metastasis from other sites. Brain tumors rank fourth as cause of death from cancer in individuals 35 to 54 years of age.

Types

Tumors of the brain may be primary, arising from tissues within the brain, or secondary, resulting from a metastasis from a malignant neoplasm elsewhere in the body. Brain tumors are generally classified according to the tissue from which they arise. If malignant, the tumor is graded according to general cancer staging procedures. Brain tumors may be classified as those arising inside the brain substance (e.g., gliomas, vascular tumors) or those arising outside the brain substance (e.g., meningiomas, cranial nerve tumors). Glioblastoma multiforme is the most common tumor, followed by meningioma and astrocytoma. More than half of the intracranial tumors are malignant; they infiltrate the brain parenchyma and are not amenable to complete surgical removal. Other tumors may be histologically benign but are located such that complete removal is not possible. Brain tumors are more commonly seen in middle-aged persons, but they may occur at any age.

Unless treated, all intracranial tumors eventually cause death from increasing tumor volume leading to increased ICP. Brain tumors rarely metastasize outside the central nervous system (CNS) because they are contained by structural (meninges) and physiologic (blood-brain) barriers. Table 54-13 compares the major intracranial tumors. An astrocytoma is shown in Fig. 54-14.

Clinical Manifestations

The clinical manifestations of intracranial tumors are generally caused by the local destructive effects of the tumor, the resulting accumulation of metabolites, the displacement of structures, the obstruction of CSF flow, and the effects of edema and increased ICP on cerebral function. The rate of growth and the

Table 54-13 Major Intracranial Tumors

Tumor	Tissue of Origin	% of Brain Tumors	Usual Locations	Malignant or Benign
Gliomas				
Astrocytoma	Supportive tissue, glial cells and astrocytes	20	White matter of frontal and temporal lobes in adults, lateral cerebellar lobes in children	Moderately malignant, grades I and II
Glioblastoma multiforme	Primitive stem cell (glioblast)	20	Cerebral hemispheres	Highly malignant and invasive, grades III and IV
Oligodendroglioma	Glial cells and dendrites	2	Cerebral hemispheres, most in frontal lobe, some in basal ganglia and cerebellum	Benign (encapsulation and calcification)
Ependymoma	Ependymal epithelium	1	Lateral and fourth ventricles in children and young adults (usual)	Benign to highly malignant, most benign and encapsulated
Medulloblastoma	Supportive tissue	1	Posterior fossa, fourth ventricle, brainstem in children	Highly malignant and invasive, metastatic to spinal cord and remote areas of brain
Meningioma	Endothelial cells, fibrous tissue elements, transitional cells, angioblasts	20	Arachnoid villi, dura, half over convexity of hemisphere and half at base of hemisphere	Benign, encapsulation outside brain substance
Acoustic neuroma (neurofibroma)	Sheath of vestibular portion of CN VIII	5	Site between pons and cerebellum	Benign or low-grade malignancy, encapsulation
Pituitary adenoma	Pituitary glandular tissue	10	Pituitary gland	Usually benign
Vascular tumors Hemangioblastoma Arteriovenous malformation	Overgrowth of arteries and veins enlarging from feeder vessels	3	Parietal cortex near middle cerebral vessels	Benign
Metastatic tumors	Lungs, breast, kidney, thyroid, prostate	8	Cerebral cortex, diencephalon	Malignant

appearance of manifestations depend on the location, size, and mitotic rate of the cells of tissue of origin. Figure 54-15 illustrates the functional areas of the cerebral cortex and can be used as a guide to correlate local manifestations with the location of the tumor.

A wide range of possible clinical manifestations are associated with brain tumors with the classic feature being progressive manifestation of clinical symptoms. In some circumstances, a slight decrease in mental acuity may be the initial symptom. If left untreated, symptoms continue to progress to mental deterioration or a dramatic event such as a seizure. A brain tumor, as the tumor expands, may also produce manifestations of increased ICP from increased tumor volume, cerebral edema, or obstruction of the CSF pathways. Finally, manifestations may clearly indicate the location of the tumor by an alteration in the function controlled by the affected area (Table 54-14).

Complications

If the tumor mass obstructs the ventricles or occludes the outlet, ventricular enlargement (hydrocephalus) can occur. Surgical treatment is needed to relieve the pressure and involves placement of a ventriculoatrial or a ventriculoperitoneal shunt. A catheter with one-way valves is placed in the lateral ventricle and then tunneled through the skin to drain cerebrospinal fluid into the right atrium or the peritoneum. Rapid decompression of intracranial pressure can cause prostration and headache that may be prevented by gradually introducing the patient to the upright position. The patient should be instructed to avoid contact sports that may result in a blow to the valve or shearing

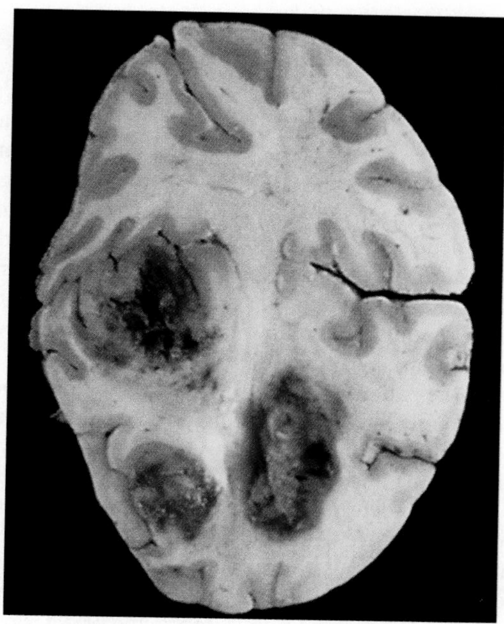

Fig. 54-14 Astrocytoma.

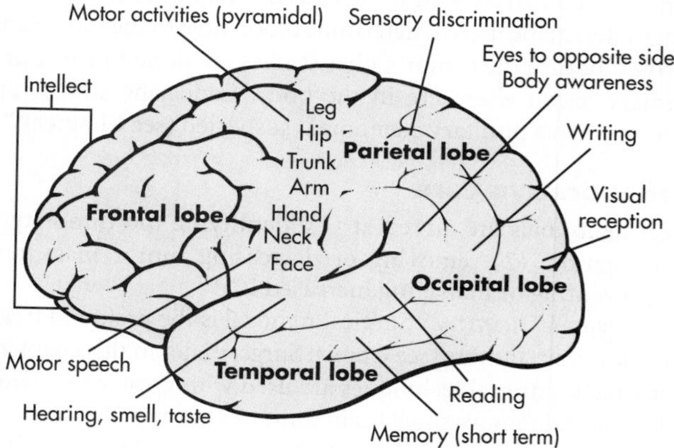

Fig. 54-15 Each area of the brain controls a particular activity.

Table 54-14 Tumor Location and Associated Presenting Symptoms

Tumor Location	Presenting Symptoms
▪ Cerebral hemisphere	
Frontal lobe (unilateral)	Unilateral hemiplegia; seizures; memory deficit; personality and judgment changes; visual disturbances
Frontal lobe (bilateral)	Symptoms associated with unilateral frontal lobe tumors; ataxic gait
Parietal lobe	Speech disturbance (if tumor is in the dominant hemisphere, inability to write, spatial disorders, unilateral neglect)
Occipital lobe	Blindness and seizures
Temporal lobe	Few symptoms; seizures, dysphagia
▪ Subcortical	Hemiplegia; other symptoms may depend on area of infiltration
▪ Meningeal tumors	Symptoms are associated with compression of the brain and depend on tumor location
▪ Metastatic tumors	Headache, nausea or vomiting because of ICP; other symptoms depend on tumor location
▪ Thalamus and sellar tumors	Headache, nausea, vision disturbances, papilledema, nystagmus occurs from an increase in ICP; diabetes insipidus may occur
▪ Fourth ventricle and cerebellar tumors	Headache, nausea, and papilledema from increased ICP; ataxic gait and changes in coordination
▪ Cerebellopontine tumors	Tinnitus and vertigo, deafness
▪ Brainstem tumors	Headache upon awakening, drowsiness, vomiting, ataxic gait, facial muscle weakness, hearing loss, dysphagia, dysarthria, "crossed eyes" or other visual changes, hemiparesis
▪ Spinal cord tumors	Depend on the nerves involved Cervical: pain, weakness or muscle wasting in arms, back, neck, or legs Thoracic area: pain accentuated with deep breathing and coughing, lack of bowel or bladder control may occur depending on tumor location

of the catheter. The physician should be notified if signs of increased ICP occur, such as decreasing level of consciousness, restlessness, headache, blurred vision, or vomiting without nausea. Signs of an infected shunt, such as high fever, persistent headache, and stiff neck, warrant investigation.

Diagnostic Studies

An extensive history and a comprehensive neurologic examination must be done in the workup of a patient with a suspected brain tumor. A careful history and physical examination may provide data with respect to location. Diagnostic studies are similar to those used for a patient with increased ICP (see Table 54-5). The sensitivity of MRI allows detection of very small tumors. Other diagnostic studies include CT scan, skull x-rays, cerebral angiography, EEG, brain scan, PET, lumbar puncture, and myelogram. CT and brain scanning are used to diagnose the location of the lesion. Newer diagnostic tools such as PET and MRI provide more reliable diagnostic information. The EEG is useful but of less importance. A lumbar puncture is seldom diagnostic and carries with it the risk of cerebral herniation. Angiography can be used to determine blood flow to the tumor and further localize the tumor. Other studies are done to rule out a primary lesion elsewhere in the body. Endocrine studies are helpful when a pituitary adenoma is suspected (see Chapter 47).

Collaborative Care

Treatment goals are aimed at (1) identifying the tumor type and location, (2) removing or decreasing tumor mass, and (3) preventing or managing increased ICP.

Surgical Therapy. Surgical removal is the preferred treatment for brain tumors (see Cranial Surgery later in this chapter). Stereotactic surgical techniques are used with greater frequency to biopsy and remove small brain tumors. However, the outcome of surgical therapy depends on the type, size, and location of the tumor. Meningiomas and oligodendrogliomas can usually be completely removed, whereas the more invasive gliomas and medulloblastomas can be only partially removed. Surgery reduces tumor mass, which decreases ICP and provides relief of symptoms with an extension of survival time. Tumors located in the deep central areas of the dominant hemisphere, the posterior corpus callosum, or the upper brainstem cause extensive neurologic damage and are considered inoperable.

Radiation and Chemotherapy. Radiation therapy lengthens survival in patients with malignant gliomas, especially when it is combined with partial surgical removal. Patients with less malignant tumors respond to radiation with a longer survival time and decreased recurrence of tumor. Cerebral edema and rapidly increasing ICP may be a complication of radiation therapy, but they can be managed with high doses of corticosteroids (dexamethasone [Decadron], prednisone, or methylprednisolone [Solu-Medrol]).

Normally the blood-brain barrier prohibits the entry of most drugs into the brain parenchyma. The most malignant tumors cause a breakdown of the blood-brain barrier in the area of the tumor, allowing chemotherapeutic agents to be used to treat the malignancy. A group of chemotherapeutic drugs called the nitrosoureas (e.g., carmustine [BCNU], lomustine [CCNU]) are particularly effective in treating brain tumors. Gliadel wafer (prolifeprosan 20 with carmustine), a biodegradable wafer implanted at the time of surgery, can deliver chemotherapy directly to the tumor site. Other drugs being used include methotrexate and procarbazine (Matulane). Two methods used to deliver chemotherapeutic drugs directly to the central nervous system are via an Ommaya reservoir and intrathecal administration. Brain tumors that cannot be totally removed may be treated with a combination of corticosteroids, surgery, radiation, and chemotherapy (see Chapter 14).

Many techniques to control and treat brain tumors are currently under investigation; these include radium implants into the tumor bed, local hyperthermia, and biologic therapy. Although progress in treatment has increased length and quality of survival of patients with gliomas, outcomes remain poor.

NURSING MANAGEMENT: INTRACRANIAL TUMOR

■ Nursing Assessment

The subjective and objective data of the patient with a brain tumor include the data the nurse collects for the unconscious patient. In addition to the assessment data listed in Fig. 54-8, the initial assessment should be structured to provide baseline data of the neurologic status and the information needed to design a realistic, individualized care plan. Areas to be assessed include the LOC and content of consciousness, motor abilities, sensory perception, integrated function (including bowel and bladder function), balance and proprioception, and the coping abilities of the patient and family. Watching a patient perform activities of daily living and listening to the patient's conversation are convenient ways to perform part of the neurologic assessment. Having the patient or the family explain the problem can be helpful in determining the patient's limitations and can also provide the nurse with information about the patient's insight into the problems. All initial data should be accurately recorded to provide a baseline for comparison to determine whether the patient's condition is improving or deteriorating.

Interview data are as important as the actual physical assessment. Questions concerning medical history, intellectual abilities and educational level, and history of nervous system infections and trauma should be asked. Determination of the presence of seizures, syncope, nausea and vomiting, pain, and headaches or other pain is important in planning care for the patient.

■ Nursing Diagnoses

Nursing diagnoses for the patient with a brain tumor may include, but are not limited to, the following:

- Altered tissue perfusion: cerebral *related to* cerebral edema
- Pain (headache) *related to* cerebral edema and increased ICP
- Self-care deficits *related to* altered neuromuscular function secondary to tumor growth and cerebral edema
- Anxiety *related to* diagnosis and treatment
- Potential complication: seizures *related to* abnormal electrical activity of the brain
- Potential complication: increased ICP *related to* presence of tumor and failure of normal compensatory mechanisms

■ Planning

The overall goals are that the patient with a brain tumor will (1) maintain normal ICP, (2) maximize neurologic functioning, (3) be free from pain and discomfort, and (4) be aware of the long-term implications with respect to prognosis and cognitive and physical functioning.

Nursing Implementation

A primary or metastatic tumor of the frontal lobe can cause behavioral and personality changes. Loss of emotional control, confusion, disorientation, memory loss, and depression may be signs of a frontal lobe lesion. These behavioral changes are often not perceived by the patient but can be disturbing and even frightening to the family. These changes can also cause a distancing to occur between the family and the patient. Assisting the family in understanding what is happening to the patient and supporting the family through this diagnostic phase are important roles for the nurse.

The confused patient with behavioral instability can be a challenge. Protecting the patient from self-harm is an important part of nursing care. At times when the patient manifests rage and aggression, the nurse must also be concerned about self-protection. Close supervision of activity, use of side rails, judicious use of restraints, padding of the rails and the area around the bed, and a calm, reassuring approach to care are all essential techniques in the care of these patients.

Perceptual problems associated with frontal lobe and parietal lobe tumors contribute to a patient's disorientation and confusion. Minimization of environmental stimuli, creation of a routine, and use of reality orientation can be incorporated into the care plan for the confused patient.

Seizures frequently occur with brain tumors. These are managed with antiseizure drugs. Seizure precautions should be instituted for the protection of the patient. Some behavioral changes seen in the patient with a brain tumor are a result of seizure disorders and can improve with control of the seizures by means of drugs (see Chapter 56).

Motor and sensory dysfunctions are problems that interfere with the activities of daily living. Alterations in mobility must be managed, and the patient should be encouraged to provide as much self-care as physically possible. Self-image often depends on the patient's ability to participate in care within the limitations of the physical deficits.

Language deficits can also occur in patients with brain tumors. Motor (expressive) or sensory (receptive) dysphasias may occur. The disturbance in communication can be frustrating for the patient and may interfere with the nurse's ability to meet the patient's needs. Attempts should be made to establish a communication system that can be used by both the patient and the staff.

Nutritional intake may be decreased because of the patient's inability to eat, loss of appetite, or loss of desire to eat. Assessing the nutritional status of the patient and ensuring adequate nutritional intake are important aspects of care. The patient may need encouragement to eat or, in some cases, may have to be fed orally, parenterally, by gastrostomy or nasogastric tube, or by total parenteral nutrition. The patient with a brain tumor who undergoes cranial surgery requires complex nursing care. This is discussed in the next section.

CRANIAL SURGERY

The cause or indication for cranial surgery may be related to a brain tumor, CNS infection (e.g., abscess), vascular abnormalities, craniocerebral trauma, epilepsy, and intractable pain (Table 54-15).

Table 54-15 Indications for Cranial Surgery

Indication	Cause	Manifestations	Procedure
Intracranial infection	Bacteria	Early findings: stiff neck, headache, fever, weakness, seizures; later findings: seizures, hemiplegia, speech disturbances, ocular disturbances, change in LOC	Excision or drainage of abscess
Hydrocephalus	Overproduction of CSF, obstruction to flow, defective reabsorption	Early findings: mental changes, disturbances in gait; later findings: memory impairment, urinary incontinence, increased tendon reflexes	Placement of ventriculoatrial or ventriculoperitoneal shunt
Intracranial tumors	Benign or malignant cell growth	Change in LOC, pupillary changes, sensory or motor deficit, papilledema, seizures, personality changes	Excision or partial resection of tumor
Intracranial bleeding	Rupture of cerebral vessels because of trauma or cardiovascular accident	Epidural: momentary unconsciousness; lucid period, then rapid deterioration; subdural: headache, seizures; pupillary changes	Surgical evacuation through burr holes or craniotomy
Skull fractures	Trauma to skull	Headache, CSF leakage, cranial nerve deficit	Debridement of fragments and necrotic tissue, elevation and realignment of bone fragments
Arteriovenous malformation	Congenital tangle of arteries and veins (frequently in middle cerebral artery)	Headache, intracranial hemorrhage, seizures, mental deterioration	Excision of malformation
Aneurysm repair	Dilation of weak area in arterial wall (usually near anterior portion of circle of Willis)	Before rupture: headache, lethargy, visual disturbance; after rupture: violent headache, decreased LOC, visual disturbances, motor deficit	Dissection and clipping of aneurysm

Table 54-16 Types of Cranial Surgery

Type	Description
▪ Burr hole	Opening into the cranium with a drill; used to remove localized fluid and blood beneath the dura
▪ Craniotomy	Opening into the cranium with removal of a bone flap and opening the dura to remove a lesion, repair a damaged area, drain blood, or relieve increased ICP
▪ Craniectomy	Excision into the cranium to cut away a bone flap
▪ Cranioplasty	Repair of a cranial defect resulting from trauma, malformation, or previous surgical procedure; artificial material used to replace damaged or lost bone
▪ Stereotaxis	Precision localization of a specific area of the brain using a frame or a frameless system based on 3-dimensional coordinates; procedure is used for biopsy, radiosurgery, or dissection
▪ Shunt procedures	Provide an alternate pathway to redirect cerebrospinal fluid from one area to another using a tube or implanted device; examples include ventriculoperitoneal shunt and Ommaya reservoir

Surgical Procedures

Various types of cranial surgical procedures are presented in Table 54-16.

Stereotactic Surgery. Stereotactic surgery is surgery targeted by three-dimensional coordinates identified through imagery (usually CT scan or MRI). These coordinates indicate where biopsy, radiosurgery, or dissection should occur. It is a procedure used frequently as part of the initial diagnostic workup. For example, stereotactic biopsy can be performed to obtain tissue samples for histologic examination. CT scan or MRI establish the sites for precise tumor sampling. With the patient under general or local anesthesia, the surgeon drills a burr hole or creates a bone flap for an entry site, and then introduces a probe and biopsy needle. Stereotactic procedures are being used with increasing frequency for removal of small brain tumors and abscesses, drainage of hematomas, ablative procedures for extrapyramidal diseases (e.g., Parkinson's), and repair of arteriovenous malformations. A major advantage of the stereotactic approach is a reduction in damage to surrounding tissue.

Stereotactic radiosurgery is a procedure that involves closed-skull destruction of an intracranial target using ionizing radiation focused with the assistance of an intracranial guiding device. The three radiosurgical techniques make use of a stereotactic Bragg peak proton beam, a linear accelerator, or a gamma knife. In the gamma knife procedure, a single, high dose of cobalt radiation is delivered to precisely targeted tumor tissue.

In combination with stereotactic procedures to identify and localize tumor sites, surgical lasers can be used to destroy tumors. Stereotactic procedures are used to identify the tumor site. Three surgical lasers are currently used: the carbon dioxide, argon, and neodymium:yttrium-aluminum-garnet (Nd:YAG) lasers. All three work by creating thermal energy, which destroys the tissue on which it is focused. Laser therapy also provides the benefit of reducing damage to surrounding tissue.

Craniotomy. Depending on the location of the pathologic condition, a craniotomy may be frontal, parietal, occipital, temporal, or a combination of any of these. A set of burr holes is drilled, and a saw is used to connect the holes to remove the bone flap. Sometimes operating microscopes are used to magnify the site. After surgery the bone flap is wired or sutured. Sometimes drains are placed to remove fluid and blood. Patients are usually cared for in a critical care unit until stable.

NURSING MANAGEMENT: CRANIAL SURGERY

▪ Nursing Assessment

The nursing assessment of the patient undergoing cranial surgery would be similar to that for the patient with increased ICP (see Nursing Management: Increased Intracranial Pressure earlier in this chapter) or that for the patient with an intracranial tumor (see Nursing Management: Intracranial Tumor earlier in this chapter).

▪ Nursing Diagnoses

Nursing diagnoses for the patient with cranial surgery may include, but are not limited to, those presented in NCP 54-2.

▪ Planning

The overall goals are that the patient with cranial surgery will (1) return to normal consciousness, (2) be free from pain and discomfort, (3) maximize neuromuscular functioning, and (4) be rehabilitated to maximum ability.

▪ Nursing Implementation

Acute Intervention. The general preoperative and postoperative nursing care for the patient undergoing cranial surgery is similar, regardless of the cause. Nursing management is presented in NCP 54-2. The patient (if conscious and coherent) and the family will be gravely concerned about the potential physical and emotional problems that can result from surgery. The uncertainty regarding prognosis and outcome requires compassionate nursing care in the preoperative period.

Preoperative teaching is important in allaying the fears of the patient and the family and also in preparing them for the postoperative period. The patient and the family should be given general information concerning the type of operation that will be performed and what can be expected immediately after the operation. Explaining that the patient's hair will be shaved to allow for better exposure and prevention of contamination may prevent unnecessary concern over this task. The head is usually shaved in the operating room after induction of anesthesia. The family should also be informed that the patient will be taken to an intensive care unit or to a special care unit after the operation.

54-2 NURSING CARE PLAN PATIENT WITH CRANIAL SURGERY

Expected Patient Outcomes	Nursing Interventions and *Rationales*
NURSING DIAGNOSIS	**Impaired gas exchange** *related to* decreased LOC and immobility *as manifested by* restlessness, irritability, abnormal ABGs.
▪ Patent airway. ▪ ABGs within normal limits. ▪ No respiratory distress.	▪ Assess all respiratory parameters q2hr for 72 hr, then every 4-8 hr *to provide a baseline for comparison to determine if breathing problem occurs.* ▪ Draw and evaluate ABGs regularly *to guide oxygen therapy and evaluate response to treatment.* ▪ Give oxygen by nasal catheter, prongs, or mechanical ventilator until ABGs are stable for at least 24-72 hr *to maintain stable cerebral oxygenation.* ▪ Encourage gentle coughing and turning and position patient on side with head slightly hyperextended if LOC is decreased *to improve ventilation, prevent atelectasis, and prevent aspiration of secretions or obstruction of airway.* ▪ Suction gently and for only <10-15 seconds duration when necessary *to minimize hypoxemia and avoid increasing ICP.* ▪ Hyperoxygenate before and after each coughing or suctioning session *to prevent hypoxia, which adversely affects cerebral perfusion.* ▪ Observe for gastric distention; insert nasogastric tube (if indicated) and maintain patency *to reduce pressure on the diaphragm and risk of aspiration.* ▪ Report any alterations in breathing patterns such as apnea or irregular and rapid ventilation *to ensure immediate medical intervention.* ▪ Be prepared for possible need for intubation *so mechanical ventilation can be started promptly if condition deteriorates.*
NURSING DIAGNOSIS	**Pain** *related to* craniotomy, position, and environmental stimuli *as manifested by* report of headache, holding head, pained expression.
▪ Decrease in complaints of pain. ▪ Expression of satisfaction with pain relief.	▪ Assess location, type, duration, degree, and severity of pain *to evaluate patient's need for and response to treatment.* ▪ Administer ordered analgesics *to decrease pain* and evaluate effects *to determine effectiveness of therapy.* ▪ Position as comfortably as possible *to relieve positional discomforts related to the location of incision.* ▪ Keep environment quiet, darken room, put cool cloth on patient's eyes *to promote comfort by reducing environmental stimuli.*
NURSING DIAGNOSIS	**Altered nutrition: less than body requirements** *related to* inability to feed self, difficulty swallowing, and decreased LOC *as manifested by* body weight 20% or more below ideal, poor muscle tone, low serum protein levels.
▪ Maintenance of weight. ▪ Normal serum protein and albumin levels.	▪ Evaluate ability to swallow *because feeding route is determined by swallowing ability.* ▪ Advance patient to high-protein, high-caloric, small, frequent feedings as tolerated *to prevent negative nitrogen balance and excessive weight loss and to prevent pressure on the diaphragm and feeling of bloating.* ▪ Feed patient if necessary *to ensure adequate nutritional intake if self-feeding is not possible.* ▪ If patient is unable to eat, use enteral tube feedings or total parenteral nutrition as ordered *to provide necessary fluids, electrolytes, calories, and protein until patient can eat.*
NURSING DIAGNOSIS	**Body image disturbance** *related to* physical appearance resulting from surgery *as manifested by* refusal to look at self or participate in self-care, crying, or anger about appearance; social withdrawal.
▪ Acceptance of temporary nature of appearance. ▪ Maintenance of normal activities.	▪ Encourage patient to express feelings about appearance *to enable patient to recognize and begin to deal with feelings.* ▪ Explain the rate of hair regrowth of ½-¾ inch/month *so patient will have realistic expectation.* ▪ Provide information about wigs or hairpieces *so patient is aware of this alternative.* ▪ Encourage the use of scarves in women and hats in men *to boost their appearance and self-esteem and minimize embarrassment.* ▪ Reassure patient about self-worth *to bolster patient's self-esteem and coping ability.*

Continued

54-2 NURSING CARE PLAN PATIENT WITH CRANIAL SURGERY—continued

Expected Patient Outcomes	Nursing Interventions and *Rationales*
NURSING DIAGNOSIS	**Sensory-perceptual alterations** *related to* altered sensory reception, transmission, or integration secondary to neurologic surgery *as manifested by* possible disorientation; altered sight, hearing, taste, or smell; decreased LOC.
▪ Maintenance of highest possible level of interaction with environment.	▪ Assess patient's ability to speak, see, hear, taste, and smell *to enable appropriate planning of care.* ▪ Orient patient to surroundings; describe surroundings when sight is impaired *to increase patient's awareness and reduce anxiety and risk of injury.* ▪ Eliminate extraneous noise *to reduce anxiety and confusion caused by sensory overload.* ▪ Provide stimulation for all senses *to aid in retraining sensory pathways to integrate reception and interpretation of stimuli.*
NURSING DIAGNOSIS	**Self-care deficits** *related to* decreased LOC, weakness, or postoperative status *as manifested by* inability or unwillingness to perform activities of daily living.
▪ All self-care needs met.	▪ Assess patient's self-care abilities *to determine level of care needed and plan appropriate interventions.* ▪ Provide for total self-care requirements of the patient, including hygiene and skin care and tube feeding or total parenteral nutrition, *to ensure that all activities of daily living needs are met.* ▪ Turn patient at least q2hr *to promote effective circulation and ventilation and to prevent skin breakdown.* ▪ Maintain indwelling catheter patency *to facilitate bladder emptying;* assess need for enema or suppository *to promote adequate bowel elimination.* ▪ Maintain range of motion of all joints *to prevent contractures.* ▪ Provide oral hygiene q2hr *to prevent stomatitis and promote comfort.* ▪ Keep patient's eyes closed or use artificial tears if unconscious or unable to blink *to prevent corneal damage.*

COLLABORATIVE PROBLEMS

Nursing Goals	Nursing Interventions and *Rationales*
POTENTIAL COMPLICATION	**Increased ICP** *related to* cerebral edema.
▪ Monitor for signs of increased ICP. ▪ Report deviations from acceptable parameters. ▪ Carry out appropriate medical and nursing interventions.	▪ Assess for signs of increased ICP (e.g., altered LOC, headache, pupil inequality, decreased respirations and pulse rate, elevated systolic blood pressure with widened pulse pressure, swelling around surgical site, elevation of bone flap) *to enable immediate reporting and initiation of treatment.* ▪ Assess neurologic function immediately on patient's return from operating room *to establish baseline parameters.* ▪ Report significant changes *to enable prompt intervention and to prevent serious complications.* ▪ Calibrate and maintain ICP monitoring equipment in functioning condition *to ensure accurate readings.* ▪ Provide aseptic care of insertion site *to prevent infection and subsequent increase in ICP from exudate.* ▪ Administer diuretics and corticosteroids as ordered *to reduce cerebral edema.* ▪ Position patient with head of bed elevated to 30 degrees *to promote venous drainage from head, reducing cerebral edema.* ▪ Avoid neck and hip flexion *to prevent venous obstruction and decrease risk of increasing intraabdominal pressure, which restricts diaphragm movement, increasing $PaCO_2$, which increases cerebral blood flow and ultimately results in cerebral edema.* ▪ Prevent constipation and straining with defecation *to prevent increased ICP caused by Valsalva's maneuver.* ▪ Manage elevated temperature *because elevated temperature increases cerebral metabolism and causes increased ICP.*

Continued

54-2 NURSING CARE PLAN PATIENT WITH CRANIAL SURGERY—continued

Expected Patient Outcomes	Nursing Interventions and *Rationales*
POTENTIAL COMPLICATION	**CSF leak from nose or ears** *related to* surgical incision.
▪ Monitor and report signs of CSF leak. ▪ Carry out appropriate medical and nursing interventions.	▪ Assess for clear or slightly yellow drainage from ears or nose *as indicators of CSF leaks, which increases risk for infection.* ▪ Test drainage for glucose or CSF ring, report to physician if positive *to confirm drainage is CSF.* ▪ Culture drainage of ears and nose *to rule out possibility of infectious drainage.* ▪ Do not plug nose or ears with cotton; use loose "snuffer" type of gauze dressing for comfort (change frequently) *to allow free drainage until injured area is repaired.* ▪ Watch for temperature elevation, irritability, headache, or nuchal rigidity and report immediately *because these are key indicators of meningitis.* ▪ Administer antibiotics if ordered *as treatment for infection.*

LOC, level of consciousness.

The primary goal of care after cranial surgery is prevention of increased ICP. The turning and positioning of the patient sometimes depends on the site of the operation. If the surgical approach is in the posterior fossa, the patient is generally kept flat or at a slight elevation (10 to 15 degrees). Lying on the back will be prevented as much as possible, and flexion of the neck will be avoided to protect the suture line. The maximum swelling in the operative area occurs within 24 to 48 hours after the surgery.

With an incision over the skull in the anterior or middle fossae, the patient will return from the operating room with the head elevated at an angle of 30 to 45 degrees. If a bone flap has been removed (craniectomy), care should be taken not to have the patient positioned on the operative side.

The dressing should be observed for color, odor, and amount of drainage. The physician should be notified immediately of any excessive bleeding or clear drainage. Checking drains for placement and assessing the area around the dressing are also important.

Frequent assessment of the neurologic status of the patient is essential during the first 48 hours. In addition to the neurologic functions, fluids, electrolyte levels, and osmolality are monitored closely to detect changes in sodium regulation, the onset of diabetes insipidus, or severe hypovolemia.

The dressing is usually in place for 3 to 5 days. Scalp care should include meticulous care of the incision to prevent wound infection. The area should be cleansed with povidone iodine (Betadine) or a similar antiseptic disinfectant. Cleansing should be followed by application of an antibiotic ointment according to procedure. Once the dressing is removed, use of an antiseptic soap for washing the scalp may also be beneficial. The psychologic impact of baldness can be alleviated by the use of a wig, turban, or cap after the incision has completely healed. For the patient who is receiving radiation, use of a sunblock and head covering should be advocated if any exposure to the sun is anticipated.

Ambulatory and Home Care. The rehabilitative potential for a patient after cranial surgery depends on the reason for the surgery, the postoperative course, and the patient's general state of health. Nursing interventions must be based on a realistic appraisal of these factors. An overall goal for the nurse is to foster independence for as long as possible and to the highest degree possible.

Specific rehabilitation potential cannot be determined until cerebral edema and increased ICP subside postoperatively. Care must be taken to maintain as much function as possible through measures such as careful positioning, meticulous skin and mouth care, regular range-of-motion exercises, bowel and bladder care, and adequate nutrition.

Referrals may be made to other specialists on the health care team. For example, the speech therapist may be helpful to the patient who has a speech problem. The needs and problems of each patient should be addressed individually because many variables affect the plan.

Mental and emotional residual deficits are often more difficult for the patient and the family to accept than are motor and sensory losses. The nurse can provide much help and support during the adjustment phase and in long-range planning.

The mental and physical deterioration of the patient, including seizures, personality disorganization, apathy, and wasting, is difficult for both family and health professionals to endure. Although progress is continuously being made to help the patient with a brain tumor by means of chemotherapy, conventional and interstitial radiation, and biologic therapies, the prognosis remains grim.

■ Evaluation

The expected outcomes are that the patient with an intracranial tumor will

- regain maximal cognitive, motor, and sensory function possible
- be free of infection
- have pain and discomfort alleviated

Table 54-17 Cerebral Inflammatory Conditions

	Bacterial Meningitis*	Encephalitis	Brain Abscess
Causative organisms	Bacteria (pneumococci, meningococci, streptococci)	Bacteria, fungi, parasites, herpes simplex virus (HSV) other viruses	Streptococci, staphylococci through bloodstream
CSF			
Pressure (normal, 60-150 mm H_2O)	Increased	Normal to slight increase with increased ICP	Increased
WBC count (normal, 0-8/μl)	>500/μl (mainly PMN)	<500/μl, PMN (early), lymphocytes (later)	25-300/μl (PMN)
Protein (normal, 15-45 mg/dl [0.15-0.45 g/L])	High	Slight increase	Normal
Glucose (normal, 45-75 mg/dl [2.5-4.2 mmol/L])	Low or absent	Normal	Low or absent
Appearance	Turbid, cloudy	Clear	Clear
Diagnostic studies	Gram's stain, smear, culture	Viral studies, MRI HSV DNA	CT scan, EEG, skull x-ray
Treatment	Antibiotics with sensitivity tests, supportive care, prevention of symptoms of ↑ ICP	Supportive care, prevention of symptoms of increased ICP, acyclovir (Zovirax) for HSV	Antibiotics, incision and drainage Supportive care

*Meningitis can also be caused by virus, yeast, and fungi.
PMN, polymorphonuclear cells; *WBC,* white blood cell.

INFLAMMATORY CONDITIONS OF THE BRAIN

Meningitis, encephalitis, and brain abscesses are the most common inflammatory conditions of the brain and spinal cord. Inflammation can be caused by bacteria, viruses, fungi, and chemicals (e.g., contrast media used in diagnostic tests or blood in the subarachnoid space) (Table 54-17). CNS infections may occur via the bloodstream, by extension from a primary site, by extension along cranial and spinal nerves, or in utero. Bacterial infections are the most common, and the organisms usually involved are *Streptococcus pneumoniae, Haemophilus influenzae, Neisseria meningitides, Staphylococcus aureus,* and *Meningococci.* The mortality rate is high, and 50% of the survivors experience long-term neurologic deficits. Bacterial meningitis carries the highest mortality rate and is considered a medical emergency.

MENINGITIS

Etiology and Pathophysiology

Meningitis is an acute inflammation of the pia mater and the arachnoid membrane surrounding the brain and the spinal cord. Therefore meningitis is always a cerebrospinal infection. The organisms usually gain entry to the CNS through the upper respiratory tract or the bloodstream, but they may enter by direct extension from penetrating wounds of the skull or through fractured sinuses in basal skull fractures.

Meningitis usually occurs in the fall, winter, or early spring and is often secondary to viral respiratory disease. Children under 6 years of age, older adults, and persons who are debilitated are more often affected than is the general population. *Streptococcus pneumoniae* causes about 30% of the infections.

The inflammatory response to the infection tends to increase CSF production, with a moderate increase in pressure. In bacterial meningitis the purulent secretion produced quickly spreads to other areas of the brain through the CSF. If this process extends into the brain parenchyma, or if a concurrent encephalitis is present, cerebral edema and increased ICP become more of a problem. All patients with meningitis must be observed closely for manifestations of increased ICP, which is thought to be a result of swelling around the dura, increased CSF volume, and endotoxins produced by the bacteria.

Clinical Manifestations

Fever, severe headache, nausea, vomiting, and nuchal rigidity (resistance to flexion of the neck) are key signs of meningitis. A positive Kernig's sign, a positive Brudzinski's sign (see Chapter 53), photophobia, a decreased LOC, and signs of increased ICP may also be present. Coma is associated with a poor prognosis and occurs in 5% to 10% of patients with bacterial meningitis. Seizures occur in 20% of all cases. With meningitis the headache becomes progressively worse and may be accompanied by vomiting and irritability. If the infecting organism is a meningococcus, a skin rash is common and petechiae may be seen.

Complications

The most common complication of meningitis is residual neurologic dysfunction. Cranial nerve dysfunction often occurs with cranial nerves III, IV, VI, VII, or VIII in bacterial meningitis. The dysfunction usually disappears within a few weeks. Hearing loss may be permanent after bacterial meningitis, but it is not a complication of viral meningitis.

Cranial nerve irritation can have serious sequelae. The optic nerve (CN II) is compressed by increased ICP. Papilledema is often present, and blindness may occur. When the oculomotor (CN III), trochlear (CN IV), and abducens (CN VI) nerves are irritated, ocular movements are affected. Ptosis, unequal pupils, and diplopia are common. Irritation of the trigeminal nerve (CN V) is evidenced by sensory losses and loss of the corneal reflex, and irritation of the facial nerve (CN VII) results in facial paresis. Irritation of the vestibulocochlear nerve (CN VIII) causes tinnitus, vertigo, and deafness.

Hemiparesis, dysphasia, and hemianopsia may also occur. These signs usually resolve over time. If resolution does not occur, a cerebral abscess, subdural empyema, subdural effusion, or persistent meningitis is suggested. Acute cerebral edema may occur with bacterial meningitis, causing seizures, CN III palsy, bradycardia, hypertensive coma, and death.

A noncommunicating hydrocephalus may occur if the exudate causes adhesions that prevent the normal flow of the CSF from the ventricles. CSF reabsorption by the arachnoid villi may also be obstructed by the exudate. Surgical implantation of a shunt is the only treatment.

A complication of meningococcal meningitis is the Waterhouse-Friderichsen syndrome. The syndrome is manifested by petechiae, disseminated intravascular coagulation, and adrenal hemorrhage. Disseminated intravascular coagulation is a serious complication of meningitis (see Chapter 29). It is the cause of death in about 1% of patients with meningitis.

Diagnostic Studies

A major diagnostic tool is examination of the CSF. Diagnosis is verified in 90% of the cases by a positive CSF culture. Variations in the CSF depend on the causative organism. Protein levels in the CSF are usually elevated and are higher in bacterial than in viral cases. Decreased CSF glucose concentration is common in bacterial meningitis and may be normal in viral meningitis. The CSF is purulent and turbid in bacterial meningitis; it may be the same or clear in viral meningitis. The predominant white blood cell type in the CSF during inflammatory disorders of the brain is polymorphonuclear cells (see Table 54-17). Specimens of blood, sputum, and nasopharyngeal secretions are taken for culture before the start of antibiotic therapy to identify the causative organism.

X-rays of the skull may demonstrate infected sinuses. CT scans are usually normal in uncomplicated meningitis. In other cases, CT scans may reveal evidence of increased ICP or hydrocephalus.

Collaborative Care

Rapid diagnosis based on history and physical examination is crucial because the patient is usually in a critical state when health care is sought. When meningitis is suspected, antibiotic therapy is instituted after the collection of specimens for cultures, even before the diagnosis is confirmed. Diagnostic measures include lumbar puncture and analysis of CSF. The fundus of the eye should be examined via ophthalmoscope for papilledema before lumbar puncture for identification of possible increased ICP.

Ampicillin, penicillin, and a third-generation cephalosporin, usually ceftriaxone (Rocephin) or cefotaxime (Claforan), are the drugs of choice for treating meningitis. These drugs are effective because of their ability to penetrate the blood-brain barrier. Collaborative care for cerebral inflammatory conditions is presented in Table 54-18.

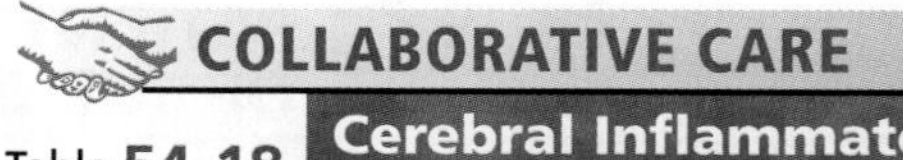

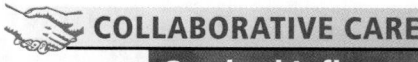

COLLABORATIVE CARE

Table 54-18 Cerebral Inflammatory Problems

Diagnostic
- History and physical examination
- Analysis of CSF
- CBC, coagulation profile, electrolyte levels, glucose, platelet count
- Routine urinalysis
- Blood cultures (twice)
- Urine specific gravity (q4hr)
- CT scan, MRI
- EEG
- Skull x-ray studies
- Brain scan

Collaborative Therapy
- Strict bed rest
- IV fluids
- Ampicillin, penicillin IV
- Cefotaxime (Claforan), ceftriaxone (Rocephin)
- Codeine for headache
- Acetaminophen or aspirin for temperature above 100.4° F (38° C)
- Hypothermia
- Clear liquids as desired or tolerated
- Phenytoin (Dilantin) IV
- Furosemide (Lasix) or mannitol for diuresis

NURSING MANAGEMENT: MENINGITIS

Nursing Assessment

Initial assessment should include vital signs, neurologic evaluation, fluid intake and output, and evaluation of lung fields and skin. Fever, severe headache, nausea, vomiting, and nuchal rigidity are common presenting symptoms in the patient with meningitis.

Nursing Diagnoses

Nursing diagnoses for the patient with meningitis may include, but are not limited to, those presented in NCP 54-3.

Planning

The overall goals are that the patient with meningitis will have (1) return to maximal neurologic functioning, (2) resolution of infection, and (3) decreased pain and discomfort.

Nursing Implementation

Health Promotion. Prevention of respiratory infections through vaccination programs for pneumococcal pneumonia and influenza should be supported by nurses. In addition, early and vigorous treatment of respiratory and ear infections is important. Persons who have close contact with anyone who has meningitis should be given prophylactic antibiotics.

Acute Intervention. The patient with meningitis is usually acutely ill. The fever is high and head pain is severe. Irritation of the cerebral cortex may result in seizures. The

54-3 NURSING CARE PLAN PATIENT WITH AN INFLAMMATORY CONDITION OF THE BRAIN

Expected Patient Outcomes	Nursing Interventions and *Rationales*
NURSING DIAGNOSIS **Sensory-perceptual alterations** *related to* decreased LOC *as manifested by* inaccurate interpretation of environment, signs of fear or anxiety, disorientation, restlessness, auditory or visual hallucinations.	
■ Minimal disorientation. ■ Lack of evidence of agitation.	■ Assess LOC *to determine extent of the problem.* ■ Administer sedative medication as ordered *to reduce fear and anxiety.* ■ Keep room quiet and lights dim; use calm, reassuring approach *to avoid stimulating or frightening the patient.* ■ Do not use restraints *to avoid increasing patient's anxiety and initiating combative behavior.* ■ Assist and support patient during uncomfortable or frightening diagnostic procedures; have family member at bedside when possible *to assist with orientation and reduce anxiety.*
NURSING DIAGNOSIS **Pain** *related to* headache, muscle and joint aches, and malaise *as manifested by* general discomfort of head, joints, and muscles; apathy; grimacing on movement.	
■ Satisfaction with pain relief. ■ Increased participation in treatment plan.	■ Administer mild analgesia as needed; assist patient to position of comfort in bed *to relieve pain.* ■ Encourage gentle range-of-motion and leg exercises *to reduce joint stiffness and promote circulation.* ■ Massage muscles as needed or requested *to promote comfort and show a caring attitude.* ■ Control environment to encourage rest *because pain can be exhausting to the patient.*
NURSING DIAGNOSIS **Ineffective management of therapeutic regimen** *related to* possible sequelae of condition *as manifested by* motor or sensory problems, activity limitations.	
■ Satisfactory management of condition by self or others.	■ Monitor for residual effects of condition such as vision, hearing, activity, and cognitive problems *to determine appropriate referrals.* ■ Inform patient and others that residual problems often improve over time *to reduce anxiety.* ■ Arrange for postdischarge care if required *so patient's needs are met.*
NURSING DIAGNOSIS **Hyperthermia** *related to* infection and abnormal temperature regulation by hypothalamus from increased ICP *as manifested by* increased temperature and chills.	
■ Normal body temperature.	■ Carry out general measures of care for patient with a fever (see NCP 11-1). ■ If prescribed, use hypothermia blanket to reduce temperature *because an elevated temperature increases brain metabolism and increases the risk of seizures or increased ICP.* ■ Reduce temperature gradually *to prevent shivering, which can cause a rebound effect and raise rather than lower the temperature.*

COLLABORATIVE PROBLEMS

Nursing Goals	Nursing Interventions and *Rationales*
POTENTIAL COMPLICATION **Seizure activity** *related to* cerebral irritation.	
■ Monitor for seizure activity. ■ Carry out appropriate medical and nursing interventions. ■ Report and record any seizure activity.	■ Monitor for seizure activity *so interventions can be initiated immediately.* ■ Keep side rails up and padded *to protect patient if a seizure occurs.* ■ Administer sedative and antiseizure medications as ordered *to control or prevent seizure activity.* ■ Reduce fever *to decrease brain's oxygen demand.* ■ Carry out interventions to treat underlying causes of inflammatory brain condition *to prevent seizure activity.*
POTENTIAL COMPLICATION **Increased ICP** *related to* presence of infectious exudate, increased production of CSF (see NCP 54-2).	

changes in mental status and LOC depend on the degree of increased ICP. Assessment of vital signs, neurologic evaluation, fluid intake and output, and evaluation of lung fields and skin should be performed at regular intervals based on the patient's condition and recorded carefully.

Head pain and neck pain secondary to movement require attention. Codeine provides some pain relief without undue sedation for most patients. The patient should be assisted to a position of comfort, often curled up with the head slightly extended. The head of the bed should be slightly elevated, when permitted after lumbar puncture. A darkened room and a cool cloth over the eyes relieve the discomfort of photophobia.

For the delirious patient, additional low lighting may be necessary to decrease hallucinations. All patients suffer some degree of mental distortion and hypersensitivity and may be frightened and misinterpret the environment. Every attempt should be made to minimize environmental stimuli and the resulting exaggerated perception. Restraints should be avoided. Padded side rails with sheets tied to the four corners to keep the patient from getting out of bed may be used to prevent injury. Arm boards, secured with multiple layers of stretch gauze (e.g., Kerlix), protect the IV infusion site. The presence of a familiar person at the bedside has a calming effect. The nurse must be efficient with care but also should project an attitude of caring and of unhurried gentleness. The use of touch and a soothing voice to give simple explanations of activities is helpful. If seizures occur, appropriate observations should be made and protective measures should be taken. Antiseizure medications such as phenytoin (Dilantin) are administered as ordered. Problems associated with increased ICP are also managed (see Increased Intracranial Pressure earlier in this chapter).

Fever must be vigorously managed because it increases cerebral edema and the frequency of seizures. In addition, neurologic damage may result from an extremely high temperature over a prolonged time. Acetaminophen or aspirin may be used to reduce fever. However, if the fever is resistant to aspirin or acetaminophen, more vigorous means are necessary. If prescribed, an automatic cooling blanket may be used to reduce high fever. Care should be taken not to reduce the temperature too rapidly because shivering may result, causing a rebound effect and increasing the temperature. The extremities should be wrapped in sheepskin, soft towels, or a blanket covered with a sheet to protect them from "frostbite." Care of the skin should be frequent to prevent breaks in the skin. If a cooling blanket is not available or desirable, tepid sponge baths with water may be effective in lowering the temperature. The skin must be protected from excessive drying and injury.

Because high fever greatly increases the metabolic rate and thus insensible fluid loss, the patient should be assessed for dehydration and adequacy of fluid intake. Diaphoresis further increases fluid losses, which should be estimated and included in an intake and output record. Replacement fluids should be calculated as 800 ml/day for respiratory losses and 100 ml for each degree of temperature above 100.4° F (38° C). Supplemental feeding to maintain adequate nutritional intake via tube or oral feedings may be necessary. The designated antibiotic schedule must be followed to maintain therapeutic blood levels. Observations should be made for side effects of the drugs used.

In most cases, meningitis no longer requires isolation, with the exception of meningococcal meningitis. However, good aseptic technique is essential to protect the patient and the nurse.

Ambulatory and Home Care. After the acute period has passed, the patient requires several weeks of convalescence before normal activities can be resumed. In this period, good nutrition should be stressed, with an emphasis on a high-protein, high-caloric diet in small, frequent feedings.

Muscle rigidity may persist in the neck and the backs of the legs. Progressive range-of-motion exercises and warm baths are useful. Activity should be gradually increased as tolerated, but adequate bed rest and sleep should be encouraged. Quiet activities that are based on an assessment of individual interests should be encouraged to prevent boredom.

Residual effects are uncommon in meningococcal meningitis, but pneumococcal meningitis can result in sequelae such as dementia, seizures, deafness, hemiplegia, and hydrocephalus. Vision, hearing, cognitive skills, and motor and sensory abilities should be assessed after recovery, with appropriate referrals as indicated. Meningitis in infancy may have "silent" neurologic sequelae, which are manifested as learning and behavior problems when the child reaches school age.

Throughout the acute and convalescent periods the nurse should be aware of the anxiety and stress experienced by individuals close to the patient.

■ Evaluation

The expected outcomes are that the patient with meningitis will

- return to maximal neurologic function possible
- be free from pain and discomfort

ENCEPHALITIS

Encephalitis is an acute inflammation of the brain and is usually caused by a virus. Many different viruses have been implicated in encephalitis, some of them associated with certain seasons of the year and endemic to certain geographic areas. Epidemic encephalitis is transmitted by ticks and mosquitoes. Nonepidemic encephalitis may occur as a complication of measles, chickenpox, or mumps.

Encephalitis is a serious, and sometimes fatal, disease. Overall mortality rate ranges from 5% to 20%, with the highest mortality rate in encephalitis caused by herpes simplex virus (HSV) and the eastern and Venezuelan equine viruses. Unfortunately, HSV encephalitis is the most common form of viral encephalitis. Cytomegalovirus encephalitis is one of the common complications in patients with acquired immunodeficiency syndrome.[31]

Manifestations resemble those of meningitis, but they have a more gradual onset. They include headache, high fever, seizures, and a change in level of consciousness.

Early diagnosis and treatment of viral encephalitis are essential for favorable outcomes. Diagnostic findings related to viral encephalitis are shown in Table 54-17. Brain imaging techniques such as MRI and PET, along with polymerase chain reaction tests for the HSV DNA levels in CSF, allow for earlier detection of viral encephalitis.[31]

Collaborative and nursing management is symptomatic and supportive. Cerebral edema is a major problem, and diuretics (mannitol) and corticosteroids (dexamethasone [Decadron]) are used to control it. The disease is characterized by diffuse

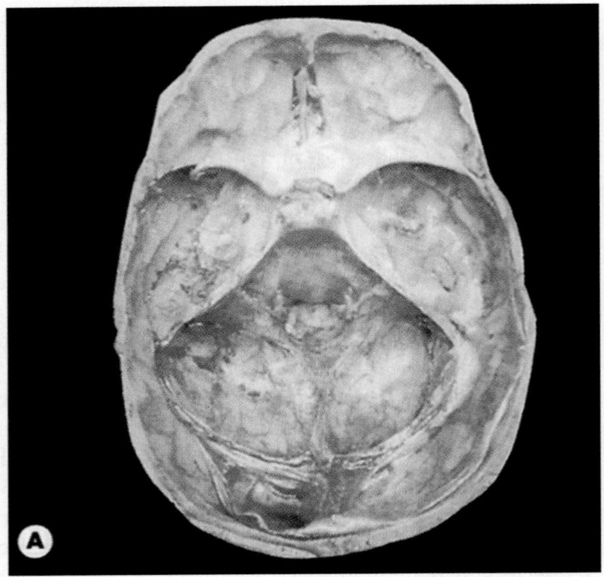

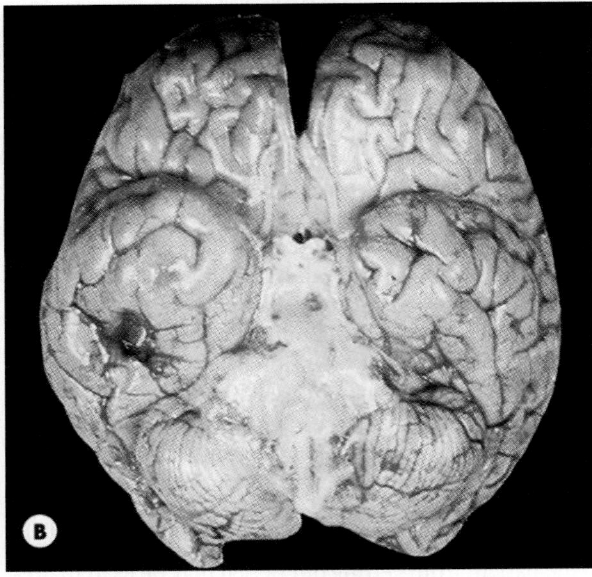

Fig. 54-16 **A,** Normal brain with most of dura intact. **B,** Brain with abscess.

CRITICAL THINKING EXERCISES

CASE STUDY

Head Injury

Patient Profile

Jason B., a 22-year-old unrestrained driver, was involved in a head-on collision. He was found at the scene of a motor vehicle accident trapped under the steering wheel of his car. He is admitted to the emergency department with a diagnosis of traumatic brain injury and open fracture of the right humerus and femur.

Subjective Data

- Paramedic reported that patient was unconscious at the scene, normotensive with Cheyne-Stokes respirations

Objective Data

At the Scene

- Slight decerebration with the left arm

In the Emergency Department

- Pupils equal, 2 mm, and fixed
- Vital signs within normal limits
- Glasgow Coma Scale = 5; ICP and CPP average 20 mm Hg and 60 mm Hg, respectively
- Fractured right femur and humerus
- Multiple lacerations and contusions

Diagnostic Studies

- Brain CT scan reveals fracture along lateral wall of right maxillary sinus, subarachnoid hemorrhage, generalized brain swelling, and slit ventricles

Critical Thinking Questions

1. What could be the cause of Mr. B.'s nonresponsive neurologic condition based on his initial clinical condition and CT scan?
2. Discuss conditions of the injury and the pathophysiologic changes that can occur from the injury in relation to Mr. B.'s neurologic status.
3. What do the signs and symptoms suggest for Mr. B.'s area of brain involvement?
4. What are the priority interventions based on the nursing assessment?
5. Write one or more appropriate nursing diagnoses based on the assessment data. Are there any collaborative problems?

NURSING RESEARCH ISSUES

1. What type of information and education do families need at each stage of recovery for the head-injured patient?
2. What are the temporal changes in brain compliance associated with mortality and poor functional outcomes?
3. Are there any age-related differences in brain compliance associated with poor outcomes?
4. What is the effect of nursing activities or interventions on intracranial pressure, cerebral perfusion pressure, cerebral blood flow, and cerebral tissue oxygenation?
5. What is the most valid noninvasive or continuous method for real-time monitoring of cerebral tissue perfusion and oxygenation?
6. What is the best method to sample cerebrospinal fluid from the ventricles without increased risk of infection?
7. Do neuromuscular blockers or other anesthetic agents (e.g., opioids, benzodiazepines) alter the patient's response to nursing care activities?
8. Do cognitive stimulation programs decrease the frequency of cognitive and behavior changes that occur after minor head injury?

damage to the nerve cells of the brain, perivascular cellular infiltration, proliferation of glial cells, and increasing cerebral edema. The sequelae of encephalitis include mental deterioration, amnesia, personality changes, and hemiparesis.

Acyclovir (Zovirax) and vidarabine (Vira-A) are used to treat encephalitis caused by HSV infection. Acyclovir has fewer side effects than vidarabine and is often the preferred treatment. Use of these antiviral agents has been shown to reduce mortality rates from 70% to 30%, although neurologic complications may not be reduced.[32] Long-term symptoms include memory impairment, epilepsy, anosmia, personality changes, behavioral abnormalities, and dysphasia. For maximal benefit, antiviral agents should be started before the onset of coma.

BRAIN ABSCESS

Brain abscess is an accumulation of pus within the brain tissue that can result from a local or a systemic infection (Fig. 54-16). Direct extension from ear, tooth, mastoid, or sinus infection is the primary cause. Other causes for brain abscess formation include septic venous thrombosis from a pulmonary infection, bacterial endocarditis, skull fracture, and a nonsterile neurologic procedure. Streptococci and staphylococci are the primary infective organisms.

Manifestations are similar to those of meningitis and encephalitis and include headache and fever. Signs of increased ICP may include drowsiness, confusion, and seizures. Focal symptoms may be present and reflect the local area of the abscess. For example, visual field defects or psychomotor seizures are common with a temporal lobe abscess, whereas an occipital abscess may be accompanied by visual impairment and hallucinations.

Antimicrobial therapy is the primary treatment for brain abscess. Other manifestations are treated symptomatically. If drug therapy is not effective, the abscess may need to be drained, or removed if it is encapsulated. In untreated cases, the mortality rate approaches 100%. Seizures occur in approximately 30% of the cases. Nursing measures are similar to those for management of meningitis or increased ICP. If surgical drainage or removal is the treatment of choice, nursing care is similar to that described under cranial surgery.

Other infections of the brain include subdural empyema, osteomyelitis of the cranial bones, epidural abscess, and venous sinus thrombosis after periorbital cellulitis.

REVIEW QUESTIONS

The number of the question corresponds to the same-numbered objective at the beginning of the chapter.

1. The nurse determines that a patient is unconscious when the patient
   a. has cerebral ischemia.
   b. responds only to painful stimuli.
   c. is unaware of self or environment.
   d. does not respond to verbal stimuli.
2. To evaluate levels of consciousness, the nurse uses the knowledge that consciousness involves
   a. adequate functioning of the autonomic nervous system.
   b. activation of a network of fibers located in the cerebral cortex.
   c. an arousal component that functions if the cerebral cortex remains intact.
   d. the ability to reason, think, feel, and react to stimuli in a purposeful manner.
3. In caring for an unconscious patient the nurse
   a. pads the side rails for safety.
   b. frequently suctions the patient to stimulate coughing.
   c. places the patient on the side with the head of bed elevated.
   d. assesses motor and sensory status of the patient every 8 hours.
4. A patient with intracranial pressure monitoring has pressure of 12 mm Hg. The nurse understands that this pressure reflects
   a. a severe decrease in cerebral perfusion pressure.
   b. a decrease in the production of cerebrospinal fluid.
   c. the loss of autoregulatory control of intracranial pressure.
   d. a normal balance between brain tissue, blood, and cerebrospinal fluid.
5. Vasogenic cerebral edema increases intracranial pressure by
   a. shifting fluid in the gray matter.
   b. changes in the endothelial lining of cerebral capillaries.
   c. leaking molecules from the intracellular fluid to the capillaries.
   d. altering the osmotic gradient flow into the intravascular component.
6. A patient with increased intracranial pressure is placed on mechanical ventilation to maintain PaO_2 at 100 mm Hg and $PaCO_2$ at 35 mm Hg. The rationale for this therapy is to
   a. increase cerebral blood flow.
   b. constrict cerebral blood vessels.
   c. remove fluid from cerebral tissues.
   d. decrease systemic blood pressure.
7. The nurse plans care for the patient with increased intracranial pressure with the knowledge that the best way to position the patient is to
   a. keep the head of the bed flat.
   b. maintain head alignment at 30 degrees.
   c. increase the head-of-bed angle to 30 degrees with patient on left side.
   d. use a continuous-rotation bed to continuously change patient position.
8. The nurse is alerted to a possible acute subdural hematoma in the patient who
   a. has a linear skull fracture crossing a major artery.
   b. has focal symptoms of brain damage with no recollection of a head injury.
   c. develops decreased level of consciousness and a headache within 48 hours of a head injury.
   d. has an immediate loss of consciousness with a brief lucid interval followed by decreasing level of consciousness.
9. During admission of a patient with a severe head injury to the emergency department, the nurse places the highest priority on assessment for
   a. patency of airway.
   b. presence of a neck injury.
   c. neurologic status with the Glasgow Coma Scale.
   d. cerebrospinal fluid leakage from the ears or nose.
10. A patient is suspected of having a cranial tumor. The signs and symptoms include memory deficits, visual disturbances, weakness of right upper and lower extremities, and personality changes. The nurse recognizes that the tumor is most likely located in the
    a. frontal lobe.
    b. parietal lobe.
    c. occipital lobe.
    d. temporal lobe.

11. The nursing management of a patient with a brain tumor includes
    a. using diversion techniques to keep the patient stimulated and motivated.
    b. discussing with the patient methods to control inappropriate behavior.
    c. assisting and supporting the family in understanding any changes in behavior.
    d. limiting self-care activities until the patient has regained maximum physical functioning.
12. The primary goal of nursing care after a craniotomy is
    a. prevention of infection.
    b. ensuring patient comfort.
    c. avoiding need for secondary surgery.
    d. preventing increased intracranial pressure.
13. During assessment of the patient with meningitis, the most critical signs and symptoms for the nurse to note are
    a. headache, fever, nuchal rigidity.
    b. irritability, headache, anorexia.
    c. headache, fever, heart palpitations.
    d. nausea, vomiting, restlessness.
14. A nursing measure that is indicated to reduce the potential for seizures and increased intracranial pressure in the patient with meningitis is
    a. administering codeine for relief of head and neck pain.
    b. controlling fever with prescribed drugs and cooling techniques.
    c. keeping the room darkened and quiet to minimize environmental stimulation.
    d. maintaining the patient on strict bed rest with the head of the bed slightly elevated.

References

1. Plum F, Posner J: *The diagnosis of stupor and coma,* ed 3, Philadelphia, 1980, FA Davis.
2. Jennett B, Teasdale G: Aspects of coma after severe head injury, *Lancet* 23:878, 1977.
3. Cushing H: *Studies in intracranial physiology and surgery,* London, 1925, Oxford University Press.
4. Go KG: The normal and pathological physiology of brain water, *Adv Tech Stand Neurosurg* 23:47, 1997.
5. Betz AL, Crockard A: Brain edema and the blood-brain barrier. In Crockard A and others, editors: *Neurosurgery: the scientific basis of clinical practice,* Boston, 1992, Blackwell Scientific.
6. Ropper AH: Coma and acutely raised intracranial pressure. In Asbury AK and others, editors: *Diseases of the nervous system: clinical neurobiology,* Philadelphia, 1992, Saunders.
7. Gilman AG: *Goodman and Gilman pharmacological basis of therapeutics,* New York, 1993, McGraw-Hill.
8. Visweswaran P, Massin EK, Dubose TD: Mannitol-induced acute renal failure, *J Am Soc Nephrol* 8:1028, 1997.
9. Prough DS, DeWitt DS: Cerebral protection. In Chernow B, editor: *The pharmacologic approach to the critically ill patient,* ed 3, Baltimore, 1994, Williams & Wilkins.
10. Cooper PR and others: Dexamethasone and severe head injury. A prospective double-blind study, *J Neurosurg* 51:307, 1979.
11. Dearden NM and others: Effect of high-dose dexamethasone on outcome from severe head injury, *J Neurosurg* 64:81, 1986.
12. Hickey JV: *Neurological and neurosurgical nursing,* ed 4, Philadelphia, 1997, Lippincott.
13. Silvestri S, Aronson S: Severe head injury: prehospital and emergency department management, *Mt Sinai J Med* 64:329, 1997.
14. Roberts P: Nutrition in the head-injured patient, *New Horizons* 3:506, 1995.
15. Kerr ME and others: Effect of short-duration hyperventilation during endotracheal suctioning on intracranial pressure in severe head injured adults, *Nurs Res* 48:195, 1997.
16. Kerr ME and others: Head injured adults: recommendations for endotracheal suctioning, *J Neurosci Nurs* 25:86, 1993.
17. Lundberg N: Continuous recording and control of ventricular fluid pressure in neurosurgical practice, *Acta Psychiatr Neurol Scand* 36:1, 1960.
18. Unterberg AW and others: Multimodal monitoring in patients with head injury: evaluation of the effects of treatment on cerebral oxygenation, *J Trauma* 42(5 suppl):S32, 1997.
19. Simmons BJ: Management of intracranial hemodynamics in the adult: a research analysis of head positioning and recommendations for clinical practice and future research, *J Neuroscience Nurs* 29:44, 1997.
20. Tillett JM and others: Effect of continuous rotational therapy on intracranial pressure in the severely brain-injured patient, *Crit Care Med* 21:1005, 1993.
21. Quigley MR and others: Defining the limits of survivorship after very severe head injury, *J Trauma* 42:7, 1997.
22. Marmarou A and others: Impact of ICP instability and hypotension on outcome in patients with severe head trauma, *J Neurosurg* 75:S59, 1991.
23. National Safety Council: *Accident facts,* Chicago, 1997, National Safety Council.
24. Sosin DM, Sniezek JE, Waxweiler RJ: Trends in death associated with brain injury, *JAMA* 278:1778, 1995.
25. Povlishock JT: Traumatic brain injury: the pathobiology of injury and repair. In Gorio A, editor: *Neuroregeneration,* New York, 1993, Raven Press.
26. Walleck C: Patients with head injury and brain dysfunction. In Clochesy JM and others, editors: *Critical care nursing,* ed 2, Philadelphia, 1997, Saunders.
27. Celli P, Fruin A, Cervoni L: Severe head trauma. Review of factors influencing the prognosis, *Minerva Chir* 52:1467, 1997.
28. Rordorf G and others: Patients in poor neurological condition after subarachnoid hemorrhage: early management and long-term outcome, *Acta Neurochir* 139:1143, 1997.
29. Acorn S, Roberts E: Head injury: impact on the wives, *J Neurosci Nurs* 24:324, 1992.
30. Landis SH and others: Cancer statistics,1998, *CA Cancer J Clin* 48:6, 1998.
31. Wildemann B and others: Quantification of herpes simplex virus type 1 DNA in cells of cerebrospinal fluid of patients with herpes simplex virus encephalitis, *Neurology* 48:1341, 1997.
32. McGrath and others: Herpes simplex encephalitis treated with acyclovir: diagnosis and long term outcomes, *J Neurol Neurosurg Psychiatry* 63:321, 1997.

Resources

American Brain Tumor Association
2720 River Road
Des Plaines, IL 60018
847-827-9910
Fax: 847-827-9918
800-886-2282
http://www.abta.org

National Brain Tumor Association
Harvard Medical School
3725 North Talman Avenue
Chicago, IL 60618
http://neurosurgery.mgh.harvard.edu/

National Head Injury Foundation
333 Turnpike Road
Southborough, MA 01772
508-485-9950

***For additional Internet resources, see the website for this book at* www.mosby.com/MERLIN/medsurg_lewis**

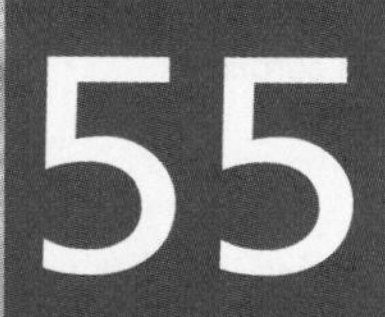

REMEMBER to check out your companion CD-ROM

55 NURSING MANAGEMENT Patient with a Stroke

Barbara Brillhart

www.mosby.com/MERLIN/medsurg_lewis

LEARNING OBJECTIVES

1. Describe the incidence of and risk factors for stroke.
2. Explain the mechanisms that affect cerebral blood flow.
3. Compare and contrast the pathophysiology of strokes caused by thrombosis, embolism, and intracranial hemorrhage.
4. Correlate the clinical manifestations of stroke with the underlying pathophysiology.
5. Describe diagnostic study abnormalities commonly found in patients with cerebrovascular accidents.
6. Describe the collaborative care, drug therapy, and dietary therapy of the stroke patient.
7. Describe the acute nursing management of the stroke patient.
8. Describe the rehabilitative nursing management of the stroke patient.
9. Explain the psychosocial impact of a stroke on the patient and family.

Cerebrovascular accident (*CVA*) (also referred to as stroke or "brain attack") is a broad term that includes a variety of disorders that influence blood flow to the brain and result in neurologic deficits. Proper functioning of the brain depends on an adequate blood supply to deliver oxygen and glucose for neuronal activity and to remove the end products of metabolism. CVAs result when there is inadequate supply of blood to the brain (cerebral ischemia) or cerebral hemorrhage within the brain. Regardless of the cause, the damaged brain no longer performs cognitive, sensory, motor, or emotional functions. The effects of the CVA may vary from minor to severe disability.

Stroke is the third most common cause of death and is the leading cause of serious, long-term disability in the United States and Canada. Strokes are considered a major public health problem in terms of mortality and morbidity; 500,000 to 600,000 persons experience CVAs annually. In the United States during 1995 there were approximately 158,000 deaths from CVA.[1] Approximately 31% of people who have an initial stroke die within 1 year. This percentage is higher among people age 65 and older. Permanent disability occurs in two thirds of the people having strokes. Although one third of individuals having a stroke die within 1 month of occurrence, 2 to 3 million people live with disability as a direct result of strokes. Rehabilitation is a realistic option for 90% of older adults who have had a stroke.

Strokes have significant economic effects on the patient, family, and community. The direct and indirect costs of strokes are estimated to be greater than $18 billion per year in the United States.[1] The majority of the cost for care of the patient who has experienced a CVA is provided by Medicare (72.8%) and Medicaid (8.7%). Self-pay (4.6%) and private insurance (1.9%) make up the rest of the financial support.[2] Disability, disruption of lives, and reduced quality of life for patients with a CVA cannot be calculated in terms of financial impact but in terms of human suffering and disruption of lives.

Reviewed by Karen March, RN, MN, CNRN, CCRN, Neuroscience Clinical Nurse Specialist, Harborview Medical Center, Seattle, Wash.

RISK FACTORS FOR STROKES

The risk factors associated with strokes can be divided into nonmodifiable and potentially modifiable. Risk for stroke increases for persons with more than one risk factor.

The nonmodifiable risk factors include gender, age, race, and heredity. The incidence of stroke is higher in men than women. The incidence of stroke increases with age until age 75. The occurrence rate in adults age 55 to 74 years is 15.1% as compared with 5.6% in those 75 years and older.[2] African-Americans experience a higher incidence of stroke that is associated with an increased incidence of hypertension. Persons with a family history of stroke or transient ischemic attacks (TIAs) are also considered at higher risk for stroke.[3]

Modifiable risk factors are those that can be potentially changed and thus reduce the risk of CVA. Lifestyle habits, including excessive alcohol consumption, cigarette smoking, obesity, diet high in fat content, and drug abuse, increase the risk for stroke. Many pathologic conditions also increase the risk for stroke and include cardiac disease, diabetes mellitus, hypertension, migraine headaches, hypercoagulability states (e.g., high serum fibrinogen levels, increased hematocrit), polycythemia, and sickle cell anemia. Approximately 9% of men and 18% of women who have had a myocardial infarction will have a stroke within 6 years. Control of hypertension is considered the most significant therapy in the prevention of strokes.[4] Women who smoke have a fivefold increased risk for

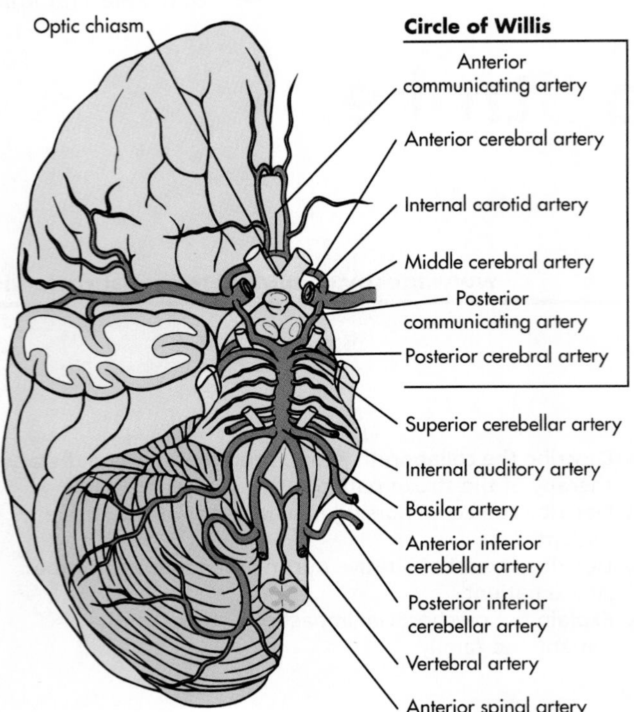

Fig. 55-1 Circle of Willis and vertebrobasilar circulation. Temporal lobes have been removed to show the course of the middle cerebral artery.

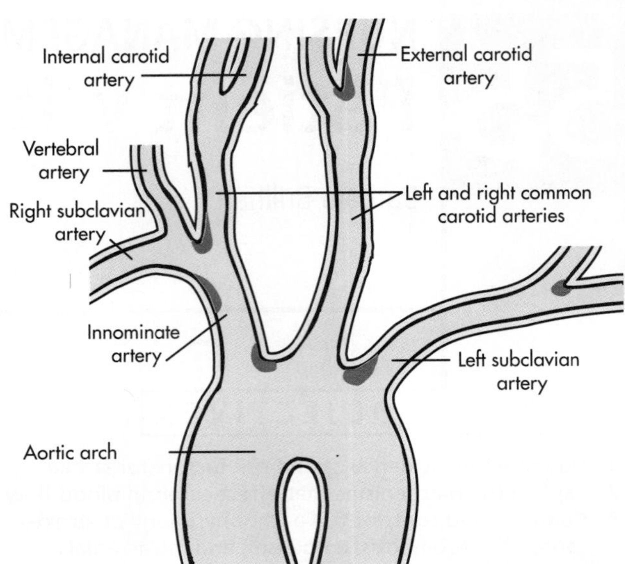

Fig. 55-2 Common sites for the development of atherosclerosis in extracranial and intracranial arteries. The main locations are just above the common carotid bifurcation (most common site) and the start of the branches from the aorta, innominate, and subclavian arteries.

stroke as compared with nonsmokers. If a woman smokes and uses estrogen-containing oral contraception, the risk for stroke increases.[5] Early treatment and management of these associated diseases and poor health habits will decrease the incidence of stroke.

ETIOLOGY AND PATHOPHYSIOLOGY

Regulation of Cerebral Blood Flow

Because neurons do not regenerate, the prevention of cerebral damage is necessary to prevent neurologic deficits. Blood flow must be maintained at 750 to 1000 ml/min (55 ml/100 g brain tissue) or 20% of the cardiac output to ensure optimal cerebral functioning. If blood flow to the brain is totally interrupted (e.g., cardiac arrest), neurologic metabolism is altered in 30 seconds, metabolism stops in 2 minutes, and cellular death occurs in 5 minutes.

The cerebrovascular system is highly adaptive. It maintains a constant blood flow to the brain in spite of significant changes in the systemic circulation. The factors that affect cerebral blood flow can be divided into extracranial and intracranial factors.

Extracranial Factors. The extracranial factors are primarily related to the circulatory system. They include systemic blood pressure, cardiac output, and viscosity of the blood. During activities of daily living (ADLs) there are great variations in local oxygen requirements. Alterations in cardiac output, vasomotor tone, and distribution of blood flow are effective in maintaining constant cerebral perfusion. The mean arterial blood pressure has to fall below 70 mm Hg or rise above 160 mm Hg before the cerebral blood flow is altered, and cardiac output has to be reduced by one third before cerebral blood flow is reduced. Changes in blood viscosity increase or decrease cerebral blood flow. Anemia increases cerebral blood flow and polycythemia reduces it.

Intracranial Factors

Metabolic factors. Metabolic alterations are important intracranial factors involved in the regulation of cerebral blood flow. Metabolic factors that result in vasodilation with restoration of blood flow toward normal include high carbon dioxide concentration and low oxygen tension. Carbon dioxide, however, is the most potent regulator of cerebral blood flow. An increase in hydrogen ion concentration also increases cerebral blood flow. Alone or in combination, these metabolic factors can maintain adequate cerebral blood flow in normal situations.

Blood vessels. The condition of the blood vessels supplying the brain also influences the cerebral blood flow (see Chapter 53). Many persons have congenital anomalies in the cerebrovascular system. These anomalies include tortuosity, coiling, kinking, and arteriovenous malformations. These congenital anomalies may interfere with cerebral blood flow and are common sites for the development of atherosclerotic diseases. Atherosclerosis from any cause increases resistance in the blood vessels and further reduces blood flow.

Collateral circulation (alternate flow to compensate for decreased blood flow) is another factor related to cerebral blood flow. Collateral circulation develops in response to a decrease in normal blood flow. The circle of Willis contains many collateral circulatory connections and is responsible for the greater part of collateral circulation (Fig. 55-1). These collateral vessels can maintain cerebral blood flow in the event of damage to the main blood supply. Individual differences in the state of the collateral circulation when a stroke occurs partly determine the degree of functional loss.

Intracranial pressure. Intracranial pressure is another factor that influences cerebral blood flow (see Chapter 54). Among

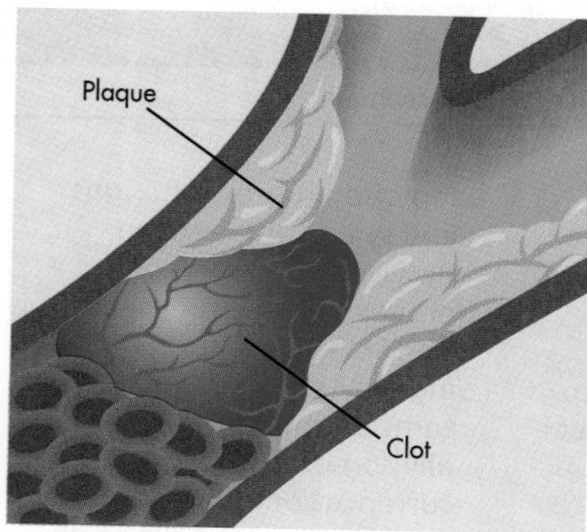

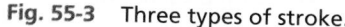

A. Thrombotic stroke. Cerebral thrombosis is a narrowing of the artery by fatty deposits called *plaque*. Plaque can cause a clot to form, which blocks the passage of blood through the artery.

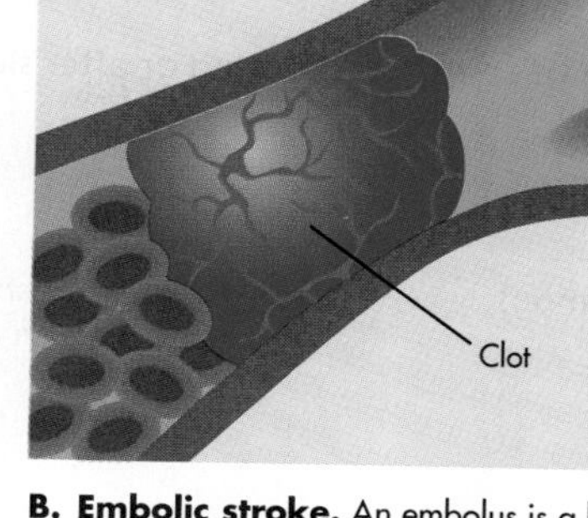

B. Embolic stroke. An embolus is a blood clot or other debris circulating in the blood. When it reaches an artery in the brain that is too narrow to pass through, it lodges there and blocks the flow of blood.

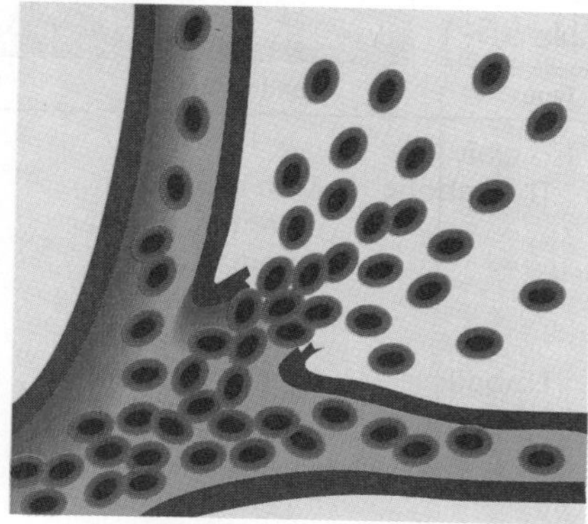

C. Hemorrhagic stroke. A burst blood vessel may allow blood to seep into and damage brain tissues until clotting shuts off the leak.

Fig. 55-3 Three types of stroke.

CULTURAL & ETHNIC CONSIDERATIONS

Cerebrovascular Disease

- A high mortality rate from CVAs exists among African-American men, possibly as a result of the high frequency of hypertension in this group.
- Ischemic strokes are twice as common among African-Americans as Caucasians.
- Hemorrhagic strokes are three times more common among African-Americans than Caucasians.

the causes of increased intracranial pressure are stroke, neoplasms, inflammation, trauma, and hydrocephalus. Increased intracranial pressure compresses the brain and reduces cerebral blood flow. Greatly reduced cerebral blood flow may result in cerebral infarction.

Both extracranial and intracranial factors may be involved in a stroke. The initial insult may be related to one or more of these factors. For example, when an intracranial hemorrhage occurs, the continuity of the vascular system is interrupted. The lost blood and cerebral edema secondary to the inflammatory process contribute to an increase in intracranial pressure. This interferes with cerebral perfusion, and carbon dioxide and hydrogen ion concentration increase, leading to a further dilation of cerebral vessels and increased intracranial pressure.

Atherosclerosis

Atherosclerosis, a common pathophysiologic process in stroke, is usually involved in the development of a thrombosis and is often implicated in strokes caused by emboli. (The role that atherosclerosis plays in the development of thrombosis and emboli is discussed in Chapter 32 and shown in Fig. 32-4.) Initially an abnormal infiltration of lipids occurs in the intima of the arteries. This fatty streak may develop into an atherosclerotic plaque. These plaques often develop where there is increased turbulence in the blood, as at the bifurcation of an artery or a tortuous area (Fig. 55-2). Turbulence may later damage the atherosclerotic plaque, resulting in a loss of intimal continuity or ulceration. Platelet and fibrin aggregate on the roughened surface. Parts of the plaque may break off and travel to a narrower distal artery. Cerebral infarction occurs at the point where the blood supply is cut off.

TYPES OF STROKE

CVAs are classified as thrombotic, embolic, or hemorrhagic strokes based on their underlying pathophysiology (Fig. 55-3). Ischemic strokes result from a decreased blood flow to the brain secondary to partial or complete occlusion of an artery. They occur much more frequently than hemorrhagic strokes. The most common types of ischemic stroke are thrombotic and embolic (Table 55-1). Hemorrhagic strokes are generally the result of spontaneous bleeding into the brain tissue itself (intracerebral or intraparenchymal hemorrhage) or into the subarachnoid space or the ventricles (subarachnoid hemorrhage).

Thrombotic Stroke

Thrombosis is the formation of a blood clot or coagulation that results in the narrowing of the lumen of a blood vessel with eventual occlusion. It is the most common cause of cerebral infarction. Two thirds of the strokes caused by thrombosis are associated with hypertension or diabetes mellitus, both of which accelerate the atherosclerotic process. Additional risk factors associated with thrombotic strokes include oral contraceptives, coagulation disorders, polycythemia vera, arteritis, chronic hypoxia, and dehydration.

Thrombosis develops readily where atheromatous plaques have already narrowed blood vessels. The thrombus results in further narrowing of the vessel lumen and ultimately hypoperfusion, infarction, and ischemia. A cascade of biochemical events occurs, including release of excitatory amino acids (e.g., glutamate, glutamine).[6] Excitatory amino acids via their direct effects on neurons may further compromise the ability of neurons to survive the ischemia and infarction.

Table 55-1 Types of Stroke

Type	Gender/Age	Warning	Time of Onset	Course/Prognosis
Ischemic				
Thrombotic	Men more than women, oldest median age	TIA (30-50% of cases)	During or after sleep	Stepwise progression, signs and symptoms develop slowly, usually some improvement, recurrence in 20-25% of survivors
Embolic	Men more than women	TIA (uncommon)	Lack of relationship to activity, sudden onset	Single event, signs and symptoms develop quickly, usually some improvement, recurrence common without aggressive treatment of underlying disease
Hemorrhagic				
Intracerebral	Slightly higher in women	Headache (25% of cases)	Activity (often)	Progression over 24 hr; poor prognosis, fatality more likely with presence of coma
Subarachnoid	Slightly higher in women, youngest median age	Headache (common)	Activity (often), sudden onset Most commonly related to head trauma	Single sudden event usually, fatality more likely with presence of coma

TIA, transient ischemic attack.

Thrombotic strokes are preceded in 30% to 50% of cases by prodromal episodes (symptoms indicating onset of disease), which occur hours to months before the stroke. The prodromal symptoms are considered TIAs and usually last 5 to 30 minutes. Prodromal episodes leave no residual deficits. Prodromal episodes include paresis (decreased strength and motion of an extremity), aphasia (disturbance of language function), paralysis, mental confusion, or visual disturbances. These symptoms suggest involvement of the carotid arteries and middle cerebral arteries. Prodromal episodes that include dizziness, diplopia (double vision), numbness, impaired vision, headaches, or dysarthria (speech difficulty) may indicate involvement of vertebral and basilar arteries (vertebrobasilar system).

The thrombotic stroke is characterized by a pattern of (1) a single attack where symptoms occur over several hours, (2) intermittent progression toward a stroke occurring over hours to days, (3) partial stroke with permanent neurologic deficits, or (4) a series of TIAs followed by a stroke with permanent neurologic deficits. The extent of the stroke depends on rapidity of onset, the size of the lesion, and the presence of collateral circulation. The typical picture of the stroke is signs and symptoms that peak in severity within 72 hours as edema increases in the infarction areas of the brain. After resolution of edema, which usually occurs within 2 weeks, there is a decrease in signs and symptoms.

In summary, the patient with a thrombotic stroke typically has some prewarning manifestations (TIAs) that may be less serious if there is collateral blood circulation and may experience decreasing symptoms as the edema is resolved.

Embolic Stroke

Cerebral embolism is the occlusion of a cerebral artery by an embolus, resulting in necrosis and edema of the area supplied by the involved blood vessel. Embolism is the second most common cause of stroke. The majority of emboli originate in the endocardial (inside) layer of the heart, with plaques or tissue breaking off from the endocardium and entering the circulation. The emboli travel to smaller vessels and become a source of obstruction at areas of vascular narrowing or bifurcation. Emboli are associated with heart conditions such as atrial fibrillation, myocardial infarction, infective endocarditis, rheumatic heart disease, valvular prostheses, and atrial septal defects. Less common causes of emboli include air, fat from long bone (femur) fractures, amniotic fluid after childbirth, and tumors.

In general, the patient with an embolic stroke commonly has a rapid occurrence of severe clinical manifestations. Embolic strokes can affect any age-group. An embolic stroke secondary to rheumatic heart disease may involve young to middle-aged adults. An embolus arising from an atherosclerotic plaque is more common in older adults. A prodromal warning is less common with embolic than with thrombotic stroke. The onset of an embolic stroke is usually sudden and may or may not be related to activity. The patient usually maintains consciousness, although a headache may develop on the side where the embolus is lodged. Prognosis is related to the amount of brain tissue deprived of its blood supply. For example, embolic strokes most commonly affect the middle cerebral artery, which is a direct continuation of the internal carotid artery. The effects of the emboli are initially characterized by severe neurologic deficits, which can be temporary if the clot breaks up and allows blood to flow. Smaller emboli then continue to obstruct smaller vessels, which in turn involve smaller portions of the brain with fewer deficits noted. The embolic stroke often occurs so rapidly that the body does not have time to accommodate with the formation of collateral circulation. Recurrence of embolic stroke is common unless the underlying cause is aggressively treated.

Intracerebral Hemorrhage Stroke

Intracerebral hemorrhage is bleeding within the brain caused by a rupture of vessels that lasts from minutes to days. Intracerebral hemorrhage is commonly caused by hypertension. Other causes of intracerebral hemorrhage include brain tumors, trauma, thrombolytic drugs, and ruptured aneurysms. Hypertension and atherosclerosis cause degenerative changes in the walls of arteries, resulting in rupture and subsequent hemorrhage. Hemorrhage commonly occurs without prodromal symptoms and during periods of activity. The extent of the symptoms varies depending on the amount and duration of the bleeding. The blood within the closed area of the brain forms a fluid mass that imposes pressure on the brain tissue. The pressure in turn displaces brain tissue and decreases blood flow to the brain, which is associated with ischemia and infarction.

The most common sites of intracerebral hemorrhage are the putamen and internal capsule (50%), central white matter, thalamus, cerebellar hemispheres, and pons. Initially, the patient experiences a severe headache with nausea and vomiting. Clinical manifestations related to putaminal and internal capsule bleeding include weakness of one side, including the face, arm, and leg; slurred speech; and deviation of the eyes. Progression of manifestations related to a severe hemorrhage include hemiplegia, fixed and dilated pupils, abnormal body posturing, and coma. Thalamic hemorrhage results in hemiplegia with more sensory than motor losses. Bleeding into the subthalamic areas of the brain leads to disturbance with vision and eye movement. Cerebellar hemorrhages are characterized by severe headache, vomiting, loss of ability to walk, dysphagia, dysarthria, and eye movement disturbances. Hemorrhage in the pons is the most serious because basic life functions (e.g., respiration) are rapidly affected. In addition, hemorrhage in the pons can be characterized by hemiplegia leading to complete paralysis, coma, abnormal body posturing, fixed pupils, hyperthermia, and death.

The prognosis of intracerebral hemorrhage strokes is poor: 70% of patients die soon after the occurrence of the stroke. If the area of bleeding is minimal, prognosis is better because the small amount of hemorrhage can be resolved. In summary, the patient with intracerebral hemorrhage has no forewarning; has rapid, severe symptoms occurring with activity; and has a poor prognosis for recovery.

Subarachnoid Hemorrhage Stroke

The causes of subarachnoid hemorrhage include aneurysms (congenital or acquired weakness and ballooning of vessels), arteriovenous malformations, trauma, and hypertension. Aneurysms within the brain affect persons from 20 to 70 years of age. They are associated with atherosclerosis, trauma, hypertension, or congenital malformations and account for approximately 30,000 new cases of subarachnoid hemorrhage annually.[7] Occasionally, hemorrhages are related to medications such as anticoagulants, thrombolytics, and sympathomimetics. The patient may exhibit prodromal symptoms if the ballooning or dilation applies pressure to brain tissue. The aneurysm may also suddenly rupture, causing rapid neurologic changes. The majority (85%) of the aneurysms are in the circle of Willis. Aneurysms may be saccular or berry aneurysms ranging from a few millimeters to 20 to 30 millimeters in size or fusiform atherosclerotic aneurysms.

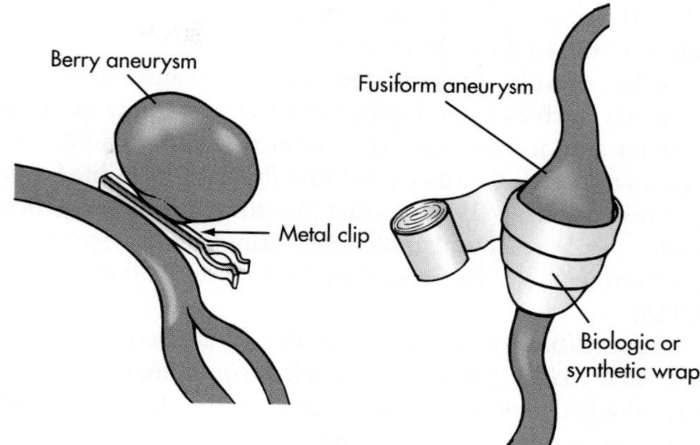

Fig. 55-4 Clipping and wrapping of aneurysms.

Headaches can be associated with a small amount of bleeding because of aneurysm leakage. Rupture of the aneurysm causes hemorrhage and pressure in the subarachnoid space, which may cause headache, lethargy, confusion, nausea, vomiting, fever, neck pain and backaches, paralysis, coma, and death.[7]

A massive hemorrhage is quantified as 30 to 50 ml of blood. Initially a clot forms at the site of a ruptured aneurysm. As the clot begins to dissolve and vasospasm subsides, the chance of renewed bleeding increases. Prognosis for patients with a subarachnoid hemorrhage is guarded because many patients (30%) experience another bleed within 2 weeks of the first occurrence. New surgical procedures, such as clipping and wrapping of aneurysms (Fig. 55-4), have decreased the death rate for these patients.

Temporal Development of Cerebrovascular Accident

The classification of temporal development of CVAs includes TIA, reversible ischemic neurologic deficit, stroke-in-evolution or progressing stroke, and completed stroke (stable stroke). Knowledge of this classification is useful in planning nursing care.

Transient Ischemic Attacks. The TIA is characterized by brief episodes of neurologic manifestations, which clear completely in less than 24 hours.[7] The neurologic deficits present with TIAs disappear leaving no residual effects. Persons experiencing TIAs fall into three categories: one third never have another TIA, one third will have more than one TIA, and one third will experience a stroke.[8]

It is thought that TIAs are a result of microemboli from atherosclerotic plaques found in extracranial arteries that lead to temporary cerebral ischemia. Patients should consider TIAs as a warning sign of progressing cerebrovascular disease. The signs and symptoms of TIAs vary according to the part of the brain affected. The anatomic location of the neurologic deficit can be identified on the basis of clinical manifestations. If the carotid system is involved, the patient may report a temporary loss of vision in one eye, a transient hemiparesis, or a sudden inability to speak. Common manifestations of TIA related to vertebrobasilar insufficiency are tinnitus, vertigo, darkened or blurred vision, diplopia, ptosis, dysarthria, dysphagia, and unilateral or bilateral numbness or weakness.

A TIA must be differentiated from other causes of cerebral ischemia, such as a developing subdural hematoma or an increasing tumor mass. Cardiac monitoring and tests often reveal an underlying cardiac condition that is responsible for the clot formation. Medications that prevent platelet aggregation, such as aspirin, dipyridamole (Persantine), and anticoagulant medications, may be prescribed for long-term therapy after a TIA.

Reversible Ischemic Neurologic Deficit. The term *reversible ischemic neurologic deficit* is sometimes used if the neurologic deficit remains after 24 hours but leaves no residual signs or symptoms after days to weeks. This is considered by some to be a completed stroke with minimal to no residual deficit.

Stroke-in-Evolution. A stroke-in-evolution, or a progressing stroke, develops over a period of hours or days. This pattern of progression is most characteristic of an enlarging intraarterial thrombus. A stepwise or intermittent progression of deterioration of neurologic findings is common. The progression occurs because ischemic tissue becomes infarcted tissue. The manifestations of stroke-in-evolution do not resolve (as compared with TIAs) and leave residual neurologic effects.

Completed Stroke. When the neurologic deficit remains unchanged over a 2- to 3-day period, the stroke is termed a *completed stroke* (stable stroke). An embolic stroke may demonstrate this characteristic from the onset. With the exception of stroke secondary to a ruptured aneurysm, a completed stroke signals readiness for more aggressive rehabilitative treatment. If a ruptured aneurysm is the suspected cause, activity may be restricted for as long as 3 to 4 weeks to reduce the possibility of rebleeding.

CLINICAL MANIFESTATIONS

A CVA ultimately affects many body functions, including neuromotor activity, elimination, intellectual function, spatial-perceptual alterations, personality and affect, sensation, and communication. The functions affected are directly related to the brain area perfused by the affected artery (Table 55-2). Manifestations related to right- and left-brain damage are shown in Fig. 55-5.

Neuromotor Function

Motor deficits are the most obvious effect of stroke. Problems associated with neuromotor function deficits include impairment of (1) mobility, (2) respiratory function, (3) swallowing and speech, (4) gag reflex, and (5) self-care abilities. The symptoms are caused by the destruction of motor neurons in the pyramidal pathway (nerve fibers from the brain and passing through the spinal cord to the motor cells). The characteristic motor deficits include loss of skilled voluntary movement (akinesia), impairment of integration of movements, alterations in muscle tone, and alterations in reflexes. The initial hyporeflexia (depressed reflexes) progresses to hyperreflexia (hyperactive reflexes) for most patients.

Motor deficits after a stroke follow characteristic patterns. Because of the pyramidal pathway crossing at the level of the medulla, a lesion on one side of the brain affects the motor function on the opposite side of the brain (contralateral). The arms and legs of the affected side may be weakened or paralyzed to different degrees depending on which part of and to what extent the cerebral circulation was compromised. A stroke affecting the middle cerebral artery leads to a greater weakness in the upper extremity than the lower extremity. The

Table 55-2 Clinical Manifestations: Specific Cerebral Artery Involvement

Middle Cerebral Artery Involvement
- Blockage of main stem
  - Contralateral paralysis (hemiplegia)
  - Contralateral anesthesia; loss of proprioception, fine touch, localization (hemiparesis)
  - Dominant hemisphere: aphasia
  - Nondominant hemisphere: neglect of opposite side, dysmetria
  - Homonymous hemianopsia, conjugate gaze paralysis

Anterior Cerebral Artery Involvement
- Occlusion of stem*
- Occlusion distal to anterior to communicating artery
  - Contralateral sensory and motor deficits of foot and leg
  - Contralateral weakness of proximal upper extremity
  - Urinary incontinence (possibly unrecognized by patient)
  - Contralateral grasp and sucking reflexes may be present
  - Apraxia
  - Personality change: flat affect, loss of spontaneity, distractibility
  - Possible cognitive impairment

Posterior Cerebral Artery Involvement†
- Thalamogeniculate branch occlusion
  - Contralateral sensory loss
  - Temporary hemiparesis
  - Homonymous hemianopsia
- Paramedian branch occlusion: central midbrain and subthalamus
  - Weber's syndrome: oculomotor nerve palsy and contralateral hemiplegia
- Cortical occlusion: temporal and occipital lobes
  - Incomplete homonymous hemianopsia
  - Dominant hemisphere: dysphasia, anomia
  - Nondominant hemisphere: disorientation
- Upper basilar occlusion (bilateral)
  - Visual disturbances (blindness, homonymous hemianopsia, visual hallucinations, apraxia of ocular movements)
  - Anomia: objects and inability to count
  - Possible memory loss

Vertebrobasilar Artery Involvement
- Bilateral motor and sensory deficits of all extremities
- Ipsilateral Horner's syndrome: miosis, ptosis, decreased sweating
- Hoarseness
- Dysphagia
- Nystagmus, diplopia, blindness
- Nausea, vomiting
- Ataxia

*There is usually no problem if the stem is occluded near the anterior communicating artery because perfusion from the opposite side is maintained.
†The site of occlusion, the origin of the basilar arteries, and the arrangement of the circle of Willis are involved in the type of deficit seen. This can occur from a thrombus or embolus.

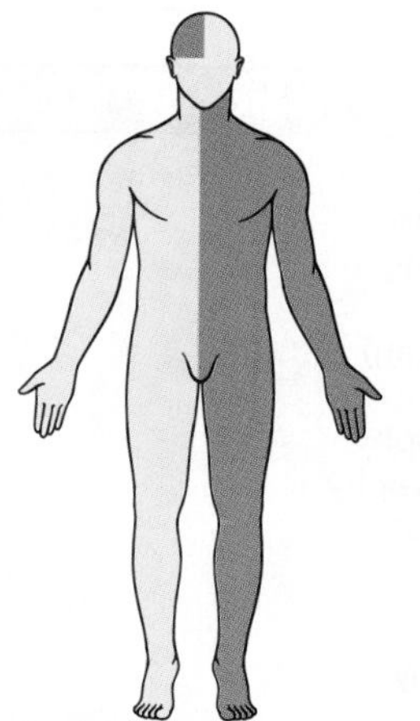

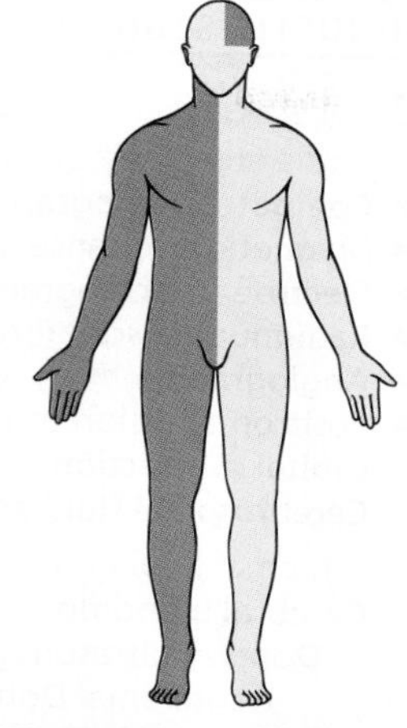

Right brain damage
(Stroke on right side of the brain)

- Paralyzed left side: hemiplegia
- Left-sided neglect
- Spatial-perceptual deficits
- Tends to deny or minimize problems
- Rapid performance, short attention span
- Impulsive, safety problems
- Impaired judgment
- Impaired time concepts

Left brain damage
(Stroke on left side of the brain)

- Paralyzed right side: hemiplegia
- Impaired speech/language aphasias
- Impaired right/left discrimination
- Slow performance, cautious
- Impaired speech/language
- Aware of deficits: depression, anxiety
- Impaired comprehension related to language, math

Fig. 55-5 Manifestations of right-sided and left-sided stroke.

affected shoulder tends to rotate internally, and the hip rotates externally. The affected foot is plantar flexed and inverted. An initial period of flaccidity may last from days to several weeks and is related to nerve damage. Spasticity of the muscles follows the flaccid stage and is related to interruption of upper motor neuron influence.

Communication

The left hemisphere is dominant for language skills in all right-handed persons and in the majority of left-handed persons. Language disorders involve the expression and comprehension of written and spoken words. The patient may experience aphasia (total loss of comprehension and use of language) when a stroke damages the dominant hemisphere of the brain. Dysphasia refers to dysfunction related to the comprehension or use of language and is due to partial disruption or loss. Patterns of dysphasia may differ as the stroke affects different portions of the brain. Dysphasias can be classified as nonfluent (minimal speech activity with slow speech that requires obvious effort) or fluent (speech is present, but contains little meaningful communication). Most dysphasias are mixed with impairment in both expression and understanding. A massive stroke may result in global aphasia, in which all communication and receptive function is lost.

Strokes affecting Wernicke's area of the brain exhibit symptoms of receptive aphasia when neither the sounds of speech nor its meaning can be understood. Damage to Wernicke's area impairs the patient's comprehension of both spoken and written language. Strokes affecting Broca's area of the brain cause expressive aphasia (difficulty in speaking and writing).

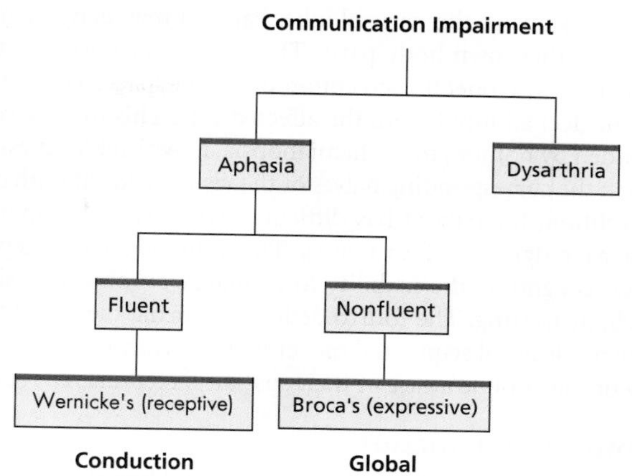

Fig. 55-6 Types of communication impairment common after stroke.

Many stroke patients also experience dysarthria, a disturbance in the muscular control of speech. Patients experience impairments with pronunciation, articulation, and phonation. Dysarthria does not affect the meaning of communication nor the comprehension of language by the patient, but it does affect the mechanics of speech. Some patients experience a combination of aphasia and dysarthria (Fig. 55-6).

Affect

Patients who have had a stroke may be unable to control their emotions. Their emotional response may be exaggerated or unpredictable. This situation is compounded by the depression associated with changes in body image and loss of function. In addition, they are frustrated related to mobility and communication problems. An example of unpredictable affect is as follows: A reserved professional engineer has returned home from the hospital following a stroke. During meals with his family, he becomes frustrated and begins to cry because of the difficulties involved in getting food into his mouth and chewing.

Intellectual Function

Both memory and judgment may be impaired as a result of stroke. These impairments are experienced with strokes affecting either side of the brain. A left-brain stroke is more likely to result in memory problems related to language. Patients with a left-brain stroke characteristically are very cautious in matters of judgment. The patient with a right-brain stroke tends to be impulsive and to move quickly. An example of behavior seen with right-brain stroke is the patient who tries to rise quickly from the wheelchair without locking the wheels or raising the foot rests. The patient with a left-brain stroke would move slowly and cautiously from the bed to the wheelchair. Patients with either type of stroke may experience difficulty in making generalizations, which interferes with their ability to learn.

Spatial-Perceptual Alterations

A stroke in the right side of the brain is more likely to cause deficits in spatial-perceptual orientation, although this can also occur with left-brain stroke. These spatial-perceptual deficits may be divided into four categories. The first is related to the patient's erroneous perception of self and illness. This deficit follows lesions of the parietal lobe. Patients may deny their illnesses or their own body parts. The second category concerns the patient's erroneous perception of self in space. The patient may neglect all input from the affected side. This may be compounded by homonymous hemianopsia, in which blindness occurs in the corresponding halves of the visual fields of both eyes. In addition, the patient has difficulty with spatial orientation, such as judgment of distances. The third spatial-perceptual deficit is agnosia, the inability to recognize an object by sight, touch, or hearing. The fourth deficit is apraxia, the inability to carry out learned sequential movements on command. Patients may or may not be aware of their spatial-perceptual alterations.

Elimination Function

Fortunately, most problems with urinary and bowel elimination occur initially and are transient. When a stroke affects one hemisphere of the brain, the prognosis for normal bladder function is excellent. The pathway between the bladder and the spinal cord remains intact, and partial sensation for bladder filling remains, as well as partial voluntary urination. Initially, the patient may experience frequency, urgency, and incontinence. Although motor control of the bowel is usually not a problem, patients are frequently constipated. Constipation is associated with immobility, weak abdominal muscles, dehydration, and diminished response to the defecation reflex. Both urinary and bowel elimination problems may also be related to the functional inabilities to express needs and inability to manage clothing.

DIAGNOSTIC STUDIES

After a stroke, various diagnostic studies are carried out in an effort to determine the cause and location of the stroke (Table 55-3). Tests are also done to guide decisions about therapeutic or surgical treatment. A computed tomography (CT) scan is the primary diagnostic test used after a stroke. It can indicate the size and location of the lesion. CT testing is also useful in differentiating between infarction and hemorrhage. Serial CT scans are often used to determine the effectiveness of treatment and to evaluate the course of healing.

Other diagnostic tests used in the diagnosis of stroke include magnetic resonance imaging (MRI), positron emission tomography (PET), and digital subtraction angiography (DSA). MRI uses a magnetic field instead of radiation to produce a picture of the brain that is similar to that of a CT scan. MRI is considered by some to be the best imaging method to differentiate hemorrhagic from nonhemorrhagic infarcts. The use of MRI in the diagnosis of stroke has increased significantly in recent years. Diffusion-weighted MRI, a more sensitive version of the MRI, shows greater sensitivity in delineating ischemic brain injury early after a stroke when CT and standard MRI may appear normal.[9]

PET shows the chemical activity of the brain and provides an excellent depiction of the extent of tissue damage after a stroke. Less active or diseased tissue appears darker than healthy, active cells. Major research efforts are aimed at perfecting this technique to aid in the diagnosis and treatment of brain disease.

DSA involves the intravenous (IV) or arterial injection of a contrast agent to produce good visualization of blood vessels in the neck and the large vessels of the circle of Willis. Intraarterial injection of contrast material has almost completely replaced IV DSA because the arterial approach requires a smaller bolus of contrast fluid and produces superior results. It is considered safer than cerebral angiography because less vascular manipulation is required. However, conventional intraarterial angiography is still needed for examination of intracranial arteries. Angiography is potentially dangerous because of the risks related to dislodging an embolus, causing vasospasm, or inducing further hemorrhage. Thus it is performed only when no other, safer test can provide the needed information.

Transcranial Doppler (TCD) ultrasonography measures the velocity of blood flow in the cerebral arteries. TCD has been shown to be effective in detecting microemboli and vasospasm. Certain neurodiagnostic tests such as skull x-rays, brain scan, lumbar puncture, and electroencephalogram (EEG) that were formerly used in the diagnosis of stroke are currently used much less. Although the skull x-ray is usually normal after a stroke, there may be a pineal shift with a massive infarction. A brain scan shows increased uptake of radioactive media in the infarcted area.

A lumbar puncture, although not performed routinely, may show a transient increase in leukocytes in the cerebrospinal fluid (CSF). The presence of blood in the CSF is indicative but not diagnostic of hemorrhage. A lumbar puncture is usually not done in the presence of increased intracranial pressure (ICP) because of the danger of herniation from a sudden decrease in pressure. An EEG may show low-voltage, slow-wave activity that is suggestive of ischemic infarction. If hemorrhage is the cause of the stroke, the EEG may show high-voltage slow waves. Arteriography can demonstrate areas of cervical and cerebrovascular occlusion, atherosclerotic plaques, and malformation of vessels. If the suspected cause of the stroke includes emboli from the heart, diagnostic cardiac tests should be done (see Table 55-3).

DIAGNOSTIC STUDIES

Table 55-3 Cerebrovascular Accident

Diagnosis of CVA, Including Extent of Involvement
- Computed tomography scan
- Magnetic resonance imaging
- Electroencephalogram
- Radionuclide scan (brain scan)
- Angiography
- Positron emission tomography
- Digital subtraction angiography
- Cerebrospinal fluid analysis*

Evaluation of Etiology of CVA
- Cerebral blood flow
  - Doppler ultrasonography
    - Transcranial Doppler
    - Carotid duplex
  - Carotid angiography
- Cardiac assessment
  - Electrocardiogram
  - Cardiac enzymes
  - Echocardiography
  - Holter monitor (evaluation of arrhythmias)

*For cerebrospinal fluid testing, a lumbar puncture is avoided if elevation of intracranial pressure is suspected.

COLLABORATIVE CARE

Prevention

Primary prevention is a priority for reducing morbidity and mortality associated with CVAs (Table 55-4). The goals of

COLLABORATIVE CARE

Table 55-4 Cerebrovascular Accident

Diagnostic*
History and physical examination

Collaborative Therapy

Prevention
- Control of hypertension
- Control of diabetes mellitus
- No smoking
- Limit alcohol intake
- Platelet inhibitors (e.g., aspirin)
- Anticoagulation therapy for patients with atrial fibrillation
- Treatment of underlying cardiac problem
- Surgical interventions for patients with aneurysms at risk of bleeding
- Carotid endarterectomy
- Transluminal angioplasty
- Extracranial-intracranial bypass

Acute Care
- Maintenance of airway
- Fluid therapy
- Ischemic (thrombotic and embolic) CVA
  - Tissue plasminogen activator (t-PA)
  - Anticoagulation
- Ischemic and hemorrhagic CVA
  - Treatment of cerebral edema
- Hemorrhagic CVA
  - Surgical decompression if indicated
- Subarachnoid hemorrhage
  - Surgical extirpation (dependent on size and location of hemorrhage)
- Embolic CVA
  - Treatment of underlying cause

*Diagnostic studies are presented in Table 55-3.

stroke prevention include health management for the well individual, management of modifiable risk factors, prevention of stroke for those with a history of TIA, and prevention of additional strokes for those who have had a CVA. Health management focuses on (1) healthy diet, (2) weight control, (3) regular exercise, (4) no smoking, (5) limiting alcohol consumption, and (6) routine health assessments. Patients with known risk factors such as diabetes mellitus, hypertension, obesity, high serum lipids, or cardiac dysfunction require close management of their illnesses. Postmenopausal women on estrogen therapy are less likely to experience a CVA as compared with women not on estrogen therapy.

Drug Therapy. Measures designed to prevent the development of a thrombus or embolus are also used in patients at risk. Low-dose aspirin is used prophylactically because of its antiplatelet effects. Studies have shown that daily aspirin use can reduce the risk of stroke in both men and women.[10] Dipyridamole (Persantine) 50 mg three times a day decreases platelet aggregation, which helps prevent thrombus and embolus formation. Daily use of platelet aggregation inhibitors such as ticlopidine (Ticlid) and clopidrogel (Plavix) has been shown to be as effective as aspirin in reducing the incidence of stroke.[11]

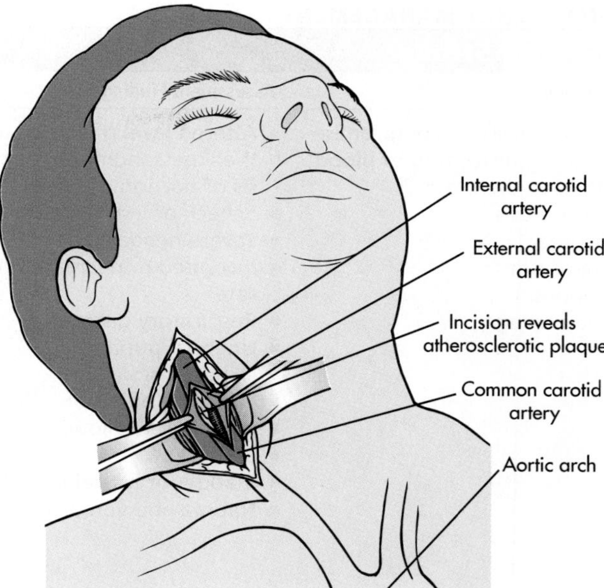

Fig. 55-7 Carotid endarterectomy. The atherosclerotic plaque in the internal carotid artery is removed to prevent impending cerebral infarction.

Surgical Therapy. Surgical interventions for the patient with TIAs from carotid disease include carotid endarterectomy (CEA), transluminal angioplasty, and extracranial-intracranial (EC-IC) bypass. In the CEA the atheromatous lesion is removed from the carotid artery to improve blood flow (Fig. 55-7). CEA surgery is associated with a reduction in stroke and vascular death.[12] This surgery is reserved for patients with occlusions of 70% to 99% of blood flow.

Transluminal angioplasty is the insertion of a balloon to open a stenosed artery to permit increased blood flow. This procedure has been used to treat patients with clinical manifestations related to stenosis in the vertebrobasilar or carotid arteries and their major branches. The risk of the angioplasty procedure is the possibility of dislodging emboli, which can travel to the brain or retina.

The EC-IC bypass is used for intracranial problems when the obstruction cannot be removed directly. The procedure usually involves anastomosing (surgically connecting) a branch of an extracranial artery to an intracranial artery just beyond an area of obstruction. Branches of the middle cerebral artery are most commonly used for the bypass surgery with the goal of increasing intracranial perfusion. Following the procedures these patients are at high risk for stroke and require close, long-term assessment and management (see Table 55-4).

Acute Care

The goals for collaborative care during the acute phase are preservation of life, prevention of further brain damage, and reduction in the level of disability. Treatment differs according to the type of stroke. Treatment also changes as the patient progresses from the acute phase to the rehabilitation phase of stroke.

The first goal is to maintain a patent airway because the airway may be compromised by decreased consciousness.[8] Interventions to maintain adequate oxygenation must be initiated immediately to prevent cerebral anoxia and permanent brain

✚EMERGENCY MANAGEMENT

Table 55-5 Stroke

Etiology	Assessment Findings	Interventions
Sudden vascular compromise causing disruption of blood flow to the brain Thrombosis Trauma Aneurysm Embolism Hemorrhage	▪ Altered level of consciousness ▪ Weakness, numbness, or paralysis of portion of body ▪ Speech or visual disturbances ▪ Severe headache ▪ Increased or decreased heart rate ▪ Respiratory distress ▪ Unequal pupils ▪ Hypertension ▪ Facial drooping on affected side ▪ Difficulty swallowing ▪ Seizures ▪ Bladder or bowel incontinence ▪ Nausea and vomiting	**Initial** ▪ Ensure patent airway. ▪ Remove dentures. ▪ Administer oxygen via nasal cannula or non-rebreather mask. ▪ Establish IV access with normal saline to maintain BP. ▪ Remove clothing. ▪ Obtain CT scan immediately. ▪ Position head midline. ▪ Elevate head of bed 30 degrees if no symptoms of shock or injury. ▪ Institute seizure precautions. ▪ Anticipate thrombolytic therapy for ischemic stroke. **Ongoing Monitoring** ▪ Monitor vital signs, level of consciousness, oxygen saturation, cardiac rhythm, Glasgow Coma Score, pupil size and reactivity. ▪ Maintain patient warmth. ▪ Reassure patient and family.

damage. Table 55-5 outlines the emergency management of the patient with a CVA. Common interventions for adequate oxygenation may include oxygen administration, artificial airway, intubation, and mechanical ventilation. The patient is monitored closely for signs of increasing neurologic deficit.

In response to both thrombotic and embolic strokes (ischemic strokes), a series of events termed the *ischemic cascade* occurs. During the initial period the ischemic area becomes discolored and soft. Around the core area of ischemia is a border zone termed *ischemic penumbra* that has marginal perfusion. The penumbra maintains function during an initial period of time following stroke, perhaps 3 to 6 hours, although the exact length is not known. If adequate blood flow is restored during the first 3 to 6 hours, the ischemic cascade is interrupted and less neurologic function will be lost. However, if the ischemic cascade is not interrupted, it continues producing neurologic deficits and disability. Therefore efforts are made to increase perfusion with the goal of reducing neurologic deficits.

Patients with ischemic strokes may be treated with hypervolemic hemodilution and volume expansion with crystalloids or colloids. The goal of treatment is to decrease blood viscosity, which promotes blood flow to the area of stroke.[7]

The fluid and electrolyte balance must be controlled carefully. The goal of fluid and electrolyte replacement generally is to keep the patient adequately hydrated to promote perfusion and decrease secondary injury. While the goal is to maintain perfusion to the brain, overhydration may further compromise perfusion by increasing cerebral edema. Adequate fluid intake during acute care via oral, IV, or tube feedings should be 1500 to 2000 ml/day.[13,14] Patients are monitored for urine output. If secretion of antidiuretic hormone (ADH) increases in response to the stroke, there is a decrease in urine output and an increase in fluid retention. IV solutions with glucose and water are avoided because these solutions are hypotonic and may further increase cerebral edema and intracranial pressure.[8] In addition, hyperglycemia may be associated with further brain damage. In general, individualized fluid and electrolyte replacement therapy decisions are based on the extent of intracranial edema, symptoms of increased intracranial pressure, central venous pressure levels, laboratory values for electrolytes, and intake and output.

Increased ICP is more likely to occur with hemorrhagic strokes, but it can occur with ischemic strokes. Increased ICP from cerebral edema usually peaks in 72 hours and may cause brain herniation. Management of increased ICP includes practices that enhance venous drainage, including elevation of head of the bed as ordered, maintenance of the head and neck in alignment, and avoidance of hip flexion. Efforts to limit cerebral tissue metabolism and thus vasodilation include avoidance of hyperthermia. Additional measures include treatment of pain, avoidance of hypervolemia, and management of constipation. Cerebrospinal fluid drainage may be used in some patients to reduce ICP. Diuretic medications, such as mannitol (Osmitrol) and furosemide (Lasix), may be used to decrease cerebral edema. Dexamethasone (Decradron, Hexadrol) may be used in patients with vasogenic cerebral edema.

A clinical pathway for care of the patient with CVA is provided on p. 1655.

Drug Therapy

Thrombolytic therapy. Recombinant tissue plasminogen activator (t-PA) is used to reestablish blood flow and prevent cell death for patients with ischemic strokes. A study by the National Institute of Neurological Disorders and Stroke (NINDS) found that patients who received IV t-PA within 3 hours of onset of stroke were 32% more likely to have minimal or no disability 3 months after the stroke.[1,15] Thrombolytic drugs such as t-PA act to produce localized fibrinolysis by binding to the fibrin in the thrombi. The lytic action of t-PA occurs as the plasminogen is converted to plasmin (fibrinolysin), whose enzymatic action digests fibrin and fibrinogen and thus lyses the clot. Because it is clot specific in its activation of the fibrinolytic

CLINICAL PATHWAY Cerebrovascular Accident

Admit Date: DRG: 14 LOS: 4 days Discharge Date: ____________

Pathway	ER—Day 1	Day 2	Day 3	Day 4
Critical Path Implemented				
Diagnostic Studies	■ CBC, sed rate ■ BMP ■ Lipid profile ■ Progressive U/A ■ PT, PTT ■ Chest x-ray ■ ECG ■ CT of head without contrast	■ PT if on Coumadin ■ Carotid duplex if indicated	■ PT if on Coumadin	■ PT if on Coumadin ■ Schedule further imaging as OP (CT, Angio, MRI)
Treatments	■ Telemetry (include ↑↓ parameters) ■ O_2____L/min via NC if indicated ■ Antiembolic stockings ■ Evaluate for high-risk pressure/ reduction therapy and place on bed	■ O_2____L/min NC→ ■ Telemetry	■ O_2____L/min NC→ ■ Consider D/C telemetry	■ D/C O_2 if appropriate for condition ■ D/C telemetry
IV/Meds	■ IV____@____cc/hr → ■ Anticoagulation/antiplatelet Rx if indicated → ■ Antihypertensives if indicated →		■ Adjust IV rate to accommodate PO/TF intake	■ Write transition orders for rehab/ECF
Consults	■ Physiatrist ■ Neurology if ind. ■ Social Services ■ Speech/language eval. ■ Dysphagia eval. ■ Nutrition services	■ PT: functional eval. ■ OT eval.: safety ■ ET: skin care		
Team Directives	( )Neuro assessment with LOC q4hr and prn; evaluate for risk for aspiration and sensorial changes. Use Glasgow Coma Scale. ( )Follow swallow program prescription to prevent aspiration. ( )Physical assessment q8hr and prn with close attention to respiratory system and skin integrity. ( )VS q4hr × 24hr, then q8hr × 24hr, then q shift and prn. ( )I & O, notify physician if UO $<$ 600 cc/24 hr. Weigh on admission. ( )Skin care bid with daily reevaluation of skin risk assessment and implementation of appropriate interventions. ( )Assist with ADLs. Obtain BSC and overhead trapeze if indicated to assist with mobility and allow independence. ( )Monitor diagnostic study results and collaborate with the care team to further individualize the plan of care. ( )Provide emotional support and assist with reducing pt/family anxiety. (sign/date/time____/____/____, ____/____/____, ____/____/____, ____/____/____			
Diet	■ NPO; transition to swallow program prescription as ordered→ →			
Activity and Safety	( )Active and passive ROM within pt's functional capability ( )Turn, cough, deep breathe q2hr; assist with IS if ordered ( )Assist with turning and positioning q2hr ( )Bed rest, elevate HOB 30° ____/____/____, ____/____/____		( )Evaluate safety measures periodically and make necessary changes as neuro status changes ( )Reinforce PT activity protocol qid ( )Proper cushioning when OOB in chair ____/____/____, ____/____/____, ____/____/____	
Teaching Patient and Family	Instruct pt/family to call staff for assistance ( )Orient to environment, person, time (frequently if needed) ( )Initiate CVA (stroke) teaching plan ( )Explain tests and procedures to pt/family ( )Explain antiplatelet/anticoagulation Rx and precautions (sign/date/time)____/____/____, ____/____/____		( )Explain potential for surgical intervention (if it exists) ( )Evaluate need for long-term teaching in smoking cessation, cholesterol control, hypertension, weight reduction ( )Teach stroke prevention strategies ____/____/____ ____/____/____	
Transition Planning	( )Initial CM/SS evaluation to determine rehab needs ( )Review advance directives ____/____/____ ____/____/____	( )Rehab placement initiated ( )Risk evaluation referrals from admission database assessment initiated ____/____/____, ____/____/____	( )Outpatient and community support agencies identified and contacted; or pt/family have means to contact once in home setting ____/____/____	

Author: Molly Metzler, RN, BSN, for Nanticoke Health Services. Licensed by the Center for Case Management, South Natick, Mass, Nanticoke Health Services.

Continued

system, it is less likely to cause hemorrhage as compared with streptokinase or urokinase.

As stated previously, t-PA treatment is most effective if administered within 3 hours of the stroke occurrence as defined by the onset of clinical manifestations. Therefore the single most important factor is timing. Patients are screened carefully before treatment initiation. This includes blood tests for coagulation disorders, recent history of GI bleeding, and a CT or MRI scan to rule out hemorrhagic stroke.

The major side effect of t-PA is cerebral hemorrhage.[1,15] During the infusion of the drug the patient's vital signs are monitored to assess for improvement or deterioration related to intracerebral hemorrhage. Control of blood pressure is critical during treatment and for 24 hours following treatment. No anticoagulants or antiplatelet drugs are administered for 24 hours after t-PA treatment.

Currently other agents are being tested for their effectiveness during the acute phase. In a limited study, prourokinase (Proact I) has been shown to enhance vessel patency in patients when given within the first 6 hours of stroke symptoms.

Platelet inhibition/anticoagulant therapy. Patients with stroke caused by thrombi and emboli (ischemic strokes) may also be treated with platelet inhibitors and anticoagulants (after the first 24 hours if treated with t-PA) to prevent the formation of more clots. Common anticoagulants include heparin and warfarin (Coumadin, Panwarfin). Platelet inhibitors include

CLINICAL PATHWAY Cerebrovascular Accident—continued

DRG: 14 LOS: 4 days

Meets Expected Outcomes (initial)	ER—Day 1	MET	NOT	Day 2	MET	NOT	Day 3	MET	NOT	Day 4	MET	NOT
Ineffective Airway Clearance: ■ RR changes ■ Inability to clear mucous secretions	■ Airway maintained____/RC ■ Suctions easily if indicated____/RC or N ■ Passive cooperation with TC and DB regimen____/N ■ PT/family understand need for cough and deep breathing q2hr____/RC or N			■ Performs C and DB exercises within limitations of function ____/RC or N ■ Pt. cooperating with pulmonary toilet regimen within functional capabilities ____/RC or N ■ Pt. using **IS** effectively ____/RC or N			■ Minimal adventitious breath sounds____/RC or N ■ Pt. able to clear mucous secretions on own, or suctions easily____/RC or N ■ Pt/family understand the need to continue **IS** after discharge or in subacute care facility____/RC or N			■ No evidence of pulmonary infection____/RC or N ■ Breath sounds clear____/RC or N ■ **IS** sent with patient on discharge____/RC or N		
Impaired Mobility: ■ Unable to perform purposeful movement ■ Hemiplegia ■ Limited ROM ■ Decreased muscle strength ■ Impaired coordination	■ Pt/family understand and cooperate with passive ROM____/N ■ Skin integrity maintained clean, dry, and protected from pressure and rubbing____/N ■ Pt.'s functional alignment maintained on air mattress or specialty bed____/N			■ Functional mobility maintained____/PT or N ■ No evidence of skin breakdown____/N or ET ■ PT program initiated and pt/family understand the importance of early intervention to recovery____/PT or N ■ Passive ROM keeping joints flexible____/PT or N			■ Pt/family understand importance of maintaining long-term therapeutic exercise regimen____/PT or N ■ Postdischarge rehab therapy arrangements in place____/CM or N ■ No evidence of thromboembolic complications evident____/N			■ Performing ADLs with assistance____/N ■ Discharge environment safe for functional capabilities, or rehab placement procured____/SS ■ Skin intact____/N or ET		
Sensory-Perceptual Alteration: ■ Altered LOC ■ Inability to communicate needs ■ Impaired memory or intellectual capacity ■ Aphasia ■ Impaired awareness of bodily functions	■ Pt/family received and understand an explanation of care regimen and safety measures in place ____/N ■ Alternate form of communication devised and functional ____/N ■ Pt. responding to frequent reorientation to environment ____/N ■ Urinary cath patient (if indicated)____/N			■ Pt/family starting to recognize physical limitations resulting from CVA____/N ■ Pt able to communicate needs ____/N ■ Sensory-perceptual changes from CVA stabilizing____/N ■ Bladder and bowel functions maintained with personal hygiene and pt's dignity in mind____/N			■ LOC stabilized____/N ■ Ability to communicate needs improving____/N ■ Pt.'s response to reorientation to environment improving____/N ■ Bladder and bowel function maintained with no S/S of infection____/N			■ LOC stabilized for transfer to rehab facility or home care ____/N ■ Communication system explained to receiving rehab agency or home caregivers____/N		
Emotional Lability: ■ Emotional outbursts ■ Inappropriate verbal and emotional responses ■ Changes in family processes from sudden-onset CVA	■ Explanation provided to family regarding inappropriate verbal and emotional responses from pt____/N ■ Family beginning to identify the need to delegate responsibilities normally performed by pt to other family members____/N			■ Family demonstrating effective coping skills with pt's inappropriateness____/N ■ Family members begin to identify their internal support systems with help from staff ____/SS or CM or N ■ Community support agencies identified for pt's transitional care____/SS or CM			■ Family activating their internal support network____/SS or CM or N ■ Family members are able to share their feelings about illness in the family with each other____/SS or CM or N ■ Community support systems discussed with pt/family____/SS or CM			■ Family actively supporting each other____/SS or CM or N ■ Family knows how to contact community support agencies after subacute care experience, or contact with appropriate agencies has been established before discharge ____/SS or CM		

Continued

Service

CM - Care management
ET - Ostomy/skin care
RC - Respiratory care
N - Nurse
PT - Physical therapy
NS - Nutrition services
RX - Pharmacist
SL - Speech/language
CCC - Primary RN clinical care coord.
SW - Social work
OT - Occupational therapy
HC - Home care
DR - Physician
Card - Cardiology
Rad - Radiology
Rehab - Cardiac, respiratory

CLINICAL PATHWAY Cerebrovascular Accident—continued

DRG: 14 LOS: 4 days

Meets Expected Outcomes (initial)	ER—Day 1	MET	NOT	Day 2	MET	NOT	Day 3	MET	NOT	Day 4	MET	NOT
Potential Nutritional Deficit: ■ Weight loss ■ Inadequate PO intake ■ Dysphagia ■ Poor muscle tone	■ Hydration/nutrition status maintained in homeostasis by IV/TF while pt unable to take or tolerate adequate PO fluids or nutrients____/NS or N			■ Weight stabilized____/NS or N ■ Pt cooperating with swallowing program prescribed to best of functional ability____/SLP or NS or N ■ Aspiration precautions explained to pt/family____/SLP or NS or N ■ Caloric and fluid needs being met____/NS or N			■ Pt. gaining strength____/NS or N ■ Weight stable____/NS or N ■ Pt/family understand aspiration precautions and know S/S of impending problems____/SLP or NS or N			■ Pt. tolerating and retaining appropriate fluid and caloric amounts to meet metabolic demands____/NS or N		
Knowledge Deficit: ■ Physiologic changes ■ Causes of CVA ■ Prevention measures ■ Rehabilitation ■ Safety measures ■ Precautions ■ Medications	■ Pt/family understand safety measures initiated____/N ■ Pt/family will understand the disease process of CVA____/N ■ Pt/family will understand some possible causes of CVA____/N			■ Pt/family will be able to understand and discuss the components of therapy for CVA____/N ■ Pt/family will understand how a CVA often leads to neurologic damage____/N			■ Pt/family will be able to identify usual impending S/S of stroke____/N ■ Pt/family will be able to identify prevention measures to reduce risk for further CVAs____/N ■ Pt/family understand medication regimen____/N			■ Pt/family know when and how to access their PCP and EMS____/N ■ Pt/family understand the importance of ongoing medical follow-up____/N		
Unmet Outcomes: (CCC Initials Required)	7-3 PM ( ) Resolved ( ) Planned /RN			7-3 PM ( ) Resolved ( ) Planned /RN			7-3 PM ( ) Resolved ( ) Planned /RN			7-3 PM ( ) Resolved ( ) Planned /RN		
	3-7 PM ( ) Resolved ( ) Planned /RN			3-7 PM ( ) Resolved ( ) Planned /RN			3-7 PM ( ) Resolved ( ) Planned /RN			3-7 PM ( ) Resolved ( ) Planned /RN		
	7-11 PM ( ) Resolved ( ) Planned /RN			7-11 PM ( ) Resolved ( ) Planned /RN			7-11 PM ( ) Resolved ( ) Planned /RN			7-11 PM ( ) Resolved ( ) Planned /RN		
	11-7 AM ( ) Resolved ( ) Planned /RN			11-7 AM ( ) Resolved ( ) Planned /RN			11-7 AM ( ) Resolved ( ) Planned /RN			11-7 AM ( ) Resolved ( ) Planned /RN		

aspirin, ticlopidine (Ticlid), clopidrogel (Plavix), and dipyridamole (Persantine).[3] IV heparin or low-molecular-weight heparin may be given in the situation of rapidly evolving strokes or strokes caused by emboli traveling from the heart. IV heparin is administered via continuous infusion, and the activated partial thromboplastin time is closely monitored.

Typically heparin is replaced by oral warfarin for long-term administration. Doses of warfarin are regulated by the results of the international normalized ratio (INR). The INR is a standardized measure of prothrombin time that adjusts for assay variations. The therapeutic dose is that which produces a value that is 2 to 3 times the normal level. Nurses must monitor the patient closely for hemorrhage or bleeding at other body sites while using anticoagulants and platelet inhibitors. A patient teaching guide for patients taking warfarin on a long-term basis is found in Table 36-15.

Anticoagulants and platelet inhibitors are contraindicated for patients with hemorrhagic strokes. The calcium channel blocker nimodipine (Nimotop) is given to patients with subarachnoid hemorrhage to decrease the effects of vasospasm and minimize tissue damage.[16] Calcium channel blockers inhibit the passage of calcium into brain cells during and after stroke. It is thought that excess intracellular calcium is harmful to brain tissue.

Acetylsalicylic acid (aspirin) is also used to prevent platelet aggregation at the site of the atherosclerotic plaque. The complications of aspirin include gastrointestinal bleeding with higher doses. Aspirin administration should be done cautiously if the patient has a history of peptic ulcer disease or is taking other anticoagulants.

Other drug therapies. Aspirin or acetaminophen (Tylenol) is given to treat hyperthermia. An elevation of as little as 1 degree of temperature can increase brain metabolism and further brain damage. The brain can tolerate hypoxia longer if the patient is hypothermic. Cooling blankets may be used cautiously to lower core temperatures. The nurse must closely monitor the patient's body temperature.

Approximately 15% of patients who experience a CVA will have seizures. Antiseizure medication, such as phenytoin (Dilantin), may be administered if seizure activity is present.[8] Prophylactic treatment with antiseizure medication is avoided unless seizure activity is present.

Investigation is ongoing to find potentially neuroprotective agents to prevent further ischemic damage in the infarcted area, including cells in the penumbra. Drugs that antagonize the action of excitatory neurotransmitters (e.g., glutamate) hold promise in the terms of protecting neurons from damage. Other agents include calcium channel blockers such as nimodipine and antagonists to nitric oxide.[15] Ultimately early treatment of stroke may involve drugs that increase blood flow and drugs that protect neurons from further ischemic damage.

Surgical Therapy. Surgical interventions for stroke include an immediate evacuation of blood occurring with strokes caused by aneurysm-induced hematomas or cerebellar hematomas larger than 3 cm. Subarachnoid hemorrhage is usually caused by a ruptured aneurysm. Approximately 20% of patients will have multiple aneurysms. Treatment of an aneurysm includes clipping the aneurysm (see Fig. 55-4) and removing the clot to prevent rebleeding into the brain.

Subarachnoid and intracerebral hemorrhage can involve bleeding into the ventricles of the brain. This situation produces hydrocephalus, which further damages brain tissue from increased intracranial pressure. The surgical procedure of ventriculostomy and drainage can give dramatic improvement in these situations.

Rehabilitation Care

After the stroke has stabilized for 12 to 24 hours, collaborative care shifts from the preservation of life to the lessening of disability and the attainment of optimal function. The patient may be evaluated by a physiatrist (a physician who specializes in physical medicine and rehabilitation). Depending on the patient's status, the patient's rehabilitation potential, and available resources, the patient may be transferred to a rehabilitation facility or unit. Other approaches for rehabilitation include outpatient therapy and home care–based rehabilitation.

As part of the long-term collaborative care after a stroke, various members of the health team may be involved in the effort to promote optimal function of the patient and the family. The exact composition of the team depends on the needs of the patient and family and the resources of the rehabilitation facility or institution (Fig. 55-8).

NURSING MANAGEMENT: STROKE

Nursing Assessment

Subjective and objective data that should be obtained from a person who has had a stroke are presented in Table 55-6. The nurse may be the initial health care professional to see a patient with a stroke. The primary assessment is focused on the cardiac and

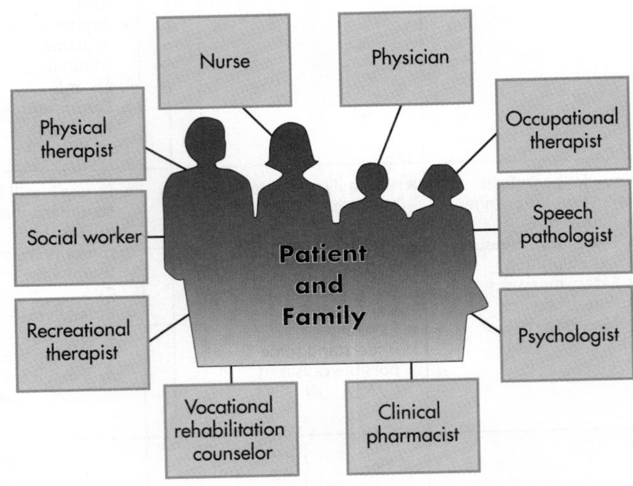

Fig. 55-8 Representative membership of the rehabilitation team.

NURSING ASSESSMENT

Table 55-6 Stroke

Subjective Data

Important Health Information

Past health history: Hypertension; previous stroke, TIA(s), aneurysm, cardiac disease (including recent myocardial infarction), arrhythmias, congestive heart failure, valvular disease, infective endocarditis; hyperlipidemia, polycythemia, diabetes, gout

Medications: Use of oral contraceptives, use of and compliance with antihypertensive and anticoagulant agents

Functional Health Patterns

Health perception–health management: Positive family history; alcohol abuse, smoking

Nutritional-metabolic: Anorexia, nausea, vomiting; dysphagia, disturbances in taste and smell

Elimination: Change in bowel and bladder patterns

Activity-exercise: Loss of movement and sensation; syncope; weakness on one side; generalized weakness, easy fatigability

Cognitive-perceptual: Numbness, tingling of one side of the body; loss of memory; alteration in speech, language, problem-solving ability; pain; headache, possibly sudden and severe (hemorrhage); visual disturbances; denial of illness

Objective Data

General

Emotional lability, lethargy, apathy or combativeness, fever

Respiratory

Loss of cough reflex, labored or irregular respirations, tachypnea, rhonchi (aspiration), airway occlusion (tongue), apnea

Cardiovascular

Hypertension, tachycardia, carotid bruit

Gastrointestinal

Loss of gag reflex, bowel incontinence, decreased or absent bowel sounds, constipation

Urinary

Urinary frequency, urgency, incontinence

Neurologic

Contralateral motor and sensory deficits, including weakness, paresis, paralysis, anesthesia; unequal pupils, hand grasps; akinesia, aphasia (expressive, receptive, global), dysarthria (slurred speech), agnosias, apraxia, visual deficits, perceptual or spatial disturbances, altered level of consciousness (drowsiness to deep coma) and Babinski's sign, decreased followed by increased deep tendon reflexes, flaccidity followed by spasticity, amnesia, ataxia, personality change, nuchal rigidity, seizures

Possible Findings

Positive CT and MRI scans showing size, location, and type of lesion; positive Doppler ultrasonography and cerebral angiography respiratory status of the patient and a brief neurologic assessment. If the patient is stable, the nursing history is obtained as follows: (1) description of the current illness with attention to initial symptoms, duration of symptoms, intermittent or continuous nature of symptoms, and changes of symptom characteristics; (2) history of similar symptoms previously experienced; (3) current medications; (4) history of associative illnesses such as hypertension; and (5) family history of stroke or cardiovascular diseases. This information would be gained through an interview of the patient, family members, significant others, or caregiver.

The secondary assessment should include a comprehensive neurologic examination of the patient. The neurologic screening examination includes the functional status of (1) level of consciousness, (2) cognition, (3) motor abilities, (4) cranial nerve function, (5) sensation, (6) proprioception, (7) cerebellar abilities, and (8) deep tendon reflexes. Serial documentation of the neurologic screening examination is essential to note progressing or diminishing status of the patient. The neurologic screen examination can be quickly evaluated and documented on a flow sheet and the Glasgow Coma Scale for ease of patient assessment.

■ Nursing Diagnoses

Nursing diagnoses for the person with a stroke may include, but are not limited to, those presented in NCP 55-1.

55-1 NURSING CARE PLAN PATIENT WITH A STROKE

Expected Patient Outcomes	Nursing Interventions and *Rationales*
NURSING DIAGNOSIS	**Altered tissue perfusion (cerebral)** *related to* decreased cerebral blood flow secondary to thrombus, embolus, hemorrhage, edema, or spasm *as manifested by* intracranial pressure (ICP) >15 mm Hg for 15 to 30 seconds or longer, decreasing Glasgow Coma Scale (GCS) score, and altered respiratory pattern.
■ ICP < 15 mm Hg. ■ Stable and improving GCS.	■ Assess ICP, level of consciousness (LOC), and breathing pattern at least hourly *to identify trends in patient's condition and to enable early notification of physician of significant changes.* ■ Administer medications as prescribed *to decrease risk of further thrombus formation.* ■ Implement measures, such as treating hypoxia, reducing pain, and maintaining patent urinary catheter, *to prevent increasing ICP.*
NURSING DIAGNOSIS	**Risk for ineffective airway clearance** *related to* inability to raise secretions.
■ Able to expectorate secretions. ■ No respiratory distress.	■ Assess for weak, ineffective cough; bronchial congestion; adventitious breath sounds; changes in color, amount, and consistency of sputum *to determine if risk factors are present.* ■ Observe for increase in pulmonary secretions, changes in color of secretions, and temperature elevation *as indicators of pulmonary infection.* ■ Auscultate lungs for breath sounds daily and as needed *to determine adequacy of respiratory excursion.* ■ Suction as needed *to remove accumulated secretions.* ■ Instruct patient and family in feeding program and emergency measures *to prevent aspiration and resultant respiratory distress.*
NURSING DIAGNOSIS	**Impaired physical mobility** *related to* generalized weakness, muscle atrophy, or paralyzed extremities *as manifested by* decreased physical activity, limited range of motion, decreased muscle strength or control.
■ Able to transfer and ambulate at maximal level of ability. ■ Able to perform activities of daily living by self or with assistance.	■ Assess and document range of motion, transfer abilities, and positioning ability *to determine extent of problem and plan appropriate interventions.* ■ Administer passive or active range-of-motion exercises to affected extremities at least tid *to prevent unnecessary muscle atrophy and contractures.* ■ Maintain alignment with support pillows and footboard according to procedures; teach and assist family and patient with positioning techniques *to prevent contractures.* ■ Follow through with techniques for activities of daily living recommended by occupational or physical therapist *to help patient incorporate teaching from specialists into daily life and activities.* ■ Encourage as much self-mobility as possible *to maintain physical activity at highest degree possible and to promote patient's sense of control.*

Continued

55-1 NURSING CARE PLAN PATIENT WITH A STROKE—continued

Expected Patient Outcomes	Nursing Interventions and *Rationales*
NURSING DIAGNOSIS	**Impaired verbal communication** *related to* residual aphasia *as manifested by* refusal or inability to speak, word-finding problems, use of inappropriate words, inability to follow verbal directions.
▪ Able to communicate effectively.	▪ Assess exact communication deficits and strengths *to determine type of communication problem and plan appropriate interventions.* ▪ Intervene as appropriate. ▪ Use short, simple questions that elicit "yes" and "no" answers; speak slowly and allow adequate time for response *to avoid overwhelming patient with verbal stimuli.* ▪ Use gestures *to support verbal cues.* ▪ Teach specific techniques *to improve speech.* ▪ Speak slowly and use visual aids such as flash cards *to avoid frustration and anger from worsening problem.*
NURSING DIAGNOSIS	**Self-care deficits** *related to* motor weakness, paralysis, and loss of ability to effectively perform activities of daily living (ADLs) *as manifested by* observation or verbal report of inability to eat, bathe, use toilet, dress, or groom independently.
▪ Able to perform ADLs by self or with assistance from family or staff.	▪ Assess and document level of self-care *to determine extent of problem and plan appropriate interventions.* ▪ Encourage independence, provide supervision or assistance as needed *to avoid development of dependency.* ▪ Follow through with techniques for ADLs recommended by occupational or physical therapist *to help patient incorporate teaching from specialists and family.*
NURSING DIAGNOSIS	**Unilateral neglect** *related to* visual field cut and sensory loss on one side of body *as manifested by* consistent inattention to stimuli on affected side.
▪ Able to bring objects into field of vision. ▪ Scanning with eyes. ▪ Expression of satisfaction with vision.	▪ Assess and document amount of visual field impairment *to determine extent of problem and plan appropriate interventions.* ▪ Teach patient to turn head and scan environment. ▪ Early in care, approach patient on unaffected side; place objects in patient's field of vision; give physical and verbal cues to aid in path finding *to compensate for visual field deficits.* ▪ Later in care, approach patient on affected side *to encourage patient to turn head.* ▪ Provide visual stimulation *to promote use of full range of visual capabilities.* ▪ Use an eye patch *to prevent diplopia.* ▪ If corneal reflex is absent, protect affected eye to prevent injury. ▪ Teach family and patient to stimulate paralyzed limbs using touch and warm and cold stimuli *to promote reintegration with the whole body.* ▪ Encourage patient to use cue cards and mirrors *as reminder to survey her or his whole body for position, cleanliness, and appropriate dress.*
NURSING DIAGNOSIS	**Altered urinary elimination** *related to* impaired impulse to void or inability to reach toilet or manage tasks of voiding *as manifested by* incontinence and flow of urine at unpredictable times.
▪ Satisfactory urinary control by natural or artificial method.	▪ Assess and record patient's continent and incontinent voidings *to determine patterns and plan appropriate interventions.* ▪ Note color and character of urine daily and as needed *to ensure early detection of urinary tract infection and to prevent highly concentrated urine.* ▪ Provide fluid intake of 2000 ml/day unless contraindicated *to foster adequate elimination of dilute urine.* ▪ If indwelling catheter is used, give perineal cleansing and catheter care every shift and as needed *to avoid infection and ensure uninterrupted urinary flow.* ▪ Offer urinal or commode q2hr and as needed *to aid in establishing regular voiding pattern.* ▪ Assure patient of your willingness to assist with urinary problem *to avoid embarrassment and to demonstrate a caring attitude.*

Continued

55-1 NURSING CARE PLAN PATIENT WITH A STROKE—continued

Expected Patient Outcomes	Nursing Interventions and *Rationales*
NURSING DIAGNOSIS **Impaired swallowing** *related to* weakness or paralysis of affected muscles *as manifested by* drooling, difficulty in swallowing, choking.	
▪ No signs or symptoms of aspiration. ▪ Able to tolerate food and fluids without choking.	▪ Assess patient *to determine ability to swallow and presence of gag reflex.* ▪ Have patient sit upright for meals and for 30 minutes afterward *to use gravity to prevent aspiration.* ▪ Teach patient to take small bites and place food in unaffected side of mouth, keep chin down, and stroke throat *to stimulate swallowing.* ▪ After patient has eaten, check oral cavity for pocketed food and teach patient and family this technique *to prevent collection and putrefaction of food and resultant risk of infection.* ▪ Give thick shakes, foods with texture, and cold foods *to facilitate swallowing and minimize danger of choking.* ▪ If problem with sputum and saliva production, avoid milk products, *which increase production of mucus and saliva.* ▪ Give oral care after meals *to promote comfort and oral health.* ▪ Notify dietician of need to change food texture or fluids as needed.
NURSING DIAGNOSIS **Self-esteem disturbance** *related to* actual or perceived loss of function *as manifested by* expression of shame or guilt, increasing dependence on others, refusal to participate in self-care.	
▪ Verbalization of feelings and concerns. ▪ Participation in appropriate socialization with family and staff. ▪ Setting of realistic goals.	▪ Encourage patient to verbalize feelings *to assess effect of stroke sequelae on self-esteem.* ▪ Spend time with patient using good listening techniques *to show a caring, concerned attitude, which fosters confidence in a relationship.* ▪ Establish achievable goals; explain all procedures and involve patient in planning goals; offer praise for every success and step of progress; involve patient as soon as possible in rehabilitation program *to promote sense of satisfaction and control and reduce frustration.* ▪ Refer for counseling or medical-psychiatric evaluation if indicated *so patient can have expert help with serious problems.*
NURSING DIAGNOSIS **Risk for ineffective management of therapeutic regimen** *related to* functional, cognitive, or communication limitations.	
▪ Patient or family will make satisfactory arrangements to have patient's needs met on a daily basis.	▪ Assess degree of functional, cognitive, or communication limitations patient is experiencing *to determine teaching plan and arrange appropriate interventions.* ▪ Teach patient and family how to treat, prevent, and monitor for problems *so early intervention is ensured.* ▪ Evaluate plan *to determine if regimen is being followed or needs to be revised based on changing patient status or circumstances.*

■ Planning

The patient, family, and nurse establish the goals of nursing care in a cooperative manner. These goals typically include that the patient will (1) maintain a stable or improved level of consciousness, (2) attain maximum physical functioning, (3) attain maximum self-care abilities and skills, (4) maintain stable body functions (e.g., bladder control), (5) maximize communication abilities, (6) maintain adequate nutrition, (7) avoid complications of stroke, and (8) maintain effective personal and family coping.

■ Nursing Implementation

Health Promotion. To reduce the incidence of stroke, the nurse should focus teaching efforts toward stroke prevention for persons with known risk (e.g., patients with TIAs, hypertension, or diabetes mellitus). The significance of other potentially modifiable risk factors for the occurrence of stroke is unclear. However, control of risk factors implicated in coronary artery disease may indirectly help prevent stroke. (For the nurse's role in management of these risk factors, see Table 32-4.) In any health care setting and for the population as a whole, nurses can play a major role in the promotion of a healthy lifestyle. An overall program to prevent events such as stroke includes the recognition that people are responsible to some degree for their own health and for the health of future generations.

Another aspect of health promotion is teaching patients about when to seek health care for symptoms. Individuals

PATIENT & FAMILY TEACHING GUIDE

Table 55-7 Warning Signs of Stroke

Patients should be taught to seek help immediately if the following symptoms are present:

- Sudden weakness or numbness of the face, arm, or leg on one side of the body
- Sudden dimness or loss of vision, particularly in one eye
- Sudden difficulty speaking or trouble understanding speech
- Sudden severe headache with no known cause
- Unexplained dizziness, unsteadiness, or sudden falls, especially with any of the other symptoms

should be taught about early symptoms associated with stroke or TIA (Table 55-7).

Acute Intervention

Respiratory system. During the acute phase following a stroke the nursing priority is the management of the respiratory system. Stroke patients are particularly vulnerable to respiratory problems. Advancing age and immobility make them particularly susceptible to atelectasis and pneumonia. These patients are at high risk for aspiration pneumonia because of impaired consciousness or dysphagia. Problems commonly seen include poor chewing and swallowing, food pouching (food remaining in the buccal cavity of the mouth), and falling back of the tongue resulting in obstruction of the airway. Enteral tube feedings also place the patient at risk for aspiration pneumonia.

Nursing interventions to support adequate respiratory function are individualized to meet the needs of the patient. An oropharyngeal airway may be used in comatose patients to hold the tongue in place, prevent airway obstruction, and make suctioning accessible. In more prolonged situations, the oropharyngeal airway is replaced by a tracheostomy. Nasopharyngeal airways provide protection and access to the airway in patients with impaired consciousness. Nursing interventions include frequent assessment of airway patency and function, suctioning, patient mobility, positioning of the patient to prevent aspiration, and encouraging deep breathing. Patients who have an unclipped aneurysm may experience rebleeding and the possibility of further ICP increases with coughing exercises. Interventions related to maintenance of airway function are described in NCP 55-1.

Neurologic system. The patient's neurologic status must be monitored closely to detect changes suggesting stroke-in-evolution, extension of the stroke, increased intracranial pressure, or recovery from stroke symptoms. The Glasgow Coma Scale is used for neurologic assessment because it contains the essential factors of level of consciousness, mental status, pupillary responses, and movement and strength of extremities. (The Glasgow Coma Scale is shown in Table 54-2.) Vital signs are also closely monitored and documented. A decreasing level of consciousness is the earliest and most sensitive sign of increasing ischemia of the brain. Data from the nursing assessment are recorded on flow sheets to permit evaluation of neurologic status by the interdisciplinary team.

Cardiovascular system. Nursing goals for the cardiovascular system are aimed at maintaining homeostasis. Many patients with stroke have decreased cardiac reserves that are due to the secondary diagnoses of cardiac diseases. Cardiac efficiency is further compromised by fluid retention, overhydration, dehydration, and blood pressure variations. Fluids are retained because of increased production of ADH and aldosterone secondary to stress. Fluid retention plus overhydration can result in fluid overload. It can also increase cerebral edema and intracranial pressure. At the same time dehydration can add to the morbidity and mortality associated with stroke. Therefore the nurse should closely monitor intake and output. IV therapy is also carefully regulated.

Nursing interventions include (1) monitoring vital signs frequently; (2) monitoring cardiac rhythms; (3) calculating intake and output, noting imbalances; (4) regulating IV infusions; (5) adjusting the fluid intake to the individual needs of the patient; (6) monitoring lung sounds for crackles and rhonchi that indicate pulmonary congestion; and (7) monitoring heart sounds for murmurs or for S_3 or S_4 heart sounds. Hy-

RESEARCH

IMPLICATIONS FOR NURSING PRACTICE

Early Recognition of Stroke

Citation Rosamond WD and others: Rapid response to stroke symptoms: the Delay in Accessing Stroke Healthcare (DASH) study, *Acad Emerg Med* 5:45, 1998.

Purpose To determine the factors that contribute to delays in seeking treatment for acute cerebral ischemic events.

Methods A prospective study was done using patients treated at the emergency department (ED) with clinical manifestations of stroke. Trained nurses using a structured interview talked with patients regarding delays in seeking health care. A total of 152 interviews were conducted.

Results and Conclusions The average delay in seeking health care from the onset of clinical manifestations to arrival at the ED for all patients with stroke-like symptoms was 3 hours with a range of 1.5 to 7.8 hours. The delay was less in those situations in which a witness first recognized that there was a serious change as compared with the patient self-identifying a problem. More rapid arrival in the ED was also associated with use of emergency medical services (EMS) by the patient. Most patients arrived within 3 hours when EMS was notified.

Implications for Nursing Practice Prompt treatment of ischemic strokes with thrombolytic drugs reduces the degree of neurologic impairment following a stroke. Therefore patients should be taught to seek health care immediately if they experience symptoms such as muscle weakness, visual disturbances, or swallowing problems. This study emphasizes the need for education of not only those at risk for a stroke but also their family members.

ETHICAL DILEMMAS

Right to Die

SITUATION

A 93-year-old woman has had three strokes in the last 20 months. They have left her partially paralyzed and in need of full-time care. She has repeatedly told her home care nurse that she would not want to live if her condition worsened. She is now hospitalized for another stroke and her prognosis is the complete loss of physical functioning. She has tried to remove the feeding tube, which causes her discomfort. Responding to repeated questions of both the nurse and physician about whether she wants them to stop treatment and let her die, she has consistently answered yes.

DISCUSSION

Patients with severe life-threatening diseases or physical conditions may express concerns about not being kept alive. Providers should document these and encourage patients to execute advance directives while they are still able to do so. This patient had no advance directives but has witnesses to her repeated statements about not wanting to live like this. Competent adults have the right to refuse treatment, even if by doing so they hasten their own death. The health care providers should determine that she is competent and then ask several differently worded questions to clarify the patient's desire to die. Consistent responses would constitute the patient's desire to cease treatment, including artificial hydration and nutrition, in order to die.

ETHICAL AND LEGAL PRINCIPLES

- Competent adults have the legal right to choose to forego life-sustaining treatment, even if by doing so they hasten their death.
- The American Medical Association and other medical and nursing organizations support the ethical appropriateness of not imposing unwanted treatment on competent adults.
- By virtue of its delivery mechanism, artificial hydration and nutrition are considered to be medical treatments rather than simply the provision of food and water. The invasive nature of feeding tubes can be the grounds on which a patient refuses to continue this treatment.

pertension is sometimes seen following a stroke as the body attempts to increase cerebral blood flow.[8]

After a stroke, the patient is at risk for deep vein thrombosis in the weak or paralyzed lower extremity. This risk is related to immobility, loss of venous tone, and decreased muscle pumping activity in the leg. The most effective prevention is to keep the patient moving. Active range-of-motion exercises should be taught if the patient has voluntary movement in the affected extremity. For the patient with hemiplegia, passive range-of-motion exercises should be done several times a day. Additional measures often used to prevent deep vein thrombosis include positioning to minimize the effects of dependent edema and the use of elastic compression gradient stockings or support hose. Intermittent pneumatic compression stockings may be ordered for bedridden patients. The nursing assessment for deep vein thrombosis includes measuring the calf and thigh daily, observing swelling of the lower extremities, noting unusual warmth of the leg, and asking the patient about pain in the calf.

Musculoskeletal system. The nursing goal for the musculoskeletal system is to maintain optimal function. This is accomplished by the prevention of joint contractures and muscular atrophy. In the acute phase, range-of-motion exercises and positioning are important nursing interventions. Passive range-of-motion exercise is begun on the first day of hospitalization. If the stroke is due to subarachnoid hemorrhage, the movement is limited to the extremities. The patient is taught to actively exercise as soon as possible. Muscle atrophy secondary to lack of innervation and activity can develop within 1 month following stroke.

The paralyzed or weak side needs special attention when the patient is positioned. Each joint should be positioned higher than the joint proximal to it to prevent dependent edema. Specific deformities on the weak or paralyzed side that are characteristic of the patient with stroke include shoulder abduction; flexion contractures of the hand, wrist, and elbow; external rotation of the hip; and plantar flexion of the foot. Subluxation of the shoulder on the affected side is common and not preventable. However, careful positioning and moving of the affected arm may prevent the development of a painful shoulder condition. Immobilization of the affected upper extremity may precipitate a painful shoulder-hand syndrome.

Nursing interventions to optimize musculoskeletal function include (1) trochanter roll at the hip to prevent external rotation, (2) hand cones (not rolled wash clothes) to prevent hand contractures, (3) arm supports with slings and lap boards to prevent shoulder displacement, (4) avoidance of pulling the patient by the arm to avoid shoulder displacement, (5) footboards or high-topped tennis shoes to prevent footdrop, and (6) hand splints to reduce spasticity. Use of a footboard for the patient with spasticity is controversial. Rather than preventing plantar flexion (footdrop), the sensory stimulation of a footboard against the bottom of the foot increases plantar flexion. Likewise, there is disagreement whether hand splints facilitate or diminish spasticity. The decision regarding the use of footboard or hand splints is made on an individual patient basis.

Integumentary system. The skin of the patient with stroke is particularly susceptible to breakdown because of loss of sensation, diminished circulation, and immobility. The problem of skin integrity is compounded by the age of the patient, poor nutrition, dehydration, edema, and incontinence. The nursing plan for prevention of skin breakdown includes (1) pressure relief by position changes, special mattresses, or wheelchair cushions; (2) good skin hygiene; (3) emollients applied to dry skin; and (4) early mobility. The ideal position change schedule is side-back-side with a maximum duration of 2 hours for any position. Nurses should position the patient on the weak or paralyzed side for only 30 minutes. If an area of redness develops and does not return to normal color within 15 minutes of pressure relief, the epidermis and dermis are damaged. The damaged area should not be massaged because this may cause additional damage. Control of pressure is the single most important factor in both the prevention and treatment of skin breakdown. Vigilance and good nursing care are required to prevent pressure sores.

Gastrointestinal system. The stress of the illness contributes to a catabolic state that can interfere with recovery. Neurologic, cardiac, and respiratory problems are considered priorities in the acute phase of stroke. However, the nutritional needs of the patient require quick assessment and treatment. The patient may be initially on IV infusions to maintain fluid and electrolyte balance, as well as for administration of medications. Patients with severe impairment may require enteral or parenteral nutrition support. As the severity of stroke varies from mild to severe, individual assessment and planning for nutrition over time are necessary.

The first oral feeding should be approached with caution because the gag reflex may be impaired. Before initiation of feeding, the gag reflex may be assessed by gently stimulating the back of the throat with a tongue blade. If a gag reflex is present, the patient will gag spontaneously. If it is absent, the feeding should be deferred and exercises to stimulate swallowing should be started. The speech therapist or the occupational therapist is usually responsible for designing this program. However, the nurse may be called on to develop the program in some clinical settings.

To assess swallowing ability, the nurse should elevate the head of the bed to an upright position (unless contraindicated) and give the patient a small amount of crushed ice or ice water to swallow. If the gag reflex is present and the patient is able to swallow safely, the nurse may proceed with the feeding.

After careful assessment of swallowing, chewing, gag reflex, and pouching, oral feedings can be initiated. Mouth care before feeding helps stimulate sensory awareness and salivation and can facilitate swallowing. The patient should remain in a high Fowler's position, preferably in a chair with the head flexed forward for the feeding and for 30 minutes following feeding. Foods should be easy to swallow and provide enough texture, temperature (warm or cold), and flavor to stimulate a swallow reflex. Crushed ice can be used as a stimulant for swallowing. The patient is instructed to swallow and then swallow again. Pureed foods are not usually the best choice because they are often bland and too smooth and at room temperature by the time the patient is fed. Thin liquids are often difficult to swallow and may promote coughing. Milk products should be avoided because they tend to increase the viscosity of mucus and increase salivation. Food should be placed on the unaffected side of the mouth. The nurse should ensure that the atmosphere is unrushed and nonstressful. Each feeding must be followed by scrupulous oral hygiene because food tends to collect on the affected side of the mouth.

The most common bowel problem for the patient who has experienced a stroke is constipation. If the patient does not have a daily or every-other-day bowel movement, the patient should be checked for an impaction. In addition, if the patient has liquid stools, the patient should also be checked for stool impaction. Depending on the patient's fluid balance status and swallowing ability, fluid intake should be 1800 to 2000 ml/day and fiber intake up to 25 g/day. Physical activity also promotes bowel function. Laxative, suppositories, or stool softeners may be ordered if the patient does not respond to increased fluid and fiber.[17] Similarly, enemas are used only if suppositories and digital stimulation are ineffective because they cause vagal stimulation and increase ICP.

Table 55-8 Communication with a Patient Who Has Aphasia

1. Decrease environmental stimuli that may be distracting and disrupting to communication efforts.
2. Treat the patient as an adult.
3. Present one thought or idea at a time.
4. Keep questions simple or ask questions that can be answered with "yes" or "no."
5. Let the person speak. Do not interrupt. Allow time for the individual to complete thoughts.
6. Make use of gestures or demonstration as an acceptable alternative form of communication. Encourage this by saying "Show me. . ." or "Point to what you want."
7. Do not pretend to understand the person if you do not. Calmly say you do not understand and encourage the use of nonverbal communication, or ask the person to write out what he or she wants.
8. Speak with normal volume and tone.
9. Give the patient time to process information and generate a response before repeating a question or statement.
10. Allow body contact (e.g., the clasp of a hand or touching) as much as possible. Realize that touching may be the only way the patient can express feelings.
11. Organize the patient's day by preparing and following a schedule (the more familiar the routine, the easier it will be for the person with aphasia).
12. Do not push communication if the person is tired or upset. Aphasia worsens with fatigue and anxiety.

Urinary system. In the acute stage of stroke, the primary urinary problem is poor bladder control, resulting in incontinence. Efforts should be made to promote normal bladder function and avoid the use of indwelling catheters. If an indwelling catheter must be used initially, it should be removed as soon as the patient is medically and neurologically stable. Long-term use of the indwelling catheter is associated with urinary tract infections and delayed bladder retraining. An intermittent catheterization program may be used for patients with urinary retention because this procedure has less incidence of urinary infections. An alternative to intermittent catheterizations is the external catheter for male patients who are incontinent of urine. External catheters will not alleviate the problem of urine retention.

The bladder retraining program consists of (1) adequate fluid intake with the majority given between 8 AM and 7 PM; (2) scheduled toileting every 2 hours using bedpan, commode, or bathroom; and (3) noting signs of restlessness because this may indicate the need for urination.

Communication. During the acute stage of stroke, the nurses' role in meeting the psychologic needs of the patient is primarily supportive. An alert patient is usually anxious because of lack of understanding about what has happened and an inability to communicate or difficulty with communication. The patient is assessed both for the ability to speak and the ability to understand communication. The patient's response to simple questions can give the nurse a guideline for structuring explanations and instructions. If the patient cannot understand

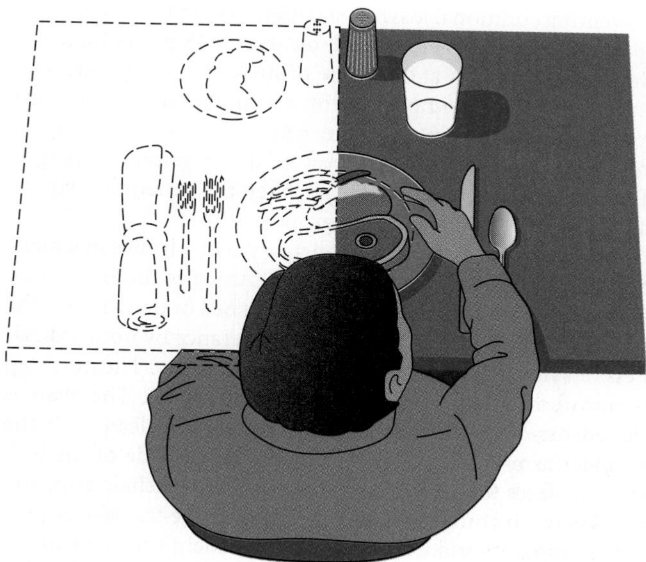

Fig. 55-9 Spatial and perceptual deficits in stroke. Perception of a patient with homonymous hemianopsia shows that food on the left side is not seen and thus is ignored.

words, gestures may be used to support verbal cues. It is helpful to speak slowly and calmly using simple words or sentences to enhance communication. The nurse must give the patient extra time to comprehend and respond to communication. The stroke patient with aphasia may easily be overwhelmed by verbal stimuli. (Guidelines for communicating with a patient who has aphasia are presented in Table 55-8.) Evaluation and treatment of language and communication deficits are often done by the speech pathologist after the patient has stabilized.

Sensory-perceptual alterations. Homonymous hemianopsia (blindness in the same half of each visual field) is a common problem after a stroke (Fig. 55-9). Persistent disregard of objects in part of the visual field should alert the nurse to this possibility. Initially, the nurse helps the patient to compensate by arranging the environment within the patient's perceptual field, such as arranging the food tray so that all foods are on the right side or the left side to accommodate for field of vision (see Fig. 55-9). Later, the patient learns to compensate for the visual defect by consciously attending or scanning the neglected side. The weak or paralyzed extremities are carefully noted for adequacy of dressing, for hygiene, and for trauma.

In the clinical situation it is often difficult to distinguish between a visual field cut and a neglect syndrome. Both problems may occur with strokes affecting either the right side or the left side of the brain. A person may be unfortunate enough to have both homonymous hemianopsia and a neglect syndrome, which increases the inattention to the weak or paralyzed side. A neglect syndrome results in decreased safety awareness and places the patient at high risk for injury. Immediately after the stroke, the nurse must anticipate potential safety hazards and provide protection from injury. Safety measures can include close observation of the patient by the nursing staff, elevating side rails, lowering the height of the bed, and video monitors. The use of restraints and soft vests is avoided because this may agitate the patient.

Other visual problems may include diplopia (double vision), loss of the corneal reflex, and ptosis (drooping eyelid), especially if the area of stroke is in the vertebrobasilar distribution. Diplopia is often treated with an eye patch. If the corneal reflex is absent, the patient is at risk for corneal abrasion and should be observed closely and protected against eye injuries. Corneal abrasion can be prevented with artificial tears or gel to keep the eyes moist. Ptosis is generally not treated because it usually does not inhibit vision.

Coping. A stroke is usually a sudden, extremely stressful event for the patient, close family members, and significant others. A stroke is often a family disease, affecting the family emotionally, socially, and financially, as well as changing roles and responsibilities within the family. An older couple may perceive the stroke as a very real threat to life and to accustomed lifestyle. Reactions to this threat vary considerably but may involve fear, apprehension, denial of the severity of stroke, depression, anger, and sorrow. During the acute phase of caring for the stroke patient and the family, nursing interventions designed to facilitate coping involve providing information and emotional support.

Explanations to the patient about what has happened and about diagnostic and therapeutic procedures should be clear and understandable. It will be particularly challenging to keep the aphasic patient adequately informed. Tone, demeanor, and touch may also be used to convey support.

The patient's family should be given a careful, detailed explanation of what has happened to the patient. However, if the family is extremely anxious and upset during the acute phase, explanations may have to be repeated at a later time. Because family members usually have not had time to prepare for the illness, they may need assistance in arranging care for family members or pets and for transportation and finances. A social services referral is often helpful.

Ambulatory and Home Care

Discharge planning. The patient is usually discharged from the acute care setting to home, an intermediate or long-term care facility, or a rehabilitation facility. Ideally, discharge planning with the patient and family starts early in the hospitalization and promotes a smooth transition from one care setting to another. The interdisciplinary team provides the guidance for the appropriate care required after discharge. If the patient requires a short- or long-term health care facility, the team can make appropriate referrals that allow time for family selection and arrangement of care. A critical factor in discharge planning is the patient's level of independence in performing ADLs. If the patient is returning home, the team can make referrals for needed equipment and services in preparation for discharge.

Nurses have an excellent opportunity to prepare the patient and family for discharge through education, demonstration and return demonstration, practice, and evaluation of self-care skills before discharge. Total care is considered in discharge planning: medications, nutrition, mobility, exercises, hygiene, and toileting. Follow-up care is carefully planned to permit continuing nursing, physical, occupational, and speech therapy, as well as medical care. Community resources should be identified to provide recreational activities, group support, spiritual assistance, respite care, adult day care, and home assistance based on the individual patient's needs.

Rehabilitation. *Rehabilitation* is the process of maximizing the patient's capabilities and resources to promote optimal functioning related to physical, mental, and social well-being. The goals of rehabilitation are to prevent deformity and maintain and improve function. Regardless of the care setting, ongoing rehabilitation is essential to maximize the patient's abilities.

The team approach to rehabilitation is used so the patient and family can benefit from the combined, expert care of the interdisciplinary team. The team must communicate and coordinate care to achieve the patient's and family's goals. The nurse is in a good position to facilitate this process and is often key to successful rehabilitation efforts. The patient's and family's participation in decision making during rehabilitation is essential to goal achievement after a stroke. The interdisciplinary team is composed of many members, including nurses, physicians, psychiatrist, physical therapist, occupational therapist, speech therapist, respiratory therapist, vocational therapist, recreational therapist, social worker, psychologist, pharmacist, and chaplains. Physical therapy focuses on mobility, progressive ambulation, transfer techniques, and equipment needed for mobility. Occupational therapy emphasizes retraining for skills of daily living such as eating, dressing, hygiene, and cooking. Occupational therapists are also skilled in cognitive and perceptual evaluation and training. Speech therapy focuses on speech, communication, cognition, and eating abilities.

Many of the nursing interventions outlined in the nursing care plan for the patient with stroke (see NCP 55-1) are initiated in the acute phase and continue throughout the rehabilitation phase of care. Some of the interventions are independent nursing actions, whereas others involve the entire rehabilitation team.

The rehabilitation nurse assesses the patient and family with attention to (1) rehabilitation potential of the patient, (2) physical status of all body systems, (3) presence of complications caused by the stroke or other chronic conditions, (4) cognitive status of the patient, (5) family resources and support, and (6) expectations of the patient and family related to the rehabilitation program.

The goals for rehabilitation of the patient with stroke are mutually set by the patient, family, nurse, and other members of the rehabilitation team. The rehabilitation goals typically include the following:

1. Learn techniques to self-monitor and maintain physical wellness
2. Demonstrate self-care skills
3. Exhibit problem-solving skills with self-care
4. Avoid complications associated with stroke
5. Establish and maintain a useful communication system
6. Maintain nutritional and hydration status
7. List community resources for equipment, supplies, and support
8. Establish flexible role behaviors to promote family cohesiveness

Musculoskeletal system. The nurse initially emphasizes the musculoskeletal functions of eating, toileting, and walking for the rehabilitation of the patient. The initial assessment consists of determining the stage of recovery of muscle function. If the muscles are still flaccid several weeks after the stroke, the prognosis for regaining function is poor and the focus of care is on preventing additional loss. Most patients begin to show signs of spasticity with exaggerated reflexes within 48 hours following the stroke. Spasticity at this phase of stroke denotes progress toward recovery. As improvement continues, small voluntary movements of the hip or shoulder may be accompanied by involuntary movements in the rest of the extremity (synergy). The final stage of recovery occurs when the patient has voluntary control of isolated muscle groups.

Interventions for musculoskeletal system advance in a manner of progressive activity. Balance training is the initial step and begins with the patient sitting up in bed or dangling on the edge of the bed. The nurse evaluates tolerance by noting dizziness or syncope caused by vasomotor instability. The next step is transferring from bed to chair or wheelchair. The chair is placed beside the bed so that the patient can lead with the stronger arm and leg. The patient sits on the side of the bed, stands, places the strong hand on the far wheelchair arm, and sits down. The nurse may either supervise the transfer or provide minimal assistance by guiding the patient's strong hand to the wheelchair arm, standing in front of the patient blocking the patient's knees with the nurse's knees to prevent knee buckling, and guiding the patient into a sitting position.

In some rehabilitation units the Bobath approach is used as a neurodevelopmental approach to mobility. The goal of the Bobath approach is to help the patient gain control over patterns of spasticity by inhibiting abnormal reflex patterns. Therapists and nurses use the Bobath approach to encourage normal muscle tone, normal movement, and promotion of bilateral function of the body. An example of the Bobath approach is to have the patient transfer into the wheelchair using the weak or paralyzed side and the stronger side to facilitate more bilateral functioning.

Supportive or assistive equipment, such as canes, walkers, and leg braces, may be needed on a short-term or long-term basis for mobility. The physical therapist usually selects and instructs the patient regarding the most appropriate supportive device(s) to meet individual needs. The nurse should incorporate physical therapy activities into the daily routine of the patient for additional practice and repetition of rehabilitation efforts.

Nutritional therapy. After the acute phase the registered dietician can assist in determining the appropriate daily caloric intake based on the patient's size, weight, and activity level. If the patient is unable to take in an adequate oral diet, enteral feedings via a nasogastric tube may be used. Most commercially prepared formulas provide about 1 calorie per milliliter. (Enteral feedings are described in Chapter 38.)

The nurse and speech therapist must assess the ability of the patient to swallow solids and fluids and adjust the diet appropriately. The registered dietician plans the diet type, texture, calorie count, and fluids to meet the patient's nutritional needs. The occupational therapist and nurse must evaluate the patient's ability to feed himself or herself and recommend assistive devices to allow for independent eating. Nurses are involved in the daily planning, implementation, and evaluation of the nutritional status of the patient.

The inability to feed oneself can be frustrating and may result in malnutrition and dehydration. Interventions to promote self-feeding include using the unaffected upper extremity to eat; employing assistive devices such as rocker knives, plate guards, and nonslip pads for dishes (Fig. 55-10); removing unnecessary items from the tray or table, which can reduce spills;

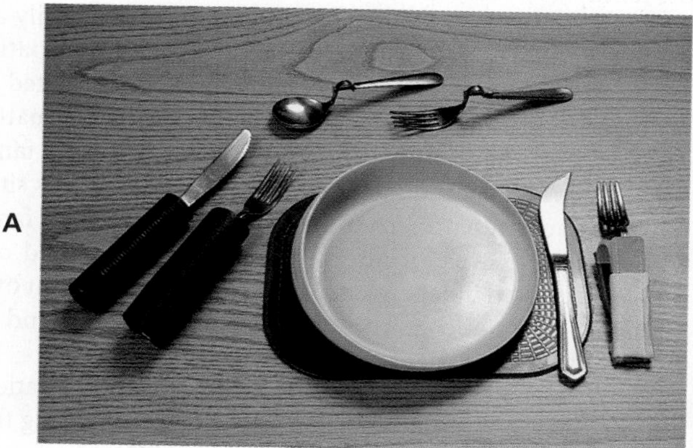

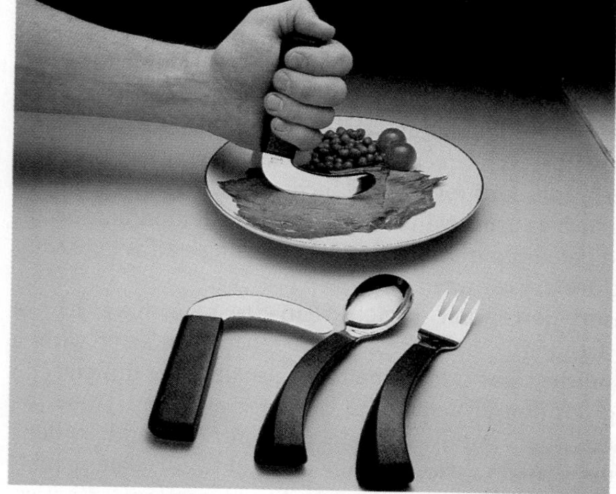

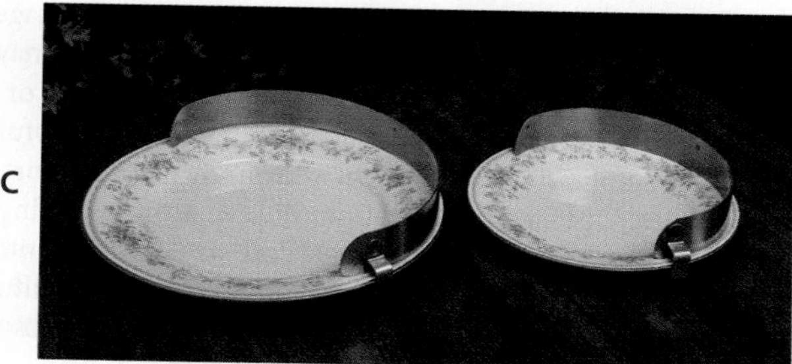

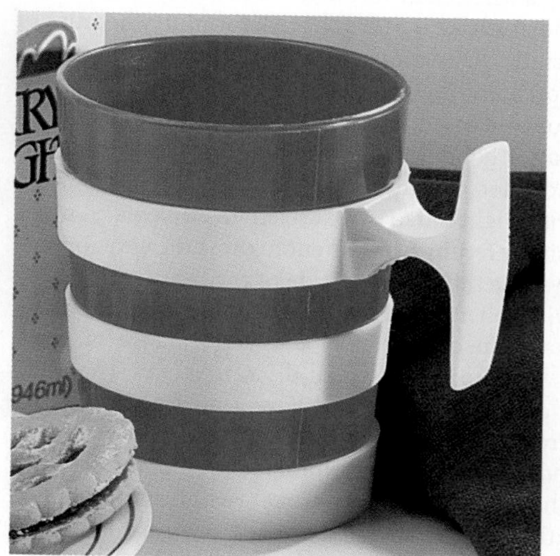

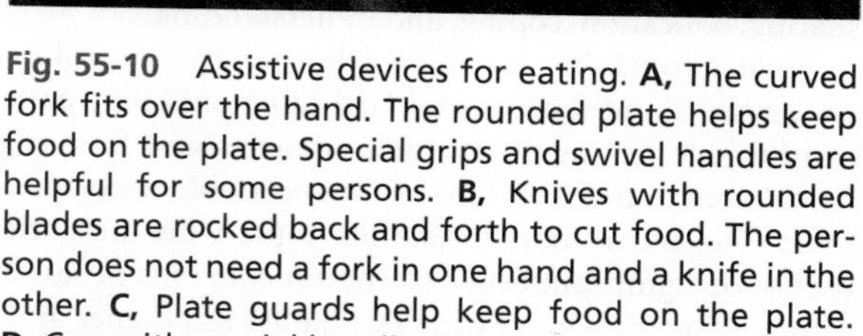

Fig. 55-10 Assistive devices for eating. **A,** The curved fork fits over the hand. The rounded plate helps keep food on the plate. Special grips and swivel handles are helpful for some persons. **B,** Knives with rounded blades are rocked back and forth to cut food. The person does not need a fork in one hand and a knife in the other. **C,** Plate guards help keep food on the plate. **D,** Cup with special handle.

and providing a nondistracting environment to decrease sensory overload and distraction. The effectiveness of the dietary program is evaluated in terms of maintenance of weight, adequate hydration, and patient satisfaction.

Elimination. A bowel management program is implemented for problems with bowel control, constipation, or incontinence. A high-fiber diet (see Table 40-9) and adequate fluid intake (2500 to 3000 ml) are usually recommended. Patients with stroke frequently have constipation, which responds to the following dietary management:

1. Fluid intake of 2500 to 3000 ml daily unless contraindicated
2. Prune juice (120 ml) or stewed prunes daily
3. Cooked fruit three times daily
4. Cooked vegetables three times daily
5. Whole-grain cereal or bread three to five times daily

The bowel management program for incontinence consists of placing the patient on the bedpan or bedside commode or taking the patient to the bathroom at a regular time daily to reestablish bowel regularity. A good time for the bowel program is 30 minutes after breakfast because eating stimulates the gastrocolic reflex and peristalsis. The time can be adjusted for individual bowel habits and preferred timing. Sitting on the commode or toilet promotes bowel elimination through both gravity and increased abdominal pressure. Stool softeners or suppositories may be ordered if the bowel program is ineffective in reestablishing bowel regularity. A glycerin suppository can be inserted 15 to 30 minutes before evacuation time to stimulate the anorectal reflex. The bisacodyl (Dulcolax) suppository is a chemical stimulant to the bowel and is used when other measures are ineffective. Ideally the suppository use is for short-term management.

Bladder function. The nurse often assists the patient with urinary difficulties or incontinence that may follow a stroke. Often the patient with stroke has functional incontinence, which is associated with communication difficulties, mobility problems, and dressing or undressing difficulties. Nursing interventions focused on urinary continence include (1) assessment for bladder distention by palpation; (2) offering the bedpan, urinal, commode, or toilet every 2 hours during waking hours and every 3 to 4 hours at night; (3) focusing the patient on the need to urinate with direct command; (4) assistance with clothing and mobility; (5) scheduling the majority of fluid intake between 7 AM and 7 PM; and (6) encouraging the usual position for urinating (standing for men and sitting for women). Short-term interventions for urinary incontinence may include indwelling catheters, intermittent catheterization, external catheters for men, or incontinent briefs. These are not long-term solutions for urinary incontinence because complications such as urinary infections or skin irritation may occur. A coordinated program by the entire nursing staff is needed to achieve urinary continence.

Sensory-perceptual system. Patients who have had a stroke frequently have perceptual deficits. Patients with a stroke on the right side of the brain usually have difficulty in judging position, distance, and rate of movement. These patients are often impulsive and impatient and tend to deny problems related to strokes. They may fail to correlate spatial-perceptual problems with the inability to perform activities, such as guiding a wheelchair through the doorway. The patient with a right-sided stroke is at higher risk for injury because of mobility difficulties. Directions for activities are best given verbally for comprehension. The task should be broken down to simple steps for ease of understanding. Environmental control such as less clutter, good lighting, and no obstacles aids in concentration and safer mobility. One-sided neglect is common for people with right-sided stroke (left hemiplegia), so the nurse may assist or remind the patient to dress the weak or paralyzed side or shave the forgotten side of the face.

Patients with a left-sided stroke (right hemiplegia) commonly are slower in organization and performance of tasks. They tend to have impaired spatial discrimination. These patients usually admit to deficits and have a fearful, anxious response to a stroke. Their behaviors are slow and cautious. Nonverbal cues and instructions are helpful for comprehension with patients who have had a left-sided stroke (right hemiplegia).

Affect. Patients who have had strokes often exhibit emotional responses that are not appropriate or typical for the situation. Patients may appear apathetic, depressed, fearful, anxious, weepy, frustrated, and angry. Some patients exhibit exaggerated mood swings, especially those with a stroke on the left side of the brain (right hemiplegia). The patient may be unable to control emotions and may suddenly burst into tears or laughter. This behavior is out of context and often is unrelated to the underlying emotional state of the patient. Nursing interventions for atypical emotional response are to (1) distract the patient who suddenly becomes emotional, (2) explain to the patient and family the reason for emotional outbursts, (3) maintain a calm environment, and (4) avoid shaming or scolding the patient during emotional outbursts.

Coping. The patient with a stroke may experience many losses, including sensory, intellectual, communicative, functional, role behavior, emotional, social, and vocational losses. The patient and family often go through the process of grief and mourning associated with the losses. Some patients experience long-term depression with symptoms such as anxiety, weight loss, loss of energy, poor appetite, and sleep disturbances.[18] In addition, the time and energy required to perform previously simple tasks can result in anger and frustration.

The patient and family need help with coping with the losses associated with stroke. The nurse may assist the coping by (1) supporting communication between the patient and family; (2) assisting with focusing on how stroke deficits will change lifestyle; (3) changing roles and responsibilities within the family; (4) being an active listener to allow the expression of fear, frustration, and anxiety; (5) including the family and patient in short- and long-term goal planning and patient care; and (6) supporting family conferences. Maladjusted dependence with inadequate coping occurs when the patient does not maintain optimal functioning for self-care, family responsibilities, decision making, or socialization. This situation can cause resentment from both the patient and family with a negative cycle of interpersonal dependency and control. Maladjusted independence occurs when the patient overestimates personal cognitive or physical capabilities and energy levels. These patients are at risk for injury.[19]

Family members must cope with three aspects of the patient's behavior: (1) recognition of behavioral changes resulting from neurologic deficits that are not changeable, (2) responses to multiple losses both by the patient and the family, and (3) behaviors that may have been reinforced during the early stages of stroke as continued dependency. The patient and family may express feelings of guilt over not living healthy lifestyles or not seeking professional help sooner. Family therapy is a helpful adjunct to rehabilitation. The patient and family need support and reassurance. Open communication, information regarding the total effects of stroke, education regarding stroke treatment, and therapy are helpful. Stroke support groups within rehabilitation facilities and in the community are helpful in terms of mutual sharing, education, coping, and understanding.

Sexual function. A patient who has had a stroke may be concerned about the loss of sexual function. Many patients are comfortable talking about their anxieties and fears regarding sexual function if the nurse is comfortable and open to the topic. The nurse may initiate the topic with the patient and spouse or significant other. Common concerns of sexual activity involving the patient with a stroke are impotence and the occurrence of another stroke during sex. Nursing interventions for sexual activity include education on (1) optional positioning of partners, (2) timing for peak energy times, and (3) patient and partner counseling.

Communication. Speech, comprehension, and language deficits are the most difficult problems for the patient and family. Speech therapists can assess and formulate a plan of care to support communication. The nurse can be a role model for communication with the patient who has aphasia. Nursing interventions that support communication include (1) frequent, meaningful communication; (2) allowing time for the patient to comprehend and answer; (3) using simple, short sentences; (4) using visual cues; (5) structuring conversation so that it permits simple answers by the patient; and (6) praising the patient honestly for improvements with speech.

Community integration. Traditionally, successful community integration following stroke may be difficult for the patient because of persistent problems with cognition, coping, physical deficits, and emotional lability that interfere with functioning. Older patients who have had a stroke often have more severe deficits and frequently experience multiple health problems. Advances in health care have resulted in an increased survival rate for patients with extensive stroke damage. Successful community integration can be redefined by the patient, family, and interdisciplinary health team as successful mobility, achievement of activities of daily living, and quality life with family and friends.

Community resources can be an asset to patients and their families. The National Stroke Association provides information, resources, referral services, and quarterly newsletters on stroke. The American Heart Association has information regarding stroke, hypertension, diet, exercise, and assistive devices. This association sponsors self-help groups in many areas. The Easter Seal Society provides wheelchairs and other assistive devices for stroke patients. Local groups can offer more daily assistance such as meals and transportation. These resources can be identified by nurse case managers, home health nurses, discharge planners, and clinical nurse specialists. (Resources are listed at the end of the chapter.)

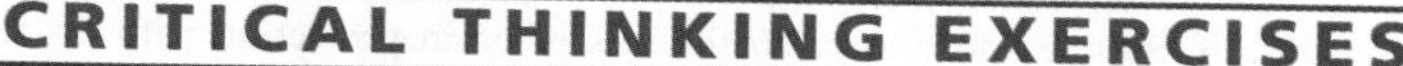

Stroke

Strokes are among the primary causes of death and disability among older adults. The highest incidence of stroke occurs among older adults. A stroke is a profound disruption for the life of an older person. The magnitude of disability and profound changes in total function can cause patients to wonder if they can ever return to their "old self." Changes in the totality of daily living require many disruptive changes because of current physical, emotional, perceptual, and cognitive deficits. Home management can be a challenge because often the patient has an elderly spouse caretaker who may also have health problems. There may be a limited number of family members (including adult children) who live in close proximity to the patient. This reduces the number of potential family caretakers. Middle-aged family members are becoming the "sandwich generation" caring for both old, ill parents and their own young families.

The nursing management of the older person who has had a stroke is a challenge. Skilled nursing care is obviously needed in the acute phase. However, the more demanding nursing challenge occurs in the rehabilitative phase in assisting the older patient to deal with residual deficits of stroke, as well as aging. These patients may become fearful and depressed because they think they may have another attack or die. The fear can become immobilizing and prevent effective rehabilitation.

There may be changes in the patient-spouse relationship. The dependency resulting from a stroke may be threatening to a previously stable marriage. The spouse may also have chronic medical problems that may affect the ability to take care of the stroke patient.

CRITICAL THINKING EXERCISES

CASE STUDY

Stroke

Patient Profile

John, a 76-year-old man, had a right-brain (left hemiplegic) stroke 2 months ago. Before the stroke, John, a retired engineer, had been an alert, involved person. He has been married for 40 years and has four adult children. He played golf and drove a car before the stroke. John has now returned home and is living with his wife. His past health history includes a 15 year history of hypertension, obesity, smokes one-half pack of cigarettes per day, moderate beer drinker, and had a myocardial infarction 5 years ago. He is eager to return to prior activity level.

Subjective Data

- Weakness in left arm and leg
- Speech difficulties, especially when tired
- Independent with ADLs
- Emotional instability and impulsive behaviors

Objective Data

Physical Examination

- Sensory impairment of the left side, especially the left hand
- Walks with a slight limp
- Slurred speech while using the phone or when fatigued
- Homonymous hemianopsia

Critical Thinking Questions

1. How does John's prior health history put him at risk for development of a stroke?
2. Are John's reported symptoms and behaviors typical of a person having a right-brain stroke?
3. How can John and his family address activity issues such as driving after the stroke?
4. What strategies might the home health nurse use to help John and his family cope with his emotional lability?
5. What lifestyle changes should John make to reduce the likelihood of another stroke?
6. How will homonymous hemianopsia affect John's hygiene, eating, driving, and golf game?
7. What factors should the nurse assess for in relation to further outpatient rehabilitation for John?
8. Based on the assessment data provided, write one or more nursing diagnoses. Are there any collaborative problems?

NURSING RESEARCH ISSUES

1. Determine the effectiveness of weight loss and stop smoking programs in reducing the incidence of strokes.
2. Examine the relationship between functional abilities and level of independence following a stroke.
3. Determine the effectiveness of nursing interventions to promote full-field visualization for patients with homonymous hemianopsia.
4. Examine the spouse-patient relationship and coping styles during the 6-month period following a stroke.
5. Examine the impact of stroke on socialization, quality of life, and loneliness.

One of the most difficult tasks in home management is helping the spouse or significant other who has to take care of the stroke patient. Living with these demands can be challenging for a younger person and can be even more so for the older spouse. The spouse may experience guilt if others try to help with care. The patient may not want anyone other than the spouse to provide care.

The nurse has the opportunity to aid the patient's and family's transition through acute hospitalization, rehabilitation, long-term care, and home care. The needs of the patient and family require continual nursing assessment, revision of interventions, and evaluation of changing health needs to optimize quality of life for the patient and family.

REVIEW QUESTIONS

The number of the question corresponds to the same-numbered objective at the beginning of the chapter.

1. Of the following patients the nurse recognizes that the one with the highest risk for a stroke is
   a. an obese 45-year-old Native-American.
   b. a 35-year-old Asian-American woman who smokes.
   c. a 32-year-old Caucasian woman on oral contraceptives.
   d. a 65-year-old African-American man with hypertension.
2. The factor related to cerebral blood flow that most often determines the extent of cerebral damage from a stroke is the
   a. amount of cardiac output.
   b. oxygen content of the blood.
   c. degree of collateral circulation.
   d. level of carbon dioxide in the blood.
3. Information provided by the patient that would help differentiate a thrombotic stroke from a hemorrhagic stroke includes
   a. a history of hypertension.
   b. a history of cardiac valvular disease.
   c. the type of early symptoms manifested.
   d. the patient's activity at the onset of symptoms.
4. A right-handed patient with hemiplegia and aphasia resulting from a stroke most likely has a lesion in the
   a. left frontal lobe.
   b. right brainstem.
   c. motor area of the right cerebrum.
   d. medial superior area of the paracentral lobule.
5. The nurse explains to the patient with a stroke who is scheduled for angiography that this test is used to determine the
   a. presence of increased ICP.
   b. site and size of the infarction.
   c. presence of blood in the CSF.
   d. patency of the cerebrovascular system.
6. A patient experiencing TIAs is scheduled for a carotid endarterectomy. The nurse explains that this procedure is done to
   a. promote cerebral blood flow to decrease cerebral edema.
   b. reduce the brain damage that occurs during a stroke-in-evolution.
   c. prevent a stroke by removing atherosclerotic plaques obstructing cerebral blood flow.
   d. provide a circulatory bypass around thrombotic plaques obstructing cranial circulation.
7. Nursing management of the patient with hemiplegia during the acute phase of a stroke includes
   a. using a footboard to prevent footdrop.
   b. positioning each joint higher than the proximal joint.
   c. performing passive range of motion on all limbs every 4 hours.
   d. maintaining the patient in a recumbent, side-lying position.
8. Bladder training in a male patient who has urinary incontinence after a stroke includes
   a. limiting fluid intake.
   b. keeping a urinal in place at all times.
   c. assisting the patient to stand to void.
   d. catheterizing the patient every 4 hours.
9. The most common response of the stroke patient to the change in body image is
   a. denial.
   b. depression.
   c. disassociation.
   d. intellectualization.

References

1. Kongable G: Code stroke: using t-PA to prevent ischemic brain injury, *AJN* 97:16BB, 1997.
2. *Statistical abstracts of the United States: the national data book,* ed 116, Washington, DC, 1996, US Department of Commerce, US Government Printing Office.
3. McCrory DC, Matchar DB: Stroke prevention: the emerging strategies, *Hosp Pract* 31:123, 1996.
4. Hennekens CH: Lessons from hypertension trials, *Am J Med* 104:50S, 1998.
5. Heinemann LA and others: Thromboembolic stroke in young women. A European case-control study on oral contraceptives, *Contraception* 57:29, 1998.
6. Sterz F and others: Possibilities of brain protection with tirilazad after cardiac arrest, *Semin Thromb Hemost* 22:105, 1996.
7. Hickey JV: *The clinical practice of neurological and neurosurgical nursing,* ed 4, Philadelphia, 1997, Lippincott.
8. Mower DA: Brain attack: treating acute ischemic CVA, *Nursing* 27:34, 1997.
9. Read SJ and others: Experience with diffusion-weighted imaging in an acute stroke unit, *Cerebrovasc Dis* 8:135, 1998.
10. Gonzalez ER: Antiplatelet therapy in atherosclerotic cardiovascular disease, *Clin Ther* 20:B18, 1998.
11. Diener HC: Antiplatelet drugs in secondary prevention of stroke, *Int J Clin Pract* 52:91, 1998.
12. Hallett JW and others: Comparison of North American Symptomatic Carotid Endarterectomy Trial and population-based outcomes for carotid endarterectomy, *J Vasc Surg* 27:845, 1998.
13. Kothari R: The biology of stroke and management of the stroke patient, *J Emerg Med Serv* 20:5, 1995.
14. Ball R: Treating stroke: new controversies in emergency care, *J Emerg Med Serv* 20:38, 1995.
15. Levine SR: Thrombolytic therapy for stroke: the new paradigm, *Hosp Pract* 32:57, 1997.
16. Moore K, Trifiletti E: Stroke: the first critical days, *RN* 57:22, 1994.
17. Hayn MA, Fisher TR: Stroke rehabilitation, *Nursing* 27:40, 1997.
18. Fowler S, Durkee CM, Webb DJ: Rehabilitating stroke patients in the acute care setting, *Medsurg Nurs* 5:327, 1996.
19. Brillhart B: Role-relationship pattern. In McCourt AE, editor: *The specialty practice of rehabilitation nursing: a core curriculum,* ed 3, Skokie, Ill, 1993, The Rehabilitation Nursing Foundation of the Association of Rehabilitation Nurses.

Resources

Academy of Aphasia (AA)
Boston Veterans Administration
Medical Center 116B
150 South Huntingdon Avenue
Boston, MA 02130
617-495-4342
http://cortex.neurology.umab.edu/academy/

American Association of Neuroscience Nurses (AANN)
218 North Jefferson Street, #204
Chicago, IL 60606
312-993-0043
http://www.aann.org/

American Brain Tumor Association
2720 River Road
Des Plaines, IL 60018
847-827-9910
800-886-2282
Fax: 847-827-9918
http://www.abta.org

Association of Rehabilitation Nurses (ARN)
4700 West Lake Avenue
Glenview, IL 60025-1485
847-375-4710
800-229-7530
Fax: 847-375-4777
http://www.rehabnurse.org/

Heart and Stroke Foundation of Canada
222 Queen Street, Suite 1402
Ottawa, Ontario K1P 5V9
CANADA
613-569-4361
Fax: 613-569-3278
http://www.hsf.ca/

Information Center for Individuals with Disabilities
Fort Point Place, First Floor
27-43 Wormwood Street
Boston, MA 02210-1606
617-727-5540

National Institute of Neurological and Communicative Disorders and Stroke
Division of Stroke and Trauma (grant applications)
Federal Building, Room 1016
7550 Wisconsin Avenue
Bethesda, MD 20892
301-496-4188

National Stroke Association
96 Inverness Drive East, Suite 1
Englewood, CO 80112-5112
303-649-9299
800-STROKES (787-6537)
Fax: 303-649-1328
http://www.stroke.org

Society for Neuroscience
11 Dupont Circle NW, Suite 500
Washington, DC 20036
202-462-6688
http://www.sfn.org/

Stroke Club International
805 12th Street
Galveston, TX 77550
409-762-1022

Stroke Foundation
898 Park Avenue
New York, NY 10021
800-367-1990

***For additional Internet resources, see the website for this book at* www.mosby.com/MERLIN/medsurg_lewis**

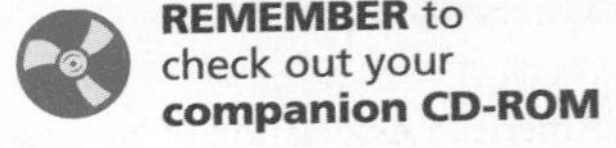

56 NURSING MANAGEMENT Chronic Neurologic Problems

Judith M. Ozuna

www.mosby.com/MERLIN/medsurg_lewis

LEARNING OBJECTIVES

1. Explain the potential impact of chronic neurologic disease on physical and psychologic well-being.
2. Compare and contrast tension-type, migraine, and cluster headaches in terms of etiology, clinical manifestations, and collaborative care and nursing management.
3. Describe the etiology, clinical manifestations, diagnostic studies, and collaborative management of epilepsy, multiple sclerosis, Parkinson's disease, and myasthenia gravis.
4. Explain the nursing role in the acute and chronic management of a patient with a chronic neurologic disease.
5. Describe the clinical manifestations and collaborative care of amyotrophic lateral sclerosis and Huntington's chorea.
6. Identify common physical complications in a patient who is immobilized by chronic neurologic disease.
7. Outline the major goals of treatment for the patient with a chronic, progressive neurologic disease.

Management of chronic neurologic diseases can be challenging for both the patient and the health care provider. Many neurologic disorders involve progressive deterioration in physical or mental capabilities, which can be devastating to the patient and the family. The patient may experience psychologic distress in the form of depression, fear, anxiety, anger, or withdrawal. This is compounded by changes in body image and self-esteem. In addition, the physical disabilities that result from degenerative diseases necessitate varying and sometimes extreme alterations in lifestyle, which add to the emotional trauma of the patient. Families are torn between their sense of obligation to care for the ill patient and the need to lead their own lives. They are simultaneously pushed and pulled by feelings of guilt, love, despair, hope, resentment, and empathy.

The challenge of chronic neurologic illness is equally great for health care providers. Many of these diseases have no cure. Therefore health care professionals can only attempt to alleviate physical symptoms, prevent complications, assist patients in maximizing self-care abilities in the face of neurologic deficits, and help them in the difficult task of adjusting to their illness. Nurses can and should greatly influence these aspects of management.

HEADACHE

Headache is probably the most common type of pain experienced by humans. Of all persons with headache, the majority have functional headaches, such as benign migraine or tension-type headaches; the remainder have organic headaches caused by significant intracranial or extracranial disease.

Not all tissues of the cranium are sensitive to pain. The pain-sensitive structures in the head include the venous sinuses, the dura (at the base of the brain near large blood vessels), cranial blood vessels, the three divisions of the trigeminal nerve (CN V), the facial nerve (CN VII), the glossopharyngeal nerve (CN IX), the vagus nerve (CN X), and the first three cervical nerves. Thus headache pain can arise from both intracranial and extracranial sources.

Headaches are classified based on the characteristics of the headache and the facial pain. The primary classifications include tension-type, migraine, and cluster headaches. Characteristics of these headaches are shown in Table 56-1. A patient may have more than one type of headache. The history and neurologic examination are diagnostic keys to determining the type of headache.

TENSION-TYPE HEADACHE

Tension-type headache is described as bilateral, dull, and nonpulsatile. Tension-type headache has been called muscle-contraction, tension, psychogenic, and rheumatic headache. It is the most common type of headache and is also considered the most difficult to treat. Tension-type headaches are often subcategorized as acute or episodic and chronic.

Etiology and Pathophysiology

It was originally thought that tension-type headache was the result of sustained and painful contraction of the muscles of the scalp and the neck. Recent evidence, however, does not support this mechanism in all patients with tension-type headaches. It

Reviewed by Patricia A. Blissett, RN, MSN, CCRN, CNRN, CCM, Staff Nurse, Neurosurgical Intensive Care Unit, Harborview Medical Center, Seattle, Wash.

Table 56-1 Comparison of Tension-type, Migraine, and Cluster Headaches

Pattern	Tension-type	Migraine	Cluster
Site	Bilateral, bandlike pressure at base of skull, in face, or in both	Unilateral (in 60%), may switch sides, commonly anterior	Unilateral, radiating up or down from one eye
Quality	Constant, squeezing tightness	Throbbing, synchronous with pulse	Severe, bone-crushing
Frequency	Cycles for several years	Periodic; cycles of several months to years	May have months or years between attacks; attacks occur in clusters: one to three times a day over a period of 4-8 wk
Duration	Intermittent for months or years	Continuous for hours or days	30 to 90 min
Time and mode of onset	Not related to time	May be preceded by prodrome; onset after awakening; gets better with sleep	Nocturnal; commonly awakens patient from sleep
Associated symptoms	Palpable neck and shoulder muscles, stiff neck, tenderness	Nausea or vomiting, edema, irritability, sweating, photophobia, prodrome of sensory, motor, or psychic phenomena; family history (in 65%)	Vasomotor symptoms such as facial flushing or pallor, unilateral lacrimation, ptosis, and rhinitis

is likely that both increased pain sensitivity and muscle factors contribute to the etiology of tension-type headaches.

Clinical Manifestations

There is no prodrome (early manifestation of impending disease) in tension-type headache. The pain is usually bilateral, occurring most often in the back of the neck. It usually does not interfere with sleep. The pain is often described as a tight, squeezing, bandlike pressure. It is sustained, chronic, dull, and persistent. The headaches may occur intermittently for weeks, months, or even years. Many patients can have a combination of migraine and tension-type headaches, with features of both headaches occurring simultaneously. Patients with migraine headaches may experience tension-type headaches between migraine attacks.

Diagnostic Studies

Careful history taking is probably the most important diagnostic tool for tension-type headache. Electromyography (EMG) may reveal sustained contraction of the neck, scalp, or facial muscles, but many patients may not show increased muscle tension with this test, even when the test is done during the actual headache. Conversely, patients with diagnosed migraine headaches may show increased muscle tension on EMG. If tension-type headache is present during physical examination, increased resistance to passive movement of the head and tenderness of the head and neck may be present.

MIGRAINE HEADACHE

Migraine headache is a benign, recurring headache characterized by unilateral or bilateral pain, a triggering event or factor, strong family history, and manifestations associated with neurologic and autonomic nervous system dysfunction. For some individuals migraine headaches begin in childhood or adolescence. A family history of migraine can be found in 65% of patients with migraine. Estimates of migraine prevalence in recent studies are about 6% in men and 15% to 18% in women.[1] Although migraine headaches have often been associated with patients who are high achievers and who suppress expressions of aggression and hostility, no single personality type describes all patients who experience migraine headache.

Etiology and Pathophysiology

In the past it was thought that migraine headaches had a vascular origin and involved the intracranial and extracranial arteries of the head. The classic theory of migraine headaches is that the prodromal or aural phase is associated with vasoconstriction and decreased blood flow. The headache phase is associated with vasodilation and increased blood flow. Although the exact etiology of migraine headaches is not known, evidence now suggests that neurologic, vascular, and chemical factors are involved.[2] The neurogenic model of migraine implies that a stimulus can trigger the trigeminovascular system (trigeminal nerve and its connections to meningeal blood vessels) resulting in inflammation of the blood vessels and vasodilation, resulting in headache. The neurotransmitter serotonin appears to play an important role in migraine headache progression.

Migraine headaches, in many cases, have no known precipitating events. However, for other patients, the headache may be precipitated or triggered by stress, excitement, bright lights, menstruation, alcohol, or certain foods such as chocolate or cheese.

The aura of migraine is associated with "spreading depression," a wave of oligemia (diminished cerebral blood flow) beginning in the occipital lobe and spreading forward in the brain at a rate of 2 to 3 mm per minute. The progression of oligemia does not correlate with blood vessel supply, so it is unlikely to be generated by the blood vessels themselves.

Clinical Manifestations

There are two major types of migraine headaches: migraine without aura (formerly called common migraine) and migraine with aura (formerly called classic migraine). Migraine without aura is the most common type of migraine headache. The prodrome is not sharply defined, and it can involve psychic disturbances, gastrointestinal upset, and changes in fluid balance. The prodrome may precede the headache phase by several hours or several days. The headache itself may last several hours or days.

Migraine with aura occurs in only 10% of migraine headache episodes. The sharply defined aura may last for 10 to 30 minutes before the start of the headache and may include sensory dysfunction (e.g., visual field defects, tingling or burning sensations, or paresthesias), motor dysfunction (e.g., weakness, paralysis), dizziness, confusion, and even loss of consciousness. The classic preheadache symptom is perception of flashing lights in one quadrant of the visual field, often termed *scintillating scotomata.* This type of migraine headache usually peaks in 1 hour and may last several hours.

Clinical manifestations that occur in migraine with and without aura are generalized edema, irritability, pallor, nausea and vomiting, and sweating. During the headache phase, patients with migraine tend to "hibernate"; that is, they seek shelter from noise, light, odors, people, and problems. The headache is described as a steady, throbbing pain that is synchronous with the pulse. Although the headache is usually unilateral, it may switch to the opposite side in another episode. The diagnosis of migraine headache is usually made from the history. The neurologic and other diagnostic examinations are often normal.

CLUSTER HEADACHE

Cluster headache is one of the most severe forms of head pain. Cluster headache occurs less frequently than migraine (the cluster headache to migraine frequency is 1:10) and is more frequent in men than in women by a ratio of 5:1. The onset is usually between 30 and 60 years of age.

Etiology and Pathophysiology

Neither the cause nor the pathophysiology of cluster headache is fully known. The vasodilation that occurs in the affected part of the face is extracranial. The trigeminal nerve is implicated in the production of pain. Activation of this nerve causes release of substance P and other vasoactive substances that cause vasodilation, stimulation of afferent pain fibers, and neurogenic inflammation with extravasation of protein and platelets in the perivascular areas. The periodicity and the clocklike regularity of cluster headache indicate a dysfunction of the biologic clock mechanisms of the hypothalamus.[3] These headaches can also be triggered by alcohol ingestion.

Clinical Manifestations

The headache has an abrupt onset, usually without a prodrome. It peaks in 5 to 10 minutes and lasts 30 to 90 minutes. It is not uncommon for this type of headache to start at night, awakening the patient after a few hours of sleep. Headaches may recur several times a day over a period of several days, with each cluster lasting 2 to 3 months. It usually affects the upper face, the periorbital region, and the forehead on one side of the face and the head. The headache may not recur for months or years. The patient may also exhibit conjunctivitis, increased lacrimation (tearing), and nasal congestion on the side of the headache. Sweating may occur on the forehead of the affected side. A partial Horner's syndrome (miosis [constriction of the pupil] and ptosis [drooping of the eyelid on the affected side]) may be seen. The headache is described as deep, steady, and penetrating but not throbbing.

Unlike the patient with migraine, who seeks isolation and quiet, the patient with a cluster headache paces the floor, cries out, does bizarre things, and resents being touched. The patient with a cluster headache does not experience the systemic manifestations that accompany a migraine headache, such as nausea or vomiting. As with migraine headaches, there are usually no complications.

DIAGNOSTIC STUDIES

Table 56-2 Patient with Headache

- Complete health history
- Clinical examination (often negative)
  - Inspect for local infections
  - Palpation for tenderness, hardened arteries, bony swellings
  - Auscultation for bruits over major arteries
- Routine laboratory studies to rule out underlying causes of headache
  - CBC
  - Electrolytes
  - Urinalysis
- CT scan of sinuses
- Special studies (e.g., CT scan, angiography, EMG, EEG, MRI)

CBC, complete blood count; *CT,* computed tomography; *EEG,* electroencephalography; *EMG,* electromyography; *MRI,* magnetic resonance imaging.

Diagnostic Studies

The diagnosis of cluster headache is primarily based on the history. However, computed tomography (CT) scan, magnetic resonance imaging (MRI), or cerebral angiography may be performed to rule out an aneurysm, tumor, or infection.

OTHER TYPES OF HEADACHES

Although tension, migraine, and cluster headaches are by far the most common types of headaches, other types of headache can also occur. These headaches may be the first symptom of a more serious illness. Headache can accompany subarachnoid hemorrhage; brain tumors; other intracranial masses; arteritis; vascular abnormalities; trigeminal neuralgia (tic douloureux); diseases of the eyes, nose, and teeth; and systemic illness (e.g., bacteremia, carbon monoxide poisoning, mountain sickness, polycythemia vera). The symptoms vary greatly. Because of the variety of causes of headache, clinical evaluation must be thorough. It should include an evaluation of personality, life adjustment, environment, and family situation, as well as a comprehensive evaluation of physical status.

Collaborative Care: Headache

If no systemic underlying disease is found, therapy is directed toward the functional type of headache. Table 56-2 outlines the general workup for a patient with headache to rule out any intracranial or extracranial disease. Table 56-3 summarizes the current therapies for symptomatic relief of common headaches. These therapies include medications, meditation, yoga, biofeedback, and muscle relaxation training.

Biofeedback involves the use of physiologic monitoring equipment to give the patient information regarding muscle tension and peripheral blood flow (skin temperature of the fingers). The patient is trained to relax the muscles and raise the finger temperature and is given reinforcement (operant conditioning) in accomplishing these physiologic alterations.

COLLABORATIVE CARE

Table 56-3 Headache

	Tension-type Headache	Migraine Headache	Cluster Headache
Diagnostic	History of neck and head tenderness, resistance to movement, EMG	History	History, thermography
Collaborative Therapy			
▪ Symptomatic	Nonnarcotic analgesics (aspirin, acetaminophen, ibuprofen) Analgesic combinations (butalbital [Fiorinal]) Muscle relaxants	Nonnarcotic analgesics (aspirin, acetaminophen, ibuprofen) Serotonin receptor agonist (sumatriptan [Imitrex], zolmitriptan [Zomig], naratriptan [Amerge], rizatriptan [Maxalt]) Alpha-adrenergic blockers (ergotamine tartrate [Ergomar]) Vasoconstrictors (isometheptene [Midrin]) Corticosteroids (dexamethasone)	Alpha-adrenergic blockers (ergotamine tartrate) Vasoconstrictors Oxygen
▪ Prophylactic	Tricyclic antidepressants (doxepin [Sinequan], amitriptyline [Elavil]) Beta-adrenergic blockers (propranolol [Inderal]) Biofeedback Muscle relaxation training Psychotherapy	Beta-adrenergic blockers (propranolol) Serotonin antagonists* (methysergide [Sansert]) Antidepressants (amitriptyline, imipramine) Calcium channel blockers (verapamil [Isoptin]) Divalproex (Depakote) Biofeedback Yoga Meditation Electric counterstimulation	Alpha-adrenergic blockers (ergotamine tartrate) Serotonin antagonists (methysergide) Corticosteroids (prednisone) Lithium Calcium channel blockers (verapamil) Divalproex (Depakote)

*Only for patients suffering from one or more severe headaches per week.
EMG, electromyography.

Acupuncture, acupressure, and hypnosis are successful innovative therapies that work well in some patients with headaches. Some patients can benefit from psychotherapy that is aimed at helping them recognize conflicts and deal with them more effectively. Treatments for tension-type headache include physical therapy (e.g., massage, hot packs, cervical collar), injection of local anesthetic into spastic muscles, and correction of faulty posture.

Drug Therapy

Tension-type headache. Drug treatment for tension-type headache usually involves a nonnarcotic analgesic (e.g., aspirin, acetaminophen) used alone or in combination with a sedative, a muscle relaxant, a tranquilizer, or codeine. However, many of these drugs have potentially dangerous side effects. The patient should be cautioned about the long-term use of aspirin and aspirin-containing drugs because they can cause gastric bleeding and coagulation abnormalities in susceptible patients. Long-term use of Fiorinal should be avoided because in addition to aspirin it contains a barbiturate (butalbital), which may be habit forming. Drugs containing acetaminophen (Tylenol, Phenaphen, Midrin) can cause kidney damage with chronic use and liver damage when combined with alcohol. Daily use of nonsteroidal antiinflammatory drugs (NSAIDs) can cause chronic daily headaches. Narcotics and benzodiazepines can cause addiction and habituation. Discontinuing an overused medication too abruptly can lead to withdrawal symptoms (analgesic rebound).

Migraine headache. Drug treatment of the acute migraine attack is aimed at terminating or decreasing the symptoms of the attack. Many people with mild or moderate migraine can obtain relief with aspirin or acetaminophen. Ergotamine (Ergomar) is often used when simple analgesics do not relieve headache. Ergotamine inhibits the reuptake of neuronally liberated norepinephrine into storage sites of the postganglionic nerve terminal of the sympathetic nervous system. This allows more norepinephrine to attach to alpha-adrenergic sites on smooth muscle in the artery wall, thereby causing prolonged vasoconstriction of cranial vessels. Ergotamine can be administered orally, sublingually, parenterally, rectally, or by inhalation. The usual dosage is 1 to 2 mg (oral or rectal) at the onset of the headache, followed by 2 mg within 1 hour. No more than 6 mg is given for any single attack. Dihydroergotamine mesylate is available as a nasal spray called Migranal. Other drugs that may relieve migraine headache include butalbital with aspirin or acetaminophen (Fiorinal, Fioricet), isometheptene with acetaminophen and dichloralphenazone (Midrin), and, in certain cases, narcotics.

Drugs that affect serotonin have been found to relieve migraine headaches. Sumatriptan (Imitrex), which is selective for vascular serotonin receptors, produces vasoconstriction and is used for the management of acute migraine headaches. In addition, sumatriptan inhibits the release of pain-producing inflammatory neuropeptides such as substance P, thus interfering with pain transmission. Sumatriptan can be given subcutaneously, orally, or nasally. It is a currently the drug of choice for acute management of migraine headaches. Newer agents that work via a serotonergic mechanism to constrict cerebral blood vessels include zolmitriptan (Zomig), naratriptan (Amerge), and rizatriptan (Maxalt). Similar to sumatriptan, these drugs can cause chest pain and are avoided in patients with heart disease.

A variety of drugs are used to prevent further tension-type and migraine attacks. Methysergide (Sansert) is an ergot alkaloid that competitively blocks serotonin receptors in the central and peripheral nervous systems. This drug has been found to be effective in the prevention of migraine headaches. However, because of side effects, including retroperitoneal, pulmonary, and cardiac fibrosis, the patient requires regular follow-up. It is recommended that a patient take a break ("drug holiday") every 4 to 6 months.

Other drugs taken daily to prevent recurrence of very severe or very frequent migraine headaches include β-adrenergic blockers (e.g., propranolol [Inderal], atenolol [Tenormin]), tricyclic antidepressants (e.g., amitriptyline [Elavil]), selective serotonin reuptake inhibitors (e.g., fluoxetine [Prozac]), calcium channel blockers (verapamil [Isoptin]), divalproex (Depakote), clonidine (Catapres), thiazides, and lithium.

Cluster headache. Because cluster headaches occur suddenly, often at night, and are not long lasting, drug therapy is not as useful as it is for the other types of headache. Prophylactic medications may include verapamil, lithium, ergotamine, divalproex (Depakote), or NSAIDs. Acute treatment of cluster headache is inhalation of 100% oxygen delivered at a rate of 7 to 9 L/min for 15 to 20 minutes, which may relieve headache by causing vasoconstriction. It can be repeated after a 5-minute rest. However, a drawback to this treatment is that the patient must have continuous access to the oxygen supply. Sumatriptan is also effective in treating acute cluster headache. Methysergide may be used prophylactically when the cluster headache recurs at a known time.

NURSING MANAGEMENT: HEADACHES

Nursing Assessment

Subjective and objective data that should be obtained from a patient with headache are presented in Table 56-4. Because the history provides the key to assessment of headache, it should include specific details of the headache itself, such as the location and type of pain, the onset, the frequency, the duration, the relation to events (emotional, psychologic, physical), and the time of day of the occurrence. Information about previous illnesses, surgery, trauma, allergies, family history, and response to medication should also be obtained. The nurse can suggest that the patient keep a diary of headache episodes with specific details. This type of record can be of great help in determining the type of headache and the precipitating events. If the patient has a history of migraine, tension-type, or cluster headaches, it is important to determine if the character, intensity, or location of the headache has changed. This may be an important clue as to the cause of the headache.

Nursing Diagnoses

Nursing diagnoses for the patient with headache may include, but are not limited to, those presented in NCP 56-1.

NURSING ASSESSMENT

Table 56-4 Headaches

Subjective Data

Important Health Information

Past health history: Hypertension, seizures, cancer, recent fall or trauma, cranial infection, craniotomy; cerebrovascular accident; asthma or allergies; mental illness; relationship of headache to overwork, stress, menstruation, exercise, food, sexual activity, travel, bright lights, or other noxious environmental stimuli

Medications: Use of hydralazine, bromides, nitroglycerin, ergotamine (withdrawal), nonsteroidal antiinflammatory drugs (in high daily doses), estrogen preparations, oral contraceptives, over-the-counter or prescription remedies

Surgery or other treatments: Craniotomy, sinus surgery, facial surgery

Functional Health Patterns

Health perception–health management: Positive family history; malaise

Nutritional-metabolic: Ingestion of alcohol, caffeine, cheese, chocolate, monosodium glutamate, aspartame, lunch meats (nitrites in cured meats), sausage, hot dogs, onions, avocados; anorexia, nausea, vomiting (migraine prodrome); unilateral lacrimation (cluster)

Activity-exercise: Vertigo, fatigue, weakness, paralysis, fainting

Sleep-rest: Insomnia

Cognitive-perceptual:

Migraine: aura; unilateral, severe, throbbing (possible switching of side) headache; visual disturbances; photophobia; phonophobia; dizziness; tingling or burning sensations

Cluster: unilateral and severe, nocturnal headache; nasal stuffiness

Tension-type: bilateral, band-like, dull and persistent, base of skull headache, neck tenderness

Self-perception–self-concept: Depression

Coping–stress tolerance: Stress, anxiety, irritability, withdrawal

Objective Data

General

Anxiety, apprehension

Integumentary

Cluster: forehead diaphoresis, pallor, unilateral facial flushing with cheek edema, conjunctivitis

Migraine: generalized edema (prodrome), pallor, diaphoresis

Neurologic

Horner's syndrome, restlessness (cluster), hemiparesis (migraine)

Musculoskeletal

Resistance of head and neck movement, nuchal rigidity (meningeal, tension-type), palpable neck and shoulder muscles (tension-type)

Possible Findings

Possible evidence of disease, deformity, or infection on brain imaging (CT, MRI), cerebral arteriogram, lumbar puncture, electroencephalogram, electromyography; nonspecific brain imaging or laboratory tests

56-1 NURSING CARE PLAN PATIENT WITH HEADACHE

Expected Patient Outcomes	Nursing Interventions and *Rationales*
NURSING DIAGNOSIS	Pain *related to* headache *as manifested by* complaint of steady, throbbing, or severe crushing pain.
▪ Reduced pain. ▪ Satisfaction with pain relief.	▪ Assess pain intensity, characteristics, location, and duration *to determine appropriate interventions.* ▪ Encourage patient to keep a pain log including associated factors or precipitators *to provide patient some control in identifying and controlling factors that may precipitate headaches.* ▪ Encourage patient to learn and use alternative therapies such as meditation, yoga, biofeedback, and muscle-relaxation techniques *to supplement drug therapy and provide the patient with some sense of control over pain.* ▪ Support patient's use of counseling or psychotherapy *to enhance stress reduction.* ▪ Administer drugs as ordered *to reduce pain.** ▪ Monitor patient following administration of pain medication *to assess drug efficacy and identify adverse drug effects.* ▪ Provide a quiet, dimly lighted environment *to reduce stimuli that may trigger headaches.* ▪ Massage head/neck/shoulder area as tolerated *to relieve muscle tension and promote relaxation.*
NURSING DIAGNOSIS	**Anxiety** *related to* lack of knowledge about headache's etiology and ways to treat it *as manifested by* increased heart rate, insomnia, feeling of helplessness.
▪ Increased psychologic comfort and decreased anxiety. ▪ Effective coping mechanisms to manage anxiety.	▪ Assess level of anxiety *to determine appropriate interventions.* ▪ Encourage patient to verbalize concerns *because this reduces anxiety.* ▪ Teach relaxation techniques and coping strategies *to promote muscle relaxation and reduce anxiety.* ▪ Explain possible etiology of patient's specific headache type *to reduce patient's fear of unknown.* ▪ Reinforce physician's explanation of diagnostic tests *to relieve concerns about cause and seriousness of headache.* ▪ Discuss the physiologic dynamics of tension/anxiety *because knowledge about how these factors influence headache can help with management.*
NURSING DIAGNOSIS	**Hopelessness** *related to* chronic pain, alteration of lifestyle, and ineffective treatment modalities *as manifested by* expressions of extreme apathy and listlessness, lack of interest in doing usual activities.
▪ Expression of confidence in ability to function despite headaches.	▪ Assess patient's degree of hopelessness *to enable appropriate planning.* ▪ Explore patient's self-treatment of pain and alterations in lifestyle *to identify appropriateness and make appropriate adjustments.* ▪ Promote verbalization of fears and concerns *to convey empathy and correct patient's misconceptions.* ▪ Assist patient in identifying support systems that can be used *to bolster hopefulness.* ▪ Initiate referrals as indicated for counseling *to continue work on feeling of hopelessness.*
NURSING DIAGNOSIS	**Sleep pattern disturbance** *related to* pain *as manifested by* inability to maintain usual sleep pattern.
▪ Use effective strategies to get to and maintain sleep. ▪ Feeling rested.	▪ Assess patient's usual sleep pattern *to determine appropriate interventions.* ▪ Reduce external stimuli *to provide a calm environment conducive to sleep.* ▪ Use massage or relaxation techniques *to facilitate relaxation and sleep.* ▪ Schedule analgesia administration *so maximum effect for headache relief will coincide with bedtime.* ▪ Medicate for pain if patient awakens with headache pain *to foster return to sleep and pain-free awakening.*

*See Table 56-3.

Planning

The overall goals are that the patient with a headache will (1) have reduced or no pain, (2) experience increased comfort and decreased anxiety, (3) demonstrate understanding of triggering events and treatment strategies, and (4) use positive coping strategies to deal with chronic pain.

Nursing Implementation

Patients with chronic headache present a great challenge to health care providers. Headaches may result from an inability to cope with daily stresses. The most effective therapy may be to help patients examine their lifestyle, recognize stressful situations, and learn to cope with them more appropriately. Precipitating factors can be identified, and ways of avoiding them can be developed. Daily exercise, relaxation periods, and socializing can be encouraged, since each can help decrease the recurrence of headache. The nurse can suggest alternative ways of handling the pain of headache through techniques such as relaxation, meditation, yoga, and self-hypnosis.

In addition to using analgesics and analgesic combination drugs for the symptomatic relief of headache, the patient should be encouraged to use relaxation techniques because they are effective in tension-type and migraine headaches. The migraine sufferer often needs a quiet, dimly lit environment. Massage and moist hot packs to the neck and head can help a patient with tension-type headaches. The patient should learn about the medications prescribed for prophylactic and symptomatic treatment of headache and should be able to describe the purpose, action, dosage, and side effects of the medication. To prevent accidental overdose, the patient should make a written note of each dose of medication or headache remedy.

For the patient whose headaches are triggered by food, dietary counseling may be provided. The patient is encouraged to eliminate foods that may provoke headaches, such as vinegar, chocolate, onions, alcohol (particularly red wine), excessive caffeine, cheese, fermented or marinated foods, monosodium glutamate, and aspartame. Active challenge and provocative testing with specific foods may be necessary to determine the specific causative agents.[4] Patients should avoid smoking and exposure to triggers such as strong perfumes, volatile solvents, and gasoline fumes. Cluster headache attacks may occur at high altitudes with low oxygen levels during air travel. Ergotamine, taken before the plane takes off, may decrease the likelihood of these attacks. A teaching guide for the patient with a headache is listed in Table 56-5.

PATIENT TEACHING GUIDE

Table 56-5 Headache

1. Avoid factors that can trigger a headache:
   - Foods containing amines (cheese, chocolate), nitrites (meats such as hot dogs), vinegar, onions, fermented or marinated foods
   - Monosodium glutamate
   - Caffeine
   - Nicotine
   - Ice cream
   - Alcohol (particularly red wine)
   - Emotional stress
   - Fatigue
   - Medications such as ergot-containing and monoamine oxidase inhibitors
2. Able to describe the purpose, action, dosage, and side effects of medications taken
3. Able to self-administer sumatriptan subcutaneously if prescribed
4. Use stress-reduction techniques such as relaxation
5. Participate in regular exercise
6. Keep a diary or calendar of headaches and possible precipitating events
7. Contact health care provider if the following occur:
   - Symptoms become more severe, last longer than usual, or are resistant to medication
   - Nausea, vomiting, change in vision, or fever occur with the headache
   - Problems with medications

Evaluation

Expected outcomes for the patient with headache are addressed in NCP 56-1.

SEIZURE DISORDERS AND EPILEPSY

A *seizure* is a paroxysmal, uncontrolled electrical discharge of neurons in the brain that interrupts normal function. Seizures are frequently symptoms of an underlying illness. They may accompany a variety of disorders, or they may occur spontaneously without any apparent cause. Seizures resulting from systemic and metabolic disturbances are not considered epilepsy if the seizures cease when the underlying problem is corrected. In the adult, metabolic disturbances that cause seizures include acidosis, electrolyte imbalances, hypoglycemia, hypoxia, alcohol and barbiturate withdrawal, dehydration, and water intoxication. Extracranial disorders that can cause seizures are heart, lung, liver, or kidney disease; systemic lupus erythematosus, diabetes mellitus; hypertension; and septicemia.

Epilepsy is a condition in which a person has spontaneously recurring seizures caused by a chronic underlying condition. Over 2 million people in the United States have epilepsy.[5] The incidence rates are high during the first year of life, decline through childhood and adolescence, plateau in middle age, and rise sharply again among the elderly.[5]

Etiology and Pathophysiology

The most common causes of epilepsy during the first 6 months of life are severe birth injury, congenital defects involving the central nervous system (CNS), infections, and inborn errors of metabolism. In patients between 2 and 20 years of age, the primary causative factors are birth injury, infection, trauma, and genetic factors. In individuals between 20 and 30 years of age, epilepsy usually occurs as the result of structural lesions, such as trauma, brain tumors, or vascular disease. After 50 years of age the primary causes of epilepsy are cerebrovascular lesions and metastatic brain tumors. Although many causes of epilepsy have been identified, three fourths of all epilepsy cases cannot be attributed to a specific cause and are considered idiopathic.

The role of heredity in the etiology of epilepsy has been difficult to determine because of the problem of separating hereditary from environmental or acquired influences. In addition, some families carry a predisposition to epilepsy in the form of an inherently low threshold to seizure-producing stimuli, such as trauma, disease, and high fever. For example, an inherently low seizure threshold may explain the reason some patients develop seizures after a head injury or similar insult, whereas others do not.

In recurring seizures (epilepsy) a group of abnormal neurons (seizure focus) seems to undergo spontaneous firing. This firing spreads by physiologic pathways to involve adjacent or distant areas of the brain. If this activity spreads to involve the whole brain, a generalized seizure occurs. The factor that causes this abnormal firing is not clear. Any stimulus that causes the cell membrane of the neuron to depolarize induces a tendency to spontaneous firing. Often the area of the brain from which the epileptic activity arises is found to have scar tissue (gliosis). The scarring is thought to interfere with the normal chemical and structural environment of the brain neurons, making them more likely to fire abnormally.

Repetitive electrical discharges from an epileptic focus in experimental animals can produce long-lasting and possibly permanent changes in neuron excitability, both locally and in distant areas of the brain. This effect is called *kindling,* and it presents an interesting and important implication for epilepsy in humans: seizures can beget more seizures. Clinical experience indicates that the longer a patient goes without good seizure control, the lower the likelihood that the seizures will be controllable. Therefore a vigorous attempt must be made to control recurring seizures.

Table 56-6 International Classification of Epileptic Seizures

Generalized Seizures (bilaterally symmetric and without local onset)
- Absence seizures, atypical absence seizures
- Myoclonic seizures
- Clonic seizures
- Tonic seizures
- Tonic-clonic seizures
- Atonic seizures

Partial Seizures (local onset)
- Simple partial seizures (no impairment of consciousness)
  - With motor symptoms
  - With somatosensory or special sensory symptoms
  - With autonomic symptoms
  - With psychic symptoms
- Complex partial seizures (impairment of consciousness)
  - Simple partial seizures with progression to impairment of consciousness
    - With no other features
    - With features of simple partial seizures
    - With automatisms
  - Impairment of consciousness at onset
    - With no other features
    - With features of simple partial seizures
    - With automatisms

Unclassified Epileptic Seizures (inadequate or incomplete data)

Modified from Commission on Classification and Terminology of the International League against Epilepsy: Proposal for revised clinical and electroencephalographic classification of epileptic seizures, *Epilepsia* 22:489, 1981.

Clinical Manifestations

The specific clinical manifestations of a seizure are determined by the site of the electrical disturbance. The preferred method of classifying epileptic seizures is the International Classification System proposed by Gastaut in 1970 and revised in 1981 (Table 56-6).[6,7] This system is based on the clinical and electroencephalographic manifestations of seizures. In this system, seizures are divided into two major classes: generalized and partial. Depending on the type, a seizure may progress through several phases, which include (1) the prodromal phase with signs or activity, which precede a seizure; (2) the aural phase with a sensory warning; (3) the ictal phase with full seizure; and (4) postictal phase, which is the period of recovery after the seizure.

Generalized Seizures. Generalized seizures are characterized by bilateral synchronous epileptic discharge in the brain from the onset of the seizure. Because the entire brain is affected at the onset of the seizures, there is no warning or aura. In most cases, the patient loses consciousness for a few seconds to several minutes.

Tonic-clonic seizures. The most common generalized seizure is the generalized tonic-clonic, or grand mal, seizure. This seizure is characterized by loss of consciousness and falling to the ground if the patient is upright, followed by stiffening of the body (tonic phase) for 10 to 20 seconds and subsequent jerking of the extremities (clonic phase) for another 30 to 40 seconds. Cyanosis, excessive salivation, tongue or cheek biting, and incontinence may accompany the seizure.

In the postictal phase the patient usually has muscle soreness, is very tired, and may sleep for several hours. Some patients may not feel normal for several hours or days after a seizure. The patient has no memory of the seizure activity.

Typical absence seizures. The absence (petit mal) seizure usually occurs only in children and rarely continues beyond adolescence. This type of seizure may cease altogether as the child matures, or it may evolve into another type of seizure. The typical clinical manifestation is a brief staring spell that lasts only a few seconds, so it often occurs unnoticed. There may be an extremely brief loss of consciousness. When untreated, the seizures may occur up to 100 times a day.

The electroencephalogram (EEG) demonstrates a 3 Hz (cycles per second) spike-and-wave pattern that is unique to this type of seizure. Absence seizures can often be precipitated by hyperventilation and flashing lights.

Atypical absence seizures. Another type of generalized seizure is the staring spell accompanied by other signs and symptoms, including brief warnings, peculiar behavior during the seizure, or confusion after the seizure. The EEG demonstrates atypical spike-and-wave patterns, usually greater or less than 3 Hz.

Other types of generalized seizures. Other generalized seizures are myoclonic and akinetic seizures. A myoclonic seizure is characterized by a sudden, excessive jerk of the body or extremities. The jerk may be forceful enough to hurl the person to the ground. These seizures are very brief and may occur in clusters. The terms *akinetic* (arrest of movement), *atonic* (loss of tone), and *astatic* (loss of balance) have been used interchangeably to describe drop attacks or falling spells. This type of seizure involves either a tonic episode or a paroxysmal loss of muscle tone and begins suddenly with the person falling to the ground. Consciousness usually returns by the time the person hits the ground, and normal activity can be resumed immediately. Patients with this type of seizure are at a great risk of head injury and often have to wear protective helmets. A less severe akinetic seizure involves brief loss of muscle tone without falling.

Partial Seizures. Partial (focal) seizures are another major class of the International Classification System. Partial seizures begin in a specific region of the cortex, as indicated by the EEG and usually by the clinical manifestations. For example, if the discharging focus is located in the medial aspect of the postcentral gyrus, the patient may experience paresthesias and tingling or numbness in the leg on the side opposite the focus. If the discharging focus is located in the part of the brain that governs a particular function, sensory, motor, cognitive, or emotional manifestations may occur.

Partial seizures may be confined to one side of the brain and remain partial or focal in nature, or they may spread to involve the entire brain, culminating in a generalized tonic-clonic seizure. Any tonic-clonic seizure that is preceded by an aura or warning is a partial seizure that generalizes secondarily. Many tonic-clonic seizures that appear to be generalized from the outset may actually be secondary generalized seizures, but the preceding partial component may be so brief that it is undetected by the patient, the observer, or even on the EEG. Unlike the primary generalized tonic-clonic seizure, the secondary generalized seizure may result in a transient residual neurologic deficit postictally. This is referred to as Todd's paralysis (focal paresis), which resolves after varying lengths of time.

Partial seizures are further divided into those with simple motor or sensory phenomena and those with complex symptoms (also called psychomotor seizures). Simple partial seizures with elementary symptoms do not involve loss of consciousness and rarely last longer than 1 minute. They may involve motor, sensory, or autonomic phenomena or a combination of these. The terms *focal motor, focal sensory,* and *jacksonian* have been used to describe seizures of the simple partial type.

Partial seizures with complex symptoms can involve a variety of behavioral, emotional, affective, and cognitive functions. The location of the discharging focus is usually in the temporal lobe, hence the term *temporal lobe seizure.* These seizures usually last longer than 1 minute and are frequently followed by a period of postictal confusion. Partial complex seizures are distinct from simple partial (focal motor, focal sensory) seizures in that they involve some alteration in consciousness. The sole manifestation of partial complex seizures may be clouding of consciousness or a confused state without any motor or sensory components. This type of attack is sometimes termed *temporal lobe absence.* There is rarely the complete loss of consciousness that is typical of the generalized absence attack, nor does the patient snap back to the preseizure state as does the patient who has had a generalized absence attack.

The most common complex partial seizure involves lip smacking and automatisms (repetitive movements that may not be appropriate). These are often called *psychomotor seizures.* The patient may continue an activity that was initiated before the seizure, such as counting out change or picking items from a grocery shelf, but after the seizure does not remember the activity performed during the seizure. Other automatisms are less organized, such as picking at clothing, fumbling with objects (real or imaginary), or simply walking away.

A variety of psychosensory symptoms may occur during a partial complex seizure, including distortions of visual or auditory sensations and vertigo. There may be alterations in memory, such as a feeling of having experienced an event before (déjá vu), or alterations in thought processes. Alterations in sexual functioning can vary from hyposexuality to hypersexuality. Many patients with temporal lobe seizures have decreased sexual drive or erectile dysfunction. However, some may experience sexual sensations during their seizures. This is because the abnormal electrical activity arises from the brain centers responsible for these sensations. Some experience increased sexual drive just after a seizure. In addition, some antiseizure medications can cause a decrease in sexual drive because of sedation. Others can cause erectile dysfunction.

Complications

Physical. *Status epilepticus* is a state in which seizures recur in rapid succession and the patient does not regain consciousness or normal function between seizures. It is the most serious complication of epilepsy and a neurologic emergency. Status epilepticus can involve any type of seizure. During repeated seizures the brain uses more energy than can be supplied. Neurons become exhausted and cease to function. Permanent brain damage may result. Tonic-clonic status epilepticus is the most dangerous because it can cause ventilatory insufficiency, hypoxemia, cardiac arrhythmias, hyperthermia, and systemic acidosis, all of which can be fatal.

Another complication of epilepsy is severe injury and even death from trauma suffered during a seizure. Patients who lose consciousness during a seizure are at greatest risk. Death can result from head injury incurred in a fall, from drowning in the bathtub, or from severe burns.

Psychosocial. Perhaps the most common complication of epilepsy is the effect it has on a patient's lifestyle. Although attitudes have improved in recent years, epilepsy still carries a social stigma. It used to be associated with supernatural powers, possession by the devil, and insanity. Today the stigma probably exists because the characteristics of seizures are in direct conflict with modern societal values of self-control, conformity, and independence. The patient with epilepsy may experience discrimination in employment and educational opportunities. Transportation may be difficult because of legal sanctions against driving in some states. The patient may develop ineffective methods of coping.

COLLABORATIVE CARE

Table 56-7 Seizures

Diagnostic
- Complete history and physical examination
  - Birth and development history
  - Significant illnesses and injuries
  - Family history
  - Febrile seizures
  - Comprehensive neurologic assessment
- Seizure history
  - Precipitating factors
  - Antecedent events
  - Seizure description (including onset, duration, frequency, postictal state)
- Diagnostic studies
  - CBC, urinalysis, electrolytes, creatinine, fasting blood glucose
  - Lumbar puncture
  - CT, MRI, PET scan
  - Electroencephalography

Collaborative Therapy
- Antiseizure medication (see Table 56-9)
- Surgery (see Table 56-10)
- Vagal nerve stimulation
- Psychosocial counseling

PET, positron emission tomography.

Diagnostic Studies

The most useful diagnostic tools are accurate and comprehensive description of the seizures and the patient's health history (Table 56-7). The EEG is a useful diagnostic adjuvant to the history but only if it shows abnormalities. Abnormal findings help determine the type of seizure and help pinpoint the seizure focus. Unfortunately, only a small percentage of patients with epilepsy have abnormal findings on the EEG the first time the test is done. EEGs may need to be repeated often, or continuous EEG monitoring may be needed to detect abnormalities. Abnormal discharges may not occur during the 30 to 40 minutes of sampling during EEG, and the test may never indicate an abnormality. It is not a definitive test. Some patients who do not have epilepsy have abnormal patterns on their EEGs, whereas many patients with epilepsy have normal EEGs.

A complete blood count, serum chemistries, studies of liver and kidney function, and urinalysis should be done to rule out metabolic disorders. A CT or MRI scan should be done in any new-onset seizure to rule out a structural lesion. Cerebral angiography and positron emission tomography (PET) may be used in selected clinical situations.

Collaborative Care

Most seizures do not require professional emergency medical care because they are self-limiting and rarely cause bodily injury. However, if status epilepticus occurs, if significant bodily harm occurs, or if the event is a first-time seizure, medical care should be sought immediately. Table 56-8 summarizes emergency care of the patient with a generalized tonic-clonic seizure, the seizure most likely to warrant professional emergency medical care.

The diagnostic and collaborative care of seizure disorders are summarized in Table 56-7.

Drug Therapy. Epilepsy is treated primarily with antiseizure medication (Table 56-9). Therapy is aimed at preventing seizures, because cure is not possible. Medications generally act by stabilizing nerve cell membranes and preventing spread of the epileptic discharge. In about 70% of the patients epilepsy is controlled by medication. The primary goal of antiseizure drug therapy is to obtain maximum seizure control with a minimum of toxic side effects. The principle of drug therapy is to begin with a single drug and increase the dosage until seizures are controlled or toxic side effects occur. Serum levels of the drug should be monitored regularly. The therapeutic range for each drug indicates the serum level above which most patients experience toxic side effects and below which most continue to have seizures. Therapeutic ranges are only guides for therapy. If the patient's seizures are well controlled with a subtherapeutic level, the drug dose need not be increased. Likewise, if a drug level is above the therapeutic range and the patient has good seizure control without toxic side effects, the drug dose need not be decreased. If seizure control is not achieved with a single drug, a second drug is added.

The primary drugs for treatment of generalized tonic-clonic and partial seizures are phenytoin (Dilantin), carbamazepine (Tegretol), phenobarbital, primidone (Mysoline), and divalproex (Depakote). The primary drugs for treatment of absence, akinetic, and myoclonic seizures are ethosuximide (Zarontin), divalproex (Depakote), and clonazepam (Klonopin).

Four new antiepileptic drugs have recently been approved by the Food and Drug Administration (FDA). Gabapentin (Neurontin), lamotrigine (Lamictal), topiramate (Topamax), and tiagabine (Gabitril) are indicated for partial seizures and for secondary generalized seizures. These drugs are currently used as adjunctive therapy.

Felbamate (Felbatol) may be used to treat patients whose seizure disorders are refractory to other medications. However, its use is limited because it can cause aplastic anemia and liver toxicity.

Table 56-9 summarizes the known interactions of the major antiseizure drugs. Because many of these drugs (e.g., phenytoin, phenobarbital, ethosuximide, lomotrigine, topiramate) have a long half-life, they can be given in once- or twice-daily doses. This increases the patient's compliance with taking medication by simplifying the drug regimen and avoiding the need to take medication at work or school. Antiseizure drugs should not be discontinued abruptly because this can precipitate seizures.

During seizure activity, phenytoin will not immediately stop the seizure. Other agents such as benzodiazepines or phenobarbital may be given during an acute seizure.

Toxic side effects of antiseizure drugs involve the CNS and include diplopia, drowsiness, ataxia, and mental slowing. Neurologic assessment for dose-related toxicity involves testing the eyes for nystagmus, hand and gait coordination, cognitive functioning, and general alertness.

EMERGENCY MANAGEMENT

Table **56-8** **Tonic-Clonic Seizures**

Etiology	Assessment Findings	Interventions
Head Trauma Epidural hematoma Subdural hematoma Intracranial hematoma Cerebral contusion Traumatic birth injury **Drug-Related Process** Overdose Withdrawal of alcohol, opioids, antiseizure drugs Ingestion, inhalation **Infectious Processes** Meningitis Septicemia **Intracranial Event** Brain tumor Subarachnoid hemorrhage Stroke Hypertensive crisis Increased ICP secondary to clogged shunt **Metabolic Imbalance** Fluid and electrolyte imbalance Hypoglycemia **Medical Disorders** Heart, liver, lung, or kidney disease Systemic lupus erythematosus **Other** Cardiac arrest Idiopathic Psychiatric disorders High fever	■ Aura—peculiar sensations that precede seizure ■ Loss of consciousness ■ Bowel and bladder incontinence ■ Tachycardia ■ Diaphoresis ■ Warm skin ■ Pallor, flushing, or cyanosis ■ *Tonic phase*—continuous muscle contractions ■ *Hypertonic phase*—extreme muscular rigidity lasting 5 to 15 seconds ■ *Clonic phase*—rigidity and relaxation alternate in rapid succession ■ *Postictal phase*—lethargy, altered level of consciousness ■ Confusion and headache ■ Repeated tonic clonic seizures for several minutes	**Initial** ■ Ensure patent airway. ■ Assist ventilations if patient does not breathe spontaneously after seizure. Anticipate need for intubation if gag reflex absent. ■ Suction as needed. ■ Stay with patient until seizure has passed. ■ Protect patient from injury during seizure. *Do not restrain.* Pad side rails. ■ Establish IV access. ■ Anticipate administration of phenobarbital, phenytoin, or benzodiazepines (Valium, Versed, Ativan) to control seizures. ■ Remove or loosen tight clothing. **Ongoing Monitoring** ■ Monitor vital signs, level of consciousness, oxygen saturation, Glasgow Coma Scale, pupil size and reactivity. ■ Reassure and orient the patient after seizure. ■ Never force an airway between a patient's clenched teeth. ■ Give dextrose for hypoglycemia.

ICP, intracranial pressure.

DRUG THERAPY

Table **56-9** **Antiseizure Drugs**

Generalized Tonic-Clonic and Partial Seizures
Phenytoin (Dilantin)
Carbamazepine (Tegretol)
Phenobarbital
Divalproex (Depakote)
Primidone (Mysoline)
Gabapentin (Neurontin)
Lamotrigine (Lamictal)
Topiramate (Topamax)
Tiagabine (Gabitril)
Absence, Akinetic, and Myoclonic Seizures
Ethosuximide (Zarontin)
Divalproex (Depakote)
Clonazepam (Klonopin)
Phenobarbital

Idiosyncratic side effects involve organs outside the CNS, including the skin (rashes), gingiva (hypertrophy), bone marrow (blood dyscrasias), liver, and kidneys. Nurses should be knowledgeable about these side effects so that patients can be informed and proper treatment can be instituted. A common idiosyncratic side effect of phenytoin is hypertrophy of the gingiva, especially in children and young adults. This can be limited by good dental hygiene, including regular toothbrushing and flossing. If gingival hypertrophy is extensive, the hypertrophied tissue may have to be surgically removed (gingivectomy), and phenytoin may have to be replaced by another antiseizure drug. Because phenytoin can also cause hirsutism in young people, other drugs are often used first.

Surgical Therapy. A significant number of patients whose epilepsy cannot be controlled with drug therapy are candidates for surgical intervention (Table 56-10). Surgery may be considered to control intractable seizures, prevent cerebral degeneration from repeated seizures, prevent toxic

Table 56-10 Surgical Procedures for Epilepsy

Type of Seizure	Surgical Procedure	Results
Complex partial seizure of temporal lobe origin	Resectioning of epileptogenic tissue	Absence of seizures 5 yr postoperatively in 55-70% of patients
Partial seizures of frontal lobe origin	Resectioning of epileptogenic tissue (if in resectable area)	Absence of seizures 5 yr postoperatively in 30-50% of patients
Generalized seizures (Lennox-Gastaut syndrome or drop attacks)	Sectioning of corpus callosum	Persistence of seizures, less violent, less frequent, less disabling events
Intractable unilateral multifocal epilepsy associated with infantile hemiplegia	Hemispherectomy or callosotomy	Reduction in seizure frequency and type, improvement in behavior

syndromes from long-term use of antiseizure drugs, and improve the quality of life.[8]

Not all types of epilepsy benefit from surgery. The benefits of surgery include cessation or reduction in frequency of the seizures. An extensive preoperative evaluation is important, including continuous EEG monitoring and other specific tests to ensure precise localization of the focal point. Before surgery is performed, three requirements must be met: (1) the diagnosis of epilepsy must be confirmed; (2) there must have been an adequate trial with drug therapy without satisfactory results; and (3) the electroclinical syndrome (type of seizure disorder) must be defined.[8]

Alternative Therapies. Biofeedback to control seizures is aimed at teaching the patient to maintain a certain brain-wave frequency that is refractory to seizure activity. This method is still in the experimental stage. Vagal nerve stimulation is a method of controlling or reducing seizures in poorly controlled patients by placement of electrodes around the left vagus nerve in the neck. An external generator is programmed to deliver intermittent electrical stimulation to the nerve. The exact mechanism of action is unknown, although the stimulation may interrupt synchronization of epileptic brain-wave activity. This method is currently used in only a small number of patients.

NURSING MANAGEMENT: SEIZURES

■ Nursing Assessment

Subjective and objective data that should be obtained from a patient with a seizure disorder are presented in Table 56-11. Data related to a specific seizure episode can be obtained from a witness.

■ Nursing Diagnoses

Nursing diagnoses for the patient with seizures may include, but are not limited to, those presented in NCP 56-2.

■ Planning

The overall goals are that the patient with seizures will (1) be free from injury during a seizure, (2) have optimal mental and physical functioning while taking antiseizure medication, and (3) have satisfactory psychosocial functioning.

■ Nursing Implementation

Health Promotion. Many cases of seizures can be prevented by promotion of general safety measures, such as the wearing of helmets in situations involving risk of head injury. Improved perinatal, labor, and delivery care have reduced fetal trauma and hypoxia and thereby have reduced brain damage leading to epilepsy. Children with fever should be treated quickly to avoid high temperatures, which may cause seizures.

The patient with epilepsy should practice good general health habits (e.g., maintaining a proper diet, getting adequate rest, and exercising). The patient should be helped to identify events or situations that precipitate the seizures and should be given suggestions for avoiding them or handling them better. Excessive alcohol intake, fatigue, and loss of sleep should be avoided, and the patient should be helped to handle stress constructively.

Acute Intervention. The nurse caring for a hospitalized patient with epilepsy or a patient who has had seizures as a result of metabolic factors has several responsibilities, including observation and treatment of the seizure, education, and psychosocial intervention.

When a seizure occurs, the nurse should carefully observe and record details of the event because the diagnosis and subsequent treatment often rest solely on the seizure description. All aspects of the seizure should be noted. What events preceded the seizure? When did the seizure occur? How long did each phase (aural [if any], ictal, postictal) last? What occurred during each phase?

Both subjective data (usually the only type of data in the aural phase) and objective data are important. Objective data should include the exact onset of the seizure (which body part was affected first and how), the course and nature of the seizure activity (loss of consciousness, tongue biting, automatisms, stiffening, jerking, total lack of muscle tone), the body parts involved and their sequence of involvement, and the presence of autonomic signs such as dilated pupils, excessive salivation, altered breathing, cyanosis, flushing, diaphoresis, or incontinence. Assessment of the postictal period should include a detailed description of the level of consciousness, vital signs, memory loss, muscle soreness, speech disorders (aphasia, dysarthria), weakness or paralysis, sleep period, and the duration of each sign or symptom.

During the seizure it is important to maintain a patent airway. This may involve supporting and protecting the head, turning the

NURSING ASSESSMENT

Table 56-11 Seizures

Subjective Data

Important Health Information

Past health history: Previous seizures, birth defects or injuries, anoxic episodes, CNS trauma, tumors, or infections; hypertension, cerebrovascular disease; metabolic disorders, alcoholism; exposure to metals and carbon monoxide; hepatic or renal failure; fever; pregnancy, systemic lupus erythematosus

Medications: Compliance with antiseizure medications; barbiturate or alcohol withdrawal; use and overdose of cocaine, amphetamines, lidocaine, theophylline, penicillin, lithium, phenothiazines, tricyclic antidepressants, benzodiazepines

Functional Health Patterns

Health perception–health management: Positive family history

Cognitive-perceptual: Headaches, aura, mood or behavioral changes before seizure; mentation changes; abdominal pain, muscle pain (postictal)

Self-perception–self-concept: Anxiety, depression; loss of self-esteem, social isolation

Sexuality-reproductive: Decreased sex drive, erectile dysfunction; increased sexual drive (postictal)

Objective Data

General

Precipitating factors, including severe metabolic acidosis or alkalosis, hyperkalemia, hypoglycemia, dehydration, or water intoxication

Integumentary

Bitten tongue, soft-tissue damage, cyanosis, diaphoresis (postictal)

Respiratory

Abnormal respiratory rate, rhythm, or depth; apnea (ictal); absent or abnormal breath sounds, possible airway occlusion

Cardiovascular

Hypertension, tachycardia or bradycardia (ictal)

Gastrointestinal

Bowel incontinence; excessive salivation

Urinary

Incontinence

Neurologic

Generalized

Tonic-clonic: loss of consciousness, muscle tightening then jerking, dilated pupils, hyperventilation, then apnea; postictal somnolence

Absence: altered consciousness (5-30 seconds), minor facial motor activity

Partial

Simple: aura, consciousness, focal sensory, motor, cognitive, or emotional phenomena (focal motor); unilateral "marching" motor seizure (jacksonian)

Complex: altered consciousness with inappropriate behaviors, automatisms, amnesia of event

Musculoskeletal

Weakness, paralysis, ataxia (postictal)

Possible Findings

Positive toxicology screen or alcohol level; altered serum electrolytes, acidosis or alkalosis, very low blood glucose level, elevated blood urea nitrogen or serum creatinine, liver function tests, ammonia; abnormal CT scan or MRI of head, lumbar puncture; epileptiform discharges on EEG

EEG, electroencephalogram.

patient to the side, loosening constrictive clothing, or easing the patient to the floor, if seated. The patient should not be restrained and no objects should be placed in the mouth. After the seizure the patient may require suctioning and oxygen may be needed.

A seizure can be a frightening experience for the patient and for others who may witness it. The nurse should assess the level of their understanding and provide information about how and why the event occurred. This is an excellent opportunity for the nurse to dispel many common misconceptions about seizures.

Ambulatory and Home Care. Prevention of recurring seizures is the major goal in the treatment of epilepsy. Because epilepsy cannot be cured, medication must be taken regularly and continuously, often for a lifetime. The nurse should ensure that the patient knows this, as well as the specifics of the medication regimen and what to do if a dose is missed. Usually the dose should be made up if the omission is remembered within 24 hours. The patient should be cautioned not to adjust medications without professional guidance because this can increase seizure frequency and even cause status epilepticus. The patient should be encouraged to report any medication side effects and to keep regular appointments with the health care provider.

Nurses play an important role in educating the patient and the patient's family. Guidelines for patient teaching are shown in Table 56-12. Nurses should teach family members and significant others the emergency management of tonic-clonic seizures (see Table 56-8). They should be reminded that it is not necessary to call an ambulance or send a person to the hospital after a single seizure unless the seizure is prolonged, another seizure immediately follows, or extensive injury has occurred.

Patients with epilepsy also experience concerns or fears related to recurrent seizures, incontinence, or loss of self-control. The nurse provides support for the patient through education and by helping to identify coping mechanisms.

Perhaps the greatest challenge that epilepsy presents to the patient is adjusting to the personal limitations imposed by the illness. Discrimination in employment is the most serious problem facing the person with epilepsy. Patients can be informed that the Rehabilitation Act of 1973 was designed to protect handicapped persons (including those with epilepsy) from discrimination in employment. For issues relating to job discrimination, patients can be referred to the State Human Rights Commission or the State Department of Vocational Rehabilitation.

A variety of other resources can be offered to the patient with epilepsy who has a specific problem. If the nurse believes that associating with others who have epilepsy would be beneficial, the patient can be referred to the local chapter of the Epilepsy Foundation (EF), a voluntary agency that offers a variety of services to patients with epilepsy. The patient who is an eligible veteran can be referred to a Department of Veterans Affairs medical center that provides comprehensive care.

56-2 NURSING CARE PLAN PATIENT WITH SEIZURES

Expected Patient Outcomes	Nursing Interventions and *Rationales*
NURSING DIAGNOSIS	**Ineffective breathing pattern** *related to* neuromuscular impairment secondary to prolonged tonic phase of seizure or during postictal period *as manifested by* abnormal respiratory rate, rhythm, or depth.
▪ Appropriate rate, rhythm, and depth of respirations.	▪ Loosen constricting clothing *to avoid restricting breathing.* ▪ Assess breathing pattern, observing for labored respiration, tachypnea, bradypnea, dyspnea, apnea, and cyanosis *to determine if problem is present and extent of problem and to initiate appropriate interventions.* ▪ Provide manual ventilation or oxygen when necessary; be prepared to assist with endotracheal intubation *to maintain adequate oxygenation and prevent hypoxia.* ▪ Insert oral airway (if indicated) only after seizure activity has ceased *to prevent mouth and teeth injury from forcing airway between clamped teeth.*
NURSING DIAGNOSIS	**Ineffective airway clearance** *related to* tracheobronchial obstruction *as manifested by* ineffective cough, inability to remove secretions, absence of or abnormal breath sounds.
▪ No airway obstruction. ▪ Clear breath sounds.	▪ Observe for signs of airway obstruction *to determine extent of problem and to plan appropriate interventions.* ▪ If vomiting occurs, turn patient's head gently to side and remove as much vomitus as possible after the seizure *to prevent aspiration of vomitus and subsequent interference with breathing.* ▪ Suction airway if necessary *to remove accumulated secretions.* ▪ Establish and maintain patent airway *to ensure adequate oxygenation.*
NURSING DIAGNOSIS	**Risk for injury** *related to* seizure activity and subsequent impaired physical mobility secondary to postictal weakness or paralysis.
▪ No injury. ▪ Verbalization of knowledge of potential for injury during seizure. ▪ Arrangement of environment to minimize risk for injury.	▪ Assess for trauma to mouth, cheek, tongue, lips; abrasions, bruises; broken bones; burns *because these injuries may occur during seizure activity.* ▪ Assess for weakness, paralysis of one side of body, ataxia, fatigue, lethargy *as potential postictal risks for injury to plan appropriate interventions.* ▪ Do not permit smoking in bed *to prevent the patient from being burned by a bed fire if a seizure occurs.* ▪ If patient anticipates a seizure may occur, assist to a safe location or position; use seizure precautions as appropriate; remove potentially harmful objects from surrounding area; gently guide arm or leg movements *to prevent injury during a seizure.* ▪ Refrain from moving or restraining patient during a seizure *to prevent bone or soft-tissue injury.* ▪ Assist in determining whether operation of a motor vehicle or dangerous machinery is appropriate for patient *to assist patient in making the appropriate choice about driving.*
NURSING DIAGNOSIS	**Ineffective individual coping** *related to* perceived loss of control and denial of diagnosis *as manifested by* verbalizations about not having epilepsy, lack of truth-telling regarding seizure frequency, noncompliant behavior.
▪ Acceptance of disorder as evidenced by using word *epilepsy* to describe illness. ▪ Acknowledgment that a seizure has occurred.	▪ Explore reasons for denial *to determine extent of problem and to plan appropriate interventions.* ▪ Implement and individualize teaching plan about causes and mechanisms of seizures, effectiveness of drugs in controlling seizures, inaccuracy of myths about epilepsy, avoidance of precipitating factors, state law regarding driving, pros and cons of medical ID tags, moderation in drinking and eating, exposure to stress, and avoidance of hazardous activities *to promote effective coping by providing facts.*

Continued

56-2 NURSING CARE PLAN PATIENT WITH SEIZURES—continued

Expected Patient Outcomes	Nursing Interventions and *Rationales*
NURSING DIAGNOSIS	**Self-esteem disturbance** *related to* diagnosis of epilepsy *as manifested by* anxiety, fear, social isolation, depression, role disturbance, altered family dynamics.
▪ Sharing of feelings about diagnosis. ▪ Identification of positive aspects about self. ▪ Appropriate interactions with others.	▪ Discuss patient's views about self in relation to seizures *to clarify effect of disease on self-concept.* ▪ Determine effect of seizures on daily activities and other activities important to patient *because major interference will likely affect self-concept.* ▪ Provide information about possible overprotection, community resources, and social stigmas that may be encountered *to improve self-concept by increasing sense of control.* ▪ Assist patient with explaining seizures and management to friends, school personnel, and employers *so these people can provide support and acceptance.* ▪ Advise patient about employment counseling and job retraining *because gainful employment usually improves self-concept.*
NURSING DIAGNOSIS	**Ineffective management of therapeutic regimen** *related to* lack of knowledge about management of epilepsy *as manifested by* verbalization of lack of knowledge, inaccurate perception of health status, noncompliance with prescribed health behavior.
▪ Optimal seizure control. ▪ Therapeutic drug levels of antiseizure medication. ▪ Compliance with therapeutic regimen.	▪ Provide education to patient and family about seizure activity and therapeutic management including diagnosis, treatment, lifestyle adjustments, and community resources *so patient and family can make necessary lifestyle modifications to manage a chronic disease.*

PATIENT & FAMILY TEACHING GUIDE

Table 56-12 Seizures

The patient with a seizure disorder should be taught the following:

1. Medications must be taken as prescribed. Any and all side effects of medications should be reported to the health care provider. When necessary, blood drawings are done to ensure that therapeutic levels are maintained.
2. Use of nondrug techniques, such as relaxation therapy and biofeedback training to potentially reduce the number of seizures.
3. Availability of resources in the community.
4. Need to wear a Medic Alert bracelet, necklace, and identification card.
5. Avoidance of excessive alcohol intake, fatigue, and loss of sleep.
6. Regular meals and snack in between if feeling shaky, faint, or hungry.

Family members should be taught the following:

1. First aid treatment of tonic-clonic seizure. It is not necessary to call ambulance or send the patient to the hospital after a single seizure unless the seizure is prolonged, another seizure immediately follows, or extensive injury has occurred.
2. During an acute seizure, it is important to protect the patient from injury. This may involve supporting and protecting the head, turning the patient to the side, loosening constrictive clothing, and easing the patient to the floor, if seated.

The patient should be informed that medical alert bracelets, necklaces, and identification cards are available through the EF, local pharmacies, or companies specializing in identification devices (e.g., Medic Alert). However, the use of these medical identification tags is optional. Some patients have found them beneficial, but others have found them to be more a burden than a help because they prefer not to be identified as having epilepsy.

Social workers and welfare agencies can help with financial problems and living arrangements. State services for individuals with developmental disabilities include assistance with job training and placement for patients whose seizures are not well controlled. Sheltered housing and funding for special needs, such as medical and psychologic evaluation and transportation, are also offered. State agencies specializing in vocational rehabilitation services can offer vocational assessment, counseling, funding for training, and assistance with job placement. They can also offer financial assistance for transportation and medical costs that are necessary for vocational rehabilitation or job maintenance. If intensive psychologic counseling is needed, the nurse can refer the patient to a community mental health center.

The patient should be encouraged to learn more about epilepsy through self-education materials. The EF provides several information pamphlets and may facilitate support groups. Many agencies that offer services to epileptic patients, as well as local chapters of EF, have these available as teaching aids.

■ Evaluation

Expected outcomes for the patient with seizures are addressed in NCP 56-2.

MULTIPLE SCLEROSIS

Multiple sclerosis (MS) is a chronic, progressive, degenerative disorder of the CNS. It is not known exactly how many people have MS. Currently it is thought that there are approximately 250,000 to 350,000 people in the United States with MS diagnosed by a physician. Approximately 200 new cases are diagnosed each week. MS is five times more prevalent in temperate climates (between 45 and 65 degrees of latitude), such as those found in the northern United States, Canada, and Europe as compared with tropical regions. Age 15 seems to be critical in terms of risk for developing the disease. For example, if a person moves from a high-risk (temperate) to a low-risk (tropical) area before the age of 15, she or he will adopt the risk (in this case, low) of the new area and vice versa.[9] MS is considered a disease of young adults, with the onset usually being between 15 and 50 years of age. Women are affected more often than men.

MS primarily affects Caucasians of northern European descent, which means that the disease is associated with certain environmental and familial factors. African-Americans and Asians have a lower incidence of MS than do Caucasians.

Etiology and Pathophysiology

The cause of MS is unknown, although research findings suggest MS is related to infectious (viral), immunologic, and genetic factors and is perpetuated as a result of intrinsic factors (e.g., faulty immunoregulation). The susceptibility to MS appears to be inherited. First-, second-, and third-degree relatives of patients with MS are at a slightly increased risk. Multiple unlinked genes confer susceptibility to MS.

The role of precipitating factors such as exposure to pathogenetic agents in the etiology of MS is controversial. It is possible that their association with MS is random and that there is no cause-and-effect relationship. Possible precipitating factors include infection, physical injury, emotional stress, excessive fatigue, pregnancy, and a poorer state of health.

MS is characterized by chronic inflammation, demyelination, and gliosis (scarring) in the CNS. The primary neuropathologic condition is an immune-mediated inflammatory demyelinating process that some believe may be triggered by a virus in genetically susceptible individuals. Activated T cells responding to environmental triggers (e.g., infection) enter the CNS in increased numbers. These T cells, in conjunction with astrocytes, disrupt the blood-brain barrier, thereby promoting the entry of other immune mediators into the CNS. These factors, in combination, damage oligodendrocytes (cells that make myelin), resulting in demyelination. Macrophages are recruited and cause further cell damage.[10] The disease process consists of loss of myelin, disappearance of oligodendrocytes, and proliferation of astrocytes. These changes result in characteristic plaque formation, or sclerosis, with plaques scattered throughout multiple regions of the CNS.

Initially the myelin sheaths of the neurons in the brain and spinal cord are attacked (Fig. 56-1, *A* and *B*). Early in the disease the myelin sheath is damaged, but the nerve fiber is not affected and nerve impulses are still transmitted (Fig. 56-1, *C*). At this point the patient may complain of a noticeable impairment of function (e.g., weakness). However, the myelin can regenerate and the symptoms disappear, resulting in a remission.

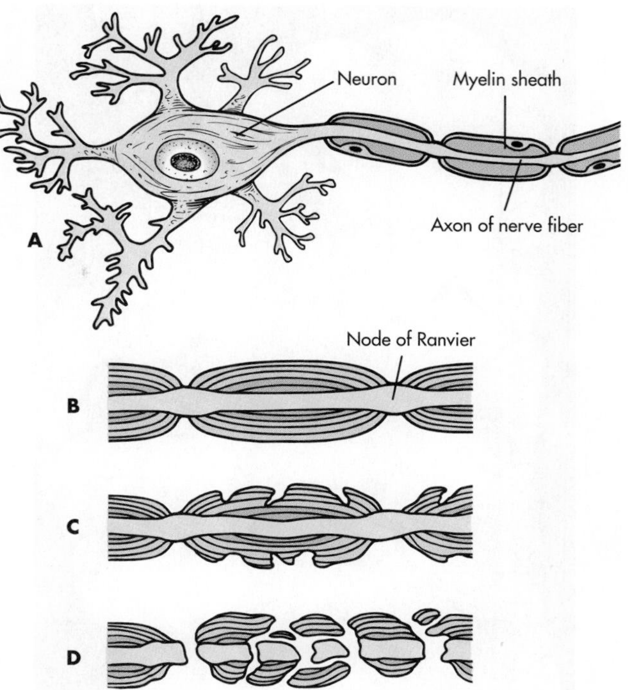

Fig. 56-1 Pathogenesis of multiple sclerosis. **A,** Normal nerve cell with myelin sheath. **B,** Normal axon. **C,** Myelin breakdown. **D,** Myelin totally disrupted; axon not functioning.

As the disease progresses, the myelin is totally disrupted, and the axon becomes involved (Fig. 56-1, *D*). Myelin is replaced by glial scar tissue, which forms hard, sclerotic plaques in multiple regions of the CNS (Fig. 56-2). Without myelin, nerve impulses slow down, and with destruction of nerve axons, impulses are totally blocked, resulting in permanent loss of function. In many chronic lesions, demyelination continues with progressive loss of nerve function.

Clinical Manifestations

Because the onset is often insidious and gradual, with vague symptoms that occur intermittently over months or years, the disease may not be diagnosed until long after the onset of the first symptom. The disease process has a spotty distribution in the CNS, so the signs and symptoms vary over time. The disease is characterized by chronic, progressive deterioration in some persons and by remissions and exacerbations in others. With repeated exacerbations, however, progressive scarring of the myelin sheath occurs, and the overall trend is progressive deterioration in neurologic function.

The clinical manifestations vary according to the areas of the CNS involved. Some patients have severe, long-lasting symptoms early in the course of the disease. Others may experience only occasional and mild symptoms for several years after onset. A classification scheme that identifies the various courses of MS has been developed.[10] *Relapsing-remitting MS* is characterized by clearly defined relapses with full recovery or with sequelae and residual deficit on recovery. *Primary-progressive MS* is characterized by disease progression from onset with occasional plateaus and temporary minor improvements. *Secondary-progressive MS* is characterized by a

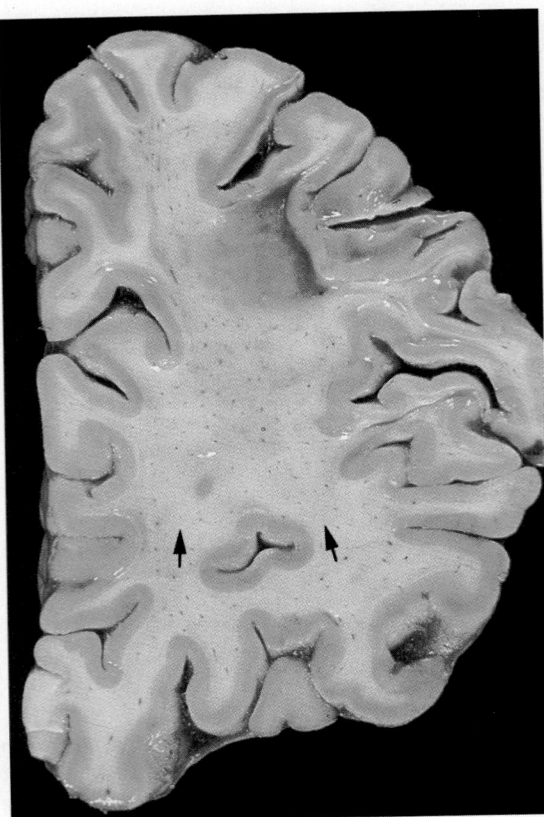

Fig. 56-2 Chronic multiple sclerosis. Demyelination plaque at gray-white junction and adjacent partially remyelinated shadow plaque *(arrow).*

relapsing-remitting initial course, followed by progression with or without occasional relapses, minor remissions, and plateaus. *Progressive-relapsing MS* is characterized by progressive disease from onset, with clear acute relapses, with or without full recovery; periods between relapses are characterized by continuing progression.

Common signs and symptoms of MS include motor, sensory, cerebellar, and emotional problems. Motor symptoms include weakness or paralysis of the limbs, trunk, or head, diplopia, scanning speech, and spasticity of the muscles that are chronically affected. Sensory symptoms include numbness and tingling and other paresthesias, patchy blindness (scotomas), blurred vision, vertigo, tinnitus, and decreased hearing. Cerebellar signs include nystagmus, ataxia, dysarthria, and dysphagia.

Bowel and bladder function can be affected if the sclerotic plaque is located in areas of the CNS that control elimination. Problems with defecation usually involve constipation rather than fecal incontinence. Urinary problems are variable. A common problem in MS patients is a spastic (uninhibited) bladder. This indicates a lesion above the second sacral nerve, which cuts off suprasegmental inhibiting influences on bladder contractility. As a result, the bladder has a small capacity for urine, and its contractions are unchecked. This is accompanied by urinary urgency and frequency and results in dribbling or incontinence. A flaccid (hypotonic) bladder indicates a lesion in the reflex arc governing bladder function. The bladder has a large capacity for urine because there is no sensation or desire to void,

COLLABORATIVE CARE

Table 56-13 Multiple Sclerosis

Diagnostic
- History and physical examination
- CSF analysis
- Evoked response testing (also called evoked potential testing, e.g., SSEP—somatosensory evoked potential; AEP—auditory evoked potential; VEP—visual evoked potential)
- CT scan
- MRI

Collaborative Therapy

Drug Therapy*
- Antiinflammatory
- Immunosuppressants
- Anticholinergics
- Cholinergics
- Muscle relaxants
- Immunomodulators

Surgical Therapy
- Thalamotomy (unmanageable tremor)
- Neurectomy, rhizotomy, cordotomy (unmanageable spasticity)

*See Table 56-14.

no pressure, and no pain. Generally, there is urinary retention, but urgency and frequency may also occur with this type of lesion. Urinary problems cannot be adequately diagnosed and treated unless urodynamic studies are done.

Sexual dysfunction occurs in many persons with MS. Physiologic erectile dysfunction may result from spinal cord involvement in men. Women may experience decreased libido, difficulty with orgasmic response, painful intercourse, and decreased vaginal lubrication. Diminished sensation can prevent a normal sexual response in both sexes. The emotional effects of chronic illness and the loss of self-esteem also contribute to loss of sexual response.

MS has no apparent effect on the course of pregnancy, labor, delivery, or lactation. Some women with MS who become pregnant experience remission or an improvement in their symptoms during the gestation period. The hormonal changes associated with pregnancy appear to affect the immune system. However, during the postpartum period women are at greater risk for exacerbation of the disease.[11]

Although intellectual functioning generally remains intact, emotional stability may be affected. Persons may experience anger, depression, or euphoria. Signs and symptoms of MS are aggravated or triggered by physical and emotional trauma, fatigue, and infection.

The average life expectancy after the onset of symptoms is more than 25 years. Death usually occurs because of infective complications (e.g., pneumonia) of immobility or because of unrelated disease; occasionally, suicide is a cause.

Diagnostic Studies

Because there is no definitive diagnostic test for MS, diagnosis is based primarily on history and clinical manifestations (Table 56-13). Certain laboratory tests are currently used as adjuncts

DRUG THERAPY

Table 56-14 Multiple Sclerosis

Drug	Symptoms Relieved	Precautions	Side Effects	Educational Needs
Corticosteroids				
ACTH Prednisone Methylprednisolone	Exacerbations	Widespread effects on many enzymes and metabolic processes, few adverse effects with use for <1 mo at a time	Edema, mental changes (euphoria), weight gain, redistribution of body fat*	Restrict salt intake. Do not abruptly stop therapy. Know drug interactions.
Immunomodulators				
Beta-interferon (Betaseron) (Avonex)	Exacerbations	Monitor CBC, blood chemistries, and liver function tests every 3 mo	Flulike symptoms, local skin reactions, depression	Learn self-injection techniques, report side effects.
Glatiramer acetate (Copaxone)	Exacerbations	No laboratory monitoring required	Local skin reactions; chest pain; weakness	Learn self-injection techniques; report side effects.
Cholinergics				
Bethanecol (Urecholine) Neostigmine (Prostigmine)	Urinary retention (flaccid bladder)	History of hypotension, cardiac dysfunction, allergies, hyperthyroidism, stomach and intestinal problems; contraindication with adrenergic drugs (antiasthmatic drugs) because of possible induction of serious asthma attack (Urecholine only)	Hypotension, diarrhea, diaphoresis, salivation, muscle weakness	Consult physician before using other drugs.
Anticholinergics				
Propantheline (Pro-Banthine) Oxybutynin (Ditropan)	Urinary frequency[†] and urgency (spastic bladder)	History of glaucoma, prostatic hypertrophy, cardiac dysfunction, intestinal obstruction	Dry mouth, blurred vision, constipation, hypertension, flushing, urinary retention (too high of dose)	Consult physician before using other drugs, especially sleeping aids, antihistamines (possibly leading to potentiated effect).
Muscle Relaxants				
Diazepam (Valium)	Spasticity	History of narrow-angle glaucoma	Drowsiness, ataxia, fatigue	Avoid driving and similar activities because of CNS-depressant effects. Be aware of addictive potential; avoid long-term use. Avoid concomitant use of phenothiazines, narcotics, barbiturates, MAO inhibitors, other antidepressants.
Baclofen (Lioresal)	Spasticity	History of hypersensitivity and renal damage, contraindication in pregnancy, possible exacerbation of seizures in patients with epilepsy	Drowsiness, weakness	Do not abruptly stop therapy (possibly leading to hallucinations). Avoid driving and similar activities because of sedative effect. Avoid use with other CNS depressants; take with food or milk.

Continued

DRUG THERAPY

Table 56-14 Multiple Sclerosis—cont'd

Drug	Symptoms Relieved	Precautions	Side Effects	Educational Needs
Dantrolene (Dantrium)	Spasticity	History of respiratory or cardiac dysfunction, possible induction of abnormal liver function or hepatitis, contraindication with estrogen therapy because of predisposition of hepatotoxicity	Drowsiness, dizziness, malaise, fatigue, diarrhea	Avoid driving. Avoid use with tranquilizers and alcohol (possibly causing photosensitivity).
Tizanidine (Zanaflex)	Spasticity	History of hypersensitivity, possible liver injury, hypotension, bradycardia	Drowsiness, dry mouth, tiredness	Use with caution in women on oral contraceptives

*See Chapter 47 for effects of long-term corticosteroid therapy.
†Urodynamic studies must be done before institution of therapy because patients with MS have multiple lesions and type of bladder dysfunction cannot be diagnosed from symptoms alone.
ACTH, adrenocorticotropic hormone; *CBC,* complete blood count; *MAO,* monoamine oxidase.

to the clinical examination. In some patients, cerebrospinal fluid (CSF) analysis may show an increase in oligoclonal immunoglobulin G (IgG). The CSF also contains a high number of lymphocytes and monocytes. Evoked responses are often delayed in persons with MS because of decreased nerve conduction from the eye and the ear to the brain. MRI scan may be helpful, because sclerotic plaques as small as 3 to 4 mm in diameter can be detected. Characteristic white-matter lesions scattered through the brain or spinal cord are evident on such a scan.

Collaborative Care

Drug Therapy. Because there is no cure for MS, collaborative care is aimed at treating the disease process and providing symptomatic relief (see Table 56-13). The disease process is treated with drugs, and the symptoms are controlled with a variety of medications and other forms of therapy. Adrenocorticotropic hormone (ACTH), methylprednisolone, and prednisone are helpful in treating acute exacerbations of the disease, probably by reducing edema and acute inflammation at the site of demyelination. However, these medications do not affect the ultimate outcome or degree of residual neurologic impairment from the exacerbation. Immunosuppressive drugs, such as azathioprine (Imuran), cyclosporine (Sandimmune), and cyclophosphamide (Cytoxan), have been shown to produce some beneficial effects in patients with severe and relapsing MS. However, the potential benefits of these drugs in patients with MS must be counterbalanced against the potentially serious side effects. Table 56-14 summarizes the drugs that are commonly used for symptomatic treatment of MS.

Interferon β-1b (Betaseron) was the first drug aimed at controlling the disease rather than the symptoms. It was approved by the FDA in 1993 for ambulatory patients with exacerbating and remitting MS. Clinical trials with subcutaneous injections every other day have shown that the drug decreases the number of relapses and the number of new lesions seen on an MRI scan.[12] Since then two more drugs have become available for controlling the disease. Interferon β-1a (Avonex) is similar to interferon β-1b in efficacy. It is given intramuscularly once a week. Glatiramer acetate (Copaxone), formerly known as copolymer-1, is unrelated to interferon, but likewise reduces the number of relapses in MS. It is given subcutaneously every day.

Surgical Therapy. Spasticity is primarily treated with muscle relaxants (antispasmodic drugs). However, surgery (e.g., neurectomy, rhizotomy, cordotomy) or dorsal-column electrical stimulation may be required. Intention tremor that becomes unmanageable with medication is sometimes treated by stereotactic surgery on the thalamus. This involves selective destruction of the ventrolateral nucleus in the thalamus.

Other Therapies. Neurologic dysfunction sometimes improves with physical therapy, speech therapy, and hypothermia, which normalizes body temperature if it is above normal. Physical therapy is important in keeping the patient as functionally active as possible. The purpose of therapy is to relieve spasticity, increase coordination, and train the patient to substitute unaffected muscles for impaired ones. An especially beneficial type of physical therapy is water exercise (Fig. 56-3). Water gives buoyancy to the body and allows the patient to perform activities that would normally be impossible. In water, a patient experiences more control over the body.

Nutritional Therapy. Various nutritional measures that have been advocated in the management of MS include megavitamin therapy (cobalamin [vitamin B_{12}], vitamin C) and diets consisting of low-fat and gluten-free food and raw vegetables. These particular dietary measures have not come into widespread use because of lack of proof of their effectiveness.

A nutritious, well-balanced diet is essential. Although there is no standard prescribed diet, a high-protein diet with supplementary vitamins is often advocated. A diet high in roughage may help relieve the problem of constipation. Vitamins are merely supplemental and not curative.

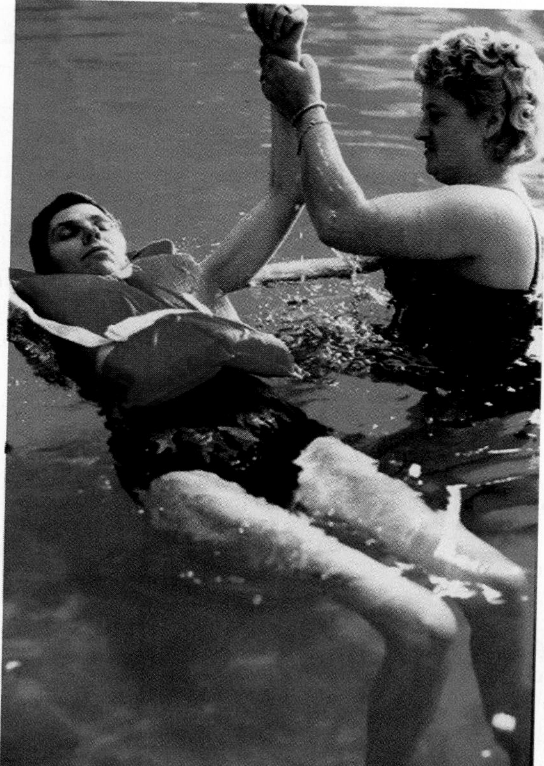

Fig. 56-3 Water therapy provides exercise and recreation for the patient with a chronic neurologic disease.

NURSING ASSESSMENT

Table 56-15 Multiple Sclerosis

Subjective Data

Important Health Information

Past health history: Recent or past viral infections or vaccinations, other recent infections, residence in cold or temperate climates, recent physical or emotional stress, pregnancy, exposure to extremes of heat and cold

Medications: Use of and compliance in taking corticosteroids, immunosuppressants, anticholinergics, antispasmodics

Functional Health Patterns

Health perception–health management: Positive family history; malaise

Nutritional-metabolic: Weight loss; difficulty in chewing, dysphagia

Elimination: Urinary frequency, urgency, dribbling or incontinence, retention; constipation

Activity-exercise: Generalized muscle weakness, muscle fatigue; tingling and numbness, ataxia (clumsiness)

Cognitive-perceptual: Eye, back, leg, joint pain; painful muscle spasms; vertigo; blurred or lost vision; diplopia; tinnitus

Sexuality-reproductive: Impotence, decreased libido

Coping–stress tolerance: Anger, depression, euphoria, social isolation

Objective Data

General

Apathy, inattentiveness

Integumentary

Pressure ulcers

Neurologic

Scanning speech, nystagmus, ataxia, tremor, spasticity, hyperreflexia, decreased hearing

Musculoskeletal

Muscular weakness, paresis, paralysis, spasms, foot dragging, dysarthria

Possible Findings

Reduction in T-suppressor cells, demyelinating lesions on MRI scans, increased IgG or oligoclonal banding in cerebrospinal fluid

NURSING MANAGEMENT: MULTIPLE SCLEROSIS

■ Nursing Assessment

Subjective and objective data that should be obtained from a person with MS are presented in Table 56-15.

■ Nursing Diagnoses

Nursing diagnoses for the patient with MS may include, but are not limited to, those presented in NCP 56-3.

■ Planning

The overall goals are that the patient with MS will (1) maximize neuromuscular function, (2) maintain independence in activities of daily living for as long as possible, (3) optimize psychosocial well-being, (4) adjust to the illness, and (5) reduce factors that precipitate exacerbations.

■ Nursing Implementation

The patient with MS should be aware of triggers that may cause exacerbations or worsening of the disease. Exacerbations of MS are triggered by exogenous events, including infection (especially upper respiratory infections), trauma, immunization, delivery after pregnancy, stress, and change in climate. Of these the best documented are upper respiratory infections, delivery, and head trauma.[13] Each person responds differently to these triggers. The nurse should help the patient identify particular triggers and develop ways to avoid them or minimize their effects.

The most common reasons for hospitalization of the patient with MS are for a diagnostic workup and treatment of an acute exacerbation. During the diagnostic phase the patient needs reassurance that even though there is a tentative diagnosis of MS, certain diagnostic studies must be done to rule out other neurologic disorders. The nurse should assist the patient in dealing with the anxiety caused by a diagnosis of a disabling illness. The patient with recently diagnosed MS may need assistance with the grieving process.

During an acute exacerbation the patient may be immobile and confined to bed for 2 to 3 weeks. The focus of nursing intervention at this phase is to prevent major complications of immobility, such as respiratory and urinary tract infections and pressure ulcers.

56-3 NURSING CARE PLAN PATIENT WITH MULTIPLE SCLEROSIS

Expected Patient Outcomes	Nursing Interventions and *Rationales*
NURSING DIAGNOSIS	**Impaired physical mobility** *related to* muscle weakness or paralysis and muscle spasticity *as manifested by* inability to ambulate, intermittent muscle spasms, pain associated with muscle spasms.
▪ Demonstration of use of adaptive devices. ▪ Maintenance of or increased strength of limbs. ▪ Decreased duration of muscle spasms.	▪ Use assistive devices as indicated *to decrease fatigue and to enhance independence, comfort, and safety.* ▪ Do active range-of-motion exercises at least twice per day *to prevent contractures and minimize muscle atrophy.* ▪ Encourage and assist with ambulation and transfer as indicated *to maintain mobility, promote independence, and provide for safety.* ▪ Change position of patient (if bedridden) at least q2hr *to prevent pressure ulcers and circulatory problems.* ▪ Administer medication as ordered *to reduce spasticity or to treat inflammatory response.* ▪ Perform stretching exercises every 6-8 hr *to relieve spasms and contracted muscles.*
NURSING DIAGNOSIS	**Self-care deficits** *related to* muscle spasticity and neuromuscular deficits *as manifested by* inability to perform some or all activities of daily living.
▪ Maximum level of functioning. ▪ Activities of daily living needs met by self or others.	▪ Assess self-care problems *to plan appropriate interventions to meet care needs.* ▪ Promote use of appropriate assistive devices *so patient can maximally participate in self-care activities with minimum fatigue.* ▪ Counsel regarding need for homemaker services *to assist in meeting patient's needs, conserving energy, and promoting independence.* ▪ Perform or assist with activities of daily living only as indicated *to promote patient's independence.* ▪ Encourage independence when appropriate *to promote patient's sense of autonomy and control.*
NURSING DIAGNOSIS	**Risk for impaired skin integrity** *related to* immobility, sensorimotor deficits, and inadequate nutrition.
▪ Intact skin.	▪ Assess skin for redness and irritation *to monitor changes in skin integrity and make appropriate plan for interventions.* ▪ Turn patient at least q2hr *to prevent pressure ulcers from developing.* ▪ Use circular massage of unreddened bony prominences with each turning *to improve circulation to these areas.* ▪ Provide high-protein diet *to promote healthy skin resistant to breakdown.* ▪ Cleanse back and buttocks if patient is incontinent *to prevent skin irritation and skin breakdown.*
NURSING DIAGNOSIS	**Sensory-perceptual alterations** *related to* visual disturbances *as manifested by* blurred vision, decreased visual acuity, visual field defects, diplopia.
▪ Satisfactory visual function for activities of daily living.	▪ Orient patient to environment *to promote safety and to compensate for visual disturbances.* ▪ Patch alternate eyes *to alleviate diplopia.* ▪ Assess visual acuity monthly *to monitor increase or decrease in vision.* ▪ Maintain safe environment (e.g., side rails up, bed in low position) *to prevent injury.* ▪ Indicate visual impairment on chart, care plan, and over bed *to communicate visual problems to health team and foster continuity of care.*
NURSING DIAGNOSIS	**Altered urinary elimination (retention)** *related to* sensorimotor deficits or inadequate fluid intake *as manifested by* posturination residual >50 ml, dribbling, bladder distention.
▪ Residual urine <50 ml. ▪ Maintenance of urinary continence.	▪ Administer cholinergic medications as ordered *to improve the muscle tone of bladder and facilitate emptying.* ▪ Follow intermittent catheterization protocol *to prevent distention or dribbling.* ▪ Use Credé maneuver or reflex stimulation (manual stimulation) *as an alternative method of emptying bladder.* ▪ Maintain fluid intake of 3000 ml/day *to dilute urine and reduce risk of urinary tract infection.* ▪ Teach patient signs and symptoms of urinary tract infection *to ensure early identification and treatment.*

Continued

56-3 NURSING CARE PLAN PATIENT WITH MULTIPLE SCLEROSIS—continued

Expected Patient Outcomes	Nursing Interventions and *Rationales*
NURSING DIAGNOSIS	**Altered urinary elimination (incontinence)** *related to* sensorimotor deficits or possible urinary tract infection *as manifested by* incontinence, urgency, frequency.
▪ Urinary continence.	▪ Administer anticholinergic medications as ordered *to reduce urinary frequency and urgency.* ▪ Initiate bladder-training program *to help restore adequate bladder function.* ▪ Provide incontinence briefs *to ensure that patient is protected and will not be embarrassed by incontinence.* ▪ Maintain fluid intake of 3000 ml/day *to promote urinary output and aid in preventing infection.*
NURSING DIAGNOSIS	**Constipation** *related to* immobility, inadequate fluid intake, improper diet, and neuromuscular impairment *as manifested by* hard stool, decreased bowel sounds, infrequent or absent bowel movements.
▪ Regular bowel evacuation.	▪ Turn patient regularly; maintain activity to individual tolerance *because mobility enhances peristalsis.* ▪ Maintain fluid intake (3000 ml/day) *to promote normal stool consistency.* ▪ Use prune juice at same time of day *because dihydroxyphenyl isatin in prune juice has a laxative effect.* ▪ Encourage high-residue diet *to improve stool consistency and promote evacuation.* ▪ Administer stool softeners and suppositories as ordered *to promote regularity by improving stool consistency.* ▪ Initiate and maintain bowel program *to foster regular bowel elimination.*
NURSING DIAGNOSIS	**Sexual dysfunction** *related to* neuromuscular deficits *as manifested by* impotence, verbalization of problem, decreased libido.
▪ Verbalization of satisfaction with expression of sexuality.	▪ Initiate sexual counseling if indicated *because not all nurses have the education required for this type of counseling.* ▪ Suggest alternative methods of achieving sexual gratification *because sexual intercourse may not be possible due to neuromuscular deficits.*
NURSING DIAGNOSIS	**Self-esteem disturbance** *related to* prolonged debilitating condition *as manifested by* feelings of inadequacy, depression, fatigue, withdrawal.
▪ Maintenance of realistic self-concept in relation to disease.	▪ Focus on remaining abilities and maintaining independence *because a major part of self-concept is the ability to perform one's role functions.* ▪ Assist patient in grieving process *because progressive losses or changes in body function may interfere with resolution of grieving process.* ▪ Encourage patient to discuss effect of MS on self-concept *to clarify issues and identify coping behaviors.* ▪ Discuss importance of maintaining social interactions *to prevent social isolation, withdrawal, and negative self-concept.*
NURSING DIAGNOSIS	**Altered family processes** *related to* changing family roles, potential financial problems, and fluctuating physical condition *as manifested by* strained family relations, ineffective communication, verbalization of financial concerns.
▪ Open communication between family and patient. ▪ Able to seek outside assistance when indicated. ▪ Maintenance of adequate care.	▪ Facilitate open communication among family members *to help family understand behaviors that may be triggered by emotional or physical effects of MS.* ▪ Promote problem solving *to enable the family to handle the issues of long-term illness.* ▪ Refer for family and financial counseling (if indicated) *to provide additional help in coping with a chronic debilitating disease.* ▪ Educate family regarding fluctuating nature of disease *because lack of knowledge about MS affects ability to cope with the changes.*

RESEARCH
IMPLICATIONS FOR NURSING PRACTICE

Health Promotion for Women with Multiple Sclerosis

Citation Stuifbergen AK, Roberts GJ: Health promotion practices of women with multiple sclerosis, *Arch Phys Med Rehabil* 78:S3, 1997.

Purpose To examine health-promoting behaviors of women with multiple sclerosis (MS). The investigators hypothesized that health-promoting behaviors influence the relationship between severity of illness and quality of life.

Methods A community-based sample of women ($n = 629$) with MS completed a series of questionnaires focused on measures of illness-related disability, health-promoting behaviors (e.g., stress management, physical activity, nutrition), and quality of life. Results were compared with a community-based group of healthy women. In addition, women with MS were grouped by clinical course (e.g., benign sensory, relapsing-remitting, progressive, severe progressive) and compared on frequency of health-promoting behaviors.

Results and Conclusions As a group women with MS scored lower on physical activity but higher on stress management and interpersonal relationships than the control group. When grouped by severity of disease, women with benign sensory and relapsing-remitting MS were more likely to engage in physical activity and spiritual growth behaviors than women with progressive MS. The course of disease affects the health-promoting behaviors that women engage in, as do the severity of symptoms.

Implications for Nursing Practice The presence of a chronic disabling condition affects the degree to which women engage in health-promoting behaviors. Symptoms such as fatigue, weakness, and incoordination can affect the desire and ability to participate in physical activity. Women with MS should be encouraged to participate in physical activities that can be performed, such as yoga, tai-chi, and other stress-reducing activities.

Patient education should focus on building general resistance to illness, including avoiding fatigue, extremes of heat and cold, and exposure to infection. The last measure involves avoiding exposure to cold climates and to people who are sick, as well as vigorous and early treatment of infection when it does occur. It is important to teach the patient to (1) achieve a good balance of exercise and rest, (2) eat nutritious and well-balanced meals, and (3) avoid the hazards of immobility (contractures and pressure sores). Patients should know their treatment regimens, the side effects of medications and how to watch for them, and drug interactions with over-the-counter medications. The patient should consult a health care provider before taking nonprescription medications.

Bladder control is a major problem for many patients with MS. While anticholinergics may be beneficial for some patients to decrease spasticity, other patients may need to be taught self-catheterization (see Chapter 43). Bowel problems, particularly constipation, occur frequently in patients with MS. Increasing the dietary fiber may help some patients achieve regularity in bowel habits.

The patient with MS and the family must make many emotional adjustments because of the unpredictability of the disease, the need to change lifestyles, and the challenge of avoiding or decreasing precipitating factors. The National Multiple Sclerosis Society and its local chapters can offer a variety of services to meet the needs of patients with MS.

■ Evaluation

Expected outcomes for the patient with MS are addressed in NCP 56-3.

PARKINSON'S DISEASE

Parkinsonism is a syndrome that consists of a slowing down in the initiation and execution of movement (bradykinesia), increased muscle tone (rigidity), tremor, and impaired postural reflexes. Parkinson's disease, a form of parkinsonism, is named after James Parkinson, who, in 1817, wrote a classic essay on "shaking palsy," a disease whose cause is still unknown today. Many other disorders resemble this disease, but their causes are known. These include drug-induced parkinsonism, postencephalitic parkinsonism, and arteriosclerotic parkinsonism. The pathophysiology of these disorders, with the exception of drug-induced parkinsonism, is the same. Damage or loss of the dopamine-producing cells of the substantia nigra in the midbrain leads to depletion, in the basal ganglia, of dopamine that influences the initiation, modulation, and completion of movement and regulates unconscious autonomic movements (see Chapter 53). In cases of drug-induced parkinsonism the dopamine receptors in the brain are blocked.

Etiology and Pathophysiology

Parkinson's disease affects about 1.5% of the population in the United States over 65 years of age.[14] The disease shows no gender, socioeconomic, or cultural preference, and symptoms most commonly occur after 50 years of age. The average age of the patient with Parkinson's disease is 65 years. There is no apparent genetic cause and no known cure. The disease rarely occurs in African-Americans.

There are many causes of parkinsonism. Encephalitis lethargica, or type A encephalitis, has been clearly associated with the onset of parkinsonism. However, the incidence of postencephalitic parkinsonism has dwindled since the 1920s, when there was a large outbreak of this infectious illness. Parkinsonism-like symptoms have occurred after intoxication with a variety of chemicals, including carbon monoxide and manganese (among copper miners) and product of meperidine-analog synthesis. Drug-induced parkinsonism can follow reserpine (Hydropres), methyldopa (Aldomet), haloperidol (Haldol), and phenothiazine (Thorazine) therapy. Although patients with cerebrovascular disease may have parkinsonism-like

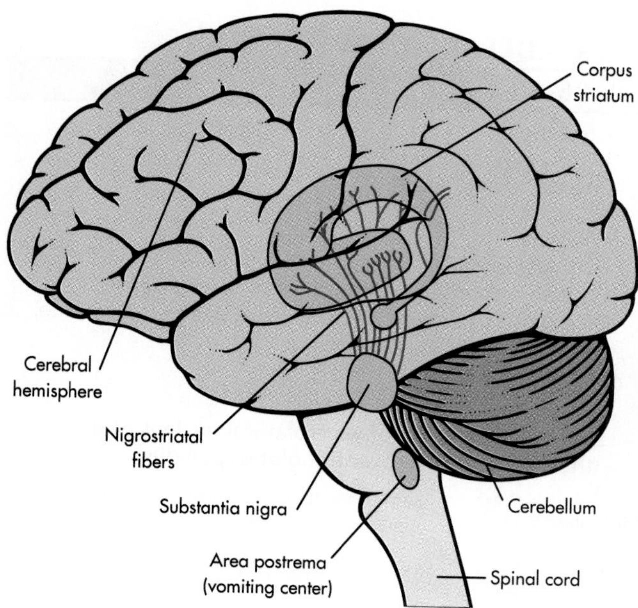

Fig. 56-4 Nigrostriatal disorders produce parkinsonism. Left-sided view of the human brain showing the substantia nigra and the corpus striatum (*shaded area*) lying deep within the cerebral hemisphere. Nerve fibers extend upward from the substantia nigra, divide into many branches, and carry dopamine to all regions of the corpus striatum.

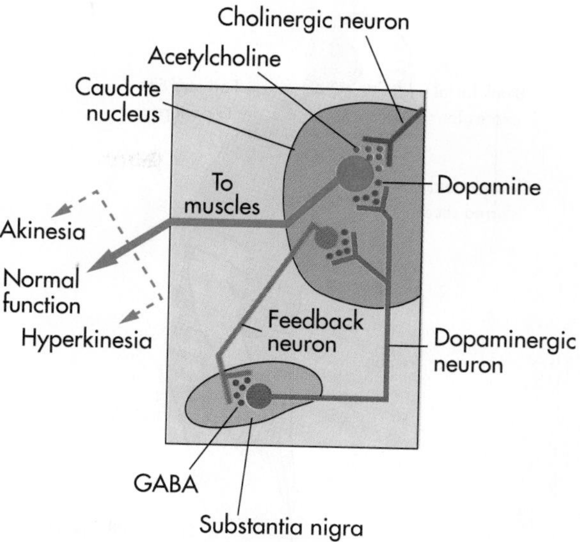

Fig. 56-5 Dopaminergic synaptic activity is mediated by dopamine. Cholinergic synaptic activity is mediated by acetylcholine. A balance between the two kinds of activity produces normal motor function. A relative excess of cholinergic activity produces akinesia and rigidity. A relative excess of dopaminergic activity produces involuntary movements. Neurons in the caudate nucleus contain gamma-aminobutyric acid (GABA) and possibly control dopaminergic neurons in the substantia nigra through a feedback pathway.

symptoms, there is little evidence that parkinsonism is caused by arteriosclerosis. Distinguishing arteriosclerosis from true Parkinson's disease is important for prognostic purposes. Patients with arteriosclerosis do not respond as well to treatment and are more likely to experience side effects of drug therapy. Most patients with parkinsonism have the degenerative or idiopathic form, for which the term *Parkinson's disease* is usually reserved.

The pathology of Parkinson's disease is associated with the degeneration of the dopamine-producing neurons in the substantia nigra of the midbrain (Figs. 56-4 and 56-5). It is hypothesized that there is normally a balance between acetylcholine (ACh) and dopamine (DA) in the basal ganglia. Any shift in the balance of activity (an increase in ACh or a decrease in DA) seems to lead to parkinsonism-like symptoms. Dopamine is a neurotransmitter that is essential for normal functioning of the extrapyramidal motor system, including control of posture, support, and voluntary motion. In Parkinson's disease the levels of DA-synthesizing enzymes and metabolites are reduced, and postmortem analysis of cross sections of the midbrain shows loss of the normal melanin pigment in the substantia nigra and loss of neurons. In addition, deficient amounts of gamma-aminobutyric acid (GABA), serotonin, and norepinephrine have been found in basal ganglia and in the substantia nigra.

Clinical Manifestations

The onset of Parkinson's disease is gradual and insidious, with a gradual progression and a prolonged course. In the beginning stages, only a mild tremor, a slight limp, or a decreased arm swing may be evident. Later in the disease the patient may have a shuffling, propulsive gait with arms flexed and loss of postural reflexes. In some patients there may be a slight change in speech patterns. None of these alone is sufficient evidence for a diagnosis of the disease.

Because there is no specific diagnostic test for Parkinson's disease, the diagnosis is based solely on the history and the clinical features. A firm diagnosis can be made only when there are at least two of the three characteristic signs of the classic triad: tremor, rigidity, and bradykinesia (slow or retarded movement). Dementia occurs in up to 40% of patients with Parkinson's disease.[15,16] The ultimate confirmation of Parkinson's disease is a positive response to antiparkinsonian medication.

Tremor. Tremor, often the first sign, may be minimal initially, so the patient is the only one who notices it. This tremor can affect handwriting, causing it to trail off, particularly toward the ends of words. Parkinsonian tremor is more prominent at rest and is aggravated by emotional stress or increased concentration. The hand tremor is described as "pill rolling" because the thumb and forefinger appear to move in a rotary fashion as if rolling a pill, coin, or other small object. Tremor can involve the diaphragm, tongue, lips, and jaw but rarely causes shaking of the head. Unfortunately, in many people a benign essential tremor has mistakenly been diagnosed as Parkinson's disease. Essential tremor occurs during voluntary movement, has a more rapid frequency than parkinsonian tremor, and is often familial.

Rigidity. Rigidity, the second sign of the triad, is the increased resistance to passive motion when the limbs are moved through their range of motion. Parkinsonian rigidity

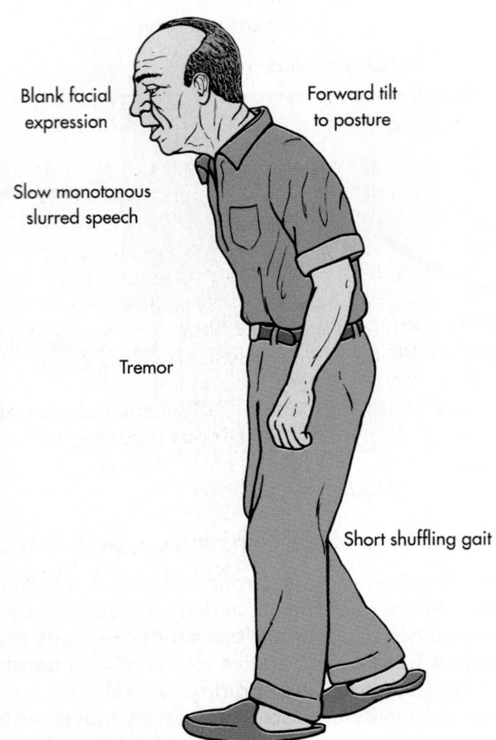

Fig. 56-6 Characteristic appearance of a patient with Parkinson's disease.

is typified by a jerky quality, as if there were intermittent catches in the movement of a cogwheel, when the joint is moved. This is termed *cogwheel rigidity.* The rigidity is caused by sustained muscle contraction and consequently elicits a complaint of muscle soreness; feeling tired and achy; or pain in the head, upper body, spine, or legs. Another consequence of rigidity is slowness of movement, because it inhibits the alternating of contraction and relaxation in opposing muscle groups (e.g., the biceps and triceps).

Bradykinesia. Bradykinesia is particularly evident in the loss of automatic movements, which is secondary to the physical and chemical alteration of the basal ganglia and related structures in the extrapyramidal portion of the CNS. In the unaffected patient, automatic movements are involuntary and occur subconsciously. They include blinking of the eyelids, swinging of the arms while walking, swallowing of saliva, self-expression with facial and hand movements, and minor movement of postural adjustment. The patient with Parkinson's disease does not execute these movements, and there is a lack of spontaneous activity. This accounts for the stooped posture, masked facies ("deadpan" expression), drooling of saliva, and shuffling gait (festination) that are characteristic of a person with this disease. In addition, there is difficulty in initiating movement. Movements such as getting out of a chair cannot be executed unless they are consciously willed.

Complications

Many of the complications of Parkinson's disease are caused by the deterioration and loss of spontaneity of movement. Swallowing may become very difficult (dysphagia) in severe cases, leading to malnutrition or aspiration. General debilitation may lead to pneumonia, urinary tract infections, and skin breakdown. Mobility is greatly decreased. The gait slows, and turning is especially difficult. The gait usually consists of rapid, short, shuffling ministeps. The posture is that of the "old man" image, with the head and trunk bent forward and the legs constantly flexed (Fig. 56-6). The lack of mobility may lead to constipation, ankle edema, and, more seriously, contractures.

Orthostatic hypotension may occur in some patients, and along with loss of postural reflexes, may result in falls or other injury. Bothersome complications include seborrhea (increased oily secretion of the sebaceous glands of the skin), dandruff, excessive sweating, conjunctivitis, difficulty in reading, insomnia, incontinence, and depression.

Many of the apparent complications of Parkinson's disease are the result of side effects of medication, particularly levodopa. Dyskinesias (e.g., fidgeting movements of limbs) and weakness and akinesia (total immobility) may cause problems. These complications become apparent after prolonged levodopa therapy.

COLLABORATIVE CARE

Table 56-16 Parkinson's Disease

Diagnostic
- History
- Physical examination
  - Tremor
  - Rigidity
  - Bradykinesia
- Positive response to antiparkinson medication*
- Ruling out of side effects of phenothiazines, reserpine, benzodiazepines, haloperidol

Collaborative Therapy
- Antiparkinson medication*
- Surgical destruction of ventrolateral nucleus of the thalamus or posteroventral globus pallidus

*See Table 56-17.

Collaborative Care

Because there is no cure for Parkinson's disease, collaborative management (Table 56-16) is aimed at relieving the symptoms.

Drug Therapy. Pharmacotherapy of Parkinson's disease is aimed at correcting an imbalance of neurotransmitters within the CNS. Antiparkinsonian drugs either enhance the release or supply of DA (dopaminergic) or antagonize or block the effects of the overactive cholinergic neurons in the striatum (anticholinergic). Levodopa with carbidopa (Sinemet) is often the first drug to be used. Levodopa is a precursor of dopamine and can cross the blood-brain barrier. It is converted to dopamine in the basal ganglia. Sinemet is the preferred medication because it also contains carbidopa, an agent that inhibits the enzyme dopa-decarboxylase in the peripheral tissues. This enzyme breaks down levodopa before it reaches the brain. The net result is that more levodopa reaches the brain, and therefore less drug is needed.

DRUG THERAPY

Table 56-17 Parkinson's Disease

Drug	Symptoms Relieved	Side Effects and Precautions
Dopaminergic		
Levodopa (L-dopa)	Bradykinesia, tremor, rigidity	Nausea, dyskinesia, hypotension, palpitations, arrhythmias; agitation, hallucinations, confusion (in older patient); avoidance of vitamin pills and diet high in vitamin B_6 (reversal of effect of levodopa); contraindicated in narrow-angle glaucoma
Levodopa/carbidopa (Sinemet)	Bradykinesia, tremor, rigidity	Less nausea but greater chance of dyskinesia, confusion, hallucinations; periodic check of BUN, AST, WBCs, Hct; contraindicated in melanoma, narrow-angle glaucoma, combination with MAO inhibitors, reserpine, methyldopa, guanethidine, antipsychotics
Bromocriptine mesylate (Parlodel)	Bradykinesia, tremor, rigidity	Orthostatic hypotension, nausea, vomiting, toxic psychosis, limb edema, phlebitis, dizziness, headache, insomnia
Pergolide (Permax)	Same as above	Same as above
Pramipexole (Mirapex)	Same as above	
Ropinirole (Requip)	Same as above	
Amantadine (Symmetrel)	Rigidity, akinesia	Nervousness, insomnia, confusion, hallucinations, dry mouth, nausea, edema, orthostatic hypotension
Anticholinergic		
Trihexyphenidyl (Artane)	Tremor	Dry mouth, blurred vision, constipation, delirium, anxiety, agitation, hallucinations; avoidance of drugs with similar actions, including over-the-counter drugs containing scopolamine or antihistamines (e.g., Sominex), antispasmodics (e.g., Donnatal, Bellergal), tricyclic antidepressants (Tofranil, Elavil, Norpramin, Vivactil)
Cycrimine (Pagitane)		
Procyclidine (Kemadrin)		
Benztropine (Cogentin)		
Biperiden (Akineton)		
Antihistamine		
Diphenhydramine (Benadryl)	Tremor, rigidity	Sedation, same precautions as for anticholinergic drugs
Orphenadrine (Disipal)		
Chlorphenoxamine (Phenoxene)		
Phenindamine (Thephorin)		
Monoamine Oxidase Inhibitor		
Selegiline (Eldepryl, Carbex)	Bradykinesia, rigidity, tremor	Similar to dopaminergic drugs

AST, aspartate aminotransferase; *BUN*, blood urea nitrogen; *Hct*, hematocrit; *MAO*, monoamine oxidase; *WBCs*, white blood cells.

During early-stage Parkinson's disease, if the symptoms are not severe, mild antiparkinsonian drugs (e.g., dopamine agonists such as bromocriptine [Parlodel] and pergolide [Permax]), can provide improvement in symptoms. Newer dopamine receptor agonists (ropinirole [Requip] and pramipexole [Mirapex]) have also been shown to be effective in improving symptoms of early Parkinson's disease.[17,18] These drugs directly stimulate dopamine receptors. When more moderate to severe symptoms are present, carbidopa/levodopa are added to the drug regimen. Other adjuvant agents include amantadine (Symmetrel), anticholinergic medications (trihexyphenidyl [Artane] or benztropine [Cogentin]), selegiline (Eldepryl, Carbex), and diphenhydramine (Benadryl).

Anticholinergic drugs are also used to manage Parkinson's disease. These drugs act by decreasing the activity of ACh and thus providing balance between cholinergic and dopaminergic actions. Antihistamines (e.g., diphenhydramine [Benadryl]) with anticholinergic properties or propanolol (e.g., long-acting Inderal) are used to manage tremors. The antiviral agent amantadine (Symmetrel) is also an effective antiparkinsonian drug. Although its exact mechanism of action is not known, amantadine promotes the release of DA from neurons. Selegiline is a monoamine oxidase (MAO) inhibitor that is sometimes used in combination with Sinemet. By inhibiting MAO, the degradative enzyme for DA, the levels of DA are increased.

Table 56-17 summarizes the drugs commonly used in Parkinson's disease, the symptoms they relieve, and their common side effects. The use of only one drug is preferred, since there are fewer side effects and the medication is easier to adjust than when several drugs are used. Excessive amounts of dopaminergic drugs can lead to paradoxic intoxication (aggravation

NURSING ASSESSMENT

Table 56-18 Parkinson's Disease

Subjective Data	Objective Data
Important Health Information *Past health history:* CNS trauma, cerebrovascular disorders, exposure to metals and carbon monoxide, encephalitis *Medication:* Use of major tranquilizers, especially haloperidol (Haldol) and phenothiazines, reserpine, methyldopa **Functional Health Patterns** *Health perception–health management:* Fatigue *Nutritional-metabolic:* Excessive salivation, dysphagia; weight loss *Elimination:* Constipation, incontinence; excessive sweating *Activity-exercise:* Difficulty in initiating movements; frequent falls; loss of dexterity; micrographia (handwriting deterioration) *Sleep-rest:* Insomnia *Cognitive-perceptual:* Diffuse pain in head, shoulders, neck, back, legs, and hips; muscle soreness and cramping *Self-perception–self-concept:* Depression; mood swings, hallucinations	**General** Blank (masked) facies, slow and monotonous speech, infrequent blinking **Integumentary** Seborrhea, dandruff; ankle edema **Cardiovascular** Postural hypotension **Gastrointestinal** Drooling **Neurologic** Tremor at rest, first in hands (pill-rolling), later in legs, arms, face, and tongue; aggravation of tremor with anxiety, absence in sleep; poor coordination; subtle dementia, impaired postural reflexes **Musculoskeletal** "Cogwheel" rigidity, dysarthria, bradykinesia, contractures, stooped posture, shuffling gait **Possible Findings** Lack of specific tests, diagnosis on basis of history and physical findings and ruling out of other diseases

rather than relief of symptoms). Anticholinergic drugs can cause impaired erection and failure of ejaculation.

Surgical Therapy. Surgical procedures are aimed at relieving symptoms (e.g., tremor, rigidity) of Parkinson's disease. Surgical procedures such as thalamotomy, thalamic stimulation, and pallidotomy are often reserved for patients who are unresponsive to drug therapy or who have developed severe motor complications.[19,20] Stereotactic thalamotomy relieves tremor and to a lesser extent rigidity. However, bradykinesia and postural instability are not improved. It involves making a lesion in a specific region of the thalamus. Bilateral posteroventral pallidotomy relieves tremor, rigidity, and bradykinesia. The procedure involves making a lesion in a specific area between the medial and lateral segments of the globus pallidus.[19] Improvements in rigidity, tremor, dyskinesia, and dystonia have been shown. Chronic thalamic electrical stimulation has been used to reduce tremor and enhance motor function.[20]

Transplantation of fetal neural tissue into the caudate nucleus in an attempt to provide viable dopamine-producing cells to the brain has had variable results.[21] Fetal adrenal brain tissue transplantation has also been used with less promising results.[22]

Nutritional Therapy. Diet is of major importance to the patient with Parkinson's disease because malnutrition and constipation can be serious consequences of inadequate nutrition. Patients who have dysphagia and bradykinesia need appetizing foods that are easily chewed and swallowed. The diet should contain adequate roughage and fruit to avoid constipation. Food should be cut into bite-sized pieces before it is served, and it should be served on a warmed plate to preserve its appeal. Eating six small meals a day may be less exhausting than eating three large meals a day. Ample time should be planned for eating to avoid frustration and encourage independence.

NURSING MANAGEMENT: PARKINSON'S DISEASE

Nursing Assessment

Subjective and objective data that should be obtained from a person with Parkinson's disease are presented in Table 56-18.

Nursing Diagnoses

Nursing diagnoses for the patient with Parkinson's disease may include, but are not limited to, those presented in NCP 56-4.

Planning

The overall goals are that the patient with Parkinson's disease will (1) maximize neurologic function, (2) maintain independence in activities of daily living for as long as possible, and (3) optimize psychosocial well-being.

Nursing Implementation

Promotion of physical exercise and a well-balanced diet are major concerns for nursing care. Exercise can limit the consequences of decreased mobility, such as muscle atrophy, contractures, and constipation. The American Parkinson's Disease Association publishes a booklet, *Home Exercises for Patients with Parkinson's Disease,* that illustrates a variety of exercises; it can be used by family members and health professionals.

A physical therapist may be consulted to design a personal exercise program aimed at strengthening specific muscles. Overall muscle tone, as well as specific exercises to strengthen the muscles involved with speaking and swallowing, should be included. Although exercise will not halt the progress of the disease, it will bring the patient's motor function to an optimal level.

Because Parkinson's disease is a chronic degenerative disorder with no acute exacerbations, nurses should note that health teaching and nursing care are directed toward maintenance of

56-4 NURSING CARE PLAN PATIENT WITH PARKINSON'S DISEASE

Expected Patient Outcomes | **Nursing Interventions and *Rationales***

NURSING DIAGNOSIS **Impaired physical mobility** *related to* rigidity, bradykinesia, and akinesia *as manifested by* difficulty in initiation of volitional movements.

Expected Patient Outcomes
- Safe ambulation.
- Maintenance of joint mobility.

Nursing Interventions and Rationales
- Assist with ambulation *to assess degree of impairment and to prevent injury.*
- Perform active range-of-motion (ROM) exercises to all extremities *to maintain joint ROM, prevent atrophy, and strengthen muscles.*
- Consult physical therapist or occupational therapist for aids *to facilitate activities of daily living (ADLs) and safe ambulation.*
- Evaluate tremor in relation to medication *to monitor patient's response and identify possible overdose.*
- Teach techniques to assist with mobility by instructing patient to step over imaginary line, rock from side to side to initiate leg movements *because these are helpful in dealing with "freezing" (akinesia) while walking.*

NURSING DIAGNOSIS **Self-care deficits** *related to* parkinsonian symptoms *as manifested by* inability to perform ADLs, need for assistive devices.

Expected Patient Outcomes
- Optimal independence in ADLs.
- Daily needs met by self or other.

Nursing Interventions and Rationales
- Encourage activities of daily living within limits of mobility *to prolong patient's independence.*
- Arrange patient's room *to facilitate optimal self-care.*
- Plan sufficient time for patient to perform self-care *because rigidity causes slowness of movement.*
- Provide assistance as needed *so patient's needs are met and frustration reduced.*
- Arrange occupational therapy consultation *to teach additional strategies for achieving ADLs and to minimize complications such as contractures.*
- Offer emotional support *to bolster patient's effort in coping with a chronic degenerative disease.*

NURSING DIAGNOSIS **Impaired verbal communication** *related to* dysarthria and tremor or bradykinesia *as manifested by* decreased amount of communication, slow and slurred speech, inability to move facial muscles, decreased tongue mobility, micrographia, inability to write.

Expected Patient Outcomes
- Development of communication method to meet needs.

Nursing Interventions and Rationales
- Allow sufficient time for communication *to reduce patient's frustration.*
- Encourage deep breaths before speaking.
- Consult speech therapist *to provide specialized guidance in care of the patient.*
- Provide alternative communication methods such as picture books or flash cards *since muscle involvement has impaired writing and speaking ability.*
- Massage patient's facial and neck muscles *to foster relaxation that can facilitate speech.*

NURSING DIAGNOSIS **Constipation** *related to* weakness of abdominal and perineal muscles, lack of exercise, and side effects of medication *as manifested by* hardened stool and decreased bowel sounds.

Expected Patient Outcomes
- Maintenance of regular bowel evacuation.

Nursing Interventions and Rationales
- Increase fluid intake to 3000 ml/day *to maintain soft stool.*
- Increase fiber in diet with every meal *to provide bulk to stool.*
- Increase mobility to tolerance *to stimulate peristalsis.*
- Give stool softeners, laxatives, suppositories as needed *to ensure regular bowel evacuation.*

NURSING DIAGNOSIS **Altered nutrition: less than body requirements** *related to* dysphagia *as manifested by* difficulty in swallowing and chewing, drooling, decreased gag reflex.

Expected Patient Outcomes
- Maintenance of satisfactory body weight.

Nursing Interventions and Rationales
- Carefully monitor swallowing ability during medication administration and mealtime *to evaluate patient's level of impairment and minimize risk of aspiration.*
- Provide soft-solid and thick-liquid diet *because these consistencies are more easily swallowed.*
- Massage patient's facial and neck muscles before meals *to reduce rigidity and enhance ability to chew and swallow.*
- Maintain patient in upright position for all meals *to reduce risk of aspiration.*
- Consult speech therapist and dietician *because they can provide specific plans to improve swallowing and intake.*

Continued

56-4 NURSING CARE PLAN PATIENT WITH PARKINSON'S DISEASE—continued

Expected Patient Outcomes	Nursing Interventions and *Rationales*
NURSING DIAGNOSIS **Altered nutrition: less than body requirements**—*continued*	
	▪ Maintain caloric counts and weekly weights *to evaluate patient's nutritional status and adjust plan if indicated.* ▪ Have suction available *to remove pooled secretions and prevent choking and aspiration.*
NURSING DIAGNOSIS **Diversional activity deficit** *related to* inability to perform usual recreational activities *as manifested by* boredom, lack of participation, restlessness, depression, hostility.	
▪ Engagement in satisfying diversional activities. ▪ Expression of acceptance of diminished capabilities.	▪ Assess patient's activity *to determine physical and emotional response to difficulties.* ▪ Determine preferred diversional activities *so individual needs are considered.* ▪ Adapt difficult activities when possible *so patient is able to continue performing activities.* ▪ Initiate new activities within patient's capabilities, such as reading, *to replace activities patient can no longer perform.* ▪ Encourage patient to discuss emotional response to decreasing capabilities *to provide opportunity to problem solve and demonstrate a caring attitude.*
NURSING DIAGNOSIS **Sleep pattern disturbance** *related to* medication side effects (e.g., hallucinations), anxiety, rigidity, and muscle discomfort *as manifested by* poor sleep history, inability to sleep uninterrupted, nightmares, vivid dreams or hallucinations, anxiety, rigidity, or muscle discomfort.	
▪ Verbalization of feeling rested on awakening.	▪ Provide quiet environment *to promote uninterrupted sleep.* ▪ Turn and position for comfort *because muscle soreness and inability to make minor postural changes as a result of bradykinesia may interfere with sleep.* ▪ Provide passive ROM exercises to extremities *to alleviate rigidity that may interfere with sleep.* ▪ Provide daytime stimulus to maintain wakefulness *to avoid excess napping, which prevents quality nighttime sleep.* ▪ Offer support if hallucinations are present *to decrease anxiety, since levodopa may produce hallucinations.* ▪ Give sleep medications as ordered *to facilitate sleep.*

good health, encouragement of independence, and avoidance of complications such as contractures.

Problems secondary to bradykinesia can be alleviated by relatively simple measures. The following are helpful hints for patients who tend to "freeze" while walking: consciously think about stepping over imaginary or real lines on the floor, drop rice kernels and step over them, rock from side to side, lift the toes when stepping, take one step backward and two steps forward. The patient should be assessed for the possibility of levodopa overdose because it is a common cause of akinesia "freezing." A brief period of dyskinesia, usually athetosis of the neck, should alert the nurse to this possibility.

Getting out of a chair can be facilitated by using an upright chair with arms and placing the back legs on small (2-inch) blocks. Other aspects of the environment can be altered. Rugs and excess furniture can be removed to avoid stumbling. An ottoman can be used to elevate the legs and avoid dependent ankle edema. Clothing can be simplified by the use of slip-on shoes and Velcro hook-and-loop fasteners or zippers on clothing, instead of buttons and hooks. An elevated toilet seat can facilitate getting on and off the toilet. The nurse should work closely with the patient's family in exploring creative adaptations that allow maximum independence and self-care.

Evaluation

Expected outcomes for the patient with Parkinson's disease are addressed in NCP 56-4.

MYASTHENIA GRAVIS

Myasthenia gravis (MG) is a disease of the neuromuscular junction characterized by the fluctuating weakness of certain skeletal muscle groups. The prevalence is estimated to be from 43 to 84 persons per million. The peak age at onset in women is 20 to 30 years. Women are affected slightly more often than men, although among patients with both thymoma and myasthenia gravis (15% of all persons with MG), the majority are men over the age of 50.

Etiology and Pathophysiology

MG is caused by an autoimmune process that results in production of antibodies directed against the ACh receptors and a reduction in the number of ACh receptor sites at the neuromuscular junction. This prevents ACh molecules from attaching and stimulating muscle contraction. Anti-ACh receptor antibodies are detectable in the serum of 70% to 85% of patients with MG. As a result of this process there is loss of muscle strength. Thymic tumors are found in about 15% of patients.

COLLABORATIVE CARE

Table 56-19 Myasthenia Gravis

Diagnostic
- Complete history
- Physical examination
  - Fatigability with prolonged upward gaze (2-3 min)
  - Muscle weakness
- EMG
- Tensilon test

Collaborative Therapy
- Drugs
  - Anticholinesterase agents
  - Corticosteroids
  - Immunosuppressive agents
- Surgery (thymectomy)
- Plasmapheresis

EMG, electromyography.

Although a viral infection is suspected as precipitating an attack, a single specific cause for all cases of MG has not been found.

Clinical Manifestations and Complications

The primary feature of MG is easy fatigability of skeletal muscle during activity. Strength is usually restored after a period of rest. The muscles most often involved are those used for moving the eyes and eyelids, chewing, swallowing, speaking, and breathing. The cell bodies of the neurons for these muscles are located in the brainstem. The muscles are generally the strongest in the morning and become exhausted with continued activity. Consequently, by the end of the day, muscle fatigue is prominent.

In more than 90% of the cases, the eyelid muscles or extraocular muscles are involved. Facial mobility and expression can be impaired. There may be difficulty in chewing and swallowing food. Speech is affected, and the voice often fades after a long conversation. The muscles of the trunk and limbs are less often affected. Of these, the proximal muscles of the neck, shoulder, and hip are more often affected than the distal muscles. No other signs of neural disorder accompany MG; there is no sensory loss, reflexes are normal, and muscle atrophy is rare.

The course of this disease is highly variable. Some patients may have short-term remissions, others may stabilize, and others may have severe, progressive involvement. Restricted ocular myasthenia, usually seen only in men, has a good prognosis. Exacerbations of MG can be precipitated by emotional stress, pregnancy, menses, secondary illness, trauma, temperature extremes, hypokalemia, ingestion of drugs with neuromuscular blocking properties, and surgery. In some cases the onset of MG occurs after one of these events.

The major complications of MG result from muscle weakness in areas that affect swallowing and breathing. Aspiration, respiratory insufficiency, and respiratory infection are the major complications. An acute exacerbation of this type is sometimes termed *myasthenic crisis.*

Diagnostic Studies

The simplest diagnostic test for myasthenia gravis is to have the patient look upward for 2 to 3 minutes. If the problem is MG, there will be an increased droop of the eyelids, so that the person can barely keep the eyes open. After a brief rest the eyes can open again. Other tests may be used if the diagnosis is still in doubt. EMG may show a decrementing response to repeated stimulation of the hand muscles, indicative of muscle fatigue. Use of pharmacologic agents may also aid in the diagnosis. The Tensilon test in a patient with MG reveals improved muscle contractility after intravenous (IV) injection of the anticholinesterase agent edrophonium chloride (Tensilon). This test also aids in the diagnosis of cholinergic crisis (secondary to overdose of neostigmine). In this condition, Tensilon does not improve muscle weakness but may actually increase it. Atropine should be readily available to counteract Tensilon effects when it is used diagnostically.

Collaborative Care

Drug Therapy. The major forms of therapy for MG are anticholinesterase drugs, alternate-day corticosteroids, immunosuppressants, and plasmapheresis (Table 56-19). Anticholinesterase drugs are used in the management of MG. Acetylcholinesterase is the enzyme responsible for the breakdown of ACh in the synaptic cleft. Thus inhibition of this enzyme by an anticholinesterase inhibitor will prolong the action of ACh and facilitate transmission of impulses at the neuromuscular junction. Neostigmine (Prostigmin) and pyridostigmine (Mestinon) are the most successful drugs of this group. Tailoring the dose to avoid a myasthenic or cholinergic crisis often presents a clinical challenge. Because of the autoimmune nature of the disorder, corticosteroids (specifically prednisone) are used to suppress immunity. Cytotoxic drugs such as azathioprine (Imuran) and cyclophosphamide (Cytoxan) may also be used for immunosuppression.

Many drugs are contraindicated or must be used with caution in patients with MG. Classes of drug that should be cautiously evaluated before use include anesthetics, antiarrhythmics, antibiotics, quinine, antipsychotics, barbiturates and sedative-hypnotics, cathartics, diuretics, narcotics, muscle relaxants, thyroid preparations, and tranquilizers.

Surgical Therapy. Because the presence of the thymus gland in the patient with MG appears to enhance the production of ACh receptor antibodies, removal of the thymus gland results in improvement in a majority of patients. Thymectomy is indicated for almost all patients with thymoma, for patients with generalized MG between the ages of puberty and about 60 years, and for patients with purely ocular MG.[23]

Other Therapies. Plasmapheresis as a therapy for MG was first reported in 1976. This procedure involves separation of plasma from blood by a machine called a cell separator, which is connected to the patient by a vascular cannula. This process removes anti-ACh receptor antibodies. Plasmapheresis can yield a short-term improvement in symptoms and is indicated for patients in crisis or in preparation for surgery when corticosteroids must be avoided. (Plasmapheresis is discussed in Chapter 12.) Intravenous IgG has been used with some success. However, there have been no large, well-controlled, randomized prospective studies of this therapy in MG.[24]

NURSING MANAGEMENT: MYASTHENIA GRAVIS

■ Nursing Assessment

The nurse can assess the severity of MG by asking the patient about fatigability, what body parts are affected, and how severely they are affected. The patient's coping abilities and

Table 56-20 Comparison of Myasthenic Crisis and Cholinergic Crisis

	Myasthenic Crisis	Cholinergic Crisis
Causes	Exacerbation of myasthenia following precipitating factors or failure to take medication as prescribed or dose of medication too low	Overdose of anticholinesterase drugs resulting in increased ACh at the receptor sites, remission (spontaneous or after thymectomy).
Differential diagnosis	Improved strength after IV administration of anticholinesterase drugs; increased weakness of skeletal muscles manifesting as ptosis, bulbar signs (e.g., difficulty in swallowing, difficulty in articulating words), or dyspnea.	Weakness within 1 hr after ingestion of anticholinesterase; increased weakness of skeletal muscles manifesting as ptosis, bulbar signs, dyspnea; effects on smooth muscle include pupillary miosis, salivation, diarrhea, nausea or vomiting, abdominal cramps, increased bronchial secretions, sweating, or lacrimation

ACh, acetycholine.

understanding of the disorder should also be assessed. Some patients become so fatigued that they are no longer able to work or even ambulate.

Objective data should include respiratory rate and depth, oxygen saturation, arterial blood gas analyses, pulmonary function tests, and evidence of respiratory distress in patients with acute myasthenic crisis. Muscle strength of all face and limb muscles should be assessed, as should swallowing, speech (volume and clarity), and cough and gag reflexes.

Nursing Diagnoses

Nursing diagnoses for the patient with MG may include, but are not limited to, the following:

- Ineffective breathing pattern *related to* intercostal muscle weakness
- Ineffective airway clearance *related to* intercostal muscle weakness and impaired cough and gag reflex
- Impaired verbal communication *related to* weakness of the larynx, lips, mouth, pharynx, and jaw
- Altered nutrition: less than body requirements *related to* impaired swallowing, weakness, and inability to prepare food or feed self
- Sensory/perceptual alterations *related to* ptosis, decreased eye movements, and dysconjugate gaze
- Activity intolerance *related to* muscle weakness and fatigability
- Body image disturbance *related to* inability to maintain usual lifestyle and role responsibilities

Planning

The overall goals are that the patient with MG will (1) have a return of normal muscle endurance, (2) avoid complications, and (3) maintain a quality of life appropriate to disease course.

Nursing Implementation

The patient with MG who is admitted to the hospital usually has a respiratory tract infection or is in an acute myasthenic crisis. Nursing care is aimed at maintaining adequate ventilation, continuing drug therapy, and watching for side effects of therapy. The nurse must be able to distinguish cholinergic from myasthenic crisis (Table 56-20), because the causes and treatment of the two conditions differ greatly.

As with other chronic illnesses, care focuses on the neurologic deficits and their impact on daily living. A balanced diet with food that can be chewed and swallowed easily should be prescribed. Semisolid foods may be easier to eat than solids or liquids. Scheduling doses of medication so that peak action is reached at mealtime may make eating less difficult. Diversional activities that require little physical effort and match the interests of the patient should be arranged. Education should focus on the importance of following the medical regimen, potential adverse reactions to specific drugs, planning activities of daily living to avoid fatigue, the availability of community resources, and the complications of the disease and therapy (crisis conditions) and what to do about them. Contact with the Myasthenia Gravis Foundation or an MG support group may be helpful and should be explored.

Evaluation

The overall expected outcomes are that the patient with MG will

- maintain optimal muscle function throughout the day
- be free from side effects of medication
- not experience complications from the disease
- maintain a quality of life appropriate to the disease course

ALZHEIMER'S DISEASE

Alzheimer's disease is a type of dementia that is characterized by progressive deterioration in memory and other aspects of cognition. Alzheimer's disease is increasingly recognized as one of the major health problems in the United States, particularly for persons over 65 years of age. It accounts for more than half of the cases of dementia (about 4 million cases). The major causes of progressive dementia are listed in Table 56-21.

Etiology and Pathophysiology

The etiology of Alzheimer's disease is still unclear, although age is the most important risk factor for developing it. Pathologic changes associated with Alzheimer's disease include neurofibrillary tangles and β-amyloid plaques in the cerebral cortex and hippocampus. The neuritic plaque is a cluster of degenerating axonal and dendritic nerve terminals that contain an abnormal protein (β-amyloid). Neurofibrillary tangles are seen in the cytoplasm of abnormal neurons (Fig. 56-7). These bundles of proteins are in the form of paired helical filaments. There is also an excessive loss of cholinergic neurons, particularly in regions essential for memory and cognition.

There has been much research on the possible genetic etiology of Alzheimer's disease. At least four chromosomes (1, 14, 19, and 21) are involved in some forms of familial Alzheimer's disease.[25] Inheritance of the apo E4 genotype (a gene responsi-

Table 56-21 Major Causes of Progressive Dementia

Senile dementia, Alzheimer type	50%
Multiinfarct (arteriosclerotic)	10%
Combination of senile dementia and multiinfarct	15%
Communicating hydrocephalus Alcoholic or posttraumatic dementia Huntington's chorea Intracranial mass lesions	15%
Uncommon or in combination with other causes Chronic drug use, Creutzfeldt-Jakob disease, metabolic disease (thyroid, liver), nutritional deficits, degenerative disease (spinocerebellar, amyotrophic lateral sclerosis, parkinsonism, multiple sclerosis, Pick's disease, Wilson's disease, epilepsy), AIDS dementia, static postanoxic dementia	10%

Modified from Andreoli TE and others: *Cecil essentials of medicine,* ed 4, Philadelphia, 1997, Saunders.
AIDS, acquired immunodeficiency syndrome.

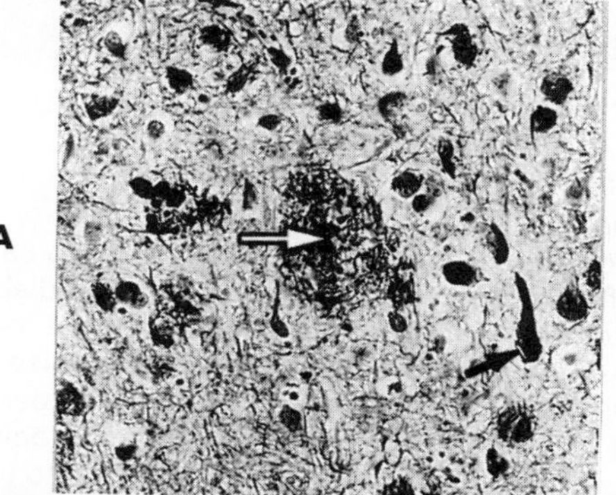
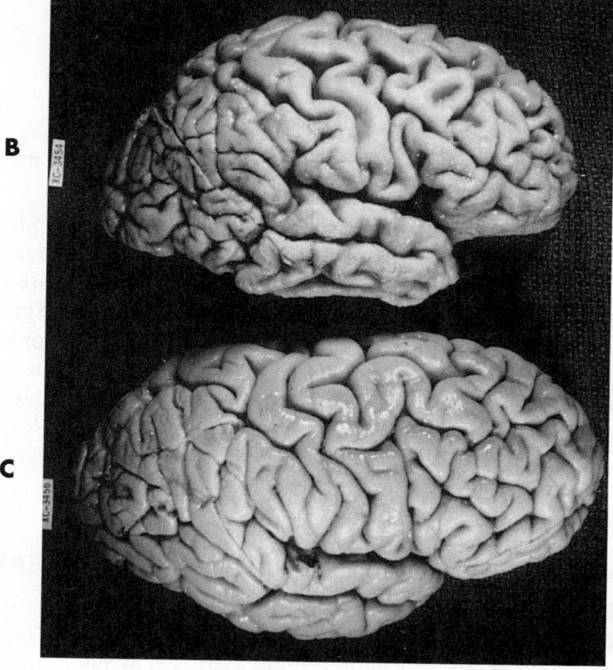

Fig. 56-7 Pathologic changes in Alzheimer's disease. **A,** Neuritic (mature) plaque with central amyloid core *(white arrow)* next to a neurofibrillary tangle *(black arrow).* **B,** Alzheimer's disease compared with **C,** age-matched and sex-matched control.

Table 56-22 Differentiation of Depression and Dementia of Alzheimer's Disease

Characteristic	Depression	Dementia
Onset	Abrupt (weeks)	Insidious
Psychiatric history	Previous depression common	Usually no history
Mental status	Pervasive dysphoria	Flattening of affect
	Normal or impaired cognition	Impaired cognition
	Variable performance	Stable performance
	Variable memory disturbance	Serious effects on memory
Sleep disturbance	Initial and early-morning insomnia	Frequent awakenings
Somatic complaints	Often multiple	Often none
Self-image	Poor	Normal
Suicidal ideation	Present	Present early in disease, then absent
Treatment	High effectiveness of antidepressants	Very limited usefulness of antidepressants
Weight loss	Yes, with appetite disturbance	Not until late in disease

ble for making apolipoprotein) is a major genetic risk factor for developing Alzheimer's disease. There are also data to suggest that estrogen protects against the development of Alzheimer's. Estrogen may also slow the progression of Alzheimer's disease in those who already have it.[26] There is also recent interest in the role of NSAIDs in reducing the risk of Alzheimer's disease. Individuals who have a history of taking NSAIDs (e.g., ibuprofen) for other indications seem to have a lower risk of developing Alzheimer's disease.[26] However, long-term use of NSAIDs is associated with gastrointestinal and kidney problems.

Clinical Manifestations

An initial sign of Alzheimer's disease is a subtle deterioration in memory. Inevitably this progresses to more profound memory loss that interferes with the patient's ability to function. Recent events and new information cannot be recalled. Some patients develop psychotic symptoms. Personal hygiene deteriorates, as does the ability to maintain attention. Later in the disease, long-term memories cannot be recalled, and patients lose the ability to recognize family members. Eventually the ability to communicate and to perform activities of daily living is lost. The progression of the deterioration, which eventually leads to death, varies but can last as long as 20 years.

Alzheimer's disease must be distinguished from depression, a clinically similar condition, because depression is potentially reversible and often responds to appropriate treatment. A careful assessment can distinguish the two clinical conditions (Table 56-22).

Diagnostic Studies

The diagnosis of Alzheimer's disease is a diagnosis of exclusion.[27] When all other possible conditions that can cause mental impairment have been ruled out and the manifestations of dementia persist, the diagnosis of Alzheimer's disease can be made. A

DRUG THERAPY

Table 56-23 Alzheimer's Disease

Manifestation	Drugs	Side Effects
Depression	Tricyclic antidepressants (e.g., nortriptyline [Aventyl, Pamelor], amitriptyline [Elavil], imipramine [Tofranil], doxepin [Sinequan])	Orthostatic hypotension, sedation, dry mouth, constipation, urinary retention, blurry vision
	Nontricyclic antidepressant (e.g., trazodone [Desyrel])	Dry mouth, sedation, confusion
Psychoses and behavioral disturbances	Neuroleptics or antipsychotics (e.g., loxapine [Loxapac], haloperidol [Haldol])	Sedation, extrapyramidal effects, orthostatic hypotension, tardive dyskinesia
	Benzodiazepines (e.g., oxazepam [Serax], diazepam [Valium])	Sedation, confusion, disinhibition with paradoxic agitation, unsteady gait, dysarthria, incoordination
Anxiety	Benzodiazepines	Same as in psychoses and behavioral disturbances
Sleep disturbances	Benzodiazepines, neuroleptics	Same as in psychoses and behavioral disturbances
Decreased memory and cognition	Tacrine (Cognex)	Liver toxicity, nausea and vomiting
	Donepezil (Aricept)	Nausea, diarrhea, insomnia

NURSING ASSESSMENT

Table 56-24 Alzheimer's Disease

Subjective Data

Important Health Information

Past health history: Repeated head trauma, exposure to metals (especially aluminum), previous CNS infection

Medication: Use of any drug to mitigate symptoms (e.g., tranquilizers, hypnotics, antidepressants, antipsychotics)

Functional Health Patterns

Health perception–health management: Positive family history; emotional lability

Nutritional-metabolic: Anorexia, malnutrition, weight loss

Elimination: Incontinence

Activity-exercise: Poor personal hygiene; gait instability, weakness; inability to perform activities of daily living

Sleep-rest: Frequent nighttime awakening, daytime napping

Cognitive-perceptual: Forgetfulness, inability to cope with complex situations, difficulty with problem solving (early signs); depression, withdrawal, suicidal ideation (early)

Objective Data

General

Disheveled appearance, agitation

Neurologic

Early: Loss of recent memory; disorientation to date and time; flat affect; lack of spontaneity; impaired abstraction, cognition, and judgment; loss of remote memory; restlessness and agitation; inability to recognize family and friends; nocturnal wandering; repetitive behavior; loss of social graces; stubbornness, paranoia, belligerence

Advanced: Aphasia, agnosia, alexia (inability to understand written language), apraxia, seizures, limb rigidity, flexor posturing

Possible Findings

Diagnosis by exclusion, cerebral cortical atrophy on CT scan, poor scores on mental status tests, hippocampal atrophy on MRI scan

CT scan or an MRI scan may show brain atrophy and enlarged ventricles in the later stages of the disease, although this finding occurs in other diseases and can also be seen in normal persons. Neuropsychologic testing can help document the degree of cognitive dysfunction in the early stages.[27] The definitive diagnosis of Alzheimer's disease can be made only at autopsy, when the presence of neurofibrillary tangles is observed.

Collaborative Care

The collaborative care of Alzheimer's disease is aimed at improving or controlling decline in cognition and controlling the undesirable symptoms that the patient may exhibit. Table 56-23 details the manifestation of symptoms, the usual drug therapy, and the possible side effects of the prescribed drugs. It is important to be aware that these drugs do not significantly alter the course of the disease.

Recently drugs that inhibit the breakdown of acetylcholine in the brain and thereby enhance cognitive function have become available. In 1993 tacrine (Cognex), an acetylcholinesterase inhibitor, was approved for Alzheimer's disease. It slows the decline in cognitive function.[26,28] However, because of liver toxicity, frequent laboratory monitoring of liver function is required. Donepezil (Aricept) is also an acetylcholinesterase inhibitor. It does not require laboratory monitoring, can be given once a day, and has been shown to either mildly improve or stabilize cognitive decline in some people with Alzheimer's disease. Both drugs are used in the early and middle stages of Alzheimer's disease. These drugs do not cure Alzheimer's disease but rather slow the progression of symptoms.

NURSING MANAGEMENT: ALZHEIMER'S DISEASE

■ Nursing Assessment

Subjective and objective data that should be obtained from a person with Alzheimer's disease are presented in Table 56-24.

■ Nursing Diagnoses

Nursing diagnoses for Alzheimer's disease may include, but are not limited to, those presented in NCP 56-5.

56-5 NURSING CARE PLAN PATIENT WITH ALZHEIMER'S DISEASE

Expected Patient Outcomes	Nursing Interventions and *Rationales*
NURSING DIAGNOSIS **Altered thought processes** *related to* effects of dementia *as manifested by* loss of memory and cognitive deficits.	
▪ Participation in care and social activities to maximum level of ability.	▪ Assess extent of cognitive deficits by direct contact with patient and information from family *to plan appropriate interventions.* ▪ Plan strategies to promote communication, increase self-esteem, and provide stimulation *to maximize patient's cognitive abilities.* ▪ Use reality orientation (early) and routine schedule *to promote memory and reduce confusion.*
NURSING DIAGNOSIS **Self-care deficits** *related to* memory deficit and neuromuscular impairment *as manifested by* inability to independently and appropriately dress, bathe, groom, or toilet.	
▪ Able to appropriately dress and groom self. ▪ Establishment of satisfactory toileting routine. ▪ Adequate nutritional intake.	▪ Assess self-care deficit and determine probable cause *to plan interventions specific to patient's unique problems.* ▪ Verbally remind (cue) patient of appropriate activity; demonstrate use of equipment (e.g., toothbrush, hairbrush, washcloth); lay out clothing daily *because memory loss impairs patient's ability to plan and complete specific sequential activities.* ▪ Continue to assess self-care capabilities and deficits, intervening when necessary, *because self-care abilities fluctuate and interventions must be revised regularly.* ▪ Toilet and change incontinence brief as scheduled *to prevent discomfort and skin excoriation and promote regularity.* ▪ Direct patient to feed self or feed patient if necessary *to ensure adequate food and fluid intake.*
NURSING DIAGNOSIS **Sleep pattern disturbance** *related to* physical discomfort, environmental changes, excessive napping *as manifested by* erratic sleep patterns, nighttime wandering, daytime sleepiness.	
▪ Reasonable periods of uninterrupted rest at appropriate times.	▪ Monitor patient's sleep pattern or get report from caregiver *to plan appropriate interventions.* ▪ Ensure that patient's physical needs are met related to bedtime (e.g., patient toileted, comfortable room temperature, quiet environment) *to prevent physical discomfort from interfering with quality sleep.* ▪ Adapt usual nightly habits such as bedtime, night-lights, warm milk *to provide as much continuity as feasible.* ▪ Reassure wakened patient and reorient in soft, soothing tone (e.g., "It's nighttime. It is time to go back to bed") *to avoid development of anxiety and fear.* ▪ Identify and initiate appropriate daytime diversional activities; plan and implement periods of physical activity during the day *because exercise reduces agitation, produces a calming effect, and promotes sleep at night.*
NURSING DIAGNOSIS **Risk for injury** *related to* impaired judgment, possible gait instability, muscle weakness, and sensory-perceptual alteration.	
▪ No injuries.	▪ Assess regularly for bruises, abrasions, broken bones, and burns *to determine presence of injury.* ▪ Monitor activity; maintain environment free from safety hazards *to decrease or prevent occurrence of injury.* ▪ Assess and record extent of physical limitation (if any) *so appropriate adjustments can be made in care routine and environment.* ▪ Provide assistance when necessary *so patient's needs are met.* ▪ Allow freedom in a safe environment *to give the patient a sense of autonomy.*

Continued

56-5 NURSING CARE PLAN PATIENT WITH ALZHEIMER'S DISEASE—continued

Expected Patient Outcomes	Nursing Interventions and *Rationales*
NURSING DIAGNOSIS	**Risk for violence: self or other-directed** *related to* sensory overload, misinterpretation of environmental stimuli, lack of appropriate coping mechanisms, and unfamiliar environment.
▪ No self-directed or other-directed physical trauma.	▪ Monitor for indicators such as acting-out behavior, verbal threats, and agitation *to identify possibility of violent behavior and initiate appropriate nursing plan.* ▪ Decrease environmental stimuli; avoid giving patient tasks that prove frustrating *to avoid triggering violent behavior.* ▪ Ensure adequate sleep and rest periods *because tiredness and exhaustion can provoke violence.* ▪ Provide opportunities for patient to vent anxiety and frustration; use distraction *to prevent these emotions from escalating to a catastrophic reaction.* ▪ Observe and document in detail any catastrophic reaction and precipitating events *so interventions can be incorporated into care plan to prevent recurrence.*
NURSING DIAGNOSIS	**Ineffective individual coping** *related to* depression in response to diagnosis of Alzheimer's disease *as manifested by* depression, withdrawal, fatigue, social isolation.
▪ Feeling valued as an individual.	▪ Assess for possibility and extent of depression *to develop appropriate interventions.* ▪ Provide opportunity for patient to verbalize feelings *to help clarify issues and show a caring attitude.* ▪ Facilitate communication between patient and family *to foster mutual understanding about relevant issues.* ▪ Provide appropriate diversional activities *to provide pleasurable activities to relieve depression.* ▪ Allow patient to make decisions regarding self-care and environment when possible *to increase sense of worth and control.* ▪ Refer for further evaluation and counseling if indicated.
NURSING DIAGNOSIS	**Risk for ineffective management of therapeutic regimen** *related to* decreasing level of cognitive functioning and memory.
▪ Care needs met by self or others as condition deteriorates.	▪ Discuss with patient need to make plans for care as condition deteriorates *to ensure patient's wishes are respected and health needs are met.* ▪ Assist patient to make lifestyle adjustments such as labeling items and ceasing driving *to compensate for changing cognitive status and to live independently as long as possible.*

Planning

The overall goals are that the patient with Alzheimer's disease will (1) maintain functional ability for as long as possible, (2) be maintained in a safe environment with a minimum of injuries, and (3) have personal care needs met.

Nursing Implementation

Because traumatic brain injury is a risk factor for developing Alzheimer's disease, the nurse should promote safety in physical activities and driving. Depression should be recognized and treated early.

Although there is no current treatment for reversing Alzheimer's disease, there is a need for ongoing monitoring of both the patient with Alzheimer's disease and the patient's caregiver. An important nursing responsibility is to work collaboratively with the patient's physician to manage symptoms effectively as they change over time (see NCP 56-5). The nurse is often responsible for teaching the caregiver to perform the many tasks that are required to manage the care of the patient with Alzheimer's disease. The nurse must consider both the patient with Alzheimer's disease and the caregiver as patients with overlapping but unique problems. To aid in identifying the many problems of the caregiver, a nursing care plan for the caregiver of a person with Alzheimer's disease is presented (NCP 56-6).

Adult day care is one of the options available to the person with Alzheimer's disease. Although programs vary in size, structure, physical environment, and degree of experience of staff, the common goals of all day care programs are to provide respite for the family and a protective environment for the patient.

The middle stage of the disease is probably the most beneficial time for adult day care when the person with Alzheimer's disease can still benefit from stimulating activities that encourage independence and decision making in a protective

56-6 NURSING CARE PLAN CAREGIVER OF THE PATIENT WITH ALZHEIMER'S DISEASE

Expected Patient Outcomes	Nursing Interventions and *Rationales*
NURSING DIAGNOSIS	**Caregiver role strain** *related to* grieving the family member's illness, change in role, and unrelieved caregiving *as manifested by* reported inadequate resources to provide care and worry about having to put the family member in a long-term care facility.
▪ Seeking of appropriate assistance by caregiver. ▪ Satisfactory care to the person with Alzheimer's disease.	▪ Assess health status of caregiver *to determine if health planning is needed.* ▪ Refer for medical evaluation when appropriate. ▪ Discuss effects of caregiving with the caregiver *to determine status of caregiver and to enable open discussion of needs.* ▪ Encourage visits from other family members or Alzheimer's support group member *to provide support and relief to caregiver as needed.* ▪ Acknowledge caregiver's fears of being unable to care for family member *to demonstrate empathy and awareness of this fear.* ▪ Provide financial or social service referrals *to assist caregiver with planning for long-term care.* ▪ Counsel and support caregiver if patient is placed in a long-term care facility *to allay guilt and reinforce services the patient now requires.*
NURSING DIAGNOSIS	**Social isolation** *related to* diminishing social relationships, behavioral problems of patient with Alzheimer's disease, and underdeveloped social support system *as manifested by* feelings of abandonment and uselessness, behavior changes, inability to make decisions or concentrate.
▪ Satisfactory contact with significant others or members of a support group.	▪ Assess past social network and diversional activities *to determine size and scope of network and personal interests.* ▪ Assess social support system of family and willingness and ability to participate in care *to develop care alternatives.* ▪ Assist in planning respite care through this system or formal community resources *to enable caregiver to continue with important activities and social contacts.* ▪ Refer to social services *for realistic appraisal of financial resources for respite care and for linkage to community resources.* ▪ Provide information regarding available support groups (e.g., Alzheimer's Association) *because these groups can meet socialization, recreational, and educational needs of caregiver.*
NURSING DIAGNOSIS	**Anxiety** *related to* uncertain outcome, perceived powerlessness, possible change in role functioning, erratic behavioral patterns of the person with Alzheimer's disease, risk for injury secondary to possible violent reactions of patient, and financial insecurity *as manifested by* tachycardia, hypertension, apprehension, helplessness, fear, irritability, forgetfulness, inability to concentrate.
▪ Decreased anxiety. ▪ Sense of control of situation.	▪ Assess past roles of patient with Alzheimer's disease and of caregiver *to determine extent of role changes required of caregiver.* ▪ Document changes in role expectations and refer to community resources or provide instruction as needed; assess knowledge of behavioral management techniques and instruct as appropriate; assist caregiver in problem-solving techniques; assist in looking at possible causes of catastrophic reactions, as well as indications of agitation that may indicate their onset, *to ensure that caregiver has skills to manage changing roles and patient status.* ▪ Refer to appropriate agencies as indicated for complete list of community resources and possible sources of financial aid *to relieve anxiety related to financial insecurity.*

Continued

56-6 NURSING CARE PLAN CAREGIVER OF THE PATIENT WITH ALZHEIMER'S DISEASE—continued

Expected Patient Outcomes	Nursing Interventions and *Rationales*
NURSING DIAGNOSIS **Altered health maintenance** *related to* unrelieved caregiving responsibilities, fatigue, and chronic stress *as manifested by* failure to care for self.	
▪ Optimal health. ▪ Appropriate health practices for age and sex.	▪ Assess physical and emotional health status of caregiver *to determine if problem is present and to plan appropriate interventions.* ▪ Collaborate with caregiver in planning interventions in major identified problem areas *to prevent further deterioration of health.* ▪ Refer for additional evaluation if indicated. ▪ Assist with planning of continued care of patient *so that caregiver's personal health needs can be pursued.* ▪ Stress need for maintaining own health *to avoid increasing the complexity of the caregiving situation.*
NURSING DIAGNOSIS **Ineffective family coping** *related to* chronic and deteriorating nature of Alzheimer's disease, feelings of helplessness and hopelessness, increasing financial hardship, and disappearing support systems *as manifested by* verbalization of lack of help and hope in caring for family members, concern over finances, deteriorating emotional and physical health of caregiver.	
▪ No evidence of inappropriate coping behaviors.	▪ Encourage family to discuss caregiving situation with one another *so consensus can be reached regarding plan of care.* ▪ Provide information on community resources such as day care, support groups, counseling, and respite care *to relieve stress and facilitate coping.* ▪ Encourage and support family in their caregiving efforts *to persons involved in a difficult situation.* ▪ Refer for assistance with financial concerns. ▪ Provide information on nature and course of Alzheimer's disease *so appropriate plans can be made for the patient based on accurate information.*

environment. The patient returns home tired, content, less frustrated, and ready to be with the family. The respite from the demands of care allows the family to be more responsive to the patient's needs.

Although adult day care may delay the transition, the demands on the caregiver eventually exceed the resources, and the person with Alzheimer's disease may be placed in a long-term care facility. Special units to care for persons with Alzheimer's disease are becoming increasingly common in long-term care settings. The nursing care needs of the patient with Alzheimer's disease change as the disease progresses, emphasizing the need for regular assessment, monitoring, and support. Regardless of the setting, the severity of the symptoms and the amount of care required intensify over time.

Patients with Alzheimer's disease are subject to acute and other chronic illnesses. Their inability to communicate health symptoms and problems places the responsibility for assessment and diagnosis on caregivers and health professionals. Hospitalization of the patient with Alzheimer's disease can be a traumatic event for both the patient and the caregiver and can precipitate a worsening of the disease.

Alzheimer's disease is a devastating disease that disrupts all aspects of personal and family life. Support groups for caregivers and family members have been formed throughout the United States to provide an atmosphere of understanding and to give current information about the disease itself and related topics such as safety, legal, ethical, and financial issues. Nurses often receive personal and professional satisfaction in participating in such support groups.

▪ Evaluation

Expected outcomes for the patient with Alzheimer's disease are addressed in NCP 56-5.

RESTLESS LEGS SYNDROME

Etiology and Pathophysiology

Restless legs syndrome (RLS) is characterized by sensory and motor abnormalities of, but not limited to, the legs. It has been estimated that between 3% and 8% of adults in the United States have RLS.[29] Although the exact cause of RLS is not known, there are epidemiologic data to support a genetic component, and it occurs in families. It has been associated with metabolic abnormalities associated with iron deficiency, uremia, or pregnancy. Up to 30% of patients receiving renal dialysis experience RLS. RLS resolves after kidney transplantation, supporting its relationship to uremia.

Clinical Manifestations

The severity of RLS ranges from infrequent minor discomfort to severe pain. Sensory symptoms often appear first and are manifested as an annoying and uncomfortable (but usually not painful) sensation in the legs. The sensation is often compared to the sensation of bugs creeping or crawling on the legs. The leg pain is localized within the calf muscles. Patients can also experience pain in the upper extremities and trunk. The discomfort occurs when the patient is sedentary and usually in the evening or at night. The pain at night can produce sleep disruptions and is often relieved by physical activity such as walking, stretching, rocking, or kicking. In the most severe cases, patients sleep only a few hours at night, resulting in daytime fatigue and disruption of the daily routine. The motor abnormalities associated with RLS consist of voluntary restlessness and stereotyped, periodic, involuntary movements. The involuntary movements usually occur during sleep. Symptoms are aggravated by fatigue. Over time, RLS advances to more frequent and more severe episodes.

Diagnostic Studies

RLS is a clinical diagnosis and is based in large part on the patient's history or the report of the bed partner related to nighttime activities. Polysomnography studies during sleep may be performed for the patient with RLS to distinguish the problem from other clinical conditions (e.g., sleep apnea) that can disturb sleep. The patient's history of diabetes mellitus and its management may provide information to determine whether paresthesias are due to peripheral neuropathy or RLS.

NURSING AND COLLABORATIVE MANAGEMENT: RESTLESS LEGS SYNDROME

The goal of collaborative management is to reduce patient discomfort and distress and to improve sleep quality. When RLS is secondary to uremia or iron deficiency, correction of these conditions will decrease symptoms. Nonpharmacologic approaches to RLS management include establishing regular sleep habits, providing adequate rest periods, encouraging exercise, and avoiding activities that cause symptoms. To promote sleep, caffeinated beverages should be avoided starting in the afternoon.

If nonpharmacologic measures fail to provide symptom relief, drug therapy may be started. The main drugs used in RLS are dopaminergic agents, opioids, and benzodiazepines. Dopaminergic agents such as carbidopa/levodopa (Sinemet) and dopamine agonists (pergolide [Permax], bromocriptine [Parlodel]) are the drugs of choice in treating RLS. These agents are effective in managing sensory and motor symptoms. Dopaminergic agents have a number of side effects, including hypotension and gastric irritation.

Opioids (e.g., oxycodone) in low doses have also been found to be effective in reducing the symptoms associated with RLS. The main side effect of opioids is constipation, so the patient may need to take a stool softener or laxative. Other agents that may be used include antiseizure medications such as gabapentin (Neurontin), divalproex (Depakote), lamotrigine (Lamictal), and carbamazepine (Tegretol).

OTHER NEUROLOGIC DISORDERS

AMYOTROPHIC LATERAL SCLEROSIS

Amyotrophic lateral sclerosis (ALS) is a rare progressive neurologic disorder characterized by loss of motor neurons. ALS usually leads to death within 2 to 6 years after diagnosis. This disease became known as Lou Gehrig's disease when the famous baseball player was stricken with it in the early 1940s. The onset is between 40 and 70 years of age, and two times as many men as women are affected.

For unknown reasons, motor neurons in the brainstem and spinal cord gradually degenerate in ALS (Fig. 56-8). The dead motor neuron cannot produce or transport vital signals to muscle. Consequently, electrical and chemical messages originating in the brain do not reach the muscles to activate them.

The primary symptoms are weakness of the upper extremities, dysarthria, and dysphagia. Muscle wasting and fasciculations result from the denervation of the muscles and lack of stimulation and use. Death usually results from respiratory infection secondary to compromised respiratory function. Unfortunately, there is no cure for ALS. Riluzole (Rilutek) was approved in 1997 to slow the progression of ALS.[30,31] This drug works to decrease the amount of glutamate (an excitatory neurotransmitter) in the brain. It was shown to delay the need for tracheostomy and to delay death by a few months in clinical trials.

The illness trajectory for ALS is devastating because the patient remains cognitively intact while wasting away. The challenge of nursing care is to support the patient's cognitive and emotional functions by facilitating communication, providing diversional activities such as reading and human companionship, and helping the person and family with advance care planning and anticipatory grieving related to loss of motor function and ultimately death.

HUNTINGTON'S DISEASE

Huntington's disease (HD) is a genetically transmitted, autosomal dominant disorder that affects both men and women of all races. The offspring of a person with this disease have a 50% risk of inheriting it. The diagnosis often occurs after the affected individual has had children. In the United States the incidence of HD is 1 in 15,000. Diagnosis in the past was based on family history and clinical symptoms. However, since the gene for HD has been discovered, one now can be tested for presence of the gene. People who are asymptomatic but who have a positive family history of HD face the dilemma of whether or not to get tested. If the test is positive, the person will develop HD, but when and to what extent the disease develops cannot be determined.

Like Parkinson's disease, the pathology of HD involves the basal ganglia and the extrapyramidal motor system. However, instead of a deficiency of DA, HD involves a deficiency of the

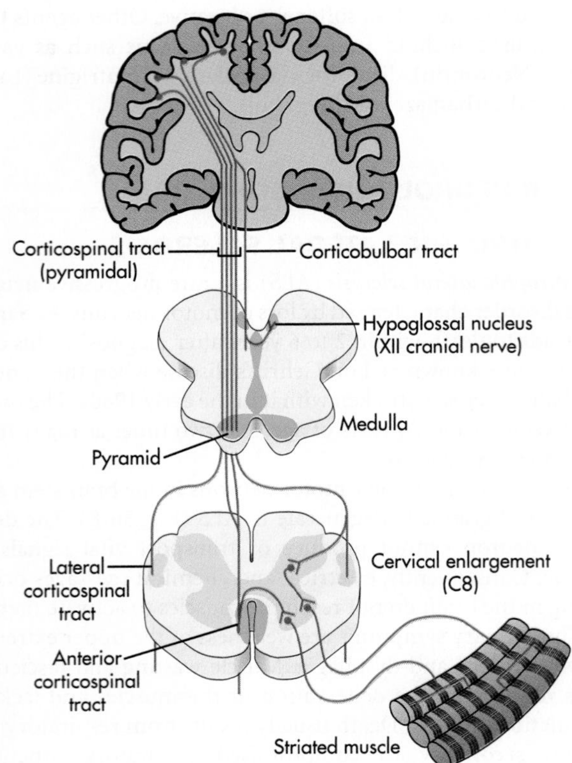

Fig. 56-8 Pathogenesis of amyotrophic lateral sclerosis. This disease is characterized by degeneration of the pyramidal tract and the motor cells in the anterior gray horns. In cases with corticobulbar involvement, the motor nuclei of cranial nerves V, VII, IX, X, XI, and XII also undergo degeneration.

neurotransmitters ACh and GABA. The net effect is an excess of DA, which leads to symptoms that are the opposite of those of parkinsonism. The clinical manifestations, the onset of which is between 35 and 45 years of age, are characterized by abnormal and excessive involuntary movements (chorea). These are writhing, twisting movements of the face, limbs, and body. The movements get worse as the disease progresses. Facial movements involving speech, chewing, and swallowing are affected and may cause aspiration and malnutrition. The gait deteriorates, and ambulation eventually becomes impossible. Perhaps the most devastating deterioration is in mental functions, which include intellectual decline, emotional lability, and psychotic behavior. Death usually occurs 10 to 20 years after the onset of symptoms.

Because there is no cure, collaborative care is palliative. Antipsychotic, antidepressant, and antichorea medications are prescribed and have some benefit. However, they do not alter the course of the disease. Surgical procedures involving transplantation of fetal striatal neural tissues are performed at some medical centers.[32] This disease presents a great challenge to health care professionals. The goal of nursing management is to provide the most comfortable environment possible for the patient and the family by maintaining physical safety, treating the physical symptoms, and providing emotional and psychologic support. Because of the choreic movements, caloric requirements are high. Patients may require as high as 4000 to 5000 calories per day to maintain body weight. As the disease progresses, meeting caloric needs becomes a greater challenge when the patient has difficulty swallowing and holding the head still. Depression and mental deterioration can also compromise nutritional intake.

CRITICAL THINKING EXERCISES

CASE STUDY

Multiple Sclerosis

Patient Profile

Ms. S., a 32-year-old Caucasian woman, born and raised in Minneapolis, was diagnosed with multiple sclerosis after an episode of numbness and tingling on the left side of her body. Two years ago she had an episode of optic neuritis in the right eye.

Subjective Data

- Difficulty seeing out of the right eye
- Numbness and tingling on the left side that worsens in hot weather
- Tires easily
- Used all sick days at work; concerned about losing her job and ability to care for 3-year-old son

Objective Data

Physical Examination

- Crying softly during interview
- Tense and anxious

Diagnostic Studies

- Prolonged visual evoked response in right eye
- MRI scan of head shows several plaques in white matter

Critical Thinking Questions

1. What is the pathogenesis of multiple sclerosis?
2. What precipitating factors for multiple sclerosis are present in Ms. S.'s life?
3. Why did it take so long for a definitive diagnosis to be made for Ms. S.?
4. What teaching plan should be developed for Ms. S.?
5. What treatment would be appropriate for Ms. S.?
6. Write one or more appropriate nursing diagnoses based on the assessment data presented. Are there any collaborative problems?

NURSING RESEARCH ISSUES

1. What kinds of physical activity can enhance functioning and well-being in patients with multiple sclerosis and Parkinson's disease?
2. How can caregivers of patients with Alzheimer's disease be helped to deal with their situation?
3. What are the most effective ways to assist patients with chronic neurologic problems to maintain a positive self-esteem?
4. What factors influence the quality of life for patients with epilepsy?
5. What can be done to promote self-efficacy in patients with chronic neurologic conditions?

REVIEW QUESTIONS

The number of the question corresponds to the same-numbered objective at the beginning of the chapter.

1. The emotional responses of the patient with a chronic neurologic disease are often
   a. symptoms of intellectual deterioration.
   b. absent in patients with cognitive impairment.
   c. a result of physical disability and changes in body image.
   d. reduced in patients who have family members to care for them.
2. The nurse plans care for the patient with a migraine headache based on the knowledge that during a migraine the patient is most likely to
   a. withdraw from stimuli.
   b. act out with bizarre behavior.
   c. seek out the company of others.
   d. experience painful facial spasms and tearing.
3. The triad of symptoms the nurse would expect to find during assessment of the patient with Parkinson's disease is
   a. spasticity, diplopia, tremor.
   b. tremor, rigidity, bradykinesia.
   c. ataxia, drowsiness, dysarthria.
   d. diplopia, tremor, bradykinesia.
4. Nursing intervention for the patient with MS is aimed at management of
   a. incontinence, tremor, seizures.
   b. chorea and mental deterioration.
   c. incontinence, depression, spasticity.
   d. intercostal muscle weakness and impaired swallowing.
5. During assessment of the patient with ALS the nurse would expect to find
   a. muscle wasting.
   b. emotional lability.
   c. mental deterioration.
   d. sensory loss in the extremities.
6. The nurse plans interventions for patients with chronic neurologic disease knowing that the most common cause of death in these patients as a result of their immobility is
   a. suicide.
   b. malnutrition.
   c. physical injury.
   d. respiratory infection.
7. A major goal of treatment for the patient with a chronic, progressive neurologic disease is
   a. reversal of pathophysiology.
   b. continuation of usual lifestyle.
   c. total remission of the disease.
   d. adjustment by patient and family to the disease.

References

1. Lipton RB, Stewart WF, Von Korff M: Burden of migraine: societal costs and therapeutic opportunities, *Neurology* 48(suppl 3):S4, 1997.
2. Goadsby PJ: Current concepts of the pathophysiology of migraine, *Neurol Clin* 15:27, 1997.
3. Kudrow L: Cluster headache and paroxysmal hemicrania. In Samuels M, Feske S, editors: *Office practice of neurology,* New York, 1996, Churchill Livingstone.
4. Blau JN: The effect of national lifestyles, *Cephalalgia* 18:23, 1998.
5. Hauser A: Epidemiology of seizure disorders and the epilepsies. In Santilli N, editor: *Managing seizure disorders,* Philadelphia, 1996, Lippincott-Raven.
6. Gastaut H: Clinical and electroencephalographical classification of epileptic seizures, *Epilepsia* 11:102, 1970.
7. Commission on Classification and Terminology of the International League Against Epilepsy: Proposal for the revised clinical and electroencephalographic classification of epileptic seizures, *Epilepsia* 22:249, 1981.
8. Behrens E and others: Surgical and neurological complications in a series of 708 epilepsy surgery procedures, *Neurosurgery* 41:1, 1997.
9. Health Information, National Institute of Neurological Disorders and Stroke, Bethesda, Md, NIH, 1998.
10. Lublin FD, Reingold SC: Defining the clinical course of multiple sclerosis, *Neurology* 46:907, 1996.
11. Confavreux C and others: Rates of pregnancy-related relapse in multiple sclerosis, *N Engl J Med* 339:285, 1998.
12. Khan OA, Hebel JR: Incidence of exacerbations in the first 90 days of treatment with recombinant human interferon beta-1b in patients with relapsing-remitting multiple sclerosis, *Ann Neurol* 44:138, 1998.
13. Edwards S and others: Clinical relapses and disease activity on magnetic resonance imaging associated with viral upper respiratory infections in multiple sclerosis, *J Neurol Neurosurg Psychiatry* 64:736, 1998.
14. Sudarsky LR: Parkinson's disease: recognition, diagnosis and management. In Samuels M, Feske S, editors: *Office practice of neurology,* New York, 1996, Churchill Livingstone.
15. Calne DB: Diagnosis and treatment of Parkinson's disease, *Hosp Pract* 30:83, 1995.
16. Scharre DW, Mahler ME: Parkinson's disease: making the diagnosis, selecting drug therapies, *Geriatrics* 49:14, 1994.
17. Schrag AE and others: The safety of ropinirole, a selective nonergoline dopamine agonist, in patients with Parkinson's disease, *Clin Neuropharmacol* 21:169, 1998.
18. Dooley M, Markham A: Pramipexole. A review of its use in the management of early and advanced Parkinson's disease, *Drugs Aging* 12:495, 1998.
19. Lozano AM, Lang AE: Pallidotomy for Parkinson's disease, *Neurosurg Clin North Am* 9:325, 1998.
20. Hariz GM and others: Assessment of ability/disability in patients treated with chronic thalamic stimulation for tremor, *Mov Disord* 13:78, 1998.
21. Lindvall O: Update on fetal transplantation: the Swedish experience, *Mov Disord* 13:83, 1998.
22. Fink JS: Transplantation in Parkinson's disease, *Artif Organs* 21:1199, 1997.
23. Urschel JD, Grewal RP: Thymectomy for myasthenia gravis, *Postgrad Med J* 74:139, 1998.
24. Lewis RA, Selwa JF, Lisak RP: Myasthenia gravis: immunological mechanisms and immunotherapy, *Ann Neurol* (suppl 1):S51, 1995.
25. Roses AD: Alzheimer's disease: the genetics of risk, *Hosp Pract* 33:51, 1997.
26. Smith AL, Whitehouse PJ: Progress in the management of Alzheimer's disease, *Hosp Pract* 34:151, 1998.
27. Adair JC: Is it Alzheimer's? *Hosp Pract* 34:35, 1998.
28. Kettl PA: Alzheimer's disease: an update, *Hosp Med* 33:12, 1997.
29. Hening WA: Restless legs syndrome: diagnosis and treatment, *Hosp Med* 33:54, 1997.
30. Miller RG: New approaches to therapy of amyotrophic lateral sclerosis, *West J Med* 168:262, 1998.
31. Riviere M and others: An analysis of extended survival in patients with amyotrophic lateral sclerosis treated with riluzole, *Arch Neurol* 55:526, 1998.
32. Kopyov OV and others: Safety of intrastriatal neurotransplantation for Huntingon's disease patients, *Exp Neurol* 149:97, 1998.

Resources

Alzheimer's Association
919 North Michigan Avenue, Suite 1000
Chicago, IL 60611-1676
312-335-8700
800-272-3900
Fax: 312-335-1110
http://www.alz.org

Alzheimer's Disease and Related Disorders Association
4709 Golf Road, Suite 1015
Skokie, IL 60076
708-933-1000

Alzheimer's Disease Education and Referral Center
ADEAR Center
PO Box 8250
Silver Spring, MD 20907-8250
800-438-4380
Fax: 301-495-3334
http://www.radiospace.com/adear.htm

Alzheimers.com
http://www.alzheimers.com/

American Association of Neuroscience Nurses (AANN)
218 North Jefferson Street, #204
Chicago, IL 60606
312-993-0043
http://www.aann.org/

Association of Rehabilitation Nurses
5700 Old Orchard Road, First Floor
Skokie, IL 60077
708-966-8673
Fax: 708-966-9418

Epilepsy Foundation
4351 Garden City Drive, 5th Floor
Landover, MD 20785-2267
301-459-3700
800-EFA-1000
Fax: 301-577-2684
http://www.efa.org

Huntington's Disease Society of America, Inc.
140 West 22nd Street, 6th Floor
New York, NY 10011-2420
212-242-1968
800-345-4372
Fax: 212-243-2443

Myasthenia Foundation
222 South Riverside Plaza
Suite 1540
Chicago, IL 60606-9524
312-258-0522
800-541-5454

National Foundation for Brain Research
1250 24th Street NW, Suite 300
Washington, DC 20037
202-293-5453
202-466-0585
http://www.brainnet.org/

National Headache Foundation
5252 Northwestern Avenue
Chicago, IL 60625
800-843-2256
Fax: 312-907-6278
http://www.headaches.org

National Institute of Neurological and Communicative Disorders and Stroke
Building 31, Room 8A52
9000 Rockville Pike
Bethesda, MD 20892
301-496-9746

National Multiple Sclerosis Society
800-Fight-MS (800-344-4867)
733 Third Avenue
New York, NY 10017
http://www.nmss.org/

National Parkinson Foundation, Inc.
1501 NW 9th Avenue/Bob Hope Road
Miami, FL 33136
305-547-6666
800-327-4545
Fax: 305-243-4403
http://www.parkinson.org

Parkinson's Disease Foundation
William Black Medical Research Building
Columbia Presbyterian Medical Center
650 West 168th Street
New York, NY 10032
212-923-4700

Restless Legs Foundation
4410 19th Street NW
Suite 201
Rochester, MN 55901-6624

For additional Internet resources, see the website for this book at www.mosby.com/MERLIN/medsurg_lewis

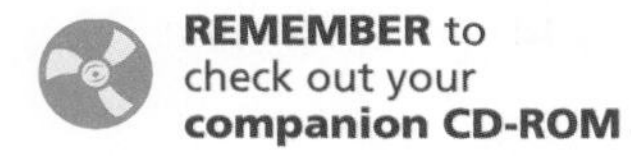

57 NURSING MANAGEMENT Peripheral Nerve and Spinal Cord Problems

Diane H. Michalec

www.mosby.com/MERLIN/medsurg_lewis

LEARNING OBJECTIVES

1. Explain the etiology, clinical manifestations, collaborative care, and nursing management of trigeminal neuralgia and Bell's palsy.
2. Explain the etiology, clinical manifestations, collaborative care, and nursing management of Guillain-Barré syndrome, botulism, tetanus, and neurosyphilis.
3. Identify the population at risk for spinal cord injuries.
4. Describe the classification of spinal cord injuries and associated clinical manifestations.
5. Describe the clinical manifestations, collaborative care, and nursing management of spinal cord shock.
6. Correlate the clinical manifestations of spinal cord injury with the level of disruption and rehabilitation potential.
7. Describe the nursing management of the major physical and psychologic problems of the patient with a spinal cord injury.
8. Explain the types, clinical manifestations, collaborative care, and nursing management of spinal cord tumors.
9. Describe the effects of spinal cord injury on the older adult population.

CRANIAL NERVE DISORDERS

Cranial nerve disorders are commonly classified as peripheral neuropathies. The 12 pairs of cranial nerves are considered the peripheral nerves of the brain. The disorders usually involve the motor or sensory (or both) branches of a single nerve (*mononeuropathies*). Causes of cranial nerve problems include tumors, trauma, infections, inflammatory processes, and idiopathic (unknown) causes. Two cranial nerve disorders are trigeminal neuralgia (tic douloureux) and acute peripheral facial paralysis (Bell's palsy).

TRIGEMINAL NEURALGIA

Etiology and Pathophysiology

Trigeminal neuralgia (tic douloureux) is a relatively uncommon cranial nerve disorder with an estimated prevalence of 155 cases per million persons.[1] It is more commonly seen in women and usually begins in the fifth or sixth decade of life, but it may occur at any age. The trigeminal nerve is the fifth cranial nerve (CN V) and has both motor and sensory branches. The sensory branches are involved in trigeminal neuralgia, primarily the maxillary and mandibular branches (Fig. 57-1).[2]

Although no specific cause has been identified, major initiating pathologic events may include nerve compression by tortuous arteries of the posterior fossa blood vessels, demyelinating plaques, herpes virus infection, infection of teeth and jaw, and a brainstem infarct.[3] The effectiveness of antiseizure drug therapy may be related to the ability of these drugs to stabilize the neuronal membrane and decrease paroxysmal afferent impulses of the nerve.[4]

Clinical Manifestations

The classic feature of trigeminal neuralgia is an abrupt onset of paroxysms of excruciating pain described as a burning, knifelike, or lightninglike shock in the lips, upper or lower gums, cheek, forehead, or side of the nose. Intense pain, twitching, grimacing, and frequent blinking and tearing of the eye occur during the acute attack (giving rise to the term *tic*). The attacks are usually brief, lasting only seconds to 2 or 3 minutes, and are generally unilateral. Recurrences are unpredictable; they may occur several times a day or weeks or months apart. After the refractory (pain-free) period, a phenomenon known as *clustering* can occur. Clustering is characterized by a cycle of pain and refractoriness that continues for hours.

The painful episodes are usually initiated by a triggering mechanism of light cutaneous stimulation at a specific point (*trigger zone*) along the distribution of the nerve branches. Precipitating stimuli include chewing, teeth brushing, a hot or cold blast of air on the face, washing the face, yawning, or even talking. Touch and tickle seem to predominate as causative triggers rather than pain or changes in temperature. As a result, the patient may eat improperly, neglect hygienic practices, wear a cloth over the face, and withdraw from interaction with other

Reviewed by Patricia A. Blissett, RN, MSN, CCRN, CNRN, CCM, Staff Nurse, Neurosurgical Intensive Care Unit, Harborview Medical Center, Seattle, Wash.

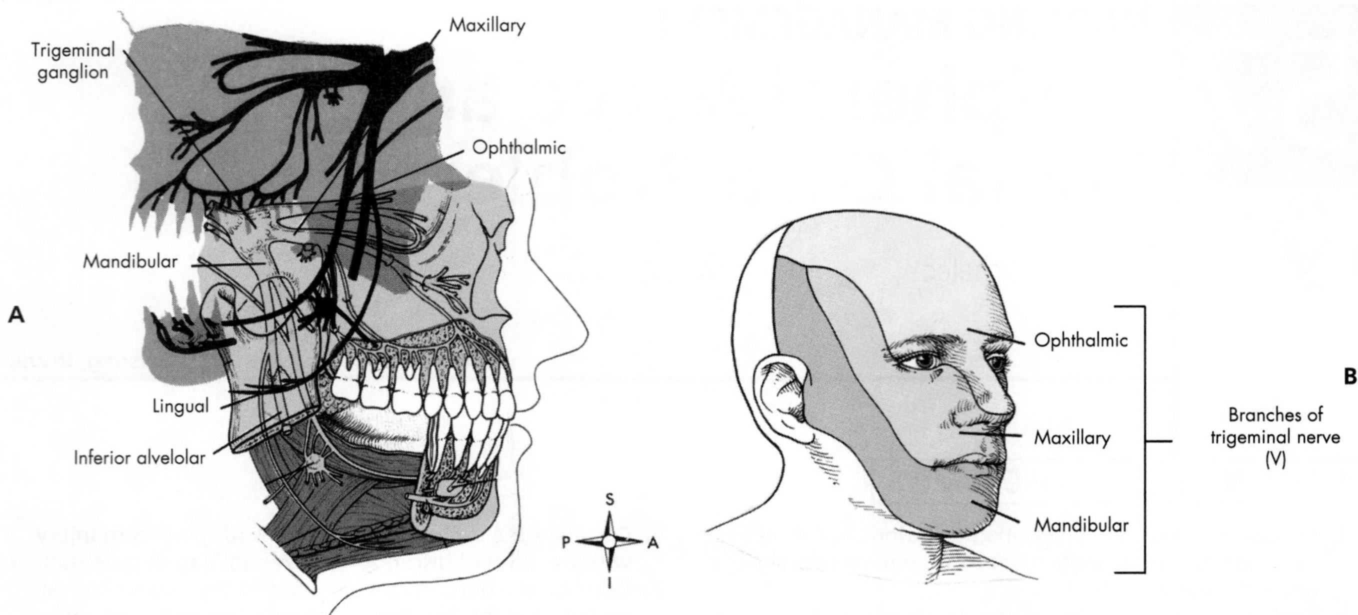

Fig. 57-1 **A,** Trigeminal (fifth cranial nerve and its three main divisions, the ophthalmic, maxillary, and mandibular nerves). **B,** Cutaneous innervation of the head.

COLLABORATIVE CARE

Table 57-1 Trigeminal Neuralgia

Diagnostic
- History and physical examination
- Brain or CT scan
- Audiologic evaluation
- EMG
- CSF analysis
- Arteriography
- Posterior myelography
- MRI

Collaborative Therapy
- Drug therapy (e.g., phenytoin [Dilantin] carbamazepine [Tegretol], valproic acid [Depakene])
- Local nerve blocking
- Biofeedback
- Surgical intervention (see Table 57-2)

CT, computed tomography; *CSF,* cerebrospinal fluid; *EMG,* electromyography; *MRI,* magnetic resonance imaging.

individuals. The patient may sleep excessively as a means of coping with the pain.

Although this condition is considered benign, the severity of the pain and the disruption of lifestyle can result in almost total physical and psychologic dysfunction or even suicide.

Diagnostic Studies

It is important to rule out other problems with similar manifestations, such as other forms of facial and cephalic neuralgias and pain arising from the sinuses, teeth, and jaws. In young patients with bilateral facial pain, a CT scan is performed to rule out any lesions or vascular abnormalities and a lumbar puncture and an MRI are done to rule out multiple sclerosis. A complete neurologic assessment is done, although results are usually normal. Once the diagnosis is made, the goal of treatment is relief of pain either medically or surgically (Tables 57-1 and 57-2).

Collaborative Care

Drug Therapy. The majority of patients obtain adequate relief through antiseizure drugs such as carbamazepine (Tegretol), phenytoin (Dilantin), and valproate (Depakene). Carbamazepine is the most commonly prescribed. These drugs may prevent an acute attack or promote a remission of symptoms, although the mechanism by which they work is not known. Side effects of carbamazepine may include bone marrow suppression leading to blood abnormalities. Therefore, routine complete blood cell (CBC) counts are required. Because drug therapy may not provide permanent pain relief, some patients may seek continued help by numerous visits to otolaryngologists or from therapies such as acupuncture and megavitamins.

Conservative Therapy. Nerve blocking with local anesthetics is another treatment possibility. Local nerve blocking results in complete anesthesia of the area supplied by the injected branches. Relief of pain is temporary, lasting from 6 to 18 months. This treatment is usually tolerated well by older adults.

Biofeedback is another strategy that may be helpful for some patients. In addition to controlling the pain, the patient may experience a strong sense of personal control by mastering the technique and altering certain body functions.

Surgical Therapy. If a conservative approach is not effective, surgical therapy is available (see Table 57-2). *Percutaneous radiofrequency rhizotomy* (electrocoagulation) and *microvascular decompression* afford the greatest relief of pain. Percutaneous radiofrequency rhizotomy consists of placing a needle into the trigeminal rootlets that are adjacent to the pons and destroying the area by means of a radiofrequency

Table 57-2 Surgical Interventions for Trigeminal Neuralgia

Procedure	Technique	Benefit
Peripheral		
Glycerol injection into one or more branches of the trigeminal nerve	Chemical ablation	Total pain relief with sparing of touch and corneal reflex
Intracranial		
Retrogasserian rhizotomy	Temporal craniotomy (sectioning of sensory root in middle cranial fossa)	Permanent anesthesia (with adeptness, corneal reflex, touch)
Suboccipital craniotomy	Sectioning of sensory root of posterior fossa	Permanent anesthesia
Percutaneous radiofrequency rhizotomy	Destruction of sensory fibers by low-voltage current	Total pain relief, sparing of touch and corneal reflex (increased risk for sensory changes)
Microvascular decompression (Jannetta procedure)	Lifting of artery pressing on nerve root in posterior fossa with wedge of sponge, leading to removal of pressure at nerve-root entry zone or removing the involved vessel	Pain relief without loss of sensation
Gamma knife radiosurgery	Technique that uses high doses of radiation focused on the trigeminal nerve root using stereotactic localization	Pain relief 1 day to 4 months posttreatment; noninvasive; no loss of sensation

current. This can result in anesthesia of the face (although some degree of sensation may be retained) or trigeminal motor weakness. Irritation or inadvertent destruction of the ophthalmic branches of the nerve can result in loss of the corneal reflex. This procedure is easily performed with minimal risk to the patient and is based on the exchange of pain for numbness. It is tolerated well by older adults and avoids a major operative procedure in the high risk patient.[5]

Microvascular decompression of the trigeminal nerve is the most commonly used procedure for neuralgia. It is accomplished by displacing and repositioning blood vessels that appear to be compressing the nerve at the root-entry zone where it exits the pons. This procedure relieves pain without residual sensory loss, but it is potentially dangerous, as is any surgery near the brainstem. Microvascular decompression has a long-term success rate equal to or superior to percutaneous procedures without the higher rate of permanent neurologic sequelae. It is a safe operation with an almost negligible mortality and low morbidity in skilled hands.[6] Approximately 30% of patients experience a recurrence of symptoms within 6 years following surgery.[4]

Glycerol rhizotomy has become more popular in the last 10 years and is preferred over percutaneous radiofrequency rhizotomy. Glycerol rhizotomy consists of an injection of glycerol through the foramen ovale into the trigeminal cistern (Fig. 57-2). Glycerol rhizotomy is a more benign procedure with less sensory loss and fewer sensory aberrations than radiofrequency rhizotomy and with comparable or better pain relief.[7]

Gamma knife radiosurgery is a surgical treatment that is now available for the treatment of trigeminal neuralgia. Radiosurgery using the gamma unit provides precise radiation of the proximal trigeminal nerve identified on high resolution imaging. This image-guided approach has been useful for both patients with persistent pain after other surgeries and as a primary surgical option.[8]

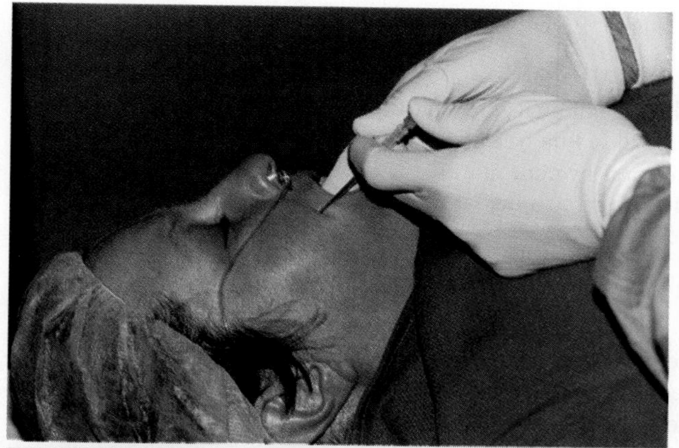
A

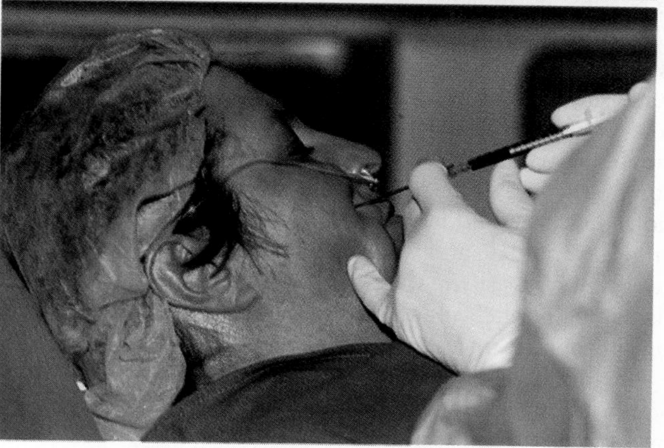
B

Fig. 57-2 **A,** Patient with trigeminal neuralgia having needle placed. **B,** Physician injecting glycerol.

NURSING MANAGEMENT: TRIGEMINAL NEURALGIA

■ Nursing Assessment

Assessment of the attacks, including the triggering factors, characteristics, frequency, and pain management techniques, helps the nurse plan for patient care. The nursing assessment should include the patient's nutritional status, hygiene (especially oral), and behavior (including withdrawal). Evaluation of the degree of pain and its effects on the patient's lifestyle, drug history, emotional state, and suicidal tendencies are other important factors.

■ Nursing Diagnoses

Nursing diagnoses for the patient with trigeminal neuralgia include, but are not limited to, the following:

- Pain *related to* inflammation or compression of the trigeminal nerve
- Altered nutrition: less than body requirements *related to* fear of triggering pain by eating or chewing
- Anxiety *related to* uncertainty of timing and initiating event of pain and uncertainty regarding effectiveness of pain-relieving treatments
- Altered oral mucous membrane *related to* unwillingness to practice oral hygiene measures secondary to potential for initiating pain
- Social isolation *related to* anxiety over pain attacks and desire to maintain nonstimulating environment

■ Planning

The overall goals are that the patient with trigeminal neuralgia will (1) be free of pain, (2) maintain adequate nutritional and oral hygiene status, (3) have minimal to no anxiety, and (4) return to normal or previous socialization and occupational activities.

■ Nursing Implementation

Health Promotion. Because the etiology of trigeminal neuralgia remains unknown, health promotion is directed at reducing recurrent episodes in those who have trigeminal neuralgia. Awareness and reduction of triggering events may be possible in some patients.

Acute Intervention. Pain relief is primarily obtained by the administration of the recommended drug therapy. The nurse should monitor the patient's response to therapy and note any side effects. Strong narcotics such as morphine should be used cautiously because of the potential for addiction over time. Alternative pain relief measures, such as biofeedback, should be explored for the patient who is not a surgical candidate and whose pain is not controlled by other therapeutic measures. Careful assessment of pain, including history, pain relief, and drug dependency, can assist in selecting appropriate interventions.

Environmental management is essential during an acute period to lessen triggering stimuli. The room should be kept at an even, moderate temperature and free of drafts. A private room is preferred during an acute period. The nurse must use care to avoid touching the patient's face or jarring the bed. Many patients prefer to carry out their own care, fearing that they will be inadvertently injured by someone else.

The nurse should instruct the patient about the importance of nutrition, hygiene, and oral care and convey understanding if previous neglect is apparent. The nurse should provide lukewarm water and soft cloths or cotton saturated with solutions not requiring rinsing for cleansing the face. A small, soft-bristled toothbrush or a warm mouthwash assist in promoting oral care. Hygiene activities are best carried out when analgesia is at its peak.

The patient will probably not engage in extensive conversation during the acute period. Alternative communication methods such as paper and pencil should be provided.

Food should be high in protein and calories and easy to chew. It should be served lukewarm and offered frequently. The diet should be individualized according to personal, cultural, and religious preferences. When oral intake is sharply reduced and the patient's nutritional status is compromised, a nasogastric tube is inserted on the unaffected side for nasogastric feedings.

The nurse is responsible for instruction related to diagnostic studies to rule out other problems, such as multiple sclerosis, dental or sinus problems, and neoplasms, and for preoperative teaching if surgery is planned. The nurse may also need to reinforce the surgeon's instructions related to postoperative expectations; appropriate teaching of postoperative activities depends on whether a craniotomy or a local procedure is planned. The patient needs to know that he or she will be awake during local procedures so that he or she can cooperate when corneal and ciliary reflexes and facial sensations are checked.

After the operation the patient's pain is compared with the preoperative level. The corneal reflex, extraocular muscles, hearing, sensation, and facial nerve function are evaluated frequently (see Chapter 53). If there is impairment of the corneal reflex, special attention must be paid to eye protection. This includes the use of artificial tears or eye shields. General postoperative nursing care after a craniotomy is appropriate if intracranial surgery is performed. (Nursing care related to craniotomy is discussed in Chapter 54.) Diet and ambulation should be increased according to the patient's progress or specific orders.

After a radiofrequency percutaneous electrocoagulation procedure, an ice pack is applied to the jaw on the operative side for 3 to 5 hours. To avoid injuring the mouth, the patient should not chew on the operative side until sensation has returned.

Ambulatory and Home Care. Regular follow-up care should be planned. The patient needs instruction regarding the dosage and side effects of medications. Although relief of pain may be complete, the patient should be encouraged to keep environmental stimuli to a moderate level and to use stress reduction methods. Herpes simplex infection (cold sores) can occur from manipulation of the gasserian ganglion. Treatment consists of antiviral agents such as acyclovir (see Chapter 22).

Long-term management after surgical intervention depends on the residual effects of the type of procedure. If anesthesia is present or the corneal reflex is altered, the patient should be taught to (1) chew on the unaffected side; (2) avoid hot foods or beverages, which can burn the mucous membranes; (3) check the oral cavity after meals to remove food particles; (4) practice meticulous oral hygiene and continue with semiannual dental visits; (5) protect the face against extremes of temperature; (6) use an electric razor; and (7) wear a protective eye shield.

The patient may have developed protective practices to prevent pain and may need counseling or psychiatric assistance in the readjustment, especially in reestablishing personal relationships. Some patients grieve the loss of the pain, especially if it had a special significance such as relieving guilt or anxiety.

Occasionally patients may have used their pain to manipulate family members and friends and may not adjust after successful relief of pain. Careful management in the rehabilitative period can prevent the patient from claiming continual pain for secondary gain (see Chapter 9).

■ Evaluation

The expected outcomes are that the patient with trigeminal neuralgia will

- report an improvement or relief from pain
- appear more comfortable and less anxious
- have normal facial sensation or expected paresthesias and anesthesias
- return to previous socialization and occupational activities

BELL'S PALSY

Etiology and Pathophysiology

Bell's palsy (peripheral facial paralysis, acute benign cranial polyneuritis) is a disorder characterized by a disruption of the motor branches of the facial nerve (CN VII) on one side of the face in the absence of any other disease such as a stroke. It can affect any age-group, but it is more commonly seen in the 20- to 60-year age range. Incidence rates in the United States are 23 cases per 100,000 persons annually.[9] Although the exact etiology is not known, there is evidence that reactivated herpes simplex virus (HSV) may be involved in the majority of cases.[10] The reactivation of the HSV causes inflammation, edema, ischemia, and eventual demyelination of the nerve, creating pain and alterations in motor and sensory function.

Bell's palsy is considered benign, with full recovery after 6 months in about 85% of patients, especially if treatment is instituted immediately. A small number of patients may have some residual effects. The remaining 15% of patients continue to be bothered by asymmetrical movement of facial muscles.[10]

Clinical Manifestations

The onset of Bell's palsy is often accompanied by an outbreak of herpes vesicles in or around the ear. Patients may complain of pain around and behind the ear. In addition, manifestations may include fever, tinnitus, and hearing deficit. The paralysis of the motor branches of the facial nerve typically results in a flaccidity of the affected side of the face, with drooping of the mouth accompanied by drooling (Fig. 57-3). An inability to close the eyelid, with an upward movement of the eyeball when closure is attempted, is also evident. A widened palpebral fissure (the opening between the eyelids), flattening of the nasolabial fold, and inability to smile, frown, or whistle are also common. Unilateral loss of taste is common. Decreased muscle movement may alter chewing ability, and although some patients may experience a loss of tearing, many patients complain of excessive tearing. The muscle weakness causes the lower lid to turn out, allowing overflow of normal tear production. Pain may be present behind the ear on the affected side, especially before the onset of paralysis. Interventions are primarily supportive until the patient has a return of function.

Complications

Complications can include psychologic withdrawal because of changes in appearance, malnutrition and dehydration, mucous membrane trauma, corneal abrasions, muscle stretching, and facial spasms and contractures.

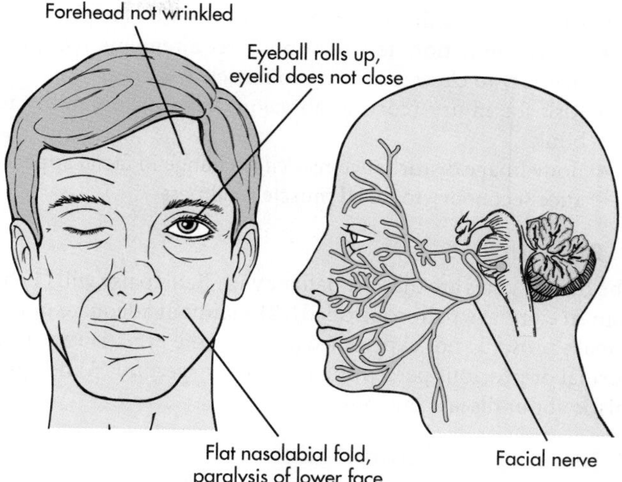

Fig. 57-3 Bell's palsy: facial characteristics.

Diagnostic Studies

The diagnosis of Bell's palsy is one of exclusion. There is no definitive test. The diagnosis and prognosis are indicated by observation of the typical pattern of onset and signs and the testing of percutaneous nerve excitability by electromyogram (EMG).

Collaborative Care

Methods of treatment for Bell's palsy include moist heat, gentle massage, and electrical stimulation of the nerve. Stimulation may maintain muscle tone and prevent atrophy. Care is primarily focused on relief of symptoms and prevention of complications.

Drug Therapy. Corticosteroids, especially prednisone, are started immediately, and the best results are obtained if corticosteroids are initiated before paralysis is complete. When the patient improves to the point that the corticosteroids are no longer necessary, they should be tapered off over a 2 week period. Usually, the corticosteroid treatment decreases the edema and pain, but mild analgesics can be used if necessary. Because the HSV is implicated in approximately 70% of cases of Bell's palsy, treatment with acyclovir (Zovirax), alone or in conjunction with prednisone, are used.[10] Newer drugs to treat HSV, including valacyclovir (Valtrex) and famciclovir (Famvir), have also been used in the management of Bell's palsy.

NURSING MANAGEMENT: BELL'S PALSY

■ Nursing Assessment

Early recognition of the possibility of Bell's palsy is important. Because HSV is a possible etiologic factor, any person who is prone to herpes simplex should be alerted to seek health care if pain occurs in or around the ear. Assessment of facial muscles for any signs of weakness should also be done (see Chapter 53). Careful recording of assessment data provides information related to the progress of the syndrome.

■ Nursing Diagnoses

The nursing diagnoses for the patient with Bell's palsy may include, but are not limited to, the following:

- Pain *related to* the inflammation of CN VII (facial)
- Altered nutrition: less than body requirements *related to* inability to chew secondary to muscle weakness
- Risk for injury (corneal abrasion) *related to* inability to blink
- Body image disturbance *related to* change in facial appearance secondary to facial muscle weakness

■ Planning

The overall goals are that the patient with Bell's palsy will (1) be pain free or have pain controlled, (2) maintain adequate nutritional status, (3) not experience injury to the eye, (4) return to normal or previous perception of body image, and (5) be optimistic about disease outcome.

■ Nursing Implementation

The patient with Bell's palsy does not usually require inpatient hospitalization. The following interventions are used throughout the course of the disease. Mild analgesics can relieve pain. Hot wet packs can reduce the discomfort of herpetic lesions, aid circulation, and relieve pain. The face should be protected from cold and drafts because trigeminal hyperesthesia may accompany the syndrome. Maintenance of good nutrition is important. The patient should be taught to chew on the unaffected side of the mouth to avoid trapping food and to enjoy the taste of food. Thorough oral hygiene must be carried out after each meal to prevent the development of parotitis, caries, and periodontal disease from accumulated residual food.

Dark glasses may be worn for protective and cosmetic reasons. Artificial tears (methylcellulose) should be instilled frequently during the day to prevent drying of the cornea. The eye should be inspected for the presence of eyelashes. Ointment and an impermeable eye shield can be used at night to retain moisture. In some patients, taping the lids closed at night may be necessary to provide protection. The patient is taught to report ocular pain, drainage, or discharge.

A facial sling may be helpful to support affected muscles, improve lip alignment, and facilitate eating. The facial sling is usually made and fitted by a physical or occupational therapist. Vigorous massage can break down tissues, but gentle upward massage has psychologic benefits even if physical effects other than the maintenance of circulation are questionable. When function begins to return, active facial exercises are performed several times a day.

The change in physical appearance as a result of Bell's palsy can be devastating. The patient must be reassured that a stroke did not occur and that chances for a full recovery are good. The patient's need for privacy should be respected, especially during meals, but the nurse's assistance in the patient's adjustment to the physical changes should not be delayed. Enlisting support from family and friends is important. It is important to share with the patient that most patients recover within about 6 weeks of the onset of symptoms.

■ Evaluation

The expected outcomes are that the patient with Bell's palsy

- will be free of pain
- will not experience any complications
- will return to previous perception of body image

POLYNEUROPATHIES

GUILLAIN-BARRÉ SYNDROME

Etiology and Pathophysiology

Guillain-Barré syndrome (Landry-Guillain-Barré-Strohl syndrome, postinfectious polyneuropathy, ascending polyneuropathic paralysis) is an acute, rapidly progressing, and potentially fatal form of polyneuritis. It affects the peripheral nervous system and results in loss of myelin (a segmental demyelination) and edema and inflammation of the affected nerves, causing a loss of neurotransmission to the periphery. With adequate supportive care, 85% of these patients recover completely from this disorder.[11]

The etiology of this disorder is unknown, but it is believed to be a cell-mediated immunologic reaction directed at the peripheral nerves. The syndrome is frequently preceded by immune system stimulation from a viral infection, trauma, surgery, viral immunizations, human immunodeficiency virus (HIV), or lymphoproliferative neoplasms. These stimuli are thought to cause an alteration in the immune system, resulting in sensitization of T lymphocytes to the patient's myelin, causing myelin damage. Demyelination occurs, and the transmission of nerve impulses is stopped or slowed down. The muscles innervated by the damaged peripheral nerves undergo denervation and atrophy. In the recovery phase, remyelination occurs slowly and returns in a proximal to distal pattern. The lymphocytes are basically normal and return to complete functioning after the illness.

The syndrome affects both genders equally and is more commonly seen in adults, although it is observed in all age-groups. Worldwide the incidence has varied from 0.4 to 1.7 cases per 100,000 persons per year. Guillain-Barré syndrome has an estimated annual cost of 2 to 3 billion dollars in the United States.[11]

Clinical Manifestations

Symptoms of Guillain-Barré syndrome usually develop 1 to 3 weeks after an upper respiratory or GI infection. Weakness of the lower extremities (evolving more or less symmetrically) occurs over hours to days to weeks, usually peaking about the fourteenth day. Distal muscles are more severely affected. *Paresthesia* (numbness and tingling) is frequent, and paralysis usually follows in the extremities. Hypotonia and areflexia are common, persistent symptoms. Objective sensory loss is variable, with deep sensitivity more affected than superficial sensations.

Autonomic nervous system dysfunction results from alterations in both the sympathetic and parasympathetic nervous systems. Autonomic disturbances are usually seen in patients with severe muscle involvement and respiratory muscle paralysis. The most dangerous autonomic dysfunctions include orthostatic hypotension, hypertension, and abnormal vagal responses (bradycardia, heart block, asystole). Other autonomic dysfunctions include bowel and bladder dysfunction, facial flushing, and diaphoresis. Patients may also have syndrome of inappropriate antidiuretic hormone (SIADH) secretion. SIADH is discussed further in Chapter 47. Progression of Guillain-Barré syndrome to include the lower brainstem involves the facial, abducens, oculomotor, hypoglossal, trigeminal, and vagus nerves (CN VII, VI, III, XII, V, and X, respectively). This involvement manifests itself through facial weakness, extraocular eye movement difficulties, dysphagia, and paresthesia of the face.

Pain is a common symptom in the patient with Guillain-Barré syndrome. The pain can be categorized as paresthesias, muscular aches and cramps, and hyperesthesias. Pain appears to be worse at night. Narcotics may be indicated for those experiencing severe pain. Pain may lead to a decrease in appetite and may interfere with sleep.

Complications

The most serious complication of this syndrome is respiratory failure, which occurs as the paralysis progresses to the nerves that innervate the thoracic area. Constant monitoring of the respiratory system by checking respiratory rate, depth, forced vital capacity, and negative inspiratory force provides information about the need for immediate intervention including intubation and mechanical ventilation. Respiratory or urinary tract infections (UTIs) may occur. Fever is generally the first sign of infection, and treatment is directed at the infecting organism. Immobility from the paralysis can cause problems such as paralytic ileus, muscle atrophy, deep vein thrombosis, pulmonary emboli, skin breakdown, orthostatic hypotension, and nutritional deficiencies.

Diagnostic Studies

Diagnosis is based primarily on the patient's history and clinical signs. Cerebrospinal fluid (CSF) is normal or has a low protein content initially, but after 7 to 10 days it shows an elevated protein level to 700 mg/dl (7 g/L) (normal protein is 15 to 45 mg/dl; 0.15 to 0.45 g/L) with a normal cell count. Electromyographic (EMG) and nerve conduction studies are markedly abnormal (reduced nerve conduction velocity) in the affected extremities.

Collaborative Care

Management is aimed at supportive care, particularly ventilatory support, during the acute phase. Plasmapheresis is used in the first 2 weeks of Guillain-Barré syndrome. In patients with severe disease treated within 2 weeks of onset, there is a distinct reduction in the length of stay, length of time on ventilator, and time required to resume walking. After 3 weeks of onset little value has been seen in plasmapheresis.[12] IV administration of high-dose immunoglobulin has also shown to be as effective as plasmapheresis and has the advantage of immediate availability and greater safety. Because of the ease of administering immunoglobulin, it is now being used more frequently than plasmapheresis. The costs of the two treatments are comparable.[11] Recovery is accelerated by early institution of plasmapheresis and IV therapy.[13] (Plasmapheresis is discussed in Chapter 12.) Corticosteroids and ACTH are used to suppress the immune response but appear to have little effect on the prognosis or duration of the disease.

Nutritional Therapy. Nutritional intake is compromised in the patient with Guillain-Barré syndrome. During the acute phase, the patient may experience difficulty swallowing because of cranial nerve involvement. Mild dysphagia can be managed by placing the patient in an upright position and flexing the head forward during feeding. For more severe dysphagia, tube feedings may be required. Patients who experience paralytic ileus or intestinal obstruction may require total parenteral nutrition. Later in the course of the disease, motor paralysis or weakness continue to affect the ability to self-feed. The patient's nutritional status, including body weight, serum albumin levels, and calorie counts, must be evaluated at regular intervals.

NURSING MANAGEMENT: GUILLAIN-BARRÉ SYNDROME

Nursing Assessment

Assessment of the patient is the most important aspect of nursing care during the acute phase. The nurse must monitor the ascending paralysis, assess respiratory function, monitor arterial blood gases (ABGs), and assess the gag, corneal, and swallowing reflexes during the routine assessment.

Monitoring blood pressure and cardiac rate and rhythm is also important during the acute phase because transient cardiac arrhythmias have been reported. Autonomic dysfunction is common and usually takes the form of bradycardia and arrhythmias. Orthostatic hypotension secondary to muscle atony may occur in severe cases. Vasopressor agents and volume expanders may be needed to treat the low blood pressure.

Nursing Diagnoses

Nursing diagnoses for the patient with Guillain-Barré syndrome may include, but are not limited to, the following:

- Inability to sustain spontaneous ventilation *related to* progression of disease process resulting in respiratory muscle paralysis
- Risk for aspiration *related to* dysphagia
- Pain *related to* paresthesias, muscle aches and cramps, and hyperesthesias
- Impaired verbal communication *related to* intubation or paralysis of the muscles of speech
- Fear *related to* uncertain outcome and seriousness of the disease
- Self-care deficits *related to* inability to use muscles to accomplish ADLs

Planning

The overall goals are that the patient with Guillain-Barré syndrome will (1) maintain adequate ventilation, (2) be free from aspiration, (3) be pain free or have pain controlled, (4) maintain an acceptable method of communication, (5) maintain adequate nutritional intake, and (6) return to usual physical functioning.

Nursing Implementation

The objective of therapy is to support body systems until the patient recovers. Respiratory failure and infection are serious threats. Monitoring the vital capacity and ABGs is essential. If the vital capacity drops to less than 800 ml (<15 ml/kg or two thirds of the patient's normal vital capacity) or the ABGs deteriorate, endotracheal intubation or tracheostomy may be done so that the patient can be mechanically ventilated (see Chapter 63). Meticulous suctioning technique is needed to prevent infection whether the patient has an endotracheal tube or tracheostomy. Thorough bronchial hygiene and chest physiotherapy help clear secretions and prevent respiratory deterioration. If fever develops, sputum cultures should be obtained to identify whether the respiratory tract is the source of the pathogen. Appropriate antibiotic therapy is then initiated.

A communication system must be established with the use of the patient's available abilities. This is extremely difficult if the disease progresses to involvement of the cranial nerves. At the peak of a severe episode the patient may be incapable of communicating. The nurse must explain all procedures before doing them and reassure the patient that muscle function will return.

Urinary retention is common for a few days. Intermittent catheterization is preferred to an indwelling catheter to avoid UTIs. However, for the acutely ill patient receiving a large volume of fluids (>2.5 L/day) indwelling catheterization may be safer to reduce overdistention of a temporarily flaccid bladder and to prevent vesicoureteral reflux. Physiotherapy is indicated early to help prevent problems related to immobility. Passive range-of-motion exercises and attention to body position help maintain function and prevent contractures. Patients who develop facial paralysis must receive meticulous eye care to avoid cornea irritation or damage (exposure keratitis).[13] Artificial tears should be instilled frequently during the day to prevent drying of the cornea. The eyes should be inspected for the presence of eyelashes. Ointment and an impermeable eye shield can be used at night to retain moisture.

Nutritional needs must be met in spite of possible problems associated with delayed gastric emptying, paralytic ileus, and potential for aspiration if the gag reflex is lost. In addition to checking for the gag reflex, nurses should note drooling and other difficulties with secretions, which may be more indicative of an inadequate gag reflex. Initially, tube feedings or parenteral nutrition may be used to ensure adequate caloric intake. Because of delayed gastric emptying, residual volumes of the feedings should be assessed at regular intervals or before feedings (see Chapter 38). Fluid and electrolyte therapy must be monitored carefully to prevent electrolyte imbalances. A bowel program should be initiated because constipation is a common problem related to diet changes, immobility, and decreased GI motility.

Throughout the course of the illness, the nurse needs to provide support and encouragement to the family and patient. Because residual problems and relapses are uncommon except in the chronic form of the disease, complete recovery can be anticipated although it is generally a slow process that takes months or years if axonal degeneration occurs.

BOTULISM

Etiology and Pathophysiology

Botulism is the most serious type of food poisoning. It is caused by GI absorption of the neurotoxin produced by *Clostridium botulinum*. This organism is found in the soil, and the spores are difficult to destroy. It can grow in any food contaminated with the spores. Improper home canning of foods is often the cause. It is thought that the neurotoxin destroys or inhibits the neurotransmission of acetylcholine at the myoneural junction, resulting in disturbed muscle innervation.

Clinical Manifestations

Symptoms are usually nausea, vomiting, and abdominal cramps, generally within 6 to 48 hours after consumption of the contaminated food. Neurologic manifestations develop rapidly over 2 to 4 days. They include difficulty in convergence of the eyes, photophobia, ptosis, paralysis of extraocular muscles, blurred vision, diplopia, dry mouth, sore throat, and difficulty in swallowing. Other manifestations include paralytic ileus, mild muscle weakness, seizures, and respiratory symptoms that can rapidly deteriorate to respiratory arrest and/or cardiac arrest. The course of the disease depends on the amount of toxin absorbed from the gut. If only a small amount is absorbed, symptoms are mild and recovery is complete. When large amounts are absorbed, death usually occurs in 4 to 8 days from circulatory failure, respiratory paralysis, or development of pulmonary complications.[14]

Because botulism is a reportable disease, local, state, and federal health agencies, particularly the Centers for Disease Control in Atlanta, must be notified.

Diagnostic Studies

Blood and CSF are obtained for studies to rule out other diseases. However, in botulism the blood and CSF results are normal.

Collaborative Care

Drug Therapy. The initial treatment of botulism is IV administration of botulinum antitoxin. Before administration of the antitoxin, an intradermal test dose for sensitivity to horse serum is given. If there are no reactions, the test dose is followed by daily doses of 50,000 units of botulism antitoxin IM until improvement begins.[11]

The GI tract is purged by laxatives, high colonic enemas, and gastric lavage to decrease the absorption of the toxin. Prophylactic penicillin may be ordered to halt the release of toxin in the GI tract.[15]

NURSING MANAGEMENT: BOTULISM

■ Nursing Implementation

Primary prevention is the goal of nursing management through educating consumers to be alert to situations that may result in botulism. Particular attention should be given to foods with a low acid content, which support germination and the production of botulin, a deadly poison. These foods include fish, vichyssoise, and peppers. All varieties of spores are destroyed by boiling for 10 minutes or maintaining a temperature of 176° F (80° C) for 30 minutes. Specific suggestions related to the preparation, storage, and use of food include the following:[11]

1. In home canning, the equipment manufacturer's directions should be followed. Only fresh fruits and vegetables (with all questionable spots removed) should be used. All containers and utensils must be cleansed, and the seal on the can or jar must be airtight. Canned foods should be stored properly in a cool, dry place.
2. A can with a swollen end should never be used; the swelling may be caused by gases from *Clostridium botulinum.*
3. If the food is forcefully expelled when a container is opened, it should be discarded immediately and the contents should not be tasted.
4. If the contents of a can look or smell bad after opening, the can should be discarded without tasting of the contents. Materials may be flushed down the toilet or disposed of in the garbage disposal if a large amount of water is used.

Nursing care during the acute illness is similar to that for Guillain-Barré syndrome. Supportive nursing interventions include rest, activities to maintain respiratory function, adequate nutrition, and prevention of loss of muscle mass. Because the recovery process is slow, the patient may develop problems related to a feeling of helplessness, boredom, and low morale.

TETANUS

Etiology and Pathophysiology

Tetanus (lockjaw) is an extremely severe polyradiculitis and polyneuritis affecting spinal and cranial nerves. It results from the effects of a potent neurotoxin released by the anaerobic bacillus *Clostridium tetani.* The toxin interferes with the function of the reflex arc by blocking of inhibitory transmitters at the presynaptic sites in the spinal cord and brainstem.[11] The spores of the bacillus are present in soil, garden mold, and manure. Thus *Clostridium tetani* enters the body through a traumatic or suppurative wound that provides an appropriate low-oxygen environment for the organisms to mature and produce toxin. Other possible sources include dental infection, injections of heroin, human and animal bites, frostbite, compound fractures, and gunshot wounds. The incubation period is usually 7 days but can range from 3 to 21 days, with symptoms frequently appearing after the original wound is healed. In general, the longer the incubation period, the milder the illness and the better the prognosis.

Worldwide the number of cases per year is estimated to be 1 million. Most victims are neonates born to unimmunized mothers in developing countries. In the United States about 100 to 200 cases occur each year and are due to infection of puncture wounds of the extremities by nails or splinters.[15] Of those reported cases the majority of patients are over the age of 59 years, suggesting inadequate immunization among older adults.[16] Mortality rates vary according to age, with infants and persons more than 50 years of age most seriously affected. Overall mortality rates range from 45% to 55%.

Clinical Manifestations

Manifestations of generalized tetanus include a feeling of stiffness in the jaw (*trismus*) or neck, slight fever, and other symptoms of general infection. Generalized tonic spasms occur because of the lack of reciprocal innervation. As the disease progresses, the neck muscles, back, abdomen, and extremities become progressively rigid. In severe forms, continuous tonic convulsions may occur with *opisthotonos* (extreme arching of the back and retraction of the head). Laryngeal and respiratory spasms cause apnea and anoxia. Additional effects are manifested by overstimulation of the sympathetic nervous system, including profuse diaphoresis, labile hypertension, episodic tachycardia, hyperthermia, and arrhythmias. The slightest noise, jarring motion, or bright light can set off the seizure. These seizures are agonizingly painful. Mortality is almost 100% in the severe form. Death is usually attributable to asphyxia or heart failure, the result of constantly recurring spasms. Residual injury, such as vertebral fracture, muscle contracture, and brain damage secondary to hypoxia, may be long-term consequences.

Collaborative Care

Serum electrolytes, CBC count, albumin, clotting factors, glucose, and ABGs are monitored. Cardiac function is monitored by electrocardiogram (ECG) and auscultation. As increasing numbers of nerve cells become involved, their inhibitory control over muscle activity decreases and symptoms develop.

Drug Therapy. The management of tetanus includes administration of tetanus toxoid booster (Td) and tetanus immune globulin (TIG) before the onset of symptoms to neutralize circulating toxins (see Table 64-8). Control of spasms is essential and is managed by deep sedation, usually with diazepam (Valium), barbiturates, or chlorpromazine (Thorazine). Chlorpromazine is also helpful in reducing hyperthermia. A 10-day course of penicillin is recommended to inhibit further growth of the organism.

Because of laryngospasm, a tracheostomy is usually performed early and the patient is maintained on mechanical ventilation. If sedation does not control seizures, skeletal muscle–paralyzing drugs such as d-tubocurarine (curare) are used. Pain is relieved by means of codeine or meperidine, often with the addition of promethazine (Phenergan). Any recognized wound should be debrided or an abscess drained. Antibiotics may be given to prevent secondary infections.

Nutrition is maintained through parenteral nutrition or nasogastric feeding. Even with the best of care, the mortality rate is 50%. Those who recover have a long convalescence that includes extensive physiotherapy.

NURSING MANAGEMENT: TETANUS

■ Nursing Implementation

Health teaching is aimed at ensuring tetanus prophylaxis, which is the most important factor influencing the incidence of this disease. Tetanus prevention and immunization protocols are summarized in Table 64-8. The patient should be taught that immediate, thorough cleansing of all wounds with soap and water is important in the prevention of tetanus. If an open wound occurs and the patient has not been immunized within 10 years, the primary care provider should be contacted so that a tetanus booster can be given.

If equine tetanus antitoxin is to be used, the patient should be tested for sensitivity. Administration of equine antitoxin is not recommended if sensitivity occurs; anaphylactic shock is potentially life threatening and desensitization is ineffective. The side effects of routine administration of the antitoxin are mild and include a sore arm, swelling at the site, and itching. Serious side effects rarely occur. Routine administration of a booster shot to an adequately immunized patient can cause arm swelling and lymphadenopathy.

Every patient should receive a written record of immunizations and be encouraged to complete the active immunization schedule. The patient's immunization history should be accurately recorded to protect the patient and care providers.

The acute nursing management of the patient with tetanus is aimed at supportive care based on the treatment of clinical manifestations. The patient should be placed in a quiet, darkened room insulated against noise. Judicious sedation should be given. Nursing care should be administered with the utmost caution to avoid triggering spasms. For example, the nurse should avoid unnecessary touching, use firm touching when necessary, avoid the use of linens to cover the patient, and maintain a slightly higher than normal ambient temperature. Nursing care related to tracheostomy and mechanical ventilation is given as appropriate. An indwelling urinary catheter may be used to prevent bladder distention and urinary reflux in the presence of spasms in the muscles of the pelvic floor. Attention must also given to skin care. The patient needs emotional support during the acute phase because the fear of death is real. The family also needs support and education.

NEUROSYPHILIS

Neurosyphilis (tertiary syphilis) is an infection of any part of the nervous system by the organism *Treponema pallidum.* It is the result of untreated or inadequately treated syphilis (see Chapter 50). The organism can invade the central nervous system (CNS) within a few months of the original infection. Except for causing some changes in the CSF, including increased white blood cells (WBCs) and protein and positive serologic reaction, the organism lies dormant for years. Untreated neurosyphilis, although not contagious, can be fatal. Penicillin therapy is effective for syphilitic meningitis, but the neurologic deficits remain.

Late neurosyphilis results from degenerative changes in the spinal cord (tabes dorsalis) and brainstem (general paresis). *Tabes dorsalis* (progressive locomotor ataxia) is characterized by vague, sharp pains in the legs; ataxia; "slapping" gait; loss of proprioception and deep tendon reflexes; and zones of hyperesthesia. *Charcot's joints,* which are characterized by enlargement, bone destruction, and hypermobility, also occur as a result of joint effusion and edema.

Dementia paralytica is an ongoing spirochetal meningoencephalitis that causes a general dissolution of mental and physical capabilities. It may mimic a number of major or minor psychoses. Management includes treatment with penicillin, symptomatic care, and protection from physical injury.

SPINAL CORD TRAUMA

Before World War II, the life expectancy for the person with a spinal cord injury ranged from months to 10 years from the onset of injury. The leading causes of death were renal failure and sepsis. Today, with improved treatment strategies (specifically, intermittent catheterization), even the very young patient with a spinal cord injury can anticipate a long life. The prognosis for life is generally only about 5 years less than for persons of the same age without spinal cord injury. The cause of premature death in the patient with quadriplegia is usually related to compromised respiratory function.

The disruption of individual growth and development, altered family dynamics, economic loss in terms of absence from work, and the high cost of rehabilitation or maintenance make spinal cord trauma a devastating problem. About 200,000 people in the United States today had traumatic spinal cord injuries and 6000 to 7000 people are newly injured each year.[17] The number of persons with spinal cord injuries living in the United States at any one time ranges from 183,000 to 203,000. The cost of spinal cord injury management is high. The average cost of care for a person with a high cervical injury is $417,067 in the first year and $74,707 in each subsequent year.[18]

Although many patients with spinal cord injuries can care for themselves with minimal assistance, a larger number are confined to nursing homes, care centers, and rehabilitation units. The loss to the workforce in terms of human potential is enormous.

Etiology and Pathophysiology

The population at risk for spinal cord injury is primarily young adult men between the ages of 15 and 30 years and those who are impulsive or risk takers in daily living. A history of numerous injuries before the cord injury is common. A high correlation exists between alcohol and drug abuse and spinal cord injury. Individuals at risk for spinal cord injury include motorcyclists, sky divers, football players, police officers, divers, and military personnel.

There has also been an increase in the number of older adult spinal cord injuries. Trauma has been called a young man's "disease," but when it happens in the older adult, trauma is often even more devastating. Besides having greater mortality, older adults with traumatic injuries as a group experience more complications than younger ones, and they are hospitalized longer. As the nation's population ages, the human and financial tolls of trauma in the elderly are certain to grow.[19] The most common causes of spinal cord injury include motor vehicle accidents, falls, gunshot wounds, and sports injuries.

Gunshot wounds is now listed as the third most common cause of spinal cord injuries in the United States. In large urban areas, gun shot wounds have recently surpassed falls as the second most common cause of spinal cord injuries.[20] The resulting spinal cord injury can be due to cord compression by bone displacement, interruption of blood supply to the cord, or traction resulting from pulling on the cord.

Initial Injury. The spinal cord is wrapped in tough layers of dura and is rarely torn or transected by direct trauma. Penetrating trauma, such as gunshot and stab wounds, can result in tearing and transection. The complete cord dissolution (previously thought to be transection) in severe trauma is related to autodestruction of the cord. Shortly after the injury, petechial hemorrhages are noted in the central gray matter of the cord. Hemorrhagic areas in the center of the spinal cord (gray matter) are grossly visible within 1 hour. Within 4 hours there may be infarction in the gray matter.[21]

Hemorrhage, edema, and metabolites act together to produce ischemia, which progresses to necrotic destruction of the cord. Figure 57-4 illustrates the cascade of events that follow spinal cord injury. The resulting hypoxia reduces the oxygen tension below the level that meets the metabolic needs of the cord. Lactate metabolites and an increase in vasoactive substances including norepinephrine, serotonin, and dopamine are noted. At high levels, these vasoactive substances cause vasospasms and hypoxia leading to subsequent necrosis. Unfortunately, the spinal cord has minimal ability to adapt to vasospasm.

By 24 hours, permanent damage has occurred because of the development of edema. Edema secondary to the inflammatory response is particularly harmful because of lack of space for tissue expansion. Therefore, resultant compression of the cord and extension of edema above and below the injury increase the ischemic damage. The end result is the same as mechanical severance of the cord.

The hemorrhagic necrosis causes the lesion to be complete after 48 hours, and any function of nerves that arise in and pass through this level is lost. Because additional edema extends the level of injury beyond the immediate level of destruction for 72 hours to 1 week, the exact extent of injury cannot be determined before that time.

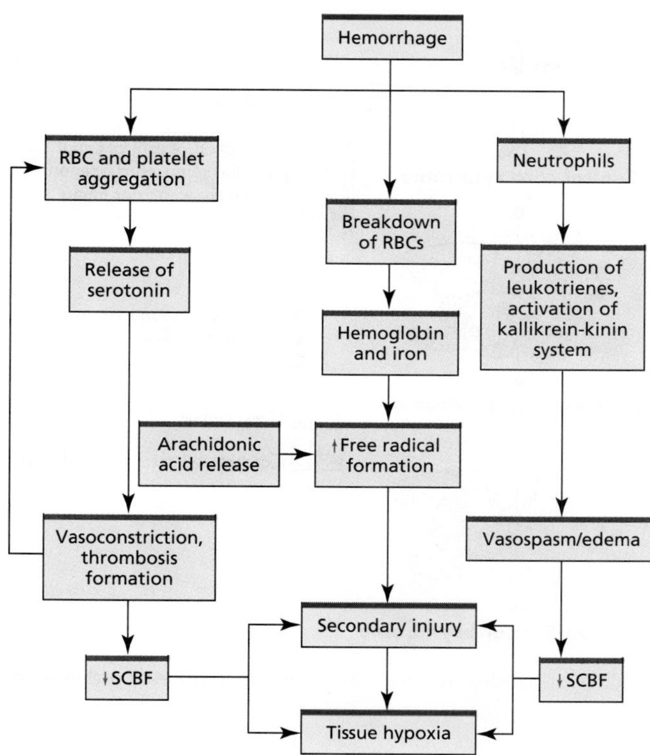

Fig. 57-4 Cascade of metabolic and cellular events that leads to spinal cord ischemia and hypoxia of secondary injury. *SCBF,* spinal cord blood flow. (Redrawn from Marciano FF and others: *BNI Quarterly* 11(2):6,1995. In McCance KL, Heuther SE: *Pathophysiology: the biologic basis for disease in adults and children,* St. Louis, 1998, Mosby.)

Spinal and Neurogenic Shock. In addition to the discrete damage at the trauma site, the entire cord below the level of the lesion fails to function, resulting in spinal shock characterized by decreased reflexes and flaccid paralysis below the level of the injury. There is complete loss of motor and sensory function below the level of the lesion. Spinal shock usually occurs at the time of injury in response to severe damage to the cord and results in immediate depression of all cord functions. This affects musculoskeletal, bowel, and bladder function. Neurogenic shock characterized by hypotension, bradycardia, and warm, dry extremities also occurs. Loss of sympathetic innervation causes peripheral vasodilation, venous pooling, and a decreased cardiac output. These effects are generally associated with a cervical or high thoracic injury.

Spinal shock generally lasts for 7 to 10 days after onset but can last from weeks to months. Indications that spinal shock has ended include spasticity, reflex emptying of the bladder, and hyperreflexia. Active rehabilitation may begin in the presence of spinal shock.

Classification of Spinal Cord Injury

Spinal cord injuries are classified by the mechanism of injury, level of injury, or degree of injury.

Mechanisms of Injury. The major mechanisms of injury are flexion, hyperextension, flexion-rotation, extension-rotation, and compression (Fig. 57-5). The flexion injury that includes dislocation is the most unstable of all injuries because the ligamentous structures that stabilize the spine are torn. This injury is most often implicated in severe neurologic deficits.

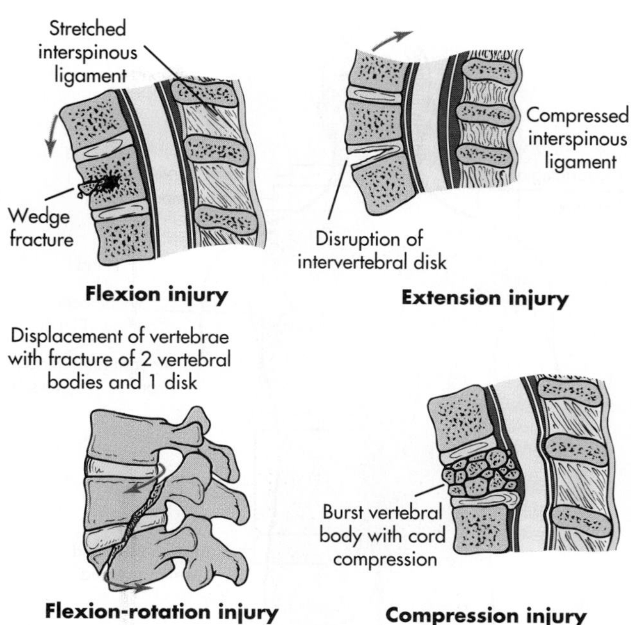

Fig. 57-5 Mechanisms of spinal injury.

Level of Injury. The level of injury may be cervical, thoracic, or lumbar. Cervical and lumbar injuries are most common because these levels are associated with the greatest flexibility and movement.

Degree of Injury. The degree of spinal cord involvement may be either complete or incomplete (partial). *Complete cord* involvement results in flaccid paralysis and total loss of sensory and motor function below the level of the lesion (injury). If the cervical cord is involved, paralysis of all four extremities (particularly the hands and forearms) occurs, resulting in quadriplegia. However, even with a cervical injury the arms are rarely completely paralyzed. If the thoracic or lumbar cord is damaged, the result is paraplegia. Figure 57-6 shows affected structures and functions at different levels of cord injury.

Incomplete cord lesion involvement (partial transection) results in a mixed loss of voluntary motor activity and sensation and leaves some tracts intact. The degree of sensory and motor loss varies depending on the level of the lesion and reflects the specific nerve tracts damaged and those spared. Four syndromes are associated with incomplete lesions: central cord syndrome, anterior cord syndrome, Brown-Séquard syndrome, and posterior cord syndrome.

Central cord syndrome. Damage in the cervical central cord is termed *central cord syndrome,* which is characterized by microscopic hemorrhage, edema of the central spinal cord, and compression on anterior horn cells (Fig. 57-7). Central cord syndrome is more common in older adults. Motor weakness is present in both the upper and lower extremities, but the weakness is much greater in the upper extremities than in the lower ones. It may change to a progressive lesion. Sensory dysfunction varies according to the site of injury or lesion. Bladder dysfunction is variable. This syndrome is frequently a result of hyperextension of an osteoarthritic spine. The extent of recovery

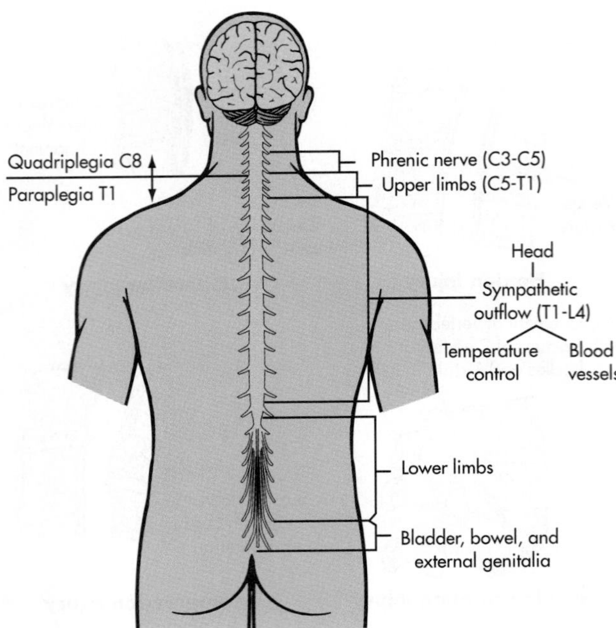

Fig. 57-6 Symptoms, degree of paralysis, and potential for rehabilitation depend on the level of the lesion.

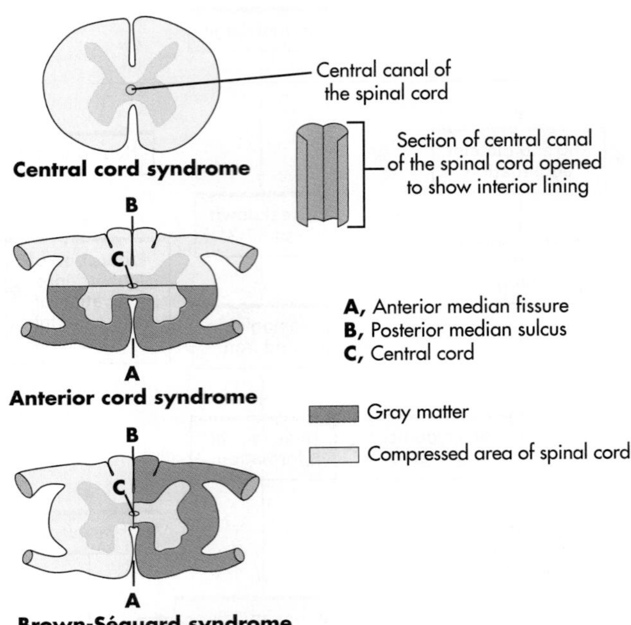

Fig. 57-7 Syndromes associated with incomplete cord lesions.

depends on the resolution of edema and the intactness of the spinal cord tracts.

Anterior cord syndrome. *Anterior cord syndrome* is characterized by injury resulting in an acute compression of the anterior portion of the spinal cord, often a flexion injury (see Fig. 57-7). The spinal cord lesion is in the anterior two thirds of the cord. Compression is usually caused by a disk or bony fragment; it may also be caused by actual destruction of the anterior cord by an anterior spinal artery occlusion caused by ischemia or thrombus. Manifestations include immediate, complete motor paralysis from the site of the injury and below. *Hypoesthesia* (decreased sensation), decreased pain sensation, and loss of temperature occur below the level of injury. Because the posterior cord tracts are not injured, sensations of touch, position, vibration, and motion remain intact. Dorsal column function is preserved. If the syndrome is caused by the compression of the anterior cord from bony fragments, surgical decompression is indicated.

Brown-Séquard syndrome. *Brown-Séquard syndrome* is a result of transection or lesion of one half of the spinal cord (see Fig. 57-7). Brown-Séquard syndrome is usually caused by penetrating injuries, such as a gunshot wound or knife or possibly an acute ruptured disk. This syndrome is characterized by a loss of motor function (paralysis) and position and vibratory sense, as well as vasomotor paralysis on the same side (ipsilateral) and below the hemisection. The opposite (contralateral) side of the hemisection has loss of pain and temperature sensation below the level of the lesion or hemisection. Fibers that carry pain and temperature cross to the opposite side of the cord immediately after entering the cord and ascend, which accounts for the described symptoms.

Posterior cord syndrome. Less commonly seen is the *posterior cord syndrome.* This syndrome is associated with cervical hyperextension trauma. It results from compression or damage to the posterior part of the spinal cord that contains the sensory neurons and position-sense capabilities. Generally the dorsal columns are damaged, resulting in loss of proprioception. However, pain, temperature sensation, and motor function below the level of the lesion remain intact.

Clinical Manifestations

The manifestations of spinal cord injury are generally the direct result of trauma that causes cord compression, ischemia, edema, and possible cord transection. Manifestations are related to the level and degree of injury. The patient with an incomplete lesion may demonstrate a mixture of symptoms. The higher the injury, the more serious the sequelae because of the proximity of the cervical cord to the medulla and brainstem. Movement and rehabilitation potential related to specific locations of the spinal cord injury are described in Table 57-3. In general, sensory function closely parallels motor function at all levels.

Immediate postinjury problems include maintaining a patent airway, adequate ventilation, and adequate circulating blood volume and preventing extension of cord damage.

Respiratory System. Cervical injury or fracture above the level of C4 presents special problems because of the total loss of respiratory muscle function. Mechanical ventilation is required to keep the patient alive. At one time the majority of these patients died at the scene of the injury, but with improved Emergency Medical Services more of these patients are surviving the initial events of their spinal cord injury. Injury or fracture below the level of C4 results in diaphragmatic breathing if the phrenic nerve is functioning. Even if the injury is below C4, spinal cord edema and hemorrhage can affect the function of the phrenic nerve and cause respiratory insufficiency. Hypoventilation almost always occurs with diaphragmatic respirations because of the decrease in vital capacity and tidal

Table 57-3 Functional Level of Spinal Cord Disruption and Rehabilitation Potential

Level of Injury	Movement Remaining	Rehabilitation Potential
Quadriplegia		
C1-C3		
Usually fatal injury, vagus nerve domination of heart, respiration, blood vessels, all organs below injury	Movement in neck and above, loss of innervation to diaphragm, absence of independent respiratory function	Ability to drive electric wheelchair equipped with portable respirator by using chin control or mouth stick, headpiece to stabilize head, lack of bowel and bladder control
C4		
Vagus nerve domination of heart, respirations, and all vessels and organs below injury	Sensation and movement above neck	Ability to drive electric wheelchair by using chin control or mouth stick, lack of bowel and bladder control
C5		
Vagus nerve domination of heart, respirations, and all vessels and organs below injury	Full neck, partial shoulder, back, biceps; gross elbow, inability to roll over or use hands; decreased respiratory reserve	Ability to drive electric wheelchair with mobile hand supports, ability to use powered hand splints (in some patients), lack of bowel and bladder control, feed self with setup and adaptive equipment
C6		
Vagus nerve domination of heart, respirations, and all vessels and organs below injury	Shoulder and upper back abduction and rotation at shoulder, full biceps to elbow flexion, wrist extension, weak grasp of thumb, decreased respiratory reserve	Ability to assist with transfer and perform some self-care, feed self with hand devices, push wheelchair on smooth, flat surface; lack of bowel and bladder control
C7-C8		
Vagus nerve domination of heart, respirations, and all vessels and organs below injury	All triceps to elbow extension, finger extensors and flexors, good grasp with some decreased strength, decreased respiratory reserve	Ability to transfer self to wheelchair, roll over and sit up in bed, push self on most surfaces, perform most self-care; independent use of wheelchair; ability to drive car with powered hand controls (in some patients); lack of bowel and bladder control
Paraplegia		
T1-T6		
Sympathetic innervation to heart, vagus nerve domination of all vessels and organs below injury	Full innervation of upper extremities, back, essential intrinsic muscles of hand; full strength and dexterity of grasp; decreased trunk stability, decreased respiratory reserve	Full independence in self-care and in wheelchair, ability to drive car with hand controls (in most patients), ability to use full body brace for exercise but not for functional ambulation, lack of bowel and bladder control
T6-T12		
Vagus nerve domination only of leg vessels, GI and genitourinary organs	Full, stable thoracic muscles and upper back; functional intercostals, resulting in increased respiratory reserve	Full independent use of wheelchair; ability to stand erect with full body brace, ambulate on crutches with swing (although gait difficult); inability to climb stairs; lack of bowel and bladder control
L1-L2		
Vagus nerve domination of leg vessels	Varying control of legs and pelvis, instability of lower back	Good sitting balance, full use of wheelchair
L3-L4		
Partial vagus nerve domination of leg vessels, GI and genitourinary organs	Quadriceps and hip flexors, absence of hamstring function, flail ankles	Completely independent ambulation with short leg braces and canes, inability to stand for long periods, bladder and bowel continence

GI, gastrointestinal.

volume, which occurs as a result of impairment of the intercostal muscles.

Cervical fractures or severe injuries cause a paralysis of abdominal musculature and frequently intercostal musculature; therefore the patient cannot cough effectively enough to remove secretions, leading to atelectasis and pneumonia. An artificial airway provides direct access for pathogens making bronchial hygiene and chest physiotherapy extremely important to reduce infection. Neurogenic pulmonary edema may occur secondary to a dramatic increase in sympathetic nervous system activity at the time of injury, which shunts blood to the lungs. In addition, pulmonary edema may occur in response to fluid overload.

Cardiovascular System. Any cord transection above the level of T5 greatly decreases the influence of the sympathetic nervous system. Bradycardia occurs as a result of the unopposed effect of the parasympathetic nervous system on the heart, and vasodilation results in hypotension. Cardiac monitoring is necessary. In marked bradycardia, appropriate medications to increase the heart rate and prevent hypoxemia are necessary. The peripheral vasodilation reduces the venous return of blood to the heart and subsequently decreases cardiac output, resulting in hypotension. IV fluids may resolve the problem, or vasopressor drugs may be required.

Urinary System. Urinary retention is a common development in acute spinal cord injuries and spinal shock. While the patient is in spinal shock the bladder is atonic and becomes overdistended. An indwelling catheter is inserted to drain the bladder. In the postacute phase the bladder can be hyperirritable, with a loss of inhibition from the brain resulting in reflex emptying. Consequently, the patient urinates small amounts frequently. However, the bladder may become distended because of inadequate emptying. Urinary retention increases the risk of infection. In addition, urinary calculi are more likely to develop in a distended bladder retaining urine. Catheterization is usually indicated. The indwelling catheter should be removed and intermittent catheterization should begin as early as possible.

Gastrointestinal System. If the cord transection has occurred above the level of T5, the primary GI problems are related to hypomotility. Decreased GI motor activity contributes to the development of paralytic ileus and gastric distention. A nasogastric tube for intermittent suctioning may relieve the gastric distention. The development of stress ulcers is common because of excessive release of hydrochloric acid in the stomach. Histamine H_2-receptor blockers, such as ranitidine (Zantac) and famotidine (Pepcid), are frequently used to prevent the occurrence of these ulcers during the initial phase. Other medications such as sucralfate (Carafate) and antacids may also be useful in prophylaxis. Intraabdominal bleeding may occur and is difficult to diagnose because no subjective signs such as pain, tenderness, and guarding are observed. Continued hypotension in spite of vigorous treatment and decreased hemoglobin and hematocrit may be indications of bleeding. Expanding girth of the abdomen may also be noted. Additional GI problems include gallstone formation, constipation, and fecal impaction.

Integumentary System. A major consequence of lack of movement is the potential for tissue breakdown in the area of denervation, which can occur quickly and can lead to major infection or sepsis. A certain degree of muscle atrophy occurs during the flaccid paralysis state, whereas contractures tend to occur during the spastic state.

Poikilothermism is the adjustment of the body temperature to the room temperature. This occurs in spinal cord injuries because the interruption of the sympathetic nervous system prevents peripheral temperature sensations from reaching the hypothalamus. Another factor is the reduction in heat generation because of minimal movement. With spinal cord disruption there is also decreased ability to sweat below the level of the lesion, which also affects the ability to regulate body temperature.

Metabolic Needs. Correcting an existing acid-base disturbance and maintaining acid-base balance promote the functions of other body systems. Nasogastric suctioning may lead to metabolic alkalosis, and decreased tissue perfusion may lead to acidosis. Electrolyte levels, including sodium and potassium, can be altered by gastric suctioning and must be monitored until suctioning is discontinued and a normal diet is resumed. A positive nitrogen balance and a high-protein diet help to prevent skin breakdown and infections and help to decrease the rate of muscle atrophy.

Peripheral Vascular Problems. Deep vein thrombosis (DVT) is a common problem accompanying spinal cord injury. It is more difficult to detect a DVT in a person with a spinal cord injury because the usual signs and symptoms such as pain, tenderness, and a positive Homans' sign will not be present.[18] Pulmonary embolism is one of the leading causes of death in patients with spinal cord injury. Techniques for assessment of DVT include Doppler examination, impedance plethysmography, and measuring leg and thigh girth.

Collaborative Care

The initial goals for the patient with a spinal cord injury are to sustain life and prevent further cord damage. Table 57-4 outlines the emergency management of the patient with a spinal cord injury. Systemic, neurogenic, and spinal cord shock must be treated. For injury at the cervical level, all body systems must be maintained until the full extent of the damage can be evaluated. Treatment of a spinal cord injury may be medical or surgical.

Collaborative care for the patient with a cervical injury is described in Table 57-5. The systemic support required by the patient is less intense for spinal cord injuries of the thoracic and lumbar vertebrae. Respiratory compromise is not as severe, and bradycardia is not a problem. Specific problems are treated symptomatically. After stabilization at the accident scene the person is transferred to a medical facility. A thorough assessment is done to specifically evaluate the degree of deficit and to establish the level and degree of injury. A history is obtained, with emphasis on how the accident occurred and the degree of disruption as perceived by the patient immediately after the accident. Assessment involves testing muscle groups rather than individual muscles. Muscle groups should be tested with and against gravity, alone and against resistance, and on both sides of the body. Spontaneous movement should be noted. The patient should be asked to move legs and then hands, spread fingers, extend wrists, and shrug shoulders. After assessment of motor status, a sensory examination including touch and pain as tested by pinprick should be carried out, starting at the toes and working upward. If time and conditions permit, position sense and vibration can also be assessed.

The types of accidents that cause spinal cord trauma can also result in head injury. The patient should therefore be assessed

EMERGENCY MANAGEMENT

Table 57-4 Spinal Cord Injury

Etiology	Assessment Findings	Interventions
Blunt Compression, flexion, extension, or rotational injuries to spinal column Motor vehicle accidents Pedestrian accidents Falls Diving **Penetrating** Stretched, torn, crushed, or lacerated spinal cord Gunshot wounds Stab wounds	▪ Pain, tenderness, deformities, or muscle spasms adjacent to vertebral column ▪ Numbness, paresthesias ▪ Alterations in sensation: temperature, light touch, deep pressure, proprioception ▪ Weakness or heaviness in limbs ▪ Weakness, paralysis, or flaccidity of muscles ▪ Spinal shock ▪ Cuts, bruises, open wounds over head, face, neck, or back ▪ Neurogenic shock: hypotension, bradycardia, dry, flushed skin ▪ Bowel and bladder incontinence ▪ Urinary retention ▪ Difficulty breathing ▪ Priapism ▪ Diminished rectal sphincter tone	**Initial** ▪ Ensure patent airway. ▪ Stabilize cervical spine. ▪ Administer oxygen via nasal cannula or non-rebreather mask. ▪ Establish IV with two large-bore catheters and infuse normal saline or lactated Ringer's solution as appropriate. ▪ Assess for other injuries. ▪ Control external bleeding. ▪ Obtain cervical spine radiographs or CT scan. ▪ Prepare for stabilization with cranial tongs and traction. ▪ Administer high-dose methylprednisolone. **Ongoing Monitoring** ▪ Monitor vital signs, level of consciousness, oxygen saturation, cardiac rhythm, urine output. ▪ Keep warm. ▪ Monitor for urinary retention, hypertension. ▪ Anticipate need for intubation if gag reflex absent.

for signs of concussion and increased intracranial pressure (see Chapter 54). In addition, a careful assessment for musculoskeletal injuries and trauma to internal organs should be performed. Because there are no muscle, bone, or visceral sensations, the only clue to internal trauma with hemorrhage may be a rapidly falling hematocrit level. Urinary output is examined for hematuria, which is also indicative of internal injuries.

An x-ray is done to document the injury. The patient must be handled carefully before and during the x-ray procedure to prevent further injury. Respiratory, cardiac, urinary, and GI functions should be monitored closely. The patient may go directly to surgery following initial immobilization and stabilization or to the intensive care unit (ICU) for monitoring and management.

Surgical Therapy. The decision to perform surgery on a patient with a spinal cord injury often depends on the preference of a particular clinician. When cord compression is certain or the neurologic disorder progresses, benefit may be seen following immediate surgery.[17] Surgery stabilizes the spinal column. Other criteria used in the decision for early surgery include (1) evidence of cord compression, (2) progressive neurologic deficit, (3) compound fracture of the vertebrae, (4) bony fragments (may dislodge and penetrate the cord), and (5) penetrating wounds of the spinal cord or surrounding structures.

The more common surgical procedures include decompression laminectomy by anterior cervical and thoracic approaches with fusion, posterior laminectomy with the use of acrylic wire mesh and fusion, and insertion of stabilizing rods (e.g., Harrington rods for the correction and stabilization of thoracic deformities). (Specific surgical and nursing interventions for these techniques are discussed in Chapter 59.)

COLLABORATIVE CARE

Table 57-5 Cervical Cord Injury

Diagnostic
Complete neurologic examination
ABGs
Electrolytes, glucose, hemoglobin, and hematocrit levels
Urinalysis
Anteroposterior, lateral, and odontoid spinal x-ray studies
CT scan
Myelography
MRI
EMG to measure evoked potentials
Collaborative Therapy
Acute Care
Immobilization of vertebral column by skeletal traction
Maintenance of heart rate (e.g., atropine) and blood pressure (e.g., dopamine [Intropin])
Methylprednisone therapy to reduce edema
Insertion of nasogastric tube and attachment to suction
Intubation (if indicated by ABGs)
Oxygen by high humidity mask
Indwelling urinary catheter
Administration of IV fluids
Ambulatory/Home Care
Stress ulcer prophylaxis
Physical therapy (range-of-motion exercises)
Occupational therapy (splints, activities of daily living training)

ABGs, arterial blood gases.

NURSING ASSESSMENT

Table 57-6 Spinal Cord Injury

Subjective Data

Important Health Information

Past health history: Motor vehicle accident, sports injury, industrial accident, gunshot or stabbing injury, falls

Functional Health Patterns

Health perception–health management: Use of alcohol or recreational drugs; risk-taking behaviors

Activity-exercise: Loss of strength, movement, and sensation below level of injury; dyspnea, inability to breathe adequately

Cognitive-perceptual: Presence of tenderness, pain at or above level of injury; numbness, tingling, burning, twitching of extremities

Coping–stress tolerance: Fear, denial, anger, depression

Objective Data

General

Poikilothermia

Integumentary

Warm, dry, flushed extremities below level of injury (spinal shock)

Respiratory

Lesions at C1 to C3: apnea, inability to cough; lesions at C4: poor cough, diaphragmatic breathing, hypoventilation; lesions at C5 to T6: decreased respiratory reserve

Cardiovascular

Lesions above T5: bradycardia, hypotension, postural hypotension, absence of vasomotor tone

Gastrointestinal

Decreased or absent bowel sounds (paralytic ileus in lesions above T5), abdominal distention, constipation, fecal incontinence, fecal impaction

Urinary

Retention (for lesions between T1, L2); flaccid bladder (acute stages); spasticity with reflex bladder emptying (later stages)

Reproductive

Priapism, loss of sexual function

Neurologic

Complete: Flaccid paralysis and anesthesia below level of injury resulting in quadriplegia (for lesions above C8) or paraplegia (for lesions below C8), hyperactive deep tendon reflexes, bilaterally positive Babinski's test

Incomplete: Mixed loss of voluntary motor activity and sensations

Musculoskeletal

Muscle atony (in flaccid state), contractures (in spastic state)

Possible Findings

Location of level and type of bony involvement on spinal x-ray: lesion, edema, compression on CT scan and MRI; positive finding on myelogram

Drug Therapy. Vasopressor agents such as dopamine (Intropin) are employed in the acute phase as adjuvants to treatment. These agents are used to maintain the mean arterial pressure at a level greater than 80 to 90 mm Hg so that perfusion to the spinal cord is improved.

The National Acute Spinal Cord Injury Study II (NASCIS II) showed that methylprednisolone (MP), when administered early, resulted in an increased recovery of neurologic function. As a result of this study, MP is a standard of care and is administered IV bolus over 15 minutes. Dosing pauses for 45 minutes and then a maintenance dose of IV MP is started and infuses over the next 23 hours. Total dosing is completed over a 24 hour time period. MP, a blocker of lipid peroxidation by-products, has been found to improve blood flow and reduce edema in the spinal cord.[22] MP produces a number of effects that may account for the overall improvement noted in the spinal cord injured patient, including reduction of posttraumatic spinal cord ischemia, improvement of energy balance, restoration of extracellular calcium, improvement of nerve impulse conduction, and repression of the release of free fatty acids from spinal cord tissues.[23] MP is now a standard of comparison for future agents.

Currently a multicenter randomized trial NASCIS III is ongoing. The three purposes of this clinical trial are to determine (1) whether 48 hours of MP is as safe or safer than 24 hours, (2) whether tirilazad (Freedox) is a safe and effective substitution for MP, and (3) more precisely define the optimum time for drug administration. Tirilazad has been studied extensively in both spinal cord injury and brain injury. It inhibits both iron-dependent and independent lipid peroxidation. In vitro studies indicate that it has a stabilizing effect on cell membranes. Animal studies are ongoing and the drug looks promising as a treatment for acute spinal cord injuries.[23]

Pharmacologic properties and drug metabolism are altered in spinal cord injury; therefore, drug interactions may occur. For example, propoxyphene (Darvon) is believed to enhance vasodilation and possibly aggravate orthostatic hypotension, as well as act as an analgesic. The result may aggravate existing problems in the neurologically disabled patient. Drug-induced sedation can also mask a decreasing level of consciousness as a result of head injury or rising CO_2 levels with hypoventilation.

Pharmacologic agents are used to treat specific autonomic dysfunctions such as GI hyperactivity, bleeding, bradycardia, orthostatic hypotension, inadequate emptying of the bladder, and autonomic dysreflexia. The nurse must observe the response to these drugs and provide specific interventions when adverse reactions are seen.

NURSING MANAGEMENT: SPINAL CORD INJURY

■ Nursing Assessment

Subjective and objective data that should be obtained from a patient with a spinal cord injury are presented in Table 57-6.

■ Nursing Diagnoses

Nursing diagnoses for the patient with a spinal cord injury depend on the severity of the injury and the level of dysfunction. The nursing diagnoses for a patient with a spinal cord injury may include, but are not limited to, those presented in NCP 57-1. The care plan presented is for a patient with a complete cervical cord injury.

57-1 NURSING CARE PLAN PATIENT WITH A SPINAL CORD INJURY*

Expected Patient Outcomes	Nursing Interventions and *Rationales*
NURSING DIAGNOSIS	**Impaired gas exchange** *related to* muscle fatigue and retained secretions *as manifested by* decreased PaO_2 content, increased $PaCO_2$ concentration, fatigue, diminished breath sounds.
▪ ABGs within normal limits. ▪ Normal chest x-ray. ▪ Clear lungs on auscultation. ▪ Absence of respiratory distress.	▪ Maintain a patent airway *to prevent respiratory arrest.* ▪ Assess all respiratory parameters initially and at least q2hr *to determine extent of problem and plan appropriate interventions.* ▪ Monitor ABGs to determine oxygenation and ventilation status. ▪ Provide aggressive pulmonary toilet, including chest physiotherapy and quad-assist coughing q4hr *to facilitate the raising of secretions.* ▪ Assess strength of cough at least q4hr *to determine adequacy for raising secretions.* ▪ Suction as necessary *to remove accumulated secretions.*
NURSING DIAGNOSIS	**Inability to sustain spontaneous ventilation** *related to* diaphragmatic fatigue or paralysis *as manifested by* dyspnea, increased use of accessory muscles, decreased PaO_2, increased $PaCO_2$.
▪ No signs of respiratory compromise.	▪ Provide chest physiotherapy *to mobilize secretions and prevent pneumonia.* ▪ Assist with application of mechanical ventilation *to support respiration.* ▪ Provide emotional support *as intubation and mechanical ventilation can be frightening.*
NURSING DIAGNOSIS	**Decreased cardiac output** *related to* venous pooling of blood and immobility *as manifested by* hypotension, tachycardia, restlessness, oliguria, decreased pulmonary artery pressures.
▪ Adequate cardiac output. ▪ Stable blood pressure and pulse. ▪ Absence of arrhythmias. ▪ No complications such as venous thrombosis or pulmonary emboli.	▪ Monitor blood pressure and pulse at least q2hr initially; monitor cardiac rhythm *as indicators of cardiac status.* ▪ Administer dopamine (Intropin) or other vasopressor agents *to maintain mean blood pressure >80 mm Hg.* ▪ Apply pneumatic compression devices to calves and/or compression gradient stockings *to prevent venous pooling and thromboemboli.* ▪ Perform range-of-motion to all extremities at least q8hr *to cause muscle contractions, which aid in venous return.* ▪ Measure pulmonary artery wedge pressure and cardiac output as ordered *to evaluate circulatory status.*
NURSING DIAGNOSIS	**Impaired skin integrity** *related to* immobility and poor tissue perfusion *as manifested by* reddened skin over bony prominences and at pin and tong sites.
▪ Intact skin. ▪ No pressure ulcers.	▪ Inspect all skin areas, especially over bony prominences, at least q2hr; observe area around pins or tongs for signs of breakdown or infection at least every shift *so interventions can be initiated promptly if a problem develops.* ▪ Turn patient at least q2hr; use kinetic treatment table or other specialty care devices as needed *to prevent development of pressure areas.* ▪ Ensure adequate nutritional intake *to maintain healthy skin resistant to breakdown.* ▪ Wash and dry patient's skin thoroughly *to prevent moisture from predisposing to skin breakdown.* ▪ Inform patient and family about risk of pressure ulcers *to empower them in participating in prevention measures.*
NURSING DIAGNOSIS	**Constipation** *related to* the injury, inadequate fluid intake, diet low in roughage, and immobility *as manifested by* lack of bowel movement for more than 2 days, decreased bowel sounds, palpable impaction, hard stool or stool incontinence.
▪ Established bowel program. ▪ Bowel movement at least every other day.	▪ Auscultate bowel sounds at least q4hr; monitor abdominal distention *to determine if peristalsis is present.* ▪ Note any nausea and vomiting *as possible indicators of paralytic ileus.* ▪ Begin bowel program as soon as bowel sounds return and include suppository every other day and stool softeners *to establish a bowel routine as quickly as possible.*

Continued

57-1 NURSING CARE PLAN PATIENT WITH A SPINAL CORD INJURY*—continued

Expected Patient Outcomes	Nursing Interventions and *Rationales*
NURSING DIAGNOSIS **Constipation**—*continued*	
	▪ Teach patient and family the bowel program *to ensure continuity of the program.* ▪ Ensure appropriate food and fluid intake *as bulk, fiber, and fluid are necessary to the success of a bowel program.*
NURSING DIAGNOSIS **Urinary retention** *related to* injury and limited fluid intake *as manifested by* lack of urine output, bladder distention, involuntary emptying of bladder (after spinal shock).	
▪ No urinary retention or infection. ▪ Able to perform self-catheterization or Credé maneuver to empty bladder.	▪ Palpate bladder every shift *as loss of autonomic and reflex control of bladder and sphincter can cause distention.* ▪ Insert indwelling catheter during acute phase *to ensure continuous flow of urine preventing kidney reflux or possible bladder rupture.* ▪ Begin intermittent catheterization program when appropriate; teach patient and family intermittent catheterization using a clean technique *to avoid long-term use of indwelling catheter with high potential for infection.* ▪ Maintain accurate intake and output records *to evaluate balance.* ▪ Encourage fluids (2-4 L/day) *to maintain high volume of dilute urine,* which aids in preventing infection. ▪ Monitor BUN and creatinine levels, urine cultures, and WBC count *to monitor kidney function and presence of infection.* ▪ Teach Credé maneuver *to supplement intermittent catheterization or use alone for more complete emptying of the bladder.*
NURSING DIAGNOSIS **Impaired physical mobility** *related to* spinal cord injury, vertebral column instability, or forced immobilization by traction *as manifested by* inability to move purposefully, limited muscle strength, impaired coordination, impaired perception of position or presence of body parts.	
▪ No complications of immobility.	▪ Assess motor and sensory function at least q4hr initially *to promptly detect deterioration of neurologic status.* ▪ Check traction to ensure that frames are secure and properly aligned and that weights are hanging freely *to ensure maintenance of vertebral column stability.* ▪ Promote good pulmonary function *as pulmonary complications are a common sequelae of immobility.* ▪ Use specialty bed or turn patient q1-2hr as ordered *to prevent prolonged pressure, which can lead to pressure ulcers.* ▪ Perform full range-of-motion to all extremities several times a day *to promote circulation and prevent contractures.* ▪ Use splints, foot boards, and trochanter rolls as appropriate *to prevent contractures and promote functional positioning.* ▪ Mobilize patient as soon as appropriate *to prevent hazards of immobility and provide encouragement to patient.*
NURSING DIAGNOSIS **Risk for autonomic dysreflexia** *related to* reflex stimulation of sympathetic nervous system.	
▪ No occurrence of autonomic dysreflexia. ▪ Receive immediate and appropriate nursing or medical interventions if autonomic dysreflexia occurs.	▪ Assess for hypertension, bradycardia, severe headache, sweating, blurred vision, flushed feeling, nasal congestion *as signs of autonomic dysreflexia.* ▪ Reduce or eliminate noxious stimuli such as fecal impaction, urinary retention, tactile stimulation, and skin lesions by appropriate interventions *to prevent occurrence of autonomic dysreflexia.* ▪ If autonomic dysreflexia occurs, check for elevated blood pressure and administer antihypertensive medication as ordered; check for and correct possible sources of irritation such as a distended bladder or bowel; elevate head of bed immediately *to prevent a rupture of cerebral blood vessels or an increase in intracranial pressure.*

Continued

57-1 NURSING CARE PLAN PATIENT WITH A SPINAL CORD INJURY*—continued

Expected Patient Outcomes	Nursing Interventions and *Rationales*
NURSING DIAGNOSIS	**Risk for autonomic dysreflexia**—*continued*
	▪ If nursing interventions do not reverse symptoms, notify physician so immediate medical interventions can be initiated *to prevent a life-threatening situation from developing.* ▪ Teach patient and family to recognize and treat autonomic dysreflexia *to reverse occurrence and prevent occurrence of status epilepticus, stroke, and possible death.*
NURSING DIAGNOSIS	**Altered nutrition: less than body requirements** *related to* increased metabolic demand and inability to eat independently *as manifested by* weight loss >5.5 lb (2.5 kg) of admission weight and decreased serum albumin or protein.
▪ Weight loss <10 lb (4.5 kg). ▪ Normal values for serum protein and albumin.	▪ Assess nutritional status on admission *to provide baseline data.* ▪ Ensure enteral feedings given as ordered during acute phase *so nutrient intake is not interrupted.* ▪ When patient is eating, encourage high-protein, high-carbohydrate, high-calorie diet with high bulk *to counteract the severe catabolism that occurs with spinal cord injury and to promote bowel function.* ▪ Keep a caloric count and weigh patient at least weekly *to evaluate nutritional plan and continue or revise as necessary.*
NURSING DIAGNOSIS	**Sexual dysfunction** *related to* inability to achieve erection or perceive pelvic sensations and lack of knowledge of alternate means of achieving sexual satisfaction *as manifested by* verbalization of problems in sexual dysfunction.
▪ Expression of satisfaction with sexual activities. ▪ Knowledgeable about variety of ways to achieve sexual expression.	▪ Establish an honest, caring relationship with patient and sexual partner *to encourage open discussion of sexual concerns.* ▪ Provide accurate information about effects of spinal cord injury on sexual functioning; encourage questions; suggest alternate methods and use of assistive devices to achieve sexual satisfaction *to provide important information to patient.* ▪ Discuss reflexogenic erection with men and vaginal lubrication techniques with women *as means of enhancing sexual satisfaction.* ▪ Refer for sexual counseling if indicated.
NURSING DIAGNOSIS	**Risk for injury** *related to* sensory deficit and lack of self-protective abilities.
▪ No injuries.	▪ Assess environment for potentially injurious situations *to plan appropriate adjustments.* ▪ Use side rails; pad side rails; turn and transfer patient carefully with adequate assistance *as means of preventing patient injury.* ▪ Teach patient to anticipate possible injurious events *to develop a prevention mentality.*
NURSING DIAGNOSIS	**Altered family processes** *related to* change in function of ill family member *as manifested by* poor communication patterns among family members, use of ineffective coping techniques (e.g., shouting, blaming, isolation), inability of family members to meet physical needs of family member.
▪ Family will maximize individual and collective strengths and meet patient's needs.	▪ Assess family dynamics related to roles and responsibilities *to determine problematic areas and strengths.* ▪ Encourage open communication among family members regarding long-term planning to meet patient's needs, including financial aspects *so ideas and concerns of all involved family members are considered.* ▪ Assist family members to understand patient's feelings *to strengthen patient's feeling of worth and support.* ▪ Assist family members to develop an action plan to meet patient's needs *to reduce sense of frustration and helplessness.* ▪ Coordinate an organized team approach *to help the patient and family cope with the complex changes.*

Continued

57-1 NURSING CARE PLAN PATIENT WITH A SPINAL CORD INJURY*—continued

Expected Patient Outcomes	Nursing Interventions and *Rationales*
NURSING DIAGNOSIS **Risk for ineffective individual coping** *related to* loss of control over bodily functions and altered lifestyle secondary to paralysis.	
▪ Verbalization of ability to cope with effects of spinal cord injury.	▪ Assess for prolonged use of inappropriate defense mechanisms, inability to accept permanence of prognosis, refusal to use available support services *to determine presence of risk factors for ineffective coping.* ▪ Offer support and acceptance of feelings; assist patient with problem solving *to bolster patient's confidence in ability to cope.* ▪ Encourage use of support systems *to discuss concerns.* ▪ Provide information *as knowledge of expectations can help patient cope with the future.* ▪ Teach patient healthy coping behaviors such as relaxation techniques to *prevent patient from practicing ineffective behaviors such as smoking, drinking, or angry outbursts.*
NURSING DIAGNOSIS **Body image disturbance** *related to* paralysis *as manifested by* expression of anger or other negative feelings, refusal to discuss changes in function, participate in social contacts, or look at body.	
▪ Expression of feelings about self. ▪ Work through feelings to adaptation.	▪ Encourage discussion of feelings *to aid patient in venting and clarifying feelings.* ▪ Allow patient to grieve *as spinal cord injury results in a real loss, which requires adjustment through grieving.* ▪ Encourage social interaction *to foster sense of returning normalcy to life.* ▪ Assist family members in supporting patient *to enhance patient's sense of worth and value as a person.* ▪ Make referral for counseling as needed.

*This care plan is suitable for a patient with a high cervical injury caused by flexion-rotation. It can be modified for patients with less severe problems.

■ Planning

The overall goals are that the patient with a spinal cord injury will (1) maintain optimal level of neurologic functioning, (2) have minimal or no complications of immobility, and (3) return to home and the community at an optimal level of functioning.

■ Nursing Implementation

Health Promotion. Nursing interventions include identification of risk populations, counseling, and education. Support of local legislation related to seat belt use in cars, helmets for motorcyclists and bicyclists, child-safety seats, and tougher penalties for drunk-driving offenses is a professional responsibility. A coordinated community program for the training of emergency personnel is essential.

Acute Intervention. High cervical injury caused by flexion-rotation is the most complex spinal cord injury and is discussed in this section. Interventions for this type of injury can be modified for patients with less severe problems.

Immobilization. Proper immobilization of the neck involves the maintenance of a neutral or extension position. Sandbags, hard cervical collars, and backboards can be used to stabilize the neck to prevent lateral rotation of the cervical spine. The body should always be correctly aligned and turning should be performed so that the patient is moved as a unit (e.g., log-rolling) to prevent movement of the spine. For cervical injuries, skeletal traction is usually provided by Crutchfield (Fig. 57-8), Vinke (Fig. 57-9), Gardner-Wells tongs, or other types of skull tongs. Traction is provided by a rope that is extended from the center of the tongs over a pulley and has weights attached at the end. Traction must be maintained at all times. One disadvantage of skull tongs is that the skull pins can be displaced. If this occurs,

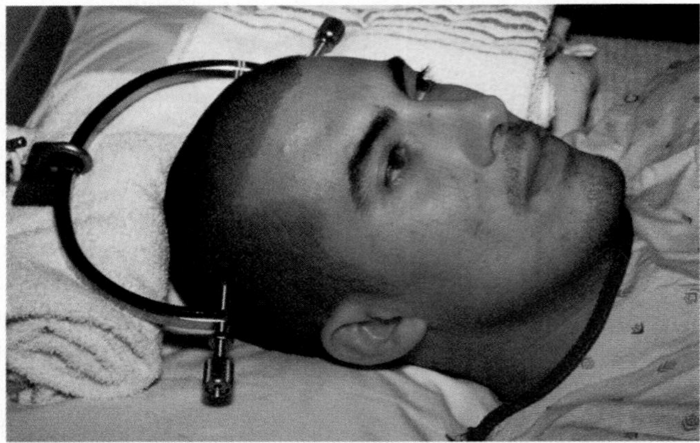

Fig. 57-8 Cervical traction is attached to tongs inserted in the skull.

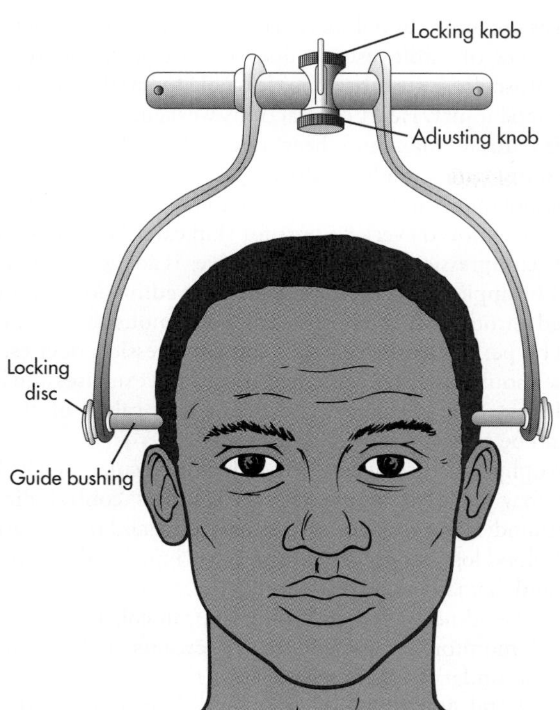

Fig. 57-9 Vinke tongs for cervical immobilization.

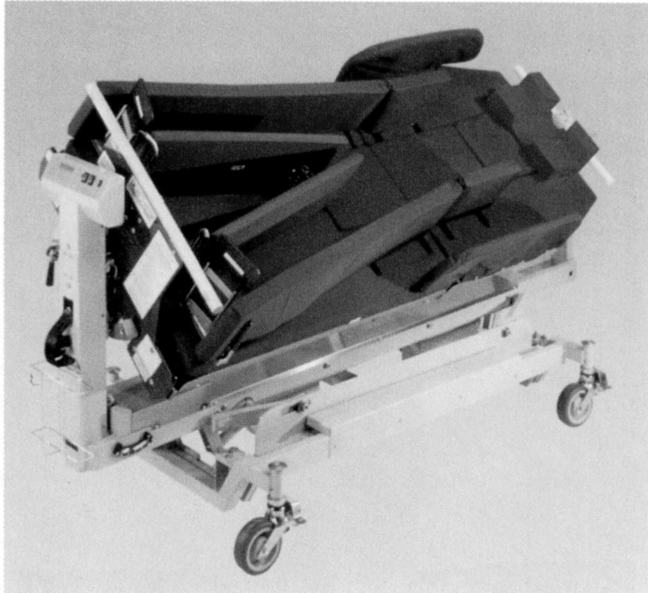

Fig. 57-10 Kinetic therapy treatment table.

the head should be held in a neutral or extended position and help should be summoned. Sandbags can be positioned to stabilize the head while the physician reinserts the tongs.

Infection at the sites of tong insertion is another potential problem. Preventive care includes cleansing the sites twice a day with normal saline solution and applying an antibiotic ointment, which acts as a mechanical barrier to the entrance of bacteria. The preventive care of insertion sites may vary depending on individual hospital standards of care.

Special frames and beds are often used in the management of the patient with a spinal cord injury. Equipment includes the Stryker frame and the Roto Rest® Delta bed (Fig. 57-10). The Stryker frame was developed in 1939 and was the first bed that afforded some benefits of mobilization. The Stryker frame bed uses a side-to-side lateral turn. The Roto Rest® Delta bed provides kinetic therapy using a continual side-to-side slow rotation 62 degrees laterally with the patient in constant motion. The bed allows a frequency of turns greater than 200 times per day. The bed is used to decrease the likelihood of pressure sores and cardiopulmonary complications. However, in some patients the turning can induce motion sickness and fear of falling out of bed when turned to the extremes. (Motion sickness is unlikely when automatic rather than manual turning is used.)

Depending on the type of injury and therapeutic interventions, the tongs and traction may be removed 2 to 4 weeks after injury. In a stable injury, halo traction may be applied. The removal of traction and application of a collar or halo traction device allows the patient to be more mobile and to begin active rehabilitation. The halo apparatus applies cervical traction by means of a jacket-like arrangement that allows greater mobility and wheelchair activity than other traction systems (Fig. 57-11).

Immobilization of the neck of the patient with a spinal cord injury prevents further injury, but the effects of immobility are profound. Meticulous skin care is critical because decreased sensation and circulation make the patient particularly susceptible to skin breakdown. Patients should be removed from backboards as soon as possible and cervical collars properly fitted or replaced with other forms of immobilization to prevent coccygeal and occipital area skin breakdown. It is important that areas under the halo vest or jacket be inspected to assess skin condition.

Respiratory dysfunction. During the first 48 hours after injury, edema may increase the level of dysfunction and respiratory distress may occur. If the patient is exhausted from labored breathing or ABGs deteriorate (indicating inadequate oxygenation), endotracheal intubation or tracheostomy and mechanical ventilation should be initiated. Respiratory arrest is a possibility that requires careful monitoring of the respiratory system and prompt action should it occur. Pneumonia and atelectasis are potential problems because of reduced vital capacity and the loss of intercostal and abdominal muscle function, resulting in diaphragmatic breathing, pooled secretions, and an ineffective cough. The older adult has a more difficult time responding to hypoxia and hypercapnia and is extremely intolerant of hypoxia caused by lack of reserve. Therefore aggressive chest physiotherapy, adequate oxygenation, and proper pain management are essential to maximize respiratory function and gas exchange.[19] Other problems include nasal stuffiness and bronchospasms.

The nurse regularly assesses (1) breath sounds, (2) ABGs, (3) tidal volume, (4) vital capacity, (5) skin color, (6) breathing patterns (especially the use of accessory muscles), (7) subjective comments about the ability to breathe, and (8) the amount and color of sputum. A PaO_2 (partial pressure of oxygen in arterial blood) above 60 mm Hg and a $PaCO_2$ (partial pressure of

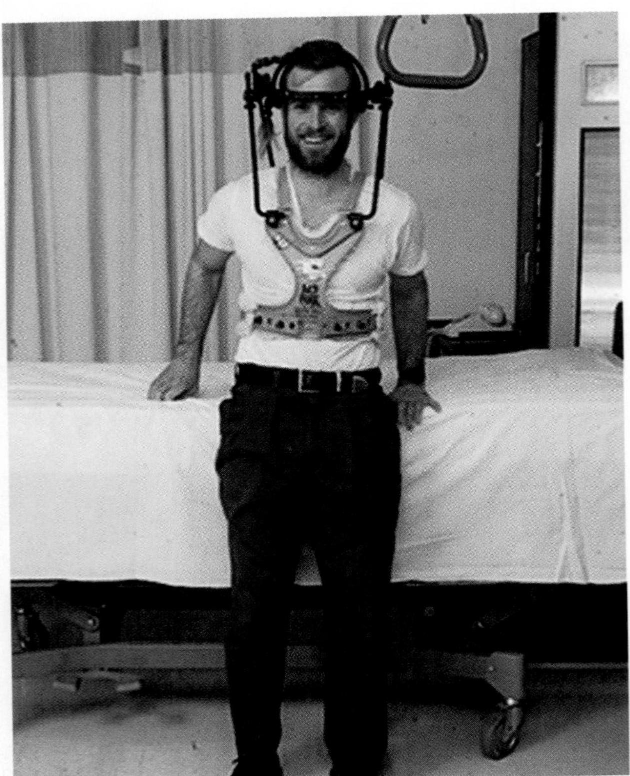

Fig. 57-11 Halo vest, Ace manufacturing design. Note the rigid shoulder straps and encompassing vest. Various vest sizes are available prefabricated. The halo ring, superstructure, and vest are magnetic resonance imaging (MRI)–compatible.

carbon dioxide in arterial blood) below 45 mm Hg are acceptable values in a patient with uncomplicated quadriplegia. The nurse should note the effect of the prone position because it can significantly reduce vital capacity and result in respiratory arrest. A patient who is unable to count to 10 out loud without taking a breath needs immediate attention.

In addition to monitoring activities, the nurse can intervene in maintaining ventilation. Oxygen is administered until ABGs stabilize. Chest physiotherapy and quad-assist coughing facilitate the raising of secretions. Quad-assist coughing stimulates the action of the ineffective abdominal muscles during the expiratory phase of a cough. The nurse places a fist or the heel of a hand between the umbilicus and xiphoid process and exerts firm pressure to the area (see Fig. 62-6). Tracheal suctioning should be performed if crackles or rhonchi are present. Incentive spirometry is an additional technique to improve the patient's respiratory status.

Cardiovascular instability. Because of unopposed vagal response, the heart rate is slowed, often to below 60 beats per minute. Any increase in vagal stimulation such as turning or suctioning can result in cardiac arrest. Loss of sympathetic tone in peripheral vessels results in chronic low blood pressure with potential postural hypotension. Lack of muscle tone to aid venous return can result in sluggish blood flow and predispose the patient to DVT.

Vital signs should be assessed frequently. If bradycardia is symptomatic, an anticholinergic medication such as atropine is administered. A temporary pacemaker may be inserted in some instances. Hypotension is managed with a vasopressor agent such as dopamine and fluid replacement. In the older adult, the prevalence of cardiovascular disease must be considered. The cardiovascular system becomes less able to handle the stress of traumatic injury. Heart contractions weaken, and cardiac output is reduced. Maximum heart rate is also reduced.[19]

Compression gradient stockings can be used to prevent thromboemboli and to promote venous return. The stockings must be removed every 8 hours for skin care. The use of pneumatic compression devices for the calves is advocated, and they must be applied as soon as possible after admission and maintained throughout the hospitalization. Venous duplex studies may be performed before applying compression devices. The nurse should also perform range-of-motion exercises and heel-cord stretching regularly. The thighs and calves of the legs should be assessed every shift for signs of DVT.

Prophylactic use of heparin or low molecular weight heparin may be used to prevent DVT unless contraindicated. Contraindications include internal bleeding and recent surgery.

If blood loss has occurred from other injuries, the hemoglobin and hematocrit levels should be monitored and blood should be administered according to protocol. The nurse also should monitor the patient for indications of hypovolemic shock secondary to hemorrhage.

Fluid and nutritional maintenance. During the first 48 to 72 hours after the injury the GI tract may stop functioning (paralytic ileus) and a nasogastric tube must be inserted. Because the patient cannot have oral intake, fluid and electrolyte needs must be carefully monitored. Specific solutions and additives are ordered based on individual requirements. Once bowel sounds are present or flatus is passed, oral food and fluids can gradually be introduced. Because of severe catabolism, a high-protein, high-calorie diet is necessary for energy and tissue repair. In patients with high cervical cord injuries, swallowing must be evaluated before starting oral feedings. If the patient is unable to resume eating, total parenteral nutrition may be started to provide nutritional support.

Increased roughage should be included to promote bowel function. Some patients experience anorexia, which can be due to psychologic depression, boredom with institutional food, or discomfort at being fed (often by a hurried nurse). Some patients have a normally small appetite. Occasionally, refusal to eat is used as a means of maintaining control over the environment because of diminished or absent body control. If the patient is not eating adequately, the cause should be thoroughly assessed. On the basis of this assessment, a contract may be made with the patient using mutual goal setting regarding the diet. This gives the patient increased control of the situation and often results in improved nutritional intake. General measures such as providing a pleasant eating environment, allowing adequate time to eat (including any self-feeding the patient can achieve), encouraging the family to bring in special foods, and planning social rewards for eating may be useful. A calorie count should be kept and the patient's daily weight recorded as a means of evaluating progress. If feasible, the patient should participate in recording calorie intake. The nurse should avoid allowing the patient's nutritional intake to become a basis for a power struggle.

Bowel and bladder management. Urine is retained because of the loss of autonomic and reflex control of the bladder and sphincter. Because there is no sensation of fullness, overdistention of the bladder can result in reflux into the kidney with eventual renal failure. Bladder overdistention may even result

RESEARCH
IMPLICATIONS FOR NURSING PRACTICE

Bowel Function Following Spinal Cord Injury

Citation Kirk PM and others: Long-term follow-up of bowel management after spinal cord injury, *SCI Nursing* 14:56, 1997.

Purpose To describe bowel management programs, the prevalence of GI complaints, the impact of neurogenic bowel on life activities, and satisfaction with bowel management in patients with spinal cord injury.

Methods A telephone survey was used to ask 171 adults with spinal cord injury a series of questions related to bowel program, bowel function, and satisfaction. The mean duration of spinal cord injury for the participants was 8.9 years and their mean age was approximately 39 years.

Results and Conclusions In this sample, the most commonly reported bowel program was chemical rectal stimulation using laxatives. The average dietary fiber intake was 6.8 g per day. During the past year 90% of sample complained of GI problems such as constipation. Overall satisfaction with their bowel program was high.

Implications for Nursing Practice Constipation remains a problem for spinal cord injury patients long after the acute phase. In the patient with a spinal cord injury, constipation is related to a number of factors related to diet, mobility, and sensory and motor changes. Patients with spinal cord injury and their families need instructions related to diet (e.g., increase fiber), fluid intake, and other options (stool softeners, chemical laxatives) to enhance bowel function.

in rupture of the bladder. Consequently, an indwelling catheter is usually inserted as soon as possible after injury. Its patency must be ensured by frequent inspection and irrigation if warranted. In some institutions a physician's order is required for this procedure. Strict aseptic technique for catheter care is essential to avoid introducing infection. After the patient is stabilized, the best means of managing long-term urinary function is assessed. Usually the patient is started on an intermittent catheterization program. The patient is often maintained on a fluid restriction of 1800 to 2000 ml per day to facilitate a bladder training program. Urinary output is monitored closely.

UTIs are a common problem. A large fluid intake and the liberal use of juices such as cranberry, grape, and apple are used to prevent infections. When used in large quantities, these juices leave an acid ash in the urine, which discourages bacterial growth. Citrus juices are used sparingly. Ascorbic acid and a urinary antiseptic such as methenamine mandelate (Mandelamine) are sometimes given. The pH of the urine should be tested daily to evaluate acidity. If the appearance or odor of the urine is suspicious, a specimen is sent for culture. Age-related changes in renal function should be considered. The older adult is more likely to develop renal calculi and older men may have prostatic hyperplasia, which may interfere with urinary flow and complicate urinary management.[19]

Constipation is generally a problem during spinal shock because no voluntary or involuntary evacuation of the bowels occurs. Suppositories are used in combination with a laxative to assist in bowel evacuation. Enemas are used only if absolutely necessary because they can overdistend the rectum and create problems for initiating an effective bowel program.

Temperature control. Because there is no vasoconstriction, piloerection, or heat loss through perspiration below the level of injury, temperature control is largely external to the patient. Therefore the nurse needs to monitor the environment closely to maintain an appropriate temperature. Body temperature needs to be monitored regularly. The patient should not be overloaded with covers or unduly exposed (such as during bathing). If an infection develops, more extensive means of temperature control, such as a cooling blanket, may be necessary.

Stress ulcers. Stress ulcers are a problem for the patient with a spinal cord injury because of the physiologic response to severe trauma, psychologic stress, and high-dose corticosteroids. Peak incidence of stress ulcers is 6 to 14 days after injury. Stool and gastric contents are tested daily for blood, and the hematocrit is observed for a slow drop. When corticosteroids are given, they should be accompanied by antacids or food. Histamine H_2-receptor blockers, such as ranitidine (Zantac) and famotidine (Pepcid), may be given prophylactically to decrease the secretion of hydrochloric acid. Upper GI bleeding may also predispose to aspiration pneumonia.

Sensory deprivation. The nurse must compensate for the patient's absent sensations to prevent sensory deprivation. This is done by stimulating the patient above the level of injury. Conversation, music, strong aromas, and interesting flavors should be a part of the nursing care plan. Prism glasses are provided so that the patient can read and watch television. Every effort should be made to prevent the patient from withdrawing from the environment.

Patients with spinal cord injury often report altered sensorium and vivid dreams during the acute phase of their treatment. Whether this is due to drugs used to manage pain and anxiety is not known. Patients may also experience disrupted sleep patterns as a result of the hospital environment or posttraumatic stress disorder.

Reflexes. Once spinal cord shock is resolved, the return of reflexes may complicate rehabilitation. Lacking control from the higher brain centers, reflexes are inappropriate and often excessive. Erections can occur from a variety of stimuli, causing embarrassment and discomfort. Spasms ranging from mild twitches to convulsive movements below the level of the lesion may also occur. This reflex activity may be interpreted by the patient or family as a return of function, and the nurse must tactfully explain the reason for the activity. The patient may be informed of the positive use of these reflexes in sexual, bowel, and bladder retraining. Spasms may be relieved with the use of warm baths, whirlpool treatments, antispasmodics, and muscle relaxants. Peak spasticity occurs after 2 years, and if it is severe, destruction of the reflexes (cordotomy) may be necessary. This procedure compromises retraining and should only be done as a last resort.

Autonomic dysreflexia. *Autonomic dysreflexia* (hyperreflexia) is a massive uncompensated cardiovascular reaction mediated by the sympathetic nervous system. It occurs in response to visceral stimulation once spinal shock is resolved in patients with spinal cord lesions above T7. The condition is a

PATIENT & FAMILY HOME CARE GUIDE

Table 57-7 Autonomic Dysreflexia

Patient and family members must know the signs and symptoms of autonomic dysreflexia so that timely intervention can occur. These include the following:

- Sudden onset of acute headache
- Elevation in blood pressure and/or reduction in pulse rate
- Flushed face and upper chest (above the level of the lesion) and pale extremities (below the level of the lesion)
- Sweating above the level of the lesion
- Nasal congestion
- Feeling of apprehension

Immediate interventions include the following:

- Raise the person to a sitting position.
- Remove the stimulus (fecal impaction, kinked urinary catheter).
- Call the primary care provider if above actions do not relieve the signs and symptoms.

Efforts to decrease the likelihood of autonomic dysreflexia include the following:

- Maintain regular bowel function.
- If manual rectal stimulation is used, local anesthetics may reduce stimulation of autonomic dysreflexia.
- Monitor urine output.
- Wear a Medic-Alert bracelet indicating a history of autonomic dysreflexia.

Source: Autonomic hyperreflexia. In *Mosby's patient teaching guides,* St Louis, 1996, Mosby.

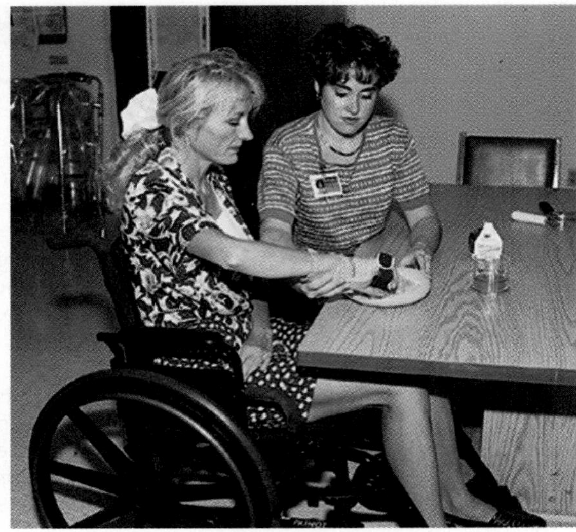

Fig. 57-12 A patient participating in occupational therapy using mobile arm supports and upper-extremity orthotics.

life-threatening situation that requires immediate resolution. If resolution does not occur, this condition can lead to status epilepticus, stroke, myocardial infarction, and even death.

The most common precipitating cause is a distended bladder or rectum, although any sensory stimulation may cause autonomic dysreflexia. Contraction of the bladder or rectum, stimulation of the skin, or stimulation of the pain receptors may also cause autonomic dysreflexia. Manifestations include hypertension (up to 300 mm Hg systolic), blurred vision, throbbing headache, marked diaphoresis above the level of the lesion, bradycardia (30 to 40 beats per minute), piloerection (erection of body hair) as a result of pilomotor spasm, nasal congestion, and nausea. It is important to measure blood pressure when a patient with a spinal cord injury complains of a headache.

The pathology of autonomic dysreflexia involves the stimulation of sensory receptors below the level of the cord lesion. The intact autonomic system below the level of the lesion responds to the stimulation with a reflex arteriolar vasoconstriction that increases blood pressure. Baroreceptors in the carotid sinus and the aorta sense the hypertension and stimulate the parasympathetic system. This results in a decrease in heart rate, but the visceral and peripheral vessels do not dilate because efferent impulses cannot pass through the cord lesion.

Nursing interventions in this serious emergency are elevation of the head of the bed 45 degrees, notification of the physician, and assessment to determine the cause. The most common cause is bladder irritation. Immediate catheterization to relieve the distention may be necessary. Catheter irrigation performed slowly and gently may open a plugged catheter, or a new catheter may be inserted. A digital rectal examination should be performed only after application of an anesthetic ointment to decrease rectal stimulation and to prevent an increase of symptoms. The nurse should remove all skin stimuli such as constrictive clothing and tight shoes. If symptoms persist after the source has been relieved, an α-adrenergic blocker or an arteriolar vasodilator may be given. Careful monitoring must continue until the vital signs stabilize.

Patient and family must be taught the causes and symptoms of autonomic dysreflexia (Table 57-7). They must understand the life-threatening nature of this dysfunction and must know how to relieve the cause.

Ambulatory and Home Care. The physiologic and psychologic rehabilitation of the person with spinal cord injury is complex and involved. With physical and psychologic care and intensive and specialized rehabilitation, the patient with a spinal cord injury learns to function at the highest level of wellness. Special rehabilitation centers are available, but patients must demonstrate adequate motivation for self-care to be admitted.

Health care providers often consider spinal cord disability to be one of the most devastating of physical disabilities. However, patients with spinal cord injury are remarkably resourceful and possess an impressive resilience. Staff members often underestimate the patient's potential for independence. Misplaced sympathy and overidentification can compromise the nurse's attempt to give the involved and complex care required by the injured person for optimal rehabilitation. Recovery is prolonged, and nurses must learn to gauge progress in inches rather than miles. Skilled, persistent care draws on every known nursing intervention until the patient achieves a maximal level of independence.

Many of the problems identified in the acute period become chronic and continue throughout life. Rehabilitation focuses on refined retraining of physiologic processes. Braces, electronic wheelchairs, and mechanical devices are used to maximize the patient's remaining function (Fig. 57-12). Patient and

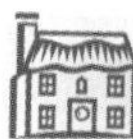

PATIENT & FAMILY HOME CARE GUIDE

Table 57-8 Halo Vest Care

The following are teaching guidelines for a patient with a halo vest:

- Inspect the pins on the halo traction ring. Report to health care provider if pins are loose or if there are signs of infection including redness, tenderness, swelling, or drainage at the insertion sites.
- Clean around pin sites carefully with hydrogen peroxide on a cotton swab. Repeat the procedure using water.
- Use alcohol swabs to cleanse pin sites of any drainage.
- Apply antibiotic ointment as prescribed.
- To provide skin care, have the patient lie down on a bed with his or her head resting on a pillow to reduce pressure on the brace. Loosen one side of the vest. Gently wash the skin under the vest with soap and water, rinse it, and then dry it thoroughly. At the same time, check the skin for pressure points, redness, swelling, bruising, or chafing. Close the open side and repeat the procedure on the opposite side.
- If the vest becomes wet or damp it can be carefully dried with a blow dryer.
- An assistive device (e.g., cane or walker) may be used to provide greater balance. Flat shoes should be worn.
- Turn the entire body, not just the head and neck, when trying to view sideways.
- In case of an emergency, keep a set of wrenches close to the halo vest at all times.
- Mark the vest strap such that consistent buckling and fit can be maintained.

Source: Halo vest care at home. In *Mosby's patient teaching guides,* St Louis, 1996, Mosby.

PATIENT & FAMILY HOME CARE GUIDE

Table 57-9 Skin Care for Patients with Spinal Cord Injuries

Skin breakdown is a potential problem following spinal cord injury. The following measures are used to decrease this possibility:

Change Position Frequently

- If in a wheelchair, lift self up and shift weight every 15 to 30 minutes.
- If in bed, a regular turning schedule (at least every 2 hours) that includes sides, back, and abdomen is encouraged to change position.
- Use special mattresses and wheelchair cushions.
- Use pillows to protect bony prominences when in bed.

Monitor Skin Condition

- Inspect skin frequently for areas of redness, swelling, and breakdown.
- Keep fingernails trimmed to avoid scratches and abrasions.
- If a wound develops, follow standard wound care management, which includes keeping wound open to air and applying treatments as prescribed.

Source: Skin care tips following spinal cord injury. In *Mosby's patient teaching guides,* St Louis, 1996, Mosby.

family teaching related to care of the halo vest are described in Table 57-8 and home care guidelines for skin care are presented in Table 57-9.

The patient with high cervical spinal cord injury has greatly increased mobility with phrenic nerve stimulators or electronic diaphragmatic pacemakers. Diaphragmatic pacemakers may allow the patient to become independent of mechanical ventilation. Today, ventilators are also reasonably portable, and ventilator-dependent quadriplegic patients can be mobile and somewhat independent. Although rehabilitation and the special equipment required are costly, many programs are funded by the state or federal governments.

If the patient can be successfully brought through the acute period, the patient's life can be fuller and richer than previously believed possible. Like other persons who have been close to death, some patients find that their lives are richer and more meaningful than before the injury. Unfortunately, other patients may not have such a positive future outlook. The nurse has a pivotal role in the coordinated efforts of the health team to influence a positive outcome.

Neurogenic bladder. Once spinal cord shock and the resulting bladder atony are resolved, the bladder is neurogenic. A neurogenic bladder is any type of bladder dysfunction related to abnormal or absent bladder innervation. It may lead to problems with residual urine, stone formation (urolithiasis), or infection, and it is often associated with progressive renal deterioration and urinary incontinence. The network of fibers of the detrusor muscle forms the muscular wall of the bladder. The trigone is a small rectangular area near the bladder neck sometimes called the *internal sphincter.* The urogenital diaphragm or baseplate encircles the urethral opening completely and is sometimes called the *external sphincter.* Depending on the lesion, a neurogenic bladder may have no reflex detrusor contractions (*areflexic, flaccid*) or may have hyperactive reflex detrusor contractions (*hyperreflexic, spastic*). Common symptoms of a neurogenic bladder include urgency, frequency, incontinence, inability to void, and characteristics of obstruction.

Neurogenic bladder can be classified according to reflex detrusor activity, intravesical filling pressure, and continence function. Types of neurogenic bladder are outlined in Table 57-10. Diagnostic and collaborative care of neurogenic bladder are described in Table 57-11. The patient with a spinal cord injury and a neurogenic bladder requires a comprehensive program to manage bladder function. The program should include the following:

1. *Diagnostic evaluation:* After the patient's overall condition is stable with evidence of neurologic reflexes, a cystometrogram, an IV pyelogram, and a urine culture are taken.
2. *Drug therapy:* Drugs to increase the strength of bladder contractions (detrusor), acidify the urine, and relax the urethral sphincter are administered.
3. *Nutrition:* A low-calcium diet (1 g/day) is advocated to reduce the possibility of kidney and bladder stones.

Table 57-10 Types of Neurogenic Bladders

Type	Characteristics	Cause	Clinical Manifestations
▪ Uninhibited	No inhibitions influence time and place of voiding	Corticospinal tract lesion; observed in CVA, multiple sclerosis, brain tumor, brain trauma	Incontinence, increased frequency, urgency
▪ Reflex	Bladder behaves as part of spinal reflex arc with no connection to brain	Lesion of motor and sensory fibers; occasionally seen in multiple sclerosis, pernicious anemia	Incontinence, urinary frequency, lack of sensation of bladder filling
▪ Autonomous	Bladder behaves autonomously, as if it were cut off from brain and spinal cord	Lesions of cauda equina, pelvic nerves, spina bifida	Incontinence, difficulty initiating micturition
▪ Motor paralysis	Bladder acts as if there were paralysis of all motor functions	Lower motor neuron lesion caused by trauma involving S2-S4	If sensory function intact, feels bladder distention and hesitancy; no control of micturition, resulting in overdistention of bladder and overflow incontinence
▪ Sensory paralysis	Bladder acts as if there were paralysis of all sensory modalities	Damage to sensory limb of bladder spinal reflex arc; seen in multiple sclerosis, diabetes mellitus, pernicious anemia	Poor bladder sensation, infrequent voiding, large residual volume

CVA, cerebrovascular accident.

COLLABORATIVE CARE

Table 57-11 Neurogenic Bladder

Diagnostic
- Neurologic examination
- Cystometrogram
- IV pyelogram
- Urine culture

Collaborative Therapy

Drug Therapy
- Increasing detrusor muscle strength (bethanechol [Urecholine])
- Acidification of urine (ascorbic acid [vitamin C])
- Urinary antiseptics (e.g., methenamine mandelate [Mandelamine])
- Relaxation of urethral sphincter

Nutrition
- Low-calcium diet (<1 g/day)
- Fluid intake at 1800-2000 ml/day

Urine Drainage
- Reflex training
- Intermittent catheterization
- Indwelling catheter
- Urinary diversion surgery

4. *Fluids:* A fluid intake of 1800 to 2000 ml per day must be maintained to prevent stone formation and to ensure adequate urine flow.
5. *Urine drainage:* The method used for urinary drainage depends on the condition of the patient; the preference of the physician, nursing staff, and patient; and the policy of the institution. Numerous drainage methods are possible, including reflex training, indwelling catheter, intermittent catheterization, and urinary diversion surgery.

Many factors are considered when selecting a bladder management strategy. These include upper extremity function, caregiver burden, and lifestyle choices.

With the return of the reflex arc, bladder function may be a reflex. However, because of the interruption in the pathways to the brain, the patient has no control over urination, which results in a bladder with a small capacity, hyperirritable detrusor muscle and sphincter, and loss of inhibition of the reflex by the brain. The patient or the nurse can use techniques such as the Credé and Valsalva maneuvers or a rectal stretch to facilitate complete emptying of the bladder. The Credé maneuver involves the exertion by the nurse or patient of downward pressure over the bladder with a pumping motion. This maneuver is only used in those patients with a lower motor neuron pattern bladder and may require a physician's order in some settings because it has the potential of stimulating autonomic dysreflexia in the patient with upper motor neuron disease. In the Valsalva maneuver, the patient inhales deeply, holds his or her breath, and bears down. The rectal stretch is the insertion of a gloved finger into the rectum, gently pulling to exert pressure on the sphincter to cause relaxation of the perineal floor. Combining the Valsalva maneuver with rectal stretch results in more complete emptying of the bladder. The patient should be regularly assessed for residual urine after reflex bladder emptying. It may take up to 3 to 5 days before residual urine is less than 100 ml. Many drugs affect urinary retention and thus should be assessed for their effects on residual volume. The ultimate goal for this technique is for the patient to not need a catheter.

The long-term use of an indwelling catheter should be carefully evaluated because of the associated high incidence of UTI, fistula formation, and diverticula. Adequate fluid intake and patency of the catheter should be ensured. The frequency of catheter changing ranges from 1 week to 1 month, depending on the type of catheter used and agency policy.

Intermittent catheterization is the recommended method of bladder management (see Chapter 43). Nursing assessment is important in selecting the time interval between catheterizations. Initially, catheterization is done every 4 hours. If less than 200 ml of urine is drained, the time interval may be extended. If 500 ml or more of urine is obtained, the time interval is shortened. An overdistended bladder can cause ischemia, which may predispose tissues to bacterial invasion and infection. Patients often experience diuresis at a regular time during a 24-hour period, which may necessitate an extra catheterization. The number of intermittent catheterizations per day is usually five or six.

Urinary diversion surgery may be necessary if the patient has repeated UTIs with renal involvement or repeated stones or if therapeutic intervention has been unsuccessful (see Table 43-19). Surgical treatment of neurogenic bladder includes bladder neck revision (sphincterotomy), bladder augmentation (augmentation cystoplasty), penile prosthesis, artificial sphincter, perineal ureterostomy, cystotomy, vesicotomy, and anterior urethral transplantation.

Bowel evacuation. Bowel evacuation needs careful management in the patient with a spinal cord injury because voluntary control of this function may be lost. The usual measures for preventing constipation include a high-fiber diet and adequate fluid intake (see Table 40-11). Patient and family teaching guidelines related to bowel management are presented in Table 57-12. However, these measures by themselves may not be adequate to stimulate evacuation. In addition, suppositories or digital stimulation by the nurse or patient may be necessary. In the patient with an upper motor neuron lesion, digital stimulation is necessary to promote defecation. Small-volume enemas and agents such as docusate sodium (Colace), bisacodyl (Dulcolax), and glycerin may also be used.

Valsalva maneuver and manual stimulation are useful in patients with lower motor neuron lesions. The Valsalva maneuver requires intact abdominal muscles, so it is used in those patients with injuries below T12. In general, a bowel movement every other day is considered adequate. However, preinjury patterns should be considered. Incontinence can result from too much stool softener or a fecal impaction.

Careful recording of bowel movements, including amount, time, and consistency, is important to the overall success of the program. Timing of defecation may also be an important factor. If bowel evacuation is planned for 30 to 60 minutes following the first meal of the day, this may enhance success by taking advantage of the gastrocolic reflex induced by eating.

Sexuality. Because the majority of patients with spinal cord injuries are men between 18 and 35 years of age, sexual rehabilitation is a major issue. It is important to remember that sexuality is an important issue regardless of the patient's age. To work with these patients, the nurse must have an awareness and an acceptance of personal sexuality, as well as knowledge of human sexual responses. When discussing sexual potential, the nurse should use scientific terminology rather than slang whenever possible. Knowledge of the level of the lesion is needed to understand the patient's potential for orgasm, erection, and fertility and the patient's capacity for sexual satisfaction (Table 57-13). All patients with spinal cord injuries generally lack perineal sensation during intercourse regardless of the type of lesion.

Reflex sexual function capability is possible if the patient has an upper motor neuron lesion. The presence of tone in the external rectal sphincter indicates an upper motor lesion. The absence of external rectal sphincter tone, bulbocavernosus reflex, or both indicates that the patient has lower motor neuron involvement and may be capable of psychogenic erection but not reflex erection. If ejaculation occurs, it may be retrograde into the bladder.

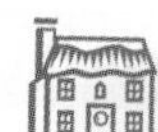

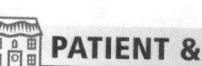

PATIENT & FAMILY HOME CARE GUIDE

Table 57-12 Bowel Management After Spinal Cord Injury

The following are teaching guidelines for a patient with a spinal cord injury:

- Optimal nutritional intake includes:
  - 3 well-balanced meals each day
  - 2 servings from the milk group
  - 2 or more servings from the meat group, including beef, pork, poultry, eggs, fish
  - 4 or more servings from the vegetable and fruit groups
  - 4 or more servings from the bread and cereal group
- Fiber intake should be approximately 20 to 30 g per day. Gradually increase amount of fiber eaten over 1 to 2 weeks.
- Three quarts of fluid per day should be consumed unless contraindicated. Water or fruit juices should be used and caffeinated beverages such as coffee, tea, and cola should be avoided. Fluid softens hard stools; caffeine stimulates fluid loss through urination.
- Foods that produce gas (e.g., beans) or upper GI upset (spicy foods) should be avoided.
- Timing: A regular schedule for bowel evacuation should be established. A good time is 30 minutes after the first meal of the day.
- Position: If possible, an upright position with feet flat on the floor or a step stool enhances bowel evacuation. Staying on the toilet, commode, or bedpan for longer than 20 to 30 minutes causes skin breakdown. Based on stability, someone may need to stay with the patient.
- Activity: Exercise is important for bowel function. In addition to improving muscle tone, it also increases GI transit time and increases appetite. Muscles should be exercised. This includes stretching, range-of-motion, and position changing.
- Drug treatment: Laxatives, including suppositories, may be necessary to stimulate a bowel movement. However, these drugs can be habit-forming and thus should only be taken when necessary. Manual stimulation of the rectum may also be helpful in initiating defecation.

Source: Bowel management at home following spinal cord injury. In *Mosby's patient teaching guides,* St Louis, 1996, Mosby.

Table **57-13** Potential for Sexual Activity in Men with Spinal Cord Injuries

Erection	Ejaculation	Orgasm
Upper Motor Neuron		
Complete		
Frequent (93%), reflexogenic only	Rare	Absent
Incomplete		
Most frequent (99%), reflexogenic (80%), reflexogenic and psychogenic (19%)	Less frequent (32%), after reflexogenic erection (74%), after psychogenic erection (26%)	Present (if ejaculation occurs)
Lower Motor Neuron		
Complete		
Infrequent (26%)	Infrequent (18%)	Present (if ejaculation occurs)
Incomplete		
Psychogenic and reflexogenic	Frequent (70%), after psychogenic and reflexogenic erections	Present (if ejaculation occurs)

The type of lesion determines the physical sexual response. Men with upper motor neuron lesions may have reflexogenic erections that are produced by reflex activity or external stimuli or that occur spontaneously. These spontaneous erections are often short lived and uncontrolled and cannot be maintained or summoned at the time of coitus. Orgasm and ejaculation are usually not possible for men with a complete upper motor neuron lesion.

Most patients with a complete lower motor neuron lesion are unable to have either psychogenic or reflexogenic erections. Patients with incomplete lower motor neuron lesions have the highest possibility of successful psychogenic erection with ejaculation, and up to 10% of these patients are fertile.

The woman of childbearing age with a spinal cord injury usually remains fertile, although orgasmic ability is lost. The injury does not affect the ability to become pregnant or to deliver normally through the birth canal.

Sexual rehabilitation for both men and women should begin informally after the acute phase of the injury has passed. Questions such as "Have you had an erection since your accident?" and "Have your menstrual periods continued since the accident?" are nonthreatening ways to introduce the topic of sexual functioning. The male patient may pose a question such as, "Can I ever be a man again?"

Open discussion with the patient is essential. This important aspect of rehabilitation should be handled by someone specially trained in sexual counseling. Unless this type of training has occurred, the nurse should not attempt to direct the plan for sexual rehabilitation.

The properly trained nurse works with the patient and partner to provide support during new relationships, with the emphasis on open communication. The nurse's educational role requires respect for every couple's personal standards of religious and cultural beliefs. Alternative methods of obtaining sexual satisfaction such as oral-genital sex (cunnilingus and fellatio) may be suggested. Explicit films (e.g., *Touching*) may also be used. This film demonstrates the sexual activities of a patient with paraplegia and a nondisabled partner. Graphics should be used cautiously because they may be too limiting or focus too much on the mechanics of sex rather than on the relationship.

Sexual activities may require more planning and be less spontaneous than before the injury. For example, an attendant may have to undress the patient and remove equipment. A relaxed atmosphere with music and perfume creates an attractive environment. Ample time for caressing, fondling, and kissing is essential. The partners should be encouraged to explore each other's erogenous areas, such as the lips, neck, and ears, which can arouse psychogenic erection or orgasm. Few demands should be made initially.

Care should be taken not to dislodge the indwelling catheter during sexual activity. If a Texas catheter is used, it should be removed before sexual activity and the patient should refrain from fluids. The bowel program should include evacuation the morning of sexual activity. The partner should be informed that an accident is always possible. The woman may need a water-soluble lubricant to supplement diminished vaginal secretions and facilitate vaginal penetration.

Menses may cease for as long as 6 months. If sexual activity is resumed, protection against an unplanned pregnancy is necessary. A normal pregnancy may be complicated by UTIs, anemia, and autonomic dysreflexia. Because uterine contractions are not felt, a precipitous delivery is always a danger. In men, fertility is reduced because of decreased number and motility of sperm and retrograde ejaculation of sperm into the bladder. For male patients desiring children, alternative methods include sperm harvesting and concentration, adoption, and artificial insemination.

Grief. Patients with spinal cord injuries are aware of the extent of injury and feel an overwhelming sense of loss. They are no longer in control and must depend on others for ADLs and for life-sustaining measures. Patients may believe that they are useless and burdens to their families. At a stage when independence is often of the greatest importance developmentally (the ages of 18 to 35 years), they are totally dependent on others.

The patient's response and recovery differ in some important aspects from those experiencing loss from amputation or terminal illness. First, regression can and does occur at different stages. Working through grief is a difficult, lifelong process with which the patient needs support and encouragement. With recent advances in rehabilitation, it is usual for the patient to be independent physically and discharged from the rehabilitation center before completion of the grief process. Another phenomenon involves that of triggering experiences, including new experiences such as marriage, that may recall earlier unresolved

Table 57-14 Mourning Process and Nursing Interventions in Spinal Cord Injury

Patient Behavior	Nursing Intervention
Shock and Denial	
Struggle for survival, complete dependence, excessive sleep, withdrawal, fantasies, unrealistic expectations	Use of meticulous nursing care. Be honest. Use simple diagrams to explain injury. Encourage patient to begin road to recovery.
Anger	
Refusal to discuss paralysis, decreased self-esteem, manipulation, hostile and abusive language	Coordinate care with patient and encourage self-care. Support family members; prevent alleviation of guilt by supporting dependency. Use humor liberally. Allow patient outbursts. Do not allow fixation on injury.
Depression	
Sadness, pessimism, anorexia, nightmares, insomnia, agitation, psychomotor retardation, "blues," suicidal preoccupation, refusal to participate in any self-care activities	Encourage family involvement and resources. Plan graded steps in rehabilitation to give success with minimal opportunity for frustration. Give cheerful and willing assistance with activities of daily living. Avoid sympathy. Use firm kindness.
Adjustment	
Planning for future, active participation in therapy, finding of personal meaning in experience and continuation of growth, return to premorbid personality	Remember that patients with spinal cord injuries have individual personalities. Balance support systems to encourage independence. Set goals with patient input. Emphasize potentials as achieved by others. Avoid use of clichés.

difficulties. Depending on the success of previous grief work, the new demand for grief work may be shortened or prolonged. The goal of recovery is related more to adjustment than to acceptance. Adjustment implies the ability to go on with living with certain limitations. Although the patient who is cooperative and accepting is easier to treat, the nurse should expect a wide fluctuation of emotions from a patient with a spinal cord injury. Depression may not be a component of the recovery process. Societal norms allow depression after severe loss and almost impose it on those confronted with death or radical lifestyle changes. However, every patient may not experience depression.

The nurse's role in grief work is to allow mourning as a component of the rehabilitation process. Table 57-14 summarizes the mourning process and appropriate nursing interventions. During the shock and denial stage the nurse reassures the patient and stresses the expertise of the entire health care team. During the anger stage, the nurse assists the patient in achievement of control over the environment, particularly by allowing the patient's input into the plan of care. The nurse should not respond to anger or manipulation or become involved in a power struggle with the patient. As self-care abilities increase, the patient's independence increases.

The patient's family also requires counseling to avoid promoting dependency in the patient through guilt or misplaced sympathy. The family is also experiencing an intense grieving process. A support group of family members and friends of patients with spinal cord injury can help increase family members' knowledge and participation in the grieving process, physical difficulties, rehabilitation plan, and the meaning of the disability in society.

During the stage of depression, the nurse must be patient, persistent, and maintain a sense of humor. Sympathy is not helpful. The patient should be treated in an adult manner and be involved in decision making about care, but the nurse must insist that the care be performed. A primary nurse relationship is helpful, but the nurse needs some relief from the intense stress of continual interaction with the patient. Staff planning and sessions in which staff members can express their feelings are helpful in providing consistency of care. To achieve the stage of adjustment, the patient needs continual support throughout the rehabilitation in the forms of acceptance, affection, and caring. The nurse must be attentive when the patient needs to talk and sensitive to needs at the various stages of the grief process.

■ Evaluation

Expected outcomes for the patient with a spinal cord injury are presented in NCP 57-1 on p. 1729.

SPINAL CORD TUMORS

Etiology and Pathophysiology

Tumors that affect the spinal cord account for 0.5% to 1% of all neoplasms. These tumors are classified as primary (arising from some component of cord, dura, nerves, or vessels) or secondary (from primary growths in the breast, thyroid, lung, kidney, and other sites). The thoracic and lumbar spine, including the sacrum, are the most commonly affected areas. Spinal cord tumors are further classified as extramedullary (outside the spinal cord), including extra- and intradural, or intramedullary (within the spinal cord) (Fig. 57-13, Table 57-15). Extramedullary tumors compose 90% of all spinal cord tumors. Neurofibromas, meningiomas, gliomas, and hemangiomas are the most frequently occurring neoplasms.

Because many of these tumors are slow growing, their symptoms stem from the mechanical effects of slow compression and irritation of nerve roots, displacement of the cord, or gradual obstruction of the vascular supply. The slowness of growth does not cause autodestruction as in traumatic lesions. Therefore complete functional restoration is possible when the tumor is removed, except with the intradural-intramedullary tumors.

Most metastatic tumors are extradural lesions.[24] Tumors that commonly metastasize to the spinal epidural space are those that spread to bone, such as carcinomas of the breast, lung, prostate, and kidney.

Clinical Manifestations

The most common early symptom of a spinal cord tumor outside the cord is pain in the back with radicular pain simulating intercostal neuralgia, angina, or herpes zoster. The location of the pain depends on the level of compression. The pain worsens with activity, coughing, straining, and lying down. Sensory disruption is later manifested by coldness, numbness, and tingling in an extremity or in several extremities, slowly progressing upward until it reaches the level of the lesion. Impaired sensation of pain, temperature, and light touch precedes a deficit in vibration and position sense that may progress to complete anesthesia. Motor weakness accompanies the sensory disturbances and consists of slowly increasing clumsiness, weakness, and spasticity. The sensory and motor disturbances are ipsilateral to the lesion. Bladder disturbances are marked by urgency with difficulty in starting the flow and progressing to retention with overflow incontinence.

Manifestations of intradural spinal tumor develop as progressive damage to the long spinal tracts, producing paralysis, sensory loss, and bladder dysfunction. Pain can be severe as a result of compression of spinal roots or vertebrae.

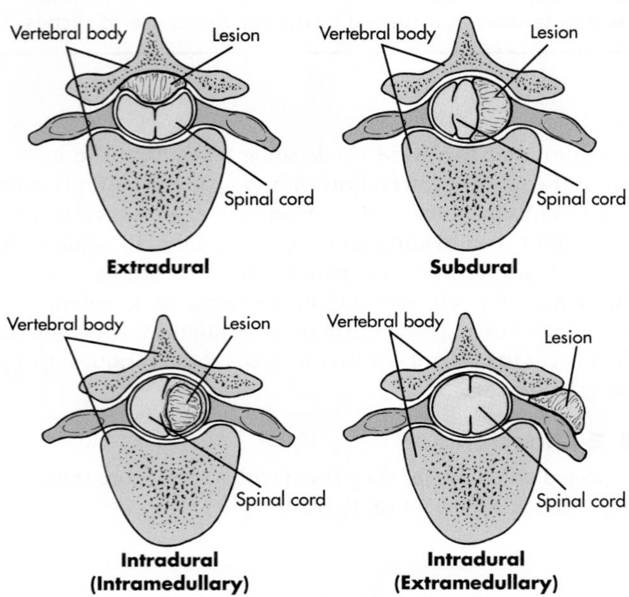

Fig. 57-13 Types of spinal cord tumors.

NURSING AND COLLABORATIVE MANAGEMENT: SPINAL CORD TUMORS

Extradural tumors are seen early on routine spinal x-rays, whereas intradural and intramedullary tumors require MRI or CT scans for detection. CSF analysis may reveal tumor cells. The cord is decompressed after removal of the tumor by a laminectomy. More than 85% of primary neoplasms are benign and can be completely resected; 90% of patients recover without residual problems.

Compression of the spinal cord is an emergency. Relief of the ischemia related to the compression is the goal of therapy. Corticosteroids are generally prescribed immediately to relieve tumor-related edema. Dexamethasone (Decadron) is usually used, often in large doses.

Treatment for nearly all spinal cord tumors is surgical removal. The exception is the metastatic tumor that is sensitive to radiation and that has caused only minimal neurologic deficits in the patient.[24] In general, tumors of the extradural or intradural-extramedullary group can be completely removed surgically. Intramedullary tumors offer a less favorable prognosis; however, exploration and removal is usually attempted.

Radiation therapy after the operation is fairly effective. Maximum permissible tissue dose is given over 6 to 8 weeks. Chemotherapy has also been used in conjunction with radiation therapy.

Relief of pain and return of function are the ultimate goals of treatment. Nurses must be aware of the neurologic status of the patient before and after treatment. Ensuring that the patient receives pain medication as needed is an important nursing responsibility. Depending on the amount of neurologic dysfunction exhibited, the patient may need to be cared for as though recovering from a spinal cord injury.

Table 57-15 Classification of Spinal Cord Tumors

Type	Incidence	Treatment	Prognosis
Extradural			
From bones of spine, in extradural space, or in paraspinal tissue	20-50% of all intraspinal tumors, mostly malignant metastatic lesions	Relief of cord pressure by surgical laminectomy, radiation, chemotherapy, or combination approach	Poor
Intradural Extramedullary			
Within dura mater outside cord	Most frequent of intradural tumors (40%), mostly benign meningiomas and neurofibromas	Complete surgical removal of tumor (if possible), partial removal followed by radiation	Usually very good if lack of damage to cord from compression
Intradural Intramedullary	Least frequent of intradural tumors (5-10%)	Partial surgical removal, radiation therapy (resulting in only temporary improvement)	Very poor

CRITICAL THINKING EXERCISES

CASE STUDY

Spinal Cord Injury

Patient Profile

Samuel D., a 25-year-old-male, is admitted to the emergency department with the diagnosis of a cervical spinal cord injury. Samuel was swimming at a neighbor's backyard pool. He dove into the shallow end, striking his head on the bottom of the pool. His friends noticed that he did not resurface and they brought him to the side of the pool. They maintained neck immobilization until the rescue crews arrived.

Subjective Data

- Is awake and alert
- Has complaints of neck pain
- Is anxious and asking why he cannot move his legs
- Is asking to see his family

Objective Data

Physical Examination

- Weak biceps movement
- No triceps movement
- Gross elbow movement present
- Decreased sensation from the shoulders down
- No bladder or bowel control
- BP 90/56; pulse 56; respirations 32 and labored

Diagnostic Studies

- X-rays revealed C5 fracture dislocation

Collaborative Care

- Placed in tongs and traction in the emergency department
- Started on methylprednisolone in the emergency department
- Admitted to intensive care unit

Critical Thinking Questions

1. What nursing activities would be a priority on Samuel D.'s arrival in the intensive care unit?
2. What physiologic problems are causing Samuel D. to have hypotension and bradycardia?
3. What would the first line of treatment be for Samuel D.'s hypotension and bradycardia?
4. What signs and symptoms would indicate respiratory distress and what physiologic problem would cause respiratory distress in Samuel D.'s injury state?
5. What can the nurse do to decrease Samuel D.'s anxiety?
6. Based on the assessment data provided, write one or more nursing diagnoses. Are there any collaborative problems?

NURSING RESEARCH ISSUES

1. What is the best method of education in the prevention of spinal cord injuries?
2. What is the best method to prevent skin breakdown?
3. What type of support or education is best for the families of patients with spinal cord injuries to help them cope with their situation?
4. What nursing interventions enhance self-care in the patient with a spinal cord injury?
5. What is the best method of preventing UTIs in the spinal cord injured patient?
6. Examine the relationship between the functional ability of spinal cord injury and quality of life.

REVIEW QUESTIONS

The number of the question corresponds to the same-numbered objective at the beginning of the chapter.

1. During assessment of the patient with trigeminal neuralgia the nurse should
   a. inspect all aspects of the mouth and teeth.
   b. lightly palpate the affected side of the face for edema.
   c. ask the patient to describe factors that initiate an episode.
   d. test for temperature and sensation perception on the face.
2. During routine assessment of a patient with Guillain-Barré syndrome the nurse finds the patient to be short of breath. The patient's respiratory distress is caused by
   a. immobility resulting from ascending paralysis.
   b. elevated protein levels in the CSF.
   c. degeneration of motor neurons in the brainstem and spinal cord.
   d. paralysis ascending to the nerves that stimulate the thoracic area.
3. The person most likely to sustain a spinal cord injury is a
   a. 35-year-old male tennis player.
   b. 75-year-old male with heart disease.
   c. 19-year-old male who rides a motorcycle.
   d. 60-year-old female with multiple sclerosis.
4. A patient is admitted to the ICU with a C7 spinal cord injury and diagnosed with Brown-Séquard syndrome. On physical examination the nurse would most likely find
   a. upper extremity weakness only.
   b. complete motor and sensory loss below C7.
   c. ipsilateral motor loss and contralateral sensory loss below C7.
   d. loss of position sense and vibration in both lower extremities.
5. A patient is admitted to the hospital with a spinal cord injury following an automobile accident. The nurse recognizes that the pathophysiology of indirect spinal cord trauma involves
   a. initial infarction of the white matter of the cord.
   b. mechanical transection of the cord by the trauma.
   c. necrotic destruction of the cord from hemorrhage and edema.
   d. release of epinephrine leading to massive vasodilation of spinal cord vessels.

6. A rehabilitation goal for the patient with an injury at the C5 level includes
   a. feeding self with hand devices.
   b. driving an electric wheelchair.
   c. assisting with transfer activities.
   d. controlling bowel and bladder functions.
7. A patient with a C7 spinal cord injury undergoing rehabilitation tells the nurse he must have the flu because he has a bad headache and nausea. The initial action of the nurse is to
   a. call the physician.
   b. check the patient's temperature.
   c. take the patient's blood pressure.
   d. palpate the patient's bladder for distention.
8. The most common early symptom of a spinal cord tumor is
   a. urinary incontinence.
   b. back pain that worsens with activity.
   c. paralysis below the level of involvement.
   d. impaired sensation of pain, temperature, and light touch.

References

1. DeMarco JK, Hesselink JR: Trigeminal neuropathy, *Neurosurg Clin N Am* 8:1, 1997.
2. Brown JA: The trigeminal complex, *Neurosurg Clin N Am* 8:1, 1997.
3. Lange DJ, Trojaburg W, Roland LP: Peripheral and cranial nerve lesion. In Rowland LP, editor: *Merritt's textbook of neurology,* ed 9, Baltimore, 1995, Williams & Wilkins.
4. MacFarlane BV and others: Chronic neuropathic pain and its control by drugs, *Pharmacol Ther* 75:1, 1997.
5. McConoghy DJ: Trigeminal neuralgia: a personal review and nursing implications, *J Neurosci Nurs* 26:85, 1994.
6. Lovely TJ, Jannetta PJ: Microvascular decompression for trigeminal neuralgia, *Neurosurg Clin N Am* 8:1, 1997.
7. Jho HD, Lunsford LD: Percutaneous retrogasserian glycerol rhizotomy, current techniques and results, *Neurosurg Clin N Am* 8:1, 1997.
8. Kondziolka D and others: Gamma knife radiosurgery for trigeminal neuralgia, *Neurosurg Clin N Am* 8:1, 1997.
9. Hashisaki GT: Medical management of Bell's palsy, *Compr Ther* 23:715, 1997.
10. Billue JS: Bell's palsy: an update on idiopathic facial paralysis, *Nurse Pract* 22:88, 1997.
11. Adams RD, Victor M, Ropper AH, editors: *Principles of neurology,* ed 6, New York, 1997, McGraw-Hill.
12. Koski CL: Guillian-Barré syndrome and chronic inflammatory demyelinating polyneuropathy: pathogenesis and treatment, *Semin Neurol* 14:123, 1994.
13. Lange DJ, Latov N, Trojabor W: Acquired neuropathies. In Rowland LP, editor: *Merritt's textbook of neurology,* ed 9, Baltimore, 1995, Williams & Wilkins.
14. Hui YH and others, editors: *Foodborne disease handbook,* New York, 1994, Marcel Dekker.
15. Miller JR: Bacterial toxins. In Rowland LP, editor: *Merritt's textbook of neurology,* ed 9, Baltimore, 1995, Williams & Wilkins.
16. Dworkin R, Leggett J: Gram positive bacillary infections and clostridial infections. In Stein JH, editor: *Internal medicine,* ed 5, St Louis, 1998, Mosby.
17. Marotta JT: Spinal injury. In Rowland LP, editor: *Merritt's textbook of neurology,* ed 9, Baltimore, 1995, Williams & Wilkins.
18. Wirtz KM, LaFavor KM, Ang R: Managing chronic spinal cord injury: issues in critical care, *Crit Care Nurse* 16:4, 1996.
19. Stamatos CA and others: Meeting the challenge of the older trauma patient, *AJN* 96:5, 1996.
20. Heary RF and others: Steroids and gun shot wounds to the spine, *Neurosurgery* 41:3, 1997.
21. Hickey JV: *The clinical practice of neurological and neurosurgical nursing,* ed 4, Philadelphia, 1997, Lippincott.
22. Segator M, Way C: Neuroprotection after spinal cord injury: state of the science, *Sci Nursing* 14:8, 1997.
23. Rhoney DH and others: New pharmacological approaches to acute spinal cord injuries, *Pharmacotherapy* 16:3, 1996.
24. McCormick PC, Fetell MR: Spinal tumors. In Rowland LP, editor: *Merritt's textbook of neurology,* ed 9, Baltimore, 1995, Williams & Wilkins.

Resources

American Association for Rehabilitation Therapy (AART)
PO Box 6412
Gulfport, MS 39506

American Association of Spinal Cord Injury Nurses (AASCIN)
75-20 Astoria Boulevard
Jackson Heights, NY 11370-1177
718-803-3782
Fax: 718-803-0414
http://www.aascin.org/default.html

American Congress of Rehabilitation Medicine
4700 W Lake Avenue
Glenview, IL 60025
847-375-4725
Fax: 847-375-4777
http://www.acrm.org/

American Paralysis/Spinal Cord Hotline
2201 Argonne Drive
Baltimore, MD 21218
800-526-3456
800-638-1733 (in Maryland)

Amyotrophic Lateral Sclerosis Association
21021 Ventura Blvd, Suite 321
Woodland Hills, CA 91364
818-990-2151
http://www.alsa.org

Guillain-Barré Syndrome Foundation International
PO Box 262
Wynnewood, PA 19096
610-667-0131
Fax: 610-667-7036
http://www.webmast.com/gbs/

Myasthenia Gravis Foundation
53 West Jackson Blvd, Suite 909
Chicago, IL 60604
800-541-5454
312-258-0522
Fax: 312-258-0461
http://www.med.unc.edu/mgfa/

National Rehabilitation Information Center
8455 Colesville Road, Suite 935
Silver Spring, MD 20910
301-588-9284
http://www.naric.com/naric/index.html

National Spinal Cord Injury Association
8300 Colesville Road, Suite 551
Silver Spring, MD 20910
301-588-6959
800-962-9629
http://www.spinalcord.org/

Paralyzed Veterans of America
801 18th Street NW
Washington, DC 20006
202-872-1300
800-424-8200 x619 or x620
202-416-7619 or 7620
http://www.pva.or

***For additional Internet resources, see the website for this book at* www.mosby.com/MERLIN/medsurg_lewis**

REMEMBER to check out your companion CD-ROM

58 NURSING ASSESSMENT Musculoskeletal System

Susan C. Ruda

www.mosby.com/MERLIN/medsurg_lewis

LEARNING OBJECTIVES

1. Describe the gross anatomic and microscopic composition of bone.
2. Explain the classification system of joints and movements at synovial joints.
3. Describe the types and structure of muscle tissue.
4. Describe the functions of cartilage, muscles, ligaments, tendons, fascia, and bursae.
5. Describe age-related changes in the musculoskeletal system and differences in assessment findings.
6. Identify the significant subjective and objective data related to the musculoskeletal system that should be obtained from a patient.
7. Describe the appropriate techniques used in the physical assessment of the musculoskeletal system.
8. Differentiate normal from abnormal findings of a physical assessment of the musculoskeletal system.
9. Describe the purpose, significance of results, and nursing responsibilities related to diagnostic studies of the musculoskeletal system.

The ability to perform complex and precise movements permits human beings to interact and adapt to the environment. Proper functioning of the musculoskeletal system makes such movements possible. The musculoskeletal system consists of bones, muscles, joints, cartilage, ligaments, tendons, fascia, and bursae.

The musculoskeletal system is particularly vulnerable to external forces. These forces can cause alteration in the structure of bone or soft connective tissue, resulting in functional disruption. The consequences may be deformity, alteration of body image, alteration in mobility, pain, or permanent disability. These problems may produce long-term health problems that interfere with activities of daily living and quality of life.

STRUCTURES AND FUNCTIONS OF THE MUSCULOSKELETAL SYSTEM

Bone

Function. The main functions of the musculoskeletal system are support, protection of vital organs, movement, blood cell production, and mineral storage.[1] Bone forms the body's supporting framework. Without this support, the body would collapse. Bone also allows the body to bear weight. The musculoskeletal system is important in protecting underlying vital organs and tissues. For example, the skull protects the brain, the vertebrae protect the spinal cord, and the rib cage protects the lungs and heart. Bones serve as a point of attachment for muscles; muscles are anchored to bones by tendons. Bone acts as a lever for muscles, and joints serve as fulcrums. Movement occurs as a result of muscle contractions applied to these levers. Bone also serves as a site for storage of inorganic minerals such as calcium and phosphorus. Cancellous bone contains hematopoietic tissue for the production of blood cells and platelets.

Gross Structure. Bone is a dynamic tissue that changes form and substance continually. It is composed of organic material (collagen) and inorganic material (calcium, phosphate). The internal and external growth and remodeling of bone are continuous processes.

Bone is classified according to structure as compact (dense) or cancellous (spongy). In compact bone, cylinder-shaped structural units (haversian systems) fit closely together, giving a dense consistency to the bone structure.[2] In cancellous bone, there are many open spaces between thin processes and networks of bone tissue. The networks are filled with either red or yellow marrow.

The anatomic structure of bone can best be visualized by the typical long bone (e.g., femur) (Fig. 58-1). Each long bone consists of an epiphysis, articular cartilage, a diaphysis, periosteum, and a medullary (marrow) cavity.

The epiphysis is located at each end of a long bone and is composed of cancellous bone. It is the location for muscle attachment and provides stability for the joint. Articular cartilage covers the ends of the bone and provides a smooth surface for joint movement.

The diaphysis is the main shaft of bone. It provides the bone with structural support and is composed of compact bone. The metaphysis is the flared area between the epiphysis and the diaphysis. During bone development it contains the growth zones. In the adult the metaphysis is joined to the epiphysis. The epiphyseal plate, or growth zone, is the cartilaginous area that

Reviewed by Dennis Ross, RN, PhD, Professor of Nursing, Castleton State College, Castleton, Vt; Nursing Faculty, Regents College, Albany, NY.

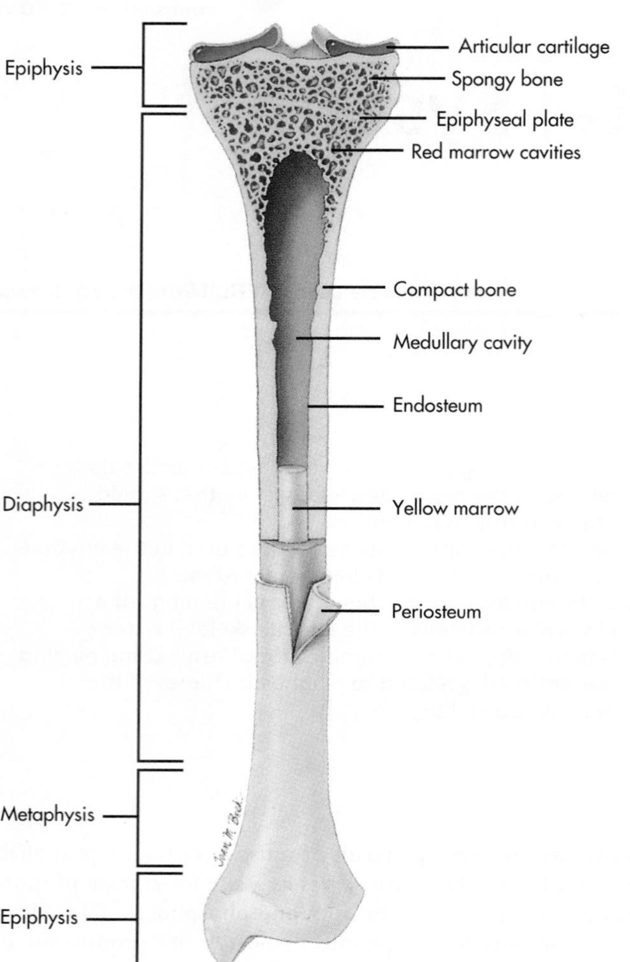

Fig. 58-1 Longitudinal section of a long bone.

actively produces bone and results in longitudinal growth in children. Injury to the epiphyseal plate in a growing child can cause significant problems, such as altered growth of the extremity. In the adult, this plate will harden to mature bone, and longitudinal growth will cease.

The periosteum is fibrous connective tissue that covers the bone. Musculotendinous fibers attach to the outer layer of the periosteum. The inner layer of the periosteum contains osteoblasts (bone-forming cells), which are essential for transverse bone growth and fracture repair.

The medullary (marrow) cavity is in the center of the diaphysis. In the adult, the medullary cavity of long bones contains yellow bone marrow, which is mainly adipose tissue. In the growing child, red bone marrow in the medullary cavity is actively involved in hematopoiesis. In the adult, hematopoiesis normally occurs only in the red bone marrow of the skull, ribs, sternum, pelvis, vertebrae, and proximal ends (epiphyses) of the humerus and femur.

Microscopic Structure. The three types of bone cells are osteoblasts, osteocytes, and osteoclasts. *Osteoblasts* synthesize organic bone matrix (collagen) and are the basic bone-forming cells. *Osteocytes* are the mature bone cells. *Osteoclasts* function in the breakdown of bone tissue and participate in bone remodeling. *Bone remodeling* is the removal of old bone by osteoclasts (resorption) and the deposition of new bone by osteoblasts (ossification). The inner layer of bone is primarily made up of osteoblasts with a few osteoclasts.

Bone is a special kind of connective tissue in which organic matter (collagen) has become mineralized. The structural unit of compact bone is the haversian system (Fig. 58-2). It consists of lamellae, which are concentric layers of calcified collagen matrix that enclose a long canal (haversian system). The main function of the haversian system is to transport blood to bone tissue. Blood vessels from the periosteum travel through Volkmann's canals to the blood vessels of the haversian system.

Osteocytes (mature bone cells) lie in small spaces termed *lacunae* between lamellae. Canaliculi (tiny canals) extend from the lacunae to connect the osteocytes to one another and to the haversian system.

Types. The skeleton consists of 206 named bones. These bones are classified according to shape as long, short, flat, or irregular.

Long bones are characterized by a central shaft (diaphysis) and two epiphyseal ends (see Fig. 58-1). Examples include the femur, humerus, and radius. Short bones are characterized by cancellous bone covered by a thin layer of compact bone. Examples include the carpals and tarsals.

Flat bones are characterized by two layers of compact bone separated by a layer of cancellous bone. Examples include the ribs, skull, scapula, and sternum. The spaces in the cancellous bone contain bone marrow. Irregular bones have a variety of shapes and sizes. Examples include the vertebrae, sacrum, and mandible.

Joints

A *joint* (articulation) is a place where two bones come together. Joints hold bones firmly together while permitting movement between them. Joints are commonly classified according to their degree of movement (Fig. 58-3).

The diarthrodial (synovial) type, the most common joint, consists of a cavity between the articular surfaces of the bones that make up the joint (Fig. 58-4). The ends of the bone are covered with articular (hyaline) cartilage. A capsule of connective tissue (the fibrous or joint capsule) joins the two bones together, forming a cavity. The capsule is lined by a synovial membrane, which secretes a thick synovial fluid to lubricate the joint and reduce friction. Types of diarthrodial joints are shown in Fig. 58-5. Structures surrounding the joint (periarticular tissues) provide support for joint function (e.g., ligaments and tendons).

Cartilage

Cartilage is a rigid connective tissue that functions to support soft tissue and provides the articular surface for joint movement. It protects underlying tissues. The cartilage that makes up the epiphyseal plate is also essential for the growth of long bones before physical maturity is reached.

Cartilage is avascular and therefore is nourished by the diffusion of material from capillaries in adjacent connective tissue. Cartilage cells are slow to reproduce because of the lack of a direct blood supply, which explains why damaged cartilage heals slowly.

The three types of cartilage tissue are hyaline, elastic, and fibrous. Hyaline cartilage, the most common, contains a moderate amount of collagen fibers. It is found in the trachea,

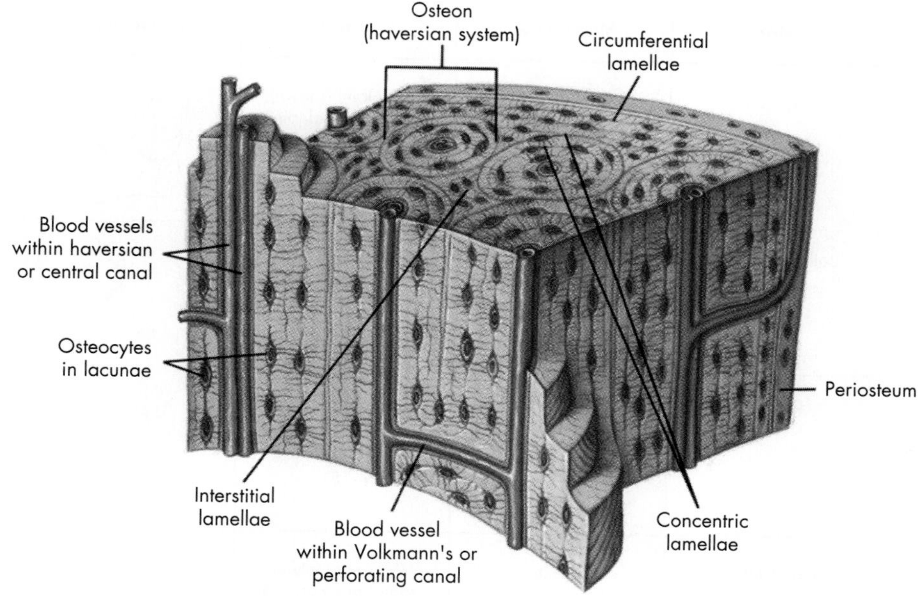

Fig. 58-2 Structure of compact bone showing haversian system.

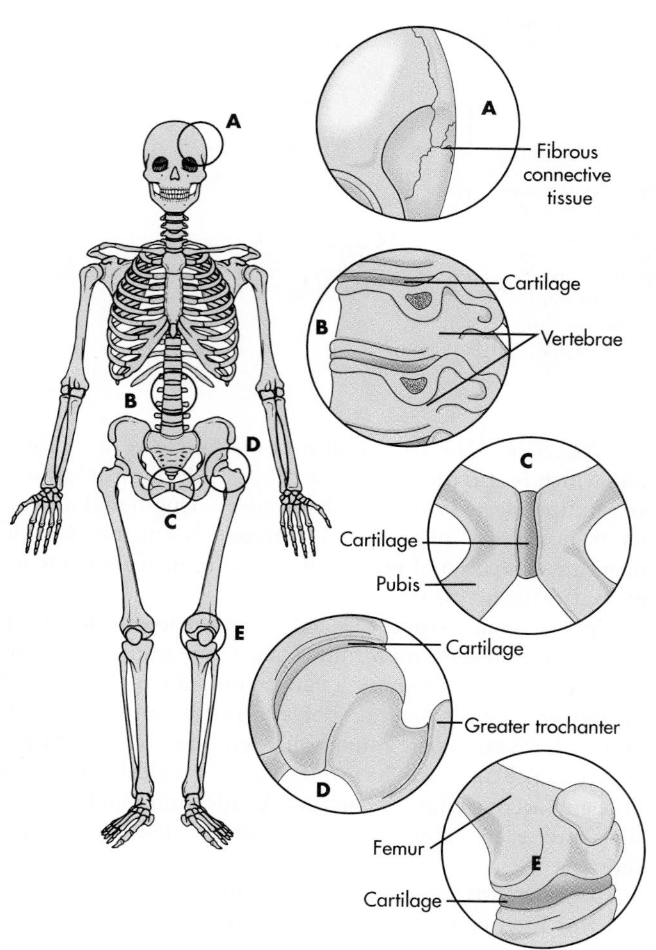

Fig. 58-3 Classification of joints. **A, B, C,** Synarthrotic (immovable) and amphiarthrotic (slightly movable) joints. **D, E,** Diarthrodial (freely movable) joints.

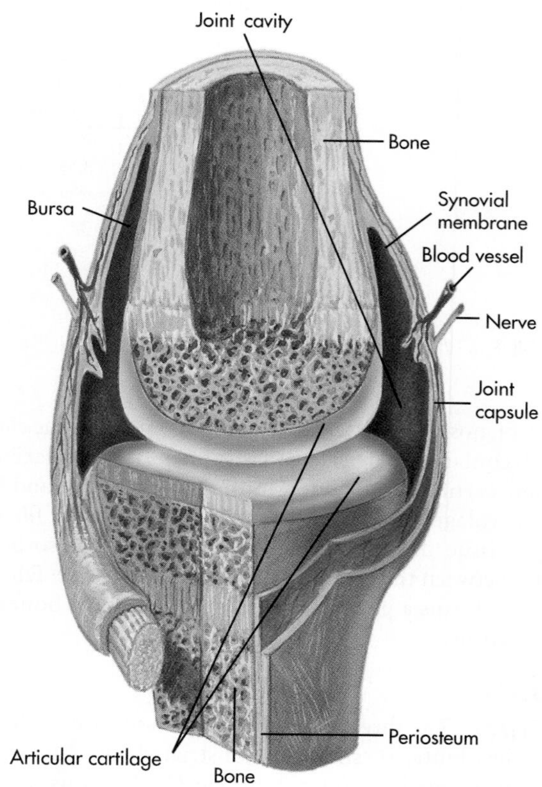

Fig. 58-4 Structure of a synovial joint.

Joint	Movement	Examples	Illustration
Hinge joint	Flexion, extension	Elbow joint (shown), interphalangeal joints, knee joint	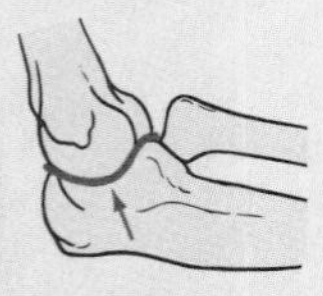
Ball and socket (spheroidal)	Flexion, extension; adduction, abduction; circumduction	Shoulder (shown), hip	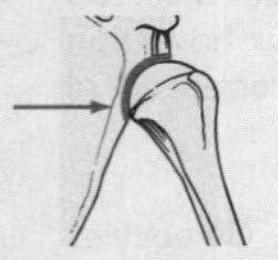
Pivot (rotary)	Rotation	Atlas-axis, proximal radioulnar joint (shown)	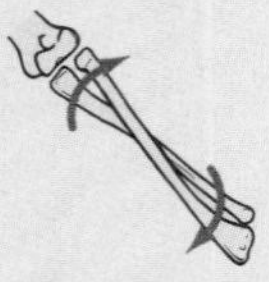
Condyloid	Flexion, extension; abduction, adduction; circumduction	Wrist joint (between radial and carpals) (shown)	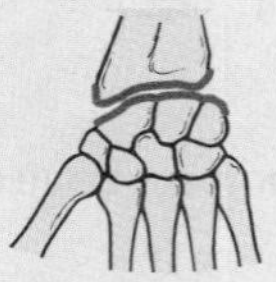
Saddle	Flexion, extension; abduction, adduction; circumduction, thumb-finger opposition	Carpometacarpal joint of thumb	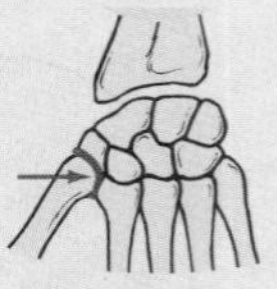
Gliding	One surface moves over another surface	Between tarsal bones, sacroiliac joint, between articular processes of vertebrae, between carpal bones (shown)	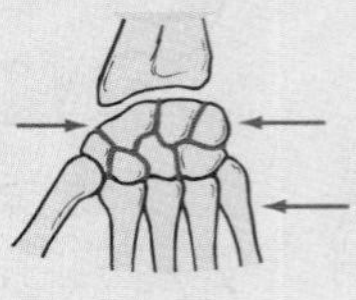

Fig. 58-5 Types of diarthrodial joints.

bronchi, nose, and articular surfaces of bones. Elastic cartilage, which contains collagen and elastic fibers, is more flexible than hyaline cartilage. It is found in the ear, epiglottis, and larynx. Fibrocartilage, which consists mostly of collagen fibers, is a tough tissue that often functions as a shock absorber. It is found between the vertebral disks and in the knee. Fibrocartilage also forms a protective cushion between the bones of the pelvic girdle.

Muscle

Types. The three types of muscle tissue are cardiac (striated, involuntary), smooth (nonstriated, involuntary), and skeletal (striated, voluntary) muscle. Cardiac muscle is found in the heart. Its contractions provide the major force for propelling blood through the circulatory system. Cardiac muscle contracts spontaneously. Smooth muscle is found in the walls of hollow structures such as airways, the gastrointestinal (GI) tract, urinary bladder, uterus, and some blood vessels. Smooth muscle contraction is modulated by neuronal and hormonal influences. Skeletal muscle requires neuronal stimulation for contraction. Skeletal muscle composes the largest mass of tissue in the body and is the focus of the following discussion.

Structure. The structural unit of muscle is the muscle cell, which is also called a muscle fiber. Skeletal muscle fibers are multinucleated cylinders that range in length and diameter from several millimeters to several centimeters. Muscle fibers are composed of myofibrils, which in turn are made up of contractile filaments.

Under a microscope, skeletal muscle shows alternating banding, which accounts for the striated appearance.[3] This appearance is due to a repeating pattern of filaments seen in the myofibrils. The sarcomere is the contractile unit of the myofibrils. Each sarcomere contains myosin (thick) filaments and actin (thin) filaments. The arrangement of the thin and thick filaments accounts for the banding. As thick and thin filaments slide past each other, the sarcomeres shorten and muscle shortens.

Contractions. Skeletal muscle contractions are responsible for the functions of posture, movement, and facial expressions. Isometric contractions increase the tension within a muscle but do not produce movement. Repeated isometric contractions make muscles grow larger and stronger. Isotonic contractions produce movement. Most contractions are a combination of tension generation (isometric) and shorten-

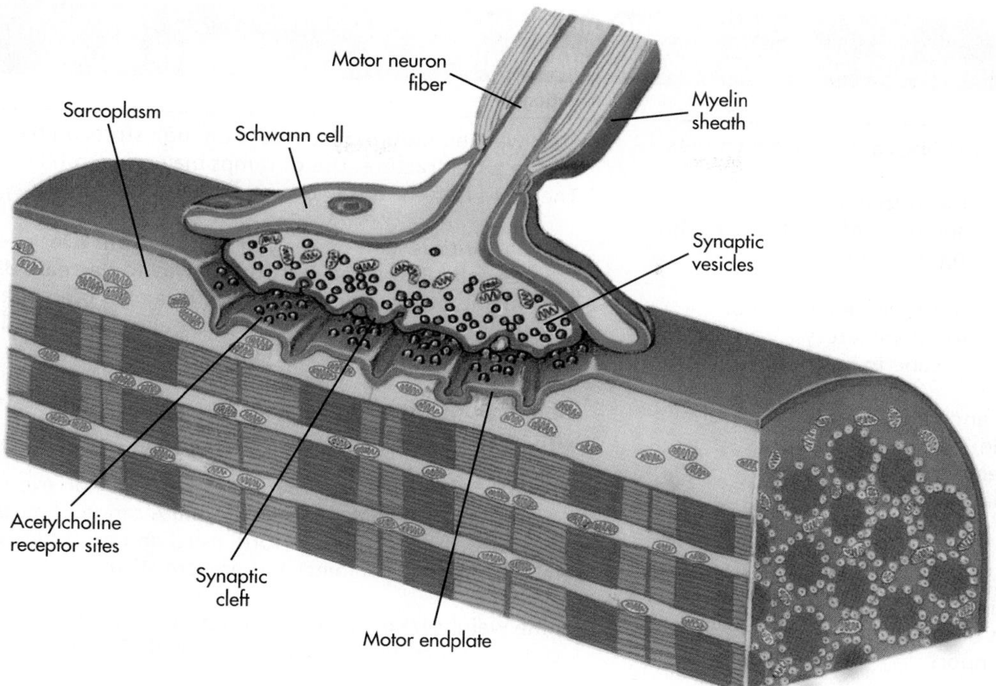

Fig. 58-6 Neuromuscular junction.

ing (isotonic). Without muscle contraction there is atrophy (decrease in size), and with increased muscle activity there is hypertrophy (increase in size).

Skeletal muscle produces other types of contractions that have little to do with functional posture and movement. They are a twitch contraction (a quick contraction in response to a single stimulus) and a tetanic contraction (a more sustained twitch).

Neuromuscular Junction. Skeletal muscles require a nerve supply in order to contract. The nerve fiber and the skeletal muscle fibers it supplies are called a *motor end plate.*[4] The junction between the axon of the nerve cell and the muscle cell it supplies is called the *myoneural* or *neuromuscular junction* (Fig. 58-6).

When acetylcholine is released from the motor end plate of the neuron, it diffuses across the neuromuscular junction and binds with receptors on the muscle fiber. In response to this stimulation, the sarcoplasmic reticulum releases calcium ions into the cytoplasm. The presence of these ions triggers the contraction in the myofibrils.

Energy Source. The energy source used in muscle fiber contractions comes from adenosine triphosphate (ATP). ATP is synthesized by cellular oxidative metabolism in numerous mitochondria located close to the myofibrils. A second energy source is creatine phosphate, which supplies phosphate to rephosphorylate ATP. Creatine phosphate is synthesized and stored in muscle tissue.

Ligaments and Tendons

Ligaments and tendons are both composed of dense, fibrous connective tissue. This type of connective tissue contains large numbers of collagen fibers that are closely packed. Tendons attach muscles to bones. They are an extension of the muscle sheath that attaches to the periosteum. Ligaments connect bones to bones at joints (e.g., the knee joint). They permit movement while providing stability.

Fibrous connective tissue has a relatively poor blood supply. Although the tissue can repair itself after injury, it is usually a slow process. For example, a sprain, which is the stretching or tearing of the ligaments, may require a long time to heal.[5]

Fascia

Fascia is the term used for layers of connective tissue. It is classified as either superficial or deep. Superficial fascia is the loose connective tissue located immediately under the skin. Deep fascia (dense, fibrous connective tissue) is found surrounding muscle, between muscles, and surrounding the bundles that bind muscles, nerves, and blood vessels together.

Fascia separates one muscle from another to permit independent muscle action. It allows gliding of one muscle over another. In addition, fascia provides strength to muscle tissues.

Bursae

Bursae are small sacs of connective tissue lined with synovial membrane and synovial fluid. They are commonly located at bone prominences such as the joint. Bursae function as cushions to relieve pressure between the moving parts and prevent friction (see Fig. 58-4). For example, they are found between the patella and the skin (prepatellar bursa), between the olecranon process and the skin (olecranon bursa), between the head of the humerus and the acromion process (subacromial bursa), and between the lower portion of the gluteus maximus muscle and the bony ischial tuberosity (submuscular bursa). Bursitis (inflammation of the bursa) may be caused by mechanical injury to the bursa or excessive use of a joint.

GERONTOLOGIC DIFFERENCES IN ASSESSMENT

Table 58-1 Prevention of Common Musculoskeletal Problems in the Older Adult

Activity	Rationale
▪ Use of ramps in buildings and at street corners instead of steps	Stair-walking motion may create enough stress on fragile bones to cause a hip fracture. Use of ramps may prevent falls.
▪ Elimination of scatter rugs in the home	These are notorious for causing falls and fractures.
▪ Response to pain and discomfort of osteoarthritis	
Resting in reclining position	Osteoarthritis is seen on x-ray of most persons over age 50 and causes pain. Rest is the most useful way to decrease discomfort.
Use of plain or enteric-coated aspirin or nonsteroidal antiinflammatory	Aspirin and other antiinflammatory drugs (as prescribed by physician) diminish inflammation of joints and reduce pain.
Use of a walker or cane to help with walking	Assistance decreases stress on inflamed joints and thus decreases discomfort. Use may prevent falls.
▪ Eating amount and kind of foods to prevent excess weight gain	Obesity adds stress to bones, which may predispose patient to osteoarthritis.
▪ Regular and frequent exercise	
Activities of daily living	Activities of daily living provide range-of-motion exercise, which should be done four times a day; 100% range of motion is not as critical as the ability to perform usual and preferred activities.
Hobbies (e.g., jigsaw puzzles, needlework, model building)	These exercise distal joints and prevent stiffness.
Walking short distances daily with shoes that give good support	Some weight-bearing exercise is essential and should be done two or three times daily. Good shoes provide for safety and promote comfort.
▪ Gradual initiation of all activities	Starting gradually promotes optimal coordination. When a patient rises slowly to a standing position, dizziness and hence falls and fractures can be prevented.

GERONTOLOGIC CONSIDERATIONS

Effects of Aging on the Musculoskeletal System

Many of the functional problems of the aging adult are due to changes of the musculoskeletal system. Many of these changes begin in early adulthood, but obvious signs of musculoskeletal impairment may not appear until later in adulthood. These alterations may affect posture, function, and gait and lead to an increase in falls. They affect the older adult's lifestyle and activities of daily living, ranging from discomfort and decreased ability to perform activities of daily living to severe, chronic pain and immobility.[6]

Numerous age-related changes affect the bones, muscles, joints, and connective tissue. The bone remodeling process is altered, resulting in increased bone resorption and decreased osteoblastic activity. These alterations in bone density are a major factor in osteoporosis (see Chapter 59). Muscle functioning declines because of a decrease in muscle mass and strength.[7] Almost 30% of the muscle mass is lost by the eighth decade of life. An age-related loss in the motor neurons that control skeletal muscle movement also occurs. Joints, tendons, and ligaments harden over time, resulting in less flexible and rigid movement.[8] Joints become stiff.

In addition to the usual musculoskeletal assessment with a particular emphasis on exercise practices, the nurse should determine the impact of age-related changes of the musculoskeletal system on the functional status of the older patient. Functional limitations that are accepted by older adults as a normal part of aging can often be halted or reversed with appropriate preventive strategies (Table 58-1). Age-related changes in the musculoskeletal system and differences in assessment findings are presented in Table 58-2.

ASSESSMENT OF THE MUSCULOSKELETAL SYSTEM

Correct diagnosis depends on an accurate patient history and a thorough examination. A musculoskeletal assessment can be made on a specific body part, as part of a general physical examination, or as an examination in itself. Judgment must be used on the basis of the patient's problem in selecting all or part of the components of the musculoskeletal history and physical examination. Accidents often result in trauma to the musculoskeletal system and require a thorough assessment. If the injury is serious or life threatening, only pertinent information related to the accident is obtained, and a complete assessment is deferred.

Complaints that should alert the nurse to obtain subjective and objective data related to the musculoskeletal system include joint or muscle pain, joint swelling, decreasing strength or function, change in size of an extremity or muscle, deformity, spasms, crepitation, changes in sensation, stiffness, and changes in gait. Health history questions presented in Table 58-3 should be asked when a musculoskeletal problem is noted.

Subjective Data

Important Health Information

Past health history. Certain illnesses are known to affect the musculoskeletal system either directly or indirectly. The patient should be questioned specifically about a history of tuberculosis, poliomyelitis, diabetes mellitus, gout, inflammatory and degenerative arthritis, hemophilia, parathyroid problems, rickets, osteomalacia, scurvy, osteomyelitis or soft tissue infection, fungal infection of the bones or joints, and neuromuscular disabilities. If the patient has a history of any of these problems, a detailed account of the illness should be obtained. In addition, the patient should be questioned about

GERONTOLOGIC DIFFERENCES IN ASSESSMENT

Table 58-2 Musculoskeletal System

Changes	Differences in Assessment Findings
Muscle	
Decreased number and diameter of muscle cells, replacement of muscle cells by fibrous connective tissue	Decreased muscle strength and bulk, abdominal protrusion, muscle flabbiness
Loss of elasticity in ligaments and cartilage	Decreased fine motor activity, decreased agility
Reduced ability to store glycogen; decreased ability to release glycogen as quick energy in times of stress	Slowed reaction times, slowing of most muscle neuronal reflexes, slowing of impulse conduction along motor units, easy fatigability
Joints	
Erosion of articular cartilage, possible direct contact between bone ends	Manifestations of osteoarthritis, joint stiffness, possible crepitation on movement of joints, pain with range-of-motion movements
Overgrowth of bone around joint margins (osteophytes)	Heberden's nodes in fingers (especially in women), limited mobility in affected joints
Loss of water from disks between vertebrae, narrowing of joint vertebral spaces	Loss of height, back pain, joint subluxation
Bone	
Decrease in bone mass	Dowager's hump (kyphosis) caused by compression of vertebral bodies Decreased height

possible sources of secondary bacterial infections, such as ears, tonsils, teeth, sinuses, or genitourinary tract, which can result in osteomyelitis.

Medications. The patient should be questioned carefully regarding prescription and over-the-counter drugs used to treat a musculoskeletal problem. Information on the reason for taking the medication, its name, the dose and frequency, length of time it was taken, its effect, and any side effects should be obtained. Specific inquiry should be made related to skeletal muscle relaxants, antirheumatoid agents, nonsteroidal antiinflammatory drugs, narcotics, and systemic corticosteroids. The patient should be questioned about GI distress or a bleeding ulcer if antiinflammatory agents have been taken.

In addition to drugs taken for treatment of a musculoskeletal problem, the patient should be questioned about drugs that can have detrimental effects on this system. These drugs include antiseizure drugs (osteomalacia), phenothiazines (gait disturbances), corticosteroids (abnormal fat distribution, avascular necrosis, and decreased bone and muscle mass), and potassium-depleting diuretics (muscle cramps and weakness). Amphetamines and caffeine intake can cause a generalized increase in motor activity. Older women should be questioned about their menopausal status, the use of hormone replacement therapy, and calcium and vitamin D supplementation.

Surgery or other treatments. Information should be obtained about hospitalizations that were necessitated by a musculoskeletal problem. The reason for the hospitalization, the date and duration, and the treatment should be carefully documented. Specifics of any surgical procedure and postoperative course should also be obtained. If there was a period of prolonged immobilization, the possible development of osteoporosis and muscle atrophy should be considered. The patient should also be questioned about emergency treatment related to musculoskeletal disorders and injuries.

Functional Health Patterns. The use of functional health patterns aids the nurse in organizing the data and formulating diagnoses based on data collected about the musculoskeletal system. Table 58-3 summarizes the health history questions to ask in relation to functional health patterns.

Health perception–health management pattern. The nurse should ask about the patient's health practices related to the musculoskeletal system, such as maintenance of a normal body weight, avoidance of excessive stress on muscles and joints, and the use of proper body mechanics when lifting objects.[9]

The patient should be specifically questioned about immunizations related to tetanus and polio. The most current date and reaction to a tuberculin skin test should also be obtained.

Food or contact allergies are of little consequence in relation to musculoskeletal problems. However, the general malaise often associated with allergic reactions may manifest in musculoskeletal stiffness and lethargy. Allergic reactions to drugs used to treat musculoskeletal problems can interfere with therapy, and an alternative treatment may have to be employed if the allergic reaction is severe.

The list of minor and major injuries of the musculoskeletal system can be extensive in the patient who is a good historian. It includes documentation of fractures, sprains, strains, and dislocations. The information should be recorded chronologically and should include the following:

1. Mechanism of the injury (twist, crush, stretch)
2. Circumstances related to the injury
3. Diagnostic evaluations
4. Methods of treatment
5. Duration of treatment
6. Current status related to the injury
7. Need for assistive devices
8. Interference with activities of daily living

A three-generation family history should be obtained related to rheumatoid arthritis, degenerative joint disease, gout, osteoporosis, and scoliosis because these problems have a familial predisposition.

Safety practices can play a role in the patient's predisposition for certain injuries and illnesses. Specific questions should be

HEALTH HISTORY

Table 58-3 Musculoskeletal System

Health Perception–Health Management Pattern
- Describe your usual daily activities.
- Do you experience any difficulties performing these activities?* Describe what you do when you experience difficulty in dressing, feeding yourself, performing basic hygiene, or maintaining your home.
- Do you use any mechanical assistive devices?* Do you have to lift heavy objects? If so, describe how you do this.
- Describe any specialized equipment you use or wear when you work or exercise that helps protect you from injury.
- What type of safety precautions do you take?
- Do you take any medications to manage your musculoskeletal problem? If so, what is/are the name(s) of the medication? When did you have your last tetanus and polio immunization? When were you last tested for tuberculosis?

Nutrition-Metabolic Pattern
- Give a 24 hr diet recall. Do you take supplemental vitamins or minerals? (Ask specifically about calcium and vitamin D supplements.)
- What is your weight? Have you had a recent change in your weight?*

Elimination Pattern
- Does your musculoskeletal problem make it difficult for you to reach the toilet in time?* Do you experience constipation related to immobility?
- Do you need any assistive devices or equipment to achieve satisfactory toileting?*

Activity-Exercise Pattern
- Do you have any limitations in your activities of daily living because of a musculoskeletal problem?*
- Describe your usual exercise pattern. Do you experience symptoms related to your musculoskeletal system before, during, or after exercising?*
- Are you able to move all your joints comfortably through full range of motion? Describe any limitations in mobility.
- Do you require assistance in moving or in doing activities of daily living?*
- Do you use any prosthetic or orthotic devices?*

Sleep-Rest Pattern
- Do you experience any difficulty sleeping because of a musculoskeletal problem?* Do you require frequent position changes at night? Why?
- Do you wake up at night because of musculoskeletal pain?*

Cognitive-Perceptual Pattern
- Describe any musculoskeletal pain you experience. How do you manage your pain?

Self-Perception–Self-Concept Pattern
- Describe how changes in your musculoskeletal system (posture, walking, muscle strength) or the ability to do certain things have affected how you feel about yourself. How have these changes affected your lifestyle?

Role-Relationship Pattern
- Do you live alone?
- Describe how your family or others assist you with your musculoskeletal problems.
- Describe the effect of your musculoskeletal problem on your work and on your social relationships.

Sexuality-Reproductive Pattern
- Describe the effect of your musculoskeletal problem on your sexual activity. How do you feel about this?

Coping–Stress Tolerance Pattern
- Describe how you deal with the problems such as pain or immobility that have resulted from your musculoskeletal problem.

Value-Belief Pattern
- Describe any cultural or religious beliefs that may influence the treatment of your musculoskeletal problem.

*If yes, describe.

asked about safety practices of the patient as they relate to the job environment, recreation, and exercise. For example, if the patient is a jogger, the type of shoes worn and the jogging surface used should be investigated. The high incidence of trauma to the musculoskeletal system requires a careful investigation in the area of safety practices. Identification of problems in this area will direct the plan for patient education.

Nutritional-metabolic pattern. The patient's recounting of a typical day's diet can provide clues to areas of nutritional concern in relation to the musculoskeletal system. Obesity predisposes people to ligamentous instability, particularly in the lower back region. It also adds stress to weight-bearing joints such as the knees and hips. The maintenance of normal weight is an important patient goal.

Abnormal nutritional states can predispose individuals to specific musculoskeletal problems such as osteoporosis, osteomalacia, and rickets. Adequate amounts of vitamins C and D, calcium, and protein are essential for a healthy, intact musculoskeletal system. The nurse should also evaluate the patient's ability to tolerate lactose in milk products.

Elimination pattern. The patient's ability to ambulate adequately to reach a toileting facility should be assessed. A musculoskeletal problem could be an etiologic factor in functional incontinence of bladder and bowel. Also, immobility secondary to a musculoskeletal problem can result in constipation. The patient should be asked if an assistive device such as an elevated toilet seat or grab bar is necessary to accomplish toileting.

Activity-exercise pattern. A detailed account of the type, duration, and frequency of activities related to exercise and recreation should be obtained and assessed regarding adequacy and predisposition to musculoskeletal problems. This information can be obtained when the patient recounts a typical day. Daily, weekend, and seasonal patterns should be compared because occasional or sporadic exercise can be more problematic than regular exercise. Many musculoskeletal problems can affect the patient's activity-exercise pattern. The nurse should question the patient about limitations of movement, pain, weakness, clumsiness, crepitus, or any change in the bones or joints that interfere with daily activities.

Extremes of activity related to occupation can affect the musculoskeletal system. A sedentary occupation does not allow for maintaining muscle flexibility and strength. Jobs that require extreme effort and use of the body for heavy lifting and pushing can result in damage to the joints and supporting structures of the body. The nurse should inquire about job-related injuries to the musculoskeletal system, the amount of time lost from work, and the treatments used.

Sleep-rest pattern. Musculoskeletal disorders might require frequent position changes at night. Discomfort may also interfere with a normal sleep pattern. The patient should be questioned about sleep patterns and how they have been altered. If the patient recounts that a musculoskeletal problem is interfering with sleep, further inquiry should be made related to the type of bedding, pillows used, sleeping partner, and sleeping positions.

Cognitive-perceptual pattern. Any pain experienced by the patient as a result of a musculoskeletal problem should be fully explored and documented. Pain assessment conducted over time can assist in determining the effectiveness of the treatment plan. The patient should be asked what measures are used at home to control pain. Other complaints that could cause a problem either directly or indirectly through pain include joint swelling, decreasing strength, and changes in sensation.

Self-perception–self-concept pattern. Many musculoskeletal problems are chronic and deforming. Such changes can have a serious impact on the patient's body image and sense of personal worth. An account of how the patient feels about these changes should be addressed by the nurse.

Role-relationship pattern. Musculoskeletal problems that affect mobility or result in a chronic pain syndrome can seriously affect the patient's roles and responsibilities, such as spouse, parent, and worker. Also, such problems can affect the ability to seek and maintain meaningful social and personal relationships. These problems should be assessed and documented during the history.

If the patient lives alone, the possibility of maintaining this living arrangement in the future should be assessed in light of the problem and rehabilitation potential. The degree of assistance from family, friends, and organized caregivers should also be determined.

Sexuality-reproductive pattern. Musculoskeletal problems and the resulting pain or potential for pain can greatly affect the patient's ability to obtain sexual satisfaction. This area must be sensitively assessed so the patient feels comfortable in relating sexual problems related to pain, movement, and positioning.

Coping–stress tolerance pattern. Mobility limitations and pain, both acute and chronic, can be serious stressors that affect the patient's coping ability. The nurse must recognize the potential for ineffective coping (both patient and family or significant other) and gather adequate data to determine if a musculoskeletal problem is causing a coping problem.

Objective Data

Physical Examination. The primary methods used in the physical examination of the musculoskeletal system include inspection and palpation. The data gathered from a careful health history will provide the nurse with clues about areas on which to concentrate the examination.

Inspection. Inspection begins during the nurse's initial contact with the patient. The nurse should observe the patient for any apparent asymmetry and for sitting and standing posture, gait, general body build, and configuration of the muscles. The nurse should be particularly aware of limitations in the patient's ability to perform normal activities such as dressing, toileting, and eating.

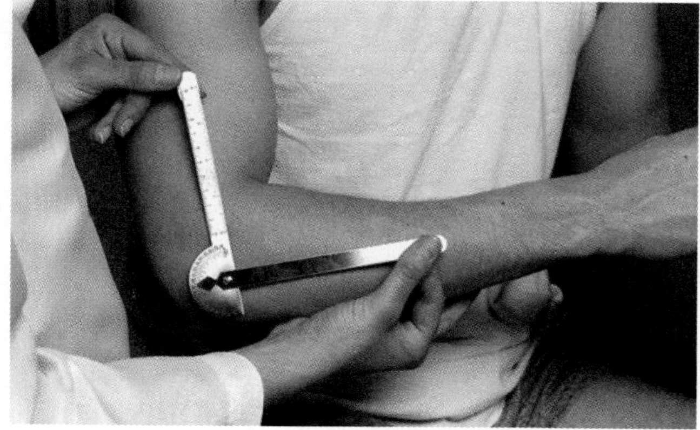

Fig. 58-7 Measurement of joint motion with a goniometer.

The condition of the skin is observed for general color, scars, or overt signs of previous injury or operations. A systematic inspection is performed starting at the head and neck and proceeding to the upper extremities, the lower extremities, and the back. Although the order is not of great importance, the regular use of a systematic approach is important to avoid missing important aspects of the examination. The nurse should specifically inspect for joint motion and asymmetry of movement, swelling, deformity, masses, and evidence of limb-length or muscle-size discrepancies. The patient's opposite body part is used for comparison when an abnormality is suspected.

Palpation. Any area that has aroused concern because of a subjective complaint or has been noted on inspection should be carefully palpated. The examiner's hands should be warm to prevent muscle spasm, which can interfere with identification of essential landmarks or soft-tissue structures. Palpation of the soft tissues, including muscles and joints, enables the examiner to evaluate skin temperature, local tenderness, swelling, and crepitation. It is important to establish the relationship of adjacent structures and to evaluate the general contour, abnormal prominences, and local landmarks. The usual sequence is to begin at the neck and proceed cephalopedally (head to toe) to examine the neck, shoulders, elbows, wrists, hands, back, hips, knees, ankles, and feet. Both superficial and deep palpation are usually performed consecutively.

Movement. When examining joint movement, the nurse must carefully evaluate passive and active range of joint motion. Normally the active and passive joint motions are similar. There are three range-of-motion categories: passive, active, and functional. Passive range of motion occurs when someone else moves the patient's joints through their range of motion. Caution is required when testing passive joint motion because of the possibility of injury to the underlying soft-tissue structures. Manipulation must cease immediately if pain or resistance is encountered. Active range of motion means the patient actively moves his or her own joints through their normal range of motion. Functional range of motion is assessed by asking the patient if the activities of daily living, such as eating and bathing independently, are performed with assistance or not at all. The patient may require an assistive device such as a cane, wheelchair, or walker, which should be noted.

Joint motion is most accurately measured by a goniometer, which measures the amount of bending or angles of the joints (Fig. 58-7). Specific degrees of range of motion of all joints are

Table 58-4 Movement at Synovial Joints

Movement	Description
Flexion	Bending of joint that decreases angle between two bones; shortening of muscle length
Extension	Bending of joint that increases angle between two bones
Hyperextension	Extension in which angle exceeds 180 degrees
Abduction	Movement of part away from midline
Adduction	Movement of part toward midline
Pronation	Turning of palm downward or sole outward
Supination	Turning of palm upward or sole inward
Circumduction	Combination of flexion, extension, abduction, and adduction resulting in circular motion of body part
Rotation	Movement about longitudinal axis
Inversion	Turning of sole inward toward midline
Eversion	Turning of sole outward away from midline

usually not measured unless a musculoskeletal problem has been identified. A less accurate but nevertheless valuable method is to compare the range of motion of one extremity with the range of motion on the opposite side. The most common movements that occur at the synovial joints are listed in Table 58-4.

Measurement. Limb length and circumferential measurement of muscle mass are often obtained when subjective problems or length discrepancies are noted. For example, leg length measurements are obtained when gait disorders are observed. Limb length is measured between two bony prominences and compared with the similar measurement of the opposite extremity. Muscle mass is measured circumferentially at the largest area of the mass. When recording measurements, the nurse should record the exact location at which the measurements were obtained (e.g., the quadriceps muscle is measured 15 cm above the patella). This informs the next examiner of the exact area to be measured and ensures consistency in future examinations.

Muscle-strength testing. The strength of individual muscles or groups of muscles is graded in performance of movements during contraction against applied resistance (Table 58-5). The examiner should instruct the patient to apply resistance to the force exerted by the examiner. For example, the examiner tries to pull the bent arm down while the patient tries to raise it. Muscle strength should also be compared with the strength of the opposite extremity. Subtle variations in muscle

Table 58-5 Muscle Strength Scale

0—No detection of muscular contraction
1—A barely detectable flicker or trace of contraction
2—Active movement of body part with elimination of gravity
3—Active movement against gravity
4—Active movement against gravity and some resistance
5—Active movement against full resistance without evident fatigue (normal muscle strength)

Table 58-6 Normal Physical Assessment of the Musculoskeletal System

Full range of motion of all joints
No joint swelling, deformity, or crepitation
Normal spinal curvatures
No tenderness on palpation of spine
No muscle atrophy or asymmetry
Muscle strength of 5

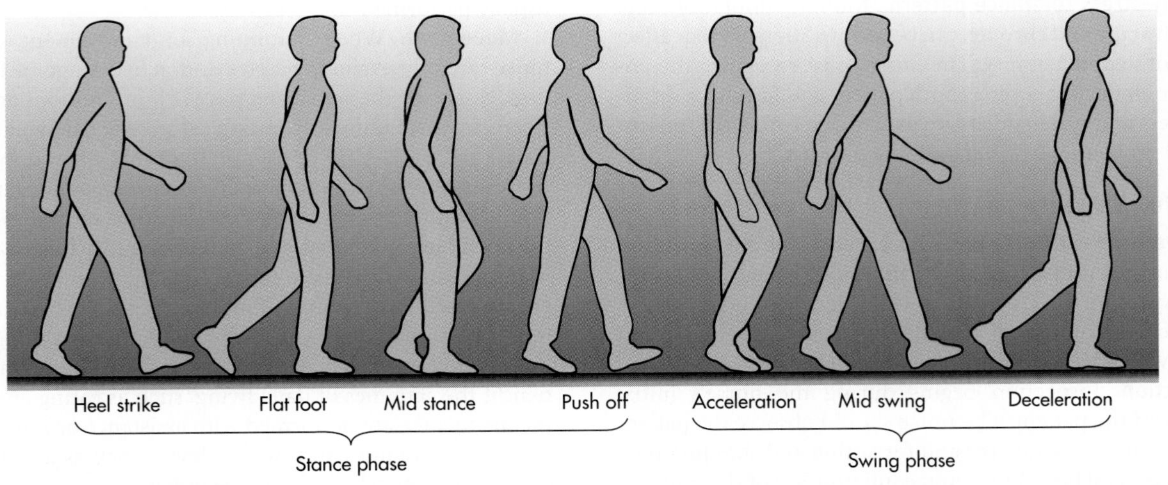

Fig. 58-8 Phases of gait. (Modified from DeLisa J, Gans B: *Rehabilitation medicine principles,* ed 2, Philadelphia, 1993, JB Lippincott.)

strength may be noted when comparing the patient's dominant side with the nondominant side.[9]

Gait. The nurse assesses gait by having the patient walk across the room and back. The normal gait is divided into two separate phases: the stance phase and the swing phase (Fig. 58-8). The two occur simultaneously: while one limb is in stance phase, the other is in swing phase. Musculoskeletal and neurologic problems can result in gait abnormalities.

Other. Assessment of reflexes is discussed in Chapter 53. Table 58-6 is an example of how to record a normal physical assessment of the musculoskeletal system. Common abnormal assessment findings of the musculoskeletal system are presented in Table 58-7.

DIAGNOSTIC STUDIES OF THE MUSCULOSKELETAL SYSTEM

Diagnostic studies provide important information to the nurse in monitoring the patient's condition and planning appropriate interventions. These studies are considered to be objective data. Table 58-8 contains diagnostic studies common to the musculoskeletal system.

Radiologic Studies

The most common diagnostic study used to assess musculoskeletal problems is an x-ray examination. Radiologic studies are important to establish the presence of a musculoskeletal problem and to follow its progress and the effectiveness of treatment.

A standard x-ray study is a film produced by the action of x-rays emitted from a cathode tube diphotosensitive surface. X-rays can be thought of as shadows of structures, particularly bony structures. Bones are more dense than other tissues and do not allow the x-ray to penetrate. The standard x-ray develops dense areas as white.

The anteroposterior and lateral views are the most commonly used standard x-ray perspectives. Because disk and cartilage structures are not visible on standard x-rays, special x-rays (diskograms, arthrograms) involving the use of contrast media can be used to visualize them.

Magnetic Resonance Imaging

Magnetic resonance imaging (MRI) is a diagnostic study that is useful in diagnosing numerous musculoskeletal disorders.

COMMON ASSESSMENT ABNORMALITIES

Table 58-7 Musculoskeletal System

Finding	Description	Possible Etiology and Significance
Ankylosis	Scarring within a joint leading to stiffness or fixation	Chronic joint inflammation
Atrophy	Wasting of muscle, characterized by decrease in circumference and flabby appearance and resulting in decrease in function and muscle tone	Prolonged disuse, contracture, immobilization, muscle denervation
Contracture	Resistance to movement of muscle or joint as result of fibrosis of supporting soft tissues	Shortening of muscle or ligament structure, tightness of soft tissue, immobilization, incorrect positioning
Crepitation	Crackling sound or grating sensation as result of friction between bones	Fracture, chronic inflammation, dislocation
Effusion	Fluid in joint possibly with swelling and pain	Trauma, especially to knee
Felon	Abscess occurring in pulp space (tissue mass) of distal phalanx of finger as a result of infection	Minor hand injury, puncture wound, laceration
Ganglion	Small, fluid-filled synovial cyst usually on dorsal surface of wrist and foot	Degeneration of connective tissue close to tendons and joints leading to formation of small cysts
Hypertrophy	Increase in size of muscle as result of enlargement of existing cells	Exercise, increased androgens, increased stimulation or use
Kyphosis (round back)	Anteroposterior or forward bending of spine with convexity of curve in posterior direction; common at thoracic and sacral levels	Poor posture, tuberculosis, chronic arthritis, growth disturbance of vertebral epiphysis, osteoporosis
Lordosis	Deformity of spine resulting in anteroposterior curvature with concavity in posterior direction; common in lumbar spine	Secondary to other deformities of spine, muscular dystrophy, obesity, flexion contracture of hip, congenital dislocation of hip
Pes planus	Flatfoot	Congenital condition, muscle paralysis, mild cerebral palsy, early muscular dystrophy
Scoliosis	Deformity resulting in lateral curvature of spine	Idiopathic or congenital condition, fracture or dislocation, osteomalacia, functional condition
Subluxation	Partial dislocation of joint	Instability of joint capsule and supporting ligaments (e.g., from trauma, arthritis)
Valgus	Angulation of bone away from midline	Alteration in gait, pain, abnormal erosion of articular cartilage
Varus	Angulation of bone toward midline	Alteration in gait, pain, abnormal erosion of articular cartilage

DIAGNOSTIC STUDIES

Table 58-8 Musculoskeletal System

Study	Description and Purpose	Nursing Responsibility
Radiologic Studies		
▪ Standard x-ray	An x-ray is taken to determine density of bone. Study evaluates structural or functional changes of bones and joints. In anteroposterior view, x-ray beam passes from front to back, allowing one-dimensional view; lateral position provides two-dimensional view.	Avoid excessive exposure of patient and self. Before procedure, remove any radiopaque objects that can interfere with results. Explain procedure to patient.
▪ Arthrogram	Study involves injection of contrast medium or air into joint cavity, which permits visualization of joint structures. Joint movement is followed with series of x-rays.	Assess patient for possible allergy to contrast medium, including iodine or seafood. Explain procedure. Prepare area to be injected aseptically.
▪ Diskogram	An x-ray of cervical or lumbar intervertebral disk is done after injection of contrast dye into nucleus pulposus. Study permits visualization of intervertebral disk abnormalities.	Same as for arthrogram. May be performed in surgery.
▪ Sinogram	An x-ray is taken after injection of contrast dye into sinus tract (deep draining wound). Study visualizes course of sinus and tissues involved.	Same as for arthrogram.
▪ Tomogram	Multiple x-ray views of body region are focused at successively deeper layers of tissue lying in predetermined planes. Study focuses on certain tissues, eliminating or blurring surrounding structures. Technique is useful in locating bone destruction, small body cavities, foreign bodies, and lesions overshadowed by opaque structures.	Inform patient that procedure is painless.
▪ Computed tomography (CT) scan	An x-ray beam is used with a computer to provide a three-dimensional picture. It is used to identify soft-tissue abnormalities, bony abnormalities, and various musculoskeletal trauma.	Inform patient that procedure is painless. Inform patient of importance of remaining still during procedure.
▪ Magnetic resonance imaging (MRI)	Radio waves and magnetic field are used to view soft tissue. Study is especially useful in the diagnosis of avascular necrosis, disk disease, tumors, osteomyelitis, ligament tears, and cartilage tears. Patient is placed inside scanning chamber. Gadolinium may be injected into a vein to enhance visualization of the structures. Open MRI does not require the patient to be placed inside a chamber.	Inform patient that it is painless. Be aware that it is contraindicated in patient with aneurysm clips, metallic implants, pacemakers, electronic devices, hearing aids, shrapnel, and extreme obesity. Ensure that patient has no metal on clothing (e.g., snaps, zippers, jewelry, credit cards). Convert IV to heparin lock. Inform patient of importance of remaining still throughout examination. Inform patients who are claustrophobic that they may experience symptoms during examination. Administer antianxiety agent (if indicated and ordered). Open MRI may be indicated for obese patient or patient with large chest and abdominal girth or severe claustrophobia. Open MRI may not be available at all facilities.
Bone Mass Measurements		
▪ Radiogrammetry, radiodensitometry	Study evaluates bone mass of metacarpals. A very low dose of radiation is used.	Explain procedure to patient. Inform patient that procedure is painless.
▪ Single-photon absorptiometry (SPA)	Low-dose radiation scanner measures mostly peripheral cortical bone at distal radius or midradius. Study is not useful for follow-up because of slow changes in cortical bone.	Same as above.

Continued

DIAGNOSTIC STUDIES

Table 58-8 Musculoskeletal System—cont'd

Study	Description and Purpose	Nursing Responsibility
Bone Mass Measurements—cont'd		
▪ Dual-photon absorptiometry (DPA)	Technique measures mixed trabecular and cortical bones at sites such as hip and lumbar spine. It can be used to calculate total body calcium concentration.	Same as above.
▪ Dual-energy x-ray absorptiometry (DEXA)	Technique measures bone mass of spine, femur, forearm, and total body. Considered to be fast and precise with low dose of radiation.	Same as above.
Radioisotope Studies		
▪ Bone scan	Technique involves injection of radioisotope (usually sodium pertechnate) that is taken up by bone. Camera scans entire body (front and back), and recording is made on paper. Degree of uptake is related to blood flow to bone. Increased uptake is seen in osteomyelitis, osteoporosis, primary and metastatic malignant lesions of bone, and with certain fractures. Decreased uptake is seen in areas of avascular necrosis.	Give calculated dose of radioisotope 2 hr before procedure. Ensure that bladder is emptied before scan. Inform patient that procedure requires 1 hr while patient lies supine and that no pain or harm will result from isotopes. Be aware that no follow-up scans are required.
Endoscopy		
▪ Arthroscopy	Study involves insertion of arthroscope into joint (usually knee) for visualization of structure and contents. It can be used for exploratory surgery (removal of loose bodies and biopsy) and for diagnosis of abnormalities of meniscus, articular cartilage, ligaments, or joint capsule. Other structures that can be visualized through the arthroscope include the shoulder, elbow, wrist, and ankle.	Inform patient that procedure is performed in operating room with strict asepsis and that either local or general anesthesia is used. After procedure, cover wound with sterile dressing. Wrap leg from midthigh to midcalf with compression dressing for 24 hr for knee arthroscopy. Instruct patient to limit activity for a few days.
Mineral Metabolism		
▪ Alkaline phosphatase	This enzyme, produced by osteoblasts of bone, is needed for mineralization of organic bone matrix. Elevated levels are found in healing fractures, bone cancers, osteoporosis, osteomalacia, and Paget's disease. *Normal:* 20-90 U/L (0.3-1.5 μkat/L).	Obtain blood samples by venipuncture. Observe venipuncture site for bleeding or hematoma formation. Inform patient that procedure does not require fasting.
▪ Calcium	Bone is primary organ for calcium storage. Calcium provides bone with rigid consistency. Decreased serum level is found in osteomalacia, renal disease, and hypoparathyroidism; increased level is found in hyperparathyroidism, some bone tumors. *Normal:* 9-11 mg/dl (2.3-2.7 mmol/L).	Same as above.
▪ Phosphorus	Amount present is indirectly related to calcium metabolism. Decreased level is found in osteomalacia; increased level is found in chronic renal disease, healing fractures, osteolytic metastatic tumor. *Normal:* 2.8-4.5 mg/dl (0.9-1.5 mmol/L).	Same as above.
Serologic Studies		
▪ Rheumatoid factor (RF)	Study assesses presence of autoantibody (rheumatoid factor) in serum. Factor is not specific for rheumatoid arthritis and is seen in other connective tissue diseases, as well as in a small percentage of normal population. *Normal:* negative or titer <1:20.	Same as above.

Continued

DIAGNOSTIC STUDIES

Table 58-8 Musculoskeletal System—cont'd

Study	Description and Purpose	Nursing Responsibility
Serologic Studies—cont'd		
▪ Erythrocyte sedimentation rate (ESR)	Study is nonspecific index of inflammation. Study measures rapidity with which red blood cells settle out of unclotted blood in 1 hr. Results are influenced by physiologic factors, as well as diseases. Elevated levels are seen with any inflammatory process (especially rheumatoid arthritis, rheumatic fever, osteomyelitis, and respiratory infections). *Normal:* <20 mm/hr. Some gender variation.	Observe venipuncture site for bleeding or hematoma formation. Inform patient that procedure does not require fasting.
▪ Lupus erythematosus (LE) cells	Lupus erythematosus cells are seen in about 80% of cases of systemic lupus erythematosus. Normally no lupus erythematosus cells are present.	Obtain blood from patient and have blood smear made on slide. Observe venipuncture site for bleeding or hematoma formation.
▪ Antinuclear antibody (ANA)	Study assesses presence of antibodies capable of destroying nucleus of body's tissue cells. Finding is positive in 95% of patients with systemic lupus erythematosus and may also be positive in individuals with scleroderma or rheumatoid arthritis and in a small percentage of normal population.	Observe venipuncture site for bleeding or hematoma formation. Inform patient that procedure does not require fasting.
▪ Anti-DNA antibody	Study detects serum antibodies that react with DNA. It is the most specific test for systemic lupus erythematosus.	Same as above.
▪ Complement	Complement, a normal body protein, is essential to both immune and inflammatory reactions. Complement components used up in these reactions are depleted. Subsequent test applied to serum yields little or no serum complement components. Complement depletions may be found in patients with rheumatoid arthritis or systemic lupus erythematosus.	Same as above.
▪ Uric acid	End product of purine metabolism is normally excreted in urine. Although not specific, levels are usually elevated in gout. *Normal:* male 4.5-6.5 mg/dl (268-387 μmol/L); female 2.5-5.5 mg/dl (149-327 μmol/L).	Same as above.
▪ C-reactive protein (CRP)	Study is used to diagnose inflammatory diseases, infections, and active widespread malignancy. CRP is synthesized by the liver and is present in large amounts in serum 18-24 hr after onset of tissue damage. *Normal:* negative.	Same as above.
▪ Human leukocyte antigen (HLA)-B27	Antigen present in disorders such as ankylosing spondylitis and variants of rheumatoid arthritis.	Same as above.
Muscle Enzymes		
▪ Creatine kinase (CK)	Highest concentration is found in skeletal muscle. Increased values are found in progressive muscular dystrophy, polymyositis, and traumatic injuries. *Normal:* men 5-55 U/L (0.1-0.9 μkat/L); women 5-35 U/L (0.01-0.6 μkat/L).	Same as above.
▪ Aldolase	Study is useful in monitoring muscular dystrophy and dermatomyositis. *Normal:* 1.0-7.5 U/L (16.7-125 nkat/L).	Same as above.

Continued

DIAGNOSTIC STUDIES

Table 58-8 Musculoskeletal System—cont'd

Study	Description and Purpose	Nursing Responsibility
Muscle Enzymes—cont'd		
▪ Aspartate aminotransferase (AST) or serum glutamic-oxaloacetic transaminase (SGOT)	Enzyme is found in skeletal muscle but is primarily an enzyme of cardiac and hepatic cells. *Normal:* 15-45 U/L (0.12-0.67 μkat/L).	Observe venipuncture site for bleeding or hematoma formation. Inform patient that procedure does not require fasting.
Invasive Procedures		
▪ Arthrocentesis	Incision or puncture of joint capsule is done to obtain samples of synovial fluid from within joint cavity or to remove excess fluid. Local anesthesia and aseptic preparation are used before needle is inserted into joint and fluid aspirated. Study is useful in diagnosis of joint inflammation.	Inform patient that procedure is usually done at bedside or in examination room. Send samples of synovial fluid to laboratory for examination (if indicated). After procedure apply compression dressing and have patient rest joint for 8-24 hr. Observe for leakage of blood or fluid on dressing.
▪ Electromyogram (EMG)	Study evaluates electrical potential associated with skeletal muscle contraction. Long, small-gauge needles are inserted into certain muscles. Needle probes are attached to leads that feed information to electromyogram machine. Recordings of electrical activity of muscle are traced on audiotransmitter, as well as on oscilloscope and recording paper. Study is useful in providing information related to lower motor neuron dysfunction and primary muscle diseases.	Inform patient that procedure is usually done in electromyogram laboratory while patient lies supine on special table. Keep patient awake to cooperate with voluntary movement. Inform patient that procedure involves some discomfort from needle insertion. Avoid administration of stimulants and sedatives 24 hr before procedure.
Miscellaneous		
▪ Thermography	Technique uses infrared detector, which measures degree of heat radiating from skin surface. Study is useful in investigation of cause of inflamed joints and in following up patient's response to antiinflammatory drug therapy.	Inform patient that procedure is painless and noninvasive.
▪ Plethysmography	Study records variations in volume and pressure of blood passing through tissues. Test is nonspecific and quantitative.	Inform patient that procedure is painless and noninvasive.
▪ Somatosensory evoked potential (SSEP)	Study evaluates evoked potential of muscle contractions. Electrodes are placed on skin and provide recordings of electrical activity of muscle. Study useful in identifying subtle dysfunction of lower motor neuron and primary muscle disease. SSEP measures nerve conduction along pathways not accessible by electromyogram. Transcutaneous or percutaneous electrodes are applied to the skin and help identify neuropathy and myopathy.	Inform patient that procedure is similar to electromyogram but does not involve needles. Electrodes are applied to the skin.

Radio waves and magnetic fields are used to construct soft-tissue and bone images. It is advantageous in determining soft-tissue disorders, including cartilage and ligament tears and herniated disks, but it also can be helpful in diagnosing bone disorders such as avascular necrosis, tumors, and multiple myeloma.

Arthroscopy

Endoscopy of the joints involves the use of an arthroscope for direct visualization of the interior of a joint cavity.[5] It is performed in the operating room under sterile conditions. After local or general anesthesia has been administered, a large-bore needle is inserted into the joint and the joint is distended with saline solution (Fig. 58-9). The arthroscope is inserted and the joint cavity is examined. Photographs or videotapes can be made through the scope, and a biopsy of the synovium or cartilage can be obtained. The procedure is particularly useful in the diagnosis of disorders of the knee and shoulder. It can also be used in procedures involving other joints, such as the wrist, elbow, and ankle. Tears in cartilage and other repairs can be made through the arthroscope (arthroscopic surgery), thus eliminating the need for a more extensive incision and surgical procedure.

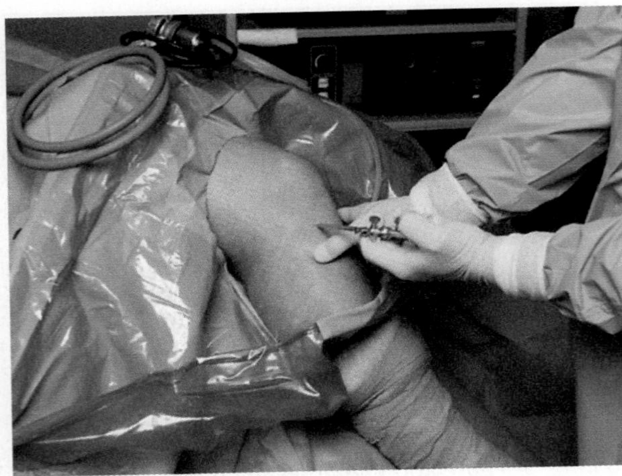

Fig. 58-9 Arthroscopy of a knee.

Arthrocentesis and Synovial Fluid Analysis

An arthrocentesis is usually performed to obtain synovial fluid for examination. It may also be used to instill medications and remove fluid from joints to relieve pain. After the skin has been cleaned, a local anesthetic is instilled. An 18-gauge or larger needle is inserted into the joint, and fluid is aspirated. The appropriate container must be readily available for laboratory analysis of the aspirated fluid. The fluid is examined grossly for volume, color, clarity, viscosity, and mucin clot formation. Normal synovial fluid is clear, light yellow, and scanty (1 to 3 ml). Fluid from a septic joint may be purulent and thick, or gray and thin. In gout the fluid may be whitish yellow. Blood may be aspirated if there is hemarthrosis because of injury. The mucin clot test indicates the character of the protein portion of the synovial fluid. Normally a white, ropelike mucin clot is formed. In an inflammatory process the clot breaks apart easily and fragments.

The fluid is examined microscopically for cell count and identification of the cells. The normal white blood cell (WBC) count is less than 200 cells/μl with fewer than 25% neutrophils and no bacteria. The WBC count and protein are increased in an inflammatory process. The presence of uric acid crystals may indicate gout.

Muscle Enzymes

Muscle enzymes are released from injured or dead muscle cells. Determinations of muscle enzyme values are used to distinguish between muscle weakness that is due to nerve innervation problems and dystrophic disease of the muscle itself. The level of enzymes reflects the progress of the disorder and the effectiveness of treatment. Aspartate aminotransferase (AST) (also known as serum glutamic-oxaloacetic transaminase[SGOT]) levels are the least sensitive indicators of muscle disease, and creatine kinase (CK) levels are the most sensitive. Enzyme levels are also helpful in determining hepatic and cardiac disease.

Serologic Studies

Approximately 85% of people with rheumatoid arthritis and related diseases have an autoantibody known as rheumatoid factor in their serum. This autoantibody is usually of the IgM class, although it may be IgG. The test used to determine the presence of this factor is the latex fixation test. Latex particles are coated with aggregated immunoglobulin G. If serum containing rheumatoid factor is mixed with these latex particles, it reacts with the latex particles and causes agglutination. An estimation of the titer is obtained by performing serial dilutions of the serum.

REVIEW QUESTIONS

The number of the question corresponds to the same-numbered objective at the beginning of the chapter.

1. The bone cells that function in the breakdown of bone tissue (resorption) are called
   a. osteoids.
   b. osteocytes.
   c. osteoclasts.
   d. osteoblasts.
2. While performing passive range of motion for a patient, the nurse puts a hinge joint through the movements of
   a. rotation.
   b. flexion and extension.
   c. flexion, extension, abduction, and adduction.
   d. flexion, extension, abduction, adduction, and circumduction.
3. The nurse teaches a patient with a leg immobilized in traction to prevent muscle atropy in the affected leg by performing
   a. twitch contractions.
   b. tetanic contractions.
   c. isotonic contractions.
   d. isometric contractions.
4. A patient with bursitis of the shoulder asks the nurse what the bursa does. The nurse's response is based on the knowledge that bursae
   a. connect bone to bone.
   b. separate muscle from muscle.
   c. lubricate joints with synovial fluid.
   d. relieve friction between moving parts.
5. The decreased agility found during assessment of the older adult is caused by the age-related change of
   a. decrease in bone mass.
   b. erosion of articular cartilage.
   c. loss of elasticity in ligaments and cartilage.
   d. decrease in number and diameter of muscle cells.
6. While obtaining subjective assessment data related to the musculoskeletal system it is particularly important for the nurse to ask about family history in the patient with
   a. osteomyelitis.
   b. osteomalacia.
   c. low back pain.
   d. rheumatoid arthritis.
7. When grading muscle strength the nurse records a score of 2 indicating
   a. active movement against gravity.
   b. a barely detectable flicker of contraction.
   c. active movement with elimination of gravity.
   d. active movement against full resistance without evident fatigue.
8. A normal assessment finding of the musculoskeletal system is
   a. muscle strength of 4.
   b. a lateral curvature of the spine.
   c. angulation of bone toward midline.
   d. simultaneous occurrence of stance and swing phase of gait.

9. A patient is scheduled for an electromyogram. The nurse explains that this diagnostic test involves
   a. placement of long, thin needles into the muscles.
   b. placement of electrodes on the skin to record electrical activity of muscles.
   c. measurement of the heat of muscle contractions radiating from the skin surface.
   d. administration of a calculated dose of radioisotope 2 hours before the procedure.

References

1. Thompson JM and others, editors: *Mosby's clinical nursing,* ed 4, St Louis, 1997, Mosby.
2. Thibodeau GA, Patton KT: *Anatomy and physiology,* ed 4, St Louis, 1999, Mosby.
3. Guyton AC, Hall JE, editors: *Textbook of medical physiology,* ed 9, Philadelphia, 1996, Saunders.
4. *Mastering geriatric care,* Springhouse, Penn, 1997, Springhouse.
5. Beare PG, Myers JL, editors: *Adult health nursing,* ed 3, St Louis, 1998, Mosby.
6. Browstein B, Bronner S, editors: *Functional movement in orthopaedic and sports physical therapy,* New York, 1997, Churchill Livingstone.
7. Lueckenotte A, editor: *Gerontologic nursing,* St Louis, 1996, Mosby.
8. Ebersole P, Hess P, editors: *Toward healthy aging,* ed 5, St Louis, 1998, Mosby.
9. Potter PA, Perry AG, editors: *Fundamentals of nursing,* ed 4, St Louis, 1997, Mosby.
10. McCance KL, Huether SE, editors: *Pathophysiology: the biologic basis for disease in adults and children,* ed 3, St Louis, 1998, Mosby.

Resources

Resources for this chapter are listed after Chapter 59 on p. 1818.

REMEMBER to check out your companion CD-ROM

59 NURSING MANAGEMENT Musculoskeletal Problems

Susan C. Ruda

www.mosby.com/MERLIN/medsurg_lewis

LEARNING OBJECTIVES

1. Explain the etiology, pathophysiology, clinical manifestations, and collaborative care of soft-tissue injuries, including strains, sprains, dislocations, subluxations, bursitis, carpal tunnel syndrome, repetitive strain injury, and muscle spasms.
2. Describe the sequential events involved in fracture healing.
3. Explain common complications associated with fracture injury and fracture healing.
4. Differentiate among open reduction, closed reduction, traction, and cast immobilization regarding purpose, complications, and nursing management.
5. Describe the neurovascular assessment of an injured extremity.
6. Describe the collaborative care and nursing management of patients with specific fractures.
7. Describe the pathophysiology, collaborative care, and nursing management of osteomyelitis.
8. Describe the indications for and collaborative care and nursing management of amputation.
9. Describe the types, pathophysiology, clinical manifestations, and collaborative care of bone cancer.
10. Differentiate between the causes and characteristics of acute and chronic low back pain.
11. Describe the conservative and surgical treatments of low back pain.
12. Describe the postoperative nursing management of a patient who has undergone spinal surgery.
13. Explain the etiology and collaborative care of common foot disorders.
14. Describe the etiology, pathophysiology, clinical manifestations, and management of metabolic bone disorders.

The most common cause of musculoskeletal problems is injury from accidents resulting in fracture, dislocations, and associated soft-tissue injuries. Although most of these injuries are not fatal, the cost in terms of pain, disability, medical expense, and lost wages is enormous. For all ages, accidents are exceeded only by heart disease, cancer, and strokes as a cause of death. Accidents are the leading cause of death in children and young adults.

The nurse has an important role in educating the public about the basic principles of safety and accident prevention. The morbidity associated with accidents can be significantly reduced if people are aware of environmental hazards, use existing safety equipment, and apply safety and traffic rules. In the industrial setting, the nurse should educate employees and employers about the use of proper safety equipment and avoidance of hazardous working situations.

In the home environment, falls account for many musculoskeletal injuries. Preventive education should be directed toward the importance of wearing shoes with functional soles and heels, avoidance of wet or slippery surfaces, careful placement of throw rugs, and removal of obstacles from the pathway of high risk individuals such as persons with gait instability or visual or cognitive impairment.

Reviewed by Dennis Ross, RN, PhD, Professor of Nursing, Castleton State College, Castleton, Vt; Nursing Faculty, Regents College, Albany, NY.

SOFT-TISSUE INJURIES

Soft-tissue injuries include sprains, strains, dislocations, and subluxation. These common injuries are usually caused by trauma. The increase in the number of people who have committed themselves to maintaining a regular fitness program or participate in sports has contributed to the increased incidence of soft-tissue injuries.[1] Common sports-related injuries are summarized in Table 59-1. Most sport injuries result from direct trauma or contusion or indirect stretch injury.[1]

SPRAINS AND STRAINS

Sprains and strains are the two most common types of injury affecting the musculoskeletal system. These injuries are usually associated with abnormal stretching or twisting forces that may occur during vigorous activities.

A *sprain* is an injury to ligamentous structures surrounding a joint, usually caused by a wrenching or twisting motion. A sprain is classified according to the amount of ligament fibers torn. A first-degree sprain involves tears of only a few fibers resulting in mild tenderness and slight swelling. A second-degree sprain is partial disruption of the involved tissue with more swelling and tenderness. A third-degree sprain is a complete tearing of the ligament. A gap in the muscle may be apparent or felt through the skin if the muscle is torn. Because these areas are rich in nerve endings, the injury can be extremely painful. The most common areas of sprains occur in the ankle

Table 59-1 Common Sports-Related Injuries

Injury	Definition	Treatment
Impingement syndrome	Entrapment of soft-tissue structures under coracoacromial arch of the shoulder	NSAIDs; rest until symptoms decrease and then gradual range-of-motion and strengthening exercises
Rotator cuff tear	Tear within muscle or ligaments of shoulder	If minor tear, rest, NSAIDs, and gradual mobilization with range-of-motion and strengthening exercises If major tear, surgical repair
Shin splints	Inflammation along tibial shaft from tearing away of tendons caused by improper shoes, overuse, or running on hard pavement	Rest, ice, NSAIDs, proper shoes; gradual increase in activity; if pain persists, x-ray should be done to rule out stress fracture of tibia
Tendinitis	Inflammation of tendon in upper or lower extremity as a result of overuse or incorrect use	Rest, ice, NSAIDs; gradual return to sport activity; protective brace (orthosis) may be necessary if symptoms recur
Ligament injury	Tearing or stretching of ligament; usually occurs as a result of direct blow; characterized by sudden pain, swelling, and instability	Rest, ice, NSAIDs; protection of affected extremity by use of brace; if symptoms persist, surgical repair may be necessary
Meniscal injury	Injury to fibrocartilage of the knee characterized by popping, clicking, or tearing sensation, swelling	Rest, ice, NSAIDs; gradual return to regular activities; if symptoms persist, surgical arthroscopy to diagnose and repair meniscal injury may be necessary

NSAIDs, nonsteroidal antiinflammatory drugs.

and wrist. A *strain* is a stretching of a muscle and its fascial sheath.

The clinical manifestations of sprains and strains are similar and include pain, edema, decrease in function, and bruising. Pain aggravated by continued use is common. Edema develops in the injured area because of minute hemorrhages within the disrupted tissues and the ensuing inflammatory response. Usually the patient will recount a history of traumatic injury, possibly of a twisting nature, or recent exercise activity.

Minor sprains and strains are usually self-limiting, with full function returning within 3 to 6 weeks. A severe sprain can result in an avulsion fracture, in which the ligament pulls loose a fragment of bone. Alternatively, the joint structure may become unstable and result in subluxation or dislocation. At the time of injury, hemarthrosis (bleeding into a joint space or cavity) or disruption of the synovial lining may occur. An acute strain may involve partial or complete rupture of a muscle.

X-rays of the affected part are usually taken to rule out a fracture or widening of the joint structure. Surgical repair may be necessary if the injury is significant enough to produce severe disruption of ligamentous or muscle structures, fracture, or dislocation.

NURSING MANAGEMENT: SPRAINS AND STRAINS

■ Nursing Implementation

Health Promotion. The use of elastic support bandages or adhesive tape wrapping before beginning a vigorous activity is thought to reduce the occurrence of sprains. However, some physicians do not support preventive wrapping or taping because it may predispose the athlete to injury. Stretching and warm-up exercises before vigorous activity significantly reduce sprains and strains.

Preconditioning exercise protects an inherently weak joint, because slow stretching is tolerated better by biologic tissues than is quick stretching. Warm-up exercises "prelengthen" potentially strained tissues by avoiding the quick stretch often encountered in sports. Warm-up exercises also increase the temperature of muscle, which increases the speed of cell metabolism and the speed of nerve impulse transmission. The increased metabolism contributes to better oxygenation of muscle fiber during work. Stretching is also thought to improve kinesthetic awareness, thus lessening the chance of uncoordinated movement.

Acute Intervention. If an injury occurs, the immediate care focuses on (1) rest and limitation of movement, (2) application of ice to the injured area, (3) compression of the involved extremity, (4) elevation of the extremity, and (5) analgesia as necessary (Table 59-2). Movement should be limited and the extremity rested as soon as pain is felt. Unless the injury is severe, prolonged rest is usually not necessary. Cold in several forms can be used to produce hypothermia to the involved part. Physiologic changes that occur in soft tissue as a result of the use of cold include vasoconstriction, reduction in transmission of nerve impulses, and reduction in conduction velocity. These changes result in analgesia and anesthesia, reduction of muscle spasm without changes in muscular strength or endurance, reduction of local edema and inflammation, and reduction of local metabolic requirements. Few unwanted side effects accompany the use of cold to treat a soft-tissue injury. Cold is most useful when applied immediately after the injury has occurred. Ice applications should not exceed 20 to 30 minutes per application, allowing a "warm-down" time of 10 to 15 minutes between applications.

Compression also helps limit swelling, which, if left uncontrolled, could lengthen healing time. An elastic compression

✚ EMERGENCY MANAGEMENT

Table 59-2 Acute Soft-Tissue Injury

Etiology	Assessment Findings	Interventions
Falls Direct blows Crush injury Motor vehicle collisions Sports injuries	■ Edema ■ Ecchymosis ■ Pain, tenderness ■ Decreased sensation with severe edema ■ Decreased pulse, coolness, and capillary refill ■ Decreased movement ■ Pallor ■ Shortening or rotation of extremity ■ Inability to bear weight when lower extremity involved ■ Decreased function with upper-extremity involvement ■ Muscle spasms	**Initial** ■ Ensure airway, breathing, and circulation. ■ Assess neurovascular status of involved limb. ■ Elevate involved limb. ■ Apply compression bandage unless dislocation present. ■ Apply ice packs to affected area. ■ Immobilize affected extremity in the position found. ■ Anticipate x-rays of injured extremity. ■ Give analgesia as necessary. ■ Administer tetanus prophylaxis if skin integrity broken. **Ongoing Monitoring** ■ Monitor for changes in neurovascular status. ■ Eliminate weight bearing when lower extremity involved. ■ Anticipate compartment pressure monitoring if neurovascular status changes.

bandage can be wrapped around the injured part. The bandage is too tight if numbness is felt in the area or there is cramping or additional pain or swelling beyond the edge of the bandage. The bandage can be left in place for 30 minutes and then removed for 15 minutes.

The injured part should be elevated above the heart level to help drain excess fluid from the area and impede further edema. The injured part should be elevated even during sleep. Mild analgesia such as aspirin, ibuprofen, or acetaminophen may be necessary to manage patient discomfort.

After the acute phase (usually lasting 24 to 48 hours), warm, moist heat can be applied to the affected part to reduce swelling and provide comfort. Heat applications should not exceed 20 to 30 minutes, allowing a "cool down" time between applications. Nonsteroidal antiinflammatory drugs (NSAIDs) may be recommended to decrease edema and pain. The patient is encouraged to use the limb provided that the joint is protected by means of casting, taping, or splinting. Movement of the joint maintains nutrition to the cartilage, and muscle contraction speeds circulation and resolution of the hematoma.

Ambulatory and Home Care. With the exception of treatment in the emergency department following the injury, sprains and strains are treated in the outpatient setting. The patient should be instructed in the use of ice and elevation for 24 to 72 hours after injury to reduce edema. The use of mild analgesics to promote comfort should be encouraged. Use of an elastic wrap may provide additional support during activity. To prevent reinjury, the patient should learn proper measures of prevention.

The physical therapist may help provide added comfort by means of specialized techniques, such as ultrasound. The therapist may also teach the patient exercises to perform to strengthen shortened muscles.

DISLOCATION AND SUBLUXATION

A *dislocation* is a severe injury of the ligamentous structures that surround a joint. It results in the complete displacement or separation of the articular surfaces of the joint. A *subluxation* is a partial or incomplete displacement of the joint surface. The clinical manifestations of a subluxation are similar to those of a dislocation but are less severe. Treatment of subluxation is similar to that of a dislocation, but subluxation requires less healing time.

Dislocations characteristically result from overwhelming forces transmitted to the joint that cause a disruption of the soft tissues surrounding the joint. The joints most frequently dislocated in the upper extremity include the thumb, elbow, and shoulder. In the lower extremity, the hip is vulnerable to dislocation occurring as a result of severe trauma, often associated with motor vehicle accidents (Fig. 59-1). The patella may dislocate because of instability of the ligaments surrounding the knee.

The most obvious clinical manifestation of a dislocation is asymmetry of the musculoskeletal contour. For example, if a hip is dislocated, the limb is shorter on the affected side. Additional manifestations include local pain, tenderness, loss of function of the injured part, and swelling of the soft tissues in the region of the joint. The major complications of a dislocated joint are open joint injuries, intraarticular fractures, fracture dislocation, avascular necrosis, and damage to adjacent neurovascular tissue.

X-ray studies are performed to determine the extent of shifting of the involved structures. The joint may also be aspirated to determine the presence of blood (hemarthrosis) or fat cells. Fat cells from the synovial fluid indicate probable intraarticular fracture.

NURSING AND COLLABORATIVE MANAGEMENT: DISLOCATION

A dislocation requires prompt attention. The longer the joint remains unreduced, the greater is the possibility of avascular necrosis (bone cell death as a result of inadequate blood supply). The hip joint is particularly susceptible to avascular necrosis. The first goal of management is to realign the dislocated

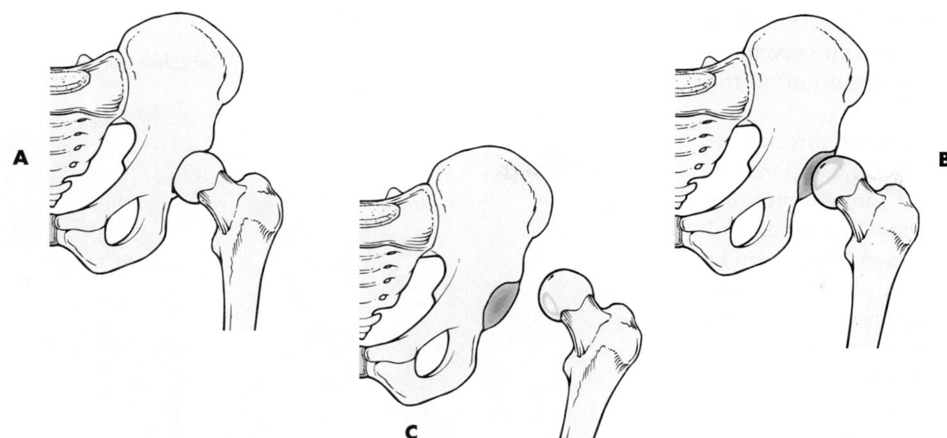

Fig. 59-1 Soft-tissue injury of the hip. A, Normal. B, Subluxation (partial dislocation). C, Dislocation.

portion of the joint in its original anatomic position. This can be accomplished by a closed reduction, which may be performed under local or general anesthesia. Anesthesia is often necessary to produce muscle relaxation so that the bones can be manipulated. In some situations, surgical open reduction may be necessary. After reduction, the extremity is usually immobilized by taping or using a sling to allow the torn ligaments and capsular tissue time to heal. Observation is indicated for the patient with a posterior sternoclavicular dislocation because delayed intrathoracic complications, such as pneumothorax or subclavian vessel injury, may occur.[2]

Nursing management of subluxation or dislocation is directed toward relief of pain and support and protection of the injured joint. After the joint has been reduced and immobilized, motion is usually restricted. A carefully regulated rehabilitation program can prevent the formation of contractures. The patient should not stretch the joint beyond its limits because the torn capsule and ligament heal in a shortened position with fibrous scar tissue that is not as strong as the original tissue. An exercise program slowly and methodically restores the joint to its original range of motion without causing another dislocation. The patient should gradually return to normal activities.

A patient who has dislocated a joint may be at greater risk to experience repeated dislocations because the joint has been weakened by shortened ligaments and scar tissue. Activity restrictions of the affected joint may be imposed to decrease the risk of repeatedly dislocating the joint.

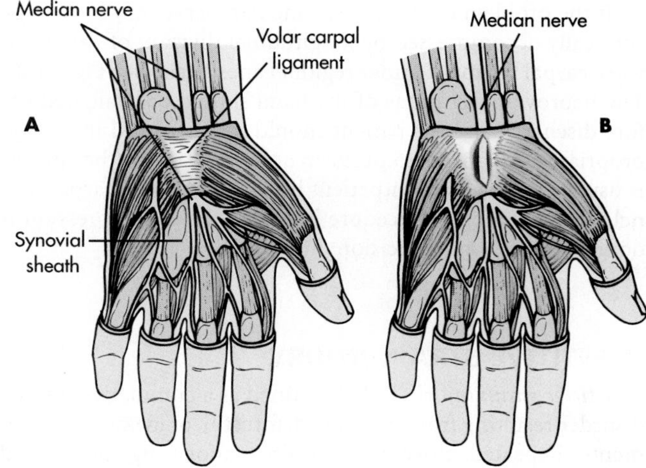

Fig. 59-2 A, Wrist structures involved in carpal tunnel syndrome. B, Decompression of median nerve.

CARPAL TUNNEL SYNDROME

Carpal tunnel syndrome is a condition caused by compression of the median nerve beneath the transverse carpal ligament within the narrow confines of the carpal tunnel located at the wrist (Fig. 59-2). This condition frequently is due to pressure from trauma or edema caused by inflammation of a tendon (tenosynovitis), neoplasm, rheumatoid synovial disease, or soft-tissue masses such as ganglia. Carpal tunnel syndrome occurs most frequently in middle-aged or postmenopausal women. This syndrome is associated with occupations that require continuous wrist movement (e.g., butchers, musicians, hair stylists, secretaries, carpenters, computer operators).

The clinical manifestations of carpal tunnel syndrome are weakness (especially of the thumb), pain and numbness, or impaired sensation in the distribution of the median nerve, and clumsiness in performing fine hand movements. Numbness and tingling may be present that awaken the patient at night. Holding the wrist in acute flexion for 60 seconds will produce tingling and numbness over the distribution of the median nerve, the palmar surface of the thumb, the index finger, the middle finger, and part of the ring finger. This is known as a positive Phalen's sign. Tapping gently over the area of the inflamed median nerve may reproduce the paresthesia. This is known as a positive Tinel's sign. In late stages there is atrophy of the thenar muscles around the base of the thumb. This syndrome can result in recurrent pain and eventual dysfunction of the hand.

NURSING AND COLLABORATIVE MANAGEMENT: CARPAL TUNNEL SYNDROME

Prevention of carpal tunnel syndrome involves educating employees and employers to identify risk factors. Adaptive devices such as wrist splints may be worn to hold the wrist in slight dorsiflexion to relieve pressure on the median nerve. Special keyboard pads that help prevent repetitive pressure on the median nerve are available for computer operators to help prevent or reduce carpal tunnel syndrome by decreasing tension on the carpal tunnel.

Collaborative care of carpal tunnel syndrome is directed toward relieving the underlying cause of the nerve compression. The early symptoms associated with carpal tunnel syndrome can usually be relieved by stopping the aggravating action and by placing the hand and wrist at rest by immobilizing them in a hand splint. If the cause is inflammation, injection of hydrocortisone directly into the carpal tunnel may provide relief. The patient's sensation may be impaired. Therefore the patient should be instructed to avoid hazards such as extreme heat because of the risk of thermal injury. Nursing care of the patient with carpal tunnel syndrome usually occurs in the office or outpatient setting. The patient may be required to consider occupational changes because of discomfort and sensory and functional changes.

If the problem continues, the median nerve may have to be surgically decompressed by longitudinal division of the transverse carpal ligament under regional anesthesia (see Fig. 59-2). The neurovascular status of the hand should be evaluated before discharge and the patient should be instructed in the appropriate assessments to perform at home because the surgery is usually done on an outpatient basis. Endoscopic carpal tunnel release is a new procedure in which the decompression is done through a small incision puncture site.

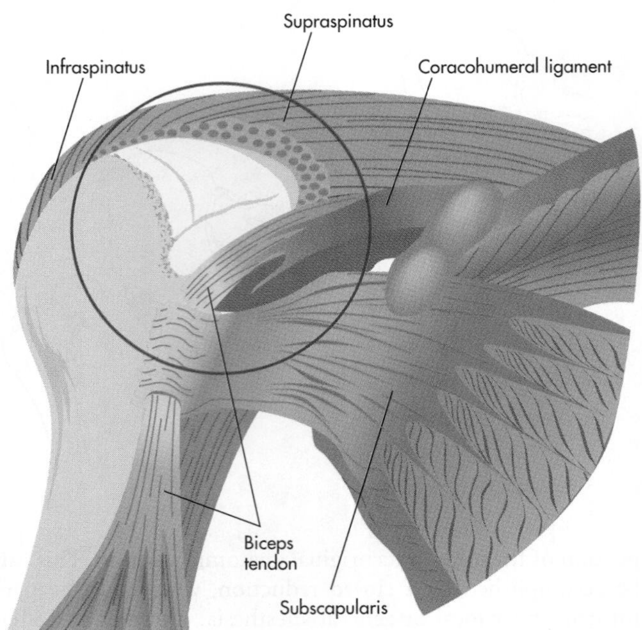

Fig. 59-3 Massive rotator cuff tear.

REPETITIVE STRAIN INJURY

Repetitive strain injury (RSI) is defined as a cumulative trauma disorder resulting from prolonged, forceful, or awkward movements. Repeated movements strain tendons, ligaments, and muscles, causing tiny tears that become inflamed. If the tissues are not given time to heal properly, scarring can occur. Blood vessels of the arms and hands may become constricted, depriving tissues of vital nutrients and causing an accumulation of factors such as lactic acid. Without intervention, tendons and muscles can deteriorate and nerves become hypersensitive. At this point even the slightest movement can cause pain.

In addition to the repetitive movements, other factors related to RSI include poor posture and positioning, ill-fitting furniture, a badly designed keyboard, and a heavy workload. The result is damage to the muscles, tendons, and nerves of the neck, shoulder, forearm, and hand. Symptoms of RSI include pain, weakness, numbness, or impairment of motor function. Persons most often affected by RSI include musicians, dancers, electricians, butchers, and, most commonly, keyboard operators.[3]

RSI is becoming a serious public health problem. Reported incidence has risen from 1% to 4% in less than 10 years. It is theorized that the increase is due to increased productivity, an increased number of women in the workforce, and a heightened awareness of RSI in the media and health care system.[4] It is expected that the number of cases of RSI will continue to increase as computers become more commonplace.

RSI can be prevented through education, ergonomics (consideration of the interaction of humans and their work environment), and appropriate job design. Once diagnosed, the treatment of RSI consists of avoidance of the precipitating activity, physical therapy, and careful use of analgesia. In most cases, the muscle and tendon damage associated with RSI cannot be surgically repaired.

ROTATOR CUFF INJURIES

The rotator cuff is a complex of four muscles in the shoulder: supraspinatus, infraspinatus, teres minor, and subscapularis. These muscles act to stabilize the humeral head in the glenoid fossa and rotate the humerus.[5]

A tear in the rotator cuff may occur as a gradual, degenerative process resulting from aging, poor posture, repetitive stress (especially overhead arm motions), or using an arm to break a fall[6] (Fig. 59-3). Young adults are more prone to experience a tear as a result of trauma such as a fall, lifting a heavy object, or throwing a ball.

Patients with a rotator cuff injury will complain of shoulder pain and cannot initiate or maintain abduction of the arm or shoulder. An X-ray alone is usually not much benefit in diagnosing a rotator cuff injury. A tear can be confirmed by arthrogram or magnetic resonance imaging (MRI).[7]

The patient may be treated conservatively with rest, ice and heat, NSAIDs, periodic corticosteroid injections into the joint, and physical therapy. If the patient does not respond to conservative treatment or if a complete tear is present, a surgical repair may be necessary. Surgical repair may be done through the arthroscope. If an extensive tear is present, open repair may be necessary. An immobilization device such as a sling or more commonly a shoulder immobilizer may be used for several weeks after surgery.[8] Exercises and physical therapy begin within a few days of surgery.

MENISCUS INJURY

The meniscus is the fibrous cartilage in the knee and other joints. Meniscus injuries are closely associated with ligament

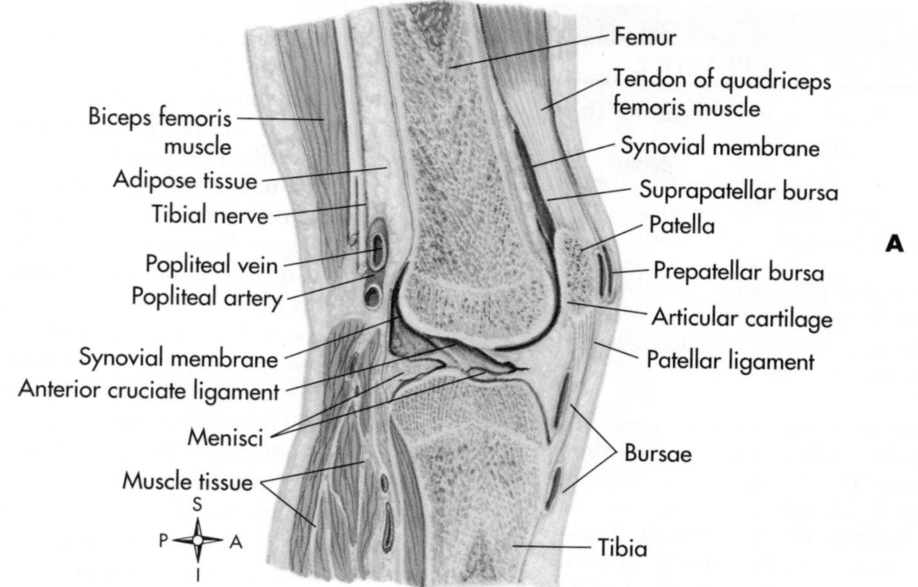

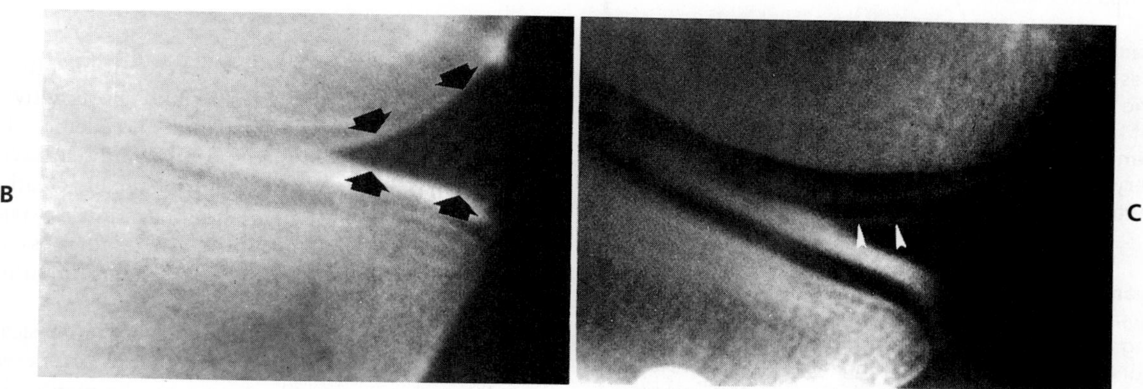

Fig. 59-4 **A,** Sagittal section through knee joint. Knee arthrogram. **B,** Normal medial meniscus. Spot film shows normal triangular shape of meniscus *(arrows)*. **C,** Linear tear of medial meniscus *(arrowheads)*.

sprains commonly occurring in athletes engaged in sports such as basketball, rugby, football, soccer, and hockey. These activities produce a rotational stress when the knee is in a flexed position and the foot is fixed. A blow to the knee can cause the meniscus to be trapped between the femoral condyles and the plateau of the tibia, resulting in a torn meniscus (Fig. 59-4). A causal relationship exists between occupations that require working in a squatting or kneeling position and meniscus injuries.

Meniscus injuries alone do not usually cause chronic edema because cartilage is avascular and aneural. However, a torn meniscus may be suspected when local tenderness or pain is reported. Pain is elicited by abduction or adduction of the leg at the knee. The usual clinical picture is a feeling by the patient that the knee is unstable and a report that the knee may click and lock periodically. Quadriceps atrophy is evident if the injury has been present for some time. Degenerative joint disease can occur if a damaged, roughened meniscus is not surgically removed.

An arthrogram or arthroscopy or both can diagnose knee problems. MRI is beneficial in confirming the diagnosis before arthroscopy is used. MRI has eliminated the use of an arthrogram as a diagnostic tool in many cases.

NURSING AND COLLABORATIVE MANAGEMENT: MENISCUS INJURY

Because meniscal injuries are commonly caused by sports-related activity, athletes should be educated about warm-up activities. Proper stretching may make the patient less prone to meniscal injury when a fall or twisting occurs. Examination of the acutely injured knee should occur within 24 hours of injury. Initial care of this type of injury involves application of ice, immobilization, and partial weight bearing with crutches. Most meniscal injuries are treated in an outpatient setting. The patient should be allowed to ambulate as tolerated. Crutches may

RESEARCH

IMPLICATIONS FOR NURSING PRACTICE

Effectiveness of Education in Patients with Total Knee Arthroplasty

Citation Lin P, Lin L, Lin J: Comparing the effectiveness of different education programs for patients with total knee arthroplasty, *Orthop Nurs* 16:43, 1997.

Purpose To compare the differences between patients having two different types of educational programs on subsequent outcomes of anxiety, knowledge level, exercise performance, and recovery.

Methods A quasi-experimental design was used. The experimental group ($n = 30$) received preadmission (outpatient) and preoperative (hospital) teaching with the control group ($n = 30$) receiving only preoperative teaching. Mean subject age was 69 years. In the preoperative and postoperative phases both groups completed questionnaires related to anxiety and knowledge about arthroplasty. Data were also collected postoperatively on regularity and accuracy of exercises performed and recovery.

Results and Conclusions There were no significant differences between the two groups in preoperative anxiety. The experimental group had a significantly higher level of knowledge and performed exercises more regularly and correctly than subjects in the control group. Recovery as evidenced by flexion of the operative knee joint was significantly higher in the experimental group.

Implications for Nursing Practice Preoperative teaching alone may not be effective in reducing anxiety and increasing patient knowledge about impending surgery. The nurse should begin teaching the patient before hospital admission with repeated preoperative instruction before surgery. The extra time allowed for learning may be especially helpful for older patients who are in an unfamiliar hospital environment. Providing teaching before hospital admission when anxiety is lower may facilitate improved patient outcomes.

be necessary. Use of an immobilizer during the first few days protects the knee.

After acute pain has decreased, gradual increases in flexion and strengthening help return the patient to full functioning. Physical therapy may be needed to help the patient strengthen muscles before returning to sport activities. Surgical repair or excision of part of the meniscus (meniscectomy) may be necessary. Frequently this can be done by arthroscopy.

Use of the laser for arthroscopy is being investigated. It is used to vaporize the exposed tissue in an area where precise cutting and ablation of tissue is needed during an arthroscopy. The value of the laser for arthroscopic surgery is undergoing clinical research.[9]

BURSITIS

Bursae are closed sacs that are lined with synovial membrane and contain a small amount of synovial fluid. They are located at sites of friction, such as between tendons, bones, and overlying joints. A bursa may become inflamed (bursitis) from repeated or excessive trauma or friction, gout, rheumatoid arthritis, or infection. The primary clinical manifestations of bursitis are warmth, pain and swelling, and limited range of motion in the affected part. Sites at which bursitis commonly occurs include the hand, knee, trochanter, shoulder, and elbow.

Attempts are made to determine and correct the cause of the bursitis. Rest is often the only treatment needed. Icing the area will decrease pain and may reduce inflammation. The affected part may be immobilized in a compression dressing or plaster splint. NSAIDs may be recommended to reduce inflammation and pain. Aspiration of the bursal fluid and injection of hydrocortisone may be necessary. If the bursa wall has become thickened and continues to interfere with normal joint function, surgical excision (bursectomy) may be necessary. For example, subacromial bursal thickening causes pain and loss of range of motion on abduction of the shoulder. Septic bursae usually require surgical drainage.

MUSCLE SPASMS

Local muscle spasms are a common condition often associated with excessive everyday activities and sports activities. Injury to a muscle results in inflammation and edema, which stimulates free nerve endings, resulting in muscle excitation and spasm. The spasms produce additional pain, creating a repetitive cycle. The clinical manifestations of muscle spasm include pain, palpable muscle mass in spasm, tenderness, diminished range of motion of the affected site, and limitation of daily activities.

A careful history should be taken and a physical examination should be performed to rule out central nervous system (CNS) problems. Muscle spasms can be managed with drug therapy, physical therapy, or both. A physical therapy program might include the use of heat or ice, supervised exercise, massage, hydrotherapy, local heat-producing applications (oil of wintergreen), ultrasound (deep heat), manipulation, and bracing. Drugs used for treatment of local muscle spasm include mild analgesics, NSAIDs, and skeletal muscle relaxants.

FRACTURES

Classification

A *fracture* is a disruption or break in the continuity of the structure of bone. Traumatic injuries account for the majority of fractures, although some fractures are secondary to a disease process (pathologic fractures). Fractures are described and classified according to (1) type (Fig. 59-5), (2) communication or noncommunication with the external environment (Fig. 59-6), and (3) location of fracture (Fig. 59-7). Fractures are also described as stable or unstable. A stable fracture occurs when some of the periosteum is intact across the fracture and either external or internal fixation has rendered the fragments stationary. Stable fractures are usually transverse, spiral, or greenstick. An unstable fracture is grossly displaced

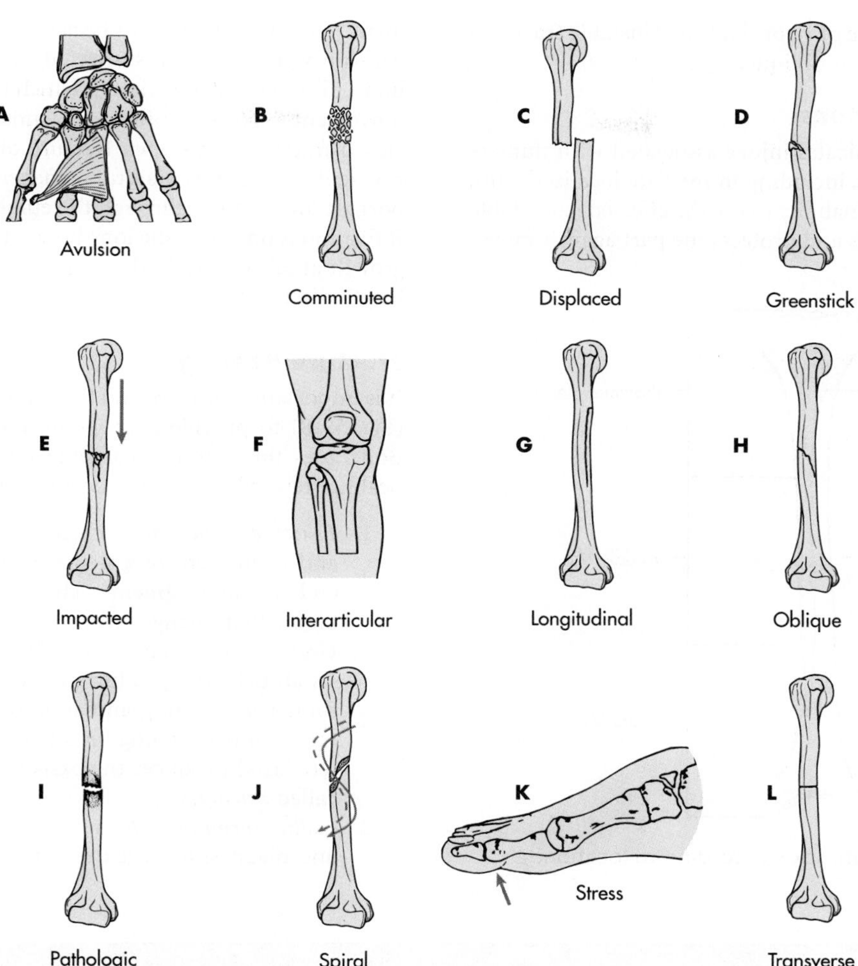

Fig. 59-5 Types of fractures. **A,** An avulsion is a fracture of bone resulting from the strong pulling effect of tendons or ligaments at the bone attachment. **B,** A comminuted fracture is a fracture with more than two fragments. The smaller fragments appear to be floating. **C,** A displaced (overriding) fracture involves a displaced fracture fragment that is overriding the other bone fragment. The periosteum is disrupted on both sides. **D,** A greenstick fracture is an incomplete fracture with one side splintered and the other side bent. **E,** An impacted fracture is a comminuted fracture in which more than two fragments are driven into each other. **F,** An interarticular fracture is a fracture extending to the articular surface of the bone. **G,** A longitudinal fracture is an incomplete fracture in which the fracture line runs along the longitudinal axis of the bone. The periosteum is not torn away from the bone. **H,** An oblique fracture is a fracture in which the line of the fracture extends in an oblique direction. **I,** A pathologic fracture is a spontaneous fracture at the site of a bone disease. **J,** A spiral fracture is a fracture in which the line of the fracture extends in a spiral direction along the shaft of the bone. **K,** A stress fracture is a fracture that occurs in normal or abnormal bone that is subject to repeated stress, such as from jogging or running. **L,** A transverse fracture is a fracture in which the line of the fracture extends across the bone shaft at a right angle to the longitudinal axis.

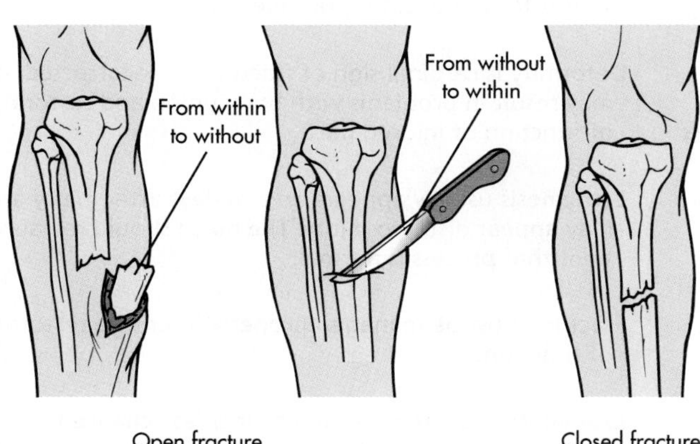

Fig. 59-6 Fracture classification according to communication.

during injury and is a site of poor fixation. Unstable fractures are usually comminuted or oblique.

Clinical Manifestations

The patient's history indicates injury associated with numerous signs and symptoms, including immediate localized pain, decreased function, and inability to use the affected part (Table 59-3). The patient guards and protects the part against movement. The fracture may not be accompanied by obvious bone deformity. If a fracture is suspected, the affected part should be immobilized in the position in which it is found. Unnecessary movement increases soft-tissue damage and may convert a closed fracture to an open fracture or involve adjacent neurovascular structures. Careful management is particularly important for fractures through the epiphyseal plate in children. If fixation is not solid, the long bone may cease its longitudinal growth at all or part of the epiphyseal plate, causing a limb-length discrepancy.

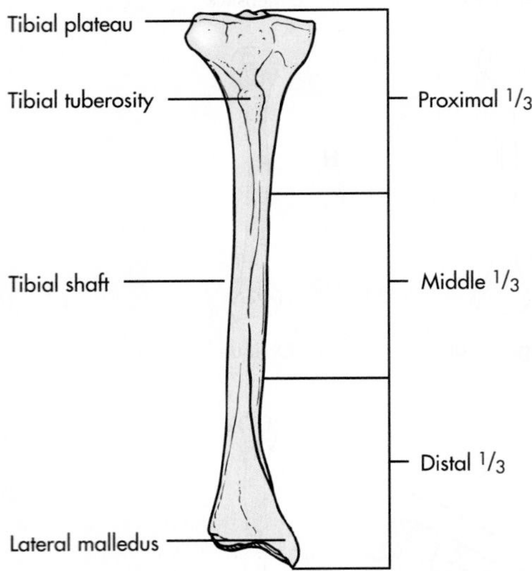

Fig. 59-7 Fracture classification according to location.

Fracture Healing

It is important to understand the principles of fracture healing (Fig. 59-8) to provide appropriate therapeutic interventions. Bone goes through a remarkable reparative process of self-healing (termed *union*) that occurs in the following stages:

1. *Fracture hematoma.* When a fracture occurs, bleeding and edema create a hematoma, which surrounds the ends of the fragments. The hematoma is extravasated blood that changes from a liquid to a semisolid clot.
2. *Granulation tissue.* During this stage active phagocytosis absorbs the products of local necrosis. The hematoma converts to granulation tissue. Granulation tissue (consisting of young blood vessels, fibroblasts, and osteoblasts) produces the basis for a new bone substance called *osteoid.*
3. *Callus formation.* As minerals (calcium, phosphorus, and magnesium) are deposited in the osteoid, it forms

Table 59-3 Clinical Manifestations of Fracture

Manifestation	Significance
Edema and Swelling	
Disruption of soft tissues or bleeding into surrounding tissues	Unchecked edema in closed space can occlude circulation and damage nerves (i.e., there is a risk of acute compartment syndrome).
Pain and Tenderness	
Muscle spasm as result of involuntary reflex action of muscle, direct tissue trauma, increased pressure on sensory nerve, movement of fracture parts	Pain and tenderness encourage splinting of fracture with reduction in motion of injured area.
Muscle Spasm	
Protective response to injury and fracture	Muscle spasms may displace nondisplaced fracture or prevent it from reducing spontaneously.
Deformity	
Abnormal position of bone as result of original forces of injury and action of muscles pulling fragment into abnormal position; seen as a loss of normal bony contours	Deformity is cardinal sign of fracture; if uncorrected, it may result in problems with bony union and restoration of function of injured part.
Ecchymosis	
Discoloration of skin as result of extravasation of blood in subcutaneous tissues	Ecchymosis usually appears several days after injury and may appear distal to injury. The nurse should reassure patient that process is normal.
Loss of Function	
Disruption of bone, preventing functional use	Fracture must be managed properly to ensure restoration of function.
Crepitation	
Grating or crunching together of bony fragments, producing palpable or audible crunching sensation	Examination of crepitation may increase chance for nonunion if bone ends are allowed to move excessively.

an unorganized network of bone that is woven about the fracture parts. Callus is primarily composed of cartilage, osteoblasts, calcium, and phosphorus. It usually begins to appear by the end of the first week after injury. Evidence of callus formation can be verified by x-ray.

4. *Ossification.* Ossification of the callus begins within 2 to 3 weeks after the fracture and continues until the fracture has healed. This stage is marked by ossification of the callus that is sufficient to prevent movement at the fracture site when the bones are gently stressed. However, the fracture is still evident on x-ray. During this stage of clinical union the patient can be converted from skeletal traction to a cast or the cast can be removed to allow limited mobility.
5. *Consolidation.* As callus continues to develop, the distance between bone fragments diminishes and eventually closes. This stage is called *consolidation,* and ossification continues. It can be equated with radiographic union.
6. *Remodeling.* Excess tissue is absorbed in the final stage of bone healing, and union is completed. Gradual return of the injured bone to its preinjury structural strength and shape occurs. Remodeling of bone is enhanced as it responds to physical stress. Initially, stress is provided through exercise. Weight bearing is gradually introduced. New bone is deposited in sites subjected to stress and resorbed at areas where there is little stress. Radiographic union occurs when there is x-ray evidence of complete bony union.

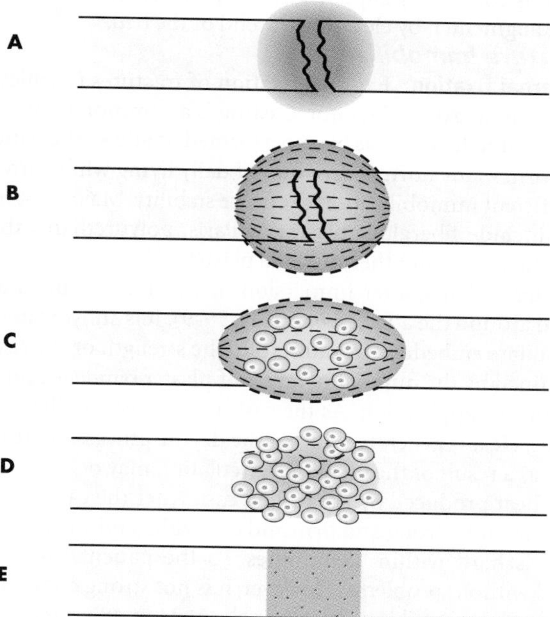

Fig. 59-8 Bone healing (schematic representation). **A,** Bleeding at broken ends of the bone with subsequent hematoma formation. **B,** Organization of hematoma into fibrous network. **C,** Invasion of osteoblasts, lengthening of collagen strands, and deposition of calcium. **D,** Callus formation: new bone is built up as osteoclasts destroy dead bone. **E,** Remodeling is accomplished as excess callus is reabsorbed and trabecular bone is laid down.

Many factors, such as age, initial displacement of the fracture, site of the fracture, and blood supply to the area, influence the time required for fracture healing to be complete. Fracture healing may not occur in the expected time (delayed union) or may not occur at all (nonunion). The ossification process is arrested by causes such as inadequate immobilization and reduction, excess movement, infection, and poor nutrition. Healing time for fractures increases with age. For example, an uncomplicated midshaft fracture of the femur heals in 3 weeks in a newborn and requires 20 weeks in an adult. Table 59-4 summarizes complications of fracture healing.

Electrical stimulation is used successfully to stimulate bone healing in some situations of nonunion or delayed union. The electric current acts by modifying cell behavior causing bone remodeling.[10] The underlying mechanism for electrically induced bone remodeling remains unknown. It is thought to be related to negative electrical fields attracting positive ions such as calcium. The electrodes are semiinvasive, noninvasive, or surgically implanted. Patient motivation and adherence to prescribed stimulator use must be high because the treatment can take up to 10 hours a day for many months.[11]

Collaborative Care

The overall goals of fracture treatment are (1) anatomic realignment of bone fragments known as reduction, (2) immobilization to maintain realignment, and (3) restoration of function of the injured part. Table 59-5 summarizes the collaborative care of fractures.

Fracture Reduction

Manipulation or closed reduction. Manipulation is a nonsurgical, manual realignment of bone fragments to their previous anatomic position. Traction and countertraction are manually applied to the bone fragments to restore position, length, and alignment. Closed reduction is usually performed under local or general anesthesia. After reduction or manipulation, the injured part is immobilized by traction, casting, external fixation, splints, or orthoses (braces) to maintain alignment until healing occurs.

Open reduction. Open reduction is the correction of bone alignment through a surgical incision. It frequently includes internal fixation of the fracture with the use of wire, screws, pins, plates, intramedullary rods, or nails. The type and location of the fracture, age of patient, and concurrent disease, as well as the result of attempted closed reduction by means of traction, may influence the decision to use open reduction. The chief disadvantages of this form of treatment are the possibility of infection and the complications associated with anesthesia.

If open reduction with internal fixation (ORIF) is used for intraarticular fractures (involving joint surfaces), early initiation of range of motion of the joint is indicated. Machines that provide continuous passive motion (CPM) to various joints are now available. Use of such machines can result in prevention of intraarticular adhesions, faster reconstruction of the subchondral (beneath cartilage) bone plate, more rapid healing of the articular cartilage, and possibly decreased incidence of later posttraumatic arthritis. If open reduction is used, early ambulation may be initiated in some instances for patients with lower-extremity fractures. Early ambulation decreases the risk of complications related to prolonged immobility while also facilitating healing with gradually increasing increments of stress.

Table 59-4 Complications of Fracture Healing

Problem	Description
Delayed union	Fracture healing progresses more slowly than expected; healing eventually occurs.
Nonunion	Fracture fails to heal properly despite treatment, resulting in fibrous union or pseudoarthrosis.
Malunion	Fracture heals in expected time but in unsatisfactory position, possibly resulting in deformity or dysfunction.
Angulation	Fracture heals in abnormal position in relation to midline of structure (type of malunion).
Pseudoarthrosis	This type of nonunion occurs at fracture site in which false joint is formed on shaft of long bones. It is a fracture site that failed to fuse (neoarthrosis). Each bone end is covered with fibrous scar tissue.
Posttraumatic osteoporosis	This condition represents loss of mineral (bone substance) as result of immobilization or disuse.
Refracture	New fracture occurs through original fracture site.
Myositis ossificans	This condition is a response to muscle hemorrhage caused by trauma. The hematoma ossifies. Response may occur in arm, elbow, and thigh.

COLLABORATIVE CARE

Table 59-5 Fractures

Diagnostic
- History and physical examination
- X-ray examination
- CT scan or MRI

Collaborative Therapy

Fracture Reduction
- Manipulation
- Open reduction
- Closed reduction
- Traction devices
  - Skin traction
  - Skeletal traction

Fracture Immobilization
- Casting
- External fixation
- Internal fixation
- Maintenance traction

Open Fractures
- Surgical debridement and irrigation
- Tetanus immunization
- Prophylactic antibiotic therapy
- Immobilization

CT, computed tomography; *MRI,* magnetic resonance imaging.

Traction. Traction devices apply a pulling force on the fractured extremity and result in realignment. The two most common types of maintenance traction are skin traction and skeletal traction. Skin traction is generally used for short-term treatment (48 to 72 hours) until skeletal traction or surgery is possible. Tape, boots, or splints are applied directly to the skin to maintain alignment, assist in reduction, and help diminish muscle spasms in the injured part. The traction weights are usually limited to 5 to 10 lb (2.3 to 4.5 kg). Skeletal traction, generally in place for longer periods of time, is used to align injured bones and joints or to treat joint contractures and congenital hip dysplasia. It provides a long-term pull that keeps the injured bones and joints aligned. To establish skeletal traction, the physician inserts a pin or wire into the bone, either partially or completely, to align and immobilize the injured body part. Weight for skeletal traction ranges from 5 to 45 lb (2.3 to 20.4 kg).

When traction is used to treat fractures, the forces are usually exerted on the distal fragment to obtain alignment with the proximal fragment. Several types of traction are used for this purpose (Table 59-6). Fracture alignment depends on the correct positioning and alignment of the patient while the traction forces remain constant. For extremity traction to be effective, forces must be pulling in the opposite direction (countertraction) to prevent the patient from sliding to the end or side of the bed. Countertraction is commonly supplied by the patient's body weight or may be augmented by elevating the end of the bed.

Fracture Immobilization

External fixation. External fixation of fractures is achieved by a cast or an external fixator. Casting is a common treatment after closed reduction has been performed. It allows the patient to perform many normal activities of daily living while providing sufficient immobilization to ensure stability. Major cast materials include fiberglass, plaster of Paris, polyurethane, thermoplastic resins, and thermolabile plastic.

Plaster of Paris, after immersion in water, is wrapped and molded around the affected part (Fig. 59-9). It is anhydrous calcium sulfate embedded in gauze roll. The strength of the cast is determined by the number of layers of plaster bandage and the technique of application. As the cast dries, it recrystallizes and hardens. Heat is generated during the drying process. Increased edema as a result of the increased circulation may occur as a result of heat produced by the drying cast. After the cast is completely dry, it is strong and firm and can withstand stresses. The plaster is hard within 15 minutes, so the patient can move around without problems. However, it is not strong enough for weight bearing until it is dry (after about 24 to 48 hours).

Thermolabile plastic (Orthoplast) and thermoplastic resins (Hexcelite) are molded to fit the torso or extremity after being heated in warm water. Polyurethane, which is formed from polyester and cotton fabric impregnated with a chemical, is water activated by immersing in cool water to start the chemical process. Casts made of this fiberglass tape are frequently used because they are lightweight and relatively waterproof and support earlier mobilization. They are appropriate in cases in

Table 59-6 Common Types of Traction

Type	Indications	Nursing Implications
Skin		
Buck's	Used for many conditions affecting hip, femur, knee, or back. It is generally used for temporary immobilization and stabilization of fractured hips or fractures of the femoral shaft. It can be unilateral or bilateral. May also be used to correct knee and hip joint contractures.	All assessments should be at least q4hr. Assess for altered neurovascular status caused by original injury or the application of the bandages used in Buck's traction. Especially note decreased peripheral vascular flow and peroneal nerve deficit by assessing for ability to dorsiflex toes and foot, and for changes in sensation in the first webspace between the great and second toes. Pressure from the elastic wrap may result in pressure necrosis, especially over bony prominences and areas prone to pressure (anterior tibial border, fibular head, both malleoli, Achilles tendon, calcaneus, and dorsum of the foot). In addition, assess for an allergic reaction to the adhesive material, rotation of the extremity, and constant traction and countertraction forces. 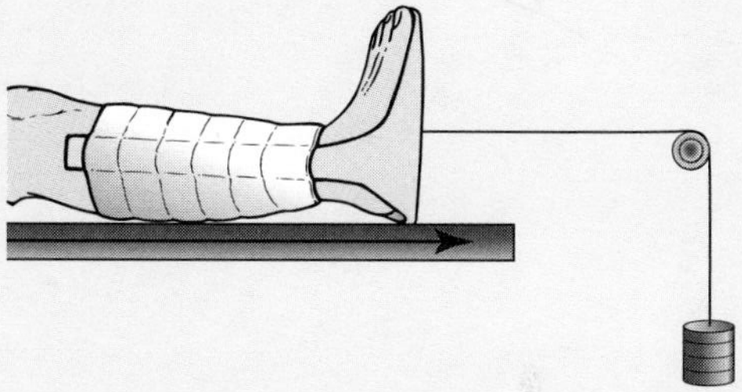
Russell's	Used for fractures of femur or hip.	Same as above. An additional area prone to pressure necrosis is the area over the hamstring tendons in the popliteal space. 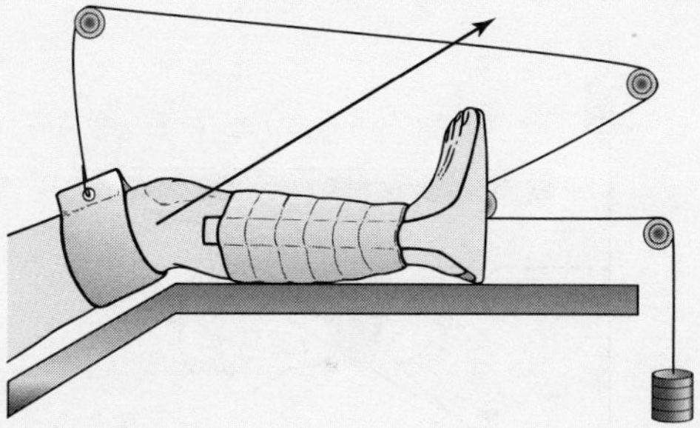
Bryant's	Used for fractures of the femur, fractures in small children, and stabilization of hip joints in children under 2 yr or 30 lb (14 kg) in weight.	Be aware that with traction in place, buttocks should just clear the mattress. Check for undue pressure over the outer head and neck of fibula, dorsum of foot, Achilles tendon, scapulae, and shoulders. Check that bandages or boot has not slipped. Be aware that these are usually removed for skin care and assessment q4hr. 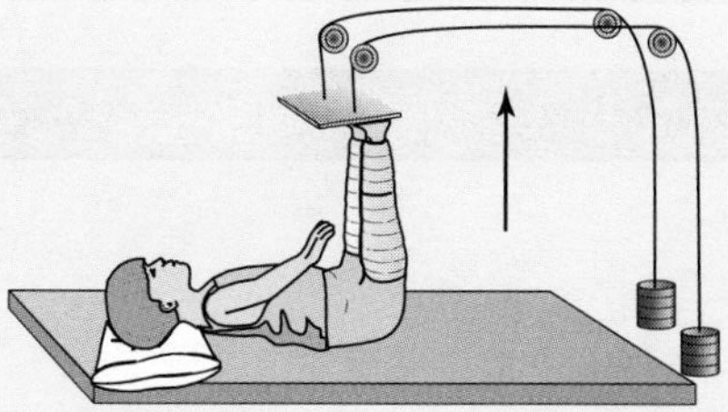

Continued

Table 59-6 Common Types of Traction—cont'd

Type	Indications	Nursing Implications
Skin—cont'd		
Pelvic belt (or girdle)	Used for sciatica, muscle spasms (low back), and minor fractures of the lower spine.	Check for security of the pelvic belt. Check frequently for skin irritation over iliac crests and in the intergluteal fold. Use measures to prevent skin breakdown. Check and adjust pelvic belt straps so that they are unrestricted and equal in length. Secure the straps with adhesive tape. Use a footboard to prevent footdrop. Maintain the correct angle of pull of the traction. Be aware that the physician orders the type of countertraction.
Pelvic sling traction	Used for pelvic fractures to provide compression for a separated pelvic girdle.	The sling should keep the pelvis just above the surface of the bed. Assess for pressure necrosis and skin irritation q4hr; especially assess for pressure over the iliac crests, intergluteal fold, and greater trochanters. Monitor for soiling of the sling and change as needed; use a fracture bedpan for toileting. Limit use of trapeze since it will reduce compressive force from the sling. Use alternating air pressure mattress or other pressure dispersing devices; provide frequent back care.
Circumferential		
Head halter	Used for soft-tissue disorders and degenerative disk disease of the cervical spine. It is not commonly used for unstable fractures of the cervical spine.	Assess for alignment with trunk, areas of local pressure over the ears and mandibular joints and under the chin and occipital area, and pain or dysfunction in the temporomandibular joint. Patients may be permitted to remove traction for meals; if not, provide a liquid or mechanical soft diet to reduce temporomandibular joint pain. Since this traction is commonly used in the home, ensure patients can demonstrate safe and effective setup, application, and use of the traction before discharge.

30°

Skeletal		
Overhead arm (90°-90°)	Commonly used for immobilization of fractures and dislocations of the upper arm and shoulder.	Be aware that the shoulder and elbow joint are maintained at 90° angles. Assess for pressure necrosis beneath the sling, especially over bony prominences. Assess distal neurovascular status; because of exposure, skin temperature may be cool and thus not indicative of decreased perfusion. Perform assessments q4hr. Inspect the pin site and perform pin site care according to hospital policy. 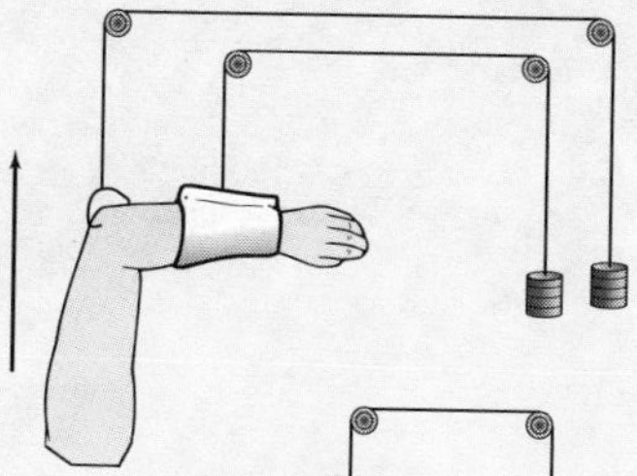
Lateral arm	Commonly used in immobilization of fractures and dislocations of the upper arm and shoulder.	Inspect the pin site and perform pin site care according to hospital policy. Assess neurovascular status. 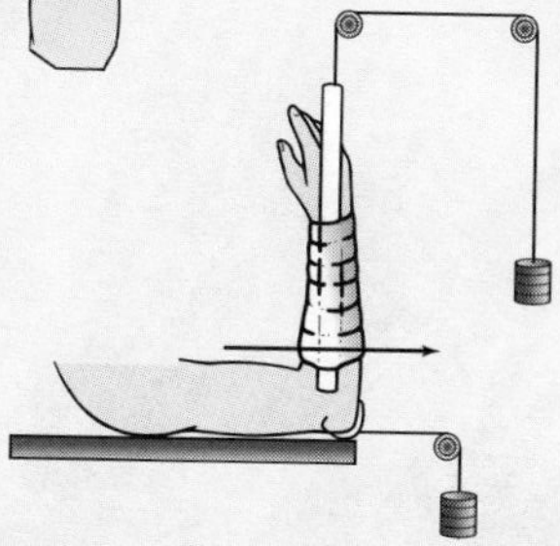
Balanced suspension traction	Used for injury or fracture of the femoral shaft of the femur, acetabulum, hip, tibia, or any combination of these.	Be aware that this traction uses half-ring Thomas splint (1) and Pearson attachment (2) and that suspension of the extremity and direct skeletal traction are applied. This allows raising of the buttocks off the bed for bedpan use and skin care without altering the line of traction. Use nursing assessments so that countertraction is maintained (e.g., position patient high in bed so that feet do not press on foot of bed, do not elevate the head of the bed >25° if it causes continual movement toward foot of the bed). Encourage self-help in patient's performance of activities of daily living, movement in bed with help of trapeze, and flexion and extension of affected foot to prevent footdrop. Assess for pressure necrosis in areas contacted by the traction, especially the greater trochanter, ischial tuberosity, hamstring tendons, fibular head, and both malleoli. Assess distal neurovascular status q4hr. Inspect the pin site and perform pin site care according to hospital policy. 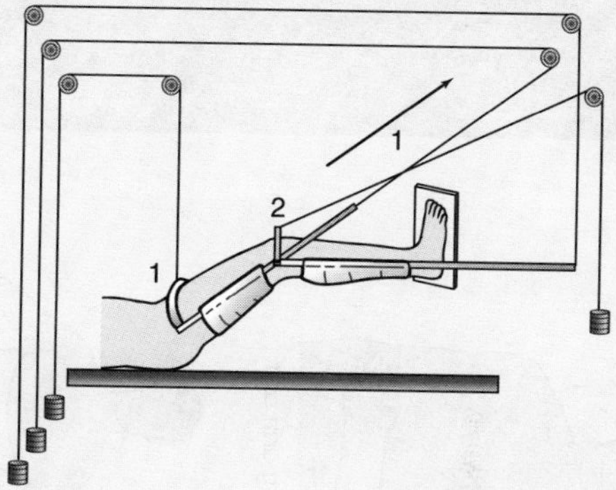

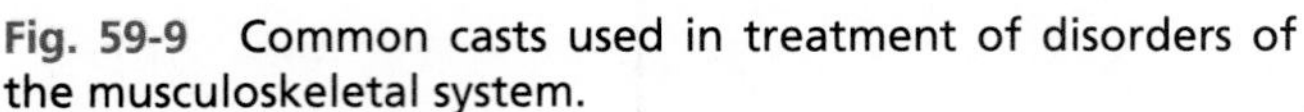

Fig. 59-9 Common casts used in treatment of disorders of the musculoskeletal system.

which severe edema is not present or when multiple cast changes are not anticipated.

An external fixator is a metallic device composed of metal pins that are inserted into the bone and attached to external rods to stabilize the fracture while it heals. It can be used to apply traction or to compress fracture fragments and to immobilize reduced fragments when the use of a cast or other traction is not appropriate. The external device holds fracture fragments in place much like surgically implanted internal devices do. The external fixator is attached directly to the bones by percutaneous pins (Fig. 59-10). Assessment for pin loosening and infection is critical. Infection signaled by exudate, redness, tenderness, and pain may require removal of the device. An external fixator used to treat fractures with associated soft-tissue trauma facilitates wound care.

External fixator devices can also be used as part of a limb-lengthening process for patients who have a significant leg-

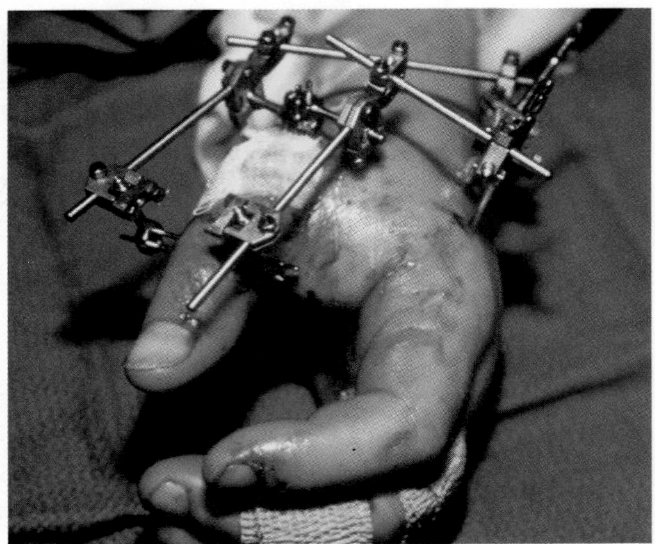

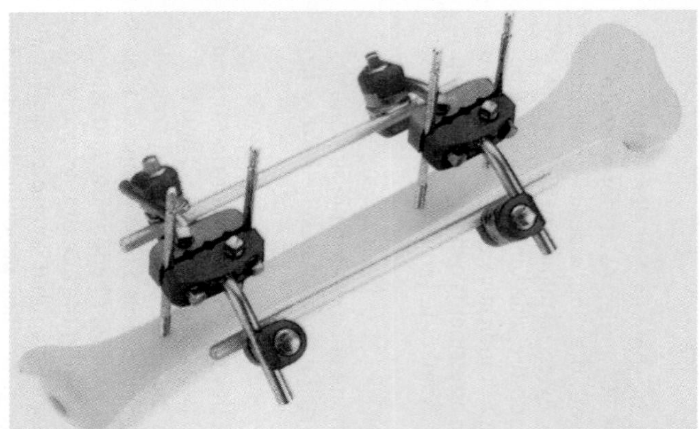

Fig. 59-10 External fixators. **A,** Mini Hoffman system in use on hand. **B,** Hoffman II on the tibia (standard system).

length discrepancy. The pins connected to these fixators are turned regularly as part of a prescribed regimen.

Types of casts (see Fig. 59-9). Immobilization of an acute fracture or soft-tissue injury of the upper extremity is frequently accomplished by use of (1) the sugar-tong splint, (2) the posterior splint, (3) the short arm cast, and (4) the long arm cast. The sugar-tong splint is typically used for acute wrist injuries or injuries that may result in significant swelling. Plaster splints are applied to the well-padded forearm, beginning at the phalangeal joints of the hand and extending up the dorsal aspect of the forearm around the distal humerus and then extending down the volar aspect of the forearm to the distal palmar crease. The splinting material is wrapped with either elastic bandage or bias stockinette. The major advantage of the sugar-tong cast and posterior splint are avoidance of the circumferential effects of a nonelastic cylinder cast, because these devices allow for swelling.

The short arm cast is frequently used for the treatment of stable wrist or metacarpal fractures. An aluminum finger splint can be fabricated into the short arm cast for concurrent treatment of phalangeal injuries. The short arm cast is a circular cast extending from the distal palmar area to the proximal forearm. This cast provides wrist immobilization and permits unrestricted elbow motion.

The long arm cast is commonly used for stable forearm or elbow fractures and unstable wrist fractures. It is similar to the short arm cast but extends to the proximal humerus, restricting motion in the wrist and elbow. Nursing measures should be directed toward supporting the extremity and reducing the effects of edema by maintaining extremity elevation with a sling. However, when a hanging arm cast is used for a proximal humerus fracture, elevation or a supportive sling are contraindicated because hanging provides traction and promotes fracture healing.

When a sling is used, the nurse must ensure that the axillary area is well padded to prevent skin maceration associated with direct skin-to-skin contact. Placement of the sling should not put undue pressure on the posterior neck. Movement of the fingers (unless contraindicated) should be encouraged to enhance the pumping action of veins to decrease edema. The nurse should also encourage the patient to actively move nonimmobilized joints of the upper extremity to prevent stiffness and contractures.

The body jacket cast is frequently used for immobilization and support for stable spine injuries of the thoracic or lumbar spine. This cast is applied around the chest and abdomen and extends from above the nipple line to the pubis. After application of the cast, the nurse must assess the patient for the development of *cast syndrome.* This condition occurs if the body cast is applied too tightly and the cast compresses the superior mesenteric artery against the duodenum. The patient generally complains of abdominal pain, abdominal pressure, nausea, and vomiting. The abdomen should be assessed for bowel sounds (a window may be left over the umbilicus). Treatment includes gastric decompression with a nasogastric tube and suction. The cast may need to be removed or split. Nursing assessment also includes observation of respiratory status, bowel and bladder function, and areas of pressure over the bony prominences, especially the iliac crest. During the time required for the cast to dry, the nurse should reposition the patient every 2 to 3 hours to promote even cast drying and to relieve pressure and discomfort.

The hip spica cast is used in treating femoral fractures, especially in children. The purpose of the hip spica cast is to immobilize the affected extremity and the trunk securely. It includes two casts joined together: (1) the body jacket cast and (2) the long leg cast. The location of the femoral fracture will determine whether the thigh of the unaffected extremity will have to be immobilized to restrict rotation of the pelvis and possible hip motion on the side of the femur fracture. The hip spica cast extends from above the nipple line to the base of the foot (single spica) and may include the opposite extremity up to an area above the knee (spica and a half) or both extremities (double spica).

The nurse should assess the patient with a hip spica cast for the same problems that are associated with the body jacket cast. During the initial drying stage the patient should not be placed in the prone position, because the cast may break. The patient should be slightly turned from side to side and supported with pillows. When the patient is repositioned, the support bar joining the thighs must never be used to assist in moving, since the bar can break and cause cast disruption. After the cast has dried, the nurse (with assistance) can turn the patient to the prone position and provide pillow support under the chest and immobilized extremity. Skin care around the cast edges and the areas not encompassed by plaster is important to prevent any pressure sores. The nurse should instruct the patient in the positioning activities required to get on and off the bedpan. A fracture bedpan may be used to provide comfort and ease the movement of getting on and off the bedpan. After the hip spica cast has dried sufficiently, the patient may be instructed in ambulation techniques by the physical therapist.

Injuries to the lower extremity are frequently immobilized by either a long leg, short leg, or cylinder cast or a Jones dressing. The usual indications for applying a long leg cast are an unstable ankle fracture, soft-tissue injuries, a fractured tibia, and knee injuries. The cast usually extends from the base of the toes to the groin and gluteal crease. The short leg cast can be used for a variety of conditions but is usually used for stable ankle and foot injuries. A cylinder cast is used for knee injuries or fractures. The cast extends from the groin to the malleoli of the ankle. A Jones dressing is composed of significant padding materials (absorption dressing and sheet wadding), anterior or posterior and lateral splints, and an elastic wrap or bias-cut stockinette. The Jones dressing, like the sugar-tong splint, is used for knee fractures or surgery when there is a risk of significant edema. After the application of a lower-extremity cast or dressing, the extremity should be elevated with pillows above the heart level for the first 24 hours. After the initial phase, the casted extremity should not be placed in a dependent position because of the possibility of excessive edema.

Initially, no weight can be put on the injured extremity. Later, a walking heel or cast shoe may be added to the cast if the patient will be allowed to bear weight and walk on the affected leg. Following cast application, the nurse should observe for signs of pressure, especially in the regions of the heel, anterior tibial border, fibular head, and malleoli.

Internal fixation. Internal fixation devices are surgically inserted at the time of realignment. Examples of internal fixation devices include pins, plates, and screws. They are biologically inert metal devices such as stainless steel, vitallium, or titanium that are used to realign and maintain bony fragments. Proper alignment is evaluated by x-ray studies at regular intervals.

Maintenance traction. Maintenance traction is initiation or continuation of traction and countertraction. A continuous pulling force can be applied directly to bone with wires and pins (skeletal traction) or can be applied indirectly by weights that are attached to the skin with slings, belts, adhesive straps, or boots (skin traction). Skin traction is usually applied directly to the extremity by adhesive material that is wrapped circumferentially with a bandage or slings, belts, or a special splint that is attached to a rope with a weight. Skin traction for extremities is applied for a short time and usually consists of not more than 7 to 10 lb (3.2 to 4.5 kg) of traction weight because of skin intolerance to pressure. Pelvic or cervical skin traction may require heavier weights applied intermittently. Skeletal traction is usually indicated when the traction forces are expected to exceed 10 lb (4.5 kg) or when traction will be used for a long time. Use of too much weight to maintain traction can result in delayed union or nonunion. The major disadvantages of skeletal traction are infection in the area of bone where the skeletal pin has been inserted and the consequences of prolonged immobility necessitated by skeletal traction.

Open fracture. An open fracture involves communication to or from the fracture through the skin, formerly termed *compound fracture.* Tetanus prevention should be ensured with tetanus toxoid or tetanus antitoxin for a patient who has not been immunized. A broad-spectrum antibiotic (such as the cephalosporins) is usually used prophylactically. A decision on whether to close the wound or leave it open is based on the degree of contamination and the time elapsed before initiation of treatment. Infection is the greatest risk of an open fracture.

The overall long-term goal of treatment is the union of the fracture and return of the patient to the preinjury level of functioning as soon as possible. Discharge planning should include referral to the appropriate human service agency for assistance in the transition to the home environment.

Drug Therapy. Patients with fractures often experience varying degrees of pain associated with muscle spasms. These spasms are caused by involuntary reflexes that result from edema following muscle injury. Muscle relaxants, such as carisoprodol (Soma), cyclobenzaprine (Flexeril), or methocarbamol (Robaxin), may be prescribed for relief of pain associated with muscle spasms.

Common side effects associated with muscle relaxants are drowsiness, lassitude, headache, weakness, fatigue, blurred vision, ataxia, and gastrointestinal upset. Hypersensitivity reactions may include skin rash or pruritus. Ingestion of large doses of muscle relaxants may cause hypotension, tachycardia, or respiratory depression. The possible habituating effects associated with long-term use and the potential for abuse must be carefully considered.

Some physicians do not advocate the use of muscle relaxants for relief of muscle spasms. Their rationale is that the reflex spasm will continue as long as the precipitating pain persists. If the pain is controlled by use of appropriate analgesia, the muscle spasms will cease.

Nutritional Therapy. Proper nutrition is an essential component of the reparative process in injured tissue. An adequate energy source is needed to promote muscle strength and tone, build endurance, and enhance ambulation and gait-training skills. The patient's dietary requirements must include ample protein (e.g., 1 g per kilogram of body weight), vitamins (especially D, B, and C), and calcium to ensure optimal soft-tissue and bone healing. Low serum protein levels and vitamin C deficiencies interfere with tissue healing. Immobility and callus formation increase calcium needs. Three well-balanced meals a day will usually provide the necessary nutrients. The well-balanced meal should be supplemented by a fluid intake of 2000 to 3000 ml/day to promote optimal bladder and bowel function. Adequate fluid and a high-fiber diet with fruits and vegetables will prevent constipation. If immobilized in a body jacket or hip spica bandage, the patient should be instructed not to overeat to avoid abdominal pressure and cramping.

NURSING MANAGEMENT: FRACTURES

Nursing Assessment

A brief history of the accident, mechanism of injury, and the position in which the victim was found can be obtained from the patient or witnesses. As soon as possible, the patient should be transported to an emergency department where a thorough assessment and treatment can be initiated (Table 59-7). Subjective and objective data that should be obtained from an individual with a fracture are presented in Table 59-8.

Special emphasis must be focused on the region distal to the site of injury. The involved extremity should be compared with the uninvolved extremity. Clinical findings must be documented before fracture treatment is initiated to avoid doubts about whether a problem discovered later was missed during the original examination or was caused by the treatment. Misdiagnosis may result from failure to consider clinical procedures as the cause of a patient's complaints.

Neurovascular Assessment. Many musculoskeletal injuries have the potential of causing neurovascular injuries. Such events as the original trauma, application of a cast or constrictive dressing, or poor positioning can cause nerve or vascular damage, usually distal to the injury. One method to use for a neurovascular assessment is to consider the five *Ps*: *pain, pulses, pallor, paresthesia,* and *paralysis.*

The nurse should carefully assess the location, quality, and intensity of the pain of the affected extremity. Pain unrelieved by medication could be an early sign of compartment syndrome. The pulses on both the affected and injured extremity should be compared to identify differences in rate or quality. A diminished or absent pulse distal to the injury can indicate vascular insufficiency.

Paresthesia (abnormal sensation, such as numbness or tingling) can be evaluated by comparing the patient's sensations above and below the injury. Comparison of the sensations felt between the injured and uninjured extremity should also be made. Changes in sensation such as decreased sensation, hypersensation, numbness, tingling, or loss of sensation may be reported by the patient.

Next, color (pallor) and temperature changes in the area of nerve distribution of the affected extremity should be assessed. Pallor or a cold extremity below the injury could indicate arterial insufficiency. A warm, bluish extremity could indicate poor venous return. Capillary refill should also be checked. A compressed nailbed should return to its original color within 3 seconds. Comparisons should be made between the injured and uninjured extremities.

The final assessment of a neurovascular assessment is to check for paralysis or decreased motor strength. Range of motion and strength can be compared between the two extremities. Reduced motion or strength in the injured extremity can alert to problems with the motor portion of the involved nerves.

Patients should be instructed to report any changes in strength, sensation, color, temperature, or pain in the fractured extremity.

Nursing Diagnoses

Nursing diagnoses for the patient with a fracture may include, but are not limited to, those presented in NCP 59-1.

Planning

The overall goals are that the patient with a fracture will (1) have no associated complications, (2) obtain satisfactory pain relief, and (3) achieve maximal rehabilitation potential.

Nursing Implementation

Health Promotion. The public should be educated to take appropriate safety precautions to prevent injuries while at home, at work, when driving, or when participating in sports. Nurses should be vocal advocates for personal actions known to reduce injuries such as regular use of seat belts,

EMERGENCY MANAGEMENT

Table 59-7 Fractured Extremity

Etiology	Assessment Findings	Interventions
Blunt Motor vehicle collision Pedestrian event Falls Direct blows Forced flexion or hyperextension Twisting forces **Penetrating** Gunshot **Other** Pathologic conditions Violent muscle contractions (seizures)	■ Deformity (loss of normal bony contours) or unnatural position of affected limb ■ Edema and ecchymosis ■ Muscle spasm ■ Tenderness and pain ■ Loss of function ■ Numbness, tingling, loss of distal pulses ■ Grating (crepitus) ■ Open wound over injured site, exposure of bone	**Initial** ■ Treat life-threatening injuries first. ■ Ensure airway, breathing, and circulation. ■ Control external bleeding with direct pressure or sterile pressure dressing. ■ Splint joints above and below fracture site. ■ Check neurovascular status distal to injury before and after splinting. ■ Elevate injured limb if possible. ■ Do *not* attempt to straighten fractured or dislocated joints. ■ Do *not* manipulate protruding bone ends. ■ Apply ice packs to affected area. ■ Obtain x-rays of affected limb. ■ Administer tetanus prophylaxis if skin integrity is violated. ■ Mark location of pulses to facilitate repeat assessment. ■ Splint fracture site, including joints above and below fracture site. **Ongoing Monitoring** ■ Monitor vital signs, level of consciousness, oxygen saturation, peripheral pulses, and pain. ■ Monitor for compartment syndrome characterized by excessive pain, pain with passive stretch, pallor, paresthesia, paralysis, pulselessness. ■ Monitor for fat embolism (dyspnea, chest pain).

NURSING ASSESSMENT

Table 59-8 Fracture

Subjective Data

Important Health Information

Past health history: Traumatic injury; long-term repetitive forces (stress fracture); bone or systemic diseases, prolonged immobility (pathologic fracture)

Medications: Use of corticosteroids (pathologic fractures); analgesics

Surgery or other treatments: First aid treatment of fracture

Functional Health Patterns

Health perception–health management: Estrogen replacement therapy, calcium supplementation

Activity-exercise: Loss of motion or weakness of affected part; muscle spasms

Cognitive-perceptual: Sudden and severe pain in affected area; numbness, tingling, loss of sensation distal to injury; chronic pain that increases with activity (stress fracture)

Objective Data

General

Apprehension, guarding of injured site

Integumentary

Skin lacerations, pallor and cool skin or bluish and warm skin distal to injury; ecchymosis, hematoma, edema at site of fracture

Cardiovascular

Reduced or absent pulse distal to injury, decreased skin temperature, delayed capillary refill

Neurologic

Paresthesias, decreased or absent sensation, hypersensation

Musculoskeletal

Restricted or lost function of affected part, local bony deformities, abnormal angulation, shortening, rotation, crepitation; muscle weakness

Possible Findings

Localization and extent of fractures on x-ray, bone scans, tomograms, CT scan, or MRI

59-1 NURSING CARE PLAN PATIENT WITH A FRACTURE

Expected Patient Outcomes	Nursing Interventions and *Rationales*
NURSING DIAGNOSIS **Risk for peripheral neurovascular dysfunction** *related to* nerve compression.	
▪ Has normal neurovascular examination.	▪ Assess for signs and symptoms of peripheral neurovascular dysfunction such as pain in affected extremity that is unrelieved by medication, paresthesias, pain on passive movement, weakness, cool temperature, pallor, diminished pulses *to ensure early recognition and intervention.* ▪ Elevate extremity above heart level *to reduce edema by promoting return circulation to heart.* (Note: If compartment syndrome is suspected, elevate extremity no higher than heart level.) ▪ Apply ice compresses as ordered *to reduce edema and provide comfort.* (Note: If compartment syndrome is suspected, remove ice because it may exacerbate decreased tissue perfusion.) ▪ Notify physician immediately if patient complains of increasing pain that is unrelieved by medication *because this may indicate neurovascular impairment, which can result in significant injury if unrelieved.* ▪ Teach patient the signs of peripheral neurovascular dysfunction *to enable patient participation in care.*
NURSING DIAGNOSIS **Pain** *related to* edema, movement of bone fragments, and muscle spasms *as manifested by* complaints of pain, guarding, moaning, crying, restlessness.	
▪ Tolerable or no pain. ▪ Satisfaction with plan for pain relief.	▪ Gently and correctly position fractured extremity *to minimize pain and prevent bone displacement.* ▪ Assess site for constriction or pressure caused by immobilization apparatus *to prevent skin or neurovascular injury.* ▪ Use a pain scale *to assess pain and evaluate effectiveness of interventions.* ▪ Give patient analgesics or muscle relaxants as indicated *to relieve pain and promote muscle relaxation.* ▪ Elevate, apply ice (if prescribed), and support affected extremity *to reduce edema and promote comfort.* ▪ Be alert for pain that is not diminished after analgesic is administered *since this may indicate an impending compartment syndrome.*
NURSING DIAGNOSIS **Risk for infection** *related to* disruption of skin integrity and presence of environmental pathogens secondary to open fracture or external fixation pins.	
▪ No evidence of wound infection.	▪ Assess fracture or pin insertion points for blistering, tenting discoloration, and drainage *as indicators of infection.* ▪ Use aseptic technique when providing pin or wound care or when performing dressing change *to prevent cross-contamination and possible introduction of infection.* ▪ Obtain culture of wound if infection is suspected *to identify infective organism.* ▪ Administer antibiotics as ordered *to provide prophylaxis or treatment of diagnosed infection.* ▪ Monitor temperature q2hr *because fever may reflect developing sepsis.*
NURSING DIAGNOSIS **Risk for impaired skin integrity** *related to* immobility and presence of cast.	
▪ No evidence of skin breakdown.	▪ Examine potential pressure areas q4hr *to assess condition of skin.* ▪ Petal cast edges *to prevent skin abrasion or cast crumbs from falling beneath the cast.* ▪ Turn patient q2hr *to reduce pressure over bony prominences.* Use special pressure mattresses for prolonged bed rest. ▪ Assess exposed skin areas of traction sites for signs of infection or irritation *because improper positioning of traction devices can cause localized pressure necrosis.* ▪ Seek medical attention if cast becomes loose *to prevent rotation, flexion, and skin abrasion.* ▪ Instruct patient not to insert items (e.g., hangers or forks) into cast to scratch self *because these may cause tissue injury.* ▪ Instruct patient to report areas of warmth, pain, burning, or moisture beneath the cast; foul odor from cast ends; or areas of new or increasing drainage on cast surfaces.

Continued

59-1 NURSING CARE PLAN PATIENT WITH A FRACTURE—continued

Expected Patient Outcomes	Nursing Interventions and *Rationales*
NURSING DIAGNOSIS	**Ineffective management of therapeutic regimen** *related to* lack of knowledge regarding muscle atrophy, exercise program, and cast care *as manifested by* questioning of long-term effect of casting and cast care, activity restrictions.
▪ Minimal loss of muscle bulk of affected extremity. ▪ Verbalization of confidence in ability to follow prescribed discharge plan.	▪ Instruct patient on home care measures related to exercise, cast care, and prevention of complications *so patient can carry out prescribed discharge plan.* ▪ Explain factors that contribute to atrophy; emphasize relationship of inactivity to muscle atrophy *so patient will exercise involved extremity to maximum allowed and will not be alarmed at appearance of extremity when cast is removed.* ▪ Provide written instructions of prescribed exercise.
NURSING DIAGNOSIS	**Impaired walking** *related to* ineffective use of crutches *as manifested by* inability to move about independently.
▪ Crutches correctly used to move about as needed.	▪ Teach gait-training principles to patient (non–weight-bearing gait status unless otherwise ordered by physician); sit with feet over edge of bed, stand with no weight on affected extremity, measure and adjust crutches *to promote mobility according to patient's abilities.* ▪ Start gait training on parallel bars *because this increases patient's confidence.* ▪ Ensure gait is compatible with weight-bearing status *to prevent malalignment.* ▪ Cooperate with physical therapist regarding exercise and gait training *to reinforce plan and to provide unified approach to patient.*

COLLABORATIVE PROBLEMS

Nursing Goals	Nursing Interventions and *Rationales*
POTENTIAL COMPLICATION	**Fat embolism** *related to* fracture of a long bone.
▪ Monitor for embolic phenomena. ▪ Report abnormal findings. ▪ Carry out appropriate medical and nursing interventions.	▪ Monitor for changes in mental status caused by hypoxemia; symptoms of acute respiratory distress syndrome such as mild agitation, confusion, chest pain, tachypnea, cyanosis, dyspnea, apprehension, tachycardia, and decreased PaO_2; and petechiae on upper trunk and axillae *to enable prompt identification and reporting to physician.* ▪ As indicated, assess oxygen saturation with oximetry and report O_2 saturation $\leq$92%. ▪ Initiate oxygen therapy if indicated. ▪ Maintain immobilization of long bone fractures *to reduce the occurrence of fat embolism.* ▪ Be alert to patient's verbalization of a feeling of impending doom *because this is frequently a premonitory sign.* ▪ Provide emergency respiratory support as needed *to prevent respiratory arrest.*

driving within posted speed limits, stretching before exercise, use of protective devices (helmets, knee, wrist, and elbow pads), and not combining drinking and driving.

Elderly patients should be encouraged to participate in moderate exercise to aid in the maintenance of muscle strength and balance. To reduce falls, their living environment should be examined to rule out the use of scatter rugs, to ensure adequate footwear and lighting, and to clear paths to bathrooms for nighttime use. The nurse should also stress the importance of adequate calcium and vitamin D intake.

Acute Intervention. Patients with fractures may be treated in an emergency department or a physician's office and released to home care, or they may require hospitalization for varying amounts of time. Specific nursing measures depend on the type of treatment used and the setting in which patients are placed.

Preoperative management. If surgical intervention is required to treat the fracture, patients will need preoperative preparation. In addition to the usual preoperative nursing measures (see Chapter 16), the nurse should inform patients of the type of immobilization device that will be used and the expected activity limitations. Patients must be assured that their needs will be met by the nursing staff until they can again meet their needs. Assurance that pain medication will be available, if needed, is often beneficial.

Proper skin preparation is an important part of preoperative preparation. The protocol for skin preparation varies among agencies and may be the responsibility of the nurse.

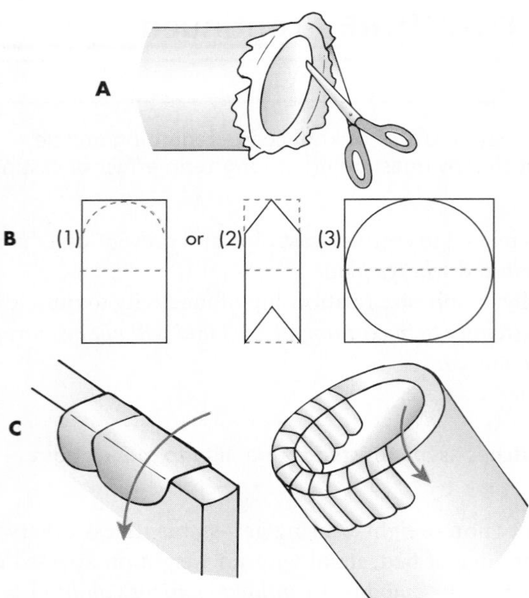

Fig. 59-11 Finishing edges of cast with waterproof adhesive strips. **A,** The cast must be thoroughly dry. The nurse trims the excess sheet wadding and stretches the stockinette over the cast edge (when possible). **B,** Several strips (petals) of waterproof adhesive tape (2-inch-wide strips for wide areas and 1-inch-wide strips for small areas, each 1 inch long) are made in advance. **C,** The uncut end of the tape is placed beneath the cast edge. Each succeeding petal overlaps the previous one by one-half inch, ensuring a smooth cast edge. A family member can help, and this can be done at home as needed.

The aim of skin preparation is to clean the skin and remove debris and hair to reduce the possibility of infection. Careful attention to this preoperative treatment can influence the postoperative course.

Postoperative management. In general, postoperative nursing care and management is directed toward monitoring vital signs and applying the general principles of postoperative nursing care (see Chapter 18). Frequent neurovascular assessments of the affected extremity are necessary to detect subtle changes. Any limitations of movement or activity related to turning, positioning, and extremity support should be monitored closely. Pain and discomfort can be minimized through proper alignment and positioning. Dressings or casts should be carefully observed for any overt signs of bleeding or drainage. A significant increase in size of the drainage area should be reported. If a wound drainage system is in place, the patency of the system and the volume of drainage should be regularly assessed. Whenever the contents of a drainage system are measured or emptied, the nurse should use sterile technique to avoid contamination. Additional nursing responsibilities depend on the type of immobilization used. A blood salvage and reinfusion system that allows for recovery and reinfusion of the patient's own blood may be used. The blood is retrieved from a joint space or cavity and the patient receives this blood in the form of an autotransfusion.[12]

Cast care. Immediately after a plaster cast is applied, there is a short period of exothermic reaction, during which heat is released from the plaster. The patient should be alerted to this occurrence, since it can increase edema. Evaporation of water and dissipation of heat from the cast can be hastened by exposing the cast to room air. A fresh cast should never be covered with a blanket because air cannot circulate and heat builds up in the cast. The patient should be turned every 2 hours to reduce continuous pressure and promote even drying of the cast. The drying process is usually complete within 24 to 72 hours. During the drying period the cast should not be subjected to any wetness, soiling, or abnormal stresses that can cause weakening or a break in the cast. It should be carefully handled by the palms of the hands rather than with the fingertips to avoid indentations that will dry and become potential pressure areas. Once the cast is thoroughly dry, the edges may need to be finished if it is rough to avoid skin irritation from rough spots or cast "crumbs" falling into the cast and causing irritation or pressure necrosis (Fig. 59-11).

Regardless of the type of material of which it is made, a cast can interfere with circulation and nerve function from being applied too tightly or because of excessive edema after application. Thus frequent neurovascular assessments of the immobilized extremity are critical. The patient must be taught about signs of cast complications so that they can be reported promptly. Elevation of the extremity above the level of the heart to promote venous return and applications of ice to control or prevent edema are measures frequently used during the initial phase of immobilization. The nurse should instruct the patient to exercise joints above and below the cast. Pulling out cast padding and scratching or placing foreign objects inside the cast is forbidden because it predisposes the patient to skin breakdown and infection.

Other measures. If the patient is immobilized as a result of the fracture, the nurse must plan care to prevent the occurrence of constipation and renal calculi. Constipation can be prevented by activity and maintenance of a high fluid intake (more than 2500 ml/day) and a diet high in bulk and roughage (fresh fruit and vegetables). If these measures are not effective in maintaining the patient's normal bowel pattern, stool softeners, laxatives, or suppositories may be necessary. Maintaining a regular time for elimination despite bed rest aids in promoting regularity.

Renal calculi can develop as a result of bone demineralization caused by immobilization. The resulting hypercalcemia causes a rise in urine pH and stone formation resulting from the precipitation of calcium. Unless contraindicated, a fluid intake of 2500 ml/day is recommended. Cranberry juice or ascorbic acid (500 mg/day) may be recommended to acidify the urine and prevent calcium precipitation. (Renal calculi are discussed in Chapter 43.)

Rapid deconditioning of the circulatory system can occur as a result of bed rest, resulting in orthostatic hypotension. Unless contraindicated, these effects can be diminished by permitting the patient to sit on the side of the bed, allowing the patient's lower limbs to dangle over the bedside, and performing standing transfers. When the patient is allowed to increase activity, careful evaluation should be made to assess for orthostatic hypotension.

Traction. The nurse is responsible for patient comfort and safety while traction is used and for ensuring proper functioning of the traction equipment. The equipment should be regularly examined for frayed ropes, loose knots, ropes out of the groove of the pulley, pulley clamps not fastened firmly to the bed frame, and weights not hanging freely.

When slings are used with traction, the nurse should inspect the skin area that is exposed in and near the sling regularly. Pressure over a bony prominence or a wrinkled area can impair blood flow, causing injury to the peripheral neurovascular structures. Skeletal traction pin sites must be observed for signs of infection. Pin site care varies according to the preference of the physician but usually includes regular removal of exudate with hydrogen peroxide, rinsing pin sites with sterile saline, drying of the area with sterile gauze, and application of antibiotic ointment.

External rotation of the hip can occur when skin traction is used on the lower extremity. The nurse can correct this position by placing a pillow, sandbag, or rolled-up drawsheet along the greater trochanteric region of the femur. When traction is used, the nurse should ensure that the patient's body is always correctly aligned. Generally, the patient should be in the center of the bed in a supine position. Incorrect alignment can result in increased pain, nonunion, or malunion.

To offset some of the problems associated with prolonged immobility, the nurse should discuss specific patient activity with the physician. If exercise is permitted, the nurse should encourage participation by the patient in a simple exercise regimen within activity restrictions. Activities that the patient should participate in include frequent position changes, range-of-motion exercises of unaffected joints, deep breathing exercises, isometric exercises, and use of the trapeze bar (if permitted) to raise oneself off the bed for linen changes and use of the bedpan. These activities should be performed several times each day.

Active exercises that move uninvolved joints through the range of motion are the preferred activity, if allowed. Frequent exercise of the trunk and extremities is an excellent stimulus to deep breathing. Active, resistive exercise (isotonic) of uninvolved extremities helps reduce deconditioning from prolonged immobility.

Ambulatory and Home Care

Cast care. Because many fractures are casted in an outpatient setting, the patient often requires only a short hospitalization or none at all. Therefore patient education is an important nursing responsibility to prevent complications. In addition to specific instructions for cast care and recognition of complications, the nurse should encourage the patient to contact the clinic or care provider should questions arise. Table 59-9 summarizes patient instructions for cast care. The nurse should validate the patient's understanding of these instructions before discharge from the clinic or hospital.

Psychosocial problems. Short-term rehabilitative goals are directed toward the transition from dependence to independence in performing simple activities of daily living and preservation or increasing strength and endurance. Long-term rehabilitative goals are aimed at preventing problems associated with musculoskeletal injury (Table 59-10). An important part of nursing care during the rehabilitative phase is assisting the patient to adjust to any problems caused by the injury (e.g., separation from family, financial impact of medical care, loss of income from inability to work). The nurse must exhibit gentleness, support, and encouragement and should actively listen to the patient's fears.

PATIENT TEACHING GUIDE

Table 59-9 Cast Care

Do Not

- Get cast wet*
- Remove any padding
- Insert any foreign object inside cast
- Bear weight on new cast for 48 hr (not all casts are made for weight bearing; check with health care provider when unsure)
- Cover cast with plastic for prolonged periods

Do

- Apply ice directly over fracture site for first 24 hr (avoid getting cast wet by keeping ice in plastic bag and protecting cast with cloth)
- Check with physician before getting cast wet†
- Dry cast thoroughly after exposure to water
  - Blot dry with towel
  - Use hair dryer on low setting until cast is thoroughly dry
- Elevate extremity above level of heart for first 48 hr
- Move joints above and below cast regularly
- Report signs of possible problems to health care provider
  - Increasing pain
  - Swelling associated with pain and discoloration of toes or fingers
  - Pain during movement
  - Burning or tingling under cast
  - Sores or foul odor under the cast
- Keep appointment to have fracture and cast checked

*Plaster of Paris cast.
†Synthetic cast.

Ambulation. The physical therapist often assumes primary responsibility for directing the patient during the strengthening phase of care. The nurse must know the overall goals of physical therapy in relation to the patient's abilities, needs, and tolerance. Mobility training and instruction in the use of assistive aids constitute one of the major areas of responsibility of the physical therapist. The patient with lower extremity dysfunction is usually started in mobility training when able to sit in bed and dangle the feet over the side. This activity should be done two or three times for 10 to 15 minutes, with the nurse assisting as necessary. As endurance increases, the patient is instructed in the techniques of transferring from bed to chair. Progressive ambulation is usually started with parallel bars and progresses to ambulatory assistive devices. When the patient begins to ambulate, the nurse must know the weight bearing allowed for the affected extremity and the correct technique if the patient is using an assistive device. There are different degrees of weight-bearing ambulation: (1) non–weight-bearing ambulation, (2) partial–weight-bearing ambulation, and (3) full–weight-bearing ambulation.

Assistive devices. Devices for ambulation range from a cane, which can relieve up to 40% of the weight normally borne by a lower limb, to a walker or crutches, which allow complete non–weight-bearing ambulation. The decision about which

Table **59-10** Problems Associated with Injury of the Musculoskeletal System

Problem	Description	Nursing Considerations
Muscle atrophy	Decreased muscle mass normally occurs as a result of disuse following prolonged immobilization.	An isometric muscle-strengthening exercise regimen within the confines of the immobilization device assists in reducing the amount of atrophy. Muscle atrophy interferes with and prolongs the rehabilitation process.
Contracture	Abnormal condition of joint characterized by flexion and fixation. Caused by atrophy and shortening of muscle fibers or by loss of normal elasticity of skin over a joint. Related to improper support and positioning of a joint.	This condition can be prevented by frequent position change, correct body alignment, and active-passive range-of-motion exercises several times a day. Contracture of a joint immobilized for a long time with a cast is common. Intervention requires gradual and progressive stretching of the muscles or ligaments in the region of the joint.
Footdrop	Plantar-flexed position of the foot (footdrop) occurs when the Achilles tendon in the ankle shortens because it has been allowed to assume an unsupported position. This may signify damage to the peroneal nerve.	Nursing management of the patient with long-term injuries must include preventive measures by supporting the foot in a neutral position. Once footdrop has developed, ambulation and gait training may be significantly hindered.
Pain	Frequently associated with fractures, edema, and muscle spasm; pain varies in intensity from mild to severe and is usually described as aching, dull, burning, throbbing, sharp, or deep.	Important causal factors of pain include incorrect positioning and alignment of the extremity, incorrect support of the extremity, sudden movement of the extremity, and immobilization device that is applied too tightly or in an incorrect position, constrictive dressings, motion occurring at the fracture site, and psychosocial factors. Pain is a valuable assessment parameter, and the underlying causes should be determined so that corrective nursing action can be taken before analgesics are administered.
Muscle spasms	Caused by involuntary muscle contraction after fracture and may last as long as several weeks. Pain associated with muscle spasms is often intense. The duration varies from several seconds to several minutes.	Nursing measures to reduce the intensity of the muscle spasms are similar to the corrective actions for pain control. The area involved in muscle spasms should not be massaged. Thermotherapy, especially heat, may reduce muscle spasm.

device is appropriate for a patient involves weighing the need for maximum stability and safety versus maneuverability, which is required in small spaces such as bathrooms and buses. The decision is made more easily by discussing with patients the requirements of their lifestyles and determining the device with which each patient feels most secure and independent.

The technique for using assistive devices varies. The involved limb is usually advanced at the same time or immediately after the advance of the device. The uninvolved limb is advanced last. In almost all cases, canes are held in the hand opposite the involved extremity.

The common gait patterns with assistive devices are the two-point gait, the four-point gait, the swing-to gait, and the swing-through gait:

- *Two-point gait.* Crutch on one side advances simultaneously with the opposite foot; gait is also used with cane ambulation.
- *Four-point gait.* A slower version of the two-point gait, each "point" is advanced separately.
- *Swing-to gait.* Both crutches are advanced together, followed by the lifting of both lower limbs to the same place; this gait is also used with walkers.
- *Swing-through gait.* This gait is similar to the swing-to gait, but the patient swings body past the crutches.

A belt should be placed around the patient's waist to provide stability during the learning stages. The nurse should discourage the patient from reaching for furniture or relying on another person for support. When there is inadequate upper limb strength or poorly fitted crutches, the patient bears weight at the axilla rather than at the hands, endangering the neurovascular bundle that passes across the axilla. If verbal coaching does not correct the problem, the patient should be kept from further ambulation until strength is adequate.

Patients who must ambulate without weight bearing require sufficient upper limb strength to lift their own weight at each step. Since the muscles of the shoulder girdle are not accustomed to this work, they require vigorous and diligent training in preparation for this task. Push-ups, pull-ups using the overhead trapeze bar, and lifting weights develop the triceps and biceps. Straight-leg raises and quadriceps-setting exercises strengthen the quadriceps.

Counseling and referrals. During the rehabilitative process the patient's family assumes an important role in the provision and follow-through of long-term care plans. The family must be instructed in the techniques of strength and endurance exercises, assistance with mobility training, and promoting activities that enhance the quality of daily living. Sexual counseling should be included in discharge planning. Unless nurses have specific preparation for sexual health counseling, they should remember that wrong answers may be more harmful than no answers. For referral purposes, nurses must know whether sexual activity is compatible with the degree of injury and whether any immobilization or support devices are necessary.

■ Evaluation

The expected outcomes for a patient with a fracture are presented in NCP 59-1.

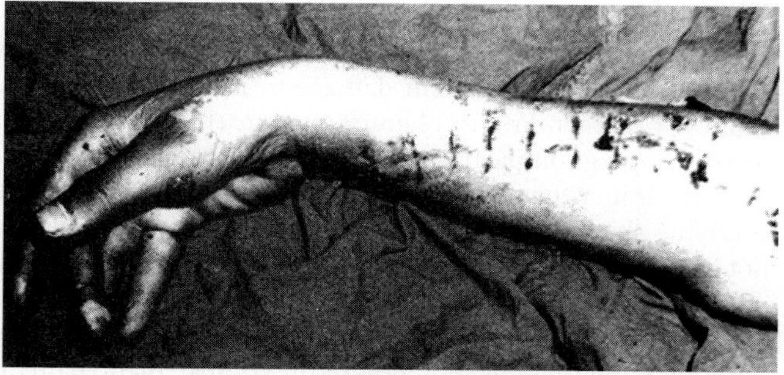

Fig. 59-12 Volkmann's ischemic contracture of the forearm following acute compartment syndrome secondary to a supracondylar fracture of the humerus. Note the incision line of an unsuccessful fasciotomy.

COMPLICATIONS OF FRACTURES

The majority of fractures heal without complications. If death occurs after a fracture, it is usually the result of damage to underlying organs and soft tissue or from complications of the fracture or immobility. Complications of fractures may be either direct or indirect. Direct complications include problems with bone union, avascular necrosis, and bone infection. Indirect complications of fractures are associated with blood vessel and nerve damage resulting in conditions such as compartment syndrome, venous thrombosis, fat embolism, and traumatic or hypovolemic shock. Although most musculoskeletal injuries are not life threatening, open fractures or fractures accompanied by severe blood loss and fractures that damage vital organs (such as the lung or bladder) are medical emergencies requiring immediate attention.

Infection

Open fractures and soft-tissue injuries have a high incidence of infection. An open fracture usually results from the impact of severe external forces. The soft-tissue injury often has more serious consequences than the fracture. Devitalized and contaminated tissue is an ideal medium for many common pathogens, including gas-forming (anaerobic) bacilli. Treatment of infections is costly in terms of extended nursing and medical care and treatment and loss of patient income. Infection may be present for a long time. (Osteomyelitis is discussed later in this chapter.)

Collaborative Care

Open fractures require surgical intervention. The wound is cleaned by extensive irrigation, usually with sterile normal saline, and any gross contaminants are mechanically removed. Contused, contaminated, and devitalized tissue such as muscle, subcutaneous fat, skin, and fragments of bone are surgically excised (debridement). The extent of the soft-tissue damage determines whether the wound will be closed at the time of surgery, whether closed suction drainage will be used, and whether skin grafting will be necessary. Depending on the location and extent of the fracture, reduction may be maintained by a cast or by traction. During surgery the open wound may be irrigated with antibiotic solution. During the postoperative phase the patient may have antibiotics administered intravenously or orally usually for 7 to 10 days. Antibiotics, in conjunction with aggressive surgical management, have greatly reduced the occurrence of infection.

Compartment Syndrome

Compartment syndrome is the compression of structures within closed compartments of the upper and lower extremities formed by fascial sheaths or bone. A closed compartment may also be created by an externally applied circumferential dressing, splint, or cast.[13] Normally there is some increase in edema as a result of soft-tissue injury in the general region of the injury. If edema continues, there may be an increase of pressure within the closed spaces of the tissue compartments. This can create sufficient pressure to obstruct circulation and cause venous occlusion, which increases edema. Eventually arterial flow is compromised, resulting in inadequate circulation to the extremity or ischemia. As ischemia continues, muscle and nerve cells are destroyed over time, and fibrotic tissue replaces the healthy tissue. Contracture and loss of function can occur. Delay in diagnosis and treatment can result in irreversible muscle and nerve ischemia.[14] This produces a functionally useless or severely impaired extremity.

Compartment syndrome is associated with fractures or extensive soft-tissue damage or crush injury in an extremity. The forearm and lower leg are the most common sites of compartment syndrome. Fractures of the distal humerus and proximal tibia are the most common fractures associated with compartment syndrome. In the upper extremity this condition is referred to as *Volkmann's ischemic contracture* (Fig. 59-12) and in the lower extremity as *anterior tibial compartment syndrome,* although the underlying pathophysiology is similar.

Although compartment syndrome is frequently associated with fractures, it should be noted that it can occur in situations when the soft tissue has been disrupted such as persons who have experienced severe burns, crush injuries, wringer injuries, venomous bites, or revascularization procedures. Prolonged pressure on a muscle compartment may occur when someone is trapped under a heavy object or a person's limb is trapped beneath the body due to an obtunded state such as drug or alcohol overdose. It has even been known to occur as the result of massive infiltration of intravenous fluids. An acute form of exertional compartment syndrome may occur after intensive exercise.[15]

Clinical Manifestations

Early recognition and treatment of compartment syndrome is essential to avoid permanent damage to muscles and nerves. This can occur within 4 to 12 hours after onset. The earliest sign of a developing compartment syndrome is progressive pain distal to the injury that is not relieved by the usual analgesics. The overlying skin may appear normal because surface vessels are not occluded. In addition to the inability to actively extend the digits, pain results from passive extension of the digits. Other symptoms that develop as the condition progresses include numbness and tingling, tenseness of the compartment, pain on passive stretch of muscle traveling through the compartment, loss of sensation, loss of function, pallor, coolness of the extremity, and diminished or absent peripheral pulses. Absence of a peripheral pulse is an ominous late sign that indicates severe disturbance of circulation. Regular neurovascular assessments should be performed on all patients with fractures, but especially those with injury of the distal humerus or proximal tibia or soft-tissue disruption in these areas.

Because of the possibility of muscle damage, urine output should be assessed. Myoglobin, released from damaged muscle cells, can be trapped in renal tubules because of its high molecular weight. Large amounts of myoglobinemia may result in acute renal failure. Common signs of myoglobinuria are (1) dark urine associated with a positive benzidine test in the absence of hematuria and (2) the manifestations associated with acute renal failure (see Chapter 44).

Collaborative Care

Prompt, accurate diagnosis of compartment syndrome is critical. Prevention or early recognition is the key. Because elevation may raise venous pressure, the extremity should not be elevated above the heart level. Similarly, ice may result in vasoconstriction and exacerbate compartment syndrome. Ice should not be used in patients with suspected compartment syndrome. It may also be necessary to remove or loosen the bandage or cast or to reduce traction weight to prevent edema formation.

Treatment is often a fasciotomy of the involved compartment. The fasciotomy is left open for several days to ensure edema formation has subsided. Infection is a potential problem following a fasciotomy.[16] Severe compartment syndrome may require amputation to decrease myoglobinemia or to replace a functionally useless extremity with a more effective prosthesis.

Venous Thrombosis

The veins of the lower extremities and pelvis are highly susceptible to thrombus formation after fracture, especially hip fracture. Precipitating factors are venous stasis caused by incorrectly applied casts or traction, local pressure on a vein, or immobility. Venous stasis is aggravated by inactivity of the muscles that normally assist in the pumping action of venous return of blood in the extremities. In addition to wearing compression gradient stockings (antiembolism hose) and using sequential compression devices, the patient should be instructed to move the fingers or toes of the affected extremity against resistance and to perform range-of-motion exercises on the unaffected lower extremities. Because of the high risk of venous thrombosis in the immobile patient, prophylactic anticoagulant medication such as aspirin, warfarin, or heparin may be ordered. Low-molecular-weight heparin (e.g., enoxaparin [Lovenox]) has recently been shown to be more effective in preventing venous thrombosis than warfarin.[17] Because it has a predictable dose response, there is no need to provide follow-up monitoring of prothrombin time. Assessment and management of venous thrombosis is discussed in Chapter 36.

Fat Embolism Syndrome

Fat embolism syndrome (FES) occurs in 0.5% to 2% of patients with fractures of long bones and up to 10% of patients with multiple fractures associated with pelvic injuries. FES is a contributory factor in many deaths associated with fractures. The fractures that most frequently cause FES are those of the femur, ribs, tibia, and pelvis. FES has also been known to occur following total joint replacement, spinal fusion, liposuction, crush injuries, and bone marrow transplantation. Two theories related to the origin of fat emboli exist. One theory suggests that fat is released from the marrow of injured bone. It is driven out by an increase in intramedullary pressure and enters the circulation through draining veins traveling to pulmonary capillaries, where it lodges. Some fat droplets traverse the capillary bed to enter systemic circulation and embolize to other organs such as the brain. The other theory postulates that catecholamines released at the time of trauma mobilize free fatty acids from the adipose tissue, causing loss of chylomicron emulsion stability. The chylomicrons form large fat globules that lodge in the lungs. This is possibly due to some biochemical change initiated by injury. The tissues of the lungs, brain, heart, kidneys, and skin are most frequently affected.

Clinical Manifestations

Early recognition of FES is crucial in preventing a potentially lethal course. Initial manifestations usually occur 24 to 48 hours after injury.[18] Severe forms have occurred within hours of injury. The fat globules transported to the lungs cause a hemorrhagic interstitial pneumonitis that produces signs and symptoms of acute respiratory distress syndrome (ARDS), such as chest pain, tachypnea, cyanosis, dyspnea, apprehension, tachycardia, and decreased partial pressure of arterial oxygen (PaO_2). All of these symptoms are caused by poor oxygen exchange. Because they are frequently the presenting symptoms, changes in the mental status as a result of hypoxemia are important to recognize. Memory loss, restlessness, confusion, elevated temperature, and headache prompt further investigation so that CNS involvement is not mistaken for alcohol withdrawal or acute head injury. The continued change in level of consciousness and petechiae located around the neck, anterior chest wall, axilla, buccal membrane, and conjunctiva of the eye help distinguish fat emboli from other problems. Petechiae result from intravascular thromboses caused by decreased oxygenation.

The clinical course of a fat embolus may be rapid and acute. Frequently the patient expresses a feeling of impending disaster. In a short time, skin color changes from pallor to cyanosis, and the patient may become comatose. No specific laboratory examinations are available to aid in the diagnosis. However, certain diagnostic abnormalities may be present. These include fat cells in the blood, urine, or sputum; a decrease of the PaO_2 to less than 60 mmHg; ST segment changes on electrocardiogram (ECG); a decrease in the platelet count and hematocrit

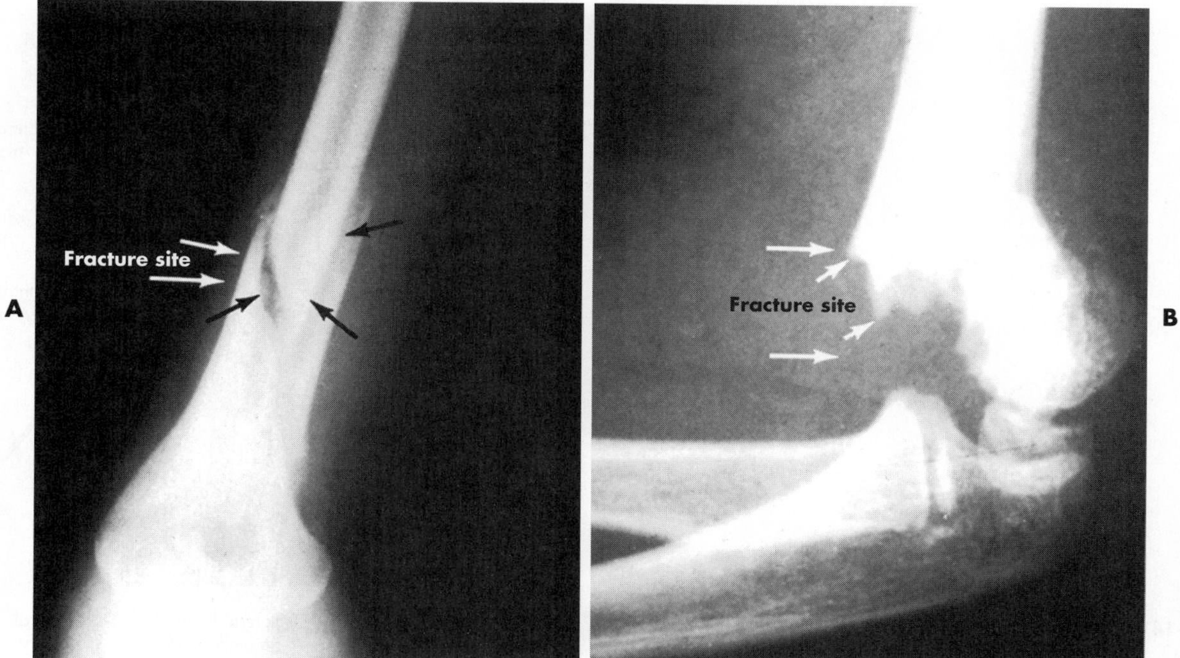

Fig. 59-13 **A,** Supracondylar fracture of the humerus. This type of injury results in the formation of a large hematoma. **B,** Fracture of distal shaft of humerus.

levels; and a prolonged prothrombin time. A chest x-ray may reveal areas of pulmonary infiltrate or multiple areas of consolidation. This is sometimes referred to as the *snowstorm effect.*

Collaborative Care

Treatment for fat embolism is directed at prevention. Careful immobilization of a long bone fracture is probably the most important factor in the prevention of fat embolism. Management of FES is essentially symptom related and supportive.[19] It includes maintaining adequate fluid intake, correction of acidosis, and replacement of any blood loss. Coughing and deep breathing should be encouraged. The patient should be repositioned as little as possible before fracture immobilization or stabilization because of the danger of dislodging more fat droplets into the general circulation. Use of corticosteroids to prevent or treat fat embolism is controversial.[20,21] Oxygen is administered to treat hypoxia. Intubation or intermittent positive pressure breathing may be considered if a satisfactory PaO_2 cannot be obtained with supplemental oxygen alone. Some patients may develop pulmonary edema, acute respiratory distress syndrome (ARDS), or both, leading to an increased mortality rate. Most patients survive FES with few sequelae.[18]

TYPES OF FRACTURES

Colles' Fracture

A *Colles' fracture* is a fracture of the distal radius and is one of the most common fractures in adults. The styloid process of the ulna may be involved as well. The injury usually occurs when the patient attempts to break a fall on an outstretched hand. This type of fracture most frequently occurs in women over age 50 whose bones are osteoporotic. The clinical manifestations of Colles' fracture are pain in the immediate area of injury, pronounced swelling, and dorsal displacement of the distal fragment (dinner-fork deformity). This may appear as a bump on the wrist. The major complication associated with a Colles' fracture is vascular insufficiency as a result of edema.

A Colles' fracture is usually managed by closed manipulation of the fracture and immobilization by either a sugar-tong splint or a long arm cast. The elbow must be immobilized to prevent wrist supination and pronation. Nursing management should include measures to prevent or reduce edema and frequent neurovascular assessment. Support and protection of the extremity should be provided, along with encouragement of active movement of the thumb and fingers. This type of movement helps reduce edema and increases venous return. The patient should be instructed to perform active movements of the shoulder to prevent stiffness or contracture.

Fracture of the Humerus

Fractures involving the shaft of the humerus are a common injury among young and middle-aged adults. The prominent clinical manifestations are an obvious displacement of the humerus shaft, shortened extremity, abnormal mobility, and pain (Fig. 59-13). The major complications associated with fracture of the humerus are radial nerve injury and vascular injury to the brachial artery as a result of laceration, transection, or spasm.

The treatment for a fracture of the humerus depends on the location and displacement of the fracture. Treatment may include a hanging arm cast, a shoulder immobilizer, or the sling and swathe, which is a type of immobilization that prevents glenohumeral movement. The swathe encircles the trunk and humerus as an additional binder. It is often used for surgical repairs and shoulder dislocation.

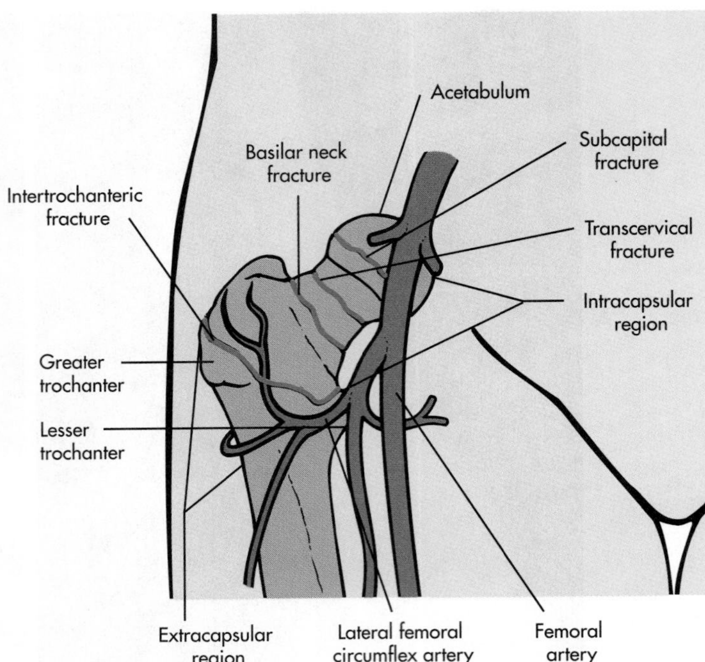

Fig. 59-14 Femur with location of various types of fracture.

When these devices are used, the head of the bed should be elevated to assist gravity in reducing the fracture. The arm should be allowed to hang freely when the patient is sitting and standing. Nursing care should include measures to protect the axilla and prevent skin maceration by placing lightly powdered absorbable dressing pads in the axilla and changing them twice daily or as needed. Skin or skeletal traction may be used for purposes of reduction and immobilization.

During the rehabilitative phase an exercise program geared toward improving strength and motion of the injured extremity is extremely important. This should include assisted motion of the hand and fingers. The shoulder can also be exercised if the fracture is stable, which prevents stiffness.

Fracture of the Pelvis

Pelvic fractures are usually caused by vehicular or skiing accidents. Older adult patients may sustain this injury from a fall. Although only a small percentage of all fractures are pelvic fractures, this type of injury accounts for 5% to 20% of the mortality rate from fractures. Preoccupation with associated injuries at the time of an accident may result in neglect of pelvic injuries. Pelvic fractures may cause serious intraabdominal injury such as colon laceration, paralytic ileus, hemorrhage, and laceration of the urethra, bladder, or colon.

Physical examination demonstrates local swelling, tenderness, deformity, unusual pelvic movement, and ecchymosis. The neurovascular status of the lower extremities and manifestations of associated injuries should be assessed. Pelvic fractures are diagnosed and classified by x-ray study. They may range from simple undisplaced fractures to more serious fracture dislocations with the potential for serious complications.

Treatment of a pelvic fracture depends on the severity of the injury. Bed rest for stable pelvic fractures is maintained from a few days to 6 weeks. More complex fractures may be treated with pelvic sling traction, skeletal traction, hip spica casts, external fixation, open reduction, or a combination of these methods. Internal fixation of a pelvic fracture may be necessary if the fracture is displaced. Extreme care in handling or moving the patient is important to prevent serious injury from a displaced fracture fragment. Because a pelvic fracture can damage other organs, assessment of bowel and urinary tract function and distal neurovascular status are important in early nursing activities for this patient.

The patient should be turned only when specifically ordered by the physician. Back care is provided while the patient is raised from the bed either by independent use of the trapeze or with adequate assistance. Weight bearing on the affected side should be avoided until healing is complete. If the pelvic fracture is undisplaced, the patient is usually allowed to ambulate using a walker or crutches to distribute the weight bearing between the upper and lower extremities.

Fracture of the Hip

Hip fractures are a common trauma in older adults. More than 250,000 hip fractures occur annually.[22] A hip fracture may be expected to occur more frequently in women than in men older than 65 years because of osteoporosis. It is estimated that 14% to 36% of patients who experience a hip fracture will die within 1 year of injury because of medical complications caused by the fracture or resulting immobility. More than 25% of the survivors lose their ability to walk independently, and 60% do not regain their preinjury level of ambulation.[23]

Fractures that occur within the capsule are called *intracapsular* fractures. Intracapsular fractures are further identified by a name taken from their specific location: (1) subcapital, (2) transcervical, and (3) basilar neck. These fractures are often associated with osteoporosis and minor trauma. *Extracapsular* fractures occur below the capsule and are termed *intertrochanteric* if they occur in a region between the greater and lesser trochanter. They are termed *subtrochanteric* if they occur in the region below the trochanter (Fig. 59-14). Extracapsular fractures are usually caused by severe direct trauma or a fall.

Clinical Manifestations

The clinical manifestations of hip fractures are external rotation, muscle spasm, shortening of the affected extremity, and severe pain and tenderness in the region of the fracture site. Displaced femoral neck fractures cause serious disruption of the blood supply to the femoral head, which can result in avascular necrosis.

Collaborative Care

Surgical repair is the preferred method of managing intracapsular and extracapsular hip fractures. Surgical treatment permits the patient to be out of bed sooner and decreases the major complications associated with immobility. In contrast, treatment with traction requires 12 to 16 weeks of immobilization for healing to occur, even if the blood supply to the region is intact. Initially the affected extremity may be temporarily immobilized by either Buck's or Russell's traction until the patient's physical condition is stabilized and surgery can be performed. Traction also helps relieve painful muscle spasms.

Intracapsular fractures are usually repaired with the use of an endoprosthesis to replace the femoral head (Fig. 59-15, *A*). Extracapsular fractures are usually pinned (Fig. 59-15, *B*). The principles of patient care for these procedures are similar.

The intracapsular fracture is slow to heal because of interruptions in blood supply. When avascular necrosis appears imminent, the surgeon may elect to resect the femoral head and neck and insert a femoral head prosthesis. A variety of devices in the form of compression screws and plates, nails, and pins are available to the surgeon for the purpose of repairing a hip fracture by pinning.

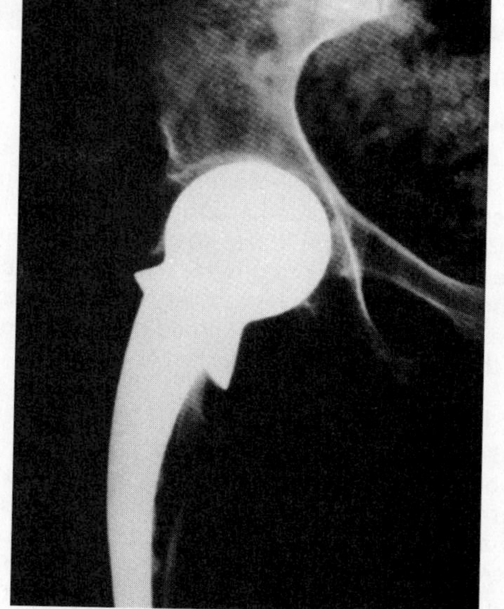

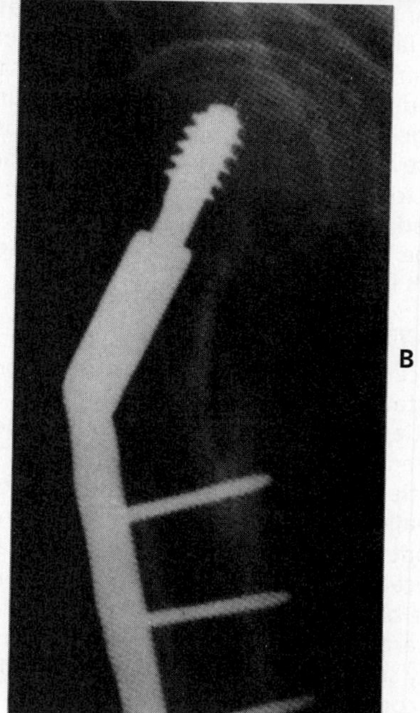

Fig. 59-15 Types of internal fixation for a hip fracture. **A,** Femoral head endoprosthesis. **B,** Type of hip compression screw with side plate.

NURSING MANAGEMENT: HIP FRACTURE

■ Preoperative Management

Because older adults are most prone to hip fractures, chronic health problems must often be considered when planning treatment. Diabetes mellitus, hypertension, cardiac decompensation, pulmonary disease, and arthritis are chronic problems that may complicate clinical status. Surgery may be delayed for a brief time until the patient's general health is stabilized.

Before surgery, severe muscle spasms can increase pain. These spasms are managed by appropriate analgesics or muscle relaxants, comfortable positioning unless contraindicated, and properly adjusted traction if it is being used.

Careful preoperative patient teaching can affect future mobility. The patient should know the method and frequency for exercising the unaffected leg and both arms. The patient should also be shown how to use the trapeze bar and the opposite side rail to assist in changing positions. Practice in getting out of bed and transferring to a chair should be discussed and demonstrated before surgery. The family should be informed about the patient's weight-bearing status after surgery. Plans for discharge should be discussed, and arrangements should be initiated well before the actual discharge date.

■ Postoperative Management

The initial postoperative management of a patient following surgical repair of hip fracture is similar to that for any older surgical patient. The nurse must monitor vital signs and intake and output, supervise respiratory activities such as deep breathing and coughing, administer pain medication cautiously, and observe the dressing and incision for signs of bleeding and infection. Specific nursing interventions for the patient with a fracture of the hip are described in NCP 59-2.

In the early postoperative period there is a potential for neurovascular impairment. The nurse should assess the patient's toes for (1) ability to move and weakness, (2) warmth and color, (3) sensation and absence of paresthesia, (4) distal pulses and capillary refill, and (5) edema, which may develop after the patient is out of bed. Edema is alleviated by elevation of the leg whenever the patient is in a chair. The pain resulting from poor

ETHICAL DILEMMAS

Premature Discharge of Patient

SITUATION

An 83-year-old patient with a total hip replacement is to be discharged from the hospital because of diagnosis-related group (DRG) standards for the number of days in the hospital. The nurse knows that the patient lives alone, has no relatives to care for him, and is unable to manage at this stage in his recovery with the limited home care available to him. Should the nurse request that the patient not be discharged at this time?

DISCUSSION

Third-party payer procedures for determining reimbursement for medical care are a means to determine reimbursement, *not* medical diagnoses. They are based on standards of medical care and pooled patient information rather than an individual patient's history and the physician's orders. In his current condition, this patient does not seem to have access to appropriate home care. If discharge planning is unable to find suitable care or to arrange transfer to an intermediate nursing facility, it would be unethical to discharge him. Both the physician and a hospital administrator should be involved in the plans for this patient to guarantee that appropriate care will be extended beyond the hospital. If it is not, the hospital might be liable for any medical consequences of the patient's inadequate care.

ETHICAL AND LEGAL PRINCIPLES

- Medicare began basing payment for short-term hospitalization on a DRG system in 1983, but not all facilities receiving Medicare reimbursement are covered under this system.
- Facilities may extend the length of stay beyond the DRG-alloted time, but the reimbursement for the patient will be reduced for the additional days.
- Medical decisions may not be ethically or legally made based on profit or reimbursement concerns. Concerns about reimbursement procedures and social policy should not be expressed in individual patient care contexts.

alignment of the affected extremity can be reduced by keeping pillows (or an abductor splint) between the knees when the patient is turning to either side. Sandbags and pillows are also used to prevent external rotation. If an endoprosthesis was placed, these patients are at risk for hip dislocation.

The physical therapist usually supervises active-assistance exercises for the affected extremity and ambulation when the surgeon permits it. Ambulation usually begins on the first or second postoperative day. The nurse should monitor the patient's ambulation status for proper crutch walking or use of the walker. The patient must be able to use crutches or a walker before discharge.

Complications associated with femoral neck fracture include nonunion, avascular necrosis, dislocation, and degenerative arthritis. As a result of an intertrochanteric fracture, the affected leg may be shortened.

If the hip fracture has been treated by insertion of a femoral head prosthesis, measures to prevent dislocation must always be used (Table 59-11). The patient and family must be fully aware of positions and activities that predispose the patient to dislocation (greater than 90 degrees of flexion, adduction, or internal rotation). Many daily activities may reproduce these positions (e.g., putting on shoes and socks, crossing the legs or feet while seated, assuming the side-lying position incorrectly, standing up or sitting down while the body is flexed relative to the chair, sitting on low seats—especially low toilet seats). Until the soft tissue surrounding the hip has healed sufficiently to stabilize the prosthesis these activities must be avoided, usually for at least 6 weeks. Sudden severe pain, a lump in the buttock, limb shortening, and external rotation indicate prosthesis dislocation. This requires a closed reduction or open reduction to realign the femoral head in the acetabulum.

In addition to teaching the patient and family how to prevent prosthesis dislocation, the nurse should (1) place a large pillow between the patient's legs when turning, (2) keep leg abductor splints on the patient except when bathing, (3) avoid extreme hip flexion, and (4) avoid turning the patient on the affected side until approved by the surgeon.

If the hip fracture is treated by pinning, dislocation precautions are not necessary. The patient is usually encouraged to be out of bed on the first postoperative day. Weight bearing on the involved extremity varies. Weight bearing of especially fragile fractures may be restricted until x-ray examination indicates adequate healing, usually within 6 to 12 weeks.

The nurse must assist both the patient and the family in adjusting to the restrictions and dependence imposed by the hip fracture. Depression can easily occur, but creative nursing care and awareness of the problem can do much to prevent it. The patient and family may need to be informed about community referral services that can assist in the postdischarge rehabilitation phase. Hospitalization averages 4 days. Patients frequently require care at a skilled nursing facility or rehabilitation facility for a few weeks before returning home. Regular follow-up care after discharge including home health nursing should be arranged. Recovery can take up to a year.[22]

Evaluation

The expected outcomes for the patient with fracture of the hip are presented in NCP 59-2.

GERONTOLOGIC CONSIDERATIONS

Hip Fracture

Factors that contribute to the occurrence of a hip fracture in older adults include a propensity to fall, inability to correct a postural imbalance, orientation of the fall, adequacy of local tissue shock absorbers (e.g., fat and muscle bulk), and underlying skeletal strength. Several factors have been identified in older persons that increase their risk of falling. These include gait and balance problems, decreased vision and hearing, decreased reflexes, orthostatic hypotension, and medication use.[23] Leading hazards of falls are loose rugs and slippery or

59-2 NURSING CARE PLAN PATIENT WITH FRACTURE OF THE HIP

Expected Patient Outcomes	Nursing Interventions and *Rationales*
NURSING DIAGNOSIS	**Pain** *related to* edema, movement of bone fragments, muscle spasms, and ineffective pain relief or comfort measures *as manifested by* guarding, moaning, crying, restlessness, rating pain as >2 on a scale of 1 through 5.
▪ Decrease in or absence of pain. ▪ Satisfaction with pain relief (rates pain as 2 or less on scale of 1 through 5).	▪ Align and position extremity and patient correctly *to reduce pressure on nerves and tissue.* ▪ Gently position or turn *to prevent muscle spasm and malalignment of bone fragments.* ▪ Maintain constant traction forces *to reduce muscle spasm and maintain alignment of bone.* ▪ Administer analgesics, nonsteroidal antiinflammatory agents, and muscle relaxants as indicated *to reduce pain, edema, and muscle spasms.* ▪ Use a pain scale to assess pain and evaluate pain-control interventions.
NURSING DIAGNOSIS	**Risk for peripheral neurovascular dysfunction** *related to* edema, concurrent injury of adjacent neurovascular structures from fracture fragment, or hematoma formation (see NCP 59-1).
NURSING DIAGNOSIS	**Impaired physical mobility** *related to* decreased muscle strength, or pain *as manifested by* inability to purposefully move, limited joint range of motion, inability to bear weight, presence of immobilization device.
▪ Sufficient muscle strength to participate in gait-training program. ▪ Optimal level of function with ambulatory assistive device.	▪ Cooperate with physical therapist in muscle-strengthening program *to maximize patient's progress in rehabilitation.* ▪ Teach and assist patient in exercise program; include resistive strengthening exercises of uninvolved lower and both upper limbs, elbow extension, shoulder depressors, and knee and hip extension *to develop strength in all extremities preparatory to initiation of ambulation.* ▪ Provide written instructions for exercises for patient to refer to as needed. ▪ Assist patient in standing at side of bed with abductor pillow (if indicated) using non–weight bearing (if indicated) on affected leg *to increase mobility.* ▪ Encourage quadriceps exercises, arm-strengthening exercises, and abdominal and gluteal contraction exercises *to develop muscle strength, which will help with rehabilitation.* ▪ Be aware that ordered weight-bearing status of involved extremity must be maintained unless changed by physician *because soft tissue surrounding hip requires about 3 to 5 months of healing to sufficiently stabilize the endoprosthesis.* ▪ Get patient out of bed and into chair, usually within 24 to 48 hours after surgery, *to reduce the complications associated with immobility.* ▪ Instruct and assist patient with transfer from bed to chair *to prevent accidental falling and improper movements, which could cause endoprosthesis dislocation or hip malalignment.*
NURSING DIAGNOSIS	**Risk for wound infection** *related to* exposure to environmental pathogens and surgical procedure.
▪ No evidence of wound infection.	▪ Assess wound site for erythema, local warmth, tenderness, edema, and drainage; monitor temperature q4hr *to identify fever as an indication of infection and initiate appropriate interventions.* ▪ Teach patient the signs and symptoms of infection and the need to promptly report them. ▪ Obtain wound culture, if indicated, *to identify infecting organism.* ▪ Administer antibiotics as ordered *for prophylaxis or to treat infection.* ▪ Use sterile technique when changing dressings or providing wound care *to minimize the risk of cross-contamination.*

Continued

59-2 NURSING CARE PLAN PATIENT WITH FRACTURE OF THE HIP—continued

Expected Patient Outcomes	Nursing Interventions and *Rationales*
NURSING DIAGNOSIS	**Ineffective management of therapeutic regimen** *related to* injury, surgery, and lack of knowledge of postdischarge care *as manifested by* verbalization of concern by patient or caregiver regarding ability to care for patient after discharge, lack of knowledge regarding postdischarge care.
▪ Verbalization by patient and family of confidence in ability to manage postdischarge care.	▪ Assess home environment *to identify needed modifications such as elevated toilet seat, height of shelves, steps, scatter rugs, low chairs.* ▪ Teach patient and family about proper ambulation, diet, medications, wound care, and physician follow-up *to reduce risk of injury, promote proper wound healing, and foster effective rehabilitation.* ▪ Inform about symptoms to report to physician such as fever, signs of wound infection, severe pain, cognitive changes *because these are indicators of complications that require prompt treatment.* ▪ Teach patient and family positions and activities to avoid such as putting on shoes and socks, crossing legs while seated, sitting on low seats *because these may cause dislocation of prosthesis.* ▪ Refer for home care as needed *because this resource can provide additional therapy and other assistance.* ▪ Provide written information that reviews preceding information and provide phone numbers to call with any questions.

COLLABORATIVE PROBLEMS

Nursing Goals	Nursing Interventions and *Rationales*
POTENTIAL COMPLICATION	**Thromboembolic complications** *related to* immobility.
▪ Monitor for thromboembolic complications. ▪ Report abnormal findings. ▪ Carry out appropriate medical and nursing interventions.	▪ Monitor for coolness, paleness, edema, and distended veins of the distal lower extremity *to detect decreased venous return.* ▪ Monitor for local warmth, edema, erythema, increased circumference, pain over the area, and systemic low-grade fever (<101° F [38° C]) *to detect thrombophlebitis.* ▪ Instruct patient in the need for fluid intake to exceed 2500 ml/day *to reduce hemoconcentration.* ▪ Apply antiembolism hose *to reduce venous pooling and promote venous return.* ▪ Provide ordered anticoagulant therapy prophylaxis (i.e., heparin, warfarin, aspirin, or low-molecular-weight heparin) as prescribed *to reduce thrombus formation.* ▪ Monitor for tachypnea, tachycardia, changes in mental status, voiced feelings of "impending doom," decreased O_2 saturation by oximetry, chest pain, dyspnea, and orthopnea *to detect thromboembolism.*

uneven surfaces. Approximately 75% of all falls occur indoors. Many falls are associated with getting in or out of a chair or bed. Falls to the side, the most common type in the frail elderly, are more likely to result in a hip fracture than a forward fall.

Two important factors influencing the amount of force imposed on the hip are the presence of energy-absorbing soft tissue over the greater trochanter and the state of leg muscle contraction at the time of the fall. Since many elderly have poor muscle tone these are important factors in the severity of a fall. Finally, elderly women often have osteoporosis and accompanying low bone density, which increases the risk of hip fracture.

Targeted interventions to reduce hip fractures in the elderly include a variety of strategies. Calcium and vitamin D supplementation, estrogen replacement, and drug therapy have been shown to decrease bone loss or increase bone density and decrease the likelihood of fracture.[24] (See section on osteoporosis later in this chapter.) Nurses must be vigilant in planning interventions for the elderly that are known to reduce the incidence of hip fracture.

FEMORAL SHAFT FRACTURE

Femoral shaft fracture is a common injury occurring particularly in young adults. Severe direct force is required to produce this injury, since the femur can bend slightly before actual fracture occurs. The force exerted to cause the fracture frequently causes damage to the adjacent soft-tissue structures. These injuries may be more serious than the bone injury. Displacement of the fracture fragments frequently results in open fracture and increased soft-tissue damage. This can result in considerable blood loss (1 to 1.5 L).

The clinical manifestations of a fracture of the femoral shaft are usually obvious. They include marked deformity and angu-

PATIENT & FAMILY TEACHING GUIDE

Table 59-11 Femoral-Head Prosthesis

Do Not

- Force hip into greater than 90 degrees of flexion*
- Force hip into adduction
- Force hip into internal rotation
- Cross legs
- Put on own shoes or stockings until 8 wk after surgery without adaptive device (e.g., long-handled shoehorn or stocking-helper)
- Sit on chairs without arms to aid rising to a standing position*

Do

- Use toilet elevator on toilet seat*
- Place chair inside shower or tub and remain seated while washing
- Use pillow between legs for first 8 wk after surgery when lying on "good" side or when supine*
- Keep hip in neutral, straight position when sitting, walking, or lying*
- Notify surgeon if severe pain, deformity, or loss of function occurs*
- Inform dentist of presence of prosthesis before dental work so that prophylactic antibiotics can be given

*These precautions may also apply after a hip pinning.

lation, shortening of the extremity, inability to move either the hip or knee, and pain. The common complications associated with fracture of the femoral shaft include fat embolism, nerve and vascular injury, and problems associated with union, open fracture, and soft-tissue damage.

Initial management is directed toward stabilization of the patient and immobilization of the fracture. Treatment may consist of skeletal traction via a tibial pin and balanced suspension traction. Traction continues for 8 to 12 weeks. The nurse must encourage the patient to perform exercises and range-of-motion activities for the uninvolved extremities and joints to discourage deconditioning. The physician determines when active exercise can be instituted on the affected extremity. When there is sufficient clinical evidence of bone union, a hip spica or long leg cast may be applied.

Internal fixation is another way to manage a femoral fracture. It is carried out with an intramedullary rod, compression plate, and screws or side plate with an intercondylar nail. Internal fixation is frequently the preferred treatment because it reduces hospital stay and the complications associated with prolonged bed rest. Other indications for internal fixation are failure to obtain satisfactory reduction by nonsurgical methods and multiple associated injuries. In some instances the surgically repaired femur may be supported by suspension traction for 3 to 4 days to prevent excessive movement of the extremity and to control rotation; non–weight-bearing gait training is then begun. Fractures associated with extensive soft-tissue injury may be treated with external fixation.

Promotion and maintenance of strength in the affected extremity usually include gluteal and quadricep isometric exercises. It is important to ensure performance of range-of-motion and strengthening exercises for all uninvolved extremities in preparation for ambulation. The patient may be immobilized in a hip spica cast and gradually progress to an articulating cast brace or may be allowed to begin non–weight-bearing activities with an ambulatory assistive device. Full weight bearing is usually restricted until there is x-ray evidence of bony union of the fracture fragments.

FRACTURE OF THE TIBIA

Although the tibia is vulnerable to injury because it lacks anterior muscle covering, strong force is required to produce a fractured tibia. As a result, soft-tissue damage, devascularization, and open fracture are frequent. Other complications associated with tibial fractures are compartment syndrome, fat embolism, problems associated with bony union, and possible infection associated with open fracture.

The recommended management for closed tibial fracture is closed reduction followed by immobilization in a long leg cast. Open reduction may be achieved with intramedullary rods or compression plate. With either method of reduction, emphasis is placed on maintaining the strength of the quadriceps.

The neurovascular status of the affected extremity must be assessed at least every 2 hours during the first 48 hours. Patients are instructed to perform active range-of-motion exercises with all uninvolved extremities, as well as exercises for the upper extremities, to build the strength required for crutch walking. When the physician has determined that the patient is ready for gait training, the patient is instructed in the principles of crutch walking. The patient may be on non–weight-bearing status for 6 to 12 weeks depending on healing. When fracture healing has progressed sufficiently, a walking heel is applied to the cast and full weight bearing is allowed.

STABLE VERTEBRAL FRACTURES

A stable fracture of the vertebral column is usually caused by motor vehicle accidents, falls, diving, or athletic injuries. A stable fracture is one in which the fracture or the fragment is not likely to move or cause spinal cord damage. This type of injury is frequently confined to the anterior element (vertebral body) of the spinal column in the lumbar region. It involves the cervical and thoracic regions less frequently. The vertebral bodies are usually protected from displacement by the intact spinal ligaments.

Most patients with spinal fractures have stable fractures and experience only brief periods of disability. However, if the ligamentous structures are significantly disrupted, dislocation of the vertebral structures may occur, resulting in instability and injury to the spinal cord (unstable fracture). These injuries may require surgery. The most serious complication of vertebral fractures is fracture displacement, which can cause damage to the spinal cord (see Chapter 57). Although stable vertebral fractures are not associated with abnormal spinal cord pathology, all spinal injuries should initially be considered unstable and potentially serious until diagnostic tests and the physician determine that the fracture is stable.

The most common injury to the vertebral body is the compression type of fracture caused by excessive vertical load, such as a severe fall on the buttocks or injury resulting from sudden flexion that forces the spine beyond its normal range of motion.

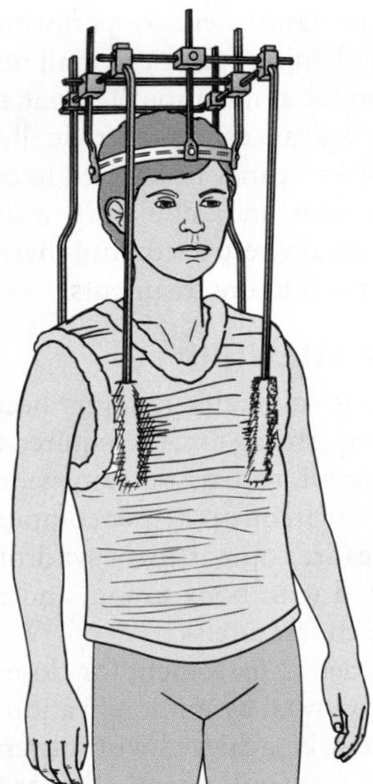

Fig. 59-16 Halo apparatus attached to a body jacket cast. It may also be attached to a brace. A halo vest can be used in treatment of a cervical spine injury or following cervical spine surgery.

The patient usually complains of pain and tenderness in the affected region of the spine. Compression fractures are associated with a gibbous deformity (flexion angulation of several vertebrae). This deformity may be noted during the physical examination. In patients with osteoporosis, several vertebral levels may be involved as evidenced by a dowager's hump (abnormal backward curvature of cervical spine). Bowel and bladder dysfunction may be an indication of an interruption of the autonomic nervous system or injury to the spinal cord.

The overall goal in management of stable fractures of a vertebral body is to keep the spine in good alignment until union has been accomplished. Many nursing interventions are aimed at assessing for the possibility of spinal cord trauma. Vital signs and bowel and bladder function should be evaluated regularly, as should the motor and sensory status of the peripheral nerves distal to the injured region. Any deterioration in the patient's neurovascular status should be promptly reported.

Treatment includes support, heat, and traction. The patient is usually placed in a standard hospital bed with firm support from the mattress or a bedboard. The aim is to support the spinal column, relax muscles, and release any compression on nerve roots. Heat and traction may be used to relieve muscle spasms resulting from the fracture. Traction may also be used to reduce and immobilize fracture fragments. A trapeze is not usually allowed because its use disrupts spinal alignment. Both an upright position and turning of the torso are prohibited. When turning, the patient should be taught to keep the spine straight by turning shoulders and pelvis together. Nursing assistance is necessary for the patient to learn how to turn in this "logrolling" fashion. Several days after the initial injury, the physician may apply a specially constructed orthotic device (e.g., Milwaukee, Jewett, or Taylor braces), a jacket cast, or a removable corset if there is no evidence of neurologic deficit.

Table 59-12 Clinical Manifestations of Facial Fractures

Fracture	Clinical Manifestation
Frontal bone	Rapid edema that may mask underlying fractures
Periorbital	Possible frontal sinus involvement, entrapment of ocular muscles
Nasal	Displacement of nasal bones, epistaxis
Zygomatic arch	Depression of zygomatic arch
Maxilla	Segmental motion of maxilla
Mandible	Dental fractures, bleeding, limited motion of mandible

If the fracture is in the cervical spine, a cervical collar may be worn by the patient. Some cervical fractures are immobilized by use of a halo vest (Fig. 59-16). This consists of a plastic jacket or cast fitted about the chest and attached to a halo that is held in place by skeletal pins inserted into the cranium. These devices immobilize the spine in the fracture area but allow patient mobility. The patient is discharged after (1) regaining ambulation skills, (2) learning care of the cast or orthotic device, and (3) learning how to cope with interferences in safety and security imposed by injury and treatment.

MAXILLOFACIAL FRACTURES

Any bone of the face can be fractured as a result of trauma. Fractures can occur as a result of collision with another person or object, fighting, or blunt trauma. The primary concern after facial injury is to establish and maintain a patent airway and to provide adequate ventilation by removal of foreign material and blood. Suctioning may be necessary. An artificial airway (tracheostomy) may be needed if a patent airway cannot be maintained. Hemorrhage is controlled by pressure packing. Cervical spine injuries are common. All patients with maxillofacial injuries should be treated as though they have a cervical injury until proven otherwise by examination and testing. Table 59-12 describes the clinical manifestations of more common facial fractures.

Concurrent soft-tissue injury often makes assessment of a facial injury difficult. Oral and maxillofacial examinations should be performed after the patient has been stabilized and any life-threatening situations have been treated. Careful assessment is made for entrapment of ocular muscles and cranial nerve involvement.

An x-ray documents the extent of the injury. Computed tomography (CT) imaging helps differentiate between bone and soft tissue and gives a more specific view of the fracture.[25]

Injury to the eye must be suspected when a facial injury occurs, particularly if the injury is near the orbit. If a global rupture is suspected the examination is stopped and a protective shield is placed over the eye until examined by the ophthalmologist. Signs of global rupture include brown tissue (iris or ciliary body) on the surface of the globe or penetrating through a laceration with an eccentric or teardrop-shaped pupil.[26] Specific treatment of a facial fracture depends on the site and extent of the fracture and the associated soft tissue injury. Immobilization or surgical stabilization may be necessary. (Mandibular fractures are discussed in Chapter 39.)

The patient who sustains a facial fracture requires sensitive nursing care, since alteration in appearance after the trauma may be drastic. Edema and discoloration subside with time, but concurrent soft-tissue injuries may result in permanent scarring. Attention to maintenance of a patent airway and adequate nutrition are ongoing concerns of the nurse throughout the recovery period. Suction should always be available to maintain a patent airway for these patients.

OSTEOMYELITIS

Etiology and Pathophysiology

Osteomyelitis is an infection of bone by direct or indirect invasion by an organism. In children, long bones are most commonly affected whereas the vertebrae are more commonly affected in adults. Direct entry results from contamination as a result of an open fracture or surgery. Indirect inoculation results from a blood-borne infection from a distant site such as teeth, infected tonsils, diabetic ulcers, or furuncles. The most common infecting organism is *Staphylococcus aureus.* Aerobic gram-negative bacteria alone or mixed with gram-positive organisms are often found.[27] The course and virulence of osteomyelitis are influenced by the blood supply to the affected bone. The widespread use of antibiotics in conjunction with surgical treatment has significantly reduced the mortality rate associated with osteomyelitis. However, the incidence and morbidity remain relatively unchanged because new, drug-resistant strains of organisms, such as methicillin-resistant *Staphylococcus aureus* (MRSA), have developed.

The indirect-entry (also called hematogenous) type of osteomyelitis most frequently affects growing bone in boys and is associated with local trauma. The most common sites of indirect-entry osteomyelitis are the long bones of the leg, although any bone can be involved.

The direct-entry type of osteomyelitis can occur at any age when there is an open wound. After gaining entrance to the bone by way of the arterial blood supply, the bacteria lodge in an area of bone in which circulation slows, usually the metaphysis. The locus of bacteria grows, resulting in an increase in pressure because of the nonexpanding container of tubular bone. This increasing pressure eventually leads to ischemia and vascular compromise. Once ischemia occurs, the bone dies. The area of devitalized bone eventually separates from the surrounding living bone, forming *sequestra.* These sequestra form havens for bacteria, and chronic osteomyelitis develops.

Once formed, a sequestrum continues to be an infected island of bone, surrounded by pus and difficult to reach by blood-borne antibiotics or leukocytes. It may enlarge and serve as a source of bacteria for spread to other sites, including the lungs and brain. Two situations are possible. The sequestrum may extrude through a defect in tubular bone; however, this is hindered by the formation of new bone laid down by the elevated periosteum called *involucrum* (Fig. 59-17). Once outside the bone, the sequestrum may revascularize and undergo removal by normal defense processes. The other possibility is surgical removal. Unless resolved naturally or surgically, the necrotic sequestrum may develop a sinus tract, resulting in chronic purulent wound drainage.

Clinical Manifestations

Acute osteomyelitis refers to the initial infection or an infection of less than 1 month in duration. The clinical manifestations of acute osteomyelitis are both systemic and local. Systemic manifestations include fever, night sweats, chills, restlessness, nausea, and malaise. Local manifestations include severe bone pain that is unrelieved by rest and worse with activity; swelling, tenderness, and warmth at infection site; and restricted movement of affected part. Later signs include drainage from sinus tracts to the skin and fracture site.

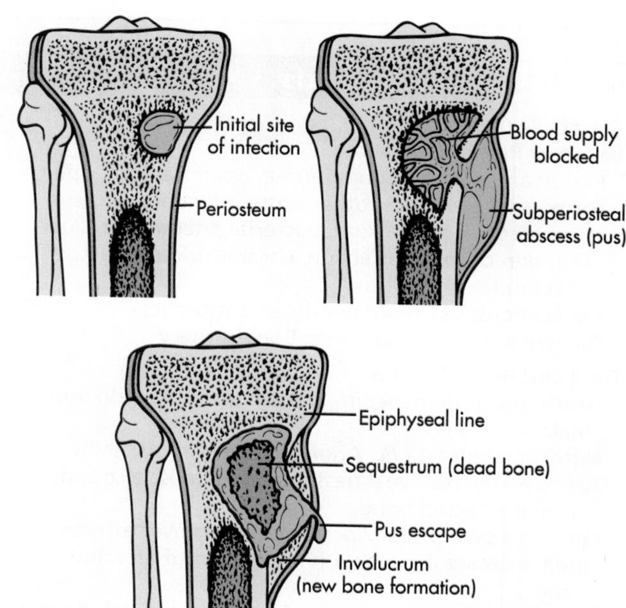

Fig. 59-17 Development of osteomyelitis infection with involucrum and sequestrum.

Chronic osteomyelitis refers to a bone infection that persists for longer than 4 weeks or an infection that has failed to respond to the initial course of antibiotic therapy. Chronic osteomyelitis can represent either a continuous, persistent problem or a process of exacerbations and quiescence. It results from inadequately treated acute osteomyelitis. Pus accumulates, causing ischemia of the bone. Over time, granulation tissue turns to scar tissue. This avascular scar tissue provides an ideal site for bacterial growth and is impenetrable to antibiotics.

Diagnostic Studies

Wound culture determines the causative organism. A bone or tissue biopsy is the definitive way to determine the causative agent. The patient's blood or sequestrum cultures are frequently positive. An elevated blood leukocyte count and sedimentation rate may also be found. Radiologic signs suggestive of osteomyelitis usually do not appear until 10 days to weeks after the appearance of clinical symptoms, by which time the disease will have progressed. Radionuclide bone scans can establish the diagnosis within 24 to 72 hours.[28] MRI and CT scans may be used to help identify the boundaries of the infection. Gallium scans and indium scans may also prove useful in some instances.

Collaborative Care

Vigorous antibiotic therapy is the treatment of choice for acute osteomyelitis, as long as ischemia has not yet occurred. Wound cultures or bone biopsy should be taken before antibiotic therapy is initiated so that the specific antibiotic therapy can be determined by sensitivity studies. If antibiotic therapy is not

NURSING ASSESSMENT

Table 59-13 Osteomyelitis

Subjective Data

Important Health Information

Past health history: Bone trauma, open fracture, open or puncture wounds, other acute infections (e.g., streptococcal sore throat, bacterial pneumonia, sinusitis, skin or tooth infection, chronic urinary tract infection)

Medications: Use of analgesics or antibiotics

Surgery or other treatments: Bone surgery

Functional Health Patterns

Health perception–health management: IV drug abuse; malaise

Nutritional-metabolic: Anorexia, weight loss; chills

Activity-exercise: Weakness, paralysis, muscle spasms around affected bone

Cognitive-perceptual: Local tenderness over affected area, increase in pain with movement of affected bone

Coping–stress tolerance: Irritability, withdrawal, dependency, anger

Objective Data

General

Restlessness; high, spiking temperature; night sweats

Integumentary

Diaphoresis; erythema, warmth, edema at infected bone

Musculoskeletal

Restricted movement; wound drainage; spontaneous fractures

Possible Findings

Leukocytosis, positive blood and wound cultures, elevated erythrocyte sedimentation rate; rarefaction with presence of sequestrum and involucrum on x-rays, radionuclide bone scans, CT, and MRI

started early in the course of the illness, surgical debridement and decompression are necessary to relieve pressure within the bone and prevent ischemia. Some type of immobilization for the affected part is usually indicated. Pathologic fractures may occur because of weakened, devitalized bone. Soft-tissue and bone healing occur slowly in the presence of infection, and subsequent deformity of the extremity may develop.

Treatment for chronic osteomyelitis includes surgical removal of poorly vascularized tissue and dead bone and extended use of antibiotics.[28] After surgical debridement of devitalized and infected tissue, the wound may be closed, and a suction irrigation system for removal of any devitalized tissues remaining in the wound area is inserted. Intermittent or constant irrigation of the affected bone with antibiotics may be initiated. Hyperbaric oxygen therapy may be used as an adjunctive therapy for chronic osteomyelitis where available, especially when associated with pressure necrosis or diabetic ulcers.

Treatment for chronic osteomyelitis previously involved an extended hospital stay for intravenous (IV) antibiotic treatment or stabilization of the patient and discharge with IV antibiotics. Most oral antibiotics have limited success rate because of poor penetration into organic bone. Ciprofloxacin (Cipro) and ofloxacin (Floxin) are effective agents for the treatment of some forms of osteomyelitis. IV antibiotics are delivered via a central venous catheter or peripherally inserted central catheter (PICC). IV antibiotic therapy may be started in the hospital and continued in the home for 4 to 6 weeks or as long as 3 to 6 months.[29]

Surgical removal of the infection may be necessary. Myocutaneous flaps or skin and bone grafting may be necessary if destruction is extensive. Antibiotic-impregnated bead chains may be surgically implanted at the time of debridement to aid in combating the infection. Infection may occur in the presence of a foreign body such as an implant or an orthopedic device such as a plate or a total joint prosthesis. It may be necessary to remove the device to effectively treat the infection.[30] Infection and bone destruction may be so extensive that amputation of the extremity may be necessary to preserve life or improve the quality of life.

NURSING MANAGEMENT: OSTEOMYELITIS

The nursing management of the patient with osteomyelitis is challenging and demanding. A prolonged hospital or long-term care facility stay may be required to ensure that adequate remission has been achieved. Extended home care with frequent home visits by nurses is currently a more common mode of therapy.

Nursing Assessment

Subjective and objective data that should be obtained from an individual with osteomyelitis are presented in Table 59-13.

Nursing Diagnoses

Nursing diagnoses for the patient with osteomyelitis may include, but are not limited to, those presented in NCP 59-3.

Planning

The overall goals are that the patient with osteomyelitis will (1) have satisfactory pain and fever control, (2) not experience any complications associated with osteomyelitis, (3) cooperate with the treatment plan, and (4) maintain a positive outlook on the outcome of the disease.

Nursing Implementation

Health Promotion. Patients with artificial implants such as a total joint replacement or metallic bone implants should be educated about methods to reduce the risk of osteomyelitis. Some physicians recommend prophylactic doses of antibiotics for procedures such as teeth cleaning, colonoscopy, or vaginal examinations.

Acute Intervention. The involved extremity should be handled carefully to avoid excessive manipulation, which increases pain and may cause pathologic fracture. Sterile dressings are used to contain the exudate from draining wounds. Besides protecting the wound area, dressings are also used as adjuncts in the mechanical debridement of devitalized tissue from the wound site when they are removed. Types of dressings used include dry, sterile dressings, dressings saturated in saline or antibiotic solution, and wet-to-dry dressings. Soiled dressings should be handled carefully to prevent cross-contamination of the wound or spread of the infection to other patients. When the dressing is changed, sterile technique is essential; it should always include sterile dressing sets, gloves, and surgical cap, gown, and mask to reduce wound contamination from external sources.

59-3 NURSING CARE PLAN PATIENT WITH OSTEOMYELITIS

Expected Patient Outcomes	Nursing Interventions and *Rationales*

NURSING DIAGNOSIS **Pain** *related to* inflammatory process secondary to infection *as manifested by* guarding, moaning, crying, restlessness, altered muscle tone, decreased activity, rating pain as >2 on a scale of 1 through 5.

Expected Patient Outcomes	Nursing Interventions and *Rationales*
■ Decrease in or absence of pain. ■ Satisfaction with pain relief.	■ Assess location and severity of pain and previous pain-relieving measures *to plan appropriate interventions.* ■ Use a pain scale *to assess pain and evaluate effectiveness of interventions.* ■ Give analgesics as indicated *to relieve pain.* ■ Instruct patient to request analgesia *before pain becomes severe.* ■ Avoid activities that increase circulation, such as exercise or application of heat, *to prevent increasing edema and subsequent pain.* ■ Use gentle handling and support when moving extremity *to reduce pain and prevent pathologic fractures.* ■ Utilize the prescribed immobilization device and maintain patient's body in correct alignment and positioning *to prevent unusual position or muscle stretching from increasing pain.* ■ Restrict ambulation or teach patient to use assistive device (e.g., crutches) *to prevent pathologic fracture, pain, and increased stress on bone.* ■ Elevate extremity *to reduce swelling and provide comfort.* ■ Instruct patient in nonpharmacologic methods of pain control such as auditory, visual, or tactile distraction; rhythmic breathing; guided imagery; thermotherapy *to augment or reduce the need for analgesics.*

NURSING DIAGNOSIS **Hyperthermia** *related to* infection *as manifested by* fever, restlessness, diaphoresis, chills.

Expected Patient Outcomes	Nursing Interventions and *Rationales*
■ Normal temperature. ■ Minimal discomfort. ■ Absence of chilling or dehydration.	■ Take temperature q4hr *to determine presence of elevated temperature and to monitor patient's response to treatment.* ■ Provide cool environment, light clothing and bedding, antipyretic drugs as ordered, and sponge bath or tub bath *to increase patient's comfort and reduce temperature.* ■ Offer fluids every hour *to prevent dehydration from insensible fluid loss.* ■ When chilled, cover with light blankets.

NURSING DIAGNOSIS **Impaired physical mobility** *related to* pain, immobilization devices, and weight-bearing limitations *as manifested by* inability or unwillingness to move purposefully within environment.

Expected Patient Outcomes	Nursing Interventions and *Rationales*
■ Consistent increase in mobility and range of motion with minimal pain or discomfort.	■ Assist patient as needed *to reduce patient's frustration with impaired mobility and prevent injury.* ■ Explain the rationale for immobilization *to foster the patient's cooperation.* ■ Increase mobility as ordered and tolerated *to maintain muscle function and strength.* ■ Provide assistive devices (e.g., pick-up stick, long-handled shoe horn, stocking helpers) *to increase independence in ADLs and activity.*

NURSING DIAGNOSIS **Ineffective management of therapeutic regimen** *related to* lack of knowledge regarding long-term management of osteomyelitis *as manifested by* verbalization of concern regarding home care by patient or family members, need to learn new knowledge or skills for home management.

Expected Patient Outcomes	Nursing Interventions and *Rationales*
■ Verbalization of confidence in self or caregiver's ability to carry out home management routine.	■ Provide information and instruction regarding wound care, aseptic technique, and dressing disposal *to reduce risk of cross-contamination and encourage wound healing.* ■ Review medication regimen including schedule, name, dosage, purpose, and side effects *because long-term antibiotic therapy is required.* ■ Stress importance of proper diet, rest, physician follow-up, and physical rehabilitation *to facilitate wound healing and reduce risk of chronic osteomyelitis.* ■ Provide written instructions about the preceding information along with a phone number to call with any questions.

Good body alignment and frequent position changes prevent complications associated with immobility and promote comfort. Flexion contracture, especially of the hip or knee, is a common sequela of osteomyelitis of the lower extremity because the patient frequently positions the affected extremity in a flexed position to promote comfort. This can cause the development of contracture, which may progress to a deformity. Footdrop can develop quickly in the lower extremity if the foot is not correctly supported. A splint is frequently applied to the involved extremity in an attempt to maintain immobilization, support, and comfort. The patient should be instructed to avoid any activities such as exercise or heat application that increase circulation and serve as stimuli to the spread of infection.

The patient should also be taught potential complications of antibiotic therapy and the need to report symptoms as early as possible. This includes hearing deficit and fluid retention associated with the aminoglycosides (e.g., tobramycin [Nebcin], neomycin) and jaundice, photosensitivity, and hepatotoxicity with cephalosporins (e.g., cefazolin [Ancef]).

Patients are frightened and discouraged because of the serious nature of the disease, systemic illness, pain, and the length and cost of treatment. Continued psychologic support is an integral part of nursing management.

Ambulatory and Home Care. With the introduction of various intermittent venous access devices, IV antibiotics can be administered to the patient in a nursing home or home setting. If at home, the patient and family must be instructed on the proper care and management of the venous access device. They must also be taught how to administer the antibiotic and the need for follow-up laboratory testing. Periodic home nursing visits provide the family with a resource on correct technique, which relieves anxiety. If there is an open wound, dressing changes may be necessary. The patient may require supplies and instruction in the technique.

If the osteomyelitis becomes chronic, patients need physical and psychologic support for a prolonged period. They may become suspicious and hostile toward the care providers when treatment plans do not effect a cure. Well-informed patients are better able to participate in decisions and cooperate in treatment plans.

■ Evaluation

The expected outcomes for the patient with osteomyelitis are presented in NCP 59-3.

AMPUTATION

During the past 20 years, major advances have been made in surgical amputation techniques, prosthetic design, and rehabilitation programs. These advances are enabling amputees to return to productive and satisfying social roles. There are an estimated 400,000 amputees in the United States, with an annual increase of 20,000. The middle and older age-groups have the highest incidence of amputation because of the effects of peripheral vascular disease, especially atherosclerosis and vascular changes related to diabetes mellitus. Traumatic injury is the usual cause for amputation in the younger adult. Amputation is required more often in persons engaged in hazardous occupations. The incidence in men is greater, since men are more often involved in such occupations. Amputation may also be indicated for certain types of bone cancer affecting an extremity (e.g., osteogenic sarcoma).

COLLABORATIVE CARE

Table 59-14 Amputation

Diagnostic
- Physical examination
  - Physical appearance of soft tissues
  - Skin temperature
  - Sensory function
  - Presence of peripheral pulses
- Arteriography
- Thermography
- Plethysmography
- Transcutaneous ultrasonic Doppler recordings

Collaborative Therapy

Medical
- Appropriate management of underlying disease process
- Stabilization of trauma victim

Surgical
- Appropriate type of amputation, leaving as long a residual limb as possible
- Residual limb management
  - Immediate prosthetic fitting
  - Delayed prosthetic fitting

Rehabilitation
- Coordination of prosthesis-fitting and gait-training activities
- Coordination of muscle-strengthening and physical therapy regimens

Clinical Indications

The clinical features that indicate the need for an amputation depend on the underlying diseases or trauma. Common indications for amputation include circulatory impairment resulting from a peripheral vascular disorder, traumatic and thermal injuries, malignant tumors, uncontrolled or widespread infection of the extremity, and congenital disorders. These conditions may manifest as loss of sensation, inadequate circulation, pallor, sweating, and local or systemic infection. Although pain is often present, it is not usually the primary reason for an amputation. The underlying problem dictates whether the amputation is performed as elective or emergency surgery.

Diagnostic Studies

The types of diagnostic studies done depend on the underlying problem that makes the amputation necessary (Table 59-14). An elevated white blood cell (WBC) count may be indicative of infection. Vascular studies such as arteriography provide information about the circulatory status of the extremity.

Collaborative Care

The potential for revascularization surgery rather than amputation can be assessed on the basis of vascular studies. If amputation is to be considered "elective," the patient's general health is carefully assessed. Chronic illnesses and infection are monitored closely. The patient and family should be helped to un-

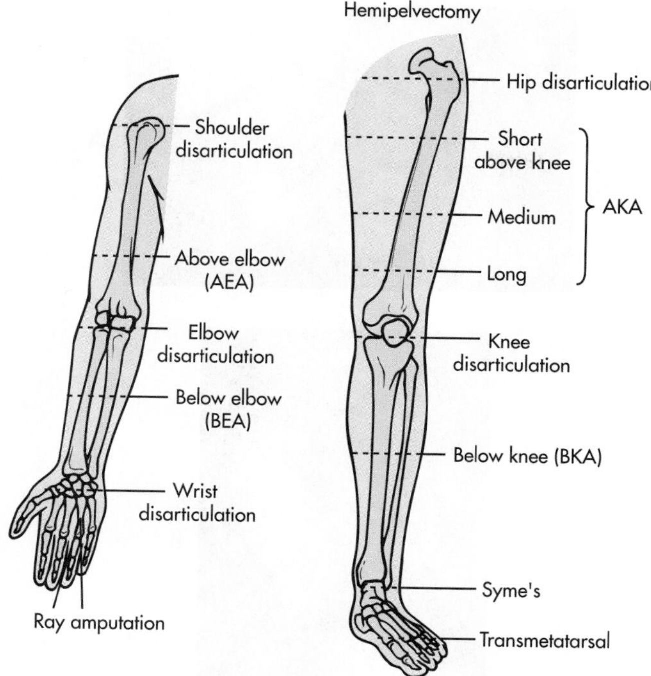

Fig. 59-18 Location and description of amputation sites of the upper and lower extremities. *AKA*, above the knee amputation.

derstand the need for the amputation and be assured that rehabilitation can result in an active, useful life. If the amputation is done on an emergency basis as a result of trauma, the management is physically and emotionally more complicated.

The goal of amputation surgery is to preserve extremity length and function while removing all infected, pathologic, or ischemic tissue. This improves the possibility of good prosthetic, cosmetic, and functional satisfaction. (Levels of amputation of upper and lower extremities are illustrated in Fig. 59-18.) The type of amputation depends on the reason for the surgery. A closed amputation is performed to create a weight-bearing residual limb (or stump); an anterior skin flap with dissected soft-tissue padding covers the bony part of the residual limb. The skin flap is sutured posteriorly so it will not be positioned in a weight-bearing area. Special care is necessary to prevent the accumulation of drainage, which can produce pressure and harbor infection. *Disarticulation* is an amputation performed through a joint. A Syme's amputation is a form of disarticulation at the ankle. An *open amputation* leaves a surface on the residual limb that is not covered with skin. This type of surgery is generally indicated for control of actual or potential infection. The wound is usually closed later by a second surgical procedure or closed by skin traction surrounding the residual limb. This type of amputation is often referred to as a *guillotine amputation.*

NURSING MANAGEMENT: AMPUTATION

■ Nursing Assessment

Preexisting illnesses must be adequately assessed since most amputations are performed because of vascular problems. Assessment of the vascular and neurologic status is an important part of this assessment process (see Chapters 30 and 53).

■ Nursing Diagnoses

Nursing diagnoses for the patient with an amputation may include, but are not limited to, the following:

- Body image disturbance *related to* amputation and impaired mobility
- Impaired skin integrity *related to* immobility and improperly fitted prosthesis
- Pain *related to* phantom limb sensation
- Impaired physical mobility *related to* amputation of lower limb

■ Planning

The overall goals are that the patient with an amputation will (1) have relief from the underlying health problem, (2) have satisfactory pain control, (3) reach maximum rehabilitation potential with the use of a prosthesis (if indicated), (4) cope with the body image changes, and (5) make satisfying lifestyle adjustments.

■ Nursing Implementation

Health Promotion. Most lower-limb amputations result from peripheral vascular disease, and most upper-limb amputations result from severe trauma. This knowledge directs patient education related to prevention of amputation. Control of causative illnesses such as peripheral vascular disease, diabetes mellitus, chronic osteomyelitis, and pressure ulcers can eliminate or delay the need for amputation. Patients with these problems should be taught to carefully examine their lower extremities daily for signs of potential problems. If the patient cannot assume this responsibility, a family member should be instructed in the procedure. Patients and their families should be instructed to report problems such as change in skin color or temperature, decrease or absence of sensation, tingling, pain, or the presence of a lesion to the health care provider.

Instruction in proper safety precautions in recreation and in the performance of hazardous work is a nursing responsibility of major importance, especially for occupational health nurses. Preventing limb mutilation and subsequent amputation is one of the serious consequences of trauma avoided through such instruction.

Acute Intervention. The nurse must recognize the tremendous psychologic and social implications of a lower-limb amputation for the patient. The disruption in body image caused by an amputation often causes a patient to go through psychologic stages similar to the grieving process of death. Allowing the patient to go through a grieving process or period of depression and recognizing it as a normal consequence of the amputation may do much to aid the patient's acceptance of the amputation. The patient's family must also be helped to work through the process to arrive at a realistic and positive attitude about the future. The reasons for an amputation and the rehabilitation potential depend on age, diagnosis, occupation, personality, resources, and support systems.

Preoperative management. Before surgery, the nurse should reinforce information the patient and family have received about the reasons for the amputation, the proposed prosthesis, and the mobility training program. In addition to the usual preoperative instructions, the patient undergoing an amputation has special education needs. To meet these needs, the nurse must know the level of amputation, the type of postsurgical dressing to be applied, and the type of prosthesis planned. The patient should receive instruction in the performance of upper-extremity exercises such as push-ups in bed or the wheelchair to promote arm strength. This is essential for later crutch walking and gait training. If possible, the nurse should instruct the patient in the technique of crutch walking and the type of gait that will be used after surgery and during gait training with the prosthesis. General postoperative nursing care should be discussed, including positioning, support, and residual limb care. If a compression bandage is to be used after surgery the patient should be instructed about its purpose and how it will be applied. If an immediate prosthesis is planned, the general ambulation program should be discussed.

The patient should be warned that she or he may feel as though the amputated limb is still present after surgery. This phenomenon, termed *phantom sensation* (a sensation of aching, tingling, or itching of the amputated limb), usually disappears but may cause patients grave concern unless they are forewarned. If pain was present in the affected limb preoperatively, the patient may experience phantom limb pain postoperatively. The patient may have feelings of coldness and heaviness or cramping, shooting, burning, or crushing pain. Often, the patient may be extremely anxious about this pain because the patient knows the limb is gone but still feels pain in it. Usually, phantom limb pain goes away in time, although it can become chronic. The pain is a real sensation to the patient and interventions should be provided for relief. As recovery and ambulation progress, phantom limb sensation usually subsides.

Postoperative management. General postoperative care for the patient who has had an amputation depends largely on the patient's general state of health, the reason for the amputation, and the patient's age. Nursing care must be individualized on the basis of these factors. For example, an older adult patient needs particularly careful monitoring of respiratory status; a victim of a motor vehicle accident may need careful neurologic monitoring.

Prevention and detection of complications are important nursing responsibilities during the postoperative period. Careful monitoring of the patient's vital signs and dressing can alert the nurse to hemorrhage in the operative area. Careful attention to sterile technique during dressing changes reduces the potential for wound infection and subsequent interruption of rehabilitation.

If an immediate postoperative prosthesis has been applied, the nurse must monitor vital signs carefully, since the surgical site is heavily covered and may not be visible. A surgical tourniquet must always be available for emergency use. If hemorrhage occurs, the surgeon should be notified immediately and efforts to control the hemorrhage should begin at once.

The surgeon must decide the type of prosthetic fitting that will be used after surgery. An immediate prosthetic fitting, often called the immediate postsurgical fitting or the immediate postoperative fitting, is done in the operating room after the amputation (Fig. 59-19). A rigid, cast-like bandage is applied around the closed residual limb with a prosthetic pylon and an ankle-foot assembly. While the patient is still anesthetized, the prosthetic pylon and ankle-foot assembly are aligned and adjusted to provide a smooth gait and to avoid excessive pressure on the residual limb area. A strap is placed on the proximal anterior surface of the rigid plaster bandage and attached to a waistband to prevent slippage. The main advantages of this device are reduction of edema and the psychologic benefit of early ambulation. A disadvantage is the inability to directly visualize the surgical site.

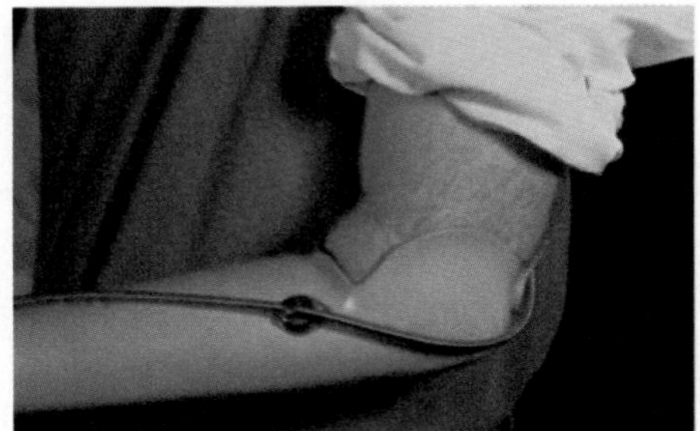

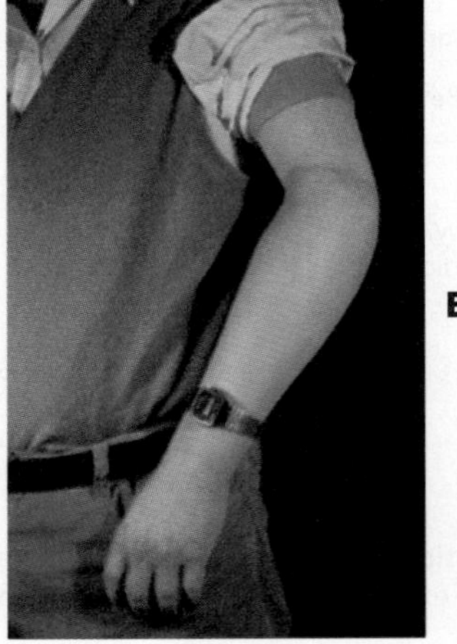

Fig. 59-19 Two types of prosthesis. **A,** Traditional fiberglass. **B,** New materials and techniques have made possible fabrication of prosthetic sockets that are light, soft, flexible, and secure.

The delayed prosthetic fitting may be the best choice for certain patients. Patients who have had amputations above the knee or below the elbow, older adults, debilitated individuals, and those with infection usually have delayed prosthetic fittings. The appropriate time for use of a prosthesis depends on satisfactory healing of the residual limb, as well as on the general condition of the patient. A temporary prosthesis may be used for partial weight bearing once the sutures are removed. Barring any problems, patients can bear full weight on permanent prostheses by approximately 3 months after amputation.

Not all patients are candidates for a prosthesis. It is important that the surgeon discuss ambulation possibilities frankly with the patient and family. The seriously ill or debilitated patient may not have the energy required to use a prosthesis. Mobility with a wheelchair may be the most realistic goal for this type of patient.

Collaborative care also includes the direction and coordination of the rehabilitation program for the amputee. Success depends on the physical and emotional health of the patient. Chronic illness and debilitation complicate aggressive rehabilitation efforts.

Flexion contractures may delay the rehabilitation process. The most common and debilitating contracture is hip flexion. Hip adduction contracture is rare. Patients should avoid sitting in a chair with hips flexed or having pillows under the surgical extremity to prevent flexion contractures. Unless specifically

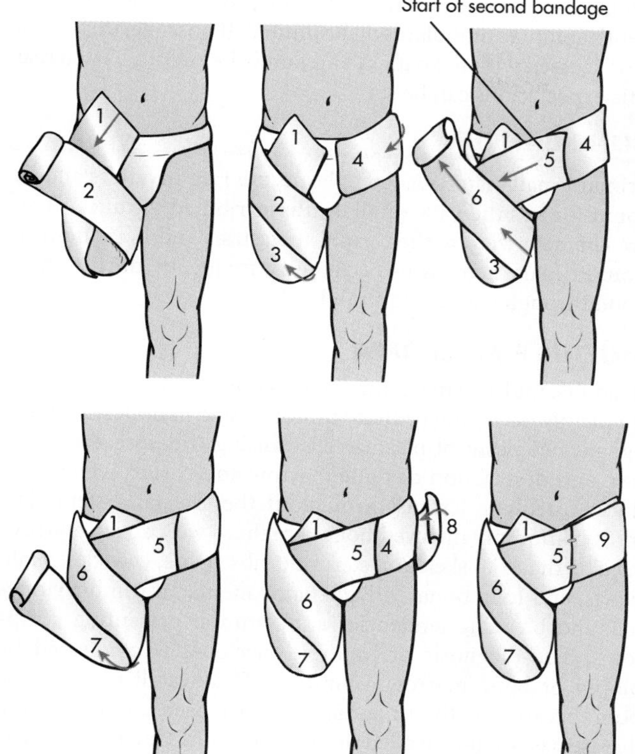

Fig. 59-20 Bandaging for the above-the-knee amputation residual limb. Figure-eight style covers progressive areas of the residual limb. Two elastic wraps are required.

PATIENT & FAMILY TEACHING GUIDE

Table 59-15 Following an Amputation

1. Inspect the residual limb daily for signs of skin irritation, especially redness and abrasion. Pay particular attention to areas prone to pressure.
2. Discontinue use of the prosthesis if an irritation develops. Have the area checked before resuming use of the prosthesis.
3. Wash residual limb thoroughly each night with warm water and a bacteriostatic soap. Rinse thoroughly and dry gently. Expose the residual limb to air for 20 minutes.
4. Do not use any substance such as lotions, alcohol, powders, or oil unless prescribed by the physician.
5. Wear only a residual limb sock that is in good condition and supplied by the prosthetist.
6. Change residual limb sock daily. Launder in a mild soap, squeeze, and lay flat to dry.
7. Use prescribed pain management techniques.
8. Perform ROM to all joints daily. Perform general strengthening exercises including the upper extremities daily.
9. Do not elevate the residual limb on a pillow.
10. Lay prone with hip extension for 30 minutes three to four times daily.

contraindicated, patients should lie on their abdomen for 30 minutes three to four times each day and position the hip in extension while prone.

Proper residual limb bandaging fosters shaping and molding for eventual prosthesis fitting (Fig. 59-20). The physician usually orders a compression bandage to be applied immediately after surgery to support the soft tissues, reduce edema, hasten healing, minimize pain, and promote residual limb shrinkage and maturation. This bandage may be an elastic roll applied to the residual limb or a residual limb shrinker, which is an elastic stocking that fits tightly over the residual limb and lower trunk area.[31]

The compression bandage is initially worn at all times except during physical therapy and bathing. The bandage is taken off and reapplied several times daily, and care is taken so that it is applied snugly but not so tight as to interfere with circulation. Shrinker bandages should be washed and changed daily. It is recommended that the patient have two residual limb shrinker bandages so one can be worn while the other is being washed. After healing has occurred, the residual limb is bandaged only when the patient is not wearing the prosthesis. The patient should be instructed to avoid dangling the residual limb over the bedside to minimize edema formation.

As the patient's overall condition improves, the nurse begins instruction in the principles and techniques of transferring from bed to chair and back. Active exercises and conditioning are essential in developing ambulation skills. The exercise regimen is normally started under the supervision of the physician and the physical therapist. The nurse must have a clear understanding of the exercise regimen to reinforce it and ensure that the exercises are performed correctly. Active range-of-motion exercises of all joints should be started as soon after surgery as the patient's pain level and medical status permit. In preparation for mobility, the patient should increase triceps and shoulder strength and lower limb support and learn balance of the altered body. The loss of the weight of a limb requires adaptation of the patient's proprioceptive mechanisms to prevent falls and frustration.

Crutch walking is started as soon as patients are physically able. If they have had immediate postsurgical fitting, orders related to weight bearing must be carefully followed to avoid disruption of the skin flap and delay of the training process. Initial periods of ambulation should not exceed 5 minutes to prevent dependent edema.

Before discharge, the patient and family need careful instruction related to residual limb care, ambulation, prevention of contractures, recognition of complications, exercise, and follow-up care. Table 59-15 outlines patient teaching following an amputation.

Ambulatory and Home Care. When the healing has occurred satisfactorily and the residual limb is well molded, the patient is ready for fitting a prosthesis. Walking with a below-the-knee prosthesis requires 40% additional energy, and an above-the-knee prosthesis requires 60% more energy. Matching a patient with a suitable prosthesis involves many factors, including age, general health, intelligence, motivation, occupation, and finances. After the physician makes the recommendation, the patient is referred to a prosthetist, who initially makes a mold of the residual limb and measures landmarks for the fabrication of the prosthesis. The molded residual limb socket allows the residual limb to fit snugly into the prosthesis. The residual limb is covered with a residual limb stocking to ensure good fit and prevent skin breakdown. The residual limb may continue to shrink, causing a loose fit, in which case a new socket has to be fabricated. The patient may need to have the prosthesis adjusted to prevent rubbing and friction between the residual limb and the socket. Excessive movement of a loose prosthesis can cause severe skin irritation and breakdown.

The prosthesis is fitted by the prosthetist, who may also train the amputee to use it. It is important for the nurse to be familiar with the training program to encourage and assist the patient. Learning to use a prosthesis is frustrating, and the patient may easily become discouraged. The nurse must continually offer support until the patient is able to manage alone.

Artificial limbs become an integral part of the patient's body image. Proper care ensures their long life and useful functioning. The patient should be instructed to clean the prosthesis socket daily with a mild soap and rinse thoroughly to remove irritants. The leather and metal parts of the prosthesis should not get wet. The patient should be encouraged to have regular maintenance of the prosthesis. Consideration of the condition of the shoe is also necessary. A badly worn shoe alters the gait and may cause damage to the prosthesis.

Referral to a community health nurse can foster optimal physical and emotional adjustment. The family should be instructed on ambulation and transfer techniques and proper residual limb care.

■ Evaluation

The expected outcomes are that the patient with an amputation will

- accept changed body image and integrate changes into lifestyle
- have no evidence of skin breakdown
- have reduction or absence of pain
- become mobile within limitations imposed by amputation

Special Considerations in Upper-Limb Amputation

The emotional implications of an upper-limb amputation are often more devastating than those for lower-limb amputation. The enforced dependency brought about by one-handedness is both frustrating and humiliating to many patients. Because most upper-extremity amputations result from trauma, the patient has also not had the opportunity to adjust psychologically to an amputation or to participate in the decision-making process.

Both immediate and delayed prosthetic fittings are possible for the below-the-elbow amputee. Prosthetic fitting is delayed for the above-the-elbow amputee. The usual functional prosthesis is the arm and hook. A cosmetic hand is available but has limited functional value. As with the lower-limb prosthesis, patient motivation and endurance are major factors toward a satisfactory outcome.

GERONTOLOGIC CONSIDERATIONS

Amputation

If a lower limb amputation has been performed on an older adult, the patient's previous ability to ambulate may affect the extent of recovery. Use of a prosthesis requires a significant amount of energy for ambulation. Older adults whose general health is weakened by disorders such as cardiac or pulmonary problems may not be candidates for prosthesis use. This patient's ability to ambulate will be limited. If possible, this should be discussed with the patient and family before surgery so realistic expectations can be set.

BONE CANCER

Primary malignant bone neoplasms are rare in adults and account for less than 1% of all deaths attributed to cancer. They are characterized by their rapid metastasis and bone destruction. Primary neoplasms occur most frequently during childhood through young adulthood.

MULTIPLE MYELOMA

In adults, multiple myeloma (plasma cell myeloma) is the most frequently occurring primary tumor arising in bone. It is a malignant neoplasm of plasma cells causing widespread infiltration and destruction of bone marrow and cortex, which produces osteolytic lesions throughout the skeletal system. The most commonly involved bones are those with active marrow, such as the axial skeleton, sternum, ribs, spine, clavicles, skull, pelvis, and long bones.[32] Back pain, anemia, thrombocytopenia, and bleeding tendencies are common presenting symptoms. The diagnosis of multiple myeloma is confirmed by biopsy or bone marrow aspiration. The overall prognosis is poor, because by the time diagnosis has been confirmed, the disease has usually invaded the axial skeleton. Chemotherapeutic treatment of multiple myeloma has limited usefulness; it is primarily directed toward suppressing plasma cell growth. Radiation therapy may be helpful in reducing pain. Corticosteroids are commonly used in conjunction with melphalan (Alkeran), vincristine (Oncovin), or doxorubicin (Adriamycin). (Multiple myeloma is also discussed in Chapter 29.)

OSTEOGENIC SARCOMA

Osteogenic sarcoma (osteosarcoma) is a primary neoplasm of bone that is extremely malignant and is characterized by rapid growth and metastasis. It usually occurs in the metaphyseal region of the long bones of the extremities, particularly in the regions of the distal femur, proximal tibia, and proximal humerus, as well as the pelvis. Osteogenic sarcoma is the most common malignant bone tumor affecting children and young adults; its highest incidence is in the 10- to 25-year-old age-group. It occurs most commonly in males. Secondary osteosarcoma is known to occur in adults over age 60 and is most commonly associated with Paget's disease.

The clinical manifestations of osteogenic sarcoma are usually associated with a past history of minor injury and gradual onset of pain and swelling, especially around the knee. The injury does not cause the neoplasm but rather serves to bring the preexisting condition to medical attention. The neoplasm grows rapidly and produces a noticeable increase in the size of the general region, which can restrict joint motion if the lesion is close to a joint structure. The diagnosis is confirmed from biopsied tissue specimens, elevation of serum alkaline phosphatase and calcium levels, x-ray, CT scan, and MRI findings.

Major advances continue to be made in the treatment of osteosarcoma. Preoperative (neoadjuvant) chemotherapy is used to decrease tumor size. As a result limb-salvage procedures, including a wide surgical resection of the tumor, are being used more frequently. Amputation may be necessary depending on the size and location of the tumor. Current use of adjunct chemotherapy following amputation has increased the projected 5-year survival rate to 60%.[33]

OSTEOCLASTOMA

True osteoclastoma (giant cell tumor) is a destructive tumor that arises in the cancellous ends of long bones in young adults. Most (98%) of these variant giant cell tumors are benign. Giant cell tumors most commonly occur between the ages of 20 and 35. The common sites are the distal ends of the femur, proximal tibia, and distal radius. The giant cell tumor is a locally destructive lesion, the growth of which extends from a few months to several years. The clinical manifestations are usually swelling, local pain, and some disturbances in joint function. X-ray evidence of giant cell tumor is variable but usually reveals local areas of bone destruction and eventual expansion of the bone ends. Treatment initially includes biopsy to establish the diagnosis, followed by surgical curettage of the lesion with bone grafting. After treatment there is a greater than 50% chance of recurrence. Recurrent giant cell tumors may subsequently make amputation necessary. Advances in chemotherapy have improved the rate of survival.

EWING'S SARCOMA

Ewing's sarcoma is the fourth most common primary malignant neoplasm of bone, occurring most frequently in male patients under the age of 30. This neoplasm is characterized by rapid growth within the medullary cavity of long bone, especially the femur, humerus, pelvis, tibia, and ribs. Metastasis occurs early, and the most frequent site is the lungs. The use of radiation, surgical excision, and chemotherapy has increased the 5-year survival rate to 70%. Common manifestations are progressive local pain, swelling, palpable soft-tissue mass, noticeable increase in size of the affected part, fever, and leukocytosis. Initially, x-rays show periosteal bone destruction. Treatment usually involves radiation therapy and wide surgical resection of the tumor or amputation. Chemotherapeutic agents commonly used are cyclophosphamide (Cytoxan), vincristine (Oncovin), ifosfamide (Ifex), and doxorubicin (Adriamycin). New chemotherapeutic techniques hold promise of improvement in survival rates. Surgical resection of the tumor has helped decrease the rate of recurrence.[34]

METASTATIC BONE LESIONS

The most common type of malignant bone tumor occurs as a result of metastasis from a primary tumor. Common sites for the primary tumor include the breast, intestinal tract, lungs, prostate, kidney, ovary, and thyroid. The metastatic bone lesion is commonly found in the vertebrae, pelvis, femur, humerus, or ribs. Pathologic fractures at the site of metastasis are common because of weakening of the involved bone.

Once a primary lesion has been identified, bone scans are often done to detect the presence of metastatic lesions before they are visible on x-ray. It is important to note that metastatic bone lesions may occur at any time (even years later) following diagnosis and possible treatment of the primary tumor. Metastasis to the bone should be suspected in any patient who has local pain to the bone and a past history of cancer. Treatment may be palliative and consists of pain management and radiation. Surgical stabilization of the fracture may be indicated if there is a fracture or pending fracture. Prognosis depends on the extent of metastasis and location.

NURSING MANAGEMENT: BONE CANCER

■ Nursing Assessment

The patient with bone cancer should be assessed for the location and severity of pain. Weakness caused by anemia and increased debility may also be noted. Swelling at the involved site and decreased joint function, depending on the tumor site, should also be monitored.

■ Nursing Diagnoses

Nursing diagnoses for the patient with bone cancer may include, but are not limited to, the following:

- Pain *related to* the disease process, inadequate pain medication, or comfort measures
- Impaired physical mobility *related to* disease process, pain, weakness, and debility
- Body image disturbance *related to* possible amputation, deformity, swelling, and effects of chemotherapy
- Anticipatory grieving *related to* poor prognosis of the disease
- Risk for injury (pathologic fracture) *related to* disease process and inadequate handling or positioning of affected body part

■ Planning

The overall goals are that the patient with bone cancer will (1) have satisfactory pain relief; (2) maintain preferred activities as long as possible; (3) demonstrate acceptance of body image changes resulting from chemotherapy, radiation, and surgery; (4) be free from injury; and (5) verbalize a realistic idea of disease progression and prognosis.

■ Nursing Implementation

Health Promotion. The nurse should teach the public to recognize the warning signs of bone cancer, including swelling, bone pain of unexplained origin, limitation of joint function, and changes in skin temperature. As with all forms of cancer, health promotion should stress the importance of periodic health examinations.

Acute Intervention. Nursing care of the patient with a malignant bone neoplasm does not differ significantly from the care given to the patient with a malignant disease of any other body system. However, special attention is required to reduce the complications associated with prolonged bed rest and to prevent pathologic fractures. The patient is often reluctant to participate in therapeutic activities because of weakness and fear of pain. Regular rest periods should be provided between activities. Careful handling of the affected extremity is important to prevent pathologic fractures. As with all forms of cancer, health promotion should stress the importance of periodic health examinations.

Ambulatory and Home Care. The nurse must be able to assist the patient in accepting the guarded prognosis associated with neoplasms of the bone. Inability to accomplish age-specific developmental tasks can increase the frustrations with this condition. General principles related to cancer nursing are applicable (see Chapter 14). Special attention is necessary for the problems of pain and dysfunction, chemotherapy, and specific surgery such as spinal cord decompression or amputation.

■ Evaluation

The expected outcomes are that the patient with bone cancer will

- have minimal to no pain
- have no falls
- have no pathologic fractures
- accept changes in body image
- have maximal functional ability

LOW BACK PAIN

Etiology and Pathophysiology

Low back pain is common and has probably affected about 80% of adults in the United States at least once during their lifetime. In industry, low back pain is responsible for more lost working hours than any other medical condition and represents one of the nation's most costly health problems. Each year about 18 million visits are made to physicians for treatment of this condition.[35]

Several risk factors are associated with low back pain, including lack of muscle tone and excess weight, poor posture, smoking, and stress. Jobs that require repetitive heavy lifting, vibration (such as a jackhammer operator), and prolonged periods of sitting are also associated with low back pain.

Pain in the lumbar region is a common problem because this area (1) bears most of the weight of the body, (2) is the most flexible region of the spinal column, (3) contains nerve roots that are vulnerable to injury or disease, and (4) has an inherently poor biomechanical structure.

Low back pain is most often due to a musculoskeletal problem. However, other causes such as metabolic, circulatory, gynecologic, urologic, or psychologic problems, which may refer pain to the lower back, must not be overlooked. The causes of low back pain of musculoskeletal origin include (1) acute lumbosacral strain, (2) instability of lumbosacral bony mechanism, (3) osteoarthritis of the lumbosacral vertebrae, (4) intervertebral disk degeneration, and (5) herniation of the intervertebral disk. Of these, the most common cause is mechanical strain of paravertebral muscles. Herniation of the nucleus pulposus is another common cause of low back pain.

Acute Low Back Pain

Acute low back pain is usually associated with some type of activity that causes undue stress on the tissues of the lower back. Often symptoms do not appear at the time of injury but develop later because of gradual increase in paravertebral muscle spasms. Few definitive diagnostic abnormalities are present with paravertebral muscle strain. The straight-leg raise test may produce pain in the lumbar area without radiation along the sciatic nerve.

Collaborative Care

If the muscle spasms are not severe, the patient may be treated on an outpatient basis with a combination of the following: (1) analgesics, (2) NSAIDs, (3) muscle relaxants (e.g., cyclobenzaprine [Flexeril]), and (4) use of a corset. A corset prevents rotation, flexion, and extension of the lower back.

If the spasms and pain are severe, a brief period of rest at home may be necessary. Since paravertebral muscle spasms are worse when the patient is upright, bed rest is the prime treatment for severe acute low back pain. Bathroom privileges are usually allowed. Bed rest is maintained until the patient can move and turn from side to side with minimal discomfort. At this time, gradually increasing activity is initiated. When the patient is comfortable on oral pain medication, a progressive physical therapy program is begun to regain mobility and strength in lower back structures.

If conservative treatment is ineffective and the cause of the pain is nerve root irritation, an epidural corticosteroid injection may be performed. A needle is inserted into the epidural space and a corticosteroid and local anesthetic are injected. Epidural corticosteroids have been shown to decrease pain, speed return of function, and improve objective neurologic signs. These injections are most effective in patients with acute rather than chronic pain and patients with radicular pain who are not candidates for surgery. Epidural injections typically consist of a series of one to three injections over a span of several days to several weeks.

NURSING ASSESSMENT

Table 59-16 Low Back Pain

Subjective Data

Important Health Information

Past health history: Acute or chronic lumbosacral strain, osteoarthritis, degenerative disk disease, obesity

Medications: Use of analgesics, muscle relaxants, nonsteroidal antiinflammatory drugs, corticosteroids, over-the-counter remedies

Surgery or other treatments: Previous back surgery, epidural corticosteroid injections

Functional Health Patterns

Health perception–health management: Smoking, lack of exercise

Nutritional-metabolic: Obesity

Activity-exercise: Poor posture, muscle spasms; activity intolerance

Elimination: Constipation

Sleep-rest: Interrupted sleep

Cognitive-perceptual: Pain in back, buttocks, or leg associated with walking, turning, straining, coughing, leg raising; numbness or tingling of legs, feet, toes

Role-relationship: Occupation requiring heavy lifting, vibrations, or extended driving

Objective Data

General

Guarded movement

Neurologic

Depressed or absent Achilles tendon reflex; positive straight-leg raise test

Musculoskeletal

Tense, tight paravertebral muscles on palpation, decreased range of motion of spine

Possible Findings

Localization of site of lesion on myelogram, CT scan, or MRI; determination of nerve irritation on electromyography

NURSING MANAGEMENT: ACUTE LOW BACK PAIN

■ Nursing Assessment

Subjective and objective data that should be obtained from the patient with low back pain are summarized in Table 59-16.

59-4 NURSING CARE PLAN PATIENT WITH LOW BACK PAIN

Expected Patient Outcomes	Nursing Interventions and *Rationales*
	Acute Management
NURSING DIAGNOSIS	**Pain** *related to* herniated nucleus pulposus, muscle spasms, and ineffective comfort measures *as manifested by* verbalization of back pain on movement, guarded movements, palpable muscle spasm, decreased physical activity, rating pain as >2 on a scale of 1 through 5.
▪ Reduction or absence of pain and muscle spasms. ▪ Expression of satisfaction with pain relief (rates pain as 2 or less on scale of 1 through 5).	▪ Assess location, severity, and circumstances of pain *to plan appropriate interventions.* ▪ Use a pain scale and evaluate pain relief interventions *to assess pain and treatment measures.* ▪ Enforce decreased activity *to reduce paravertebral muscle spasms and resulting pain.* ▪ Keep head of bed elevated 20 degrees and knee of bed flexed *to promote comfort by reducing stress on lower back muscles.* ▪ Maintain pelvic traction, correctly aligned, as ordered *to reduce muscle spasm.* ▪ Apply moist heat or ice to lower back *to reduce pain and muscle spasm.* ▪ Administer analgesics, nonsteroidal antiinflammatory drugs, or muscle relaxants as ordered; document effect *to promote comfort and evaluate effectiveness.*
NURSING DIAGNOSIS	**Impaired physical mobility** *related to* pain *as manifested by* limited active joint range of motion (ROM), movement restrictions, muscle spasms.
▪ Unrestricted gait. ▪ Ambulation within normal limits. ▪ Resumption of previous level of mobility. ▪ Performance of prescribed exercises.	▪ Have patient perform ROM and muscle-strengthening exercises daily *to strengthen the supporting muscles and maintain all joints in normal ROM.* ▪ Start ambulation program and progress with assistance *to promote gradual and progressive return to previous mobility level.* ▪ Avoid having patient bend, sit, or lift *to prevent back strain and increased pain.* ▪ Report leg or back pain and change in sensation *because these are indicators of severe lumbosacral intravertebral pressure and sciatic nerve involvement.* ▪ Provide written instructions that describe each exercise and activity and a phone number to call with any questions.
	Chronic Management
NURSING DIAGNOSIS	**Chronic pain** *related to* progression of problem *as manifested by* verbal report or evidence of pain longer than 6 months in duration.
▪ Development of effective methods of managing pain. ▪ Expression of satisfaction with pain control measures.	▪ Assess variety and effectiveness of pain management techniques *to determine extent of problem and develop appropriate interventions.* ▪ Use a pain scale *to assess pain and to evaluate pain control interventions.* ▪ Instruct patient and family about home care and alternative methods of pain control, including use of heat, transcutaneous electrical nerve stimulation, and massage, *to provide information about supplementary methods of pain management.* ▪ Avoid strenuous activities, *which increase pain.* ▪ Assist in identifying activities that exacerbate pain *to make adjustments in lifestyle so that pain is reduced.*
NURSING DIAGNOSIS	**Ineffective individual coping** *related to* effects of chronic pain on lifestyle *as manifested by* verbalization of inability to cope, irritability, tension, inability to meet role expectations, altered participation in social events, ineffective or inappropriate use of defense mechanisms.
▪ Return to previous levels of work and lifestyle or successfully adapt to lifestyle changes.	▪ Explain factors that may contribute to development of maladaptive coping behavior *to communicate information and a caring attitude.* ▪ Explain how to develop therapeutic coping skills and activities that enhance self-esteem and social interaction *to foster effective coping behaviors and adjustment to chronic pain condition.* ▪ Discuss chronic nature of pain and need for lifestyle adjustments to patient *to avoid repeated and demoralizing attempts to eliminate pain.*

Continued

59-4 NURSING CARE PLAN PATIENT WITH LOW BACK PAIN—continued

Expected Patient Outcomes	Nursing Interventions and *Rationales*
NURSING DIAGNOSIS	**Ineffective management of therapeutic regimen** *related to* lack of knowledge regarding posture, exercises, body mechanics, and weight reduction *as manifested by* lack of necessary knowledge to participate in treatment plan, inadequate understanding or inaccurate follow-through of previous instructions.
▪ Use of proper body mechanics at all times. ▪ Maintenance of weight within normal limits. ▪ Maintenance of activity and ambulation appropriate to age and state of health.	▪ Assess body mechanics *to identify incorrect techniques and intervene appropriately.* ▪ Instruct patient on proper body mechanics and use of firm mattress or bedboard *to reduce risk of reinjury, provide back support, and maintain proper body alignment.* ▪ Assess for decreasing muscle strength *to identify complications and modify care plan.* ▪ Refer to physical therapist for low back exercises *to develop abdominal and paravertebral muscle strength to provide increased support.* ▪ Encourage activity and ambulation within limitations *to maintain physical mobility and minimize sick-role behaviors.* ▪ Teach about weight reduction or refer to dietician if indicated *because increased abdominal weight puts strain on low back.*
NURSING DIAGNOSIS	**Body image disturbance** *related to* impaired mobility and chronic pain *as manifested by* negative statements about body, change in social involvement or relationships, statements of hopelessness.
▪ Positive self-image.	▪ Provide psychologic support, active listening, and encouragement *to prevent development of negative body image.* ▪ Assist patient in becoming as independent as possible *to prevent assumption of sick role.* ▪ Refer to local support groups or psychologic evaluation *to provide therapeutic adjustment.*

■ Nursing Diagnoses

Nursing diagnoses for the patient with low back pain may include, but are not limited to, those presented in NCP 59-4.

■ Planning

The overall goals are that the patient with low back pain will (1) have satisfactory pain relief, (2) avoid constipation secondary to medication and immobility, (3) learn back-sparing practices, and (4) return to previous level of activity within prescribed restrictions.

■ Nursing Implementation

Health Promotion. The nurse is a significant role model and teacher for patients with low back problems. As a role model, the nurse should use proper body mechanics at all times. This should be a primary consideration when teaching patients and care providers transfer and turning techniques. The nurse should assess the patient's use of body mechanics and offer advice when activities that could produce back strain are used (Table 59-17).

Some health care providers refer patients with back pain to a program called "Back School." It is a formal program usually taught by health professionals such as physicians, nurses, and physical therapists. It is designed to teach the patient how to minimize back pain and avoid repeat episodes of low back pain. Tips for prevention of back injury are listed in Table 59-17. Exercises to strengthen the back are presented in Table 59-18.

Patients are also advised to maintain appropriate body weight. Excess body weight places extra stress on the lower

PATIENT TEACHING GUIDE

Table 59-17 Low Back Problems

Do Not
- Lean forward without bending knees
- Lift anything above level of elbows
- Stand in one position for prolonged time
- Sleep on abdomen or on back or side with legs out straight
- Exercise without consulting health care provider if having severe pain
- Exceed prescribed amount and type of exercises without consulting health care provider

Do
- Prevent lower back from straining forward by placing a foot on a step or stool during prolonged standing
- Sleep in a side-lying position with knees and hips bent
- Sleep on back with a lift under knees and legs or on back with 10-inch-high pillow under knees to flex hips and knees
- Sit in a chair with knees higher than hips and support arms on chair or knees
- Exercise 15 min in the morning and 15 min in the evening regularly; begin exercises with a 2- or 3-min warm-up period by moving arms and legs, by alternately relaxing and tightening muscles; exercise slowly with smooth movements as directed by a physical therapist
- Avoid chilling during and after exercising
- Maintain appropriate body weight
- Use a lumbar roll or pillow for sitting

PATIENT TEACHING GUIDE

Table 59-18 Back Exercises

Knee-to-chest lift (to stretch hip, buttocks, lower back muscles)
- Lie on back on the floor with knees bent and feet flat on floor.
- Draw both knees up to chest.
- Place both hands around knees and pull them firmly against chest. Hold for 30 seconds.
- Lower legs and return to starting position.
- Repeat 5-10 times.

Simple leg lift
- Lie flat on back on floor with left knee bent and left foot flat on floor.
- Raise right leg as high as comfortably possible.
- Hold for 5 counts.
- Slowly return leg to floor.
- Bend right knee and put right foot flat on floor.
- Raise left leg and hold for 5 counts.
- Repeat 5-10 times for each leg.

Double leg lift
- Lie flat on back.
- Slowly lift legs until feet are 12 inches from the floor.
- Keep legs straight and hold this position for 10 counts.
- Lower legs to floor.
- Repeat 5 times.

Pelvic tilt
- Lie flat on back on floor with knees bent and feet flat on the floor.
- Firmly tighten your buttock muscles.
- Hold for 5 counts.
- Relax buttocks.
- Repeat 5-10 times.
- Be sure to keep lower back flat against floor.

Half sit-ups (to strengthen abdominal muscles)
- Lie flat on floor on back with knees bent, feet flat on floor, and hands on chest.
- Slowly raise head and neck to top of chest.
- Reach both hands forward and place them on knees.
- Hold for 5 counts.
- Return to starting position.
- Repeat 5-10 times.

Elbow props (to extend lower back)
- Lie face down with your arms beside your body and your head turned to one side.
- Stay in this position for 2-5 minutes, making sure that you relax completely.
- Remain face down and prop yourself on your elbows.
- Hold this position for 2-3 minutes.
- Return to starting position and relax for 1 minute.
- Repeat 5-10 times.

Hip tilts
- Lie flat on back with knees bent.
- Slowly bend legs and hips to one side as far as possible.
- Bend to other side.
- Repeat 5 times.

Toe touches
- Stand straight and relaxed.
- Lower head and body and try to touch floor with fingertips.
- Keep knees straight.
- Do not jerk or lunge toward floor.
- Bend only as far as you can.
- Repeat 5 times.

From Canobbio MM: *Mosby's handbook of patient teaching,* St Louis, 1996, Mosby.

back and weakens the abdominal muscles that support the lower back.

The position assumed while sleeping is also important in preventing low back pain. Sleeping in a prone position should be avoided because it produces excessive lumbar lordosis, placing excessive stress on the lower back. A firm mattress is recommended. The patient should sleep in either a supine or side-lying position with the knees and hips flexed to prevent unnecessary pressure on support muscles, ligamentous structures, and lumbosacral joints. Patients should be educated about the necessity to avoid or cease smoking. Nicotine has been shown to decrease circulation to the disks, and a causal relationship exists between smoking and some types of low back pain.[36,37]

Acute Intervention. The primary nursing responsibilities in acute low back pain are to assist the patient to maintain activity limitations, promote comfort, and educate the patient about the health problem and appropriate exercises. Other nursing interventions are summarized in NCP 59-4. Use of analgesics, nonsteroidal antiinflammatory agents, thermotherapy (ice and heat), and muscle relaxants to promote comfort is incorporated into the plan of care.

Muscle stretching and strengthening exercises may be part of the management plan. Although the actual exercises are often taught by the physical therapist, it is the nurse's responsibility to ensure that the patient understands the type and frequency of exercise prescribed, as well as the rationale for the program.

Ambulatory and Home Care. The goal of management is to make an episode of acute low back pain an isolated incident. If the lumbosacral mechanism is unstable, repeated episodes can be anticipated. The lumbosacral spine may be unable to meet the demands placed on it without strain because of factors such as obesity, poor posture, poor muscular support, advancing age, or local trauma. Intervention is aimed at strengthening the supporting muscles by exercise and the use of a corset to limit extremes of movement. In addition, weight reduction decreases the mechanical demands on the lower back.

Persistent use of poor body mechanics may result in repeated episodes of low back pain. If the strain is work related, occupational counseling may be necessary. The frustration, pain, and disability imposed on the patient with low back pain require emotional support and understanding care by the nurse.

■ Evaluation

The expected outcomes for the patient with low back pain are presented in NCP 59-4.

Chronic Low Back Pain

Etiology and Pathophysiology

The causes of chronic low back pain include degenerative disk disease, lack of physical exercise, prior injury, obesity, structural and postural abnormalities, and systemic disease. Structural degeneration of the intervertebral disk results in degenerative disk disease manifested by low back pain. This degeneration can also occur in the cervical spine area. The degeneration results in intervertebral narrowing and a lessening of the efficiency of the intervertebral disks in acting as shock absorbers. This inefficiency causes small tears in the annulus fibrosis, which predisposes the patient to herniated nucleus pulposus. As the stresses on the degenerated disk continue and eventually exceed the strength of the disk, herniation of the intervertebral disk may result. Nuclear material from the intervertebral disk herniates and may compress or place tension on a cervical lumbar or sacral spinal nerve root (Fig. 59-21).

Clinical Manifestations

The most common feature of a lumbar herniated intervertebral disk is back pain with associated buttock and leg pain along the distribution of the sciatic nerve (radiculopathy). (Specific manifestations based on the level of lumbar disk herniation are summarized in Table 59-19.) The straight-leg raise test may be positive. Back or leg pain may be reproduced by raising the leg and flexing the foot at 90 degrees. Low back pain from other causes may not be accompanied by leg pain.

Reflexes may be depressed or absent, depending on the spinal nerve root involved. Paresthesia or muscle weakness in the legs, feet, or toes may be reported by the patient. If the disk ruptures in the cervical area, the clinical manifestations are stiff neck, shoulder pain radiating to the hand, and paresthesias and sensory disturbances of the hand.

Diagnostic Studies

X-rays are done to note any structural defects. A myelogram, MRI, or CT scan is helpful in localizing the site of herniation. A diskogram may be necessary if other methods of diagnosis are unsuccessful. An electromyogram (EMG) of the extremities can be performed to determine the severity of nerve irritation caused by herniation or to rule out other pathology such as peripheral neuropathy.

Collaborative Care

Degenerative disk disease is managed conservatively with rest, limitation of extremes of spinal movement (corset), local heat or ice, ultrasound, transcutaneous electrical nerve stimulation (TENS), and NSAIDs. If herniation of the disk occurs, more aggressive treatment may be indicated (Table 59-20). Conservative treatment sometimes results in a healing over of the herniated area with a decrease in the pain of nerve root irritation. Muscle relaxants may be used to decrease muscle spasms. Once the symptoms subside, back strengthening exercises are begun. The patient should be educated in principles of good body mechanics. Extremes of flexion and torsion are strongly discouraged. Most patients with herniated disks recover with a conservative treatment plan. However, if conservative treatment is unsuccessful, radiculopathy becomes progressively worse, or there is documented loss of bowel or bladder control (cauda equina), surgery may be indicated.

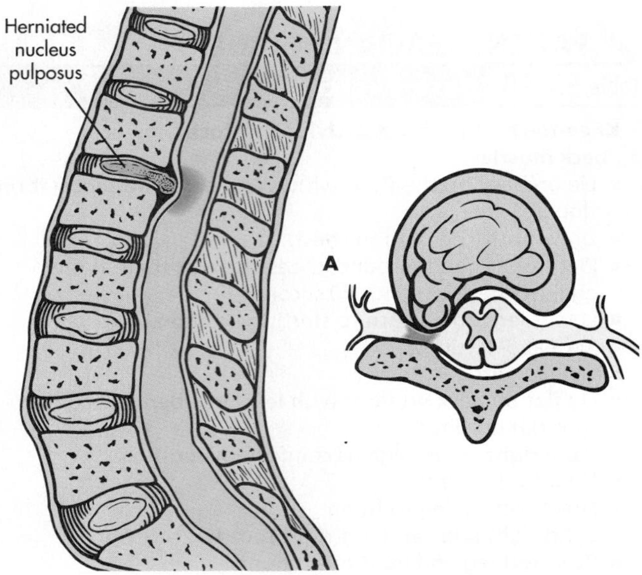

Fig. 59-21 Compression of spinal cord caused by herniation of nucleus pulposus into spinal cord. **A,** Pressure on nerves as they leave the spinal canal.

Surgical Therapy. A *percutaneous laser diskectomy* is a surgical procedure using a tube that is passed through the retroperitoneal soft tissues to the lateral border of the disk with the aid of fluoroscopy. Laserization is performed to the herniated portion of the disk.[38] Small stab wounds are used, and minimal blood loss occurs during the procedure. The long-term effects of this procedure are being investigated.

A *diskectomy* is another type of surgical procedure that may be performed to decompress the nerve root.[39] It involves the partial removal of the lamina to allow access to the intervertebral disk. *Microsurgical diskectomy* is a version of the standard diskectomy in which the surgeon uses a microscope to allow better visualization of the disk and disk space during surgery to aid in the removal of the herniated portion.

The traditional and most common procedure performed is a *laminectomy.* It involves the surgical excision of part of the posterior arch of the vertebra (referred to as the lamina) to gain access to part or all of the protruding disk to remove it.

A *spinal fusion* may be performed if an unstable bony mechanism is present. The spine is stabilized by creating an ankylo-

Table 59-19 Neurologic Assessment of Herniated Intervertebral Disk*

Intervertebral Level	Subjective Pain	Affected Reflex	Motor Function	Sensation
L3-L4	Back to buttocks to posterior thigh to inner calf	Patellar	Quadriceps, anterior tibialis	Inner aspect of lower leg, anterior part of thigh
L4-L5	Back to buttocks to dorsum of foot and big toe	None	Anterior tibialis, extensor halucis longus, gluteus medius	Dorsum of foot and big toe
L5-S1	Back to buttocks to sole of foot and heel	Achilles	Gastrocnemius, hamstring, gluteus maximus	Heel and lateral foot

*A disk herniation can involve pressure on more than one nerve root.

COLLABORATIVE CARE

Table 59-20 Herniated Intervertebral Disk

Diagnostic
- History
- Physical examination with emphasis on neurologic deficits and straight-leg raising
- CT scan
- MRI
- Myelogram
- Diskogram
- EMG
- Somatosensory evoked potential

Collaborative Therapy

Conservative
- Restricted activity
- Medication
  - Analgesics
  - Nonsteroidal antiinflammatory drugs
  - Muscle relaxants (e.g., cyclobenzaprine [Flexeril])
- Diathermy
- Thermotherapy
- Physical therapy

Surgical
- Laminectomy with or without spinal fusion
- Diskectomy
- Percutaneous lateral diskectomy
- Spinal fusion with or without instrumentation

EMG, electromyogram.

sis (fusion) of contiguous vertebrae with a bone graft from the patient's fibula or iliac crest or donated bone. If vertebral instability exists, metal fixation with rods, plates, or screws may be implanted at the time of spinal surgery to provide more stability and decrease vertebral motion.

NURSING MANAGEMENT: SPINAL SURGERY

Patients who have undergone spinal surgery require vigilant postoperative care. Nursing implementation is aimed at maintaining proper alignment of the spine at all times until healing has occurred. Flat bed rest may be maintained for 1 to 2 days depending on the extent of surgery. Logrolling patients when turning is essential to maintain proper body alignment. Pillows can be used under the thighs of each leg when supine and between the legs when in side-lying positions to provide comfort and ensure alignment.

Severe muscle spasms in the surgical area can be managed with medication and with correct turning and positioning. The patient often fears turning or any movement that increases pain by straining the surgical area. The nurse must offer reassurance to the patient that the proper technique is being used to maintain body alignment. Sufficient staff should be available to move the patient without undue pain or strain on staff members or the patient.

Because the spinal canal may be entered during surgery, there is potential for spinal fluid leakage. Severe headache or leakage of cerebrospinal fluid (CSF) on the dressing should be reported immediately. CSF appears as clear or slightly yellow drainage on the dressing. It has a high glucose concentration and will be positive for glucose when a dipstick test is done. The amount and characteristics of drainage should be noted.

Frequent monitoring of peripheral neurologic signs of the extremities is a routine postoperative nursing responsibility after spinal surgery. Movement of arms and legs and assessment of sensation should be unchanged when compared with the preoperative status. Table 59-21 summarizes a lumbar laminectomy

Table 59-21 Postoperative Assessment Following Lumbar Surgery

Sensation*
Assess sensation of extremities for paresthesia in all appropriate neurotomes.

Movement*
Assess ability to move all extremities.

Muscle Strength*
Assess for any weakness of the extremities.

Wound
Assess dressing for drainage and note amount, color, characteristics.

Pain
Document location of the pain.
Ask patient to rate the pain on a scale of 1 to 5, with 1 being no pain and 5 being worst pain.
Evaluate pain after analgesia has been administered.

*Postoperative findings should be compared with preoperative assessments. It is not unusual for the patient to continue to experience these symptoms after surgery. Symptoms gradually decrease over several months.

assessment appropriate for the patient who has undergone back surgery. These assessments are repeated every 2 to 4 hours during the first 48 hours after surgery, and findings are compared with the preoperative assessment. Paresthesias, such as numbness and tingling, may not be relieved immediately after surgery. Any new muscle weakness or paresthesias should be documented and reported to the surgeon immediately.

Paralytic ileus and interference with bowel function may occur for several days and may manifest as nausea, abdominal distention, and constipation. The nurse should assess whether the patient is passing flatus, has bowel sounds in all quadrants, and has a flat, soft abdomen.

Adequate bladder emptying may be altered because of activity restrictions, narcotics, or anesthesia. If allowed by the surgeon, men should be encouraged to dangle or stand to urinate. Patients should use the commode or ambulate to the bathroom when allowed to promote adequate emptying of the bladder. The nurse should ensure that privacy is maintained. It is necessary to clarify whether the patient can be allowed up to the bathroom without the corset or brace. Intermittent catheterization or an indwelling catheter may be necessary for patients who have difficulty urinating.

Loss of sphincter tone or bladder tone may be indicative of nerve damage. Incontinence or difficulty evacuating the bowel or bladder must be monitored closely and reported to the surgeon.

Activity prescriptions vary with surgeons, but the patient who has had spinal surgery usually ambulates early in the postoperative period. It is a nursing responsibility to know the specific orders related to activity for any patient.

In addition to the nursing care appropriate for a patient who has had a laminectomy, there are other nursing responsibilities if the patient has also had a spinal fusion. Because a bone graft is usually involved, the postoperative healing time is prolonged compared with that of a laminectomy. Immobilization over an extended time may be necessary. A rigid orthosis (thoracic-lumbar-sacral orthosis or chairback brace) is often used during the period of immobilization. Some surgeons require that the patient be taught to put it on and take it off by logrolling in bed, whereas others allow their patients to apply the brace in a sitting or standing position. The nurse should verify the preferred method before initiating this activity. The extended immobilization required by a spinal fusion carries with it all the potential problems related to this inactive state.

In addition to the primary surgical site, the donor site for the bone graft must be regularly assessed. The posterior iliac crest is the most commonly used donor site, although a rib or fibula may also be used. The donor site usually causes greater postoperative pain than the fused area. The donor site is bandaged with a pressure dressing to prevent excessive bleeding. If the donor site is the fibula, neurovascular assessments of the extremity are a postoperative nursing responsibility. Any restrictions on activity such as exercise should be clarified with the physician.

As the bone graft heals, the patient must adjust to the permanent immobility at the graft or fusion site. Instruction in proper body mechanics is essential and should be evaluated during the hospital stay.

The patient should be instructed to avoid sitting or standing for prolonged periods. Activities that should be encouraged include walking, lying down, and shifting weight from one foot to the other when standing. The patient should learn to mentally think through an activity before starting any potentially injurious task such as bending, lifting, or stooping. Any twisting movement of the spine is contraindicated. The thighs and knees, rather than the back, should be used to absorb the shock of activity and movement. A firm mattress or bedboard is essential.

NECK PAIN

Causes of neck pain are similar to those of the low back. Patients have symptoms of neck pain and possible pain radiating into the arm and hand. They also may have weakness or paresthesia of the arm and hand. Diagnosing the cause of neck pain is done by x-ray, MRI, CT scan, and myelogram. An EMG of the upper extremities is done to diagnose cervical radiculopathy.

Types of surgery done on the neck are similar to those done on the lower back with the exception that either posterior or anterior approaches may be used. These include a diskectomy, laminectomy, and spinal fusion. If surgery is done on the cervical spine, the nurse must be alert for symptoms of spinal cord edema such as respiratory distress and a worsening neurologic status of the upper extremities. After surgery, the patient's neck is immobilized in either a soft or hard cervical collar.

COMMON FOOT PROBLEMS

The foot is the platform that provides support for the weight of the body and absorbs considerable shock in ambulation. It is a complicated structure composed of bony structures, muscles, tendons, and ligaments. It can be affected by (1) congenital conditions, (2) structural weakness, (3) traumatic injuries, and (4) systemic conditions such as diabetes mellitus and rheumatoid arthritis. Abnormalities of the foot affect over 80 million persons in the United States. Much of the pain, deformity, and disability associated with foot disorders can be directly attributed to or accentuated by improperly fitting shoes, which cause crowding and angulation of the toes and inhibition of the normal movement of foot muscles. The purposes of footwear are to (1) provide support, foot stability, protection, shock absorption, and a foundation for orthoses; (2) increase friction with the walking surface; and (3) treat foot abnormalities. (Table 59-22 summarizes common foot problems and their treatment.)

NURSING MANAGEMENT: COMMON FOOT PROBLEMS

Health Promotion. Well-constructed and properly fitted shoes are essential for healthy, pain-free feet. Fashion styles, especially for women, often influence selection of footwear instead of considerations of comfort and support. Patient education should stress the importance of having a shoe that conforms to the foot rather than to current fashion trends. The shoe must be long enough and wide enough to prevent crowding of the toes and forcing of the great toe into a position of hallux valgus. At the metatarsal head the width of the shoe should be sufficient to allow free movement of the foot muscles and permit bending of the toes. The shank of the shoe should be rigid enough to give optimal support. The height of the heel should be realistic in relation to the purpose for which the shoe is worn. Ideally, the heel of the shoe should not rise more than 1 inch higher than the forefoot support.

Table 59-22 Common Foot Problems

Disorder	Definition	Treatment
Common Disorders		
Forefoot		
Hallux valgus (bunion)	Painful deformity of great toe consisting of lateral angulation of great toe toward second toe, bony enlargement of medial side of first metatarsal head, and formation of bursa or callus over bony enlargement	Conservative treatment includes wearing shoes with wide forefoot or "bunion pocket" and use of bunion pads to relieve pressure on bursal sac. Surgical treatment is removal of bursal sac and bony enlargement and correction of lateral angulation of great toe; may include temporary or permanent internal fixation.
Hallux rigidus	Painful stiffness of first metatarsophalangeal joint caused by osteoarthritis or local trauma	Conservative treatment includes intraarticular corticosteroids and passive manual stretching of first metatarsophalangeal joint. A shoe with a stiff sole decreases pain in the joint during walking. Surgical treatment is joint fusion or arthroplasty with silicone rubber implant.
Hammertoe	Deformity of second through fifth toes, including dorsiflexion of metatarsophalangeal joint, plantar flexion of proximal interphalangeal joint, and callus on dorsum of proximal interphalangeal joint and end of involved toe; complaints related to hammertoe include burning on bottom of foot and pain and difficulty in walking when wearing shoes	Conservative treatment consists of passive manual stretching of proximal interphalangeal joint and use of metatarsal arch support. Surgical correction consists of resection of base of middle phalanx and head of proximal phalanx and bringing raw bone ends together. Kirschner wire maintains straight position.
Morton's neuroma (Morton's toe or plantar neuroma)	Neuroma in web space between third and fourth metatarsal heads, causing sharp, sudden attacks of pain and burning sensations	Surgical excision is the usual treatment.
Midfoot		
Pes planus (flatfoot)	Loss of metatarsal arch causing pain in foot or leg	Symptoms are relieved by use of resilient longitudinal arch supports. Surgical treatment consists of triple arthrodesis or fusion of subtalar joint.
Pes cavus	Elevation of longitudinal arch of foot resulting from contracture of plantar fascia or bony deformity of arch	Treatment is manipulation and casting (in patients younger than 6 yr of age); surgical correction is necessary if it interferes with ambulation (in patients older than 6 yr of age).
Hindfoot		
Painful heels	Complaint of heel pain with weight bearing, common cause of plantar bursitis or calcaneal spur in adult	Corticosteroids are injected locally into inflamed bursa and sponge rubber heel cushion is used; surgical excision of bursa or spur is performed.
Local Problems		
Corn	Localized thickening of skin caused by continual pressure over bony prominences, especially metatarsal head, frequently causing localized pain	Corn is softened with warm water or preparations containing salicylic acid and trimmed with razor blade or scalpel. Pressure on bony prominences caused by shoes is relieved.
Soft corn	Painful lesion caused by bony prominence of one toe pressing against adjacent toe; usual location in web space between toes; softness caused by secretions keeping web space relatively moist.	Pain is relieved by placing cotton between toes to separate them. Surgical treatment is excision of projecting bone spur (if present).
Callus	Similar formation to corn but covering of wider area and usual location on weight-bearing part of foot	Same as for corn.
Plantar wart	Painful papillomatous growth caused by virus that may occur on any part of skin on sole of foot	Excision with electrocoagulation or surgical removal is done; ultrasound may also be used.

Acute Intervention. Many foot problems require surgery. When surgery is performed, the foot is usually immobilized by a bulky dressing, short leg cast, slipper (plaster) cast, or a platform "shoe" that fits over the dressing and has a rigid sole (known as a bunion boot). The foot should be elevated with the heel off the bed to help reduce discomfort and prevent edema. The neurovascular status should be assessed frequently during the immediate postoperative period. Depending on the type of surgery, pins or wires may extend through the toes, or a protective splint that extends over the end of the foot may be in place. Care must be taken not to jar these devices and cause pain. The devices may interfere with or preclude assessment for movement. The nurse should be aware that sensation may be difficult to evaluate, since postoperative pain can interfere with the patient's ability to differentiate pain caused by the surgical procedure from pain resulting from nerve pressure or circulatory impairment.

The type and extent of surgery determine the degree of ambulation allowed. Crutches or canes may be necessary. The patient may experience pain or a throbbing sensation when starting ambulation. The nurse should reinforce instructions given by the physical therapist and ensure that the patient does not develop a faulty gait pattern such as walking on the heels in an attempt to avoid excessive pain or pressure. The nurse must reinforce the importance of walking with an erect posture and with proper weight distribution. Dysfunction of gait or continued pain should be reported to the physician. The nurse should instruct the patient on the importance of frequent rest periods with the foot elevated.

Ambulatory and Home Care. Foot care should include daily hygienic care and the wearing of clean stockings. Stockings should be long enough to avoid wrinkling and the development of pressure areas. Trimming toenails straight across helps prevent ingrown toenails and reduces the possibility of infection. Persons with impaired circulation or diabetes mellitus require detailed instruction to prevent serious complications associated with blisters, pressure areas, and infections (see Table 46-25 for guidelines for foot care).

GERONTOLOGIC CONSIDERATIONS

Foot Problems

The older adult is prone to developing foot problems because of poor circulation, atherosclerosis, and decreased sensation in the lower extremities. This is especially a problem for older patients with diabetes mellitus. A patient may develop an open wound but not feel it because of altered sensation. This may be the result of peripheral vascular disease or diabetic neuropathy. Older adults should be instructed to inspect their feet daily and report any open wounds or breaks in the skin to their physician. If left untreated, wounds may become infected, lead to osteomyelitis, and require surgical debridement. If infection becomes widespread, amputation may be necessary.

METABOLIC BONE DISEASES

Normal bone metabolism is dependent on adequate intake, absorption, and use of calcium, phosphorus, protein, and vitamins. When there is dysfunction in any of these critical factors, generalized reduction of bone mass may result.

OSTEOMALACIA

Osteomalacia is an uncommon disorder of adult bone associated with vitamin D deficiency, resulting in decalcification and softening of bone. This disease is the same as rickets in children except that the epiphyseal growth plates are closed in the adult. Vitamin D is required for the absorption of calcium from the intestines. Insufficient vitamin D intake can interfere with the normal mineralization of bone, causing failure or insufficient calcification of bone, which results in softening of bone, bone pain, and deformities. Etiologic factors in the development of osteomalacia include lack of exposure to ultraviolet rays, gastrointestinal malabsorption, extensive burns, chronic diarrhea, pregnancy, kidney disease, and medications such as phenytoin (Dilantin).

The most common clinical feature of osteomalacia is persistent skeletal pain, especially while bearing weight. Other clinical manifestations include low back pain, progressive muscular weakness, weight loss, and progressive deformities of the spine (kyphosis) or extremities. Fractures are common and demonstrate delayed healing when they occur.

Laboratory findings commonly associated with osteomalacia are decreased serum calcium or phosphorus levels and elevated serum alkaline phosphatase. X-ray examination may demonstrate the effects of generalized bone demineralization, especially loss of calcium in the bones of the pelvis and the presence of associated bone deformity. Looser's transformation zones (ribbons of decalcification in bone found on x-ray) are diagnostic of osteomalacia. Significant osteomalacia may exist without demonstrable x-ray changes.

Collaborative care of osteomalacia is directed toward correction of the underlying cause. Vitamin D (cholecalciferol) is usually supplemented, and the patient often shows a dramatic response. Calcium or phosphorus intake may also be supplemented.

OSTEOPOROSIS

Osteoporosis, or porous bone, is a condition characterized by low bone mass and structural deterioration of bone tissue, leading to increased bone fragility. This metabolic bone disease is the major cause of fractures (especially hip, spine, and wrist) in postmenopausal women and older adults in general.[40] Osteoporosis is increasing in incidence because more people are surviving to an older age. At least 25 to 35 million persons in the United States have some degree of osteoporosis, and with the projected increase in life expectancy, this number is expected to grow. In the United States, the total cost of osteoporosis in terms of medical care, nursing home fees, and loss of income is estimated to exceed 10 billion dollars.[40,41]

Osteoporosis is eight times more common in women than in men for several reasons: (1) women tend to have lower calcium intake than men throughout their lives (men between 15 and 50 years of age consume twice as much calcium as women); (2) women have less bone mass because of their generally smaller frame; (3) resorption begins at an earlier age in women and is accelerated at menopause; (4) pregnancy and breastfeeding deplete a woman's skeletal reserve unless calcium intake is adequate; and (5) longevity increases the likelihood of osteoporosis, and women live longer than men. Although osteoporosis is more common in women than men, it is important to realize that men can also develop osteoporosis.

CULTURAL & ETHNIC CONSIDERATIONS

Osteoporosis

- Caucasian and Asian-American women have a higher incidence of osteoporosis than African-American women.
- African-American women have 10% more bone mass than non–African-American women.
- Postmenopausal women are at the highest risk regardless of cultural background or ethnic group.

Etiology and Pathophysiology

Risk factors for osteoporosis are female gender, increasing age, family history of osteoporosis, Caucasian or Asian race, small stature, anorexia, oophorectomy, sedentary lifestyle, and insufficient dietary calcium.[42] Increased risk is associated with cigarette smoking and alcoholism, and decreased risk is associated with adequate physical activity and fluoride and vitamin D ingestion (risk factors for osteoporosis are listed in Table 59-23). Family history is the predominant risk factor in men.

Peak bone mass (maximum bone tissue) is achieved during adolescence. It is determined by a combination of four major factors: hereditary, nutrition, exercise, and hormone function. Heredity may be responsible for up to 70% of peak bone mass. Bone loss from midlife (age 35 to 40 years) onward is inevitable, but the rate of loss varies. At menopause, women experience rapid bone loss with reduced rates after 8 to 10 years.[43]

Bone is continually being deposited by osteoblasts and resorbed by osteoclasts, a process called remodeling. Normally the rates of bone deposition and resorption are equal to each other so that the total bone mass remains constant. In osteoporosis, bone resorption exceeds bone deposition. Although resorption affects the entire skeletal system, osteoporosis occurs most commonly in the bones of the spine, hips, and wrists. Over time, wedging and fractures of the vertebrae produce gradual loss of height and a humped back known as dowager's hump or kyphosis. The usual first signs are back pain or spontaneous fractures. The loss of bone substance causes the bone to become mechanically weakened and prone to either spontaneous fractures or fractures from minimal trauma.

Specific diseases associated with osteoporosis include intestinal malabsorption, kidney disease, rheumatoid arthritis, advanced alcoholism, cirrhosis of the liver, and diabetes mellitus. Many medications can contribute to bone loss, including corticosteroids, antiseizure drugs (phenytoin [Dilantin]), aluminum-containing antacids, heparin, isoniazid (INH), and tetracycline.[44] At the time a medicine is prescribed, the patient should be informed of this possible side effect. Long-term corticosteroid use is a major contributor to osteoporosis. When a corticosteroid is taken, there is a disproportionate loss of trabecular or cancellous bone.

Genetic factors influence bone mass. A genetic marker, the vitamin D receptor (VDR) gene, has been linked to bone density. The VDR gene is responsible for constructing the receptors that assist cells to use vitamin D, a vitamin important to bone and calcium metabolism. Persons with a specific VDR genotype may have significantly lower bone density. This relationship remains under investigation.[45] Identification of a person's genotype could allow targeted interventions at an early age for persons genetically at risk for the development of osteoporosis.

Table 59-23 Risk Factors for Osteoporosis

- Female gender
- Thin, small framed
- Family history of osteoporosis
- Diet low in calcium
- Caucasian or Asian-American
- Excessive use of alcohol
- Cigarette smoking
- An inactive lifestyle
- Long-term use of corticosteroids, thyroid replacements, or antiseizure medications
- Postmenopausal, including early or surgically induced menopause
- History of anorexia nervosa or bulimia, chronic liver disease, or malabsorption

From National Osteoporosis Foundation: *Position paper: current perspectives on diagnosis, prevention, and treatment of osteoporosis,* Washington, DC, 1995, The Foundation.

Clinical Manifestations

Osteoporosis is often called the "silent disease" because bone loss occurs without symptoms. People may not know they have osteoporosis until their bones become so weak that a sudden strain, bump, or fall causes a hip, vertebral, or wrist fracture. Collapsed vertebrae may initially be manifested as back pain, loss of height, or spinal deformities such as kyphosis or severely stooped posture.

Diagnostic Studies

Osteoporosis often goes unnoticed because it cannot be detected by conventional x-ray until more than 25% to 40% of calcium in the bone is lost. Serum calcium, phosphorus, and alkaline phosphatase levels usually are normal, although alkaline phosphatase may be elevated after a fracture. Bone minimal density (BMD) measurements are used to measure the bone density. BMD assesses the mass of bone per unit volume, or how tightly the bone is packed. (BMD measurements are presented in Table 58-8.) One of the most common studies is dual-energy x-ray absorptiometry (DEXA), which measures bone density in the spine, hips, and forearm (the most common sites of fractures resulting from osteoporosis). DEXA studies are also useful to evaluate changes in bone density over time and to assess the effectiveness of treatment.

NURSING AND COLLABORATIVE MANAGEMENT: OSTEOPOROSIS

Collaborative care of osteoporosis focuses on proper nutrition, calcium supplementation, exercise, and medication (Table 59-24). Prevention and treatment of osteoporosis focuses on adequate calcium intake (1000 mg/day in premenopausal women and postmenopausal women taking estrogen, and 1500 mg/day in postmenopausal women who are not receiving supplemental estrogen). If dietary intake of calcium is inadequate, supplemental calcium should be taken.[46] Foods that are high in

COLLABORATIVE CARE

Table 59-24 Osteoporosis

Diagnostic
- History and physical examination
- Serum calcium, phosphorus, and alkaline phosphatase
- Bone mineral densitometry

Collaborative Therapy
- Calcium supplements (see Table 59-26)
- Vitamin D supplements
- Diet high in calcium (see Table 59-25)
- Exercise program
- Estrogen replacement therapy
- Calcitonin
- Biphosphonates
  - Etidronate (Didronel)
  - Alendronate (Fosamax)
- Raloxifene (Evista)

calcium content include whole and skim milk, yogurt, turnip greens, cottage cheese, ice cream, sardines, and spinach (Table 59-25). The amount of elemental calcium varies in different calcium preparations (Table 59-26). Calcium supplementation inhibits age-related bone loss; however, no new bone is formed.

Vitamin D is important in calcium absorption and function and may have a role in bone formation. Most people get enough vitamin D from the diet or naturally through synthesis in the skin from exposure to sunlight. However, supplemental vitamin D (400 to 800 IU) may be recommended for older adults, those who are homebound, and those who get minimal sun exposure. Many calcium supplements also have vitamin D.

Moderate amounts of exercise are important to build up and maintain bone mass. Exercise also increases muscle strength, coordination, and balance. The best exercises are weight-bearing exercises that force an individual to work against gravity. These exercises include walking, hiking, weight training, stair climbing, tennis, and dancing. Walking is preferred to high-impact aerobics or running, both of which may put too much stress on the bones of patients with osteoporosis.

Cigarette smoking and excess alcohol intake are risk factors for osteoporosis. Regular consumption of 2 to 3 ounces of alcohol a day may increase the degree of osteoporosis, even in young men and women. Patients should be instructed to quit smoking and cut down on alcohol intake to decrease the likelihood of losing bone mass.

Although loss of bone cannot be significantly reversed, further loss can be prevented if the patient follows a regimen of calcium and vitamin D supplementation, exercise, estrogen replacement, and alendronate (Fosamax) or raloxifene (Evista), if indicated. Efforts should be made to keep patients with osteoporosis ambulatory to prevent further loss of bone substance as a result of immobility. Treatment also involves protecting areas of potential pathologic fractures; for example, a corset can be used to prevent vertebral collapse.

Drug Therapy. Estrogen replacement therapy after menopause is used to prevent osteoporosis. Although the exact mechanism for the protective function of estrogen is not known, it is believed that estrogen inhibits osteoclast activity, leading to decreased bone resorption and preventing both cortical and trabecular bone loss. Estrogen replacement therapy is most effective when combined with calcium. The greatest benefit of estrogen is probably in the first 10 years after menopause. Transdermal estrogen treatment has been shown to be effective in the treatment of postmenopausal women with established osteoporosis. (See Chapter 51 for further discussion of estrogen replacement therapy.)

Calcitonin is secreted by the thyroid gland and inhibits osteoclastic bone resorption by directly interacting with active

NUTRITIONAL THERAPY

Table 59-25 Sources of Calcium

Food	Calcium (mg)
1 cup milk	
Buttermilk	285
Chocolate	284
Whole	291
Low-fat	300
Skim	302
Half and half	254
Evaporated, canned	657
Egg nog	330
1 oz cheese	
American	174
Blue	150
Brie	52
Camembert	110
Cheddar	130
Cottage	130
Mozzarella	207
Parmesan	390
Swiss	272
8 oz yogurt	415
1 cup ice cream	176
Soft serve	272
3 oz seafood	
Salmon	167
Sardines with bones	372
Shrimp	98
Oysters	113
1 med stalk cooked broccoli	158
1 cup cooked spinach	200
1 cup cooked mustard greens	193
1 cup turnip greens	252
1 cup cooked collard greens with stems	289
1 cup bok choy	250
1 cup kale	206
Bonus Sources	
1 cup almonds	304
1 cup hazelnuts	240
1 tbs blackstrap molasses	137
Poor Sources	
Egg	28
1 cup cabbage	44
1 oz cream cheese	23
3 oz beef, pork, poultry	10
Apple, banana	10
½ grapefruit	20
1 med potato	14
1 med carrot	14
¼ head lettuce	27

Table 59-26 Elemental Calcium Content of Various Oral Calcium Preparations

Calcium Preparation	Elemental Calcium Content
Calcium carbonate (Tums 500)	500 mg/tablet
Calcium carbonate + 5 μg vitamin D_2 (Os-Cal 250)	250 mg/tablet
Calcium gluconate	40 mg/500 mg
Calcium carbonate	400 mg/g
Calcium lactate	80 mg/600 mg
Calcium citrate	40 mg/300 mg

osteoclasts. Calcitonin (Calcimar) is available as intramuscular, subcutaneous, and intranasal forms. The nasal form is easy to administer, and patients should be taught to alternate nostrils daily. Nasal dryness and irritation are the most frequent side effects. Administration of the intramuscular or subcutaneous form of the medication at night has been shown to decrease the side effects of nausea and facial flushing. Nausea does not occur with the nasal spray. When calcitonin is used, calcium supplementation is necessary to prevent secondary hyperparathyroidism.[42]

Biphosphonates inhibit osteoclast-mediated bone resorption, thereby increasing bone mineral density and total bone mass.[44] This group of drugs includes etidronate (Didronel), alendronate (Fosamax), pamidronate (Aredia), risendronate (Actonel), clodronate (Bonefos), and tiludronate (Skelid). The most commonly used biphosphonate drug in treating osteoporosis is alendronate. Patients should be instructed on the proper administration of alendronate to aid in its absorption. It should be taken after rising in the morning with a full glass of water. The patient should not eat or drink anything for 30 minutes after taking it. The patient should also be instructed not to lie down after taking the medication. These precautions have been proven to decrease gastrointestinal side effects (especially esophageal irritation) and increase absorption.

Another type of drug used in treating osteoporosis is selective estrogen receptor modulators, such as raloxifene (Evista). This drug mimics the effect of estrogen on bone by reducing bone resorption without stimulating the tissues of the breast or uterus. Raloxifene in postmenopausal women significantly increases bone mineral density.[47] The most commonly reported side effects are leg cramps and hot flashes. Unlike estrogen, it does not relieve menopausal symptoms or have a cardiovascular protective function.

Medical management of patients receiving corticosteroids includes prescribing the lowest possible dose of the drug, as well as calcium and vitamin D supplementation and estrogen replacement in postmenopausal women. If osteopenia is evident on bone densitometry, treatment with bisphosphonate agents, such as alendronate (Fosamax), should be considered.

PAGET'S DISEASE

Paget's disease (osteitis deformans) is a skeletal bone disorder in which there is excessive bone resorption followed by replacement of normal marrow by vascular, fibrous connective tissue and new bone that is larger, disorganized, and weaker. It occurs most often after the fourth decade of life and most commonly in men. It is characterized by deformities of bone caused by unexplained abnormal focal remodeling and resorption of bone, fibrotic changes, and remodeling with structurally uneven bone. The regions of the skeleton commonly affected are the pelvis, long bones, spine, ribs, sternum, and cranium. The cause of Paget's disease is unknown, although a viral etiology has been proposed.[48]

In milder forms of Paget's disease, patients may remain free of symptoms, and the disease may be discovered incidentally on x-ray or serum chemistry. The initial clinical manifestations are usually insidious development of skeletal pain (which may progress to severe intractable pain), complaints of fatigue, and progressive development of a waddling gait. Patients may complain that they are becoming shorter or that their heads are becoming larger. Serum alkaline phosphatase levels are markedly elevated in advanced forms of the disease. X-rays may demonstrate that the normal contour of the affected bone is curved and the bone cortex is thickened, especially the weight-bearing bones and cranium. Pathologic fracture is the most common complication of Paget's disease and may be the first indication of the disease. Other complications include malignant osteosarcoma, fibrosarcoma, and benign giant cell tumors.

Collaborative care of Paget's disease is usually limited to symptomatic and supportive care and correction of secondary deformities by either surgical implementation or braces. Bone resorption, relief of acute symptoms, and lowering the serum alkaline phosphatase levels may be significantly influenced by the administration of calcitonin, which inhibits osteoclastic activity. Response to calcitonin therapy is not permanent and often stops when therapy is discontinued.[48] Biphosphonates, such as alendronate (Fosamax), tiludronate (Skelid), risedronate (Actonel) and pamidronate (Aredia), are nonhormonal agents that are effective in reducing the bone resorption in Paget's disease.[48] Radiation therapy and local surgical procedures such as periosteal stripping may be used for the control of the patient's pain.

A firm mattress should be used to provide back support and to relieve pain. The patient may be required to wear a corset or light brace to relieve back pain and provide support when in the upright position. The patient should be proficient in the correct application of such devices and know how to regularly examine areas of the skin for friction damage. Activities such as lifting and twisting should be discouraged. Good body mechanics are essential. Analgesics and muscle relaxants may be administered to relieve pain. A properly balanced nutritional program is important in the management of metabolic disorders of bone, especially pertaining to vitamin D, calcium, and protein, which are necessary to ensure the availability of the components for bone formation. Prevention measures such as patient education, use of an assistive device, and environmental changes should be actively pursued to prevent falls and subsequent fractures.

GERONTOLOGIC CONSIDERATIONS

Metabolic Bone Diseases

Osteoporosis and Paget's disease are common in older adults. Patients should be instructed in proper nutritional management to prevent further bone loss such as that occurring from osteoporosis.

Because metabolic bone disorders increase the possibility of pathologic fractures, the nurse must use extreme caution when the patient is turned or moved. It is important to keep the

CRITICAL THINKING EXERCISES

CASE STUDY

Osteoporosis

Patient Profile

Mrs. Green is a 52-year-old cafeteria worker who had a total hysterectomy and salpingo-oophorectomy for removal of a benign ovarian cyst 3 years ago.

Subjective Data

- Experiences chronic, mild lumbar pain and tenderness that radiates to her right hip and the lateral thigh
- Had a stress fracture in wrist 6 months ago
- Regular walking offers some relief
- Reports no noticeable loss of height
- Has maternal history of osteoporosis
- On corticosteroids past 6 years for Addison's disease
- Drinks socially—two alcoholic beverages per day
- Dislikes dairy products

Objective Data

- Is Asian-American, 5 ft 6 in tall, 116 lb

Diagnostic Studies

- Bone mass/density tests show decreased bone mineral density at spine and hip
- Laboratory tests reveal normal serum calcium, phosphorus, and alkaline phosphatase levels

Collaborative and Nursing Management

- Conjugated equinine estrogen—0.625 mg PO daily
- Alendronate (Fosamax)—10 mg PO daily
- Calcium supplements—1200 mg PO daily
- Increase calcium intake from food
- Reduce alcohol intake
- Maintain regular exercise program

Critical Thinking Questions

1. What risk factors made Mrs. Green prone to develop osteoporosis?
2. Why does regular exercise help Mrs. Green's symptoms?
3. What is the purpose of prescribing estrogen replacement for Mrs. Green?
4. What educational teaching should the nurse provide to Mrs. Green regarding alendronate?
5. How might the nurse assist Mrs. Green in increasing her intake of calcium?
6. Based on the assessment data presented, write one or more nursing diagnoses. Are there any collaborative problems?

NURSING RESEARCH ISSUES

1. What is the most effective technique of providing pin care for a patient in skeletal traction?
2. What body image and self-concept issues does a patient who has undergone an amputation experience?
3. Are casual and weekend athletes using proper protective gear to prevent injury? How compliant are these individuals?
4. Have postoperative orthopedic complications (e.g., deep vein thrombosis, dislocations) increased with shorter length of hospital stay?
5. Do nurses' pain medication–dispensing behaviors change in relation to the orthopedic patient's mental status: alert (able to communicate needs) versus demented (unable to communicate needs)?
6. What home health nursing interventions are most effective for increasing mobility in the patient recovering from a hip fracture?
7. Do nurses recognize the signs and symptoms of fat embolism and acute compartment syndrome?
8. What factors are important for the nurse to address in helping an adolescent female increase her calcium intake?

patient as active as possible to retard demineralization of bone resulting from disuse or extended immobilization. A supervised exercise program is an essential part of the treatment program. If the patient's condition permits, ambulation without causing fatigue must be encouraged.

REVIEW QUESTIONS

The number of the question corresponds to the same-numbered objective at the beginning of the chapter.

1. The nurse suspects an ankle sprain when a patient at the urgent care center
   a. is hit by another soccer player on the field.
   b. has ankle pain after running a 10-mile race.
   c. drops a 10 lb weight on his lower leg at the health club.
   d. has a twisting injury while running bases during a baseball game.
2. The nurse explains to a patient with a distal tibial fracture returning for a 3-week checkup that healing is indicated by
   a. callus formation.
   b. complete union of bone.
   c. presence of granulation tissue.
   d. formation of a hematoma at the fracture site.
3. A patient with a stable, closed fracture of the humerus caused by trauma to the arm has a temporary splint with bulky padding applied with an elastic bandage. The nurse suspects compartment syndrome and notifies the physician when the patient experiences
   a. pain at the fracture site.
   b. increasing edema of the limb.
   c. muscle spasms of the lower arm.
   d. pain when the nurse passively extends the fingers.
4. A patient with a comminuted fracture of the femur is to have an open reduction with internal fixation (ORIF) of the fracture. The nurse explains that ORIF is indicated when
   a. a cast would be too large to provide normal mobility.
   b. the patient is able to tolerate long-term immobilization.
   c. adequate alignment cannot be obtained by other methods.
   d. the patient cannot tolerate the discomfort of a closed reduction.

5. An indication of a neurovascular problem noted during assessment of the patient with a fracture is
   a. exaggeration of extremity movement.
   b. petechiae on the head and upper thorax.
   c. purulent drainage at the site of an open fracture.
   d. decreased sensation distal to the fracture site.
6. A patient with symphysis pubis and pelvic rami fractures should be monitored for
   a. sudden thirst.
   b. changes in urinary output.
   c. a palpable lump in the buttock.
   d. sudden decrease in blood pressure.
7. A patient with osteomyelitis is treated with surgical debridement followed by continuous irrigation of the affected bone with antibiotics. In responding to the patient who asks why oral or IV antibiotics cannot be used alone, the nurse explains that
   a. the irrigation is necessary to wash out dead tissue and pus from the infected area.
   b. the ischemia and bone death associated with osteomyelitis is frequently impenetrable to most antibiotics carried by the blood.
   c. there are not effective oral or IV antibiotics to treat *S. aureus,* the most common cause of osteomyelitis.
   d. an irrigation can penetrate involucrum created by the infection and prevent bacterial seeding to other tissue.
8. During the postoperative period, the patient with an above-the-knee amputation should be instructed that the residual limb should not be routinely elevated because
   a. the flexed position can promote hip flexion contracture.
   b. this position reduces the development of phantom pain.
   c. this position promotes clot formation at the incision site and thigh.
   d. unnecessary movement of the extremity can cause wound dehiscence.
9. A patient with an osteogenic sarcoma of the left femur has a nursing diagnosis of risk for injury: pathologic fracture related to bone tissue changes. The nursing management of this patient is primarily directed toward
   a. preventing pain.
   b. relieving edema.
   c. increasing physical mobility.
   d. supporting and positioning the leg.
10. In identifying people at risk for back injuries the nurse recognizes that the person at greatest risk for low back pain is a
   a. long-distance truck driver.
   b. 100 lb aerobics instructor.
   c. 62-year-old widow who walks daily.
   d. 25-year-old newborn nursery nurse.
11. The primary nursing responsibility in caring for a patient with acute low back pain associated with severe pain and muscle spasms is
   a. positioning the patient on the abdomen with the legs extended.
   b. teaching exercises such as straight-leg raises to decrease pain.
   c. providing pain medication to promote exercise and ambulation.
   d. assisting the patient to maintain activity restrictions with a gradual increase in activity.
12. In caring for the patient after a spinal fusion, the nurse recognizes that interventions for this surgery differ from a simple laminectomy in that
   a. body alignment is maintained by the fusion procedure.
   b. earlier ambulation is permitted because the spine is more stabilized.
   c. the donor site for the bone graft may be more painful than the spinal incision.
   d. teaching regarding body mechanics and prevention of future back injuries is not as critical.
13. Before discharge from the same-day surgery unit, the nurse instructs the patient who has had a surgical correction of bilateral hallux valgus to
   a. rest frequently with the feet elevated.
   b. soak the feet in warm water several times a day.
   c. walk primarily on the heels to relieve pressure on the toes.
   d. expect the feet to be numb for several days postoperatively.
14. The nurse advises the patient with early osteoporosis to
   a. lose weight.
   b. stop smoking.
   c. eat a high-protein diet.
   d. start swimming for exercise.

References

1. Best TM: Soft tissue injuries and muscle tears, *Clin Sports Med* 16:419, 1997.
2. Jobe FW and others, editors: *Operative techniques in upper extremity sports injuries,* St Louis, 1996, Mosby.
3. English CJ and others: Relations between upper limb soft tissue disorders and repetitive movements at work, *Am J Ind Med* 27:75, 1995.
4. Brogmus GE, Sorock GS, Webster BS: Recent trends in work-related cumulative trauma disorders of the upper extremities in the United States: an evaluation of possible reasons, *J Environ Med* 38:401, 1996.
*5. Heveron B, Kaempffe FA: Tears of the rotator cuff, *Orthop Nurs* 14:38, 1995.
6. Mayo Clinic: Rotator cuff injuries, *Mayo Clin Health Lett* 16:1, 1998.
7. Guckel C, Nidecker A: Diagnosis of tears in rotator cuff injuries, *Eur J Radiol* 25:168, 1997.
8. McFarland EG and others: Shoulder immobilization devices, *Orthop Nurs* 16:66, 1997.
9. Verdonk R: Alternative treatments for meniscal injuries, *J Bone Joint Surg Br* 79:866, 1997.
10. Scott G, King JB: A prospective double-blind trial of electrical capacitive coupling in the treatment of non-union of long bones, *J Bone Joint Surg* 76A:820, 1994.
11. Brighton CT and others: Tibial nonunion treated with direct current, capacitive coupling of bone graft, *Clin Orthop Relat Res* 321:223, 1995.
12. Salmond SW, Mooney NE, Verdisco LA, editors: *NAON core curriculum for orthopaedic nursing,* ed 3, Pitman, NJ, 1996, Anthony Jannetti.
13. Wilson SC and others: A simple method to measure compartment pressures using an intravenous catheter, *Orthopedics* 20:403, 1997.
14. Resnick D, Goergen T, Pathria M: Traumatic, iatrogenic, and neurogenic diseases. In Resnick D, editor: *Bone and joint imaging,* ed 2, Philadelphia, 1996, Saunders.
15. Gwynne DP, Theis J: Acute compartment syndrome due to closed muscle rupture, *Aust N Z J Surg* 67:227, 1997.
16. Thelan L and others, editors: *Critical care nursing diagnosis and management,* ed 3, St Louis, 1998, Mosby.
17. Colwell CW and others: Efficacy and safety of enoxaparin versus unfractionated heparin for prevention of deep venous thrombosis after elective knee arthroplasty, *Clin Orthop Relat Res* 321:19, 1995.
18. Johnson MJ, Lucas GL: Fat embolism syndrome, *Orthopedics* 19:41, 1996.
19. Hager CA, Brncick N: Fat embolism syndrome: a complication of orthopaedic trauma, *Orthop Nurs* 17:41, 1998.
20. Richards RR: Fat embolism syndrome, *Can J Surg* 40:334, 1997.
21. Bulger EM and others: Fat embolism syndrome: A 10-year review, *Arch Surg* 132:435, 1997.
22. Mayo Clinic: Hip fractures, *Mayo Clin Health Lett* 16:2, 1998.
23. Ebersole P, Hess P, editors: *Toward healthy aging: human needs and nursing response,* ed 5, St Louis, 1998, Mosby.
24. Reichel W, editor: *Care of the elderly: clinical aspects of aging,* ed 4, Baltimore, 1995, Williams & Wilkins.

25. Magee D: *Orthopedic physical assessment,* ed 3, Philadelphia, 1997, Saunders.
26. Feliciano DV, Moore EE, Mattox KL, editors: *Trauma,* ed 3, Stamford, Conn, 1996, Appleton & Lange.
27. Reese RE, Betts RF, editors: *A practical approach to infectious diseases,* ed 4, Boston, 1996, Little, Brown.
28. Hellman D: Arthritis and musculoskeletal disorders. In Tierney L, McPhee S, Papadakis M, editors: *Medical diagnosis and treatment,* ed 36, Stanford, Conn, 1997, Appleton & Lange.
29. Keen J, Swearingen P: *Critical care nursing consultant,* St Louis, 1997, Mosby.
30. Mourad L: Alterations of musculoskeletal function. In McCance KL, Huether SE, editors: *Pathophysiology: the biologic basis for disease in adults and children,* ed 3, St Louis, 1998, Mosby.
31. Yetzer EA: Helping the patient through the experience of an amputation, *Orthop Nurs* 15:45, 1996.
32. Wiernik PH and others, editors: *Neoplastic diseases of the blood,* ed 3, New York, 1996, Churchill Livingstone.
33. Vander Griend RA: Osteosarcoma and its variants, *Orthop Clin North Am* 27:575, 1996.
34. Vlasak R, Sim FH: Ewing's sarcoma, *Orthop Clin North Am* 27:591, 1996.
35. Kuritzky L: Steps in the management of low back pain, *Hosp Pract* 31:109, 1996.
36. Chase J: Outpatient management of low back pain, *Orthop Nurs* 11:11, 1992.
37. Leboeuf-Yde C, Yashin A, Lauritzen T: Does smoking cause low back pain? Results from a population-based study, *J Manipulative Physiol Ther* 19:99, 1996.
38. Nerubay J, Caspi I, Levinkopf M: Percutaneous carbon dioxide laser nucleolysis with 2- to 5-year followup, *Clin Orthop Relat Res* 337:45, 1997.
39. Bigos S, Nordin M, Leger D: Treatment of the acutely injured worker. In Nordin M, Andersson G, Pope M, editors: *Musculoskeletal disorders in the work place, principles and practice,* St Louis, 1997, Mosby.
*40. Hunt AH: The relationship between height change and bone mineral density, *Orthop Nurs* 15:57, 1996.
41. Kessenich CR, Rosen CJ: Vitamin D and bone status in elderly women, *Orthop Nurs* 15:67, 1996.
42. Kessenich C: Preventing and managing osteoporosis, *AJN* 97:16B, 1997.
43. Tucci JR and others: Effect of three years of oral alendronate treatment in postmenopausal women with osteoporosis, *Am J Med* 101:488, 1996.
44. Jackson R: Forestalling fracture in osteoporosis, *Hosp Pract* 32:77, 1997.
45. Vandevyver C and others: Influence of the vitamin D receptor gene alleles on bone mineral density in postmenopausal and osteoporotic women, *J Bone Mineral Res* 12:241, 1997.
46. Barzel U: Osteoporosis: taking a fresh look, *Hosp Pract* 31:59, 1996.
47. Balfour JA and others: Raloxifene, *Drugs Aging* 12:335, 1998.
48. Weinstein R: Advances in the treatment of Paget's bone disease, *Hosp Pract* 32:63, 1997.

*Nursing research-based article.

Resources

American Academy of Orthopedic Surgeons
6300 North River Road
Rosemont, IL 60018-4262
847-823-7186
800-346-AAOS
Fax: 847-823-8125
http://www.aaos.org

American College of Sports Medicine
PO Box 1440
401 W Michigan Street
Indianapolis, IN 46202
317-637-9200
Fax: 317-634-7817
http://www.acsm.org

Amputees In Motion
PO Box 2703
Escondido, CA 92033
619-454-9300
http://www.usinter.net/wasa/sandiego1.html

Calcium Information Center
Clinical Nutrition and Research Unit
Division of Nephrology, Hypertension, and Clinical Pharmacology
Oregon Health Sciences University
3314 SW U.S. Veterans Hospital Road
Portland, OR 97201
800-321-2681

Muscular Dystrophy Association
3561 East Sunrise Avenue
Tucson, AZ 85718
602-529-2000
http://www.mdausa.org/

National Amputation Foundation
38-40 Church St
Malverne, NY 11565
516-887-3600
http://www.va.gov/vso/naf.htm

National Arthritis/Musculoskeletal and Skin Diseases Information Clearinghouse
9000 Rockville Pike
Bethesda, MD 20892-2350
800-283-7800
http://www.nih.gov/niams/

National Association of Orthopaedic Nurses, Inc. (NAON)
East Holly Avenue
Box 56
Pitman, NJ 08071-0056
609-256-2310
Fax: 609-589-7463
naon@mail.ajj.com
http://naon.inurse.com

National Easter Seal Society
70 East Lake Street
Chicago, IL 60601
312-726-6200
http://www.easter-seals.org

National Fibromyalgia Research Association
PO Box 500
Salem, OR 97302
http://www.teleport.com/~nfra/

National Osteoporosis Foundation
1150—17th Street NW, Suite 500
Washington, DC 20036-4603
202-223-2226
800-223-9994
http://www.nof.org/

Older Women's League
666 Eleventh Street SW, Suite 700
Washington, DC 20001
202-783-6686
800-TAKE-OWL
http://www.womenconnect.com/

***For additional Internet resources, see the website for this book at* www.mosby.com/MERLIN/medsurg_lewis**

REMEMBER to check out your **companion CD-ROM**

60 NURSING MANAGEMENT Arthritis and Connective Tissue Diseases

Melissa Bush

www.mosby.com/MERLIN/medsurg_lewis

LEARNING OBJECTIVES

1. Describe the pathophysiology, clinical manifestations, and collaborative care of osteoarthritis, rheumatoid arthritis, gout, systemic lupus erythematosus, and systemic sclerosis.
2. Describe the clinical manifestations and management of juvenile rheumatoid arthritis, human leukocyte antigen–associated rheumatic diseases, septic arthritis, polymyositis, dermatomyositis, and fibromyalgia.
3. Compare and contrast the sequence of events leading to joint destruction in osteoarthritis and rheumatoid arthritis.
4. Compare and contrast osteoarthritis with rheumatoid arthritis related to clinical manifestations, treatment, and prognosis.
5. Identify the nursing management of arthritis and related rheumatic disorders.
6. Describe the types of reconstructive surgery associated with arthritis and related rheumatic disorders.
7. Identify the preoperative and postoperative teaching and collaborative care of the patient having reconstructive surgery associated with arthritis and related rheumatic disorders.
8. Describe the drug therapy and related nursing considerations associated with arthritis and related rheumatic disorders.
9. Identify psychologic and sociocultural issues of the patient with rheumatic disease and the appropriate nursing strategies that meet these needs.
10. Identify the importance of the interdisciplinary team approach to comprehensive management of rheumatic disorders.

OSTEOARTHRITIS

Osteoarthritis (OA), also known as *degenerative joint disease* (DJD), is a slowly progressive disorder of articulating joints, particularly weight-bearing joints, and is characterized by degeneration of articular cartilage. The damage from OA is confined to the joints and surrounding tissues. Clinical manifestations include joint pain, stiffness, and limited range of motion (ROM). Radiographically, the disease is characterized by joint-space narrowing, subchondral sclerosis, and osteophyte (bony outgrowth) formation. There is a wide spectrum of disease severity, ranging from annoying and uncomfortable symptoms to significantly disabling disease.

The most significant risk factor for OA is age. It is estimated that nearly one third of all adults have x-ray evidence of degenerative joint disease, with the incidence increasing to 60% to 80% by age 60. Because only one half of these adults experience significant symptoms, joint pain and functional disability should not be considered a normal finding in aging persons. OA is generally distributed throughout the peripheral and central joints.[2]

Reviewed by Debra A. Bancroft, RN, MSN, FNP-C, Nurse Practitioner, Rheumatic Disease Center, Milwaukee, Wisc; and Sharon G. Childs, RN, MS, CRNP, CS, CEN, ONC, Orthopedic Clinical Specialist, Johns Hopkins Hospital, Assistant Professor, Johns Hopkins University, Baltimore, Md.

Etiology and Pathophysiology

OA may occur as a primary idiopathic or secondary disorder.[1] The cause of primary OA is unknown. Although both primary and secondary OA are influenced by multiple factors (e.g., metabolic, mechanical, genetic, chemical), secondary OA has an identifiable precipitating event, such as previous trauma, fractures, infection, or congenital deformities, that is believed to predispose the person to later degenerative changes.

Degenerative changes over time cause the normally smooth, white, translucent joint cartilage to become yellow and opaque, with rough surfaces and areas of malacia (softening). As the layers of cartilage become thinner, bony surfaces are drawn closer together. As the cartilage breaks down, fissures may appear and fragments of cartilage become loose. Inflammation of the synovial membrane secondary to cartilage breakdown may follow. As the articular surface becomes totally denuded of cartilage, subchondral bone increases in density and becomes sclerotic (eburnated). New bone outgrowths (osteophytes) are formed at joint margins and at the attachment sites of ligaments and tendons.

There are several possible causes for cartilage deterioration, which is an active process. The enzyme hyaluronidase, which is

CULTURAL & ETHNIC CONSIDERATIONS

Arthritis and Connective Tissue Disorders

- Systemic lupus erythematosus is more common among African-American women than Caucasian women.
- Ankylosing spondylitis is more common and disease presentation is more severe in Caucasians than in non-Caucasians.
- Osteoarthritis is more common in Native-Americans than Caucasians.

normally found in the synovial fluid, may be responsible for digestion of proteoglycans via cracks in the surface layer of articular cartilage. Another possible cause is that inadequate nutrition of the cartilage may result in cartilage degeneration. Because cartilage is avascular, nutrients are provided by the synovial fluid. DNA synthesis, which is normally absent in adult articular cartilage, is active in OA tissue and appears to be directly proportional to disease severity.[3]

Specific predisposing factors such as excessive use of or stress on a joint have been identified as accelerating osteoarthritic changes (e.g., in the knees of football players and the feet and ankles of ballet dancers). Genetic factors influence the development of Heberden's nodes, which involve a single autosomal gene, dominant in women and recessive in men. (Heberden's nodes are discussed later.)

Other factors that influence the development of OA include congenital structural defects (e.g., Legg-Calvé-Perthes disease [osteochrondritis of head of femur in children]), metabolic disturbances (e.g., diabetes mellitus, acromegaly), repeated intraarticular hemorrhage (e.g., hemophilia), neuropathic arthropathies (Charcot's joints), and inflammatory and septic arthritis.

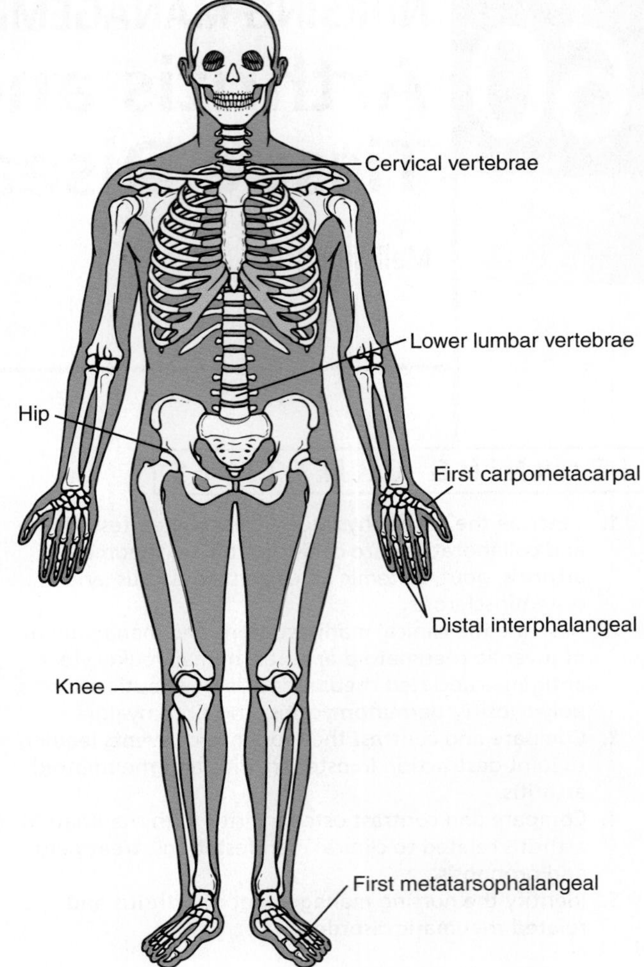

Fig. 60-1 Joints most frequently involved in osteoarthritis.

Clinical Manifestations

Systemic. Systemic manifestations, such as fatigue or fever, are not present in OA. Other organ involvement is absent as well, which is an important differentiation between OA and inflammatory joint disorders such as rheumatoid arthritis.[4]

Joints. Articular manifestations are related to the particular joint involved. The patient has pain on motion and weight bearing that is generally relieved by rest. In advanced disease, sleep may be disrupted by joint pain. As cartilage (which does not contain nerve endings) is worn away, direct irritation and pressure occur on the nerves of subchondral bone. Pain is most often caused by swelling and stretching of soft tissue structures surrounding the joint and not by the arthritic joint itself. Increasing pain is accompanied by progressive loss of function. Overall body coordination and posture may be affected as a result of the pain and loss of mobility.

Unlike pain, which is typically provoked by activity, joint stiffness occurs after periods of rest or static position. The symptoms related to OA are often aggravated by rising humidity and falling barometric pressure. Crepitation (grating sensation caused by the rubbing together of abnormal joint surfaces) on motion and malalignment of the extremity may be noted on physical examination. Advanced disease is characterized by gross deformity and subluxation (partial dislocation) caused by deterioration of cartilage, collapse of subchondral bone, and extensive bony overgrowth.

Joints are usually affected asymmetrically. The joints most frequently involved are the distal and proximal interphalangeal joints of the fingers, first carpometacarpal joint, hips, knees, first metatarsophalangeal joint, and lower lumbar and cervical vertebrae (Fig. 60-1). Degenerative changes are rarely seen in metacarpophalangeal joints, elbows, or shoulders.

Nodules. Heberden's nodes are another common manifestation of OA, particularly in women with primary OA. These nodes are reactive bony overgrowths located at the distal interphalangeal joints (Fig. 60-2). Heberden's nodes are palpable protuberances that are often associated with flexion and lateral deviation of the distal phalanx, occur more frequently in women, and tend to appear in families. Bouchard's nodes, seen less commonly in OA, involve the proximal interphalangeal joints.

Heberden's nodes and Bouchard's nodes may cause redness, swelling, tenderness, and aching. They often begin in one finger and spread to others. Although there is usually no significant loss of function caused by the bony enlargements, the patient is often distressed by the resulting disfigurement of the hands. Little can be done to prevent the occurrence of these nodes.

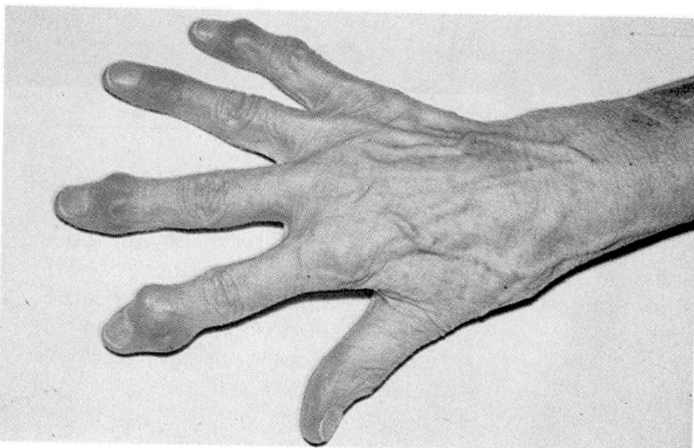

Fig. 60-2 Heberden's nodes.

Hips. OA of the hips may be extremely disabling. Congenital or structural abnormalities are frequent causes. This problem occurs more frequently in men than in women and may be unilateral or bilateral. Hip pain may be perceived as pain in the groin, buttock, or medial side of the thigh or knee, so the patient may find it difficult to localize the problem correctly. Pain on motion or on weight bearing may become progressively severe, and pain on rest may ensue. Sitting down is difficult, as is rising from a chair when the hips are lower than the knees. The patient learns to sit in a high seat with firm support and arm rests. Eventually, loss of ROM is significant, with pronounced limitation of extension and internal rotation.

Knees. Softening of the posterior surface of the patella (chondromalacia patellae) is seen most commonly in young people. Degeneration of the weight-bearing surfaces of the femoral and tibial condyles is usually seen in older women and is associated with limitation of motion, crepitus, and flexion deformity. Obesity has been implicated in OA of the knee in women, which is possibly the result of mechanical stress.

Vertebral Column. OA in the spine may produce localized symptoms of stiffness and pain. Degenerative disease of the intervertebral disks results as the nucleus pulposus deteriorates, becoming brittle and inelastic. Herniation of the degenerating nucleus most often occurs posteriorly or laterally, compressing a nerve root and causing muscle spasm or radicular pain. Another type of OA of the vertebral column involves development of degenerative disease of the intervertebral (apophyseal) joints, which generally follows disk disease by a number of years. Marginal osteophytes (spurs) also appear at vertebral attachments of the anulus, periosteum, and longitudinal ligaments. These osteophytes may fuse and limit ROM, or they may press against intervertebral foramina, producing symptoms of nerve root compression. Although rare, osteophyte formation in the posterior aspect of the cervical spine may produce vascular compression on the vertebrobasilar arteriole system producing insufficiency, resulting in intermittent dizziness, visual disturbances, headaches, and ataxia.

Diagnostic Studies

In late OA disease, x-rays show joint space narrowing, bony sclerosis, spur formation, and subluxation in some cases. X-ray changes do not always correlate with the degree of pain experienced by the patient. The patient may be completely free of symptoms, despite significant radiologic joint space narrowing. Conversely, some patients have severe pain with only moderate x-ray changes. No specific laboratory abnormalities are useful in the diagnosis of OA. The erythrocyte sedimentation rate (ESR) is normal except in instances of erosive OA, when moderate ESR elevation may be noted. Synovial fluid aspirated from an involved joint may be increased in volume but is clear yellow and viscous. Analysis of the fluid reveals little or no sign of inflammation.

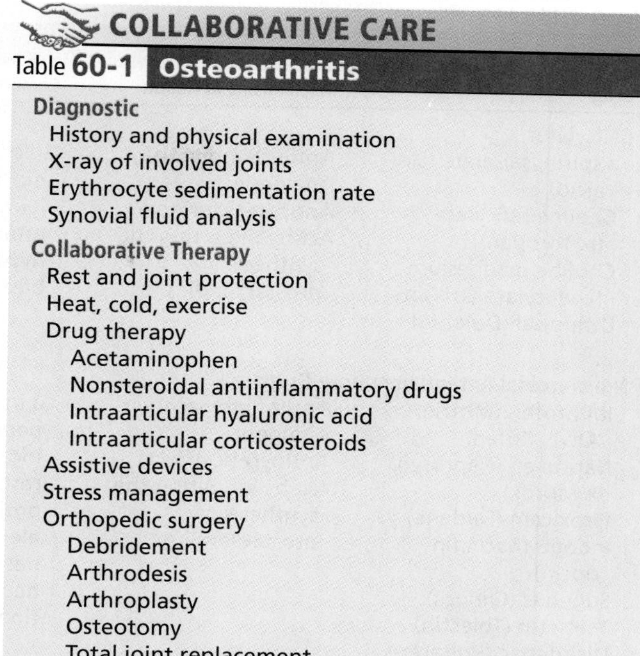

COLLABORATIVE CARE

Table 60-1 Osteoarthritis

Diagnostic
- History and physical examination
- X-ray of involved joints
- Erythrocyte sedimentation rate
- Synovial fluid analysis

Collaborative Therapy
- Rest and joint protection
- Heat, cold, exercise
- Drug therapy
  - Acetaminophen
  - Nonsteroidal antiinflammatory drugs
  - Intraarticular hyaluronic acid
  - Intraarticular corticosteroids
- Assistive devices
- Stress management
- Orthopedic surgery
  - Debridement
  - Arthrodesis
  - Arthroplasty
  - Osteotomy
  - Total joint replacement

Collaborative Care

There is no specific treatment for OA. Therapy is aimed at pain control, prevention of progression and disability, and restoration of joint function (Table 60-1). Once the diagnosis is confirmed, the patient should be assured that OA is likely to remain confined to a few joints and does not generally cause crippling. However, if joint destruction is extensive and pain is severe, surgery may be an option. Possible surgical procedures are listed in Table 60-1.

Drug Therapy. New guidelines for the management of OA were developed in 1995.[5,6] First-line therapy starts with acetaminophen 1 g up to four times daily. Topical agents such as capsaicin cream may be used alone or in conjunction with acetaminophen. This cream, made from chili peppers, causes depletion of substance P from nerve endings, thus blocking pain signals to the brain. Various strengths are available and must be used regularly for maximal effect. A generally short-lived burning sensation may accompany initial use. If response to these methods is suboptimal, low-dose ibuprofen (Motrin, Advil) 400 mg up to four times daily or nonacetylated salicylates are subsequently used.

Second-line therapy used in OA consists of nonsteroidal antiinflammatory drugs (NSAIDs) at full doses (Table 60-2). NSAIDs block the production of prostaglandins from arachidonic acid by inhibiting the production of cyclooxygenase (COX) (see Fig. 11-7). Concerns have been raised regarding

DRUG THERAPY

Table 60-2 Rheumatic Disorders

Drug	Mechanisms of Action	Common Side Effects	Nursing Considerations
Salicylates			
Aspirin, salsalate (Disalcid) Choline salicylate (Arthropan) Choline magnesium trisalicylate (Trilisate) Diflunisal (Dolobid)	Antiinflammatory Analgesic Antipyretic effect Act by inhibiting the synthesis of prostaglandins*	GI irritation (ulcer and hemorrhage), hypersensitivity, salicylism (nausea, tinnitus, dizziness, hyperpnea), prolonged bleeding time	When drug is taken for antiinflammatory effect, discontinue if pain decreases. Administer drug with food, milk, antacids as prescribed, or full glass of water or use enteric-coated aspirin. Report signs of bleeding (e.g, tarry stool, bruising, petechiae, melena).
Nonsteroidal Antiinflammatory Drugs			
Ibuprofen (Motrin, Advil, Rufen) Naproxen (Naprosyn, Anaprox) Piroxicam (Feldene) Indomethacin (Indocin) Sulindac (Clinoril) Tolmetin (Tolectin) Diclofenac (Voltaren) Meclofenamate (Meclomen) Celecoxib (Celebrex)[†] Rofecoxib (Vioxx)[†]	Antiinflammatory Analgesic Antipyretic effect Act by inhibiting the synthesis of prostaglandins*	GI irritation, including dyspepsia, nausea and vomiting, GI bleeding, dizziness, rash, headache, tinnitus, prolonged bleeding time, elevated serum transaminases, drug-induced nephrotoxicity, exacerbation of asthma	Administer drug with food, milk, or antacids as prescribed. Report signs of bleeding, edema, skin rashes, persistent headaches, or visual disturbances. Monitor elevations in BP.
Nonnarcotic Analgesics			
Acetaminophen (Tylenol)	Analgesic Antipyretic effect	Rash, urticaria, hepatotoxicity, leukopenia	Advise patient that concomitant use of alcohol may cause liver damage. Teach patient not to exceed recommended dosage.
Capsaicin cream (Zostrix, Capzacin P)	Topical analgesic, depletes substance P from nerve endings thereby interrupting pain signals to the brain	Localized burning sensation, erythema	Must be used regularly over time for maximal effect. Aloe vera cream may moderate burning sensation. Fatty substance such as butter or milk will deactivate action of cream. Available in several strengths.
Tramadol (Ultram)	Analgesic, centrally acting, binds to opioid receptors	Dizziness, nausea, constipation, headache, GI bleeding, somnolence, vomiting, pruritus, dyspepsia	Not recommended with concomitant MAO inhibitors. Advise patient to make position changes slowly, because orthostatic hypotension may occur. May potentiate seizure risk with MAO inhibitors, tricyclics, or neuroleptics. Administer with antiemetic to prevent nausea and vomiting.
Narcotic Analgesics			
Propoxyphene with acetaminophen or aspirin (Darvocet, Darvon) Codeine with acetaminophen or aspirin (Tylenol #3 or #4, Empirin #3 or #4) Hydrocodone with acetaminophen or aspirin (Lorcet, Lortab, Vicodin) Oxycodone with acetaminophen or aspirin (Oxycontin, Percodan, Percocet, Tylox)	Analgesic	Constipation, arrhythmias, dizziness, sedation, nausea, headache, vomiting, rash; respiratory depression or hepatotoxicity with overdosage	Advise patient regarding potential for constipation. Report signs of bleeding with products containing aspirin. Monitor CBC and liver function tests. Administer with antiemetic if nausea occurs. Teach patient and family to report any CNS or respiratory changes.

Continued

DRUG THERAPY

Table 60-2 Rheumatic Disorders—cont'd

Drug	Mechanisms of Action	Common Side Effects	Nursing Considerations
Corticosteroids			
Intraarticular Injections			
Methylprednisolone acetate (Depo-Medrol) Triamcinolone (Aristospan)	Antiinflammatory Analgesic Act by inhibiting the synthesis of prostaglandins*	Local osteoporosis, tendon rupture, and neuropathic arthropathy from repeated injection. Possibility of local infection.	Use strict aseptic technique as joint fluid is removed and corticosteroids are injected. Inform patient that joint may feel worse immediately after injection. Inform patient that improvement lasts weeks to months after injection and that weight bearing should be minimized for 2-6 wk after injection.
Systemic			
Hydrocortisone sodium succinate (Solu-Cortef) Methylprednisolone succinate sodium (Solu-Medrol) Dexamethasone (Decadron) Prednisone Triamcinolone (Aristocort)	Antiinflammatory Analgesic	Cushing's syndrome, including fluid retention, GI irritation, osteoporosis, insomnia, hypertension, psychosis, diabetes mellitus, acne, menstrual irregularities, hirsutism, risk of infection, bruising	Use only when symptoms persist with less potent antiinflammatory drugs or in life-threatening situations. Administer for limited time only, tapering dose slowly. Be aware that exacerbation of symptoms occurs with abrupt withdrawal. Monitor blood pressure, weight, CBC, and potassium. Limit sodium intake. Report signs of infection. Instruct patient to report corticosteroid use to surgeon or dentist to avoid postoperative adrenal insufficiency.
Immunosuppressive Agents			
Azathioprine (Imuran)	Acts as an immunosuppressant by inhibiting purine metabolism and decreasing DNA, RNA, and protein	GI irritation and ulceration, alopecia, oral lesions, dermatitis, blood dyscrasia, bone marrow depression, general increase in susceptibility to infection	Be aware of teratogenic potential that cautions against use for children or women of childbearing age. Monitor CBC, platelets, and urinalysis values. Be aware that drug should be used with great caution in patients with hepatic or renal impairment and should not be used in patients with a history of malignant tumors.
Cyclophosphamide (Cytoxan)	Acts as an immunosuppressant by crosslinking DNA and RNA strands and inhibiting the synthesis of protein	GI irritation and ulceration, alopecia, oral lesions, dermatitis, blood dyscrasia, bone marrow depression, oncogenicity, hemorrhagic cystitis, sterility	Be aware that therapy is limited to patients not responsive to conventional therapy. Monitor CBC, platelets, and urinalysis values. Be aware of teratogenic potential that cautions against use for children or women of childbearing age. Inform patient that contraception should be used during therapy. Use usually limited to treatment of rheumatoid vasculitis.
Cyclosporine (Sandimmune, Neoral)	Acts as an immunosuppressant by inhibiting T lymphocytes	Hypertension, tremor, hepatotoxicity, nephrotoxicity, hyperkalemia, increased susceptibility to infection, nausea, and vomiting	Be aware drug should be used with caution in patients with hepatic or renal impairment. Monitor CBC and liver function tests. Administer with meals for GI upset.

Continued

DRUG THERAPY

Table 60-2 Rheumatic Disorders—cont'd

Drug	Mechanisms of Action	Common Side Effects	Nursing Considerations
Immunosuppressive Agents—cont'd			
Methotrexate (Rheumatrex)	Acts as an immunosuppressant by inhibiting the metabolism of folic acid, thus inhibiting the synthesis of RNA and DNA	GI irritation, photosensitivity, oral lesions, hepatic toxicity, blood dyscrasia, infertility	Monitor CBC, liver function tests, and serum creatinine. Instruct patient to avoid alcoholic beverages and report signs of jaundice. Be aware of teratogenic potential that cautions against use for children or women of childbearing age. Inform patient that contraception should be used during and 3 mo after treatment.
Sulfasalazine (Azulfidine)	Acts as an antiinflammatory/immunosuppressant by causing release of adenosine at sites of inflammation thereby increasing secretion of IL-10 and decreasing T cell function	Rash, yellow-orange skin color, neutropenia, thrombocytopenia, fever, GI irritation, dizziness, photosensitivity, headache, myelosuppression	Monitor CBC and liver function tests. Avoid sun exposure. Also used in patient with inflammatory bowel conditions.
Remission-Inducing Agents			
Chrysotherapy Parenteral Gold sodium thiomalate (Myochrysine) Aurothioglucose (Solganal) Oral Auranofin (Ridaura)	Unknown, inflammatory-suppressive effect, possibly due to inhibition of macrophage function, complement activation, and prostaglandin synthesis	Parenteral: Dermatitis, pruritus, stomatitis, blood dyscrasia, nephrotoxicity, diarrhea Oral: Less toxic than parenteral; GI irritation, mucocutaneous, hematopoietic system, and kidney complications	Parenteral: Test blood and urine regularly. Check urine for blood and protein before each dose and delay injection until negative. Mix drug well and give deep intramuscular injection in buttocks. Inform patient that symptomatic improvement is not expected for 3-6 mo and that therapy may be continued indefinitely. Oral: Institute new oral therapy with bulking agents. Do not taper oral dosage; be aware that laboratory testing is less frequent with oral drug. Instruct women to not become pregnant while receiving chrysotherapy. Less toxic and less effective than parenteral gold.
Antimalarials Chloroquine (Aralen) Hydroxychloroquine (Plaquenil)	Unknown, but it has the ability to bind and alter DNA-modifying effect	Nausea, abdominal discomfort, rash, asymptomatic retinopathy, corneal opacity, headache, dizziness, blood dyscrasia	Inform patient that ophthalmologic examination including slit-lamp studies is required every 6-12 mo. Instruct patient to take drug with meals, milk, or antacid as prescribed, to report all skin eruptions and visual disturbances, and to avoid excessive sun exposure. Monitor CBC and liver enzyme values periodically. Instruct patient to discuss condition with physician before pregnancy and breastfeeding.

Continued

possible negative effects of long-term NSAID treatment on cartilage metabolism, particularly in older patients. Gastrointestinal (GI) side effects also commonly occur with the use of NSAIDs. This has led to use of misoprostol (Cytotec) to prevent NSAID-induced GI effects. Arthrotec, a combination of misoprostol and the NSAID diclofenac (Voltaren), is available. Newer NSAIDs offer the advantage of a once- or twice-daily regimen, which improves compliance (see Table 60-2 for a list of drugs used in the management of OA). When given in equivalent antiinflammatory dosages, all NSAIDs are comparable in efficacy but vary widely in cost. Individual responses and side effects of NSAIDs are variable. Aspirin, no longer

DRUG THERAPY

Table 60-2 Rheumatic Disorders—cont'd

Drug	Mechanisms of Action	Common Side Effects	Nursing Considerations
Remission-Inducing Agents—cont'd			
Penicillamine (Cuprimine, Depen)	Unknown, disease-modifying effect	Blood dyscrasias, glomerulonephropathy, myasthenia gravis, rashes, GI irritation, diarrhea, pruritus	Give drug on empty stomach before meals (not with). Monitor CBC, urinalysis, and liver function values. Report fever, sore throat, chills, bruising, or bleeding. Be aware that drug is contraindicated with gold therapy. Instruct women to not become pregnant while taking drug.
Tetracyclines (minocycline, doxycycline)	Unclear, possibly antiinflammatory, immunomodulatory, and chondroprotective effects in addition to antibacterial properties.	GI irritation, rash, photosensitivity, blood dyscrasias, hepatotoxicity	Monitor renal and liver function tests in long-term use. May increase digoxin levels. Antacids, iron, zinc, calcium, and magnesium reduce absorption.

*See Fig. 11-7.
†Cyclooxygenase—two inhibitors that are less likely to cause GI problems than traditional NSAIDs.
CBC, complete blood count; *IL,* interleukin; *MAO,* monoamine oxidase.

common in treatment, should not be used in combination with NSAIDs because both inhibit platelet function and prolong bleeding time.

A new generation of NSAIDs, COX-2 inhibitors, has recently been approved by the FDA. These drugs include celecoxib (Celebrex) and rofecoxib (Vioxx). They work by inhibiting cyclooxygenase-2 (COX-2) without affecting cyclooxygenase-1 (COX-1), an enzyme that primarily protects the stomach lining. Traditional NSAIDs are nonspecific inhibitors of both COX-1 and COX-2. The major advantage of COX-2 inhibitors as compared to traditional NSAIDs is that they are less likely to cause GI problems, such as ulcers and bleeding.

Intraarticular injections of corticosteroids are used to treat a symptomatic flare of OA. Systemic use of corticosteroids should be avoided because they may accelerate the disease process. The use of oral glucosamine sulfate and chondroitin sulfate as dietary supplements has become popular among individuals with OA.[7] However, concerns remain that well-controlled studies of significant length have not been done. These agents are not currently recommended by the Arthritis Foundation.

A newly approved treatment for OA of the knee uses intraarticular injections of synthetic and naturally occurring hyaluronic acid derivatives (Orthovisc, Synvisc, Artz, and Hyalgan). Although the exact mechanisms of action are unknown, these compounds appear to have some antiinflammatory benefits and a short-term lubricant effect.[7] In addition, an analgesic effect may be possible through the direct buffering effect of hyaluronic acid on synovial nerve endings, and a stimulating effect on synovial lining cells may produce normal hyaluronic acid.

Nutritional Therapy. There is no specific diet for OA except one that maintains optimal health. If a patient is overweight, a weight-reduction program becomes an important part of the total treatment plan. Body weight is magnified five times through the hips and three times through the knees. The additional strain of extra pounds can greatly increase pain and loss of function in OA. Furthermore, heavy thighs lead to malalignment at the knee, increasing wear on the medial aspect. (Chapter 38 discusses ways to assist the patient in attaining and maintaining a healthy body weight.)

NURSING MANAGEMENT: OSTEOARTHRITIS

■ Nursing Assessment

Nursing assessment of the patient with OA should include careful documentation of the nature, location, severity, and frequency of joint pain and stiffness. The extent to which these symptoms affect the patient's ability to perform activities of daily living should also be assessed. Successful and unsuccessful pain-relieving practices should be noted. Physical examination of the affected joint or joints includes assessment of tenderness, swelling, limitation of movement, and crepitation. It is useful to compare the involved joint with the same joint on the opposite side of the body if that joint is not affected.

■ Nursing Diagnoses

Nursing diagnoses for the patient with OA may include, but are not limited to, the following:

- Pain *related to* physical activity and lack of knowledge of pain self-management techniques
- Sleep pattern disturbance *related to* pain
- Impaired physical mobility *related to* weakness, stiffness, or pain on ambulation
- Self-care deficits *related to* joint deformity and pain with activity
- Altered nutrition: more than body requirements *related to* intake in excess of energy output
- Self-esteem disturbance *related to* changing social and work roles

PATIENT & FAMILY TEACHING GUIDE

Table 60-3 Joint Protection and Energy Conservation

- Maintain good posture and proper body mechanics.
- Maintain normal weight.
- Use assistive devices, if indicated.
- Avoid positions of deviation and stress.
- Find less stressful ways to perform tasks.
- Avoid tasks that cause pain.
- Develop organizing and pacing techniques.
- Avoid forceful repetitive movements.

Planning

The overall goals are that the patient with OA will (1) balance rest and activity; (2) use joint-protection measures (Table 60-3) to improve activity tolerance; (3) modify the home and work environment to include work-saving and joint-protecting assistive devices; (4) use pharmacologic and nonpharmacologic pain management techniques to achieve satisfactory pain control (see Chapter 9); and (5) perform ROM, muscle-strengthening, and aerobic exercise regularly.

Nursing Implementation

Health Promotion. Prevention of primary OA is not possible. However, preventive education may include elimination of excessive strain on joints by reduction of occupational and recreational hazards and nutritional counseling for weight reduction. Community education may include proper body mechanics of lifting and good posture. Athletic instruction and physical fitness programs should include safety measures that protect and reduce trauma to the joint structures. Congenital conditions, such as Legg-Calvé-Perthes disease, that are known to predispose to the development of OA should be treated promptly.

Acute Intervention. The person with OA is most troubled by pain, stiffness, limitation of function, and the frustration of coping with these physical difficulties on a daily basis. The older adult may believe that OA is an inevitable part of the aging process and that nothing can be done to ease the discomfort and related disability.

Usually a patient with OA is treated on an outpatient basis by a team of arthritis professionals including a personal physician or rheumatologist, a nurse, an occupational therapist, and a physical therapist. Health assessment questionnaires are helpful tools to pinpoint areas of difficulty for the patient with arthritis and target those areas for which specific interventions can then be developed.[8] These questionnaires may also be updated periodically to monitor the effectiveness of therapy. Hospitalization is usually necessary only if joint surgery or osteotomy is planned.

Medications are administered for the relief of pain and inflammation, if present. Nonpharmacologic pain management includes massage, application of heat (thermal packs) and cold (ice packs), relaxation, and guided imagery. Once an acute flare has subsided, a physical therapist can provide valuable assistance in planning an exercise program.

The hospital or home health nurse or family should assist the patient with activities of daily living as necessary and help the patient plan rest periods during the day. The patient needs sufficient time to move stiff, painful joints, especially when arising in the morning or after any period of sustained inactivity. Proper body alignment should be maintained at all times.

Patient education related to OA is an important nursing responsibility that should be carried out regardless of the care setting. Teaching should include information about the nature and treatment of the disease, pain management, correct posture and body mechanics, correct use of assistive devices such as a cane or walker, principles of joint protection and energy conservation (see Table 60-3), and a therapeutic exercise program. Home management goals must be individualized to meet the patient's needs, and family and social support should be included in goal setting and education.

Ambulatory and Home Care. After the diagnosis of OA and the initial educational efforts have been completed, the nurse should assist the patient in developing long-term strategies in managing the disease. The patient should be assured that OA is a localized disease and that severe deforming arthritis is not the usual course.

Safety measures in the home and work environment are important. These measures include removing scatter rugs, providing rails at stairs and bathtub, using night-lights, and wearing well-fitting supportive shoes. Assistive devices such as canes, walkers, elevated toilet seats, and grab bars reduce joint load and promote safety.

Splints may be prescribed to rest and stabilize painful or inflamed joints. Soft collars or cervical traction may be used at home for cervical OA. Stiff, painful hands can be relieved by warm-water soaking, contrast baths, or paraffin.[9] If swelling is more diffuse, stretch gloves can be worn at night to provide relief. Sexual counseling helps the patient and significant other to enjoy physical closeness by learning to adapt positions, alter timing, and increase awareness of partner's needs. Analgesics may be helpful when taken before activities.

Management of the chronic pain and loss of function of affected joints continue to be a primary concern. Nonpharmacologic techniques such as meditation, relaxation, and transcutaneous electric nerve stimulation (TENS) are particularly suited to chronic pain management (see Chapter 9). The nurse should be open to helping the patient and family to develop creative new approaches to pain relief. The practice of tai chi, for example, can increase mobility through gentle stretching and provides a calming effect with its focus on breathing and emotional centering. Nursing interventions should assist the patient and family to overcome feelings of helplessness and encourage active participation in managing chronic symptoms. The correct combination of joint protection, exercise (range of motion, isotonic, and isometric), heat or cold therapy, and medication can restore self-esteem and improve physical functioning. An aerobic exercise program, such as walking or aerobic aquatics, is also important.[10]

Evaluation

The expected outcomes are that the patient with osteoarthritis will

- experience adequate amounts of rest and activity
- use joint protection and energy conservation measures
- achieve satisfactory pain control
- maintain joint flexibility and muscle strength through ROM, aquatic, or aerobic exercises

RHEUMATOID ARTHRITIS

Rheumatoid arthritis (RA) is a chronic, systemic disease characterized by recurrent inflammation of the diarthrodial joints and related structures. It is frequently accompanied by a variety of extraarticular manifestations, such as rheumatoid nodules, arteritis, neuropathy, scleritis, pericarditis, lymphadenopathy, and splenomegaly.[11] RA is characterized by periods of remission and exacerbation of disease activity. The course of illness varies, ranging from episodes of illness separated by periods of remission to a more continuous, progressive disease.[12] Mortality rates are higher with severe disease.[13]

Of the approximately 6 million Americans who have RA, 75% are women. Although RA can occur at any age, it most often occurs in women of childbearing age.[14] There are no geographic or ethnic predispositions. RA is considered a significant national health problem in terms of its potential for chronic disability.

Etiology and Pathophysiology

The cause of RA is unknown. Whether a single causative factor is responsible or multiple factors are involved is unclear. Several etiologies are possible:

1. *Infection.* Research continues to probe the possibility of specific infectious pathogens, such as Epstein-Barr virus, parvovirus, and mycobacteria, which may trigger the process.
2. *Autoimmunity.* Although no virus particles have been identified, it is likely that an antigenic stimulus such as a virus leads to the formation of an abnormal immunoglobulin G (IgG). RA is characterized by the presence of autoantibodies against this abnormal IgG. The autoantibodies to this altered IgG are termed *rheumatoid factors*, and they combine with IgG to form immune complexes that deposit in the joints, blood vessels, and pleura. Complement is activated and an inflammatory response results (see Chapter 11). Neutrophils are attracted to the site of inflammation and release proteolytic enzymes that can damage articular cartilage and basement membranes of blood vessels and pleura.

   Joint changes are characterized by chronic inflammation with the presence of inflammatory cells and mediators. The infiltrating macrophages are activated and release a variety of cytokines, including interleukin-1 and interleukin-6, tumor necrosis factor (TNF), and colony-stimulating factor[15] (see Table 12-4). The activity of these cytokines accounts for many of the features of rheumatoid synovitis, including the synovial tissue inflammation, synovial proliferation, cartilage and bone damage, and systemic manifestations of RA.
3. *Genetic factors.* Certain familial factors may influence the expression of the disease. An increased prevalence of a human leukocyte antigen (HLA) known as the HLA-DR4 occurs in 65% of persons with RA. Persons in this group seem to experience a particularly crippling form of the disease. It is possible that the presence of this HLA and perhaps other genetic factors increase genetic susceptibility to an unidentified environmental antigen, such as a virus, which may then initiate the disease process (see Chapter 12).
4. *Other factors.* Metabolic and biochemical abnormalities, nutritional and environmental factors, and occupational and psychosocial influences may play a part in the cause or expression of the disease, but their contribution is entirely speculative.

The pathogenesis of RA is more clearly understood than its etiology. If unarrested, the disease progresses through four stages:

1. *First stage.* The unknown etiologic factor initiates joint inflammation, or synovitis, with swelling of the synovial lining membrane and production of excess synovial fluid.
2. *Second stage.* Pannus (inflammatory granulation tissue) is formed at the juncture of the synovium and cartilage. This extends over the surface of the articular cartilage and eventually invades the joint capsule and subchondral bone.
3. *Third stage.* Tough fibrous connective tissue replaces pannus, occluding the joint space. Fibrous ankylosis results in decreased joint motion, malalignment, and deformity.
4. *Fourth stage.* As fibrous tissue calcifies, bony ankylosis may result in total joint immobilization.

Clinical Manifestations

Joints. RA typically develops insidiously. Nonspecific manifestations such as fatigue, anorexia, weight loss, and generalized stiffness may precede the onset of arthritic complaints. The stiffness becomes more localized after weeks to months. Some patients report a history of a precipitating stressful event such as infection, work stress, physical exertion, childbirth, surgery, or emotional upset. However, there is no scientific evidence to correlate these events with the onset of RA.

Specific articular involvement is manifested clinically by pain, stiffness, limitation of motion, and signs of inflammation (heat, swelling, and tenderness). Joint symptoms are generally bilaterally symmetric and frequently affect small joints of the hands (proximal interphalangeal and metacarpophalangeal) and feet (metatarsophalangeal), as well as larger peripheral joints, including wrists, elbows, shoulders, knees, hips, ankles, and jaw. The cervical spine may be affected, but the axial spine is generally spared. Early shoulder involvement is common in the older adult. Table 60-4 compares the manifestations of RA and OA.

The patient characteristically has joint stiffness on arising in the morning and after periods of inactivity. This morning stiffness may last for 30 minutes to several hours or more, depending on disease activity. Metacarpal and proximal interphalangeal joints are typically swollen. The fingers may become spindle shaped from synovial hypertrophy and thickening of the joint capsule (Fig. 60-3). Joints become tender, painful, and warm to the touch. The pain is more pronounced on motion, varies in intensity, and may not be proportional to the degree of inflammation. Tenosynovitis frequently affects the extensor and flexor tendons around the wrists, producing manifestations of carpal tunnel syndrome and making it difficult to grasp objects.

As disease activity progresses, inflammation and fibrosis of the joint capsule and supporting structures may lead to deformity and disability. Atrophy of muscles and destruction of tendons around the joint cause one articular surface to slip past the

Table 60-4 Comparison of Rheumatoid Arthritis and Osteoarthritis

Parameter	Rheumatoid Arthritis	Osteoarthritis
Age	Young and middle-aged	Usually >40 yr of age
Gender	Female more often than male	Same incidence
Weight	Weight loss	Usually overweight
Illness	Systemic manifestations	Local joint manifestations
Affected joints	PIPs, MCPs, MTPs, wrists, elbows, shoulders, knees, hips, cervical spine Usually bilateral	DIPs, first CMCs, thumbs, first MTPs, knees, spine, hips; asymmetric, one or more joints
Effusions	Common	Uncommon
Nodules	Present	Heberden's nodes
Synovial fluid	Inflammatory	Noninflammatory
X-rays	Osteoporosis, narrowing, erosions	Osteophytes, subchondral cysts, sclerosis
Anemia	Common	Uncommon
Rheumatoid factor	Positive	Negative
Sedimentation rate	Elevated	Normal except in erosive osteoarthritis

CMC, carpometacarpal; *DIP,* distal interphalangeal; *MCP,* metacarpophalangeal; *MTP,* metatarsophalangeal; *PIP,* proximal interphalangeal.

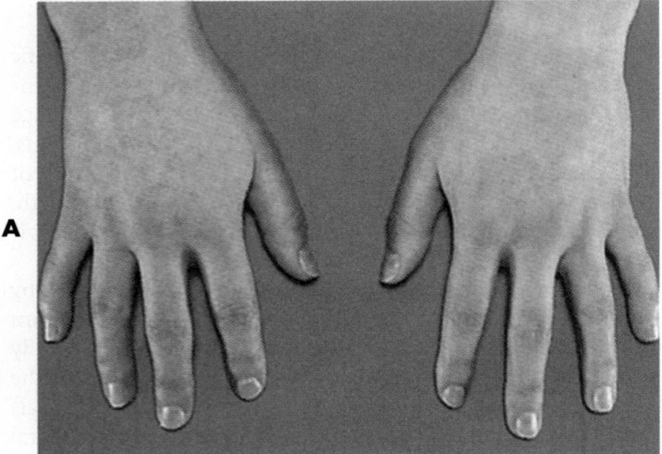

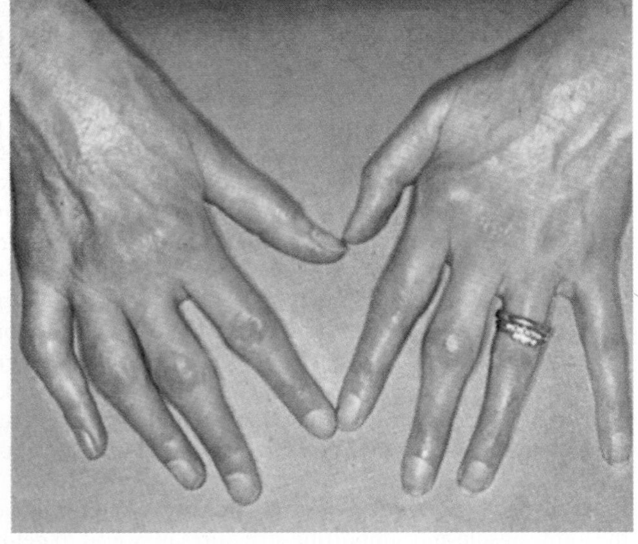

Fig. 60-3 Rheumatoid arthritis of the hand. **A,** Early stage. **B,** Moderate involvement.

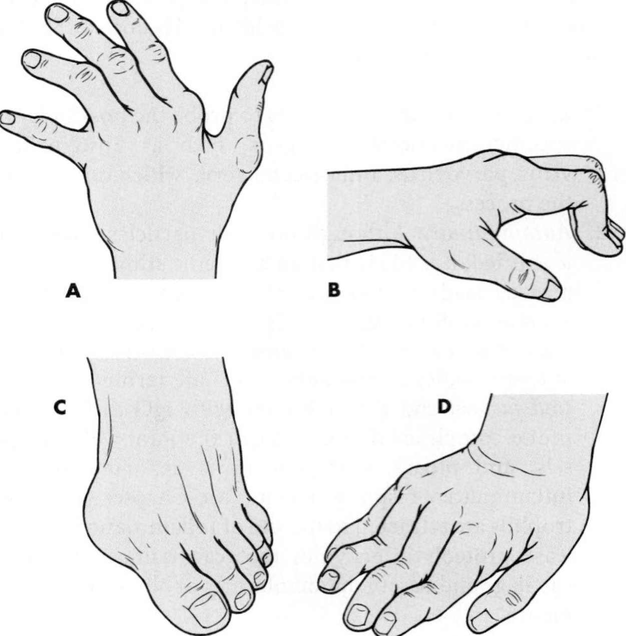

Fig. 60-4 Typical deformities of rheumatoid arthritis. **A,** Ulnar drift. **B,** Boutonnière deformity. **C,** Hallux valgus. **D,** Swan-neck deformity.

other (subluxation). Typical deformities of the hand include ulnar drift, swan-neck, and boutonnière deformities (Fig. 60-4). Metatarsal-head subluxation and hallux valgus (bunion) may cause pain and walking disability.

Extraarticular Manifestations. Rheumatoid nodules are present in 25% to 50% of all people with RA and are probably the most common extraarticular finding. Small-vessel vasculitis is considered to be the initiating event in the formation of these nodules. The nodules appear subcutaneously as firm, nontender masses and are usually found on olecranon bursae or along the extensor surface of the forearm. Nodules at the base of the spine and back of the head are common in older adults. Nodules develop insidiously and can persist or regress spontaneously. They are usually not removed because of the high probability of recurrence unless they are signifi-

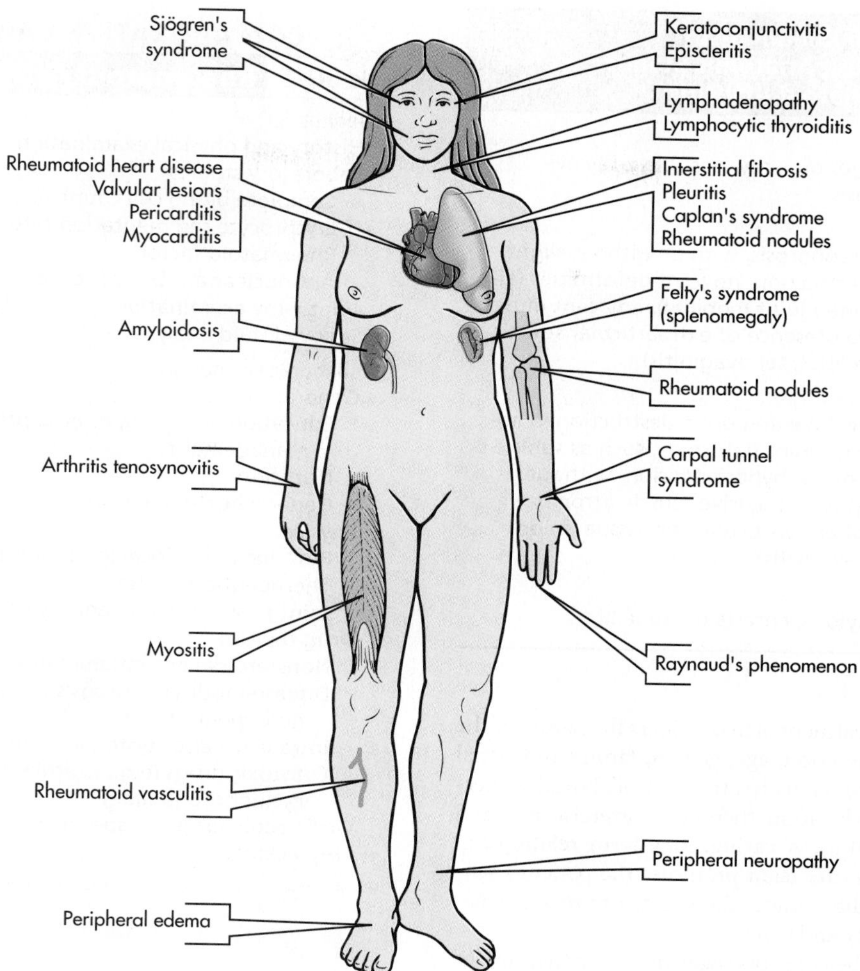

Fig. 60-5 Extraarticular manifestations of rheumatoid arthritis.

cantly disabling. Nodules may also appear on the eye or lungs; these indicate active disease and a poor prognosis.

Vasculitis (inflammation of blood vessels) may be responsible for a variety of systemic complications, including peripheral neuropathy, myopathy, cardiopulmonary involvement, and ischemic ulcerations of the skin. Figure 60-5 shows extraarticular manifestations of RA.

Complications

Potential complications of RA include infection, osteoporosis, and amyloidosis. Spinal cord compression may occur from instability of articulations in the cervical spine.

Diagnostic Studies

Although no single laboratory test is conclusive, several findings are helpful in diagnosing RA in conjunction with the history and physical examination.[16] Moderate anemia is common. The erythrocyte sedimentation rate (ESR) is elevated in 85% of patients and is useful in monitoring the response to therapy. Serum rheumatoid factor is present in titers greater than 1:160 in nearly 80% of individuals with RA. Antinuclear antibody and lupus cell tests may be positive in a smaller percentage of patients.

Synovial fluid analysis may show increased volume and turbidity but decreased viscosity of the fluid. The white blood cell (WBC) count of synovial fluid is elevated (often as high as 30,000/μl [30×10^9/L]) and consists predominantly of neutrophils. Inflammatory changes in the synovium can be confirmed by tissue biopsy.

X-ray findings (which are not specifically diagnostic) may reveal only bone demineralization and soft-tissue swelling during the early stage of the disease. Later, narrowing of the joint space, destruction of articular cartilage, erosion, subluxation, and deformity are present. Malalignment and ankylosis occur in advanced disease. Table 60-5 describes the anatomic stages of RA.

Collaborative Care

Care of the patient with RA begins with a comprehensive program of drug therapy and education. Physical comfort is promoted by NSAIDs and rest. The patient and family are educated about the disease process and home management strategies. Compliance with drug therapy includes correct administration, reporting of side effects, and frequent medical and laboratory follow-up visits. Physical therapy maintains joint motion and muscle strength. Occupational therapy develops upper-extremity function and encourages joint protection through the use of splinting, pacing techniques, and assistive devices.

Table 60-5 American Rheumatism Association Anatomic Stages of Rheumatoid Arthritis

Stage I—Early
No destructive changes on x-ray, possible x-ray evidence of osteoporosis

Stage II—Moderate
X-ray evidence of osteoporosis, with or without slight bone or cartilage destruction, no joint deformities (although possibly limited joint mobility), adjacent muscle atrophy, possible presence of extraarticular soft tissue lesions (e.g., nodules, tenovaginitis)

Stage III—Severe
X-ray evidence of cartilage and bone destruction in addition to osteoporosis; joint deformity, such as subluxation, ulnar deviation, or hyperextension, without fibrous or bony ankylosis; extensive muscle atrophy; possible presence of extraarticular soft tissue lesions (e.g., nodules, tenosynovitis)

Stage IV—Terminal
Fibrous or bony ankylosis, criteria of stage III

An individualized treatment plan considers the nature of the disease activity, joint function, age, gender, family and social roles, and response to previous treatment. Collaborative therapy generally includes education, therapeutic exercise, rest, and drug therapy (Table 60-6). A caring, long-term relationship with an arthritis health care team promotes the patient's self-esteem and hope and discourages the use of unproven remedies, which waste money and time.

Drug Therapy. The concepts regarding drug therapy for RA have changed considerably in recent years. In the past, patients were maintained on high doses of aspirin or NSAIDs for several years until there was x-ray evidence of characteristic bone erosions. Now a more aggressive drug therapy approach that is initiated earlier is more common because the erosive, destructive process begins within the first 2 years of disease.

Many rheumatologists are now using a disease-modifying agent (such as methotrexate) early in the course of the disease. A disease-modifying agent is a drug that has the potential to lessen the permanent effects of RA such as joint deformity. The damaging effects of the disease may be prevented or postponed by this plan. The exact time to introduce a disease-modifying drug varies among clinicians. Some start treatment when the patient has been symptomatic for only a few weeks. Others prefer to wait several months until the diagnosis is confirmed by x-ray and laboratory findings or the patient has sustained symptomatic arthritis. At this time there is no way to differentiate patients with mild disease from the larger group whose disease may be relentlessly progressive.[17] The least toxic agent, alone or in combination, that is likely to be effective is usually the drug chosen for initial therapy. Table 60-2 lists drugs commonly used in the treatment of RA.

For patients with mild disease, hydroxychloroquine (Plaquenil) is often prescribed initially. It is one of the safest of the disease-modifying drugs. The most common side effects of this drug are nausea, abdominal discomfort, and rash. The possibility of rare, irreversible retinal degeneration caused by deposition of this drug in the pigment layer of the retina requires ophthalmologic examination before therapy and at 6-month intervals. A low dose of prednisone may be given with or instead of hydroxychloroquine.

COLLABORATIVE CARE

Table 60-6 Rheumatoid Arthritis

Diagnostic
- History and physical examination
- Laboratory studies
  - Complete blood cell count
  - Erythrocyte sedimentation rate
  - Rheumatoid factor
  - Antinuclear antibody profile
- Joint x-ray examination
- Synovial fluid analysis

Collaborative Therapy
- General
  - Education, including disease process and management
  - Nutrition
  - General health measures
- Physical
  - Rest, including local joint, systemic, and emotional
  - Therapeutic exercise
  - Joint protection and energy conservation
- Drug therapy
  - Nonsteroidal antiinflammatory drugs
  - Disease-modifying drugs such as hydroxychloroquine, gold, penicillamine
  - Intraarticular or systemic corticosteroids
  - Cytotoxic drugs (e.g., azathioprine, methotrexate, cyclophosphamide)
- Orthopedic surgery, especially reconstructive joint replacement

Corticosteroid therapy can be used to aid in symptom control. Intraarticular injections are administered for a flare-up of the disease in one or two joints. Pain in the joint may increase for 1 to 2 days after injection because of the irritation by the medication. Alternatively, intramuscular injections of methylprednisolone (Solu-Medrol), for example, may be useful if several joints are affected. Pain and swelling are usually relieved for 1 to 6 weeks.

Bridge therapy (5 to 10 mg orally of the prescribed corticosteroid daily for 4 to 6 weeks) is used until one of the longer-acting drugs, such as hydroxychloroquine, gold, or D-penicillamine (Cuprimine), has been used long enough to suppress disease activity. Burst corticosteroid therapy, used for a severe articular flare, consists of high-dose (e.g., 40 to 60 mg) corticosteroids, which are then quickly tapered in 7 to 14 days. Pulse therapy (Solu-Medrol, at dosages of no more than 1 g per day intravenously for 3 days) is used to achieve fast control of inflammation and results in fewer side effects over the long term as a result of taking a smaller daily dose. Regardless of the regimen, high-dose or long-term corticosteroid therapy carries a high risk of drug dependency and serious side effects (see Chapter 47).

For patients with moderate to severe disease with symmetric joint involvement and a positive rheumatoid factor assay, a more aggressive drug regimen may be initiated. Usually methotrexate is the first drug of choice. The rapid antiinflammatory effect of methotrexate reduces clinical symptoms in days to weeks. Side effects include bone marrow suppression and hepatotoxicity. Methotrexate therapy requires frequent laboratory monitoring, including CBC and chemistry panel. A sustained, nonprogressive cough may be related to methotrexate therapy and should be evaluated with pulmonary function testing.[18] Avoidance of alcohol is often advised because it can increase the toxicity of methotrexate and confound liver enzyme elevations.

Gold therapy may be considered for patients who do not respond to methotrexate. Gold has an antiinflammatory action and may decrease phagocytosis and lysosomal activity.[19] It is usually given in a weekly injection for 5 months, then biweekly or monthly to sustain the clinical effects. Although the serious side effects of proteinuria and cytopenia are uncommon, gold therapy often causes minor side effects, such as skin rashes, mouth sores, and GI problems, particularly diarrhea.

Azathioprine (Imuran) or D-penicillamine (Cuprimine) may be used if the patient does not respond to either methotrexate or gold therapy. Azathioprine and penicillamine may cause mild pancytopenia.

There is increased interest in combination therapy to treat RA, although it is still somewhat controversial. Combinations include methotrexate plus sulfasalazine (Azulfidine) and hydroxychloroquine plus sulfasalazine, among others.[20] Multiple agents may provide a synergistic effect and more adequately control symptoms.

Although new drug regimens are being used with increasing frequency, aspirin and NSAIDs are still commonly used. Aspirin is often used in high dosages of 4 to 6 g per day (10 to 18 tablets) in divided doses to obtain a blood level of 15 to 30 mg/dl. Enteric-coated aspirin is absorbed in the small intestine and is often used to prevent gastric irritation. Enteric-coated tablets have a special covering to prevent them from disintegrating in the stomach and may require higher doses than regular tablets. The ability to obtain serum salicylate levels, unavailable with other NSAIDs, is helpful in individualizing treatment programs and evaluating compliance.

NSAIDs have antiinflammatory, analgesic, and antipyretic properties. Although many NSAIDs are potent inhibitors of inflammation, they do not appear to alter the natural history of RA. Although some relief from NSAIDs may be noted within days of the start of treatment, it takes approximately 2 to 3 weeks for full effectiveness to be demonstrated. NSAIDs may be used when patients are intolerant to high doses of aspirin. NSAIDs that are taken only once or twice a day may improve patient compliance.

There are significant but subtle differences in the mechanisms of action, effectiveness in various diseases, and other properties of the different NSAIDs. The unpredictable differences in effectiveness in various patients make it worthwhile to try different NSAIDs if the first drug does not work satisfactorily in a given patient. NSAIDs are often used in conjunction with disease-modifying drugs for their antiinflammatory effect.

The newer generation of NSAIDs, Cox-2 inhibitors, are effective in RA as well as OA. These include celecoxib (Celebrex) and rofecoxib (Vioxx) (see p. 1825).

Relatively new drugs used in the treatment of RA include leflunomide (Arava) and etanercept (Enbrel). Leflunomide inhibits the proliferation of activated lymphocytes, which are linked to the inflammation and pathophysiology of RA. Leflunomide slows joint deterioration and is well tolerated by patients. Leflunomide is contraindicated in pregnant women or women of childbearing age who are not using reliable birth control methods.

Etanercept is a biologically engineered copy (using recombinant DNA technology) of the tumor necrosis factor (TNF) cell receptor. This soluble TNF receptor binds to TNF in circulation before TNF can bind to its cell surface receptor. TNF, a naturally occurring cytokine, once bound to its cell receptor promotes inflammation. This drug is given two times per week as a subsutaneous injection. Etanercept may be especially effective in patients who have not responded to other therapies.

Nutritional Therapy. There is no special diet for RA. However, balanced nutrition is important. The fatigue, pain, depression, limited endurance, and limitation of mobility that may accompany RA may interfere with the patient's appetite and ability to shop for and prepare food, resulting in weight loss. The occupational therapist may help the patient to modify the home environment and to use assistive devices to make food preparation easier. Although patients are vulnerable to fad claims for improvement through health foods and vitamins, there is little credible research evidence for their use.

Corticosteroid therapy or immobility secondary to pain may result in unwanted weight gain. A sensible weight loss program consisting of balanced nutrition and exercise reduces stress on arthritic joints. Limited sodium intake may help minimize fluid gain caused by sodium retention. Corticosteroids also increase the appetite, resulting in a higher caloric intake. Even the most compliant patient becomes distressed as Cushing's syndrome signs and symptoms, such as moon face and redistribution of fatty tissue to the trunk, change the body's appearance. The patient must be encouraged to continue a balanced diet and not to alter corticosteroid dose or stop therapy abruptly. Weight slowly adjusts to normal several months after cessation of therapy.

GERONTOLOGIC CONSIDERATIONS

Arthritis

The prevalence of rheumatic disease in older adults is high, and the disease is accompanied by problems unique to this age-group. The most problematic areas related to rheumatic disease in older adults include the following:

1. The high incidence of OA expected in older adults often keeps the clinician from considering the presence of other rheumatic diseases.
2. Age alone causes changes in serologic profiles, making interpretation of laboratory values such as rheumatoid factors and sedimentation rates more difficult.
3. Multidrug regimens common to the older adult can result in iatrogenic arthritis.
4. Nonorganic musculoskeletal pain syndromes and weakness may be related to depressive reactions and physical inactivity.
5. Rheumatic diseases, such as systemic lupus erythematosus, that commonly manifest in younger adults can occur in older adults, but often in milder form.
6. Residual effects of rheumatic disease are present for long periods and must be managed.

Aging brings many physical and metabolic changes that may increase the older patient's sensitivity to both the therapeutic and toxic effects of some drugs. The use of NSAIDs with a

NURSING ASSESSMENT

Table 60-7 Rheumatoid Arthritis

Subjective Data

Important Health Information

Past health history: Epstein-Barr or other viral infections; presence of precipitating factors such as emotional upset, infections, overwork, childbirth, surgery; pattern of remissions and exacerbations

Medications: Use of aspirin, NSAIDs, corticosteroids, gold salts, penicillamine

Surgery or other treatments: Any joint surgery

Health Patterns

Health perception–health management: Positive family history for rheumatoid arthritis, malaise, ability to comply with therapeutic regimen

Nutritional-metabolic: Anorexia, weight loss; dry mucous membranes of mouth and pharynx

Activity-exercise: Morning stiffness and joint swelling, muscle weakness, difficulty walking, fatigue

Cognitive-perceptual: Paresthesias of hands and feet; numbness, tingling, loss of sensation; symmetric joint pain and aching that increases with motion or stress on joint

Objective Data

General

Lymphadenopathy, fever

Integumentary

Keratoconjunctivitis; subcutaneous rheumatoid nodules on forearm, elbows; skin ulcers; shiny, taut skin over involved joints; peripheral edema

Cardiovascular

Symmetric pallor and cyanosis of fingers (Raynaud's phenomenon); distant heart sounds, murmurs, arrhythmias (rheumatoid heart disease)

Respiratory

Chronic bronchitis, tuberculosis, histoplasmosis, fibrosing alveolitis

Gastrointestinal

Splenomegaly (Felty's syndrome)

Musculoskeletal

Symmetric joint involvement with swelling, erythema, heat, tenderness, and deformities; enlargement of proximal phalangeal and metacarpophalangeal joints; limitation of joint movement; muscle contractures, muscle atrophy

Possible Findings

Positive rheumatoid factor, elevated ESR, anemia; increased WBC in synovial fluid; evidence of osteoporosis, joint space narrowing, and bony erosion and deformity on x-ray

ESR, erythrocyte sedimentation rate.

shorter half-life requiring more frequent dosing may produce fewer side effects in the older patient with altered drug metabolism. The common occurrence of polypharmacy makes the use of multidrug therapy in RA particularly problematic in the older adult because of the increased likelihood of untoward drug interactions. Particular care should be taken when the older adult takes NSAIDs because of their increased propensity for side effects, particularly GI and renal toxicity. If such therapy is necessary, a cytoprotective agent such as misoprostol (Cytotec) should be considered.[21] The frequency of taking medication and the complexity of the drug regimen should be simplified as much as possible to increase compliance in the older adult, particularly for the patient without regular assistance.

A major concern of treatment in the older patient relates to the use of corticosteroid therapy. Corticosteroid-induced osteopenia adds to the problem of age-related and inactivity-related osteoporosis and can increase the occurrence of pathologic fractures, especially compression fractures of vertebrae. Corticosteroid-induced myopathy can be minimized or prevented by an age-appropriate exercise program. Although important for all age-groups, an adequate support system for the older adult is a critical factor in compliance with the management program, which should include nutritional planning, exercise, general health maintenance, and appropriate pharmacotherapy.

NURSING MANAGEMENT: RHEUMATOID ARTHRITIS

■ Nursing Assessment

Subjective and objective data that should be obtained from the patient with RA are presented in Table 60-7.

■ Nursing Diagnoses

Nursing diagnoses for the patient with RA may include, but are not limited to, those presented in NCP 60-1.

■ Planning

The overall goals are that the patient with RA will (1) have satisfactory pain relief, (2) have minimal loss of functional ability of the affected joints, (3) participate in planning and carrying out the therapeutic regimen, (4) maintain a positive self-image, and (5) perform self-care to the maximum amount possible.

■ Nursing Implementation

Health Promotion. Prevention of RA is not possible at this time. However, community education programs should include information concerning the symptoms of RA to promote early diagnosis and treatment. Many publications for the public are available through the Arthritis Foundation (see Resources at end of this chapter).

Acute Intervention. The primary objectives in the management of RA are reduction of inflammation, relief of pain, preservation of joint function, and prevention or correction of joint deformity. These may be approached by a comprehensive program of daily antiinflammatory medication, rest, joint protection, therapeutic heat, exercise, and thorough patient and family teaching. The nurse is an integral member of the health team, working closely with the physician, physical and occupational therapists, and social worker to restore function and to help the patient make lifestyle adjustments to chronic illness (Fig. 60-6).

The newly diagnosed patient with RA may be hospitalized for control of acute inflammation, evaluation of systemic in-

60-1 NURSING CARE PLAN PATIENT WITH RHEUMATOID ARTHRITIS

Expected Patient Outcomes	Nursing Interventions and *Rationales*
NURSING DIAGNOSIS	**Chronic pain** *related to* joint inflammation, overuse of joint, and ineffective pain or comfort measures *as manifested by* complaints of pain and limited joint function; hot, swollen, painful joints of more than 6 months duration.
▪ Decreased pain, swelling, and erythema of joints.	▪ Assess location, severity, and precipitators of pain *to plan appropriate interventions.* ▪ Encourage decreased activity, increased rest, and supportive resting splints for affected joints *to decrease stress on joints and resulting pain during acute flare-ups of disease.* ▪ Teach self-administration of antiinflammatory medications as prescribed, including names, actions, side effects, dose, and administration of prescribed drugs. ▪ Use relaxation techniques *to reduce physical and emotional stress;* protective techniques *that limit stress to joints;* and nonpharmacologic pain strategies (e.g., heat or cold application, meditation, massage) *to reduce pain.*
NURSING DIAGNOSIS	**Impaired physical mobility** *related to* joint pain, stiffness, and deformity *as manifested by* limitation of joint motion, strength, and endurance; inability to perform routine activities of daily living.
▪ Increased ROM and function. ▪ Decreased stiffness. ▪ Ability to perform activities of daily living. ▪ Minimal deformity.	▪ Apply moist heat to affected joints (e.g., paraffin bath, hot packs, warm shower) *to relieve stiffness and increase mobility.* ▪ Encourage ROM exercises *to prevent unnecessary mobility restriction;* reduce frequency if pain and swelling are present *to prevent joint destruction when active disease is present.* ▪ Schedule morning care and procedures later in the day *after morning stiffness subsides.* ▪ Teach patient to use assistive devices *to promote independence.* ▪ Encourage flexibility, strengthening, and conditioning exercises in water or on land *to increase joint motion, flexibility, muscle strength, and endurance.* ▪ Instruct patient on correct application of resting splints, selection of properly fitting footwear, maintenance of proper posture and body alignment, and selection and use of assistive devices *to prevent or limit joint deformity.*
NURSING DIAGNOSIS	**Fatigue** *related to* exacerbation of disease activity, anemia, drug side effects, sleep disturbance, or depression *as manifested by* verbilization of overwhelming lack of energy and decreased activity tolerance.
▪ Improved stamina and endurance. ▪ Better quality of sleep. ▪ Good eating habits.	▪ Assess causative factors and degree of fatigue *to plan appropriate activities.* ▪ Balance activity with rest periods. ▪ Encourage regular general physical exercise such as walking, bicycling, or swimming to patient's level of tolerance *to prevent deconditioning and foster a positive attitude.* ▪ Teach energy conservation techniques *to enable continued activity.* ▪ Review nutrition and sleep patterns *to determine if adjustments could prevent fatigue.*
NURSING DIAGNOSIS	**Body image disturbance** *related to* chronic disease activity, long-term treatment, deformities, stiffness, and inability to perform usual activities *as manifested by* social withdrawal, flat affect, altered self-concept, reduced sexual interest.
▪ Acceptance of body changes. ▪ Maintenance of interest in life.	▪ Allow patient to express feelings about disease *to determine extent of problems and plan appropriate interventions.* ▪ Offer psychologic support to patient and family *to prevent unnecessary or excessive emotional response to disease.* ▪ Provide sexual counseling *because sexual problems and concerns can have a serious impact on body image.* ▪ Reassure patient of self-worth *so a positive body image is fostered in spite of distressing physical manifestations.*

Continued

60-1 NURSING CARE PLAN PATIENT WITH RHEUMATOID ARTHRITIS—continued

Expected Patient Outcomes	Nursing Interventions and *Rationales*
NURSING DIAGNOSIS	**Ineffective management of therapeutic regimen** *related to* complexity of chronic health problem, pain, and fatigue *as manifested by* questioning management plan, self-doubt about ability to manage disease, ability to perform activities for only short periods.
▪ Expression of increased confidence in ability to manage disease. ▪ Ability to describe treatment plan. ▪ Expression of satisfaction with pain and fatigue management.	▪ Assess patient's knowledge of disease *to plan appropriate interventions.* ▪ Include patient's family members in discussion of disease management *to increase their sense of control and to increase patient's sense of support.* ▪ Evaluate patient's understanding through verbalization and demonstration *to ensure correct understanding of disease management.* ▪ Focus on patient's problems of pain and fatigue *because these are major deterrents to successful disease management and must be addressed.* ▪ Assist patient to recognize need for ongoing therapy and to resist false advertising and unproven remedies *so only proven methods of treatment will be used.*
NURSING DIAGNOSIS	**Altered family processes** *related to* patient's inability to function secondary to chronic illness and complexity of treatment regimen *as manifested by* changes in family, social, and occupational roles; dysfunctional family dynamics.
▪ Successful adjustment to disease activity by patient and family. ▪ Vocational rehabilitation or modification.	▪ Help patient and family identify appropriate coping strategies *to foster adjustment to changes in function and role responsibilities.* ▪ Refer patient to community vocational centers *for work adjustment or retraining.* ▪ Encourage professional family counseling *because unresolved serious family problems can interfere with successful disease management.*
NURSING DIAGNOSIS	**Self-care deficits** *related to* disease progression, weakness, and contracture *as manifested by* inability to perform activities of daily living (ADLs).
▪ Completion of ADLs independently or with assistance. ▪ Expression of satisfaction with how self-care needs are met.	▪ Assess patient's ability to perform ADLs *to plan appropriate interventions.* ▪ Assist patient with ADLs as necessary *to ensure all needs are met.* ▪ Provide assistive devices or refer to occupational therapist where appropriate *to compensate for contractures and weakness so patient can perform as many self-care activities as possible.* ▪ Encourage patient to pace activities *to foster maximum independence with minimal fatigue.*

volvement, and comprehensive education by the health team. Hospitalization may also be necessary for patients with extraarticular complications or advanced disease requiring reconstructive surgery for disabling deformities.

Nursing intervention begins with a careful assessment of physical needs (joint pain, swelling, ROM, and general health status), psychosocial needs (family support, sexual satisfaction, emotional stress, financial constraints, vocation and career limitations), and environmental needs (transportation, home or work modifications). After the identification of problems and potential problems, a carefully planned program for rehabilitation and education can be coordinated by the nurse for the health care team.

Suppression of inflammation is most effectively achieved through the administration of antiinflammatory or disease-modifying agents. Careful attention to timing sustains a therapeutic level and reduces early-morning stiffness. Education centers around the action and side effects of each drug prescribed and the importance of laboratory monitoring when necessary. Many patients with RA are taking several different drugs. The nurse must make the drug regimen as clear and simple as possible. High-dose intravenous (IV) corticosteroids (pulse therapy) require careful observation for changes in blood pressure, peripheral edema, and signs of congestive heart failure.

Nonpharmacologic relief of pain may include the use of therapeutic heat and cold, rest, relaxation techniques, joint protection (see Tables 60-3 and 60-8), biofeedback (see Chapter 8), transcutaneous electrical nerve stimulation (see Chapter 9), and hypnosis. Assessment for individual differences and preference allows the nurse to help the patient and family set goals that promote optimal comfort.

Lightweight splints are sometimes used to rest an inflamed joint and prevent deformity from muscle spasms and contractures. These splints should be removed, skin care given, ROM exercises performed, and splints reapplied as prescribed. The occupational therapist may help identify self-help devices that can assist in activities of daily living.

Morning care and procedures should be planned around the patient's morning stiffness. Sitting or standing in a warm shower, sitting in a tub with warm towels around the shoulders, or simply soaking the hands in a basin of warm water may help

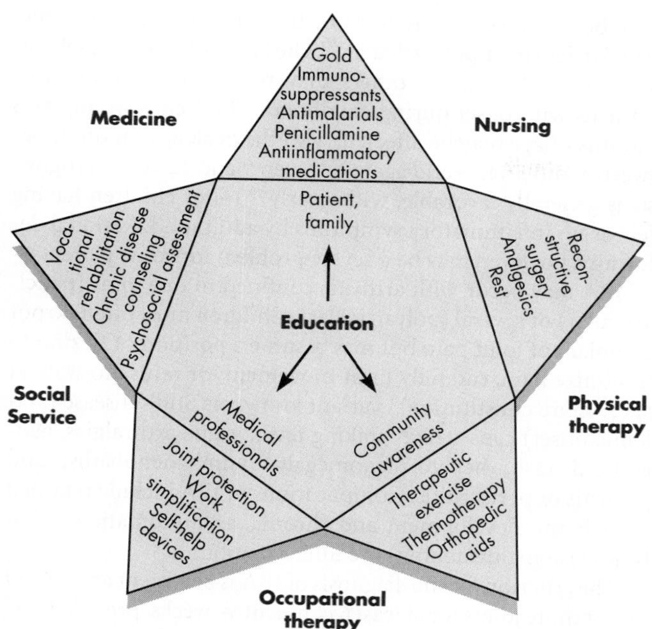

Fig. 60-6 Team approach to the management of rheumatoid arthritis.

PATIENT TEACHING GUIDE

Table 60-8 Protection of Small Joints

1. Avoid positions of deformity.
   - Press water from a sponge instead of wringing.
2. Use strongest joint available for any task.
   - When rising from chair, push with palms rather than fingers.
   - Carry laundry basket in both arms rather than with fingers.
3. Distribute weight over many joints instead of stressing a few.
   - Slide objects instead of lifting them.
   - Hold packages close to body for support.
4. Change positions frequently.
   - Do not hold book or grip steering wheel for long periods without resting.
   - Avoid grasping pencil or cutting vegetables with knife for extended periods.
5. Avoid repetitious movements.
   - Do not knit for long periods.
   - Rest between rooms when vacuuming.
6. Modify chores to avoid stress on joints.
   - Avoid heavy tasks.
   - Sit on stool instead of standing.

relieve joint stiffness and allow the patient to more comfortably perform activities of daily living. Careful skin care should be offered, particularly if the patient is confined to bed.

The professional nurse acts as liaison between the patient, family, and other members of the health team, coordinating services and evaluating the patient's understanding of the total home management program (see NCP 60-1).

Ambulatory and Home Care

Rest. Regularly scheduled rest periods alternated with activity throughout the day help relieve fatigue and pain and minimize excessive weight bearing.[22] The amount of rest necessary varies according to the severity of the disease and each patient's limitations. Total bed rest is rarely necessary and should be avoided to prevent stiffness and immobility. Even a patient with mild disease may require daytime rest in addition to 8 to 10 hours of sleep at night. The nurse should help the patient identify ways to modify daily activities because overexertion can lead to fatigue and a flare-up in disease activity. For instance, the patient may tolerate meal preparation more easily if the patient sits on a high stool in front of the sink. Patients should rest before becoming exhausted. The nurse should assist the patient to pace activities and set priorities on the basis of realistic goals.

Good body alignment while resting is important. A firm mattress or bedboard should be used. Positions of extension should be encouraged, and positions of flexion should be avoided. Lying prone for half an hour twice daily is recommended. Pillows should never be placed under the knees. A small, flat pillow may be used under the head and shoulders. Splints and casts may be helpful in maintaining proper alignment and promoting rest, especially when joint inflammation is present.

Joint protection. Protecting joints from stress is an important part of the therapeutic regimen for RA. Nursing intervention includes helping the patient identify ways to modify tasks. Each patient must learn less stressful ways that put less stress on joints to accomplish routine activities. The emphasis is on changing the way the task is done and on work simplification techniques.

Energy conservation requires careful planning. Work should be done in short periods with scheduled rest breaks to avoid fatigue (pacing). Chores should be spread through the week rather than concentrated (e.g., all cleaning should not be done on the weekend). Activities should be organized to avoid running up and down stairs. Carts should be used to carry things. Materials used often should be stored in a convenient, easily reached area. Time-saving and joint-protective devices (e.g., electric can opener) should be used if possible. Chores should be delegated to other family members.

The nurse should instruct the patient with arthritis to protect the small joints from stress. Assessment of the patient's performance of tasks at work, in the hospital, and in the home identifies activities that must be revised. Joint-saving activities should be reinforced. Table 60-8 lists sample activities that protect small joints.

Patient independence may be increased by occupational therapy training with assistive devices that help simplify tasks, such as built-up utensils, buttonhooks, modified drawer handles, lightweight plastic dishes, and raised toilet seats. Wearing shoes with Velcro fasteners and clothing with buttons or a zipper down the front instead of the back makes dressing easier. A cane or a walker offers support and relief of pain when walking. A platform-wheeled walker minimizes strain on the small joints of the hands and wrists. The Arthritis Foundation offers many programs to assist people with rheumatologic disorders and is an excellent resource for additional suggestions related to self-care.[23]

Daily heat and exercise. Heat and cold therapy help relieve stiffness, pain, and muscle spasm. Application of ice may be beneficial in an acute episode ("flare"), and moist heat appears to offer better relief of chronic stiffness. Superficial heat sources such as heating pads, moist hot packs, paraffin baths, whirlpool baths, and warm baths or showers relieve stiffness before therapeutic exercises. The modality should be selected according to disease severity, ease of application, and cost. Cold therapy effectively relieves joint and muscle pain. Easy home applications include plastic bags of frozen vegetables (peas or corn), which can easily mold around the shoulder, wrists, or knees, or "icing" the skin proximally or distally to a painful joint with ice cubes or small paper cups of frozen water. Heat and cold can be used as often as desired as long as the heat application does not exceed 20 minutes at one time and the cold application does not exceed 10 to 15 minutes at one time.[24] The nurse should alert the patient to the possibility of a burn, especially if a heat-producing liniment is used with another external heat device.

Individualized exercise is an integral part of the treatment plan. This program is usually developed by a physical therapist and includes exercises to improve flexibility, strength, and endurance. The nurse should reinforce compliance with the program and ensure that the exercises are being done correctly. Inadequate joint movement can result in progressive joint immobility and muscle weakness; overaggressive exercise can result in increased pain, inflammation, and joint damage.

Gentle ROM exercises are usually done daily to keep the joints functional. The nurse should emphasize that usual daily activities do not provide adequate exercise to maintain joint motion. Careful adherence to the prescribed exercise program should be a prime goal of the teaching program. The patient should have the opportunity to practice the exercises with supervision. Warm-water (78° to 86° F [25° to 30° C]) aquatic exercises allow easier ROM because of the buoyancy of the water.[25] Aerobic conditioning programs have been shown to improve the physical fitness levels of patients with arthritis. During an acute inflammatory episode, exercise should be limited to one or two repetitions of ROM.

Psychologic support. Self-management and adherence to an individualized home program are contingent on a thorough understanding of RA, the nature and course of the disease, and the objectives of treatment. In addition, the patient's perception of the disease and value system must be considered. Chronic pain or loss of function may make the patient vulnerable to fad claims of false advertising and unproven remedies.

A treatment program tailored to individual problems and lifestyle increases adherence. The nurse can help the patient recognize common fears and concerns faced by all people living with a chronic illness. Evaluation of the family support system is important. The patient is constantly threatened by problems of limited function and fatigue, loss of self-esteem, altered body image, and fear of disability and deformity. Alterations in sexuality should be discussed. Financial planning may be necessary. Community resources such as a home care nurse, homemaker services, and vocational rehabilitation may be considered. Self-help groups are beneficial for some patients. Self-management classes are available in many communities.

JUVENILE RHEUMATOID ARTHRITIS

Juvenile rheumatoid arthritis (JRA), a major rheumatic disease of youth, is defined as RA beginning before 16 years of age. It may be classified on the basis of the type of onset: systemic, pauciarticular, or polyarticular.[26] The last form most closely resembles adult RA; the others may represent other types of arthritis with onset during childhood. Children as young as 6 months of age may be affected, with the peak ages at onset between 1 and 5 years and again between 9 and 12 years. Prognosis is generally favorable, with nearly 70% of children having few or no inflammatory symptoms by adulthood. Residual deformity, however, may be a severe problem for some patients.

JRA may occur with arthritis confined to one joint (pauciarticular) or several (polyarticular). Children most often do not complain of joint pain but may assume a position of flexion to minimize pain, carefully limit movement, or refuse to walk at all. A more constitutional variant known as Still's disease (systemic onset) causes high-spiking fever, vague arthralgias, generalized rash, hepatosplenomegaly, lymphadenopathy, and pleuritis or pericarditis. Complications of JRA include retarded growth and development and chronic, asymptomatic (and at times vision-threatening) eye inflammation.

The criterion for the diagnosis of JRA is persistent arthritis of one or more joints for at least 6 consecutive weeks, provided certain other similar disorders are ruled out. High-spiking fever, generalized lymphadenopathy, and splenomegaly are more common in children than in adults with RA. Leukocytosis is common, whereas rheumatoid factor is present in only 15% of those affected. NSAIDs suppress inflammation in the majority of cases. Chrysotherapy (treatment with gold salts) can be used for arthritis unresponsive to NSAIDs. Corticosteroids are avoided when possible because of their effect on growth.

Nursing intervention requires an individualized written home program with emphasis on compliance. The family is best counseled about the course and prognosis of their child's arthritis according to the onset classification. Daily participation in a planned physical training program encourages full ROM and muscle strengthening and does not strain affected joints. Swimming, bicycling, and dance therapy are better than running, jumping, and kicking. Growth and development should be documented. Slit-lamp ophthalmologic examinations must be done routinely for those children at highest risk for developing ocular complications.

The school nurse should be involved in the child's care. Early-morning classes and stair climbing may be difficult for the child with arthritis. Parents are encouraged to treat the child as normally as possible, avoiding infantilizing or overprotecting. An experienced multidisciplinary health care team can help the child and family meet the challenges of social and personality development. A family-oriented rather than a child-oriented approach is critical for the optimal management of JRA.

DISEASES ASSOCIATED WITH HLA-B27

An unusually high frequency of HLA-B27 is found in patients with ankylosing spondylitis, psoriatic arthritis, and Reiter's syndrome, known as the seronegative spondyloarthritides.[27] (Human leukocyte antigens [HLA] and their relationship to autoimmune diseases are discussed in Chapter 12.) The common characteristics of the spondyloarthropathies are (1) predilection for involvement of sacroiliac joints and spine; (2) oligoarticular asymmetric arthritis; (3) enthesopathy (e.g., plantar fasciitis, Achilles tendinitis); (4) absence of rheumatoid factor and autoantibodies; (5) extraarticular disease in characteristic sites (e.g., eye, heart, skin, mucous membranes); (6) male predominance; and (7) a strong association with the HLA antigen B27.[28] Detection of this marker is an important aid to early diagnosis of these diseases.

ANKYLOSING SPONDYLITIS

Ankylosing spondylitis (AS) is a chronic inflammatory disease that primarily affects the sacroiliac joints, apophyseal and costovertebral joints of the spine, and adjacent soft tissues. Approximately 90% of Caucasian patients with AS are positive for HLA-B27. The disease typically appears in adolescence or young adulthood.

AS is prevalent in both sexes, with progressive disease more common in men. Because women tend to have more peripheral joint involvement, the diagnosis is often delayed or missed.[29] There appears to be a definite familial tendency, and the disease is unusual in African-Americans.

Etiology and Pathophysiology

The cause of AS is unknown. Genetic predisposition appears to play an important role in the disease pathogenesis, but the precise mechanisms are unknown. Environmental factors and infectious agents are also suspected. Inflammation in joints and adjacent tissue causes the formation of granulation tissue and eroding vertebral margins, resulting in spondylitis. Calcification tends to follow the inflammation process, leading to bony ankylosis.

Clinical Manifestations and Complications

The patient typically has lower back pain, stiffness, and limitation of motion that is worse during the night and in the morning but improves with mild activity. General constitutional features such as fever, fatigue, anorexia, and weight loss are rarely present. Other symptoms depend on the stage of the disease and include arthritis of the shoulders, hips, and knees and occasional ocular inflammation (iritis).

Involvement of costovertebral joints leads to a decrease in chest expansion. Advancing kyphosis leads to a bent-over posture, and compensating hip-flexion contractures may occur. There is pronounced impairment of neck motion in all directions. Extraskeletal involvement may include iritis, aortic valvular regurgitation, and apical pulmonary fibrosis.

Diagnostic Studies

Changes on x-rays may not become apparent for months to years after the onset of symptoms. When abnormalities are present, they include sacroiliac joints that show pseudowidening of the joint space and later obliteration with ankylosis. New bone formation (syndesmophytes) may be spotty or generalized (classic "bamboo spine"). ESR, alkaline phosphatase, and creatine kinase (CK) levels are usually elevated. Tissue typing is positive for HLA-B27 in the majority of patients.

Collaborative Care

Prevention of AS is not possible. However, families with diagnosed HLA-B27–positive rheumatic diseases should be alert to signs of low back pain and arthritis symptoms so early treatment can be initiated.

Care of the patient is aimed at maintaining maximal skeletal mobility. Proper posture is important in all activities. Although drugs do not halt the progression of the disease, NSAIDs, such as diclofenac (Voltaren) and indomethacin (Indocin), can reduce inflammation, which makes proper posture easier. Disease-modifying agents such as sulfasalazine (Azulfidine) or methotrexate are sometimes used to control symptoms and delay disease progression. Surgery to correct extreme flexion deformities may be performed in certain cases. A total hip replacement is done for patients with crippling hip ankylosis.

NURSING MANAGEMENT: ANKYLOSING SPONDYLITIS

Nursing responsibilities for the patient with AS include education about the nature of the disease and principles of therapy. A home management program consists of local heat and exercise and proper use of medications. Baseline ROM including chest expansion (using breathing exercises) should be assessed by the nurse. Smoking cessation should be a goal because the risk for lung complications is increased in those with reduced chest expansion. Pain should be managed by appropriate medication, heat, massage, and gentle exercise. Application of moist heat should be followed by ROM exercises and daily chest expansion and deep-breathing exercises. A continuing physical therapy program incorporating gentle, graded stretching and strengthening exercises preserves ROM and improves thoracolumbar flexion and extension. Excessive physical exertion during periods of active inflammation should be discouraged. Proper positioning at rest is essential. The mattress should be firm, and pillows must be avoided. The patient should sleep on the back and avoid positions that encourage flexion deformity. Postural training emphasizes avoiding forward flexion (e.g., leaning over a desk); heavy lifting; and prolonged walking, standing, or sitting. Sports that facilitate natural stretching, such as swimming and racquet games, should be encouraged. Family counseling and vocational rehabilitation are important.

PSORIATIC ARTHRITIS

Psoriatic arthritis can be defined as an association of clinically apparent psoriasis with inflammatory polyarthritis. Psoriatic skin changes may precede or follow articular symptoms. Approximately 10% to 15% of persons with psoriasis have such an arthritis, which is generally mild, with intermittent flare-ups affecting only a few peripheral joints. However, a severe erosive form is also seen. Certain x-ray findings such as asymmetric distribution and resorption of tufts of the distal phalanges of hands, feet, and metatarsal bones help distinguish psoriatic arthritis from RA. Patients with psoriasis are likely to get spondylitis, which is associated with an 80% frequency of HLA-B27 positivity. Hyperuricemia often accompanies the disease. Forms of treatment include splinting, joint protection, and physical therapy. Although gold therapy has recently been used with success for the treatment of psoriatic arthritis, methotrexate continues to be one of the most effective agents for both cutaneous and articular manifestations.

REITER'S SYNDROME

Reiter's syndrome is a self-limiting disease associated with arthritis, urethritis, conjunctivitis, and mucocutaneous lesions.

Although the exact etiology is unknown, Reiter's syndrome appears to be a reactive arthritis after certain enteric (e.g., *Shigella*) or venereal (e.g., *Chlamydia trachomatis*) infections. The disease usually affects males, and 85% of patients with Reiter's syndrome are positive for HLA-B27, which provides evidence for a genetic predisposition. Few other laboratory abnormalities occur, although the ESR may be elevated.

The arthritis of Reiter's syndrome tends to be asymmetric, frequently involving the weight-bearing joints of the lower extremities and sometimes the lower part of the back. Arthralgias usually begin 1 to 3 weeks after the appearance of the initial infection. The full attack may be accompanied by fever and other constitutional complaints, including anorexia with considerable weight loss, and may prove highly debilitating. Soft-tissue manifestations commonly include Achilles tendinitis.

Prognosis is favorable, with most patients recovering after 2 to 16 weeks. Joints heal completely, and many patients have complete remission with full joint function. About one half of the patients, however, have recurring acute attacks; others follow a chronic course, having continued synovitis and progression of x-ray changes closely resembling those of AS. Progressive disease may result in major disability. Treatment is symptomatic, and joint inflammation is treated with NSAIDs.

SEPTIC ARTHRITIS

Septic arthritis (infectious or bacterial arthritis) is caused by invasion of the joint cavity with microorganisms. Various bacteria are commonly responsible, including *Staphylococcus aureus, Streptococcus hemolyticus, Diplococcus pneumoniae*, and *Neisseria gonorrhoeae*. Factors increasing the risk of such infections include previous joint trauma or arthritic disease, diseases of decreased host resistance such as leukemia and diabetes mellitus, treatment with corticosteroids or immunosuppressive drugs, and serious chronic illness. Infants, young children, and older adults appear to be more frequently affected, with the exception of gonococcal arthritis, which affects sexually active young adults. A site of active infection is often responsible for bacteremia (microorganisms reaching the bloodstream), leading to hematogenous seeding of joints.

Inflammation of the joint cavity causes severe pain, erythema, and swelling of one or several joints. Large joints, such as the knee and the hip, are most frequently involved. Fever or shaking chills often accompany articular symptoms because bacterial entry into a joint is usually by the hematogenous route from a primary site of infection. Precise diagnosis is made by aspiration of the joint and culture of the synovial fluid. Blood cultures for aerobic and anaerobic organisms should be obtained.

Septic arthritis is a medical emergency that requires prompt diagnosis and treatment to prevent joint destruction. Parenteral antibiotic administration is maintained until there are no clinical signs of active synovitis or inflammation in the joint fluid. Infections may respond to treatment within 2 weeks or take as long as 4 to 8 weeks, depending on the causative organism. Open surgical drainage may be required.

Nursing intervention includes assessment and monitoring of joint inflammation, pain, and fever. Immobilization of affected joints to control pain is often achieved by resting splints or traction. Gentle ROM exercises should be done. Strict aseptic technique should be used during assistance with joint aspiration procedures. The necessity of antibiotics should be explained, and the importance of their continued use should be stressed. Support should be offered to the patient requiring repeated arthrocentesis or operative drainage. The extent of joint damage is generally related to the invading microorganism and the time between infection onset and initiation of effective treatment.

LYME DISEASE

Lyme disease is a spirochetal infection caused by *Borrelia burgdorferi* and transmitted by the bite of an infected tick. It was first identified in 1975 in Lyme, Connecticut, after an unusual clustering of arthritis in children.[30] It is the most common vector-borne disease in the United States.[31] The tick is no bigger than a poppy seed and typically feeds on mice, dogs, cats, cows, horses, raccoons, deer, and humans. Wild animals do not exhibit the illness, but clinical Lyme disease does occur in domestic animals. The peak season for human infection is during the summer months.

The most characteristic clinical symptom is a skin lesion, erythema migrans (EM), which occurs at the site of the tick bite in 80% of patients. This lesion begins as a red macule or papule that slowly expands to form a large round lesion with a bright red border and central clearing. The EM lesion is often accompanied by other acute symptoms, such as fever, chills, headache, stiff neck, and migratory joint and muscle pain. If not treated, Lyme disease can progress in several weeks or months to (1) severe arthritis; (2) atrioventricular conduction defects, bradycardia, or myocarditis; and (3) neurologic abnormalities, including meningitis, facial palsy, and radiculoneuropathy.

Diagnosis is based on clinical manifestations, history of exposure in an endemic area, and a positive serologic test for *B. burgdorferi*. Other illnesses are frequently misdiagnosed as Lyme disease, particularly chronic fatigue syndrome and fibromyalgia. Serologic testing for antibodies to *B. burgdorferi* is available. Most U.S. cases occur in three endemic areas: along the northeastern coast from Maryland to Massachusetts; in the midwestern states of Wisconsin and Minnesota; and along the northwestern coast of northern California and Oregon.

Active lesions can be treated with antibiotic therapy. Oral doxycycline or amoxicillin is often effective in early-stage infection and in prevention of later stages of the disease. More diffuse infection may require 20 to 30 days of therapy. Intravenous ceftriaxone (Rocephin) is used for cardiac or neurologic abnormalities. Lyme disease arthritis usually responds to oral antibiotic therapy. However, in genetically susceptible persons, chronic arthritis of the knees may not respond to either oral or IV antibiotics. It usually resolves eventually, although it may take several years. LYMErix is a new vaccine for Lyme disease that was recently approved by the FDA.[32] The vaccine is given in three doses over a two-month period. This vaccine is recommended for individuals at high risk. Patient education for the prevention of Lyme disease in endemic areas is outlined in Table 60-9.

HUMAN IMMUNODEFICIENCY VIRUS INFECTION AND ARTHRITIS

A variety of inflammatory arthritis conditions have been reported in the presence of human immunodeficiency virus (HIV) infection.[33,34] The pathogenesis of these disorders is unknown. With suppression of the $CD4^+$ lymphocytes, oppor-

PATIENT & FAMILY TEACHING GUIDE

Table 60-9 Prevention of Lyme Disease (Endemic Areas)

- Avoid walking through tall grasses and low brush.
- Mow grass and remove brush along paths, buildings, and campsites.
- Move woodpiles and bird feeders away from house.
- Wear long pants or nylon tights of tightly woven, light-colored fabric so that ticks can be easily seen.
- Tuck pants into boots or long socks, tuck long-sleeved shirts into pants, and wear closed shoes when hiking.
- Check often for ticks crawling from legs to open skin.
- Thoroughly inspect and wash clothes.
- Spray insect repellent containing DEET on skin or permethrin on clothes, especially on lower extremities.
- Have pets wear tick collars, inspect them often, and do not allow them on furniture or beds.
- Remove attached ticks with tweezers (not fingers). Grasp tick's mouth parts as close to skin as possible and gently pull straight out. Do not twist or jerk.
- Dispose of tick in alcohol or flush down toilet. Do not crush with fingers.
- Wash bitten area with soap and water and apply antiseptic. Wash hands.
- See a doctor immediately if flulike symptoms or "bull's-eye" rash appears within a few weeks after removal of tick.

DEET, NN, diethyl-M-toluamide.

tunistic organisms cause infectious arthritis, osteomyelitis, and polymyositis. RA and SLE generally improve as immunodeficiency develops. However, rheumatic diseases associated with HLA-B27 appear to become more severe in HIV-infected patients. For example, progressive, erosive upper-extremity joint disease occurs in Reiter's syndrome, and psoriatic arthritis exhibits a generalized, pustular rash. A Sjögren's-type syndrome, diffuse infiltrative lymphocytosis syndrome, has been identified as a response to HIV infection in children and adults with specific HLA typing. Vasculitis may be responsible for unexplained multisystem disease, arthritis, or fever of unknown origin in HIV-infected patients. Antirheumatic therapy may be effective for short periods but may impair cellular immunity and promote exacerbations of underlying infections.

GOUT

Gout is characterized by recurrent attacks of acute arthritis in association with increased levels of serum uric acid. It may be classified as primary or secondary. In primary gout a hereditary error of purine metabolism leads to the overproduction or retention of uric acid. Secondary gout may be related to another acquired disorder (Table 60-10) or may be the result of medications known to inhibit uric acid excretion. Secondary gout may also be caused by medications that increase the rate of cell death, such as the chemotherapeutic agents used in treating leukemia.

Primary gout occurs predominantly (90%) in middle-aged men, with almost no incidence in premenopausal women. Frequency of hyperuricemia is increased in the families of patients with primary gout. Although some races have been identified as having a low incidence of gout, people of the same race living in another country may exhibit higher mean serum uric acid levels, indicating that both genetic and environmental factors contribute to the etiology.

Table 60-10 Associated Conditions Leading to Hyperuricemia

Acidosis or ketosis
Alcoholism
Atherosclerosis
Cytotoxic drugs
Diabetes mellitus
Drug-induced renal impairment
Hyperlipidemia
Hypertension
Intrinsic renal disease
Malignant disease
Myeloproliferative disorders
Obesity
Sickle cell anemia

Etiology and Pathophysiology

Uric acid is the major end product of the catabolism of purines and is primarily excreted by the kidneys. Thus hyperuricemia may be the result of increased purine synthesis, decreased renal excretion, or both. About half the patients with primary gout can be shown to produce excessive amounts of uric acid. Folklore has long associated excesses of food and drink with acute attacks of gouty arthritis. Although high dietary intake of purine alone has relatively little effect on uric acid levels, it is clear that hyperuricemia may result from prolonged fasting or excessive alcohol drinking because of increased production of keto acids, which then inhibit normal renal excretion of uric acid.

Clinical Manifestations and Complications

In the acute phase, gouty arthritis may occur in one or more joints but usually less than four. Affected joints may appear dusky or cyanotic and are extremely tender. Inflammation of the great toe (podagra) is most commonly the initial involvement and occurs in 75% of all patients. Other joints affected are the midtarsal, ankle, knee, and wrist joints and the olecranon bursa. Acute gouty arthritis is usually precipitated by events such as trauma, surgery, alcohol ingestion, or systemic infection. Onset of symptoms is usually rapid, with swelling and pain peaking within several hours, often accompanied by low-grade fever. Individual attacks usually subside, treated or untreated, in 2 to 10 days. The affected joint returns entirely to normal, and patients are often free of symptoms between attacks.

Chronic gout is characterized by multiple joint involvement and deposits of sodium urate crystals called *tophi.* These are typically seen in the synovium, subchondral bone, olecranon bursa, and vertebrae; along tendons; and in the skin and cartilage (Fig. 60-7). Tophi are rarely present at the time of the initial attack and are generally noted only many years after the onset of disease.

The severity of gouty arthritis is variable. The clinical course may consist of infrequent mild attacks or multiple severe

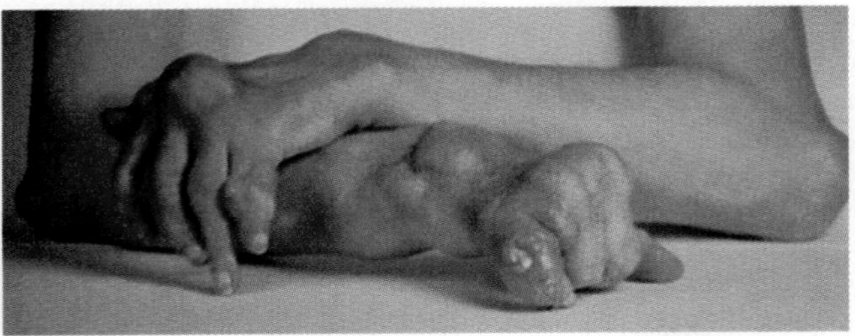

Fig. 60-7 Tophaceous gout. (Reprinted from the Clinical Slide Collection on the Rheumatic Diseases, copyright 1991, 1995, 1997. Used by permission of the American College of Rheumatology. In Seidel HM and others: *Mosby's guide to physical examination,* ed 4, St. Louis, 1999, Mosby.)

episodes associated with a slowly progressive disability. In general, the higher the serum uric acid level, the earlier the appearance of tophi and the greater the tendency toward more frequent and severe episodes of acute gout. An elevated serum uric acid alone does not indicate gout, even when joint symptoms are present, because high serum uric acid levels are found in a variety of diseases. Gout can be diagnosed unequivocally only when urate crystals are found in joint fluid.

Chronic inflammation may result in joint deformity. Destruction of the cartilage may predispose the joint to secondary OA. Tophaceous deposits may be large and unsightly and may perforate overlying skin, producing draining sinuses that often become secondarily infected. Excessive uric acid excretion may lead to kidney or urinary tract stone formation. Pyelonephritis associated with intrarenal sodium urate deposits and obstruction may contribute to renal disease.

Diagnostic Studies

The diagnosis can be established by finding monosodium urate monohydrate crystals in the synovial fluid of an inflamed joint or tophus. In another goutlike syndrome, termed *pseudogout,* nonurate (calcium pyrophosphate dihydrate) crystals are identified in synovial fluid analysis. Serum uric acid levels are almost always elevated to 8 mg/dl (476 (mol/L) or higher. Specimens for 24-hour urine uric acid levels are obtained to control for daily fluctuations in urate concentrations and are important in determining whether the patient undersecretes or overproduces uric acid. Hyperuricemia is not specifically diagnostic of gout because increased levels may be related to a variety of drugs or may exist as a totally asymptomatic abnormality in the general population.

Collaborative Care

Care of the patient with gout (Table 60-11) has several goals. The first is to terminate an acute attack. This is accomplished by the use of an antiinflammatory agent such as colchicine. Future attacks are prevented by a maintenance dose of colchicine, weight reduction if necessary, avoidance of alcohol and high-purine foods, and the use of drugs to reduce the serum urate concentration. Treatment is also aimed at preventing the formation of uric acid kidney stones and other associated conditions such as hypertriglyceridemia and hypertension.

Drug Therapy. Acute gouty arthritis is treated with one of three types of antiinflammatory agents: colchicine, NSAIDs, or corticosteroids. Corticosteroids should be reserved for cases in which colchicine and NSAIDs are contraindicated or ineffective.

COLLABORATIVE CARE

Table 60-11 Gout

Diagnostic
- History and physical examination
- Family history of gout
- Presence of monosodium urate monohydrate crystals in synovial fluid
- Elevated serum uric acid levels
- Elevated 24 hr urine for uric acid levels

Collaborative Therapy
- Joint immobilization
- Local application of heat or cold
- Joint aspiration and intraarticular corticosteroids
- Drug therapy
  - Nonsteroidal antiinflammatory drugs
  - Colchicine
  - Probenecid (Benemid)
  - Allopurinol (Zyloprim)
- Dietary avoidance of food/fluids with high purine content (e.g., anchovies, liver, wine/beer)

Although medication does not prevent recurrent attacks of gout, it can control its symptoms in 75% of gout attacks, particularly with prompt treatment. Oral administration of colchicine generally produces dramatic pain relief within 24 to 48 hours. Colchicine has diagnostic merit in that a good response to treatment gives further evidence for the diagnosis of gout. Prophylactic doses of colchicine reduce the frequency of attacks but do not alter the serum uric acid level.

For many years the standard therapy for hyperuricemia has been a uricosuric drug (e.g., probenecid [Benemid]), which acts by increasing urinary uric acid excretion through inhibiting tubular reabsorption of urates. Aspirin inactivates the effect of uricosurics, resulting in urate retention, and should be avoided while patients are taking probenecid and other uricosuric drugs. Acetaminophen can be used safely if analgesia is required.

Adequate urine volume must be maintained to prevent precipitation of uric acid in the renal tubules. Allopurinol (Zyloprim), which blocks the production of uric acid, may control the serum level and is particularly useful in patients with uric acid stones or renal impairment, in whom uricosuric drugs may be ineffective or dangerous. Regardless of which drug or combination of drugs is prescribed, it is essential that the concentration of serum uric acid be checked regularly to monitor the effectiveness of treatment.

Nutritional Therapy. Dietary restrictions may include limiting the use of alcohol and of foods high in purine (see Table 43-11). However, medication can generally control the situation without necessitating these limitations. Obese patients should be instructed in a carefully planned weight-reduction program.

NURSING MANAGEMENT: GOUT

Acute gouty arthritis may be prevented by maintenance of the serum uric acid at normal levels. Nursing intervention is directed at supportive care of the inflamed joints. Bed rest may be appropriate, with affected joints properly immobilized. The limitation of motion and degree of pain should be assessed. Treatment effectiveness should be documented. Special care is taken to avoid causing pain to an inflamed joint by careless handling. Involvement of a lower extremity may require use of a cradle or footboard to protect the painful area from the weight of bedclothes.

The patient and the family should understand that hyperuricemia and gouty arthritis are chronic problems that can be controlled with careful adherence to a treatment program.[35] Thorough explanations should be given concerning the importance of drug therapy and the need for periodic determination of blood uric acid levels. The patient should be able to demonstrate knowledge of precipitating factors that may cause an attack, including overindulgence in the intake of calories, purines, and alcohol; starvation (fasting); medication use (e.g., aspirin, diuretics); and major medical events (e.g., surgery, myocardial infarction).

SYSTEMIC LUPUS ERYTHEMATOSUS

Systemic lupus erythematosus (SLE) is a chronic multisystem inflammatory disease of connective tissue that often involves the skin, joints, serous membranes (pleura, pericardium), kidneys, hematologic system, and central nervous system (CNS).[36] SLE is characterized by its variability within and among persons, with a chronic unpredictable course of exacerbations of disease activity alternating with periods of remission. The clinical presentation of SLE ranges from a mild to a serious illness, with a tendency to acute exacerbations precipitated by several factors. Individuals with SLE can now live a normal life span.

The true incidence of SLE is unknown, but the rate appears to be increasing. It is unknown whether this increase is a reflection of heightened diagnostic awareness or a true increase in frequency.[37] The general prevalence of SLE is approximately 1 in 2100. Women have a higher incidence of SLE than men. The disease occurs three times more often in African-American than in Caucasian women.[38] Because of the difficulty in diagnosing SLE, the incidence and prevalence of the disease may be much higher than statistics indicate.

Etiology and Pathophysiology

The etiology of SLE is unknown. However, factors implicated in the etiology of SLE include genetic predisposition, sex hormones, race, environmental factors (e.g., ultraviolet radiation, drugs, chemicals), viruses and infections, stress, and immunologic abnormalities. SLE is a disorder of immunoregulation. Autoimmune reactions are directed against constituents of the cell nucleus, particularly DNA. In SLE, autoantibodies are produced against nuclear antigens (DNA, histones, ribonucleoproteins, and nucleolar factors), cytoplasmic antigens (ribosomal and cardiolipin), and blood cell surface antigens (WBCs, red blood cells [RBCs], and platelets). When autoantibodies bind to their specific antigens, complement activation occurs. Accumulation of immune complexes within the blood vessel walls and subsequent complement activation leads to a condition called lupus vasculitis. The ensuing ischemia within the blood vessel walls gradually leads to the thickening of the internal lining, fibrinoid degeneration, and thrombus formation. The specific manifestations of SLE depend on which cell types or organs are involved.

The overaggressive antibody response is related to B cell hyperactivity accompanied by multiple abnormalities in immunoregulation. Examples of these include decreased T-suppressor cells and diminished interleukin-2 production.[39]

Although studies have shown the importance of heredity in the development and expression of SLE, the susceptibility genes are largely unknown.[40] The major histocompatibility complexes HLA-DR2, HLA-DR3, and HLA-DR4 show significant associations with SLE.

Hormones are known to play a role in the etiology of SLE. A disproportionate number of females have SLE. In addition, there is a tendency for the disease to worsen in the immediate postpartum period. Healthy women are more immunologically reactive than healthy men because estrogens enhance immune reactivity, whereas androgens suppress it. It is thought that estrogens produce their effect through their impact on suppressor T cells, which normally regulate B cell reactivity. In the absence of the T cell regulatory function, the antibody production by the B cells continues.[41] In addition, it has been determined that the type of lymphocytes varies between women and men. Women have slightly higher proportions of T-helper cells (which increase immune reactivity) and lower proportions of T-suppressor cells (which decrease immune reactivity) than men.[42] These factors may contribute to a woman's increased potential for acquiring autoimmune diseases. Onset or exacerbation of disease symptoms sometimes occurs after the onset of menarche, with the use of oral contraceptives, and during and after pregnancy.

SLE may also be precipitated or aggravated by certain drugs such as procainamide (Pronestyl), hydralazine (Apresoline), and a number of antiseizure agents. Sulfonamides (e.g., Bactrim) should not be used in patients with SLE because they can cause a flare-up of the condition. Oral contraceptives may also aggravate the disease and should be used cautiously. Some foods, such as alfalfa sprouts, celery, parsley, and shiitake or reishi mushrooms, should be avoided for the same reason.

Clinical Manifestations and Complications

SLE is extremely variable in its severity, ranging from a relatively mild disorder to a rapidly progressive one affecting many organ systems (Fig. 60-8). There is no characteristic pattern of progressive organ involvement, nor is it predictable which systems may become affected. Theoretically, any organ can be affected by the accumulation of the circulating immune complexes. However, cutaneous and muscle tissue, the lining of the lungs, the heart, nervous tissue, and the kidneys are most commonly affected. SLE is characterized by alternating periods of remission and exacerbation. General constitutional complaints include fever, weight loss, arthralgia, and excessive fatigue and may precede an exacerbation of disease activity.

Dermatologic Manifestations. The most common cutaneous feature of SLE is an erythematous rash that can occur on the face, neck, and extremities. The classic butterfly rash, which is distributed across the bridge of the nose and cheeks, occurs in about 40% of patients (Fig. 60-9). The rash may appear as discoid (coin-like) lesions or as a diffuse maculopapular rash; it may occur anywhere on the body but is

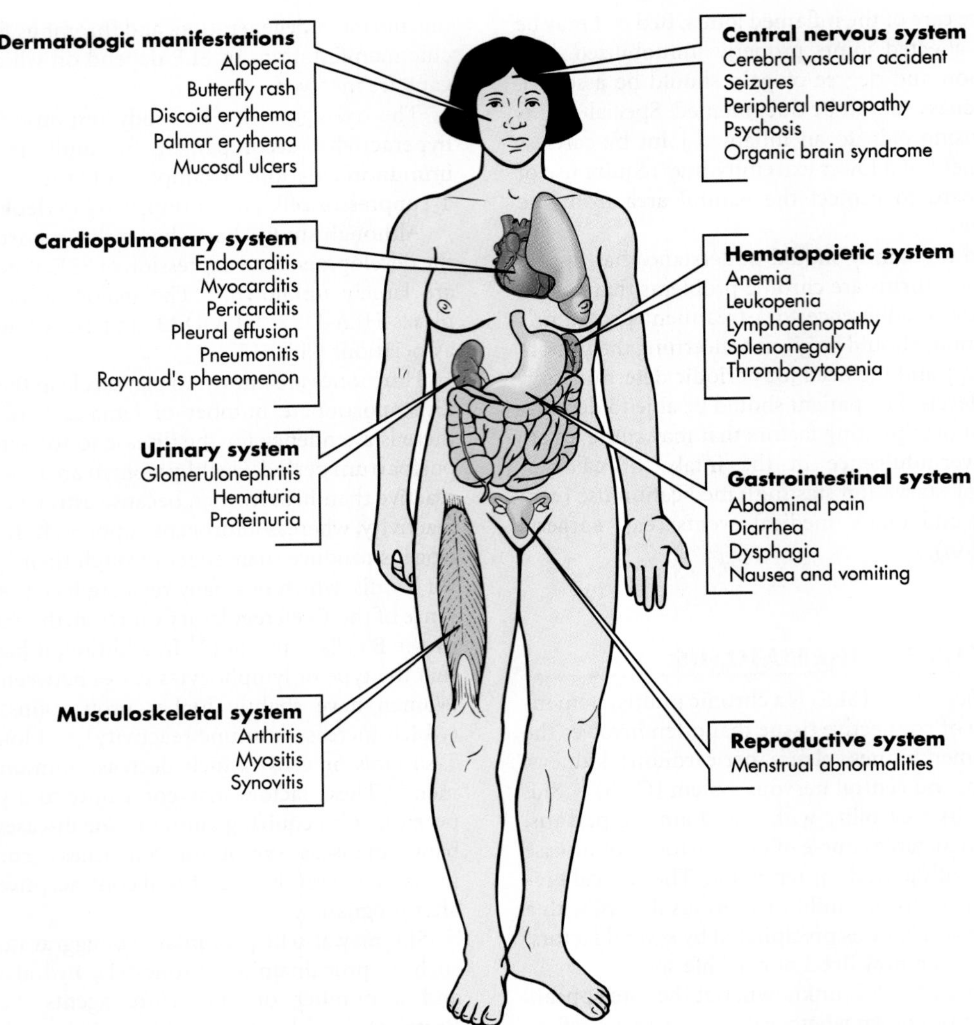

Fig. 60-8 Multisystem involvement in systemic lupus erythematosus.

most frequently seen on the face and chest. A small number of patients have persistent lesions, photosensitivity, and mild systemic disease. This syndrome is referred to as *subacute cutaneous lupus.*[43]

Exposure to sunlight and to other sources of ultraviolet radiation can cause a severe skin reaction and may precipitate a flare-up of disease activity in persons who are photosensitive.[44] Ulcers of the oral or nasopharyngeal membranes occur in up to one third of patients with SLE. Transient diffuse or patchy hair loss (alopecia) is common, with or without underlying scalp lesions. The hair may grow back during remission. The scalp becomes dry, scaly, and atrophied.

Musculoskeletal Problems. Polyarthralgia with morning stiffness is often the patient's first complaint and may precede the onset of multisystem disease by many years. Arthritis occurs in 95% of all patients with SLE at some time in the disease course. Joint symptoms are typically migratory, producing pain without objective signs of inflammation. Lupus-related arthritis is generally nonerosive, but it may cause deformities such as swan-neck appearance of the hands, ulnar deviation, and subluxation with hyperlaxity of the joints. Only about 15% to 35% of SLE patients test positive for rheumatoid factor.[45]

Cardiopulmonary Problems. Pericarditis is present in nearly one fourth of patients with SLE and is usually associated with myocardial disease. Patients treated with corticosteroids have a higher incidence of atherosclerosis. Pleurisy with or without effusion is seen in nearly 50% of patients at some time during the illness, and pulmonary function studies are abnormal in 90%. Raynaud's phenomenon occurs in 20% of patients. Cardiovascular involvement is an ominous sign of advanced disease and contributes significantly to the morbidity and mortality seen in SLE.

Renal Problems. Clinical evidence of renal involvement is present in nearly one half of patients with SLE and includes microscopic hematuria, excessive cellular casts in the urine sediment, proteinuria, and elevation of serum creatinine level. Kidney involvement varies in degree but may eventually end in renal failure. Regardless of whether renal manifestations are evident, nearly all patients with SLE show renal histologic abnormalities in renal biopsy studies or autopsy results. Lupus nephritis is the leading cause of death in SLE.[46]

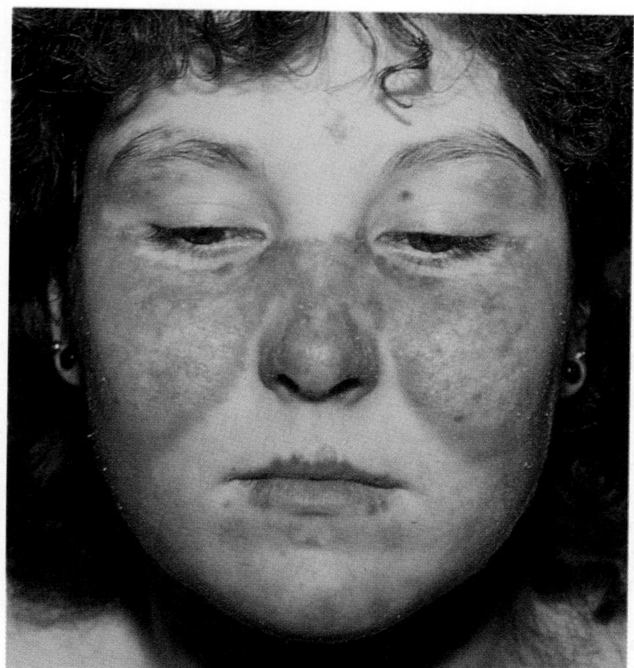

Fig. 60-9 Butterfly rash of systemic lupus erythematosus.

Table **60-12** Criteria for Diagnosis of Systemic Lupus Erythematosus*
Malar rash
Discoid rash
Photosensitivity
Oral ulcers
Arthritis: nonerosive, involvement of two or more joints
Serositis: pleuritis or pericarditis
Renal disorder: proteinuria or cellular casts in urine
Neurologic disorder: seizures or psychosis
Hematologic disorder: hemolytic anemia, leukopenia, lymphopenia, or thrombocytopenia
Immunologic disorder: positive lupus cell preparation; anti-DNA antibody or antibody to Sm nuclear antigen; false-positive serologic tests for syphilis
Antinuclear antibodies

*A person is classified as having SLE if four or more of the criteria are present, serially or simultaneously, during any interval of observation. Revised criteria by a subcommittee of the American College of Rheumatology are used for the purpose of *classification* in population surveys, *not* for the diagnosis of individual patients.
Sm, Smith.

Clinical factors, including blood pressure, urinalysis, serum creatinine levels, serum complement levels, and autoantibodies to DNA, should be monitored carefully and frequently over prolonged periods because renal involvement in the early stages is usually asymptomatic.

Central Nervous System Problems. CNS involvement ranks close behind kidney disease and infection as a leading cause of death in SLE. Seizures are the most common neurologic manifestation and occur in as many as 15% of patients with SLE by the time of diagnosis. They are generally controlled by corticosteroids or antiseizure therapy.

Organic brain syndrome, another recognized CNS manifestation of SLE, may result from the deposition of immune complexes within brain tissue. It is characterized by disordered thought processes, disorientation, memory deficits, and psychiatric symptoms such as severe depression and psychosis. Recovery from organic brain disease is expected, although some residual impairment may result. Occasionally a cerebrovascular accident (stroke) or aseptic meningitis may be attributable to SLE. It is difficult to differentiate neuropsychiatric SLE from non-SLE neurologic problems.

Hematologic Problems. The formation of antibodies against blood cells, such as erythrocytes, leukocytes, thrombocytes, and coagulation factors, is one of the most common features of SLE. Anemia (98%), mild leukopenia (80%), and thrombocytopenia (36%) are often present.[47] Some patients show a tendency to bleed whereas others show a tendency toward blood clots. In addition, SLE patients have positive antinuclear antibodies.

Infection. Patients with SLE appear to have increased susceptibility to infections, possibly related to defects in their ability to phagocytize invading bacteria, deficiencies in production of antibodies, and the immunosuppressive effect of many antiinflammatory drugs. Infection, a major cause of death, has an incidence of 30%. Pneumonia is most common. Fever should be considered serious because it may indicate an underlying infectious process rather than lupus activity alone. However, it is not unusual for patients with SLE to have low-grade fevers of 99° to 100° F (37.2° to 37.8° C).

Diagnostic Studies

The diagnosis of SLE is based on the history, physical examination, and laboratory findings (Table 60-12). A variety of abnormalities may be present in the blood, including elevated ESR, increased gamma-globulin levels, anemia, decreased WBC and platelet counts, electrocardiogram (ECG) or chest x-ray evidence of pericarditis or pleural effusion, and a false-positive serologic test for syphilis. Abnormalities in urine sediment (cellular casts, proteinuria), reduced serum complement levels (C3 and CH 50), and tissue specimens demonstrating changes compatible with SLE are other confirmatory findings.

The lupus erythematosus cell prep is the presence of neutrophils with phagocytized inclusions of IgG antibody to DNA. It is a nonspecific test for SLE and is positive in other rheumatologic diseases.

Antinuclear antibodies (ANA), autoantibodies against nuclear antigens, have been detected in 99% of persons with SLE. Although extremely sensitive, ANA is not specific for SLE because it is present in 5% of normal persons and 38% of all persons more than 60 years of age. Anti-DNA is found most commonly in SLE and is rarely seen in other rheumatic diseases. Anti-Sm antibody, an antibody to the Smith nuclear antigen, is a definitive serologic marker for SLE and is not demonstrated in other rheumatic diseases.[48] About 15% to 35% of SLE patients test positive for rheumatoid factor.[45]

Collaborative Care

The rate of spontaneous remission in SLE is high. Corticosteroids remain the mainstay for treatment of severe illness. Their use should be reserved for acute generalized exacerbation

COLLABORATIVE CARE

Table 60-13 Systemic Lupus Erythematosus

Diagnostic
- History and physical examination
- Lupus cell preparation
- Antibodies
  - Anti-DNA antibody
  - Anti-Sm antibody
  - Antinuclear antibody (ANA)
- Complete blood cell count
- Urinalysis
- X-ray of affected joints
- Chest x-ray
- Complement levels (CH50, C3)
- ECG

Collaborative Therapy
- NSAIDs
- Antimalarials (e.g., hydroxychloroquine [Plaquenil])
- Corticosteroids for exacerbations and severe disease
- Immunosuppressive drugs
  - Cyclophosphamide (Cytoxan)
  - Azathioprine (Imuran)

Sm antibody, Smith antibody.

or serious organ involvement, although a reduced maintenance dosage is sometimes used. Immunosuppressive drugs may be used for symptoms that are resistant to or to reduce the need for long-term corticosteroid therapy (Table 60-13). Efficacy of treatment is most appropriately monitored by serial serum complement levels and anti-DNA titers. Simpler and less costly tests such as ESR or C-reactive protein levels may also help in monitoring treatment effectiveness.

An improving prognosis of SLE may be the result of earlier diagnosis, prompt recognition of serious organ involvement, and better therapeutic regimens. Survival is influenced by several factors, including age, race, gender, socioeconomic status, accompanying morbid conditions, and severity of disease. For example, childhood-onset SLE accounts for nearly 20% of all cases and has a higher incidence of lupus nephritis (up to 80%) than in other age-groups.

Drug Therapy. Medications are prescribed to suppress inflammation and the immune system. The type of medication used depends almost entirely on disease activity. Aspirin or other NSAIDs may reduce mild symptoms such as fever and arthritic complaints. GI upset and tinnitus should be reported. Antimalarial drugs, such as hydroxychloroquine (Plaquenil), may be used to improve skin and musculoskeletal problems, but eye examinations must be scheduled periodically during this therapy because visual loss is a rare but a serious side effect.[49] Topical corticosteroid preparations and intralesional corticosteroid injections are effective treatments for skin lesions.

Corticosteroids are potent antiinflammatory medications used for acute generalized exacerbations of SLE and for the treatment of serious involvement of vital organs, including hematologic abnormalities. As clinical and laboratory values improve, the dosages are gradually tapered.

Patient teaching must include indications for use and proper administration of corticosteroids and possible side effects (see Chapter 47). The patient should understand that abrupt cessation may precipitate recurrence of disease activity. Immunosuppressive drug therapy such as azathioprine (Imuran) and cyclophosphamide (Cytoxan) is often used in life-threatening situations for symptoms unresponsive to more conservative treatment. Close monitoring is necessary to minimize drug toxicity.

NURSING MANAGEMENT: SYSTEMIC LUPUS ERYTHEMATOSUS

Nursing Assessment

As in the majority of rheumatic diseases, the chronic and unpredictable nature of SLE presents many challenges to the patient and family. The physical, psychologic, and sociocultural problems associated with the long-term management of SLE require the varied approaches and skills of the multidisciplinary health care team.

Subjective and objective data that should be obtained from a patient with SLE are presented in Table 60-14. The extent to which pain and fatigue influence activities of daily living must be evaluated. A developmental approach focuses on age-appropriate educational and counseling issues, such as personal relationships, family planning, occupational responsibilities, and recreational activities.

Nursing Diagnoses

Nursing diagnoses for the patient with SLE may include, but are not limited to, those presented in NCP 60-2.

Planning

The overall goals are that the patient with systemic lupus erythematosus will (1) have satisfactory pain relief, (2) comply with therapeutic regimen to achieve maximum symptom management, (3) avoid activities that induce disease exacerbation, and (4) maintain a positive self-image.

Nursing Implementation

Health Promotion. Prevention of SLE is not possible at this time. Education of health professionals and the community may promote a clearer understanding of the disease and earlier diagnosis and treatment.

Acute Intervention. During an exacerbation, patients may become abruptly and dramatically ill. Nursing intervention includes accurately recording the severity of symptoms and documenting the response to therapy. Fever pattern, joint inflammation, limitation of motion, location and degree of discomfort, and fatigability should be specifically assessed. The patient's weight and fluid intake and output should be monitored because of the fluid-retention effect of corticosteroids and the possibility of renal failure. Collection of 24-hour urine samples for protein and creatinine clearance may be ordered. The nurse should observe for signs of bleeding that result from drug therapy, such as pallor, skin bruising, petechiae, or tarry stools.

NURSING ASSESSMENT

Table 60-14 Systemic Lupus Erythematosus

Subjective Data

Important Health Information

Past health history: Exposure to ultraviolet radiation, drugs, chemicals, viral infections; physical or psychologic stress; states of increased estrogen activity, including early onset of menarche, pregnancy, and postpartum period; pattern of remissions and exacerbations

Medications: Use of oral contraceptives, procainamide (Pronestyl), hydralazine (Apresoline), isoniazid (INH), antiseizure drugs, antibiotics (possibly precipitating symptoms of SLE); corticosteroids, NSAIDs

Functional Health Patterns

Health perception–health management: Family history of SLE or immunologic disorders; frequent infections; malaise

Nutritional-metabolic: Weight loss, oral and nasal ulcers; nausea and vomiting; xerostomia (salivary gland dryness), dysphagia; photosensitivity with rash; frequent infections

Elimination: Decreased urine output; diarrhea or constipation

Activity-exercise: Morning stiffness; joint swelling and deformity; shortness of breath, dyspnea; excessive fatigue

Sleep-rest: Insomnia

Cognitive-perceptual: Visual disturbances; vertigo; headache; polyarthralgia; chest pain (pericardial, pleuritic); abdominal pain; joint pain; pain, throbbing, coldness of fingers with numbness and tingling

Sexuality-reproductive: Amenorrhea, irregular menstrual periods

Coping–stress tolerance: Depression, withdrawal

Objective Data

General

Fever, lymphadenopathy, periorbital edema

Integumentary

Alopecia; dry, scaly scalp; keratoconjunctivitis, malar "butterfly" rash, palmar or discoid erythema, urticaria, periungal erythema, purpura, or petechiae; leg ulcers

Respiratory

Pleural friction rub, decreased breath sounds

Cardiovascular

Vasculitis; pericardial friction rub; hypertension, edema, arrhythmias, murmurs; bilateral, symmetric pallor and cyanosis of fingers (Raynaud's phenomenon)

Gastrointestinal

Oral and pharyngeal ulcers; splenomegaly

Neurologic

Facial weakness, peripheral neuropathies, papilledema, dysarthria, confusion, hallucination, disorientation, psychosis, seizures, aphasia, hemiparesis

Musculoskeletal

Myopathy, myositis, arthritis

Possible Findings

Positive lupus cell preparation, elevated ANA titers, presence of anti-DNA, Sm-nuclear, and antinuclear antibodies; decreased T-suppressor lymphocyte count, elevated gamma globulin; anemia, leukopenia, thrombocytopenia; increased erythrocyte sedimentation rate; increased serum creatinine; proteinuria, microscopic hematuria, cellular casts in urine; pericarditis or pleural effusion evident on chest x-ray

ANA, antinuclear antibody

Careful assessment of neurologic status includes observation for visual disturbances, headaches, personality changes, seizures, and forgetfulness. Psychosis may indicate CNS disease or may be the effect of corticosteroid therapy. Irritation of the nerves of the extremities (peripheral neuropathy) may produce numbness, tingling, and weakness of the hands and feet. Less frequently a stroke may result.

The nurse must explain the nature of the disease and modes of therapy and prepare the patient for numerous diagnostic procedures. Emotional support for the patient and family is essential.

Ambulatory and Home Care. Nursing interventions must emphasize health teaching and home management. The patient must understand that even perfect adherence to the treatment plan is not a guarantee against exacerbation because the course of the disease is unpredictable. However, a variety of factors may encourage exacerbation, such as fatigue, sun exposure, emotional stress, infection, drugs, and surgery. Nursing interventions should be directed toward assisting the patient and family to eliminate or minimize exposure to precipitating factors (Table 60-15). Patient understanding and cooperation are important to this goal.

Lupus and pregnancy. For the best outcome for the female patient with SLE, pregnancy should be planned with the cooperation of the primary physician and obstetrician at a point when the disease activity is minimal.[50] Only women with serious renal, cardiac, or CNS involvement should be counseled against pregnancy. Exacerbation is common during the postpartum period. Therapeutic abortion offers the same risk of postdelivery exacerbation as carrying the fetus to term.

Fetal risks include increased rates of miscarriage, prematurity, and stillbirth. Neonatal lupus, an uncommon occurrence, is characterized by rash, transient lupus antibodies, or congenital complete heart block. The presence of antiphospholipid antibodies in the mother may be predictive of placental insufficiency and thrombosis and have been correlated with repeated miscarriage and intrauterine fetal death. Regular clinical and laboratory monitoring is essential for the pregnant woman with SLE.

Psychosocial issues. The patient with SLE confronts many psychosocial issues. Disease onset may be vague, and SLE is often undiagnosed for long periods of time. The nurse should counsel the patient and family that SLE has a good prognosis for the majority of persons. Men are often embarrassed that they have a "woman's disease." Families are anxious about hereditary aspects and want to know whether their children will also have SLE. Many couples require pregnancy and sexual counseling. Individuals making decisions about marriage and

60-2 NURSING CARE PLAN PATIENT WITH SYSTEMIC LUPUS ERYTHEMATOSUS

Expected Patient Outcomes	Nursing Interventions and *Rationales*
NURSING DIAGNOSIS **Fatigue** *related to* disease process *as manifested by* lack of energy, inability to maintain usual routine.	
■ Completion of priority activities. ■ Pacing of activities. ■ Verbalization of having more energy.	■ Analyze energy level patterns *to plan daily activities.* ■ Assist patient to prioritize activities *to establish preferred daily routine.* ■ Teach energy conservation techniques such as sitting at kitchen sink, enlisting aid of others *to accomplish as much as possible with a minimum of energy expenditure.** ■ Include family in planning *to increase patient's sense of support and family's understanding of patient's disease and related problems.* ■ Teach patient techniques such as meditation, yoga *to provide patient with stress-reducing strategies.* ■ Encourage patient to rest regularly and as needed *to temporarily reverse effect of fatigue.*
NURSING DIAGNOSIS **Pain** *related to* disease process and inadequate comfort measures *as manifested by* complaints of joint pain, lack of relief from pain-relieving measures; reduction of activity to avoid exacerbating pain.	
■ Expression of satisfaction with pain relief measures. ■ Performance of activities of daily living without pain.	■ Assess pain location and severity *to plan appropriate interventions.* ■ Administer analgesia as ordered and monitor effect; teach joint protection measures; apply heat or cold as individually determined *to relieve pain.* ■ Use nonpharmacologic pain interventions such as relaxation and visual imagery *to replace or supplement analgesics.*
NURSING DIAGNOSIS **Body image disturbance** *related to* changes in physical appearance *as manifested by* verbalization of dissatisfaction with physical appearance, lack of participation in hygiene and grooming practices.	
■ Increased self-interest and participation in self-care. ■ Expression of positive comments about self.	■ Discuss realistic expectations of physical changes *to help patient make plans to maximize physical assets and minimize problematic areas.* ■ Encourage interest in hygiene and grooming and teach ways to use cosmetics creatively *because these activities improve body image and sense of control.* ■ Encourage discussion about feelings and positive attributes *to reduce patient's sense of isolation and poor body image and redirect self-focus to positive attributes.*
NURSING DIAGNOSIS **Impaired skin integrity** *related to* photosensitivity, skin rash, and alopecia *as manifested by* rash anywhere on body, butterfly rash on face, hair loss, areas of ulceration on fingertips.	
■ Limitation of direct exposure to sun and use of sunscreens. ■ No open skin lesions. ■ Strategies to cope with alopecia.	■ Assess and monitor location and progression of rash *to plan appropriate interventions.* ■ Administer medications and apply ointments as ordered *to control skin manifestations.* ■ Keep skin clean and dry *to avoid secondary infections.* ■ Avoid unprescribed ointments *because these often exacerbate existing conditions.* ■ Discuss need to limit direct sun exposure and use of sunscreens and sun-protective clothing when outdoors *because sun exacerbates skin and systemic manifestations.*
NURSING DIAGNOSIS **Activity intolerance** *related to* arthralgia, weakness, and fatigue *as manifested by* inability or unwillingness to ambulate or engage in physical activity, dyspnea, abnormal response to activity (e.g., increased pulse, respiratory rate).	
■ Expression of satisfaction with activity pattern. ■ Pacing of activities to match level of tolerance.	■ Monitor vital signs when ambulating *because an increasing pulse and respiratory rate may indicate a need to allow patient to rest.* ■ Pace activities and allow periods of rest between activities *to promote recuperation and to foster maximum participation in activities.* ■ Encourage patient to assist in setting activity schedule *to allow patient a sense of control and to foster cooperation with the plan.* ■ Provide bed rest during exacerbation *to conserve energy for vital activities.* ■ Provide ROM exercises q4hr to unaffected joints *to prevent development of stiffness and contractures.* ■ Encourage use of assistive devices *to minimize energy expenditure.*

Continued

60-2 NURSING CARE PLAN PATIENT WITH SYSTEMIC LUPUS ERYTHEMATOSUS—continued

Expected Patient Outcomes	Nursing Interventions and *Rationales*
NURSING DIAGNOSIS	**Altered nutrition: less than body requirements** *related to* anorexia, fatigue, oral ulcerations, and side effects of medication *as manifested by* weight loss, poor appetite, inability or unwillingness to eat adequate food to meet nutritional requirements.
■ Maintenance of weight. ■ Intake of sufficient quantity and quality of food to meet daily needs.	■ Assess food preferences and include them in meal planning when possible *to promote adequate intake and patient's sense of control.* ■ Offer small, frequent meals *to foster adequate intake by reducing fatigue and bloating associated with larger meals.* ■ Provide oral hygiene before and after meals *to increase patient comfort and prevent causing or exacerbating oral ulcerations.* ■ Monitor pertinent laboratory values such as hemoglobin, electrolytes, and protein levels *because lowered levels can indicate inadequate intake.* ■ Encourage family to bring in favorite foods *to increase patient's intake and as a gesture of love and caring.*
NURSING DIAGNOSIS	**Ineffective management of therapeutic regimen** *related to* lack of knowledge of long-term management of disease *as manifested by* questions about SLE or incorrect answers to questions by patient or family, use of unproven remedies.
■ Expression of confidence in ability to manage SLE over time and in home environment.	■ Teach patient about disease process, including chronic management, *to increase probability of successful long-term management.* ■ Include family in teaching activities *to provide caregivers support during exacerbation and increase their sense of involvement.* ■ Discuss need to wear Medic Alert bracelet *to alert uninformed health care providers in time of emergency.* ■ Teach patient to report signs and symptoms of complications such as fever, edema, decreased urine output, chest pain, and dyspnea *to ensure early intervention.* ■ Inform patient of availability of assistance from Lupus Foundation and Arthritis Foundation *to provide additional sources of information and support.*

*See Tables 60-3 and 60-8.

PATIENT & FAMILY TEACHING GUIDE
Table 60-15 Systemic Lupus Erythematosus

1. Education on the disease process
2. Names of medications and actions, side effects, dosage, and administration
3. Energy-conservation and pacing techniques
4. Daily heat and exercise program (for arthralgia)
5. Avoidance of physical and emotional stress, overexposure to ultraviolet light, and unnecessary exposure to infection
6. Regular medical and laboratory follow-up
7. Marital counseling, if necessary
8. Referral resources to community and health care agencies

careers worry about how SLE will interfere with their plans. The nurse may have to educate teachers, employers, and co-workers.

The obvious physical effects of skin rashes, discoid lesions, and alopecia may cause social isolation for the patient with SLE, yet pain and fatigue are cited most frequently as interfering with quality of life. Friends and relatives are confused by the patient's complaints of transient joint pain and overwhelming fatigue. Pacing techniques and relaxation therapy can help keep the patient actively involved. Daily planning should include recreational and occupational activities. Children and young adults find sun restrictions and physical limitations particularly difficult to follow. SLE may also have a negative effect on the patient's self-esteem and body image.[51] Nursing interventions should assist the patient in developing and accomplishing reasonable goals toward improving mobility, energy levels, and self-esteem.[52]

■ Evaluation

The expected outcomes for the patient with SLE are presented in NCP 60-2.

SYSTEMIC SCLEROSIS

Systemic sclerosis (SS), or *scleroderma,* is a disorder of connective tissue characterized by fibrotic, degenerative, and occasion-

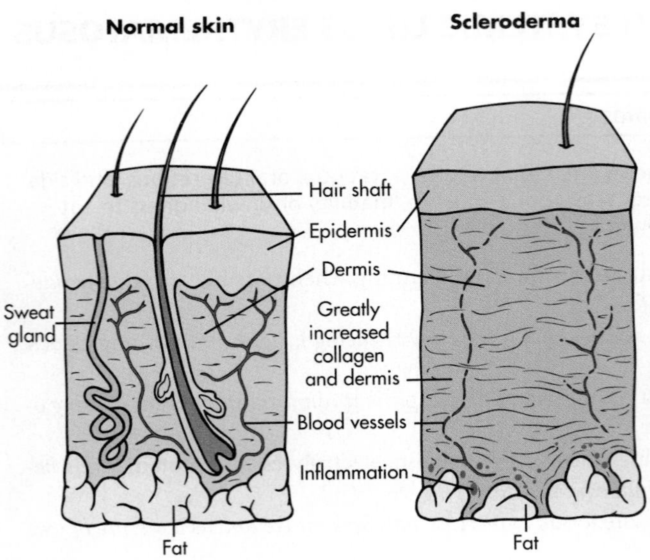

Fig. 60-10 Scleroderma skin changes.

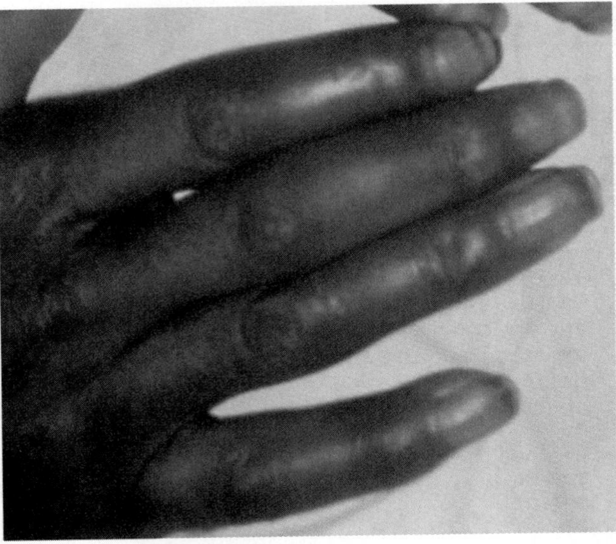

Fig. 60-11 Hand of a patient with systemic sclerosis showing sclerodactyly.

ally inflammatory changes in the skin, blood vessels, synovium, skeletal muscle, and internal organs. Skin thickening and tightening are the cardinal features. The disease may range from a diffuse cutaneous thickening with rapidly progressive and fatal visceral involvement to a more benign variant called CREST syndrome (*c*alcinosis, *R*aynaud's phenomenon, *e*sophageal hypomotility, *s*clerodactyly [skin change of the fingers], and *t*elangiectasia [macule-like angioma on the skin]).[53] (Raynaud's phenomenon is explained in Chapter 36.)

SS affects women three times more frequently than men, with the female-to-male ratio increasing to 15:1 during the childbearing years. SS has been reported in all races but is more common in African-Americans than Caucasians. Although symptoms may begin at any time, the usual age at onset is between 30 and 50 years. SS affects approximately 250,000 people in the United States.

The disease course of SS is variable. Persons with CREST syndrome have limited disability and the longest survival rates, although they are at higher risk for pulmonary hypertension. Myocardial and renal involvement adversely affect the outcome in diffuse disease.

Etiology and Pathophysiology

The exact cause of SS remains unclear. Possible links include environmental toxin exposure to vinyl chloride, epoxy resins, and trichloroethylene. Occupational silica dust exposure has been associated with an increased incidence of systemic sclerosis.[54] Vibrational tool exposure may be another factor involved in the development of this disorder. Collagen, the protein that gives normal skin its strength and elasticity, is overproduced (Fig. 60-10). Widespread systemic disease may be the result of primary vessel injury or immune dysregulation. Disruption of the cell is followed by platelet aggregation, myointimal cell proliferation, and fibrosis. Proliferation of collagen disrupts the normal functioning of internal organs, such as the lungs, kidney, heart, and GI tract.

Clinical Manifestations

Raynaud's Phenomenon. Raynaud's phenomenon (paroxysmal vasospasm of the digits) occurs in nearly 98% of patients with SS and is the most common initial complaint in CREST syndrome. Patients have diminished blood flow to the fingers and toes on exposure to cold (blanching or white phase), followed by cyanosis as hemoglobin releases oxygen to the tissues (blue phase), and then erythema on rewarming (red phase). The color changes are often accompanied by numbness and tingling. Raynaud's phenomenon may precede the onset of systemic disease by months, years, or even decades.

Skin and Joint Changes. Symmetric painless swelling or thickening of the skin of the fingers and hands may progress to diffuse scleroderma of the trunk. In CREST syndrome skin thickening is generally limited to the fingers and face. The skin loses elasticity and becomes taut and shiny, producing the typical expressionless facies with tightly pursed lips. The hands may be affected by sclerodactyly in which the fingers are in a semiflexed position, with tightened skin to the wrist (Fig. 60-11). Polyarthralgias and morning stiffness may be early symptoms. Tendon friction rubs may be present.

Internal Organ Involvement. Esophageal hypomotility causes frequent reflux of gastric acid, causing heartburn and substernal dysphagia for solid foods. If swallowing becomes difficult, the patient often decreases food intake and loses weight. GI complaints also include abdominal distention, diarrhea, malodorous floating stools (malabsorption syndrome) as a result of small-bowel disease, and constipation secondary to colonic involvement.

Lung involvement includes pleural thickening, pulmonary fibrosis, and pulmonary function abnormalities. Pulmonary hypertension is seen almost exclusively in CREST syndrome.

Primary heart disease consists of pericarditis, pericardial effusion, and cardiac arrhythmias. Myocardial fibrosis resulting in congestive failure occurs most frequently in those persons with diffuse SS.

COLLABORATIVE CARE

Table 60-16 Systemic Sclerosis

Diagnostic
History and physical examination
Antinuclear antibody titers
Nail-bed capillary microscopy
X-rays of chest, hands
Upper or lower GI series (or both)
Skin or visceral biopsy
Urinalysis (proteinuria, hematuria, casts)
Collaborative Therapy
Vasodilator drugs
Calcium channel blockers
Reserpine (Serpasil)
Antiinflammatory drugs
Aspirin
NSAIDs
Penicillamine (Cuprimine)
Corticosteroids
Antihypertensive drugs
Physical therapy

Renal disease is a major cause of death in SS. Malignant arterial hypertension associated with rapidly progressive and irreversible renal insufficiency is often present. Recent improvements in dialysis, bilateral nephrectomy in patients with uncontrollable hypertension, and kidney transplantation have offered some hope to patients with renal failure.

Diagnostic Studies

Blood studies may reveal a mildly elevated ESR and occasionally hypergammaglobinemia. The presence of ANA is observed in almost all persons with SS. Autoantibody Scl-70 has been reported in diffuse SS; anticentromere antibody is associated with the CREST syndrome. Nail-bed capillary microscopy characteristically shows capillary loop dilation with limited disease and dilation with avascular areas in patients with diffuse disease.[55] If renal involvement is present, urinalysis may show proteinuria, microscopic hematuria, and casts. X-ray evidence of subcutaneous calcification, digital tuft resorption, distal esophageal hypomotility, or bilateral pulmonary fibrosis is diagnostic of SS. Pulmonary function studies reveal decreased vital capacity. Skin biopsy shows dermal collagen thickening, condensation, or homogenization.

Collaborative Care

The collaborative care of SS (Table 60-16) offers no specific treatment with long-term effects. Care is directed toward attempts to prevent or treat secondary complications of involved organs. Various drugs such as antiinflammatory agents, D-penicillamine (Cuprimine), minocycline, and colchicine have been used with varying degrees of success.

Physical therapy helps maintain joint mobility and preserve muscle strength. Occupational therapy assists the patient in maintaining functional abilities. Gastroesophageal reflux may be treated by antacids and periodic dilation of the esophagus. (Gastroesophageal reflux is discussed in Chapter 39.)

Drug Therapy. No specific drugs or combination of drugs has been proven effective as treatment for SS. Corticosteroids are generally reserved for patients with myositis or overlap syndromes (e.g., mixed connective tissue disease). D-penicillamine increases the solubility of dermal collagen and may cause thinning of the skin, but it has many side effects. Minocycline may improve symptoms, particularly collagen thickening. Colchicine is being used to inhibit the accumulation of collagen, but evidence is still insufficient to prove its therapeutic worth. The use of immunosuppressive agents is under investigation.

Raynaud's phenomenon can be treated with supportive measures, including oral (e.g., niacin) or topical vasodilating drugs (e.g., nitroglycerin ointment) applied to fingers and toes. However, calcium channel blockers (nifedipine [Adalat, Procardia] and diltiazem [Cardizem]) are the treatment of choice for Raynaud's phenomenon.[56] Reserpine (Serpasil), an adrenergic blocking agent, increases blood flow to the fingers. Iloprost, a prostaglandin that promotes vasodilation, is also used to treat Raynaud's phenonomen in SS.[57]

Infected ulcers of the fingertips may be treated by soaking with hyaluronidase and using bacterial antibiotic ointment. Joint symptoms may be relieved by aspirin and other NSAIDs. Antacids and H_2 receptor antagonists (e.g., cimetidine [Tagamet]) may be useful for heartburn. Combinations of antihypertensive medications, including hydralazine (Apresoline), minoxidil (Loniten), captopril (Capoten), propranolol (Inderal), and methyldopa (Aldomet), have been used in the treatment of hypertension.

NURSING MANAGEMENT: SYSTEMIC SCLEROSIS

Because prevention is not possible, nursing intervention often begins during a hospitalization for diagnostic purposes. Vital signs, weight, intake and output, respiratory function, and joint ROM should be assessed daily as indicated by specific symptoms to plan appropriate care. Emotional stress and a cold environment may aggravate Raynaud's phenomenon. Patients with SS should not have finger-stick blood testing done because of compromised circulation and poor healing of the fingers. Diagnostic studies should be thoroughly explained. The nurse can help the patient resolve feelings of helplessness by providing information about the illness and encouraging active participation in planning care.

Health teaching is a major nursing concern as the patient and family begin to live with this disease. Obvious changes in the face and hands lead to poor self-image and loss of mobility and function. The patient must actively carry out therapeutic exercises at home. The nurse should reinforce heat therapy, the use of assistive devices, and organization of activities to preserve strength and reduce disability.

Hands and feet should be protected from cold exposure and possible burns or cuts that might heal slowly. Smoking should be avoided because of its vasoconstricting effect. Signs of infection should be reported. Lotions may help alleviate skin dryness and cracking, but they must be rubbed in for an unusually long time because of the thickness of the skin.

Dysphagia may be reduced by eating small, frequent meals, chewing carefully and slowly, and drinking fluids. Heartburn may be minimized by using antacids 45 to 60 minutes after each meal and by sitting upright for 30 to 45 minutes after eating. Using additional pillows or raising the head of the bed on blocks may help reduce nocturnal gastroesophageal reflux.

Job modifications are often necessary because stair climbing, typing, writing, and cold exposure may pose particular problems. The patient may become socially withdrawn as skin tightening alters the appearance of the face and hands. Some people must wear gloves to protect fingertip ulcers and to provide extra warmth. Sensitive areas on fingertips resulting from ulcers or calcinosis may require padded utensils or special assistive devices to reduce discomfort. Dining out may become a socially embarrassing event because the patient's small mouth, difficulty swallowing, and reflux make eating less enjoyable. Daily oral hygiene must be emphasized, or neglect may lead to increased tooth and gingival problems. The patient needs a dentist who is familiar with SS and can deal with a small oral aperture. Psychologic support reduces stress and may positively influence peripheral motor response. Biofeedback training and relaxation techniques can reduce tension, improve sleeping habits, and raise the temperature of the fingers and toes.

Sexual dysfunction resulting from body changes, pain, muscular weakness, limited mobility, decreased self-esteem, and decreased vaginal secretions may require sensitive counseling by the nurse. Specific suggestions based on individual patient assessment should be offered.[58]

POLYMYOSITIS AND DERMATOMYOSITIS

Polymyositis and *dermatomyositis* are diffuse inflammatory myopathies of striated muscle, producing symmetric weakness usually most severe in the proximal muscles (e.g., trunk, shoulders, and hips). These disorders occur twice as frequently in women as in men. Onset of the disease occurs most frequently in the fifth and sixth decades of life. The incidence is slightly greater than that of muscular dystrophy in adults. Some cases of myositis are associated with an underlying malignant disease. In this situation the myositis is a paraneoplastic syndrome.

Etiology and Pathophysiology

The exact cause of polymyositis and dermatomyositis is unknown. Theories include the presence of an infectious agent, a hypersensitivity response, and cell-mediated immune system abnormalities.

Clinical Manifestations and Complications

Muscular. The patient usually experiences an insidious onset of proximal muscle weakness over a period of several months, primarily of the shoulders, neck, and pelvic girdle. The patient may have difficulty rising from a chair or bathtub, climbing stairs, combing the hair, or reaching into a high cupboard. Neck muscles may become so weak that the patient is unable to raise the head from the pillow. Muscle discomfort or tenderness is uncommon. Muscle examination reveals an inability to move against resistance or even gravity. Weak pharyngeal muscles may produce dysphagia and dysphonia (nasal or hoarse voice).

Dermal. The typical skin rash appears as a dusky erythema of the face, neck, shoulders, anterior part of the chest, upper part of the back, and arms and occurs in nearly 40% of patients with muscular disease. A heliotrope (lavender hue) rash over the eyelids and periorbital edema are nearly pathognomonic for dermatomyositis.[59] The rash is prominent on the extensor surfaces of the forearms, elbows, knuckles, periungual areas, knees, and ankles. A scaly, red, often raised rash on the knuckles is the Gottron's rash of dermatomyositis, which may easily be confused with that of psoriasis or seborrheic dermatitis. Hyperemia and telangiectasias are often present at the nail beds.

Other Manifestations. Nearly half of the patients with polymyositis have mild or transient arthritis and Raynaud's phenomenon. "Cotton-wool" patches can occur in the retina. Calcinosis, contractures, and muscle atrophy may occur with advanced disease. Aspiration pneumonia may result from weak pharyngeal muscles. Childhood dermatomyositis appears to have a more progressive, crippling course. Dermatomyositis diagnosed in men older than 40 years of age is more frequently associated with concurrent malignant disease. In severe cases, deglutition impairment and cardiorespiratory complications, such as pulmonary fibrosis and conduction defects, contribute to mortality.

Diagnostic Studies

Elevations in serum muscle enzymes (creatine kinase, aldolase, and aspartate aminotransferase) are valuable in determining the diagnosis and response to treatment. Circulating autoantibodies designated anti-Jo (antibodies to histidyl tRNA synthetase) are now recognized to be highly disease specific in patients with inflammatory myopathies.[60] Elevation of ESR is expected with active disease. The electromyogram shows polyphasic, short-duration potentials, fibrillation, and positive-spike waves. Muscle biopsy reveals necrosis, degeneration, regeneration, and interstitial chronic inflammatory cell infiltration (primarily lymphocytes).

Collaborative Care

Polymyositis and dermatomyositis can be treated with some success by the use of corticosteroids and, occasionally, immunosuppressive drugs. Improvement is generally achieved with prompt institution of corticosteroid therapy, and dosage is usually reduced as clinical improvement is noted. Relapses are common. Topical corticosteroids may be applied to the skin rash. Patients who respond poorly to corticosteroids may improve with immunosuppressives (e.g., intermittent IV or daily oral cyclophosphamide [Cytoxan]). Corticosteroid therapy may cause potassium to be released from damaged muscle cells and to be lost in the urine. Supplemental dietary potassium (e.g., from orange juice, bananas) is encouraged. Corticosteroid-induced myopathy may complicate long-term therapy. Immunosuppressive agents such as methotrexate, azathioprine (Imuran), and cyclophosphamide are used for their corticosteroid-sparing effect, allowing functional improvement with reduction in corticosteroid dosage.

Physical therapy can be helpful and should be tailored to the activity of the disease. Massage and passive movement are appropriate during active disease, with more aggressive exercises reserved for periods when disease activity is minimal, as evidenced by low serum enzyme levels.

A careful search for possible malignant lesions should be undertaken for the patient more than 40 years of age. If malignant disease is found, it should be treated appropriately. Complete remission of dermatomyositis may occur if the malignant lesion is removed.

NURSING MANAGEMENT: POLYMYOSITIS AND DERMATOMYOSITIS

Although prevention is not possible, greater recognition of polymyositis and its insidious onset resembling muscular dystrophy may favorably influence prognosis by more rapid diagnosis and institution of therapy.

Nursing interventions should include assessment of muscular weakness and limitation of motion. The nurse should maintain the patient on bed rest and assist the patient with activities of daily living when extreme weakness is present. Special attention is provided at mealtime to prevent aspiration. The nature of the disease and modes of therapy should be thoroughly reviewed, and the diagnostic tests should be explained. Understanding that the benefits of therapy are often delayed is important; for example, weakness may increase during the first few weeks of corticosteroid therapy.

The patient should have a thorough understanding of the chronic nature of this disorder, the usefulness and the side effects of all prescribed medications, and the importance of regular medical care and serial laboratory testing. The nurse should provide guidelines for conserving energy by means of organizing activities and pacing techniques. Daily ROM exercises are encouraged to prevent contractures. When active inflammation is not evident, muscle-strengthening (repetitive) exercises may be started. Home care will be necessary during the acute phase of polymyositis because profound muscle weakness renders the patient unable to carry out activities of daily living. Homemaker services, visiting nurses, and family caregivers are needed to assist the patient in routine hygiene, meal preparation and eating, and ambulation.

OVERLAPPING FORMS OF CONNECTIVE TISSUE DISEASE

Patients having a combination of clinical features of several rheumatic diseases are described as having *overlapping* or *mixed connective tissue disease.* Although this combination was believed to be a distinct clinical disorder, follow-up revealed evolution primarily to SLE or SS. This early undifferentiated or transitional form of connective tissue disease has a typical serologic pattern, including high titer of speckled pattern of ANA (a type of ANA), high levels of antibody to ribonuclease-sensitive extractable nuclear antibody, and autoantibodies to ribonucleoprotein.

SJÖGREN'S SYNDROME

Sjögren's syndrome is characterized by autoantibodies to two protein-RNA complexes termed *SS-A/Ro* and *SS-B/La.* The clinical manifestations are caused by inflammation and dysfunction of the exocrine glands, particularly the salivary and lacrimal glands.[61]

More than 90% of the patients are women, and half have RA or another connective tissue disease. Dry mouth can complicate the differential diagnosis in older women. Decreased tearing leads to a "gritty" sensation in the eyes, burning, and photosensitivity. Dry mouth produces buccal membrane fissures, dysphagia, and frequent dental caries. Dry nasal and respiratory passages are common and can result in a cough. Often the parotid glands are enlarged. Other exocrine glands may also be affected; for example, vaginal dryness may lead to dyspareunia.

Histologic study reveals lymphocyte infiltration of salivary and lacrimal glands, but the disease may become more generalized and involve lymph nodes, bone marrow, and visceral organs (pseudolymphoma). Extraglandular proliferation may become frankly malignant (e.g., lymphoma). Rheumatoid and antinuclear factors are present in the majority of patients. Anemia, leukopenia, hypergammaglobulinemia, and elevated ESR are usually found.

Ophthalmologic examination (Schirmer's test), salivary flow rates, and lower lip biopsy of minor salivary glands confirm the diagnosis. The treatment is symptomatic, including (1) instillation of artificial tears as often as necessary to maintain adequate hydration and lubrication, (2) surgical punctal occlusion, and (3) increased fluids with meals. Dental hygiene is important. Pilocarpine (Salagen) can be used to treat symptoms of dry mouth. Increased humidity at home may reduce respiratory infections. Vaginal lubrication with a water-soluble product such as K-Y jelly may increase comfort during intercourse. Corticosteroids and immunosuppressive drugs are indicated for treatment of pseudolymphoma.

FIBROMYALGIA

Fibromyalgia (FM) is a musculoskeletal chronic pain syndrome of unknown etiology.[62] It is characterized by fatigue, stiffness, myalgias, arthralgias, headaches, irritable bowel syndrome, and sleep disturbance. Temporomandibular joint dysfunction, premenstrual symptoms, and mitral valve prolapse may also accompany the disorder. Cognitive disturbances such as memory problems ("brain fog") or difficulty concentrating are common. Depression, anxiety, and feelings of hopelessness often result because of the chronic nature of FM. There is a 50% association of FM and irritable bowel syndrome.[63] FM is seen most commonly in women, with the highest incidence occurring in women age 50 years and older.[63]

Although the etiology and pathogenesis of FM are not known, clinicians have speculated that the syndrome is a result of referred pain from deep structures (pain amplification), a pain-spasm cycle, repetitive stress to the muscle, or reactivation of a latent virus.[64] It is known that FM has a powerful stress-related component that needs attention for long-lasting resolution.

The diagnosis of FM is made by the presence of typical symptoms and the location of *tender points.* Eighteen points, tender in normal people, have been identified that are hypersensitive in persons with FM. The diagnostic criterion for FM is a history of widespread pain and the presence of at least 11 consistent tender points on digital palpation.[65] FM may be localized to a specific region of the body (often termed *myofascial pain*) or generalized with migratory tender points. Myofascial pain most often involves the posterior neck, low back, shoulders, and chest.

The treatment of FM is symptomatic and requires a high level of patient motivation. The nurse can play a key role in educating the patient to be an active participant in the therapeutic regimen. Pain, aching, and tenderness can be helped by rest, and NSAIDs are effective for some patients. Stress, fatigue, and sleep disturbances can be helped by low-dose tricyclic antidepressants (e.g., amitriptyline [Elavil], imipramine [Tofranil], or

RESEARCH
IMPLICATIONS FOR NURSING PRACTICE

Health of Women with Fibromyalgia

Citation Schaefer KM: Health patterns of women with fibromyalgia, *J Adv Nurs* 26:565, 1997.

Purpose To improve understanding of fibromyalgia from the perspective of women who are living with this disease.

Methods The sample included eight women diagnosed with fibromyalgia ranging in age from 27 to 46 years old. Women completed a health diary for 3 months related to how they were living with their fibromyalgia on a daily basis. Demographic information was also collected.

Results and Conclusions Aches and pains were the most common symptom patterns. For most women pain was the worst when the weather was damp or cool. All women used complementary approaches to supplement care with relaxation and heat the most effective. Narrative data from diaries revealed six qualitative themes: (1) pain as mental and physical, (2) fear of pain interferes with ability to do things, (3) suffering results from doing things out of the ordinary, (4) knowing oneself helps control illness, (5) stress affects how one feels, and (6) doing pleasant things helps ease discomfort.

Implications for Nursing Practice Patient diaries can help identify disease symptom patterns and assist the nurse in developing helpful interventions. Diaries can also empower patients by giving back some control over their disease. Patients can anticipate times when they will feel worse and learn what interventions help most. Complementary approaches to pain management should be offered and reinforced by the health care team. The nurse should support the uniqueness of each woman's experience in living with this disease.

trazodone [Desyrel]), muscle relaxants, stress management and stress-reduction techniques, deep relaxation, and a healthful diet. Zolpidem (Ambien) is useful in more recalcitrant cases of sleep disturbance, and clonazepam (Klonopin) may help restless legs syndrome, but both can be habit forming. Selective serotonin reuptake inhibitor antidepressants (e.g., paroxetine [Paxil] and sertraline [Zoloft]) may alleviate pain and fatigue. Participation in a safe, moderate exercise program (e.g., swimming, walking) is one of the most beneficial approaches for reducing FM symptoms. In addition, gentle stretching exercises, yoga, massage therapy, or tai chi may be helpful.

Many parameters of FM except morning stiffness improve on cyclobenzaprine (Flexeril), a muscle relaxant that is a tricyclic derivative. Opioids are rarely used because of the addiction potential. Tramadol (Ultram) acts at the same receptor sites as narcotic analgesics but is thought to have less addiction potential. Subcutaneous injections of lidocaine, cortisone, or both, or even sterile saline, directly into tender points may temporarily relieve pain, but risks are associated with this invasive procedure.

Because of the chronic nature of FM and the need to maintain an ongoing rehabilitation program, the patient with FM needs consistent support from the nurse and other members of the health care team. The most successful treatment approaches combine physical fitness, stress-reduction programs, and psychologic counseling (individual or group).

COMMON JOINT SURGICAL PROCEDURES

Surgery plays an important role in the treatment and rehabilitation of patients with various forms of arthritis, conditions related to trauma, and other painful conditions resulting in functional disability. Joint replacement surgery is the most common orthopedic operation performed on older adults. Significant advances in the field of reconstructive surgery have resulted in improvements in prosthetic design, materials, and surgical techniques that provide significant relief of pain and deformity and improve function and joint motion for patients with arthritis.

Indications

Surgery is aimed at relieving pain, improving joint motion, correcting deformity and malalignment, reducing vertical loads and shear stresses, and removing intraarticular causes of erosion. Pain is one of the primary reasons for joint surgery. In addition to the effects of chronic pain on the physical and emotional well-being of the patient, any movement of the painful joint is often avoided. If this lack of movement is not corrected, contraction with permanent limitation of motion often occurs. Limitation of motion at any joint can be demonstrated on physical examination and by joint-space narrowing on radiologic examination.

There may also be a slow loss of cartilage in affected joints, which may be related to loss of motion. Synovitis can cause tendon damage, resulting in rupture or subluxation of the joint and subsequent loss of function. Continuing disease activity may cause loss of cartilage and bony surface and result in mechanical barriers to movement requiring surgical intervention.

Types of Joint Surgeries

Synovectomy. Synovectomy (removal of synovial membrane) is used as a prophylactic measure and as a palliative treatment of RA. Removal of synovial membrane, thought to be the location of the basic pathologic changes in joint destruction, helps prevent further progression of joint damage. A synovectomy is best performed early in the disease process to prevent serious destruction of joint surfaces. Removal of the thickened synovium prevents extension of the inflammatory process into the adjacent cartilage, ligaments, and tendons.

It is impossible to surgically remove all the synovium in a joint. The underlying disease process is still present and will again affect the regenerating synovium. However, the disease appears to be milder after synovectomy, and definite improvement in pain, weight bearing, and ROM can be expected. Common sites for this surgery include the elbow, wrist, and fingers. Synovectomy in the knee is done less frequently because knee joint replacement techniques are usually used.

Osteotomy. An osteotomy is performed by removing or adding a wedge or slice of bone to change its alignment and shift weight bearing, thereby correcting deformity and relieving pain. Cervical osteotomy may be used to correct defor-

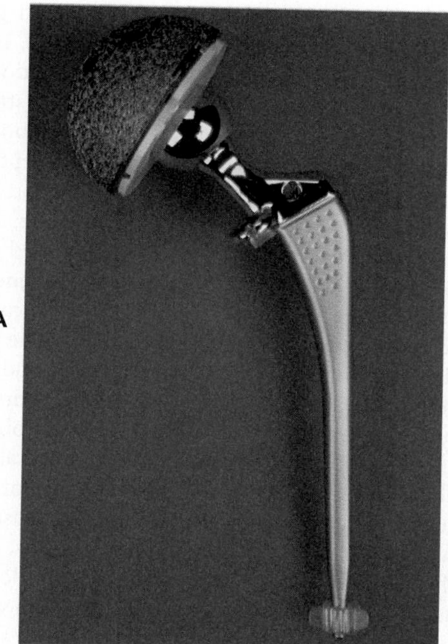

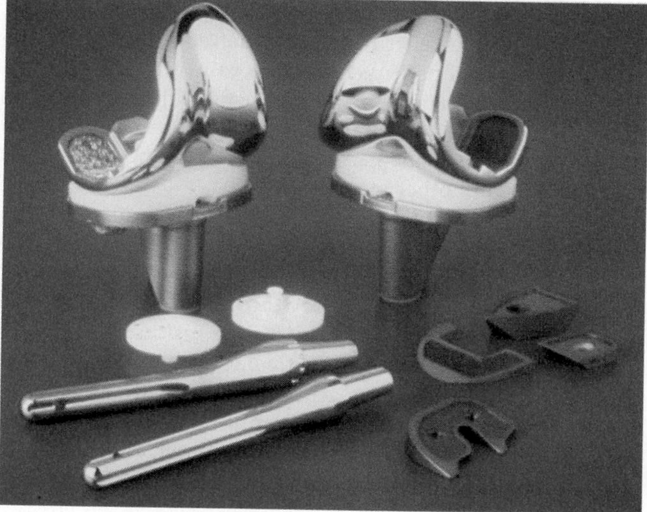

Fig. 60-12 Total joint replacements. **A**, Hip. **B**, Knee.

mity in some patients with ankylosing spondylitis. A halo and body jacket are worn until fusion occurs (3 or 4 months). Subtrochanteric or femoral osteotomy may provide some relief of pain and improve motion in selected patients with hip osteoarthritis. Osteotomy has proven ineffective in patients with inflammatory joint disease. Osteotomy of the knee provides relief of pain in selected patients, but advanced joint destruction is usually corrected by joint replacement surgery. The postoperative care is similar to the treatment of an internal fixation of a fracture at a comparable site (see Chapter 59). The osteotomy is usually fixed by internal wires, screws and plates, bone grafts, or an external fixator.

Debridement. *Debridement* is the removal of degenerative debris such as loose bodies, osteophytes, joint debris, and degenerated menisci from a joint. This procedure is usually performed on the knee or the shoulder using a fiberoptic arthroscope. A compression dressing is applied postoperatively.

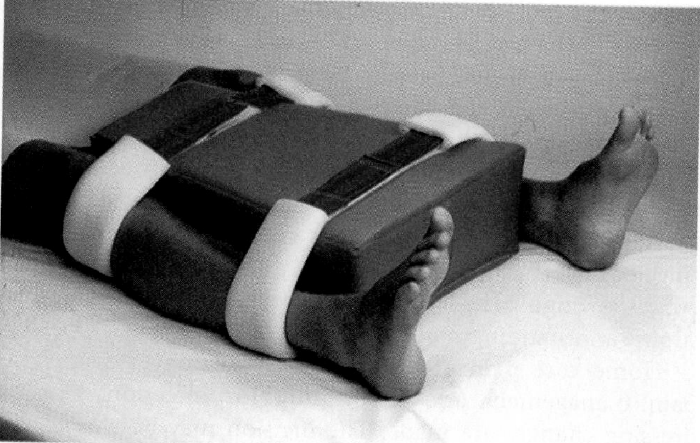

Fig. 60-13 Maintaining postoperative abduction following total hip replacement.

Weight bearing is permitted following knee arthroscopy. Because this is done as an outpatient procedure, patient education includes monitoring for signs of infection, managing pain, and restricting excessive activity for 24 to 48 hours.

Arthroplasty. *Arthroplasty* is the reconstruction or replacement of a joint. This surgical procedure is performed to relieve pain, improve or maintain ROM, and correct deformity—conditions that can result from OA, RA, avascular necrosis, congenital deformities or dislocations, and other systemic problems. There are several types of arthroplasty, including replacement of part of a joint, surgical reshaping of the bones of the joints, and total joint replacement. Innovative procedures and prosthetic devices offer exciting possibilities for reconstructive joint surgery (Fig. 60-12). Replacement arthroplasty is available for the elbow, shoulder, phalangeal joint of the finger, hip, knee, ankle, and foot.[66]

Hip. Total hip replacement is undoubtedly the most important advancement in reconstructive surgery of the twentieth century and has provided significant relief of pain and improvement of function for patients with arthritis. Hip reconstruction is frequently used in the treatment of patients with RA and OA, as well as for fractures of the hip.

Implants are often "cemented" in place with polymethylmethacrylate, which bonds to the bone. With time, a significant number of femoral components loosen and require revision. Because of this risk, total hip replacement is recommended for less active, older adults. More recently, "cementless" arthroplasties have been used. They provide long-term implant stability by facilitating biologic ingrowth of new bone tissue into the porous surface coating of the prosthesis. A patient with a high activity potential and a life expectancy of 25 years or more is an excellent candidate for an uncemented prosthesis.

In both types of arthroplasties, extremes of internal rotation, adduction, and 90-degree flexion of the hip must be avoided for 4 to 6 weeks postoperatively. A foam abduction pillow is sometimes placed between the legs to prevent dislocation of the new joint (Fig. 60-13). Elevated toilet seats and platforms under chairs at home are necessary. Tub baths and driving a car are not allowed for 4 to 6 weeks. An occupational therapist may teach the patient to use assistive devices such as reach bars ("reachers") to avoid bending over to pick something off the floor, long-handled shoehorns, or sock pullers. The knees must be kept apart; the patient must never cross the legs or twist to reach behind. Physical therapy is initiated 1 day postoperatively with ambulation and weight bearing with a walker for cemented prosthesis and partial weight bearing on the operative side for uncemented prosthesis.

Exercises are designed to restore strength and muscle tone in the hip muscles essential to improved function and range of motion. These include quadriceps setting, gluteal muscle setting, leg raises in supine and prone positions, and abduction exercises (swinging the leg out but never crossing midline) from supine and standing positions.

Home care management includes nursing assessment of pain management and monitoring for infection. Periodic dressing changes are made. The incision may be closed with metal staples, which are removed at the surgeon's office. Prothrombin times will be drawn weekly and anticoagulation adjusted accordingly if warfarin is used. Enoxaparin (Lovenox), a low-molecular-weight heparin, is administered subcutaneously and can be given at home by the patient or family member. An advantage of enoxaparin is that it does not require daily blood monitoring of the patient's coagulation status. The patient should be instructed to use prophylactic antibiotics before dental appointments or procedures that might put the patient at risk for bacteremia.

A physical therapist will assess range of motion, ambulation, and compliance with the exercise regimen.[67] The patient will gradually increase the number of repetitions of exercises, add weights to ankles, swim, and may eventually use a stationary bicycle to tone quadriceps and improve cardiovascular fitness. High-impact exercises and sports, such as jogging and tennis, may loosen the implant and should be avoided. The elderly adult may require rehabilitation at an extended care facility until able to function independently.

A clinical pathway for care of the patient with primary total hip replacement is provided on p. 1855.

Knee. Unremitting pain and instability as a result of severe destructive deterioration of the knee joint is the main indication for knee arthroplasty. The presence of osteoporosis may necessitate bone grafting to augment defects and to correct bone deficiencies. Either part or all of the knee joint may be replaced with a metal and plastic prosthetic device. A compression dressing is used to immobilize the knee in extension immediately after the operation. This is removed before discharge and may be replaced with a knee immobilizer or posterior plastic shell, which maintains extension during ambulation and at rest for about 4 weeks.

Great emphasis is placed on postoperative exercising, and dislocation is not a problem. Isometric quadricep setting begins the first day after surgery. The patient progresses to straight-leg raises and gentle ROM to increase muscle strength and obtain 90-degree knee flexion. Active flexion exercises through the use of a passive-motion machine postoperatively promotes earlier joint mobility and shortens hospitalization. Full weight bearing is begun before discharge. An active home exercise program involves progressive ROM, muscle strengthening, and stationary bicycle exercising.

Finger joints. A silicone rubber arthroplastic device is used to help restore function in the fingers of the patient with RA. The goal of hand surgery is primarily to restore function related to grasp, pinch, stability, and strength rather than to correct cosmetic deformity. The metacarpophalangeal and proximal interphalangeal joints are most commonly involved. Ulnar deviation is often present, which results in severe functional limitations of the hand. Before surgery the patient is instructed in hand exercises, including flexion, extension, abduction, and adduction of the fingers. Postoperatively, the hand is kept elevated with a bulky dressing in place. The operative area and the hand should be checked for sensation, temperature, pulse, and signs of infection. Once the dressing is removed, a guided splinting program is initiated. The success of the surgery depends largely on the postoperative treatment plan, which is often carried out under the direction of an occupational therapist. The patient is discharged with splints to use while sleeping and hand exercises to perform for 10 to 12 weeks at least three to four times a day. The patient is also instructed to avoid lifting heavy objects.

Elbows and shoulders. Although available, total replacement of elbow and shoulder joints is not as common as other forms of arthroplasty. Shoulder replacements are used in patients with severe pain because of RA, OA, necrosis, or an old trauma. The shoulder replacement is usually considered if the patient has adequate surrounding muscle strength and bone stock. If joint replacement is necessary for both elbow and shoulder, the elbow is usually done first because a severely painful elbow interferes with the shoulder rehabilitation program.

Significant pain relief has been achieved following arthoplasty, with 90% of patients having no pain at rest or minimal pain with activity. Functional improvements have resulted in better hygiene and increased ability to perform activities of daily living in most patients. Rehabilitation is longer and more difficult than with other joint surgeries.

Arthrodesis. Arthrodesis is the surgical fusion of a joint. This procedure is indicated only if articular surfaces are too severely damaged or infected to allow joint replacement or for reconstructive surgery failures. Arthrodesis relieves pain and provides a stable but immobile joint. The fusion is usually accomplished by removal of the articular hyaline cartilage and the addition of bone grafts across the joint surface. The affected joint must be immobilized until bone healing has occurred. Common areas of fusion are the wrist, ankle, cervical spine, lumbar spine, and the metatarsophalangeal joint of the great toe.

Complications of Joint Surgery

Infection is a serious complication of joint surgery, particularly joint replacement surgery. The most common causative organisms are gram-positive aerobic streptococci and staphylococci. Infection almost always leads to pain and loosening of the prosthesis, generally requiring extensive surgery. Efforts to reduce the incidence of infection include the use of specially designed hypersterile operating rooms with laminar air flow and prophylactic antibiotic administration.

Deep vein thrombosis is another potentially serious complication after selected joint surgeries, particularly those involving the lower extremities. Prophylaxis such as aspirin, warfarin, or pneumatic compression of the legs is usually instituted. Patients may be followed postoperatively with venous Doppler ultrasound to detect proximal deep vein thrombosis, the source of most pulmonary emboli. The peak incidence of pulmonary embolus is bimodal, occurring on the fourth and fourteenth postoperative day.

CLINICAL PATHWAY Primary Total Hip

MR
Patient Name
Diagnosis
Procedure
Procedure Data

____

Function	Activity	PreOp ___/___	Or Day ___/___	PostOp #1___/___	Post Day #2___/___	PostOp #3___/___
Hemostasis Thromboembolic Prophylaxis	Lab Work	PT/CBC, U/A Type and cross one unit PRBC (send 10 cc clot)	PT at 4 P.M. Heme Panel *(See Left Side Panel)	PT at 6 A.M. Heme Panel*	PT at 6 A.M. Heme Panel*	PT at 6 A.M. Heme Panel*
Heme Panel Hgb/Hct and Total **WBC w/o DIFF Hgb/Hct RBC Indices Total WBC W/DIFF Quant. Platelets**	Assessment	Assess for transfusion Assess for sequential compression device if cannot anticoagulate	Assess for transfusion **Criteria** < 11 anticipate blood loss with autogolous unit expiration < 10 active bleeding anticipated mod/massive bleeding marginal cardiac reserve/ O_2 capacity < 9 above criteria suspected bone marrow suppression < 8 MD discretion	Assess for transfusion See Criteria	Assess for transfusion See Criteria	Assess for transfusion See Criteria
	Medications	No NSAIDs 10-14 days preop	If on Coumadin maintain INR at 1.5-2.0 or low-molecular-weight heparin 30 mg SC bid No NSAIDs	If on Coumadin adjust to protime or low-molecular-weight heparin 30 mg SC bid NO NSAIDs	In on Coumadin adjust to protime or low-molecular-weight heparin 30 mg SC bid NO NSAIDs	If on Coumadin adjust to protime or low-molecular-weight heparin 30 mg SC bid NO NSAIDs
	Treatments	Measure for thigh-high TEDS and tape to chart for OR	APPLY TEDS	APPLY TEDS	APPLY TEDS	APPLY TEDS
	Education	Anticoagulant instructions		Anticoagulant Instructions		
	Clinical Outcomes			No DVT or PE, stable Hgb and Hct No hemorrhagic complications	No DVT or PE, stable Hgb and Hct No hemorrhagic complications	No DVT or PE, stable Hgb and Hct No hemorrhagic complications
Pain Management	Assessment		Pain assessment q4hr while awake	Pain assessment q4hr while awake	Pain assessment q4hr while awake	Pain assessment q4hr while awake
	Medication		If motor deficit, contact anesthesia to evaluate. If inadequate pain relief, contact anesthesia to adjust dose PCA (if no epidural)	If motor deficit, contact anesthesia to evaluate D/C epidural/PCA after afternoon PT session Start oral meds q4hr around the clock	Oral meds q4hr after PM PT Change oral meds to prn	Oral meds q4hr Change oral meds to prn
	Clinical Outcomes		Adequate pain relief (pain scale score____)	Adequate pain relief (self-report scale)	Adequate pain relief (self-report scale)	Adequate pain relief (self-report scale)
Wound Management	Assessment			Wound drainage	Wound drainage	Wound drainage
	Treatment			Service to D/C drain and collection devices when clotted or <100 cc in 8 hr for 2 shifts Surgical service to change OR dressing	Change dressing daily and prn if excessive drainage	Change dressing daily and prn if excessive drainage
	Medications	Ancef (Use Vancomycin if allergic PCN)	Start Ancef IV in OR 1 hour before incision then Ancef 1 g q8hr × 3 doses (Vancomycin if allergic to PCN)	Keflex PO if Foley is continued Septra DS if PCN allergic	Keflex PO if Foley is continued Septra DS if PCN allergic	
	Clinical Outcomes		No hematoma/dehiscence/infection	No hematoma/dehiscence/ infection	No hematoma/dehiscence/infection	No hematoma/dehiscence/infection Wound dry and intact Afrebile (Temp <100.0)

From Rush-Presbyterian St. Luke's Medical Center.

Continued

CLINICAL PATHWAY Primary Total Hip—continued

Function	Activity	PreOp ___/___	Or Day ___/___	PostOp #1___/___	Post Day #2___/___	PostOp #3___/___
General	Test	CXR, ECG if > 40 yr old SMA 18, hepatitis B profile if no autologous blood donation				
	Consults	Internal medicine consult CRC for discharge assessment				
	Medications		Compazine in PAR	Colace QAM Compazine PRN for nausea	Colace QAM Compazine PRN for nausea	Colace QAM Compazine PRN for nausea
	Assessments		Skin assessment, I & O q8hr, VS q4hr Circulation and neuro checks q2hr × 8 hr then q4hr × 4 hr	Skin assessment, I & O q8hr, VS q4hr Circulation and neuro checks q4hr	Skin assessment, I & O q8hr, VS q8hr Circulation and neuro checks q8hr	Skin assessment, I & O q8hr, VS q8hr Circulation and neuro checks q8hr
	Treatments		Introduce Inspiratory spirometer Encourage pt to use spirometer q1hr	Inspiratory spirometer q1hr	Inspiratory spirometer q4hr	Inspiratory spirometer q4hr
	Diet	NPO	Administer IV fluids as ordered Clear liquid diet as tolerated	Change IV to heplock Advance diet	D/C heplock after antibiotics completed General diet	General diet
	Elimination		Order raised toilet seat if 5′4″ or taller Foley with epidural	Prune juice prn D/C Foley 4-6 hr after epidural D/C	Prune juice prn Fleet enema prn	Prune juice prn Fleet enema prn
	Education	Preop standards of care	Reinforce hip precautions			
	Clinical Outcomes		Braden Score > 17 No IV restarts needed	Braden Score >17	Braden Score >17	Braden Score > 17 Tolerate general diet Chest clear to auscultation Voids freely
	Discharge Planning		Nursing to notify CRC for discharge assessment	CRC to review case		CRC to make home arrangements for: Blood draws for PT Physical therapy and other services PRN Transfer to outside rehabilitation facility or ECF on selected patients
Rehabilitation	Consults		PT (physical therapy) OT (occupational therapy)	Physical med and rehab consults on selected pts		OT to see patient before discharge
	Assessments			Pain assessment pre–physical therapy	Pain assessment pre–physical therapy	Pain assessment pre–physical therapy
	Treatments		Regular pillow for abduction Hip flexion not exceed 90 degrees No adduction of operated leg No internal rotation of operated leg	Regular pillow for abduction Hip flexion not to exceed 90 degrees No adduction of operated leg No internal rotation of operated leg	Regular pillow for abduction Hip flexion not to exceed 90 degrees No adduction of operated leg No internal rotation of operated leg	Regular pillow for abduction Hip flexion not to exceed 90 degrees No adduction of operated leg No internal rotation of operated leg
	Activity		Trapeze on bed Dangle at bedside late PM	Bathroom, chair, and ambulation when approved by PT For cemented or hybrid THR: - WBAT - crutches or walker For cementless THR: - touchdown weight bearing For all THR: - active/passive abduction per surgical protocol On nursing unit - Assist with ADLs PRN - Up to chair for dinner	Bathroom, chair, and ambulation when approved by PT Move trapeze to end of bed after PM PT session On unit Up to chair for dinner Ambulate in hallway with assistive device in accordance with PT note	Bathroom, chair, and ambulation when approved by PT On unit Up to chair for dinner Ambulate in hallway with assistive device
	Education	Hip precautions Home preparation for discharge	Reinforce postop teaching with patient and family	Transfer techniques		Home exercise program Hip precautions
	Clinical Outcomes	No hip dislocation	No hip dislocation Patient tolerates activities	Pain control adequate to participate in PT No hip dislocation Patient tolerates activities	Pain control adequate to participate in PT No hip dislocation Patient tolerates activities	Pain control adequate to participate in PT No hip dislocation Independent gait with appropriate device Independent transfers

Collaborative Care

Preoperative Management. As surgical techniques and care improve, more patients with chronic diseases such as RA are being considered as surgical candidates. The primary goal of preoperative assessment is to identify risk factors associated with postoperative complications so that nursing strategies can be implemented that promote optimal positive outcomes. A careful history will include previous medical diagnosis and complications such as diabetes and thrombophlebitis, pain tolerance and management preferences, current functional status and expectations following surgery, and level of social support and home care needs after discharge. The patient should be free from evidence of infection and acute joint inflammation. If lower-extremity surgery is planned, upper extremity muscle strength and joint function are assessed to determine the type of assistive devices needed postoperatively for ambulation and activities of daily living. Preoperative education informs the patient and family of the expected hospital course and postoperative management at home and readies them for a lifestyle that is compatible with the intrinsic capabilities of the prosthetic components so that prosthesis longevity can be maximized.

Postoperative Management. Postoperatively, a neurovascular assessment of the affected extremity is done to assess nerve function and circulatory status. Anticoagulation therapy, analgesia, and parenteral antibiotics are administered. In general, the affected joint is exercised and ambulation is encouraged as early as possible to prevent complications of immobility. Specific protocols vary according to patient, type of prosthesis, and surgeon preference.

The hospital stay after arthroplasty is about 3 to 5 days depending on the patient's course and need for physical therapy. Physical therapy and ambulation enhance mobility, build muscle strength, and reduce the risk of thrombus formation. If the patient is on Coumadin, therapy starts on the day of surgery and continues for 3 weeks with a prothrombin time (PT) done twice weekly. For those on enoxaparin, therapy starts 24 to 36 hours after surgery and continues for 3 weeks postoperatively. Daily monitoring of the patient's coagulation status is not necessary with enoxaparin therapy. The decision to use Coumadin or enoxaparin depends on many factors, including the patient's age and overall state of health.

60-3 NURSING CARE PLAN PATIENT WITH JOINT REPLACEMENT SURGERY

Expected Patient Outcomes	Nursing Interventions and *Rationales*
	Acute Intervention
NURSING DIAGNOSIS	**Impaired physical mobility** *related to* pain, stiffness, and surgical procedure *as manifested by* difficulty in ambulating, inability to participate in physical rehabilitation, guarded movement.
▪ Functional ROM of joint.	▪ Assess effect of surgery on patient's mobility *to plan appropriate interventions.* ▪ Maintain proper positioning *to prevent dislocation or other complications.* ▪ Begin exercise program as directed *to minimize mobility impairment and stiffness.* ▪ Collaborate with physical and occupational therapist *to increase patient compliance and promote continuity of exercise.* ▪ Give pain medication before exercise *to decrease discomfort from exercise and increase patient participation.*
NURSING DIAGNOSIS	**Self-care deficits** *related to* restrictions imposed by joint surgery, pain, weakness *as manifested by* inability to perform part or all of activities of daily living (ADLs).
▪ ADLs met satisfactorily by patient or caregivers.	▪ Assess patient's ability to perform ADLs *to plan appropriate assistance.* ▪ Assist as necessary *to ensure all basic needs are met.* ▪ Assure patient of your willingness to assist with ADLs postoperatively *to relieve anxiety related to feelings of helplessness.* ▪ Assure patient that self-care abilities will be resumed with time *to decrease anxiety over dependency.*
NURSING DIAGNOSIS	**Ineffective management of therapeutic regimen** *related to* lack of knowledge of follow-up care *as manifested by* expression of concern with ability to care for self after discharge, frequent questioning about follow-up care, lack of plan for follow-up care.
▪ Confidence in ability to manage self-care after discharge and to make necessary lifestyle changes.	▪ Instruct patient on usual follow-up protocol, including activity limitations, medications, follow-up visit, signs of infection, and dislocation, *to prepare patient for self-care and decision making.* ▪ Assist patient to identify activities that require modification *so appropriate modification can be made.* ▪ Refer for vocational counseling *so expert guidance is available if necessary.* ▪ Initiate a nurse referral *to monitor the long-term exercise program at home.*

Continued

60-3 NURSING CARE PLAN PATIENT WITH JOINT REPLACEMENT SURGERY —continued

Expected Patient Outcomes	Nursing Interventions and *Rationales*
NURSING DIAGNOSIS	**Risk for peripheral neurovascular dysfunction** *related to* edema and dislocated prosthesis.
▪ Palpable peripheral pulses. ▪ Warm extremities.	▪ Assess nerve and circulatory status q1hr first 24 hr, then every 2-4 hr *to determine if problem is present so treatment can be initiated promptly.* ▪ Notify surgeon immediately if abnormalities are noted *so interventions are started without delay.* ▪ Initiate measures such as cold packs and elevation of affected part *to minimize edema.* ▪ Carry out measures to prevent dislocation *because this can be a cause of neurovascular dysfunction.* ▪ Teach patient to report signs of neurovascular dysfunction such as paresthesia, coldness, pallor, excessive pain, swelling of affected extremity or body area *so treatment is not delayed.*

COLLABORATIVE PROBLEMS

Nursing Goals	Nursing Interventions and *Rationales*
POTENTIAL COMPLICATION	**Dislocation of prosthesis** *related to* improper movement or activity.
▪ Monitor and report signs of joint dislocation. ▪ Carry out appropriate medical and nursing interventions.	▪ Monitor for pain in affected joint, loss of function, shortening or malalignment of extremity *to determine if dislocation has occurred.* ▪ Instruct patient on safe positions and activities; use assistive devices (e.g., raised toilet seat) as indicated *to avoid extremes of movement, which can cause dislocation.* ▪ Reinforce instructions of physical therapists *to foster confidence in plan and prevent misunderstanding.* ▪ Teach signs of dislocation to report (e.g., pain, loss of function, deformity) *so treatment is initiated promptly.*
POTENTIAL COMPLICATION	**Thrombophlebitis** *related to* surgery and immobilization.
▪ Monitor and report signs of thrombosis. ▪ Carry out appropriate medical and nursing interventions.	▪ Monitor for redness, swelling, and tenderness or pain of the extremity *to recognize and report signs of thrombophlebitis.* ▪ Apply elastic compression stockings and instruct patient to perform isotonic exercises such as quadriceps setting, ankle rolling, and pushing on footboard *to promote circulation and prevent clot formation.* ▪ Provide adequate parenteral and oral fluids *to prevent dehydration and thrombus formation.* ▪ Instruct the patient in the importance of home exercise *to prevent venous stasis.* ▪ Instruct the patient and caregivers in the proper administration and follow-up of oral anticoagulation medications *to prevent side effects of under- or over-anticoagulation.*

NURSING MANAGEMENT: JOINT SURGERY

The nursing management of the patient undergoing joint surgery begins with preoperative teaching and realistic goal setting. It is important that the patient understands and accepts the limitations of the proposed surgery and realizes that it will not remove the underlying disease process. Postoperative procedures such as turning, deep breathing, use of bedpan and bedside commode, and use of abductor pillows should be explained and opportunities for practice provided. The patient should be reassured that pain relief will be available. Patient-controlled analgesia such as intravenous ketorolac (Toradol) and morphine sulfate can be helpful postoperatively, as can intramuscular ketorolac. A preoperative visit from a physical therapist allows practice of postoperative exercises and measurement for crutches or other assistive devices. The spirit of respect and cooperation displayed between the physical therapist and the nurse can do much to reassure an anxious patient.

Discharge planning begins immediately. The duration of the hospital stay and the expected postoperative events should be discussed so that the patient and family can plan ahead. The home environment should be assessed for safety (e.g., presence of scatter rugs and electrical cords) and accessibility. (Are the bathroom and bedroom on the first floor? Are door frames wide enough to accommodate a walker?) Social support must be assessed. Is a friend or family member available to assist the patient in the home? Will the patient require homemaker or meal services? The elderly patient may need the rehabilitation services of an extended care facility for a few weeks postoperatively to progressively develop independent living skills. Specific nursing interventions related to joint surgery are summarized in NCP 60-3.

Patient teaching includes instructions on reporting complications, including infection (e.g., fever, increased pain, drainage) and dislocation of the prosthesis (pain, loss of function, shortening or malalignment of an extremity). The home

CRITICAL THINKING EXERCISES

CASE STUDY

Systemic Lupus Erythematosus

Patient Profile

Nicole is a 30-year-old married woman who is seen at the rheumatology clinic following a recent 2-week vacation to Australia.

Subjective Data

- Works in a flower shop
- Complains of migratory joint pain, overwhelming fatigue, and a facial rash
- Is 6 months pregnant
- Has Raynaud's phenomenon when she works in the refrigerator room stocking flowers
- Had episode of pleurisy at age 21
- Fears something is horribly wrong with her
- Is afraid to take medication because of pregnancy

Objective Data

Physical Examination

- Malar rash
- Swelling of third and fourth metacarpophalangeal joints of both hands
- Dry, scaly scalp
- Pain on motion of both wrists, shoulders, and knees with no obvious swelling

Diagnostic Studies

- WBC count 4000/μl (4×10^9/L)
- Platelets 100,000/μl (150×10^9/L)
- Complement (C3) 60 mg/dl (0.6 g/L)
- Positive ANA and antiphospholipid antibodies

Collaborative Care

- Diagnosed with systemic lupus erythematosus
- Started on prednisone 10 mg daily

Critical Thinking Questions

1. How might the nurse explain the pathophysiology of systemic lupus erythematosus to Nicole?
2. How might the vacation have influenced the symptoms that she is currently experiencing?
3. What are some home and work modifications that the nurse can suggest to Nicole that will reduce her symptoms?
4. Discuss the types of prenatal and postpartal considerations essential in caring for Nicole.
5. What other sources of information regarding systemic lupus erythematosus might the nurse suggest to Nicole and her family?
6. Based on the assessment data presented, write one or more nursing diagnoses. Are there any collaborative problems?

NURSING RESEARCH ISSUES

1. What is the relationship between social support systems and quality of life for people with SLE?
2. What are the needs of the family when the patient is diagnosed with SLE?
3. Is gender a factor in the experience of arthritic pain?
4. What are effective measures that the nurse can institute to improve patient compliance with arthritis home management programs?
5. Are the coping strategies of younger patients diagnosed with systemic sclerosis different from those of older patients?

care nurse acts as the liaison between the patient and the surgeon, monitoring for postoperative complications, assessing comfort and ROM, and facilitating improvements in functional performance.

REVIEW QUESTIONS

The number of the question corresponds to the same-numbered objective at the beginning of the chapter.

1. In teaching a patient with SLE about the disorder the nurse uses the knowledge that the pathophysiology of SLE includes
   a. production of autoantibodies directed against constituents of cellular DNA.
   b. an autoimmune reaction resulting in degeneration, necrosis, and fibrosis of muscle fibers.
   c. deposition in tissues of immune complexes formed from IgG autoantibodies reacting with IgG.
   d. chronic inflammation and cytokine activity, which results in synovial proliferation and cartilage and bone damage.
2. An important nursing intervention in caring for the patient with ankylosing spondylitis is to teach the patient
   a. thoracic stretching and ROM exercises to prevent deformity.
   b. to sleep on the side with the legs flexed and supported with pillows.
   c. to prevent enteric and venereal infections that precipitate recurring attacks.
   d. that continuous therapeutic blood levels of nonsteroidal antiinflammatory drugs can limit the progression of the disease.
3. In assessing the joints of a patient with rheumatoid arthritis the nurse understands that the joints are damaged by
   a. the development of Heberden's nodes in the joint capsule.
   b. the deterioration of cartilage by the enzyme hyaluronidase.
   c. invasion of pannus into the joint capsule and subchondral bone.
   d. bony ankylosis following inflammation of the joints in HLA-B27–positive individuals.

4. Assessment data noted by the nurse in the patient with osteoarthritis commonly include
   a. elevated ESR.
   b. significant morning stiffness.
   c. progressive joint pain with activity.
   d. symmetric swelling of metacarpophalangeal joints.
5. When teaching the patient with arthritis the nurse should instruct the patient to
   a. avoid foods high in fat and calories.
   b. use cold applications to increase mobility in stiff joints.
   c. balance regularly scheduled rest periods with periods of activity.
   d. prevent any movement of affected joints during an acute inflammatory attack.
6. A patient with rheumatoid arthritis is scheduled for an arthroplasty. The nurse explains that the purpose of this procedure is to
   a. fuse a joint and reduce pain.
   b. prevent further joint damage.
   c. assess the extent of joint damage.
   d. replace the joint and improve function.
7. The nurse teaches a patient recovering from a total hip replacement that it is important to avoid
   a. sleeping on the abdomen.
   b. sitting with the legs crossed.
   c. abduction exercises of the affected leg.
   d. bearing weight on the affected leg for 6 weeks.
8. The nurse planning education for the patient with rheumatoid arthritis who is on multiple drug therapy includes information related to the need to
   a. use aspirin only on a prn basis for pain relief.
   b. use birth control during and 3 months following gold therapy.
   c. have frequent laboratory monitoring while taking methotrexate.
   d. stop taking any corticosteroids as soon as symptoms are relieved.
9. A patient with SLE has a nursing diagnosis of body image disturbance related to change in physical appearance. An appropriate nursing intervention for the patient is to
   a. discourage the patient from talking about her appearance.
   b. teach the patient creative uses of cosmetics in hygiene and grooming.
   c. enlist the support of family members to reassure the patient that she is valued.
   d. refer the patient for sexual counseling since sexual problems affect body image.
10. The most effective way to manage the health care needs of the patient with arthritis is to
    a. provide round-the-clock nursing care.
    b. let the family take over the patient's workload.
    c. explore the patient's spiritual response to pain.
    d. endorse the skills of a multidisciplinary health care team.

References

1. Hellmann D: Arthritis and musculoskeletal disorders. In Tierney L and others, editors: *Current medical diagnosis and treatment,* ed 36, Stamford, Conn, 1997, Appleton & Lange.
2. McCance K, Huether S: *Pathophysiology: biologic basis for disease in adults and children,* ed 3, St Louis, 1998, Mosby.
3. Kraus VB: Pathogenesis and treatment of osteoarthritis, *Med Clin North Am* 81:1, 1997.
4. Greidinger EL, Hellman DB: Arthritis: what to emphasize on the rheumatologic exam, *Consultant* 35:1609, 1995.
5. Griffin MR and others: Practical management of osteoarthritis: integration of pharmacologic and non-pharmacologic measures, *Arch Fam Med* 4:1049, 1995.
6. Hochberg MC, Altman RD, Brandt KD: Guidelines for the medical management of osteoarthritis, *Arthritis Rheum* 38:11, 1995.
7. Lozada CJ, Altman RD: Chondroprotection in osteoarthritis, *Bull Rheum Dis* 46:7, 1997.
8. McDowell I, Newell C: *Measuring health: a guide to rating scales and questionnaires,* ed 2, New York, 1996, Oxford University Press.
9. Torburn L: Principles of rehabilitation, *Prim Care* 23:2, 1996.
10. Stein MC, Griffin MR, Brandt KD: Osteoarthritis. In Wegener S and others, editors: *Clinical care in the rheumatic diseases,* Atlanta, 1996, American College of Rheumatology.
11. O'Dell JR, Pischel KD, Weinblatt M: Rheumatoid arthritis: what's new in treatment, *Patient Care* 31:5, 1997.
12. Ross C: A comparison of osteoarthritis and rheumatoid arthritis: diagnosis and treatment, *Nurse Pract* 22:9, 1997.
13. Callahan LF, Pincus T: Mortality in rheumatic diseases, *Arthritis Care Res* 8:229, 1995.
14. Mayo Clinic: Rheumatoid arthritis, *Mayo Clin Health Lett* 15:6, 1997.
15. Ali H and others: Mechanisms of inflammation and leukocyte activation, *Med Clin North Am* 81:1, 1997.
16. Dearborn JT, Jergesen HE: The evaluation and initial management of arthritis, *Prim Care* 23:2, 1996.
17. Lipsky PE, Jain R: Treatment of rheumatoid arthritis, *Med Clin North Am* 81:1, 1997.
18. Schnabel A and others: Sustained cough in methotrexate therapy for rheumatoid arthritis, *Clin Rheumatol* 15:277, 1996.
19. Skidmore-Roth L: *Nursing drug reference,* St Louis, 1998, Mosby.
20. O'Dell JR and others: Treatment of rheumatoid arthritis with methotrexate alone, sulfasalazine, and hydroxychloroquine or a combination of all three medications, *N Engl J Med* 334:20, 1996.
21. Silverstein FE and others: Misoprostol reduces serious gastrointestinal complications in patients with rheumatoid arthritis receiving nonsteroidal antiinflammatory drugs, *Ann Intern Med* 123:241, 1995.
22. Pigg JS: Rheumatoid arthritis: how allied health professionals can help, *J Musculoskel Med* 12:2, 1995.
23. Boutaugh MC, Brady TJ: Quality of life programs of the Arthritis Foundation, *Orthop Nurs* 15:5, 1996.
24. Veeser PI, editor: Patient education: treating arthritis, *Nurse Pract* 22:4, 1997.
25. Hall J and others: A randomized and controlled trial of hydrotherapy in rheumatoid arthritis, *Arthritis Care Res* 9:3, 1996.
26. Erlandson M: Rheumatic diseases in childhood. In Wegener S and others, editors: *Clinical care in the rheumatic diseases,* Atlanta, 1996, American College of Rheumatology.
27. Halverson PB: The spondyloarthropathies, *Orthop Nurs* 16:4, 1997.
28. Khan MA: Ankylosing spondylitis: clinical features. In Klippel JH, Dieppe PA, editors: *Rheumatology,* St Louis, 1995, Mosby.
29. Wollenhaupt J, Hoffmann A: HLA-B27 associated diseases. In Zierhut M, Thiel HJ, editors: *Immunology of the joint and the eye,* Boston, 1996, Butterworth Heinemann.
30. Verdon ME, Sigal LH: Recognition and management of Lyme disease, *Am Fam Physician* 56:2, 1997.
31. Schlesinger P: Lyme disease: an update, *Hospital Medicine* 34:26, 1998.
32. Jancin B: Give Lyme disease vaccine over a 2-month period, *Skin and Allergy News* 30:10, 1998.
33. Itescu S: Rheumatic aspects of acquired immunodeficiency syndrome, *Curr Opin Rheumatol* 8:4, 1996.
34. Gomez-Reino JJ, Carreira PE: Inflammation and HIV infection: a friendly connection, *Lancet* 348(suppl II):24, 1996.
35. Calin A: Managing hyperuricemia and gout: challenges and pitfalls, *J Musculoskel Med* 12:2, 1995.
36. Pisetsky DS, Gilkeson G, St Clair EW: Systemic lupus erythematosus: diagnosis and treatment, *Med Clin North Am* 81:1, 1997.
37. Ward MM, Pyun E, Studensk S: Long-term survival in systemic lupus erythematosus, *Arthritis Rheum* 38:2, 1995.
38. Howser RL: Nursing care of a patient with lupus cerebritis, *DCCN* 15:5, 1996.
39. Llorente L and others: Dysregulation of interleukin-10 production in relatives of patients with systemic lupus erythematous, *Arthritis Rheum* 40:8, 1997.
40. Tsao B and others: The genetic basis of systemic lupus erythematosus, *Proc Assoc Am Physicians* 110:113, 1998.

41. Clark J and others: B-lymphocyte hyperactivity in families of patients with systemic lupus erythematosus, *J Autoimmun* 9:59, 1996.
42. Petri M: Systemic lupus erythematosus. In Rich RR, editor: *Clinical immunology: principles and practice,* St Louis, 1996, Mosby.
43. Wallace DJ, Metzger AL: Systemic lupus erythematosus: clinical aspects and treatment. In Koopman WJ, editor: *Arthritis and allied conditions,* ed 13, Baltimore, 1997, Williams & Wilkins.
44. Tebbe B, Orfanos CE: Epidemiology and social impact of skin disease in lupus erythematosus, *Lupus* 6:96, 1997.
45. Peter JB, Reyes HR: *Use and interpretation of tests in rheumatology,* Santa Monica, 1996, Specialty Laboratories.
46. Lefkowith JB, Gilkeson GS: Nephritogenic autoantibodies in lupus, *Arthritis Rheum* 39:6, 1996.
47. Panush RS, Schur PH: Is it lupus? *Bull Rheum Dis* 46:6, 1997.
48. Sanchez-Guerrero J and others: Utility of anti-SM, anti-RNP, anti-Ro/SS-A and anti-La/SS-B (extractable nuclear antigens) detected by enzyme-linked immunosorbent assay for the diagnosis of systemic lupus erythematosus, *Arthritis Rheum* 39:6, 1996.
49. Levy GD and others: Incidence of hydroxychloroquine retinopathy in 1207 patients in a large multicenter outpatient practice, *Arthritis Rheum* 40:8, 1997.
50. Wallace DJ, Metzger AL: Systemic lupus erythematosus. In Koopman WJ, editor: *Arthritis and allied conditions,* ed 13, Baltimore, 1997, Williams & Wilkins.
51. Failla S and others: Adjustment of women with systemic lupus erythematosus, *Appl Nurs Res* 9:2, 1996.
52. Kostyak LR: Systemic lupus erythematosus. In Goreczny AJ, editor: *Handbook of health and rehabilitation psychology,* New York, 1995, Plenum Press.
53. Mitchell H, Bolster MB, LeRoy EC: Scleroderma and related conditions, *Med Clin North Am* 81:1, 1997.
54. Seibold JR: Connective tissue diseases characterized by fibrosis. In Kelley WN and others, editors: *Textbook of rheumatology,* ed 5, Philadelphia, 1997, Saunders.
55. Casale R, Buonocore M, Matucci-Cerinic M: Systemic sclerosis (scleroderma): an integrated challenge in rehabilitation, *Arch Phys Med Rehab* 78:7, 1997.
56. Pope J: Treatment of systemic sclerosis, *Rheum Dis Clin North Am* 22:893, 1996.
57. Kremer JM: Nutrition and rheumatic diseases. In Kelley WN and others, editors: *Textbook of rheumatology,* ed 5, Philadelphia, 1997, Saunders.
58. Dale KG: Intimacy and rheumatic diseases, *Rehabil Nurs* 21:1, 1996.
59. Wortmann RL: Inflammatory diseases of muscle and other myopathies. In Kelley WN and others, editors: *Textbook of rheumatology,* ed 5, Philadelphia, 1997, Saunders.
60. Vazquez-Abad D, Rothfield NF: Sensitivity and specificity of anti-Jo-1 antibodies in autoimmune diseases with myositis, *Arthritis Rheum* 39:2, 1996.
61. Manthorpe R, Asmussen K, Oxholm P: Primary Sjögren's syndrome: diagnostic criteria, clinical features, and disease activity, *J Rheumatol Suppl* 24:50, 1997.
62. Boisset-Pioro MH, Esdaile JM, Fitzcharles MA: Sexual and physical abuse in women with fibromyalgia syndrome, *Arthritis Rheum* 38:2, 1995.
63. Gordon S, Morrison C: Fibromyalgia and its primary care implications, *Medsurg Nurs* 7:207, 1998.
64. Wolfe F and others: The prevalence and characteristics of fibromyalgia in the general population, *Arthritis Rheum* 38:19, 1995.
65. Yunus MB: Fibromyalgia syndrome: blueprint for a reliable diagnosis, *Consultant* 36:1260, 1996.
66. Brewster N, Lewis P: Joint replacement for arthritis, *Aust Fam Physician* 27:21, 1998.
67. Enloe LF and others: Total hip and knee replacement treatment programs: a report using consensus, *J Orthop Sports Phys Ther* 23:3, 1996.

Resources

Arthritis Foundation
1330 West Peachtree Street
Atlanta, GA 30309
404-872-7100
800-283-7800
http://www.arthritis.org/

Association of Rheumatology Health Professionals
American College of Rheumatology
1800 Century Place, Suite 250
Atlanta, GA 30345
404-633-3777
Fax: 404-633-1870
http://www.rheumatology.org/arhp/

Lupus Foundation of America, Inc.
1300 Piccard Drive, Suite 200
Rockville, MD 20850-4303
301-670-9292
800-558-0121
http://internet-plaza.net/lupus/

National Arthritis and Musculoskeletal and Skin Diseases
Information Clearinghouse
National Institutes of Health
1 AMS Circle
Bethesda, MD 20892-3675
301-495-4484
Fax: 301-587-4352
http://www.nih.gov/niams/healthinfo/info.htm

Scleroderma Foundation, Inc.
89 Newbury Street, Suite 201
Danvers, MA 01923
978-750-4499
800-722-HOPE
Fax: 978-750-9902
http://www.scleroderma.org/

Scleroderma International Foundation
1725 York Avenue, #29F
New York, NY 10128
212-427-7040

Scleroderma Research Foundation
Pueblo Medical Commons
2320 Bath Street, Suite 307
Santa Barbara, CA 93105
800-441-CURE
http://www.srfcure.org/

Spondylitis Association of America
511 N. La Cienega, Suite 216
Los Angeles, CA 90048
800-777-8189
http://www.spondylitis.org/jas.htm

United Scleroderma Foundation
PO Box 399
Watsonville, CA 95077
800-722-4673
408-728-2202

***For additional Internet resources, see the website for this book at* www.mosby.com/MERLIN/medsurg_lewis**

SECTION

12

NURSING CARE IN SPECIALIZED SETTINGS

SECTION OUTLINE

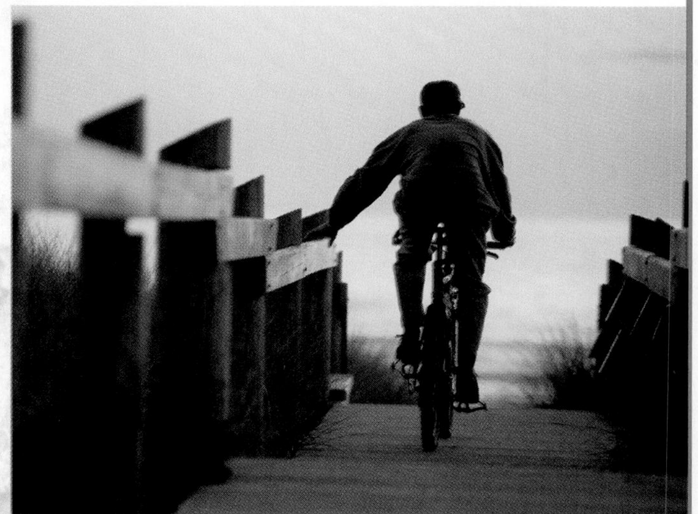

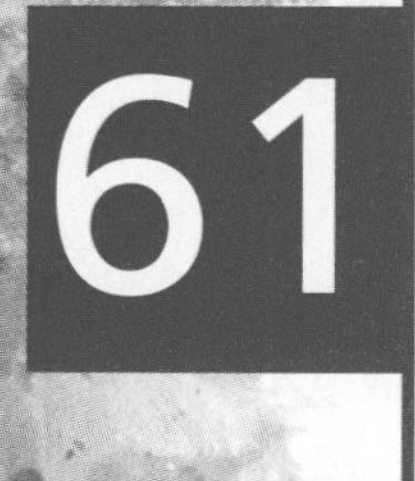

REMEMBER to check out your companion CD-ROM

61 NURSING MANAGEMENT Shock and Multiple Organ Dysfunction Syndrome

Julie M. Dax & Cynthia L. Hermey

www.mosby.com/MERLIN/medsurg_lewis

LEARNING OBJECTIVES

1. Define shock.
2. Differentiate among the three major classifications of shock in relationship to cause and precipitating factors.
3. Describe the pathophysiology and clinical manifestations of shock, systemic inflammatory response syndrome, and multiple organ dysfunction syndrome.
4. Describe the effects of shock, systemic inflammatory response syndrome, and multiple organ dysfunction syndrome on the major body systems.
5. Compare the collaborative care, drug therapy, and nursing management of patients with the different types of shock.
6. Discuss the nursing management of the patient with multiple organ dysfunction syndrome.

Shock, systemic inflammatory response syndrome (SIRS), and multiple organ dysfunction syndrome (MODS) are serious and interrelated complications. Shock is a complex pathophysiologic process that often leads to the development of SIRS and MODS (Fig. 61-1). This chapter provides a comprehensive overview of shock and then a discussion of SIRS and MODS.

SHOCK

Shock is a clinical syndrome characterized by an inadequate supply of oxygen and nutrients to cells from impaired tissue perfusion. Shock has many signs and symptoms and may be precipitated by a variety of etiologic factors. Although the cause and initial presentation of various types of shock differ, the physiologic responses to cellular hypoxia are the same, leading to the same sequence of events if shock is not recognized and treated early.[1] The challenge is to recognize early manifestations of impending shock and intervene quickly and appropriately to prevent further progression to MODS or death.

It is important to note that shock cannot be defined solely in terms of hypotension, because shock may be manifested in the absence of hypotension. Conversely, hypotension may occur in the absence of shock.

The morbidity and mortality rates associated with shock are extremely difficult to determine. It is estimated that the financial impact of patients in shock is between 10 and 20 billion dollars annually. For all types of shock, older adults have a greater mortality rate than younger adults. Sepsis has increased by 137% in the last decade and is the thirteenth leading cause of death, the tenth leading cause of death in the elderly, and the most common cause of death in critical care units. The mortality rate related to sepsis remains between 40% and 60%. It is predicted that the incidence and mortality rate of sepsis will continue to increase over the coming years as more immunocompromised patients enter the health care system.[2,3]

Although the intensive care unit (ICU) may be the only environment where a critically ill patient can be sustained, it is an environment in which there is a high risk for infection and an increasing prevalence of multidrug-resistant microorganisms. It is a major nursing responsibility to institute the highest standards of asepsis in caring for patients who are vulnerable to infection, especially immunocompromised patients.

CLASSIFICATION OF SHOCK

Although there have been many attempts to classify shock, none has been totally satisfactory. Table 61-1 presents one classification system that lists common types of shock and precipitating factors. This classification is based on the three primary mechanisms responsible for adequate circulation: (1) vascular tone (distributive shock), (2) the ability of the heart to pump (cardiogenic shock), and (3) intravascular volume (hypovolemic shock). In all shock states, the etiology should be considered because each shock state has its own specific causes. Patients may have more than one form of shock simultaneously. For example, hypovolemic shock and septic shock may coexist. Table 61-2 compares the hemodynamic effects of the three types of shock. (Hemodynamic monitoring is discussed in Chapter 63.)

Reviewed by Rebecca Fruge, RN, MN, Clinical Nurse Specialist and Coordinator, English Trimester Nursing Program, InterAmerican University–Metropolitan Campus, San Juan, Puerto Rico; and Susan B. Stillwell, RN, MSN, Clinical Associate Professor, College of Nursing, Arizona State University, Tempe, Ariz.

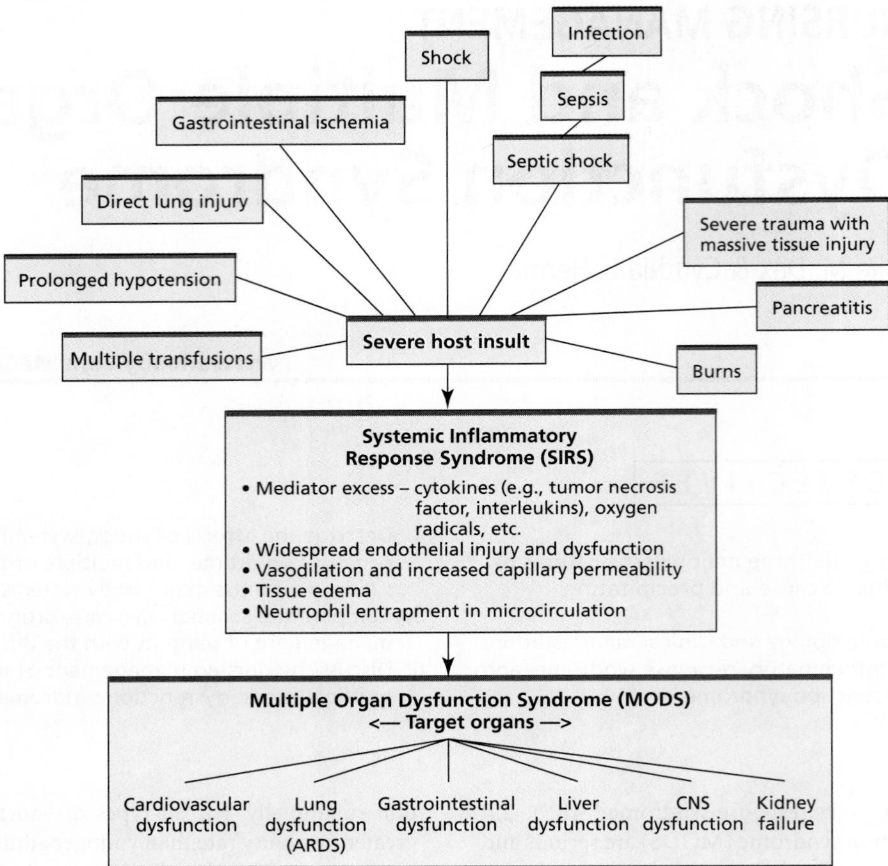

Fig. 61-1 Relationship of shock, systemic inflammatory response syndrome, and multiple organ dysfunction syndrome. *ARDS,* acute respiratory distress syndrome; *CNS,* central nervous system.

Table 61-1 Classification and Precipitating Factors of Shock

Distributive Shock

Neurogenic Shock
- Injury and disease to the spinal cord at or above T_6
- Spinal anesthesia, deep general anesthesia, or epidural block
- Vasomotor center depression (severe pain, drugs, hypoglycemia)

Septic Shock
- Infection (urinary tract, respiratory tract, septic abortion, postpartum, invasive procedures [especially urologic procedures], and indwelling lines and catheters)
- At-risk patients: older adults, patients with chronic diseases (diabetes, cancer, HIV/AIDS), patients receiving immunosuppressive therapy, malnourished or debilitated patients

Anaphylactic Shock
- Contrast media
- Drugs (especially antimicrobials)
- Insect bites/stings
- Anesthetic agents
- Foods/food additives
- Vaccines
- Environmental agents (pet dander, molds, pollens)

Hypovolemic Shock

Absolute Hypovolemia
- Loss of whole blood (hemorrhage from trauma or surgery, GI bleeding)
- Loss of plasma (burn injuries)
- Loss of other body fluids (vomiting, diarrhea, excessive use of diuretics or laxatives, diaphoresis, diabetes insipidus, diabetic ketoacidosis)

Relative Hypovolemia
- Pooling of blood (ascites, peritonitis, bowel obstruction)
- Internal bleeding (fracture of long bones, ruptured spleen, hemothorax, severe pancreatitis, femoral arterial punctures, or catheters in patients on anticoagulant therapy)
- Massive vasodilation (as can occur in conditions that cause distributive shock)

Cardiogenic Shock
- Primary ventricular dysfunction (acute myocardial infarction, cardiac surgery)
- Arrhythmias
- Structural problems (septal rupture, papillary muscle rupture, ventricular aneurysm, cardiomyopathy)
- Obstructive causes (pericardial tamponade, pericardial diseases, tension pneumothorax, acute valvular damage, pulmonary embolism)

AIDS, acquired immunodeficiency syndrome; *HIV,* human immunodeficiency virus.

Table 61-2 Hemodynamic Effects of Shock, Systemic Inflammatory Response Syndrome, and Multiple Organ Dysfunction Syndrome

Type	HR	Pulse Pressure	BP	SVR	PVR	CVP	PAP	PAWP	CO	SvO_2
Hypovolemic shock	↑	↓	↓	↑	↑	↓	↓	↓	↓	↓
Cardiogenic shock	↑	↓	↓	↑	↑	≈ ↑	↑	↑	↓	↓
Anaphylactic shock	↑	↓	↓	↓	≈ ↑	↓	↓	↓	↓	↓
Neurogenic shock	↓	↓	↓	↓	≈	↓	↓	↓	↓	↓
Septic shock	↑	↓	↓	↓	≈ ↑	↓	↑ ≈ ↓	↓	↑	↑ ≈ ↓
SIRS	↑	≈	≈	↓	≈ ↑	↓	↑ ≈ ↓	↓	↑	↑ ≈ ↓
MODS	↑	≈	≈	↓	↑	↓	↑ ≈ ↓	↓ ≈ ↑	↓	↑

KEY: ↓ decrease; ↑ increase; ≈ no change.
NOTE: Hemodynamic effects in some illnesses are quite variable. The hemodynamic findings in MODS depend on the system failing.
BP, blood pressure; *CO,* cardiac output; *CVP,* central venous pressure; *HR,* heart rate; *MODS,* multiple organ dysfunction syndrome; *PAP,* pulmonary artery pressure; *PAWP,* pulmonary artery wedge pressure; *PVR,* pulmonary vascular resistance; *SIRS,* systemic inflammatory response syndrome; *SvO_2,* mixed venous oxygen saturation; *SVR,* systemic vascular resistance.

Distributive Shock

Distributive shock includes three types of shock: neurogenic, septic, and anaphylactic. In distributive shock, relative hypovolemia occurs when vasodilation increases the size of the vascular space and results in altered distribution of the blood volume rather than actual loss of volume. This type of shock is often complicated by loss of intravascular fluid from increased capillary permeability, resulting in decreased blood flow to tissues. In distributive shock, there is no change in the blood volume but rather a decrease in the vascular tone.

Neurogenic Shock. Neurogenic shock is caused by massive vasodilation without compensation as a result of impairment of autonomic nervous system function and loss of sympathetic vasoconstrictor tone in the vascular smooth muscle. This massive vasodilation causes pooling of the blood in the venous vasculature, decreased venous return to the heart, decreased cardiac output (CO), and eventually inadequate tissue perfusion (Fig. 61-2). Typically, the patient with neurogenic shock has hypotension and bradycardia. Hypotension is the result of the vasodilation, and the decreased heart rate (HR) is caused by the increased vagal tone from the now unopposed parasympathetic nervous system.

Several precipitating factors can lead to neurogenic shock (see Table 61-1). Disease or injury to the spinal cord above or at the T6 level is the most common cause because transmission of sympathetic nerve impulses to peripheral blood vessels is interrupted. After spinal cord injury, neurogenic shock (sometimes called spinal shock) can last from hours to weeks. (Spinal shock is discussed in Chapter 57.)

Spinal anesthesia can also block the transmission of impulses from the sympathetic nervous system. Depression of the vasomotor center of the medulla as a result of drugs can also decrease vasoconstrictor tone of peripheral blood vessels.

Septic Shock. The definitions and clinical indicators related to the septic-SIRS continuum are presented in Table 61-3. Bacteria, fungi, parasites, viruses, and other causes may cause infection leading to sepsis. Sepsis is SIRS caused by an infection; SIRS is a systemic inflammatory response to a variety of causes, including burn injury, trauma, and pancreatitis (see Fig. 61-1). Severe sepsis is sepsis that is accompanied by organ dysfunction. Septic shock is sepsis with hypotension despite adequate fluid resuscitation.[4]

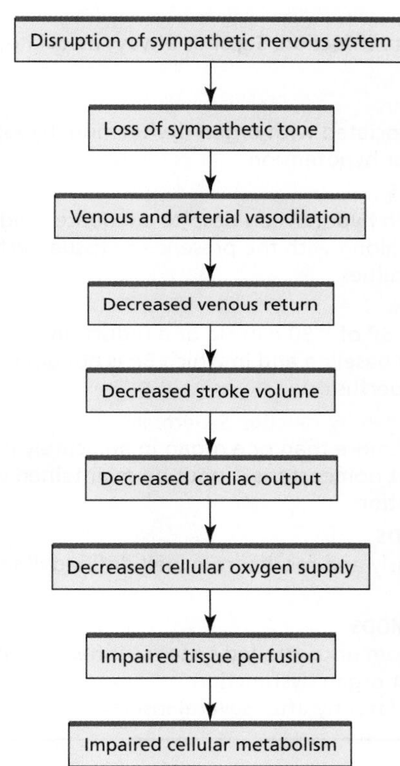

Fig. 61-2 The pathophysiology of neurogenic shock.

Sepsis is most commonly caused by gram-negative bacteria but is increasingly occurring secondary to staphylococcal, streptococcal, fungal, and protozoan infections. Toxic shock syndrome is an example of gram-positive shock resulting from *Staphylococcus aureus.* (Toxic shock syndrome is discussed in Chapter 51.) Causes of septic shock are listed in Table 61-1.

Gram-negative bacteria are responsible for more than one half of the cases of septic shock.[5] When gram-negative bacteremia occurs, endotoxin, a component of the gram-negative bacteria cell wall, triggers a cascade of host inflammatory responses that produce the major detrimental effects seen in

Table 61-3 Definitions of Terms Related to Sepsis and Organ Failure

Infection
Disease caused by invasion of body by pathogenic organisms.

Bacteremia
Presence of viable bacteria in the blood. Demonstrated by positive blood culture.

Systemic Inflammatory Response Syndrome (SIRS)
Systemic inflammatory response to a variety of insults. Manifested by two or more of the following:
- Temperature >100.4° F (38° C) or <97° F (36° C)
- Heart rate >90 beats/min
- Respiratory rate >20 breaths/min or $PaCO_2$ <32 mm Hg
- White blood cell count >12,000 cells/μl or <4000 cells/μl or >10% immature (band) neutrophils

Sepsis
SIRS due to infection. Sepsis is always associated with SIRS.

Severe Sepsis
Sepsis associated with organ dysfunction, hypoperfusion, or hypotension.

Septic Shock
Sepsis with hypotension despite adequate fluid resuscitation along with the presence of tissue perfusion abnormalities.

Hypotension
A systolic BP of <90 mm Hg or a reduction of >40 mm Hg from baseline and in which BP is not adequate for normal perfusion.

Multiple Organ Dysfunction Syndrome
Failure of more than one organ in an acutely ill patient such that homeostasis cannot be maintained without intervention.

Primary MODS
Occurs early and results from well-defined illness or injury.

Secondary MODS
Results from uncontrolled systemic inflammation with resultant organ dysfunction.
Develops latently after several insults.

sepsis. (A comparable cell-wall substance from gram-positive bacteria or fungi can similarly trigger this cascade.[2]) When endotoxin binds to monocytes and macrophages, it stimulates the release of mediators, including tumor necrosis factor (TNF) and interleukin-1 (IL-1). These mediators stimulate the release or activation of other mediators, including platelet-activating factor (PAF), prostaglandins, leukotrienes, thromboxane A_2, kinins, and complement[6] (Table 61-4). These factors are responsible for widespread vasodilation and increased capillary permeability, resulting in decreased systemic vascular resistance (SVR) and normal or high CO because of the decreased peripheral resistance (Fig. 61-3). Endotoxins cause the release of histamine, which results in increased capillary permeability and further decreases circulating blood volume.[7]

Myocardial depressant factor works together with TNF, PAF, and other mediators to suppress myocardial contractility. Myocardial depression is almost always present despite an initial rise in CO.

The clinical presentation of septic shock is often subtle, especially in the older, debilitated, or malnourished patient. The blood pressure (BP) is usually low, but the skin is warm and dry because of the vasodilation. In the early stage of septic shock, the patient may have urine output of up to 100 ml/hr.

The survivors of septic shock typically have resolved their high CO and low SVR in the first 24 hours. Cardiovascular parameters that are associated with a high mortality rate include persistent elevation in both HR and CO with low SVR and refractory hypotension for more than 24 hours.

Septic shock is more common among older persons, who often have debilitating chronic diseases and weakened immune systems. The increased longevity of patients with complex, chronic diseases has increased the number of patients who are at risk for developing severe infection and subsequent complications. The rise in the incidence of sepsis is largely due to advances in health care and technology and the rise in the number of immunocompromised patients.

Anaphylactic Shock. Anaphylactic shock is an acute and life-threatening allergic reaction. It is an immediate hypersensitivity reaction that causes massive vasodilation and increased capillary permeability, causing microvascular leakage throughout the body. Anaphylactic shock can lead to respiratory failure, as a result of laryngeal edema or severe bronchospasm, and circulatory failure, as a result of massive vasodilation.[8] (Anaphylactic shock is discussed in Chapter 12.) Generally, the severity of an anaphylactic reaction is directly related to how rapid the onset of symptoms occurs.

A patient can develop a severe allergic reaction, possibly leading to anaphylactic shock, after ingesting or being injected with an antigen to which the person has previously been sensitized. Parenteral administration of an antigen is the route most likely to cause anaphylaxis. However, oral, topical, and inhalation routes of administration of an antigen have been known to cause anaphylactic reactions. Examples of substances that can cause anaphylactic shock are listed in Table 61-1.

Hypovolemic Shock

Hypovolemic shock occurs when there is a loss of intravascular fluid volume. In hypovolemic shock the volume is inadequate to fill the vascular space. Loss of intravascular volume can be divided into absolute causes and relative causes (see Table 61-1). The external loss of fluid from the body is defined as *absolute hypovolemia.* Internal fluid shifting from the intravascular to the extravascular space (interstitial, intracellular, or cavitary space) is defined as *relative hypovolemia.*

In hypovolemic shock the vascular compartment has not changed, but the volume of blood or plasma has decreased. Loss of fluid results in decreased venous return to the heart, decreased stroke volume, decreased CO, circulatory insufficiency, and eventually inadequate tissue perfusion (Fig. 61-4). In hypovolemic shock there is no decrease in the pumping ability of the heart or dilation of the vascular space. The fluid that is lost may be either whole blood, plasma, or water and electrolytes.

In relative hypovolemia, fluid has not left the body, but has shifted out of the intravascular space and is unavailable for cir-

Table 61-4 Mediators of Sepsis, Systemic Inflammatory Response Syndrome, and Multiple Organ Dysfunction Syndrome

Mediator	Action
Endotoxin (component of gram-negative bacterial cell wall)	Stimulation of monocytes, macrophages, and neutrophils to produce cytokines
Interleukin-1	Vasodilation, increased capillary permeability
Tumor necrosis factor	Endothelial injury, vasodilation, increased capillary permeability
Hageman factor	Activation of intrinsic clotting system
Prekallikrein	Production of bradykinin
Bradykinin	Vasodilation, increased capillary permeability, leukocyte chemotaxis
Complement components C3a, C5a	Neutrophil aggregation, release of toxic oxygen radicals, histamine release, vasodilation, increased capillary permeability
Prostaglandins	Vasodilation, decreased platelet aggregation
Platelet activating factor	Platelet aggregation with resultant microvascular stasis; decreased renal perfusion, decreased coronary blood flow, decreased cardiac output
Histamine	Vasodilation, increased capillary permeability
Catecholamines	Inotropic stimulation; altered regional blood flow; increased blood glucose
Cortisol	Gluconeogenesis, hyperglycemia
Myocardial depressant factor	Decreased cardiac contractility and output

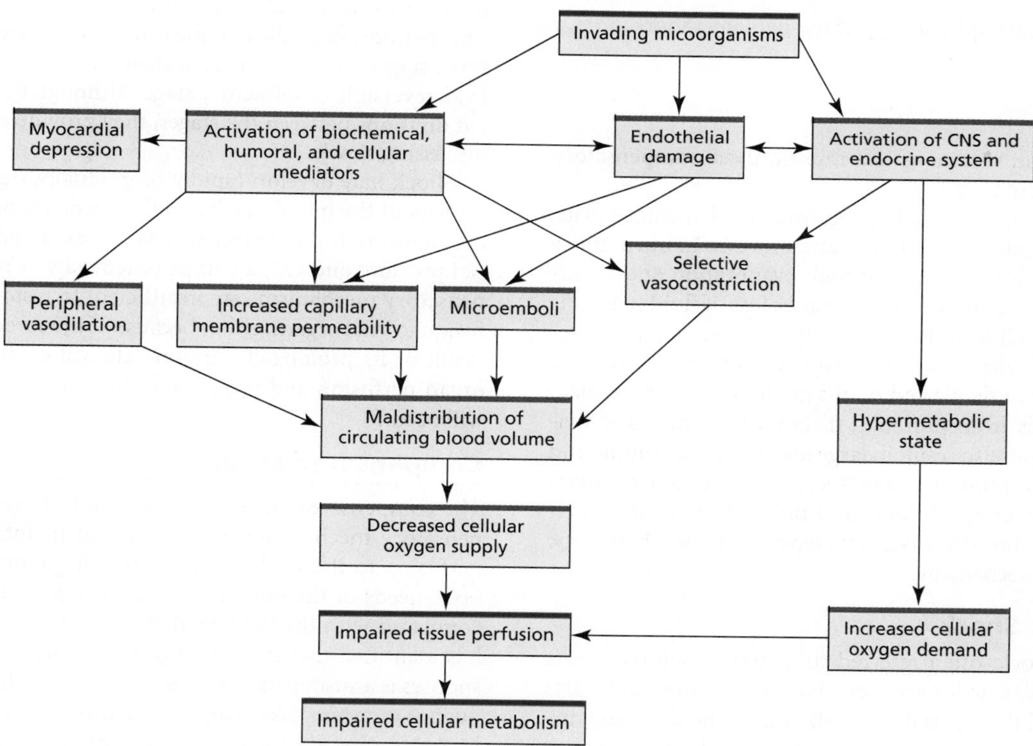

Fig. 61-3 The pathophysiology of septic shock.

culation. Increased capillary permeability can cause pooling of fluid in the interstitial or intracavitary spaces (third spacing). This loss of fluid from the intravascular space causes increased viscosity of the blood and sludging of blood components (microsludging). This, in turn, can block capillaries and venous return, as well as contribute to an increased SVR and decreased tissue perfusion. In addition, the loss of intravascular volume will decrease venous return to the heart and cardiac output.

The most common cause of absolute hypovolemia is hemorrhage (an excessive loss of whole blood). The amount of blood loss that results in shock depends on the efficiency of a person's compensatory mechanisms and the rapidity of blood loss. A healthy adult can compensate for a sudden loss of up to 15% (750 ml in a 70 kg man, 500 ml in a 60 kg woman) of the total blood volume, primarily using sympathetic nervous system–mediated vasoconstriction. However, if greater than

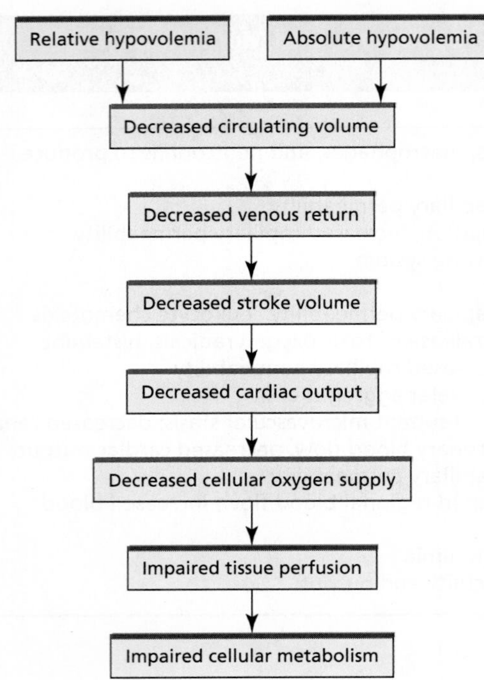

Fig. 61-4 The pathophysiology of hypovolemic shock.

15% of the blood volume is lost rapidly, these compensatory mechanisms begin to fail.

Other common causes of hypovolemic shock include burns, loss of gastrointestinal (GI) fluids, and diuresis. In burn injury there is a direct loss of fluid through evaporation and an increased capillary permeability that causes loss of fluid to the interstitial spaces. GI fluid losses usually occur secondary to severe vomiting, diarrhea, or excessive drainage from a nasogastric tube or fistula and results in a loss of water and electrolytes. Diuresis from diuretics, diabetes insipidus, and diabetes mellitus may also result in large losses of fluid volume and electrolytes. Susceptibility to shock as a result of these factors is generally related to age. Infants and the elderly are at highest risk because of the decreased efficiency of their physiologic compensatory mechanisms.

Cardiogenic Shock

Cardiogenic shock, often referred to as pump failure, occurs when the heart can no longer pump blood efficiently to all parts of the body and the CO is decreased. There is no decreased intravascular volume or vasodilation. Conversely, the vascular space vasoconstricts and further decreases the CO.

Cardiogenic shock is usually the result of left ventricular dysfunction. However, the right ventricle can also be involved. Damage to the ventricles, especially the left, results in failure of the pumping chambers and blood backs up. In right ventricular dysfunction, blood is backed up into the systemic circulation. Left ventricular dysfunction (1) results in decreased cardiac output to the systemic circulation and (2) causes blood to back up into the pulmonary circulation, resulting in pulmonary congestion (Fig. 61-5). A vicious cycle develops as the SVR increases in response to the decreased CO. The failing heart now has to pump harder against a higher systemic resistance.

The most common cause of cardiogenic shock is an acute myocardial infarction (MI). Cardiogenic shock occurs when at least 40% of the left ventricular myocardium has been damaged by infarction.[5] This damage to the myocardium can occur after one massive MI, or it may be cumulative as a result of several smaller MIs occurring over a period of time. With the infarcted muscle, there is a decrease in myocardial compliance and therefore a decrease in contractility. Thus decreased functioning of the left ventricle occurs, as evidenced by decreased CO and BP. There is then less arterial pressure to perfuse the coronary arteries. This continued decrease in coronary perfusion causes increased ischemia of the myocardium, leading to a larger infarction, less contractility, arrhythmias, and metabolic acidosis. These conditions further reduce the effective functioning of the left ventricle.

Other causes of cardiogenic shock are listed in Table 61-1. Regardless of the cause, the extent of pump failure depends on the degree of heart muscle impairment and the adequacy of compensatory mechanisms.

STAGES OF SHOCK

Shock is a dynamic event in which several different processes may be occurring at the same time. In addition, the patient may progress toward death or toward recovery over widely varying time periods. Regardless of the cause, shock can be divided into three stages: (1) compensated stage, (2) progressive stage, and (3) irreversible or refractory stage. Although there are no clear-cut divisions between the stages, they provide a framework for discussing shock.

Shock may develop rapidly or gradually, depending on the severity of the initial insult and the adequacy of compensatory mechanisms. If these mechanisms can maintain adequate arterial pressure and CO, a compensated stage is reached. If compensatory mechanisms are insufficient to restore effective perfusion to vital organs, either because of the severity of the initial insult or its prolonged duration, clinical evidence of reduced organ perfusion and progression through the stages of shock will occur.[9]

Compensated Stage

The compensated stage is the reversible stage in which compensatory mechanisms are effective in maintaining adequate perfusion to the vital organs. In this stage, most of the metabolic needs of the body continue to be met. The stage can be compared with the fight-or-flight response in which the body has identified that it is in danger. The end result of these responses is a sustained stress response. The pathophysiologic sequence of events occurring during this stage is detailed in Fig. 61-6. If promptly treated, the patient will recover with no or minimal organ damage.

Pathophysiology

Regardless of the cause of shock, the body attempts to compensate for a decrease in tissue perfusion in a variety of ways. First, a reduction in mean arterial pressure will inhibit baroreceptor activity, resulting in stimulation of the vasomotor center in the medulla, causing activation of the sympathetic nervous system and release of epinephrine from the medulla and norepinephrine from nerve endings. Stimulation of alpha-adrenergic receptors causes selective peripheral vasoconstriction. Blood flow to the heart and brain is maintained, and blood flow to the

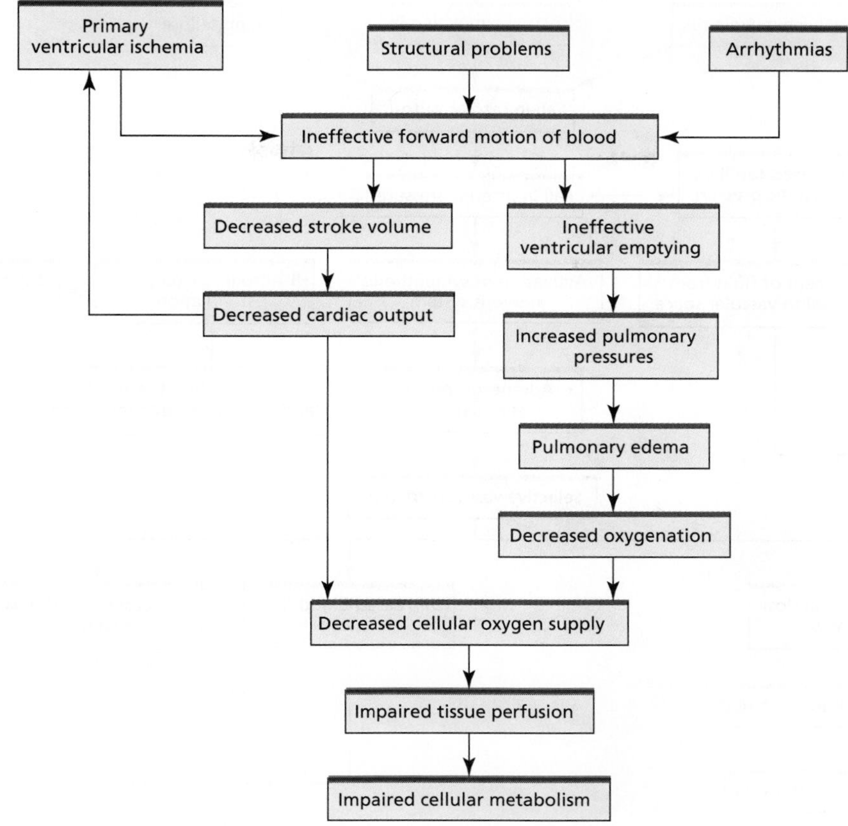

Fig. 61-5 The pathophysiology of cardiogenic shock.

kidneys, GI tract, lungs, muscles, and skin is decreased. Beta-adrenergic receptor stimulation causes a mild increase in HR and force of myocardial contraction, resulting in increased CO. This sympathetic stimulation also causes dilation of the coronary arteries, increasing the O_2 delivery to the myocardium, which now has an increased oxygen demand from the increase in heart rate and contractility.

The decrease in blood flow to the kidneys stimulates the release of renin into the blood where it activates angiotensinogen to produce angiotensin I, which is then converted to angiotensin II (see Fig. 42-6). Angiotensin is a strong vasoconstrictor, causing arterial and venous constriction. The net result is increased venous return to the heart and an increase in BP. Angiotensin also stimulates the adrenal cortex to release aldosterone, which results in sodium reabsorption by the kidneys. The increased sodium raises the serum osmolarity and stimulates the release of antidiuretic hormone (ADH). (ADH is also released when there is decreased blood flow to the posterior pituitary.) The action of ADH results in increased water reabsorption by the kidneys, increased blood volume, and increased venous return to the heart.

A decrease in arterial pressure also causes a similar decrease in capillary hydrostatic pressure. When the hydrostatic pressure no longer exceeds the colloidal osmotic pressure, fluid moves from the interstitial space to the intravascular space. This fluid shift may add sufficient volume to the vascular space to maintain normal arterial pressure without the aid of other compensatory mechanisms.

Venous return is increased by the combination of vasoconstriction and hormonal changes. Increased venous return, as well as increased HR and myocardial contractility, results in increased CO, maintenance of BP, and adequate tissue perfusion.

Clinical Manifestations

The clinical manifestations of the compensated stage of shock may be subtle and can be easily overlooked (Table 61-5). One of the most reliable signs of the compensatory stage is the patient's level of consciousness. Subtle changes in sensorium, usually in the form of restlessness, irritability, or apprehension, are frequently observed and are probably caused by hypoxia of brain cells. Sedation at this time may be contraindicated because it may mask important neurologic signs.

During this stage, the resting supine BP may be slightly decreased or normal for the patient. For this reason, the BP may not be a useful indicator at this stage. However, a narrowing of the pulse pressure (difference between systolic and diastolic blood pressure) is a classic sign of compensatory shock. Orthostatic hypotension (a decrease in systolic BP of at least 15 mm Hg when a patient is raised from a flat position to an upright, sitting position [90 degrees]) is significant and indicates absolute or relative volume depletion.

The heart rate in the compensatory stage is moderately increased. The pulse is likely to be bounding (in septic shock) or thready because of peripheral vasoconstriction. Respirations increase in rate and depth in an attempt to compensate for decreased cardiac output, resulting in respiratory alkalosis. Urine output may begin to decrease because of reduced renal perfusion and the action of ADH. Because of extravascular volume depletion and decreased secretion of saliva secondary to peripheral vasoconstriction, the patient may complain of thirst.

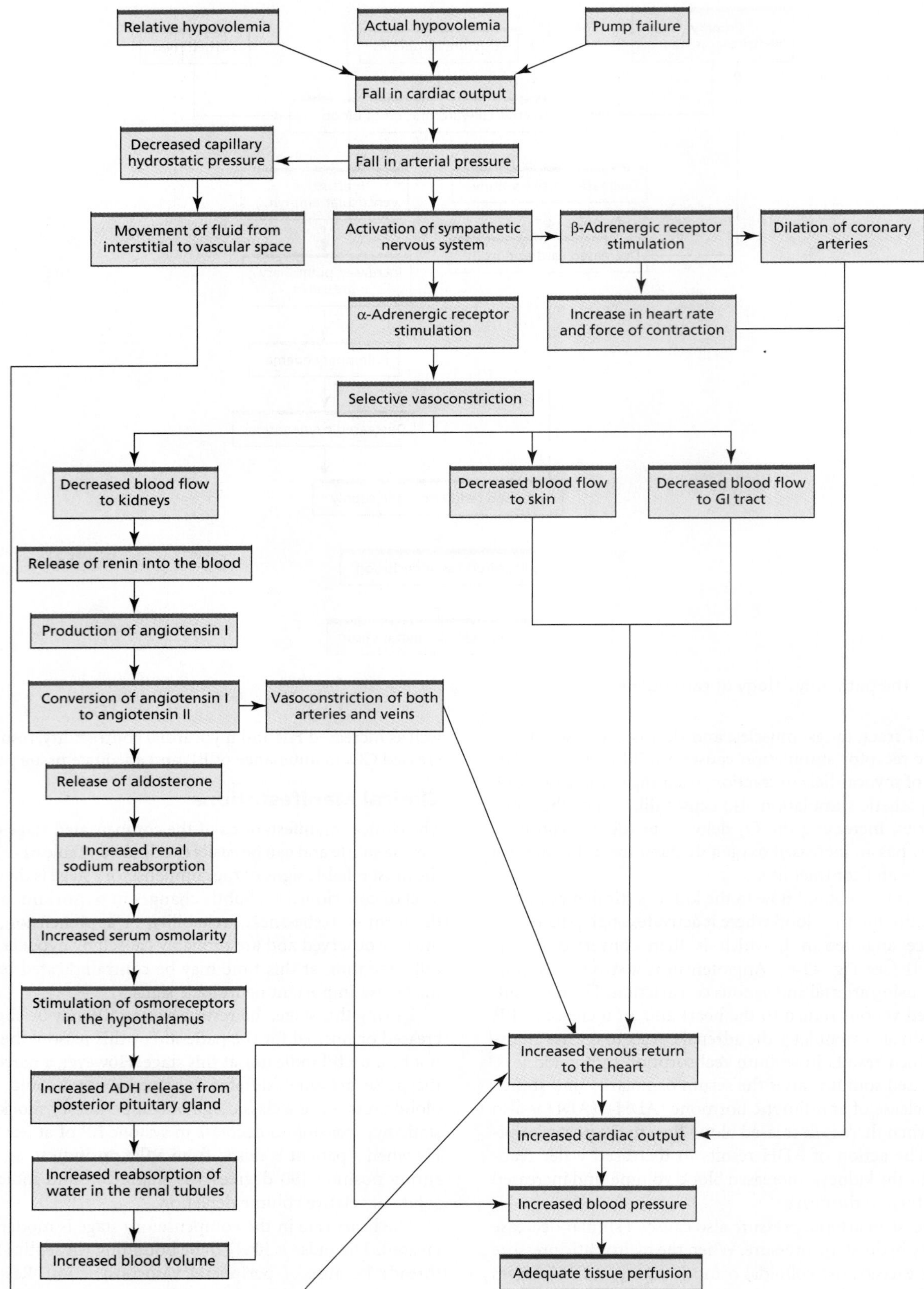

Fig. 61-6 Compensated stage: reversible stage during which compensatory mechanisms are effective and homeostasis is maintained.

Table 61-5 Clinical Manifestations Correlated with Stage of Shock

Clinical Manifestations	Compensated Stage	Progressive Stage	Irreversible or Refractory Stage
Neurologic Status			
Level of consciousness	Restlessness, irritability, and apprehension	Listlessness or agitation; apathy, confusion, alteration or decrease in response to painful stimuli	Unconsciousness, absent reflexes likely
Orientation	Oriented, verbal	Orientation possible, slowed speech	Confusion and disorientation with slurred, incoherent speech
Cardiovascular Status			
Heart rate	Increased (20 beats/min above patient's normal)	Tachycardia (rate of >100 beats/min), often irregular	Slow and irregular
Peripheral pulses	Bounding (septic shock) or thready	Weak, thready, may be absent	Absent
Blood Pressure			
Systolic	Normal or slight decrease	Hypotension <90 mm Hg with decrease in pulse pressure	Falling to unobtainable
Diastolic	Normal or slight increase	Falling	Approaching zero
Respiratory Status			
Rate	Greater than patient's normal rate	Rapid (>20/min)	Slow
Depth	Deeper than normal	Shallow	Shallow with irregular rhythm such as Cheyne-Stokes or Biot's respirations
Renal Status			
Urine output	Slight decrease but within normal limits	Oliguria (<0.5 ml/kg/hr) with increase in specific gravity	≤18 ml/hr, progressing to anuria with proteinuria
General Status			
Appearance of skin	Pale and cool (warm and flushed in septic shock)	Cold and clammy, cyanosis possible	Cold, clammy, cyanotic, and mottled
Body temperature	Decrease, normal, or increase	Usually subnormal (subnormal or elevated in sepsis)	Significant decrease
Degree of thirst	Normal or slight increase	Marked increase	Severe increase if patient conscious
Bowel sounds	Normal or hypoactive	Hypoactive or absent	Absent

The skin will be cool and pale (except in sepsis where the skin may be warm and dry). Bowel sounds will often be hypoactive because of decreased peristalsis, and abdominal distention can occur.

Associated with the sympathetic nervous system response is the secretion of large amounts of catecholamines from the adrenal medulla. Catecholamines enhance the cellular metabolism of the brain and heart. Catecholamines also stimulate the liver to undergo glycogenolysis, releasing its glycogen stores in the form of glucose. In addition, the pancreatic release of insulin is suppressed. Therefore the brain, which does not require insulin for glucose utilization, has large quantities of glucose available for metabolism.

Progressive Stage

During the progressive stage of shock, compensatory mechanisms are becoming ineffective and may even be detrimental to the patient. The pathophysiologic sequence of events occurring during this stage is outlined in Fig. 61-7. Aggressive management is necessary at this stage to reverse the shock state. Impaired cell function, altered capillary dynamics, and altered systemic circulation are the hallmarks of this stage.

Pathophysiology

When shock is not detected and the precipitating cause is not corrected during the earlier stages, a massive sympathetic nervous system response occurs. Profound vasoconstriction of most vascular beds occurs with some peripheral vessels possibly becoming totally occluded. Renal ischemia leads to further activation of the renin-angiotensin mechanism, causing even more pronounced vasoconstriction. Despite the attempt of the body to increase CO by increasing the heart rate and myocardial contractility, there is a net decrease in CO. This decreased CO and profound peripheral vasoconstriction lead to tissue hypoxia, which causes the cells to undergo anaerobic metabolism. A by-product of anaerobic cellular metabolism is lactic acid production. Metabolic acidosis results from the accumulation of lactic acid and impaired renal excretion of acids. As the shock state progresses, the rise in the lactic acid level will often correlate with the severity of the shock state. Severe acidosis (pH less

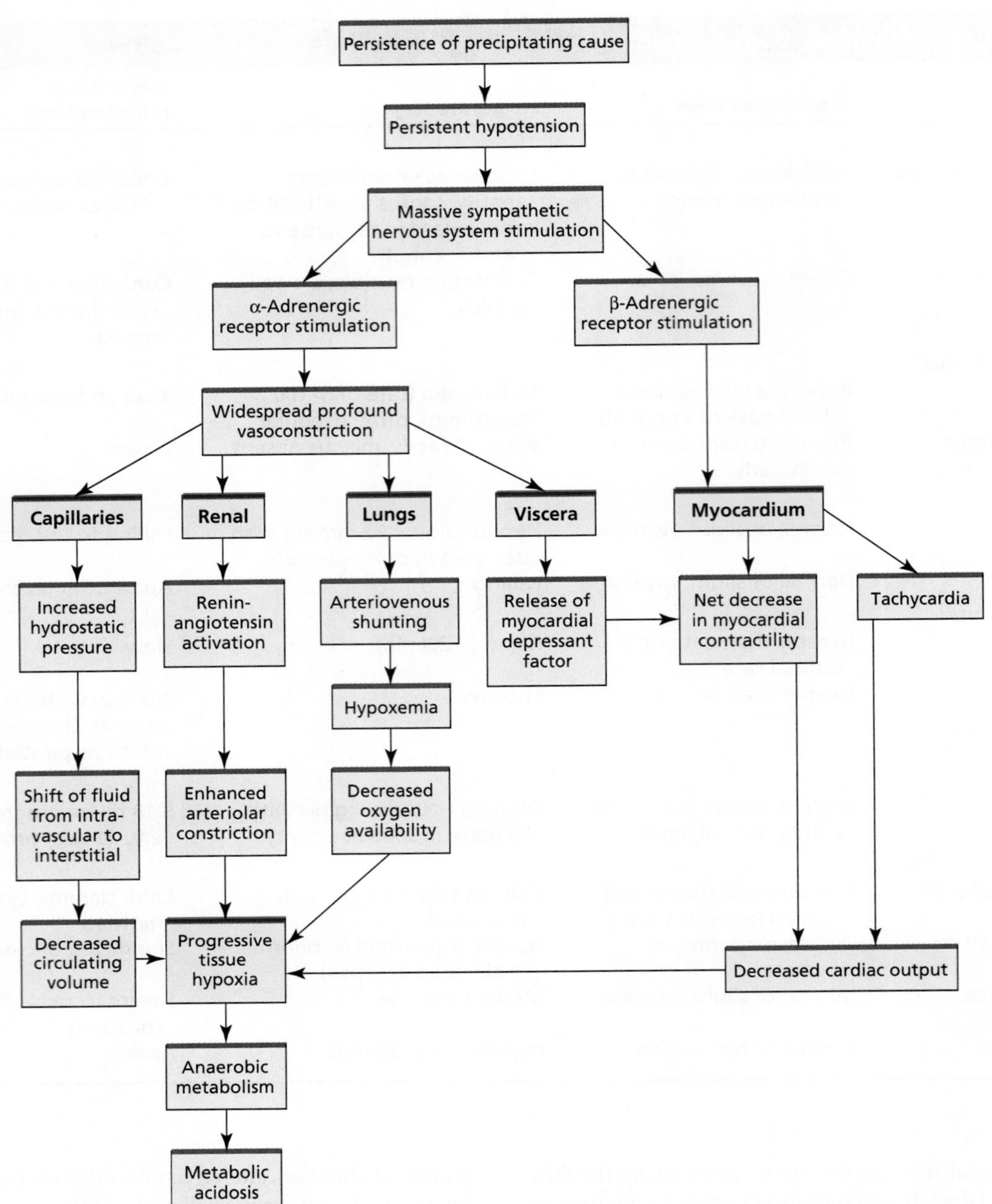

Fig. 61-7 Progressive stage: compensatory mechanisms are becoming ineffective and fail to maintain perfusion to vital organs.

than 7.20) has a direct depressant effect on cardiac function by impairing calcium metabolism within myocardial cells.

Clinical Manifestations

The clinical manifestations of the progressive stage of shock are presented in Table 61-5. The patient demonstrates listlessness, apathy, and confusion. A decreased response to painful stimuli may be observed.

When the BP begins to fall, the patient is no longer in compensated shock. Regardless of the previous normal BP, a systolic pressure below 80 mm Hg or a reduction of greater than 25% in the hypertensive patient is considered to be significant, as well as the increasingly narrow pulse pressure. The narrowed pulse pressure is indicative of decreased stroke volume caused by a decrease in systolic pressure. Because of the severe peripheral vasoconstriction, BPs taken with cuff pressures are likely to be inaccurate. Therefore intraarterial monitoring may be used to provide more reliable pressure readings.

Tachycardia is more evident during this stage of shock, and the pulse is weak and thready. However, older adults and patients who are receiving beta-adrenergic blockers may show little change in their heart rate. Other cardiovascular effects of shock during the progressive stage are shown in Table 61-5.

Respirations increase in rate in an attempt to compensate for tissue hypoxia and metabolic acidosis. Urine output decreases and may fall below 0.5 ml/kg per hour, indicating inadequate renal perfusion, which can lead to acute renal failure. The lips and oral mucosa are dry, and the patient may continue to complain of thirst. The skin is cold, pale, and clammy, with slow capillary refill. There may be cyanosis

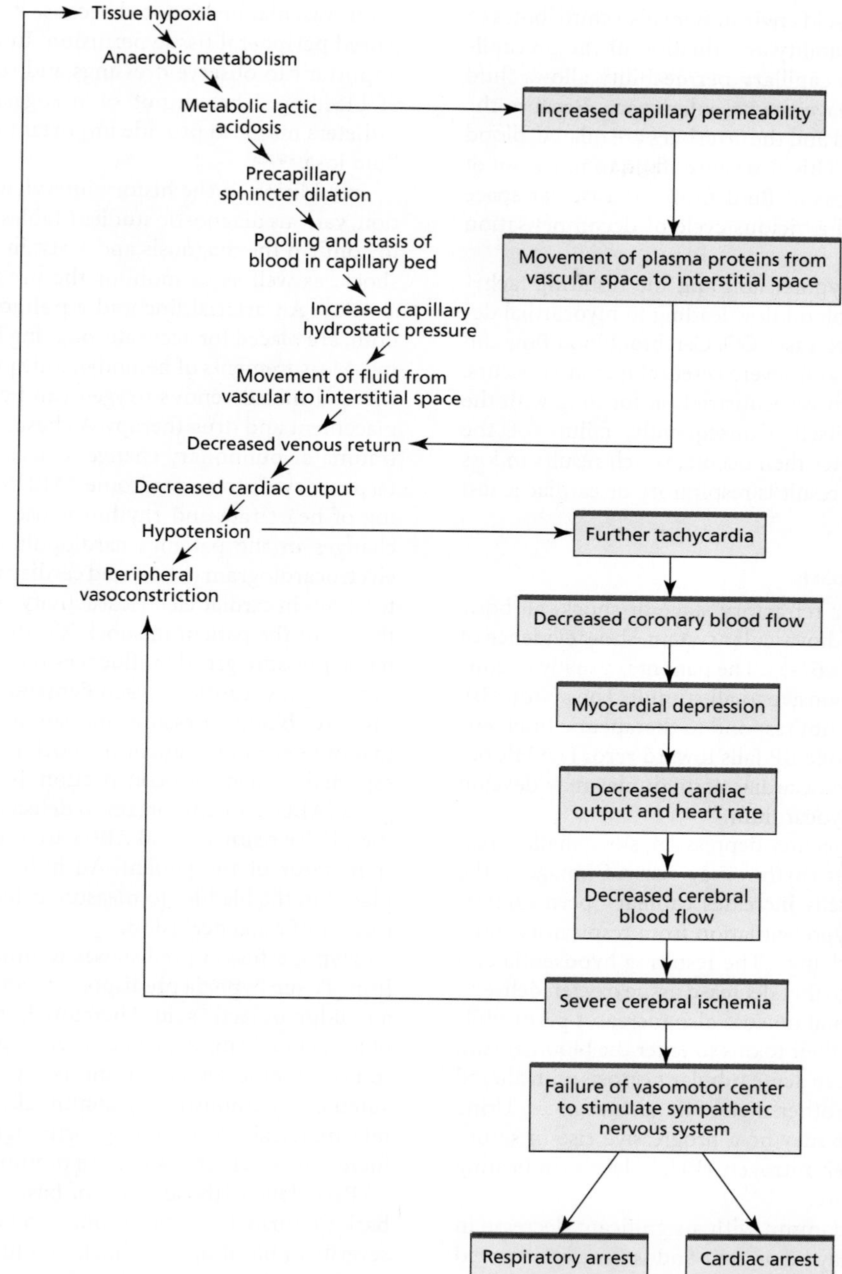

Fig. 61-8 Irreversible or refractory stage: compensatory mechanisms are not functioning or are totally ineffective, leading to multiple organ dysfunction syndrome.

caused by tissue hypoxia. Body temperature is usually low, except in septic shock.

Irreversible or Refractory Stage

The irreversible or refractory stage of shock is the stage during which compensatory mechanisms are either nonfunctioning or totally ineffective. Cellular necrosis and MODS may occur. Attempts to restore the BP have failed, and death becomes imminent. Occasionally patients may be resuscitated from this stage, only to die 7 to 14 days later as a result of the massive cellular death related to MODS.

Pathophysiology

As shock progresses, the sympathetic nervous system activity can no longer compensate to maintain homeostasis. Thus one of the major compensatory mechanisms has failed. There is pooling and sludging of the blood because of the lack of vasomotor tone. Thrombosis of the small blood vessels occurs. Increased vascular permeability and oliguria also occur.

Tissue hypoxia resulting from peripheral vasoconstriction and decreased CO makes it necessary for cells to continue to metabolize anaerobically (Fig. 61-8). The accumulation of lactic acid and other acid metabolites in the body's tissues contributes to cell death. The acid environment also contributes to increased capillary permeability and dilation of the precapillary sphincters. Increased capillary permeability allows fluid and plasma proteins to leave the vascular space. Because the venules remain constricted and the arterioles are dilated, blood pools in the capillary bed. This also causes fluid to move out of the vascular space. The loss of fluid from the vascular space leads to hypotension, and a vicious cycle of decompensation ensues.

As shock progresses, hypotension and the resulting tachycardia decrease coronary blood flow leading to myocardial depression, which further decreases CO. Cerebral blood flow can no longer be maintained, and severe cerebral ischemia occurs. The body cannot maintain vasoconstriction for long with the vicious cycle repeating itself. Consequently, failure of the medullary vasomotor center then occurs, which results in loss of sympathetic tone. The result is respiratory or cardiac arrest and death.

Clinical Manifestations

During the irreversible or refractory stage of shock, all body systems, especially the cardiovascular system, show evidence of decompensation (see Table 61-5). The patient is usually unconscious and may be unresponsive to all stimuli. The systolic BP continues to fall and does not respond to therapeutic interventions to raise it. The diastolic BP falls toward zero. The HR becomes progressively slower. Cardiac arrhythmias may develop because of an ischemic myocardium.

Because of respiratory center depression, slow, shallow respirations with an irregular rhythm may occur. Damage to the pulmonary endothelial cells increases capillary permeability. Pulmonary edema and hypoventilation from respiratory muscle fatigue impair gas exchange. The resulting hypoxemia and respiratory acidosis will further decrease tissue oxygen delivery.

Ischemia of the intestinal mucosa also increases permeability, allowing bacteria and their toxins to enter the bloodstream. Renal ischemia may result in acute tubular necrosis with altered fluid and electrolyte and other metabolic disturbances. Urine output is minimal. There may be a progressive rise in serum creatinine and blood urea nitrogen (BUN) levels, indicating some degree of renal failure.

The skin is cold and clammy, with a significant decrease in temperature. Cyanosis may be present and is usually observed in the lips, mucous membranes, and nail beds. However, it may be more obvious in the palms, soles, and palpebral conjunctiva (inside the eyelid) of dark-skinned patients.

DIAGNOSTIC STUDIES

The history and physical examination provide initial clues leading to a diagnosis of shock and identifying the person at high risk for shock. A history of a recent event that may be associated with shock (e.g., trauma, infection, crushing chest pain, pancreatitis) is significant. Changes in sensorium and a decreased level of consciousness reported by others also are important considerations. During the physical examination, it is important to observe for the clinical manifestations of shock. Of particular importance is the immediate overall impression of central nervous system (CNS) function, which is a measure of cerebral perfusion. Also, the status of the cutaneous vascular bed is noted because it may be indicative of impaired peripheral tissue perfusion. In the surgical patient it is important to observe dressings and tubes for the appearance of bleeding. The output of nasogastric tubes and urinary catheters may also provide important clues as to the source of fluid loss.

In addition to the history interview and physical examination, various diagnostic studies (Tables 61-6 and 61-7) are used to confirm the diagnosis and assist in identifying the cause of shock, as well as to monitor the progression and severity of shock.[10] An arterial line and a pulmonary artery catheter, or both, are placed for accurate, ongoing hemodynamic monitoring. Measurements of hemodynamic pressures, flows, and arterial and mixed venous oxygen can be used to guide fluid replacement and drug therapy. A chest x-ray may reveal thoracic trauma or pulmonary changes consistent with shock or acute respiratory distress syndrome (ARDS). Continuous monitoring of heart rate and rhythm is useful for early detection of changes in the patient's cardiopulmonary status. A 12-lead electrocardiogram (ECG) and cardiac monitor may indicate alterations in cardiac electrical activity. Accurate measurement of the BP of the patient in shock is critical, since the level of systemic pressure greatly influences the adequacy of tissue blood flow and myocardial oxygen demands. Auscultatory and noninvasive blood pressure measurements with a sphygmomanometer in the patient in shock may be grossly inaccurate, especially when vasoconstriction is present. Arterial blood gases (ABGs) are important to detect any acid-base abnormalities. Pulse oximetry and ABGs are used to assess the oxygenation status of the patient. An indwelling urinary catheter is placed in the bladder to measure urine output, which is an indicator of renal perfusion.

Hypoperfusion predisposes to impaired oxidative metabolism. Tissue hypoxia predisposes to anaerobic metabolism with a buildup of lactic acid. Therefore lactate is a marker of anaerobic metabolism. A lactate level of greater than 3 mEq/L (3 mmol/L) indicates significant hypoperfusion. Sequential measurements demonstrating continually decreasing levels of lactate are usually a good prognostic sign, whereas high stable or increasing levels are usually an ominous sign.

Base deficit (the amount of base needed to correct the pH back to normal) has been found to be a good indicator of the severity of bleeding and shock in trauma patients. Base deficits may be tracked to assess the effectiveness of therapy.

GENERAL COLLABORATIVE CARE: SHOCK

The critical factor in management of shock is early recognition and treatment (see Table 61-7). Prompt intervention can alter the shock process and prevent the development of the refractory stage and death.[10] Successful management of shock depends on the ability to do the following:

1. Identify the patient at high risk for shock
2. Diagnose shock swiftly and accurately
3. Eliminate or treat the primary cause
4. Initiate therapy to correct pathologic changes, modify the systemic response, and enhance tissue perfusion
5. Protect target organs from dysfunction
6. Provide supportive care

DIAGNOSTIC STUDIES

Table 61-6 Abnormalities in Shock and Multiple Organ Dysfunction Syndrome

Diagnostic Study	Abnormal Finding	Significance of Abnormality
Blood		
Red blood cell count, hematocrit, hemoglobin	Normal	■ Remains within normal limits in shock because of relative hypovolemia and pump failure and in hemorrhagic shock before fluid restoration
	Decreased	■ Decreases in hemorrhagic shock after fluid resuscitation when fluids other than blood are used
	Increased	■ Increases in nonhemorrhagic shock as a result of actual hypovolemia because fluid lost does not contain erythrocytes
DIC screen		
Fibrin split products	Increased	■ Acute DIC can develop within hours to days after an initial assault on the body (i.e., shock)
Fibrinogen level	Decreased	
Platelet count	Decreased	
PTT and PT	Prolonged	
Thrombin time	Increased	
D-dimer	Increased	
BUN	Increased	■ Indicates impaired kidney function caused by hypoperfusion as a result of severe vasoconstriction or occurs secondary to catabolism of cells (e.g., trauma)
Serum creatinine	Increased	■ Indicates impaired kidney function caused by hypoperfusion as a result of severe vasoconstriction; is more sensitive indicator of renal function than BUN
Blood glucose	Increased	■ Occurs in early shock because of breakdown of liver glycogen to glucose in response to sympathetic nervous system stimulation
	Decreased	■ Occurs because of depleted glycogen stores with hepatocellular dysfunction possible as shock progresses
Serum electrolytes		
Sodium	Increased	■ Occurs early in shock because of increased secretion of aldosterone, causing renal retention of sodium
	Decreased	■ May occur iatrogenically when excess hypotonic fluid is administered after fluid loss
Potassium	Increased	■ Occurs when cellular death liberates intracellular potassium; also occurs in acute renal failure and in the presence of acidosis
	Decreased	■ Occurs early in shock because of increased secretion of aldosterone, causing renal excretion of potassium
Calcium	Decreased	■ Sometimes occurs after rapid infusion of large amounts of citrated blood; also occurs secondary to respiratory alkalosis of early shock
	Increased	■ Occurs secondary to lactic acidosis, permitting increased ionization of calcium
Arterial blood gases	Respiratory alkalosis	■ Occurs early in shock secondary to hyperventilation
	Metabolic acidosis	■ Occurs later in shock when organic acids, such as lactic acid, accumulate in blood from anaerobic metabolism
Base deficit	>−6	■ Indicates acid production secondary to hypoperfusion
Blood cultures	Growth of organisms	■ May grow organisms in patients who are in septic shock
Lactate	Increased	■ Usually increases once significant hypoperfusion has occurred with impaired oxygen utilization at the cellular level
Liver enzymes (AST, ALT, LDH)	Increased	■ Elevations confirm liver cell destruction in progressive stage of shock
Urine		
Specific gravity	Increased	■ Occurs secondary to the action of ADH
	Fixed at 1.010	■ Occurs in renal failure

ADH, antidiuretic hormone; *ALT,* alanine aminotransferase; *AST,* aspartate aminotransferase; *BUN,* blood urea nitrogen; *DIC,* disseminated intravascular coagulation; *LDH,* lactate dehydrogenase; *PT,* prothrombin time; *PTT,* partial thromboplastin time.

COLLABORATIVE CARE

Table 61-7 Shock

Diagnostic

- History and physical examination
- Diagnostic studies (see Table 61-6)
- Placement of CVP, pulmonary artery catheter, arterial line (as indicated)
- Chest x-ray
- Twelve-lead ECG and cardiac monitor
- Identification of precipitating cause (if possible)

Collaborative Therapy

General Measures

- Establishment of a patent airway and administration of oxygen; careful monitoring of oxygenation
- Intubation and mechanical ventilation
- Placement of peripheral IV lines with large-gauge catheters
- Stabilization of BP with fluid replacement (blood, blood products, colloids, crystalloids, or autotransfusion) or drug therapy (see Table 61-10)
- Treatment of cardiac arrhythmias
- Placement of indwelling urinary catheter
- Nutritional support (enteral or parenteral nutrition)
- Emotional support of patient and family

Specific Measures

Hypovolemic Shock

- Control of bleeding (surgery, if indicated)
- Reduction of fluid loss from vomiting, diarrhea, and diuresis
- Volume replacement and blood/blood products (if necessary)
- Discontinue thrombolytics and anticoagulants (as indicated)

Cardiogenic Shock

- Correction of arrhythmias
- Cardiac catheterization with coronary angioplasty or stenting
- Administration of inotropic agents (e.g., dopamine [Intropin]) to increase cardiac contractility
- Careful fluid administration if patient is volume depleted (monitor PAWP)
- Reduction of workload of heart by decreasing afterload with vasodilator drugs (e.g., nitroglycerin)
- IABP to increase coronary perfusion and decrease afterload (if indicated)
- Use of ventricular assist device
- Emergency cardiac surgery or cardiac transplantation

Distributive Shock

Neurogenic Shock

- Treatment according to cause (e.g., pain relief, management of hypoxemia)
- Correction of underlying cause (if possible)
- Careful administration of fluid
- Administration of dopamine for hypotension and bradycardia (as indicated)
- Administration of phenylephrine (Neo-Synephrine) or norepinephrine (Levophed) to increase SVR

Anaphylactic Shock

- Maintenance of patent airway
- Administration of epinephrine for vasoconstriction, bronchodilation, and block histamine
- Administration of fluid
- Administration of inhaled albuterol (Proventil) for bronchodilation (aminophylline if ineffective)
- Administration of aerosolized epinephrine for laryngeal edema
- Administration of diphenhydramine (Benadryl) to counteract effects of histamine
- Administration of vasopressors (e.g., norepinephrine [Levophed]) as indicated

Septic Shock

- Administration of fluid
- Collection of cultures to identify organism
- Use of vasopressors (e.g., norepinephrine [Levophed]) to support BP as indicated
- Administration of appropriate antibiotics
- Control of temperature

CVP, central venous pressure; *ECG,* electrocardiogram; *IABP,* intraaortic balloon pump; *PAWP,* pulmonary artery wedge pressure; *SVR,* systemic vascular resistance.

Emergency care of the patient in shock is important and greatly increases the patient's chance of survival. The emergency care of the patient in shock is presented in Table 61-8.

The patient should be treated in an ICU and have continuous ECG and hemodynamic monitoring. A general goal is to maintain the mean arterial BP greater than 60 mm Hg.

Oxygen and Ventilatory Assistance

Management of shock begins by ensuring that the patient has an adequate airway. This may be accomplished solely by hyperextension of the neck (unless contraindicated by possibility of spinal cord injury). Placement of an endotracheal (ET) tube may be necessary. The patient requires mechanical ventilation to provide adequate ventilation and to decrease the work of breathing. In addition, it is essential that the patient in shock receive sufficient supplemental oxygen to maintain oxygen saturation above 90% or arterial oxygen pressure (PaO_2) at 60 mm Hg or higher and to avoid hypoxemia.

Oxygen delivery is dependent on CO, hemoglobin, oxygenation saturation of hemoglobin, mean arterial pressure, and circulating blood volume. Methods to optimize oxygen delivery include increasing the cardiac output (with drug therapy, fluid replacement), increasing the hemoglobin (with blood products), and increasing the oxygen saturation (supplemental oxygen, mechanical ventilation as necessary). Mean arterial pressure and circulating blood volume are optimized by fluid replacement and drugs. Oxygen utilization is decreased by sedation and analgesics and using antipyretics in hyperthermic patients. Nursing care must be provided as gently as possible and spaced out to provide recovery between interventions.

Patient Position

In terms of the patient's cardiovascular status, the recommended position for the treatment of shock (after neck and spine injuries have been ruled out) is supine with the legs elevated to an angle of 45 degrees. The trunk should be horizon-

EMERGENCY MANAGEMENT

Table **61-8** **Shock**

Etiology*	Assessment Findings	Interventions
Surgical Postoperative bleeding Ruptured ectopic pregnancy or ovarian cyst Ruptured organ/vessel Gastrointestinal bleeding Esophageal varices Vaginal bleeding Aortic dissection **Medical** Myocardial infarction Dehydration Addisonian crisis Diabetes insipidus Sepsis Diabetes mellitus Pulmonary embolus **Trauma** Ruptured or lacerated vessel or organ Fractures Multisystem or multiorgan injury	■ Decreased level of consciousness ■ Restlessness ■ Anxiety ■ Weakness ■ Rapid, weak, thready pulse ■ Arrhythmia ■ Hypotension ■ Narrowed pulse pressure ■ Cool, clammy skin (warm skin in sepsis) ■ Tachypnea, dyspnea, or shallow, irregular respirations ■ Decreased oxygen saturation ■ Extreme thirst ■ Nausea and vomiting ■ Chills ■ Feeling of impending doom ■ Pallor ■ Cyanosis ■ Obvious hemorrhage or injury ■ Temperature elevation (in sepsis)	**Initial** ■ Establish and maintain patent airway. ■ Administer high-flow oxygen (100%) by non-rebreather mask. ■ Anticipate need for intubation. ■ Stabilize cervical spine as appropriate. ■ Establish IV access with two large-bore catheters and begin fluid resuscitation with crystalloids (lactated Ringer's, normal saline). ■ Control external bleeding with direct pressure or pressure dressing. ■ Assess for life-threatening injuries (e.g., hemothorax, cardiac tamponade, liver laceration, pelvic fractures.) ■ Consider vasopressor therapy only after hypovolemia has been corrected. ■ Insert an indwelling urinary catheter and nasogastric tube. ■ Treat arrhythmias. **Ongoing Monitoring** ■ Monitor vital signs, level of consciousness, cardiac rhythm, oxygen saturation, and urine output.

*Other etiologies of shock are listed in Table 61-1.

tal, the head at the level of the chest, and the knees straight. The Trendelenburg's (head-down) position should be avoided in shock because it may (1) initiate aortic and carotid sinus reflexes, causing impaired cerebral blood flow and decreased jugular venous outflow; (2) cause the abdominal organs to press against the diaphragm, thus limiting respiratory excursion and contributing to respiratory distress; (3) decrease filling of the coronary arteries, causing myocardial ischemia; and (4) cause an increase in intracranial pressure in the presence of a head injury. Pneumatic antishock garments should also be avoided because they can increase pressure on the abdomen and decrease diaphragm excursion.

Fluid Replacement

Because shock (with the exception of cardiogenic shock) almost always involves a decreased effective circulating blood volume, the cornerstone of shock therapy is volume expansion by intravenous (IV) administration of appropriate fluids, either crystalloids, colloids, blood products, or a combination[11] (Table 61-9). At least two large-gauge IV catheters should be inserted immediately into large, easily accessible arm veins before severe vasoconstriction occurs and IV access becomes difficult. Crystalloids are electrolyte solutions that are either hypotonic, hypertonic, or isotonic relative to plasma. However, in the critically ill patient approximately two thirds of the volume will diffuse out of the vascular space because of increased capillary permeability and reduced oncotic pressure. Therefore large amounts of crystalloids are needed for adequate volume replacement.[12] Because of the expansion of the interstitial space following large amounts of crystalloid administration, the development of systemic edema is common.

Colloids usually remain in the intravascular space because of the size of the molecules. The osmotic pressure of these solutions draws fluid into the intravascular space, expanding the intravascular volume. Colloids are extremely effective volume expanders. Colloids are used in the treatment of shock when plasma protein loss is excessive, as in burn shock and peritonitis.

It is important to replace blood with blood or blood products to maintain the hemoglobin for promoting the delivery of oxygen to the tissues to occur. If needed, packed cells or whole blood is administered as soon as available once blood loss has been stopped. The patient's hemoglobin should be used as a guide for blood administration, because 1 U will raise the hemoglobin level about 1 g/dl. (Blood transfusions are discussed in Chapter 29.)

The choice of fluid for volume expansion remains controversial. Neither crystalloids nor colloids are the perfect fluid replacement. However, it is generally accepted that isotonic crystalloids, such as normal saline, are used in the initial resuscitation of shock.[13] Lactated Ringer's solution should be used cautiously in all shock situations because the lactate levels will increase further, and the failing liver cannot convert lactate to bicarbonate. Furthermore, several medications and all blood products are incompatible with lactated Ringer's solution. Crystalloids may be the only fluid used in volume replacement when neither blood nor serum proteins have been lost, as in shock resulting from GI fluid loss. Fluid replacement in cardiogenic shock should be done cautiously, and

RESEARCH
IMPLICATIONS FOR NURSING PRACTICE

Use of Trendelenburg's Position

Citation Ostrow CL: Use of the Trendelenburg position by critical care nurses: Trendelenburg survey, *Am J Crit Care* 6:172, 1997.

Purpose To assess the degree of use of the Trendelenburg's position by critical care nurses, the clinical uses of this position, and the sources of knowledge and beliefs of nurses about the efficacy of the position.

Methods A survey was mailed to 1000 nurses whose names were randomly selected from the membership list of the American Association of Critical Care Nurses. The survey consisted of 17 questions about the frequency of use of the Trendelenburg's position and the reasons for use.

Results and Conclusions The return rate was 49.4%. Ninety-nine percent of the respondents had used the Trendelenburg's position, and 80% had used the modified Trendelenburg's position, mostly for treatment of hypotension. Most used this intervention as an independent nursing action, and most learned about these positions from their nursing education, nurse colleagues, supervisors, and physicians. Eighty percent of the respondents believed that use of the Trendelenburg's position improves hypotension almost always or sometimes.

Implications for Nursing Practice According to this study, the use of the Trendelenburg's position in critical care nursing is widespread. However, there is no scientific evidence indicating that changing a patient's body position to the Trendelenburg's position (head lower than feet) or the modified Trendelenburg's position (only the legs elevated) significantly improves blood pressure or low cardiac output. The results of this study provide evidence that tradition-based therapy still underlies some interventions used in the care of critically ill patients and that some nurses may be relying on an outdated knowledge base that is not supported by the current literature.

colloids should not be used because of the osmotic pull of fluid into the vascular space, further decreasing the ability of the heart to pump. The amount and type of fluid given are based on the patient's response to treatment. This can be assessed by observing the BP, pulse, urine output, skin perfusion, lung sounds, hemodynamic parameters, and sensorium.

Ideally fluid replacement should be monitored with a pulmonary artery catheter to determine the pulmonary artery wedge pressure (PAWP) and the CO. The physical assessment of the patient is an important indicator of the patient's fluid status. Complications of excessive volume replacement, such as pulmonary edema and postresuscitation hypertension, can be treated with diuretics. If the patient does not have a pulmonary artery catheter, a urine output of 1 ml/kg per hour will usually indicate adequate fluid replacement. If, after fluid replacement, the cardiac output is still low, an inotropic agent with vasopressor activity such as dopamine (Intropin) or a vasopressor such as norepinephrine (Levophed) should be administered. Dobutamine (Dobutrex) is an inotropic agent with no vasopressor activity and could be added after adequate vasoconstriction has occurred.

The patient who has sustained a major hemorrhage requires rapid, massive fluid volume and blood replacement, which can exceed the patient's normal blood volume. Complications of massive volume infusion include hypothermia (from cold blood) and coagulopathy (from hemodilution of clotting factors). All blood products and IV solutions should be warmed to prevent hypothermia. Commercial devices are available that warm solutions, as well as provide pumps for rapid infusion. Clotting factor values (see Table 61-6) should be closely monitored.

Acid-Base Imbalance

Frequent monitoring of ABGs allows the physician to prescribe therapy to correct acid-base imbalances. This may be accomplished through the use of fluid administration and mechanical ventilation. Lactic acidosis resolves rapidly once circulating blood volume has been restored. Sodium bicarbonate is used only when the pH is below 7.20. At this point inotropic and vasopressor drugs are ineffective because of the profound acidosis.

Cardiac Arrhythmias

Arrhythmias may cause rapid, profound shock. As a general rule, prompt treatment of the arrhythmia will abolish the shock. Treatment of cardiac arrhythmias is discussed in Chapter 34.

COLLABORATIVE CARE: SPECIFIC TYPES OF SHOCK

In addition to general management of shock, there are specific interventions for different types of shock (see Table 61-7).

Hypovolemic Shock

The major treatment priority for hypovolemic shock is rapid fluid volume replacement. Each patient must be carefully monitored during fluid administration. The patient has probably received adequate volume replacement when the CO, hemoglobin, ABGs, and BP return to the acceptable range and urine output is at least 0.5 ml/kg per hour. Blood and blood products are needed for hemorrhagic shock. Autotransfusion (collection and administration of patient's own blood) may be used in patients with hemorrhage from trauma, especially chest trauma. Because control of bleeding is essential, surgical intervention may be required.

Cardiogenic Shock

The first goal in the management of cardiogenic shock is early restoration of coronary artery blood flow to the myocardium. Cardiac catheterization with coronary angioplasty or stenting is performed as soon as possible. Catheterization may also reveal the extent of myocardial compromise and may unmask surgically treatable mechanical lesions (e.g., septal rupture, papillary muscle rupture). Thrombolytic therapy may be used if cardiac catheterization is unavailable or delayed.

The intraaortic balloon pump (IABP) is a circulatory assist device that is inserted into the femoral, axillary, or subclavian

Table 61-9 Fluid Therapy in Shock and Multiple Organ Dysfunction Syndrome

Fluid Type	Mechanism of Action	Type of Shock	Nursing Implications
Crystalloids			
Isotonic ▪ 0.9% NaCl ▪ Lactated Ringer's (LR)	Fluid primarily remains in the intravascular space, increasing intravascular volume	Used for initial volume replacement in most types of shock	Monitor patient closely for circulatory overload. LR should not be used in patients with liver failure.
Hypertonic ▪ Hypertonic saline (3%)	Draws intracellular and interstitial fluid into the intravascular space, increasing intravascular volume	Hypertonic saline may be indicated for shock from hemorrhage or burns	Carefully monitor serum sodium levels and serum osmolarity.
Colloids (Plasma Volume Expanders)			
▪ Human serum albumin (5%, 25%)	Can increase intravascular volume up to five times within 30-60 minutes	All types of shock except cardiogenic	Monitor for circulatory overload. Mild side effects of chills, fever, and urticaria may develop. More expensive than other colloids.
▪ Plasma protein fraction	Has albumin as primary component; similar action to that of albumin	All types of shock	May cause greater hypersensitivity reactions than albumin.
▪ Hetastarch (Hespan)	Made from starch and acts as volume expander and is at least as effective as albumin; can exert osmotic effect for up to 36 hours	All types of shock	May be 50% less costly than albumin. Use cautiously in patients with congestive heart failure, renal failure, or bleeding disorders (because of anticoagulant effect).
▪ Dextran Dextran 40 Dextran 70	Hyperosmotic glucose polymer; similar degrees of volume expansion with dextran 40 and dextran 70; longer duration of action with dextran 70	Limited use because of side effects including reducing platelet adhesion, diluting clotting factors	Increases risk of bleeding. Important to monitor patient for allergic reactions and acute renal failure.
Blood			
▪ Whole blood/packed cells	Replaces blood loss, increases oxygen-carrying capability, improves oxygenation of tissues	All types of shock if hemoglobin is <12 g/dl (120 g/L)	Same precautions as any blood administration (see Chapter 29).

artery and placed in the aorta, just distal to the aortic arch (see Chapter 63). The goal of this intervention is to decrease the systemic vascular resistance and thus left ventricular workload, while increasing diastolic pressure resulting in increased coronary and cerebral blood flow. Another type of circulatory assist device is a ventricular assist device (VAD). Ventricular assist devices may be used on a temporary basis for the cardiogenic shock patient or as a bridge while awaiting cardiac transplantation if the treatable lesion cannot be repaired immediately. (IABPs and VADs are discussed in Chapter 63.) Cardiac transplantation is an option for a small and select group of patients with cardiogenic shock.

Cardiogenic shock requires hemodynamic monitoring. If the patient is volume depleted, fluid is replaced cautiously. The goal of drug therapy is to increase cardiac contractility while decreasing afterload and thus the workload of the heart. Inotropic and vasodilator agents (Table 61-10) are commonly used. In addition, diuretics used to decrease preload are indicated if the patient is volume overloaded, and arrhythmias should be aggressively treated.

Septic Shock

In septic shock, the source of infection must be identified and treated with antimicrobial therapy, surgical drainage, or both. The specific organisms causing septic shock are frequently not identified when patients have this illness. Therefore broad-spectrum, antimicrobial therapy must be instituted until the specific organisms are identified through culture and sensitivity testing. Usually two broad-spectrum antibiotics, including an aminoglycoside, are used.[2]

Rapid infusion of large amounts of fluid, including both crystalloids and colloids, are used in treating septic shock. Hemodynamic monitoring of pulmonary artery pressure (PAP), PAWP, and CO is often necessary because of the increased risk

DRUG THERAPY

Table 61-10 Shock and Multiple Organ Dysfunction Syndrome

Drug	Mechanism of Action	Type of Shock	Nursing Implications
Sympathomimetics*			
Dobutamine (Dobutrex)	Primarily stimulates β_1-adrenergic receptors with minimal β_2 and α-adrenergic effects. Increases myocardial contractility. Causes mild vasodilation, decreasing SVR.	Cardiogenic shock in absence of profound hypotension (<80 mm Hg systolic).	Do not give with sodium bicarbonate. Observe for hypotension, arrhythmias, and tachycardia at higher doses.
Dopamine (Intropin)	Is precursor of epinephrine and norepinephrine. Has dose-dependent actions. Stimulates α- and β-adrenergic receptors, causing peripheral vaso-constriction and positive inotropic effect. Increases renal perfusion at low doses only.	All types of shock, especially with decreased SVR; often used with nitroglycerin for cardiogenic shock.	Administer drug through central venous catheter or large peripheral vein (infiltration may cause tissue damage). Monitor for hypotension, tachycardia, and arrhythmias. Be aware that intravascular volume should be adequate.
Epinephrine (Adrenalin)	Stimulates α- and β-adrenergic receptors. Counteracts effects of histamine. Causes bronchodilation and peripheral vasoconstriction, elevating BP. Positive inotropic effect.	All types of shock; drug of choice for anaphylactic shock.	Observe for cardiac arrhythmias, dyspnea, and pulmonary edema.
Norepinephrine (Levophed)	Stimulates α-and β-adrenergic receptors, causing marked vasoconstriction, as well as inotropic and chronotropic effects.	All types, especially shock from decreased SVR. Reserved for patients with hypotension unresponsive to fluids and dopamine.	Best administered through a central venous line. Closely monitor rapid fluctuations in BP and urine output (severe decrease in renal perfusion may occur). Be aware that drug may also cause reflex bradycardia.
Phenylephrine (Neo-Synephrine)	Predominately stimulates α-adrenergic receptors, causing vasoconstriction.	Shock resulting from relative hypovolemia, neurogenic shock.	Observe for reflex bradycardia and ventricular ectopy.
Phosphodiesterase Inhibitor			
Milrinone (Primacor)	Produces inotropic action, increasing CO. Directly relaxes vascular smooth muscles, decreasing preload and afterload.	Cardiogenic shock unresponsive to initial drug therapy.	An initial bolus is administered before beginning the continuous IV infusion. Monitor for arrhythmias and hypotension.
Vasodilators			
Nitroglycerin (Tridil, Nitrol)	Primarily acts as venous vasodilator. Dilates veins and arteries at higher doses.	Cardiogenic shock, with inotropic agent.	Monitor BP carefully. Observe for reflex tachycardia. Be aware that headache is common. Use non-PVC tubing and glass bottle to prevent drug absorption.
Nitroprusside (Nipride)	Acts as a potent vasodilator on veins and arteries. May increase or decrease CO depending on the extent of preload and afterload reduction.	Primarily cardiogenic shock with increased SVR and preload and afterload; decreased CO, with inotropic drug, such as dopamine.	Closely monitor for hypotension and reflex tachycardia. Administer only with D_5W and protect solution from light. Be aware that thiocyanate toxicity and cyanide poisoning may occur when used for >72 hr.
Morphine sulfate	Is narcotic analgesic and acts as potent venodilator (decreases preload) with some arterial dilation (decreased afterload)	Primarily cardiogenic shock (to decrease preload).	Monitor carefully for hypotension and respiratory depression. Have naloxone (Narcan) at bedside.

Continued

DRUG THERAPY

Table 61-10 Shock and Multiple Organ Dysfunction Syndrome—cont'd

Drug	Mechanism of Action	Type of Shock	Nursing Implications
Corticosteroids			
Dexamethasone (Decadron) Hydrocortisone (Solu-Cortef) Methyl-prednisolone (Solu-Medrol)	Inhibit inflammatory process, stabilizes lysosomal membranes, reduces capillary permeability, reduces release of chemical mediators in the septic process, and promotes sodium retention.	Serious cases of anaphylactic shock; adrenal insufficiency.	Monitor patient for GI bleeding and hypotension. Be aware that these drugs may make control of diabetes difficult and may cause slow wound healing and predisposition to infection.

*All sympathomimetic drugs are incompatible with sodium bicarbonate.

for multiple system involvement with shock. Therefore these patients have an increased risk of developing fluid overload and cardiac failure. Assessment is important because subtle changes can rapidly occur, and the patient's condition can rapidly deteriorate. If tissue perfusion is inadequate, inotropic and vasopressor drugs (primarily dopamine or norepinephrine) are indicated to improve the blood flow and oxygen delivery.

Antibiotics may not be effective once septic shock has developed, because the harmful effects of the endotoxins and mediators continue even after the bacteria are dead. The current antibiotic therapy for septic shock reverses the effects in only some of the patients. Currently, research is being done using human monoclonal antibodies against various mediators of septic shock. These include antibodies to TNF, endotoxin, and IL-1.[2] To date results have been disappointing. Research is also being conducted regarding the use of continuous renal replacement therapy in removing the endotoxins and mediators from the bloodstream mechanically. (Renal replacement therapies are discussed in Chapter 44.)

Anaphylactic Shock

Full-blown anaphylactic shock is dramatic, and immediate drug intervention is required. Epinephrine is the drug of choice to treat anaphylactic shock. It causes peripheral vasoconstriction and bronchodilation and blocks the effect of histamine. Attention to the airway is important, because the patient can quickly develop respiratory failure from laryngeal edema or bronchoconstriction. Nebulized bronchodilators (e.g., albuterol [Proventil]) are highly effective. Aerosolized epinephrine can be used to treat laryngeal edema. Aminophylline may also be used when bronchoconstriction is severe. Endotracheal intubation or tracheostomy may be necessary to maintain a patent airway. Hypotension results from the leakage of fluid out of the intravascular space as a result of increased vascular permeability and peripheral vasodilation. Aggressive fluid replacement (usually with colloids) is necessary. Diphenhydramine (Benadryl) is used to counteract the effects of massive histamine release. However, it is not effective for the life-threatening vasodilation or bronchoconstriction. Corticosteroids may be administered if hypotension persists.

Neurogenic Shock

Neurogenic shock has multiple causes, and therefore the treatment varies. Fluid replacement for blood pressure maintenance and tissue perfusion is extremely important. Careful monitoring of the patient during fluid administration is important to prevent the patient from developing pulmonary edema as a result of volume overload. Sympathomimetic and vasopressor drug therapy may be indicated to increase BP through vasoconstriction and to increase heart rate.

Drug Therapy: Shock

The primary purpose of drugs used in the treatment of shock is correction of the poor tissue perfusion. These drugs are administered intravenously. Drugs used in the treatment of shock are presented in Table 61-10.

Sympathomimetic Drugs. Many of the drugs used in the treatment of shock have an effect on the sympathetic nervous system. Drugs that mimic the action of the sympathetic nervous system are termed *sympathomimetic.* The effects of these drugs are mediated through action of the α-adrenergic or β-adrenergic receptors. The various drugs differ in their relative α-adrenergic and β-adrenergic effects. (Table 31-1 discusses sympathetic nervous system receptors.)

Many of the sympathomimetic drugs cause peripheral vasoconstriction and are referred to as vasopressor drugs (e.g., epinephrine, norepinephrine). At high doses these vasopressor drugs have the potential to cause severe peripheral vasoconstriction and to further jeopardize tissue perfusion, either directly or indirectly. The increased SVR increases the workload of the heart and can be detrimental to a patient in cardiogenic shock, causing further myocardial damage. Use of vasopressor drugs is generally reserved for patients who have been unresponsive to other therapy. Adequate volume replacement must be administered before the use of any vasopressor drug, because peripheral vasoconstrictor effects in patients with low blood volume cause further reduction in tissue perfusion.

The goals of vasopressor therapy are to achieve and maintain a mean arterial blood pressure of 70 to 80 mm Hg, which ensures improved perfusion to key organs. The sympathomimetic drug of choice for cardiogenic shock is norepinephrine if the systolic BP is less than 70 mm Hg; dobutamine is added when the systolic BP is greater than 90 mm Hg.[14] Norepinephrine and dopamine are the drugs of choice for hypovolemic shock and distributive shock.

Vasodilator Drugs. Some patients in shock show evidence of excessive vasoconstriction and poor tissue perfusion in spite of volume replacement and normal or even high systemic pressures. This is especially true of patients in cardiogenic shock. Although generalized sympathetic vasoconstriction is a useful compensatory mechanism for maintaining systemic pressure, excessive constriction can reduce tissue blood flow and increase the workload of the heart. The rationale for using vasodilator therapy for a patient in shock is to break the deleterious cycle in which widespread vasoconstriction causes a decrease in CO and BP, resulting in further sympathetic-induced vasoconstriction.

The goal of vasodilator therapy, as in vasopressor therapy, is to maintain a mean arterial blood pressure of 70 to 80 mm Hg. It is also important to closely monitor PAP and mean arterial pressure so that fluid administration can be increased or the dose of the vasodilating drug decreased if a serious fall in BP occurs. The vasodilator agent most often used for the patient in cardiogenic shock is nitroglycerin. In noncardiogenic shock vasodilation may be enhanced with nitroprusside (Nipride).

Corticosteroids. IV corticosteroids may be helpful in anaphylactic shock if significant symptoms continue after 1 to 2 hours of aggressive therapy. Although corticosteroids do not have an effect in neurogenic shock, methylprednisolone is used in spinal cord injury to prevent secondary spinal cord damage caused by the release of chemical mediators (see Chapter 57). Corticosteroids are not used in the treatment of other types of shock except in patients with suspected adrenal insufficiency. The use of these immunosuppressant agents may actually increase the incidence of secondary infections in patients with septic shock.[2]

Antibiotics. Antibiotics are always used in the treatment of septic shock. Susceptibility to infection is increased in all patients with prolonged shock of nonseptic etiology. Broad-spectrum prophylactic antibiotic therapy may be indicated because of the high prevalence of nosocomial organisms in critical care units. Methods to prevent nosocomial infections include hand washing, aseptic technique when managing invasive lines and tubes, instituting enteral feeding as soon as possible, elevating the head of the bed to prevent gastric reflux of enteral feedings to the lung, and frequent mouth care. Before antibiotic therapy is begun, specimens of the blood, urine, wound exudate, and sputum should be obtained for culture and sensitivity studies. The organisms that most frequently cause septic shock are gram-negative bacteria. Antibiotic therapy should never be delayed. Unless appropriate antibiotics are started within 24 hours of the beginning of shock, the mortality rate is greatly increased.

Nutritional Therapy: Shock

Protein-calorie malnutrition is one of the primary manifestations of hypermetabolism in shock. Nutrition is vital to decreasing morbidity. Some type of nutrition should be implemented within the first 24 hours. Generally, parenteral feeding is used only if enteral feedings have failed, are contraindicated, or fail to meet the patient's caloric requirements. (Total parenteral nutrition and enteral tube feedings are discussed in Chapter 38.) The patient is started on a continuous drip of very small amounts of enteral feeding. Early enteral feedings are thought to enhance perfusion of the GI tract and prevent translocation of gut bacteria.[15]

A patient in shock should be weighed daily on the same scale at the same time of day. If the patient experiences a significant weight loss, dehydration should be ruled out before additional calories are provided parenterally. Large weight gains are common because of third spacing of fluids. Therefore daily weights may function more as an indicator of fluid status than caloric needs and balance. Serum protein, nitrogen balance, BUN, serum glucose, and serum electrolytes are all used to assess nutritional status.

NURSING MANAGEMENT: SHOCK

■ Nursing Assessment

Subjective and objective data that should be obtained from a person with shock are presented in Table 61-11. Initial assessment of the patient in shock, or impending shock, need not be extensive. The assessment should focus on the evaluation of the indicators of tissue perfusion, including level of consciousness, skin, vital signs, and urine output. Although a continual decline in the patient's level of consciousness indicates a further reduction in cerebral blood flow and a worsening of the shock state, some patients in shock may remain fully conscious. As shock progresses, severe arterial vasoconstriction continues to decrease perfusion to the skin and kidneys. Therefore the skin becomes colder and mottled and the urine output declines to eventual anuria. The BP may not be a reliable indicator of the severity of shock. Changes from the baseline vital signs are important to evaluate and document.

■ Planning

The overall goals are that the patient in shock will have (1) adequate tissue perfusion, (2) normal BP for the patient, (3) return of organ function, and (4) no complications related to shock.

■ Nursing Diagnoses

Nursing diagnoses for the patient with shock may include, but are not limited to, those presented in NCP 61-1.

■ Nursing Implementation

Health Promotion. It is important for nurses to become involved in the prevention of shock. To prevent shock, the nurse must first identify persons who are at risk. In general, the very old; the very young; persons with chronic, debilitating disease; and the immunocompromised are at an increased risk. More specifically, any person who sustains surgical or accidental trauma is at high risk of shock resulting from hemorrhage, spinal cord injury, burn injury, and the conditions listed in Table 61-1.

Any patient who is at risk for decreased oxygen delivery or tissue hypoxia is at risk for the development of shock. Implementation of the nursing process is essential to help prevent shock after a susceptible individual has been identified. A thorough baseline nursing assessment and frequent ongoing assessments to monitor and detect changes in the patient's condition are the initial nursing actions. Identification of pertinent nursing diagnoses, implementation of appropriate nursing interventions, and evaluation of these actions should follow. Health education is important to prevent the onset of diseases that may result in shock. For example, regular exercise and cessation of smoking may help decrease the risk of MI.

A person with an acute MI, especially an anterior wall MI, is at risk for cardiogenic shock. All patients with symptoms of angina or MI should be encouraged to seek medical attention immediately. The primary goal for the patient with an acute MI is to limit the size of the infarction. This is done by attempting

NURSING ASSESSMENT

Table 61-11 Shock and Multiple Organ Dysfunction Syndrome

Subjective Data

Important Health Information

Past health history: MI, pulmonary embolism, infection, spinal cord injury, hemorrhage, trauma, burns, diabetes mellitus, dehydration, congestive heart failure, valvular dysfunction, pancreatitis, intestinal obstruction, use of tampons, severe reaction to insect bites or stings or blood products

Medications: Severe reaction to any drugs, vaccines, contrast dye, general anesthesia; drug overdose (including insulin); immunosuppressive agents

Surgery or other treatments: Any major surgical procedure, especially involving extensive blood or fluid loss

Functional Health Patterns

Nutritional-metabolic: Thirst, nausea, vomiting, abdominal cramps; chills

Activity-exercise: Weakness, dizziness, fainting, palpitations, dyspnea, productive or nonproductive cough

Elimination: Decreased urinary output, diaphoresis

Cognitive-perceptual: Pruritus; chest pain

Coping–stress tolerance: Apprehension, anxiety, irritability

Objective Data

General

Normal, decreased, or increased (septic shock) body temperature; external evidence of bleeding

Integumentary

Pale, cool, moist skin or warm, flushed skin (septic and anaphylactic shock); dry lips and mucosa; urticaria, rash, and angioedema (anaphylaxis); cyanosis (late)

Respiratory

Rapid, deep respirations, may progress to slow, shallow, irregular respirations; wheezes, crackles, absence of breath sounds, choking, coughing (anaphylaxis)

Cardiovascular

Tachycardia with weak, thready pulse, may progress to slow, irregular pulse with pulse deficit; orthostatic hypotension, narrowing pulse pressure, progressive hypotension; slow capillary refill; flat neck veins (except in cardiogenic shock); abnormal heart sounds; arrhythmias

Gastrointestinal

Diminished or absent bowel sounds

Urinary

Progressive decrease in urinary output

Neurologic

Irritability, restlessness progressing to lethargy, agitation, stupor, coma; slurred speech progressing to disoriented, incoherent speech; decreased response to painful stimuli and absence of reflexes; pupils normal size progressing to dilation and minimal or absent response to light

Possible Findings

Altered serum electrolytes, decreased hemoglobin and hematocrit, leukocytosis, hypoxemia, and hypocapnia or hypercapnia; respiratory alkalosis and metabolic acidosis; increased creatinine and BUN; increased cardiac enzymes (cardiogenic); elevated liver enzymes; elevated lactate levels; positive wound, blood, and body fluid cultures; abnormal chest and abdominal x-rays and ECG

to increase coronary artery perfusion and decrease the workload of the heart through rest, drug therapy, thrombolytic therapy, and coronary artery angioplasty.

A person with a severe allergy to such substances as drugs, shellfish, and insect bites may develop anaphylactic shock. The risk of anaphylactic shock can be decreased if the patient is carefully questioned about allergies before administering a new drug (even if the patient has received this drug in the past) or before undergoing a diagnostic procedure involving the use of an IV dye. Patients with severe allergies should wear a Medic Alert tag and report their allergies to their health care providers. These patients should also be instructed about the availability of special kits that contain equipment and medication for the treatment of acute hypersensitivity reactions.

Careful monitoring of fluid balance can help prevent hypovolemic shock. Intake and output, daily body weights, and drainage from wounds and tubes must be carefully calculated and documented. Immediate control of hemorrhage is essential.

An immunocompromised person may develop an opportunistic infection that may rapidly develop into shock. A patient who is at risk of sepsis must be carefully monitored for signs of infection. Limitation of portals of entry into the body, including IV lines and indwelling catheters, is important. Aseptic technique must be used with all invasive procedures.[16] Frequent hand washing is essential. Care must be taken to clean all equipment and other items that are used on more than one patient.

Acute Intervention. The nursing role in the acute stages of shock involves (1) monitoring the patient's ongoing physical and emotional status to detect subtle changes in the patient's condition, (2) planning and implementing nursing interventions and therapy, (3) evaluating the patient's response to therapy, and (4) providing emotional support to the patient and significant others. Nursing responsibilities also include judging when it is necessary to alert other health team members to changes in the patient's status that may require reevaluation of treatment. Therefore reassessment, as often as the patient's condition warrants it, is important (see NCP 61-1).

As care is begun, it is essential for the nurse to obtain the following brief history from the patient or another knowledgeable person:

1. Description of the events leading to the shock condition
2. Time of onset and duration of symptoms
3. Health history, especially medications and allergies
4. Care received before hospital admission
5. Date of last tetanus immunization, if shock is a result of trauma
6. Patient's religious faith
7. Presence of Medic Alert tag

Neurologic status. Neurologic checks, including orientation and level of consciousness, should be performed at least every hour. The patient's neurologic status is the best indicator

61-1 NURSING CARE PLAN PATIENT IN SHOCK

Expected Patient Outcomes	Nursing Interventions and *Rationales*
NURSING DIAGNOSIS	**Decreased cardiac output** *related to* shock state *as manifested by* increased diastolic, decreased systolic BP; postural hypotension; tachycardia; weak, thready pulse; flat neck veins; low CVP and PAWP; thirst and dry mucous membranes; urinary output <0.5 ml/kg/hr; altered mentation; arrhythmias; tachypnea; hypoxemia; pallor or cyanosis; cool, clammy skin.
▪ Normal BP (for patient). ▪ HR 60-110 beats/min and regular. ▪ Strong peripheral pulses. ▪ Normal CVP (1-8 mm Hg) and PAWP (6-12 mm Hg). ▪ Warm, dry, pink skin. ▪ Urinary output >0.5 ml/kg/hr. ▪ Normal mentation. ▪ Respiratory rate >12 and <20 breaths/min. ▪ $SaO_2 \geq 90\%$.	▪ Monitor vital signs, CVP, pulmonary artery pressures every 15 min to 1 hr *to monitor patient's status and detect fluid deficits or excesses.* ▪ Administer crystalloids, colloids, or blood *to restore blood and fluid volume to maintain perfusion of vital organs.* Assess response. ▪ Titrate drug therapy (as indicated) to support BP *to maintain perfusion.* ▪ Record accurate intake and output of vital organs *to monitor fluid balance status.* ▪ Monitor laboratory and x-ray findings *to evaluate patient's response to treatment.* ▪ Keep patient at normal body temperature *to prevent an increase in metabolic need for O_2 and increased CO_2 production.* ▪ Administer oxygen *to keep $SaO_2 \geq 90\%$.*
NURSING DIAGNOSIS	**Fear and anxiety** *related to* severity of condition *as manifested by* verbalization of anxiety about condition and fear of death, or withdrawal with no communication; restlessness; sleeplessness; increase in heart and respiratory rate.
▪ Verbalization of anxieties and fears. ▪ Verbalization of reduced anxiety.	▪ Acknowledge expressed fear and anxiety *to validate patient's feelings.* ▪ Demonstrate concern and respect for patient. ▪ Try to draw out patient if withdrawn *to encourage verbalization and discussion of fears.* ▪ Seek out significant other's perception of situation *to enlist help.* ▪ Maintain calm and reassuring demeanor and environment *to reduce patient's anxieties and oxygen need.* ▪ Explain interventions, patient status, and equipment simply and honestly *to reduce patient's fear of the unknown and assist patient in making informed decisions.* ▪ Teach simple relaxation techniques *to aid in stress reduction.*

COLLABORATIVE PROBLEMS

Nursing Goals	Nursing Interventions and *Rationales*
POTENTIAL COMPLICATION	Organ ischemia/dysfunction *related to* decreased tissue perfusion.
NEUROLOGIC ISCHEMIA/DYSFUNCTION	
▪ Monitor for signs of neurologic ischemia. ▪ Report deviations from acceptable parameters. ▪ Carry out medical and nursing interventions.	▪ Perform neurologic assessment every hour including assessment of changes in mentation or level of consciousness *to provide information regarding status of cerebral blood flow.* ▪ Record and report any changes *to guide selection of appropriate interventions.* ▪ Closely observe and protect confused patient from injury *to prevent falls and accidents.* ▪ Take measures to minimize noise *to control sensory input and allow for rest.*
RENAL ISCHEMIA/DYSFUNCTION	
▪ Monitor for signs of renal ischemia. ▪ Report deviations from acceptable parameters. ▪ Carry out medical and nursing interventions.	▪ Monitor for urine output <0.5 ml/kg/hr, increase in urine specific gravity, elevation in serum BUN and creatinine, abnormal serum electrolytes, low urine sodium, protein and blood in urine, metabolic acidosis *to assess renal function.* ▪ Insert indwelling catheter *to accurately measure urinary output.* ▪ Take daily weights *to monitor fluid status and evaluate renal function.* ▪ Administer fluids and drug therapy as ordered and assess results *to maintain adequate renal perfusion.* ▪ Monitor signs and symptoms of fluid overload *to identify a possible complication of overtreatment.*

Continued

61-1 NURSING CARE PLAN PATIENT IN SHOCK—continued

Nursing Goals	Nursing Interventions and *Rationales*
GASTROINTESTINAL ISCHEMIA/DYSFUNCTION	
▪ Monitor for signs of GI ischemia. ▪ Report deviations from acceptable parameters. ▪ Carry out medical and nursing interventions.	▪ Monitor for presence of abdominal pain, distention, nausea, vomiting, anorexia, diarrhea, thirst, absent or diminished bowel sounds *to assess GI status.* ▪ Monitor bowel sounds q4hr. ▪ Measure intake and output *to determine fluid balance.* ▪ Initiate parenteral or enteral nutrition as soon as possible.
PERIPHERAL VASCULAR ISCHEMIA/DYSFUNCTION	
▪ Monitor for signs of peripheral vascular ischemia. ▪ Report deviations from acceptable parameters. ▪ Carry out appropriate medical and nursing interventions.	▪ Monitor for presence of cool, pale, or cyanotic extremities; diminished or absent peripheral pulses; pain, tingling, or numbness in extremities; necrotic or gangrenous extremities; poor capillary refill *as indicators of peripheral vascular ischemia.* ▪ Report any changes in peripheral perfusion *so treatment can be initiated promptly.* ▪ Prevent pressure ulcers *because they can develop quickly when immobility is combined with tissue ischemia.* ▪ Keep patient warm and dry *to promote comfort and prevent vasoconstriction.*
RESPIRATORY ISCHEMIA/DYSFUNCTION	
▪ Monitor for signs of respiratory distress. ▪ Report deviations from acceptable parameters. ▪ Carry out appropriate medical and nursing interventions.	▪ Monitor for the following: altered respiratory rate and depth, dyspnea, use of accessory muscles, cyanosis, adventitious breath sounds, cough, abnormal chest x-ray *to assess for respiratory distress.* ▪ Initiate oxygen and maintain $SaO_2 \geq 90\%$ *to ensure adequate oxygenation.* ▪ Monitor ABGs *to evaluate gas exchange in the lungs and acid-base balance.* ▪ Auscultate and record breath sounds q1-2hr to determine presence of crackles, wheezes, and decreased or unequal breath sounds *as indicators of impaired respirations.* ▪ Assist patient to deep breathe *to open up alveoli and improve gas exchange.* ▪ Suction as needed *to remove secretions patient cannot remove independently.* ▪ Maintain patent airway and prepare for possible mechanical ventilation.

CVP, central venous pressure; *PAWP,* pulmonary artery wedge pressure.

of cerebral blood flow. The nurse should be alert to clinical manifestations that may indicate neurologic involvement, such as changes in behavior, restlessness, overalertness, blurred vision, agitation, confusion, and paresthesias.

Attempts should be made to orient the patient to time, place, person, and situation. If the patient is in an ICU, orientation to the environment is particularly important. Measures such as minimizing noise and light levels should be taken to control sensory input. A day-night cycle of activity and rest should be maintained as much as possible. Sensory overload and disruption of the patient's diurnal cycle may contribute to an altered neurologic status, especially if the patient is elderly.

Cardiovascular status. Much of the therapy for shock is based on information about the patient's cardiovascular status. Until the patient is stable, the heart rate, BP, central venous pressure (CVP), and pulmonary artery pressures (if available) should be determined every 15 minutes. (Hemodynamic monitoring is discussed in Chapter 63.) Once the patient is stable, the PAWP should be obtained only as often as needed to avoid complications associated with balloon inflation. The PAWP most accurately reflects left ventricular function, especially in the presence of lung problems (e.g., pulmonary embolism, chronic lung disease) when the pulmonary artery pressure is often elevated. Trends in pulmonary artery pressures and other hemodynamic parameters are more important than the individual numbers themselves. In addition, care should be taken to avoid dependence on these numbers. It should be remembered that direct physical assessment of the patient is extremely valuable.

The patient's ECG should be continuously monitored to detect arrhythmias that may result from the shock itself or the medications used in treatment. Heart sounds should be assessed for quality and the presence of an S_3 or S_4 sound or murmurs. The presence of an S_3 sound in an adult usually indicates heart failure. The frequency of this monitoring is decreased as the patient's condition improves.

In addition to carrying out these measures, which are necessary to monitor the patient's cardiovascular status, the nurse must administer the prescribed therapy that is designed to correct the patient's impaired cardiovascular status. The response to fluid and medication administration must be assessed every 15 minutes. Appropriate adjustments should be made as needed. After the patient is stable, medications are slowly weaned.

Respiratory status. The respiratory status of the patient in shock must be frequently assessed to ensure adequate oxygenation and early detection of respiratory complications, as well as to provide data regarding the patient's acid-base status. The rate, depth, and rhythm of respirations are initially monitored every 15 to 30 minutes. Increased rate and depth provide information regarding the patient's attempts to correct metabolic acidosis. Breath sounds should be assessed every hour for the development of crackles, which can indicate the presence of fluid buildup in the lungs.

Pulse oximetry, a noninvasive method, is used to continuously monitor oxygen saturation. Pulse oximetry consists of a microprocessor and a probe that attaches to the patient's ear, finger, toe, or nose. Pulse oximetry using a finger or toe may not be accurate in an advanced shock state because of poor peripheral circulation. In this situation, the ear or nose should be used to increase accuracy. ABGs provide definitive information on oxygenation status and acid-base balance. Initial interpretation of ABGs is often the nurse's responsibility. A PaO_2 below 60 mm Hg (in the absence of chronic lung disease) indicates the presence of hypoxemia and the need for the administration of higher oxygen concentrations or for a different method of oxygen administration. A low $PaCO_2$ in the presence of a low pH and a low bicarbonate level indicates that the patient's hyperventilation is attempting to compensate for the metabolic acidosis. A rising $PaCO_2$ in the presence of a persistently low pH indicates the need for intubation and mechanical ventilation.

Most patients in shock will be intubated and on mechanical ventilation. Maintaining a patent airway and monitoring for ventilator-related complications are important. (Mechanical ventilation is discussed in Chapter 63.)

Renal status. Hourly measurements of urinary output are essential in assessment of the adequacy of renal perfusion. An indwelling catheter is inserted to facilitate measurements. Urine output of less than 0.5 ml/kg per hour may indicate inadequate perfusion of the kidneys. BUN and serum creatinine determinations are used as guides to assess renal function. Serum creatinine is a better indicator of renal function because BUN levels can be influenced by the catabolic state of the patient.

Body temperature and skin changes. In the presence of an elevated or subnormal temperature, tympanic or pulmonary arterial temperatures should be obtained hourly. If normal, the temperature should be monitored only every 4 hours. The patient should be kept comfortably warm with the use of light covers and the control of environmental temperature. If the patient's temperature rises above 101.5° F (38.6° C), this condition may be treated with medication such as acetaminophen suppositories, tepid sponge baths, removal of some covers, or a hypothermia blanket (in some situations). Nonsteroidal antiinflammatory drugs (e.g., ibuprofen) decrease body temperature. It is important to treat a fever (greater than 101.5° F [38.6° C]) because an elevated temperature and shivering cause an increased metabolic need for oxygen and increased carbon dioxide production.

Skin color should be assessed for pallor, flushing, and cyanosis. Diaphoresis or piloerection should be noted. In addition, the rapidity of capillary refill should be assessed as an indicator of peripheral perfusion.

Gastrointestinal status. Bowel sounds should be auscultated at least every 4 hours, and abdominal distention should be assessed. Serial measurements of abdominal girth may be indicated. If a nasogastric tube is used, the drainage should be measured as part of the fluid output and tested for occult blood. If the patient has a bowel movement, the stool should be checked for occult blood.

Personal hygiene. Hygiene is especially important to the patient in shock because impaired tissue perfusion predisposes to infection and skin breakdown. However, bathing and other nursing measures must be carried out judiciously because a patient in shock has major problems with oxygen delivery to tissues. Nursing measures must be performed with the least fatiguing method possible and spaced to allow adequate recovery. Using an alternating-pressure or other special foam mattress, turning the patient every 1 to 2 hours, and positioning the patient in good body alignment help prevent pressure ulcer formation. The patient in shock frequently is hemodynamically unstable, and repositioning may result in a worsening of vital signs. The nurse must use clinical judgment in determining priorities of care. Passive ROM should be performed three to four times per day to maintain joint mobility if the patient can tolerate it.

Oral care for the patient in shock is essential because mouth breathing is common and mucous membranes may be dry in the volume-depleted patient. In addition, the intubated patient usually has difficulty swallowing, resulting in pooled secretions in the mouth. A water-soluble lubricant applied to the lips prevents drying and cracking. Moist swabbing of the tongue and oral mucosa with saline solution or diluted mouthwash is also beneficial. Lemon glycerin swabs should not be used because they can cause drying of the mucosa.

Emotional support. The effects of the patient's anxiety and fear in the face of this critical, life-threatening situation are frequently overlooked or underestimated. Anxiety and fear may aggravate respiratory distress and increase catecholamine secretion. It is important for the nurse to remember that compassionate understanding is as essential as scientific and technical expertise in the total care of a patient in shock.

In planning and implementing the nursing care of the patient in shock, the nurse should assess the patient's anxiety. Medication to decrease anxiety is a common mode of therapy. However, in some shock situations, sedation may be contraindicated. Continuous infusions of a benzodiazepine (e.g., lorazepam [Ativan]), a narcotic (e.g., morphine), and occasionally a neuromuscular blocking agent (e.g., vecuronium [Norcuron]) are extremely helpful in decreasing pain, anxiety, and oxygen utilization.

The nurse should talk to the patient, even if the patient is intubated or appears comatose. If the intubated patient is capable of writing, a magic slate or a pencil and paper should be provided. The patient should also receive simple explanations of procedures before they are carried out, as well as information regarding the current plan of care and its rationale. If the patient asks questions about progress and prognosis, simple and honest answers should be given.

Privacy should be provided as much as possible, but the patient should be assured that assistance is readily available should it be required. The call bell should be in reach. In addition, joking and "kidding around" among health care personnel should be kept to a minimum or occur where the patient and family cannot hear it. This type of behavior can often lead the patient to believe that staff members are having too much fun to be available to provide adequate care. Furthermore, conversations about the patient should not take place where the patient can overhear them. Such conversations can constitute a violation of the patient's confidentiality or may be misinterpreted in a way that causes the patient unnecessary distress. Hearing is often the last sense to go, and even if the patient cannot respond, he or she may still be able to hear.

Many patients desire the comfort of a priest, rabbi, or minister. The nurse should offer to call a member of the clergy rather than wait for the patient or family to express a wish for spiritual counseling.

Family and significant others have a therapeutic effect on the patient. To perform this role, they need support and comfort. Family and significant others (1) link the patient to the outside world, (2) facilitate decision making and advise the patient, (3) assist with activities of daily living, and (4) provide safe, caring, familiar relationships for the patient.[17]

The family primarily needs to be kept informed of the patient's condition with reassurance that capable, compassionate personnel are taking care of their loved one. If possible, the same nurse should continue to care for the patient to decrease anxiety, avoid confusing contradictions, and increase trust. Should the prognosis become increasingly grave, the patient's family should be given support when making difficult decisions regarding continuation of life support. The nursing staff must support the family's decisions and facilitate realism. Family members and friends should be shown where they can wait and where a telephone can be found.

Family time with the patient should be facilitated rather than hindered, provided this time is perceived as a comfort by the patient. The nurse should explain in simple terms the purpose of tubes and machines surrounding the patient, and the family should be informed of what they may and may not touch. They should be encouraged to touch their loved one and to perform simple comfort measures. Privacy should be ensured as much as possible. The patient is much more likely to receive comfort from a loved one than from the nurse.

Ambulatory and Home Care. Rehabilitation of the patient in shock necessitates prevention or early treatment of complications and correction of the precipitating cause. The nurse should continue to assess the patient for indications of complications throughout the recovery period. These complications include such problems as chronic renal failure following acute tubular necrosis or the development of fibrotic lung disease as a result of ARDS (see Chapters 44 and 62).

■ Evaluation

Expected outcomes for the patient with shock are addressed in NCP 61-1.

SYSTEMIC INFLAMMATORY RESPONSE SYNDROME AND MULTIPLE ORGAN DYSFUNCTION SYNDROME

Systemic inflammatory response syndrome (SIRS) is an abnormal host response to a variety of insults and is characterized by generalized inflammation in organs remote from the initial insult. Normally the inflammatory process is contained within a confined environment. (Inflammation is discussed in Chapter 11.) If the inflammation is not contained, SIRS (a widespread systemic inflammatory response) occurs that is deleterious to organ function.[18] Clinical conditions that predispose to SIRS are presented in Fig. 61-1. When SIRS is the result of infection, the term *sepsis* is used.

Multiple organ dysfunction syndrome (MODS) results from SIRS and is a progressive failure of more than one organ. Transition from the hypermetabolic state of SIRS to clinically defined MODS does not occur in a clear-cut manner because these two entities represent a continuum. In addition, it is difficult to measure organ dysfunction in its early stage. Furthermore, not all patients with SIRS develop MODS.

In MODS, organ dysfunction can be a direct result of the insult (primary MODS) or can manifest latently secondary to a widespread systemic inflammation and involve organs not directly affected in the initial insult (secondary MODS). Examples of primary MODS include the immediate consequences of trauma (e.g., pulmonary contusion, aspiration or inhalation injury). A common cause of secondary MODS is sepsis. Patients can experience both primary and secondary MODS.[5]

Etiology and Pathophysiology

Initiating Events. Bacteria are common causes and can release toxins that initiate the systemic inflammatory response. Exotoxins are released from certain bacteria (e.g., *S. aureus* and *Clostridium perfringens*). Endotoxins originate from the cell walls of gram-negative bacteria (e.g., *Escherichia coli, Pseudomonas*). These substances often have direct toxic effects and can activate cellular and humoral immune responses, and ultimately cause sepsis, SIRS, or MODS. Other clinical conditions that predispose to SIRS and MODS are presented in Fig. 61-1.

Whatever the stimulus, the cause of SIRS and MODS seems to be an uncontrollable systemic inflammatory response mediated by a variety of factors (see Table 61-4). Activation of one mediator leads to activation of another.[19]

When the inflammatory process is not controlled, consequences may occur that can lead to SIRS and MODS. These include activation of inflammatory cells and release of mediators, direct damage to the vascular endothelium, and hypermetabolism. During SIRS endothelial cells are common targets for white blood cell–derived mediators, which cause endothelial destruction and increased vascular permeability. Inflammatory mediators causing endothelial damage include endotoxin, TNF, IL-1, PAF, and many others (see Table 61-4). Organ perfusion may be compromised by hypotension, microemboli, or redistributed or shunted blood flow. Cellular metabolism may be impaired even if adequate oxygen is delivered.

Organ and Metabolic Dysfunction. The lungs are highly vulnerable to mediator-induced injury and are generally the first organ system affected in SIRS and MODS. Acute lung injury manifests as ARDS and generally occurs 1 to 3 days after the initial injury. (ARDS is discussed in Chapter 62.) ARDS is accompanied by a hypermetabolic response.

Cardiovascular changes include myocardial depression and vasodilation. Vasodilation results in decreased systemic vascular resistance (decreased afterload) and decreased blood pressure. The baroreceptor reflex causes release of inotropic (increasing force of contraction) and chronotropic (increasing heart rate) factors that enhance cardiac output. For a while, blood pressure may be maintained but at a higher heart rate and cardiac output. Increases in capillary permeability result in shifting of albumin and fluid from the vascular space, which further diminishes preload. The patient is warm and tachycardic with a high cardiac output and a low systemic vascular resistance. Mixed venous oxygen saturation may be abnormally high because the patient is perfusing areas not consuming much oxygen (e.g., skin, nonworking muscle) while other areas may have blood shunted away from them. Eventually, either perfusion of vital organs becomes insufficient or the cells are unable to use oxygen and their function is compromised. As MODS progresses, cardiac failure develops.

Neurologic dysfunction commonly manifests as mental changes with SIRS and MODS. Acute alteration in mental status can be an early sign of SIRS. The patient may become confused and agitated, combative, disoriented, lethargic, or comatose. These changes may be due to hypoxemia or impaired perfusion. Mediators may damage neuronal tissue directly or indirectly via capillary leakage and related tissue damage. This in turn may produce cerebral edema resulting in increased intracranial pressure.

Peripheral neurologic dysfunction also occurs in patients with MODS, possibly from edema and hypoxia of the peripheral nerves. Clinical findings may be obvious (e.g., severe weakness) or subtle (e.g., difficulty weaning from mechanical ventilation).

Renal failure may result from prerenal causes (impaired perfusion) or from direct damage to renal tubular cells (acute tubular necrosis [ATN]). The frequent use of nephrotoxic drugs (see Table 42-2) for critically ill patients also increases the risk of ATN.

Failure of the coagulation system manifests as disseminated intravascular coagulation (DIC). DIC results in simultaneous microvascular clotting and bleeding because of the depletion of clotting factors and platelets and excessive fibrinolysis. (DIC is discussed in Chapter 29.)

Initially leukocytosis generally occurs. This is especially true if MODS is caused by an infectious agent. Hematopoiesis is impaired, causing anemia, leukopenia, and thrombocytopenia.

Impaired GI circulation may diminish motility, causing paralytic ileus. The GI system is extremely vulnerable to ischemia. Hypoperfusion damages the normal GI mucosa. Following injury the potential for translocation of GI luminal bacteria into the systemic circulation is thought to be increased.[15] This mechanism may be a source of additional activators (e.g., bacteria and endotoxin). Mucosal ischemia results in an increased incidence of gastric and duodenal ulcer formation, and places the patient at risk for GI bleeding.

Liver dysfunction may result in clinical evidence of bleeding, jaundice, hypoglycemia, and lactic acidosis. The patient develops hypoproteinemia because of a shift in the liver activity toward production of acute phase proteins. The serum level of liver enzymes is increased because of ischemic hepatitis, and the prothrombin time is prolonged.

Metabolic changes are pronounced. SIRS and MODS trigger a hypermetabolic response. Glycogen stores are rapidly converted to glucose. Catecholamines and glucocorticoids result in hyperglycemia and insulin resistance. Once glycogen is gone, amino acids are converted to glucose, depleting protein stores. Fatty acids are mobilized for fuel. The net result is a catabolic state, and lean body mass is lost. If hepatic insufficiency is severe, hypoglycemia occurs. Serum protein and albumin levels are generally low because of the catabolic state, leakage of these substances across capillary membranes, and altered liver production.

Electrolyte imbalances, which are common, are related to hormonal and metabolic changes and fluid shifts. These changes exacerbate mental status changes, neuromuscular dysfunction, and cardiac arrhythmias. Antidiuretic hormone results in water retention and hyponatremia. Aldosterone increases urinary potassium loss, and the patient becomes hypokalemic. Catecholamines cause potassium to move into the cell, increasing hypokalemia. Hypokalemia is associated with arrhythmias and muscle weakness. Metabolic acidosis results from impaired tissue perfusion, hypoxia, and a shift to anaerobic metabolism with a related increase in hydrogen ion production. Progressive renal dysfunction also causes an increase in metabolic acidosis. Hypocalcemia, hypomagnesemia, and hypophosphatemia are common.

Clinical Manifestations of SIRS and MODS

The clinical manifestations and laboratory findings of SIRS include the following:

1. Temperature greater than 100.4° F (38° C) or less than 97° F (36° C)
2. Heart rate greater than 90 beats per minute
3. Respiratory rate greater than 20 breaths per minute or $PaCO_2$ less than 32 mm Hg
4. White blood cell count greater than 12,000 cells/μl or less than 4000 cells/μl or greater than 10% immature (band) neutrophils

SIRS is present when two or more of these four clinical manifestations are present (see Table 61-3). The patient may also demonstrate hypotension, confusion, hyperglycemia, and thrombocytopenia. Manifestations range from mild signs and symptoms to circulatory collapse.

Early signs and symptoms of SIRS vary widely. Most patients initially have mild restlessness or confusion, hyperthermia, tachycardia, some increase in fluid requirements, tachypnea with mild respiratory alkalosis, oliguria with reduced responsiveness to diuretics, abdominal distention, and hyperglycemia or increased glucose requirements.

In fully developed sepsis or SIRS the patient appears acutely sick and unstable. Confusion worsens to lethargy or stupor. Cardiac output is greatly increased, the heart rate is rapid, and the skin is warm. Although large volumes of fluid are required to maintain preload, cardiac output tends to be low because of third spacing. Maintaining blood pressure requires volume expansion and vasoactive and cardiotonic drugs. Mixed venous oxygen saturation may be increased because of failure to effi-

Table 61-12 Clinical Evidence of Organ Dysfunction

Cardiovascular Failure
- Heart rate <55 beats/min
- Mean arterial pressure <50 mm Hg or systolic blood pressure <60 mm Hg
- Ventricular tachycardia or fibrillation
- Cardiac index <2.0 L/min/m^2
- Serum pH <7.25 with a $PaCO_2$ <50 mm Hg

Respiratory Failure
- Severe dyspnea
- Respiratory rate <6 or >50 breaths/min
- Chest x-ray with decreased lung volumes and bilateral diffuse patchy infiltrates
- $PaCO_2$ ≥50 mm Hg
- Crackles, wheezes
- PaO_2/FIO_2 <200
- Ventilatory dependence >72 hr

Renal Failure
- Urine output <0.5 ml/kg/hr
- BUN ≥100 mg/dl (35.7 mmol/L)
- Serum creatinine ≥3.5 mg/dl (309 μmol/L)

Central Nervous System Failure
- Glasgow Coma Scale ≤6 (in absence of sedation)
- Hypothermia or hyperthermia
- Cardiovascular failure
- Respiratory depression

Hematologic Failure
- White blood cell count ≤1000/μl (1×10^9/L)
- Platelets ≤20,000/μl (20×10^9/L)
- Hematocrit ≤ 20% (.20)
- Bleeding studies prolonged

Hepatic Failure
- Presence of both of the following:
  - Serum bilirubin ≥6 mg/dl (102.6 μmol/L)
  - Prothrombin time >4 sec over control in the absence of systemic anticoagulation

Pancreatic Failure
- Elevated serum lipase and amylase
- Elevated serum glucose (often resistant to insulin administration)

Gastrointestinal Failure
- Mucosal erosion on endoscopy
- Perforation
- Upper or lower GI bleeding
- Diarrhea
- Paralytic ileus

BUN, blood urea nitrogen; *FIO_2,* fraction of inspired O_2; *$PaCO_2$,* partial arterial pressure of CO_2; *PaO_2,* partial arterial pressure of O_2.

ciently distribute blood to working organs. The patient is tachypneic, hypocapneic, and possibly hypoxemic, especially if ARDS develops. There is oliguria progressing to renal failure. The GI tract, especially the stomach and colon, is adynamic, and enteral feedings are poorly tolerated. Stress ulceration may occur. As the liver is compromised, bilirubin levels increase and the patient may appear jaundiced. The prothrombin time is prolonged. The patient may develop thrombocytopenia progressing to DIC. Stress-related hormones are high, resulting in increased catabolism and hyperglycemia.

Table 61-13 Progression of Multiple Organ Dysfunction Syndrome*

Days after Precipitating Event or Insult

1-4 Days
- Low grade fever
- Tachycardia
- Dyspnea
- Altered mental status
- Hyperdynamic/hypermetabolic state
- Lungs first to fail—acute respiratory distress syndrome

6-10 Days
- Hyperdynamic/hypermetabolic state increases
- Bacteremia
- Signs of liver and renal failure

10-14 Days
- Liver and renal failure more severe
- Gastrointestinal system fails
- Cardiovascular collapse

15-21 Days
- Multiple organ dysfunction syndrome

21-28 Days
- Death occurs

*This is a possible sequence of events.

In advanced SIRS and MODS, the patient is unstable and appears close to death. The patient may lose consciousness. Vasopressors and inotropic agents are needed to maintain blood pressure. The patient will be grossly edematous (anasarca). Mixed venous oxygen saturation may rise because of problems with tissue oxygen delivery or may fall if the patient has severe arterial hypoxemia. The patient may be hypercapneic despite aggressive ventilation and have a combined metabolic and respiratory acidosis. The patient may become anuric and require renal replacement therapy. Liver enzyme and bilirubin levels increase. Lactic acidosis worsens. Coagulopathy becomes impossible to correct.

Multiple organs can fail. Criteria for organ system failure are presented in Table 61-12. A prototype progression of MODS is presented in Table 61-13.

NURSING AND COLLABORATIVE MANAGEMENT: SIRS AND MODS

The prognosis of SIRS and MODS is poor, with estimated mortality rates at 90% to 95% when three or more organs fail.[3] Therefore the most important goal is to prevent the development of SIRS and MODS.[19] An important component of the nursing role is vigilant assessment to detect early signs of deterioration or organ dysfunction.

Collaborative care for patients with SIRS or MODS focuses on (1) prevention and treatment of infection, (2) maintenance of tissue oxygenation, (3) nutritional and metabolic support, and (4) appropriate support of individual failing organs.

■ Prevention and Treatment of Infection

Aggressive avoidance, early detection, and prompt treatment of infection are important to eliminate the source of inflammation. If there is an infection, it is important to quickly di-

ETHICAL DILEMMAS

Entitlement to Treatment

SITUATION

A 35-year-old European tourist had a hang gliding accident while touring the United States. He was taken to the regional trauma center for treatment of internal injuries, loss of blood, and severe pelvic fractures. He has become septic with a rare organism, is now in renal failure, and has acute respiratory distress syndrome. Despite a 5% to 6% chance of survival, his wife and parents want all possible measures to be taken.

DISCUSSION

The patient, who is not a U.S. resident or citizen, intentionally participated in a (potentially) dangerous activity when he had no insurance coverage. According to federal law, a patient may not be refused admission to an emergency department for acute care. His family believes that his condition entitles him to treatment. His overall prognosis is grim, but his individual condition can be treated with modern technology and expensive drug therapy. There is still a question about the futility of continuing his treatment. The hospital may be left with an enormous uncompensated bill for this patient whether or not he survives. Many hospitals suffer the same dilemma with U.S. residents and citizens who are unable to pay for their treatment.

ETHICAL AND LEGAL PRINCIPLES

- Under the Emergency Medical Treatment and Labor Act (also known as COBRA), hospitals receiving federal money under Medicaid and Medicare must provide emergency screening and treatment in order to stabilize a patient before transferring to another facility.
- The Hill-Burton Act requires states to provide sufficient hospitals and necessary services for those unable to pay.
- Medically futile treatment need not be offered by the hospital. If the family or patient demands obviously futile treatment, the medical team should seek clarification of the goals of such treatment (i.e., recovery, survival, continuing biologic existence, nonabandonment of the patient.) There is no legal right to require medical treatment in cases where the treatment goals cannot be met.

agnose it. Sometimes infections may be difficult to identify. Known infections should be treated with specific agents. If the organism is not known, therapy should begin with broad-spectrum antibiotics and then changed to indicated antibiotics when the organism is identified. Early, aggressive surgery is recommended to remove necrotic tissue (e.g., early debridement of burn tissue) that may provide a culture medium for microorganisms. Aggressive pulmonary management, including early ambulation, can decrease infection. Strict asepsis can decrease infections related to intraarterial lines, endotracheal tubes, urinary catheters, IV lines, and other invasive procedures.

Patients may become infected even when infection control procedures are stringent. Critically ill patients may infect themselves. For example, bacterial contamination of the respiratory tract and development of pneumonia can result from colonization of GI tract bacteria. In some cases infections are thought to be due to systemic invasion by GI bacteria, which are able to penetrate the mucosal barrier following ischemia of the GI tract. Selective decontamination of the GI tract and pharynx has been used to reduce infection but does not alter morbidity or mortality rates from MODS. Another approach to this problem is to institute early enteral feedings, which may enhance perfusion of the GI tract. The induction and maintenance of enteral feedings improves the GI mucosal barrier and decreases the incidence of bacterial and endotoxin translocation.[15,20]

■ Maintenance of Tissue Oxygenation

Hypoperfusion and resultant hypoxemia frequently occur in patients with SIRS or MODS. These patients have greater O_2 needs and decreased O_2 supply to the tissues. Interventions that decrease O_2 demand and increase O_2 delivery are essential. Decreasing O_2 demand may be accomplished by sedation, mechanical ventilation, analgesia, and rest. Oxygen delivery may be increased by maintenance of a normal hematocrit and PaO_2, positive end-expiratory pressure, increasing preload or myocardial contractility to enhance cardiac output, or reducing afterload to increase cardiac output. Throughout treatment, the ICU nurse must assess the intensity of symptoms, stability of the patient, and potential for recovery. The nurse should discuss the treatment progress with the patient and family.

■ Nutritional and Metabolic Needs

Hypermetabolism in SIRS or MODS can result in profound weight loss, cachexia, and organ failure. Protein-calorie malnutrition is one of the primary manifestations of hypermetabolism and MODS. Total energy expenditure is increased 1.5 to 2.0 times the normal metabolic rate. Plasma transferrin and prealbumin levels are monitored to indicate hepatic protein synthesis.

The goal of nutritional support is to preserve organ function. Providing adequate nutrition decreases morbidity and mortality rates in patients with SIRS and MODS. The enteral route is preferable to parenteral nutrition and may limit bacterial translocation. If the enteral route cannot be used, parenteral nutrition is used. (Enteral and parenteral nutrition are discussed in Chapter 38.)

■ Support of Failing Organs

Support of any failing organ is a primary goal of therapy. The patient with ARDS requires oxygen therapy and mechanical ventilation (see Chapter 62). DIC should be treated appropriately (see Chapter 29). Renal failure may require renal replacement therapy (see Chapter 44). Continuous renal replacement therapy is better tolerated than dialysis, especially in a patient with hemodynamic instability.

■ Research in SIRS and MODS

Monoclonal antibodies and antagonists have been developed against a number of different mediators, including TNF, endotoxin, IL-1, PAF, and bradykinin. Preliminary results have not been encouraging. Thus continued research with this approach will be necessary before effective clinical therapy becomes available to control sepsis or an excessive inflammatory response.[19,21]

CRITICAL THINKING EXERCISES

CASE STUDY

Shock

Patient Profile

Mr. S., a 25-year-old man, was an unrestrained driver involved in a motor vehicle crash. He was found face down 15 feet from his car. There were no passengers. The windshield was broken and the car was found up against a tree. Mr. S. was found conscious and moaning. He was taken to the emergency department (ED).

Subjective Data

- States that he cannot breathe
- Complains of abdominal pain

Objective Data

Physical Examination

- Cardiovascular: BP 84/70; apical pulse 120 but no radial or brachial pulses palpable; carotid pulse present but weak
- Lungs: respiratory rate 35/min; labored breathing with severe respiratory distress; asymmetric chest wall movement; absence of breath sounds on left side
- Abdomen: slightly distended and painful to palpation

Diagnostic Studies

- Chest x-ray: hemopneumothorax and rib fractures on left side
- Hematocrit: 28%

Collaborative Care

- In the ED, placement of chest tube, which drained bright red blood

Surgical Procedure

- Splenectomy
- Repair of torn thoracic artery

Critical Thinking Questions

1. What type of shock was present in Mr. S.? What clinical manifestations did he display?
2. What were the causes of Mr. S.'s shock? What are other causes of this type of shock?
3. What are the initial nursing responsibilities for Mr. S.?
4. What continual nursing assessment parameters are essential for this patient?
5. Based on the assessment data presented, write one or more nursing diagnoses. Are there any collaborative problems?

NURSING RESEARCH ISSUES

1. What is the patient's ability to understand what is being said and happening as the shock state worsens?
2. Compare the cognitive status of patients in different stages of shock.
3. What nursing measures can be implemented to conserve oxygen and decrease oxygen utilization in patients with shock or MODS?
4. What patient positions improve oxygenation and circulatory status?
5. Compare the accuracy of blood pressure monitoring devices to detect the blood pressure changes in shock: invasive arterial monitoring compared with noninvasive devices.

REVIEW QUESTIONS

The number of the question corresponds to the same-numbered objective at the beginning of the chapter.

1. *Shock* is best defined as
   a. cardiovascular collapse.
   b. loss of sympathetic tone.
   c. inadequate tissue perfusion.
   d. blood pressure less than 90 mm Hg systolic.
2. A 78-year-old man has confusion and temperature of 104° F (40° C). He is a diabetic with purulent drainage from his right great toe. His hemodynamic findings are BP 90/40; HR 110; respiratory rate 42 and shallow; CO 6L/min; and PAWP 4 mm Hg. This patient's presentation of symptoms is most likely indicative of
   a. septic shock.
   b. hypovolemic shock.
   c. cardiogenic shock.
   d. anaphylactic shock.
3. A patient in shock is very pale and has a falling blood pressure with tachycardia; a weak, thready pulse; and shallow respirations at a rate of 24 per minute. The nurse recognizes that the patient is in
   a. the compensated phase of shock.
   b. the progressive phase of shock.
   c. the refractory phase of shock.
   d. multiple organ dysfunction syndrome.
4. The effect that shock has on the body includes
   a. sympathetic nervous system activation that results in stimulation of adrenergic receptors.
   b. massive vasoconstriction in the heart and brain that causes stimulation of the renin-angiotensin system.
   c. a heart rate that is usually slow and irregular in the compensatory stage because of parasympathetic nervous stimulation.
   d. decreased tissue perfusion that causes the cells to undergo aerobic metabolism, leading to the development of lactic acidosis.
5. Appropriate treatment modalities for the management of cardiogenic shock include
   a. dopamine to increase myocardial contractility.
   b. corticosteroids to stabilize the cell wall in the infarcted area.
   c. vasopressors to increase systemic vascular resistance.
   d. plasma volume expanders such as albumin to decrease an elevated preload.

6. The most accurate assessment parameters for the nurse to use to determine adequate tissue perfusion in the patient with MODS are
   a. blood pressure, pulse, and respirations.
   b. breath sounds, blood pressure, and body temperature.
   c. pulse pressure, level of consciousness, and pupillary response.
   d. level of consciousness, urine output, and skin color and temperature.

References

1. Hill KA, Suter RE: Shock: recognition and care, *JEMS* 21:38, 1996.
2. Sundaresan R, Sheagren JN: Current understanding and treatment of sepsis, *Infect Med* 12:261, 1995.
3. Wadhwa J, Sood R: Multiple organ dysfunction syndrome, *Natl Med J India* 10:277, 1997.
4. Members of the American College of Chest Physicians/Society of Critical Care Medicine Consensus Conference Committee: Definitions for sepsis and organ failure and guidelines for the use of innovative therapies in sepsis, *Crit Care Med* 20:864, 1992.
5. Thelan LA and others: *Critical care nursing: diagnosis and management,* ed 3, St Louis, 1998, Mosby.
6. Koch T: Origin and mediators involved in sepsis and the systemic inflammatory response syndrome, *Kidney Int (Suppl)* 64:S66, 1998.
7. Bone RC, Grodzin CJ, Balk RA: Sepsis: a new hypothesis for pathogenesis of the disease process, *Chest* 112:235, 1997.
8. James JM: Anaphylaxis: multiple etiologies—focused therapy, *J Ark Med Soc* 93:281, 1996.
9. Fink M: Shock: an overview. In Rippe J and others: *Intensive care medicine,* ed 3, Boston, 1996, Little, Brown.
10. Pearl RG: Treatment of shock—1998, *Anesth Analg* (suppl):75, 1998.
11. Kreimeier U, Peter K: Strategies of volume therapy in sepsis and systemic inflammatory response syndrome, *Kidney Int (Suppl)* 64:S75, 1998.
12. Conte MA: Fluid resuscitation in the trauma patient, *CRNA* 8:31, 1997.
13. Sandrock J: Treating traumatic hypovolemia: which fluid to choose? *Nursing* 98:32cc1, 1998.
14. Marino PL: The ICU book, ed 2, Baltimore, 1998, Williams & Wilkins.
15. Lemaire LC and others: Bacterial translocation in multiple organ failure: cause or epiphenomenon still unproven, *Br J Surg* 84:1340, 1997.
16. Tasota FJ and others: Protecting ICU patients from nosocomial infections: practical measures for favorable outcomes, *Crit Care Nurse* 18:54, 1998.
17. Leske JS: Needs of relatives of critically ill patients: a follow-up, *Heart Lung* 15:189, 1990.
18. Nystrom PO: The systemic inflammatory response syndrome: definitions and aetiology, *J Antimicrob Chemother* 41(suppl A):1, 1998.
19. Baue AE: Multiple organ failure, multiple organ dysfunction syndrome, and systemic inflammatory response syndrome, *Arch Surg* 132:703, 1997.
20. Campbell IT: Can body composition in multiple organ failure be favorably influenced by feeding? *Nutrition* 13(suppl):79S, 1997.
21. Horn KD: Evolving strategies in the treatment of sepsis and systemic inflammatory response syndrome (SIRS), *Q J Med* 91:265, 1998.

Resources

Resources for this chapter are listed after Chapter 63 on p. 1957.

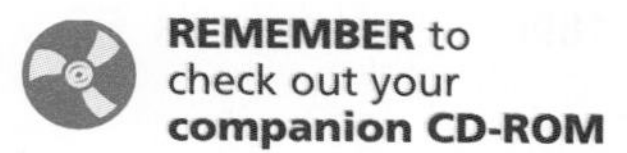

62 NURSING MANAGEMENT Respiratory Failure

Patricia J. Davies & Leslie A. Hoffman

www.mosby.com/MERLIN/medsurg_lewis

LEARNING OBJECTIVES

1. Explain the physiologic mechanisms that result in hypoxemic or hypercapnic respiratory failure, including acute respiratory distress syndrome (ARDS).
2. Differentiate between early and late clinical manifestations of respiratory failure.
3. Describe the nursing and collaborative management of the patient with hypoxemic or hypercapnic respiratory failure.
4. Describe nursing and collaborative management for the patient with ARDS.
5. Identify complications that may result from acute respiratory failure and measures to prevent or reverse these complications.

ACUTE RESPIRATORY FAILURE

The major function of the respiratory system is gas exchange, which involves the transfer of oxygen (O_2) and carbon dioxide (CO_2) between the atmosphere and the blood (Fig. 62-1). Respiratory failure results when one or both of these gas-exchanging functions are inadequate. For example, insufficient O_2 is transferred to the blood or inadequate CO_2 is removed from the lungs. Inadequate O_2 transfer results in hypoxemia, which is manifested by a decrease in arterial O_2 tension (PaO_2) and a decrease in arterial O_2 saturation (SaO_2). Insufficient CO_2 removal results in hypercapnia, which is manifested by an increase in arterial CO_2 tension ($PaCO_2$).[1] Changes in PaO_2, $PaCO_2$, and SaO_2 can be assessed using arterial blood gases. Pulse oximetry can be used to measure SaO_2 (see Chapter 24). Respiratory failure is not a disease; it is a condition that occurs as a result of one or more diseases involving the lungs or other body systems (Tables 62-1 and 62-2).

Respiratory failure can be classified as hypoxemic or hypercapnic (Fig. 62-2). Hypoxemic respiratory failure is also referred to as oxygenation failure because the primary problem is inadequate O_2 transfer.[1] Although no universal definition exists, hypoxemic respiratory failure is commonly defined as a PaO_2 of 60 mm Hg or less when the patient is receiving an inspired O_2 concentration of 60% or greater. This definition incorporates two important concepts: (1) the PaO_2 is at a level that indicates danger of inadequate O_2 saturation of hemoglobin; and (2) this PaO_2 level exists despite administration of supplemental O_2 at a percentage (60%) that is about three times that in room air (21%).

Hypercapnic respiratory failure is also referred to as ventilatory failure because the primary problem is insufficient CO_2 removal. Hypercapnic respiratory failure is commonly defined as a $PaCO_2$ above normal (greater than 45 mm Hg) in combination with acidemia (pH less than 7.35). This definition incorporates three important concepts: (1) the $PaCO_2$ is higher than normal; (2) there is evidence of the body's inability to compensate for this increase (acidemia); and (3) the pH is at a level where a further decrease may lead to severe acid-base imbalance. (See Chapter 15 for a discussion of acid-base balance.) Many patients experience both hypoxemic and hypercapnic respiratory failure.

Etiology and Pathophysiology

Hypoxemic Respiratory Failure. Common diseases and conditions that cause hypoxemic respiratory failure are listed in Table 62-1. Four physiologic mechanisms may cause hypoxemia and subsequent hypoxemic respiratory failure: (1) mismatch between ventilation ($\dot{V}$) and perfusion ($\dot{Q}$), commonly referred to as $\dot{V}/\dot{Q}$ mismatch; (2) shunt; (3) diffusion limitation; and (4) hypoventilation. The most common causes are $\dot{V}/\dot{Q}$ mismatch and shunt.[1,2]

$\dot{V}/\dot{Q}$ mismatch. In the normal lung, the volume of blood perfusing the lungs each minute (4 to 5 L) is approximately equal to the amount of fresh gas that reaches the alveoli each minute (4 to 5 L). In a perfectly matched system, each portion of the lung would receive about 1 ml of air for each 1 ml of blood flow. This match of ventilation and perfusion would result in a $\dot{V}/\dot{Q}$ ratio of 1:1 (e.g., 1 ml of air per 1 ml of blood), which is expressed as $\dot{V}/\dot{Q} = 1$. Ventilation is ideally matched with perfusion.[3]

Reviewed by Susan B. Stillwell, RN, MSN, Clinical Associate Professor, College of Nursing, Arizona State University, Tempe, Ariz; and Janet T. Crimlisk, RN, MS, NP, CS, Pulmonary Clinical Nurse Specialist, Adult Nurse Practitioner, Boston Medical Center, Boston, Mass.

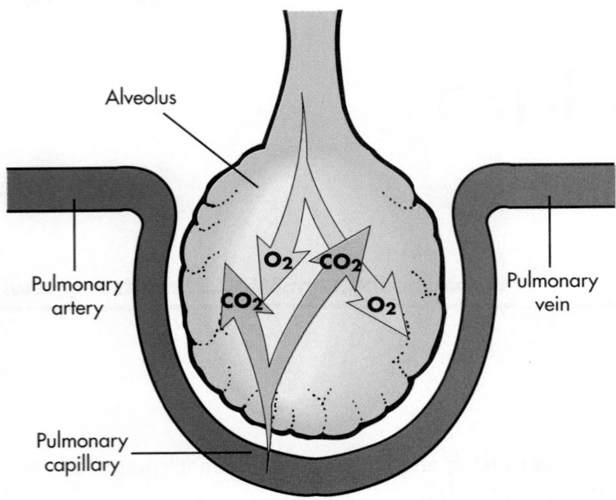

Fig. 62-1 Normal gas exchange unit in the lung.

Glossary Of Abbreviations

ARTERIAL BLOOD MONITORING

ABGs	Arterial blood gases
pH	Negative log of the free hydrogen ion $[H^+]$
PaO_2	Partial pressure of oxygen in arterial blood
$PaCO_2$	Partial pressure of carbon dioxide in arterial blood
SaO_2	Oxygen saturation in arterial blood measured by ABGs
SpO_2	Oxygen saturation in arterial blood measured by pulse oximetry

OXYGEN AND LUNG FUNCTION MONITORING

FIO_2	Fraction of inspired oxygen concentration
FRC	Functional residual capacity (volume of air in lung at end of expiration)
PEEP	Positive end-expiratory pressure (pressure in lungs at end of expiration)
PEFR	Peak expiratory flow rate (maximum airflow during a forced expiration)
$\dot{V}/\dot{Q}$	Ventilation/perfusion ratio (relationship of ventilation to perfusion in the lungs)
V_E	Minute ventilation (product of tidal volume times respiratory rate)
V_T	Tidal volume (volume of air inspired with each breath)

Although this example presumes that ventilation and perfusion are ideally matched in all areas of the lung, this situation does not normally exist. Although there is overall matching of ventilation to perfusion within the normal lung, there is some regional mismatch. At the lung apex, $\dot{V}/\dot{Q}$ ratios are greater than 1 (more ventilation than perfusion). At the lung base, $\dot{V}/\dot{Q}$ ratios are less than 1 (less ventilation than perfusion). The net effect is a close overall match, since changes at the lung apex balance changes at the base (Fig. 62-3, p. 1898).

Table 62-1 Types of Respiratory Failure and Common Causes

Hypoxemic Respiratory Failure*	Hypercapnic Respiratory Failure*
Respiratory System	**Respiratory System**
Acute respiratory distress syndrome	Asthma
Respiratory distress syndrome of the newborn	COPD
Pneumonia	Cystic fibrosis
Cardiac System	**Central Nervous System**
Cardiogenic pulmonary edema	Brainstem infarction
Pulmonary Vascular System	Sedative and narcotic overdose
Massive pulmonary embolism (e.g., thrombus emboli or fat emboli)	Severe head injury
	Chest Wall
	Flail chest
	Kyphoscoliosis
	Massive obesity
	Neuromuscular System
	Amyotrophic lateral sclerosis
	Phrenic nerve injury
	Cervical cord injury
	Guillain-Barré syndrome
	Poliomyelitis
	Muscular dystrophy
	Multiple sclerosis

*This list is not all inclusive.
COPD, chronic obstructive pulmonary disease.

Many diseases and conditions alter overall $\dot{V}/\dot{Q}$ matching and thus cause $\dot{V}/\dot{Q}$ mismatch (Fig. 62-4, p. 1899). The most common are those in which increased secretions are present in the airways (e.g., chronic obstructive pulmonary disease [COPD]) or alveoli (e.g., pneumonia) or when bronchospasm is present (e.g., asthma). $\dot{V}/\dot{Q}$ mismatch may also result when alveoli collapse (atelectasis). In these conditions, secretions or bronchospasm limit airflow (ventilation) to alveoli but have no effect on blood flow (perfusion) to the gas exchange units. The consequence is $\dot{V}/\dot{Q}$ mismatch. A pulmonary embolus causes the opposite change. The embolus limits blood flow but has no effect on airflow to the alveoli, again causing $\dot{V}/\dot{Q}$ mismatch. O_2 therapy is usually effective in reversing hypoxemia caused by $\dot{V}/\dot{Q}$ mismatch because not all gas exchange units are affected. O_2 therapy increases the PaO_2 in blood leaving normal gas exchange units, thus causing a higher than normal PaO_2. The well-oxygenated blood mixes with poorly oxygenated blood, raising the overall PaO_2 of blood leaving the lungs.

Shunt. Shunt occurs when blood exits the heart without being exposed to O_2. A shunt can be viewed as an extreme $\dot{V}/\dot{Q}$ mismatch (see Fig. 62-4). There are two types of shunt: anatomic and intrapulmonary. An anatomic shunt occurs when blood passes through an anatomic channel in the heart (e.g., a ventricular septal defect or a patent ductus arteriosus) and therefore does not pass through the lungs. An intrapulmonary shunt occurs when blood flows through the pulmonary capillaries without participating in gas exchange. Intrapulmonary shunt is seen in conditions in which the alveoli fill with fluid (e.g., acute respiratory distress syndrome [ARDS]

Table 62-2 Predisposing Factors for Acute Respiratory Failure

Predisposing Factors	Mechanisms of Respiratory Failure
Airways and Alveoli	
Acute respiratory distress syndrome	Direct lung injury from aspiration of gastric contents, diffuse infection, near-drowning, toxic gas inhalation, or airway contusion. Indirect lung injury from sepsis syndrome, severe nonthoracic trauma, or cardiopulmonary bypass. Fluid enters the interstitial space and, ultimately, the alveoli markedly impairing gas exchange. The result is an initial ↓ in PaO_2 and later ↑ in $PaCO_2$.
Asthma	Bronchospasm escalates in severity rather than responding to therapy. Bronchospasm, edema of the bronchial mucosa, and plugging of small airways with secretions greatly reduce airflow. Work of breathing increases, causing respiratory muscle fatigue. ↓ PaO_2 and ↑ $PaCO_2$.
Chronic obstructive pulmonary disease	Alveoli are destroyed by protease-antiprotease imbalance or respiratory infection or an exacerbation of COPD escalates in severity rather than responding to therapy. Secretions obstruct airflow. Work of breathing increases and causes respiratory muscle fatigue. ↓ PaO_2 and ↑ $PaCO_2$.
Cystic fibrosis	Abnormal Na^+ and Cl^- transport produces secretions that are viscous, poorly cleared, and therefore a foci for infection. Over time the airways become clogged with viscous, purulent, often greenish-colored sputum. Secretions obstruct airflow. Repeated infections destroy alveoli. Work of breathing increases, causing respiratory muscle fatigue. ↓ PaO_2 and ↑ $PaCO_2$.
Central Nervous System	
Narcotic or other drug overdose	Respirations slowed by drug effect. Insufficient CO_2 is excreted, resulting in an increase in $PaCO_2$.
Brainstem infarction, head injury	Medulla cannot alter respiratory rate in response to change in $PaCO_2$
Chest Wall	
Flail chest	Fractures prevent normal rib cage expansion resulting in inadequate gas exchange.
Kyphoscoliosis	Change in spinal configuration compresses the lungs and prevents normal expansion of the chest wall.
Massive obesity	Weight of the chest and abdominal contents prevents normal rib cage movement.
Neuromuscular Conditions	
Cervical cord injury, phrenic nerve injury	Neural control is lost preventing use of the diaphragm, the major muscle of respiration. As a consequence, the patient inspires a smaller tidal volume, which predisposes to ↑ $PaCO_2$.
Amyotrophic lateral sclerosis (ALS), Guillain-Barré, muscular dystrophy, multiple sclerosis, poliomyelitis	Respiratory muscle weakness or paralysis occurs preventing normal CO_2 excretion. Dysfunction may be slowly progressive (muscular dystrophy, multiple sclerosis), progressive with no potential of recovery (ALS), rapid with good expectation of recovery (Guillain-Barré), or stable for extended periods of time (poliomyelitis).

and pulmonary edema).[1] O_2 therapy may be ineffective in increasing the PaO_2 if hypoxemia is due to shunt because (1) blood passes from the right to the left side of the heart without passing through the lungs (anatomic shunt); or (2) the alveoli are filled with fluid, which prevents gas exchange (intrapulmonary shunt). Patients with shunt are usually more hypoxemic than patients with $\dot{V}/\dot{Q}$ mismatch, and they may require mechanical ventilation to improve gas exchange.

Diffusion limitation. Diffusion limitation occurs when gas exchange across the alveolar-capillary membrane is compromised by a process that thickens or destroys the membrane (Fig. 62-5). Pulmonary capillary blood flow may be reduced as a result of obstruction or destruction of vessels such as severe emphysema or recurrent pulmonary emboli. Some diseases cause the alveolar-capillary membrane to become thicker (fibrotic), which slows gas transport. These diseases include pulmonary fibrosis, interstitial lung disease, and ARDS. Diffusion limitation is more likely to cause hypoxemia during exercise than at rest. During exercise, blood moves more rapidly through the lungs. Because transit time is increased, red blood cells are in the lungs for a shorter time, decreasing the time for diffusion of O_2 across the alveolar-capillary membrane. The classical sign of diffusion limitation is hypoxemia that is present during exercise but not at rest.

Alveolar hypoventilation. Alveolar hypoventilation is a generalized decrease in ventilation that results in an increase in the $PaCO_2$ and a consequent decrease in PaO_2. Hypoventilation may be the result of lung disease, central nervous system (CNS) disease, chest wall dysfunction, or neuromuscular disease. Although alveolar hypoventilation is primarily a mechanism of hypercapnic respiratory failure, it is mentioned here because it can cause hypoxemia.

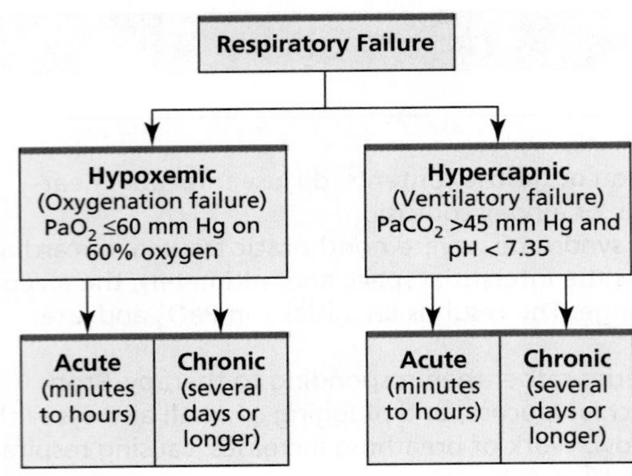

Fig. 62-2 Classification of respiratory failure.

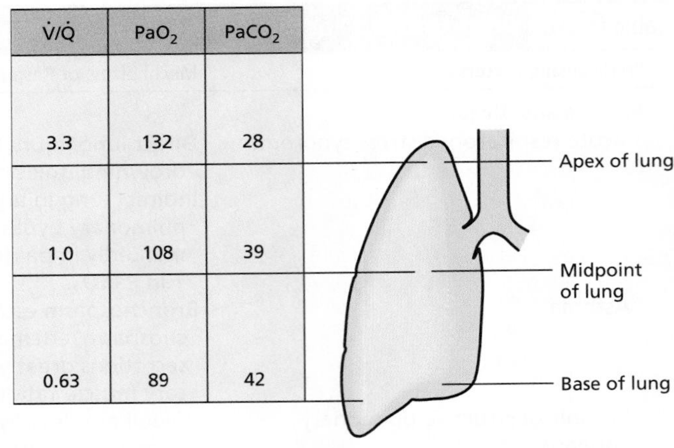

Fig. 62-3 Regional $\dot{V}/\dot{Q}$ differences in the normal lung. At the lung apex, the $\dot{V}/\dot{Q}$ ratio is 3.3, at the midpoint 1.0, and at the base 0.63. This difference causes the PaO_2 to be higher at the apex of the lung and lower at the base. Values for $PaCO_2$ are the opposite (i.e., lower at the apex and higher at the base). Blood that exits the lung is a mixture of these values.

Interrelationship of mechanisms. Frequently, hypoxemic respiratory failure is caused by a combination of two or more of the following: $\dot{V}/\dot{Q}$ mismatch, shunting, diffusion limitation, and hypoventilation. The patient with acute respiratory failure secondary to pneumonia may have a combination of $\dot{V}/\dot{Q}$ mismatch and shunt because the inflammation, edema, and hypersecretion of exudate within the bronchioles and terminal respiratory units obstruct the airways ($\dot{V}/\dot{Q}$ mismatch) and fill the alveoli with exudate (shunt). The patient with cardiogenic pulmonary edema or ARDS may have a combination of shunt and $\dot{V}/\dot{Q}$ mismatch because some alveoli are completely filled with fluid from edema (shunt) and others are partially filled with fluid ($\dot{V}/\dot{Q}$ mismatch).

Hypercapnic Respiratory Failure. Hypercapnic respiratory failure results from an imbalance between ventilatory supply and ventilatory demand. Ventilatory supply is the maximum ventilation (gas flow in and out of the lungs) that the patient can sustain without developing respiratory muscle fatigue. Ventilatory demand is the amount of ventilation needed to keep the $PaCO_2$ within normal limits. Normally, ventilatory supply far exceeds ventilatory demand. As a consequence, individuals with normal lung function can engage in strenuous exercise, which greatly increases CO_2 production without an elevation in $PaCO_2$. Patients with lung disease do not have this advantage. However, considerable dysfunction is typically present before ventilatory demand exceeds ventilatory supply.

When ventilatory demand exceeds ventilatory supply, the $PaCO_2$ can no longer be sustained within normal limits and hypercapnia occurs. Hypercapnia reflects substantial lung dysfunction.[1] Hypercapnic respiratory failure is sometimes called pump failure because the primary problem is the inability of the respiratory system to expel (pump out) sufficient CO_2 to maintain a normal $PaCO_2$. Hypercapnic respiratory failure may also be described as acute on chronic respiratory failure since the episode of respiratory failure represents an acute decompensation in a patient whose underlying lung function has deteriorated to the point that some degree of decompensation is always present (chronic respiratory insufficiency).

Many different diseases can cause a limitation in ventilatory supply (see Tables 62-1 and 62-2). These diseases can be grouped into four categories: (1) abnormalities of the airways and alveoli, (2) abnormalities of the CNS, (3) abnormalities of the chest wall, and (4) neuromuscular conditions.[1]

Airways and alveoli. Patients with asthma, emphysema, chronic bronchitis, and cystic fibrosis are at high risk for hypercapnic respiratory failure because the underlying pathophysiology of these conditions results in airflow obstruction and air trapping.

Central nervous system. A variety of problems may suppress the drive to breathe. A common example is an overdose of a narcotic or other respiratory depressant drug. A brainstem infarction or severe head injury may also interfere with normal function of the respiratory center in the medulla. Patients with these conditions are at risk for respiratory failure because the medulla does not alter the respiratory rate in response to a change in $PaCO_2$.

Chest wall. A variety of conditions may prevent normal movement of the chest wall and hence limit lung expansion. In patients with flail chest, fractures prevent the rib cage from expanding normally. In patients with kyphoscoliosis, the change in spinal configuration compresses the lungs and prevents normal expansion of the chest wall. In patients with massive obesity, the weight of the chest and abdominal contents may limit lung expansion. Patients with these conditions are at risk for respiratory failure because these dysfunctions limit lung expansion or diaphragmatic movement and consequently gas exchange.

Neuromuscular conditions. Various types of neuromuscular diseases may result in respiratory muscle weakness or paralysis (see Table 62-1). Patients with these conditions are at risk for respiratory failure because the respiratory muscles are weakened or paralyzed as a consequence of the underlying neuromuscular condition. Therefore they are unable to maintain normal $PaCO_2$ levels.

Ventilatory failure with normal lung function. In three of these categories (CNS, chest wall, neuromuscular conditions), respiratory failure may occur despite the presence of normal lungs. Respiratory failure occurs because the medulla, respiratory muscles, or chest wall is not functioning normally. The patient may have no damage to lung tissue but may be unable to inspire a tidal volume sufficient to expel CO_2 from the lungs.

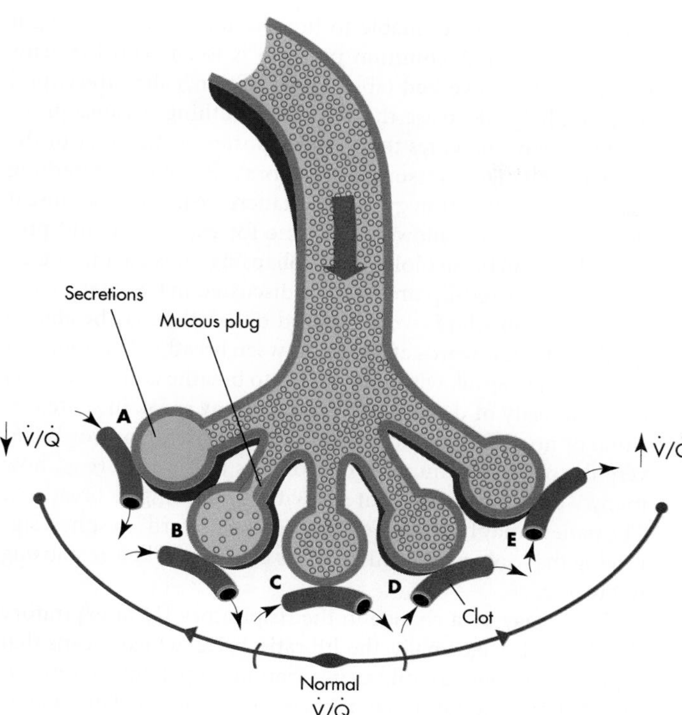

Fig. 62-4 Range of ventilation to perfusion ($\dot{V}/\dot{Q}$) relationships. *A* = absolute shunt, no ventilation because of fluid filling the alveoli; *B* = $\dot{V}/\dot{Q}$ mismatch, ventilation partially compromised by mucus in the airway; *C* = normal lung unit; *D* = $\dot{V}/\dot{Q}$ mismatch, perfusion partially compromised by emboli obstructing blood flow; *E* = dead space, no perfusion because of obstruction of the pulmonary capillary.

Tissue Oxygen Needs. It is important to remember that even though the definition of respiratory failure is determined by the PaO_2 and $PaCO_2$, the major threat of respiratory failure is inability to meet tissue O_2 needs. This inability may occur as a result of inadequate tissue O_2 delivery or because the tissues are unable to use the O_2 delivered to them. Tissue O_2 delivery is determined by the amount of O_2 carried in the hemoglobin, as well as cardiac output. Therefore respiratory failure places the patient at greater risk if there is coexisting cardiac problems or anemia. Failure of O_2 utilization most commonly occurs as a result of septic shock. In this situation, adequate O_2 may be delivered to the tissues, but an abnormally high amount of O_2 returns in the venous blood indicating that it is not being extracted at the tissue level. (Shock is discussed in Chapter 61.)

Clinical Manifestations

Respiratory failure may develop suddenly (minutes or hours) or gradually (several days or longer). A sudden decrease in PaO_2 or a rapid rise in $PaCO_2$ implies a serious condition, which can rapidly become a life-threatening emergency. An example is the patient with asthma who develops severe bronchospasm and a marked decrease in airflow, resulting in a respiratory arrest. A more gradual change in PaO_2 and $PaCO_2$ is better tolerated because compensation can occur. An example is the patient with COPD who develops a progressive increase in $PaCO_2$ over several days following the onset of a respiratory infection. Because the change occurred over several days, there is time for renal compensation (e.g., retention of bicarbonate),

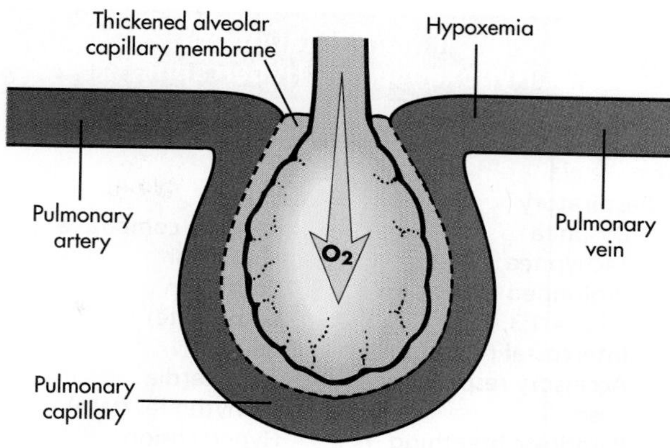

Fig. 62-5 Diffusion limitation. Exchange of CO_2 and O_2 cannot occur because of the thickened alveolar-capillary membrane.

which will minimize the change in pH. The patient has compensated respiratory acidosis.[4] (See Chapter 15 for a discussion of renal compensation for acid-base disorders.)

Manifestations of respiratory failure are related to the extent of change in PaO_2 or $PaCO_2$, the rapidity of change (acute versus chronic), and the ability to compensate to overcome this change. When the patient's compensatory mechanisms fail, respiratory failure occurs. Because clinical manifestations are variable, it is important to monitor arterial blood gas (ABG) values or use pulse oximetry to evaluate the extent of change. However, these cannot substitute for clinical assessment.

The nurse may detect manifestations of respiratory failure that are specific (arise from the respiratory system) or nonspecific (arise from other body systems) (Table 62-3). An understanding of the significance of these manifestations is critical to the ability to detect the onset of respiratory failure and effectiveness of treatment.

Restlessness, confusion, and combative behavior suggest inadequate delivery of O_2 to the brain. Such changes are seen early because the brain is highly sensitive to a decrease in O_2 delivery. Tachycardia and mild hypertension are also early signs. Such changes indicate an attempt by the heart to compensate for decreased O_2 delivery. A severe morning headache suggests that hypercapnia may have occurred during the night. At night the respiratory rate is slower and less $PaCO_2$ may be removed by the lungs. Rapid, shallow breaths suggest that the tidal volume may be inadequate to remove CO_2 from the lungs. Cyanosis is an unreliable indicator of hypoxemia and is a late sign of respiratory failure because it does not occur until hypoxemia is severe (PaO_2 45 mm Hg or less).

Hypoxemia versus Hypoxia. Hypoxemia occurs when the amount of O_2 in arterial blood is less than the normal value (see Chapter 24 for normal values). Hypoxia occurs when the PaO_2 has fallen sufficiently to cause signs and symptoms of inadequate oxygenation (see Table 62-3). Hypoxemia can lead to hypoxia if not corrected. If hypoxia or hypoxemia is severe, the cells must shift from aerobic to anaerobic metabolism. Anaerobic metabolism uses more fuel and produces less energy and is less efficient than aerobic metabolism. The waste product of anaerobic metabolism, lactic acid, is more difficult to remove from the body than CO_2 because lactic acid has to be buffered with sodium bicarbonate. When the body does not have adequate amounts of sodium bicarbonate

Table 62-3 Clinical Manifestations of Hypoxemia and Hypercapnia*

Specific	Nonspecific
Hypoxemia	
Respiratory	**Cerebral**
Dyspnea	Restless, combative behavior
Tachypnea	Confusion
Prolonged expiration (I:E = 1:3, 1:4)	Coma (late)
Intercostal retraction	**Cardiac**
Accessory respiratory use	Tachycardia
Paradoxic breathing (late)	Arrhythmias (late)
Cyanosis (late)	Hypertension
↓ SpO_2 (<80%)	Hypotension (late)
	Other
	Fatigue
	Unable to speak without pausing to breathe
Hypercapnia	
Respiratory	**Cerebral**
Dyspnea	Morning headache
↓ Respiratory rate or rapid rate with shallow respirations	Disorientation
↓ Tidal volume	Progressive somnolence
↓ Minute ventilation	Coma (late)
	Cardiac
	Arrhythmias
	Neuromuscular
	Muscle weakness
	Tremor, seizures (late)
	Other
	Pursed-lip breathing
	Use of tripod position

*List is not all inclusive.

to buffer the lactic acid produced by anaerobic metabolism, metabolic acidosis and cell death occur.

Hypoxia and metabolic acidosis have adverse effects on the vital organs, especially the heart and CNS. The heart tries to compensate for the decreased O_2 level in the blood by increasing the heart rate and cardiac output. As the PaO_2 decreases and acidosis increases, the heart muscle may be unable to function and arrhythmias may occur, resulting in a further decrease in PaO_2. Permanent brain damage may occur because of O_2 deprivation. Renal function may also be impaired, and sodium retention, edema formation, acute tubular necrosis, and uremia may occur. Gastrointestinal system alterations include tissue ischemia, increased permeability of the intestinal wall, and possible translocation of bacteria into the circulation.

Specific Clinical Manifestations The patient may have a rapid, shallow breathing pattern or a respiratory rate that is slower than normal. Both changes predispose to insufficient CO_2 removal. The patient may increase the respiratory rate in an effort to blow off accumulated CO_2. This breathing pattern requires a substantial amount of work and predisposes to respiratory muscle fatigue. A change from a rapid rate to a slower rate in a patient in acute respiratory distress suggests tiring and the possibility of respiratory arrest.

The position that the patient assumes is an indication of the effort associated with breathing. The patient may be able to lie down (mild distress), be able to lie down but prefer to sit (moderate distress), or be unable to breathe unless sitting upright (severe distress). A common position is to sit with the arms propped on the overbed table. This position, called the tripod position, helps decrease the work of breathing because propping the arms increases the anterior-posterior diameter of the chest and changes pressure in the thorax. Pursed-lip breathing may be used. This strategy causes an increase in SaO_2 because it slows respirations, allows more time for expiration, and prevents the small bronchioles from collapsing, thus facilitating air exchange. (Pursed-lip breathing is discussed in Chapter 27.)

The person who is working hard to breathe may be able to speak only a few words at a time between breaths. The ability of the patient to speak without pausing to breathe is an indication of the severity of dyspnea. The patient may speak in sentences (mild or no distress), phrases (moderate distress), or words (severe distress). The number of words is also a clue (e.g., how many words can the patient say without pausing to breathe?). The patient may have "three-word" or "two-word" dyspnea, signifying that only two or three words can be said before pausing to breathe.

There may be a change in the inspiratory (I) to expiratory (E) (I:E) ratio. Normally, the I:E ratio is 1:2, which means that expiration is twice as long as inspiration. In patients in respiratory distress, the ratio may increase to 1:3 or 1:4. This change signifies airflow obstruction and that more time is required to empty the lungs.

The nurse may observe retraction (inward movement) of the intercostal spaces or the supraclavicular area and use of the accessory muscles during inspiration or expiration. Use of the accessory muscles signifies moderate distress. Paradoxic breathing indicates severe distress. Normally, the thorax and abdomen move outward on inspiration and inward on exhalation. During paradoxic breathing, the abdomen and chest move in the opposite manner—outward during exhalation and inward during inspiration. Paradoxic breathing results from maximal use of the accessory muscles of respiration. The patient may be diaphoretic from the work associated with breathing.

The nurse's assessment may result in early detection of manifestations associated with respiratory insufficiency, allowing therapy to be instituted before the patient experiences respiratory failure. Patients with end-stage (severe) chronic lung disease may have low PaO_2 values or elevated $PaCO_2$ levels as their "normal" baseline. It is especially important to monitor specific and nonspecific signs of respiratory failure in patients with COPD because a small change can cause significant decompensation (see Table 62-3). Any deterioration in mental status, such as combative behavior, confusion, or decreased level of consciousness, should be reported immediately since this change may indicate the onset of rapid deterioration in clinical status and the need for mechanical ventilation.

Diagnostic Studies

The most common diagnostic study used to determine respiratory failure is ABGs.[5] ABG analysis is used to determine the levels of $PaCO_2$, PaO_2, and blood pH. An indwelling catheter may be inserted into an artery for monitoring pressures. This arterial line can be used to obtain frequent arterial blood gases. Pulse oximetry is frequently used for monitoring of oxygenation status, but in respiratory failure, ABGs are necessary to obtain both oxygenation (PaO_2) and ventilation ($PaCO_2$) status.

NURSING ASSESSMENT

Table 62-4 Acute Respiratory Failure

Subjective Data

Important Health Information

Past health history: Chronic lung disease; previous hospitalizations related to lung disease; thoracic or spinal cord trauma; extreme obesity, altered consciousness

Medications: Use of oxygen, inhalers, home nebulization, over-the-counter medications; immunosuppressant therapy, CNS depressants

Surgery or other treatments: Previous intubation and mechanical ventilation; recent thoracic or abdominal surgery

Functional Health Patterns

Health perception–health management: Smoking (pack-years)

Nutritional-metabolic: Anorexia, bloatedness, heartburn; weight gain or loss; decreased appetite; diaphoresis

Activity-exercise: Fatigue, dizziness; dyspnea at rest or with activity, wheezing, cough (productive or nonproductive); sputum (volume, color, viscosity); palpitations, swollen feet

Sleep-rest: Changes in sleep pattern

Cognitive-perceptual: Headache, chest pain or tightness

Coping–stress tolerance: Anxiety, depression

Objective Data

General

Restlessness, agitation

Integumentary

Pale, cool, clammy skin or warm flushed skin; peripheral and central cyanosis; peripheral dependent edema

Respiratory

Shallow, increased respirations progressing to decreased rate; use of accessory muscles with evidence of retractions, altered I/E ratio; increased diaphragmatic excursion or asymmetric chest expansion; asynchronous respirations; tactile fremitus, crepitus, or deviated trachea on palpation; resonant, hyperresonant, or dull percussion note; absent, diminished, or adventitious breath sounds; bronchial or bronchovesicular sounds heard in other than normal location, inspiratory stridor, pleural friction rub

Cardiovascular

Tachycardia progressing to bradycardia, arrhythmias, extra heart sounds (S_3, S_4); bounding pulse; hypertension progressing to hypotension; pulsus paradoxus; jugular vein distention; pedal edema

Gastrointestinal

Abdominal distention with tympany; ascites, epigastric tenderness, hepatojugular reflex

Neurologic

Somnolence, confusion, slurred speech, tremors, seizures, coma; asterixis, decreased deep tendon reflexes; papilledema

Possible Findings

$\uparrow\downarrow$ pH, $\uparrow\downarrow$ $PaCO_2$, $\downarrow$ PaO_2, $\downarrow$ SaO_2, $\downarrow$ PEFR, $\downarrow$ tidal volume, $\downarrow$ forced vital capacity, $\downarrow$ minute ventilation, $\downarrow$ negative inspiratory force; altered values of serum electrolytes, hemoglobin, and hematocrit; abnormal findings on chest x-ray; abnormal pulmonary artery and pulmonary artery wedge pressures

Other diagnostic studies that may be done include a chest x-ray, complete blood cell count, serum electrolytes, urinalysis, and electrocardiogram (ECG). Cultures of the sputum and blood are obtained as necessary to determine sources of possible infection. If pulmonary embolus is suspected, a ventilation/perfusion ($\dot{V}/\dot{Q}$) lung scan or pulmonary angiography may be done. Although not commonly done in acute situations, pulmonary function tests may be performed.

In severe respiratory failure, measurement of cardiac output and mixed venous blood gases by a pulmonary artery catheter (see Chapter 63) is important in determining the amount of blood flow to tissues and the response to treatment. Pulmonary artery, pulmonary artery wedge, and left atrial pressures are monitored to determine whether the accumulation of fluid in the lungs is the result of cardiac or pulmonary problems. These parameters also are monitored to determine the response of the lung and heart to hypoxemia and the patient's response to therapy. (Hemodynamic monitoring is discussed in detail in Chapter 63.)

NURSING AND COLLABORATIVE MANAGEMENT: ACUTE RESPIRATORY FAILURE

Because many different problems cause respiratory failure, specific care of these patients varies. This section will discuss general assessment and collaborative care measures that apply to patients with acute respiratory failure. In acute care settings there is often an overlap of function between nursing and other members of the health care team.

Nursing Assessment

Subjective and objective data that should be obtained from the patient with acute respiratory failure are presented in Table 62-4.

Nursing Diagnoses

Nursing diagnoses for the patient with acute respiratory failure include, but are not limited to, those presented in NCP 62-1.

Planning

The overall goals are that the patient in acute respiratory failure will have (1) ABG values within the patient's baseline, (2) baseline breath sounds, (3) no dyspnea or dyspnea at patient's baseline, and (4) effective cough and ability to clear secretions.

Respiratory Therapy

The major goals of respiratory care for acute respiratory failure include maintaining adequate oxygenation and ventilation. This goal is accomplished through cooperative efforts of the medical, nursing, and respiratory care team. The therapy used includes O_2 therapy, mobilization of secretions, and positive pressure ventilation (Table 62-5).

62-1 NURSING CARE PLAN PATIENT WITH ACUTE RESPIRATORY FAILURE*

Expected Patient Outcomes	Nursing Interventions and *Rationales*
NURSING DIAGNOSIS	**Ineffective airway clearance** *related to* excessive secretions, decreased level of consciousness, presence of an artificial airway, neuromuscular dysfunction, and pain *as manifested by* difficulty in expectorating sputum, presence of rhonchi or crackles, ineffective or absent cough.
▪ No abnormal breath sounds (e.g., rhonchi, crackles). ▪ Normal baseline breath sounds. ▪ Presence of effective cough. ▪ Easy expectoration of sputum.	▪ Assess patient's ability to cough *to determine need for assistance in secretion removal.* ▪ Implement assistive coughing strategies *to promote secretion removal.* ▪ Position patient with head of bed elevated at least 45 degrees or in the tripod position *to promote maximal chest expansion and cough effects.* ▪ Humidify O_2 if over 3 L/min *to prevent drying of the mucosa.* ▪ Perform tracheobronchial suctioning if cough is ineffective or if artificial airway is present *to remove secretions and improve oxygenation.* ▪ Perform chest physiotherapy *to enhance removal of secretions.* ▪ Splint any abdominal or chest incision with pillow *to reduce pain and allow for improved inspiratory efforts.* ▪ Turn every 2 hours *to prevent stasis of secretions and promote optimal ventilation.* ▪ Ensure adequate fluid intake of 2-3 L/day *to liquefy secretions.* ▪ Administer prescribed routine and as needed bronchodilator and mucolytic medications *to promote better airflow and secretion removal.*
NURSING DIAGNOSIS	**Ineffective breathing pattern** *related to* neuromuscular impairment of respirations, pain, anxiety, decreased level of consciousness, respiratory muscle fatigue, and bronchospasm *as manifested by* respiratory rate <12 or >24 breaths/min, alterated I/E ratio, irregular breathing pattern, use of accessory muscles, asynchronous thoracoabdominal movement, wheezing, apnea.
▪ Respiratory rate, depth, and rhythm within normal limits for patient. ▪ Synchronous thoracoabdominal movement. ▪ Use of accessory muscles appropriate for level of activity.	▪ Monitor for increased or decreased respiratory rate, periods of apnea, decreased inspiratory depth, and alternating rocking movement between chest and abdomen *to assess for presence of inability to sustain ventilation.* ▪ Position patient with head of bed elevated at least 45 degrees or in a tripod position *to promote diaphragmatic excursion.* ▪ Place oral or nasal airway and Ambu bag at the bedside *because airway support may be needed in the event of severely impaired ventilation or apnea.* ▪ Provide comfort measures (e.g., analgesics, positioning) *to reduce anxiety and promote patient cooperation.* ▪ Anticipate the need for possible application of NIPPV or intubation with mechanical ventilation *to maintain adequate oxygenation and ventilation.*
NURSING DIAGNOSIS	**Risk for fluid volume excess** *related to* increases in peripheral or pulmonary fluid.
▪ Normal breath sounds. ▪ Decreased or absent peripheral edema. ▪ Normal pulmonary artery or pulmonary artery wedge pressures.	▪ Assess for manifestations of fluid volume excess such as abnormal breath sounds (crackles), weight gain, jugular venous distention, peripheral or sacral edema *to identify if problem is present.* ▪ Monitor fluid status by I & O measurements, daily weights, and pulmonary artery or pulmonary artery wedge pressures *to monitor for changes in systemic fluid volume.* ▪ Restrict fluid intake and administer diuretics as ordered *to prevent or reduce fluid overload.*
NURSING DIAGNOSIS	**Anxiety** *related to* dyspnea, intubation, severity of illness, loss of personal control and uncertain outcome *as manifested by* increased heart rate, respiratory rate, and blood pressure; agitation, restlessness; verbalization of anxiety.
▪ Decreased anxiety. ▪ Relaxed demeanor. ▪ Increased sense of personal control. ▪ Verbalization of hopeful attitude toward outcome.	▪ Perform interventions in a calm, assured manner *to decrease patient's anxiety.* ▪ Reassure patient of competence of caregivers *to encourage patient relaxation.* ▪ Answer questions simply and honestly *to provide patient with needed information for decision making.* ▪ Teach and demonstrate to patient relaxation techniques of slow pursed-lip breathing, progressive relaxation, and guided imagery *to promote restoration of control over breathing.* ▪ Administer and evaluate effectiveness of any prescribed antianxiety medication.

Continued

62-1 NURSING CARE PLAN PATIENT WITH ACUTE RESPIRATORY FAILURE* —continued

Expected Patient Outcomes	Nursing Interventions and *Rationales*
NURSING DIAGNOSIS	**Impaired gas exchange** *related to* alveolar hypoventilation, intrapulmonary shunting, $\dot{V}/\dot{Q}$ mismatch, and diffusion impairment *as manifested by* hypoxemia or hypercapnia.
▪ PaO_2 and $PaCO_2$ within normal ranges for patient. ▪ Normal breath sounds.	▪ Monitor for clinical manifestations of hypoxemia and hypercapnia *to detect systemic manifestations of decreased oxygen and increased carbon dioxide.* ▪ Administer oxygen as ordered *to increase PaO_2 and SaO_2 levels.* ▪ Monitor ABGs for PaO_2 below 60 mm Hg, SaO_2 below 90%, and $PaCO_2$ above 50 mm Hg *to assess pulmonary gas exchange.* ▪ Place the patient on continuous pulse oximetry *to assess for increases or decreases in blood oxygen levels.* ▪ Monitor the apical heart rate for irregular rhythm, tachycardia, bradycardia, and cardiac arrhythmias on the cardiac monitor *because hypoxemia may precipitate cardiac arrhythmias.* ▪ Teach and encourage pursed-lip breathing *to improve gas exchange.* ▪ Anticipate the need for ventilatory support *to improve oxygenation and ventilation status.* ▪ Withhold sedative drugs unless discussed with physician *because they can depress respirations.* ▪ Administer narcotic antagonists (e.g., naloxone [Narcan]) as ordered *to reverse respiratory depression resulting from narcotic administration.*
NURSING DIAGNOSIS	**Altered nutrition: less than body requirements** *related to* poor appetite, shortness of breath, presence of artificial airway, decreased energy level, and increased caloric requirements *as manifested by* weight loss, weakness, muscle wasting, dehydration, poor muscle tone, poor skin integrity.
▪ Maintenance of weight or weight gain. ▪ Serum albumin and protein within normal ranges.	▪ Provide high-protein, high-calorie, enteral or parenteral nutrition as ordered *to meet increased nutritional requirements.* ▪ If able to take nutrition orally, provide six small meals per day *to decrease oxygen energy expenditure during digestion.* ▪ Provide between-meal nutritional supplements *to maintain adequate caloric intake.* ▪ Maintain the ordered oxygen delivery device during meals *to prevent shortness of breath and blood oxygen desaturation while eating.* ▪ Monitor for signs of CO_2 increase with parenteral nutrition *because carbohydrates may increase CO_2 levels in patients with hypercapnia.*

*The nursing care for the patient on mechanical ventilation is presented in NCP 63-2 and discussed in Chapter 63.
NIPPV, noninvasive positive pressure ventilation.

Oxygen Therapy. The primary goal of O_2 therapy is to correct hypoxemia. If hypoxemia is secondary to $\dot{V}/\dot{Q}$ mismatch, supplemental O_2 administered at 1 to 3 L/min by nasal cannula or 24% to 32% by simple face mask should improve the PaO_2 and SaO_2. Hypoxemia secondary to an intrapulmonary shunt is usually not responsive to high O_2 concentrations and the patient will usually require positive pressure ventilation (PPV). PPV offers a means of providing O_2 therapy, decreasing the work of breathing, and reducing respiratory muscle fatigue. In addition, the positive pressure may assist in opening collapsed airways and decreasing shunt. (Mechanical ventilation is discussed in Chapter 63.)

The type of O_2 delivery system chosen for the patient in acute respiratory failure should (1) be tolerated by the patient, since anxiety caused by feelings of claustrophobia related to the face mask or dyspnea may prompt the patient to remove the O_2 device; and (2) maintain a PaO_2 at 55 to 60 mm Hg or more and SaO_2 at 90% or more at the lowest O_2 concentration possible. High O_2 concentrations eliminate the nitrogen normally present in the alveoli, causing instability and atelectasis. O_2 toxicity, a condition that results in fibrotic changes in the alveoli, may also occur. In intubated patients, exposure to 60% or greater O_2 for longer than 48 hours poses a significant risk for O_2 toxicity. In nonintubated patients, the risk is less clear. (O_2 delivery devices are discussed in Chapter 27.)

Additional risks of O_2 therapy are specific to the patient with chronic hypercapnia such as the patient with COPD. Chronic hypercapnia may blunt the response of chemoreceptors in the medulla, a condition termed *CO_2 narcosis.* In this situation, respirations are stimulated by hypoxia. If the PaO_2 is

COLLABORATIVE CARE

Table 62-5 Acute Respiratory Failure

Diagnostic
- History and physical examination
- Arterial blood gases
- Pulse oximetry
- Chest x-ray
- CBC
- Serum electrolytes and urinalysis
- ECG
- Blood and sputum cultures (if indicated)
- PAP, PAWP, LAP

Collaborative Therapy

Respiratory Therapy
- O_2 therapy
- Mobilization of secretions
  - Effective coughing
  - Hydration/humidification
  - Chest physical therapy
  - Airway suctioning
- Positive pressure ventilation
  - Noninvasive positive pressure ventilation
  - Intubation with mechanical ventilation

Drug Therapy
- Relief of bronchospasm (e.g., metaproterenol [Alupent])
- Reduction of airway inflammation (corticosteroids)
- Reduction of pulmonary congestion (e.g., furosemide [Lasix])
- Treatment of pulmonary infections
- Reduction of severe anxiety and restlessness (e.g., lorazepam [Ativan])

Medical Supportive Therapy
- Management of the underlying cause of respiratory failure
- Maintenance of adequate cardiac output
- Maintenance of adequate hemoglobin concentration

Nutritional Therapy
- Parenteral nutrition support
- Enteral nutrition support

CBC, complete blood count; *LAP*, left atrial pressure; *PAP*, pulmonary artery pressure; *PAWP*, pulmonary artery wedge pressure.

suddenly increased, the patient will no longer be hypoxemic, will have no stimulus to breathe, and may experience a respiratory arrest. Patients with chronic hypercapnia should receive O_2 through a low-flow device such as a nasal cannula at 1 to 2 L/min or a Venturi mask at 24% to 28%. They should be closely monitored for changes in mental status and respiratory rate, and ABG results, until their PaO_2 level has reached their normal value.

Mobilization of Secretions. Retained pulmonary secretions may cause or exacerbate acute respiratory failure by blocking movement of O_2 into the alveoli and pulmonary capillary blood. Secretions can be mobilized through effective coughing, adequate hydration and humidification, chest physical therapy, and suctioning.

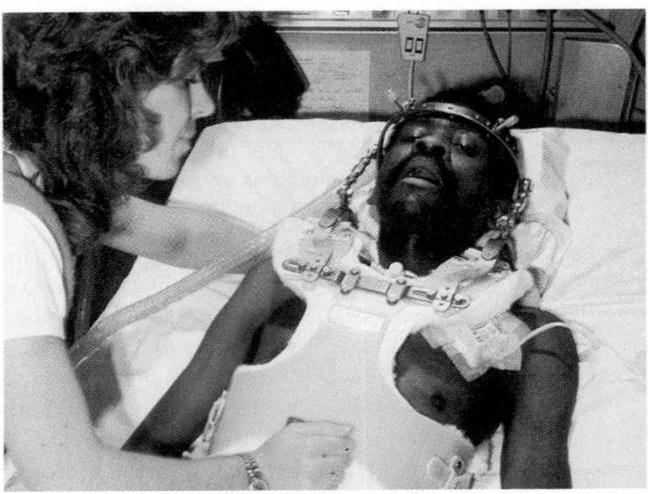

Fig. 62-6 Augmented cough. Augmented coughing is performed by placing the hand on the abdominal musculature below the xiphoid process. As the patient ends a deep inspiration and begins the expiration, the hand should be moved forcefully downward, increasing abdominal pressure, resulting in a forceful cough.

Effective coughing and positioning. If secretions are obstructing the airway, the patient should be encouraged to cough. The patient with a neuromuscular weakness, from the disease or exhaustion, may not be able to generate sufficient airway pressures to produce an effective cough. Augmented coughing (quad coughing) may be of benefit to these patients. Augmented coughing is performed by placing the palm of the hand or hands on the abdomen below the xiphoid process (Fig. 62-6). As the patient ends a deep inspiration and begins the expiration, the hands should be moved forcefully downward, increasing abdominal pressure and facilitating the cough. This measure helps increase expiratory flow and thereby facilitate secretion clearance.

Some patients may benefit from therapeutic cough techniques. Huff coughing is a series of coughs performed while saying the word "huff." This technique prevents the glottis from closing during the cough. Patients with COPD generate higher flow rates with a huff cough than is possible with a normal cough. The huff cough is effective in clearing only the central airways, but it may assist in moving secretions upward. The staged cough also assists secretion mobilization. To perform the staged cough, the patient sits in a chair, breathes three or four times in and out through the mouth, and coughs while bending forward and pressing a pillow inward against the diaphragm.

Positioning the patient either by elevating the head of the bed to at least 45 degrees or by using a reclining chair or chair bed may help maximize thoracic expansion, thereby decreasing dyspnea and improving secretion mobilization. A sitting position improves pulmonary function and assists in venous pooling. Lateral or side-lying positioning may be used in patients with disease involving only one lung. This position, termed *down with the good lung*, allows for improved $\dot{V}/\dot{Q}$ matching in the affected lung. The patient should be side lying if there is any possibility that the tongue will obstruct the airway or that aspiration may occur. An oral or nasal airway should be kept at the bedside for use if necessary.

Hydration and humidification. Thick and viscous secretions are difficult to raise and should be thinned. Adequate fluid intake (2 to 3 L per day) is necessary to keep secretions thin and easy to expel. If the patient is unable to take sufficient fluids orally, intravenous (IV) hydration will be used. An appropriate humidification device is an adjunct in secretion management. Aerosols of sterile normal saline, administered by a nebulizer, may be used to liquefy secretions. Aerosol therapy may induce bronchospasm and severe coughing causing a decreased PaO_2. Mucolytic agents such as nebulized acetylcysteine (Mucomyst) mixed with a bronchodilator may be used to thin secretions but as a side effect may also cause airway erythema and bronchospasm. Therefore it is used only in special situations.

Chest physical therapy. Chest physical therapy is indicated in patients who produce more than 30 ml of sputum per day. If tolerated, postural drainage, percussion, and vibration to the affected lung segments may assist in moving secretions to the larger airways where they may be removed by coughing or suctioning. Because positioning may affect oxygenation, patients may not tolerate head-down or lateral positioning because of extreme dyspnea or hypoxemia caused by $\dot{V}/\dot{Q}$ mismatch. (Chest physical therapy is discussed in Chapter 27.)

Airway suctioning. If the patient is unable to expectorate secretions, nasopharyngeal, oropharyngeal, or nasotracheal suctioning (blind suctioning without a tracheal tube in place) is indicated. Suctioning through an artificial airway, such as endotracheal or tracheostomy tubes, may also be performed (see Chapters 25 and 63). A mini-tracheostomy (or mini-trach) may be used to suction patients who have difficulty mobilizing secretions and when blind suctioning is difficult or ineffective. The mini-trach is a 4 mm indwelling plastic cuffless cannula inserted through the cricothyroid membrane. It is used to instill sterile normal saline solution to elicit a cough and to perform suctioning with a no. 10 French catheter. Contraindications for a mini-trach include an absent gag reflex, history of aspiration, and the need for long-term mechanical ventilation.[6]

Positive Pressure Ventilation. If intensive measures fail to improve ventilation and oxygenation and the patient continues to exhibit manifestations of acute respiratory failure, ventilatory assistance may be initiated. PPV may be provided invasively through endotracheal or nasotracheal intubation or noninvasively through a nasal or face mask. Patients who require PPV are typically cared for in a critical care unit. (See Chapter 63 for a discussion of artificial airways and mechanical ventilation.)

Noninvasive positive pressure ventilation (NIPPV) may be used as a treatment for patients with acute or chronic respiratory failure.[7,8] During NIPPV a mask is placed over the patient's nose or nose and mouth and the patient breathes spontaneously while PPV is delivered (Fig. 62-7). With NIPPV it is possible to decrease the work of breathing without the need for endotracheal intubation. Bilevel positive airway pressure (BiPAP® Ventilatory Support System) is a form of NIPPV in which different positive pressure levels are set for inspiration and expiration (see Fig. 62-7). Continuous positive airway pressure (CPAP) is another form of NIPPV in which a constant positive pressure is delivered to the airway during inspiration and expiration.

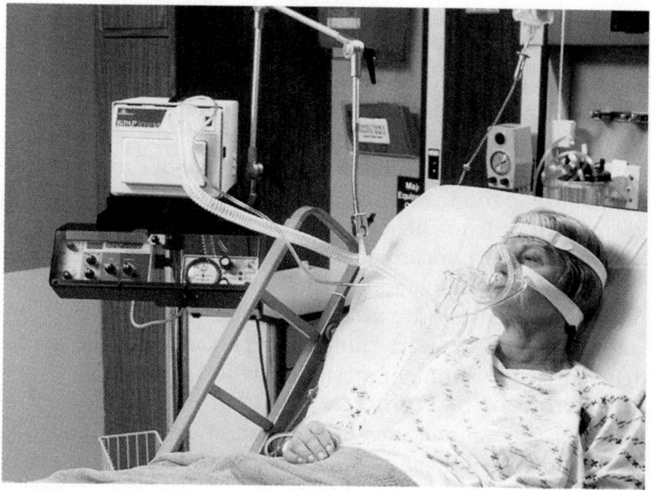

Fig. 62-7 Noninvasive bilevel positive pressure ventilation. A mask is placed over the nose or nose and mouth. Positive pressure from a mechanical ventilator assists the patient's breathing efforts, decreasing the work of breathing.

NIPPV is most useful in managing chronic respiratory failure in patients with chest wall and neuromuscular disease (see Table 62-1). NIPPV has been used in patients with hypoxemic respiratory failure (ARDS, cardiogenic pulmonary edema), but with less success. NIPPV may also be used for patients who refuse endotracheal intubation but still desire some palliative ventilatory support (e.g., patients with end-stage COPD).[9] NIPPV is not appropriate for the patient who has absent respirations, excessive secretions, a decreased level of consciousness, high O_2 requirements, facial trauma, or hemodynamic instability.

Drug Therapy

Goals of drug therapy for patients in acute respiratory failure include relief of bronchospasm, reduction of airway inflammation and pulmonary congestion, treatment of pulmonary infection, and reduction of severe anxiety and restlessness.

Relief of Bronchospasm. Alveolar ventilation will be increased with relief of bronchospasm. Short-acting bronchodilators, such as metaproterenol (Alupent) and albuterol (Ventolin), are frequently administered to reverse bronchospasm using either a handheld nebulizer or a metered-dose inhaler with a spacer.[10] In acute bronchospasm these drugs may be given at 30- to 60-minute intervals until it can be determined that a response is occurring. If severe bronchospasm continues, IV aminophylline may be administered. The bronchodilator effects of these medications can sometimes cause a worsening of arterial hypoxemia by redistributing the inspired gas to areas of decreased perfusion. Administering the bronchodilator with an O_2-enriched gas mixture usually alleviates this effect. (See Chapter 27 for nursing management related to bronchodilators.)

Reduction of Airway Inflammation. Corticosteroids may be used in conjunction with bronchodilating agents when bronchospasm and inflammation are present. Inhaled corticosteroids are not used for acute respiratory failure, because they require 4 to 5 days before optimum therapeutic effects are seen. However, IV corticosteroids (e.g., methylprednisolone) have an immediate onset of action.

Reduction of Pulmonary Congestion. Pulmonary interstitial fluid can occur as a consequence of direct or indirect injury to the alveolar capillary membrane (e.g., ARDS) or from right or left ventricular failure, and therefore can be either cardiac or noncardiac in origin. The result is decreased alveolar ventilation and hypoxemia. IV diuretics (e.g., furosemide [Lasix]) are used to decrease the pulmonary congestion caused by heart failure. Digitalis may also be used if left ventricular failure or atrial fibrillation is present.

Treatment of Pulmonary Infections. Pulmonary infections (pneumonia, acute bronchitis) result in excessive mucus production and inflamed, fluid-filled, or collapsed alveoli. Alveoli that are fluid filled or collapsed cannot participate in gas exchange. Pulmonary infections can either cause or exacerbate acute respiratory failure. IV antibiotics are frequently administered to inhibit bacterial growth. Chest x-rays are performed to determine the location and extent of a suspected infectious process. Sputum cultures are used to determine the type of organisms causing the infection and their sensitivity to antimicrobial medications.

Reduction of Severe Anxiety and Restlessness. Anxiety, restlessness, and agitation result from cerebral hypoxia. In addition, fear caused by the inability to breathe and a sense of loss of control may exacerbate anxiety. Agitation and anxiety increase O_2 consumption, which may worsen the degree of hypoxemia. Several nursing strategies can assist the patient in reducing the level of anxiety (see NCP 62-1).

Low-dose sedation (e.g., lorazepam [Ativan]) may be used to decrease anxiety because continued agitation will increase the patient's work of breathing and therefore O_2 consumption. Patients receiving any sedative medication must be monitored for respiratory depression. In the critical care setting sedation and neuromuscular paralysis are commonly used for severely restless and agitated patients in acute respiratory failure who breathe asynchronously with mechanical ventilation. These medications inhibit patient breathing efforts and patient awareness of surroundings, thereby allowing the ventilator to provide optimum ventilation.

Medical Supportive Therapy

Therapeutic goals and interventions to maximize O_2 delivery and treat the underlying cause of the respiratory failure are essential to improving the patient's oxygenation and ventilation status. The primary goal is to treat the underlying cause of the respiratory failure.[11] Other goals include maintaining an adequate cardiac output and hemoglobin concentration.

Treating the Underlying Cause. Interventions are directed toward reversing the disease process that resulted in the development of acute respiratory failure. Patients with hypoventilation can be diagnosed and treated rapidly. Patients with $\dot{V}/\dot{Q}$ mismatch, shunting, or diffusion limitation are managed differently depending on the underlying cause. In all patient situations, monitoring treatment effects and ABG results is a continuous process.

Maintaining Adequate Cardiac Output. Cardiac output reflects the blood flow reaching the tissues. Blood pressure is an important indicator of the adequacy of cardiac output. Usually a systolic blood pressure of at least 90 mm Hg is adequate to maintain perfusion to the vital organs. (See Chapter 30 for a discussion of cardiac output.) If the systolic blood pressure is at least 90 mm Hg, changes in mental status may be attributed to the level of O_2 and CO_2 rather than decreased cerebral perfusion. Decreased cardiac output is treated by administration of IV fluids, medications, or both. (See Chapter 61 for a discussion of drugs used in decreased cardiac output and shock.)

Maintaining Adequate Hemoglobin Concentration. Hemoglobin is the primary carrier when delivering O_2 to the tissues. If the patient is anemic, tissue O_2 delivery will be compromised. A hemoglobin concentration of 9 to 10 g/dl (90 to 100 g/L) or greater typically ensures adequate O_2 saturation of the hemoglobin. The patient should be monitored for sites of blood loss and transfused with packed red blood cells if an adequate hemoglobin concentration cannot be maintained.

Nutritional Therapy

Maintenance of protein and energy stores is especially important in patients who experience acute respiratory failure because nutritional depletion causes a loss of muscle mass, including the respiratory muscles, and may prolong recovery. During the acute manifestations of respiratory failure, the risk of aspiration typically prevents oral nutritional intake. Enteral or parenteral nutrition may therefore be administered. When the acute manifestations subside, the patient may resume oral intake as tolerated.

Evaluation

The expected outcomes for the patient with acute respiratory failure are presented in NCP 62-1.

GERONTOLOGIC CONSIDERATIONS

Respiratory Failure

Older adults are at higher risk of developing respiratory failure because of the reduction in ventilatory capacity that accompanies aging, especially if other risk factors are present. In older adults, the PaO_2 falls further and the $PaCO_2$ rises to a higher level before the respiratory system is stimulated to alter the rate and depth of breathing. This delayed response predisposes to the development of respiratory failure.

ACUTE RESPIRATORY DISTRESS SYNDROME

ARDS is a sudden and progressive form of acute respiratory failure in which the alveolar capillary membrane becomes damaged and more permeable to intravascular fluid (Fig. 62-8). The alveoli fill with fluid, resulting in severe dyspnea, hypoxemia refractory to supplemental O_2, reduced lung compliance, and diffuse pulmonary infiltrates.

The incidence of ARDS in the United States is estimated at more than 150,000 cases annually. Despite supportive therapy, the mortality rate from ARDS is approximately 50%. Patients who have both gram-negative septic shock and ARDS have a mortality rate of 70% to 90%.[12]

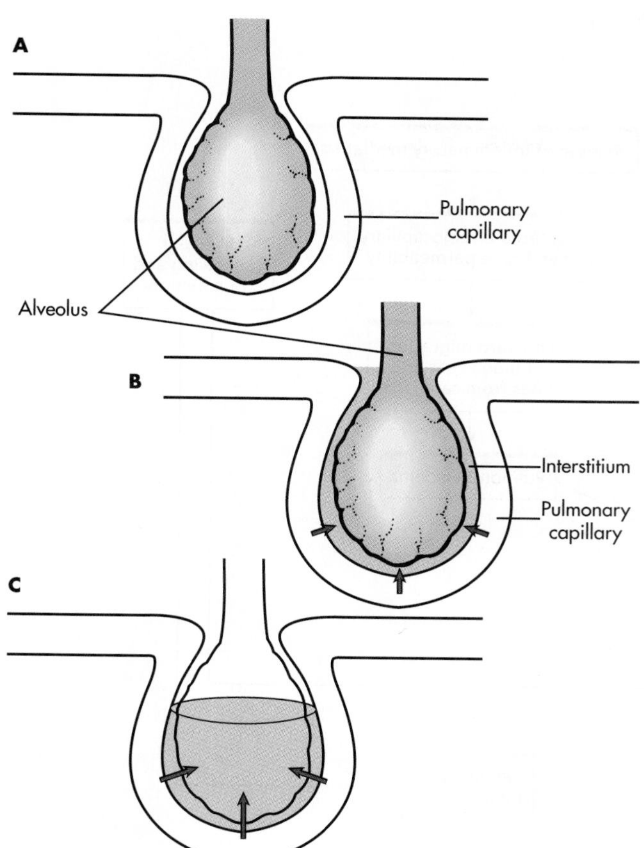

Fig. 62-8 Stages of edema formation in acute respiratory distress syndrome. **A,** Normal alveolus and pulmonary capillary. **B,** Interstitial edema occurs with increased flow of fluid into the interstitial space. **C,** Alveolar edema occurs when the fluid crosses the blood-gas barrier.

Table 62-6 Conditions Predisposing to Acute Respiratory Distress Syndrome

Direct Lung Injury
Aspiration of gastric contents or other substances
Near-drowning
Inhalation of toxic substances
Viral/bacterial pneumonia
Chest trauma
Embolism: fat, air, amniotic fluid
Oxygen toxicity
Radiation pneumonitis
Indirect Lung Injury
Sepsis (especially gram-negative infection)
Severe pancreatitis
Multiple blood transfusions
Multiple trauma/fractures
Severe head injury
Disseminated intravascular coagulation
Shock states
Nonpulmonary systemic diseases
Cardiopulmonary bypass
Anaphylaxis
Narcotic drug abuse

Etiology and Pathophysiology

Table 62-6 lists conditions that predispose patients to the development of ARDS. The two risk factors most commonly associated with ARDS are gram-negative septic shock and aspiration of gastric contents. Patients with multiple risk factors are 3 to 4 times more likely to develop ARDS.[13]

Direct lung injury may cause ARDS (Fig. 62-9), or ARDS may develop as a consequence of the systemic inflammatory response syndrome (SIRS) (see Fig. 61-1). SIRS may have an infectious or a noninfectious etiology and is characterized by widespread inflammation or clinical responses to inflammation following a variety of physiologic insults, including severe trauma, gut ischemia, injury to the lung, and sepsis.[14] ARDS may also develop as a consequence of multiple organ dysfunction syndrome (MODS). MODS results from organ system dysfunction that progressively increases in severity and ultimately results in multisystem organ failure. (SIRS and MODS are discussed in Chapter 61.)

An exact cause for the damage to the alveolar-capillary membrane is not known. However, the pathophysiologic changes of ARDS are thought to be due to stimulation of the inflammatory and immune systems, which causes an attraction of neutrophils to the pulmonary interstitium.[15] The neutrophils cause a release of biochemical, humoral, and cellular mediators (Table 62-7) that produce changes in the lung, including increased pulmonary capillary membrane permeability, destruction of elastin and collagen, formation of pulmonary microemboli, and pulmonary artery vasoconstriction (see Fig. 62-9). (These mediators are discussed in Chapters 11 and 12.)

The pathophysiologic changes in ARDS are divided into three phases: (1) injury or exudative phase, (2) reparative or proliferative phase, and (3) fibrotic phase.

Injury or Exudative Phase. The injury or exudative phase occurs approximately 1 to 7 days (usually 24 to 48 hours) after the initial direct lung injury or host insult. Neutrophils adhere to the pulmonary microcirculation, causing damage to the vascular endothelium and increased capillary permeability. In the earliest phase of injury, there is engorgement of the peribronchial and perivascular interstitial space, which produces interstitial edema. Next, fluid from the interstitial space crosses the alveolar epithelium and enters the alveolar space. Intrapulmonary shunt develops because the alveoli fill with fluid and blood passing through them cannot be oxygenated (see Figs. 62-4 and 62-8).

Alveolar type I and type II cells (which produce surfactant) are damaged by the changes caused by ARDS. This damage, in addition to further fluid and protein accumulation, results in surfactant dysfunction. The function of surfactant is to maintain alveolar stability by decreasing alveolar surface tension and preventing alveolar collapse. Decreased synthesis and inactivation of surfactant causes the alveoli to become unstable and collapse (atelectasis). Widespread atelectasis further decreases lung compliance, compromises gas exchange, and contributes to hypoxemia.

Also during this stage, hyaline begins to line the alveolar membrane. These hyaline membranes are thought to result from the exudation of high-molecular-weight substances (particularly fibrinogen) in the edema fluid. Hyaline membranes

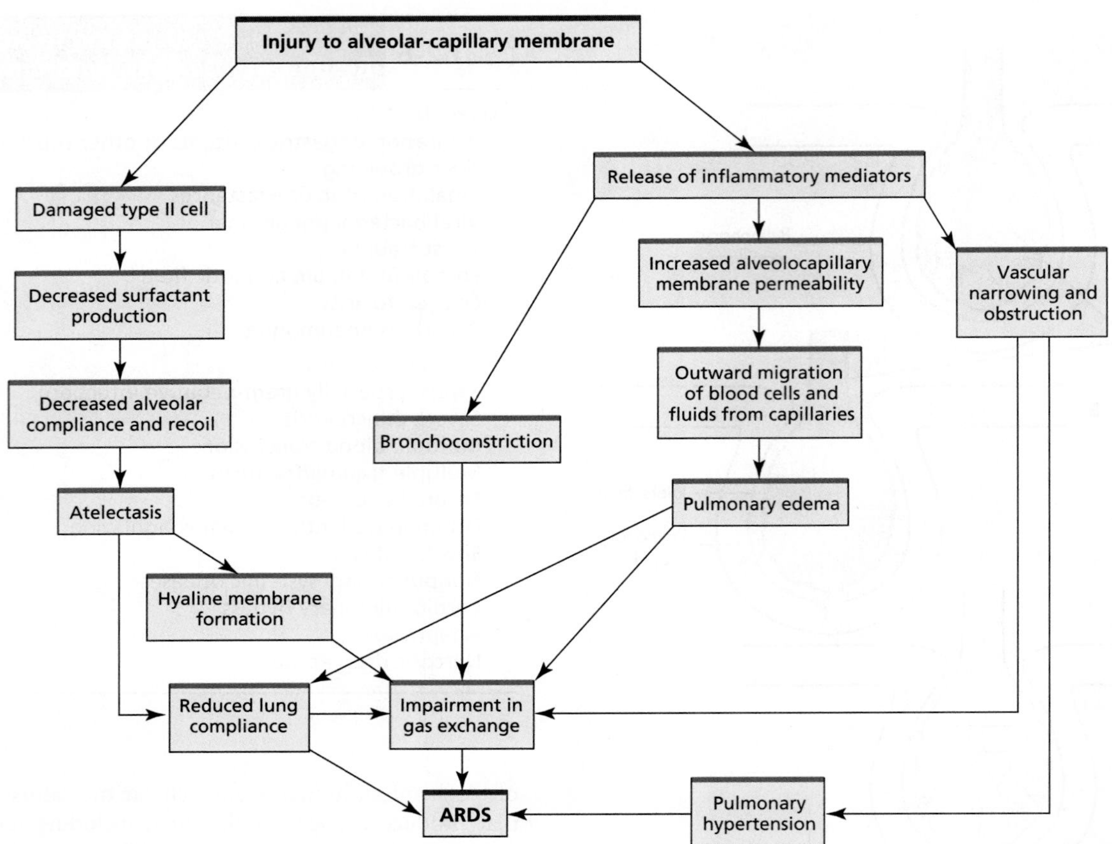

Fig. 62-9 Pathophysiology of ARDS.

Table 62-7 Mediators of Acute Lung Injury

Complement component C5a
Neutrophil products, including proteases and O_2 radicals
Monocyte and macrophage products, including tumor necrosis factor, interleukin-1, and colony-stimulating factor
Arachidonic acid metabolites, including prostaglandins and leukotrienes
Coagulation products, including kallikreins, kinins, fibrin degradation products, and plasminogen-activating factor
Histamine
Serotonin
Endotoxin
Elastase
Collagenase

contribute to the development of fibrosis and atelectasis, leading to a decrease in gas exchange capability and lung compliance.

The primary pathophysiologic changes that characterize the injury or exudative phase of ARDS are interstitial and alveolar edema (noncardiogenic pulmonary edema) and atelectasis.[16] Severe $\dot{V}/\dot{Q}$ mismatch and shunting of pulmonary capillary blood result in hypoxemia unresponsive to increasing concentrations of O_2 (refractory hypoxemia). Diffusion limitation, caused by hyaline membrane formation, further contributes to the severity of the hypoxemia. As the lungs become less compliant because of decreased surfactant, pulmonary edema, and atelectasis, the patient must generate higher airway pressures to inflate "stiff" lungs. Reduced lung compliance greatly increases the patient's work of breathing.

Hypoxemia and the stimulation of juxtacapillary receptors in the stiff lung parenchyma (J reflex) initially cause an increase in respiratory rate and decrease in tidal volume. This breathing pattern increases CO_2 removal, producing respiratory alkalosis. Cardiac output increases in response to hypoxemia, a compensatory effect to increase pulmonary blood flow. However, as atelectasis, pulmonary edema, and pulmonary shunt increase, compensation fails, and hypoventilation, decreased cardiac output, and decreased tissue O_2 perfusion eventually occur.

Reparative or Proliferative Phase. The reparative or proliferative phase begins 1 to 2 weeks after the initial lung injury. During this phase, there is an influx of granulocytes, monocytes, and lymphocytes and fibroblast proliferation as part of the inflammatory response. The injured lung has an immense regenerative capacity after acute lung injury. The proliferative phase is complete when the diseased lung becomes characterized by dense, fibrous tissue. Increased pulmonary vascular resistance and pulmonary hypertension may occur in this stage because the presence of fibroblasts and inflammatory cells obliterate the pulmonary vasculature. Lung compliance continues to decrease as a result of interstitial fibrosis. Hypoxemia worsens because of the thickened alveolar membrane, causing diffusion limitation and shunting. If the

Table 62-8 Diagnostic Findings in Acute Respiratory Distress Syndrome

Hypoxemia
PaO_2 <50 mm Hg on FIO_2 >40% with PEEP >5 cm H_2O
Chest X-ray
New bilateral interstitial and alveolar infiltrates
Pulmonary Artery Wedge Pressure
≤18 mm Hg and no evidence of heart failure
Predisposing Condition
Identification of a predisposing condition for ARDS within 48 hours of clinical manifestations

reparative phase persists, widespread fibrosis results. If the proliferative phase is arrested, the lesions resolve.

Fibrotic Phase. The fibrotic phase occurs approximately 2 to 3 weeks after the initial lung injury. This phase is also called the chronic or late phase of ARDS. By this time the lung is completely remodeled by sparsely collagenous and fibrous tissues. There is diffuse scarring and fibrosis, resulting in decreased lung compliance. In addition, the surface area for gas exchange is significantly reduced because the interstitium is fibrotic, and therefore hypoxemia continues. Pulmonary hypertension results from pulmonary vascular obliteration and fibrosis.

Clinical Progression

Progression of ARDS varies among patients. Some persons survive the acute phase of lung injury; pulmonary edema resolves and complete recovery occurs in a few days. The chance for survival is poor in patients who enter the fibrotic (chronic or late) stage, which requires long-term mechanical ventilation. It is not known why injured lungs repair and recover in some patients, and in others ARDS progresses. Several factors seem to be important in determining the course of ARDS, including the nature of the initial injury, extent and severity of coexisting diseases, and the pulmonary complications.

Clinical Manifestations

The initial presentation of ARDS is often insidious. At the time of the initial injury, and for several hours to 1 to 2 days afterward, the patient may not experience respiratory symptoms, or the patient may exhibit only dyspnea, tachypnea, cough, and restlessness. Chest auscultation may be normal or reveal fine, scattered crackles. ABGs usually indicate mild hypoxemia and respiratory alkalosis caused by hyperventilation. Respiratory alkalosis results from hypoxemia and the stimulation of juxtacapillary receptors. The chest x-ray may be normal or exhibit evidence of minimal scattered interstitial infiltrates. Edema may not show on the x-ray until there is a 30% increase in fluid content in the lung.

As ARDS progresses, symptoms worsen because of increased fluid accumulation and decreased lung compliance. Respiratory discomfort becomes evident as the work of breathing increases. Tachypnea and intercostal and suprasternal retractions may be present. Pulmonary function tests in ARDS reveal decreased compliance and decreased lung volumes, particularly a decreased functional residual capacity (FRC). Tachycardia, diaphoresis, changes in sensorium with decreased mentation, cyanosis, and pallor may be present. Chest auscultation usually reveals scattered to diffuse crackles and rhonchi. The chest x-ray demonstrates diffuse and extensive bilateral interstitial and alveolar infiltrates. A pulmonary artery catheter may be inserted. Pulmonary artery wedge pressure does not increase in ARDS since the cause is noncardiogenic (not related to cardiac function). Pulmonary edema that is caused by cardiac dysfunction will cause an increase in pulmonary artery wedge pressure.

Table 62-9 Complications Associated with Acute Respiratory Distress Syndrome

Infection	**Renal complications**
Nosocomial pneumonia	Acute renal failure
Catheter-related infection	**Cardiac complications**
Sepsis (bacteremia)	Arrhythmias
Respiratory complications	Decreased cardiac output
Pulmonary emboli	**Hematologic complications**
Pulmonary barotrauma (e.g., pneumothorax, pneumomediastinum, subcutaneous emphysema)	Anemia
O_2 toxicity	Thrombocytopenia
Pulmonary fibrosis	Disseminated intravascular coagulation
Gastrointestinal complications	**ET intubation complications**
Stress ulceration and hemorrhage	Laryngeal ulceration
Paralytic ileus	Tracheal ulceration
Pneumoperitoneum	Tracheal malacia
	Tracheal stenosis

Refractory hypoxemia, despite increased FIO_2 by mask, cannula, or endotracheal tube, is a hallmark of ARDS. ABGs may initially demonstrate a normal or decreased $PaCO_2$ despite severe dyspnea and hypoxemia. Hypercapnia signifies that hypoventilation is occurring, and the patient is no longer able to maintain the level of ventilation needed to provide optimum gas exchange.

As ARDS progresses it is associated with profound respiratory distress requiring endotracheal intubation and PPV. The chest x-ray is often termed *whiteout* or *white lung,* because consolidation and coalescing infiltrates are widespread throughout the lungs, leaving few recognizable air spaces. Pleural effusions may also be present. Severe hypoxemia, hypercapnia, and metabolic acidosis, with symptoms of target organ or tissue hypoxia, may ensue if prompt therapy is not instituted.

No precise criteria define ARDS. ARDS is considered to be present if the patient has hypoxemia, a chest x-ray with new bilateral interstitial or alveolar infiltrates, a pulmonary artery wedge pressure of 18 mm Hg or less or no evidence of heart failure, and a predisposing condition consistent for ARDS within 48 hours of clinical manifestations (Table 62-8).

Complications

Complications may develop as a result of ARDS itself or its treatment. (Table 62-9 lists the common complications of

COLLABORATIVE CARE

Table 62-10 Acute Respiratory Distress Syndrome

Diagnostic*
Collaborative Therapy
Respiratory Therapy
- O_2 administration
- Prone positioning
- Medical ventilation with PEEP

Supportive Therapy
- Identification and treatment of underlying cause
- Hemodynamic monitoring
- Inotropic/vasopressor medications
  - Dopamine (Intropin)
  - Dobutamine (Dobutrex)
- Diuretics
- Intravenous fluid administration

*See Table 62-8.

ARDS.) The major cause of death in ARDS is MODS, often accompanied by sepsis. The organs most commonly involved are the kidneys, liver, and heart. The systems most often involved are the CNS, hematologic, and gastrointestinal systems.

Nosocomial Pneumonia. A frequent complication of acute respiratory failure is nosocomial pneumonia, occurring in 20% of mechanically ventilated patients, and in as many as 68% of patients with ARDS. Risk factors include impaired host defenses, contaminated medical equipment, invasive monitoring devices, aspiration of gastrointestinal contents, and colonization of the respiratory tract. Strategies to prevent nosocomial pneumonia include infection control measures (e.g., strict hand washing and sterile technique during endotracheal suctioning) and elevating the head of the bed more than 30 degrees to prevent aspiration. (See Chapter 26 for discussion of pneumonia.)

Barotrauma. Barotrauma or volutrauma may result from rupture of overdistended alveoli during mechanical ventilation. The high peak airway pressures that may be required in patients with ARDS predispose to this complication. Barotrauma results in the presence of alveolar air in locations where it is not usually found. This can lead to pulmonary interstitial emphysema, pneumothorax, subcutaneous emphysema, pneumoperitoneum, pneumomediastinum, and tension pneumothorax. (See Chapter 26 for discussion of pneumothorax.) To avoid barotrauma, the patient with ARDS is sometimes ventilated with smaller tidal volumes, resulting in higher $PaCO_2$. This method of mechanical ventilation is termed *permissive hypercapnia* because the $PaCO_2$ is allowed (permitted) to rise above normal limits.

Stress Ulcers. Critically ill patients with acute respiratory failure are at high risk for stress ulcers. Bleeding from stress ulcers occurs in 30% of patients with ARDS who require PPV, a higher incidence than other causes of acute respiratory failure. Management strategies include correction of predisposing conditions such as hypotension, shock, and acidosis. Prophylactic management includes antacids, histamine-receptor blockers (e.g., cimetidine [Tagemet] or ranitidine [Zantac]), sucralfate, and enteral nutrition.

Renal Failure. Renal failure can occur from decreased renal tissue oxygenation as a result of hypotension, hypoxemia, or hypercapnia. Renal failure may also be caused by administration of nephrotoxic drugs (e.g., aminoglycosides), which are used to treat infections associated with ARDS.

NURSING AND COLLABORATIVE MANAGEMENT: ACUTE RESPIRATORY DISTRESS SYNDROME

The collaborative care for acute respiratory failure (see Table 62-4) is applicable to ARDS. The following section discusses additional collaborative care measures for the patient with ARDS (Table 62-10). Patients with ARDS are commonly cared for in critical care units. The nursing care plan for acute respiratory failure (see NCP 62-1) is applicable to patients with acute respiratory failure.

Nursing Assessment

Because ARDS causes acute respiratory failure, the subjective and objective data that should be obtained from a person with ARDS are the same as that for acute respiratory failure (see Table 62-4.) Abnormal findings on physical examination are indications that ARDS has progressed beyond the initial stages.

Nursing Diagnoses

Nursing diagnoses for the patient with ARDS may include, but are not limited to, those described for acute respiratory failure (see NCP 62-1).

Planning

The overall goals are that the patient with ARDS will have (1) PaO_2 within limits of normal for age or baseline values, (2) SaO_2 greater than 90%, (3) patent airway, and (4) clear lungs on auscultation.

Respiratory Therapy

Oxygen Administration. The primary goal of O_2 therapy is to correct hypoxemia. O_2 administered via a simple face mask or nasal cannula is usually inadequate to treat refractory hypoxemia. Masks with high-flow systems that deliver higher O_2 concentrations are initially used to maximize O_2 delivery. SpO_2 is continuously monitored to assess the effectiveness of O_2 therapy. The general standard for O_2 administration is to give the patient the lowest concentration that results in a PaO_2 of 60 mm Hg or greater. When the FIO_2 exceeds 60% for more than 48 hours, the risk for O_2 toxicity increases. Patients with ARDS commonly need intubation with mechanical ventilation because the PaO_2 cannot otherwise be maintained at acceptable levels.

Mechanical Ventilation. Endotracheal intubation and mechanical ventilation provide additional respiratory support. However, even with these interventions it may be necessary to maintain the FIO_2 at 60% or greater to maintain the PaO_2 at 60 mm Hg or greater. During mechanical ventilation, it is common to apply positive end-expiratory pressure (PEEP) at 5 cm H_2O to compensate for loss of glottic function caused by the presence of the endotracheal tube.[17] In patients with ARDS, additional PEEP is often used. PEEP is a ventilatory maneuver that applies positive pressure to the airway and lungs at the end of exhalation. Without PEEP, pressure in the chest becomes equal to atmospheric pressure (zero) at the end of exhalation. When PEEP is applied, the lung is kept partially expanded, which prevents the alveoli from totally collapsing. PEEP is typically applied in 3 to 5 cm H_2O increments until oxygenation is adequate with FIO_2 of 60% or less. The mechanism of action of PEEP is related to its ability to increase FRC and recruit (open up) collapsed alveoli. PEEP may improve $\dot{V}/\dot{Q}$ in respiratory units that collapse at low airway pressures, allowing the FIO_2 to be lowered.[18]

If hypoxemic failure persists in spite of high levels of PEEP, alternative modes and therapies may be used. These include pressure support ventilation, pressure release ventilation, pressure control ventilation, inverse ratio ventilation, high frequency ventilation, and permissive hypercapnia (low tidal volumes that allow $PaCO_2$ to increase slowly, maintaining normal pH and low airway pressures). (See Chapter 63 for a discussion of mechanical ventilation.) Extracorporeal membrane oxygenation (ECMO) and extracorporeal CO_2 removal ($ECCO_2R$) pass blood across a gas-exchanging membrane outside the body and then return oxygenated blood back to the body. $ECCO_2R$ with low-frequency PPV allows the lung to heal while the lung is not functional.

Prone Positioning. Some patients with ARDS demonstrate a marked improvement in PaO_2 when turned from the supine to prone position (e.g., PaO_2 70 mm Hg supine, PaO_2 90 mm Hg prone) with no change in inspired O_2 concentration. The response may be sufficient to allow a reduction in inspired O_2 concentration or PEEP.

In the early phases of ARDS, edema fluid moves freely throughout the lung. Because of gravity, this fluid pools in dependent regions of the lung. As a consequence, some alveoli are fluid filled (dependent areas), whereas others are air filled (nondependent areas). In addition, when the patient is supine the heart and mediastinal contents place more pressure on the lungs than in the prone position, which changes pleural pressure and predisposes to atelectasis. If the patient is turned from supine to prone, air-filled, nonatelectatic alveoli in the dorsal (upper) portion of the lung become dependent. Perfusion may be better matched to ventilation, causing less $\dot{V}/\dot{Q}$ mismatch. Not all patients respond to prone positioning with an increase in PaO_2, and there is no reliable way of predicting who will respond. Prone positioning is typically reserved for patients with refractory hypoxemia who do not respond to other strategies to increase PaO_2.[19,20] When this positioning is used, there must be a plan in place for immediate positioning for cardiopulmonary resuscitation in the event of a cardiac arrest.

■ Medical Supportive Therapy

Maintenance of Cardiac Output and Tissue Perfusion. Patients on PPV and PEEP frequently experience decreased cardiac output. One cause is decreased venous return, which results from the PEEP-induced increase in intrathoracic pressure. Cardiac output may also be decreased by impaired contractility and decreased preload. Continuous hemodynamic monitoring is essential to detect these changes and titrate therapy. An arterial catheter is inserted to permit continuous monitoring of blood pressure and to withdraw blood for ABGs. A pulmonary artery catheter is normally inserted to allow monitoring of pulmonary artery pressure and pulmonary artery wedge pressures (which indicate the fluid status of the left side of the heart) and cardiac output. If the cardiac output falls, it may be necessary to administer crystalloid fluids or colloid solutions or to lower PEEP. Use of inotropic drugs such as dobutamine (Dobutrex) or dopamine (Intropin) may also be necessary. (See Chapter 63 for discussion of hemodynamic monitoring.)

The hemoglobin level is usually kept at levels of more than 9 to 10 g/dl (90 to 100 g/L) with an oxygen saturation of 90% or greater (when PaO_2 is more than 60 mm Hg). Packed red blood cells may be administered to increase O_2-carrying capacity of the blood.

Maintenance of Fluid Balance. Maintenance of fluid balance is precarious in the patient with ARDS. Leaky capillaries increase fluid in the lungs and cause pulmonary edema. At the same time, the patient may be volume depleted and therefore prone to hypotension and decreased cardiac output from mechanical ventilation and PEEP. Controversy exists as to the benefits of fluid replacement with crystalloids versus colloids. Critics of colloid replacement believe that proteins of colloid fluid may leak into the pulmonary interstitium, exacerbating the movement of proteinaceous fluid into the alveoli. Advocates of colloid replacement believe that colloids help keep fluid from leaking into the alveoli. The pulmonary artery wedge pressure is kept as low as possible without impairing cardiac output. The patient is usually placed on mild fluid restriction, and diuretics are used as necessary. Pulmonary artery wedge pressures, intake and output, and daily weights are monitored to assess the patient's fluid status.

■ Evaluation

The expected outcomes for the patient with ARDS are similar to those for a patient with acute respiratory failure and are presented in NCP 62-1.

Trends and Research in ARDS Management

Pharmacologic agents to treat ARDS have been researched extensively. Monoclonal antibodies are being studied for their effects in binding endotoxin and interleukins, thus limiting or preventing mediator-induced damage to the alveolar capillary endothelium. Prostaglandin E_1 (PGE_1), a vasodilator, is being studied for its use in decreasing systemic and pulmonary vascular resistance.[21] Inhaled nitric oxide (NO) is another vasodilator currently being studied for its effects on decreasing pulmonary artery pressure and improving oxygenation.[22,23] Surfactant (a lipid-protein complex produced by alveolar type II cells), which decreases surface tension and maintains lung compliance, is also being used in ARDS.[24] Surfactant replacement therapy has been effective in respiratory distress syndrome in infants. The use of partial liquid ventilation in the ARDS patient on mechanical ventilation is under investigation. A liquid fluorocarbon is instilled into the lung. This liquid keeps the alveoli open and has a high carrying capacity for O_2. Both actions help improve O_2 movement across the alveolus into the pulmonary blood.[25]

The use of corticosteroids in the acute phase of ARDS has not proven beneficial. However, the use of corticosteroids in the chronic phases of ARDS may be indicated if the patient is not responding to conventional treatment.[26]

CRITICAL THINKING EXERCISES

CASE STUDY

Acute Respiratory Distress Syndrome

Patient Profile

Mr. J. is a 35-year-old man who was admitted 32 hours ago to a general surgical unit after surgery for multiple gunshot wounds in the abdomen. The surgical procedure involved extensive abdominal surgery to repair a perforated colon, remove bullets, and repair a torn mesenteric artery. During transport to the hospital and during surgery his systolic blood pressure dropped to 70 mm Hg. Ten units of packed red blood cells and 6 L of normal saline were administered intravenously to restore blood loss and volume. He is receiving 60% oxygen through an aerosol face mask. He is being monitored with a cardiac monitor and pulse oximeter. He has a central intravenous catheter in place and is receiving 0.9% normal saline intravenously at 125 ml per hour. A urinary catheter is in place.

Subjective Data

- Complains of shortness of breath, inability to lie flat, and diffuse abdominal pain

Objective Data

Physical Assessment

- General: alert, well-nourished man who appears restless and anxious; head of bed elevated 45 degrees; skin cool with moderate diaphoresis
- Respiratory: no accessory muscle use, retraction, paradoxic breathing; respiratory rate 28 breaths/min; SpO_2 88%; fine crackles at lung bases
- Cardiovascular: blood pressure 100/60 mm Hg; cardiac monitor shows sinus tachycardia at 120 beats/min, which correlates with his apical pulse rate; temperature 101° F (38° C) orally
- Gastrointestinal: surgical dressing dry and intact; sharp pain on palpation over incisional area
- Urologic: urinary catheter draining concentrated urine

Diagnostic Findings

- Chest x-ray shows scattered interstitial infiltrates compatible with an ARDS pattern as interpreted by the radiologist

Critical Thinking Questions

1. How does the pathophysiology of ARDS predispose to the development of refractory hypoxemia?
2. What clinical manifestations does Mr. J. exhibit that support a diagnosis of ARDS?
3. What are the possible causes of ARDS in Mr. J.?
4. What are the possible complications Mr. J. is at risk for developing secondary to ARDS?
5. What respiratory care interventions might be implemented to improve Mr. J's hypoxemia?
6. Based on the assessment data presented, write one or more appropriate nursing diagnoses. Are there any collaborative problems?

REVIEW QUESTIONS

The number of the question corresponds to the same-numbered objective at the beginning of the chapter.

1. Hypercapnic respiratory failure can be caused by
   a. ARDS.
   b. asthma.
   c. pneumonia.
   d. pulmonary emboli.
2. An early sign of acute respiratory failure is
   a. restlessness.
   b. coma.
   c. cyanosis.
   d. paradoxic breathing.
3. The oxygen delivery system chosen for the patient in acute respiratory failure should
   a. always be a low-flow device, such as a nasal cannula.
   b. correct the PaO_2 to a normal level as quickly as possible.
   c. administer positive pressure ventilation to prevent CO_2 narcosis.
   d. maintain the PaO_2 at 55 to 60 mm Hg or greater at the lowest O_2 concentration possible.
4. The most common early clinical manifestations of ARDS that the nurse may observe are
   a. dyspnea and tachypnea.
   b. hypotension and tachycardia.
   c. cyanosis and apprehension.
   d. respiratory distress and frothy sputum.
5. Maintenance of fluid balance in the patient with ARDS involves
   a. hydration using colloids.
   b. administration of surfactant.
   c. mild fluid restriction and diuretics as necessary.
   d. keeping the hemoglobin at levels of 15 to 16 g/dl (150 to 160 g/L).

References

1. Grippi MA: Respiratory failure: an overview. In Fishman AP and others, editors: *Fishman's pulmonary diseases and disorders,* ed 3, New York, 1998, McGraw-Hill.
2. Pierson DJ: Normal and abnormal oxygenation: physiology and clinical syndromes, *Respir Care* 38:587, 1993.
3. Misasi R, Keyes JL: Matching and mismatching ventilation and perfusion in the lung, *Crit Care Nurse* 16:23, 1996.
4. Panettieri RA, Murray RK: *Chronic obstructive pulmonary disease.* In Fishman AP, editor: *Pulmonary diseases and disorders: companion handbook,* ed 3, New York, 1998, McGraw-Hill.
5. Syabbalo N: Measurement and interpretation of arterial blood gases, *Br J Clin Pract* 51:173, 1997.
6. Callaghan SP and others: Minitracheostomy: an alternative to "blind" endotracheal suctioning, *DCCN* 13:38, 1994.
7. Clark HE, Wilcox PG: Noninvasive positive pressure ventilation in acute respiratory failure or chronic obstructive pulmonary disease, *Lung* 175:143, 1997.
8. Abou-Shala N, Meduri U: Noninvasive mechanical ventilation in patients with acute respiratory failure, *Crit Care Med* 24:705, 1996.

9. Freichels T: Palliative ventilatory support: use of noninvasive positive pressure ventilation in terminal respiratory insufficiency, *Am J Crit Care* 3:6, 1994.
10. Karpel JP and others: Emergency treatment of acute asthma with albuterol metered-dose inhaler plus holding chamber, *Chest* 112:348, 1997.
11. Zuege DJ, Whitelaw WA: Management of acute respiratory failure in chronic obstructive pulmonary disease, *Curr Opin Pulmonary Med* 3:190, 1997.
12. *American Lung Association fact sheet,* New York, *ARDS,* 1997, American Lung Association.
13. Volman K: Adult respiratory distress syndrome mediators on the run, *Crit Care Nurs Clin North Am* 6:2, 1994.
14. Luce JM: Acute lung injury and the acute respiratory distress syndrome, *Crit Care Med* 26:369, 1998.
15. Shanley TP, Warner RL, Ward PA: The role of cytokines and adhesion molecules in the development of inflammatory injury, *Molecular Medicine Today* 1:40, 1995.
16. Thelan LA and others: *Critical care nursing: diagnosis and management,* ed 3, St Louis, 1998, Mosby.
17. Cawley MJ and others: Mechanical ventilation and pharmacologic strategies for acute respiratory distress syndrome, *Pharmacotherapy* 18:140, 1998.
18. Moore FA, Haenel JB: Ventilatory strategies for acute respiratory failure, *Am J Surg* 173:53, 1997.
19. Volman K: Prone positioning for the ARDS patient, *DCCN* 16:4, 1997.
20. Shapiro R, Broccard A: Patient positioning in respiratory disease, *Clinical Pulmonary Medicine* 4:45, 1997.
21. Lackmann B, Heulitt M: New therapies in respiratory failure, *Controversies in Critical Care* 3:2, 1997.
22. Kalweit S: Inhaled nitric oxide in the ICU, *Crit Care Nurse* 17:26, 1997.
23. Kalweit S: Inhaled nitric oxide in the ICU, *Crit Care Nurse* 17:26, 1998.
24. Baudouin SV: Surfactant medication for acute respiratory distress syndrome, *Thorax* 52(suppl 3):S9, 1997.
25. Dirkes S: Liquid ventilation: new frontiers in the treatment of ARDS, *Crit Care Nurse* 16:53, 1996.
26. Honig EG, Ingram RH: Acute respiratory distress syndrome. In Fauci and others, editors: *Harrison's principles of internal medicine,* ed 14, New York, 1998, McGraw-Hill.

Resources

Resources for this chapter are listed after Chapter 63 on p. 1957.

REMEMBER to check out your companion CD-ROM

63 NURSING MANAGEMENT Critical Care

Eleanor F. Bond & Julie Dax

www.mosby.com/MERLIN/medsurg_lewis

LEARNING OBJECTIVES

1. Describe the critical care unit.
2. Describe the critical care nurse.
3. Identify common problems and needs of patients in critical care units and related nursing management.
4. Identify common problems and needs of families of patients in critical care units and related nursing management.
5. Describe the principles of hemodynamic monitoring and related nursing management.
6. Describe the types, indications, potential complications, and nursing management of ventricular assist devices.
7. Describe the purpose, indications, and function of intra-aortic balloon pumps and related nursing management.
8. Describe the types and potential complications of endotracheal intubation.
9. Discuss the nursing management of the patient who requires endotracheal intubation.
10. Describe the indications for and modes of mechanical ventilation and related nursing management.
11. Describe the principles of intracranial pressure monitoring.
12. Identify strategies for management of patients with increased intracranial pressure.

CRITICAL CARE NURSING

Critical Care Units

Critical care units or intensive care units are designed to meet the special needs of acutely and critically ill patients. The concept of clustering the most acutely ill is not new. Florence Nightingale recommended grouping acutely ill patients together.[1] During poliomyelitis and tuberculosis pandemics in the middle of the twentieth century, special units were established, equipped with technical equipment to manage the airway and ventilate the patient, and staffed by specialized care providers. During World War II and the Vietnam War, trauma units were developed for battle casualties.

In the 1960s technologic developments allowed for more accessible monitoring of the electrocardiogram (ECG), arterial and central venous pressures, and arterial blood gases. Coronary care units were developed for patients with acute myocardial infarction. In these units patients were continually monitored for cardiac arrhythmias. Nurses followed protocols to aggressively manage arrhythmias. By the 1970s the intensive care unit (ICU) was a standard component of most general hospitals. Since that time, technical advances have continued at a rapid pace, bringing improved monitoring capabilities and new strategies to manage life-threatening problems.

The term *critical care nursing* is often used interchangeably with the term *ICU nursing.* The critical care nurse is responsible for diagnosing life-threatening conditions and instituting appropriate treatment. Technology and equipment available in the ICU are extensive and continually evolving. In ICUs the capability exists to continuously monitor ECG, blood pressure, cardiac output, ventilation, intracranial pressure, oxygenation, and temperature. More advanced monitoring devices allow for the measurement of stroke volume, ejection fraction, end-tidal carbon dioxide, and oxygen consumption. Patients may be receiving continual support from mechanical ventilators, ventricular assist devices, or dialysis machines. A typical critical care patient unit is illustrated in Fig. 63-1. Some common abbreviations used in ICUs are given in Table 63-1.

Critical Care Nurse

The critical care nurse cares for patients and the families of patients with acute and unstable physiologic problems in an environment equipped for technically advanced methods of assessing and managing patient problems. The American Association of Critical Care Nurses (AACN) defines *critical care nursing* as that specialty dealing with human responses to life-threatening problems. Critical care nursing requires knowledge of physiology, pathophysiology, pharmacology, and the ability to use advanced technology to accurately measure physiologic parameters. The nurse provides ongoing assessment and early recognition and management of complications while fostering healing and recovery. Appropriate actions by an astute nurse can prevent complications. The nurse must also be able to provide psychologic support to the patient and the family. To be effective the critical care nurse must be able to communicate clearly and work as a team member.

Reviewed by Susan B. Stillwell, RN, MSN, Clinical Associate Professor, College of Nursing, Arizona State University, Tempe, Ariz.

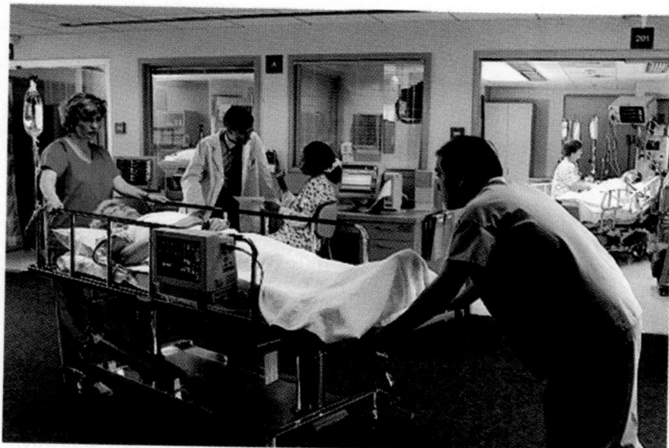

Fig. 63-1 Typical intensive care unit.

Nursing practice in the ICU often follows a primary care model with the patient cared for by a limited group of nurses who become thoroughly familiar with the patient's condition and the needs of the patient and the family. The ICU nurse spends most working hours near the patient's bedside. Specialization in ICU nursing usually requires formal training and mentored clinical practice, which is usually followed by an internship.

Certification in critical care nursing (CCRN) is offered by the AACN Certification Corporation. The designation requires registered nurse certification, clinical experience, and successful completion of a written test. Additional experience and testing or education are required for recertification. CCRN certification designates competency and not advanced practice. It does not require a master's degree and is not a basis for prescriptive authority.

Advanced practice critical care nurses generally have a graduate (master's or doctorate) degree. These nurses are employed as patient and staff educators, consultants, administrators, researchers, or practitioners. The critical care clinical nurse specialist role traditionally includes aspects of each of these role components. An important emerging role is the acute care nurse practitioner. These master's-prepared nurses provide advanced, comprehensive care to selected critically ill patients and their families. The acute care nurse practitioner is prepared to conduct comprehensive health assessments, order and interpret diagnostic tests, diagnose and treat health problems and disease-related symptoms, prescribe and evaluate drugs and treatments, and coordinate care during transitions in settings. They may practice independently (e.g., providing comprehensive care to the chronically critically ill) or collaboratively (e.g., providing symptom management in conjunction with physician specialists).

Critical Care Patient

A patient is generally admitted to the ICU for one of three reasons. First, the patient may be physiologically unstable, requiring advanced and sophisticated clinical judgments by the nurse or physician. Second, the patient may be at risk for serious complications and require frequent and often invasive physical assessment. Third, the patient may require intensive and complicated nursing support such as the use of life support technology and invasive monitoring equipment such as ventricular assist devices, mechanical ventilation, renal dialysis, and hemodynamic monitoring.

Table 63-1 Abbreviations Commonly Used in the Intensive Care Unit

Abbreviation	Term
ABP	Arterial blood pressure
CI	Cardiac index
CO	Cardiac output
CVP	Central venous pressure
FIO_2	Fraction of inspired oxygen
IABP	Intraaortic balloon pump
MAP	Mean arterial pressure
MRB	Manual resuscitation bag
PA	Pulmonary artery
PAS, PAD	PA systolic (pressure), PA diastolic (pressure)
PAWP	Pulmonary artery wedge pressure
PVR	Pulmonary vascular resistance
SpO_2	Percent oxygen saturation of hemoglobin measured by pulse oximetry
SvO_2	Percent oxygen saturation of hemoglobin in mixed venous blood (i.e., in the PA)
SV	Stroke volume
SVR	Systemic vascular resistance
VAD	Ventricular assist device

ICU patients can be clustered by disease condition (e.g., neurology) or age-group (e.g., pediatrics). ICU patients are sometimes clustered by acuity (e.g., acute and unstable versus technology dependent but stable). The patient with myocardial ischemia or infarction or respiratory distress is commonly treated in the ICU, as is the patient with acute neurologic impairment, after cardiac surgery, or after major organ transplantation. Trauma ICUs treat the critically injured. The patient with a medical emergency (e.g., sepsis, diabetic ketoacidosis, drug overdoses, poisonings, thyroid, adrenal, or hematologic crises) is often treated in a medical ICU. The patient with a serious underlying condition may be monitored in the ICU while receiving care for unrelated conditions. The patient who is not expected to recover is not treated in an ICU. The ICU should not be used to treat the patient in a persistent coma, nor should ICU care be used to prolong the natural process of death.

Despite the emphasis on caring for the patient who can survive, death is common in ICU patients. A review of British adult ICU admissions (excluding patients with burns or cardiac surgery) showed that 32.5% of patients died in the hospital.[2] Similar rates were reported in Canada.[3] Nonsurvivors were older and had longer ICU stays. However, even patients at relatively low risk such as those with asthma and drug overdoses had high death rates (greater than 10%). Often death occurred following transfer from ICU to the general hospital units, suggesting a need for caution and coordination of care in transferring patients from ICUs.

Progressive care units have recently been established as a graded option, intermediate between the ICU and the general hospital ward.[4] Generally patients in the progressive care unit are at risk for serious complications, but their risk is lower than that of ICU patients. Patients may require cardiac telemetry monitoring or slow weaning from mechanical ventilation. Progressive care units offer an opportunity to reduce health care costs and provide a calmer and quieter care environment.

Common Problems of Critical Care Patients. The patient admitted into the ICU is at risk for complications and special problems. Invasive devices carry a risk of infection, particularly in the immunocompromised patient. Sepsis and multiple organ dysfunction syndrome may follow (see Chapter 61). Other special problems for ICU patients include anxiety, dependency, impaired communication, sensory-perceptual problems, and sleep difficulties.

Anxiety. Patients commonly find the ICU frightening. Frequently patients are at risk of dying and fear death. Many patients and families feel uncomfortable in the ICU environment with its equipment, high noise and light levels, and intense pace of activity. Pain and sleeplessness enhance anxiety, as do immobilization, loss of control, and impaired communication.[5] Some patients become acutely stressed by the ICU experience and others experience chronic posttraumatic stress disorder (PTSD), characterized by intrusive memories, irritability, and difficulty concentrating. In one study 25% of patients treated in the ICU for acute respiratory distress syndrome experienced PTSD.[6] Patients experienced PTSD even when they could not remember details of the ICU experience.

The nurse can assist the patient and family with their feelings of anxiety by encouraging them to express concerns, ask questions, and state their needs. The nurse should explain equipment and procedures. The nurse may be able to structure the patient's surrounding environment in a way that may decrease anxiety. For example, family members can be encouraged to bring in photographs and personal items. Flexible visiting schedules may diminish the patient's anxiety.[5] Judicious use of sedation may blunt some of the acute and chronic stress-related conditions.

Dependency. Patients in the ICU commonly are unable to perform self-care activities such as eating, bathing, and oral hygiene. The patient may lack control over bodily functions such as elimination and breathing. The patient is frequently dependent on the nursing staff for access to food, liquids, the bedpan, and other needed items. In addition, the ICU patient is frequently connected to equipment and placed on bed rest. The degree of dependency experienced by an ICU patient can be distressing. Although the highest priority is the safety of the patient, the nurse should provide as much autonomy as the patient's condition allows. Family members can be taught to assist the patient with activities of daily living.

Impaired communication. Inability to communicate can be a distressing problem for the patient who may be unable to speak because of the use of paralyzing drugs or an endotracheal tube. As part of any procedure the nurse should explain what will happen or is happening to the patient. When the patient cannot speak, the nurse should explore alternative methods of communication, including the use of devices such as picture boards, notepads, magic slates, or computer keyboards. When speaking with the patient, the nurse should look directly at the patient and use hand gestures when appropriate.

Nonverbal communication is important. The ICU is characterized by high levels of procedure-related touch and decreased affection-related or comfort-related touch. Patients have different levels of tolerance for being touched, possibly related to cultural background and personal history. It may be appropriate to provide comforting touch with ongoing evaluation of the patient's response. Often the ICU nurse encourages the family to touch and talk with the patient.

Sensory-perceptual problems. Transient sensory-perceptual changes are common in ICU patients. Approximately 50% of patients treated in the ICU experience decreased orientation and impaired cognition.[7] The combination of changes in mentation (e.g., hallucinations, delusions) and behavior (e.g., shouting, hitting) has been inappropriately labeled *ICU psychosis.* The patient is not psychotic, but is suffering from delirium and may demonstrate confusion, irritability, and inappropriate behavior.[8] Factors predisposing the patient to sensory-perceptual changes include sleep deprivation, anxiety, sensory overload, stress, and many drugs. Physical conditions such as hypoxemia and electrolyte disturbances can produce similar symptoms, including confusion and irritability. Potassium, calcium, and magnesium imbalances are common in the critically ill patient, and each can result in altered cognition.

The task of the ICU nurse is to identify predisposing factors, whether they be physiologic, psychologic, or environmental, and attempt to improve the patient's mental clarity and cooperation with therapy. Helpful strategies include correction of contributing oxygenation, perfusion, and electrolyte problems. The use of clocks and calendars may help the patient remain oriented. Although symptoms may be managed pharmacologically with a sedative, hypnotic, or psychotropic (e.g., haloperidol [Haldol]) medication, these drugs may decrease the patient's ability to interact with family members. This may deprive patients and families of what may be the short and precious time remaining to discuss intimate and important issues.

Sensory overload can also result in patient distress and anxiety. Noise levels are particularly high in the ICU.[9] The "meaning" of a noise may determine its stressfulness with meaningful noise being less stressful. The nurse can limit noise and assist the patient in understanding noises that cannot be prevented. Conversation is a particularly stressful noise, especially when the discussion concerns the patient and is conducted in the presence of, but without participation from, the patient. The nurse can eliminate this source of stress by identifying better places for discussing the patient and by including the patient in the discussion. The nurse can also limit noise levels directly by muting phones, setting alarms appropriate to the patient's condition, and eliminating unnecessary alarms. For example, the nurse should silence the blood pressure alarms while manipulating invasive lines, and then reactivate the alarms when the procedures are complete. Similarly, ventilator alarms should be transiently silenced during endotracheal suctioning. Overhead paging should be limited in patient care areas. Music should be played only if it comforts the patient.

Sleep problems. Nearly all ICU patients experience serious sleep disturbances.[10] Patients may have difficulty falling asleep or have disrupted sleep because of frequent monitoring or treatment procedures.[11,12] Drugs such as sedatives and hypnotics may result in disturbed sleep patterns, including reductions in slow wave and rapid eye movement (REM) sleep.[13] Sleep disturbance is a significant stressor in the ICU, contributing to impaired cognition and possibly affecting recovery. The ICU nurse can structure the environment to promote patient sleep. Strategies include clustering activities, scheduling rest, making physiologic measurements without changing the patient's position, limiting noise, and promoting comfort and relaxation.

Issues Related to Family Members

When someone becomes critically ill, loved ones and family should not be forgotten. Family members play a valuable role in recovery and should be considered as members of the health care team. They can contribute to the patient's well-being by doing the following:[14]

1. Providing a link to the patient's personal life (e.g., news of family, friends, and job) to which the nurse has no access
2. Advising the patient in health care decisions because they know the patient better than the nursing staff
3. Helping with activities of daily living (e.g., bathing, oral suctioning)
4. Having a positive, loving, and caring presence

To be effective in caring for their loved one, family members need guidance and support from the nurse. The experience of having a friend or family member in the ICU is physically and emotionally difficult. Families of the critically ill are usually anxious about the patient's condition and prognosis. They have concerns regarding the patient's pain and other discomforts. They may question the quality of care that the patient is receiving. In addition, it is common for families to experience anxiety regarding the financial issues related to planning and providing care in the next phases of the illness. The family will typically be experiencing disruption of their daily routines to support the patient. They may be far from their own home, routines, and supportive friends and family members. During these difficult times, they are often asked to make critical decisions.

Lack of information is a source of anxiety for the family.[15] The nurse should assess the family's understanding of the patient's status, goals, treatments, and prognosis and provide information as appropriate. The first time the family member visits it is important for the nurse to prepare the family member for the experience by briefly describing the patient's appearance, condition, treatments, tubes, and equipment. Families should be told what to expect regarding the environment (sounds, noise, odors). It is helpful if the nurse can accompany the family members as they enter the room. They should be encouraged to participate in the patient's care. The nurse should observe the responses of both the patient and family. Sometimes the family may cease to be therapeutic and may tire the patient who is reluctant to tell them to leave. Another problem may be a family member whose own needs are neglected because of a sense of obligation to stay with the patient. The nurse should ensure that the patient's needs are being met and intervene with the family as needed. Family members who are exhausted, sleep deprived, anxious, and fearful are in no position to provide support to the patient. Rather than a rigid open or closed visiting policy, each patient should have a plan tailored to the patient's and family's needs.

The family needs information about the way in which the patient's care is managed and decisions are made. The family should have the opportunity to be involved in decision making. The family should also be invited to meet the health care team members, including physicians, dietician, respiratory therapist, social worker, and physical therapist. The nurse should evaluate the appropriateness of including family members in multidisciplinary care conferences. It helps family members to accept and cope with problems if they observe that providers are caring and competent, decisions are deliberate, and they themselves have the opportunity to help shape the course of care.

While working with families, the ICU nurse should assess the response of the family to the stress. Their feelings should be acknowledged and accepted. They should be supported in their decisions. Institutional support personnel, such as chaplains, social workers, and psychologists, may be helpful in assisting the family and patient to adjust. The extent to which the family is involved and supported will in turn affect the patient's clinical course in the ICU.

HEMODYNAMIC MONITORING

Hemodynamic monitoring refers to measurement of pressure, flow, and oxygenation of blood within the cardiovascular system. Both invasive (internally placed devices) and noninvasive (external devices) measurements are made in the ICU. Values commonly measured include systemic and pulmonary arterial pressures, central venous pressure (CVP), pulmonary artery wedge pressure (PAWP), cardiac output, and oxygen saturation of the hemoglobin of arterial blood (SaO_2) and mixed venous blood (SvO_2). From these measurements the clinician calculates several values, including the resistance of the systemic and pulmonary arterial vasculature and oxygen content, delivery, and consumption. When these data are integrated with clinical assessment data, the nurse can derive a better picture of the patient's hemodynamic status and the effect of therapy. It is important that all measures be made with attention to technical aspects. False or inaccurate data are potentially misleading and thus dangerous.

Hemodynamic Terminology

Cardiac Output. *Cardiac output* (CO) is the volume of blood pumped by the heart in 1 minute. Although minor beat-to-beat changes may occur, generally the left and right ventricles pump the same volume. The volume pumped with each heartbeat is the *stroke volume.* Stroke volume times heart rate equals CO. Blood pressure, the force exerted by blood on the vessel wall, is determined by CO and the forces opposing blood flow. The opposition to blood flow offered by the vessels is called *systemic vascular resistance* or *pulmonary vascular resistance.* Stroke volume (and thus CO and blood pressure) is determined by preload, afterload, and contractility (see Chapters 30 and 31). Understanding these concepts and relationships is essential for the ICU nurse. In addition, the nurse must understand the effects of manipulation of each of these variables. Normal values for hemodynamic variables are given in Table 63-2.

Preload. *Preload* is the volume within a cardiac chamber at the end of diastole. Unfortunately, chamber volumes are difficult to obtain. Instead, various pressures are used to estimate volume. Left ventricular preload is called *left ventricular end-diastolic pressure.* PAWP, a measure of pulmonary capillary pressure, reflects left ventricular end-diastolic pressure under normal conditions (i.e., when there is no mitral valve pathology, intracardiac defect, or arrhythmia). CVP, measured in the right atrium or in the vena cava close to the heart, is the right ventricular preload or right ventricular end-diastolic pressure when there is no tricuspid valve pathology.

Table 63-2 Hemodynamic Parameters at Rest

Indicators	Normal Range
Preload	
Right atrial pressure (RAP) or central venous pressure (CVP)	2-8 mm Hg
Pulmonary artery wedge pressure (PAWP) or left atrial pressure (LAP)	6-12 mm Hg
Pulmonary artery diastolic pressure	4-12 mm Hg
Afterload	
Pulmonary vascular resistance (PVR) = (mean pulmonary artery pressure [PAP] − mean pulmonary artery wedge pressure [PAWP]) × 80/cardiac output	<250 dyne sec/cm^5
Pulmonary vascular resistance index (PVRI) × 80 = pulmonary vascular resistance (PVR) × body surface area	160-380 dyne sec m^2/cm^5
Systemic vascular resistance (SVR) = (mean arterial pressure − central venous pressure) × 80/cardiac output	800-1200 dyne sec/cm^5
Systemic vascular resistance index (SVRI)=(systemic vascular resistance) × body surface area	1970-2390 dyne sec m^2/cm^5
Mean arterial pressure (MAP) = diastolic blood pressure + ⅓ pulse pressure*	70-105 mm Hg
Mean pulmonary artery pressure (PAP) = pulmonary artery diastolic pressure + ⅓ pulmonary artery pulse pressure*	10-20 mm Hg
Other	
Stroke volume = (cardiac output × 1000)/heart rate	60-150 ml/beat
Stroke volume index = (cardiac index × 1000)/heart rate	30-65 ml/beat/m^2
Heart rate	60-100 beats/min
Cardiac output = stroke volume × heart rate	4-8 L/min
Cardiac index = cardiac output/body surface area	2.2-4.0 L/min/m^2
Arterial hemoglobin oxygen saturation	92-99%
Mixed venous hemoglobin oxygen saturation	60-80%

*This formula is an approximation because it does not take into consideration the heart rate. The monitor looks at the area under the pressure curve, as well as the heart rate, to calculate MAP and PAP.

The effects of preload are based on muscle fiber length. The greater the stretch of the heart muscle at the end of diastole, the greater the force of the next contraction. As preload increases, force generated in the following contraction increases, thus stroke volume and CO increase. The greater the preload, the greater the myocardial (heart muscle) stretch, and the greater the oxygen requirement of the myocardium. Hence, increases in CO via increased preload require increased delivery of oxygen to the myocardium. It should be remembered that the change in stroke volume with preload comes about because of stretching of the heart muscle. However, the clinical measurement made is not a direct measurement of the muscle length; the measurement made is pressure at the time of the peak stretch (end-diastole). The pressure indirectly indicates the amount of stretch and the volume. The pressure is also important because it indicates pressure in the blood vessels of the lung or in the blood returning to the heart. Preload can be increased by fluid administration and decreased by diuresis.

Afterload. *Afterload* refers to the forces opposing ventricular ejection. These forces include systemic arterial pressure, the resistance offered by the aortic valve, and the mass and density of the blood to be moved. Clinically, although the measures fail to include all the components of afterload, systemic vascular resistance and arterial pressure are indices of left ventricular afterload. Similarly, pulmonary vascular resistance and pulmonary arterial pressure are indices of right ventricular afterload. Increased afterload results in a decreased CO. CO can be increased by decreasing afterload (i.e., decreasing forces opposing contraction). When afterload is reduced, myocardial oxygen needs are decreased. Thus CO is increased and myocardial oxygen requirements are decreased. Therapies directed at reducing afterload are used in the management of heart failure (see Chapter 33).

Contractility. *Contractility* describes the strength of contraction. Contractility is said to increase when preload is not changed, yet the heart contracts more forcefully. Contractility is increased by epinephrine, norepinephrine, isoproterenol (Isuprel), dopamine, dobutamine (Dobutrex), digitalis-like drugs, calcium, and milrinone (Primacor). These agents are termed *positive inotropes.* Contractility is diminished by *negative inotropes,* such as acidosis and certain drugs (e.g., barbiturates, alcohol, procainamide [Pronestyl], calcium channel blockers, beta-adrenergic blockers). Increased contractility results in increased stroke volume and increased myocardial oxygen requirements. There are no direct clinical measures of cardiac contractility. To indirectly determine contractility, the ICU nurse measures the patient's preload (PAWP) and CO and graphs the results. If preload, heart rate, and afterload remain constant, yet CO changes, contractility is altered. Contractility is diminished in the failing heart.

Vascular Resistance. Systemic vascular resistance (SVR) is the resistance of the systemic vascular bed. Pulmonary vascular resistance (PVR) is the resistance of the pulmonary vascular bed. SVR and PVR are calculated as indicated in Table 63-2.

Principles of Invasive Pressure Monitoring

Invasive lines are commonly used in the ICU to measure systemic and pulmonary blood pressures. Components of a typical invasive arterial pressure monitoring system are illustrated

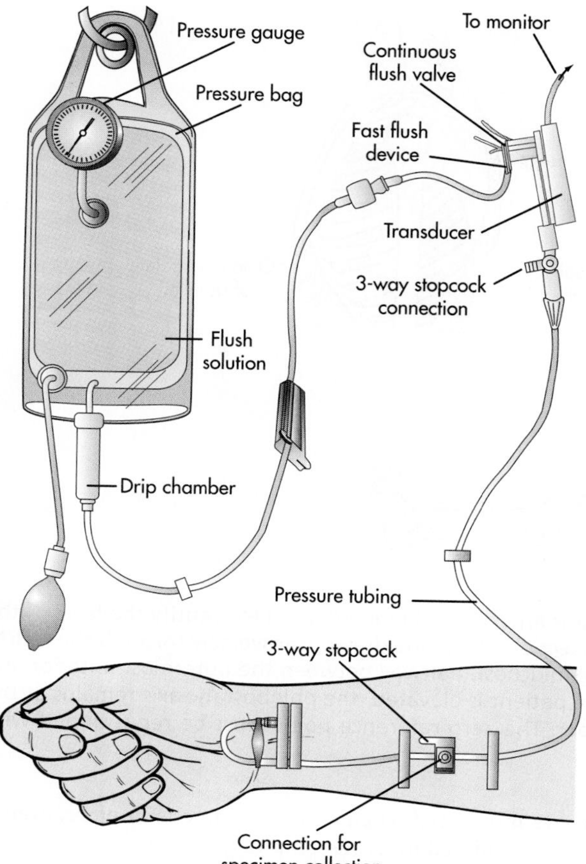

Fig. 63-2 Components of a pressure monitoring system. The cannula, shown entering the radial artery, is connected via pressure (nondistensible) tubing to the transducer. The transducer converts the pressure wave into an electronic signal. The transducer is wired to the electronic monitoring system, which amplifies, conditions, displays, and records the signal. Stopcocks are inserted into the line for specimen withdrawal and for referencing and zero-balancing procedures. A flush system consisting of a pressurized bag of intravenous fluid, tubing, and a flush device is inserted into the line. The flush system provides continuous slow (approximately 3 ml hourly) flushing and provides a mechanism for fast flushing of lines. All items except the electronic monitoring system are commonly disposable equipment.

in Fig. 63-2. Catheter, pressure tubing, flush system, and usually the transducer are disposable.

To accurately measure pressure, equipment must be referenced and zero balanced and dynamic response characteristics optimized. Referencing means positioning the monitoring equipment so that the zero reference point is at the vertical level of the left atrium of the heart. The port of the stopcock nearest the transducer is usually the zero reference for the transducer. To place this level with the left atrium, the nurse uses an external landmark, the phlebostatic axis. To identify the phlebostatic axis, two imaginary planes are drawn with the patient supine (Fig. 63-3). One plane is midchest, halfway between the outermost anterior and posterior surfaces. The second plane is transverse through the fourth intercostal space at the sternum. The phlebostatic axis is the intersection of the two planes. Once the phlebostatic axis is identified, it is marked on the patient's chest with a permanent marker. The port of the stopcock nearest the transducer is positioned level with the phlebostatic axis.

Zeroing confirms that when pressure within the system is zero, the equipment reads zero. Most transducers in common current use are disposable and have little zero drift; thus once-per-shift zeroing is recommended.

Optimizing dynamic response characteristics involves checking that the equipment reproduces without distortion a signal that changes rapidly. Optimizing dynamic response characteristics is performed once per shift. It involves checking that the equipment reproduces a distortion-free signal.

In addition to performing these procedures each shift, they are repeated each time a major component in the monitoring system is changed, the recording system is moved, or unusual readings are obtained.

Steps in measuring pressure with an invasive line are given in Table 63-3. Pressure measurements can be obtained from both digital and printed analog outputs, but accurate readings are best obtained from a printed pressure tracing at the end-expiration point. Initial readings are made with the patient flat. Unless the patient's blood pressure is extremely sensitive to orthostatic changes, values at modest degrees of backrest elevation (up to 30 degrees) are generally equivalent to measurements with the patient flat.[16] After confirming that values are similar whether the backrest is flat or slightly elevated, subsequent measurements can be made with the backrest slightly elevated. Thus it is not necessary to reposition the patient for each pressure reading. However, it is necessary to move the zero reference stopcock to keep it positioned at the phlebostatic axis. Consistent landmarks for the left atrium have not been identified for the side-lying position. Thus pressures are not obtained in side-lying positions.

Types of Invasive Pressure Monitoring

Arterial Blood Pressure. Continuous arterial pressure monitoring is indicated for patients experiencing hypotension or increased intracranial pressure, receiving vasoactive drugs (e.g., sodium nitroprusside, dopamine [Intropin]), or requiring frequent arterial blood sampling (e.g., for arterial blood gases [ABGs]). A 20-gauge, 1.5 in (3.8 cm) plastic catheter is typically used to cannulate a peripheral artery such as the radial, brachial, dorsalis pedis, or femoral. The catheter can be inserted percutaneously or via cutdown. It is important that the insertion site be immobilized by an arm board so that the catheter line is not dislodged and lines are not kinked.

Measurements. The nurse can use the arterial line to obtain systolic, diastolic, and mean blood pressure (Fig. 63-4). The arterial waveform provides useful information. In heart failure, the systolic upstroke may be slower. In volume depletion, systolic pressure varies greatly with mechanical ventilation, diminishing during inspiration. In severe congestive heart failure, systolic amplitude does not vary with ventilation. With arrhythmias it is useful to observe simultaneous ECG and pressure tracings. Arrhythmias that significantly diminish arterial pressure are more urgent than those that cause only a slight decrease in systolic amplitude.

Complications. Arterial lines carry the risk of hemorrhage, infection, thrombus formation, and distal circulatory occlusion. Hemorrhage is most likely to occur when the

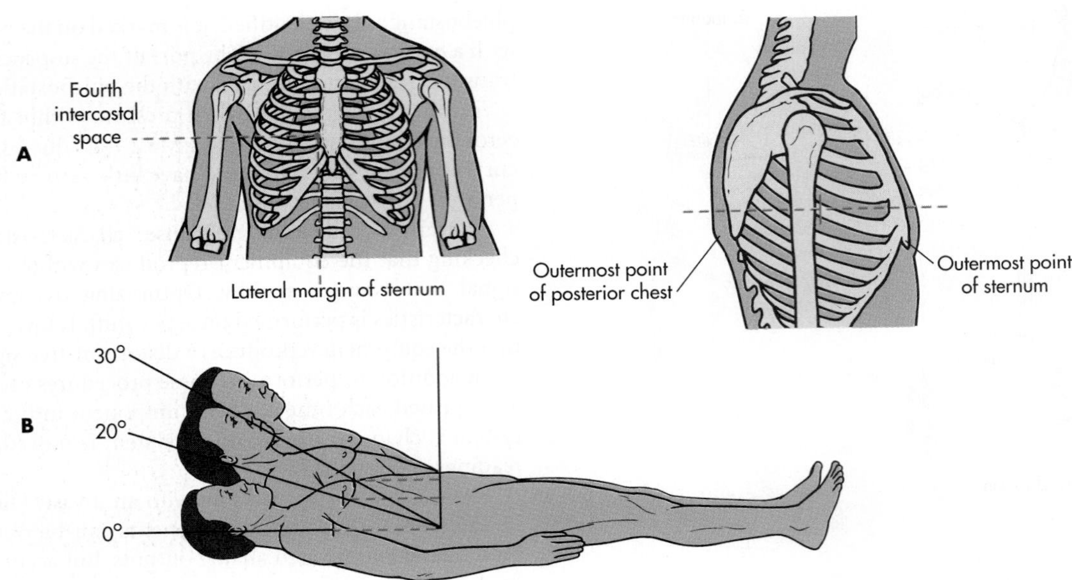

Fig. 63-3 Identification of the phlebostatic axis. **A,** The phlebostatic axis is an external landmark used to identify the level of the atrium in the supine patient. The phlebostatic axis is defined as the intersection of a plane drawn transversely through the fourth intercostal space at the sternum and a frontal plane drawn through the midchest, halfway between the outermost anterior and outermost posterior points of the chest. **B,** As the backrest of the supine patient is elevated, the phlebostatic axis remains at the same anatomic location, becoming progressively elevated from the floor. The zero reference point must be repositioned with changes in backrest elevation to keep it at the phlebostatic level.

Table 63-3 Measurement of Blood Pressure with Invasive Lines

1. Explain the procedure to the patient.
2. Inactivate the high-pressure and low-pressure alarms for the duration of the procedure.
3. Identify and mark the phlebostatic axis on the patient's chest (mid–anterior-posterior chest at the fourth intercostal space [see Fig. 63-3]).
4. Position the patient supine and flat, or if appropriate, elevated up to 30°.
5. Confirm that the zero reference (port of the stopcock nearest the transducer) is placed at the level of the phlebostatic axis. It may be helpful to use a carpenter's level.
6. Observe the monitor tracing and assess the quality of the tracing. Check dynamic response.
7. Obtain an analog printout, if available, and measure the pressures of interest at end expiration. If no printout is available, freeze the tracing on the oscilloscope screen and use the cursor to measure the pressures at end expiration.
8. Reset the high-pressure and low-pressure alarms.
9. Record the pressure measurements promptly, including (if available) the printout marked to identify the points read.

catheter becomes dislodged or the line becomes disconnected. To avoid this serious complication, the nurse uses Luer-Lok connections and always activates (and records activation of) the low-pressure alarm. Thus if the pressure in the line falls (as it would when the line is disconnected), an alarm sounds immediately, allowing prompt repair of the problem. Pressure is always monitored when an arterial line is in place, even if the line was placed for ABG sampling.

Infection is a risk with any invasive line. The nurse should inspect the insertion site for inflammation and exudate and monitor the patient for signs of systemic infection. When infection occurs, the catheter, tubing, flushing apparatus, and transducers must be changed.

Circulatory impairment can result from formation of a thrombus around the catheter, release of an embolus, spasm, or occlusion of the circulation by the catheter. Before inserting a line into the radial artery, Allen's test should be performed to confirm that ulnar circulation is sufficient to sustain the hand. In this test, pressure is applied to the radial and ulnar arteries simultaneously. The patient is instructed to open and close the hand repeatedly. The hand should blanch. The nurse then releases the pressure on the ulnar artery while compressing the radial artery. If pinkness fails to return within 6 seconds, the ulnar artery is insufficient, indicating that the radial artery should not be used for line insertion.

Once the catheter is inserted, the nurse should evaluate the circulation distal to the arterial insertion site hourly. The limb with compromised arterial flow will appear cool and pale, with capillary refill greater than 3 seconds. There may be symptoms of neurologic impairment, such as tingling or paresthesia. Circulatory impairment can result in loss of a limb and is an emergency. In addition, the nurse should maintain the continuous flush irrigation system.

Pulmonary Artery Flow-Directed Catheter. Pulmonary artery (PA) pressure monitoring is used to guide acute-phase management in patients with complicated cardiac and intravascular volume problems (Table 63-4). PA diastolic (PAD) pressure and PAWP are sensitive indicators of fluid volume status and cardiac function. PAD pressure and

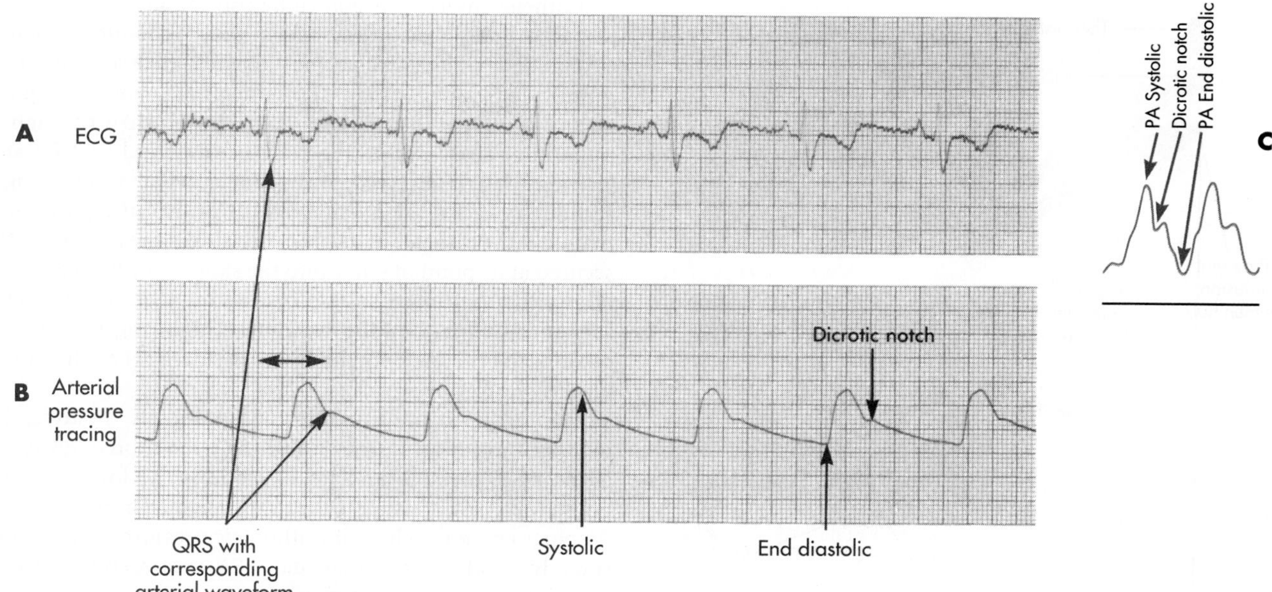

Fig. 63-4 **A,** Simultaneously recorded electrocardiogram tracing and **B,** systemic arterial pressure tracing. **C,** Pulmonary artery waveform. Systolic pressure is the peak pressure. The dicrotic notch indicates aortic valve closure. Diastolic pressure is the lowest value before contraction. Mean pressure is the average pressure over time calculated by the monitoring equipment. *PA,* pulmonary artery.

Table 63-4 Clinical Indications for Pulmonary Artery Catheterization

- Acute respiratory distress syndrome
- Acute respiratory failure in patients with chronic obstructive pulmonary disease
- Cardiac tamponade
- Cardiogenic or noncardiogenic pulmonary edema
- Complex fluid imbalance (burns, sepsis)
- Evaluation of circulatory syndromes (mitral valve regurgitation and intraventricular shunts)
- Intraaortic balloon support
- Myocardial infarction with left ventricular failure or cardiogenic shock
- Perioperative fluid imbalance in high risk patients
- Septic and hypovolemic shock
- Vasoactive pharmacologic support

PAWP are increased in fluid volume overload and heart failure. They are decreased with volume deficit. Fluid therapy based on PA pressure allows restoration of fluid balance while avoiding overcorrection of the problem. Monitoring PA pressures can allow precise therapeutic manipulation of preload, which allows CO to be maintained without placing the patient at risk for pulmonary edema.

A PA flow-directed catheter (e.g., Swan-Ganz) is used to measure PA pressures, including PAWP. The standard PA catheter is no. 7 French, 43 in (110 cm) long, with four lumens (Fig. 63-5). When properly positioned, the distal lumen (catheter tip) is within the pulmonary artery (Fig. 63-6). This lumen is used to monitor PA pressures and withdraw mixed venous blood specimens (e.g., to evaluate oxygen saturation). The distal lumen is surrounded by a balloon connected to an external valve via a second lumen. Balloon inflation has two purposes: (1) to allow moving blood to float the catheter forward and (2) to allow PAWP measurement. The third and fourth lumens are proximal, with exit ports in the right atrium. These are used for measurement of CVP, infusion of fluid and drugs, injection of fluid for CO determination, and withdrawal of blood specimens. The larger of the two proximal lumens is used for blood specimen collection. Often, when the patient is receiving total parenteral nutrition (TPN), the smaller proximal lumen is reserved for TPN infusion and is not interrupted for blood testing or injections. A thermistor located near the distal tip is wired to an external connector. The thermistor allows monitoring of core temperature and is used in the thermodilution method of measuring CO.

In addition to these relatively standard and common features of the PA flow-directed catheter, catheters with other features are available. One modification is the inclusion of an atrial electrode, useful in recording the atrial ECG or pacing the heart. Another common modification is inclusion of a fiberoptic sensor in the distal tip that detects mixed venous oxygen saturation. Another type of catheter provides continuous measurement of right ventricular volume and ejection fraction, while another catheter provides continuous CO monitoring. The pulmonary artery catheter sheath usually has a side port that serves as another intravenous line. Most catheters also have a plastic "sleeve" connected to the sheath, which permits manipulation of the catheter without breaking sterility.

Pulmonary artery catheter insertion. Before pulmonary artery catheter insertion, the nurse notes the patient's electrolyte, acid-base, oxygenation, and coagulation status. Imbalances such as hypokalemia, hypomagnesemia, hypoxemia, or acidosis can make the heart more irritable and increase the risk of ventricular arrhythmia during catheter insertion. Coagulopathy increases the risk of hemorrhage. The nurse prepares

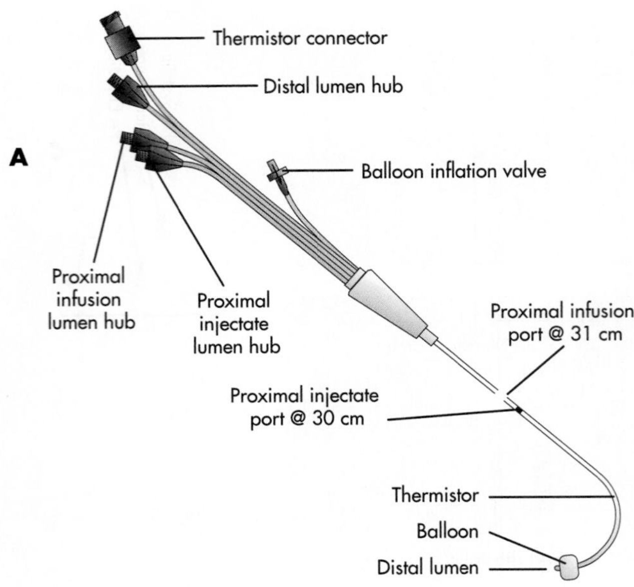

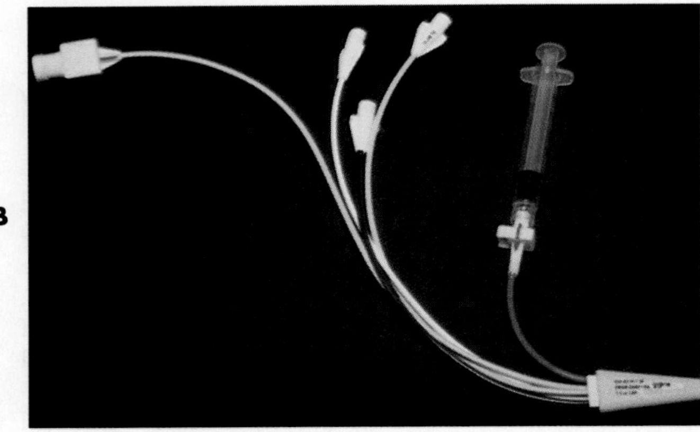

Fig. 63-5 Venous infusion port pulmonary artery (PA) catheter. **A,** The illustrated catheter has four lumens. When properly positioned, the distal lumen exit port is in the PA and the proximal lumen ports are in the right atrium. The distal and one of the proximal ports are used to measure PA and central venous pressures, respectively. A balloon surrounds the catheter near the distal end. The balloon inflation valve is used to inflate the balloon with air to allow reading of the pulmonary artery wedge pressure. A thermistor located near the distal tip senses PA temperature and is used to measure thermodilution cardiac output when solution cooler than body temperature is injected into a proximal port. **B,** Actual catheter.

for the procedure by preparing the monitor, cables, and flush and infusion solutions. The system is zero referenced to the phlebostatic axis. The patient is prepared for the procedure by explaining what will happen, and informed consent is obtained. The patient is positioned supine with the head of the bed tilted downward if tolerated.

The PA catheter is inserted through a sheath percutaneously into a deep peripheral vein using surgical asepsis. Venous cutdown is rarely required. Internal jugular, subclavian, antecubital, or femoral veins are acceptable insertion sites. The line is then advanced through the venous system to the heart.

Catheter insertion is guided by continuously observing the distal port (catheter tip) waveform on the monitor. When the tip reaches the right atrium, the balloon is inflated with the recommended volume of air. The catheter is floated through the tricuspid valve into the right ventricle and then through the pulmonic valve and into the PA. Once a typical PAWP tracing (see Fig. 63-6) is observed, the balloon is deflated. Following insertion, a chest x-ray is obtained to confirm the position. To maintain the catheter in its proper position, the catheter is then secured at its point of entry into the skin. An occlusive dressing is applied and changed according to unit protocol. It is necessary to monitor the ECG continuously during insertion because of the risk for arrhythmias, particularly when the catheter reaches the right ventricle.

Pulmonary artery pressure measurements. Systolic, diastolic, and mean pressures are routinely monitored. PA systolic is the peak pressure and PA diastolic is the lowest pressure point. Mean PA pressure is the time-weighted average. Because PA ports are in the chest, intrathoracic pressures alter PA pressure. To produce consistent data, PA measurements are obtained at the end of expiration.

The measurement of PAWP is obtained by slowly inflating the balloon with 1.5 ml of air while observing the distal lumen pressure tracing. Before inflation the pressure tracing visualized on the monitor looks like an arterial tracing, with a systolic peak, dicrotic notch, and then the diastolic low point. As the line becomes "wedged," the tracing changes shape and amplitude. The typical wedged waveform is characterized by two small waves, the A and V waves. The A wave indicates atrial contraction. The A wave is followed by the X descent, indicating atrial relaxation. Then the V wave is seen during the interval between the T and P waves of the ECG. The V wave indicates venous inflow into the atrium when the mitral valve is closed and the ventricle is contracting. The V wave is followed by the Y descent, indicating the emptying of the atrium when the mitral valve opens and ventricular filling.

When the tracing changes from arterial to atrial, the catheter is said to be wedged and PAWP is measured at the end of expiration. When measuring the wedge pressure, the balloon should be inflated for less than four respiratory cycles. There is danger of rupture of the pulmonary artery if the balloon is inflated too long or if the catheter migrates distally into a smaller vessel. This is suspected when less than 1.25 ml is needed to wedge the tracing, or an "overwedge" tracing is obtained. Readings should be acquired from an analog strip pressure recording, and the strip should be placed into the patient's record. If a printout of the tracing is not available, the readings should be taken from the monitor using the cursor.

Central venous or right atrial pressure measurement. CVP is a measurement of right ventricular preload. It can be measured with a PA catheter using one of the proximal lumens. Occasionally a CVP line may be placed. CVP is measured as a mean pressure at the end of expiration. CVP waveforms (Fig. 63-7) are similar to PAWP waveforms. Although the PA diastolic pressure and PAWP are more sensitive indicators of fluid volume status, CVP also reflects fluid volume problems. An elevated CVP indicates right ventricular failure or volume overload. A low CVP indicates hypovolemia.

Thermodilution cardiac output measurement. CO is frequently monitored in patients with hemodynamic instability.

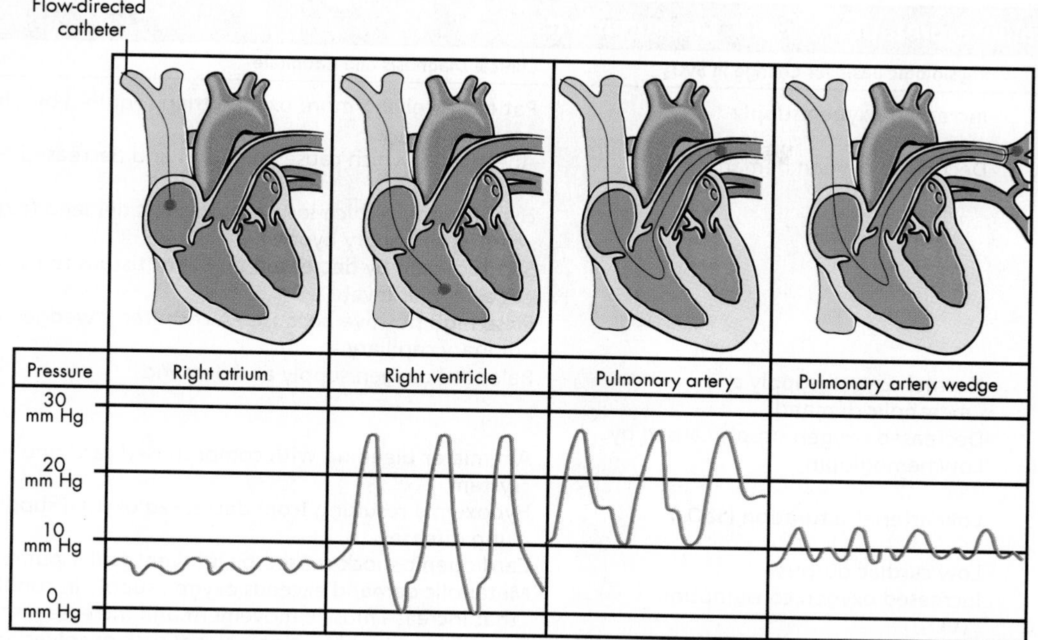

Fig. 63-6 Position of the pulmonary artery flow-directed catheter during progressive stages of insertion with corresponding pressure waveforms.

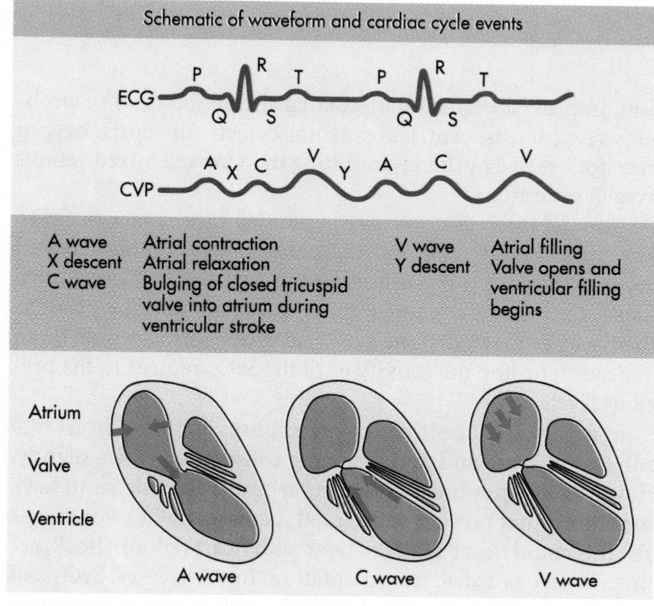

Fig. 63-7 Cardiac events that produce the CVP waveform with A, C, and V waves. A wave represents atrial contraction. X descent represents atrial relaxation. C wave represents the bulging of the closed tricuspid valve into the right atrium during ventricular systole. V wave represents atrial filling. Y descent represents opening of the tricuspid valve and filling of the ventricle.

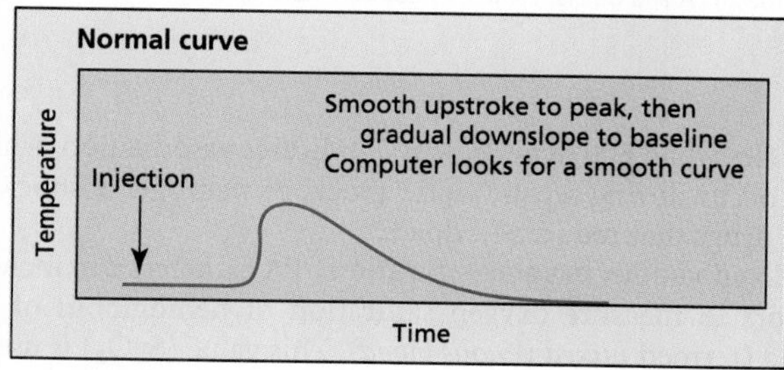

Fig. 63-8 Normal cardiac output curve. Cardiac output is calculated from the temperature change in the pulmonary artery when a fixed volume of a cool solution is injected into the proximal port in the right atrium. The nurse should visualize the curve and make sure that it is smooth. The larger the curve, the smaller the cardiac output.

Normal resting CO is 4 to 8 L per minute and varies with body size. Cardiac index (CI) is CO divided by body surface area. Cardiac index can be compared among individuals of varying body sizes. The normal cardiac index is 2.2 to 4.0 L/min/m^2. The CO is decreased in conditions such as hypovolemia, cardiogenic shock, and heart failure. Under normal conditions, CO increases with exercise. Increases in CO at rest indicate a hyperdynamic state seen with fever or sepsis.

The PA catheter is commonly used to measure CO by thermodilution. With this technique, a known amount of solution (saline or 5% dextrose in water) of known temperature (room temperature or chilled) is injected rapidly into the right atrial lumen of the PA catheter. The drop in blood temperature is detected by a thermistor embedded in the catheter tip in the pulmonary artery. The CO computer is programmed to calculate the CO from the temperature waveform. The larger the curve, the smaller the CO (Fig. 63-8).

SVR can be calculated each time CO is measured. The formula for calculating SVR is shown in Table 63-2. Normal SVR is 800 to 1200 dyne sec/cm^5. Increased SVR indicates vasoconstriction from shock, increased release or administration of epinephrine or norepinephrine, or left ventricular failure. A low

Table 63-5 Clinical Interpretation of SvO_2 Measurements

SvO_2 Measurement	Physiologic Basis for Change in SvO_2	Clinical Diagnosis and Rationale
High SvO_2 (80-95%)	Increased oxygen supply	Patient receiving more oxygen than required by clinical condition
	Decreased oxygen demand	Anesthesia, which causes sedation and decreased muscle movement.
		Hypothermia, which lowers metabolic demand (e.g., with cardiopulmonary bypass)
		Sepsis caused by decreased ability of tissues to use oxygen at a cellular level
		False high positive because PA catheter is wedged in a pulmonary capillary
Normal SvO_2 (60-80%)	Normal oxygen supply and metabolic demand	Balanced oxygen supply and demand
Low SvO_2 (less than 60%)	Decreased oxygen supply caused by:	
	Low hemoglobin	Anemia or bleeding with compromised cardiopulmonary system
	Low arterial saturation (SaO_2)	Hypoxemia resulting from decreased oxygen supply or lung disease
	Low cardiac output	Cardiogenic shock caused by left ventricular pump failure
	Increased oxygen consumption (VO_2)	Metabolic demand exceeds oxygen supply in conditions that increase muscle movement and increase metabolic rate, including physiologic states such as shivering, seizures, and hyperthermia and nursing interventions such as obtaining bedscale weight and turning

From Thelan LA and others, editors: *Critical care nursing: diagnosis and management*, ed 3, St Louis, 1998, Mosby.

SVR (less than 800 dyne sec/cm^5) indicates vasodilation, which may occur during sepsis, septic shock, or neurogenic shock or with drugs that reduce afterload.

Mixed venous oxygen saturation. PA catheters can include sensors to measure oxygen saturation of hemoglobin of PA blood (termed *mixed venous blood*). This value (SvO_2) is useful in determining the adequacy of tissue oxygenation. SvO_2 reflects the dynamic balance between oxygenation of the arterial blood, tissue perfusion, and tissue oxygen consumption. SvO_2, when considered in conjunction with the arterial oxygen saturation, is useful in analyzing hemodynamic status and response to treatments or activities (Table 63-5). Normal SvO_2 at rest is 60% to 80%.

Sustained decreases and increases in SvO_2 must be analyzed carefully. Decreased SvO_2 may indicate decreased arterial oxygenation, low CO, low hemoglobin, or increased oxygen consumption. If the SvO_2 falls, the nurse determines which of these four factors has changed. The nurse can observe for a change in arterial oxygenation by monitoring pulse oximetry or ABG analysis. Tissue perfusion can be grossly assessed by noting CO and organ function indicators (mentation, urine output, skin color). If arterial oxygenation, hemoglobin, and tissue perfusion are unchanged, a fall in SvO_2 indicates increased oxygen consumption, which could result from an increased metabolic rate, pain, movement, or fever. If oxygen consumption increases without a comparable increase in CO, more oxygen is extracted from the blood and SvO_2 falls. Similarly, when CO falls but arterial oxygenation and oxygen consumption are unchanged, the SvO_2 falls.

Increased SvO_2 is also clinically significant and may indicate a clinical improvement (e.g., increased arterial oxygen saturation, improved perfusion, decreased metabolic rate) or problems (e.g., sepsis, ventricular septal defect). In sepsis, oxygen may not be used optimally, resulting in increased mixed venous oxygen saturation.

Nursing interventions may be guided by changes in SvO_2. The nurse might note that the patient's heart rate increased moderately during repositioning but that the SvO_2 remained stable. In this case the nurse might conclude that the position change was tolerated. If the SvO_2 had dropped, this would be an indication to stop the activity until the SvO_2 returns to the previous level.

In many cases as activity or metabolism increases, heart rate and CO increase and SvO_2 remains constant or varies slightly. However, it is not uncommon for critically ill patients to have conditions that prevent substantial increases in CO. For example, this could occur in the patient with heart failure, shock, arrhythmias, or cardiac transplantation. In these cases, SvO_2 can provide a useful indicator of the balance between oxygen consumption and perfusion.

Complications with pulmonary artery catheters. Like arterial catheters, PA catheters are associated with an increased risk of thrombus and embolus formation, and the PA catheter is continuously flushed with a slow infusion of saline solution to prevent thrombus formation. If a thrombus begins to form, the waveform appears blunted.

Infection and sepsis are serious problems associated with PA catheters. Careful surgical asepsis for insertion and maintenance of the catheter and tubing line is mandatory to prevent infection. The skin is cleaned according to unit procedure, usually with an iodine preparation. The insertion site is covered with a sterile occlusive dressing. The nurse should monitor the patient for local and systemic signs of infection (e.g., redness and exudate at the insertion site, fever, increased white blood cell count). The PA catheter must be removed if there are local or systemic signs of infection. To reduce the risk of infection, PA catheters should not be left in place any longer than necessary.

Air embolus is another risk associated with PA catheters. Air embolus can be caused by balloon rupture or by injection of air into the lumen of a ruptured balloon. The nurse decreases the risk of embolus by injecting only the prescribed volume of air into the balloon. Catheters are checked for balloon leak before insertion; defective catheters are not used. If the nurse observes that the catheter cannot be wedged or that injected air does not flow back into the syringe, the catheter should be so labeled and the physician notified. The nurse should use Luer-Lok connections on all pressure line connections. For lines that are used to monitor pressure, the nurse sets the low alarm limit to activate if the pressure in the line drops substantially. Any time the line must be opened to change the apparatus, the nurse closes the line to the patient via clamping or stopcocks.

The patient with a PA catheter is at risk for pulmonary infarction or PA rupture from the following causes: (1) the balloon may rupture, releasing fragments that could embolize; (2) balloon inflation may obstruct blood flow; (3) the catheter may advance into a wedge position, obstructing blood flow; and (4) a thrombus could form and embolize. To reduce the risk of pulmonary infarction and rupture, the balloon must never be inflated with more than 1.5 ml. The balloon must not be left inflated for more than four breaths (except during insertion). PA pressure waveforms are monitored continuously for evidence of catheter occlusion, dislocation, or spontaneous wedging. The pressure tracing will be blunted if the catheter starts to be occluded. The pressure tracing will appear wedged if the PA catheter advances and becomes spontaneously wedged. In each of these cases, the catheter must be immediately repositioned.

Ventricular arrhythmias can occur during PA catheter insertion or removal or if the tip migrates back from the PA to the right ventricle. The catheter should be repositioned, usually by the physician.

Noninvasive Arterial Oxygenation Monitoring. Pulse oximetry is a noninvasive and continuous method of determining arterial oxygenation. Oxygenated and reduced (desaturated) hemoglobin absorb light differently. The pulse oximeter estimates the arterial oxygen saturation by detecting the differences in the light absorption by the two forms of hemoglobin. A light-emitting diode (LED) in the probe tip emits light at two specific wavelengths. The light is transmitted through the capillary bed of a finger or earlobe to a photodetector. Arterial hemoglobin is normally 95% to 100% saturated with oxygen.

A common use for pulse oximetry is to determine the effectiveness of oxygen therapy. By continuously monitoring with the pulse oximeter, there is less need for ABG sampling. Decreased arterial saturation indicates inadequate oxygenation of the blood in the pulmonary capillaries. This may be corrected by increasing the fraction of inspired oxygen (FIO_2). Similarly, the nurse uses the pulse oximeter to monitor how the patient tolerates a decreased FIO_2. Continuous monitoring of oxygenation is also useful to monitor the patient's response to changes in position and treatments. For example, the nurse might note that arterial saturation falls when the patient is positioned in a left lateral recumbent position. The nurse could then plan position changes that pose less risk for the patient.

Pulse oximetry may be inaccurate in the setting of (1) vasoconstriction from hypoperfusion or hypothermia, (2) patient movement, or (3) bright ambient light. Placing the probe on the earlobe or bridge of the nose may solve the problem of hypoperfusion. Obtaining readings only during rest will solve the second problem. Covering the probe with a towel will solve the third problem.

NURSING MANAGEMENT: HEMODYNAMIC MONITORING

Assessment of hemodynamic status requires integration of data from many sources and comparison of the data over time. Observations include the patient's general appearance, skin color, vital signs, and organ function. The nurse should begin with the patient's general appearance. Does the patient appear weak, tired, exhausted? There may be too little cardiac reserve to sustain minimum activity. Changing skin color or temperature may indicate decreased CO. If the patient is bleeding and developing shock, blood pressure might initially be relatively stable, yet the patient may become increasingly pale and cool from peripheral vasoconstriction. The nurse can confirm suspicion of impending shock by noting the SVR, which would increase in these circumstances. Conversely, the patient may remain warm and pink yet develop tachycardia and blood pressure instability. These features are characteristic of septic shock. The suspicion can be confirmed with measurements of CO, which would initially increase with septic shock, and of SVR, which would decrease.

The heart rate is often a useful indicator of the hemodynamic state. As tissue perfusion becomes compromised, heart rate increases. Although heart rates of 100 beats per minute are common among stressed, compromised, critically ill patients, further increases in heart rate may indicate compromised perfusion. In patients in whom heart rate cannot increase, such as those with atrioventricular block, the SvO_2 can be a useful indicator of impending compromise.

In addition to high technology measurements available to the ICU nurse, simple observations may provide useful insights into the patient's hemodynamic status. Mental clarity may reflect cerebral perfusion. Urine output may reflect renal perfusion. The patient with diminished gastrointestinal perfusion may develop hypoactive or absent bowel sounds and may have nausea and vomiting when gastrointestinal motility is impaired by a lack of perfusion. By carefully monitoring the patient, the astute nurse is able to recognize early clues and manage problems before they escalate.

CIRCULATORY ASSIST DEVICES

Mechanical circulatory assist devices, such as the intraaortic balloon pump (IABP) and left ventricular assist device (VAD), are used to decrease cardiac work and improve organ perfusion in patients with heart failure when conventional drug therapy is no longer adequate. The type of device used depends on the extent and nature of the myocardial problem and the

Table 63-6 Indications and Contraindications for the Intraaortic Balloon Pump

Indications
- Unstable angina (when medications have failed)
- Severe cardiac disease as a bridge to cardiac transplant
- Acute myocardial infarction with any of the following:*
  - Ventricular aneurysm accompanied by ventricular arrhythmias
  - Acute ventricular septal defect
  - Acute mitral valve regurgitation
  - Cardiogenic shock
  - Continuing chest pain
- Preoperative, intraoperative, and postoperative open heart surgery (e.g., aneurysectomy, revascularization, or valve replacement); often used to wean from cardiopulmonary bypass

Contraindications
- Irreversible brain damage
- Terminal or untreatable diseases of any major organ system
- Ruptured or dissecting aortic or thoracic aneurysm
- Generalized peripheral vascular disease (may prevent placement of balloon)
- Incompetent aortic valve (considered an *absolute* contraindication)

*Allows time for emergency angiography and corrective cardiac surgery to be performed.

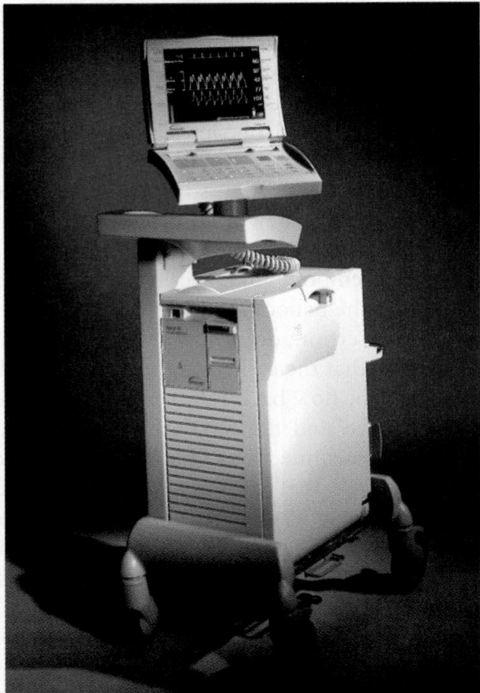

Fig. 63-9 Intraaortic balloon pump machine.

capabilities of the institution and staff. Circulatory assist devices provide interim support in three types of situations: (1) the left ventricle requires support while recovering from acute injury; (2) the heart requires surgical repair (e.g., a ruptured septum) but the patient must be stabilized and preparations made for the procedure; and (3) the patient in end-stage heart failure awaits cardiac transplantation. All circulatory assist devices decrease left ventricular workload, increase myocardial perfusion, and augment circulation. The most commonly used device is the IABP, and thus most ICU nurses encounter patients receiving IABP support. Several types of VADs are available, and additional devices are under development.

Intraaortic Balloon Pump

The IABP provides temporary circulatory assistance to the compromised heart by reducing afterload (via reduction in systolic pressure) and augmenting the aortic diastolic pressure. Table 63-6 lists clinical conditions for which the IABP is used. The IABP consists of a sausage-shaped balloon, a pump that inflates and deflates the balloon, control devices for synchronizing the balloon inflation to the cardiac cycle, and fail-safe devices (Figs. 63-9 and 63-10). The balloon is inserted percutaneously or surgically into the femoral artery, advanced toward the heart, and positioned in the descending thoracic aorta just below the left subclavian artery. Following placement, the position is confirmed with an x-ray. A pneumatic device cyclically fills the balloon with helium during diastole and deflates it just before systole. The ECG is used to trigger deflation on the R wave and inflation on the T wave. The arterial pressure tracing is used to refine timing. IABP support is referred to as *counterpulsation* because the timing of balloon inflation is opposite to ventricular contraction.

Effects of Counterpulsation. The balloon is rapidly inflated at the start of diastole, immediately after aortic valve closure, partially occluding the aorta (see Fig. 63-10). Displaced blood is forced forward into the extremities and back into the coronary arteries and main branches of the aortic arch. Diastolic arterial pressure rises (diastolic augmentation), increasing coronary artery perfusion pressure and perfusion of vital organs. The rise in coronary artery perfusion pressure causes an increase in blood flow to the myocardium. The balloon is rapidly deflated just before systole. The suddenly created vacuum causes aortic pressure to drop. With aortic resistance to left ventricular ejection reduced (reduced afterload), the left ventricle empties more easily and completely. As with other types of afterload reduction, the stroke volume increases, yet the myocardial oxygen consumption decreases. Hemodynamic effects of the IABP are summarized in Table 63-7.

Complications with Intraaortic Balloon Pumps. Complications are common with the IABP.[17-19] Vascular injuries such as dislodging of plaque, arterial dissection, and compromised distal extremity circulation are common, occurring in 3% to 65% of cases. Thrombus and embolus formation add to the risk of distal circulatory compromise. Peripheral nerve damage can occur, particularly when a cutdown is performed for insertion. To reduce these risks, hourly neurovascular assessment is necessary. Because the balloon pumping can cause physical destruction of platelets, mild thrombocytopenia is common and coagulation status indicators are monitored. Displacement of the balloon can occlude the left subclavian, renal, or mesenteric arteries. Patients on IABP therapy are prone to infection, as is any patient with invasive lines. Insertion site infection or sepsis caused by an unknown source necessitates catheter removal.

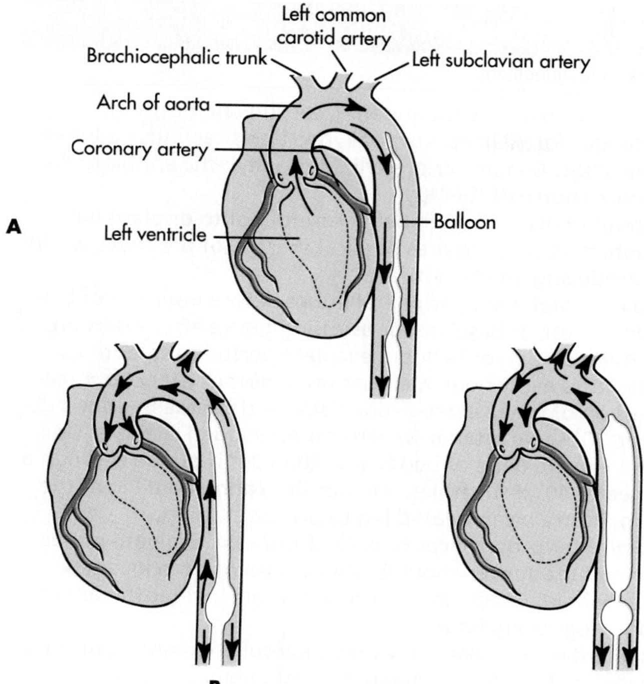

Fig. 63-10 Intraaortic balloon pump. **A,** During systole the balloon is deflated, which facilitates ejection of the blood into the periphery where systemic arterial resistance vessels are perfused. **B,** In early diastole, the balloon begins to inflate. **C,** In late diastole, the balloon is totally inflated, which augments aortic pressure and increases the coronary perfusion pressure with the end result of increased coronary and cerebral blood flow.

Table 63-7 Hemodynamic Effects of Intraaortic Balloon Pumps

Hemodynamic Effects of Intraaortic Balloon Pumps
Effects of Inflation During Diastole
Increased diastolic pressure (may exceed systolic pressure)
Increased pressure in the aortic root during diastole
Increased coronary perfusion pressure
Improved oxygen delivery to the myocardium
Decreased angina pain
Decreased electrocardiographic evidence of ischemia
Decreased ventricular ectopy
Effects of Deflation During Systole
Decreased afterload
Decreased peak systolic pressure
Decreased myocardial oxygen consumption
Increased stroke volume, possibly associated with:
Improved sensorium
Warmed skin
Increased urine output
Decreased heart rate
Increased forward flow of blood, decreasing preload
Decreased PA pressures, including PAWP
Decreased crackles

Mechanical complications are rare but may occur. Improper timing of balloon inflation may cause increased afterload, decreased CO, myocardial ischemia, and increased myocardial oxygen use and must be immediately corrected by the nurse. If the balloon develops a leak, the catheter must be changed immediately to avoid a gas embolus. Signs of a leak include less effective augmentation and blood backing up into the catheter. A malfunction of the balloon or console triggers fail-safe alarms and automatic shutdown of the unit.

The patient with an IABP is relatively immobile, limited to side-lying or supine positions with the head of the bed elevated no more than 30 to 40 degrees. The leg in which the catheter is inserted must not be flexed at the hip. The patient may be receiving ventilatory support and will likely have multiple invasive lines that increase the challenge of comfortable positioning. The patient may experience sleeplessness and anxiety. Adequate sedation, pain relief, skin care, and comfort measures are required.

As the patient improves, he or she is "weaned" from the IABP; that is, circulatory support provided by the IABP is gradually reduced. Weaning involves reducing the pumping to every second or third beat or decreasing augmentation pressure until the IABP catheter is removed. Even if the patient is stable without IABP, pumping is continued every third or fourth beat until the line is removed. This reduces the risk of thrombus formation around the catheter. Detailed, frequent hemodynamic assessment continues to be required during the weaning phase.

NURSING MANAGEMENT: INTRAAORTIC BALLOON PUMP

The patient with an IABP requires highly skilled nursing care. Detailed cardiovascular assessment, including measurement of vital signs, hemodynamic pressures, CO, cardiac auscultation, and cardiac rhythm evaluation, is performed frequently. Assessments of myocardial ischemia (indicated by T-wave inversion, ST segment changes, chest pain) skin color and temperature, mentation, urine output, and bowel sounds are also performed at regular intervals. It is expected that with continuing IABP treatment these parameters should improve. Nursing management of IABP complications is presented in Table 63-8.

Ventricular Assist Devices

The VAD provides longer-term support for the failing heart (usually days to months) and allows more mobility than the IABP. There are several types of VAD. VADs work by being inserted into the path of the flowing blood to augment or replace the ventricle. For example, a typical arrangement would shunt the blood from the left atrium or ventricle into the VAD and then into the aorta. Other arrangements allow biventricular support. The types of VAD are listed in Table 63-9. A typical VAD is illustrated in Fig. 63-11.

Failure to wean from cardiopulmonary bypass after surgery has been the primary indicator for VAD support. Increasingly the VAD is used to support patients with ventricular failure caused by myocardial infarction and patients awaiting cardiac transplantation. A VAD is a temporary device with the capability to partially or totally support circulation until the heart recovers or a donor heart can be obtained. Cannula sites depend on the type of device used. For support of the right side of the heart, the right atrium and PA are cannulated. The left

Table **63-8** Nursing Management: Potential Complications of the Intraaortic Balloon Pump

Potential Complication	Nursing Management
Site infection from invasive lines	Use strict aseptic technique for insertion and dressing changes for all lines. Cover all insertion sites with occlusive dressings. Administer prescribed prophylactic antibiotic for entire course of therapy.
Pneumonia associated with immobilization	Reposition patient q2hr, being careful not to displace balloon. If patient requires physical therapy of the chest, avoid introducing an ECG artifact.
Arterial trauma caused by insertion or displacement of balloon	Evaluate and mark peripheral pulses before insertion of balloon to use as baseline for assessing pulses after insertion. After insertion of balloon, evaluate perfusion to both extremities every hour. Measure urine output every hour (occlusion of renal arteries causes severe decrease in urine output). Observe arterial waveforms for sudden changes. Do not elevate head of bed higher than 30° if placed through a sheath; 40° if sheathless. Do not flex cannulated leg at the hip. Restrain cannulated leg to prevent flexion.
Thromboembolism caused by trauma, balloon obstruction of blood flow distal to catheter	Administer prophylactic heparin if ordered. Evaluate pulses, urine output every hour. Evaluate level of consciousness every hour. Check circulation, sensation, and movement in both legs every hour.
Hematologic complications caused by platelet aggregation along the balloon (decrease in platelets possible)	Administer Rheomacrodex (low-molecular-weight dextran) if ordered. Monitor coagulation status, hematocrit, and platelet count.
Hemorrhage from insertion site	Check site for bleeding every hour. Observe vital signs for hypovolemia with each vital sign check

Table **63-9** Ventricular Assist Devices

Type	Example	Use	Description
Centrifugal	Biomedicus	Univentricular or biventricular support	Blood is diverted to a cone-shaped pump head where blades rotate and propel blood back through return cannula via continuous (nonpulsatile) flow
Rotary	Hemopump	LV support	A propeller housed in the LV cannula draws blood from the LV and propels it into the aorta
Pneumatic	Thoratec	Univentricular or biventricular support	External pulsatile pump that uses a pressurized air sac to eject blood through outflow cannula
	Abiomed BVS 5000	Univentricular or biventricular support	A two-chamber external pump with bladders that fill by gravity; blood pumps are positioned at a level relative to the patient
	TCI Heartmate	LVAD	A pneumatically driven, totally implantable pump with external drive console
Electric	Novacor	LVAD	An electrically driven pulsatile pump that is implanted in an upper abdominal quadrant
	TCI Heartmate Vented Electric	LVAD	Totally implantable pump, powered by two 12-volt batteries or a direct power source
Cardiopulmonary support	Bard CPS	Emergency resuscitation (e.g., supported angioplasty)	Femoral-femoral bypass; venous blood delivered to centrifugal pump that passes through normothermic heat exchanger to membrane oxygenator and back to patient

Modified from Thelan LA and others, editors: *Critical care nursing: diagnosis and management,* ed 3, St Louis, 1998, Mosby.
LA, left atrium; *LV,* left ventricle; *LVAD,* left ventricular assist device; *PA,* pulmonary artery; *RA,* right atrium; *RVAD,* right ventricular assist device.

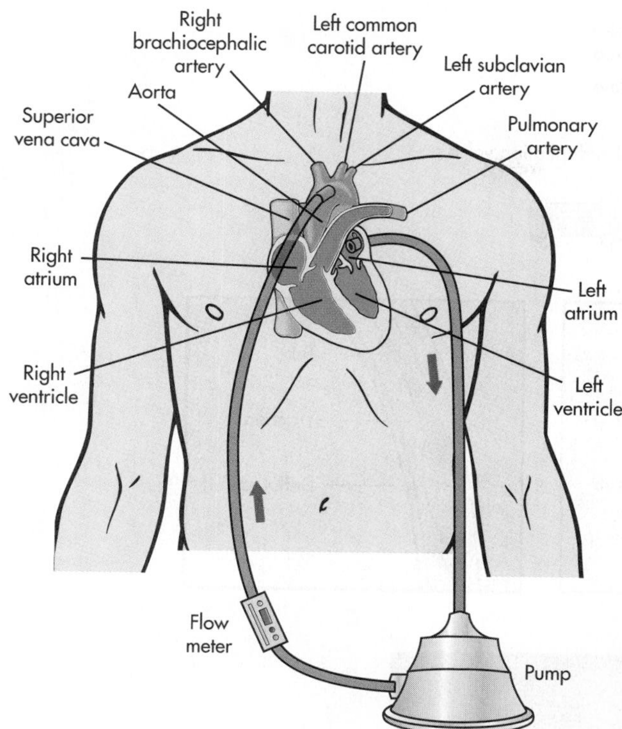

Fig. 63-11 Schematic diagram of a left ventricular assist device.

ventricular apex can be cannulated for left ventricular devices. Cannulation may occur at the bedside with femoral percutaneous technique or femoral cutdown. Direct cannulation of the atria and great vessels occurs in the operating room through a sternotomy.

Patient selection is critical. Three groups are recognized as potential candidates: (1) postcardiotomy patients, (2) those awaiting cardiac transplantation, and (3) patients with acute myocardial infarction in cardiogenic shock. Exclusion criteria include (1) significant aortic valve insufficiency, (2) major cerebrovascular accident, (3) body surface area less than 1.5 m^2, (4) sepsis, (5) life-limiting comorbid conditions (such as chronic renal failure, metastatic cancer, severe hepatic disease), and (6) comorbid conditions that would pose technical difficulties (coagulopathy, blood dyscrasia, certain infectious diseases, severe pulmonary disease).[20] Device selection depends on the institution and physician approval to use investigational or Food and Drug Administration (FDA)–approved devices.

Nursing care of the patient with a VAD is similar to that of the patient with an IABP. The patient is observed for bleeding, cardiac tamponade, ventricular failure, infection, arrhythmias, renal failure, hemolysis, and thromboembolism. The patient requires nutritional support. Unlike the patient with an IABP, who must remain in bed with limited position change, the patient with VAD is usually mobile and requires an activity plan.

Ideally, patients with VAD recover either through ventricular improvement or transplantation. However, many patients do die. Both the patient and family require psychologic support. Nursing care should include the family as much as possible. Other members of the health care team, such as social workers or clergy, should be notified to help the family and friends.

When the ventricle improves or transplantation occurs, the patient is taken to the operating room where the VAD is removed. Cannula sites are packed and wounds are closed. Usual wound care is followed after the patient is returned to the ICU.

The results of mechanical circulatory assist device use have been encouraging. With the development of new mechanical pumps that will act as biologic donor hearts and as cardiac replacements, nursing care will be a challenge.

ARTIFICIAL AIRWAYS

The patient in the ICU often requires mechanical assistance to maintain airway patency. An artificial airway is created by inserting a tube into the trachea, bypassing upper airway and laryngeal structures. A tube is placed into the trachea via the mouth or nose past the larynx (endotracheal [ET] intubation) or through the neck structures (tracheostomy). ET intubation is more common in ICU patients. It can be performed quickly without taking the patient to surgery. Tracheostomy is accomplished surgically and is used when the need for an artificial airway is more long term. Endotracheal tubes are illustrated in Fig. 63-12. Tracheostomies are discussed in Chapter 25 and illustrated in Fig. 25-6.

Indications for an artificial airway are to (1) prevent or relieve upper airway obstruction, (2) decrease aspiration when the patient lacks airway protection reflexes, (3) facilitate secretion removal when the patient cannot effectively clear the airway, and (4) provide a closed system for positive pressure mechanical ventilation. The patient who requires an artificial airway is often in acute respiratory distress and may have an altered level of consciousness.

Endotracheal Tubes

Endotracheal intubation can be performed by inserting the tube into the trachea through the mouth (oral intubation) or through the nose (nasal intubation). In oral intubation the endotracheal tube is passed through the mouth and vocal cords and into the trachea with the aid of a laryngoscope or bronchoscope. In nasal intubation, insertion is performed by manipulating the tube through the nose, nasopharynx, and vocal cords.

Oral ET intubation is the procedure of choice for most emergencies because the airway can be secured rapidly. Compared with the nasal route, a larger-diameter tube can be used for oral intubation. With a larger-bore tube, work of breathing is reduced because there is less airway resistance. It is easier to remove secretions and perform fiberoptic bronchoscopy if needed.

There are disadvantages of oral ET intubation. It is difficult to place an oral tube if head and neck mobility are limited. Salivation is increased and swallowing is difficult. A bite block or oral airway is used to stop the patient from biting and kinking the tube. The tube and bite block are taped to the face. Mouth care is a challenge. Finally, the larger tubes used in oral intubation are associated with laryngeal trauma and subglottic stenosis, particularly in smaller individuals (women).

Nasal ET intubation is sometimes preferred because it is more stable than the oral tube and more difficult to dislodge. It can be placed "blindly," that is, without visualizing the larynx, and thus is indicated when head and neck manipulation is risky. The nasal tube may be uncomfortable for some patients

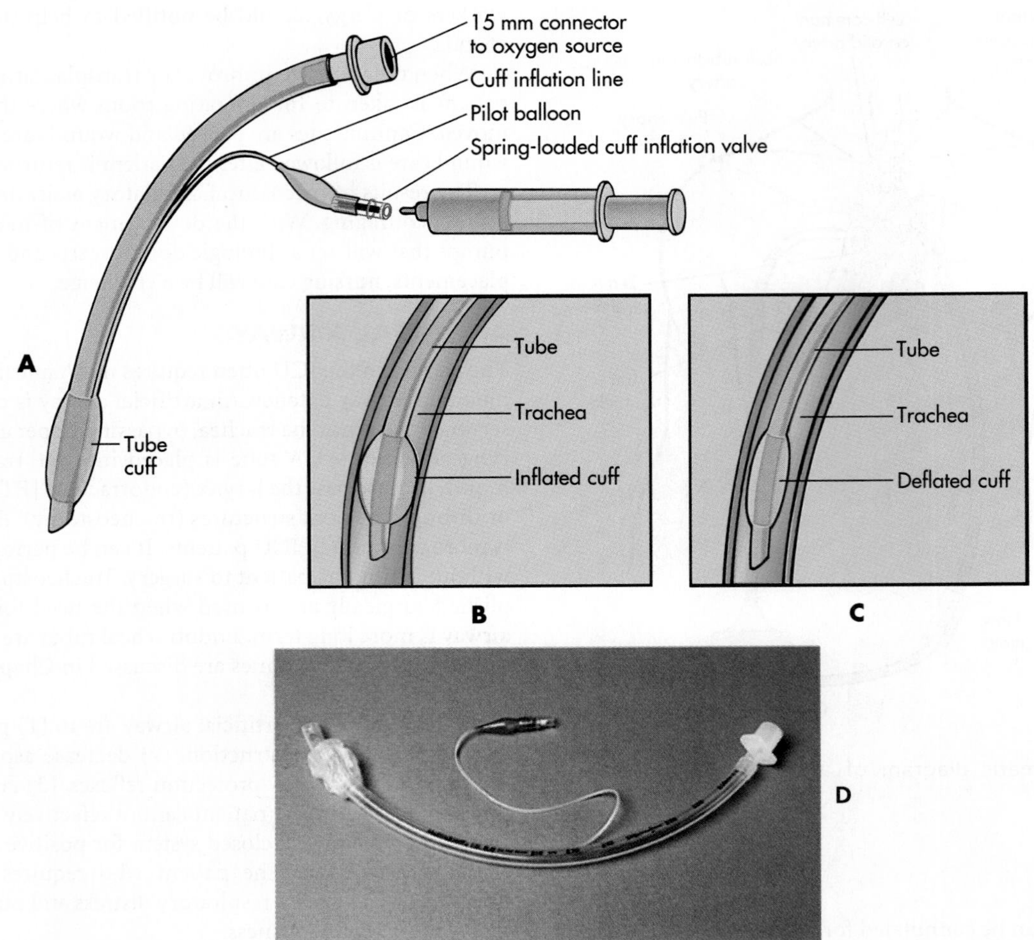

Fig. 63-12 Endotracheal tube. **A,** Parts of an endotracheal tube. **B,** Tube in place with the cuff inflated. **C,** Tube in place with the cuff deflated. **D,** Photo of tube before placement.

because it presses on the septum, whereas others may prefer it because there is no need for a bite block and mouth care is more easily accomplished. However, nasal ET tubes are more subject to kinking than oral tubes; the work of breathing is greater because the longer, narrower tube offers more airflow resistance; and suctioning and secretion removal are more difficult. Nasal tubes have been linked with increased sinus infection incidence, which may be a source of sepsis.[21]

Tracheostomy Tubes

Tracheostomy tubes are used if the artificial airway will be needed for a long time (more than 4 to 6 weeks). Upper airway damage is minimized and patient comfort maximized when a tracheostomy is performed early in the course of treatment. The patient may be able to eat and to speak with some types of tracheostomy tubes. Secretion removal is easier and the work of breathing less than with ET intubation. There is debate regarding when to perform a tracheotomy in the patient with an ET tube. The situation varies with the patient, physician, and institution. Some institutions use ET intubation in patients for up to 6 weeks without harmful sequelae. Tracheostomy tubes and related nursing management are discussed in Chapter 25. Types of tracheostomy tubes are listed in Table 25-5 and illustrated in Fig. 25-6.

Endotracheal Intubation Procedures

Before intubation, the nurse should ensure that the patient is properly oxygenated. The nurse should explain why ET intubation is necessary, the procedure involved, and sensations (gagging, a feeling of suffocation) that may be experienced during the procedure. The nurse should also explain that because of the inflated cuff, it will not be possible to talk when the tube is in place, but speech will be possible after the tube is removed.

The nurse should assemble and check the equipment to be used during the procedure, remove the patient's dentures or partial plates, and administer medication as ordered. Premedication varies, depending on the patient's health status. In the operating room, premedication may include intravenous barbiturates (to induce sleep) and a neuromuscular blocking agent. In ICUs, premedication often includes a topical anesthetic spray such as 4% lidocaine. A sedative-hypnotic and amnestic (e.g., midazolam [Versed]) is used if the patient is agitated, disoriented, or combative. A rapid-onset narcotic such as fentanyl (Sublimaze) may be used to blunt the pain of laryngoscopy and intubation. A paralytic drug such as succinylcholine [Anectine] may be used to prevent movement. Atropine may be used to limit secretions. In emergency situations, intubation is commonly performed without premedication because the patient may be unconscious.

If oral intubation is selected, the patient is positioned so that the mouth, pharynx, and trachea are in relatively direct alignment. The patient is placed supine with the head extended and the neck flexed ("sniffing position"). The head must not hang over the edge of the bed. The lower jaw is held forward. The person performing the procedure (usually a physician or nurse practitioner) uses a laryngoscope to visualize the vocal cords and pass the ET tube through the mouth over the vocal cords into the trachea. Nasal intubation can be accomplished blindly without the patient moving the head and neck. For nasal intubation it may be helpful to have the patient extrude the tongue. The patient is preoxygenated with 100% oxygen via a manual resuscitation bag (MRB). Each insertion attempt is limited to 30 seconds. Pulse oximetry is helpful during intubation to assess hypoxemia.

Following tube insertion, the cuff is inflated, placement confirmed, and the tube secured. The nurse must immediately auscultate the chest to confirm bilateral breath sounds and observe to confirm bilateral chest expansion. The tube is secured with tape and bite block as needed. A chest x-ray is immediately obtained to confirm tube placement at 3 to 5 cm above the carina in the adult, about halfway between the vocal cords and carina. This position allows the patient to move the neck without dislodging the tube or causing it to enter the right mainstem bronchus.

Once proper positioning is confirmed with x-ray, the tube is marked where it exits the nose or mouth ("exit mark") and securely fixed in position. The tubing is cut to remove excess. To fix the oral tube in position, a bite block is used. Adhesive tape is placed on each cheek. A second, longer piece of tape is placed over the first piece; the free ends are split and wrapped around the tube and bite block. The bottom tape remains in place, and only the top piece is changed if necessary. The nasal tube is similarly taped to the side of the cheeks. In the event of facial injuries, it is possible to use ties made of umbilical tape rather than adhesive tape to secure the nasal tube. Several commercial devices are available to assist in securing ET tubes.

Following intubation, the patient might require suctioning. Oral suctioning is almost always needed because the patient cannot swallow normally. Tracheal suctioning may be needed because few patients can cough with sufficient vigor. Following intubation, the nurse should auscultate over the central airways. Coarse rhonchi suggest that secretions are present, which should be removed by suctioning or coughing (see Table 63-11).

The ET tube is connected either to humidified air, oxygen, or a mechanical ventilator. ABGs should be sampled 10 to 20 minutes after intubation to determine oxygenation and ventilation status. ABG values are reviewed and used to guide oxygenation and ventilation changes. Pulse oximetry provides useful continuous monitoring of arterial oxygenation.

NURSING MANAGEMENT: ARTIFICIAL AIRWAY

Nursing responsibilities for the patient with an artificial airway include (1) maintaining correct tube placement, (2) maintaining proper cuff inflation, (3) maintaining and monitoring ventilation status (includes oxygenation and acid-base status), (4) maintaining tube patency, (5) assessing for complicatons, (6) providing mouth care and rotating the tube placement, and (7) fostering comfort and communication. Nursing care for the patient with an artificial airway is presented in NCP 63-1.

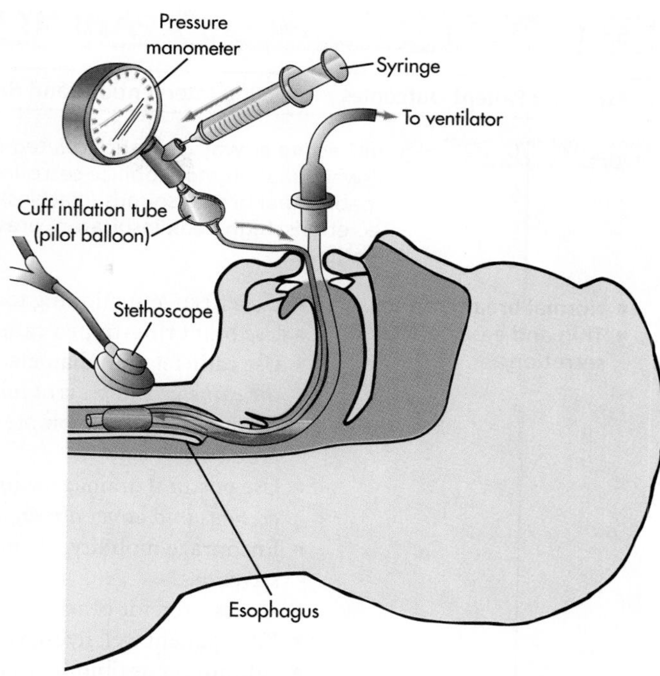

Fig. 63-13 Technique to inflate cuff and check cuff pressure. The cuff is inflated until no leak is heard at peak inspiratory pressure (end of ventilator inspiration). A stethoscope is then placed over the trachea or, for spontaneously breathing patients, after a deep breath or inhalation with a manual resuscitation bag. A manometer is used to verify that the pressure is within the recommended range (<20 mm Hg).

Maintaining Correct Tube Placement

The nurse must monitor and maintain tube placement. If the ET tube is not inserted to a sufficient depth, the tube can be dislodged from the trachea and terminate in the pharynx or enter the esophagus. If the tube is inserted too deeply, it can enter the right mainstem bronchus with the result that only the right lung receives ventilation. The nurse monitors tube position by confirming that the exit mark on the tube remains at the point of exit from the body. The nurse observes for symmetric rise and fall of both sides of the chest and auscultates to confirm bilateral breath sounds. If the ET tube is not positioned properly, this is an emergency. The nurse stays with the patient, maintains the airway, supports ventilation, and secures the appropriate assistance to immediately reposition the tube. It may be necessary to ventilate the patient with a manual resuscitation bag (MRB). If a malpositioned tube is not repositioned, no oxygen will be delivered to the lungs or the entire tidal volume will be delivered to one lung, placing the patient at risk for pneumothorax.

Maintaining Proper Cuff Inflation

The cuff is an inflatable, pliable sleeve encircling the outer wall of the ET tube. The inflated cuff stabilizes and seals the ET tube within the trachea. It prevents escape of ventilating gases. However, the cuff can cause pressure damage to the trachea wall. To avoid damage, the cuff is inflated a minimal amount and pressure in the cuff is measured and monitored. Normal capillary perfusion is estimated at 30 mm Hg. To ensure adequate tracheal perfusion, cuff pressure is kept well below this level, not to exceed 20 mm Hg (Fig. 63-13).

63-1 NURSING CARE PLAN PATIENT WITH AN ARTIFICIAL AIRWAY*

Expected Patient Outcomes	Nursing Interventions and *Rationales*
NURSING DIAGNOSIS	**Ineffective airway clearance** *related to* presence of artificial airway, accumulation of secretions in airways, inability to mobilize secretions and drying of mucous membranes *as manifested by* presence of abnormal breath sounds (crackles), frequent or absent cough, presence of thick or copious secretions, high peak inspiratory pressures on ventilator or frequent high-pressure alarm sounds on ventilator.
■ Normal breath sounds. ■ Thin and easily removed secretions.	■ Use effective suctioning technique (see Table 63-11) *to prevent tissue damage.* ■ Use blunt ring-tipped catheters *to diminish trauma to trachea and bronchi.* ■ Use catheter with diameter <½ tube diameter *to allow space for air to move in or out around the catheter and prevent lung collapse.* ■ Limit negative suction pressure (−80 to −120 mm Hg) *to prevent excess buildup of negative pressure.* ■ Use postural drainage, vibration, and percussion maneuvers when indicated *to help move secretions into larger airways.* ■ Encourage mobility; change patient's position at least q2hr as tolerated *to prevent pooling of secretions.* ■ Assess need for other measures *to facilitate liquefication and mobilization of secretions.* ■ Keep patient well hydrated; provide warm (98.6° F [37° C]) humidified gases for ventilation. ■ Administer antibiotics as prescribed *to treat infection.* ■ Administer aerosolized bronchodilators (if indicated) *to treat bronchospasm and reduce bronchial narrowing.* ■ Auscultate breath sounds q2-4hr *to monitor effectiveness of interventions.*
NURSING DIAGNOSIS	**Risk for infection** *related to* exposure to pathogens and loss of normal protective barrier to infection.
■ No evidence of infection. ■ Negative sputum cultures.	■ Observe for change in color, quantity, odor, and viscosity of sputum; difficulty in suctioning secretions; increase in cough; fever; chills; diaphoresis; abnormal breath sounds (e.g., crackles, wheezing); tachycardia; deterioration of ABGs; flushing of skin; elevated WBC count; evidence of infiltrate or atelectasis on chest x-ray; positive sputum cultures *to determine if infection is present or developing.* ■ Obtain sputum culture and order sensitivity test if secretions become purulent or tenacious, change color, or become odorous *to diagnose infectious agent.* ■ Keep head of bed elevated (especially if receiving enteral nutrition) *to prevent aspiration.* ■ Keep ventilator tubing cleared of condensed water *to eliminate source of infection.* ■ Use sterile technique with suctioning (see Table 63-11) *to reduce the risk of infection.* ■ Suction oropharynx *to remove pooled secretions.*
NURSING DIAGNOSIS	**Risk for injury** *related to* suctioning, potential for aspiration of gastric secretions, right mainstem intubation, esophageal intubation, accidental extubation, mechanical obstruction or kinking of ET tube, and irritation from artificial airway.
■ Maintenance of tube alignment. ■ No accidental extubation. ■ No aspiration. ■ No gastric contents in trachea. ■ No tracheal trauma.	■ Assess for progressive hypoxemia, tachycardia, tachypnea, increase in BP, cyanosis, absent or unilateral breath sounds, dyspnea *to identify signs of ineffective ventilation.* ■ Monitor for inability to ventilate patient with ventilation bag, inability to introduce suction catheter into ET tube, misplacement of ET tube on chest x-ray, high peak airway pressures and frequent high airway pressure alarms, aspiration of gastric contents, frequent suctioning *as indicators of ineffective respirations.* ■ Use bite block or oral airway *to keep patient from biting tube and obstructing tube opening.* ■ Move patient with care if connected to ventilator *to avoid traction on ET tube from ventilator tubing.*

Continued

63-1 NURSING CARE PLAN PATIENT WITH AN ARTIFICIAL AIRWAY*—continued

Expected Patient Outcomes	Nursing Interventions and *Rationales*
NURSING DIAGNOSIS **Risk for injury** —*continued*	
	▪ Mark tube with india ink or indelible marker at teeth, gums, or nose insertion point *as indicator of proper positioning.* ▪ Auscultate breath sounds immediately after intubation, q4hr, and as needed *to ensure correct placement and effective ventilation.* ▪ Ensure that chest x-ray is done immediately after intubation and whenever serious question of tube position arises *to validate correct placement.* ▪ Restrain patient with wrist restraints *to prevent inadvertent extubation.*
NURSING DIAGNOSIS **Risk for aspiration** *related to* presence of artificial airway.	
▪ No occurrence of aspiration.	▪ Elevate head of bed and keep cuff inflated during tube feedings or while patient is eating *to prevent aspiration.* ▪ Use small-bore feeding tubes for enteral nutrition *to minimize pressure on esophagus.* ▪ Add food coloring to feedings *to make identification of aspiration easier.* ▪ If patient is eating, encourage anteflexion of head *to open esophagus wider.* ▪ Position patient in side-lying position (never flat on back) *if danger of aspiration is high.*
NURSING DIAGNOSIS **Altered oral mucous membrane** *related to* tissue trauma caused by presence of artificial airway, dry mouth, increased oral secretions, or frequent mechanical stimulation with suction catheter *as manifested by* presence of red, shiny, edematous mucosa of mouth; stomatitis; coated or encrusted oral ulcers.	
▪ Pink, moist, intact mucous membranes. ▪ Absence of lesions, crusts, hard debris.	▪ With bite block or oral airway removed, gently brush mouth and teeth with toothbrush, toothette, or swab with normal saline every 2 hours while awake *to provide comfort and to maintain integrity of oral mucosa.* ▪ Apply lubricant to lips *to protect lips from drying.* ▪ Maintain ventilator thermostat at 98.6° F (37° C) *to ensure that adequate humidity and warmth are being applied by mechanical ventilator or O_2 source.* ▪ Check cascade water level on ventilator *to ensure that respiratory gases are continually humidified.*
NURSING DIAGNOSIS **Risk for ineffective breathing pattern** *related to* possible upper airway damage secondary to cuffed ET tube.	
▪ Maintenance of normal integrity of upper airway structures. ▪ Able to phonate and swallow adequately within 1 week after extubation.	▪ Monitor for tachypnea, tachycardia, decreased breath sounds, inspiratory stridor, use of accessory muscles, inability to phonate, hoarseness, sore throat, cough, swallowing difficulties after extubation *to identify signs of ineffective breathing pattern.* ▪ Use smallest-diameter ET tube that will support effective ventilation *to minimize tracheal trauma.* ▪ Use only low-pressure cuffs for intubation *to minimize tracheal and laryngeal damage.* ▪ Use minimal leak or minimal occluding volume (MOV) technique and cuff pressures of $<$20 mm Hg (or 27 cm H_2O) *to prevent tracheal dilation, which may lead to esophageal compression, causing aspiration and difficulty in swallowing.* ▪ Stabilize tube, tubing, and patient's head when turning *to prevent tracheal tissue trauma.* ▪ Deflate cuff when mechanical ventilator not required for ventilation *to relieve pressure on the trachea.* ▪ Immediately after extubation, monitor patient closely *for signs of respiratory distress secondary to laryngeal edema and other signs of upper airway damage.*

Continued

63-1 NURSING CARE PLAN PATIENT WITH AN ARTIFICIAL AIRWAY*—continued

Expected Patient Outcomes	Nursing Interventions and *Rationales*
NURSING DIAGNOSIS **Impaired verbal communication** *related to* inability to speak secondary to intubation *as manifested by* inability to speak.	
■ Effective method of communicating basic needs.	■ Provide patient with paper and pencil, magic slate, alphabet board, symptom board, or computer *to have an alternative means of communication.* ■ Learn to read patient's body language, facial expression, and signals *to ease patient's efforts to communicate.* ■ Attempt to anticipate patient's needs *to decrease frustration.* ■ Provide easily accessible call light or bell *to enable patient to call for assistance.* ■ Explain temporary nature of problem and that patient will have no vocalization with ET tube in place and will be hoarse after intubation *to inform patient and relieve anxiety.* ■ Acknowledge that inability to speak can be frustrating *to empathize with patient.* ■ Instruct family in effective strategies for communication with patient.
NURSING DIAGNOSIS **Altered nutrition: less than body requirements** *related to* possible inability to take nourishment orally, increased caloric demands secondary to clinical condition, and need for mechanical ventilation *as manifested by* loss of more than 10% of body weight (see NCP 62-1 for nursing interventions related to this diagnosis).	

*Nursing care plan for the patient with a tracheostomy is presented in NCP 25-5.

Most cuffs are inflated by injecting air into the fine-bore tubing leading to the cuff. If an air leak is heard, the nurse adds air to the cuff following the minimal occluding volume technique, outlined in the next paragraph. The nurse measures and records cuff pressure after intubation and once every 8 hours to confirm that the cuff is properly inflated.

The steps in cuff inflation are as follows: (1) inflate the cuff to minimal occluding volume (MOV) by adding air until no leak is heard at peak inspiratory pressure (end of ventilator inspiration) when a stethoscope is placed over the trachea; (2) for the spontaneously breathing patient, inflate until no sound is heard after a deep breath or after inhalation with an MRB; (3) use a manometer to verify that cuff pressure is less than 20 mm Hg; and (4) record cuff pressure value in the chart. See Table 63-10 for nursing management of endotracheal tubes and monitoring of cuff pressure.

■ Maintaining and Monitoring Ventilation and Oxygenation

The patient with an ET tube is vigilantly monitored for adequate oxygenation status by monitoring ABGs, clinical condition, and oximetry of arterial or mixed venous blood. Periodic ABGs are analyzed to give objective information regarding oxygenation. In addition, the nurse monitors for clinical signs of hypoxemia, such as dusky skin coloring, confusion, irritability, and cardiac arrhythmias. Continuous pulse oximeter (SpO_2) detects hypoxemia and is especially helpful in the patient with low hemoglobin who is unlikely to become dusky or with a dark complexion, and at night when room lighting is low. SpO_2 greater than 95% is generally desired. Lower values are expected in patients with obstructive pulmonary disease. PA catheters with a device to monitor oxygen saturation of the mixed venous blood hemoglobin in the pulmonary artery (SvO_2) can give an indirect indication about the patient's oxygenation status. A drop in SvO_2 may indicate a drop in arterial oxygenation, CO, or oxygen demand. Mixed venous values are observed for a substantial drop in value.

Indicators of ventilation include arterial PCO_2, end-tidal PCO_2 (capnography), and clinical assessment data. Arterial PCO_2 is the best indicator of alveolar hypoventilation (elevated PCO_2, respiratory acidosis) or hyperventilation (low PCO_2, respiratory alkalosis). The PCO_2 at the end of expiration in the normal patient is equivalent to the arterial PCO_2 and can indicate ventilation status. However, in patients with unusually large dead space, unusually prolonged expiration, or serious mismatch between ventilation and perfusion, capnography is inaccurate. The patient who is hyperventilating will be breathing rapidly and deeply and may experience circumoral and peripheral numbness and tingling. The patient who is hypoventilating will be breathing shallowly or slowly and may appear dusky.

■ Maintaining Tube Patency by Suctioning

Suctioning an ET or tracheostomy tube is performed to remove secretions from the central airways. The procedure is performed as needed and not routinely. Dyspnea, increased ventilator peak-inspiratory pressures, activation of the ventilator pressure alarm, and noisy or gurgling respirations suggest the presence of secretions. Auscultation of coarse rhonchi over the central airways confirms the presence of secretions. Peripheral crackles are not an indication for suctioning. Suctioning has been suggested as a means of inducing a cough, but this is not recommended.[22]

When the presence of secretions is confirmed, the nurse encourages the patient to move the secretions by coughing. The patient may be able to expel the secretions or advance them into the ET tube for removal. If the secretions cannot be moved or expelled by the patient, suctioning is indicated. Coughing will be induced if the suction catheter touches the carina. Two recommended procedures for suctioning the patient with an artificial airway are described in Table 63-11.

Table 63-10 Characteristics and Nursing Management of Endotracheal Tubes

Characteristics	Nursing Management
When properly inflated, low-pressure, high-volume cuff distributes cuff pressure over large area, minimizing pressure on tracheal wall.	▪ Inflate the cuff to MOV by slowly injecting air into the cuff until no leak is heard at peak inspiratory pressure (end of ventilator inspiration), when a stethoscope is placed over the trachea (Fig. 63-13). If the patient is breathing spontaneously, inflate cuff until no sound is heard after deep breath or during inhalation with MRB. Verify pressure is within accepted range with a manometer. Record value in chart. ▪ Monitor and record cuff pressure q8hr using above technique. Cuff pressure should be ≤20 mm Hg or ≤25 cm H_2O to allow adequate tracheal capillary perfusion. If needed, remove or add air to the pilot tubing using a syringe and stopcock. Afterward, verify cuff pressure is within accepted range with manometer. ▪ Report inability to keep the cuff inflated or need to use progressively larger volumes of air to keep cuff inflated. Potential causes include tracheal dilation at the cuff site or a crack or slow leak in the housing of the one-way inflation valve. If the leak is caused by tracheal dilation, the physician may intubate the patient with a larger tube. Cracks in the inflation valve may be temporarily managed by clamping the small-bore tubing with a hemostat. The tube should be changed within 24 hr. ▪ Assess for signs of respiratory distress when a fenestrated cannula is first used. If this occurs, the cap should be removed, the inner cannula replaced, and the cuff reinflated. ▪ Monitor cuff pressure q8hr as noted above.

Table 63-11 Suctioning Procedures for a Patient on a Mechanical Ventilator

General Measures

1. Wash hands.
2. Apply eye protection (shield or goggles) and clean (nonsterile) glove to nonsterile hand.
3. Explain procedure, purpose, and sensations to patient.
4. Prepare all equipment:
   Check negative suction pressure (usual range between –80 and –120 mm Hg).
   Pour sterile normal saline solution into sterile container.
   Turn on O_2 flow to bag ventilator to 15 L.
   Place manual resuscitation bag (MRB) on bed.
   Open suction catheter and glove packages. Suction catheter should be no wider than half the diameter of artificial airway.

One-Person Method

1. Pause ventilator alarms.
2. Disconnect patient from ventilator.
3. Preoxygenate with 100% O_2* and hyperventilate patient with MRB or ventilator breaths 3-6 times (done before and after suctioning).
4. Connect patient to ventilator.
5. Put on sterile glove and pick up catheter with sterile hand.
6. Connect catheter to suction tubing, using sterile hand for catheter and nonsterile hand for suction tubing.
7. Disconnect patient from ventilator.
8. Using nonsterile hand, stabilize artificial airway and hold catheter suction regulator.
9. Insert catheter gently, swiftly, and without suction with sterile hand.
10. When resistance is met, pull back catheter 1-2 cm without suction.
11. Begin depressing suction vacuum regulator in an on-off (intermittent) fashion with nonsterile hand while rotating catheter in sterile hand between thumb and forefinger.
12. Swiftly remove catheter. Each suctioning pass should not exceed 15 sec.
13. Rinse catheter in sterile saline between suctioning passes as necessary.
14. With nonsterile hand, reconnect patient to ventilator.
15. Depress manual breath or sigh button (if activated) on ventilator to hyperventilate or ventilate patient.†
16. Let patient equilibrate for 30 sec to 1 min or as needed.
17. Rinse catheter with sterile normal saline solution.
18. Repeat procedure as needed.
19. Place patient back on ventilator.
20. Suction oropharynx.
21. Discard catheter.
22. Hyperventilate and oxygenate via MRB or ventilator for three to six breaths.
23. Assess patient's tolerance to suctioning (continuous observation of the patient during entire suctioning procedure is necessary).
24. Confirm that ventilator alarms are reactivated.

Two-Person Method

1. First person hyperventilates and preoxygenates before, between, and after suctions; stabilizes airway.
2. Second person suctions as in one-person method.

*Use O_2 concentration of 60% or less for patients with chronic hypercapnia who are breathing spontaneously.
†As nurse becomes more adept at suctioning, bag ventilation may be done with nonsterile hand between suctioning passes. Ideally, it is better for two persons to be present during suctioning so one person can bag ventilate the patient while the other person does the suctioning. (One nurse with one hand on the bag ventilator can generate up to 800 ml and with two hands up to 1000 ml.)

Complications associated with suctioning include hypoxemia, arrhythmias, mucosal damage, pneumothorax, contamination and infection, retained secretions, discomfort, and anxiety. Hypoxemia occurs when oxygen-enriched gas is sucked from the lungs along with secretions. Other causes of hypoxemia include irritation-induced bronchospasm and microatelectasis resulting from aspiration of intrapulmonary air. Arterial oxygen tension may be reduced by 10 to 39 mm Hg with ET suctioning.[23]

Hypoxemia is prevented by preoxygenation, postoxygenation, hyperinflation, and limiting each suction pass to 10 to 15 seconds. If pulse oximetry is used, SpO_2 can be assessed throughout the suctioning procedure. Saturations greater than 95% are desired. If SvO_2 monitoring is available, it provides an indirect indication about the patient's oxygenation status. During suctioning, the patient is observed for tachycardia, arrhythmias, hypertension, diaphoresis, and pallor or graying of mucous membranes. If these occur, the patient should be ventilated with an MRB or placed back on the ventilator until equilibration occurs before another suction pass is attempted. In spontaneously breathing patients with chronic hypercapnia (e.g., patients with chronic obstructive pulmonary disease [COPD]) an MRB with 35% to 60% oxygen is used. The patient is assessed to confirm spontaneous ventilation after the suctioning procedure. There is some evidence that patients are more stable hemodynamically when ventilator-delivered preoxygenation is used.[23]

Causes of cardiac arrhythmias during suctioning include hypoxemia resulting in myocardial hypoxia, vagal stimulation caused by tracheal irritation, and sympathetic nervous system stimulation caused by anxiety, discomfort, or pain. Arrhythmias include tachycardia; bradycardia; premature atrial, junctional, or ventricular beats; and asystole. Suctioning should be halted if serious arrhythmias develop. The patient should be slowly ventilated via MRB with 100% oxygen until the arrhythmia subsides. Excessive suctioning should be avoided in patients with hypoxemia or bradycardia.

Tracheal mucosal damage may occur because of excessive suction pressures, overly vigorous catheter insertion, and the characteristics of the suction catheter itself. The presence of blood streaks or tissue shreds in aspirated mucus indicates that mucosal damage has occurred. Mucosal damage increases the risk of infection. Trauma to the mucosa can be prevented by the following precautions:

1. Use blunt or ring-tipped catheters with side holes.
2. Lubricate the catheter tip with sterile saline solution.
3. Stabilize the ET tube throughout the procedure.
4. Insert the catheter gently and quickly without suction.
5. Limit negative suction to −80 to −120 mm Hg.
6. Withdraw catheter 1 to 2 cm before applying suction (to prevent adhering to mucosa).
7. Apply intermittent suction as the catheter is removed.
8. Gently rotate the catheter during removal.

Although rare, pneumothorax can occur when a large catheter is inserted into a small-diameter artificial airway. If there is inadequate space for air to move in or out around the catheter, the lung may collapse or microatelectasis may occur when vacuum is applied. To prevent this, the suction catheter should not occupy more than half the internal diameter of the tube being suctioned. Suction should be maintained at −80 to −120 mm Hg. Intermittent suction should be used when removing the catheter.

Secretions may be thick and difficult to suction because of inadequate hydration, inadequate humidification, infection, or inaccessibility of the left mainstem bronchus or lower airways. Chest physical therapy and having the patient turn and cough before suctioning may help move secretions into larger airways. If the patient is inadequately hydrated, oral or intravenous fluids should be administered. If the airway is inadequately humidified, the inspired gases should be prewarmed to body temperature and hydrated with sterile water. If infection causes thick mucus, the patient should be placed on appropriate antibiotics.

The patient may experience anxiety during suctioning because of the inability to breathe, choking, or not knowing what to expect. An explanation should precede each suctioning. The patient should be told that breathing will be impossible for a short period but that the patient will soon be connected to oxygen and receive ventilation. The patient should be told that suctioning often stimulates coughing. If the patient has severe coughing during suctioning, ventilation should be done with slow, small-volume breaths using the MRB. Large volumes of air are avoided because they may overdistend the lungs and reflexly stimulate further coughing episodes. The patient with an incision or who has sustained trauma may experience pain during suctioning when coughing is induced. This patient should be premedicated with narcotics and incisions splinted before suctioning.

Closed tracheal suctioning (CTS), in which a suction catheter is enclosed in a plastic sleeve connected directly to the patient's artificial airway and ventilator, is used in many ICUs (Fig. 63-14). With CTS, suctioning can be accomplished without disconnecting the ventilator or opening the system. The nurse follows the usual suctioning procedures by preoxygenating the patient, then activating the suction during inspiration. CTS is designed to prevent loss of positive end-expiratory pressure (PEEP) and minimize hypoxemia during suctioning. There is some cost saving related to decreased need for suction sets and less opportunity for external contamination using this system. Staff members are protected from the patient's secretions, and suctioning can be performed more quickly.

Mouth Care and Endotracheal Tube Repositioning

Meticulous care is required to prevent skin breakdown or pressure sores on the lips and tongue as a result of adhesive tape or pressure from the tube, bite block, or tube holder. For the orally intubated patient, the outer layer of adhesive tape is removed every shift and the tube is moved to the other side of the mouth. The tube must be retaped to the cheeks and not to the jaw. If the jaw moves, the ET tube will also move, causing tracheal irritation and possibly damage. If a tube holder is used, the straps can be loosened, the area under the straps massaged, and the straps reapplied. Mouth care and shaving can be done at this time. Because ET tube position may change during mouth care, whenever the tube is untaped, during repositioning, or when the straps are adjusted, two nurses are needed for these procedures. The presence of bilateral breath sounds should always be confirmed after completion of any of these procedures.

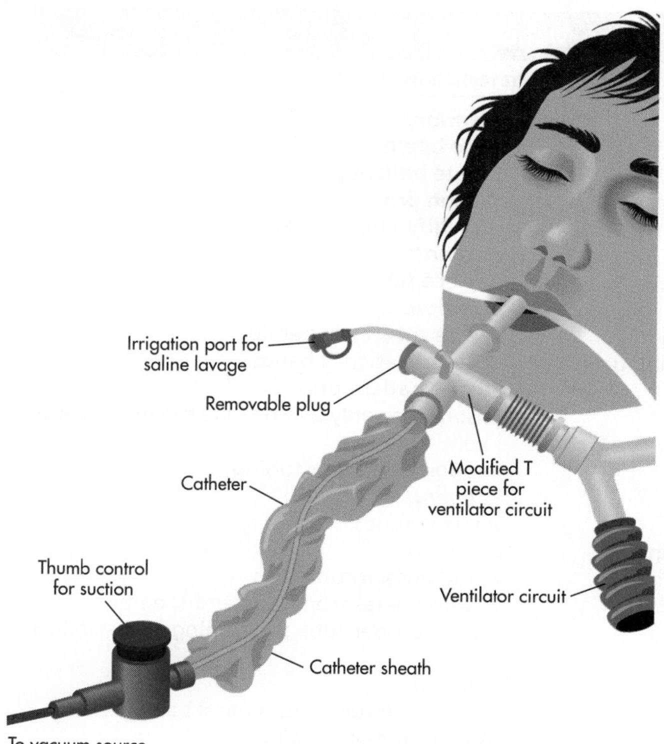

Fig. 63-14 Closed tracheal suction system.

Because the patient's mouth is always open when an oral ET tube is in place, lips and mouth should be moistened with saline or water swabs to prevent mucosal drying. Mouth care, including cleaning of teeth and gums, should be performed every 4 to 8 hours as a comfort measure and to prevent injury to the gums and plaque accumulation. Mouthwash containing alcohol should not be used because these preparations dry the mucosa, predisposing it to cracking and creating sites for infection.

■ Fostering Comfort and Communication

The discomfort associated with ET intubation and mechanical ventilation may make it necessary to sedate the patient or administer an analgesic until the ET tube is no longer required.

Communicating with the intubated patient can be a frustrating experience. To communicate more effectively, the nurse should have available a variety of methods. A magic slate or pad and pencil should be provided if the patient can use her or his hands. Additional options for communication include an alphabet board, flash cards, photo boards, lip reading, and hand signals.

Extubation

Extubation (tube removal) should be performed as soon as possible. The health care team should assess the patient's status each day to determine whether (1) the underlying condition has improved so that intubation is no longer required, (2) spontaneous respiration can be maintained without the ventilator, and (3) the patient can cough, clear secretions, and protect the airway.

Extubation should be attempted only by trained persons. Once the tube is removed, the patient is encouraged to cough to clear secretions. The mouth is suctioned and humidified oxygen is administered through a face mask. The patient is observed at frequent intervals for signs of laryngospasm (e.g., stridor, dyspnea) and respiratory distress (e.g., restlessness, irritability, tachycardia, tachypnea). A pulse oximeter should be used to monitor oxygen saturation. If the patient cannot tolerate extubation, immediate reintubation may be necessary.

Complications of Endotracheal Intubation

The major complications of ET intubation result from injury to the hypopharynx, larynx, and trachea and are related to the pressure exerted on upper airway structures by the tube and cuff. Improper tube placement, aspiration, oral and nasal pressure sores, and accidental extubation are also potential problems. Table 63-12 summarizes complications seen in patients with ET tubes.

Improper Tube Placement and Accidental Extubation. Improper tube placement is a potential hazard of ET intubation. If the tube is not inserted deeply enough, the cuff can damage the larynx or the tube can slip out of the trachea. If the tube is inserted too deeply, it might extend into the right mainstem bronchus, resulting in the ventilation of the right lung only. It is also possible with too deep a tube placement that the distal orifice could rest against the carina or tracheal wall, causing airway obstruction.

A chest x-ray should be taken immediately after intubation and whenever there is a question of improper ET tube placement. The tube should be repositioned as needed by a health care provider who is able to reintubate if necessary. The ET tube tip should be seen on chest x-ray at least 2 cm above the carina. Chest auscultation should be done immediately after intubation and before securing the tube to determine the presence of bilateral equal breath sounds. Auscultation of breath sounds is performed regularly at least every 4 hours. The tube must be well secured to prevent slipping or accidental extubation. Accidental extubation can be a catastrophic event. The nurse is responsible for preventing its occurrence through the use of soft wrist restraints and sedation. It is wise to mark the tube with india ink at the teeth or nose level or note the centimeter mark closest to the teeth or nose level and chart it on the care plan or flowchart. This mark provides a quick reference point to check proper tube placement.

The ET tube should not extend more than 1.5 to 2 in (3.8 to 5 cm) out of the patient's nose or mouth because the added length can cause additional pressure to be exerted on structures. Once ET tube position has been verified by chest x-ray, the tube can be cut and the adapter reapplied.

Aspiration. Aspiration is a potential hazard for the patient with an ET tube. The ET tube passes through the epiglottis, splinting it open. Thus the intubated patient cannot protect the airway from aspiration. The cuff cannot totally prevent the trickle of oral or gastric secretions into the trachea. Furthermore, secretions accumulate above the cuff. When the cuff is deflated those secretions move into the lungs. Oral intubation increases salivation yet swallowing is difficult, so the mouth must be suctioned frequently. The posterior pharynx should always be suctioned before cuff deflation. This may be performed by the patient with a Yankauer (tonsil-tip) suction catheter. Other factors causing aspiration

Table **63-12** **Complications of Endotracheal Tubes and Nursing Management**

Complications	Causes	Prevention/Treatment
■ Tube obstruction	Patient biting tube Tube kinking during repositioning Cuff herniation Dried secretions, blood, or lubricant Tissue from tumor Trauma Foreign body	*Prevention:* Place bite block. Sedate patient prn. Suction prn. Humidify inspired gases. *Treatment:* Replace tube.
■ Tube displacement	Movement of patient's head Movement of tube by patient's tongue Traction on tube from ventilator tubing Self-extubation	*Prevention:* Secure tube to upper lip. Restrain patient's hands. Sedate patient prn. Ensure that only 2 in of tube extend beyond lip. Support ventilator tubing. *Treatment:* Replace tube.
■ Sinusitis and nasal injury	Obstruction of paranasal sinus drainage Pressure necrosis of nares	*Prevention:* Avoid nasal intubations. Cushion nares from tube and tape/ties. Ensure proper tube positioning and stabilization. *Treatment:* Remove all tubes from nasal passages. Administer antibiotics.
■ Tracheoesophageal fistula	Pressure necrosis of posterior tracheal wall resulting from overinflated cuff and rigid nasogastric tube	*Prevention:* Stabilize airway. Inflate cuff with minimal amount of air necessary. Monitor cuff pressures q8hr. Use small-bore feeding tube for enteral feeding. *Treatment:* Position cuff of tube distal to fistula. Place gastrostomy tube for enteral feedings. Place esophageal tube for secretion clearance proximal to fistula.
■ Mucosal lesions	Pressure at tube and mucosal interface	*Prevention:* Inflate cuff with minimal amount of air necessary. Monitor cuff pressures q8hr. Use appropriate size tube. *Treatment:* May resolve spontaneously. Perform surgical intervention.
■ Laryngeal or tracheal stenosis	Injury to area from end of tube or cuff, resulting in scar tissue formation and narrowing of airway	*Prevention:* Inflate cuff with minimal amount of air necessary. Monitor cuff pressures q8hr. Suction area above cuff frequently. *Treatment:* Perform tracheostomy. Place laryngeal stent. Perform surgical repair.
■ Cricoid abscess	Mucosal injury with bacterial invasion	*Prevention:* Inflate cuff with minimal amount of air necessary. Monitor cuff pressures q8hr. Suction area above cuff frequently. *Treatment:* Perform incision and drainage of area. Administer antibiotics.

From Thelan LA and others, editors: *Critical care nursing: diagnosis and management,* ed 3, St Louis, 1998, Mosby.

Table 63-13 Indicators for Mechanical Ventilation and Weaning

	Measurement and Significance	Normal Values*	Mechanical Ventilation Indicated*	Weaning Feasible*
Tests of Ventilatory Reserve or Mechanical Ability				
VT	Amount of air exchanged during normal breathing at rest	7-9 ml/kg	<5 ml/kg	>5 ml/kg
Respiratory rate per minute		12-20	<10 or >35	12-20
Forced vital capacity (FVC)	Maximal inspiration and then measurement of air during maximal forced expiration; determination of whether patient can sigh deeply enough to avoid atelectasis; best indicator of ventilatory reserve; patient's cooperation necessary	65-75 ml/kg	<10-15 ml/kg	>10-15 ml/kg
Peak inspiratory pressure, negative inspiratory force	Complete occlusion of anaeroid manometer attached to airway or mouth for 10-20 sec while negative inspiratory efforts of patient noted; useful index of neuromuscular strength; less patient cooperation necessary	−75 to −100 cm H_2O	>−25 cm H_2O	<−20 cm H_2O
Forced expiratory volume in 1 sec (FEV_1)	Volume of air measured in first second of exhalation of forced vital capacity maneuver; use in patients with COPD to determine degree of obstruction	50-60 ml/kg	<10 ml/kg	>16 ml/kg
Resting minute ventilation	Multiplication of tidal volume by respiratory rate for 1 min, general indication of patient's total ventilation	5-10 L/min	>10 L/min	<10 L/min
VD/VT	Estimation from VT; accurate calculation requiring $PaCO_2$ and partial pressure of CO_2 in mixed expired gas; measurement of portion of each breath that does not participate in gas exchange; indication of lungs' efficiency in removing CO_2	0.25-0.40	>0.6	<0.5-0.6
$PaCO_2$	Indication of lungs' efficiency in removing CO_2 and reflection of body's acid-base status	35-45 mm Hg	>55 mm Hg (acute)	<45 mm Hg
Tests of Oxygenation Capability				
PaO_2/FIO_2	Provision of evidence of lung's ability to oxygenate arterial blood; couples PO_2 with amount of oxygen given	350-400	<200	>300

*These parameters are only guidelines and must be related to the individual patient's status (e.g., patients with severe COPD may have a normal $PaCO_2$ of 60 mm Hg and values lower than normal for FEV_1, VC, MV, and maximal voluntary ventilation).
COPD, chronic obstructive pulmonary disease.

include cuff leak, tracheal distention, and tracheoesophageal fistula. The patient with an ET tube is at risk for aspiration of gastric contents. Even when the cuff is inflated, the nurse must take precautions to avoid emesis, which can lead to aspiration. The head of the bed should be elevated when the patient is receiving tube feedings.

MECHANICAL VENTILATION

Mechanical ventilation is the process by which room air or oxygen-enriched air is moved into and out of the lungs mechanically. Mechanical ventilation is not curative. It is a means of supporting patients until they recover the ability to breathe independently. Indications for mechanical ventilation are listed in Table 63-13.

Patients with chronic pulmonary disease who are managed by pulmonary health care specialists on a continuous, long-term basis and their families should be given the opportunity to decide the issue of mechanical ventilation before terminal respiratory disease develops. Other patients with chronic disease should also be encouraged to discuss the subject. It is much easier for the physician, patient, and family to decide not to institute ventilatory support initially than it is to remove the support system once it has been initiated. The decision to use mechanical ventilation must be made carefully, respecting the informed wishes of the patient and family.

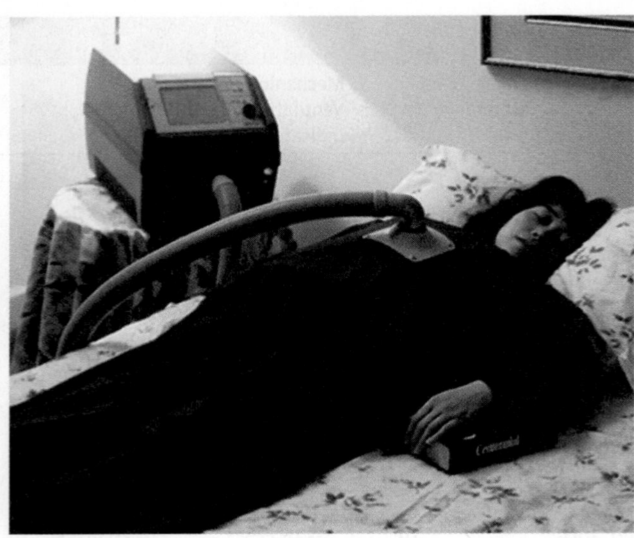

Fig. 63-15 Negative pressure ventilator.

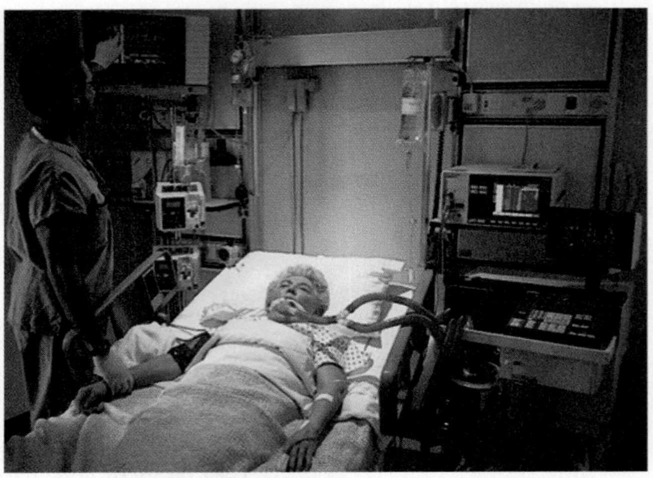

Fig. 63-16 Patient receiving mechanical ventilation.

Types of Mechanical Ventilators

There are two major types of mechanical ventilators: negative pressure and positive pressure ventilators.

Negative Pressure Ventilators. Negative pressure ventilators are composed of chambers that encase the chest or body and surround it with intermittent subatmospheric or negative pressure. Intermittent negative pressure around the chest wall causes the chest to be pulled outward. This reduces intrathoracic pressure. Air rushes in via the upper airway, which is outside the sealed chamber. Expiration is passive; the machine cycles off, allowing chest retraction. This type of ventilation is similar to normal ventilation in that inspiration is produced by decreased intrathoracic pressures and expiration is passive. An artificial airway is not required.

Negative pressure ventilators include the Poncho (Puritan Bennett, Emerson) and Pulmowrap (Lifecare). These ventilators are made of a flexible nylon cover that fits over the head, ties at the neck with drawstrings, and fastens to the arms or wrists and upper legs with elastic (Fig. 63-15).

New developments in negative pressure ventilation enable both control and assist-control ventilation modes. Lightweight, portable negative pressure ventilators are used in the home for patients with neuromuscular diseases, central nervous system (CNS) disorders, diseases and injuries of the spinal cord, and severe COPD. Negative pressure ventilators are not used extensively for acutely ill patients. However, because cardiac output is enhanced and not diminished during inspiration, negative pressure ventilation has been used successfully in those with heart disease.[26]

Positive Pressure Ventilators. Positive pressure ventilation is the primary method used with acutely ill patients. During inspiration the ventilator pushes air into the lungs under positive pressure. Unlike spontaneous ventilation, intrathoracic pressure is raised during lung inflation rather than lowered. Expiration occurs passively as in normal expiration. The three types of positive pressure ventilators are (1) volume-cycled or volume-limited ventilators, (2) time-cycled or time-limited ventilators, and (3) pressure-cycled or pressure-limited ventilators. Each type is classified by the physical parameter that ends the inspiratory cycle. Mechanical ventilators are illustrated in Figs. 63-16 and 17.

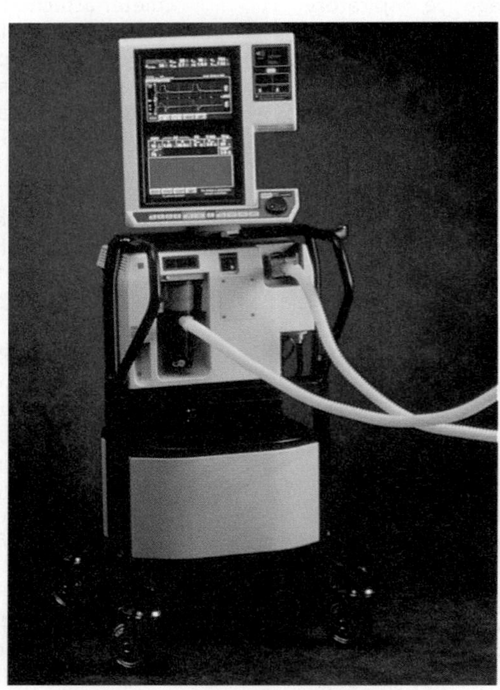

Fig. 63-17 Typical positive pressure ventilator.

Volume-cycled or volume-limited ventilators. Volume-cycled ventilators are the most common type used for intubated adults. Inspiration is terminated when a preset volume of gas is delivered through the ventilator circuit. Volume-cycled ventilators have built-in pressure-limiting valves to prevent excess pressure in the lungs. Once the pressure limit is reached, the remainder of the tidal volume is vented to the outside air. With volume-cycled ventilators, volume delivery remains constant despite lung resistance and compliance changes (unlike pressure-cycled ventilators). Inspired oxygen concentration remains consistent. An example is the Siemens Servo 900. Some ventilators (e.g., Monoghan 225) can be adapted to function as pressure-cycled, time-cycled, or volume-cycled ventilators.

Table **63-14** Settings of Mechanical Ventilation

Parameter	Description
Respiratory rate (f)	Number of breaths the ventilator delivers per minute; usual setting is 4-20 breaths/min
Tidal volume (V_T)	Volume of gas delivered to patient during each ventilator breath; usual volume is 5-15 ml/kg
Oxygen concentration (FIO_2)	Fraction of inspired oxygen delivered to patient; may be set between 21% and 100%; usually adjusted to maintain PaO_2 level greater than 60 mm Hg or SaO_2 level greater than 90%
I:E ratio	Duration of inspiration to duration of expiration; usual setting is 1:2 to 1:1.5 unless IRV is desired
Flow rate	Speed with which the tidal volume is delivered; usual setting is 40-100 L/min
Sensitivity/trigger	Determines the amount of effort the patient must generate to initiate a ventilator breath; it may be set for pressure triggering or flow triggering; usual setting for a pressure trigger is 0.5-1.5 cm H_2O below baseline pressure and for a flow trigger is 1-3 L/min below baseline flow
Pressure limit	Regulates the maximal pressure the ventilator can generate to deliver the tidal volume; when the pressure limit is reached, the ventilator terminates the breath and spills the undelivered volume into the atmosphere; usual setting is 10-20 cm H_2O above peak inspiratory pressure

From Thelan LA and others, editors: *Critical care nursing: diagnosis and management*, ed 3, St Louis, 1998, Mosby.
IRV, inverse ratio ventilation.

Time-cycled or time-limited ventilators. Time-cycled ventilators terminate inspiration and switch to expiration at a preset time. The amount of gas delivered with each breath (tidal volume) is regulated by adjusting inspiratory duration and flow rate of the pressurized gas. The tidal volume and inspiratory pressure delivered to the patient may vary from breath to breath. The Siemans 900-C is an example of a time-cycled ventilator for adults. Time-cycled ventilators have fail-safe pressure limits beyond which the ventilator ceases to push gas into the lungs, thus preventing lung overdistention and barotrauma.

Pressure-cycled or pressure-limited ventilators. Pressure-cycled ventilators terminate inspiration when a preselected airway pressure is achieved. The volume of gas delivered to the patient and duration of delivery vary according to airway resistance, pulmonary compliance, and ventilator circuit integrity. When there is obstruction (such as secretions) or when the patient breathes out of synchrony with the ventilator, the pressure limit is reached quickly and the volume of gas delivered is small. Because tidal volume is dependent on the airway resistance, tidal volume is checked frequently when the patient is receiving pressure-cycled mechanical ventilation. Pressure-cycled ventilators are common in acute care. They are indicated in patients at risk for barotrauma and are also used for home therapy, for short-term ventilation, or in a patient whose lungs are relatively free of diseases involving altered resistance and compliance.

Settings of Mechanical Ventilators

Mechanical ventilator settings regulate the rate, depth, and other characteristics of ventilation (Table 63-14). Settings are based on the patient's status (ABGs, body weight, level of consciousness, muscle strength). The ventilator is tuned as finely as possible to match the patient's ventilatory pattern. Settings are evaluated and adjusted frequently until the patient achieves optimal ventilation. Some settings serve as a fail-safe, alerting staff to problems with ventilation. It is important that the nurse ensure and document that all ventilator alarms are turned on at all times. Alarms sense potentially dangerous situations of mechanical malfunction, apnea, or patient asynchrony with the ventilator. On many ventilators the alarms can be temporarily bypassed or silenced for up to 2 minutes for suctioning or testing. After that period of time, the alarm system automatically becomes functional again.

Modes of Volume-Cycled Ventilation

The term *mode* refers to the manner in which the breath is initiated and the volume controlled, either by the mechanical ventilator or the patient. Mode is selected based on the patient's ventilatory status, including respiratory drive and ABGs. The three basic modes of mechanical ventilation are (1) controlled mechanical ventilation (CMV), (2) assist-control ventilation (ACV), and (3) synchronized intermittent mandatory ventilation (SIMV). These modes are compared in Table 63-15.

Controlled Mechanical Ventilation. With CMV, breaths are delivered regularly and independent of the patient's ventilatory efforts. Although CMV is infrequently used, it is used when the patient has no drive to breathe (e.g., the anesthetized patient) or is unable to breathe spontaneously (e.g., the paralyzed patient). With CMV the normal processes of regulation of ventilation are not operating. Thus the patient's ability to adjust ventilation to changing demands has been lost.

Assist-Control Mechanical Ventilation. With ACV, the ventilator is set so that it delivers a preset tidal volume at a preset frequency, but the patient is able to initiate a breath by attempting to inhale. The ventilator senses a decrease in intrathoracic pressure and then delivers the preset tidal volume. The patient can ventilate faster than the preset rate but not slower. This mode has the advantage of allowing the patient some control over ventilation while providing support. ACV is used in patients with a variety of conditions, including neuromuscular disorders (e.g., Guillain-Barré syndrome), pulmonary edema, and acute respiratory distress syndrome. The

Table 63-15 Modes of Mechanical Ventilation

Description	Advantages	Disadvantages	Uses
Controlled Mechanical Ventilation (CMV)			
Machine delivers preset number of breaths/min at preset volume. Patient cannot trigger breathing.	Breathing is totally controlled by ventilator.	Does not allow patient to initiate breathing or respiratory rate to change with varying patient needs. Airway pressure always positive during inspiration, compromising venous return. Provides limited use of respiratory muscles.	Apnea secondary to brain damage, respiratory muscle paralysis, drug overdose, sedation
Assist-Control Ventilation (ACV)			
Delivery of breath is triggered by inspiratory effort of patient after preselected time interval has elapsed. If patient fails to initiate breathing, ventilator cycles as in controlled ventilation.	Patient can initiate own breathing, use respiratory muscles, and alter respiratory rate according to need. Intrathoracic pressure decreases transiently before inspiratory phase, decreasing the venous return and suppression of cardiac output.	Problems of overventilation and underventilation are possible and can occur in anxious patients or in those with low lung compliance.	Wide range of situations in which patients are spontaneously breathing but have ventilatory failure or gas exchange inefficiency
Synchronized Intermittent Mandatory Ventilation (SIMV)			
Patient breathes spontaneously at own V_T and rate. Ventilator is synchronized to patient's ventilatory rate. Machine set to give certain number of breaths and is triggered by patient's inspiration.	Ventilator does not compete with patient's breathing.	Allows maintenance of even minor spontaneous excursions. Respiratory muscles remain in use. Ventilator augments patient's own efforts.	Wide range of situations in which patients need ventilatory support, method of weaning

patient with ACV mode has the potential for hypoventilation and hyperventilation. The spontaneously breathing patient can easily be overventilated, resulting in hyperventilation. If the volume or minimum rate is set low and the patient is apneic or weak, the patient will be hypoventilated. Thus these patients require vigilant assessment and monitoring of ventilatory status, including ABGs. It is important that the amount of negative pressure required to initiate a breath is appropriate to the patient's condition. If it is too difficult to initiate a breath, the work of breathing is increased. If it is too easy, the patient will be at risk for overventilation and respiratory alkalosis.

Synchronized Intermittent Mandatory Ventilation. With SIMV, the ventilator delivers a preset tidal volume at a preset frequency in synchrony with the patient's spontaneous breathing. Between ventilator-delivered breaths, the patient is able to breathe spontaneously through the ventilator circuit. Thus the patient receives the preset inspired oxygen concentration during the spontaneous breaths but self-regulates the rate and depth of those breaths. This mode of ventilation differs from ACV, in which all breaths are of the same preset volume. SIMV is the most common mode of ventilatory support. It is used during continuous ventilation and during weaning from the ventilator. Potential benefits of SIMV include avoidance of respiratory alkalosis, minimizing the patient "fighting" the ventilator, lower mean airway pressure, more uniform intrapulmonary gas distribution, and prevention of muscle atrophy.[25]

SIMV has advantages over other modes with respect to cardiovascular effects. Spontaneous inspiration decreases intrathoracic pressure, reduces mean intrathoracic pressure, and enhances venous blood return to the heart. Thus the patient with an extracellular fluid volume deficit is better able to maintain CO. Because of the lower mean intrathoracic pressure, higher levels of PEEP may be used with SIMV than with other modes of volume-controlled ventilation.

Weaning patients from ventilators can be accomplished using SIMV. Instead of abruptly removing patients from ventilators and letting them breathe totally on their own, SIMV allows a smooth transition to spontaneous ventilation by gradually decreasing the ventilator rate as patients assume an increasing percentage of the total work of breathing.

There are disadvantages with SIMV. If spontaneous breathing decreases when the rate is low, ventilation might not be adequately supported. Low-rate SIMV should be used only in patients with regular, spontaneous breathing. Weaning with SIMV demands close monitoring and may take longer because the rate of breathing is gradually reduced. Patients being weaned with SIMV may become fatigued, especially during the night.

Other Ventilatory Maneuvers

Positive End-Expiratory Pressure. PEEP is a ventilatory maneuver in which positive pressure is applied to the airway during exhalation. Normally during exhalation airway pressure drops to zero, and exhalation occurs passively. With PEEP exhalation remains passive, but pressure falls to a preset level greater than zero, often 3 to 20 cm H_2O. With PEEP lung volume during expiration and between breaths is greater than normal. Thus PEEP increases functional residual capacity (FRC). This often improves oxygenation. The mechanisms by which PEEP increases FRC and oxygenation include increased distention of already patent alveoli, prevention of alveolar collapse, and aeration of previously collapsed alveoli.[25] PEEP often allows the fraction of inspired oxygen (FIO_2) to be reduced, thus lowering the risk of oxygen toxicity.

PEEP is prescribed in increments of 2 to 5 cm H_2O. The amount of PEEP selected is determined by the amount that improves oxygenation without decreasing blood pressure and CO. This is termed *best* or *optimal PEEP.* Often 5 cm H_2O PEEP (so-called physiologic PEEP) is used prophylactically to replace the glottic mechanism, help maintain a normal FRC, and prevent alveolar collapse. Clinical studies vary regarding the benefits of physiologic PEEP. PEEP of 5 cm H_2O is also used for patients with a history of alveolar collapse during weaning. PEEP has demonstrated improvements in gas exchange, vital capacity, and inspiratory force when used during weaning.

Inspiratory pressure increases when expiratory pressure is added. The most common mode of PEEP delivery is with SIMV. The decreased mean airway pressure that occurs during spontaneous breathing is enough to prevent some of the adverse effects produced by the increased pressures.

In general, the major purpose of PEEP is to maintain adequate oxygenation while limiting risk of oxygen toxicity. PEEP is also used to prevent atelectasis. PEEP is thought to be useful in pulmonary edema, providing a counterpressure opposing fluid extravasation. PEEP is indicated in lungs with diffuse disease, severe hypoxemia unresponsive to FIO_2 greater than 0.5 (50% oxygen), and loss of compliance or stiffness. The classic indication for PEEP therapy is acute respiratory distress syndrome (ARDS) characterized by a reduced FRC and hypoxemia that is refractory to oxygen therapy. PEEP is generally contraindicated or used with extreme caution in patients with highly compliant lungs (e.g., COPD), unilateral or nonuniform disease, hypovolemia, and low CO. In these situations the adverse effects of PEEP may outweigh any benefits.

Continuous Positive Airway Pressure. Continuous positive airway pressure (CPAP) is the use of PEEP in a spontaneously breathing patient. With CPAP there is a constant flow of gas at a rate greater than the patient's spontaneous inspiratory flow rate. Thus the patient's airway pressure never falls to zero. For example, if CPAP is 5 cm H_2O, during exhalation airway pressure is 5 cm H_2O; during inspiration, 1 to 2 cm H_2O of negative pressure is generated, reducing airway pressure to 3 or 4 cm H_2O. The patient receiving SIMV with PEEP receives CPAP when breathing spontaneously. CPAP is often used in infants. It is also commonly used in the treatment of obstructive sleep apnea. CPAP can be administered by a tight-fitting mask or an ET or tracheal tube. CPAP increases work of breathing because the patient must forcibly exhale against the CPAP.

Pressure Support Ventilation. With pressure support ventilation (PSV), positive pressure is applied to the airway only during inspiration and is used in conjunction with the patient's spontaneous respirations. A preset level of positive airway pressure is selected so that the gas flow rate is greater than the patient's inspiratory flow rate. As the patient initiates a breath, the machine senses the spontaneous effort and supplies a rapid flow of gas, supporting the inspiratory effort. With PSV the patient determines inspiratory length, flow rate, and respiratory rate. Tidal volume depends on the pressure level and airway compliance. PSV is used with continuous ventilation and is especially helpful in combination with SIMV during weaning. PSV is not used as a sole ventilatory support during acute respiratory failure because of the risk of hypoventilation. Advantages to PSV include increased patient comfort, decreased work of breathing (because inspiratory efforts are augmented), decreased oxygen consumption (because inspiratory work is reduced), and increased endurance conditioning (because the patient is exercising respiratory muscles).[26]

Inverse-Ratio Ventilation. With inverse-ratio ventilation (IRV), inspiration is prolonged and expiration shortened. The I/E ratio is the ratio of duration of inspiration (I) to the duration of expiration (E). This value is normally less than 1. With IRV the I/E ratio approaches 1. With IRV a prolonged positive pressure is applied, increasing inspiratory time. IRV progressively expands collapsed alveoli. The short expiratory time has a PEEP-like effect, preventing alveolar collapse. Because IRV imposes a nonphysiologic breathing pattern, the patient requires sedation or paralysis. IRV is indicated for patients with ARDS who continue to have refractory hypoxemia despite a PEEP of 15 cm H_2O or more. Not all patients with poor oxygenation respond to IRV.

High-Frequency Ventilation. High-frequency ventilation (HFV) involves delivery of a small tidal volume (usually 1 to 5 ml/kg body weight) at rapid respiratory rates (100 to 300 breaths per minute). HFV can minimize some complications attributed to conventional mechanical ventilation because mean airway pressure is lower. Use of HFV is limited to severely ill patients. HFV is used in patients with bronchopleural fistulas because lower peak airway pressures can prevent worsening of this condition. Some patients with ARDS and acute respiratory failure may benefit from HFV, although results of clinical trials do not indicate many advantages or improvement in mortality rates over conventional forms of mechanical ventilation. HFV is more commonly used in neonatal patients.

Complications of Mechanical Ventilation

Although mechanical ventilation may be essential to maintain ventilation and oxygenation, it can cause adverse effects. It is often difficult to distinguish complications of mechanical ventilation from the underlying disease.

Cardiovascular System. Positive pressure mechanical ventilation can cause circulatory problems because of transmission of increased mean airway pressure to the thoracic cavity. With increased intrathoracic pressure, thoracic vessels are compressed. This results in decreased venous return to the heart, decreased left ventricular end-diastolic volume (preload), decreased CO, and lowered blood pressure. Mean airway pressure is further increased with PEEP.

If the lungs are noncompliant (as in ARDS), airway pressures are not as easily transmitted to the heart and blood vessels. Thus effects of mechanical ventilation on CO are reduced. Conversely, with compliant lungs (e.g., emphysema), there is increased danger of transmission of high airway pressures and CO may decrease.

Compromise of venous return by positive pressure ventilation is exaggerated by hypovolemia (e.g., hemorrhage, multiple trauma) and decreased venous tone (e.g., sepsis, spinal shock). Restoration and maintenance of the circulating blood volume is important in minimizing cardiovascular complications.

Some studies have found improved cardiac performance after the initiation of mechanical ventilation in patients with poor left ventricular function.[27] It is postulated that positive pressure ventilation decreases right-sided heart preload by its increase in intrathoracic pressure. The increased airway pressure may restrict left ventricular filling by mechanical compression. These effects may improve the failing left ventricle by optimizing ventricular end-diastolic volume.

Sodium and Water Balance. Progressive fluid retention often occurs after 48 to 72 hours of mechanical ventilation. Positive pressure ventilation, especially with PEEP, is associated with decreased urinary output and increased sodium retention. Fluid balance changes may be due to decreased CO, which in turn results in diminished renal perfusion. Renin release is stimulated, which increases aldosterone secretion and subsequent sodium and water retention. It is also possible that pressure changes within the thorax are associated with decreased release of atrial natriuretic peptide, also causing sodium retention. Mild water retention is also associated with mechanical ventilation. There is less insensible water loss via the airway, because inspired gases are saturated with water at body temperature. In addition, as with all stressed patients, release of antidiuretic hormone may be increased, causing water retention.

Pulmonary System

Barotrauma. As lung inflation pressures increase, risk of pneumothorax, pneumomediastinum, and subcutaneous emphysema increases. Patients with compliant lungs (e.g., COPD) are at greater risk because the increased airway pressure readily distends the lungs and may rupture alveoli or emphysematous blebs. Patients with stiff lungs (e.g., ARDS), who are given high inspiratory pressures and high levels of PEEP, and patients with suppurative lung abscesses resulting from necrotizing organisms (e.g., staphylococci) are also susceptible to barotrauma.

Air can escape into the pleural space from alveoli or interstitium, accumulate, and become trapped. Pleural pressure increases and collapses the lung, causing pneumothorax. (Clinical manifestations of pneumothorax are discussed in Chapter 26.) The lung receives air during inspiration but cannot expel it during expiration. Respiratory bronchioles are larger on inspiration than expiration. They may close on expiration, and air becomes trapped. With positive pressure breathing, a simple pneumothorax can become a life-threatening tension pneumothorax. With tension pneumothorax, the mediastinum and contralateral lung are compressed, compromising CO. Immediate treatment of the pneumothorax is required.

Pneumomediastinum usually begins with rupture of alveoli into the lung interstitium; progressive air movement then occurs into the mediastinum and subcutaneous neck tissue. This is commonly followed by pneumothorax. Occurrence of new, unexplained subcutaneous air is an indication for immediate chest x-ray. Pneumomediastinum and subcutaneous emphysema in the neck may be too small to be detected radiographically or clinically before the development of a pneumothorax.

Subcutaneous emphysema may occur after a tracheotomy as a result of leakage of air around the surgical site, or it may occur around the site of a chest tube for pneumothorax. In the latter case, subcutaneous emphysema is usually caused by the passage of gas from the pleural space into the chest tube wound, indicating that the space is not being adequately drained. Chest tube patency must be maintained to prevent a further increase in the pneumothorax.

Alveolar hypoventilation. Hypoventilation can be caused by inappropriate ventilator settings, leakage of air from the ventilator tubing or around the ET tube or tracheostomy cuff, lung secretions or obstruction, and low ventilation/perfusion ratio. Low tidal volume or respiratory rate decreases minute ventilation, causing hypoventilation. A leaking cuff or tubings that are not secured may cause air leakage, lowering the delivered tidal volume. Too low a SIMV rate in a patient who is unable to produce adequate spontaneous ventilation causes hypoventilation, respiratory acidosis, and additional problems related to acidosis such as cardiac arrhythmias. Excess lung secretions can cause hypoventilation. This can be alleviated by turning the patient every 1 to 2 hours, providing chest physical therapy to lung areas with increased secretions, encouraging deep breathing and coughing, and suctioning as needed. Atelectasis may develop. Increasing the tidal volume, adding small increments of PEEP, and sighing the patient lessens the likelihood of atelectasis. Frequent position change also helps.

Alveolar hyperventilation. Respiratory alkalosis can occur if the rate or tidal volume is set too high (mechanical overventilation) or if the patient receiving assisted ventilation is hyperventilating. Hyperventilation means that the $PaCO_2$ tension is less than 35 mm Hg. The patient or the ventilator is blowing off CO_2 too rapidly.

It is easy to overventilate a patient on mechanical ventilation. Particularly at risk is the patient with chronic alveolar hypoventilation and CO_2 retention (e.g., the COPD patient). This patient may have a chronic arterial CO_2 elevation and compensatory bicarbonate retention by the kidneys. When the patient is ventilated, the patient's "normal" rather than standard normal values should be the therapeutic goal. If the COPD patient is returned to a standard normal arterial CO_2 tension, the patient will develop alkalosis because of the retained bicarbonate. Such a patient could move from compensated acidosis to serious metabolic alkalosis. The presence of alkalosis makes weaning from the ventilator difficult. Alkalosis, especially if the onset is abrupt, can have additional serious consequences, including hypokalemia and hypocalcemia, predisposing the patient to arrhythmias. Neuromuscular irritability, seizures, coma, and death can occur.

To prevent alkalosis, mechanical ventilation should be initiated and should remain at a level that will not dramatically lower the arterial CO_2 level ($PaCO_2$). ABGs must be assessed 15 to 30 minutes after mechanical ventilation begins and after each ventilator change, serially thereafter, and whenever changes in the patient's clinical status occur. The $PaCO_2$ tension should be gradually lowered only to the patient's baseline (before acute illness) level. Usually patients with COPD on the ventilator do better with a short inspiratory and longer expiratory time.

If the hyperventilation is spontaneous, it is important to determine the cause and treat it. Causes might include hypoxemia, pain, fear, anxiety, or compensation for metabolic acidosis. Patients who fight the ventilator or breathe out of synchrony may be anxious or in pain. If the patient is anxious and fearful, sitting with the patient and verbally coaching the patient to breathe with the ventilator may help. If these measures fail, manually bagging the patient slowly with the MRB connected to an oxygen source may slow breathing enough to bring it in synchrony with the ventilator. The patient may require morphine, lorazepam (Ativan), or other sedatives.

Ventilator-associated pneumonia. Ventilator-associated pneumonia (VAP) is common because normal upper airway defenses have been bypassed by the ET or tracheostomy tube, increasing the patient's risk for infection. In addition, poor nutritional state, immobility, and the underlying disease process (e.g., immunosuppression, organ failure) make the patient more prone to infection.

In patients receiving prolonged mechanical ventilation, sputum cultures often grow gram-negative bacteria such as *Pseudomonas, Serratia,* and *Klebsiella.* These are abundant in the hospital environment and the patient's gastrointestinal tract. Organisms can spread in a number of ways, including contaminated respiratory equipment, inadequate hand washing, adverse environmental factors such as poor room ventilation and high traffic flow, and decreased patient ability to cough and clear secretions. Colonization of the oropharynx tract by gram-negative organisms is a predisposing factor in the development of gram-negative pneumonia.

Infection can be minimized by using strict aseptic technique while suctioning or handling the artificial airway. Frequent hand washing is imperative. The nurse should wear latex or other impermeable gloves when in contact with the patient or equipment and change gloves between procedures (such as bathing the patient and administering an intravenous medication).

Oral and nasal care are important, as well as frequent turning to promote mobilization of secretions. Condensation collecting in the ventilator tubing should be drained away from the patient as it collects. Instillation of normal saline into the endotracheal tube, a common practice thought to facilitate the removal of secretions with suctioning, is to be discouraged. It is not effective and may actually wash microbes lining the ET tube back into the lungs.

Keeping the head of the bed elevated, especially in patients receiving tube feedings, may help decrease aspiration. Frequent suctioning of the oropharynx will remove pooled secretions. A new type of ET tube is available that has a port above the vocal cords. Suction to the port is thought to evacuate pooled secretions and could reduce aspiration. Chest physical therapy, adequate humidification of inspired gases, and sterile suctioning may help prevent infection by eliminating secretion accumulation.

Clinical evidence suggesting VAP includes fever, elevated white blood cell count, purulent sputum, sputum odor, auscultation that reveals crackles or rhonchi, and pulmonary infiltrates noted on chest x-ray. The patient is treated with antibiotics after appropriate cultures are taken by tracheal suctioning or bronchoscopy and when infection is evident.

Neurologic System. In patients with head injury, positive pressure ventilation, especially with PEEP, can impair cerebral blood flow. This is related to increased intrathoracic positive pressure impeding venous drainage from the head, as evidenced by jugular venous distention. As a result of the impaired venous return and increase in cerebral volume, the patient may exhibit increases in intracranial pressure. Elevating the head of the bed may decrease the effects of PEEP.

Gastrointestinal System. Patients receiving mechanical ventilation are often stressed because of serious illness, immobility, and discomforts associated with the ventilator. Thus the ventilated patient is at risk for developing stress ulcers and gastrointestinal (GI) bleeding. Patients with a preexisting ulcer or those receiving corticosteroid therapy are at an especially increased risk. Direct visualization of the stomach via endoscopy demonstrates that gastric and duodenal mucosal changes occur in many critically ill patients. Any kind of circulatory compromise, including reduction of CO caused by mechanical ventilation, may contribute to ischemia of the intestinal mucosa and possibly increase the risk of translocation of GI bacteria.[28]

Prophylactic administration of antacids to maintain a gastric pH greater than 5 and enteral tube feedings reduce the occurrence of upper GI bleeding. Specially designed feeding tubes with a pH-sensitive probe allow for the measurement of gastric pH. Other methods of assessment include checking the pH of gastric aspirates. Prophylactic use of histamine H_2-receptor blockers (cimetidine [Tagamet] and ranitidine [Zantac]), administered intravenously or orally, decrease gastric acidity and diminish the risk of stress ulcer and hemorrhage.

Gastric and bowel dilation may occur as a result of gas accumulation in the GI tract mainly by being swallowed into the stomach. The irritation of an artificial airway may cause excessive air swallowing and subsequent gastric dilation. Gastric or bowel dilation may put pressure on the vena cava, decrease CO, and prohibit adequate diaphragmatic excursion during spontaneous breathing. Elevation of the diaphragm as a result of paralytic ileus or bowel dilation leads to compression of the lower lobes of the lungs, which may cause atelectasis and compromise respiratory function. Decompression of the stomach can be accomplished by the insertion of a nasogastric tube. Some clinicians routinely insert nasogastric tubes prophylactically when mechanical ventilation is initiated. A nasogastric tube may also be inserted to decrease aspiration if the patient is in danger of vomiting.

Immobility, sedation, circulatory impairment, decreased oral intake, use of opioid pain medications, and stress contribute to decreased peristalsis. The patient's inability to exhale against a closed glottis may make defecation difficult. As a result the ventilated patient could be predisposed to constipation. With the early use of enteral nutrition, constipation is usually not a problem.

Musculoskeletal System. Maintenance of muscle strength and prevention of the problems associated with immobility are important. Exercise tolerance is enhanced by adequate analgesia and adequate nutrition. Progressive ambulation of patients receiving long-term ventilation can be attained without interruption of mechanical ventilation. The ventilator can be pushed around the room, or the patient can be ventilated with an oxygenated MRB while ambulating. Passive and active exercises, consisting of movements to maintain muscle tone in the upper and lower extremities, should be done in bed. Simple maneuvers such as leg lifts, knee bends, quadriceps setting, or arm circles are appropriate. Prevention of contractures, pressure ulcers, footdrop, and external rotation of the hip and legs by proper positioning is important.

Psychologic Effects. The patient receiving mechanical ventilation may experience physical and emotional stress. In addition to the problems related to critical care patients discussed at the beginning of this chapter, the patient on a mechanical ventilator is unable to speak, eat, move, or breathe normally. Tubes and machines may cause pain, fear, and anxiety. Ordinary functions such as eating, elimination, and coughing are complicated.

Patients receiving mechanical ventilation usually require some type of sedation (e.g., propofol [Diprivan]) or paralyzing agent (e.g., pancuronium [Pavulon]) to facilitate optimal ventilation. Before initiating sedation or paralysis in the mechanically ventilated patient who is agitated, it is important to assess for the cause of agitation. Common problems that can result in patient agitation include ET tube malposition, pain, hypoxemia, pulmonary embolism, drug reaction, and emotional distress. The treatment should be explained to the patient. If the patient is paralyzed, the nurse should remember that the patient can hear, see, think, and feel. Sedative and pain medications are commonly administered as continuous infusions and must be given if neuromuscular blocking agents are used. Many patients have few memories of their time in the ICU, whereas others remember in vivid detail. Although appearing to be asleep, sedated, or paralyzed, patients may be aware of their surroundings and should always be addressed as though awake.

It is important that the patient have a means to communicate. This may be as simple as eye blinking or head motion, or a computer, paper and pencil, an alphabet, word or picture boards, or a magic slate might be provided if the patient does not require wrist restraints. In some instances tracheostomy tubes that allow speech can be used. The nurse should be attuned to the patient's body language and facial expressions, but this should not be allowed to substitute for providing the patient an opportunity for verbal expression if at all possible.

Measures to make the ventilated patient's environment more restful include efficient scheduling of care to reduce interruptions and a calm, reassuring approach. Especially helpful to the patient is the presence of a loved one or significant family member. This person may have a calming, restful effect on the patient by merely being in the room. The nurse should assess family members and recruit those who have a therapeutic role.

The patient receiving long-term ventilation should be moved to an area with a window to better appreciate night and day and the outside world. Even if the patient is unable to converse, the patient should be addressed. The nurse should discuss the patient's interests and explain in simple terms what the different tubes and equipment are and what progress is being made. Reassuring the patient honestly about progress and allowing the patient as much control as possible may ease the frustration of dependence. Deciding when to bathe or wash hair, which direction to turn, or what to eat may be the patient's only way of maintaining control.

Machine Malfunction or Disconnection. Mechanical ventilators may malfunction or become disconnected. When turned on and operative, alarms alert the nurse to problems. Most deaths from accidental ventilator disconnections occur while the alarm is turned off, and most accidental disconnections in critical care settings are discovered by alarm activation. The most frequent site for disconnection is between the tracheal tube and the adapter. The nurse should ascertain that alarms are set at all times and should chart that this is the case. Alarms should be paused (not inactivated) during suctioning or removal from the ventilator. If alert, the patient should be provided a call bell to bring attention to problems. Connections should be pushed together and then twisted to secure more tightly. The patient's bedside should be arranged so that an MRB with tubing sufficient to reach the patient is set up and functional at all times. Before placing the patient in a chair, the nurse should make sure that the MRB is accessible and functional and that the tubing will reach the patient in the event of an emergency. Although most institutions have emergency generators in the event of a power failure, the nurse should always consider the possibility that power will fail and have a plan for manually ventilating all the patients who are dependent on a ventilator.

Nutritional Therapy: Patient Receiving Mechanical Ventilation

Mechanical ventilation and the hypermetabolism associated with critical illness can contribute to inadequate nutrition. Presence of an ET tube eliminates the normal route for eating. Although patients who are nasotracheally intubated may be allowed liquid and semiliquid feedings orally, it is difficult to ingest sufficient calories, protein, and fat. A patient with a tracheostomy can eat normally once the stoma has healed. When a tracheostomy tube is present, the patient should tilt the head slightly forward to facilitate swallowing and to prevent aspiration. Often, soft foods (e.g., puddings, ice cream) are more easily swallowed than liquids.

Patients likely to be without food for 3 to 5 days should have a nutritional program initiated. Inadequate nutrition makes the patient receiving prolonged mechanical ventilation more prone to poor oxygen transport secondary to anemia and to poor tolerance of minimal exercise. Disuse of respiratory muscles and poor nutrition result in decreased respiratory muscle strength. In addition, the hypermetabolism associated with critical illness, trauma, and surgery and the presence of anxiety, pain, and increased work of breathing greatly increase caloric expenditure. Serum protein levels (e.g., transferrin, prealbumin) are usually decreased. Inadequate nutrition can delay weaning, decrease the speed of recovery, and decrease resistance to infection. Enteral feeding is the preferred method to meet caloric needs.

A concern regarding the nutritional support of patients on mechanical ventilation is the carbohydrate content of the diet. Metabolism of carbohydrates results in high levels of CO_2 production. The resulting CO_2 load results in a higher required minute ventilation. This in turn can cause an unnecessary increased effort to breathe. Decreasing carbohydrate content in the diet lowers CO_2 production. Preparations such as Pulmocare, which are high in protein and fat but low in carbohydrate content, may be beneficial in ventilated patients. A dietician can provide useful consultation for the ventilated patient.

The ventilated patient receiving enteral feedings should have the head of the bed elevated. A soft, flexible, small-bore feeding tube should be used. When the tube is initially placed, the position of the tube is verified by x-ray. (Procedures for tube feedings are discussed in Chapter 38.)

Tube feedings should be stopped for at least 30 minutes before placing the patient in a head-down position for postural drainage. Residuals should be checked periodically. Elevated residuals indicate that the feeding is not moving through the GI system. Other indications of feeding problems include bloating, nausea, vomiting, and abdominal distention. The tube feeding should be temporarily stopped and the physician notified. The patient must be observed closely for signs of hypoglycemia if the tube feedings are discontinued for long periods of time. Food coloring in the feedings can help identify the presence of feedings in secretions suctioned from the trachea. The presence of a positive glucose reaction on a dipstick of tracheal secretions may indicate aspiration of feedings into the trachea. If there is evidence that aspiration may have occurred, the tube feeding should be stopped immediately and the physician notified.

Manual Resuscitation Bag and Suction Equipment

All patients receiving mechanical ventilation should have an MRB along with a mask attached to oxygen and suctioning equipment ready and available at the bedside. The MRB should contain a reservoir to sequester oxygen so that oxygen concentrations of 90% to 95% can be delivered. The slower the bag is deflated and inflated, the higher the oxygen concentration that will be delivered. The Ambu (air mask bag unit) is a well-known self-inflatable bag. This unit consists of a bag fitted to a face mask or a tracheal tube attachment. In the event the patient self-extubates, ventilation is maintained with the MRB and mask.

Weaning from Mechanical Ventilation

The process of reducing ventilator support and resuming spontaneous ventilation is termed *weaning*. Weaning may be of varying length, ranging from a few hours in postoperative open heart patients to weeks in the patient with chronic pulmonary disease. Patients likely to require prolonged mechanical ventilation generally are those with underlying lung disease who develop respiratory failure because of surgical procedure, trauma, or infection. Preparations for weaning begin well in advance of the event. These preparations include maintaining nutrition, fluid-electrolyte and acid-base balances, CO, pulmonary, and psychologic status.

Readiness for weaning depends on many factors.[29] Criteria vary, depending on prior lung status and ventilatory reserve. For weaning to be successful, the patient should be as stable as possible. Respiratory parameters should demonstrate a patent airway, adequate ventilatory muscle strength, and an effective cough. Oxygenation should be adequate, and the lungs should be reasonably clear on auscultation and chest x-ray. It is important to have an alert, well-rested patient relatively free from pain who will readily take deep breaths to obtain optimum alveolar ventilation and prevent atelectasis. This does not mean complete withdrawal from sedatives or analgesics. Instead, medications should be titrated to relieve pain without causing excessive drowsiness.

A variety of weaning methods are available, and no one method is superior. All methods can be delivered with the patient remaining connected to the ventilator circuit. The patient on SIMV can have the ventilator breath frequency gradually reduced as the patient's ventilatory status permits. CPAP or PSV can be added to SIMV. Another method involves PSV, CPAP, or both delivered without SIMV. PSV is thought to provide gentle, slow respiratory muscle conditioning and may be especially beneficial for patients who are deconditioned or have cardiac problems. Some patients may be weaned by simply providing humidified oxygen (T-piece or flowby method).

The patient might be allowed spontaneous ventilation for 10 minutes each hour and receive ventilator support for 50 minutes, with the ratio of spontaneous ventilation to ventilation support gradually increasing. Regardless of method used, it is important to allow the patient's respiratory muscles adequate rest between weaning trials. Once the respiratory muscles become fatigued, they may require 12 to 24 hours to recover.

With all methods, patients usually require a 10% increase in FIO_2 to maintain arterial oxygen tension. This is because tidal volume usually drops with spontaneous respiration, and carbon dioxide tension may increase. Weaning is usually carried out during the day, with the patient ventilated at night until there is sufficient spontaneous ventilation without excess fatigue.

The patient being weaned should be provided continuing psychologic support. The weaning process should be explained and the patient informed of progress. The patient should be placed in a sitting or semirecumbent position and made comfortable. Respiratory parameters are measured to provide a baseline with which serial determinations can be compared. The tidal volume, respiratory rate, negative inspiratory force, and vital capacity are measured. ABGs are drawn at baseline and at specified intervals during weaning.

The patient must be monitored closely for signs of respiratory distress, including shallow breathing, use of accessory respiratory muscles, restlessness, tiring, somnolence, tachycardia, decrease or increase in blood pressure, tachypnea or bradypnea, ECG changes, drop in SpO_2, and secretion buildup with a need for frequent suctioning. Statements from the patient regarding weaning tolerance are important.

When the patient is ready for extubation, the mouth and oropharynx should be thoroughly suctioned and the cuff deflated. An oxygen mask or cannula should be set up and ready for use. The patient should be told to expect to cough when the tube is removed. The nurse should be prepared to manage copious secretions. Once the patient has been extubated and stabilized with oxygen delivered by mask or nasal cannula, care of the mouth and nares should be provided. ABGs are obtained 20 to 30 minutes after extubation. The patient must be monitored for respiratory distress caused by the underlying lung problems and also because laryngeal or tracheal edema may develop. Manifestations of laryngeal and tracheal edema include symptoms of acute upper airway obstruction. Measures to ensure pulmonary toilet (e.g., coughing, deep breathing, turning, and suctioning [if necessary]) must be continued.

Home Mechanical Ventilation

Mechanical ventilators are no longer limited to the ICU, but are now a part of home health care. Families can be taught to care for the person receiving mechanical ventilation as an alternative to prolonged hospitalization.[30,31] The emphasis on controlling hospital health care costs has increased the early discharge of patients and the need to provide highly technical care such as mechanical ventilation in home settings.

Home mechanical ventilation has several advantages. Having the patient in the home eliminates the strain that the hospital setting may impose on family dynamics. The feeling of helplessness by family members when they first hear about the necessity for long-term mechanical ventilation is frequently countered by the ability of the family to participate fully in the patient's care in the home setting. At home the patient may be able to participate more in activities of daily living around a more individualized schedule and, because of the smaller size of the home ventilator, be more mobile.[32] Another advantage of home mechanical ventilation is the reduction in the patient's risk of nosocomial infection. Disadvantages include problems related to reimbursement, equipment, caregiving, and the complex needs of these patients. Ventilated patients are usually dependent, requiring extensive nursing care. In one study it was found that an average of 8 hours of care per day was required.[30] Disposable products may be nonreimbursable. Financial resources must be carefully assessed when arranging home mechanical ventilation. Another disadvantage of home mechanical ventilation is its potential impact on the family. Family members may seem enthusiastic about caring for their loved one in the home but may be motivated by guilt. They may lack understanding of the potential sacrifices they may have to make financially and in time and commitment.

Both negative pressure and positive pressure (volume) ventilators can be used in the home. Negative pressure ventilators are frequently the ventilator of choice because they do not require an artificial airway and are less complicated to use. Small, portable volume ventilators that can be attached to a wheelchair or placed on a bedside table are available. Settings and alarms on these ventilators are similar to the larger ones used in ICUs. Some home ventilators have IMV capability.

NURSING MANAGEMENT: MECHANICAL VENTILATION

Nursing management of the patient receiving mechanical ventilation is presented in NCP 63-2.

INTRACRANIAL PRESSURE MONITORING

Intracranial pressure (ICP) is the hydrostatic force measured in the brain cerebrospinal fluid (CSF) compartment. ICP may become elevated because of head trauma, stroke, subarachnoid hemorrhage, brain tumor, inflammation, or brain tissue damage from other causes (see Table 54-4). Any patient who becomes acutely unconscious, regardless of the cause, is managed as if there were actual or potential increased ICP. Patients with or at risk for elevated ICP are usually cared for in an ICU and often receive invasive ICP monitoring. As with other invasive ICU measures, ICP monitoring is provided to those who may benefit from treatment and in whom the underlying process is thought to be self-limiting. Patients with irreversible pathology or advanced neurologic decline caused by primary or metastatic lesions usually do not receive ICP monitoring. Nursing management goals in elevated ICP include preservation of function, early identification of neurologic changes, and prevention of complications. Patients may require intensive physical care and emotional support.

Increased Intracranial Pressure

ICP is important because it influences cerebral perfusion. When evaluating cerebral perfusion, it is important to consider systemic blood pressure, ICP, blood flow, vascular resistance, and blood volume. Mean arterial pressure (MAP) provides the driving force for brain blood flow. ICP, reflecting the pressure within the brain tissue and CSF, opposes blood flow. Thus cerebral perfusion pressure (CPP), which equals MAP minus ICP, is the clinically relevant variable that must be considered. Cerebral blood flow, expressed in milliliters of blood per minute, must be maintained at a relatively high rate because of the high and continuing metabolic needs of brain tissue. Cerebral vascular resistance, generated by the arterioles within the cranium, links CPP and blood flow as follows:

$$\text{CPP} = \text{Flow} \times \text{Resistance}$$

The volume of blood within the cranium (intracranial blood volume) is important because it affects ICP. Cerebral blood flow and increased intracranial pressure are discussed in Chapter 54.

Elevated ICP is clinically significant because it diminishes CPP, causing brain ischemia or infarction. Also, brain structures can be compressed and damaged or irreversibly destroyed. Death can occur. High ICP causes herniation of brain tissue, that is, extrusion into abnormal spaces. Cerebral hemispheres can shift across the midline. Brainstem and cerebral hemispheres can herniate through the tentorium cerebelli. The cerebellum can herniate through the foramen magnum (tonsillar herniation; herniation is discussed in further detail in Chapter 54). These complications are generally fatal.

A slow increase in ICP, as with an enlarging brain tumor, is tolerated better than a rapid increase, as in primary brain injury. If an elevated pressure is evenly distributed throughout the brain, it is better tolerated. Crucial to preservation of tissue is preservation of cerebral blood flow. With slower, distributed rises in ICP, blood flow tends to be preserved.

CPP is useful in evaluating brain blood flow. Normal CPP is 70 to 100 mm Hg. At least 50 to 60 mm Hg is necessary for adequate cerebral perfusion. CPP less than 50 mm Hg is associated with ischemia and neuronal death. It is of paramount importance to maintain MAP when ICP is elevated. It should be remembered that CPP might not reflect perfusion pressure in all parts of the brain. There may be local areas of swelling and compression. Thus a higher CPP may be needed for these patients to prevent localized tissue damage.

Intracranial Pressure Measurement and Line Management

Technical Apparatus. ICP monitoring is used regularly to guide therapy in patients with suspected increased ICP. Some invasive ICP monitoring systems are similar to invasive blood pressure monitoring systems in that a fluid-filled tube couples

63-2 NURSING CARE PLAN PATIENT ON MECHANICAL VENTILATION

Expected Patient Outcomes	Nursing Interventions and *Rationales*
NURSING DIAGNOSIS **Risk for injury** *related to* possible machine malfunction, accidental disconnection, inability to breathe unassisted, asynchrony with ventilator, and settings unsuitable to maintain adequate ventilation.	
▪ ABGs within normal range for patient. ▪ Early detection of signs and symptoms of decreased PaO_2 and increased $PaCO_2$. ▪ Breathe synchronously with ventilator. ▪ Early detection, correction, or prevention of complications associated with mechanical malfunction or disconnection.	▪ Monitor for risk factors such as hypoxemia, hypercapnia, tachycardia, tachypnea, increase in BP, agitation, confusion, headache, lethargy, cyanosis; respiratory pattern asynchronous with machine's pattern of ventilation; machine malfunction or disconnection *to determine presence of risk factors and plan for intervention.* ▪ Begin mechanical ventilation slowly (especially in patients with COPD); lower $PaCO_2$ only to patient's baseline level *to prevent alkalosis, especially in patient with compensated respiratory acidosis.* ▪ Assess patient for possible causes of hyperventilation such as retained secretions, hypoxemia, pain, fear, and anxiety. ▪ Check ventilator settings (FIO_2, respiratory rate, tidal volume, O_2 flow rate, PEEP, airway pressure, thermistor temperature, and I:E ratio) *to determine if appropriate to clinical situation.* ▪ Keep manual resuscitation bag connected to O_2 source at bedside *for use in case of an emergency.* ▪ If patient is fighting ventilation, slowly bag for three to six breaths and verbally coach patient to breathe *to help synchronize patient with ventilator.* ▪ Determine and treat cause of asynchrony. ▪ Turn all alarms on; pause but do not turn off alarms during suctioning and disconnections. ▪ Respond immediately to alarm *because potentially dangerous situations of mechanical malfunction or patient asynchrony with the ventilator may be present.* ▪ Check cuff for leaks *to prevent loss of ventilation gas and to prevent aspiration of oral secretions.* ▪ Monitor ventilator tubing q1-2hr for condensed water and drain when water present *to prevent aspiration of accumulated fluid.*
NURSING DIAGNOSIS **Decreased cardiac output** *related to* impeded venous return by positive pressure ventilation *as manifested by* decreased BP, increased heart rate, decreased urine output, presence of arrhythmias, mental confusion.	
▪ BP and cardiac output within normal range. ▪ Adequate urinary output.	▪ Monitor vital signs and level of consciousness q2-4hr. ▪ Observe and monitor for clinical manifestations of decreased cardiac output *to identify decreased venous return to the heart, decreased left ventricular end-diastolic volume, and lowered blood pressure.* ▪ Monitor direct measurement of cardiac output by thermodilution, especially when >10 cm H_2O PEEP is used *to anticipate need for plasma expanders, vasopressors, and IV fluids as ordered because hemodynamic complications of decreased venous return induced by positive pressure ventilation are exaggerated by hypovolemia.*
NURSING DIAGNOSIS **Ineffective airway clearance** *related to* presence of artificial airway, problems with positioning, accumulation of secretions, and immobility *as manifested by* presence of abnormal breath sounds, absent cough, presence of thick or copious secretions.	
▪ Normal breath sounds. ▪ Thin and easily removed secretions.	▪ Change patient's position q2hr *to prevent pooling of secretions in the lungs.* ▪ Have patient cough and, if feasible, deep breathe q2hr *to remove secretions and to prevent hypoventilation.* ▪ Perform tracheobronchial suctioning *to remove retained secretions and improve oxygenation.* ▪ Auscultate breath sounds q2-4hr *to monitor effectiveness of interventions.*

Continued

63-2 NURSING CARE PLAN PATIENT ON MECHANICAL VENTILATION —continued

Expected Patient Outcomes	Nursing Interventions and *Rationales*
NURSING DIAGNOSIS	**Impaired physical mobility** *related to* restricted movement *as manifested by* inability to perform active range-of-motion exercise.
▪ Normal range of motion of joints.	▪ Perform active and passive range-of-motion exercises (e.g., leg lifts, knee bends, quadriceps setting, arm circles) *to maintain patient's joint and muscle functioning and improve circulation.* ▪ Prevent contractures and external rotation of hips by proper positioning *to prevent musculoskeletal complications resulting from bed rest.* ▪ Use footboard, high-top sneakers, and frequent foot flexion *to prevent footdrop.* ▪ Provide progressive ambulation for patients receiving long-term ventilation *to prevent "pulmonary crippling."*
NURSING DIAGNOSIS	**Anxiety** *related to* diagnosis and clinical condition, pain, possible machine malfunction or disconnection, inability to communicate, ICU environment, possibility of death, and fear of suffocation and choking *as manifested by* expression of feelings of anxiety, anxious appearance, rigid body posture.
▪ Communication of feelings and anxieties. ▪ Absent or manageable anxiety level.	▪ Assess patient's behavior for clues of handling stressful situation *to determine a plan for interventions.* ▪ Give simple, honest explanations regarding care and progress *to foster a realistic understanding and help patient make informed decisions.* ▪ When possible, allow patient to make decisions regarding all aspects of care *to increase patient's sense of control.* ▪ Provide for diversion and occupational therapy as needed and tolerated *to relieve anxiety.* ▪ Refer to psychiatric clinical nurse specialist, psychiatrist, or hospital chaplain when appropriate *to offer additional counseling and support.* ▪ Be available to family; offer support and help *to lessen their anxiety and increase their cooperation.*
NURSING DIAGNOSIS	**Sleep pattern disturbance** *related to* frequent awakenings, anxiety, depression, and ICU environment *as manifested by* insomnia, restlessness, irritability, disorientation, morning headaches.
▪ Rested on awakening. ▪ Minimal number of awakenings for treatments.	▪ Perform bedtime preparations (e.g., wash patient's face and hands, rub back, provide oral care) *to promote relaxation and facilitate sleep.* ▪ Turn off lights at night *to preserve usual sleep-wake cycle.* ▪ Provide drug therapy intervention as ordered *to promote sleep.* ▪ Provide relaxation techniques and tapes *to promote relaxation.* ▪ Schedule activities so that patient gets at least 2 hours of uninterrupted time to sleep.
NURSING DIAGNOSIS	**Dysfunctional ventilatory weaning response** *related to* too-rapid pacing of the weaning process, insufficient knowledge of the weaning process, and anxiety *as manifested by* restlessness, tachypnea, fatigue, increased blood pressure, shallow breathing, use of accessory muscles, tachycardia, skin color changes (e.g., pallor or cyanosis), agitation.
▪ Achievement of progressive weaning goals. ▪ Remain extubated. ▪ Communication of increased comfort during weaning. ▪ Less tired from work of weaning.	▪ Assess respiratory parameters (e.g., inspiratory effort, minute ventilation, vital capacity, effective cough) *to determine patient's weaning ability.* ▪ Explain the weaning process *so patient understands what is expected.* ▪ Jointly negotiate progressive weaning goals *to involve patient in establishing the plan.* ▪ Adopt a weaning pace that will ensure success and minimize setbacks *to maintain patient confidence.* ▪ Draw ABGs at specified periods during the weaning *to monitor patient's ventilatory status.* ▪ Deflate cuff totally or partially during weaning *since tracheal tubes add to airway resistance.* ▪ Monitor for respiratory distress and place patient back on ventilator if observed *to ensure adequate ventilation.* ▪ If the weaning process is discontinued, explain rationale and revised plan to patient *to minimize frustration and disappointment and enhance cooperation.*

Continued

63-2 NURSING CARE PLAN PATIENT ON MECHANICAL VENTILATION —continued

Expected Patient Outcomes	Nursing Interventions and *Rationales*

NURSING DIAGNOSIS **Risk for infection** *related to* exposure to environmental pathogens, presence of artificial airway, decreased resistance secondary to debilitated state and prolonged immobility.*

NURSING DIAGNOSIS **Altered nutrition: less than body requirements** *related to* inability to take in nourishment orally and increased caloric demands secondary to clinical condition and need for mechanical ventilation *as manifested by* loss of 10% of body weight.†

COLLABORATIVE PROBLEMS

Nursing Goals	Nursing Interventions and *Rationales*

POTENTIAL COMPLICATION **Gastric distention** *related to* improper ET tube placement, GI bleeding, or ileus.

Nursing Goals	Nursing Interventions and *Rationales*
▪ Performance of abdominal assessment. ▪ Report deviations from expected findings.	▪ Assess for abdominal distention, tympany, and bowel sounds and measure abdominal girth *to detect signs of bowel dilation.* ▪ Test stools and gastric drainage for occult blood *since the patient is at risk of developing stress ulcers and GI bleeding.* ▪ Check for gastric air on chest x-ray. ▪ Administer antacids, H_2-receptor blocker, and tube feedings as ordered *to reduce the occurrence of GI bleeding and to decrease the acidity of gastric secretions.* ▪ If abdominal distention is present, elevate head of bed to allow for optimal diaphragmatic excursion. ▪ Obtain order and place nasogastric tube or, if present, confirm patency by irrigating *to relieve gastric tension.* ▪ Confirm correct position of nasogastric tube *to prevent aspiration and the accumulation of GI fluids.*

POTENTIAL COMPLICATION **Pneumothorax or pneumomediastinum** *related to* barotrauma caused by positive pressure ventilation.

Nursing Goals	Nursing Interventions and *Rationales*
▪ Monitor for signs of pneumothorax. ▪ Report positive findings. ▪ Carry out appropriate medical and nursing interventions.	▪ Observe for sudden increase (by 5 cm H_2O or more) in peak inspiratory pressure, sudden patient agitation or coughing, frequent activation of high-pressure alarm, decrease in static and effective compliance, palpable subcutaneous emphysema over neck and anterior chest areas, deterioration in ABGs and BP, decrease or absence of breath sounds, hyperresonance on percussion; pneumothorax on chest x-ray *to detect signs of pneumothorax.* ▪ Bag ventilate with O_2 using tidal volume *to reduce airway pressures until a chest tube can be inserted.* ▪ Notify physician and set up for chest tube insertion immediately *because pneumothorax can convert to a life-threatening tension pneumothorax.* ▪ Check and record ventilator settings q2hr. ▪ Record level of peak inspiratory pressure to establish baseline data *to evaluate changes in lung compliance.*‡

*Interventions for this nursing diagnosis are presented in the nursing care plan for the patient with an artificial airway (NCP 63-1).
†Interventions for this nursing diagnosis are presented in the nursing care plan for the patient with acute respiratory failure (NCP 62-1).
‡This assessment is especially important in patients receiving PEEP because they are at more risk of barotrauma.
PAD, pulmonary artery pressure—diastolic; *PAS,* pulmonary artery pressure—systolic; *PAWP,* pulmonary artery wedge pressure.

an internal space to an external transducer. Devices include intraventricular catheters, subarachnoid bolts or screws, and subdural catheters (Fig. 63-18). Table 63-16 outlines advantages and disadvantages of such devices. As with fluid-coupled blood pressure monitoring systems, signals can be distorted by excessive tube length or bubbles in the line. In these systems, the transducer is external and its position must remain constant with respect to the patient's head to produce pressures that can be compared.

With a second type of technology, the sensor is placed within the cranium. For example, with the fiberoptic catheter the transducer is within the catheter tip. Other, less commonly used transducers include pneumatic systems and intracranial strain gauges. These systems produce excellent quality waveforms and

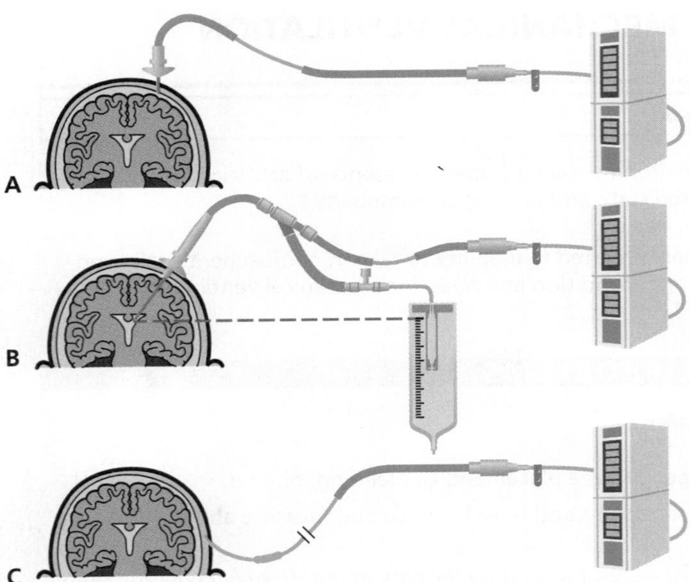

Fig. 63-18 **A,** Subarachnoid pressure monitoring system. **B,** Ventricular pressure monitoring system. **C,** Subdural placement of a sensor.

do not require repositioning with patient movement. They usually cannot be rezeroed.

Infection is a serious consideration with ICP monitoring. Rates are highest in fluid-coupled systems, with reports ranging from 1% to 22% of patients developing infections.[33] Prophylactic systemic antibiotics such as nafcillin (Unipen), cephalothin (Keflin), and gentamicin (Garamycin) have been administered with mixed results.[34]

Intracranial Pressure Waveform. ICP should be measured at end expiration as a mean pressure. The strip recording should be inserted into the record at least every 4 hours. The normal ICP waveform is shaped somewhat like an arterial pressure tracing (Fig. 63-19), although the pressures are in a much lower range. This is because arterial pressure is transmitted to the choroid plexus and then to the CSF in the ventricular and subarachnoid spaces. When the waveform is monitored so that components in synchrony with the cardiac cycle can be visualized, three peaks are noted:

- P1: initial peak, reflecting transmission of systolic arterial pressure from the choroid plexus
- P2: "tidal wave" ends in the dicrotic notch
- P3: third wave follows the dicrotic notch and may reflect venous pressure

Table 63-16 Comparison of Intracranial Pressure Monitoring Systems

System	Description	Advantages	Disadvantages
Ventricular catheter	External transducer system; soft, radiopaque Silastic tube inserted via stylet, usually through a twist drill hole into anterior horn of lateral ventricle of nondominant hemisphere	Accurate (can level and zero) CSF can be tapped to reduce ICP and sample CSF Compliance can be tested Contrast media can be inserted for diagnostic tests	Infection risk Hemorrhage risk Difficult to place in patient with small ventricles or intracranial shift Transducer must be repositioned with head movement
Subarachnoid screw or bolt	External transducer system; hollow metal shaft or screw, threaded at one end; threaded end is inserted through a hole drilled into bone through dura into subarachnoid space; placed over frontal area of nondominant hemisphere so that same site can be used for subsequent placement of ventricular catheter if needed.	Simple insertion procedure Useful if ventricle is small or shifted No disruption of neuron tissue of brain Less risk of infection, hemorrhage	Leaks can limit accuracy Obstruction by blood or brain tissue can distort readings Some risk of infection (less than ventriculostomy) Intact skull is required Not useful for draining CSF Not useful for compliance testing If made of metal, patient cannot have MRI performed Transducer must be repositioned with head motion
Fiberoptic devices	Intracranial transducer system; catheter consists of a mobile mirrored diaphragm; fiberoptic signal is bounced off diaphragm and sensed by another fiberoptic cable within the same catheter; usually has CSF sampling port; can be placed into ventricle, subdural, subarachnoid space, or brain parenchyma	Versatile regarding site Insertion possible through subarachnoid bolt Irrigation not necessary Detailed, artifact-free waveform produced If intraventricular, CSF can be tapped to reduce ICP and sample CSF No need to modify equipment with head movement	Catheter fragile Once positioned, rezeroing not possible Unique monitoring system required (but couples to most oscilloscopes) Expensive

CSF, cerebrospinal fluid; *ICP,* intracranial pressure; *MRI,* magnetic resonance imaging.

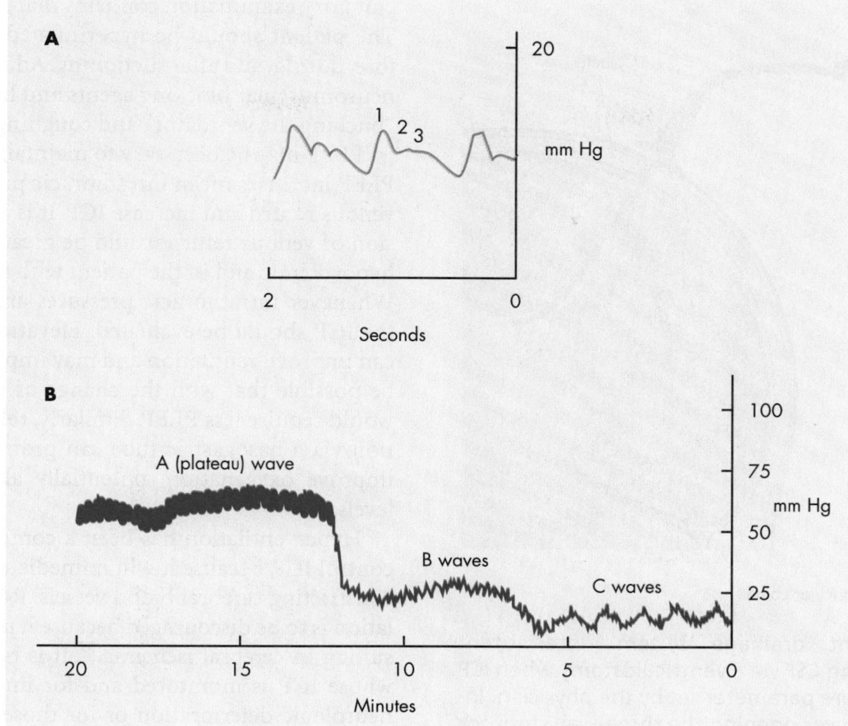

Fig. 63-19 **A,** Intracranial pressure (ICP) waveform as noted on a fast time scale recording. *1, 2, 3* indicate P1, P2, P3 (see text). **B,** Pathologic ICP waves as noted on a slow time scale recording.

Three types of pathologic waves might be seen when ICP is elevated (see Fig. 63-19). Visualization of these requires monitoring with a slowly moving strip recorder.

- A waves: Plateau waves seen with ICP elevations of 50 to 100 mm Hg; last 5 to 20 min; associated with a fall in CPP to less than 40 mm Hg; associated with severe cerebral ischemia; signal a neurologic emergency and must be treated promptly to avoid irreversible brain damage
- B waves: sharp, rhythmic pressure elevations of 20 to 40 mm Hg; frequency of one per 30 to 120 seconds; seen with changes in the respiratory pattern; may be precursors of A waves
- C waves: transient rhythmic pressure elevations of less than 20 mm Hg; frequency of one every 4 to 8 minutes; significance not determined

It is important that the nurse monitor ICP waveform, as well as mean pressure. It has been noted that when the height of P2 is higher than P1, the intracranial space may be noncompliant and the patient is at risk for development of elevated ICP.[35] The patient must be monitored for pathologic waves. In addition to noting pressure measurements and waveform morphology, it is important to consider the rate at which changes occur and the patient's clinical condition. It is important to note that neurologic deterioration might not occur until ICP elevation is pronounced and sustained.[34,35] If A or B waves are noted, the physician must be informed immediately.

In fluid-coupled systems, the waveform should be inspected for damping, which could indicate the presence of bubbles in the line or that the line is obstructed with tissue or blood clots. Inaccurate ICP readings can be caused by CSF leaks around the monitoring device, obstruction of the intraventricular catheter or bolt, difference in the height of the bolt and the transducer, kinks in the tubing, and Valsalva's maneuver.

Cerebrospinal Fluid Drainage. With the ventricular catheter and certain fiberoptic systems, it is possible to control ICP by removing CSF. To do this, a Y-connector or stopcock is inserted in the line (Fig. 63-20). A closed system should be used to decrease infection risk. ICP and drainage volume are controlled by the height of the drainage bag or drip chamber relative to the patient reference point. Typically, a point 15 cm above the ear canal is selected as a reference point. Raising the system diminishes drainage; lowering the system increases drainage volume. Careful monitoring of volume of CSF drained is essential, keeping in mind that normal adult CSF production is about 20 to 30 ml per hour, with a total CSF volume of 90 to 150 ml within the ventricles and subarachnoid space. The amount of fluid to be drained, frequency of drainage, and the height of the highest point in the system should be ordered by the physician.

Ventricular collapse, a major complication of this type of drainage system, occurs when fluid is removed too rapidly. Another complication of rapid decompression is development of a subdural hematoma. To ensure that fluid is not removed too rapidly, intermittent drainage with close observation is used. With this method the line typically is opened only to drain when ICP reaches a preset level and then closed when ICP drops.

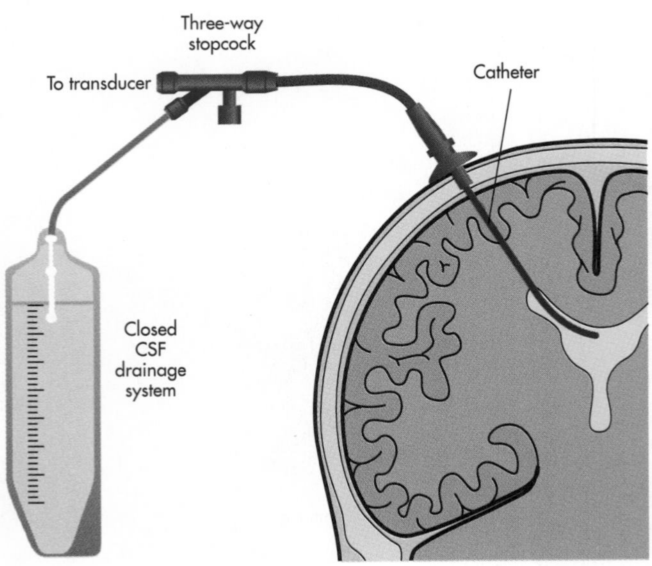

Fig. 63-20 Intermittent drainage system. Intermittent drainage involves draining CSF via a ventriculostomy when ICP exceeds the upper pressure parameter set by the physician. Intermittent drainage involves opening the three-way stopcock to allow CSF to flow into the drainage bag for brief periods (30 to 120 seconds) until the pressure is below the upper pressure parameters.

NURSING AND COLLABORATIVE MANAGEMENT: INCREASED INTRACRANIAL PRESSURE

Care of the patient with actual or potential increased ICP is similar to that described for the patient with primary brain injury or the unconscious patient (see Chapter 54). Specific therapies are directed at maintaining CPP through manipulating ICP and MAP. Therapies to decrease ICP include CSF drainage, diuresis, oxygenation, neuromuscular blockade, and positioning. Therapies to maintain MAP include fluid resuscitation, positioning, and vasopressors. Intensive monitoring is required, including vital signs, heart rate and rhythm, ventilation, oxygenation, fluid balance, mental status and level of consciousness, ICP, CPP, cranial nerve function, peripheral movement, and sensation.

■ Oxygenation and Ventilation

Patients with elevated ICP or compromised CPP are likely to have a reduced level of consciousness with inadequate ventilatory effort and airway maintenance. Measures taken early in the patient's care include airway control by ET intubation and mechanical ventilation to ensure adequate oxygenation and breathing. Arterial oxygen tensions greater than 100 mm Hg are recommended.

The ET tube must be secured without ties around the neck. Neck ties impede venous return, thus elevating ICP. In patients with normal ICP, ET suctioning is usually well tolerated. In patients with elevated ICP, suctioning can lead to dangerous ICP increases. Three factors associated with suctioning might contribute to ICP elevation: hypercapnia, hypoxemia, and stress. Suctioning should be performed in all patients only when auscultatory examination confirms that suctioning is necessary.[36] The patient should be hyperinflated and preoxygenated before, during, and after suctioning. Additional measures include neuromuscular blocking agents and heavy sedation to prevent "bucking the ventilator" and coughing during suctioning.

PEEP may be necessary to maintain oxygenation. However, PEEP increases mean intrathoracic pressure, so it may impede venous return and increase ICP. It is anticipated that suppression of venous return would be greatest in the patient who is hypovolemic and in the patient with a highly compliant chest. Whenever intrathoracic pressures are changed, the effect on the ICP should be evaluated. Elevation of the bed 30 degrees can improve ventilation and may improve oxygenation. It may be possible that with the change of bed position the patient would require less PEEP. Similarly, relief of abdominal distention via a nasogastric tube can promote lung expansion and improve oxygenation, potentially allowing decreased PEEP levels.

Hyperventilation has been a commonly used treatment to control ICP, because it will immediately decrease ICP by vasoconstricting cerebral blood vessels. Routine use of hyperventilation is to be discouraged because it is possible to overdo it, resulting in cerebral ischemia.[37] It is best used only in patients whose ICP is monitored and for immediate management of neurologic deterioration or for those who do not respond to sedation, paralysis, CSF drainage, and diuresis.[38]

■ Cerebrospinal Fluid Drainage

CSF drainage is an early intervention. However, it can be used only if the ICP device includes an intraventricular catheter. Patients with acute ICP elevation have their CSF drained intermittently when the ICP reaches a specified limit (e.g., 15 mm Hg). The requirement for increasing frequency of CSF drainage is considered a sign of worsening neurologic status.

■ Volume Resuscitation

Volume resuscitation is important in the patient with increased ICP. Hypotension has been identified as a major factor in elevated ICP because it decreases blood pressure and thus CPP. Intravenous fluids are infused to maintain the CPP at greater than 70 mm Hg. Normally a MAP of 90 mm Hg would be judged adequate. However, if the ICP is over 20 mm Hg, the CPP will be less than 70 mm Hg. If fluid infusion is ineffective, vasoactive agents such as norepinephrine (Levophed), dopamine (Intropin), or phenylephrine (Neo-Synephrine) may be used. Pulmonary artery or at least CVP monitoring is used to monitor fluid management. The patient with underlying hypertension presents a special problem because a higher MAP may be required. In this case a higher CPP is the goal of therapy.

■ Diuresis

Diuresis is a cornerstone in the treatment of increased ICP. Osmotic diuresis pulls water out of brain tissue into the systemic circulation and then fluid is removed by the kidneys. Mannitol is the agent most commonly used. Bolus doses are thought to be more effective than continuous infusions because a continuous infusion is thought to encourage accumulation of mannitol in the brain, which could cause a reverse osmotic shift and increase swelling and ICP. When using diuretics, care must be taken to prevent a drop in CPP through volume loss. Serum osmolality and sodium must also be monitored.[39]

Sedation

Sedation, pain control, and sometimes neuromuscular blockers are used to control surges in ICP associated with agitation, ventilator asynchrony, and coughing. This therapy also prevents patients who are confused and combative from seriously harming themselves by self-extubation or pulling out lines and catheters. Therapy is usually maintained by continuous infusions of the various agents. A problem with this therapy is the loss of clinical markers for changes in neurologic status. Some clinicians prefer propofol (Diprivan) as a sedative because it is rapidly dissipated once discontinued, and the underlying level of neurologic functioning can be rapidly determined, with the patient then being quickly resedated if needed.

Long-term use of these agents can lead to problems. Prolonged neuromuscular blocker use is associated with a risk of significant residual muscle weakness, and effects from toxicity are poorly understood. Patients on neuromuscular blockers should be closely monitored for achievement of therapeutic effect with the minimal amount of drug necessary. If the patient requires narcotic and sedative administration, gradual weaning of the drugs is needed to prevent withdrawal.[40]

The ultimate in sedation is achieved through the use of barbiturate coma. This treatment is used only when the patient is refractory to other previously mentioned therapies. Barbiturates can reduce cerebral metabolism by as much as 50%, causing a significant reduction in cerebral blood flow. The patient's electroencephalogram is monitored continuously. Problems associated with this therapy include hypotension, hypothermia, and a possible risk for infection because of immune suppression.

Temperature Control

Temperature control is important. Hypothermia is induced in some patients to control cerebral metabolic rate and thereby control cerebral blood flow. An elevated temperature will increase cerebral metabolic rate by as much as 7% for each degree centigrade. Elevations in temperature should be reduced in the patient with elevated ICP by means of antipyretics. Cooling blankets can induce shivering, which may require additional medications to control.

Positioning

Positioning can affect ICP. Usually patients are placed in a semirecumbent position (30 to 45 degrees) to facilitate jugular venous drainage. Additionally, the head should be maintained in midline position to prevent kinking of the blood vessels, and the ET tube should not be taped circumferentially, because it could restrict venous drainage. However, elevating the head of the bed could lower CPP. Therefore patients who have a reduced CPP may respond better to being flat. Trendelenburg's position should be avoided because it could increase ICP by impeding venous drainage.

CRITICAL THINKING EXERCISES

CASE STUDY

Critical Care and Mechanical Ventilation

Patient Profile

Mr. R., a 55-year-old man, was found lying on the street by the police. He was unconscious on admission and has not regained consciousness. He has an endotracheal tube in place and is receiving mechanical ventilation. It is 24 hours after admission.

Subjective Data

- None; is unresponsive to painful stimuli

Objective Data

- Blood pressure 100/75; heart rate 120; temperature 102° F (38.8° C); SpO2 98%
- CVP 3 mm Hg
- Purulent secretions from ET tube
- Breath sounds: many rhonchi bilaterally, decreased breath sounds on the right

Diagnostic Studies

- Chest x-ray reveals right lower lung consolidation
- ABGs: pH 7.48, PaO_2 100 mm Hg, $PaCO_2$ 30 mm Hg, HCO_3^- 22 mEq/L

Collaborative Care

- Ventilator settings: assist control at 14 breaths per minute; tidal volume 900 cc; FIO_2 0.6
- Enteral nutrition at 25 ml/hr via small-bore feeding tube
- Indwelling urinary catheter to bedside drainage
- Chest physical therapy every 4 hours
- Gentamycin (Garamycin) 80 mg IV q8hr
- Ceftriaxone (Rocephin) 1 g IV q12hr
- D_5NS with KCl 20 mEq/L at 100 ml/hr

Critical Thinking Questions

1. What are two reasons for intubation and mechanical ventilation in Mr. R.?
2. What do Mr R.'s ABGs demonstrate, and what ventilator setting(s) should be changed and why?
3. What is his PaO_2/FIO_2 ratio, and what does it signify?
4. How can the nurse decrease Mr. R.'s chances of aspiration?
5. What clinical signs would the nurse expect to see if Mr. R.'s condition worsens?
6. What clinical signs would the nurse expect to see if Mr. R.'s pulmonary condition improves?
7. As Mr. R. begins to regain consciousness, what psychosocial aspects of his care will change and why?
8. Given Mr. R.'s vital signs, what effect might be expected if he were placed on 10 cm of PEEP and why?
9. Based on the assessment data presented, write one or more appropriate nursing diagnoses. Are there any collaborative problems?

Table **63-17** Cross-References to Other Critical Care Content

Topic	Discussed in Chapter
Acute congestive heart failure	33
Acute myocardial infarction	32
Acute respiratory distress syndrome	62
Acute respiratory failure	62
Advanced cardiac life support	34
Burns	23
Cardiac arrhythmias	34
Cardiac pacemakers	34
Cardiac surgery	33
Cardiopulmonary resuscitation	34
Emergencies	64
Head injury	54
Multiple organ dysfunction syndrome	61
Oxygen delivery	27
Pulmonary edema	33
Renal dialysis	44
Shock	61
Systemic inflammatory response syndrome	61
Total parenteral nutrition	38
Tracheostomy	25
Trauma	64

Environmental Control

Controlling the patient's environment and exercising judgment in nursing interventions have been shown to affect ICP. Each patient should be managed individually by observing the effects of nursing interventions and tailoring care accordingly. Suctioning, turning, and painful procedures are all possible factors that increase ICP. The nurse should space interventions that have an adverse effect and allow the patient's ICP to recover between nursing interventions. The nurse should watch the patient's ICP and hemodynamic parameters for changes when family members interact with the patient. Those individuals with a soothing effect should be included in simple care and comfort measures. Noise, lighting, and other noxious stimuli (identified at the beginning of this chapter) should be controlled. Conversation in the patient's room should not be loud. The nurse should speak quietly and address comments to the patient as though the patient were awake and participating in his or her care.

OTHER CRITICAL CARE CONTENT

Table 63-17 lists additional critical care content presented in other chapters of this text.

REVIEW QUESTIONS

The number of the question corresponds to the same-numbered objective at the beginning of the chapter.

1. The critical care unit is
   a. the best place for dying patients to be cared for.
   b. a special care unit found only in large metropolitan hospitals.
   c. where all patients requiring mechanical ventilation must be placed.
   d. best used for patients who have sustained (or are at risk for) life-threatening illness or injury.
2. Certification in critical care nursing by the American Association of Critical Care Nurses indicates that a nurse
   a. is master's prepared to provide advanced critical care.
   b. has demonstrated clinical competency in caring for critically ill patients.
   c. is an advanced practice nurse specialist in the care of acutely ill patients.
   d. may practice independently to provide symptom management for the critically ill.
3. An appropriate nursing intervention for the patient with delirium in the ICU is
   a. using tranquilizers to establish normal sleep patterns.
   b. identifying the factors contributing to the patient's confusion and irritability.
   c. sedating the patient with psychotropic drugs to protect the patient from harmful behaviors.
   d. silencing all alarms, overhead paging, and conversations around the patient.
4. The critical care nurse recognizes that an ideal plan for family involvement includes
   a. a family member at the bedside at all times.
   b. allowing family at the bedside at preset, brief intervals.
   c. an individually devised plan with family involved with care and comfort measures.
   d. prohibition of visiting in the ICU because the environment is too threatening to visitors.
5. To establish hemodynamic monitoring for a patient, the nurse zeros
   a. pressure monitoring systems to the level of the catheter tip.
   b. cardiac output monitoring systems to the level of the left ventricle.
   c. pressure monitoring systems to the level of the left atrium, identified as the phlebostatic axis.
   d. pressure monitoring systems to the level of the right atrium, identified as the midaxillary line.
6. A patient with a ventricular assist device (VAD) is assessed for complications that include
   a. bleeding.
   b. cardiogenic shock.
   c. aortic valve insufficiency.
   d. severe pulmonary disease.
7. The hemodynamic changes the nurse expects to find after successful initiation of an intraaortic balloon pump in a patient in cardiogenic shock include
   a. ↓ PAWP and ↑ CO.
   b. ↓ CVP and ↑ right atrial pressure.
   c. ↓ SVR and ↓ stroke volume.
   d. ↑ diastolic BP and ↓ systolic BP.
8. When caring for a patient with an endotracheal tube, the nurse is assessing for the development of
   a. accidental extubation.
   b. a negative inspiratory force.
   c. increased intracranial pressure.
   d. positive end-expiratory pressure.
9. The nursing management of a patient with an artificial airway includes
   a. routine suctioning of the tube at least every 2 hours.
   b. observing for cardiac arrhythmias during suctioning.
   c. maintaining endotracheal tube cuff pressure at 30 cm H_2O.
   d. preventing tube dislodgment by limiting mouth care to lubrication of the lips.
10. The nurse monitors the patient with positive pressure mechanical ventilation for
    a. paralytic ileus because pressure on the abdominal contents affects bowel motility.

b. diuresis and sodium depletion because of increased release of atrial natriuretic peptide.
c. signs of cardiovascular insufficiency because pressure in the chest impedes venous return.
d. respiratory acidosis in a patient with COPD because of alveolar hyperventilation and increased PaO_2 levels.

11. In a patient with intracranial pressure monitoring the nurse identifies a normal waveform as
    a. plateau waves.
    b. a P3 wave following the dicrotic notch.
    c. sharp, rhythmic elevations of 20 to 40 mm Hg lasting 30 seconds to 2 minutes.
    d. rhythmic pressure elevations of less than 20 mm Hg at a frequency of one every 4 to 8 minutes.
12. While caring for a patient with increased intracranial pressure the nurse recognizes that
    a. the MAP should be maintained below 60 mm Hg.
    b. hypoxemia decreases cerebral blood volume and ICP.
    c. ICP may be decreased by draining cerebrospinal fluid.
    d. the head should be flexed to the right to facilitate venous return from the head.

References

1. Nightingale F: *Notes on hospitals,* ed 3, Longman, 1863, Roberts-Green.
2. Goldhill DR, Summer A: Outcome of intensive care patients in a group of British intensive care units, *Crit Care Med* 26:1337, 1998.
3. Wong DT and others: Evaluation of predictive ability of APACHE II system and hospital outcome in Canadian intensive care unit patients, *Crit Care Med* 23: 1175, 1995.
4. Nasraway SA and others: American College of Critical Care Medicine of the Society of Critical Care Medicine. Guidelines on admission and discharge for adult intermediate care units, *Crit Care Med* 26: 607, 1998.
5. Clark S, Fontaine D, Simpson T: Recognition, assessment, and treatment of anxiety in the critical care setting, *Crit Care Nurse* 14(suppl):2, 1994.
6. Schelling G and others: Health-related quality of life and posttraumatic stress disorder in survivors of the acute respiratory distress syndrome, *Crit Care Med* 26:651,1998.
7. Tess MM: Acute confusional states in critically ill patients: a review, *J Neurosci Nurs* 23:398, 1991.
8. Geary S: Intensive care unit psychosis revisited: understanding and managing delirium in the critical care setting, *Crit Care Nurs Q* 17:51, 1994.
9. Kahn DM and others: Identification and modification of environmental noise in an ICU setting, *Chest* 114:535, 1998.
10. Fontaine DK: Measurement of nocturnal sleep patterns in trauma patients, *Heart Lung* 18:402, 1989.
11. Meyer TJ and others: Adverse environmental conditions in the respiratory and medical ICU settings, *Chest* 105:1211, 1994.
12. Richards KC, Bairnsfather L: A description of night sleep patterns in the critical care unit, *Heart Lung* 17:35, 1988.
13. Grozinger M, Kogel P, Roschke J: Effects of lorazepam on the automatic online evaluation of sleep EEG data in healthy volunteers, *Pharmacopsychiatry* 31:55, 1998.
14. Simpson T: The family as a source of support for the critically ill adult, *AACN Clin Issues Crit Care Nurs* 2:229, 1991.
15. Daly K and others: The effect of two nursing interventions on families of ICU patients, *Clin Nurs Res* 3:414, 1994.
16. Woods SL, Grose BL, Laurent-Bopp D: Effect of backrest position on pulmonary artery pressures in acutely ill patients, *Cardiovasc Nurs* 18:19, 1982.
17. Davidson J and others: Intra-aortic balloon pump: indications and complications, *J Natl Med Assoc* 90:137, 1998.
18. Busch T and others: Vascular complications related to intraaortic balloon counterpulsation: an analysis of ten years experience, *Thorac Cardiovasc Surg* 45:55, 1997.
19. Tatar H and others: Vascular complications of intraaortic balloon pumping: unsheathed versus sheathed insertion, *Ann Thorac Surg* 55:1518, 1993.
20. Oz MC and others: Screening scale predicts patients successfully receiving long-term implantable left ventricular assist devices, *Circulation* 92:II169, 1995.
21. Antonelli M and others: A comparison of noninvasive positive-pressure ventilation and conventional mechanical ventilation in patients with acute respiratory failure, *N Engl J Med* 339:429, 1998.
22. Luce JM, Pierson DJ, Tyler ML: *Intensive respiratory care,* Philadelphia, 1993, Saunders.
*23. Stone KS: Ventilator versus manual resuscitation bag as the method for delivering hyperoxygenation before endotracheal suctioning, *AACN Clin Issues Crit Care Nurs* 1:289, 1990.
24. Shekerdemian LS and others: Cardiopulmonary interactions after Fontan operations: augmentation of cardiac output using negative pressure ventilation, *Circulation* 96:3934, 1997.
25. Sassoon CS: Positive pressure ventilation: alternate modes, *Chest* 100:1421, 1991.
26. Burns SM: Advances in ventilator therapy, *Focus Crit Care* 17:227, 1990.
27. Wright SE, Heffner JE: Positive pressure mechanical ventilation augments left ventricular function in acute mitral regurgitation, *Chest* 102:1625, 1992.
28. Schoeffel U and others: The influence of ischemic bowel wall damage on translocation, inflammatory response, and clinical course, *Am J Surg* 174:39, 1997.
29. Daly BJ, Thomas D, Dyer MA: Procedures used in withdrawal of mechanical ventilation, *Am J Crit Care* 5:331, 1996.
*30. Sevick MA and others: Home-based ventilator-dependent patients: measurement of the emotional aspects of home caregiving, *Heart Lung* 23:269, 1994.
*31. Smith CE and others: Caregiver learning needs and reactions to managing home mechanical ventilation, *Heart Lung* 23:157, 1994.
32. Czarnik B: Home care for the patient receiving mechanical ventilation, *Home Healthc Nurse* 15:777, 1997.
33. Doyle DJ, Mark PWS: Analysis of intracranial pressure, *J Clin Monit* 8:81, 1992.
34. Hickey JV: Intracranial pressure: theory and management of increased intracranial pressure. In Hickey JV, editor: *The clinical practice of neurological and neurosurgical nursing,* ed 4, Philadelphia, 1997, Lippincott.
35. McNair ND: Intracranial pressure monitoring. In Clochesy J and others, editors: *Critical care nursing,* ed 2, Philadelphia, 1996, Saunders.
36. Kerr ME and others: Head-injured adults: recommendations for endotracheal suctioning, *J Neurosci Nurs* 25:86, 1993.
*37. Kerr ME, Brucia J: Hyperventilation in the head injured patient: an effective treatment modality? *Heart Lung* 22:516, 1993.
38. Bullock R and others: Guidelines for the management of severe head injury, Brain Trauma Foundation, *Eur J Emerg Med* 3:109, 1996.
39. Bullock R: Mannitol and other diuretics in severe neurotrauma, *New Horizons* 3:448, 1995.
40. Prielapp RC, Coursin DB: Sedative and neuromuscular blocking drug use in critically ill patients with head injuries, *New Horizons* 3:456, 1995.

*Nursing research-based articles.

Resources

American Association of Critical Care Nurses (AACN)
One Civic Plaza, Suite 330
Newport Beach, CA 92660
714-644-9310
http://www.aacn.org

Anesthesia and Critical Care Website
University of Chicago
5841 S. Maryland
MC 4028
Chicago, IL 60637
773-702-6700
Fax: 773-702-3535
http://dacc.uchicago.edu/

For additional Internet resources, see the website for this book at www.mosby.com/MERLIN/medsurg_lewis

REMEMBER to check out your companion CD-ROM

64 NURSING MANAGEMENT Emergency Care Situations

Lorene Newberry

www.mosby.com/MERLIN/medsurg_lewis

LEARNING OBJECTIVES

1. Describe the sequential steps in the assessment of a patient in an emergency situation.
2. Explain the pathophysiology, assessment, and collaborative care of select environmental emergencies related to thermoregulation, near drowning, and animal bites.
3. Discuss the pathophysiology, assessment, and collaborative care of select toxicologic emergencies.

Most patients with life-threatening or potentially life-threatening problems enter the hospital through the emergency department (ED). Visits to the ED have increased significantly because of the lack of health insurance, increased violence, and inability to access health care. Emergency nurses care for patients of all ages and with a variety of problems. However, some EDs specialize in certain patient populations or conditions, such as pediatric ED or chest pain ED.

Specific emergency management of patients with various medical, surgical, and traumatic emergencies are presented throughout this book where the disorders are discussed. Tables that highlight emergency management of specific problems are presented throughout the book. Table 64-1 lists each emergency management table by title, number, and page location. This chapter focuses on initial assessment and management of the trauma patient and emergency conditions not addressed elsewhere in this book, including heat- and cold-related emergencies, near drowning, bites, stings, and poisonings.

CARE OF THE EMERGENCY PATIENT

Recognition of life-threatening illness or injury is one of the most important aspects of emergency care. Before a diagnosis can be made, recognition of dangerous clinical signs and symptoms with initiation of interventions to reverse or prevent a crisis is essential. This process begins with the first patient contact. The emergency nurse is usually confronted with multiple patients who have a variety of problems. Prompt identification of patients requiring immediate treatment and determination of appropriate treatment area are essential in a busy ED.[1]

A triage system identifies and categorizes patients so the most critical are treated first. *Triage* is a French word meaning "to sort."[2] The process is based on the premise that patients with a threat to life, vision, or limb should be treated before other patients. The ED may use a system of words, color coding, numbers for triage acuity, or the ED may use international codes (Table 64-2).

The emergency nurse must complete an initial assessment to determine the presence of actual or potential threats to life and then rapidly initiate interventions appropriate for the patient's condition.[3] A history is obtained simultaneously. A systematic approach to the initial patient assessment decreases the time required to identify potential threats and minimizes the risk of missing a life-threatening condition. Two systematic approaches, a primary and secondary survey, were initially developed for use with the trauma patient, but these can be easily applied to assessment of any emergency patient.

PRIMARY SURVEY

The primary survey (Table 64-3) focuses on airway, breathing, and circulation and serves to identify life-threatening problems so that appropriate interventions can be initiated.[4] Life-threatening problems related to the airway (Table 64-4), breathing (Table 64-5), or circulation (Table 64-6) may be identified during the primary survey and appropriate interventions started immediately.

A = Airway with Cervical Spine Immobilization

Nearly all immediate trauma deaths occur because of airway obstruction. Saliva, bloody secretions, vomitus, direct trauma, laryngeal trauma, facial trauma, fractures, and the tongue can obstruct the airway. Medical patients at risk for airway compromise include those who have seizures, near drowning, anaphylaxis, foreign body obstruction, or are in cardiopulmonary arrest. If an airway is not maintained, obstruction of air flow occurs and hypoxia, acidosis, and death result.

Signs and symptoms of a compromised airway are presented in Table 64-4. Airway maintenance should progress rapidly from the least to the most invasive method. Treatment

Reviewed by Darlene F. Schelper, RN, MSN, CEN, RNC, Clinical Nurse Educator of Emergency Services, Hershey Medical Center, Penn State Geisinger Health System, Hershey, Penn.

includes suctioning of secretions, jaw thrust maneuver (avoiding hyperextension of the neck) (Fig. 64-1, p. 1962), insertion of a nasopharyngeal or oropharyngeal airway (will cause gag if patient is conscious), forward sitting position if no cervical spine injuries are present, and intubation. If unable to intubate because of airway obstruction, an emergency surgical cricothyrotomy or tracheotomy should be performed (see Chapter 25).

Any patient with significant upper torso injuries or face, head, or neck trauma should always be suspected of cervical spine trauma. The cervical spine must be kept in alignment and immobilized during assessment of the airway. The cervical spine is immobilized with a stiff immobilization collar, soft rolls are taped to a backboard on either side of the head, and the patient's forehead is taped to the backboard. Sandbags should not be used because the weight of the bags could move the head if the patient must be turned.

B = Breathing

Adequate air flow through the upper airway does not ensure adequate ventilation. Breathing alterations are caused by many conditions, including fractured ribs, pneumothorax, penetrating injury, allergic reactions, pulmonary emboli, and asthma attacks (see Table 64-5). Every injured or ill patient has an increased metabolic and oxygen demand and should have supplemental oxygen. Life-threatening conditions such as tension pneumothorax, open pneumothorax, and flail chest can compromise ventilation. Treatment for a nonbreathing patient includes bag valve mask ventilation with 100% oxygen, intubation, and treatment of the underlying cause.

C = Circulation

An effective circulatory system includes the heart, intact blood vessels, and adequate blood volume. (Life-threatening circulation problems are presented in Table 64-6.) Uncontrolled bleeding places a person at risk for hemorrhagic shock. The patient's carotid or femoral pulse should be checked because peripheral pulses may be absent as a result of direct injury or vasoconstriction. Delayed capillary refill (longer than 3 seconds) and altered mental status are the most significant signs of shock. Care must be taken when evaluating capillary refill in cold environments because cold delays refill.

IV lines are inserted into veins in the upper extremities unless contraindicated, such as in a massive fracture or an injury that affects limb circulation. Two large-gauge IV catheters should be inserted and aggressive fluid resuscitation initiated using lactated Ringer's solution or normal saline. Direct pressure with a sterile dressing should be applied to obvious bleeding sites. Blood samples are obtained for a type and crossmatch; electrolyte, glucose, blood urea nitrogen, and creatinine levels; complete blood cell count; and coagulation studies. Blood samples may also be obtained for alcohol or drug levels or liver or cardiac enzyme levels. The patient should be monitored by electrocardiogram (ECG) for arrhythmias. Type-specific packed red blood cells should be administered if needed.

✚EMERGENCY MANAGEMENT

Table 64-1 Emergency Management Tables

Table 64-2 Triage Acuity Systems

	Emergent	Urgent	Nonurgent	Expectant
Colors	Red	Yellow	Green	Black
Numbers	Priority I	Priority II	Priority III	Priority 0
Urgency	Life-threatening; needs immediate attention	Needs treatment in 20 minutes to 2 hours	Can wait hours or days	Dying or dead
Example	Trauma, chest pain, respiratory distress, chemicals in the eyes, arm or leg amputation, shock	Fever >104° F (40° C), diastolic blood pressure >130 mm Hg, kidney stone, simple fracture	Sprain, minor laceration, flulike symptoms, rash, chronic headache	Massive head trauma, cardiopulmonary arrest

Table 64-3 Primary Survey of an Emergency Patient

Assessment	Intervention
Airway with Cervical Spine ■ Clear and open airway ■ Assess for obstructed airway ■ Assess for respiratory distress ■ Check for loose teeth or foreign objects ■ Assess for bleeding, vomitus, or edema	■ Suction ■ Jaw thrust ■ Nasal or oral airway, endotracheal tube, cricothyrotomy ■ Cervical spine immobilization using collar, backboard, soft rolls; tape forehead
Breathing ■ Assess ventilation Look for chest movements associated with breathing Note use of accessory muscles or abdominal muscles Listen for air being expired through nose and mouth Feel for air being expelled ■ Observe and count respiratory rate ■ Note color of nail beds, mucous membranes, skin ■ Auscultate lungs ■ Assess for jugular venous distention and position of trachea	■ Ventilate with bag-valve mask with 100% O_2 ■ Prepare to intubate if respiratory arrest ■ Have suction available ■ Give supplemental oxygen via appropriate delivery system ■ If head trauma, hyperventilate with 100% O_2 ■ If absent breath sounds, perform needle thoracostomy and prepare for chest tube insertion
Circulation ■ Check carotid or femoral pulse ■ Assess color, temperature, and moisture of skin ■ Assess level of consciousness ■ Check capillary refill ■ Assess for external bleeding	■ If absent pulse, begin chest compressions ■ If shock symptoms or hypotensive, start IVs with at least two large-bore (14-16 gauge) IV catheters with normal saline or lactated Ringer's solution ■ Administer blood products if ordered ■ Consider autotransfusion if isolated chest trauma ■ Obtain blood samples for type and crossmatch ■ Control bleeding with direct pressure
Disability ■ Assess level of consciousness ■ Assess response to verbal and painful stimuli ■ Assess extremity movement (all four) ■ Perform Glasgow Coma Scale (Table 54-2) ■ Check pupil response to light	■ Periodically reassess level of consciousness

Table 64-4 Life-Threatening Airway Problems

Problem	Signs and Symptoms	Interventions
Airway obstruction (complete or partial)	■ Dyspnea, labored respirations ■ Decreased or no air movement ■ Cyanosis ■ Presence of foreign body in airway ■ Trauma to face or neck	Airway opening maneuvers ■ Jaw thrust ■ Chin lift ■ Suction Airway adjuncts ■ Nasal airway ■ Oral airway ■ Endotracheal tube (ET) Surgical airway ■ Cricothyrotomy ■ Tracheostomy
Inhalation injury	■ History of enclosed space fire, unconsciousness, or exposure to heavy smoke ■ Dyspnea ■ Wheezing, rhonchi, crackles ■ Hoarseness ■ Singed facial or nasal hairs ■ Carbonaceous sputum ■ Burns to face or neck	■ Provide high-flow oxygen (100%) via non-rebreather mask or bag-valve device ■ Prepare for endotracheal intubation as soon as possible

From Kidd PS, Stuart P: *Mosby's emergency nursing reference,* St Louis, 1996, Mosby.

Table 64-5 Life-Threatening Breathing Problems

Problem	Signs and Symptoms	Interventions
Tension pneumothorax	■ Dyspnea, labored respirations ■ Decreased or absent breath sounds on affected side ■ Unilateral chest rise and fall ■ Tracheal deviation away from affected side ■ Cyanosis ■ Jugular venous distention ■ Tachycardia and hypotension ■ History of chest trauma or mechanical ventilation	■ Provide high-flow oxygen (100%) via non-rebreather mask or bag-valve device ■ Rapid chest decompression by needle thoracostomy on affected side ■ Chest tube placement on affected side
Pneumothorax	■ Dyspnea, labored respirations ■ Decreased or absent breath sounds on affected side ■ May have unilateral chest rise and fall ■ May have visible wound to chest or back ■ History of chest trauma	■ Provide high-flow oxygen (100%) via non-rebreather mask or bag-valve device ■ Chest tube placement on affected side ■ Place occlusive dressing over any open chest wound and secure on three sides with tape
Hemothorax	■ Dyspnea, labored respirations ■ Decreased or absent breath sounds on affected side ■ May have unilateral chest rise and fall ■ Tachycardia and hypotension ■ May have visible wound to chest or back ■ History of chest trauma (usually penetrating)	■ Provide high-flow oxygen (100%) via non-rebreather mask or bag-valve device ■ Chest tube placement on affected side ■ Consider autotransfusion
Sucking chest wound	■ Dyspnea, labored respirations ■ Visible, sucking wound to chest or back ■ Decreased or absent breath sounds on affected side	■ Provide high-flow oxygen (100%) via non-rebreather mask or bag-valve device ■ Cover wound with occlusive dressing and secure on 3 sides with tape ■ Watch for signs of tension pneumothorax and remove dressing during exhalation if they are noted
Flail chest	■ Dyspnea, labored respirations ■ Paradoxical chest wall movement ■ Chest pain ■ Tachycardia	■ Provide high-flow oxygen (100%) via non-rebreather mask or bag-valve device ■ Prepare for intubation and mechanical ventilation

Modified from Kidd PS, Stuart P: *Mosby's emergency nursing reference,* St Louis, 1996, Mosby.

Table 64-6 Life-Threatening Circulation Problems

Problem	Signs and Symptoms	Interventions
External hemorrhage	■ Obvious bleeding site	■ Direct pressure ■ Elevation of extremity
Shock	■ Tachycardia ■ Weak, thready pulses ■ Cool, pale, clammy skin ■ Tachypnea ■ Altered mental status ■ Delayed capillary refill ■ Oliguria or anuria	■ Provide high-flow oxygen (100%) via non-rebreather mask or bag-valve device ■ Place two large-bore IV lines with warm isotonic crystalloid solution (lactated Ringer's or 0.9% NaCl) ■ Administer fluid bolus (2 L in adults) ■ Prepare to administer blood

From Kidd PS, Stuart P: *Mosby's emergency nursing reference,* St Louis, 1996, Mosby.

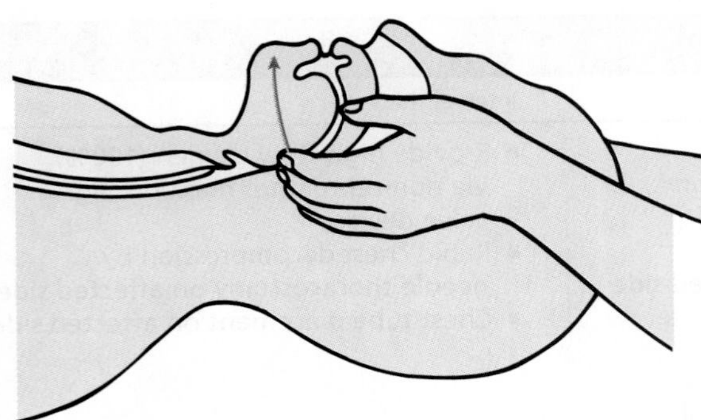

Fig. 64-1 Jaw-thrust maneuver is the only widely recommended procedure for use on an unconscious patient with possible neck or spinal injuries. The patient should be lying supine with the rescuer kneeling at the top of the head. The rescuer should carefully reach forward and gently place one hand on each side of the patient's chin at the lateral angles of the lower jaw. The patient's head should be stabilized with the rescuer's forearms, then the jaw pushed forward while pressure is applied with the index fingers.

D = Disability

A brief neurologic examination should follow the primary survey. Level of consciousness and pupil size and reactivity to light should be assessed. A simple mnemonic to remember is AVPU: A = alert, V = responds to verbal stimuli, P = responds to painful stimuli, and U = unresponsive. Extremities should be observed for spontaneous movement and assessed for sensation. A Glasgow Coma Scale score is calculated (see Chapter 54, Table 54-2).

E = Expose

All trauma patients should have their clothes removed so that a thorough physical assessment can be performed. The patient should be covered with warm blankets to prevent hypothermia.

SECONDARY SURVEY

The secondary survey should not be done until the primary survey is complete. During the primary survey, life-threatening airway, breathing, or circulation problems are corrected as quickly as possible. Once this has been accomplished, a secondary survey is initiated. The secondary survey involves obtaining a history, identifying all injuries, and performing a head-to-toe assessment, including an evaluation of the patient's back (Table 64-7).

F = Fahrenheit

The patient is kept warm with warm IV fluids, warm blankets, and overhead warming lights. Trauma patients and ill medical patients are at risk for hypothermia caused by hypovolemia and environmental exposure.

G = Get Vital Signs

A complete set of vital signs, including blood pressure, heart rate, respiratory rate, temperature, and oxygen saturation, should be obtained after the patient is exposed. The patient's heart rate and rhythm should be monitored.

H = History and Head-to-Toe Assessment

The history of the incident, accident, or illness provides clues to the cause of the crisis and suggests specific assessment needs.

The patient may be unable to give a history, but family, friends, and witnesses can frequently provide information. An experienced ED team can complete a history within 5 minutes of the patient's arrival. If the patient is emergently ill, a thorough history is obtained from the friends or family after the patient is taken to the treatment area. The history should include the following questions:

1. What is the chief complaint? What caused the person to seek attention?
2. How long ago did the accident or incident occur? How long ago did the patient become ill?
3. Where did the accident or incident occur? Where did the patient become ill?
4. Describe the accident, incident, or illness. How did it happen? Details of the incident are extremely important because the mechanism can indicate specific injuries. For example, a front seat passenger with a lap belt may have a head injury from hitting the windshield; knee, femur, or hip fractures or dislocation from striking the dashboard; and an abdominal injury from the lap belt. If other victims were dead at the scene, the patient has a high chance of significant injury.

   Patients who jump from buildings or bridges may have bilateral calcaneal fractures, bilateral wrist fractures, lumbar spine compression fractures, and be at risk for aortic tears. Older patients who have climbed ladders and fallen may have had a cerebrovascular accident or myocardial infarction that led to the fall. Bullets can ricochet in the body if they strike bone. It is essential to determine the number of shots fired and to look for entry and exit wounds. A patient shot in the abdomen may have a bullet lodged in the right shoulder. The bullet trajectory may have gone through the liver and lung en route to the shoulder.
5. What has happened since the onset of the illness or injury?
   a. Has the patient been moved?
   b. What emergency care was started at the scene of the incident?
   c. What are the patient's subjective complaints?
   d. What are witnesses' (if any) descriptions of the patient's behavior since the onset?
6. What is the patient's health care history? The mnemonic AMPLE assists the nurse in remembering what to ask:

   A Allergies
   M Medications (current medications that the patient is taking)
   P Past health history (especially cardiac and respiratory conditions and diabetes), pregnancy status
   L Last meal
   E Events preceding illness or injury

Head, Neck, and Face. The patient should be assessed for general appearance, skin color, and temperature. The eyes should be evaluated for extraocular movements. A disconjugate gaze is an indication of neurologic damage. Raccoon eyes or periorbital ecchymosis is usually caused by a basilar skull fracture. The tympanic membranes and external canal are checked for blood and cerebrospinal fluid. Drainage from the ear should not be stopped.

The throat and airway are assessed for bruising, foreign bodies, bleeding, edema, loose or missing teeth, difficulty swal-

Table 64-7 Secondary Survey of an Emergency Patient

Parameter	Assessment
Expose	■ Remove clothing for adequate examination.
Fahrenheit	■ Keep patient warm with warm blankets, IV fluids, overhead lights
Get Vital Signs	■ Blood pressure ■ Pulse, cardiac rhythm ■ Respiratory rate and effort ■ Temperature ■ Oxygen saturation ■ Urinary catheter if not contraindicated ■ Gastric tube ■ Laboratory studies for presenting condition
History and Head-to-Toe Assessment	
History	■ Length of time since incident occurred ■ Accident type, location, and patient's position in accident ■ Description of accident, incident, or illness ■ Allergies ■ Medications ■ Past health history, pregnancy ■ Last meal ■ Events leading to accident, incident, or illness
Head, Neck, Face	■ Examine face and scalp for lacerations, bone or soft tissue deformity, tenderness, bleeding, and foreign objects ■ Examine eyes, ears, nose, and mouth for bleeding, foreign bodies, drainage, pain, deformity, ecchymosis, lacerations ■ Examine head for depressions of cranial or facial bones, contusions, hematomas, areas of softness, bony crepitus ■ Examine neck for stiffness, pain in cervical vertebrae, tracheal deviation, distended neck veins, bleeding, edema, difficulty swallowing, bruising, subcutaneous emphysema, bony crepitus
Chest	■ Rate, depth, and character of breathing ■ Anterior and posterior chest wall movement ■ Palpate for bony crepitus, subcutaneous emphysema ■ Use of accessory muscles ■ External signs of injury: petechiae, bleeding, cyanosis, bruises, abrasions, lacerations, old scars
Abdomen and Pelvis	■ Symmetry of external abdominal wall and bony structures ■ External signs of injury: bruising, abrasions, lacerations, punctures ■ Assess for masses, guarding, femoral pulses ■ Type and location of pain ■ Bowel sounds ■ Rigidity or distention of abdomen ■ Assess genitalia for blood at the meatus, priapism, ecchymosis, rectal bleeding, anal sphincter tone
Extremities	■ Signs of external injury: deformity, ecchymosis, abrasions, lacerations, swelling ■ Pain ■ Movement and strength in arms and legs ■ Sensation in each limb ■ Color skin ■ Presence and quality of peripheral pulses
Back	■ Log-roll and inspect and palpate back for deformity, bleeding, lacerations, bruising

lowing, movement of the palate, and ability to open the mouth. Neck examination includes palpation and visualization of the trachea to determine that it is in the midline. A deviated trachea may signal a life-threatening tension pneumothorax. Subcutaneous emphysema may indicate laryngotracheal disruption. A stiff or painful cervical spine area may signify a fracture of a cervical vertebra. The cervical spine *must* be protected using a rigid collar, backboard, towel rolls or other soft rolls on either side of the head, and the forehead should be taped to the backboard.

Chest. The chest is examined for paradoxical chest movements and large sucking chest wounds. The sternum, clavicles, and ribs are palpated for deformity and point tenderness. The chest is assessed for pain on palpation, respiratory distress, decreased breath sounds, distant heart sounds, and distended neck veins. In addition to tension pneumothorax and open

Table 64-8 Prophylaxis Against Tetanus in Wound Management

History of Tetanus Toxoid (Doses)	Type of Wound			
	Tetanus-Prone Wound		Non–Tetanus-Prone Wound	
	Td	TIG*	Td	TIG
Unknown to fewer than three	Yes	Yes	Yes	No
Three or more†	No‡	No	No§	No

*When TIG and Td are administered concurrently, separate sites and syringes must be used.
†If only three doses of fluid toxoid have been received, a fourth dose of toxoid, preferably absorbed toxoid, should be given.
‡Yes, if more than 5 years since last dose.
§Yes, if more than 10 years since last dose.
Td, tetanus and diphtheria toxoid absorbed (for adult use); *TIG,* tetanus immunoglobulin (human).

pneumothorax, the patient should be evaluated for rib fractures, pulmonary contusion, myocardial contusion, and simple pneumothorax. A 12-lead ECG should be obtained, particularly on an older patient or a patient with suspected heart disease. The ECG should be done to detect arrhythmias (e.g., bradycardia).

Abdomen and Pelvis. The abdomen is more difficult to assess. Frequent evaluation for subtle changes in the abdominal examination is essential. Blunt trauma can be caused by motor vehicle collisions and assaults. Penetrating trauma tends to injure specific organs. Decreased bowel sounds may indicate a temporary paralytic ileus. Bowel sounds in the chest may indicate a diaphragmatic rupture. The abdomen is percussed for gastric distention and peritoneal irritation. A dull sound indicates blood or fluid. The pelvis is gently palpated. If pain is elicited, it may indicate a pelvic fracture. The genitalia are inspected for bleeding and obvious injuries. A rectal examination is performed to check for blood, a high-riding prostate, and loss of sphincter tone.

Extremities. The upper and lower extremities are assessed. Injured extremities are splinted above and below the injury to decrease further soft tissue injury and pain. Grossly deformed, pulseless extremities should be realigned and splinted. Pulses are checked before and after movement of an extremity. The extremities are palpated for point tenderness, crepitus, and abnormal movements. Injured extremities should be elevated and ice packs applied. Prophylactic antibiotics are administered for open fractures. Patients with fractures should receive analgesia.

Back. The trauma patient should always be turned (using spinal precautions) to inspect the back. The back is inspected for ecchymosis, abrasions, puncture wounds, cuts, and obvious deformities. The entire spine is palpated for misalignment, deformity, and pain.

INTERVENTION AND EVALUATION

Regardless of the patient's chief complaint, a thorough assessment and an accurate history are critical in an emergency situation. Once the secondary survey is complete, all findings are recorded. Additional interventions may include placement of a nasogastric tube to decrease gastric distention. The contents of the nasogastric drainage should be checked for blood. A nasogastric tube should not be placed in the nares in a patient suspected of having a basilar skull fracture because the tube might enter the brain; rather, it should be placed orally. An indwelling catheter is inserted and urinary output monitored. Urine output should be at least 0.5 ml/kg/hr. An indwelling catheter should not be inserted if a urethral tear is suspected. Patients with pelvic injuries, blood at the meatus, or men with high-riding prostates are at risk for a urethral tear. A urethrogram should be obtained before a catheter is inserted. The urine should be checked for blood and a urine pregnancy test performed on women. All trauma patients should receive tetanus prophylaxis if the tetanus status is unknown (Table 64-8).

Depending on the patient's injuries, the patient is transported for diagnostic tests such as a CT scan, x-ray, or MRI or admitted to a general or intensive care unit. The emergency nurse is responsible for monitoring the trauma patient during transport and notifying the trauma team should the patient's condition change from baseline.

DEATH IN THE EMERGENCY DEPARTMENT

Unfortunately, there are a number of emergency patients who do not benefit from the skill, expertise, and technology available in the ED. It is important for the emergency nurse to be able to deal with feelings about sudden death so that the nurse can help families and significant others begin the grieving process.

The emergency nurse should recognize the importance of certain hospital rituals in preparing the bereaved to grieve, such as collecting the belongings, arranging for an autopsy, viewing the body, and making mortuary arrangements. The death must seem real so that the significant others can begin to grieve and accept the death. The emergency nurse cannot afford to forget the surviving loved ones after a death in the ED. Family members may benefit from observing resuscitation of a loved one. Should a family member request to be present, it is essential that a member of the team explain care rendered and be available to answer questions.

ENVIRONMENTAL EMERGENCIES

Increased interest in outdoor activities such as running, hiking, cycling, skiing, sailing, and swimming has increased the number of environmental emergencies seen in the ED. Illness or injury may be caused by the activity, exposure to weather, or attack from various animals. Specific environmental emergencies discussed include heat stress and cold stress, drowning and near drowning, bites, and stings.

HEAT-RELATED EMERGENCIES

Brief exposure to intense heat or prolonged exposure to less intense heat leads to heat stress when thermoregulatory mechanisms such as sweating, vasodilation, and increased respirations cannot compensate for exposure to increased ambient

ETHICAL DILEMMAS

Brain Death

SITUATION

The emergency nurse receives a radio call from emergency medical technicians about a young male who has been involved in a motorcycle crash. The patient was not wearing a helmet and has a large open skull fracture with obvious gray matter oozing from the area. Transport from the accident scene was delayed by 45 minutes as a result of downed power lines. En route to the hospital the patient experiences cardiopulmonary arrest. Estimated arrival at the hospital is an additional 45 minutes as a result of severe weather. EMS personnel request permission to stop resuscitation efforts.

DISCUSSION

Degree of trauma and extent of brain damage in this patient has been complicated by delay in providing basic life support. Description of the patient's injuries associated with cardiopulmonary arrest suggest brain death. There is a slight chance that the patient's heart can be resuscitated; however, the likelihood that the patient's brain will survive is minuscule. A hospital is not obligated to continue futile medical care for a brain dead patient who cannot survive even with mechanical intervention.

ETHICAL AND LEGAL PRINCIPLES

The definition of brain death was originally made in 1968 by a Harvard Medical School ad hoc committee in response to technology that kept the heart and lungs functioning—even without brainstem activity.

- When a brain dead patient is maintained on mechanical support, the heart and lungs eventually cease functioning. It is medically futile to continue treatment of a brain dead patient.
- Brain death criteria do not address patients in a permanent vegetative state or anencephalic infants, since the brainstem in these patients is adequate to maintain function of the heart and lungs.

Table 64-9 Risk Factors for Heat-Related Emergencies

Age
Elderly
Infants
Environmental Conditions
High environmental temperature
High relative humidity
Low wind
Preexisting Illness
Cardiovascular disease
Previous stroke or other CNS lesion
Obesity
Diabetes
Cystic fibrosis
Skin disorders (e.g., large burn scars)
Prescription Drugs
Anticholinergics
Phenothiazines
Butyrophenones
Tricyclic antidepressants
Antihistamines
Antispasmodics
Diuretics
Antiparkinsonian drugs
β-Adrenergic blockers
Street Drugs
Lysergic acid diethylamide (LSD)
Jimsonweed
Amphetamines
Phencyclidine (PCP)
Alcohol

From Newberry L, editor: *Sheehy's emergency principles and practice,* ed 4, St Louis, 1998, Mosby.

temperatures.[5] Ambient temperature is a product of environmental temperature and humidity. (See Chapter 11 for discussion of thermoregulation.) Strenuous activities in hot or humid environments, clothing that interferes with perspiration, high fevers, and preexisting illnesses predispose individuals to heat stress (Table 64-9). Effects can be mild (heat rash and heat edema) or severe (heat exhaustion and heat stroke). Heat stress is a leading cause of death in athletes. Specific heat emergencies are heat rash, heat edema, heat cramps, heat syncope, heat exhaustion, and heat stroke (Table 64-10).

Heat rash (miliaria or prickly heat) is a fine, red, papular rash that occurs on the torso, neck, and skin folds.[6] The rash occurs when sweat ducts are obstructed and become inflamed so sweat excretion does not occur. The rash usually occurs in warm weather, but has also been reported in cold weather as a result of clothing.

Heat syncope is associated with prolonged standing and heat exposure. Manifestations include dizziness, orthostatic hypotension, and syncope. Inadequate vasomotor tone associated with aging place the elderly at greater risk for heat syncope.

Heat edema is characterized by swelling of the hands, feet, and ankles, usually in nonacclimatized individuals as a result of prolonged standing or sitting. Swelling usually resolves in days with rest, elevation, and support hose. Diuretics are not recommended as this condition is self-limiting and requires no additional treatment.

Heat cramps are severe cramps in large muscle groups fatigued by heavy work. Cramps are brief, intense, and tend to occur during rest after exercise or heavy labor. Nausea, tachycardia, pallor, weakness, and profuse diaphoresis are often present. The condition is seen most often in healthy, acclimated athletes with adequate fluid intake. Profuse sweating and ingestion of water or other salt-poor solutions deplete sodium and lead to hyponatremia. Cramps resolve rapidly with rest and oral or parenteral replacement of sodium and water. Elevation, gentle massage, and analgesia minimize pain associated with heat cramps. The patient should avoid strenuous activity for 12 hours after discharge. Education should emphasize salt replacement during strenuous exercise in hot, humid environments. Commercially prepared electrolyte solutions such as Gatorade, Powerade, and All Sport are recommended.

EMERGENCY MANAGEMENT

Table 64-10 Hyperthermia

Etiology	Assessment Findings	Interventions
Environmental Lack of acclimatization Prolonged exposure to extreme temperatures Hot tubs Physical exertion **Trauma** Head injury **Metabolic** Thyrotoxicosis Diabetes Dehydration **Drugs** Sympathomimetic drugs β-Adrenergic blockers Diuretics Cocaine Alcohol Antihistamines Tranquilizers **Other** Cardiovascular disease CNS lesions	**Heat Rash** ▪ Rash on torso, neck, skin folds **Heat Edema** ▪ Edema of hands, feet, ankles **Heat Cramps** ▪ Severe muscle contractions **Heat Syncope** ▪ Syncope ▪ Dizziness ▪ Hypotension **Heat Exhaustion** ▪ Fatigue, weakness ▪ Profuse sweating ▪ Anxiety, irritability ▪ Headache ▪ Nausea and vomiting ▪ Hypotension ▪ Tachycardia ▪ Weak, thready pulse ▪ Hypotension ▪ Cold, clammy skin ▪ Altered level of consciousness ▪ Rectal temperature ≥104° F (40° C) **Heat Stroke** ▪ Headache ▪ Chills ▪ Nausea, vomiting ▪ Ataxia ▪ Hot, dry skin ▪ Altered mental status ▪ Hypotension ▪ Tachycardia ▪ Seizures ▪ Coma ▪ Rectal temperature >105° F (40.6° C)	**Initial** ▪ Ensure patent airway. ▪ Refer to text for treatment of heat rash, heat edema, heat cramps, and heat syncope. ▪ Establish IV access and begin rapid fluid replacement for significant heat injury. ▪ Remove patient's clothing and begin cooling procedures by placing wet sheets over patient with ice packs in groin, neck, and torso. ▪ Obtain serum electrolytes, ECG, and CBC. ▪ Insert urinary catheter. ▪ Cool rapidly. Use cooling blanket if temperature does not decrease with evaporative measures. **Ongoing Monitoring** ▪ Monitor vital signs, level of consciousness, cardiac rhythm, oxygen saturation, electrolytes, and urinary output. ▪ Monitor urine for development of myoglobinuria secondary to muscle breakdown.

Heat Exhaustion

Prolonged exposure to heat over hours or days leads to heat exhaustion, a clinical syndrome characterized by fatigue, lightheadedness, nausea, vomiting, diarrhea, and feelings of impending doom (see Table 64-10). Tachypnea, hypotension, tachycardia, elevated body temperature, dilated pupils, mild confusion, ashen color, and profuse diaphoresis are also present. Orthostatic hypotension and mild to severe temperature elevation (98.6° F to 105° F [37° C to 40.6° C]) are due to dehydration.[7] Heat exhaustion usually occurs in individuals engaged in strenuous activity in hot, humid weather, but it also occurs in sedentary individuals.

Treatment begins with placement of the patient in a cool area and removal of constrictive clothing. Oral fluid and electrolyte replacement is initiated unless the patient is nauseated. Salt tablets are not recommended because of potential gastric irritation and hypernatremia. A 0.9% normal saline solution is initiated intravenously when oral solutions are not tolerated. An initial fluid bolus may be used to correct hypotension. However, fluid replacement should be correlated to clinical and laboratory parameters. A moist sheet placed over the patient decreases core temperature through evaporative heat loss. Hospital admission is considered for the elderly, chronically ill, or those who do not improve within 3 to 4 hours.

Heat Stroke

Heat stroke, the most serious form of heat stress, is common when excessive environmental temperature and high humidity occur over 3 or more days. Table 64-9 lists risk factors for heat-related emergencies, especially heat stroke. Increased sweating, vasodilation, and increased respiratory rate (the body's attempt to lower temperature) deplete fluids and electrolytes. Eventually, sweat glands stop functioning, so core temperature increases rapidly. The patient presents with core temperature greater than 105° F (40.6°C), altered mentation, absence of perspiration, and circulatory collapse. The skin is hot, dry, and ashen. The brain is extremely sensitive to thermal injuries so a range of neurologic symptoms occur, such as hallucinations, loss of muscle coordination, and combativeness. Cerebral edema and hemorrhage may occur as a result of direct thermal injury to the brain and decreased cerebral blood flow.

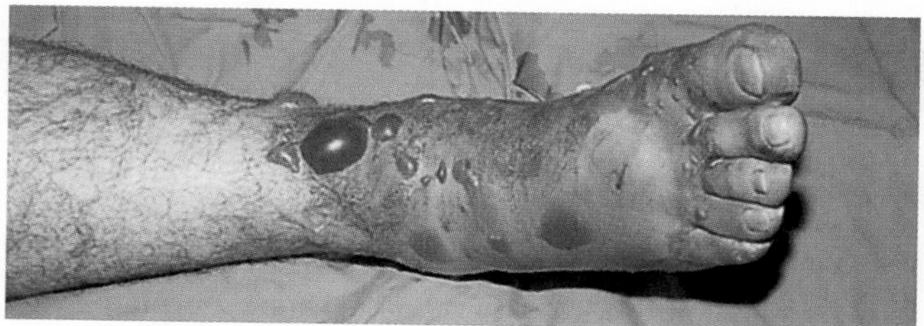

Fig. 64-2 Edema and blister formation 24 hours after frostbite injury occurring in an area covered by a tightly fitted boot.

Mortality with heat stroke approaches 70%.[8] Prognosis is related to age, health, and length of exposure. Older adults and individuals with diabetes mellitus, chronic renal disease, cardiovascular disease, pulmonary disease, or other physiologic compromise are particularly vulnerable.

Collaborative Care

Treatment of heat stroke focuses on rapid reduction of core temperature and treatment of subsequent complications. Administration of 100% oxygen compensates for the patient's hypermetabolic state. Intubation and ventilation with a bag valve mask may be required. Hypovolemia is usually not present. Therefore fluid resuscitation with 1 to 2 L of 0.9% normal saline solution over the first 4 hours is usually adequate. Lactated Ringer's solution is not recommended because the ischemic liver cannot metabolize lactate to bicarbonate.

Conventional cooling methods include tepid water mist, fans, and ice packs to the head, groin, axillae, and neck. Ice baths, alcohol rubs, and antipyretics should not be used. More aggressive cooling techniques are implemented when conventional techniques fail. Ice water immersion is not recommended, since the massive peripheral vasoconstriction that occurs can interfere with cooling. Cooling blankets are used. However, cooling from wet skin is 25 times more effective than cooling from dry skin.[9] Ice water lavage, cold water peritoneal dialysis, and cardiopulmonary bypass are used in extreme cases of hyperthermia.

Cooling efforts are complicated by shivering, since associated muscle activity increases core temperature. Chlorpromazine (Thorazine) IV is the drug of choice to suppress shivers. Aggressive temperature reduction should continue until core temperature reaches 102° F (38.8°C). Additional therapy includes corticosteroid therapy with methylprednisolone for cerebral edema and mannitol when urinary output is less than 0.5ml/kg/hr. Antipyretics are not recommended. Muscle breakdown associated with hypothermia leads to myoglobinuria, which places the kidneys at risk. Therefore urine should be carefully monitored for color, amount, pH, and hemoglobin.

COLD-RELATED EMERGENCIES

Cold injuries may be localized (frostbite) or systemic (hypothermia). Contributing factors include age, duration of exposure, environmental temperature, preexisting conditions (e.g., diabetes), medications that suppress shivering (narcotics, heroin, psychotropic agents, and antiemetics), and alcohol intoxication, which causes peripheral vasodilation, increases sensations of warmth, and depresses shivering. Smokers have an increased risk of cold-related injury as a result of the vasoconstrictive effects of nicotine.

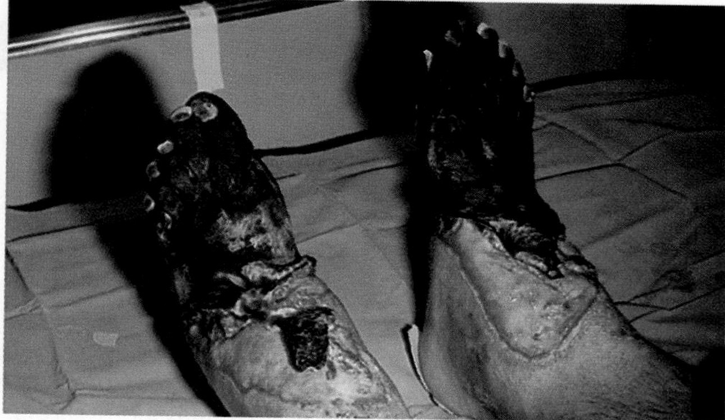

Fig. 64-3 Gangrenous necrosis 6 weeks after the frostbite injury shown in Fig. 64-2.

Frostbite

Peripheral vasoconstriction in response to cold exposure decreases blood flow. Average cutaneous blood flow in a 70-kg person is 200 to 250 ml/min. Heat stress increases this rate to as much as 7000 ml/min, whereas cold-related vasoconstriction may decrease cutaneous blood flow to ≤50 ml/min. As cellular temperature decreases and ice crystals form in intracellular spaces, intracellular sodium and chloride increase, the cell membrane is destroyed, and organelles are damaged. Depth of frostbite is the result of ambient temperature, length of exposure, type and condition (wet or dry) of clothing, and contact with metal surfaces. Other factors that affect severity include skin color (dark-skinned people are more prone to frostbite), lack of acclimatization, previous episodes, exhaustion, and poor peripheral vascular status.[10]

Superficial frostbite involves skin and subcutaneous tissue, usually the ears, nose, fingers, and toes. The skin is pale, waxy, and feels crunchy and frozen. The patient may complain of tingling, numbness, or a burning sensation. Injured tissue is easily damaged so the area should be handled carefully and never squeezed, massaged, or scrubbed. Clothing and jewelry should be removed because they may constrict the extremity and decrease circulation. The affected area should be elevated and warm soaks (104°-110° F [40°-43° C]) applied. The nurse should not attempt to warm the area by application of snow or ice or use of flame. The patient often experiences a warm, stinging sensation as tissue thaws. Blisters form within a few hours (Fig. 64-2). The blisters should be debrided and a sterile dressing applied. Heavy blankets and clothing should be avoided as friction and weight can lead to sloughing of damaged tissue. Rewarming is extremely painful. Residual pain may last weeks or even years. Analgesia should be administered and tetanus prophylaxis should be given as appropriate (see Table 64-8). The patient should be evaluated for systemic hypothermia.

Deep frostbite involves muscle, bone, and tendon. The skin is white, hard, and insensitive to touch. The area has the appearance of deep thermal injury with mottling gradually progressing to gangrene (Fig. 64-3). The affected extremity is submersed in a circulating water bath (104° F to 108° F [40° C to

+EMERGENCY MANAGEMENT

Table 64-11 Hypothermia

Etiology	Assessment Findings	Interventions
Environmental Prolonged exposure to cold Prolonged immersion Excessive perspiration Inadequate clothing for environmental temperature **Physiologic** Head injury Hypoglycemia **Iatrogenic** Cold IV fluids Blood administration Inadequate warming in the ED or surgery **Other** Drugs Ethanol	▪ Shivering ▪ Sleepiness ▪ Apathy ▪ Listlessness, areflexia ▪ Coma ▪ Cyanosis ▪ Decreased respiratory rate, pulse rate, temperature, blood pressure ▪ Blue, white, or frozen extremities ▪ Arrhythmias: bradycardia, asystole, ventricular fibrillation ▪ Intoxication ▪ History of exposure	**Initial** ▪ Remove patient from cold environment. ▪ Ensure patent airway. ▪ Administer oxygen via nasal cannula or non-rebreather mask. ▪ Establish IV access with two large-bore catheters and infuse warmed normal saline or lactated Ringer's solution. ▪ Assess for other injuries. ▪ Remove patient's wet clothing and apply warm blankets. ▪ Initiate passive warming with warm humidified oxygen. ▪ Keep patient's head covered with warm, dry towels, or stocking cap. ▪ Warm slowly (1° C/hr) to avoid cardiac irritability from sudden return of cold blood to the heart. ▪ Treat patient gently to avoid increased cardiac irritability. ▪ Do not rub areas of suspected frostbite. ▪ Anticipate intubation for diminished or absent gag reflex. ▪ Anticipate aggressive rewarming techniques if patient does not respond to warm blankets, warm IV fluids, and warmed humidified oxygen. Techniques include warm gastric lavage, thoracotomy, cardiopulmonary bypass, peritoneal lavage, esophageal rewarming, pleural rewarming, and bladder lavage. **Ongoing Monitoring** ▪ Monitor vital signs, level of consciousness, oxygen saturation, cardiac rhythm, temperature. ▪ Loss of ability to shiver indicates severe hypothermia. ▪ Do not give IM medications.

42° C]) until distal flush occurs. Significant edema may begin within 3 hours, with blistering in 6 hours to days. Parenteral analgesia is required in severe frostbite because of the pain associated with tissue thawing. Amputation may be required if the injured area is untreated or treatment is unsuccessful. The patient is admitted to the hospital for observation over 24 to 48 hours with bed rest, elevation of the injured part, and prophylactic antibiotics if the wound is at risk for infection.

Hypothermia

Environmental exposure to freezing temperatures, cold winds, and wet, damp terrain in the presence of physical exhaustion, inadequate clothing, and/or inexperience predispose individuals to hypothermia. Near drowning and water immersion are also associated with hypothermia. The elderly are more prone to hypothermia resulting from decreased mobility, diminished energy reserves, decreased basal metabolic rate, decreased shivering response, decreased sensory perception, chronic medical conditions, and medications that alter body defenses. Hypothermia mimics cerebral or metabolic disturbances causing ataxia, confusion, and withdrawal, so the patient may be misdiagnosed.

Hypothermia, defined as a core temperature less than 95° F (35°C), occurs when heat produced by the body cannot compensate for heat lost to the environment. Fifty-five to sixty percent of all body heat is lost as radiant energy with the greatest loss from the head, thorax, and with each breath.[11] Peripheral vasoconstriction is the body's first attempt to conserve heat. Wet clothing increases evaporative heat loss five times greater than normal and immersion in cold water increases heat loss by a factor of 25. Wind increases heat loss by lowering environmental temperature through conduction. The body produces heat largely through caloric intake. As cold temperatures persist, shivering and movement are the body's only mechanisms for producing heat. Death usually occurs when core temperature falls below 78° F (25.6° C). However, survival has been reported at a core temperature of 64° F (17° C).

Core temperature below 87° F (30.5° C) is severe and potentially life-threatening. Assessment findings in hypothermia are variable and dependent on core temperature (Table 64-11).[11] Patients with *mild hypothermia* (90° F to 95° F [33° C to 35° C]) have shivering, lethargy, confusion, rational to irrational behavior, and minor heart rate changes. Shivering disappears at temperatures less than 92° F (32° C). *Moderate*

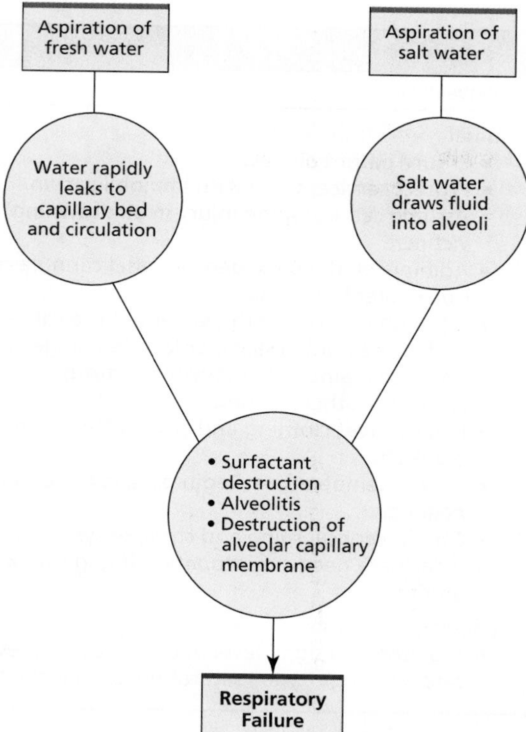

Fig. 64-4 Pulmonary effects of water aspiration.

hypothermia (87° F to 90° F [31° C to 33° C]) causes rigidity, bradycardia, slowed respiratory rate, blood pressure obtainable only by Doppler, metabolic and respiratory acidosis, and hypovolemia.

As core temperature drops by 18° F (10° C), basal metabolic rate decreases two or three times. The cold myocardium is extremely irritable so any movement can precipitate ventricular fibrillation. Decreased renal blood flow decreases glomerular filtration rate, which impairs water reabsorption and leads to dehydration. The hematocrit increases as intravascular volume decreases. Cold blood becomes thick and acts as a thrombus, placing the patient at risk for stroke, myocardial infarction, pulmonary emboli, acute tubular necrosis, and renal failure. Decreased blood flow leads to lactic acid accumulation from anaerobic metabolism and subsequent metabolic acidosis.

Profound hypothermia (<87° F [30.5° C]) makes the person appear dead. Metabolic rate, heart rate, and respirations are so slow they may be difficult to detect. Reflexes are absent and the pupils fixed and dilated. Profound bradycardia, asystole, or ventricular fibrillation may be present. Every effort is made to warm the patient to ≥90° F (32° C) before the person is pronounced dead. The cause of death is usually refractory ventricular fibrillation.

Collaborative Care

Treatment of hypothermia focuses on rewarming the patient, correcting dehydration and acidosis, maintaining patent airway, and treating cardiac arrhythmias (see Table 64-11). *Passive rewarming* is used for mild hypothermia. The patient is moved to a warm, dry place, damp clothing removed, and warm blankets placed on the patient. Gentle handling is essential to prevent stimulation of the cold myocardium.

Active external rewarming with warming blankets, radiant heat lamps, hot water bottles, and hot water baths are used for moderate hypothermia. The patient should be closely monitored for marked vasodilation and hypotension. *Active core rewarming* refers to heat applied directly to the core. Techniques include heated, humidified oxygen 105° F to 115° F (40.5° C to 46.1° C) and installation of heated fluids via IV infusions, bladder lavage, gastric lavage, peritoneal dialysis, hemodialysis, heart-lung bypass, and mediastinal lavage via thoracotomy.

The patient with hypothermia is at risk for ventricular fibrillation when core temperature falls below 82° F (28° C). Ventricular fibrillation does not respond to conventional therapy at low core temperatures, so only one defibrillation attempt is recommended. Only essential IV medications are given; no IM injections are given because of poor perfusion and drug absorption.

Core temperature should be carefully monitored during rewarming procedures. Warming places the patient at risk for rewarming shock, a drop in core temperature, which occurs as cold peripheral blood returns to the central circulation. Rewarming should be discontinued once the core temperature reaches 93° F (34° C). The temperature should not be increased more than 1° C per hour. Fluid resuscitation using warmed IV fluids should be correlated to hemodynamic and respiratory status.

Discharge teaching focuses on teaching the patient how to avoid future problems. Essential information includes dressing in layers for cold weather, covering the head, carrying high-carbohydrate foods for extra calories, and developing a plan for survival should an accident occur. Homeless individuals should be sheltered until fully recovered.

DROWNING AND NEAR DROWNING

Drowning accounts for approximately 9000 deaths annually in the United States with an additional 50,000 near drowning cases reported. Drowning is the third leading cause of death, with 40% of the victims under 5 years of age. Drowning occurs five times more often in men.[11] Alcohol is a significant factor in 60% of all adolescent drownings.

Drowning is death from suffocation after submersion in water or other fluid medium. *Near drowning* is defined as survival from potential drowning. *Immersion syndrome* occurs with immersion in cold water, which leads to stimulation of the vagus nerve and potentially fatal arrhythmias.

Death from drowning is caused by hypoxia secondary to aspiration or airway obstruction. The majority of all drowning victims aspirate water into the pulmonary tree and develop pulmonary edema. Those victims that do not aspirate fluid develop intense bronchospasm and airway obstruction, the cause of death in dry drowning. Regardless of what fluid is aspirated into the pulmonary tree, the ultimate result is pulmonary edema. The osmotic gradient caused by aspirated fluid causes fluid imbalances in the body. Hypotonic fresh water is rapidly absorbed into the circulatory system through the alveoli. Fresh water may be contaminated with chlorine, mud, and algae, causing the breakdown of lung surfactant, fluid seepage, and pulmonary edema. Hypertonic salt water draws fluid from adjacent capillaries into interstitial tissue and the alveoli causing hemoconcentration and hypovolemia. Figure 64-4 shows the pulmonary effects of water aspiration.

EMERGENCY MANAGEMENT

Table 64-12 Near Drowning

Etiology	Assessment Findings	Interventions
Exhaustion while swimming Loss of control or support in water Entrapment or entanglement with objects in water Loss of ability to move secondary to cervical spine injury Poor judgment resulting from alcohol or drugs Seizure while in water	**Pulmonary** ■ Ineffective breathing ■ Dyspnea ■ Respiratory distress ■ Respiratory arrest ■ Crackles, rhonchi ■ Cough with pink-frothy sputum **Cardiac** ■ Tachycardia ■ Bradycardia ■ Arrhythmia ■ Cardiac arrest **Other** ■ Panic ■ Exhaustion ■ Coma ■ Cervical spine injury ■ Hypothermia	**Initial** ■ Ensure patent airway. ■ Protect cervical spine with immobilization. ■ Assume cervical spine injury in all drowning victims. ■ Administer 100% oxygen via nasal cannula or non-rebreather mask. ■ Establish IV access with two large-bore catheters and infuse normal saline or lactated Ringer's solution to maintain hemodynamic status. ■ Assess for other injuries. ■ Remove wet clothing and cover with warm blankets. ■ Obtain temperature. Begin passive rewarming if needed. ■ Obtain cervical spine and chest x-rays. ■ Anticipate need for intubation if gag reflex is absent. **Ongoing Monitoring** ■ Monitor vital signs, level of consciousness, respiratory status, oxygen saturation, cardiac rhythm.

The body attempts to compensate for hypoxia by shunting blood to the lungs, which increases pulmonary pressures and worsens the respiratory status. More and more blood is shunted through alveoli. However, the blood is not adequately oxygenated so the hypoxemia worsens. Anaerobic metabolism develops, which leads to metabolic acidosis.

The assessment findings of a patient with near drowning are listed in Table 64-12. Core temperature may be slightly elevated or below normal depending on water temperature.

Near drowning victims have recovered with no long-term effects after being submerged in cold water up to 40 minutes.[12,13] Aggressive resuscitation efforts and the mammalian diving reflex improve survival.[14] Cold water lowers the body's metabolic rate and oxygen demand. The mammalian diving reflex causes apnea, bradycardia, peripheral vasoconstriction, and further decreases metabolic rate. Blood flow is redistributed to the heart, lungs, and brain.

Collaborative Care

Treatment focuses on correcting hypoxia, acid-base imbalances, and fluid imbalances; supporting basic physiologic functions; and rewarming when hypothermia is present. Initial evaluation involves assessment of airway, cervical spine, breathing, and circulation. Other interventions are listed in Table 64-12.

Mechanical ventilation with positive end-expiratory pressure or continuous positive airway pressure may be used to improve gas exchange across the alveolar-capillary membrane when significant pulmonary edema is present. Ventilation and oxygenation are the primary techniques used to treat acidosis. Mannitol or furosemide (Lasix) may be given to decrease free water and treat cerebral edema.

Deterioration in neurologic status suggests cerebral edema, increased hypoxia, or profound acidosis. Near drowning victims may also have head injuries that cause prolonged alterations in level of consciousness. All victims of near drowning should be observed in a hospital for a minimum of 4 to 6 hours. Delayed pulmonary edema (also called secondary drowning), pneumonia, and cerebral edema have been reported in patients who were essentially free of symptoms immediately after the near drowning episode.

Education needs to focus on water safety and minimizing the risks for drowning. Swimming pool gates should be locked, life jackets should be used on all water craft, including inner tubes and rafts, and water survival skills, that is, swimming lessons, should be a priority. The dangers of combining alcohol and drugs with swimming and other water sports should be taught.

BITES AND STINGS

Animals, spiders, and insects cause injury and even death by biting or stinging. Morbidity is a result of either direct tissue damage or lethal toxins. Direct tissue damage is a product of animal size, characteristics of the animal's teeth, and strength of the jaw. Tissue may be lacerated, crushed, or chewed while toxins released through teeth, fangs, stingers, spines, or tentacles have local or systemic effects. Mortality associated with animal bites is due to blood loss, allergic reactions, or lethal toxins. Injuries caused by insects, spiders, scorpions, ticks, snakes, dogs, cats, rodents, and humans are described below.

Hymenoptera Stings

The *Hymenoptera* family includes bees, yellow jackets, hornets, and wasps. Stings can cause mild discomfort or life-threatening anaphylaxis. Venom may be cytotoxic, hemolytic, allergenic, or vasoactive. Symptoms may begin immediately or be delayed up to 48 hours. Reactions are more severe with multiple stings. Most hymenopterans sting repeatedly. However, the honeybee stings only once, usually leaving the stinger in the skin so that release of venom continues. A scraping motion with a fingernail, knife, or needle is recommended for removing the stinger. Tweezers squeeze the stinger and cause more venom release.

Manifestations vary from stinging, burning, swelling, and itching to edema, headache, fever, syncope, malaise, nausea, vomiting, wheezing, bronchospasm, laryngeal edema, and hypotension. Treatment depends on the severity of the reaction. Mild reactions are treated with elevation, cool compresses, antipruritic lotions, and oral antihistamines. Rings, watches, and restrictive clothing are removed. More severe reactions require IM or IV antihistamines (diphenhydramine [Benadryl]), SC epinephrine (0.3 to 0.5 ml 1:1000), and corticosteroids. Allergic reactions and anaphylaxis are discussed in Chapter 12.

Spider Bites (Arachnid)

Although there are 20,000 species of venomous spiders in the world, only 50 species cause illness. Two venomous spiders found in the United States are the black widow spider and the brown recluse spider. Their venom can cause a localized reaction or systemic anaphylaxis. Tarantulas appear more dangerous than they are, as their bite causes only localized stinging and pain. Other types of spiders release venom when they bite and may cause allergic reactions in some individuals, but they are not considered poisonous.

Black Widow Spiders. *Black widow spiders* have a black body with a bright red hourglass shape on the abdomen. The spider is usually found in damp, cool places under rocks or in woodpiles. The black widow spider venom is neurotoxic. The patient has a tiny, red bite mark associated with pain out of proportion to the size of the bite. Systemic reactions develop over 24 to 48 hours and include nausea, vomiting, elevated temperature, diaphoresis, respiratory distress, hypertension, headache, syncope, and weakness. Symptoms usually peak 2 to 3 hours after onset; however, muscle spasms and hypertension can recur for 12 to 24 hours. Chest and abdominal pain, seizures, and shock can also occur. Bites on the lower body cause abdominal rigidity whereas bites on the upper body lead to chest, back, and shoulder rigidity. A black widow spider bite is not prominent and can be easily missed. Patients not aware of the bite can be misdiagnosed, since symptoms mimic a perforated ulcer, appendicitis, pancreatitis, or other abdominal emergency.

Treatment includes cooling the area to slow the action of the neurotoxin. The wound should be cleaned and tetanus prophylaxis given as appropriate. Muscle spasms are treated with calcium gluconate, methocarbamol (Robaxin), or diazepam (Valium). Severe pain may require narcotic analgesia. Antivenin is used for severe reactions, young children, or adults with hypertension or cardiac disease.

Brown Recluse Spiders. *Brown recluse spiders* are usually found in dark areas such as garages, closets, and boxes. The spider, common in the southeastern, south central, and southwestern United States, is a light brown color with a characteristic dark brown fiddle shape that extends from the eyes down the back. The venom is cytotoxic, so local tissue effects can be dramatic. Stinging, burning, and itching start almost immediately with severe pain several hours later. A bleb (blister), bluish ring around the bite, and erythema eventually progress to necrosis by the third or fourth day. An open sore may persist for days or even weeks. Systemic manifestations, although rare, include fever, myalgia, rash, hemolysis, petechia, joint pain, seizures, shock, hemorrhage, and pulmonary edema. Hemolysis may lead to hemoglobinuria, renal failure, and death.

Treatment depends on severity of the reaction. Treatment is necessary when there is bleb or bullae formation, intense pain, and signs of rapidly progressive ischemia and necrosis. Initial interventions include cool compresses, elevation, and resting of the affected extremity. Analgesia, tetanus prophylaxis, antihistamines, corticosteroids, and antibiotics for prevention of secondary infection may also be required. Surgical debridement with grafting is necessary for some patients. Dapsone, a polymorphonuclear leukocyte inhibitor, has been used for patients with deep crater wounds. Patients with systemic manifestations are hospitalized and monitored for hemolysis, disseminated intravascular clotting, and acute renal failure.

Tick Bites

Ticks inhabit various parts of the country, but they are most common in the Rocky Mountain region and the Northwest. Emergencies associated with tick bites include Rocky Mountain spotted fever, Lyme disease, and tick paralysis. Disease is caused by an infected tick or by the release of neurotoxin. Ticks release a neurotoxic venom as long as the tick head is attached to the body. Therefore, removal of the attached tick is essential for effective treatment. Forceps may be used to safely remove the tick by grasping at the point of entry and pulling upward in a steady motion. Covering the tick with alcohol, mineral oil, petroleum jelly or ether causes the tick to release from the skin. These methods work because the tick breathes through the skin in which they are embedded.

Rocky Mountain spotted fever, caused by *Rickettsia rickettsii,* has an incubation period of 2 to 14 days. A pink, macular rash appears on the palms, wrists, soles, feet, and ankles within 10 days of exposure. Other symptoms include fever, chills, malaise, myalgias, and headache. Treatment is antibiotic therapy.

Lyme disease is the most common arthropod-borne disease in the United States, with 12,000 to 16,000 new cases reported each year.[15] Symptoms appear within 3 to 30 days of exposure to the spirochete *Borrelia burgdorferi,* found on the *Ixodes* tick. Lyme disease occurs most often in the northeastern, north central, and mid-Atlantic regions.[16] The initial stage of this disease is characterized by flulike symptoms and a characteristic bull's eye rash—an expanding circular area of redness of 5 cm diameter or more. Neurologic, cardiac, and musculoskeletal problems such as meningitis, hepatitis, neuropathies, and cardiomyopathies occur days or weeks later. Chronic arthritis and peripheral radiculopathy characterize later stages of the disease, which lasts months or years. Treatment includes antibiotic therapy; however, controversy exists over what the most effective regimen should be. (Lyme disease is discussed in Chapter 60.)

Tick paralysis occurs 5 to 7 days after exposure to the wood tick or dog tick. Classic symptoms are flaccid ascending paralysis, which develops over 1 to 2 days. Without tick removal, the patient dies as respiratory muscles become paralyzed. Tick removal leads to return of muscle movement, usually within 48 to 72 hours.

Snakebite

Only 375 of the 3000 species of snakes in the world are poisonous. Poisonous snakes indigenous to the United States are

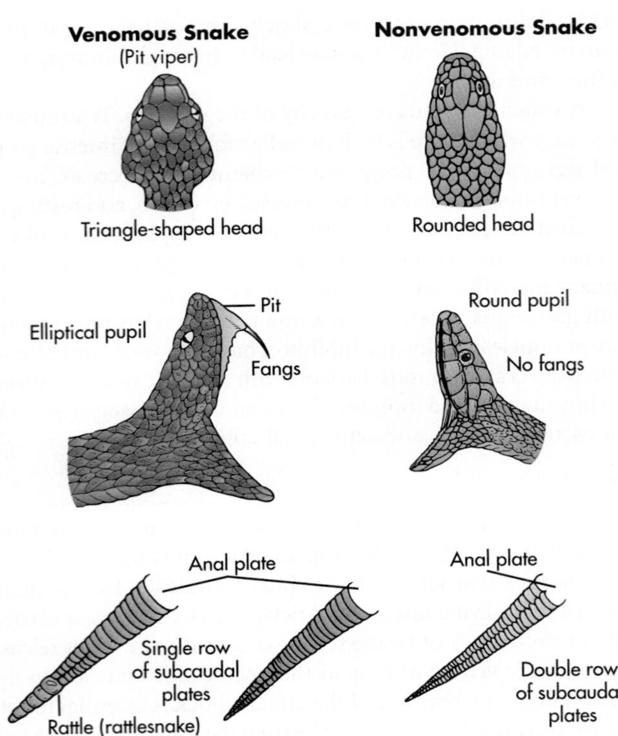

Fig. 64-5 Venomous and nonvenomous snakes.

members of the *Crotalid* and *Elapid* family. *Crotalids,* or pit vipers, include rattlesnakes, copperheads, and water moccasins. Coral snakes belong to the *Elapid* family. Other poisonous snakes in the *Elapid* family not indigenous to the United States are the cobra and the mamba. Figure 64-5 highlights differences between poisonous and nonpoisonous snakes.

Venom from the pit viper is hemolytic, whereas coral snake venom is neurotoxic. Envenomation occurs in approximately 75% to 80% of all snakebites. If swelling does not occur within 30 minutes after the bite, envenomation is unlikely. Local reaction is characterized by 1 or 2 fang marks associated with pain, bruising, edema within 36 hours of injury, petechiae, ecchymosis, and erythema. Loss of function and necrosis of the affected limb may occur 16 to 36 hours after the bite. Systemic reactions include nausea and vomiting, dizziness, tachycardia, muscle fasciculations, gastrointestinal bleeding, and respiratory problems. The patient may experience a metallic or rubber taste. Neurologic symptoms such as constricted pupils, drowsiness, weakness, fasciculations, muscle weakness, and seizures occur with neurotoxic venom. Life-threatening problems associated with systemic envenomation include severe hemorrhage, renal failure, and hypovolemic shock.

Treatment focuses on preventing the spread of venom (Table 64-13). Rings, watches, and restrictive clothing should be removed, and then the affected limb should be immobilized at the level of the heart. Ice and tourniquets are not recommended. Incision of the wound is controversial. If done within 3 minutes of injury, 25% to 30% of the venom may be removed. Caffeine, alcohol, and smoking increase the spread of venom and should be avoided.

ED management includes vascular access with a large gauge catheter and administration of crystalloids to maintain blood pressure. Diagnostic tests include complete blood count, urinalysis, coagulation studies, blood urea nitrogen, creatinine, creatine kinase, and electrolytes. Other measures include assessment of extremity swelling, usually through documentation of circumference every 30 to 60 minutes. Pain should be treated with acetaminophen. Aspirin and nonsteroidal antiinflammatory drugs should be avoided because they may cause bleeding; narcotics may cause respiratory depression. Tetanus prophylaxis should be administered as needed (see Table 64-8). Secondary infection caused by microorganisms in the snake's mouth or other contaminants may require antibiotic therapy. Debridement or fasciotomy is necessary in some patients. Antivenin therapy is used only for life-threatening envenomation because of the high incidence of allergic reactions.[17] A skin test is done before administration of antivenin. The amount of antivenin required depends on the amount of envenomation (Table 64-14). Incomplete dosage is the most common cause of treatment failure so antivenin is administered until symptoms subside. Serum sickness develops in most patients who receive more than 10 vials of antivenin. (Serum sickness is described in Chapter 12.)

Animal Bites

Approximately 500,000 to 2 million animal bites are reported each year in the United States. Children are at greatest risk. The most significant problems associated with animal bites are infection and mechanical destruction of the skin, muscle, tendons, blood vessels, and bone. The bite may cause a simple laceration or be associated with crush injury, puncture wound, or tearing or avulsion of tissue. The severity of injury depends on animal size, victim size, and anatomical location of the bite. Dog bites account for 75% to 90% of reported cases whereas domestic cats are the cause in 10%.[18] Wild or domestic rodents are ranked behind cats and dogs as the third most frequent offenders in reported animal bites. Bite injury secondary to humans, squirrels, ferrets, monkeys, lions, tigers, horses, cows, sheep, goats, camels, and swine also occur. Skull fractures have been reported after camel bites.

Cat bites cause a greater incidence of infection than dog bites. *Pasteurella multocida* occurs in the majority of healthy cats. Cat bites cause deep puncture wounds that can involve tendons and joint capsules. Septic arthritis, osteomyelitis, and tenosynovitis have been reported in cat bites.

Dog bites usually occur on the extremities; however, facial bites are common in small children. Most victims own the dogs that bite them. Dog bites may involve significant tissue damage, with fatalities reported, usually in children. Skull fractures with intracranial injury and death occur in children less than 2 years old. Disfiguring wounds of the face should be evaluated by a plastic surgeon.

Collaborative Care

Treatment of animal bites includes cleaning and irrigation with copious amounts of saline, debridement, tetanus prophylaxis, and analgesics as needed. Prophylactic antibiotics are used for human bites and animal bites at risk for infection such as wounds over joints, those greater than 6 to 12 hours old, puncture wounds, and bites of the hand or foot. Individuals at greatest risk of infection are infants, older adults, immunosup-

EMERGENCY MANAGEMENT

Table 64-13 Snakebite

Etiology	Assessment Findings	Interventions
Pit Vipers Rattlesnake Copperhead Water moccasin **Other** Coral snake	■ Fang marks ■ Progressive swelling at site ■ Nausea and vomiting ■ Headache ■ Dizziness ■ Paresthesia ■ Burning pain ■ Ecchymosis, erythema ■ Decreased distal pulses ■ Respiratory compromise ■ Muscular weakness, paralysis ■ Pit viper venom is hemolytic and can be neurotoxic. ■ Severity of injury is due to amount of envenomation.	**Initial** ■ Ensure airway, breathing, and circulation. ■ Reassure patient to decrease panic. ■ Immobilize affected part at heart level. ■ Reduce physical activity. ■ Remove rings, bracelets, and other constricting items on the bitten extremity. ■ Do not put injured part in ice or apply ice packs. ■ Administer oxygen via nasal cannula or non-rebreather mask. ■ Establish IV access in unaffected limb with two large-bore catheters and infuse normal saline. ■ Obtain clotting studies, CBC, electrolytes, BUN, serum creatinine, creatine kinase, urinalysis, and type and crossmatch. ■ Anticipate administration of antivenin. ■ Administer tetanus prophylaxis as appropriate. **Ongoing Monitoring** ■ Monitor vital signs, level of consciousness, oxygen saturation, cardiac rhythm. ■ Monitor for respiratory compromise or hemorrhage.

Table 64-14 Antivenin Snakebite Treatment

Envenomation	Signs and Symptoms	Number of Vials of Antivenin*
None	Fang marks, no local swelling, hemorrhage, or paresthesia	No antivenin. Tetanus prophylaxis, observation
Minimal	Fang marks, local swelling of hands or feet, no systemic reactions	3-5 vials
Moderate	Fang marks, progressive swelling beyond bite, mild systemic reaction	6-10 vials
Severe	Multiple fang marks, progressive swelling, pronounced systemic reaction, hypotension, twitching, clotting abnormalities	15+ vials

*Depends on type of snakebite, body surface area, and age. Skin testing should be done before injection of antivenin.

pressed patients, alcoholics, diabetics, and people taking corticosteroids. Puncture wounds are left open while lacerations are loosely sutured.

Consideration of rabies prophylaxis is an essential component in management of animal bites. Rabies is caused by a neurotoxic virus found in the saliva of some mammals. The condition is fatal in humans. Approximately 35,000 deaths are reported worldwide with one or two cases in the United States.[19] Rabies exposure should be considered if an animal attack was not provoked, involved a wild animal, or involved a domestic animal not immunized against rabies. Rabies prophylaxis is always given when the animal cannot be found or the bite is caused by a carnivorous wild animal. Approximately 25,000 persons receive rabies prophylaxis each year in the United States. Rabies prophylaxis uses an initial injection of rabies immune globulin (RIG) to provide passive immunity, and a series of five injections of human diploid cell vaccine (HDCV) on days 0, 3, 7, 14, and 28 is used to provide active immunity. Dosage is based on the patient's weight.

Human Bites

Human bites carry a high risk of infection from oral bacterial flora, most commonly *Staphylococci aureus* and streptococci. Human bites can cause more tissue destruction than other animal bites. Hands, fingers, and noses are the most common sites of injury with infection rates greatest in wounds of the hands. Boxer's fracture, fracture of the fifth metacarpal, is often associated with an open wound when the knuckles impact teeth. The human jaw has great crushing ability causing laceration, puncture, crush injury, soft tissue tearing, and even amputation. More than 40 potential pathogens found in the human mouth account for an infection rate of approximately 50% in cases where victims did not seek medical intervention within 24 hours of injury.

Initial treatment includes cleaning with copious irrigation, debridement, prophylactic antibiotics, and tetanus prophylaxis. Wounds over joints are splinted; however, initial closure is reserved only for facial wounds. The patient is admitted for IV antibiotic therapy when an infection is present. There is an increased incidence of cellulitis, osteomyelitis, and septic arthritis in these patients. Human bites must be reported to the police in some states.

POISONINGS

A poison is any chemical that harms the body. More than 1 million cases of poisonings occur each year in the United States. Poisonings can be accidental, occupational, recreational, or intentional.[20] Natural or manufactured toxins can be ingested, inhaled, injected, splashed in the eye, or absorbed through the skin. Common poisons are reviewed in Table 64-15. Other poisonings related to the use of illegal drugs such as amphetamines, narcotics, and hallucinogens are discussed in Chapter 10. Poisoning may also be due to toxic plants or contaminated foods. (Food poisoning is discussed in Chapter 39.)

Severity of the poisoning depends on type, concentration, and route of exposure. Toxins can affect every tissue of the body, so symptoms can be seen in any body system. Specific management of toxins involves decreasing absorption, enhancing elimination, and implementation of toxin-specific interventions.

Options for decreasing absorption of poisons include emesis, gastric lavage, activated charcoal, dermal cleansing, and eye irrigation. Ipecac (15 to 45 ml for adults) followed by 250 to 500 ml water is used to induce emesis. This process is most effective if used within 1 hour of ingestion. Use of Ipecac has lost favor over the past decade for a variety of reasons. Onset of action is delayed and unpredictable, overall rate of drug return is low, and Ipecac is not effective with drugs that are rapidly absorbed such as alcohol.[21] Other problems associated with induced emesis include fluid losses, electrolyte abnormalities, and acid-base disturbances secondary to protracted vomiting.

Table 64-15 Common Poisons

Poison	Manifestations	Treatment
▪ Acetaminophen (Tylenol)	Nausea and vomiting, anorexia, malaise, diaphoresis, liver abnormalities	Activated charcoal, *N*-acetylcysteine
▪ Acids and alkalis *Acids:* toilet bowl cleaners, antirust compounds; *alkalis:* drain cleaners, dishwashing detergents, ammonia	Excess salivation, dysphagia, epigastric pain, pneumonitis, burns of mouth, esophagus, and stomach	Immediate dilution (water, milk), corticosteroids (for alkali burns), contraindication for induced vomiting
▪ Aspirin and aspirin-containing medications	Increased respiratory rate, respiratory alkalosis, headache, vertigo, tinnitus, sweating, nausea, electrolyte imbalances	Gastric lavage, activated charcoal, alkaline diuresis, supportive care
▪ Bleaches	Irritation of lips, mouth, and eyes, superficial injury to esophagus; chemical pneumonia and pulmonary edema	Washing of exposed skin and eyes, dilution with water and milk, gastric lavage, prevention of vomiting and aspiration
▪ Carbon monoxide	Dyspnea, headache, tachypnea, confusion, impaired judgment, cyanosis, respiratory depression	Removal from source, administration of 100% oxygen
▪ Cyanide	Headache, faintness, vertigo, tachycardia, hypertension, nausea and vomiting, almond odor to breath	Amyl nitrate, sodium nitrate, sodium thiosulfate, oxygen
▪ Ethylene glycol	Sweet aromatic odor to breath, nausea and vomiting, slurred speech, ataxia, lethargy, respiratory depression	Gastric lavage, activated charcoal, supportive care
▪ Iron	Vomiting (often bloody), diarrhea (often bloody), fever, hyperglycemia, lethargy, hypotension, seizures, coma	Gastric lavage, chelation therapy (deferoxamine)
▪ Nonsteroidal antiinflammatory drugs	Gastroenteritis, abdominal pain, drowsiness, nystagmus, hepatic damage	Gastric lavage, activated charcoal, cathartics
▪ Tricyclic antidepressants (e.g., amitriptyline, imipramine)	In low doses: anticholinergic effects, agitation, hypertension, tachycardia; in high doses: central nervous system depression, respiratory depression, seizures, hypotension	Activated charcoal, gastric lavage, supportive care, contraindication for induced emesis
▪ Alcohol, barbiturates, benzodiazepines, cocaine, hallucinogens, stimulants	See Chapter 10	See Chapter 10

Gastric lavage involves oral insertion of a large diameter (36F to 40F) gastric tube for installation of copious amounts of saline. The head of the bed should be elevated or the patient placed on the side to prevent aspiration. Patients with an altered level of consciousness or diminished gag reflex are intubated before lavage. Lavage is contraindicated in patients who ingested caustic agents. Problems associated with lavage include epistaxis, esophageal perforation, and aspiration.

The most effective intervention for management of poisonings is administration of activated charcoal orally or via a gastric tube. Toxins adhere to charcoal and are excreted through the GI tract rather than absorbed into the portal circulation. Adults receive 50 to 100 g of charcoal. Activated charcoal can absorb a number of poisons from the GI tract, but it does not absorb ethanol, alkali, iron, boric acid, lithium, methanol, or cyanide. Contraindications to charcoal administration are diminished bowel sounds, ileus, ingestion of a substance poorly absorbed by charcoal, or previous administration of *N*-acetylcysteine (NAC). Charcoal inactivates NAC, the antidote used for acetaminophen toxicity.

Dermal and ocular decontamination involve removal of toxins from eyes and skin using copious amounts of water. With the exception of mustard gas, most toxins can be safely removed with water. Water mixes with mustard gas and releases chlorine gas. As a general rule, dry substances should be brushed from the skin and clothing before water is used. Powdered lime should not be removed with water; it should just be brushed off. Protective clothing (gloves, gowns, and goggles) should be worn for decontamination to prevent secondary exposure. Decontamination procedures are usually done by those specially trained in hazardous material decontamination before the patient arrives at the hospital. Decontamination takes priority over all interventions except basic life support techniques.

Elimination is increased through administration of cathartics, whole-bowel irrigation, repeat-dose activated charcoal, forced diuresis, hemodialysis, charcoal hemoperfusion, oxygen inhalation, surgical removal, and administration of chelating agents. Cathartics such as sorbitol, magnesium citrate, or magnesium sulfate are given together with activated charcoal to stimulate intestinal motility and increase elimination. Multiple doses of cathartics should be avoided because of potentially fatal electrolyte abnormalities. Whole bowel irrigation involves administration of an isotonic polyethylene glycol and electrolyte solution (GoLYTELY) to flush heavy metals, enteric coated medications, or slowly dissolving tablets. This process is also effective for swallowed objects such as cocaine-filled balloons or condoms.

Repeat-dose activated charcoal (administration of charcoal every 2 to 4 hours) is indicated for theophylline, phenobarbital, salicylates, antidepressants, and carbamazepine (Tegretol).[22] Forced diuresis is used for removal of ethanol, methanol, isopropyl alcohol, and ethylene glycol. Large amounts of IV saline are infused to flush toxins through the kidneys. Mannitol or furosemide (Lasix) may be used to enhance the process. Hemodialysis and hemoperfusion are used for patients when ingestion is associated with severe acidosis.

Other interventions include alkalinization and antidote administration. Sodium bicarbonate administration raises the pH ($\geq$7.5), which is particularly effective for phenobarbital and salicylates. Vitamin C may be added to IV fluids to enhance excretion of amphetamines and quinidine. A limited number of true antidotes are available and many of these recommended agents are themselves toxic.

Education for toxic emergencies focuses on how the poisoning occurred. Patients who experience poisoning because of a suicide attempt or related to substance abuse should be evaluated by a mental health counselor and then admitted for alcohol or drug detoxification or scheduled for follow-up with a mental health professional. Poisoning related to an occupational hazard should be evaluated by the Department of Occupational Safety and Health Administration.

CRITICAL THINKING EXERCISES

CASE STUDY

Trauma

Patient Profile

A 42-year-old male trauma patient is brought to the ED in an ambulance. He was the driver in a motor vehicle collision and was not wearing a seat belt. The passenger in the car was dead at the scene. The paramedics stated that there was significant damage to the car on the passenger side.

Subjective Data

- Is awake
- Complains of shortness of breath and abdominal pain

Objective Data

Physical Examination

- 4-cm head laceration
- Badly deformed right lower leg without pulses
- Unequal pupils
- Decreased breath sounds on left side of chest
- Asymmetric chest movement
- Vital signs: BP 90/40, HR 130 beats/min, respiratory rate 36 breaths/min
- O_2 saturation 82%

Critical Thinking Questions

1. What life-threatening injury does this patient probably have?
2. What is the priority of care?
3. What intervention is needed immediately?
4. What other interventions should the nurse consider?
5. How should the nurse approach the family?
6. Based on assessment data presented, write one or more nursing diagnoses. Are there any collaborative problems?

REVIEW QUESTIONS

The number of the question corresponds to the same-numbered objective at the beginning of the chapter.

1. During triage of patients in an emergency department, the person that the nurse should treat first is
   a. A 2-year-old child with scalp laceration who is awake and crying
   b. An 85-year-old woman with crushing chest pain who is pale and diaphoretic
   c. A 32-year-old complaining of recent onset of fever, aches, and chills after a camping trip
   d. A 34-year-old woman who has raspy breathing and facial and neck edema from a wasp sting
2. An elderly male arrives at the ED disoriented, breathing rapidly, and has hot, dry skin. The priority for treatment is to
   a. Assess his airway, breathing, and circulation
   b. Obtain a detailed medical history from his family
   c. Determine the kind of insurance he has before treating him
   d. Start oxygen administration and have the ED physician see him
3. Which of the following interventions is most effective in decreasing absorption of an ingested poison?
   a. Gastric lavage
   b. Ipecac administration
   c. Activated charcoal
   d. Milk dilution

References

1. Kelly SJ: *Pediatric emergency nursing,* ed 2, Norwalk, Conn, 1994, Appleton & Lange.
2. Rund DA, Rausch TS: *Triage,* St Louis, 1981, Mosby.
3. Brackin JE. In Newberry L, editor: *Sheehy's emergency nursing principles and practice,* St Louis, 1998, Mosby.
4. Kidd PS, Sturt P: *Mosby's emergency nursing reference,* St Louis, 1996, Mosby.
5. Tintinalli JE, Ruiz E, Krome RL, editors: *Emergency medicine: a comprehensive study guide,* ed 4, New York, 1996, McGraw-Hill.
6. Davis LL: Environmental heat-related illnesses, *MEDSURG Nurs* 6:3, 1997.
7. Morris J. In Newberry L, editor: *Sheehy's emergency nursing principles and practice,* St Louis, 1998, Mosby.
8. Simon HB: Hyperthermia and heatstroke, *Hosp Pract* 29:65, 1994.
9. Rosen P, Barkin R: *Emergency medicine concepts and clinical practice,* ed 4, St Louis, 1998, Mosby.
10. Auerbach P, Geehr E: *Management of wilderness and environmental emergencies,* ed 3, St Louis, 1995, Mosby.
11. Emergency Nurses Association: *Emergency nursing core curriculum,* ed 5, Philadelphia, 1999, WB Saunders.
12. Glankler DM: Caring for the victim of near drowning, *Crit Care Nurse* 13:25, 1993.
13. Siebake H and others: Survival after 40 minutes submersion without cerebral sequelae, *Lancet* 1:1275, 1975.
14. DeBoer SL: Neurologic outcomes after near drowning, *Crit Care Nurse* 17:4, 1997.
15. Massachusetts Medical Society: Lyme disease—United States, 1995, *MMWR* 45:481, 1996.
16. Briant C, Roye K, Hutscher AH: Pericarditis as a manifestation of Lyme disease, *J Emerg Nurs* 23:525, 1997.
17. Soski JE: *Snakebite assessment and treatment in the eastern United States,* ed 2, Midway, Fla, 1994, Snakebite Publishing.
18. Strange G, Towns D: Environmental emergencies. In Strange GR and others, editors: *Pediatric emergency medicine: a comprehensive study guide,* New York, 1996, McGraw-Hill.
19. Chonel BB: The modern epidemiological aspects of rabies in the world, *Comp Immunol Microbiol Infect Dis* 16:11, 1993.
20. Kitt S and others: *Emergency nursing: a physiologic and clinical perspective,* ed 2, Philadelphia, 1995, WB Saunders.
21. Criddle LM. In Newberry L, editor: *Sheehy's emergency nursing principles and practice,* St Louis, 1998, Mosby.
22. Johnson D and others: Effect of multiple-dose activated charcoal on the clearance of high-dose intravenous aspirin in a porcine model, *Ann Emerg Med* 26:671, 1995.

Resources

American Association of Emergency Physicians
PO Box 81020
Chicago, IL 60681-0020
800-449-4237
fax: 312-819-1103
http://www.aep.org

American College of Emergency Physicians
PO Box 619911
Dallas, TX 75261-9911
972-550-0911
800-798-1822
fax: 972-580-2816
http://www.acep.org

American Red Cross
8111 Gatehouse Road, 6th Floor
Falls Church, VA 22042
703-206-7090
800-HELP-NOW
http://www.redcross.org

American Trauma Society
8903 Presidential Parkway, Suite 512
Upper Marlboro, MD 20772
301-420-4189
800-556-7890
http://www.amtrauma.org/

Emergency Nurses Association
216 Higgins Road
Park Ridge, IL 60068-5736
708-698-9400
fax: 708-698-9406
http://www.ena.org/

On Emergency Medicine
http://nj5.injersey.com/~pscott/

***For additional Internet resources, see the website for this book at* www.mosby.com/MERLIN/medsurg_lewis**

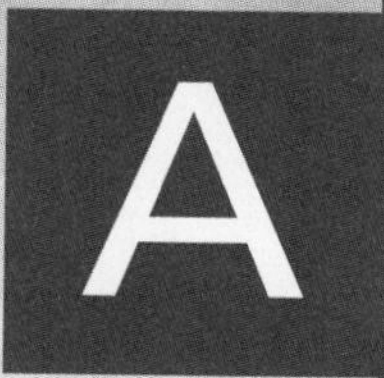

Nursing Diagnoses

ALPHABETICAL LISTING

Activity Intolerance
Activity Intolerance, Risk for
Adaptive Capacity: Intracranial, Decreased
Adjustment, Impaired
Airway Clearance, Ineffective
Anxiety
Aspiration, Risk for
Body Image Disturbance
Breastfeeding, Effective
Breastfeeding, Ineffective
Breastfeeding, Interrupted
Breathing Pattern, Ineffective
Cardiac Output, Decreased
Caregiver Role Strain
Caregiver Role Strain, Risk for
Communication, Impaired Verbal
Confusion, Acute
Confusion, Chronic
Constipation
Constipation, Colonic
Constipation, Perceived
Constipation, Risk for
Coping, Defensive
Coping, Ineffective Community
Coping, Ineffective Individual
Coping, Potential for Enhanced Community
Death Anxiety
Decisional Conflict
Denial, Ineffective
Dentition, Altered
Development, Risk for Altered
Diarrhea
Disuse Syndrome, Risk for
Diversional Activity Deficit
Dysreflexia
Dysreflexia, Risk for Autonomic
Energy Field Disturbance
Environmental Interpretation Syndrome, Impaired
Failure to Thrive, Adult
Family Coping, Ineffective: Compromised
Family Coping, Ineffective: Disabling
Family Coping: Potential for Growth
Family Processes, Altered
Family Processes, Altered: Alcoholism
Fatigue
Fear
Fluid Volume Deficit
Fluid Volume Deficit, Risk for
Fluid Volume Excess
Fluid Volume Imbalance, Risk for
Gas Exchange, Impaired
Grieving, Anticipatory
Grieving, Dysfunctional
Growth, Altered: Risk for
Growth and Development, Altered
Health Maintenance, Altered
Health-Seeking Behaviors (Specify)
Home Maintenance Management, Impaired
Hopelessness
Hyperthermia
Hypothermia
Incontinence, Bowel
Incontinence, Functional Urinary
Incontinence, Reflex Urinary
Incontinence, Risk for Urinary Urge
Incontinence, Stress
Incontinence, Total
Incontinence, Urge
Infant Behavior: Disorganized
Infant Behavior, Disorganized: Risk for
Infant Behavior, Potential for Enhanced Organized
Infant Feeding Pattern, Ineffective
Infection, Risk for
Injury, Risk for
Knowledge Deficit
Latex Allergy Response
Latex Allergy Response, Risk for
Loneliness, Risk for
Management of Therapeutic Regimen, Effective: Individual
Management of Therapeutic Regimen, Ineffective: Community
Management of Therapeutic Regimen, Ineffective: Families
Management of Therapeutic Regimen, Ineffective: Individuals
Memory, Impaired
Mobility, Impaired: Bed
Mobility, Impaired: Physical
Mobility, Impaired: Wheelchair
Nausea
Noncompliance
Nutrition, Altered: Less than Body Requirements
Nutrition, Altered: More than Body Requirements
Nutrition, Altered: Risk for More Than Body Requirements
Oral Mucous Membrane, Altered
Pain
Pain, Chronic
Parent/Infant/Child Attachment, Risk for Altered
Parental Role Conflict
Parenting, Altered
Parenting, Altered: Risk for
Perioperative Positioning Injury, Risk for
Peripheral Neurovascular Dysfunction, Risk for
Personal Identity Disturbance
Poisoning, Risk for
Post-Trauma Syndrome
Post-Trauma Syndrome, Risk for
Powerlessness
Protection, Altered
Rape Trauma Syndrome
Rape Trauma Syndrome: Compound Reaction
Rape Trauma Syndrome: Silent Reaction
Relocation Stress Syndrome
Role Performance, Altered
Self-Care Deficit, Bathing/Hygiene
Self-Care Deficit, Dressing/Grooming
Self-Care Deficit, Feeding
Self-Care Deficit, Toileting
Self-Esteem, Chronic Low
Self-Esteem Disturbance
Self-Esteem, Situational Low
Self-Mutilation, Risk for
Sensory/Perceptual Alterations (Specify: Visual, Auditory, Kinesthetic, Gustatory, Tactile, Olfactory)
Sexual Dysfunction
Sexuality Patterns, Altered

Skin Integrity, Impaired
Skin Integrity, Impaired: Risk for
Sleep Deprivation
Sleep Pattern Disturbance
Social Interaction, Impaired
Social Isolation
Sorrow, Chronic
Spiritual Distress (Distress of the Human Spirit)
Spiritual Distress, Risk for
Spiritual Well-Being, Potential for Enhanced
Suffocation, Risk for
Surgical Recovery, Delayed
Swallowing, Impaired
Temperature, Risk for Altered Body
Thermoregulation, Ineffective
Thought Processes, Altered
Tissue Integrity, Impaired
Tissue Perfusion, Altered (Specify Type: Renal, Cerebral, Cardiopulmonary, Gastrointestinal, Peripheral)
Transfer Ability, Impaired
Trauma, Risk for
Unilateral Neglect
Urinary Elimination, Altered
Urinary Retention
Ventilation, Inability to Sustain Spontaneous
Ventilatory Weaning Response, Dysfunctional
Violence, Risk for: Directed at Others
Violence, Risk for: Self-Directed
Walking, Impaired

GROUPED BY FUNCTIONAL HEALTH PATTERNS

HEALTH PERCEPTION–HEALTH MANAGEMENT PATTERN

Development, Altered: Risk for
Energy Field Disturbance
Growth, Altered: Risk for
Health Maintenance, Altered
Health-Seeking Behaviors
Infection, Risk for
Injury, Risk for
Management of Therapeutic Regimen, Ineffective (Community)
Management of Therapeutic Regimen, Ineffective (Family)
Management of Therapeutic Regimen, Ineffective
Noncompliance
Poisoning, Risk for
Protection, Altered
Suffocation, Risk for
Surgical Recovery, Delayed
Trauma, Risk for

NUTRITIONAL-METABOLIC PATTERN

Aspiration, Risk for
Breastfeeding, Effective
Breastfeeding, Ineffective
Breastfeeding, Interrupted
Dentition, Altered
Fluid Volume Deficit
Fluid Volume Deficit, Risk for
Fluid Volume Excess
Fluid Volume Imbalance, Risk for
Hyperthermia
Hypothermia
Infant Feeding Pattern, Ineffective
Latex Allergy Response
Latex Allergy Response, Risk for
Nausea
Nutrition, Altered: Less than Body Requirements
Nutrition, Altered: More than Body Requirements
Nutrition, Altered: Risk for More than Body Requirements
Oral Mucous Membrane, Altered
Skin Integrity, Impaired
Skin Integrity, Impaired: Risk for
Swallowing, Impaired
Temperature, Risk for Altered Body
Thermoregulation, Ineffective
Tissue Integrity, Impaired

ELIMINATION PATTERN

Constipation
Constipation, Colonic
Constipation, Perceived
Constipation, Risk for
Diarrhea
Incontinence, Bowel
Incontinence, Functional Urinary
Incontinence, Reflex Urinary
Incontinence, Stress
Incontinence, Total
Incontinence, Urge
Urinary Elimination, Altered
Urinary Retention

ACTIVITY-EXERCISE PATTERN

Activity Intolerance
Activity Intolerance, Risk for
Airway Clearance, Ineffective
Breathing Pattern, Ineffective
Cardiac Output, Decreased
Disuse Syndrome, Risk for
Diversional Activity Deficit
Dysreflexia
Dysreflexia, Risk for Autonomic
Energy Field Disturbance
Failure to Thrive
Fatigue
Gas Exchange, Impaired
Growth and Development, Altered
Home Maintenance Management, Impaired
Infant Behavior, Disorganized
Infant Behavior, Potential for Enhanced Organized
Infant Behavior, Risk for Disorganized
Mobility, Impaired: Bed, Physical, Wheelchair
Perioperative Positioning Injury, Risk for
Peripheral Neurovascular Dysfunction, Risk for
Self-Care Deficit, Bathing/Hygiene
Self-Care Deficit, Dressing/Grooming
Self-Care Deficit, Feeding
Self-Care Deficit, Toileting
Surgical Recovery, Delayed
Tissue Perfusion, Altered
Transfer Ability, Impaired
Ventilation, Inability to Sustain
Ventilatory Weaning Response, Dysfunctional
Walking, Impaired

SLEEP-REST PATTERN

Sleep Deprivation
Sleep Pattern Disturbance

COGNITIVE-PERCEPTUAL PATTERN

Adaptive Capacity, Decreased, Intracranial
Confusion, Acute
Confusion, Chronic
Decisional Conflict
Environmental Interpretation Syndrome, Impaired
Knowledge Deficit
Memory, Impaired
Nausea
Pain
Pain, Chronic
Sensory-Perceptual Alterations
Thought Processes, Altered
Unilateral Neglect

SELF-PERCEPTION–SELF-CONCEPT PATTERN

Anxiety
Body Image Disturbance
Death Anxiety
Fear
Hopelessness
Personal Identity Disturbance
Powerlessness
Self-Esteem, Chronic Low
Self-Esteem Disturbance
Self-Esteem, Situational Low
Self-Mutilation, Risk for

ROLE-RELATIONSHIP PATTERN

Caregiver Role Strain
Caregiver Role Strain, Risk for
Communication, Impaired Verbal

Family Processes, Altered
Grieving, Anticipatory
Grieving, Dysfunctional
Parental Role Conflict
Parenting, Altered
Parenting, Altered: Risk for
Relocation Stress Syndrome
Role Performance, Altered
Social Interaction, Impaired
Social Isolation
Violence, Risk for: Directed at Others
Violence, Risk for: Self-Directed

SEXUALITY-REPRODUCTIVE PATTERN

Rape Trauma Syndrome
Rape Trauma Syndrome: Compound Reaction
Rape Trauma Syndrome: Silent Reaction
Sexual Dysfunction
Sexuality Patterns, Altered

COPING–STRESS-TOLERANCE PATTERN

Adjustment, Impaired
Coping, Defensive
Coping, Ineffective Community
Coping, Ineffective Individual
Coping, Potential for Enhanced Community
Denial, Ineffective
Failure to Thrive, Adult
Family Coping, Ineffective: Compromised
Family Coping, Ineffective: Disabling
Family Coping: Potential for Growth
Post-Trauma Syndrome
Post-Trauma Syndrome, Risk for
Sorrow, Chronic

VALUE-BELIEF PATTERN

Spiritual Distress (Distress of Human Spirit)
Spiritual Well-Being, Potential for Enhanced

Modified from *NANDA nursing diagnosis: definitions and classification 1999-2000,* North America Nursing Diagnosis Association; and Gordon M: *Manual of nursing diagnoses,* St Louis, 1997, Mosby.

B Laboratory Values

Cecilia C. Dail, Sally Sperry Steen, and Lee Danielson

The tables in this appendix list some of the most common tests, their normal values, and possible etiologies of abnormal values. Laboratory values may vary with different techniques or different laboratories. Possible etiologies are presented in alphabetic order. Abbreviations appearing in the tables are defined as follows:

$<$ = less than
$>$ = greater than
L = liter
mEq = milliequivalent
ml = milliliter
dl = deciliter
mm Hg = millimeter of mercury
fl = femtoliter
mm = millimeter
g = gram
mg = millogram (10^{-3})
μg = microgram (one millionth of a gram) (10^{-6})
ng = nanogram (one billionth of a gram) (10^{-9})
pg = picogram (one trillionth of a gram) (10^{-12})
μU = microunit
μl = microliter
IU = international unit
mOsm = milliosmole
U = unit
mmol = millimole
μmol = micromole
nmol = nanomole
pmol = picomole
kPa = kilopascal
μkat = microkatal

Table B-1 Serum, Plasma, and Whole Blood Chemistries

Test	Normal Values: Conventional Units	Normal Values: SI Units	Possible Etiology: Higher	Possible Etiology: Lower
Acetone			Diabetic ketoacidosis, high-fat diet, low-carbohydrate diet, starvation	
Quantitative	0.3-2.0 mg/dl	52-344 μmol/L		
Qualitative	Negative	Negative		
Albumin	3.5-5.0 g/dl	35-50 g/L	Dehydration	Chronic liver disease, malabsorption, malnutrition, nephrotic syndrome, pregnancy
Aldolase	1.0-7.5 U/L	0.02-0.13 μkat/L	Skeletal muscle disease	Renal disease
α-1-Antitrypsin	78-200 mg/dl	0.78-2.0 g/L	Acute and chronic inflammation, arthritis, stress syndrome	Chronic lung disease (early onset), malnutrition, nephrotic syndrome
α-1-Fetoprotein	<15 ng/ml	<15 μg/L	Cancer of testes and ovaries, carcinoma of liver	
Ammonia	30-70 μg/dl	17.6-41.1 μmol/L	Severe liver disease	
Amylase	0-130 U/L (method dependent)	0-2.17 μkat/L	Acute and chronic pancreatitis, mumps (salivary gland disease), perforated ulcers	Acute alcoholism, cirrhosis of liver, extensive destruction of pancreas
Ascorbic acid	0.4-1.5 mg/dl	23-85 μmol/L	Excessive ingestion of vitamin C	Connective tissue disorders, hepatic disease, renal disease, rheumatic fever, vitamin C deficiency
Bicarbonate	20-30 mEq/L	20-30 mmol/L	Compensated respiratory acidosis, metabolic alkalosis	Compensated respiratory alkalosis, metabolic acidosis
Bilirubin			Biliary obstruction, impaired liver function, hemolytic anemia, pernicious anemia, prolonged fasting	
Total	0.2-1.3 mg/dl	3.4-22.0 μmol/L		
Indirect	0.1-1.0 mg/dl	1.7-17.0 μmol/L		
Direct	0.1-0.3 mg/dl	1.7-5.1 μmol/L		
Blood gases*				
Arterial pH	7.35-7.45	Same as conventional units	Alkalosis	Acidosis
Venous pH	7.35-7.45	Same as conventional units		
Arterial PCO_2	35-45 mm Hg	4.67-6.00 kPa	Compensated metabolic alkalosis	Compensated metabolic acidosis
Venous PCO_2	42-52 mm Hg	5.60-6.93 kPa	Respiratory acidosis	Respiratory alkalosis
Arterial PO_2	75-100 mm Hg	10.0-13.33 kPa	Administration of high concentration of oxygen	Chronic lung disease, decreased cardiac output
Venous PO_2	30-50 mm Hg	4.0-6.67 kPa		
Calcium	9-11 mg/dl (4.5-5.5 mEq/L)	2.25-2.74 mmol/L	Acute osteoporosis, hyperparathyroidism, vitamin D intoxication, multiple myeloma	Acute pancreatitis, hypoparathyroidism, liver disease, malabsorption syndrome, renal failure, vitamin D deficiency

Continued

Table B-1 Serum, Plasma, and Whole Blood Chemistries—cont'd

Test	Normal Values: Conventional Units	Normal Values: SI Units	Possible Etiology: Higher	Possible Etiology: Lower
Calcium, ionized	4-4.6 mg/dl (2-2.3 mEq/L	1.0-1.15 mmol/L		
Carbon dioxide (CO_2 content)	20-30 mEq/L	20-30 mmol/L	Same as bicarbonate	
Carotene	10-85 μg/dl	0.19-1.58 μmol/L	Cystic fibrosis, hypothyroidism, pancreatic insufficiency	Dietary deficiency, malabsorption disorders
Chloride	95-105 mEq/L	95-105 mmol/L	Metabolic acidosis, respiratory alkalosis, corticosteroid therapy, uremia	Addison's disease, diarrhea, metabolic alkalosis, respiratory acidosis, vomiting
Cholesterol	140-200 mg/dl (age dependent)	3.6-5.2 mmol/L	Biliary obstruction, hypothyroidism, idiopathic hypercholesterolemia, renal disease, uncontrolled diabetes	Extensive liver disease, hyperthyroidism, malnutrition, corticosteroid therapy
HDL (high-density lipoproteins)				
Male	>45 mg/dl	>1.2 mmol/L		
Female	>55 mg/dl	>1.4 mmol/L		
LDL (low-density lipoproteins)	<130 mg/dl	<3.4 mmol/L		
Cholinesterase (RBC)	0.65-1.00 pH	Same as conventional units	Exercise	Acute infections, insecticide intoxication, liver disease, muscular dystrophy
Pseudocholinesterase (plasma)	5-12 U/ml	Same as conventional units		
Copper	80-150 μg/dl	12.6-23.6 μmol/L	Cirrhosis, female on contraceptives	Wilson's disease
Cortisol	8 AM: 5-25 μg/dl 8 PM: <10 μg/dl	0.14-0.69 μmol/L <0.28 μmol/L	Cushing's syndrome, pancreatitis, stress	Adrenal insufficiency, panhypopituitary states
Creatine	0.2-1.0 mg/dl	15.3-76.3 μmol/L	Active rheumatoid arthritis, biliary obstruction, hyperthyroidism, renal disorders, severe muscle disease	Diabetes mellitus
Creatine kinase (CK)			Musculoskeletal injury or disease, myocardial infarction, severe myocarditis, exercise, numerous intramuscular injections, brain damage	
Male	15-105 U/L	0.26-1.79 μkat/L		
Female	10-80 U/L	0.17-1.36 μkat/L		
CK-MB (CK-2)	0-9 U/L	<0.1 μkat/L	Acute myocardial infarction	
Creatinine	0.5-1.5 mg/dl	44-133 μmol/L	Severe renal disease	
Ferritin (serum)			Sideroblastic anemia, Anemia of chronic disease (infection, inflammation, liver disease)	Iron deficiency anemia
Male	20-300 ng/ml	20-300 μg/L		
Female	10-120 ng/ml	10-120 μg/L		
Folic acid (folate)	3-25 ng/ml	7-57 nmol/L	Hypothyroidism	Alcoholism, hemolytic anemia, inadequate diet, malabsorption syndrome, megaloblastic anemia
Gamma-glutamyl transpeptidase (GGT)	0-30 U/L	0-0.5 μkat/L		Liver disease, infectious mononucleosis

Continued

Table B-1 Serum, Plasma, and Whole Blood Chemistries—cont'd

Test	Normal Values		Possible Etiology	
	Conventional Units	SI Units	Higher	Lower
Glucose, fasting	70-120 mg/dl	3.89-6.66 mmol/L	Acute stress, cerebral lesions, Cushing's disease, diabetes mellitus, hyperthyroidism, pancreatic insufficiency	Addison's disease, hepatic disease, hypothyroidism, insulin overdosage, pancreatic tumor, pituitary hypofunction, postgastrectomy dumping syndrome
Glucose tolerance (GTT)			Diabetes mellitus	Hyperinsulinism
Fasting	70-120 mg/dl	3.89-6.66 mmol/L		
30 min	30-60 mg/dl above fasting	1.67-3.33 mmol/L		
60 min	20-50 mg/dl above fasting	1.11-2.78 mmol/L		
120 min	5-15 mg/dl above fasting	0.28-0.83 mmol/L		
180 min	Fasting level or lower	Fasting level or lower		
Haptoglobin	26-185 mg/dl	260-1850 mg/L	Infectious and inflammatory processes, malignant neoplasms	Hemolytic anemia, mononucleosis, toxoplasmosis, chronic liver disease
Insulin	4-24 μU/ml	29-172 pmol/L	Acromegaly, adenoma of islet cells, untreated mild case of type 2 diabetes	Diabetes mellitus, obesity
Iron, total	50-150 μg/dl	9.0-26.9 μmol/L	Excessive RBC destruction	Iron-deficiency anemia, anemia of chronic disease
Iron-binding capacity	250-410 μg/dl	45-73 μmol/L	Iron-deficient state, oral contraceptives, polycythemia	Cancer, chronic infections, pernicious anemia, uremia
Lactic acid	5-20 μg/dl	0.56-2.2 mmol/L	Acidosis, congestive heart failure, shock	
Lactic dehydrogenase (LDH)	50-150 U/L	0.83-2.5 μkat/L	Congestive heart failure, hemolytic disorders, hepatitis, metastatic cancer of liver, myocardial infarction, pernicious anemia, pulmonary embolus, skeletal muscle damage	
Lactic dehydrogenase isoenzymes				
LDH_1	20-35%	0.20-0.35	Myocardial infarction, pernicious anemia	
LDH_2	30-40%	0.30-0.40	Pulmonary embolus, sickle cell crisis	
LDH_3	15-25%	0.15-0.25	Malignant lymphoma, pulmonary embolus	
LDH_4	0-10%	0-0.10	Lupus erythematosus, pulmonary infarction	
LDH_5	4-12%	0.04-0.12	Congestive heart failure, hepatitis, pulmonary embolus and infarction, skeletal muscle damage	

Continued

Table B-1 Serum, Plasma, and Whole Blood Chemistries—cont'd

Test	Normal Values		Possible Etiology	
	Conventional Units	SI Units	Higher	Lower
Lipase	0-160 U/L	0-2.66 μkat/L	Acute pancreatitis, hepatic disorders, perforated peptic ulcer	
Magnesium	1.5-2.5 mEq/L	0.62-1.03 mmol/L	Addison's disease, hypothyroidism, renal failure	Chronic alcoholism, hyperparathyroidism, hyperthyroidism, hypoparathyroidism, severe malabsorption
Osmolality	285-295 mOsm/kg	285-295 mmol/kg	Chronic renal disease, diabetes mellitus	Addison's disease, diuretic therapy
Oxygen saturation (arterial)	95-98%	0.95-0.98 saturated	Polycythemia	Anemia, cardiac decompensation, respiratory disorders
pH	See blood gases			
Phenylalanine	0-2 mg/dl	0-121 μmol/L	Phenylketonuria	
Phosphatase, acid	0-5.5 U/L	0-90 nkat/L	Advanced Paget's disease, cancer of prostate, hyperparathyroidism	
Phosphatase, alkaline	30-120 U/L	0.5-2.0 μkat/L	Bone diseases, marked hyperparathyroidism, obstruction of biliary system, rickets	Excessive vitamin D ingestion, hypothyroidism, milk-alkali syndrome
Phosphorus, inorganic	2.8-4.5 mg/dl	0.90-1.45 mmol/L	Healing fractures, hypoparathyroidism, renal disease, vitamin D intoxication	Diabetes mellitus, hyperparathyroidism, vitamin D deficiency
Potassium	3.5-5.5 mEq/L	3.5-5.5 mmol/L	Addison's disease, diabetic ketosis, massive tissue destruction, renal failure	Cushing's syndrome, diarrhea (severe), diuretic therapy, gastrointestinal fistula, pyloric obstruction, starvation, vomiting
Prostate-specific antigen (PSA)	<4 ng/mL	<4 μg/L	Prostate cancer	
Proteins			Burns, cirrhosis (globulin fraction), dehydration	Congenital agammaglobulinemia, liver disease, malabsorption
Total	6.0-8.0 g/dl	60-80 g/L		
Albumin	3.5-5.0 g/dl	35-50 g/L		
Globulin	2-3.5 g/dl	20-35 g/L		
Albumin/globulin ratio	1.5:1-2.5:1	Same as conventional units	Multiple myeloma (globulin fraction), shock, vomiting	Malnutrition, nephrotic syndrome, proteinuria, renal disease, severe burns
Renin			Renal hypertension, volume decrease (e.g., hemorrhage)	Increased salt intake, primary aldosteronism
Supine position	1.4-2.9 ng/ml/hr	0.39-0.81 ng/L·sec		
Upright position	0.4-4.5 ng/ml/hr	0.11-1.25 ng/L·sec		
Sodium	135-145 mEq/L	135-145 mmol/L	Dehydration, impaired renal function, primary aldosteronism, corticosteroid therapy	Addison's disease, diabetic ketoacidosis, diuretic therapy, excessive loss from gastrointestinal tract, excessive perspiration, water intoxication

Continued

Table B-1 Serum, Plasma, and Whole Blood Chemistries—cont'd

Test	Normal Values		Possible Etiology	
	Conventional Units	SI Units	Higher	Lower
Testosterone				
Male	300-1200 ng/dl	10.4-41.6 nmol/L		Hypofunction of testes
Female	25-90 ng/dl	0.87-3.1 nmol/L	Polycystic ovary, virilizing tumors	
T_4 (thyroxine), total	5-12 μg/dl	64-154 nmol/L	Hyperthyroidism, thyroiditis	Cretinism, hypothyroidism, myxedema
T_4 (thyroxine), free	0.8-2.3 ng/dl	10-30 pmol/L		
T_3 uptake	25-35%	0.25-0.35	Hyperthyroidism, metastatic neoplasms	Hypothyroidism, pregnancy
T_3 (triiodothyronine)	110-230 ng/dl	1.7-3.5 nmol/L	Hyperthyroidism	Hypothyroidism
Thyroid-stimulating hormone (TSH)	0.3-5.4 μU/ml	0.3-5.4 mU/L	Myxedema, primary hypothyroidism, Graves' disease	Secondary hypothyroidism
Transaminases				
Serum glutamicoxaloacetic (SGOT) or aspartate aminotransferase (AST)	7-40 U/L	0.12-0.67 μkat/L	Liver disease, myocardial infarction, pulmonary infarction, acute hepatitis	
Serum glutamate pyruvate (SGPT) or alanine aminotransferase (ALT)	5-36 U/L	0.08-0.6 μkat/L	Liver disease, shock	
Triglycerides	40-150 mg/dl	0.45-1.69 mmol/L	Diabetes mellitus, hyperlipidemia, hypothyroidism, liver disease	Malnutrition
Urea nitrogen (BUN)	10-30 mg/dl	1.8-7.1 mmol/L	Increase in protein catabolism (fever, stress), renal disease, urinary tract infection	Malnutrition, severe liver damage
Uric acid			Gout, gross tissue destruction, high-protein weight reduction diet, leukemia, renal failure, eclampsia	Administration of uricosuric drugs
Male	4.5-6.5 mg/dl	149-327 μmol/L		
Female	2.5-5.5 mg/dl	268-387 μmol/L		
Vitamin A	15-60 μg/dl	0.52-2.09 μmol/L	Excess ingestion of vitamin A	Vitamin A deficiency
Vitamin B_{12}	200-1000 pg/ml	148-738 pmol/L	Chronic myeloid leukemia	Strict vegetarianism, malabsorption syndrome, pernicious anemia, total or partial gastrectomy
Zinc	50-150 μg/dl	7.6-22.9 μmol/L		Alcoholic cirrhosis

*Because arterial blood gases are influenced by altitude, the value for PO_2 decreases as altitude increases. The lower value is normal for an altitude of 1 mile.
RBC, red blood cell.

Table **B-2** Hematology

Test	Normal Values: Conventional Units	Normal Values: SI Units	Possible Etiology: Higher	Possible Etiology: Lower
Bleeding time (Simplate)	3.0-9.5 min	180-570 sec	Defective platelet function, thrombocytopenia, von Willebrand's disease, aspirin ingestion, vascular disease	
Activated partial thromboplastin time (APTT)	30-45 sec*	Same as conventional units	Deficiency of factors I, II, V, VIII, IX and X, XI, XII; hemophilia, liver disease, heparin therapy	
Prothrombin time (Protime, PT)	10-14 sec*	Same as conventional units	Warfarin therapy, deficiency of factors I, II, V, VII, and X, vitamin K deficiency, liver disease	
Fibrinogen	200-400 mg/dl	2.0-4.0 g/L	Burns (after first 36 hr), inflammatory disease	Burns (during first 36 hr), DIC, severe liver disease
Fibrin split (degradation) products	<10 μg/ml	Same as conventional units	Acute DIC, massive hemorrhage, primary fibrinolysis	
D-Dimer	Negative	Negative	DIC, myocardial infarction, deep vein thrombosis, unstable angina	
Erythrocyte count† (altitude dependent)			Dehydration, high altitudes, polycythemia vera, severe diarrhea	Anemia, leukemia, posthemorrhage
Male	$4.5\text{-}6.0 \times 10^6/\mu L$	$4.5\text{-}6.0 \times 10^{12}/L$		
Female	$4.0\text{-}5.0 \times 10^6/\mu L$	$4.0\text{-}5.0 \times 10^{12}/L$		
Mean corpuscular volume (MCV)	82-98 fl	Same as conventional units	Macrocytic anemia	Microcytic anemia
Mean corpuscular hemoglobin (MCH)	27-33 pg	Same as conventional units	Macrocytic anemia	Microcytic anemia
Mean corpuscular hemoglobin concentration (MCHC)	32-36%	0.32-0.36	Spherocytosis	Hypochromic anemia
Erythrocyte sedimentation rate (ESR), Westergren			Moderate increase: acute hepatitis, myocardial infarction; rheumatoid arthritis; marked increase: acute and severe bacterial infections, malignancies, pelvic inflammatory disease	Malaria Severe liver disease Sickle cell anemia
Male <50 yr	<15 mm/hr	Same as conventional units		
Male >50 yr	<20 mm/hr			
Female <50 yr	<20 mm/hr	Same as conventional units		
Female >50 yr	<30 mm/hr			

Continued

Table B-2 Hematology—cont'd

Test	Normal Values: Conventional Units	Normal Values: SI Units	Possible Etiology: Higher	Possible Etiology: Lower
Hematocrit (altitude dependent)†			Dehydration, high altitudes, polycythemia	Anemia, hemorrhage, overhydration
Male	40-54%	0.40-0.54		
Female	38-47%	0.38-0.47		
Hemoglobin (altitude dependent)†				
Male	13.5-18.0 g/dl	135-180 g/L	COPD, high altitudes, polycythemia	Anemia, hemorrhage
Female	12.0-16.0 g/dl	120-160 g/L		
Hemoglobin, glycosylated	4.0-6.0%	Same as conventional units	Poorly controlled diabetes mellitus	Sickle cell Chronic renal failure Pregnancy
Red cell distribution width (RDW)	10.2-14.5%	Same as conventional therapy		Anisocytosis, macrocytic anemia, microcytic anemia
Platelet count (thrombocytes)	150-400 × $10^3/\mu l$	150-400 × $10^9/L$	Acute infections, chronic granulocytic leukemia, chronic pancreatitis, cirrhosis, collagen disorders, polycythemia, postsplenectomy	Acute leukemia, DIC, thrombocytopenic purpura
Reticulocyte count (manual)	0.5-1.5% of RBC	Same	Hemolytic anemia, polycythemia vera	Hypoproliferative anemia, macrocytic anemia, microcytic anemia
White blood cell count†	4.0-11.0 × $10^3/\mu l$	4.0-11.0 × $10^9/L$	Inflammatory and infectious processes, leukemia	Aplastic anemia, side effects of chemotherapy and irradiation
WBC differential				
Segmented neutrophils	50-70%	0.50-0.70	Bacterial infections, collagen diseases, Hodgkin's disease	Aplastic anemia, viral infections
Band neutrophils	0-8%	0-0.08	Acute infections	
Lymphocytes	20-40%	0.20-0.40	Chronic infections, lymphocytic leukemia, mononucleosis, viral infections	Corticosteroid therapy, whole body irradiation
Monocytes	4-8%	0.04-0.08	Chronic inflammatory disorders, malaria, monocytic leukemia, acute infections, Hodgkin's disease	
Eosinophils	0-4%	0-0.04	Allergic reactions, eosinophilic and chronic granulocytic leukemia, parasitic disorders, Hodgkin's disease	Corticosteroid therapy
Basophils	0-2%	0-0.02	Hyperthyroidism, ulcerative colitis, myeloproliferative diseases	Hyperthyroidism, stress
Sickle cell solubility test	Negative	Negative	Sickle cell anemia	

*Values depend on reagent and instrumentation used.
†Components of complete blood count (CBC).
COPD, chronic obstructive pulmonary disease; *DIC,* disseminated intravascular coagulation; *WBC,* white blood cell.

Table B-3 Serology-Immunology

Test	Normal Values		Possible Etiology	
	Conventional Units	SI Units	Higher	Lower
Antinuclear antibody (ANA)	Negative or titer <1:10	Same as conventional units	Chronic hepatitis, rheumatoid arthritis, scleroderma, systemic lupus erythematosus	
Anti-DNA antibody	Negative or titer <1:10 or <20% binding	Same as conventional units	Systemic lupus erythematosus	
Anti-RNP	Negative	Negative	Mixed connective tissue disease, rheumatoid arthritis, systemic lupus erythematosus, Sjögren's syndrome, scleroderma	
Anti-Sm (Smith)	Negative	Negative	Systemic lupus erythematosus	
Antistreptolysin-O (ASO)	≤166 Todd units or ≤1:85	Same as conventional units	Acute glomerulonephritis, rheumatic fever, streptococcal infection	
C-reactive protein (CRP)	Negative or ≤1.2 mg/dl	Same as conventional units	Acute infections, any inflammatory condition, widespread malignancy	
Carcinoembryonic antigen (CEA)	≤2.5 ng/ml	≤2.5 μg/L	Carcinoma of colon, liver, pancreas; chronic cigarette smoking; inflammatory bowel disease; other cancers	
Complement components				Acute glomerulonephritis, systemic lupus erythematosus, rheumatoid arthritis, subacute bacterial endocarditis, serum sickness
C1q	11-21 mg/dl	0.11-0.21 g/L		
C3	80-180 mg/dl	0.8-1.8 g/L		
C4	15-50 mg/dl	0.15-0.5 g/L		
Direct antihuman globulin test (DAT) or direct Coombs	Negative	Negative	Acquired hemolytic anemia, hemolytic disease of the newborn, drug reactions, transfusion reactions	
Fluorescent treponemal antibody absorption (FTAAbs)	Nonreactive	Negative	Syphilis	

Continued

Table B-3 Serology-Immunology—cont'd

Test	Normal Values: Conventional Units	Normal Values: SI Units	Possible Etiology: Higher	Possible Etiology: Lower
Hepatitis A antibody	Negative	Negative	Hepatitis A	
Hepatitis B surface antigen (HB_sAg)	Negative	Negative	Hepatitis B	
Hepatitis C antibody	Negative	Negative	Hepatitis C	
Immunoglobulin				
IgA	90-400 mg/dl	0.9-4.0 g/L	IgA myeloma, chronic liver disease, chronic infection, rheumatoid arthritis, autoimmune disorders	Burns, hereditary telangiectasia, malabsorption syndromes
IgD	0.5-12 mg/dl	5-120 mg/L	Chronic infection, connective tissue disease	
IgE	<1 mg/dl	<10 mg/L	Anaphylactic shock, atopic disease (allergies), parasite infections	
IgG	650-1800 mg/dl	6.5-18.0 g/L	Infections—acute and chronic, hepatitis, IgG monoclonal gammopathy, systemic lupus erythematosus	Congenital deficiencies, acquired deficiencies, nephrotic syndromes, burns, immunosuppression
IgM	55-300 mg/dl	0.5-3.0 g/L	Acute infections, rheumatoid arthritis, liver disease	Congenital and acquired antibody deficiencies, lymphocytic leukemia, protein-losing enteropathies
Monospot or monotest	Negative	Negative	Infectious mononucleosis	
Rheumatoid factor (RA factor)	Negative or titer <1:20	Same as conventional units	Rheumatoid arthritis, Sjögren's syndrome, systemic lupus erythematosus	
RPR	Nonreactive	Same as conventional units	Syphilis, systemic lupus erythematosus, rheumatoid arthritis, leprosy, malaria, febrile diseases, IV drug abuse	
VDRL	Nonreactive	Same as conventional units	Syphilis	
Thyroid antibodies	≤1:10 titer	Same as conventional units	Hashimoto's thyroiditis, thyroid carcinoma, early hypothyroidism, pernicious anemia, systemic lupus erythematosus, Graves' disease	

CSF, colony-stimulating factor; *RNP,* ribonuclear protein; *RPR,* rapid plasma reagin test; *VDRL,* Venereal Disease Research Laboratory test.

Table B-4 Urine Chemistry

Test	Specimen	Normal Values: Conventional Units	Normal Values: SI Units	Possible Etiology: Higher	Possible Etiology: Lower
Acetone	Random	Negative	Negative	Diabetes mellitus, high-fat and low-carbohydrate diets, starvation states	
Aldosterone	24 hr	1-80 μg/day (depends on urinary sodium)	2.7-222 nmol/day	Primary aldosteronism: adrenocortical tumors; secondary aldosteronism: cardiac failure, cirrhosis, large dose of ACTH, salt depletion	ACTH deficiency, Addison's disease, corticosteroid therapy
Amylase	24 hr	1-17 U/hr	Same as conventional units	Acute pancreatitis	
Bence Jones protein	Random	Negative	Negative	Multiple myeloma, biliary duct obstruction	
Bilirubin	Random	Negative	Negative	Hepatitis	
Calcium	24 hr	100-250 mg/day	2.5-6.3 mmol/day	Bone tumor, hyperparathyroidism, milk-alkali syndrome	Hypoparathyroidism, malabsorption of calcium and vitamin D
Catecholamines	24 hr			Pheochromocytoma, progressive muscular dystrophy, heart failure	
Epinephrine		<20 μg/day	<118 nmol/day		
Norepinephrine		<100 μg/day	<591 nmol/day		
Chloride	24 hr	110-250 mEq/day	110-250 mmol/day	Addison's disease	Burns, excess perspiration, vomiting, diarrhea, menstruation
Copper	24 hr	<30 μg/day	<0.5 μmol/day	Cirrhosis, Wilson's disease	
Coproporphyrin	24 hr	50-200 μg/day	76-305 nmol/day	Lead poisoning, oral contraceptive use, poliomyelitis	
Creatine	24 hr	<100 mg/day	<763 μmol/day	Carcinoma of liver, hyperthyroidism, diabetes, Addison's disease, infections, burns, muscular dystrophy, skeletal muscle atrophy	Hypothyroidism
Creatinine	24 hr	0.8-2.0 g/day	7.1-17.7 mmol/day	Anemia, leukemia, muscular atrophy, salmonellae	Renal disease
Creatinine clearance	24 hr	85-135 ml/min	1.42-2.25 ml/sec		Renal disease
Estrogens	24 hr				
Female				Gonadal or adrenal tumor	Agenesis of ovaries, endocrine disturbance, ovarian dysfunction, menopause
Ovulation peak		28-100 μg/day	104-370 nmol/day		
Luteal peak		22-80 μg/day	81-296 nmol/day		
Pregnancy		Up to 45,000 μg/day	Up to 166,455 nmol/day		
Menopause		1.4-19.6 μg/day	5.2-72.5 nmol/day		
Male		5-18 μg/day	18-67 nmol/day		
Glucose	Random	Negative	Negative	Diabetes mellitus, low renal threshold for glucose resorption, physiologic stress, pituitary disorders	

Continued

Table B-4 Urine Chemistry—cont'd

Test	Normal Values			Possible Etiology	
	Specimen	Conventional Units	SI Units	Higher	Lower
Hemoglobin	Random	Negative	Negative	Extensive burns, glomerulonephritis, hemolytic anemias, hemolytic transfusion reaction	
5-Hydroxyindoleacetic acid (5-HIAA)	24 hr	2-9 mg/day	10.5-47.1 μmol/day	Malignant carcinoid syndrome	
Ketone bodies	24 hr	20-50 mg/day	0.34-0.86 mmol/day	Marked ketonuria	
Lead	24 hr	<100 μg/day	<0.48 μmol/day	Lead poisoning	
Metanephrine	24 hr	<1.3 mg/day	<7.1 μmol/day	Pheochromocytoma	
Myoglobin	Random	Negative	Negative	Crushing injuries, electric injuries, extreme physical exertion	
pH	Random	4.0-8.0	Same as conventional units	Chronic renal failure, compensatory phase of alkalosis, salicylate intoxication, vegetarian diet	Compensatory phase of acidosis, dehydration, emphysema
Phenylpyruvic acid	Random	Negative	Negative	Phenylketonuria	
Phosphorus, inorganic	24 hr	0.9-1.3 g/day	29-42 mmol/day	Fever, hypoparathyroidism, nervous exhaustion, rickets, tuberculosis	Acute infections, nephritis
Porphobilinogen	Random 24 hr	Negative <2.0 mg/day	Negative <9 μmol/day	Acute intermittent porphyria, liver disorders	
Protein (dipstick)	Random	Negative	Negative	Congestive heart failure, nephritis, nephrosis, physiologic stress	
Protein (quantitative)	24 hr	<150 mg/day	<0.15 g/day	Cardiac failure, inflammatory processes of urinary tract, nephritis, nephrosis, toxemia of pregnancy	
Sodium	24 hr	40-250 mEq/day	40-250 mmol/day	Acute tubular necrosis	Hyponatremia
Specific gravity	Random	1.003-1.030	Same as conventional units	Albuminuria, dehydration, glycosuria	Diabetes insipidus
Titratable acidity	24 hr	20-50 mEq/day	Same as conventional units	Metabolic acidosis	Metabolic alkalosis
Uric acid	24 hr	250-750 mg/day	1.5-4.5 mmol/day	Gout, leukemia	Nephritis
Urobilinogen	24 hr Random	0.5-4.0 EU/day <1.0 Erhlich unit	Same as conventional units Same as conventional units	Hemolytic disease, hepatic parenchymal cell damage, liver disease	Complete obstruction of bile duct
Uroporphyrins	Random	Random	Same as conventional units	Porphyria	
Vanillylmandelic acid	24 hr	1-8 mg/day 1.5-7 μg/mg creatine	5-40 μmol/day	Pheochromocytoma	

ACTH, adrenocorticotropic hormone; *EU,* Ehrlich unit.

Table B-5 Gastric Analysis

Test	Normal Values: Conventional Units	Normal Values: SI Units	Possible Etiology: Higher	Possible Etiology: Lower
Basal				
Free hydrochloric acid	0.30 mEq/L	Same as conventional units	Hypermotility of stomach	Pernicious anemia
Total acidity	15-45 mEq/L	Same as conventional units	Gastric and duodenal ulcers, Zollinger-Ellison syndrome	Gastric carcinoma, severe gastritis
Poststimulation				
Free hydrochloric acid	10-130 mEq/L	Same as conventional units		
Total acidity	20-150 mEq/L	Same as conventional units		

Table B-6 Fecal Analysis

Test	Normal Values: Conventional Units	Normal Values: SI Units	Possible Etiology: Higher	Possible Etiology: Lower
Fecal fat	<6 g/24 hr	Same as conventional units	Chronic pancreatic disease, obstruction of common bile duct, malabsorption syndrome	
Urobilinogen	30-220 mg/100 g of stool	51-372 μmol/100 g of stool	Hemolytic anemias	Complete biliary obstruction
Mucus	Negative	Negative	Mucous colitis, spastic constipation	
Pus	Negative	Negative	Chronic bacillary dysentery, chronic ulcerative colitis, localized abscesses	
Blood*	Negative	Negative	Anal fissures, hemorrhoids, malignant tumor, peptic ulcer, inflammatory bowel disease	
Color				
Brown			Various color depending on diet	
Clay			Biliary obstruction or presence of barium sulfate	
Tarry			More than 100 ml of blood in gastrointestinal tract	
Red			Blood in large intestine	
Black			Blood in upper gastrointestinal tract or iron medication	

*Ingestion of meat may produce false-positive results. Patient may be placed on a meat-free diet for 3 days before the test.

Table B-7 Cereobrospinal Fluid Analysis

	Normal Values		Possible Etiology	
Test	**Conventional Units**	**SI Units**	**Higher**	**Lower**
Pressure	60-150 mm H_20	Same as conventional units	Hemorrhage, intracranial tumor, meningitis	Head injury, spinal tumor, subdural hematoma
Blood	Negative	Negative	Intracranial hemorrhage	
Cell count (age dependent)				
WBC	0-5 cells/μl	0.5×10^6/L	Inflammation or infections of CNS	
RBC	0	0×10^6/L		
Chloride	100-130 mEq/L	100-130 mmol/L	Uremia	Bacterial infections of CNS (meningitis, encephalitis)
Glucose	40-75 mg/dl	2.5-4.2 mmol/L	Diabetes mellitus, viral infections of CNS	Bacterial infections and tuberculosis of CNS
Protein				
Lumbar	15-45 mg/dl	0.15-0.45 g/L	Guillain-Barré syndrome, poliomyelitis, traumatic tap	
Cisternal	15-25 mg/dl	0.15-0.25 g/L	Syphilis of CNS	
Ventricular	5-15 mg/dl	0.05-0.15 g/L	Acute meningitis, brain tumor, chronic CNS infections, multiple sclerosis	

CNS, central nervous system.

Table B-8 Toxicology of Common Drugs

Drug	Therapeutic Level		Toxic Level	
	Conventional Units	SI Units	Conventional Units	SI Units
Acetaminophen (Tylenol)	0.2-0.6 mg/dl	13-40 μmol/L	>5 mg/dl	>330 μmol/L
Barbiturates				
Short acting	1-2 mg/dl	Dependent on composition of mixture	>5 mg/dl	
Intermediate acting	1-5 mg/dl		>10 mg/dl	
Long acting	15-35 mg/dl		>40 mg/dl	
Carbon monoxide (carboxyhemoglobin)				
Normal values	<5% saturation of hemoglobin	<0.05	Symptoms with >20% saturation	>0.20
Urban nonsmokers	<5% saturation of hemoglobin	<0.05		
Rural nonsmokers	0.5-2% saturation of hemoglobin	0.005-0.02		
Smokers	5-9% saturation of hemoglobin	0.05-0.09		
Heavy smokers	>9% saturation of hemoglobin	>0.09		
Chlordiazepoxide (Librium)	0.05-5.0 mg/L	2-17 μmol/L	>10 mg/L	>33 μmol/L
Chlorpromazine (Thorazine)	0.5 μg/ml	1.6 μmol/L	>2.0 μg/ml	>6.3 μmol/L
Diazepam (Valium)	0.10-0.25 mg/L	0.35-0.88 μmol/L	>1.0 mg/L ≥2.0 mg/L (lethal)	>3.5 μmol/L
Digitalis preparations				
Digoxin	0.8-2.4 ng/ml	1.0-3.1 nmol/L	>2.5 ng/ml	>2.6 nmol/L
Digitoxin	14-30 ng/ml	18-39 nmol/L	>30 ng/ml	>39 nmol/L
Dilantin	10-20 mg/L	40-80 μmol/L	>30 mg/L	>120 μmol/L
Gentamicin (Garamycin)				
Peak	4-10 mg/L	9-22 μmol/L	>10 mg/L	>22 μmol/L
Trough	<2 mg/L	<4 mmol/L	>2 mg/L	>4 μmol/L
Propranolol (Inderal)	50-100 ng/ml	192-386 nmol/L	>200 ng/ml	>771 nmol/L
Salicylates	10-20 mg/dl	0.724-1.45 mmol/L	>20 mg/dl	>1.45 mmol/L
Alcohol (ethanol)*			>60 mg/dl (lethal)	>4.34 mmol/L

*See Table 10-10.

C Answer Key to Review Questions

Chapter 1
1. d
2. c
3. d
4. c
5. b
6. c
7. b
8. b

Chapter 2
1. d
2. d
3. b
4. a

Chapter 3
1. d
2. d
3. b
4. d
5. a
6. c

Chapter 4
1. a
2. a
3. c
4. b
5. d
6. b
7. c
8. c
9. a
10 b
11. a
12. c

Chapter 5
1. d
2. c
3. a
4. b
5. c
6. b

Chapter 6
1. c
2. b
3. c
4. d
5. e
6. c
7. b
8. a

Chapter 7
1. b
2. a
3. a
4. c
5. d
6. d
7. a
8. d

Chapter 8
1. b
2. c
3. a
4. a
5. c
6. c
7. c
8. d
9. b

Chapter 9
1. b
2. c
3. c
4. c
5. b
6. b
7. c
8. b
9. d

Chapter 10
1. a
2. d
3. c
4. b
5. b
6. b
7. d
8. c
9. c
10. d
11. b
12. b

Chapter 11
1. b
2. a
3. b
4. d
5. b
6. b
7. d
8. c
9. d

Chapter 12
1. b
2. b
3. c
4. a
5. d
6. a
7. d
8. b
9. c
10. d
11. a
12. a

Chapter 13
1. a
2. b
3. d
4. a
5. c
6. d
7. c
8. a
9. c

Chapter 14
1. b
2. d
3. d
4. a
5. d
6. b
7. c
8. b
9. c
10. d
11. b
12. c
13. c
14. d
15. d
16. a

Chapter 15
1. c
2. a

3a. d
3b. b
3c. c
3d. c
3e. a
3f. b
3g. c

4. a

Chapter 16
1. d
2. c
3. c
4. a
5. b
6. c
7. a
8. d

Chapter 17
1. c
2. c
3. c
4. a
5. d

6. d
7. c
8. b
9. c

Chapter 18

1. d
2. b
3. d
4. a
5. c
6. a

Chapter 19

1. c
2. d
3. c
4. a
5. c
6. d
7. a

Chapter 20

1. b
2. d
3. c
4. c
5. d
6. b
7. a
8. a
9. a
10. b
11. b

Chapter 21

1. c
2. a
3. c
4. a
5. d
6. a
7. c
8. a
9. a

Chapter 22

1. b
2. a
3. d
4. a
5. d
6. d
7. c
8. b
9. d
10. a
11. c

Chapter 23

1. c
2. a
3. c
4. d
5. c
6. c
7. b
8. a
9. b
10. b
11. b

Chapter 24

1. a
2. c
3. a
4. b
5. b
6. c
7. c
8. a
9. d
10. a
11. d

Chapter 25

1. a
2. b
3. a
4. c
5. b
6. d
7. a
8. d

Chapter 26

1. a
2. d
3. c
4. a
5. c
6. d
7. c
8. d
9. c
10. a
11. c
12. d
13. c
14. b

Chapter 27

1. a
2. a
3. b
4. d
5. c
6. c
7. d

Chapter 28

1. b
2. c
3. b
4. a
5. a
6. c
7. a
8. b

Chapter 29

1. a
2. b
3. d
4. c
5. c
6. a
7. a
8. c
9. c
10. d
11. d
12. c
13. c
14. a
15. c
16. d
17. d

Chapter 30

1. c
2. c
3. d
4. d
5. b
6. d
7. a
8. b
9. c
10. a
11. b

Chapter 31

1. d
2. b
3. d
4. b
5. d
6. d
7. a
8. b

Chapter 32

1. c
2. a
3. a
4. b
5. c
6. c
7. c
8. b
9. c

Chapter 33

1. b
2. b
3. a
4. a
5. b
6. b
7. a

Chapter 34

1. d
2. b
3. d
4. a
5. a
6. c
7. b
8. d

Chapter 35

1. a
2. b
3. a
4. a
5. c
6. c
7. b
8. c
9. c
10. b

Chapter 36

1. a
2. c
3. c
4. c
5. b
6. a
7. c
8. b
9. a
10. d
11. d
12. c

Chapter 37

1. d
2. b
3. b
4. a
5. c
6. c
7. b
8. a
9. b

Chapter 38

1. c
2. d
3. a
4. c
5. b
6. a
7. d
8. d

Chapter 39

1. a
2. d
3. a
4. c
5. d
6. c
7. c
8. c
9. b
10. c
11. a
12. d
13. a
14. d
15. b

Chapter 40

1. d
2. a
3. c
4. b
5. b
6. d
7. c
8. d
9. a
10. a
11. a
12. b
13. b
14. c
15. a
16. c

Chapter 41

1. d
2. b
3. b
4. b
5. d
6. a
7. d
8. d
9. c
10. c
11. b

Chapter 42

1. d
2. b
3. d
4. b
5. a
6. a
7. b
8. d

Chapter 43

1. d
2. a
3. b
4. a
5. d
6. a
7. d
8. d
9. b
10. a
11. b
12. d

Chapter 44

1. b
2. a
3. c
4. c
5. d
6. c
7. d
8. c
9. a
10. d
11. b

Chapter 45

1. b
2. c
3. a
4. d
5. a
6. c
7. d
8. c
9. a

Chapter 46

1. b
2. d
3. c
4. c
5. d
6. d
7. c

Chapter 47

1. b
2. b
3. c
4. a
5. d
6. d
7. d
8. a
9. c

Chapter 48

1. c
2. c
3. d
4. b
5. d
6. b
7. a
8. b

Chapter 49

1. d
2. d
3. c
4. a
5. c
6. c
7. d
8. b

Chapter 50

1. c
2. a
3. c
4. d
5. d
6. c
7. a

Chapter 51

1. d
2. b
3. c
4. d
5. d
6. c
7. a
8. c
9. d
10. c
11. b
12. b
13. c
14. a
15. d

Chapter 52

1. b
2. d
3. b
4. a
5. c
6. b
7. c

Chapter 53

1. c
2. a
3. d
4. c
5. d
6. c
7. d
8. a
9. c
10. a
11. b

Chapter 54

1. c
2. d
3. c
4. d
5. b
6. b
7. b
8. c
9. a
10. a
11. c
12. d
13. a
14. b

Chapter 55

1. d
2. c
3. d
4. a
5. d
6. c
7. b
8. c
9. b

Chapter 56

1. c
2. a
3. b
4. c
5. a
6. d
7. d

Chapter 57

1. c
2. d
3. c
4. c
5. c
6. b
7. c
8. b

Chapter 58

1. c
2. b
3. d
4. d
5. c
6. d
7. c
8. d
9. a

Chapter 59

1. d
2. b
3. d
4. c
5. d
6. b
7. b
8. a
9. d
10. a
11. d
12. c
13. a
14. b

Chapter 60

1. a
2. a
3. c
4. c
5. c
6. d
7. b
8. c
9. b
10. d

Chapter 61

1. c
2. a
3. b
4. a
5. a
6. d

Chapter 62

1. b
2. a
3. d
4. a
5. c

Chapter 63

1. d
2. b
3. b
4. c
5. c
6. b
7. a
8. a
9. b
10. c
11. b
12. c

Chapter 64

1. d
2. a
3. c

ILLUSTRATION CREDITS

Chapter 1

1-3, From Potter PA, Perry AG: *Fundamentals of nursing: concepts, process, and practice,* ed 4, St Louis, 1997, Mosby.

Chapter 2

2-1, 2-2, 2-3, 2-4, From Potter PA, Perry AG: *Fundamentals of nursing: concepts, process, and practice,* ed 4, St Louis, 1997, Mosby.

Chapter 3

3-1, 3-3, 3-7, 3-8, 3-9, Courtesy CLG Photographics, St Louis; 3-4, from Potter PA, Perry AG: *Basic nursing,* ed 4, St Louis, 1997, Mosby; 3-5, from Sorrentino SA: *Nursing assistants*, St Louis, 1996, Mosby.

Chapter 4

4-1, US Bureau of Census; 4-2, 4-5, 4-9, from Sorrentino SA: *Nursing assistants,* St Louis, 1996, Mosby; 4-3, 4-7, 4-8, 4-10, courtesy CLG Photographics, St Louis; 4-4, from Wilson SF, Thompson JM: *Respiratory disorders,* St Louis, 1995, Mosby; 4-6, redrawn from Benzon J: Approaching drug regimens with a therapeutic dose of suspicion, *Geriatr Nurs* 12:4, 1991, p. 1813.

Chapter 5

5-1, From Thompson JM, Wilson SF: *Health assessment for nursing practice,* St Louis, 1996, Mosby.

Chapter 6

6-1, Reprinted from *Patient Educ Couns*, vol 27, Boise L and others: *Facing chronic illness: the family support model and its benefits,* p 76, 1996, with permission from Elsevier Science.

Chapter 8

8-1, 8-2, 8-3, 8-5, 8-6, 8-7, Courtesy CLG Photographics, St Louis.

Chapter 9

9-17, Courtesy CLG Photographics, St Louis.

Chapter 10

10-4, 10-5, Courtesy CLG Photographics, St Louis.

Chapter 11

11-2, Courtesy Cameron Bangs, MD. In Auerbach PS, editor: *Wilderness medicine: management of wilderness and environmental emergencies,* ed 3, St Louis, 1995, Mosby; 11-10, courtesy Molnlyche Health Care, Eddystone, Pa. In Potter PA, Perry AG: *Fundamentals of nursing: concepts, process, and practice*, ed 4, St Louis, 1997, Mosby; 11-11, from Habif TP: *Clinical dermatology: a color guide to diagnosis and therapy,* ed 2, St Louis, 1992, Mosby; 11-12, from Potter PA, Perry AG: *Fundamentals of nursing: concepts, process, and practice,* ed 4, St Louis, 1997, Mosby.

Chapter 13

13-6, 13-7, From Grimes DE, Grimes RM: *AIDS and HIV infection*, St Louis, 1994, Mosby; 13-8, from the Centers for Disease Control. Courtesy Jonathan WM Gold, MD, New York, NY; 13-9, from Seidel HM and others: *Mosby's guide to physical examination,* ed 4, St Louis, 1999, Mosby. Courtesy Douglas A. Jabs, MD, the Wilmer Ophthalmological Institute, The Johns Hopkins University and Hospital, Baltimore.

Chapter 14

14-4, Modified from DeVita VT, Helman S, Rosenberg SA, editors: *Cancer: principles and practice of oncology,* Philadelphia, 1997, Lippincott-Raven; 14-19, modified from Krakoff IH: Systemic treatment of cancer, *CA Cancer J Clin* 46:134, 1996; 14-22, courtesy Pharmacia Deltec, Inc, St Paul, Minn; 14-23, courtesy Strato/Infusaid, Inc, Norwood, Mass; 14-24, data from The World Health Organization, 1990.

Chapter 16

16-1, 16-3, 16-4, Courtesy Rush-Presbyterian St Luke's Medical Center, Chicago, Ill; 16-2, courtesy Swedish American Hospital, Rockford, Ill; 16-5, courtesy St Joseph Hospital, Albuquerque, NM.

Chapter 17

17-1, Courtesy Greg McVicar; 17-2, from Potter PA, Perry AG: *Basic nursing,* ed 3, St Louis, 1995, Mosby; 17-3, courtesy Spacelabs Medical, Redmond, Wash; 17-5, courtesy of The Methodist Hospital, Houston, Texas. Photograph by Donna Dahms, RN, CNOR; 17-6, courtesy of ConMed, Englewood, Colo; 17-7, 17-8, from Litwack K: *Post anesthesia care nursing,* ed 2, St Louis, 1995, Mosby; 17-10, from Meeker MH, Rothrock JC: *Alexander's care of the patient in surgery,* ed 11, St Louis, 1999, Mosby.

Chapter 18

18-1, Courtesy Rush-Presbyterian St Luke's Medical Center, Chicago, Ill.

Chapter 19

19-1, From Seeley R, Stephens T, Tate P: *Anatomy and physiology,* ed 3, New York, 1995, McGraw-Hill; 19-3, from Thibodeau GA, Patton KT: *Anatomy and physiology*, ed 4, St Louis, 1999, Mosby; 19-8, from Seeley R, Stephens T, Tate P: *Anatomy and physiology,* ed 2, New York, 1992, McGraw-Hill, Marcia J. Dohrmann, artist; 19-9, from Seidel HM and others: *Mosby's guide to physical examination,* ed 4, St Louis, 1999, Mosby; 19-11, courtesy Medical Records Subcommittee of the University of Iowa Hospitals and Clinics, Iowa City, Iowa.

Chapter 20

20-8, 20-10, Courtesy CLG Photographics, Inc, St Louis.

Chapter 21

21-1, From Thibodeau GA, Patton KT: *Anatomy and physiology,* ed 4, St Louis, 1999, Mosby; 21-3A, 21-3B, from Habif TP: *Clinical dermatology: a color guide to diagnosis and therapy,* ed 3, St Louis, 1996, Mosby.

Chapter 22

22-2, 22-3, 22-5, 22-6, 22-7, From Habif TP: *Clinical dermatology: a color guide to diagnosis and therapy,* ed 3, St Louis, 1996, Mosby; 22-4, from US Centers for Disease Control; 22-8, from Potter PA, Perry AG: *Basic nursing; a critical thinking approach,* ed 4, St Louis, 1999, Mosby, courtesy Laurel Wiersma, RN, MSN, Clinical Nurse Specialist, Barnes Hospital, St Louis; 22-9, from Potter PA, Perry AG: *Fundamentals of nursing: concepts, process, and practice,* ed 4, St Louis, 1997, Mosby. Courtesy ConvaTec.

Chapter 24

24-1, Redrawn from Price SA, Wilson LM: *Pathophysiology: clinical concepts of disease processes,* ed 5, St Louis, 1997, Mosby; 24-2, 24-3, from Thompson JM and others: *Clinical nursing,* ed 4, St Louis, 1997, Mosby; 24-4A, from Bone RC and others, editors: *Pulmonary and critical care medicine,* vol 1, St Louis, 1993, Mosby; 24-4B, from Staub NC, Albertine KH: Anatomy of the lungs. In Murray JF, Nadel JA, editors: *Textbook of respiratory medicine,* ed 2, Philadelphia, 1994, Saunders; 24-8A, redrawn from *Principles of pulse oximetry,* Nellcor, Inc, Haywood, Calif; 24-8B, from Potter PA, Perry AG: *Fundamentals of nursing: concepts, process, and practice,* ed 4, St Louis, 1997, Mosby; 24-10, redrawn from Wilkins RL and others: *Clinical assessment in respiratory care,* ed 3, St Louis, 1995, Mosby; 24-12, modified from Thompson JM and others: *Clinical nursing,* ed 4, St Louis, 1997, Mosby; 24-14, from Beare PG, Myers JL: *Adult health nursing,* ed 3, St Louis, 1998, Mosby; 24-15A, courtesy Olympus America, Melville, NY; 24-15B, from Meduri GU and others: Protected bronchoalveolar lavage, *Am Respir Dis* 143:855, 1991; 24-16, redrawn from Du Bois RM, Clarke SW: *Fiberoptic bronchoscopy in diagnosis and management,* Orlando, Fla, 1987, Grune & Stratton.

Chapter 25

25-4, Courtesy Robert Margulies, Miami. From Smolley LA: How to help patients with obstructive sleep apnea, *J Respir Dis* 11:723, 1990; 25-5, courtesy Respironics, Inc, Murrysville, Pa; 25-11, courtesy Passy-Muir, Inc, Irvine, Calif; 25-13, from the American Cancer Society; 25-16, Courtesy CLG Photographics, St Louis.

Chapter 26

26-2C, 26-4, From Damjanov I, Linder J: *Anderson's pathology,* ed 10, St Louis, 1996, Mosby; courtesy CLG Photographics, Inc, St Louis; 26-10, courtesy of Deknatel, Inc, Fall River, Mass.

Chapter 27

27-3, Redrawn from Price SA, Wilson LM: *Pathophysiology: clinical concepts of disease processes,* ed 5, St Louis, 1997, Mosby; 27-10A and B, from Potter PA, Perry AG: *Fundamentals of nursing: concepts, process, and practice,* ed 4, St Louis, 1997, Mosby; 27-13, courtesy Nellcor Puritan Bennett, Inc.

Chapter 28

28-1, Micrograph copyright 1994 Dennis Kunkel, PhD, Micro Vision, Kailua, Hawaii. In McCance KL, Huether SE: *Pathophysiology: the biologic basis for disease in adults and children,* ed 3, St Louis, 1998, Mosby; 28-3, from Erlandson S, Magney J: *Color atlas of histology,* St Louis, 1992, Mosby. In McCance KL, Huether SE: *Pathophysiology: the biologic basis for disease in adults and children,* ed 3, St Louis, 1998, Mosby.

Chapter 29

29-4, Redrawn from Raven PH, Johnson GB: *Biology,* ed 2, St Louis, 1991, Mosby; 29-5, redrawn from McCance KL, Huether SE: *Pathophysiology: the biologic basis for disease in adults and children,* ed 3, St Louis, 1998, Mosby; 29-8, from Bingham BJG, Hawke M, Kwok P: *Atlas of clinical otolaryngology,* St Louis, 1992, Mosby; 29-12, 29-13, reprinted from Groenwald SL, Frogge MH, Goodman J, editors: *Cancer nursing: principles and practice*, Boston, 1993, Jones & Bartlett.

Chapter 30

30-1, 30-3, Modified from Price SA, Wilson LM: *Pathophysiology: clinical concepts of disease processes,* ed 5, St Louis, 1997, Mosby; 30-5, 30-9, 30-12, modified from Kinney M and others: *Comprehensive cardiac care,* ed 8, St Louis, 1996, Mosby; 30-14, modified from Kinney M and others: *Comprehensive cardiac care,* ed 7, St Louis, 1991, Mosby.

Chapter 31

31-1, Redrawn from West JB: *Physiological basis of medical practice,* ed 12, Baltimore, 1991, Williams & Wilkins; 31-3, from Kissane JM: *Anderson's pathology,* ed 9, 1990, St Louis, Mosby; 31-4, 31-5, from US Department of Health and Human Services: *The sixth report of the Joint National Committee on Detection, Evaluation, and Treatment of High Blood Pressure (JNC-VI),* Washington, DC, 1997, National Institutes of Health.

Chapter 32

32-1, Courtesy National Center for Health Statistics and the American Heart Association; 32-8, modified and reprinted with permission from Matrisciano L, Alspach JG: Unstable angina: an overview, *Critical care nurses* 12:31, 1992; 32-10, from *Heart Disease and Stroke* 2:199, 1993, Copyright American Heart Association; 32-11, from *Heart Disease and Stroke* 2:201, 1993, Copyright American Heart Association; 32-12, 32-13, courtesy of Mayo Clinic, Rochester, Minn.

Chapter 33

33-1, Redrawn from McCance KL, Huether SE: *Pathophysiology: the biologic basis for disease in adults and children,* ed 3, St Louis, 1998, Mosby; 33-2, 33-4, redrawn from Thelan LA and others: *Textbook of critical care nursing: diagnosis and management,* ed 3, St Louis, 1998, Mosby; 33-3, 33-5, from Stevens A, Lowe J: *Pathology,* St Louis, 1995, Mosby.

Chapter 34

34-2, From Goldberger AL, Goldberger E: *Clinical electrocardiography: a simplified approach,* ed 6, St Louis, 1999, Mosby; 34-4, 34-7, 34-10, 34-12, from Thelan LA and others: *Textbook of critical care nursing: diagnosis and management,* ed 3, St Louis, 1998, Mosby; 34-6, 34-11B, 34-19, from Conover MB: *Understanding electrocardiography, arrhythmias, and the 12-lead ECG,* ed 7, St Louis, 1996, Mosby; 34-11A, 34-13, 34-14, 34-15, 34-20, from Conover MB: *Understanding electrocardiography, arrhythmias, and the 12-lead ECG,* ed 6, St Louis, 1992, Mosby; 34-21, 34-27, courtesy Physio-Control Corporation, Redmond, Wash; 34-24A, 34-25, courtesy Medtronic, Inc., Minneapolis, Minn.

Chapter 35

35-2, From Kissane JM: *Anderson's pathology,* ed 9, St Louis, 1990, Mosby; 35-4, from Anderson WAD, Scotti TM: *Synopsis of pathology,* ed 10, St Louis, 1980, Mosby; 35-5, from Guzetta CE, Dossey BM: *Cardiovascular nursing: holistic practice,* St Louis, 1992, Mosby; 35-6, redrawn from Lorell BH, Braunwald E: *Pericardial disease in heart disease: a textbook of cardiovascular medicine,* ed 3, Philadelphia, 1998, Saunders; 35-7, 35-10, 35-11B, from Stevens A, Lowe J: *Pathology,* St Louis, 1995, Mosby; 35-9, 35-11A, from McCance KL, Huether SE: *Pathophysiology: the biologic basis for disease in adults and children,* ed 3, St Louis, 1998, Mosby; 35-12, redrawn from Block PC: Balloon valvuloplasty, *Cardiol Consult* 9:4, 1988; 35-13, from Nichols L and others: Percutaneous aortic valvuloplasty procedure and implications for nursing, *Heart Lung* 18:357, 1989; 35-14A, courtesy St Jude Medical, Inc, St Paul, Minn. All rights reserved; 35-14B, courtesy Medtronic, Inc, Minneapolis, Minn; 35-14C, courtesy American Red Cross Tissue Services and Baxter Healthcare Corporation. CardioVascular Group, Santa Ana, Calif.

Chapter 36

36-1, Courtesy Jo Menzoian, Boston, Mass; 36-3, from Damjanov I, Linder J, editors: *Anderson's pathology,* ed 10, St Louis, 1996, Mosby; 36-8, courtesy FW LoGerfo, Boston, Mass; 36-9, 36-10, 36-13, from Kamal A, Brockelhurst JC: *Color atlas of geriatric medicine,* ed 2, 1991, Mosby–Year Book–Europe; 36-12, from Lofgren KA: Varicose veins. In Haimovici H, editor: *Vascular surgery: principles and techniques,* New York, 1976, McGraw-Hill.

Chapter 37

37-1, 37-3, From Thibodeau GA, Patton KT: *Anatomy and physiology,* ed 4, St Louis, 1999, Mosby; 37-9, from Doughty DB, Jackson DB: *Gastrointestinal disorders,* St Louis, 1993, Mosby.

Chapter 38

38-1, From *Human nutrition information service: making health food choices*, Washington, DC, 1993, USDA; 38-2, redrawn from Mahan LK, Arlin M: *Krause's food, nutrition, and diet therapy,* ed 4, 1992, Saunders; 38-7, copyright 1978 by George A. Bray, MD; 38-8, from Fortunato N, McCullough S: *Plastic and reconstructive surgery,* St Louis, 1998, Mosby.

Chapter 39

39-1, From Thibodeau GA, Patton KT: *Anatomy and physiology,* ed 4, St Louis, 1999, Mosby; 39-3, from Murray PR and others: *Medical microbiology*, ed 2, St Louis, 1994, Mosby; 39-4, courtesy RA Weinstein, Denver, CO; 39-6, 39-10, 39-12, 39-17, redrawn from Price SA, Wilson LM: *Pathophysiology: clinical concepts of disease processes,* ed 5, St Louis, 1997, Mosby; 39-8, from Doughty DB, Jackson DB: *Gastrointestinal disorders,* St Louis, 1993, Mosby; 39-13, from McCance KL, Huether SE: *Pathophysiology: the biologic basis for disease in adults and children*, ed 3, St Louis, 1998, Mosby; 39-14, from Damjanov I, Linder J, editors: *Anderson's pathology,* ed 10, St Louis, 1996, Mosby. In McCance KL, Huether SE: *Pathophysiology: the biologic basis for disease in adults and children,* ed 3, St Louis, 1998, Mosby; 39-17, redrawn from Price SA, Wilson LM: *Pathophysiology: clinical concepts of disease processes,* ed 5, St. Louis, Mosby.

Chapter 40

40-2, From Damjanov I, Linder J, editors: *Anderson's pathology,* ed 10, St Louis, 1996, Mosby; 40-5, 40-15, from Stevens A, Lowe J: *Pathology,* London, 1995, Mosby; 40-8, from McCance KL, Huether SE: *Pathophysiology: the biologic basis for disease in adults and children*, ed 3, St Louis, 1998, Mosby. Courtesy David Bjorkman, MD, University of Utah School of Medicine, Department of Gastroenterology; 40-10, from McCance KL, Huether SE: *Pathophysiology: the biologic basis for disease in adults and children*, ed 3, St Louis, 1998, Mosby; 40-12, redrawn from Meeker MH, Rothrock JC: *Alexander's care of the patient in surgery,* ed 9, St Louis, 1991, Mosby; 40-13, redrawn from Hampton BG, Bryant RA: *Ostomies and continent diversions,* St Louis, 1992, Mosby.

Chapter 41

41-1, From Kamal A, Brockelhurst JC: *Color atlas of geriatric medicine,* ed 3, St Louis, 1991, Mosby–Year Book–Europe; 41-4, from Damjanov I, Linder J, editors: *Anderson's pathology,* ed 10, St Louis, 1996, Mosby; 41-6, adapted from Doughty DB, Jackson DB: *Gastrointestinal disorders,* St Louis, 1993, Mosby; 41-11, 41-13, 41-15, from Stevens A, Lowe J: *Pathology,* London, 1995, Mosby.

Chapter 42

42-7, From Brundage DJ: *Renal disorders,* St Louis, 1992, Mosby; 42-8, from Price S, Wilson L: *Pathophysiology: clinical concepts of disease processes,* ed 5, St Louis, 1997, Mosby; 42-10, courtesy Circon Corporation, Santa Barbara, Calif.

Chapter 43

43-3, 43-5, Courtesy Harborview Medical Center, University of Washington, Seattle; 43-6, From Brundage DJ: *Renal disorders,* St Louis, 1992, Mosby; 43-9, 43-11, 43-12, courtesy Lynda Brubacher, Virginia Mason Hospital, Seattle.

Chapter 44

44-2, From United States Data System, Washington, DC, 1998, Dept of Health and Human Services; 44-7, 44-8, 44-9, 44-10, copyright 1994 Baxter Healthcare Corp; 44-12A, courtesy Quinton Instrument Co, Seattle; 44-14, modified from Thelan L, Davie JK, Urden JD: *Textbook of critical care nursing: diagnosis and management,* ed 3, St Louis, 1998, Mosby; 44-15, copyright Baxter Healthcare Corporation.

Chapter 45

45-1, 45-3, 45-4, From Thibodeau GA, Patton KT: *Anatomy and physiology,* ed 4, St Louis, 1999, Mosby; 45-6, from McCance KL, Huether SE: *Pathophysiology: the biologic basis for disease in adults and children,* ed 3, St Louis, 1998, Mosby; 45-9, from Seeley R, Stephens T, Tate P: *Anatomy and physiology,* ed 3, New York, 1995, McGraw-Hill, Carlyn Iverson, artist; 45-10, from Thompson JM, Wilson SF: *Health assessment for nursing practice,* St Louis, 1996, Mosby.

Chapter 46

46-3, From *Diabetes mellitus*, Indianapolis, Eli Lilly, Inc; 46-4, 46-5, from American Diabetes Association: *Maximizing the role of nutrition in diabetes management*, Alexandria, Va, American Diabetes Association, 1994; 46-10, 46-12, redrawn from McCance KL, Huether SE: *Pathophysiology: the biologic basis for disease in adults and children,* ed 3, St Louis, 1998, Mosby; 46-13, from Thelan L, Davie JK, Urden JD: *Textbook of critical care nursing: diagnosis and management,* ed 3, St Louis, 1998, Mosby.

Chapter 47

47-1, Courtesy Linda Haas, Seattle; 47-3, redrawn from Thelan L, Davie JK, Urden JD: *Textbook of critical care nursing: diagnosis and management,* ed 2, St Louis, 1994, Mosby; 47-4, 47-5, redrawn from Thelan L, Davie JK, Urden JD: *Textbook of critical care nursing: diagnosis and management,* ed 3, St Louis, 1998, Mosby; 47-6, redrawn from Seidel HM and others: *Mosby's guide to physical examination,* ed 4, St Louis, 1999, Mosby; 47-7, from Besser GM, Cudworth AG: *Clinical endocrinology: an illustrated text,* London, 1987, Gower Medical Publishing; 47-8, from Williams GH, Dluhy RG: *Diseases of the adrenal cortex.* In Isselbacher K and others, editors: *Harrison's principles of internal medicine,* ed 14, St Louis, 1998, Mosby.

Chapter 48

48-1, 48-5, From Seeley R, Stephens T, Tate P: *Anatomy and physiology,* ed 2, New York, 1992, McGraw-Hill; 48-3, 48-6, from Thibodeau GA, Patton KT: *Anatomy and physiology,* ed 4, St Louis, 1999, Mosby; 48-8, from Seeley R, Stephens T, Tate P: *Anatomy and physiology,* ed 3, New York, 1995, McGraw-Hill.

Chapter 49

49-2, From Powell DE, Stelling CB: *The diagnosis and detection of breast disease*, St Louis, 1993, Mosby; 49-5, from Fortunato N, McCullough SM: *Plastic and reconstructive surgery*, St Louis, 1998, Mosby. Courtesy Brian W. Davies, MD; 49-6, modified from Beare PG, Myers JL: *Adult health nursing*, ed 3, St Louis, 1998, Mosby, and Fortunato N, McCullough SM: *Plastic and reconstructive surgery*, St Louis, 1998, Mosby.

Chapter 50

50-4, 50-5, Courtesy USPHS, Washington, DC; 50-6, 50-7, reproduced with permission of Glaxo Wellcome, Inc, Research Triangle Park, NC.

Chapter 51

51-1, From Gowan ADT, Hodge C, Callender R: *Gynecology illustrated*, ed 3, New York, 1985, Churchill Livingstone; 51-4, from Bobak I, Jensen M, Zalar M: *Maternity and gynecologic care,* ed 5, St Louis, 1993, Mosby; 51-6, from Mishell DR and others: *Comprehensive gynecology,* ed 3, St Louis, 1997, Mosby; 51-7, redrawn from Novak ER, Woodruff JD, editors: *Novak's gynecologic and obstetric pathology*, ed 6, Philadelphia, 1967, Saunders. In McCance KL, Huether SE: *Pathophysiology: the biologic basis for disease in adults and children,* ed 3, St Louis, 1998, Mosby; 51-8, 51-12, redrawn from Seidel HM and others: *Mosby's guide to physical examination,* ed 4, St Louis, 1999, Mosby; 51-9, from Phipps WJ, Sands JK, Marek JF: *Medical-surgical nursing: concepts and clinical practice,* ed 6, St Louis, 1999, Mosby; 51-11, from Seidel HM and others: *Mosby's guide to physical examination,* ed 3, St Louis, 1995, Mosby.

Chapter 52

52-5, From Seidel HM and others: *Mosby's guide to physical examination,* ed 4, St Louis, 1999, Mosby, modified from Burroughs-Wellcome Co, 1989; 52-7, courtesy of *Mayo Clinic Health Letter* with permission from Mayo Foundation for Medical Education and Research, Rochester.

Chapter 53

53-1, 53-4, 53-5, 53-10, 53-11, 53-14, 53-15, 53-20, From Thibodeau GA, Patton KT: *Anatomy and physiology,* ed 4, St Louis, 1999, Mosby; 53-6, 53-13, from Seeley R, Stephens T, Tate P: *Anatomy and physiology,* ed 3, New York, 1995, McGraw-Hill; 53-12, from McCance KL, Huether SE: *Pathophysiology: the biologic basis for disease in adults and children,* ed 3, St Louis, 1998, Mosby; 53-19A, from Elkin MK, Perry AG, Potter PA: *Nursing interventions and clinical skills*, ed 2, St Louis, 1999, Mosby; 53-19B, from Chipps E, Clanin N, Campbell V: *Neurologic disorders*, St Louis, 1992, Mosby.

Chapter 54

54-1, From Wong J, Wong S, Dempster JK: Care of the unconscious patient: a problem-oriented approach, *Am Assoc Neurosci Nurses* 16:145, 1984; 54-5, redrawn from McCance KL, Huether SE: *Pathophysiology: the biologic basis for disease in adults and children,* ed 3, St Louis, 1998, Mosby; 54-7, from Thelan LA and others: *Textbook of critical care nursing: diagnosis and management,* ed 2, St Louis, 1994, Mosby; 54-8, redrawn from Kinney MR and others, editors: *AACN's clinical reference for critical care nursing,* St Louis, 1993, Mosby; 54-11, redrawn from Barker E: *Neuroscience nursing,* St Louis, 1994, Mosby; 54-12, from Bingham BJG, Hawke M, Kwok P: *Clinical atlas of otolaryngology,* St Louis, 1992, Mosby; 54-13, from Price SA, Wilson LM: *Pathophysiology: clinical concepts of disease processes,* ed 5, St Louis, 1997, Mosby; 54-14, from Okazaki H, Scheithauer BW: *Atlas of neuropathology,* Gower Medical Publishing, 1988; 54-16, from Perkin GD and others: *Atlas of clinical neurology,* ed 2, London, 1993, Wolfe Publishing.

Chapter 55

55-8, Modified from Hoeman SP: *Rehabilitation nursing,* ed 2, St Louis, 1995, Mosby; 55-10A-C, courtesy Sammons Preston.

Chapter 56

56-2, 56-7, From Damjanov I, Linder J, editors: *Anderson's pathology,* ed 10, St Louis, 1996, Mosby; 56-5, from McCance KL, Huether SE: *Pathophysiology: the biologic basis for disease in adults and children,* ed 3, St Louis, 1998, Mosby; 56-6, redrawn from Rudy E: *Advanced neurological and neurosurgical nursing,* St Louis, 1984, Mosby; 56-8, redrawn from Barker E: *Neuroscience nursing,* St Louis, 1994, Mosby.

Chapter 57

57-1, From Thibodeau GA, Patton KT: *Anatomy and physiology,* ed 4, St Louis, 1999, Mosby; 57-2, courtesy Joe Rothrock, Media, Pa; 57-3, redrawn from Chipps E, Clanin N, Campbell V: *Neurologic disorders,* St Louis, 1992, Mosby; 57-4, redrawn from Marciano FF and others: *BNI Q* 11:6, 1995. In McCance KL, Huether SE: *Pathophysiology: the biologic basis for disease in adults and* children, ed 3, St Louis, 1998, Mosby; 57-8, courtesy Michael S Clement, MD, Mesa, Ariz; 57-9, 57-13, from Barker E: *Neuroscience nursing,* St Louis, 1994, Mosby; 57-10, courtesy Kinetic Concepts, Inc, San Antonio, Texas; 57-11, courtesy Acromed Corporation, Cleveland; 57-12, courtesy CLG Photographics, St Louis.

Chapter 58

58-1, 58-4, 58-6, From Thibodeau GA, Patton KT: *Anatomy and physiology,* ed 4, St Louis, 1999, Mosby; 58-2, from Seeley R, Stephens T, Tate P: *Anatomy and physiology,* ed 3, New York, 1995, McGraw-Hill; 58-7, 58-9, from Mourad LA: *Orthopedic disorders,* St Louis, 1991, Mosby; 58-8, modified from De Lisa J, Gans B: *Rehabilitation medicine principles,* ed 2, Philadelphia, 1993, JB Lippincott.

Chapter 59

59-1, Redrawn from Price SA, Wilson LM: *Pathophysiology: clinical concepts of disease processes,* ed 5, St Louis, 1997, Mosby; 59-2, 59-15, from Thompson J and others: *Mosby's manual of clinical nursing,* ed 4, St Louis, 1997, Mosby; 59-3, Jobe FW and others, editors: *Operative techniques in upper extremity sports injuries,* St Louis, 1996, Mosby; 59-4, from Thibodeau GA, Patton KT: *Anatomy and physiology,* ed 4, St Louis, 1999, Mosby; 59-8, redrawn from Long BC, Phipps WJ, Cassmeyer VL: *Medical-surgical nursing: a nursing process approach,* St Louis, 1993, Mosby; 59-10, courtesy Howmedica, Inc; 59-17, redrawn from Mourad L: *Orthopedic disorders,* St Louis, 1992, Mosby; 59-19, from Hunter JM and others: *Rehabilitation of the hand,* ed 4, St Louis, 1995, Mosby.

Chapter 60

60-2, From Kamal A, Brockelhurst JC: *Color atlas of geriatric medicine*, ed 2, St Louis, 1991, Mosby. In *Mosby's medical, nursing, and allied health dictionary*, ed 5, 1998, Mosby; 60-3, from Shipley M: *A colour atlas of rheumatology,* ed 3, London, 1993, Mosby–Year Book–Europe; 60-7, reprinted from the Clinical Slide Collection on the Rheumatic Diseases, copyright 1991, 1995, 1997. Used by permission of the American College of Rheumatology. In Seidel HM and others: *Mosby's guide to physical examination,* ed 4, St Louis, 1999, Mosby; 60-9, from Habif TP: *Clinical dermatology: a color guide to diagnosis and therapy*, ed 3, St Louis, 1996, Mosby; 60-11, from Zitelli BJ, Davis HW: *Atlas of pediatric physical diagnosis,* ed 3, St Louis, 1997, Mosby–Wolfe; 60-12, 60-13, courtesy Zimmer, Inc, Warsaw, Ind.

Chapter 61

61-2, 61-3, 61-4, 61-5, From Thelan LA and others: *Critical care nursing: diagnosis and management,* ed 3, St Louis, 1998, Mosby.

Chapter 62

62-6, From Richmond TS: The patient with a cervical spinal cord injury, *Focus on critical care* 12:27, 1985; 62-7, Courtesy Respironics, Inc, Pittsburgh.

Chapter 63

63-1, 63-16, Courtesy Spacelabs Medical, Redmond, Wash; 63-2, redrawn from Gardner PE: *Hemodynamic pressure monitoring*, Redmond, Wash, 1994, Spacelabs Medical; 63-3, redrawn from Flynn JBM, Bruce NP: *Introduction to critical care skills,* St Louis, 1993, Mosby; 63-4, 63-6, 63-7, 63-11, 63-20, from Thelan LA and others, editors: *Critical care nursing: diagnosis and management,* ed 3, St Louis, 1998, Mosby; 63-5, courtesy Edwards Critical Care Division, Baxter Healthcare Corporation, Santa Ana, Calif; 63-9, courtesy Datascope Corporation, Fairfield, NJ; 63-12A, from Beare PG, Myers JL: *Adult health nursing,* ed 3, St Louis, 1998, Mosby; 63-14, from Sills JR: *Respiratory care certification guide: the complete review resource for the entry level exam*, ed 2, St Louis, 1994, Mosby. In Thelan LA and others, editors: *Critical care nursing: diagnosis and management*, ed 3, St Louis, 1998, Mosby; 63-15, courtesy Lifecare, Westminster, Colo; 63-17, courtesy Mallinckrodt, Inc, Carlsbad, Calif; 63-18, courtesy Camino Laboratories, San Diego.

Chapter 64

64-2, 64-3, Courtesy Cameron Bangs, MD, from Auerbach P, editor: *Wilderness medicine: management of wilderness and environmental emergencies,* ed 3, St Louis, 1995, Mosby; 64-5, redrawn from Rosen P and others: *Emergency medicine,* vol 1, ed 2, St Louis, 1988, Mosby.

INDEX

A

Note: Disorder names are in **bold face.** Entries in **bold face** indicate main discussions. Page numbers followed by *f*, *t*, and *b* indicate figures, tables, or boxed material, respectively.

Note: Disorder names are in **bold face.** Entries in **bold face** indicate main discussions. Page numbers followed by *f*, *t*, and *b* indicate figures, tables, or boxed material, respectively.

Note: Disorder names are in **bold face.** Entries in **bold face** indicate main discussions. Page numbers followed by *f*, *t*, and *b* indicate figures, tables, or boxed material, respectively.

Note: Disorder names are in **bold face.** Entries in **bold face** indicate main discussions. Page numbers followed by *f*, *t*, and *b* indicate figures, tables, or boxed material, respectively.

Note: Disorder names are in **bold face.** Entries in **bold face** indicate main discussions. Page numbers followed by *f*, *t*, and *b* indicate figures, tables, or boxed material, respectively.

Note: Disorder names are in **bold face.** Entries in **bold face** indicate main discussions. Page numbers followed by *f*, *t*, and *b* indicate figures, tables, or boxed material, respectively.

Note: Disorder names are in **bold face.** Entries in **bold face** indicate main discussions. Page numbers followed by *f, t,* and *b* indicate figures, tables, or boxed material, respectively.

Note: Disorder names are in **bold face**. Entries in **bold face** indicate main discussions. Page numbers followed by *f*, *t*, and *b* indicate figures, tables, or boxed material, respectively.

Note: Disorder names are in **bold face.** Entries in **bold face** indicate main discussions. Page numbers followed by *f*, *t*, and *b* indicate figures, tables, or boxed material, respectively.

Note: Disorder names are in **bold face.** Entries in **bold face** indicate main discussions. Page numbers followed by *f*, *t*, and *b* indicate figures, tables, or boxed material, respectively.

Note: Disorder names are in **bold face.** Entries in **bold face** indicate main discussions. Page numbers followed by *f, t,* and *b* indicate figures, tables, or boxed material, respectively.

Note: Disorder names are in **bold face.** Entries in **bold face** indicate main discussions. Page numbers followed by *f, t,* and *b* indicate figures, tables, or boxed material, respectively.

D

Note: Disorder names are in **bold face.** Entries in **bold face** indicate main discussions. Page numbers followed by *f, t,* and *b* indicate figures, tables, or boxed material, respectively.

E

Note: Disorder names are in **bold face.** Entries in **bold face** indicate main discussions. Page numbers followed by *f*, *t*, and *b* indicate figures, tables, or boxed material, respectively.

Note: Disorder names are in **bold face.** Entries in **bold face** indicate main discussions. Page numbers followed by *f*, *t*, and *b* indicate figures, tables, or boxed material, respectively.

F

Note: Disorder names are in **bold face.** Entries in **bold face** indicate main discussions. Page numbers followed by *f*, *t*, and *b* indicate figures, tables, or boxed material, respectively.

Note: Disorder names are in **bold face.** Entries in **bold face** indicate main discussions. Page numbers followed by *f, t,* and *b* indicate figures, tables, or boxed material, respectively.

Note: Disorder names are in **bold face.** Entries in **bold face** indicate main discussions. Page numbers followed by *f*, *t*, and *b* indicate figures, tables, or boxed material, respectively.

H

Note: Disorder names are in **bold face.** Entries in **bold face** indicate main discussions. Page numbers followed by *f, t,* and *b* indicate figures, tables, or boxed material, respectively.

Note: Disorder names are in **bold face.** Entries in **bold face** indicate main discussions. Page numbers followed by *f*, *t*, and *b* indicate figures, tables, or boxed material, respectively.

Note: Disorder names are in **bold face.** Entries in **bold face** indicate main discussions. Page numbers followed by *f*, *t*, and *b* indicate figures, tables, or boxed material, respectively.

I

Note: Disorder names are in **bold face.** Entries in **bold face** indicate main discussions. Page numbers followed by *f*, *t*, and *b* indicate figures, tables, or boxed material, respectively.

Note: Disorder names are in **bold face.** Entries in **bold face** indicate main discussions. Page numbers followed by *f*, *t*, and *b* indicate figures, tables, or boxed material, respectively.

J

K

Note: Disorder names are in **bold face.** Entries in **bold face** indicate main discussions. Page numbers followed by *f*, *t*, and *b* indicate figures, tables, or boxed material, respectively.

L

Note: Disorder names are in **bold face.** Entries in **bold face** indicate main discussions. Page numbers followed by *f*, *t*, and *b* indicate figures, tables, or boxed material, respectively.

M

Note: Disorder names are in **bold face.** Entries in **bold face** indicate main discussions. Page numbers followed by *f*, *t*, and *b* indicate figures, tables, or boxed material, respectively.

Note: Disorder names are in **bold face.** Entries in **bold face** indicate main discussions. Page numbers followed by *f*, *t*, and *b* indicate figures, tables, or boxed material, respectively.

N

Note: Disorder names are in **bold face.** Entries in **bold face** indicate main discussions. Page numbers followed by *f, t,* and *b* indicate figures, tables, or boxed material, respectively.

Note: Disorder names are in **bold face.** Entries in **bold face** indicate main discussions. Page numbers followed by *f, t,* and *b* indicate figures, tables, or boxed material, respectively.

O

Note: Disorder names are in **bold face.** Entries in **bold face** indicate main discussions. Page numbers followed by *f*, *t*, and *b* indicate figures, tables, or boxed material, respectively.

P

Note: Disorder names are in **bold face.** Entries in **bold face** indicate main discussions. Page numbers followed by *f*, *t*, and *b* indicate figures, tables, or boxed material, respectively.

Note: Disorder names are in **bold face.** Entries in **bold face** indicate main discussions. Page numbers followed by *f, t,* and *b* indicate figures, tables, or boxed material, respectively.

Note: Disorder names are in **bold face.** Entries in **bold face** indicate main discussions. Page numbers followed by *f*, *t*, and *b* indicate figures, tables, or boxed material, respectively.

Note: Disorder names are in **bold face.** Entries in **bold face** indicate main discussions. Page numbers followed by *f*, *t*, and *b* indicate figures, tables, or boxed material, respectively.

Q

R

Note: Disorder names are in **bold face.** Entries in **bold face** indicate main discussions. Page numbers followed by *f*, *t*, and *b* indicate figures, tables, or boxed material, respectively.

Note: Disorder names are in **bold face.** Entries in **bold face** indicate main discussions. Page numbers followed by *f*, *t*, and *b* indicate figures, tables, or boxed material, respectively.

S

Note: Disorder names are in **bold face.** Entries in **bold face** indicate main discussions. Page numbers followed by *f, t,* and *b* indicate figures, tables, or boxed material, respectively.

Note: Disorder names are in **bold face.** Entries in **bold face** indicate main discussions. Page numbers followed by *f*, *t*, and *b* indicate figures, tables, or boxed material, respectively.

Note: Disorder names are in **bold face.** Entries in **bold face** indicate main discussions. Page numbers followed by *f, t,* and *b* indicate figures, tables, or boxed material, respectively.

Note: Disorder names are in **bold face.** Entries in **bold face** indicate main discussions. Page numbers followed by *f*, *t*, and *b* indicate figures, tables, or boxed material, respectively.

T

Note: Disorder names are in **bold face.** Entries in **bold face** indicate main discussions. Page numbers followed by *f*, *t*, and *b* indicate figures, tables, or boxed material, respectively.

Note: Disorder names are in **bold face.** Entries in **bold face** indicate main discussions. Page numbers followed by *f, t,* and *b* indicate figures, tables, or boxed material, respectively.

U

Note: Disorder names are in **bold face.** Entries in **bold face** indicate main discussions. Page numbers followed by *f*, *t*, and *b* indicate figures, tables, or boxed material, respectively.

Note: Disorder names are in **bold face.** Entries in **bold face** indicate main discussions. Page numbers followed by *f*, *t*, and *b* indicate figures, tables, or boxed material, respectively.

W

X

Y

Z

Note: Disorder names are in **bold face.** Entries in **bold face** indicate main discussions. Page numbers followed by *f*, *t*, and *b* indicate figures, tables, or boxed material, respectively.

CLINICAL PATHWAYS

NUTRITIONAL THERAPY

PATIENT TEACHING GUIDES

PATIENT AND FAMILY HOME CARE GUIDES

PATIENT AND FAMILY TEACHING GUIDES

NURSING CARE PLANS

NURSING CARE PLANS—cont'd

CRITICAL THINKING EXERCISES

CULTURAL AND ETHNIC CONSIDERATIONS

GERONTOLOGIC DIFFERENCES IN ASSESSMENT/EFFECTS OF AGING